FOURTH EDITION

MEDICAL-SURGICAL NURSING

Assessment and Management of Clinical Problems

Research Implications—cont'd

Clinical Pathways

Gerontologic Differences in Assessment

Nursing Assessment

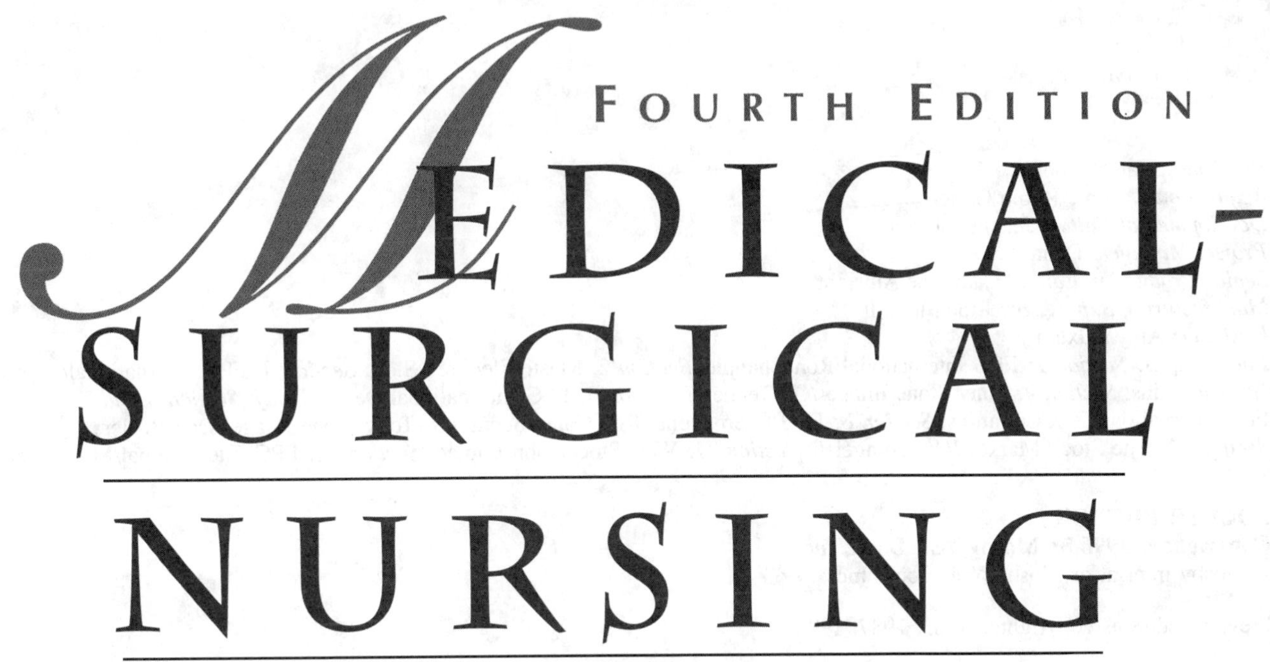

FOURTH EDITION MEDICAL-SURGICAL NURSING

Assessment and Management of Clinical Problems

Sharon Mantik Lewis, RN, PhD, FAAN
Professor, College of Nursing
Research Associate Professor
Department of Pathology
School of Medicine
University of New Mexico
Albuquerque, New Mexico

Idolia Cox Collier, RNCS, DNSc
Associate Professor, College of Nursing
University of New Mexico
Albuquerque, New Mexico

Margaret M. Heitkemper, RN, PhD, FAAN
Professor
Department of Biobehavioral
Nursing and Health Systems
School of Nursing
University of Washington
Seattle, Washington

with 1260 illustrations

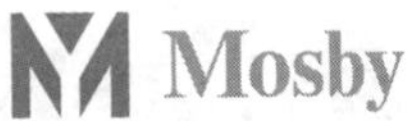

St. Louis Baltimore Boston Carlsbad Chicago Naples New York Philadelphia Portland
London Madrid Mexico City Singapore Sydney Tokyo Toronto Wiesbaden

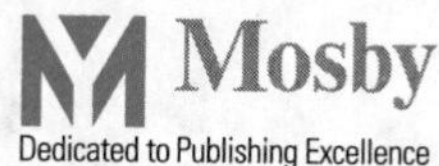

Dedicated to Publishing Excellence

A Times Mirror Company

Publisher: Nancy Coon
Acquisitions Editor: Robin Carter
Developmental Editor: Jeanne Allison
Project Manager: Dana Peick
Senior Production Editor: Catherine Albright
Manufacturing Supervisor: Linda Ierardi
Designer: Amy Buxton
Photographs: Section 1: FPG International/Ron Chapple; *Section 2:* Masterfile/Greg Stott; *Section 3:* FPG International/Jim Cummins; *Section 4:* Tony Stone Images/Oli Tennent; *Section 5:* FPG International/Denise Cody; *Section 6 and 7:* FPG International/Jim Cummins; *Section 8:* FPG International/Rob Gage; *Section 9:* Tony Stone Images/Dan Bosler; *Section 10:* The Stock Market/John Feingersh; *Section 11:* West Stock/John Laptad; *Section 12:* FPG International/Mark Scott

FOURTH EDITION

Printed in the United States of America
Composition by Carlisle Communications, Ltd.
Illustration by DesignPointe Communications, Inc.
Printing by Rand McNally

Mosby-Year Book, Inc.
11830 Westline Industrial Drive
St. Louis, Missouri 63146

Library of Congress Cataloging-in-Publication Data

Medical-surgical nursing : assessment and management of clinical problems / [edited by] Sharon Mantik Lewis, Idolia Cox Collier, Margaret M. Heitkemper. -- 4th ed.
p. cm.
Includes bibliographical references and index.
ISBN 0-8151-5301-5 (alk. paper)
1. Nursing. 2. Surgical nursing. I. Lewis, Sharon Mantik. II. Collier, Idolia Cox. III. Heitkemper, Margaret M. (Margaret McLean)
[DNLM: 1. Nursing Care. 2. Nursing Assessment. 3. Surgical Nursing. WY 100 M489 1996]
RT41.M488 1996
610.73—dc20
DNLM/DLC
for Library of Congress

95-30732
CIP

95 96 97 98 99 / 9 8 7 6 5 4 3 2 1

About the Authors

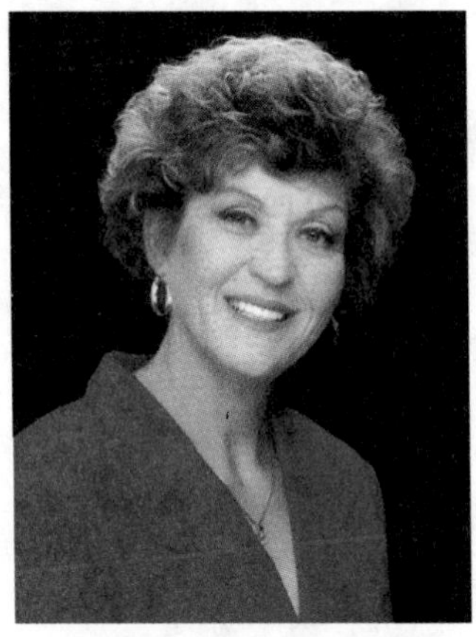

Sharon Mantik Lewis, RN, PhD, FAAN

Sharon Lewis received her Bachelor of Science in nursing from the University of Wisconsin-Madison, Master of Science in nursing with a minor in biologic sciences from the University of Colorado-Denver, and PhD in immunology from the Department of Pathology at the University of New Mexico School of Medicine. She had a 2-year postdoctoral fellowship from the National Kidney Foundation. Her 25 years of teaching experience include inservice education and teaching in associate degree, baccalaureate, and masters degree programs in Maryland, Illinois, Wisconsin, and New Mexico. Favorite teaching areas are pathophysiology, immunology, and renal failure. She has been actively involved in clinical research for the last 15 years, investigating altered immune responses in patients with chronic renal failure and other chronic illnesses.

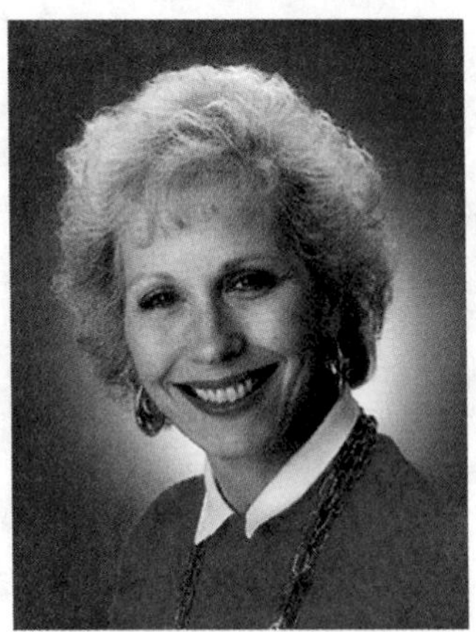

Idolia Cox Collier, RNCS, DNSc

Idolia Cox Collier received her Bachelor of Science in nursing from Marquette University, Master of Science in nursing from Loyola University, and Doctor of Science in nursing from the University of California, San Francisco. She has twelve years of experience as a staff nurse. Her 20 years of teaching experience include teaching at Loyola University and the University of New Mexico at the graduate and undergraduate levels. She is the author of a nursing diagnoses reference book also published by Mosby. Her primary area of interest is gerontology, and she has completed research on the functional status of the elderly.

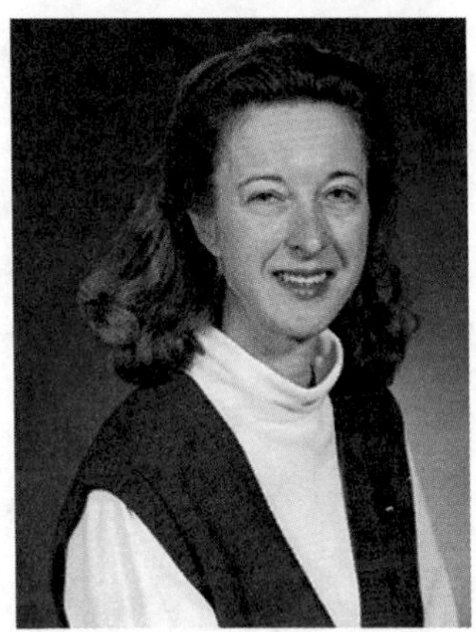

Margaret McLean Heitkemper, RN, PhD, FAAN

Margaret Heitkemper received her Bachelor of Science in nursing from Seattle University, Master of Science in gerontologic nursing from the University of Washington, and PhD in physiology and biophysics from the University of Illinois. She was a research associate on an NIH research grant project related to problems with enteral nutrition, where she developed an interest in gastrointestinal problems. She has experience as a staff nurse and has worked in an acute geriatric care facility associated with Rush–St. Luke's Presbyterian Medical Center. Since 1981, she has been on the faculty at the University of Washington where she teaches at all levels—undergraduate and graduate. She currently teaches medical-surgical nursing theory and pharmacology for nurses.

CONTRIBUTORS

Charlotte R. Abbink, RN, PhD, Former Associate Professor, University of New Mexico College of Nursing, Albuquerque, New Mexico

Judith Barrows, RN, MSN, CCRN, Instructor/ Consultant, Nursing Staff Development Department, Cape Cod Hospital, Hyannis, Massachusetts

Patricia Bates, RN, BSN, CURN, Urology Staff Nurse, West Interstate Medical Office, Kaiser-Permanente, Portland, Oregon

Darlene Batson, RN, CRNA, BSEd, Chief Certified Registered Nurse Anesthetist, Lovelace Medical Center, Albuquerque, New Mexico

Catherine M. Bender, RN, PhD, Assistant Professor, University of Pittsburgh School of Nursing, Pittsburgh, Pennsylvania

Eleanor F. Bond, RN, PhD, Associate Professor, Department of Biobehavioral Nursing and Health Systems, University of Washington, Seattle, Washington

Lucy Bradley-Springer, RN, PhD, Assistant Professor, University of New Mexico School of Medicine; Co-Director, New Mexico AIDS Education and Training Center, Albuquerque, New Mexico

Lynda Sawchuk, ARNP, CETN, Enterostomal Therapy Nurse, Virginia Mason Medical Center, Seattle, Washington

Gayle Ziegler Casterline, RN, MSN, Research Associate, Department of Pediatrics, University of Texas Medical School, Houston Health Sciences Center, University of Texas, Houston, Texas

Ceil Dail, BS, MT (ASCP), CLS, Instructor, Medical Laboratory Sciences, Department of Pathology, School of Medicine, University of New Mexico, Albuquerque, New Mexico

Jeanne Doyle, RN, BS, Executive Director, Society for Vascular Nursing, Norwood, Massachusetts

Ellen Stoetzner Duke, RN, MSN, Instructor of Nursing, Stephen F. Austin State University, Nacogdoches, Texas

Laura Dulski, RNC, MSN, Teaching Assistant, Rush College of Nursing, Chicago, Illinois

Patsy L. Orth Duphorne, RN, MN, Assistant Professor, University of New Mexico College of Nursing, Albuquerque, New Mexico

Tana Durnbaugh, RNCS, EdD, Professor, School of Nursing, College of Lake County, Grayslake, Illinois

Rachel Elrod, RN, MS, Professor, Nursing, Front Range Community College, Westminster, Colorado; Faculty member, University of Phoenix, Colorado Campus

Lori Finlay, MS, APRN, CCRN, Nurse Practitioner, Utah Heart Clinic, Salt Lake City, Utah

Jane M. Georges, RN, PhD, Assistant Professor, College of Nursing, Ohio State University, Columbus, Ohio

Kate Goldblum, RN, CS, CRNO, MSN, Clinical Specialist—Ophthalmology, Albuquerque, New Mexico

Linda Griego, RN, MSN, CCRN, Cardiovascular Clinical Nurse Specialist, Presbyterian Hospital, Albuquerque, New Mexico

Linda Haas, RN, PhD, CDE, Endocrinology Clinical Nurse Specialist, Seattle VA Medical Center, Seattle, Washington

Mary Ann House-Fancher, RN, ARNP, MSN, CCRN, Nurse Practitioner, Thoracic Surgery, Shands Hospital, University of Florida, Gainesville, Florida

Margaret McLean Heitkemper, RN, PhD, FAAN, Professor, Department of Biobehavioral Nursing and Health Systems, University of Washington, Seattle, Washington

Patricia Ann Hercules, RN, MS, Manager, Department of Nursing Education, The Methodist Hospital, Houston, Texas

Leslie A. Hoffman, RN, PhD, FAAN, Professor of Nursing, Chair, Department of Acute/Tertiary Care, University of Pittsburgh School of Nursing, Pittsburgh, Pennsylvania

Mima M. Horne, RN, MS, CDE, Diabetes Clinical Nurse Specialist, New Hanover Regional Medical Center, Wilmington, North Carolina; Adjunct Lecturer, School of Nursing, University of North Carolina, Wilmington, North Carolina

Carolyn Johns, RN, MS, CANP, Cardiology Nurse Practitioner, Lovelace Medical Center, Albuquerque, New Mexico

The Reverend Barbara Gail Jorelman, BA, MDiv, President, New Mexico Health Decisions, Albuquerque, New Mexico

Mary E. Kerr, RN, PhD, Assistant Professor, University of Pittsburgh School of Nursing, Pittsburgh, Pennsylvania

Cindy Knipe, RN, Nursing Manager, Adult Burn Unit, Indiana University Medical Center, Wishard Health Services, Indianapolis, Indiana

Nancy Stoetzner Kupper, RN, MSN, Associate Professor, Tarrant County Junior College, Arlington, Texas

Adele A. Large, RN, MSN, CCRN, Case Manager, Medicine, University of Pittsburgh Medical Center, Pittsburgh, Pennsylvania

Eileen Leach, RN, MPH, Director of Clinical Investigations, Roche Laboratories, Hoffman–La Roche, Nutley, New Jersey; Associate in Dermatology, Columbia University, New York, New York

Sharon L. Lewis, RN, PhD, FAAN, Professor, College of Nursing; Research Associate Professor, Department of Pathology, University of New Mexico, Albuquerque, New Mexico

Phyllis Lisanti, RN, PhD, Clinical Assistant Professor, Undergraduate Program Director, Division of Nursing, New York University, New York, New York

Kim Litwack-Saleh, RN, PhD, CPAN, Associate Professor, College of Nursing, University of New Mexico, Albuquerque, New Mexico

Janice Luft, BSN, MSN, OB/GYN Nurse Practitioner, University of California—San Francisco, Mt. Zion Faculty Practice, San Francisco, California

Nancy MacMullen, RNC, PhD, Assistant Professor, Rush College of Nursing, Chicago, Illinois

Jan Manzetti, RN, PhD, CRNP, Coordinator of Cardiothoracic Transplantation, University of Pittsburgh Medical Center, Pittsburgh, Pennsylvania

Patricia Bargo McCarley, RN, BSN, CNN, Nurse Manager/Administrator, Medical Center, Dialysis Clinic, Inc., Nashville, Tennessee

Katheryn E. McCash, RNC, MSN, Lecturer, College of Nursing, University of New Mexico, Albuquerque, New Mexico

Cindy Meredith, RN, MSN, Urology Nurse Consultant, University of Michigan, Flint, Michigan

Diane Michalec, RN, MSN, Patient Care Manager, Trauma/Neuro ICU, University of Pittsburgh Medical Center, Pittsburgh, Pennsylvania

Joyce Tremper Mitchell, RN, MS, NS, CPHQ, Assistant Chief, Quality Management Section, Veterans Affairs Medical Center, Tucson, Arizona

Christina M. Mumma, RN, PhD, CRRN, Associate Professor, University of Alaska, Anchorage, Alaska

Judy Ozuna, RN, MN, Clinical Nurse Specialist, Veterans Affairs Medical Center, Seattle, Washington

Kathryn A. Patterson, RN, CNM, PhD, Associate Professor, University of Hawaii School of Nursing, Honolulu, Hawaii

Susan C. Ruda, RN, MS, ONC, Clinical Nurse Specialist, Parkview Orthopaedic Group, Palos Heights, Illinois

Diane Rudolphi, RN, MS, Staff Nurse, Union Hospital, Elkton, Maryland

Anne Marie Ruszkowski, RN, BSN, Director of Nursing, Department of Dermatology, Columbia University, New York, New York

Kathleen C. Solotkin, RN, BSN, Trauma Nurse Coordinator, Indiana University, Wishard Regional Trauma Center, Indianapolis, Indiana

Roberta Strohl, RN, MN, OCN, Clinical Nurse Specialist, Department of Radiation Oncology, University of Maryland, Baltimore, Maryland

Dee Trottier, RN, BSN, Clinical Research Nurse, Olsten Kimberly Quality Care, Portage, Michigan

Virginia Valentine, RN, MS, CDE, Clinical Nurse Specialist—Diabetes, University of New Mexico, Health Sciences Center, Albuquerque, New Mexico

Trisch Van Sciver, RN, MS, PCNS, CFNP, Nurse Practitioner, Lovelace Health Systems, Albuquerque, New Mexico

Kristi Vaughn, RN, MN, Clinical Nurse Specialist/Case Management, Emergency Department, Oregon Health Sciences University, Portland, Oregon

Cynthia L. Vorpahl, RN, MSN, OCN, Customer Service Manager, Vitas Hospice, Houston, Texas

Pam Becker Weilitz, RN, MSN, CS, Manager, Nursing Care Delivery, Barnes and Jewish Hospitals, BJC Health System, St. Louis, Missouri

Una Elizabeth Westfall, RN, PhD, Associate Professor, Department of Adult Health and Illness, Oregon Health Sciences University, School of Nursing, Portland, Oregon

Joan Stehle Werner, RN, DNS, Professor, Department of Adult Health Nursing, University of Wisconsin–Eau Claire, Eau Claire, Wisconsin

Marie Bakitas Whedon, RN, MSN, OCN, Hematology/Oncology Clinical Nurse Specialist, Dartmouth Hitchcock Medical Center, Lebanon, New Hampshire

Diana Wilkie, Associate Professor, Department of Biobehavioral Nursing and Health Systems, American Cancer Society Professor of Oncology Nursing, University of Washington, Seattle, Washington

Joyce Yasko, RN, PhD, FAAN, Associate Director, University of Pittsburgh Cancer Institute, Pittsburgh, Pennsylvania

REVIEWERS

Barbara Albertson, RN, MN
Seattle, Washington

Jane Blackwell, RN, DNSc, CNM
Toledo, Ohio

Patricia Lidbetter Bradley, RN, MEd, MSN
Ste. Anne de Bellevue, Quebec

Diane Britt, RN, MN, CS, CDE
Seattle, Washington

Mary C. Brucker, RN, DNSc, CNM
Dallas, Texas

Richard Buhrer, RN, MN, CRRN
Seattle, Washington

Janet Crimlisk, RN, MSN, CS
Boston, Massachusetts

Julie Dax, RN, MSN
Albuquerque, New Mexico

Kathleen Dietz-Lovett, RN, MA, MS
Marstons Mills, Massachusetts

Carol Dolan, RN, MSN, OCN
Albuquerque, New Mexico

Katie Drake-Speer, RN, MSN
Tuskegee, Alabama

Tana Durnbaugh, EdD, RNCS
Grayslake, Illinois

Mary Beth Egloff-Parr, RN, MSN, CCRN
San Diego, California

Susan Fairchild, RN, MSN, CNOR, CS, Doctoral Candidate-EdD
Pembroke Pines, Florida

Mary Ann Faucher, RN, MS, MPH
Dallas, Texas

Florencetta Hayes Gibson, RN, MEd, MSN
Monroe, Louisiana

Eileen Grass, RN, MSN
Albuquerque, New Mexico

Mikel Gray, RN, PhD, CURN, CCCN
Louisville, Kentucky

Pauline McKinney Green, RN, PhD
Washington, District of Columbia

Peggi Guenter, RN, PhD, CNSN
Philadelphia, Pennsylvania

Jim Halloran, RN, MSN, OCN, ANP
Houston, Texas

Jacqueline Helt, RN, BSN
New York, New York

Kathryn Hennessy, RN, MS, CNSN
Northbrook, Illinois

Kay A. Herth, RN, PhD, FAAN
Statesboro, Georgia

Mary Jo Holechek, RN, MS, CNN
Baltimore, Maryland

Linda Janusek, RN, PhD
Maywood, Illinois

Judy Knighton, RN, MScN
Toronto, Ontario

Hilary Lipe, RN, MN
Seattle, Washington

Karen March, RN, MN
Seattle, Washington

Deborah L. Martin, RN, MN
Austin, Texas

Sandi Martin, RN, BSN, CCRN
Salt Lake City, Utah

Donna McCarthy, RN, PhD
Madison, Wisconsin

Lora McGuire, RN, MS
Joliet, Illinois

Gail D'Eramo Melkus, RN, EdD, CDE, ANP
New Haven, Connecticut

Mary Merchant, RN, MSN
Charleston, South Carolina

Jim Mulchay, RN, BA, CRNA
Ft. Lauderdale, Florida

Joan Murphy, RN, MS, EdD in Progress
Utica, New York

Mary Lou Muwaswes, RN, MS
San Francisco, California

Madeline Naegle, RN, PhD, FAAN
New York, New York

Janice Smith Pigg, RN, MS
Milwaukee, Wisconsin

Mary F. Rodts, RN, MS, ONC
Chicago, Illinois

Roberta Ronayne, RN, BScN(ed), MSc(A)
Ottawa, Ontario

Linda Schakenbach, RN, MSN, CS, CCRN
Annandale, Virginia

Darlene Schelper, RN, MSN, CEN
Albuquerque, New Mexico

Kay D. Sedler, RN, MN, CNM
Albuquerque, New Mexico

Juli Shea, RN, MSN, CCRN
Starr, South Carolina

Sandra Somma, RN, BSN
New Haven, Connecticut

Marilyn Sommers, RN, PhD
Cincinnati, Ohio

Susan Stillwell, RN, MSN
Shaker Heights, Ohio

Sharon Walker, RN, MSN, CCRN, CNRN
Albuquerque, New Mexico

Sally Weiss, RN, MSN
Pembroke Pines, Florida

Norma Jean Weldy, BS, MS
Goshen, Indiana

Donna Wilson, RN, RRT, MSN
New York, New York

To the profession of nursing
and
to the important people in our lives

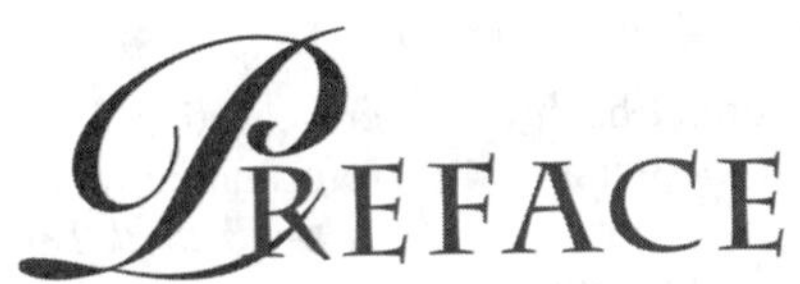

The knowledge base on which nurses make decisions changes rapidly. To accommodate these changes, we have prepared a revised, updated, and expanded edition of *Medical-Surgical Nursing: Assessment and Management of Clinical Problems.*

The strengths of the first three editions have been retained, including the use of the nursing process as an organizational theme for nursing management and a commitment to support the role of nurses on the health care team. Numerous new features have been added to address some of the rapid changes in practice. Contributors have again been selected for their acknowledged excellence in specific content areas; one or more specialists in the subject area has thoroughly reviewed each chapter to increase accuracy. The editors have undertaken final rewriting and editing to achieve internal consistency. All efforts were directed to building on the strengths of the previous edition and preparing an even more effective new edition.

ORGANIZATION

Content is organized into two major divisions. The first division (Section One: Chapters 1 through 8) discusses general nursing concepts related to adult patients. We have intentionally omitted material typically covered in nursing fundamentals textbooks to avoid overlap in content and keep the book at a manageable length. The second division (Sections Two through Nine: Chapters 9 through 62) presents nursing assessment and the nursing role in management of medical-surgical problems.

To promote the reader's understanding of the body as an integrated whole, we have grouped the various body systems to reflect their interrelated functions. Each section is organized around two main themes: assessment and management. Chapters dealing with the first theme, *assessment of a body system,* include a discussion of the following:

1. A brief review of anatomy and physiology focusing on information that will promote understanding of nursing care.
2. Health history and noninvasive physical assessment skills to expand the data base on which decisions are made.
3. Common diagnostic studies, expected results, and related nursing responsibilities to provide easily accessible information.

The second theme is the *nursing role in management* of the various diseases and disorders of body systems. Chapters embracing this theme focus on the significance and pathophysiologic bases of the diseases and disorders, clinical manifestations, and diagnostic study results. In addition, each chapter presents a concise discussion of the usual therapeutic and nursing management for major diseases and disorders. The nursing management sections are organized into nursing assessment, nursing diagnoses, planning, and nursing implementation. Levels of care continue to be the organizational theme for nursing implementation, enabling the nurse to provide care related to the following:

1. Health promotion and maintenance
2. Acute intervention
3. Chronic and home care

This unique and functional approach is used in discussing nursing management of all major health problems.

SPECIAL FEATURES

We have added many new features to this edition to address trends in nursing practice and to increase the overall appeal of the book.

■ *Color* The addition of color is used throughout for both functionality and visual enhancement. Color has been used in headings to make content easier to locate, in tables and boxes to draw attention to special topics, in figures for clarity, and in pedagogy for emphasis. The use of color—a first in medical-surgical nursing texts—is an important addition because it will more fully engage students in the content.

■ *Gerontology* The fourth edition offers expanded content devoted to the older adult in both the assessment and management chapters. Each assessment chapter has a table highlighting gerontologic differences in physical assessment findings. A chapter on gerontology has been added. This focus on gerontology reflects the changing population demographics related to the increasing number of older adults. Gerontologic content is denoted with a symbol for emphasis.

■ *Nursing Management* Content has been expanded in all areas related to nursing management of health problems. Phases of the nursing process have been delineated more specifically in this edition and include greatly expanded content on problem-specific nursing diagnoses. The theoretic background for the nursing process and its specific components are presented in Chapters 1 and 4. Defining characteristics for nursing diagnoses and rationales for nursing interventions have been added to all nursing care plans. Each of the more than 80 nursing care plans in this edition includes nursing diagnoses, defining characteristics, nursing interventions, rationales, planning and outcome criteria, and collaborative problems.

■ *Nursing Assessment* Nursing assessment tables are divided into subjective and objective data. The presentation of subjective data has been revised using functional health patterns in both the assessment chapters and in the nursing assessment tables.

■ *Key Assessment Questions* These highlighted nursing assessment tables identify key questions to ask patients related to a specific disease. These tables appear in each assessment chapter and are indicated with a symbol.

■ *Common Assessment Abnormalities* These tables also appear in each assessment chapter to alert the nurse to frequently encountered assessment abnormalities. These tables are indicated with a symbol.

■ *Nursing Research* Nursing research boxes in the management chapters present relevant nursing research studies. These research boxes assist the learner in incorporating results from nursing research studies into clinical practice. Nursing research issues at the ends of management chapters present possible research questions that could be used for research studies. Nursing research-based articles in the references and bibliographies are marked with asterisks.

■ *Cultural and Ethnic Considerations* Cultural and ethnic information is highlighted in boxes where appropriate. In addition, this material is integrated throughout the text in relevant areas. This content has been expanded to highlight important issues related to the nursing care of various ethnic populations.

■ *Ethical Dilemmas* Ethical dilemma boxes have been added to management chapters to help the readers focus on bioethical principles. To promote decision-making skills, each box presents a discussion of ethical and legal principles.

■ *Clinical Pathways* Examples of clinical pathways for major diseases and disorders are presented throughout the text to show how hospitals are implementing collaborative management.

■ *Emergency Management* Emergency management tables, denoted with ✚, outline treatment of health problems most likely to require emergency intervention.

■ *Nutritional Management* Nutritional management tables, marked with a △ symbol, summarize nutritional interventions for patients with specific conditions.

■ *Critical Care* A new chapter on critical care has been added to provide timely information on this specialty practice area that is of increasing importance to medical-surgical nursing students.

LEARNING AIDS

We have also added or revised numerous new learning aids for this edition.

■ *Learning Objectives and Review Questions* Learning objectives precede each chapter to focus on essential content, and multiple-choice review questions follow each chapter to enable the reader to assess mastery of the content. An answer key for the review questions is found in the appendix.

■ *Case Study with Critical Thinking Challenges* Each management chapter concludes with a case study with critical thinking questions. The case studies have been reformatted to guide critical thinking.

■ *Critical Thinking Content* To promote the development of clinical decision-making skills, we have provided critical thinking content in the following areas: ethical dilemmas, nursing research issues, and case studies. This content is identified with a symbol.

■ *Tables and Figures* The authors recognize that learning occurs in a variety of ways. This book intentionally addresses both the verbally-oriented and the visually-oriented learner. Accordingly, the authors use both approaches and have selected many tables and over 700 color figures to supplement the text.

ANCILLARIES

Accompanying the fourth edition is an enhanced ancillary package.

■ *Clinical Companion to Medical-Surgical Nursing* This portable clinical handbook includes approximately 250 medical-surgical conditions and associated outcomes, nursing diagnoses, and management.

■ *Transparency Acetates* Illustrations reproduced as transparency acetates make the book's most informative figures available for use in the classroom.

■ *Instructor's Resource Manual* The new Instructor's Resource Manual provides key terms, chapter outlines with suggested teaching strategies, case studies with critical thinking questions, and the content from the Study Guide.

■ *Study Guide* This extensive guide presents review questions and worksheets in a variety of formats. Case studies with critical thinking questions are also included.

■ *Test Bank* A completely new Test Bank is bound in a printed manual. The Test Bank is also available in IBM- and Macintosh-computerized versions. The bank contains over 1000 questions. Twenty-five percent of the questions are based on case studies and 75% are independent questions. The test questions are coded for correct answer, cognitive level, step in the nursing process, and NCLEX application.

ACKNOWLEDGMENTS

The editors are especially grateful to many people at Mosby-Year Book who assisted with this major revision effort. In particular, we wish to thank the team of Robin Carter, Jeanne Allison, Dana Peick, Catherine Albright, Dottie Martin, and Amy Buxton. In addition, we want to thank the marketing team of Joyce Owen, Tim Griswold, and Bob Boehringer.

Our persevering typists have earned our special thanks and include Loretta Campbell and Christa Cooper. Kay McCash provided invaluable assistance as a consultant on nursing diagnoses and revision of the nursing care plans. Pat O'Brien worked diligently on the Test Bank and provided excellent new material for the Study Guide and the Instructor's Resource Manual.

We are particularly grateful to the nurses and student nurses who have put their faith in our book to assist them on their path to excellence. The increasing use of this book throughout the United States and Canada has been gratifying. We are grateful to the many users who have shared their comments and suggestions on the previous editions.

We also wish to thank our contributors and reviewers for their conscientious attention to detail throughout the revision process. Their commitment to nursing kept them at their tasks until the job was done. We sincerely hope that this book will assist both students and clinicians in practicing truly professional nursing.

Sharon Lewis Idolia Cox Collier Margaret McLean Heitkemper

Publisher's Note

The publication of this book represents a landmark in Mosby's publishing history. This textbook is our first four-color book manufactured by going direct from disk to printing plate, without using film. This electronic process is a revolutionary change in the printing technology of textbooks and is likely to become a standard practice in the industry.

CONTENTS

Section One

GENERAL CONCEPTS of NURSING PRACTICE

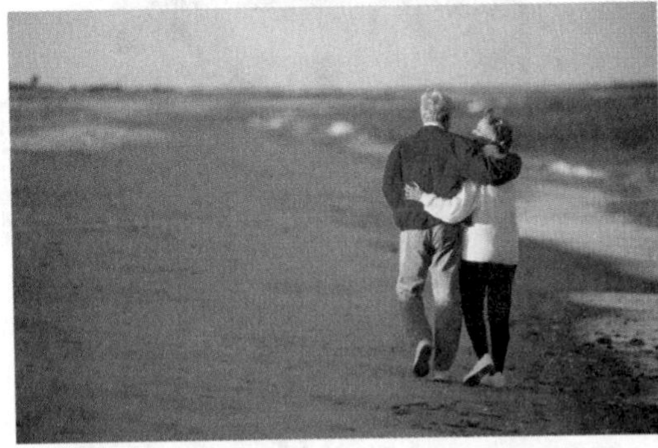

Section Two

PATHOLOGIC MECHANISMS of DISEASES

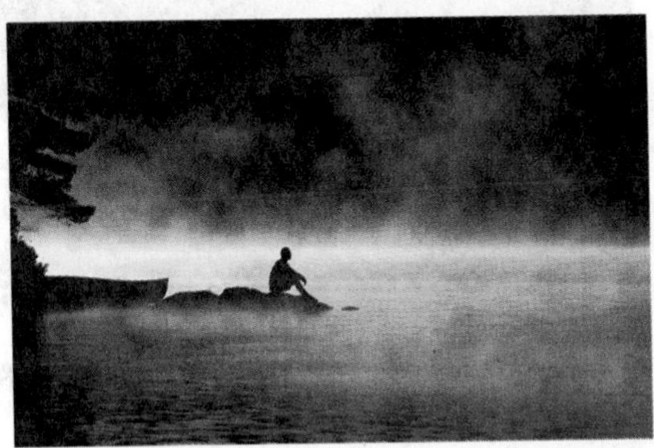

Section Three

The Surgical Experience

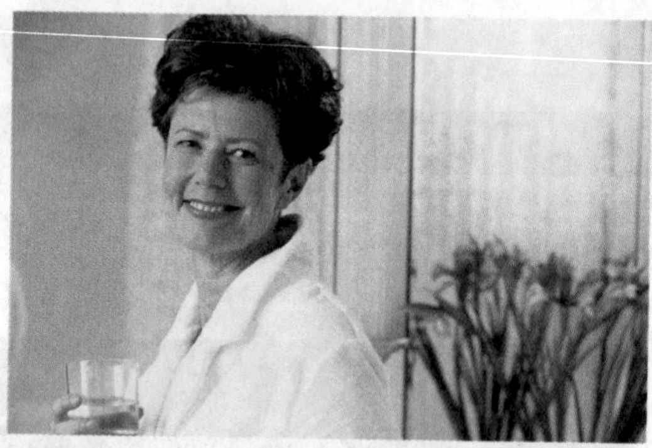

Section Four

Problems Related *to* Altered Sensory Input

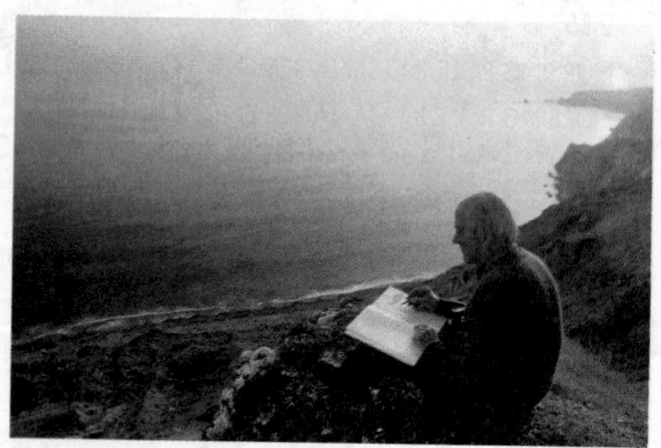

Section Five

Problems *of* Oxygenation: Ventilation

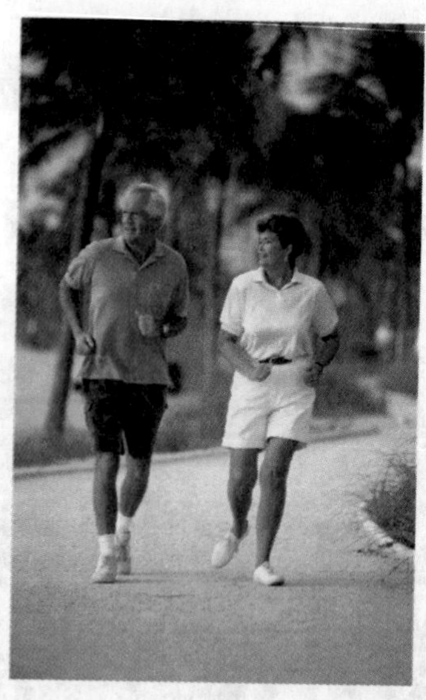

Section Six

PROBLEMS *of* OXYGENATION: TRANSPORT

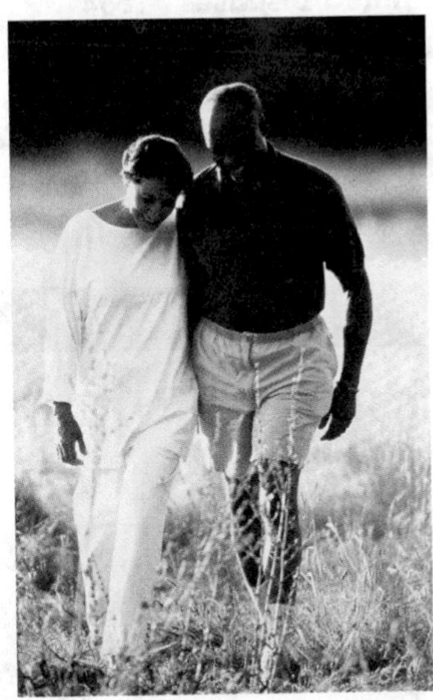

Section Seven

PROBLEMS *of* OXYGENATION: PERFUSION

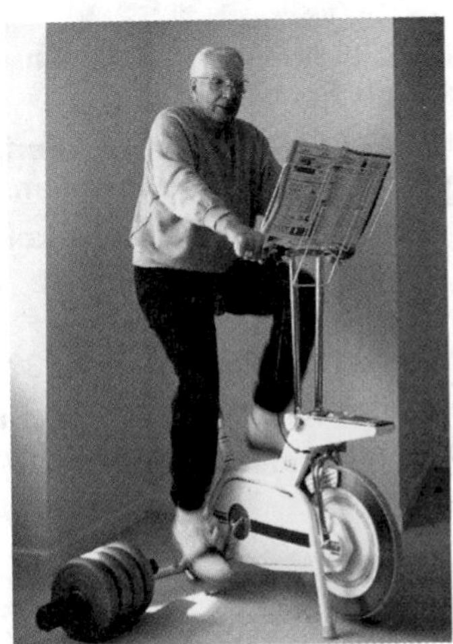

Section Eight

PROBLEMS *of* INGESTION, DIGESTION, ABSORPTION, *and* ELIMINATION

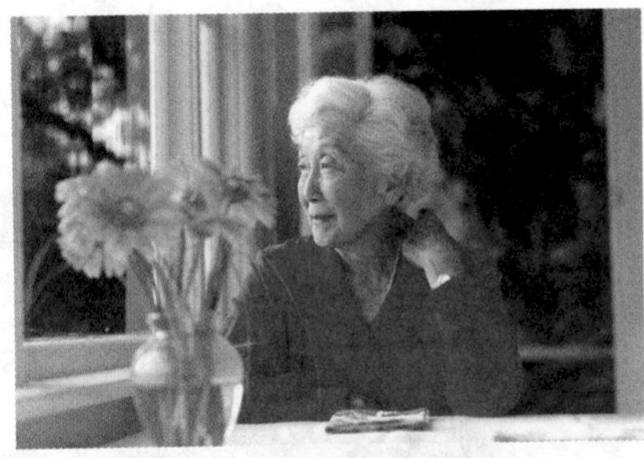

Section Nine

PROBLEMS of URINARY FUNCTION

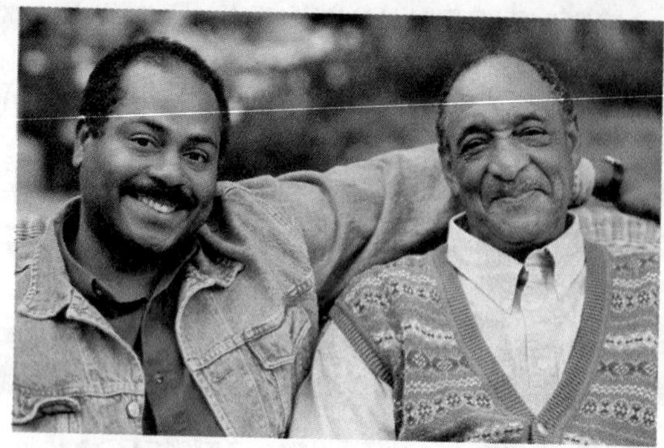

Section Ten

PROBLEMS RELATED to REGULATORY MECHANISMS

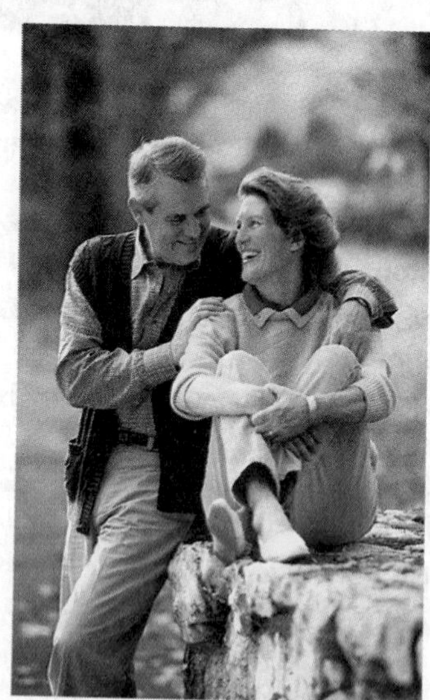

Section Eleven

PROBLEMS RELATED to MOVEMENT and COORDINATION

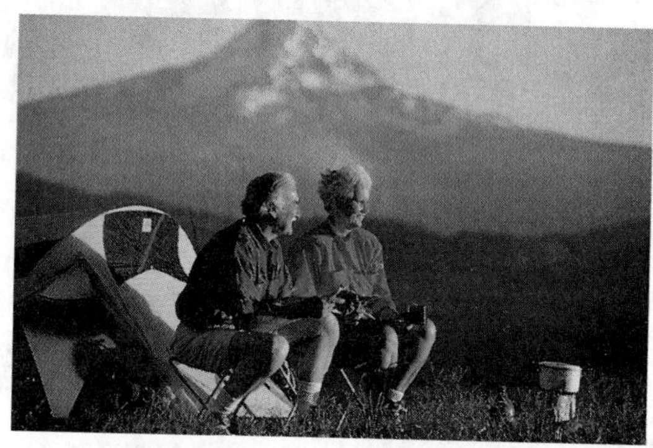

Section Twelve

NURSING CARE *in* SPECIALIZED SETTINGS

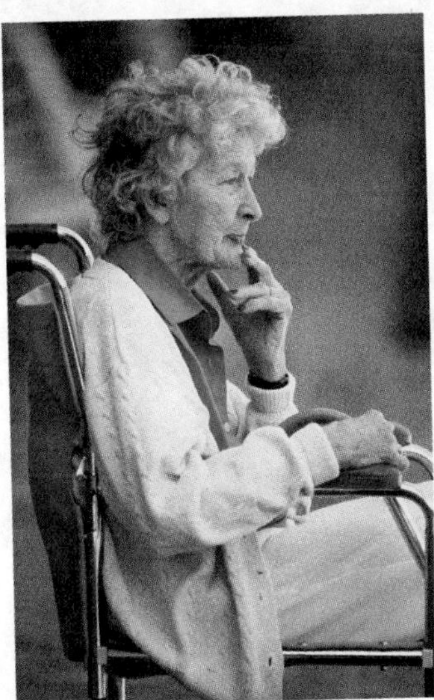

Appendixes

DETAILED CONTENTS

Section One

GENERAL CONCEPTS *of* NURSING PRACTICE

Section Two

PATHOLOGIC MECHANISMS *of* DISEASES

Section Three

THE SURGICAL EXPERIENCE

Section Four

PROBLEMS RELATED *to* ALTERED SENSORY INPUT

Section Seven

PROBLEMS *of* OXYGENATION: PERFUSION

Section Eight

PROBLEMS *of* INGESTION, DIGESTION, ABSORPTION, *and* ELIMINATION

Section Nine

PROBLEMS *of* URINARY FUNCTION

Section Ten

PROBLEMS RELATED *to* REGULATORY MECHANISMS

Section Twelve

NURSING CARE *in* SPECIALIZED SETTINGS

General Concepts of Nursing Practice

Section One

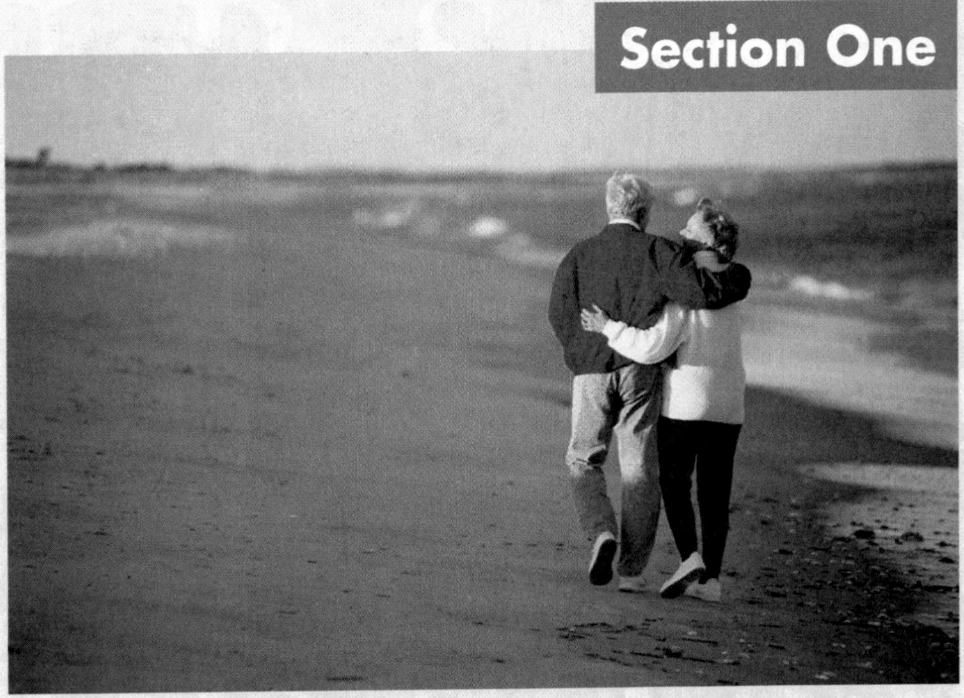

Chapter 1

GENERAL CONCEPTS

Nursing Process

Katheryn Ellen McCash

Learning Objectives

1. Describe the basic focus of the domain of nursing.
2. Distinguish among the independent, dependent, and collaborative functions of nursing practice.
3. Describe the five phases of the nursing process.
4. Differentiate between subjective and objective data.
5. Describe factors that affect success in obtaining accurate information during an interview.
6. Differentiate between the process of making a nursing diagnosis and a nursing diagnosis as a form of diagnostic nomenclature.
7. Describe the criteria for writing patient goals.
8. Identify the types of interventions a nurse can use to implement the plan.
9. Identify the places in the nursing process where evaluation is appropriate.
10. Describe the importance of documentation to the nursing process.

The nursing process is a framework used by the nurse to organize thinking about the health care needs of individuals, families, and communities and to organize and deliver nursing care. Once learned, the nursing process becomes an inherent part of nursing care and is actualized in the unique style of each nurse.

NURSING YESTERDAY AND TODAY

In primitive times, there was no distinction between nursing and medicine. The sick and injured were merely cared for by those with nurturant instincts.[1] In more recent times, society has tried to differentiate between nursing and medical practice. However, even today there is not a clear delineation in the public view between nursing and medical practice.

Nurses deal with "the diagnosis and treatment of human responses to actual or potential health problems,"[2] whereas medicine is primarily concerned with the diagnosis and treatment of illness or injury. The emphasis for nursing is the *response* of an individual or group to an actual or potential health problem rather than to the disease process itself. For example, in caring for a person with a fractured hip, the nurse focuses on the self-care restrictions and the effects of immobility and pain. The surgeon is concerned with the type of surgery and prosthesis to use in doing the surgical repair.

Nursing's Territory

Many modern theorists such as Neuman, Orem, and Rodgers are attempting to precisely define nursing's domain.[3] Although much work is needed in testing nursing theories, many of the current issues in nursing today were concerns of Florence Nightingale. In 1893 she addressed holistic health when she emphasized that one must nurse the whole person rather than the disease.[4] Current emphases in nursing practice, such as health maintenance and promotion, health teaching, family and community nursing, establishment of trust, use of good communication skills, and stress reduction techniques, were all an integral part of nursing as defined by Florence Nightingale.[5]

In the 1960s the popular health care delivery system was the team concept in which each member of the team (physician, dietician, nurse) carried out a particular contribution to patient care in isolation. Fragmentation of care occurred as nurses and health care workers descended on the patient to complete their designated tasks. Nursing professionals were not satisfied with this system of fragmented care. Furthermore, changing needs of patients, a longer life span, and more leisure time have contributed to the changing role of nursing. Primary nursing care is once again seen as a means to deliver quality health care. Primary nursing care is a continuous and coordinated

---

Reviewed by Pauline McKinney Green, RN, PhD, Assistant Professor, Howard University College of Nursing, Washington, DC.

nursing process in which a primary nurse ensures that all the basic needs of the patient are met on a 24-hour basis.[6]

Managed care is a new health care delivery concept that evolved from the health care reform movement of the 1990s.[7] Interdisciplinary cooperation, as well as renewed appreciation of joint contributions of various disciplines, is the current trend. As a member of this interdisciplinary effort, the nurse case manager follows the patient from admission to the unit, through discharge, and back home in an effort to achieve optimal outcomes.

Expanded Roles

Today, those in the health care system also speak of expanded roles for nurses. These roles emphasize health assessment, diagnosis, and treatment of conditions previously considered only within the physician's domain. Examples of the expanded roles are clinical nurse specialist, nurse practitioner, nurse midwife, and nurse anesthesiologist. These nurses may work in hospitals, but they also may work in a variety of settings such as clinics, schools, and industry. A closer look at nursing history indicates that, rather than expanding into totally new areas, nurses are merely reclaiming old territory once held.

Nurses have always assessed their patients' health status. Today, however, as a result of scientific and technologic advances, there are new methods available requiring new equipment and skills. Today, nurses are asserting their right to learn and apply skills that enhance their abilities to determine health status. By increasing their assessment skills, nurses increase their data base on which they make sound judgments. The stethoscope was at one time the private domain of the chief physician. Today, no one questions whether the nurse should use this instrument in patient care activities.

By expanding their scientific understanding of pathophysiology, psychopathology, pharmacology, and biochemistry, nurses are better able to understand the scientific basis of assessment findings that indicate various levels of health or disease. Incorporating the sciences and humanities into nursing education has broadened and deepened the knowledge base of nursing practice. Nurses continuously face the challenge of keeping current with developments in science and technology.

Scientific and technologic advances have made an impact on health care and care of the sick. In response to these advances, nursing is in a state of evolution. In its attempt to keep pace, nursing would do well to remember what the Queen in *Through the Looking Glass* said to Alice[8]:

> Now *here*, you see, it takes all the running *you* can do to keep in the same place. If you want to get somewhere else, you must run at least twice as fast as that.

Increasing emphasis on accountability, assertiveness, persistence, risk taking, and decision making are essential if nursing is to "get somewhere else."

Definitions of Nursing

A basic question revolves around how the profession of nursing views itself. Several well-known definitions of nursing indicate that a basic theme of health, illness, and caring has existed since Florence Nightingale. Two such examples are:

> The unique function of the nurse is to assist the individual, sick or well, in the performance of those activities contributing to health or its recovery (or to peaceful death) that he would perform unaided if he had the necessary strength, will, or knowledge. And to do this in such a way as to help him gain independence as rapidly as possible.[9]

> Nursing is putting the patient in the best condition for nature to act.[4]

In this textbook the American Nurses Association's definition of nursing is used:

> Nursing is the diagnosis and treatment of human responses to actual and potential health problems.[10]

Nursing's View of Humanity

Nursing's view of humanity must be considered when describing nursing. Although different terms have been used, there is widespread agreement among nursing theorists that an individual has physiologic (or biophysical), psychologic (or emotional), sociocultural (or interpersonal), spiritual, and environmental components or dimensions. In this text the human individual is considered "a biopsychosocial being in constant interaction with a changing environment."[11] The individual is composed of dimensions that are not, in actuality, separate entities but are interrelated. Thus a problem in one dimension generally affects one or more of the other dimensions. Psychologic anxiety, for instance, affects the autonomic nervous system, a part of the biophysical dimension.

Growth and development are influenced by interactions with others. No two individuals are exactly alike. No one individual remains the same from moment to moment. Therefore each individual has value as an irreplaceable member of humanity. Inherent in this individuality is the right to develop unique potentials according to a personal value system to the extent that the exercise of this right does not deny it to others.

The behavior of the individual is meaningful and oriented toward fulfilling needs and coping with environmental stresses. At times, however, the individual needs assistance to meet these needs and to cope successfully.

THE NURSING PROCESS

Nursing accomplishes its goal of assisting others to resolve actual or potential problems by the use of the nursing process. The nursing process is a method of organizing thought processes for clinical decision making and problem solving.[12] Using the nursing process, the nurse can focus on the unique *responses* of patients to actual or potential health problems. The nursing process is actualized by means of the cognitive (thinking, reasoning), psychomotor (doing), and affective (feelings, values) skills and abilities used by the nurse to plan care for a patient.[13]

Phases of the Nursing Process

The nursing process consists of five phases: assessment, diagnosis, planning, implementation, and evaluation (Fig.1-1). However, numerous other terms or phrases are used in nursing to describe the steps of the nursing process (see Table 1-1). *Assessment* involves collecting subjective and objective information about the patient. The *diagnosis* phase involves analyzing the information, drawing conclusions from the information, and labeling the human response. *Planning* consists of setting goals with the patient, when feasible, and determining strategies for accomplishing the goals. *Implementation* is the plan set in action. *Evaluation* is the analysis of the effectiveness of the assessment, diagnosis, planning, and implementation phases.

Interrelatedness of Phases

The five phases of the nursing process do not occur in isolation from one another. For example, nurses may gather data about the wound condition (assessment) as they change the soiled dressing (implementation.) There is, however, a basic order to the nursing process, beginning with assessment. This provides the data on which to base the plan. A judgment about the nature of the assessment data follows immediately. Implementation follows a careful plan based on the nursing diagnosis. Evaluation continues throughout the cycle. This continuous evaluation provides feedback on the effectiveness of the plan or the need for revision. Revision may be needed in the data collection method, the diagnosis, the goals, the plan, or the intervention method. Once begun, the nursing process is not only continuous but also cyclic in nature. There is no limit to the number of times the cycle can be reinitiated. Application of the nursing process requires sound knowledge of the physical and behavioral sciences and a repertoire of intellectual, interpersonal, and technical skills.

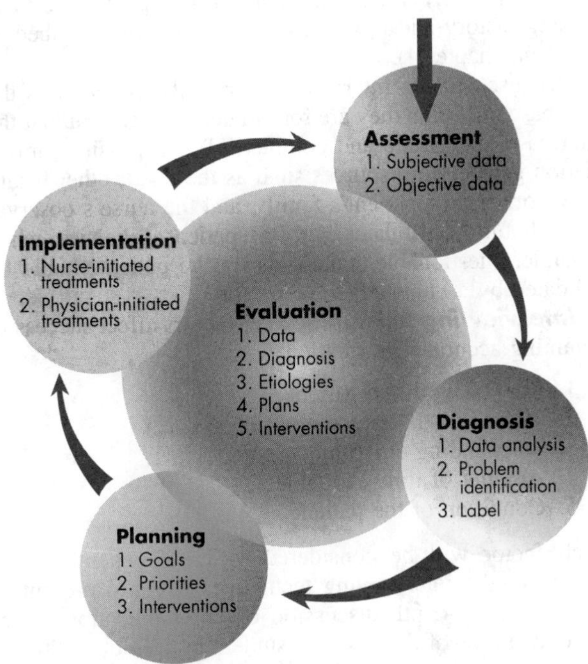

Fig. 1-1 The nursing process.

The nursing profession and the medical profession use a problem-solving process in caring for a patient. The uniqueness of nursing's problem-solving approach stems from the goals of nursing and the means of accomplishing these goals. A comparison of the goals of medicine and nursing is made in Table 1-2.

Independent and Collaborative Functions

Nursing practice has independent, dependent, and collaborative functions. As the profession becomes more autonomous, nurse-initiated (independent) interventions, such as health teaching, counseling, and other measures that assist

Table 1-1 Commonly Used Terms for Components of the Nursing Process

Assessment Phase	
	Data collection
	Data gathering
	Assessment
	Collection of information
	History and physical examination
Diagnosis Phase	
Step I:	Data analysis
	Assessment
	Judgment
	Decision making
	Clustering information
	Determination of strengths and weaknesses
	Determination of unmet needs
	Determination of assets and limitations
Step II:	Nursing diagnosis
	Problem identification
	Etiology determination
	Determining etiology of problem
	Labeling the problem
	Naming the problem
Planning Phase	
Step I:	Priority setting
Step II:	Expected outcome determined
	Goal setting
	Objective setting, subgoals
	Desired behaviors
Step III:	Planning interventions
	Planning nursing actions
	Nursing orders
	Planning strategies of care
Implementation	
	Application
	Intervention
	Nursing care
	Implementation
Evaluation	
	Reassessment
	Audit

Table 1-2 Comparison of Primary Goals: Nursing and Medicine

Nursing	Medicine
▪ Determines responses to health problems, level of wellness, and need for assistance	Determines etiology of illness or injury
▪ Provides physical care, emotional care, teaching, guidance, and counseling	Provides medical treatments and surgery
▪ Interventions aimed at assisting the patient to meet his own needs	Interventions aimed at preventing and curing injury or illness

the patient in meeting basic needs, are carried out to manage the nursing diagnosis.[14]

When a nurse carries out medical orders, the nurse functions dependently. Physician-initiated functions may include administering medications, performing or assisting with certain medical treatments, and assisting with diagnostic tests and procedures. The exact lines are often determined by individual state and agency policies. The nurse's role in most cases is one of "interdependence and coparticipation" with the patient and other health team members.

In the collaborative role, the nurse is primarily responsible for monitoring for possible or actual complications and for treating the patient to prevent or manage the complication. In this role the nurse may use either physician-prescribed or nurse-prescribed interventions.

In general, the nurse is expected to have the following intellectual, interpersonal, and technical skills:

Administrative	Leadership and management
Analytic	Physical examination
Communication	Improvisation
Counseling and referral	Psychosocial assessment
Creativity	Recording and reporting
Decision making	Research
Diagnostic	Teaching
Group leadership	Technical
Health assessment	Therapeutic
History taking	

Some or all of these skills are used during the various phases of the nursing process.

ASSESSMENT PHASE

Data Collection

A sound data base is the foundation for the entire nursing process. Collection of data is a prerequisite to diagnosis, planning, and intervention. A human being as a biopsychosocial being has needs and problems in all dimensions: biophysical, psychologic, sociocultural, spiritual, and environmental. A nursing diagnosis made without supporting data in all dimensions can lead to incorrect conclusions and depersonalized care. For example, a hospitalized patient who does not sleep all night may be mistakenly diagnosed as having a sleep-pattern disturbance. In fact the patient may have worked nights his entire adult life, and it is normal for him to be awake at night. Information concerning his sleeping habits is necessary to individualize his care so that he does not routinely receive a sleep medication at 10 PM. The importance of assessment to the process of clinical decision making cannot be overemphasized. The use of a nursing data base is recommended to facilitate the collection of data. Chapter 4 provides a detailed discussion of the nursing data base.

Subjective and Objective Data. A sound data base includes subjective and objective data. *Subjective data* are what the patient or family members tell you spontaneously or in response to direct questioning. *Objective data* are what the nurse and other members of the health team gather directly by methods such as measurement, inspection, palpation, percussion, and auscultation. This data can be verified by others. The patient's chart, diagnostic tests, and other health team members also provide additional useful subjective and objective data. An easy way to remember the common abbreviations, "S" and "O," is the following:

S = Subjective statements
O = Objective observations

In the initial assessment phase, most of the subjective data are obtained through the nursing history. However, while interviewing, the nurse also observes the patient's general appearance and nonverbal behavior. These observations provide some objective data. The majority of the objective data is obtained through physical examination of the patient. The nurse continues to obtain subjective data as the patient makes statements during the examination procedures, especially regarding pain during palpation. (The nursing history and physical examination are described in detail in Chapter 4).

Because nursing interventions are only as sound as the data base on which they are formulated, it is critical that the data base is accurate and complete. When possible, information gained from sources such as the chart, other health care workers, the patient's family, and the nurse's observations should be validated with the patient. Likewise, when possible, questionable statements by the patient should be validated by a knowledgeable person.

Interviewing Skills. Several factors affect success in obtaining accurate information:

1. Rapport with the patient
2. Timing of the interview
3. Surrounding environment
4. Amount of time available
5. Condition of the patient

Each factor will be considered as basic generalizations related to the interviewing techniques that are presented. Because an in-depth discussion of communication is beyond the scope of this text, the student in need of additional information is encouraged to refer to a specialty book on this topic.

First, the nurse should identify herself and explain the purpose of the interview. The patient should be informed about what information is needed and why. The patient cannot be expected to discuss personal health concerns with a caregiver without first receiving a sound reason. Seemingly nonpersonal questions posed by the nurse may be perceived by the patient as private information.

An interview should begin with easily answered, impersonal questions. As rapport is established, the nurse can advance to more personal questions. The nurse's comfort level with the topic, as well as a genuine concern for the patient, promotes rapport. The nurse needs to know the reason certain information is necessary and must have insight into personal attitudes and feelings about asking personal questions.

The nurse should listen to rather than anticipate the patient's comments. A nurse who is mentally planning how to respond to the patient cannot listen to what is being said. While listening, the nurse should closely observe the patient, noting any incongruency between verbal and nonverbal behaviors. Before beginning a purposeful interview, the nurse should take time to hear the patient's concerns. This not only helps establish rapport but can also provide important additional information. It is neither necessary nor wise to strictly adhere to a rigid interviewing format because much psychosocial data are obtained as the individual is allowed time to share concerns. Open-ended questions that foster discussion will provide the most information. In contrast, closed questions can be answered by a "yes" or "no" or by a short statement. Asking a patient to "Tell me about your pain," would elicit more information than a closed question, such as "Are you in pain?" The nurse should always give the patient sufficient time to answer.

The number and rapidity of questions asked during the history interview can give the patient a sense of urgency that discourages communication. The nurse should select words carefully, on the basis of the patient's apparent ability to understand. Underestimating or overestimating a patient's ability to comprehend the questions can negatively affect communication. The purpose is an interview, not an interrogation. It is important to use simple language. The nurse should never assume that the patient understands but should look for nonverbal and verbal clues and ask the patient to request clarification of unfamiliar terms.

The time of the interview should be carefully selected. Pain, fear, fatigue, anxiety, and other stressors associated with illness are examples of situations that should alert the nurse to defer an interview until a more appropriate time. A calm, comfortable patient is more likely to share information.

Careful attention should be directed to the environment. If necessary, the environment should be altered to make it more conducive to sharing information. For example, the nurse should provide privacy, close the door to eliminate distractions, and change the lighting or temperature in the room as necessary for the patient's age and condition. The patient's and nurse's attention are required for an interaction to be successful. The patient should be informed of the approximate amount of time the interview will take. The amount of time should be realistic, considering the nurse's responsibilities and the patient's condition. If additional time is required, the patient should be consulted for a suitable time. When possible the patient and nurse should be at the same eye level to reduce the possibility of the patient feeling dominated by the nurse; the nurse should avoid standing when the patient is lying in bed.

The patient's condition must be a primary concern when planning a data-gathering session. If acutely ill, the patient will be unable to expend energy on noncritical questions. Other sources of information such as old charts, family members, or friends may be used in such a situation. The nurse must be attuned to the patient's priorities when directing an interview. For instance, the nurse may want to focus on the learning needs of a preoperative patient, whereas the patient may only care to discuss how the pain will be managed postoperatively.

DIAGNOSIS PHASE

Data Analysis and Problem Identification

The diagnostic phase begins with the clustering of information and ends with an evaluative judgment about a patient's health status. This evaluative judgment is reached after analysis of the assessment data. Analysis involves sorting through and organizing or clustering the information and determining unmet needs, as well as patient strengths. The findings are then compared with documented norms to determine whether anything is interfering or could interfere with the patient's needs or ability to maintain his usual health pattern.

After a thorough analysis of all available information, one of two possible conclusions results. Either there are no problems that require nursing intervention, or the patient needs nursing assistance to solve a potential or actual problem. The final conclusions about the problems are the diagnoses.

Nursing Diagnosis

The term *nursing diagnosis* has many different meanings. To some it merely connotes the identification of a health problem. More commonly, a nursing diagnosis is viewed as the conclusion about an identified cluster of signs and symptoms. The diagnosis is generally expressed as concisely as possible according to specific guidelines.

Diagnosis is the act of identifying and labeling human responses to actual or potential health problems or stressors. Throughout this book, the term *nursing diagnosis* will mean (1) the process of identifying actual and potential health problems and (2) the label or concise statement that describes "a clinical judgment about an individual, family, or community response to actual or potential health problems and life processes. Nursing diagnoses provide the basis for the selection of nursing interventions to achieve outcomes for which the nurse is accountable."[15] The human responses identified, however, frequently result from the disease process. For example, a patient may have the medical diagnosis of chronic obstructive pulmonary disease (COPD). However, the nursing diagnosis will focus on how the COPD affects daily functioning (e.g., activity intolerance related to imbalance between oxygen supply and demand).

There are a number of other terms or situations that are not nursing diagnoses but are often mislabeled as such.[16] These include the following:

Medical pathologic conditions (coronary artery disease)
Diagnostic tests or studies (upper gastrointestinal series)
Equipment (nasogastric tube)
Signs (restlessness)
Symptoms (fatigue)
Surgical procedures (hysterectomy)
Treatments (pressure ulcer care)
Therapeutic goals (perform own oral care)
Nursing problems (difficult to turn)
Therapeutic needs (needs more rest)
Staff problems (Mr. Jones is too demanding)

Collaborative problems are potential or actual complications of disease or treatment that nurses treat with other health care providers, most frequently physicians.[16] A look at the primary goals of nursing (Table 1-2) helps in differentiating between nursing and medical diagnoses.

North American Nursing Diagnosis Association. Nursing is moving toward a common language for classifying patients' responses or problems. The identification and development of a classification system of nursing diagnoses formally began in 1973 when Kristine Gebbie and Mary Ann Lavin of St. Louis University called the First National Conference on Classification of Nursing Diagnosis. National Conferences have been held regularly since 1973.

Since the Fifth National Conference, the National Group for the Classification of Nursing Diagnosis has evolved into a formal organization and has been renamed the North American Nursing Diagnosis Association (NANDA). The two main purposes of NANDA are to develop a diagnostic classification system (taxonomy) and to identify and approve nursing diagnoses. A list of diagnoses accepted by NANDA for clinical testing is found in Appendix A.

The accepted diagnoses are evolving as research results are interpreted. In addition, the current NANDA list is not complete. The nurse may encounter diagnoses in clinical practice that are not cited on the list. Nurses are encouraged to submit refinements of accepted diagnoses and new submissions to NANDA.* A two-part statement is acceptable if the signs and symptoms data are easily accessible to other nurses caring for the patient through such means as the nursing history or progress note. Use of a three-part statement is recommended during the learning process. The terminology from the NANDA list of accepted nursing diagnoses will be used in this text.

Diagnostic Process

Nursing diagnostic statements are acceptable when written as two-part or three-part statements. When written as a three-part statement, the problem-etiology-signs and symptoms (PES) format is used.[17]

Problem (P): A brief statement of the patient's potential or actual health problem
Etiology (E): A brief description of the probable cause of the problem; contributing or related factors
Signs and symptoms (S): A list of the cluster of the objective and subjective data that lead the nurse to pinpoint a problem; major or minor defining characteristics

It is important to remember that gathering the "S" comes first in the diagnostic process, even though the format has been described as PES.

Identifying the Problem. The NANDA list of accepted nursing diagnoses has been grouped using Gordon's 11 functional patterns (see Appendix A). This framework is extremely useful when analyzing the data for actual, at risk, and possible nursing diagnoses. Clinically relevant cues are clustered together. Clustered data are analyzed to generate diagnostic hypotheses. These hypotheses may include nursing diagnoses and collaborative problems.

However, the nurse should not force a problem to fit accepted terminology. At times the nurse may need to use a new word or phrase that should then be used consistently with the same problem.

It is also important not to state an untreatable condition, instead of the patient's underlying problem, as the "P" statement. "Inability to turn related to traction" is not treatable as such, whereas "risk for altered skin integrity related to effects of traction or immobility" is treatable.

Etiology. The etiology of a nursing diagnosis should be included in the diagnostic statement and separated from the defining characteristics. Taking time to refine the problem with its proper etiology directs the nurse to the correct interventions. Interventions are planned to manage the problem by directing nursing efforts toward the etiology. The etiology can be a pathophysiologic, maturational, situational, or treatment-related factor.[16] The etiology is written after the diagnostic label. These two components are separated by the statement "related to." For example, a correctly written nursing diagnosis might be, "Feeding self-care deficit related to upper limb weakness." The etiology directs the nurse to select the appropriate interventions to modify the factor of lower limb weakness. When the etiology is not included in the diagnosis, the nurse is not able to plan the correct intervention to treat the specific cause of the problem. When possible, the etiology should be validated with the patient. When the etiology is unknown, the statement reads, "related to unknown etiology."

Multiple etiologies become more common as expertise in the use of nursing diagnoses increases. There is often no single cause of a problem. Most nursing diagnoses presented in the general nursing care plans of this book contain multiple etiologies. They can be used as a checklist of possible related factors to be considered when determining the nursing diagnosis specific to an individual patient.

Signs and Symptoms. Defining characteristics are signs and symptoms commonly associated with a nursing

*NANDA, c/o NURSECOM, 1211 Locust St., Philadelphia, PA 19107-63104.

diagnosis. Major defining characteristics have been identified for most actual nursing diagnoses by NANDA publications. At least one major defining characteristic must be present to have an actual nursing diagnosis. Minor defining characteristics have also been identified and are suggestive as evidence of a possible nursing diagnosis. The signs and symptoms are included in the diagnostic statement using the phrase "... as manifested by." A correctly written nursing diagnostic statement would be, "Feeding self-care deficit related to upper limb weakness as manifested by inability to bring food to mouth."

PLANNING PHASE

Priority Setting

After the nursing diagnoses and collaborative problems are identified, the nurse must decide on the urgency of intervention needed. Diagnoses of the highest priority require immediate intervention. Those of lower priority can be addressed at a later time. When setting priorities, the nurse should first intervene for life-threatening problems involving airway, breathing, or circulation.

Maslow's hierarchy of needs also acts as a useful guide in determining priorities. These needs include physical, safety, love and belonging, esteem, and self-actualization.[18] As in climbing a mountain, the lower level must be reached before a higher level can be attained.

Another guideline in setting priorities is to determine the patient's perception of what is important. When the patient's priorities are not congruent with the actual situation, the nurse may need to give explanations or do some teaching to help the patient understand the need to do one thing before another. Often it is more efficient to meet the patient's priority need before moving on to other priorities.

Another suggestion is to identify nursing diagnoses that may be managed simultaneously. For example, the nurse may assess the condition of a pressure ulcer (impaired skin integrity) while giving morning care (bathing self-care deficit).

Identified priorities change as a patient's level of wellness fluctuates. For example, the patient's highest priority in the morning may be a need for information about diabetes because he is going home and must care for himself. During the teaching session, the patient shows signs of a hypoglycemic reaction. The nurse would interrupt the teaching session to provide a glass of orange juice to avoid a worsening of the patient's condition. Risk problems may have a higher priority than existing (actual) problems.

Goal Setting

After priorities are established, long-term and short-term goals need to be set (Fig. 1-2). Once goals are set, the nurse can then set outcome criteria, which will assist in the evaluation of nursing interventions. Although the ultimate goal for the patient is to maintain or attain a state of dynamic equilibrium at the highest possible level of wellness, the setting of more specific goals, both short-term and long-term, is necessary for systematic evaluation of the patient's progress. Short-term goals can be met relatively quickly (i.e., in less than a week). Long-term goals may take weeks or months to achieve. In today's acute-care setting where the length of stay is often short, there is a predominance of short-term goals. Long-term goals may be addressed by a community-based nurse. Short-term goals may also be small steps toward achieving a long-term goal. For example, a short-term goal may be, "Mr. Smith will ambulate with crutches 1 day postoperatively," whereas a long-term goal may be, "Mr. Smith will ambulate unassisted by discharge."

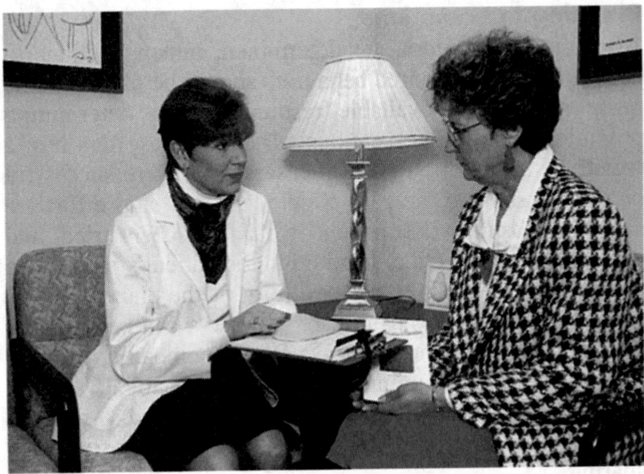

Fig. 1-2 Cooperation between the patient and the nurse is necessary in setting goals.

Thus goals must be worded as expected outcomes and with enough specificity so that everyone caring for the patient will be able to agree whether the goals have been achieved. Writing the goals in terms of desired, measurable behaviors and specifying a date when the expected outcome should be accomplished facilitates this process. To be worthwhile, written short-term goals should fit the following criteria:

1. Realistic and achievable
2. Measurable, observable, behavioral
3. Patient-centered (the patient's expected outcome)
4. Time-designated (by end of shift)
5. Mutually set

Short-term goals can serve as motivators for the patient and nurse, especially when a long-term goal takes significant time and effort to reach or when the patient is poorly motivated. For example, for the nursing diagnosis, "altered health maintenance related to lack of knowledge regarding oral hygiene," the long-term goal for the patient is to attain healthy gums and teeth. Short-term goals may be that after teaching sessions the patient does the following:

1. Demonstrates proper brushing technique after each meal
2. Demonstrates proper flossing of teeth before going to bed at night
3. Permanently refrains from chewing gum containing sugar
4. Visits the dentist by 11-9

Planning Interventions

After outcome criteria are determined, nursing actions to accomplish these desired behaviors should be planned. The nurse should use available resources when determining possible nursing interventions. The patient often has a wealth of information about measures that were successful or unsuccessful in the past. Significant time and effort are saved by asking the patient what has been tried and discarded as ineffective. In addition the patient's family can be consulted regarding the feasibility of the plan.

Other nurses and health care providers can be valuable sources for intervention ideas. Because members of the health team share common goals for the patient, sharing ideas to reach these goals should be encouraged. A patient-centered conference is an effective way to foster such sharing.

Literature and research provide valuable suggestions and information that can facilitate the process of determining a means to accomplish the goals. The nurse needs to foster the use of a research-based approach to interventions.

Sound knowledge, good judgment, and decision-making ability are required to effectively choose the interventions the nurse will use. Interventions should be based on sound rationales from the behavioral and physical sciences. In addition, the nurse must use ingenuity, intuition, creativity, and past experience when tailoring a plan to meet a patient's needs. The benefits of the intervention must outweigh the disadvantages. Factors such as availability of help, equipment, time, money, and other resources must also be considered. As in the case of goal determination, when the patient is able, the final selection of strategies remains the prerogative of the patient.

When recording the plan on the chart or Kardex, the nurse needs to be specific. Specificity enables everyone concerned with the patient to understand precisely what is to be accomplished. The plan should be tailored to meet each patient's needs and should note particulars, such as how, when, how long, how often, where, by whom, and with what. For example, "Wound care qid," is not an adequate plan. The following plan communicates much more: "The nurse (who) is to irrigate the leg wound (where) with 200 ml normal saline (with what) @ 9-1-5-9 (how often)." These specific, individualized interventions may be called *nursing orders*.

IMPLEMENTATION PHASE

Carrying out a specific, individualized plan constitutes the implementation phase. The planned activities that the nurse performs to accomplish the implementation phase are called *nursing interventions*. The nurse may carry out the interventions or designate others who are qualified to intervene (Fig. 1-3).

A nursing intervention is any direct action that a nurse performs (or designates others to perform) on behalf of a patient. These actions include nurse-initiated treatments resulting from nursing diagnoses; physician-initiated treatments resulting from medical diagnoses; and daily, essential activities that the patient cannot perform independently.

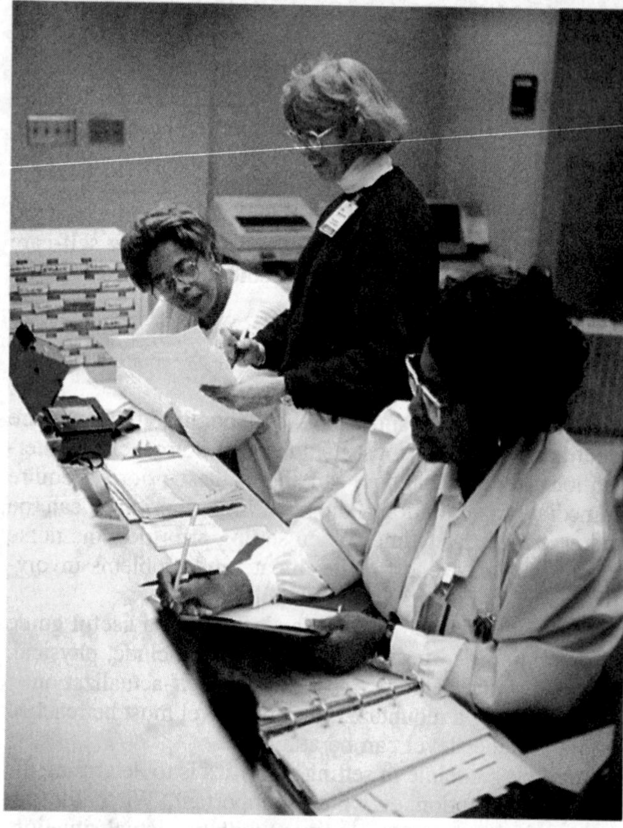

Fig. 1-3 Even though the nurse may designate another health care worker to implement a nursing activity, the nurse maintains responsibility for the patient's welfare.

When choosing an intervention, the nurse considers the following:

1. Appropriateness of the nursing diagnosis
2. Research base associated with the intervention
3. Feasibility of successfully implementing the intervention
4. Acceptability of the intervention to the patient
5. Capability of the nurse[14]

There are a variety of nursing interventions from which to choose. Examples include:

1. Directly performing an activity for a patient
2. Assisting the patient
3. Supervising the patient and family
4. Teaching
5. Counseling
6. Monitoring[14]

Throughout the implementation phase the nurse must evaluate the effectiveness of the method chosen to implement the plan. For example, the nurse may determine that the nursing assistant caring for a patient with a mastectomy should not continue to be the person who implements the patient's exercise plan. Perhaps the patient is more depressed than anticipated and would benefit from contact with a nurse who is knowledgeable about changes in body image and sensitive to patient cues that may indicate body image disturbance. The exercise plan might essentially remain the same, but the implementor of the plan would be different and would use different skills to carry out the plan. Referrals to other professionals may also be made when the nurse anticipates that expertise in specialized areas will help the patient.

EVALUATION PHASE

The diagram of the nursing process (Fig. 1-1) indicates that all phases must be evaluated. Evaluation not only occurs after implementation of the plan but is ongoing throughout the process.

The nurse evaluates whether sufficient assessment data have been obtained to allow a nursing diagnosis to be made. The diagnosis is, in turn, evaluated for accuracy. For example, was the pain actually related to the wound itself or related to pressure from a constricting dressing?

Next the nurse evaluates whether the outcome criteria and interventions are realistic and achievable. If not, a new plan should be formulated. This may involve revision of goals and interventions. Consideration must be given to whether the plan should be maintained, modified, totally revised, or discontinued in light of the patient's status.

The effectiveness of each intervention and its contribution to progress toward the goal are also evaluated. In addition, the nurse considers whether a different method of implementation of the same plan will provide better results.

Documentation

It is critical that the patient's progress be documented in a systematic way. Many documentation methods are used, depending on personal preference and agency policy. One method of evaluating and recording patient progress is the problem-oriented progress note, referred to as the subjective-objective-assessment-plan (SOAP) method. This type of progress note is problem-specific and incorporates the components described in Table 1-3. In some institutions, SOAP notes constitute the "Nurses' Notes" portion of the nurses' charting.

Table 1-3 Components of a Problem-Oriented Progress Note

	Explanation
Subjective (S)	Information supplied by patient or knowledgeable other
Objective (O)	Information obtained by nurse directly by observation or measurement, from patient records, or through diagnostic studies
Assessment (A)	Tentative conclusion or diagnosis based on subjective and objective data
Plan (P)	Specific interventions related to a problem or diagnosis considering diagnostic, therapeutic, and patient education needs

The process of SOAP documentation is as follows:

1. Additional subjective and objective data are gathered concerning the area of concern.
2. Based on old and new data, an assessment of the patient's progress toward the goal and the effectiveness of each intervention is made.
3. Based on the reassessment of the situation, the initial plan is maintained, revised, or discontinued.

For example, the diagnosis is risk for infection related to traumatized tissue secondary to surgery. Wound is more painful today is "S." Elevated temperature of 103°, facial grimacing, and dressing saturated with purulent drainage is "O." Risk for wound infection is "A." Notify surgeon, take temperature q2hr, and reinforce dressing is "P."

Other methods of documentation include the clinical pathway method, FOCUS charting, and charting by exception. The *clinical (critical) pathway* is a guide specifically designed to direct the health care team in the daily care goals for select health care problems. It includes a care plan, interventions specific for each day of hospitalization, and a documentation tool.[7]

The clinical pathway is part of a total clinical system that organizes and sequences the caregiving process at the patient level to better achieve quality and cost outcomes.[5] It is a cyclic process organized for specific case types by all related health care departments. The case types selected for developing clinical pathways are usually those that occur in high volume and are highly predictable.

The clinical pathway describes the care required of a patient at specific times in the treatment. A multidisciplinary approach moves the patient toward desired outcomes within an estimated length of stay. The exact contents and format of these clinical pathways varies among institutions. Numerous samples of clinical pathways are presented in this textbook for major health problems.

FOCUS charting is a method of documentation that structures the nurse's note according to the focus of the note, such as a sign or symptom, a condition, or a nursing diagnosis.[19] *Charting by exception* is a shorthand method for documenting normal findings and routine care based on clearly defined standards of practice and predetermined criteria for nursing assessments and interventions.[20]

WRITTEN CARE PLANS

An individualized nursing care plan is recorded to facilitate continuity of care and to help avoid duplication of services. When kept as a permanent part of the patient's chart, the care plan can aid in the evaluation of nursing care. It also documents the patient's nursing care requirements and directs nursing care. Generally only the more unusual or unexpected problems are addressed in the care plan. Predictable routine problems experienced by many patients with the same diagnosis should be planned for but not necessarily recorded on the care plan. These routine problems are covered by unit policies or protocols.

Sometimes the care plan is written in pencil so that the outdated interventions can be erased; the current plan remains, avoiding confusion. However, this method should

NURSING CARE PLAN Sample

Planning: Outcome Criteria	Nursing Interventions and Rationales
➤ **NURSING DIAGNOSIS**	Pain *related to* surgical incision and localized pressure and edema *as manifested by* verbalization of pain, isolation, withdrawal
Verbalize satisfaction with pain relief.	Assess degree of pain *to plan appropriate intervention.* Administer analgesics as needed *to relieve pain.* Assess and document effectiveness. Encourage patient to avoid sudden movements *that increase pain.* Do not position patient on operative side *to avoid accumulation of fluid and subsequent increase in pain.*

not be used without some kind of permanent record of the plan, because the nurse also needs a source of information on which interventions were unsuccessful to avoid repeating them. The permanent care plan is considered a part of the legal medical record. Some nurses use a "highlighter" pen over completed or changed items, leaving current plans readable in ink while preserving a record of outdated care plans.

Institutions continually experiment with various methods of recording the care plan, and there are many formats available. An example of the format for a nursing care plan for the patient undergoing ear surgery is shown above.

Some institutions write the care plan in ink and retain the entire plan as a part of the patient's record. This kind of care plan often has a column for evaluation, where comments are recorded on the progress toward the outcome criteria and the effectiveness of the interventions.

Standardized care plans are often used as guides for routine nursing care and for developing individualized care plans. The care plans throughout this book are general or standardized. This type of plan lists nursing actions, or broad interventions, that are applicable to any number of patients having the particular problem. When planning individualized care, a standardized care plan should be personalized and made specific based on the unique needs of the patient.

SUMMARY

Nursing roles continually evolve as our society changes and we learn to apply new technology. Although nursing is defined in different ways, the various definitions of nursing have commonalities of health, illness, and caring.

Nursing care is provided through the application of the nursing process: assessment, diagnosis, planning, implementation, and evaluation. Assessment involves collecting data by chart review, performing an interview, and providing a nursing history and physical. Good interviewing skills are essential for obtaining these data. The nurse's skill at collecting subjective and objective data affects the quality of the data base.

There are two major steps to the diagnosis phase: data analysis and nursing diagnosis (or problem identification). The planning phase also has three major steps: priority setting, goal formulation, and planning interventions. The plan of action must be founded on a sound data base. Implementation, the actual carrying out of the plan, may be performed by the nurse or by someone whom the nurse designates. It continues throughout the nursing process.

Several methods of record keeping are used to promote continuity of patient care and facilitate the nursing process. These documentation methods include SOAP charting, critical pathway method, FOCUS charting, and charting by exception.

The nursing process requires the use of analytic thinking skills. It differs from medicine's problem-solving approach in its goals and the means of accomplishing its goals. Knowledge of the physical and behavioral sciences and specific skills such as critical thinking, teaching, counseling, and technical skills are required to apply the nursing process. Through the systematic use of the nursing process, nursing can best accomplish its goal of assisting others to maintain or attain optimal health.

REVIEW QUESTIONS

The number of the question corresponds to the same-numbered objective at the beginning of the chapter.

1. The focus of nursing is on
   a. diagnosis.
   b. treatment.
   c. human response.
   d. etiology.
2. An example of an independent nursing intervention is
   a. administering medication per physician's order.
   b. starting an intravenous fluid.
   c. administering blood.
   d. applying lotion to dry skin.
3. The phases of the nursing process are
   a. assessment, problem solving, diagnosis, evaluation.
   b. subjective, objective, assessment, plan.
   c. assessment, diagnosis, planning, implementation, evaluation.
   d. problem identification, goal setting, intervention, evaluation.
4. Which type of data is exemplified by a patient who describes his feelings about the impending surgery?
   a. Subjective
   b. Objective
   c. Invalid
   d. Irrelevant

5. Rapport is established in an interview by
   a. explaining your role and the purpose of the interview.
   b. telling stories to relieve tension.
   c. keeping the patient distracted from environmental noises.
   d. using humor to lighten the patient's concerns.

6. Which of the following would be considered a nursing diagnosis?
   a. Needs suctioning
   b. Sleep pattern disturbance
   c. Diabetes
   d. Restlessness

7. A patient goal should be
   a. patient-oriented and measurable.
   b. nurse-focused.
   c. a broad statement open to individual interpretation.
   d. determined by the nurse regardless of patient input.

8. Which of the following is a type of nursing intervention?
   a. Diagnostic tests
   b. Performing surgical procedure
   c. Health teaching
   d. Administering medication

9. The main purpose of the evaluation phase of the nursing process is to
   a. identify effectiveness of interventions and progress toward goal.
   b. assess the patient's strengths.
   c. implement new nursing strategies.
   d. describe new nursing diagnoses.

10. The primary purpose of the nurse documenting all steps of the nursing process is
   a. communication with physicians.
   b. for reimbursement of nursing services.
   c. to provide a record of the nursing plan, its implementation, and the patient's response.
   d. to maintain quality of care.

REFERENCES

1. Goodnow M: *Outlines of nursing history,* ed 6, Philadelphia, 1938, WB Saunders.
2. American Nurses' Association, Congress for Nursing Practice: *Nursing: a social policy statement,* Kansas City, MO, 1980, The Association.
3. Fawcett J: *Analysis and evaluation of nursing theories,* Philadelphia, 1993, FA Davis.
4. Nightingale F: *Notes on nursing: what it is and what it is not,* facsimile edition, Philadelphia, 1946, JB Lippincott.
5. Bower F, Bevis E: *Fundamentals of nursing practice,* St Louis, 1979, Mosby.
6. Manthey M: Can primary nursing survive? *Am J Nurs* 88:644, 1988.
7. Mosher C and others: Upgrading practice with critical pathways, *Am J Nurs* 92:41, 1992.
8. Carroll L: *Alice's adventures in wonderland and through the looking glass,* New York, 1973, Collier Books.
9. Henderson V: *The nature of nursing,* New York, 1966, Macmillan Publishing.
10. American Nurses' Association: *Standards of practice,* Kansas City, MO, 1973, The Association.
11. Roy S: *The Roy adaptation model, the definitive statement,* Norwalk, CT, 1991, Appleton & Lange.
12. Doenges M, Moorhouse M: *Nurse's pocket guide: nursing diagnosis with interventions,* Philadelphia, 1991, FA Davis.
13. Cox H and others: *Clinical applications of nursing diagnosis: adult, child, women's, psychiatric, gerontic and home health considerations,* ed 2, Philadelphia, 1993, FA Davis.
14. Bulechek G, McCloskey J: *Nursing interventions classification,* St Louis, 1992, Mosby.
15. North American Nursing Diagnosis Association: *Nursing diagnoses: definitions and classifications,* Philadelphia, 1994, North American Nursing Diagnosis Association.
16. Carpenito L: *Nursing diagnosis: application to clinical practice,* ed 5, Philadelphia, 1995, JB Lippincott.
17. Gordon M: *Nursing diagnosis: process and application,* ed 3, St Louis, 1994, Mosby.
18. Maslow A: *Motivation and personality,* New York, 1954, Harper & Row.
19. Lampe S: *Focus charting: a patient-centered approach,* Minneapolis, 1988, Creative Nursing Management.
20. Murphy J, Burke L: Charting by exception, a more efficient way to document, *Nurs* 20:65, 1990.

Chapter 2

GENERAL CONCEPTS

Adult Development and the Impact of Disruption

Charlotte R. Abbink

Learning Objectives

1. Explain the major concepts in the adult developmental theories proposed by Erikson, Peck, Havighurst, and Levinson.
2. Compare and contrast the disengagement, activity, and identity continuity psychosocial aging theories.
3. Describe the major psychodynamic concerns of young, middle, and older adults in terms of self-concept, concept of death, intellectual processes, and sexuality.
4. List the major family developmental tasks for young, middle, and older adults.
5. Compare the community activities of young, middle, and older adults in terms of work, leisure, and civic participation.
6. Describe important health maintenance concerns for young, middle, and older adults related to changes resulting from the process of aging.
7. Describe the impact of illness on young, middle, and older adults related to their developmental status.

WHY CONSIDER DEVELOPMENTAL STAGES?

For many nurses and nursing students, the first and sometimes only mental picture when reading the words "developmental stages" is of children. However, the entire human life span is a dynamic sequence of biologic, psychologic, and social changes that occur in predictable patterns. Like childhood, adulthood can be divided into developmental stages, although adult stages have not been as comprehensively described or studied as childhood stages.

The following discussion of adulthood describes predictable patterns in adult growth and development. Understanding these patterns gives the nurse insight into what may be happening in a patient's life at given points in the life cycle. Assessing growth and developmental status is as crucial in planning appropriate nursing care for an adult as it is for a child. Nursing care is superficial and incomplete if it separates the experiences of illness from what the patient is experiencing in all other areas of life.

Although predictable developmental patterns exist, caution must be used in imposing these patterns on a patient before first validating the unique developmental processes the patient is experiencing. For example, the nurse cannot determine that an unmarried young adult is not mastering the intimacy tasks until a complete developmental assessment is made and validated. The nurse also must be sensitive to the impact culture has on developmental expectations and norms. Developmental theories do not necessarily fit universally across all cultures, although they have underlying assumptions that are applicable to most of Western society.

CONCEPTUAL APPROACHES TO ADULT DEVELOPMENT

Theorists have proposed models for understanding adult development based on the following premises:

1. Adult development continues to occur in definable, predictable, and sequential patterns.
2. Critical periods occur throughout the life span when physical and psychosocial growth undergoes reorganization.
3. In each stage of development, there are certain normative activities or tasks to be accomplished.
4. Mastering the tasks of preceding stages is fundamental to transition and mastery of tasks in future stages.

The adult development models of Erikson, Peck, Levinson, and Havighurst use this stage approach. Table 2-1 summarizes the adult developmental stages according to these theorists.

Reviewed by Tana Durnbaugh, RNCS, EdD, Professor, College of Lake County, Elgin, IL.

Table 2-1 Adult Developmental Stage Theories

Theorist	Young Adulthood	Middle Adulthood	Older Adulthood
■ Erikson	Intimacy versus isolation	Generativity versus self-absorption	Ego integrity versus despair
■ Peck		Valuing wisdom versus physical power Socializing versus sexualizing relationships Emotional flexibility versus emotional impoverishment Mental flexibility versus mental rigidity	Ego differentiation versus work role preoccupation Body transcendence versus body preoccupation Ego transcendence versus ego preoccupation
■ Havighurst	Mate selection and marriage adjustments Establishing family and child rearing Home management Occupation launching Beginning civic responsibility	Launching teenage children Maturing relationship with spouse Adjusting to aging parents Career and occupational maturity Adult social and civic responsibility Developing leisure activities Adjusting to physiologic changes	Adjusting to health decline Adjusting to retirement Adjusting to social role changes Establishing satisfactory living arrangements Adjusting to death of spouse
■ Levinson	Early adult transition Entering the adult world Thirties transition Settling down	Midlife transition Payoff years	

Erikson's Theory: Psychosocial Developmental Conflicts

Erikson views personality development as resulting from the confrontations between ego and social milieu.[1] He identifies points in the life cycle when specific developmental conflicts become paramount because a person's capacities or experiences dictate that a major self-adjustment and adjustment to the environment must be made. In the process of making this adjustment, the individual moves toward one of two opposing positions, such as toward intimacy or toward isolation. When a person successfully masters a core conflict (such as intimacy), the negative sense (isolation) remains as a dynamic counterpart and may be demonstrated in new situations in which this conflict needs to be mastered again at a higher level. Although critical times for mastery of each core conflict exist, all conflicts are present throughout the life span. For example, autonomy is especially important to a toddler; however, adolescents striving for identity need some independent space, and older adults frequently suffer loss of autonomy when limitations are placed on their decision-making prerogatives.

Intimacy Versus Isolation. In Erikson's model, the young adult task is *intimacy* (Fig. 2-1). This involves fusing self-identity with the identities of others in friendships, for causes or creative efforts, or in close personal relationships, including sexual union. Intimacy requires a degree of commitment that necessitates sacrifice, compromise, and self-abandonment for the benefit of others. The young adult who avoids making this commitment to others, fearing the loss of self-identity, will experience a sense of isolation and, consequently, self-absorption.

Generativity Versus Stagnation. During middle adulthood, the primary task is *generativity.* Generative adults are concerned with establishing the next generation by nurturing and guiding either their children or other young people. A sense of productivity in work and creativity in living are also important components of this task. This core conflict probably arises out of an altruistic need to leave some mark that will make the world a better place in which to live. If generativity does not occur, adults experience a sense of stagnation and turn inward, becoming self-preoccupied and overly concerned with physical and psychologic health needs. The focus of self-absorbed people on physical changes of middle age may result in either invalidism or inappropriate youthfulness in an attempt to stay young. Regression to an obsessive need for pseudointimacy may occur, which may be expressed through affairs with younger members of the opposite sex.

Ego Integrity Versus Despair. Older adulthood is a time for reviewing the past and rearranging the "photo album of life." This bringing together of all the previous life stages should result in a sense of wholeness, purpose, and a life well lived, or a sense of *ego integrity,* according to Erikson. When a person accepts and approves of a unique life, death also can be accepted as a meaningful part of life. However, if the life review is laden with opportunities missed or wrong directions taken, a sense of despair arises. At this point the person knows life is too short to

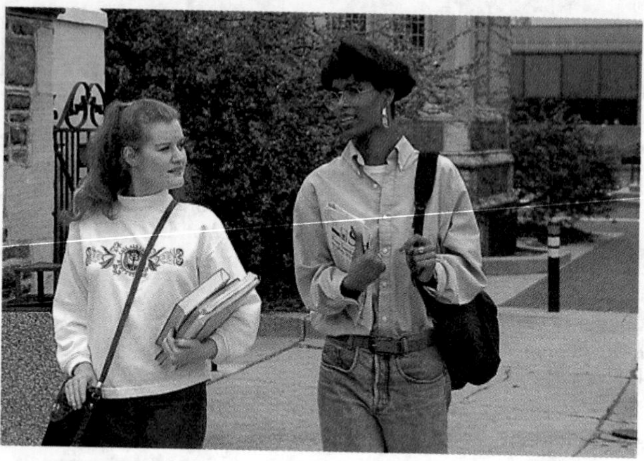

Fig. 2-1 The building of friendships is an important task for young adults.

correct the failures. Death is faced with anxiety because it steals away the chance to make changes. In this last stage of ego integrity versus despair, each person must face adjustments and come to a final conflict resolution that is the product of all previous developmental conflict resolutions.

Peck's Theory: Developmental Tasks

Building on Erikson's work, Robert Peck has further defined psychosocial tasks of middle and older adulthood.[2]

Middle Adult Tasks. Peck identifies four tasks relevant to middle adulthood. The first two tasks, *valuing wisdom versus physical power* and *socializing versus sexualizing relationships,* reflect the biologic changes of middle age. With a general decline in physical and sexual functioning, the middle-aged adult's self-esteem can suffer if it is heavily based on these attributes. However, judgmental abilities tend to increase with experience, so valuing the use of one's "head" becomes a positive alternative for maintaining esteem. The progression to a socializing relationship is appropriate as sexual motivations decline. This allows a love relationship to focus on total personalities and companionship rather than sexual performance.

Tasks three and four, *emotional flexibility versus emotional impoverishment* and *mental flexibility versus mental rigidity,* arise from the need for adjusting to life changes and new events that occur in the middle years. When children leave home, parents die, jobs change, and friends die or move away, adults must be flexible enough to shift attachments and reinvest emotions in other people and pursuits. People also need the mental flexibility to allow for new solutions to life problems, rather than being dogmatic and governed by past experiences or judgments.

Older Adult Tasks. Peck delineates three tasks for older adulthood. The first, *ego differentiation versus work preoccupation,* is important for maintaining a sense of self-esteem after retirement. This is achieved by reassigning the value of the work role to other roles and dimensions of life. The task of *body transcendence versus body preoccupation* involves recognizing physical decline but rising above aches and pains so that happiness is not defined by physical well-being. This task is exemplified by the person who experiences suffering but retains a zest and pleasure in life. The final task of old age, *ego transcendence versus ego preoccupation,* is very similar to Erikson's ego-integrity task. It denotes an ability to accept personal death without fear. It is neither a denial nor a passive resignation to death but an acceptance that moves the individual to be actively and emotionally involved in a legacy that continues. In contrast, the ego-preoccupied individual becomes mired in the thought of personal death, unable to let go of life and immediate gratification.

Havighurst's Theory: Developmental Tasks

Havighurst has also proposed specific developmental tasks for each life stage.[3] (See Table 2-1 for the list of tasks. The listed order does not imply hierarchic arrangement.) Like Erikson, he contends that there are optimal points in life to master these tasks and that current mastery is contingent on having successfully mastered the tasks of previous life stages. Unlike Erikson and Peck, who focus on individual developmental tasks, Havighurst includes family-oriented tasks that are significant to individual development.

Levinson's Theory: Evolution of Life Structures

Levinson and colleagues describe sequential eras in adult life that originally were identified with men. More recently, he has found that women go through the same sequences. However, women may have more difficulty planning a life course if the themes of family and career are viewed as mutually exclusive choices.[4] Levinson's basic concept, *individual life structure,* is the pattern of a given life at any point in time.[5] Life structure is formed by the interactions of self-system (for example, judgments, motives, and values), the social and cultural context of life (such as family, ethnicity, religion, occupation, and social events such as war), and the particular set of roles a person assumes (for example, husband or wife, worker, and friend). When any component changes, the life structure must reorganize (Fig. 2-2). Levinson considers some aspects of life structure, such as family and occupation, as central because they hold great significance to the individual; other aspects are peripheral because they are less critical and more fluid.

Life structure is dynamic, with predictable changes occurring as the individual moves through life. There are four major periods in adult life: early adulthood (age 20 to 40), middle adulthood (age 40 to 60), late adulthood (age 60 to 80), and late-late adulthood (beyond 80). Within each period the individual experiences alternating times of transition and stability in life structure. *Transitions* are a time of evaluating and making changes that permit growth and redirection of life toward identified goals and values. *Stable times* are those times for building on changes while maintaining an intact life structure to focus on the goals and values of that life period.

Early Adult Transition. The first transition is the *early adult transition,* which occurs between the ages of 18 and 22. The major concerns of this time are to terminate or modify existing life structures and to make preliminary adult choices that move an individual toward new life

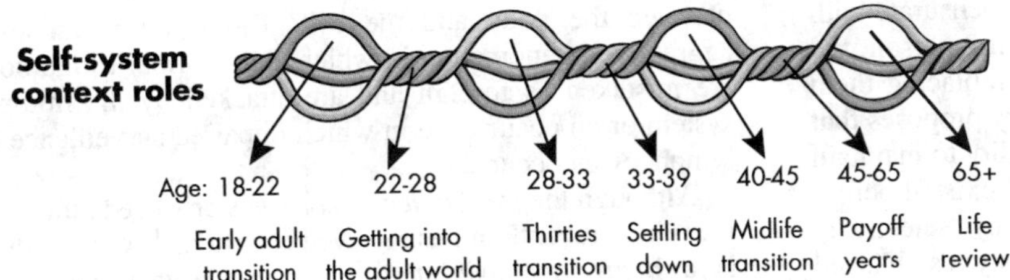

Fig. 2-2 An individual's life structure. According to Levinson's theory, life structure may be seen as a "life rope" in which the interacting strands are taken apart and individually reviewed during transition periods and are then rewoven in stable periods.

structures, consolidating an initial adult identity. This transition includes breaking away from the family of origin; making an initial career choice; establishing new intimate relationships; and selecting personal goals, values, and a lifestyle (Fig. 2-3).

Entering the Adult World. From ages 22 to 28, the young adult is *entering the adult world.* This is a time to grasp onto the adult world by doing what "should be done" as defined by external models such as family, peers, culture, and media. Concurrently, the young adult is working out a balance between building on previous choices and exploring alternative opportunities to avoid cementing the future prematurely. Because of this exploring, the occupational choices and relationships that are being established at this time may have a transient quality.

The Thirties Transition. The transition experienced between ages 28 and 33 may bring enrichment or dramatic changes to the life structure of the twenties. Previous commitments made to a mate, career, friends, and goals are evaluated with greater realism and a focus on self-directed decisions rather than external-directed decisions. Single persons may consider marriage, unhappy marriages may terminate, childless couples may conceive or adopt, and careers may be left or reconfirmed with new vigor.

Settling Down. During the thirties, there is a calm period referred to as *settling down.* This is a time of investing in those areas of life that are of primary importance, for example, family, work, friends, and community.

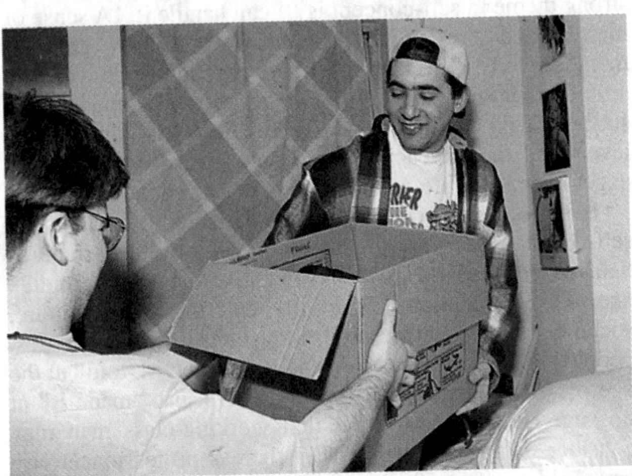

Fig. 2-3 The move from home to college is an external sign of the early adult transition.

During this time, establishing a place in society as a full-fledged adult is important so that an individual can advance and attain the goals that have been set. There is a striving toward exerting authority and gaining status and recognition with respect to and reward from others.

Midlife Transition. The *midlife transition,* occurring between ages 40 and 45, is the gateway into middle adulthood. This usually involves a profound reappraisal of life goals and values, with a concurrent emotional upheaval. Self-identity and authenticity are questioned and stripped of the illusions of young adulthood. All life structures are renegotiated, including marriage, friendships, occupation, and social roles. Time is realigned relative to the amount of time left to live. For some individuals, this transition results in a continuation of the previous lifestyle, but with new confirmation and enthusiasm for the current life structure. For others, there are varying degrees of change and, in some cases, dramatic reorganization of life structures. For example, a person may return to school to complete previously aborted educational plans.

The Payoff Years. As middle adults emerge from the transitional stage, having reorganized or reaffirmed the direction of life, they enter a time that may be very satisfying and creative. Ages 45 to 65 become the *payoff years* when people experience a time of maximum influence, heightened self-perception, self-approval, and self-direction. Middle adults can demonstrate wisdom and sound judgment as well as vision and innovation. Levinson projects that beyond middle age there is a continued growth process involving transition and stability based on previous life structures.

Psychosocial Aging Theories

Because developmental theories are least explicit about the later years of life, other theoretic approaches have been taken to explain the processes of aging. The *disengagement theory* proposes that successful psychosocial aging is characterized by a reciprocal decline in the involvement of the individual with society and society with the individual.[6] The criticism of this theory has focused on the proposition that disengagement is intrinsic and therefore a norm for successful aging. Disengagement will vary in older people depending on factors such as health, abilities, previous lifestyle, and personality type. Contrasting with disengagement, the *activity theory* maintains that continued productivity and social interaction are necessary for successful aging.[7] Although forms of activity may need to change because of reductions in physical health and strength, the level of activity with society should be commensurate with lifelong patterns. To remain engaged, the aging person will compensate for lost roles and activities by replacing them with new ones. The *identity continuity theory* proposes that adaptation to aging is correlated with the ability to maintain the same behavior patterns and lifestyle that existed before old age.[8] This continuity is maintained by selectively attending to those things that fit previously established behavioral patterns. However, in the present change-oriented society, maintaining consistencies in lifestyle is increasingly difficult.

Biologic Aging Theories

No single set of theories can describe the multidimensional process of aging. Some of the biologic theories that have been proposed are discussed below.

The *somatic mutation* and *intrinsic mutagenesis* theories postulate that aging is a result of lifelong genetic damage.[9] This damage may include the progressive accumulation of faulty copying in dividing cells or the accumulation of errors in information-containing molecules. According to somatic mutation theory, body cells develop spontaneous mutations in the same way germ cells do. These mutations are presumably a result of lifelong background radiation of various types. Subsequent cell divisions perpetuate the mutations until organs become inefficient and ultimately fail. The intrinsic mutagenesis theory suggests that the increase in mutational cells occurs because of a breakdown of genetic regulatory mechanisms. The basic premise is that the regulatory capacity of the human genetic constitution diminishes throughout life, and thus more mutations occur with aging that will ultimately result in functional failure. Although both theories are attractive, little evidence exists to support or deny them.

The *neuroaging theory* proposes that aging occurs because of functional decrements in neurons and associated hormones.[10] It suggests that neural and endocrine changes may be pacemakers for many cellular and physiologic aspects of aging. This approach relates aging to the organism's loss of responsiveness of neuroendocrine tissue to various signals. In some cases this is a result of a loss of receptors, but in others, it is caused by changes in neurotransmission beyond the receptors. An important focus of this theory is the functional changes of the hypothalamic-pituitary system, which are accompanied by a decline in functional capacity in all systems.

The *immunologic theory* proposes declining functional capacity of the immune system as the basis for the aging process.[7] It suggests that aging is not a passive wearing out of systems but an active self-destruction mediated by the immune system. This theory is based on observing an age-associated decline in T-cell functioning, accompanied by a decreased resistance and an increase in autoimmune diseases with aging. Whether the immunologic changes are genetically determined, regulated by environment, or influenced by endocrine factors remains to be defined. However, some studies of cell division suggest that the cells of the immune system become more diversified with age and demonstrate a progressive loss of self-regulatory patterns between the body and the cell. The result is an auto-aggressive phenomenon in which cells normal to the body are mistaken as foreign and are attacked by the immune system or an occurrence in which impaired surveillance by lymphocytes occurs.

Although the *free radical theory* was proposed almost 30 years ago, recently it has received attention.[11] A free radical is a highly reactive atom or molecule that carries an unpaired electron and thus seeks to combine with another molecule. The most common free radicals in humans are oxygen molecules. Free radicals are natural by-products of many normal cellular processes. They also are created by such environmental factors as tobacco smoke and radiation. This theory hypothesizes that free radicals alter basic genetic material, affect cellular integrity, and reduce cellular function and regeneration mechanisms.

Extensive research is being done on the use of antioxidants to combine with and inactivate free radicals. The antioxidant vitamins are E and C, as well as betacarotene. Optimal doses of these vitamins have not been agreed upon. These vitamins seem to be protective against several health problems associated with aging, such as oral esophageal and reproductive cancer, coronary artery disease, and cataracts. Antioxidants may even delay some effects of aging.[11] Further research will clarify the role of antioxidants and aging.

PSYCHODYNAMIC ISSUES OF ADULTHOOD

Psychodynamic issues arise from confrontation between inner development and the demands of the social world. People continually try to find a comfortable fit between themselves and their world, attempting to integrate their sense of who they are and who they are becoming.

Self-Concept

Self-concept and self-esteem are interdependent constructs. *Self-concept* may be defined as the totality of ideas people hold about themselves, and *self-esteem* is self-evaluation, that is, satisfaction or dissatisfaction with these ideas.

Young Adulthood. During the young adult years, a strong theme in self-concept is "I can handle it." A sense of mastery and self-control over life events and the environment prevails. The actions of young adults convey the attitude that self-will and boldness are the components of success. This confidence is a reflection of the high energy levels and the increasing power and control young adults experience over life when moving out of adolescence.

Middle Adulthood. During the middle adult years, self-concept may vary greatly, depending on the perceived balance between positive and negative aspects of middle age. This perception is partially determined by culture, social class, personality, and health status. In some cultures, people are programmed to consider themselves "old" at the age of 40; in other groups, people have just "made it" at this age. It has been found that working-class men may consider themselves old at 40, whereas professionals perceive old as after 70. Some middle-age people have "the time of their life," with an increased sense of self-approval because of peak family and career investments in terms of power, prestige, and income and continued good health. In contrast, if people experience a decline in career or health, self-esteem may also decline.

The sense of self-control continues into middle age; however, during middle adulthood, people recognize the finiteness of life and shift to a more realistic appraisal of the limits of self-will. Recognizing that willpower alone does not overcome life circumstances, people become aware that help and advice from others can be valuable rather than allowing it to threaten self-esteem. With this new insight regarding self-will, middle-age adults may also reevaluate a personal spiritual position, determining that placing trust in God is not a crutch for the weak personality but a desire for living beyond human finiteness (Fig. 2-4).

Older Adulthood. Although self-concept is usually stable from middle age to old age, it is not static. Life events experienced with aging (poor health, loss of income, loss of roles, isolation, relocation, and institutionalization) all serve to decrease the older adult's sense of control and may threaten self-esteem. However, it has been found that older people have compensatory mechanisms to offset some threats brought on by aging changes. A paradox exists in that age perception decreases with age. Older adults may think of age peers as old, according to social stereotypes attributed to older people. However, they may not perceive themselves as old and will refuse to respond to the suggestions of others that they are aging or need help or care. Another compensatory mechanism is that many older adults retain their middle-age self-concepts by thinking of themselves in their former roles. A retired farmer still may think of himself as a farmer, or a school teacher as a teacher. Maintaining a consistent sense of self, making decisions, and managing life are clearly important to well-being at this stage of life. Autonomy and dignity are essential elements to an older adult's positive self-esteem.

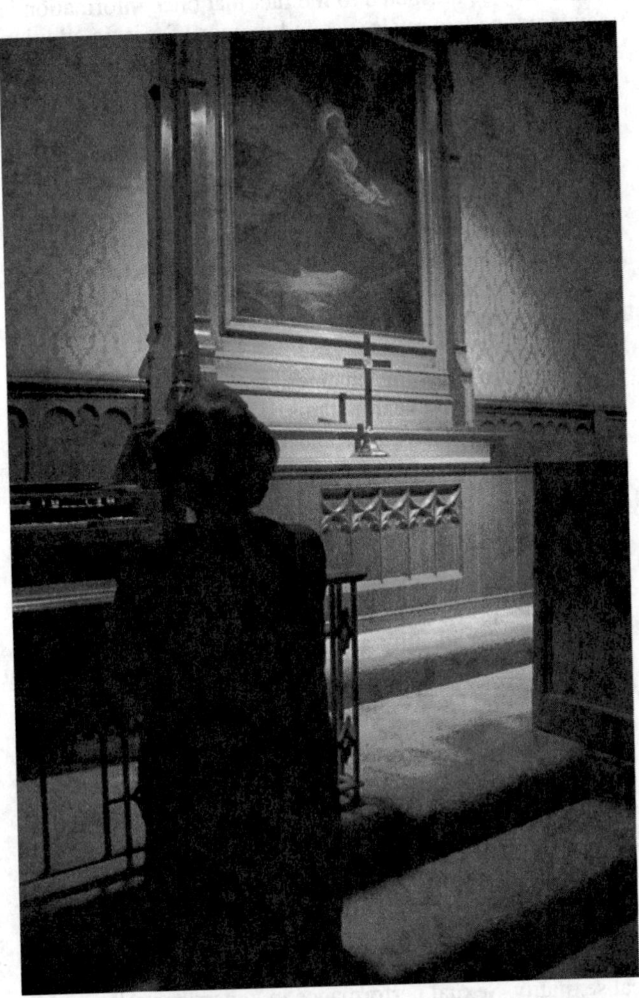

Fig. 2-4 An increasing awareness of spiritual needs often occurs in the middle years.

Conception of Death and Dying

Death is more than a biologic event; it is also a social phenomenon. It has been conceptualized as a life course or "career" with a social stage and a terminal stage.[12]

The *social stage of death* begins early in life with an awareness of finitude. However, this recognition is not salient to most people until later in life (most theorists suggesting it occurs at midlife or later). A heightened awareness of one's mortality is associated with the social experiences of death such as death of age peers, attainment of parent's age at death, and personal deterioration in social activity, mobility, and physical and mental functioning. Awareness of finitude comes not only from within but from society by subtle—and not so subtle—messages that the older person does not have enough future to deserve a major investment of the resources of others.

Anticipated losses associated with death include not only the cessation of relationships but also loss of the future and ability to complete projects and plans. Studies have shown that when asked to report anticipated important future events in life, older persons project a more limited time frame than did younger persons. They also were less likely to indicate that their activities would change if they knew they would die in 6 months.[13] Because of a heightened awareness of finitude, older persons often engage in social reminiscence with others. This talking about the past brings the past and present together as an integrated whole life. Success in legitimating life and death is associated with satisfaction and finding meaning in death.

The *terminal stage of dying* occurs with the news that one "is dying." People facing death confront the task of making sense of death itself. Factors such as culture, religion, race, and socioeconomic status are important in determining the meaning of death. Kubler-Ross described five stages of coping with the dying process: denial, anger, bargaining, depression, and acceptance. These stages have not been empirically demonstrated to be serial or to represent a universal psychologic process. Because her sample represented mostly young and middle-age adults, the results may not be generalizable to older persons. The assumption that people instinctively fear death and respond with anger and bargaining may be a more common reaction for younger rather than older adults. Comparative data indicate a growing evidence that the fear of death diminishes with advancing age.[12] Older adult communal settings and hospice settings, where people are frequently reminded of death, facilitate the development of social conventions to deal routinely with death.

Mental Functioning

Intelligence. Traditionally it has been held that intelligence declines after age 30. However, longitudinal research indicates that intellectual abilities can be improved or at least sustained until late adulthood.[14] Much of the observed intellectual losses in persons as old as the 80s and 90s occurs primarily in unfamiliar, complex, or stressful situations. In the months before death an older adult's intellectual abilities may decrease sharply. This change is part of a complex phenomenon called *terminal decline.*

The patterns of change in adult intelligence vary with the specific mental abilities measured (Table 2-2). *Fluid intelligence* consists of those abilities that are related to neurologic development and includes associative power, memory, figural relationships, and visual-motor flexibility. Because of degenerative neurologic changes, fluid intelligence may decline during middle age. *Crystallized intelligence* consists of those abilities that arise out of experience and the accumulation of learning and includes verbal comprehension, formal reasoning, and general information. Crystallized intelligence improves with age.

Several environmental and individual variables such as education, social class, illness, personality, and motivation affect adult intelligence. Generally, individuals who have above-average IQs as young adults, who have obtained more years of formal education, and who have continued to use intellectual processes demonstrate greater increases in intelligence throughout adulthood.[14]

Nurses must recognize that speed in mental functioning may be a major problem for older adults. Because of central nervous system decline and sensory deficits such as poor eyesight, some older persons have trouble with quick thinking and quick performance. Older people perform equally as well as younger people when time is not a factor. Because of this, any teaching or skills practice should be planned carefully to allow the older patient adequate time for comprehension and performance without the pressure of hurrying.

Memory. Although many middle adults fear becoming forgetful, no real decline in memory has been demonstrated until old age. *Short-term memory* deteriorates first. This refers to immediate recall that requires information retention for a few seconds to a few minutes. An example is remembering how to dial an unfamiliar phone number after having read it in the phone book. The decline in short-term memory may be related to neurotransmission interference or temporary storage integration problems. Because neurotransmission is slower, older adults become vulnerable to interference from other stimuli, which impede acquisition and storage of information. Thus information cannot be retrieved later because it was inadequately registered. This short-term memory problem can have significant effects on the learning process, because learning new material often requires speed in acquisition, comprehension, and registration.

Long-term memory seems resistant to aging. It is often noted that older adults can describe in minute detail past life events yet forget recent ones. This recall ability for past events may be attributed to the fact that once information is registered, people retain a sound memory for it. In addition it is likely that the memory for past events is consolidated firmly because the details have been previously recalled and rehearsed by the person.

Another memory difficulty in older adults is the inability to recall specifics after recognizing a person or a place. For example, a grandmother may recognize her grandchild but call him by another family member's name. In this case she has placed the child in the family and recognized the person but cannot recall the name. This problem seems to be in the retrieval process rather than in the registration of information.

In addition to aging changes, the memory of an older adult is affected by health status, drugs, education, amount of stimulation, motivation, and the meaningfulness of the material.

Table 2-2 Effects of Aging on Adult Mental Functioning

Function	Effect of Aging
Fluid intelligence	Declines during middle age
Crystallized intelligence	Improves
Vocabulary and verbal reasoning	Improves
Spatial perception	Constant or improves
Synthesis of new information	Declines during middle age
Mental performance speed	Declines during middle age
Short-term recall memory	Declines during old age
Long-term recall memory	Constant

Sexuality

Sexuality is a broad concept that incorporates physiologic characteristics, attitudes, values, and behaviors related to gender perceptions. The task of developing a compatibility between gender identity and self-expression of sex-related roles is vital to self-concept integration during adulthood. This is an ongoing task that pervades practically all aspects of adult life, including mate selection, career choices, friendships, and all forms of self-expression.

Young Adulthood. For the young adult, gender identity and sexual relationships are primary concerns in achieving a sexual self-concept and sense of intimacy. Although intimacy transcends a sexual relationship to include affiliative sharing, for the sexually active young adult intimacy usually is established by commitment to a relationship that includes an expression of affection and physical sexuality. Sexual performance in a marriage relationship represents more than physical pleasure. It becomes an expression of caring and closeness, which helps the couple find satisfaction in sharing their work, play, childbearing, and child-rearing activities. It has been found that young couples who are satisfied with their sexual relationship most often are satisfied with their overall marriage and vice versa.

For some, a homosexual relationship provides a feeling of intimacy and comfort. As in heterosexual individuals, homosexual men and women vary greatly in their emotional and social adjustments. The increased incidence of human immunodeficiency virus (HIV) infections appears to have caused a reconsideration in the lifestyles of those homosexuals who were accustomed to multiple partners.

Young adults are in the prime of physical and reproductive performance. Many of their biosocial concerns center around sexual activity, including cyclic changes in sexual arousal and orgasm, use and selection of contraceptives, sexual changes with pregnancy and postpartum, abortion, infertility, and sexually transmitted diseases. It has been found that the peak sexual drive and responsiveness in men occurs during the late teens and early twenties, whereas this peak occurs between the ages of 30 and 45 in women. However, most healthy adults maintain a strong sex drive beyond the age of 70.

Middle Adulthood. During the middle years both men and women experience hormonal declines that produce physiologic changes affecting sexual desire and responsiveness. However, more important than the physiologic changes are the psychologic expectations related to these changes. It has been found that menopausal and postmenopausal women have fewer fears and negative feelings about the effects of menopause on their sexuality than young adult women. Rather than experiencing a decline in sexual capacity, postmenopausal women frequently experience an increased libido and greater enjoyment. With the male climacteric, the decline in testosterone may result in a decreased libido and a slower sexual arousal and climax, but these changes do not necessarily lessen the pleasure of sexual intercourse.

Factors normally more important than hormonal changes that negatively affect sexual activity in the middle years include monotony in a repetitious sexual pattern, boredom with a relationship, career and economic preoccupation, mental and physical fatigue, excessive eating or drinking, and fear of sexual failure. Becoming a victim to the myth that a youthful body is equated with sexual desirability and potency also negatively affects sexual activity. Middle-age adults are at risk for the potential onset of chronic illnesses that may affect libido. Also they may be taking a variety of prescribed drugs that can reduce sexual responsiveness.

Sexual activity continues to be an important part of middle-age adult life. Satisfaction with sexual life in the middle years is not as related to frequency of intercourse as it is to vitality in the relationship and enjoyment derived from all sexual experiences in younger years.

Older Adulthood. Although our society attributes sexlessness to the older adult, people are sexual beings throughout their lives. Most studies attest to continued sexual activity well into the last decades of life for men and women who have been sexually active as young and middle adults. Physical changes in the sexual organs should not be considered as biologic limiters of sexual activity, nor should they reduce the satisfaction experienced by sexual partners. The most important criteria for remaining sexually active in older adulthood are a receptive partner, reasonable physical health, and a positive attitude about regular sexual activity.

Because society has been slow to recognize the sexual needs of older adults and because most older adults have been socialized not to talk about sex, identifying and intervening in sex-related problems is difficult for caregivers. It has been suggested that sex education programs be developed for older adults to inform them of normal changes and to help them cope with unmet sexual needs and with social and familial attitudes about continued sexual activity.

Intimacy. In a broad context, *intimacy* incorporates the concept of attachment or seeking a relationship in which an individual can maintain contact or proximity to the object of attachment. From this perspective, intimacy is a need that is manifest from conception to death and does not decrease in intensity or significance throughout adulthood. Intimacy is maintained physically by touching, stroking, patting, hugging, kissing, and through sexual intercourse. It is maintained emotionally by sharing joys, sorrows, affection, ideas, and values.

Throughout life, touch plays an important role in receiving and expressing intimacy. However, as hearing and sight decline with age, reaching out to touch becomes an even more important way to make intimate physical contact. Elderly people often attempt to touch and be touched by others to experience some sense of physical closeness. The response to their touch communicates a message of acceptance or nonacceptance that may never have been expressed verbally.

The need for expressing physical intimacy in behaviors having sexual connotations often is disregarded for older adults. Although these expressions are accepted as normal in younger adults, they may be viewed with disdain and disapproval or as an amusing and childish behavior when expressed by older people. This disregard is seen in some institutional structures and policies. Many nursing homes provide little opportunity for expression of sexual needs. Private rooms and locked doors often are neither provided nor respected. Older adult couples may be segregated and placed on separate men's and women's units or, if in the same room, may have single beds. Is it any wonder that an older person, who for years has shared a bed with a spouse, becomes disoriented at night and wanders or gets into bed with someone else? The youth-oriented society has developed skewed ideas about appropriate sexual behavior in older adults and, as a result, has placed severe restrictions on intimate relationships during old age.

SOCIAL PROCESSES IN ADULTHOOD

Adulthood is lived out in a social context with major developmental tasks being determined by the interaction of individuals with their social systems. Adult social concerns primarily involve the family, work and leisure, and community responsibilities.

Family and Adult Development

Throughout life the family is the major socializing institution for its members. A global survey of people representing 70 nations found that family life is overwhelmingly the greatest source of satisfaction and happiness for most people.[15] The family is a focal source for adults in meeting their needs for emotional security, belonging, love, companionship, esteem, and approval from others. The process of family development reflects the developmental changes occurring in the adult members. (See Table 2-3 for a summary of family tasks during adulthood.)

Young Adulthood. Emancipation from the family of origin is the first family task of young adulthood. This usually occurs as a gradual process that includes physical, economic, and emotional independence from parents. However, emancipation is not the end of a relationship with the family but rather the first step to establishing an interdependent adult relationship between young adults and their parents.

Often concurrent with emancipation from the family of origin, the young adult establishes a new family system in which roles, relationships, and expectations are being determined. This usually includes adjusting to an intimate relationship requiring a high level of communication and compromise and adapting to the predictable crises of childbearing. Stress frequently is high in the emerging young adult family because of the multiplicity of changing relationships and structures. Also, the work trajectories for both husband and wife often are launched and new outside demands are placed on adult family members. Because of these changes the emerging family easily may become dysfunctional. This is reflected in the fact that the highest divorce rate occurs during the first 3 to 5 years of marriage for young adults under the age of 30.

Following the initial family transition, young adults move into a more stable, comfortable family life period. Commitment to the success of the family is high, and there is less turmoil with children, who are usually now in middle childhood. Couples without children also find this to be a time for strengthening relationships with one another and their social group.

Middle Adulthood. Middle adults find themselves caught in the "family sandwich" between the needs of their children and their aging parents. Family life can be stressful because it is a complex chore to concurrently work through a midlife identity transition, the identity confusion of teenagers, and the redefinition of family roles and relationships in both the family of origin and the family of marriage and parenthood.

Disenchantment with the marital relationship frequently is experienced by middle-age adults. Research has demonstrated that married couples are satisfied least with each other when they are between the ages of 40 and 50. There are multiple contributing factors to this dissatisfaction. A husband or wife may be preoccupied or confused about occupational goals and blame the spouse for personal dissatisfaction. Some middle-age adults may feel that self-development needs were sacrificed for a spouse's job and the family. Also, the financial and emotional strain of adolescent children may come between a husband and wife. Although the divorce rate is not as high during middle adulthood as during early young adulthood, it does increase again during the years shortly after children leave home.

Middle-age couples who recommit themselves to their spouses and a continuing marriage find marital satisfaction frequently hits a new high. Although much discussion has been heard about the crisis of the "empty nest," many middle-age men and women experience a new sense both of self and of unity as a couple after the children leave home. They again define their relationship as lovers and companions rather than as parents. In many ways the postparental years become the payoff for investing in a mutual relationship with shared problems and joys, if the couple survives the trials of the midlife marriage.

During middle age, adults often begin to appreciate their parents and understand the problems of older people in a new way. When the aging parent is in good health and is basically self-reliant, the parent-child relationship is usually characterized by a friendship that is satisfactory to both. If aging parents are confronted with problems, such as inadequate finances, ill health, or death of a spouse, that make it impossible for them to remain independent, the parent-child relationship and roles may be restructured. A difficult and sometimes necessary role reversal occurs when a middle-age child must become a parent to the parent. This requires giving up feelings of dependency on the parent and assum-

Table 2-3 Family Tasks in Adult Development

Young Adulthood	Middle Adulthood	Older Adulthood
Emancipating from family of origin Establishing interdependent adult relationship with parents Selecting mate and adjusting to intimate relationship Adapting family system to demands of childbearing Finding balance to family, work, and social demands	Assisting teenage children to become responsible adults Restructuring relationship with spouse as children leave home Restructuring relationship with aging parents Adjusting to death of parents Defining roles and responsibilities of grandparent	Establishing satisfactory living arrangements with limited income Restructuring family roles and responsibilities after retirement Adapting living arrangements to meet problems caused by physical decline Adjusting to death of spouse

ing an uncomfortable authority role, which the older adult parent may find difficult to relinquish. The manner in which the middle-age adult responds to the parent's dependency needs will be determined by the previous relationship, available resources, and other responsibilities of the middle-age adult. Eventually, many middle-age adults must deal with their feelings about the death of parents. Although little has been done to study the family changes at this time, becoming a member of the family's oldest generation (because of the death of parents) is an important phase in family life.

Grandparenting. An increasing number of adults today become grandparents during middle adulthood (Fig. 2-5). This new social role may have a positive or negative impact on the grandparent's self-esteem. To some it is met with excitement and anticipation; for others it represents "growing old," which conflicts with how the grandparent wants to feel. Birth of children to teenagers also may spark unwelcome early transitions to grandparenthood. Because teenage parents often are unwilling or unable to assume the responsibilities of parenthood, many grandparents are becoming the primary caregivers to their young grandchildren. This family arrangement can cause significant physical and emotional stress to grandparents in middle adulthood.

Older Adulthood. The onset of this final period in family life generally is considered to be marked by retirement and poses new and unique developmental tasks for the aging family. The first task is to establish satisfactory living arrangements within a limited income, considering the role changes brought on by retirement and the physical incapacities of aging. In terms of living arrangements, most older adults live in their own households[16] (see Table 2-4). In a recent survey, 87% of the elderly preferred independent living in their own homes rather than living with children.[16] However, contact with children is frequent; 73% of older adults have at least one child living less than 30 minutes away, and 77% have contact with a child each week.[17] For older adults who are in relatively good health and have an adequate income, living in their own homes rather than with family members allows them to maintain a sense of privacy, competency, and independence (Fig. 2-6).

Table 2-4 Living Arrangements for Persons More Than 65 Years of Age (1992)

	Percentage of Men	Percentage of Women
Living in household	99.7	99.8
Living alone	16.3	41.8
Spouse present	73.8	39.8
Living with someone else	9.6	18.0
Not in household (e.g., institutions)	0.3	0.2

From US Bureau of Census, Current Population Reports: *Statistical abstract of the United States*, 1993, Washington, DC.

The ability to adjust family responsibilities and routines is an important part of the adaptation a couple must make following retirement. Schedules and activities are readjusted, and a retiree frequently will turn to family members to meet self-esteem needs that previously were met by the referent work group.

Loss of spouse. The loss of a spouse is a crisis at any stage in life. The reaction to a spouse's death may vary, depending on how compatible the relationship was; the circumstances of the death; the available support systems, including family and religious beliefs; the physiologic independence of the survivor; and the adequacy of financial resources. Although the degree of marital happiness varies for older adults, couples who have had a long marriage generally have established an interdependent symbiotic relationship that gives them a great deal of pleasure during their later years.

Developing a new social identity and adjusting living arrangements are major tasks of adjusting to the loss of a spouse. For many, this is a time when they are socially

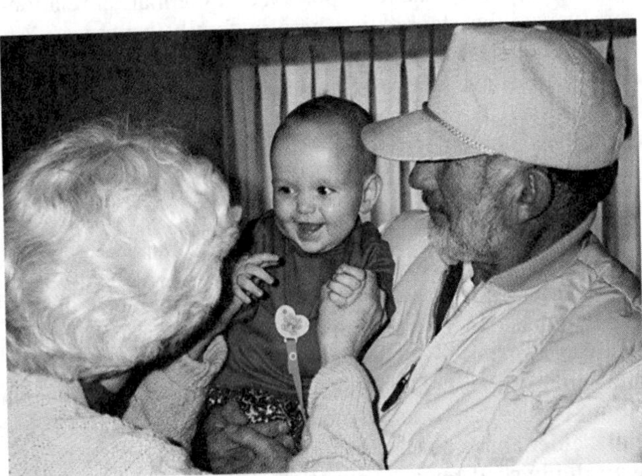

Fig. 2-5 The active grandparent plays a positive role in the lives of the child and the grandchild.

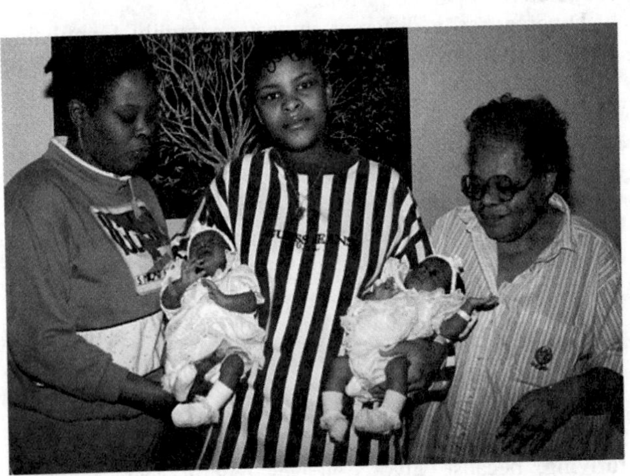

Fig. 2-6 This four-generation family demonstrates that the child of an older grandparent may also be a grandparent.

marooned unless they actively seek activities in which they can participate without a spouse. Some older adults choose to move in with family members; others move to smaller apartments, mobile homes, or a community for older adults. In any case, relocation may be an additional trauma.

Remarriage is an alternative to living alone or to living with children or friends. Many older adults remarry for companionship, and although there is the danger of idealizing the deceased mate and making unrealistic comparisons with the new spouse, most of these remarriages are happy.

Singlehood and Single Parenting. Single adults include the never-married, separated, divorced, and those who have lost a spouse. Some people choose not to marry or remarry because of personal freedom and development; career goals; family responsibilities to parents, siblings, or children; ill health; or the inability to find a compatible mate. Those who prefer to remain single value their roles and contributions to society. They do not see the unmarried state as a period of waiting.

A change in the traditional American family is the single-parent family. Often, single parenting results from divorce or death of the spouse. However, some single persons choose to have children by adoption, artificial insemination, surrogate parenting, or pregnancy. A major stress for a single parent is playing all the roles of mother and father that are necessary for discipline and socialization of the child. Some of this role overload may be relieved by joint child custody in the case of divorce and by other members of the extended family. Downward economic mobility is a frequent problem faced by the single-parent mother.

Divorce. Divorce is the major disrupter of families. Multiple social and individual factors contribute to family dissolution. With divorce there are a myriad of membership roles and boundaries that must be restructured. Because the family structure is permanently altered, family members must learn new ways of functioning and interacting to accomplish family tasks. Terminating the marital relationship is difficult, particularly when the couple must maintain cooperative coparenting roles.

Divorce has a different impact on family functioning depending on the family life cycle stage. It is a source of personal crisis for all family members and, as such, affects their physical and mental health status. Loss and grieving can be complicated because divorce often is associated with feelings of guilt and a sense of social failure. Developmentally, it requires that a reorientation process be started. Each family member must make adjustments in self-identity and establish new social roles. This process usually is harder for middle-age and older adults who terminate long marriages, because life patterns and the incorporation of a spouse into personal identity have been well established. Research indicates that the process of postdivorce restabilization takes at least 2 to 3 years. However, this does not mean that after this restabilization the individuals are happy and thriving, because divorce leaves painful scars for both children and adults. Although between two thirds and three fourths of those who divorce will remarry, the high divorce rate for remarried couples suggests that these marriages often are under enormous pressure.[18]

Stepfamilies. It is predicted that by the year 2000 remarried families with stepchildren will outnumber other family forms.[19] Stepfamilies (also referred to as blended or reconstituted families) have unique family dynamics. Complex relationships may lead to ambiguous roles and expectations for family members as they rework old relationships and establish new ones. Major characteristics of reconstituted families include: (1) virtually all members have sustained a primary relationship loss, (2) the marital and family life cycles may be incongruent with individuals' life cycles, (3) children and adults bring expectations from previous family experiences, (4) some parent-child relationships predate the marriage relationship, (5) there may be a living biologic parent elsewhere, (6) children may be members of more than one household, and (7) the stepparent may have no legal relationship with the stepchildren.[19] In addition to the usual family tasks, stepfamilies must make the transition from a previous family identity to a stepfamily identity. The family emotional process in this transition includes struggling with fears about investing in the new relationships and may involve dealing with hostile responses of the children, extended families, and ex-spouse. Making a successful transition includes having mourned the previous losses, setting realistic expectations for the new family, negotiating different developmental needs, developing a strongly unified couple and "parenting coalition," enhancing the previously existing parent-child bonds, developing new steprelationships including between stepsiblings, developing a sense of membership in a new family unit, establishing new rituals and traditions, and establishing cooperative relationships between separate households and accepting continual shifts in composition.

When assessing a stepfamily's functioning, the blended family must be evaluated in its own family structure, recognizing that norms vary among the different stepfamily structural types. Major issues related to stepfamily functioning and integration include marital bonding, stepparent-child roles, and the presence of a mutual child. Research is equivocal on the relative importance of the marital relationship versus the steprelationships in family happiness. Although couples may decide to have a mutual child to confirm the new marriage, enhance unity, and strengthen stepfamily relationships, research does not strongly document these outcomes.[20] Support, information, and literature are available through The Stepfamily Association of America, Inc., 215 Centennial Mall South, Suite 212, Lincoln, NE 68508.

Family Violence. Dysfunctional family behavior may be manifested by violence toward any member that is perceived as dependent or a source of frustration. There are five types of family violence: spousal, child, elder, parent, and sibling abuse. Only recently have elder, parent, and sibling abuse been acknowledged in the literature. Typically, elder abuse occurs in families where an elderly parent with diminished physical functioning is being cared for in the home of one of the children.[21] Studies that have examined parent abuse report that mothers were most likely to be the victims of adolescent sons.[21] Abusive adolescents usually are recipients of abuse and have friends who assaulted their parents. Most domestic violence is related to social stress in families. Often the violent family is socially isolated. Although domestic violence is more common in lower socioeconomic families, it is not confined to that group. Extensive research has addressed factors that are associated with family violence. It is clear that the causes are multidimensional and include intergenerational transmission of violence, social stress and isolation, financial strain, personality problems, psychopathology, and drug abuse. Maladaptive coping, inadequate communication, and dysfunctional role performance all may lead to family conflicts that end in violence.

Community Life in Adulthood

Participating in community life is a major developmental task of adulthood. Personal and family well-being strongly depends on successful interactions with the community through work, leisure, and civic participation.

Work and Young Adulthood. Work provides more than the financial means to support a standard of living. It becomes a salient feature of personal identity and self-concept. Launching a career is the first point in the work cycle and occurs in young adulthood for most men and women. This entry point confronts the young adult with many potentially stressful role adjustments on the job and within the family. The interactions of family and work life cycles become more complex in a two-career family in which husband and wife are seeking career advancements.

Work and the Middle-age Career Clock. The second major occupational crisis occurs during middle age when people assess whether they are "on time" or "behind time" according to their personal career clock (Fig. 2-7). With the perspective of time until retirement, occupational goals often need to be revised toward more realistic expectations.

Because the middle-age adult is frequently at the peak of job performance, work may become the pivot around which all relationships and activities are ordered. Because the job is so central, job stresses and dissatisfaction can have profound effects on physical and mental health. Also, the person who develops health problems that impede the ability to work or threaten career timing will experience less job satisfaction, thus producing a vicious, stressful cycle. Frequently, nurses must help middle-age patients adjust to job restrictions created by hospitalization and medical regimens.

Retirement. Retirement is the third major event in the occupation cycle. The significant issues adults must face with retirement include a lower income, which can have profound effects on lifestyle; a loss of work role and associated relationships, which are part of the individual's personal identity and social status; a readjustment of time and restructuring of daily activities; a change in family roles and arrangements; and the psychologic mark of old age, which increases awareness of the aging process. However, with improved retirement benefits and better pension plans, more individuals are choosing to retire early.

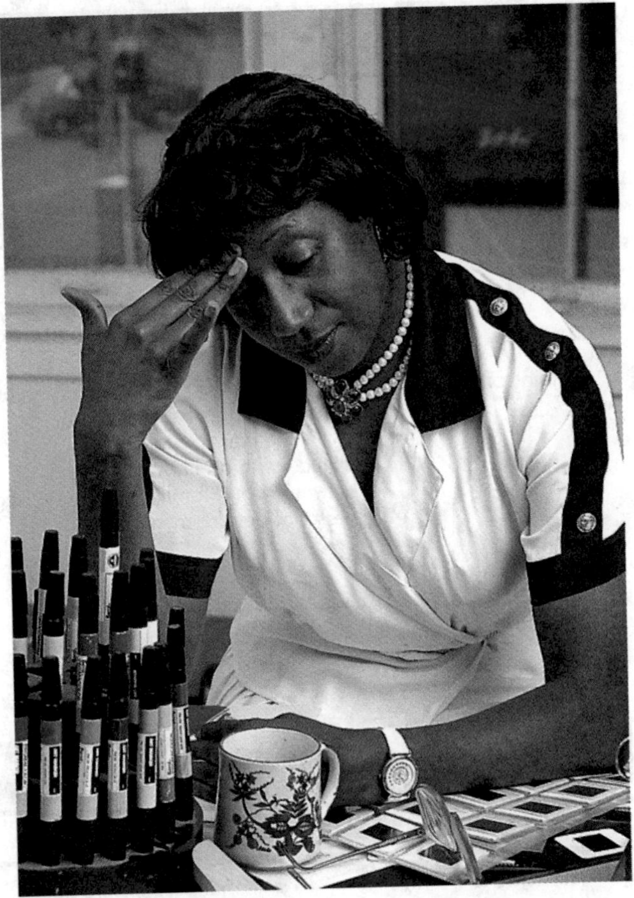

Fig. 2-7 The middle-age woman may experience the same career clock as a man because of economic concerns and increased life choices.

They view retirement as a reward for past productivity and an opportunity to pursue new goals and satisfy previously unmet needs.

The transition from employed to retired is less stressful when the person has planned comprehensively for retirement. Gerontologic nurses should play significant roles in preparing patients for the predictable stresses that occur with retirement and thus lessen some of the potential crises of this major life change. Table 2-5 further describes the work cycle.

Leisure During Adulthood

The concept of leisure is becoming more important in society. It is of interest not only to the retiree but also to young and middle-age adults who are experiencing more nonwork time and need to determine how to spend this time in a satisfying manner. In general, the amount of available leisure time increases as an individual moves from young adulthood to retirement (Table 2-6). During any life stage, occupational choice and leisure are interdependent. The job heavily influences the amount of leisure time available in addition to the financial resources and the physical and mental energy left for leisure activities.

Table 2-5 Work Cycle

Work	Young Adulthood	Middle Adulthood	Older Adulthood
▪ Focus	Career launch	Midlife career crisis	Retirement
▪ Expectations	Reorganization of time Job role adjustments Family role adjustments	Measurement of accomplishments against goals Revision of unrealistic career goals with the perspective of time until retirement If desired, change of jobs or careers before it is "too late"	Reorganization of time and daily activities Family role adjustments Establishment of referent group other than co-workers
▪ Major problems	Expectations for job not standard congruent with reality "Now is the time to make it" attitude with an imbalance between work, family, and personal development needs	Sense of occupational failure and frustration if unable to give up idealistic young adult goals and set realistic current goals Ego deflation with being at the "entry level" of a new career when changing careers at midlife	Lowered income and standard of living Loss of self-esteem if unable to transfer status from the work role to other roles Psychologic mark of old age

Table 2-6 Adult Leisure Time

	Young Adulthood	Middle Adulthood	Older Adulthood
▪ Time factor	Minimal pure leisure time because of holding second job or going to school and working full time	Increasing amounts of available time because of usually greater occupational stability and less time spent on child-rearing activities	Possibly too much available time
▪ Cost factor	Financial resources limiting time spent and type of leisure activities pursued	More money available for leisure because of higher earning power	Reduced and fixed incomes limiting activities Reduction of cost of leisure activities for retired citizens because of government programs
▪ General types of leisure	Activities that sustain marital and family closeness such as family outings and home entertainment Activities with other young families Activities with same-sex friends such as sports and arts and crafts	Less home-centered activities because of greater freedom; traveling, going out with friends Activities that are less physically demanding and do not require quick reflexes Activities oriented toward health maintenance; swimming, jogging, exercising	Activities enjoyed during middle adulthood if health and finances permit Creative arts and crafts and recreational activities such as cards and dancing Activities with family members and friends Volunteer services such as Foster Grandparents

Young Adulthood. Young adults often have busy schedules with little time for leisure. Attempts to balance work, school, family responsibilities, and leisure often result in frustration. The forms of leisure they engage in are affected by personal interests and social factors, including marriage and parenting roles, new friendships, occupational choices, and financial resources.

Middle Adulthood. The leisure patterns in middle adulthood change slightly from young adulthood because of physical and social changes in this stage of life. The use of leisure time is an important concern for middle-age adults because they are beginning to prepare for retirement. During this time they can develop interests that can continue into the retirement years and bridge the gap from the working life to full-time leisure.

Older Adulthood. Older adults tend to continue to fill their time with the leisure activities they enjoyed in middle age as long as their health and finances remain adequate. However, as more older adults have opportunities to participate in a variety of programs such as those provided by senior centers, they can increase their scope of activities and do things they have never tried before. Government programs at federal, state, and local levels as well as private enterprise have joined to help provide and make leisure activities more accessible to older people. The Older American Act has established funds and programs such as multipurpose senior citizens' centers, which provide a variety of activities including classes, recreational activities, arrangements for discount tickets for entertainment programs and travel, and special education programs.

Older adults use their leisure time in self-oriented activities, and they also contribute much to society through volunteer services. Volunteering provides older adults with an opportunity to share their talents and to participate in meaningful activities that fill a need in society.

With continued aging and decline in health, older people may engage in more homebound solitary activities, such as relaxing in a rocking chair, thinking, daydreaming, people watching, and patting a pet. In general, the leisure activities of older adults are determined by their health, previous activities, money, and current expectations about what they can do (Fig. 2-8).

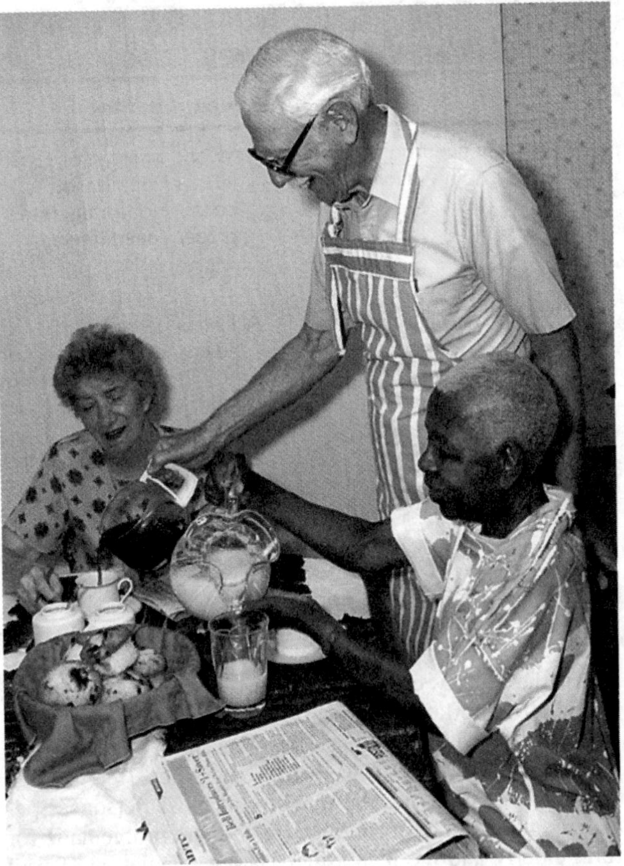

Fig. 2-8 Good friends and pleasant activities help fill the lives of active older adults.

Civic Participation

Participation in the community through civic and government organizations, church groups, professional groups, and special interest groups begins in young adulthood, peaks in middle adulthood, and generally declines during older adulthood. Because young adults are involved with the commitments of establishing an overall lifestyle, including a family, career, and friendships, their time and energy are limited for consistent participation in community activities.

Although society is youth oriented, the control is held by middle-age and older adults. This becomes apparent when examining the ages of individuals who are in high decision-making positions at all levels of government and private enterprise. Middle-age adults not only participate in more community and professional activities, they also have developed the expertise and leadership qualities to participate at higher organizational levels. The increase in political activism among middle-age women has become especially prominent because of their successful election attempts. In general, middle-age men and women are at the peak of their influence and responsibility for the affairs of society in local, national, and international arenas. Older people who have been active in their communities usually will remain active as long as their health and income permit.

With the growing population of older adults, various forms of retirement communities have arisen. These include communities with private homes, condominiums, apartment complexes, and recreational vehicles in organized private campgrounds for retired people. Older adults who live in these communities become involved with all aspects of their community's life. Older adults also remain politically active and organize for their own causes, in groups such as the American Association of Retired Persons, National Council of Senior Citizens, and the Gray Panthers. Most politicians recognize the political strength of older adults as a group because of their organizations and the fact that they vote. Table 2-7 further describes civic activities.

Transportation programs to meet the needs of the elderly are a necessary support for community-based activities.

Table 2-7 Civic Participation in Adulthood

	Young Adulthood	Middle Adulthood	Older Adulthood
▪ Factors encouraging or discouraging involvement	Time and energy for civic involvement limited because of family and career commitments	Concern for future of society fostering civic participation as a priority	Available time, resources, and special interest causes encouraging civic participation Declining health reducing ability to participate
▪ Type of participation	Activities perceived as having direct bearing on day-to-day lives, such as labor unions, PTA, church activities Participation usually at the local level	Increased political and professional activity Leadership and decision-making positions at all levels of government and private enterprise	Civic involvements begun during the middle adult years continuing Retirement community activities Political involvement, including political action groups that promote legislation for causes of special interest to older adults

When the elderly can no longer drive, they must rely on special transportation systems because most mass transit systems pose physical obstacles that limit accessibility. Passage of the Americans with Disabilities Act has the potential of improving the mobility of older persons. Specialized transportation continues to be more problematic for rural elderly and the increasingly larger population of frail elderly over the age of 85.

PHYSIOLOGIC PROCESSES IN ADULTHOOD

Having a healthy body is truly an asset and can be a major factor in having positive or negative feelings.

Physiologic Changes During Adulthood

The young adult body is generally at its peak of health and performance. Although the physical changes associated with aging are beginning at this time, the effects are not yet great enough to require attention. Extrinsic factors such as accidents and physical stressors such as lack of sleep and substance abuse are the most common source of disabling biophysical problems in young adults.

Structural and functional body changes that were unnoticed in young adulthood may begin to be apparent during middle age. The rate and expression of physiologic aging changes are highly individual. Frequently, changes in physical appearance such as dry skin, wrinkles, thinning and graying hair, and inches on the waist and hips are the first noticeable clues of aging. Sometime during the middle years, most adults notice that muscle strength and agility are declining, but, on a day-to-day basis, most people make small compensations that minimize the effects of these changes. Although the middle-age individual is aware of these signs of aging, changes in the vital organs are often going on unnoticed. Because these changes involve aging rather than a pathologic process, they begin insidiously in young adulthood, become more apparent in middle adulthood, and culminate in death, when the body can no longer compensate for or adapt to the changes.

Although many older people remain vigorous beyond the age of 80, the general decline in all systems and a reduction of normally functioning cells caused by aging decrease the older person's overall ability to withstand and adapt to physical or emotional stress. When one system is placed under stress, there is a domino effect; without the ability to compensate, all systems may collapse. Thus, maintaining physical and emotional integrity in the older person can be precarious. For a more complete discussion of physiologic changes resulting from the aging process, see Table 3-2.

Considerations for Health Maintenance

Young Adulthood. Although the young adult years are a time of generally good physical and emotional health, the young adult lifestyle may hold potential health hazards. Accidents, acquired immunodeficiency syndrome (AIDS), substance abuse, sleep deprivation, inactivity, obesity, exposure to environmental and occupational hazards, and stress-related illnesses such as ulcers, depression, and suicide are important health problems during this time of life. Chronic illnesses such as hypertension, coronary artery disease, and diabetes may have their onset in young adulthood without being known to the young adult but become serious health threats later.

Middle Adulthood. The middle-age lifestyle should be assessed for areas that are detrimental to health. With a decline in strength and stamina, daily exercise is essential; however, sporadic weekend exercise or competitive physical overexertion can lead to injury (Fig. 2-9). Reducing caloric intake often is necessary to prevent weight gain. This may be difficult, particularly for middle-age adults whose social and business lifestyles encourage overindulgence at dinners and parties. Life pressures frequently

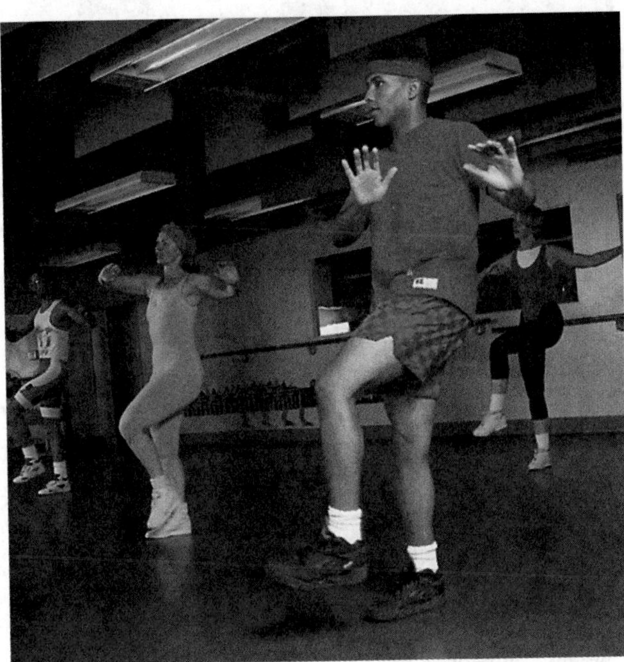

Fig. 2-9 Both young and middle-age adults are subject to injuries associated with sporadic activity.

mount during middle age, and a variety of substances may be used and overconsumed to cope, including cigarettes, alcohol, food, and tranquilizers. Rather than relying on these, the individual may need assistance to deal with the sources of pressure.

Middle-age adults need to be encouraged to seek routine medical and dental examinations directed toward disease prevention and early treatment of problems. Healthy People 2000 recommends annual dental and biannual physical examinations for healthy middle-age adults.[22] The American Cancer Society also recommends Pap smears every 3 years, unless estrogen therapy or oral contraceptives are being used, and yearly mammography after the age of 40 for women with a family history of breast cancer. After the age of 50, mammography is recommended yearly when the woman is asymptomatic. Nurses have a fundamental role in health maintenance care by educating and promoting self-care responsibility among middle-age adults.

Although many middle-age adults feel they are in the prime of life, a rising incidence of chronic illnesses is associated with middle age. In addition to those that continue into middle age from young adulthood, some major health concerns are heart and vascular disease, cancer, liver cirrhosis, diabetes, and sexual dysfunctions.

Older Adulthood. An estimated 86% of the population over 65 has one or more chronic conditions with varying degrees of disability.[23] The health problems of older people reflect past health and lifestyle influences. The major problems include chronic or recurrent conditions from earlier adult stages, chronic brain syndrome, degenerative bone and joint diseases, malnutrition, acute and chronic respiratory diseases, renal diseases, drug-induced problems, and mental disorders.

The health of older adults is influenced not only by pathophysiologic disease processes but also by the process of aging. Although the aging process cannot be stopped, the effects can be reduced by good health habits, including proper nutrition, activity and rest, safety, and correct drug usage.

Stress of Illness During Adulthood

Illness is a situational crisis that can disrupt adult life at any time. The extent of the disruption may vary from a minor annoyance to a complete lifestyle change. The significance that "being ill" holds for an individual is determined by multiple variables: the type of illness and its perceived threat, the personality type, socioeconomic resources, family or significant other support, and possible restrictions on current lifestyle or structure. With Levinson's model, the impact of illness will differ depending on whether the individual is in a transitional or stable period of development. During stable periods when life generally is going smoothly, people have more energy to cope with illness. In contrast, there is less energy to cope with illness during the transitional periods as a result of the changes made in overall life structure. In addition, illness and its potential effects add new variables to consider in the restructuring process. Because transitional stages represent a time of uncertainty, role changes, and anxiety, the individual is also more vulnerable to becoming ill. Conversely, the stable periods, which are typically times of commitment, confidence, and success, foster health. Also, the presence of illness, either personal illness or illness in a significant other, can trigger movement from a stable period into a transitional stage. This characteristically may be seen in the midlife transition during which an illness can initiate the "time left" thinking that is fundamental to the profound reassessment of life at this time.

Illness of an individual member may also pose a developmental threat to the family's integrity. The nurse must consider the family as a unit of care, identifying family needs and supporting family strengths and positive coping mechanisms.

Young Adulthood. The most frequent acute conditions in young adults are minor accidents, drug abuse, respiratory infections, influenza, gastroenteritis, urinary tract infections, and minor surgery. These conditions may be developmentally significant to young adults for several reasons. First, with the hectic schedules of young adults, an acute minor illness is annoying because of disruption in life activities. With an acute disability, young adults may know that the effects are short term; however, they may be impatient with the healing process and concerned that long-term problems will result. Family rearrangements can be stressful, especially when hospitalization is required. Also, hospitalization is frustrating because of forced dependency and limitations posed by treatment regimens. Maintaining control is important for young adults; consequently, they need to be informed and involved with decisions about care. Young adults generally are motivated strongly toward recuperation to resume life activities.

Although chronic conditions are not common in young adulthood, they can occur. Disabilities caused by accidents, multiple sclerosis, rheumatoid arthritis, AIDS, and cancer are the common long-term conditions facing by young adults. Chronic illness and disability in young adulthood strike at the core of developmental tasks and can result in delayed development. With the onset of chronic illness or disability, the threat to the young adult's independence may precipitate multiple crises when personal, family, and career goals need to change. The nurse must identify and direct nursing interventions toward potential developmental problems in the areas of identity reorganization; establishment of independence; reorganization of intimate relationships and family structure; and launching of a chosen career.

Middle Adulthood. The characteristics of acute illness are much the same in middle adulthood as in young adulthood. However, recuperative power in middle adulthood slows. Injuries and acute conditions that were resolved rapidly in young adulthood may have a longer recovery period and are more likely to become chronic problems.

Chronic conditions during middle age interfere with the individual's sense of generativity. This task requires outward-directed concerns and activities. Long-term recurrent illness often forces an inferiority that can lead to physical and psychologic self-absorption. When middle-age adults develop a chronic illness or disability, they may feel unable to influence their destiny, let alone influence and provide for others. The impact on generativity includes changes in family, job, and community involvement.

With the onset of chronic illness in middle age, established family roles are often forced to change. The psychologic trauma of these role changes is caused by the strong emotional component to roles, which is based on the value placed on a role as a part of self-identity and the vested power the role holds. The nurse should be perceptive to the potential for family dysfunction and should serve as a resource to the entire family, helping them to seek counseling and therapy as necessary.

Career or occupational orientation may need to change as a result of chronic illness. This is stressful particularly during the middle years because it confounds the career timing and readjustment of goals that occur with the midlife occupational crisis. When the illness is severely disruptive, the person may need to change occupations or jobs or may need to face an early forced retirement. Both these options may be a source of great stress and a threat to generativity because of occupational regression or being denied the gratification that comes from closing a career with the feeling of a job well done.

Older Adulthood. The distinction between acute and chronic illness in older adults is less precise, because acute conditions may become chronic or may be an exacerbation of chronic problems. However, acute problems such as gastroenteritis, primary pneumonia, removable tumors, and noncomplicated accidental injuries can have a short course with complete recovery. The difficulties such illnesses pose for older adults are the added stress to a body system and a decreased physiologic and psychologic ability to compensate for stress. The ability to perform self-care is an important problem for older adults when an acute illness occurs. If the person lives alone or with a frail spouse or housemate and does not have adequate support systems, an acute illness can precipitate a life disorganization that results in a move from the home and toward dependency.

When an older adult is hospitalized, many situations occur that threaten ego integrity and cause the hospitalization to be a very disorganizing experience. Normally, new situations and environments often produce anxiety, and, when combined with the stress of being sick, the unfamiliar becomes confusing. When giving care the nurse needs to carefully orient and reorient the older adult to the hospital environment. Also, allowing the older adult patient to keep personal belongings visible and in reach will help maintain a sense of orientation, as well as reduce the depersonalized feeling that accompanies hospitalization. Nursing care should be paced to allow older adult patients an opportunity to participate without hurrying; as a result they can maintain control and have time to understand and cooperate with what is being done.

Family situations are an important concern in caring for the hospitalized older adult. The nurse must recognize when role reversals are occurring between an older parent and the adult children. Children who have problems with this reversal may respond by withdrawing or by becoming overprotective and smothering. In either case the parent's self-worth is threatened. The nurse also should be perceptive to other family concerns of the hospitalized older adult such as worry over a spouse being home alone or concern for pets and plants or household maintenance if the patient lives alone.

Chronic conditions are common health problems that older adults learn to manage. Part of this process includes incorporating the accoutrements of aging such as canes, wheelchairs, dentures, and hearing aids into a healthy self-esteem. Chronic conditions also have social implications if the illness imposes an involuntary disengagement process. When this occurs, transcending the physical problems is increasingly difficult. The social isolation that is experienced may reduce self-esteem and the physical and emotional strength needed to cope with the stresses of disease and aging.

REVIEW QUESTIONS

The number of the question corresponds to the same-numbered objective at the beginning of the chapter.

1. Levinson's developmental stages are based on
   a. biologic changes during adulthood.
   b. adjustments of self and social environment.
   c. changes in the individual life structure.
   d. instinctual energies and drives.

2. Identity continuity theory
   a. is a developmental stage theory.
   b. suggests that middle-age life patterns are important to aging adaptation.

c. assumes that older adults cannot adapt to the changes brought on by aging.
d. is appropriate only for healthy elderly whose identity is not threatened.

3. Reminiscence about the past is

a. a way to avoid dealing with the present and future.
b. an idle pastime.
c. a part of the process of preparing for death.
d. satisfying only if the past has been positive.

4. The most likely cause of stress in a typical young adult family is

a. role reversal in caring for aging parents.
b. health problems that threaten the career timetable.
c. identity confusion of the adult family members.
d. multiplicity of changing relationships and social demands.

5. Community activities and civic participation are

a. of little interest to adults who have retired.
b. more important to middle adults than to young adults.
c. focused on broad societal concerns in young adulthood.
d. focused on personal and family concerns in young adulthood.

6. Health maintenance during middle adulthood should be directed toward

a. halting the physiologic aging changes.
b. preventing illnesses due to lifestyle.
c. preparing for the inevitable physical decline.
d. maintaining stamina and strength at a young adult level.

7. For the elderly adult, hospitalization can be a disorganizing experience resulting in confusion because

a. poor ego integrity is characteristic of this age group.
b. restricted activity results in boredom.
c. hospitalization forces self-absorption.
d. unfamiliar, stressful surroundings can cause loss of control.

REFERENCES

1. Erikson E: *Childhood and society,* ed 2, New York, 1963, WW Norton.
2. Peck RC: Psychological developments in the second half of life. In Neugarten BL, editor: *Middle-age and aging: a reader in social psychology,* Chicago, 1986, University of Chicago Press.
3. Havighurst RJ: *Developmental tasks and education,* ed 3, New York, 1973, David McKay.
4. Levinson DJ: Toward a conception of the adult life course. In Smelser NJ and Erikson EH, editors: *Themes of work and love in adulthood,* Cambridge, Mass, 1980, Harvard University Press.
5. Levinson DJ: *The seasons of a man's life,* New York, 1978, Alfred A Knopf.
6. Cummings E, Henry WE: *Growing old: the process of disengagement,* New York, 1961, Basic Books.
7. Kart CS: *The realities of aging: an introduction to gerontology,* ed 3, Boston, 1990, Allyn & Bacon.
8. Atchley RC: A continuity theory of normal aging, *Gerontologist* 29:183, 1989.
9. Birren JE, Bengston V: *Emergent theories of aging,* New York, 1988, Springer Publishing.
10. Kane RL, Ouslander JG, Abrass IB: *Essentials of clinical geriatrics,* ed 2, New York, 1989, McGraw-Hill.
11. Our vitamin prescription: the big four, *University of California at Berkeley Wellness Letter,* 4:1, 1994.
12. Marshall V, Levy J: Aging and dying. In Binstock RH, George LK, editors: *Handbook of aging and the social sciences,* ed 3, San Diego, 1990, Academic Press.
13. Kart CS, Metress ES: Death and dying. In Kart CS, editor: *The realities of aging: an introduction to gerontology,* ed 3, Boston, 1990, Allyn & Bacon.
14. Schaie KW: Intellectual development in adulthood. In Birren J, Schaie KW, editors: *Handbook of the psychology of aging,* ed 3, San Diego, 1990, Academic Press.
15. Gallup GH: Human needs and satisfaction: a global survey, *Public Opinion Q* 40:459, 1976.
16. American Association of Retired Persons: *Home equity conversion for the elderly: an analysis for lenders,* Washington, DC, 1989, The Association.
17. Schick FL, editor: *Statistical handbook on aging Americans,* Phoenix, 1986, Oryx Press.
18. Glick PC: The family life style and social change, *Family Relations* 38:123, 1989.
19. Visher EB, Visher JS: Dynamics of successful stepfamilies, *Journal of Divorce and Remarriage* 14:3, 1990.
20. Hobart M: Stepparents' contentment with their stepchild: does a joint biological child make a difference? Unpublished thesis: University of New Mexico, 1994.
21. Steinmetz SK: Family violence: past, present and future. In Sussman MB, Steinmetz SK: *Handbook of marriage and the family,* New York, 1987, Plenum Press.
22. US Department of Health and Human Services, Office of Disease Prevention and Health Promotion: *Healthy people 2000: national health promotion and disease prevention objectives,* Washington, DC, 1979, US Government Printing Office, pub No 017-001-00473, 1990.
23. American Cancer Society: Cancer facts and figures—1994, Atlanta, GA, 1994, The Society.

Chapter 3

GENERAL CONCEPTS

Gerontologic Considerations

Tana Durnbaugh

Learning Objectives

1. Describe the unique role of nursing in assisting the older adult to meet health care needs.
2. Describe the impact of older adults on the health care system.
3. Describe clinical manifestations related to specific age-related physiologic changes.
4. Describe the nursing interventions and needs of special populations of older adults.
5. Identify the effects of culture on aging.
6. Identify differences in health status and disease manifestation between the older and younger adult.
7. List adaptations to the nursing process that the nurse must make when caring for the older adult.
8. Identify the role of the nurse in health screening and promotion and disease prevention for the older adult.
9. Describe the tasks of the chronically ill older adult and the nursing behaviors needed to assist in the accomplishment of each.
10. Describe common problems of the older adult related to hospitalization and acute illness.
11. Identify the role of the nurse in assisting the older adult with selected care problems.
12. Describe social support alternatives for the older adult.
13. Identify care alternatives to meet patient-specific needs of the older adult.
14. Identify the legal and ethical issues of common concern to the nurse and the older adult.

GERONTOLOGIC NURSING

Care of the older adult is based on the specialty body of knowledge of gerontologic nursing. The nurse approaches the patient with a whole-person (physical, psychologic, socioeconomic) perspective. The actions of the nurse skilled in the care of the older adults directly affect the health status of the older adult patient.

In 1987 standards were set by the American Nurses Association that established quality indicators for the nursing care of the older adult.[1] These standards are summarized below. The professional nurse should develop the following knowledge and skills:

1. Recognition of age-related changes
2. Assessment skills to determine health status, including functional abilities
3. Recognition of special-needs populations, including frail elderly, minorities, and institutionalized elderly
4. Ability to establish therapeutic relationships with the older adult and the family
5. Ability to teach the older adult and his family about measures to restore and promote health
6. Ability to refer the older adult to appropriate gerontologic community resources

This chapter presents information specific to the older adult that will assist the medical-surgical nurse in his care. Additional information about developmental issues related to the older adult is discussed in Chapter 2.

Older adults make up 40% to 60% of a hospital's inpatient census.[2] Therefore gerontologic considerations present challenges to nurses that require skilled assessment and creative adaptations of nursing interventions. Complex health problems that often follow atypical patterns require critical thinking and careful problem solving.

ATTITUDES TOWARD AGING

Who is old? The answer to this question often depends on the age and attitude of the respondent. It is important that the nurse maintains the position that aging is normal and is not related to disease. Age is a date in time and is influenced by many factors, including emotional and physical health, developmental stage, socioeconomic status, culture, and ethnicity.

Reviewed by Kay A. Herth, RN, FAAN, PhD, Professor and Chair, Department of Nursing, Georgia Southern University, Statesboro, GA.

As people age, they are exposed to more and different life experiences. The accumulation of these differences makes older adults more diverse than any other age group.[3] As the nurse assesses the older adult, it is important to consider this diversity. The nurse should assess the patient for perceptions of age. Older adults with poor health report a higher perceived age and lower sense of psychologic well-being.[4] Age is important, but it may not be the most relevant data for determining appropriate care of an individual patient.

Myths and stereotypes about aging, found throughout society, are supported by media reports of needy, problematic older adults. Myths and stereotypes regarding aging provide the basis of commonly held misconceptions that may lead to errors in assessments and unnecessary limitations to interventions. For example, if the nurse thinks all old people are rigid, new ideas will not be presented to the patient.

Ageism is a negative attitude based on age. It leads to discrimination in the care given to the older adult. The nurse who demonstrates negative attitudes may fear her own aging process or be misinformed about aging and the health care needs of the older adult. The nurse may benefit from gaining knowledge about normal aging, increasing contact with the healthy, independent older adult, and participating in simulation life experiences of the older adult. The older adult exposed to ageism may see oneself in a negative manner.

TRENDS IN HEALTH CARE

The rapid growth of the oldest population group has had an impact on nursing care. In the last two decades the older adult population (those 65 years of age and older) has grown twice as fast as the rest of the population. This growth is expected to continue into the next century (Fig. 3-1). Several factors have led to this incre-ase. The large post-World War II immigrant population has now grown older. Common diseases of the early 1900s, such as influenza and diarrhea, that killed many older adults are now less common.

People born today have a life expectancy 26 years longer than those born in 1900. The U.S. Census Bureau predicts life expectancy to continue to increase for both men and women. The life expectancy of women in the United States is 79.6 years, and for men it is 72.7 years. For Canadian women it is 78 years and for Canadian men it is 71 years. In both the United States and Canada, 12% of the Caucasian population is 65 years of age and older. In the United States, only 8% of African-Americans and 3.5% of all Hispanic- Americans are older than 65.[5,6]

The most rapidly increasing population age group is composed of those persons 85 years of age and older. The terms *young-old* (55 to 75 years of age) and *old-old* (75 years of age and older) were introduced in 1978.[7] These two groups represent chronologic ranges that often present different characteristics and needs. The term *frail elderly* has been suggested to represent those 75 years of age and older with a variety of ongoing and accumulating health concerns.[8] The nurse should increase self-awareness of the variability among the older population groups: healthy young-old, healthy old-old, and frail elderly.

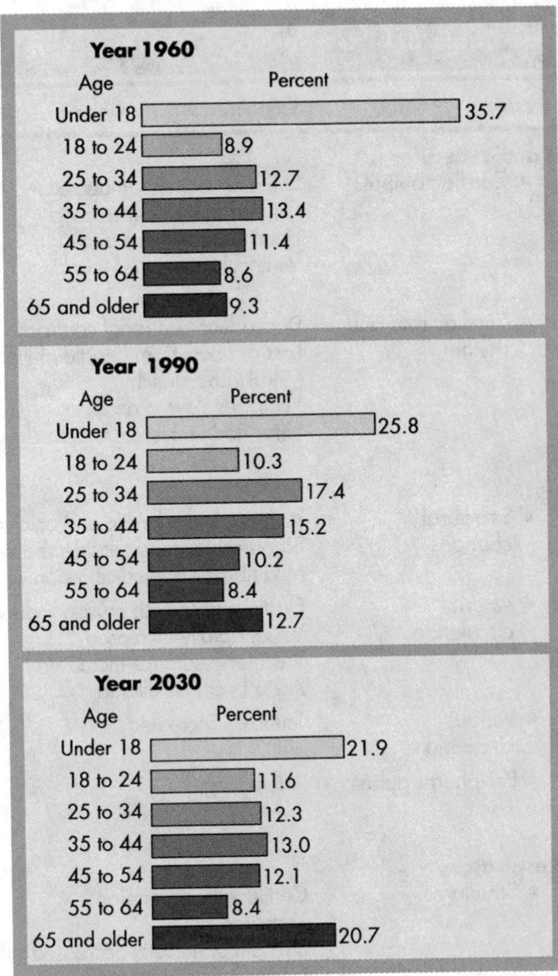

Fig. 3-1 Age distribution of total U.S. population.

Age-Related Changes

Age-related changes affect every body system. These changes are normal and occur as people age. However, the age at which specific changes become evident differs from person to person and within the same person. For instance, a person may have gray hair at age 45 but relatively unwrinkled skin at age 80. The nurse should assess for these age-related changes. Nursing diagnoses can be identified from these normal aging changes and their effect on functional ability. Table 3-1 presents the age-related changes and associated clinical manifestations.

SPECIAL POPULATIONS

Older Adult Women

For the aging woman, the impact of an aging body and being a woman is considered a double jeopardy. Women are often discriminated against for being older and female. Table 3-2 lists numerous factors that have had a significant negative impact on the health of the older woman. Gender-

Table 3-1 Gerontologic Differences in Assessment

System	Expected Aging Changes	Clinical Manifestations
Cardiovascular		
▪ Cardiac output	Force of contraction decreased Fat and collagen increased Heart muscle decreased Ventricular wall thickened	Myocardial oxygen demand increased Stroke volume and CO decreased Fatigue, shortness of breath, tachycardia occur Blood flow to vital organs and periphery decreased
▪ Cardiac rate and rhythm	Dependence on atrial contraction increased Loss of fibers from bundle of His Mitral valve stretching Ventricles slow to relax Sinus node pacemaker cells decreased	HR slow to increase with stress Decrease in maximum HR (e.g., 80-year-old person, 120 bpm; 20-year-old person, 200 bpm) Possible AV block Resting HR constant Recovery time from tachycardia prolonged Premature beats increased
▪ Structural changes	Aortic valves sclerotic and calcified Baroreceptor sensitivity decreased Mild fibrosis and calcification of valves	Diastolic murmur present in 50% of older patients Heart position landmarks change
▪ Arterial circulation	Elastin and smooth muscle reduced Vessel rigidity increased Vascular resistance increased Aorta becomes dilated	Modest increase in systolic BP (160/90) Rigid arteries contribute to coronary artery and peripheral vascular disease
▪ Venous circulation	Tortuosity increased	Inflamed, painful, or cordlike varicosities
▪ Peripheral pulses	Arteries rigid	Pulses weaker but equal Circulation slowed to periphery Cold feet and hands
Respiratory		
▪ Structures	Cartilage degeneration Vertebrae rigid Strength of muscles decreased Ciliary action decreased Respiratory muscles atrophy Thoracic wall increased ridigity	Kyphosis Anterior-posterior diameter increased Use of accessory muscles decreased Chest rigid and barrel-shaped Respiratory excursion decreased Cough and deep breathing diminished
▪ Change in ventilation and perfusion	Pulmonary vascular bed decreased Alveoli decreased Thickened alveolar walls Elastic recoil decreased Residual lung volume increased	Lung compliance decreased Total lung volume not changed Vital capacity decreased Residual volume increased Mucus thickens PaO_2 and oxygen saturation decreased Hyperresonance
▪ Ventilation control	Response to hypoxia and hypercarbia decreased	Response to stress decreased Ability to maintain acid-base balance decreased Rate 12-24/min
Integumentary		
▪ Skin	Collagen and subcutaneous fat decreased Sweat glands decreased Epidermal cell turnover slowed Skin tissue fluid decreased Capillary fragility increased Pigment cells decreased Sebaceous gland activity decreased Sensory receptors decreased Thresholds for touch, vibration, heat, pain increased	Skin less elastic Wrinkles and folds increased Extremity fat lost; fat on trunk increased Skin heals slowly Skin dry Skin tears and bruises easily Skin color uneven Multiple senile lentigines Normal skin lesions increased Ability to respond to heat and cold decreased Ability to feel light touch decreased Cutaneous pain sensitivity declines

continued

Table 3-1 Gerontologic Differences in Assessment—cont'd

System	Expected Aging Changes	Clinical Manifestations
Integumentary—cont'd		
▪ Hair	Melanin decreased Germ center and hair follicle decreased	Gray or white hair Hair quantity decreased and thinner Scalp, pubic, axillary hair decreased Facial hair on men decreased Facial hair on women increased
▪ Nails	Blood supply to nail bed decreased Longitudinal striations increased	Growth slowed Nails thickened and brittle Split easily Potential for fungal infection increased
Urinary		
▪ Structural changes in kidney	Renal mass decreased Number of functioning glomeruli decreased Glomerular filtration rate decreased Renal plasma flow decreased	Protein in urine increased Potential for dehydration Creatinine clearance decreased Serum creatinine and BUN increased Excretion of toxins and drugs decreased Nocturia increased
▪ Bladder	Bladder smooth muscle and elastic tissue decreased	Capacity decreased Less control: stress incontinence
▪ Micturition	Sphincter control decreased	Frequency, urgency, and nocturia increased
Reproductive		
▪ Male structures	Prostatic enlargement Testicular volume decreased Sperm count decreased Seminal vesicles atrophy Serum testosterone constant Estrogen level increased	Sexual response less intense Longer to achieve erection Erection maintained without ejaculation Force of ejaculation decreased
▪ Female structures	Estradiol, prolactin, progesterone diminished Size of ovaries, uterus, cervix, fallopian tubes, labia decreased Associated glands and epithelium atrophied Elasticity in the pelvic area decreased Breast tissue decreased Vaginal pH becomes alkaline	Responses to changing hormone levels altered Cervical, vaginal secretions dry Intensity of sexual response gradually decreased Potential for vaginal infections increased Potential for vaginal and uterine prolapse increased
Gastrointestinal		
▪ Oral cavity	Dentine decreased Gingival retraction Bone density lost Papillae of tongue decreased Taste threshold for salt and sugar increased Salivary secretions decreased	Taste changes Potential loss of teeth Gingivitis Bleeding gums and dry mouth Oral mucosa dry
▪ Esophagus	Lower esophageal sphincter relaxed Tone and motility decreased	Epigastric distress Dysphagia Potential for hiatal hernia and aspiration
▪ Stomach	Gastric mucosa atrophy Hydrochloric acid production decreased	Food intolerance
▪ Small intestine	Intestinal villae decreased Enzyme secretions decreased Motility decreased	Absorption of nutrients diminished Absorption of fat-soluble vitamins delayed
▪ Large intestine	Blood flow decreased Motility decreased Sensation to defecation decreased	Potential for constipation and fecal impaction
▪ Pancreas	Pancreatic ducts distend Lipase production decreased Pancreatic reserve impaired	Impaired fat absorption Decreased glucose tolerance
	Number and size of cells decreased Hepatic protein synthesis impaired	Lower border extends past costal margin

continued

Table 3-1 Gerontologic Differences in Assessment—cont'd

System	Expected Aging Changes	Clinical Manifestations
Musculoskeletal		
▪ Skeleton	Intervertebral discs narrowed Cartilage of nose and ears increased	Height diminished 1-4 in (2.5-10 cm) Nose and ears lengthen Kyphosis Pelvis wider
▪ Bone	Cortical and trabecular bone decreased	Bone resorption exceeds bone formation Potential for osteoporotic falls and fractures
▪ Muscles	Number of muscle fibers decreased Muscle fibers atrophy Muscle regeneration slowed Contraction time and latency period prolonged Flexion of joints increased Ligaments stiffening Sclerosis of tendons Tendon flexor reflexes decreased	Strength decreased Agility decreased Rigidity in neck, shoulders, hips, and knees increased Potential restless leg syndrome
▪ Joints	Cartilage erosion Calcium deposits increased Water in cartilage decreased	Mobility decreased ROM limited Potential osteoarthritis
Nervous		
▪ Structure	Loss of neurons in brain and spinal cord Brain size decreased Dendrites atrophy Major neurotransmitters decreased	Conduction of nerve impulses slowed Peripheral nerve function lost Reaction time decreased Response time precise and slowed Potential for altered balance, vertigo, syncope Postural hypotension increased Proprioception diminished Sensory input decreased EEG Alpha waves decreased
▪ Sleep	Deep sleep decreased REM sleep decreased	Difficulty remembering dreams Difficulty falling asleep Periods of wakefulness increased Sleeptime averages 6 hr
Visual		
▪ Eye structure	Orbital fat lost Eyebrows and eyelashes gray Elasticity of eyelid muscles decreased Tear production decreased	Eyes sunken Eyes dry Potential ectropion and entropion Potential conjunctivitis
▪ Cornea	Corneal sensitivity decreased Corneal reflex decreased Arcus senilis	Potential corneal abrasion
▪ Ciliary	Aqueous humor secretion decreased Ciliary muscle atrophy	Ability of lens to accommodate declines Potential presbyopia Peripheral vision decreased
▪ Lens	Less elastic, more dense Blue-green color discrimination decreased	Lens yellow and opaque Less ability to adapt to light and dark Tolerance to glare decreased Incidence of cataracts increased Night vision impaired
▪ Iris and pupil	Pigment lost Smaller Vitreous gel debris increased	Visual acuity decreased Pupils appear constricted Floaters
Auditory		
▪ Structure	Hairs in external auditory canals of males increased Ceruminal glands decreased	Cerumen more dry Potential conductive hearing loss

continued

Table 3-1 Gerontologic Differences in Assessment—cont'd

System	Expected Aging Changes	Clinical Manifestations
Auditory—cont'd		
▪ Middle ear	Middle ear long joints degenerate Ear drum thickens	Sound conduction decreased
▪ Inner ear	Vestibular structures decline Hair cells lost Cochlea atrophies Organ of Corti atrophies	Sensitivity to high tones: "s," "t," "f," "g" decreased Understanding of speech decreased Discrimination of background voice decreased Equilibrium-balance deficits Potential for tinnitus
Immune System	Secretory immunoglobulin (IgA) declines Thymus gland involuted Thymopoietin decreased Lymphoid tissue decreased Stem cells impaired Antibody production impaired T lymphocytes decreased Autoantibodies increased	Potential increase for infection on mucosal surfaces Impaired cell-mediated immune response Malignancy incidence increased Response to acute infection reduced Potential recurrence of latent herpes zoster and tuberculosis Autoimmune disease increased

AV, Atrioventricular; *BP,* blood pressure; *bpm,* beats per minute; *BUN,* blood urea nitrogen; *CO,* cardiac output; *EEG,* electroencephalogram; *HR,* heart rate; *REM,* rapid eye movement; *ROM,* range of motion.

Table 3-2 Factors Negatively Affecting Health of Older Women

1. A disproportionately higher number of women than men live in poverty.
2. Minority women have the highest poverty rates.
3. Lack of formal work experience of older women leads to low incomes.
4. More older women rely on social security as a major source of income than men.
5. Older women more frequently live alone than men.
6. Traditional caregiving and homemaking roles increase women's economic insecurity.
7. Older women have less access to health insurance.
8. Older women have a higher incidence of chronic health problems, such as arthritis, hypertension, strokes, and diabetes.
9. Older women who are married are likely to be caregivers for ill husbands.

Compiled from Hooyman NR, Kujak HA: Populations at risk: older women. In *Social Gerontology,* ed 3, Boston, 1993, Allyn and Bacon.

based inequities in health care can be seen in the emphasis on (1) Medicare coverage of acute care conditions that occur more frequently in men, such as coronary artery disease; (2) high out-of-pocket costs for depression, arthritis, and hypertension, which occur more often in women; (3) lack of research on diseases for which women are at risk, such as breast cancer; (4) less aggressive diagnostic work-up for anxiety, depression, and cardiac disease in women.[9]

The nurse is in an excellent position to be an advocate for health equity for the older woman in the health care system. Advocacy organizations, such as the Older Women's League (OWL), can be helpful in this process.

Cognitively Impaired Older Adults

For the majority of healthy older adults, there is no noticeable decline in mental abilities. The older adult may experience a memory lapse or benign forgetfulness that is significantly different from cognitive impairment (Table 3-3).

The older adult who is forgetful should be encouraged to use memory aids, to attempt recall in a calm and quiet environment, and to actively engage in memory improvement techniques. Memory aids include clocks, calendars, notes, marked pill boxes, safety alarms on stoves, and identity necklaces or bracelets. Memory techniques include word association, mental imaging, and mnemonics.

Declining physical health is an important factor that influences cognitive impairment. The older adult who experiences sensory loss, cardiovascular disease, or hypertension shows a decline in cognitive functioning. Although intelligence quotient (IQ) is important, the nurse needs to assess functional use of information. An appropriate cognitive assessment includes functional ability, memory recall, orientation, use of judgment, and appropriate emotional state. The use of standard mental status examinations and behavioral descriptions provide data for determining cognitive status. The three most common cognitive problems of the elderly are compared in Table 3-4. (See Chapter 56 for a discussion of Alzheimer's disease.)

Rural Older Adults

Approximately one half of all persons 65 years and older live in nonmetropolitan areas. The older adult tends to move to these areas because living costs are reduced, communities are less complex, and crime is less common.

Table 3-3 Forgetfulness Versus Cognitive Impairment

Benign—Forgetfulness	Pathology—Cognitive Loss
Forgets, then remembers	Forgets important people
When item is lost, mental retracing occurs	Unable to mentally retrace
Forgets unimportant events	Forgets entire recent events
Forgets long-ago events	Forgets events minutes ago
Uses reminders and notes	Cannot use reminders consistently
Oriented to self as a person	May be disoriented to self
May repeat stories over time	Repeats same question in a short time

Modified from Gwyther L: *Care of Alzheimer's patients: a manual for nursing home staff,* American Health Care Association, 1985.

Table 3-4 A Comparison of the Clinical Features of Acute Confusion, Dementia, and Depression

Feature	Acute Confusion (Delirium)	Dementia	Depression
Onset	Rapid, often at night	Usually insidious	Coincides with life changes; often abrupt
Course	Fluctuates, worse at night; lucid intervals	Long; symptoms progressive yet relatively stable over time	Diurnal effects, typically worse in the morning; situational fluctuations
Progression	Abrupt	Slow but even	Variable, rapid-slow but uneven
Duration	Hours to less than 1 month	Months to years	At least 2 weeks, but can be several months to years
Awareness	Reduced	Clear	Clear
Alertness	Fluctuates, lethargic or hypervigilant	Generally normal	Normal
Orientation	Fluctuates in severity, generally impaired	May be impaired	Selective disorientation
Memory	Recent and immediate impaired	Recent and remote impaired	Selective or patchy impairment, "islands" of intact memory
Thinking	Disorganized, distorted, fragmented; slow or accelerated incoherent speech	Difficulty with abstraction, thoughts impoverished, judgment impaired, words difficult to find	Intact but with themes of hopelessness, helplessness, or self-deprecation
Perception	Distorted; illusions, delusions, and hallucinations	Misperceptions often present; delusions and hallucinations absent except in severe cases	
Psychomotor behavior	Variable; hypokinetic, hyperkinetic, or mixed	Normal, may have apraxia	Variable; psychomotor retardation or agitation
Sleep-wake cycle	Disturbed, cycle reversed	Fragmented	Disturbed, often early morning awakening
Mental status testing	Distracted from task; poor performance; improves when patient recovers	Frequent "near miss" answers, struggles with test, great effort to find an appropriate reply; consistently poor performances	Frequent "don't know" answers, little effort, frequently gives up, indifferent

Statistically, the rural older adult is most frequently Caucasian, male, married, and has a higher poverty rate.[10]

Because of geographic isolation and a higher poverty level, the rural older adult is highly stressed by changing financial resources and declining self-care abilities.[11] Although the rural older adult fears dependence on others, symptoms of ill health are greater than those found in urban peers. These concerns may be related to two factors: the rural older adult is less likely to engage in health-promoting activities, and the rural community is underserved by health care workers.[12]

The nurse working with the rural older adult needs to clearly define the lifestyle values and practices of rural life. Health care providers should consider transportation as a possible barrier to service. Alternate service approaches such as videotapes, radio, and church social events should be used to promote healthful practices or to conduct health screening. Innovative models of nursing practice need to be developed to assist the rural older adult.

Frail Older Adults

The old-old population (75 years of age and older) is steadily increasing in number. Since the 1960s this group has increased 250%. The old-old adult is usually a widowed woman dependent on family or kinship support. Many have outlived children, spouses, and siblings. The old-old adult is often characterized as a hardy, elite survivor. Because the old-old adult has lived so long, she may have become the family icon, the symbol of family tradition and legacy. Approximately one fourth are in nursing homes or other institutions. In this old-old population, ethnic group members often live with extended family and often continue to speak their native language.

The old-old adult has difficulty coping with declining functional abilities and decreasing daily energy. When stressful life events (such as the death of a pet) and daily strain (such as caring for an ill spouse) occur, the old-old individual often cannot alleviate the effects of stress and, as a result, may become ill.

The frail older adult is at particular risk for malnutrition. Malnutrition is related to sociopsychologic factors such as living alone, depression, and low income. Physical factors such as declining cognitive status, inadequate dental care, sensory limitation, physical fatigue, and limited mobility also add to the risk of malnutrition. Because many frail older adults have therapeutic diets and multiple drug regimens, their nutritional state may be altered. It is important for the nurse to monitor the frail older adult for adequate calorie, protein, iron, calcium, and vitamin D intake.

The acronym *SCALES* can remind the nurse to assess important nutritional indicators: (*Sadness*) mood change, high *Cholesterol,* low *Albumin, Loss* or gain of weight, *Eating* problems, or *Shopping* and food preparation problems. Once the older adult's nutritional needs are identified, common interventions include home-delivered meals, dietary supplements, food stamps, dental referrals, and vitamin supplements.

The frail older adult considers his health to be fair with specific deficits in activities of daily living (ADLs).[13] Common health problems of the frail older adult include mobility limitations, sensory impairment, cognitive decline, falls, and increasing frailty.

The nurse should remember that the frail older adult tires easily, has little physical reserve, and is at risk for disability, elder abuse, and institutionalization. This older adult is dependent on a delicate network of family, individual, and social support that should be respected and supported.

Sick Older Adults

The older adult population has a higher rate of hospitalization, homecare, day surgery, and physician visits than any other group. Eighty percent of all older adults have at least one chronic disease. The older adult is more likely than the adult in a younger age group to have days of restricted activity as a result of acute illness. Although health status refers to acute and chronic illness, it also includes an individual's level of daily functioning. *Functional health* includes ADLs, such as bathing, dressing, eating, toileting, and transfer. Instrumental ADLs, such as using a telephone, shopping, preparing food, housekeeping, doing laundry, arranging transportation, taking medication, and handling finances, are also included in functional health assessment.

As age increases, a pattern of declining functional health and increasing disability is seen. The nurse caring for the older adult can advocate accurate comprehensive assessment in which health and disease states are diagnosed accurately and can actively teach health promotion strategies.

Disease in the older adult is often difficult to accurately diagnose. The older adult tends to underreport symptoms and to treat these symptoms by altering functional status. The older adult eats less, sleeps more, or "walks it out." The older adult often attributes a new symptom to "old age" and will ignore it.

Disease in the older adult may vary greatly, based on age-related individual change. As one disease is treated, another may be affected. For example, the use of an anticholinergic medication may cause urinary retention. In the older adult, diseases are atypical, and complaints of "aching in the joint" may actually be a broken hip. Silent asymptomatic pathology is frequently seen. Cardiac disease may be diagnosed when the patient is being treated for a urinary tract infection. Pathologies with similar symptoms are often confused. Depression may be mistreated as dementia. A cascade disease pattern may occur. An example is the patient who experiences insomnia, treats the condition with a hypnotic medication, becomes lethargic and confused, falls, and breaks a hip.

ETHNICITY AND AGING

The older adult who identifies with a certain ethnic group presents a particular challenge to the nurse (Fig. 3-2). Ethnic identity can be determined by asking these questions:

1. Does this person identify with an ethnic or racial group?
2. Do others identify this person with an ethnic or racial group?
3. Does this person show behavioral patterns that are unique to the ethnic group?

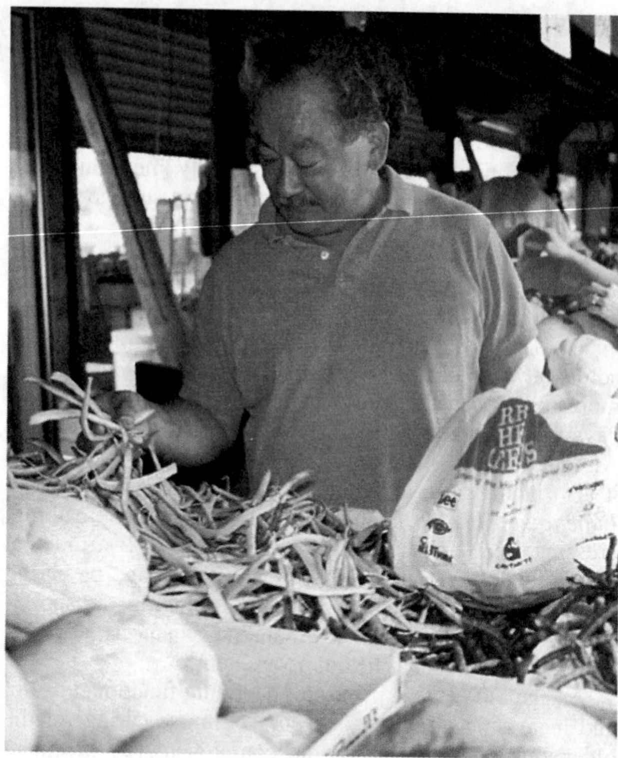
Fig. 3-2 Ethnic elders need special consideration.

Ethnic identity is often found in certain religious groups, nations, and minorities. As American society changes, ethnic institutions and neighborhoods may be altered. For the older adult with strong ethnic roots, the loss of friends who speak the "mother tongue," the loss of the church that supports social ethnic activities, and the loss of stores that carry desired ethnic foods may present situational crises that emphasize and diminish a sense of self-worth and personhood. This loss of self is increased when children and others deny or ignore ethnic practices and behaviors. Support for the ethnic older adult is most frequently found in family, religious practices, and isolated geographic or community ethnic clusters.

The ethnic older adult is faced with specific problems. Because the ethnic older adult often lives in older neighborhoods, physical security and personal safety related to high crime rates become a concern. Because the individual with an ethnic identity often has a disproportionately low income, Medicare deductibles or medications needed to treat chronic illnesses may not be affordable.

For the nurse to be effective with the ethnic older adult, a sense of respect and clear communication is critical. The nurse must identify self-behaviors that could be interpreted as noncaring or disrespectful, such as a refusal to allow a patient to display an item considered important for healing. Nursing interventions to assist in meeting the needs of the ethnic older adult are described in Table 3-5. Questions to ask the ethnic older adult about health-related practices include:

Table 3-5 Nursing Interventions to Assist in Meeting the Needs of Ethnic Older Adults

1. Identify health practices, rituals, and food patterns that are central to an ethnic identity.
2. Identify stereotypic attitudes in the ethnic older adult that interfere with multiethnic group participation.
3. Inform ethnic older adult about services available.
4. Support the ethnic older adult who is fearful about traveling outside the accepted neighborhood for services.
5. Advocate for ethnic older adult to receive services that provide special attention to language limitations and cultural health practices.
6. Use strategies specific to an ethnic group. For example, African-Americans may respond to themes like "do it for your loved ones." Asians may respond to fear of dependency themes.
7. Learn about services and programs that focus on specific ethnic groups. Examples include home-meal services that serve ethnic foods or nursing homes that include specific ethnic or religious preferences.

1. What makes people ill?
2. When do you know someone is sick?
3. What helps people get better?
4. Who can assist people to get well?
5. Do you believe this will help you get well?

American culture is changing. For some older adults, ethnic identity is also changing. The nurse should not assume that ethnic identity is or is not of value to the patient and the patient's family. The nurse must assess each older adult's ethnic orientation.[14,15]

NURSING PROCESS AND THE OLDER ADULT

Establishing a Therapeutic Environment

The older adult may face a developing health problem with fear and anxiety. Health workers may be perceived as helpful while institutions are perceived as negative, potentially harmful places. The nurse can communicate a sense of concern and care by careful use of direct and simple statements, appropriate eye contact, direct touch, and gentle humor. These actions assist the older adult to relax in this stressful situation.

Before beginning the interview the nurse should attend to primary needs first, ensuring that the patient is pain-free and does not need to urinate. All assistive devices such as glasses and hearing aids should be in place. The interview should be short so the patient is not fatigued. The interviewer should allow adequate time for response to questions. The older adult and caregiver should be interviewed separately, unless the patient is cognitively impaired or specifically requests the caregiver's presence. Medical history may be lengthy. The nurse must determine what is relevant information. Old medical records should be obtained and available for review.

Assessment

As with all age groups, assessment of the older adult provides the data base for the rest of the nursing process. The focus of a geriatric assessment is to determine appropriate interventions to maintain and enhance the functional abilities of the older adult. Cure is often not possible because of the complexity and chronicity of the health problems that commonly affect the older adult. Consequently, the nurse directs the planning and implementation of those actions that assist the older adult in remaining as functionally independent as possible.

Elements in a comprehensive assessment include a history using a functional health pattern format (see Chapter 4), physical assessment, assessment of ADLs and instrumental activities of daily living (IADLs), mental status evaluation, and a social-environmental assessment. Evaluation of mental status is particularly important for the older adult because results often determine the patient's potential for independent living. Evaluation of the results of a comprehensive assessment helps to determine the service and placement needs of the older adult patient. A good match between needs and services should be the goal of a geriatric assessment.

Clinical assessment should be based on instruments specific to the older adult population (Table 3-6). Interpretation of laboratory results can be problematic because many values change with age, and parameters are not well defined for the older adult, particularly the old-old patient.[16,17] The healthy adult may have age-related changes that may be considered abnormal in a younger population but are normal for an older adult. An appropriate reference book should be consulted for the correct ranges of laboratory values for the older adult. The nurse is in an important position to recognize and correct inaccurate interpretation of laboratory tests.

The comprehensive geriatric assessment is often conducted at a Geriatric Evaluation Unit (GEU) by an interdisciplinary geriatric assessment team. The interdisciplinary team may include many disciplines, but the minimum components include the nurse, the physician, and the social worker. After the assessment is complete, the interdisciplinary team meets with the patient and family to present the team's findings and recommendations. These assessment centers are often affiliated with large medical complexes.

Diagnosis

With few exceptions the same nursing diagnoses apply to the older adult as to a younger person. Often, however, the etiology and defining characteristics are related to age and unique to the older adult. Table 3-7 lists nursing diagnoses

Table 3-6 Geriatric Assessment Instruments

Area of Concern	Example of Assessment Instrument	What Is Tested
Mental status	Folstein Mini-Mental State[1]	Tests orientation, memory, attention, language, recall Low score = cognitive impairment-general
Mood state	Geriatric Depression Scale[2]	30 affective items test for depression
Functional ability	Katz Index of Activities of Daily Living[3]	Tests bathing, dressing, toileting, transfer, continence, feeding Coded as: Independent—Assistance—Dependent
Functional ability	Lawton Instrumental Activities of Daily Living[4]	Tests telephone usage, traveling, shopping, meal preparation, housework, medication, money Coded as: Independent—Assistance—Dependent
Dementia indicators	Set Test[5]	Tests ability to name up to 10 items in 4 sets: Fruits, Animals, Colors, Towns (*FACT*) Score maximum = 40
Social support	Zarit Burden Interview[6]	Tests for feelings of burden in caregiving
Alcohol usage	CAGE[7]	Tests for alcohol abuse 4 items; response of yes in 2 or more = problem
Falls assessment	Get Up and Go Test[8]	Tests balance and sway as risk for fall

1. Folstein MF, Folstein SE, McHugh PR: Mini-mental state: a practical method for grading the cognitive state of patients for the clinician, *J Psychiatr Res* 12:189, 1975.
2. Yesavage JA, Brink TL: Development and validation of a geriatric depression screening scale: a preliminary paper, *J Psychiatr Res* 17:41, 1983.
3. Katz S and others: Studies of illness in the aged. The index of ADL: a standardized measure of biological and psychological function, *JAMA* 185:914, 1963.
4. Lawton H, Brody E: Assessment of older people: self-maintaining and instrumental activities of daily living, *Gerontologist* 9:179, 1969.
5. Isaacs B, Kennie AT: The Set Test as an aid to the detection of dementia in old people, *Br J Psychiatry* 123:467,1973.
6. Zarit SH: Relatives of impaired elderly: correlates of feelings of burden, *Gerontologist* 20:699, 1980.
7. Mayfield D, Mcleod G, Hall P: The CAGE questionnaire: validation of a new alcoholism screening instrument, *Am J Psychiatry* 131:10, 1974.
8. Mathias S, Nayok U, Isaacs B: Balance in elderly patients: the "get up and go" test, *Arch Phys Med Rehabil* 67:387, 1986.

Table 3-7 Nursing Diagnoses Associated with Age-Related Physiologic Changes

Cardiovascular System
Decreased cardiac output
Activity intolerance
Fatigue
Respiratory System
Ineffective breathing pattern
Impaired gas exchange
Ineffective airway clearance
Risk for respiratory infection
Risk for aspiration
Integumentary System
Impaired skin integrity
Urinary System
Fluid volume deficit
Altered pattern of urinary elimination
Reproductive System
Altered sexuality pattern
Body image disturbance
Sexual dysfunction
Gastrointestinal System
Altered nutrition
Constipation
Alteration in oral mucous membranes
Musculoskeletal System
Risk for injury and falls
Self-care deficit
Pain
Impaired physical mobility
Nervous System
Altered thought processes
Sensory-perceptual alterations
Sleep pattern disturbance
Hypothermia
Hyperthermia
Senses
Sensory perceptual alteration
Body image disturbance
Impaired verbal communication
Social isolation
Immune System
Risk for infection

that are commonly associated with specific age-related changes. The identification and management of nursing diagnoses result in improved patient function and quality patient care for the older adult.

Planning

When setting goals with the older adult, it is helpful to identify the strengths and abilities that the patient demonstrates. Personal characteristics such as hardiness, persistence, and the ability to laugh and learn are positive factors in goal setting. Caregivers should be included in goal development. In contrast, the older adult who perceives increasing dependence and learned helplessness as an appropriate response may be resistant to self-care. Priority goals for the older adult may be gaining a sense of control, feeling safe, and reducing stress.

Table 3-8 Evaluating Nursing Care for Older Adults

Evaluation questions may include the following:

1. Is there an identifiable change in ADLs, IADLs, mental status, or disease signs and symptoms?
2. Does the patient identify a better health state?
3. Does the patient think the treatment is helpful?
4. Do the patient and caregiver think the care is worth the time and cost?
5. Can the nurse document positive changes that support interventions?
6. Does change adequately meet the required mandates for reimbursement?

ADLs, Activities of daily living; *IADLs*, instrumental activities of daily living.

Implementation

When carrying out a plan of action, the nurse may need to modify the approach and techniques used on the basis of the physical and mental status of the elderly patient. Small body size, common in the frail older adult, may necessitate the use of smaller pediatric equipment. Bone and joint changes often require transfer assistance, altered positioning, and use of gait belts and lift devices. The older adult with declining energy reserves requires extra rest periods alternated with short periods of exertion. A slower approach, restricted scheduling, and the use of a bedside commode or other adaptive equipment may be necessary.

Cognitive impairment, if present, requires the nurse to offer careful explanations and a calm approach to avoid producing anxiety and resistance in the patient. Depression can result in apathy and poor cooperation with the treatment plan.

Evaluation

The evaluation phase of the nursing process is similar for all patients. Evaluation is ongoing throughout the nursing process. The results of evaluation direct the nurse to continue the plan of care or revise as indicated. Often the change in health status is not as dramatic in the older adult as it is in the younger patient. Because of this, the nurse needs to be cautious in changing plans prematurely.

When evaluating nursing care with the older adult, the nurse should focus on functional improvement, rather than cure. Useful questions to consider when evaluating the plan of care for an older adult are included in Table 3-8.

TEACHING OLDER ADULTS

The nurse is involved in teaching the older adult self-care practices to enhance health and modify disease processes (Fig. 3-3). The older adult presents the following challenges to learning: (1) time needed to learn is increased, (2) new learning needs to relate to the patient's actual experience,

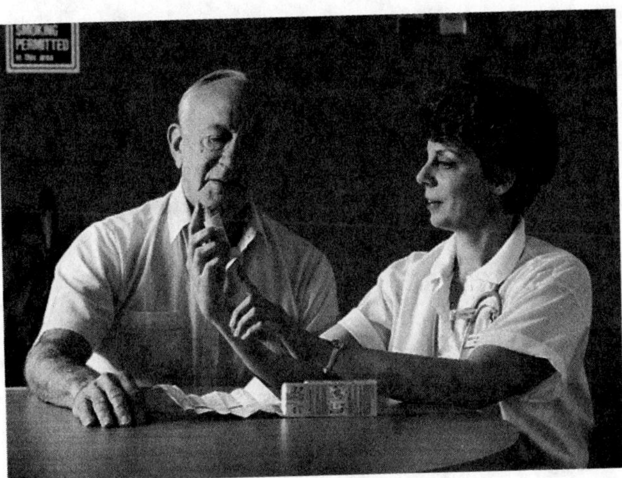

Fig. 3-3 Careful patient teaching increases the possibility of successful discharge of the older adult patient.

(3) anxiety and distractions decrease learning, (4) lack of risk taking and cautiousness decrease motivation to learn, and (5) sensory-perceptual deficits and cognitive decline require modified teaching techniques.

Specific approaches that increase the level of learning in the older adult include (1) the use of peer educators, (2) the use of simplicity and repetition, and (3) the support of the belief that change in behavior is both helpful and worth the effort of increased learning.[18]

HEALTH PROMOTION AND SCREENING

Health promotion and prevention of health problems in the older adult are focused in three areas: reduction in diseases and problems, increased participation in health promotion activities, and increased targeted services that reduce health hazards. These goals are central to three major health initiatives currently guiding services for the older adult: (1) *The Healthy People 2000* national health objectives, (2) the recommendations of the U.S. Preventive Services Task Force Guide to Clinical Preventive Services, and (3) the Nutrition Screening Initiative.[19,20,21]

The nurse places a high value on health promotion and positive health behaviors. Programs have been successfully developed for screening for chronic health conditions, smoking cessation, geriatric foot care, vision and hearing screening, stress reduction, exercise programs, medication usage, crime prevention, and home hazards assessment. The nurse can carry out and teach the older adult about the need for specific preventive services.

Health promotion and prevention can be included in nursing interventions at any location or level where the nurse and the older adult interact. The nurse can use health promotion activities to strengthen self-care, to increase personal responsibility for health, and to increase independent functioning that will enhance the well-being of the older adult.[22]

The nurse interested in older adult health promotion can contact the organizations listed below:

National Center for Health Promotion
National Council on the Aging
600 Maryland Avenue, SW
West Wing 100
Washington, DC 20024

Health Promotion Interest Group
Gerontological Society of America
1275 K Street, NW
Suite 350
Washington, DC 20005-4006

CHRONIC ILLNESS

Although the U.S. health care system is dominated by an acute illness focus, daily living with chronic illness is a reality for many older adults. Although persons of all ages have chronic health problems, chronic illness is most common in the older adult. Eighty-five percent of persons 65 years of age and older have at least one chronic condition. The ten most common chronic conditions present in the older adult are visual impairment, diabetes, cataracts, heart disease, hearing impairment, hypertension, arthritis, orthopedic impairment, varicose veins, and chronic sinusitis.[23]

Often, chronic illness is composed of multiple health problems that have a protracted, unpredictable course. Diagnosis and an acute phase of a chronic illness are often managed in a hospital. All other phases of a chronic illness are usually managed at home. The management of a chronic illness can profoundly affect the lives and identities of the patient, caregiver, and family.

Tasks required for daily living with chronic illness are defined.[24] These include (1) preventing and managing crisis, (2) carrying out prescribed regimens, (3) controlling symptoms, (4) reordering time, (5) adjusting to changes in the course of the disease, (6) preventing social isolation, and (7) attempting to normalize interactions with others.

Both the patient and the nurse must practice behaviors different from that required of patients with an acute illness if the older adult is to accomplish the tasks associated with a chronic disease.

GERIATRIC REHABILITATION

Older adults make up 40% of the disabled population yet receive only 10% of all services. Rehabilitation interventions are focused toward adapting to or recovering from disability. With proper training, assistive equipment, and attendant personal care, the patient with disabilities can often live an independent life. For the younger disabled adult, the approach of personal attendant care with a focus on independent living stimulated the 1990 Americans with Disabilities Act. Advocates suggest that the elimination of environmental barriers allows the disabled to function normally in society. The older adult, primarily through Medicare reimbursement, receives rehabilitative assistance through postincident, inpatient rehabilitation (limited days), and home care programs. These health care services are extensions of medical services. Reliance on unpaid family caregivers and a focus on patient limitations restrict the rehabilitation potential for the older adult.[25]

The nurse needs to understand physical disability in the older adult. The older person with cerebral vascular disease, arthritis, and coronary artery disease has a risk of becoming functionally limited within 4 years. Hip fracture, amputation, and stroke occur at higher rates in the older adult population. These disabilities lead to increased mortality, decreased life span, and increased rates of institutionalization. Reducing residual disability through geriatric rehabilitation is important to the quality of life of the older adult.

Rehabilitation of the older adult is influenced by several factors. First, the older patient shows greater initial variability in functional capacity than an adult at any other age. Preexisting problems associated with reaction time, visual acuity, fine motor ability, physical strength, cognitive function, and motivation affect the rehabilitation potential of the older adult.

Also, the older adult often loses functioning because of inactivity and immobility. This deconditioning can occur as a result of unstable acute medical conditions, environmental barriers that limit mobility, and a lack of motivation to stay in condition. The effect of inactivity clearly leads to "use it or lose it" consequences. The older adult can improve flexibility, strength, and aerobic capacity even into very old age. The nurse must use passive and active range-of-motion exercises with all older adults to prevent deconditioning and subsequent functional decline.

Lastly, the goal of geriatric rehabilitation is to strive for maximal function and physical capabilities considering the individual's current health status. When a patient demonstrates suboptimal health, the nurse screens and evaluates for risk behaviors. For example, a woman with a history of osteoporosis should be given a fall-risk appraisal, or the older adult diabetic patient should receive a geriatric foot assessment.

Rehabilitation is directed at preventing permanent disability. Therefore, rehabilitation interventions emphasize four areas: (1) functional activity to increase capacity and mobility, (2) balance improvement, (3) good nutrition, and (4) social and emotional support.

Often the older adult has specific fears and anxieties related to falling and fatigue. The older adult is limited in the rehabilitation process by sensory-perceptual deficits, other disease states, slowed cognition, poor nutrition, and funding problems. Disability can be diminished by using appropriate assistive devices and adapting the environment to support function. Supportive and concerned caregivers are critical to the success of these modifications. Nurse and caregiver encouragement, support, and acceptance assist the older adult in remaining motivated for the hard work of rehabilitation.[26]

HOSPITALIZATION AND ACUTE ILLNESS

Frequently the hospital is the first point of contact for the older adult and the formal health care system. Approximately 20% of all Medicare recipients are hospitalized annually. The hospitalized older adult is often experiencing multisystem failure. Illnesses that most commonly result in hospitalization include heart dysrhythmias, heart failure, cerebral vascular accidents, fluid and electrolyte imbalances, dehydration, hyponatremia, pneumonia, and hip fractures.[27] The complexity of the acute situation often results in a loss of the whole-person perspective and focuses care on the diseased part. Because the nurse provides an integrated approach, care that is individualized and helpful to the older adult can be reestablished.

The outcome of hospitalization for the older adult varies. Of particular concern are the problems of high surgical risk, acute confusional state, nosocomial infection, and premature discharge with an unstable condition.

High Surgical Risk

Age-related body changes, chronic illness, and declining physical reserve place the older adult at increased surgical risk. Other key factors that increase surgical risk include age older than 75 years, emergency operations, use of spinal anesthesia, and thrombolytic complications. The risk of surgery should be balanced against the benefit and appropriateness of surgery for the older adult patient. (See Chapters 14, 15, and 16 for additional surgical considerations for the older adult.)

Acute Confusional State

The sudden onset of an acute confusional state (delirium) occurs in 18% to 38% of hospitalized older adults.[28] Although delirium is usually a transient condition that lasts from 1 to 7 days, research indicates some delirium symptoms may persist up to discharge. Delirium is one of the most frequent consequences of unscheduled surgery because the older adult has not been stabilized physically or prepared emotionally. The patient who experiences delirium will exhibit a decline in ADL capacity.[29]

Nosocomial Infection

Nosocomial infections occur at higher rates in older adults. For the old-old patient, the rate is two to five times the rate of a younger person. Age-related changes of decreased immunocompetence, the presence of pathologic conditions, and an increase in disability all contribute to higher infection rates. Infections common to the older adult include pneumonia, urinary tract infections, and skin infections.[30] Tuberculosis is disproportionately high in the older adult population.[31] These infections often have atypical presentations showing cognitive and behavioral changes before alterations occur in laboratory values or temperature.

Hospital Discharge

At the time of hospital discharge, 15% to 93% of older adults are considered to be in an unstable condition. The frail older adult and the oldest-old patient are particularly vulnerable. Most of these patients are discharged under Medicare regulations that specify a registered nurse or qualified person develop a plan to evaluate discharge. The discharge plan should be periodically reassessed, and caregivers and patients must be counseled to prepare the patient for posthospital care.

The nurse can use screening inventories, such as Blaylock's Discharge Planning Risk Assessment Screen, to identify at-risk patients.[32] The postdischarge assistance needed by high risk patients includes bathing, taking medications, housekeeping, shopping, preparing meals, and making satisfactory transportation arrangements.[33] Risk of unstable discharge increases in the patient who experiences greater length of stay and who is dependent for meals.[34] Early hospital discharge is most successful when patients have had little change in functional status or are returning to a place with a high level of assistance, such as a nursing home.[35]

Nursing Role in Hospital Care

When caring for the hospitalized older adult, both patient and caregivers are assisted when the nurse performs the following:

1. Identifies the frail and old-old patients at risk for the iatrogenic effects of hospitalization.
2. Considers discharge needs early in the hospital stay, especially assistance with ADLs, IADLs, and medications.
3. Encourages the development and use of interdisciplinary teams, special care units, and individuals who focus on the special needs of gerontologic patients.[36]
4. Develops standard protocols to screen for at-risk conditions commonly present in the hospitalized older adult patient, such as urinary tract infection and delirium.
5. Advocates for referral of the patient to appropriate community-based formal care services.

GENERAL CARE CONSIDERATIONS

Environmental Considerations

As people age, the environment in which they live can be adapted to increase safety and comfort. Uncluttered floor space, railings, increased lighting and nightlights, and clearly-marked stair edges are some of the easiest and most practical adaptations.

The older adult in an inpatient or long-term care setting needs a thorough orientation to the environment. The nurse should repeatedly reassure the patient that he is safe and attempt to answer all questions. The unit should foster patient orientation by displaying large print clocks, avoiding complex or visually confusing wall designs, clearly designating doors, and using simple bed and nurse-call controls. Lighting should be adequate while avoiding glare. Beds should be close to the floor with four siderails that can be modified to individual needs. Environments that provide consistent caregivers and an established daily routine assist the older adult patient.

Assistive Devices

The use of assistive devices should be considered as an intervention for the older adult. Many older adults use or could benefit from the use of assistive devices such as dentures, glasses, hearing aids, walkers, wheelchairs, adult briefs or protectors, adaptive utensils, elevated toilet seats, and skin protective devices. These tools and devices should be included in the patient's care plan when appropriate. The nurse is in a position to assure the correct and consistent use of these devices.

Pain Management

The older adult does not often ask for pain relief. When pain is a known complication of a particular condition, the nurse should offer pain medication at regular intervals. Pain assessment in the elderly may be complicated by cognitive decline, sensory-perceptual deficits, and age-related changes. The use of verbal and visual pain scales can assist in correct assessment. For the patient with ongoing pain, a pain diary may be helpful in identifying activities that relieve or increase pain.[37] Because the older adult may believe that pain is something that must be endured, creative methods may be developed to deal with it. The nurse should ask the patient to describe techniques used to reduce pain. People use change in body position, heat, exercise, distraction, and rest to deal with pain. Mental imaging, positive thinking, and prayer and other spiritual interventions are also used. Poor pain management may lead to reduced socialization, limited mobility, impaired posture, sleep disturbances, depression, anxiety, and constipation.[38,39] (See Chapter 6 for additional discussion of pain.)

Medication Use

Medication usage in the older adult requires thorough and regular assessment and care planning. The use and abuse of medication by the older adult is supported by the following facts:

1. The older adult woman may take as many as six prescription drugs and three or more over-the-counter medications at the same time.
2. The oldest-old patient takes an average of 12 prescribed medications.
3. The frequency of adverse drug reactions increases as the number of prescribed drugs increases.
4. Twelve percent of older adult hospital admissions occur because of drug reactions.
5. Upon discharge from a hospital, more than 25% of all older adults receive at least six prescriptions.[40]

Age-related changes alter the pharmacodynamics and pharmacokinetics of drugs. Drug-drug, drug-food, and drug-disease interactions all influence the absorption, distribution, and excretion of drugs. Figure 3-4 illustrates the effect of drug use on the aging body.

In addition to changes in the metabolism of drugs, the older adult may have difficulty as a result of cognitive decline, altered sensory perceptions, limited hand mobility, and the high cost of many prescriptions. Common medication errors made by the older adult includes (1) forgetting to take drugs, (2) failing to understand instructions or the importance of drug treatment, (3) taking over-the-counter drugs, (4) taking out-of-date drugs, (5) taking drugs prescribed for someone else, and (6) refusing to take medication because of undesirable side effects such as nausea and impotence. Polypharmacy, overdose, and addiction to prescription drugs are recognized as major causes of illness in the older adult.

To accurately assess drug use and knowledge, many nurses ask their older adult patients to bring to the health

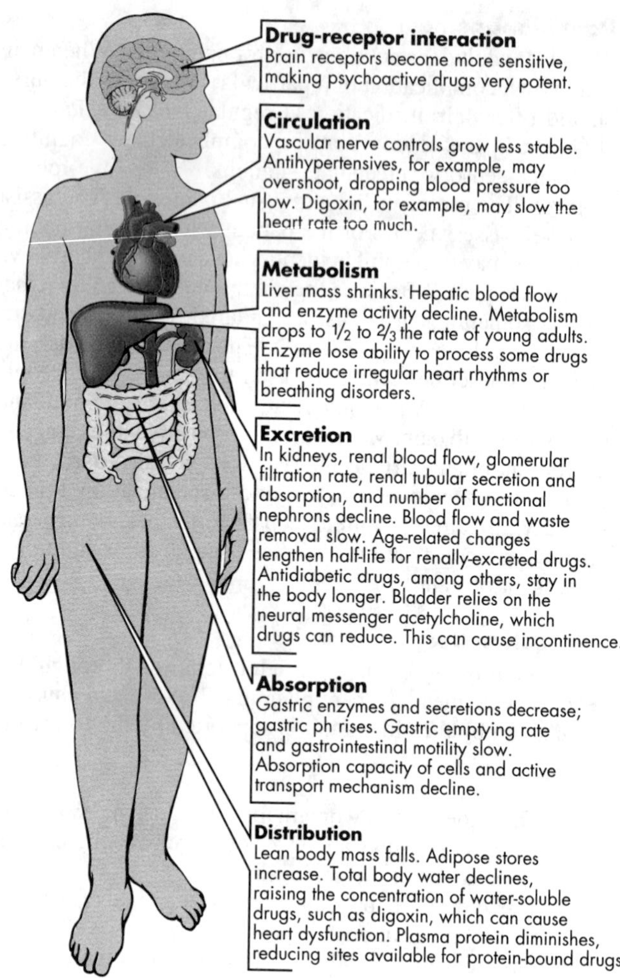

Fig. 3-4 Aging body and drug use.

care appointment all medications (both over-the-counter and prescription) that they take regularly or occasionally. The nurse can then accurately assess *all* medications the older adult is taking, including drugs that the patient may have omitted or thought unimportant. Additional nursing interventions to assist the older adult in following a safe medication routine are listed in Table 3-9.

Depression

Depression, seen in 12% to 25% of community-based elderly, is the most common emotional problem of the older adult. Rates of depressive symptoms in institutionalized older adults are high. Although depressive symptoms occur frequently, marked mood alteration is not common. Depression in the older adult tends to arise from a loss of self-esteem and to be related to life situations such as loss of a spouse or retirement. Symptoms such as hypochondriac complaints, insomnia, lethargy, agitation, decreased memory, and inability to concentrate are common. Feelings of guilt are seldom present with depression in the older adult.

Late-life depression is often accompanied by physical illness. It is important that assessment includes physical examination and laboratory testing for physical disorders that may have symptoms similar to depression. Diseases of concern are thyroid disorders and vitamin deficiencies. The older adult who exhibits depressive symptoms should be encouraged to seek treatment.

Because a patient often feels unworthy and may withdraw and become isolated, the nurse may need to seek the support of the family to assist in helping the older adult seek treatment. The depressed older adult who is involved in caregiving should seek respite and reevaluate the caregiving role.

Older adults commit 17% of all suicides. The nurse should take seriously comments such as "ending this life." Suicide precautions should be followed. The low-income older man who is divorced or widowed with a history of substance abuse is at greatest risk for suicide.

Table 3-9 Nursing Interventions Related to the Uses of Medications by Older Adults

1. Emphasize medications that are essential.
2. Attempt to reduce medication usage that is not essential for minor symptoms.
3. Screen medication usage using a standard assessment tool—including over-the-counter drugs, eye and ear drops, antihistamines, and cough syrups.
4. Assess alcohol usage.
5. Encourage the use of written or medication-reminder systems.
6. Monitor medication dosage strength; normally the strength should be 30-50% less than that of the younger person.
7. Encourage the use of one pharmacy.
8. Work with physicians and pharmacists to establish routine drug profiles on all older adult patients.
9. Advocate (with drug companies) for low-income prescription support services and dosage routines that are simple once-a-day time-release forms.

Nutritional Management

Maintaining adequate nutrition can be a problem for the older adult for physical and social reasons. Physiologically, food may be less appealing with the decline in taste and smell, and chewing is more difficult with dentures or loss of teeth. Swallowing and digestive problems may also result because of a decrease in saliva, gastric motility, and enzyme production. Socially, if a person eats alone, snacking on quick foods is easier than preparing meals. The lack of transportation or access to a grocery store, the inability to see the merchandise, and poverty may be additional factors in poor nutrition. However, obesity may be a problem for some older adults. Normally this problem has arisen earlier in adulthood and continues because of difficulty in changing lifelong eating patterns.

The nurse can have the patient keep a 3-day dietary history. Analysis of this record is helpful in determining dietary adequacy. When appropriate the nurse can arrange for transportation to a senior meal site or delivery of home meals. Attention to and correction of the many reasons for poor nutrition in the elderly person is an important nursing responsibility.

Sleep

Adequacy of sleep is often a concern of the older adult because of changed sleep patterns. Older people no longer experience stage IV deep sleep and are easily aroused. As a result they have difficulty maintaining prolonged sleep. Although the demand for sleep decreases with age, older adults may be disturbed by insomnia and complain that they spend more time in bed but still feel tired. Frequently, the older person prefers to spread sleep throughout 24 hours with short naps that provide adequate rest. Often, assurance from the nurse that this type of sleep pattern is adequate and normal for the patient's age will relieve anxiety concerning sleep. Many times a later bedtime will promote a better night's sleep and a feeling of being refreshed upon awakening.

Safety

Environmental safety is crucial in the health maintenance of the older person. With normal sensory changes, slowed reaction time, decreased thermal and pain sensitivity, changes in gait and balance, and medication effects, the older adult is prone to accidents. Most accidents occur in or around the home. Falls, motor vehicle accidents, and fires are the common causes of accidental death in older adults.[41] Another environmental problem arises from an impaired thermoregulating system that cannot adapt to extremes in environmental temperatures. The body of an older adult can neither conserve nor dissipate heat efficiently. Therefore both hypothermia and heat prostration occur more readily. This age group accounts for the majority of mortality statistics during severe cold spells and heat waves.

The nurse can provide valuable counsel regarding environmental changes, which may improve safety for the older adult. Measures such as stronger lighting, colored step strips, tub and toilet grab bars, and stairway handrails can be effective in "safety-proofing" the living quarters of the older adult. The nurse can also advocate for home fire alarms.

Behavioral Management

When patient behaviors such as agitation, anxiety, resisting care, and wandering become problematic, the nurse needs to plan nursing interventions carefully. Initially the patient's physical status needs to be assessed. The patient should be checked for changes in vital signs, urinary patterns, or constipation, which could be responsible. Disruptive behaviors can be interrupted and redirected by encouraging the patient to participate in activities such as stacking papers, singing, playing music, exercising, or walking with the nurse.

When the patient is agitated by the environment, either the patient or the stimulus should be moved. The patient can be assisted to call family members if it is reassuring. When a patient resists or pulls tubes or dressings, these items can be covered with stretch tube gauze or removed from the visual field.[42] The older adult with behavioral problems should be reassured that the nurse is present to keep him safe. Reality orientation can be used to orient to time, place, and person. The confused or agitated patient should not be asked challenging "why" questions. If the patient cannot verbalize distress, his mood should be validated. The patient's emotional state should be closely observed. The patient's statement can be rephrased to validate its meaning.

When dealing with the difficult patient, the nurse's frustration should be acknowledged. The nurse should not threaten to restrain the patient or call the physician. A calming family member can be requested to stay with the patient until the person becomes more calm. The patient should be monitored frequently, and all interventions should be documented.[43]

Use of Restraints

Chemical and physical restraints should be a last resort in the care of the older patient. The nurse should clearly document restraint use and the behaviors that require this intervention. Research indicates that nurses are unclear about the use of restraint measures.[44] It is not appropriate to use restraints on a patient whom the nurse assumes will fall or on the patient who demonstrates irritating behaviors such as calling out.[45] The use of restraints makes care more time consuming and complex. Restraints do not reduce falls but do increase potential patient confusion and the severity of injury when falls occur. Restraint alternatives require vigilant, creative nursing care. Restraint alternatives include wedge cushions, low beds, body props, and bed alarm signaling devices.[46] The nurse can avoid chemical restraint by using early interventions as discussed in the section on behavioral management.

Elder Abuse

Elder abuse occurs in approximately 4% of the general older adult population and 10% of impaired older adults. The abuse is seldom reported to authorities even though it shows a repetitive pattern. The typical victim is an older woman with at least one limitation in ADLs. Most of these women are widowed, Caucasian, low income, and dependent on the abuser for some aspect of care. Elder abuse is often associated with substance abuse, caregiver strain, and depression. The lack of reporting abuse may be related to the older adult's feeling of vulnerability, lack of self-worth, impaired cognitive functioning, and sense of isolation.

Elder abuse can occur in a variety of forms (Table 3-10). Self-neglect is also a form of elder abuse when the older adult is no longer competent to perform self-care or when the older adult has severe psychologic impairments.

In assessing elder abuse the nurse needs to understand the legal limits of practice within state mandates. With a competent, older adult victim, the nurse may be limited in intervention because of patient resistance. In some situations health care workers are seen as interferences and opportunists. There are several elder abuse assessment instruments that include basic information, signs of maltreatment, severity of signs, and response of abuser.[47] If the nurse suspects abuse, an appropriate assessment protocol should be carried out, and consultation should be obtained based on agency policy. Follow-up actions for the nurse

Table 3-10 Types of Elder Abuse

Type	Example
Violation of individual rights	Lack of privacy; unwanted visitors
Exploitation	Taking a social security check or property
Physical abuse	Shaking or hitting
Psychologic neglect	Isolating or locking the person in a room
Psychologic abuse	Swearing at person; displaying threatening behavior
Physical neglect	Not providing correct medications or proper physical care

may include consultation with adult protective services and potential court testimony. In most situations, nurses are mandated to report abuse.

SOCIAL SUPPORT AND THE OLDER ADULT

Social support for the older adult occurs at three levels. Family and kinship relations are the first and preferred providers of social support. Second, a semiformal level of support is found in clubs, churches, neighborhoods, and senior citizen centers. Last, the older adult may be linked to a formal system of social welfare agencies, health facilities, and government support. Generally the nurse is part of the formal support system.

Caregivers

Generally more than 80% of care is provided by a family caregiver who lives with the patient. A caregiver is usually a married woman who is often old herself, has chronic diseases and disabilities, and is often poor. Ethnic background influences the type of caregiving network. Italian, Polish, Irish, and African-American people most commonly use extended family networks for caregiving.[48,49]

A caregiver provides supervision, direct care, and coordinates services. The tasks of caregiving include (1) assisting with ADL and IADL, (2) providing emotional and social support, and (3) managing health care.

Caregiver Problems. Caregiver concerns change as the intensity of the caregiving role changes. For example, a caregiver may need to adjust work schedules to accommodate patient health care appointments, or the caregiver may need to be available to monitor the cognitively impaired patient's safety 24 hours a day.

Common problems facing the caregiver include the following: (1) a lack of understanding of the time and energy needed for caregiving; (2) a lack of information about specific tasks of caregiving, such as bathing or medication administration; (3) a lack of respite or relief from caregiving; (4) an inability to meet personal self-care needs, such as socialization and rest; (5) conflict in the family unit related to decisions about caregiving; and (6) financial depletion of resources as a result of a caregiver's inability to work and the increased cost of health care.[50,51]

The intensity and complexity of caregiving places the caregiver at risk for high levels of stress; the caregiver may develop a sense of being overwhelmed with feelings of inadequacy, powerlessness, and depression.[52] Although most older adults deny loneliness even when they spend much time alone, the caregiver often lacks sufficient social exchange. The primary caregiver is often at risk for social isolation; the burden of caregiving separates the individual from others who provide social, emotional, and interactional involvement. Time commitments, fatigue, and, at times, socially inappropriate behaviors of the dependent older adult contribute to social isolation. The socially isolated caregiver needs to be identified, and plans should be designed to meet the needs for social support and exchange.

The burden of caregiving may result in the nursing diagnosis of caregiver strain. The escalating incidence of caregiving sets the stage for increased incidences of elder abuse. Physical, financial, psychologic, or sexual abuse and neglect may occur in families ill equipped to handle caregiving. The nurse should assess the caregiver and the patient for the possibility of caregiver strain and elder abuse.

Emotional Problems of Caregivers. The stress of caregiving may result in emotional problems such as depression, anger, and resentment and feelings of hopelessness and powerlessness. The nurse should consider the caregiver as a patient and plan behaviors to reduce caregiver strain. The nurse should communicate a sense of empathy to the caregiver while allowing discussion about the burdens and joys of caregiving. The caregiver can be taught about age-related changes and diseases and specific caregiving techniques. Attendance at a support group should be encouraged by the nurse. The nurse can also assist the caregiver in seeking help from the formal social support system regarding matters such as respite care, housing, health coverage, and finances. Finally, the nurse should monitor the caregiver for indications of declining health, emotional distress, and caregiver strain.[53,54]

Older Adult Network

A network of services supports the older adult both in the community and in health care facilities. Most older adults are involved in at least one social or governmental service. This is true in both Canada and the United States. To understand the older adult situation, the nurse should know the government structures that fund and regulate the older adult programs.

In the United States the Department of Health and Human Services is the responsible federal agency for many older adult programs. In 1958 interest in the older citizen inspired the formation of the President's Council on Aging. From this beginning the Administration on Aging (AOA) has evolved. The general goal of AOA is to include older people wherever programs exist by cooperating and consulting with other agencies or organizations. There are several major grant programs under AOA. Title III of the Older Americans Act funds comprehensive, community-based service systems. Title IV funds the training of persons who are employed or preparing for employment in the field of aging. Funding from the AOA is funneled to state and local area agencies on aging.

Concurrent with the founding of AOA was the establishment of the White House Conferences on Aging, a forum for issue debate and policy recommendation. These conferences, held approximately every 10 years, have fostered decision making at a grass roots level for the good of older adults. Older adult delegates from all over the United States represent their home communities.

The legislative action that has evolved from this process is dramatic. At the 1951 exploratory conference the AOA had its roots. As a result of the 1961 conference, legislative action included the Older Americans Act, Medicare, Medicaid, and the Age Discrimination Act. From the 1972 conference the National Nutrition Program and Multipurpose Senior Centers were developed. In later conferences the federal, state, and local networks on aging were established, and the National Institute on Aging was designed. More than a dozen federal agencies are involved in programs for the elderly.

In Canada the Department of National Health and Welfare is the responsible federal agency for many older adult programs. The policies of the Federal and Provincial Governments cannot be easily separated. Policy often results in an intermingling of activities through shared jurisdiction and cost sharing. This shared role has been changing during the last 30 years. Before 1950 the provincial government's responsibility ended with assistance to the aged poor. Since that time a wide range of federal and provincial programs have evolved. The role of the government has changed from that of regulator to provider.[55]

Medicare

Almost all Americans older than 65 years of age have Medicare coverage. Medicare also covers persons who receive social security disability benefits and persons with end-stage renal disease. Medicare is designed for acute illness care. Reimbursement is based on daily documentation that indicates a patient is improving in function. This nursing documentation process is complex and critical for adequate reimbursement. Medicare is composed of two parts, A and B. Part A covers inpatient hospital care. Medicare A pays reasonable charges on the basis of the diagnosis, not on the length of stay. Skilled nursing facility care in a hospital or long-term care facility is paid if the stay results in an improved or rehabilitated condition. These skilled nursing benefit days are limited. The percentage of coverage changes each year. Medicare A pays for home care if it requires skilled nursing or rehabilitation intervention and is needed on a part-time basis. The patient must be homebound. Durable medical equipment used daily is covered, but home safety equipment is not. Hospice care is covered under Medicare A. When hospice care is elected, the patient no longer qualifies for the condition to be treated in the standard Medicare program.

Part B covers outpatient treatment and physician's services. Medicare B is voluntary and has a monthly premium and an annual deductible before payment begins.

Medicare does not cover long-term nursing home care, custodial ADLs or IADLs care, dental care or dentures, preventative health care, prescription drugs, routine foot care, hearing aids, or eye glasses. These costs plus the Medicare deductible costs explain the reason most older adults pay for 50% of all acquired health care costs yearly.[56]

General Support Services

Services for the older adult in the United States and Canada include hospital and medical benefits, community-based services, long-term institutional care, house and shelter assistance, transportation, employment programs, and income maintenance and support. These services are diverse and complex. Eligibility is limited and requires a subtle understanding of the rules. The older adult is often too frail, undereducated, or uninformed about these services to evaluate eligibility.

The nurse can assist the elderly patient and the caregiver by acknowledging the complexity of the health care system and empathizing with anger and frustration about regulations that seem unfair or inadequate. The nurse can assist the older adult to access the appropriate service or refer the patient to a case manager or other health care expert when appropriate.

CARE ALTERNATIVES FOR OLDER ADULTS

Housing

Most older adults are aging in place. Most do not move or return to the geographic location of childhood when health becomes frail. The community becomes important to the older adult as an environment that is safe from crime and accidents. The older adult needs privacy and companionship, as well as a sense of belonging. The community needs to be accessible. The older adult may need housing assistance through property tax relief, assistance with home repair, and fuel payment. A variety of subsidized, low-income housing arrangements are available for the older adult.

For the older adult who chooses to remain in the home as functional abilities decline, home adaptations and modifications can be made. Homes can be made wheelchair accessible. Lighting can be increased and adjusted. Safety devices can be installed in bathrooms and kitchens. Alarms and assistive listening devices can be used.

Retirement communities may be an option for some older adults (Fig. 3-5). These communities are age-segregated, self-contained developments and provide social activities, security, and recreational facilities. When retirement communities offer expanded health care and social support services, including nursing home care, they become Continuing Care Retirement Communities (CCRC). The CCRC requires an entrance fee and monthly fees for continuing care.

Congregate housing provides services to the older adult at two levels—independent and assisted living. Independent living facilities provide housing and congregate meals but no supervision. Assisted-living homes, also called "board and care homes," provide housing, meals, and 24-hour protective oversight. Other home maintenance and care services can be purchased from these facilities.

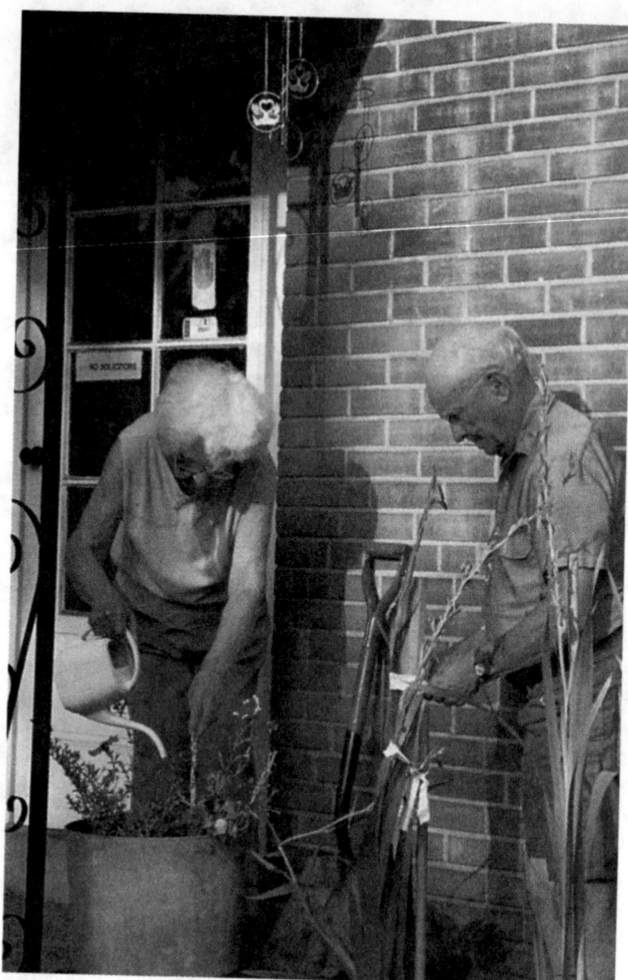

Fig. 3-5 This older couple works together to stay in their home.

Creative housing options are being developed by home sharing, the use of "granny flats," and apartment rentals in established older homes. The nurse can play a role in meeting the housing needs of the older adult by identifying housing preferences and by advocating community housing changes that create a safe, liveable community.

Community-Based Older Adults with Special Needs

Older adults with special care needs include homeless persons, persons who need constant assistance with ADLs, persons who are home bound, and persons who can no longer live at home. The older adult may be served by adult day care, home health care, and nursing home care.

Homeless Older Adults. In areas where homelessness is increasing, the older adult is at additional risk because many aging network services are not designed to reach out to homeless persons. It is estimated that between 14% and 50% of homeless persons are older adults (Fig. 3-6). Street surveys suggest that most older homeless people are transient men. The older homeless person is less likely to use shelters or meal sites. The low-income older adult often becomes homeless because of a lack of affordable housing. Key factors that are associated with homelessness include (1) having a low income, (2) reduced cognitive capacity, and (3) living alone.[57] Nursing home placement is often an alternative to homelessness. Fear of institutionalization may explain the reason the older homeless adult does not use shelter and meal site services.

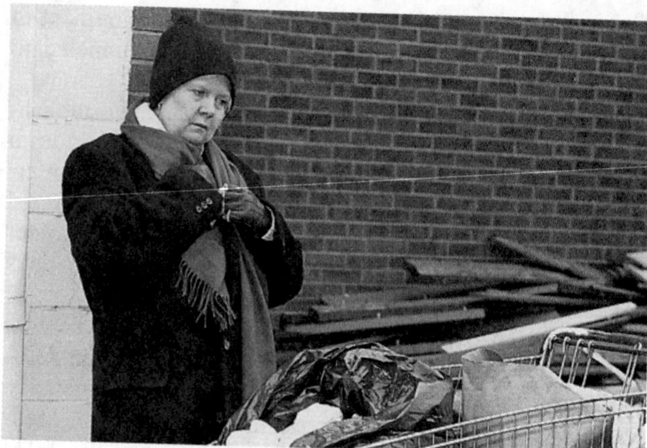

Fig. 3-6 Elderly homeless person.

Research on older shelter users indicated more than 80% are alcoholic, 43% have pulmonary disease, and 80% have multiple chronic diseases. Usually these people had been on the street more than 4 years yet have had fewer health problems related to exposure and trauma than their younger peers.[58]

The older homeless person needs affordable housing. When cognitively impaired and alone, the older person needs financial management assistance. Solutions to the problem of homelessness among the elderly require more research and intervention studies.

Adult Day Care Programs. Adult day care (ADC) programs provide daily supervision, social activities, and ADLs assistance for two major groups of older adults—persons who are cognitively impaired and persons who have ADLs management problems. The services offered in the ADC programs are based on patient needs. Restorative programs for persons with problems of ADLs management offer health monitoring, therapeutic activities, one-to-one ADLs training, individualized care planning, and personal care services. Programs designed for the cognitively impaired offer therapeutic recreation, support for family, family counseling, and social involvement. Patient characteristics in the cognitively impaired group include a high number of persons with Alzheimer's disease. In this group, incontinence is a common problem. Patient characteristics in the restorative care group include a large number of wheelchair users, problems with incontinence, and some depression.[59]

Day-care centers provide relief to the caregiver, allow continued employment for the caregiver, and delay institutionalization for the patient. Centers are regulated and standards are set by the state. Costs are $25 to $50 per day and are not covered by Medicare. Adult day care is tax deductible as dependent care. Appropriate placement in a day-care program that matches the patient's needs is important. The nurse can assist by knowing the available day-care services and assessing the needs of the patient. The nurse is then in a position to aid the patient and family in making a good placement decision. The caregiver and the patient are often uninformed about day care and its services as an alternative care option.

Home Health Care. Home health care can be a cost-effective care alternative for the older adult patient who is homebound, has health needs that are intermittent or acute, and has supportive caregiver involvement. Home health care is not an alternative for the patient in need of 24-hour ADLs assistance or continuous safety supervision. Home health care services require physician recommendation and skilled nursing care for Medicare reimbursement. Unless these requirements are met, assistance by a home health aide for ADLs management or assistance by a homemaker for IADLs management will not be paid by Medicare.

Home care is usually given to the patient requiring home medical treatments (intravenous [IV] therapy, catheters, colostomy, injections, dressings). More than one third of home care patients need assistance in three or more ADLs. The use of home care increases as disability increases. Home care is used more frequently in states that provide state-funded home care and in urban areas. The use of home care is linked to income—the higher the income, the more likely is the use. African-American and Hispanic persons are less likely to use home care. It is unclear if this is a preference or a result of a lack of access to the service. Most home care is informal and provided by the caregiver.[60] In some situations home care may be purchased from untrained immigrant groups or trained assistive personnel. This unregulated situation, "the caregiver underground," can lead to caregiver exploitation, patient abuse or neglect, and unsafe care. The family and patient are often desperate for low-cost assistance. The nurse should identify these situations and clearly explain the limitations and cost of formal regulated caregiving.

Nursing Home Care

Nursing home care is a placement alternative for the older adult who can no longer live alone, who needs continuous supervision, who has three or more ADLs disabilities, or who is frail. The nursing home patient is usually a woman, widowed, and 80 years of age or older. Only 5% of older adults reside in nursing homes at any one time. However, 23% of the oldest-old adults are in nursing homes.

The cost of nursing home care is high. These costs are paid privately for 50% of all patients and by state-funded public assistance programs (Medicaid) for 40% of all patients. This public assistance support for nursing home care accounts for more than 50% of all Medicaid care costs. When nursing home patients receive Medicaid, they contribute all their personal income to pay their expenses, except for a small amount per month kept as a personal needs allowance.[61]

Services Provided. Nursing homes are part of the long-term care structure. Nursing homes provide 24-hour care each day including ADLs assistance, skilled nursing care, health monitoring, medical care, activity therapy, and social support services. Nursing homes are state licensed and regulated by the Departments of Health and Public Assistance. The nursing home can offer special services including a Medicare rehabilitation unit, dementia unit, ventilator-dependent unit, behavioral management unit, and respite care. Depending on the other services provided, nursing homes can be regulated by other agencies. Nursing homes that participate in skilled Medicare programs or Medicaid reimbursement programs must meet the requirements established by the 1987 Omnibus Reconciliation Act (OBRA '87). This legislation impacted nursing homes in five areas. First, the patient is now prescreened for appropriate placement. The patient who has developmental disabilities or mental illnesses cannot be commingled with disabled adults 18 years of age or older. Treatment programs must be in place for each patient group. Second, to qualify for reimbursement, the patient's level of care must be skilled. Most older adult nursing home patients need assistance with three or more ADLs areas. Third, the nursing home must establish treatment options and standards of care appropriate to patient needs. Fourth, the facility must monitor patient outcomes and develop a quality assurance program. Fifth, the patient must be assessed using the federally developed Resident Assessment Instrument (RAI).[62]

Nursing Role. The nurse is a vitally important worker in the long-term care setting. The registered nurse must assess each patient using the RAI process. This assessment process is designed to search for and identify the 18 most common nursing home patient problems or areas of need (Table 3-11). From this assessment a patient care plan is developed by the interdisciplinary team to respond to each identified area of concern. Most nursing home patients have seven to nine areas "triggered" by the assessment.

In addition to patient assessment, the nurse who works in a nursing home has responsibilities specific to this setting. The nursing home nurse must work with and supervise assistive personnel, primarily nursing assistants. This nurse documents the highly mandated and regulatory standards. This nurse participates in interdisciplinary care planning that directly affects patient care and outcomes.

Table 3-11 Most Common Problems or Need Areas of Nursing Home Patients

Delirium	Activities
Cognitive	Falls
Visual function	Nutritional status
Communication	Feeding tubes
Rehabilitation potential	Dehydration
Urinary incontinence	Dental care
Psychosocial well-being	Pressure ulcers
Mood state	Psychotropic drug use
Behavior problems	Physical restraints

Finally, the nursing home nurse plans for the diverse needs of the older adult that can be positively affected by appropriate nursing interventions.

Placement Issues. Three factors appear to precipitate nursing home placement. They are (1) rapid patient deterioration, (2) caregiver inability to continue care as a result of "burnout"—too much and too long, and (3) an alteration in or loss of family support system. Physical changes of confusion, incontinence, or a major health event, such as a stroke, can accelerate placement.[63]

The conflicts and fears faced by the family and patient make nursing home placement a transition time. Common fears caregivers express include the following:

1. The process of admission will be resisted by the patient.
2. The level of care given by staff will be insufficient.
3. The patient will be lonely.
4. The financing of nursing care will not be adequate.[64]

This time of disruption is increased by the physical relocation of the patient. Research indicates the process of physical relocation results in adverse health effects for the older adult.[65] The crisis of relocation syndrome should be anticipated by the nurse, and appropriate interventions to reduce the relocation impact should be used. Whenever possible the older adult should be involved in the decision to move and should be fully informed about the location. The caregiver can share information, pictures, or a videotape of the new location. New health personnel can send a welcome message. Upon arrival the new patient can be greeted with a flower and a staff member to orient the older adult. To bridge the relocation the new patient can be "buddied" with a seasoned patient.

The satisfied nursing home patient tends to show a variety of behaviors indicating adjustment. The patient is assertive and self-reliant; keeps active, follows a routine, keeps mentally involved, and is sociable; and maintains family interaction and shows a level of acceptance. The satisfied patient also expresses a determined, positive perspective. The satisfied patient uses coping strategies that increase control and management of her life.[66] The nurse can encourage and enable the use of these strategies for the nursing home patient.

Case Management

Matching older adult social support services to the needs of the older adult is complex. For family members who live out of town and cannot provide direct caregiving, the use of a case manager may be helpful. This is a new and developing role that the nurse is well suited to assume. The case manager supervises and manages care to ensure continuity of care for the older adult. The process of locating and organizing older adult services is time consuming. The use of the Elder Care Locator program (800-677-1116), a national telephone resource for older adult services, is available toll free. A written directory of nationwide services (A National Eldercare Directory of Information and Referral) is available from the National Association of Area Agencies on Aging (202-296-8130) for $30.

LEGAL AND ETHICAL ISSUES

Patient Concerns

Legal assistance is a concern for many older adults. Legal concerns center on advance directives, estate planning, taxation issues, and appeals for denied services and advance directives. Legal aid is available to the low-income older adult by contacting a local multipurpose senior center (Fig. 3-7). This service is supported by funds authorized through Title III of the Older Americans Act.

Advance directives are mandated upon admission to a health care facility by the Patient Self-Determination Act of 1991. There are primarily two types—a living will and a durable power of attorney for health. A living will is a directive that permits an individual to direct his health care in the event of a terminal or irreversible condition. Most living wills direct that in the event of a terminal illness, extraordinary medical care should not be initiated or should be withdrawn so that the process of dying will not be artificially prolonged.[67] A living will is directive but not legally binding. A durable power of attorney for health is another form of advance directive that designates another person to voice health care decisions when the patient is unable to do so personally. A durable power of attorney for health is directive and legally binding. In most states it includes the naming of an individual to carry out directives when the patient cannot make choices.[68] Discussion of estate planning, taxation issues, and appeals for denied services is beyond the scope of this text.

Nursing Concerns

The nurse who works with the older adult identifies areas of ethical concern that influence practice. This nurse identifies that these issues center around the following: (1) to restrain or not restrain and (2) to evaluate the patient's ability to make decisions.[69] The physician identifies ethical concerns related to (1) resuscitation, (2) treatment of infections, (3) issues of nutrition and hydration, and (4) transfer to more intensive treatment units.[70]

These situations are often complex and emotionally charged. The nurse can assist the patient, family, and other

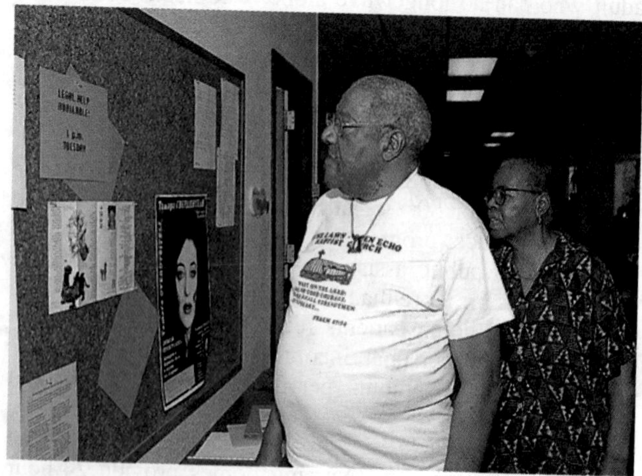

Fig. 3-7 Bulletin board at a senior center showing time legal help is available.

health care workers by acknowledging when an ethical dilemma is present, by keeping current on the ethical implications of new biotechnology, and by advocating for an institutional ethics committee to help in the decision making process.

REVIEW QUESTIONS

The number of the question corresponds to the same-numbered objective at the beginning of the chapter.

1. The standards for gerontologic nursing were set by the
a. Gerontological Society of America.
b. American Nurses Association.
c. Gerontological Nursing Association.
d. National League for Nursing.

2. The most rapidly increasing population group is
a. children less than 1 year.
b. teenagers from 16 to 19.
c. persons from ages 50 to 65.
d. persons older than 85.

3. All of the following age-related skin changes are expected *except*
a. decreased sensory receptors.
b. increased capillary fragility.
c. increased sweat glands.
d. slowed epidermal cell turnover.

4. The onset of dementia could be described as
a. chronic, generally insidious.
b. acute, subacute depending on cause.
c. coincidental with life changes.
d. acute to prolonged, depending on cause.

5. Appropriate nursing interventions to use with a person with an ethnic identity include all of the following *except*
a. using an interpreter when necessary.
b. excluding all ethnic food from a special diet.
c. supporting harmless health rituals.
d. informing the patient about ethnic support services.

6. When the older adult has disease, it would be *unusual* for which of the following to occur?
a. A pattern that overlaps other chronic diseases
b. The patient considers the problem to be a normal part of aging
c. A subtle, silent beginning
d. The symptom manifestation is similar to younger patients

7. An important adaptation to make in assessing an older adult is to
a. omit a reproductive history.
b. have the caregiver present.
c. allow sufficient time for responses.
d. avoid asking embarrassing questions.

8. The recommended counsel to an older adult related to reducing influenza and pneumonia deaths is
a. to receive pneumococcal vaccine every 10 years.
b. to receive pneumococcal vaccine annually.
c. to receive influenza vaccine annually.
d. to receive influenza vaccine once in life.

9. An important nursing action helpful to a chronically ill older adult is
a. avoiding discussion about future lifestyle changes.
b. assuring the patient that the condition is stable.
c. encouraging the patient to "fight" the disease as long as possible.
d. treating the patient as a competent manager of the disease.

10. Major problems related to hospitalization of the older adult include all of the following *except*
a. sudden onset of dementia.
b. unstable condition at discharge.
c. nosocomial infection.
d. increased surgical risk.

11. When assessing pain in the older adult, the nurse should
a. rely on the patient's verbal report.
b. offer pain medication every 3 hours.
c. assume the patient is exaggerating the amount of pain.
d. use a visual pain scale.

12. An important fact the nurse should know about the caregiver is that the caregiver
a. usually does not live with the patient.
b. is generally strong and in good health.
c. is usually a family member.
d. is usually a single daughter.

13. Adult day care generally provides all of the following services to the older adult *except*
a. physical therapy.
b. personal care services.
c. social activities.
d. health monitoring.

14. A living will is an advanced directive that
a. is legally binding.
b. allows a person to direct her health care in the event of terminal illness.
c. encourages the use of artificial means to prolong life.
d. designates who can act for the patient when the patient is unable to do so personally.

REFERENCES

1. Task force to revise a statement on the scope of gerontological nursing practice and standards of gerontological nursing practice, Kansas City, 1987, The American Nurses' Association.
2. Myers DL: Gerontologic nursing and the national gerontological nursing association, *Geriatr Nurs* 14:101, 1993.
3. Neugarten B: Adult personality: toward a psychology of the life cycle. In Neugarten B, editor: *Middle age and aging,* Chicago, 1968, University of Chicago Press.
*4. Smith MA and others: Age and health perception among elderly blacks, *J Gerontol Nurs* 17:13, 1991.
5. Schneider EL, Guralnik JM: The aging of America: impact on health care costs, *JAMA* 263:17, 1990.
6. The elderly in Ontario: an agenda for the '80s: task force on aging, 1-44, 1981.
7. Neugarten B: The future and the young-old. In Jarvik LF, editor: *Aging into the 21st century: middle ages today,* New York, 1978, Gardner Press.
8. Burke MM, Walsh MB: *Gerontologic nursing: care of the frail elderly,* St Louis, 1992, Mosby.

9. Demond J: Older women: social policies and health care, *J Gerontol Nurs* 10:5, 1993.
10. McLaughlin DK, Jensen L: Poverty among older Americans: the plight of non-metropolitan elders, *J Gerontol* 48:544, 1993.
11. Johnson JE and others: Research considerations: stress and perceived health status in the rural elderly, *J Gerontol Nurs* 10:25, 1993.
12. Salomom MP, Nelson GM, Rous SG: The continuum of care revisited: a rural perspective, *Gerontologist* 33:658, 1993.
13. Roberts BL, Dunkle R, Hauj M: Physical, psychologic, and social resources as moderators of the relationship of stress to mental health of the very old, *J Gerontol* 49:535, 1994.
14. Gelfand A: *Aging and ethnicity*, New York, 1994, Springer Publishing.
15. White EC: *The black women's health book*, Seattle, 1994, Seal Publishing.
16. Melillo KD: Interpretation of abnormal laboratory values in older adults: Part I, *J Gerontol Nurs* 1:39, 1993.
17. Melillo KD: Interpretation of abnormal laboratory values in older adults: Part II, *J Gerontol Nurs* 2:35, 1993.
18. Dellasya C and others: Nursing process: teaching elderly clients, *J Gerontol Nurs* 20:31, 1994.
19. US Department of Health and Human Services, Office of Disease Prevention and Health Promotion: *Healthy people 2000: national health promotion and disease prevention objectives*, Washington DC, 1990, US Government Printing Office, Pub No 017-001-00473.
20. US preventive services task force: *Guide to clinical preventive services: an assessment of the effectiveness of 169 initiatives*, Baltimore, 1989, Williams and Wilkins.
21. Report of nutrition screening I: *Toward a common view*, Nutrition Screening Initiative, Washington DC, 1991.
22. Walker SN: Health promotion and aging: the time is now, *J Gerontol Nurs* 17:4, 1991.
23. Guralnik JM, Semonsick EM: Physical disability in older Americans, *J Gerontol* 48:3, 1993.
24. Strauss A, Corbin JM: *Shaping a new health care system: the explosion of chronic illness as a catalyst for change*, San Francisco, 1988, Jossey-Bass.
25. Simon-Rusinowitz L, Hofland BF: Adapting a disability approach to home care services for older adults, *Gerontologist* 33:159, 1993.
26. Bottomley JM: Principles and practice in geriatric rehabilitation. In Satin DG: *The clinical care of the aged person*, New York, 1994, Oxford University Press.
27. May DS and others: Surveillance of major causes of hospitalization among the elderly, United States, 1988, *Morbidity and Mortality Weekly Report* 40:7, 1991.
*28. Rockwood K: The occurrence and duration of symptoms in elderly patients with delirium, *J Gerontol* 48:M162, 1993.
*29. Murray AM and others: Acute delirium and functional decline in the hospitalized elderly patient, *J Gerontol* 48:M181, 1993.
30. Fraser D: Patient assessment: infection in the elderly, *J Gerontol Nurs* 7:5, 1993.
31. Lancaster E: Tuberculosis comeback, *J Gerontol Nurs* 19:16, 1993.
*32. Wilson EB and others: Take a fresh look at discharge planning, *J Geriatr Nurs* 1:23, 1991.
33. Schaefer AL and others: Are they ready? Discharge planning for older surgical patients, *J Gerontol Nurs* 16:16, 1990.
*34. Blaylock A, Cason CL: Discharge planning: predicting patient's needs, *J Gerontol Nurs* 18:5, 1992.
*35. Ensberg MD and others: Identifying elderly patients for early discharge after hospitalization for hip fracture, *J Gerontol* 48:M187, 1993.
*36. Carty AES, Day SS: Interdisciplinary care: effect in acute hospital setting, *J Gerontol Nurs* 3:22, 1993.
37. Herr KA, Mobily PR: Complexities of pain assessment in the elderly, *J Gerontol Nurs* 17:12, 1991.
38. Ferrell BR, Ferrell BA: Easing the pain, *Geriatr Nurs* 7:175, 1990.
*39. Hopland SL: Elder beliefs, blocks to pain management, *J Gerontol Nurs* 18:19, 1992.
40. Carruth AK, Boss BJ: Adverse drug effect: more than they bargained for, *J Gerontol Nurs* 16:27, 1992.
41. Williams B: Prescribing for older patients, *Practitioner* 3:260, 1993.
42. Salerno C: Alternatives to restraints, *Geriatr Nurs* 3:63, 1992.
43. Scanland SG, Emershaw LE: Reality orientation and validation therapy, *J Gerontol Nurs* 6:7, 1993.
44. Houston KA, Lach HW: Restraints: how do you score? *Geriatr Nurs* 9:23, 1990.
45. Kayser-Jones J: Culture, environment and restraints: a conceptual model for research and practice, *J Gerontol Nurs* 11:13, 1992.
46. Kallmann SL, Denine-Flynn M, Blackburn DM: Comfort, safety, and independence: restraint release and its challenge, *Geriatr Nurs* 5:143, 1992.
47. Fulmer T, Birkenhauer D: Elder mistreatment assessment as a part of everyday practice, *J Gerontol Nurs*, 3:42, 1992.
*48. Beach DL: Gerontological caregiving: analysis of family experience, *J Gerontol Nurs* 12:35, 1993.
49. Lawton MP and others: The dynamics of caregiving for a demented elder among black and white families, *J Gerontol* 47:S156, 1992.
*50. Haley WE, Clair JM, Saulsberry K: Family caregiver satisfaction with medical care of their demented relatives, *Gerontologist* 32:219, 1992.
*51. Mui AC: Caregiver strain among black and white daughter caregivers: a role theory perspective, *Gerontologist* 32:203, 1992.
*52. Rosenthal CJ, Sulman J, Marshall V: Depressive symptoms in family caregivers of long-stay patients, *Gerontologist* 33:249, 1993.
53. Hardy VL, Riffle KL: Support for caregivers of dependent elderly, *Geriatr Nurs* 14:161, 1993.
54. Gallienne RL and others: Alzheimer's caregivers psychosocial support via computer networks, *J Gerontol Nurs* 12:15, 1993.
55. Shulman N, Marshall V: *The aging of urban Canada, aging in Canada: social perspectives*, Ontario, 1980, Fitzhenry and Whiteside.
56. Lifkowitz D, Monheit A: *Health insurance, use of health services, and health care expenditures*, AHCPR Oyb No 92-0017, National medical expenditure survey research findings 12, Agency for Health Care Policy and Research, Rockville, MD, 1991, Public Health Service.
*57. Keigher SM, Greenblatt S: Housing emergencies and the ecology of homelessness among the urban elderly, *Gerontologist* 32:457, 1992.
*58. Blakiney B: Old, homeless, and sick, *Geriatr Nurs* 10:221, 1991.
*59. Conrad KG and others: Classification of adult day care: a cluster analyses of services and activities, *J Gerontol* 48:S112, 1993.
60. Kemper P: The use of formal and informal home care by the disabled elderly, HSR: *Health Serv Res* 24:10, 1992.
61. Health Care Financing Administration, Department of Health and Human Services, task force on long-term health care policies: *Fact sheet on long-term care*, 4:1, 1987.
62. Congress passes quality care bill: major reforms become law at last, *Quality Care Advocate*, 1:1, 1988.

*63. Retsenas J: Triggers to nursing home placement, *Geriatr Nurs* 9:235, 1991.
*64. VanAuken E: Crisis intervention: elders awaiting placement in an acute care facility, *J Gerontol Nurs* 17:30, 1991.
*65. Sorrells VL: Nursing home fears, *Geriatr Nurs* 9:237, 1991.
66. Daley OE: Women's strategies for living in a nursing home, *J Gerontol Nurs* 9:5, 1993.
67. Burke M, Walsh M: *Gerontological nursing: care of the frail elderly,* St Louis, 1992, Mosby.
68. Pokala C: Understanding the patient self-determination act, *J Gerontol Nurs* 3:47, 1992.
69. Pacer G, Miller P: The development of ethical thought in long-term care, *J Gerontol Nurs* 17:28, 1991.
70. Lund M, Wei FF: Speaking out on ethics, *Geriatr Nurs* 9:233, 1990.

---

*Nursing research-based articles.

Chapter 4

NURSING ASSESSMENT

Nursing History and Physical Examination

Katheryn Ellen McCash

Learning Objectives

1. Explain the purpose, components, and techniques related to the patient history interview and physical examination.
2. Obtain a nursing history using a functional health pattern format.
3. Describe the appropriate use and techniques of inspection, palpation, percussion, and auscultation.
4. Identify the equipment needed to perform a physical examination.
5. Describe the indications, purposes, and components of the branching or regional examination.
6. Record a nursing history and physical examination using a standard format.

The patient history interview and physical examination are part of the assessment phase of the nursing process. This information provides a data base about a patient's health, including potential and actual health problems, on which the other phases of the nursing process are based.[1] Numerous formats exist for taking histories in the various health care settings. These histories are described as *medical history* and *nursing history.*

Both subjective and objective information are collected. A nursing history provides subjective data about the state of the patient's health. Subjective data are supplied by the patient either as spontaneously offered information or as a response to direct questioning by the nurse. Knowledgeable others, such as family members and caregivers, can also contribute subjective data about the patient. The *general survey* statement provides a comprehensive descriptive statement about the patient. The *physical examination* provides objective data related to the health status of the patient. Objective data are gathered by the nurse through inspection, palpation, percussion, and auscultation. Additional sources of objective data include the findings of other health care providers and the results of diagnostic studies.

INTERVIEWING CONSIDERATIONS

Effective communication is a key factor in the interview process. Establishing a relationship and obtaining information are the goals of communication. Nurses should remember that individuals communicate not only through language but in their manner of dress, gestures, and body language. Sitting with arms crossed and a downward gaze is an example of body language that suggests an unwillingness to communicate.

Collection of data assists the examiner and the patient in identifying health problems as well as patient strengths and resources. The nurse can use the data to identify areas where the patient may be unable to meet personal needs and therefore require nursing assistance. The patient perceives this encounter as an indication of how the health care system will provide assistance. A direct interview technique, which is more structured, is used to collect factual, easily categorized information. Closed questions such as, "Have you had surgery before?" that require brief, specific responses are used.[2]

The amount of time needed to complete a nursing history may vary with the format used and the experience of the nurse. It may be completed in one or several sessions, depending on the setting and the patient. In the case of an older adult patient with a low energy level, several short sessions may need to be scheduled. Allowing time for the patient to volunteer information about particular areas of concern enables the nurse to work with the patient to identify existing and potential health problems. When a patient is unable to provide the necessary data (e.g., is unconscious or aphasic), the nurse should ask the person who has assumed responsibility for the patient's welfare to provide as much information as possible.

Reviewed by Joan Murphy, RN, MS, Associate Professor, Utica College of Syracuse University, Utica, NY.

Before beginning the nursing history interview, the nurse should explain to the patient that the purpose of a detailed history is to collect information that will provide a health profile for comprehensive health care, including health maintenance and promotion. This detailed information is collected during entry into the health care system, and, subsequently, only updates are needed. The nurse should explain that personal and social data are needed to individualize the plan of care. This explanation is necessary because the patient may not be accustomed to sharing personal information and may need to know the purpose of such questioning. The nurse should assure the patient that all information will be kept confidential.

A nursing history form indicates *what to ask* not *how to ask it.* In addition to understanding the principles of effective communication, each nurse must develop a personal style of relating to patients. Although no single style fits all people, wording specific questions in certain ways will increase the probability of eliciting the needed information. Ease at asking questions, particularly those related to sensitive areas such as sexual functioning and income, comes with experience. Videotaping and reviewing the health history interview is an effective method to use in evaluating communication techniques and identifying areas in need of improvement.

To obtain accurate social and personal information, the nurse must communicate acceptance of the patient as an individual. When asking sensitive questions, the nurse can communicate the acceptance or normalcy of behaviors by prefacing questions with phrases such as "most people" or "frequently." For example, stating, "Most people have sexual concerns; do you have any you would like to discuss?" shows the patient that a particular situation may not be unique to him. Another method of putting the patient at ease is to word the question so that an affirmative answer appears expected. An example of this technique is to ask "What do you like to drink at a party?" instead of "Do you drink?" "How often do you drink alcohol?" is another way of obtaining information related to alcohol intake. These questions are open-ended, encouraging the patient to speak freely and showing concern for what worries the patient most.[3]

The nurse needs to judge the reliability of the patient as an historian. An older adult may give a false impression about her mental status because of a prolonged response time or visual and hearing impairment. The complexity and long duration of health problems also make it difficult for an older adult to be an accurate, orderly historian.

It is important that the nurse determine the patient's priority concerns and expectations from the present encounter. Often there is a lack of congruency between the priorities of the patient and the nurse. For example, the priority for the nurse might be to get a consent form signed, whereas the patient is interested only in getting relief from his pain. Until the patient's priority need is met, the nurse will probably be unsuccessful in meeting her priority goal.

The amount of information that should be collected on initial contact with the patient is a nursing judgment based on the patient, the problem, and the setting. Interviews with older adult patients, patients with long-term chronic disease, and emergency room admissions are examples of situations in which the nurse must use this judgment. The nurse may choose to ask only those questions that are pertinent to a specific problem and to defer the complete history interview until a more appropriate time.

Table 4-1 Medical History Format

Demographic data	Past health history
Chief complaint	Family health history
History of present illness	Review of systems

MEDICAL HISTORY

The nurse and physician use different formats and analyze the data differently because of each discipline's different focus. A medical history is a standard format designed to collect data to be used primarily by the physician to diagnose a health problem (Table 4-1). However, much information from this history also is used by nurses and other health care providers. In an inpatient setting, members of the medical team (physician, resident, and medical student) usually collect the medical history. In other settings, such as clinics and physicians' offices, the nurse may be primarily responsible for collecting the medical history.

NURSING HISTORY—SUBJECTIVE DATA

A nursing history has a different focus than a medical history. Nursing is concerned with "the diagnosis and treatment of human responses to actual or potential health problems."[4] During a nursing history interview the nurse needs to ask questions that elicit information related to individual responses to actual or potential problems. Information obtained from this questioning will provide the necessary data to support the identification of nursing diagnoses.

The format used in this text for gathering a nursing history is based on a patient's functional health patterns (Table 4-2). Gordon has described an assessment format, which specifies functional areas that are collected regardless of the conceptual framework being used.[1] Analysis of each functional health pattern facilitates the nursing diagnosis process. The format is designed to gather information systematically to determine the presence of actual, risk, or possible nursing diagnoses. Subjective data are collected related to each functional health pattern. Objective data are collected using a systems approach.

At any time during the history interview or physical examination the patient may relate a symptom such as pain, fatigue, or weakness. Because symptoms are directly experienced by the patient and not observable to the nurse, the symptom must be investigated. Table 4-3 lists eight areas that should be investigated if a symptom is present. The information that is obtained may help determine the cause of the symptom. For example, if a patient states that he has "pain in his leg at times," the provider may obtain and record the following information:

Table 4-2 Nursing History: Functional Health Pattern Format

DEMOGRAPHIC DATA
Name, address, age, occupation

IMPORTANT HEALTH INFORMATION
Past health history
Medications
Surgery or other treatments

FUNCTIONAL HEALTH PATTERNS

Health Perception–Health Management Pattern
1. Reason for visit?
2. General state of health?
3. Any colds in past year?
4. Most important things done to keep healthy? Breast self-exam? Testicular self-exam? Other routine screening?
5. Health compliance problems?
6. Cause of illness? Action taken? Results?
7. Things important to you while here?
8. Family health history?
9. Illness and injury risk factors: use of cigarettes, alcohol, drugs?
10. Allergies? Immunizations?

Nutritional-Metabolic Pattern
1. Typical daily food intake (describe)? Supplements?
2. Typical daily fluid intake (describe)?
3. Weight loss or gain (amount, time span)?
4. Desired weight?
5. Appetite?
6. Food or eating: Discomfort? Diet restrictions?
7. Appetite?
8. Heal well or poorly?
9. Skin problems: lesions? dryness?
10. Dental problems?
11. Change in appetite with anxiety?
12. Food preferences?
13. Food allergies?

Elimination Pattern
1. Bowel elimination pattern (describe): Frequency? Character? Discomfort? Laxatives? Enemas?
2. Urinary elimination pattern (describe): Frequency? Problem in control? Diuretics?
3. Any external devices?
4. Excess perspiration? Odor problems? Itching?

Activity-Exercise Pattern
1. Sufficient energy for desired or required activities?
2. Exercise pattern? Type? Regularity?
3. Spare time (leisure) activities?
4. Dyspnea? Chest pain? Palpitations? Stiffness? Aching? Weakness?
5. Perceived ability for (code for level):
   Feeding ______ Cooking ______
   Grooming ______ Bed mobility ______
   Bathing ______ Home maintenance ______
   General mobility ______ Dressing ______
   Toileting ______ Shopping ______

Sleep-Rest Pattern
1. Generally rested and ready for daily activities after sleep?
2. Sleep onset problems? Aids? Dreams (nightmares)? Early awakening?
3. Usual sleep rituals?
4. Usual sleep pattern?

Cognitive-Perceptual Pattern
1. Hearing difficulty? Aid?
2. Vision? Wear glasses? Last checked?
3. Any change in taste? Any change in smell?
4. Any recent change in memory?
5. Easiest way to learn things?
6. Any discomfort? Pain? How managed?
7. Ability to communicate?
8. Understanding of illness?
9. Understanding of treatments?

Self-Perception–Self-Concept Pattern
1. Self-description? Self-perception?
2. Effect of illness on self-image?
3. Relieving factors?

Role-Relationship Pattern
1. Live alone? Family? Family structure diagram?
2. Difficult family problems?
3. Family problem solving?
4. Family dependence on you for things? How managing?
5. Family's and others' feelings about illness/hospitalization?*
6. Problems with children? Difficulty handling?*
7. Belong to social groups? Have close friends? Feel lonely (frequency)?
8. Work satisfaction (school)? Income sufficient for needs?*
9. Feel part of or isolated to neighborhood where living?

Sexuality-Reproductive Pattern
1. Any changes or problems in sexual relations?*
2. Effect of illness?
3. Use of contraceptives? Problems?
4. When menstruation started? Last menstrual period? Menstrual problems? Para? Gravida?†
5. Effect of present condition or treatment on sexuality?
6. Sexually transmitted diseases?

Coping–Stress Tolerance Pattern
1. Tense a lot of the time? What helps? Use any medicines, drugs, alcohol?
2. Have someone to confide in? Available to you now?
3. Recent life changes?
4. Problem-solving techniques? Effective?

Value-Belief Pattern
1. Satisfied with life?
2. Religion important in your life?
3. Conflict between treatment and beliefs?

Other
1. Other important issues?
2. Questions?

Functional Levels Code
Level 0: Full self-care
Level I: Requires use of equipment or device
Level II: Requires assistance or supervision from another person
Level III: Is dependent and does not participate

Modified from Fuller J, Schaller-Ayers J: *Health assessment, a nursing approach*, ed 2, Philadelphia, 1994, JB Lippincott.
*If appropriate.
†For women.

Table 4-3 Investigation of a Symptom

Location	
Ask:	"Where do you feel it? Where is it located?"
Record:	Region of the body Local or radiating, superficial or deep
Quality	
Ask:	"What does it (feel, look) like?"
Record:	The patient's analogy (e.g., "Like being burned")
Quantity	
Ask:	"How often do you have this feeling? How bad is it? How much is it? How big is it?"
Record:	Frequency (mild, moderate, severe), volume, size, extent, number
Chronology	
Ask:	"When was the first time it occurred? Any particular time of day, week, month, or year?"
Record:	Time of onset, duration, periodicity and frequency, course of symptoms
Setting	
Ask:	"Where are you when this occurs? What are you doing?"
Record:	Where patient is when symptom occurs, what patient is doing, if symptom is related to anything
Aggravating or Alleviating Factors	
Ask:	"What makes it better? Worse? Is there any activity that seems to cause it? What have you done for it? Did it help? Was there some reason you didn't do anything about it?"
Record:	Influence of physical and emotional activities, patient's attempts to alleviate (or treat) the symptom
Associated Manifestations	
Ask:	"What other things do you see or feel when it occurs? Has it affected your appetite? Elimination? Sleeping?"
Record:	Other symptoms
Meaning of the Symptom to the Patient	
Ask:	"How has it affected your life? Why have you sought care now? What do you think may be the cause?"
Record:	Patient's statements about the effect of the symptom and the cause of the symptom

Has right midcalf pain *(location)*, described as "like being stabbed with a knife" *(quality)*. Pain is so severe that it is not possible for the patient to continue walking *(quantity)*. Onset is abrupt, lasting for 1 to 2 minutes; it occurs once or twice daily, and it last occurred on 5/5/95 *(chronology)*. Generally occurs at work when climbing stairs after lunch, but last occurred when cutting lawn *(setting)*. Pain is alleviated by rest for 2 to 3 minutes. The patient has been salting his food "more heavily" than he used to, but "it doesn't help" *(alleviating factor)*. Leg pain is at times accompanied by chest pain that causes some nausea *(associated manifestations)*. The patient has not altered his lifestyle because of the intermittent pain. He thinks it is caused by "muscle cramps from lack of salt" *(personal meaning)*.

Important Health Information

Important health information provides an overview of past and present medical conditions and treatments. Past health history, medications, and surgery or other treatments are included in this part of the history.

Past Health History. The *past health history* provides information about the patient's prior state of health. The patient is specifically asked about major childhood and adult illnesses, injuries, hospitalizations, operations, therapeutic regimens, travel, habits, and the use of supportive devices. Specific questioning is more effective than simply asking if the patient has had any illness or health problems in the past.

Medications. Specific details related to past or present medications are obtained. This includes the use of prescription or over-the-counter medications. Examples of specific medications to ask about include steroids, birth control pills, antibiotics, diuretics, aspirin, antacids, and laxatives. Older adult patients, in particular, need to be questioned about medication routines. Changes in absorption, metabolism, reaction to, and elimination of drugs, as well as surgery and concurrent disease, make drug-related concerns a serious potential problem for older adults.[5]

Surgery or Other Treatments. All injuries, hospitalizations, and surgeries are recorded along with the date of the event, the treatment, and the outcome (whether the problem was completely resolved). Blood transfusions received by the patient also are noted.

Functional Health Patterns

The nurse assesses the patient's functional patterns *(strengths)*, dysfunctional health patterns *(nursing diagnoses)*, and potential dysfunctional patterns *(risk conditions)*. Use of the functional health pattern framework for assessment assists the nurse in differentiating between areas for independent nursing intervention and areas requiring collaboration or referral. Table 4-4 presents an overview of the content usually included in each functional health pattern.

Health Perception–Health Management Pattern. Assessment of the health perception–health management functional health pattern focuses on the patient's perceived level of health and well-being and on personal practices for

Table 4-4 Overview of Functional Health Patterns

Health Perception–Health Management Pattern
- Description of health (usual); description of present illness (onset, course, treatment)
- Relevance of health to activities
- Preventive measures, general health care behavior
- Previous hospitalizations, expectations of this hospitalization
- Potential self-care problems

Nutritional-Metabolic Pattern
- Usual food and fluid intake; appetite
- Daily eating times
- Recent weight change and reason
- Food restrictions or preferences, food supplements
- Swallowing, chewing, eating problems, food allergies
- Skin lesions and general ability to heal
- Condition of skin, hair, nails, mucous membranes, and teeth
- Temperature, pulse, respiration, height, weight

Elimination Pattern

Bowel
- Usual time, frequency, color, consistency
- Assistive devices (laxatives, suppositories, enemas)
- Constipation, diarrhea

Bladder
- Usual frequency
- Problems with dysuria or polyuria
- Assistive devices

Skin condition
- Color, temperature
- Turgor, lesions, edema, pruritus

Activity-Exercise Pattern
- Exercise, activity, leisure, and recreation patterns
- Limitations in activities of daily living

Sleep-Rest Pattern
- Usual sleep routine, sleep pattern
- Perception of quality and quantity

Cognitive-Perceptual Pattern
- Sensory adequacy—hearing, sight, smell, touch, taste
- Prosthetic devices (glasses, hearing aids)
- Pain
- Problems with vertigo
- Heat or cold sensitivity
- Language, understanding, memory abilities

Self-Perception–Self-Concept Pattern
- Self-description
- Effects of illness on self
- Perception, body image, identity, self-esteem
- Posture, eye contact, voice and speech patterns

Role-Relationship Pattern
- Life roles and responsibilities
- Satisfaction or dissatisfaction in family, work, and social relationships

Sexuality-Reproductive Pattern
- Sexuality patterns and satisfaction or dissatisfaction with
- Adequacy of sexual knowledge
- Reproductive state (female—premenopausal or postmenopausal)

Coping–Stress Tolerance Pattern
- General coping strategies
- Stress tolerance, stress reduction behaviors
- Support systems
- Ability to manage situations

Value-Belief Pattern
- Values, goals, beliefs that are basis for decisions
- Value or belief conflict
- Spiritual practices

maintaining health. This includes preventive screening activities, such as breast and testicular examinations; colorectal cancer, hypertension, and cardiac-risk factor screening; and Papanicolaou's (Pap) test.

The questions for this pattern also seek to identify risk factors by obtaining a family history, history of health habits (e.g., smoking, alcohol, and drug use), and exposure to environmental hazards.

There are several ways to identify the patient's perceived level of health and well-being. First, when questioning the patient, the nurse determines the patient's feelings of effectiveness at staying healthy by asking what helps and what hinders.

Next, the patient is asked to describe personal health and any concerns about it. This information should be recorded in the patient's own words. It often is useful to determine whether the patient considers his health to be excellent, good, fair, or poor.

In addition, the patient is asked about a family history of major problems, such as cardiovascular disease, hypertension, cancer, diabetes mellitus, psychiatric illness, and genetic disorders. Information about sexual abuse, violence, and drug and alcohol abuse should also be obtained. The patient should be asked about immunization history as well as allergies. One of the objectives in this pattern is to identify any preventive measures used by the patient to promote personal health.

If the patient is hospitalized, expectations of this hospitalization should be determined. A description of the patient's understanding of the current health problem, including a description of its onset, course, and treatment, should be obtained. Determining what the patient does when not well is important. These questions elicit information about a patient's knowledge of the health problem, awareness of what should be done, and ability to use appropriate resources to manage the problem.

The nurse also assesses the patient's developmental stage in this pattern. This ensures that care appropriate for the developmental capabilities of the patient is planned.

Nutritional-Metabolic Pattern. The processes of ingestion, digestion, absorption, transport, and metabolism are assessed in this pattern. A 24-hour dietary recall should be obtained from the patient. From this information the nurse can evaluate the quantity and quality of foods and fluids consumed. If a problem is identified, the nurse may request that the patient keep a 3-day food diary for a more careful analysis of dietary intake. Questions regarding weight gain, weight loss, and energy level should be asked to evaluate metabolism.

The impact of psychologic factors such as depression, anxiety, and self-concept on nutrition is assessed. For example, "How is your appetite affected by anxiety?" is an appropriate question. Sociocultural factors such as food budget, who prepares the meals, and food preferences are also assessed.

Determining how the patient's present condition has interfered with eating and appetite is important. If the patient's present condition has produced symptoms such as nausea, gas, or pain, the effect of these symptoms on appetite should be determined. Food allergies and the need for a special or restricted diet should be noted. The person's knowledge of nutrition can be determined by asking specific questions such as, "Tell me how many fruits and vegetables you eat a day." "Give me an example of your usual intake of meat." "How well do you heal from a wound?"

Elimination Pattern. The nurse assesses bowel, bladder, and skin function in this pattern. The nurse asks about the frequency of bowel and bladder activity. A description of consistency, amount, color, and aroma should be elicited. The patient should be asked if loss of control or pain are associated with defecating or urinating. If laxatives or enemas are used, the frequency, type, and results should be noted. If any collecting devices are used, such as catheter or colostomy equipment, the nurse asks about their care.

The skin is also assessed in this pattern in terms of its excretory function. The patient should be asked about the condition of his skin, the presence of any lesions, and whether edema or pruritus are problematic.

Activity-Exercise Pattern. The patient's usual pattern of exercise, activity, leisure, and recreation is assessed by the nurse. The patient should be questioned about his ability to perform activities of daily living. Table 4-2 includes the grading scale for self-care abilities under the activity-exercise pattern. If the patient is unable to perform activities of daily living, such as toileting, eating, and moving independently, the specific problems that limit an activity should be noted. Chest pain, dyspnea, dizziness, claudication, musculoskeletal pain, fatigue, and weakness are problems that commonly result in some degree of self-care deficit.

Sleep-Rest Pattern. This pattern describes the patient's pattern of sleep, rest, and relaxation in a 24-hour period. The individual's perception of the effectiveness of sleep and relaxation is pertinent. This information can be elicited by asking, "Do you feel rested when you wake up?" Most people take sleep for granted unless they have a problem with sleeping.

The patient's usual activities related to bedtime and the usual sleep pattern should be determined. Particular routines, position, and environmental factors used to foster sleep should also be elicited.

Cognitive-Perceptual Pattern. Assessment of this pattern involves a description of all senses (vision, hearing, taste, touch, and smell) and the cognitive functions such as communication, memory, and decision making. The patient should be asked about any sensory deficits that affect the ability to perform activities of daily living. Routine eye care, including the date of the last examination, should be elicited. Ways in which the patient compensates for any sensory-perceptual problems should be discussed and noted. The patient should be asked how he communicates best and about his understanding of his illness and treatments. This information is used by the nurse in planning for patient education.

Also, pain is assessed in this pattern. See Chapter 6 for details on pain assessment.

Self-Perception–Self-Concept Pattern. This pattern describes the patient's self-concept, which is critical in determining the way the person interacts with others. Included are attitudes about self, perception of personal abilities, body image, and general sense of worth.[6]

The nurse should ask the patient for a self-description and how the health condition affects self-attitude. Nurses should avoid making value judgments about how people perceive themselves. What concerns the patient about a personal situation may differ from what concerns the nurse. For example, the patient may feel cheated by the system when denied disability benefits. The nurse may feel the patient was not eligible for the benefit.

Role-Relationship Pattern. This pattern describes the roles and relationships of the patient, including major responsibilities. It also examines the patient's self-evaluation of his performance of the expected behaviors related to these roles.

The patient should be asked to describe family, social, and work relationships. The nurse should determine if patterns in these relationships are satisfactory or if strain is evident. The nurse should note the patient's feelings about his role in these relationships and the effect the present condition has on his role and relationship.

Sexuality-Reproductive Pattern. This pattern describes satisfaction or dissatisfaction with personal sexuality and describes the reproductive pattern. Assessing this pattern is important because many illnesses, surgical procedures, and medications affect sexual function. A patient's sexual and reproductive concerns may be expressed, teaching needs and treatable problems may be identified, and normal growth and development may be monitored through information obtained in this pattern.

The interview should be appropriate to the sex, age, and developmental stage of the patient. For example, a 60-year-old widowed female patient might be asked if she has any problems related to her genital area, as these may occur in postmenopausal women. However, a 25-year-old single male patient might be asked about his knowledge and use of condoms.

Obtaining information related to sexuality often is difficult for the inexperienced nurse. However, a beginning nurse, with no advanced education or experience related to sexual issues, can take a health history and screen for sexual function and dysfunction. Based on the complexity of the problem, this nurse may be able to provide limited intervention or refer the patient to a more experienced professional.

Specifically, the nurse should determine if there is a lack of knowledge in relation to sexuality and reproduction. Whether the patient perceives a problem in the area of sexuality should also be determined. The effect of the patient's present condition or treatment on personal sexuality should be noted.

Coping-Stress Tolerance Pattern. This pattern describes the general coping pattern and the effectiveness of the coping mechanisms. Assessment of this pattern involves analyzing the specific stressors or problems that confront the patient, the patient's perception of the stressor, and the patient's response to the stressor.

The major losses or changes experienced by the patient in the previous year are important to document. Current major stressors confronting the patient are also important. The strategies used by the patient to deal with stressors and relieve tension should be noted. The person on whom the patient can rely when problems arise should be recorded.

Value-Belief Pattern. This pattern describes the values, goals, and beliefs (including spiritual) that guide health-related choices.[1] The patient's ethnic background and the effects of culture and beliefs on health practices should be noted. The patient's beliefs about health and illness should be documented. The patient's wishes about continuation of religious practices and the use of religious articles should be noted and honored. The possibility of a conflict in values or beliefs can be determined by asking a question such as, "Does your plan of care cause any conflict in your value or belief system?"

OBJECTIVE DATA

General Survey

Following the nursing history interview, a *general survey* statement is made. The general survey is a statement of the provider's general impression of a patient, including behavioral observations. This initial survey is considered a scanning procedure and begins with the provider's first encounter with the patient and continues during the health history interview.

Although the provider may include other data that seem pertinent, the major areas usually included in the general survey statement are (1) body features, (2) state of consciousness and arousal, (3) speech, (4) body movements, (5) obvious physical signs, (6) nutritional status, and (7) behavior. Vital signs, height, and weight are often included in the general survey statement. Observations of these areas provide the data for the general survey statement. The following is a sample of a general survey statement:

> Mrs. H. is a 34-year-old Hispanic woman, BP 130/84/80, P 88, R 18. No distinguishing body features. Alert but anxious. Speech rapid with trailing thoughts. Wringing hands and shuffling feet during interview. Skin flushed, hands clammy. Overweight relative to height. Sits with eyes downcast and shoulders slumped and avoids eye contact.

Physical Examination

The *physical examination* is the systematic assessment of the physical and mental status of a patient and is considered objective data. It is observable data that are not distorted by the patient's perception.[7] During the physical examination, additional subjective data may be obtained from the patient. This may occur as a result of direct questioning by the nurse in response to a finding or as a result of the patient remembering a forgotten piece of information.

Throughout the history, any *positive findings* are explored using the same criteria as the investigation of a symptom (Table 4-3). A positive finding indicates that the patient has or had the particular problem or symptom under discussion. For example, if the patient answers "yes" to a question about chest pain, it is a positive finding. Relevant information about this problem should then be gathered.

Negative findings may also be significant. A negative finding is the absence of a symptom usually associated with a problem. For example, peripheral edema is common with congestive heart failure. If edema is not present in a patient with congestive heart failure, this should be specifically noted as "no peripheral edema." Another type of negative finding is the absence of usual health promotion practices. Lack of tetanus immunization is an example of a negative finding that should be recorded.

Types. There are two types of physical examinations: the screening physical examination and the branching or regional examination. The *screening physical examination* is performed for screening situations, health surveillance, and health maintenance purposes. It is an organized, purposeful check of major body systems to detect any possible problems. If a problem is detected in the course of the screening physical examination, a more detailed branching examination of the involved system should be done.

A *branching* or *regional examination* is a more detailed assessment of a particular body system. The patient's clinical manifestations should alert the nurse to the appropriate branching examination. For example, abdominal pain indicates the need to do a branching examination of the abdomen. Some problems necessitate more than one branching examination. A complaint of headache indicates the need to do musculoskeletal, neurologic, head and neck, and psychiatric examinations.

Techniques. Four major techniques are used in performing the physical examination: inspection, palpation, percussion, and auscultation.

Inspection. Inspection is the visual examination of a part or region of the body to assess normal conditions or deviations from normal. Inspection is more than just looking. This technique is deliberate, systematic, and focused. The nurse needs to compare what is seen with the known, generally visible characteristics of the body part being inspected. For example, most 30-year-old men have hair on their legs. Absence of hair may indicate a vascular problem and signals the need for further investigation. This same absence of hair in a 70-year-old man may represent a normal skin change of aging.

Palpation. Palpation is the examination of the body through the use of touch. The use of light and deep palpation can yield information related to masses, pulsations, organ enlargement, tenderness or pain, swelling, muscular spasm or rigidity, elasticity, vibration of voice sounds, crepitus, moisture, and differences in texture.[8] The nurse will learn that different parts of the hand are more sensitive for specific assessments. For example, the tips of the fingers are used to palpate lymph nodes, the dorsa of hands and fingers are used to assess temperatures, and the palmar surface is best suited for feeling vibrations (Fig. 4-1).

Percussion. Percussion is an assessment technique involving the production of sound to obtain information about the underlying area. The percussion sound may be produced directly or indirectly. Direct percussion is performed by directly tapping the body with one or two fingers to elicit a sound. Indirect or mediated percussion is the more common percussion technique. The middle finger (pleximeter) of the nondominant hand is placed firmly against the body surface. The tip of the middle finger of the dominant hand (plexor) strikes the distal phalanx of the pleximeter finger (Fig. 4-2). A relaxed wrist and rapid strike produce the best sounds. The sounds and the vibrations produced are evaluated relative to the underlying structures. Deviation from an expected sound may indicate a problem. For example, the usual percussion sound in the right lower quadrant of the abdomen is tympany. Dullness in this area may indicate a problem and the need to be investigated. (Specific percussion sounds of various body parts and regions are discussed in the appropriate assessment chapters.)

Auscultation. Auscultation is the listening to sounds produced by the body to assess normal conditions and deviations from normal. Auscultation is usually indirect, using a stethoscope to amplify sounds (Fig. 4-3). The bell of the stethoscope is more sensitive to low-pitched sounds. The diaphragm of the stethoscope is more sensitive to high-pitched sounds. Auscultation is particularly useful in evaluating sounds from the heart, lungs, abdomen, and vascular system. (Specific auscultatory sounds are discussed in the appropriate assessment chapters.)

Not all assessment techniques are appropriate for all body parts and systems. The nurse will learn which technique to use to elicit the most information. The physical

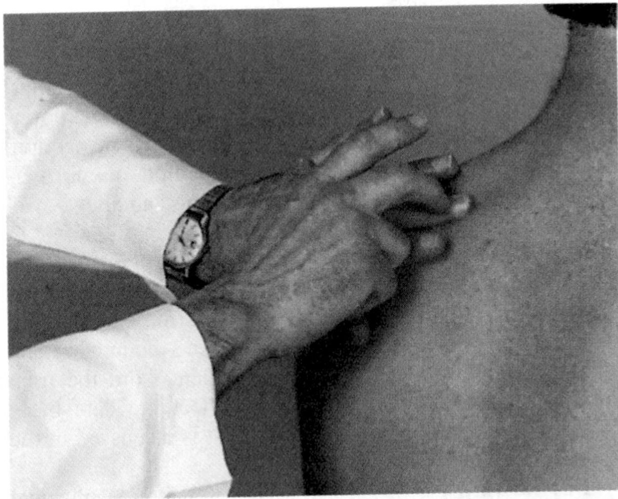

Fig. 4-2 Percussion technique: tapping the interphalangeal joint. Only the middle finger of the nondominant hand should be in contact with the skin surface.

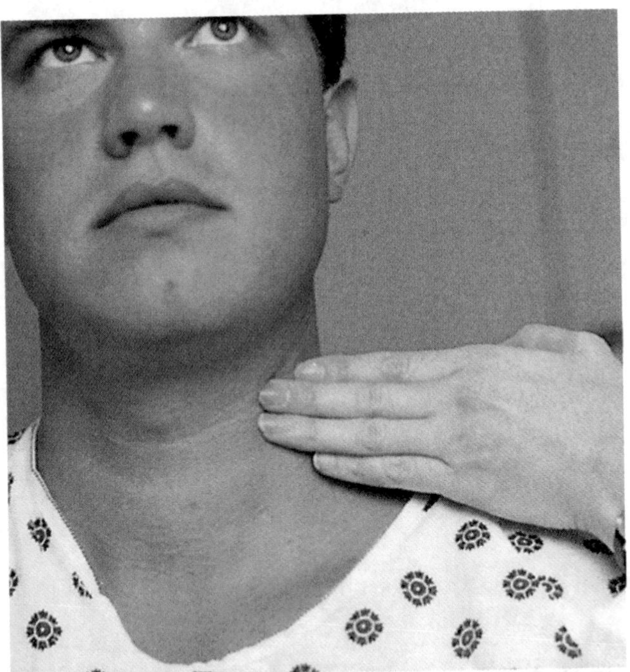

Fig. 4-1 Palpation is the examination of the body through the use of touch.

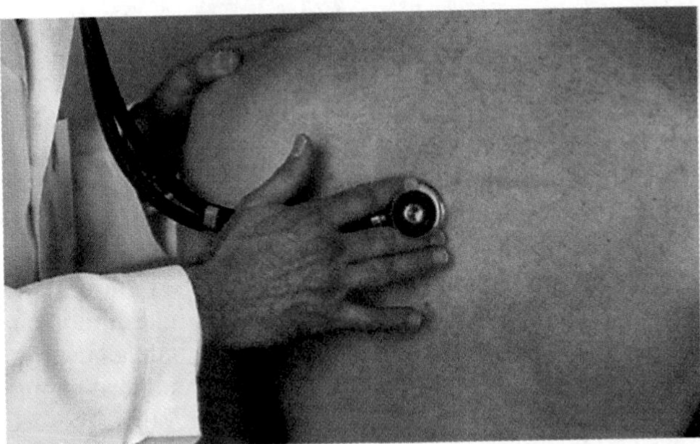

Fig. 4-3 Auscultation is listening to sounds produced by the body to assess normal conditions and deviations from normal.

Table 4-5 Equipment for Screening Physical Examination

Stethoscope (with bell and diaphragm, tubing 15-18 in [38-46 cm])
Wristwatch (with second hand)
Blood pressure cuff
Ophthalmoscope/otoscope set
Eye chart (wall chart or Snellen pocket eye card)
Pocket flashlight
Tongue blades
Cotton balls
Percussion hammer
Tuning fork
Alcohol swabs
Patient gown
Paper cup with water
Examining table or bed

assessment techniques are usually performed in the sequence of inspection, palpation, percussion, and auscultation. The only exception to this sequence is for the abdominal examination. In this situation the sequence is inspection, auscultation, percussion, and palpation. Palpation and percussion of the abdomen before auscultation can alter bowel sounds and produce false findings.

Equipment. The equipment needed for the screening physical should be easily accessible during the examination (Table 4-5). Organizing equipment before the examination saves the time and energy of the patient and the nurse. Lack of organization can discourage the patient from the trust and confidence the nurse needs to collect the data base. (The use of specific pieces of equipment is discussed in the appropriate assessment chapters.)

Developing a System. The screening physical should be performed systematically and efficiently. Explanations should be given to the patient as the examination proceeds. The factors to be considered are the nurse's efficiency, and the patient's comfort, safety, and privacy. The examiner is less likely to forget a procedure, a step in the sequence, or a portion of the body if the same sequence is followed every time. Table 4-6 presents an outline for the screening physical examination that is organized, logical, and complete. Adaptations of the physical examinations often are useful for the older adult patient who may have age-related problems such as decreased mobility, limited energy, and perceptual changes.[9] An outline listing some of the useful adaptations is found in Table 4-7.

Recording the Screening Physical Examination. Only abnormal findings should be recorded during the actual examination. This prevents needless interruptions in the examination to write lengthy normal findings. At the conclusion of the examination, the nurse should combine the normal and abnormal findings in a carefully recorded physical examination. Table 4-8 is an example of how to record a screening physical on a healthy adult. Table 3-1, Gerontologic Differences in Assessment, and the age-related assessment findings in each assessment chapter are helpful references in recording age-related assessment differences.

PROBLEM IDENTIFICATION AND NURSING DIAGNOSES

After completing the history interview and physical examination, the nurse is ready to develop a list of *nursing diagnoses* and collaborative problems. Figure 4-4 illustrates the problem identification phase of the nursing process.

Nursing diagnoses are health-related problems that are managed primarily by nursing care. (Chapter 1 explains the process of establishing nursing diagnoses.)

In this text, nursing diagnoses are presented in two formats. For major health problems, a full nursing care plan has been developed. The nursing diagnosis statement is presented first and includes the problem, etiologic statement, and defining characteristics. Outcome criteria are identified, which can be used to evaluate if the goal has been achieved. Specific nursing interventions that address the nursing diagnosis including rationale are then specified.

For less common health problems, the nursing diagnoses are listed under the Nursing Diagnosis heading. In either case, appropriate nursing interventions are discussed under the Nursing Management heading.

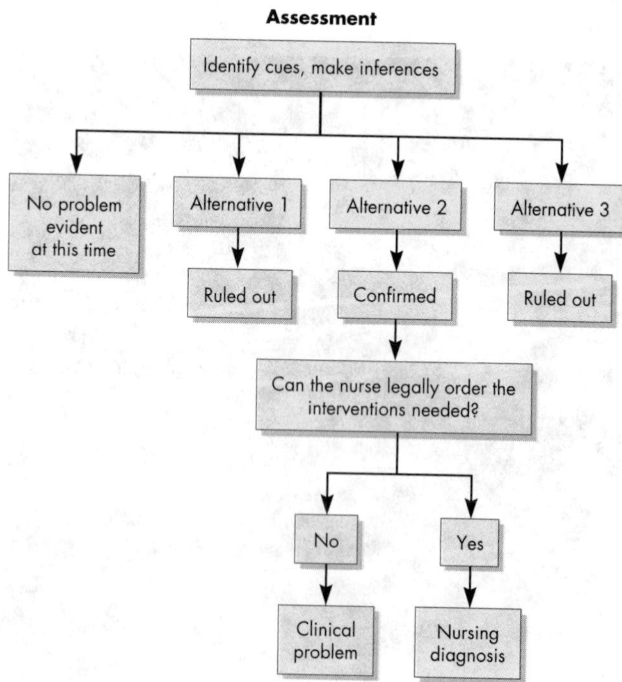

Fig. 4-4 Problem identification phase of the nursing process.

Table 4-6 Outline for Screening Physical Examination

1. General Survey

Observe general state of health (patient is seated)

- Body features
- State of consciousness and arousal
- Speech
- Body movements
- Physical signs
- Nutritional status
- Stature

2. Vital Signs

Record vital signs:

- Blood pressure
- Radial pulse
- Respiration

Record height and weight

3. Integumentary System

Inspect and palpate skin for the following:

- Color
- Lesions
- Scars
- Bruises
- Edema
- Moisture
- Texture
- Temperature
- Turgor
- Vascularity

Inspect and palpate nails for the following:

- Color
- Lesions
- Size
- Flexibility
- Shape
- Angle

4. Head and Neck

Inspect and palpate head for the following:

- Shape and symmetry of skull
- Masses
- Tenderness
- Hair
- Scalp
- Skin
- Temporal arteries
- Temporomandibular joint
- Sensory (CN V, light touch, pain)
- Motor (CN VII, shows teeth, purses lips, raises eyebrows)
- Looks up, wrinkles forehead (CN VII)
- Raises shoulders against resistance (CN XI)

Inspect and palpate eyes for the following:

- Visual acuity
- Eyebrows
- Position and movement of eyelids
- Visual fields
- Extraocular movements (CN III, IV, VI)
- Cornea, sclera, conjunctiva
- Pupillary response
- Red reflex
- Eyeball tension

Inspect and palpate ears for the following:

- Placement
- Pinna
- Auditory acuity (Weber's or Rinne, whispered voice, ticking watch)
- Mastoid process
- Auditory canal
- Tympanic membrane

Inspect and palpate nose and sinuses for the following:

- External nose
  - Shape
  - Blockage
- Internal nose
  - Patency of nasal passages
  - Shape
  - Turbinates or polyps
  - Discharge
- Discharge
- Frontal and maxillary sinuses

Inspect and palpate mouth for the following:

- Lips (symmetry, lesions, color)
- Buccal mucosa (Stensen's and Wharton's ducts)
- Teeth (absence, state of repair, color)
- Gums
- Tongue for strength (asymmetry, ability to stick out tongue, side to side, fasciculations)
- Palates
- Tonsils and pillars
- Uvular elevation (CN IX)
- Posterior pharynx
- Gag reflex (CN X)
- Jaw strength (CN XI)
- Moisture
- Color
- Floor of mouth

Inspect and palpate (occasionally auscultate) neck for the following:

- Skin (vascularity and visible pulsations)
- Symmetry
- Postural alignment
- Range of motion
- Pulses (carotid)
- Midline structure (trachea, thyroid gland, cartilage)
- Lymph nodes (preauricular, postauricular, occipital, mandibular, tonsillar, submental, anterior and posterior cervical, infraclavicular, supraclavicular)

Inspect neurologic status:

- Motor status observations
  - Gait
  - Toe walk
  - Heel walk
  - Drift
- Coordination
  - Finger to nose
  - Romberg's sign
- Spine (scoliosis)

continued

Table 4-6 Outline for Screening Physical Examination—cont'd

5. Extremities

Observe size and shape, symmetry and deformity, involuntary movements

Inspect and palpate arms, fingers, wrists, elbows, shoulders for the following:

Strength
Range of motion
Crepitus
Joint pain
Swelling
Fluid

Test reflexes:

Biceps
Triceps
Brachioradialis
Patellar
Achilles
Plantar

Inspect and palpate legs for the following:

Strength of hips
Edema
Hair distribution
Pulses (dorsalis pedis, posterior tibialis)

6. Posterior Thorax

Inspect for muscular development, respiratory movement, approximation of AP diameter

Palpate for symmetry of respiratory movement, tenderness of CVA, spinous processes, tumors or swelling, tactile fremitus
Percuss for pulmonary resonance
Auscultate for breath sounds

7. Anterior Thorax

Assess breasts for configuration, symmetry, dimpling of skin
Assess nipples for rash, direction, inversion, retraction
Initiate teaching or review of breast self-exam
Perform upright examination
Inspect for PMI, other precordial pulsations
Palpate for thrills, lifts, heaves, tenderness over precordium
Inspect neck for venous distention, pulsations, waves
Palpate axillae
Inspect, neck palpate, check breasts for discharge (patient is supine)
Complete teaching of breast self-examination
Auscultate for rate and rhythm, character of S_1 and S_2; S_1 and S_2 in the aortic, pulmonic, Erb's point, tricuspid, mitral areas; bruits at carotid, epigastrium; breath sounds at RML

8. Abdomen

Inspect for scars, shape, symmetry, bulging, muscular development, position and condition of umbilicus, movements (respiratory, pulsations, presence of peristaltic waves)
Auscultate for peristalsis, femoral bruits
Percuss border of liver, all quadrants
Palpate to confirm positive findings; check liver (size, surface contour, tenderness); spleen; kidney (size, contour, consistency, tenderness, mobility); urinary bladder (distention); femoral pulses; inguinofemoral nodes

9. Completion of Examinations of Extremities

Observe the following:

Range of motion of hips, ankles, feet
Crepitus
Joint pain
Swelling
Fluid
Muscle development
Coordination (heel to skin)
Homan's sign
Proprioception (position sense of great toe)

10. Genitalia*

Male external genitalia

Inspect penis, noting hair distribution, prepuce, glans, urethral meatus, scars, ulcers, eruptions, structural alterations
Inspect epidermis of perineum, rectum
Inspect skin of scrotum; palpate for descended testes, masses, pain

Female external genitalia

Inspect hair distribution; mons pubis, labia (minora and majora); urethral meatus; Bartholin's, urethral, Skene's glands (may also be palpated, if indicated); introitus
Assess for presence of cystocele, rectocele, prolapse (patient bears down)
Inspect perineum, rectum

AP, Anteroposterior; *CVA,* costovertebral angle; *PMI,* point of maximal impulse; *RML,* right middle lobe.
*If the nurse has the appropriate training, the speculum and bimanual examination of women and the prostate gland examination of men should be performed after this inspection.

Table 4-7 Adaptations in Physical Assessment Techniques for Older Adult Patient

General Approach
Keep patient warm and comfortable, because loss of subcutaneous fat decreases ability to stay warm. Adapt positioning to physical limitations. Avoid unnecessary changes in position. Perform as many activities as possible in the position of comfort for the patient.

Skin
Handle with care because of fragility and loss of subcutaneous fat.

Head and Neck
Provide a quiet environment free from distraction because of patient's sensory deficits (e.g., decreased vision, touch, hearing).

Extremities
Use nonvigorous movements and reinforcement techniques. Avoid having patient hop on one foot or perform deep knee bends because of patient's limited range of motion of the extremities, decreased reflexes, and diminished sense of balance.

Thorax
Adapt examination for changes due to decrease in force of expiration, weakened cough reflex, and shortness of breath.

Abdomen
Be cautious in palpating patient's liver, because it is easily palpated with increased size. The older adult patient may have diminished pain perception in abdominal wall.

Genitalia
Use a well-lubricated, smaller speculum for vaginal examination because dryness and atrophy of the female genitalia may cause discomfort.

Table 4-8 Recording a Screening Physical Examination

Patient's Name ____________________
Age ______

General Status
Well-nourished, well-hydrated, well-developed Caucasian (woman) or (man) in NAD, appears stated age, looks pleasant, smiles readily, speech clear and evenly paced; is alert and oriented × 3; cooperative, calm

Skin
Clear ō lesions, warm and dry, trunk warmer than extremities, turgor returns quickly, no ↑ vascularity, no varicose veins

Nails
Well-groomed, round 160-degree angle s̄ lesions, nail beds pink, nails flexible

Hair
Thick, brown, shiny, normal (male, female) distribution

Head
Normocephalic, sinuses nontender

Eyes
Visual fields intact on gross confrontation
VA: OD 20/20
OS 20/20
OU 20/20
s̄ glasses
EOM: Intact on all gazes s̄ ptosis, nystagmus
Fundi: Red reflex present bilat no opacities, fundi WNLs
Pupils: PERRLA, negative cover and uncover tests, negative Hirschberg test

Ears
Pinna intact, in proper alignment; external canal patent; small amount cerumen present; TMs intact; pearly gray LM, LR visible, not bulging; Rinne: AC>BC; Weber's: does not lateralize, whisper heard at 3 ft

Nose
Patent bilaterally; turbinates pink, no swelling

Mouth
Moist and pink, soft and hard palates intact, uvula rises midline on "ahh," 24 teeth present and in good repair

Throat
Tonsils surgically removed, no redness

Tongue
Moist, pink, size appropriate for mouth

Neck
Supple, s̄ masses, s̄ bruits, lymph nodes nonpalpable and nontender
Thyroid: Palpable, smooth, not enlarged
ROM: Full, intact, strong
Trachea: Midline, nontender

Breasts
Soft, nonpendulous, s̄ venous pattern, s̄ dimpling, puckering
Nipples: s̄ inversion, point in same direction, areola dark and symmetric, no discharge, no masses, nontender

Axilla
Hair present, shaved, no lesions, nontender

Lungs
No increase in AP diameter, resp rate 18, reg rhythm, no ↑ in tactile fremitus, no tenderness, lungs resonant throughout, diaphragmatic excursion 4 cm bilaterally, lung fields clear throughout

Heart
Rate 82, reg rate and rhythm; no lifts, heaves
PMI: 5th ICS at MCL; L nonpalpable; nonpalpable thrills
S_1, S_2 louder, softer in appropriate locations; no S_3, S_4; no murmurs, rubs, clicks
Carotid, femoral, pedal, and radial pulses present; equal, strong bilaterally

continued

Table 4-8 Recording a Screening Physical Examination—cont'd

Abdomen
No pulsations visible, rounded, active bowel sounds, no bruits or CVA tenderness, no palpable masses

Liver
Edge palpable, smooth, nontender; approx 9 cm in size

Spleen
Nonpalpable, nontender

Neurologic System
Cranial nerves I-XII intact
Motor (drift, toe stand) intact
Coord (FN, Romberg) intact
Reflexes: See diagram
Sensation (touch, vibration, prop) intact
Grading Scale
0 No response
1+ Diminished
2+ Normal
3+ Increased
4+ Hyperactive

Musculoskeletal System
Well developed, no muscle wasting; s̄ crepitus, nodules, swelling
ROM: Full, intact, and equal bilaterally; no scoliosis
Strength: Equal, strong bilaterally
Gait: Walks erect 2-foot steps, arms swinging at side s̄ staggering

Female Genitalia
External genitalia: No swelling, redness, tenderness in BUS; normal hair distribution, no cysts, rectocele
Vagina: No lesions, discharge; pink
Cervix: Os closed; no lesions, erosions, nontender
Uterus: Small, firm, nontender; pink
Adnexa: No enlargement; nontender
Rectovaginal: Sphincter intact; confirms above findings

Male Genitalia
Normal male hair distribution
Penis: Urethral opening patent; no redness, swelling, discharge; no lesions, structural alterations
Scrotum: Testes descended; no redness, masses, tenderness
Rectal: No lesions, redness; sphincter intact; prostate small, nontender

Psychologic Status
Affect appropriate; eye contact
Orientation: Oriented × 3—time, place, person
Mood: Pleasant, appropriate
Thought content: Intelligent, coherent
Memory: Remote and recent intact
Serial sevens: Not done or intact

Signature ______________________

AC>BC, Air conduction greater than bone conduction; *AP*, anteroposterior; *BUS*, Bartholin's gland, urethral meatus, Skene's duct; *coord*, coordination; *CVA*, costovertebral angle; *EOM*, extraocular movements; *FN*, finger to nose; *LM*, landmarks; *LR*, light reflex; *MCL*, midclavicular line; *NAD*, no acute distress; *PERRLA*, pupils equal, round, reactive to light and accommodation; *PMI*, point of maximal impulse; *prop*, proprioception; *ROM*, range of motion; *s̄*, without; *TM*, tympanic membrane; *VA*, visual acuity; *WNL*, within normal limits.

REVIEW QUESTIONS

The number of the question corresponds to the same-numbered objective at the beginning of the chapter.

1. The nursing history provides information to assist the nurse in
a. diagnosing a medical problem.
b. more accurately identifying nursing diagnoses.
c. admitting the patient to the hospital.
d. validating the medical history.

2. The patient's information about leg pain would be placed in which of the following functional health patterns?
a. Health perception–health management
b. Sleep-rest
c. Cognitive-perceptual
d. Coping–stress tolerance

3. Examination of the body through the use of touch is called
a. inspection.
b. palpation.
c. percussion.
d. auscultation.

4. The proper length for a stethoscope is
a. 10 inches (25 cm).
b. 15 inches (38 cm).
c. 22 inches (56 cm).
d. 25 inches (64 cm).

5. A branching examination is an examination of
a. a region of the body.
b. the four extremities.
c. mental status.
d. a system of the body.

6. In a screening history and physical, the first information to record is the
a. health history.
b. problem list.
c. general survey.
d. physical examination.

REFERENCES

1. Gordon M: *Nursing diagnosis: process and application*, ed 3, St Louis, 1994, Mosby.
2. Wilkinson J: *Nursing process in action*, Redwood City, CA, 1992, Addison-Wesley.

3. Bowers A, Thompson J: *Clinical manual of health assessment,* ed 4, St Louis, 1992, Mosby.
4. American Nurses' Association, Congress for Nursing Practice: *Nursing: a social policy statement,* Kansas City, MO, 1980, The Association.
5. Carnevali D, Patrick M: *Nursing management for the elderly,* ed 3, Philadelphia, 1993, JB Lippincott.
6. Fuller J, Schaller-Ayers J: *Health assessment: a nursing approach,* ed 2, Philadelphia, 1994, JB Lippincott.
7. Hickey P: *Nursing process handbook,* St Louis, 1990, Mosby.
8. Weber J: *Health assessment,* ed 2, Philadelphia, 1993, JB Lippincott.
9. Ebersole P, Hess P: *Toward healthy aging,* ed 3, St Louis, 1990, Mosby.

Chapter 5

NURSING ASSESSMENT AND ROLE IN MANAGEMENT

Stress

Joan Stehle Werner

Learning Objectives

1. Define stressor, stress, demands, primary appraisal, secondary appraisal, coping, and adaptation.
2. Describe the three stages of Selye's general adaptation syndrome.
3. Describe the role of cognitive appraisal in the stress process.
4. Describe the role of the nervous and endocrine systems in the stress process.
5. Describe the effects of stress on the immune system.
6. Describe the coping behaviors used by a patient experiencing stress.
7. List the variables that may influence the response to stress.
8. Describe the nursing assessment and management of a patient experiencing stress.

Interest in the study of stress has intensified as investigators have begun to identify its role in relation to physical and emotional health. Most contemporary approaches to the study of stress have been influenced by three different but complementary stress theories. The first theory conceptualizes stress as a *response* to an environmental stressor. This theory was first proposed by Selye, who identified *stress* as a nonspecific response of the body to any demand made upon it.[1] Selye referred to these stress-inducing demands as *stressors.* Stressors can be physical or emotional and pleasant or unpleasant, as long as they require the individual to adapt (Table 5-1). In response to either physical (e.g., burns) or psychologic (e.g., death of a loved one) stressors, a series of physiologic changes occur. Selye called this pattern of responses the *general adaptation syndrome* (GAS).

A second stress theory views stress as a *stimulus* that causes a response. This theory originated with Holmes, Rahe, and Masuda who developed a tool (Table 5-2) to assess the effects of life changes on health.[2,3] *Life changes* are defined as conditions ranging from minor violations of the law to death of a loved one. The major assumption of this theory is that frequent life changes make people more vulnerable to illness (Table 5-3).

A third stress theory focuses on person-environment transactions and is referred to as the *transaction* or *interaction* theory.[4] A proponent of this theory is Lazarus, who emphasized the role of *cognitive appraisal* in assessing stressful situations and selecting coping options. Lazarus and Folkman defined *psychologic stress* as a particular relationship between the person and the environment that is appraised by the person as taxing or exceeding his resources and endangering his well-being.[5] These three stress theories are discussed in more detail in this chapter.

STRESS AS A RESPONSE

Historically, Selye's early research using animals supported his theory that stressors from different sources produce a similar physical response pattern. He called these physical responses to stress the *general adaptation syndrome* (GAS). The GAS is composed of three stages: *alarm reaction, stage of resistance,* and *stage of exhaustion.* Stressors are also likely to result in a local response called *local adap-*

Table 5-1 Examples of Stressors

Physical	Emotional
Noise	Diagnosis of cancer
Amphetamines	Promotion at work
Burns	Watching a loved one die
Running a marathon	Failing an examination
Infectious diseases	Financial loss
Pain	Winning a beauty contest

Reviewed by Linda Janusek, RN, PhD, Associate Professor, Loyola University, Chicago, IL.

Table 5-2 Social Readjustment Rating Scale

No.	Life Event	Mean Value
1	Death of spouse	100
2	Divorce	73
3	Marital separation from mate	65
4	Detention in jail or other institution	63
5	Death of a close family member	63
6	Major personal injury or illness	53
7	Marriage	50
8	Being fired at work	47
9	Marital reconciliation with mate	45
10	Retirement from work	45
11	Major change in health of a family member	44
12	Pregnancy	40
13	Sexual difficulties	39
14	Gaining a new family member (e.g., through birth, adoption, moving in)	39
15	Major business readjustment (e.g., merger, reorganization, bankruptcy)	39
16	Major change in financial state (e.g., a lot worse off or a lot better than usual)	38
17	Death of a close friend	37
18	Changing to different line of work	36
19	Major change in number of arguments with spouse (e.g., either a lot more or a lot less than usual regarding child-rearing, personal habits)	35
20	Taking out a mortgage or loan for a major purchase (e.g., for a home, business)	31
21	Foreclosure on a mortgage or loan	30
22	Major change in responsibilities at work (e.g., promotion, demotion, lateral transfer)	29
23	Son or daughter leaving home (e.g., marriage, attending college)	29
24	Trouble with in-laws	29
25	Outstanding personal achievement	28
26	Spouse beginning or ceasing work outside the home	26
27	Beginning or ceasing normal schooling	26
28	Major change in living conditions (e.g., building a new home, remodeling, deterioration of home or neighborhood)	25
29	Revision of personal habits (e.g., dress, manners, associations)	24
30	Trouble with boss	23
31	Major change in working hours or conditions	20
32	Change in residence	20
33	Changing to a new school	20
34	Major change in usual type or amount of recreation	19
35	Major change in church activities (e.g., a lot more or a lot less than usual)	19
36	Major change in social activities (e.g., clubs, dancing, movies, visiting)	18
37	Taking out a mortgage or loan for a lesser purchase (e.g., for a car, TV, freezer)	17
38	Major change in sleeping habits (a lot more or a lot less sleep, or change in part of day when asleep)	16
39	Major change in number of family get-togethers (e.g., a lot more or a lot less than usual)	15
40	Major change in eating habits (a lot more or a lot less food intake, or very different meal hours or surroundings)	15
41	Vacation	13
42	Christmas	12
43	Minor violation of law (e.g., traffic tickets, jaywalking, disturbing the peace)	11

Modified from Holmes TH, Rahe RH: Social readjustment rating scale, *J Psychosom Res* 11:216, 1967.

tation syndrome (LAS). Once the stressor or stimulus is integrated into the central nervous system (CNS), multiple responses occur because of activation of the hypothalamic-pituitary-adrenal axis and autonomic nervous system. The nature of these responses, in which the stimulus and its effects successively cause changes in the nervous, endocrine, and immune systems, is fundamental to understanding the physiologic and behavioral changes that occur in an individual experiencing stress.

Stage of Alarm Reaction

The first stage of the stress response is the alarm reaction of the GAS, in which the individual perceives a stressor physically or mentally, and the "*fight-or-flight*" response is ini-

Table 5-3 Life Change Units and Incidence of Major Illness*

Number	Amount of Change	Incidence of Major Illness
0-149	Insignificant	Minimal
150-199	Mild	33%
200-299	Moderate	50%
300+	Major	80%

Modified from Holmes T, Rahe E: The social readjustment rating scale, *J Psychosom Res* 11:213, 1967.
*This table describes the amount of stress as measured by LCUs (life change units), followed by the statistical incidence of disease according to the number of LCUs. The chance of illness is based on the number of LCUs during 1 to 2 years.

tiated. When the stressor is of sufficient intensity to threaten the steady state of the individual, it requires a reallocation of energy so that adaptation can occur. This temporarily decreases the individual's resistance and may even result in disease or death if the stress is prolonged and severe.

Physical signs and symptoms of the alarm reaction are generally those of sympathetic nervous system stimulation. These signs include increased blood pressure, increased heart and respiratory rate, decreased gastrointestinal (GI) motility, pupil dilatation, and increased perspiration. The patient may complain of such symptoms as increased anxiety, nausea, and anorexia.

Stage of Resistance

Ideally the individual quickly moves from the alarm reaction to the stage of resistance in which physiologic forces are mobilized to increase the resistance to stress. At this time adaptation may occur, involving modification of the external and internal environments. Resistance is high at this time as compared with the normal state. The amount of resistance varies among individuals, depending on the level of physical functioning, coping abilities, and total number and intensity of stressors experienced. For example, a person who has been exercising regularly and is physically fit will have greater ability to adapt to the stress of emergency surgery than a person who is deconditioned and leads a sedentary lifestyle.

Although few overt physical signs and symptoms occur in this stage as compared with the alarm stage, the person is expending energy in an attempt to adapt. This adaptive energy is limited by the resources of the individual. When resources are adequate, the patient may successfully recover from a stressor such as surgery and return to a normal coping state. If adaptation does not occur, the person may move to the next phase of the GAS, which is the stage of exhaustion.

Stage of Exhaustion

The stage of exhaustion is the final stage of the GAS. It occurs when all the energy for adaptation has been expended. Physical symptoms of the alarm reaction may briefly reappear in a final effort by the body to survive. This is exemplified by a terminally ill person who becomes alert and has stronger vital signs shortly before death. The individual in the stage of exhaustion usually becomes ill and may die if assistance from outside sources is not available. This stage can often be reversed by external sources of adaptive energy, such as medication, blood transfusions, or psychotherapy.

Refinements in Selye's Stress Theory

Selye's work addressed the importance of conditioning factors that may affect the stress response. These internal conditioning factors include age, genetic makeup, and previous experience with the stressors, and external conditioning factors such as diet and climate.[6] Selye coined the term *eustress* to refer to stress associated with positive events such as winning a tennis match. However, he never fully explained the health consequences of eustress versus stress. This relationship is currently under investigation by others.

Selye's description of stress focuses on the physiologic changes of the nervous, immune, and endocrine systems that occur as an organism responds to a specific stressor. In his original work, Selye described a triad of responses including (1) adrenocortical activation, (2) thymic involution, and (3) GI ulceration. His work indicates that there is a predictable uniform pattern in the physiologic responses to various stressors. This emphasis is due in part to the fact that Selye used animal models that exhibited a predictable response. As stress researchers began to study humans, the individual variations in responses became apparent.

Human research supports different patterns of physiologic responses that occur during stress.[7] Illustrating this view is an early classic study conducted by Lacey and Lacey in 1958.[8] These investigators subjected 42 participants to four mild stressors. Stressors included (1) the cold pressor test, in which one arm is placed in ice water; (2) anticipating the cold pressor test; (3) a mental math problem; and (4) a test of word fluency. A number of physiologic stress responses were assessed. These findings indicate substantial variability in blood pressure, heart rate, pulse pressure, and other measures among subjects in response to the same stressor. The investigators labeled these individual physiologic responses as *individual response stereotypy.* Thus stressors are likely to produce complex and varying profiles of hormonal and tissue changes in different individuals. This may help explain why a variety of the diseases or disorders of adaptation exist (Table 5-4).

STRESS AS A STIMULUS

Life Events

Another approach to the study of stress is to view stress as a stimulus or event that results in a disrupted response. Stress defined in this way is similar to Selye's definition of stressor. Historically this approach stems from attempts to develop questionnaires to measure stress in terms of life changes or life events.[2,3] Two such questionnaires are the

Table 5-4 Examples of Disorders and Diseases of Adaptation

Angina	Impotence
Carpal tunnel syndrome	Insomnia
Depression	Irritable bowel syndrome
Dyspepsia	Low back pain
Eating disorders	Myocardial infarction
Fatigue	Sexual dysfunction
Headaches	Ulcers
Hypertension	

Table 5-5 Examples of Daily Hassles

Misplacing or losing things	Chronic pain
Inconsiderate smokers	Inadequate financial resources
Planning meals	Job dissatisfaction
Concerns about job security	Caring for disabled child
Difficulties with friends	Marital problems
Waiting	

Social Readjustment Rating Scale (SRRS) (see Table 5-2) and the Schedule of Recent Experiences (SRE). Life events questionnaires such as the SRRS and the SRE were developed in an attempt to numerically weight the impact (stress) of various life changes (e.g., death of a spouse, financial changes). A life event is regarded as stressful if it is associated with some adaptive or coping behavior on the part of the involved individual.[3] Each event, whether desirable or not, is indicative of or requires a significant change in the ongoing life pattern of the individual.

It was originally theorized that the more stressful life events occurring throughout a specific period of time, the greater the vulnerability to illness. Of particular interest was the research that reported an association between the number and intensity of life events and the resulting probability of physical and emotional illness following the events (see Table 5-3).[9] Although several studies have shown statistically significant relationships between stressful life events and illness onset, these relationships are often weak. Findings contrary to these studies have also been reported.[10] Life-events scaling has raised methodologic issues regarding additional factors (e.g., age, perception, previous experiences, health) that must be taken into account when considering life events.

Refinements in the Stress as a Stimulus Theory

Factors that affect an individual's response to life events include cultural influences, personality, clustering of events, biologic variables, socioeconomic status, timing, and interpersonal support systems. Another important factor is the issue of outcomes. Often, disease outcomes (biologic processes and disease diagnoses) are confused with illness outcomes (total effect of the disease on an individual), leading to inconclusive results.[10] These factors indicate the importance of using a holistic approach when assessing the patient.

Hardiness and Sense of Coherence. An interesting aspect of research focused on life events is the identification of some individuals who experience high scores in terms of life-events changes but do not succumb to illness. Kobasa and others have described *hardiness* as a mediating factor in the stress-illness relationship.[11,12] The hardy person has (1) a clear sense of personal values and goals, (2) a strong tendency toward interaction with the environment, (3) a sense of meaningfulness, and (4) an internal rather than external locus of control.

Sense of coherence (SOC), a closely related concept to hardiness, has been defined and developed by Antonovsky.[13] It has been shown that SOC is a more powerful mediator of stress and illness than hardiness.[14] In general, SOC refers to how an individual sees the world and one's life in it. It is a personality characteristic or coping style rather than a response to a specific situation. The three components of SOC are *comprehensibility* (stimuli derived from one's internal and external environments are structured, predictable, and explicable), *manageability* (resources are available to meet the demands posed by these stimuli), and *meaningfulness* (demands are challenges worthy of investment and engagement). An individual with a strong SOC has an enduring tendency to see one's life as ordered, predictable, and manageable.

Hassles and Uplifts. Daily-hassle scores have been found to be an important supplement to the life events approach in predicting health and illness outcomes related to the impact of a stressor. *Daily hassles* are experiences and conditions of daily living that have been appraised as salient and harmful or threatening to an individual's well-being.[15] The frequency and intensity of daily hassles have a stronger relationship with somatic illness than the life-events scale.[5] Items addressed on the daily hassles scale (Table 5-5) reflect the content areas of work, family, social activities, environment, practical considerations, finances, and health.[16]

As an adjunct to hassles, *uplifts* are defined as positive experiences that are likely to occur in everyday life.[5] This concept seems comparable with the eustress described earlier by Selye. Further investigation is needed to determine the effects of positive experiences on health outcomes.

STRESS AS A TRANSACTION

Appraisal

In contrast to theories of stress as a response or stimulus, Lazarus' theory focuses on the person-environment transaction and the cognitive appraisal of demands and coping options.[5] A multitude of internal and external data are received at the neurocognitive level. Lazarus proposed that these data are interpreted during the process of cognitive appraisal. *Appraisal* is a judgment process that includes recognizing the degree of *demands,* or stressors, placed on

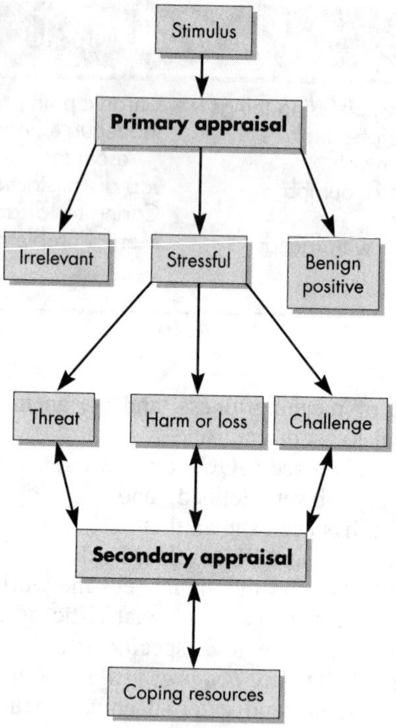

Stimulus
Primary appraisal
Irrelevant
Stressful
Benign positive
Threat
Harm or loss
Challenge
Secondary appraisal
Coping resources

Fig. 5-1 Cognitive appraisal process.

the individual (Fig. 5-1). The appraisal process also involves the recognition of available resources or options that help when dealing with potential or actual demands.

During *primary appraisal,* demands are assessed according to the possible impact on the individual's well-being. Demands can be judged as irrelevant, benign-positive, or stressful. If demands are appraised as stressful, they can be classified as representing harm or loss, threat, or challenge. *Harm* or *loss demands* involve actual damage, and *threat demands* involve anticipated harm or loss. *Challenge demands* differ from threat and harm or loss demands because they are viewed as a potential for personal gain or growth. For example, hiking in the wilderness may place demands on the individual that will provide an opportunity to test and exhibit strength and endurance.

Therefore, stress is a situation in which *demands* exceed the individual's adaptive resources. If an adaptive response to these demands does not occur, negative consequences will result.[17]

Secondary appraisal refers to the process of recognizing the coping resources and options that are available. Primary and secondary appraisal often occur simultaneously and interact with each other in determining stress. *Cognitive reappraisal* is the process of continuously relabeling cognitive appraisals. Certain factors influence the labeling of appraisals.[5] Situational factors include the intensity of the external demands, the immediacy of the expected impact, and ambiguity. Person-related factors include motivational characteristics, belief systems, and intellectual resources and skills.

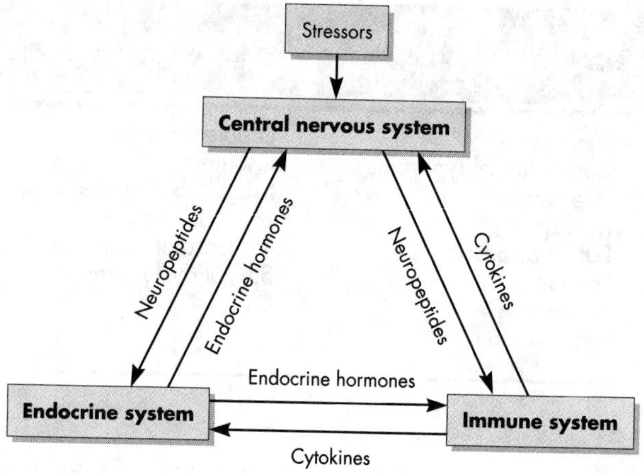

Fig. 5-2 Neurochemical links among the nervous, endocrine, and immune systems. The communication among these three systems is bidirectional.

Theoretic Summary

The role of perception is the key to understanding the difference between the three major stress theories presented. In Selye's stress response theory, all demands are stressors with the capacity to elicit the GAS. Conditioning factors in individuals influence the stress response. In the life-change theory, perceived stressfulness of the event is not considered because each individual receives the same score for a certain stressor. In the Lazarus transaction theory, the cognitive appraisal process determines whether the demands will be assessed as stressful. Through cognitive appraisal, individuals experience different outcomes in dealing with demands, not only because of conditioning factors, but also as a result of how the demand is perceived and labeled during the person-stressor interaction. An event that is stressful to one individual may not be stressful to another.

PHYSIOLOGIC RESPONSE TO STRESS

To simplify the description of the physiologic response to stress, the following discussion is divided into the roles of the nervous system, the endocrine system, and the immune system. However, these systems are interrelated, and thus the ultimate responses of the person to stress reflect the integration of the three systems (Fig. 5-2). Understanding the physiologic changes associated with stress will help provide the foundation for the assessment of the patient experiencing stress and the implications for health outcomes.

Nervous System

Stressors, or demands, may be physical, psychologic, or social. The body will respond physiologically to both actual and symbolic stressors. The complex process by which an event is perceived as a stressor and by which the body responds is not fully understood. The hypothalamus participates in both the emotional and physiologic response to

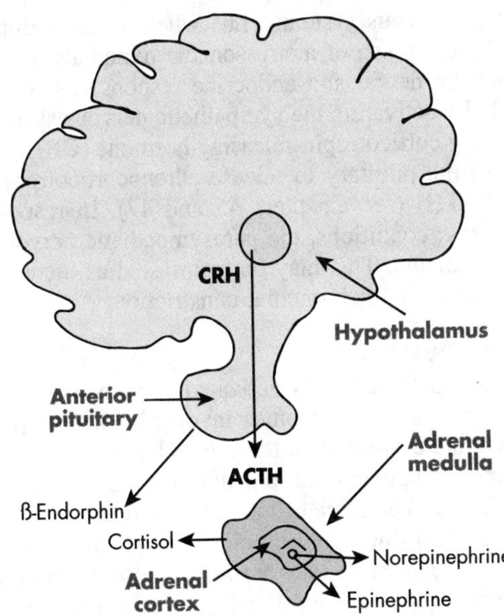

Fig. 5-3 Hypothalamic-pituitary-adrenal axis. *ACTH,* Adrenocorticotropic hormone; *CRH,* Corticotropin-releasing hormone.

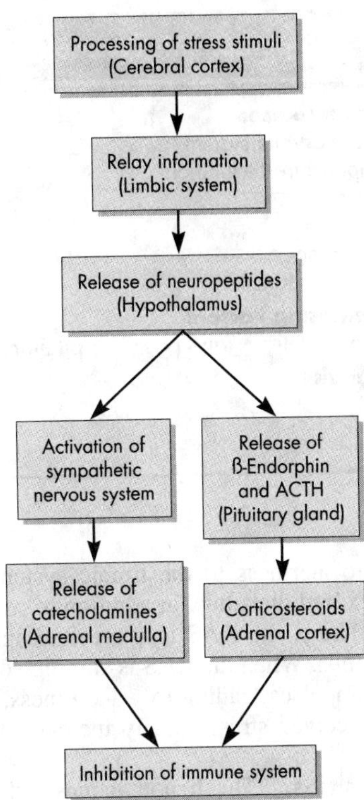

Fig. 5-4 The cerebral cortex processes stressful stimuli and relays the information via the limbic system to the hypothalamus. Corticotropin-releasing hormone (CRH) stimulates the release of adrenocorticotropic hormone (ACTH) from the pituitary gland. ACTH stimulates the adrenal cortex to release corticosteroids. The sympathetic nervous system is also stimulated, resulting in the release of epinephrine and norepinephrine.

stressors. This control is significant because most stressors precipitate an emotional reaction. In addition to the hypothalamus, other parts of the CNS including the cerebral cortex, limbic system, and reticular formation are involved in the neural control of emotions and the physiologic responses to stress (Figs. 5-3 and 5-4). The functions of these structures are closely interrelated.

Cerebral Cortex. After an external event has occurred, afferent input is sent to the cerebral cortex via sensory impulses from the peripheral nervous system including the eyes and the ears. For example, the pressure of a restraint on an arm or leg that is applied too tightly will act as a stressor. Afferent impulses that travel to the cortex from the periphery via the spinal cord (spinothalamic pathways) also activate the reticular formation in the area of the brainstem. The reticular formation then relays input to the thalamus and from the thalamus to the cerebral cortex. This network of neurons, which is involved with arousal and consciousness, is called the *reticular activating system* (RAS). The RAS functions to maintain wakefulness and alertness.

The somatic, auditory, and visual associative areas of the cerebral cortex receive input from the peripheral sensory fibers and then interpret it. The prefrontal area serves to reduce the speed of the associative functions so that the person has time to evaluate the information in light of past experiences and future consequences (primary and secondary appraisal) and to plan a course of action. All these functions are involved in the perception of a stressor.

The temporal lobes of the cerebral cortex contain the auditory association areas, which when stimulated, produce the sensation of fear. Stimulation of the temporal lobes can result in sounds that seem louder or softer, visual displays that seem nearer or farther, and experiences that seem familiar or strange. These effects modify the perception of stress.

Limbic System. The limbic system, which lies in the inner midportion of the brain near the base, includes the *septum, cingulate gyrus, amygdala, hippocampus,* and anterior nuclei of the *thalamus.* (The hypothalamus is located in the center of these structures but is not considered a part of the limbic system.) The function of the limbic system is thought to be primarily involved with emotions and behavior. When these structures are stimulated, emotions, feelings, and behaviors can occur that ensure survival and self-preservation, such as feeding, sociability, and sexuality. The cerebral cortex and limbic systems interact to serve the experiential and executive functions of emotion. Endorphins are found in structures of the limbic system and in the thalamus, brain, and spinal cord. They are known to reduce the perception of painful stimuli. Endogenous opioids have also been shown to increase in response to stress in the absence of pain.

Reticular Formation. The reticular formation is located between the lower end of the brainstem and the thalamus. It contains the RAS, which sends impulses

Table 5-6 Hypothalamic Functions

Coordinates Impulses
Autonomic nervous system
Body temperature regulation
Food intake
Water balance
Urine formation
Cardiovascular function
Secretes Releasing Factors
Regulation of anterior and posterior pituitary hormones
Affects Behavior
Emotion
Alertness

contributing to alertness to the limbic system and to the cerebral cortex and thalamus. In addition to receiving input from the periphery, the RAS also receives impulses from the hypothalamus. When the RAS is stimulated, it increases its output of impulses leading to wakefulness. Both physiologic and perceived stress usually increase the degree of wakefulness.

Hypothalamus. The hypothalamus, which lies just above the pituitary gland, has many functions (Table 5-6). The hypothalamus receives information regarding traumatic stimuli via the spinothalamic pathway, pressure-sensitive input from the baroreceptors via the brainstem, and emotional stimuli via the limbic system. Because the hypothalamus secretes peptide hormones and factors that regulate the release of hormones by the anterior pituitary, it is central to the connection between the nervous and endocrine systems in responding to stress (see Fig. 5-3).

In addition, the hypothalamus regulates the function of both the sympathetic and parasympathetic branches of the autonomic nervous system. Thus when an individual perceives the existence of a stressor, the hypothalamus mediates both the neural and endocrine responses. It does this primarily by activating the sympathetic nervous system and by releasing corticotropin-releasing hormone (CRH), which stimulates the pituitary to release adrenocorticotropic hormone (ACTH) (see Chapters 45 and 47). In response to certain stress conditions, the parasympathetic nervous system is stimulated. This may be manifested as increased GI motility, flushing, or bronchial constriction.

Endocrine System

Once the hypothalamus is activated in response to stress, the endocrine system becomes involved. The sympathetic nervous system stimulates the adrenal medulla to release the hormones epinephrine and norepinephrine (catecholamines). The effect of catecholamines and the sympathetic nervous system, including the adrenal medulla, is referred to as the *sympathoadrenal* response. These hormones prepare the body for the "fight-or-flight" response (Fig. 5-5). This response is activated by physical stressors such as hypovolemia and hypoxia and emotional states, particularly anger, excitement, and fear.[18] Catecholamines can be measured in the blood or urine; as a result, numerous research studies have used blood and urine catecholamine measurements to determine the impact of various stressors.

The hypothalamus releases CRH, which stimulates the anterior pituitary to release *proopiomelanocortin* (POMC). Both ACTH and endorphin are derived from POMC. ACTH, in turn, stimulates the adrenal cortex to synthesize and secrete glucocorticoids and, to a lesser degree, aldosterone and androgens. Glucocorticoids, in particular cortisol, are essential for the stress response. Cortisol produces a number of physiologic effects that include increasing blood glucose levels, potentiating the action of catecholamines on blood vessels, and inhibiting the inflammatory response. Aldosterone acts to increase sodium reabsorption in the

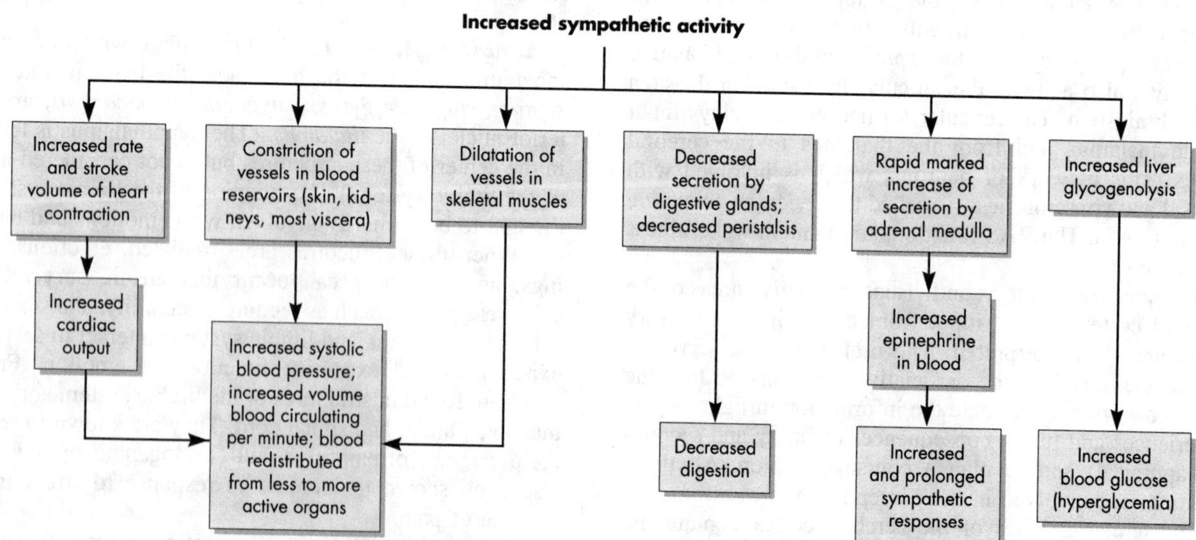

Fig. 5-5 Alarm reaction responses resulting from increased sympathetic activity. Note that these are the responses commonly referred to as the "fight-or-flight" reaction.

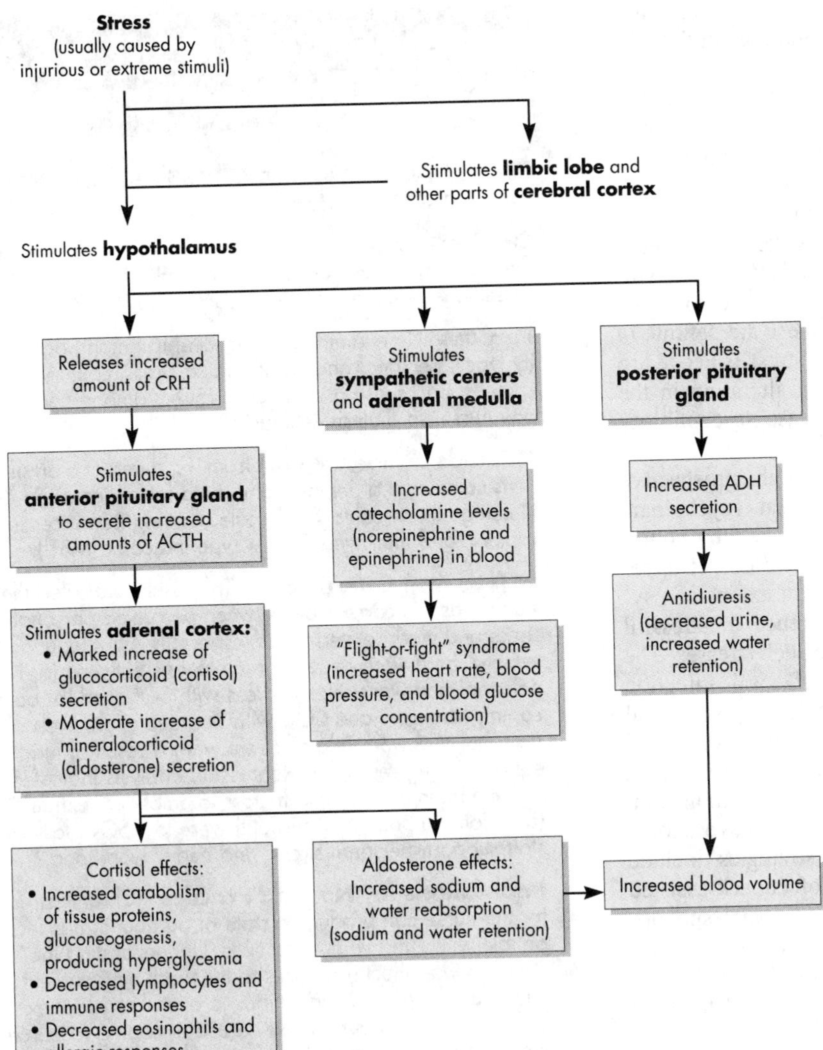

Fig. 5-6 Current concepts of the stress syndrome. *ACTH,* Adrenocorticotropin hormone; *ADH,* antidiuretic hormone; *CRH,* corticotropin-releasing hormone.

kidney tubules and, as a result, increases extracellular fluid (ECF). This hypothalamic-pituitary-adrenal system, termed the *conservation-withdrawal* system, is activated by acute and chronic stress situations and depression.[18] During stress, neural stimulation of the posterior pituitary results in the secretion of antidiuretic hormone (ADH), which also promotes water reabsorption by the distal and collecting tubules of the kidney.

Stimulation of both the adrenal medulla and cortex results in an increased blood glucose level. This elevation provides the additional fuel for the increased metabolism needed for fighting or fleeing. The increased cardiac output (resulting from the increased heart rate and increased ECF), increased blood glucose levels, and increased metabolic rate make the physical responses possible. In addition, dilatation of skeletal muscle blood vessels and resulting increased blood supply to the large muscles and the brain provide for quick movement and increased alertness. The increased blood volume (from increased ECF and the shunting of blood from the GI system) and increased clotting time function to help maintain adequate circulation to vital organs in case of traumatic blood loss. These responses to stress illustrate the complexity and interrelated nature of the processes involved (Fig. 5-6).

The physiologic responses to stressors seem better suited to persons living in a primitive society than in the industrialized societies of today. Because of social conventions, many of the physiologic responses to stress are internalized and produce wear and tear on the body. As a result, many diseases (the diseases of adaptation) experienced by modern people are considered maladaptations to stress.

Immune System

Recently there has been a major focus on understanding the potential impact of stress on immune function. Negative stressors lead to alterations in immune function in humans through processes involving the hypothalamic-pituitary-adrenal axis and the autonomic nervous system that affect immune function (see Fig. 5-4). In return, the immune system also affects endocrine and CNS responses (see Fig. 5-2). Both corticosteroids and catecholamines are known to suppress immune function. Interleukin-1 (which is released by activated macrophages), one type of cytokine, may directly stimulate the release of ACTH and thus initiate the stress response.

There is now a large body of literature that documents a relationship between stress and illness. The overall evidence points in the direction of stress-induced immunosuppression. Multiple studies have shown that both acute and chronic stress can affect immune function, including decreased number and function of natural killer cells, altered lymphocyte proliferation, decreased production of cytokines by lymphocytes, and decreased phagocytosis by neutrophils and monocytes.[19] Although these are definite *in vitro* findings, it is not known how much stress is needed to cause these changes or how much of an alteration in the immune system is necessary before disease susceptibility occurs.

Recently a well-designed and thorough prospective study demonstrated a relationship between psychologic stress and the common cold.[20] In this study healthy volunteers were inoculated intranasally with low doses of upper respiratory viruses. The subjects underwent extensive psychologic testing to determine the occurrence of stressful events in their lives and their reactions to such stresses. The results indicated that both the rates of viral infection (assessed by viral isolation and serologic response) and clinical colds (identified by signs and symptoms) increased with the rate of psychologic stress. This study substantiated that psychologic stress may predispose to the common cold.

Strategies to enhance immunocompetence have shown increases in immune function. These strategies include relaxation and imagery techniques, biofeedback-assisted relaxation strategies, humor, exercise, and social support. An important study in this area showed that patients with metastatic breast cancer who were involved in a weekly support group lived longer (on an average of 18 months) than patients in the control group.[21]

IDENTIFYING STRESSORS OR DEMANDS

Work-Related Stressors

The nurse should become familiar with the types of stressors experienced by various populations and individuals in particular circumstances. For example, work-related stressors are common.[22,23] Some demands are intrinsic to the job, such as poor working conditions, work overload, and time pressures. Other demands stem from the individual's role in the organization (role conflict), career development (overpromotion or underpromotion), relationships at work (difficulties in delegating responsibilities), and the organizational climate (restrictions on behavior). The extensive research on these factors and their effects validates inclusion of occupation and work experience as essential factors in assessment.[24]

Nurses and student nurses have been extensively studied as groups experiencing high levels of stress and burnout. Stressors such as heavy work load, lack of adequate rewards, and lack of participation in decision making have been identified in various practice settings. Knowledge of these stressors is important if nurses do not want to become victims of stress and burnout in the work environment.[25]

RESEARCH

IMPLICATIONS FOR NURSING PRACTICE

PERSONAL AND WORK STRESS AND BURNOUT IN DIALYSIS NURSES

Citation Lewis SL and others: Personality, stress, coping, and sense of coherence among nephrology nurses in dialysis settings, *Am Nephr Nurs Assoc J* 21:325-336, 1994.

Purpose To examine the relationship among personality types, personal and work-related stress, coping resources, and sense of coherence (SOC) among nephrology nurses in dialysis settings.

Methods Nurses (n = 49) from 13 different dialysis units completed a demographic data form, Perceived and Nursing Stress scales, SOC scale, Coping Resources Inventory, and the Myers-Briggs Type Indicator (MBTI).

Results and Conclusions The results indicated there was a positive correlation between perceived personal stress and work-related stress, especially work load. Conversely, there were negative correlations between (a) both personal and work-related stress with SOC and (b) both coping resources and SOC with burnout. High levels of personal and work-related stress were a result of inadequate coping resources. Regression analysis indicated that the main contributing factors to emotional exhaustion (a major component of burnout) were low SOC, lack of staff support, personal stress, and heavy work load.

Implications for Nursing Practice Chronic stress for the nurse can produce a state of burnout that is incompatible with effective nursing care. Understanding the stressors that affect responses to the work environment will allow for successful interventions to alter the risk of exhaustion and burnout. Increased use of coping resources would facilitate the nurse's management of personal and work-related stressors.

Illness-Related Stressors

Another major source of stress relates to illness experienced by a patient, which often causes stress for family members as well as the patient. The nurse needs to assess what aspects of the illness are the most stressful for the patient. These may include such factors as physical health, job responsibilities, finances, and children. This information is valuable because it gives the nurse the patient's perspective on stressors.

Although the nurse and patient generally agree on what stressors are experienced by the patient, the nurse generally rates all items as significantly more stressful than the patient does.[26] These findings emphasize the need for understanding the patient's perception of the situation.

A hospital stress rating scale has been developed based on stressors identified by medical-surgical patients.[27] The five most stressful events in descending order of stressfulness included (1) the possibility of losing sight, (2) the anticipated diagnosis of cancer, (3) the possibility of losing

Table 5-7 Examples of Coping Resources

Coping Resources in the Person	
Health, Energy, Morale	***Problem-solving Skills***
Robust health	Collection of information
High energy level	Identification of problem
High morale	Generation of alternatives
Positive Beliefs	***Social Skills***
Self-efficacy	Communication skills
Spiritual faith	Compatibility
Coping Resources in the Environment	
Social Networks	***Utilitarian Resources***
Family members	Finances
Co-workers	Instructional manuals
Social contacts	Social agencies

a kidney or other organ, (4) knowing the illness is serious, and (5) the possibility of losing one's sense of hearing.[28]

In a recent study the hospital stressors of patients with acquired immunodeficiency syndrome (AIDS) were identified. Major stressors for all patients were in the areas of loss of independence, separation from significant others, and medication problems.[29] Knowledge of these and other stressors can further assist the nurse in identifying potential and actual sources of stress during hospitalization for a similar group of patients.

COPING

The concept of *coping* has been defined as constantly changing cognitive and behavioral efforts to manage specific external or internal demands that are appraised as taxing or exceeding the resources of the person.[5] Defense processes, such as denial, may also be included as coping processes, since both defensive and coping processes intertwine and are intrinsic to the psychologic integrity of the individual.[30] *Coping resources,* defined as characteristics or actions drawn on to manage stress (Table 5-7), include factors in the person or environment that encompass categories such as (1) health, energy, and morale; (2) positive beliefs; (3) problem-solving skills; (4) social skills; (5) social networks; and (6) material resources.

Coping efforts function broadly in two ways, as *problem-solving* (problem-focused) and *emotion-regulating* (emotion-focused) efforts (Table 5-8). As an individual attempts to deal with demands (internal or environmental) or obstacles that create the demands, the person is said to be using the problem-focused coping efforts. When the individual's effort is concentrated on methods of regulating the emotional response to the problem, the person is said to be using the emotion-focused coping efforts. For example, a patient with diabetes mellitus who learns to give injections is engaged in problem-focused coping. This patient is using emotion-focused coping when the distress of being diagnosed with diabetes is lessened by the thought that it would be worse if the diagnosis had been cancer. Combinations of emotion-focused and problem-focused coping can be used.

As an individual begins to deal with a stressor, modes of coping may include the following:

Table 5-8 Examples of Demands and Coping

Demands	Coping
Being diagnosed with diabetes	Attending diabetic education classes (P-S) Taking a short vacation (E-R)
Failing an examination	Obtaining a tutor (P-S) Having dinner with friends (E-R)
Being told that more work will be required as part of the job	Learning to use a word processor (P-S) Venting negative feelings about paperwork to spouse (E-R)
Being notified of an appointment for an IRS audit	Reviewing tax records with accountant (P-S) Practicing deep breathing exercises (E-R)
Giving a public speech for the first time	Practicing in front of family members (P-S) Jogging the morning of the speech (E-R)

E-R, Emotion-regulating efforts; *P-S,* problem-solving skills.

1. Information seeking (gathering data about the problem and possible solutions to the problem)
2. Direct actions (performing concrete acts to alter self or environment)
3. Inhibition of action (refraining from any action)
4. Intrapsychic processes (reappraising the situation; initiating cognitive activity aimed at improving feelings)
5. Turning to others (obtaining social support)
6. Escaping or avoiding

The choice of coping strategies depends on various factors. Variables that affect an individual's choice of coping strategies include degrees of uncertainty, threat, or helplessness, and the presence of conflict.[31] If uncertainty is high, direct action is less likely to be selected as a coping strategy. If the degree of appraised threat is severe, more primitive coping modes such as panic are more likely to occur. In the presence of conflict, an individual may not be able to take direct actions. Helplessness promotes immobilization. The strategy chosen may also be influenced by the outcome of the cognitive appraisal that categorizes the stressor as harm or loss, threat, or challenge.

Specific strategies labeled as *coping activities* or *processes* have been identified by studying groups of individuals assumed to be dealing with specific stressors.[32] In a study of women with cancer, four problem-focused coping modes were identified: (1) bargaining, (2) focusing on the positive, (3) social support, and 4) concentrated efforts. Three emotion-focused coping processes were also determined: (1) wishful thinking, (2) detachment, and (3) acceptance. The emotion-focused strategies of detachment and wishful thinking and the problem-focused strategy of focusing on the positive were shown to significantly affect various types of emotional distress. Detachment and focusing on the positive helped to mitigate distress, whereas wishful thinking increased emotional distress.[33]

Most of the research to date has focused on types of coping strategies. Findings about which coping strategies are the most beneficial or adaptive are inconclusive.

NURSING MANAGEMENT

STRESS

Nursing Assessment

The patient faces an array of potential stressors, or demands, that can have health consequences. The nurse needs to be aware of situations that are likely to result in stress and must also assess the patient's appraisal of the situation. In addition to the stress itself, specific coping mechanisms have health consequences and therefore must be included in the assessment.

Although the manifestations of stress may vary from person to person, the nurse should assess the patient for the signs and symptoms of the stress response that occur as a result of changes in the nervous, endocrine, and immune systems (see Chapters 50, 45, and 10, respectively).

Three major areas are important in assessment of stress. These areas provide the nurse with a useful guide in the assessment process. The areas include *demands, human responses to stress,* and *coping.*

Demands. Stressors, or demands, on the patient may include major life changes, events, or situations, such as changes in family constellation or daily hassles the patient is experiencing. Demands may be categorized as external (environmental) or internal (e.g., perceived tasks, goals, and commitments). Internal demands may also include physical demands resulting from disease or injury. In addition, the number of simultaneous demands, the duration of these demands, and previous experience with similar demands should be assessed. Specific assessment guides for particular types of patients are also available.

Primary appraisal or perception of the demands should be assessed. Demands may be categorized as representing harm or loss, threat, or challenge. Family responses to demands on the patient should also be assessed.[34]

Human Responses to Stress. Physiologic effects of demands that are appraised as stressful are mediated primarily via the sympathetic nervous system and the hypothalamic-pituitary-adrenal system. Responses such as increased heart rate, increased blood pressure, loss of appetite, sweating, and dilated pupils are included. In addition, the patient may exhibit some of the diseases of adaptation (see Table 5-4).

Behavioral human responses include observable actions and cognitions of the patient. Behavioral effects may include responses such as accident proneness, impaired speech, anxiety, crying, and shouting. Behavior in other aspects of life such as occupation may include absenteeism or tardiness at work, lowered productivity, and job dissatisfaction. Observable cognitive responses include self-reports of excessive demand, inability to make decisions, and forgetfulness. Some of these responses may also be apparent in significant others.

Coping. Secondary appraisal by the patient, or the patient's evaluation of coping resources and options, should be assessed. Resources such as supportive family members, adequate finances, and the ability to solve problems are examples of positive resources (see Table 5-7).

Coping strategies include cognitive and behavioral efforts to meet demands. The use and effectiveness of problem-focused and emotion-focused coping efforts should be addressed (see Table 5-8). These efforts may be categorized as direct action, avoidance of action, seeking information, defense mechanisms, and seeking assistance of others. The probability that a certain coping strategy will bring about the desired result is another important aspect to be assessed.[31]

Table 5-9 Nursing Diagnoses in Coping-Stress Tolerance Pattern

Impaired adjustment
Caregiver role strain
Ineffective individual coping
  Defensive coping
  Ineffective denial
Ineffective family coping: compromised
Ineffective family coping: disabled
Family coping: potential for growth
Posttrauma response
Relocation stress syndrome
Risk for self-harm
Risk for violence

Nursing Diagnoses

The importance of stress and coping to the nurse is shown by the amount of attention these concepts have received related to nursing diagnoses. A coping-stress-tolerance pattern has been identified as 1 of 11 functional health patterns.[35] This pattern includes the diagnoses presented in Table 5-9. Assessment of the health pattern results in a description of the coping-stress-tolerance patterns of a patient. Stressors can be identified at the individual or family level.

Two specific nursing diagnoses have been identified related to stress: ineffective individual coping and ineffective family coping. *Ineffective individual coping* is defined as an inability to manage internal or environmental stressors appropriately as a result of inadequate resources (physical, psychologic, behavioral, or cognitive). Potential etiologies include disruption of emotional bonds, unsatisfactory support system, sensory overload, and inadequate psychologic resources.[35] *Ineffective family coping: compromised* refers to the usually supportive primary person (family member or close friend) providing insufficient, ineffective, or compromised support, comfort, assistance, or encouragement, which may be needed by the patient to manage or master adaptive tasks related to health challenge.[35]

Table 5-10 Conditioning Factors Altering the Stress Response

Age	Personality
Nutrition	Circadian rhythms
Heredity	Previous experiences
Social support	Socioeconomic status
Health	Financial resources

Nursing Implementation

The first step in managing stress is to become aware of its presence. This includes identifying and expressing stressful feelings. The role of the nurse is to facilitate and enhance the processes of coping and adaptation. Nursing interventions depend on the severity of the stress experience or demand. In the multiple trauma patient, the person expends energy in an attempt to physically survive. The nurse's efforts are directed to life-supporting interventions and to the inclusion of approaches aimed at the reduction of additional stressors to the patient. For example, the multiple trauma patient is much less likely to adapt or recover if faced with additional stressors such as sleep deprivation or an infection.

The importance of cognitive appraisal in the stress experience should prompt the nurse to assess if changes in the way the patient perceives and labels particular events or situations (cognitive reappraisal) are possible. Some experts also propose that the nurse consider the positive effects that result from successfully meeting stressful demands. Greater emphasis should also be placed on the part of cultural values and beliefs enhancing or constraining various coping options.

Since dealing with physical, social, and psychologic demands is an integral part of daily experiences, the coping behaviors that are used should be adaptive and should not be a source of additional stress to the individual. Generalizing about which coping strategies are the most adaptive is not yet possible. However, in evaluating coping behaviors, the nurse should look at the short-term outcomes (i.e., the impact of the strategy on the reduction or mastery of the demands and the regulation of the emotional response) and the long-term outcomes that relate to health, morale, and social and psychologic functioning.

Conditioning factors affect the response to various stressors (Table 5-10). Resistance to stress can be increased with a healthy lifestyle. Some behaviors seem to promote and maintain health. These include the following:

1. Sleeping regularly 7 to 8 hours per night
2. Eating breakfast
3. Eating regular meals with minimal or no snacking
4. Eating moderately to maintain an ideal weight
5. Exercising moderately
6. Drinking alcohol moderately
7. Not smoking (best if have never smoked)

These behaviors help people maintain good health regardless of sex, age, and economic status. These behaviors are also cumulative; that is, the greater the number of these factors habitually practiced by the individual, the better the health.

Good mental health practices are important for good health as well. These practices primarily result in a realistic, positive self-conception, and the ability to solve problems.

Stress-reducing activities can be incorporated into nursing practice. The activities suggested can also be viewed as conditioning factors, because the patient is developing a sense of control with an increase in self-esteem as the practices are incorporated into daily activities. A sense of control is an important mediator in the stress process.[36]

The nurse can assume a primary role in planning stress-reducing interventions. Specific stress-reducing activities within the scope of nursing practice (some of which may require additional training) include relaxation training, cognitive reappraisal, music therapy, exercise, decisional control, massage, and humor (Table 5-11). Specific relaxation strategies are presented in Table 6-11.

Table 5-11 Examples of Stress Management Techniques

Techniques	Descriptions
Progressive relaxation	Self-taught or instructor-directed exercise that involves learning to contract and relax muscles in a systematic way, beginning with the face and ending with the feet. The exercise may be combined with breathing exercises that focus on inner self.
Guided imagery	Purposeful use of one's imagination to achieve relaxation and control. An individual concentrates on images and mentally pictures oneself in the scene.
Thought stopping	Self-directed behavioral approach used to gain control of self-defeating thoughts. When these thoughts occur, the individual stops the thought process and focuses on conscious relaxation.
Exercise	Regular exercise, especially aerobic movement, results in improved circulation, increased release of endorphins, and an enhanced sense of well-being.
Humor	Humor in the form of laughter, cartoons, funny movies, riddles, audiocassettes, comic books, and joke books can be used for both the nurse and patient.
Assertive behavior	Open, honest sharing of feelings, desires, and opinions in a controlled way. The individual who has control over one's life is less subject to stress.
Social support	This may take the form of organized support and self-help groups, relationships with family and friends, and professional help.

CRITICAL THINKING EXERCISES

CASE STUDY

STRESS DURING HOSPITALIZATION

Patient Profile

Mr. R. Ranson, a 20-year-old college student and starting basketball guard, was admitted for an emergency appendectomy the night before his basketball team entered the final playoffs.

Subjective Data

- Has exertional asthma that has been controlled with medication
- Has primarily been eating pizza, doughnuts, and drinking coffee and sodas
- Does not want his family or friends to visit

Critical Thinking Questions

1. Explain the physiologic changes that would be expected in Mr. Ranson during the first 24 hours postoperatively as a result of the demand of surgery.
2. Explain how Mr. Ranson's previous diet may affect his current adaptability.
3. What physiologic and psychologic stressors can be identified or predicted in Mr. Ranson's situation? Describe the possible effects of these stressors on his asthma.
4. What factors will Mr. Ranson's secondary appraisal process focus on?
5. What specific nursing interventions can be included in Mr. Ranson's management that will enhance his adaptability?
6. Based on the assessment data provided, write one or more nursing diagnosis. Are there any collaborative problems?

In summary, a knowledge of stress and coping theories provides the nurse with useful concepts that are applicable to all phases of the nursing process. Keeping abreast of the current research on this topic is a challenge. The models and concepts proposed are useful to the nurse who chooses to establish a research- and theory-based practice that recognizes the relationships among stress, coping, and health. The nurse should recognize when the patient or family needs to be referred to a professional with advanced training in counseling.

REVIEW QUESTIONS

The number of the question corresponds to the same-numbered objective at the beginning of the chapter.

1. Choose the false statement regarding stress.
   a. It occurs when demands exceed the adaptive resources of an individual.
   b. It occurs only as a result of physiologic stressors.
   c. What is stressful to one individual may not be stressful to another.
   d. It may result from a perceived threat.

2. All the following statements are true about the GAS *except*
   a. it was first defined by Selye and involves stages.
   b. it involves the central and autonomic nervous systems and the pituitary and adrenal glands.
   c. symptoms of the stage of resistance are caused by stimulation of the sympathetic nervous system.
   d. symptoms of the stage of exhaustion may initially mimic those of the stage of alarm reaction.

3. All the following statements regarding cognitive appraisal are true *except* it is a judgment process that
   a. occurs on a cognitive level.
   b. recognizes the degree of demands placed on the individual.
   c. occurs only during perceived threats.
   d. recognizes available resources.

4. When an individual perceives the existence of a stressor, the response is mediated by the part of the CNS called the
   a. hypothalamus.
   b. reticular formation.
   c. limbic system.
   d. temporal lobes.

5. The part of the nervous system that connects it to the endocrine system is the
   a. hypothalamus.
   b. cerebral cortex.
   c. reticular formation.
   d. limbic system.

6. Choose the false statement regarding coping behaviors.
   a. Coping behaviors may include efforts to regulate emotion.
   b. Some coping behaviors are problem-focused efforts.
   c. Denial is a form of coping.
   d. If uncertainty is high, direct action is usually the selected coping strategy.

7. All the following statements regarding hardiness are true *except*
   a. it involves having a clear sense of goals.
   b. it involves having an external rather than internal locus of control.
   c. there is a strong tendency toward interaction with the environment.
   d. the person has a sense of meaningfulness.

8. Examples of the signs and symptoms exhibited by the patient experiencing stress include all *except*

a. anxiety.
b. forgetfulness.
c. decreased blood pressure.
d. impaired speech.

REFERENCES

1. Selye H: The stress concept: past, present, and future. In Cooper CL, editor: *Stress research: issues for the eighties,* New York, 1983, John Wiley & Sons.
2. Holmes T, Masuda M: Magnitude estimations of social readjustments, *J Psychosom Res* 11:219, 1966.
3. Holmes T, Rahe R: The social readjustment rating scale, *J Psychosom Res* 12:213, 1967.
4. Derogatis LR, Coons H: Self-report measures of stress. In Goldberger L, Breznitz S, editors: *Handbook of stress: theoretical and clinical aspects,* ed 2, New York, 1993, Free Press.
5. Lazarus R, Folkman S: *Stress, appraisal, and coping,* New York, 1984, Springer.
6. Selye H: *The stress of life,* New York, 1956, McGraw-Hill.
7. Calabrese JR, Wilde C: Alterations in immunocompetence during stress: a medical perspective. In Plotnikoff N and others, editors: *Stress and immunity,* Boca Raton, FL, 1991, CRC Press.
8. Lacey JI, Lacey BC: Verification and extension of the principle of autonomic response stereotype, *Am J Psychol* 71:50, 1958.
9. Holmes TH, Masuda M: Life change and illness susceptibility. In Dohrenwend BA, Dohrenwend BP, editors: *Stressful life events: their nature and effects,* New York, 1974, John Wiley & Sons.
10. Leventhal H, Tomarken A: Stress and illness: perspectives from health psychology. In Kasl SV, Cooper CL, editors: *Stress and health: issues in research methodology,* New York, 1978, John Wiley & Sons.
11. Kobasa SC: Stressful life events, personality, and health: an inquiry into hardiness, *J Pers Soc Psychol* 37:2, 1979.
12. Ouellette SC: Inquiries into hardiness. In Goldberger L, Breznitz S, editors: *Handbook of stress: theoretical and clinical aspects,* ed 2, New York, 1993, Free Press.
13. Antonovsky AA: *Unraveling the mystery of health: how people manage stress and stay well,* San Francisco, 1987, Jossey-Bass.
14. Williams SJ: The relationship among stress, hardiness, sense of coherence and illness in critical care nurses, *Medical Psychotherapy* 3:171, 1990.
15. Lazarus RS: Puzzles in the study of daily hassles, *J Behav Med* 7:376, 1984.
16. Kanner AD and others: Comparison of two modes of stress measurement: daily hassles and uplifts versus major life events, *J Behav Med* 4:1, 1981.
17. Lazarus RS, Launier R: Stress-related transactions between person and environment. In Pervin LA, Lewis M, editors: *Perspectives in international psychology,* New York, 1978, Plenum.
18. O'Leary A: Stress, emotion, and human function, *Psychol Bull* 108:363, 1990.
19. Herbert TB, Cohen S: Stress and immunity in humans, *Psychosom Med* 55:364, 1993.
20. Cohen S and others: Psychological stress and susceptibility to the common cold, *N Engl J Med* 325:606, 1991.
21. Spiegel D and others: Effect of psychosocial treatment on survival of patients with metastatic breast cancer, *Lancet* 2:881, 1989.
22. Holt RR: Occupational stress. In Goldberger L, Breznitz S, editors: *Handbook of stress: theoretical and clinical aspects,* ed 2, New York, 1993, Free Press.
23. Karasek R, Theorell T: *Health work: stress, productivity, and the reconstruction of working life,* New York, 1990, Basic Books.
24. Repetti RL: The effects of work load and the social environment at work on health. In Goldberger L, Breznitz S, editors: *Handbook of stress: theoretical and clinical aspects,* ed 2, New York, 1993, Free Press.
25. Pines AM: Burnout. In Goldberger L, Breznitz S, editors: *Handbook of stress: theoretical and clinical aspects,* ed 2, New York, 1993, Free Press.
26. Werner JS: Stressors and health outcomes: synthesis of nursing research, 1980-1990. In Barnfather JS, Lyon BL, editors: *Stress and coping: State of the science and implications for nursing theory, research, and practice,* Indianapolis, 1993, Sigma Theta Tau Center Press.
27. Volicer BJ: Perceived stress levels of events associated with the experience of hospitalization: development and testing of a measurement tool, *Nurs Res* 22:491, 1973.
28. Volicer BJ, Bohannon MW: A hospital stress rating scale, *Nurs Res* 24:352, 1975.
29. Van Servellen G, Lewis CE, Leake B: The stresses of hospitalization among AIDS patients on integrated and special care units, *Int J Nurs Stud* 27:235, 1990.
30. Jalowiec A: Revision and testing of the Jalowiec Coping Scale. Proceedings of the thirteenth annual conference of the Midwest Nursing Research Society 13:150, 1989.
31. Moos RH, Schaefer J: Coping resources and processes: current concepts and measures. In Goldberger L, Breznitz S, editors: *Handbook of stress: theoretical and clinical aspects,* ed 2, New York, 1993, Free Press.
32. Taylor SE, Aspinwall L: Coping with chronic illness. In Goldberger L, Breznitz S, editors: *Handbook of stress: theoretical and clinical aspects,* ed 2, New York, 1993, Free Press.
33. Mishel MH, Sorenson D: Revision of the ways of coping checklist for a clinical population, *West J Nurs Res* 15:59, 1993.
34. Halm MA and others: Behavioral responses of family members during critical illness, *Clin Nurs Res* 2:414, 1993.
35. Carpenito LJ: *Nursing diagnosis: application to clinical practice,* ed 6, Philadelphia, 1995, Lippincott.
36. Wallston KA: Assessment of control in health care settings. In Steptoe A, Appels A, editors: *Stress, personal control, and health,* New York, 1989, John Wiley & Sons.

Chapter 6

NURSING ASSESSMENT AND ROLE IN MANAGEMENT

Pain

Diana J. Wilkie   Barbara J. Boss

Learning Objectives

1. Describe the basic neural mechanisms of acute pain.
2. Describe the mechanisms of pain modulation.
3. Differentiate among the different types of pain.
4. Describe individual factors that affect the pain experience.
5. Describe subjective and objective data that should be obtained when a pain assessment is conducted.
6. Describe therapeutic pain management techniques.
7. Describe the nursing management of the patient experiencing pain.

Pain is a complex, multidimensional phenomenon. The understanding of this phenomenon is evolving as research is conducted by scientists from many disciplines, including nursing. Increased knowledge provides health care professionals with many strategies for pain management. In choosing the most effective strategy, it is important to approach the patient experiencing pain from a holistic perspective. This chapter summarizes current knowledge about pain and pain management to enable the nurse to collaborate with other health care professionals in the assessment and management of pain.

DEFINITIONS OF PAIN

Pain is defined as whatever the person experiencing the pain says it is, existing whenever the person says it does.[1] This clinical definition recognizes pain as a personal, private experience. Scientists at the International Association for the Study of Pain (IASP) have proposed another definition. This definition states that pain is an unpleasant sensory and emotional experience associated with actual or potential tissue damage, or it is described in terms of such damage.[2] It is important to note that both definitions indicate that pain is a subjective experience.

The first definition, however, does not allow the nurse to adequately distinguish between the statement "I have pain in my heart" made by a person who has just experienced the loss of a loved one and by a person who is experiencing angina related to cardiac disease. In both situations the nurse using the clinical definition would diagnose chest pain but would not be correct in providing pain medications to the first person without further assessment. Appropriate interventions for these two people should be quite different and based on further assessment. If the IASP definition of pain is used to guide practice, the nurse is less likely to provide inappropriate interventions to these two people. The nurse would investigate the patient's statement and would consider the potential for the stimulus to cause tissue damage. This consideration would stimulate further assessment to determine the cause of the problem and, from that information, appropriate therapy would be initiated.

In considering the IASP definition, it is also important to note that not all potentially tissue damaging (noxious) stimuli result in pain. For this reason, it is critical for the nurse to differentiate pain from nociception. *Nociception* is the activation of the primary afferent nerves with peripheral terminals (free nerve endings) that respond differently to noxious (tissue damaging) stimuli. Nociceptors function primarily to sense and transmit pain signals. Nociception may or may not be perceived as pain, depending on a complex interaction within the nociceptive pathways. If nociceptive stimuli are blocked, pain is not perceived.

Finally, it is important to distinguish pain or nociception from suffering. *Suffering* is the state of severe distress associated with events that threaten the intactness of the person.[3] Suffering is an emotion. It is important to recognize that pain and suffering are not the same phenomenon. The person who complained of pain in the heart because of the death of a loved one is suffering rather than experiencing pain as it is defined by the IASP. It is clear that three conditions could exist where suffering occurs in the presence of pain, suffering occurs when pain is not present, and pain occurs when suffering is not present. For example, the woman awaiting breast biopsy may suffer because of anticipated loss of her breast. After the biopsy, she may have

Reviewed by Lora McGuire, RN, MS, Nursing Instructor, Joliet Junior College, Joliet, IL.

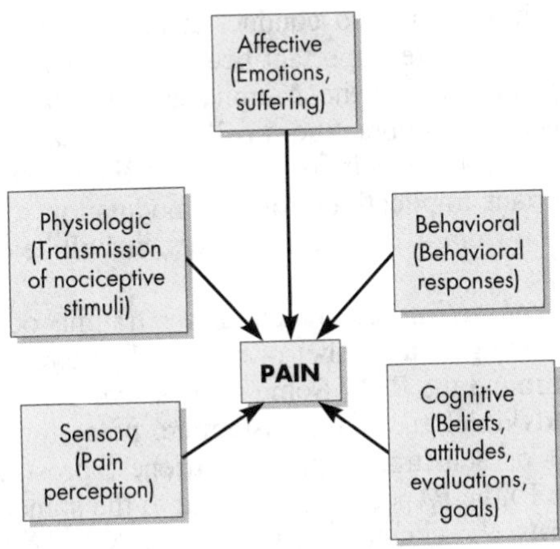

Fig. 6-1 The five components of pain.

pain without suffering if the biopsy is negative or pain with suffering if the biopsy is positive for malignancy. Interventions aimed at relieving pain and suffering may have some commonalities, but clearly some interventions for suffering will be inadequate for pain just as some interventions for pain are inadequate for suffering. Therefore, it is crucial to correctly diagnose alterations in comfort that are caused by pain and alterations in comfort that result from suffering. It also is important to use the correct term when referring to pain and suffering and to not interchange them. Pain, not suffering, is the focus of this chapter.

MAGNITUDE OF THE PAIN PROBLEM

Pain is one of the most common reasons patients seek health care. Approximately 15% to 20% of all Americans annually have acute pain, about 25% to 30% have chronic pain,[4] and 40% to 80% of the 1,200,000 Americans with cancer have pain.[5] A significant number of people with pain are disabled by their pain, resulting in a serious economic problem in society as well as a major health problem. Adding to the problems of patients with acute pain, especially cancer pain, is a tendency for physicians to prescribe small, insufficient doses of analgesics to control the pain. Also, nurses tend to routinely administer the smallest prescribed dose when a range of doses is prescribed.[6] Such practices do little to provide relief from unremitting pain.

DIMENSIONS OF PAIN

As a multidimensional phenomenon, pain consists of five components: **a**ffective, **b**ehavioral, **c**ognitive, **s**ensory, and **p**hysiologic[7] (Fig. 6-1). For simplicity, these components have been described as the ABCs of pain.[8] The emotions related to the pain (***a**ffective component*), the behavioral responses to the pain (***b**ehavioral component*), and the beliefs, attitudes, evaluations, and goals about the pain (***c**ognitive component*) control how pain is perceived (***s**ensory component*) by altering transmission of nociceptive stimuli to the brain (***p**hysiologic component*). Therefore each dimension is important in the assessment and management of pain. Pain results from complex interactions among these dimensions and can be understood by considering first

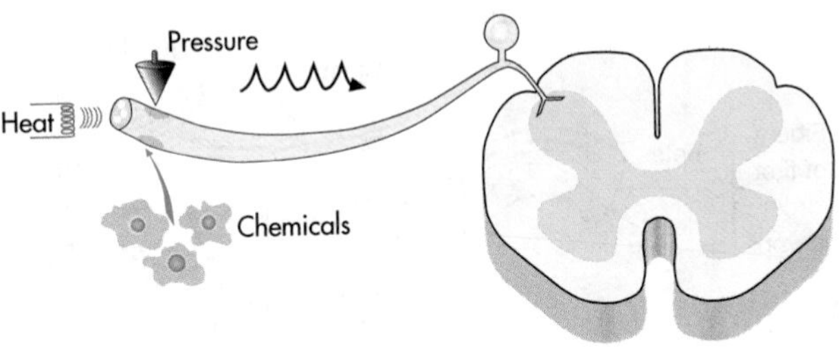

Fig. 6-2 Peripheral terminals are sensitive to direct heat, mechanical pressure, and chemicals released in response to tissue damage.

the physiologic and then the sensory, affective, behavioral, and cognitive dimensions.

Physiologic Dimension of Pain*

Understanding the physiologic dimension of pain requires knowledge of neural anatomy and physiology. Neural mechanisms by which pain is perceived involve a process. This pain process is composed of four major steps: transduction, transmission, perception, and modulation. Transduction and transmission involve processing nociceptive stimuli, and, depending on the amount of modulation occurring, a nociceptive stimuli may or may not be perceived as pain. If there is no perception of nociception, there is no pain. Perception and modulation are crucial to the sensation of pain.

Transduction. The first step of the pain process is transduction. *Transduction* is conversion of a mechanic, thermal, or chemical stimulus into a neuronal action potential[9] (Fig. 6-2). Peripheral nerve fibers are stimulated by noxious pressure, heat, or chemical forces. These forces trigger an action potential causing the nerve fiber to become activated. The noxious impulse is transmitted to the central nervous system (CNS). It is easily understood how pressure or heat that is great enough to injure tissue can activate nerve fibers. It may be less clear, however, how chemicals influence generation of an action potential. Therefore chemical transduction will be described.

Types of peripheral nerve fibers. In understanding transduction of chemical nociceptive stimuli, it is helpful to consider the environment around the peripheral nerve fiber. Each nerve fiber is surrounded by its own microenvironment. Peripheral nerve fibers, which conduct nociceptive signals, commonly are called bare nerve endings or free nerve endings. More specifically, these nerve fibers are *A-delta* and *C fibers* and are known as *primary afferent nociceptors* (PANs).[10] These fibers extend through the dorsal root ganglia along with the A-alpha (sensory muscle), A-beta (sensory skin), and sympathetic afferent fibers, into the dorsal horn of the spinal cord where various connections are made (Fig. 6-3). The A-alpha and A-beta fibers transmit the sensation of light pressure to deep muscles, soft touch to skin, and vibration. A-delta fibers are

*Parts of this section are copyrighted material by DJ Wilkie, 1994.

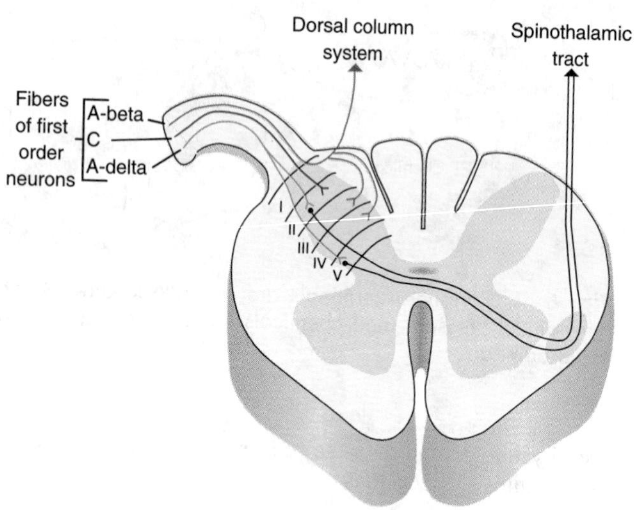

Fig. 6-3 Dorsal root nociceptive afferents.

particularly sensitive to sharp, pointed stimulation. This type of pain is typically well localized and of relatively short duration. C fibers are associated with dull, aching, or burning sensations. This pain is characterized by its diffuse nature, slow onset, and relatively long duration.

Figure 6-3 shows that A-beta fibers also make connections (synapses) in the spinal dorsal horn close to synapses of the A-delta and C fibers. This dorsal horn connection means that input from touch fibers can enter the spinal cord and synapse or communicate with cells carrying nociceptive input, a fact important to nonpharmacologic management of pain, as will be discussed later.

Different fibers have different characteristics (Table 6-1). A-alpha and A-beta fibers are large and enclosed by myelin sheaths. Because of the myelin sheath and axon size, A-alpha and A-beta fibers conduct at a rapid rate. A-delta fibers are smaller fibers also with myelin sheaths. Because of their smaller size, A-delta fibers conduct at a slower rate than the larger A-alpha and A-beta fibers. C fibers, in comparison, are the smallest fibers and are unmyelinated. C fibers occur singly or in clusters and conduct at the slowest rate. The conduction rates are important because information carried to the spinal cord by the A-alpha and A-beta fibers will communicate with dorsal horn cells sooner than will information carried by A-delta or C fibers. This conduction rate has important implications for the modulation of noxious information from A-delta and C fibers, as will be discussed later.

Table 6-1 Characteristics of Peripheral Nerve Fibers

Type of Fiber	Size	Myelinization	Conduction Velocity*
A-alpha	Large	Myelinated	Rapid
A-beta	Large	Myelinated	Rapid
A-delta	Small	Myelinated	Medium
C	Smallest	Not myelinated	Slow

*The conduction rates are important because information carried to the spinal cord by the larger, myelinated nerve fibers will communicate with dorsal horn cells sooner than will information carried by the smaller, unmyelinated fibers.

Chemical activation. When tissue trauma occurs and cells are damaged, a number of chemicals are released into the area around the PAN. Some of these chemicals activate (e.g., bradykinin, serotonin, histamine, potassium, norepinephrine) or sensitize (e.g., leukotrienes, prostaglandins, substance P) the PAN to send a signal to the spinal cord. In other words, the chemicals cause the PAN to be excitable and fire an action potential toward the spinal cord. Several details are helpful in fully understanding this process.

When cells are damaged, phospholipids are liberated and can be converted to arachidonic acid, which is then oxidized by two different pathways. The lipoxygenase pathway leads to the production of leukotrienes. The cyclooxygenase pathway leads to the production of prostaglandins (Fig. 6-4). Leukotrienes and prostaglandins sensitize the PAN to be activated by a smaller stimulus than when these chemicals are not present near the PAN. For example, light pressure is not perceived as painful in normal conditions, but sometimes is considered painful if leukotrienes or prostaglandins are present near the PAN.

Therefore, blocking leukotriene and prostaglandin synthesis can improve pain management when tissue damage is

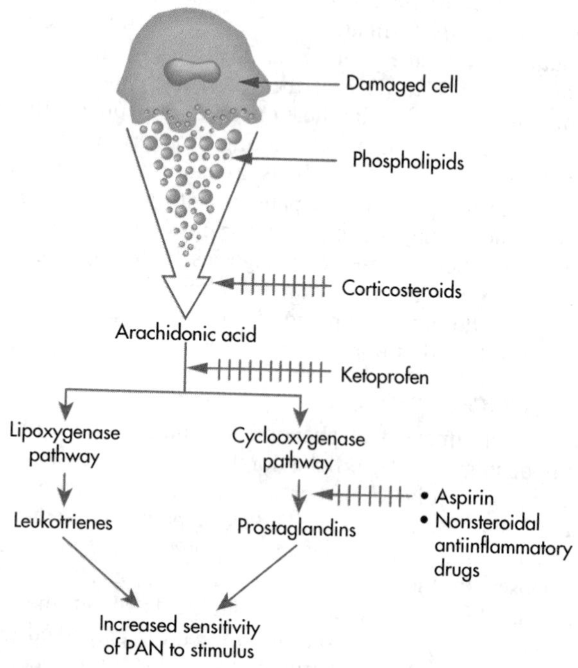

Fig. 6-4 Schematic representation of two pathways that lead to the production of chemicals that cause the peripheral afferent nociceptors (PAN) to be more easily excited. Drugs that block the synthesis of these chemicals are also shown.

known or suspected. For example, a specific inhibitor of leukotrienes is not yet approved for clinical use, but ketoprophen, a nonsteroidal antiinflammatory drug (NSAID), appears to have some effect in blocking leukotriene synthesis.[11,12] Aspirin and other NSAIDs block prostaglandin synthesis, and most interfere with platelet aggregation. Corticosteroids act earlier in the cascade by preventing the production of arachidonic acid, effectively inhibiting the synthesis of both leukotrienes and prostaglandins. When these drugs are present in a condition of tissue damage, a larger stimulus is required to produce transduction of the PAN than when these drugs are not present.

When cells are injured, many other chemicals leak out of the cell or are released into the intracellular space as part of the inflammatory response. These chemicals also activate the PAN. For example, potassium and histamine exude from damaged cells, and bradykinin is produced from the activation of the clotting system.[13] Other chemicals are released from platelets (e.g., serotonin) or mast cells (e.g., histamine). The presence of any one of these chemicals near the PAN will cause the PAN to be activated (transduced) to fire an action potential. These chemicals also act in combination to sensitize the PAN, enabling it to fire with a lower stimulus than usual. Few drugs inhibit the excitatory actions of these chemicals; antihistamine drugs are the exception. Anthihistamines interfere with the excitatory action of histamine by blocking histamine receptors. Antihistamine drugs are usually considered adjuvant drugs in pain management.

If the PAN is activated and fires an action potential, the PAN itself releases chemicals, one of which is substance P. Substance P is stored in the distal terminals of the PAN and, when released, sensitizes the PAN, dilates nearby blood vessels with subsequent production of edema, and causes release of histamine from mast cells.[4]

Finally, activation of the autonomic nervous system (ANS) contributes to PAN transduction through release of norepinephrine and prostaglandins. Norepinephrine activates a PAN upon contact, if the PAN has been injured.[14] Therefore, emotional responses mediated by the ANS can increase pain through physiologic mechanisms.

Therapies to prevent transduction. A number of chemicals that are produced or released around the PAN can sensitize or activate it directly and indirectly through secondary processes. If any or all of these chemicals can be eliminated or inhibited, the PAN is transduced less often or a larger stimulus is needed to produce transduction. A number of nonopioid analgesics (e.g., acetaminophen, acetylsalicylic acid, NSAIDs) inhibit these chemicals. Drugs that block production or release of these chemicals can be powerful analgesics and are often the first drugs used in pain management.

People with pain often engage in behaviors that limit PAN transduction. For example, if a certain movement routinely produces pain, a person will avoid that movement. Guarding and immobilization of the injured body area are common methods of preventing pain onset.[15,16] One way a patient might guard against pain is to wear loose, unrestrictive clothing when light touch produces pain. Use of a foot cradle is another way to remove the pressure of a sheet or blanket when the weight causes pain. Use of a cane, walker, or back brace are examples of methods a person with a back injury might use to prevent PAN transduction. Immobilization through use of these devices prevents movement-induced vertebral flexion, a common source of pain in people with cancer or back injuries. However, pain control behaviors may have harmful effects. For example, long-term immobilization can increase the risk that the person will develop a pressure ulcer. Behavioral methods of pain control can supplement drugs that also prevent transduction.

Nonpharmacologic and pharmacologic methods of reducing ANS activation can be important analgesic methods. For example, reducing fear, anger, and anxiety through behavioral methods, theoretically, can reduce activation of the PAN. Anxiolytic agents also can reduce transduction of the PAN by reducing ANS activation.

Transmission. Once the PAN has been transduced, the neuronal action potential must be transmitted to and through the CNS before pain is perceived. Three steps are involved in nociceptive signal transmission: projection to the CNS, processing within the dorsal horn of the spinal cord, and transmission to the brain (i.e., through the brainstem and the thalamus to the cortex). Each step in the transmission process is important in pain perception.

Projection to the central nervous system. When the PAN terminal is transduced, the PAN membrane becomes depolarized, sodium enters the cell, and potassium exits the cell to generate an action potential. The action potential rapidly spreads along the neuron, more rapidly for myelinated than unmyelinated axons. The transmission of the action potential along the entire length of the neuron is necessary for the cell to deliver the nociceptive signal to cells in the spinal cord.

The action potential can be inhibited, however, if the ion channels are inactivated. Drugs known as membrane stabilizers inactivate the sodium channels and disrupt the transmission of the action potential along the PAN axon.[17] Some adjuvant drugs, such as local anesthetics (e.g., lidocaine, bupivacaine, tocainide, mexiletine) and anticonvulsant drugs (e.g., phenytoin, carbamazepine, clonazepam), prevent transmission via this type of mechanism. In diluted concentrations, local anesthetics are effective in blocking small fiber transmission without affecting nonpainful sensation or motor function. Larger concentrations of local anesthetics are required to block larger fibers.

It is important to understand that one nerve cell extends the entire distance from the periphery to the dorsal horn of the spinal cord with no synapses. For example, an afferent fiber from the great toe travels from the toe through the fifth lumbar nerve root into the spinal cord; this is one cell. Once generated, an action potential travels all the way to the spinal cord. The message conveyed in the action potential will be transmitted to the dorsal horn of the spinal cord unless it is blocked by a sodium channel inhibitor or disrupted by a lesion at the central terminal of the fiber (e.g., by a dorsal root entry zone [DREZ] lesion). For this reason, the importance of altering the PAN environment and sensitivity of the PAN at the distal end of the peripheral

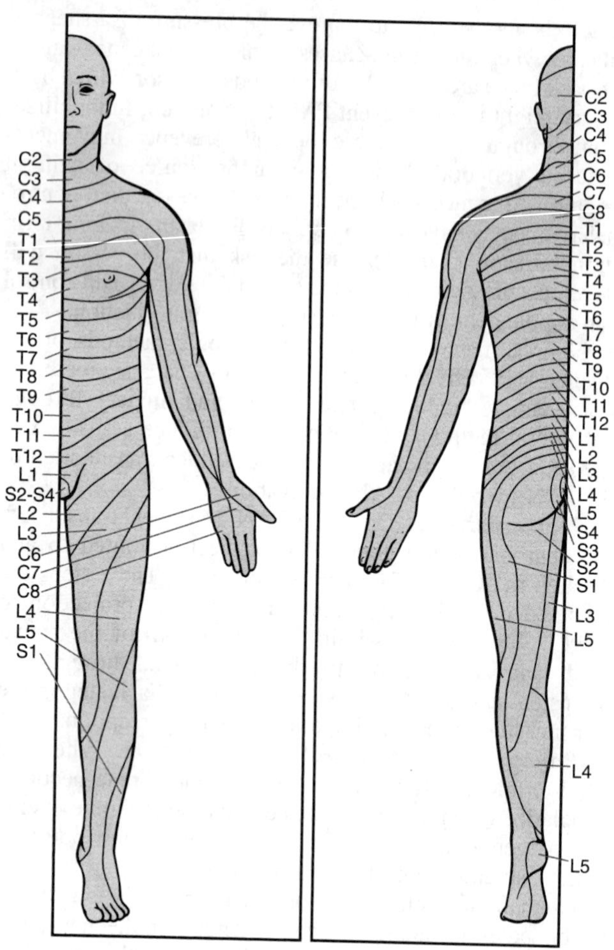

Fig. 6-5 Spinal dermatomes representing organized sensory input carried via specific spinal nerve roots. *C*, cervical; *L*, lumbar; *S*, sacral; *T*, thoracic.

fiber is a central issue; once the first nerve cell in the pain process has fired an action potential, the message will be transmitted to the spinal cord.

The A-alpha, A-beta, A-delta, and C fibers extend from the peripheral tissues through the dorsal root ganglia to the dorsal horn of the spinal cord (see Fig. 6-3). The manner in which nerve fibers enter the spinal cord is central to the notion of spinal dermatomes (Fig. 6-5). Each nerve root innervates a specific segment of the body, sometimes far removed from the area in which the nerve enters the spinal cord. Although fibers enter the spinal segment associated with the nerve root in which they travel to the spinal cord, the A-delta and C fibers send dendrites up toward the brain or downward for two to four spinal segments. Therefore, one fiber can communicate with as many as nine spinal segments. The innervation expanse is important when transcutaneous electrical nerve stimulators (TENS) are used to block transmission of nociceptive stimuli. If, in positioning TENS electrodes, the full range of spinal segments innervated by a single nerve cell is not considered, pain may not be blocked.

Dorsal horn processing. Once the nociceptive signal arrives in the CNS, it is processed within the dorsal horn of the spinal cord. This processing includes releasing neurotransmitters from the PAN into the synaptic cleft and binding neurotransmitters to receptors on nearby cell bodies and dendrites of cells that may be located elsewhere in the dorsal horn. Some of these PAN neurotransmitters produce activation when bound to receptors whereas others inhibit activation of nearby cells. Cells excited by PAN input release other neurotransmitters, which increases the complexity of the neurochemical communication occurring within the dorsal horn. The effects of the complex neurotransmitter release can facilitate or inhibit transmission of nociceptive stimuli.

The complex neurotransmitter release and binding involve several different types of cells located in the dorsal horn. Areas within the gray matter of the spinal cord are represented by laminae numbered I through X; the dorsal horn is represented by laminae I to V. Cells that receive nociceptive input are located in lamina I (projection cells), lamina II (some projection cells and interneurons), and lamina V (wide dynamic range neurons, most of which are projection cells). All of the cells are important to propagation of the nociceptive signal from the spinal cord to the brain.

Most *projection cells* send axons to the brain on the opposite side of the body. They receive excitatory and inhibitory messages, the net sum of which determines whether the PAN message will be transmitted to the brain.

Interneurons can be either excitatory or inhibitory. They communicate with other lamina II cells, located within one or two spinal segments, and with dendrites from cells located in laminae I, III, IV, and V. The concept of excitatory and inhibitory interneurons is important because it helps to explain why some nonpharmacologic therapies are effective. Although the exact mechanisms have not been determined, it is known that stimulation of large sensory fibers (A-beta) can have an inhibitory effect on cells that project nociceptive signals to the brain. TENS and massage are examples of methods by which rapidly conducting large fibers can be activated. Application of heat or cold are examples of methods by which smaller, less rapidly conducting fibers can be activated by nonnoxious stimuli. All of these methods are known to inhibit transmission of nociceptive stimuli. A person with pain, or a family member of a person with pain, will engage in activities (rubbing, massaging, applying heat or cold) that are known to activate large or small fibers for the purpose of reducing pain intensity. Additionally, TENS has been effective in the treatment of pain via similar mechanisms.[18]

Wide dynamic range (WDR) neurons receive input from noxious stimuli primarily carried by A-delta and C fiber afferents (especially from viscera), nonnoxious stimuli from A-beta fibers, and indirect input from dendritic projections into laminae I, II, III, and IV.[10] Most lamina V neurons project to the brainstem and to the thalamus.

Discovery that WDR neurons receive input from noxious as well as innocuous stimuli from distant areas provides a neural explanation for *referred pain.* Input from nociceptive fibers and A-beta fibers converge on the WDR neuron, and, when the message is transmitted to the brain, the originating location is poorly localized. Pain is therefore perceived in the body part presumably innervated by the

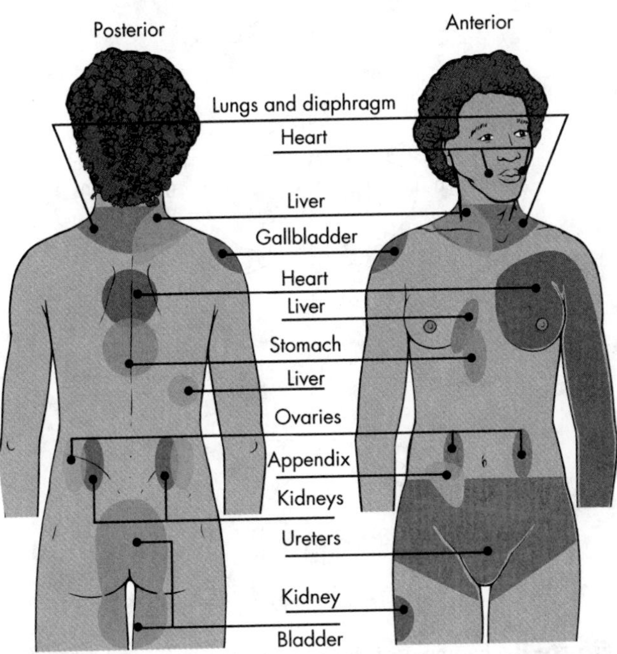

Fig. 6-6 Typical areas of referred pain.

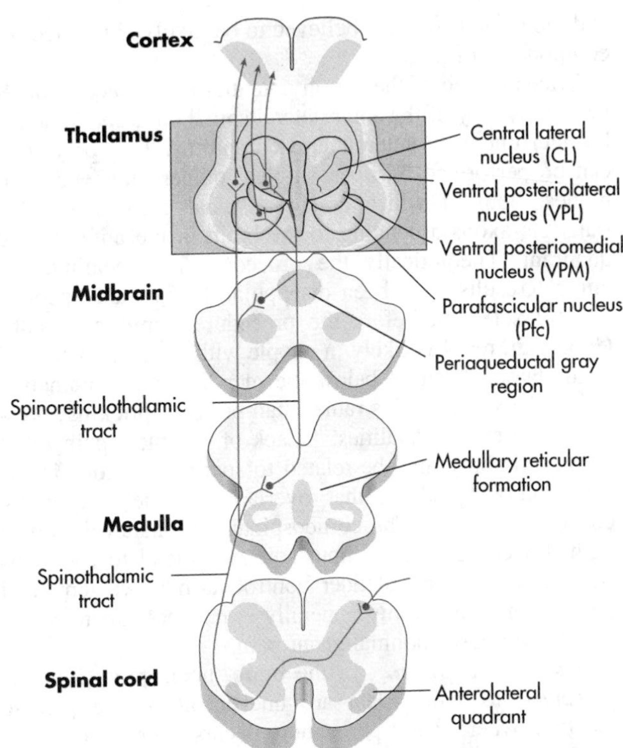

Fig. 6-7 Nociceptive pathways and synaptic connections of selected pain pathways.

A-beta fiber rather than from the visceral A-delta or C fibers. The concept of referred pain must be considered when interpreting the location of pain reported by the person with injury to or disease involving visceral organs. The location of the tumor may be quite distant from the pain location reported by the patient (Fig. 6-6). For example, pain from liver disease is located in the right upper abdominal quadrant, but it frequently is referred to the anterior and posterior neck region and to a posterior flank area. If referred pain is not considered when evaluating a pain location report, therapy could be misdirected.

An important concept related to neural mechanisms of pain is *neural plasticity*.[19] Repetitive transmission of PAN nociceptive signals to the dorsal horn results in several changes in dorsal horn processing, including enlargement of the receptive field of a peripheral neuron, activation of receptors normally inactive, 'wind-up' with a progressively increased response to noxious stimuli, and allodynia (pain evoked by light tactile stimulation).[13,19,20]

N-methyl-D-aspartate (NMDA) and non–NMDA receptors have been implicated in the changes observed in dorsal horn processing.[19] The NMDA receptors are enabled once the neuron has been depolarized. Along with subsequent changes in calcium channel conduction, they produce profound alterations in neural processing of afferent stimuli that can persist for long periods of time. For this reason, an important goal of therapy is to prevent pain and avoid adverse neural plasticity. Although research is being conducted to develop NMDA antagonist drugs for clinical use, the only NMDA antagonist currently available is ketamine, a drug occasionally used in anesthesia.

Pain Pathways

Transmission to the brain. With adequate summation (net excitatory effects) on projection cells, nociceptive stimuli are communicated to the third-order neuron, primarily in the thalamus and several other areas of the brain. Fibers of dorsal horn projection cells enter the brain through several pathways, including the (1) spinothalamic tract (STT), (2) spinoreticular tract (SRT), (3) spinomesencephalic tract (SMT), (4) spinocervical tract, (5) second-order dorsal column tract (SDCT), and (6) spinohypothalamic tract.[4] The anterolateral quadrant of the spinal white matter contains all but the SDCT, which traverses in the dorsal column pathway.[20] The nociceptive pathways and synaptic connections of each of these pathways are summarized in Fig. 6-7.

Generally, the STT and SRT are the best understood pathways. The STT segregates into medial and lateral branches near the thalamus with the medial branch terminating in the medial thalamus and the lateral branch terminating in the lateral thalamus (see Fig. 6-7). The lateral branch is also known as the neospinothalamic pathway, and the medial branch is also known as the paleospinothalamic pathway or the paramedian pathway. The paleospinothalamic pathway also sends a collateral to the reticular formation and appears functionally similar to the SRT.[20]

Each of four distinct thalamic nuclei, which receive nociceptive input from the spinal cord, has distinct projections to the cerebral cortex (see Fig. 6-7).[4] The primary somatosensory cortex has neurons responding selectively to nociceptive input. Additionally, the frontal cortex is known to receive projections from the central lateral and submedial thalamic nuclei.[20] The somatosensory cortex is believed to be important for interpretation of sensory aspects of pain, and the frontal cortex is believed to be involved in affective components of pain.

Transmission of the action potential in the second-order neuron by way of the anterolateral spinal cord quadrant can be interrupted by anterolateral cordotomy. This procedure can be performed by open surgical or percutaneous techniques, both of which create a spinal cord lesion that transects axons ascending to the brain in the anterolateral quadrant. Theoretically the procedure is appealing, but clinical results have been disappointing for many people. Careful selection before the procedure improves results. Good pain relief is likely in people with pain characterized by unilateral location below the mandible and lancinating (or toothache) qualities rather than burning, pricking, pressure, or crawling qualities.[20] Lack of complete pain relief with cordotomy may be related to sparing of axons in the anterolateral quadrant that overlap into the descending corticospinal tract. The corticospinal neurons are involved with descending motor input and are crucial to functions such as bowel and bladder control, arm movement, and ambulation. Cordotomy generally is not recommended for people who have nonmalignant pain.

Pain Perception. In the brain, nociceptive input is perceived as pain. Data are unclear as to the precise location where pain perception occurs. Perception may occur in the thalamus or in the cerebrum. Recent evidence implicates the posterior sector of the anterior cingulate cortex in pain perception.[21] It is known that the brain is necessary for pain perception; hence no brain, no pain. Until it is understood clearly where pain is perceived, prudent nursing practice involves treatment of any noxious stimulus as potentially painful, even in the comatose person who does not respond to noxious stimuli. Lack of a behavioral response to a noxious stimulus does *not* indicate that the person lacks pain perception. It is crucial for the nurse to provide pain therapies to the person with any nociceptive input, even though the person cannot report pain perception or show behaviors indicative of pain.

Modulation. Transmission of nociceptive stimuli and pain perception can be changed by descending (efferent) modulatory mechanisms (Fig. 6-8). Modulation may include both inhibition as well as enhancement of nociceptive stimuli.[22] The firing pattern of specific cells in the rostral ventral medulla may be associated with the inhibition of nociception, but other cells may permit transmission of the nociceptive information.[22] Enhancement of nociceptor transduction has been described in previous sections.

Several centers, including the periventricular and periaqueductal gray, rostral ventral medulla, and spinal cord are involved in generating analgesia or inhibition of nociceptive stimuli.[22] Afferent input to the descending pain modulating system is less well known, but certainly hypothalamic and amygdala inputs are involved as is possibly the frontal cortex.

Descending inhibition of pain occurs through a complex circuit involving a number of receptor systems, such as mu, delta, and kappa opioid; $alpha_2$ adrenergic; serotonin (5-hydroxytryptamine); adenosine; gamma aminobutyric acid (GABA); neuropeptide Y; calcitonin; somatostatin; and neurotensin receptors.[13] Although serotonin, $alpha_2$ agonists, and opioids are known to inhibit nociceptive cells in the spinal dorsal horn, the role of the neurochemicals in each of the CNS pain modulation areas is not fully known.

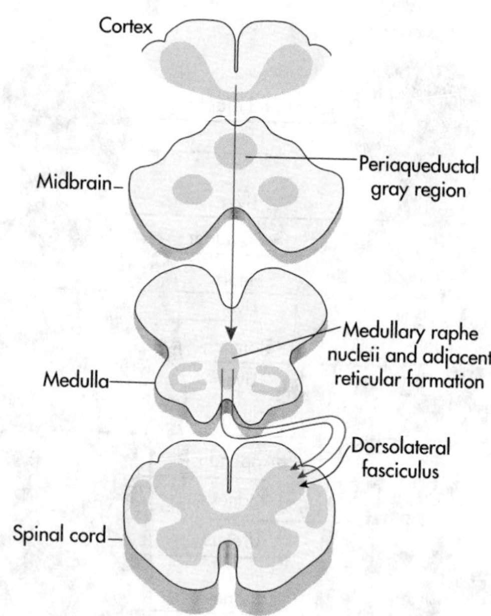

Fig. 6-8 Example of the descending pain-modulation system at receptors in the dorsal horn of the spinal cord.

Figure 6-9 provides a summary of the descending inhibitory mechanisms. Once nociceptive information is perceived as pain, inhibition can occur at any of the synapses in the ascending pathways. A well studied and important inhibitory synapse is in the spinal dorsal horn. For example, serotonin, norepinephrine, and enkephalin are released by descending fibers and inhibit release of neurotransmitters, thereby diminishing excitation of projection cells. The inhibitory neurotransmitters successfully prevent the PAN from communicating its information about the nociceptive stimuli to the second-order neuron, and pain is blocked even though the PAN has been transduced and has transmitted an action potential to the spinal cord. If the PAN action potential does not result in release of sufficient neurotransmitters to communicate the signal to the projection cell, pain is blocked.

Mimicking or Enhancing Modulation

Many drug and nondrug therapies provide pain relief through actions involving the descending pain inhibition mechanisms. Opioids, tricyclic antidepressants, $alpha_2$ agonists, placebos, counterirritation, hypnosis, imagery, and distraction act as mechanisms to mimic or enhance descending inhibitory systems. When these therapies are combined with methods that influence PAN transduction and transmission, impressive analgesia can be obtained (Fig. 6-10).

Opioids mimic the descending inhibitory system by binding to endogenous endorphin receptors (mu, delta, kappa) in the brain, brainstem, and spinal cord. Opioids act by hyperpolarizing the cell membrane and thereby inhibiting

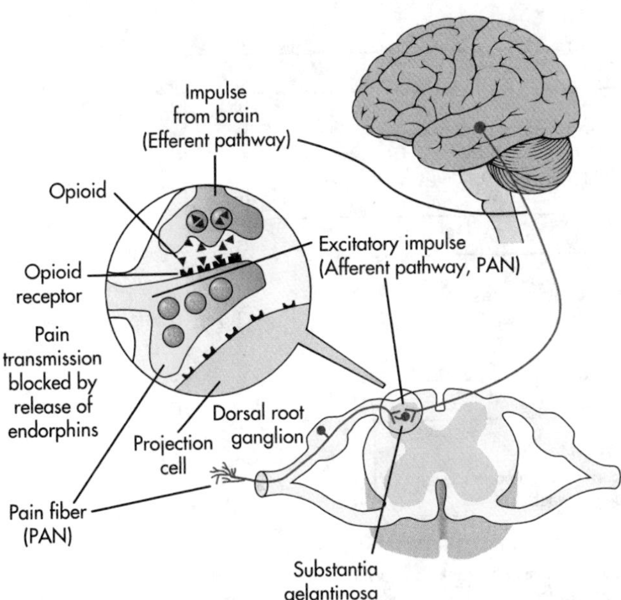

Fig. 6-9 Descending pathway and endorphin response. The biologic receptors of the enkephalins and endorphins are located close to pain receptors in the peripheral primary afferent nociceptor (PAN), ascending, and descending pain pathways.

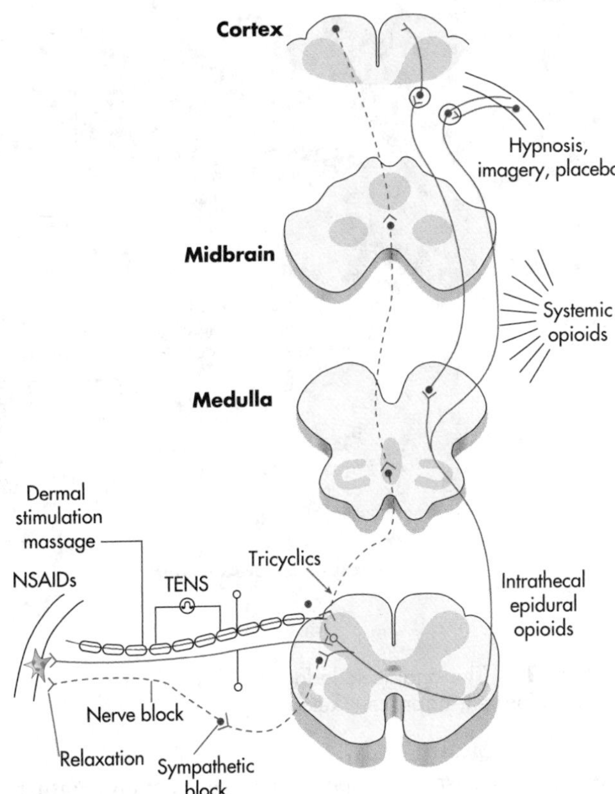

Fig. 6-10 The sites of commonly used pharmacologic and nonpharmacologic analgesic therapies. *NSAIDs,* Nonsteroidal antiinflammatory drugs; *TENS,* transcutaneous electrical nerve stimulation.

generation of an action potential.[13] Opioids effectively inhibit A-delta and C fibers, but are less effective in the wind-up state described previously. Administered intrathecally in small volumes, opioids exert powerful analgesic action at spinal cord synapses with limited rostral spread. In contrast, opioids delivered by the epidural route exert action not only at spinal cord sites, but also brain sites because a substantial portion of the dose is absorbed by epidural blood vessels. Opioids administered systemically (oral, transdermal, rectal, vaginal, subcutaneous, intramuscular, or intravenous) cross the blood-brain barrier, enter the cerebrospinal fluid, and bind to opioid receptors throughout the brain and the spinal cord. The effects, side effects, and doses of analgesics required to produce analgesia differ based on the route of administration. This is due, in part, to the fact that opioid-receptor access varies by administration route.

In comparison to opioids, tricyclic antidepressant drugs enhance the descending pain inhibitory system by preventing cellular re-uptake of serotonin and norepinephrine. These neurotransmitters typically are released from the cell and are rapidly taken back up by the cell or stored for re-release.[20] Rapid re-uptake limits the time serotonin and norepinephrine are available for receptor binding and inhibits transmission of nociceptive signals. Tricyclic antidepressants, which have moderate serotonin effects and weak to potent norepinephrine effects, are classified as adjuvant analgesics according to the World Health Organization (WHO) Analgesic Ladder (Fig. 6-11).

Alpha$_2$ adrenergic agonists (e.g., clonidine), calcitonin, somatostatin, and baclofen are other agents known to provide analgesia. The exact location where these agents act is known for some drugs but not others. Although not specifically mentioned by the WHO, these agents could be classified as adjuvant drugs.

The exact mechanisms by which some nonpharmacologic therapies exert analgesia is not known. It has been demonstrated, however, that *placebo response* probably is mediated by endogenous opioid systems. The placebo somehow causes the individual to mobilize endogenous opioids. Placebo response can be reversed by naloxone (Narcan), indicating that its mechanism involves endogenous opioid systems.[23] It is possible that other nonpharmacologic therapies, such as counterirritation, hypnosis, imagery, and distraction also act via endogenous opioid or possibly nonopioid inhibitory systems.

Affective, Behavioral, and Cognitive Dimensions of Pain

Because of the complex neural mechanisms of nociceptive processing, pain is perceived as a multidimensional sensory and affective experience to which there are cognitive and behavioral responses. The sensory component is the recognition of the sensation as painful. Sensory-pain elements include *location*, *intensity*, *quality*, and *pattern*. Persons with pain easily report these four sensory-pain elements. Based on knowledge about the pain process, information about these elements provided by the person with the pain

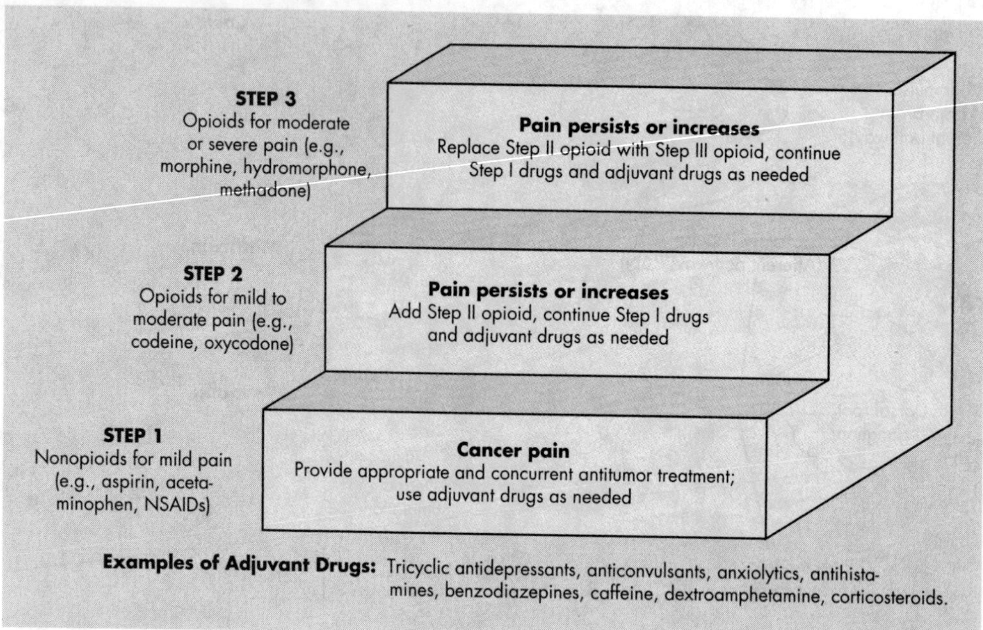

Fig. 6-11 The analgesic ladder proposed by the World Health Organization. *NSAIDs,* Nonsteroidal antiinflammatory drugs (e.g., ibuprofen, naproxen, ketorolac).

can be indispensable to appropriate pain therapy. Furthermore, the person with pain is the most appropriate expert on the effectiveness of prescribed therapy to modulate the pain process and block pain perception.

Sensory pain is affected not only by activation of nociceptors but also by affective, behavioral, and cognitive components of the pain. Pain is a subjective experience that varies from person to person.

The *affective component* of pain refers to the feelings and emotions that affect the experience of pain. A patient with unrelieved pain often has concurrent emotional responses, such as anger, fear, depression, and anxiety, that can increase ANS release of norepinephrine and thereby intensify the pain sensation. In addition, simultaneous emotions such as joy may decrease the amount of pain perceived by persons with pain. Evaluation of emotions that activate or control ANS discharge can help to determine the amount of suffering experienced by patients. This is important because suffering is treated differently than pain. For example, opioids are not effective for suffering but can be the treatment of choice for pain. Antidepressant and antianxiety drugs, as well as active listening and relaxation techniques, may be useful in the treatment of suffering.

The *behavioral component* of pain refers to the actions and posturing of a patient to express the pain or to control the pain. Pain control behaviors are those that reduce pain, prevent pain onset, reduce pain duration, and help the patient to tolerate the pain. For example, watching television or talking with friends, staff, or family members helps to distract patients from the pain and can be effective in helping to control pain.[15,16] How the patient complies with or adjusts analgesic therapy plans is also an important aspect of the patient's pain behavior. Pain may interfere with usual behaviors that bring the patient joy and satisfaction. Inability to perform activities because of pain has been associated with increased negative emotions, such as anxiety.[15]

Table 6-2 Important Sensory Pain Components

Location	Place on the body where pain is felt
Intensity	Amount of pain felt
Quality	How the pain feels to the patient
Pattern	When it starts, how long it lasts

The *cognitive component* of pain refers to the meanings, beliefs, attitudes, past experiences, and expectations about the illness or disease (e.g., cancer) and about the pain that influence the patient's response to pain therapy. A patient's goal for and expectations about pain relief and treatment outcomes are crucial to understanding cognitive aspects of pain. Goals of treatment, however, must be realistic and attainable given the patient, health care providers, and environment. Determining the optimal goal (usually 0 pain) as well as the goal with which the patient will be satisfied (usually 1 to 4 on a 0 to 10 scale) helps to evaluate progress toward pain relief. Level of consciousness (sedation level), dementia, memory of past pain, source of motivation (internal versus external locus of control), and cognitive resources to cope with the pain can dramatically influence the pain the person experiences.

Summary of Pain Process. The pain process includes neural mechanisms related to transduction, transmis-

RESEARCH

Implications for Nursing Practice

PERCEIVED CONTROL OVER PAIN IN THE PATIENT WITH CHRONIC NONMALIGNANT PAIN

Citation Wells N: Perceived control over pain: relation to stress and disability, *Res Nurs Health* 17:295-302, 1994.

Purpose To examine the relationship between perceived control and distress and disability in the patient with chronic pain.

Methods Descriptive study using patients (n = 71) with chronic nonmalignant pain. Global and situational beliefs about control over pain and outcome measures of distress and disability were measured at initial evaluations. Daily pain ratings were recorded over a one-week period.

Results and Conclusions After controlling for pain intensity, the control belief subscales explained a significant amount of variance in distress and disability. These findings provide support for cognitive modulation of the distress and disability associated with chronic nonmalignant pain.

Implications for Nursing Practice Knowledge of the specific control beliefs that a patient holds can guide the types of interventions that are used. Use of this knowledge could help the nurse plan a patient-specific, focused treatment package based on the individual's situation and control beliefs.

sion, perception, and modulation (Fig. 6-12). These mechanisms represent complex, not fully understood systems, but begin to explain the tremendous variability in pain reported by persons experiencing similar degrees of tissue damage. The idea for these mechanisms was previously described in 1965 by the Gate Control Theory of pain, which emphasizes that the outcome of activation of nociceptive receptors is not totally predictable. The amount of pain perceived by a patient may vary tremendously depending on the context of the situation. The context of the situation may include other physiologic, sensory, affective, cognitive, or behavioral variables, the effects of which cannot be physiologically measured today.

Gerontologic Considerations

The effects of aging on the pain process may be confounded in an older adult who has a chronic illness that affects the nervous system. An older person who is well instructed in use of pain measurement tools and without diseases (e.g., diabetes) affecting the nervous system tends to report pain intensity similar to a younger person.[24] In the presence of decreased sensation associated with peripheral nerve disease (e.g., diabetic neuropathy), however, an elderly person is not likely to sense pain. Older age is associated with chronic health problems, increased risk for musculoskeletal pain, depression, and limitations in activities of daily living. Increased pain intensity has been noted in older individuals, particularly when adequate treatment is not provided for chronic and recurrent pain. Treatment of pain in the older adult is as likely to be successful as that for a younger person.[24]

A condition that would produce acute pain in some younger people may remain virtually undetected in some older people until complications occur. For example, an older person experiencing a myocardial infarction may complain of excess gas, an upset stomach, or extreme fatigue rather than the crushing chest pain identified by a younger adult. In this situation, the complication of congestive heart failure may be the first indicator of the older individual's primary problem. It is important to recognize, however, that pain is the most frequent presenting symptom of acute myocardial infarction in both older and younger patients. The frequency of silent myocardial infarctions in older adults has been overestimated.[24]

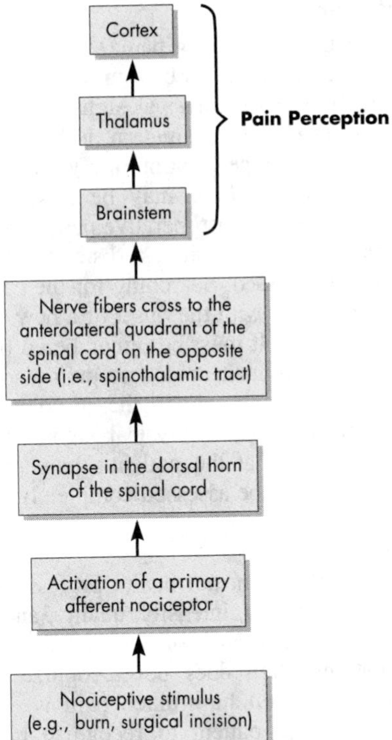

Fig. 6-12 Mechanism of acute pain.

ASSESSMENT OF PAIN

The goals of pain assessment are to identify the etiology of the pain; to understand the patient's sensory, affective, behavioral, and cognitive pain experience for the purpose of implementing pain management techniques; and to identify the patient's goal for therapy and resources for self-management of the pain. Often it is the nurse who is responsible for gathering and documenting assessment data.

Etiology of Pain

When a patient is experiencing pain, the cause of the pain should be sought so that it can be removed if possible. The nurse should observe for physical signs of the source of pain, including trauma, inflammation, ischemia, distention (especially of a viscus), perforation of a viscus, and muscle spasm. In many cases there may be a secondary pain source. For example, the postoperative patient may have, in addition to the surgical incision, a distended bladder that needs to be decompressed. Searching for the cause of pain is especially important with the onset of a new or recurrent episode of acute pain. It must be remembered that persons with chronic nonmalignant or cancer pain also may have related or unrelated acute pain. If the etiology of the pain cannot be determined from physical signs or diagnostic tests, it is important that the patient's pain report is not dismissed. Pain should be assessed completely and treated.

Pain Expert

The person with the pain, not health professionals, is the expert about the location, intensity, quality, and pattern of the pain as well as the degree of pain relief obtained from therapy. A patient often does not recognize that health professionals cannot tell how much pain is experienced. The nurse assists the patient to recognize his expertise about the pain and that, when the expertise is shared in partnership with health professionals, better pain management can be obtained. Empowering the patient to be an active partner in reporting information about the pain is an important nursing therapy.

A patient with pain does not always know *how* to report the pain to health professionals. The nurse has an important role in helping the patient by conducting nursing pain assessments.

Type of Pain. Persons from different racial or cultural backgrounds are consistent about the level of stimulus that is perceived as painful; pain threshold does not vary in persons without tissue damage.[27] The amount of pain that is tolerated (pain tolerance) by a person, however, varies tremendously among different individuals, probably because of variability in pain modulation.[22] The etiology of the pain may dramatically influence the affective, behavioral, and cognitive responses, and therefore the pain experience.

Types of pain experienced by patients include acute, chronic nonmalignant, or malignant pain. *Acute pain* occurs abruptly after an injury or disease, persists until healing occurs, and often is intensified by anxiety or fear. Acute pain consistently increases during wound care, ambulation, coughing, and deep breathing. If acute pain is not effectively managed, it may progress to a chronic state.

Chronic pain lasts for a prolonged period of time, and its cause is not amenable to specific treatment.[2] It is associated with prolonged tissue pathology or pain that persists beyond the normal healing period for an acute injury or disease. There may be abnormalities in the peripheral nervous system or CNS that result in persistent pain long after the original injury has healed. Many times the abnormalities are not detectable with current diagnostic techniques. Depression, frustration, and fear related to chronic pain are not uncommon.

Malignant pain is a third type of pain with recurrent, acute pain episodes, persistent chronic pain, or both acute and persistent pain associated with a progressive malignant-type process. The etiology of malignant pain is resistant to cure, and the pain may be described as intractable. The patient with malignant pain often describes it as all-consuming and interfering with mood, family relationships, and quality of life. Examples of causes of malignant pain are arthritis or cancer. A patient may have one pain type or combinations of the pain types.[5]

Assessment Process

The nature of pain is efficiently assessed by a three-step process.[8] The steps provide a method by which to triage the information collected based on the patient's condition and ability to share his expertise about the pain.

The *first step* is to assess the sensory components of pain. In critical situations such as in the emergency department, postanesthesia recovery room, critical care unit, or other critical care areas, each patient should be questioned about pain location and intensity. Vital signs and gross body activities often are used to assess pain. However, changes in these indicators are difficult to attribute specifically to the pain or pain therapy because of the number of therapies used in critical situations. Vital signs used in isolation are unreliable indicators of the amount of pain experienced by a patient.[25] Abnormally high values may be an indicator of increased pain, but normal or low values may also be present when a patient has excruciating pain. *Pain reporting is the single best measure of pain.* Research indicates that even critically ill patients can provide reports about the location and intensity of their pain.[26]

Sensory components of *every* pain assessment in *noncritical situations* include location, intensity, quality, and pattern of the pain. Each component is briefly discussed considering the type of pain.

For the person with acute pain, the *location* of pain draws attention to a new injury or process and may indicate damage to deep structures. A patient with chronic pain may be able to pinpoint a specific location. However, it is common for a patient with chronic pain to locate the pain in several areas. A patient with cancer pain also may have pain in multiple sites of the body, usually two to four sites, but up to 14 sites have been reported.[16] Location helps to identify the site and spinal dermatome where there is injury or tumor. For example, back pain frequently is felt by the patient with cancer months before sensory or bladder dysfunction would indicate that tumor growth has caused compression of the spinal cord, an oncologic emergency usually treated with immediate radiation therapy.

A new pathologic condition must be ruled out when there is a sudden increase in pain *intensity.* Pain treatment, however, should not be withheld pending comprehensive evaluation of the patient. The nurse should ask the question, "Will the differential diagnosis or medical treatment be altered if pain is obscured by pain therapy?" If not, there is not ethical reason not to provide pain treatment. It is also important to evaluate how intense the pain is when it is best (lowest intensity) and when it is worst (highest intensity). Wide variation in pain intensity and analgesic requirements may exist between patients despite similar tissue damage and type of injury, procedure, or disease process. The reason for the variation is not clearly understood, but probably represents variation in modulation of nociceptive stimuli. The intensity of chronic pain can range from 0 to 10, just like acute or cancer pain. Patients with pain may not use the term *pain* to refer to mild or small amounts of pain; they save the word *pain* to refer to the strong or really tough sensation.[27] Level of pain intensity can be used to select appropriate analgesic medications. Optimal pain therapy is possible when it is guided by measurement and documentation of the pain intensity.

Quality is how the pain feels to the patient. Quality of acute, chronic, and cancer pain provides information regarding the nature of the pain. For example, a burning, hypersensitive area or a sharp, shooting pain may indicate nerve damage. Patients frequently use words such as aching, burning, gnawing, heavy, sharp, shooting, stabbing, tender, throbbing, exhausting, sickening, terrifying, tiring, intense, unbearable, nagging, tight, or torturing to describe how their pain feels. The quality characteristics combined with the location can be used to select adjuvant analgesic agents to help control pain. Some types of pain respond to treatment with certain drugs (i.e., burning pain often responds to tricyclic antidepressants; shooting pain often responds to phenytoin or carbamazepine).[5]

Pain onset (when it starts) and duration (how long it lasts) are components of pain *pattern.* Acute pain consistently increases during wound care, ambulation, coughing and deep breathing. Acute pain associated with surgery or injury tends to diminish over time with recovery as tissues heal. Like chronic and cancer pain, acute pain often increases at night. A patient may have pain all the time (constant pain around-the-clock), incident or procedural pain (pain with movement or specific procedures [e.g., lumbar punctures]), or breakthrough pain (pain that returns before the regularly scheduled analgesic dose). Pain pattern can be used to determine the appropriate dosing schedule and medication preparation (immediate release versus long acting). Return of pain before the end of analgesic duration of a drug suggests the need for an increased amount of drug or more frequent dosing intervals (dosing frequency). Determining the pattern of pain is useful in guiding pain therapy.

After the sensory components of pain have been assessed, it is important to provide therapy for the pain. If pain relief is not at the level expected following therapy, the second step of the assessment process should be undertaken.

The *second step* of the pain assessment is begun if the expected level of pain relief is not obtained by the patient. The second step includes comprehensive assessment of pain difficult to manage in noncritical situations. In addition to the sensory components, a comprehensive pain assessment includes evaluation of the affective, behavioral, and cognitive aspects of pain. The nurse conducts a comprehensive pain assessment when initial pain treatments do not provide the anticipated pain relief.

The *third step* of the pain assessment process is providing follow-up assessments. The nurse assesses the sensory components of pain (location, intensity, quality, and pattern) when initial care is provided to the patient. Additionally, pain intensity is reassessed at the analgesic action onset, peak, and duration time points until pain relief has been stabilized. Pain intensity values at onset indicate initiation of analgesic effect; at peak they determine maximum relief obtained; and at duration of action they reveal length of analgesic effect. These pieces of information can be used to convince the physician to alter dose, interval, or drug if pain relief is not obtained. The nurse evaluates pain at rest, with activity, and when pain procedures are performed (e.g., when wound care is provided). Also, assessment of the highest pain intensity, lowest pain intensity, and present pain intensity provides a perspective on how the pain fluctuates with time. Each new pain, particularly unexpected, intense pain, needs to be evaluated promptly. Follow-up assessment of chronic nonmalignant pain and cancer should be conducted regularly to ensure that pain relief is continuous.

Measurement of Pain

A common belief is that pain cannot be measured but can be assessed. Assessment has been defined as the act of determining the importance, size, or value of something. In contrast, measurement is the act or process of applying a metric to gauge something. Because pain is a subjective phenomenon, many health professionals believe that pain cannot be measured; it can only be assessed. Other subjective phenomena, however, are considered to be measurable. For example, vision is a subjective phenomenon, yet a metric can be applied to determine visual acuity (e.g., Snellen Eye Chart) and ability to see color. The concept of measuring pain can be applied in a similar fashion by using valid and reliable metrics (tools) for components of the pain experience.

Many tools are available to measure the sensory components of pain (location, intensity, quality, and pattern). Fewer tools are available to measure the affective, behavioral, and cognitive pain components in clinical practice. Therefore nurses can measure pain location, intensity, quality, and pattern and assess affective, behavioral, and cognitive pain components until valid and reliable measures become available for these components.

There is no one best tool to measure sensory pain components, although some are easier to use than others. The nurse should choose a tool and use it consistently. If multiple tools are used in a clinical setting, it is important to communicate which tool has been used when measurement information is communicated to colleagues. The patient and family need to understand the pain measurement tool that is used to ensure a valid measurement. If the agency does not have a specific pain assessment tool, the following are suggested because they have been tested for validity, reliability, feasibility, and include instructions for use.

Pain Location. Pain location can be determined by using a drawing of the body and having the patient mark all the areas where pain is felt (Fig. 6-13). Another method is to ask the patient to point to the places where pain is felt, and the nurse can document those places on either a body outline or descriptively in the medical record and on the

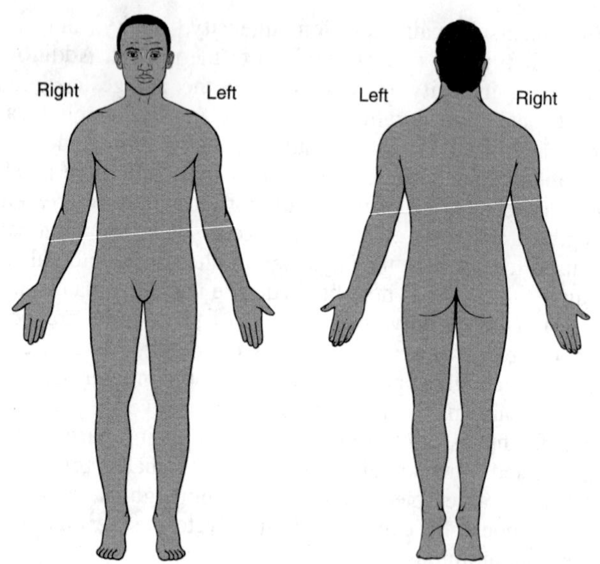

Fig. 6-13 Body outline—a method of documenting pain location. The patient is instructed to place a mark on the figures to indicate all the currently painful places. The patient is also instructed to indicate where the pain is generally located.

care plan. New pain sites should be reported, since they may signal complications.

Pain Intensity. Pain intensity can be measured using the numbers 0 through 10 as a scale to report the pain magnitude.[26] A patient may not intuitively know how to use numbers to measure pain. The script shown in Table 6-3 has been useful even with children as young as 8 years[28] and with elderly patients.[15] The use of a pain scale is also very effective in monitoring the effects of pain treatment.

The visual analog scale is a variation of the verbal scale. It usually consists of a straight line that represents a continuum of pain intensity. Verbal anchors—no pain to the worst pain possible—are placed at either end of the scale (Fig. 6-14). The length of the line may vary, but it is most commonly set at 4 inches (10 cm).

Pain intensity scales can also be used to help a patient identify a goal for pain therapy. The patient can be asked what amount of pain is desired (usually 0 or a small number) and what is acceptable (often a higher number than what is desired). This information is useful to both the patient and the nurse in planning and evaluating pain interventions.

Pain Quality. Pain quality is measured using a verbal descriptor list, such as the words listed in Table 6-4.[28] These words represent those most commonly used to describe the quality of pain and are derived from a more comprehensive list included in the McGill Pain Questionnaire.[29] The patient is asked to select the word or words that best describe the pain. If the patient has pain in more than one site, often several words per group will be selected, and the patient will indicate that some words describe one pain site and the other words describe another pain site. The number of the words selected are counted with a possible score of 0 to 19. Research indicates that complex pain quality, as reflected by a higher score, is associated with increased patient attempts to engage in pain control behaviors.[15]

Table 6-3 Standardized Instructions for Using the Pain Intensity Number Scale

"I need to know how much pain you have. Because I can't feel your pain, I want you to use a scale to let me know how much pain you have right now. The numbers between 0 and 10 represent *all* the pain a person could have. Zero means no pain and 10 means pain as bad as it could be. You can use *any* number between 0 and 10 to let me know how much pain you have right now. **Call** your pain a number between 0 and 10, so I will know the intensity of the pain you feel now."

Note: Use the phrase **"call your pain"** rather than **"rate your pain"** because patients have difficulty knowing what is expected of them when asked to rate their pain. They easily **"call"** their pain a number.

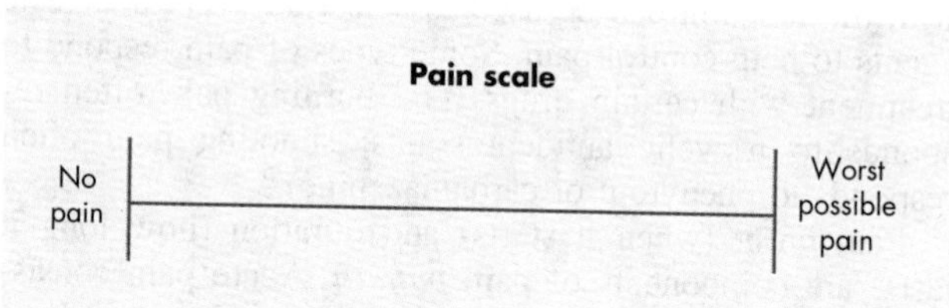

Fig. 6-14 Visual analog scale for measuring pain intensity.

Pain Pattern. Pain pattern is measured by the use of words listed in Table 6-5 to describe how the pain changes with time. The patient is asked to describe the pain as variations of constant, intermittent, or transient in pattern. The patient is also asked the date or time that the pain started and how long the pain lasts to measure the onset and duration of a painful episode. Figure 6-15 shows another method for the patient to document how the pain changes with time depending on activity level and other factors.

The complex nature of pain can be better understood through the use of standardized assessment tools. Use of these tools also helps to make the pain less abstract for the patient. When pain is a more concrete experience, the patient often feels empowered to cope with it and seek help to obtain pain relief.

Documentation of Pain

Pain assessment information should be documented in a part of the medical record that is easy to access by all health care providers, such as on the bedside vital signs form.[30] Even the best pain measurement or assessment conducted by one nurse is of limited value, unless the information is shared with other nurses and health professionals responsible for the care of the patient with pain. Until standardized documentation forms are available in all health care institutions, the progress notes and flow sheets can be used to document pain measurement information. There are usually blank sections on flow sheets that can be modified

Table 6-4 Pain Quality Descriptors Most Commonly Used to Describe Pain

Some of the words below describe your **present** pain. Circle **only** those words that best describe it.

1	2
Throbbing	Tiring
Shooting	Exhausting
Stabbing	Sickening
Sharp	Terrifying
Gnawing	Torturing
Burning	**3**
Aching	Nagging
Tender	Annoying
Heavy	Intense
Tight	Unbearable

From Wilkie DJ and others: Use of the McGill Pain Questionnaire to measure pain: a meta-analysis, *Nurs Res* 39:36, 1990.

Table 6-5 Pain Pattern Descriptors from the McGill Pain Questionnaire

How does your pain change with time? Circle the words you would use to describe the pattern of your pain.

1	2	3
Continuous	Rhythmic	Brief
Steady	Periodic	Momentary
Constant	Intermittent	Transient

From Melzack R: The McGill Pain Questionnaire: major properties and scoring methods, *Pain* 1:277, 1975.

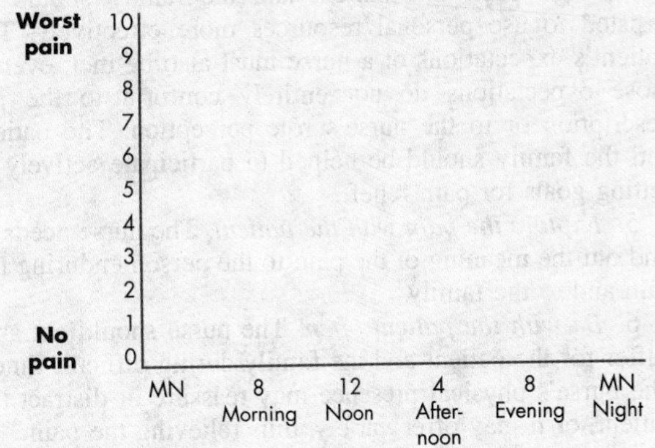

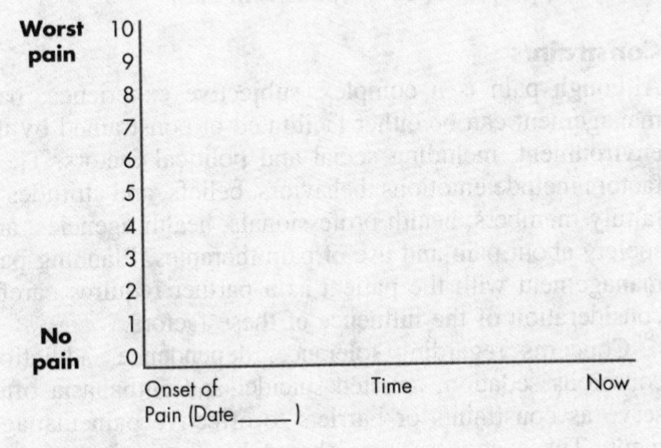

Fig. 6-15 A method for the tracking of pain over time.

to document the area and number of pain sites, intensity numbers, number of pain quality words selected, and the type of pain pattern words selected by the patient.

NURSING MANAGEMENT

PAIN

The nurse directs or participates in many of the pain-relieving strategies discussed in this chapter. The extent of the nurse's involvement depends on the unique factors associated with the patient, the setting, and the problem responsible for the pain.

A critical element in the nursing management of a patient with a pain syndrome is the establishment of a trusting relationship and a good rapport with the patient and the family. The patient and the family need to know that the nurse considers the pain significant and understands that pain may totally disrupt a person's life. The nurse's goal is to help the patient cope with the pain by using medications and techniques to help with relaxation, comfort, sense of aloneness and isolation, and protection from depersonalization; and the nurse will help the patient maintain or regain control over the environment. A priority for the nurse caring for a patient with pain is to let it be known that the nurse believes the person has pain and to explain some of the physiologic mechanisms of pain.

Nursing actions that promote the establishment of an effective relationship with the person who is experiencing pain and with the family should include the following:

1. *Believe the patient.* The patient needs to be able to trust the nurse to believe in the pain's existence. This message can be conveyed verbally to the patient by saying "I know you are in pain." The nurse may need to help the family believe the patient.

2. *Clarify responsibilities in pain relief.* Discuss what the nurse is going to do, and what the patient and the family are expected to do.

3. *Respect the patient's response to pain.* The nurse should accept the right of the patient to respond to the pain in the necessary manner. The family also needs help in this

area. The patient may need help to accept the response to the pain; the behavior may be less than is expected by the patient and the family.

4. *Collaborate with the patient.* The patient should be encouraged to use coping techniques that have been effective in the past. The patient and the family should be assisted to use personal resources more effectively. The patient's expectations of a nurse must also be met, even if those expectations do not entirely conform to the job description or to the nurse's role perception. The patient and the family should be helped to participate actively in setting goals for pain relief.

5. *Explore the pain with the patient.* The nurse needs to find out the meaning of the pain to the person enduring the pain and to the family.

6. *Be with the patient often.* The nurse should act as a buffer for the patient and the family during difficult times. The nurse's physical presence may reassure or distract the patient, or it may offer variety, thus relieving the pain.

Because pain has such a pervasive impact on the lives of the patient and family, many possible nursing diagnoses need to be considered. Table 6-6 lists nursing diagnoses that may be appropriate for the patient in pain.

Constraints

Although pain is a complex, subjective experience, pain management can be either facilitated or constrained by the environment, including social and political factors. These factors include emotions, behaviors, beliefs, and attitudes of family members, health professionals, health agencies, and society about pain and use of pain therapies. Planning pain management with the patient as a partner requires careful consideration of the influence of these factors.

Concerns regarding tolerance, dependence, addiction, conscious sedation, assisted suicide, and euthanasia often serve as constraints or barriers to effective pain management. These concerns are shared by the patient, family members, and health care providers. It is important that the nurse understand and be able to explain the differences among these various concepts.

Tolerance. Tolerance occurs with chronic exposure to a variety of drugs. In the case of opioids, tolerance is characterized by the need for an increased opioid dose to maintain the same degree of analgesia. Every patient does not experience tolerance. The need for an increase in the analgesic dose may reflect other factors, such as disease progression (e.g., cancer progression), or a new pathologic condition (e.g., pulmonary embolus), rather than tolerance. The patient's reports of increased pain should not be ignored; the increased pain should be treated while the cause is pursued. One of the ways tolerance is managed is by drug titration to balance desired effects and side effects to maintain patient comfort. Other approaches include changing to another drug in the same class or adding a nonopioid drug such as ibuprofen. It is important to note that there is no ceiling effect (increased dosing provides additional pain relief) for opioid-agonist drugs. As tolerance increases, doses can be increased; the largest dose noted in the literature has been 1654 mg intravenous morphine per hour.[31]

Table 6-6 Possible Nursing Diagnoses for the Patient with Pain

Activity intolerance	Risk for self-harm
Altered family processes	Hopelessness
Anxiety	Ineffective individual coping
Chronic pain	Pain
Constipation	Powerlessness
Fear	Sleep pattern disturbance
Risk for altered thought processes	

Dependence. Dependence is an expected physiologic response to ongoing exposure to pharmacologic agents that can produce a withdrawal syndrome when exposure is abruptly stopped. Withdrawal from opioids is characterized by symptoms such as chills alternating with hot flashes, salivation, sweating, runny nose, anxiety, irritability, insomnia, abdominal cramps, vomiting, and diarrhea when the drug dosage is markedly decreased or abruptly discontinued[32] (Table 6-7). Dependence appears to be highly individualized. Some patients will gradually decrease pain medication use as the pain decreases. Other patients require a tapering schedule. For example, to withdraw a patient from morphine, the 24-hour dose is calculated and decreased by 50%. Of this decreased amount, 25% is given every 6 hours. After 2 days, the daily dose is reduced by an additional 25% every 2 days until the 24-hour oral dose is 30 mg per day. The morphine is then discontinued.[33]

Addiction. Addiction is a psychologic condition characterized by a drive to obtain and take substances for other than the prescribed therapeutic value. Research findings suggest that less than 0.1% of patients who receive analgesics as a part of their medical treatment regimen become addicted.[34] In populations of patients with a substance abuse history, this percentage may be higher. A previous or present substance abuse problem can be identified during the initial pain assessment. Two examples of behavior suggestive of an addicted patient are receiving pain medications from multiple physicians, and reporting that pain prescriptions have been lost or stolen. Other types of behavior may be incorrectly interpreted as signs of addiction, such as clock-watching by the person undertreated for the pain. Addiction cannot be verified in the person with pain until the etiology of the pain has been eliminated, physical dependence has been eliminated through detoxification, and the patient seeks and takes the substance again. The patient who is physically dependent on the drug will seek and take the drug but may not be addicted. Often the term addiction is inappropriately applied to a patient, and the label can be a barrier to pain relief for that person. It is important for the nurse to recognize that opioid tolerance and physical dependence are expected with long-term opioid treatment and should not be confused with addiction.[35]

Table 6-7 Withdrawal Syndrome from Short-acting Opioids

	Early Responses (6-12 hr)	Late Responses (48-72 hr)
Psychosocial	Anxiety Irritability	Excitation
Secretions	Lacrimation Rhinorrhea Diaphoresis	Diarrhea
Other	Yawning Piloerection Shaking chills Dilated pupils Anorexia Tremor	Restlessness Fever Nausea and vomiting Abdominal cramps Hypertension Tachycardia Insomnia

Conscious Sedation. Conscious sedation implies that the patient can respond to verbal and physical stimuli when sedatives are used. The American Nurses Association (ANA) has established practice guidelines for the role of the registered nurse in the management of patients receiving intravenous (IV) conscious sedation for short-term therapeutic, diagnostic, or surgical procedures.[36] It is crucial to understand that, although analgesics may produce sedation as a side effect, sedatives generally do not produce analgesia.

Assisted Suicide and Euthanasia. It is not uncommon for the health professional, patient, and family members to be concerned that the effect of providing sufficient medication to relieve pain will precipitate the death of a terminally ill person. When large doses of opioids are required to control pain, a physician will often worry about prescribing and the nurse hesitate to administer a dose that could be considered euthanasia or that may be associated with assisting the patient to commit suicide. Relieving pain, even if it hastens the death of a terminally ill person, is considered the ethical and moral obligation of the professional nurse; it is not euthanasia or assisted-suicide.[37] When consistent with the patient's wishes, the position of the ANA is: "Nurses should not hesitate to use full and effective doses of pain medication for the proper management of pain in the dying patient. The increasing titration of medication to achieve adequate symptom control, even at the expense of life, thus hastening death, is ethically justified".[37] Relief of pain, not death, is the objective of the intervention.

PHARMACOLOGIC MANAGEMENT OF PAIN

In 1986 WHO proposed that clinicians use analgesic medications via a systematic plan (Fig. 6-11).[38] The systematic plan calls for concurrent treatment of the cause of the pain when possible and use of a three-step ladder approach. If pain persists or increases, drugs from the next step are used to control the pain. For chronic nonmalignant pain and cancer pain, drug use is recommended from the bottom of the ladder to the top (i.e., up the ladder from Step 1 to Step 2 to Step 3). For acute pain, the steps can be reversed in order from the top step to the bottom step (i.e., down the ladder from Step 3 to Step 2 to Step 1) as recovery occurs.

Although a physician or advanced practitioner prescribes the drugs, it is usually the nurse's responsibility to evaluate the effectiveness and side effects of prescribed medications. It is also a nursing responsibility to communicate the effectiveness of the medication regimen to the prescriber and suggest changes when appropriate.

It is important that the nurse understands the concept of equianalgesic dose. *Equianalgesic dose* refers to a dose of one analgesic that is equivalent in pain-relieving effects to another analgesic. This equivalence permits substitution of medications to relieve the pain and avoid possible adverse effects of one of the drugs. The tables describing Step 1, 2, and 3 drugs have columns indicating the approximate equivalent analgesic dose of common drugs of each class (see Tables 6-8, 6-9, 6-10, and 6-11).

Analgesic Ladder

Step 1 Drugs. When pain is mild, Step 1 nonopioid drugs, aspirin and other salicylates, other nonsteroidal antiinflammatory drugs (NSAIDs), or acetaminophen are used with or without adjuvant drugs to control the pain. Step 1 drugs can be very effective for pain; they provide adequate analgesia until death for 27% of patients with mild to moderate cancer pain.[39] Aspirin-like drugs and NSAIDs provide analgesia by blocking prostaglandin synthesis. Acetaminophen does not block this synthesis but instead produces pain relief through central mechanisms, which are not clearly understood. Pharmacokinetics of common Step 1 drugs are listed in Table 6-8.

Many of these drugs are available over-the-counter (OTC) without prescription. This means that a patient can use them without any type of medical supervision. Although effective for alleviation of mild pain, OTCs can cause serious problems related to drug interactions, side effects, and overdose.[39]

Adjuvant drugs have been shown to provide analgesia, but traditionally have not been used as analgesics. Adjuvant drugs act in many different ways. Some are central and some are peripheral, but adjuvant drugs work differently than acetaminophen, aspirin, NSAIDs, or opioids. Therefore it is a rational approach to combine selected adjuvants (e.g., tricyclic antidepressants and anxiolytics) with Step 1 drugs and continue the adjuvants when moving to Step 2 or Step 3 drugs. Pharmacokinetics of common adjuvant drugs are listed in Table 6-9.

Step 2 Drugs. When pain is moderate in intensity or mild but persistent with Step 1 drugs, Step 2 drugs are indicated. Codeine, oxycodone, propoxyphene, pentazocine, and hydrocodone are examples of Step 2 opioid drugs. Thirty-two percent of patients with cancer pain can have pain relief with Step 2 opioids until death.[40] When progressing up to Step 2, it is important to continue Step 1 drugs, including the adjuvants. If drugs with acetaminophen (Percocet or Vicodin) are used at Step 2, however, it is important

Table 6-8 Step 1 Analgesics: Pharmacokinetics

Generic Drug (Trade Drug)	Typical Dose (Maximum Dose)	Approximate Equivalent	Onset Effect (min)	Peak Effect (min)	Duration Effect (hr)
■ Acetaminophen (Tylenol, Tempra, others)	600 mg PO 600 mg PR (4000-6000 mg/day)	Aspirin 600 mg	30	60	3-4
■ Acetylsalicylic acid (aspirin)	600 mg PO 600 mg PR (5200 mg/day)	Morphine 2 mg IM	30	60	3-4
■ Ibuprophen (Motrin, Advil, others)	200 mg PO (3200 mg/day)	Aspirin 650 mg	30	60-120	4
■ Choline magnesium trisalicylate (Trilisate)	2000-3000 mg PO (3000 mg/day)		5-30	60-180	3-6
■ Diflunisal (Dolobid)	500 mg PO (1500 mg/day)	Aspirin 650 mg	60	120-180	8-12
■ Ketoprofen (Orudis)	25 mg PO (300 mg/day)	Aspirin 650 mg	30	30-120	6
■ Naproxen (Naprosyn)	250 mg PO (1250 mg/day)	Aspirin 650 mg	60	120-240	6-8
■ Ketorolac tromethamine (Toradol)	30-60 mg IM initially (150 mg IM for 1 day, then 120 mg IM/day)	Morphine 6-12 mg IM	10	60	3-6
■ Piroxicam (Feldene)	20 mg/day		60	180-300	>12
■ Sulindac (Clinoril)	200 mg/day		1-2 days	60-120	Unknown
■ Indomethacin (Indocin)	25 mg PO (100 mg/day)	Aspirin 650 mg	60	60-120	4

IM, Intramuscular; *IV*, intravenous; *PO*, oral; *PR*, rectal.

to stop the Step 1 acetaminophen because more than 4000 mg of acetaminophen per day can be toxic to the liver.

Step 2 drugs bind to opioid receptors in the CNS and perhaps on the peripheral nerves to block transmission of nociceptive signals. There are several subtypes of opioid receptors, which are found in differing proportions throughout the nervous system. Mu, delta, and kappa receptors are associated with analgesia. Some opioids bind to receptors and produce an effect at some but not all of the receptors. Agonist opioids, such as oxycodone and hydrocodone, are believed to bind to mu, delta, and kappa receptors and produce effects at each receptor. Agonists fit into a receptor site, "turn on" the site, and the drug effect occurs. Agonist-antagonist opioids, such as pentazocine, bind to mu and kappa receptors and produce an effect at the kappa receptor (agonist) but block the drug's effect at the mu receptors (antagonist). Partial agonist drugs bind to opioid receptors but produce a submaximal bodily response.

Drugs classified as agonist-antagonists or partial agonists have an analgesic ceiling (larger doses do not produce greater analgesic effects) and can produce a withdrawal syndrome if used in a patient physically dependent on agonist drugs. In contrast, agonist drugs do not have an analgesic ceiling. A drug acting as an antagonist binds to a receptor site without activating it. This binding blocks other drugs or neurotransmitters from activating the site. An antagonist can also dislodge an agonist from its receptor site, counteracting the agonist's effects. Naloxone is an example of an opioid antagonist (Fig. 6-16). Table 6-10 lists the classifications of commonly prescribed Step 2 opioid drugs.

Step 3 Drugs. Step 3 drugs are recommended for moderate to severe pain or when Step 2 drugs do not produce effective pain relief. Step 3 drugs include opioid drugs, such as morphine, hydromorphone, and methadone. Meperidine could be considered a Step 3 opioid, but the high incidence of neurotoxicity (e.g., seizures) associated with its metabolite, normeperidine, limits its use.[33] Use of meperidine is contraindicated for more than 2 days or in large doses (more than 600 mg per 24 hours). Approximately 35% of patients with cancer require step 3 opioids to effectively manage their pain.[40] Step 3 drugs produce a desired effect—analgesia—by binding to opioid receptors in the CNS and perhaps the peripheral nervous system. Pharmacokinetics of Step 3 opioids are listed in Table 6-11.

Recommended Drug and Route

Morphine has been recommended as the drug of choice for the patient with pain and oral administration as the route of choice.[35,38,42] Intramuscular (IM) opioid administration produces pain on injection and unreliable pain relief because of

Table 6-9 Step 1 Adjuvant Drugs: Pharmacokinetics

Generic Drug (Trade Drug)	Approximate Daily Dose	Onset Effect	Peak Effect	Duration Effect (hr)
▪ Carbamazepine (Tegretol, Epitol)	200-1600 mg PO	8-72 hr	2-12	Unknown
▪ Phenytoin (Dilantin)	300-500 mg PO	2-24 hr	1.5-3	6-12
▪ Amitriptyline (Elavil and others)	10-150 mg PO	3-4 days	1-2 wks	days-wks
▪ Doxepin (Sinequan, Adapin)	25-150 mg PO	3-4 days	1-2 wks	days-wks
▪ Imipramine (Tofranil and others)	20-100 mg PO	60 min	2-6 wks	wks
▪ Trazodone (Desyrel and others)	75-225 mg PO	2 wks	2-4 wks	wks
▪ Hydroxyzine (Vistaril, Atarax, and others)	300-450 mg IM	15-30 min	2-4 hr	4-6 hr
▪ Lidocaine	5 mg/kg IV	2 min	2 min	10-20 min
▪ Mexiletine (Mexitil)	200-400 mg PO	30-120 min	2-3 hr	8-12 hr
▪ Tocainide (Tonocard)	20 mg/kg PO	30-60 min	0.5-2 hr	8-12 hr
▪ Dexamethasone (Decadron and others)	16-96 mg PO/IV	2-4 days	1-2 hr	2.75 days
▪ Dextroamphetamine (Dexedrine and others)	10-15 mg PO	1-2 hr	Unknown	2-10 hr
▪ Methylphenidate (Methidate, Ritalin)	10-15 mg PO	Unknown	1-3 hr	4-6 hr

CNS, Central nervous system; *IM*, intramuscular; *IV*, intravenous; *PO*, oral; *PR*, rectal.

variable drug absorption. Novel administration routes for opioid drugs, such as epidural, intrathecal, transdermal, and transmucosal, have been developed but achieving pain relief by these routes is generally more expensive than by the oral route. In cancer pain management, federal guidelines recommend that these routes be used only when oral administration is not possible.[35] Morphine is a very effective drug; however, recent evidence raises questions about its use as the drug of choice when high doses are used and for use in the patient with compromised renal function.[43] High-dose morphine administered orally or intrathecally has been associated with hyperalgesia (exaggerated pain sensation) and myoclonus (severe muscle spasm).[44,45] Also, it has been shown recently that the hepatic-formed morphine metabolite, M-6-glucuronide (M-6G), is pharmacologically active with analgesic and side-effect properties, crosses the blood-brain barrier, and accumulates when renal function is impaired, as is reflected by elevated blood urea nitrogen (BUN) and serum creatinine concentrations.[43] Hydromorphone, methadone, or fentanyl are examples of opioids that may be used by the person with compromised renal function.

Administration Routes

Oral. Many opioids are available in oral preparations, such as liquid and tablet formulations. Equianalgesic doses for oral opioids are larger than for doses administered IM or IV (see Table 6-11). The reason larger doses are required is related to the first-pass effect of hepatic metabolism. This means that oral opioids are absorbed from the GI tract into the portal circulation and shunted to the liver. Partial metabolism in the liver occurs before the drug enters systemic circulation and becomes available to cross the blood-brain barrier and access CNS opioid receptors to produce analgesia. Oral opioids are as effective as parenteral opioids if the dose administered is sufficiently large based on the concept of first-pass metabolism. In general, the oral route is preferred.

Transmucosal: sublingual. Opioids administered under the tongue and absorbed into systemic circulation are exempt from the first-pass effect. Although morphine is commonly administered to persons with cancer pain via the sublingual route, little of the drug is absorbed from the sublingual tissue.[46] Most probably, morphine administered sublingually is dissolved in saliva and swallowed, making its properties similar to oral morphine. In contrast, fentanyl and buprenorphine are readily absorbed from the sublingual tissue. A fentanyl preparation is available as a premedication before surgery and for use in monitored anesthesia care.[47] Sublingual delivery systems for buprenorphine are under investigation.

Transmucosal: transnasal. When the patient is not able to tolerate oral opioids, the transnasal route may be an alternative delivery method that allows rapid absorption by the nasal mucosa blood vessels. Currently, butorphanol is the only commercially available transnasal opioid, but

Table 6-10 Step 2 Analgesics: Pharmacokinetics

Generic Drug (Trade Drug)	Typical Dose (Maximum Dose)	Approximate Equivalent	Onset Effect (min)	Peak Effect (min)	Duration Effect (hr)
Step 2 Opioid-Agonist Drugs					
▪ Codeine	30-60 mg PO (200 mg PO)	Aspirin 650 mg Morphine 10 mg IM	30-45	20-120	4
	15-60 mg IM	Morphine 10 mg IM	10-30	30-60	4
▪ Oxycodone (Roxicodone, w/aspirin-Percodan, w/acetaminophen-Percocet)	5 mg PO (30 mg PO)	Codeine 60 mg PO Morphine 10 mg IM	10-15	60	3-4
▪ Hydrocodone (Vicodin, Lortab, Lorcet, and others)	5 mg PO (30 mg PO)	Morphine 10 mg IM	10-30	3-60	4-6
▪ Meperidine (Demerol, Pethidine)	50 mg PO (300 mg PO)	Aspirin 650 mg Morphine 10 mg IM Demerol 75 mg IM	15	60-90	2-4
	75 mg IM	Morphine 10 mg IM	10-15	30-60	2-4
	50 mg IV	Morphine 10 mg IM	1	5-7	2-3
▪ Propoxyphene HCl (Darvon, Dolene);	65 mg PO	Aspirin 600 mg	15-60	120	4-6
Propoxyphene napsylate (w/aspirin-Darvon-N, w/acetaminophen-Darvocet-N)	100 mg PO	Aspirin 600 mg			
Step 2 Agonist-Antagonist Drugs					
▪ Pentazocine HCl (Talwin)	60 mg IM	Morphine 10 mg IM	15-20	30-60	2-3
	30 mg PO (180 mg PO)	Aspirin 600 mg Morphine 10 mg IM or Talwin 60 mg IM	15-30	60-90	3

IM, Intramuscular; *IV*, intravenous; *PO*, oral.

several agents are being investigated. It is classified as an agonist-antagonist, which limits its use in patients dependent on agonist opioids. Acute headache is the type of pain for which this drug is indicated.

Transmucosal: rectal. The rectal route is often overlooked but is particularly useful when the patient cannot take an analgesic by mouth. Rectal suppositories that are effective for pain relief include hydromorphone (Dilaudid), oxymorphone (Numorphan), and morphine.

Transdermal. Fentanyl also is available as a transdermal patch system for application to nonhairy skin. This delivery system is useful for the patient who cannot tolerate oral analgesic medications. Absorption from the patch is slow. Therefore, transdermal fentanyl is not suitable for rapid dose titration but can be effective if the patient's pain is stable and the dose required to control it is known.[48]

Currently, creams and lotions containing 10% trolamine salicylate (Aspercreme, Myoflex cream) are available. These agents have been recommended by the manufacturers for joint and muscle pain. Although no sensation is experienced when they are applied at or near the pain source, the aspirin-like substance is absorbed locally. This route of administration avoids gastric irritation, but the other side effects of high-dose salicylate are not necessarily prevented.

Ointments, lotions, gels, liniments, and balms (most of which are OTC products), are sometimes applied to the skin to achieve pain relief. Although these agents contain various substances, two common ingredients are menthol and methyl salicylate (wintergreen oil). The salicylate component is absorbed from the skin. On application, these agents usually produce a strong hot or cold sensation and should not be used after massage or a heat treatment when blood vessels are already dilated. Skin testing is advisable when the patient has not used the particular agent before, since the strengths of the agents vary and different intensities of sensation are produced. Relief of pain is reported for muscle pain, joint pain, headache, and visceral pain associated with gas, distention, and endometriosis.

Other topical analgesic agents, such as capsaicin (Zostrix), and local anesthetic agents, such as lidocaine and prilocaine (Emla), also provide analgesia. Capsaicin has been useful in controlling pain associated with postherpetic neuralgia, diabetic neuropathy, and arthritis. Emla is useful for control of pain associated with venipunctures, ulcer

Table 6-11 Step 3 Analgesics: Pharmacokinetics

Generic Drug (Trade Drug)	Typical Dose	Approximate Equivalent	Onset Effect (min)	Peak Effect (min)	Duration Effect (hr)
Step 3 Agonist Drugs					
■ Morphine sulfate	30 mg PO	Morphine 10 mg IM	20-60	120	4-5
Immediate release tablets and liquids	30 mg PR	Morphine 10 mg IM			
Sustained release (MS Contin, Oramorph SR)	30 mg PO	Morphine 10 mg IM		210	8-12
Injectable (Astramorph PF, Duramorph, Infumorph)	10 mg IM	Morphine 10 mg IM	10-30	60	4-5
	5 mg IV	Morphine 10 mg IM	5	20	2-4
■ Methadone (Dolophine)	20 mg PO	Morphine 10 mg IM	30-60	90-120	4-6
		Methadone 10 mg IM			
	10 mg IM	Morphine 10 mg IM	10-20	60-120	4-5
	5 mg IV	Morphine 10 mg IM	5	15-30	3-4
■ Hydromorphone (Dilaudid)	7.5 mg PO	Morphine 10 mg IM	30	90-120	4
	3 mg PR	Hydromorphone 1.5 mg IM	15-30	30-90	4-5
	1.5 mg IM	Morphine 10 mg IM	15	30-60	4-5
	1 mg IV	Morphine 10 mg IM	10-15	15-30	2-3
■ Oxymorphone (Numorphan)	1 mg IM	Morphine 10 mg IM	10-15	30-90	3-6
	0.5 mg IV	Morphine 10 mg IM	5-10	15-30	3-4
	10 mg PR	Oxymorphone 1 mg IM	15-30	60	3-6
■ Levorphanol (Levo-Dromoran)	4 mg PO	Morphine 10 mg IM	10-60	90-120	4-5
		Levorphanol 2 mg IM		60	4-5
	2 mg IM	Morphine 10 mg IM	10-15	15	3-4
	1 mg IV	Morphine 10 mg IM			
■ Fentanyl (Sublimaze, Duragesic)	0.1 mg IM	Morphine 10 mg IM	7-15	20-30	1-2
	25-50 µg/hr transdermal	Morphine 30 mg sustained-release q8hr	6 hr	12-24 hr	72
Step 3 Agonist-Antagonist Drugs					
■ Butorphanol (Stadol); see pentazocine	2 mg IM	Morphine 10 mg IM	10-30	30-60	3-4
	2 mg IV	Morphine 10 mg IM	2-3	30	2-4
■ Nalbuphine (Nubain); see pentazocine	10 mg IM	Morphine 10 mg IM	15	60	3-6
	10 mg IV	Pentazocine 60 mg IM	2-3	30	3-4
■ Dezocine (Dalgan)	10 mg IM	Morphine 10 mg IM	30	60-120	3-6
Step 3 Partial Agonist Drugs					
■ Buprenorphine (Buprenex)	0.4 mg IM	Morphine 10 mg IM	15	60	6

IM, Intramuscular; *IV*, intravenous; *PO*, oral; *PR*, rectal.

debridement, and postherpetic neuralgia. The area to which Emla is applied should be covered with a plastic wrap for 30 to 60 minutes before beginning a painful procedure.

Infusions

Subcutaneous, Intravenous, Epidural, and Intrathecal Routes. These routes are used for administration of continuous infusions of analgesic medications. A continuous infusion technique provides a relatively stable plasma or cerebrospinal fluid (CSF) concentration. The portion of the total analgesic requirement administered as a continuous infusion typically depends on the patient's situation. It is important to provide a loading dose (a dose that provides comfort) before starting a continuous infusion. This loading is accomplished by giving a bolus equivalent to the hourly dose of the medication to be used in the continuous infusion. To manage the patient on a continuous infusion

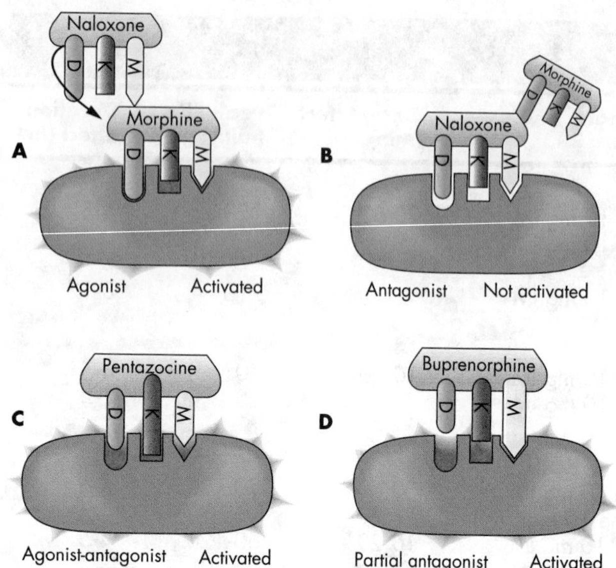

Fig. 6-16 Opioid receptor subtypes. ***A,*** Agonist action; ***B,*** antagonist action; ***C,*** agonist-antagonist action; ***D,*** partial agonist action. *M,* Mu receptor; *K,* kappa receptor; *D,* delta receptor.

alone suggests there is no fluctuation in the pain; this is unusual, since continuous infusion plus bolus injections are more common. Pain unrelieved by the continuous infusion needs to be reevaluated and appropriate treatment instituted. If the patient requires frequent additional doses of medication for pain relief, and the pain is not expected to diminish abruptly, the continuous infusion may need to be adjusted upward.

PATIENT-CONTROLLED ANALGESIA. Another type of delivery system is patient-controlled analgesia (PCA), or demand analgesia. In patient-controlled analgesia, a dose of opioid is delivered when the patient decides a dose is needed. PCA may be accomplished using oral medications or an infusion system in which the patient pushes a button to receive a bolus infusion of an analgesic into the subcutaneous tissue, a vein, or the epidural or intrathecal spaces. Ability to deliver a dose when needed places the patient in control and eliminates waiting for medication to be brought and given. Infusion pumps, however, deliver the drug only as frequently as the preset interval allows. PCA has rapidly gained acceptance for use in the management of acute and cancer pain. The addition of a continuous infusion to a PCA regimen will improve nighttime pain relief and promote sleep, since PCA administration naturally decreases at night because the patient is sleeping and cannot self-administer doses.

Use of PCA begins with patient education. The patient needs to understand the mechanics of getting a medication dose as well as how to titrate the medication to achieve good pain relief. The patient needs to be guided to take another dose when pain intensity is greater than the patient's desired pain intensity goal (a cognitive aspect of pain). The effectiveness of the initial PCA programming must be assessed. If the patient reports pain that is intolerable, the nurse can request an order to give the patient bolus doses (load) until comfort is achieved. The nurse can then make adjustments in the PCA settings. A routine order for the loading process is: give 1.5 to 2 times the PCA dose, evaluate pain relief at the time peak analgesic effect is expected (specific for each drug and route), and repeat the loading dose if the pain is unrelieved. This process should be continued until the patient reports either comfort or unacceptable side effects. If there are no orders for management of breakthrough pain (pain unrelieved by the prescribed pain management regimen), the patient's report of breakthrough pain needs to be communicated to the physician for a change in the orders. In a patient whose pain is steady and predictable, the majority of the patient's requirements can be met with a background infusion plus an occasional bolus (e.g., once an hour).

If the patient experiences side effects or toxic effects of PCA therapy, the specific symptom (e.g., nausea) should be treated. Ineffective symptom relief may require either a dose adjustment or an alternate drug. It is crucial to remember that when a patient sleeps medication cannot be self-administered, and the patient may awaken in pain and require increased nursing attention and substantial time to regain pain relief.

To make a smooth transition from infusion PCA to oral medications, it may be helpful to start the oral regimen before discontinuing the PCA or at least to give the first oral dose at the time PCA is discontinued. Another method is to replace the continuous infusion and a portion of the PCA dose requirement with an around-the-clock, equally potent oral medication while continuing the PCA for another 24 hours.[33] When there is a transition in the pain management plan, a consistent approach to the assessment of pain is vital to pain relief.

OTHER INJECTIONS AND INFUSIONS. Intraspinal (epidural, intrathecal, or regional) opioid therapy is extremely effective. Epidural analgesia has demonstrated effectiveness in the management of acute, chronic nonmalignant, and cancer pain.[49] Epidural catheters may be surgically implanted or placed percutaneously (through a needle). Although the lumbar region is the most common site of placement, epidural catheters may be placed at any point along the neuroaxis (cervical, thoracic, lumbar, or caudal). When choosing the epidural opioid dose, the site of pain in relation to the position of the epidural catheter and the age of the patient is considered. An elderly patient may be more sensitive to epidural opioids because of slowed or altered metabolism and excretion. There is great variability in response to given doses. Timing, frequency, and type of the assessment (e.g., sensory and motor effects) depend on the drug being delivered. Inadequate pain relief should be treated. Opioids with diluted concentrations (0.125% or less) of local anesthetics, such as bupivacaine, are examples of drugs used epidurally. Fentanyl is the ideal drug for treatment of breakthrough pain because of its rapid onset (5 minutes) and short duration of action (4 to 8 hours). Epidural drugs may be given as an intermittent bolus injection or as a continuous infusion.

The ANA has established practice guidelines for the role of the registered nurse in management of the patient receiving analgesia by catheter techniques. Prompt recognition and treatment of side effects and complications are necessary, and meticulous catheter care is required. The patient's skin needs to be assessed regularly and frequent position changes made to prevent skin breakdown if a local anesthetic is used because it can cause altered sensation with numbing. Intrathecal (into the CSF) administration and monitoring guidelines are similar to epidural administration. Doses administered, however, are much lower because the entire dose reaches the spinal cord (i.e., is not influenced by the dura and high vascularity of the epidural space). Other regional sites for infusions of local anesthetics or analgesics include the brachial plexus, celiac plexus, lumbar sympathetic chain, and along a nerve. This type of infusion has been used for both acute and chronic pain. The drug concentration varies with each patient. The anesthetic or analgesic agent is usually delivered in 300 ml of normal saline solution with an infusion rate adjusted to the degree of pain and to the physiologic responses to the medication, such as hypotension, bradycardia, or respiratory depression, during the first 24 hours. After that time, the dosage is gradually titrated downward.

Side Effects of Step 2 and Step 3 Drugs. In addition to producing analgesia, Step 2 and Step 3 drugs produce side effects, such as constipation, sedation, nausea, vomiting, itching, and respiratory depression. *Constipation* is common when repeated opioid doses are administered. It is necessary to prevent this type of constipation by giving laxatives (e.g., senna) and stool softeners (e.g., docusate sodium) early in the course of opioid therapy. Stool softeners alone are insufficient to overcome the constipating, physiologic effects of opioids on opioid receptors in the GI tract (stomach; small and large intestines). For example, laxatives should be started immediately if long-term treatment is expected in chronic and cancer pain or if frequent doses are required to control acute pain. Intractable constipation has been treated effectively with oral naloxone (Narcan).[50]

Sedation can be effectively treated with stimulants (caffeine, dextroamphetamine, methylphenidate). Metoclopramide, transdermal scopolamine, hydroxyzine, or a phenothiazine antiemetic can be used to treat opioid-related *nausea and vomiting*. Metoclopramide is particularly effective when a patient complains of gastric fullness, since opioids delay gastric emptying and this effect is reversed by metoclopramide. An antihistamine or a low-dose opioid antagonist (e.g., naloxone) can be used to treat *itching*.

Respiratory depression is rare when opioids are titrated to analgesic effect. A patient who is awake does not succumb to respiratory depression.[33] A patient is most at risk for respiratory depression when asleep. For this reason, it is important to observe rate and depth of respirations of the sleeping patient for 3 to 4 hours past the expected time for peak blood concentrations based on the route of administration. If severe respiratory depression occurs and stimulation of the patient (calling and shaking patient) does not reverse the somnolence or increase the respiratory rate and depth, naloxone (0.4 mg in 10 ml saline) in 0.5 ml increments every 2 minutes can be administered.[33] The naloxone dose should be titrated to avoid precipitation of profound withdrawal, seizures, and severe pain.

Titration

One of the most important aspects of using the WHO Analgesic Ladder is to titrate the analgesic dose to effect. *Analgesic titration* is dose adjustment based on decision making about the adequacy of analgesic effect versus the side effects produced. For example, a patient titrates to effect when using a prescription, such as Percodan 1 to 2 tablets every 3 to 4 hours as needed. The patient makes a decision 3 hours after 1 tablet was taken by evaluating how much pain relief was obtained. If the patient continues to have good pain relief, another Percodan would not be taken. If very little pain relief was obtained, the patient would take 2 tablets and after an additional 3 hours evaluate if more tablets should be taken at that time or at 4 hours. A patient with constant pain relieved by 2 tablets for 4 hours could effectively manage the pain by scheduling the Percodan to be taken around-the-clock every 4 hours.

In clinical settings, the nurse assists the patient to make decisions about titrating analgesics. Titration requires pain assessment to evaluate the desired effect of the analgesic and the side effects produced by the analgesic. There is no set amount of an opioid that will produce pain relief for every patient; the right dose is the dose that works and helps the patient achieve the pain intensity goal. Application of professional knowledge helps the nurse, in collaboration or partnership with the patient, to determine the appropriate opioid dose. Morphine 0.05 to 0.1 mg/kg IV can be used as a formula to determine the size of the dose to begin titration.[30,35] Skillful titration results in the optimal dose of an analgesic being given and helps the nurse to identify conditions when additional or alternative drugs might be helpful. Consultation with the physician provides the patient with the appropriate prescription to effectively continue dose titration.

Timing Analgesics

A preventive approach to pain is crucial. A patient should be medicated before painful procedures and activities that can be expected to produce pain. If these procedures or activities are planned so that they occur when the patient's analgesic has reached its peak effectiveness, the pain will be decreased and the patient's ability to participate will be increased. Moreover, if the patient is medicated before the pain begins to increase rather than once it has become severe, far less medication is required. This action may minimize the drug's side effects, which often are barriers to effective pain relief. The patient and the family should be taught when to ask for pain medication. Administration may also be time-controlled, with the medication given on a set schedule regardless of the presence or absence of pain.

NONPHARMACOLOGIC MANAGEMENT OF PAIN

In addition to the pharmacologic analgesics described, a number of nonpharmacologic strategies provide analgesia and can be used alone or in combination with pain medications. Use of nonpharmacologic pain management strategies can reduce the dose of an analgesic required to control pain and thereby minimize side effects of drug therapy. Some strategies are believed to alter ascending nociceptive input or stimulate descending pain modulation mechanisms. Exact mechanisms by which most of the nonpharmacologic strategies provide analgesia are not known at this time, but the theoretic rationales for many nonpharmacologic strategies have been discussed as part of the physiologic dimension of pain. Categorizing the nonpharmacologic pain relief methods as physical or cognitive-behavioral strategies is a helpful way of considering the potential mechanisms by which they provide pain relief.

Physical Pain Relief Strategies

Physical methods of producing analgesia include invasive and noninvasive techniques. The nurse can prescribe and administer many of the noninvasive therapies and can monitor and provide patient education when invasive techniques are prescribed by the physician.

Noninvasive Pain Relief Strategies

Positioning. Institution of preventive measures to minimize joint and muscle stiffness is important to the pain-management regimen, especially when the patient immobilizes or guards painful body parts in an attempt to control the pain. Establishment of a passive range-of-motion program and, if not contraindicated by the patient's condition, an active exercise regimen for the patient can reduce joint and muscle stiffness. These strategies are particularly beneficial when timed to coincide with the peak analgesic effect of the drug therapy. The exercise program reduces the stiffness and helps to release any muscle spasms that may be present. Both patient and family should be taught the exercise regimen. The patient should be encouraged to move about as much as possible within the medically prescribed activity order.

The nurse must also prevent painful complications that result from immobility, including pressure ulcers, contractures, and thrombophlebitis. Because pain can be intensified by distention of an internal organ, constipation should be prevented by ensuring that the patient is mobilized as soon as possible and given laxatives as necessary. Because urinary retention can cause or increase pain, intake and output should be monitored and the bladder percussed to assess the degree of distention. An indwelling catheter, if present, should be checked frequently to ensure patency and free flow of urine. The patient should be helped to identify the precipitating physical factors that cause pain. Measures to prevent the pain should then be instituted and taught to the patient and family.

Pain management must include methods to promote rest and sleep. The person deprived of rapid-eye-movement sleep and deep sleep (phases III and IV) becomes irritable and fatigued and has an increased sensitivity to pain. The patient must be allowed to sleep undisturbed for at least 2 hours at a time. Comfort measures, analgesics and hypnotics, and relaxation techniques should be used as appropriate to promote sleep.

Dermal stimulation. Dermal (cutaneous) stimulation to produce analgesia is defined as noninjurious stimulation of the patient's skin for the purpose of pain relief.[1] Dermal stimulation may be provided by the patient or someone else. Dermal stimulation methods differ in relation to convenience, cost, need for a physician's prescription, precautions, contraindications, and the availability of trained health care professionals who may provide the intervention. A major difference from the patient's perspective is that the various methods produce different sensations.

Application of *pressure* is an instinctual response to pain. An injured part is reflexively clutched and pressure is applied. Dermal stimulation that uses a pressure method harnesses this automatic response in a deliberate fashion. Pressure may be applied with the fingertips, the ball of the thumb, knuckles, heel of the hand, entire hand, or both hands. Occasionally a hard but smooth object, such as a sandbag, may be used to apply pressure. Pressure applied to a trigger point is effective in some instances. A *trigger point* is a small hyperirritable area with a taut band in the muscle or connective tissue, often just below the skin, that causes pain when it is stimulated sufficiently.[51] Trigger points may be present in the painful area or at a point distant from the actual pain. There is a strong association between trigger points and acupuncture points for pain.[1] Although pressure on a trigger point may produce a dull, aching discomfort, continued pressure may relieve the pain. Certified massage therapists are trained in these techniques.

Acupressure is a specific pressure technique that involves application of pressure, massage, or both to specified points on the skin. These points are the same as the traditional acupuncture points. Pressure is applied with the thumb, the tip of the index finger, or the palm of the hand.

Massage of an injured body part with rubbing is also an instinctual response. This response can be deliberately tapped to manage pain. Many massage techniques exist. Examples include moving the hands or fingers over the skin slowly or briskly with long strokes or in circles (superficial massage) or applying firm pressure to the skin to maintain contact while massaging the underlying tissues (deep massage) (Fig. 6-17). Specific massage techniques are involved

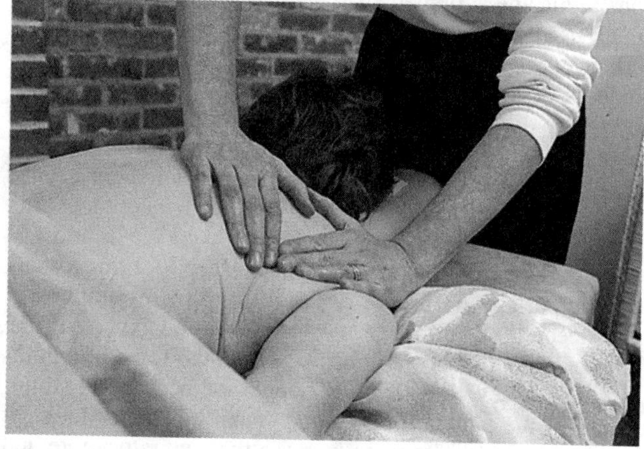

Fig. 6-17 A back rub is a time-honored method of providing deep massage.

in some forms of acupressure and in trigger point massage. Cold massage to trigger points is also used.[52]

The application of *cutaneous vibration* and high-frequency energy, such as by ultrasound, short-wave and long-wave diathermy, and microwave, is used to provide pain relief.[53] The pain relief may be immediate, or it may require several minutes to occur. The duration of the pain relief is highly variable. Many different vibration devices exist, varying in size and shape to meet individual needs. A physician's prescription is not necessary for the purchase of a vibratory device. Cutaneous vibration is often done in an outpatient physical therapy department.

TENS involves the delivery of an electric current through electrodes applied to the skin surface over the painful region, at trigger points, or over a peripheral nerve. Pain relief with TENS has been reported in low-back pain, cervical (neck) syndrome, arthritis, sciatica, tic douloureux, postherpetic neuralgia, peripheral nerve injuries, brachial plexus injuries, stump and phantom limb pain, and during childbirth labor.[18] During the actual application of TENS, acute postoperative pain is reduced. Postoperative pulmonary and GI tract complications can also be minimized with the use of TENS. Pain relief after discontinuance of TENS varies.

A TENS system consists of two or more electrodes connected by lead wires to a small, battery-operated stimulator (Fig. 6-18). Most stimulators may be worn and used 24 hours a day. The system can also be disassembled for intermittent use by detaching the stimulator and wires while leaving the electrodes in place. A physician's order is required to initiate this therapy.

Physical therapists often apply the TENS, but application and patient education can be done by a nurse. Experimentation with different stimulators, different electrode placements, and different frequency settings is often necessary to achieve therapeutic results with TENS. If one stimulator is not effective in providing pain relief, another should be tried. Multiple sites of stimulation, based on spinal dermatomes, may also be tried during successive trials to determine the most effective site for pain modulation.

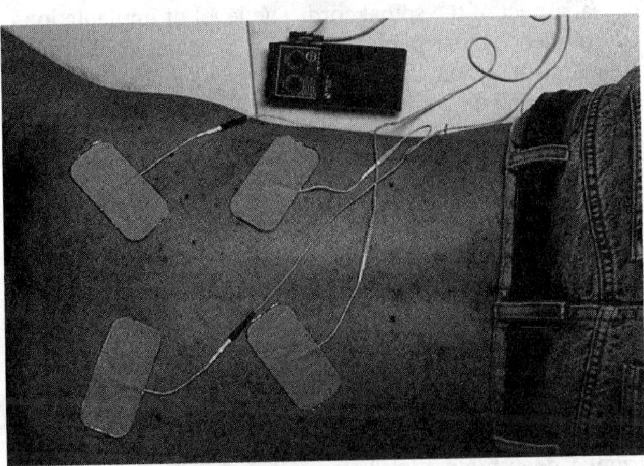

Fig. 6-18 Initial TENS treatment being given by physical therapy department to assess value in pain relief.

Conventional (high-frequency) TENS units that use alternating currents set at a rate of 40 to 400 Hz (cycles per second) typically produce rapid analgesia (within 20 minutes).[18] The person receiving high-frequency TENS experiences paresthesias (subjective sensation of numbness or tingling) during the treatments. The voltage and the rate of stimulation are altered according to the patient's response to the paresthesias.

Contraindications for the use of TENS are not firmly established. TENS is not currently recommended for patients with cardiac pacemakers or with a history of myocardial ischemia or dysrhythmias. TENS is not applied over a pregnant uterus, broken skin, or anesthetic areas; in areas of the carotid sinuses, or laryngeal and pharyngeal muscles; or in the eyes.

Heat therapy is the application of either moist or dry heat to the skin. Heat therapy can be either superficial or deep. Superficial dry heat can be applied by means of an electrical device, such as a heating pad, a heat cradle, or a gooseneck or infrared lamp, or by nonelectric means, such as hot-water bottles and exposure to the sun. Superficial moist heat can be obtained nonelectrically from hydrocollator (moist heat) packs, soaks, showers, baths, whirlpools, and Hubbard tanks and by wrapping the body part in plastic to trap body heat. Electric heating pads designed to provide moist heat are also available. Physical therapy departments provide deep-heat therapy through such techniques as short-wave diathermy, microwave diathermy, and ultrasound therapy. Heat therapy generally involves intermittent applications of heat for short periods of time (5 minutes for acute pain and 20 to 30 minutes for chronic pain), but some therapy methods, such as trapping of body heat, may be continued for prolonged periods or may be continuous.[53]

Cold therapy involves the application of either moist or dry cold to the skin. Dry cold can be applied by means of an ice bag, moist cold by means of towels soaked in ice water, cold hydrocollator packs, or immersion in a bath or under running cold water. Icing, with ice cubes or blocks of ice made to resemble Popsicles, is another technique used for pain relief. Ice massage is a technique combining cold therapy and massage; the ice is applied evenly over the area of pain with slow up-and-down strokes for 10 to 30 minutes. Physical therapists sometimes use ethyl chloride or "vasocoolant" sprays as part of a cold-therapy regimen.

Cold therapy is used for a variety of painful conditions, including posttraumatic pain and postoperative pain (especially following orthopedic procedures) and with bursitis, osteomyelitis, and muscle spasms. In addition, contrast baths (alternating hot and cold applications) and hydrotherapy used in conjunction with relaxation, passive movement exercises, and breathing exercises may be used to treat pain.

GUIDELINES FOR DERMAL STIMULATION. Any type of dermal stimulation should initially be of moderate intensity and then increased or decreased to achieve optimal pain relief. The most effective intensity for dermal stimulation is slightly less than the intensity that produces discomfort in persons with normal skin—frequently a stimulation of slightly above moderate intensity.[18,53] Dermal stimulation may be continuous or intermittent. The duration of most cutaneous stimulation is 10 to 30 minutes; however, ice massage rarely lasts longer than 10 minutes. Cold therapy is contraindicated in the person with hypersensitivity to cold. When firm pressure is applied to trigger points or acupuncture points, steady pressure is usually not maintained more than a few seconds. The frequency of dermal stimulation should be determined by how long the pain relief lasts following stimulation. When the pain recurs, the dermal stimulation is reapplied. An arbitrary schedule (such as tid or qid) may be established in an institutional setting. On an outpatient basis, dermal stimulation that requires professional supervision is scheduled by appointment, usually with a physical therapy department. Continuous application of most dermal stimulation methods is impractical. If the patient needs continuous stimulation to achieve pain relief, TENS or a menthol product may be the most practical solution.

Generally, dermal stimulation is applied directly over the painful area, around the painful site, or just proximal and distal to the painful area. Another possible area of stimulation is over peripheral nerves that innervate the painful area. This type of stimulation is most readily accomplished by TENS. Contralateral stimulation may be necessary when a painful area is too sensitive to be directly stimulated or when the painful area is not accessible because of a covering. The reason for the effectiveness of contralateral stimulation is not known. Contralateral stimulation is also used with phantom limb pain. If contralateral stimulation is unacceptable, unrelated areas can be stimulated. Use of cutaneous stimulation techniques must be individualized to the patient and the particular type of pain. The patient may have strong preferences regarding the type of dermal stimulation used and the area to be stimulated. Individual concerns are cost, convenience, intensity of stimulation, and duration of stimulation.

Many different persons may be able to administer the dermal stimulation techniques. The nurse, physical therapists, certified massage therapists, the patient, and family members may be able to perform the prescribed technique. Often, the patient and family members can be taught the effective technique after the therapy has been initiated by a trained person. Some of the techniques require purchasing or renting equipment (e.g., TENS) or using a physical therapy department (e.g., ultrasound). Some treatments are covered by insurance although others are not. The practical aspects of dermal stimulation must be considered if this method of treatment is to provide long-term relief.

Invasive Pain Relief Strategies

Acupuncture. Acupuncture involves the insertion of needles at specified cutaneous sites. The needles are activated by hand or by low-voltage electric current (Fig. 6-19). Onset of analgesia may not be immediate, but once the endogenous opioids have been mobilized, the technique's pain-relieving capacities extend beyond the period of actual stimulation. It is unknown at this time if acupuncture analgesia is superior to placebo analgesia or other types of hyperstimulation procedures.[18] Extensive education is necessary to become certified to perform acupuncture.

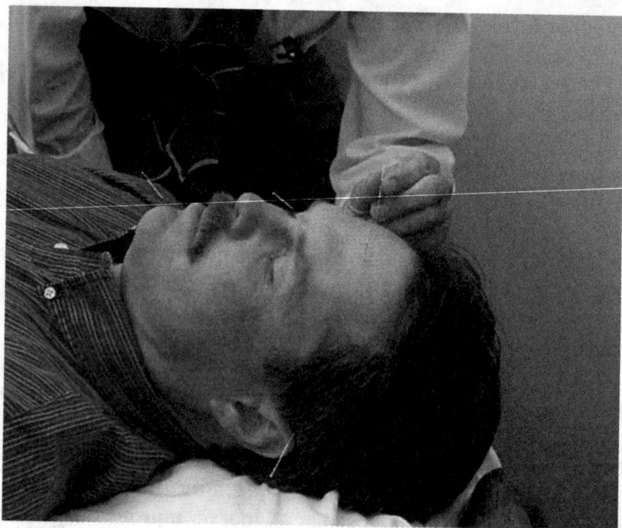

Fig. 6-19 Acupuncture.

Percutaneous electrical nerve stimulation. Deeper peripheral tissues can be stimulated through *percutaneous electrical nerve stimulation* or acupuncture. Percutaneous electrical nerve stimulation is a preliminary step designed to evaluate the potential usefulness of a permanently implanted device. It is accomplished by inserting a needle, to which a stimulator is attached, near a large peripheral or spinal nerve. The amount of electric current is regulated to provide maximum pain relief. If the percutaneous stimulation successfully reduces the patient's pain, a permanent peripheral nerve stimulator is surgically implanted. A special electrode is placed around the nerve, and an internal receiver is implanted subcutaneously at waist level on the anterior chest wall. The patient activates the receiver by means of a special transmitter and antenna as is needed for optimal pain relief.[51]

Dorsal cord or deep brain stimulation. CNS stimulation can be achieved through *dorsal cord stimulation* or *deep brain stimulation.*[54,55] Dorsal cord stimulation is an alternative pain-management technique to percutaneous electrical nerve stimulation when the pain involves large areas, such as the lower extremities or the back. During a laminectomy, electrodes are implanted intradurally in the dorsal aspect of the spinal cord. The level of implantation is determined by the pain location. A receiver is implanted subcutaneously on the anterior chest wall at waist level. The antenna and the transmitter system are similar to those used in permanent peripheral nerve stimulation.

Electrical stimulation of certain regions of the brain, including areas of the frontal lobes, thalamus, midbrain, lower brain stem, caudate nucleus of the basal ganglion, and internal capsule, produces long-lasting analgesia. Motor function, affect, and other behavior responses are unaffected. At least two pain-modulating systems are involved. In the periventricular gray system, the release of enkephalin is hypothesized to activate neurons that exert an inhibitory action on small pain afferents. Pain syndromes responsive to morphine are treated with periaqueductal and periventricular deep brain stimulation. Central pain is best treated with internal capsule and lateral thalamus stimulation, although the mechanism of action is unclear. Some patients respond only to stimulation of all four sites.[54]

Nerve blocks. Nerve blocks are used to reduce pain by temporarily or permanently interrupting transmission of nociceptive input by application of local anesthetics or neurolytic agents. Initially, temporary nerve blocks with local anesthetics are used to isolate the involved pain pathway and to determine the possible effectiveness of a permanent blocking procedure for the particular individual. Typically, the local anesthetic effects last for only a few hours. The effects of neurolytic agents such as alcohol or phenol last for weeks to months; therefore these agents are used for a more long-lasting effect.

Nerve blocks have been a successful pain-management technique for more localized chronic pain states, such as peripheral vascular disease, trigeminal neuralgia, causalgia, and some cancer pain. A nerve block was formerly considered advantageous in managing localized pain caused by malignancy and in debilitated patients who could not withstand a surgical procedure for pain relief. This use is currently being reevaluated in view of the increasing life expectancy of persons being treated for malignancies and the availability of other therapeutic modalities.

Neurosurgical interventions. Neurosurgical interventions are accomplished by surgical resection or thermocoagulation, including radiofrequency coagulation. Interventions that destroy the sensory division of a peripheral or spinal nerve are classified as neurectomies, rhizotomies, and sympathectomies. Neurosurgical procedures that ablate the lateral spinothalamic tract are classified as cordotomies if the tract is interrupted in the spinal cord, or tractotomies if the interruption is in the medulla or the midbrain of the brain stem. Figure 6-20 identifies the sites of neurosurgical procedures for pain relief. Surgical resection of the lateral spinothalamic tract is rare today because a percutaneous approach is available. Both cordotomy and tractotomy can be performed with the aid of local anesthesia by a percutaneous technique in which the pain fibers are isolated by fluoroscopy and a radio-frequency lesion is created.

Neurosurgical interventions involving the thalamus or frontal lobe region of the brain are carried out through a stereotactic procedure. Long electrodes or other probes are inserted deep into the brain tissue and positioned by the use of external points or landmarks of the skull. The tissue is destroyed by thermocoagulation or other means.

Intractable pain may be controlled by surgery, such as a pituitary resection. This type of procedure is used only for severe, intractable pain that does not respond to other therapeutic measures. Ablative procedures are less frequently used today because of the availability of good analgesic methods to control pain.

Cognitive-Behavioral Therapies

Techniques to alter the affective, cognitive, and behavioral components of pain include a variety of cognitive strategies and behavioral approaches. Many cognitive-behavioral techniques elicit emotions, behaviors, and thoughts that are incompatible with pain. For example, relaxation is incompatible with muscle tension. Thinking or talking about a scenic view is incompatible with thinking about pain. Rhythmic breathing is incompatible with the holding one's breath and gasping that are associated with pain. Eliciting behaviors that are incompatible with pain is part of the nursing management of the patient experiencing pain. Preserving the patient's energy for enjoyable activities is also important. The nurse must first identify the activities that are most important or pleasurable for the patient. Together they must find ways for the patient to carry out these activities by reorganizing priorities and schedules and perhaps changing some rules and regulations. Providing periods of rest and sleep may also be necessary to conserve the energy needed for those activities the patient considers important.

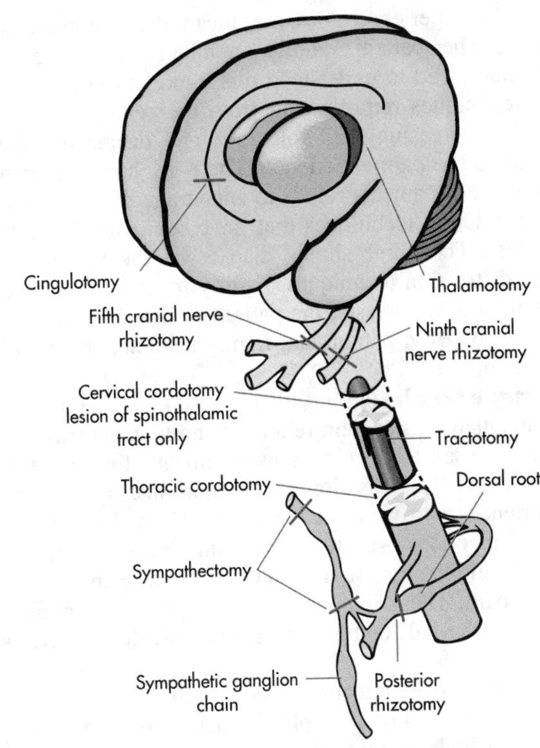

Fig. 6-20 Sites of neurosurgical procedures for pain relief.

Anticipatory Guidance. The patient should be prepared as much as possible regarding pain experiences. This is referred to as *anticipatory guidance.* Preparing the patient for what to expect allows the nurse to help reduce anxiety and clarify misinformation and misinterpretation. Knowing what to expect helps the patient cope. In the anticipatory phase of the pain experience some anxiety mobilizes the development of coping strategies. This is an important point when the nurse is dealing with a patient who is to have a painful experience. Such a patient cannot be reassured that there will be little or no pain, but instead must be helped to identify ways to cope with the expected pain.

Distraction. Distraction involves redirection of attention on something away from the pain. The distraction stimuli may be external events, internal activities, or bodily sensations. Distraction techniques help the patient cope with the pain being experienced. When assisting the patient to use cognitive strategies, the nurse must remember that the patient's ability to use distraction effectively to decrease the pain experience does not mean that the pain is not severe. The patient, family members, and health care personnel need to understand this important point. Distraction techniques remove pain from the center of attention, thereby increasing pain tolerance and decreasing the response to the pain experience. The pain, however, is real.

Part of the nurse's role is to encourage the patient to use the distraction techniques that have been found helpful in the past. The nurse should also assist the patient to use these distraction techniques. Family members also need to be taught how to assist the patient to use these techniques effectively. Both patient and family need support in adopting them.

Imagery. Imagery is the purposeful or therapeutic use of imagination. For pain relief the individual's own imagination is used to develop sensory images that focus away from the pain sensation and emphasize other sensory experiences and pleasant memories. Guided imagery provides a mental substitute for the pain. Specific images have been developed for use in pain relief to bring about removal of the pain. These include the techniques of breathing out the pain, the ball of healing energy, and the healthy body image.[1]

Another imagery technique is to use images in the course of conversation. For example, the patient is helped to "pretend your body is a puppet on a string," "let your body go limp all over," or "try to feel like a limp dishrag." To explain a therapeutic measure, the nurse may tell the patient that "this will loosen the knots you describe in the back of your neck," "this is stretching out the back muscles to stop the spasms," "the heat is melting away the pain," or "the heat is driving away the pain." Use of images the patient has used to describe the pain may be particularly effective.

A similar imagery technique is brief instruction. The patient is told to "think of the sensation as unusual, not painful," "concentrate on other things," "think of your hand as dull and insensitive," or "think of your hand as a wax hand or a rubber hand and not really part of your body."[1]

Images that suggest a return to health are also helpful. They increase therapeutic physiologic functioning. Examples of such images are "the food is supplying nutrients to repair the damaged tissues," or "the heat is bringing increased blood flow to the area to cleanse the tissues and carry away the wastes."

The nurse should use imagery in conversation with the patient. Then the nurse should assist the patient with imaging by encouraging the patient to relive past events and asking for a detailed description of a pleasant event or scene. If the patient focuses on only one sensory modality—for example, what the mountain looked like—the nurse should ask about other sensory modalities, such as sound, smell, or temperature. Involving multiple senses helps reinforce the image. The technique can also be taught to family members.

A patient, especially a child, is often more accepting of the use of imagery than is the health care professional. A nurse might be reluctant to teach patients these techniques for fear of disapproval from physicians or other nurses, or because the techniques seem "unscientific." However, research findings support the relationship between imagery and alpha brain wave activity associated with relaxation and sleep.

Hypnosis. Hypnosis is a state of altered consciousness characterized by extreme responsiveness to suggestion. Through hypnosis the patient is separated from the analytic and judgmental component of the thought processes so that acceptance of suggestion is possible. Hypnosis is induced artificially in a subject by means of verbal suggestion from the hypnotist or by the subject's concentration on some object. Although it requires training, hypnosis can be used successfully for a person whose pain syndrome involves a strong affective component, including a person with cancer pain.[56] This technique decreases tension by reducing fear and anxiety and by enhancing the person's optimism and sense of well-being. Hypnotic suggestion can also be used to induce analgesia, for sensory-imagery conditioning, and to induce a relaxation state.

Conscious Suggestion. Conscious suggestion, which involves the use of voice and carefully chosen words to help the conscious and aware person relax, may be effectively used to assist the person in pain. Conscious suggestion, unlike hypnosis, uses suggestion with the conscious alert person. The first step is a disarming statement that seems likely to have come from the patient's own mouth. For example, "You want yourself to relax, don't you?" The suggestions are subtle. The first statement is positive, but it always implies a subtle command, "you want to." The emphasis is on the "you want to, don't you?" This is followed with more suggestions. For example, "You are going to let yourself relax, aren't you?" Therefore with conscious suggestion, the nurse sells relaxation to the patient.

Conditioning. Certain pain-relief measures result in relief frequently enough for *classic conditioning* to take place. The nurse can help the patient benefit from this phenomenon by deliberately pairing relief methods. For example, the nurse should teach a relaxation technique to be used each time a pain medication is given. One result of this is the additive effect gained from two measures used simultaneously.

Behavior modification (*operant conditioning*) is based on the principle that the frequency of a behavior may be increased or decreased by the use of reinforcement. Positive reinforcement results in an increase in the frequency of the behavior. The nurse can use behavior modification by giving praise and attention to the patient who is willing to try new pain relief methods or who engages in behaviors incompatible with pain. The patient's attempts to progress toward recovery should be praised and noticed. Silence or ignoring nonbeneficial behavior is also important. The family should be taught to provide positive reinforcement, ignore nonbeneficial behavior, and use silence.

Stress inoculation training involves a three-stage approach to behavioral change. First, the meaning of the clinical manifestations is taught. Secondly, the patient is taught coping strategies that are incompatible with the pain experience and pain behavior. Finally, the patient is taught how to use this new knowledge and awareness in the pain situation. The nurse participates in all phases of stress inoculation training, assisting the patient to progress through the stages.

In behavioral programs, the nurse assesses and documents pain behaviors in the patient and family. In addition, the nurse works with the patient on medication regimens. The nurse plays a major role in reinforcing "well" behaviors and promoting attendance at prescribed therapies, exercise, and other beneficial assignments. The primary goal of behavioral programs is to reduce the number and frequency of pain behaviors by means of medication management, exercise, and family retraining. Baseline data about medication use, activity level, and patient-family interactions are collected. Medication intake is systematically reduced and converted to the oral route. The liquid form often is used. A program of scheduled activity is initiated. The exercise regimen starts at baseline or less and is gradually increased along with recreational activities. Family retraining is directed toward assisting family members to identify ways by which they reinforce pain behaviors and then teaching family members alternate ways of interacting. Other management techniques used in behavioral programs may include hypnosis, biofeedback, vocational counseling, and marital therapy.

Relaxation. The positive effects of relaxation include reducing the effects of stress, decreasing acute anxiety, distracting from the pain, alleviating skeletal muscle tension or contraction, producing a state of increased susceptibility to suggestions of comfort, combating fatigue, facilitating sleep, and enhancing the effectiveness of other pain-relief measures.[30,35] Elicitation of the relaxation response requires a quiet environment, a comfortable position, and a mental device as a focus of concentration (e.g., a word, a sound, the heartbeat, or the person's breathing). Relaxation strategies include deep-breathing regimens, heartbeat breathing, music, slow and rhythmic breathing, and progressive relaxation exercises with a trainer (Table 6-12).

Relaxation techniques are used in autogenic training, biofeedback, meditation, yoga, Zen practices, imagery, and hypnosis. *Autogenic training* involves learning to self-regulate bodily functions, such as heart rate, breathing rate, blood flow, and muscle tension. *Biofeedback* uses a monitoring device, such as an electrocardiograph (ECG), electroencephalograph (EEG), or electromyelograph (EMG), to provide the patient with information about a physiologic function that is not normally available. The physiologic signal itself is transformed, amplified, and then displayed on a monitor or by means of an auditory feedback system. With this increased awareness of the physiologic state and with special training, the individual can learn to modify a particular physiologic state (e.g., reduce heart rate and muscle tension or increase peripheral circulation). Biofeedback includes aspects of distraction and relaxation strategies and produces a sense of control over the pain. Biofeedback has been used to treat chronic pain syndromes with a stress-related component. Several types of biofeedback training have been used in pain management: EMG feedback has been used for muscle-contraction (traction) headache; EEG feedback trains the person to produce alpha brain wave activity, which is believed to be incompatible with the experiencing of pain. Finger temperature feedback is used for migraine. When the patient learns to increase peripheral circulation, sympathetic nervous system activity in the cranial blood vessels is decreased. Temporal artery pulse amplitude feedback is also used to treat migraine by teaching the person to reduce temporal artery dilatation.

MULTIDISCIPLINARY PAIN-MANAGEMENT PROGRAMS

Therapeutic techniques to manage pain syndromes are generally directed at altering either the physiologic-sensory or the affective, behavioral, and cognitive components of pain. Comprehensive, holistic pain-management programs use a multidisciplinary approach including a combination of techniques directed at all components of pain. Most comprehensive pain-management programs began in the early 1970s. This approach involves comprehensive assessment and problem identification by an interdisciplinary team. The treatment plan includes elimination of unnecessary drug dependence, therapeutic measures to reduce the pain, physical rehabilitation, psychologic rehabilitation for the patient and family, and the return of control over the pain-management program to the patient. A comprehensive multidisciplinary pain assessment and pain profile, along with a complete physical and laboratory evaluation, are the first steps.

Generally, treatment is aimed at achieving maximum mobilization and relief of pain with the use of physical and psychologic treatment techniques. Physical reconditioning is initiated slowly. A sound and reasonably vigorous exercise program is gradually established. Physical treatment modalities may include massage, pressure, heat therapy- ,cold therapy, vibration, TENS, and acupuncture. An equally important component of chronic pain management is psychotherapy and cognitive-behavioral approaches. The patient is taught skills to help cope with the pain while cognitive restructuring is addressed. Biofeedback training is often used. Psychologic counseling for both the patient and the family is a critical component. A person who has been in pain for a prolonged time may have markedly altered interpersonal relationships and communication patterns with family, friends, and health care personnel. The chronic stress of the pain may have left the person's life in shambles. Most authorities recommend an intensive program of psychologic therapy over a short time, dealing with issues in the present, rather than the more traditional prolonged therapy.

In a holistic pain-management program, the patient learns to draw on inner resources and to assume responsibility for practicing skills that will help to cope with the pain. The person is helped to use family and significant others effectively. The patient learns to manage the pain.

The nurse is an important member of the multidisciplinary pain-management team. The nurse acts as planner, educator, patient advocate, interpreter, and supporter of the patient in pain and the families. Because pain can be present in any patient in a wide variety of care settings—home, hospital, clinic—the nurse must be knowledgeable

Table 6-12 Relaxation Strategies

Rhythmic Breathing*

1. Provide a quiet environment.
2. Help the patient get comfortable by elevating the legs with the knees bent (relaxing the leg, back, and abdominal muscles) or supporting the neck with a pillow. Check to see that arms and legs are not crossed.
3. Instruct patient to close eyes and to breathe in and out slowly, saying, "Breathe in, 2, 3, 4; breathe out, 2, 3, 4."
4. Once rhythmic breathing is established, instruct patient to listen to your voice, and with a low and steady voice, instruct patient to do the following:

   Breathe in and out slowly and deeply.
   Try to breathe from the abdomen.
   Feel more relaxed with each exhalation.
   Try to identify your own special feeling of relaxation (e.g., light and weightless or very heavy).
   While you are breathing, let your imagination take you to a place you remember as peaceful and pleasant; look around, listen to the sounds, feel the air, notice the smells.
   When you are ready to end this relaxation exercise, count silently from 1 to 3; on 1, move your lower body; on 2, move your upper body; on 3, breathe in deeply, open your eyes, and while breathing out slowly, say silently: "I am relaxed and alert." Stretch as if just waking up.

Progressive Relaxation*

1. Follow steps 1, 2, and 3 of rhythmic breathing.
2. Once patient is breathing slowly and comfortably, instruct patient to focus with each exhalation on a particular area of the body, starting with the feet, tensing and then relaxing them, while *feeling* the part relax.
3. Instruct patient to tense and then relax the calves, knees, and so on.

Relaxation by Sensory Pacing

1. Follow steps 1 and 2 of rhythmic breathing.
2. Instruct patient to slowly repeat and finish either in a low voice or to self each of the following sentences:

   Now I am aware of seeing . . .
   Now I am aware of feeling . . .
   Now I am aware of hearing . . .

   Instruct patient to repeat and complete each sentence 4 times, then 3 times, then twice, and finally once.
3. Instruct patient to allow the eyes to close when they feel heavy.

Relaxation by Color Exchange

1. Follow steps 1, 2, and 3 of rhythmic breathing.
2. Instruct patient to notice any tension, tightness, aches, or pains in the body and to give that sensation the first color that comes to mind.
3. Instruct patient to breathe in pure white light from the universe and send the light to the tense or painful place in the body, letting the white light surround the color of the discomfort.
4. Instruct patient to exhale the color of the discomfort and let the white light take its place.
5. Instruct patient to continue breathing in the white light and exhaling the color of the discomfort, allowing the white light to fill the entire body and bring about a sense of peace, well-being, and energy.

Modified Autogenic Relaxation

1. Follow steps 1, 2, and 3 of rhythmic breathing.
2. Instruct patient to repeat each of the following phrases to self 4 times, saying the first part of the phrase while breathing in for 2 to 3 sec, holding the breath for 2 to 3 sec, then saying the last part of the phrase while breathing out for 2 to 3 sec:

Breathing in	*Breathing out*
I am	relaxed
My arm and legs	are heavy and warm
My heartbeat	is calm and regular
My breathing	is free and easy
My abdomen	is loose and warm
My forehead	is cool
My mind	is quiet and still

Relaxing with Music

1. Provide patient with a tape recorder and headset.
2. Ask patient to select a favorite cassette of slow, quiet music.
3. Instruct patient to get into a comfortable position (either sitting or lying down but with arms and legs uncrossed) and to close eyes and listen to the music through the headset.
4. Instruct patient to imagine floating or drifting with the music while listening.

Rhythmic Massage

1. Massage near the area of pain in a circular, firm manner.
2. Avoid tender, red, or swollen areas.

*In conditioning of a relaxation response, a "signal breath" involving deep inhalation through the nose and forceful exhalation through the mouth is the key. This signal breath precedes and follows each run through the exercise.

about current therapies and flexible in trying new approaches to pain management.

Evaluation of the Pain-Management Plan

In acute and chronic pain situations, the nurse should evaluate the effectiveness of the pain-relief measures taken by the patient, nurses, and other health care personnel. The judgments about effectiveness are made by comparing the patient's self-report of pain location, intensity, quality, and pattern, and affective, behavioral, and cognitive responses before the intervention with additional reports and responses after the intervention. Both subjective and objective data enter into the evaluation, but it must be remembered that the patient is the final judge.

If the patient says that the relief measures are not adequate, the nurse should reassess the pain and also consider the following questions:[1]

1. Are a variety of pain-relief measures being used? (If not, additional measures should be added.)
2. Are the pain-relief measures being used before the pain becomes severe? (If not, an anticipatory analgesia regimen should be implemented.)
3. Is what the patient believes will be effective included in the pain-management protocol? (If not, the reasons should be determined.) Can classic conditioning be used if the patient cannot keep receiving what is perceived as most effective?
4. Is the patient willing and able to be a more active participant in the pain management? (If not, the reasons should be determined.) How can the patient be helped to become more active?
5. Can the patient be encouraged to try the pain-relief measure one or two more times, especially if some additional measures are implemented? A revised pain-management plan should then be formulated and implemented.

NEEDS OF CAREGIVERS

Working with the patient who is experiencing pain generates stress in the nurse as well as in other health care personnel. Pain, like death, is one of the most universally frightening experiences, not only for those experiencing it but also for those witnessing it. The patient's fear of the pain and feelings of powerlessness to control the pain elicit an awareness of the nurse's own vulnerability and limitations. Fear and a sense of powerlessness may be evoked. These affective experiences and the stress they engender may elicit defense mechanisms and inappropriate coping behaviors, such as alienation from or avoidance of the patient and the family and denial of the severity of the pain experience or of the fact that the patient has any pain at all.

The nurse working with the patient experiencing pain needs self-insight and value clarification. The nurse needs peer group involvement, not only to assist with value clarification but to offer support, guidance, and perhaps counseling on an ongoing informal and formal basis. In addition, consultation from experts in the area of pain management may be necessary. The nurse also needs ongoing in-service or continuing education to correct the myths and misconceptions that prevail about pain and pain management, such as the exaggerated fears of addicting the patient, which often results in the withholding of pain medication. Another educational need of the nurse is to keep abreast of the rapidly expanding knowledge in the area of pain and pain management and to acquire additional skills in this area.

Family teaching and the family-nurse relationships are extremely important. Assessment of the family and friends and their interaction with the patient is essential in the presence of a pain syndrome. Relationships are often inappropriate and stressful. Nursing interventions to teach the family and friends and to provide information on more effective coping techniques for themselves as well as strategies to help the patient are essential.

CRITICAL THINKING EXERCISES

CASE STUDY

PAIN

Patient Profile

Mrs. C. is a 280-pound (112 kg) 48-year-old African-American woman admitted for an incision and drainage of a right renal abscess.

Subjective Data

- RN for 20 years
- Lives alone
- Desires 0 pain during therapy but will accept 1-2 on a 0-10 scale
- Reports incision area pain as a 2-3 between dressing changes and as a 10 during dressing changes
- States sharp, pulling pain persists 1-2 hr after dressing change
- Reports pain between dressing changes controlled by 2 Percocet tablets
- Reports morphine 2 mg IV barely touches pain during dressing changes

Objective Data

- Requires qid dry to dry dressing changes
- Morphine 4-15 mg IV every 1-2 hr

Critical Thinking Questions

1. Initially, what dose of IV morphine should be given?
2. Describe the assessment data that supports the dose selected in question 1.
3. How long should the nurse wait after the IV morphine dose to begin the dressing change?
4. If an initial dose of 6 mg IV morphine reduces the pain to a 6 mid-dressing change, what nursing action is indicated?
5. What dose should be administered for subsequent dressing changes?
6. What additional pain therapies might the nurse plan to help Mrs. C through the dressing change?
7. Based on the data presented, write one or more appropriate nursing diagnosis. Are there any collaborative problems?

NURSING RESEARCH ISSUES

1. Does a person with acute, chronic nonmalignant, or cancer pain spontaneously tell others about the pain?
2. What information (location, intensity, quality, pattern) does the patient with pain tell others?
3. What is the most effective and efficient way to overcome misconceptions the patient has about addiction, dependence, and tolerance to opioid drugs?
4. Based on the patient's usual methods of coping with pain, what nonpharmacologic pain-management strategies are most effective in promoting pain relief?
5. What is the onset of action, peak action, and duration of action for specific nonpharmacologic pain-management strategies?

REVIEW QUESTIONS

The number of the question corresponds to the same-numbered objective at the beginning of the chapter.

1. The slowest fibers for pain conduction are the
   a. C fibers.
   b. A-alpha fibers.
   c. A-beta fibers.
   d. delta fibers.

2. Drugs that are considered as adjuvant analgesics according to the WHO Analgesic Ladder include
   a. nonopioid analgesics.
   b. tricyclic antidepressants.
   c. agonist-antagonist drugs.
   d. opioid-agonist drugs.

3. Acute pain is characterized by all of the following *except*
   a. it occurs abruptly.
   b. it is intensified by fear.
   c. it is not amenable to specific treatment.
   d. it persists until healing occurs.

4. All of the following affect the pain experience *except*
   a. emotional state.
   b. pain tolerance.
   c. pain intensity.
   d. size of thalamus.

5. An activity appropriate for the nurse during the pain assessment process is to
   a. conduct a comprehensive pain assessment.
   b. assess critical sensory components.
   c. provide appropriate treatment.
   d. teach the patient about pain therapies.

6. The recommended route of administration for morphine is

a. IM.
b. oral.
c. IV.
d. sublingual.

7. An important nursing responsibility related to pain is to

a. assume responsibility for eliminating the patient's pain.
b. believe what the patient says about the pain.
c. help the patient appear to not be in pain.
d. leave the patient alone to rest.

REFERENCES

1. McCaffery M, Beebe A: *Pain: a clinical manual for nursing practice,* St Louis, 1989, Mosby.
2. Merskey H, Bogduk N: *Classification of chronic pain: descriptions of chronic pain syndromes and definitions of pain terms,* Seattle, 1994, IASP Press.
3. Cassell EJ: The relationship between pain and suffering. In Hill CS, Fields WS, editors: *Advances in pain research and therapy,* ed 11, New York, 1989, Raven Press.
4. Bonica JJ, editor: *The management of pain,* ed 2, Philadelphia, 1990, Lea & Febiger.
5. Kelly JB, Payne R: Pain syndromes in the cancer patient. *Neurol Clin* 9:937, 1991.

*6. Maxam-Moore VV, Wilkie DJ, Woods SL: Analgesics for cardiac surgery patients in critical care: describing current practice, *Am J Crit Care* 3:31, 1994.

7. Ahles TA, Blanchard EB, Ruckdeschel JC: The multidimensional nature of cancer-related pain, *Pain* 17:277, 1983.
8. Wilkie DJ, Olsson GL, Metcalf CL: *Essentials of pain management; a nursing handbook,* Seattle, 1993, Optioncare.
9. Wall PD: Introduction. In Wall PD, Melzack R, editors: *Textbook of pain,* ed 2, New York, 1989, Churchill Livingston.
10. Besson JM, Chaouch A: Peripheral and spinal mechanisms of nociception, *Physiol Rev* 67:67, 1987.
11. Kanter TG: New strategies for the use of anti-inflammatory agents. In Dubner R, Gebhart GF, Bond MR, editors: *Proceedings of the Vth world congress on pain, pain research and clinical management,* ed 3, New York, 1988, Elsevier.
12. Stambaugh J, Drew J: A double-blind parallel evaluation of the efficacy of a single dose of ketoprofen in cancer pain, *J Clin Pharmacol* 28:S39, 1988.
13. Yaksh TL: The spinal pharmacology of anomalous pain processing. In Casey KL, editor: *Pain and central nervous system disease: the central pain syndromes,* New York, 1991, Raven Press.
14. Sato J, Perl ER: Adrenergic excitation of cutaneous pain receptors induced by peripheral nerve injury, *Science* 251:1608, 1991.

*15. Wilkie DJ and others: Behavior of patients with lung cancer: description and associations with oncologic and pain variables, *Pain* 51:231, 1992.

*16. Wilkie DJ and others: Cancer pain control behaviors: description and correlation with pain intensity, *Oncol Nurs Forum* 15:723, 1988.

17. Woolf CJ, Wiesenfield-Hallin Z: The systemic administration of local anaesthetics produce a selective depression of C-afferent fiber evoked activity in the spinal cord, *Pain* 23:361, 1985.
18. Woolf CJ, Thompson JW: Stimulation-induced analgesia: transcutaneous electrical nerve stimulation (TENS) and vibration. In Wall PD, Melzack R, editors: *Textbook of pain,* ed 3, New York, 1994, Churchill Livingston.
19. Woolf CJ: The dorsal horn: state-dependent sensory processing and the generation of pain. In Wall PD, Melzack R, editors: *Textbook of pain,* ed 3, New York, 1994, Churchill Livingstone.
20. Fields HL: *Pain,* New York, McGraw-Hill, 1987.
21. Talbot JD and others: Multiple representations of pain in human cerebral cortex, *Science* 251:1355, 1991.
22. Fields HL, Basbaum AL: Central nervous system mechanisms of pain modulation. In Wall PD, Melzack R, editors: *Textbook of pain,* ed 3, New York, Churchill Livingstone, 1994.
23. Levine JD, Gordon NC, Fields HL: The mechanism of placebo analgesia, *Lancet* 2:654, 1978.
24. Harkins SW and others: Geriatric pain. In Wall PD, Melzack R, editors: *Textbook of pain,* ed 3, New York, Churchill Livingstone, 1994.
25. McCaffery M, Ferrell BR: How vital are vital signs? *Nurs* 22:42, 1992.
26. Puntillo KA, Wilkie DJ: The assessment of pain in the critically ill. In Puntillo KA, editor: *Pain in the critically ill: assessment and management,* Rockville, MD, 1991, Aspen.

*27. Gaston-Johansson F, Albert M, Fagan E: Similarities in pain descriptions of four different ethnic-culture groups, *J Pain Symptom Manage* 5:94, 1990.

*28. Tesler MD and others: The word-graphic rating scale as a measure of children's and adolescents' pain intensity, *Res Nurs Health* 14:361, 1991.

29. Melzack R: The McGill pain questionnaire: major properties and scoring methods, *Pain* 1:277, 1975.
30. Agency for Health Care Policy and Research: *Clinical practice guideline. Acute pain management: operative or medical procedures and trauma.* Rockville, MD, 1992, US Department of Health and Human Services.
31. Miser AW and others: Prospective study of continuous intravenous and subcutaneous morphine infusion for therapy-related or cancer-related pain in children and young adults with cancer, *Clin J Pain* 2:101, 1986.
32. Miaskowski C: Current concepts in the assessment and management of cancer-related pain, *Medsurg Nurs* 2:113, 1993.
33. American Pain Society: *Principles of analgesic use in the treatment of acute pain and chronic cancer pain: a concise guide to medical practice,* ed 3, Skokie, IL, 1992.
34. Porter J, Jick H: Addiction rare in patients treated with narcotics, *N Engl J Med* 302:123, 1980.
35. Agency for Health Care Policy and Research: *Clinical practice guideline. Management of cancer pain.* Rockville, MD, 1994 US Department of Health and Human Services.
36. American Nurses Association: Position statement on the role of the registered nurse (RN) in the management of analgesia by catheter techniques (epidural, intrathecal, intrapleural, or peripheral nerve catheters), Washington, DC, 1990, The Association.
37. American Nurses Association: Compendium of position statements on the nurse's role in end-of-life decisions, Washington, DC, 1992, The Association.
38. World Health Organization: *Cancer pain relief,* Geneva, 1986, World Health Organization.
39. Nurse's guide to OTC analgesics, *Nursing* 93:66, 1993.
40. Wilkie DJ: Pharmacological management of cancer pain: summary-of-the-science, *JNCI* 85:1117, 1993.
41. Blake GJ: Close-up on opioid receptor subtypes, *Nursing* 95:55, 1995.
42. World Health Organization: *Cancer pain relief and palliative care,* Geneva, 1990, World Health Organization.
43. Portenoy RK and others: Plasma morphine and morphine-6-glucuronide during chronic morphine therapy for cancer pain: plasma profiles, steady-state concentrations, and the consequences of renal failure, *Pain* 47:13, 1991.

44. Glare P and others: A pilot study of the side effects of morphine sulfate in advanced cancer. 1st Congress of the European Association for Palliative Care, Abstract Book, Paris, October 17-19, 1990.
45. De Conno F and others: Hyperalgesia and myoclonus with intrathecal infusion of high-dose morphine, *Pain* 47:337, 1991.
46. Weinberg DS and others: Sublingual absorption of selected opioid analgesics, *Clin Pharmacol Ther* 44:335, 1988.
47. Streisand JB: OTFC: a new opioid delivery system, *APS Bulletin* 4:1, 1994.
48. Portenoy RK and others: Transdermal fentanyl for cancer pain: repeated dose pharmacokinetics, *Anesthesiology* 23:207, 1993.
49. Naber L, Jones G, Halm M: Epidural analgesia for effective pain control, *Crit Care Nurse* 17:69, 1994.
50. Culpepper-Morgan JA and others: Treatment of opioid-induced constipation with oral naloxone: a pilot study, *Clin Pharmacol Ther* 52:90, 1992.
51. King MF, Jacob PA: Special procedures. In Carroll D, Bowsher D, editors, *Pain management and nursing care,* Oxford, 1993, Butterworth-Heinemann.
52. Charman RA: Physiotherapy for the relief of pain. In Carroll D, Bowsher D, editors, *Pain management and nursing care,* Oxford, 1993, Butterworth-Heinemann.
53. Lehmann JF, de Lateur B: Ultrasound, shortwave, microwave, laser, superficial heat and cold in the treatment of pain. In Wall PD, Melzack R, editors, *Textbook of pain,* ed 3, New York, 1994, Churchill Livingstone.
54. Krainick FU, Thoden U: Spinal cord stimulation. In Wall PD, Melzack R, editors, *Textbook of pain,* ed 3, New York, 1994, Churchill Livingstone.
55. Young RF, Rinaldi PC: Brain stimulation for relief of chronic pain. In Wall PD, Melzack R, editors, *Textbook of pain,* ed 3, New York, 1994, Churchill Livingstone.
56. Spira JL, Spiegel J: Hypnosis and related techniques in pain management. In Turk DC, Feldman CS, editors: *Noninvasive approaches to pain management in the terminally ill,* New York, 1992, Haworth Press.

*Nursing-research based articles.

Chapter 7

NURSING ROLE IN MANAGEMENT
Shock

Judith J. Barrows

Learning Objectives

1. Define the shock syndrome.
2. Differentiate among the three major classifications of shock related to cause and precipitating factors.
3. Describe the pathophysiology and clinical manifestations of the shock syndrome.
4. Describe the effects of shock on the major body systems.
5. Compare the therapeutic and pharmacologic management of the patient with the different types of shock.
6. Discuss the nursing management of the patient in shock.

SHOCK SYNDROME

Shock is a clinical syndrome resulting in decreased blood flow to body tissues causing cellular dysfunction and eventual organ failure.[1] Regardless of the cause of shock, the end result is inadequate supply of oxygen and nutrients to body cells from *impaired tissue perfusion.* Shock is a complex group of signs and symptoms that may be precipitated by a variety of etiologic factors. It is important to note that shock cannot be defined solely in terms of hypotension, because the shock syndrome may be manifested in the absence of hypotension. Conversely, hypotension may occur in the absence of shock.

Significance

Once shock occurs, multiple organ dysfunction syndrome (MODS), with a very high mortality rate, can develop rapidly.[1] (MODS is discussed in Chapter 61). Although the morbidity and mortality rates associated with shock are extremely difficult to determine, some estimates have been reported. For example, an estimate of the annual incidence of sepsis in the United States is 400,000 cases with 200,000 of these cases progressing to septic shock.[2] The mortality rates from severe sepsis and septic shock have changed little over the past several decades. The mortality rate of septic shock is 40% to 60%.[3] Septic shock is the most common cause of death in intensive care units in the United States. The estimated incidence of acute anaphylactic reactions is one out of every 2700 hospitalized patients.[4] Despite current therapeutic measures, most studies indicate a high mortality rate for cardiogenic shock. In-hospital fatality rates range from 70% to 100%. The 5-year survival rate is only 40% for the few hospital survivors.[5] In hypovolemic shock, the mortality rate is directly affected by the amount of time from injury and blood loss to the initiation of volume replacement.[6] For all types of shock, the elderly population has a greater mortality rate than other age groups.[6]

Classification of Shock

Although there have been many attempts to classify shock, none have been totally satisfactory. Table 7-1 presents one classification system, listing common types of shock and precipitating factors. This classification is based on a consideration of defects in the three primary mechanisms responsible for adequate circulation: (1) vascular tone *(distributive shock),* (2) the ability of the heart to act as a pump *(cardiogenic shock),* and (3) intravascular volume *(hypovolemic shock).* Patients may have more than one form of shock simultaneously. For example, hypovolemic and septic shock may coexist.

Table 7-2 compares the hemodynamic effects of the three types of shock. Hemodynamic monitoring is discussed in Chapter 61.

Distributive Shock. Distributive shock includes three types of shock: neurogenic, septic, and anaphylactic. In distributive shock, relative hypovolemia occurs when vasodilatation increases the size of the vascular space and results in altered distribution of the blood volume rather than actual loss of volume. This type of shock is often complicated by loss of intravascular fluid from increased

---

Reviewed by Marilyn Sawyer Sommers, RN, PhD, Assistant Professor, College of Nursing and Health and Staff Nurse, Surgical Intensive Care Unit, University of Cincinnati Medical Center, Cincinnati, OH; Sharon Walker, RN, MSN, CCRN, CNRN, Clinical Nurse Specialist-ICU/CCU, Lovelace Health System, Albuquerque, NM; and Julie Dax, RN, MSN, Nurse Educator, Adult Intensive Care Units, University of New Mexico Hospital, Albuquerque, NM.

Table 7-1 Classification and Precipitating Factors of Shock

Distributive Shock

Neurogenic Shock

Injury and disease to the spinal cord
Spinal anesthesia, deep general anesthesia, or epidural block
Vasomotor center depression (e.g., severe pain, drugs, hypoglycemia, emotional stress)

Septic Shock

Infection (e.g., urinary tract, respiratory tract, postabortion, postpartum, caused by invasive procedures [especially urologic procedures] and indwelling lines and catheters)
Compromised patients, including older adults, patients with chronic disease (e.g., diabetes, cancer, acquired immunodeficiency syndrome), patients receiving immunosuppressive therapy, malnourished or debilitated patients

Anaphylactic Shock

Drugs (especially penicillin)
Insect bites/stings
Contrast media
Blood transfusions
Anesthetic agents
Foods
Vaccines

Cardiogenic Shock

Myocardial infarction (most common cause)
Dysrhythmias
Severe congestive heart failure
Cardiomyopathy
Obstructive causes, including pericardial tamponade, pericardial diseases, tension pneumothorax, acute valvular damage, pulmonary embolism

Hypovolemic Shock

External Fluid Losses

Hemorrhage (most common cause)
Burns
Excessive use of diuretics
Loss of gastrointestinal fluid (vomiting, diarrhea, fistulas, nasogastric suctioning)
Diabetes insipidus
Diabetic ketoacidosis
Profound diaphoresis

Internal Fluid Shifts

Pooling of blood in the interstitial spaces (ascites, peritonitis, bowel obstruction)
Internal bleeding (fracture of long bones, ruptured spleen, hemothorax, severe pancreatitis, femoral arterial punctures or catheters in patients on anticoagulant therapy)

capillary permeability. In distributive shock there is no change in the blood volume but rather a decrease in the vascular tone.

Neurogenic shock. Neurogenic shock, an uncommon and often transitory disorder, is caused by massive vasodilatation as a result of loss of sympathetic vasoconstrictor tone in the vascular smooth muscles and impairment of autonomic function. The massive vasodilatation causes pooling of blood in the venous vasculature, decreased venous return to the heart, decreased cardiac output (CO), and, eventually, inadequate tissue perfusion. Typically, the patient with neurogenic shock will develop hypotension and bradycardia. Hypotension is a result of the vasodilatation, and the decreased heart rate (HR) is caused by the increased vagal tone from the now unopposed parasympathetic nervous system.

There are several precipitating factors that can lead to neurogenic shock (see Table 7-1). Disease or injury to the spinal cord can interrupt transmission of sympathetic nerve impulses to peripheral blood vessels. After a spinal cord injury, neurogenic shock usually lasts from hours to weeks.[7] Spinal anesthesia can also block the transmission of impulses from the sympathetic nervous system. Depression of the vasomotor center of the medulla as a result of drugs, fear, severe pain, or hypoglycemia can also decrease vasoconstrictor tone of peripheral blood vessels.

Septic shock. Septic shock is most commonly caused by gram-negative bacteria, although many patients with septic shock never have positive blood cultures.[8] Septic shock can also occur secondary to staphylococcal, streptococci, fungal, and protozoan (e.g., *Pneumocystis carinii*) infections.

When gram-negative bacteremia occurs, it appears that endotoxin, a component of the gram-negative bacteria cell walls, triggers a cascade of host inflammatory responses and is responsible for the major detrimental effects. When endotoxin binds to monocytes and macrophages, it stimulates the release of tumor necrosis factor (TNF) and interleukin-1 (IL-1). These mediators stimulate the release and/or activation of other mediators, including platelet-activating factor (PAF), prostaglandins, leukotrienes, thromboxane A_2, kinins, and complement. These factors are responsible for widespread vasodilatation and increased capillary permeability, resulting in decreased systemic vascular resistance and normal or high CO as a result of the decreased peripheral resistance. In addition, endotoxins cause the release of histamine, which results in increased capillary permeability and further decreases circulating blood volume.

The clinical presentation of this type of shock is often subtle, especially in the older, debilitated, or malnourished patient. The blood pressure (BP) is usually low, but the skin is often warm and dry because of the vasodilatation. In the early stage of septic shock the patient may have polyuria, up to 100 ml per hour.[9]

Myocardial depressant substance works together with TNF, PAF, and other mediators to suppress myocardial function. Myocardial depression is almost always present despite an initial rise in CO.[10] Hemodynamic stability is further compromised by endothelial factors such as endothelin-1, an intense vasoconstrictor, and endothelium-derived relaxing factor (nitric oxide), which is a vasodilator.

The terms "warm," or early shock, and "cold," or late shock, should not be used. The distinct stages of septic shock are not as evident as once thought to be; high CO with low systemic vascular resistance (SVR) is likely to be

Table 7-2 Hemodynamic Effects of Shock

Type of Shock	Cardiac Output	Central Venous Pressure	Systemic Vascular Resistance	Pulmonary Artery Pressure*	Pulmonary Capillary Wedge Pressure*
Hypovolemic	↓	↓	↑	↓	↓
Cardiogenic	↓	↑ or nl	↑	↑	↑
Anaphylactic	↑ or nl	↓	↓	↓ or nl	↓ or nl
Septic					
Early	↑ or nl	↓	↓	↓	↓
Late	↓ or ↑	↓ or ↑	↓ or ↑	↑	↓ or ↑
Neurogenic	↓	↓	↓	↓	↓

nl, Normal.
*Pulmonary pressures are explained in Chapter 61.

found throughout a patient's course of septic shock if the patient is receiving adequate fluid. Survivors of septic shock typically have resolved their high CO and low SVR in the first 24 hours. Cardiovascular parameters, which are associated with a high mortality in septic patients, include persistent elevation in both heart rate and CO with low SVR and refractory hypotension for more than 24 hours.[11]

The longevity of patients with complex, chronic diseases has increased the number of patients who are at risk for developing severe infection and subsequent complications. The rise in the incidence of gram-negative sepsis is largely a result of advances in health care and technology and the rise in the number of immunocompromised patients.[11] Septic shock is more common in neonates and infants who have underdeveloped immune defenses and in the older population who often have debilitating chronic diseases and weakened immune systems. Table 7-1 lists causes of septic shock.

Anaphylactic shock. Anaphylaxis is an acute and potentially life-threatening allergic reaction. It is an immediate hypersensitivity reaction characterized by dilatation of arterioles and capillaries and increased capillary permeability, causing microvascular leakage throughout the body. Anaphylactic shock can result in respiratory failure as a result of laryngeal edema or severe bronchospasm, and circulatory failure resulting from vasodilatation. (Anaphylactic shock is discussed in Chapter 10.) Generally the severity of an anaphylactic reaction is directly related to how rapidly the onset of symptoms occurs.[4]

A patient can develop a severe allergic reaction, possibly leading to anaphylactic shock, after ingesting or being injected with an antigen to which the person has previously been sensitized. Parenteral administration of an antigen is the route most likely to cause anaphylaxis. However, oral, topical, and inhalation routes of administration of an antigen have been known to cause anaphylactic reactions.[4] Examples of foreign substances that can act as antigens are listed in Table 7-1.

Hypovolemic Shock. Hypovolemic shock occurs when there is an actual loss of intravascular fluid volume. Loss of intravascular volume can be due to either actual external fluid loss (*actual hypovolemia*) or internal fluid shifts from the intravascular space to the interstitial or intracellular spaces (*relative hypovolemia*). Loss of fluid results in decreased venous return to the heart, decreased stroke volume, decreased CO, circulatory insufficiency, and eventually inadequate tissue perfusion. In hypovolemic shock there is no decrease in the pumping ability of the heart or dilatation of the vascular space. The fluid that is lost may be either whole blood, plasma, or water and electrolytes.

In relative hypovolemia (e.g., burn injury), the fluid has not left the body, but has shifted from the intravascular space and is unavailable for circulation. Increased capillary permeability can cause pooling of fluid in the interstitial spaces. Plasma is the primary fluid lost from the vascular space in burn injuries (see Chapter 21). Because of increased vascular permeability, there is a rapid shift of plasma from the vascular space to the interstitial space. The greater the burn area, the greater the quantity of plasma lost. This loss of plasma from the intravascular space causes increased viscosity of the blood and sludging of blood components. The latter also contributes to increased SVR and decreased tissue perfusion.

The most common cause of external fluid loss is hemorrhage (an excessive loss of whole blood). The amount of blood loss that results in the shock syndrome depends on the efficiency of a person's compensatory mechanisms. A healthy adult can compensate for a sudden loss of 10% of total blood volume, primarily using sympathetic-mediated vasoconstriction. However, if 20% to 25% of the blood volume is lost rapidly, the compensatory mechanisms usually begin to fail. Hemorrhagic shock frequently occurs after trauma and is secondary to such problems as bleeding esophageal varices or a ruptured aortic aneurysm. It can also occur as a result of a surgical procedure, delivery of a baby, or coagulation disorders.

Another common cause of hypovolemic shock is loss of gastrointestinal (GI) fluids. GI fluid losses usually occur secondary to severe vomiting, diarrhea, or excessive drainage from a nasogastric tube or fistula and result in a loss of water and electrolytes. Susceptibility to shock as a result of these factors is generally related to age. Infants and older adults are at highest risk because of the decreased efficiency of their physiologic compensatory mechanisms.

Cardiogenic Shock. Cardiogenic shock, often referred to as *pump failure,* occurs when the heart can no longer pump blood efficiently to all parts of the body and when CO is decreased. There is no decreased intravascular volume or vasodilatation of the vascular space. Cardiogenic shock is usually the result of left ventricular dysfunction. However, the right ventricle can also be involved. The ventricles are the pumping chambers of the heart and when either one fails, blood backs up. In right ventricular dysfunction, the blood is backed up into the systemic circulation. Left ventricular dysfunction causes blood to back up into the pulmonary system causing pulmonary congestion and decreased CO to the systemic circulation. A vicious cycle develops as the SVR increases in response to the decreased CO. The failing heart now has to pump harder against this higher systemic resistance.

The major cause of cardiogenic shock is extensive myocardial necrosis caused by a myocardial infarction (MI). Cardiogenic shock occurs when at least 40% to 45% of the left ventricular myocardium has been damaged by infarction.[12] This damage to the myocardium can be a result of more than one MI, occurring over a period of time. With the infarction there is a decrease in myocardial compliance and, therefore, a decrease in contractility. Thus decreased functioning of the left ventricle occurs, as evidenced by decreased CO and BP. Consequently there is less arterial pressure to perfuse the coronary arteries. This continued decrease in coronary perfusion causes increased ischemia of the myocardium leading to a larger infarction, less contractility, dysrhythmias, and metabolic acidosis. These conditions further reduce the effective functioning of the left ventricle.

Other causes of cardiogenic shock include cardiomyopathy, cardiac dysrhythmias that impair the efficiency of myocardial contractions, and congestive heart failure (see Chapter 32). Cardiogenic shock can also occur when there is sudden obstruction of blood flow as a result of such factors as cardiac tamponade, tension pneumothorax, acute valvular dysfunction, and pulmonary embolism. In addition, cardiogenic shock may develop as a result of ventricular septal defect or rupture of the ventricular wall. Regardless of the cause, the extent of pump failure depends on the degree of heart muscle impairment and the adequacy of compensatory mechanisms.

Stages of Shock

Shock is a dynamic event in which several different processes may be occurring at the same time. In addition, a patient may progress toward death or toward normal homeostatic functioning over widely varying time periods. The shock syndrome can be divided into four stages: (1) initial stage, (2) compensatory stage, (3) progressive stage, and (4) irreversible or refractory stage. Although there are no clear cut divisions between the stages, they provide a framework for discussing the shock syndrome.

The shock syndrome may develop rapidly or gradually, depending on the severity of the initial insult and the adequacy of compensatory mechanisms. If these mechanisms can maintain adequate arterial pressure and CO, a compensatory stage is reached. If compensatory mechanisms are insufficient to restore effective perfusion to vital organs, either because of the initial insult or its prolonged duration, clinical evidence of reduced organ perfusion and progressive or irreversible shock will be apparent.

Initial Stage. During the initial stage no clinical signs or symptoms are present; however, changes are occurring at the cellular level. In most patients with shock, CO and tissue perfusion are reduced, resulting in decreased delivery of oxygen and other nutrients to the cells. At this stage, aerobic metabolism is decreased, anaerobic metabolism is increased, and excess lactic acid is produced.[13] Septic shock is characterized by increased CO and low SVR.

Compensatory Stage. The compensatory stage is the reversible stage in which compensatory mechanisms are effective in maintaining adequate perfusion to the vital organs. In this stage, most of the metabolic needs of the body continue to be met. The pathophysiologic sequence of events occurring during this stage is detailed in Fig. 7-1.

Pathophysiology. Regardless of the cause of shock, the body attempts to compensate for a decrease in tissue perfusion in a variety of ways. First, a decrease in arterial pressure causes a similar decrease in capillary hydrostatic pressure. When the hydrostatic pressure no longer exceeds the colloidal osmotic pressure, fluid moves from the interstitial space to the intravascular space. This process is sometimes called *autotransfusion.* It may add sufficient volume to the vascular space to maintain normal arterial pressure without the aid of other compensatory mechanisms.

A reduction in mean arterial pressure will inhibit baroreceptor activity, resulting in stimulation of the vasomotor center in the medulla, causing activation of the sympathetic nervous system and release of epinephrine and norepinephrine (see Table 30-1). Stimulation of α_1-adrenergic receptors causes selective peripheral vasoconstriction. Blood flow to the heart and brain is maintained, whereas blood flow to the kidneys, gastrointestinal (GI) tract, lungs, muscles, and skin is decreased. β-adrenergic receptor stimulation causes a mild increase in HR and force of contraction, resulting in increased CO. This sympathetic stimulation also causes dilatation of the coronary arteries, resulting in an increase in oxygen to the myocardium, which now has an increased oxygen demand as a result of the increase in HR and contractility.

The decrease in blood flow to the kidneys stimulates the release of renin into the blood. In the bloodstream, renin activates angiotensinogen to produce angiotensin I, which then circulates to the lungs where it is converted to angiotensin II (see Fig. 42-6). Angiotensin is a strong vasoconstrictor, resulting in arterial and venous constriction. The net result is increased venous return to the heart and an increase in BP. Angiotensin also stimulates the adrenal cortex to release aldosterone, which results in sodium reabsorption by the kidneys. The increased sodium reabsorption raises the serum osmolarity and stimulates the release of antidiuretic hormone (ADH). (ADH is also

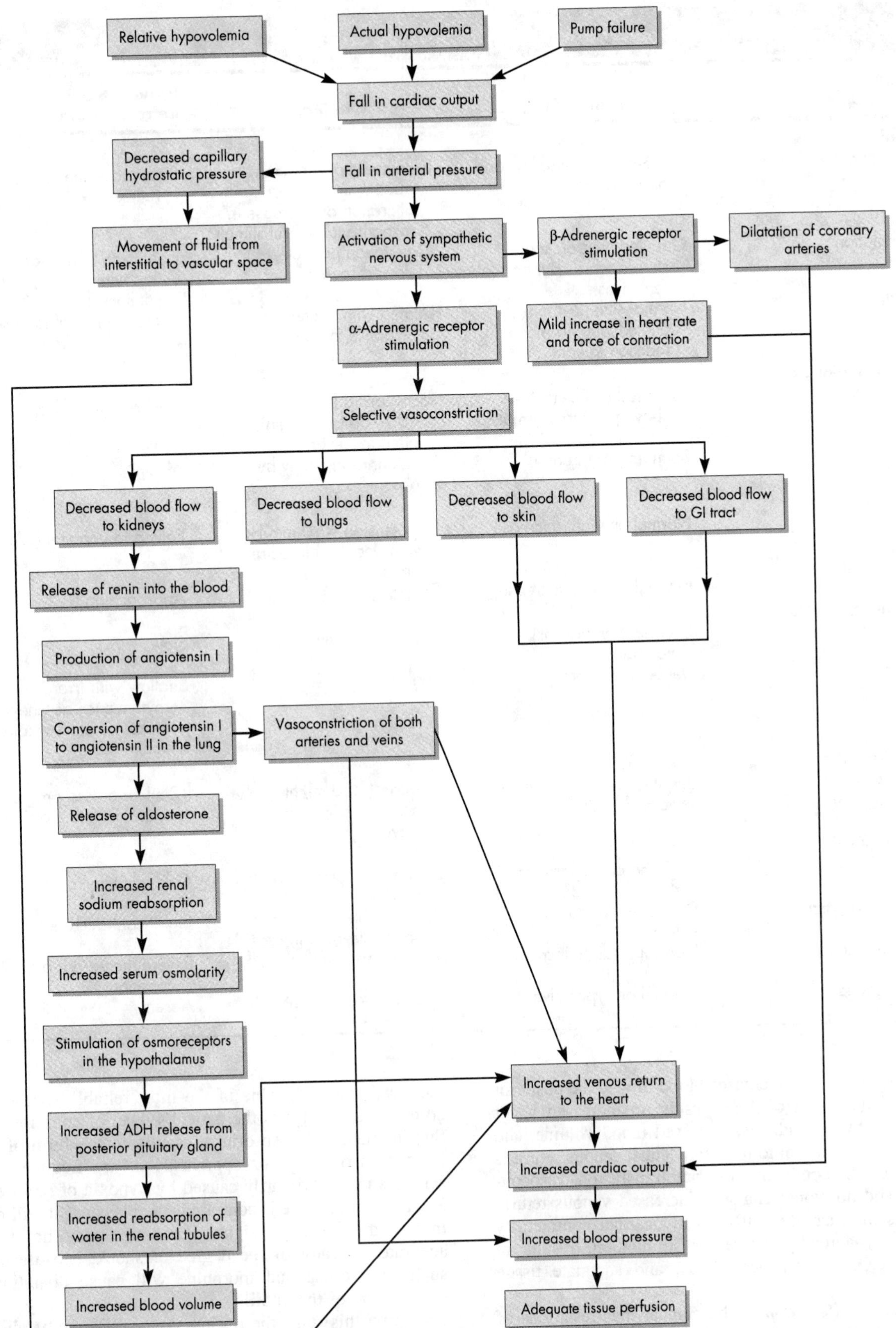

Fig. 7-1 Compensatory stage: reversible stage during which compensatory mechanisms are effective and homeostasis is maintained. *ADH*, Antidiuretic hormone; *GI*, gastrointestinal.

Table 7-3 Clinical Manifestations Correlated with Severity of Shock

Clinical Manifestations	Compensatory Stage	Progressive Stage	Irreversible or Refractory Stage
Neurologic Status			
Level of consciousness	Restlessness, irritability, and apprehension	Listlessness or agitation; apathy, confusion, alteration or decrease in response to painful stimuli	Unconsciousness, absent reflexes likely
Orientation	Oriented, verbal, some slurred words but normal sentences	Orientation possible, slowed speech	Confusion and disorientation with slurred, incoherent speech
Pupils	Normal size (2-4 mm) or dilated with normal reaction to light	Dilated with decreased response to light	Dilated, minimal to absent response to light
Cardiovascular Status			
Heart rate	Increased (20 beats/min above patient's normal rate)	Tachycardia (rate of 100-150 beats/min), often irregular	Slow and irregular
Peripheral pulses	Bounding or thready	Weak, thready, may be absent	Absent
Blood Pressure			
Systolic	Normal or slight decrease	Hypotension <90 mm Hg with decrease in pulse pressure	Falling to unobtainable
Diastolic	Normal or slight increase	Falling	Approaching 0
Respiratory Status			
Rate	Greater than patient's normal rate	Rapid, >20/min	Slow
Depth	Deeper than normal	Shallow	Shallow with irregular rhythm such as Cheyne-Stokes or Biot's respirations
Renal Status			
Urine output	Slight decrease but within normal limits	Oliguria (<20 ml/hr) with increase in specific gravity	18 ml/hr or less, progressing to anuria with proteinuria
General Status			
Appearance of skin	Pale and cool (warm and flushed in septic shock)	Cold and clammy, cyanosis possible	Cold, clammy, cyanotic, and mottled
Body temperature	Decrease, normal, or increase	Usually subnormal (subnormal or elevated in sepsis)	Significant decrease
Degree of thirst	Normal or slight increase	Marked increase	Severe increase if patient conscious
Bowel sounds	Normal or hypoactive	Hypoactive or absent	Absent

released when there is decreased blood flow to the posterior pituitary.) The action of ADH results in increased water reabsorption by the kidneys, increased blood volume, and increased venous return to the heart. Thus, venous return is increased by the combination of autotransfusion, vasoconstriction, and hormonal changes. Increased venous return, as well as the increased HR and myocardial contractility caused by β-adrenergic receptor stimulation, results in increased CO, maintenance of BP, and adequate tissue perfusion.

Clinical manifestations. The clinical manifestations of the compensatory stage may be subtle and can be overlooked (Table 7-3). One of the most reliable signs of the compensatory stage is the patient's level of consciousness. Subtle changes in sensorium, usually in the form of restlessness, irritability, or apprehension, are frequently observed and are primarily caused by hypoxia of brain cells. Sedation at this time is contraindicated because it will mask important neurologic signs. Pupil size may not be an accurate indicator of the degree of shock, because drugs such as atropine and morphine will cause dilatation or constriction of the pupil.

During this stage the resting supine BP may be slightly elevated, slightly decreased, or normal for the patient. For this reason the BP may not be a useful indicator at this stage. Orthostatic hypotension (a decrease in systolic BP of at least 15 mm Hg when a patient is raised from a flat position to an elevation of 90 degrees or standing) is significant and indicates absolute or relative volume depletion.

The HR in the compensatory stage is moderately increased. The pulse may be bounding or thready, depending on the stroke volume and the degree of peripheral vasoconstriction. Respirations increase in rate and depth in an attempt to compensate for tissue hypoxia, resulting in respiratory alkalosis. Urine output may begin to decrease because of reduced renal perfusion as a result of vasoconstriction. Because of extravascular volume depletion, the patient may complain of thirst. In addition, thirst may be caused by decreased secretion of saliva secondary to peripheral vasoconstriction. Vasoconstriction in the skin will result in cool and pale extremities. An exception is septic shock, in which the skin may be warm and dry. The body temperature at this stage will be slightly decreased except in septic shock, in which it may be elevated. Bowel sounds will often be hypoactive because of decreased peristalsis as a result of reduced blood flow to the GI system.

Progressive Stage. During the progressive stage of shock compensatory mechanisms are becoming ineffective and may even be detrimental to the patient. The pathophysiologic sequence of events occurring during this stage is outlined in Fig. 7-2. Aggressive management is necessary at this stage to reverse the shock state.

Pathophysiology. When shock is not detected and the precipitating cause is not corrected during the earlier stages, a massive sympathetic nervous system response occurs. Profound vasoconstriction of most vascular beds occurs with some peripheral vessels possibly becoming totally occluded. Renal ischemia leads to activation of the renin-angiotensin mechanism, causing even more pronounced vasoconstriction. Despite the attempt of the body to increase CO by increasing the HR and myocardial contractility, there is a net decrease in CO. This decreased CO and profound peripheral vasoconstriction lead to tissue hypoxia, which causes the cells to undergo anaerobic metabolism. A by-product of anaerobic cellular metabolism is lactic acid production. Metabolic acidosis results from the accumulation of lactic acid and impaired renal excretion of acids. As the shock state progresses, the rise in the lactic acid level will often correlate with the severity of the shock state. Acidosis has a direct depressant effect on cardiac function by impairing calcium metabolism within myocardial cells.

Associated with the sympathetic nervous system response is the secretion of large amounts of catecholamines from the adrenal medulla. Catecholamines enhance the cellular metabolism of the brain and heart. Catecholamines also stimulate the liver to undergo glycogenolysis, releasing its glycogen stores in the form of glucose. In addition, the pancreatic release of insulin is suppressed. Therefore the brain, which does not require insulin for glucose utilization, has large quantities of glucose available for metabolism.

Clinical manifestations. The manifestations of the intermediate or progressive stage of shock are presented in Table 7-3. The patient demonstrates listlessness, apathy, and confusion. In addition, a decreased response to painful stimuli may be observed.

When the BP begins to fall, the patient is no longer in compensatory shock. Regardless of the previous normal BP, a systolic pressure below 80 mm Hg should be regarded as a danger signal. It is important to remember that a hypertensive patient does not often initially display a pressure this low. A guide for determining hypotension is a reduction in BP greater than 25% of the baseline level for the patient. In addition to hypotension, a narrowed pulse pressure (difference between systolic and diastolic BP) is often present. This finding indicates decreased stroke volume from a decrease in systolic pressure and a normal or elevated diastolic pressure. Since cuff pressures are likely to be inaccurate during this stage of shock because of the severe peripheral vasoconstriction, intraarterial monitoring may be used to provide more reliable pressure readings.

Tachycardia is evident during this stage of shock, and the pulse is weak and thready. Older adults and patients who are receiving β-adrenergic blocking drugs may be an exception and show little HR change. Other cardiovascular effects of shock during the progressive stage are shown in Table 7-3.

Respirations increase in rate in an attempt to compensate for tissue hypoxia and metabolic acidosis. However, the respirations become more shallow as the patient begins to tire and weaken. Urine output decreases and may fall below 0.5 ml/kg/hr, indicating inadequate renal perfusion, which can lead to renal failure. The lips and mucosa are dry, and the patient may continue to complain of thirst. The skin is cold, pale, and clammy, with slow capillary refill noted. There may be cyanosis caused by tissue hypoxia. Body temperature is usually subnormal.

Irreversible or Refractory Stage. Irreversible or refractory stage of shock is the stage during which compensatory mechanisms are either nonfunctioning or totally ineffective. Cellular necrosis and MODS may occur. Attempts to restore the BP have failed, and death is imminent.

Pathophysiology. As shock progresses, the sympathetic nervous system activity can no longer compensate to maintain homeostasis. Thus one of the major compensatory mechanisms has failed. There is pooling and sludging of blood because of the lack of vasomotor tone. Thrombosis of the small blood vessels also occurs.

Tissue hypoxia resulting from peripheral vasoconstriction and decreased CO makes it necessary for cells to metabolize anaerobically (Fig. 7-3). The accumulation of lactic acid and other acid metabolites in the body's tissues contributes to cell death. The acid environment also causes increased capillary permeability and dilatation of the precapillary sphincters. Increased capillary permeability allows fluid and plasma proteins to leave the vascular space. Because the venous end of the capillaries remains constricted and the arterial end is dilated, blood pools in the capillary bed. This also causes fluid to move out of the vascular space. The loss of fluid from the vascular space leads to hypotension, which causes further peripheral vasoconstriction, and a vicious cycle of decompensation ensues.

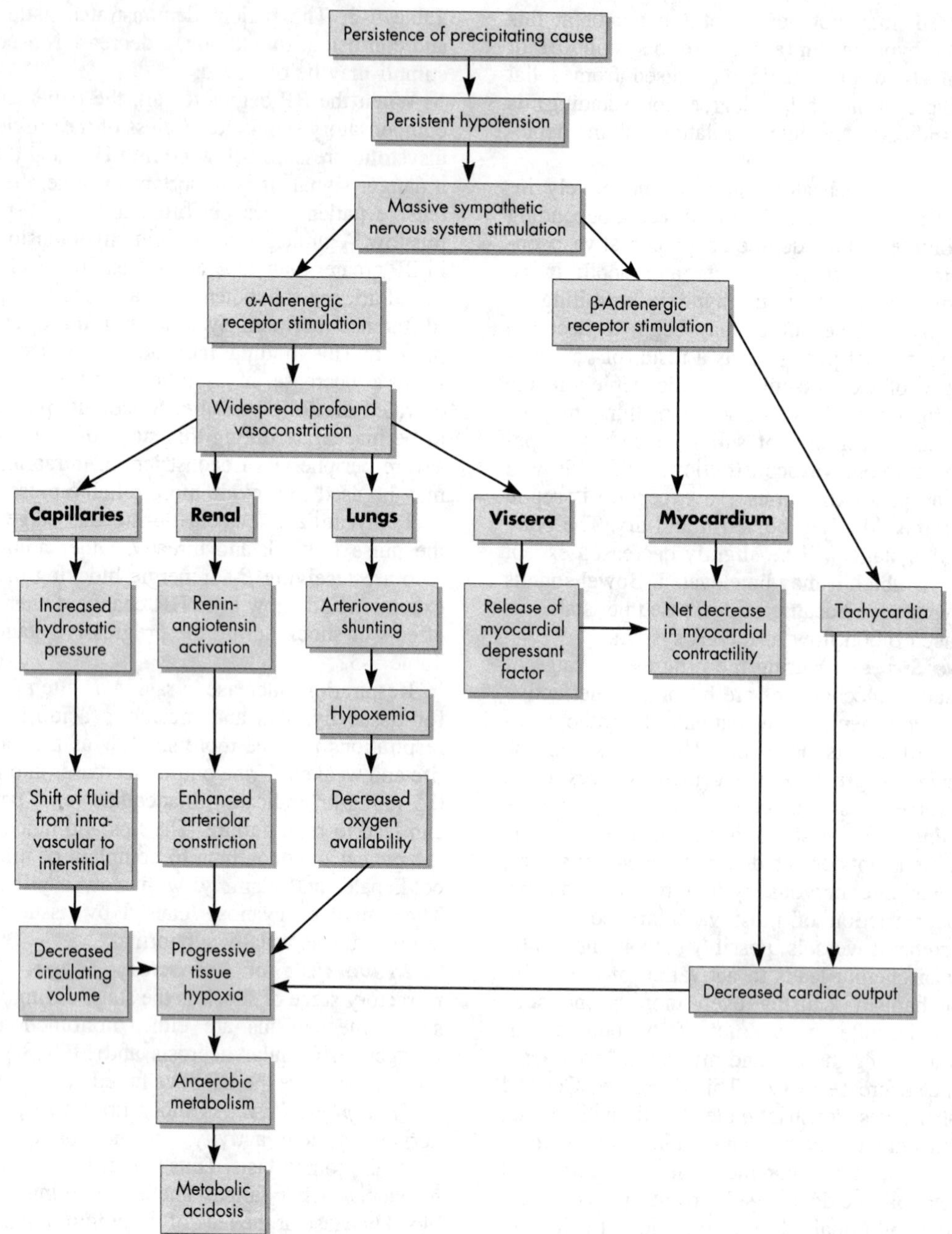

Fig. 7-2 Progressive stage: compensatory mechanisms are becoming ineffective and fail to maintain perfusion to vital organs.

As shock progresses, hypotension and the resulting tachycardia decrease coronary blood flow leading to myocardial depression, which further decreases CO. Cerebral blood flow can no longer be maintained and severe cerebral ischemia occurs. The body cannot maintain vasoconstriction for long with the vicious cycle repeating itself. Consequently, failure of the medullary vasomotor center occurs, which results in loss of sympathetic tone. The result is respiratory or cardiac arrest and death.[13]

Clinical manifestations. During the late or irreversible stage of shock, all body systems, especially the cardiovascular system, show evidence of decompensation (Table 7-3). The patient is usually unconscious and may be unresponsive to all stimuli. The systolic BP continues to fall and may not respond to therapeutic measures to raise it. The diastolic blood pressure falls toward 0. The HR becomes progressively slower. The pulse is weak, and a pulse deficit may be present. Cardiac dysrhythmias may develop because of an ischemic myocardium and increased serum potassium levels from the release of potassium from the dead cells.

Because of respiratory center depression, there are likely to be slow, shallow respirations with an irregular rhythm

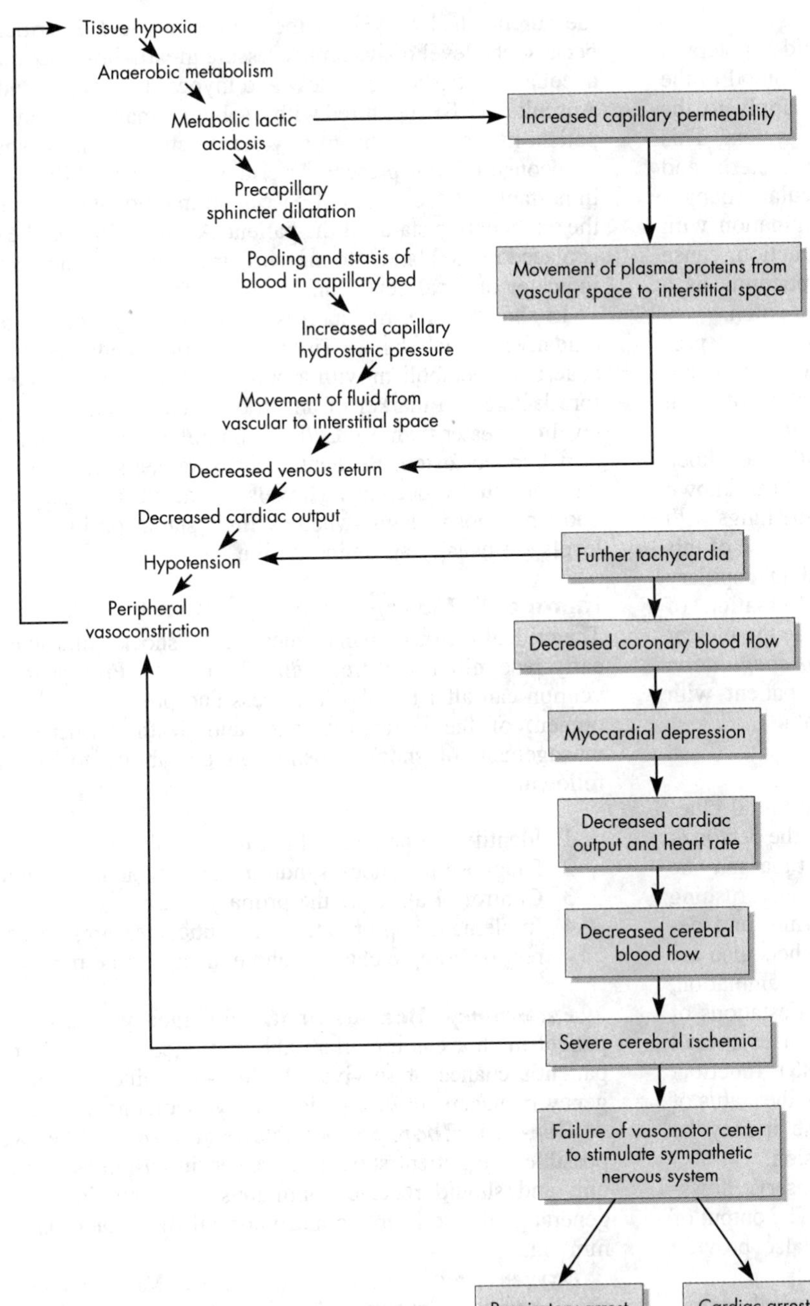

Fig. 7-3 Irreversible or refractory stage: compensatory mechanisms are not functioning or are totally ineffective leading to multiple organ dysfunction syndrome (MODS).

and sometimes Cheyne-Stokes respirations. If the patient is in an intensive care unit, intubation and mechanical ventilation will usually be used. Damage to the pulmonary endothelial cells increases capillary permeability and interstitial and alveolar edema, and hemorrhage and impaired gas exchange may occur. The resulting hypoxemia and respiratory acidosis will further decrease tissue O_2 delivery.

Ischemia of the intestinal mucosa also increases permeability, allowing bacteria and their toxins to enter the bloodstream and causing sepsis. Renal ischemia may result in acute tubular necrosis with altered fluid and electrolyte and other metabolic disturbances. Urine output is minimal, and there may be a progressive rise in serum creatinine and blood urea nitrogen (BUN) levels, indicating some degree of acute renal failure.

The skin is cold and clammy, with a significant decrease in temperature. (In septic shock, the patient's body temperature may be either elevated or subnormal, depending on the age and clinical condition of the patient.) Cyanosis may be present and is usually observed in the lips, mucous membranes, and nail beds. However, it may be more obvious in the palms, soles, and palpebral conjunctiva (inside the eyelid) of dark-skinned patients.

Complications of Shock

Infection may be a complication of shock and a potential cause of the shock syndrome. The shunting of blood to the vital organs results in a decreased nutrient supply to the various parts of the mononuclear phagocyte system. This may decrease the body's ability to remove bacteria and their endotoxins from the blood. The vascular changes resulting in hypoxia to the intestine, in combination with the depressed monocytes and macrophage function, cause patients to be particularly susceptible to septicemia as a result of gram-negative bacteria present in the colon.

A variety of other complications may result from prolonged or severe shock. *Acute tubular necrosis* may occur when impaired renal perfusion causes destruction of renal tubules (see Chapter 44). *Acute respiratory distress syndrome* (ARDS) is frequently associated with the shock syndrome. Although no one specific factor has been known to cause ARDS, a period of hypoperfusion to the lungs with resulting pulmonary hypotension is a common cause of this syndrome (see Chapter 26). Stasis of blood in capillary beds and intravascular clotting from the formation of microthrombi and platelet aggregates predispose the patient to a disorder called *disseminated intravascular coagulation* (DIC) (see Chapter 28), particularly in the patient with septic shock. Finally, shock may result in death.

Diagnostic Studies

The history and physical examination provide initial clues leading to a diagnosis of shock and identifying the person at high risk for shock. A history of a recent event that may be associated with shock (e.g., trauma, infection, crushing chest pain) is significant. Changes in sensorium and decreased levels of consciousness reported by others also are important considerations. During the physical examination, it is important to observe for the clinical manifestations of shock. Of particular importance is the immediate overall impression of central nervous system (CNS) function, which is a measure of cerebral perfusion. Also, the status of the cutaneous vascular bed is noted, because it may be indicative of impaired peripheral tissue perfusion.

In the surgical patient it is important to observe dressings and tubes for the appearance of bleeding. The output of nasogastric tubes and urinary catheters may also provide important clues as to the source of fluid loss.

In addition to the history interview and physical examination, various diagnostic studies (see Tables 7-4 and 7-5) are used to confirm the diagnosis and assist in identifying the cause of shock, as well as to monitor the progression and severity of shock. An arterial line and a pulmonary artery catheter (see Chapter 61), or both, are placed for accurate, ongoing hemodynamic monitoring. Measurements of hemodynamic pressures, flows, and arterial and mixed venous oxygen can be used to guide fluid replacement and drug management. A chest x-ray may reveal thoracic trauma or pulmonary changes consistent with shock. Continuous monitoring of HR and heart rhythm is useful for early detection of changes in the patient's cardiopulmonary status. A 12-lead electrocardiogram (ECG) or cardiac monitor may indicate alterations in cardiac electrical activity. Accurate measurement of the BP of the patient in shock is critical, because the level of systemic pressure greatly influences the adequacy of tissue blood flow and myocardial O_2 demands. Auscultatory BP measured with a sphygmomanometer in the patient in shock may be grossly inaccurate, especially when vasoconstriction is present. Arterial blood gases (ABGs) are important to detect any acid-base abnormalities and to assess the oxygenation status of the patient. An indwelling catheter is placed in the bladder to measure urine output, which is an indicator of renal perfusion.

In shock tissue, hypoperfusion predisposes to impaired oxidative metabolism. Tissue hypoxia predisposes to anaerobic metabolism with a buildup of lactic acid. Therefore lactate is a marker of anaerobic metabolism. A lactate level of greater than 3 mEq/L (3 mmol/L) indicates significant hypoperfusion. Sequential measurements demonstrating continually decreasing levels of lactate are usually a good prognostic sign, whereas high stable or increasing levels are usually an ominous sign.

Therapeutic Management

The critical factor in management of the shock syndrome is early recognition and treatment (Table 7-5). Prompt intervention can alter the shock process and prevent the development of the refractory stage and death.[12] Successful management of shock depends on the ability to do the following:

1. Identify the patient at high risk for shock
2. Diagnose the shock syndrome swiftly and accurately
3. Control or alleviate the primary cause
4. Implement appropriate therapeutic measures to correct pathologic changes and enhance tissue perfusion

Emergency Management. Emergency care of the patient in shock is important and may increase greatly the patient's chance of survival. Table 7-6 outlines the emergency management of a patient in hypovolemic shock.

General Therapeutic Management. Whenever possible, the patient should be treated in an intensive care unit and should receive continuous ECG monitoring. A general goal is to keep the mean arterial BP greater than 60 mm Hg.

Oxygen and ventilatory assistance. Management of shock begins by ensuring that the patient has an adequate airway (see Table 7-5). This may be accomplished solely by hyperextension of the neck (unless contraindicated by possibility of spinal cord injury). Placement of an oral airway or endotracheal (ET) intubation may be necessary. The patient may require mechanical ventilation to decrease ventilatory effort. In addition, it is essential that the patient in shock receives sufficient supplemental oxygen (usually via nasal prongs or a mask) to maintain oxygen saturation of >90%, an arterial oxygen pressure (PaO_2) of 60 mm Hg or higher, and to avoid hypoxemia.

Patient position. In terms of the patient's cardiovascular status, the recommended position for the treatment of shock (after chest x-rays have ruled out neck and spine injuries), is supine with the legs elevated to an angle of 45 degrees. The

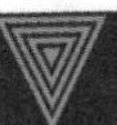

Table 7-4 Diagnostic Studies: Abnormalities in Shock Syndrome

Diagnostic Study	Abnormal Finding	Significance of Abnormality
Blood		
Red blood cell count, hematocrit, hemoglobin	Normal	▪ Remains within normal limits in shock because of relative hypovolemia and pump failure and in hemorrhagic shock before fluid restoration
	Decreased	▪ Decreases in hemorrhagic shock after fluid resuscitation when fluids other than blood are used
	Increased	▪ Increases in nonhemorrhagic shock from actual hypovolemia, because lost fluid does not contain erythrocytes
DIC screen		
Fibrin split products	Increased	▪ Acute DIC can develop within hours to days after an initial assault on the body (i.e., shock)
Fibrinogen level	Decreased	
Platelet count	Decreased	
PTT and PT	Prolonged	
Thrombin time	Increased	
D-Dimer	Increased	
Erythrocyte sedimentation rate	Increased	▪ Is nonspecific; increases are in response to tissue injury
BUN	Increased	▪ May indicate impaired kidney function from hypoperfusion as a result of severe vasoconstriction or occurs secondary to catabolism of cells (e.g., trauma)
Serum creatinine	Increased	▪ Usually indicates impaired kidney function from hypoperfusion as a result of severe vasoconstriction; is more sensitive indicator of renal function than BUN
Blood glucose	Increased	▪ Occurs in early shock because of release of liver glycogen stores in response to sympathetic stimulation
	Decreased	▪ Occurs because of depleted glycogen stores with hepatocellular dysfunction possible as shock progresses
Serum electrolytes		
Sodium	Increased	▪ Occurs early in shock because of increased secretion of aldosterone, causing renal retention of sodium
	Decreased	▪ May occur iatrogenically when excess hypotonic fluid is administered after fluid loss
Potassium	Increased	▪ Occurs when cellular death liberates intracellular potassium; also occurs in acute renal failure and in the presence of acidosis
	Decreased	▪ Occurs early in shock because of increased secretion of aldosterone, causing renal excretion of potassium
Calcium	Decreased	▪ Sometimes occurs after rapid infusion of large amounts of citrated blood; also occurs secondary to respiratory alkalosis of early shock
	Increased	▪ Occurs secondary to lactic acidosis, permitting increased ionization of calcium
Arterial blood gases	Respiratory alkalosis	▪ Occurs early in shock secondary to hyperventilation
	Metabolic acidosis	▪ Occurs later in shock when organic acids, such as lactic acid, accumulate in blood from anaerobic metabolism
Blood cultures	Growth of organism	▪ May grow organisms in the patient who is in septic shock
Lactate	Increased	▪ Usually increases once significant hypoperfusion has occurred with impaired oxygen use at the cellular level
Liver enzymes (AST, ALT, LDH)	Increased	▪ Elevations confirm liver cell destruction in progressive stage of shock
Urine		
Specific gravity	Increased	▪ Occurs secondary to the action of ADH
	Fixed at 1.010	▪ Occurs in renal failure

ADH, Antidiuretic hormone; *ALT*, alanine aminotransferase; *AST*, aspartate aminotransferase; *BUN*, blood urea nitrogen; *DIC*, disseminated intravascular coagulation; *LDH*, lactate dehydrogenase; *PT*, prothrombin time; *PTT*, partial thromboplastin time.

Table 7-5 Therapeutic Management: Shock Syndrome

Diagnostic
- History and physical examination
- Diagnostic studies*
- Placement of CVP or pulmonary artery catheter, as indicated
- Chest x-ray
- Twelve-lead ECG and cardiac monitor
- Identification of cause of shock (if possible)

Therapeutic

General Measures
- Establishment of a patent airway and administration of oxygen (ventilatory assistance with endotracheal intubation, if indicated); careful monitoring of oxygenation
- Placement of peripheral intravenous lines with large gauge catheters
- Fluid placement
  - Typing and crossmatching for packed cells and administration of blood or blood components, as indicated
  - Crystalloids (balanced electrolyte solutions)
  - Colloids (plasma volume expanders)
  - Autotransfusion
- Stabilization of BP (fluids and vasopressor agents, if indicated)
- Placement of indwelling urinary catheter
- Correction of acid-base imbalance as indicated by arterial blood gases
- Pharmacologic therapy†
- Treatment of cardiac dysrhythmias
- Emotional support of patient and family
- Nutritional support

Specific Measures

Hypovolemic Shock
- Control of bleeding, as indicated
- Surgery, if indicated
- Reduction of fluid loss from vomiting, diarrhea, and diuresis
- Volume replacement and blood, if necessary
- Discontinue thrombolytics and anticoagulants, as indicated

Cardiogenic Shock‡
- Administration of inotropic agents to increase cardiac contractility
- Careful fluid administration if patient volume depleted (monitor PCWP)
- Correction of dysrhythmias
- Reduction of work load of heart by decreasing afterload with vasodilator drugs
- Intraaortic balloon pump to increase coronary perfusion and decrease afterload, as indicated
- Thrombolytic therapy or coronary angioplasty, if indicated
- Use of ventricular assist device
- Emergency cardiac surgery (e.g., coronary artery revascularization, valve replacement, repair of ventricular aneurysm if indicated)
- Cardiac transplantation (select few)

Distributive Shock
- Septic shock
  - Collection of cultures to identify organism
  - Administration of appropriate antibiotics
  - Administration of fluid
  - Use of vasopressors to support BP, as indicated
- Anaphylactic shock
  - Maintenance of open airway
  - Administration of epinephrine for vasoconstriction and bronchodilatation
  - Administration of diphenhydramine to counteract effects of histamine
  - Administration of aminophylline for bronchodilatation
  - Use of vasopressors, as indicated
  - Administration of fluid
- Neurogenic shock
  - Treatment according to cause (i.e., pain relief, management of hypoxemia)
  - Correction of underlying cause, if possible
  - Careful administration of fluid
  - Administration of dopamine for hypotension and bradycardia, as indicated

BP, Blood pressure; *CVP,* central venous pressure; *ECG,* electrocardiogram; *PCWP,* pulmonary capillary wedge pressure.
*See Table 7-4.
†See Table 7-8.
‡See Chapter 32.

trunk should be horizontal, the head at the level of the chest, and the knees straight. The Trendelenburg (head-down) position should be avoided in shock because it may (1) initiate aortic and carotid sinus reflexes, causing impaired cerebral blood flow and decreased jugular venous outflow, (2) cause the abdominal organs to press against the diaphragm, thus limiting respiratory excursion and possibly contributing to respiratory distress, (3) decrease filling of the coronary arteries, causing myocardial ischemia, and (4) cause an increase in intracranial pressure in the presence of a head injury.

Fluid replacement. Because shock (with the possible exception of cardiogenic shock) almost always involves a decreased effective circulating blood volume, the cornerstone of shock therapy is expansion of that volume by the intravenous (IV) administration of appropriate fluids, either crystalloids, colloids, or blood products, or a combination (Table 7-7). At least two large-gauge IV catheters should be inserted immediately before severe vasoconstriction occurs and intravenous access becomes difficult. Crystalloids are electrolyte solutions that are either hypotonic, hypertonic,

RESEARCH

IMPLICATIONS FOR NURSING PRACTICE

ACCURACY OF FINGERSTICK GLUCOSE VALUES

Citation Sylvain HF and others: Accuracy of fingerstick glucose values in shock patients, *Am J Critical Care* 4:44-48, 1995.

Purpose Determine the accuracy of fingerstick blood glucose measurements in patients with shock.

Methods Results obtained from three methods of glucose analysis (fingerstick blood glucose, venous blood bedside analysis, and venous blood laboratory analysis) were examined on 38 patients from inpatient medical and surgical critical care units or the emergency department of a large hospital.

Results and Conclusions Analysis of the mean glucose values showed that the laboratory values were significantly higher than the fingerstick glucose values. There were no significant differences between the mean values of the laboratory glucose determinations and the bedside venous glucose values. These results indicate that fingerstick glucose measurements are inaccurate in patients with inadequate tissue perfusion.

Implications for Nursing Practice Critical care nurses often choose the method of blood collection for bedside glucose analysis. Based on the results of this study, these nurses should not use fingerstick blood samples for bedside glucose analysis in patients who may have inadequate tissue perfusion.

or isotonic relative to the plasma. However, in the critically ill patient approximately two thirds of the volume will diffuse out of the vascular space because of increased capillary permeability and reduced oncotic pressure.[14] Therefore large amounts of crystalloids are needed for adequate volume replacement. Because of the expansion of the interstitial space following large amounts of crystalloid administration, the development of systemic edema is common.[15]

Colloids primarily remain in the intravascular space because of the size of the molecules. The osmotic pressure of these solutions draws fluid into the intravascular space, expanding the intravascular volume. Colloids are extremely effective volume expanders; however, none are ideal. Each colloid has significant toxicities that must be considered.[16] Colloids are used in the treatment of shock when plasma protein loss is excessive, as in burn shock and peritonitis. If needed, packed cells are administered as soon as available, after they have been typed and cross matched. The patient's hematocrit value can be used as a guide for blood administration, because one unit of packed cells will raise the hematocrit level 2 to 4 points. (Blood transfusions are discussed in Chapter 28.)

The choice of fluid for volume expansion remains controversial. Neither crystalloids nor colloids are the perfect fluid replacement. However, it is generally accepted that isotonic crystalloids (e.g., lactated Ringer's solution or

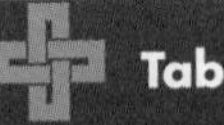

Table 7-6 Emergency Management: Hypovolemic Shock

Possible Etiologies

Major trauma resulting in multiple or serious injuries that are associated with blood or fluid loss, esophageal varices, postoperative bleeding

Possible Assessment Findings

Decreased level of consciousness
Restlessness, anxiety, weakness
Rapid, weak, thready pulse
Hypotension
Cool, clammy skin
Tachypnea, dyspnea, or shallow irregular respirations
Extreme thirst
Nausea and vomiting
Chills
Feeling of impending doom

Management

- Establish and maintain airway; anticipate need for intubation if respiratory distress is evident.
- Administer high flow humidified O_2 (100%) by nonrebreather mask.
- Maintain cervical spine precautions, if indicated.
- Monitor vital signs, level of consciousness, and cardiac rhythm.
- Establish IV access with two large gauge catheters and administer IV fluids.
- Assess for external bleeding sites and apply pressure dressing; consider use of pneumatic antishock garment (PASG) to control bleeding, if indicated.
- Assess for life-threatening injuries (e.g., hemothorax, cardiac tamponade, liver laceration, pelvic fractures).
- Insert an indwelling catheter and nasogastric tube, if indicated.

0.9% saline) are used in the initial resuscitation from shock as a result of hemorrhage. If liver failure is present, lactated Ringer's solution should be avoided because the liver cannot convert lactate to bicarbonate. Crystalloids may be the only fluid used in volume replacement when neither blood nor serum proteins have been lost, as in shock resulting from GI fluid loss or cardiogenic shock. The amount and type of fluid given are based on the patient's need. This can be assessed by observing BP, pulse rate, urine output, skin perfusion, and presence and location of adventitious breath sounds.

Ideally, fluid replacement should be monitored with a pulmonary artery catheter to determine the pulmonary capillary wedge pressure (PCWP) and the CO. The physical assessment of the patient is an important indicator of the patient's fluid status. Complications of excessive volume replacement, such as pulmonary edema and postresuscitation hypertension, can be treated with diuretics. If the patient does not have a pulmonary artery catheter, a urine output of 1 ml/kg per hour will usually indicate adequate fluid replacement. If the CO is still low after fluid replace-

Table 7-7 Types of Fluid Therapy

Type of Fluid	Mechanism of Action	Type of Shock	Nursing Implications
Crystalloids			
Isotonic 0.9% saline (NS), lactated Ringer's (LR)	Fluid primarily remains in the intravascular space, increasing intravascular volume	Used for initial volume replacement in most types of shock	Important to monitor patient closely for circulatory overload; LR should not be used in patients with liver failure
Hypertonic D_5NS hypertonic saline: 3%	Draws intracellular and interstitial fluid into the intravascular space, increasing intravascular volume	Hypertonic saline may be indicated for shock as a result of hemorrhage or burns	Necessary to carefully monitor serum Na levels and serum osmolarity
Hypotonic .45% NS, .33% NS, D_5W	Rapid diffusion of this fluid out of the intravascular space and into cells and interstitial space	Not indicated for shock because pulls fluid out of the intravascular space; indicated for cellular dehydration	D_5W becomes hypotonic once the body uses up the dextrose
Colloids (Plasma Volume Expanders)			
Human serum albumin 5%, 25%	Can increase intravascular volume up to 5 times its volume within 30-60 min	All types of shock except cardiogenic	Patient should be monitored for circulatory overload; mild side effects of chills, fever, and urticaria may develop; more expensive than other colloids
Dextran Dextran 40, Dextran 70	Has similar degrees of volume expansion with Dextran 40 and Dextran 70; have longer duration of action with Dextran 70	Limited use because of potentially serious side effects	Agent alters clotting factors and has antiplatelet effect; important to monitor patient closely for hypersensitivity reactions and acute renal failure
Plasma protein fraction	Has albumin as primary component, and similar action to that of albumin	All types of shock	Drug may cause greater hypersensitivity reactions than albumin
Hetastarch	Acts as volume expander and is at least as effective as albumin	All types of shock	Drug may be 50% less costly than albumin; should be used cautiously with patient with congestive heart failure, renal failure, or bleeding disorder because of anticoagulant effect

ment, an inotropic agent, such as dopamine or dobutamine, or a vasopressor, such as high-dose dopamine, levarterenol (Levophed), or phenylephrine, should be administered (see section on Pharmacologic Management).

The patient who has sustained a major hemorrhage requires massive fluid volume and blood replacement, which can exceed the patient's normal blood volume. Complications of massive volume infusion include hypothermia (from cold blood) and coagulopathy (from hemodilution of clotting factors). All blood products and IV solutions should be warmed to prevent hypothermia. Devices that warm solutions as well as provide pumps for rapid infusion are commercially available.

Acid-base imbalance. Frequent monitoring of ABGs allows the physician to prescribe therapy to correct acid-base imbalances. This may be accomplished through the use of ventilatory assistance or, rarely, by the infusion of IV sodium bicarbonate. When a mechanical ventilator is used to correct acid-base imbalances, it is sometimes necessary to administer a paralyzing drug, such as pancuronium (Pavulon), vecuronium (Norcuron), or atracurium (Tracrium), especially if the patient is competing with the ventilator. This allows better control of the rate and depth of respirations by the ventilator.

Cardiac dysrhythmias. Methods of treating cardiac dysrhythmias are detailed in Chapter 33.

Specific Therapeutic Management. In addition to general management of shock, each type of shock has specific interventions (see Table 7-5).

Hypovolemic shock. A major treatment priority for hypovolemic shock is volume replacement. Each patient must be carefully monitored during fluid administration. The patient has probably received adequate volume replacement when his pulse pressure and HR return to the normal range and urine output is at least 0.5 ml/kg per hour.[17] Blood and blood products are needed for hemorrhagic shock. Because control of bleeding is essential, surgical intervention may be required.

The pneumatic antishock garment (PASG) may be helpful in controlling internal and external hemorrhage below the diaphragm by applying direct pressure and thereby stopping the bleeding. The ability of the PASG to raise the blood pressure is thought to be a result of the increase in systemic vascular resistance. The use of PASG is controversial, but may be indicated for severe pelvic fractures associated with continuing blood loss or abdominal trauma with serious hypovolemia while the patient is transported to a hospital or operating room. The major complication results from rapid deflation before restoration of adequate intravascular volume (Fig. 7-4). The PASG should not be deflated until the patient is either in the operating room or in a controlled situation with experienced personnel. Volume replacement is administered to maintain the BP because the pressure in the PASG is gradually decreased over 30 to 60 minutes. Contraindications to the use of PASG include pulmonary edema, heart failure, intrathoracic bleeding, and diaphragmatic rupture.

Cardiogenic shock. Cardiogenic shock requires careful fluid replacement guided by hemodynamic monitoring if the patient is volume depleted. Relative hypovolemia, resulting in decreased venous return (preload), is present in up to 20% of patients with cardiogenic shock.[5] The goal of drug therapy is to increase cardiac contractility while decreasing afterload, and thus the work load of the heart. Inotropic and vasodilator agents (Table 7-8) are commonly used. In addition, diuretics used to decrease preload are indicated if the patient is volume overloaded. Drug therapy alone has not significantly decreased the mortality of cardiogenic shock. The intraaortic balloon pump (IABP) is often used in addition to drug therapy. The IABP is a counterpulsation device that is inserted into the femoral, axillary, or subclavian artery and placed in the aorta, just distal to the aortic arch (see Chapter 61). The goal of this intervention is to decrease the systemic vascular resistance and thus left ventricular work load, while increasing diastolic pressure resulting in increased coronary and cerebral blood flow.

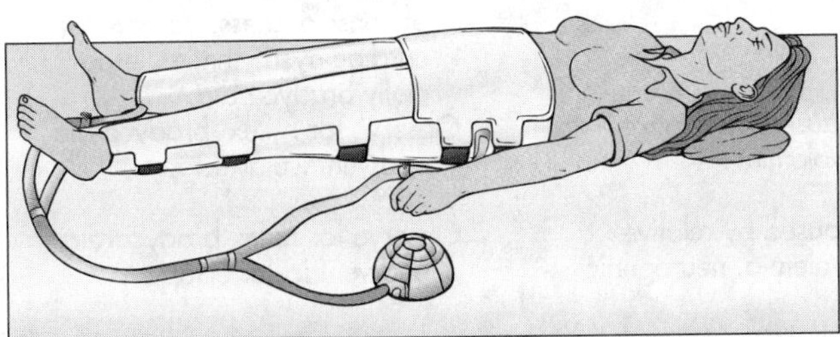

Fig. 7-4 Pneumatic antishock garment (PASG) is a one-piece garment placed over the patient's legs and abdomen. When the PASG is inflated, pelvic fractures are stabilized and the vessels in the legs and abdomen are compressed, which controls bleeding. PASG may be indicated in the emergency management of shock related to pelvic fractures with ongoing hemorrhage and abdominal injuries with significant hypovolemia.

Other goals for management of cardiogenic shock include early restoration of blood flow to the affected coronary arteries by using thrombolytic therapy and surgical correction of any mechanical complication related to the acute MI that may be contributing to the cardiogenic shock (e.g., papillary muscle rupture with mitral regurgitation and ventricular septal defect).[18] Emergency coronary artery bypass graft surgery and coronary artery angioplasty are other approaches used to treat patients with acute cardiogenic shock. Ventricular assist devices (VAD) may be used on a temporary basis for the cardiogenic shock patient or as a bridge while awaiting cardiac transplantation. Cardiac transplantation is an option for a small and select group of patients with cardiogenic shock.[5]

Septic shock. First, the source of infection must be identified and treated with antimicrobial therapy or surgical drainage, or both.[19] The specific organisms causing septic shock frequently are not identified initially in a patient with this illness. Therefore, broad-sprectrum, antimicrobial therapy must be instituted that will be effective until the specific organisms are identified through culture and sensitivity. Usually two broad spectrum antibiotics, including an aminoglycoside, are used.

Rapid infusion of large amounts of fluid, including both crystalloids and colloids, are used in treating septic shock. Hemodynamic monitoring of the PAP and PCWP often is necessary because of the multiple system involvement with shock. Therefore, the patient has an increased risk to develop fluid overload and cardiac failure. Assessment is important because subtle changes can rapidly occur, and the patient's condition can quickly deteriorate. If tissue perfusion is inadequate, inotropic drugs (primarily dopamine) are indicated to improve the patient's circulatory status. If dopamine does not raise the mean arterial pressure, vasopressor drugs (e.g., norepinephrine [Levophed]) are used.

Antibiotics may not be effective once septic shock has developed, because the harmful effects of the endotoxins continue after the bacteria are dead. The current therapy for septic shock reverses the effects in only 50% or less of the patients. Currently, research is being done using human monoclonal antibodies against various mediators of septic shock. These include antibodies to TNF, endotoxin, and IL-1.[20]

Refractory hypotension and MODS are two of the major causes of mortality in septic shock. Support of dysfunctional organ systems is an important therapeutic goal. The patient with ARDS requires O_2 therapy and mechanical ventilation (see Chapter 26). DIC should be treated appropriately (see Chapter 28). Renal failure may require dialysis therapy (see Chapter 44).

Table 7-8 Drugs Used in the Treatment of Shock

Drug	Mechanism of Action	Type of Shock	Nursing Implications
Sympathomimetics*			
Dobutamine (Dobutrex)	Primarily stimulates β_1 receptors with minimal β_2- and α-adrenergic effects; increases myocardial contractility without inducing marked tachycardia; causes mild vasodilatation, decreasing SVR.	Cardiogenic shock in absence of profound hypotension (<80 mm Hg systolic).	Do not give with sodium bicarbonate; observe for hypotension, dysrhythmias, and tachycardia at higher doses.
Dopamine (Intropin)	Is precursor of epinephrine and norepinephrine; has dose-dependent actions. Stimulates α- and β-adrenergic receptors, causing peripheral vasoconstriction and positive inotropic effect. Increases renal perfusion at low doses only.	All types of shock, especially in patients with oliguria (low dose) or with decreased SVR; often with nitroprusside for cardiogenic shock.	Administer drug through central venous catheter or large peripheral vein (infiltration may cause tissue damage); monitor for hypotension, tachycardia, and dysrhythmias; be aware that intravascular volume should be adequate
Epinephrine (Adrenalin)	Stimulates α and β receptors. Counteracts effects of histamine. Causes bronchodilatation and peripheral vasoconstriction, elevating BP. Positive inotropic effect.	All types of shock. Drug of choice for anaphylactic shock.	Observe for cardiac dysrhythmias, dyspnea, pulmonary edema, and severe headaches.
Isoproterenol (Isuprel)	Stimulates β-adrenergic receptors, causing vasodilatation and marked inotropic and chronotropic effects.	Shock with accompanying bradycardia unresponsive to atropine.	Observe for ventricular dysrhythmias and extreme tachycardia (increased rate increases oxygen demands).
Levarterenol (Levophed)	Stimulates α-adrenergic and β-adrenergic receptors, causing marked vasoconstriction as well as inotropic and chronotropic effects.	All types, especially shock caused by decreased SVR; usually reserved for patients with hypotension unresponsive to fluids and dopamine.	Be aware that drug is best administered through a central venous line and, if infiltration occurs, is sometimes given with phentolamine to prevent excessive vasoconstriction and tissue sloughing; closely monitor rapid fluctuations in BP; closely monitor urine output (severe decrease in renal perfusion may occur); be aware that drug may also cause reflex bradycardia.
Metaraminol (Aramine)	Stimulates α and β receptors, causing marked vasoconstriction; causes inotropic effects in some patients.	Shock caused by relative hypovolemia.	Observe for reflex bradycardia, oliguria, and decreased level of consciousness.Observe for cardiac dysrhythmias, especially bradycardia.
Methoxamine (Vasoxyl)	Stimulates α-adrenergic receptors, causing vasoconstriction.	Shock caused by relative hypovolemia.	Observe for reflex bradycardia and ventricular ectopy.
Phenylephrine (Neo-Synephrine)	Predominantly stimulates α receptors, causing vasoconstriction.	Shock caused by relative hypovolemia, neurogenic shock.	Observe for reflex bradycardia and ventricular ectopy.

continued

Table 7-8 Drugs Used in the Treatment of Shock—cont'd

Drug	Mechanism of Action	Type of Shock	Nursing Implications
Phosphodiesterase Inhibitor			
Amrinone (Inocor) Milrinone (Primacor)	Produces inotropic action, increasing CO; directly relaxes vascular smooth muscles, decreasing preload and afterload.	May be indicated for patients with cardiogenic shock unresponsive to initial drug therapy.	An initial bolus is administered before beginning the continuous IV infusion; monitor for dysrhythmias and hypotension.
Vasodilators			
Nitroglycerin (Tridil)	Primarily acts as venous vasodilator; dilates veins and arteries at higher doses.	Cardiogenic shock, with inotropic agent.	Monitor BP carefully; observe for reflex tachycardia; be aware that headache is common; use non-PVC tubing and glass bottle to prevent drug absorption.
Sodium nitroprusside (Nipride)	Acts as a potent vasodilator on veins and arteries; may increase or decrease CO depending on the extent of preload and afterload reduction.	Primarily cardiogenic shock with increased SVR and preload and afterload; decreased CO, with inotropic drug, such as dopamine.	Closely monitor for hypotension and reflex tachycardia; administer only with D_5W and protect solution from light; be aware that thiocyanate toxicity and cyanide poisoning may occur when used for >72 hr.
Phentolamine (Regitine)	Acts as an α-adrenergic blocking agent with no depressent effects on myocardial contractility.	Primarily cardiogenic shock.	Monitor for adequacy of fluid replacement as action of drug can cause a rapid decrease in cardiac filling pressure.
Morphine sulfate	Is narcotic analgesic and acts as potent venodilator (decreases preload) with some arterial dilatation (decreases afterload)	Primarily cardiogenic shock (to decrease preload).	Monitor carefully for hypotension and respiratorydepression; have Narcan at bedside.
Corticosteroids			
Dexamethasone (Decadron) Hydrocortisone (Solu-Cortef) Methylprednisolone (Solu-Medrol)	Inhibits inflammatory process, stabilizes lysosomal membranes, reduces capillary permeability, reduces release of chemical mediators in the septic process, and promotes sodium retention.	Serious cases of anaphylactic shock; adrenal insufficiency.	Monitor patient for GI bleeding and hypotension; be aware that these drugs may make control of diabetes difficult and may cause slow wound healing and predisposition to infection.

BP, Blood pressure; *CO,* cardiac output; *GI,* gastrointestinal; *SVR,* systemic vascular resistance.
*All sympathomimetic drugs are incompatible with sodium bicarbonate.

Anaphylactic shock. Full-blown anaphylactic shock is dramatic, and immediate drug intervention is required. The primary drug is epinephrine, which causes peripheral vasoconstriction and bronchodilatation. Attention to the airway is important, because the patient can quickly develop respiratory failure from the bronchoconstriction. Aminophylline also is used when bronchoconstriction is severe. Endotracheal intubation or tracheostomy may be necessary to maintain a patent airway. Hypotension results from the leakage of fluid out of the intravascular space as a result of increased vascular permeability. Fluid replacement is necessary. Diphenhydramine (Benadryl) is used to counteract the effects of histamine. However, it is not effective for the life-threatening vasodilatation or bronchoconstriction. Steroids may be administered, but their effect is not immediate.

Neurogenic shock. Neurogenic shock has multiple causes, and therefore the treatment varies. Fluid replacement for blood pressure maintenance and tissue perfusion continues to be important. Careful monitoring of the patient during fluid administration is important to prevent the development of pulmonary edema as a result of volume overload. Sympathomimetic drug therapy may be indicated to increase BP through vasoconstriction and to increase HR.

Pharmacologic Management of Shock

The primary purpose of drugs used in the treatment of shock is correction of the poor tissue perfusion. These drugs are administered intravenously. Drugs used in the treatment of shock are presented in Table 7-8.

Sympathomimetic Drugs. Many of the drugs used in the treatment of shock have an effect on the sympathetic nervous system. Drugs that mimic the action of the sympathetic nervous system are called *sympathomimetic drugs*. The effects of these drugs are mediated through action on the α-adrenergic- or β-adrenergic receptors. The various drugs differ in their relative α and β effects. Activation of myocardial-β receptors increases HR and contractility.

Many of the sympathomimetic drugs cause peripheral vasoconstriction and are referred to as *vasopressor drugs* (e.g., epinephrine and norepinephrine). At high doses these vasopressor drugs have the potential to cause severe peripheral vasoconstriction and to further jeopardize tissue perfusion, either directly or indirectly. The increased SVR increases the work load of the heart and can be detrimental to a patient in cardiogenic shock, causing further myocardial damage. Use of vasopressor drugs is reserved for patients who have been unresponsive to other therapy. Adequate volume replacement must be administered before the use of any vasopressor drug, since peripheral vasoconstrictor effects in low-volume states can be detrimental to tissue perfusion.

The goal of vasopressor therapy is to achieve and maintain a mean arterial BP of 70 to 80 mm Hg and improve tissue perfusion. This ensures adequate blood flow to all organs. The sympathomimetic drugs of choice for shock are norepinephrine (levarterenol [Levophed]) and dopamine.

Vasodilator Drugs. Some patients in shock show evidence of excessive vasoconstriction and poor tissue perfusion in spite of volume replacement and normal or high systemic pressures. Although generalized sympathetic vasoconstriction is a useful compensatory mechanism for maintaining systemic pressure, excessive constriction can reduce tissue blood flow. The rationale for using vasodilator therapy for a patient in shock is to break the deleterious cycle in which widespread vasoconstriction causes a decrease in CO and BP, resulting in further sympathetic-induced vasoconstriction.

The goal in vasodilator therapy, as in vasopressor therapy, is to maintain a mean BP of 70 to 80 mm Hg. Also, it is important to closely monitor pulmonary artery pressures and arterial pressure so that fluid administration can be increased or the dose of the vasodilator drug decreased if a serious fall in blood pressure occurs. The vasodilator agents most often used for the patient in shock are nitroprusside and phentolamine.

Corticosteroids. IV corticosteroid therapy may be helpful in anaphylactic shock if significant symptoms continue after 1 to 2 hours of aggressive therapy.[4] Steroids may prevent the delayed symptoms that are thought to be caused by the release of chemical mediators. Because of the lack of evidence of beneficial effects, steroids are not used in the treatment of septic shock except in patients with suspected adrenal insufficiency or for specific indications.[3]

Antibiotics. Susceptibility to infection is increased in all patients with prolonged shock of nonseptic etiology. Broad-spectrum prophylactic antibiotic therapy may be indicated. Antibiotics are always used in the treatment of septic shock. Before antibiotic therapy is begun, specimens of blood, urine, wound exudate, and sputum should be obtained for bacteriologic culture and sensitivity studies. If possible, the anatomic sites of origin of the infection should be identified to ensure that the most likely etiologic agent can be predicted. The organisms that most frequently cause septic shock are gram negative. Antibiotic therapy should never be delayed. Unless appropriate antibiotics are started within 24 hours of the beginning of shock, the mortality rate is increased greatly.

Factors to consider in the initial selection of antibiotics for the patient are as follows:

1. Broad-spectrum antibiotics are needed because culture and sensitivity study reports are not yet available.
2. The serum half life of drugs may be increased because of renal or hepatic insufficiency.
3. Some antibiotics are nephrotoxic or hepatotoxic; renal and liver function need to be monitored when these drugs are used.

Nutritional Management

During the acute phase of the shock syndrome, the patient receives nothing by mouth because the GI tract is not adequately perfused. As recovery begins, nutrition plays an important role in limiting morbidity. Since anorexia is almost universally present, parenteral or enteral feeding often is used. Enteral tube feeding via a feeding pump is commonly the initial method of supplying nutrition. Parenteral feeding is generally adopted only if tube feedings are contraindicated or if they fail to meet the patient's caloric requirements. (Total parenteral nutrition and enteral tube feedings are discussed in Chapter 37.)

A patient in shock should be weighed daily (on the same scale at the same time of day) to determine whether caloric needs are being met. If the patient experiences a significant weight loss, dehydration should be ruled out before additional calories are provided parenterally. Measurements of BUN levels also provide pertinent data, because falling levels may indicate overhydration or malnutrition.

NURSING MANAGEMENT

SHOCK

Nursing Assessment

Subjective and objective data that should be obtained from a person with shock are presented in Table 7-9. Initial assessment of the patient in shock, or impending shock, need not be extensive. The assessment should focus on the evaluation of the indicators of tissue perfusion: level of consciousness, skin, vital signs, and urine output.[8] Although a continual decline in the patient's level of consciousness indicates a further reduction in cerebral blood

Table 7-9 Nursing Assessment: Shock

Subjective Data

Important Health Information

Past health history: Myocardial infarction, pulmonary embolism, infection, spinal cord injury, hemorrhage, trauma, burns, diabetes, dehydration, congestive heart failure, valvular dysfunction, pancreatitis, intestinal obstruction, use of tampons, severe reaction to insect bites or stings or blood products

Medications: Severe reaction to any drugs, vaccines, contrast dye, general anesthesia; drug overdose (including insulin)

Surgery and other treatments: Any major surgical procedure, especially involving blood loss

Functional Health Patterns

Nutritional-metabolic: Thirst, nausea, vomiting, abdominal cramps; urticaria and pruritis (anaphylactic shock); diaphoresis; chills

Elimination: Decreased urinary output

Activity-exercise: Weakness, dizziness, restlessness, fainting, palpitations, chest pain, dyspnea, productive or nonproductive cough

Objective Data

Neurologic

Initially: Restlessness, anxiety

Later: Altered mentation, lethargy, stupor, coma

Cardiovascular

Tachycardia; hypotension; weak, thready pulse; flat neck veins (except in cardiogenic shock); abnormal heart sounds; dysrhythmias

Integumentary

Pale, cool, moist skin or warm, flushed skin (septic and anaphylactic shock); cyanosis (later shock); urticaria, rash, and angioedema (anaphylaxis)

Urinary

Decreased urinary output

Respiratory

Tachypnea; wheezing, crackles, absence of breath sounds, choking, coughing (anaphylaxis)

Gastrointestinal

Vomiting, hyperactive or diminished bowel sounds

General

Fever (septic), normal or subnormal temperature (other types of shock). Presence of blood in tubes or on dressings.

Possible Findings

Altered serum electrolytes, decreased hemoglobin and hematocrit, leukocytosis, hypoxemia, and hypocapnia; respiratory alkalosis and metabolic acidosis; elevated BUN and cardiac enzymes (cardiogenic); elevated liver enzymes; elevated lactate levels; positive wound, blood, and body fluid cultures; abnormal chest and abdominal x-rays and ECG

BUN, Blood urea nitrogen; *ECG,* electrocardiogram.

flow and a worsening of the shock state, some patients in shock may remain fully conscious. As shock progresses, severe arterial vasoconstriction continues to decrease perfusion to the skin and kidneys. Therefore the skin becomes colder and more mottled and the urine output declines to eventual anuria. The BP may not be a reliable indicator of the severity of the shock state. Changes from the baseline vital signs are important to evaluate and document.

Planning

The overall goals are that the patient in shock will have (1) adequate tissue perfusion, (2) normal BP for the patient, and (3) no complications related to shock.

Nursing Diagnoses

Nursing diagnoses are determined when the problem and etiologic factors are supported by the clinical data. Nursing diagnoses related to shock may include, but are not limited to, those presented in the nursing care plan for the patient in shock.

Nursing Implementation

Health Promotion and Maintenance. It is important for nurses to become involved in the prevention of the shock state. To prevent shock, the nurse must first identify persons who are at risk. In general, the very old, the very young, and persons who have chronic, debilitating diseases are at an increased risk for shock. More specifically, any person who sustains surgical or accidental trauma is at high risk of shock resulting from hemorrhage, spinal cord injury, burn injuries, and the conditions listed in Table 7-1. A person with diabetes whose disease is not well controlled or who does not adhere to therapy may go into shock. A person with an acute MI, especially anterior, is at risk for cardiogenic shock. A person with a severe allergy to such substances as drugs, shellfish, and insect bites may also develop shock.

Implementation of the nursing process is essential to help prevent shock after a susceptible individual has been identified. A thorough baseline nursing assessment with frequent ongoing assessments to monitor and detect changes in the patient's condition are the initial nursing actions. Identification of pertinent nursing diagnoses, implementation of appropriate nursing interventions, and evaluation of these actions should follow. All patients with symptoms of angina or MI should be encouraged to seek medical attention immediately. The primary goal for the patient with an acute MI is to limit the size of the infarction. This is done by attempting to increase coronary artery perfusion and decrease the work load of the heart through rest, drug therapy, thrombolytic therapy, and other procedures (e.g., coronary artery angioplasty, IABP).

Careful monitoring of fluid balance can help prevent hypovolemic shock. Intake and output, daily body weights, and drainage from wounds and tubes must be carefully calculated and documented. Immediate control of hemorrhage is essential. A patient who is at risk of sepsis must be carefully monitored for signs of infection. Limitation of portals of entry into the body, including IVs and indwelling catheters, is important. Aseptic technique must be used with all procedures. Frequent handwashing is essential.

The risk of anaphylactic shock can be decreased if the patient is carefully questioned about allergies before administering a new drug or antibiotics (even if the patient has

NURSING CARE PLAN Patient in Hypovolemic Shock

Planning: Outcome Criteria	*Nursing Interventions and Rationales*
➤ **NURSING DIAGNOSIS**	Decreased cardiac output *related to* absolute or relative hypovolemia *as manifested by* increased diastolic, decreased systolic BP; postural hypotension; tachycardia; weak, thready pulse; flat neck veins; low CVP and PCWP; thirst and dry mucous membranes; falling urinary output <0.5 ml/kg/hr; altered mentation; dysrhythmias; tachypnea; hypoxemia; pallor or cyanosis; cool, clammy skin
Normal BP (for patient); HR 60-110 bpm; strong peripheral pulses; normal CVP (1-8 mm Hg) and PCWP (6-12 mm Hg); warm, dry, pink skin; urinary output >30 ml/hr; normal mentation; no dysrhythmias; respiratory rate >12 and <20; Sa02 > 90%; return of laboratory findings and x-ray films to baseline.	Monitor vital signs, CVP, pulmonary artery pressures every 15 min to 1 hr *to monitor patient's status and detect fluid deficits.* Administer crystalloids and colloids *to restore blood and fluid volume* and sympathomimetics to support BP *to maintain perfusion of vital organs.* Assess response. Maintain peripheral IV line and central IV line *to ensure ready access to the vascular system for both plasma expanders and other medications.* Record accurate intake and output to help detect fluid imbalances. Obtain weight daily *to monitor fluid volume changes through daily weight changes.* Monitor laboratory and x-ray findings *to evaluate patient's response to treatment.* Keep patient warm *to prevent an increase in metabolic need for O_2 and increased CO_2 production.* Administer oxygen *to keep SaO_2 >90%.*
➤ **NURSING DIAGNOSIS**	Fear and anxiety *related to* severity of condition, perceived threat of death, and family distress *as manifested by* verbalization of anxiety about condition and fear of death to family, staff, or withdrawal with no communication; facial, muscle tension; restlessness; voice and hand tremors; sleeplessness; tense, narrowed focus of attention; diaphoresis; increase in heart and respiratory rate
Verbalization of anxieties and fears; more relaxed appearance; verbalization of reduced anxiety; appropriate questions being asked; reduction in heart and respiratory rate; ability to relax, sleep; return of sense of humor; less tense appearance.	Acknowledge expressed fear and anxiety *to validate patient's feelings.* Demonstrate concern, respect for patient. Encourage verbalization and discussion of fears if patient is withdrawn. Seek out significant other's perception of situation *to enlist help.* Maintain calm and reassuring demeanor and environment *to reduce patient's anxieties and oxygen need.* Explain interventions, patient status, and equipment simply and honestly *to reduce patient's fear of the unknown and assist patient in making informed decisions.* Assess level of understanding. Keep call bell within easy reach *to increase sense of support and staff availability.* Teach simple relaxation techniques *to aid in stress reduction.* Check on patient and family frequently. Use humor if appropriate *to reduce anxiety.*

COLLABORATIVE PROBLEMS

Nursing Goals	*Nursing Interventions and Rationales*
➤ **POTENTIAL COMPLICATION**	Organ ischemia or dysfunction related to decreased tissue perfusion
Neurologic ischemia or dysfunction	
Monitor for signs of neurologic ischemia. Report deviations from acceptable parameters.	Perform hourly neurologic assessment including assessment of changes in mentation or level of consciousness to provide information regarding status of cerebral blood flow. Record and report any changes to guide in selecting appropriate interventions. Question patient about headache and paresthesias to assess patient's subjective complaints. Observe patient closely and protect confused patient from injury with soft restraints as needed. Keep side rails up at all times to keep patient from falling out of bed as a result of confused state. Take measures to minimize noise to control sensory input.
Renal ischemia or dysfunction	
Monitor for signs of renal ischemia, report deviations from acceptable parameters, and carry out medical and nursing interventions.	Monitor for urine output <.5 ml/kg/hr, increase in urine specific gravity, elevation in BUN and creatinine, abnormal serum electrolytes, low urine sodium, protein and blood in urine, metabolic acidosis *to assess renal function.* Insert indwelling catheter *to accurately measure urinary output.* Take weight daily *to monitor fluid status and evaluate renal function.* Administer fluids and sympathomimetics as ordered and assess results *to maintain adequate renal perfusion.* Watch for fluid overload *to identify a possible complication of overtreating the hypovolemia.*

continued

NURSING CARE PLAN Patient in Hypovolemic Shock—cont'd

COLLABORATIVE PROBLEMS

Nursing Goals	Nursing Interventions and Rationales
Gastrointestinal ischemia or dysfunction	
Monitor for signs of GI ischemia and report deviations from acceptable parameters.	Monitor for presence of abdominal pain, distention, nausea, vomiting, anorexia, diarrhea, thirst, constipation, absent or diminished bowel sounds *to assess GI status.* Keep patient on NPO status *to prevent accumulation of fluid secondary to GI inactivity.* Monitor bowel sounds q2-4 hr. Check stools and emesis for blood *as possible source of hypovolemia.* Measure intake and output *to determine fluid balance.* Maintain adequate hydration *to help restore normal blood and fluid volume.*
Peripheral vascular ischemia or dysfunction	
Monitor for signs of peripheral vascular ischemia and report deviations from acceptable parameters.	Monitor for presence of cool, pale, or cyanotic extremities; diminished or absent peripheral pulses; pain, tingling, or numbness in extremities; necrotic or gangrenous extremities; poor capillary refill *as indicators of peripheral vascular ischemia.* Assess for color, warmth, and size of extremities *as deviations from expected can result from peripheral vascular ischemia.* Watch for pressure sores *which can develop quickly when immobility is combined with tissue ischemia.* Keep patient warm and dry *to promote comfort and prevent vasoconstriction.* Report any changes in peripheral perfusion such as prolonged capillary refill or cool extremities *so treatment can be initiated promptly.* Avoid restrictive clothing and stockings *which impede peripheral circulation.*
Respiratory ischemia or dysfunction	
Monitor for signs of respiratory distress, report deviations from acceptable parameters, and perform appropriate treatments, and carry out appropriate medical and nursing interventions.	Monitor for the following: *Early:* Rapid ($>$20/min), deep respirations; *late:* rapid (30-40/min), shallow respirations, dyspnea, use of accessory muscles, cyanosis, adventitious breath sounds and cough, abnormal chest x-ray; *early:* respiratory alkalosis ($\downarrow$PaCO2, $\uparrow$pH), *normal or low PaO2; late:* metabolic acidosis ($\downarrow$pH, $\downarrow$HCO3) and hypoxemia ($\downarrow$PaO2) *to assess for respiratory distress.* Initiate oxygen and maintain SaO2 $\geq$90% *to ensure adequate oxygenation.* Monitor ABGs *to evaluate gas exchange in the lungs and acid-base balance.* Auscultate and record breath sounds q1-2 hr *to determine presence of* crackles, wheezes, and decreased or unequal breath sounds *as indicators of impaired respirations.* Report any abnormal findings. Assist patient to cough and deep breathe *to open up alveoli and improve gas exchange.* Suction as needed *to remove secretions patient cannot remove independently.* Keep head of bed slightly elevated *to minimize respiratory effort.* Obtain chest x-ray as ordered *to assess presence of lung pathology.* Monitor skin and mucous membranes for cyanosis *as cyanosis indicates inadequate oxygenation.* Assess respiratory rate, depth, and pattern *as indicators of respiratory status.* Maintain patent airway and prepare for mechanical ventilation.

ABGs, Arterial blood gases; *BP,* blood pressure; *BUN,* blood urea nitrogen; *CVP,* central venous pressure; *GI,* gastrointestinal; *PCWP,* pulmonary capillary wedge pressure.

received this drug in the past) or before undergoing a diagnostic procedure involving the use of an IV dye. Before and during blood administration, the nurse should carefully follow hospital procedure. Two nurses should check the blood before administration, and the patient should be closely monitored for signs of reaction during the entire transfusion. Patients who have severe allergies should wear a Medic-Alert tag and report their allergies to their health care providers. These patients should also be instructed about the availability of special kits that contain equipment and medication for the treatment of acute hypersensitivity reactions. Early immobilization of spinal cord injuries can help prevent neurogenic shock. In addition, health education is important to prevent the onset of diseases that may result in shock. For example, regular exercise and cessation of smoking may help decrease the risk of MI.

Acute Intervention. The nursing role in the acute stages of shock involves monitoring the patient's ongoing physical and emotional status to detect subtle changes in the patient's condition, planning and implementing nursing interventions and therapy, evaluating the patient's response to therapy, and providing emotional support to the patient and significant others. Nursing responsibilities also include judging when it is necessary to alert other health team members to changes in the patient's status that may require reevaluation of treatment. Therefore, reassessment, as often as the patient's condition warrants it, is important. (Nursing care plan for the patient in shock is presented on p. 136.)

As care is begun, it is essential for the nurse to obtain the following brief history from the patient or another knowledgeable person:

1. Description of the events leading to the shock condition
2. Time of onset and duration of symptoms
3. Health history, especially medications and allergies
4. Care received before hospital admission
5. Date of last tetanus immunization, if shock is a result of trauma
6. Patient's religious faith
7. Presence of Medic-Alert tag

Neurologic status. Neurologic checks, including pupillary response, orientation, and level of consciousness, should be performed at least every hour. The patient's neurologic status is the best indicator of cerebral blood flow. The nurse should be alert to clinical manifestations that may indicate neurologic involvement, such as changes in behavior, restlessness, overalertness, blurred vision, agitation, confusion, and paresthesias.

Attempts should be made to orient the patient to time, place, person, and situation. If the patient is in an intensive care unit, orientation to the environment is particularly important. Measures such as minimizing noise and light levels should be taken to control sensory input. A day-night cycle of activity and rest should be maintained as much as possible. Sensory overload and disruption of the patient's diurnal cycle may contribute to an altered neurologic status, especially if the patient is elderly.

Cardiovascular status. Much of the therapy for shock is based on information about the patient's cardiovascular status. Until the patient is stable, the HR, BP, central venous pressure (CVP), and pulmonary artery pressures (if available) should be determined every 5 to 15 minutes. (Hemodynamic monitoring is discussed in Chapter 61). Once the patient is stable, the PCWP should be obtained only as often as needed to avoid complications associated with balloon inflation. The PCWP most accurately reflects left ventricular function, especially in the presence of lung problems (e.g., pulmonary embolism or chronic lung disease) when the pulmonary artery pressure often is elevated. Trends in pulmonary artery pressures are more important than the individual numbers themselves. In addition, care should be taken to avoid dependence on these numbers, because direct physical assessment of the patient is extremely valuable.

The patient's ECG should be monitored continuously to detect dysrhythmias that may result from the shock or from medications used in treating the shock. The rate and quality of peripheral and apical pulses should be compared every 15 to 30 minutes, and heart sounds should be assessed for quality and the presence of an S_3 or S_4, or murmurs. The presence of an S_3 in an adult usually indicates heart failure. The frequency of this monitoring is decreased as the patient's condition improves.

In addition to carrying out these measures, which are necessary to monitor the patient's cardiovascular status, the nurse must administer the prescribed therapy that is designed to correct the patient's impaired cardiovascular status.

Respiratory status. The respiratory status of the patient in shock must be frequently assessed to ensure adequate oxygenation and early detection of respiratory complications, as well as to provide data regarding the patient's acid-base status. The rate, depth, and rhythm of respirations are initially monitored every 15 minutes. Increased rate and depth provide information regarding the patient's attempts to correct metabolic acidosis. Chest sounds should be assessed every hour for the development of crackles, which can indicate the presence of fluid buildup in the lungs.

Pulse oximetry, a noninvasive method, is used to continuously monitor oxygen saturation. Pulse oximetry consists of a microprocessor and a probe that attaches to the patient's ear, finger, toe, or nose. ABGs provide definitive information on oxygenation status and acid-base balance. Initial interpretation of ABGs is often the nurse's responsibility. A PaO_2 below 60 mm Hg (in the absence of chronic lung disease) indicates the presence of hypoxemia and the need for the administration of higher oxygen concentrations or for a different method of oxygen administration. A low $PaCO_2$ in the presence of a low pH and a low or normal bicarbonate level indicates that the patient's hyperventilation is compensating for the metabolic acidosis. A rising $PaCO_2$ in the presence of a persistently low pH indicates the need for intubation and ventilatory assistance.

Renal status. Hourly measurements of urinary output are essential in assessment of the adequacy of renal perfusion. An indwelling catheter is inserted to facilitate measurements. Urine output of less than 0.5 ml/kg per hour may indicate inadequate perfusion of the kidneys. The nurse should be sure that blood is drawn daily for BUN and serum creatinine determinations and should alert the physician if elevations in these values occur. Serum creatinine is a better indicator of renal function because BUN levels can be influenced by the catabolic state of the patient.

Body temperature and skin changes. In the presence of an elevated or subnormal temperature, tympanic or pulmonary arterial temperatures should be obtained hourly. If normal, the temperature needs to be monitored only every 4 hours. The patient should be kept comfortably warm with the use of light covers and the control of environmental temperature. If the patient's temperature rises above 101.5° F (38.6° C), this condition may be treated with medication such as acetaminophen suppositories, tepid sponge baths, removal of some covers, or a hypothermia blanket. It is important to avoid an elevated temperature and shivering because both cause an increased metabolic need for oxygen and increased carbon dioxide production.

Skin color should be assessed for pallor, flushing, and cyanosis. Diaphoresis or piloerection should be noted. In addition, the rapidity of capillary refill should be assessed as an indicator of peripheral perfusion.

Gastrointestinal status. Bowel sounds should be auscultated at least every 8 hours and abdominal distention should be assessed through percussion. Serial measurements of abdominal girth may be indicated. If a nasogastric tube is used, the drainage should be measured as part of the fluid output and tested for occult blood. If the patient has a bowel movement, the stool should be checked for occult blood.

Personal hygiene. Hygiene is especially important to the patient in shock because impaired tissue perfusion predisposes to infection and skin breakdown. However, bathing and other nursing measures must be carried out judiciously because a patient in shock has major problems with oxygen delivery to tissues. Nursing measures must be performed with the least fatiguing method possible and spaced to allow adequate recovery. Using an alternating-pressure or special foam mattress, turning the patient every 1 to 2 hours, and positioning the patient in good body alignment help prevent pressure ulcer formation. The patient in shock frequently is hemodynamically unstable, and repositioning may result in a worsening of vital signs. The nurse must use clinical judgment in determining priorities of care.

Oral care for the patient in shock is essential because mouth breathing is common and mucous membranes may be dry in the volume-depleted patient. In addition, the intubated patient usually has difficulty swallowing, resulting in pooled secretions in the mouth. A water-soluble lubricant applied to the lips prevents drying and cracking. Moist swabbing of the tongue and oral mucosa with saline solution or diluted mouthwash is also beneficial. Lemon and glycerin swabs should not be used because they can cause drying of the mucosa.

Emotional support. The effects of the patient's anxiety and fear in the face of this critical, life-threatening situation are frequently overlooked or underestimated. Anxiety and fear may aggravate respiratory distress and increase catecholamine secretion. It is important for the nurse to remember that compassionate understanding is as essential as scientific and technical expertise in the total care of a patient in shock.

In planning and implementing the nursing care of the patient in shock, the nurse should assess the patient's anxiety. Medication to decrease anxiety may seem to be the simplest mode of therapy. However, in some shock situations, sedation may be contraindicated.

The nurse should talk to the patient, even if the patient is intubated or appears comatose. If the intubated patient is capable of writing, a magic slate or a pencil and paper should be provided. The patient should also receive simple explanations of procedures before they are carried out, as well as information regarding the current plan of care and its rationale. If the patient asks questions about progress and prognosis, simple and honest answers should be given.

Privacy should be provided as much as possible, but the patient should be assured that assistance is readily available should it be required. The call bell should be in reach. In addition, joking, teasing, and "kidding around" among health care personnel should be kept to a minimum or occur where the patient cannot hear it. This sort of behavior can often lead the patient to believe that staff members are having too much fun to be available to provide adequate care. Furthermore, conversations about the patient should not take place where the patient can overhear them. Such conversations can constitute a violation of the patient's confidence or may be misinterpreted in a way that causes the patient unnecessary distress.

Finally, many patients desire the comfort of a priest, rabbi, or minister. The nurse should offer to call a member of the clergy rather than wait for the patient or the family to express a wish for spiritual counseling.

Also, the patient's family and significant others need support and comfort. The family primarily wants to be kept informed of the patient's condition and needs reassurance that capable personnel are taking care of their loved one. If possible, the same person should continue to serve as the patient's nurse to decrease anxiety and avoid confusing contradictions. Family members and friends should be shown where they can wait and where a telephone can be found. Directions to the restrooms and to the hospital cafeteria are also appropriate.

Visits with the patient should be facilitated rather than hindered, provided the visits are perceived as a comfort by the patient. The nurse should explain in simple terms the purpose of the tubes and machines surrounding the patient, and the family should be informed of what they may and may not touch. Privacy should be ensured as much as possible. The family should be instructed to avoid tiring the patient.

Chronic and Home Management. Rehabilitation of the patient in shock necessitates prevention or early treatment of complications and correction of the precipitating cause. The nurse should continue to assess the patient for indications of complications throughout the recovery period. These complications include such problems as chronic renal failure after acute tubular necrosis or the development of fibrotic lung disease as a result of ARDS (see Chapters 44 and 26).

CRITICAL THINKING EXERCISES

CASE STUDY

HYPOVOLEMIC SHOCK

Patient Profile

Mr. S., a 25-year-old man, was an unrestrained driver involved in a motor vehicle accident. He was found face down 15 feet from his car. There were no other passengers in his car. The windshield was broken and the car was found up against a tree. Mr. S. was found conscious and moaning, and he was taken to the emergency department.

Subjective Data

- States that he cannot breathe
- Complains of abdominal pain

Objective Data

Physical Examination

- Circulation: BP 84/70; apical pulse 120 but no radial or brachial pulses palpable; carotid pulse present but weak.
- Lungs: Respiratory rate 35/min; labored breathing with severe respiratory distress; asymmetric chest wall movement; absence of breath sounds on right side.
- Abdomen: Slightly distended and painful to palpation.

Diagnostic Studies

- Peritoneal lavage positive for blood
- Hematocrit: 28%.

Therapeutic Management

In the ER, placement of chest tube, which drained bright red blood

Surgical Procedure

- Splenectomy
- Repair of torn thoracic artery

Critical Thinking Questions

1. What type of shock was present in Mr. S., and what clinical manifestations did he display?
2. What were the causes of Mr. S.'s shock? What are other causes of this type of shock?
3. What are the initial nursing responsibilities for Mr. S.?
4. What continual nursing assessment parameters are essential for this patient?
5. Based on the assessment data presented, write one or more nursing diagnoses. Are there any collaborative problems?

NURSING RESEARCH ISSUES

1. Compare the accuracy of blood pressure monitoring devices to detect the blood pressure changes in shock: invasive arterial monitoring compared with noninvasive devices.
2. How can the nurse's ability to identify changes in the patient's level of consciousness be enhanced in a patient with hypovolemic shock?
3. What is the patient's ability to understand what is being said and what is happening as the shock state worsens?
4. Compare the cognitive status of patients in different stages of shock.

REVIEW QUESTIONS

The number of the question corresponds to the same-numbered objective at the beginning of the chapter.

1. Shock is best defined as
   a. blood pressure less than 90 mm Hg systolic.
   b. loss of sympathetic tone.
   c. inadequate tissue perfusion.
   d. cardiovascular collapse.

2. A 78-year-old man has confusion and a temperature of 104° F (40° C). He is a diabetic with purulent drainage from his right great toe. His hemodynamic findings are: B/P 70/40; HR 110; respiratory rate 42 and shallow; CO 9L/min; and PCWP 4 mm Hg. This patient's symptoms are most likely indicative of which type of shock?
   a. Anaphylactic
   b. Hypovolemic
   c. Cardiogenic
   d. Septic

3. Which of the following events occurs during the compensatory stage of shock?
   a. Movement of fluid into the interstitial space
   b. Activation of the renin-angiotensin system
   c. Myocardial depression
   d. Severe vasoconstriction

4. Which statement is *true* about the effect that shock has on the body?

a. Sympathetic nervous system activation results in stimulation of adrenergic receptors.
b. Massive vasoconstriction in the heart and brain causes stimulation of the renin-angiotensin system.
c. The HR is usually slow and irregular in the compensatory stage as a result of parasympathetic stimulation.
d. Decreased tissue perfusion causes the cells to undergo aerobic metabolism, which leads to the development of lactic acidosis.

5. Appropriate treatment modalities for the management of cardiogenic shock include all of the following *except*

a. dopamine to increase myocardial contractility.
b. corticosteroids to stablize the cell wall in the infarcted area.
c. diuretics to decrease an elevated preload.
d. nitroprusside to decrease systemic vascular resistance.

6. The most accurate assessment parameters for the nurse to use to determine adequate tissue perfusion in the shock patient include

a. blood pressure, pulse, and respirations.
b. level of consciousness, urine output, and skin color and temperature.
c. pulse pressure, level of consciousness, and pupillary response.
d. breath sounds, blood pressure, and body temperature.

REFERENCES

1. Rice V: Shock, a clinical syndrome: an update, part 1: an overview of shock, *Crit Care Nurse* 11:20, 1991.
2. Klein D, Witek-Janusek L: Advances in immunotherapy of sepsis, *Dimensions Crit Care Nursing* 11:75, 1992.
3. Rackow E, Astiz M: Pathophysiology and treatment of septic shock, *JAMA* 266:548, 1991.
4. Sim T: Anaphylaxis: how to manage and prevent this medical emergency, *Postgrad Med J* 92:277, 1992.
5. Alpert J, Becker R: Mechanisms and management of cardiogenic shock, *Crit Care Clin* 9:205, 1993.
6. Teba L and others: Understanding circulatory shock, *Postgrad Med* 91:121, 1992.
7. Laskowski-Jones L: Acute SCI: how to minimize the damage, *Am J Nurs* 93:23, 1993.
8. Glauser MP and others: Pathogenesis and potential strategies for prevention and treatment of septic shock: an update. *Clin Infect Dis* 18:S205, 1994.
9. Rice V: Shock, a clinical syndrome: an update, part 4: nursing care of the shock patient, *Crit Care Nurse* 11:28, 1991.
10. Murray M, Kumar M: Sepsis and septic shock, *Postgrad Med* 90:199, 1991.
11. Hazinski M and others: Epidemiology, pathophysiology and clinical presentation of gram-negative sepsis, *Am J Crit Care* 2:224, 1993.
12. Alspach G, editor: *Core curriculum for critical care nursing*, ed 4, Philadelphia, 1991, WB Saunders.
13. Rice V: Shock, a clinical syndrome: an update, part 2: the stages of shock, *Crit Care Nurse* 11:74, 1991.
14. Fiddian-Green RG and others: Goals for resuscitation, *Crit Care Med* 21:525, 1993.
15. Imm A, Carlson R: Fluid resuscitation in circulatory shock, *Crit Care Clin* 9:313, 1993.
16. Griffel M, Kaufman B: Pharmacology of colloids and crystalloids, *Crit Care Clin* 8:235, 1992.
17. Sommers M: Fluid resuscitation following multiple trauma, *Crit Care Nurse* 10:74, 1990.
18. Goldenberg I: Nonpharmacologic management of cardiac arrest and cardiogenic shock, *Chest* 102:596S, 1992.
19. Natanson C and others: Selected treatment strategies for septic shock based on proposed mechanisms of pathogenesis, *Ann Intern Med* 120:771, 1994.
20. Jafari HS, McCracken GH: Sepsis and septic shock: a review for clinicians, *Pediatr Infect Dis J* 11:739, 1992.

Chapter 8

NURSING ROLE IN MANAGEMENT

Substance Abuse and Dependence

Phyllis Lisanti   Patsy L. Orth Duphorne

Learning Objectives

1. Explain how the models of addiction influence treatment.
2. Define addiction, abuse, craving, loss of control, dependence, tolerance, withdrawal, abstinence, detoxification, and relapse.
3. List common characteristics of substance abuse.
4. Describe the process of addiction.
5. List criteria for classification and diagnoses of substance abuse and substance dependence.
6. Recognize signs and symptoms of abuse and dependence on stimulant, depressant, and hallucinogenic drugs.
7. Describe the nursing management of a patient who experiences intoxication, toxic reactions, or withdrawal from stimulants, depressants, or hallucinogens.
8. Describe primary, secondary, and tertiary prevention activities aimed at different patterns of substance abuse.
9. Identify health promotion strategies to prevent substance abuse that the nurse can use in a variety of settings.
10. List nursing diagnoses related to substance abuse.
11. Discuss the long-term problems of a patient with substance abuse problems and related nursing management.
12. Discuss substance abuse problems of an older adult.
13. Describe factors that contribute to the problem of chemical dependence among nurses.

The increased prevalence of substance abuse poses a threat to the health and welfare of many populations throughout the world. Recreational drugs (e.g., cocaine, heroin) play a major role in crime and corruption. Abuse of prescription drugs and alcohol places a heavy burden on health resources because of the associated medical problems.

Individuals who abuse substances typically use the health care system more than non–substance-abusing individuals do, both for acute and chronic problems.[1,2] It is estimated that approximately 30% of all patients hospitalized in general acute care settings abuse or are dependent on alcohol.[3] Among hospitalized older adults, the prevalence of alcoholism is as high as 20%.[4]

The abuse of other drugs such as marijuana, inhalants, and hallucinogens is not as well documented, but it is known that they are responsible for significant use of health resources. Intravenous (IV) drug use is the second leading cause of human immunodeficiency virus (HIV) infection. Cocaine is used regularly by more than 5 million Americans and is responsible for a sixfold increase in emergency department-related visits since 1983.[5]

Nurses, employed in a variety of health care settings, are in key positions to identify patients who are abusing or addicted to substances. This chapter addresses the nurse's role in identifying and managing the substance-abusing patient in a variety of medical-surgical care settings. Promotion of health and long-term care of the chronic substance abuser is also addressed.

OVERVIEW OF SUBSTANCE ABUSE

Models of Addiction

Models are useful in directing treatment and planning prevention, education, and research activities. Theories and research related to alcohol use are the basis for the development of most of the models that have been applied to substance abuse. The *disease* or *medical model* focuses on addiction as an illness and removes the element of blame from the addict. The *biopsychosocial model* integrates current research findings and promotes a holistic approach. The *public health model* expands the focus of concern to the community and implies a multifaceted approach to the problem. Specific information on these and other models of addiction is presented in Table 8-1.

Reviewed by Madeline A. Naegle, RN, PhD, FAAN, Associate Professor, Division of Nursing, School of Education; and the Project Director of Substance Abuse Education in Nursing (SAEN), New York University, New York, NY.

Table 8-1 Models of Addiction

Model	Causal Factors	Treatment Focus	Nursing Implications
Medical/Disease Substance abuse is a chronic, progressive problem.	Biochemical differences (e.g., metabolic abnormalities), genetic predisposition	Physical symptoms Related illnesses Control of progression Intervention for drug treament, rehabilitation, abstinence, relapse	Identify signs and symptoms. Recognize related illnesses. Educate about stages, including relapse. Refer for treatment and support groups.
Psychodynamic Addiction develops as a function of intrapsychic or interpersonal needs or as emotional and mental problems.	Personality disorder Neurosis Depression Anxiety Family dysfunction	Psychotherapy Group therapy Family therapy	Assist in increasing self-esteem, communication skills, and coping and social skills. Assess emotional problems; refer for treatment.
Biopsychosocial Addiction is a multi-dimensional problem and not the result of a single factor.	Biologic Psychologic Social	Comprehensive—based on role of family, culture, and society in problem and solution	Assess all dimensions. Include family. Help to build social support network. Assist to increase functioning, healthy lifestyle.
Social Learning Addiction is a mal-adaptive habit of learned behavior.	Skill deficits Expectancies (relief of tension) Poor modeling	Cognitive therapy Behavioral therapy Skill training Self-control training	Teach coping and assertive-ness skills. Identify antecedents ("trig-gers"). Link triggers with conse-quences. Encourage self-responsibility. Provide positive reinforce-ment of healthy coping. Guide relapse prevention.
Sociocultural Addiction reflects conflicts and issues in society.	Role strain Family problems Socioeconomic conditions Rituals, practices, taboos Unclear cultural norms Changing cultures Mixed social messages	Traditions, values, beliefs Peer pressure Role and job satisfaction Separation from family	Support tradition. Clarify norms. Increase awareness of mixed messages. Assist in increasing problem-solving skills. Address codependency issues. Empower to make healthy choices.
Public Health Addiction is based on interactions of host, agent, and environment.	*Host:* high risk, drug dependence in families, psychologic conflict *Agent:* type of drug, frequency of use, route of administration, availability *Environment:* family, friends, community resources, media, socioeconomic factors	Multifaceted (medical, emotional, and social problems) Risk appraisal Genetic counseling Self-control training Social action and responsibility	Assess risk factors Provide information and assist with developing coping skills. Support lifestyle changes.

Table 8-2 Terminology of Substance Abuse

Term	Definition
▪ Substance	Drug, chemical, or biologic entity is self-administered.
▪ Habituation	Pattern of repeated drug use that exists in the absence of an actual physical need for the drug. There is no desire for increased use. There may be withdrawal manifestations.
▪ Misuse	Drugs are used for purposes other than those for which they are intended. Misuse is common among people, especially the elderly, who self-medicate for a variety of reasons.
▪ Abuse	Drug use patterns that lie outside the limits acceptable by society and that impact negatively on psychologic, physiologic, and social functioning of an individual. Drug abuse may be combined with misuse.
▪ Dependence	Reliance on a substance that has reached the level that absence of it will cause an impairment in function.
Psychologic	Compulsive need to experience pleasurable response from the substance exists.
Physical	An altered physiologic state from prolonged substance use exists; regular use is necessary to prevent withdrawal.
▪ Tolerance	Decreased effect of a substance that results from repeated exposure. It is possible to develop cross-tolerance to other substances in same category.
▪ Withdrawal	Constellation of physiologic and psychologic responses that occur when there is abrupt cessation or reduced intake of a substance on which an individual is dependent or when the effect is counteracted by a specific antagonist.
▪ Addiction	Compulsive substance use that exists for both physical and psychologic reasons.
Dual	Simultaneous dependence on substances that have similar effects, such as barbiturates and alcohol, exists.
Mixed	Dependence is on more than one substance not necessarily similar in effects, such as alcohol and cocaine.
▪ Craving	Subjective need for a substance develops, usually experienced after decreased use or abstinence.
▪ Abstinence	Refrain from substance use.
▪ Detoxification	The substance and its effects are removed from the individual's body.
▪ Relapse	Readdiction occurs during rehabilitation period.
▪ Binge	Large quantities of a substance are consumed on occasion to the point of excess.

Terminology of Substance Abuse

Commonly used terms in the diagnosis and treatment of substance abuse are presented in Table 8-2. These terms are applicable to all abused substances, including those substances intended to be helpful such as prescribed and over-the-counter medications.

Patterns of Substance Use and Abuse

There are various patterns of substance use and abuse with a growing tendency among substance abusers to take a variety of drugs simultaneously. These patterns are presented within the prevention framework in Fig. 8-1.

Different types of multiple drug use may include mixed addiction, dual addiction, or cross-tolerance. *Mixed addiction* occurs when an individual alternates the use of one class of drugs with another to alleviate or counteract the effects of the original drug (e.g., alternate use of "uppers" like cocaine with "downers" like alcohol or heroin). *Dual addiction* refers to the use of drugs that have similar effects (e.g., alcohol and barbiturates). This term has also been used to indicate an addiction to more than one drug. *Cross-tolerance* is a type of dependence that occurs after tolerance has developed for one drug (e.g., diazepam [Valium] or chlordiazepoxide [Librium]), and the use of other drugs in the same class precipitates similar effects of tolerance (e.g., meperidine [Demerol] or morphine).

Risk Factors Associated with Substance Abuse

Although numerous studies have focused on the problem of substance abuse, the cause (or causes) remains unknown or unclear. Substance abuse is a multidimensional phenomenon with no single etiology. However, there is a variety of factors that increase an individual's vulnerability or risk to developing problems of substance abuse. Several risk factors are discussed below. Table 8-3 presents risk factors related to alcoholism.

Availability and Encouragement. Advertising campaigns make many chemical substances, such as alcohol and nicotine, seem appealing and socially acceptable. Sedatives and antianxiety agents are prescribed excessively for a variety of reasons. The combination of availability and media influence is thought to contribute to substance use and abuse. Peer pressure, particularly among adolescents and young adults, is also a strong motivator.

Adverse Social Conditions. Poverty, unemployment, discrimination, homelessness, and lack of social and educational opportunities contribute to high rates of substance abuse. Some individuals may abuse substances as a

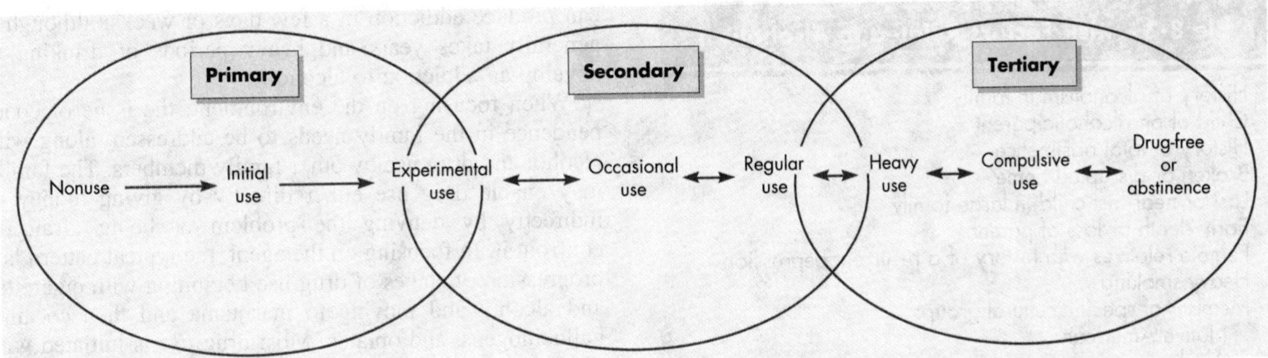

Fig. 8-1 Drug use patterns and prevention framework. Experimental use is usually short-term and no pattern of abuse develops. The occasional user may use a substance for social or recreational purposes for pleasure or diversion. The regular user abuses substances on a daily basis. In heavy use increased amounts of the substance are used extending over a long-term period. The compulsive user has lost control and has become addicted; there is continued abuse of the substance despite adverse consequences. The ultimate goal is that the substance abuser is drug-free or abstinent.

MYTHS ABOUT SUBSTANCE ABUSE

Myths	Truths
Narcotic users are sociopaths who frequently commit murder, rape, and other crimes of violence while under the influence of drugs.	Narcotic users, alone or in groups, prefer a quiet, secluded place where they can enjoy the drugs' effects in peace and quiet.
Narcotic parties are characterized by highly stimulating sexual activities.	Narcotics reduce sexual drives.
Drug addicts are easily distinguished from other people by their appearance and behavior.	It is often difficult for police and medical experts to identify a user without specific medical tests or interviews.
Professional pushers hang around schools and street corners waiting to introduce innocent victims to narcotics.	Individuals are generally introduced to the use of narcotics through their friends.
Marijuana use inevitably leads to a dependence on heroin.	Marijuana does not usually produce physical dependence; it can lead to emotional dependence, which can be equally habit-forming. Most heroin dependence started with marijuana or pills.
Users can control casual use of narcotics without becoming dependent.	No one can predict at which point an individual can or will lose control. The occasional user is highly vulnerable to becoming addicted.
Beer drinkers do not become alcoholics. Only people who drink "hard" liquor become alcoholics.	Any form of alcohol, if frequently consumed in large quantities over a period of years, may lead to alcoholism.

means of coping with adverse conditions. It is also possible that the adverse social conditions may result from substance abuse.

Biologic or Genetic Factors. There may be biologic or genetic factors that contribute to substance abuse. It is well known that substance abuse occurs in families. It is debated whether these influences are environmental or biologic. However, family studies have shown that a genetic predisposition is an important factor in the development of alcoholism.

Psychologic Influence. Although research findings do not support an "addictive personality," certain personality dispositions may contribute to the development of substance abuse. Substances may be used to reduce uncomfortable states of anxiety, stress, and depression for these individuals. Psychodynamic factors, which may be associated with substance abuse, include anxiety or panic disorders, a basic depressive personality (particularly in women), risk-taking personality, impulsivity, intolerance to frustration, poor judgment, and antisocial behaviors.

Table 8-3 Risk Factors Related to Alcoholism

History of alcoholism in family
Child of an alcoholic parent
History of total abstinence
Broken or disrupted home
Last or near last child in large family
Early death or loss of parent
Female relatives with history of a recurrent depression
Heavy smoking
Member of specific cultural groups
Native American
Alaskan natives

Disabilities. Physically disabled individuals have a rate twice as high as the general population for alcoholism and problems with other substances. A high percentage of people with disabilities suffer from low self-esteem, chronic medical problems, a history of reliance on prescription medication, and a high incidence of depression.[6] All of these factors contribute to an increased risk for substance abuse.

Developmental Influence. Parents are important role models for their children's emotional and behavioral growth and development. An individual who sustains some form of parental loss (through death, divorce, or abandonment) may be predisposed to substance abuse problems. The inability of some parents to develop satisfying emotional relationships with their children also increases the risk for substance abuse. Children of substance-abusing parents are at a greater risk for becoming substance abusers.

Addictive Process

The length of time required to move from casual use to dependence is a function of many factors related to the host, agent, and environment (Fig. 8-2). The type of drug, frequency of use, amount of drug used, route of administration, health of the user, and support for drug use from friends or family members (*enabling*) affect the development of an addiction. Repeated IV use of heroin or cocaine can produce addiction in a few days or weeks, although it generally takes years and heavy periods of drinking to develop an addiction to alcohol.

When focusing on the environment, the issue of codependence in the family needs to be addressed, along with alcohol and drug use by other family members. The family may enable drug use either directly by giving money or indirectly by denying the problem or being afraid to confront it. In focusing on the agent, the typical pattern is a progression of stages of drug use beginning with cigarettes and alcohol and moving to marijuana and then cocaine, hallucinogens, and opiates. Most drug use is initiated with the involvement of at least one legal drug.

The process of addiction may be thought of as a cycle that is self-reinforcing (Fig. 8-3). Interruptions in the cycle occur because of inaccessibility of the substance, decrease in the amount used, attempts to control drug use, or entry into treatment. These factors may precipitate withdrawal symptoms in the physically dependent individual. Rapid reinstatement of the cycle occurs when the individual relapses.

Characteristics of Addictions. Substance abusers have certain common characteristics (Table 8-4). These characteristics may influence the initiation or maintenance of patterns of abuse and dependence. The nurse needs to recognize the importance of these features in contributing to the complex problems of addiction.

Classification

Medical diagnoses of addictions are based on the criteria of the American Psychiatric Association in the *Diagnostic and*

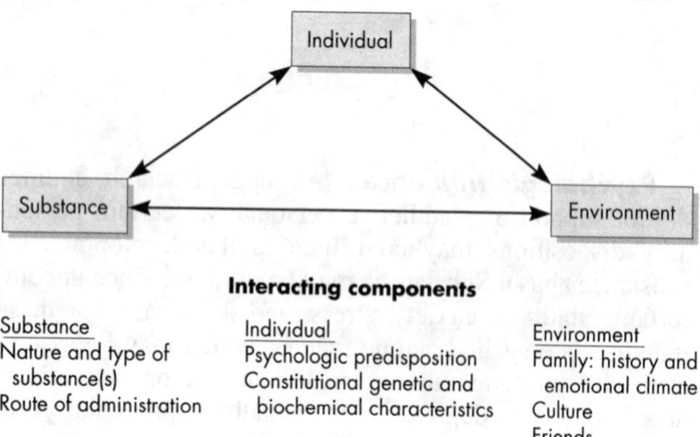

Fig. 8-2 Factors involved in the development of addiction.

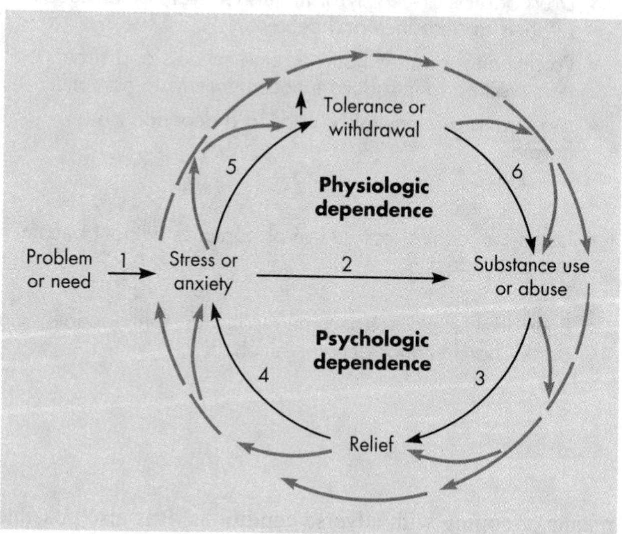

Fig. 8-3 The addictive cycle. *Step 1,* The problem or need arouses stress or anxiety and is dealt with through substance use. *Steps 2 to 4,* The cycle of substance use, relief, and recurring stress or anxiety is repeated until psychologic dependence is established. Interruping the cycle brings about anxiety but not physical symptoms. *Steps 5 to 6,* Physiologic dependence usually follows psychologic dependence. Withdrawal symptoms follow abstinence. Interruptions in the cycle are indicated by a *broken line.*

Statistical Manual of Mental Disorders (DSM-IV). The DSM-IV classification for substance-related disorders includes two categories—*substance use disorders* and *substance-induced mental disorders.* The former refers to patterns of abuse and dependence associated with maladaptive behavioral changes (Table 8-5). The latter refers to the primary central nervous system (CNS) effects of intoxication, withdrawal, delirium, anxiety disorder, psychotic disorder with delusions or hallucinations, sleep disorder, persisting perception disorder, sexual dysfunction, and mood disorder. Criteria for the diagnosis of alcoholism have also been compiled by the National Council on Alcoholism. Major and minor clinical, physiologic, behavioral, and laboratory indicators of alcoholism are identified and differentiated among early, middle, and late stages.

Table 8-4 Common Characteristics of Substance Abusers

Excessive and compulsive use
Impulsive behaviors
Powerful immediate reinforcement
Feelings of depression, helplessness, dependence
Defenses, including denial, projection, manipulation
Low frustration tolerance
Poor body image, low self-esteem
Tendency to relapse
Family dysfunction
Lack of social support (unrelated to drug use)
Chronic or terminal illness related to abuse patterns (e.g., cirrhosis)

STIMULANTS

The two most frequently used stimulants are nicotine and caffeine. However, amphetamines and cocaine are the stimulants that lead to the most serious types of abuse. The most potent stimulant of natural origin is cocaine.

Nicotine (Tobacco Abuse)

Characteristics. Nicotine, an alkaloid found in tobacco, is the component of tobacco that causes dependence. Smoking is the most common form of substance abuse in the United States and Canada. Nicotine has a much greater potential for the development of dependence than alcohol.

Table 8-5 Diagnostic Criteria for Psychoactive Substance Dependence and Abuse

Criteria for Substance Dependence

A maladaptive pattern of substance use, leading to clinically significant impairment or distress, as manifested by three (or more) of the following, occurring at any time in the same 12-mo period.

1. Tolerance, as defined by
   a. a need for markedly increased amounts of the substance to achieve intoxication or desired effect, or
   b. markedly diminished effect with continued use of the same amount of the substance.
2. Withdrawal, as manifested by
   a. the characteristic withdrawal syndrome for the substance (refer to Criteria A and B of the criterion sets for withdrawal from the specific substances), or
   b. the same (or a closely related) substance is taken to relieve or avoid withdrawal symptoms.
3. The substance is often taken in larger amounts or over a longer period than was intended.
4. There is a persistent desire or unsuccessful efforts to cut down or control substance use.
5. A great deal of time is spent in activities necessary to obtain the substance (e.g., visiting multiple doctors or driving long distances), to use the substance (e.g., chain-smoking), or to recover from its effects.
6. Important social, occupational, or recreational activities are given up or reduced because of substance use.
7. The substance use is continued despite knowledge of having a persistent or recurrent physical or psychologic problem that is likely to have been caused or exacerbated by the substance (e.g., current cocaine use despite recognition of cocaine-induced depression or continued drinking despite recognition that an ulcer was made worse by alcohol consumption).

Criteria for Substance Abuse

A. A maladaptive pattern of substance use leading to clinically significant impairment or distress, as manifested by one (or more) of the following, occurring within a 12-mo period:
   1. Recurrent substance use results in a failure to fulfill major role obligations at work, school, or home (e.g., repeated absences or poor work performance related to substance use; substance-related absences, suspensions, or expulsions from school; neglect of children or household).
   2. Recurrent substance use exists in situations in which it is physically hazardous (e.g., driving an automobile or operating a machine when impaired by substance use).
   3. Recurrent substance-related legal problems develop (e.g., arrests for substance-related disorderly conduct).
   4. Substance use continues despite having persistent or recurrent social or interpersonal problems caused or exacerbated by the effects of the substance (e.g., arguments with spouse about consequences of intoxication, physical fights).

B. The symptoms have never met the criteria for Substance Dependence for this class of substance.

Modified from American Psychiatric Association: *Diagnostic and statistical manual of mental disorders,* ed 4, Washington, DC, 1994, American Psychiatric Association.

The trends in smoking have varied over the past 10 years, but the percentage of smokers appears to be decreasing. The percentage of female smokers has not decreased as much as that of male smokers. In 1993 the effects of smoking cost $50 billion in medical care with 54% of this cost spent on hospitalization. More than 400,000 people each year die as a result of smoking.[7] These figures do not take into account the indirect costs of smoking, such as loss of productivity because of illness, economic loss from an early death, injuries caused by fires, or treatment for the effects of second-hand smoke.

Smoking is the predominant form of tobacco abuse. Other forms include chewing a plug of tobacco or snuffing tobacco powder intranasally. Since a greater number of harmful substances are released during the smoking process, more attention has been focused on cigarette smoking. Pipe and cigar smokers usually puff and do not inhale; therefore they are considered to be at lower risk than cigarette smokers for developing health problems. Occupations involving smoke or dust increase the risk of illness and early death in a person who also smokes. Teenagers who are most likely to smoke include those whose parents, siblings, or friends smoke.

Passive or involuntary smoking occurs under conditions of heavy smoking and poor ventilation when nonsmokers inhale the by-products of tobacco smoke. Young children and people with respiratory or cardiovascular diseases are at greatest risk for developing illnesses from passive smoking. Federal, state, and local agencies have attempted to address the rights of nonsmokers by mandating nonsmoking areas in public places and smoke-free workplaces and hospitals.

Effects of Use. Smoking is a powerful self-reinforcing behavior. It decreases stress and tension, which is important in both the initiation and the continuation of this behavior. Tobacco contains more than 100 known chemical compounds, including at least 15 known carcinogens and a number of hydrocarbons or solvents that may cause death. Three of the most damaging substances are nicotine, carbon monoxide, and tar.

Nicotine is a mild stimulant that has no therapeutic value. It has a unique biphasic effect on the peripheral system and the CNS. It initially acts as a stimulant, followed by a depressant effect, which may be associated with fatigue. The amount or dose of nicotine varies with the form and method of ingestion. The effects of nicotine appear to be dose related. Nicotine is absorbed through the lungs in smoking, through the buccal mucosa in chewing, and through the nasal mucosa in snuffing. When taken by these routes, nicotine initially bypasses the liver and goes directly to the brain and other parts of the body. The effects of smoking are listed in Table 8-6.

The strong psychologic dependency associated with nicotine abuse is supported by the fact that it acts on the brain within seconds of use. Physiologic dependence occurs with regular heavy use and is evidenced by increased tolerance and withdrawal symptoms following attempts to stop smoking. Withdrawal symptoms may occur within the first few hours after stopping, peak in 24 to 48 hours, and may last from several days to a month. Symptoms may include craving, restlessness, decreased ability to concentrate, hyperirritability, headache, insomnia, anxiety, drowsiness, decreased blood pressure and heart rate, and an initial increased appetite that may not be permanent.

Table 8-6 Effects of Smoking (Nicotine-related)*

Raised arousal level
Decreased attention to extraneous stimuli
Decreased muscle tone
Stress reduction
Performance enhancement
Fine tremor (nicotine tremor)
Shortness of breath
Decreased appetite
Antidiuretic effect
Decreased aggressiveness

*Found in varying degrees in nicotine users.

All tobacco smoke contains carbon monoxide. When the smoke is inhaled, the carbon monoxide combines with hemoglobin and prevents the hemoglobin from carrying oxygen. This decreased oxygenation of blood may explain the smoker's shortness of breath during exertion.

Tar contains several hundred chemicals, some of which are carcinogenic. The small particles of tar are trapped inside the lung where they damage the tissue.

Smoking has an adverse effect on the development of the fetus, the infant's survival, and long-term effects on the child. There is an increased risk for spontaneous abortion, impaired fetal growth, stillbirth, premature birth, and neonatal death. Newborns of mothers who smoked during pregnancy tend to have a lower birth weight and a smaller head circumference and tend to be shorter. Nicotine crosses the placental barrier to the fetal bloodstream, directly affecting the fetus. Symptoms of hyperactivity in children may be associated with smoking during pregnancy.

Complications. A major concern related to smoking involves accidental death resulting because of fires from careless habits, especially smoking in bed. Smoking predisposes a person to respiratory disease (especially chronic obstructive pulmonary disease), cardiovascular disease, and increased incidence of cancer of the mouth, throat, lungs, urinary bladder, pancreas, and kidney. The incidence of cancer of the mouth, throat, larynx, and stomach is higher for cigar and pipe smokers than for nonsmokers. There also appears to be an association between smoking and the development of peptic ulcers and cirrhosis of the liver. Women over age 35 who smoke and take birth control pills have an increased risk of hemorrhage, especially cerebral hemorrhage.

Therapeutic Management. Pharmacologic aids to control symptoms of nicotine withdrawal include nicotine gum (Nicorette) and, more recently, a nicotine transdermal system or patches (Habitrol, Nicoderm, Prostep), which are available only by prescription. In general, gradual reduction in nicotine is usually less effective over the long term than

RESEARCH

Implications for Nursing Practice

NICOTINE PATCH FOR SMOKING CESSATION

Citation Imperial Cancer Research Fund General Practice Research Group: Effectiveness of a nicotine patch in helping people stop smoking: results of a randomized trial in general practice, *BMJ* 306:1304-1308, 1993.

Purpose To assess the effectiveness of 12-week treatment with a 24-hour transdermal nicotine patch in helping heavy smokers to stop smoking

Methods Double-blind placebo controlled, randomized trial involved 1686 heavy smokers, ages 25-64 years, with a mean cigarette consumption of 24 per day and mean duration of smoking of 25 years. Salivary cotinine determinations were used to confirm smoking cessation. The treatment period lasted 12 weeks.

Results and Conclusions Cessation of smoking was confirmed in 19.4% of the patients using the nicotine patch and 11.7% using the placebo. The most significant adverse effect of the patch was local skin irritation. Nicotine patches were effective in promoting smoking cessation. However, the extent to which this effect can be sustained cannot be assessed until long-term results are evaluated.

Implications for Nursing Practice Nicotine withdrawal symptoms make it difficult for heavy smokers to stop smoking. Nicotine replacement in chewing gum and patches reduces withdrawal symptoms. The cessation rate in the placebo group indicates the importance of nursing support. As evidenced in this study, nursing support is an integral part of promoting smoking cessation.

abrupt cessation, or the "cold turkey" method. Formal or community-based behavioral smoking cessation programs that promote alternate tension relieving and leisure activities are valuable aids to the nicotine-dependent person.

Caffeine Abuse

Characteristics. Caffeine use is integral to American culture. As a result of mass marketing, coffee is promoted for use to wake up in the morning and to enhance work performance during the day. Although its acceptance as a social drug implies it has few negative effects on health, caffeine has many significant physiologic effects.

Approximately 80% of adults and 30% of youths (ages 12 to 17 years) use coffee. Adults and youths have similar rates (60%) in the consumption of tea. One cup of coffee contains approximately 100 to 150 mg of caffeine, which is considered a therapeutic dose. The content of caffeine in tea varies according to how it is brewed. A cup of tea averages 60 to 75 mg caffeine, and a glass of cola averages 40 to 60 mg caffeine.

Caffeine is a xanthine derivative that occurs naturally in a number of plants such as coffee beans, tea leaves, cocoa, and cola nuts. It is also found in medications such as No Doz, Vivarin, Excedrin, Vanquish, Anacin, Bromo–Seltzer, cold preparations, appetite suppressants, and prescription medications.

Table 8-7 Effects of Caffeine*

Increased alertness and thinking
Increased respirations
Relaxation of smooth visceral muscles
Decreased peristalsis
Possible interference with REM and deep sleep
Increased speed of motor tasks
Increased myocardial contractions
Increased heart rate
Diuresis
Jitteriness
Nervousness
Gastrointestinal upset

REM, Rapid eye movements.
*Found in varying degrees in caffeine users.

Effects of Use. Caffeine is one of the most widely used stimulant drugs in the world. It is a relatively weak CNS stimulant. It also relaxes smooth muscles, promotes vasodilatation, is a diuretic, constricts cerebral arteries, enhances contraction of skeletal muscles, and is a myocardial stimulant. Caffeine is absorbed by the gastrointestinal (GI) tract and is rapidly distributed throughout the body. Peak blood plasma levels occur within 30 minutes after ingestion. Stimulant effects may last from 3 to 5 hours. Caffeine crosses the placenta and is also secreted in the milk of lactating women.

The effects of caffeine are listed in Table 8-7. Some of the physiologic actions help to explain caffeine's effectiveness in increasing work output and prolonging the time one can perform physically exhausting work. The effects of caffeine are dose-related. Oral doses of 200 mg (two cups of coffee) can elevate mood, produce insomnia, increase irritability, cause anxiety, or offset fatigue. Heavy doses of 500 mg or more are known to cause tachycardia and respiratory stimulation. Caffeine may be useful in reversing respiratory depression in cases of drug overdose. Ingestion of a lethal dose is extremely rare but could occur with caffeine-containing drugs or the oral ingestion of 10 g (70 to 100 cups of coffee).

Caffeine interferes with sleep by increasing sleep onset time, decreasing dreaming (rapid eye movement [REM]) sleep, and decreasing deep sleep time. Coffee taken in the evening is more likely to have adverse effects on light users than on regular or heavy users (five to six cups or more per day). Coffee taken in the morning by regular or heavy users is required to avoid morning tiredness and irritability.

Tolerance to caffeine's stimulant effects develops slowly but may be overcome by increasing the amount consumed. Physical and psychologic dependence have been found with chronic heavy use (more than five cups per day). The most common and best substantiated withdrawal symptoms are headache, irritability, and nervousness. They occur within 12 to 24 hours, peak at 20 to 48 hours, and last for about 1 week. Other effects of withdrawal include sleepiness and feelings of decreased contentment that may be mistaken for depression.

Complications. Caffeine is contraindicated in the patient with glaucoma. It can significantly raise the intraocular pressure when the glaucoma is uncontrolled, resulting in a caffeine-induced headache.

Toxic effects of caffeine include ringing in the ears, flashes of light, insomnia, increased sensitivity, tachycardia, dysrhythmias, and hypotension. In heavy coffee drinkers, blood lipid levels may be increased, which may lead to an increased incidence of angina and myocardial infarction. Habitual users are reported to have slightly higher blood pressure, increased basal metabolic rates, and increased blood glucose levels. In high doses, caffeine influences behavior patterns and may precipitate anxiety states.

Amphetamines

Characteristics. Amphetamines, developed in the 1930s as a substitute for ephedrine, were found to be potent bronchodilators and useful in inhalers. The drug also has been found to be effective in the treatment of narcolepsy. Currently, methylphenidate (Ritalin) is primarily used in the treatment of attention-deficit hyperactivity disorder in children, and phenmetrazine (Preludin) is used as an appetite suppressant.

The amphetamine group includes amphetamine (Benzedrine), dextroamphetamine (Dexedrine), and methamphetamine (Desoxyn), also known as *speed.* Phenmetrazine and methylphenidate are also stimulants that may be abused. Other drugs in this category are benzphetamine (Didrex), diethylpropion (Tenuate), fenfluramine (Pondimin), mazindol (Sanorex), phendimetrazine (Anorex, Adphen), and phentermine (Fastin, Ionamin), which are used as anorectic drugs.

As amphetamine use has become more tightly controlled through prescriptions, "look-alike" pills that are identical in appearance and illicit methamphetamine (e.g., "crank," "crystal") have become popular. Recently, "act-alikes," less potent forms with no resemblance to amphetamines, have appeared in states prohibiting look-alikes. Use of crank and "ice," a smokable form of methamphetamine, has increased in some parts of the country.

Effects of Use. Amphetamines act by stimulating the sympathetic nervous system. Manifestations initially begin with feelings of euphoria and excitement and continue with effects on the cardiovascular and respiratory systems. These drugs result in excess catecholamine release that leads to a "fight or flight" reaction.

The primary effects of stimulants are listed in Table 8-8 and include dilated pupils, diaphoresis, smooth-muscle relaxation, and an increase in metabolic rate. Initial use results in increased alertness or concentration, improved performance, relief of fatigue, or weight control. The user comes to rely on the euphoric effects and the feeling of power. These drugs may also lead to unpleasant feelings of irritability, fear, and anxiety. Increased doses tend to precipitate rapid mood swings, hallucinations, racing thoughts, feelings of being out of control, aggression, and compulsive or meaningless behaviors.

Amphetamines are primarily taken orally; peak effects occur within 2 to 3 hours with complete elimination occurring within 2 days.[8] Effects are generally intensified by IV injection of the drug, which produces a "rush" or "flash," an almost immediate intense burst of energy. Frequent or heavy IV use may lead to a psychosis that mimics schizophrenia or mania. Smoking these drugs produces a similar instantaneous effect and is believed to be the most rapid, intense response route. Intranasal ingestion *(snorting)* has the longest effect because of local constriction of blood vessels.[9]

Tolerance to these drugs develops rapidly and leads to intense craving, even in the absence of euphoria. Physical dependence has been recognized but is characterized more by psychologic manifestations than physical ones. Certain mental abnormalities may develop as a result of high doses. Early signs include *bruxism* (grinding of teeth), touching and picking the face and extremities, repetitious movements, suspiciousness, and a sense of being watched.

Complications. Toxic reactions to stimulants are usually dose-related and include increased levels of stimulation, sometimes described as "overamping," which may culminate in massive overdose and death. Reactions to high doses are paranoia with auditory and visual hallucinations. A sublethal overdose is recognized by symptoms of headache, dizziness, agitation, hostility, tremor, panic, flushed skin, chest pain with palpitations, diaphoresis, vomiting, and abdominal cramps. Without medical intervention, death may occur as the result of seizures, cardiovascular collapse, and hyperthermia. Physical exertion increases the risk of toxicity and may contribute to sudden death even when moderate amounts of the drug are used.

Stimulant withdrawal is characterized by depression, irritability, anxiety, fatigue, insomnia or hypersomnia, or psychomotor agitation. Symptoms peak in about 2 to 4 days. Suicidal thoughts, anxiety, and extreme tension may persist for weeks or months.

Therapeutic Management. Patients generally seek treatment for complications such as panic reactions or temporary psychosis related to intoxication, overdose, or withdrawal. Overdose has also been termed *acute poisoning.* Primary features of amphetamine intoxication are maladaptive behavioral changes such as fighting, manifestations of grandiosity, hypervigilance, psychomotor agitation, impaired judgment, and social or occupational dysfunction. Physical symptoms may include dilated pupils, elevated blood pressure, tachycardia, perspiration or chills, and nausea and vomiting. Agitation is usually the first symptom, and it can develop rapidly into a potentially fatal condition. Other symptoms may be decreased appetite, sleep disorders, chest pain, tremors, delirium, dizziness, respiratory paralysis, and cardiac dysrhythmias.

Amphetamine intoxication may be self-limiting within 24 hours. Treatment is directed toward symptoms and support. Acute intoxication requires careful observation to prevent symptoms from developing into a medical emer-

Table 8-8 Effects of Frequently Abused Drugs

Drug	Psychologic Effects	Physiologic Effects	Effects of Overdose	Withdrawal Syndrome
Stimulants Cocaine, amphetamines, methylphenidate, phenmetrazine, other stimulants	Elation, psychomotor agitation, grandiosity, talkativeness, ↑ alertness, mood swings	Dilated pupils, ↑ blood pressure, ↑ TPR, diaphoresis, nausea, vomiting, insomnia, loss of appetite	Agitation, ↑ body temperature, hallucinations, convulsions, possible death	Severely depressed mood, prolonged sleep, apathy, irritability, disorientation
Depressants Chloral hydrate, barbiturates, methaqualone, benzodiazepines, alcohol	Disorientation, euphoria, emotional lability, ↑ sexual and aggressive drives with intoxication (↓ with increased doses), talkativeness	Slurred speech, staggering, constricted pupils, ↓ respirations, sedation, nausea	Shallow respirations, cold and clammy skin, weak and rapid pulse, coma, possible death	Anxiety, insomnia, tremors, delirium, convulsions, possible death
Narcotics Opium, morphine, codeine, heroin, methadone, other narcotics	Euphoria, ↓ sexual and aggressive drives	↓ Respiratory rate, nausea, "nodding out," insensitivity to pain, constricted pupils	Slow and shallow breathing, clammy skin, constricted pupils, coma, possible death	Watery eyes, runny nose, yawning, loss of appetite, tremors, panic, chills and sweating, cramps, nausea
Hallucinogens LSD, psilocybin, mescaline, peyote, amphetamine variants, phencyclidine	Hallucinations, illusions, altered body and time perception, mood swings, suspiciousness, confusion, anxiety, panic, intense emotions, depersonalization	Lack of coordination, dilated pupils, ↑ blood pressure, tremors, blurred vision, nausea, dizziness, weaknesses, ↓ response to pain	More prolonged episodes, possibly resembling psychotic states	NA
Cannabis Marijuana, tetrahydrocannabinol, hashish	Euphoria, impaired memory and attention, relaxation, poor judgment, apathy, abrupt mood changes, slowed time sensation	↑ Appetite, tachycardia, reddened eyes	Fatigue, paranoia; hallucinogen-like psychotic state (at very high doses)	Insomnia, hyperactivity (rare syndrome)
Inhalants Glues, aerosols, cleaning solutions, nail polish removers, lighter fluids, paints and paint thinners, other petroleum products, halothane, nitrous oxide, amyl nitrite, butyl nitrite	Giddiness, lightheadedness, decreased inhibitions, floating sensation, illusions, clouding of thoughts, drowsiness, amnesia	Eye irritation, sensitivity to light, double vision, ringing in ears, irritation in lining of nose and mouth, cough, nausea, vomiting, diarrhea, faint heart beat, cardiac irregularities or dysrhythmias	Anxiety, mental impairment, depressed respiration, cardiac dysrhythmias, sudden death	No clinically relevant syndrome, development of tolerance likely at high doses

LSD, Lysergic acid diethylamide; *NA*, no data available; *TPR*, temperature, pulse, respirations.

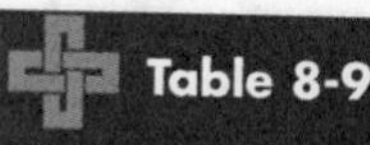

Table 8-9 Emergency Management: Drug Overdose

Possible Etiology
Ingestion, inhalation, or injection of drugs either accidentally or intentionally

Possible Assessment Findings
Aggressive behavior
Agitation
Disorientation
Lethargy
Stupor
Hallucinations
Depression
Slurred speech
Pinpoint pupils
Seizures
Needle tracks
Cold, clammy skin
Rapid, weak pulse
Slow or rapid shallow respirations
Cardiac or respiratory arrest

Management
- Establish and maintain airway.
- Anticipate need for intubation if respiratory distress evident.
- Establish IV access.
- Obtain information about substance: name, route, when taken, period of time taken, amount taken.
- Obtain a health history including drug use and allergies.
- Assess level of consciousness.
- Monitor vital signs including temperature.
- Perform a 12-lead ECG and then continue to monitor with ECG.
- Use measures to decrease systemic absorption (if appropriate), including:
  gastric lavage
  induced emesis (e.g., ipecac)
  absorbents (e.g., activated charcoal)
  induced diarrhea (e.g., magnesium)
  antidote

ECG, Electrocardiogram; *IV*, intravenous.

gency. Emergency management of drug overdose is presented in Table 8-9.

Management of withdrawal involves assessment and monitoring of symptoms with particular attention to suicidal thoughts and complications from multiple drug use. The primary goals are to control symptoms, decrease craving, and establish a basis for recovery. Specific approaches to managing withdrawal include providing active support, encouraging adequate nutrition (including vitamin supplements), maintaining adequate fluid balance, recommending aerobic exercise if there are no medical contraindications, and teaching relaxation techniques and measures to promote sleep. Drugs that may be helpful during this period include dopaminergic agents, including amantadine, bromocriptine, and levodopa to decrease craving; neuroleptics or some benzodiazepines to relieve "crash" symptoms; and antidepressants, such as desipramine (Norpramin), imipramine (Tofranil), or trazodone (Desyrel), to prevent relapse.

Cocaine

Characteristics. Cocaine is extracted from the leaves of the coca plant. It is now the most abused major stimulant in the United States. Approximately 5 to 6 million Americans use cocaine on a regular basis, and more than 25 million Americans have used the substance.[10] Use of cocaine continues to increase in the United States and Canada. The prevalence of the use of cocaine has been surpassed by the widespread use of "crack," a cocaine alkaloid that gets its name from the popping sound the crystals make when heated. Crack has grown in popularity with adolescents because it is inexpensive, readily available, easy to use, and has an increased purity over cocaine.

Effects of Use. Cocaine is a potent stimulant of the central nervous, cardiovascular, and respiratory systems and has potentially fatal effects (Table 8-10). The most common route of administration is intranasally, although it may be used parenterally, orally, vaginally, sublingually, and rectally; it may also be smoked. The most rapid routes of administration are via IV and inhalation. When taken IV or inhaled, cocaine's effects are felt within 1 minute and last about 20 minutes.

Addiction can develop from any route of administration. Collapse and scarring of the veins at the injection site may occur as a result of "shooting up." With intranasal use, the nasal septum and mucosa may be damaged, leading to nasal sores, decreased olfaction, chronic sinusitis, perforation, and collapse of the nose or septal necrosis. Cocaine "runny nose" or chronic rhinitis is common with long-term intranasal use. Frequent sniffing and increased susceptibility to upper respiratory infections are common symptoms of cocaine abuse.[11]

Users who experience personality changes are described as being "coked out." Anxiety, restlessness, and extreme irritability may signal the onset of a toxic psychosis. Cocaine psychosis is characterized by tactile hallucinations of bugs crawling under the skin *(formication)* and scratches on arms, legs, or chest, which may indicate attempts to dig out the bugs. This psychosis is shorter in duration than the psychosis observed with amphetamine abuse.

Crack in the form of chips, chunks, or rocks is the most potent form of the drug and produces the most dramatic "high" and the most rapid addiction. Because crack is inhaled, it is absorbed more rapidly (2 to 3 seconds) as a result of the larger surface area in the lungs compared with that of the nasal mucosa. Consequently, crack produces a more intense effect and withdrawal. Pulmonary damage from smoking crack may be evident with black or dark brown sputum.

Complications. Complications are directly related to the route of administration, type of cocaine, dose, and individual vulnerabilities. They may include cellulitis, wound abscess, hepatitis, HIV infection, seizures, myocardial ischemia and infarction, cardiac dysrhythmias, sudden cardiac death, rhabdomyolysis (skeletal muscle injury), acute renal

Table 8-10 Effects of Cocaine Use

	Early Effects	Long-term Effects
■ Central nervous system	Excitation, euphoria, restlessness, talkativeness	Depression, hallucinations, tremors, visual disturbances, dysarthria, seizure activity, headaches, insomnia, stroke
■ Cardiovascular system	Tachycardia, hypertension, angina, dysrhythmias, palpitations	Ventricular dysrhythmias, hypotension, congestive heart failure, myocardial infarction, cardiomyopathy
■ Respiratory system	Increased respiratory rate, dyspnea, chest pain, epistaxis	Chronic cough, inflamed throat, congestion of lungs, brown or black sputum production, pneumonia, respiratory distress or arrest, pulmonary edema, rhinorrhea, rhinitis, erosion and perforation of the nasal septum
■ Sexuality	Heightened sexual desire, delayed orgasm and ejaculation; women may have difficulty achieving orgasm.	Difficulty in maintaining erection and ejaculation, loss of interest in sexual activity; women may develop aberrant sexual behavior
■ Gastrointestinal system	Decreased appetite	Dehydration, weight loss, nausea, intestinal ischemia may cause gangrene
■ Emotions	Behavior changes or mood swings	Depression or suicidal thoughts

failure, acute respiratory distress, pulmonary edema, asthma, abruptio placentae, premature onset of labor, and bilateral loss of eyebrow and eyelash hair (from inhalation of hot vapors).

The infant whose mother used cocaine during pregnancy is at higher risk for intrauterine growth retardation, lower birth weight, smaller head circumference, decreased length, lower Apgar scores, neurobehavioral impairment, some congenital abnormalities, and sudden infant death syndrome.[12,13]

Acute cocaine toxicity may be manifested by forceful cardiac palpitations with feelings of impending doom, tachycardia, hypertension, myocardial ischemia or infarction, seizures, hallucinations, confusion, paranoia, aggressive behavior, and fever. An overdose is an exaggerated version of the classic physical and psychologic response to cocaine use.

Frequent causes of death associated with cocaine abuse include cerebral hemorrhage, respiratory failure, and cardiovascular collapse. There is no margin of safety with the use of cocaine, and there is no antidote for toxicity. Repeated use appears to lower the level of toxicity, especially for seizures.

Overdose occurs more frequently with IV use, smoking "freebase," or "body packing." Freebasing is the process of extracting the alkaloid form from cocaine hydrochloride, producing crack and rock. Freebase can be smoked in a cigarette with tobacco or heated and inhaled through a water pipe. Body packing is a form of smuggling packets of cocaine in the intestines. If the packets burst, a toxic reaction and death occur unless immediate medical intervention is available.

Therapeutic Management. Cocaine abuse and dependence have become growing concerns in emergency departments and drug treatment programs. The picture of the addict may be complicated by the cocaine abuser's frequent use of alcohol, marijuana, or heroin. The addict may use drugs such as chlordiazepoxide (Librium), diazepam (Valium), lorazepam (Ativan), or alprazolam (Xanax) to minimize unpleasant effects of withdrawal. Cocaine combined with heroin is called *speedball,* and cocaine combined with phencyclidine hydrochloride (PCP) is called *space base.* One of the most dangerous combinations is cocaine and alcohol because it increases the risk of liver injury.

An individual who is addicted to cocaine does not initially seek treatment for drug abuse but rather for problems with sleep, appetite, depression, sinusitis, respiratory infections, chest pain, or migrainelike headaches. Specific clues that should alert the nurse to cocaine abuse or dependence are included in Table 8-10. A patient is usually hesitant to admit to illegal drug use. The importance of providing an accurate drug history, which will be kept confidential, needs to be understood. Questions about drug use patterns need to be stated in a direct, nonjudgmental manner.

Management of cocaine intoxication is presented in Table 8-11 and the nursing care plan on p. 155. Overdose and withdrawal are handled in the same manner as amphetamines. Nursing management involves closely monitoring the neurologic status, level of consciousness, and breathing in addition to continuous physical assessment.

There is growing concern and recognition of the role of cocaine in both accidental and violent crime-related trauma. A large number of trauma victims may be under the influence of cocaine and need to be carefully assessed for signs and symptoms of overdose, withdrawal, and medical

RESEARCH

IMPLICATIONS FOR NURSING PRACTICE

GENDER DIFFERENCES IN CRACK COCAINE USE

Citation Henderson DJ, Boyd C, Mieczkowski T: Gender, relationships, and crack cocaine: a content analysis, *Res Nurs Health* 17:265-272, 1994.

Purpose To explore the context in which women abuse crack and to describe how this use differs from crack abuse by men

Methods Data from open-ended, structured interviews with 46 predominantly African-American women (*N* = 23) and men (*N* = 23) were compared using content analysis. This study was a secondary analysis of a larger descriptive study of crack abuse in adults.

Results and Conclusions Women were more likely to begin, use, and maintain their use of crack in the context of more intimate relationships with the opposite sex. Men were more likely to begin their use with male friends and associates and to maintain drug use with income from jobs and selling drugs. Overall relationships (both sexual and familial) were a more prominent aspect of crack use for women, whereas entrepreneurship was more important for men.

Implications for Nursing Practice The findings of this study have implications for the treatment and prevention of crack abuse, particularly in women. For a woman, the ability to initially resist crack or to stop once she is using heavily must be considered in the context of her relationships with men. The addictive qualities of the drug are compounded by the emotional and psychologic components of intimate relationships.

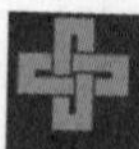

Table 8-11 Emergency Management: Acute Cocaine Toxicity

Possible Etiology

Intranasal, parenteral, oral, vaginal, rectal, or sublingual administration of large doses of cocaine

Possible Assessment Findings

Cardiovascular manifestations: Cardiac palpitations with feelings of impending doom, tachycardia, hypertension, dysrhythmias, myocardial ischemia or infarction
Euphoria, agitation, combativeness
Seizures
Hallucinations, confusion, paranoia
Fever

Management

- Establish and maintain airway.
- Anticipate need for intubation if respiratory distress evident.
- Establish IV access and give IV fluid replacement.
- Administer:
  - lidocaine or propranolol IV for ventricular dysrhythmias
  - midazolam IV for agitation
  - haloperidol IV for psychosis
  - diazepam or lorazepam IV for seizures
  - naloxone IV for CNS depression
  - propranolol or labetalol for hypertension and tachycardia
- Do a 12-lead ECG, and maintain ECG monitoring.
- Be prepared to perform CPR or defibrillation.
- Monitor vital signs including level of consciousness.
- Obtain medical history including drug use.

CNS, Central nervous system; *CPR,* cardiopulmonary resuscitation; *ECG,* electrocardiogram; *IV,* intravenous.

complications that could lead to adverse interactions with drugs used in the management of pain or administration of anesthesia. During the surgical recovery period, the nurse should be alert for the patient who may exhibit signs and symptoms of drug interactions with pain medications or anesthesia or who may exhibit symptoms of withdrawal.[14]

Engaging an individual who is addicted to cocaine in treatment is difficult because of the intense craving for the drug and a strong denial that cocaine is addicting or that the individual cannot control it. Often various forms of leverage such as family threats, loss of job or professional license, legal action, or major health consequences provide sufficient motivation for an individual to enter a treatment program. Although many drug abusers can be effectively treated in outpatient programs, inpatient programs should be recommended for some. A structured inpatient program may be desirable during early recovery to provide a support system until the individual is able to develop coping skills and resources to resist drug use and begin working toward a drug-free lifestyle.

DEPRESSANTS

Drugs categorized as depressants have common psychologic effects and the ability to produce sedation and other major depressant effects. Drugs in this category include sedative-hypnotics, alcohol, and opioid narcotics (Table 8-12). Antipsychotics are not considered CNS depressants and are not physically addictive. They are seldom used to produce a state of euphoria.

With the exception of alcohol and some federally regulated drugs, most CNS depressants are medically useful. They can be used for relief of anxiety, insomnia, pain, symptoms of withdrawal from alcohol, or as anticonvulsants or anesthetic agents. These drugs are also widely recognized for their abuse potential, which leads to rapid tolerance, dependence, and medical emergencies involving overdoses and withdrawal.

Alcohol is a major depressant and the most widely used substance in this category. It is frequently used in combination with barbiturates or benzodiazepines, as well as with stimulants and hallucinogens. Depressants have been used frequently with stimulants to produce an upper-downer effect or to "mellow out" the effect of stimulants.

NURSING CARE PLAN Patient with Cocaine Toxicity

Planning: Outcome Criteria	*Nursing Interventions and Rationales*
➤ **NURSING DIAGNOSIS**	Anxiety *related to* increased CNS stimulation *as manifested by* increased pulse rate, palpitations, hyperventilation, talkativeness, fearfulness, irritability, emotional lability, tremors, chest pains, confusion, disorientation, paranoia-type psychosis, or feelings of losing control or going crazy
Have decreased physiologic and psychologic manifestations of anxiety; discuss feelings of anxiety, dread, and helplessness; acknowledge toxic effects of cocaine.	Continuously monitor vital signs *to detect indicators of effects of cocaine and subsequent anxiety.* Explain procedures *to reduce patient's agitation and to increase cooperation.* Provide safe, secure environment *to prevent anxiety related to unfamiliar or threatening events.* Reduce level of anxiety with comfort measures and medications, if indicated; use calm approach *to facilitate reduction in CNS stimulation.* Decrease stimuli (if possible) *to decrease delusions and agitation.* Reinforce reality orientation because *disorientation and confusion increase anxiety.*
➤ **NURSING DIAGNOSIS**	Total self-care deficit *related to* extreme CNS stimulation progressing to CNS depression *as manifested by* self-feeding, self-bathing, self-dressing, or self-toileting deficits or inability to perform any self-care activities
Have care needs met by self or others to patient's satisfaction; have increasing ability to meet personal care needs.	Assess self-care deficits *to initiate appropriate treatment plan.* Provide assistance as needed and explain procedures *to meet patient's care requirements.* Monitor vital signs *to identify patient's response to care activities.* As patient recovers, reassess ability to participate in self-care *to make appropriate changes in care plan and to allow as much self-care as possible.* Refer to occupational therapist *to relearn skills, if indicated.* Provide opportunities for self-care and hope of recovery to previous level of functioning *to motivate patient to accept increasing amount of responsibility for care.*
➤ **NURSING DIAGNOSIS**	Fluid volume deficit *related to* diaphoresis and hypermetabolic state *as manifested by* dry throat, thirst, decreased urinary output, fluid loss greater than intake, dry skin and mucous membranes, decreased skin turgor, nausea, vomiting, confusion, dizziness, diaphoresis, hemorrhage, hyperthermia, increased pulse rate
Have no manifestations of dehydration, maintain intake of at least 1500 ml/day (oral fluids) and output of at least 1000 to 1500 ml/day; have vital signs and laboratory work within normal limits; have clear sensorium, absence of vomiting, hemorrhage, diarrhea.	Monitor fluid intake and output *to plan for adequate fluid replacement.* Assess for dehydration *to ensure early identification and treatment.* Start IV lines with large-bore needles for one or more fluid resuscitations with normal saline and lactated Ringer's solution *for rapid infusion of large volume of fluid.* Monitor vital signs *because decreasing BP and increasing pulse and respiratory rate can indicate hypovolemia.* Monitor serum electrolytes, creatinine, BUN, urine and serum osmolalities, hematocrit, and hemoglobin levels *to identify hypovolemia and dehydration.* Consider additional fluid losses associated with vomiting, diarrhea, fever *to increase the accuracy of monitoring output.* Give sips of 5% glucose solution *to meet some of patient's requirements for both calories and fluid.*
➤ **NURSING DIAGNOSIS**	Situational low self-esteem *related to* addictive behavior or cocaine abuse *as manifested by* self-destructive behavior associated with cocaine abuse, isolation, negative self-talk, anger, despair, powerlessness, helplessness, sadness, depression, self-neglect, apathy, denial, noncompliance with treatment
Express feelings of self-worth, identify positive aspects of self, express positive outlook for future; be able to analyze own behavior associated with cocaine abuse and its consequences.	Assess emotional status *to determine patient's perception of situation and to plan appropriate interventions.* Assist patient in identifying and expressing feelings *to enable patient to begin to accept responsibility for self.* Provide support and reassurance for short-term improvement and eventual recovery *to instill motivation and a sense of hope.* Support use of effective coping mechanisms to deal with crisis *to reinforce new behaviors.* Assist patient in identifying responsibility and control in situations *because these insights are necessary before dealing with an addiction.* Assist patient in management of specific problems (e.g., hospitalization, depression) *because patient may be incapable of managing these problems during crisis.* Refer to treatment program, counseling, support group, or other resources *because these are often required to provide patient new skills and hope.*

continued

NURSING CARE PLAN Patient with Cocaine Toxicity—cont'd

Planning: Outcome Criteria	Nursing Interventions and Rationales
➤ NURSING DIAGNOSIS	Risk for self-directed violence *related to* cocaine abuse
Abstain from further drug use; seek treatment for cocaine abuse; develop effective coping mechanisms in handling stress; demonstrate no apparent risk of self-harm.	Assess risk for self-destruction as evidenced by compulsive focus of attention on cocaine, low self-esteem, hopelessness, acute agitation, depression, suicidal thoughts, poor impulse control, helplessness, lack of support systems, hallucinations, and proneness to violence *to initiate appropriate plan of care.* Assist patient in building self-esteem with caring, emphatic approach *as improved self-esteem will decrease impulse for self-destruction.* Assess support systems *as possible resources in preventing self-destructive behavior.* Assist patient in contacting members of support systems *as patient may not be motivated to do so independently.* Help patient develop positive coping mechanisms *to replace previously practiced self-destructive negative coping strategies.* Initiate health teaching and referral for treatment or counseling when crisis is resolved *to ensure knowledge of positive health practices and adequate assistance with follow-up planning.*
➤ NURSING DIAGNOSIS	Risk for altered health maintenance *related to* practices of behaviors and activities associated with cocaine use
Maintain long-term abstinence from cocaine; participate in recovery program that encourages a drug-free lifestyle.	Assess patient's lifestyle *to determine activities that are likely to result in relapse.* Assist patient to make specific plans *to avoid such activities.* Encourage appropriate inpatient or outpatient treatment *to meet patient's specific treatment needs.* Teach patient early warning signs *to prevent relapse.* Assist patient in learning positive ways to deal with stress and to live a balanced lifestyle *to reduce need to use drugs.*

COLLABORATIVE PROBLEMS

Nursing Goals	Nursing Interventions and Rationales
➤ POTENTIAL COMPLICATIONS	Neurologic, cardiovascular, and respiratory problems *related to* the direct toxic action of cocaine on tissues and its potentiation of the effects of norepinephrine and epinephrine.
Monitor neurologic, cardiovascular, and respiratory functions; report abnormal findings; initiate appropriate medical and nursing interventions.	Assess for neurologic, cardiovascular, and respiratory problems such as compromised vital signs, seizures, altered levels of consciousness and motor activity, dysrhythmias, vascular collapse, cerebral vascular accident, congestive heart failure, hypoxia, acute respiratory distress syndrome, or cardiopulmonary arrest *to initiate immediate medical and nursing interventions, if indicated.* Monitor neurologic status, including level of consciousness *to identify signs of CNS stimulation or depression.* Take seizure precautions *because cocaine poisoning can precipitate seizures.* Provide airway management and ventilation support *to treat respiratory failure.* Continuously monitor vital signs *as an indicator of carciovascular complications.* Keep open IV lines *to provide immediate access to vascular system for IV fluids or medications.* Administer medications aggressively (as indicated) *to treat specific problems.* Put patient in 30-degree Trendelenburg position when indicated *to treat hypotension.* Employ cardiac life support measures (if indicated) *to treat cardiac or respiratory arrest.*

BP, Blood pressure; *BUN*, blood urea nitrogen; *CNS*, central nervous system; *IV*, intravenous.

Sedative-Hypnotics

Characteristics. Chloral hydrate and paraldehyde were two of the earliest drugs in this category used for their sedating effects. They were generally replaced when barbiturates were introduced. The barbiturates are frequently responsible for accidental overdoses and are often used to commit suicide, especially in combination with alcohol. Benzodiazepines are considered more selective as antianxiety agents with less drowsiness and a larger margin of safety than the barbiturates. Chlordiazepoxide (Librium), diazepam (Valium), and alprazolam (Xanax) have been the most commonly used benzodiazepines.

Two patterns of abuse and dependence have been recognized with sedative-hypnotic drugs. The first pattern begins

Table 8-12 Depressants

Sedative-Hypnotic Drugs	**Alcohol**
Chloral hydrate	Ethanol
Barbiturates	Methanol
Amobarbital (Amytal)*	Ethylene glycol
Butabarbital (Butisol)*	Isopropyl alcohol
Talbutal (Lotusate)*	**Narcotics**
Pentobarbital (Nembutal)†	Opiate
Secobarbital (Seconal)†	Opium
Phenobarbital (Luminal)‡	Morphine
Benzodiazepines	Codeine
Lorazepam (Ativan)*	Heroin
Flurazepam (Dalmane)‡	Hydrocodone (Hycodan)
Diazepam (Valium)‡	Hydromorphone (Dilaudid)
Chlordiazepoxide (Librium)‡	Meperidine (Demerol)
Alprazolam (Xanax)*	Methadone (Dolophine)
Oxazepam (Serax)*	Oxymorphone (Numorphan)
Chlorazepate (Tranxene)‡	Fentanyl (Sublimaze)
Midazolam (Versed)†	Pentazocine (Talwin)
Triazolam (Halcion)†	Oxycodone (Percodan)
Halazepam (Paxipam)‡	Propoxyphene (Darvon)
Temazepam (Restoril)*	Acetaminophen with oxycodone (Tylox)
Methaqualone (Quaalude, Parest, Sopor)	
Glutethimide (Doriden)	
Meprobamate (Equanil, Miltown)	
Methyprylon (Noludar)	
Ethchlorvynol (Placidyl)	

*Intermediate acting.
†Short acting.
‡Long acting.

with prescription use of the drug for the treatment of anxiety or insomnia. Subsequently, the patient increases the dose and frequency of use without medical advice or indication. The second and more common pattern involves illegal sources, which often begins with intermittent use by teenagers or young adults at parties and leads to daily use and rapid tolerance.

Effects of Use. Sedative-hypnotic drugs act primarily on the CNS by depressing cardiac and respiratory function. They are largely metabolized in the liver and excreted in the urine. The effects of this group of drugs are dose related. With low doses, sedation and calming effects occur; with high doses, they act as hypnotics, and sleep is induced. They decrease the time needed to fall asleep and increase total sleep time but decrease the amount of REM sleep or dream sleep. Excessive amounts produce an initial euphoria and a state of intoxication similar to alcohol intoxication, including impaired judgment, slurred speech, and loss of motor coordination.

Tolerance develops rapidly with a narrow margin of safety between intoxicating effects and lethal dose. Accidental overdoses may occur because of differences in tolerance levels. Tolerance develops to the sedative effects, requiring higher doses to achieve euphoria. The tolerance may not develop to the brainstem-depressant effects, so an increased dose may trigger hypotension and respiratory depression, resulting in death.

The benzodiazepines affect the limbic system and decrease anxiety without producing sedation at low doses. Although they are believed to have a wide margin of safety, they are not without adverse reactions, including rebound anxiety and insomnia with short-acting drugs and confusion and memory loss with long-acting drugs. Benzodiazepines should be used cautiously in individuals who are older, who have organic brain disorders, or who are taking substances such as narcotics, antidepressants, antipsychotics, antihypertensives, antihistamines, other sedative-hypnotic drugs, or alcohol.

Complications. The symptoms of mild to moderate overdose are similar to those of alcohol intoxication. The signs of severe overdose include coma; cold, clammy skin; weak, rapid pulse; and slow, rapid, shallow respirations. Death may result from cardiac or respiratory arrest.

Manifestations of withdrawal from benzodiazepines include nausea and vomiting, muscle cramps, diaphoresis, increased sensitivity to light and sound, anxiety, dysphoria, tachycardia, hypertension, convulsions, and coarse tremors of the hands, tongue, and eyelids. The withdrawal syndrome may be a medical emergency, since it may progress from minor symptoms within the first 24 hours and lead to convulsions, delirium, psychoses, and respiratory and cardiac arrest. Symptoms of major withdrawal peak on the second or third day for short-acting barbiturates, benzodiazepines, and meprobamate and on the seventh or eighth day for long-acting drugs.

Therapeutic Management. There are no known antagonists to counteract the effects of these drugs. Emergency life support measures must be taken in cases of overdose. In addition to the symptoms associated with overdose and withdrawal, there can be complications associated with the route of administration. These may include cellulitis, vascular complications, hepatitis, endocarditis, pneumonia, bacterial infections, and HIV infection.

Treatment of a drug dependent individual must include a gradual withdrawal of the drug. Most individuals who have been abusing large amounts of these drugs need to be hospitalized to safely manage symptoms of withdrawal. Nursing management includes ensuring safety, preventing injury, and halting the progression of symptoms. Specific nursing approaches include careful monitoring of vital signs and levels of consciousness and providing reassurance and orientation as needed. The patient who has overdosed must be treated aggressively and may require dialysis to decrease the drug level and to prevent irreversible CNS depressant effects and death. It is important to avoid the use of any CNS stimulants in the treatment of overdose.

Alcohol

Characteristics. Millions of people worldwide are dependent on alcohol. The degree of dependence varies, but all either feel that they have to drink or have a physical need to do so. It is estimated that 65% to 70% of Americans use alcohol, and that more than 10 million are alcohol-dependent.[15] Additionally, 10 million more Americans are

Table 8-13 Blood Alcohol Concentration and Related Effects

BAC (mg%)*	Psychophysiologic Effect
20	Light and moderate drinkers begin to feel some effects. Approximate BAC is reached after one drink.†
40	Most people begin to feel relaxed.
60	Judgment is mildly impaired. People are less able to make rational decisions about their capabilities (e.g., driving skills)
80	Definite impairment of muscle coordination and driving skills occurs. Person is legally drunk in some states.
100	Clear deterioration of reaction time and control is observed. Person is legally drunk in most states.
120	Vomiting occurs unless this level is reached slowly.
150	Balance and movement are impaired. Equivalent of one-half pint of whiskey is circulating in the bloodstream
300	Many people lose consciousness.
400	Most people lose consciousness, and some die.
450	Breathing stops; person eventually dies.

*Blood alcohol concentration (BAC) is generally recorded in milligrams of alcohol per deciliter (mg/dl) of blood, or milligrams percent (mg%). BAC is determined by how much alcohol is consumed, how fast it is consumed, and the person's weight.
†One drink is 12 oz of beer, 5 oz of wine, or 1 oz of distilled spirits, which provide the same amount of alcohol.

subject to the negative consequences of alcohol abuse including automobile accidents, arrests, violence, occupational injuries, and negative effects on job performances. Almost one half of all fatal motor vehicle accidents are alcohol-related, and as many as 37% of all emergency department trauma admissions involve alcohol use.[16] These dramatic statistics indicate that the nurse must become knowledgeable about the acute and chronic effects of alcohol use and able to recognize the subtle cues of alcohol abuse.

Alcoholism is currently viewed as a chronic, progressive, potentially fatal disease if left untreated. Numerous factors appear to be interrelated in the development of alcohol abuse. Currently, there are no clearcut explanations for its development. Alcohol dependence may be related to a combination of factors including genetic and biologic factors, psychosocial factors, and cultural-environmental background (see Table 8-3).

There are several patterns of alcohol abuse and dependence: 1) large amounts daily, 2) large amounts on weekends, and 3) binge drinking for weeks or months with periods of sobriety. Alcohol dependence generally occurs over a period of years and may be preceded by heavy social drinking and progress to abuse accompanied by multiple medical and social problems.

CULTURAL & ETHNIC Considerations

ALCOHOLISM

- Native Americans have a high prevalence of alcoholism.
- Asian-Americans have a low prevalence of alcoholism.
- Mortality rates related to alcoholism are high among Native Americans.

Effects of Use. Alcohol affects almost all cells of the body and depresses all areas and functions of the CNS. Alcohol requires no digestion because it is absorbed directly from the stomach and the small intestine. Alcohol is almost completely metabolized in the body and has a slow oxidation rate. The absorption rate can be decreased by food in the stomach, especially protein and fats or plain water mixed with alcohol. The rate is increased by mixing alcohol with soda water or by strong emotions. When large amounts are ingested, 10% to 15% may be eliminated unchanged from the kidneys, lungs, and skin.

The liver is the site of oxidation. The alcohol dehydrogenase system breaks down alcohol. If the enzymes are blocked or unable to work, acetaldehyde builds up in the system, and a disulfiram ethanol reaction, or "Antabuse" reaction, occurs. The rate of oxidation is approximately one drink per hour (7 g equals 7 ml of 100% alcohol). Alcohol (5% to 15%) is also excreted directly through the lungs, perspiration, and urine.

Alcohol's effects are directly proportional to the blood alcohol concentration (BAC). Because alcohol is evenly distributed in the body through the bloodstream, the BAC can be correlated with psychophysiologic effects on the body. Alcohol has a biphasic effect; at low doses it acts as a behavioral stimulant, and at high doses it acts as a depressant. Alcohol may be measured within 15 to 20 minutes of ingestion, peaks in 60 to 90 minutes, and is excreted in 12 to 24 hours. BAC is affected by the amount consumed, drinking rate, body size and composition (percentage of fat content), drink concentration, and hormones. For the nonalcoholic drinker, the BAC is fairly predictable. At higher levels of BAC, there is a narrow margin of safety between anesthesia and death (Table 8-13). The relationship between BAC and behavior is thought to be different in a person who has developed tolerance to alcohol and its effects. This individual is commonly able to drink large amounts without obvious impairment and perform complex tasks without problems at BAC levels several times higher

Table 8-14 Effects of Chronic Alcohol Abuse

Body Systems	Effects
▪ Central nervous system	Alcoholic dementia; Wernicke's encephalopathy (confusion, nystagmus, paralysis of ocular muscles, ataxia); Korsakoff's psychosis (confabulation, amnesic disorder); impairment of cognitive function, psychomotor skills, abstract thinking, and memory; depression, attention deficit, labile moods, seizures, sleep disturbances
▪ Peripheral nervous system	Peripheral neuropathy including pain, paresthesias, weakness
▪ Immune system	Increased risk for tuberculosis and viral infections; increased risk for cancer of oral cavity, pharynx, esophagus, liver, colon, rectum, and possibly breast
▪ Hematologic system	Bone marrow depression, anemia, leukopenia, thrombocytopenia, blood clotting abnormalities
▪ Musculoskeletal system	Painful, tender swelling of large muscle groups; painless progressive muscle weakness and wasting; osteoporosis
▪ Cardiovascular system	Elevated pulse and BP, decreased exercise tolerance, cardiomyopathy (irreversible), increased risk for hemorrhagic stroke, coronary artery disease, hypertension, sudden cardiac death
▪ Liver	Steatosis (reversible)—nausea, vomiting, hepatomegaly; alcoholic hepatitis (reversible)—anorexia, nausea, vomiting, fever, chills, abdominal pain; cirrhosis; cancer
▪ Gastrointestinal system	Gastritis, peptic ulcer, esophagitis, esophageal varices, enteritis, colitis, Mallory-Weiss syndrome, pancreatitis
▪ Nutrition	Decreased appetite, indigestion, malabsorption, vitamin deficiencies
▪ Kidneys	Diuretic effect from inhibition of antidiuretic hormone
▪ Endocrine and reproductive systems	Altered gonadal function, testicular atrophy, decreased beard growth, decreased libido, diminished sperm count, gynecomastia, glucose intolerance
▪ Integumentary system	Palmar erythema, spider angiomas, rosacea, rhinophyma

BP, Blood pressure.

than levels that would produce obvious impairment in the nontolerant drinker.

Drug interactions with alcohol. The interaction of other substances with alcohol may produce four different effects--antagonistic, additive, synergistic, and cross-tolerant. *Antagonistic* effects occur when the effect of either substance is blocked or decreased. These effects are seen with the antialcohols (e.g., Antabuse), some hypoglycemics, and some antibiotics. The disulfiram-ethanol reaction occurs within 5 to 10 minutes of drinking alcohol in the individual taking Antabuse. It may produce flushing, headache, bounding pulse, diaphoresis, nausea, vomiting, and vasomotor collapse with orthostatic hypotension.

Additive effects are enhanced effects of two substances that equal the combined effects of both substances. Drugs that interact with alcohol in this manner include antihypertensives, antihistamines, marijuana, antianginals (nitrates), and analgesics (salicylates). Alcohol taken with aspirin may exacerbate GI bleeding. Cardiovascular drugs and alcohol may cause digitalis toxicity. Alcohol and nitrates may lead to postural hypotension, faintness, and loss of consciousness.

Synergistic effects are the most dangerous because the combined effects of the two drugs are multiplied. Substances that interact in this manner with alcohol include the barbiturates, benzodiazepines, meprobamate, chloral hydrate, paraldehyde, narcotics, and anesthetics. Most of these substances potentiate depressant effects and often lead to respiratory failure and death. Alcohol may produce either a synergistic or an antagonistic effect when used with antidepressants.

Cross-tolerance is increased sensitivity to the effects of other substances in similar drug categories. Once sensitized to certain drugs, a greater amount of those drugs is required to obtain the same effect. Alcohol is cross-tolerant to other depressants, including opiates, anticonvulsants, and anesthetics. Acute intoxication increases the effects of anticonvulsants and anticoagulants, and long-term alcohol use decreases the effects of anticonvulsants and anticoagulants.

Complications. Alcohol has a direct or indirect effect on every organ and system within the body (Table 8-14). Alcohol may cause mental confusion and memory problems and a number of alcohol-associated mental disorders, including Wernicke-Korsakoff syndrome. Wernicke's encephalopathy causes early symptoms of vomiting, nystagmus, difficulty concentrating, polyneuropathy, and a sense of unreality. It is reversible with the administration of thiamine, but it may progress to Korsakoff's psychosis (alcohol amnestic disorder), coma, and death. Korsakoff's psychosis is irreversible and involves an inability to recall or assimilate new information but is not accompanied by dementia or delirium.

Intoxication is evident with increasing BAC. It may be mild, moderate, or severe, and it may result in coma. Intoxication is also evident in behavioral and physical changes. Behavioral changes include aggressiveness, impaired judgment, impaired attention, irritability, euphoria, depression, and emotional lability. Physical signs include slurred speech, incoordination, unsteady gait, nystagmus, and flushed face. Long-term alcoholics are able to mask the signs because of developed tolerance.

Major indicators of alcoholism are physical diseases related to alcohol use (e.g., cirrhosis), alcohol withdrawal, physical tolerance, loss of control, and continued abusive drinking despite known hazards. A *blackout* (period for which an individual has no memory but was conscious) is an early sign of abuse and a probable sign of alcoholism. Psychologic signs of alcoholism include depression, frequent references to drinking, drinking to relieve negative feelings or physical or social discomforts, and the use of defense mechanisms, such as denial, projection, rationalization, "all-or-nothing" thinking, and avoidance to minimize the consequences and to maintain the drinking behavior. Behavioral signs associated with alcoholism reflect impaired functioning in the areas of family relationships, employment, and legal or social situations. As the disease progresses, the individual becomes more focused on drinking activities to the exclusion of everything else.

Alcohol withdrawal is a state of hyperactivity and irritability in response to a marked decrease in consumption or cessation of alcohol use after periods of frequent or prolonged heavy drinking. Hangovers, which appear early in alcohol use, are replaced by symptoms of withdrawal. Four characteristic signs of withdrawal are gross tremors, grand mal seizures, hallucinations, and delirium tremens (DTs).

Most alcoholics experience a mild or minor withdrawal syndrome in the first 8 to 12 hours after the last drink, peak at 24 to 48 hours, and may last up to 5 days. The symptoms are manifestations of hyperactivity resulting from a rebound from the depressant effects of alcohol. Characteristic symptoms include tremulousness, anxiety, increased heart rate, increased blood pressure, sweating, nausea, hyperreflexia, and insomnia. These manifestations vary in intensity and will depend on the severity of the alcoholic problem and general physical condition of the patient.

An alcohol withdrawal seizure is most likely to occur 7 to 48 hours after the last drink and is grand mal in nature. Alcohol withdrawal delirium or DTs is considered a major withdrawal symptom occurring from 30 to 120 hours after the last drink. This is a serious complication and may be life threatening.[17] Delirium components include disorientation, visual or auditory hallucinations, and increased hyperactivity without seizures. Death may be caused by hyperthermia, peripheral vascular collapse, or cardiac failure.

Assessment of Alcoholism. Early recognition and identification of the patient with alcohol-related problems are critical to successful treatment outcomes. The nurse must be aware of the wide range of signs and symptoms of alcohol abuse and dependence. A quick assessment for possible alcohol-related emergency conditions is essential for all patients, regardless of age or condition, and particularly for accident or trauma victims. A thorough psychosocial assessment must be done, when indicated, and it should cover drinking history and current health and social problems. It is essential to obtain information about current and past alcohol and substance use patterns including nicotine.

Table 8-15 The CAGE Questionnaire*

C	Have you ever felt you should **C**ut down on your drinking?
A	Have people **A**nnoyed you by criticizing your drinking?
G	Have you ever felt bad or **G**uilty about your drinking?
E	Have you ever had a drink first thing in the morning to steady your nerves or get rid of a hangover (**E**ye-opener)?

From Mayfield D and others: The CAGE questionnaire: validation of a new alcoholism screening instrument, *Am J Psychiatry* 131:1121, 1974.
*A score of two or three "yes" responses strongly suggests alcoholism.

The way in which the nurse poses questions and the nonverbal messages conveyed about alcohol and substance use can affect a patient's willingness to respond. The nurse must use an open and nonjudgmental approach and stress the importance of having an accurate alcohol and drug history for the health care team to provide effective care and prevent any unexpected complications.

A patient's use of denial should not be viewed as a major roadblock but as an opportunity for the nurse to provide the patient with new information about the condition and the effects and consequences of alcohol use. Denial may be circumvented by asking indirect questions such as, "How often has drinking caused you a problem?" instead of "Do you have a problem with drinking?"

Some useful screening tools include the Alcohol Use Disorders Identification Test (AUDIT) (a 10-item questionnaire to identify early-stage problem drinkers)[18], the CAGE questionnaire (a four-item mnemonic tool), and the Short Michigan Alcoholism Screening Test (MAST) (a 13-item tool) (Tables 8-15 and 8-16).

Laboratory tests that may provide evidence of alcoholism are liver function tests and a complete blood count. Liver function tests include γ-glutamyltransferase (GGT), aspartate aminotransaminase (AST), alanine aminotransaminase (ALT), and alkaline phosphatase.

Therapeutic Management. Initial treatment is aimed at detoxification and stabilization of the patient's condition. The most frequent emergency problems related to alcohol are accidents and toxic reactions. Toxic reactions occur as the result of combining alcohol with another drug and may lead to respiratory and circulatory arrest without adequate intervention. Naloxone (Narcan), an opiate antagonist, may be given if opiates have been used with alcohol. Toxicology screening identifies types of drugs (including alcohol) and levels present. Methanol (wood alcohol), ethylene glycol (antifreeze), and isopropyl alcohol (rubbing alcohol) may be found in accidental overdoses or suicide attempts involving the homeless, older adults, children, or poor individuals.

Table 8-16 Short Michigan Alcoholism Screen Test

1. Do you feel you are a normal drinker? (By normal, do you drink less than or as much as most other people.) (No)*	No ____	Yes ____
2. Does your wife, husband, a parent, or other near relative ever worry or complain about your drinking? (Yes)	No ____	Yes ____
3. Do you ever feel guilty about your drinking? (Yes)	No ____	Yes ____
4. Do friends or relatives think you are a normal drinker? (No)	No ____	Yes ____
5. Are you able to stop drinking when you want to? (No)	No ____	Yes ____
6. Have you ever attended a meeting of Alcoholics Anonymous? (Yes)	No ____	Yes ____
7. Has drinking ever created problems between you and your wife, husband, a parent, or other near relative? (Yes)	No ____	Yes ____
8. Have you ever gotten into trouble at work because of drinking? (Yes)	No ____	Yes ____
9. Have you ever neglected your obligations, your family, or your work for 2 or more days in a row because you were drinking? (Yes)	No ____	Yes ____
10. Have you ever gone to anyone for help about your drinking? (Yes)	No ____	Yes ____
11. Have you ever been in a hospital because of your drinking? (Yes)	No ____	Yes ____
12. Have you ever been arrested for drunken driving, driving while intoxicated, or driving under the influence of alcohol? (Yes)	No ____	Yes ____
13. Have you ever been arrested, even for a few hours, because of other drunken behavior? (Yes)	No ____	Yes ____

From Selzer M, Vinokur A, van Roojen L: A self-administered short alcoholism screening test (SMAST), *J Stud Alcohol* 38:86, 1975.
*Alcoholism-indicating responses appear in parentheses.
Scoring: 0-1, nonalcholic; 2, possibly alcoholic; 3 or more, alcoholic.

Alcohol intoxication. Acute alcohol intoxication may present as an emergency. It is important to obtain an accurate history and assess for injuries, trauma, diseases, and hypoglycemia. The basic principles of *A*irway, *B*reathing, and *C*irculation need to be implemented. Vital signs and level of consciousness need to be monitored. Generally, the pulse rate is normal in uncomplicated intoxication but elevated in withdrawal. Hypotension may be a sign of occult bleeding. The patient who is hypoglycemic should be given thiamine before receiving dextrose to prevent Wernicke's encephalopathy. Seizures may occur and are managed with an anticonvulsant. It is critical to continue assessments until the BAC has decreased to at least 100 mg% and until any associated disorders or injuries have been ruled out. A satisfactory BAC is usually reached within 6 to 8 hours.

Alcohol withdrawal. Alcohol withdrawal or detoxification is the first step in the management of the disease. The goals of treatment for withdrawal are to prevent the progression of symptoms, to provide for the patient's safety and comfort and to engage the patient in long-term treatment. The patient needs to be carefully assessed because alcohol withdrawal may be life-threatening. Most of the life-threatening conditions occur during the first few days of withdrawal. Generally, acute withdrawal lasts for 3 to 5 days.

An individual who is experiencing withdrawal may also be suffering from other illnesses, underlying conditions, or trauma. The most common severe manifestations are hallucinations and grand mal seizures. The progression of withdrawal to DTs can be prevented by prompt early treatment. A quiet, calm environment is important to prevent exacerbation of symptoms. The use of restraints, IVs, and side rails should be avoided whenever possible. Supportive care is needed to ensure adequate rest and nutrition. It is important not to overhydrate the patient, particularly if the patient has renal or cardiac disease, because overhydration can lead to sudden dysrhythmias. The majority of patients improve without medical treatment. The nursing care for the patient in withdrawal is presented in the nursing care plan on p. 162.

Medications may be useful in decreasing symptoms, increasing levels of comfort, and decreasing the risk of convulsions and DTs. Benzodiazepines are the most effective agents in preventing and treating alcohol withdrawal seizures and DTs. Other agents may include β-adrenergic blockers (atenolol), clonidine, and calcium channel blockers. The patient who is intoxicated with rising BACs should not be given other depressants because of their additive effects. Inadequate treatment of alcohol withdrawal may precipitate more severe stages of withdrawal.

Rehabilitation. Although cessation of drinking is the short-term goal that is accomplished through detoxification and the withdrawal process, rehabilitation and prolonged abstinence are the primary long-term goals. The aim of intervention is to assist the patient to see the adverse consequences of drinking and to make appropriate lifestyle changes. The earlier an individual engages in treatment, the greater are the chances of a more complete recovery. A formal intervention process may be planned and implemented if an individual's situation is critical and if that person is unwilling or unable to recognize a problem with alcohol. This consists of a planned meeting by concerned friends, family, and co-workers who confront the individual with their observations and how the drinking behavior has affected them personally; they insist that the individual enter treatment.

NURSING CARE PLAN Patient in Alcohol Withdrawal

Planning: Outcome Criteria	Nursing Interventions and Rationales
➤ **NURSING DIAGNOSIS**	Risk for injury *related to* sensorimotor deficits, seizure activity, and confusion
Have no falls or injuries; decrease in tremors and psychomotor activity; no seizures.	Assess for risk factors such as impaired mobility (e.g., unsteady gait), sensory deficits, tremors, impaired judgment, disorientation, seizure activity *to plan appropriate preventive measures.* Assess for signs of injury such as lacerations, bruises, or burns *to treat appropriately.* Monitor vital signs frequently, especially increased pulse rate *because prompt recognition of extreme autonomic nervous system response is necessary for early intervention.* Use side rails; assist with walking and personal hygiene *to prevent injury and assure maintenance of personal hygiene.* Provide support and reassurance *to reduce anxiety and increase cooperation.* Use seizure precautions *to prevent injury.* Administer benzodiazepines *to control autonomic hyperactivity,* vitamins *to reduce neurologic complications* (e.g., Wernicke's encephalopathy), and anticonvulsants as ordered *to prevent seizures.*
➤ **NURSING DIAGNOSIS**	Sensory and perceptual alterations *related to* sensory overload *as manifested by* inaccurate interpretation of environmental stimuli, disorientation to time, place, or person, anxiety, fearful, auditory or visual hallucinations
Have no hallucinations; be oriented to person, place, time.	Assess patient's orientation to reality *to determine appropriate interventions.* Provide quiet, well-lit environment *to reduce external stimuli.* Orient to nurse and environment with each contact; use calm, matter-of-fact approach; explain procedures and what is expected *to assist in reality orientation.* Do not reinforce fears or hallucinations by agreeing or disagreeing *as this does not facilitate reality orientation.* Present reality clearly with "I" statements *to reduce confusion.* Administer benzodiazepines if ordered *to reduce CNS stimulation.*
➤ **NURSING DIAGNOSIS**	Sleep pattern disturbance *related to* increased CNS stimulation *as manifested by* feelings of fear, restlessness, agitation, hallucinations, mood alterations, fatigue, dozing, difficulty falling or remaining asleep
Able to describe factors that prevent or inhibit sleep; use techniques to induce or maintain sleep; have normal sleep patterns and rested feeling after sleep.	Monitor sleep pattern *to individualize interventions to patient's unique problems.* Identify contributing factors *so they may be corrected when possible.* Reduce or eliminate environmental stimuli (lights, noise) and interruptions *to promote restful environment.* Provide comfort measures including bedtime routine, bathing, snacks, massage, music, and reading *to promote sleep and show a caring attitude.* Assist with relaxation activities (e.g., walking; rhythmic, deep breathing), *to encourage sleep by decreasing agitation and anxiety through light physical exertion.* Decrease potential for injury during sleep (e.g., use night lights, low bed) *as confusion and disorientation lead to dangerous consequences.*
➤ **NURSING DIAGNOSIS**	Risk for violence *related to* withdrawal from alcohol and accompanying depression
Exhibit no self-destructive or violent behavior; maintain control over behavior; accept help; use effective coping mechanisms to handle stress.	Assess level of risk as evidenced by feelings of fear, suicidal or homicidal thoughts, hallucinations, environmental misperceptions, poor impulse control, and panic *to assure early recognition of violence potential and plan appropriate interventions.* Provide safe environment on the basis of risk level, including informing staff of risk *to prevent injury to self or others.* Use medications or restraints if necessary *to prevent escalation of activity to violence.* Communicate expectation of need to maintain control of behavior (no harm to self or others) in clear, simple language *so patient can compare present behavior with expected behavior.* Express concern and hope that patient will feel better; provide reassurance that feelings are temporary *to communicate a caring attitude and reduce anxiety.*
➤ **NURSING DIAGNOSIS**	Risk for ineffective breathing pattern *related to* alcohol toxicity, airway obstruction, complicating respiratory diseases
Maintain effective breathing; have no indications of hypoxia.	Monitor respiratory rate, depth, and pattern *so appropriate interventions may be taken.* Place patient on side and in semi-Fowler's position *to reduce possibility of aspiration and to enhance lung expansion by lowering diaphragm.* Monitor effects of medications given for withdrawal *to detect respiratory depression.* Encourage coughing and deep breathing *to prevent complications of hypoventilation.* Administer supplemental oxygen *to treat hypoxia.*

CNS, Central nervous system.

A variety of inpatient and outpatient treatment programs are available. There is no evidence that inpatient programs are more effective than outpatient programs. The needs of each patient should be matched to the particular goals and approaches of a treatment program.

Aftercare services are important to sustain the individual in recovery. These services may include family counseling, group meetings, support groups, and individual counseling. The family and the work environment are critical in assisting individuals in recovery to return to healthy patterns of functioning. A number of drugs have been used as adjuncts in aftercare programs, including agents that repress the desire to drink, such as bromocriptine and naltrexone, and agents that prevent drinking by causing aversive consequences when alcohol is consumed, such as disulfiram (Antabuse). (Antabuse is discussed earlier in this chapter).

Alcoholics Anonymous (AA) has been successful in assisting individuals to achieve an alcohol-free life. AA is based on the 12 steps (Table 8-17) and is designed to help the individual cope with problems. The individual focuses on self-assessment and positive thinking. The group support is a key element in the success of AA. Alateen is available for teenagers and Al-Anon for families and friends of alcoholics.

Surgery and the alcoholic. Special precautions must be taken for the patient who is intoxicated or alcohol dependent and requires surgery[19] (Table 8-18). Alcoholic shock as a cause of decreased pulse and high BAC may be overlooked in an accident victim. Many persons are undiagnosed as alcoholics at the time of admission for surgery. Health problems such as malnutrition, dehydration, and infection may need to be treated before surgery can be performed. The patient who is alcohol dependent but currently has no BAC usually requires an increased level of anesthesia because of cross-tolerance. The intoxicated individual needs a decreased level of anesthesia because of the synergistic effect of the alcohol present in the system.

Whenever possible, surgery is postponed until the BAC is less than 200 mg%. In individuals with a BAC over 150 mg% a synergistic effect occurs with anesthesia. A patient with a BAC over 250 mg% presents a significantly increased surgical risk and mortality rate. Acute withdrawal and DTs may be triggered by surgery and the cessation of alcohol consumption. Surgery should be delayed for at least 48 to 72 hours, if possible, or IV alcohol may be given to avoid this reaction if immediate surgery is required. Alcohol interferes with pulmonary function and may be associated with increased incidence of hepatic dysfunction, poor wound healing, and metabolic abnormalities that can affect the outcome of surgery. Vital signs, including body temperature, must be closely monitored to identify signs of withdrawal, possible infections, and respiratory or cardiac problems.

Table 8-17 The Twelve Steps of Alcoholics Anonymous

1. We admitted we were powerless over alcohol—that our lives had become unmanageable.
2. We came to believe that a Power greater than ourselves could restore us to sanity.
3. We made a decision to turn our wills and our lives over to the care of God as we understood Him.
4. We made a searching and fearless moral inventory of ourselves.
5. We admitted to God, to ourselves, and to another human being the exact nature of our wrongs.
6. We were entirely ready to have God remove all these defects of character.
7. We humbly asked Him to remove our shortcomings.
8. We made a list of all persons we had harmed, and became willing to make amends to them all.
9. We made direct amends to such people whenever possible, except when to do so would injure them or others.
10. We continued to take personal inventory and, when we were wrong, promptly admitted it.
11. We sought through prayer and meditation to improve our conscious contact with God as we understood Him, praying only for knowledge of His will for us and the power to carry that out.
12. Having had a spiritual awakening as the result of these steps, we tried to carry this message to alcoholics, and to practice these principles in all our affairs.

From Alcoholics Anonymous: *The Twelve Steps of Alcoholics Anonymous,* New York, 1939, Works Publishers.

Table 8-18 Considerations for Alcohol-Abusing Patient Undergoing Surgery

- Standard amounts of anesthetic and analgesic medication may not be sufficient if patient is cross-tolerant.
- Increased doses of pain medication may be required if patient is cross-tolerant.
- Anesthetic agents may have a prolonged sedative effect if the patient has liver dysfunction. This situation requires an extended observation period.
- Patients have an increased susceptibility to cardiac and respiratory depression.
- Patients have an increased risk for bleeding, postoperative complications, and infection.
- Withdrawal from substances may be delayed for up to 5 days because of cross-tolerance with anesthetics and pain medications.
- Dosage of pain medications must be reduced gradually.

Opiates

Characteristics. Opium is a natural poppy extract. Nonsynthetic narcotics that are alkaloids of opium include morphine and codeine. Thebaine is a major alkaloid of another variety of poppy and is converted to codeine, hydrocodone, oxycodone, oxymorphone, nalbuphine, naloxone, and the Bentley compounds. Semisynthetic narcotics include heroin, hydromorphone (Dilaudid), and oxycodone. Synthetic narcotics include meperidine (Demerol), methadone, and propoxyphene (Darvon). Narcotic antagonists include naloxone (Narcan) and nalorphine (Nalline).

Pure heroin addiction is rare. Heroin addicts usually also abuse alcohol and other nonopiate drugs. Over the past 20 years a shift in patterns of IV drug abuse from heroin to cocaine has occurred.

Abusers in medical settings are usually individuals who are middle class, females, and individuals with chronic pain who are frequently on more than one prescription drug. Health care professionals have the highest rate of abuse of analgesics of any middle-class population. Job stresses, interference of work with family life, long hours, and availability of drugs are considered contributing factors.

Effects of Use. Opiates are CNS depressants and are detoxified in the liver and excreted in urine and bile. Most of the metabolites, with the exception of methadone, are excreted in 24 to 48 hours.

Narcotics are the most effective medicines for relief of intense pain, cough suppression (antitussives), and treatment of intestinal disorders such as colic and diarrhea. As drugs of abuse, they are sniffed, smoked, or self-administered by subcutaneous ("skin-popping") or IV ("mainlining") injection (Fig. 8-4).

Heroin is rapidly converted to morphine in the body. Hydromorphone is shorter acting and more sedating than morphine, and 2 to 8 times as potent. Percodan is aspirin plus oxycodone.

Methadone abuse commonly causes overdose. It is as potent as morphine, but methadone addiction occurs at a lower level and has longer-lasting effects. Methadone does not produce sedation; it is a powerful antitussive and spasmolytic. Propoxyphene (Darvon), related to methadone, is less addicting and less effective as an analgesic.

The primary effects of narcotics are analgesia, drowsiness, changes in mood, and, at high doses, clouding of mental functioning. Relief of suffering may provide a short-term euphoria. However, initial effects are frequently unpleasant. Effects include constriction of the pupils, reduced vision, apathy, decreased physical activity, constipation, nausea, vomiting, and even respiratory depression. There is usually no loss of motor coordination or slurred speech as observed in use of other depressants. IV use usually causes a "kick" or "rush" of feelings in the lower abdomen, along with warm skin flushing, an intoxicated feeling, euphoria, and decreased respiratory rate, peristalsis, and pupil size. Narcotics lead to a rapid tolerance and physical dependence after short-term use.

The signs of opiate intoxication may be seen within 2 to 5 minutes of IV use, beginning with euphoria and progressing to lethargy, somnolence, apathy, and dysphoria. Pupil constriction is present unless anoxia occurs with severe overdose, which leads to pupil dilatation. Unintentional overdose frequently occurs with recreational use of narcotics because of the unpredictability in potency and purity. Some narcotic overdoses may be actual suicide attempts. Signs of overdose are presented in Table 8-9.

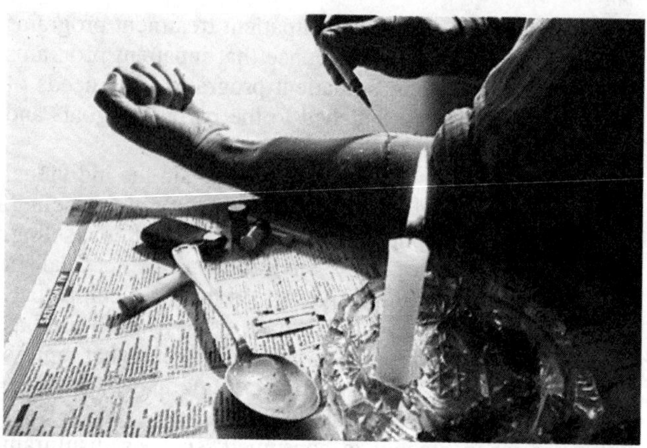

Fig. 8-4 Shooting up. Sharing needles and syringes and other contaminated "works" has increased the spread of human immunodeficiency virus.

Withdrawal from opiates occurs with decreased amounts or cessation of the drug after prolonged moderate to heavy use. The administration of an antagonist (e.g., naloxone) will trigger withdrawal symptoms in dependent individuals. Manifestations of withdrawal include craving, nausea or vomiting, muscle aches, lacrimation or rhinorrhea, pupillary dilatation, piloerection ("gooseflesh"), perspiration, diarrhea, yawning, fever, or insomnia. Generally within 12 hours of the last dose there is physical discomfort followed by a restless sleep, "flulike" symptoms, and craving. The onset of withdrawal begins at the time of the next usual dose and ranges from 4 to 6 hours for heroin to 1 day or longer for methadone. The kicking movements sometimes observed in a patient in withdrawal are responsible for the phrase "kicking the habit." The individual may be suicidal during withdrawal.

The severity of withdrawal is related to the degree of dependence, but it usually runs its course in 96 hours. Symptoms may recur for 6 to 8 months. Physical dependence may not always indicate drug abuse. The patient who receives therapeutic doses of narcotics may develop tolerance and dependence. However, when most medical conditions are resolved, the opiate is no longer desired.

Complications. Medical complications are linked with the routes of administration. Street heroin, which is often cut with quinine, has vasodilator effects when given IV and may lead to tetanus and tissue abscesses if administered subcutaneously. Heroin users have been found to have a higher incidence of infections, especially those associated with needle use. Drug use tends to reduce safe sex practices, which also increases the risk of contracting HIV.

Table 8-19 Hallucinogens

Substance	Street Names	Administration
▪ Marijuana (leaves of the *Cannibas sativa* plant), THC, hashish (resin of the cannibis plant)	Pot, grass, hemp, reefer, tea, weed, gage, Mary Jane, Acapulco gold, Panama red, hash	Oral, sniffed, smoked ("tokes"—inhalations)
▪ LSD	Acid, trips, big D, sugar cubes, 25, instant Zen	Oral, injected
▪ Psilocybin	Magic mushrooms	Oral
▪ DMT, *N,N*-dimethyltryptamine	AMT, businessman's high, businessman's trip or lunch	Injected, smoked
▪ Morning glory seeds	Pearly gates, flying saucers, heavenly blue	Oral
▪ Mescaline (peyote)	Mesc, white light, blue caps, pink wedge, big chief, cactus, button tops	Oral, injected
▪ 25-dimethoxy-4-methylamphetamine	STP, DOM	Oral
▪ Ketamine hydrochloride	Green, 1980 supergrass (when used with marijuana, it is called K, jet, superacid, purple mauve, special LA coke, special C)	Smoked, injected
▪ Methyl-3, 4-methylenedioxyamphetamine	MDA, love drug	Oral
▪ Phencyclidine hydrochloride (Sernyl)	PCP, hog, elephant tranquilizer, horse tranks, angel dust (when sprinkled on leaves such as mint or parsley, it is known as crystal joints, superweek, angel hair, CJ, or KJ)	Snorted, smoked, oral, injected
▪ Solvents such as airplane glue, automobile paint, gasoline, paint thinners		Sniffed

DMT, Dimethyltryptamine; *LSD,* lysergic acid diethylamide; *THC,* tetrahydrocannabinol.

Other complications that are associated with opiate addiction include hepatitis, gastric ulcers, dysrhythmias, endocarditis, anemias, electrolyte abnormalities, bone and joint infections, kidney failure, muscle destruction, pneumonia, lung abscesses, tuberculosis, bronchospasm and wheezing, stroke, lymphadenopathy, abnormal sexual function, and depression.

Therapeutic Management. The short-term prognosis for narcotic addicts is poor because of high relapse rates. The long-term prognosis is better because addicts in their 30s and 40s tend to burn out or stop drug use.

Overdose of opiates can precipitate a medical emergency (see Table 8-9). Laboratory analysis is performed to identify the drug ingested. A narcotic antagonist such as naloxone, nalorphine, or levallorphan should be given before any irreversible brain anoxia develops. Prophylactic tetanus immunizations are often given. If a suicide attempt is suspected, the individual should be evaluated by a trained professional before discharge.

Treatment of withdrawal is related to symptoms and may not require any medication. One of the goals of treatment for an opiate addict is to assist in maintaining a relative comfort level so the patient is more likely to consider entering a rehabilitation program.

Methadone is a federally regulated synthetic narcotic that may be used in detoxification and maintenance programs for heroin addicts. Methadone maintenance is supportive therapy that is most effective when provided in addition to education and counseling programs. Methadone has been beneficial for some individuals and is the most effective method of decreasing the risk of heroin use and the most promising available treatment for IV narcotic users seeking treatment.

HALLUCINOGENS

A number of psychoactive substances that are either natural or synthetic act to produce a change in level of consciousness, alter mood, and induce hallucinations. These drugs are classified as hallucinogens (Table 8-19).

Cannabis

Characteristics. The cannabis group includes substances with psychoactive ingredients derived from the cannabis or hemp plant, or chemically similar synthetic substances. The three drugs of this group that are most commonly found in the United States and Canada are marijuana, hashish, and hashish oil. Many chemicals or cannabinoids are synthesized from the Cannabis *sativa* plant. Tetrahydrocannabinol (THC) is believed to be responsible for most of the psychoactive effects. Marijuana, which is derived from the dried leaves and flowering tops of the cannabis plant, is a less potent source of THC than hashish, which is a rich resinous secretion of the plant. Hashish oil, a dark viscous extraction of the plant, has a much higher percent of THC. A drop or two of hashish oil on a cigarette has the same effect as a marijuana "joint."

THC has been used to treat tetanus, migraine, postpartum psychoses, insomnia, and opium addiction. Although a number of potential benefits have been reported, the only established uses are for resistant glaucoma and for the control of nausea from cancer chemotherapy.

Patterns of use vary from occasional to long-term, habitual use. Generally it is the first illegal drug that is used by young people, with the exception of alcohol. Peer influence is considered the strongest predictor of use. Occasional users are more common, and they tend to smoke in groups. Daily use may lead to compulsive or all-day, everyday use.

Effects of Use. The mechanism of action of cannabis is uncertain. It is metabolized in the liver, is fat-soluble, stored in body fats, and has a half-life of 7 to 8 days. It is excreted as metabolites in feces and urine. Metabolites may be detectable days to weeks after brief exposure to marijuana. Marijuana is usually smoked, and peak plasma level occurs within 10 minutes. The most prominent effects occur in 20 to 30 minutes, and intoxication lasts from 2 to 3 hours. Tolerance of many effects occurs. Physiologic dependence does not usually develop with long-term heavy use. A mild cross-tolerance to alcohol develops. Marijuana has low toxicity, and there are no known lethal doses with its use.

The most commonly affected organs appear to be the brain, cardiovascular system, and lungs. Most changes are reversible. Signs of intoxication include euphoria, anxiety, suspiciousness or paranoid ideation, sensation of slowed time, impaired judgment, social withdrawal, redness of conjunctiva, increased appetite for sweets, dry mouth, and tachycardia. Problems of habitual users include impaired short-term memory, visual hallucinations (from high doses), decreased motor coordination, tremors, increased heart and respiratory rates, increased sexual arousal, and sleepiness. Marijuana use may precipitate seizures in persons with epilepsy, psychotic episodes in persons with schizophrenia, and ketoacidosis in persons with diabetes mellitus.

Acute problems range from anxiety reactions to panic attacks or psychotic episodes. Panic attacks usually occur in the first-time user who is not familiar with the drug or its effects. Symptoms of panic attacks include extreme anxiety, fear of losing control or going crazy, and fear of physical illness. Flashbacks, or the reexperiencing of intense drug episodes, are time limited and involve a change in perception of time or a feeling of slowed thinking.

Medical problems associated with marijuana use are generally mild and transient. More serious potential problems have been reported with heavy use. These include bronchitis, increased rates of precancerous lesions in the lungs, sinusitis, pharyngitis, acute memory impairment, increased risk of cardiac problems for individuals with heart disease, depression of the immune system, and alterations in the reproductive and endocrine systems.

Therapeutic Management. Acute reactions, including intoxication and withdrawal, are usually mild and time limited. An individual may be treated for toxic reactions to a combination of drugs that includes marijuana or may seek treatment for panic reactions. Most therapeutic approaches depend on the characteristics and severity of symptoms. Treatment is directed toward relief of symptoms, and the administration of drugs is avoided if possible. It is important for the nurse to perform a physical examination, a toxicology screen, and a thorough history. The approach is basically the same for treating panic, flashbacks, and toxic reactions. The main interventions are to provide support and reassurance to the patient by explaining what is happening. The patient should understand that the level of intoxication may fluctuate over several days as metabolites are released.

An individual with cannabis intoxication or other acute problems related to cannabis use is seldom hospitalized and may be assisted in recovery by providing a quiet environment and adequate support and reassurance. A long-term user may seek treatment for annoying symptoms rather than drug use. A long-term user may need assistance in achieving abstinence and may experience changes in mental functioning, alertness, memory, and motivation. As with other drug use, maintaining abstinence usually involves changes in values, lifestyles, and friends.

Lysergic Acid Diethylamide, Dimethyltryptamine, Mescaline, and Related Substances

Characteristics. Hallucinogens may be natural (such as peyote) or synthetically produced (such as lysergic acid diethylamide [LSD]). Peyote or mescaline are plant products of cacti and psilocybin from fungi. Most of these substances are taken orally and introduced to adolescents by experimentation among peer groups. Some individuals find the experience unpleasant and stop use; others continue to use the drug episodically. Few individuals use these drugs daily. These drugs interfere with the ability to function effectively. Therefore with these drugs, abuse is observed more commonly than is actual dependence.

Effects of Use. The mechanism of action of these substances is unknown. Tolerance develops rapidly with recurrent use, which necessitates use of larger doses, but tolerance disappears after use is stopped. Cross-tolerance may be found for most of the hallucinogens, including LSD, mescaline, and psilocybin, but does not extend to marijuana. Psychologic dependence occurs with hallucinogens, but no significant withdrawal syndrome indicating physiologic dependence is evident.

These drugs produce a change in the level of consciousness and distort the perception of reality. Senses of time, distance, and direction may be disrupted. Vivid psychedelic effects occur that sharpen senses and distort stimuli, including altered body images. The individual may "hear" colors and "see" sounds (*synesthesia*). Illusions, visual hallucinations, and delusions are frequently observed with higher doses but may occur at low doses.

Hallucinogenic drugs produce a state of excitement of the CNS that alters mood and causes either euphoria or depression. Euphoria is usually present. If depression occurs and is severe, a mood disorder may develop and a suicide attempt may be made. Impaired thinking, problem solving, and judgment are common and can lead to impulsive acts and accidents. Acute anxiety, restlessness, and sleeplessness are also common. Most symptoms of use are related to sensory perception changes and psychologic effects. Physical symptoms reflect sympathetic nervous system stimulation, including dilated pupils, flushed face, fine tremors, increased blood pressure, elevated blood glucose levels, increased body temperature, blurred vision, tachycardia, palpitations, diaphoresis, and incoordination.

Hallucinogen intoxication or hallucinosis includes perceptual changes. As with other types of hallucinogens, the response of the user is heavily influenced by the dose, the expectation of the user, the individual's personality, and the setting of use. Fear of losing one's mind or paranoid thoughts may occur and may lead (in some cases) to a delusional disorder or to an acute psychotic disorder. The onset of symptoms of hallucinosis usually occurs within 1 hour of use and may last from 8 to 12 hours for LSD or from 1 hour to 3 days with other hallucinogens.

Mild and transitory flashbacks are common after hallucinogen use, but only severe forms are given the diagnosis of posthallucinogen perception disorder. In addition to hallucinations, other kinds of flashbacks may include feelings of depersonalization or recurrent distress. These experiences include intensified colors, flashes of color, false perceptions of movement, or halos around objects. Such reactions may be triggered by entering a darkened area, falling asleep, use of cannabis or phenothiazines, or an acute physical or personal crisis.

Therapeutic Management. Emergency problems most commonly related to abuse of LSD-type drugs are panic reactions, flashbacks, and toxic reactions. Panic reactions are a type of "bad trip" generally experienced by individuals with limited previous exposure to these drugs. The emotional dysphoria lasts for the duration of the drug's action. Treatment approaches are directed toward providing reassurance to the user, educating and orienting the user, and providing consistent verbal contact in a supportive and nonthreatening environment. Hospitalization and medications are generally not necessary. An antianxiety drug such as diazepam or chlordiazepoxide may be given if needed. A careful drug and psychosocial history are important in identifying concurrent alcohol or drug use or psychiatric problems. Because many hallucinogens are not what they claim to be, users may not know what substances they have taken.

Flashbacks are generally approached in the same manner. It is important that the use of marijuana, antihistamines, and stimulants be avoided in the treatment of flashbacks. Toxic reactions usually have a rapid onset and clear within 24 hours except for reactions to 2.5-dimethoxy-4-methylamphetamine (DOM) or PCP. Approaches follow the same outline that is used for panic reactions, with close monitoring of vital signs and airway, breathing, and circulation (ABC) to deal with life-threatening emergencies such as convulsions and hyperthermia. A physical assessment that includes a neurologic examination should be done. Any psychosis or organic brain syndrome is treated symptomatically until it is resolved or until an underlying problem is identified.

NURSING MANAGEMENT

SUBSTANCE ABUSE

Nursing Assessment

The nurse must be alert to the subtle and overt cues of substance use (Table 8-20) and the implications for nursing management. Early recognition and identification of a patient with substance-related problems is crucial to successful treatment outcomes.[20] The nurse must recognize patient behaviors that influence the history taking such as manipulation, denial, impulsiveness, avoidance, underreporting or minimizing substance use, giving inaccurate information, and inaccurate self-reporting. These behaviors are not uncommon in substance-abusing patients.

Table 8-20 Symptoms and Behaviors That May Suggest Dependence on Substances

- Trauma secondary to falls, auto accidents, fights, and burns
- Fatigue
- Insomnia
- Headaches
- Vague physical complaints
- Sexual dysfunction, decreased libido, erectile dysfunction
- Anorexia, weight loss
- Seizure disorder
- Appearance older than stated age
- Problems in areas of life function
  - Frequent job changes
  - Marital conflict, separation, or divorce
  - Work-related accidents, tardiness, absenteeism
  - Legal problems, including arrest
  - Social isolation, estrangement from friends or family
- Driving while intoxicated (more than one citation suggests dependence)
- Leisure activities that involve alcohol or other drugs
- Financial problems, including those related to spending for substances
- Failure of standard doses of sedatives to have a therapeutic effect
- Changes in mood, especially before and after visiting hours
- Overabundant use of mouthwash or toiletries
- Frequent references to alcohol or alcohol use indicating a preoccupation with the importance of alcohol in the patient's life

If the nurse is to obtain an accurate and thorough patient assessment, there are certain essential nursing behaviors which can facilitate the patient's accurate self-disclosure. The nurse must be aware of personal feelings and attitudes about substance abuse. An addicted patient can evoke hostility from a health care worker. Some health professionals may view the substance-abusing patient as emotionally weak and irresponsible. Such an individual is frequently seen as not contributing to society or as one who inflicts harm on society and drains social and economic resources. An addicted patient can elicit strong emotional responses at a time when help is needed.[21] It is important for the nurse to be aware of negative feelings that may be communicated to the patient. The nurse may also fail to recognize signs and symptoms of abuse in a patient or co-worker who does not fit the stereotype of the addict.

During assessment the nurse must (1) facilitate privacy and avoid or minimize interruptions, (2) stress the importance of an accurate and thorough substance use history to provide appropriate care and prevent complications, and (3) be aware of the concerns of the substance-abusing patient. Such a patient is fearful and distressed over loss of control of self-medicating and is concerned that withdrawal may not be treated or will be treated inadequately. There may also be concerns that the health professional will report the patient to legal authorities.

The nurse must be knowledgeable about manifestations of abuse. The nurse must have a high suspicion index to accurately and promptly identify the substance-abusing patient. A brief assessment of substance-related emergency conditions is essential for any patient newly admitted, regardless of age or condition and especially for a trauma or accident patient. A thorough health assessment must also be done and should always include a history of alcohol and other substance use. It is necessary to obtain current and past substance use information and patterns. Inquiries should be made about recreational drugs, over-the-counter drugs, alcohol, nicotine, and prescription drugs. A thorough and accurate history and assessment are the basis for diagnosis and planning for appropriate intervention. The data are necessary to avoid withdrawal syndromes or drug interactions that may be life threatening.

Nursing Diagnoses

Nursing diagnoses assist nurses in the organization and management of patient problems. Specific nursing diagnoses are useful in caring for an individual who has problems related to substance abuse. Several relevant nursing diagnoses have been identified (Table 8-21). Nursing diagnoses related to the individual with a substance abuse problem are also presented in the nursing care plan on p. 169.

Planning

The overall goals are that the patient with a substance abuse problem will abstain from the use of addicting substances, cooperate with the proposed treatment plan, make appropriate lifestyle adjustments to support abstinence, and practice healthy lifestyle behaviors to foster good health.

Table 8-21 Nursing Diagnoses Related to Substance Abuse

Acute confusion
Altered family process: alcoholism
Altered nutrition: less than bodily requirements
Altered thought processes
Anxiety and fear
Chronic low self-esteem
Decreased cardiac output
Impaired environmental interpretation syndrome
Ineffective breathing pattern
Ineffective family coping
Ineffective individual coping
Powerlessness
Risk for infection
Risk for injury
Risk for violence: self-directed or directed at others
Self-care deficit (specify)
Self-esteem disturbance
Sensory-perceptual alterations (specify)
Sexual dysfunction
Sleep pattern disturbance

Nursing Implementation

Health Promotion and Maintenance. Patterns of substance use may be viewed within a prevention framework (see Fig. 8-1). As patterns of dependence become firmly established, an individual has less chance for reversing these patterns without treatment and rehabilitation for addiction. The nurse needs to use this information when assessing patterns of substance use to initiate appropriate intervention strategies.

Primary prevention. The focus of primary prevention is health promotion. Nursing management related to primary prevention of substance use and abuse includes teaching and counseling for nonusers and minimal users.[22] Primary prevention includes activities to prevent the occurrence of a problem. The nurse can be educator, resource person, role model, and agent of change. Education about the immediate effects of substances on the body, the long-term effects of substance use, and the effects of experimentation and continued use should target risk groups such as preadolescents, women, and older adults.

Age-appropriate education is essential for the adolescent and the young adult because experimentation with various drugs and initial drinking and smoking behaviors frequently begin during these developmental years (see Fig. 8-1). The nurse needs to provide health teaching in both formal and informal settings. When history and physical examinations are performed, the nurse should be alert to opportunities for teaching. Young people need to see and hear about consequences of substance abuse and understand how these can relate to their personal lives.

A nurse who works with these age groups must be knowledgeable of risk factors associated with substance abuse and subtle cues indicating risk-taking behaviors. The nurse also needs to promote health in women of child-

NURSING CARE PLAN Patient with Substance Abuse Problem

Planning: Outcome Criteria	*Nursing Interventions and Rationales*
➤ **NURSING DIAGNOSIS**	Ineffective denial *related to* refusal to acknowledge substance abuse or dependency *as manifested by* delay in seeking or refusal of health care to detriment of health; lack of perception of personal relevance of symptoms or danger; self-treatment; minimization of symptoms; denial of impact of disease and its affects on life; blaming others for problems; use of rationalization or intellectualization.
Able to explain psychologic and physiologic effects of alcohol and drug use; admit alcohol or drug abuse problem; express sense of hope; use alternative positive coping mechanisms to relieve stress; recognize need for continued treatment.	Help patient focus on the present and not on the reasons for the problem *to avoid wasting time with past causes and to foster focusing on present plan.* Assist patient in identifying and altering patterns of substance abuse (e.g., explain health consequences) *to assist patient to develop new patterns of coping.* Do *not* argue about whether patient is an "alcoholic" or "abuser" or allow patient to use blame of others, rationalization, or intellectualization *to confront maladptive defense mechanisms.* Assist patient in identifying effect of substance abuse on life and significant others (i.e., motivation to stop abuse) *to identify possible motivators for ceasing substance abuse.* Help patient to express effects in acceptable manner *to foster development of insight on behavior and consequences.* Assist patient to improve self-esteem, *because low self-esteem is a common characteristic of the substance abuser.* Instill a sense of hope, *as hopelessness is discouraging and may inhibit recovery.* Assist patient in resocialization and building support system, including self-help groups (e.g., Alcoholics Anonymous, Narcotics Anonymous) *to provide patient with a new and healthier support system.* Initiate referral as indicated *because the emotional problems often associated with substance abuse may be beyond the scope of a nurse without special training.*
➤ **NURSING DIAGNOSIS**	Altered health maintenance *related to* lack of knowledge of progression of alcoholism and its effects and relapse prevention *as manifested by* inappropriate use of alcohol and other drugs; inaccurate knowledge or lack of knowledge of signs and symptoms of alcoholism, nature of disease, effect on body; repeated relapses; inability to maintain sobriety
Recognize signs and symptoms of disease; know warning signs of relapse; have plan for seeking help at first sign of relapse; abstain from alcohol, participate in support groups regularly.	Provide educational information to patient and family about alcoholism (e.g., development, effects, and consequences) *to enable them to be informed and to encourage active participation in treatment.* Teach early warning signs of relapse *so immediate intervention is possible.* Assist patient in rehearsing responses to stressful situations or triggers to substance abuse *to facilitate effective coping and prevent relapse.* Provide names of resources to call for help *to expand patient's support system.* Support abstinence and participation in support groups (e.g., Alcoholics Anonymous), *as these groups are known to be helpful in maintaining sobriety.* Refer to treatment program or counseling (if indicated) *to foster ongoing treatment.*
➤ **NURSING DIAGNOSIS**	Ineffective individual coping *related to* lack of knowledge of problem-solving and assertiveness skills *as manifested by* inappropriate use of alcohol and other drugs; inability to problem solve, depression, suicidal thoughts, association of anger or guilt with managing stressors
Experience decrease in depression; have increase in expression of thoughts and feelings, problem-solving ability, and assertiveness.	Assist patient to express negative thoughts and feelings (sadness, hopelessness, anger, guilt) *to clarify thoughts and begin problem-solving process.* Assess degree of depression and suicidal or homicidal thoughts or poor impulse control *to determine degree of danger to self or others.* Make referral if indicated *as some problems may be beyond the scope of the nurse.* Discuss alternative coping strategies such as anticipation of stressful events, development of problem-solving and assertiveness skills *so patient will be aware of healthier coping strategies to meet life stresses.* Assist patient in practicing assertive responses to stressful situations *to develop confidence in ability to use alternative ways of responding to stress.*

continued

NURSING CARE PLAN Patient with Substance Abuse Problem—cont'd

Planning: Outcome Criteria	Nursing Interventions and Rationales
➤ **NURSING DIAGNOSIS**	Altered nutrition: less than bodily requirements *related to* history of poor nutrition and malabsorption secondary to alcoholism *as manifested by* body weight below normal for height and age, poor skin turgor, sunken eyeballs, hair loss, low serum albumin and hemoglobin
Steadily gain weight until proper weight achieved; have no signs or symptoms of malnutrition.	Monitor patient's weight, albumin, and prealbumin *to determine extent of problem and plan appropriate interventions.* Encourage patient to abstain from alcohol *because it interferes with absorption and utilization of nutrients.* Provide frequent, small nourishing meals *to improve caloric intake and enhance tolerance of food.* Teach patient to take vitamins, including thiamine, *to correct deficiencies and reduce neurologic complications.* Explain need for NPO status if gastritis or bleeding are present *to reduce gastric stimulation.*
➤ **NURSING DIAGNOSIS**	Ineffective family coping: disabiling *related to* alcohol or drug abuse problem *as manifested by* disparaging comments, abusive treatment and neglect, and general intolerance of affected family member
Identify need to establish effective communication and living skills with family.	Assess coping patterns of patient and individual family members *to determine extent of problem.* Foster discussion of family coping patterns and explore relationship problems *to increase awareness of need for long-term family counseling.* Explore abusive treatment *identify need for immediate intervention.* Refer patient and family to qualified counselor, since a specialist is required to treat this complex problem.

NPO, Nothing by mouth.

Table 8-22 Health Promotion Strategies Related to Substance Abuse

- Recognition of nurse's attitudes, beliefs, and values related to addiction
- Assessment of nurse's patterns of substance use
- Teaching patient and family about substance abuse
- Education of public, nurses, and co-workers about substance use
- Identification of individual at risk
- Identification of early signs and symptoms of substance abuse
- Initiation of activities to effect social change

bearing age, as the health risks of substance use apply to both the pregnant woman and the developing fetus. Health-promotion strategies are listed in Table 8-22.

Secondary prevention. Secondary prevention includes activities aimed at early detection and intervention. Nurses in all health care settings are responsible for education, case finding, and early intervention for substance-related problems. In acute care settings nurses encounter patients who are substance dependent in emergency departments, trauma units, burn units, operating and recovery rooms, orthopedic units, general medical-surgical units, critical care units, and ambulatory care settings. It is estimated that 10% to 45% of adults hospitalized on units other than chemical dependency and psychiatric units meet the criteria for alcohol dependence or abuse. Health care providers must be alert to the prevalence of alcohol and other substance abuse problems in patients and co-workers. The nurse's role is to provide early detection through screening, support early intervention and treatment through referral, and facilitate the development of substance-free alternatives. Education and early treatment may improve the health outcomes and prevent or reduce long-term complications of substance abuse. Examples of secondary prevention include health screening clinics and peer or employee assistance programs.

Tertiary prevention. Tertiary prevention targets the individual who has already been identified as having a substance abuse problem. Tertiary prevention includes activities directed at controlling and monitoring the problem and minimizing the long-term effects of the disease. Following the delivery of acute care, the nurse has the responsibility and opportunity for interventions to motivate the patient to obtain treatment and initiate recovery from the addiction.

Addiction is a health problem that is chronic in nature and associated with relapses. The nurse must acknowledge this and educate the patient about the need to identify precipitating factors or triggers of substance use and relapse. An important concept is *abstinence* (refraining from using the problematic substance). It requires a conscious commitment not to use drugs and to initiate lifestyle changes that protect against persons, places, and circumstances that induce or contribute to drug use. Examples of tertiary prevention include symptom management, health education, support groups (e.g., Alcoholics Anonymous), and relapse prevention programs. Relapse prevention is a behavioral approach that identifies environmental cues that trigger relapses. It assists the recovering individual in the development of coping strategies and increased personal confidence (self-efficacy) for managing high-risk situations.

Acute Intervention. Acute care situations related to substance abuse involve overdose, intoxication, and withdrawal. The management of these problems related to the specific substances is discussed earlier in this chapter.

In general, withdrawal signs and symptoms are somewhat opposite in nature from the direct effects of the drug. Withdrawal from all classes of drugs is similar in producing symptoms of acute anxiety and protracted depression. Withdrawal from CNS depressants, including alcohol, is the most dangerous withdrawal situation. Abrupt withdrawal may be life threatening. Management is symptomatic and includes a gradual reduction in dosage. Although withdrawal from narcotics is the least life threatening, symptoms are dramatic, temporarily disabling, and painful. Methadone is often recommended for treating withdrawal, but any opiate may be administered. Symptoms of withdrawal may be reduced by administering the drug of choice in decreasing amounts over 2 weeks. Nonopiates may also be administered for detoxification and include clonidine (Catapres) and benzodiazepines.

Management of a drug overdose depends on the substance involved. Specific interventions are addressed in previous sections of this chapter. Drug overdose can be accidental or intentional. Accidental overdose usually involves only one substance, whereas intentional overdose is more likely to involve multiple substances and result in a complex and potentially confusing clinical picture.[23] The first priority of care in overdose is always the patient's ABC (see Table 8-9). After the patient is stable, a thorough history and physical examination must be completed.[24] When the patient is unwilling or unable to give a history, the patient's significant others should be questioned. A patient who intentionally overdoses should not be allowed to return home until seen by a psychiatric professional.

Another acute situation is the substance abuser who needs surgery. Because of the substance abuse problem, this individual is more likely to have accidents and injuries that require surgery. Special nursing considerations for the substance-abusing patient undergoing surgery are presented in Table 8-18.

Pain management for the substance-abusing patient can be challenging. The nurse needs to consider the issue of cross-tolerance and that the therapeutic doses of pain medication for a nonaddicted patient may not be adequate for a substance-abusing patient. Another issue to consider is whether the patient is actually experiencing pain or just wants the medication to relieve a craving or prevent withdrawal symptoms. Although the nurse can ask the patient to rate the pain, the existence and severity of pain is based on the patient's perception. The nurse needs to evaluate the pain as objectively as possible and accept and respect the patient's report of pain as an indication of the patient's experience.[25] Another factor to consider is that the acute medical-surgical problem must be managed first and the patient safely detoxified. Rehabilitation and treatment for problems with substance abuse are not realistic goals when an acute condition exists.

Chronic and Home Management. Before rehabilitation is considered, all acute medical-surgical problems must be resolved. The patient must recognize and show initial understanding of the substance problem and be willing to accept long-term treatment. Outcomes are more positive when the nurse can work closely with the family and significant others, as well as the substance-abusing patient in planning long-term care. Rehabilitation may be available for the patient in private or public psychiatric hospitals or in facilities specifically designed to meet the health care needs of the substance-abusing patient. It is important that a multidisciplinary team of nurses, physicians, social workers, and recreational therapists collaborate with the patient in planning care and in providing a therapeutic environment. The patient may progress from hospitalization to halfway houses, therapeutic communities, or other community-based programs.

Halfway houses serve as transitional settings in which the patient develops independence from the structured treatment of the hospital setting. The independence from a structured treatment program promotes opportunities to learn to handle stresses and conflicts experienced in everyday life using the resources of the treatment system before returning to the community and home.

Therapeutic communities such as Phoenix House and Daytop Village were founded for the treatment of abuse of substances other than alcohol. These communities are run mostly by former addicts or residents. An interdisciplinary staff of professionals supports the work of the residents while providing consultation and serving as resource persons.

Alternatives to inpatient hospitalization include outpatient treatment and day and evening treatment programs. These programs provide many of the services described but meet the varying needs of many patients. Day programs may meet the needs of the patient who is not quite ready to return to work but still needs self-help meetings, therapy sessions, and other counseling services. For the individual who is able to return to work but continues to need self-help meetings, therapy, and other social services, evening programs are available.

Treatment modalities for the substance-abusing patient include self-help groups, counseling and psychotherapy, pharmacotherapy, and professional peer groups. Self-help groups are usually based on 12-step programs and include AA, Cocaine Anonymous, and Narcotics Anonymous. Counseling and psychotherapy are helpful approaches for both the substance-abusing individual and family.[26] These approaches are thought to be more effective when combined with self-help groups.

Pharmacologic approaches include the use of disulfiram (Antabuse) for the alcoholic patient and the use of methadone in the treatment of opiate dependence. Antabuse, an alcohol antagonist or antialcohol, may be given orally over

Table 8-23 Warning Signs of Relapse
Apprehension about well-being
Defensiveness and denial
Loneliness and isolation
Periods of confusion and restlessness
Readiness to anger
Irregular eating and sleeping habits
Feelings of powerlessness, helplessness, depression
Development of "don't care" attitude
Wishful thinking and fantasizing
Loss of daily structure

an extended period of time, up to 1 year. Antabuse cannot be given to a patient with serious medical problems such as diabetes, cirrhosis, hypertension, and heart disease. If alcohol is in the system, the use of Antabuse may result in facial flushing, palpitations, rapid heart rate, difficulty in breathing, a possible serious drop in blood pressure, and nausea and vomiting. The patient must be taught about the effects of Antabuse, its purpose, and the very unpleasant reaction that will occur if alcohol in any form is ingested.

Methadone is used both for detoxification and maintenance to help the patient develop a lifestyle free of street drugs and to improve family and job functioning, improve health, and decrease legal problems. The drug is administered in an oral liquid once a day at a licensed clinic or designated center; weekend doses are taken by the patient at home.

Complete abstinence from drugs is important, because the use of another drug can trigger craving for the abused substance and result in relapse because of paired associations. The nurse needs to be alert for signs of relapse (Table 8-23). Relapse prevention is an essential component of any recovery program and includes behavioral, cognitive, educational, and self-control techniques. The individual needs to identify specific increased risk situations that are likely to lead to drug use and to practice ways to avoid or deal with these situations. Conditioned urges and drug cravings should be consistently extinguished by substituting other activities for drug use. Negative consequences of the drugs should be recalled to counteract distorted memories of the drug euphoria. Temporary relapses need to be viewed as learning opportunities to minimize feelings of failure and to assist the patient to continue with abstinence. The nurse can guide the patient in learning stress management techniques for promoting a healthy lifestyle.

SPECIAL POPULATIONS WITH SUBSTANCE ABUSE PROBLEMS

Gerontologic Considerations

Patterns of substance use in older persons are considerably different from other population groups. The elderly, more than any other age group, have the highest use of over-the-counter (OTC) and prescription drugs. These medications and preparations are used to ease the many discomforts that accompany chronic conditions in the older person. The simultaneous use of OTC drugs, prescription drugs, and alcohol occurs in many older adults. In the acute care setting, the prevalence of alcoholism is estimated to be as high as 20% in individuals over age 65, with higher rates occurring in nursing homes and psychiatric settings.[27] Illegal drug use is minimal in the elderly except for long-term addicts. However, it is expected that this pattern may change given the drug-using patterns now seen in the middle-aged population.

The most commonly used OTC drugs are analgesics; laxatives and antidiarrheals; vitamins, minerals and iron; antacids; sedatives; cold and cough medications; antiemetics; hemorrhoidal preparations; and ophthalmic preparations. Among the most frequently prescribed drugs are anxiolytics, sedatives, hypnotics, and analgesics, as well as those prescribed for multiple chronic conditions (e.g., hypertension, chronic obstructive pulmonary disease).

An individual with a long history of heavy alcohol consumption and abuse often demonstrates complications as changes associated with aging occur. An individual with no prior history of alcoholism may begin drinking heavily later in life as a result of stressful life changes (late-onset alcoholism). Daily drinking is more common among the elderly than binge drinking.

Losses associated with aging pose stressful adjustments. These losses include deaths of friends and spouse, retirement, relocation to new communities or supervised care facilities, lifestyle changes resulting from economic constraints, and declining health including hearing and vision losses. Maladaptive drug-using patterns may emerge as attempts to cope with perceived life stresses or as possible passive suicide attempts.

The adverse effects of interaction of alcohol and other drugs are increased with aging. Ethanol may accelerate or inhibit the metabolism of other drugs. When taken with alcohol, sedative-hypnotic drugs, minor tranquilizers, and CNS depressants have additive and synergistic effects, to which the older person is particularly sensitive. Other changes include impaired drug absorption, reduced blood circulation, and declining metabolic and excretion rates.

The interaction of physiologic and psychologic effects and drug actions results in behavioral patterns particular to the older patient. These include both acute and chronic responses to drug intake. Drug-induced memory deficits may precipitate drug misuse. Social problems, particularly isolation secondary to intoxication, may occur. Confusion, disorientation, delirium, memory loss, and neuromuscular problems are effects of the interaction of alcohol, drug misuse, and normal aging. Substance abuse problems in the elderly do not present a clear picture. Nonspecific indicators of alcohol abuse may include malnutrition, falls, frequent accidents, incontinence, decreased attention to self-care, mood swings, depression, confusion, and uncharacteristic reactions to prescribed medication.[28]

Interventions targeted at substance abuse by the older adult include recognizing alcoholism as a separate chronic illness, treating the person in familiar places, using therapies known to be helpful with older people (e.g., socialization), and peer groups. A simple tool for recognizing alcohol problems in older adults is HEAT. Questions include: *H*ow do you use alcohol? Have you ever thought you used alcohol to *E*xcess? Has *A*nyone else ever thought you used too much? Have you ever had any *T*rouble resulting from your use? Positive responses to any question should be followed up.[29] Therapy must be aimed at identifying and reducing environmental stressors that may trigger alcohol and drug use. The basic needs of food and shelter must be adequately met. Home visits provide a good source of direct assessment data.

Patient education for the older adult includes teaching about the desired effects, possible side effects, and appropriate storage of prescribed and OTC medications. The patient's knowledge of medications that are currently being taken (both prescription and OTC) needs to be assessed. The patient should be advised to use only one pharmacy because many pharmacies maintain a medication profile, which may avoid problems with drug interactions. The patient should be advised not to drink alcohol when using prescribed medications and OTC drugs. Family members and significant others need to be informed about the medication regimen, drug interactions, and the effects of alcohol on drugs.

Chemical Dependence in Nurses

Because of widespread denial and the "conspiracy of silence," chemical dependence in nurses has not been addressed as a professional issue until the past decade.[30] The American Nurses' Association responded to nurses' need for help by passing a resolution in 1982 that advocates rehabilitation for nurses who are chemically dependent and the establishment of assistance programs by state nurses' associations.

The National Nurses' Society on Addictions (NNSA) produced a position paper on impaired nurses, established a national network of resources, and created a model diversion program to assist states in developing programs. The goals of these programs are to protect the safety of the public, to maintain the integrity of the profession, and to ensure that the nurse is offered the possibility of treatment and rehabilitation before the license to practice is revoked or the job is terminated. Essential components of these programs include education, intervention, referral to appropriate treatment, monitoring of recovery, and support for reentry into practice. Types of programs include diversion programs associated with the state board of nursing, which allow nurses to maintain their licenses and practice while being monitored through recovery, state nurses' association peer assistance programs, and employee assistance programs.

The prevalence of chemical dependence among nurses is unknown. A number of contributing factors have been identified, including the caretaker mentality, which is a characteristic of codependency. Nurses with addictive problems frequently operate with a number of false perceptions and beliefs, such as taking drugs solves problems, or knowledge of drugs provides immunity to drug problems.

Nurses frequently lack the knowledge and understanding of addiction and the ability to recognize early behavioral clues. Nursing education may not adequately provide knowledge of prevention strategies, interventions, advances in research and treatment, or the skills needed to work with patients (or co-workers) with substance abuse problems. Many nurses' working knowledge is based on public stereotypes and clinical experiences with difficult alcohol and drug abusers.

Signs and symptoms of chemical dependence related to work performance may be apparent by changes in personality and behavior, job performance, and attendance. Nurses often *enable* chemical dependence to continue among coworkers by covering their mistakes or tardiness, excusing another nurse's behavior, repeatedly helping someone complete an assignment, or simply ignoring obvious signs and

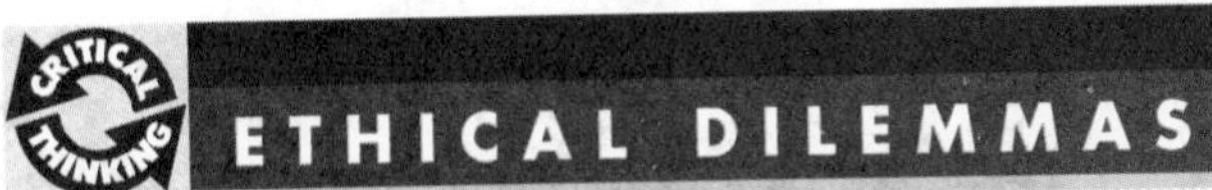

IMPAIRED PROVIDERS

Situation The nurses in the geriatric unit know that one of their colleagues has undergone treatment for prescription drug addiction. She seemed to be doing well until recently when she has been totally focused on her marital separation and subsequent divorce. Her colleagues suspect that she is using drugs again and worry that it will affect her patients' care. How should they handle this situation?

Discussion These nurses have responsibilities to their patients, colleagues, and profession. Knowing their colleague's history of drug problems, they have been especially concerned about her. Reporting her to the administration may cost her job and license. However, her patients may be endangered by her carelessness and inability to function in a crisis. If the nurses agree not to report her, they would be in collusion with her and might be held legally liable for any harm she causes to patients. These nurses will also be damaging the profession by putting a colleague's interests before their duty to their patients. These nurses have the responsibility of confronting their colleague personally, as well as reporting her to the state board of nursing. They can help by getting her the assistance she needs, not be covering for her and hoping that she will not harm patients.

ETHICAL AND LEGAL PRINCIPLES

- In cases of impaired nurses, whistle-blowing is protected under most state boards of nursing. Anonymous contacts with the board may be possible, especially if the reporting nurse is concerned about retaliation.
- Nurses have a duty to be loyal to their colleagues. However, they also have a professional obligation to protect the safety of patients who might be adversely affected by the incompetence of any health care professional.
- Nonmaleficence, not doing harm and protecting from harm, is a primary ethical principle. According to the American Nurses' Association Code, one's primary loyalty is to patients.

CRITICAL THINKING EXERCISES

CASE STUDY

COCAINE TOXICITY

Patient Profile

Mr. C. is a 34-year-old man who was admitted to the emergency department with chest pain, tachycardia, dizziness, nausea, and severe migrainelike headache.

Subjective Data

- Is extremely nervous and irritable
- Thinks he is having a heart attack
- Admits that he was at a party earlier in the evening drinking alcohol, smoking pot, and snorting cocaine
- Noted a change in personality including irritability and restlessness
- Experienced an increased need for cocaine in the past few months

Objective Data

Physical Examination

- Appears pale and diaphoretic
- Has tremors
- BP 210/110, pulse 100 bpm, respiratory rate 30/minute

Critical Thinking Questions

1. What other information is needed to assess Mr. C.'s condition?
2. How should questions regarding these areas be addressed?
3. What other clues should the nurse be alert for in assessing his drug use?
4. What emergency conditions need to be carefully monitored?
5. What nursing interventions are appropriate?
6. What is the best way to approach Mr. C. to engage him in a treatment program?
7. Based on the assessment data presented, write one or more nursing diagnoses. Are there any collaborative problems?

symptoms (see the Ethical Dilemmas box on p. 173). Helping chemically dependent nurses requires sharing observations and concerns with the nurse and supervisor to provide the means for rehabilitation. Caring about the nurse who is in trouble because of drug and alcohol abuse may be a painful process for the co-worker. It involves self-awareness, confrontation, patience, support, and belief in the nurse's recovery. The nurse who has travelled the road to recovery and regained control can offer insight to other nurses and hope for those whose lives and health have been affected by unhealthy patterns of drug and alcohol use.

REVIEW QUESTIONS

The number of the question corresponds to the same-numbered objective at the beginning of the chapter.

1. The disease model of addiction directs the nurse to
   a. recognize related illnesses.
   b. assess emotional problems.
   c. support traditions, values, and beliefs.
   d. assess stigma of "addict" label.

2. A pattern of abnormal or pathologic use resulting in physical, emotional, or social impairment is known as
   a. abuse.
   b. dependence.
   c. tolerance.
   d. loss of control.

3. One of the most compelling reasons leading to continued drug use is
   a. poor body image.
   b. powerful immediate gratification.
   c. family dysfunction.
   d. poor social skills.

4. Interruptions in the addictive cycle after the development of tolerance generally precipitate
   a. loss of control.
   b. decreased tolerance.
   c. withdrawal symptoms.
   d. no change in condition.

5. A withdrawal syndrome that is characterized by stomach cramps, diaphoresis, goose flesh, rhinorrhea, anxiety, and restlessness is associated with dependence on

a. stimulants.
b. alcohol.
c. narcotics.
d. cannabis.

6. Pain management of patients with drug-related problems requires the nurse to

a. thoroughly assess pain.
b. induce withdrawal.
c. avoid narcotics.
d. provide patient-controlled analgesia.

7. The key to an initial effective nursing intervention in case management of a patient with problems associated with drug use is

a. offering education on addiction.
b. providing a quiet, nonstimulating atmosphere.
c. carrying out an accurate nonjudgmental assessment.
d. assisting with reality orientation.

8. Secondary prevention activities are aimed at

a. early identification and intervention in a health problem.
b. collective action to influence social policy and develop social responsibility.
c. control and monitoring of addicted persons.
d. prevention of relapse for recovering persons.

9. The nurse's assessment of personal patterns of drug use is a health promotion strategy that supports the nurse's role as

a. educator.
b. resource.
c. case finder.
d. change agent.

10. A nursing diagnosis that represents a biologic response and that is frequently used with the addicted patient is

a. self-care deficit.
b. ineffective denial.
c. social isolation.
d. fear.

11. The trauma patient, particularly one with violent crime-related injuries, should be assessed for use of which of these?

a. Cannabis
b. Cocaine
c. LSD
d. Codeine

12. Which statement is true about older adults?

a. Older adults consume more alcohol than younger adults.
b. Older adults experience a less severe alcohol withdrawal than do younger adults.
c. Older adults have the highest use of over-the-counter drugs of all age groups.
d. Older adults seldom experience cognitive impairment with alcohol abuse.

13. Factors contributing to chemical dependence among nurses include all of the following *except*

a. caretaker mentality.
b. belief that drugs solve problems.
c. lack of knowledge of addiction.
d. recognition of early behavioral clues.

REFERENCES

1. Hareford T: Overview of epidemiology with applications to alcohol research, NIAAA, *Alcohol World Health and Res* 16:177, 1992.
2. Frances R, Miller S, editors: *Clinical textbook of addictive disorders,* New York, 1991, Guilford Press.
3. Tweed S: Identifying the alcoholic patient. In Zerwekh J, editor: Nursing interventions for addicted patients, *Nurs Clin North Am* 24:13, 1989.
4. Adams W and others: Alcoholic-related hospitalizations of elderly people, *JAMA* 270:1222, 1993.
5. Haverkos J and others: Complications of drug misuse, *Curr Opin Psychiatry* 4:454, 1991.
6. People with disabilities are at high risk for alcohol and other drug problems, *Addictions Nursing Network* 3:79, 1991.
7. National Medical Expenditure Survey, Centers for Disease Control, 1993.
8. Ray O, Ksir C: *Drugs, society, and human behavior,* ed 5, St Louis, 1990, Mosby.
9. Schuckit MA: *Drug and alcohol abuse: a clinical guide to diagnosis and treatment,* ed 3, New York, 1989, Plenum Publishing.
10. Kloner RA and others: The effects of acute and chronic cocaine use in the heart, *Circulation* 85:407, 1992.
11. Verderber A, Fitzsimmons L, Shively M: Cocaine abuse, *J Cardiovas Nurs* 6:43, 1992.
12. Neuspiel DR and others: Maternal cocaine use and infant behavior, *Neurotoxicol Teratol* 13:229, 1992.
13. Lynch M, McKeon VA: Cocaine use during pregnancy: research findings and clinical implications, *J Obstet Gynecol Neonatal Nurs* 19:285, 1990.
14. Rogers EJ: Postanesthesia care of the cocaine abuser, *Post Anesth Nurs* 6:102, 1991.
15. Arria A, Van Thiel D: The epidemiology of alcohol-related chronic disease, NIAAA, *Alcohol World Health and Res* 16:209, 1992.
16. Sawyers-Sommer M: Alcohol intoxication and multiple trauma: A catastrophic combination, *Med-Surg Q* 1:1, 1992.
17. Compton M: Nursing care in acute intoxication. In Naegle M, editor: *Substance Abuse Education in Nursing,* NLN New York, 1991, Pub No. 15-2463.
18. Nilssen O, Cone H: Screening patients for alcohol problems in primary health care settings, *Alcohol Health World* 18:136, 1994.
19. Tucker C: Adult pain and substance abuse in surgical patients, *J Neurosci Nurs,* 22:339, 1990.
20. Rassool GH: Nursing and substance misuse: responding to the challenge, *J Adv Nurs* 18:1401, 1993.
21. Allen K: Current morale issues that impede the caregiving process of substance abuse/addictions nurses, *Issues in Mental Health Nurs* 14:293, 1993.
22. Beebe GC: Efficacy of a substance abuse primary prevention skills conference for nurses, *J Contin Ed Nurs* 23:231, 1992.
23. Weinman SA: Emergency management of drug overdose, *Crit Care Nurs* 13:45, 1993.
24. Soloway RA: Street-smart advice on treating drug overdoses, *Am J Nurs,* 93:9, 1993.
25. McCaffery M, Vourakis C: Assessment and relief of pain in chemically dependent patients, *Orthop Nurs* 11:13, 1992.

26. Walsh JH: The substance-abusing family: consideration for nursing research, *J Pediatr Nurs* 6:49, 1991.
27. Adams W and others: Alcohol-related hospitalizations of elderly people, *JAMA* 270:1222, 1993.
28. Mathwig G, D'Arcangelo J: Drug misuse and dependence in the elderly, Naegle M, editor: *Substance abuse education in nursing*, vol. II, National League for Nursing, Pub. No. 15-2463, 1992.
29. Willenbring ML: Organic mental disorders associated with heavy drinking and alcohol dependence, *Clin Geriatr Med* 4:882, 1988.
30. Wheeler B: Addressing substance abuse within nursing, *J Nurs Adm* 22:8, 1992.

SECTION I BIBLIOGRAPHY

Books

Alfaro R: *Applying nursing diagnosis and nursing process*, ed 2, Philadelphia, 1990, JB Lippincott.

Barnfather JS, Lyon BL, editors: *Stress and coping: State of the science and implications for nursing theory, research, and practice*, Indianapolis, 1993, Sigma Theta Tau Center Press.

Burrell L, editor: *Adult nursing in hospital and community settings*, Norwalk, CT, 1992, Appleton and Lange.

Carnevalie DL, Patrick M: *Nursing management for the elderly*, ed 3, Philadelphia, 1993, JB Lippincott.

Carpentino L: *Nursing diagnosis: application to clinical practice*, ed 5, Philadelphia, 1993, JB Lippincott.

Chentiz WC, Stone JT, Salisbury SA: *Clinical gerontological nursing*, Philadelphia, 1991, WB Saunders.

Ebersole P, Hess P, editors: *Toward healthy aging: human needs and nursing response*, St Louis, 1994, Mosby.

Eliopoulos C: *Gerontological nursing*, ed 3, Philadelphia, 1993, JB Lippincott.

Eliopoulos C: *Health assessment of the older adult*, ed 2, Redwood City, CA, 1990, Addison-Wesley.

Goldberger L, Breznitz S, editors: *Handbook of stress: Theoretical and clinical aspects*, New York, 1993, Free Press.

Gordon M, editor: *Nursing diagnosis: process and application*, ed 3, New York, 1994, McGraw-Hill.

Grimes J, Burns E: *Health assessment in nursing practice*, ed 3, Boston, 1992, Jones & Bartlett.

Hellman S, Hellman LH: *Medicare and medigaps*, Newberry Park, CA, 1991, Sage.

Kinny J: *Clinical manual of substance abuse*, Philadelphia, 1991, Mosby.

Lazarus RS: *Emotion and adaptation*, New York, 1991, Oxford University Press.

Lazarus RS, Folkman S: *Stress, appraisal, and coping*, New York, 1984, Springer Publishing.

Lubkin IM: *Chronic illness: impact and interventions*, Boston, 1990, Jones and Bartlett.

Malasanos L and others: *Health assessment*, ed 4, St. Louis, 1990, Mosby.

Maslow A: *Motivation and personality*, New York, 1954, Harper & Row.

Morton P: *Health assessment in nursing*, ed 2, Springhouse, PA, 1993, Springhouse Corp.

NIDA Research Monograph, Acute cocaine intoxication: current methods of treatment. In Sorer H, editor: NIDA Research Monograph 12, PHS, USDHHS Pub. No. 93-3498, 1993.

NIDA Research Monograph 102, Anabolic steroid abuse. In Lin G, Erinoff L, editors: USDHHS DHHS, Pub. No. 90-1720, 1990.

NIDA Research Monograph, Cardiovascular toxicity of cocaine: Underlying mechanisms. In Thadani P, editor: NIDA Research Monograph 108, PHS, USDHHS, Pub. No. 91-1767, 1991.

NIDA Research Monograph, Drugs of abuse: Chemistry, pharmacology, immunology, and AIDS. In Pham P, Rice K, editors: Research Monograph 96, USDHHS, Pub. No. 90-1676, 1990.

Parker V, Edmonds S, Robinson V: *A change for the better: how to make communities more responsive to older residents*, American Association of Retired Persons, 1991.

Pastalan LE: *Aging in place: the role of housing and support services*, New York, 1990, Haworth Press.

Plotnikoff N and others: *Stress and immunity*, Boca Raton, 1991, CRC Press.

Slaikey KA: *Crises intervention: a handbook for practice and research*, Boston, 1990, Allyn and Bacon.

Sundeen SJ, Stuart GW, Rankin E: *Nurse-client interaction: implementing the nursing process*, ed 5, St. Louis, 1994, Mosby.

Thompson JM, Bowers AC: *Health assessment: an illustrated pocket guide*, ed 4, St. Louis, 1992, Mosby.

US Senate Special Committee on Aging: Developments in aging: 1990, vol 1, Washington DC, US Government Printing Office, 1991.

Wykle ML, Kahana E, Kowal J, editors: *Stress and health among the elderly*, New York, 1992, Springer Publishing

Yurick AG and others: *The aged person and the nursing process*, ed 3, East Norwalk, CT, 1990, Appleton-Century-Crofts.

Journals

Ade-Redder L, Kaplan L: Marriage, spousal caregiving, and a husband's move to a nursing home, *J Gerontol Nurs* 10:13, 1993.

Algase DL: A century of progress: today's strategies for responding to wandering behavior, *J Gerontol Nurs* 11:28, 1992.

Ali NS: Promoting safe use of multiple medications by elderly persons, *Geriat Nurs* 13:157, 1992.

American Nurse Hypnotherapy Association Quarterly Report. Pain and suffering are not synonymous: It is important that both be addressed, *Transcending* 1:4, 1992.

Baldwin B: Family caregiving: trends and forecasts, *Geriat Nurs* 11:172, 1990.

*Bennett SJ: Relationships among selected antecedent variables and coping effectiveness in postmyocardial infarction patients, *Res Nurs Health* 16:131, 1993.

Bezon J: Approaching drug regimens with a therapeutic dose of suspicion, *Geriat Nurs* 7:180, 1991.

Biggs AG: Family caregiver versus nursing assessments of elderly self-care abilities, *J Gerontol Nurs* 16:11, 1990.

Boult C and others: Chronic conditions that lead to functional limitations in the elderly, *J Gerontol: Medical Services* 49:M28, 1994.

Bowman AM: Relationship of anxiety to development of postoperative delirium, *J Gerontol Nurs* 18:24, 1992.

Cassetta RA: RN's fight for recognition of women's health issues, *Am Nurse* 2:1, 1994.

Chrischilles EA, Wallace RB: Nonsteroidal antiinflammatory drugs and blood pressure in an elderly population, *J Gerontol: Medical Sciences* 48:M91, 1993.

*Craft MJ and others: Behavioral responses of family members during critical illness, *Clin Nurs Res* 2:414, 1993.

*D'Avanzo CE, Frye B, Froman R: Stress in Cambodian refugee families, *Image* 26:101, 1994.

Davidhizar R: Understanding powerlessness in family member caregivers of the chronically ill, *Geriat Nurs* 3:66, 1992.

Davidhizar R, Schearer R: Humor: no geriatric nurse should be without it, *Geriat Nurs* 9:276, 1992.

Dubiel D: Action stat! Cocaine overdose, *Nursing* 20:33, 1990.

Ettinger NA, Albin RJ: A review of the respiratory effects of smoking cocaine, *Am J Med* 87:664, 1989.

Fletcher K: Restraints should be a last resort, *RN* 53:52, 1990.

Foreman MD, Grabowski R: Diagnostic dilemma: cognitive impairment in the elderly, *J Gerontol Nurs* 18:5, 1992.

Gordis E: Children of alcoholics: are they different? *Alcohol Alert* 9, PH 228, NIAAA, July, 1990.

Gordis E: The genetics of alcoholism, *Alcohol Alert* 18, PH 328, Oct, 1992.

Gould MT: Nursing home elderly: social-environmental factors, *J Gerontol Nurs* 8:13, 1992.

Griffin MM: Caring for caregivers: a nursing role in a corporate setting, *Geriat Nurs* 7:200, 1993.

Hahn K, Wietor G: Helpful tools for medication screening, *Geriat Nurs* 13:160, 1992.

Haight BL: Putting OBRA into practice, *J Gerontol Nurs* 10:43, 1992.

Hallal JC: Back pain with postmenopausal osteoporosis and vertebral fractures, *Geriat Nurs* 12:285, 1991.

Hawranik PA: Clinical possibility: preventing health problems after the age of 65, *J Gerontol Nurs* 17:201, 1991.

*Heidrich SM: The relationship between physical health and psychological well-being in elderly women: a developmental perspective, *Res Nurs Health* 16:123, 1993.

Heine C: Community issues on the holistic care of the elderly, *Holistic Nurs Pract* 7:53, 1992.

Herbert TB, Cohen S: Stress and immunity in humans: A meta-analytic review, *Psychosom Med,* 55:364, 1993.

*Hines-Martin VP: A research review: family caregivers of the chronically ill-African-American elderly, *J Gerontol Nurs* 18:25, 1992.

Huggins B: Trauma physiology, *Nurs Clin North Am* 25:1, 1990.

*Hunter S: Adult day care: promoting quality of life for the elderly, *J Gerontol Nurs* 18:17, 1992.

Imm A, Carlson RW: Fluid resuscitation in circulatory shock, *Crit Care Clin* 9:313, 1993.

Johnson JE: Health-care practices of the rural aged, *J Gerontol Nurs* 17:15, 1991.

Kane RL: The implications of assessment, *J Gerontol* 48:27, 1993.

*Lowery BJ: Psychological stress, denial and myocardial infarction outcomes, *Image* 23:51, 1991.

Lund M: Conflicts in ethics–is giving pain relief always right? *Geriat Nur* 3:83, 1990.

McCaffery M, Vourakis C: Assessment and relief of pain in chemically dependent patients, *Orthop Nurs* 11:12, 1992.

Miller C: When medication harms as well as helps, *Geriat Nurs* 11:30, 1990.

*Miller P and others: Stressors and stress management 1 month after myocardial infarction, *Rehabil Nurs,* 15:306, 1990.

*Mishel MH, Sorenson D: Revision of the Ways of Coping Checklist for a clinical population, *West J Nurs Res* 15:59, 1993.

More JF, Johnson JE: Over-the-counter drug use by the rural elderly, *Geriat Nurs* 7:190, 1993.

*Moss MS and others: Time use of caregivers of impaired elders before and after institutionalization, *J Gerontol* 48:S102, 1993.

O'Leary A: Stress, emotion, and human function, *Psychol Bull* 108:363, 1990.

Palmieri DT: Adverse effects of medications in the elderly, *J Gerontol Nurs* 17:32, 1991.

Pfister-Menoque K: Embracing patient compliance: a guide for nurses, *Geriat Nurs* 5:124, 1993.

Roberto KA and others: Provider/client views: health-care needs of the rural elderly, *J Gerontol Nurs* 18:31, 1992.

Roberts BL, Dunkle R, Haug M: Physical, psychological, and social resources as moderators of the relationship of stress to mental health of the very old, *J Gerontol:* Social Sciences 49:535, 1994.

Roberts SS: A marker gene for alcoholism? *J NIH Res* 2:25, 1990.

Robinson L: Stress and anxiety, *Nurs Clin North Am* 25:935, 1990.

Schank MJ, Lough MA: Profile: frail elderly women maintaining independence, *J Adv Nurs* 15:674, 1990.

*Schirm V, Fennel S: Nurse empathy to caregivers of chronically ill elders, *J Gerontol Nurs* 17:18, 1991.

Schoemick L, Katz P, Beam T: The many guises of infection, *Geriat Nurs* 9:223, 1991.

Shauler C and others: Clinical considerations: surrogate decision making for hospitalized elders, *J Gerontol Nurs* 6:5, 1992.

Smart R, Mann R: Alcohol and the epidemiology of liver cirrhosis, NIAAA, *Alcohol World Health and Research* 16:217, 1992.

*Smits MW, Kee CC: Correlates of self-care among the independent elderly, *J Gerontol Nurs* 9:13, 1992.

Strong V, Newfeld A: Adult day care programs, a source for respite, *J Gerontol Nurs* 16:16, 1990.

Tappen RM, Beckerman A: Multiproblem older adults in acute care, *J Gerontol Nurs* 11:38, 1993.

*Thebodeau J: Caring for a parent: a phenomenologic inquiry, *Nurs Outlook* 41:15, 1993.

Theis SL: Using previous knowledge to teach elderly clients, *J Gerontol Nurs* 17:34, 1991.

Vortherms RC: Clinically improving communication through touch, *J Gerontol Nurs* 17:6, 1991.

*Weinrick SP, Boyd M: Education in the elderly: adapting and evaluating teaching tools, *J Gerontol Nurs* 18:15, 1992.

Wilson EB and others: Take a fresh look at discharge planning, *Geriat Nurs* 1:23, 1991.

*Younger JB: Development and testing of the mastery of stress instrument, *Nurs Res,* 42:68, 1993.

*Nursing research-based articles.

Organizations

Alcohol, Drug Abuse, and Mental Health Administration
Public Health Service
5600 Fishers Lane
Rockville, MD 20857

Alcoholics Anonymous
General Service Office
Grand Central Station
Box 459
New York, NY 10164-0459

American Red Cross
National Headquarters
17 and D Streets, NW
Washington, DC 20006

American Society of Pain Management Nurses
11512 Allecingie Parkway
Richmond, VA 23235
804-378-0072
FAX: 804-379-1386

Cocaine Anonymous World Services
3740 Overland Avenue, Suite G
Los Angeles, CA 90034

Cocaine/Crack Action Helpline
1-800-888-9383

Crack Abuse 24-Hour Hotline
1-800-444-9999

Drug and Alcohol Nursing Association, Inc.
660 Lonely Cottage Drive
Upper Black Eddy, PA 18972-9313
610-847-5396
FAX: 610-847-5063

Drugs Anonymous
P.O. Box 473
Ansonia Station
New York, NY 10023

Institute of Addiction Awareness
31878 Del Obispo #118, Suite 433
San Juan Capistrano, CA 92675
Phone/FAX: 714-830-4866

National Consortium of Chemical Dependency Nurses
1720 Willow Creek Circle, Suite 519
Eugene, OR 97402
800-876-2236
FAX: 503-485-7372

National Council on Alcoholism
12 West 21st Street
New York, NY 10010

National Gerontological Nursing Association
7250 Parkway Drive, Suite 510
Hanover, MD 21076
800-723-0560

National Nurses Society on Addictions
5700 Old Orchard Road, First floor
Skokie, IL 60077

North American Nursing Diagnosis Association
1211 Locust Street
Philadelphia, PA 19107
215-545-8105
800-647-9002
FAX: 215-545-8107

AHCPR Guidelines

Guides developed and published by The Agency for Health Care Policy and Research (AHCPR). The Patient Guides are available in English and Spanish. The guidelines can be obtained by writing to: Center for Research Dissemination and Liaison, AHCPR Clearinghouse, P.O. Box 8547, Silver Spring, MD 20907, or by calling 1-800-358-9295. The Guidelines are as follows:

Acute pain management: operative or medical procedures and trauma. Clinical Practice Guideline. AHCPR Pub. No. 92-0032.

Acute pain management in adults: operative procedures. Quick Reference Guide for Clinicians. AHCPR Pub. No. 92-0019.

Pathologic Mechanisms of Diseases

Section Two

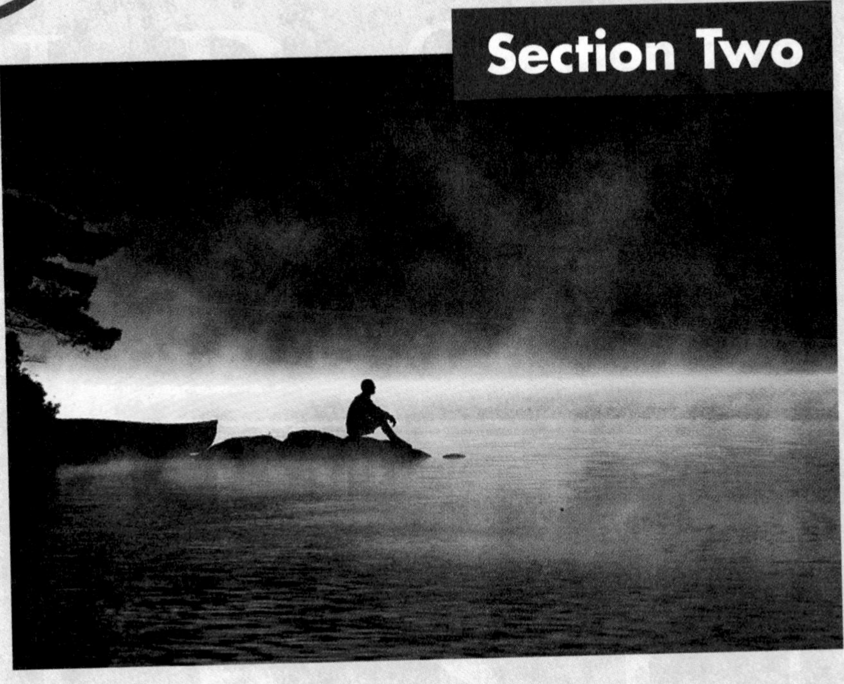

Chapter 9

NURSING ROLE IN MANAGEMENT

Cell Injury and Inflammation

Sharon L. Lewis

Learning Objectives

1. Describe the structures and functions of the normal cell.
2. Explain the cellular adaptive mechanisms to sublethal injury.
3. Describe the causes and mechanisms of lethal cell injury.
4. Differentiate among types of cell necrosis.
5. Describe the components and functions of the mononuclear phagocyte system.
6. Describe the inflammatory response, including vascular and cellular responses and exudate formation.
7. Explain local and systemic manifestations of inflammation and their physiologic bases.
8. Differentiate among healing by primary, secondary, and tertiary intention.
9. Describe the factors that delay wound healing and common complications of wound healing.
10. Describe the pharmacologic, dietary, and nursing management of inflammation.

The major work of the body occurs at the cellular level in the form of chemical reactions. Each cell has a specific function and, together with other cells, makes up body tissues, organs, and systems. Cellular reactions synthesize new products for growth and energy and break down used products. Understanding the structure and function of an individual cell is necessary to comprehend the functioning of body tissues, organs, and systems.

The cell's response to adverse conditions depends on its ability to adapt to these changes. Adaptations include responses such as atrophy, hypertrophy, degeneration, inflammation, regeneration, and repair. When the cell fails to adapt, it undergoes a series of changes that can result in cell death (necrosis) and eventually tissue death.

THE HUMAN CELL

Cell Structure

The cell is the basic unit of structure in any living organism (Fig. 9-1). Each cell is surrounded by a semipermeable plasma membrane. The two basic parts of a cell are the cytoplasm and the nucleus.

Cytoplasm. Cytoplasm is composed of viscous protoplasm, which consists of water, protein, lipid, carbohydrate, and inorganic solutes. *Organelles* located within the cytoplasm perform cellular functions, which are shown in Table 9-1.

Nucleus. A nucleus is present in all cells that can divide and consists mainly of *chromosomes.* (The tangled threads of chromosomes found when the cell is not actively dividing are called *chromatin.*) There are 23 pairs of chromosomes in human somatic cells. The basic unit of the chromosome is the *gene. Deoxyribonucleic acid* (DNA) is the building block of the gene. The sequence of nucleotides of the large, complex DNA molecule is the genetic information, which is the hereditary unit of the cell. DNA also directs the synthesis of specific proteins by the cell (Fig. 9-2), thus determining its special characteristics.

Ribonucleic acid (RNA) is also found in the nucleus. It transmits the information from DNA in the nucleus to ribosomes in the cytoplasm. Ribosomes are the site of protein synthesis of the cell. The protein products may be used for cellular metabolism (e.g., enzymes) or secreted for use in other parts of the body (e.g., insulin).

Cellular Functions

The basic functions of cells include the following:

1. *Transport of metabolites:* Transport of metabolites is the movement of substances such as electrolytes across the cell membrane actively or passively or with the assistance of a carrier.

2. *Metabolism:* The two phases of metabolism are *anabolism* and *catabolism.* Both occur within the cells. In

Reviewed by Donna McCarthy, RN, PhD, Associate Professor, School of Nursing, University of Wisconsin, Madison, WI.

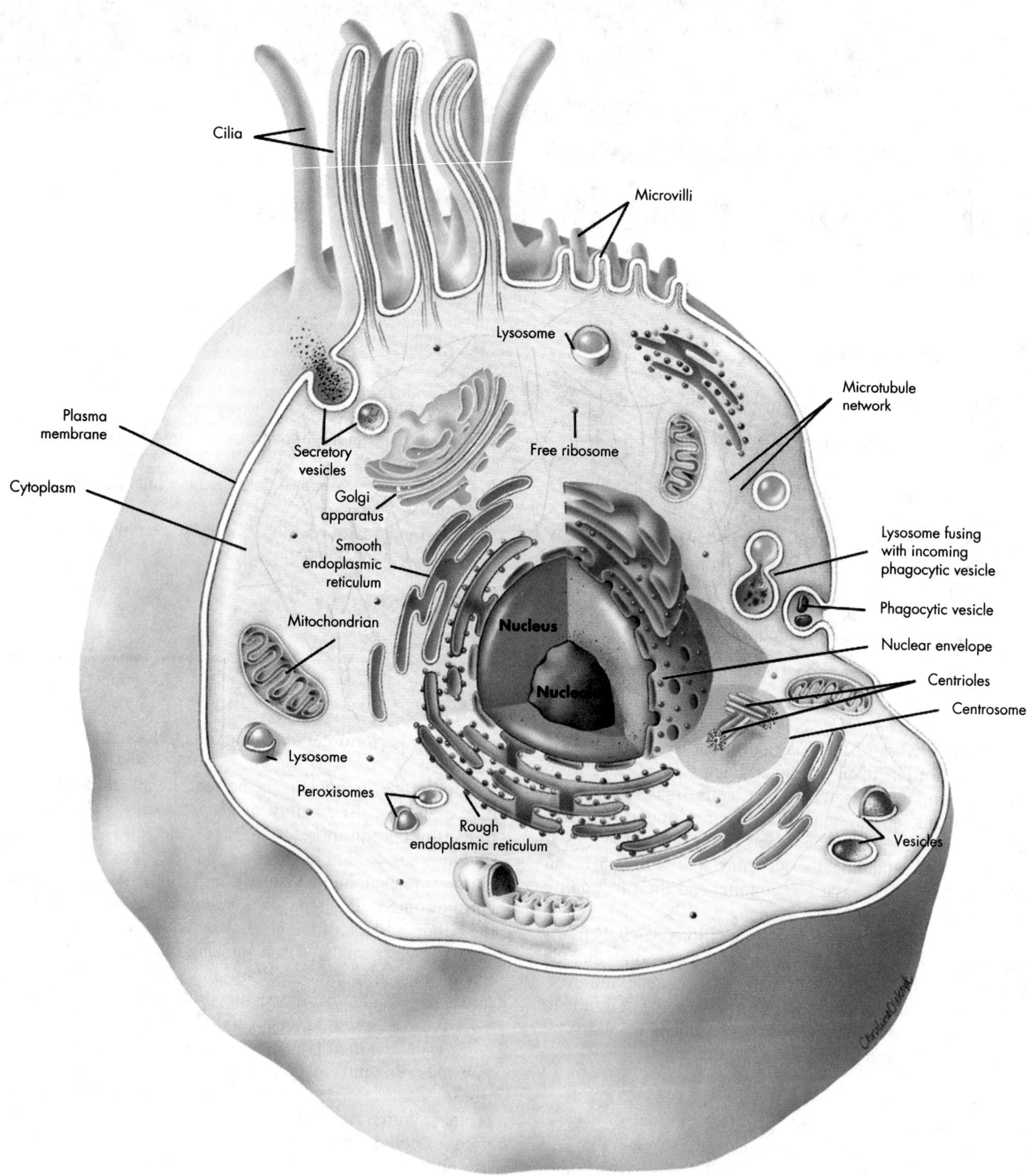

Fig. 9-1 Human cell and organelles.

the *anabolic phase,* simpler compounds are converted into larger compounds (e.g., amino acids into proteins). In the *catabolic phase* these larger compounds are broken down into simpler compounds and the energy necessary for cell function is obtained.

3. *Movement:* Many body cells, especially muscle cells, work together in a coordinated manner to permit body movement.

4. *Conduction:* Conduction is transmission of a stimulus from one part of the body to another. Transmission of a

Table 9-1 Composition and Function of Cell Organelles

Organelle	Composition	Function
▪ Nucleus	DNA	Control system of cell, site of cellular reproduction
	RNA	Site for RNA synthesis
	Nucleolus	Transmittal of information to ribosomes
▪ Endoplasmic reticulum*	Network of tubular structures	Communication between nucleus cytoplasm, cell membrane; lipid and steroid synthesis; bile conjugation; detoxification of unnecessary cell substances; protein synthesis
▪ Ribosomes	Granules of RNA held together by protein, which may merge into clumps (polyribosomes)	Protein synthesis
▪ Golgi complex	Flattened collection of tubules and vesicles	Packaging of proteins (hormones and enzymes) that are stored as secretion granules for later release from cell, packaging of newly synthesized lipids
▪ Mitochondria	Layered cristae (folds) formed into small, oval bodies	Powerhouse of cell, production of ATP, cellular respiration
▪ Lysosome	Membrane-surrounded sac containing enzymes	Release of hydrolytic enzymes on contact with phagocytized material to degrade it
▪ Centrosome	Pair of centrioles	Spindle formation during cell division

ATP, Adenosine triphosphate; *DNA*, deoxyribonucleic acid; *RNA*, ribonucleic acid.
*Includes smooth endoplasmic reticulum (SER), or agranular, and rough endoplasmic reticulum (RER), or granular.

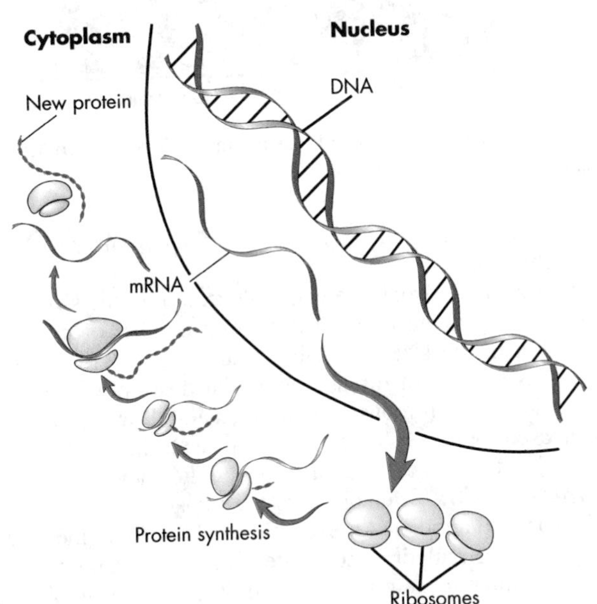

Fig. 9-2 Protein synthesis directed by DNA. Messenger RNA (mRNA) transmits message from DNA to ribosomes in cytoplasm where proteins are synthesized.

nerve impulse through nerve and muscle cells and passage of heat and sound waves through parts of the body are examples of conduction.

5. *Absorption:* Absorption is the movement of a substance through a cell membrane. An example is glucose absorption by the lining cells of the gastrointestinal (GI) tract.

6. *Body protection:* Certain cells of the body, such as the epithelial cells of the epidermis, protect the body against injury from penetration or abrasion. Other cells, such as white blood cells (WBCs), protect the body against invading agents by means of the inflammatory and immune responses.

7. *Reproduction:* New cells are necessary for replacement of aged cells and for growth of the body. *Mitosis* (cell division) is the process by which cells replace themselves. Some cells, such as neurons and muscle cells, are not capable of mitosis.

TISSUE TYPES

Cells similar in structure and function are organized to form tissues. The four types of tissue are epithelial, connective, muscular, and nervous. Table 9-2 presents examples of the various tissue types and their regenerative ability.

CELL INJURY

Cell injury can be sublethal or lethal. *Sublethal* injury alters function without causing cell death. The changes caused by

Table 9-2 Major Tissue Types

Tissue Type	Regenerative Ability
Epithelial	
Skin, linings of blood vessels, mucous membranes	Cells readily divide and regenerate
Connective Tissue	
Bone	Active tissue heals rapidly
Cartilage	Regeneration possible but slow
Tendons and ligaments	Regeneration possible but slow
Blood	Cells actively regenerate
Muscle	
Smooth	Regeneration usually possible (particularly in GI tract)
Cardiac	Damaged muscle replaced by connective tissue
Skeletal	Connective tissue replaces severely damaged muscle; some regeneration in moderately damaged muscle occurs
Nerve	
Neuron	Cells do not divide; cells regenerate only if cell body not injured
Glial	Cells regenerate; scar tissue often formed when neurons are damaged.

GI, Gastrointestinal.

this type of injury are potentially reversible if the injurious stimulus is removed. *Lethal* injury is an irreversible process that causes cell death.

Cell Adaptation to Sublethal Injury

Cell adaptations to sublethal injuries are common and are part of many physiologic and disease processes. For example, prolonged exposure to sunlight stimulates melanin production and thus provides protection of deeper skin layers by tanning the skin. Lack of muscular activity can lead to atrophy and decreased muscle tone. Adaptive processes of the cell include hypertrophy, hyperplasia, atrophy, and metaplasia (Fig. 9-3). Other responses that are considered maladaptive are dysplasia and anaplasia.

Hypertrophy. Hypertrophy refers to an increase in the size of cells without cell division. For example, a pregnant uterus enlarges from hormonal stimulation. The heart of a person with severe hypertension enlarges to compensate for the increased resistance to its pumping action. Muscle hypertrophy results from an increase in the size of muscle fibers as would occur in an individual who does weight training.

Hyperplasia. Hyperplasia refers to the actual increase in the number of cells. This process is reversible when the stimulus is removed. The female breast experiences hyperplasia during lactation. Hyperplasia of the liver may replace damaged liver tissue.

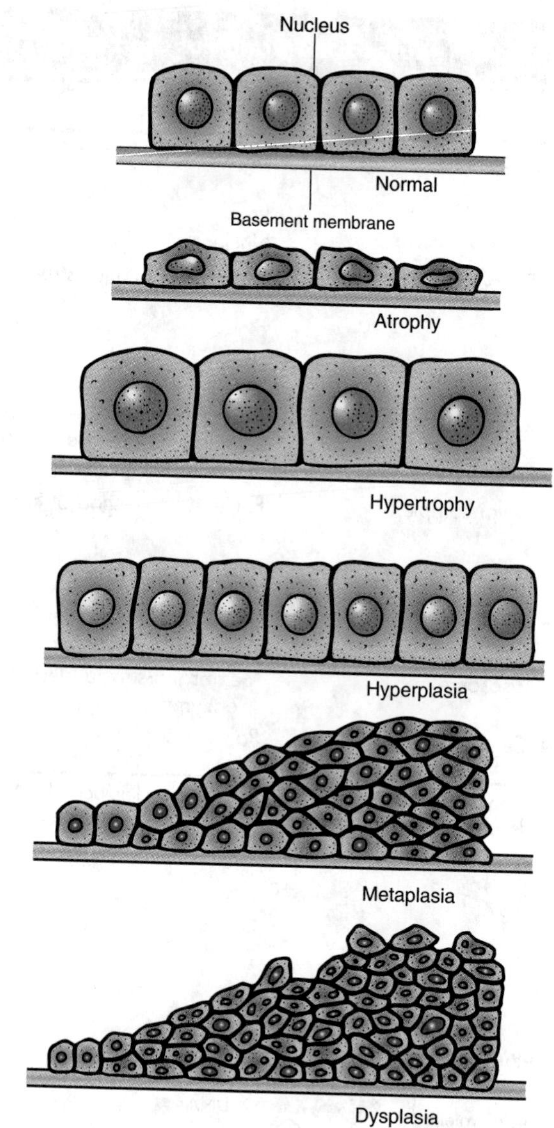

Fig. 9-3 Adaptive alterations in simple cuboidal epithelial cells.

Atrophy. Atrophy refers to a decrease in the size of a tissue or organ caused by a decreased number of cells or reduction in the size of the individual cells. It frequently occurs as a result of disease (muscular dystrophy), lack of blood supply (thrombus formation), natural aging process (decreased breast size after menopause), inactivity (decreased muscle size), and nutritional deficiency.

Metaplasia. Metaplasia is the transformation of one cell type into another. An example of physiologic metaplasia is when circulating monocytes change to macrophages as they migrate into inflamed tissues. An example of pathophysiologic metaplasia is when the normal pseudostratified columnar epithelium of the bronchi changes to squamous epithelium in response to chronic cigarette smoking.

Table 9-3 Causes of Lethal Cell Injury

Cause	Effect on Cell
Physical agents	
▪ Heat	Denaturation of protein, acceleration of metabolic reactions
▪ Cold	Decreased blood flow from vasoconstriction, slowed metabolic reactions, thrombosis of blood vessels, freezing of cell content that forms crystals and can burst cell
▪ Radiation	Alteration of cell structure and activity, alteration of enzyme systems, mutations
▪ Electrothermal injury	Interruption of neural conduction, fibrillation of cardiac muscle, coagulative necrosis of skin and skeletal muscle
▪ Mechanical trauma	Transfer of excess kinetic energy to cells causing rupture of cells, blood vessels, tissue; examples include: *Abrasion:* scraping of skin or mucous membrane *Laceration:* severing of vessels and tissue *Contusion (bruise):* crushing of tissue cells causing hemorrhage into skin *Puncture:* piercing of body structure or organ *Incision:* surgical cutting
Chemical injury	Alteration of cell metabolism, interference with normal enzymatic action within cells
Microbial injury	
▪ Viruses	Taking over of cell metabolism and synthesis of new particles that may cause cell rupture, cumulative effect possibly producing clinical disease
▪ Bacteria*	Destruction of cell membrane or cell nucleus, production of lethal toxins
Ischemic injury	Compromised cell metabolism, acute or gradual cell death
Immunologic†	
▪ Antigen-antibody response	Release of substances (histamine, complement) that can injure and damage cells
▪ Autoimmune	Activation of complement, which destroys normal cells and produces inflammation
Neoplastic growth	Cell destruction from abnormal and uncontrolled cell growth
Normal substances (e.g. digestive enzymes, uric acid)	Release into abdomen causing peritonitis, crystallization of excess accumulation in joints and renal tissue

*Bacteria are commonly classified as gram-negative or gram-positive.
†See Chapter 10 for a more detailed discussion.

Dysplasia. Dysplasia is an abnormal differentiation of dividing cells resulting in changes in the size, shape, and appearance of the cells. Minor dysplasia is found in some areas of inflammation. Dysplasia is potentially reversible if the stimulus is removed. Frequently, dysplasia can be a precursor of malignancy as in cervical dysplasia.

Anaplasia. Anaplasia is cell differentiation to a more immature or embryonic form. Malignant tumors are often characterized by anaplastic cell growth.

Causes of Lethal Cell Injury

Many different agents and factors can cause lethal cell injury (Table 9-3). The mechanism of actual cell death varies. Examples include deterioration of the nucleus, such as *pyknosis* (nuclear condensation and shrinking) and *karyolysis* (dissolution of nucleus and contents), disruption of cell metabolism, and rupture of the cell membrane.

Microbial invasion frequently, but not always, results in cell injury and death. Infection occurs when *pathogens* (microorganisms capable of producing disease) invade and multiply in body tissues. (Common viruses and bacteria that cause diseases in humans are listed in Tables 9-4 and 9-5.) *Opportunistic* organisms are microorganisms that are not usually considered pathogens. However, they may cause infection if the resistance of the host is decreased from events such as immunosuppression, trauma, or illness.

Cell Necrosis

Necrosis is the death of cells within a living organism. Different types of necrosis tend to occur in different organs or tissues (Table 9-6).

DEFENSE AGAINST INJURY

To protect against injury and infection, the body has various defense mechanisms. These defense mechanisms are (1) the skin and mucous membranes, which is the first line of defense (see Chapter 19); (2) the mononuclear phagocyte system; (3) the inflammatory response; and (4) the immune system (see Chapter 10).

Table 9-4 Common Viruses Causing Disease

Type	Disease Caused
▪ Adenoviruses	Upper respiratory tract infection, pneumonia
▪ Arbovirus	Syndrome of fever, malaise, headache, myalgia; aseptic meningitis; encephalitis
▪ Coronavirus	Upper respiratory tract infection
▪ Coxsackie viruses A and B	Upper respiratory tract infection, gastroenteritis, acute myocarditis, aseptic meningitis
▪ Echoviruses	Upper respiratory tract infection, gastroenteritis, aseptic meningitis
▪ Hepatitis	
A	Viral hepatitis
B	Viral hepatitis
C	Viral hepatitis
▪ Herpesviruses	
Varicella-zoster	Chickenpox; shingles
Herpes simplex	
Type 1	Herpes labialis ("fever blisters"), genital herpes infection
Type 2	Genital herpes infection
Epstein-Barr	Mononucleosis, Burkitt's lymphoma (possibly)
Cytomegalovirus (CMV)	Pneumonia in immunosuppressed individuals, infectious mononucleosis-like syndrome
▪ Human immunodeficiency virus (HIV)	HIV infection, acquired immunodeficiency syndrome (AIDS)
▪ Influenza A, B, C	Upper respiratory tract infection
▪ Mumps	Parotitis, orchitis in postpubertal males
▪ Papovavirus	Warts
▪ Parainfluenza 1-4	Upper respiratory tract infection
▪ Parvovirus	Gastroenteritis
▪ Poliovirus	Poliomyelitis
▪ Pox viruses	Smallpox
▪ Reoviruses 1, 2, 3	Upper respiratory tract infection
▪ Respiratory syncytial virus	Gastroenteritis, respiratory tract infection
▪ Rhabdovirus	Rabies
▪ Rhinovirus	Upper respiratory tract infection, pneumonia
▪ Rotaviruses	Gastroenteritis
▪ Rubella	German measles
▪ Rubeola	Measles

Table 9-5 Common Bacteria Causing Disease

Type	Diseases Caused
▪ Clostridia	
C. tetani	Tetanus (lockjaw)
C. botulinum	Food poisoning with progressive muscle paralysis
▪ *Corynebacterium diphtheriae*	Diphtheria
▪ *Escherichia coli*	Urinary tract infections, peritonitis
▪ *Haemophilus* organisms	
H. influenzae	Nasopharyngitis, meningitis, pneumonia
H. pertussis	Whooping cough
▪ *Helicobacter pylori*	Peptic ulcers
▪ *Klebsiella-Enterobacter* organisms	Urinary tract infections, peritonitis, pneumonia
▪ *Legionella pneumophila*	Pneumonia (Legionnaire's disease)
▪ Mycobacteria	
M. tuberculosis	Tuberculosis
M. leprae	Leprosy (Hansen's disease)
▪ Neisseriae	
N. meningitidis	Meningococcemia, meningitis
N. gonorrhoeae	Gonorrhea, pelvic inflammatory disease
▪ *Proteus* species	Urinary tract infections, peritonitis
▪ *Pseudomonas aeruginosa*	Urinary tract infections, meningitis
▪ *Salmonella* species	
S. typhi	Typhoid fever
Other *Salmonella* organisms	Food poisoning, gastroenteritis
▪ *Shigella* species	Shigellosis, diarrhea with abdominal pain and fever (dysentery)
▪ *Staphylococcus aureus*	Skin infections, pneumonia, urinary tract infections, acute osteomyelitis, toxic shock syndrome
▪ Streptococci	
S. pyogenes (group A B-hemolytic streptococci)	Pharyngitis, scarlet fever, rheumatic fever, acute glomerulonephritis, erysipelas, pneumonia
S. pyogenes (group B B-hemolytic streptococci)	Urinary tract infections
S. pneumoniae	Pneumococcal pneumonia
S. viridans	Bacterial endocarditis
S. faecalis	Genitourinary infection, infection of surgical wounds
▪ *Treponema pallidum*	Syphilis

Table 9-6 Types of Necrosis

Type	Description
■ Coagulative necrosis	Necrotic cells maintain their outline. Lytic enzymes are somewhat inhibited. Proteins are denatured. Enzymes lose their function. Commonly caused by a lack of blood supply.
■ Liquefactive necrosis	Necrotic cells rapidly disappear as lytic enzymes digest tissues. This type commonly occurs in the brain where the supply of lytic enzymes is abundant.
■ Caseous necrosis	Necrotic cells disintegrate, but cell fragments remain for long periods of time. This type is called caseous (cheeselike) necrosis because of its crumbly appearance. It is frequently found in tuberculosis of the lung.
■ Gangrenous necrosis	Necrotic cells result from severe hypoxia and subsequent ischemic injury, which is common after impaired circulation in the lower legs. Dry gangrene refers to the dry, shriveled, darkened area (Fig. 9-4), and wet gangrene refers to the liquefied underlying necrotic tissue.

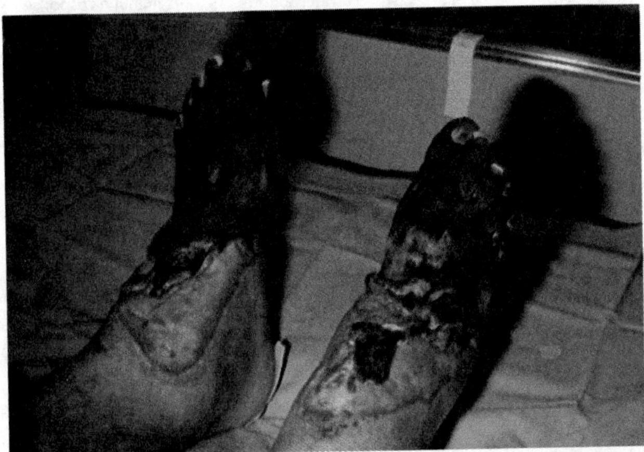

Fig. 9-4 Gangrene of the toes.

Table 9-7 Location and Name of Macrophages*

Location	Name
Connective tissue	Histiocytes
Liver	Kupffer cells
Lung	Alveolar macrophages
Spleen	Free and fixed macrophages
Bone marrow	Fixed macrophages
Lymph nodes	Free and fixed macrophages
Bone tissue	Osteoclasts
Central nervous system	Microglial cells
Peritoneal cavity	Peritoneal macrophages
Pleural cavity	Pleural macrophages
Skin	Histiocyte, Langerhans' cells
Synovium	Type A cells

*In addition, monocytes become macrophages once they leave the blood and enter the tissues.

Mononuclear Phagocyte System

The mononuclear phagocyte system (MPS) consists of monocytes and macrophages and their precursor cells. In the past, the MPS system was called the *reticuloendothelial system* (RES). However, it is not a body system with distinctly defined tissues and organs. Rather, it consists of phagocytic cells located in various tissues and organs (Table 9-7). The phagocytic cells are either *fixed* or *free* (mobile). The macrophages of the liver, spleen, bone marrow, lungs, and lymph nodes are fixed phagocytes. The monocytes (in blood) and the macrophages found in connective tissue, known as *histiocytes,* are mobile or wandering phagocytes.

Monocytes and macrophages originate in the bone marrow. Monocytes spend a few days in the blood and then enter tissues and change into macrophages. Tissue macrophages are larger and more phagocytic than monocytes.

The functions of the macrophage system include recognition and phagocytosis of foreign material such as microorganisms, removal of old or damaged cells from circulation, and participation in the immune response (see Chapter 10).

Inflammatory Response

The inflammatory response is a sequential reaction to cell injury. It neutralizes the inflammatory agent, removes necrotic materials, and establishes an environment suitable for healing and repair. The term *inflammation* is often but incorrectly used as a synonym for the term *infection.* Inflammation is always present with infection, but infection is not always present with inflammation. An infection involves invasion of tissues or cells by microorganisms such as bacteria, fungi, and viruses. In contrast, inflammation can also be caused by nonliving agents such as heat, radiation, and trauma (see Table 9-3). If infection is also present, it is from a superimposed invasion of microorganisms.

The mechanism of inflammation is basically the same regardless of the injuring agent. The intensity of the response depends on the extent and severity of injury and on the reactive capacity of the victim. The inflammatory response

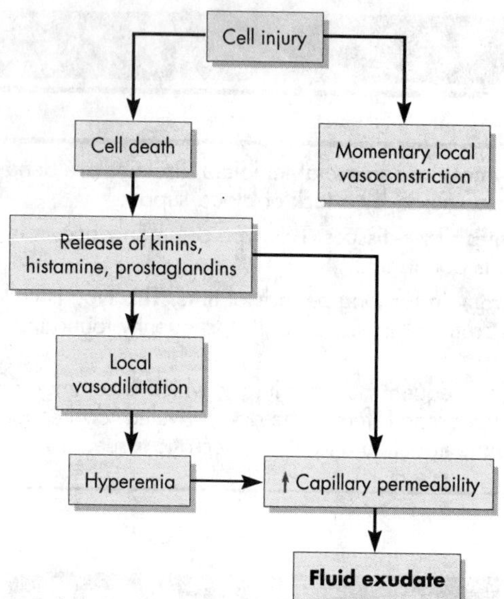

Fig. 9-5 Vascular response in inflammation.

can be divided into a vascular response, cellular response, formation of exudate, and healing.

Vascular Response. After cell injury, capillaries in the area briefly undergo vasoconstriction. After release of histamine and other chemicals by the injured cells, the vessels dilate. This vasodilatation results in *hyperemia* (increased blood supply), which raises filtration pressure. Vasodilatation and the effect of chemical mediators also make the capillaries more permeable. Movement of fluid from capillaries into tissue spaces is thus facilitated. Initially composed of serous fluid, this *inflammatory exudate* later contains plasma proteins, primarily albumin. The proteins exert oncotic pressure that further draws fluid from blood vessels. The tissue becomes edematous. This response is illustrated in Fig. 9-5.

As the plasma protein fibrinogen leaves the blood, it is activated to *fibrin* by the products of the injured cells. Fibrin strengthens a blood clot formed by platelets. In tissue the clot functions to trap bacteria, to prevent their spread, and to serve as a framework for the healing process.

Cellular Response. The cellular response to injury is illustrated in Fig. 9-6. The blood flow through capillaries in the area slows as fluid is lost and viscosity increases. Neutrophils and monocytes move to the inner surface of the capillaries (*margination*) and then, in ameboid fashion, through the capillary wall (*diapedesis*) to the site of injury (Fig. 9-7).

Chemotaxis is the directional migration of WBCs along a concentration gradient of chemoattractant. Chemotaxis is the mechanism for ensuring accumulation of neutrophils and monocytes at the focus of injury. Chemotactic factors include bacterial-derived chemotactic factors, complement-derived chemotactic factor (C5a), lipid-derived chemotactic factors (leukotriene B_4, 5-HETE, platelet-activating factor), platelet-derived chemotactic factors, and coagulation-related chemotactic factors.

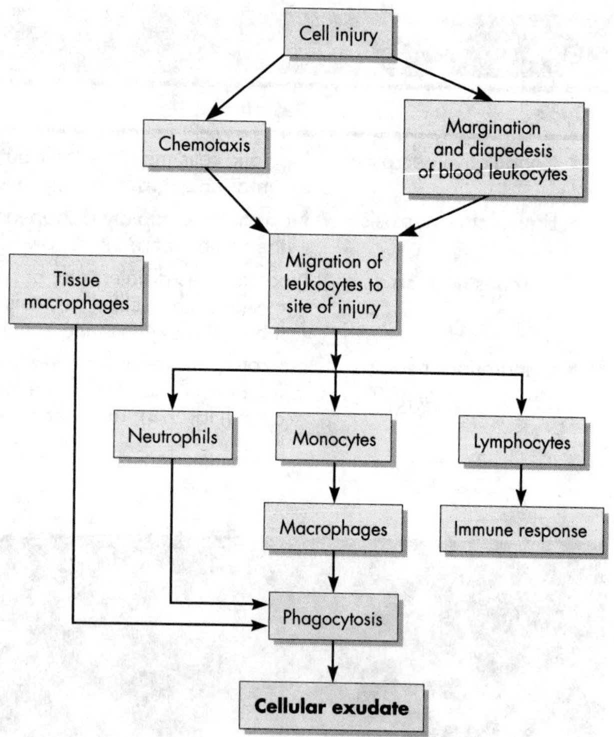

Fig. 9-6 Cellular response in inflammation.

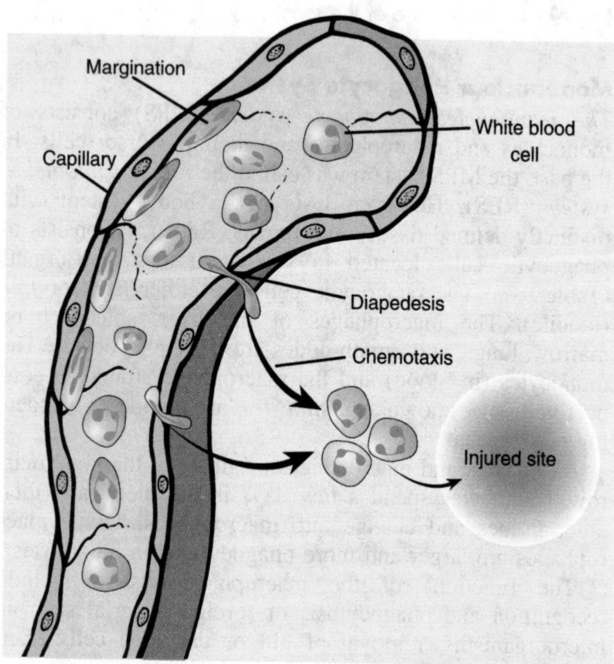

Fig. 9-7 Margination, diapedesis, and chemotaxis of white blood cells.

Neutrophils. Neutrophils are the first leukocytes to arrive (usually in 6 to 12 hours). They phagocytize bacteria, other foreign material, and damaged cells. With their short life span (24 to 48 hours), dead neutrophils soon accumulate. In time the mixture of dead neutrophils, digested bacteria, and other cell debris accumulate as a creamy substance known as *pus.*

To keep up with the demand for neutrophils, the bone marrow releases more neutrophils into circulation. This results in an elevated WBC count (especially the neutrophil count). Sometimes the demand for neutrophils increases to the extent that the bone marrow releases immature forms of neutrophils (*bands*) into circulation. (Mature neutrophils are called *segmented neutrophils*). The finding of increased numbers of band neutrophils in circulation is called a *shift to the left.*

Monocytes. Monocytes are the second type of phagocytic cells that migrate from circulating blood. On entering the tissue spaces, monocytes transform into macrophages. Together with the tissue macrophages, these macrophages assist in phagocytosis of the inflammatory debris. The macrophage role is important in cleaning the area before healing can occur. Macrophages have a long life span; they can multiply and may stay in the damaged tissues for weeks. These long-lived cells are important in orchestrating the healing process.

In some cases, macrophages perform tasks other than phagocytosis. They may accumulate and fuse to form a multinucleated *giant cell.* The giant cell serves to wall off infection. The accumulation of macrophages may lead to nodule formation (*granulomata*). A classic example of this process occurs with the tubercle bacillus in the lung. While the bacillus is walled off, a chronic state of inflammation exists. The granuloma formed is a cavity of necrotic tissue.

Lymphocytes. Lymphocytes arrive later at the site of injury. Their primary role is related to humoral and cell-mediated immunity (see Chapter 10).

Eosinophils and basophils. Eosinophils and basophils have a more selective role in inflammation. Eosinophils are released in large quantities during an allergic reaction. They are involved in phagocytosis of the allergen-antibody complex. The histamine and heparin that basophils carry in their granules are released during inflammation. Histamine is a potent vasodilator.

Chemical Mediators. Mediators of the inflammatory response are presented in Table 9-8.

Complement system. The complement system is a major mediator of the inflammatory response. Major functions of the complement system are enhanced phagocytosis, increased vascular permeability, chemotaxis, and cellular lysis. All of these activities are important in the inflammatory response.

When activated, the components occur in the sequential order of C1, C4, C2, C3, C5, C6, C7, C8, and C9 (Fig. 9-8). The numbering reflects the order of their discovery. Some components have subparts designated by lowercase letters, such as C3a, C3b, and C5a. The primary pathway for activation of the complement system is through fixation of component C1 to an antigen-antibody complex. The immunoglobulins IgG and IgM are responsible for fixing comple-

Table 9-8 Mediators of Inflammation

Mediator	Source	Mechanisms of Action
■ Histamine	Stored in granules of basophils, mast cells, platelets	Causes vasodilatation and increased vascular permeability by stimulating contraction of endothelial cells and creating widened gaps between cells
■ Serotonin	Stored in platelets, mast cells	Causes vasodilatation and increased vascular permeability by stimulating contraction of endothelial cells and creating widened gaps between cells; stimulates smooth muscle contraction
■ Kinins (e.g., bradykinin)	Produced from precursor factor kininogen as a result of activation of Hageman factor (XII) of clotting system	Cause contraction of smooth muscle and dilatation of blood vessels; result in stimulation of pain
■ Complement components (C3a, C4a, C5a)	Anaphylatoxic agents generated from complement pathway activation	Stimulate histamine release; stimulate chemotaxis
■ Fibrinopeptides	Produced from activation of the clotting system	Increase vascular permeability; stimulate chemotaxis for neutrophils
■ Prostaglandins and leukotrienes	Produced from arachidonic acid (Fig. 9-9)	PGE_1 and PGE_2 cause vasodilation; LTB_4 stimulates chemotaxis
■ Lymphokines	For information on lymphokines, see Table 10-4.	

LT, Leukotrienes; *PG*, prostaglandin.

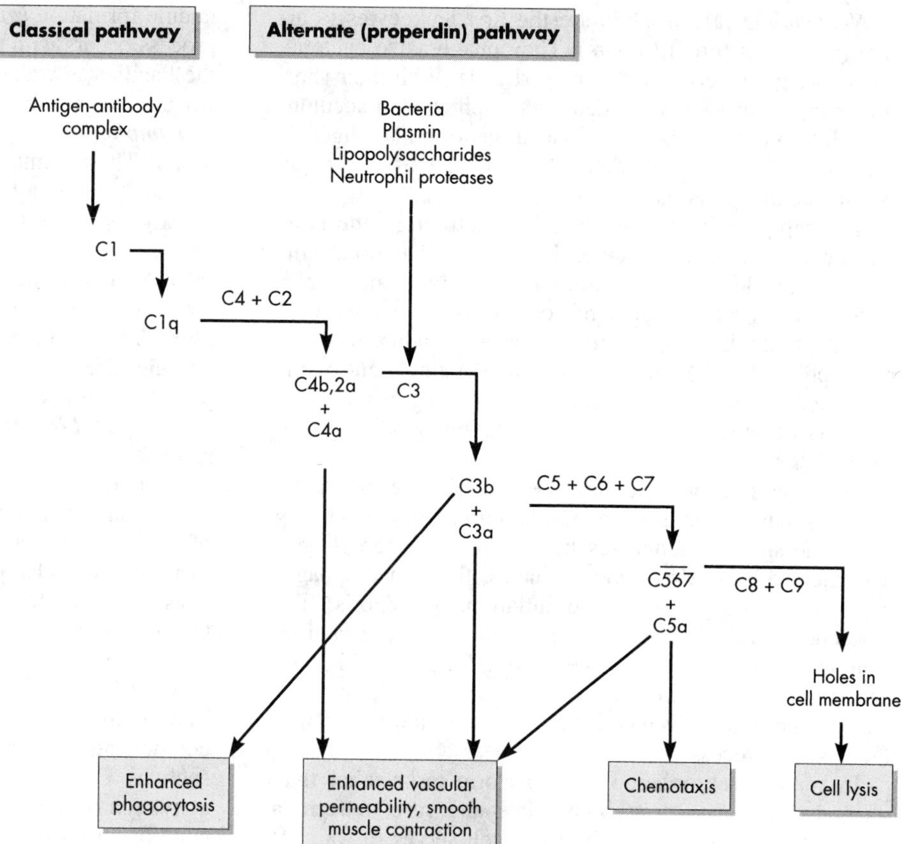

Fig. 9-8 Sequential activation and biologic effects of the complement system.

ment. Each activated complex can act on the next component, creating a cascade effect.

An alternate pathway, the *properdin pathway,* exists in which C3 is activated without prior antigen-antibody fixation. Bacterial products, lipopolysaccharides, plasmin, and neutrophil proteases can stimulate the complement sequence at the C3 level with activation of C5 through C9.

Complement increases phagocytosis through opsonization and chemotaxis. Opsonization occurs when the antigen, in combination with complement factor C3b and immunoglobulin, sticks to the surface of phagocytic cells. This leads to more rapid phagocytosis. In addition, complement component C5a promotes chemotaxis.

The components C3a, C5a, and C4a are called *anaphylatoxins,* which bind to receptors on mast cells and basophils thus triggering histamine release. Histamine causes smooth muscle contraction and an increase in vascular permeability.

The entire complement sequence of C1 to C9 must be activated for cell lysis to occur. The final component (C8, C9) acts on the cell surface causing rupture of the cell membrane and lysis. Bacteria, red blood cells (RBCs), and nucleated cells are susceptible to the lysis.

Prostaglandins and leukotrienes. Prostaglandins (PGs) are substances that can be synthesized from the phospholipids of cell membranes of most body tissues, including blood cells. On stimulation by chemotactic factors or phagocytosis or after cell injury, phospholipids can be converted to arachidonic acid (a 20-carbon polyunsaturated fatty acid), which is then oxidized by two different pathways (Fig. 9-9).

The *cyclooxygenase* metabolic pathway leads to the production of PGs of the E, I, and F series and thromboxanes (formed on activation of platelets). PGs of the E and I series are potent vasodilators and inhibit platelet and neutrophil aggregation. PGE_2 can also sensitize pain receptors to arousal by stimuli that would normally be painless. PGE_2 is also a potent pyrogen, acting on the temperature-regulating area of the hypothalamus. Thromboxane A_2 is a potent vasoconstrictor and platelet-aggregating agent. PGs are generally considered proinflammatory, contributing to increased blood flow, edema, and pain. Metabolism of arachidonic acid by the *lipoxygenase* pathway leads to the production of leukotrienes (LT). LTB_4 is a potent chemotactic factor. LTC_4, LTD_4, and LTE_4 form the slow-reacting substance of anaphylaxis (SRS-A), which constricts smooth muscles of bronchi and increases blood vessel permeability.

Drugs that inhibit PG synthesis are useful clinically. Nonsteroidal antiinflammatory drugs (NSAIDs), one type of these drugs, are a prototype drug treatment for many acute and chronic inflammatory conditions. Acetylsalicylic acid (ASA) blocks platelet aggregation; it also has antiinflammatory action. Prostacyclin (PGI_2) has been used to prevent platelet deposition in extracorporeal systems, such as hemodialysis and heart-lung bypass oxygenators. Another group of drugs that inhibit PGs are corticosteroids.

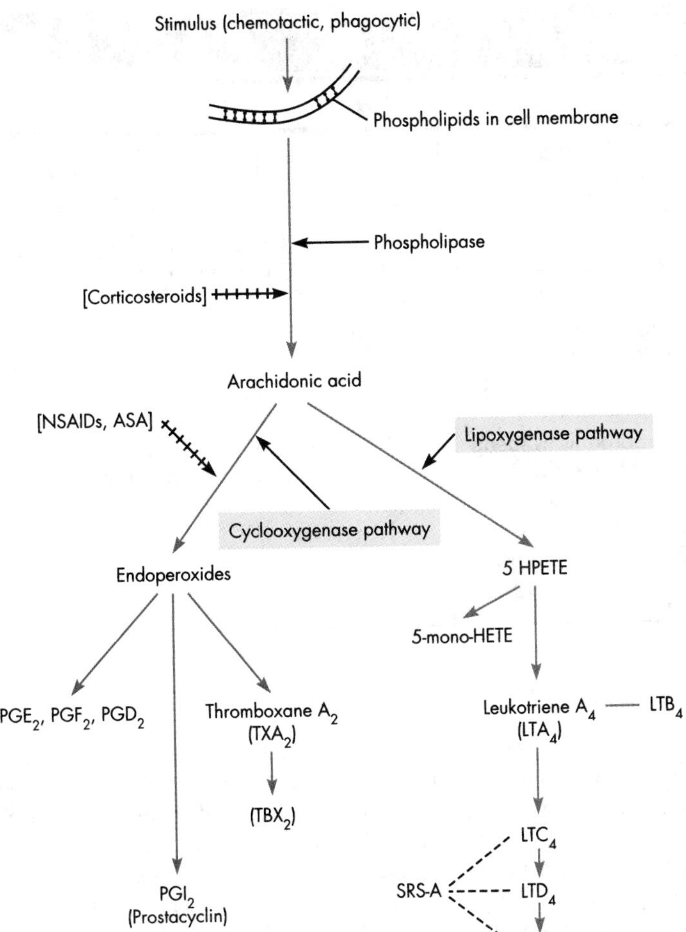

Fig. 9-9 Pathway of arachidonic acid oxygenation and generation of prostaglandins and leukotrienes. Corticosteroids, nonsteroidal antiinflammatory drugs (NSAIDs), and acetylsalicylic acid (ASA) act to inhibit various steps in this pathway. LTC_4, LTD_4, and LTE_4 form the slow-reacting substance of anaphylaxis (SRSA), an important mediator of allergic responses, by causing bronchoconstriction and increased vascular permeability.

They are valuable in the treatment of asthma because they inhibit leukotriene production and thus prevent bronchoconstriction. (Other mediators of the inflammatory response are described in Table 9-8.)

Exudate Formation. Exudate is formed from the fluid and the cells that move to the site of injury. The nature and quantity of exudate depend on the type and severity of the injury and the tissues involved (Table 9-9).

Healing. Normally, inflammation is followed by healing (see p. 193). If the cause of the inflammation is not effectively removed, the inflammation becomes chronic.

Clinical Manifestations. The *local response* to inflammation includes the manifestations of redness, heat, pain, swelling, and loss of function (Table 9-10).

Systemic manifestations of inflammation include leukocytosis with a shift to the left, malaise, nausea and anorexia, increased pulse and respiratory rate, and fever.

Leukocytosis results from the increased release of leukocytes from the bone marrow. An increase in the circulating number of one or more types of leukocytes may be found. Inflammatory reactions are accompanied by the vaguely defined constitutional symptoms of malaise, nausea, anorexia, and fatigue. The causes of these systemic changes are poorly understood but are probably the result of the production of factors released from stimulated WBCs. Collectively, these factors are called cytokines and function as intercellular messengers. Two of these cytokines, interleukin-1 (IL-1) and tumor necrosis factor (TNF), are released from mononuclear phagocyte cells and are important in causing the constitutional manifestations of inflammation, as well as inducing the production of fever. An increase in pulse and respiration follows the rise in metabolism as a result of an increase in body temperature.

Fever. Fever is caused by the cytokine IL-1, which acts as an endogenous pyrogen. It stimulates the release of another cytokine, IL-6, in the anterior hypothalamus. These ILs act on the temperature-regulating center in the hypothalamus to raise the core body temperature[1] (Fig. 9-10). Prostaglandins such as PGE_2 act directly to increase the thermostatic set point. The hypothalamus then activates the autonomic nervous system to stimulate increased muscle tone and shivering and decreased perspiration and blood flow to the periphery. Epinephrine release from the adrenal medulla increases the metabolic rate. The net result is fever.

With the thermostat fixed at a higher-than-normal temperature, the rate of heat production is increased until the

Table 9-9 Types of Inflammatory Exudate

Type	Description	Examples
▪ Serous	Serous exudate results from outpouring of fluid that has low cell and protein content; it is seen in early stages of inflammation or when injury is mild.	Skin blisters, pleural effusion
▪ Catarrhal	Catarrhal exudate is found in tissues where cells produce mucus. Mucus production is accelerated by inflammatory response.	Runny nose associated with upper respiratory tract infection
▪ Fibrinous	Fibrinous exudate occurs with increasing vascular permeability and fibrinogen leakage into interstitial spaces. Excessive amounts of fibrin coating tissue surfaces may cause them to adhere.	Adhesions
▪ Purulent (pus)	Purulent exudate consists of WBCs, microorganisms (dead and alive), liquefied dead cells, and other debris.	Furuncle (boil), abscess, cellulitis (diffuse inflammation in connective tissue)
▪ Hemorrhagic	Hemorrhagic exudate results from rupture or necrosis of blood vessel walls; it consists of RBCs that escape into tissue.	Hematoma

RBC, Red blood cell; *WBC,* white blood cell.

Table 9-10 Local Manifestations of Inflammation

Manifestations	Cause
▪ Redness (rubor)	Hyperemia from vasodilatation
▪ Heat (calor)	Increased metabolism at inflammatory site
▪ Pain (dolor)	Change in pH; change in local ionic concentration; nerve stimulation by chemicals (e.g., histamine, prostaglandins); pressure from fluid exudate
▪ Swelling (tumor)	Fluid shift to interstitial spaces; fluid exudate accumulation
▪ Loss of function (functio laesa)	Swelling and pain

body temperature reaches the new set point. As the set point is raised, the hypothalamus signals an increase in heat production and conservation to raise the body temperature to the new level. At this point the individual feels chilled and shivers. The shivering response is the body's method of raising the body's temperature until the new set point is attained. This seeming paradox is quite dramatic: the body is hot yet an individual piles on blankets and may go to bed to get warm. When the circulating body temperature reaches the set point of the core body temperature, the chills and warmth-seeking behavior ceases.[2] The febrile response is classified into four stages (Table 9-11).

IL-1 and the fever it triggers activate the body's defense mechanisms. Beneficial aspects of fever include increased killing of microorganisms, increased phagocytosis by neutrophils, and increased proliferation of T cells.[3] Higher body temperatures may also enhance the activity of interferon, the body's natural virus-fighting substance (see Chapter 10).

Types of Inflammation. The basic types of inflammation are acute, subacute, and chronic. In *acute inflammation* the healing occurs in 2 to 3 weeks and usually leaves no residual damage. Neutrophils are the predominant cell type. A *subacute inflammation* has the features of the acute process but lasts longer. For example, infective endocarditis is a smoldering infection with acute inflammation, but it persists throughout weeks or months (see Chapter 34).

Chronic inflammation lasts for weeks, months, or even years. The injurious agent persists or repeatedly injures tissue. The predominant cell types are lymphocytes, plasma cells, and macrophages. Examples of chronic inflammation include rheumatoid arthritis and tuberculosis. Tuberculosis is a type of chronic granulomatous inflammation.

A chronic inflammatory process is debilitating and can be devastating. The prolongation and chronicity of any inflammation may be the result of an alteration in the immune response.

THE HEALING PROCESS

The final phase of the inflammatory response is healing. Healing includes the two major components of regeneration and repair. *Regeneration* is the replacement of lost cells and tissues with cells of the same type. *Repair* is healing as a result of lost cells being replaced by connective tissue. Repair is the more common type of healing and usually results in scar formation.

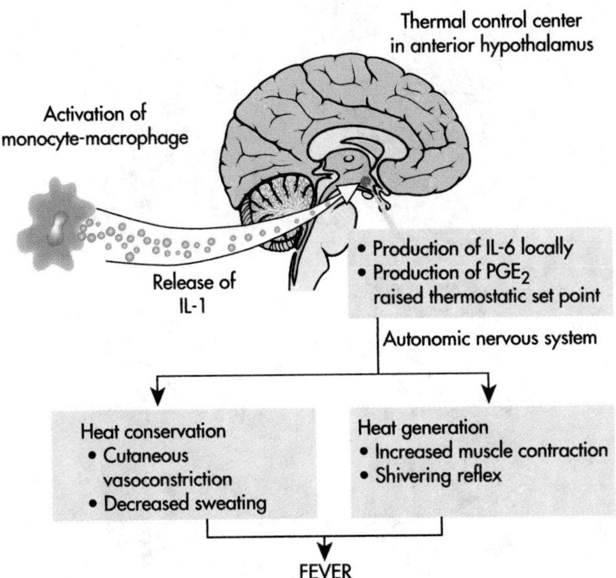

Fig. 9-10 When monocytes and macrophages are activated, they secrete interleukin-1 (IL-1), which reaches the hypothalamic thermoregulatory center by the arterial blood supply. Interleukin-6 (IL-6) release is stimulated, and it promotes the synthesis and secretion of prostaglandins in the anterior hypothalamus. Prostaglandins increase the thermostatic set point, and the autonomic nervous system is stimulated, resulting in shivering, muscle contraction, and peripheral vasoconstriction.

Table 9-11 Stages of the Febrile Response

Stage	Characteristics
▪ Prodromal	Nonspecific complaints such as mild headache, fatigue, general malaise, muscle aches
▪ Chill	Cutaneous vasoconstriction, "goose pimples," pale skin; feeling of being cold; generalized, shaking chill; shivering causing body to reach new temperature set by control center in hypothalamus
▪ Flush	Sensation of warmth throughout body; cutaneous vasodilatation; warming and flushing of skin
▪ Defervescence	Sweating; decrease in body temperature

Regeneration

The ability of cells to regenerate depends on the cell type (see Table 9-2). *Labile cells,* such as cells of the skin, lymphoid organs, bone marrow, and mucous membranes of the GI, urinary, and reproductive tracts, divide constantly. Injury to these organs is followed by rapid regeneration.

Stable cells retain their ability to regenerate but do so only if the organ is injured. Examples of stable cells are liver, pancreas, kidney, and bone cells.

Permanent cells do not regenerate. Examples of these cells are neurons of the central nervous system (CNS) and cardiac muscle cells. Damage to heart muscle or CNS neurons leads to permanent loss. Healing will occur by repair with scar tissue.

Repair

Repair is a more complex process than regeneration. Most injuries heal by connective tissue repair. Repair healing occurs by primary, secondary, or tertiary intention (Fig. 9-11).

Primary Intention. Primary intention healing takes place when wound margins are neatly approximated, such as in a surgical incision. A continuum of processes is associated with primary healing (Table 9-12). These processes include three phases.

Initial phase. The initial phase lasts for 3 to 5 days. The edges of the incision are first aligned and sutured in place. The incision area fills with blood from the cut blood vessels, and blood clots form. An acute inflammatory reaction occurs because of the exudate and necrotic cells. The area of injury is composed of fibrin clots, erythrocytes, neutrophils (both dead and dying), and other debris. Macrophages ingest and digest cellular debris, fibrin fragments, and RBCs. Extracellular enzymes derived from macrophages and neutrophils help to digest fibrin. As the wound debris is removed, the fibrin clot serves as a meshwork for future capillary growth and migration of epithelial cells.

Granulation phase. The granulation (fibroplasia) phase is the second step and lasts from 5 days to 4 weeks. The components of granulation tissue include proliferating fibroblasts; proliferating capillary sprouts (angioblasts); various types of WBCs; exudate; and loose, semifluid, ground substance.

Fibroblasts are immature connective tissue cells that migrate into the healing site and secrete collagen. In time the collagen is organized and restructured to strengthen the healing site. At this stage it is called *fibrous* or *scar tissue.*

During the granulation phase the wound is pink and vascular. Numerous red granules (young budding capillaries) are present. At this point the wound is friable, has an anesthetic quality, and is resistant to infection.

Surface epithelium at the wound edges begins to regenerate. In a few days a thin layer of epithelium migrates across the wound surface. The epithelium thickens and begins to mature, and the wound now closely resembles the adjacent skin. In a superficial wound, reepithelialization may take 3 to 5 days.

Scar contraction and maturation phase. The scar contraction and maturation phase overlaps with the granulation phase. It may begin 7 days after the injury and continue for several months. Collagen fibers are further organized, and the remodeling process occurs. Fibroblasts disappear as the wound becomes stronger. The active movement of the myofibroblasts causes contraction of the healing area, helping to close the defect and bring the skin edges closer together. A

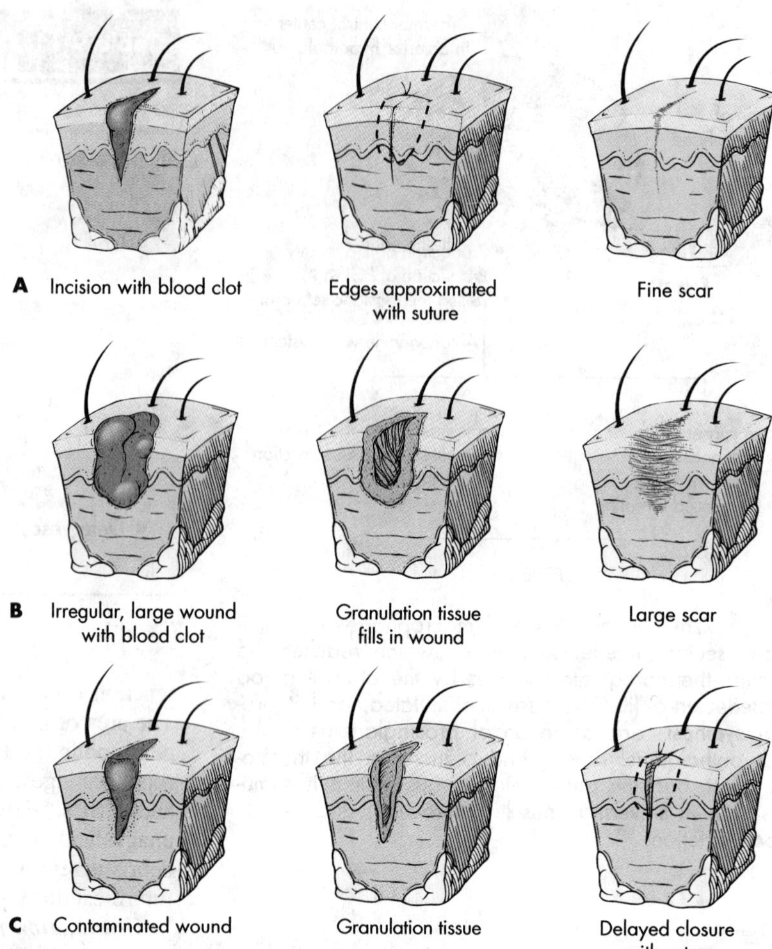

Fig. 9-11 Types of wound healing. ***A,*** Primary intention. ***B,*** Secondary intention. ***C,*** Tertiary intention.

mature scar is then formed. In contrast to granulation tissue, a mature scar is virtually avascular and pale, and it may be more painful at this phase than in the granulation phase.

Secondary Intention. Wounds that occur from trauma, ulceration, and infection and have large amounts of exudate and wide, irregular wound margins may not have edges that can be approximated. The inflammatory reaction may be greater than in primary healing. This results in more debris, cells, and exudate. The debris may have to be cleaned away (*debrided*) before healing can take place.

In some instances a primary incision may become infected, creating additional inflammation. The wound may reopen, and healing by secondary intention takes place.

The process of healing by secondary intention is essentially the same as by primary healing. The major differences are the greater defect and the gaping wound edges. Healing and granulation take place from the edges inward and from the bottom of the wound upward until the defect is filled. There is more granulation tissue, and the result is a much larger scar.

Wound classification. The red-yellow-black concept is sometimes used to describe open wounds. This concept is based on the color of the open wound (red, yellow, black) rather than on the depth of tissue destruction (Table 9-13). It can be applied to any wound allowed to heal by secondary intention, including surgically induced wounds left to heal without skin closure because of a risk for infection. A wound may have two or three colors at the same time. In this situation the wound is classified according to the least-desirable color present.

Table 9-12 Phases in Primary Intention Healing

Phase	Activity
▪ Initial (3 to 5 days)	Approximation of incision edges; migration of epithelial cells; clot serving as meshwork for starting capillary growth
▪ Granulation (5 days to 4 weeks)	Migration of fibroblasts; secretion of collagen; abundance of capillary buds; fragility of wound
▪ Scar contracture (7 days to several months)	Remodeling of collagen; strengthening of scar

Table 9-13 Red-Yellow-Black Concept of Wound Care

Red Wound	Yellow Wound	Black Wound
Characteristics		
Traumatic or surgical wound, possible presence of serosanguineous drainage, pink to bright or dark red healing or chronic wounds with granulating tissue	Presence of slough or soft necrotic tissue, liquid to semiliquid slough with exudate ranging from creamy ivory to yellow-green	Black, gray, or brown adherent necrotic tissue; possible presence of pus
Purpose of Treatment		
Protection and gentle atraumatic cleansing	Wound cleansing to remove nonviable tissue and absorb excess drainage	Debridement of eschar and nonviable tissue
Dressings and Therapy		
Transparent film dressing (e.g., Tegaderm, Opsite), hydrocolloid dressing (e.g., Duoderm), hydrogels (e.g., Vigilon), gauze dressing with antimicrobial ointment or solution, Telfa dressing with antibiotic ointment	Wound irrigations, hydrotherapy in conjunction with wet-to-dry dressings, moist gauze dressing with or without antibiotic or antimicrobial agent, hydrocolloidal dressing, hydrogel covered with gauze, absorption dressing (e.g., Debrisan beads, paste)	Topical enzyme debridement, surgical debridement, hydrotherapy, chemical debridement (e.g., Dakin's solution), moist gauze dressing, hydrogel covered with gauze, absorption dressing covered with gauze

Table 9-14 Factors Delaying Wound Healing

Factor	Effect on Wound Healing
■ Nutritional deficiencies	
Vitamin C	Delays formation of collagen fibers and capillary development
Protein	Decreases supply of amino acids for tissue repair
Zinc	Impairs epithelialization
■ Inadequate blood supply	Decreases supply of nutrients to injured area, decreases removal of exudative debris, inhibits inflammatory response
■ Corticosteroid drugs	Impair phagocytosis by WBCs, inhibit fibroblast proliferation and function, depress formation of granulation tissue, inhibit wound contraction
■ Infection	Increases inflammatory response and tissue destruction
■ Mechanical friction on wound	Destroys granulation tissue, prevents apposition of wound edges
■ Advanced age	Slows collagen synthesis by fibroblasts, impairs circulation, requires longer time for epithelialization of skin, alters phagocytic and immune responses
■ Obesity	Decreases blood supply in fatty tissue
■ Diabetes mellitus	Decreases collagen synthesis, retards early capillary growth, impairs phagocytosis (result of hyperglycemia)
■ Poor general health	Causes generalized absence of factors necessary to promote wound healing
■ Anemia	Supplies less oxygen at tissue level

WBCs, White blood cells.

Tertiary Intention. Tertiary intention (delayed primary intention) occurs with delayed suturing of a wound in which two layers of granulation tissue are sutured together. This occurs when a contaminated wound is left open and sutured closed after the infection is controlled. It also occurs when a primary wound becomes infected, is opened, is allowed to granulate, and is then sutured. Tertiary intention results in a larger and deeper scar than primary or secondary intention.

Delay of Healing

In a healthy person, wounds heal at a normal, predictable rate. Little can be done to accelerate this process. However, some factors delay wound healing. These are summarized in Table 9-14.

Complications of Healing

The shape and location of the wound determine how well the wound will heal. Complications result from interference

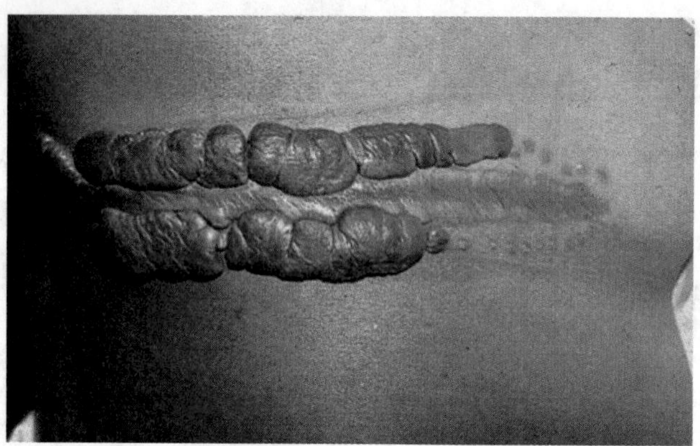

Fig. 9-12 Keloid formation resulting from suture wounds.

with wound healing. These factors may include poor nutrition, decreased blood supply, tissue trauma, denervation, and infection. Complications that may result include hypertrophic scars and keloids, contracture, dehiscence, excess granulation tissue, adhesions, and major organ dysfunction.

Hypertrophic Scars and Keloid Formation. Hypertrophic scars and keloid formation occur when the body produces an excess of collagen tissue. A hypertrophic scar is inappropriately large, red, raised, and hard. However, it remains confined to the wound edges and regresses in time. In contrast, a keloid is an even greater protrusion of scar tissue that extends beyond the wound edges and may assume tumorlike masses (Fig. 9-12). In addition, keloids are permanent, without any tendency to subside. The patient with keloids often complains of tenderness, pain, and hyperesthesia, particularly in the early stages of development. A predisposition to keloid formation is thought to be hereditary and occurs more often in dark-skinned people, particularly African-Americans. Neither complication is life-threatening, but both can have serious cosmetic implications.

Contracture. Wound contraction is necessary for healing. This process may become abnormal when there is excessive contraction resulting in deformity or contracture. A shortening of muscle or scar tissue results from excessive fibrous formation, especially if the wound is near a joint. Contracture frequently occurs in burns in which a great loss of skin and subcutaneous tissue occurs (see Chapter 21).

Dehiscence. Dehiscence is the separation and disruption of previously joined wound edges. It usually occurs when a primary healing site bursts. There are two possible causes of dehiscence. First, an infection may cause an inflammatory process. Second, the granulation tissue may not be strong enough to withstand the forces imposed on the wound. *Evisceration* occurs when wound edges separate to the extent that intestinal contents protrude through the wound.

Excess Granulation Tissue. Excess granulation tissue, or "proud flesh," protrudes above the surface of the healing wound. If the granulation tissue is cauterized or cut off, healing continues in a normal manner.

Adhesions. Adhesions are bands of scar tissue between or around organs. Adhesions may occur in the abdominal cavity or between the lungs and pleura. Adhesions in the abdomen may cause an intestinal obstruction. Adhesions between the lungs and pleura require *decortication,* or stripping of pleura, to permit normal ventilation.

Major Organ Dysfunction. Major organ dysfunction results when an acute inflammation of any organ, such as the heart, kidney, or brain, occurs. The resulting scar tissue causes an alteration in the physiologic function of the organ. The scar tissue "patch" will never function like the original tissue.

THERAPEUTIC MANAGEMENT

The actual therapeutic management of injury and inflammation is highly variable. It depends on the causative agent, the degree of injury, and the patient's condition. Superficial skin injuries may only need cleansing. Deeper skin wounds can be closed by suturing the edges together. Adhesive strips may be used instead of sutures. If the wound is contaminated, it needs to be converted into a clean wound before healing can occur normally. Surgical debridement of a wound that has multiple fragments or devitalized tissue may be necessary. If the source of injury or inflammation is an internal organ (e.g., appendix, ruptured spleen), surgical removal of the organ is the treatment of choice.

Pharmacologic Management

Pharmacologic agents are used in all types of inflammation. Drugs are used to decrease the inflammatory response (antiinflammatory agents) and destroy the infectious agent (antibiotics) (Table 9-15). Antihistamine drugs may also be used to inhibit the action of histamine. (Antihistamines are discussed in Chapter 10).

Nutritional Management

There are special nutritional measures to consider to facilitate wound healing. A high fluid intake is needed to replace fluid loss from perspiration and exudate formation. An increased metabolic rate intensifies water loss. There is a 7% increase in metabolism for every 1° F increase in temperature above 100° F (37.8° C) or a 13% increase for every 1° C increase.

A diet high in protein, carbohydrate, and vitamins with moderate fat intake is necessary to promote healing. *Protein* is needed to correct the negative nitrogen balance resulting from the increased metabolic rate. Protein is also necessary for synthesis of immune factors, leukocytes, fibroblasts, and collagen. *Carbohydrate* is needed for the increased metabolic energy required in inflammation and healing. If there is a carbohydrate deficit, the body will break down protein for the needed energy. *Fats* are also a necessary component in the diet to help in the synthesis of fatty acids and triglycerides, which are part of the cellular membrane. *Vitamin C* is needed for capillary synthesis, capillary formation, and resistance to infection. The *B-complex vitamins* are necessary as coenzymes for many metabolic reactions. If a vitamin B deficiency develops, a disruption of protein, fat, and carbohydrate metabolism will occur. *Vitamin A* is also needed in healing because it aids in the process of epithelialization. It increases collagen synthesis and tensile strength of the healing wound.

Table 9-15 Pharmacologic Agents Used to Treat Inflammation

Drug	Mechanisms of Action
Antipyretic Drugs	
Salicylates (aspirin)	Lower temperature by action on heat-regulating center in hypothalamus, resulting in peripheral dilatation and heat loss; interfere with formation and release of PGs; selectively depress CNS
Acetaminophen (Tylenol)	Lowers temperature by action in heat-regulating center in hypothalamus
NSAIDs (e.g., ibuprofen [Motrin, Advil])	Inhibit synthesis of PGs
Antiinflammatory Drugs	
Salicylates	Inhibit synthesis of PGs, reduce capillary permeability
Corticosteroids	Interfere with tissue granulation, induce immunosuppressive effects (decreased synthesis of lymphocytes), prevent liberation of lysosomes
NSAIDs (e.g., ibuprofen [Motrin], piroxicam [Feldene])	Inhibit synthesis of PGs
Antibiotic and Antimicrobial Drugs	
Penicillin	Interferes with formation of bacteria cell wall, is bacteriostatic and bactericidal
Cephalosporins	Interfere with formation of bacteria cell wall, are bactericidal
Erythromycin	Inhibits synthesis of bacterial protein, is bacteriostatic
Tetracycline	Inhibit synthesis of bacterial protein, is bacteriostatic
Aminoglycosides	Inhibit synthesis of bacterial protein, are bactericidal
Sulfonamides	Interfere with incorporation of PABA into folic acid, are bacteriostatic
Vitamins	
Vitamin A	Accelerates epithelialization
Vitamin B complex	Acts as coenzymes
Vitamin C	Assists in synthesis of collagen and angiogenesis
Vitamin D	Facilitates calcium absorption

CNS, Central nervous system; *NSAIDs*, nonsteroidal antiinflammatory drugs; *PABA*, paraaminobenzoic acid; *PG*, prostaglandin.

NURSING MANAGEMENT

INFLAMMATION

Health Promotion and Maintenance

The best management of inflammation is the prevention of infection, trauma, surgery, and contact with potentially harmful agents. This is not always possible. A simple mosquito bite causes an inflammatory response. Because occasional injury is inevitable, concerted efforts to combat inflammation are needed.

Adequate nutrition is essential so that the body has the necessary factors to promote healing when injury occurs. Individuals at risk for wound-healing problems are those with malabsorption problems (e.g., Crohn's disease, GI surgery, liver disease), deficient intake or high energy demands (e.g., malignancy, major trauma or surgery, sepsis, fever), and diabetes. An individual should always be considered at risk for wound-healing problems if the following have occurred: (1) loss of 20% or more of total body weight in the preceding 6 months or (2) 10% loss of total body weight in the preceding 2 months.[4]

Early recognition of manifestations of inflammation is necessary so that appropriate treatment can begin. This may be rest, pharmacologic treatment, or specific treatment of the injured site. Immediate treatment may prevent the extension and complications of inflammation.

Acute Intervention

Observation and Vital Signs. The ability to recognize the clinical manifestations of inflammation is important. In the individual who is immunosuppressed (e.g., taking corticosteroids or receiving chemotherapy), the classical manifestations of inflammation may be masked. In this individual, early symptoms of inflammation may be malaise or "just not feeling well."

Observation and recording of wound healing are essential. The consistency, color, and odor of any drainage should be recorded and reported if abnormal for the situation. *Staphylococcus* and *Pseudomonas* species are common organisms that cause purulent, draining wounds.

Vital signs are important to note with any inflammation and especially when an infectious process is present. When infection is present, temperature may rise, and pulse and respiration rates may increase. If a wound infection develops in a postoperative patient, vital signs will show a change in 3 to 5 days after surgery.

Fever. The most important aspect of fever management should be determining its cause.[5] Although fever is usually regarded as harmful, an increase in body temperature is an important host defense mechanism. In the seventeenth century, Thomas Sydenham noted that "fever is a mighty engine which nature brings into the world for the

NURSING CARE PLAN Patient with a Fever

Planning: Outcome Criteria	Nursing Interventions and Rationales
➤ **NURSING DIAGNOSIS**	Altered comfort: *related to* temperature alteration secondary to infection *as manifested by* increased body temperature, malaise, increased heart and respiratory rate, and increased white blood cell (WBC) count
Have body temperature below 100° F (37.8° C).	Assess patient's temperature q2-4hr *to monitor temperature.* Administer antipyretic drugs q3-4hr if ordered; keep environmental temperature at 70° F (21.1° C); avoid heavy layers of clothing or bed covers *to aid in lowering body temperature.* Give tepid sponge baths after antipyretic therapy *to reduce temperature through evaporation and to bring the temperature down more rapidly.* Use skin lotion *to prevent drying.* Change linen frequently if patient is diaphoretic *to prevent chilling and subsequent rise in body temperature from muscular activity.* Implement appropriate measures *to treat cause of fever.*
➤ **NURSING DIAGNOSIS**	Risk for fluid volume deficit *related to* increased metabolic rate, diaphoresis, and decreased oral intake
Have no signs of dehydration.	Assess for rapid respirations and pulse; damp skin, clothing, and bed clothes; unwillingness or inability to ingest fluids; signs of dehydration such as dry lips and tongue; poor skin turgor; and sunken eyes *to determine risk for or presence of fluid volume deficit.* Encourage fluid intake to 3-4 L/day if tolerated *to replace fluid lost as a result of fever and diaphoresis.* Monitor vital signs q2-4hr *as increasing pulse and respirations and decreasing blood pressure can indicate hypovolemia.* Administer intravenous (IV) fluids if necessary *to replace fluid loss if oral intake is inadequate.* Monitor intake and output accurately; give careful estimate of insensible losses *to evaluate need for replacement.*
➤ **NURSING DIAGNOSIS**	Risk for altered nutrition: less than body requirements *related to* increased caloric need secondary to increased metabolic rate and decreased oral intake
Have no weight loss.	Assess intake and monitor weight daily *to determine risk for or presence of problem.* Give high-caloric, high-protein, easily digested food and fluids *to maximize intake and minimize energy expense.* Help patient balance activity and rest to conserve energy *to ensure preferred activities can be accomplished and fatigue can be avoided.* Monitor alternate method of nutritional intake such as enteral or parenteral nutrition *if patient unable to maintain adequate intake.*

conquest of her enemies."[6] Steps are frequently taken to lower body temperature to relieve the anxiety of the patient and medical personnel. Because fever usually does little harm, imposes no great discomfort, and may benefit host defense mechanisms, antipyretic drugs are rarely essential to patient welfare.[2] Moderate fevers (up to 103° F [39.5° C]) usually produce few problems in most patients. However, if the patient is very young or very old, is extremely uncomfortable, or has a significant medical problem (e.g., severe cardiopulmonary disease, brain injury), the use of antipyretics should be considered.

Fever (especially if greater than 104° F [40° C]) can be damaging to body cells, and delirium and convulsions can occur. At temperatures greater than 105.8° F (41° C), regulation by the hypothalamic temperature control center becomes impaired, and damage can occur to the internal structures of many cells, including those in the brain.

Several drugs are commonly used to lower the body temperature set point in the hypothalamus. Aspirin specifically blocks PG synthesis in the hypothalamus and elsewhere in the body. Acetaminophen acts on the heat-regulating center in the hypothalamus. Some NSAIDS (e.g., ibuprofen [Motrin, Advil]) have antipyretic effects (Fig. 9-9). Corticosteroids are antipyretic through the dual mechanisms of inhibiting IL-1 production and preventing PG synthesis. The action of these drugs results in dilatation of superficial blood vessels, increased skin temperatures, and sweating.

Antipyretics should be given "around-the-clock" to prevent acute swings in temperature. Chills may be evoked or perpetuated by the intermittent administration of antipyretics. These agents cause a sharp decrease in temperature. When the antipyretic wears off, the body may initiate a compensatory involuntary muscular contraction (i.e., chill) to raise the body temperature back up to its previous level. This unpleasant side effect of antipyretic drugs can be prevented by administering these agents regularly and frequently at 2- to 4-hour intervals. Although sponge baths increase evaporative heat loss, there is no evidence that they decrease the body temperature unless antipyretic medications have been given to lower the set point; otherwise, the body will initiate compensatory mechanisms (i.e., shivering) to restore body heat. The same principle applies to the use of cooling blankets; they are most effective in lowering body temperature when the set point has also been lowered. The nursing care of the patient with a fever is presented in the nursing care plan on p. 198.

Rest and Immobilization. Rest and immobilization of the inflamed area promote healing by decreasing the inflammatory process, assisting in the repair process, and decreasing metabolic needs. Immobilization with a cast, splint, or bandage lessens wound debris and the possibility of hemorrhage. The repair process is facilitated by allowing fibrin and collagen to form across the wound edges with little disruption. Rest helps the body better use its nutrients and oxygen for the healing process.

Elevation. Elevating the injured extremity will reduce the edema at the inflammatory site and increase venous return. Elevation helps reduce pain and improve the circulation of blood, which provides the oxygen and nutrients needed for healing.

Oxygenation. Adequate oxygenation of the inflamed area is essential because oxygen promotes the differentiation of fibroblasts and collagen synthesis. Oxygen is also essential for cell growth and division. A person with arterial disease, hypovolemia, or hypotension is at greatest risk for infection and may benefit from oxygen administration.

Heat and Cold. Application of heat and cold are controversial interventions. Cold application is usually appropriate at the time of the initial trauma to cause vasoconstriction. This decreases swelling, pain, and congestion from increased metabolism in the area of inflammation. Heat may be used later (e.g., after 24 to 48 hours) to promote healing by increasing the circulation to the inflamed site and subsequent removal of debris. Heat is also used to localize the inflammatory agents. Warm, moist heat may help débride the wound site if necrotic material is present.

Wound Management. The type of wound management and dressings required depend on the type, extent, and characteristics of the wound.[7] The purposes of wound management include cleaning a dirty, infected wound to prepare it for healing and protecting a clean wound until it can heal normally. Emergency care of the patient with a skin wound is presented in Table 20-8. Pressure ulcers are discussed in Chapter 20.

For wounds that heal by primary intention, it is common to cover the incision with a dry, sterile dressing that is removed as soon as the drainage stops or in 2 to 3 days. Medicated sprays that form a transparent film on the skin may be used for dressings on a clean incision or injury. Sometimes a surgeon will leave a surgical wound uncovered.

Wound healing management by secondary intention can be described as the red-yellow-black concept of wound care (see Table 9-13).[8] Types of wound dressings are presented in Table 9-16.

Red wound. A red wound can be a superficial wound if it is clean and pink in appearance. Examples include skin tears, pressure necrosis sores (stage 2), partial-thickness or second-degree burns, and wounds created surgically that are allowed to heal by secondary intention. The purpose of treatment is protection of the wound and gentle cleansing (if indicated). Clean wounds that are granulating and reepithelializing should be kept slightly moist and protected from further trauma until they heal naturally. A dressing material that keeps the wound surface clean and slightly moist is optimal to promote epithelialization. Transparent adhesive semipermeable dressings (e.g., Opsite, Tegaderm) are occlusive dressings that are permeable to oxygen.[9] Antimicrobials such as bacitracin, neomycin, and povidone-iodine ointment can be used for application on clean wounds, which are then usually covered with a sterile dressing. Unnecessary manipulation during dressing changes may destroy new granulation tissue and break down fibrin formation.

Yellow wound. After the black eschar is removed, a yellow wound results. This type of wound can also result from surgical or traumatic injuries. The moist environment resulting from wound drainage creates an ideal situation for bacterial growth. The purpose of treatment is continual cleansing to remove nonviable tissue and to absorb excessive drainage. A type of dressing used in yellow wounds is absorption dressings (e.g., Debrisan), which absorb exudate and cleanse the wound surface.[9] The absorption dressings work by drawing excess drainage from the wound surface. After these preparations are saturated with exudate, they should be removed by washing with sterile saline or water. The amount of wound secretions determines the number of dressing changes (usually two to three daily).

Hydrocolloid dressings such as Duoderm are also used to treat yellow wounds. The inner part of these dressings interacts with the exudate, forming a hydrated gel over the wound. When the dressing is removed, the gel separates and stays over the wound, thus preventing damage to newly formed tissue. These types of dressings are designed to be left in place for up to 7 days or until leakage occurs around the dressing.

Black wound. A black wound is covered with thick necrotic tissue (*eschar*). Examples of black wounds include full-thickness or third-degree burns, pressure necrosis sores (stages 3 or 4), and gangrenous ulcers. The risk of wound infection increases in proportion to the amount of necrotic tissue present. The immediate treatment is debridement of the eschar and nonviable tissue. The debridement method used depends on the amount of debris and the condition of the wound tissue. There are three approaches to debridement:

1. *Surgical debridement:* This method is indicated when large amounts of nonviable tissue are present.
2. *Mechanical debridement:* This method is used when minimal debris is present. A common form of mechanical

Table 9-16 Types of Wound Dressings

Type	Description	Examples
Gauze	Provides absorption of exudate. Supports debridement if applied and kept moist. Can be used to maintain moist wound surface. Can be used as filler dressings in sinus tracts.	
Nonadherent dressings	Woven or nonwoven dressings may be impregnated with saline, petrolatum, or antimicrobials. Minimally absorbent.	Telfa Exu-Dry Vaseline gauze Xeroform
Transparent adhesive	Semipermeable membrane that permits gaseous exchange between wound bed and environment. Minimally absorbent so fluid environment is created in presence of exudate. Bacteria do not penetrate membrane.	Opsite Biocclusive Tegaderm Acu-Derm Polyskin Blisterfilm
Hydrocolloid	Occlusive dressing does not allow O_2 to diffuse from atmosphere to wound bed. Occlusion does not interfere with wound healing. Not used in infected wounds. Supports débridement and prevents secondary infections. Available in powder, wafer, and paste form.	DuoDerm Restore Intact Intrasite Tegasorb Ultec
Foam	Nonadherent wafers that have absorptive capacity. Have limited permeability and are not totally occlusive. Supports débridement in exudative wounds.	Allevyn Lyofoam Synthaderm Epilock
Absorption dressing	Large volumes of exudate can be absorbed. Supports débridement. Maintains moist wound surface. Placed into wounds and can obliterate dead space. Made up of dextranomer beads, copolymer starches, and calcium alginate.	Bard Absorption Hydragan Sorbsan Kaltostat Duoderm Paste Debrisan Sorbsan
Hydrogel	Débridement because of moisturizing effects. Maintains moist wound surface. Provides limited absorption of exudate. Available as sheet dressings and as granules.	Vigilon Elasto Gel Intrasite Gel Geliperm

debridement is wet-to-dry dressings in which open-mesh gauze is moistened with normal saline or an antimicrobial solution, packed on or into the wound surface, and allowed to dry. Wound debris adheres to the dressing. When the dressing is removed, the coarse debris is entrapped in the gauze. Topical antimicrobials and antibactericidals used on wet-to-dry dressings include povidone-iodine (Betadine), Dakin's solution (sodium hypochlorite), hydrogen peroxide (H_2O_2), and chlorhexidine (Hibiclens). Topical antimicrobials should be used with caution in wound care, because they can damage healing tissue (e.g., H_2O_2 damages new epithelium). Semiocclusive or occlusive dressings (Table 9-16) may be used to promote eschar softening by autolysis. These types of dressings are used in open wounds with minimal necrotic debris and no contamination. Another method of mechanical debridement is wound irrigation. This method may be appropriate when wounds are contaminated. However, irrigation should be used with caution because high pressure can interfere with fibroblast formation and macrophage function.

3. *Enzymatic debridement:* This method uses agents such as sutilains (Travase) in conjunction with normal, saline-moistened dressings. These enzyme products may be indicated for fragile and extremely sensitive wounds with minimal debris.

Infection Control. The nurse and the patient must scrupulously follow aseptic procedures for keeping the wound free from infection. The patient should not be allowed to touch a recently injured area. The patient's environment should be as free as possible from contamination from items introduced by roommates and visitors. Antibiotics may be administered prophylactically to some patients. If an infection develops, a culture and sensitivity test should be done to determine the most effective antibiotic for the specific organism.

Table 9-17 Occupational Health and Safety Administration (OSHA) Requirements for Personal Protective Apparel to Minimize Exposure to Bloodborne Pathogens*

Equipment	Indications for Use	Must Be
▪ Gloves	When contact with infectious material is likely During all vascular procedures Before contact with mucous membranes and nonintact skin	Suitable for task: general patient care, sterile surgical procedures Individualized: various sizes, hypoallergenic, powderless
▪ Clothing (gowns, aprons, shoe covers, hats, hoods)	When splattering of clothing with body substances is likely	Suitable for task: prevent blood, infectious materials from penetrating and reaching employee's skin or clothes
▪ Facial protection (masks, face shields, eyewear including glasses with side shields, goggles)	When splattering, splashing, or spraying of eyes, nose, or mouth with blood or other potentially infectious body substances is likely	Effective: in preventing infectious material from penetrating around or under barriers

From Occupational Safety and Health Administration: *Federal Register* 56:64003-64182, 1991.
*All personal protective equipment must be conveniently located, accessible and provided free to employee. Employer is responsible for purchasing, repairing, and laundering as appropriate.

OSHA guidelines. The Occupational Safety and Health Administration (OSHA) policy on preventing occupational transmission of blood-borne pathogens was implemented in 1992.[10] The ruling mandated that employers provide at-risk employees with appropriate personal protective equipment (PPE). The nurse needs to minimize or eliminate exposure to infectious material. When that is not possible, appropriate PPE must be selected. These include gloves, clothing, and facial protection (Table 9-17). Appropriate PPE will vary depending on the situation.

Infection precautions. If the patient develops an infection that is considered a risk to others, infection precautions may be needed. The purpose of these precautions is to prevent the spread of the infection. Four systems that are commonly used are: (1) Category-specific Precautions, (2) Disease-specific Precautions, (3) Universal Precautions, and (4) Body Substance Isolation. *Category-specific Precautions* are recommended to prevent transmission of the most infectious diseases in each category (e.g., respiratory isolation, enteric isolation). This system frequently means more isolation precautions than necessary are required to prevent transmission of a certain organism. *Disease-specific Precautions* handle each infectious disease or condition separately. With this system, it is possible to list only those precautions necessary to interrupt transmission of the specific organism. *Universal Precautions* recommend that blood and body fluid precautions be consistently used for all patients, regardless of blood-borne infection status. Universal Precautions are intended to prevent parenteral, mucous membrane, and nonintact skin exposure of health care workers to blood-borne pathogens. In addition, immunization with hepatitis B vaccine is recommended as an important adjunct to universal precautions for health care workers who are exposed to blood and blood products. The *Body Substance Isolation* (BSI) system was first described in 1984 and revised in 1990.[11] It is intended to reduce nosocomial transmission of infectious agents among patients and to reduce the risk of transmission of infectious agents to health care personnel. Table 9-18 compares the four systems of infectious precautions.

In 1995 the Centers for Disease Control and Prevention (CDC) drafted new guidelines for isolation precautions. The 1995 draft guidelines contain two levels of precautions (Table 9-19): *Standard Precautions,* which are designed for the care of all patients in hospitals regardless of their diagnosis or presumed infection status, and *Transmission-based Precautions,* which are used for patients known to be or suspected of being infected with epidemiologically important pathogens that can be transmitted by airborne or droplet transmission or by contact with dry skin or contaminated surfaces.

The 1995 Standard Precautions system synthesizes the major features of Universal Precautions and Body Substances Isolation and applies to (1) blood; (2) all body fluids, secretions, and excretions regardless of whether they contain visible blood; (3) nonintact skin; and (4) mucous membranes. Standard Precautions are designed to reduce the risk of transmission of microorganisms from both recognized and unrecognized sources of infection in hospitals.

Transmission-based precautions are designed for patients documented or suspected to be infected with highly transmissable or epidemiologically important pathogens for which additional precautions beyond Standard Precautions are needed to interrupt transmission in hospitals. The three types of Transmission-based Precautions include *airborne precautions, droplet precautions,* and *contact precautions.* They may be combined together for diseases that have multiple routes of transmission. When used either by themselves or in combination these precautions are used in addition to Standard Precautions. Transmission-based Precautions replace the Category-specific and Disease-specific systems.

Table 9-18 Comparison of Four Systems for Infection Precautions*

Situation	Category-specific; CDC, 1983	Disease-specific; CDC, 1983	Body Substance Isolation; Lynch, Jackson et al., 1984-1990	Universal Precautions; CDC, Revised 1988
▪ Patient is known to have hepatitis B or C, HIV infection, or other blood-borne diseases.	The category of blood and body fluid precautions was replaced by *Universal Precautions* in 1987 (revised in 1988).	See *Universal Precautions*, revised 1988.	*Gloves.* Use clean gloves before contact with mucous membranes, nonintact skin, and moist body substance. *Gown or plastic apron.* Use if soiling is likely. *Private room.* Use if personal hygiene is poor. *Mask and eye protection.* Use if splashing is likely. *Trash and linen.* Bag securely to prevent leakage.	*Gloves.* Use for contact with blood and body fluids epidemiologically associated with transmission of blood-borne organisms or other bloody body fluids. *Other protective barriers.* Use to reduce risk of exposure to blood or bloody body fluids. *Trash and linen.* Bag securely to prevent leakage.
▪ Patient is diagnosed with enteric disease (e.g., salmonellosis).	Enteric precautions: Use gloves for contact with feces, gown if soiling is likely, private room if personal hygiene is poor, sign on door—"Enteric Precautions."	See named disease in CDC guidelines 1983 (similar to enteric precautions); post sign on door.	Use same precautions as above.	*Universal Precautions* do not apply to feces unless visibly bloody.
▪ Patient is known to be colonized or infected with MRSA.	Contact isolation: Use gloves for touching infective material, masks if close to patient, gowns if soiling is likely. Private room is indicated; post sign on door—"Contact Isolation."	See named disease in CDC guideline, 1983 (similar to contact isolation); post sign on door.	Use same precautions as above.	*Universal Precautions* do not apply except as above.

Modified from Jackson MM, Lynch P.: An attempt to make an issue less murky: a comparison of four systems for infection precautions, *Infect Control Hosp Epidemiol* 12:448, 1991.
CDC, Centers for Disease Control and Prevention; *HIV,* human immunodeficiency virus; *MRSA,* methicillin-resistant *Staph aureus.*
*The strategies that are characteristic of each system of infection precautions are consistently applied in the same fashion for other diagnosed or undiagnosed infections.

All hospitals are encouraged to review and consider adoption of Standard Precautions and Transmission-based Precautions and discontinue use of the older forms of isolation precautions. The CDC offers hospitals the option of modifying the recommendations according to their needs and circumstances and as directed by federal, state, or local regulations. For example, OSHA's requirements are still operable, and all facilities are required to comply with these provisions. The CDC's 1995 Standard Precautions incorporate all requirements of OSHA's Bloodborne Pathogens Standard.

Reverse isolation. A low WBC count and depressed immune responses (e.g., in patient undergoing cancer chemotherapy, patient with neutropenia, or patient with leukemia or lymphoma) may indicate a need for another type of isolation called *reverse* (*protective*) isolation. The purpose of reverse isolation is to protect the vulnerable patient from environmental sources of infection. Institutional policies related to reverse isolation should be followed when the patient's condition warrants this intervention. (Reverse isolation is discussed in Chapter 28.)

Table 9-19 CDC Recommendations for Isolation Precautions in Health Care Facilities*

	Standard Precautions	Transmission-based Precautions: Airborne	Transmission-based Precautions: Droplet	Transmission-based Precautions: Contact
▪ When to use	All patients	Use in addition to Standard Precautions for patient known to be or suspected of being infected with microorganisms transmitted by airborne droplet (e.g., measles, varicella, tuberculosis).	Use in addition to Standard Precautions for patient known to be or suspected of being infected with microorganisms transmitted by droplets (e.g., *Hemophilus influenza, Neisseria meningitidis, Streptococcus pneumoniae,* Mycoplasma pneumonia).	Use in addition to Standard Precautions for specified patient known to be or suspected of being infected with epidemiologically important microorganisms that can be transmitted by direct contact with patient (e.g., enteric pathogens, multidrug-resistant bacteria, *Staphylococcus aureus, Clostridium difficile,* herpes simplex.)
▪ Handwashing	Wash hands after touching blood, body fluids, secretions, excretions, and contaminated items, regardless of whether gloves are worn; wash hands immediately after gloves are removed, between patient contacts, and to prevent transfer of microorganisms to other patients or environments.	Same as Standard Precautions.	Same as Standard Precautions.	Same as Standard Precautions.
▪ Gloves	Wear nonsterile gloves when touching bood, body fluids, secretions, excretions, and contaminated items; put on clean gloves just before touching mucous membranes and nonintact skin; remove gloves promptly after use, before touching noncomtaminated items, environmental surfaces, or going to another patient.	Same as Standard Precautions.	Same as Standard Precautions.	In addition to glove use as described in Standard Precautions, wear gloves whenever providing direct patient care or having hand contact with potentially contaminated surfaces or items in patient's environment.

continued

Table 9-19 CDC Recommendations for Isolation Precautions in Health Care Facilities*—cont'd

	Standard Precautions	Transmission-based Precautions: Airborne	Transmission-based Precautions: Droplet	Transmission-based Precautions: Contact
■ Mask, eye protection, face shield	Wear mask and eye protection or face shield to protect mucous membranes of eyes, nose, and mouth during procedures and patient care activities likely to generate spashes or sprays of blood, body fluids, secretions, and excretions.	In addition to Standard Precautions, wear respiratory protection when entering room of patient known to have or suspected of having tuberculosis.	In addition to Standard Precautions, wear a mask when working within 3 ft of patient.	Same as Standard Precautions.
■ Gown	Wear clean, nonsterile gown to protect skin and prevent soiling of clothing during procedures and patient care activities likely to generate spashes or sprays of blood, body fluids, secretions, or excretions, or to cause soiling of clothing; remove gown promptly when tasks are completed; wash hands.	Same as Standard Precautions.	Same as Standard Precautions.	Wear clean, nonsterile gown if substantial contact is anticipated with patient, surfaces, or items in environment; wear gown if patient is incontinent, has diarrhea, an ileostomy, colostomy, or uncontained wound drainage; remove gown carefully when tasks are completed, wash hands.
■ Linen	Handle, transport, and process used linen in manner that prevents skin and mucous membrane exposure, contamination of clothing, and environmental soiling.	Same as Standard Precautions.	Same as Standard Precautions.	Same as Standard Precautions.
■ Patient transport		Limit movement and transport of patient from room to essential purposes only; if transport or movement is necessary, minimize patient dispersal of droplet nuclei by placing surgical mask on patient, if possible.	Limit movement and transport of patient from room to essential purposes only; if transport or movement is necessary, minimize patient dispersal of droplet nuclei by masking patient, if possible.	Limit movement and transport of patient from room to essential purposes only; if transport is necessary, ensure that precautions are maintained to minimize contamination of environmental surfaces or equipment.

*A complete listing of recommendations is published in the Federal Register 59:214:55552, November 7, 1994.

Psychologic Implications. The patient may be distressed at the thought or sight of an incision or wound because of fear of scarring or disfigurement. Drainage from a wound often causes increased alarm. The patient needs to understand the healing process and the normal changes that occur as the wound heals. When a nurse is changing a dressing, inappropriate facial expressions can alert the patient to problems with the wound or the nurse's ability to care for it. Wrinkling of the nose by the nurse may convey disgust to the patient. A nurse should also be careful not to focus on the wound to the extent that the patient is not treated as a total person.

Chronic and Home Management

Wound healing may not be complete for 4 to 6 weeks or longer. Adequate rest and good nutrition should be continued throughout this time. Physical and emotional stresss-hould be minimal. Observing the wound for complications such as contractures, adhesions, and secondary infection is important during the rehabilitative stage.

Medications will often be taken for a period of time after recovery from the acute infection. Drug-specific side effects and adverse effects should be reviewed with the patient; the patient should be instructed to contact the health care provider if any of these effects occur. Awareness of the necessity to continue the drugs for the specified time is an important point to teach the patient. For example, a patient who is instructed to take an antibiotic for 10 days may stop taking the medication after 5 days because of decreased or absent symptoms. However, the organism may not be entirely eliminated, and it may increase in number and virulence if the medication is not continued. The organism may also become resistant to the antibiotic in this situation.

The patient or caregiver may also need instruction in some areas of personal care, including changing dressings and caring for the wound. Manifestations of abnormal wound healing should be taught so that the patient can report any findings to the health care provider.

CRITICAL THINKING EXERCISES

CASE STUDY

INJURY AND INFLAMMATION

Patient Profile

Roger, a 20-year-old man, was admitted to the hospital emergency department with burns estimated to be second degree that involved his face, neck, and upper trunk. He also had a lacerated right leg. His injuries occurred about 24 hours earlier.

Subjective Data

- Complains of slightly hoarse voice and irritated throat
- States that he tried to treat himself because he does not have health insurance
- Has been coughing up sooty sputum
- Has been a model for athletic clothing

Objective Data

Physical Examination

Leg wound is gaping and looks infected, temperature is 101.1° F (38.4° C)

X-ray

Reveals a fractured tibia

Laboratory

WBC count 26,400/µl (26.4×10^9/L) with 80% neutrophils (10% bands)

Critical Thinking Questions

1. What clinical manifestations of inflammation did Roger exhibit, and what are their pathophysiologic mechanisms?
2. What type of exudate formation did he develop?
3. What is the basis for the development of the temperature?
4. What is the significance of his WBC count and differential?
5. Because his wound was deep, primary tissue healing was not possible. How would you expect healing to take place?
6. What problems might Roger have with self-concept or body image? What concerns or problems might a nurse have in caring for Roger?
7. Based on the assessment data provided, write one or more appropriate nursing diagnoses. Are there any collaborative problems?

REVIEW QUESTIONS

The number of the question corresponds to the same-numbered objective at the beginning of the chapter.

1. What is the function of DNA?
   a. Transmiting all genetic information
   b. Determining the occurrence of cell division
   c. Building RNA
   d. Regulating the sequence of genes on chromosomes

2. Physiologic hyperplasia is commonly found in
   a. the bronchi of a chronic cigarette smoker.
   b. a distended urinary bladder.
   c. the female breast during lactation.
   d. an enlarged myocardium in congestive heart failure.

3. Which of the following describes a mechanism of cell death?
   a. Cytoplasm becomes more granular
   b. Rupture of cell membrane
   c. Increase in size of cell
   d. Embryonic differentiation

4. Which of the following is a common cause of coagulation necrosis?
   a. Autophagocytosis
   b. Granulomatous inflammation
   c. Lack of blood supply
   d. Malignant brain tumor

5. A major function of the mononuclear phagocyte system is to
   a. stimulate fibrin formation.
   b. synthesize neutrophils.
   c. release histamine.
   d. phagocytize foreign material.

6. Which of these best describes inflammation?
   a. An antigen-antibody reaction
   b. A sequential reaction to cell injury
   c. A secondary defense mechanism
   d. A detrimental defense mechanism of body

7. Which of the following are local manifestations of inflammation?
   a. Contractures and adhesions
   b. Pain and ulceration
   c. Boil and cyanosis
   d. Swelling and loss of function

8. Wound healing by primary intention involves all the following *except*
   a. abundant collagen formation.
   b. an inflammatory reaction.
   c. regenerating epithelium.
   d. blood clot formation.

9. Contractures frequently occur after burn healing because of
   a. weakness of connective tissue.
   b. lack of adequate blood supply.
   c. excess fibrous tissue formation.
   d. secondary infection.

10. Rest and immobilization are important measures of acute care for wound healing because
   a. the production of leukocytes will be decreased.
   b. they will prevent an inflammatory response.
   c. they are known mechanisms to increase the rate of healing.
   d. they increase the body's production of corticosteroids.

REFERENCES

1. Kluger MJ: Cytokines and the pathogenesis of fever, *Physiologist* 37:A28, 1994.
2. Letizia M, Janusek L: The self-defense mechanism of fever, *Medsurg Nurs* 3:373, 1994.
3. Lewis SL: Fever: thermal regulation and alterations in end-stage renal patients, *ANNA J* 19:13, 1992.
4. Meser MS: Wound care, *Crit Care Nurs Q* 11:17, 1989.
5. Holtzclaw BJ: Monitoring body temperture, *AACN Clinical Issues* 4:44, 1993.
6. Atkins E: Fever: its history, cause and function, *Yale J Biol Med* 55:283-289, 1982.
7. Krasner D: The 12 commandments of wound care, *Nursing* 22:34, 1992.
8. Stotts NA: Seeing red and yellow and black: the three-color concept of wound care, *Nurs* 20:59, 1990.
9. Motta GJ: How moisture-retentive dressings promote healing, *Nurs* 23:26, 1993.
10. Eggleston B: Infection control update, *Nurs* 24:70, 1994.
11. Lynch P and others: Implementing and evaluating a system of generic infection precautions: body substance isolation, *Am J Infect Control* 18:1, 1990.

Chapter 10

NURSING ROLE IN MANAGEMENT

Altered Immune Responses

Sharon L. Lewis

Learning Objectives

1. Describe the functions and components of the immune system.
2. Differentiate between natural and acquired immunity.
3. Compare and contrast humoral and cell-mediated immunity regarding lymphocytes involved, types of reactions, and effects on antigens.
4. Identify the five types of immunoglobulins and their characteristics.
5. Differentiate among the four types of hypersensitivity reactions in terms of immunologic mechanisms and disease manifestations.
6. Identify the clinical manifestations and emergency treatment of a systemic anaphylactic reaction.
7. Describe the assessment and management of a patient with chronic allergies.
8. Describe the pharmacologic management of the patient with allergies.
9. Describe the etiologic factors, clinical manifestations, and treatment modalities of autoimmune diseases.
10. Explain the relationship between the human leukocyte antigen (HLA) system and certain diseases.
11. Describe the etiologic factors, categories, and treatment of immunodeficiency disorders.

The human body has always had to protect itself from invasion by microorganisms. A complex defense system has evolved to withstand these constant attacks. The defense system in humans consists of a nonspecific inflammatory response (including phagocytosis) and a specific immune response (humoral immunity and cell-mediated immunity). (The inflammatory response is discussed in Chapter 9.)

Immunocompetence exists when the body's immune system can identify and inactivate or destroy foreign substances. When the immune system is incompetent or underresponsive, immunodeficiency diseases and malignancies occur. When the immune system overreacts, hypersensitivity disorders such as allergies and autoimmune diseases occur.

NORMAL IMMUNE RESPONSE

Immunity

Immunity is a state of responsiveness to invading organisms and foreign or tumor protein. Immune responses serve three functions (Table 10-1):

1. *Defense:* The body resists invasions by microorganisms and prevents infection from developing by attacking foreign antigens and pathogens.
2. *Homeostasis:* Damaged cellular substances are digested and removed. Through this mechanism the specific cell types remain uniform and unchanged.
3. *Surveillance:* Mutations continually arise in the body but are normally recognized as foreign cells and destroyed.

Properties of the Immune Response

The immune system has three important properties that make its protection diverse and long-lasting. They are the following:

1. *Specificity:* When a foreign antigen (substance capable of stimulating an immune response) enters the body, a series of cellular changes occur. These changes result in the formation of a specific antibody or sensitized lymphocyte that attaches to the specific antigen.
2. *Memory:* The immune system has the unique ability to remember the antigen. Therefore, a secondary immune response is faster and stronger.
3. *Self-recognition:* Because there frequently is little difference between the body's own proteins and foreign proteins, the body must distinguish between the two. When the body fails to recognize self-proteins, autoantibodies develop, leading to tissue destruction.

Types of Immunity. Immunity is classified as *natural* or *acquired*. Natural immunity exists in a person without prior

---

Reviewed by Donna McCarthy, RN, PhD, Associate Professor, School of Nursing, University of Wisconsin, Madison, WI.

Table 10-1 Functions of the Immune System

Function	Adaptive Response	Maladaptive Response	
		Hyper	**Hypo**
Defense	Destruction of viruses, bacteria, fungi	Allergic disorders	Immunodeficiency disorders
Homeostasis	Removal of damaged cells	Autoimmune diseases	—
Surveillance	Removal of mutated cells	—	Malignant diseases

Table 10-2 Types of Acquired Specific Immunity

Acquisition of Immunity	Protection
Active	
Natural	
Natural contact with antigen through clinical or subclinical infection; for example, recovery from childhood diseases (e.g., chickenpox, measles, mumps)	***Development*** Develops slowly; protective levels reached in few weeks ***Duration*** Long-term, often lifetime ***Spectrum*** Specific to antigen contacted
Artificial	
Immunization with antigen, (e.g., immunization with live or killed vaccines, toxoid immunization)	***Development*** Develops slowly; protective levels reached in few weeks ***Duration*** Several years; extended protection with "booster" doses ***Spectrum*** Specific to antigen targeted by immunization
Passive	
Natural	
Transplacental and colostrum transfer from mother to child (e.g., maternal immunoglobulins in neonate)	***Development*** Immediate ***Duration*** Temporary; several months ***Spectrum*** All antigens to which source has immunity
Artificial	
Injection of serum from immune human or animal (e.g., injection of pooled human γ-globulin)	***Development*** Immediate ***Duration*** Temporary; several weeks ***Spectrum*** All antigens to which source has immunity

contact with an antigen. It may be related to a species, race, or genetic tendency. Acquired immunity is the development of immunity, either actively or passively (Table 10-2).

Active acquired immunity. Active acquired immunity results from the invasion of the body by microorganisms and subsequent development of antibodies and sensitized lymphocytes. With each reinvasion of the microorganisms, the body responds more rapidly and vigorously to fight off the invader. Active acquired immunity may result naturally from a disease or artificially through inoculation of a less virulent antigen (e.g., immunizations). Because antibodies are synthesized, immunity takes time to develop but is long-lasting.

Passive acquired immunity. Passive acquired immunity implies that the host receives antibodies to an antigen rather than synthesizing them. This may take place naturally through the transfer of immunoglobulins across the placental membrane from mother to fetus. Artificial passive acquired immunity occurs through injection with γ-globulin (serum antibodies). The benefit of this immunity is its immediate effect. Unfortunately, passive immunity is short-lived, since the host did not synthesize the antibodies and consequently does not retain memory cells for the antigen.

Antigens

An *antigen* is a substance that elicits an immune response. Most antigens are composed of protein. However, other substances such as large-size polysaccharides, lipoproteins, and nucleic acids can act as antigens. All of the body's cells have antigens on their surface that are unique to that person and enable the body to recognize self. The immune system becomes "tolerant" to the body's own molecules and therefore is nonresponsive to self.

Most foreign antigens are not chemically pure substances but rather have multiple antigenic determinants with which antibodies can combine. Small variations in cell surface antigens will elicit an immune response. This is the basis of transplant rejection if the donor organ is not a perfect match with the recipient.

Haptens are low molecular weight substances that by themselves are harmless. However, they can form complexes with larger molecules that are antigenic. An immune response can be generated to multiple parts of the complex. Once antibodies are produced, future exposure to the hapten alone can elicit an immune response. Common haptens include dust, animal danders, drugs, and industrial chemicals. Immune responses to haptens are the basis for many common allergies.

Physical or chemical damage to cell membranes may expose other cell structures to the immune system. The "new" antigens can stimulate the immune system to react against the body's own tissues. This process results in autoimmunity.

Components of the Immune System

Lymphoid organs function in production of lymphocytes, one of the essential cells of the immune response. The mononuclear phagocyte system (discussed in Chapter 9) is also involved in the production of a normal immune response.

Lymphoid Organs. The lymphoid system is composed of central and peripheral lymphoid organs. The *central lymphoid organs* are the thymus gland and bone marrow. The *peripheral lymphoid organs* are the tonsils; gut-, genital-, bronchial-, and skin-associated lymphoid tissues; lymph nodes; and spleen (Fig. 10-1).

Lymphocytes are produced in the bone marrow and eventually migrate to the peripheral organs. The thymus is important in the differentiation and maturation of T lymphocytes and is therefore essential for a cell-mediated immune response. During childhood the gland is large. The gland shrinks with age and is a collection of reticular fibers, lymphocytes, and connective tissue in older persons.

Lymphoid tissue is found in the submucosa of the respiratory (bronchial-associated), genitourinary (genital-associated), and gastrointestinal (gut-associated) tracts. This tissue protects the body surface from external microorganisms. The tonsils are a typical example of lymphoid tissue.

The skin-associated lymph tissue primarily consists of lymphocytes and Langerhans cells (a type of resident macrophage) found in the epidermis of skin. When Langerhans cells are depleted, the skin can neither initiate an immune response nor support a skin-localized delayed hypersensitivity response.

When antigens are introduced into the body, they may be carried by the bloodstream or lymph channels to regional *lymph nodes*. The antigens interact with B and T lymphocytes and macrophages in the lymph node. The two important functions of lymph nodes are (1) filtration of foreign material brought to the site and (2) circulation of lymphocytes.

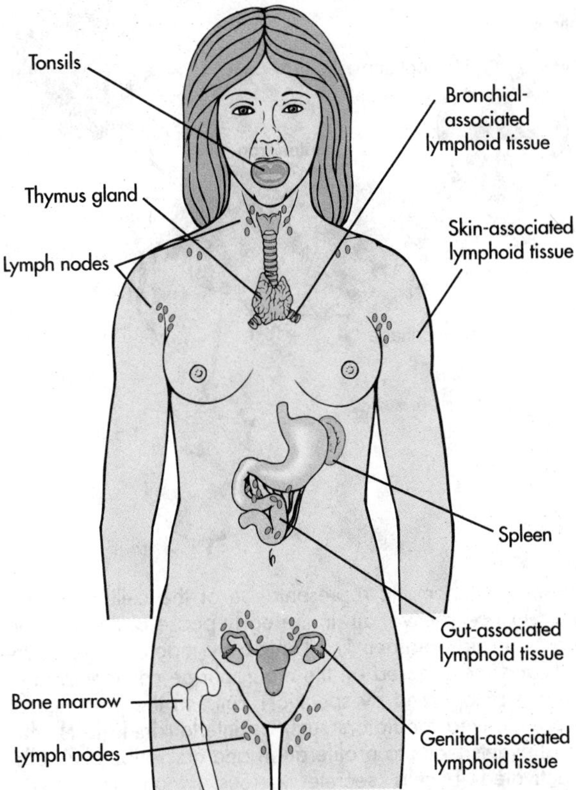

Fig. 10-1 Organs of the immune system.

The spleen is important as the primary site for filtering foreign substances from the blood. It consists of two kinds of tissue: *white pulp* containing B and T lymphocytes and *red pulp* containing erythrocytes. Macrophages line the pulp and sinuses of the spleen. If the spleen is removed in children, it can predispose them to life-threatening septicemia.

Mononuclear Phagocyte System. The mononuclear phagocyte system includes monocytes in the blood and macrophages found throughout the body. (See Chapter 9 for a more complete description.) Mononuclear phagocytes have a critical role in the immune system. They are responsible for capturing, processing, and presenting the antigen to the lymphocytes. This stimulates a humoral or cell-mediated immune response. Capturing is accomplished through phagocytosis. The macrophage-bound antigen, which is highly immunogenic, is presented to circulating T or B lymphocytes and thus triggers an immune response (Fig. 10-2).

Lymphocyte Production

Lymphocytes arise from undifferentiated stem cells in the fetal liver and later from the bone marrow (Fig. 10-3). Lymphocytes differentiate into B and T lymphocytes.

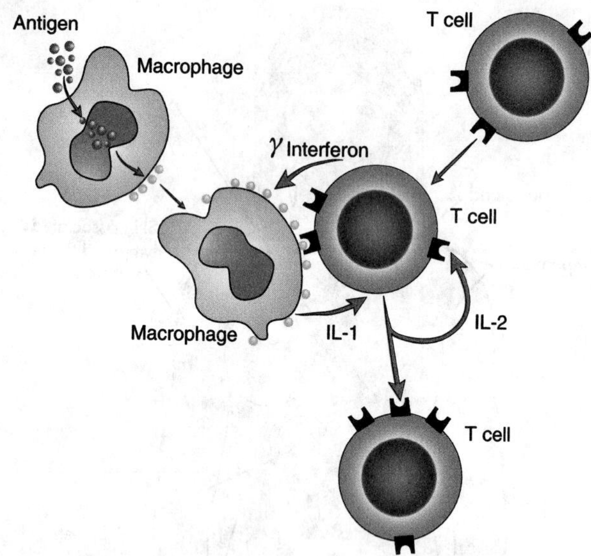

Fig. 10-2 Schematic representation of the cellular events involved in T-cell activation. In the early phase of the immune response, foreign antigen is taken up by macrophages, processed, and reexpressed on the macrophage cell membrane, where it is recognized by specific T cells. In the presence of monocyte-derived mediators such as interleukin-1 (IL-1), this series of events leads to proliferation and activation of T cells. The activated T cells secrete various lymphokines (e.g., interleukin-2 [IL-2], γ-interferon) that mediate responses involving lymphocytes and mononuclear phagocytes.

In birds, B lymphocytes (bursa-equivalent or thymus-independent cells) mature under the influence of the bursa of Fabricius. However, this lymphoid organ does not exist in humans. The bursa-equivalent tissue in humans is the bone marrow.

Cells that migrate from the bone marrow to the thymus differentiate into T lymphocytes (thymus-dependent cells). The thymus secretes hormones, including thymosin, that stimulate the maturation and differentiation of T lymphocytes. T cells compose 70% to 80% of the circulating lymphocytes and are primarily responsible for immunity to intracellular viruses, tumor cells, and fungi. These T cells live from a few months to the life span of an individual and account for long-term immunity.

Humoral Immunity

Humoral immunity consists of antibody-mediated immunity. *Humoral* comes from the Greek word humor, which means body fluid. Antibodies are proteins found in plasma, and therefore the term humoral immunity. Production of antibodies (immunoglobulins) is an essential component in a humoral immune response. Immunoglobulins are composed of amino acids arranged on two light and two heavy polypeptide chains. Differences in the heavy chain configuration differentiate the five classes of immunoglobulins, which are IgG, IgA, IgM, IgD, and IgE. Each class of immunoglobulins has specific characteristics (Table 10-3).

Humoral Immune Response. When a pathogen (especially bacteria) enters the body, it may encounter a B lymphocyte specific for antigens on that bacterial cell wall. In addition, a monocyte/macrophage may phagocytize the bacteria and present its antigens to a B lymphocyte. The B lymphocyte recognizes the antigen because it has receptors

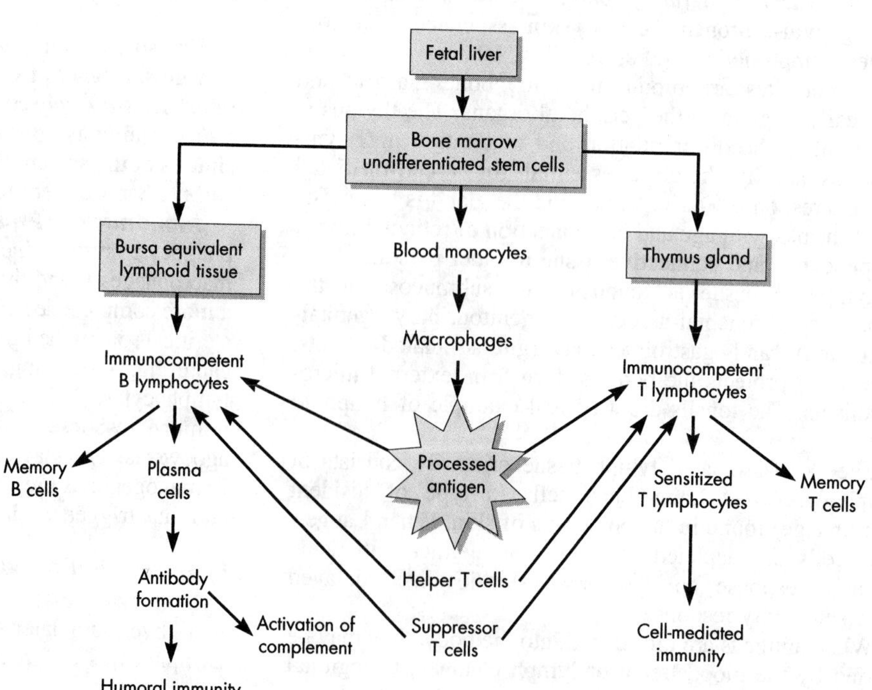

Fig. 10-3 Relationships and functions of macrophages, B lymphocytes, and T lymphocytes in an immune response.

Table 10-3 Characteristics of Immunoglobulins

Class	Relative Serum Concentration(%)	Location	Characteristics
IgG	76	Plasma, interstitial fluid	Is only immunoglobulin that crosses placenta Fixes complement Is responsible for secondary immune response
IgA	15	Body secretions, including tears, saliva, breast milk, colostrum	Lines mucous membranes and protects body surfaces
IgM	8	Plasma	Fixes complement Is responsible for primary immune response Provides specific antitoxin action when combined with IgG Forms antibodies to ABO blood antigens
IgD	1	Plasma	Is present on lymphocyte surface Assists in the differentiation of B lymphocytes
IgE	0.002	Plasma, interstitial fluids, exocrine secretions	Causes symptoms of allergic reactions Fixes to mast cells and basophils Assists in defense against parasitic infections

on its cell surface specific for that antigen. When the antigen comes in contact with the cell surface receptor, the B cell becomes activated, and most B cells will differentiate into plasma cells (see Fig. 10-3). The mature plasma cell secretes immunoglobulins. Some stimulated B lymphocytes remain as memory cells.

The *primary immune response* is evident 4 to 8 days after initial exposure to the antigen (Fig. 10-4). IgM is the first type of antibody formed. Because of the large size of the IgM molecule, this immunoglobulin is confined to the intravascular space. As the immune response progresses, IgG is produced and can move from intravascular to extravascular spaces.

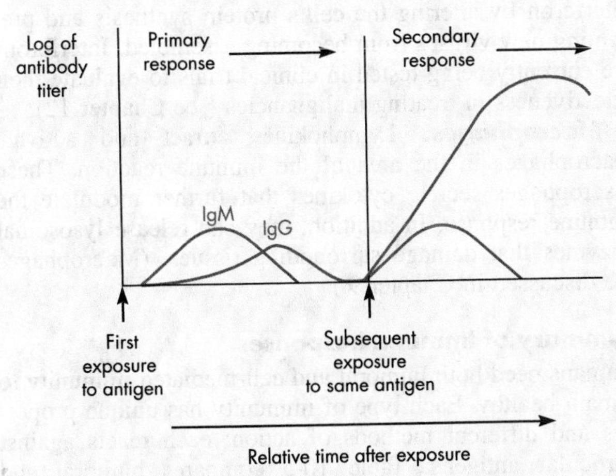

Fig. 10-4 Primary and secondary immune responses. The introduction of antigen induces a response dominated by two classes of immunoglobulins, IgM and IgG. IgM predominates in the primary response, with some IgG appearing later. After the host's immune system is primed, another challenge with the same antigen induces the secondary response, in which some IgM and large amounts of IgG are produced.

When the individual is exposed to the antigen the second time, a *secondary antibody response* occurs. This response occurs faster (1 to 2 days), is stronger, and lasts for a longer time than a primary response. Memory cells account for the memory of the first exposure to the antigen and the more rapid production of antibodies. IgG is the primary antibody found in a secondary immune response.

During gestation, the fetus has some immunity to protect against in utero infections. However, the lymph nodes and spleen are underdeveloped in the neonate. Fortunately, IgG crosses the placental membrane and provides the newborn with passive acquired immunity for at least 3 months. Infants may also get some passive immunity from IgA in breast milk and colostrum. By 9 months of age, a baby's IgM level is at a normal concentration and the lymph nodes and spleen are well-developed.

Antigen-Antibody Interactions. Antigen-antibody interactions result in elimination or destruction of the antigen. The five kinds of interactions are the following:

1. *Precipitation:* Soluble antigens combine with antibodies to form a lattice formation of insoluble complexes that precipitate.
2. *Agglutination:* Particulate antigens (e.g., red blood cells [RBCs]) may combine with antibodies to form clumps.
3. *Opsonization:* Bacteria are coated with molecules that allow them to be recognized and ingested by neutrophils and monocytes. The opsonization mechanism involves IgG and complement-derived C3b. Opsonized particles attach to receptors on the surface of neutrophils and monocytes.
4. *Lysis:* Lysis occurs after complement acts on the cell membrane of the antigen to cause rupture and leakage of cell contents. (The complement system is discussed in Chapter 9.)

5. *Neutralization:* Antibodies neutralize some toxins released from bacteria. The mononuclear phagocyte system phagocytizes the antigen-antibody complex and removes it from the body.

Cell-Mediated Immunity

The immune response may involve interactions of the cells of the immune system with the antigen. These interactions are called *cell-mediated immunity*. Although these reactions were initially considered to be mediated by T cells, several cell types and factors are involved in cell-mediated immunity. The cell types involved include T lymphocytes, macrophages, and natural killer cells. Cell-mediated immunity is of primary importance in (1) immunity against pathogens that survive inside of cells including viruses and some bacteria (e.g., *Mycobacterium*); (2) fungal infections; (3) rejection of transplanted tissues; (4) contact hypersensitivity reactions; and (5) tumor immunity.

T Lymphocytes. T lymphocytes can be categorized into T-cytotoxic, T-helper, and T-suppressor cells. Antigenic characteristics of white blood cells (WBCs) have now been classified using monoclonal antibodies. These antigens are classified as *clusters of differentiation* or CD antigens. Many types of WBCs, especially lymphocytes, are referred to by their CD designations.

T-cytotoxic cells. T-cytotoxic (CD3) cells are involved in attacking antigens on the cell membrane of foreign pathogens and releasing cytolytic substances that destroy the pathogen. These cells have antigen specificity and are sensitized by exposure to the antigen. Similar to B lymphocytes, some sensitized T cells do not attack the antigen but remain as memory T cells. As in the humoral immune response, a second exposure to the antigen will result in a more intense and rapid cell-mediated immune response.

T-helper and T-suppressor cells. T-helper (CD4) cells and T-suppressor (CD8) cells are involved in the regulation of the humoral antibody response and cell-mediated immunity, providing a positive and a negative signal, respectively. These two cell types are often referred to as *immunoregulatory* cells. With many autoimmune diseases the number of T-suppressor cells decreases in proportion to the number of T-helper cells, thus resulting in an overaggressive immune response. The human immunodeficiency virus (HIV) invades T-helper cells, thus decreasing their number and function. Therefore individuals with HIV infection do not mount an aggressive immune response and are at an increased risk for opportunistic infections and malignancies.

Natural Killer Cells. Natural killer (NK) cells are also involved in cell-mediated immunity. These cells are not T or B cells and have granules in the cytoplasm. Thus they are often referred to as *large granular lymphocytes.* NK cells do not require prior sensitization for their generation. These cells are involved in nonspecific killing of virally transformed cells, transplanted grafts, resistance to some infections, and tumor rejection. They have a significant role in immune surveillance for malignant cell changes.

Cytokines. The immune response involves complex interactions of T cells, B cells, monocytes, and neutrophils. These interactions depend on *cytokines* (soluble factors secreted by these cells) acting as messengers between the cell types. These cytokines can be classified as *lymphokines* (secreted by lymphocytes) and *monokines* (secreted by monocytes or macrophages). Cytokines instruct cells to alter their proliferation, differentiation, secretion, or activity. There are currently at least 60 different cytokines and they can be classified into distinct categories. Some of these cytokines are listed in Table 10-4.

In general, the interleukins and colony-stimulating factors act as immunomodulatory and growth-regulating factors for hematopoietic cells. The interferons are antiviral and immunomodulatory.[1]

Cytokines have a beneficial role in hematopoiesis and immune function. They can also have detrimental effects in inflammation, autoimmunity, and infection. Cytokines such as erythropoietin (see Chapter 44), colony-stimulating factors (see Chapters 12 and 28), interferons (see Chapters 12 and 41), and interleukin-2 (see Chapter 12) are used clinically either to stimulate hematopoiesis or to modulate tumor immunity. In addition, inhibitors of cytokines such as tumor necrosis factor and interleukin-1 are being used in clinical trials as antiinflammatory agents.

Interferon. Interferon, one type of lymphokine, was identified in 1957 as a substance that helps the body's natural defenses attack tumors and viruses. Three types of interferon have now been identified (see Table 10-4). In addition to their direct antiviral properties, interferons have immunoregulatory functions (e.g., enhancement of NK cell production and activation as well as inhibition of tumor cell growth).

Interferon is not directly antiviral but produces an antiviral effect in cells by reacting with them and inducing the formation of a second protein called *antiviral protein* (Fig. 10-5). This protein mediates the antiviral action of interferon by altering the cell's protein synthesis and preventing new viruses from becoming assembled. Interferons are currently being tested in clinical trials to evaluate their effectiveness in treating malignancies (see Chapter 12).

Macrophages. Lymphokines attract and activate macrophages in the area of the immune reaction. These macrophages secrete cytokines that further modulate the immune response. In addition, they can release lysosomal enzymes that damage surrounding tissues. (Macrophages are discussed in Chapter 9.)

Summary of Immune Responses

Humans need both humoral and cell-mediated immunity to remain healthy. Each type of immunity has unique properties and different methods of action; each reacts against particular antigens. Table 10-5 compares humoral and cell-mediated immunity.

Effects of Aging on the Immune System

With advancing age there is a decline in the immune system (Table 10-6). The primary clinical evidence for this immunosenescence is the high incidence of tumors in older adults. A greater susceptibility also occurs to infections (such as influenza and pneumonia) from pathogens that an

Table 10-4 Cytokines

Type	Primary Functions
Interleukins (IL)	
IL-1	Augments the immune response; inflammatory mediator; activates T cells; activates phagocytes; promotes prostaglandin production; induces a fever
IL-2	Activates T lymphocytes and NK cells; promotes growth and proliferation of T cells
IL-3 (multi-CSF)	Hematopoietic growth factor for hematopoietic precursor cells
IL-4	Growth factor for T cells, B cells, and mast cells; macrophage-activating factor; upregulates humoral immune response
IL-5	Promotes growth and proliferation of B cells
IL-6	B-cell stimulatory and differentiation factor; promotes hematopoiesis, enhances the inflammatory response
IL-7	Promotes growth of T and B cells
IL-8 (also known as neutrophil-activating protein)	Triggers chemotactic activity of neutrophils and lymphocytes; activates neutrophils
IL-9	T-cell and mast-cell growth factor; supports maturation of erythroid progenitors
IL-10	Inhibits proliferation of helper T cells; induces HLA antigen expression; upregulates the humoral immune response
IL-11	Is a multifunctional regulator of hematopoiesis and lymphopoiesis
IL-12	Stimulates T cells to make γ-interferon, activates NK cells
IL-13	Affects differentiation and function of monocytes and macrophages, generally suppressing cytotoxic functions
Interferons	
α-interferon	Provides antiviral protection; activates NK cells
β-interferon	Provides antiviral protection
γ-interferon	Activates macrophages; stimulates NK cell activity; inhibits proliferation of neoplastic cells; promotes B-cell differentiation
Tumor necrosis factor (TNF)	Promotes the immune and inflammatory responses; kills tumor cells
Colony-stimulating factors (CSF)	
Granulocyte colony-stimulating factor (G-CSF)	Promotes the proliferation and differentiation of neutrophils
Granulocyte macrophage colony-stimulating factor (GM-CSF)	Supports the growth of granulocytes and monocytes; activates neutrophils
Macrophage colony-stimulating factor (M-CSF)	Promotes the proliferation and differentiation of monocytes and macrophages
Erythropoietin (EPO)	Stimulates erythroid progenitor cells to produce red blood cells

HLA, human leukocyte antigen; *NK*, natural killer.

older person has been relatively immunocompetent against earlier in life.[2]

Aging does not affect all aspects of the immune system. The bone marrow is relatively unaffected by increasing age. However, aging has a pronounced effect on the thymus, which involutes proportionally to aging. This involution is probably a primary cause of immunosenescence. Both T and B cells show deficiencies in activation, transit time through the cell cycle, and subsequent differentiation. The most significant alterations seem to involve T cells. As thymic output of T cells diminishes, the differentiation of T cells in peripheral lymphoid structures increases. Consequently, there is an accumulation of memory cells rather than new precursor cells responsive to previously unencountered antigens.[3]

Delayed hypersensitivity response, as determined by skin testing with injected antigens, is frequently decreased or absent in older adults. This altered response reflects *anergy* (immunodeficient condition characterized by lack of or diminished reaction to an antigen or group of antigens). The clinical consequences of a decline in cell-mediated immunity are evident. Anergic responses to delayed hypersensitivity skin tests in older adults are related to an increased risk of cancer mortality as well as mortality in general.[2]

ALTERED IMMUNE RESPONSE

The immune system normally reacts protectively against the presence of foreign antigens. However, sometimes the response is overreactive and results in tissue damage. This is called a *hypersensitivity reaction*. A type of hypersensitivity response occurs when the body fails to recognize self-proteins and reacts against its own protein. Tissue damage resulting from this mechanism is called *autoimmunity*. Finally, tissue damage may occur if the immune system is deficient. The immunodeficiency state may be primary or secondary to other diseases.

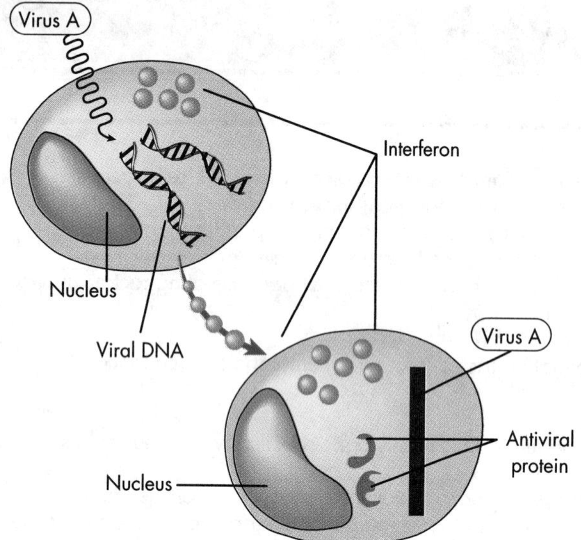

Fig. 10-5 Mechanism of action of interferon. Virus A attacks a cell. The cell begins to synthesize viral DNA and interferon. Interferon serves as an intercellular messenger. Interferon induces the production of antiviral proteins. Virus A is not able to replicate in the cell.

Table 10-5 Comparison of Humoral Immunity and Cell-Mediated Immunity

Characteristics	Humoral Immunity	Cell-Mediated Immunity
Cells involved	B lymphocytes	T lymphocytes, macrophages
Products	Antibodies	Sensitized T cells, lymphokines
Memory cells	Present	Present
Reaction	Immediate	Delayed
Protection	Bacteria Viruses (extracellular) Respiratory and gastrointestinal pathogens	Fungus Viruses (intracellular) Chronic infectious agents Tumor cells
Examples	Anaphylactic shock Atopic diseases Transfusion reaction Neutralization of exotoxins Bacterial infections	Tuberculosis Fungal infections Contact dermatitis Graft rejection Destruction of cancer cells

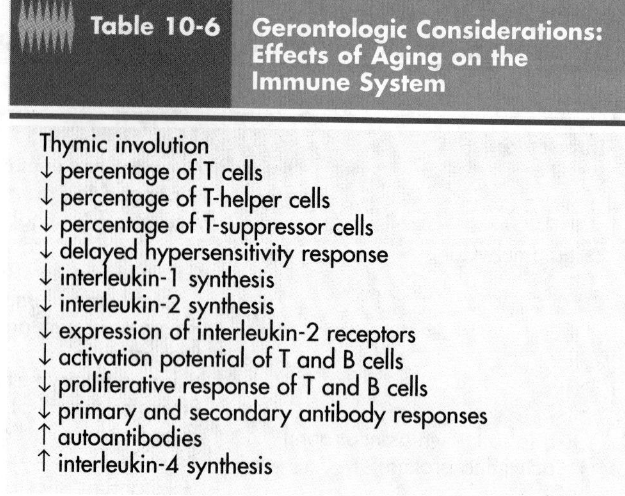
Table 10-6 Gerontologic Considerations: Effects of Aging on the Immune System

Thymic involution
↓ percentage of T cells
↓ percentage of T-helper cells
↓ percentage of T-suppressor cells
↓ delayed hypersensitivity response
↓ interleukin-1 synthesis
↓ interleukin-2 synthesis
↓ expression of interleukin-2 receptors
↓ activation potential of T and B cells
↓ proliferative response of T and B cells
↓ primary and secondary antibody responses
↑ autoantibodies
↑ interleukin-4 synthesis

Hypersensitivity Reactions

Classification of hypersensitivity reactions may be done according to the source of the antigen, time sequence (immediate or delayed), or the basic immunologic mechanisms causing the injury (Gell and Coombs classification). The Gell and Coombs classification is the most comprehensive. Basically, four types of hypersensitivity reactions exist. Types I, II, and III are immediate and are examples of humoral immunity. Type IV is a delayed hypersensitivity reaction and is related to cell-mediated immunity. Table 10-7 presents a summary of the four types of hypersensitivity reactions.

Type I: Anaphylactoid Reactions. Anaphylactoid reactions are type I reactions that occur *only* in susceptible persons who are highly sensitized to specific allergens. IgE antibodies, produced in response to the allergen, have a characteristic property of attaching to mast cells and basophils (see Fig. 25-2). Within these cells are granules containing potent chemical mediators (histamine, serotonin, slow-reacting substance of anaphylaxis [SRS-A], eosinophil chemotactic factor-anaphylaxis [ECF-A], kinins, and bradykinin). (Leukotriene components [LTC_4, LTD_4, and LTE_4] of slow-reacting substance of SRS-A are presented in Chapter 9 and Fig. 9-9.) On the first exposure to the allergen, IgE antibodies are produced. On any subsequent exposures, the allergen links with the IgE bound to mast cells or basophils and triggers degranulation of the cells. In this process, mediators are released, which then attack target organs, causing clinical allergy symptoms (Fig. 10-6). These effects include smooth muscle contraction, increased vascular permeability, vasodilatation, hypotension, increased secretion of mucus, and itching. Fortunately, the mediators are short-acting and their effects are reversible. (The mediators and their effects are summarized in Table 10-8.)

A genetic predisposition for the development of allergic diseases exists. The capacity to become sensitized to an allergen appears to be the inherited trait rather than the

Table 10-7 Types of Hypersensitivity Reactions

	Type I Anaphylactic	Type II Cytotoxic	Type III Immune-complex-mediated	Type IV Delayed-hypersensitivity
Antigen	Exogenous pollen, food, drugs, dust	Cell surface of RBC Basement membrane	Extracellular fungal, viral, bacterial	Intracellular or extracellular
Antibody involved	IgE	IgG IgM IgA	IgG IgM IgA	None
Complement involved	No	Yes	Yes	No
Mediators of injury	Histamine SRS-A	Complement lysis Neutrophils	Neutrophils Complement lysis	Lymphokines T-cytotoxic cells Monocytes/ macrophages Lysosomal enzymes
Examples	Allergic rhinitis Asthma	Transfusion reaction Goodpasture's syndrome	Serum sickness Systemic lupus erythematosus Rheumatoid arthritis	Contact dermatitis Tumor rejection Transplant rejection
Skin test	Wheal and flare	None	Erythema and edema in 3-8 hr	Erythema and edema in 24-48 hr (e.g., TB test)

RBC, Red blood cell; *SRS-A,* slow-reacting substance of anaphylaxis; *TB,* tuberculosis.

specific allergic disorder. For example, a father with asthma may have a son who has allergic rhinitis.[4]

The clinical manifestations of an anaphylactoid reaction depend on whether the mediators remain local or become systemic or whether they affect particular organs. When the mediators remain localized, a cutaneous response called the *wheal-and-flare reaction* occurs. This reaction is characterized by a pale wheal containing edematous fluid surrounded by a red flare from the hyperemia. The reaction occurs in minutes or hours and is usually not dangerous. A classic example of a wheal-and-flare reaction is the mosquito bite. The reaction serves a diagnostic purpose as a means of demonstrating allergic reactions to specific allergens during skin tests.

Common allergic reactions include anaphylactic shock (anaphylaxis), allergic asthma, allergic rhinitis, atopic dermatitis, urticaria, and angioedema.

Anaphylactic shock. Anaphylactic shock (anaphylaxis) occurs when mediators are released systemically (e.g., after injection of a drug or after an insect sting). The reaction occurs within minutes and is life-threatening because of airway obstruction and vascular collapse. The target organs affected are seen in Fig. 10-7. Initial symptoms include edema and itching at the site of the exposure to the allergen. Within minutes, shock manifested by rapid, weak pulse; hypotension; dilated pupils; dyspnea; and cyanosis may occur. This is compounded by bronchial edema and angioedema. Death will occur if emergency treatment is not initiated. Some of the important allergens leading to anaphylactic shock in hypersensitive persons are listed in Table 10-9.

Atopic reactions. An estimated 20% of the population is *atopic,* an inherited tendency to become sensitive to environmental allergens.[4] The atopic diseases that can result are allergic rhinitis, asthma, atopic dermatitis, urticaria, and angioedema.

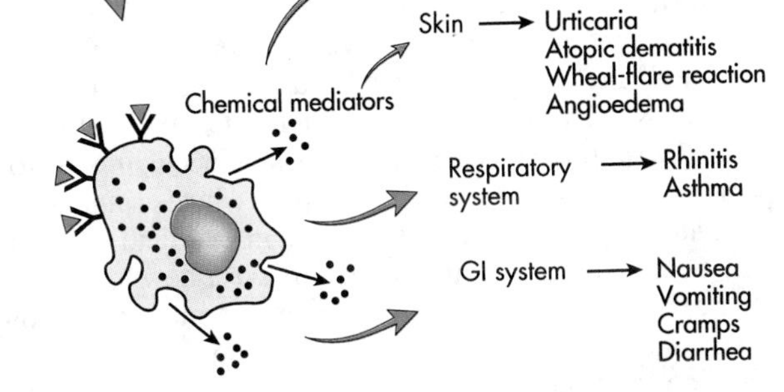

Fig. 10-6 Steps in an allergic type I reaction. *GI,* Gastrointestinal.

Table 10-8 Chemical Mediators of Allergic Response

Source and Storage	Biologic Activity	Pathologic Outcomes
Histamine		
Mast cell and basophil granules	Increases vascular permeability; constricts smooth muscle; stimulates irritant receptors	Edema of airways and larynx; bronchial constriction; urticaria, angioedema, pruritus; nausea, vomiting, diarrhea; shock
Leukotrienes		
Metabolites of arachidonic acid by lipoxygenase pathway*	Constrict bronchial smooth muscle; increase vascular permeability	Bronchial constriction; enhanced effect of histamine on smooth muscle
Prostaglandins		
Metabolites of arachidonic acid by cyclooxygenase pathway	Stimulate vasodilatation; constrict smooth muscle	Wheal-and-flare reaction on skin; hypotension; bronchospasm
Platelet-Activating Factor		
Mast cell	Aggregates platelets; stimulates vasodilatation	Increase in pulmonary artery pressure; systemic hypotension
Kinins		
Kininogen	Stimulate slow, sustained smooth muscle contraction; increase vascular permeability; stimulate secretion of mucus; stimulate pain receptors	Angioedema with painful swelling; bronchial constriction
Serotonin		
Platelets	Increases vascular permeability; stimulates smooth muscle contraction	Mucosal edema; bronchial constriction
Eosinophil Chemotactic Factor		
Mast cells	Promotes chemotaxis of eosinophils	Influx of eosinophils
Anaphylatoxins		
C3a, C4a, C5a from complement activation	Stimulate histamine release	Same as for histamine

*See Fig. 9-9.

Allergic rhinitis or *hay fever* is the most common type I hypersensitivity reaction. It may occur year-round (perennial allergic rhinitis), or it may be seasonal (seasonal allergic rhinitis). Airborne substances are the primary cause of allergic rhinitis. Perennial allergic rhinitis may be caused by dust, molds, and animal dander. Seasonal allergic rhinitis is commonly caused by trees, weeds, or grasses.[5] The target areas affected are the conjunctiva of the eyes and the mucosa of the upper respiratory tract. Symptoms include nasal discharge; sneezing; lacrimation; mucosal swelling with airway obstruction; and pruritus around the eyes, nose, throat, and mouth. (Treatment of allergic rhinitis is discussed in Chapter 23.)

Many patients with *asthma* have an allergic component to their disease. These patients frequently have a history of atopic disorders (e.g., infantile eczema, allergic rhinitis, or food intolerances). In asthma, SRS-A and histamine are primarily responsible for action on the bronchioles (see Fig. 25-2). These mediators produce bronchial smooth muscle constriction, excessive secretion of viscoid mucus, edema of the mucous membranes of the bronchi, and decreased lung compliance. Because of these physiologic alterations, patients manifest dyspnea, wheezing, coughing, tightness in the chest, and thick sputum. (Pathophysiology and management of asthma are discussed in Chapter 25.)

Atopic dermatitis is a chronic, inherited skin disorder characterized by exacerbations and remissions. It is caused by several environmental allergens that are difficult to identify. Children with infantile eczema frequently have allergic respiratory disorders, although the relationship between the two is not fully understood. Although patients with atopic dermatitis have elevated IgE levels and positive skin tests, the histopathologic features do not represent the typical, localized wheal-and-flare type I reactions. The skin lesions are more generalized and involve vasodilation of blood vessels, resulting in interstitial edema with vesicle formation (Fig. 10-8). (Dermatitis is discussed in Chapter 20.)

Urticaria (hives) is a cutaneous lesion occurring in atopic persons. It is characterized by transient wheals (pink, raised, edematous, pruritic areas) that vary in size and shape and may occur throughout the body. Urticaria develops rapidly after exposure to an allergen and may last minutes or hours. Histamine causes localized vasodilatation (erythema), transudation of fluid (wheal), and stimulation of local axon reflexes (flaring). Internal urticaria is characterized by edema in internal organs. Histamine is also responsible for

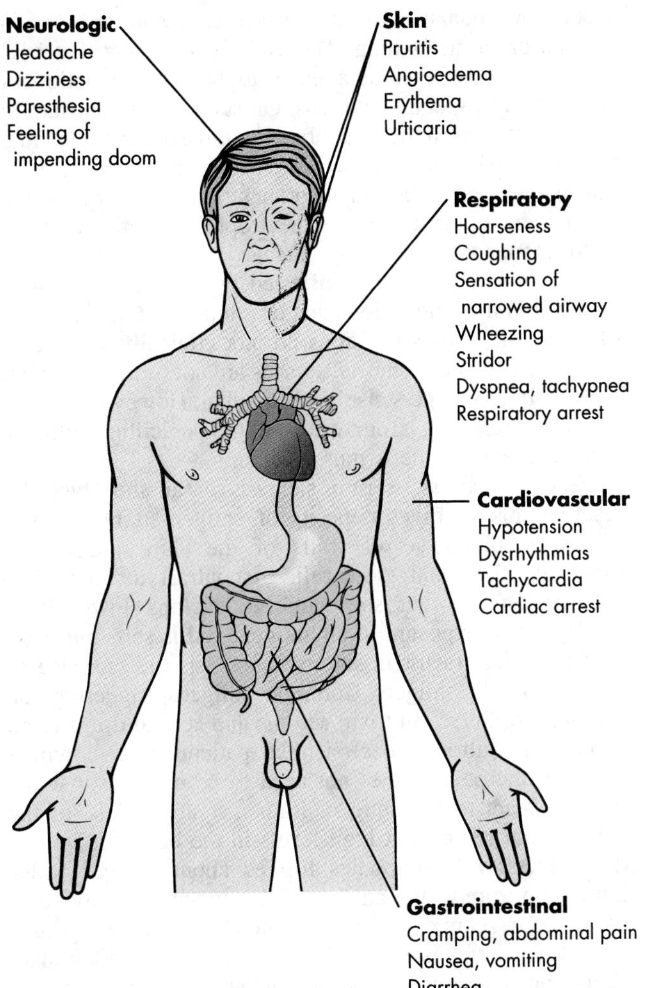

Fig. 10-7 Clinical manifestations of a systemic anaphylactic reaction.

Table 10-9 Allergens Causing Anaphylactic Shock

Drugs	
Penicillins	Sulfonamides
Insulins	Aspirin
Tetracycline	Local anesthetics
Chemotherapeutic agents	Cephalosporins
Nonsteroidal antiinflammatory agents	
Insect Venoms	
Hymenoptera*	
Foods	
Eggs	Milk
Nuts	Peanuts
Shellfish	Fish
Chocolate	Strawberries
Animal Serums	
Tetanus antitoxin	Rabies antitoxin
Diphtheria antitoxin	Snake venom antitoxin
Treatment Measures	
Blood products (whole blood and components)	Iodine-contrast media dye for IVP or angiogram test
Allergenic extracts in hyposensitization therapy	

IVP, Intravenous pyelography.
*Wasps, hornets, yellow jackets, bumblebees, and ants.

the numbness and pruritus associated with the lesions. (Urticaria is discussed in Chapter 20.)

Angioedema is a localized cutaneous lesion similar to urticaria but involving deeper layers of the skin and the submucosa. The principal areas of involvement include the eyelids, lips, tongue, larynx, hands, feet, gastrointestinal (GI) tract, and genitalia. Swelling usually occurs in only one area at a time. Dilatation and engorgement of the capillaries secondary to release of histamine cause the diffuse swelling. Welts are not apparent as in urticaria; the outer skin appears normal or has a reddish hue. The lesions may burn, sting, or itch and can cause acute pain if in the GI tract. The swelling may occur suddenly or over several hours and it usually lasts for 24 hours.

Type II: Cytotoxic and Cytolytic Reactions. Cytotoxic and cytolytic reactions are type II hypersensitivity reactions involving the direct binding of IgG, IgM, or IgA antibodies to an antigen on the cell surface. Antigen-antibody complexes activate the complement system, which mediates the reaction. Cellular tissue is destroyed in one of two ways: (1) activation of the complement cascade resulting in cytolysis, and (2) enhanced phagocytosis from complement fixation.

Target cells frequently destroyed in type II reactions are erythrocytes, platelets, and leukocytes. Some of the antigens involved are the ABO blood group, Rh factor, and drug haptens such as chloramphenicol. Pathophysiologic disorders characteristic of type II reactions include ABO incompatibility transfusion reaction, Rh incompatibility transfusion reaction, autoimmune and drug-related hemolytic anemias, leukopenias, thrombocytopenias, erythroblastosis fetalis (hemolytic disease of the newborn), and Goodpasture's syndrome. The tissue damage usually occurs rapidly.

Hemolytic transfusion reactions. A classic type II reaction occurs when a recipient receives ABO-incompatible blood from a donor. Naturally acquired antibodies to antigens of the ABO blood group are within the recipient's serum but are not present on the erythrocyte membranes (see Table 27-8). For example, a person with type A blood has anti-B antibodies, a person with type B blood has anti-A antibodies, a person with type AB blood has no antibodies, and a person with type O blood has both anti-A and anti-B antibodies.

If the recipient is transfused with incompatible blood, antibodies immediately coat the foreign erythrocytes, causing agglutination (clumping). The clumping of cells blocks small blood vessels in the body and depletes the clotting factors, leading to bleeding. Within hours, neutrophils and macrophages phagocytize the agglutinated cells. As complement is fixed to the antigen, cytolysis occurs. Cellular lysis

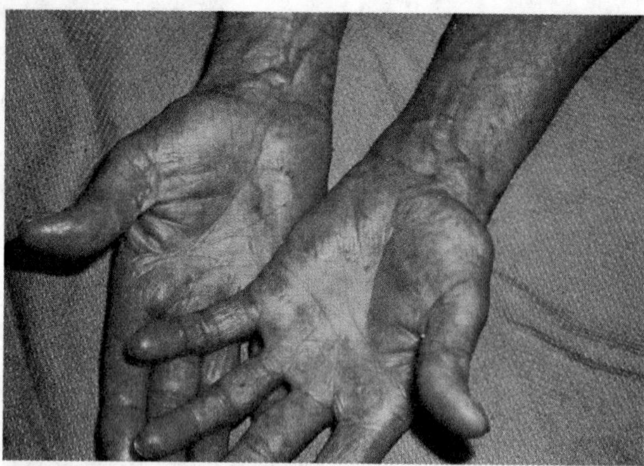

Fig. 10-8 Chronic lesions of atopic dermatitits on the hands of a woman; erythema, crusts, and cracks are evident.

causes the release of hemoglobin into the urine and plasma. In addition, a cytotoxic reaction causes vascular spasms in the kidney, which further block the renal tubules. Acute renal failure can result from the hemoglobinuria. (Blood transfusions are discussed in Chapter 28.)

Goodpasture's syndrome. Goodpasture's syndrome is a rare disorder involving the lungs and kidneys. An antibody-mediated autoimmune reaction occurs with the glomerular and alveolar basement membranes. The circulating antibodies combine with tissue antigen to activate complement, which causes deposits of IgG to form along the basement membranes of the lungs or kidney. This reaction may result in pulmonary hemorrhage and glomerulonephritis. The disease is usually rapidly progressive and fatal. Corticosteroids may induce temporary remission but will not prevent death. Plasmapheresis offers the most hope. (Goodpasture's syndrome is discussed in more detail in Chapter 43.)

Type III: Immune-Complex Reactions. Tissue damage in immune-complex reactions, which are type III reactions, occurs secondary to antigen-antibody complexes. Soluble antigens combine with immunoglobulins of the IgG and IgM classes to form complexes that are too small to be effectively removed by the mononuclear phagocyte system. Therefore the complexes deposit in tissue or small blood vessels. They cause the fixation of complement and the release of chemotactic factors that lead to inflammation and destruction of the involved tissue.

Type III reactions may be local or systemic and immediate or delayed. The clinical manifestations depend on the number of complexes and the location in the body. Common sites for deposit are the kidneys, skin, joints, and blood vessels. Severe type III reactions are associated with autoimmune disorders such as systemic lupus erythematosus, acute glomerulonephritis, and rheumatoid arthritis. Two classic disorders that illustrate type III reactions are the Arthus reaction and serum sickness.

Arthus reaction. The Arthus reaction is a localized inflammatory response resulting from antigen-antibody complexes deposited in the small vessels of the skin. It may occur from inhalation of dust or spores, resulting in pneumonitis or farmer's lung. The underlying defect that triggers an Arthus reaction appears to be the production of excess IgG to specific antigens. On subsequent exposure to soluble antigens, antigen-antibody complexes form, leading to a type III reaction. Because of the chemotactic substances released by complement, neutrophils infiltrate to the site of the complex. These neutrophils are the primary factor responsible for tissue damage.

Arthus reactions are manifested by edematous, hemorrhagic, and necrotic lesions that develop over 6 to 12 hours. Most classic Arthus reactions are not clinically significant because strong antigenic substances are not ordinarily given repeatedly to a hypersensitive individual. However, allergic vasculitis resulting from drugs (e.g., penicillin, sulfonamides) resembles the Arthus reaction.

Serum sickness. Serum sickness is another type III reaction that involves deposits of antigen-antibody complexes in blood vessel walls of the skin, joints, and especially the renal glomeruli. In contrast to an Arthus reaction, this disorder is systemic. It develops slowly, 10 to 14 days after exposure to an antigen, and is self-limiting.

The critical factor in serum sickness is the presence of excess soluble antigen. Common antigens triggering the reaction are horse antitoxin serums and certain drugs (e.g., penicillins, sulfonamides). Unlike patients with a type I reaction, the person does not need to be previously sensitized to react to the antigen. Rather, a single dose of the antigen that remains at high levels in the body for several days reacts with antibodies formed about 2 weeks after initial exposure to the antigen. The antigen-antibody complex then triggers complement to deposit in vessels, resulting in an intravascular inflammation. The predominant signs and symptoms of serum sickness are urticaria, angioedema, fever, muscle soreness, malaise, lymphadenopathy, joint pain, polyarthritis, and nephritis.

Fortunately, serum sickness reactions from the use of horse antitoxin serum can be avoided by using human serums. However, watching for drug sensitivities is still critical. The actual treatment of serum sickness depends on the severity of the reaction. For mild reactions, aspirin is prescribed for the fever and arthritis, and antihistamines are given for urticaria and angioedema. Corticosteroids are prescribed for more severe reactions, especially when renal or neurologic changes are present.

Type IV: Delayed Hypersensitivity Reactions. A delayed hypersensitivity reaction—a type IV reaction—is also called a *cell-mediated immune response*. However, a cell-mediated response is a protective mechanism; tissue damage occurs in delayed hypersensitivity reactions.

The tissue damage in a type IV reaction does not occur in the presence of antibodies or complement. Rather, sensitized T lymphocytes attack antigens or release lymphokines. Some of these lymphokines attract macrophages into the area. The macrophages and enzymes released by them are responsible for most of the tissue destruction. The delayed hypersensitivity response takes 24 to 48 hours for a reaction to occur.

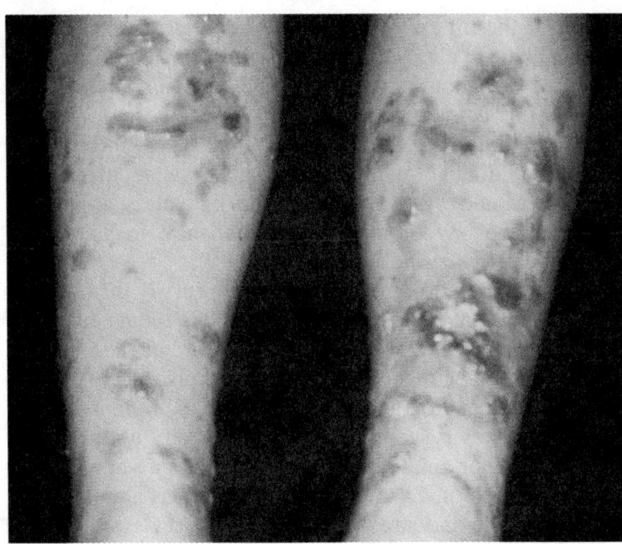

Fig. 10-9 Acute contact dermatitis on lower extremities. Note the edema, erythema, papules, bullae, and weeping vesicles.

Clinical examples of a delayed hypersensitivity reaction include contact dermatitis; hypersensitivity reactions to bacterial, fungal, and viral infections; and transplant rejections. Some drug sensitivity reactions also fit this category.

Contact dermatitis. *Allergic contact dermatitis* is an example of a delayed hypersensitivity reaction involving the skin. The reaction occurs when the skin is exposed to haptens. The haptens easily penetrate the skin to combine with epidermal proteins. The hapten-carrier substance then becomes antigenic. Over a period of 7 to 14 days, memory cells form to the antigen. On subsequent exposure to the hapten, a sensitized person develops eczematous skin lesions within 48 hours. The most common haptens encountered are metal compounds (e.g., nickel, mercury); rubber compounds; catechols present in poison ivy, poison oak, and sumac; cosmetics; and some dyes.

In acute contact dermatitis the skin lesions appear erythematous and edematous and are covered with papules, vesicles, and bullae (Fig. 10-9). The involved area is very pruritic but may also burn or sting. When contact dermatitis becomes chronic, the lesions resemble atopic dermatitis because they are thickened, scaly, and lichenified. The main difference between contact dermatitis and atopic dermatitis is that contact dermatitis is localized and restricted to the area exposed to the allergens, and atopic dermatitis is widespread.

Microbial hypersensitivity reactions. Although cell-mediated immunity plays an important defensive role in destroying viruses, bacteria, and fungi, delayed hypersensitivity reactions do occur as the surrounding tissue is damaged. Examples of infectious delayed hypersensitivity reactions include skin rashes of measles and smallpox, lesions of leprosy and herpes simplex virus, and the generalized toxemia and caseous necrosis with tuberculosis.

The classic example of a bacterial cell-mediated immune reaction is the body's defense against the tubercle bacillus. Tuberculosis results from invasion of lung tissue by highly resistant tubercle bacillus. The organism itself does not directly damage the lung tissue and may live in the host for some time before symptoms appear. However, antigenic material released from the tubercle bacilli reacts with T lymphocytes over time, initiating a cell-mediated response. The resulting lymphocytotoxicity causes extensive caseous necrosis of the lung.

After the initial cell-mediated reaction, memory cells persist, so subsequent contact with the tubercle bacillus or an extract of purified protein from the organism causes a delayed hypersensitivity reaction. This is the basis for the purified protein derivative (PPD) tuberculosis skin test read 48 to 72 hours after the injection. (Tuberculosis is discussed in Chapter 24.)

Transplant rejection. Rejection of organs occurs by cell-mediated immunity if the donor organ does not perfectly match the recipient's human leukocyte antigens, also called *histocompatibility antigens*. The rejection can be prevented by closely matching ABO, Rh, and HLA antigens between donor and recipient. Unfortunately, many different HLA antigens exist, and a perfect match is nearly impossible unless the tissue is from oneself or an identical twin.

Graft rejection is a complicated process that involves sensitized T lymphocytes (see Fig. 44-18). If the tissue is mismatched, sensitized T lymphocytes arrive at regional lymph nodes within 6 to 10 days. The clinical signs of rejection appear in about 14 days when sensitized T lymphocytes attack the graft. At this time the vascularization stops and the tissue becomes necrosed. Common manifestations of transplant rejection include fever, malaise, localized graft tenderness, hypertension, leukocytosis, elevated sedimentation rate, and elevated enzyme studies.

Drugs that interfere with cell-mediated immune responses are given to recipients of transplanted organs. (Some of the agents used are summarized in Table 44-11.) Unfortunately, the use of immunosuppressant drugs can result in major complications including increased susceptibility to infection, increased risk of developing cancer, and graft-versus-host disease.

ALLERGIC DISORDERS

Although an alteration of the immune system may be manifested in many ways, allergies or type I hypersensitivity reactions are seen most frequently.

Assessment

For a thorough assessment of a patient with allergies, a complete data base must be obtained. This consists of a comprehensive patient history, physical examination, diagnostic workup, and skin testing for allergens.

Health History. A comprehensive history that covers family allergies, past and present allergies, and social and environmental factors is essential. The information may be obtained from the patient or the patient's caregiver.

LATEX ALLERGIES

Citation Mendyka BE and others. Latex hypersensitivity: an iatrogenic and occupational risk. *Am J Critical Care* 3:198-201, 1994.

Background Anaphylactic reactons to latex rubber have increased dramatically over the past several years. Before 1988 most of the allergic reactions to latex were described as delayed hypersensitivity reactions, usually in the form of contact dermatitis. The prevalence of latex allergies in health care workers ranges from 2.8% to 12%. The increased incidence is related to the use of latex gloves to prevent the spread of infectious diseases.

Problem Type I anaphylactic reaction is a systemic response characterized by local or systemic urticaria, rhinitis, conjunctivitis, bronchospasm, and cardiovascular collapse (see Fig. 10-7). Type IV delayed hypersensitivity response (contact dermatitis) is characterized by erythema, pruritis, scaling, vesicles, and papules. The most common denonminators in latex allergic reactions include frequent contact with latex and a history of allergies. Latex is present in many products including tracheal tubes, O_2 masks, urinary catheters, diaphragms, condoms, feeding nipples, intraaortic balloons, colostomy pouches, barium enema tips, and gloves.

Implications for Nursing Practice A thorough health history and history of any allergies should be collected on all patients with any complaints of latex contact symptoms. Latex-sensitive individuals should wear a Medic-Alert bracelet and carry an epinephrine kit. Nurses should be alert for the possible occurrence of latex sensitivities in their patients.

Family history, including information about atopic reactions in relatives, is especially important in identifying high-risk patients. The specific disorder, clinical manifestations, and treatments prescribed should be assessed.

Past and present allergies must be noted. Identifying the allergens that may have triggered a reaction is essential to control allergic reactions. Table 10-10 lists four major categories of allergens that should be evaluated. Determination of the time of year that an allergic reaction occurs can be a clue to a seasonal allergen. Information should also be obtained about any over-the-counter or prescription medications used to treat the allergies.

In addition to identification of the allergen, information about the clinical manifestations and course of allergic reaction should be obtained. If the patient is a woman, assessment of symptoms during pregnancy, menstruation, or menopause may be important.

Social and environmental factors, especially the physical environment, are very important. Questions about pets, trees, and plants on property; pollutants in the air; and cooling and heating systems in the home and workplace can provide valuable information about allergens. In addition, a daily or weekly food diary with a description of any untoward reactions is important. Of particular interest is a screening for any reaction to medication. Finally, questions about the patient's lifestyle and stress level should be reviewed in connection with the appearance of allergic symptoms.

Physical Examination. A comprehensive head-to-toe physical examination should be given to a patient with allergies, with particular attention focused on the site of the allergic manifestations. A comprehensive assessment that includes subjective and objective data should be obtained from the patient (Table 10-11).

Diagnostic Studies

Many specialized immunologic techniques can be performed to detect abnormalities of lymphocytes, eosinophils, and immunoglobulins. A complete blood count (CBC) and blood serology tests are commonly done.

A CBC with white blood cell (WBC) differential is required with an absolute lymphocyte count and eosinophil count. Cellular immunodeficiency is diagnosed if the lymphocyte count is below $1200/\mu l$ ($1.2 \times 10^9/L$). T- and B-cell quantification is used to diagnose immunodeficiency syndromes. The eosinophil count is elevated with type I hypersensitivity reactions involving IgE immunoglobulins. Serum IgE level is also generally elevated in type I hypersensitivity reactions and serves as a diagnostic indicator of atopic diseases. Radioallergosorbent test (RAST) is an in vitro diagnostic test for IgE antibodies to an allergen. The RAST involves the measurement of IgE with a specific

Table 10-10 Categories of Allergens

Inhalants	Contactants	Ingestants	Injectables
Pollens	Plants	Food	Drugs
Molds	Drugs	Food additives	Vaccines
Spores	Metals	Drugs	Insect stings
Animal dander	Cosmetics		
House dust	Dyes		
Mites	Fibers		
	Various chemicals		

Table 10-11 Nursing Assessment: Allergies

Subjective Data
Important Health Information
Past health history: Recurrent respiratory problems; seasonal exacerbations; unusual reactions to insect bites or stings; past and present allergies
Medications: Unusual reactions to any drugs or medication; use of over-the-counter medication, use of medications for allegies
Functional Health Patterns
Health perception–health management: Family history of allergies, malaise, fatigue
Nutritional-metabolic: Food intolerances; vomiting; itching
Elimination: Abdominal cramps; diarrhea
Activity-exercise: Hoarseness; cough; dyspnea
Role-relationship: Environmental factors, including pets
Objective Data
Integumentary
Rashes (note symmetry and location); dryness; scaliness; irritations; scratches; urticaria
Respiratory
Wheezing; stridor
EENT
Eyes: Allergic shiners; conjunctivitis; lacrimation; rubbing or excessive blinking; styes
Ears: Diminished hearing; immobile or scarred tympanic membranes
Nose: Allergic salute; nasal polyps; nasal voice; nose twitching; rhinitis; pale, boggy mucous membranes; sniffling; sneezing; swollen nasal passages; recurrent nosebleeds
Throat: Continual throat clearing; swollen lips or tongue; red throat; orofacial and dental deformities; mouth wrinkling with facial grimaces; palpable neck lymph nodes
Possible findings
Eosinophilia; elevated serum IgE levels; positive skin tests; abnormal chest and sinus x-rays

antigen. Although expensive, it is safe but less sensitive than skin tests for detecting allergens.

Sputum, nasal, and bronchial secretions also may be tested for the presence of eosinophils. If asthma is suspected, pulmonary function tests for vital capacity, forced expiratory volume, and maximum midexpiratory flow rates are helpful.

Skin Tests. Skin testing is generally used to confirm specific sensitivity in patients with atopic disease after the history has suggested possible allergens for testing.

Procedure. Skin testing may be done by one of two methods: (1) a cutaneous scratch or prick or (2) an intracutaneous injection. The areas of the body usually used in testing are the arms and back. Allergen extracts are applied to the skin in rows with a corresponding control site opposite the test site. Saline or another diluent is applied to the control site. In the *scratch test* the epidermal skin layer is scratched with a lancet and the allergen extract is applied at the site. The *prick test* involves placing a drop of allergen extract on the skin and then piercing the underlying epidermis with a needle. In the *intracutaneous method* the allergen extract is injected intradermally in rows, usually on the arm. Since the allergic reaction is more severe with this method, the test is used only for persons who did not react to cutaneous methods.

Results. If the person is hypersensitive to the allergen, a positive reaction will occur within minutes after insertion in the skin and may last for 8 to 12 hours. A positive reaction is manifested by a local wheal-and-flare response. The size of the positive reaction does not always correlate with the severity of allergy symptoms. False-positive and false-negative results may occur. Negative results from skin testing do not necessarily mean the person does not have an allergic disorder, and positive results do not necessarily mean that the allergen was causing the clinical manifestations. Positive results imply that the person is sensitized to that allergen. Therefore, correlating skin test results with the patient's history is very important.

Precautions. A highly sensitive person is always at risk for developing an anaphylactic reaction to skin tests. Therefore, a patient should never be left alone during the testing period. Sometimes skin testing is completely contraindicated and the RAST test is used. If a severe reaction does occur with a cutaneous test, the extract is immediately removed and antiinflammatory topical cream is applied to the site. For intracutaneous testing, the arm is used so that a tourniquet can be applied during a severe reaction. A subcutaneous injection of epinephrine may also be necessary.

Therapeutic Management

After an allergic disorder is diagnosed, the therapeutic treatment is aimed at reducing exposure to the offending allergen, treating the symptoms, and desensitizing the person through immunotherapy. All health care workers must be prepared for the rare but life-threatening anaphylactic reaction, which requires immediate medical and nursing interventions. It is extremely important that all of a patient's allergies are listed on the chart, the nursing care plan, and the medication record.

Anaphylaxis. Anaphylactic reactions occur suddenly in hypersensitive patients after exposure to the offending allergen. They may occur following parenteral injection of drugs (especially antibiotics) and insect stings. The cardinal principle in therapeutic management is *speed* in (1) recognition of signs and symptoms of an anaphylactic reaction, (2) maintenance of a patent airway, (3) prevention of spread of the allergen by using a tourniquet, (4) administration of drugs, and (5) treatment for shock. Table 10-12 summarizes the emergency treatment of anaphylactic shock.

Mild symptoms such as pruritis and urticaria can be controlled by administration of 0.2 to 0.5 ml epinephrine, diluted 1:1000, given subcutaneously every 20 minutes according to the physician's orders or a hospital emergency drug protocol. An intravenous infusion should be initiated to provide a route for administration of 5 ml epinephrine, diluted 1:10,000, at 5- to 10-minute intervals; volume

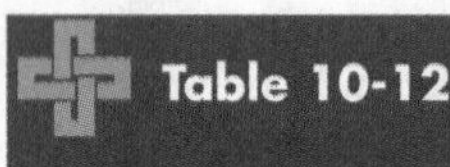

Table 10-12 Emergency Management: Anaphylactic Shock

Possible Etiologies
Injection, inhalation, ingestion of a substance that produces a profound allergic response (see Table 10-9)
Possible Assessment Findings
See Fig. 10-7.
Management
- Establish and maintain airway.
- When possible, apply tourniquet to decrease blood flow from source of antigen; remove stinger if an insect sting; remove tourniquet every 15 min.
- Administer epinephrine 1:1000, 0.2-0.5 ml subcutaneously with repeated doses at 20-min intervals for mild symptoms.
- Administer epinephrine 1:10,000, 5 ml IV at 5-10 min intervals for severe symptoms.
- Place patient in a recumbent position; elevate legs; keep patient warm; provide oxygen.
- Administer diphenhydramine (Benadryl) IM or IV.
- Maintain blood pressure with fluids, volume expanders, vasopressors (e.g., dopamine [Intropin], levarterenol [Levophed]).
- If wheezing is present, administer aminophylline IV.

IM, Intramuscular; *IV*, intravenous.

expanders; and vasopressor agents such as dopamine if intractable hypotension occurs.

Oxygen via a nasal catheter or intermittent positive pressure breathing of oxygen with isoproterenol (Isuprel) may be helpful. Endotracheal intubation or a tracheostomy is mandatory for O_2 delivery if progressive hypoxia exists. Other agents are used, including an antihistamine such as diphenhydramine (Benadryl) intravenously or intramuscularly for urticaria and angioedema and aminophylline intravenously for bronchospasm. Intravenous corticosteroids are not effective for the acute event but may be used for persistent bronchospasm and hypotension.

Hypovolemic shock may occur because of the loss of intravascular fluid into interstitial spaces. Peripheral vasoconstriction and stimulation of the sympathetic nervous system occur to compensate for the fluid shift. However, unless shock is treated early, the body will no longer be able to compensate, and irreversible tissue damage will occur, leading to death. (Hypovolemic shock is discussed in Chapter 7.)

Chronic Allergies. Most allergic reactions are chronic and are characterized by remissions and exacerbations of symptoms. Treatment focuses on identification and control of allergens, relief of symptoms through pharmacologic interventions, and hyposensitization of a patient to an offending allergen.

Allergen recognition and control. The nurse plays an important role in helping the patient make lifestyle adjustments so that there is minimal exposure to offending allergens. The nurse must reinforce that, even with drug therapy and immunotherapy, the patient will never be desensitized or completely symptom-free. The nurse can initiate various preventive measures that will help control the allergic symptoms.

Of primary importance is the need to identify the offending allergen. Sometimes this is done through skin testing. In the case of food allergies, an elimination diet is valuable. If an allergic reaction occurs, all food eaten should be eliminated and gradually reintroduced one at a time until the offending food is detected. In the case of infants with a strong family history of atopic disorders, new solid foods should be introduced one at a time.

Many allergic reactions, especially asthma and urticaria, may be aggravated by fatigue and emotional stress. The nurse can be instrumental in initiating a stress management program with the patient. Relaxation techniques can be practiced when the patient comes for frequent immunotherapy treatments.

Sometimes control of allergic symptoms requires environmental control, including changing an occupation, moving to a different climate, or giving up a favorite pet. In the case of airborne allergens, sleeping in an air-conditioned room, damp dusting daily, and wearing a mask outdoors may be helpful.

If the allergen is a drug, the patient should be instructed to avoid the drug. The patient also has the responsibility to make the drug intolerance well known to all health care providers. The patient should wear a medical-alert bracelet listing the particular drug allergy and have the offending drug listed on all medical and dental records.

For a patient allergic to insect stings, commercial bee-sting kits containing preinjectable epinephrine and a tourniquet are available. The nurse has the responsibility to instruct the patient about the technique of applying the tourniquet and self-injecting the subcutaneous epinephrine. This patient also should wear medical-alert bracelets and carry bee-sting kits whenever going outdoors.

Pharmacologic Management. The major categories of drugs used for symptomatic relief of chronic allergic disorders include antihistamines, sympathomimetic/decongestant drugs, corticosteroids, antipruritic drugs, and mast cell stabilizing drugs. Many of these drugs may be obtained over-the-counter and are often misused by patients.[6]

Antihistamines. Antihistamines are the best drugs for treatment of allergic rhinitis and urticaria (Table 10-13). They are less effective for severe allergic reactions. The drugs may be given intravenously or orally, applied topically, inhaled, or used as a nasal spray. They act by competing with histamine for H_1-receptor sites and thus blocking the effect of histamine. Best results are achieved if they are taken immediately after allergy signs and symptoms appear. Antihistamines are effective antagonists of edema and pruritus but relatively ineffective in preventing bronchoconstriction. With seasonal rhinitis, antihistamines should be taken during peak pollen seasons.

A number of side effects are associated with antihistamines, especially drowsiness, sedation, and disturbed coor-

Table 10-13 Common Drugs Used for Treatment of Allergic Rhinitis

Generic Name	Trade Name
Antihistamines	
Diphenhydramine	Benadryl
Azatadine maleate	Optimine
Carbinoxamine maleate	Clistin Histadyl
Triprolidine	Actidil
Brompheniramine maleate	Dimetane
Chlorpheniramine maleate	Coricidin, Chlor-Trimeton, Teldrin
Clemastine	Tavist
Terfenadine*	Seldane
Astemizole*	Hismanal
Loratadine*	Claritin
Decongestants	
Pseudoephedrine	Sudafed
Phenylephrine	Neo-Synephrine,
Oxymetazoline	Alconefrin, Sinex, Afrin, Dristan
Antihistamine/ Decongestant	
Clemastine/ phenylpropanolamine	Tavist D
Triprolidine/ pseudoephedrine	Actifed
Brompheniramine/ phenylpropanolamine	Dimetapp
Chlorpheniramine/ pseudoephedrine	Novafed A
Corticosteroids	
Nasal inhalers	
Beclomethasone	Beconase, Vancenase
Flunisolide	Nasalide
Mast-Cell Stabilizer	
Cromolyn	Intal, Nasalcrom, Rynacrom
Nedocromil	Tilade
Antipruritics	
Diphenhydramine	Benadryl
$ZnCO_3$	Calamine lotion
Methdilazine	Tacaryl

*Nonsedating.

dination. Therefore, patients should be cautioned about driving and operating machinery. Other side effects include dryness of mouth, GI upset, blurred vision, and dizziness.

Because of the difficulties with side effects, a new generation of antihistamines has been developed. Terfenadine (Seldane), astemizole (Hismanal), and loratadine (Claritin) do not readily cross the blood-brain barrier. Therefore, the central nervous system depression and anticholinergic side effects seen with other types of antihistamines are not frequently observed with these newer antihistamines. In addition, these drugs require administration only 1 or 2 times per day.

Sympathomimetic/decongestant drugs. The major sympathomimetic drug is epinephrine (Adrenalin), which is the drug of choice to treat an anaphylactic reaction. Epinephrine is a hormone produced by the adrenal medulla that stimulates α- and β-adrenergic receptors. Stimulation of the α receptors causes vasoconstriction of peripheral blood vessels. β-Receptor stimulation relaxes bronchial smooth muscle spasms. These drugs also act directly on mast cells to stabilize them against further degranulation. The action of epinephrine lasts only a few minutes. The drug must be given parenterally (usually subcutaneously).

Several specific, minor sympathomimetic drugs differ from epinephrine because they can be taken orally or nasally and last for several hours. Included in this category are phenylephrine (Neo-Synephrine) and pseudoephedrine (Sudafed). The minor sympathomimetic drugs are used primarily to treat allergic rhinitis. The action of these drugs includes nasal decongestion, reduction in nasal edema, elevation of blood pressure, and cardiac stimulation.

Of the drugs used in the management of chronic allergy patients, phenylephrine and pseudoephedrine are abused most frequently. Because these drugs may be bought over the counter, patients tend to overmedicate themselves. *Rhinitis medicamentosa*, a rebound effect in which nasal mucosa becomes more edematous and congested after medicating, may develop from the local overuse of nasal sprays containing ephedrine.

Corticosteroids. Nasal corticosteroid sprays are very effective in relieving the symptoms of allergic rhinitis (see Chapter 23 and Table 23-2).

Antipruritic drugs. Topically applied antipruritic drugs are most effective when the skin is not broken. These drugs protect the skin and provide relief from itching. Common over-the-counter drugs include calamine lotion, coal tar solutions, and camphor. Menthol and phenol may be added to other lotions to produce an antipruritic effect. Some more potent drugs that require a prescription include methdilazine (Tacaryl) and trimeprazine (Temaril). These drugs should be used with great caution because of the associated risk of agranulocytosis.

Mast cell–stabilizing drugs. Cromolyn (Intal, Nasalcrom, Rynacrom) and nedocromil (Tilade) are mast cell–stabilizing agents that inhibit the release of histamines, leukotrienes, and other agents from the mast cell after antigen-IgE interaction. They are available as an inhalant nebulizer solution, a nasal spray, or oral pill. They are used in the management of asthma (see Chapter 25) and treatment of allergic rhinitis (see Chapter 23). An important feature of these drugs is a very low incidence of side effects.

Immunotherapy. Immunotherapy is the recommended treatment for control of allergic symptoms when the allergen cannot be avoided and drug therapy is not effective. Immunotherapy is absolutely indicated only in individuals with anaphylactic reactions to insect venom. It involves administration of small titers of an allergen extract in increasing strengths until hyposensitivity to the specific allergen is achieved. For best results the patient should continue to avoid the offending allergen whenever possible because complete desensitization is impossible.

Mechanism of action. IgE immunoglobulin level is elevated in atopic individuals. When IgE combines with an allergen in a hypersensitive person, a reaction occurs, releasing histamine in various body tissues. Allergens more readily combine with IgG immunogobulin than with other immunoglobulins. Therefore, immunotherapy involves injecting allergen extracts that will stimulate increased IgG levels. The binding of IgG to allergen-reactive sites interferes with allergen binding to mast cell-bound IgE, preventing mast cell degranulation, and thus reduces the number of reactions that cause tissue damage. The goal of long-term immunotherapy is to keep "blocking" IgG levels high. In addition, allergen-specific T-suppressor cells develop in individuals receiving immunotherapy.

Method of administration. Immunotherapy involves the subcutaneous injection of titrated amounts of allergen extracts biweekly or weekly. The dose is small at first and is increased slowly until a maintenance dosage is reached. The maintenance dosage is given every 2 to 8 weeks for several years. For patients with severe allergies or sensitivity to insect stings, maintenance therapy is continued indefinitely. Best results are achieved when immunotherapy is administered throughout the year.

NURSING MANAGEMENT
IMMUNOTHERAPY

The nurse is often primarily responsible for giving immunotherapy. Adverse reactions should always be anticipated, especially when opening a new-strength vial, after a previous reaction, or after a missed dose. Early signs and symptoms indicative of a systemic reaction include pruritus, urticaria, sneezing, laryngeal edema, and hypotension. Emergency measures for anaphylactic shock should be initiated immediately. A local reaction should be described according to the degree of redness and swelling at the injection site. If the area is greater than the size of a nickel in a child or a fifty-cent piece in an adult, the reaction should be reported to the physician so that the allergen dosage may be decreased.

Immunotherapy always carries the risk of a severe anaphylactic reaction. Therefore, a physician, emergency equipment, and essential drugs should be available whenever injections are given. Important emergency equipment includes an oropharyngeal airway, laryngoscope, endotracheal tubes, oxygen, tourniquet, intravenous therapy equipment and fluids, and a cardiac monitor with a defibrillator. The essential drugs are epinephrine in an injectable syringe, antihistamines, corticosteroids, and vasopressor drugs.

Record keeping must be accurate and can be invaluable in preventing an adverse reaction to the allergen extract. Before giving an injection, the nurse should check the patient's name with the name on the vial. Next, the vial strength, amount of last dose, date of last dose, and any reaction information should be screened.

The physician should be consulted about the amount of allergen to administer whenever a previous severe reaction has occurred or the patient has missed the previous appointment. The dosage will have to be adjusted before administering the next dose.

The nurse should always administer the allergen extract in an extremity away from a joint so that a tourniquet can be applied for a severe reaction. The site should be rotated for each injection. The nurse must aspirate for blood before giving an injection to ensure that the allergen extract is not injected into a blood vessel. An injection directly into the bloodstream can potentiate an anaphylactic reaction. After the injection is given, the patient should be carefully observed for 20 minutes because systemic reactions are most likely to occur immediately. However, the patient should be warned that a delayed reaction can occur as long as 24 hours later.

AUTOIMMUNE PHENOMENA

Autoimmunity is a state of responsiveness to certain self-proteins; the immune system no longer differentiates self from nonself with respect to these substances. For some unknown reason, immune cells that are normally unresponsive (tolerant to self-antigens) are activated. Both T and B cells have the ability for tolerance to self-antigens. Therefore, an alteration in T cells alone or in both B cells and T cells can produce autoantibodies and autosensitized T cells to cause pathophysiologic tissue damage. The particular autoimmune disease manifested depends on which self-antigen is involved.[7]

Theories of Causation

The cause of autoimmune diseases is still unknown. Age plays some role, since the number of circulating autoantibodies increases in persons over age 50. It appears that no one theory is conclusive. A combination of etiologic factors may be involved.

Forbidden Clone Theory. Maturing lymphocytes in the central lymphoid organs encounter self-antigens during embryogenesis and, as lymphocytes reactive against self-antigens develop, their clones are prevented or forbidden from maturing. Autoimmunity may result from the survival of a forbidden clone and its proliferation later in life. These clones may become reactive against the body's own tissue, resulting in an autoimmune process.

Sequestered Antigen Theory. During embryonic development (when immune tolerance develops), certain tissues are normally separated or sequestered from the circulatory and lymph systems. These tissues include the lens of the eye, the thyroid, the testes, and the central nervous system. If later trauma, infection, or chemical exposure results in the cells' release into circulation, these cells will not be recognized as "self" and an autoimmune response will occur. Examples of this reaction include Hashimoto's thyroiditis and autoantibody formation against sperm after vasectomy and cardiac muscle after myocardial infarction.

Tissue Injury/Infections Theory. After severe trauma, necrosis, radiation, drugs, and infections, the body tissue is sometimes altered so that the body no longer recognizes it as "self." An example of this is hemolytic anemia secondary to methyldopa (Aldomet) administration.

Viral infections can cause an alteration of tissues that are not normally antigenic. There is some evidence that viruses may be involved in the development of multiple sclerosis and Type I diabetes mellitus.

Cross-reacting Antigen Theory. Autoimmunity sometimes develops because of the close structural resemblance between the body's own antigens and foreign antigens. The antibodies synthesized in response to the foreign invasion cross-react with healthy tissue. This appears to be the cause of rheumatic heart disease. Antibodies developed against group A β-hemolytic streptococcus cross-react with heart muscle, heart valves, and synovial membrane, causing tissue damage.

Genetic Instruction Theory. For an unknown reason the genetic instruction for antibody production is altered. There appears to be a genetic predisposition to develop autoimmune diseases within some families. Most of the research work in this area correlates certain HLA types with an autoimmune condition (discussed later in this chapter).

Diminished T-Suppressor Cell Function Theory. Decreased levels of T-suppressor cells have been noted in individuals with autoimmune disease. Suppressor cells are short-lived and may become less numerous with aging. The incidence of autoantibodies increases with age, presumably because atrophy of the thymus results in a decreased ability to produce new T-suppressor cells. If T-suppressor cells are decreased, immunoregulation is altered and antibody levels or T-cell responses are increased.

Autoimmune Diseases

Generally, autoimmune diseases are grouped according to *organ-specific* and *systemic* diseases. (See Table 10-14 for a summary of autoimmune diseases.)

Table 10-14 Autoimmune Diseases

Disease	Autoantigen	Comments
Systemic Diseases		
Systemic lupus erythematosus	DNA, DNA proteins	Circulating antinuclear antibodies attack DNA
Rheumatoid arthritis	IgG	Rheumatoid factor is an IgM that reacts with IgG
Progressive systemic sclerosis or scleroderma	DNA proteins	See Chapter 60
Mixed connective tissue disease	DNA proteins	See Chapter 60
Organ-Specific Diseases		
Blood		
Autoimmune hemolytic anemia	RBC surface	Drugs and trauma may alter the RBC surface antigens
Immune thrombocytopenic purpura	Platelet surface	See Chapter 28
Central nervous system		
Multiple sclerosis	Myelin sheath around nervous tissue	Possibly triggered by a viral infection; T-helper cells appear uncontrolled because of very reduced levels of T-suppressor cells
Guillain-Barré syndrome	Myelin sheath	Peripheral nerve damage
Muscle		
Myasthenia gravis	Muscle cells and thymus cells	See Chapter 56
Heart		
Rheumatic fever	Cross-reactive streptoccocal antigens	Occurs secondary to strep throat infection
Endocrine system		
Addison's disease	Adrenal cell	See Chapter 47
Thyroiditis	Thyroid cell surface	See Chapter 47
Hypothyroidism	Thyroid globulin	See Chapter 47
Type I diabetes mellitus	Islet cell antigens	See Chapter 46
Gastrointestinal tract		
Pernicious anemia	Intrinsic factor of parietal cells	See Chapter 28
Ulcerative colitis	Colon mucosal cells	See Chapter 40
Kidney		
Goodpasture's syndrome	Glomerular basement membrane	See Chapter 43
Glomerulonephritis	Cross-reactive streptococcal antigens	See Chapter 43
Liver		
Primary biliary cirrhosis	Mitochondria	See Chapter 41
Chronic active hepatitis	Virally infected liver cells	See Chapter 41
Eye		
Uveitis	Uvea	See Chapter 18

RBC, Red blood cell.

Autoimmune Hemolytic Anemia. Autoimmune hemolytic anemia is an organ-specific disease involving the erythrocytes. The autoimmune disease may be primary or secondary to other diseases such as systemic lupus erythematosus and lymphocytic leukemia. Regardless of the cause, the immune response is similar. The cause is unknown, but drugs and viruses may alter the antigenic structure of the erythrocyte membrane, making it more susceptible to hemolysis. In addition, some people appear to have a genetically determined susceptibility to form autoantibodies. Patients with hemolytic anemia present signs and symptoms of pallor, fatigue, fever, jaundice, splenomegaly, and hepatomegaly. (Hemolytic anemia is discussed in Chapter 28).

Systemic Lupus Erythematosus. Systemic lupus erythematosus is a classic example of a systemic autoimmune disease characterized by damage to multiple organs. It occurs most frequently in women ages 20 to 40 years. The etiology is unknown, but there appears to be a loss of self-tolerance for the body's own DNA antigens. Viruses, drugs, and genetic factors are believed to affect the self-tolerance.

Systemic lupus erythematosus meets the criteria of an autoimmune disease. Laboratory analysis reveals (1) elevated serum immunoglobulins because of hyperactive humoral immunity, (2) defective T-cell function, (3) deposition of antigen-antibody complexes in small blood vessels of various target organs, and (4) low serum-complement levels.

In systemic lupus erythematosus, tissue injury appears to be the result of the formation of antinuclear antibodies. For some reason (possibly a viral infection), the cell membrane is damaged and DNA is released into the systemic circulation where it is viewed as "nonself." This DNA is normally sequestered inside the nucleus of cells. On release into circulation the DNA antigen reacts with an antibody. Some antibodies are involved in immune complex formation, and others may cause damage directly. Once the complexes are deposited, complement is activated and further damages the tissue, especially the renal glomerulus. (Systemic lupus erythematosus is discussed in more detail in Chapter 60.)

Apheresis

Apheresis is the use of a procedure to separate components of the blood followed by the removal of one or more of these components. Compound words are used to describe any particular apheresis procedure, depending on the blood components being collected. *Cytapheresis* is a general term for cell separation and removal. *Leukocytapheresis* is a general term indicating the removal of WBCs and is used in chronic myelogenous leukemia to remove high numbers of leukemic cells. *Lymphocytapheresis* is used to decrease high lymphocyte counts in individuals with chronic lymphocytic leukemia. *Plasmapheresis* is the removal of plasma. When plasma is removed, it is replaced by substitution fluids such as saline or albumin. Therefore the term *plasma exchange* more accurately describes this procedure, although both terms are used simultaneously.[8]

Plasmapheresis has been used to treat antibody- or immune complex–mediated diseases such as systemic lupus erythematosus, rapidly progressive glomerulonephritis, Goodpasture's syndrome, myasthenia gravis, thrombocytopenic purpura, rheumatoid arthritis, and Guillain-Barré syndrome. Apheresis procedures are also done on healthy donors to obtain plasma and selected blood components to administer as replacement therapy for patients.

The rationale for performing therapeutic plasmapheresis in autoimmune disorders is to remove pathologic substances present in plasma. Many disorders for which plasmapheresis is being used are characterized by circulating autoantibodies (usually of the IgG class) and antigen-antibody complexes. Immunosuppressive therapy has been used to prevent recovery of IgG production, and plasmapheresis has been used to prevent antibody rebound.

In addition to removing antibodies and antigen-antibody complexes, plasmapheresis may also remove inflammatory mediators (such as complement) that are responsible for tissue damage. In the treatment of systemic lupus erythematosus, plasmapheresis is reserved for the patient in an acute attack who is unresponsive to conventional therapy. Plasmapheresis seems to lower the level of DNA antibodies and immune complexes, allowing the mononuclear phagocyte system to take control of removing immune complexes.

The procedure involves removal of whole blood through a needle inserted in one arm and circulation of the blood through a cell separator. Inside the separator the blood is divided into plasma and its cellular components by centrifugation or membrane filtration. A needle is inserted into the opposite arm for return of the blood to the patient. Plasma, platelets, WBCs, or RBCs can be separated selectively. The undesirable component is removed, and the remainder is returned to the patient. The plasma is generally replaced with normal saline, lactated Ringer's solution, fresh frozen plasma, plasma protein fractions, or albumin. When blood is manually removed, only 500 ml may be taken at one time. However, with the use of apheresis procedures, over 4 L of plasma can be pheresed in 2 to 3 hours.

As with administration of other blood products, nurses need to be aware of side effects associated with plasmapheresis. The most common complications are hypotension and citrate toxicity. Hypotension is usually the result of vasovagal reaction or transient volume changes. Citrate is used as an anticoagulant and may cause hypocalcemia, which may manifest as headache, paresthesias, and dizziness. Other complications that may arise are hepatitis (especially when fresh frozen plasma is used as replacement fluid), infections, depletion of coagulation factors, and electrolyte imbalances.[9]

Human Leukocyte Antigen System

The HLA system consists of a series of linked genes that occur together on the sixth chromosome in humans. The products of these genes include the cell membrane antigens of the HLA series. Because of its importance in the study of tissue matching in transplant rejection, the chromosomal region incorporating the HLA genes is referred to as the *major histocompatibility complex*. The genes determining the products recognized as the HLA-A, HLA-B, HLA-C,

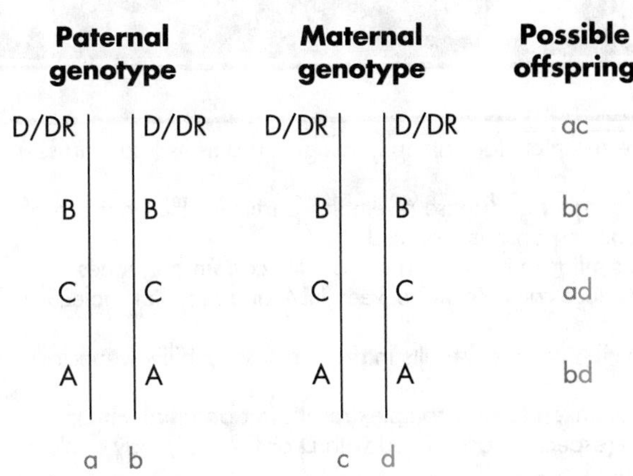

Fig. 10-10 Patterns of HLA inheritance. The two haplotypes of the father are labeled *a* and *b* and the haplotypes of the mother are labeled *c* and *d*. Each child inherits two haplotypes, one from each parent. Therefore, only four combinations—*ac, bc, ad,* and *bd*—are possible, and 25% of the offspring will have identical HLA haplotypes.

HLA-D, and HLA-DR antigens are clustered together (Fig. 10-10). HLA antigens are present on all nucleated cells and platelets.

A very important characteristic of HLA genes is that they are highly polymorphic. Each HLA locus has many possible alleles (antigens). The specific allele is identified by a number. For example, a person could be A6, B7, C8, D1, DR7. With many alleles possible at each HLA locus, many combinations exist. Each person has two antigens for each locus. Both antigens of a locus are expressed independently (i.e., they are codominant). The entire set of A, B, C, D, and DR antigens located on one chromosome is called a *haplotype*. A complete set of antigens located on a chromosome is usually inherited as a unit (haplotype). Figure 10-10 illustrates the inheritance of HLA haplotypes in a family.

Because of the polymorphic nature of the HLA system, it is an ideal marker for genetic studies. This characteristic also makes it a useful tool in settling paternity disputes. The frequencies of HLA antigens vary considerably among different races. For example, HLA-B8 is relatively high in American Caucasians, but is very low in Native American and Japanese persons.

HLA and Disease Associations. The early interest in HLA was stimulated by its potential role in matching donors and recipients of organ transplants. (Its role in transplantation is discussed in Chapter 44.) During the last few years, interest in the association between HLA and disease has grown (Table 10-15). Some very strong associations between HLA type and susceptibility to certain diseases have been demonstrated (Table 10-16). The discovery of HLA associations with certain diseases is a major breakthrough in understanding the genetic bases of these diseases. It is now known that at least part of the genetic bases of HLA-associated diseases lies in the HLA region, but the actual mechanism or mechanisms involved in these associations are still unknown. Various hypotheses have been proposed and these are briefly described in Table 10-17.

Diseases showing strong associations with A, B, and C antigens involve T-cytotoxic cells, whereas diseases strongly associated with DR antigens involve T-helper or T-suppressor lymphocytes. For example, DR-associated factors are thought to convey susceptibility to insulin-dependent diabetes mellitus. One hypothesis is that a virus infects the pancreatic islet cells of a DR3-positive person. The DR3 molecules on macrophages or other cells present the virus to T-helper cells. The

Table 10-15 Characteristics of Diseases Showing HLA Associations

1. Hereditary or familial tendencies
2. Immune or autoimmune features
3. Poorly understood etiology and pathophysiology
4. Subacute or chronic course
5. Little or no effect on reproductive capacity
6. Association with HLA-B or HLA-DR loci

Table 10-16 HLA Types and Disease Associations

Disease	HLA Type
Acute anterior uveitis	B27
Addison's disease	DR3
Ankylosing spondylitis	B27
Celiac disease	DR3 DR7 B8
Chronic active hepatitis	B8 DR3
Dermatitis herpetiformis	DR3
Diabetes mellitus, type I	DR3
Goodpasture's syndrome	DR2
Graves' disease	B35 DR3
Hashimoto's thyroiditis	DR3
Idiopathic hemochromatosis	A3
Multiple sclerosis	DR2
Myasthenia gravis	B8 DR3
Narcolepsy	DR2
Reiter's syndrome	B27
Rheumatoid arthritis	DR3 DR4
Sjögren's syndrome	B8 DW3
Systemic lupus erythematosus	B8 DW3

Table 10-17 Explanations for HLA and Disease Association

Mechanism	Description
Receptor theory	HLA antigens act as cell-surface receptors for pathophysiologic organisms (e.g., viruses) that cause disease
Molecular mimicry	Molecular structure of infectious agent of disease resembles particular HLA antigen of host so closely that no immune response is mounted
Interaction of HLA molecules with nonimmunologic factors	HLA molecules have structures similar to those on receptors for certain hormones (e.g, insulin, glucagon) that cause competition between HLA and receptor molecules for hormones
Involvement of genes closely linked with HLA complex	Specific disease gene linked to HLA complex results in disease susceptibility (especially with B locus)
	Immune response gene or genes linked to HLA complex results in abnormal immune response to specific antigens (especially associated with D or DR loci); may explain relationship with autoimmune diseases

Table 10-18 Primary Immunodeficiency Disorders

Disorder	Affected Cells	Genetic Basis
▪ Chronic granulomatous disease	PMN, monocytes	Sex-linked
▪ Job's syndrome	PMN, monocytes	
▪ Bruton's X-linked hypogammaglobulinemia	B	Sex-linked
▪ Common variable hypogammaglobulinemia	B	
▪ Selective IgA, IgM, or IgG deficiency	B	Some sex-linked
▪ DiGeorge's syndrome (thymic hypoplasia)	T	
▪ Severe combined immunodeficiency disease	Stem, B, T	Sex-linked
▪ Ataxia telangiectasia	B, T	Autosomal recessive
▪ Wiskott-Aldrich syndrome	B, T	Sex-linked
▪ Graft-versus-host disease	B, T	
▪ Acquired immunodeficiency syndrome	T	

T-helper cells, in turn, activate T-cytotoxic cells, resulting in destruction of virus-infected pancreatic islet cells. The person experiences loss of insulin-producing cells.

The association between HLA and certain diseases is presently of little practical clinical importance. Nevertheless, there is promise for the development of clinical applications in the future. For example, with certain autoimmune diseases it may be possible to identify members of a family at greatest risk for developing the same or a related autoimmune disease. These persons would need close medical supervision, preventive measures implemented (if possible), and early diagnosis and treatment instituted to prevent chronic complications.

IMMUNODEFICIENCY DISORDERS

When the immune system does not adequately protect the body, an *immunodeficient* state exists. The immunodeficiency disorders involve an impairment of one or more immune mechanisms, which include (1) phagocytosis, (2) humoral response, (3) cell-mediated response, (4) complement, and (5) a combined humoral and cell-mediated deficiency. Immunodeficiency disorders are *primary* if the immune cells are improperly developed or absent and *secondary* if an interference with the immune system develops. Primary immunodeficiency disorders are rare and often serious, whereas secondary disorders are more common and less severe.

Primary Immunodeficiency Disorders

The basic categories of primary immunodeficiency disorders include (1) phagocytic defects, (2) B-cell deficiency, (3) T-cell deficiency, and (4) a combined B- and T-cell deficiency (Table 10-18).

Hypogammaglobulinemia. The defect in B cells can range from the complete absence of all immunoglobulin classes (*agammaglobulinemia*) to a defect in only one immunoglobulin class. *Hypogammaglobulinemia* refers to a decreased level of the circulating immunoglobulins. The disorder may be congenital or acquired. *Congenital hypogammaglobulinemia (Bruton's disease)* is a rare sex-linked recessive disorder that occurs only in males. It is characterized by a deficiency of B cells and immunoglobulins and an intact thymus gland and normal T-cell immune response. The disorder usually first manifests in the infant at approximately 3 months of age when the IgG antibody from the mother is depleted and the infant develops recurrent respiratory tract and pyrogenic bacterial infections.

Acquired hypogammaglobulinemia (common variable hypogammaglobulinemia) is a more common disorder that is characterized by the presence of T and B cells but no plasma cells. There appears to be a defect in differentiation of B cells to plasma cells. A possible cause of acquired hypogammaglobulinemia is an abundance of T-suppressor cells that suppress B-cell maturation into plasma cells. The disorder resembles Bruton's disease except that the recurrent bacterial infections (primarily of the respiratory tract) do not occur until patients are 15 to 35 years of age. The treatment includes γ-globulin injections or transfusions of plasma.

DiGeorge's Syndrome. DiGeorge's syndrome (also known as congenital thymic hypoplasia) is a condition in which neither the thymus nor parathyroid gland develops. B-cell function is normal, but T-cell function is absent. The disorder manifests as recurrent viral, fungal, and protozoan infections; inability to reject allografts; and inability to react in a delayed hypersensitivity skin test. Symptoms of oral candidiasis and chronic diarrhea develop in the first year of life. Microscopically, no thymus-dependent areas in the spleen or lymph nodes are seen. Because T-helper cells are missing, the circulation levels of some antibodies may also be reduced. Hypocalcemic tetany is also present due to the absence of the parathyroid gland. Treatment consists of administration of calcium and a fetal thymus transplant. A fetal thymus gland (from a fetus less than 14 weeks' gestational age) can be locally implanted intramuscularly or minced and injected intraperitoneally. Once it is in place, mature T cells are produced.

Severe Combined Immunodeficiency Disease. This condition includes a group of inherited disorders in which B- and T-cell functions are abnormal. The most common form of severe combined immunodeficiency disease is sex-linked Swiss type agammaglobulinemia. The etiology of the disorder is unknown but seems to represent a bone marrow stem defect or a failure in normal development of thymus and bursa-equivalent tissue. Microscopically, the thymus gland is hypoplastic and lymph nodes contain no B and T cells. The disorder manifests as severe viral, bacterial, fungal, or protozoan infections that occur within the first 2 years of life. Treatment consists of controlling the infection with antibiotics and placing the patient in protective isolation. Histocompatible bone marrow transplants have been somewhat successful. Other treatments include thymus transplant, γ-globulin injections, fetal liver transplant, and administration of thymic epithelium. Even with treatment the prognosis is guarded.

Secondary Immunodeficiency Disorders

Some of the important factors that may cause secondary immunodeficiency disorders are listed in Table 10-19. Drug-induced immunosuppression is the most common. Immunosuppressive therapy is prescribed for patients to treat autoimmune disorders and to prevent transplant rejection. In addition, immunosuppression is a serious side effect

Table 10-19 Causes of Secondary Immunodeficiency

Drug-induced	Surgery and trauma
Antineoplastic agents	Infections
Corticosteroids	Burns
Stress	Chronic renal failure
Age	Diabetes
Infants	Alcoholic cirrhosis
Older adults	Systemic lupus erythematosus
Malnutrition	Anesthesia
Dietary deficiency	Malignancies
Cirrhosis	Acquired immunodeficiency syndrome
Cancer cachexia	
Radiation	

of cytotoxic drugs used in cancer chemotherapy. Generalized leukopenia often results, leading to a decreased humoral and cell-mediated response. Therefore, secondary infections are common in immunosuppressed patients. (Refer to Table 44-10 for a summary of the specific actions of the various drugs on the immune system.)

Stress alters the immune response. This response involves communication among the nervous, endocrine, and immune systems (see Chapter 5).

A hypofunctional state of the immune system exists in young children and older adults. Laboratory studies have demonstrated that immunoglobulin levels decrease with age and therefore lead to a suppressed humoral immune response in older adults. Thymic involution occurs in senescence along with decreased numbers of T cells. The incidence of malignancies and autoimmune diseases increases with aging and may be related to immunologic deterioration.

Malnutrition alters cell-mediated immune responses. When protein is deficient over a prolonged period, atrophy of the thymus gland occurs and lymphoid tissue decreases. In addition, an increased susceptibility to infections always exists.

Irradiation destroys lymphocytes either directly or through depletion of stem cells. As the radiation dose is increased, more bone marrow atrophies, leading to severe pancytopenia and severe suppression of immune function.

Surgical removal of lymph nodes, thymus, or spleen can suppress the immune response. Splenectomy in children is especially dangerous and may lead to septicemia from simple respiratory infections.

Hodgkin's disease greatly impairs the cell-mediated immune response, and patients may die from severe viral or fungal infections (Hodgkin's disease is discussed in Chapter 28). Viruses, especially rubella, may cause immunodeficiency by direct cytotoxic damage to lymphoid cells. Systemic infections can place such a demand on the immune system that resistance to a secondary or subsequent infection is impaired.

Graft-versus-Host Disease

Graft-versus-host (GVH) disease occurs when an immunoincompetent (immunodeficient) patient is transfused or transplanted with immunocompetent cells. A GVH response may result from the infusion of any blood product containing viable lymphocytes, such as in therapeutic blood transfusions; and from the transplantation of fetal thymus, fetal liver, or bone marrow. Unlike most other transplantation situations, the host's rejection of the graft is not as serious as the graft's rejection of the host.

The GVH response may have its onset 7 to 30 days following infusion of viable lymphocytes. Once the reaction is started, little can be done to modify its course. The exact mechanism involved in this reaction is not completely understood. However, it involves donor T cells attacking and destroying vulnerable host cells.

The target organs for the GVH phenomenon are the skin, gut, and liver. The skin disease may be a maculopapular rash, which can progress to a generalized erythema with bullous formation and desquamation. The liver disease may range from mild jaundice to hepatic coma. The intestinal disease may be manifested by mild to severe diarrhea, severe abdominal pain, and malabsorption. The biggest problem with GVH disease is infection, with different types of infections seen in different periods. Bacterial and fungal infections predominate immediately after transplantation when granulocytopenia exists. The development of interstitial pneumonitis is the predominant later problem. There is no adequate treatment of GVH disease once it is established. Although corticosteroids are often used, they enhance the susceptibility to infection. The use of methotrexate and cyclosporine have been most effective as preventive rather than treatment measures. Radiation of blood products before they are administered is another measure to prevent T-cell replication.

IMMUNE-RELATED DISEASES

Mononucleosis

Mononucleosis, often referred to as "mono" or the "kissing disease," is a benign, self-limiting disease characterized by lymph node enlargement, lymphocytosis, and elevated temperature. The peak incidence of mononucleosis occurs between 14 and 18 years of age. It may occur in isolated cases or in epidemics. Although benign, the disease may incapacitate patients because of the extreme fatigue associated with it.

Etiology and Pathophysiology. Mononucleosis is caused by the Epstein-Barr virus (EBV), a type of herpesvirus, which is primarily transmitted in saliva. The virus grows productively in B lymphocytes and oropharyngeal epithelial cells. Once exposed, susceptible patients manifest symptoms of disease after a 4- to 8-week incubation period. Symptoms evolve gradually, intensifying as the disease becomes apparent. After causing mononucleosis, the EBV may lie dormant in lymphocytes and other lymphatic tissue. The virus can be shed for up to 18 months following primary infection.[10]

In the United States and Canada 50% of the population have experienced a primary EBV infection by adolescence. These early infections are usually mild, nonspecific, and clinically inapparent. By adulthood, most individuals are EBV-seropositive.

Clinical Manifestations. Prodromal symptoms of headache, fatigue, malaise, chills, puffy eyelids, anorexia, and a distaste for smoking cigarettes may occur. As the disease becomes more acute, most patients have a triad of symptoms, including fever, painful lymph node enlargement (especially cervical, axillary, and groin nodes), and sore throat. The sore throat may be severe enough to cause dysphagia. If the spleen is enlarged by massive lymphocyte infiltration, pain will occur in the left upper quadrant.

Infectious mononucleosis is a self-limiting disease in the majority of cases, rarely lasting more than 2 to 3 weeks. The most persistent symptom is malaise. It is rare for significant complications to develop from mononucleosis. The problems that may occur include pneumonia, neurologic changes (e.g., encephalitis), splenic rupture, hepatitis, thrombocytopenia, hemolytic anemia, airway obstruction, myocarditis, and pericarditis.

Diagnostic Studies. Initially the WBC and differential cell counts are normal, but within a week a leukocytosis (WBC $>$20,000 μl [20×10^9/L]) will occur. There is a rise in lymphocytes and monocytes, with 10% to 20% atypical lymphocytes, which are predominantly activated T lymphocytes. Heterophil antibodies are found in the majority of individuals. The "monospot" test, which uses a commercial kit to assay these antibodies, is available and easily performed. Antibodies to EBV can also be measured. The presence of IgM antibodies to EBV is diagnostic of a primary EBV infection. Liver function studies may be used to ascertain whether any liver involvement exists. Since β-hemolytic streptococci can be isolated from the throat in up to 30% of patients with mononucleosis, isolation of this organism does not rule out the diagnosis of mononucleosis.

THERAPEUTIC AND NURSING MANAGEMENT

MONONUCLEOSIS

There is no specific therapeutic protocol for patients with mononucleosis. Patients need to rest for 2 to 3 weeks and get adequate nutrition and fluids. Fever and sore throat can be treated with acetaminophen. Isolation procedures are not required because mononucleosis is minimally contagious in adults. Antibiotics have not proved useful unless the throat culture is positive for β-hemolytic streptococci. Corticosteroids may be used to treat airway obstruction, hemolytic anemia, and thrombocytopenia. Recovery is gradual and malaise may occur intermittently for some time.

Nursing interventions are most appropriate when the disease is actually present. Helping the patient comply with the prescribed rest may prove challenging if fatigue is negligible. Saline solution mouthwashes may ease sore throat pain. The nurse needs to be observant for the development of complications. For the patient with splenomegaly, the nurse must emphasize the need to avoid any possible activities that can lead to splenic rupture. For example, the patient should avoid Valsalva's maneuver with bowel movements, and abdominal trauma from lifting or from sports must be avoided until the splenic enlargement resolves.

The need for ongoing care after mononucleosis is uncommon. After 2 to 3 weeks, the patient can usually return to a normal lifestyle. If mononucleosis occurs in older adults, complications may be more common and complete disease resolution may take longer.

Chronic Fatigue Syndrome

Chronic fatigue syndrome is a disorder characterized by debilitating fatigue and a variety of associated complaints (Table 10-20). The first major criterion is the new onset of severe and debilitating fatigue present for at least 6 months. The second major criterion is the absence of an identifiable etiology for the fatigue. Patients with chronic fatigue syndrome are twice as likely to be women as men and are generally ages 25 to 45 years. Its prevalence is difficult to determine.

Etiology and Pathophysiology. Despite numerous attempts to determine the etiology and pathology of chronic fatigue syndrome, the precise mechanisms remain unknown. However, there are many theories about the etiology of chronic fatigue syndrome. It is often postinfectious, frequently follows a viral infection, and is associated with immune alterations. A dysfunction may exist in the hypothalamus-pituitary-adrenal axis. Several viruses have been investigated as etiologic agents, including herpesviruses (e.g., EBV, cytomegalovirus), retroviruses, and enteroviruses. Antibody titers to many infectious agents are elevated in patients with chronic fatigue syndrome. It is known that viruses can precipitate the syndrome, but whether they can cause the long-term features is unknown.[11]

Immune alterations that have been shown to occur with chronic fatigue syndrome include decreased immunoglobulin production in vitro, altered NK cell activity, decreased lymphocyte proliferation, increased CD4/CD8 ratio, and increased percentage of activated T cells.[12] However, these alterations do not occur in all patients and have not been shown to correlate with the severity of the disease.

Neuroendocrine function may be altered in chronic fatigue syndrome. There may be reduced production of corticotropin-releasing hormone in the hypothalamus. Serum cortisol levels are low and adrenocorticotropic hormone levels are correspondingly high. These changes could cause decreased energy and altered mood states in patient with chronic fatigue syndrome.[13]

Because mild to moderate depression occurs in about 70% of these patients, it has been proposed that chronic fatigue syndrome is a psychiatric disorder. However, it is difficult to determine if depression is a cause or an effect of debilitating chronic fatigue.[12]

Clinical Manifestations. The typical case of chronic fatigue syndrome arises suddenly in a previously active, healthy individual. An unremarkable flulike illness or other acute stress is often identified as a triggering event. Unbearable fatigue is the problem that causes the patient to seek health care. Associated symptoms (see Table 10-20) may fluctuate in intensity over time.

The patient may become angry and frustrated with the inability of physicians to diagnose a problem. The disorder may have a major impact on work and family responsibilities. Some individuals may even need help with activities of daily living.

Diagnostic Studies. Physical examination and diagnostic studies can be used to rule out other possible causes of the patient's symptoms. No laboratory test can diagnose chronic fatigue syndrome or measure its severity. In general, it remains a diagnosis of exclusion.

Table 10-20 Chronic Fatigue Syndrome: Centers for Disease Control Case Definition

Both major criteria and either ≥ six minor symptom criteria plus ≥ two minor physical criteria or ≥ eight symptom criteria must be present to fulfill the case definition.

Major criteria

1. Persistent or relapsing fatigue or easy fatigability for greater than 6 months
2. Exclusion of other chronic conditions, including preexisting psychiatric disease

Minor criteria

Symptoms

1. Fever
2. Sore throat
3. Lymph node pain
4. Unexplained generalized muscle weakness
5. Myalgia
6. Prolonged generalized fatigue following exercise
7. New, generalized headaches
8. Migratory noninflammatory arthralgias
9. Neuropsychologic symptoms
10. Sleep disturbance
11. Patient's description of symptoms as acute or subacute onset

Physical findings

1. Fever
2. Nonexudative pharyngitis
3. Palpable or tender lymph nodes

NURSING MANAGEMENT

CHRONIC FATIGUE SYNDROME

Because there is no definitive treatment for chronic fatigue syndrome, supportive management is essential.[14] The patient should be informed about what is known about the disease and all complaints should be taken seriously. Nonsteroidal anti-inflammatory drugs can be used to treat headaches, muscle and joint aches, and fever. Antihistamines and decongestants can be used to treat allergic symptoms. Nonsedating antidepressants can improve mood and sleep disorders.

Total rest is not advised because it can potentiate the self-image of being an invalid. On the other hand, strenuous exertion can exacerbate the exhaustion. Therefore it is important to plan a carefully graduated exercise program. Behavioral therapy may be used to promote a positive outlook as well as improve overall disability, fatigue, and other symptoms.

Chronic fatigue syndrome does not appear to progress. Although most patients recover or at least improve over time, they suffer from substantial occupational and psychosocial impairments and loss, including the social pressure and isolation from being characterized as lazy or crazy.

NEW TECHNOLOGIES IN IMMUNOLOGY

Hybridoma Technology: Monoclonal Antibodies

Monoclonal antibodies are homogeneous populations of identical antibody molecules produced by specialized tissue cell culture lines. The procedure uses cell fusion techniques and standard in vitro tissue culture systems (Fig. 10-11). The two essential biologic components are immunized mice or rats and myeloma tumor cell lines, which are of lymphoid origin. Single antibody-forming cells (lymphocytes) from rodents previously immunized with antigen are fused with myeloma cells to create hybrid cells with properties of both parent cell types. The hybrids have an unlimited capacity to grow similar to that of the myeloma parent cell. The hybrids produce the single type of antibody molecule that they inherited from the normal, antibody-forming parent cell. Hybrid cells derived in this way can produce unlimited quantities of specific antibodies. With appropriate selection techniques, producing monoclonal antibodies to virtually any antigen is possible. Because the monoclonal antibodies are a completely homogeneous population, their use incurs fewer problems than conventional polyclonal antisera. Because most antigens have multiple antigenic determinants that stimulate B lymphocytes to proliferate, most humoral immune responses are polyclonal with multiple antibodies produced.

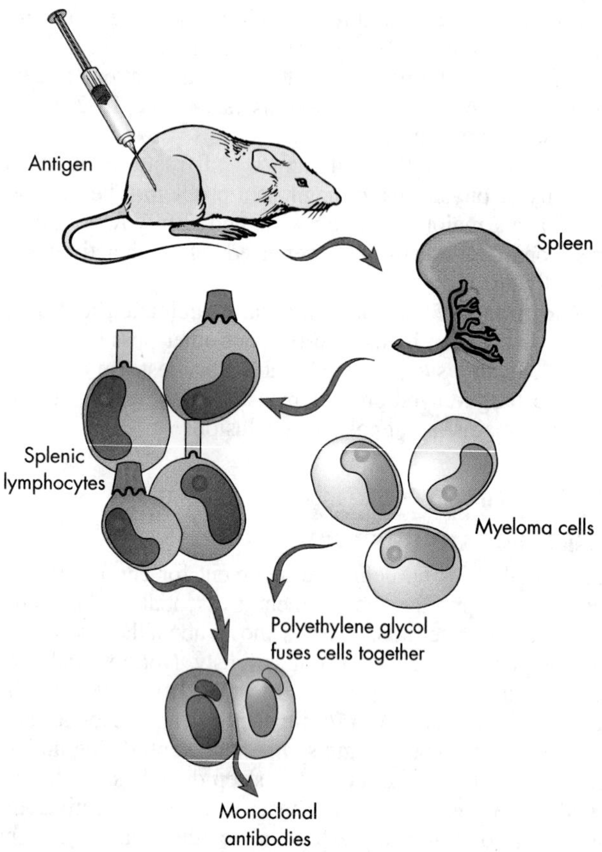

Fig. 10-11 Monoclonal antibodies are identical antibodies made by clones of a single antibody-producing cell. The target antigen is injected into a mouse. The spleen cells, which contain plasma cells, are harvested and fused with myeloma cells using polyethylene glycol. The fused cells, or hybridomas, are then cloned. A clone can secrete monoclonal antibodies over a long period of time.

Monoclonal antibodies are finding wide application in many areas of medicine and biologic science.[15] Thousands of monoclonal antibodies have been made against many different types of antigens. Monoclonal antibodies have begun to replace conventional antibodies in blood banking and are used in the identification of organisms in the bacteriology laboratory. Monoclonal antibodies have also been extensively used in radioimmunoassays to measure serum levels of various substances (e.g., parathyroid hormone). They have been very useful in quantitating types of WBCs and subgroups of lymphocytes. They are also used in the diagnosis of leukemia. More recently, monoclonal antibodies have been used in the treatment of malignancies (see Chapter 12). They have been used to treat transplant rejection episodes (see Chapter 44), purge bone marrow of tumor cells in bone marrow transplants, and remove mature T cells that cause GVH disease in bone marrow transplants.

A major limitation of these monoclonal antibodies is that they are mouse antibodies and therefore can elicit an antibody response by the host against the foreign agent. Recently, human hybridomas have been produced using human myelomas. These hybrids synthesize human monoclonals and are therefore advantageous for in vivo use in diagnosis and therapy.

Recombinant DNA Technology

Recombinant DNA technology, a form of genetic engineering, involves taking segments of DNA from one type of organism and combining them with genes of a second organism (Fig. 10-12). When the cell divides, the DNA is transcribed and a specific protein coded by the DNA is made. In this way relatively simple organisms such as *E. coli*, yeast, or mammalian tissue culture cells can be used to make large quantities of human proteins, including hormones (e.g., insulin) and cytokines.

A facet of recombinant DNA technology involves gene therapy which can be used to replace defective or missing genes with normal genes. Using recombinant DNA methods, a normal gene can be inserted into a human chromosome to counteract the effects of a missing or abnormal gene. The first approved gene therapy trials involved children with severe combined immunodeficiency disease caused by adenosine deaminase deficiency. T lymphocytes from these children were obtained and the missing gene was inserted into these T cells. The new T cells were then reinjected into the children's bloodstreams. The gene signaled the cells to produce the missing enzyme, and these children developed a functioning immune system. The success of these efforts has led scientists to try gene therapy for a variety of other genetic disorders including cystic fibrosis.

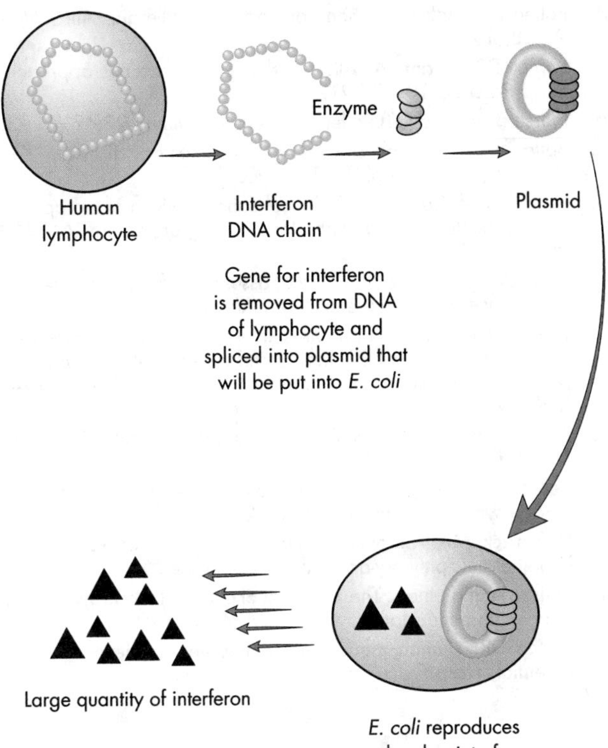

Fig. 10-12 Mass production of interferon by recombinant gene technology.

The application of gene therapy in embryonic development is controversial. By inserting genes into the embryo, all body cells could be altered, including the germ cells. The genetic composition of the embryo would be changed as would be all future offspring.

Polymerase Chain Reaction

The use of recombinant DNA techniques to clone DNA sequences can take a great deal of time (days to weeks). When rapid genetic diagnosis is necessary, polymerase chain reaction (PCR) can provide a way to make many copies of a DNA sequence in only a few hours. PCR involves the artificial replication of a DNA sequence. The DNA strands can be separated to form new templates that are used for replication.

PCR is used extensively in forensic medicine to identify DNA of criminal suspects by using samples from blood, hair, and semen. PCR can also be used as a confirmatory test in HIV testing. This is especially important when an infant of a mother who is HIV-antibody positive also tests HIV positive. In this situation it is unknown if the antibodies from the infant's blood are from the baby or the mother. PCR techniques can be used on the baby's lymphocytes to determine whether the baby is infected with HIV.

REVIEW QUESTIONS

The number of the question corresponds to the same-numbered objective at the beginning of the chapter.

1. Which of the following is not a component of the immune system?
   a. Spleen
   b. Thymus
   c. Bone marrow
   d. Connective tissue

2. Administration of the MMR (mumps, measles, rubella) vaccine is done to promote which type of immunity?
   a. Active natural immunity
   b. Passive natural immunity
   c. Passive artificial immunity
   d. Active artificial immunity

3. All the following statements are characteristic of cell-mediated immunity except
   a. effective in fighting fungal infections.
   b. response occurs within minutes.
   c. surveys the body for invasion by tumor cells.
   d. sensitized lymphocytes directly attack antigens.

4. The reason newborns are protected for the first 3 months of life from bacterial infections is because of the maternal transmission of
   a. IgG.
   b. IgA.
   c. IgM.
   d. IgE.

5. In a type I hypersensitivity reaction, the primary immunologic disorder appears to be
   a. binding of IgG to an antigen on a cell surface.
   b. deposit of antigen-antibody complexes in small vessels.
   c. release of lymphokines to interact with specific antigens.
   d. release of chemical mediators from IgE-bound mast cells.

6. The treatment of choice for an acute anaphylactic reaction is
   a. theophylline (Aminophylline).
   b. diphenhydramine (Benadryl).
   c. epinephrine (Adrenalin).
   d. corticosteroids (Solu-Cortef).

7. All the following are true about skin testing except
   a. a positive reaction is manifested by a wheal-and-flare reaction.
   b. a highly sensitive person may develop an anaphylactic reaction.
   c. the preferred site for intracutaneous testing is the back.
   d. it may be done to determine initial titer of allergen extracts.

8. Antihistamines are most effectively used in treating
   a. systemic lupus erythematosus.
   b. intrinsic asthma.
   c. allergic rhinitis.
   d. anaphylactic shock.

9. Autoimmunity is defined as a phenomenon involving
   a. production of endotoxins that destroy B lymphocytes.
   b. inability to differentiate self from nonself.
   c. overproduction of reagin antibody.
   d. depression of the immune response.

10. Association between HLA antigens and diseases is most commonly found in what disease conditions?
   a. Infectious diseases
   b. Autoimmune disorders
   c. Neurologic diseases
   d. Malignancies

11. Congenital hypogammaglobulinemia is characterized by all the following *except*
   a. deficiency of T lymphocytes.
   b. recurrent otitis media infections.
   c. symptoms manifest after age 3 months.
   d. sex-linked recessive disorder.

REFERENCES

1. Goodnough LT and others: Indications and guidelines for the use of hematopoietic growth factors, *Transfusion* 33:944, 1993.
2. Ben-Yehuda A, Weksler ME: Host resistance and the immune system, *Clin Geriatr Med* 8:701, 1992.
3. Miller RA: Aging and immune function: cellular and biochemical analyses, *Exp Gerontol* 29:21, 1994.
4. Patten BC, Holt JA: When your patient is allergic, *Am J Nurs* 92:58, 1992.
5. Engler DB, Grant JA: Allergic rhinitis: a practical approach, *Hosp Pract* 26:105, 1991.
6. Nurse's guide to OTC allergy products, *Nursing* 23:67, 1993.
7. Boitard C: Pathophysiology of autoimmune disease, *Klin Wochenschr* 68(Suppl 21):1, 1990.
8. Price CA, McCarley PB: Technical considerations of therapeutic plasma exchange as a nephrology nursing procedure, *ANNA J* 20:41, 1993.
9. Price CA, McCarley PB: Physical assessment for patients receiving therapeutic plasma exchange, *ANNA J* 21:149, 1994.
10. Schooley RT: Epstein-Barr virus infections including infectious mononucleosis. In Isselbacher KJ and others, editors: *Harrison's principles of internal medicine,* ed 13, New York, 1994, McGraw-Hill.
11. Ablashi DV: Viral studies of chronic fatigue syndrome, *Clin Infect Dis* 18 (Suppl 1):S117, 1994.
12. Bearn J, Wessely S: Neurobiological aspects of the chronic fatigue syndrome, *Eur J Clin Invest* 24:79, 1994.
13. Demitrack MA: Chronic fatigue syndrome: a disease of the hypothalamic-pituitary-adrenal axis? *Ann Med* 26:1, 1994.
14. Wilson A and others: The treatment of chronic fatigue syndrome: science and speculation, *Am J Med 96:544, 1994.*
15. Burton DR: Human monoclonal antibodies: achievement and potential, *Hosp Pract* 27:67, 1992.

Chapter 11

NURSING ROLE IN MANAGEMENT

Human Immunodeficiency Virus Infection

Lucy Bradley-Springer

Learning Objectives

1. Discuss the pathophysiology of human immunodeficiency virus (HIV) infection.
2. List the modes of transmission for HIV and the variables involved in the transmission of HIV.
3. Describe the spectrum of HIV infection.
4. List the diagnostic criteria for acquired immunodeficiency syndrome (AIDS).
5. Describe opportunistic diseases that occur in AIDS.
6. Describe the methods of testing for HIV infection.
7. Describe the therapeutic management of HIV infection.
8. Discuss the nursing management of HIV-infected patients.

In 1981 public health officials in the United States recognized a new disease that eventually became known as acquired immunodeficiency syndrome (AIDS). It is now known that AIDS is the final phase of a chronic, progressive immune function disorder caused by human immunodeficiency virus (HIV). Unlike most of the world where HIV has been predominantly transmitted through heterosexual activity, the epidemic in the United States, Canada, and Western Europe was originally observed in the male homosexual community. However, the epidemic was never confined to this group, and increasing numbers of cases are occurring in men, women, and children from all races, ethnicities, communities, and sexual orientations.[1]

SIGNIFICANCE OF PROBLEM

By the end of 1994 there were more than 426,000 cases of AIDS and over 271,000 AIDS-related deaths had been reported in the United States. At least 1 million people in the United States are estimated to be infected with HIV. In the United States the fastest-growing groups of people with HIV and AIDS are women and adolescents. Of the more than 58,000 cases of AIDS that have been reported in women since 1981, 24% of those cases were reported in 1994. During that same time, 17% of the more than 18,000 cumulative AIDS cases were reported in people 13 to 25 years of age.[2] AIDS in the United States is not only changing along the lines of gender and age; it is also becoming an increasing problem for people of color, people who live in poverty, and people who live in rural areas.

Globally, HIV is even more devastating, with a worldwide estimate of more than 10 million infected people. By the year 2000 it is estimated that 30 million[3] to 110 million[4] people throughout the world will be infected with HIV.

TRANSMISSION OF HIV

HIV is a fragile virus that can be transmitted only under specific conditions. It is transmitted from human to human through infected blood, semen, vaginal secretions, and breast milk. If these infected fluids are introduced into an uninfected person's body, the potential for transmission occurs. Transmission of HIV has occurred through sexual intercourse with an infected partner; internalized contact with HIV-infected blood or blood products; and perinatal transmission during pregnancy, at the time of delivery, or through breast milk.[5]

An HIV-infected individual can transmit HIV to others starting a few days after initial infection. After that the ability to transmit HIV is lifelong. HIV has no noninfectious state. Transmission of HIV is subject to the same requirements as other microorganisms. That is, a sufficient amount of the infectious agent must be introduced through an appropriate portal of entry into a susceptible host. Duration and frequency of contact, quantity of inoculant, virulence of the organism, and host immune defense capability all affect whether infection will actually occur after exposure.

Reviewed by James Halloran, RN, MSN, OCN, ANP, HIV Clinical Nurse Specialist, University of Texas School of Public Health, Houston, TX.

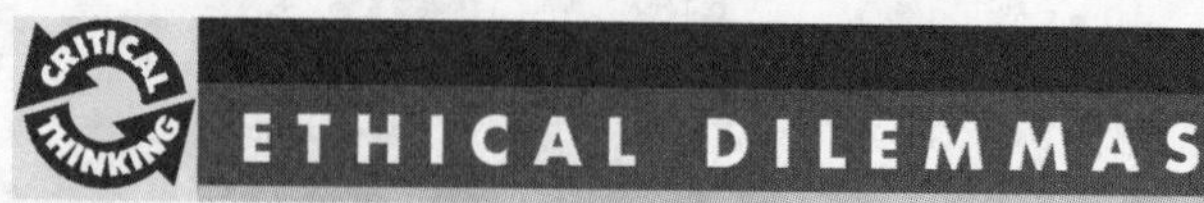

DUTY TO TREAT

Situation A nurse on a medical unit has just discovered that a patient with respiratory problems is HIV-infected. The nurse is concerned about contact with this patient and his bodily fluids, and she requests not to be assigned to his care. The nurse believes that she has her own family to support and protect.

Discussion A nurse's professional obligation to treat patients in need transcends concerns about the diseases or conditions of those patients. As infectious disease health care providers often note, it is not the known HIV-infected patient who is of concern, but the patient whose HIV or infectious status is *not* known that presents the greatest risk to health care providers. If a nurse's primary concern is personal safety, the nurse needs to reexamine her commitment to the profession. This patient can provide valuable lessons in issues related to infectious disease control, stereotyping patients, and understanding the dedication of health care providers.

ETHICAL AND LEGAL PRINCIPLES

- The Rehabilitation Act of 1973 and the Americans with Disabilities Act prohibit discrimination against the handicapped and disabled. People who are HIV-infected or who have AIDS are included under these acts.
- Refusal to treat or care for people who are HIV-infected or have AIDS, when that refusal is not based on medical judgment, is as unethical as discrimination against any person based on race or gender or other characteristic.
- Health care professionals may not pick and choose their patients if they are true to their oaths to provide care to all those in need.

The viral load in the blood, semen, vaginal secretions, or breast milk of the "donor" is an important variable. In HIV infection, large amounts of the virus are detected in the blood during the first 2 to 6 months after initial infection and again during the late stages of the disease[6] (see Fig. 11-3). During these periods, unprotected sexual or blood exposure to an infected individual becomes more risky, although HIV can be transmitted during all phases of the disease.

HIV is not spread casually; it cannot be transmitted through hugging, kissing, shaking hands, sharing eating utensils, or attending school with an HIV-infected person. It is not transmitted through tears, saliva, or sweat. In addition, there is no evidence that the virus can be transmitted by insects.[5] Repeated studies have failed to demonstrate transmission of the virus by respiratory droplets, enteric routes, or casual encounters in any setting.[7] The health care worker has a low occupational risk of acquiring the virus, even with needle-stick injury.[8,9]

Sexual Transmission

Sexual contact with an HIV-infected partner is the most common method of transmission. Sexual activity provides an opportunity for contact with semen, vaginal secretions, and blood. Although male homosexuals initially accounted for most cases of HIV in the United States, heterosexual transmission is becoming more prevalent, and it is now the most common method of infection in women. The most important variable is whether HIV is present in one of the sexual partners and not whether the couple is homosexual or heterosexual.

The most risky form of sexual intercourse is unprotected anal intercourse. Although many people associate anal intercourse exclusively with homosexual men, many heterosexual couples also use this form of sexual expression. Anal intercourse frequently results in trauma to the rectal mucosa, although this is not necessary for HIV transmission. Rectal trauma increases the likelihood of HIV infection (and all other sexually transmitted diseases) because tearing of the mucous membrane provides a portal of entry for the virus.

During any form of sexual intercourse (anal, vaginal, oral), the risk of infection is considerably greater for the receptive partner, although infection can also be transmitted to an inserting partner. This increased risk occurs because the receiver has prolonged contact with the semen. This may explain why women are more easily infected than men during heterosexual intercourse.[10] Having a large number of different sexual partners has been associated with HIV infection,[11] but an increasing prevalence of HIV infections in the population makes the number of sexual partners less of a factor. Sexual intercourse with one partner who is HIV-infected creates a risk, whereas sexual intercourse with multiple uninfected partners results in no risk. Sexual activities that involve blood, such as during menstruation or as a result of trauma to tissues, also increase the risk of transmission.

Contact with Blood and Blood Products

HIV is transmitted by exposure to contaminated blood through the accidental or intentional sharing of injection equipment. Sharing equipment to inject drugs is a major means of transmission for both sexes in many large metropolitan areas, and used equipment is becoming more common in smaller cities and rural areas. However, it is important to remember that equipment used to inject drugs such as insulin, vitamin B_{12}, and clotting factors, as well as nonnarcotic drugs such as steroids and amphetamines, are also contaminated after use. It does not matter what substance has been injected. Used equipment is potentially contaminated with HIV and should not be shared.

In the United States transfusion of infected blood and blood products has caused 2% of adult AIDS cases and 7% of pediatric AIDS cases.[2] In 1985 routine screening of blood donors was implemented to identify individuals at risk and to test the blood for the presence of HIV antibodies, thereby improving the safety of the blood supply. As a result of blood transfusions, HIV infection is now unlikely but still possible because blood donated during the window period will not be positive for HIV antibodies on testing.

No new cases of HIV related to the use of clotting factors are expected in the United States because these products are now treated with heat or chemicals to kill the virus.

HIV has been transmitted to health care workers after exposure to HIV-infected fluids through percutaneous injury and into open wounds on the skin and mucous membranes. The greatest risk for occupational transmission of HIV occurs through puncture wounds.[8] The risk of infection after a needle-stick exposure to HIV-infected blood is 0.3% to 0.4%. The risk is higher (approximately 1%) if the exposure is caused by a blood-filled, hollow-bore needle. Solid-bore needles and needles that are not blood-filled (such as those that have been used for intramuscular or subcutaneous injections) create less risk.[9] Splash exposures of blood on skin with an open lesion also present risk.

Perinatal Transmission

Transmission from an HIV-infected mother to an infant can occur during pregnancy, at the time of delivery, or after birth through breast feeding.[12] Studies have found that 9% to 25% of infants born to HIV-infected women will be born with HIV.[13,14] This means that 75% to 91% of these infants will *not* be infected. A study in Zaire found that infants whose HIV-infected mothers did not demonstrate specific markers for immune deficiency had only a 7% rate of infection, whereas those infants whose mothers showed significant immune dysfunction (indicating more advanced disease) were infected 71% of the time.[15] A recent study in the United States showed that treating HIV-infected pregnant women and their infants with zidovudine (ZDV, AZT, Retrovir) significantly decreased the rate of perinatal transmission.[16] This information is helpful when counseling the HIV-infected person who is struggling with difficult decisions related to reproduction.[17]

Diagnosis of HIV in an infant can be problematic. *All* infants born to HIV-infected mothers will be positive on the HIV antibody test because maternal antibodies cross the placental barrier. In the absence of symptoms the ability to detect infection in the infant may be delayed as long as 15 months. This is a problem for parents who may delay bonding or make hasty decisions related to adoption. Earlier diagnosis of HIV infection can sometimes be made if the infant develops symptoms or if diagnostic procedures such as polymerase chain reaction (PCR) or viral culture are used to determine the presence of HIV.

Among children with AIDS in the United States who are less than 13 years of age, 88% were infected at birth.[2] AIDS is now the ninth leading cause of death among children ages 1 to 4,[18] and this statistic may rise if research and treatment access are limited. Emerging data about the outcomes of perinatally infected children show that most of these children live longer than initially expected. One longitudinal study of 529 perinatally infected children found a median survival time of 96.2 months, with 49.5% still living at age 9.[19]

PATHOPHYSIOLOGY

HIV is a ribonucleic acid (RNA) virus (Fig. 11-1) that was discovered in 1983. RNA viruses are called retroviruses

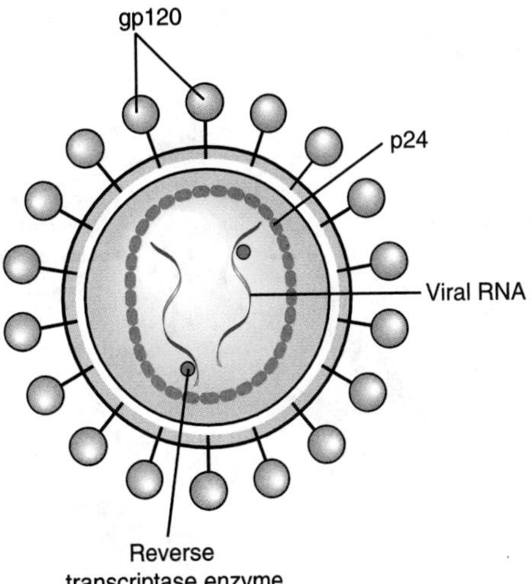

Fig. 11-1 Human immunodeficiency virus (HIV) is surrounded by an envelope of proteins (including gp120) that contains a core of viral RNA and proteins (including p24).

because they replicate in a "backward" manner, going from RNA to deoxyribonucleic acid (DNA). Like all viruses, HIV is an obligate parasite; it cannot replicate unless it is inside a living cell. HIV can enter a cell when the gp120 "knobs" on the viral envelope bind to specific CD4 receptors on the cell's surface (Fig. 11-2). Once bound, the genetic material of the virus enters the cell. In the cell, viral RNA is transcribed into a single strand of viral DNA with the assistance of reverse transcriptase, an enzyme made by HIV. The strand replicates itself, becoming double-stranded viral DNA. At this point the viral DNA can enter the cell's nucleus and splice itself into the genome, becoming a permanent part of the cell's genetic structure. Because all genetic material replicates during cellular division, all daughter cells will also be infected. Now that the genome contains viral DNA, the cell's genetic codes can direct the cell to make more HIV.

Initial infection with HIV results in a viremia during which large amounts of the virus can be isolated in the blood. A prolonged period in which HIV is not readily found in the blood follows within a few weeks or months (Fig. 11-3). During this time, which may last 10 to 12 years, there are few clinical symptoms. It was initially thought that this phase represented a period of biologic and clinical latency and that viral replication was minimal. However, recent studies demonstrate that this is probably not true and that HIV replication continues to occur, especially in the lymph tissue.

In a normal immune response, foreign antigens interact with B cells, which initiate the process of antibody development, and with T cells, which initiate a cellular immune response. In the initial stages of HIV infection these cells respond and function normally. B cells make HIV-specific antibodies that are effective in reducing viral loads in the blood, and activated T cells respond to the site of viruses trapped in the lymph nodes.

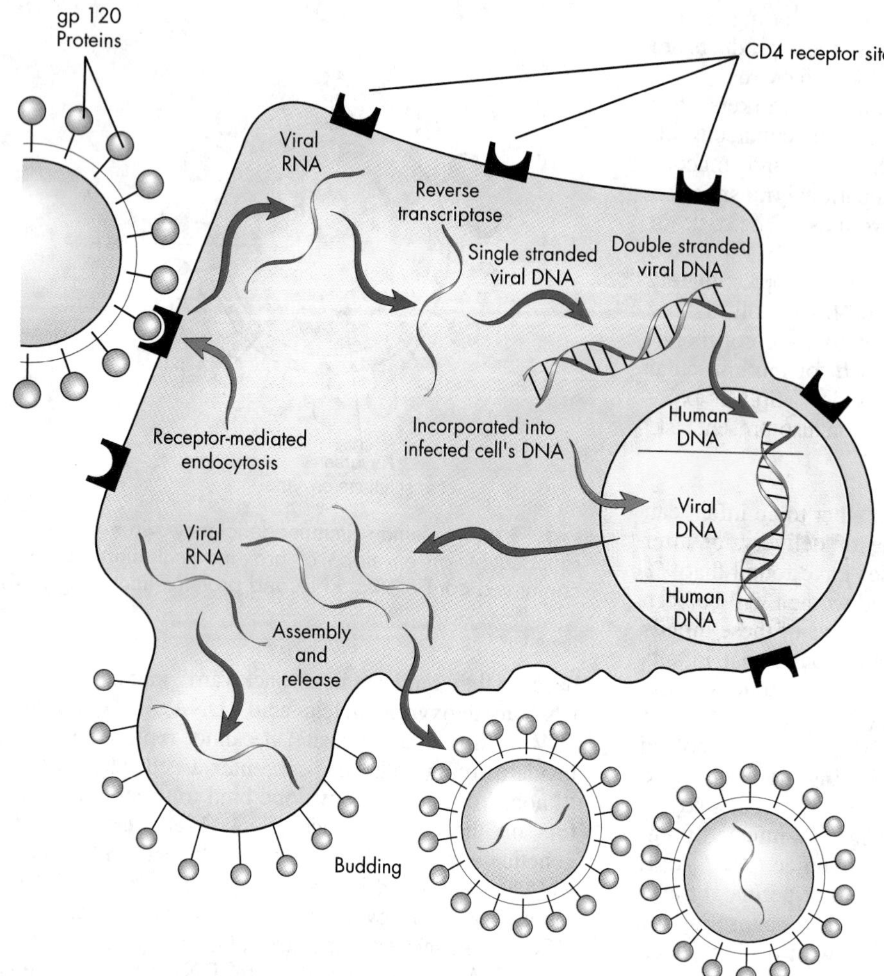

Fig. 11-2 Human immunodeficiency virus (HIV) has gp120 proteins that attach to the CD4 receptors on the surface of $CD4^+$ lymphocytes. The virus then enters the cell, produces viral DNA, and incorporates itself into the cellular genome, causing permanent cellular infection and allowing the production of new virions. New viruses leave the cell through a budding process that ultimately leads to cellular distraction.

HIV can infect several types of human cells, including monocytes and macrophages, lymphocytes, astrocytes, and oligodendrocytes. Immune dysfunction results predominantly from the dysregulation and destruction of T-helper cells, or $CD4^+$ lymphocytes. These cells are targeted because they have more CD4 receptors on their surfaces than other cells. The $CD4^+$ lymphocyte plays a pivotal role in the ability of the immune system to recognize and defend against foreign invaders. An adult normally has 800 to 1200 $CD4^+$ lymphocytes per microliter (μl) of blood. Generally the immune system remains healthy with more than 500 $CD4^+$ lymphocytes/μl; minor immune problems occur when the count drops to 200 to 499 $CD4^+$ lymphocytes/μl; and severe problems develop with less than 200 $CD4^+$ lymphocytes/μl.

Activated $CD4^+$ lymphocytes provide an ideal target for HIV. These cells are attracted to the site of concentrated HIV in the lymph nodes where they are exposed to infection through viral contact with the CD4 receptors. Once infected the activated cells support viral replication and assist in spreading or seeding the infection throughout the lymph system. Lymphoid tissue thus becomes an early reservoir for HIV, promoting active replication even during periods of clinical latency. Eventually, HIV causes significant degenerative changes of the lymph system. This is an important development because an altered lymph system allows viral particles to spill over into the blood, a factor in disease progression, and represents significant impairment of the immune system's ability to respond to new infections.[20] Although HIV infection can lead to abnormal B-cell function, the predominant clinical manifestations reflect severe deficiencies in the cell-mediated immune response.

Several mechanisms by which HIV destroys $CD4^+$ lymphocytes have been identified. Viral replication includes a process of budding that results in increased permeability of the cell's membrane and an eventual loss of cellular integrity (see Fig. 11-2). Another destructive mechanism occurs when infected cells fuse with other cells. This fusion process continues until a number of cells, some of which may not be infected, combine into a large multinucleated mass called a *syncytium*. Syncytial formation kills all affected cells. A third process of destruction is initiated by the infected person's immune system and the antibodies that are produced against HIV. Infected cells display viral protein (gp120) on their surfaces, which can be detected by circulating antibodies. These antibodies bind to the cell-surface viral proteins and activate the complement system, which ultimately promotes lysis of the infected cells.[6] In HIV infection a point is eventually reached where so many $CD4^+$ lymphocytes are destroyed that there are not enough

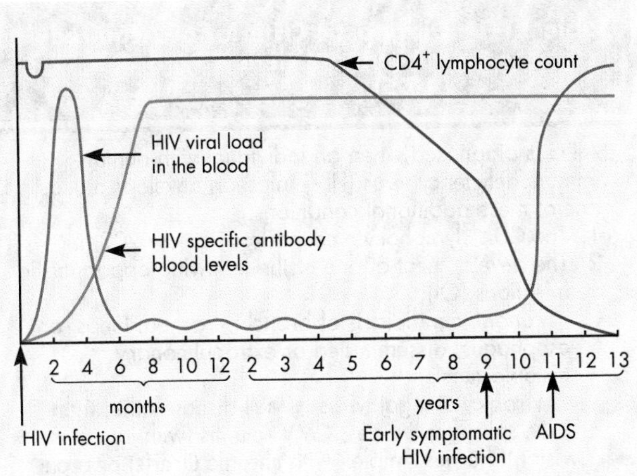

Fig. 11-3 Viral load in the blood and CD4+ lymphocyte counts over the spectrum of human immunodeficiency virus (HIV) infection. *AIDS*, Acquired immunodeficiency syndrome.

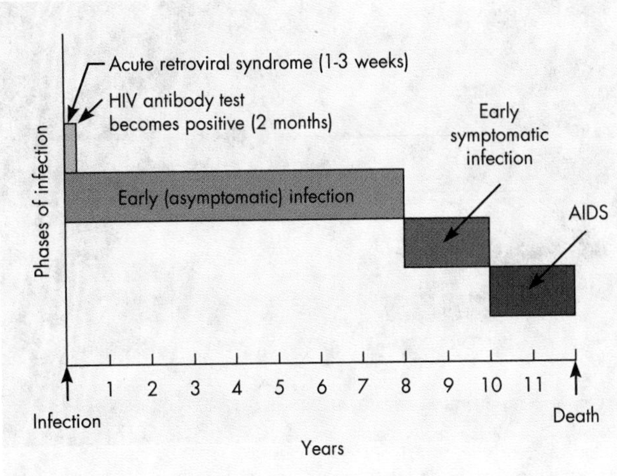

Fig. 11-4 Timeline for the spectrum of human immunodeficiency virus (HIV) infection. The timeline represents the course of the illness from time of infection to clinical manifestations of disease. *AIDS*, Acquired immunodeficiency syndrome.

to regulate immune responses (see Fig. 11-3). This sets the stage for the development of life-threatening illnesses.

HIV can also infect monocytes by attaching to CD4 receptors that are present on certain subsets of the cells or by phagocytic ingestion. Infected monocytes move into body tissues where they differentiate into macrophages. Although HIV replicates in infected macrophages, no external budding occurs. This allows the cell to remain intact while becoming an "HIV factory." A local inflammatory process may cause the infected macrophage to rupture, distributing newly formed HIV into surrounding tissue. Tissues in the skin, lymph nodes, lungs, central nervous system (CNS), and possibly the bone marrow have been directly infected in this manner.[21]

SPECTRUM OF HIV INFECTION

The typical course of HIV infection follows the pattern shown in Fig. 11-4. It is important to remember that HIV follows a highly individualized course. The information depicted in Fig. 11-4 represents median time intervals and usual disease progression, but this timeline cannot be used to predict an individual's life span after HIV infection.

Acute Retroviral Syndrome

The development of HIV-specific antibodies, or seroconversion, is frequently accompanied by a flulike or mononucleosis-like syndrome of fever, pharyngitis, headache, malaise, nausea, and a diffuse rash. These symptoms, called acute retroviral syndrome, generally occur 1 to 3 weeks after initial infection and last for 1 to 2 weeks, although some of the symptoms may persist for several months.[22] CD4+ lymphocyte counts will fall temporarily during this syndrome but will quickly return to baseline. This temporary decrease is a typically healthy immune response to acute illness. In most people the acute retroviral symptoms are mild and may be mistaken for a cold or flu. In a few people, aseptic meningitis may develop.

Early Infection

The median time between HIV infection and a diagnosis of AIDS is 10 or more years. During this time, CD4+ lymphocyte counts remain normal or only slightly decreased. An HIV-infected person remains generally healthy during early infection, but vague symptoms, including fatigue, headaches, low-grade fevers, and night sweats, may occur. Demyelinating peripheral neuropathies, which resemble Guillain-Barré syndrome, may also develop during this time.[23]

Because most of the symptoms during early infection are vague and nonspecific for HIV, a person may remain unaware of infection during this "asymptomatic phase." During this time, an infected person may continue customary activities, which may include risky sexual and drug-using behaviors. This creates a public health problem because an infected person can transmit HIV to others, even without having symptoms. These activities also contribute to personal health problems because an unidentified infected person has no motivation to seek health care or to move toward healthy life changes, which could beneficially alter the quality and quantity of life.

Early Symptomatic Disease

Toward the end of the asymptomatic phase and before a diagnosis of AIDS, the CD4+ lymphocyte count drops below 500 to 600 cells per μl, and early symptomatic disease develops. This early phase was initially called AIDS-related complex (ARC), a term that is no longer useful.

Early symptoms can include constitutional problems such as persistent fevers, recurrent drenching night sweats, chronic diarrhea, headaches, and fatigue. These symptoms may be severe enough to interrupt normal routines. Other problems that may occur at this time include localized infections, lymphadenopathy, and neurologic manifestations.

The most common early infection associated with HIV is oral candidiasis, or thrush, a fungal infection that rarely causes problems in the healthy adult. Other infections that

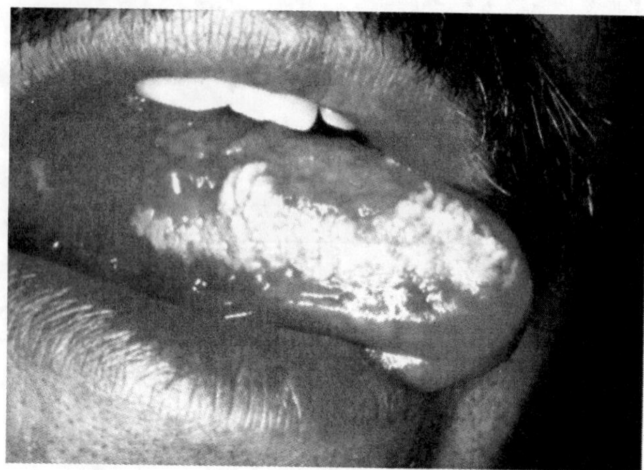

Fig. 11-5 Hairy leukoplakia on tongue.

can occur at this time include shingles (caused by the *Varicella zoster* virus), persistent vaginal yeast infections, and outbreaks of oral or genital herpes. Oral hairy leukoplakia, an Epstein-Barr virus infection that causes painless, white raised lesions on the lateral aspect of the tongue, can also occur at this point (Fig. 11-5). Oral lesions such as those seen in candidiasis and hairy leukoplakia may provide the earliest indications of HIV infection and are prognostic indicators of disease progression.[24]

As the disease progresses, an infected individual may develop persistent generalized lymphadenopathy (PGL). PGL is defined as two or more enlarged lymph nodes, 1 cm or larger, located in places other than the inginal areas, that persist for at least 3 months. PGL may continue for several years before further progression of HIV disease occurs.

Neurologic manifestations can occur at any time during the spectrum of HIV infection but may become more problematic during this phase. Approximately 10% of individuals develop neurologic problems as the first manifestation of HIV, and as many as 90% of HIV-infected people will eventually develop neurologic symptoms.[25] Common neurologic problems include headaches, aseptic meningitis, cranial nerve palsies, myopathies, and painful peripheral neuropathies that may be related to HIV, opportunistic diseases, or side effects of medications.[23]

AIDS

A diagnosis of AIDS cannot be made until the HIV-infected patient meets case definition criteria established by the Centers for Disease Control and Prevention (CDC).[26] These criteria (Table 11-1) are more likely to occur when the immune system becomes severely compromised. As the disease progresses the $CD4^+$ lymphocyte count decreases, and the ratio of CD4 to CD8 cells (T-helper cells to T-suppressor cells), which is usually approximately 2:1, gradually reverses, resulting in more T-suppressor cells than T-helper cells. There is an increase in the amount of HIV that can be detected in the blood by tests such as the p24 antigen assay, PCR, and viral cultures. Markers for disease progression include assays for beta-2 microglobulin and neopterin, which provide nonspecific indicators of immune activity. There may be decreases in white blood cell (WBC) count and the percent of lymphocytes. Delayed hypersensitivity skin reactions are decreased or absent.[27]

Table 11-1 Diagnostic Criteria for Acquired Immunodeficiency Syndrome (AIDS)*

AIDS is diagnosed when an individual with human immunodeficiency virus (HIV) infection develops at least one of these additional conditions:

1. The $CD4^+$ lymphocyte count drops below 200/μl.
2. The development of one of the following opportunistic infections (OI):
   Fungal: candidiasis of bronchi, trachea, lungs, or esophagus; disseminated or extrapulmonary histoplasmosis
   Viral: cytomegalovirus (CMV) disease other than liver, spleen, or nodes; CMV retinitis (with loss of vision); herpes simplex with chronic ulcer(s) or bronchitis, pneumonitis, or esophagitis; progressive multifocal leukoencephalopathy (PML); extrapulmonary cryptococcosis
   Protozoal: disseminated or extrapulmonary coccidioidomycosis, toxoplasmosis of the brain,
   Pneumocystis carinii pneumonia (PCP), chronic intestinal isosporiasis; chronic intestinal crytosporidiosis
   Bacterial: Mycobacterium tuberculosis (any site); any disseminated or extrapulmonary *Mycobacterium*, including *Mycobacterium avium* complex or *Mycobacterium kansasii;* recurrent pneumonia; recurrent Salmonella septicemia
3. The development of one of the following opportunistic cancers: invasive cervical cancer, Kaposi's sarcoma (KS), Burkitt's lymphoma, immunoblastic lymphoma, or primary lymphoma of the brain
4. Wasting syndrome—defined as a loss of 10% or more of ideal body mass
5. The development of dementia

*Modified from Centers for Disease Control and Prevention (CDC): Recommendations and Reports: 1993 revised classification system for HIV infection and expanded surveillance case definition *for AIDS* among adolescents and adults, *MMWR* 41(RR-17):1, December 18, 1992.

The median time for survival after a diagnosis of AIDS is 2 years, but this varies greatly. Some people with AIDS live 6 or more years, whereas others survive only a few months. There is also a wide variation in morbidity. Some people with AIDS are severely ill and have to be considered terminal, whereas others are able to continue their routines despite having to make lifestyle changes to obtain ongoing health care and to deal with symptoms such as fatigue. There is also a roller coaster effect in which the patient can feel well one day and terrible the next. Advances in the treatment and diagnosis of HIV infection, opportunistic diseases, and constitutional symptoms have increased survival times, but AIDS fatality rates remain high.

Opportunistic Diseases. Opportunistic diseases are aggressive diseases that would not have occurred in the presence of a functioning immune system. As HIV infection progresses the immune system becomes increasingly

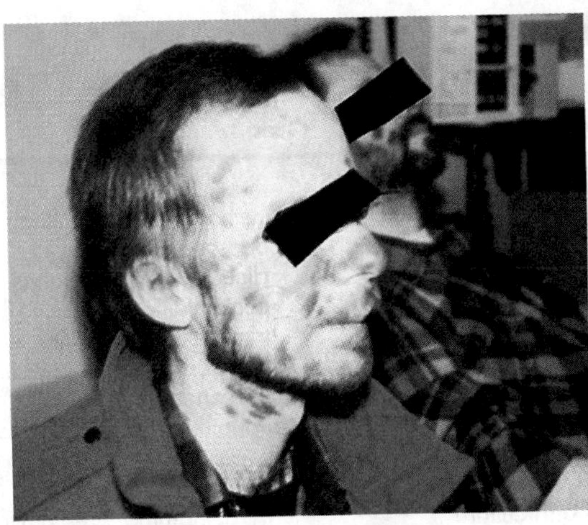

Fig. 11-6 Kaposi's sarcoma on face.

more compromised and less functional. Numerous infections, a variety of malignancies, and wasting and dementia result from this impairment. A common malignancy is Kaposi's sarcoma (Fig. 11-6). Organisms that are nonvirulent or cause limited or localized diseases in an immunocompetent individual can cause severe, debilitating, disseminated, and life-threatening opportunistic infections in persons with AIDS. Table 11-2 lists the major opportunistic diseases and their clinical manifestations, diagnoses, and potential treatments.

DIAGNOSTIC STUDIES

The most useful screening tests for HIV are those that detect the HIV-specific antibody. The major problem with these tests is the delay of 3 weeks to 6 months after infection before detectable antibody is produced (Fig. 11-3). This creates a "window period" during which an infected individual will not test HIV-antibody positive. HIV-antibody screening is generally done in the following sequence:

1. A highly sensitive enzyme immunoassay (EIA) or enzyme-linked immunosorbent assay (ELISA) is done initially to detect serum antibodies that bind to HIV antigens in test plates. Blood samples that are negative on this test are reported as negative.
2. If the blood is EIA reactive, the test is repeated.
3. If the blood is repeatedly EIA reactive, a more specific confirming test such as the Western blot (WB) or immunofluorescence assay (IFA) is done. The WB is done using purified HIV antigens electrophoresed on gels. These are incubated with serum samples. If antibody in the serum is present, it can be detected. IFA is used to identify HIV in infected cells. Infected cells are treated with a fluorescent antibody against p17 or p24 antigen and examined using a fluorescent microscope.
4. Blood that is reactive in all three steps is reported as HIV-antibody positive.
5. Tests with indeterminant results are repeated at a later date. Consistently indeterminant results require the use of PCR, viral culture, and other diagnostic measures.

Special tests, including PCR and viral culture, can be done to diagnose HIV infection. PCR analyzes DNA extracted from lymphocytes and HIV from serum using an *in vitro* amplification procedure. A cell-culture system can be used to grow viruses from infected lymphocytes. Because these tests are expensive and difficult to do, they are usually not used for screening purposes. These tests may be done in situations where the index of suspicion is high and antibody tests are negative. These procedures may also facilitate diagnosis of perinatal infection, which is complicated by the presence of maternal antibodies in the infant.

The progression of HIV infection is frequently monitored by $CD4^+$ lymphocyte counts. As the disease progresses, there is usually a decrease in the number of $CD4^+$ lymphocyte cells.

Hematologic abnormalities are common in HIV infections and may be caused by HIV, opportunistic diseases, or complications of drug or radiation therapy. A decreased WBC count is often seen, usually with concomitant absolute lymphopenia. Thrombocytopenia may be caused by antiplatelet antibodies. Anemia is related to the chronic disease process and a common adverse effect of antiretroviral agents.

Minor alterations in liver function tests are not uncommon. Early identification of hepatitis B and hepatitis C viral infections is important because these infections may have a more serious course in the patient with HIV infection.

THERAPEUTIC MANAGEMENT

Therapeutic management of the HIV-infected patient focuses on monitoring HIV disease progression and immune function, preventing the development of opportunistic diseases, initiating and monitoring antiretroviral therapy, detecting and treating opportunistic diseases, managing symptoms, and preventing complications of treatment. Ongoing assessment and nurse-patient interactions are required to accomplish these objectives. See Table 11-3 for a summary of assessment parameters that need to be accomplished during the initial and subsequent visits.

The initial visit provides an opportunity to gather baseline data and to establish rapport. In addition to the parameters noted in Table 11-3, the initial visit should include a complete history and physical examination, including an immunization history and psychosocial and dietary evaluations. Findings from the history and assessment help to determine the patient's needs. This is a good time to begin patient education related to the spectrum of HIV disease, treatments, preventing transmission to others, improving immune health, family planning, and contraception. Patient input should be used to develop a plan of care, and necessary referrals can be made. However, it is important to remember that the person newly diagnosed with HIV may be in a state of shock or denial and unable to retain or synthesize information. If case reports are required by the state health department they should be completed at this time.

Pharmacologic Management

A number of opportunistic diseases and debilitating problems associated with HIV can be delayed or prevented

Table 11-2 Common Opportunistic Diseases Associated with Acquired Immunodeficiency Syndrome

Organism or Disease	Clinical Manifestations	Diagnostic Tests	Treatment
Respiratory System			
Pneumocystis carinii pneumonia (PCP)	Fever, night sweats, nonproductive cough, progressive shortness of breath	Chest x-ray, induced sputum for culture, bronchoalveolar lavage	Trimethoprim-sulfamethoxazole, dapsone+ trimethoprim, clindamycin, atovaquone, pentamidine, steroids, trimetrexate, and folinic acid
Cryptococcus species	Pneumonia, fever, cough, malaise	Sputum culture, serum antigen assay	Amphotericin B, fluconazole, itroconazole
Histoplasma capsulatum	Pneumonia, fever, cough	Sputum culture, serum antigen assay	Amphotericin B, itroconazole
Mycobacterium tuberculosis	Productive cough, fever, night sweats	Chest x-ray, sputum for AFB stain and culture	INH, ethambutol, rifampin, pyrazinamide, streptomycin
Coccidioides immitis	Fever, weight loss, cough	Sputum culture, serology	Amphotericin B, fluconazole, itroconazole, ketoconazole
Herpes simplex (type 1) (HSV1)	Vesicular eruptions on tracheobronchial mucosa	Viral culture	Acyclovir
Kaposi's sarcoma	Dyspnea	Chest x-ray, biopsy	Chemotherapy, radiation
Integumentary System			
HSV1	Vesicular eruptions on mouth	Viral culture	Acyclovir, foscarnet
Herpes simplex (type 2) (HSV2)	Vesicular eruptions around perianal area	Viral culture	Acyclovir, foscarnet
Varicella-zoster virus (VZV)	Shingles: erythematous macules, rash, pain, pruritis	Viral culture	Acyclovir, foscarnet
Kaposi's sarcoma	Firm, flat, raised, or nodular, hyperpigmented, multicentric lesions	Biopsy of lesions	Radiation, chemotherapy, alpha interferon
Bacillary angiomatosis	Erythematous papules and nodules	Biopsy of lesions	Erythromycin, doxycycline
Eye			
Cytomegalovirus (CMV) retinitis	Lesions on the retina, blurred vision, loss of vision, painless	Ophthalmoscopic examination	Ganciclovir, foscarnet
HSV1	Blurred vision, corneal lesions, acute retinal necrosis	Ophthalmoscopic examination	Acyclovir, foscarnet
VZV	Ocular lesions, acute retinal necrosis	Ophthalmoscopic examination	Acyclovir, foscarnet

continued

through the use of prophylactic interventions. Prophylactic medications have contributed to the decreased morbidity and mortality associated with HIV infection during the past several years. Therefore they are recommended according to established parameters (Table 11-4).[28]

Four drugs have now been approved to treat HIV infection (Table 11-5). All of these agents are nucleoside analogs. They each block reverse transcriptase, an enzyme required for HIV replication. The result is a slowing of the disease process rather than a cure. None of these drugs kill HIV, and it appears that HIV can become refractory to these drugs. Zidovudine (ZDV, AZT, Retrovir) is recommended as initial therapy when the $CD4^+$ lymphocyte count drops below 500/μl. Clinicians can switch to one of the other drugs if side effects are intolerable or if the $CD4^+$ lymphocyte count falls. Combination therapy is also used. A number of antiretroviral agents are currently in the process of development. New drugs will allow greater flexibility in the therapeutic management and control of HIV.

Probably the most difficult aspect of the medical management of HIV is dealing with the many opportunistic diseases that develop as the immune system degenerates. Although it is usually impossible to totally eradicate these diseases, there are treatments that can control disease progression. However, these treatments must continue during the life of the patient, or the diseases will return. Advances in the diagnosis and treatment of opportunistic diseases have contributed significantly to increased life expectancy. Table 11-2 presents possible treatments for common opportunistic diseases in the HIV-infected individuals.

Table 11-2 Common Opportunistic Diseases Associated with AIDS—cont'd

Organism or Disease	Clinical Manifestations	Diagnostic Tests	Treatment
Gastrointestinal System			
Cryptosporidium muris	Watery diarrhea, abdominal pain, weight loss, nausea	Stool examination	Antidiarrheals, paromomycin, azithromycin, atovaquone
CMV	Stomatitis, esophagitis, gastritis, colitis, bloody diarrhea, pain, weight loss	Endoscopic visualization, culture, biopsy; rule out other causes	Ganciclovir, foscarnet
HSV1	Vesicular eruptions on tongue, buccal, pharyngeal, or perioral esophageal mucosa	Viral culture	Acyclovir, foscarnet
Candida albicans	Whitish-yellow patches in mouth, esophagus, GI tract	Microscopic examination of scraping from lesion	Nystatin, clotrimazole, ketoconazole, fluconazole, itroconazole, Amphotericin B
Mycobacterium avium complex (MAC)	Watery diarrhea, weight loss	Small bowel biopsy with AFB stain and culture	Rifabutin, clarithromycin, rifampin, clofamizine, amikacin, ciprofloxacin, ethambutol, azithromycin
Isospora belli	Diarrhea, weight loss, nausea, abdominal pain	Stool examination	Trimethoprim-sulfamethoxazole, pyrimethamine + folic acid
Salmonella	Gastroenteritis, fever, diarrhea	Blood and stool culture	Ampicillin, amoxicillin, ciprofloxacin, trimethoprim-sulfamethoxazole
Kaposi's sarcoma	Diarrhea, hyperpigmented lesions of mouth and GI tract	GI series, biopsy	Radiation, chemotherapy
Non-Hodgkin's lymphoma	Abdominal pain, fever, night sweats, weight loss	Lymph node biopsy	Chemotherapy
Neurologic System			
Toxoplasma gondii	Cognitive dysfunction, motor impairment, fever, headache, seizures	MRI, CT scan, toxoplasma serology	Pyrimethamine + folic acid, sulfadiazine, clindamycin, azithromycin, clarithromycin
JC papovavirus	Progressive multifocal leukoencephalopathy (PML), mental and motor declines	MRI, CT scan, brain biopsy	Zidovudine may help
Cryptococcal meningitis	Cognitive impairment, motor dysfunction, fever, seizures	CT scan, serum antigen test, CSF analysis	Amphotericin B, 5-flucytosine, fluconazole, itronconazole
CNS lymphomas	Cognitive dysfunction, motor impairment, aphasia, seizures, personality changes, headache	MRI, CT scan	Radiation, chemotherapy
AIDS-dementia complex (ADC)	Insidious onset of progressive dementia	CT scan	Zidovudine may help

AFB, Acid-fast bacteria; *CNS*, central nervous system; *CSF*, cerebrospinal fluid; *CT*, computed tomography; *GI*, gastrointestinal; *INH*, inhalation; *MRI*, magnetic resonance imaging.

Vaccine Development

Early in the HIV epidemic there was optimism that an HIV vaccine would be quickly developed.[29] Despite considerable research and development, a vaccine still eludes scientists, and there is no hope for an effective preventive vaccine in the near future. The problems that impede vaccine development are numerous. Because HIV is an intracellular pathogen, it can hide from circulating immune factors. HIV, like most viruses, also mutates rapidly; consequently, the infected individual quickly develops a number of HIV variants that may not all respond to a simple vaccine. A major problem is that the correlates of protective immunity for HIV are unknown. Antibody development after other types of vaccination usually indicates immunity, but the HIV-infected patient produces an antibody that does not prevent active infection or confer immunity. In addition, HIV is frequently transmitted through mucosal routes; therefore a successful vaccine would need to induce mucosal and systemic protection.[30]

There are also social, ethical, and economic issues related to vaccination. Because there is no known animal model for HIV, vaccine efficacy can be established only through human testing. How will volunteers be recruited? How will true protection be determined? Will volunteers be

Table 11-3 Baseline and Follow-Up Assessment Parameters in the Patient with Human Immunodeficiency Virus Infection

Parameters	Initial Visit	CD4 >500	CD4 <500	CD4 <200	CD4 <100
Office visit	Follow-up in 2 wk	q3-6 mo	q2-3 mo	q1-2 mo	prn
CBC with differential and platelet count	✓	q3-6 mo	q2-3 mo	q1-2 mo	prn
Chemistry panel (SMA 12, 14, or 20)	✓	q3-6 mo	q2-3 mo	q1-2 mo	prn
Amylase		Monthly if patient is on didanosine			
RPR or VDRL	✓	Annually as long as sexually active			
CD4⁺ lymphocyte count	✓	q3-6 mo	q2-3 mo	q2-3 mo	prn
β-2 microglobulin, p24 antigen, neopterin	✓				
Hepatitis B serology	✓				
Toxoplasma and CMV serologies (IgG)	✓			✓	
AFB, blood culture				✓	✓
Chest x-ray	✓			✓	prn
PPD skin test by Mantoux method with anergy panel of at least 2 controls	✓	If negative without anergy at baseline, repeat annually until anergic; q6 mo in high prevalence areas			
Family planning/contraception	✓	With each visit as needed			
Pelvic with Pap or colposcopy	✓	Annual	q6 mo	q6 mo/prn	q6 mo/prn
Mammogram	✓	Annually			
Eye examination by ophthalmologic consult	✓	Annual	Annual	q6 mo	q4-6 mo
Dental examination and prophylaxis	Oral examination at each visit; dental care q3-6 mo for cleaning and preventive treatment as needed				
Antiretroviral medications		Discuss early	Encourage if symptomatic	Encourage	

Modified from Bradley-Springer LA, Fendrick R: *HIV instant instructor cards,* El Paso, TX, 1994, Skidmore-Roth.
AFB, Acid-fast bacilli; *CBC,* complete blood count; *CMV,* cytomegalovirus; *HIV,* human immunodeficiency virus; *PPD,* purified protein derivative; *prn,* as needed; *RPR,* rapid plasma reagin; *SMA,* sequential multiple analyzer; *VDRL,* Venereal Disease Research Laboratories.

exposed to HIV after immunization to see who gets infected? HIV is a worldwide problem with developing countries bearing the brunt of the epidemic. Is it possible to develop a vaccine that can be widely distributed in a short amount of time at an acceptable cost?[30,31]

In spite of the overwhelming nature of these issues, considerable research is in progress to develop an HIV vaccine. Vaccines in various stages of development have been tested in animals, and a few have progressed to human trials. Work is not limited to prevention vaccines. Investigations are also progressing on vaccines that boost HIV-specific host immune responses for use in infected patients.[30] However, authorities warn that the development of a successful vaccine will not replace current prevention methods, based on education and elimination of risky behaviors, because no vaccine is likely to be 100% effective.[30,31]

Nutritional Management

The major HIV-related nutritional problems are decreased nutrient intake, malabsorption, and metabolic disturbances.[32] These problems can be caused by HIV infection itself, opportunistic diseases, therapeutic interventions, and psychosocial issues. Intake of nutrients in HIV is negatively affected by a number of variables. HIV-related fatigue, malaise, anorexia, and nausea decrease energy and interest in food. Opportunistic diseases result in painful mouth and esophageal lesions that can make chewing and swallowing difficult. Opportunistic diseases also contribute to nausea, anorexia, and respiratory distress. Commonly ordered medications frequently cause mouth sores, fatigue, nausea, confusion, or taste changes. Intake problems are compounded by psychosocial issues related to loss of social support (e.g., assistance in shopping and food preparation) and lack of economic resources and anxiety, depression, grief, and confusion. Infectious processes cause a hypermetabolic state and the need for increased nutrient intake at a time when intake is decreasing, creating a negative nutritional balance.

HIV-wasting syndrome is a common problem experienced in the later stages of HIV disease. HIV infection contributes to wasting and wasting hastens the negative immune consequences of HIV infection. Wasting contributes to delayed recovery from infection, impaired wound healing, increased risk of secondary infection, impaired cardiopulmonary function,[33] and early death.[34]

HIV infection depletes nutritional reserves that are required to protect the patient from opportunistic disease. Early and ongoing attention to nutritional status and the maintenance of weight is clearly an important issue for the patient with HIV infection (Table 11-6). The difficulty is that causes of and problems related to malnutrition are inextricably intertwined.

PREVENTION OF HIV INFECTION

Although there is no vaccine, HIV transmission and new cases of HIV are preventable. Specific protective behaviors

Table 11-4 Prophylactic Interventions for Patients with Human Immunodeficiency Virus Infection

Problem	Prophylactic Interventions	Comments
▪ Pneumococcal pneumonia	Pneumococcal vaccine	Provide as soon as possible during course of infection; antibody response is optimal when $CD4^+$ cells are >350/μl.
▪ Hepatitis B virus (HBV)	Hepatitis B vaccine series; screen and vaccinate those who show no evidence of previous HBV infection	Provide as soon as possible during course of infection; encourage vaccine in injecting drug users, sexually active gay men, and sex partners or household contacts of HBV-infected individuals.
▪ Herpes simplex virus (HSV) 1 and 2	Low-dose acyclovir therapy may be initiated if prompt treatment of outbreaks is not sufficient for control	Provide ongoing assessment and intervention.
▪ Pulmonary tuberculosis	Treat if PPD is >5 mm reactive or if patient is anergic or at risk. INH for 12 mo. Consider directly observed therapy. (Clinical disease requires treatment with 4 or more drugs.)	Rule out active or extrapulmonary disease, which requires multidrug therapy; remember that a negative PPD in the presence of HIV does not exclude a diagnosis of tuberculosis; provide ongoing assessment and intervention.
▪ Wasting	Nutritional support and education should be initiated as soon as HIV infection is diagnosed.	Provide ongoing assessment and intervention.
▪ *Pneumocystis carinii* pneumonia (PCP)	Trimethoprim-sulfamethoxazole (TMP-SMX) (drug of choice) or dapsone or pentamidine per inhalation	Initiate when $CD4^+$ cells go below 200/μl; offer TMP-SMX to any patient with a history of PCP, regardless of $CD4^+$ cell count; oral drugs that provide systemic effect are preferred.
▪ *Mycobacterium avium* complex (MAC)	Rifabutin	Initiate when $CD4^+$ cells go below 100/μl; Rifabutin has caused dose-related uveitis (above 600 mg/day), which is reversible with drug withdrawal or dose reduction.
▪ Toxoplasmosis	Trimethoprim-sulfamethoxazole (TMP-SMX) or dapsone with pyrimethamine and folinic acid	Initiate when $CD4^+$ cells go below 100/μl.

HIV, Human immunodeficiency virus; *INH,* inhalation; *PPD,* purified protein derivative.

have been known and recommended since the middle 1980s. These behaviors are crucial for control of the epidemic. Prevention techniques can be divided into *safe* activities (those that eliminate risk) and *risk-reducing* activities (those that decrease risk but do not eliminate it). Prevention methods must be used consistently and correctly if they are going to be effective.

Decreasing Risks Related to Sexual Intercourse

Safe activities eliminate the risk of exposure to HIV in semen and vaginal secretions. Abstaining from all sexual activity is the most effective way to accomplish this goal. Additional options maintain safety for those who do not wish to abstain. Limiting sexual behavior to activities in which the mouth, penis, vagina, or rectum does not come into contact with the partner's mouth, penis, vagina, or rectum is safe because there is no contact with blood, semen, or vaginal secretions. These activities may include massage, masturbation, mutual masturbation, telephone sex, or many other activities that meet the requirements. Insertive sex is considered to be safe only in a mutually monogamous relationship with a partner who is not infected or at risk of becoming infected with HIV. The problem with mutual monogamy is that both partners have to follow all of the rules all of the time. Unfortunately, there are a number of cases of HIV infection that occurred in individuals who were not aware that their partner had not remained monogamous.

Risk-reducing sexual activities decrease the risk of contact with HIV through the use of barriers. Barriers should be used when engaging in sexual activity with a partner whose HIV status is not definitely known or with a partner who is known to be HIV-infected. The most commonly used barrier is the male condom (Fig. 11-7). Condoms are not 100% effective, but when used correctly and consistently, they are highly effective in preventing the transmission of HIV.[35,36] Major points for correct condom use include the following:

1. Do not use a condom if the expiration date has passed or if the package looks worn or punctured.

2. Only use condoms that are made out of latex or polyurethane. "Natural skin" condoms have pores that are large enough for HIV to penetrate.

Table 11-5 Antiretroviral Agents Used for Patients with Human Immunodeficiency Virus Infection

Drug and Dosage	Adverse Effects	Comments
Zidovudine (AZT, ZDV, Retrovir)—200 mg orally 3 times/day or 100 mg orally 5 times/day; if intolerant, use 300-400 mg daily by mouth in divided doses	Fatigue, malaise, headache, rash, nausea, insomnia, myalgia, confusion, agitation, seizures; bone marrow suppression, anemia, granulocytopenia, thrombocytopenia; hepatomegaly; initial constitutional symptoms usually resolve in a few weeks	Drug of choice to initiate therapy; recommend when CD4 count <500/μl; encourage when CD4 count <200/μl, anemia can be treated with transfusions or erythropoietin (EPO); consider granulocyte colony-stimulating factor (G-CSF) to treat granulocytopenia.
Didanosine (ddI, Videx)—by weight: >60 kg-200 mg orally 2 times/day <60 kg-125 mg orally 2 times/day	Pancreatitis, painful peripheral neuropathy (dose related and reversible), nausea, abdominal pain, diarrhea, rash, hyperglycemia, hyperuricemia, hepatic failure, headache, insomnia, seizures, thrombocytopenia	Use with patients who fail or who are intolerant to zidovudine; dosage must be provided in 2 tablets to ensure adequate buffer for absorption; tablets must be chewed or dissolved and administered on empty stomach 2 hr apart from drugs whose absorption is impaired by buffer; avoid use of alcohol, H_2 antagonists, antacids, and omeprazole.
Zalcitabine (ddC, HIVID)—by weight: >30 kg-0.75 mg orally 3 times/day <30 mg-0.375 mg orally 3 times/day	Painful peripheral neuropathy (dose related and reversible); rash, oral or esophageal ulcers, pancreatitis, seizures, nausea, diarrhea, fatigue; elevations in alanine and asparate aminotransferases; cardiomyopathy, headache	Although not as effective as zidovudine, can be used as monotherapy for patients who fail or who are intolerant to zidovudine; may also be used in combination with zidovudine.
Stavudine (d4T, Zerit)—by weight: >60 kg-40 mg orally 2 times/day <60 kg-30 mg orally 2 times/day	Painful peripheral neuropathy; elevations in alanine and asparate aminotransferases; anemia, headache, rash, abdominal pain, diarrhea, nausea, vomiting, myalgia	Use for patients intolerant to other antiretroviral agents; may eventually be recommended for combination therapy.
Combination therapy: zidovudine with didanosine or zidovudine with zalcitabine	Dose dependent—additive toxicities may occur if both drugs are used in regular doses; if doses are decreased there may be some relief from side effects; alternating regimens allow "drug holidays" that may improve ability to tolerate adverse effects	Generally not used as first line therapy; combinations (either concomitant or sequential) may be added as disease progresses or as drugs become refractory.

Modified from Goldschmidt RH, Dong BJ: Current report—HIV: Treatment of AIDS and HIV-related conditions—1994, *Am Board of Fam Prac* 7:155, 1994.
AZT, Azidothymidine; *HIV*, human immunodeficiency virus.

3. The condom must be placed on the erect penis before any contact is made with the partner's mouth, vagina, or rectum to prevent exposure to preejaculatory secretions that may contain HIV.
4. Lubricants used in conjunction with condoms must be water soluble. Oil-based lubricants can weaken the latex and increase the risk of tearing or breaking. Nonlubricated, flavored condoms can provide protection during oral intercourse.
5. A new condom must be used for every act of intercourse.
6. Nonoxynol 9, a chemical found in spermicidal preparations, has shown some viricidal activity. It can be used in conjunction with condoms to provide additional protection. However, allergic reactions to nonoxynol 9 can cause genital itching, redness, and discomfort, which can lead to lesions on the penis and mucous membranes of the vagina and rectum. The user who notes these reactions should cleanse the affected areas and discontinue use of the spermicide.
7. The penis and condom should be removed from the partner's body immediately after ejaculation and before the erection is lost. This prevents semen leakage from the condom around a flaccid penis.

Other barriers include female condoms and latex, or dental, dams. Female condoms consist of a vinyl sheath with two springform rings. The smaller ring is inserted into the vagina and holds the condom in place internally. The larger ring surrounds the opening to the condom. It functions to keep the condom in place externally while protecting the external genitalia (Fig. 11-8). Use can be complicated, so careful instructions are required. Squares of latex (available from dental supply sources) or plastic wrapping paper

Table 11-6 Nutritional Management: Human Immunodeficiency Virus Infection

Dietary Recommendation	Intervention
Diarrhea	
Lactose-free, low-fat, low-fiber, and high-potassium foods	Avoid dairy products, red meat, margarine, butter, eggs, dried beans, peas, raw fruits and vegetables. Cooked or canned fruits and vegetables will provide needed vitamins. Encourage potassium-rich foods such as bananas and apricot nectar. Discontinue foods, nutritional supplements, and medications that may make diarrhea worse (e.g., Ensure, antacids, stool softeners). Avoid gas-producing foods. Serve warm, not hot, foods. Plan small, frequent meals. Drink plenty of fluids between meals.
Constipation	
High-fiber foods	Eat fruits and vegetables (e.g., beans, peas) and cereal and whole wheat breads. Gradually increase fiber. Drink plenty of fluids. Exercise.
Nausea and Vomiting	
Low-fat foods	Avoid dairy products and red meat. Plan small, frequent meals. Prepare nonodorous foods. Eat dry, salty foods. Serve food cold or at room temperature. Drink liquids between meals. Avoid gas-producing, greasy, spicy foods. Eat slowly in a relaxed atmosphere. Rest after meals with head elevated. Offer antiemetics 30 min before meals.
Candidiasis	
Soft or pureed foods	Serve moist foods. Drink plenty of fluids. Avoid acidic and spicy foods. Use straw and tilt head back and forth when drinking. To decrease discomfort, eat soft diet, such as puddings and yogurt.
Fever	
High-calorie, high-protein foods	Use nutritional supplements. Increase fluid intake.
Altered Taste	
Diet as tolerated	Try herbs and spices. Marinate meat, poultry, and fish. Serve food cold or at room temperature. Drink plenty of fluids. Add salt or sugar. Introduce alternative protein sources.
Anemia	
High-iron foods	Eat red meat, organ meats, and raisins. Drink orange juice when taking iron supplements to facilitate absorption.
Fatigue	
High-calorie foods	Cook in large quantities and freeze in meal-size packets. Use microwave and convenience foods. Use easy-to-fix snack foods. Encourage social support system to assist with meal planning and preparation. Provide in-home homemaker services. Access community Meals-on-Wheels programs.

can be used to cover the external genitalia during oral sexual activity.

Decreasing Risks Related to Drug Use

Recreational or illicit drug use is harmful. It can cause immune suppression, malnutrition, and psychosocial problems. However, drug use itself does not cause HIV infection. The major risks of HIV are related to sharing injecting equipment and having unsafe sexual experiences while under the influence of drugs. The basic rules are (1) do not use drugs; (2) if drugs are used, do not share equipment; and (3) do not have sexual intercourse when under the influence of any drug (including alcohol) that impairs decision-making ability.

The safest mechanism is to abstain from drugs. This is not a viable alternative for the user who chooses not to quit or for the user who has no access to drug treatment services. The risk of HIV for these individuals can be eliminated if they can find alternatives to injecting. Other routes of drug administration such as smoking, snorting, or ingesting are less risky because they remove the risk of exposure to blood through injecting equipment. Risk can also be eliminated if the user does not share injecting equipment. Injecting equipment includes needles, syringes, cookers (spoons or bottle caps used to mix the drug), cotton, and rinse water. None of this equipment should be shared. Of course, the safest tactic is for the user to have ready access to sterile equipment. Some communities are now instituting needle and syringe exchange programs to provide sterile equipment to users. Opposition to these programs is supported by the fear that ready access to injecting supplies will increase drug use. However, studies have shown that in communities where exchange programs have been established, drug use does not increase, and rates of HIV infection are controlled.[37]

Cleaning equipment before use is a risk-reducing activity. It decreases the risk for those who must share equipment. To clean used equipment, rinse the used needle and

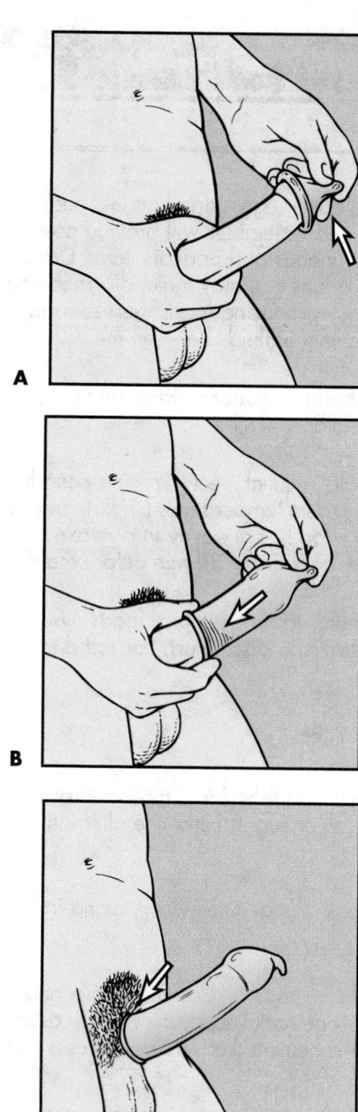

Fig. 11-7 Proper placement of the male condom. ***A,*** The condom is placed over the glans of the erect penis being careful to squeeze air out of the reservoir. ***B*** and ***C,*** The condom is then rolled down the shaft of the penis to the hairline.

syringe twice with tap water, then fill the syringe with full-strength household bleach, shake for 30 seconds, squirt bleach out, and repeat the bleaching process; then rinse equipment twice with tap water. This process takes time and may be difficult for a person in drug withdrawal.

Decreasing Risks at Work

The risk of infection from occupational exposure to HIV is small but real. The CDC and the Occupational Safety and Health Administration (OSHA) have instituted policies to assure that employees are protected from exposure to blood and other potentially infectious fluids.[38] Precautions for the prevention of blood-borne disease are discussed in Chapter 9. Precautions have been shown to decrease the risk of direct contact with blood and body fluids.[39] Decreasing the risk of contact should logically decrease the risk of infection with all blood-borne pathogens. However, should exposure to HIV-infected fluids occur, protocols now exist for postexposure prophylaxis with zidovudine (ZDV, AZT, Retrovir).[8] It is not known whether taking zidovudine after an exposure actually decreases the risk of HIV infection. Definitive data will be difficult to collect because of the low risk.[9] It is essential to report potential occupational exposures so appropriate follow-up care can be provided.

Other Methods to Reduce Risk

It is important to encourage the individual at risk for HIV to be tested. An individual found to be infected can be educated and counseled to prevent further transmissions of the virus. The HIV-infected person should be instructed not to give blood, donate organs, or donate semen for artificial insemination; not to share razors, toothbrushes, or other household items that may contain blood or other body fluids; to avoid infecting sexual and needle-sharing partners; and to consider using birth control measures to avoid spreading the virus to infants.

NURSING MANAGEMENT

HIV INFECTION

Nursing Assessment

Subjective and objective data that should be obtained from an individual who has HIV infection are presented in Table 11-7. Ongoing nursing assessment is essential because early recognition and treatment of problems can be life saving. Soliciting a complete history can help the nurse avoid missing any specific areas. However, a thorough systems review is also needed because of the interactive nature of problems related to HIV infection.

Nursing Diagnoses

Nursing diagnoses are determined when the problem and etiologic factors are supported by clinical data. The nursing diagnoses related to HIV infection include, but are not limited to, those presented in the following Nursing Care Plan.

Planning

The overall goals of a patient with HIV infection are (1) to have adequate nutritional status; (2) to have minimal to no problems with opportunistic disease; (3) not to transmit HIV virus to others; (4) to maintain or develop healthy, supportive relationships; (5) to come to terms with issues related to disease, death, and spirituality; and (6) to maintain usual activities and productivity for as long as possible. Goals will change as HIV disease progresses and disabilities develop.

Nursing Implementation

Health Promotion and Maintenance. As with most chronic conditions, disease prevention and health promotion are the most effective health care strategies.[40]

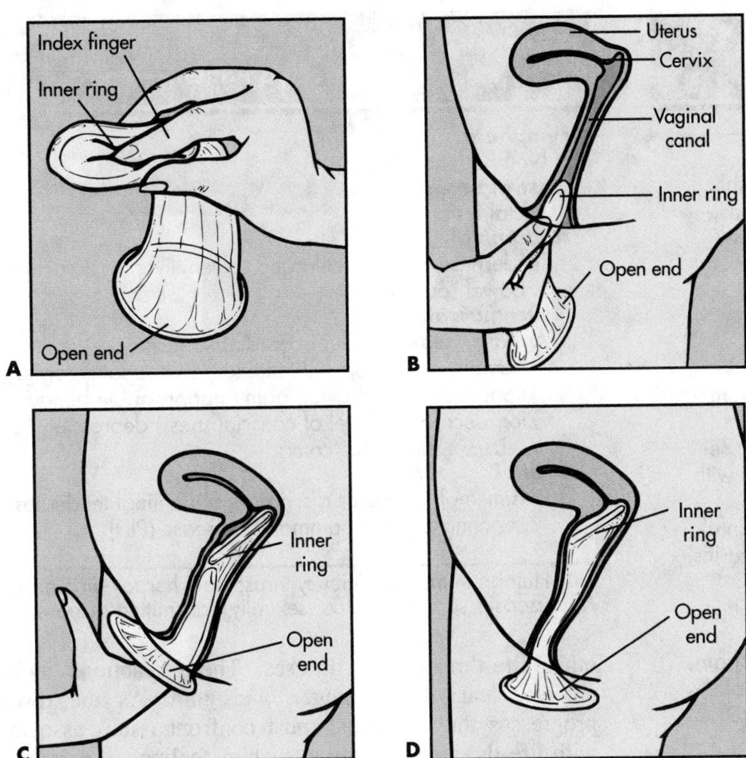

Fig. 11-8 Proper placement of the female condom. ***A,*** Inner ring is squeezed for insertion. ***B,*** Sheath is inserted similarly to a tampon. ***C,*** Inner ring is pushed up as far as it can go with index finger. ***D,*** The condom is in place.

Table 11-8 (see p. 255) presents a synopsis of nursing goals, assessment, and interventions at each level of nursing care. The initial nursing focus is to prevent infection. In the absence of a vaccination, education and behavioral change are the only effective tools for prevention. Educational messages should be specific to the patient's need, culturally sensitive, and age specific. The nurse is an excellent resource for this type of education but must be comfortable with and knowledgeable of sensitive topics such as sexuality and drug use (see section on Prevention of HIV).

The nurse should also encourage early detection of HIV infection. Testing for HIV (see section on Diagnostic Studies) is an important part of the public health response to HIV. A patient will not get tested, however, unless there is a perceived need for testing and a feeling of safety in doing so. The nurse can help the patient assess the risks by asking some basic questions.

1. Have you ever had a transfusion or used clotting factors? Was it before 1985?
2. Have you ever shared needles, syringes, or other injecting equipment with anyone?
3. Have you ever had a sexual experience in which your penis, vagina, rectum, or mouth came into contact with another person's penis, vagina, rectum, or mouth?

These questions are the minimum needed to initiate a risk assessment. They should be modified to meet the needs of the patient and the situation. Positive responses to any of these questions require a more in-depth exploration of the issues. The nurse should be prepared to refer the patient to centers that provide testing and counseling services. All testing for HIV should be accompanied by pretest and posttest counseling. Testing sessions are excellent opportunities for risk assessment and education. Table 11-9 summarizes the basic components of counseling related to HIV testing (see p. 256).

Acute Intervention. Early intervention after detection of HIV infection can promote health and limit or delay disability. Because the course of HIV is extremely variable, assessment attains primary importance.[41,42] Nursing interventions will be based on and tailored to patient needs noted during assessment. The nursing assessment in HIV disease should focus on the early detection of constitutional symptoms, opportunistic diseases, and psychosocial problems. (See Table 11-7 for information on nursing assessment.)

HIV-disease progression may be delayed by promoting a healthy immune system. Useful interventions for the HIV-infected patient include the following:

1. Nutritional changes that maintain lean body mass, increase weight, and assure appropriate levels of vitamins and micronutrients
2. Smoking and drug use cessation interventions
3. Moderation or elimination of alcohol intake
4. Regular exercise
5. Stress reduction
6. Avoiding exposure to new infectious agents
7. Mental health counseling
8. Involvement in support groups

Reactions to a positive HIV-antibody test are similar to the reactions of the person who is diagnosed with cancer or

Table 11-7 Nursing Assessment: HIV-Infected Patient

Subjective Data

Important Health Information

Past health history: Route of infection, hepatitis, other STDs, frequent viral infections, parasitic infections, tuberculosis, alcohol and drug use, foreign travel

Medications: Use of immunosuppressive drugs

Functional Health Patterns

Health perception–health management: Chronic fatigue, malaise

Nutritional-metabolic: Unexplained weight loss, low-grade fevers, night sweats; anorexia, nausea, vomiting; oral lesions, bleeding, ulcerations; abdominal cramping; lesions of lips, mouth, tongue, throat; sensitivity to acidic, salty, or spicy foods, problems with teeth and gums, difficulty swallowing; bleeding gums; skin rashes or color changes, lesions (painful or non-painful), blisters; nonhealing wounds, pruritis

Elimination: Persistent diarrhea; painful urination

Activity-exercise: Muscle weakness, difficulty walking; cough, shortness of breath

Cognitive-perceptual: Headaches, stiff neck, chest pain, rectal pain, retrosternal pain; blurred vision, photophobia, loss of vision, diplopia; confusion, forgetfulness, attention deficit, changes in mental status, memory loss; hearing impairment; personality changes; paresthesias; hypersensitivity in feet

Sexuality-reproductive: Lesions on genitalia (internal or external), pruritis or burning in vagina, painful sexual intercourse, changes in menstruation, vaginal or penile discharge

Objective Data

General

Vital signs, weight, general status, diaphoresis

Eyes

Presence of exudate, retinal lesions or hemorrhage, papilledema

Oral

Presence of a variety of mouth lesions including blisters (HSV), white-gray patches (candida), painless white lesions on lateral aspect of the tongue (hairy leukoplakia), discolorations (KS), gingivitis, tooth decay or loosening, variety of other lesions

Neck

Enlarged lymph nodes, nuchal rigidity

Throat

Redness or white patchy lesions

Integumentary

Observe integrity and turgor; general appearance; presence of lesions, eruptions, discoloration; enlarged lymph nodes, bruises, cyanosis, dryness, delayed wound healing, alopecia

Respiratory

Presence of crackles, dyspnea, cough (may be productive or nonproductive), wheezing, tachypnea, intercostal retractions

continued

Table 11-7 Nursing Assessment: HIV-Infected Patient—cont'd

Lymphatic

Lymphadenopathy

Gastrointestinal

Rectal lesions

Abdominal

Tenderness, masses, enlarged spleen/liver, hyperactive bowel sounds

Neuromuscular

Aphasia, ataxia, lack of coordination, sensory loss, tremors, slurred speech, memory loss, apathy, agitation, social withdrawal, pain, inappropriate behavior, decreasing level of consciousness, depression, seizures, paralysis, coma

Genital

Presence of lesions or discharge, abdominal tenderness denoting pelvic inflammatory disease (PID)

HIV, Human immunodeficiency virus; *HSV,* herpes simplex virus; *KS,* Kaposi's sarcoma; *STDs,* sexually transmitted diseases.

other life-threatening illnesses. These reactions include anxiety, fear, denial, anger, and guilt. As the disease progresses the individual must confront issues associated with life-threatening illness, such as feelings of powerlessness, social isolation, depression, grief, altered self-concept, thoughts of suicide, and the possibility of impending death.

The nurse needs to help the patient gain control. Facilitating empowerment is particularly important because the individual with HIV infection often experiences losses, including an overwhelming feeling of loss of control. Empowerment is facilitated by education and honest discussions about the patient's health status.

The patient should be taught to recognize clinical manifestations that may indicate progression of the disease to ensure that prompt medical care is initiated. Early manifestations that need to be reported include unexplained weight loss, night sweats, diarrhea, persistent fever, swollen lymph nodes, oral hairy leukoplakia, oral candidiasis, and persistent vaginal yeast infections. The patient should be given as much information as needed to make decisions about health care. These decisions will then dictate the appropriate medical and nursing interventions.

Nursing care becomes more complicated as the patient's immune system deteriorates and new problems arise to compound existing difficulties. Nursing care for the HIV-infected patient with symptomatic disease is presented in the nursing care plan on p. 251. The focus is usually on quality-of-life issues and caring rather than on cure issues.[43]

When opportunistic diseases develop, symptomatic nursing care, education, and emotional support are necessary. For example, an acute case of *Pneumocystis carinii* pneumonia (PCP) (Fig. 11-9, p. 257) requires intensive nursing intervention. Nursing care includes monitoring the respiratory status, administering medications and oxygen, positioning the patient to facilitate breathing, guiding relaxation exercises to decrease anxiety, promoting nutritional support, and conserving energy to decrease oxygen demand. Because

(Text continued on p. 256.)

NURSING CARE PLAN Patient with Symptomatic HIV Infection and AIDS

Planning: Outcome Criteria	*Nursing Interventions and Rationales*
➤ **NURSING DIAGNOSIS**	Chronic and acute pain *related to* peripheral neuropathies; generalized arthralgia and myalgia; pneumonia; headache; lymphadenopathy; opportunistic infections; tumor invasion; lack of knowledge of pain control measures; oral, vaginal, or perianal excoriation; and diagnostic or medical procedures *as manifested by* complaint of pain, assumption of protective posture, withdrawal, increased pulse and respiratory rate, and facial grimacing
Verbalize ability to cope with level of pain; notify nurse when relief from medications is not obtained; use alternate methods of pain relief; exert personal control over pain and relief measures.	Respond immediately to complaints of pain *to demonstrate concern for patient's comfort and welfare.* Encourage patient to describe pain episodes *to identify factors associated with pain.* Encourage patient to actively participate in planning for pain control *to enhance self-control and compliance with care plan.* Teach and encourage the use of alternate methods of pain relief such as massage, visualization, relaxation, distraction, and touching *to alter pain perception.* Assess need for medications *to plan appropriate intervention.* Administer analgesics early in the pain episode *to reduce patient anxiety and decrease pain.* Encourage use of nonsteroidal antiinflammatory agents *to potentiate effects of analgesics.* Assist patient to titrate pain medications *to allow patient control for optimal relief.*
➤ **NURSING DIAGNOSIS**	Anxiety *related to* multiple physical, social, and economic changes and losses; fear of death and dying; lack of knowledge of patient and family about disease process, transmission and prevention, medications and their side effects, alternative treatment modalities, and available community resources *as manifested by* frequent and multiple questions asked about the course and treatment of the disease; appearance of agitation, decreased verbalization, and discomfort
Verbalize understanding of HIV infection and AIDS; display knowledge of action and side effects of drugs; use appropriate community resources; verbalize feeling less anxious.	Assess anxiety levels and sources *to initiate patient development of coping methods.* Provide calm, accepting, and open atmosphere *that facilitates patient willingness to discuss difficult issues.* Provide accurate information about HIV and its signs and symptoms, treatments, medications, and transmission *to ensure patient and family ability to make informed decisions.* Provide lists and explanations of community resources, and offer to contact community-based organizations *to ensure appropriate use of available resources.* Educate patient and family about signs of opportunistic infections and malignancies *to ensure early recognition and treatment.* Teach about action and common side effects of medications; provide written list of medications with times, dosages, and possible side effects *to promote safe drug use.*
➤ **NURSING DIAGNOSIS**	Altered thought processes *related to* hypoxemia, fever, neurologic changes, dehydration, drug and alcohol use, electrolyte imbalance, problems with vision or hearing, opportunistic infections or malignancies, side effects of medications, and stress *as manifested by* inappropriate responses, disorientation, confusion, personality changes
Be oriented to person, place, time; participate in daily care as able; minimize safety hazards and daily life problems caused by altered thought processes.	Monitor onset and progression of confusion *to assess baseline and promote safety.* Monitor WBC count, temperature, ABGs, and fluid balance *to assist in determining cause of problem.* Teach stress reduction techniques *to reduce increasing confusion.* Speak in simple, short sentences and provide written instructions *to promote understanding and orientation.* Instruct caregiver in memory cues (calendar, clock, log) *to enhance reality orientation by use of commonly recognized items.* Control environmental stimuli *to avoid overstimulation.* Discuss need for 24-hr care as mental status deteriorates *to ensure that long-term care can be planned.*

continued

NURSING CARE PLAN Patient with Symptomatic HIV Infection and AIDS—cont'd

Planning: Outcome Criteria	Nursing Interventions and Rationales
➤ **NURSING DIAGNOSIS**	Altered nutrition less than body requirements *related to* opportunistic infections, oral lesions, anorexia, nausea and vomiting, diarrhea, impaired swallowing, esophagitis, catabolism, side effects to medications, fever, malabsorption, fatigue, social and economic factors, depression, and lack of knowledge regarding appropriate anabolic diet *as manifested by* weight loss, wasting, weakness
Increase nutritional intake of high protein and high caloric foods; have improved skin turgor and improved condition of skin, hair, nails, and mucous membranes; verbalize satisfaction with diet; maintain weight.	Begin early nutrition education and counseling *to initiate dietary changes, encourage weight gain, and prevent malnutrition to enhance immune function.* Monitor weight, intake and output of food, and caloric intake *to determine adequacy of intake.* Encourage daily intake of 40-45 kcal/kg and 1-1.5 g/kg of protein *to reduce catabolism.* Teach patient to prepare and store food properly *to decrease possibility of opportunistic infections from food.* Assess need for financial and social assistance to obtain or prepare food and provide referrals as needed *to allow for appropriate assistance.* Provide oral care before and after meals *to minimize unpleasant taste, prevent oral infections, and provide comfort.* Administer antiemetics before meals *to reduce nausea.*
➤ **NURSING DIAGNOSIS**	Activity intolerance *related to* chronic HIV infection, opportunistic diseases, stress, anemia, malnutrition, diarrhea, side effects of therapy, fever, electrolyte imbalance, insomnia *as manifested* by fatigue, weakness, lassitude, pallor, diaphoresis, dyspnea, or dizziness on exertion
Identify factors that contribute to fatigue; plan activities and pace for activity capabilities; use assistive devices; verbalize increased energy levels.	Minimize factors that contribute to fatigue *to increase energy reserves.* Teach energy conservation measures and the use of assistive devices *to increase safety and decrease energy expenditure.* Assist in development of 24-hr plan that sets priorities *to decrease anxiety and unnecessary energy utilization.* Provide for periods of rest after meals and fatiguing activities *to restore energy reserves.*
➤ **NURSING DIAGNOSIS**	Self-care deficit *related to* motor and cognitive deficits, fatigue, weakness, exercise intolerance, and emotional reactions to illness *as manifested by* inability to perform ADLs
Perform self-care activities as able; accept care from others when necessary; express satisfaction with care.	Assess functional ability *to determine need for assistance.* Appropriately set realistic goals and pace *to prevent frustration.* Instruct and supervise caregivers in physical care *because patient is comforted by competent caregivers.* Provide emotional support to patient and significant others *to assist with adjustments.* Refer to physical or occupational therapy as indicated *to enhance physical strength and motivation.* Provide information about community resources and initiate referrals as appropriate *to provide for episodic and long-term support.*
➤ **NURSING DIAGNOSIS**	Hyperthermia *related to* HIV and other infectious processes, dehydration, and drug reaction *as manifested by* fever, diaphoresis, chills, tachycardia
Be afebrile; verbalize feeling comfortable.	Monitor vital signs and level of dehydration *to assist with early recognition of problem onset and to evaluate efficacy of treatment.* Administer antipyretics *to assist in temperature reduction.* Evaluate need for cooling measures such as ice packs, tepid baths, cooling blanket *to assist in temperature reduction via heat dissipation.* Encourage fluid intake *to maintain hydration.* Bathe and change linens as needed *to promote comfort and evaluate skin integrity.*
➤ **NURSING DIAGNOSIS**	Diarrhea *related to* opportunistic infections, malignancy of the GI tract, adverse medication reaction, lactose intolerance, and tube feeding intolerance *as manifested by* frequent diarrheal stools, cramping, dehydration
Return to usual bowel pattern; decreased number of stools per day; return to a balanced intake and output of foods; no skin breakdown; moist mucous membranes and adequate hydration.	Monitor elimination pattern, bowel sounds, intake and output, stool cultures and skin condition *to allow early recognition of problems.* Treat causes of diarrhea and administer antimotility agents *to decrease number of stools.* Recommend low-residue, high-protein, high-calorie diet *to decrease gastrointestinal motility and maintain nutritional status.* Encourage oral fluids (e.g. juices, broths, water), and administer intravenous fluids as needed *to prevent dehydration.* Cleanse and dry rectal area after each bowel movement; apply petroleum jelly or ointment containing lanolin or petrolatum *to prevent skin breakdown.* Assist with sitz baths for perianal excoriation *to provide comfort.*

continued

NURSING CARE PLAN Patient with Symptomatic HIV Infection and AIDS—cont'd

Planning: Outcome Criteria	*Nursing Interventions and Rationales*
➤ **NURSING DIAGNOSIS**	Impaired gas exchange *related to* pulmonary infection or malignancy, increased secretions, hypoxemia, decreased air exchange, decreased tidal volume, anemia, exercise intolerance, ineffective or severe cough, anxiety and pain *as manifested by* dyspnea, tachypnea, cyanosis, wheezing, cough, inability to raise secretions, use of accessory muscles
Express less discomfort with breathing; have decreased symptoms of dyspnea and air hunger; expectorate secretions; identify causes of respiratory distress; develop coping mechanisms.	Monitor respiratory rate, breathing patterns, breath sounds and ABGs *to detect respiratory complications.* Administer antibiotics, antitussives, and expectorants *to treat underlying problem, provide comfort, and assist with removal of secretions.* Suction as indicated *to clear airway and improve ventilation.* Monitor use and effectiveness of therapies such as oxygen, mechanical ventilation, humidification, chest tubes, and medications *to evaluate effect.* Encourage deep breathing, effective coughing, ambulation, postural drainage *to prevent stasis of secretions.* Encourage fluid intake *to prevent dehydration and to assist in liquefication of secretions.* Teach positioning *to facilitate breathing.* Teach relaxation techniques *to decrease anxiety.*
➤ **NURSING DIAGNOSIS**	Impaired skin integrity *related to* prolonged immobility, poor nutritional status, edema, incontinence, diarrhea, and opportunistic infections such as herpes simplex *as manifested by* presence of broken, draining skin areas, excoriation, skin lesions, tenderness, reddened areas
Have no areas of skin breakdown; verbalize no discomfort related to skin.	Assess and monitor skin *to establish baseline and identify changes early.* Encourage mobility and adequate nutrition and fluids *to prevent skin problems.* Leave dry lesions open to air *to promote healing.* Clean draining lesions with soap and water and pat dry. Apply normal saline dressing *to dry draining lesion, relieve itching, suppress inflammation, and debride.* Apply topical antibiotic such as polymyxin B, bacitracin, or neomycin and nonadhering dressing *to treat and prevent infection, to promote healing, and to prevent trauma.* Provide immediate care after incontinent episodes *to prevent or limit excoriation and breakdown.*
➤ **NURSING DIAGNOSIS**	Altered oral mucous membranes *related to* oral infection or neoplasm, malnutrition, dehydration, and drug or radiation therapy *as manifested by* mucocutaneous lesions, mucositis, painful oral lesions, periodontal disease, dry mouth
Have decreased or no areas of oral mucous membrane breakdown; be able to perform oral hygiene; verbalize decreased symptoms and pain.	Monitor status of oral mucosa *to establish baseline and recognize problems early.* Encourage patient to get dental prophylaxis every 3 mo *to learn good oral hygiene, promote healthy mouth, and enhance early detection of problems.* Administer antiinfective agents and topical anesthetics *to promote healing and comfort.* Give oral hygiene before topical antifungal use *to remove secretions and provide clean surface for medication.* Scrub gums gently with soft toothbrush or toothette 3 to 4 times a day; rinse mouth with saline solution or non–alcohol-containing mouthwash *to prevent trauma, promote comfort, and reduce spread of lesions.*
➤ **NURSING DIAGNOSIS**	Risk for secondary infection *related to* immunosuppression; neutropenia secondary to medication, treatment, or infection; lack of knowledge regarding infection control; and impaired skin integrity
Remain free of opportunistic infections; identify ways to reduce risk of opportunistic infections.	Monitor for signs of infection such as fever, fatigue, and swollen lymph nodes *so early intervention can be initiated.* Monitor vital signs and laboratory tests *to identify signs of infection.* Encourage ambulation, adequate fluids, and optimal nutrition *to promote immune health and decrease risk of infection.* Inform patient not to clean cat litter boxes and not to eat foods that could be spoiled or drink unpasteurized milk *to avoid possible exposure to pathogens.* Assess medication regimen *to determine if it is causing low WBC counts.* Wash hands before caring for patient *to prevent nosocomial infection.* Teach infection control measures to patient, visitors, and family *to prevent secondary infection.* Teach patient to monitor for and report signs of infection *to promote early detection.*

continued

NURSING CARE PLAN Patient with Symptomatic HIV Infection and AIDS—cont'd

Planning: Outcome Criteria	Nursing Interventions and Rationales
➤ **NURSING DIAGNOSIS**	Anticipatory grieving *related to* diagnosis of potentially terminal illness *as manifested by* verbalizations of sorrow, grief, loss; withdrawal, crying
Share grief and loss feelings with caregivers.	Establish a caring relationship with patient and family *so that the nurse is considered a part of the support system.* Inquire if patient desires clergy visit *to provide additional support.* Encourage development of helpful coping strategies such as use of support groups and use of diversional activities *to enlarge support system.*
➤ **NURSING DIAGNOSIS**	Risk for infection transmission *related to* lack of knowledge, skills, or use of prophylactic measures
Verbalize knowledge of facts related to risk factors, transmission, and prevention techniques; correctly disinfect injection equipment; demonstrate correct condom use; use appropriate infection control measures; verbalize willingness to use safety measures.	Teach facts about risky behaviors and risk-reduction measures *to reduce the possibility of infecting others.* Use teaching techniques such as role playing and return demonstrations *to promote confidence in skills.* Discuss use of contraceptive measures or medication interventions *to prevent or reduce potential infection of infant.* Provide information about community resources *to give support and encouragement in lifestyle changes.* Instruct patient and caregivers on infection control measures *to reduce anxiety and encourage protection from blood and body fluids.* Supervise caregivers' ability to comply with recommendations on infection control *to assess need for further education and assistance.* Provide written, specific instructions for caregivers in home *to provide reinforcement for learning.*
➤ **NURSING DIAGNOSIS**	Impaired social interaction *related to* fear of AIDS by general population, guilt, stigma, impaired body image, and presence of terminal illness *as manifested by* inadequate support system, hopelessness, social isolation, depression
Verbalize satisfaction with social interactions and support system.	Provide a supportive environment *to enhance patient's feelings of self-worth.* Teach others about HIV infection and modes of transmission *to decrease fear.* Plan meaningful interactions and diversional activities *to increase patient's motivation and decrease social isolation.* Refer to counseling, support groups, and community resources *to provide social and emotional supports.*
➤ **NURSING DIAGNOSIS**	Caregiver role strain *related to* long-term care of debilitated patient *as manifested by* verbalization of difficulty performing caregiving activities, depression, anger, fatigue.
Express satisfaction with caregiver role; verbalize decreased anxiety and fatigue.	Encourage caregiver to identify other people to assist in care of patient *to provide alternative resources and relief from responsibility.* Allow caregiver to share feelings in a safe environment *to assure that these feelings are typical and do not mean that the caregiver is "bad."* Assist caregiver in identifying activities in which assistance is needed *to acknowledge that the caregiver needs assistance and to allow support from others.* Teach caregiver stress-management techniques such as deep breathing and relaxation *to relieve stress and develop healthy coping strategies.* Encourage caregiver to attend appropriate local support group *to provide emotional support and education.* Assess caregiver's health *to monitor effects of long-term stress and suggest follow-up if necessary.* Encourage caregiver to interact as fully as possible with patient *to enhance commitment, feelings of accomplishment, and closure.*

ABGs, Arterial blood gases; *ADLs,* activities of daily living; *AIDS,* acquired immunodeficiency syndrome; *GI,* gastrointestinal; *HIV,* human immunodeficiency virus; *WBC,* white blood cell.

Table 11-8 Nursing Activities in Human Immunodeficiency Virus Disease

Levels of Care and Goals	Assessment	Interventions
Health Promotion and Maintenance ▪ Prevention of HIV infection ▪ Early detection of HIV infection	*Risk factors:* What behaviors or social, physical, emotional, pathologic, and immune factors place patient at risk? Does patient need to be tested?	Educate, including knowledge, attitudes and behaviors with an emphasis on risk reduction to: General population—cover general information Individual patient—specific to assessed need Empower patient to take control of prevention measures Provide HIV-antibody testing with pretest and posttest counseling
Acute Intervention ▪ Promotion of health and limitation of disability ▪ Successful management of problems caused by HIV infection	*Physical health:* Is patient experiencing problems? *Mental health status:* How is the patient coping? *Resources:* Does the patient have family and social support? Is patient accessing community services? Is money and insurance a problem? Does patient have access to spiritual support?	Provide case management Educate regarding HIV, the spectrum of infection, options for care, signs and symptoms for which to watch Educate regarding immune enhancement and harm reduction Refer to needed resources Establish long-term, trusting relationship with patient, family, and significant others Provide emotional and spiritual support Provide care during acute exacerbations—recognition of life-threatening developments, life support, rapid intervention with treatments and medications, patient and family emotional support during crisis, comfort and hygiene needs Develop resources for legal needs—discrimination prevention, wills and powers of attorney, child care wishes Empower patient to identify needs, direct care, seek services
Chronic and Home Management ▪ Maximizing quality of life ▪ Resolution of life and death issues	*Physical health:* Are new symptoms developing? Is patient experiencing drug side effects or interactions? *Mental health status:* How is patient coping? What adjustment have been made? *Finances:* Can patient maintain health care and basic standards of living? *Family, social, and community supports:* Are these supports available? Is patient using supports in an effective manner? *Spirituality issues:* Does patient desire support from an established religious organization? Are spirituality issues private and personal? What assistance does patient need?	Continue case management Educate regarding treatment options Empower patient to continue to direct care and to make desires known to family members and significant others Continue physical care for chronic disease process—treatments, medications, comfort and hygiene needs Support patient and family and significant others in a trusting relationship Refer to resources that will assist in identified needs Promote health maintenance measures Assist with end-of-life issues—resuscitation orders, funeral plans, estate planning, child care continuation

HIV, Human immunodeficiency virus.

Table 11-9 Pretest and Posttest Counseling Associated with HIV-Antibody Testing

General Guidelines

People who test for HIV are frequently fearful of the test results; therefore the nurse should provide the following:
- Establish rapport with the patient.
- Assess patient's ability to understand counseling.
- Determine the patient's ability to access support systems.

Explain the following benefits of testing:
- Testing provides an opportunity for education that can decrease the risk of new infections.
- Infected patient can be referred for early intervention and support programs.

Discuss the following negative aspects of testing:
- Breaches of confidentiality have led to discrimination.
- A positive test affects all aspects of the patient's life (personal, social, economic) and can raise difficult emotions (anger, anxiety, guilt, thoughts of suicide).

Pretest Counseling
- Determine the patient's risk factors and when the last risk occurred. Counseling should be individualized according to these parameters.
- Provide education to decrease future risk of exposure.
- Provide education that will help the patient protect sex and drug-sharing partners.
- Discuss problems related to the delay between infection and an accurate test.
  Testing will need to be repeated at intervals for 6 mo after each possible exposure.
  Discuss the need to abstain from further risky behaviors during that interval.
  Discuss the need to protect partners during that interval.
- Discuss the possibility of false negative tests, which are most likely to occur during the window period.
- Explain that a positive test shows *HIV infection* and not *AIDS*.
- Explain that the test *does not establish immunity*, regardless of the results.
- Assess support systems; provide telephone numbers and resources as needed.
- Discuss patient's personally anticipated responses to test results (positive and negative).
- Outline assistance that will be offered if the test is positive.

Posttest Counseling

If the test is negative, reinforce pretest counseling and prevention education. Remind patient that test needs to be repeated at intervals for 6 mo after the most recent exposure risk.

If the test is positive, understand that the patient may be in shock and not hear what is said.
- Provide resources for medical and emotional support, and help the patient get immediate assistance.
- Evaluate suicide risk and follow up as needed.
- Determine need to test others who have had risky contact with the patient.
- Discuss retesting to verify results. This tactic supports hope for the patient, but more importantly, it keeps the patient in the system. While waiting for the second test result, the patient has time to think about and adjust to the possibility of being HIV infected.
- Encourage optimism.
  Remind patient that treatments are available.
  Review health habits that can improve the immune system.
  Arrange for patient to speak to HIV-infected people who are willing to share and assist the newly diagnosed patient during the transition period.
  Reinforce that an HIV-positive test means that the patient is infected, but a positive test does not necessarily mean that the patient has AIDS.

Modified from Bradley-Springer LA, Fendrick R: *HIV instant instructor cards*, El Paso, TX, 1994, Skidmore-Roth.
AIDS, Acquired immunodeficiency syndrome; *HIV*, human immunodeficiency virus.

a high mortality rate is associated with the disease, emotional support for the patient and caregiver is particularly important.

Diarrhea is often a long-term problem. Nursing management includes recommending dietary interventions, encouraging fluid intake to prevent dehydration, instructing the patient about skin care, and managing excoriation around the perianal area. The nurse can recommend the use of incontinence products to prevent soiling of the clothes. In addition, the nurse should assess for factors that may trigger the diarrhea, such as anxiety, medications, or lactose intolerance. Relaxation techniques and alterations in the diet may provide some relief.

Wasting occurs in many people as death approaches. The patient with wasting syndrome begins to take on the physical appearance of a frail, older adult as emaciation occurs; hair turns gray and becomes thinner, posture slumps, and gait becomes unsteady. Caring for the person with wasting is a tremendous nursing challenge. Interventions include diet modifications, enteral supplements (either orally or through gastric tubes), or intravenous (IV) nutrition.[44] Wasting causes disturbances in self-concept and

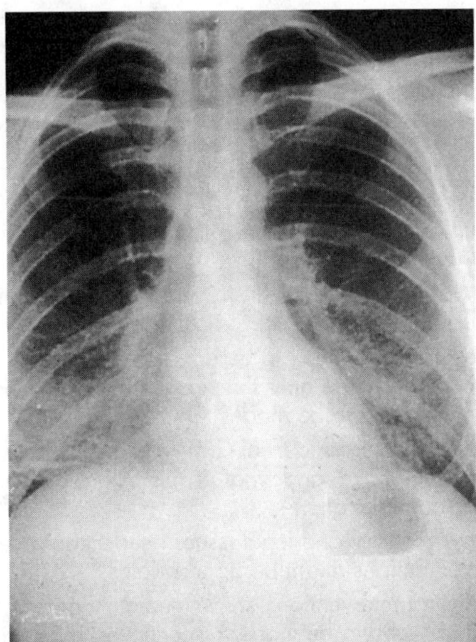

Fig. 11-9 Pulmonary pneumocystosis. Chest x-ray shows interstitial infiltrates as the result of *Pneumocystis carinii* pneumonia.

self-image. Useful interventions include creating an atmosphere of acceptance and reassurance, encouraging a focus on past accomplishments and personal strengths, and facilitating the use of positive affirmations.

AIDS-dementia complex (ADC), caused by HIV infection in the brain, is a common neurologic disorder associated with HIV. Similar symptoms may result from other CNS problems caused by lymphoma, toxoplasmosis, cytomegalovirus (CMV), herpes simplex virus type I and II, (HSV1 and HSV2), progressive multifocal encephalopathy, cryptococcus, dehydration, or side effects of medications. Dementia symptoms are sometimes reversible if a treatable cause is diagnosed. Treatable causes include dehydration, depression, toxoplasmosis, and side effects of medications.

Clinical manifestations of ADC include cognitive, behavioral, and motor abnormalities. Symptoms of ADC include decreased ability to concentrate, apathy, depression, social withdrawal, personality changes, confusion, hallucinations, and slowed response rates. ADC can progress to coma. Nursing interventions are focused on patient safety and caregiver support.

Chronic and Home Management. The complexity of HIV disease is related to its chronic nature. The HIV-infected person shares the problems experienced by all individuals with chronic diseases, but these problems are exacerbated by trauma related to the physical deterioration and social constructs surrounding HIV. Chronic diseases have no cure, continue for life, cause increasing physical disability and dysfunction, and ultimately contribute to morbidity and mortality. These dismal facts are compounded by a health care system that prefers to deal with those acute problems that respond rapidly to technologic and chemical intervention.[45]

Chronic diseases are characterized by acute exacerbations of cyclical problems that compound each other.[45] This is especially true in HIV disease where infections, cancers, debility, and social problems interact synergistically to tax the patient's ability to cope.

Chronic diseases may also be characterized by negative social attitudes that stigmatize the patient as being weak-willed or immoral for having the disease.[45] In HIV this

RESEARCH

Implications for Nursing Practice

HOME CARE NEEDS IN THE ADVANCED STAGES OF HIV DISEASE

Citation Hurley PM, Ungavarski PJ: Home health care needs of adults living with HIV disease/AIDS in New York City, *J Assoc Nurses in AIDS Care* 5:33-40, 1994.

Purpose Identify home health care needs of the adult in the advanced stages of HIV infection.

Methods Retrospective study of charts from 244 HIV-infected patients who had been discharged from a large home health care agency in New York. The sample was selected in a stratified random procedure that assured a percentage of female cases that correlated with the overall female case rate for the agency. The sample consisted of 75 women and 169 men. The chart review was structured around a data collection form that had been developed by a panel of experts. Data collection was performed by three professional nurses who achieved an interrater reliability of 85%. Information was collected in demographics, medical diagnoses and orders, and nursing admission assessment.

Results and Conclusions Demographic data revealed a poor, urban, ethnic minority population predominantly less than 40 years of age. Most of the people lived in private apartments or homes, and half lived alone. An additional 21%, mostly women, lived with children. These data revealed the dependence of the sample on home care providers. Frequently observed patient problems included dyspnea, weakness, fatigue, pain, ataxia, cough, skin lesions, and memory deficts. In addition, the review revealed problems with finances; inadequate nutrition; inability to comply with medication and treatment regimens; inadequate support systems; lack of physical facilities for cleanliness, food storage, and cooking; and drug, alcohol, and tobacco use. The findings suggest that the HIV-infected patient needs assistance to deal with a wide range of physical, psychosocial, and environmental problems.

Implications for Nursing Practice HIV infection, especially in advancing stages, is a complex problem that affects all aspects of the patient's life. Home health care has become a preferred option for many patients for personal comfort and financial reasons. However, home care must provide for all of the patient's needs, and this may require intensive nursing effort. Nursing assessment, collaboration, case management, and intervention will increasingly require creative and sensitive problem solving for the HIV-infected patient who receives care at home.

CRITICAL THINKING EXERCISES

CASE STUDY

HIV INFECTION

Patient Profile

Susan, a 35-year-old single mother, was admitted to the hospital with AIDS and CMV retinitis, which was diagnosed 2 days ago.

Subjective Data

Initially seen by a doctor 6 years ago for retrosternal pain and dysphagia that was diagnosed as esophageal candidiasis

- Had positive HIV antibody test at that time
- Married 11 years ago to Jim, who was a former IV drug user and recently died from complications related to AIDS
- Has two children, ages 6 and 8, who are both HIV-antibody negative
- Experiences fatigue and oral and vaginal candidiasis
- Expresses concern about welfare of children who are at home with her sister

Objective Data

Physical Examination

- 5′6″ (168 cm) tall, 100 lb (45.5 kg), temp 99.8° F (37.7° C)

Laboratory Studies

- $CD4^+$ lymphocyte count - 185/μl
- Hematocrit 30%

Therapeutic Management

- Insertion of central venous catheter to be used for CMV antiviral therapy at home
- Didanosine and trimethoprim-sulfamethoxazole (TMP-SMX)

Critical Thinking Questions

1. Why was Susan's initial medical problem unusual for a young, healthy woman?
2. Why is Susan taking TMP-SMX, and what are common side effects?
3. What teaching will need to be done before Susan is allowed to return home after this hospitalization? What referrals will need to be made?
4. What drugs are used to treat CMV retinitis? What side effects do they have, and what problems are associated with their administration?
5. What psychosocial and legal issues need to be assessed? What interventions might be appropriate?
6. What nursing interventions are immediately appropriate? What plans need to be made for continued nursing care after discharge?
7. Based on the assessment data presented, write one or more appropriate nursing diagnoses. Are there any collaborative problems?

NURSING RESEARCH ISSUES

1. What type of oral hygiene protocols provide the best relief for the HIV-infected patient with oral lesions?
2. What measures can the nurse use that will positively affect the self-esteem of patients with HIV infection?
3. Does a weight gain of 20 to 30 pounds in asymptomatic patients with HIV infection improve survival?
4. What effect do relaxation techniques have on pain relief in patients with HIV infection?
5. What are the psychosocial variables that influence the ability of the family and significant other to adapt to HIV infection in a loved one?
6. What procedures, techniques, or equipment can decrease the nurse's risk of exposure to blood in a health care setting?

stigma is compounded by several factors. The HIV-infected person may be seen as lacking control over urges to have sex or use drugs. It is then easy to jump to the conclusion that they brought the disease on themselves and, therefore, somehow deserve to be sick. The behaviors associated with HIV infection are frequently viewed as immoral (e.g., homosexuality, having many sexual partners) and are sometimes illegal (e.g., injecting heroin, prostitution). The fact that an infected individual can transmit the virus to others further entrenches the negative, stigmatizing social conception of HIV. Social stigmatization allows discrimination in all facets of life. HIV-infected persons have lost jobs, families, homes, and insurance because of such discrimination, even though some forms of discrimination are currently illegal in the United States because of the Americans with Disabilities Act (ADA).[46]

The chronic nature of HIV infection causes consequences seen in all such diseases: familial stress, social isolation, dependence, frustration, lowered self-image, andeconomic pressures.[45] One observation is that all of these variables may have contributed to the patient's infection in the first place. Low self-esteem, searching for social contact, frustration, and economic difficulties are all contributors to drug use and risky sexual behaviors.

Nursing interventions at every stage of HIV disease can be instrumental in improving the quality and quantity of the patient's life. The nurse who emphasizes a holistic and individualized approach to care is well suited to and capable of providing optimal care to the HIV-infected patient. A nurse already possesses most of the knowledge and skills needed to make a difference in the lives of the person affected with HIV. These skills should be applied in a compassionate and safe manner for all patients, especially those with HIV disease.

REVIEW QUESTIONS

The number of the question corresponds to the same-numbered objective at the beginning of the chapter.

1. Which of the following statements is *not* true?
   a. HIV replication occurs predominantly in B lymphocytes in lymph nodes.
   b. HIV affects the immune system predominantly through destruction of $CD4^+$ lymphocytes.
   c. During the initial phases of HIV infection, the B cells produce HIV-specific antibodies.
   d. HIV-induced syncytial formation causes the destruction of cells that may not be HIV infected.

2. Which of the following is *not* a documented route of transmission for HIV?
   a. Sharing contaminated injection equipment
   b. Breast feeding from an HIV-infected mother
   c. Being born to an HIV-infected mother
   d. Using blood clotting factor produced in 1994

3. In which of the following manners does HIV disease progress?
   a. Asymptomatic disease, AIDS, acute retroviral reaction, latent chronic disease
   b. Seroconversion illness, latent disease, AIDS, ARC
   c. Acute retroviral syndrome, early infection, early symptomatic infection, AIDS
   d. AIDS, acute viral loading, stage of chronicity, terminal phase

4. Diagnostic criteria for AIDS include all of the following *except*
   a. a $CD4^+$ lymphocyte count $>500/\mu l$.
   b. the development of *Pneumocystis carinii* pneumonia.
   c. a diagnosis of Kaposi's sarcoma.
   d. the development of wasting syndrome.

5. Which of the following statements regarding opportunistic diseases in HIV disease is accurate?
   a. Opportunistic diseases usually occur one at a time.
   b. Opportunistic diseases are curable with appropriate pharmacologic treatment.
   c. Opportunistic diseases occur in the presence of immunosuppression.
   d. Opportunistic diseases are generally slow to develop and progress.

6. Testing for HIV infection generally involves
   a. laboratory analysis of blood to detect HIV antigen.
   b. laboratory analysis of blood to detect HIV antibodies.
   c. analysis of lymphocytes for the presence of HIV RNA.
   d. electrophorectic analysis of HIV antigen in plasma.

7. Therapeutic management of HIV consists of
   a. using antiretroviral drugs to cure acute infection.
   b. prevention of opportunistic diseases and constitutional problems.
   c. radiation and surgery to inhibit HIV replication in lymph nodes.
   d. antiretroviral medications to treat opportunistic diseases.

8. Nursing management of HIV disease includes all of the following *except*
   a. a focus on preventing the transmission of HIV.
   b. interventions to decrease or eliminate constitutional symptoms.
   c. implementing isolation procedures on all HIV-infected patients.
   d. providing support for the anger, guilt, and loss experienced by the patient's family and friends.

REFERENCES

1. Agency for Health Care Policy and Research: *Evaluation and management of early HIV infection,* Rockville, MD, Pub # 94-0572, 1994, US Department of Health and Human Services.
2. US Department of Health and Human Services, Centers for Disease Control and Prevention (CDC): *HIV/AIDS surveillance report,* US HIV and AIDS cases reported through December 1994, 6(2), 1995.
3. Global programme on AIDS: Current and future dimensions of HIV/AIDS pandemic, A capsule summary, Geneva, 1992, World Health Organization (WHO).
4. Mann J, Tarantola DJM, Netter TW, editors: *A global report: AIDS in the world,* Cambridge, MA, 1992, Harvard University Press.
5. CDC HIV/AIDS Prevention Fact Sheet, Facts about the human immunodeficiency virus and its transmission, Atlanta, Centers for Disease Control and Prevention (CDC): February 1993.
6. Redfield RR, Burke DS: HIV infection: the clinical picture, *Sci Am* 259:70, 1988.
7. AIDS Working Group: Casual contact and the risk of HIV infection. APHA/SIA Report 1, 1988, American Public Health Association.
8. Henderson DK, Beekman SE, Gerberding J: Post-exposure antiviral chemoprophylaxis following occupational exposure to the human immunodeficiency virus, *AIDS Updates* 3:1, 1990.
9. Health care worker occupational exposure to HIV, *International AIDS Society—USA Newsletter* 2:1,1994.
10. Padian NS, Shiboski SC, Jewell NP: Female-to-male transmission of human immunodeficiency virus, *JAMA* 266:1664, 1991.
11. Curran JW and others: Epidemiology of HIV infection and AIDS in the United States, *Science* 239:610, 1988.
12. Nokes KM: HIV infection in women. In Flaskerud JH, Ungvarski, PJ, editors: *HIV/AIDS: a guide to nursing care,* ed 2, Philadelphia, 1992, Saunders.
13. European Collaborative Study: Children born to women with HIV-1 infection: natural history and risk of transmission, *Lancet* 337:253, 1991.
14. Halsey NA and others, and CDS/JHS AIDS Project Team: Transmission of HIV-1 infections from mothers to infants in Haiti: impact on childhood mortality and malnutrition, *JAMA* 264:2088, 1990.
15. St Louis ME and others: Risk for perinatal HIV-1 transmission according to maternal immunologic, virologic, and placental factors, *JAMA* 269:2853, 1993.
16. Antiviral briefs: ZDV reduces maternal transmission, *AIDS Patient Care* 8:164, 1994.

17. Bradley-Springer L: Reproductive decision making in the age of AIDS, *Image* 26:241, 1994.
18. Stratton P, Mofenson LM, Willoughby AD: Human immunodeficiency virus infection in pregnant women under care at AIDS clinical trials centers in the United States, *Obstetrics and Gynecology* 79:364, 1992.
19. Tovo PA and others, and the Italian Register for HIV infection in children: Prognostic factors and survival in children with perinatal HIV-1 infection, *Lancet* 339:1249, 1992.
20. Pantaleo G, Fauci AS: HIV-1 infection in the lymphoid organs: a model of disease development, *Journal of NIH Research* 5:68, 1993.
21. Connor RJ, Ho DD: Etiology of AIDS: biology of human retroviruses. In Devita VT, Hellman S, Rosenberg SA, editors: *AIDS: etiology, diagnosis, treatment, and prevention,* ed 3, Philadelphia, 1992, Lippincott.
22. Volberding PA: Clinical spectrum of HIV disease. In Devita VT, Hellman S, Rosenberg SA, editors: *AIDS: etiology, diagnosis, treatment, and prevention,* ed 3, Philadelphia, 1992, Lippincott.
23. Mudge-Grout CL: *Immunologic disorders,* 1992, St Louis, Mosby.
24. Katz MH and others: Progression to AIDS in HIV-infected homosexual and bisexual men with oral candidiasis and hairy leukoplakia: results from three San Francisco epidemiological cohorts, *AIDS* 6:95, 1992.
25. Scherer P: How HIV attacks the peripheral nervous system, *Am J Nurs* 90:67, 1990.
26. Centers for Disease Control and Prevention (CDC): Recommendations and Reports: 1993 revised classification system for HIV infection and expanded surveillance case definition for AIDS among adolescents and adults, *MMWR* 41:1, 1992.
27. Grady C, Vogel S: Laboratory methods for diagnosing and monitoring HIV infection, *J Assoc Nurses AIDS Care* 4:11, 1993.
28. Bartlett JG: *The John Hopkins Hospital guide to medical care of patients with HIV infection,* ed 4, Baltimore, 1994, Williams and Wilkins.
29. Caldwell M: The long shot, *Discover* 14:60, 1993.
30. Haynes BF: Scientific and social issues of human immunodeficiency virus vaccine development, *Science* 260:1279, 1993.
31. Merson MH: Slowing the spread of HIV: agenda for the 1990s, *Science* 260:1266, 1993.
32. Hoyt MJ, Staats JA: Wasting and malnutrition in patients with HIV/AIDS, *J Assoc Nurses AIDS Care* 2:16, 1991.
33. Weaver K: Reversible malnutrition in AIDS, *Am J Nurs* 91:25, 1991.
34. Kotler DP and others: Magnitude of body-cell-mass depletion and the timing of death from wasting in AIDS, *Am J Clin Nutr* 50:444, 1989.
35. Carey RF and others: Effectiveness of latex condoms as a barrier to human immunodeficiency virus-sized particles under conditions of simulated use, *Sex Transm Dis* 19:230, 1992.
36. Roper WL, Peterson HB, Curran JW: Commentary: condoms and HIV/STD prevention—clarifying the message, *Am J Public Health* 83:501, 1993.
37. Springer E: Effective AIDS prevention with active drug users: the harm reduction model. In Shernoff M, editor: *Counseling chemically dependent people with HIV illness,* New York, 1991, Harrington Park Press.
38. Occupational exposure to bloodborne pathogens: final rule, *Federal Register* 235:64175, 1991.
39. Wong ES and others: Are universal precautions effective in reducing the number of occupational exposures among health care workers? A prospective study of physicians on a medical service, *JAMA* 265:1123, 1991.
40. Pender NJ: *Health promotion in nursing practice,* ed 2, Norwalk, 1987, Appleton and Lange.
41. Ungvarski PJ: Nursing management of the adult patient, In Flaskerud, JH, Ungvarski, PJ, editors: *HIV/AIDS: a guide to nursing care,* ed 2, Philadelphia, 1992, Saunders.
42. Thompson JM and others: *Mosby's clinical nursing,* ed 3, St Louis, 1993, Mosby.
*43. Ragsdale D, Kotarba JA, Morrow JR: Quality of life of hospitalized persons with AIDS, *Image* 24:259, 1992.
44. Task Force on Nutrition Support in AIDS: Guidelines for nutrition support, *Nutrition* 5:39, 1989.
*45. Thorne SC: *Negotiating health care: the social context of chronic illness,* Newbury Park, 1993, Sage Publications.
46. The Americans with Disabilities Act, 42 U.S.C. s. 1201 et seq. (1992 and 1994).

---

*Nursing research-based articles.

Chapter 12

NURSING ROLE IN MANAGEMENT

Cancer

Catherine M. Bender **Joyce M. Yasko** **Roberta A. Strohl***

Learning Objectives

1. Describe the prevalence and incidence of cancer in the United States.
2. Describe the processes involved in the biology of cancer.
3. Differentiate the three phases of the development of cancer.
4. Describe the role of the immune system related to cancer.
5. Describe the use of the classification systems for cancer.
6. Explain the role of the nurse in the prevention and detection of cancer.
7. Explain the use of surgery, radiation therapy, chemotherapy, and biologic response modifier therapy in the treatment of cancer.
8. Differentiate between external beam radiation and brachytherapy.
9. Identify the classifications of chemotherapeutic agents and methods of administration.
10. Describe the effects of radiation therapy and chemotherapy on normal tissues.
11. Identify the types and effects of biologic response modifiers.
12. Describe the nursing management of the patient receiving radiation therapy, chemotherapy, and biologic response modifiers.
13. Describe the nutritional management of the patient with cancer.
14. Explain the role of the nurse related to unproven methods of cancer treatment.
15. Describe the complications that can occur in advanced cancer.
16. Describe the appropriate psychologic support of the patient with cancer and the family.

SIGNIFICANCE

It is believed that all multicellular organisms have the potential to develop cancer at some point in their lifetime. Hippocrates coined the word *carcinoma,* meaning a tumor that spreads and destroys the host. However, Galen was the first to describe cancer as being crablike in nature.

Cancer is a group of more than 200 diseases characterized by unregulated growth of cells. It can occur in persons of all ages and all races and is a major health problem in the United States. An estimated 30% of Americans now living will experience cancer at some point in their lives. The overall incidence of cancer has been steadily increasing since 1970. It is estimated that cancer (excluding nonmelanoma skin cancer and carcinoma in situ) would be diagnosed in 1,252,000 persons in 1995.[1] Some cancers, such as cancer of the stomach, uterus, and rectum, have decreased in incidence in recent times whereas others, such as cancer of the lung, colon, prostate, breast, and bladder, have increased in incidence.[2] A most notable increase in the incidence of melanoma is occurring at a rate of 3.4% per year.[1] Differences are noted in the incidence of certain cancers in men and women (Table 12-1).

Considerable progress has been made in controlling cancer for long periods of time. More than 8 million Americans alive today have a history of cancer; in 5 million of these the cancer was initially diagnosed 5 or more years ago. Many of these 5 million persons now show *no evidence of disease* (NED). NED usually means that the person has remained free of disease and has the same life expectancy as a person who has never had cancer.[1] This term is frequently substituted for the term *cured,* which is used cautiously because of the slow-developing nature of some forms of cancer.

Cancer is the second most common cause of death in the United States (heart disease is the most common). One of every five deaths is caused by cancer, with one half of these deaths occurring before the age of 65. The death rate as a result of cancer is leveling off or decreasing except for an

Reviewed by Carol Dolan, RN, MSN, OCN, Manager and Director, Nursing Services, University of New Mexico Cancer Research and Treatment Center, Albuquerque, NM.

*Contributed section on Radiation Therapy.

Table 12-1 Cancer Incidence by Site and Sex in 1994*

Male		Female	
Type	**Percentage**	**Type**	**Percentage**
Prostate	32	Breast	32
Lung	16	Colon or rectum	13
Colon or rectum	12	Lung	13
Urinary tract	9	Uterus	8
Leukemia or lymphoma	7	Leukemia or lymphoma	6

*Excluding basal and squamous cell skin cancers and carcinoma in situ.

Table 12-2 Estimates of Cancer Deaths by Site and Sex in 1994*

Male		Female	
Type	**Percentage**	**Type**	**Percentage**
Lung	33	Lung	23
Colon or rectum	10	Breast	18
Prostate	13	Colon or rectum	11
Leukemia or lymphoma	8	Leukemia or lymphoma	8

From Cancer Statistics 1994, American Cancer Society, 1994.
*Excluding basal and squamous cell skin cancers and carcinoma in situ.

increasing rate of deaths from lung cancer in women (Table 12-2). In 1994 over 500,000 Americans died from cancer. The cancer incidence and death rate are higher in African-Americans than in Caucasians. This rate is especially higher among African-American males. Most of the differences in cancer rates between African-Americans and Caucasians are attributed to environmental and social rather than biologic factors.[1]

Statistics cannot reveal the physiologic, psychologic, and sociologic impact of cancer. Cancer is known to be the most feared of all diseases, feared far more than heart disease. The word *cancer* is viewed as being synonymous with death, pain, disfigurement, and dependency. However, attitudes toward cancer do not fit today's status of the treatment and control of cancer. Education of health professionals and the public is essential if current attitudes surrounding cancer and cancer care are to become more positive and realistic.

BIOLOGY OF CANCER

Cancer is a group of many diseases of multiple causes that can arise in any cell of the body capable of evading regulatory controls over proliferation and differentiation. Two major dysfunctions present in the process of cancer are *defective cellular proliferation* (growth) and *defective cellular differentiation.*

Defect in Cellular Proliferation

Normally, most tissues of the human adult contain a population of predetermined, undifferentiated cells known as stem cells. Predetermined means that the stem cells of a particular tissue will ultimately differentiate and become mature, functioning cells of that tissue and only that tissue.

Cell proliferation originates in the stem cell and begins when the stem cell enters the cell cycle (Fig. 12-1). The time from the birth of a new cell to the time the cell divides into two identical cells is called the *generation time* of the cell. A mature cell continues to function until it degenerates and dies. At any time, there are cells at various stages of the cell cycle in all body tissues.

All cells of a tissue are controlled by an intracellular mechanism that determines when cellular proliferation is necessary. Under normal conditions, a state of dynamic equilibrium is constantly maintained (i.e., cellular proliferation equals cellular degeneration or death). The process of cellular division and proliferation is activated only in the presence of cellular degeneration or death. Cellular proliferation will also occur if the body has a physiologic need for more cells. For example, a normal increase in white blood cell (WBC) count occurs in the presence of infection.

Another explanation for the phenomenon of proliferation control of normal cells is *contact inhibition.* Normal cells respect the boundaries and territory of the cells surrounding them. They will not invade a territory that is not their own. The neighboring cells are thought to inhibit cellular growth through the physical contact of the surrounding cell membranes.

The rate of normal cellular proliferation (from the time of cellular birth to the time of cellular death) differs in each body tissue. In some tissues, such as bone marrow, hair follicles, and epithelial lining of the gastrointestinal (GI) tract, the rate of cellular proliferation is rapid. In other tissues, such as myocardium, brain, and cartilage, the rate of cellular proliferation is much slower. In fact, in adulthood the proliferation rate of these cells is so slow that it is barely perceptible.

Cancer cells usually proliferate in the manner and at the same rate of the normal cells of the tissue from which they arise. However, cancer cells respond differently than normal cells to the intracellular signals that regulate the state of dynamic equilibrium. Cancer cells divide indiscriminately and haphazardly. Sometimes they produce more than two cells at the time of mitosis. The loss of intracellular control of proliferation may be a result of a mutation of the stem cells.[3] The stem cells are viewed as the target or the origin of cancer development. The deoxyribonucleic acid (DNA) of the stem cell is substituted or permanently rearranged. When this happens the stem cell is mutated and has the potential to become malignant. It will usually proliferate at the rate of the tissue of origin, and some subpopulations can promote tumor progression to generate malignant cells (i.e., cells with invasive and metastatic potential). The stem cell theory of cancer development is not complete, because it

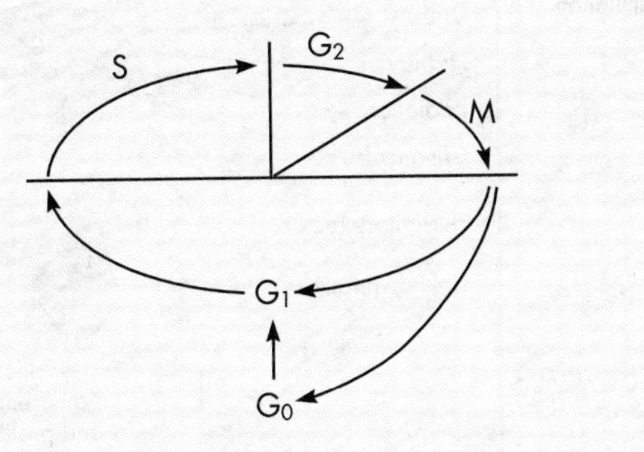

Fig. 12-1 Cell life cycle and metabolic activity. Generation time is the period from *M* phase to *M* phase. Cells not in the cycle, but capable of division, are in the resting phase (G_0). *DNA,* Deoxyribonucleic acid; *RNA,* ribonucleic acid.

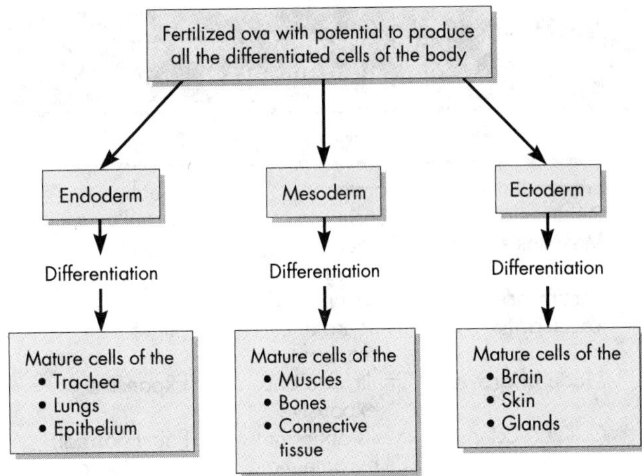

Fig. 12-2 Normal cellular differentiation.

has been noted that malignant stem cells can differentiate to form normal tissue cells.[3]

A common misconception regarding the characteristics of cancer cells is that the rate of proliferation is more rapid than that of any normal body cell. In most situations, cancer cells proliferate at the same rate as the normal cells of the tissue from which they originate. The difference is that proliferation of the cancer cells is indiscriminate and continuous. In this way, with each cell division creating two or more offspring cells, there is continuous growth of a tumor mass: 1→2→4→8→16 and so on. This is referred to as the *pyramid* effect. The time required for a tumor mass to double in size is known as its *doubling time*.

Cancer cells grown in tissue culture are also characterized by loss of contact inhibition. These cells have no regard for cellular boundaries and will grow on top of one another and also on top of or between normal cells.

Defect in Cellular Differentiation

Cellular differentiation is normally an orderly process that progresses from a state of immaturity to a state of maturity. Because all body cells are derived from the fertilized ova, all cells have the potential to perform all body functions. As cells differentiate, this potential is repressed and the mature cell is capable of performing only specific functions (Fig. 12-2).

With cellular differentiation there is a stable and orderly phasing out of cellular potential. Under normal conditions the differentiated cell is stable and will not differentiate (that is, revert to a previous undifferentiated state).

The exact mechanism that controls cellular differentiation and proliferation is not completely understood. Genes that are important regulators of these normal cellular processes are the *cellular oncogenes* or *protooncogenes*. Mutations that alter the expression of genes or their products can activate protooncogenes to function as *oncogenes* (tumor-inducing genes) by inducing mitosis but inhibiting differentiation of the cell.

The protooncogene has been described as the genetic lock that keeps the cell in its mature functioning state. When this lock is "unlocked," as may occur through exposure to *carcinogens* (agents that cause cancer) or oncogenic viruses, genetic alterations and mutations occur. The abilities and properties that the cell had in fetal development are again expressed. Although oncogenes and oncogenic products contribute to normal cell function, oncogenes interfere with normal cell expression under some conditions, causing the cell to become malignant. This cell regains a fetal appearance and function. For example, some cancer cells produce new proteins, such as those characteristic of the embryonic and fetal periods of life. These proteins located on the cell membrane include carcinoembryonic antigen and alpha-fetoprotein (AFP). They can be detected in human blood by laboratory studies (see later section on Role of the Immune System). Other cancer cells, such as oat-cell carcinoma of the lung, produce hormones (see later section on Complications Resulting from Cancer) that are ordinarily produced by cells arising from the same germ cell layer as the tumor cells.

Tumors can be classified as *benign* or *malignant*. In general, benign neoplasms are well differentiated, and malignant neoplasms range from well differentiated to undifferentiated. The ability of malignant tumor cells to invade and metastasize is the major difference between benign and malignant cells. Other differences between benign and malignant cells are presented in Table 12-3.

Development of Cancer

The following is a theoretic model of the development of cancer. The cause and development of each type of cancer are likely to be multifactorial. It is not known how many tumors have a chemical, environmental, genetic, immunologic, or viral origin. Cancers may arise spontaneously from causes that are, thus far, unexplained.

Table 12-3 Comparison of Benign and Malignant Tumors

Characteristic	Malignant Tumor	Benign Tumor
Encapsulated	Rarely	Usually
Differentiated	Poorly	Partially
Metastasis	Frequently present	Absent
Recurrence	Frequent	Rare
Vascularity	Moderate to marked	Slight
Mode of growth	Infiltrative and expansive	Expansive
Cell characteristics	Cells abnormal, become more unlike parent cells	Fairly normal; similar to parent cells

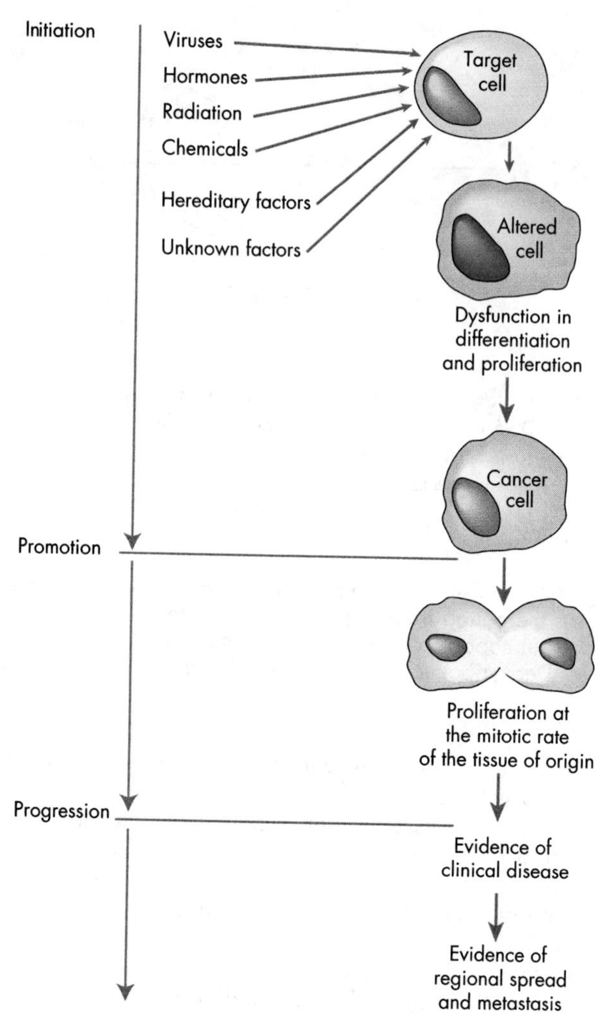

Fig. 12-3 Process of cancer development.

It is a common belief that the development of cancer is a rapid, haphazard event. However, the natural history of cancer is an orderly process comprising several stages and occurring over a period of time. These stages include *initiation, promotion,* and *progression* (Fig. 12-3).

Initiation. The first stage, *initiation,* is an irreversible alteration in the cell's genetic structure resulting from the action of a chemical, physical, or biologic agent. This altered cell has the potential for developing into a clone of neoplastic cells.[4] Most carcinogens (agents capable of producing these cellular alterations) are detoxified by protective enzymes and are harmlessly excreted. If this protective mechanism fails, carcinogens enter the cell's nucleus and may irreversibly bind to DNA. DNA repair is possible. However, if repair does not occur before cell division, the cell will replicate into daughter cells, each with the same genetic alteration.[4]

Carcinogens may be chemical, physical, or genetic in nature. Common characteristics of carcinogens are that their effects in the stage of initiation are irreversible and additive. In addition, there exists no known threshold below which their effects are not exhibited.

Chemical carcinogens. Chemicals were identified as cancer-causing agents in the latter part of the eighteenth century when Percival Pott noted that chimney sweeps, especially those with poor personal hygiene, had a higher incidence of cancer of the scrotum associated with exposure to soot residues in chimneys. As the years passed, more chemical agents were identified as actual and potential carcinogens as evidence indicated that persons exposed to certain chemicals over a period of time had a greater incidence of certain cancers than others. The long latency period from the time of exposure to the development of cancer makes it difficult to identify cancer-causing chemicals. Also, those chemicals that cause cancer in animals may or may not cause the same specific cancer in humans. Some chemicals are cancer causative in their environmental form, but others must first undergo certain metabolic changes. Chemical carcinogens thought to cause cancer in humans are listed in Table 12-4.

Certain drugs have also been identified as carcinogens (Table 12-5). Drugs that are capable of interacting with DNA (e.g., alkylating agents), as well as immunosuppressive agents, have the potential to cause neoplasms in humans. The use of alkylating agents (e.g., cyclophosphamide and nitrogen mustard), either alone or in combination with radiation therapy, has been associated with an increased incidence of acute myelogenous leukemia in persons treated for Hodgkin's disease, non-Hodgkin's lymphomas, and multiple myeloma. These secondary leukemias are relatively refractory to induction of remission with combination chemotherapy. Secondary leukemia has also been observed in persons who have undergone transplant surgery and who have taken immunosuppressive drugs.

The administration of estrogens to women has also been linked to the development of cancer. Although the use of estrogen as an oral contraceptive has not been shown to increase a woman's risk of developing cancer, the use of estrogen replacement therapy has been associated with the development of endometrial cancer. Additionally, the past

Table 12-4 Chemical Carcinogens

Carcinogen	Associated Neoplasm
Cigarette smoke	Lung, upper respiratory tract, bladder, cervix, and other cancers
Asbestos	Mesothelioma, lung
Acrylonitrile	Lung, colon, prostate
Arsenic	Skin, lung, liver
Benzene	Leukemia
Cadmium	Prostate, kidney
Chromium compounds	Lung
Nickel	Lung, nasal sinuses
Uranium	Lung
Aflatoxin	Liver
Nitrites	Stomach
Chloromethyl ethers	Lung
Isopropyl oil	Nasal sinuses
Benzidine	Bladder
Vinyl chloride	Angiosarcoma of liver
Radiation	Numerous locations
Polycyclic hydrocarbons	Lung, skin
Mustard gas	Lung

administration of diethylstilbestrol (DES) as an attempt to prevent miscarriages has an increased risk for the development of vaginal cancers in female offspring exposed to DES in utero.[4]

Chemical carcinogens associated with lifestyle have also been identified. For example, dietary factors have been demonstrated to play a role in the development of cancer. Persons who are overweight have a higher incidence of certain malignant conditions, such as breast and colon cancer. Although evidence does not support dietary factors as capable of genetic alteration, their role is believed to be one of tumor promotion.[2]

Physical carcinogens. Three classifications of physical carcinogens exist: (1) ionizing radiation, (2) ultraviolet (UV) radiation, and (3) foreign bodies. Since the turn of the century, it has been known that ionizing radiation can cause cancer in almost any human body tissue. Presently, the dose of radiation that causes cancer is not known, and there is considerable debate surrounding the effect of exposure to low-dose radiation over a period of time.[2] When cells are exposed to a source of radiation, damage occurs to one or both strands of DNA. Certain malignancies have been correlated with radiation as a carcinogenic agent:

1. Leukemia, lymphoma, thyroid cancer, and other cancers increased in incidence in the general population of Hiroshima and Nagasaki after the atomic bomb explosions.
2. A higher incidence of bone cancer occurs in persons exposed to radiation in certain occupations, such as radiologists, radiation chemists, and uranium miners.
3. Thyroid cancer has a higher incidence in those persons who have received radiation to the head and neck area for treatment of a variety of disorders, such as acne, tonsillitis, sore throat, or enlarged thyroid gland.

Table 12-5 Cancers Related to Drug Exposures in Humans

Drug	Associated Neoplasm
Radioisotopes	
Phosphorus (^{32}P)	Acute leukemia
Radium, mesothorium	Osteosarcoma and sinus carcinoma
Thorotrast	Hemangioendothelioma of liver
Immunosuppressive Agents	
Antilymphocyte serum Antimetabolites Alkylating agents Corticosteroids	Reticulum-cell sarcoma, epithelial cancer of skin and viscera, acute myelogenous leukemia
Azathioprine	Lymphoma, reticulum cell carcinoma, skin cancer Kaposi's sarcoma
Cytotoxic Drugs	
Phenylalanine mustard	Bladder cancer
Cyclophosphamide	Acute myelogenous leukemia
Hormones	
Synthetic estrogens	
Prenatal	Vaginal and cervical adenocarcinoma (clear-cell type)
Postnatal	Endometrial carcinoma (adenosquamous type)
Androgenic-anabolic steroids	Hepatocellular carcinoma
Diethylstilbesterol (DES)	Vaginal cancer
Others	
Arsenic	Skin, liver cancer
Phenacetin-containing drugs	Renal pelvis carcinoma
Coal for ointments	Skin cancer
Diphenylhydantoin(?)	Lymphoma
Chloramphenicol(?)	Leukemia
Amphetamines(?)	Hodgkin's disease

4. A higher incidence of childhood cancer occurs in children exposed to radiation during fetal life.

UV radiation has long been associated with squamous or basal cell carcinoma of the skin. Skin cancer is the most common type of cancer among Caucasians in the United States. Of concern is the relatively recent increase in the incidence of melanoma, a skin cancer that is much less responsive to treatment. It is the second most rapidly increasing cancer in the United States.[1] Although the cause of melanoma is probably multifactorial, mounting evidence suggests that UV radiation secondary to sunlight exposure is linked to the development of melanoma.[5]

Foreign bodies that are not biodegradable, such as asbestos fibers and Bakelite disc and cellophane implants, can induce the development of cancer by stimulating reactions to constant tissue damage such as scar formation, thus increasing the probability of neoplastic formations. The exact mechanism of this neoplastic transformation is as yet unknown. However, in general, the greater the surface area of the foreign body, the greater the probability of neoplastic transformation.

Certain DNA and ribonucleic acid (RNA) viruses, termed *oncogenic,* can transform the cells they infect and induce malignant transformation. Viruses have been identified as causative agents of cancer in animals and humans. One cancer found in human beings, Burkitt's lymphoma, has consistently shown evidence of the presence of the Epstein-Barr virus (EBV) in vitro.[4] This virus is also present in infectious mononucleosis, but the explanation of why an infectious disease develops in some persons and a lymphoma in others is not known. Persons with acquired immunodeficiency syndrome (AIDS), which is caused by a virus, have a high incidence of Kaposi's sarcoma (see Chapter 11). Other viruses that have been linked to the development of cancer include hepatitis B virus, associated with hepatocellular carcinoma, and human papillomavirus, which is believed to be capable of inducing lesions that progress to squamous cell carcinomas, such as cervical cancers.[4]

Genetic susceptibility. In actuality, none of the specific types of cancer are considered hereditary in the Mendelian sense. However, what is inherited in relatively few cases is a strong predisposition to cancer. An example of such an inherited predisposing condition is familial polyposis coli. The incidence of carcinoma of the colon in persons with such a syndrome is 1000 times the average incidence. Several preneoplastic syndromes can be inherited and can increase the probability of certain cancers. Xeroderma pigmentosum is a preneoplastic syndrome that can be a precursor of certain skin cancers, especially with exposure to sunlight.

"Cancer families" have also been identified in which several family members develop one or several specific cancers at an early age. The specific cancers usually involve the colon and uterus. Multiple-site cancers or cancers that occur at an early age are thought to have a genetic link. The occurrence of cancer in these instances is probably a result of inherited chromosomal abnormalities.

For many years scientists have searched for genetic patterns in the most common cancer sites. A few patterns that have emerged include:

1. The incidence of postmenopausal breast cancer is three times higher and the incidence of premenopausal breast cancer is five times higher in women with a family history of this disease. Breast cancer is rare in Asian women and common in Caucasian women.
2. The incidence of lung cancer is greater in smokers with a family history of this disease than in smokers without a family history of the disease.
3. The incidence of leukemia is greater in an identical twin of a person with the disease.
4. Neuroblastoma occurs with increased frequency among siblings.

Promotion. A single alteration of the genetic structure of the cell is not sufficient to result in cancer. At least one more mutation must occur in cells in which a mutation has already occurred. The chances of this occurring, given the billions of cells in the human body, seem highly unlikely. However, the odds of cancer development are increased with the presence of promoting agents.[2] *Promotion,* the second stage in the development of cancer, is characterized by the reversible proliferation of the altered, initiated cells and, consequently, with an increase in the initiated cell population, the likelihood of a second cell mutation is increased.

An important distinction between initiation and promotion is that the activity of promoters is reversible. This is a key concept in cancer prevention. Promoting factors include such agents as dietary fat, obesity, cigarette smoking, and alcohol consumption (Table 12-6). Prolonged stress

Table 12-6 Factors Promoting Cancer Development

Factor	Effect
Age	↑ Incidence of cancer in the young and in persons >55 yr of age
Hormones	↑ Progression of endometrial cancer in the presence of estrogen ↓ Progression of certain cancers with removal of the thyroid, adrenals, ovaries, and pituitary gland
Coping potential	↑ Progression of cancer in person with inadequate coping who exhibits feelings of hopelessness, helplessness, and being out of control (not scientifically proven at the present time)
Dietary fat, high-caloric intake	↑ Incidence and progession of cancer in persons ≥25% their recommended weight ↑ Incidence and progression of breast and gallbladder cancers in the presence of a high-fat diet ↑ Incidence and progression of colon cancer in the presence of a low-fiber diet ↑ Progression of cancer in persons with protein deficiency
Cigarette smoke	↑ Incidence of bronchogenic, esophageal, and bladder cancers
Alchoholic beverages	↑ Incidence of oral, liver, and esophageal cancers
Combination of alcohol consumption and cigarette smoke	↑ Incidence of head, neck, esophageal, and bladder cancers

may also be a promoter. (For a complete discussion of stress, see Chapter 5.) The withdrawal of these factors can reduce the risk of neoplastic formation. This characteristic is giving new insight into the existence of threshold doses for promoters below which these agents cannot exert their effects.

Several promoting agents exert activity against specific types of body tissues or organs. Therefore these agents tend to promote specific kinds of cancer. For example, cigarette smoke is a promoting agent in bronchogenic carcinoma and, in conjunction with alcohol intake, promotes esophageal and bladder cancer. Some carcinogens (complete carcinogens) are capable of both initiating and promoting the development of cancer. Cigarette smoke is an example of a complete carcinogen capable of initiating and promoting cancer.

A period of time, ranging from 1½ to 40 years, elapses between the initial genetic alteration and the actual clinical evidence of cancer. This period, called the *latent period,* is now theorized to comprise both the initiation and the promotion stages in the natural history of cancer.[2] The variation in the length of time that elapses before the cancer becomes clinically evident is associated with the mitotic rate of the tissue of origin and environmental factors.

For the disease process to become clinically evident, the cells must reach a critical mass. A 1 cm tumor (the size usually detectable by palpation) contains 1 billion cancer cells. A 0.5 cm tumor is the smallest that can be detected by current diagnostic measures, such as magnetic resonance imaging (MRI).

Progression. Progression is the final stage in the natural history of a cancer. This stage is characterized by increased growth rate of the tumor, as well as by increased invasiveness and metastasis. Certain biochemical and morphological alterations also take place during this stage, enabling the tumor to survive and thrive in this primary environment and throughout the process of metastasis.

One possible result of genetic change is that tumor cells begin to produce their own growth factor. The growth of the primary tumor may cause damage within the organ, thus causing the release of growth factor. As the tumor increases in size, it develops its own blood supply. The process of the formation of blood vessels within the tumor itself is called *tumor angiogenesis*. As the tumor grows, it can begin to mechanically invade surrounding tissues, growing into those areas of least resistance.[6]

A unique and tragic characteristic of malignant tumor cells is their ability to *metastasize* or spread to distant parts of the body. Some cancers metastasize early in the process of development (e.g., premenopausal breast cancer), whereas others spread regionally and rarely metastasize (e.g., glioblastoma multiforme and basal cell carcinoma of the skin). Certain cancers seem to have an affinity for a particular tissue or organ as a site of metastasis; other cancers are unpredictable in their pattern of metastasis. Certain cancers ("seed") require a particular site for proliferation ("soil"). The most frequent sites of metastasis are the lungs, brain, bone, and liver. Most metastatic lesions are multiple and widely disseminated, but a few cancers such as adenocarcinoma of the kidney usually produce a single metastatic lesion.

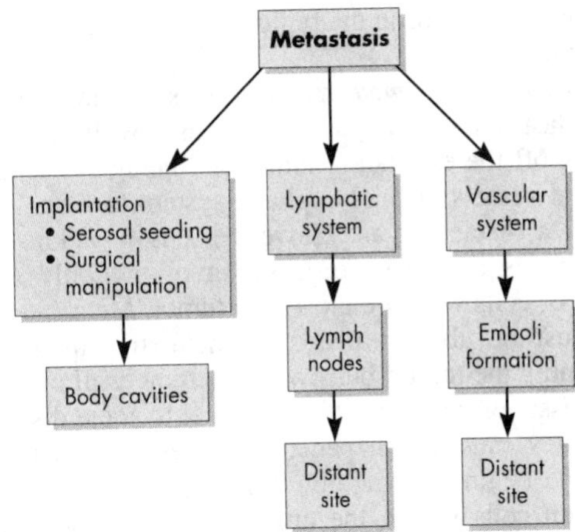

Fig. 12-4 Routes of metastasis.

Metastasis can occur via the vascular system, lymphatic system, and process of implantation (Fig. 12-4).

Vascular spread. Metastasis via the vascular system occurs in a variety of ways:

1. Proliferating cancer cells in draining lymph nodes may enter a large collecting lymphatic vessel, such as the thoracic duct, that empties into the larger veins leading to the heart.
2. Surrounding tissue may be invaded from the primary site of the cancer cells. The cancer cells penetrate the blood vessels and are released into the bloodstream.
3. Cancer cell aggregates are trapped in the small capillaries of the tissues and organs.
4. Through the secretion of *proteolytic enzymes*, cancer cells penetrate the walls of the capillary and enter the adjacent tissue where they begin to proliferate.

Lymphatic spread. Lymphatic spread occurs in a manner similar to vascular spread. Lymphatic vessels drain all interstitial fluid spaces in the body, conducting particles and fluid into lymph nodes. Cancer cells that break free from tissue or invade a lymph vessel almost always become trapped in the meshwork in the draining lymph node. If these cancer cells proliferate, the result is *lymphadenopathy* (abnormal enlargement of the lymph nodes). Continued proliferation may result in the release of cancer cells into the lymph vessel leading from the lymph node to the next lymph node up the chain.

Clinically, prognosis is best when there is no detectable spread to the lymph nodes in the region of the primary tumor. The prognosis becomes poorer when lymph nodes are involved. In reality, the spread of cancer cells to distant sites is likely to occur via the lymphatic and vascular systems concurrently. This theory is based on the fact that there are numerous interconnections between these systems.[7]

Implantation. Implantation may occur when cancer cells become embedded along the serosal surfaces of body organs, such as the peritoneal cavity or the pleural cavity. During surgical procedures, implantation may also occur in the primary organ or in the regional area if the environment is suitable.

Mechanisms of metastasis. It was formerly believed that metastasis was a passive process, with tumor cells breaking off the expanding tumor and being swept through the blood vessels or the lymphatic system to a final resting place in a distant organ. However, it is now known that metastasis is an active process, involving only a small number of cells within the original tumor. Metastatic tumor cells must be able to penetrate the extracellular matrix surrounding the tumor, burrow through the wall of a nearby blood vessel or lymph canal, and travel to some distant site, where they must again penetrate a vessel or canal wall, settle, and begin to grow into a new tumor.

Certain cells within the primary tumor possess unique attributes that facilitate the process of metastasis. These cells have decreased cell to cell adhesion in comparison with normal cells. This property equips these cancer cells with the mobility needed to move to the exterior of the primary tumor and to move within other vascular and organ structures. Some cancer cells produce proteolytic enzymes or proteases that are capable of destroying the basement membrane (a tough barrier surrounding tissues and blood vessels) of not only the tumor itself, but also of blood vessels, muscles, and nerves, and most epithelial boundaries.[6] These properties permit cancer cells to break away from the primary tumor, invade surrounding vasculature, and ultimately travel to distant organ sites.

Many cancer cells do not survive the process of metastasis. These cells can be destroyed by mechanical trauma from turbulent blood flow, inadequate oxygenation, or circulating immune cells. However, those metastatic cells that do survive must create an environment in the distant site that is conducive to their growth and development. This growth and development is facilitated by the production of a vascular supply within the metastatic site. Vascularization is critical to the supply of nutrients to the metastatic tumor and to the removal of waste products. Vascularization of the metastatic site is facilitated by tumor angiogenesis factor produced by the cancer cells.[8,9]

It is clear that an individual metastasis develops from a single cell or a group of identical cells (clone). However, as the metastatic site develops, the cells quickly become more heterogeneous. This change occurs as a result of spontaneous genetic mutations that take place in the tumor cells. The heterogeneous nature of the cells in the metastatic tumor makes it difficult to treat. Surgical removal of metastatic tumors is of value only if there is a small number of tumors. Some cells of heterogeneous, metastatic tumors have the ability to become resistant to chemotherapy and radiation therapy. Biologic response modifiers are a promising form of therapy because research indicates that tumor cells do not develop resistance to this type of therapy.

Role of the Immune System

This section is limited to a discussion of the role of the immune system in the recognition and destruction of tumor cells. (For a detailed discussion of immune system function, see Chapter 10.)

Both the normal and abnormal cell have a complex array of antigenic determinants (markers) on the surface of the cell membrane and within the cell itself. These antigenic determinants differ from one cell type to another. When foreign cells are transplanted from one individual to another individual, these antigenic determinants elicit an immunologic response. This is the basis for rejection of a transplanted organ.

Some cancer cells have changes on their cell surface antigens as a result of malignant transformation. These antigens are called *tumor-associated antigens* (TAA) (Fig. 12-5). TAA are antigens found on tumor cells and undetected on the cells of a normal adult, but they may be found on normal cells under special circumstances (e.g., fetal antigens that are normally expressed during embryonic development). In addition to the retrogenetic expression of oncofetal antigens, TAA may result from mutations in the cell's DNA (e.g., by chemical carcinogens) or the expression of new genetic material introduced by a virus (e.g., oncogenic DNA or RNA viruses).[10]

It is believed that one of the functions of the immune system is to respond to TAA. The response of the immune system to antigens of the malignant cells is called *immunologic surveillance*. Lymphocytes continually check cell surface antigens and detect and destroy cells with abnormal or altered antigenic determinants. It has been proposed that malignant transformation occurs continuously and that the malignant cells are destroyed by the immune response. (The immune system is discussed in Chapter 10.) Under most circumstances, immune surveillance will prevent these transformed cells from developing into clinically detectable tumors.[11]

Virtually every cell type involved in normal immune responses and every effector function used to inactivate or remove antigens has been demonstrated in immune responses to tumors. These immune responses involve cytotoxic T cells, natural killer cells, macrophages, and B lymphocytes.

Cytotoxic T cells are thought to play a dominant role in resisting tumor growth. These cells are capable of killing tumor cells. T cells are also important in the production of lymphokines (e.g., interleukin-2 [IL-2] and γ-interferon), which stimulate T cells, natural killer cells, B cells, and macrophages.

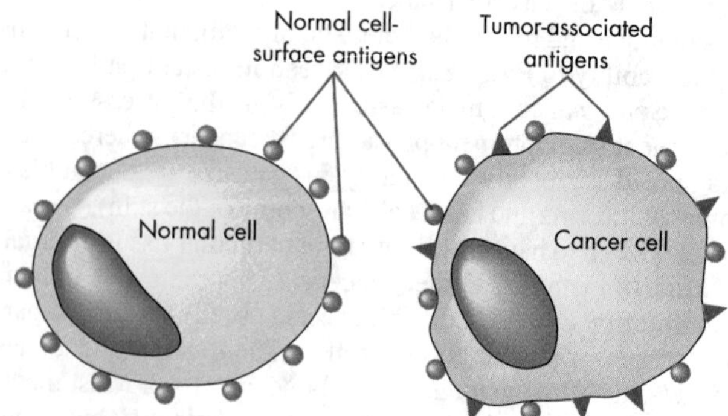

Fig. 12-5 Tumor-associated antigens appear on the cell surface of malignant cells.

Natural killer (NK) *cells* are able to directly lyse tumor cells spontaneously without any prior sensitization. These cells are stimulated by γ-interferon and IL-2 (released from T cells), resulting in increased cytotoxic activity.

Monocytes and *macrophages* have several important roles in tumor immunity (Fig. 12-6). Macrophages can be activated by γ-interferon (produced by T cells) to become nonspecifically lytic for tumor cells. Macrophages also secrete cytokines including (1) IL-1,[10] (2) α-interferon, (3) tumor necrosis factor (TNF), and (4) colony-stimulating factors. The release of IL-1, coupled with the presentation of the processed antigen, stimulates T-lymphocyte activation and production. α-Interferon augments the killing ability of NK cells. TNF causes hemorrhagic necrosis of tumors and exerts cytocidal or cytostatic actions against tumor cells. Colony-stimulating factors regulate the production of various blood cells in the bone marrow and stimulate the function of various WBCs.

B lymphocytes can produce specific antibodies that bind to tumor cells and can kill these cells by complement fixation and lysis (see Chapter 9). These antibodies are often detectable in the serum and saliva of the patient. In some persons, antibodies that are apparently specific for both the person's own tumor and a similar tumor in other persons have been found.[11]

Certain groups of people have a higher incidence of cancer than the general population. Cancer occurs in approximately 10% of children with congenital immunodeficiencies. These cancers are derived primarily from cells of the lymphoid system. The person who receives high doses of immunosuppressive drugs has an 80- to 100-fold increased risk of developing cancer. The types of cancer found in immunosuppressed persons are primarily epithelial or lymphoid. These findings are mostly reported in patients treated with immunosuppressive agents for organ transplantation, in patients with autoimmune diseases such as rheumatoid arthritis and systemic lupus erythematosus, and in patients with human immunodeficiency virus (HIV) infection.[10]

Other groups at an increased risk of cancer include very young persons and older adults. In the very young person the immune system is immature. The incidence of cancer increases dramatically in persons 40 to 60 years of age; the reasons for this are not known. It is possible that the immunologic surveillance system of the older adult works less effectively. It is also known that the thymus undergoes involution and atrophy with aging. In addition, the functional efficiency of T cells decreases with aging.

Escape Mechanisms from Immunologic Surveillance. Tumor development has often been called *immunologic escape*. In many persons with cancer there is evidence of an active immunologic response, and yet the tumor survives. Theoretic explanations for immunologic escape that have been proposed follow.

Sneaking through. The process of sneaking through is thought to occur when the cell-surface antigens are weak. Cancer cells in the early phase of growth may not excite an immunologic response because the transformed cell-surface markers are of low antigenicity. By the time the immune system is alerted, the cancer is well established and too large for the immune system to destroy.

Antigenic modulation. The malignant cell has the ability to change or lose antigenic determinants during or after a response by the immune system. The cell may then express a new set of antigens. This process is known as *antigenic modulation*. The new set of antigens on the malignant cell fails to adequately stimulate the immune system.

Overwhelming antigen exposure. Cancers may escape attack by flooding the body with tumor antigen. The antigens bind to specific antibodies or to receptors on lymphocytes and prevent them from recognizing and destroying the cancer cells. The excess of antigens paralyzes the host immune system, enhancing tumor growth.

Blocking factors. Blocking factors can prevent the attack of the TAA by T lymphocytes. For example, blocking antibodies may bind with TAA and prevent their recognition by T cells (Fig. 12-7). Another possibility is that free antigen produced and released by the malignant cell may bind with the T cell and prevent it from recognizing the

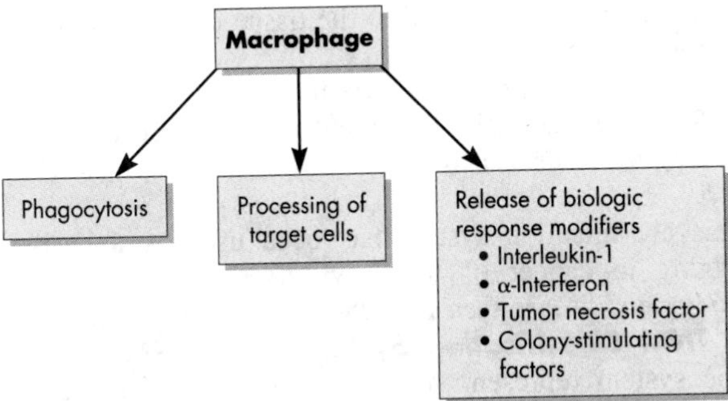

Fig. 12-6 Macrophage functioning in response to malignant target cells.

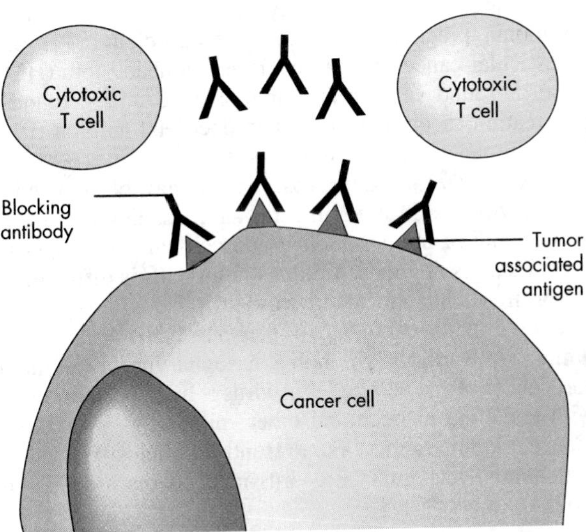

Fig. 12-7 Blocking antibodies prevent T cells from interacting with tumor-associated antigens and from destroying malignant cells.

malignant cell. These blocking factors related to the immune system can actually enhance tumor growth. This is known as *immunologic enhancement.*

Oncofetal Antigens. Oncofetal antigens, also called *carcinofetal antigens*, represent a type of tumor antigen. They are found on both the surfaces and inside of cancer cells, as well as fetal cells. These antigens are an expression of the shift of cancerous cells to a more immature metabolic pathway, an expression usually associated with embryonic or fetal periods of life. The reappearance of fetal antigens in malignant disease is not well understood, but it is believed to occur as a result of the cell regaining the cellular potential that it once had.

Examples of oncofetal antigens are carcinoembryonic antigen (CEA) and AFP. CEA is found on the surfaces of cancer cells derived from the GI tract and from normal cells from the fetal gut, liver, and pancreas. Normally, it disappears during the last 3 months of fetal life. CEA was originally isolated from colon cancer cells. However, elevated CEA levels have also been found in nonmalignant conditions (e.g., cirrhosis of the liver, ulcerative colitis, and heavy smoking). Presently, the major value of CEA is its use as an indicator of the success of cancer treatment. For example, the persistence of elevated preoperative CEA titers after surgery indicates that the tumor is not completely removed. A rise in CEA levels after chemotherapy or radiation therapy may indicate recurrence or spread of the cancer.

AFP is produced by malignant liver cells, as well as fetal liver cells. AFP levels have also been found to be elevated in some cases of testicular carcinoma, viral hepatitis, and nonmalignant liver disorders. AFP has diagnostic value in primary cancer of the liver (hepatoma), but it is also produced when metastatic liver growth occurs. The detection of AFP is of value in tumor detection and determination of tumor progression.

Other examples of oncofetal antigens currently being studied are fetal sulfated glycopeptide found in gastric carcinoma, pregnancy-specific β_1-glycoprotein (SP_1) found in testicular cancer, human chorionic gonadotropin (HCG), CA-125 found in ovarian carcinoma, CA-19-9 found in pancreatic cancer, and pancreatic oncofetal antigen (POA) found in pancreatic and lung cancers.

Virus-induced Antigens. TAA may be induced by certain viruses. In experimental animals, DNA and RNA viruses induce unique nuclear and cell-surface antigens in cells. Establishing these findings in humans is difficult. The DNA viruses include adenovirus and various herpesviruses. The three major candidates for human DNA virus-induced tumors are Burkitt's lymphoma, nasopharyngeal carcinoma, and cancer of the cervix. RNA viruses have been correlated with leukemia in mice and other animals, as well as with mouse mammary tumors. Presently, conclusive evidence that human leukemia is a virus-induced disease does not exist.[2]

CLASSIFICATION OF CANCER

Tumors can be classified according to *anatomic site, histologic analysis* (grading), and *extent of disease* (staging).

Tumor classification systems are intended to provide a standardized way (1) to communicate the status of the cancer to all members of the health care team, (2) to assist in determining the most effective treatment plan, (3) to evaluate the treatment plan, (4) to serve as a factor in determining the prognosis, and (5) to compare like groups for statistical purposes.

Anatomic Site Classification

In the anatomic classification of tumors, the tumor is identified by the tissue of origin, the anatomic site, and the behavior of the tumor (i.e., benign or malignant) (Table 12-7). *Carcinomas* originate from embryonal ectoderm (skin and glands) and endoderm (mucous membrane linings of the respiratory tract, GI tract, and genitourinary (GU) tract). *Sarcomas* originate from embryonal mesoderm (connective tissue, muscle, bone, and fat). *Lymphomas and leukemias* originate from the hematopoietic system.

Histologic Analysis Classification

In histologic grading of tumors, the appearance of cells and the degree of differentiation are evaluated. For many tumor cells, four grades are used:

Grade I: Cells differ slightly from normal cells (mild dysplasia) and are well differentiated.

Grade II: Cells are more abnormal (moderate dysplasia) and moderately differentiated.

Grade III: Cells are very abnormal (severe dysplasia) and poorly differentiated.

Grade IV: Cells are immature and primitive (anaplasia) and undifferentiated; cell of origin is difficult to determine.

Extent of Disease Classification

The extent of disease classification is often called *staging*. This classification system is based on a description of the extent of the disease rather than on cell appearance. Although there are similarities in the staging of cancers, there are many differences based on a thorough knowledge of the natural history of each specific type of cancer.

Clinical Staging. The clinical staging classification system determines the extent of the disease process of cancer by stages:

Stage 0: Cancer in situ

Stage I: Tumor limited to the tissue of origin; localized tumor growth

Stage II: Limited local spread

Stage III: Extensive local and regional spread

Stage IV: Metastasis

This classification system has been used as a basis for staging in cancer of the cervix (see Table 51-12) and Hodgkin's disease (see Fig. 28-14).

TNM Classification System. The TNM classification system represents the standardization of the clinical staging of cancer by the International Union Against Cancer (IUCC). This classification system (Table 12-8) is used to determine the extent of the disease process of cancer

Table 12-7 Anatomic Classification of Tumors

Site	Benign	Malignant
Epithelial Tissue Tumors*	**-oma**	**-carcinoma**
Surface epithelium	Papilloma	Carcinoma
Glandular epithelium	Adenoma	Adenocarcinoma
Connective Tissue Tumors†	**-oma**	**-sarcoma**
Fibrous tissue	Fibroma	Fibrosarcoma
Cartilage	Chondroma	Chondrosarcoma
Striated muscle	Rhabdomyoma	Rhabdomyosarcoma
Bone	Osteoma	Osteosarcoma
Nervous Tissue Tumors‡	**-oma**	**-oma**
Meninges	Meningioma	Meningeal sarcoma
Nerve cells	Ganglioneuroma	Neuroblastoma
Hematopoietic Tissue Tumors	—	
Lymphoid tissue		Hodgkin's disease, malignant lymphoma
Plasma cells		Multiple myeloma
Bone marrow		Lymphocytic and myelogenous leukemia

*Body surfaces, lining of body cavities, and glandular stuctures.
†Supporting tissue, fibrotic tissues, and blood vessels.
‡Brain nerves and retina.

Table 12-8 TNM Classification System

Primary Tumor (T)
- T_0 No evidence of primary tumor
- T_{is} Carcinoma in situ
- $T_{1\text{-}4}$ Ascending degrees of increase in tumor size and involvement

Regional Lymph Nodes (N)
- N_0 No evidence of disease in lymph nodes
- $N_{1\text{-}4}$ Ascending degrees of nodal involvement
- N_x Regional lymph nodes unable to be assessed clinically

Distant Metastases (M)
- M_0 No evidence of distant metastases
- $M_{1\text{-}4}$ Ascending degrees of metastatic involvement of the host, including distant nodes

according to three parameters: tumor size (T), degree of regional spread to the lymph nodes (N), and absence of metastasis (M). (This system has been applied to cancer of the breast in Chapter 49.)

Staging of the disease can be done initially and at several intervals. Clinical diagnostic staging is done at the time of diagnosis to determine the most effective treatment plan. Examples of diagnostic studies that may be performed to assess for spread of disease include bone and liver scans, ultrasonography, computerized tomography (CT) scans, and MRI.

Surgical evaluative staging is used to describe the extent of the disease process after biopsy or surgical exploration. For example, a laparotomy and a splenectomy may be performed in staging of Hodgkin's disease. During a staging laparotomy, areas of lymph node biopsy and margins of any masses may be marked with metal clips. These clips are used as markers when radiotherapy is used as a treatment modality.

Postsurgical treatment pathologic staging is used after pathologic examination of the surgical specimen. The presence of residual tumor should be recorded at this time. The stages are R_0 (no residual tumor), R_1 (microscopic residual tumor), and R_2 (macroscopic residual tumor).

After the extent of the disease is determined, the stage classification is not changed. The original description of the extent of the tumor remains part of the original record. If additional treatment is needed, or if treatment fails, retreatment staging is done to determine the extent of the disease process at the time of retreatment.

Carcinoma in situ is a commonly used term in classification of cancer. It is defined as a lesion with all the histologic features of cancer except invasion. If left untreated, carcinoma in situ will eventually become invasive.

In addition to tumor classification systems, there are also classification systems used to describe the status of the patient with cancer. The status of the patient is recorded at the time of diagnosis, treatment, and retreatment, and at each follow-up examination. The Karnofsky performance scale is an example of a method used to evaluate the performance status of the patient (Table 12-9).

PREVENTION AND DETECTION OF CANCER

The nurse plays a prominent role in the prevention and detection of cancer. Early detection and prompt treatment are directly responsible for the increased survival rate in the patient with cancer. One important aspect is to educate the public to do the following:

1. Reduce or avoid exposure to known or suspected carcinogens and cancer-promoting agents.

Table 12-9 Karnofsky Performance Scale

100	Normal; no complaints; no evidence of disease
90	Ability to carry on normal activity; minor signs or symptoms of disease
80	Normal activity with effort; some signs or symptoms of disease
70	Ability to care for self; inability to carry on normal activity or do active work
60	Occasional assistance necessary but ability to care for most needs
50	Considerable assistance and frequent medical care necessary
40	Disabled; special care and assistance necessary
30	Severely disabled; indication for hospitalization although death not imminent
20	Very sick; hospitalization necessary; active supportive treatment necessary
10	Moribund; fatal processes progressing rapidly
0	Dead

2. Eat a balanced diet that includes vegetables (green, yellow, and orange), fresh fruits, whole grains, adequate amounts of fiber, and low levels of fats and preservatives.
3. Participate in a regular exercise regimen.
4. Obtain adequate, consistent periods of rest (at least 6 to 8 hours per night).
5. Have a health examination on a consistent basis that includes a health history, a physical examination, and specific diagnostic tests for common cancers in accordance with the guidelines published by the American Cancer Society[12] (Table 12-10).
6. Eliminate, reduce, or change the perceptions of stressors and enhance the ability to positively cope with stressors.
7. Enjoy consistent periods of relaxation and leisure.
8. Know the seven warning signs of cancer as identified by the American Cancer Society (Table 12-11).
9. Learn and practice self-examination (e.g., breast self-examination and testicular examination).
10. Seek immediate medical care if cancer is suspected. Early detection of cancer has a positive impact on prognosis.

When the public is educated regarding the disease process of cancer, care should be taken to minimize the fear that surrounds the diagnosis of cancer. Tactics that increase fear should never be used. The facts should be taught in an accurate, low-key manner at the level of the learner. The goal of public education is to motivate the learner to change the pattern of behavior as necessary to achieve and maintain an optimal state of health. The nurse can play a significant role in meeting this goal. Although the general public must be taught, those who are at an increased risk of cancer are the target population for effective cancer control (see Table 12-10). The nurse can have a definite impact in convincing people that a change in lifestyle patterns will have a positive influence on health. If the nurse is to have a significant impact, the challenge needs to be recognized and strategies must be developed to teach cancer control effectively.

Diagnosis of Cancer

When a patient is admitted to a health care agency with the possible diagnosis of cancer, it is a stressful time for the patient and the family. The patient typically undergoes several days of diagnostic studies. During this time the fear of the unknown is often more stressful than ultimately being told of a positive diagnosis of cancer.

During the time the patient is waiting for the results of the diagnostic studies, the nurse needs to be available to actively listen to the patient's concerns. False reassurance that everything will be all right is inappropriate and is an effective way to shut off further communication with the patient. During this time of high anxiety the patient may need repeated explanations regarding the diagnostic workup. Explanations should include as much information as needed by the patient and the family; the information should be given in clear, understandable terms and should be reinforced as necessary.

A diagnostic plan for the person in whom cancer is suspected includes health history, identification of risk factors, physical examination, and specific diagnostic studies. (The specifics of the health history and the screening physical examination are presented in Chapter 4.)

The health history includes particular emphasis on risk factors, such as family history of cancer, exposure to or use of known carcinogens (e.g., cigarette smoking and exposure to occupational pollutants or chemicals), diseases characterized by chronic inflammation (e.g., ulcerative colitis), and drug ingestion (e.g., hormone therapy). Other important information relates to dietary habits, ingestion of alcohol, lifestyle, and patterns and degree of coping with perceived stressors.

The physical examination should be thorough, and particular attention should be given to the respiratory system, the GI system (including colon, rectum, and liver), the lymphatic system (including the spleen), the breasts, the skin, the reproductive system of the male (testicles, prostate gland) and of the female (cervix, uterus, ovary), and the musculoskeletal and neurologic systems.

Diagnostic studies to be performed will depend on the suspected primary or metastatic site(s) of the cancer. (Specific procedures as they relate to each body system are discussed in the respective assessment chapters.) Examples of studies that may be included in the process of diagnosing cancer include the following:

1. Cytology studies (e.g., Pap smear)
2. Chest x-ray
3. Complete blood count
4. Proctoscopic examination
5. Liver function studies
6. Radiographic studies (e.g., mammogram)

Table 12-10 Screening for Specific Cancer Sites

High-Risk Profile	Screening	Medium- and Low-Risk Profile	Screening
Lung Cancer			
History of 20 pack-years of smoking (1 pack a day for 20 yr); exposure to airborne carcinogens, especially asbestos, uranium, hydrocarbons; age range 40-80 yr; chronic lung disease	Early detection method not available; annual chest x-ray (advised by some physicians); observation by patient for change in respiratory status; increased frequency of infections and change in cough, sputum, breathing, voice	History of less than 20 pack-years of smoking, nonsmokers, former smokers after 10 yr	Early detection method not available
Colon and Rectal Cancer			
History of familial polyposis, ulcerative colitis, Crohn's disease; personal or family history of colon or rectal cancer; diet high in fat and low in fiber; age range 40-75 yr	Blood test on stools every year after age 50 and digital rectal examination annually after age 40; sigmoidoscopic examination (preferably flexible) every 3-5 yr after age 50, observation by patient for changes in bowel pattern: diarrhea, constipation, pain, flatus, black tarry stools, bleeding	Persons with no known risk factors	Guaiac test on stools and digital rectal examination annually after age 40; sigmoidoscopy as a baseline at age 50; after two normal examinations, repeated proctosigmoidoscopic examination every 3-5 yr
Prostatic Cancer			
Presence of prostatic hyperplasia, presence of prostatic infection, African-American, increased risk with age	Digital rectal examination at age 40 and annually thereafter and prostate specific antigen blood test every year; on men aged 50 and older observation by patient for dysuria, blood in urine, difficulty in producing stream of urine	Presence of one risk factor, excluding age	Digital rectal examination and prostate specific antigen blood test annually after age 50
Cervical Cancer			
Early intercourse (before age 20) with multiple partners, poor personal hygiene, history of herpesvirus type II infection, cervical dysplasia	Pap test and pelvic examination every year for those who are or have been sexually active or who have reached age 18; colposcopy if suspicious area is noted; observation by patient for abnormal vaginal bleeding or discharge, pain or bleeding with sexual intercourse	No known risk factors	Pap test and pelvic examination every year after age 18; after 3 or more normal examinations in a row, at least every 3 yr; Pap test may be performed less frequently at the discretion of the physician

continued

7. Radioisotope scans (liver, brain, bone, lung)
8. CT scan
9. MRI
10. Presence of oncofetal antigens such as CEA and AFP
11. Bone marrow examination (if a hematolymphoid malignancy is suspected)
12. Lymphangiography (if a lymphoid cancer is suspected)
13. Biopsy

Biopsy. The biopsy procedure is the definitive means of diagnosing cancer. It involves the histologic examination by a pathologist of a piece of tissue from the suspicious area. A biopsy is essential in planning a treatment regimen for the patient. A biopsy will determine whether the tissue is benign or malignant, the anatomic tissue from which the tumor arises, and the degree of cellular differentiation of the cancer cells present in the tumor.

The procedure may be a needle biopsy, an incisional biopsy, or an excisional biopsy. A *needle biopsy* specimen

Table 12-10 Screening for Specific Cancer Sites—cont'd

High-Risk Profile	Screening	Medium- and Low-Risk Profile	Screening
Endometrial Cancer			
Infertility, ovarian dysfunction, obesity, uterine bleeding, estrogen therapy over long period of time, diabetes, age range 30-80 yr	Pap test every year; pelvic examination every year; endometrial biopsy every year for women at menopause and at risk; observation by patient for abnormal uterine bleeding, pain, change in menstrual pattern	Presence of one risk factor, excluding estrogen therapy, over long period of time	Pap test and pelvic examination
Skin Cancer			
Prolonged exposure to sun; previous radiation exposure; fair, thin skin; positive family history of dysplastic nevus syndrome (DNS)	Self-examination monthly with suspicious lesions evaluated promptly; physical examination every year; observation by patient for sore that does not heal, change in wart or mole	Presence of one risk factor, excluding prolonged exposure to sun	Self-examination, physical examination each year
Breast Cancer			
Caucasian, early menarche, late menopause, fibrocystic breast disease, infertility, more than age 30 for first pregnancy, personal history of breast cancer, mother or sister with history of breast cancer, obesity, age range 35-65 yr	Monthly breast self-examination; breast examination by health professional every 3 yr for women age 20-40 and every year after age 40; baseline mammogram at age 40, every 1-2 yr between ages 40 and 49, and every year after age 50; observation by patient for lump or thickening discharge from nipple, pain in breast	Excluding family history of breast cancer, fewer than two risk factors	Monthly breast self-examination; breast examination by health professional every 3 yr for women age 18-39 and every year after age 39; baseline mammogram at age 40, every 1-2 yr between ages 40 and 49, and every year after age 50; observation by patient for lump or thickening discharge

Based on the American Cancer Society 1995 Recommendations.[12] Cancer Facts & Figures American Cancer Society January 1995.

Table 12-11 Seven Warning Signs of Cancer

C hange in bowel or bladder habits
A sore that does not heal
U nusual bleeding or discharge from any body orifice
T hickening or a lump in the breast or elsewhere
I ndigestion or difficulty in swallowing
O bvious change in a wart or mole
N agging cough or hoarseness

can be obtained by aspiration (e.g., bone marrow aspiration) or by the use of a large-bore needle. These needles are used in obtaining samples of prostate gland, breast, liver, and kidney tissues.

Incisional biopsy performed with a scalpel or dermal punch is a common technique used for obtaining a tissue sample for making a diagnosis of cancer. The premise that incisional biopsy may contribute to the spread of cancer has not been proven.

Excisional biopsy involves removal of the entire tumor. It is usually used for small tumors (smaller than 2 cm), skin lesions, intestinal polyps, and breast tumors. This procedure can be considered therapeutic, as well as diagnostic. Often when a tumor is not easily accessible, a major surgical procedure (laparotomy, thoracotomy, craniotomy) is necessary to obtain a piece of the tumor tissue. Biopsy specimens of the GI, respiratory, and GU systems can usually be obtained by endoscopic procedures.

TREATMENT

Goals and Modalities

The goal of cancer treatment is *cure, control*, or *palliation* (Fig. 12-8). Factors that determine the treatment modality are the cell type of the cancer, the location and size of the tumor, and the extent of the disease. The physiologic and psychologic status and the expressed needs of the patient also have an important part in determining the treatment

CULTURAL & ETHNIC *Considerations*

CANCER

- African-Americans have a higher incidence of cancer than Caucasians.
- Death rates related to cancer are higher for African-Americans than Caucasians.
- Native Americans have a lower incidence of cancer than any other group in the United States but have the poorest survival rate when they do get cancer.

plan. These factors influence the modalities chosen for treatment and the length of time the treatment is administered.

When caring for the patient with cancer, the nurse should know the goals of the treatment plan to appropriately communicate with and support the patient. When *cure* is the goal, it is expected that after treatment the patient will be free of disease and will have a normal life span. Many kinds of cancer have the potential to go into permanent remission with an initial course of treatment or with treatment that extends for several weeks, months, or years. Basal cell carcinoma of the skin is usually cured by surgical removal of the lesion or by several weeks of radiation therapy. Acute lymphocytic leukemia (ALL) in children has the potential for cure. The treatment plan for ALL includes the administration of several chemotherapy drugs on a scheduled basis over a time span of 6 months to several years. Some forms of testicular cancer are also treated for cure.

Until a few years ago, a 5-year disease-free period was thought to be indicative of a cancer cure. This is not true for all cancers. The patient with a tumor that has a rapid mitotic rate (e.g., testicular cancer) is considered in remission if cancer is not detected in a 2-year time span. The patient with a tumor that has a slower mitotic rate (e.g., postmenopausal breast cancer) needs 20 or more disease-free years before she can be considered cured of cancer.

Control is the goal of the treatment plan for many cancers considered to be chronic. The patient undergoes the initial course of therapy and is continued on maintenance therapy for a period of time or is followed closely so that early signs and symptoms of recurrence can be detected. These cancers are usually not cured, but they are controlled by therapy for long periods of time. They are controlled in a manner similar to other chronic illnesses, such as diabetes mellitus, chronic lung disease, and congestive heart failure. An example of this type of cancer is chronic lymphocytic leukemia (see Chapter 28).

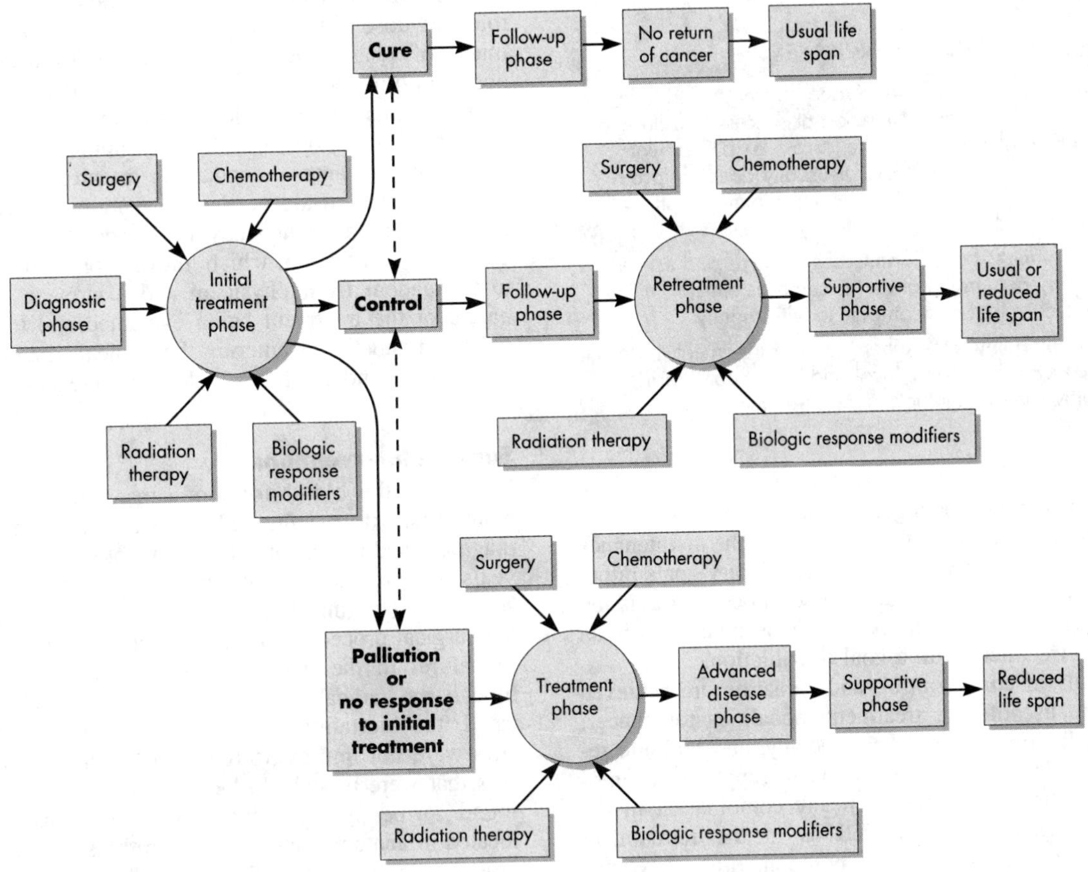

Fig. 12-8 Goals of cancer treatment.

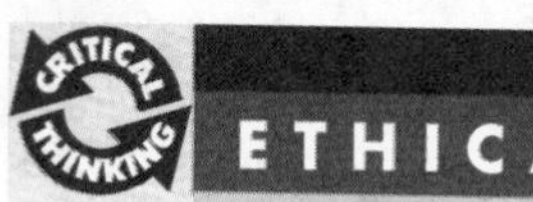

ETHICAL DILEMMAS

MEDICAL FUTILITY

Situation An intensive care nurse is approached by the family of a 65-year-old patient who questions why their mother is not receiving chemotherapy for the tumor surrounding her esophagus. The family also wants to make certain that she will be resuscitated should her heart stop. They are aware of the diagnosis that she may have less than a year to live.

Discussion If the patient is competent, she should be told her diagnosis and prognosis. If the patient is not competent and has no advance directives, the family must be consulted about both the diagnosis and the prognosis. If the patient wants life support measures instituted, including resuscitation, she must be given the range of treatment alternatives, as well as information about hospice care. A crucial piece of information is whether chemotherapy would extend her life or improve the quality of her life. If it would not affect her life span or her quality of life, chemotherapy can be considered a medically futile treatment and need not be offered or provided. When a medically futile treatment is requested or demanded by a patient or a patient's family, the health professional must be very clear in the explanations about why it is believed to be inappropriate. The patient and family are always free to seek additional medical consultation or to transfer care to another physician or hospital.

ETHICAL AND LEGAL PRINCIPLES

- Definitions of *medically futile* range from medically inappropriate to a small likelihood of success to failure to achieve intended results in the last 95 of 100 similar cases. The health care provider usually does not provide the patient and the family with treatment options that are considered to be medically futile.
- *Scientific futility,* based on medical records and scientific experience, may not be the same as *ethical futility,* which is care that is incompatible with dignity.
- Patient autonomy allows the refusal of treatment. It does not, however, have an ethical and legal counterpart that allows the patient to demand treatment.

Palliation can also be a goal of the treatment plan. With this treatment goal, relief of symptoms and the maintenance of a satisfactory quality of life are the primary goals rather than cure or control of the disease process. Radiation therapy given to relieve the pain of bone metastasis is an example of treatment with a goal of palliation.

The goals of cure, control, and palliation are achieved through the use of four treatment modalities for cancer: surgery, radiation therapy, chemotherapy, and biologic response modifiers. Surgery, radiation therapy, and chemotherapy can be used alone or in any combination in the initial treatment phase, as well as in the retreatment phase(s) of cancer. Biologic response modifiers are currently being investigated for use alone or in combination with other treatment modalities.

For many cancers, two or more of the treatment modalities are used to achieve the goal of cure or control for a long period of time. Table 12-12 gives examples of the use of the treatment modalities to achieve cure or control of the disease process of cancer.

Clinical Trials

A clinical trial is a research study conducted with patients and is usually designed with the intent of evaluating new treatments. The evaluation of treatments in cancer research begins in the laboratory and with animal studies. From these studies, those treatments determined to be most effective, with reasonable levels of toxicity, are further evaluated in a series of studies on patients with cancer. New drugs or treatments, evaluated for the first time in human beings, usually go through three phases:

Phase I clinical trials: Determine dosage and route of administration of an agent and assess potential toxicities.

Phase II clinical trials: Evaluate the effect of a particular treatment on various types of cancer.

Phase III clinical trials: Compare the new treatment with standard therapy to determine which is more effective and which is associated with less morbidity.

Phase I clinical trials of biologic response modifiers may be further delineated into phase I-A and phase I-B. Phase I-A clinical trials investigate the toxicity and maximum-tolerated dose of the biologic response modifier agent. The intent of phase I-B clinical trials is to determine the optimum biologic response modifying dose.

The rights of the patient who participates in clinical trials are closely guarded by institutional review boards (IRBs) in each agency conducting research. IRBs not only review clinical trials at their inception but continue to review and monitor the study until its completion. Informed consent is a process in which information is fully disclosed to the patient by a physician and a nurse regarding the nature of the treatment being evaluated and the potential risks and benefits of entering the clinical trial. The patient must understand that he may elect to leave a clinical trial at any time.

Surgical Interventions

Surgery is the oldest form of cancer treatment, and for many years it was the only effective method of cancer diagnosis and treatment. The treatment of choice for many years was to remove the cancer and as much of the surrounding normal tissue as possible. Therefore most of the surgical procedures used were considered to be radical in nature. In the mid-1950s it was observed that even though the radical procedures were technically sophisticated, the mortality rates associated with certain cancer sites were not improving (e.g., breast cancer). Many cancers that were thought to be local disease processes were found to be systemic diseases with metastatic lesions located in anatomic sites other than the site of the primary disease. On analysis of these findings, it became obvious

Table 12-12 Treatment Modalities Used in Cancer

Original Cancer	Surgery	Radiotherapy	Chemotherapy	Biologic Response Modifiers
▪ Breast (Stage I)	P	Adj, I	Adj, I	I
▪ Ovary (Stage I)	P	Adj, I	Adj, I	I
▪ Uterine cervix (Stage II)	P	P	I	ND
▪ Lung				
Small (oat) cell	NU	Adj, I	P	I
Adenocarcinoma	P	Adj	I	I
▪ Gastrointestinal				
Colon	P	Adj	Adj, I	I
Stomach	P	Adj	Adj	I
▪ Melanoma (Stage I)	P	I	I	I
▪ Head and neck	P	P	I	I
▪ Testes seminoma (Stage I)	P	P	Adj	ND
▪ Prostate	P	Alt	I	I
▪ Kidney	P	Adj, I	I	I
▪ Brain	P	Alt, I	I	I
▪ Lymphomas				
Hodgkin's disease				
Stage I	NU	P	Adj	ND
Stage III	NU	Alt	P	ND

Adj, Adjuvant therapy used after localized tumor is treated by a primary method; routine use is not considered essential. *Alt,* An alternate, although less commonly used, method of primary treament for which data are already available indicating results equivalent to more common approaches. *I,* Investigational. The role in treatment is under examination in controlled clinical trials. Either a new approach to treatment or an older approach, which in the absence of sufficient data to support its frequent use, is being evaluated in controlled clinical trials. *ND,* No data are available to evaluate this form of treatment. *NU,* No use in the primary treatment program. Control rate of the tumor in question may be sufficiently high with other forms of treatment to preclude the testing of this modality. *P,* Considered an integral part of standard primary treatment programs.

that surgery alone, regardless of the extent of the procedure, was not an effective treatment for every type of cancer. Currently, surgery plays several roles in the diagnosis and treatment of cancer (Fig. 12-9).

Cure and Control. Several principles are applicable when surgery is used to cure or control the disease process of cancer:

1. Cancer that arises from a tissue with a slow rate of cellular proliferation or replication is the most amenable to surgical treatment.
2. A margin of normal tissue must surround the tumor at the time of resection.
3. Only as much tissue as necessary is removed, and adjuvant therapy is used. The current trend among health care professionals is toward less radical surgery.
4. Preventive measures are used to reduce the surgical seeding of cancer cells.
5. The usual sites of regional spread may be surgically removed.

Examples of surgical procedures used for cure or control of cancer include radical neck dissection, lumpectomy, mastectomy, pneumonectomy, orchiectomy, thyroidectomy, and bowel resection.

A *debulking procedure* may be used if the tumor cannot be completely removed (e.g., attached to a vital organ). When this occurs, as much tumor as possible is removed, and the patient may be given chemotherapy or radiation therapy. This type of surgical procedure makes the adjuvant therapy more effective.

Supportive Care. Surgical procedures can also be used to provide supportive care throughout the disease process of cancer. Examples of supportive surgical procedures include the following:

1. Insertion of feeding tubes in the esophagus or stomach
2. Creation of a colostomy to allow a rectal abscess to heal
3. Suprapubic cystostomy for the patient with advanced prostatic cancer

Palliation of Symptoms. When cure or control of cancer is no longer possible, the quality of life must be maintained at the highest possible level for the longest possible period of time. Examples of surgical procedures performed for palliative care include the following:

1. Cordotomy or rhizotomy for relief of pain (see Chapter 6)

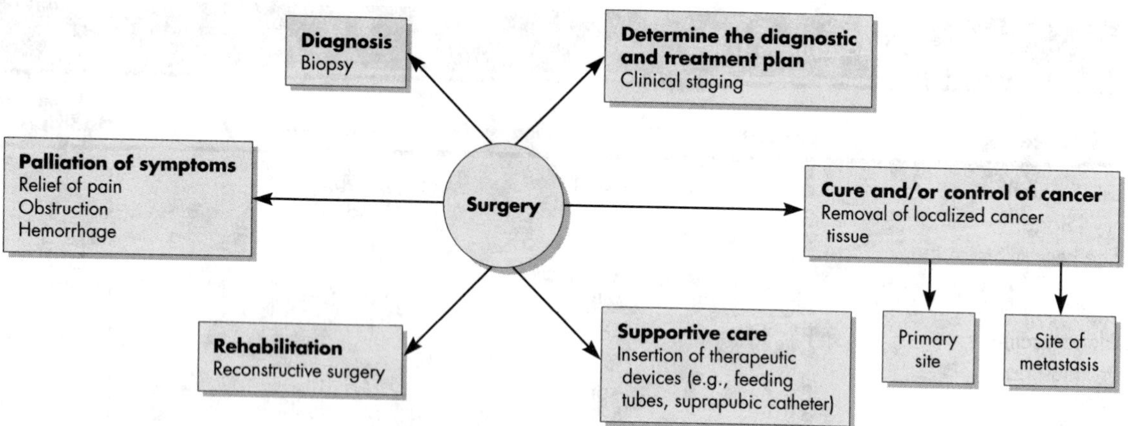

Fig. 12-9 Role of surgery in the treatment of cancer.

2. Colostomy for the relief of a bowel obstruction (see Chapter 40)
3. Laminectomy for the relief of a spinal cord compression (see Chapter 57)

Rehabilitative Management. Cancer surgery often mutilates and produces a change in the body image. It is often difficult for the patient to cope with this while attempting to maintain usual lifestyle patterns. As the treatment for certain cancers becomes more effective, the length of time the patient must live with an alteration created by surgery will be increased. If quality of life is to be maintained, the body image must be one that the patient is able to accept and cope with on a daily basis. A greater emphasis has been placed on the rehabilitative role of surgery in cancer care to increase the quality of life. Mammoplasty after a mastectomy is an example of a rehabilitative surgical procedure. The new appliances and the care of ostomies are other major focuses of rehabilitative management.

A nursing challenge is to assist the patient to think of cancer as a chronic rather than a terminal illness. Many people with chronic illnesses, such as arthritis and diabetes mellitus, learn to cope with their disease and have a high quality of life. This is also the goal for the person with cancer.

Radiation Therapy

Radiation therapy is a local treatment modality for cancer. It is one of the oldest methods of cancer treatment. From the time that Wilhelm Röntgen discovered x-rays in 1895, the Curies discovered radium in 1898, and Henri Becquerel discovered radioactivity in 1896, the role of radiation in the management of cancers has been explored. Early radiation workers, unaware of the properties of these materials, often handled radioactive sources unprotected. These workers experienced skin desquamation and developed carcinomas of the fingers. Marie and Pierre Curie both developed leukemia related to radiation exposure.[13,14]

These experiences led scientists to explore the use of radiation to treat tumors. The correlation made was that if radiation resulted in the destruction of the highly mitotic skin cells of workers it could be used in a controlled way to prevent the continued growth of highly mitotic cancer cells. Early therapeutic use of radiation was hampered by inadequate equipment and lack of knowledge of the effects of radiation on cancer and normal tissues. It was not until the 1960s that highly sophisticated equipment and treatment planning facilitated the delivery of adequate radiation doses to tumors and tolerable doses to normal tissues.[15] It is estimated in current practice that up to 60% of all persons with cancer will receive radiation therapy at some point in the treatment of their disease.

Effects of Radiation. Radiation is the emission and distribution of energy through space or a material medium. The energy produced by radiation, when absorbed into tissue, produces ionization and excitation. This local energy is sufficient to break chemical bonds in DNA, which leads to a biologic effect. The major target of the radiation effect is DNA. The ionization that occurs eventually causes damage to DNA, which renders cells incapable of surviving mitosis. Loss of proliferative capacity yields cellular death at the time of division. Cellular death is dependent on the cell going through its mitotic cycle. Thus death occurs at different rates for different cell types. This is true for both normal cells and cancer cells. However, cancer cells are more likely to be dividing because of the loss of control of cellular division. Furthermore these cells are unable to repair the radiation damage to DNA. Therefore cancer cells are more likely to be permanently damaged by cumulative doses of radiation. Normal tissues are usually able to recover from radiation damage if therapeutic doses are kept within certain ranges.[16]

Cellular death and tissue reactions. Cellular death related to radiation is defined as an irreversible loss of proliferative capacity. Cells may undergo several mitoses and then die. A cell that retains its proliferative capacity is a clonogenic cell because it is able to produce new clones or colonies of similar cells. Local control of a cancer occurs after radiation if the cells that remain are nonclonogenic.

Cellular sensitivity to radiation varies throughout the cell cycle with cells being most sensitive in the M and G_2

Table 12-13 Tumor Radiosensitivity

High Radiosensitivity	Moderate Radiosensitivity	Mild Radiosensitivity	Poor Radiosensitivity
Ovarian dysgerminoma Testicular seminoma Hodgkin's disease Non-Hodgkin's lymphoma Wilms' tumor Neuroblastoma	Skin carcinoma Oropharyngeal carcinoma Esophageal carcinoma Breast adenocarcinoma Uterine and cervical carcinoma Prostate carcinoma Bladder carcinoma	Soft tissue sarcomas (e.g., chondrosarcoma) Gastric adenocarcinoma Renal adenocarcinoma Colon adenocarcinoma	Osteosarcoma Malignant melanoma Malignant gliomas Testicular nonseminoma

phases and least sensitive during the S or synthesis phase (see Fig. 12-1). Cells treated during the M and G_2 phase of the cell cycle are more likely to suffer lethal damage. The damage to DNA in cells that are not in the M phase will be expressed when division occurs.

The amount of time that is required for the manifestation of radiation damage is determined by the mitotic rate of the tissue. Sufficient cells within the tissue must be killed to establish a noticeable effect. This is true in both normal and cancer cells. The time for this process to occur is measured in hours for intestinal epithelium and bone marrow and in months for slowly proliferating tissues such as the kidney and lung. In nonproliferating tissues such as nerves, the damage may take years to be expressed.[16,17,18]

Normal cells within the radiation field will also be affected by treatment. For each normal cell type there is a maximally tolerated radiation dose. Administration of radiation above the maximally tolerated doses results in limited ability of normal cells to recover from damage and potentially irreversible side effects. Treatment planning and computerized dosimetry assure that normal tissue tolerance is not exceeded.[19]

The manifestation of side effects of radiation therapy may be divided into phases. Acute effects occur during treatment and for up to 6 months following the completion of radiation therapy. Subacute effects occur in the next 6 months following the completion of radiation therapy, and late effects occur 1 year and beyond. The severity of acute effects does not predict the occurrence of late effects.[19,20]

Actively proliferating tissue, such as GI mucosa, esophageal and oropharyngeal mucosa, and bone marrow, exhibit early, acute responses to radiation therapy. Cartilage, bone, kidney, and central and peripheral nervous tissue manifest subacute or late responses. Tumors derived from proliferating cell types, such as lymphomas and leukemias, exhibit a rapid response to therapy at relatively low doses. These are mitotically active cells yielding a rapid expression of radiation damage. Tumors derived from more slowly growing cell types, such as rhabdomyosarcoma and leiomyosarcoma, take a higher dose of radiation and a longer period of time to respond because the mitotic rate of the tumor is slower, and many tumor cells must attempt mitosis for the damage to be expressed. Table 12-13 describes the relative radiosensitivity of a variety of tumors. In responsive tumors, even a large tumor burden will be affected by therapy. (Figures 12-10*A*, 12-10*B*, and 12-10*C* are of a patient with Hodgkin's disease before therapy and 6 years after therapy.) In less responsive tumors a large tumor burden may result in a slower and perhaps incomplete response. Late effects of radiation therapy are partially related to vascular changes that decrease circulation to tissues and lead to depletion of target cells, such as Schwann cells in peripheral nerves, tubule epithelium in the kidney, and oligodendrocytes in the central nervous system (CNS).[19,20]

Simulation and Treatment. Simulation is a part of radiation treatment planning used to determine the optimal method in which to treat a patient. The patient lies on a table in the treatment position. Under fluoroscopy the critical normal structures that will be included in the treatment field or portal are identified. A film is taken to verify the field, and marks are placed on the skin so that the field can be reproduced on a daily basis. Figures 12-11 and 12-12 illustrate the simulator and a simulation film. Computerized dosimetry using CT scanning is used to produce a treatment plan that delivers the maximum amount of radiation to the tumor within the acceptable dose to normal tissue.[21]

External radiation. Radiation treatment can be given by external beam radiation therapy (teletherapy), which is the most common form of treatment delivery. In this treatment the patient lies on the treatment couch and is exposed to radiation from the treatment machine (Fig. 12-13). The patient is never radioactive during this treatment.

Internal radiation. Another radiation delivery system is *brachytherapy*. This means "close" treatment and consists of the implantation or insertion of radioactive materials directly into the tumor or in close proximity to the tumor. An implant may be temporary with the source placed into a catheter or tube inserted into the tumor area and left in place for several days. This method is commonly used for tumors of the head and neck and gynecologic malignancies. Implants, such as prostate implants, may also be permanent with insertion of radioactive seeds into tumors. Figures 12-14 and 12-15 illustrate the applicator and a simulation film of a gynecologic implant. Brachytherapy is used in the clinical situation where the tumor dose needs to be high to eradicate the tumor. However, this dose is too high for the tolerance of nearby normal tissues. The sources used in

A

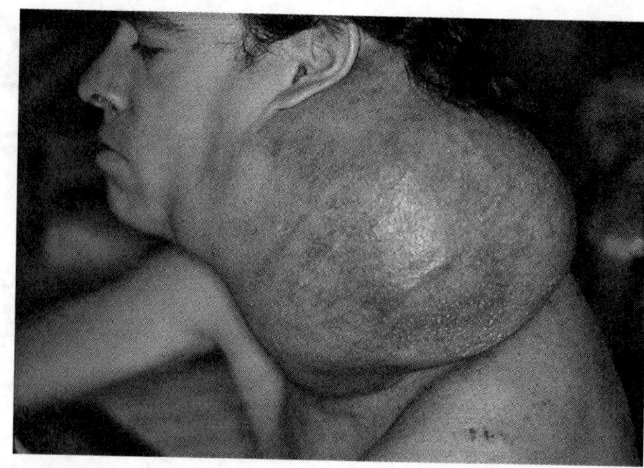

B

Fig. 12-10 ***A, B,*** Patient with Hodgkin's disease before radiation therapy.

C

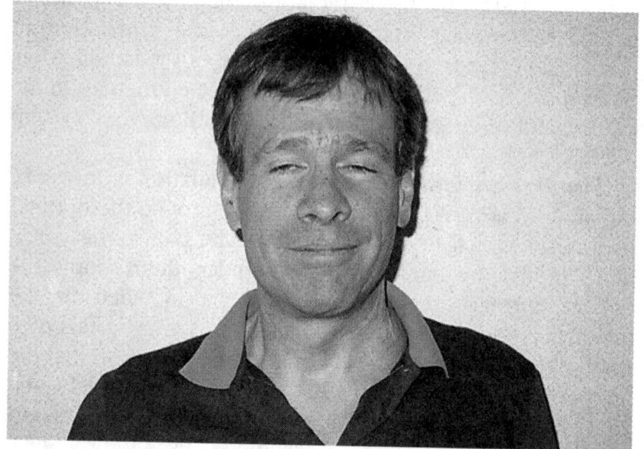

Fig. 12-10 ***C,*** Patient 6 years after radiation therapy.

brachytherapy are not as energetic or penetrating as those used in the external beam machines and thus deliver most of the dose locally. Often external beam radiation and brachytherapy will be used in combination.

Caring for the person with an implant requires that the nurse be aware that the patient is radioactive. If a patient has a temporary implant, the patient is radioactive during the time the source is in place. If the patient has a permanent implant, the radioactive exposure to the outside and others is low, and the patient may be discharged with precautions. For example, the person with a permanent radioactive I^{125} seed implant for prostate cancer may be told to double flush the toilet and not to allow children to sit on his lap for a specified period of time after the implant.

The principles of *time, distance,* and *shielding* are used when caring for the person with an implant. Nursing care should be organized so that a limited amount of time is spent with the patient. The patient should be prepared for the implant before the procedure and be aware of time limitations. The radiation safety officer will indicate how much time at a specific distance can be spent with the patient. This is determined by the dose delivered by the implant. Because the source is nonpenetrating, small differences in distance are critical. Only care that must be delivered near the source, such as checking placement of the implant, is performed in close proximity. Shielding, if available, should be used, and no care should be delivered without wearing a film badge. This badge will indicate any radiation exposure. The film badge should not be shared, should not be worn other than at work, and should be returned according to the agency's protocol.

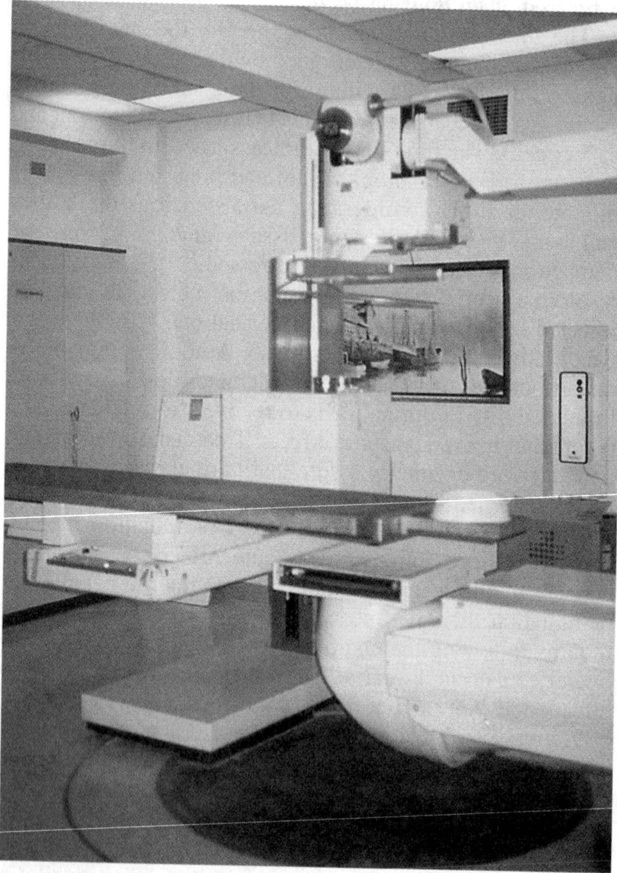

Fig. 12-11 Radiation simulator.

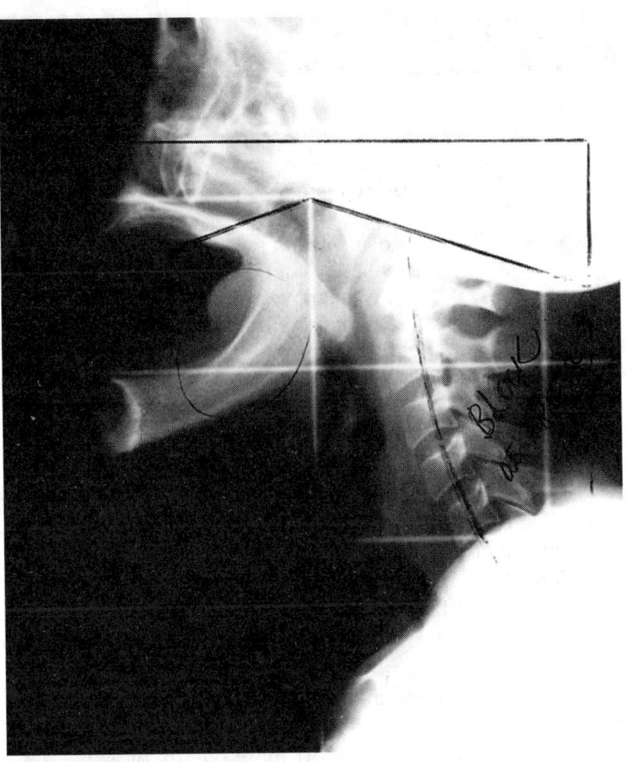

Fig. 12-12 Radiation simulation film.

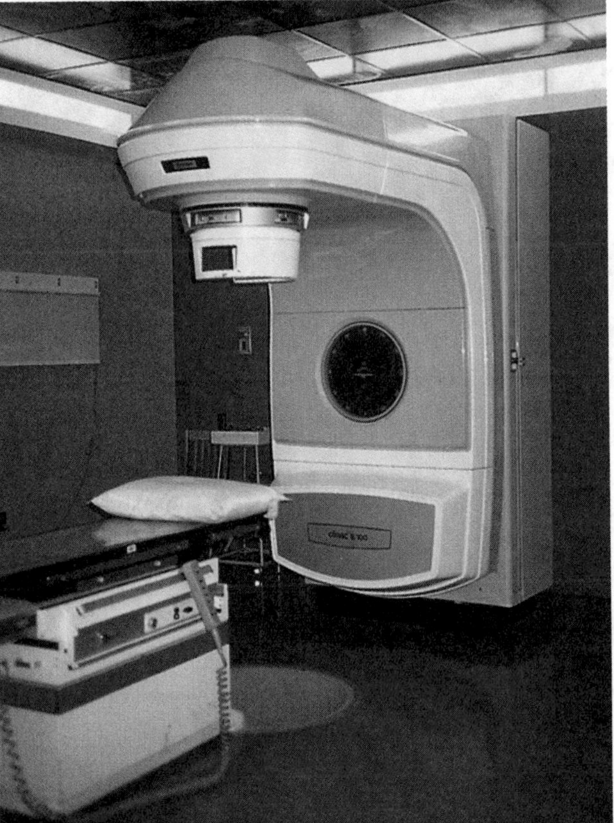

Fig. 12-13 Radiation treatment machine.

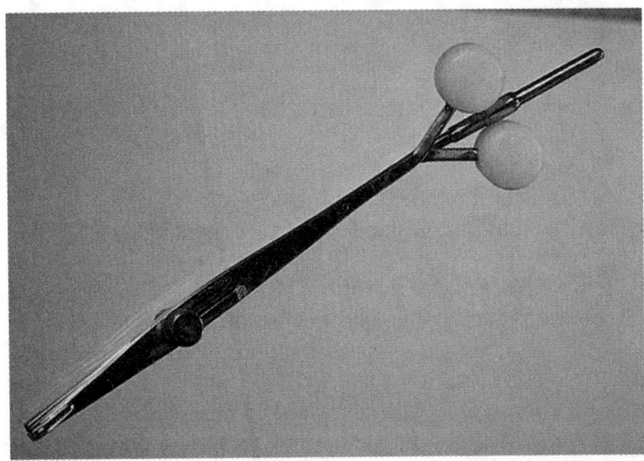

Fig. 12-14 Applicator for gynecologic implant.

Measurement of Radiation. Several different units are used to measure radiation (Table 12-14). Grays and centigrays are the units currently used in clinical practice.

Goals of Radiation Treatment. The goals of radiation therapy are cure, control, or palliation. To accomplish these treatment goals, radiation therapy can be used alone or as an adjuvant treatment modality in combination with surgery, chemotherapy, and biologic response modifiers.

Cure is the goal when radiation therapy is used alone as a curative modality for treating patients with basal cell carcinoma of the skin, tumors confined to the vocal cords, and Stage I or IIA Hodgkin's disease. Radiation therapy can be combined with surgery and chemotherapy to cure certain cancers such as (1) Stage IIB, IIIA, and IIIB Hodgkin's disease in combination with chemotherapy; (2) Wilms' tumor in combination with surgery and chemotherapy; (3) Ewing's sarcoma in combination with chemotherapy; (4) head and neck cancer in combination with surgery and chemotherapy; and (5) Stage I and II breast cancer.

Control of the disease process of cancer for a period of time is considered to be a reasonable goal in some situations. Initial treatment is offered at the time of diagnosis, and additional treatment is instituted each time symptoms of disease recur. Most patients enjoy a satisfactory quality of life during the symptom-free period. Radiation therapy can be combined with surgery to further enhance the local control of cancer. It can be given preoperatively to reduce the size of the tumor so that it can be more easily resected, or it can be given postoperatively to destroy any remaining tumor cells. Intraoperative radiation therapy is now being given at some research centers. In this procedure, radiation is administered directly to the site of the tumor during surgery.

Inoperable tumors can be treated with radiation therapy. These tumors are large and have extended regionally. An example of an inoperable cancer treated for control with radiation therapy is oat-cell cancer of the lung.

Palliation is often the goal of radiation therapy. The patient can be treated to control the distressing symptoms that are occurring as a result of the disease process. Tumors

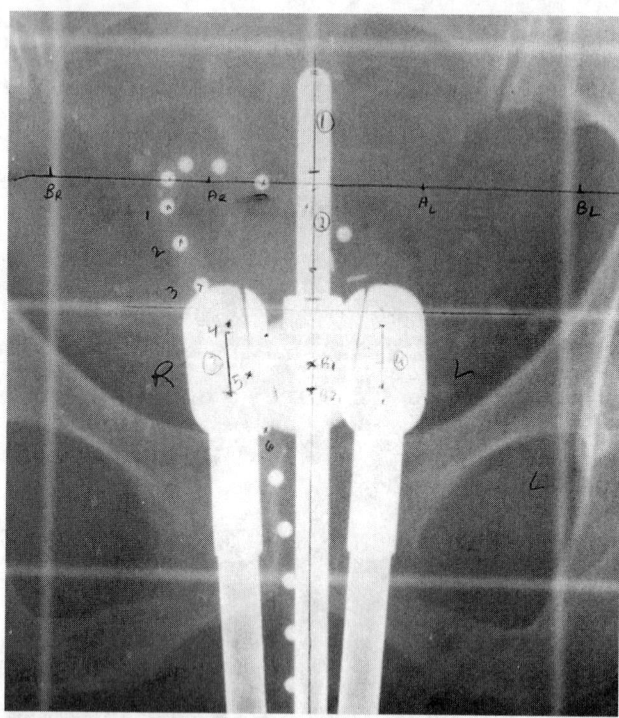

Fig. 12-15 Simulation film of a gynecologic implant.

Table 12-14 Measurement of Radiation

Unit	Definition
Curie (Ci)	A measure of the number of atoms of a particular radioisotope that disintegrate in 1 sec
Röntgen (R)	A measure of the radiation required to produce a standard number of ions in air; a unit of exposure to radiation
Rad	Measurement of radiation dosage absorbed by the tissues
Rem	Measurement of the biologic effectiveness of various forms of radiation on the human cell (1 rem = 1 rad)
Gray (Gy)	100 rads = 1 Gy

can be reduced in size to relieve symptoms such as pain and obstruction. Examples of the use of radiation therapy for palliation include the relief of:

1. Pain associated with bone metastasis
2. Pain and neurologic symptoms associated with brain metastasis
3. Spinal cord compression
4. Intestinal obstruction
5. Superior vena cava obstruction
6. Bronchial or tracheal obstruction
7. Bleeding (e.g., bladder and intrabronchial).

Side Effects of Radiation Therapy. Common side effects of radiation therapy are presented in Table 12-15. Fatigue, anorexia, bone marrow suppression, skin reactions, and mucosal reactions, as well as pulmonary, GI, and reproduction effects, are discussed in this section.

Fatigue. Fatigue is a commonly reported side effect of radiation therapy. The pathophysiologic mechanisms that result in radiation-induced fatigue are unclear, because it is not believed to be a result of loss of the cell's proliferative ability. Delay in the cell cycle may partially explain the fatigue. Accumulation of metabolites from the destruction of cells during treatment is another probable cause. The metabolites include lactate, hydrogen ions, and other end products of cellular destruction and result in decreased muscle strength. Alterations in energy production in the patient with cancer may also result from cachexia, anorexia, fever, and infection. Fatigue generally begins during the third to fourth week of treatment, persists after treatment ends, and then gradually subsides. Factors such as weight loss, anemia, depression, and other symptoms exacerbate the sensation of fatigue.

MANAGEMENT OF FATIGUE. The patient needs to recognize that fatigue is an expected side effect of radiation therapy. Otherwise the patient may interpret fatigue as a sign that the treatment is not effective and that the cancer must be spreading. A patient may report more energy on some days than on others. Encouraging the individual to identify days or times during the day when feeling better may allow the patient to remain more active. Resting before activity and having others assist with work or home management may be necessary. Ignoring the fatigue or overstressing the body when fatigue is tolerable leads to an increase in symptoms. Maintaining nutritional status and managing other symptoms also ameliorate the problem. Walking programs are a way of keeping the patient active. Most patients are able to participate in walking programs.[22] Fatigue is one symptom that shows improvement during walking programs. The ability to remain active has been shown to improve mood and avoid the debilitating cycle of fatigue-depression-fatigue that can occur.

Anorexia. Anorexia may develop as a general reaction to treatment. The mechanisms for anorexia are also unclear, but several theories exist. Macrophages release TNF and IL-1 in an attempt to fight the cancer. Both TNF and IL-1 have an anorectic effect. As tumors are destroyed by therapy, it is proposed that increased levels of these factors may be released into the system and cross the blood-brain barrier, exerting an influence on the satiety center. Large tumors produce more of these factors, thus resulting in the cachexia seen in advanced cancer. In addition, treatment to the head and neck and GI areas exacerbate eating difficulties. Anorexia peaks at about 4 weeks of treatment and seems to resolve more quickly than fatigue when treatment ends.

MANAGEMENT OF ANOREXIA. The patient with anorexia will need to be monitored carefully during treatment to ensure that weight loss does not become excessive. At least twice weekly, body weight should be obtained. The individual may assume responsibility for weighing once a return demonstration indicates the patient is able to do so

Table 12-15 Problems Caused by Radiation Therapy and Chemotherapy

Problem	Etiology and Comments
Gastrointestinal System	
Dryness of the mucous membranes of the mouth	When salivary glands are located in the radiation treatment field, they are frequently damaged. This may be a permanent side effect of radiation therapy, and it can be quite disturbing because it is difficult to eat, swallow, and talk when the mucous membranes are dry. Artificial saliva is available.
Stomatitis and mucositis	This problem occurs when epithelial cells of the oral mucosa and intraoral soft tissue structures are destroyed by chemotherapy or radiation therapy. These cells are extremely sensitive because of their normal high cell turnover rate. Mucositis can precipitate complications of infection and hemorrhage.
Esophagitis	Inflammation and ulceration of mucous membranes of esophagus as a result of rapid cell destruction occur as a side effect of chemotherapy and radiation therapy to the area of the neck, chest, and back.
Nausea and vomiting	The vomiting center in the brain is stimulated by products of cellular breakdown that occur in response to chemotherapy and radiation therapy. The drugs used in chemotherapy also stimulate the vomiting center. Destruction of the epithelial lining of the gastrointestinal tract occurs in response to chemotherapy and radiation therapy to chest, abdomen, and back. A strong psychologic impact is associated with nausea and vomiting and the high stress level associated with cancer and cancer treatment.
Anorexia	Site-specific side effects of radiation therapy—dry mouth, mucositis, esophagitis, nausea, vomiting, and diarrhea occur. Side effects of chemotherapy include nausea, vomiting, stomatitis, esophagitis, and diarrhea. Fatigue, pain, and infection are present. Alteration in the sensation of taste occurs when tumors release waste products into the bloodstream. Psychologic and social impact of cancer and cancer therapy result in an increased level of stress and changes in the usual lifestyle pattern.
Altered taste sensation	Destruction of the taste buds in the treatment field occurs with radiation therapy. The amount of taste alteration or loss depends on the radiation dosage and the extent of the treatment field. Complete loss of taste often occurs. Taste changes may be a permanent outcome of therapy. Waste products occur in response to cellular destruction from radiation therapy and chemotherapy. These waste products are thought to be responsible for alterations in taste sensation. Reduction in the amount of saliva occurs because of the location of the salivary glands in the treatment field. Food must be in solution to be tasted.
Diarrhea	Denuding of the epithelial lining of the small intestines occurs as a side effect of chemotherapy and radiation therapy to the abdomen or the lower back.
Constipation	Dysfunction of the autonomic nervous system from neurotoxic effects of plant alkaloids (vincristine, vinblastine) occurs.
Hepatotoxicity	Toxic effects of certain chemotherapy drugs such as methotrexate, mitomycin, 6-MP, and cytosine arabinoside are present.
Hematopoietic System	
Anemia	Depressant effect on bone marrow function occurs because of chemotherapy and radiation therapy. Malignant infiltration of bone marrow by cancer occurs. Ulceration, necrosis, and bleeding of neoplastic growth occur.
Leukopenia	Depressant effect on bone marrow activity is present as a result of chemotherapy and radiation therapy. The effect is especially significant because of the short life span of white blood cells. Infection is the most frequent cause of morbidity and death in the patient with cancer. Usual sites of infection are the respiratory and genitourinary systems.
Thrombocytopenia	Depressant effect on bone marrow function is present as a result of chemotherapy and radiation therapy. Malignant infiltration of the bone marrow occurs. Abnormal destruction of circulating platelets is present. When the platelet count is less than 20,000/μl, spontaneous bleeding can occur.
Integumentary System	
Alopecia	Alopecia occurs as a side effect of some chemotherapy agents and radiation therapy to the skull. Hair loss that occurs in response to chemotherapy is usually temporary, and hair loss that occurs in response to radiation therapy is usually permanent. The hair begins to fall out during the first week of therapy, and this may progress to complete hair loss.
Skin reactions	Extravasation of vesicant chemotherapeutic drugs (e.g., doxorubicin) given intravenously causes severe necrosis of tissues exposed to the drug.

continued

Table 12-15 Problems Caused by Radiation Therapy and Chemotherapy—cont'd

Problem	Etiology and Comments
Genitourinary Tract	
Cystitis	This problem occurs when the epithelial cells of the lining of the bladder are destroyed as a side effect of chemotherapy (e.g., cyclophosphamide) and as a side effect of radiation therapy when the bladder is located in the treatment field. Clinical manifestations of urgency, frequency, and hematuria are present.
Reproductive dysfunction	This problem occurs as a result of the effect of chemotherapy on the cells of the testes or ova or as a result of the effects of radiation therapy when the cells of the testes or ova are located in the treatment field. Symptoms of cancer and cancer therapy include fatigue, diarrhea, nausea, vomiting, anxiety, fear, and pain.
Nephrotoxicity	Necrosis of proximal renal tubules is present as a result of an accumulation of drugs (e.g., cisplatin) in the kidney.
Nervous System	
Increased intracranial pressure	This problem may result from radiation edema in the central nervous system. This phenomenon is not well understood but is easily controlled with steroids and pain medication.
Peripheral neuropathy	Paresthesias, areflexia, skeletal muscle weakness, and smooth muscle dysfunction (e.g., paralytic ileus, constipation) can occur as a side effect of the plant alkaloids (e.g., vinblastine, vincristine) and cisplatin.
Respiratory System	
Pneumonitis	When the lungs are located in the treatment field, radiation pneumonitis may develop 2-3 mo after the start of treatment. It is characterized by a dry, hacking cough, fever, and exertional dyspnea. After 6-12 mo, fibrosis will occur and will be persistently evident on x-ray. The patient with fibrosis is more susceptible to respiratory infection. This problem can also occur as a result of chemotherapy (e.g., bleomycin, busulfan).
Cardiovascular System	
Pericarditis and myocarditis	This problem is an infrequent complication when the chest wall is radiated. It may occur up to 1 yr after treatment.
Cardiotoxicity	Chemotherapeutic agents such as doxorubicin and daunorubicin can cause nonspecific electrical changes (i.e., low voltage) and rapidly progressive heart failure. The drug therapy needs to be modified if these effects occur.
Biochemical	
Hyperuricemia	An increase in uric acid levels occurs because of cell destruction by chemotherapy. This problem can cause a secondary form of gout.
Hypomagnesemia	This problem occurs with cisplatin therapy.
Psychoemotional	
Fatigue	Increase in the metabolic rate occurs when cancer is present with resultant increase in the amount of energy used. Destruction of cancer cells and normal cells by chemotherapy and radiation therapy occurs with the release of waste products into the bloodstream. Increase in anabolic processes of cellular proliferation and differentiation is necessary to repair the normal cells and tissue destroyed by chemotherapy and radiation therapy.
Pain	Compression or infiltration of the blood vessels, the lymphatic vessels, and the nerves occurs. Obstruction of the gastrointestinal or genitourinary system occurs. Inflammation, ulceration, or necrosis of the tissues or organs is present. Fear, anxiety, and depression are experienced in response to the diagnosis and treatment of cancer.

accurately. Laboratory values such as serum prealbumin and albumin need to be monitored. Small frequent meals of high protein, high calorie foods are better tolerated than large meals. Family members need to be supported if they are in the position of assisting the patient to eat. Anger and frustration related to the entire cancer trajectory often seem to find expression in arguments related to eating. Nutritional supplements are indicated if anorexia is severe or other factors contribute to difficulty in eating. The role of megestrol acetate as treatment for cancer-induced anorexia is under investigation.[23] This progesterone was found to be useful in the management of breast cancer with the side effect of significant weight gain related to increased appetite.

Bone Marrow Suppression. Bone marrow within the treatment field will be affected by radiation at a rate commensurate with the turnover rate of cells. WBCs are affected within a week, platelets in 2 to 3 weeks, and red blood cells (RBC) in 2 to 3 months. The degree of the acute effect is determined by the amount of proliferating bone marrow tissue in the treatment field. In the adult about 40% of active marrow is in the pelvis, and 25% is in the thoracic and lumbar vertebrae. When the marrow is irradiated, eradication of blood cells occurs within the treatment field. As a consequence, the nonirradiated marrow becomes active in an attempt to compensate.

The experience of immunosuppression is not clinically as significant a problem in radiation as it is in the patient receiving certain chemotherapeutic agents. Combination radiation and chemotherapy may cause precipitous drops in WBC, RBC, and platelet counts as does radiation following chemotherapy when bone marrow reserves are limited. Blood counts, including WBC, RBC, and platelets, in these individuals must be closely monitored. Bleeding and infection as consequences of immunosuppression are rare when radiation therapy is delivered alone.

If anemia occurs and the hemoglobin level drops below 10 g/dl (100g/L), the patient may require blood transfusions. Radiation therapy is more effective against well-oxygenated cells. Therefore there is a concern that a hemoglobin level below 10 g/dl (100 g/L) does not provide for adequate oxygenation of cells in the treatment field.

Skin Reactions. Skin reactions develop within the radiation field. The skin-sparing property of modern radiation equipment limits the severity of these reactions. Both acute and chronic changes occur in the skin. Although the skin reaction begins as early as the first treatment, it is usually transitory at first. Erythema may develop 1 to 24 hours after a single treatment. The true radiation reaction usually begins later at a dose of approximately 800 cGy. The skin cells are mitotically active and exhibit early response to treatment. Erythema is an acute response followed by desquamation. Cells become dark before they slough off because radiation stimulates the melanocytes. The basal cells of the epidermis begin to peel. A dry desquamation results when cells are shed. This dry reaction occurs when cells are shed at a rate that allows new cells to be available to replace the lost cells (Fig. 12-16). If the rate of cellular sloughing is faster than the ability of the new epidermal cells to replace dead cells, a wet desquamation occurs with exposure of the dermis and oozing of serum (Fig. 12-17). Surviving cells will form islands of new cells that eventually grow together to repair the damage. The effect of megavoltage radiation on the dermis may be greater than in the epidermis with fibroblasts exhibiting nuclear swelling. Skin reactions are particularly evident in areas subjected to pressure such as behind the ear, in gluteal folds, perineum, breast, collar line, and bony prominences.

Late effects in the skin are related to the total radiation dose. The epidermis in the field is thinner and smoother than nonradiated skin and may be unable to form pigment. The skin in the treated area may contain no hair and few or no sweat or sebaceous glands. This thin epidermis will be more subject to damage from trauma, and wound healing is delayed. Late reactions in the dermis may lead to fibrosis and fibrous hyperplasia in vessels with resultant telangiectasia. These are the dilated spidery vessels that may be seen in the treated area.[24]

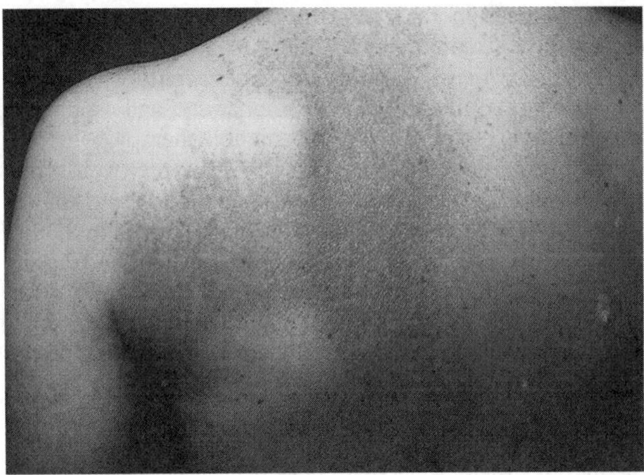

Fig. 12-16 Dry desquamation.

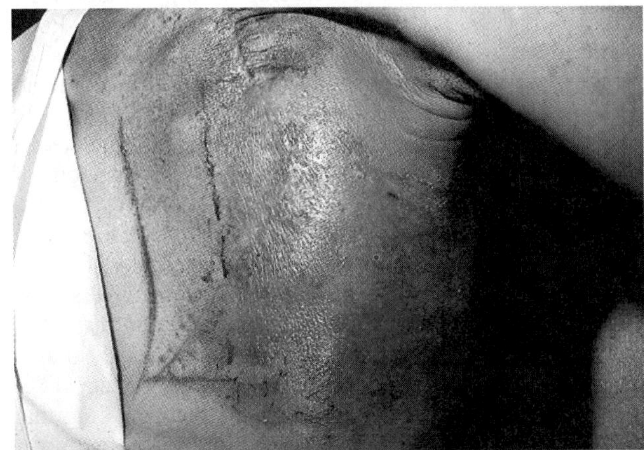

Fig. 12-17 Wet desquamation.

Management of Skin Reactions. Although there is a lack of consistency in protocols for the management of radiated skin in terms of products used, there are basic principles of skin care. Dry reactions are uncomfortable and result in pruritus. Wet reactions result in discomfort and drainage. Dry skin needs to be lubricated with a nonirritating lotion or solution that contains no metal, alcohol, perfume, or additives that irritate the skin. Wet reactions need to be kept clean and protected from further damage. Prevention of infection and facilitation of wound healing are the therapeutic goals. Even in the patient who is immunosuppressed, the development of infections within the radiated field is extremely rare.

Irradiated skin should be protected from extremes of temperature to prevent trauma. Heating pads, ice packs, and hot water bottles cannot be used in the treatment field. Constricting garments, rubbing, harsh chemicals, and deodorants may also traumatize the skin and should be avoided. The use of corticosteroids and hydrogen peroxide remains controversial because of their interference with wound healing. Because protocols vary widely, the guidelines presented in Table 12-16 should be clarified with the department of radiotherapy before being instituted.

Oral, oropharynx, and esophageal reactions. The mucosal linings of the oral cavity, oropharynx, and esophagus are sensitive to the effects of radiation therapy. Mucosal epithelium in the buccal mucosa is lost by the twelfth day of treatment. Desquamation develops first on the soft palate followed by the hypopharynx, vallecula, floor of the mouth, cheeks, medial aspect of the mandible, laryngeal surface of the epiglottis, interarytenoid area, base of the tongue, vocal cords, and the dorsum of the tongue. Capillary engorgement, edema, and leukocyte infiltration characterize the acute reaction. These changes arise in both external beam and brachytherapy treatments. Salivary glands may swell acutely from interstitial edema and duct obstruction after the first treatment. A decrease in salivary flow with resultant xerostomia (dry mouth) occurs during therapy. Serous acini appear to be more severely damaged than mucous acini, leaving saliva thick and ropey. This thick saliva is less able to perform the functions of cleansing teeth and moistening food so that the taste receptors can be stimulated. Food needs to be dissolved in saliva to be tasted. Taste loss is progressive during therapy, and, by the end of treatment, patients often report that all food has lost its flavor. With radiation doses of 3000 cGy, the patient can barely detect a sucrose solution equivalent in sweetness to 25 teaspoons of sugar.[25]

MANAGEMENT OF ORAL, OROPHARYNGEAL, AND ESOPHAGEAL REACTIONS. The oral cavity and esophageal effects of radiotherapy have the potential to compromise nutritional status. Oral assessment and meticulous intervention are essential to prevent infection and to facilitate nutritional intake. Difficulty swallowing, which characterizes esophageal reactions, further impedes eating. Patients report feeling that they have a "lump" as they swallow and that "foods get stuck." The individual with head and neck cancer often begins therapy in a compromised nutritional state related to poor eating habits associated with alcohol and tobacco abuse. All of these factors make the patient extremely vulnerable to malnutrition. Common side effects experienced by the individual with head and neck cancer include fatigue, loss of taste, anorexia, sore throat, cough, and changes in saliva.[25]

The patient needs to be taught to examine the oral cavity. The mucous membranes, characteristics of saliva, and ability to swallow need to be assessed. Oral care includes pretreatment evaluation by a dentist to perform all necessary dental work before the initiation of treatment. The patient should also be taught how to perform oral care and be fitted with fluoride trays to use during treatment. Compliance to this protocol significantly reduces the risk of radiation caries, which develop as a result of loss of saliva. These dental caries are extremely damaging to the teeth, resulting in the need for extraction. Saliva substitutes are available and may be offered to patients although many find that drinking large amounts of water has an equivalent effect. Oral care should be performed at least before and after each meal and at bedtime. A saline solution of one teaspoon of salt in a liter of water is an effective cleansing

Table 12-16 Nursing Management of Radiation Skin Reactions

1. Gently cleanse the skin in the treatment field using a mild soap (Ivory, Dove), tepid water, a soft cloth, and a gentle patting motion. Rinse thoroughly and pat dry.
2. Apply nonmedicated, nonperfumed, moisturizing lotion or creams, such as baby lotion, oil, aloe gel, or cream to alleviate dry skin. This substance must be gently cleansed from the treatment field before each treatment and reapplied. (Note: Care differs from institution to institution.) Dusting with cornstarch may reduce itching.
3. Cleanse the area involved with half-strength hydrogen peroxide and normal saline solution if a level III reaction is present. The solution is best applied with an irrigating syringe to avoid friction. Rinse the area with saline solution. Expose the area to air as often as possible. If copious drainage is present, nonadhesive absorbent dressings are warranted, and they must be changed as soon as they become wet. Observe the area daily for signs of infection.
4. Instruct the patient to avoid wearing tight-fitting clothing such as brassieres, girdles, and belts over the treatment field.
5. Instruct the patient to avoid wearing harsh fabrics, such as wool and corduroy. A light-weight cotton garment is best. If possible, expose the treatment field to air.
6. Instruct the patient to use gentle detergents such as Dreft and Ivory Snow to wash clothing that will come in contact with the treatment field.
7. Instruct the patient to avoid direct exposure to the sun. If the treatment field is in an area that is exposed to the sun, protective clothing such as a wide-brimmed hat should be worn during exposure to the sun.
8. Avoid all sources of heat (hot water bottles, heating pads, and sun lamps) on the treatment field.
9. Avoid exposing the treatment field to cold temperatures (ice bags or cold weather).
10. Instruct the patient to avoid swimming in salt water or in chlorinated pools during the time of treatment.
11. Instruct the patient to avoid the use of all medication, deodorants, perfumes, powders, or cosmetics on the skin in the treatment field. Tape, dressings, and adhesive bandages should also be avoided unless permitted by the radiation therapist. Avoid shaving the hair in the treatment field.
12. Sensitive skin must continue to be protected after the treatment is completed. Teach the patient to do the following:
    a. Avoid direct exposure to the sun. A sunscreen agent and protective clothing must be worn if the potential of exposure to the sun is present.
    b. Use an electric razor if shaving is necessary in the treatment field.

agent. One teaspoon of sodium bicarbonate may be added to the oral care solution to decrease odor, alleviate pain, and dissolve mucin. Tooth brushing and flossing are critical unless contraindicated by decreased platelet counts. This is rarely seen when radiation is used alone, but it may be a concern with combined modality therapy.

Alleviation of mucositis or pain in the throat can be achieved by systemic analgesics and antibiotics, as well as coating agents, which include antacids and sucralfate suspension. Combinations of coating and analgesic compounds may be used. Antacids, diphenhydramine (Benadryl), and viscous xylocaine have been mixed in equal proportions to use as a component of oral care. The solutions may be swallowed to alleviate esophagitis. Any coating solution must be cleansed and not allowed to build up on the mucosa where it could serve as a medium for infection. Infection, particularly with *Candida,* can occur in individuals receiving head and neck radiation. The incidence increases dramatically in protocols using concomitant chemotherapy with agents such as bleomycin. Oral nystatin, ketoconazole, fluconazole, or clotrimazole may be prescribed.[25,26]

Feedings of soft, nonirritating high protein and high caloric foods should be offered frequently throughout the day. Extremes of temperature, as well as tobacco and alcohol, should be avoided. Nutritional supplements as an adjunct to meals and fluid intake must be encouraged. The patient should be weighed several times each week to assure that excessive amounts of weight have not been lost. The individual who is an alcoholic often lacks a social support system that fosters good nutrition. Families are an integral part of the health care team. As taste loss increases, the family's role in assisting the patient to eat becomes increasingly critical. If family members are not available, alternative avenues of support such as volunteers and home aides are indicated.[26]

Pulmonary effects. The effects of radiation on the lung include both acute and late reactions. Radiation doses in the lung are actually magnified because there is no reduction of the dose through tissue. Treatment planning limits the amount of radiation dose to the lung. When the lungs are irradiated, there is damage to the alveolar type II pneumocyte, which is the cell that produces surfactant. Surfactant is a phospholipid substance that decreases surface tension and prevents alveolar collapse. When exposed to radiation, these cells initially secrete more surfactant in response to injury. Later, the gradual decrease in surfactant leads to a tendency toward alveolar collapse, which accentuates lung damage. Damage to the lung results in dyspnea and cough. Pneumonitis is the acute reaction related to blistering of capillary endothelial cells, platelet thrombi, and luminal obstruction. This reaction is often asymptomatic although an increase in cough, fever, and night sweats may occur. Infiltrates that conform to the shape of the radiation field are evident on chest x-ray. The symptomatic individual may require corticosteroids that provide relief, but symptoms may reappear precipitously when these drugs are withdrawn abruptly. Furthermore, corticosteroids do not prevent the development of fibrosis. Bronchodilators, expectorants, bed rest, and oxygen are preferable to steroids.

One to three months after treatment, alveolar cells begin to slough with exudation and the accumulation of fluid in interstitial spaces. Fibrosis develops 3 to 6 months after treatment with sclerosis of alveolar walls and loss of pulmonary function. With small radiation treatment doses the fibrosis that results is usually not clinically significant.

Management of Pulmonary Effects. The pulmonary effects of radiation are frightening to the patient because they may involve an exacerbation of the symptoms that precipitated the cancer diagnosis. Cough and dyspnea may increase. The cough becomes more productive as alveoli that had been blocked are opened as the tumor responds to treatment. As treatment continues, the cough becomes dry as the mucosa begins to be altered by the radiation. Cough suppressants may be indicated at night.

Oxygen, if prescribed for symptomatic pneumonitis, must be used judiciously if the patient has chronic obstructive pulmonary disease (see Chapter 25). The patient may mistakenly believe that increasing oxygen flow is an appropriate response to treat increasing dyspnea. Other symptoms reported by individuals receiving chest radiation include fatigue, skin irritation, anorexia, and sore throat. If the patient experiences dyspnea, anxiety may be pronounced. Lying flat on the treatment table and being alone in the room potentiate anxiety. Teaching must be reinforced frequently with the family present because the patient often forgets what has been told. Alleviation of obstruction reduces anxiety and dyspnea.[27]

Gastrointestinal effects. The mucosa of the GI tract is highly proliferative with surface cells being replaced every 2 to 6 days. Radiation alters gastric secretion by direct injury to cells. Radiation gastritis is evident after the first week of therapy with hyperemia, microscopic hemorrhage, and exudation. The secretion of mucus, hydrochloric acid, and pepsin decreases with further treatment. The intestinal mucosa is one of the most radiosensitive tissues. Reepithelization occurs within 96 hours following destruction of the mucosa. Nausea, vomiting, and diarrhea result from radiation of the GI tissue. Malabsorption of protein, fats, and carbohydrates occurs. Excessive bile salts entering the intestine may also lead to diarrhea. Cholestyramine may be indicated as an antidiarrheal because it binds with bile salts.[28]

Management of Gastrointestinal Effects. Nausea and vomiting are early reactions of radiation to the GI tract, occurring as soon as after the first treatment. The etiology of GI reactions may be related to stimulation of serotonin receptors in the GI tract, which then stimulate the chemoreceptor trigger zone and the vomiting center in the brain. Further GI irritation is related to cellular death. Prophylactic administration of antiemetics 1 hour before treatment is recommended. The patient may find that eating a light meal of nonirritating food before treatment is also helpful. The development of anticipatory nausea and vomiting can occur in the patient receiving radiation. This conditioned response develops over time in the individual who has unrelieved nausea and vomiting. As the patient repeatedly experiences these symptoms, a framework of cues is created associated with nausea and vomiting to the point that encountering the cues even without receiving treatment may precipitate nausea and vomiting. In some individuals this response persists after treatment ends. This type of reaction does not develop in the patient who does not experience posttreatment vomiting, which underscores the necessity for prophylactic treatment.

The patient experiencing nausea and vomiting must be assessed for signs and symptoms of dehydration and alkalosis. Fluid intake is recorded to assure that an adequate volume is being consumed and retained. Nausea and vomiting are usually successfully managed when conventional radiation doses and field sizes are used.

Diarrhea is a reaction of the bowel to radiation. The small bowel is extremely sensitive and does not tolerate significant radiation doses. Treating the patient with a full bladder may serve to move the small bowel out of the treatment field. The malabsorption of bile salts, as well as the irritation of the bowel wall, contribute to the development of diarrhea that occurs when abdominal and pelvic fields are radiated. Nonirritating diets and low residue diets, as well as antidiarrheals and antispasmodics, are recommended. Lukewarm sitz baths may alleviate discomfort and cleanse the rectal area. The rectal mucosa must be kept clean and dry to maintain mucosal integrity. The patient should record the number and character of stools per day. Adequate food and fluid intake promote healing and mucosal integrity. Meticulous perianal care is essential. Systemic analgesia is warranted for the painful skin irritations that may develop.

Reproductive effects. The effects of radiation on the ovary and testes are determined by the dose delivered. The testes are very sensitive to radiation, and protection of the testicles is achieved whenever possible. Doses of 15 to 30 cGy temporarily decrease the sperm count with aspermia at 35 to 230 cGy. In some cases, 200 cGy may result in permanent aspermia. The patient receiving 300 to 600 cGy either recovers in 2 to 5 years or not at all. Pretreatment status may be a significant factor as a low sperm count and loss of motility are seen in individuals with testicular cancer and Hodgkin's disease before any therapy. Combined modality treatment or prior chemotherapy with alkylating agents enhances and prolongs the effects of radiation on the testes. When radiation is used alone with conventional doses and appropriate shielding, testicular recovery often occurs.[29]

Compromise of reproductive function in men may also result from erectile dysfunction following pelvic radiation and related vascular and neurologic effects. The incidence of erectile dysfunction with radiation is reportedly less than with non–nerve-sparing surgery. Brachytherapy for prostate cancer further decreases this risk.

The radiation dose necessary to induce ovarian failure changes with age. Permanent cessation of menses occurs in 95% of women less than 40 years of age at 500 to 1000 cGy and at 375 cGy in women more than 40. Unlike the testes, there is no avenue for repair of ovarian function. The ovaries are shielded whenever possible. If exploratory laparotomies are performed in women with Hodgkin's disease, the ovaries may be moved out of the radiation field.[29]

Other factors that influence reproductive or sexual functioning in women include reactions in the cervix and endometrium. These tissues withstand a high radiation dose with minimal sequelae, accounting for the ability to treat endometrial and cervical cancer with high external and brachytherapy doses. Acute reactions such as tenderness, irritation, and loss of lubrication compromise sexual activity. Late effects of combined internal and external therapy include vaginal shortening related to fibrosis and loss of elasticity and lubrication.

MANAGEMENT OF REPRODUCTIVE EFFECTS. The patient and his partner require information about the expected effects of treatment relative to reproductive issues. Potential infertility can be a significant consequence for the individual, and counseling may be indicated. Specific suggestions to manage side effects that have an impact on sexual functioning include using a water-soluble vaginal lubrication and a vaginal dilator after pelvic radiation. The nurse must be able to encourage discussion of issues related to sexuality, to offer specific suggestions, and to make referrals for ongoing counseling when indicated.

Coping with Radiation Therapy. Assisting the patient to cope with the anxieties of receiving radiation is an essential component of the nursing role. The necessity of coming for treatment five times per week forces the individual to confront the cancer on an almost daily basis.[31] The demands on the patient and the family and the disruption of normal activities created by the treatment schedule are difficult to handle. In conjunction with the social worker, the nurse needs to assist with planning for transportation with available resources such as the American Cancer Society, churches, and community resources.

Anxiety is almost always present in the patient receiving therapy. The uncertainties regarding treatment and the fears of receiving radiation are most evident at the beginning of therapy. Anxiety continues to be a factor at the end of treatment when outcomes are still unknown. Anxiety may increase in some patients when treatment ends. The patient needs to realize that he will be followed and that support is ongoing. The impact of radiation on the quality of life of the patient undergoing therapy may be minimized with information and support. The patient may find that relaxation techniques and humor can be used to lessen anxiety. The nurse should encourage the appropriate use of humor. Research on the long-term effects, both physical and emotional, on the quality of life of the individual receiving radiation is needed.[32]

The nurse plays an important role in the management of the individual receiving radiation therapy. Patient education and symptom management allow the individual to cope with therapy while maintaining the highest possible quality of life.

Chemotherapy

Chemotherapy is the systemic treatment of cancer with chemicals (drugs). In the 1940s chemotherapy was in its infancy. Nitrogen mustard, a chemical warfare agent used in World War II, was used in the treatment of acute leukemia, and a folic acid antimetabolite (5-FU) was found

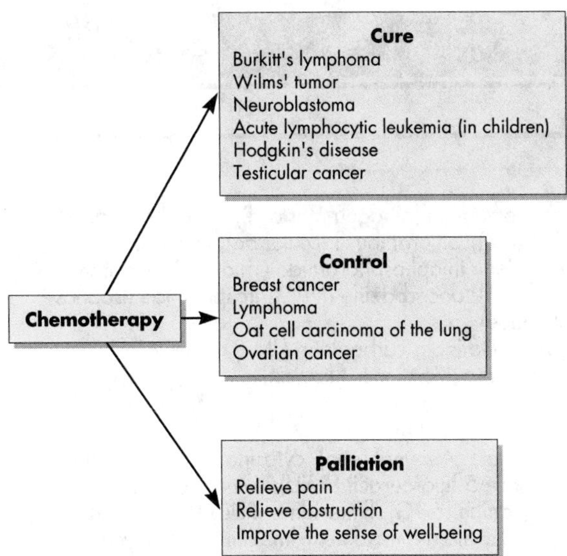

Fig. 12-18 Goals of chemotherapy.

to have antitumor activity. In the 1950s considerable experimentation with single-drug therapy began. In the 1960s the emphasis was on the development and use of combination chemotherapy. In the 1970s chemotherapy was established as an effective treatment modality for cancer. By the 1980s clinical studies looked at the effect of high doses of chemotherapy used in the treatment of cancers previously resistant to therapy. Chemotherapy is now used in the treatment of many solid tumors, and it is the primary therapy for leukemias and some lymphomas. Chemotherapy has gone from a palliative, "last-ditch effort" treatment modality to one that can cure certain cancers, control other cancers for long periods of time, and offer palliative relief of symptoms when cure or control no longer is possible[33] (Fig. 12-18).

Effect on Cells. The effect of chemotherapy is at the cellular level. All cells (cancer cells and normal cells) enter the cell cycle for replication and proliferation (see Fig. 12-1). The effects of the chemotherapeutic agents are described in relationship to the cell cycle. The two major categories of chemotherapeutic drugs are *cell cycle-nonspecific* and *cell cycle-specific*.

Cell cycle-nonspecific chemotherapeutic drugs have their effect on the cells that are in the process of cellular replication and proliferation, as well as on the cells that are in the resting phase (G_0).

Cell cycle-specific chemotherapeutic drugs have their effect on cells that are in the process of cellular replication or proliferation (G_1, S_1, G_2, or M). The cell cycle-specific chemotherapeutic drugs can be categorized more specifically into *phase-specific* chemotherapeutic agents. These drugs are effective at only one specific phase of the cell cycle.

Cell cycle-specific and cell cycle-nonspecific agents are often administered in combination with one another. The aim of this approach is to promote a better response using agents that function by differing mechanisms.

The goal of chemotherapy is to reduce the number of cancer cells present in the primary tumor site(s) and metastatic tumor site(s). Several factors will determine the response of cancer cells to chemotherapy:

1. Mitotic rate of the tissue from which the tumor arises. The more rapid the mitotic rate, the greater the response to chemotherapy. Chemotherapy is the treatment of choice for acute leukemia, choriocarcinoma of the placenta, Wilms' tumor (used in conjunction with surgery), and neuroblastoma. These cancer cells have a rapid rate of cellular proliferation.
2. Size of the tumor. The smaller the number of cancer cells, the greater the response to chemotherapy.
3. Age of the tumor. The younger the tumor, the greater the response to chemotherapy. Younger tumors have a greater percentage of proliferating cells.
4. Location of the tumor. Certain anatomic sites provide a protected environment from the effects of chemotherapy. For example, only a few drugs (nitrosoureas and bleomycin) cross the blood-brain barrier.
5. Presence of resistant tumor cells. Mutation of cancer cells within the tumor mass can result in variant cells that are resistant to chemotherapy. Resistance can also occur because of the biochemical inability of some cancer cells to convert the drug to its active form.
6. Physiologic and psychologic status of the host. A state of optimum health and a positive attitude will allow the patient to better withstand aggressive chemotherapy.

When the cancer first begins to grow, most of the cells are actively dividing. As the tumor increases in size, more and more cells become inactive and convert to a resting state (G_0). Since most chemotherapeutic agents are most effective against dividing cells, cells can escape death by staying in the G_0 phase. The main problem in cancer chemotherapy is the presence of drug-resistant resting and noncycling cells.

One method to prevent the existence of drug-resistant tumor cells is the use of high-dose chemotherapy. The aim of this approach is to maximize the effects of the drug at the cellular level before the problem of resistance occurs. An example of high-dose chemotherapy is the use of cytarabine (ara-C) for the treatment of leukemia. The standard dose of this agent is 100 mg/m^2. However, the intensified regimen of this agent includes a dose of 3 g/m^2.

Classification of Chemotherapeutic Drugs. Chemotherapeutic drugs are categorized or classified according to their structure and mechanisms of action (Table 12-17 and Fig. 12-19). Each drug in a particular classification has many similarities, but major differences in the drugs are also evident.

Methods of Administration. Chemotherapy can be administered by several routes (Table 12-18). The oral and intravenous (IV) routes are the most common. One of the major concerns with the IV administration of antineoplastic drugs is possible irritation of the vessel wall by the drug or, even worse, *extravasation* (infiltration of drugs into tissues surrounding the infusion site) causing local tissue damage.

Table 12-17 Classification of Chemotherapeutic Drugs

Mechanisms of Action	Examples
Alkyating Agents	
Cell-cycle nonspecific	
■ Damage DNA by causing breaks in the double-strand helix (similar to the effect of radiation therapy); if repair does not occur, cells will die immediately (cytocidal) or when they attempt to divide (cytostatic).	Mechlorethamine (nitrogen mustard), cyclophosphamide (Cytoxan), Chlorambucil (Leukeran), melphalan (Alkeran), triethylene thiophosphoramide (Thiotepa), busulfan (Myleran), dacarbazine (DTIC), ifosphamide (Isophosphamide)
■ Have heavy metal effect on DNA.	Cisplatin (Platinol), carboplatin (JM-8, CBDCA)
■ Suppress mitosis at interphase.	Procarbazine (Matulane, Natulan)
Antimetabolites	
Cell-cycle specific	
■ Interfere with synthesis of DNA by mimicking certain essential cellular metabolites that the cell incorporates into synthesis of DNA; cells will die immediately (cytocidal).	Methotrexate (Amethopterin), cytosine arabinoside (ara-C, Cytosar), 5-fluorouracil (5-FU), 6-mercaptopurine (6-MP), thioguanine (6-TG), floxuridine (FUDR), vidarabine (Vira-A), 5-azacitdine, hexamethylmelamine, deoxycoformycin (DCF, Pentrostatin), fludarabine
Antitumor Antibiotics	
Cell-cycle nonspecific	
■ Modify function of DNA and interferes with transcription of RNA; cells will die immediately (cytocidal) or when they attempt to divide (cytostatic).	Doxorubicin (Adriamycin), bleomycin (Blenoxane), mitomycin (Mutamycin), daunorubicin (Daunomycin), Actinomycin D, idarubicin, plicamycin (Mithracin)
Plant Alkaloids	
Cell-cycle specific	
■ Interrupt cellular replication in mitosis at metaphase; cells will die immediately (cytocidal).	Vinblastine (Velban), vincristine (Oncovin), Etoposide (VePesid), Taxol, Vindesine
Nitrosureas	
Cell-cycle nonspecific	
■ Have similar effect to alkylating agents and also block specific enzymes needed for the synthesis of purine; cells will die immediately (cytocidal) or when they attempt to divide (cytostatic).	Carmustine (BCNU), lomustine (CCNU), semustine (Methyl CCNU), streptozotocin (STZ), chlorozotozin (DCNU)
Corticosteroids	
Cell-cycle nonspecific	
■ Disrupt the cell membrane and inhibit synthesis of protein; decrease circulating lymphocytes; inhibit mitosis; depress immune system; increase feeling of well-being.	Prednisone (Merticorten), dexamethasone (Decadron)
Hormones	
Cell-cycle nonspecific	
■ Stimulate the process of cellular differentiation; metastatic lesions are less able to survive in unfavorable environment; decrease the process of cellular proliferation.	Androgens (testosterone, fluoxymesterone [Halotestine]), estrogens (diethylstilbestrol [DES]), progestins (Provera, Delalutin, Megace)
Miscellaneous	
■ Destroy exogenous supply of L-asparagine, which is needed for cellular proliferation; normal cells can synthesize but cannot be synthesized by cancer cells.	L-Asparaginase (Elspar)
■ Have effect on DNA similar to alkylating agents; also blocks incorporation of thymidine into DNA.	Hydroxyurea (Hydrea)
■ Antiestrogens are used in breast cancer.	Tamoxifen (Nolvadex)
■ Antiadrenal drug blocks adrenal steroid production.	Aminoglutethimide (Cytadren)
■ Produce single and double strand breaks in DNA.	Amasacrine (m-AMSA)

DNA, Deoxyribonucleic acid; *RNA*, ribonucleic acid.

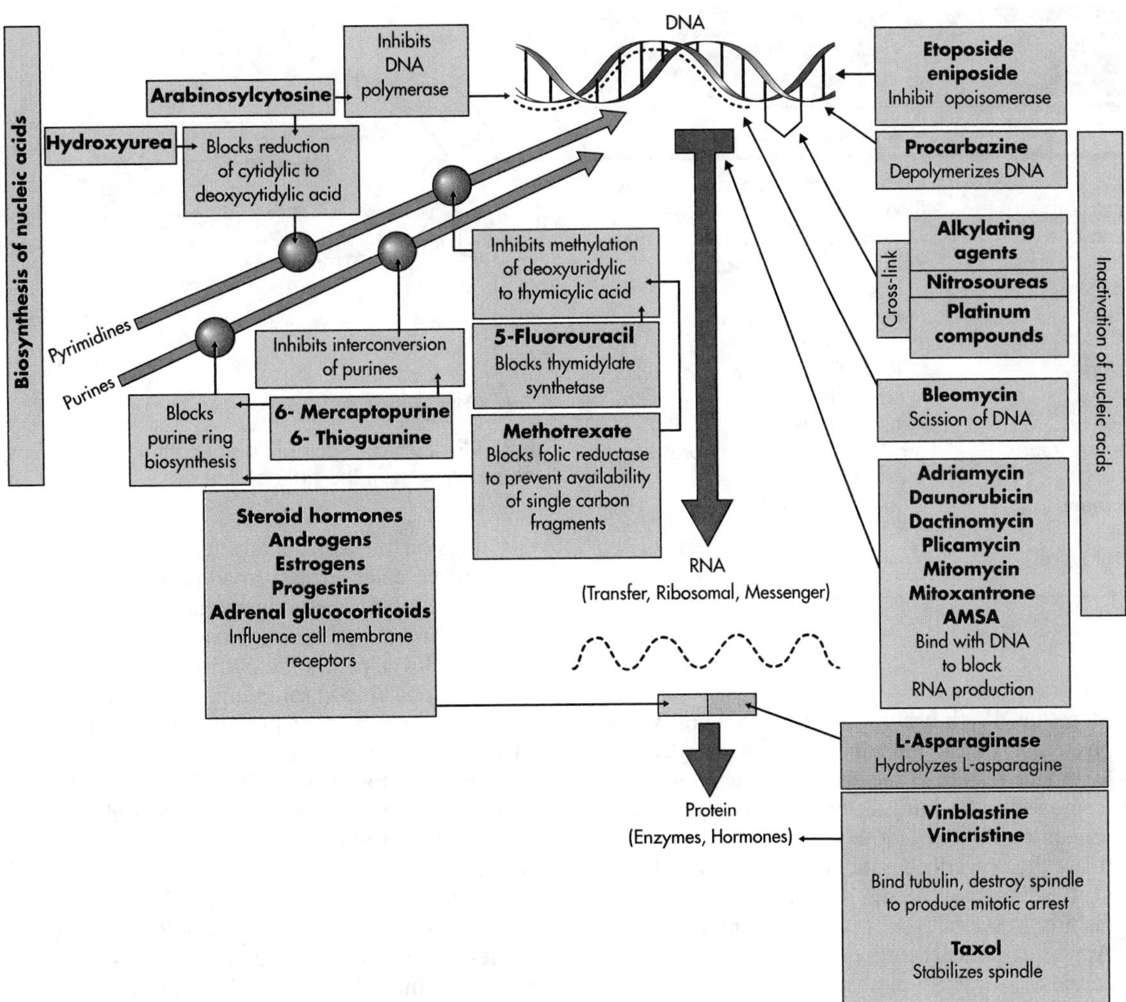

Fig. 12-19 Actions of chemotherapeutic agents.

Many chemotherapeutic drugs are *vesicants*—agents that when accidentally infiltrated into the skin cause severe local tissue breakdown and necrosis. Some guidelines to promote safe use of the chemotherapeutic drugs by IV administration follow:

1. Know specifics about the safe administration of chemotherapy.
2. Start an IV infusion of normal saline solution or 5% dextrose in water or saline solution with a small-lumen short needle or catheter. Ensure that recent venipunctures have not been performed proximal to the IV site. Avoid using an arm that has poor lymphatic drainage or that has previously received radiation therapy.
3. Select a vein that is large enough to promote infusion without irritating the intima of the vein. When a vesicant is administered, avoid the veins in the hand, wrist, and antecubital area.
4. Instruct the patient to immediately report any changes in sensation, especially burning or stinging pain.
5. Check for a blood return before infusing the chemotherapeutic drug. However, a blood return does not always indicate an intact vein.
6. If more than one drug is to be administered, give the vesicant agents first, when the vein is at its optimum integrity. (Note: This method is controversial. Some believe that vesicants should be administered last or given between two nonvesicants.)
7. Slowly push those drugs that are to be given by the push or bolus method. Give in small increments (0.5 to 1.0 ml). Pause 30 to 60 seconds after each increment, and allow the IV infusion to flush the vein; check blood return, and again gently push 0.5 to 1.0 ml of the medication. Repeat until the medication has been given and allow the IV infusion to flush the vein for several minutes.
8. Avoid continuous peripheral IV infusions of vesicant agents. If given peripherally, the administration of a vesicant agent must be monitored directly at all times.
9. Stop the IV infusion immediately if the patient complains of a burning or stinging pain or if an infiltration is suspected. If the drug is an irritant, check for blood return and, if present, continue to administer the drug. If it is a vesicant, stop the infusion and begin appropriate extravasation procedures.

Table 12-18 Methods of Chemotherapy Administration

Method	Examples
Oral	Cyclophosphamide
Intramuscular	Bleomycin
Intravenous	Doxorubicin, vincristine
Intracavitary (pleural, peritoneal)	Radioisotopes, alkylating agents
Intrathecal	Methotrexate, cytosine arabinoside
Intraarterial	DTIC, 5-FU, methotrexate, floxuridine
Perfusion	Alkylating agents
Continuous infusion	5-FU, methotrexate, cytosine arabinoside
Subcutaneous	Cytosine arabinoside
Topical	5-FU cream
Intraperitoneal	Methotrexate, 5-FU

10. If extravasation occurs:
    a. Stop the IV infusion immediately; notify the physician, or use the standing written orders for treatment related to the specific vesicant agent.
    b. Remove the IV infusion tubing and aspirate any remaining drug with a new syringe.
    c. Inject the prescribed antidote (if one is available) in the infusion needle or in a "pincushion" fashion in the skin surrounding the needle site.
    d. Apply a topical corticosteroid cream, if prescribed.
    e. Elevate the site.
    f. Apply cold compresses for the first 24 to 48 hours unless a *Vinca* alkaloid has been infiltrated; heat is applied following extravasation of Vinca alkaloids.
    g. Document the extravasation.
    h. Observe site at designated intervals.
    i. A plastic surgeon may be consulted, depending on the extent of anticipated damage.

Pain is the cardinal symptom of extravasation, although extravasation has been known to occur without causing pain. Swelling, redness, and the presence of vesicles on the skin are other early signs of extravasation. After a few days, the tissue may begin to ulcerate and necrose. The process has the potential to progress to a deep, wide crater that often warrants closure with skin grafts. If infection occurs, this is a serious problem that may be life threatening.

Chemotherapy can also be administered by means of a *vascular access device*. Vascular access devices are placed in large vessels (venous or arterial) and permit frequent, continuous, or intermittent administration of chemotherapy and other products, thus avoiding multiple punctures for vascular access. These devices are indicated in instances of limited vascular access, intensive chemotherapy, continuous infusion of vesicant agents, and projected long-term need for vascular access. In addition to their usefulness in administration of chemotherapeutic agents, vascular access devices can be used to administer additional fluids, such as blood products, parenteral nutrition, and other medications, and for venous blood sampling. The advantages of vascular access devices are that they provide for rapid dilution of chemotherapy, decreased incidence of extravasation, and reduced need for venipuncture. Three major types of vascular access devices include Silastic right atrial catheters, implanted infusion ports, and infusion (external and implanted) pumps.

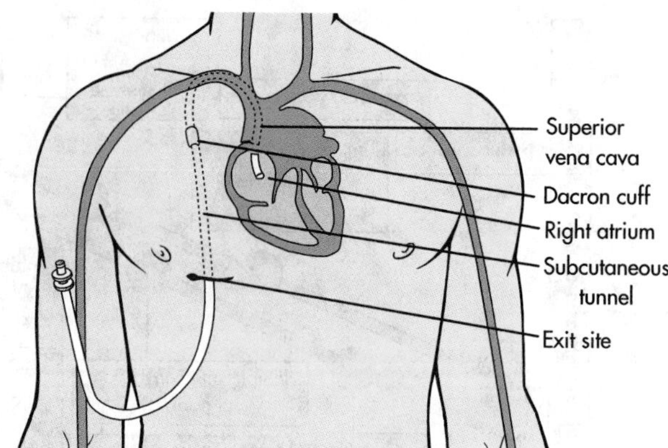

Fig. 12-20 Silastic right atrial catheter placement. Note tip of the catheter in the right atrium.

Silastic right atrial catheters. Silastic right atrial catheters (Hickman, Specialty Access Products, and Raaf) are single-, double-, or triple-lumen catheters approximately 90 cm in length with internal diameters ranging from 1 to 2 mm (Fig. 12-20). These catheters are inserted with the aid of local or general anesthesia through a central vein with the tip resting in the right atrium of the heart. The other end of the catheter is tunneled through subcutaneous tissue and exits through a separate incision on the chest or abdominal wall. A Dacron cuff on the catheter serves to stabilize the catheter and may also decrease the incidence of infection. Care requirements include cap change, cleansing, heparin flush, and dressing change. The exact frequency and procedures for these requirements vary from institution to institution. Reported complications with these catheters include occlusion, sepsis, bleeding, venous thrombosis, technical problems, and local infection at the exit site.

The Groshong catheter is a distinct type of tunneled central venous catheter. The unique features of this catheter are the existence of a pressure-sensitive valve near the distal end, which precludes the need for heparin flushing and clamping, and its placement 2 to 3 cm above the right atrium in the superior vena cava.

Peripherally inserted central venous catheters and midline catheters. Peripherally inserted central venous catheters (PICCs) (e.g., C-PICS, Per-Q-Cath, Intracath, L-CATH, Ven-A-Cath, Viggio Hydrocath, and Groshong PICC) and midline catheters (MLCs) (e.g., Landmark Midline Catheter and L-CATH) are nontunneled, polymer cath-

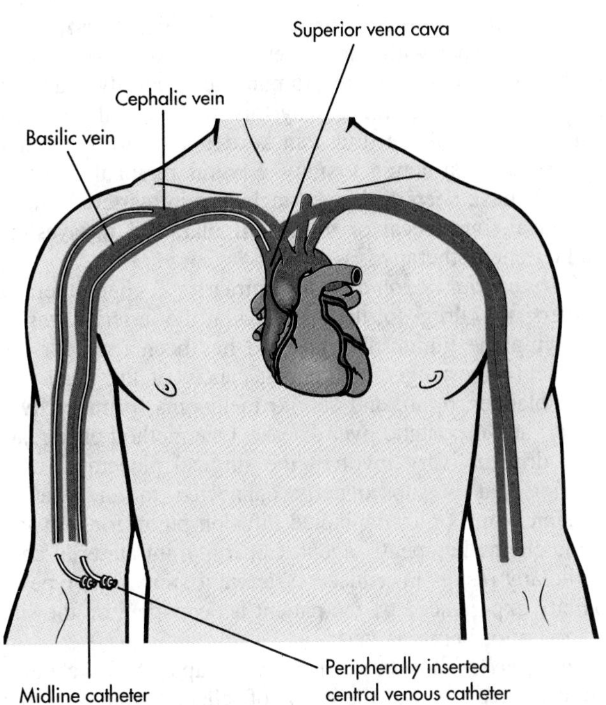

Fig. 12-21 Placement of peripherally inserted central venous catheter (PICC) and midline catheter (MLC).

eters that are primarily used in cancer care for immediate central venous access or when the need for infusion therapy is beyond the capacity of the patient's existing, long-term venous access device[34] (Fig. 12-21). These catheters are used for short-term IV therapy, frequent administration of blood products, and intermittent or continuous drug infusions. These catheters are placed by a physician or a specially trained nurse.

PICC lines are inserted at the antecubital fossa and advanced to a position in the peripheral venous system or into one of the vessels that ultimately enters the superior vena cava. These lines are up to 60 cm in length with gauges ranging from 24 to 16. They can be in place for up to 6 months. The technique for placement of a PICC line involves insertion of the catheter through a needle with the use of a guide wire or forceps to advance the line.

MLC lines are catheters that are placed between the antecubital fossa and the head of the clavicle. These catheters are shorter than PICC lines (15 to 20 cm) with the tip resting in the larger vessels of the upper arm. PICC lines can be used for this purpose. However, specific MLCs have been developed (Landmark Midline Catheter and L-Cath). MLCs are made of an elastomeric hydrogel that becomes approximately 50 times softer approximately 2 hours following insertion because of contact with body fluids. As a result, the gauge of the catheter increases and the length of the line increases. The MLC can be placed above or below the antecubital fossa. Following venipuncture, the needle is withdrawn into a tube, and the catheter is advanced using a catheter advancement tab.

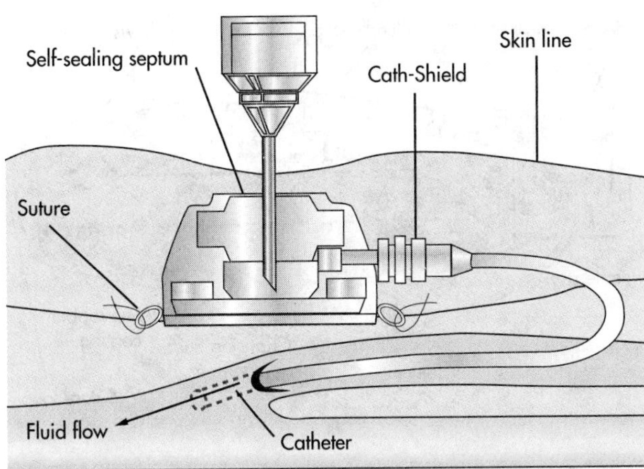

Fig. 12-22 Cross section of implantable port displaying access of the port with the Huber needle. Note the deflected point of the Huber needle, which prevents coring of the port's septum.

Complications of PICC and MLC lines include catheter occlusion and phlebitis. Urokinase can be used to lyse obstructions. If phlebitis occurs, it usually appears within 7 to 10 days following insertion. Signs of phlebitis include redness, edema, and tenderness along the track of the catheter line. The catheter should be removed, and the tip of the catheter must be cultured. The arm in which a PICC or MLC is in place should not be used for blood pressures or blood drawing.[34]

Implanted infusion ports. Implanted infusion ports (Hickman Port, Port-A-Cath, Infusaid MicroPort, Norport LS, Lifeport, and Groshong Port) consist of a central venous catheter connected to an implanted subcutaneous injection port (Fig. 12-22). The catheter is placed into the desired vein and the other end is connected to a port that is surgically implanted in a subcutaneous pocket on the chest wall. The port consists of a metal sheath with a self-sealing silicone septum. It is accessed via the septum by means of a special Huber-point needle that has a deflected tip to prevent coring of the septum. Care requirements include dressing change, cleansing, and flushing. Complications attributed to implanted infusion ports include clotting, catheter migration, infection, bleeding, thrombosis, air embolism, and infection at the exit site or in the pocket.

Infusion pumps. Infusion pumps are used in cancer treatment primarily for the continuous infusion of chemotherapy by IV, subcutaneous, intraarterial, and epidural routes. Infusion pumps can be worn externally or implanted surgically. The various types of external infusion pumps (Autosyringe, Cormed, Infumed 200, Deltec- Pharmacia, Pancreatec, Travenol Infusor) differ in terms of their mechanisms of action, components, and capabilities.

Implanted infusion pumps (Infusaid and Medtronics) are used primarily for intraarterial administration of chemotherapy (Fig. 12-23). This approach permits continuous infusion of the chemotherapeutic agent directly to the area

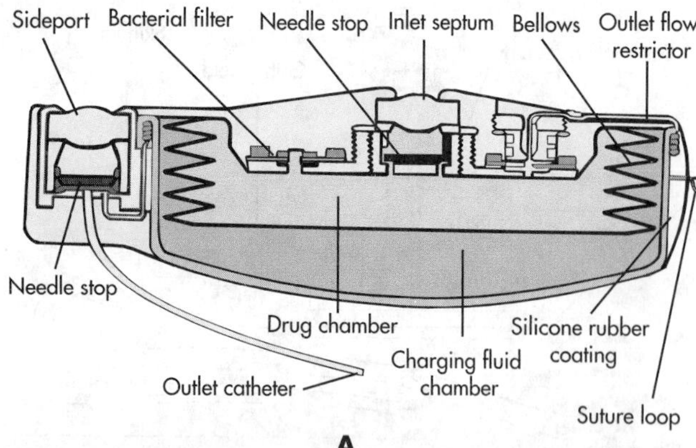

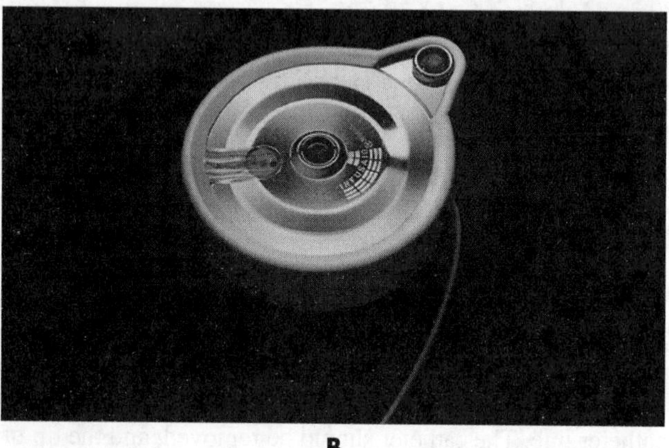

Fig. 12-23 ***A,*** Cross section of the implantable pump displaying its two chambers: the drug chamber *(inner)* and the charging fluid chamber *(outer)*. As the drug chamber is filled, the bellows expand, compressing the charging fluid in the outer chamber. The resulting increased pressure in the outer chamber forces the drug through a membrane filter and preset flow restrictor, thus ensuring a nearly constant flow. ***B,*** Infusaid pump.

of the tumor while sparing the patient the systemic effects of the drug. The most common use of this method of chemotherapy administration has been hepatic artery infusion in the treatment of liver metastasis, usually from primary colon cancer.

Implanted pumps also consist of a catheter that is threaded into the designated artery. The catheter is attached to a pump apparatus that consists of two chambers: an inner chamber that serves as the drug reservoir and an outer chamber that contains vapor pressure providing a source of power for the pump. The pump is implanted surgically in a subcutaneous pocket. Access to the pump is via a silicone septum with a Huber-point needle. Complications that have been associated with implanted infusion pumps include infection, thrombosis, clotting of the catheter, and pump malfunction.

Other access devices used in the treatment of the person with cancer include the Tenckhoff catheter used in the administration of intraperitoneal chemotherapy and the Ommaya reservoir, which delivers agents directly to the central nervous system (CNS).

Regional Chemotherapy Administration. Regional treatment with chemotherapy involves the delivery of the drug directly to the tumor site. The advantage of administering chemotherapy by this method is that higher concentrations of the drug can be delivered to the tumor with reduced systemic toxicity. Several regional delivery methods have been developed including intraarterial, intraperitoneal, intrathecal or intraventricular, and intravesical bladder chemotherapy.[35]

Intraarterial chemotherapy. Intraarterial chemotherapy delivers the drug to the tumor via the arterial vessel supplying the tumor. This method has been used for the treatment of osteogenic sarcoma; cancer of the head and neck, bladder, brain, and cervix; melanoma; primary liver cancer; and metastatic liver disease. One method of intraarterial drug delivery involves the surgical placement of a catheter that is subsequently connected to an external infusion pump or an implanted infusion pump for infusion of the chemotherapeutic agent. Generally, intraarterial chemotherapy results in reduced systemic toxicity. The type of toxicity experienced by the patient is dependent on the site of the tumor being treated.[35]

Intraperitoneal chemotherapy. Intraperitoneal chemotherapy involves the delivery of chemotherapy to the peritoneal cavity for treatment of peritoneal metastases from primary colon and ovarian cancers, mesothelioma, and malignant ascites. Temporary silastic catheters (Tenckhoff, Hickman, and Groshong) are percutaneously or surgically placed into the peritoneal cavity for short-term administration of chemotherapy. Alternatively, an implanted port can be used to administer chemotherapy intraperitoneally. Chemotherapy is generally infused into the peritoneum in 1 to 2 liters of fluid and allowed to "dwell" in the peritoneum for a period of 1 to 4 hours. Following the "dwell time," the fluid is usually drained from the peritoneum. Complications of peritoneal chemotherapy include abdominal pain; catheter occlusion, dislodgement, and migration; and infection.[35]

Intrathecal or intraventricular chemotherapy. Cancers that metastasize to the CNS, most commonly breast, lung, GI, leukemia, and lymphoma, are difficult to treat because the blood-brain barrier often prevents distribution of chemotherapy to this area. One method used to treat metastasis to the CNS is intrathecal chemotherapy. This method involves a lumbar puncture and injection of chemotherapy through the dura and arachnoid and into the subarachnoid space. However, this method has resulted in incomplete distribution of the drug in the CNS, particularly to the cisternal and ventricular areas.

To ensure more uniform distribution of chemotherapy to the cisternal and ventricular areas, an Ommaya reservoir is often inserted. An Ommaya reservoir is a silastic, dome-shaped disc with an extension catheter that is surgically implanted through the cranium into a lateral ventricle. In addition to more consistent drug distribution, the Ommaya reservoir precludes the use of repeated, painful lumbar punctures. Complications of intrathecal or intraventricular chemotherapy include headache, nausea, vomiting, fever, and nuchal rigidity.

Intravesical bladder chemotherapy. The patient with superficial transitional cell cancer of the bladder often has recurrent disease following traditional surgical therapy. Instillation of chemotherapy into the bladder promotes destruction of cancer cells and reduces the incidence of recurrent disease. Additional benefits of this therapy include reduced urinary and sexual dysfunction. The chemotherapeutic agent is instilled into the bladder via a urinary catheter and retained between 1 and 3 hours. Complications of this therapy include dysuria, urinary frequency, hematuria, and bladder spasms.[35]

Effects of Chemotherapy on Normal Tissues. Chemotherapeutic agents cannot selectively distinguish between normal cells and cancer cells. When normal cells are destroyed, the patient experiences certain signs and symptoms that are the expected side effects or toxic effects of chemotherapy. Effects of chemotherapy are caused by destruction of cells with a rapid rate of cellular proliferation (Table 12-19); response of the body to the products of cellular destruction (cellular waste products in circulation may cause fatigue, anorexia, and taste alterations); and specific drug toxicities (Table 12-20).

The adverse effects of these drugs can be classified as acute, delayed, or chronic. Acute toxicity includes vomiting, allergic reactions, and dysrhythmias. Delayed effects include mucositis, alopecia, and bone marrow depression. Mucositis can result in mouth sores, gastritis, and diarrhea. Chronic toxicities involve damage to organs such as the heart, liver, kidneys, and lungs.

Treatment Plan. When chemotherapy is used in the treatment of cancer, several drugs are usually given in combination. Today, single-drug chemotherapy is rarely chosen for a treatment plan. The drugs given are carefully selected to most effectively kill the cancer cells while allowing the normal cells to repair themselves and proliferate. The dose of each drug is carefully calculated according to the body weight or the body surface area of the patient being treated. The choice of the drugs selected to be given together to treat a particular cancer is based on the following principles of combination chemotherapy:

Table 12-19 Cells with Rapid Rate of Proliferation

Cells and Generation Time	Effect of Cell Destruction
Bone marrow stem cell, 6-24 hr	Myelosuppression; infection, bleeding, anemia
Neutrophils, 12 hr	Leukopenia, infection
Epithelial cells lining the gastrointestinal tract, 12-24 hr	Anorexia, stomatitis, esophagitis, nausea and vomiting, diarrhea
Cells of the hair follicle, 24 hr	Alopecia
Ova or testes, 24-36 hr	Reproductive dysfunction

1. The drugs used in the treatment plan are effective against the cancer being treated.
2. When drugs are given in combination, a synergistic effect occurs.
3. The combination includes drugs that are cycle specific and cycle nonspecific and drugs that have different mechanisms of action.
4. The combination includes drugs that have different toxic side effects.
5. The combination includes drugs whose nadir occurs at different time intervals. The *nadir* is the lowest level of the peripheral blood cell counts (particularly WBC) that occurs secondary to bone marrow depression. The nadir of most drugs ranges from 7 to 28 days, with recovery in 21 to 28 days after administration of chemotherapy.

The MOPP protocol, the first combination protocol for the treatment of Hodgkin's disease, is an example of a combination chemotherapy treatment regimen:

Nitrogen mustard (M)
Cycle nonspecific
Alkylating agent
Toxic side effects: myelosuppression, nausea, vomiting, alopecia
Nadir: 7 to 14 days
Oncovin (O)
Phase specific
Plant alkaloid
Toxic side effects: neurotoxicity, alopecia
Nadir: unknown
Procarbazine (P)
Cycle specific
Monoamine oxidase (MAO) inhibitor
Toxic side effects: myelosuppression, nausea, vomiting
Nadir: 2 to 8 weeks
Prednisone (P)
Toxic side effects: steroid effects
Nadir: unknown

The agents in this drug protocol differ in mechanisms of action, toxic side effects, and nadir, but the combination is synergistic in nature and effectively destroys the cancer cells present in the early stages of Hodgkin's disease.

The drugs are given according to a specific schedule that includes a time of drug administration and a time of rest from drug administration. The rest period is necessary to allow the normal body cells that have been destroyed to proliferate and repair the damaged tissue. The example in Table 12-21 describes a typical MOPP schedule. This drug schedule is repeated a specific number of times. Most chemotherapy treatment plans extend for 6 months or longer. The patient is evaluated before the administration of each course of chemotherapy to determine whether the normal cells have proliferated to a sufficient degree.

Often the most difficult decision to make is when to stop the administration of chemotherapy. The patient is evaluated according to the following criteria:

Table 12-20 Toxic Side Effects of Chemotherapy

Chemotherapeutic Agent	Myelosuppression	Mucositis	Nausea and Vomiting	Alopecia	Vesicant (V)/ Irritant (I)	Allergic Reaction	Other Specific Toxicities
Actinomycin D (Cosmegen)	+	+	+	+	+(V)	0	Diarrhea
Amsacrine (m-AMSA)	+	0	+	0	+(V)	0	Flulike syndrome, venoocclusive disease, hepatotoxicity
5-Azacytidine	+	+	+	0	0	0	Hepatotoxicity
Bleomycin (Blenoxane)	±	+	±	+	0	+	Pulmonary toxicity, skin rash
Busulfan (Myleran)	+	0	±	0	0	0	Pulmonary fibrosis
Carboplatin (CBDCA)	+	0	+	0	0	0	Pigmentation at injection site, hepatotoxicity, neurotoxicity, renal toxicity, pulmonary toxicity
Carmustine (BCNU)	+	+	+	0	+(I)	0	Hepatotoxicity
Chlorambucil (Leukeran)	+	0	±	0	0	0	
Chlorodeoxyadenosine	+	0	0	0	0	0	Neurotoxocity, renal toxicity
Cisplatin (Platinol)	+	0	+	0	0	+	Nephrotoxocity, peripheral neuropathy, ototoxicity
Cyclophosphamide (Cytoxan)	+	0	+	+	0	0	Sterile hemorrhagic cystitis, heart failure
Cytosine arabinoside (Cytosar, ara-C)	+	+	+	+	0	0	Hepatotoxicity
Dacarbazine (DTIC)	+	0	+	0	+ (I)	+	Hypotension
Daunorubicin (Daunomycin)	+	+	+	+	+ (V)	0	Cardiotoxicity, hepatotoxicity
Deoxycoformycin (DCF, Pentostatin)	+	0	+	0	0	0	Neurotoxicity, hepatotoxicity renal toxicity,
Diethystilbestrol (DES)	0	0	+	0	0	0	Congestive heart failure
Doxorubicin (Adriamycin)	+	+	+	+	+ (V)	0	Cardiotoxicity, diarrhea
Etoposide (VePesid)	+	0	+	+	+(I)	±	Hepatotoxicity, neurotoxicity, hypotension
Floxuridine (FUDR)	+	+	+	+	0	0	Diarrhea, rash
5-Fluorouracil	+	+	±	±	0	0	Diarrhea photosensitivity
Fluoxymesterone (Halotestin)	0	0	+	0	0	0	Masculinization
Hexamethylmelamine (HXM, HMM)	+	0	+	±	0	0	Peripheral neuropathy
Hydroxyurea (Hydrea)	+	+	+	+	0	0	
Idarubicin	+	+	+	+	0	0	Cardiomyopathy

continued

Table 12-20 Toxic Side Effects of Chemotherapy—cont'd

Chemotherapeutic Agent	Myelo-suppression	Mucositis	Nausea and Vomiting	Alopecia	Vesicant (V)/ Irritant (I)	Allergic Reaction	Other Specific Toxicities
Iphosphamide (Isophosphamide)	±	0	±	+	0	0	Hematuria, neurotoxicity, hemorrhagic cystitis
L-Asparaginase (Elspar)	0	0	+	0	0	+	Major organ failure
Lomustine (CCNU)	+	+	+	±	0	0	Hepatotoxicity
Melphalan (Alkeran)	+	±	±	0	0	0	
Mechlorethamine (nitrogen mustard)	+	0	+	+	+ (V)	0	
6-Mercaptopurine (6-MP)	+	+	+	0	0	0	Hepatotoxicity
Methotrexate (MTX, Amethopterin)	+	+	±	±	0	0	Nephrotoxicity
Mithramycin (Mithracin)	+	+	+	0	+(V)	0	Hemorrhagic tendency
Mitomycin (Mutamycin)	+	+	+	+	+(V)	0	Nephrotoxicity, pulmonary toxicity
Mitozantrone (DHAD)	+	+	+	+	0	0	Drug fever, diarrhea, increased liver enzymes
Oxymetholone (Androl-50)	0	0	+	0	0	0	Hepatotoxicity
Piperzinedione	+	0	+	0	+(V)	0	
Plicamycin (Mithracin)	±	±	+	0	+(I)	0	Hepatotoxicity, nephrotoxicity, facial flushing, neurotoxicity
Prednisolone	0	0	0	0	0	0	Steroid side effects
Prednisone	0	0	0	0	0	0	Steroid side effects
Procarbazine hydrochloride (Matulane)	+	±	+	0	0	0	Monoamine oxidase inhibitor
Semustine (Methyl CCNU)	+	+	+	0	0	0	
Streptozotocin (SRZ, Zanosar)	+	0	+	±	+(I)	0	Nephrotoxicity
Tamoxifen (Nolvadex)	±	0	+	0	0	0	
Paclitaxel (Taxol)	+	0	+	±	0	±	Sensory neuropathy
6-Thioguanine (6-TG)	+	+	+	0	0	0	Hepatotoxicity
Uracil mustard	+	0	+	±	0	0	
Vinblastine (Velban)	+	+	+	±	+(V)	0	Neurotoxicity
Vincristine (Oncovin)	0	0	0	+	+(V)	0	Neurotoxicity
VP-16	+	0	+	+	0	+	Hypotension

+, Common; ±, infrequent; 0, uncommon.

1. Complete remission. Complete absence of all evidence of cancer and a return to the usual performance status occur; the duration of a complete remission must exceed 1 month.
2. Partial remission. Regression of 50% or more of the disease process without evidence of progression and with subjective improvement is noted. The duration of a partial remission is usually several months.
3. Improvement. Regression of 25% to 50% of the disease process with subjective improvement is noted.
4. No response. Regression of 25% or less of the disease with no subjective improvement is noted.
5. Progression. Progression of the disease process is noted.

With a complete remission that has extended for a time, the chemotherapy is usually discontinued, and the patient is

Table 12-21 MOPP Chemotherapeutic Drug Schedule

Drug	Days 1	2	3	4	5	6	7	8	9	10	11	12	13	14	15-28
Nitrogen mustard (intravenous administration)	↔							↔							*
Oncovin (intravenous administration)	↔							↔							
Procarbazine (oral administration)	←													→	
Prednisone (oral administration)	←													→	

*No drugs given.

evaluated at frequent intervals. When partial remission or improvement occurs, the same treatment plan or a revised treatment plan is followed over a long period (several years), and the patient is evaluated frequently. No response or progression of disease warrants a change in the treatment plan or a decision to use treatment for palliation.

Safe Preparation, Administration, and Disposal of Chemotherapeutic Agents. An important issue in cancer care is that working with antineoplastic agents may be hazardous for health professionals. It is suspected that the person preparing or giving chemotherapy may absorb the drug through inhalation of particles when reconstituting a powder in an open ampule and through skin contact. There may also be some risk in handling the vomitus and excreta of persons receiving chemotherapy. At present, data regarding health risks for the professional working with chemotherapy are not conclusive.

The only well-known hazard associated with chemotherapy is that of cutaneous reactions following skin contact with certain drugs including BCNU (Carmustine), mechlorethamine (nitrogen mustard), doxorubicin (Adriamycin), and other vesicants. The literature accompanying these drugs specifically cautions against skin and eye contact to prevent possible skin reactions and corneal damage.

Guidelines for the safe handling of chemotherapeutic agents have been developed by the United States Occupational Safety and Health Administration (OSHA) and the Oncology Nursing Society. These guidelines are summarized in Table 12-22.

NURSING MANAGEMENT

PATIENT RECEIVING CHEMOTHERAPY

The role of the nurse in cancer chemotherapy has greatly expanded during the past decade. Regardless of the health care agency setting, the nurse will meet the individual who is receiving or who has received chemotherapy. One of the most important responsibilities of the nurse is that of differentiating between toxic effects of the drug and progression of the malignant process. The nurse also needs to differentiate between tolerable side effects and acute toxic effects of chemotherapeutic agents. For example, nausea and vomiting are expected and controllable side effects of many drugs. However, if paresthesia occurs with the use of vincristine or signs of heart failure appear with the use of doxorubicin, these serious reactions need to be reported to the physician so that drug dosages can be modified or discontinued. Some toxicities associated with chemotherapy may not be reversible. For example, ototoxicity may be an irreversible effect of cisplatin therapy, especially at higher doses. Periodic testing of hearing may be necessary to monitor for this toxicity. Specific nursing measures related to problems associated with chemotherapy are presented in the nursing care plan for the patient with cancer on p. 300.

Nausea and vomiting are the most commonly observed GI side effects. Vomiting may occur within 1 hour of administration and may last for 24 hours or more. Several antiemetic drugs are available (see Chapter 39 and Table 39-1). Metoclopramide (Reglan), ondansetron (Zofran), granisetron (Kytril), and dexamethasone (Decadron) have also been used to decrease nausea and vomiting caused by chemotherapy. Nursing management related to nausea and vomiting is presented in the nursing care plan for the patient with cancer.

Results of laboratory studies of the patient who is receiving chemotherapy should be monitored. Particular attention should be given to the WBC, platelet, and RBC counts. If the WBC count falls to less than 2000 per μl ($2 \times 10^9/L$), the drug regimen may need to be modified or discontinued. Every possible measure needs to be taken to prevent infections in a patient with leukopenia (see nursing care plan on neutropenia in Chapter 28). If the platelet count falls to less than 50,000 per μl ($50 \times 10^9/L$), the patient must be assessed for any signs of bleeding, and measures should be taken to prevent bleeding (see the nursing care plan on thrombocytopenia in Chapter 28). Platelet transfusions may be necessary. RBC transfusions may also be indicated for treatment of symptomatic anemia. However, anemia is an uncommon problem in the patient receiving chemotherapy.[36]

Uric acid and creatinine levels are usually monitored weekly. Optimum hydration is important to prevent uric acid crystals from causing obstructive uropathy. Allopurinol is often administered as a prophylactic measure if extensive cell breakdown is expected. Other diagnostic monitoring depends on the type of drug. For example, an electrocardiogram (ECG) is performed, and cardiac ejection fractions are measured to monitor the potential cardiotoxic effects of doxorubicin and daunorubicin.

Table 12-22 Guidelines for Safe Handling of Chemotherapeutic Agents

Preparation
- Prepare all chemotherapeutic agents in a central area and under a Class II vertical laminar-flow biologic safety cabinet, vented to the outside.
- Agents should be prepared by a pharmacist, who should do the following:
  - Wear a disposable, protective gown with long sleeves and elastic cuffs and disposable, surgical, latex gloves
  - Place a disposable, plastic-backed liner on work surface
  - Post hazardous warning signs in the mixing area
  - Avoid puncturing gloves or inoculating self
  - Use Luer-Lok fittings where possible
  - Vent all vials
  - Wrap gauze around neck of ampule when opening
  - Prime tubing under safety cabinet
  - Place all exposed waste in an approved disposal container

Administration and Exposure to Excreta and Vomitus During Administration
- Wear disposable latex surgical gloves.
- Wear gown and mask if desired (remains controversial).
- Place a disposable, plastic-backed liner under patient's extremity.

Disposal
- Place all disposable items (needles, syringes, vials, and ampules) coming in contact with antineoplastic agents in an approved leak-proof container.
- Discard waste containers in an approved incinerator.
- Place contaminated linen in an approved container; linen must be washed separately.

Spills
- Wear disposable, surgical, latex gloves.
- Wear disposable gown with elastic cuffs.
- Use "spill kits" containing all materials necessary for proper handling.

Personnel Recommendations
- Teach all persons likely to be exposed to antineoplastic agents or excreta the necessary precautions.
- Prevent contact of pregnant or lactating women with chemotherapeutic agents.
- Distribute work load to minimize employee exposure to chemotherapeutic agents.
- Provide periodic health screening for exposed persons.
- Document patterns of exposure.

Patient Education

Education of the patient is an extremely important part of the nurse's role related to chemotherapy. To decrease the fear and anxiety often associated with chemotherapy, the patient must be told what to expect during a course of treatment. The patient's attitude toward treatment should be explored so that any misconception or fear can be discussed. The patient needs to be told of the possible side effects of chemotherapy that may be experienced during treatment. This may be a discouraging revelation. Therefore good nursing judgment is essential to determine the amount of information the patient can assimilate. The patient must be reassured that this is a temporary situation and that she should be feeling better within a few weeks after chemotherapy is discontinued. The patient should also be informed that supportive care (e.g., antiemetics and antidiarrheals) will be provided as needed.

Management of Hair Loss

Many emotions are experienced and expressed when hair loss occurs including anger, grief, embarrassment, and fear. For some persons, the loss of hair is one of the most stressful events experienced during the course of the illness. Alopecia caused by the administration of chemotherapeutic agents is usually reversible. The degree and duration of hair loss depend on the dose of the chemotherapeutic agent, the duration of the treatment, and the nutritional status of the patient. Sometimes the hair begins to grow back while the patient is still receiving chemotherapeutic agents, but generally the hair cells do not grow back until the agents are discontinued. Often the new hair has a different color and texture than the hair that was lost.

Hair loss caused by certain chemotherapeutic drugs (e.g., cyclophosphamide and doxorubicin) administered by the bolus IV route can be minimized or prevented by the use of a scalp sphygmomanometer, a tourniquet, and hypothermia. The scalp tourniquet or sphygmomanometer is applied around the hairline to decrease the blood flow through the superficial scalp arteries before, during, and for 20 minutes after infusion of the drug. (This technique protects hair follicles from high concentrations of cytotoxic drugs.) When the sphygmomanometer is used, the cuff should never be more than 70 mm Hg above the normal systolic blood pressure to prevent tissue damage. When hypothermia is used, the hypothermic agent is applied at least 10 minutes before and during infusion and for 20 to 30 minutes after infusion of the chemotherapeutic agent. Several more sophisticated devices (Cryogel bags, Thermocirculator, Chemocap, Kold Kap) have been developed and provide vasoconstriction by pressure and hypothermia. The degree of protection against hair loss varies with the individual patient and with the drug administered.

Scalp tourniquets and hypothermia should not be used for the patient undergoing chemotherapy for hematopoietic cancer or brain tumors. When these devices are used, chemotherapeutic agents may be prevented from reaching the cancer cells circulating in the vascular system of the scalp, and these cancer cells are thus protected from the effects of the chemotherapeutic agents. Other nursing interventions for dealing with alopecia are presented in the nursing care plan.

Counseling Regarding Sexual and Reproductive Function

Sexual dysfunction may be manifested as temporary or permanent sterility, disruption in the menstrual cycle, temporary or permanent impotence, or chromosomal damage leading to possible genetic mutation. The patient should be instructed to use an effective means of birth control during

NURSING CARE PLAN Patient with Cancer*

Planning: Outcome Criteria	Nursing Interventions and Rationales
➤ NURSING DIAGNOSIS	Altered nutrition: less than body requirements *related to* anorexia, nausea, and vomiting *as manifested by* reported or observed inadequate food intake relative to minimum daily requirements with or without weight loss; fatigue
Maintain body weight and adequate energy for activities of daily living (ADLS); increase oral intake of high calorie food.	Avoid punitive or judgmental statements about food intake or weight loss *to avoid the nurse taking an adversarial role.* Administer antiemetic protocols as prescribed to *minimize GI effects.* Evaluate efficacy of drug, dose, and time administered. Maintain a quiet, restful environment *to avoid triggering nausea or vomiting and to allow for maximum rest.* Modify diet to include bland, lukewarm, high-calorie, high-protein foods *to prevent triggering vomiting and provide additional calories.* Try small, frequent feedings rather than fewer large meals *to facilitate gastric emptying and prevent early satiety.* Teach patient to eat and drink slowly *to allow patient to enjoy the taste and to prevent bloating.* Offer patient chewing gum, warm lemon-lime soda pop, cola syrup, sour candy, soda crackers, tepid tea, or anything patient associates with a positive outcome *to stimulate salivation.* Remove all sights, sounds, or smells that have the potential for initiating nausea, such as an emesis basin and unpleasant odors. Use techniques such as relaxation response and distraction. Provide a well-balanced diet that includes all food groups with increased protein-calorie intake *to promote positive nitrogen balance.* Provide a small amount of food every few hours. Gently encourage patient to eat, but avoid nagging *to prevent establishing a negative meal environment.* Teach patient what to eat rather than stressing the fact that more food should be eaten. (Home-prepared items are often more appealing.) Set realistic goals for consumption *to prevent repeated failure.* Avoid foods that are gas forming, such as salads, cabbage, broccoli, fruits, and beer, *which can promote nausea and a sense of fullness.* Serve all foods attractively and in a pleasant environment *to stimulate appetite.* Teach patient to sip the nutritional supplement slowly between meals to *avoid bloating.*
➤ NURSING DIAGNOSIS	Ineffective management of therapeutic regimen *related to* lack of knowledge of long-term management of cancer *as manifested by* frequent questions by patient and caregiver regarding self-care, treatment, and side effects; observed inability of patient and caregiver to manage technical aspects of long-term care
Patient and caregiver express confidence in ability to manage long-term care; demonstrate adequate knowledge base to provide self-care.	Determine knowledge and technical skills needed by patient and caregiver *to plan needed instruction.* Assess current level of knowledge and skill *to determine abilities of patient and caregiver to perform tasks correctly.* Teach required knowledge and skill. Provide opportunity for follow-up evaluation and teaching *to increase patient and caregiver confidence and assure correct performance of tasks.*

continued

the time of chemotherapy or radiation therapy and for up to 2 years after treatment. This is necessary to avoid birth defects as a result of chromosomal damage, to allow the sperm count to return to normal, and to determine the expected prognosis of the patient. Sexual or genetic counseling is necessary before the conception of a child to determine the risk of chromosomal damage.

Sexual relations can be continued in the usual patterns during and after treatment if an effective method of birth control is used. It may be necessary to alter the time of day chosen for sexual relations if fatigue is a problem. Early morning may be the time the patient feels most rested.

Denuding of the epithelial lining of the vagina may result in inflammation, edema, and ulceration. Sexual intercourse should be avoided if mucositis or ulceration is present. Sitz baths or sitting in a tub of warm water will provide some degree of comfort. A steroid-based cream available by prescription may also provide comfort. A water-based lubricant may be used at the time of intercourse to increase vaginal lubrication, which is necessary to prevent trauma to the vaginal lining and to prevent discomfort or pain.

The patient should be encouraged to use other forms of physical contact to obtain sexual pleasure during the period of disruption in sexual functioning. Hugging, caressing, touching, and quiet talking can provide sexual pleasure when sexual intercourse is not possible. The patient's partner must be included in all teaching and counseling sessions to be fully informed of the temporary or permanent changes in the patient's sexual functioning. Both patient

NURSING CARE PLAN Patient with Cancer*—cont'd

Planning: Outcome Criteria	*Nursing Interventions and Rationales*
➤ **NURSING DIAGNOSIS**	Altered oral mucous membranes *related to* chemotherapy and oral cavity radiation *as manifested by* verbalization or signs of pain or discomfort in oral mucous membranes, decreased or lack of saliva, coated tongue, xerostomia (dry mouth), halitosis, edema of membranes; hyperemia, oral lesions; ulcers, desquamation, vesicles, hemorrhagic gingivitis, leukoplakia, stomatitis, dysphagia
Patient has no oral pain, no infections in the oral mucosa, and no break in integrity of oral mucosa.	Assess oral mucosa daily. Teach patient to inspect oral cavity *as stomatitis usually occurs 4-14 days after treatment begins.* Remove dentures at night *to avoid further irritation.* Observe for dryness, redness, and white or yellow membrane and the presence of any breaks in integrity of tissues. If patient wears dentures, assess *to determine whether the dentures fit properly.* Distinguish stomatitis from candidiasis and other oral problems, such as xerostomia and herpes *so appropriate treatment is used.* Maintain good oral hygiene. Use mouthwashes of baking soda, baking soda and saline, or normal saline solution q2hr *to provide comfort.* Use soft-bristle toothbrushes, sponge-tipped applicators, or an irrigation syringe as cleansing agents *to prevent trauma.* Avoid the use of lemon and glycerin swabs for mouth care *because they increase dryness and irritation.* Apply topical anesthetics, such as viscous Xylocaine or oxethazaine, as ordered *to provide pain relief.* Modify diet to avoid hot, spicy, acidic foods *to avoid irritation.* Discourage use of irritants such as tobacco and alcohol. Encourage drinking water or other liquids at frequent intervals throughout the day or encourage use of an artificial saliva *to keep mucous membranes moist.* Apply a small amount of petroleum jelly, baby oil, or cocoa butter to the lips regularly *to promote comfort and prevent dryness.*
➤ **NURSING DIAGNOSIS**	Fatigue *related to* the effects of cancer or treatment *as manifested by* verbal report of fatigue or weakness, exertional discomfort or dyspnea; abnormal responses to activity such as increased heart rate or blood pressure or electrocardiographic changes reflecting ischemia or dysrhythmias
Maintain satisfactory activity level relative to phase of treatment.	Inform patient that fatigue is an expected side effect of therapy and that it usually begins during the first week of therapy, reaches its peak in 2 wk, continues, and then gradually disappears 2-4 wk after treatment has ended. Encourage patient to rest when fatigued, to maintain usual lifestyle patterns as closely as possible, and to pace activities in accordance with energy level *because rest periods are essential to conserve energy.* Monitor fatigue level *to determine deviations from expected pattern.*
➤ **NURSING DIAGNOSIS**	Ineffective individual coping *related to* depression secondary to diagnosis and treatment, uncertain outcome, disruption in lifestyle, and financial burden of illness *as manifested by* verbalized or observed inability to manage affective component of diagnosis and resulting symptoms; threats or attempts to commit suicide; concerns over financial implications of disease
Demonstrate appropriate response to problems; seek and accept outside support and assistance.	Have patient direct own care when possible *to encourage patient independence.* Provide information *to allow patient to make informed choices regarding treatment regime and plan of care.* Facilitate communication between patient and family *to foster a supportive network.* Assess and mobilize patient's support system. Refer patient to social services for financial assistance if appropriate *to provide additional resources.* Assess need for further counseling.

continued

and partner must understand that adjustments in sexual functioning patterns will take time, patience, and understanding.

Late Effects of Radiation and Chemotherapy

Cancer survivors are achieving long-term remission and survival rates because of advancements in treatment modalities. However, these forms of therapy (especially radiation and chemotherapy) may produce long-term sequelae known as *physiologic late effects* that occur months to years after cessation of therapy. Every body system can be affected to some extent by chemotherapy and radiation therapy. The effects of radiation on the body's tissues are caused by cellular hypoplasia of stem cells and alterations in the fine vasculature and fibroconnective tissues. In addition to the acute toxicities, chemotherapy can have long-

NURSING CARE PLAN Patient with Cancer*—cont'd

Planning: Outcome Criteria | **Nursing Interventions and Rationales**

➤ NURSING DIAGNOSIS Body-image disturbance *related to* hair loss, disfiguring surgery, and weight loss *as manifested by* expressions of concern with changes in body; refusal to interact with visitors; isolation; frequent crying; refusal to care for self or to look in mirror

Planning: Outcome Criteria	Nursing Interventions and Rationales
Verbalize acceptance of changes in body appearance and function.	Provide psychologic support, and prepare patient for expected hair loss *to lessen shock of event when it occurs.* Encourage patient to select a wig and begin to wear it before hair loss begins and to wear a scarf or turban *to conceal hair loss.* Use a mild, protein-based shampoo, cream rinse, and hair conditioner every 4-7 days *to avoid drying remaining hair.* Avoid excessive shampooing, brushing, and combing of hair *to reduce hair loss.* Avoid use of electric hair dryers, curlers, curling rods, and hair spray *to minimize scalp irritation and decrease hair loss.* When administering drugs that induce alopecia, reduce or occlude blood flow to hair follicles by using ice packs, scalp tourniquets, or scalp sphygmomanometers (see text) *to reduce the amount of drug reaching hair follicles.* Help patient select clothing and colors that minimize weight loss and effects of disfiguring surgery. Assure patient that value as a person is not associated with external appearance. Discuss expected physical changes with family members, and advise them of ways to assist patient with acceptance *to prepare the family and foster family relationships.*

➤ NURSING DIAGNOSIS Altered family processes *related to* cancer diagnosis of family member as *manifested by* observed communication problems among family members; lack of family support related to physical, emotional, and spiritual needs of patient

Planning: Outcome Criteria	Nursing Interventions and Rationales
Family members communicate about patient and cooperate in care of patient; family will seek outside help when needed.	Assess family structure and support system *to determine amount and quality of support available to patient.* Teach needed skills to family members. Provide opportunity for discussion of caregiving and emotional implications of role changes *to promote verbalization of feelings and shared understanding of problems.* Assist family members to set realistic expectations for patient and themselves. Provide guidance on course of disease and anticipated outcome *so anticipatory planning can be accomplished.*

➤ NURSING DIAGNOSIS Risk for infection *related to* leukopenia, depressed immune system, and multiple exposures to microorganisms.†

COLLABORATIVE PROBLEMS

➤ POTENTIAL COMPLICATION Hyperuricemia *related to* chemotherapy.

Nursing Goals	Nursing Interventions and Rationales
Monitor for signs of hyperuricemia, report deviations from acceptable parameters, and carry out medical and nursing interventions.	Monitor for high level of uric acid excretion in urine, high serum uric acid, obstructive uropathy, decreased urine output, nausea and vomiting, and lethargy. Record intake and output every shift *to determine fluid balance.* Encourage fluids *to prevent uric acid crystals from causing obstruction.* Evaluate blood urea nitrogen (BUN) and serum creatinine levels *to identify early changes in renal function.* Administer allopurinol (Zyloprim) as ordered *to reduce endogenous uric acid production.*

➤ POTENTIAL COMPLICATION Bleeding *related to* thrombocytopenia‡

*Only nursing diagnoses that apply to all types of cancer are included in this care plan.
† See the nursing care plan on thrombocytopenia in Chapter 28.
‡ See the nursing care plan on neutropenia in Chapter 28.

Table 12-23 Possible Late Effects of Radiation and Chemotherapy

Body System	Effects
■ Cardiac	Chronic cardiomyopathy Myocardial fibrosis
■ Pulmonary	Diffuse alveolar damage Pneumonitis Fibrosis
■ Gastrointestinal	Hepatotoxicity Enteritis Esophagitis Fistula formation
■ Renal and urologic	Nephrotoxicity Nephritis Hemorrhagic cystitis Acute tubular necrosis
■ Neurologic	Neuropathy Autonomic nervous system disorders Hearing loss Myelopathy Necrotizing leukoencephalopathy
■ Endocrine	Gonadal impairment Ovarian destruction Infertility Disturbances in sexual functioning

term effects related to the loss of cells' proliferative reserve capacity. The additive effects of multiagent chemotherapy before, during, or after a course of radiotherapy can significantly increase the resulting physiologic late effects. Some physiologic late effects of radiation and chemotherapy are summarized in Table 12-23.

The cancer survivor may also be at risk for leukemias and other secondary malignancies resulting from therapy for the primary cancer. However, the potential risk for developing a second malignancy does not contraindicate the use of cancer treatment; the overall risk of developing neoplastic complications is low, and the latency period may be long.

The cancer treatments most frequently implicated in causing secondary malignancy are the alkylating chemotherapeutic agents and high-dose radiation, which can induce cancers at the exposure site. The exact mechanism of oncogenesis of radiation and chemotherapy remains unclear. It could be related to interactions between immunosuppressive factors, direct cellular damage, and carcinogenic effects along with other environmental carcinogens.

Acute leukemias occurring as secondary malignancies have been most widely reported after treatment for Hodgkin's disease, but they also occur in survivors of ovarian, lung, and breast cancers. Secondary malignancies other than leukemias include multiple myeloma after radiation therapy for breast cancer; non-Hodgkin's lymphoma after treatment for Hodgkin's disease; and cancers of the bladder, kidney, and ureters after the use of cyclophosphamide. Radiation therapy for breast, lung, ovarian, uterine, and thyroid cancers, non-Hodgkin's lymphoma, and Hodgkin's disease has been linked to secondary osteosarcoma of the rib, scapula, clavicle, humerus, sternum, ilium, and pelvis. Fibrosarcomas have been reported several years after radiation therapy for astrocytoma, glioblastoma, and pituitary adenoma. Unfortunately, secondary malignancies are resistant to therapy.

Biologic Response Modifiers

Biologic response modifiers (BRMs) are agents that modify the relationship between the host and the tumor by altering the biologic response of the host to the tumor cells. Three categories of BRMs exist: (1) agents that have direct antitumor effects; (2) agents that restore, augment, or modulate host immune system mechanisms; and (3) agents that have other biologic effects, such as interfering with the cancer cells' ability to metastasize or differentiate.[37]

Although the use of most BRMs in the treatment of cancer is in investigational stages, knowledge and experience with these agents are rapidly gaining with increased understanding of the immune system, advancements in molecular biology, development of monoclonal antibodies, and modern technologic equipment. Current clinical studies with BRMs are being conducted to investigate their effectiveness as single agents; in combination with other BRMs; and with other treatment modalities such as chemotherapy, radiotherapy, and surgery.

Interferons. Interferons are naturally occurring complex proteins of which there are three types: (1) α- interferon, produced by lymphocytes and macrophages; (2) β-interferon produced by fibroblasts and macrophages; and (3) γ-interferon produced by T lymphocytes. Interferons are cytokines that have antiviral, antiproliferative, and immunomodulatory properties (see Table 10-4). The antiviral activity of interferons was first identified in 1957. Interferons protect cells infected by viruses from attack by other viruses, and they inhibit replication of viral DNA (see Fig. 10-5). The antiproliferative effects of interferons are not completely understood. However, they have been shown to inhibit DNA and protein synthesis in tumor cells and to stimulate the expression of tumor-associated antigens on tumor cell surfaces, thus increasing the potential for an immune response against the tumor cell. Interferons modulate the immune response by their direct interaction with lymphocytes and monocytes or macrophages. They are also capable of mediating the function of other cytokines such as IL-2 and TNF and enhancing the antigenic expression in some tumor types. Interferons have also been shown to increase the cytotoxic activity and killing potential of NK cells.[37]

Because of the protein nature of interferons, they cannot be administered orally. Therefore they are administered IV, intramuscularly (IM), and subcutaneously. To date, the best dose, route, and frequency of administration have not been determined. In addition, α-interferon is made by different pharmaceutical companies such as interferon alfa-2A (Roferon-A) made by Roche and interferon alfa-2B (Intron A) made by Schering. It is important to stress to the patient that these different brands of interferon are not interchangeable. If the patient begins to take one form of interferon, the brand of interferon being taken must not be changed unless recommended by their physician.

Clinical studies have demonstrated some effectiveness in the use of interferon to treat hematologic malignancies. α-interferon has been approved by the Food and Drug Administration (FDA) for the treatment of hairy-cell leukemia, Kaposi's sarcoma (KS), and genital warts (caused by papilloma virus). Interferons have also demonstrated effectiveness in the treatment of renal cell carcinoma, chronic myelogenous leukemia, T-cell lymphomas, malignant melanoma, multiple myeloma, ovarian carcinoma, and carcinoid tumors. Clinical trials continue to investigate the use of interferons to treat other malignancies.

Interleukins. The ILs are a family of BRMs that perform a variety of functions. They include agents such as IL-1, IL-2, IL-3, IL-4, IL-6, IL-7, and IL-10. Little is known about the biologic function of many of the ILs, and currently, most of the ILs are in the clinical or preclinical phases of development for potential use in the treatment of cancer and other diseases. However, IL-2 has been approved by the FDA for the treatment of metastatic renal cell carcinoma.

IL-2 is a cytokine produced by T lymphocytes that was first identified as an agent capable of stimulating division of T lymphocytes. It was later found to activate NK cells and *lymphokine-activated killer* (LAK) *cells.* Activated NK cells make up part of a group of cytotoxic lymphocytes that mediate lymphokine-activated killing. IL-2 also stimulates the release of other cytokines, including γ-interferon, TNF, IL-1, and IL-6.

IL-2 has been administered in clinical trials by various means, including IV bolus, continuous infusion, subcutaneous injection, and peritoneal infusion. The agent has been administered alone, in combination with chemotherapeutic agents, and with LAK cells.

Clinical trials are currently investigating the most effective approach to the administration of IL-2. One approach involves the adoptive transfer of LAK cells to the patient. It is based on the ability of IL-2 to activate LAK cells. This process involves the following:

1. Infusion of IL-2 to increase the number of lymphocytes
2. Lymphopheresis—a mechanical process designed to remove the lymphocytes from circulation
3. Incubation of the host lymphocytes with IL-2 in vitro to generate LAK cells
4. Reinfusion of the cultured lymphocytes to the host as LAK cells, which are capable of lysing tumor cells resistant to NK cells without affecting normal cells
5. Simultaneous administration of IL-2

Positive clinical responses with IL-2 and LAK cells have been reported in patients with metastatic renal cell cancer and malignant melanoma.

Another approach to the use of IL-2 involves the isolation of lymphocytes from the tumor itself. These cells, known as *tumor-infiltrating lymphocytes* (TIL), are a subpopulation of lymphocytes that can be cultured with IL-2 and then reinfused into the patient. TIL cells have been found to be more tumoricidal than LAK cells.

In addition to its use with LAK and TIL cells, IL-2 has been administered alone or in conjunction with other lymphokines such as α-, β-, and γ-interferon and TNF. Research on uses of IL-2 in cancer therapy is continuing.[38]

Monoclonal Antibodies. Monoclonal antibodies are antibodies or immunoglobulins produced by B lymphocytes that are capable of binding to specific target cells, including tumor cells. Various monoclonal antibodies (MoAbs) are currently being investigated for diagnostic and treatment capabilities. (Hybridoma technology for the production of MoAbs is described in Chapter 10.) The diagnostic use of MoAbs is primarily for the imaging of tumors to locate areas of metastatic disease and for radioimmunoassays and enzyme-linked immunoassays in laboratory studies.

MoAbs have also demonstrated limited effectiveness in treating cancers such as lymphomas, acute and chronic lymphocytic leukemias, T-cell leukemia, gastric and colon cancer, and melanoma. Clinical studies are investigating the use of MoAbs alone (unconjugated) or in combination with other agents (immunoconjugates) such as radioisotopes, toxins, chemotherapeutic agents, and other BRMs. The goal of this approach is for the antibody to deliver the immunoconjugate directly to the targeted cancer cells for their ultimate destruction. MoAbs are administered by the infusion method.

There is a risk, although rare, of anaphylaxis associated with the administration of MoAbs. This potential exists because most MoAbs are produced by mouse lymphocytes and, thus, represent a foreign protein to the human body. Onset of anaphylaxis can occur within 5 minutes of administration and can be a life-threatening event. Administration of the MoAb should be stopped immediately, an emergency code called, and epinephrine 1 mg IV (1:10,000 solution in 10 ml prefilled syringe) should be administered over 5 minutes.[38] (See Chapter 10 for a discussion of nursing management of anaphylaxis).

Tumor Necrosis Factor. TNF is a cytokine produced by macrophages, and it ultimately binds to specific receptors located on cell membranes. TNF is toxic to tumor cells by exerting a necrotizing effect. TNF also activates cells of the immune system, as in increased neutrophil and T- and B-cell activity. Significantly, TNF is known to attack tumor cells while preserving normal cells.

In clinical trials, TNF has been administered by continuous IV infusion, IV bolus, IM, subcutaneous, and intratumor methods. Studies have been conducted to test the efficacy of this BRM in the treatment of ovarian and renal cancers and melanoma. These studies are investigating the potential use of this agent alone or in combination with other therapies, such as chemotherapy.[38]

Colony-stimulating Factors. Colony-stimulating factors (CSFs) are a group of glycoproteins, produced by various cells that stimulate production, maturation, regulation, and activation of cells of the hematologic system. After release, CSFs attach to receptors on the cell surface of peripheral blood cells and hematopoietic precursors (precursors of mature blood cells). CSFs then stimulate cellular production, maturation, release from the bone marrow, and bactericidal ability and other activities. Various CSFs have been isolated. These include granulocyte-CSF (G-CSF), granulocyte-macrophage-CSF (GM-CSF), and macrophage-CSF (M-CSF or CSF-1). IL-3, also called multi-CSF, is a multipotential stimulator of hematopoietic stem cells. IL-3 has been shown to stimulate the growth of neutrophils, monocytes, eosinophils, basophils, and platelet cell lines.

There are a number of potential clinical uses of CSFs. They may hasten recovery from bone marrow depression after standard and high-dose chemotherapy and bone marrow transplantation. Clinically, CSFs can be used to prevent bone marrow suppression associated with chemotherapy administration, or they can be used therapeutically to treat this complication of therapy. These functions are important because neutropenia in the patient with cancer is a major cause of morbidity and mortality.[39] These agents may also be used to strengthen host defenses against infection and malignancy. Finally, CSFs may act as differentiating and recruiting agents in preleukemia and leukemia.

G-CSF was the first CSF to be approved by the FDA. It stimulates the production and function of neutrophil granulocytes. G-CSF can be administered subcutaneously or by IV infusion. The most commonly reported side effect of G-CSF therapy is bone pain, which occurs most often in the lower back, pelvis, and sternum. This pain generally develops at the time the neutrophil count begins to recover and lasts for about 24 hours. The pain associated with G-CSF therapy is usually relieved with nonnarcotic analgesics.[39]

GM-CSF was approved by the FDA in 1991 for the management of neutropenia associated with bone marrow transplantation. It stimulates the production and function of granulocytes, monocytes, and macrophages. In addition, GM-CSF stimulates these cells to produce cytokines. GM-CSF can be administered either subcutaneously or by IV infusion.[39]

Toxic and Side Effects of Biologic Response Modifier Therapy. The administration of one BRM usually induces the endogenous release of other BRMs. The release and action of these BRMs results in systemic immune and inflammatory responses. The toxicities and side effects of BRMs are related to dose and schedule. Table 12-24 summarizes the potential side effects associated with specific BRMs. Common side effects include constitutional flulike symptoms, including headache, fever, chills, myalgias, fatigue, malaise, weakness, anorexia, and nausea. With interferons the flulike symptoms almost invariably appear. Acetaminophen administered every 4 hours, as prescribed, often reduces the severity of the flulike syndrome. The patient is commonly premedicated with acetaminophen in an attempt to prevent or decrease the intensity of these symptoms.[38] In addition, large amounts of fluids help to decrease the symptoms.

Tachycardia and orthostatic hypotension are also commonly reported. TNF and IL-2 can cause capillary leak syndrome, which can result in pulmonary edema. Other toxic and side effects may involve the CNS, the renal and hepatic systems, and the cardiovascular system. These effects are found particularly with interferons and IL-2.

NURSING MANAGEMENT

PATIENT RECEIVING BIOLOGIC RESPONSE MODIFIERS

Some problems experienced by the patient receiving BRMs are quite different from those observed with more traditional forms of cancer therapy. For example, capillary leak syndrome and pulmonary edema, observed with high doses of IL-2, are problems that require critical care nursing. These critical care requirements are new to many oncology nurses. Other problems, such as bone marrow depression and fatigue, are more familiar but exist at different levels of severity than those customarily associated with other forms of cancer therapy. Bone marrow depression occurring with BRM administration is generally more transient and less severe than that observed with chemotherapy. Fatigue associated with BRM therapy can be so severe that it can constitute a dose-limiting toxicity.

Nursing interventions for flulike syndrome include the administration of acetaminophen before treatment and every 4 hours after treatment. Intravenous meperidine has been used to control the severe chills associated with some BRMs. Other nursing measures include monitoring of vital signs and temperature, planning for periods of rest for the patient, and assisting with activities of daily living (ADLs).

A wide range of neurologic deficits have been observed with interferon and IL-2 therapy. The nature and extent of these problems have not been completely elucidated. However, these problems are understandably frightening to the patient and the family, who must be taught to observe for neurologic problems (e.g., confusion, memory loss, difficulty making decisions, insomnia), report their occurrence, and institute appropriate safety and support measures.[40]

Bone Marrow Transplantation

Bone marrow transplantation is a treatment option for some patients with cancer. Two types of bone marrow transplantation are performed. Both require the use of high-dose chemotherapy or total body radiation aimed at complete eradication of the patient's bone marrow. Subsequently, bone marrow is infused into the patient.

In *allogeneic marrow transplantation* the infused bone marrow is acquired from a donor who has been determined to be closely matched to the recipient in terms of tissue typing. This type of transplantation is used in the treatment of leukemias, lymphomas, and aplastic anemia. The goal of allogeneic transplantation is the engraftment and subsequent normal proliferation and differentiation of the donated marrow in the host. In *autologous marrow transplantation* patients receive their own bone marrow. The aim of this approach is to enable patients to receive intensive

Table 12-24 Side Effects of Biologic Response Modifier Therapy

Biologic Response Modifier	Flulike Syndrome	Central Nervous System	Renal and Hepatic	Gastro-intestinal	Hematologic	Cardiovascular and Pulmonary	Integu-mentary	Endocrine	Miscellaneous
■ Interferon	Fever, chills, malaise, fatigue	Impaired concentration and memory, confusion, lethargy, somnolence, seizures	Proteinuria, increased AST and ALT levels	Nausea, vomiting, diarrhea, anorexia	Leukopenia, thrombocytopenia, anemia	Hypotension, tachycardia, dysrhythmia, myocardial ischemia	Alopecia, irritation at injection site, skin and nail changes		Photophobia
■ Interleukin-2	Fever, chills, malaise	Disorientation, impaired concentration and memory, somnolence, severe anxiety, agitation	Oliguria; anuria; azotemia; increased BUN, serum creatinine, serum bilirubin, and liver enzymes; hypoalbuminemia; hepatomegaly	Nausea, vomiting, anorexia, diarrhea, stomatitis	Anemia, thrombocytopenia	Capillary leak syndrome, hypotension, tachycardia, dysrhythmias, myocardial ischemia, rare myocardial infarction, pulmonary congestion	Diffuse, pruritic, erythematous rash	Hypothyroidism; increased ACTH, cortisol, prolactin, growth hormone, and acute phase proteins	
■ Granulocyte–colony-stimulating factor	Fever, chills, myalgias, headache						Generalized rash	Generalized rash	Bone pain
■ Granulocyte macrophage–colony-stimulating factor	Fever, chills, myalgias, headache, fatigue				Leukocytosis, eosinophilia	Dyspnea	Facial flushing, generalized rash, inflammation at injection site		Bone pain, fluid retention
■ Tumor necrosis factor	Fever, chills, headache	Confusion, seizures, aphasia	Increased bilirubin, AST, and alkaline phosphatase	Nausea, vomiting, anorexia, diarrhea	Granulocytopenia, thrombocytopenia, increased circulating monocytes	Hypotension, hypertension, supraventricular dysrhythmias	Inflammation at injection site	Increased triglycerides, decreased cholesterol	
■ Monoclonal antibodies	Fever, chills, malaise, fatigue					Dyspnea, hypotension	Generalized erythema, urticaria, pruritus		Anaphylaxis

ACTH, Adrenocorticotropic hormone; *ALT*, alanine aminotransferase; *AST*, aspartate aminotransferase; *BUN*, blood urea nitrogen.

Table 12-25 Nutritional Management: Protein Foods with High Biologic Value

Milk

Whole milk (1 cup) = 9 g protein

Double-strength milk—1 quart of whole milk plus 1 cup of dried skim milk blended and chilled: 1 cup = 14 g protein

Milk shake—1 cup of ice cream plus 1 cup of milk = 15 g protein, 416 calories

Use evaporated milk, double-strength milk, or half-and-half to make casseroles, hot cereals, sauces, gravies, puddings, milk shakes, and soups.

Yogurt (regular and frozen)—check labels and purchase brand with highest protein content: 1 cup = 10 g protein

Eggs

Egg = 6 g protein

Eggnog (1 cup) = 15.5 g protein

Add eggs to salads, casseroles, and sauces. Deviled eggs are especially well tolerated.

Desserts that contain eggs include angel food cake, sponge cake, custard, and cheesecake.

Cheese

Cottage	½ cup	15 g protein
American	1 slice	3 g protein
Cheddar	1 slice	6 g protein
Cream	1 tbsp	1 g protein

Use cheese in a sandwich or as a snack.

Add cheese to salads, casseroles, sauces, and baked potatoes.

Cheesecake is usually a welcome treat.

Cheese spread with crackers is a wholesome snack that can be made and stored in the refrigerator for easy accessibility.

Meat, Poultry, Fish

Beef	3 oz	approx. 21 g protein
Pork	3 oz	approx. 19 g protein
Chicken	½ breast	approx. 26 g protein
Fish	3 oz	approx. 30 g protein
Tuna fish	6½ oz	approx. 44.5 g protein

Add meat, poultry, and fish to salads, casseroles, and sandwiches.

Add strained and junior baby meats to soups and casseroles.

Cocktail weiners or deviled ham on crackers are wholesome snacks. These snacks can be made and stored in the refrigerator for easy accessibility.

chemotherapy or radiation while supporting them with their own bone marrow. Chapter 28 contains a complete discussion of bone marrow transplantation.

Table 12-26 High-Caloric Foods

Food	Amount	Calories
Mayonnaise	1 tbs	= 101 cal
Butter or margarine	1 tsp	= 35 cal
Sour cream	1 tbs	= 72 cal
Peanut butter	1 tbs	= 94 cal
Whipped cream	1 tbs	= 53 cal
Corn oil	1 tbs	= 119 cal
Jelly	1 tbs	= 49 cal
Ice cream	1 cup	= 256 cal
Honey	1 tbs	= 64 cal

Nutritional Management of Cancer

Nutritional problems that most frequently occur in the patient with cancer are malnutrition, anorexia, altered taste sensation, nausea, vomiting, diarrhea, stomatitis, and mucositis. These problems can be caused by a combination of many factors including drug toxicity, effects of radiation therapy, tumor involvement, recent surgery, emotional distress, or difficulty with ingestion or digestion of food. If the patient is inadequately nourished, the normal cells will not be able to recover from the effects of therapy, and the immune system will be depressed because of depletion of protein stores.

Malnutrition. The patient with cancer usually experiences protein and calorie malnutrition characterized by fat and muscle depletion. (Assessment of the degree of malnutrition is discussed in Chapter 37.) Foods suggested for increasing the protein intake to facilitate repair and regeneration of cells are presented in Table 12-25. High-caloric foods that provide energy and minimize weight loss are presented in Table 12-26. A sample high-caloric, high-protein diet is presented in Table 37-13.

The nurse should suggest the need for a nutritional supplement to the physician as soon as a 5% weight loss is noted or if the patient has the potential for protein and caloric malnutrition. Albumin and prealbumin levels should be monitored. Once a 10-pound (4.5 kg) weight loss occurs, it is difficult to maintain the nutritional status. The patient can be taught to use nutritional supplements in place of milk when cooking or baking. Foods to which nutritional supplements can be easily added include scrambled eggs, pudding, custard, mashed potatoes, cereal, and cream sauces. Packages of "Instant Breakfast" can be used as indicated or sprinkled on cereals, desserts, and casseroles.

If the malnutrition cannot be treated with dietary intake, it may be necessary to use enteral or parenteral nutrition as an adjunct nutritional measure. (Enteral and parenteral nutrition are discussed in Chapter 37.)

Anorexia. It is important to realize that the anorexia experienced by the patient with cancer is a challenging problem. An intervention may be effective one day and ineffective the next. Continual assessment and intervention are necessary to successfully manage this problem. The nurse must develop the philosophy that something can be done to prevent or minimize anorexia, evaluate each intervention, and continue to use those interventions that have been successful in the past. Some suggestions are presented in the nursing care plan for the patient with cancer on p. 300.

Altered Taste Sensation. It is theorized that cancer cells release substances that resemble amino acids and stimulate the bitter taste buds. The patient may also experience an alteration in the sweet taste sensation, as well as in the sour and salty taste sensations. Meat may also taste bitter to the patient. At this time the physiologic basis of these varied taste alterations is unknown. Other causes of altered taste sensation are presented in Table 12-15.

The patient with an altered taste problem should be instructed to avoid foods that are disliked. Frequently the patient may feel compelled to eat certain foods because those foods are believed to be beneficial. The patient can be taught to experiment with spices and other seasoning agents in an attempt to mask the taste alterations that are occurring. Lemon juice, onion, mint, basil, and fruit juice marinades may improve the taste of certain meats and fish. Bacon bits, onion, and pieces of ham may enhance the taste of vegetables. An additional amount of a spice or seasoning agent is usually not an effective way to enhance the taste.

Unproven Methods of Cancer Treatment

Unproven methods of cancer treatment, sometimes referred to as *cancer quackery*, are as old as the disease itself. Cancer quackery is defined as the intentional misrepresentation or misapplication of measures that delay or impede the entry of the patient into the health care system for treatment. Today, cancer quackery is a multimillion-dollar business in the United States. Fear appears to be the major factor that motivates a patient to seek "miracle cures." Other factors include an impatience with the progress of the present cancer treatment, the need to exercise control over daily life, the impersonal approach of health care workers, a need for hope when terminal illness is a reality, a lack of information on methods that are proven versus those that are not, and the suspicion that the health care system is not providing the most effective treatment plan available.[41]

The major hazard of cancer quackery is that it delays or prevents the patient from receiving proven methods of cancer diagnosis and treatment. This delay may make the difference between cure or control and terminal illness. The nurse can play a significant role in preventing or minimizing the use of cancer quackery by doing the following:

1. Provide the patient with accurate information concerning the benefits of the proven methods of cancer treatment.
2. Inform the American Cancer Society, the local medical association, the health department, and the local consumer protection office when it is learned that the patient is being approached by persons promoting unproven methods of cancer treatment.
3. Discuss the fallacies of the unproven methods of cancer treatment with the patient and the family.

The current methods of cancer quackery include chemicals and drugs, dietary alterations, occult techniques, and mechanical devices.

Chemicals and Drugs. Two drugs that have been associated with cancer quackery are krebiozin (the "wonder" drug of the 1950s and 1960s) and Laetrile (the "wonder" drug of the 1970s and 1980s). A National Cancer Institute study on a large number of patients who used krebiozin failed to demonstrate any anticancer effects of this drug. Chemical analysis revealed that the major ingredient of krebiozin is mineral oil with minute amounts of creatine and amyl alcohol.

Laetrile, also known as vitamin B_{17} and Cyto H-3, has been actively used as a treatment for cancer for the past 25 to 30 years. The active ingredient of Laetrile is hydrogen cyanide, and it is derived from apricot or peach pits. It is available in parenteral and tablet form; the parenteral form contains 30 to 40 times as much cyanide as the oral form. There is no evidence of an anticancer effect of this drug.

Since Laetrile is frequently used by the patient with cancer and, until recently, has been thought of as a harmless drug, the nurse must be aware of the possible toxic effects that may be experienced. The cyanide content of Laetrile is released in the presence of hydrolyzine β-glucosidase enzymes. These enzymes are present in raw fruits and vegetables, such as lettuce, mushrooms, green peppers, celery, and sweet almonds. When these foods are eaten after the ingestion of Laetrile, cyanide intoxication may occur. The bacteria of the intestinal tract are also thought to contain this enzyme. When the cyanide is released, it inhibits cellular respiration, and the resulting hypoxia produces symptoms such as dizziness, nausea or vomiting, hypotension, and shock. Because the drug is not controlled by the FDA, many impurities may exist that have the potential for causing systemic bacterial, viral, and fungal infections.

Dietary Alterations. Books that propose cures for cancer enumerate the foods to eat and to avoid, offer special recipes, and usually recommend the use of an expensive blender to ensure the proper potency of the food mixture. Examples of nutritional alterations that have been used are eating raw foods; fasting for long periods of time; following the grape diet, the carrot juice diet, or the coffee and Coke diet; and using coffee, buttermilk, or yogurt enemas while on a special diet. None of these diets has been found effective in treating cancer. Nutritional alterations can have a profound effect on the patient with cancer, because a great amount of protein and many calories are needed to maintain weight and prevent a negative nitrogen balance.

Occult Techniques. The most commonly used occult form of cancer quackery is "psychic surgery." This surgery is performed by a healer without an incision. The patient comes to the healer with the problem, has the healing surgery, and leaves believing that the tumor has been removed. During the surgery the area where the problem exists is massaged and rubbed with animal blood. At some point the patient is shown a piece of animal tissue and is told that it is the diseased tissue or organ. This tissue is thrown away, the massage with blood continues, and the patient is told that the tumor is gone and the cancer is cured.

Mechanical Devices. Mechanical devices are an old form of cancer quackery that have recently lost their popularity. These devices are usually nothing more than light bulbs, vibrators, low-voltage generators, dials, and knobs. The patient is told to place the device on or in front of the area of cancer for a certain amount of time each day, and the device will destroy the cancer.

Supportive Care. One of the greatest assets of cancer quackery is the emotional support given to the patient and the patient's family. This factor should demonstrate to the nurse the need to provide psychologic support, caring, and active listening to the cancer patient and the family. The nurse needs to be available, listen, and counsel the patient during times when side effects are being experienced, when treatment is not effective, and when the patient is experiencing fear, anger, and depression.

If the patient chooses an unproven method of cancer treatment, the nurse needs to support the patient and assume a nonjudgmental attitude. The nurse should attempt to persuade the patient to continue the proven treatment plan and to maintain the nutritional status while using an unproven method of cancer treatment. Belief in the treatment may provide a placebo effect that may offer some benefits. It is important that all doors remain open to the patient so that a return to the health care system can be made without feelings of fear or guilt.

COMPLICATIONS RESULTING FROM CANCER

The patient may develop complications related to the continual growth of the malignancy or the side effects of treatment.

Infection

Infection is a frequent cause of death in the patient with cancer. The usual sites of infection include the lungs, GU system, mouth, rectum, peritoneal cavity, and blood (septicemia). Infection occurs as a result of the ulceration and necrosis caused by the tumor, compression by the tumor of vital organs, and the state of neutropenia caused by the disease process or the treatment of cancer. Fungi and gram-negative bacteria are the usual causative organisms.

Many patients are neutropenic when an infection develops. In these individuals, infection may cause significant morbidity and may be rapidly fatal if not treated promptly. The classic manifestations of infection are not often present in a patient with neutropenia and a depressed immune system.

Paraneoplastic Syndrome

Paraneoplastic syndrome includes all the physiologic effects that occur as the result of the release of certain hormones by cancer cells in the primary and metastatic sites. Hormone secretion from cancer cells arising from tissues that do not normally release this hormone is caused by the process of cellular depression. This process allows the stored potential of all cells to become evident. Paraneoplastic syndrome can occur during all phases of the cancer process, but it is commonly associated with the advanced illness phase. The most common paraneoplastic syndromes include the following:

1. Syndrome of inappropriate antidiuretic hormone (SIADH) caused by cancer cells located in the lung, pancreas, or prostate gland that produce antidiuretic hormone (ADH)
2. Secretion of adrenocorticotropic hormone (ACTH) by a tumor of the lung, thymus, pancreas, thyroid, stomach, or ovary
3. Secretion of insulin by a tumor of the pancreas, liver, adrenal gland, stomach, or ovary
4. Hypercalcemia occurs when a parathyroid hormone-like substance is secreted by the cancer cells and is most frequently found in patients with lung, breast, kidney, colon, or thyroid cancer

Hypercalcemia

Hypercalcemia is a serious electrolyte disorder that occurs in the cancer patient. In addition to paraneoplastic syndrome, hypercalcemia may also occur in tumors characterized by extensive bone involvement, such as multiple myeloma and bony metastasis. Hypercalcemia may also result from immobilization with or without metastasis. Serum levels of calcium in excess of 12 mg/dl (3 mmol/L) can be life threatening. Chronic hypercalcemia can result in nephrocalcinosis and irreversible renal failure. The long-term treatment of hypercalcemia is aimed at the primary disease. Acute hypercalcemia is treated by hydration (3 L/day), diuretic (particularly loop diuretics) administration, and plicamycin (formerly mithramycin [Mithracin]) if the patient has severe symptoms. Other pharmacologic interventions that may be used to inhibit bone resorption include etidronate disodium (Didronel), pamidronate (Aredia), calcitonin, and oral phosphates.

Superior Vena Cava Syndrome

Superior vena cava syndrome results from obstruction of the superior vena cava by a tumor. The clinical manifestations include facial edema, periorbital edema, distention of veins of the neck and chest, headache, and convulsions. The presence of a mediastinal mass is often visible on chest x-ray. The most common causes are Hodgkin's disease, non-Hodgkin's lymphoma, and lung cancer. Superior vena cava syndrome is considered a serious medical problem, and management usually involves radiation therapy to the site of obstruction and treatment of the primary tumor. *Hemorrhage* can be caused by the presence of thrombocytopenia, tumor invasion of a blood vessel causing the vessel to rupture, or the development of an ulcer. Petechiae, epistaxis, hematuria, and melena may signal the possibility of an impending major hemorrhage. The usual sites of massive hemorrhage are the brain, the GI tract, and the major vessels of the neck, lungs, and peritoneal cavity. Disseminated intravascular coagulation (DIC) can also occur in the person with cancer. It is because of the release of thromboplastic substances from cancer cells. (DIC is discussed in Chapter 28.)

Infarction and Organ Failure

Infarction occurs as a result of the formation of thrombi composed of tumor cells. When the thrombi occlude vessels in major body organs, they cause necrosis of vital organ tissue. The major sites of infarction are the lung, heart, and brain. Organ failure is the result of primary or metastatic disease involvement of a vital organ, such as the brain, liver, kidney, or lung. The involvement is sufficient to cause physiologic dysfunction, organ failure, or death.

Spinal Cord Compression

Spinal cord compression is a result of the presence of a malignant tumor in the epidural space of the spinal cord. The most common primary tumors that produce this problem are breast, lung, prostate, GI, melanoma, and renal tumors. Lymphomas also pose a risk if diseased lymph tissue invades the epidural space. The manifestations are back pain that is intense, localized, and persistent, accompanied by vertebral tenderness and aggravated by the Valsalva maneuver; motor weakness and dysfunction; sensory paresthesia and loss; and autonomic dysfunction. Radiation therapy is used for the patient with slowly progressive neurologic deficits and radiosensitive tumors. Surgery is usually recommended for the patient with rapidly progressive neurologic signs, especially if the tumors are relatively radioresistant.

PSYCHOLOGIC SUPPORT

Psychologic support of the patient is an important aspect of cancer care. Because of the effectiveness of cancer treatment, many patients with cancer are cured or their disease is controlled for long periods of time. In light of this trend in cancer treatment, emphasis must be placed on maintaining an optimal quality of life after the diagnosis of cancer. A positive attitude of patient, family, and caregivers toward cancer and cancer treatment has a significant positive impact on the quality of life the patient experiences. A positive attitude may also influence the prognosis of the patient with cancer.

The diagnosis of cancer is viewed by most persons as a crisis. The most common fears experienced by the patient with cancer include disfigurement, dependency, pain, emaciation, financial depletion, abandonment, and death.

To cope with these fears, the patient with cancer will use and experience different behavioral patterns: shock, anger, denial, bargaining, depression, helplessness, hopelessness, rationalization, acceptance, and intellectualization. These behavioral patterns may occur at any time during the process of cancer. However, some patterns appear to occur more frequently or at a greater intensity at certain specific stages of the disease process. The following factors may determine how the patient will cope with the diagnosis of cancer:

1. Ability to cope with stressful events in the past (e.g., loss of job, major disappointment). By simply asking how the patient has coped with stressful events, the nurse can gain an understanding of the patient's coping patterns, the effectiveness of the usual coping patterns, and the usual coping time framework.
2. Availability of significant others. The patient who has effective support systems tends to cope more effectively than the patient who does not have a meaningful, available support system.
3. Ability to express feelings and concerns. The patient who is able to express feelings and needs and who seeks and asks for help appears to cope more effectively than the patient who internalizes feelings and needs.
4. Age at the time of diagnosis. Age determines the coping strategies to a great degree. For example, a young mother with cancer may have concerns that differ from those of a 70-year-old woman with cancer.
5. Extent of disease. Cure or control of the disease process is usually easier to cope with than the reality of terminal illness.
6. Disruption of body image. Disruption of the body image (e.g., radical neck dissection, alopecia, mastectomy) may intensify the psychologic impact of cancer.
7. Presence of symptoms. Symptoms such as fatigue, nausea, diarrhea, and pain may intensify the psychologic impact of cancer.
8. Past experience with cancer. If past experiences with cancer have been negative, the patient will probably view the present status as negative.
9. Attitude associated with the cancer. A patient who feels in control and has a positive attitude about cancer and cancer treatment is better able to cope with the diagnosis and treatment of cancer than the patient who feels hopeless, helpless, and out of control.

To facilitate the development of a hopeful attitude about cancer and to support the patient and the family during the various stages of the process of cancer, the nurse should do the following:

1. Be available and continue to be available, especially during difficult times.
2. Exhibit a caring attitude.
3. Listen actively to fears and concerns.
4. Provide relief from distressing symptoms.
5. Provide essential information regarding cancer and cancer care.
6. Maintain a relationship based on trust and confidence; open, honest, and caring in the approach.
7. Use touch to exhibit caring. A squeeze of the hand or a hug may at times be more effective than words.
8. Assist the patient in setting realistic, reachable short-term and long-term goals.
9. Assist the patient in maintaining usual lifestyle patterns.
10. Maintain hope, which is the key to effective cancer care. Hope varies, depending on the status of the patient—hope that the symptoms are not serious, hope that the treatment is curative, hope for independence, hope for relief of pain, hope for a longer life, or hope for a peaceful death. Hope provides control over what is occurring and is the basis of a positive attitude toward cancer and cancer care.

Most patients with advanced cancer know that they are dying. Attempts at circumventing the truth are usually recognized by the patient and cause feelings of distrust and hostility toward the person who makes such attempts. Honesty and openness are the best approaches. Most patients will surprise caregivers by expressing relief at a will-

RESEARCH

IMPLICATIONS FOR NURSING PRACTICE

CANCER PAIN

Citation Arathuzik D: Effects of cognitive-behavioral strategies on pain in cancer patients, *Cancer Nurs* 17: 207-214, 1994.

Purpose To examine the effects of a combination of cognitive and behavioral nursing interventions on pain control and mood in breast cancer patients with metastasis who were experiencing physical pain

Methods Patients (n = 24) with metastatic breast cancer who were experiencing physical pain were randomly assigned to a control group, to a treatment group that received relaxation and visualization training, or to a treatment group that received relaxation, visualization, and cognitive coping skills training. Measures of pain intensity, pain distress, pain control, ability to decrease pain, and mood were assessed pretreatment and posttreatment.

Results and Conclusions Significant differences were found between the treatment groups and the control group in the ability of the interventions to decrease pain. There were no significant differences in pain intensity or distress or mood among the groups. These cognitive-behavioral interventions (relaxation, visualization, and cognitive coping skills) could be useful clinical nursing interventions for selected cancer patients experiencing physical pain.

Implications for Nursing Practice Pain experienced by the cancer patient is one of the most significant nursing care challenges. Cognitive and behavioral coping strategies for pain perception and pain control can assist the nurse in planning and implementing effective nursing interventions for the cancer patient suffering from pain. Effective nursing interventions to decrease pain could potentially enhance the quality of life for the cancer patient.

ingness to discuss what is foremost in their minds, their imminent death.

Organizations and journals available as resources for the nurse are listed in the bibliography at the end of this section. In many cities, there are local units of the American Cancer Society that provide a wide variety of services.

Management of Cancer Pain

Between 30% and 75% of persons with cancer experience moderate to severe pain depending on the stage of the disease, despite the fact that studies have shown cancer pain can be well managed in up to 90% of patients.[42] Pain is most common in the patient with bone disease, but cancer-related conditions such as decubitus ulcers, cancer therapy, and pain related to the cancer itself also contribute significantly to the patient's pain experience.

Because data such as vital signs and patient behaviors are not reliable indicators of pain, especially long-standing, chronic pain, it is *essential* that every patient with cancer be assessed for pain by first asking the question "Do you have pain?" If the patient's self report is affirmative, further data are obtained and documented initially and at regular intervals on the location and intensity of the pain, what it feels like, and how it is relieved. Patterns of change also should be assessed. The patient report should *always* be believed and accepted as the primary source of assessment data. Table 12-27 presents assessment questions that may facilitate this data collection.

Table 12-27 Essential Components of Cancer Pain Assessment and Relevant Assessment Questions

Location	Where is the pain? (There may be more than one place.)
Intensity	How bad is the pain? (See Chapter 6 for rating scales.)
Quality	What does the pain feel like? (See Chapter 6 for descriptors.)
Pattern	Has the pain changed? What makes the pain better or worse?
Relief Measures	What do you do to control your pain? Are medications used? Does the relief measure help much? How much?

Modified from Agency for Health Care Policy and Research: *Patient Guide, Clinical Practice Guideline, Managing Cancer Pain,* Rockville, MD, 1994, US Department of Health and Human Services.

Pharmaceutical interventions, including nonsteroidal antiinflammatory drugs (NSAIDs), opioids, and adjuvant pain medications, should be used following the World Health Organization (WHO) Analgesic Ladder (Fig. 12-24). Analgesic medications should be given on a regular schedule, around the clock, with additional doses as needed for breakthrough pain.[42] Oral administration of the medication is preferred. It is important to remember that with opioid drugs such as morphine the appropriate dose is whatever is necessary to control the pain with the least side effects. Principles of patient-controlled analgesia should also be followed.[42] Fear of addiction is not warranted but must be addressed as part of patient education issues relevant to pain control, because fear of addiction is a significant barrier to appropriate pain management. (Additional strategies to relieve pain are discussed in Chapter 6).

Hospice Care

A hospice is not a place but a concept of care that provides compassion, concern, support, and skilled professional care for the dying. Hospice care seeks to enhance the remaining time for the person who is living with a dying body. The term *hospice* is derived from a medieval word that means a place of shelter for people on a difficult journey. The hospice concept of care has existed in England for many years. During the 1970s the idea took hold in the United States, and by the end of the decade, every state had existing hospice programs.

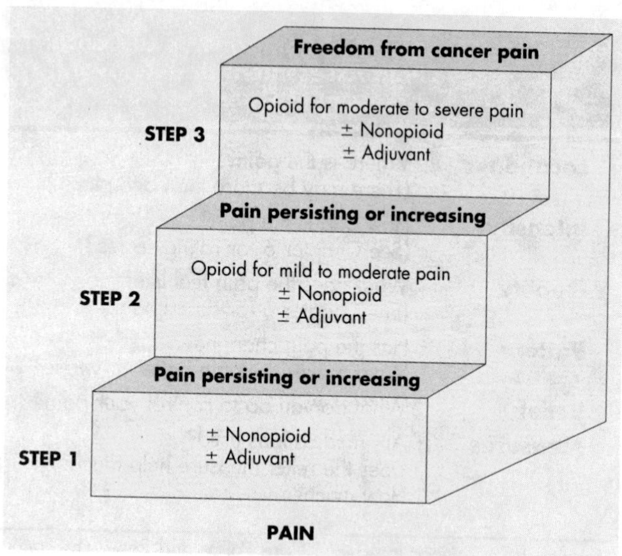

Fig. 12-24 The World Health Organization (WHO) three-step analgesic ladder.

The National Hospice Organization has defined hospice as a centrally administered program of palliative and supportive services that provides physical, psychologic, social, and spiritual care for the dying person and the family. Services are provided by a medically supervised, interdisciplinary team of professionals and volunteers.

Hospice programs are organized under a variety of models. Some are based in hospitals or in home health agencies, whereas others are freestanding or community-based, volunteer-intensive programs. The National Hospice Organization annually publishes a directory that lists hospice programs in the United States. The directory not only provides the name, address, and phone number of the hospice, but it also provides its organizational type, the scope of its services, and the geographic service area.

Admission to a hospice program is on the basis of patient and family need. Home care is provided on a part-time, intermittent, regularly scheduled, or on-call basis. Hospice services are available on a 24-hour basis 7 days a week to provide help to the patient and family in the home. Some hospice programs also have an inpatient unit in a hospital. Usually the inhospital units have been deinstitutionalized to make the atmosphere as free and homelike as possible. Staff and volunteers are available to the patient and family. A multidisciplinary team approach provides holistic personal care.

Bereavement care is a natural extension of the hospice structure. Because the patient and family are the focus of hospice care, providing grief support to family members or to significant others after the death of the patient is incorporated into the organizational structure and into the treatment plans. The objective of a bereavement program is to provide support and to assist survivors in the transition to a life without the deceased person.

Regulation and Reimbursement. A great deal of controversy surrounds the increasing bureaucratization of the U.S. hospice movement. New sources of financial reimbursement for the benefit of the patient now exist that were unheard of only 5 years ago.

Section 122 of the Tax Equity and Fiscal Responsibility Act of 1982 created the hospice Medicare benefit. In addition to the usual services covered by Medicare, the hospice benefit also covers drugs and BRMs for home use; home care service (including continuous care), whether or not the patient is homebound; counseling; bereavement; and homemaker services. The Medicare benefit is available to the patient through certified hospice programs.

There has been an increase in third-party payers in providing hospice-care benefits. These payers have added to the regulations and requirements to which hospice programs are obligated. In addition, at least half of all states currently have hospice-licensing regulations and laws in existence or in the planning stages.

Philosophy of Hospice Care. There is often a point in terminal disease when curative treatment is no longer possible. It is at this time that the hospice philosophy of promoting the quality of life and providing palliative care is appropriate. Palliative care controls symptoms and provides comfort, but it does not cure. Palliative care does not prolong life, but it does provide comfort.

Hospice care represents a return to previous times when the dying individual was allowed to remain and die at home, if possible, surrounded by familiar sights, sounds, and smells and by the love of those who care. The hospice exists to provide support and care for the person in the last phases of incurable diseases so that the person might live as fully and as comfortably as possible.

Initially, hospice programs were primarily volunteer programs of love and goodwill; the hospice of today is a health care program faced with a myriad of ethical and legal issues. Some of the issues include nonresuscitation orders, artificial feeding and hydration, the debate concerning "killing" or "letting die," and the right to truth and self-determination. Time will tell whether hospice is greater than the ethical and legal issues it faces.

Differences Between Traditional and Hospice Care. Hospice care differs from traditional care in a number of ways. The goals of traditional hospital and medical care are to treat and cure disease, prolong life, use all appropriate technology, and treat pain with limited, well-defined amounts of medication. Traditional medical care views death as a failure of treatment.

In hospice care, the patient and the family are the focus of care. Preparation for dying is a task with which the family and the patient must deal. Hospice provides a milieu in which this is more easily accomplished. Hospice recognizes dying as a normal process. It neither hastens nor postpones death. Hospice exists in the hope and belief that, through appropriate care and the promotion of a caring community sensitive to needs, the patient and family may be free to attain a degree of mental and spiritual preparation for a satisfactory death.

Hospice care is not technology oriented. Instead it is intensive personal care that provides skilled bedside nursing and focuses attention on the emotional, social, spiritual,

CRITICAL THINKING EXERCISES

CASE STUDY

CANCER

Patient Profile

Ms. L. is a 32-year-old woman who is scheduled for radiation treatment following a lumpectomy (surgical removal of malignant tumor in her breast).

Subjective Data

- Expresses a great deal of fear and anxiety about radiation therapy
- Believes she should have had a mastectomy; therefore, she would not have needed radiation
- States that no one has told her about what to expect related to radiation therapy
- Has two young children at home and is concerned about their care

Critical Thinking Questions

1. What are potential side effects of radiation therapy to the chest?
2. What are appropriate nursing interventions to control these side effects?
3. What should Ms. L. be taught about skin care in the treatment field?
4. How should she be helped to reduce her anxiety and fear about beginning radiation therapy?
5. Based on the assessment data provided, write one or more appropriate nursing diagnoses. Are there any collaborative problems?

NURSING RESEARCH ISSUES

1. Do patients who have been successfully treated for cancer with radiation or chemotherapy know about the late effects of treatment?
2. What is the quality of life for patients 5 or more years following successful radiation therapy?
3. What are the most challenging or difficult problems encountered by hospice nurses?
4. Is there a difference in quality of life between the patient receiving traditional chemotherapy as compared with the patient receiving BRMs?
5. Can relaxation strategies, such as guided imagery, decrease the side effects associated with chemotherapy?
6. Why do some individuals choose nontraditional methods of cancer treatment?

and familial aspects of the patient. Hospice offers little opportunity to do things *to* the patient but offers great opportunity to do things *with* the patient and family.[43]

Pain is a common concern with the terminally ill patient. In hospice, pain is considered a total experience rather than a physiologic event. Adequate medication, usually opioids, is used to provide relief. The prn order for pain is not found in hospice. Analgesia is routinely given in an attempt to eliminate the pain and, more importantly, to prevent its recurrence and to erase the memory of pain. Attention is also given to the other factors that contribute to pain or to its increasing intensity, such as fear, loneliness, anxiety, insomnia, spiritual doubts or concerns, financial concerns, and depression.

When the patient dies, the hospice team continues to follow the family and significant others through the bereavement period. The hospice team makes itself available to aid survivors through the grief period.

Support groups are available to hospice staff and volunteers. Crises and grief result in varying forms of stress for caregivers. To give to the patient and family, the staff and volunteers must also have a means to be nourished and refreshed. Various means of stress relief are used by different hospices. Professionally assisted groups, informal rap sessions, flexible time schedules, and additional time off for the hospice worker are a few ways to decrease stress. The needs of the caregiver must be considered important, or the care receiver will receive less of what is needed.

REVIEW QUESTIONS

The number of the question corresponds to the same-numbered objective at the beginning of the chapter.

1. Which type of cancer is increasing in incidence?
   a. Uterine cancer
   b. Esophageal cancer
   c. Stomach cancer
   d. Lung cancer

2. Cancer is a name for a large group of diseases, all of which are characterized by
   a. cell growth that escapes normal control.
   b. rapid, explosive proliferation of cells.
   c. production of toxins that alter cells.
   d. a long and painful course.

3. A characteristic of the stage of progression in the development of cancer is
a. mutation of stem cells.
b. continual steady growth facilitated by promoting factors.
c. proliferation of cancer cells in spite of host-control mechanisms.
d. oncogenic viral transformation of target cells.

4. The primary protective role of the immune system related to malignant cells is
a. immunologic surveillance.
b. immunologic enhancement.
c. antigenic blindfolding.
d. antigenic modulation.

5. The primary difference between benign and malignant neoplasms is
a. the rate of cell proliferation.
b. the requirements for cellular nutrients.
c. the characteristics of tissue invasiveness.
d. the site of the malignant tumor.

6. Important nursing roles related to prevention and detection of cancer include all the following *except*
a. teaching people self-examination of breast and testicles.
b. instructing people to eat low-fiber, refined-carbohydrate diets.
c. instructing people on methods to increase capacity to cope with stress.
d. teaching people to obtain regular health care.

7. The only definitive means of diagnosing cancer is by
a. radiologic study.
b. culture.
c. chemical testing.
d. biopsy.

8. All of the following are true of the acute effects of radiation therapy *except* they
a. can occur during the radiation treatments.
b. affect actively proliferating tissues in the treatment field.
c. are partially related to vascular changes in the area of the treatment field.
d. affect GI mucosa because of its rapid mitotic rates.

9. Which of the following sets of drug classifications and examples are incorrect?
a. Alkylating agent—nitrogen mustard
b. Antibiotic—actinomycin D
c. Antimetabolite—5-fluorouracil
d. Plant alkaloid—L-asparaginase

10. Stomatitis, a common side effect of chemotherapeutic agents, occurs because the
a. general health of the patient with cancer is poor.
b. rapidly dividing cells of the mucous membranes of the mouth are being destroyed.
c. chemotherapeutic drugs have an external, local, and irritating effect.
d. site of the malignancy is near the oral cavity.

11. Radiation precautions on the clinical unit must be observed by the nurse caring for the patient
a. who is receiving supervoltage radiation therapy for lung cancer.
b. who has ingested radioactive iodine for diagnostic brain scan.
c. who is having cobalt teletherapy for esophageal cancer.
d. who has implanted radium needles in the breast.

12. Which of the following is not characteristic of BRMs?
a. No side or toxic effects
b. Augment the body's natural defenses
c. Most therapies are still under investigation
d. Monoclonal antibodies can be made to be antigen specific

13. The most common nutritional problems found in cancer patients include all the following *except*
a. malnutrition.
b. anorexia.
c. altered taste sensation.
d. hypernatremia.

14. If a patient decides to take Laetrile, the nurse should inform the patient that
a. foods with hydrolyzine β-glucosidase enzymes should be avoided.
b. chemotherapy and Laetrile should not be taken simultaneously.
c. a pulmonary fungal infection will probably develop.
d. buttermilk should be ingested simultaneously to avoid toxic effects.

15. Paraneoplastic syndrome that occurs in certain types of cancer is primarily caused by
a. invasiveness of cancer cells.
b. gram-negative septicemia.
c. ectopic hormonal production.
d. autoimmune reaction.

REFERENCES

1. Wingo PA, Tong T, Bolden S: Cancer Statistics, 1995, *CA* 45:1, 1995.
2. DeVita VT, Helman S, Rosenberg SA, editors: *Cancer: principles and practice of oncology,* Philadelphia, 1993, Lippincott.
3. Gallucci BB: Cancer biology: molecular and cellular aspects. In Baird SB, editor: *Cancer nursing,* Philadelphia, 1991, Saunders.
4. Mettlin C, Mirand AL: The causes of cancer. In Baird SB, editor: *Cancer nursing,* Philadelphia, 1991, Saunders.
5. Morton DL and others: Malignant melanoma. In Holland JF and others, editors: *Cancer medicine,* ed 3, Philadelphia, 1993, Lea & Febiger.
6. Dudjak LA: Cancer metastasis, *Sem Oncol Nurs* 8:40, 1992.
7. Kim YS, Liotta LA, Kohn EC: Cancer invasion and metastasis, *Hosp Pract* 28:92, 1993.
8. Marx JL: How cancer cells spread in the body, *Science* 244:147, 1989.
9. Hubbard SM, Liotta LA: The biology of metastases. In Baird SB, editor: *Cancer nursing,* Philadelphia, 1991, Saunders.
10. Appelbaum JW: The role of the immune system in the pathogenesis of cancer. *Semin Oncol Nursing* 8:51, 1992.

11. Workman ML, Ellerhorst-Ryan J, Hargrave-Koertge V: *Nursing care of the immunocompromised patient,* Philadelphia, 1993, Saunders.

12. Cancer-related checkups: If you're between 18 and 39: if you're 40 or over, Atlanta, 1993, American Cancer Society Publication.

13. Perez C, Brady L: Preface. In Perez C, Brady L, editors: *Principles and practice of radiation oncology,* ed 27, Philadelphia, 1992, Lippincott.

14. Kaplan H: Historic milestones in radiobiology and radiation therapy, *Semin Oncol* 4:479, 1979.

15. Stein J: Some observations of the history of irradiation therapy, *Endocur Hyperthermia Oncology* 1:59, 1985.

16. Withers HR: Biological basis of radiation therapy for cancer, *Lancet* 339:156, 1992.

17. Chapman J, Allalunis-Turner M: Cellular and molecular targets in normal tissue radiation injury. In Gutin P, Leibel SL, Sheline G, editors: *Radiation injury to the central nervous system,* NY, 1991, Raven Press.

18. Walden T, Farzaneh N: Biochemical response of normal tissues to ionizing radiation. In Gutin P, Leibel S, Sheline G, editors: *Radiation injury to the central nervous system,* NY, 1991, Raven Press.

19. Withers HR: Biologic basis of radiation therapy. In Perez C, Brady L, editors: *Principles and practice of radiation oncology,* ed 27, Philadelphia, 1992, Lippincott.

20. Phillips T: Early and late effects of radiation on normal tissues. In Gutin P, Leibel S, Sheline G, editors: *Radiation injury to the central nervous system,* New York, 1991, Raven Press.

21. Hilderly L, Dow K: Radiation oncology. In Baird S, McCorkle R, Grant M, editors: *Cancer nursing: a comprehensive textbook,* Philadelphia, 1991, Saunders.

*22. Winningham M: Walking program for people with cancer: getting started, *Cancer Nurs* 4:270, 1991.

23. Bruera E: Current pharmacological management of anorexia in cancer patients, *Oncology* 6:125, 1991.

24. Chahbazian C: The skin. In Moss W, Cox J, editors: *Radiation oncology: rationale, technique, results,* ed 6, St Louis, 1989, Mosby.

25. Marcial V: The oral cavity and oropharynx. In Moss W, Cox J, editors: *Radiation oncology: rationale, technique, results,* ed 6, St Louis, 1989, Mosby.

26. Iwamoto R: Alterations in oral status. In Baird S, McCorkle R, Grant M, editors: *Cancer nursing: a comprehensive textbook,* Philadelphia, 1991, Saunders.

27. Gift A: Dyspnea, *Nurs Clin North Am* 24:955, 1990.

28. Fernandez-Banares F and others: Acute effects of abdominopelvic irradiation on the orocecal transit time: its relation to clinical symptoms and bile salt and lactose malabsorption, *Am J Gastroenterol* 86:1771, 1991.

29. Damewood M, Grochow L: Prospects for fertility after chemotherapy for neoplastic disease, *Fertil Steril* 45:443, 1986.

30. Dembo A: The ovary. In Moss W, Cox J, editors: *Radiation oncology: rationale, techniques,* results, ed 6, St Louis, 1989, Mosby.

*31. Oberst M and others: Self-care burden, stress appraisal, and mood among persons receiving radiotherapy, *Cancer Nurs* 14:71, 1991.

*32. Christman N: Uncertainty and adjustment during radiotherapy, *Nurs Res* 39:17, 1990.

33. Krakoff IH: Cancer chemotherapeutic and biologic agents. *CA Cancer J Clin* 41:264, 1991.

34. Meares C: PICC and MLC lines: options worth exploring, *Nursing* 22:52, 1992.

35. Goodman M: Delivery of cancer chemotherapy. In Baird SB, McCorkle R, Grant M, editors: *Cancer nursing: a comprehensive textbook,* Philadelphia, 1991, Saunders.

36. Maxwell MB, Maher KE: Chemotherapy-induced myelosuppression, *Semin Oncol Nurs* 8:113, 1992.

37. Dudjak LA, Yasko JM: Biological response modifier therapy. In Yasko JM, Dudjak LA, editors: *Biological response modifier therapy: symptom management,* 1990, Park Row Publishers for the Cetus Corporation.

38. Jassak PF: Biotherapy. In Groenwald SL and others, editors: *Cancer nursing: principles and practice,* ed 3, Boston, 1993, Jones and Bartlett.

39. Haeuber D: Future strategies in the control of myelosuppresion: the use of colony stimulating factors, *Oncol Nurs Forum* 18:16, 1991.

40. Bender, CM: Cognitive dysfunction associated with biological response modifier therapy, *Oncol Nurs Forum* 21:515, 1994.

41. Henke-Yarbro C: Questionable methods of cancer therapy. In Groenwald SL and others, editors: *Cancer nursing: principles and practice,* Boston, 1993, Jones and Bartlett.

42. Agency for Health Care Policy and Research (AHCPR): Clinical practice guidelines, management of cancer pain, Rockville, MD, US Department of Health and Human Services, 1994.

*43. Degner LF, Gow CM, Thompson LA: Critical nursing behaviors in care for the dying, *Cancer Nurs* 14:246, 1991.

---

*Nursing research-based articles.

Chapter 13

NURSING ROLE IN MANAGEMENT

Fluid, Electrolyte, and Acid-Base Imbalances

Mima M. Horne

Learning Objectives

1. Identify the major fluid compartments and the electrolytes in each compartment.
2. Describe the mechanisms controlling fluid and electrolyte movement.
3. Describe the mechanisms and causes of extracellular fluid (ECF) shifts.
4. Explain the physiologic mechanisms that regulate fluid and electrolyte balance.
5. Describe the common causes, clinical manifestations, and therapeutic and nursing management of fluid and electrolyte imbalances.
6. Describe pH and the mechanisms that regulate acid-base balance.
7. Describe the common causes, pathophysiology, compensatory mechanisms, and clinical manifestations of respiratory and metabolic acidosis and alkalosis.
8. Identify the significant assessment data and common abnormal assessment findings related to fluid and electrolyte imbalances.
9. Compare and contrast the types of solutions available for fluid and electrolyte therapy, including tonicity and indications for use.

HOMEOSTASIS

The cells that make up body tissues exist in a chemically constant but physiologically dynamic internal environment. Physiologic processes function to regulate this environment so that responses to stimuli minimally affect the body. The chemical consistency achieved through fluid, electrolyte, and acid-base balance is essential to the maintenance of homeostasis. *Homeostasis* is the term used to describe the ability to maintain internal balance in the presence of external stressors.[1]

As long as life exists, the body is affected by stressors. Stressors such as disease and injury alter the normal balance. A stress state is produced by failure to satisfy a psychologic or physiologic need. Homeostatic compensatory mechanisms participate in the adjustment to stressors so that the body efficiently and effectively reestablishes a steady state.

The homeostatic mechanisms that regulate fluid and electrolyte balance represent an interaction between chemical and physiologic processes. The challenge to the health care professional is to understand how these processes control fluid and electrolyte movement and concentrations in the body. This knowledge is essential to understand not only the pathophysiologic effects of diseases but also how treatments affect this delicate balance.

WATER CONTENT OF THE BODY

Water is the primary component of all body fluids. It is the solvent used to transport nutrients to cells and to remove waste products produced by cellular metabolism. Temperature regulation is assisted by evaporation of water on the body's surface.

Variations

The adult human body is approximately 60% water. The water content varies with gender, body mass, and age. Men generally have a greater water content because they have more lean body mass than women. Adipose tissue contains less water than an equivalent amount of muscle tissue. Age also influences the body's water content (Fig. 13-1). In the older adult, body water content averages 45% to 55% of body weight. In the infant, water content is 70% to 80% of the body weight. Therefore the young are at risk for fluid problems because of a greater percentage of their body weight is water. Older adults are at risk because they have less fluid reserve. Both the very young and very old have a decreased ability to compensate for fluid loss.

Reviewed by Norma Jean Weldy, BS, MS, Professor of Nursing Emerita, Goshen College, Goshen, IN.

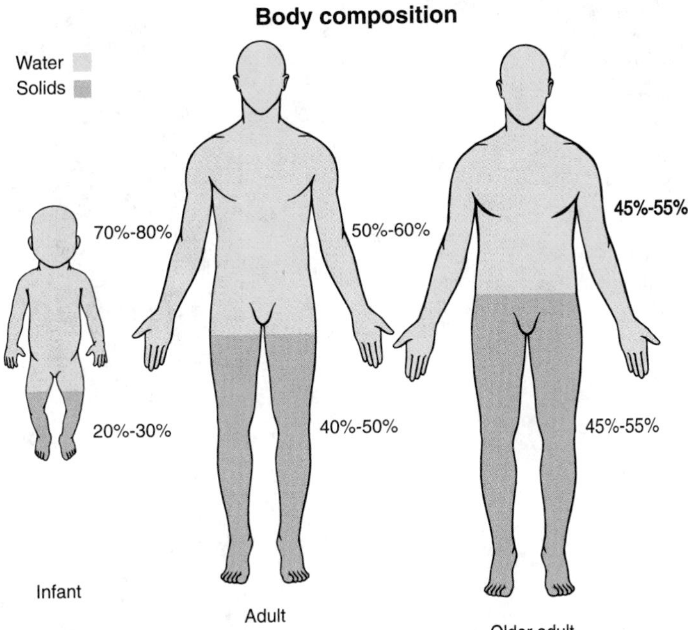

Fig. 13-1 Changes in body water content correlated with age.

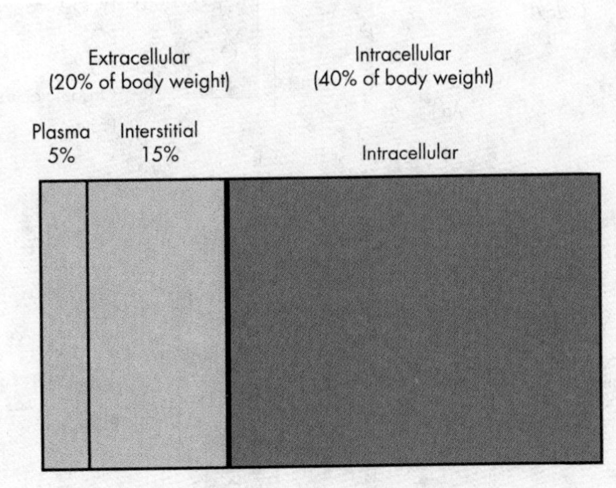

Fig. 13-2 Fluid compartments in the body.

Body Fluid Compartments

The two major fluid compartments in the body are *intracellular* and *extracellular* (Fig. 13-2). Intracellular fluid (ICF) is located in cells and constitutes approximately 40% of body weight or 70% of the total body water. Extracellular fluid (ECF) constitutes about 20% of body weight or 30% of total body water. ECF consists of interstitial (between cells), intravascular (plasma), cerebrospinal, and intraocular fluid, as well as secretions of the gastrointestinal (GI) tract. Sometimes the term *transcellular* (a product of secretion and diffusion from cells) is used to refer to cerebrospinal fluid, intraocular fluid, and GI secretions.

Fluid spacing is a term used to classify the distribution of body water. *First spacing* is a normal distribution of fluid in both the extracellular and intracellular compartments. *Second spacing* refers to an excess accumulation of interstitial fluid (edema). *Third spacing* occurs when fluid accumulates in areas that normally have no fluid or only a minimum amount of fluid. Examples of third spacing are ascites, sequestration of fluid in the bowel with peritonitis, and edema associated with burns. Third spacing is a concern because it takes fluid away from the normal fluid compartments and may produce hypovolemia.

Calculation of Fluid Gain or Loss

One liter of water weighs 2.2 lbs (1 kg). If a patient drank 240 ml of fluid, weight gain would be 0.5 lb (0.24 kg). A patient under diuretic therapy with no dietary changes who loses 2 kg in 24 hours has experienced a fluid loss of approximately 2 L. A sudden weight change is the best indicator of fluid volume loss or gain.

ELECTROLYTES

Electrolytes are substances whose molecules dissociate or split into ions when placed in water. *Ions* are electrically charged particles. *Cations* are positively charged ions. Examples include sodium (Na^+), potassium (K^+), calcium (Ca^{2+}), and magnesium (Mg^{2+}) ions. *Anions* are negatively charged ions. Examples include bicarbonate (HCO_3^-), chloride (Cl^-), and phosphate (PO_4^{3-}) ions. The ionic charge is termed *valence*. Cations and anions combine according to their valence. (Terminology related to body fluid chemistry is presented in Table 13-1.)

Measurement

The concentration of electrolytes can be expressed in milligrams per deciliter (mg/dl), millimoles per liter (mmol/L),

Table 13-1 Terminology Related to Body Fluid Chemistry

Anion	Ion that carries a negative charge
Cation	Ion that carries a positive charge
Electrolyte	Substance that dissociates in solution into ions (charged particles); a molecule of sodium chloride (NaCl) in solution becomes Na^+ and Cl^-
Nonelectrolyte	Substance that does not dissociate into ions in solution; examples include glucose and urea
Osmolality	A measure of the total solute concentration per kilogram of solvent
Osmolarity	A measure of the total solute concentration per liter of solution
Solute	Substance that is dissolved in a solvent
Solution	Homogeneous mixture of solutes dissolved in a solvent
Solvent	Substance that is capable of dissolving a solute (liquid or gas)
Valence	The degree of combining power of an ion

or milliequivalents per liter (mEq/L). The international standard for measuring electrolytes is mmol/L. The combining power of electrolytes is measured in mEq/L. For sodium ion (Na^+), 2.3 mg/dl (or 23 mg/L), 1 mmol/L, and 1mEq/L all refer to the same concentration of sodium. Milliequivalents equal millimoles multiplied by the valence of the ion:

$$\text{mEq/L} = \text{mmol/L} \times \text{valence}$$

The weight of an electrolyte gives no direct information regarding the number of ions or the number of charges carried by an electrolyte. Because milliequivalents express the chemical combining power of an electrolyte, ions combine milliequivalent for milliequivalent and not millimole for millimole. For example, 1 mEq (1mmol) of sodium combines with 1 mEq (1 mmol) of chloride, and 1 mEq (0.5 mmol) of calcium combines with 1 mEq (1 mmol) of chloride.

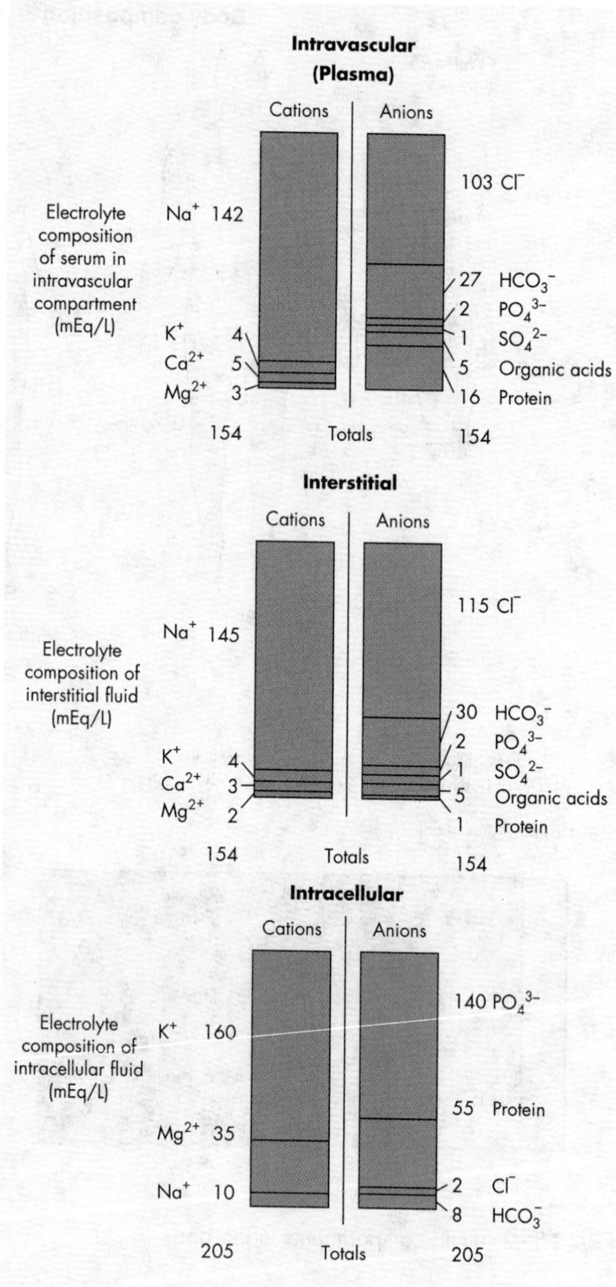

Fig. 13-3 Electrolyte content of fluid compartments.

Electrolyte Composition of Fluid Compartments

The electrolytes found in the ECF and ICF are essentially the same. However, their concentrations vary greatly between the compartments (Fig. 13-3). The primary intracellular cation is potassium, and the primary extracellular cation is sodium. The primary intracellular anion is phosphate, and the primary extracellular anion is chloride. The main difference between plasma fluid and interstitial fluid is a higher concentration of protein in the plasma.

Functions

The roles of electrolytes in cellular function include the following:

1. Regulation of water distribution
2. Transmission of nerve impulses
3. Contraction of muscle
4. Generation of adenosine triphosphate (ATP)
5. Regulation of acid-base balance
6. Clotting of blood

MECHANISMS CONTROLLING FLUID AND ELECTROLYTE MOVEMENT

Many different processes control the movement of fluid and electrolytes between the intracellular and extracellular spaces.

These processes include simple diffusion, facilitated diffusion, active transport, osmosis, hydrostatic pressure, and oncotic pressure.

Diffusion

Diffusion is the movement of molecules from an area of high concentration to one of low concentration (Fig. 13-4). It occurs in liquids, gases, and solids. Net movement of molecules stops when the concentrations are equal in both areas. The membrane separating the two areas must be permeable to the diffusing substance for the process to occur. These molecules move without external energy. Diffusion is an efficient mechanism for the movement of molecules in and out of cells.

Facilitated Diffusion

Because of the composition of cellular membranes, some molecules diffuse slowly into the cell. However, when they are combined with a specific carrier molecule, the rate of diffusion accelerates. Like simple diffusion, *facilitated diffusion* moves molecules from an area of high concentration to one of low concentration. Glucose transport into the cell is an example of facilitated diffusion. The hormone insulin increases the rate of facilitated diffusion of glucose in most tissues.

Active Transport

Active transport is a process in which molecules move in the absence of a favorable diffusion gradient. External energy is required for this process because molecules are being moved against a concentration gradient. The concentrations of sodium and potassium differ greatly intracellularly and extracellularly (see Fig. 13-3). By active transport, sodium moves out of the cell and potassium moves in to maintain this concentration difference (Fig. 13-5). The energy source for the sodium-potassium pump is ATP, which is produced in the mitochondria.

Osmosis

Osmosis, a special type of diffusion, is the flow of water between two compartments separated by a membrane permeable to water but not to a solute. Water moves through the membrane from an area of low solute concentration to an area of high solute concentration (Fig. 13-6); that is, water moves from the compartment that is more dilute (has more water) to the side that is more concentrated (has less water). The semipermeable membrane prevents movement of solute particles. Osmosis requires no outside energy sources and stops when concentration differences disappear. In addition to diffusion, osmosis is very important for maintaining the chemical stability of body cells.

Osmotic pressure, or *force,* is a term used to describe the movement of water by the process of osmosis. It can be described as a "pulling" of water. Osmotic pressure is an important factor in the movement of water between fluid compartments. Osmolarity and osmolality both measure

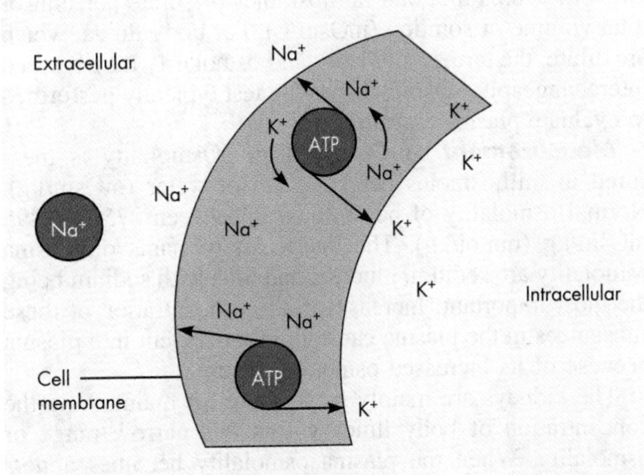

Fig. 13-5 Sodium-potassium pump. As sodium diffuses into the cell and potassium out of the cell, an active transport system supplied with energy delivers sodium back to the extracellular compartment and potassium to the intracellular compartment. *ATP,* Adenosine triphosphate.

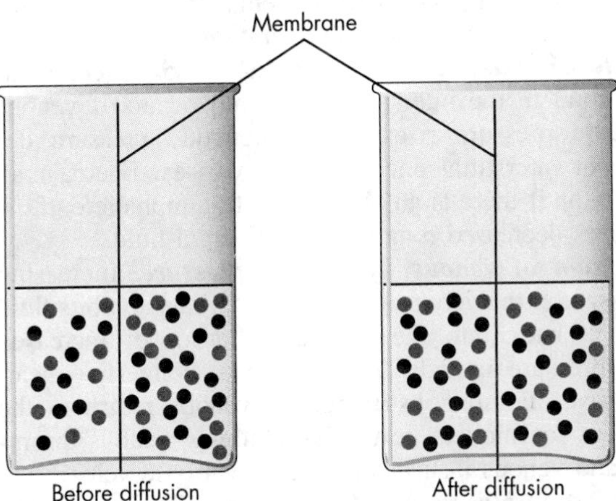

Fig. 13-4 Diffusion is the movement of molecules from an area of high concentration to an area of low concentration.

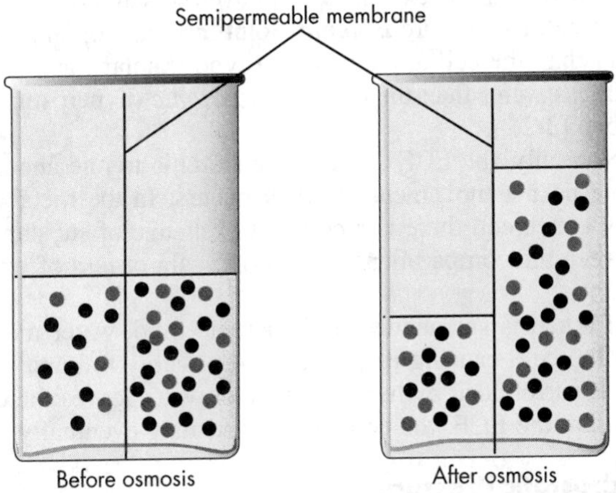

Fig. 13-6 Osmosis is the process of water movement through a semipermeable membrane from an area of low solute concentration to an area of high solute concentration.

Table 13-2 Definitions of Tonicity

Tonicity	Osmolality	Effect on Cell Size
Hypotonic	Less than 270 mOsm/kg (mmol/kg)	Swelling
Isotonic	275-295 mOsm/kg (mmol/kg)	None
Hypertonic	More than 300 mOsm/kg (mmol/kg)	Shrinking

osmotic pressure. *Osmolality* measures the osmotic force of solute per unit of weight of solvent (mOsm/kg or mmol/kg). Osmotic force is measured in units of milliosmoles. *Osmolarity* measures the total milliosmoles of solute per unit of total volume of solution (mOsm/L). For body fluids, which are dilute, the terms osmolality and osmolarity may be used interchangeably.[2] Osmolality is the test typically performed to evaluate plasma and urine.

Measurement of Osmolality. Osmolality is measured in milliosmoles per kilogram of water (mOsm/kg). Normal osmolality of body fluids is between 275 and 295 mOsm/kg (mmol/kg). The major determinants of plasma osmolality are sodium, glucose, and urea with sodium being the most important. Increases in the concentration of these substances in the plasma cause fluid movement into plasma because of its increased osmotic pressure.

The kidneys are mainly responsible for maintaining the concentration of body fluids within this narrow range of osmolality. When the plasma osmolality becomes abnormal, changes in the level of antidiuretic hormone (ADH) cause the kidneys to conserve or increase the excretion of water to return the osmolality to normal. The osmolality of urine may range from 100 to 1300 mOsm/kg (mmol/kg).

Osmotic Movement of Fluids. Cells are affected by the osmolality of the fluid that surrounds them. When fluids are added to the body, those that have the same osmolality as the cell interior are *isotonic.* Solutions that contain more water than the cell are *hypotonic* (hypoosmolar), and those with less water than the cell are *hypertonic* (hyperosmolar) (Table 13-2).

Normally, the ECF and ICF are isotonic to one another; hence no net movement of water occurs. In the metabolically active cell there is a constant exchange of substances between the compartments, but no net gain or loss of water occurs.

If a cell is surrounded by hypotonic fluid, water moves into the cell, causing it to swell and possibly to burst. If a cell is surrounded by hypertonic fluid, water leaves the cell to dilute the ECF; the cell shrinks and may eventually die.

Hydrostatic Pressure

Hydrostatic pressure is the force exerted by a fluid against the walls of its container. The heart is a main component in generating pressure in blood vessels. Hydrostatic pressure in the vascular system gradually decreases as the blood moves through the arteries until it is about 40 mm Hg at the arterial end of a capillary. Because of the size of the capillary bed and fluid movement into the interstitium, the pressure decreases to about 10 mm Hg at the venous end of the vessel. Hydrostatic pressure is the major force that moves water out of the vascular system at the capillary level.

Oncotic Pressure

Oncotic pressure (colloidal osmotic pressure) is osmotic pressure exerted by colloids in solution. In plasma, protein molecules attract water and contribute to the total osmotic pressure in the vascular system. Unlike electrolytes, the large molecular size prevents proteins from leaving the vascular space through pores in capillary walls. Plasma oncotic pressure is approximately 25 mm Hg. Some proteins are found in the interstitial space, and they exert an oncotic pressure of approximately 1 mm Hg.

FLUID MOVEMENT IN CAPILLARIES

There is normal movement of fluid between the capillary and the interstitium. The amount and direction of movement are determined by the interaction of (1) capillary hydrostatic pressure, (2) plasma oncotic pressure, (3) interstitial hydrostatic pressure, and (4) interstitial oncotic pressure.

Capillary hydrostatic pressure and interstitial oncotic pressure influence the movement of water *out of* the capillary. Plasma oncotic pressure and interstitial hydrostatic pressure attract and bring fluid *into* the capillary. At the arterial end of the capillary (Fig. 13-7), capillary hydrostatic pressure exceeds plasma oncotic pressure, and fluid is moved into the interstitium. Capillary hydrostatic pressure is lower than plasma oncotic pressure at the venous end of the capillary, and fluid is drawn back into the capillary by plasma proteins.

Fluid Shifts

If capillary or interstitial pressures are altered, fluid may abnormally shift from one compartment to another. Clinically, the two shifts of fluid seen most often are plasma-to-interstitial, seen in persons with edema; and interstitial-to-plasma, seen in persons with dehydration.

Shifts of Plasma to Interstitial Fluid. Accumulation of fluid in the interstitium (edema) occurs if venous hydrostatic pressure rises, plasma oncotic pressure decreases, or interstitial oncotic pressure rises. Edema may also develop if there is an obstruction to lymphatic outflow that causes decreased removal of interstitial fluid.

Elevation of venous hydrostatic pressure. Increasing the pressure at the venous end of the capillary inhibits fluid movement back into the capillary. Causes of increased venous pressure include fluid overload, congestive heart failure, liver failure, obstruction of venous return to the heart (e.g., tourniquets, restrictive clothing, venous thrombosis), and venous insufficiency (e.g., varicose veins).

Decrease in plasma oncotic pressure. Fluid remains in the interstitium if the plasma oncotic pressure is too low to draw fluid back into the capillary. Decreased oncotic pres-

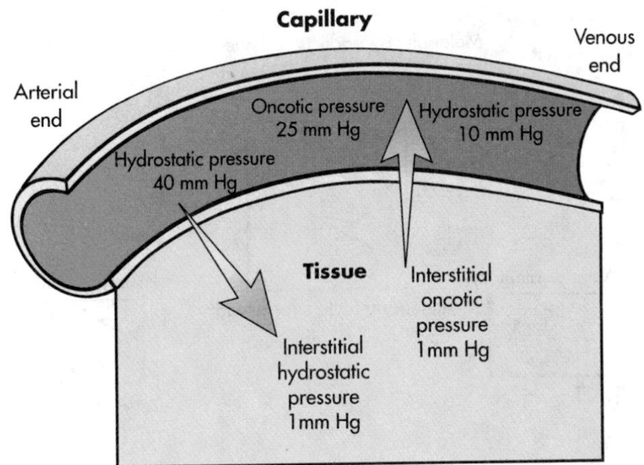

Fig. 13-7 Dynamics of fluid exchange between the capillary and the tissue. An equilibrium exists between forces filtering fluid out of the capillary and forces absorbing fluid back into the capillary. Note that the hydrostatic pressure is greater at the arterial end of the capillary than the venous end. The net effect of pressures at the arterial end of the capillary causes a movement of fluid into the tissue. At the venous end of the capillary there is net movement of fluid back into the capillary.

sure can result from excessive protein loss (nephrotic syndrome), deficient protein synthesis (liver disease), and deficient protein intake (malnutrition).

Elevation of interstitial oncotic pressure. Trauma, burns, and inflammation can damage capillary walls and allow plasma proteins to accumulate in the interstitium. The resultant increased interstitial oncotic pressure draws fluid into the interstitium and retains it there.

Shifts of Interstitial Fluid to Plasma. Fluid moves from the interstitium in abnormally large quantities whenever there is an increase in the plasma osmotic-oncotic pressure. This is often therapeutically induced by the administration of colloids, dextran, mannitol, or hypertonic solutions.

Increasing the tissue hydrostatic pressure is another way of causing a shift of fluid into plasma. The wearing of elastic wraps or hose to decrease peripheral edema is a therapeutic use of this concept.

Hypovolemic shock acutely decreases the hydrostatic pressure at the arterial and the venous ends of the capillary, causing a rapid movement of interstitial fluid into plasma. The resultant increase in vascular volume is a way to temporarily compensate for the problem.

FLUID MOVEMENT BETWEEN THE EXTRACELLULAR FLUID AND INTRACELLULAR FLUID

Changes in the osmolality of the ECF cause changes in the volume of the water in the cells. Increased ECF osmolality (hyperosmolality) results in a shift of water out of the cells until equilibrium between the two compartments is reached. Hyperosmolality occurs when there is an increase in the ECF sodium or glucose levels. Conditions associated with ECF hyperosmolality present neurologic symptoms caused by altered central nervous system (CNS) function as brain cells shrink. Decreased ECF osmolality (hypoosmolality) develops as the result of gain or retention of excess water. Again, the primary symptoms are neurologic as a result of brain cell swelling as water shifts into the cells.

REGULATION OF FLUID AND ELECTROLYTES

Hypothalamic Regulation

Water ingestion in the conscious patient is regulated by the thirst receptors located in the hypothalamus. The thirst mechanism is stimulated by hypotension and increased serum osmolality. An intact thirst mechanism is critical because it is the primary protection against the development of hyperosmolality. The patient who cannot recognize or act on the sensation of thirst is at risk for fluid deficit and hyperosmolality. The sensitivity of the thirst mechanism decreases in the elderly patient.

The desire to consume fluids is also affected by social and psychologic factors not related to fluid balance. A dry mouth will cause the patient to drink, even when there is no measurable body water deficit. Water ingestion will equal water excretion in the individual who has free access to water, a normal thirst and ADH mechanism, and normally functioning kidneys.

Pituitary Regulation

The posterior pituitary releases ADH, which regulates water retention by the kidneys. The distal tubules and collecting ducts in the kidneys respond to ADH by becoming more permeable to water so that water is reabsorbed into the blood and not excreted. Normally an increase in plasma osmolality or a decrease in circulating volume will stimulate ADH secretion. When there is a normal plasma osmolality and normal circulating plasma volume, continued ADH secretion is called *syndrome of inappropriate antidiuretic hormone* (SIADH) (see Chapter 47). Causes of SIADH include stress, trauma, tumors, surgery, ventilation with a positive-pressure ventilator, and certain drugs. The inappropriate ADH causes water retention, which produces a decrease in plasma osmolality below the normal value and an increase in urine osmolality with a decrease in volume.

Reduction in the release or action of ADH produces diabetes insipidus (see Chapter 47). A copious amount of dilute urine is excreted because the renal tubules and collecting ducts do not appropriately reabsorb water. The patient with diabetes insipidus exhibits extreme polyuria and, if alert, polydipsia. Symptoms of dehydration and hypernatremia develop if the water losses are not adequately replaced.

Adrenal Cortical Regulation

ECF volume is maintained by a combination of hormonal influences. ADH affects only water reabsorption. Hormones released by the adrenal cortex help regulate both water and electrolytes. Two groups of hormones secreted by the adrenal cortex include glucocorticoids and mineralocorticoids. The glucocorticoids primarily have an antiinflamma-

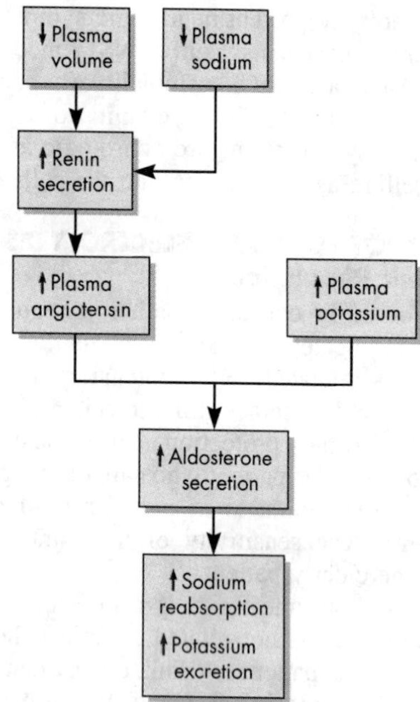

Fig. 13-8 Influences of aldosterone secretion.

tory effect and increase serum glucose levels, whereas the mineralocorticoids (e.g., aldosterone) enhance sodium retention and potassium excretion (Fig. 13-8). When sodium is reabsorbed, water follows as a result of osmotic changes.

Cortisol is the most common example of a naturally occurring adrenocorticosteroid. In large doses, cortisol has both glucocorticoid (antiinflammatory) and mineralocorticoid (sodium-retention) properties. The adrenocortical hormone cortisol is secreted whenever the body experiences stress. Many body systems, including fluid and electrolyte balance, are affected by stress (Fig. 13-9).

Aldosterone is the naturally occurring mineralocorticoid with the most potent sodium-retention and potassium-excreting capability. The secretion of aldosterone is stimulated by a decrease in plasma volume, renal perfusion, or serum sodium. The kidneys respond by secreting renin into the plasma. Angiotensinogen produced in the liver and normally found in blood is acted on by the renin to form angiotensin I, which converts to angiotensin II, which stimulates the adrenal cortex to secrete aldosterone (Fig. 13-8). An increase in plasma potassium directly stimulates the adrenal cortex to secrete aldosterone.

Renal Regulation

The primary organs for regulating fluid and electrolyte balance are the kidneys (see Chapter 42). The kidneys regulate water balance through adjustments in urine volume. Similarly, urinary excretion of most electrolytes is adjusted so that a balance is maintained between overall intake and output. The total plasma volume is filtered by the kidneys many times each day. In the average adult the kidney reabsorbs 99% of this filtrate, producing approximately 1.5 L of urine per day. As the filtrate moves through

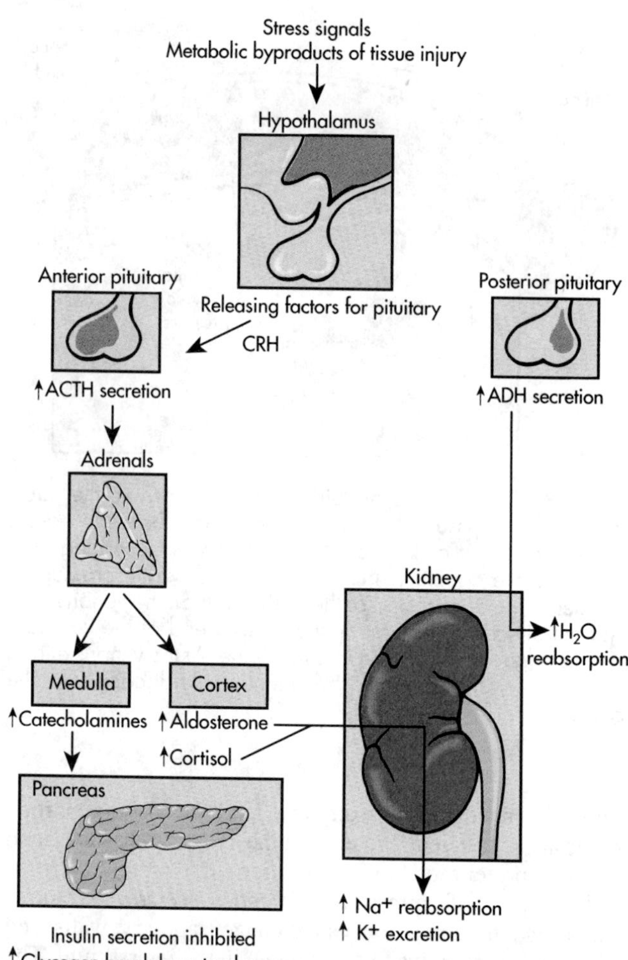

Fig. 13-9 Effects of stress on fluid and electrolyte balance. *ACTH*, Adrenocorticotropic hormone; *ADH*, antidiuretic hormone; *CRH*, corticotropin releasing hormone.

the renal tubule, selective reabsorption of water and electrolytes and secretion of electrolytes result in the production of urine that is greatly different in composition and concentration than the plasma. This process helps maintain normal plasma osmolality, electrolyte balance, blood volume, and acid-base balance. The renal tubules are the site for the hormonal action of ADH and aldosterone.

With severely impaired renal function, the kidneys cannot maintain fluid and electrolyte balance. This condition results in edema, potassium and phosphorus retention, acidosis, and other electrolyte imbalances (see Chapter 44). Renal function is typically decreased in the elderly person, placing the patient at increased risk for fluid and electrolyte imbalances. In particular, the ability to concentrate urine may be reduced in the older adult.[3]

Gastrointestinal Regulation

Daily water intake and output are between 2000 and 3000 ml (Table 13-3). The gastrointestinal tract accounts for most

Table 13-3 Normal Fluid Balance in the Adult

Intake	
Fluids	1200 ml
Solid food	1000 ml
Water from oxidation	300 ml
	2500 ml
Output	
Insensible loss (skin and lungs)	900 ml
In feces	100 ml
Urine	1500 ml
	2500 ml

Table 13-4 Normal Serum Electrolyte Values

Anions	Normal Value
Bicarbonate (HCO_3^-)	20-30 mEq/L (20-30 mmol/L)
Chloride (Cl^-)	96-106 mEq/L (96-106 mmol/L)
Phosphate (PO_4^{3-})	2.8-4.5 mg/dl (0.90-1.45 mmol/L)
Protein	6-8 g/dl (60-80 g/L)

Cations	Normal Value
Potassium (K^+)	3.5-5.5 mEq/L (3.5-5.5 mmol/L)
Magnesium (Mg^{2+})	1.5-2.5 mEq/L (0.75-1.25 mmol/L)
Sodium (Na^+)	135-145 mEq/L (135-145 mmol/L)
Calcium (Ca^{2+})	9-11 mg/dl 4.5-5.5 mEq/L (2.25-2.75 mmol/L)

of the water intake. Water intake includes fluids, water from food metabolism, and water present in solid foods. Lean meat is approximately 70% water, whereas the water content of many fruits and vegetables approaches 100%.

Most of the body water is excreted by the kidneys. A small amount of water is eliminated by the GI tract in feces.

Insensible Water Loss

Insensible water loss, which is unavoidable vaporization from the lungs and skin, assists in regulating body temperature. Normally, about 900 ml per day is lost. The amount of water loss is increased by accelerated body metabolism, which occurs with increased body temperature and exercise.

Insensible perspiration should not be confused with the vaporization of water excreted by sweat glands. Only water is lost by insensible perspiration. Excessive sweating (perspiration) caused by fever or high environmental temperatures may lead to large losses of water and electrolytes.

FLUID AND ELECTROLYTE IMBALANCES

Fluid and electrolyte imbalances occur to some degree in most patients with a major illness or injury because illness disrupts the normal homeostatic mechanism. Some fluid and electrolyte imbalances are directly caused by illness or disease (e.g., burns, congestive heart failure). At other times, therapeutic measures (e.g., intravenous fluid replacement, diuretics) cause or contribute to fluid and electrolyte imbalances.

The imbalances are commonly classified as *deficits* or *excesses*. Each imbalance is discussed separately. (For normal values, see Table 13-4.) In actual clinical situations, more than one imbalance found in the same patient is common. For example, a patient with prolonged nasogastric suction will lose Na^+, K^+, H^+, and Cl^-. These imbalances may result in a deficiency of both sodium and potassium, as well as metabolic alkalosis and fluid volume deficit.

SODIUM AND VOLUME IMBALANCES

Sodium plays a major role in maintaining the concentration and volume of the ECF. Sodium is the main cation of the ECF and the primary determinant of ECF osmolality. Sodium imbalances are typically associated with parallel changes in osmolality. Because of its impact on osmolality, sodium affects the water distribution between the ECF and the ICF. Sodium is also important in the generation and transmission of nerve impulses and the regulation of acid-base balance. Serum sodium is measured in milliequivalents per liter (mEq/L) or millimoles per liter (mmol/L).

The GI tract absorbs sodium from foods. Typically, daily intake of sodium far exceeds the body's daily requirements. Sodium leaves the body through urine, sweat, and feces. The kidneys are the primary regulator of sodium balance. Urinary excretion of excess sodium is adjusted in part through the action of aldosterone. The kidneys regulate the ECF concentration of sodium by excreting or retaining water under the influence of ADH. The serum sodium level reflects the ratio of sodium to water, not necessarily the loss or gain of sodium. Thus changes in the serum sodium level may reflect either a primary water imbalance, primary sodium imbalance, or a combination of the two. Sodium imbalances are typically associated with imbalances in ECF volume (Figs. 13-10 and 13-11).

Hypernatremia

Common causes of hypernatremia are listed in Table 13-5. An elevated serum sodium may occur with water loss or sodium gain. Because sodium is the major determinant of the ECF osmolality, hypernatremia causes hyperosmolality. In turn, hyperosmolality causes a shift of water out of the cells, which leads to cellular dehydration.

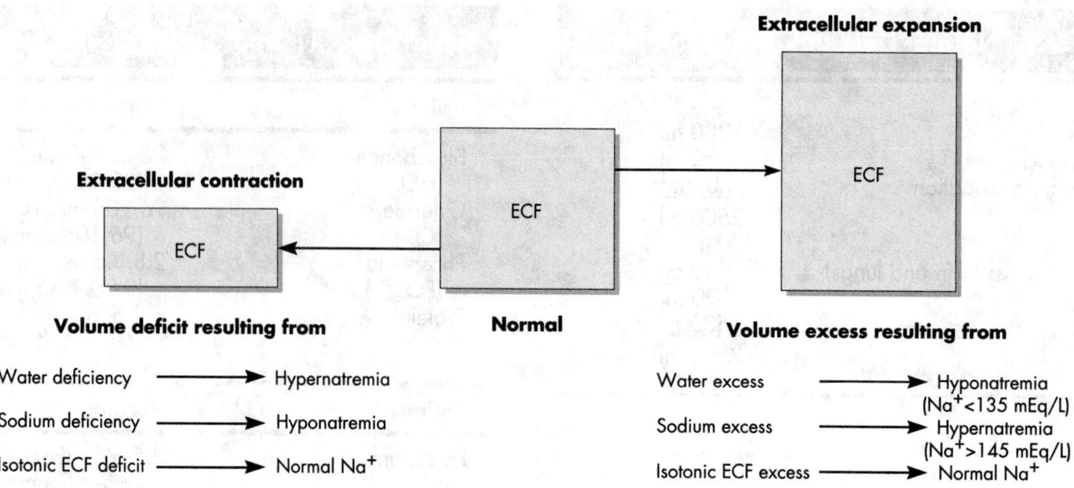

Fig. 13-10 Differential assessment of extracellular fluid (ECF) volume.

As discussed earlier, the primary protection against the development of hyperosmolality is thirst. As the plasma osmolality increases, the thirst center in the hypothalamus is stimulated, and the individual seeks fluids. Although increased release of ADH is another important protective response to hypernatremia, thirst provides the ultimate defense.[1]

Hypernatremia is not a problem in an alert person who has access to water, is able to swallow, and can sense thirst. Water deficiency is often the result of an impaired level of consciousness or an inability to obtain fluids. The infant is at risk because of an inability to adequately express thirst. Often the older adult, especially if ill, does not drink enough fluids because of a reduction in the sensitivity of the thirst center and an inability to access water.

Several clinical states can produce water loss and hypernatremia. A deficiency in the synthesis or a release of ADH from the posterior pituitary gland (central diabetes insipidus) or a decrease in kidney responsiveness to ADH (nephrogenic diabetes insipidus) can result in profound diuresis resulting in a water deficit and hypernatremia. More common causes include concentrated tube feedings used in unconscious patients and osmotic diuresis, which

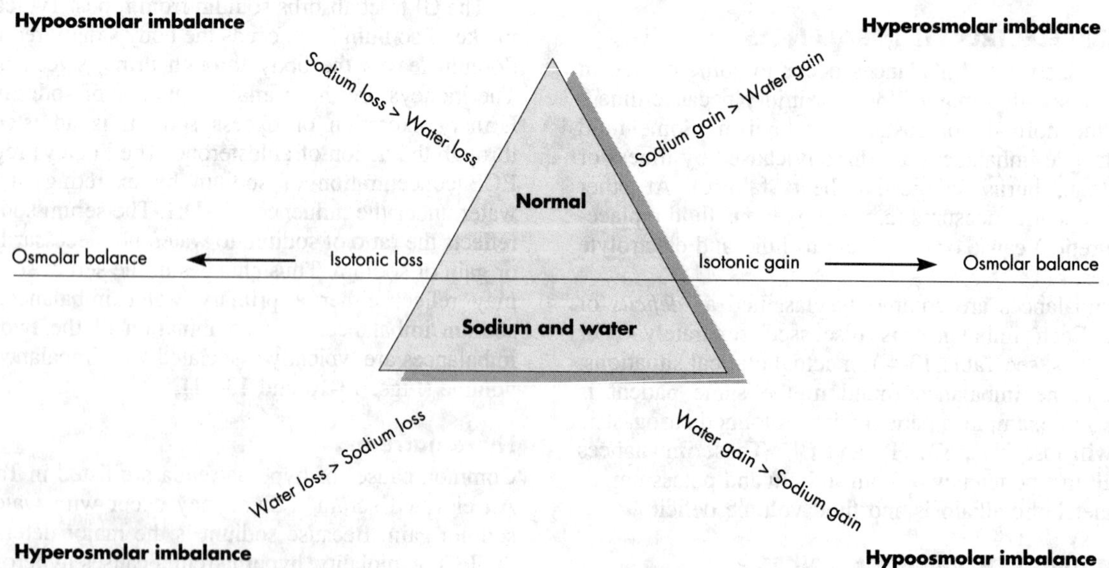

Fig. 13-11 Isotonic gains and losses affect mainly the extracellular fluid (ECF) compartment with little or no water movement into the cells. Hypertonic imbalances cause water to move from inside the cell into the ECF to dilute the concentrated sodium, causing cell shrinkage. Hypotonic imbalances cause water to move into the cell, causing cell swelling.

Table 13-5 Sodium Imbalances: Causes and Clinical Manifestations

Hyponatremia (Na^+ <135mEq/L [mmol/L])	Hypernatremia (Na^+ >145mEq/L [mmol/L])
Causes	
Sodium Loss	***Water Loss***
GI losses: Diarrhea, vomiting, fistulas, NG suction	Increased insensible water loss or perspiration (high fever, heatstroke)
Renal losses: Diuretics, adrenal insufficiency, Na^+ wasting renal disease	Diabetes insipidus
Skin losses: Burns, wound drainage	Osmotic diuresis
Water Gain	***Sodium Gain***
SIADH	IV hypertonic NaCl
Congestive heart failure	IV sodium bicarbonate
Excessive hypotonic IV fluids	IV excessive isotonic NaCl
Primary polydipsia	Primary aldosteronism
	Saltwater near drowning
Clinical Manifestations	
Decreased ECF Volume (Sodium Loss)	***Decreased ECF Volume (Water Loss)***
Irritability, apprehension, confusion	Intense thirst, dry, swollen tongue
Postural hypotension	Restlessness, agitation, twitching
Tachycardia	Seizures, coma
Rapid, thready pulse	Weakness
Decreased CVP	Postural hypotension, decreased CVP
Decreased jugular venous filling	Weight loss
Nausea, vomiting	
Dry mucous membranes	
Weight loss	
Tremors, seizures, coma	
Normal or Increased ECF Volume (Water Gain)	***Normal or Increased ECF Volume (Sodium Gain)***
Headache, lassitude, apathy, weakness, confusion	Intense thirst
Nausea, vomiting	Restlessness, agitation, twitching
Weight gain	Seizures, coma
Increased blood pressure, increased CVP	Flushed skin
Muscle spasms, convulsions, coma	Weight gain
	Peripheral and pulmonary edema
	Increased blood pressures, increased CVP

CVP, Central venous pressure; *ECF*, extracellular fluid; *GI*, gastrointestinal; *IV*, intravenous; *NG*, nasogastric; *SIADH*, syndrome of inappropriate antidiuretic hormone.

occurs with hyperglycemia (uncontrolled diabetes mellitus) or after the administration of osmotic diuretics (mannitol). Other causes include insensible loss with high fever and diarrhea in infants. Excessive sweating without water replacement also leads to hypernatremia.

Sodium intake in excess of water intake can also result in hypernatremia. Examples of sodium gain include intravenous administration of hypertonic saline or sodium bicarbonate, use of sodium-containing medications, excessive oral intake of sodium (ingestion of sea water), or primary aldosteronism caused by a tumor of the adrenal glands.

The clinical manifestations of hypernatremia are listed in Table 13-5. Symptoms are primarily the result of changes in the plasma osmolality that lead to changes in the volume of cellular water. Dehydration of cerebral cells leads to neurologic manifestations such as intense thirst, lethargy, agitation, seizures, and even coma. Sodium excess also has a direct effect on the irritability and conduction of nerve cells, causing them to be more easily excited. Patients with hypernatremia will also exhibit the symptoms of any accompanying volume imbalance.

Therapeutic Management. The goal of treatment in hypernatremia that is caused by either water loss or sodium gain is to treat the underlying cause. In primary water deficit the continued water loss must be prevented, and water replacement must be provided. If oral fluids cannot be ingested, intravenous solutions of 5% dextrose in water or hypotonic saline may be given initially. Serum sodium levels must be reduced gradually to prevent too rapid a shift of water back into the cells.

The goal of treatment for sodium excess is to dilute the sodium concentration and to promote excretion of the excess sodium. Intravenous solutions of 5% dextrose in water are usually given in combination with diuretics. Sodium intake will also be restricted. See Chapter 47 for specific treatment of diabetes insipidus.

Hyponatremia

Hyponatremia may result from loss of sodium containing fluids or from water excess. Hyponatremia causes hypoosmolality with a shift of water into the cells.

Common causes of hyponatremia caused by water excess are inappropriate use of sodium-free or hypotonic intravenous (IV) fluids especially after surgery or major trauma, after unchecked fluid intake in patients with renal failure, or with psychiatric disorders associated with excessive water intake. SIADH will result in dilutional hyponatremia caused by abnormal retention of water. Refer to Chapter 47 for a discussion of the causes of SIADH.

Losses of sodium-rich body fluids (caused by abnormal GI tract, kidney, or skin losses) alone will not result in hyponatremia because these are either isotonic or hypotonic fluids; that is, sodium is lost with an equal or greater proportion of water. However, the physiologic response to this volume loss (i.e., release of ADH and thirst) can lead to the development of hyponatremia as a result of retention of water.[4]

Clinical manifestations of water excess include rapid weight gain, decreased hematocrit, and increased central venous pressure (CVP). Neurologic symptoms develop with hyponatremia that is caused by a reduction in the plasma osmolality with a shift of water into brain cells. The clinical manifestations of hyponatremia are listed in Table 13-5.

Therapeutic Management. In hyponatremia that is caused by water excess, fluid restriction is often all that is needed to treat the problem. If severe symptoms (convulsions) develop, small amounts of intravenous hypertonic saline solution (3% NaCl) are given to restore the serum sodium level while the body is returning to a normal water balance. Treatment of hyponatremia associated with abnormal fluid loss includes fluid replacement with sodium-containing solutions. Replacing losses with commercially available oral rehydration fluids containing electrolytes instead of water may help prevent the development of hyponatremia.

Extracellular Fluid Volume Imbalances

ECF volume deficit (hypovolemia) and *ECF volume excess* (hypervolemia) are commonly occurring clinical conditions (Table 13-6). ECF fluid volume imbalances are typically accompanied by one or more electrolyte imbalances. As previously discussed, volume imbalances are often associated with changes in the serum sodium level. Fluid volume deficit can occur with abnormal loss of body fluids (e.g., diarrhea, fistula drainage, hemorrhage), decreased intake, or a plasma-to-interstitial fluid shift. Fluid volume excess may result from excessive intake of fluids, abnormal retention of fluids (e.g., congestive heart failure, renal failure), or interstitial-to-plasma fluid shift. Although shifts in fluid between the plasma and interstitium do not alter the overall volume of the ECF, these shifts do result in changes in the clinically important intravascular volume.

Therapeutic Management. The goal of treatment for fluid volume deficit is to correct the underlying cause and to replace both water and electrolytes. Balanced IV solutions, such as lactated Ringer's solution, are usually given. Isotonic sodium chloride is used when rapid volume replacement is indicated. Blood is administered when volume loss is due to blood loss.

Table 13-6 Causes of ECF Volume Imbalances

ECF Volume Deficit	ECF Volume Excess
Increased Loss	**Increased Retention**
Vomiting	Congestive heart failure
Diarrhea	Cushing's syndrome
Fistula drainage	Chronic liver disease with portal hypertension
GI tract suction	Long-term use of corticosteroids
Excessive sweating	Renal failure
Fever	
Third-space fluid shifts (e.g., burns, intestinal obstruction)	
Overuse of diuretics	
Hemorrhage	
Decreased Intake	**Increased Intake**
Nausea	Rare with adequate renal function
Anorexia	Excessive IV administration of fluids
Inability to drink	
Inability to obtain water	

ECF, Extracellular fluid; *GI,* gastrointestinal; *IV,* intravenous.

The goal of treatment for fluid volume excess is removal of sodium and water without producing abnormal changes in the electrolyte composition or osmolality of ECF. The primary cause needs to be identified and treated. Intravenous therapy is usually not indicated for this type of fluid imbalance. Diuretics and fluid restriction are the primary forms of therapy. Restricton of sodium intake may also be indicated. If the fluid excess leads to ascites or pleural effusion, an abdominal paracentesis or thoracentesis may be necessary.

NURSING MANAGEMENT

SODIUM AND VOLUME IMBALANCES

Nursing Diagnoses

Nursing diagnoses and collaborative problems specific to the patient with various fluid and sodium imbalances include, but are not limited to, the following:

Extracellular fluid volume excess

- ECF volume excess related to increased sodium and water retention
- Risk for impaired skin integrity related to edema
- Body image disturbance related to altered body appearance secondary to edema
- Potential complications: pulmonary edema, ascites

Extracellular fluid volume deficit

- Fluid volume deficit related to excessive ECF losses or decreased fluid intake
- Potential complication: hypovolemic shock

Hypernatremia

Risk for injury related to altered sensorium and seizures secondary to abnormal CNS function

Hyponatremia

Risk for injury related to altered sensorium and decreased loss of consciousness secondary to abnormal CNS function

Nursing Implementation

Intake and Output. The use of 24-hour intake and output records gives valuable information regarding fluid and electrolyte problems. Sources of excessive intake or fluid losses can be identified on a properly recorded intake-and-output flowsheet. Intake should include oral, intravenous and tube feedings, and retained irrigants. Output includes urine, excess perspiration, wound or tube drainage, vomitus, and diarrhea. Fluid loss from wounds and perspiration should be estimated. Urine specific gravity measurements can be done. Readings of greater than 1.025 indicate a concentrated urine, whereas those of less than 1.010 indicate a dilute urine.

Vital Signs. Signs and symptoms of ECF volume excess and deficit are reflected in changes in blood pressure, heart rate, respiratory rate, central venous pressure (CVP) readings, and lung sounds. In fluid volume excess, tachycardia secondary to sympathetic CNS stimulation occurs. The pulse is rapid and bounding. Because of the expanded intravascular volume, the pulse is not easily obliterated. The respiratory rate is increased. Blood pressure is usually elevated secondary to the increased volume, along with CVP. With pulmonary congestion and edema, the patient will experience shortness of breath, and moist crackles will be heard.

In fluid volume deficit, vital signs are similar to those seen in shock. Compensatory mechanisms for a decrease in intravascular volume include sympathetic CNS stimulation of the heart and peripheral vasoconstriction. Stimulation of the heart increases heart rate and, combined with vasoconstriction, maintains blood pressure within normal limits. If vasoconstriction and tachycardia provide inadequate compensation, hypotension occurs secondary to the reduced volume. Because of reduced intravascular volume, the pulse is weak, thready, and easily obliterated. The decreased volume is also reflected in a lowered CVP. Respiratory rate increases as a result of decreased tissue perfusion and hypoxia.

Neurologic Changes. Changes in neurologic function may occur with sodium and water imbalances. With increased water volume and hyponatremia, water moves by osmosis into the brain cells. Alternatively, decreased water volume and hypernatremia cause water to shift out of the cerebral cells with resultant shrinkage.

Assessment of neurologic function includes evaluation of (1) the level of consciousness, which includes responses to verbal and painful stimuli and the determination of a person's orientation to time, place, and person; (2) pupillary response to light and equality of pupil size; and (3) voluntary movement of the extremities, degree of muscle strength, and reflexes.

Daily Weights. Accurate daily weights provide the best bedside measurement of volume status. An increase of 1 kg is equal to 1000 ml fluid retention (provided the person has maintained usual dietary intake or has not been on NPO status). However, weight changes can be relied on only if obtained under standardized conditions. An accurate weight requires the patient to be weighed at the same time every day and on the same carefully calibrated scale. Excess clothing and bedding should be removed and all drainage bags should be emptied before the weighing. If bulky dressings or tubes are present, which may not necessarily be used every day, a notation regarding these variables should be recorded on the flowsheet or nursing notes.

Skin Assessment and Care. Clues to fluid volume deficit and excess can be detected by inspection of the skin. Skin should be examined for turgor and mobility. Normally a fold of skin, when pinched, will readily move and, on release, will rapidly return to its former position. Skin areas over the sternum, abdomen, and anterior forearm are the usual sites for evaluation of tissue turgor (Fig. 13-12).

In fluid volume deficit, skin turgor is diminished; there is a lag in the pinched skin fold's return to its original state. The skin may be cool and moist if there is sympathetic vasoconstriction to compensate for the decreased fluid volume. Mild hypovolemia usually does not stimulate this compensatory response; consequently, the skin will be warm and dry. Volume deficit may also cause the skin to appear dry and wrinkled. These signs may be difficult to evaluate in the older adult because the patient's skin may be normally dry, wrinkled, and nonelastic.

Skin that is edematous may feel cool because of fluid accumulation and a decrease in blood flow secondary to the pressure of the fluid. The fluid can also stretch the skin causing it to feel taut and hard. *Edema* is assessed by pressing

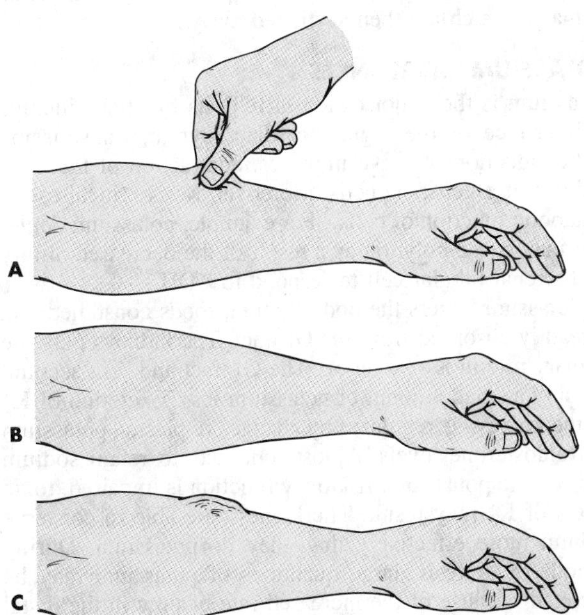

Fig. 13-12 Assessment of skin turgor. ***A*** and ***B***, When normal skin is pinched, it resumes shape in seconds. ***C***, If the skin remains wrinkled for 20 to 30 seconds, the patient has poor skin turgor.

with a thumb or forefinger over the edematous area. A grading scale is used to standardize the description if an indentation (ranging from 1+ [slight, 2 mm indentation] to 4+ [pitting, 8 mm indentation]) remains when pressure is released. The areas to be evaluated for edema are those where soft tissues overlie a bone. Skin areas over the tibia, fibula, and sacrum are the preferred sites.

Good skin care for the person with fluid volume excess or deficit is important. Edematous tissues need to be protected from extremes of heat and cold, prolonged pressure, and trauma. Frequent skin care and changes in position will protect the patient from skin breakdown. Elevation of edematous extremities helps promote venous return. Dehydrated skin needs frequent care without the use of soap. The application of moisturizing creams or oils will increase moisture retention and stimulate circulation.

Other Nursing Measures. The rates of infusion of intravenous fluid solutions should be carefully monitored. Attempts to "catch up" should be approached with extreme caution, particularly when large volumes of fluid or certain electrolytes are involved. This is especially true in patients with cardiac, renal, or neurologic problems. The nurse needs to encourage and often assist the older or debilitated patient to maintain an adequate oral intake. Patients receiving tube feedings need supplementary water added to their enteral formula.

The patient with nasogastric suction should not be allowed to drink water because it will increase the loss of electrolytes. Occasionally the patient may be given small amounts of ice chips to suck. A nasogastric tube should always be irrigated with isotonic saline solution and not with water. Water causes diffusion of electrolytes into the stomach, which are then suctioned away.

POTASSIUM IMBALANCES

Potassium is the major cation in ICF. Its functions include maintenance of the regular cardiac rhythm, transmission and conduction of nerve impulses, contraction of muscles, and use of glucose by cells. Moreover, K^+ is critical to the metabolic function of cells.[5] For example, potassium depletion may cause polyuria as a result of the decreased ability of the renal tubular cell to respond to ADH.

Potassium enters the body through foods consumed and is readily absorbed from the GI tract. The kidneys play the primary role in K^+ excretion. The GI tract and skin account for only a small amount of potassium loss. Excretion of K^+ by the kidneys is regulated by changes in plasma potassium and aldosterone levels. Aldosterone acts to retain sodium and excrete potassium. If kidney function is impaired, toxic levels of K^+ may result. The kidneys are able to conserve sodium more effectively than they do potassium. During periods of diuresis, large quantities of potassium may be excreted because of the increased rate of flow in the distal renal tubule.

The vast majority of the body's K^+ is located in the cells. The distribution of K^+ between the cells and ECF will affect potassium balance. Factors that maintain normal distribution include the sodium-potassium pump, insulin, catecholamines, and the plasma K^+ level. Factors that may adversely affect distribution include extracellular pH, cell breakdown, and certain chronic diseases. The laboratory measurement of potassium determines the amount of potassium in serum and reflects the ECF concentration. Because ECF potassium is only a small portion of total body potassium, it is only an indirect indicator of the level of intracellular K^+. Causes of potassium imbalance are presented in Table 13-7.

Hyperkalemia

Hyperkalemia may develop after massive cell destruction (e.g., burns or a crush injury), rapid transfusion of aged blood, and massive catabolic states (e.g., severe infections) that result in the release of intracellular K^+ into the ECF. Increased intake or decreased excretion (renal failure) of potassium also elevates serum potassium levels. Metabolic acidosis causes a shift of K^+ from the ICF to the ECF as hydrogen ions move into the cell and K^+ exits. The resultant hyperkalemia is corrected either by increased renal excretion of K^+ or by correction of the acidosis. Acute insulin deficiency (uncontrolled diabetes mellitus) will also cause a shift of K^+ out of the cells. Adrenal insufficiency leads to retention of K^+ in the serum because of aldosterone deficiency.

Clinical Manifestations. Hyperkalemia initially increases cell excitability but eventually produces muscle weakness because of persistent neuromuscular depolarization. Cardiac cells demonstrate the most clinically significant changes with potassium imbalances because of changes in cardiac conduction. Figure 13-13 illustrates the electrocardiographic (ECG) effects of hypokalemia and hyperkalemia. Clinical manifestations of hyperkalemia include cardiac dysrhythmias, muscle twitching, seizures, cramping pain, and diarrhea. Other clinical manifestations are listed in Table 13-7.

THERAPEUTIC AND NURSING MANAGEMENT

HYPERKALEMIA

Nursing Diagnoses

Nursing diagnoses and collaborative problems specific to the patient with hyperkalemia include, but are not limited to, the following:

- Risk for injury related to muscle twitching and seizures
- Potential complication: dysrhythmias

Nursing Implementation

Treatment of hyperkalemia consists of the following:

1. Decrease in dietary sources of potassium (see Table 44-8)
2. Administration of IV sodium bicarbonate
3. Administration of calcium gluconate
4. IV infusion of glucose and insulin
5. Use of cation exchange resin (Kayexalate)
6. Dialysis

Table 13-7 Potassium Imbalances: Causes and Clinical Manifestations

Hypokalemia (K^+ <3.5 mEg/L [mmol/L])	Hyperkalemia (K^+ >5.5 mEg/L [mmol/L])
Causes	
Vomiting	Renal failure
Diarrhea	Early stage of burns
Potent diuretics	Adrenal insufficiency
Aldosterone-producing tumor	Massive crushing injury
Potassium-free IV solutions	Excess IV administration of K^+
Recovery phase of diabetic acidosis	Metabolic acidosis
Fistulas	
Metabolic alkalosis	
Anorexia	
Starvation	
Malnutrition	
Appearance	
Drowsiness	No specific findings
Behavior	
Confusion	No alteration in mentation
Irritability	Irritability
Lethargy	
Depression	
Cardiovascular	
ECG changes	ECG changes
ST depression	Peaked T waves
T wave inversion *or* flattening	PR interval prolongation
	Disappearance of P wave
U waves	Widening of QRS
Cardiovascular—cont'd	
Bradycardia, first- and second-degree heart block, atrial dysrhythmias	Complete heart block
	Ectopic beats
	Ventricular fibrillation → ventricular standstill
PVCs, especially for patients on digitalis	
Postural hypotension	
Gastrointestinal	
Anorexia, nausea	Nausea
Paralytic ileus	Vomiting
Constipation	Cramping pain
	Diarrhea
Neuromuscular	
Hyporeflexia	Twitching
Muscle weakness→paralysis	Seizures
	Paresthesias
Muscle cramps and paresthesias	Paralysis when severe
Urinary Findings	
Urinary output ↑	Urine potassium ↑
Specific gravity ↓	
May have decreased output because of urinary retention	
Serum Values	
Serum potassium ↓	Serum potassium ↑
pH ↑	pH ↓

ECG, Electrocardiogram; *IV*, intravenous; *PVC*, premature ventricular contractions.

Sodium bicarbonate corrects acidosis and facilitates potassium movement into the ICF. Calcium stabilizes cell membranes and antagonizes the effect of potassium on the heart. Glucose and insulin infusion may be used in the acute management of symptomatic hyperkalemia because insulin enhances the movement of potassium into the cell. Kayexalate binds potassium in exchange for sodium, and the resin is excreted in feces (see Chapter 44). Hemodialysis is the most effective means of removing potassium from the body.

Hypokalemia

Hypokalemia (low serum potassium) can result from loss of potassium in intestinal tract fluids, excretion in urine, or a shift of potassium from the ECF to the ICF. Metabolic alkalosis causes potassium to move intracellularly in exchange for hydrogen ions. This type of hypokalemia will usually correct itself with treatment of the alkalosis.

Hypokalemia is often associated with the treatment of diabetic ketoacidosis because of a combination of factors, including an increased urinary loss of potassium and a shift of potassium into cells with the administration of insulin and correction of acidosis. When glucose and insulin move intracellularly, potassium moves with them, thus decreasing the ECF potassium. Causes of hypokalemia (reflecting a decrease in total body potassium) include diuretic therapy, increased aldosterone secretion, stress, and GI tract losses from diarrhea, vomiting, and ileostomy drainage.

Extreme malnutrition and starvation can also cause hypokalemia by decreasing potassium intake. Anabolic states of cell repair lower extracellular potassium as it moves into the cell.

Clinical Manifestations. Hypokalemia enhances automaticity and delays repolarization of cardiac cells. The net result of these changes is an increased risk of dysrhythmias. Hypokalemia has been implicated in some cases of sudden cardiac death in persons with compromised cardiac function. Muscle weakness and paralysis may also occur with hypokalemia. The likelihood of symptoms is related to the level of hypokalemia and how quickly it developed. Clinical manifestations are presented in Table 13-7.

THERAPEUTIC AND NURSING MANAGEMENT

HYPOKALEMIA

Nursing Diagnoses

Nursing diagnoses and collaborative problems specific to the patient with hypokalemia include, but are not limited to, the following:

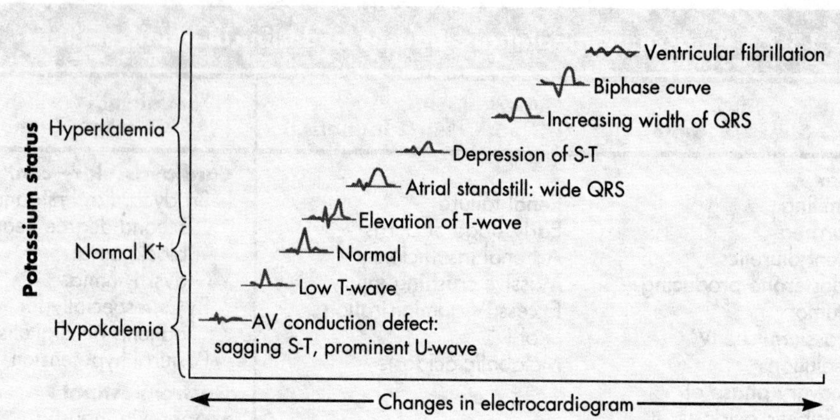

Fig. 13-13 Electrocardiogram changes associated with alterations in potassium status.

- Risk for injury related to muscle weakness and hyporeflexia
- Potential complication: dysrhythmias

Nursing Implementation

Hypokalemia is treated by giving potassium chloride supplements and increasing dietary intake of potassium. Potassium chloride (KCl) supplements can be given orally or intravenously. Except in severe deficiencies, KCl is never given unless there is urine output of at least 0.5 ml/kg body weight per hour. KCl supplements added to IV solutions should never exceed 60 mEq/L. The preferred level is 40 mEq/L. The rate of IV administration of KCl should not exceed 10 to 20 mEq per hour to prevent hyperkalemia and cardiac arrest. When given intravenously, potassium may cause pain in the area of the vein where it is entering. Central IV lines should be used when rapid correction of hypokalemia is necessary. Potassium may also be replaced with potassium phosphate.

The patient who is taking diuretics (especially thiazide and loop diuretics) should be aware of the need to increase dietary potassium intake (Table 44-8). It may be necessary for the patient to take oral KCl supplements or salt substitutes that contain potassium. The patient should be taught which foods are high in potassium. The patient should also be instructed to recognize the clinical manifestations of hypokalemia and to report them to the health care provider. If a patient is also taking digitalis preparations, the serum potassium level must be closely monitored because hypokalemia enhances the action of digitalis.

CALCIUM IMBALANCES

Calcium is obtained from ingested foods. However, only about 30% is absorbed in the gastrointestinal tract. More than 99% of the body's calcium is combined with phosphorus and concentrated in the skeletal system. Bones serve as a readily available store of calcium. Thus wide variations in serum calcium levels are avoided. Usually the amount of calcium and phosphorus found in the serum has an inverse relationship; that is, as one increases, the other decreases. The functions of calcium include transmission of nerve impulses, cardiac contractions, blood clotting, formation of teeth and bone, and muscle contraction.

Calcium is present in the serum in three forms: free or ionized, bound to protein (primarily albumin), and complexed with phosphate, citrate, or carbonate. The ionized form is the biologically active form. Approximately one half of the total serum calcium is ionized.

Calcium is typically measured in mg/dl. As usually reported, serum calcium levels reflect the total calcium level (all three forms), although ionized calcium levels may be reported.[6] The levels listed in Table 13-8 reflect total calcium levels. Changes in serum pH will alter the level of ionized calcium without altering the total calcium level. Acidosis decreases calcium binding, leading to more ionized calcium, and alkalosis increases calcium binding. Alterations in serum albumin levels affect interpretation of total calcium levels. Low albumin levels result in a drop in the total calcium level, although the level of ionized calcium usually does not change.

Calcium balance depends on the proper functioning of three hormones: vitamin D, parathyroid hormone (PTH), and calcitonin. Vitamin D is formed through the action of ultraviolet (UV) rays on a precursor found in the skin or is ingested in the diet. Vitamin D is important for absorption of calcium from the gastrointestinal tract.

PTH is produced by the parathyroid gland. Its production and release are stimulated by low serum calcium levels. PTH increases bone resorption (movement of calcium out of bones), increases GI absorption of calcium, and increases renal tubule reabsorption of calcium.

Calcitonin is produced by the thyroid gland and is stimulated by high serum calcium levels. It opposes the action of PTH and thus lowers the serum calcium level by decreasing GI absorption, increasing bone mineralization, and promoting renal excretion. Causes of calcium imbalances are listed in Table 13-8.

Hypercalcemia

Hypercalcemia is most commonly associated with malignancy, with or without skeletal metastasis, multiple myeloma, hyperparathyroidism, vitamin D overdose, and prolonged immobilization.[7] Hypercalcemia rarely occurs from increased calcium intake (e.g., ingestion of antacids containing calcium or excessive administration during cardiac arrest).

Table 13-8 Calcium Imbalances: Causes and Clinical Manifestations

	Hypocalcemia (<9 mg/dl [2.25 mmol/L])	Hypercalcemia (>11 mg/dl [2.75 mmol/L])
Causes	Acute pancreatitis Primary hypoparathyroidism Steatorrhea Generalized peritonitis Chronic renal failure Vitamin D deficiency Surgical removal of parathyroids Excess administration of citrated blood Diuretic therapy Alcoholism Malabsorption Total parenteral nutrition	Excess milk-product ingestion Hyperparathyroidism Prolonged immobilization Multiple myeloma Thyrotoxicosis Vitamin D excess
Appearance	Tonic and clonic convulsions	Lethargy Weight loss Dehydration
Behavior	Personality changes Depression Irritability Easy fatigability Anxiety Confusion	Decreased intellectual function Malaise Confusion Psychosis Coma Increased thirst Impaired memory Fatigue
Musculoskeletal	Bone pain Fractures Rickets	Bone pain Fractures Pseudogout
Cardiovascular	Electrocardiogram changes Prolonged QT Dysrhythmias	Electrocardiogram changes Depressed T waves Shortened QT interval Hypertension Cardiac arrest
Gastrointestinal	Colicky discomfort Diarrhea	Anorexia Nausea Constipation Paralytic ileus
Neuromuscular	Hyperreflexia Muscle cramps Numbness and tingling in extremities Carpopedal spasms Chvostek's sign Trousseau's sign Seizures Tetany	Decreased muscle strength Depressed reflexes
Respiratory	Laryngeal spasm Respiratory arrest	Hypoventilation
Urinary Findings	No specific findings	Increased urinary output
Serum Values	Overcorrection of acid pH (may precipitate symptomatic hypocalcemia) ↓Serum albumin (patient may not have symptoms despite decreased Ca^{2+})	

Clinical Manifestations. Excess serum calcium causes decreased memory span, confusion, disorientation, fatigue, muscle weakness, constipation, and cardiac dysrhythmias (Table 13-8.)

THERAPEUTIC AND NURSING MANAGEMENT

HYPERCALCEMIA

Nursing Diagnoses

Nursing diagnoses and collaborative problems specific to the patient with hypercalcemia include, but are not limited to, the following:

- Risk for injury related to neuromuscular and sensorium changes
- Potential complication: dysrhythmias

Nursing Implementation

The basic treatment of hypercalcemia is promotion of excretion of calcium in urine by administration of a loop diuretic (furosemide or ethacrynic acid) and hydration of the patient with normal saline infusions. In hypercalcemia the patient needs to drink 3000 ml to 4000 ml of fluid daily to promote the renal excretion of calcium and to decrease the possibility of renal calculi formation.

Synthetic calcitonin can also be administered to lower serum calcium levels. Plicamycin (formerly called mithramycin), a cytotoxic antibiotic, inhibits bone resorption and thus lowers the serum calcium level. A diet low in calcium may be prescribed. Mobilization with weight-bearing activity is encouraged to enhance bone mineralization. In hypercalcemia associated with malignancy the drug of choice is pamidronate (Aredia), which inhibits the activity of osteoclasts.

Hypocalcemia

Any condition that causes a decrease in the production of PTH may result in the development of hypocalcemia. This condition may occur with surgical removal of a portion of or injury to the parathyroid glands during thyroid or neck surgery. Acute pancreatitis is another potential cause of hypocalcemia. The patient who receives multiple blood transfusions can become hypocalcemic because the citrate used to anticoagulate the blood binds with the calcium. Hypocalcemia can also occur if the diet is low in calcium or if there is increased loss of calcium with laxative abuse and malabsorption syndromes. Sudden alkalosis may result in symptomatic hypocalcemia despite a normal total serum calcium level because of a reduction in the level of ionized calcium. (See Table 13-8 for the clinical manifestations and etiologies of hypocalcemia.)

Clinical Manifestations. Because calcium is essential for conduction of nerve impulses and muscle contraction, procedures that evaluate neuromuscular irritability are useful for assessing a low serum calcium level. *Trousseau's sign* refers to carpal spasms induced by inflating a blood pressure cuff on the arm (Fig. 13-14). The blood pressure cuff is inflated above the systolic pressure. Carpal spasms become evident within 3 minutes if hypocalcemia is present. *Chvostek's sign* is contraction of facial muscles in response to a tap over the facial nerve in front of the ear (Fig. 13-14), and it also indicates hypocalcemia with latent tetany.

Tetany refers to the increased neuroexcitability and sustained muscle contraction associated with hypocalcemia. Manifestations of impending tetany include positive Chvostek's and Trousseau's signs (Fig. 13-14), laryngeal stridor, dysphagia, and numbness and tingling around the mouth or in the extremities. Other clinical manifestations of hypocalcemia are listed in Table 13-8.

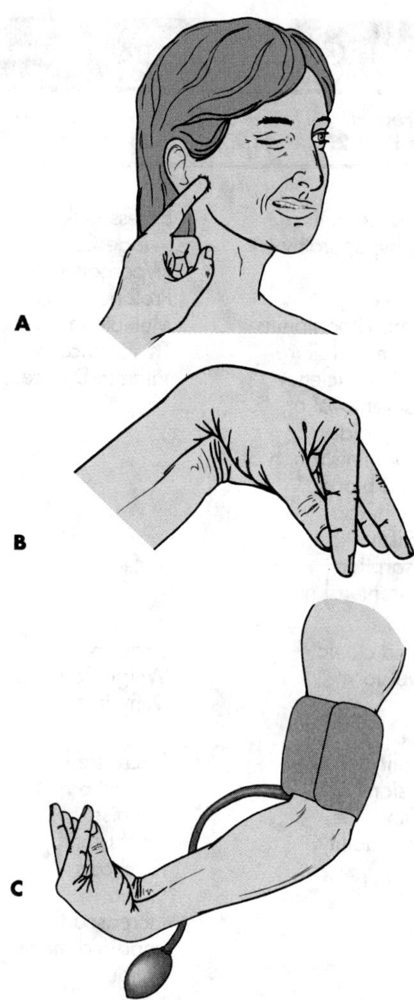

Fig. 13-14 Tests for hypocalcemia. ***A,*** Chvostek's sign is a contraction of facial muscles in response to a light tap over the facial nerve in front of the ear. ***B,*** Trousseau's sign is a carpal spasm induced by ***C,*** inflating a blood pressure cuff above the systolic pressure for a few minutes.

THERAPEUTIC AND NURSING MANAGEMENT

HYPOCALCEMIA

Nursing Diagnoses

Nursing diagnoses and collaborative problems specific to the patient with hypocalcemia include, but are not limited to, the following:

- Risk for injury related to tetany and seizures
- Potential complications: fracture, respiratory arrest

Nursing Implementation

Hypocalcemia is managed as an emergency, particularly if laryngeal spasms and respiratory arrest are imminent. Any patient who has had thyroid or neck surgery must be observed closely for manifestations of hypocalcemia. The primary goal in treatment of hypocalcemia is aimed at treating the cause. Hypocalcemia can be treated with oral or IV calcium supplements. Calcium carbonate (oral) and calcium gluconate IV are commonly used as supplements. Care must be taken because infiltration of IV calcium can cause sloughing of the tissue. Calcium is not given intramuscularly (IM) because it will precipitate in the muscle. A diet high in calcium-rich foods may be ordered along with vitamin D supplements for the patient with hypocalcemia. Synthetic PTH (parathormone) can also be given.

Phosphate Imbalances

Phosphorus is a primary anion in the ICF and is essential to the function of muscle, red blood cells, and the nervous system. It is deposited with calcium for bone and tooth structure. It is also involved in the acid-base buffering system, in the mitochondrial energy production of ATP, in cellular uptake and use of glucose, and as an intermediary in the metabolism of carbohydrates, proteins, and fats.

Maintenance of normal phosphate balance requires adequate renal functioning because the kidneys are the major route of phosphate excretion. A small amount is lost in the feces. A reciprocal relationship exists between phosphorus and calcium in that a high serum phosphate level tends to cause a low calcium concentration in the serum.

Table 13-9 Causes of Phosphate Imbalances

Hypophosphatemia	Hyperphosphatemia
Malabsorption syndrome Nutritional recovery syndrome Glucose administration Hyperalimentation Alcohol withdrawal Phosphate-binding antacids Diabetic ketoacidosis Respiratory alkalosis	Renal failure Chemotherapeutic agents Enemas containing phosphorus (e.g., Fleet's) Excessive ingestion (e.g., milk, phosphate-containing laxatives) Large vitamin D intake Hypoparathyroidism

Hyperphosphatemia. The major condition that can lead to hyperphosphatemia is acute or chronic renal failure that results in an altered ability of the kidneys to excrete phosphate. Other causes include chemotherapy for certain malignancies (lymphomas), excessive ingestion of milk or phosphate-containing laxatives, and large intakes of vitamin D that increase GI absorption of phosphorus (Table 13-9).

Clinical manifestations of hyperphosphatemia primarily relate to metastatic calcium-phosphate precipitates. Ordinarily, calcium and phosphate are deposited only in bone. However, an increased serum phosphate concentration along with calcium precipitates readily, and calcified deposits can occur in soft tissue such as joints, arteries, skin, kidneys, and cornea (see Chapter 44). Other manifestations of hyperphosphatemia are neuromuscular irritability and tetany, which are related to the low serum calcium levels often associated with high serum phosphate levels.

Management of hyperphosphatemia is aimed at identifying and treating the underlying cause. Ingestion of foods and fluids high in phosphorus (e.g., dairy products) should be restricted. Adequate hydration and correction of hypocalcemic conditions can enhance the renal excretion of phosphate. For the patient with renal failure, measures to reduce serum phosphate levels include phosphate-binding agents or gels and dietary phosphate restrictions (see Chapter 44).

Hypophosphatemia. Hypophosphatemia (low serum phosphate) is seen in the patient who is malnourished or has malabsorption syndromes. Other causes include alcohol withdrawal, parenteral nutrition with inadequate phosphorus replacement, use of phosphate-binding antacids, and nutritional recovery syndrome (refeeding after starvation). During the anabolic phase of metabolism, an influx of phosphorus into the cells occurs. Table 13-9 lists causes of phosphorus imbalances.

Most clinical manifestations of hypophosphatemia relate to a deficiency of ATP or 2,3-diphosphoglycerate (2,3-DPG), an enzyme in red blood cells. Both conditions result in impaired cellular energy resources and oxygen delivery to tissues. Hemolytic anemia may occur because of the fragility of the red blood cells. Acute manifestations include

Table 13-10 Causes of Magnesium Imbalances

Hypomagnesemia	Hypermagnesemia
Diarrhea Vomiting Chronic alcoholism Impaired gastrointestinal absorption Malabsorption syndrome Prolonged malnutrition Large urine outputs Nasogastric suction Diabetic ketoacidosis Hyperaldosteronism	Renal failure (especially if patient is given magnesium products) Excessive administration of magnesium for treatment of eclampsia Adrenal insufficiency

CNS depression, confusion, and other mental changes. Other manifestations include muscle weakness and pain, dysrhythmias, and cardiomyopathy.

Management of a mild phosphorus deficiency may involve oral supplementation (e.g., Neutra-Phos) and ingestion of foods high in phosphorus (e.g., dairy products). Severe hypophosphatemia can be serious and requires IV administration of sodium phosphate or potassium phosphate. Frequent monitoring of serum phosphate levels is necessary to guide intravenous therapy. Sudden symptomatic hypocalcemia, secondary to increased calcium phosphorus binding, is a potential complication of IV phosphorus administration.[8]

Magnesium Imbalances

Magnesium is the second most abundant intracellular cation. It functions as a coenzyme in the metabolism of carbohydrates and protein. It is also involved in metabolism of cellular nucleic acid and proteins. Regulation of magnesium is not well understood, but many of the factors that regulate calcium balance (e.g., PTH, vitamin D) influence magnesium balance. About 50% to 60% of the body's magnesium is contained in bone. The kidneys are the primary route of magnesium excretion. Causes of magnesium imbalances are listed in Table 13-10.

Neuromuscular excitability is profoundly affected by alterations in serum magnesium. Hypomagnesemia (a low serum magnesium level) produces neuromuscular and CNS hyperirritability. Additionally, diets low in magnesium are believed to be a risk factor for hypertension, cardiac dysrhythmias, ischemic heart disease, and sudden cardiac death.[9] Decreased intracellular magnesium levels may contribute to the hypertension, abnormal glucose tolerance, and insulin resistance common in diabetes.[10] A high serum magnesium level (hypermagnesemia) depresses neuromuscular and CNS functions.

Hypermagnesemia. Hypermagnesemia usually occurs only with an increase in magnesium intake accompanied by renal insufficiency or failure. A patient with chronic renal failure who ingests products containing magnesium (e.g., Maalox, milk of magnesia) will have a problem with excess magnesium. Magnesium excess could develop in the pregnant woman who receives magnesium sulfate for the management of eclampsia.

Initial clinical manifestations of a mildly elevated serum magnesium concentration include lethargy, drowsiness, and nausea and vomiting. As the levels of serum magnesium increase, deep tendon reflexes are lost, followed by somnolence; then respiratory and, ultimately, cardiac arrest can occur.

Management of hypermagnesemia should focus on prevention. Persons with renal failure should not take magnesium-containing medication. The emergency treatment of hypermagnesemia is IV administration of calcium chloride or calcium gluconate to physiologically oppose the effects of the magnesium on cardiac muscle. Promoting urinary excretion with fluid will decrease serum magnesium. The patient with impaired renal function will require dialysis because the kidneys are the major route of excretion for magnesium.

Hypomagnesemia. Hypomagnesemia tends to develop gradually. Prolonged IV feeding without magnesium supplementation and excessive losses of fluids from the GI tract are potential causes. The most common cause is chronic alcoholism. The significant clinical manifestations include confusion, hyperactive deep tendon reflexes, tremors, and convulsions. Magnesium deficiency also predisposes to cardiac dysrhythmias. Clinically, hypomagnesemia resembles hypocalcemia and may contribute to the development of hypocalcemia. Hypomagnesemia may also be associated with hypokalemia that does not respond well to potassium replacement. This occurs because intracellular magnesium is critical to normal function of the sodium-potassium pump.

Mild magnesium deficiencies can be treated with oral supplements and increased dietary intake of foods high in magnesium (e.g., green vegetables, nuts, bananas, oranges, peanut butter, chocolate). If the condition is severe, parenteral IV or IM magnesium (e.g., magnesium sulfate) should be administered. Too rapid administration of magnesium can lead to cardiac or respiratory arrest.

Protein Imbalances

Plasma proteins, particularly albumin, are a significant determinant of plasma volume. Because of their large molecular size, they remain in the vascular space and contribute to the colloidal oncotic pressure. Causes of protein imbalances are listed in Table 13-11.

Hypoproteinemia can occur over time. Causes related to intake are anorexia, malnutrition, starvation, fad dieting, and poorly balanced vegetarian diets. Poor absorption of protein can occur in certain GI malabsorptive diseases. Protein can shift out of the intravascular space with inflammation. Increased breakdown of proteins occurs with elevated basal metabolic rates and catabolic states, such as fever, infection, and certain malignancies. Increased use of protein occurs with cell growth and repair after surgical wounds or burns. Hemorrhage with loss of red blood cells can be a cause of protein deficit. The kidneys can lose large amounts of protein, especially albumin, in nephrotic syndrome.

Table 13-11 Causes of Protein Imbalances

Hypoproteinemia	Hyperproteinemia
Decreased food intake	Dehydration
Starvation	Hemoconcentration
Diseased liver	
Massive burns	
Loss of albumin in renal disease	
Major infection	

Clinical manifestations of protein deficit include edema (from decreased oncotic pressure), slow healing, anorexia, fatigue, anemia, and muscle loss that results from the breakdown of body tissue to meet the body's need for protein. Ascites is an example of third-space shifting that may develop with hypoproteinemia.

Management of protein deficit includes providing a high-carbohydrate, high-protein diet and dietary protein supplements. If the patient cannot meet the needs for protein orally, enteral nutrition or total parenteral nutrition may be used. (Protein-calorie malnutrition is discussed in Chapter 37.)

Hyperproteinemia is rare, but it can occur with dehydration and hemoconcentration.

ACID-BASE IMBALANCES

Hydrogen Ion Concentration

The acidity or alkalinity of a solution depends on its hydrogen ion (H^+) concentration. An increase in H^+ concentration leads to acidity; a decrease leads to alkalinity. (Definitions related to acid-base balance are presented in Table 13-12.)

Despite the fact that acids are produced by the body daily, the hydrogen ion concentration of body fluids is small (0.0004 mEq/L). This tiny amount is maintained within a narrow range to ensure optimal cellular function. Hydrogen ion concentration is usually expressed as a negative logarithm (symbolized as pH) rather than in milliequivalents. The use of the negative logarithm means that the lower the pH, the higher the hydrogen ion concentration. In contrast to a pH of 7, a pH of 8 represents a tenfold decrease in hydrogen ion concentration.

The pH of a chemical solution may range from 1 to 14. A solution with a pH of 7 is considered neutral. An acid solution has a pH less than 7, and an alkaline solution has a pH greater than 7. Blood is slightly alkaline (pH 7.35 to 7.45); yet if it drops below 7.35, the person has *acidosis,* even though the blood may never become truly acidic. If the blood pH is greater than 7.45, the person has *alkalosis* (Fig. 13-15). The pH of blood is computed through the use of the Henderson-Hasselbalch equation (Table 13-13). This equation demonstrates that the pH level is determined by the ratio of base (bicarbonate) to acid (carbonic acid). A 20 to 1 relationship must exist to maintain the pH within a normal range.

Table 13-12 Terms in Acid-Base Physiology

Term	Definition
Acid	Donor of hydrogen ions (H^+); separation of an acid into hydrogen ion and its accompanying anion in solution
Acidemia	Signifying an arterial blood pH of less than 7.35
Acidosis	Process that adds acid or eliminates base from body fluids
Alkalemia	Signifying an arterial blood pH of more than 7.45
Alkalosis	Process that adds base or eliminates acid from body fluids
Base	Acceptor of hydrogen ions; chemical combining of acid and base when hydrogen ions are added to a solution containing a base; bicarbonate (HCO_3^-) most abundant base in body fluids
Buffer	Substance that reacts with an acid or base to prevent a large change in pH
pH	Negative logarithm of the hydrogen ion concentration

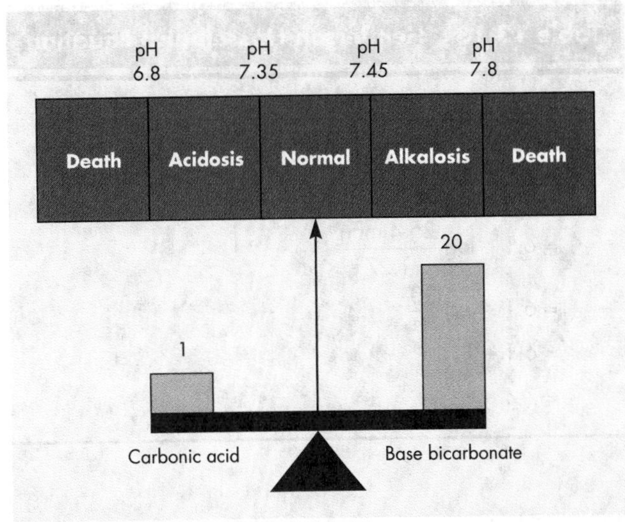

Fig. 13-15 The normal range of plasma pH is 7.35 to 7.45. A normal pH is maintained by a ratio of 1 part carbonic acid to 20 parts base bicarbonate.

Acid-Base Regulation

The body's metabolic processes constantly produce acids. These acids must be neutralized and excreted to maintain acid-base balance.

Normally the body has three mechanisms by which it regulates acid-base balance to maintain the arterial pH between 7.35 and 7.45. These mechanisms are the buffer systems, the respiratory system, and the renal system.

The regulatory mechanisms react at different speeds. Buffers react immediately; the respiratory system responds in minutes and reaches maximum effectiveness in hours; the renal response takes 2 to 3 days to respond maximally, but the kidneys can maintain balance for a long period of time.

Buffer System. The buffer system is the fastest-acting system and the primary regulator of acid-base balance. Buffers act chemically to change strong acids into weaker acids or to bind acids to neutralize their effect. The buffers in the body include carbonic acid-bicarbonate, monohydrogen-dihydrogen phosphate, intracellular and plasma proteins, and hemoglobin.

A buffer consists of a weakly ionized acid or a base and its salt. The mechanisms of buffering function to minimize the effect of acids on blood pH until they can be excreted from the body. The carbonic acid (H_2CO_3)-bicarbonate (HCO_3^-) buffer system neutralizes hydrochloric acid (HCl) in the following manner:

$$\underset{\text{strong acid}}{H^+Cl^-} + \underset{\text{strong base}}{Na^+HCO_3^-} \rightarrow \underset{\text{salt}}{NaCl} + \underset{\text{weak acid}}{H_2CO_3}$$

In this way, HCl is prevented from making a large change in the solution's pH, and more H_2CO_3 is formed. The carbonic acid, in turn, is broken down to H_2O and CO_2. The CO_2 is excreted by the lungs. In this process the buffer system maintains the 20:1 ratio between bicarbonate and carbonic acid and the normal pH.

The phosphate buffer system is composed of sodium and other cations in combination with $H_2PO_4^+$ and HPO_4^{2-}. This buffer system acts in the same manner as the bicarbonate system. Strong acids are neutralized to form a weak acid of sodium biphosphate, which can be excreted in the urine, and sodium chloride: $Na_2HPO_4 + HCl \rightarrow NaCl + NaH_2PO_4$. When a strong base is added to the system, it is neutralized to form a weak base and H_2O:

$$NaOH + NaH_2PO_4 \rightarrow Na_2HPO_4 + H_2O.$$

Intracellular and extracellular proteins are an effective buffering system throughout the body. The protein buffering system acts like the bicarbonate system. Some of the amino acids of proteins contain free acid radicals, –COOH, which can dissociate into CO_2 and H. Other amino acids have basic radicals, $-NH_3OH$, which can dissociate into NH_3 and OH that can combine with a hydrogen ion to form H_2O.

Using the "chloride shift" mechanism, hemoglobin regulates pH by shifting chloride in and out of red blood cells in exchange for bicarbonate. This shift is regulated by the level of oxygen in blood.

The cell can also act as a buffer by shifting hydrogen in and out of the cell. With an accumulation of H^+ in the ECF, the intracellular compartment can accept hydrogen in exchange for another cation (e.g., sodium or potassium).

The body buffers an acid load better than it neutralizes base excess. Buffers cannot maintain pH without the adequate functioning of the respiratory and renal systems.

Respiratory System. The lungs excrete carbon dioxide and water, which are by-products of cellular metabolism. When released into circulation, CO_2 enters red blood cells and combines with H_2O to form H_2CO_3. The carbonic acid dissociates into hydrogen ions and bicarbonate. The

Table 13-13 Henderson-Hasselbalch Equation

$$pH = pK\ (\text{constant}) + \log \frac{\text{base}}{\text{acid}}$$
$$= 6.1 + \log \frac{HCO_3^-\ (\text{renal})}{H_2CO_3\ (\text{lung})}$$
$$= 6.1 + \log \frac{25.4\ \text{mEq}}{1.27}$$
$$= 6.1 + \log \frac{20}{1}$$
$$= 6.1 + 1.3$$
$$= 7.4$$

free hydrogen is buffered by hemoglobin molecules, and the bicarbonate diffuses into the plasma. In the pulmonary capillaries, this process is reversed, and CO_2 is formed and excreted by the lungs. The overall reversible reaction is expressed as the following:

$$CO_2 + H_2O \leftrightharpoons H_2CO_3 \leftrightharpoons H^+ + HCO_3^-$$

The amount of CO_2 in the blood directly relates to carbonic acid concentration and subsequently to hydrogen ion concentration. With increased respirations, less CO_2 remains in the blood. This leads to less carbonic acid and fewer H^+ ions. With decreased respirations, more CO_2 remains in the blood. This leads to increased carbonic acid and more hydrogen ions.

The rate of excretion of CO_2 is controlled by the respiratory center in the medulla of the brain. If increased amounts of CO_2 or hydrogen ions are present, the respiratory center stimulates an increased rate and depth of breathing. Respirations are inhibited if the center senses low H^+ or CO_2 levels.

As a compensatory mechanism the respiratory system acts on the CO_2 + H_2O side of the reaction by altering the rate and depth of breathing to "blow off" or "retain" carbon dioxide. If a respiratory problem is the cause of an acid-base imbalance (e.g., respiratory failure), the respiratory system loses its ability to correct a pH alteration.

Renal System. Under normal conditions the kidneys reabsorb and conserve all of the bicarbonate they filter. The kidneys can generate additional bicarbonate and eliminate excess hydrogen ions as compensation for acidosis. The three mechanisms of acid elimination include (1) secretion of small amounts of free hydrogen into the renal tubule, (2) combination of hydrogen ions with ammonia (NH_3) to form ammonium (NH_4^+), and (3) excretion of weak acids.

The body depends on the kidneys to excrete a portion of the acid produced by cellular metabolism. Thus the kidneys normally excrete an acidic urine (average pH equals 6). They are able to act on the H^+ + HCO_3^- side of the reaction. As a compensatory mechanism, the pH of the urine can decrease to 4 and increase to 8. If the renal system is the cause of an acid-base imbalance (e.g., renal failure), it loses its ability to correct a pH alteration. In the patient with renal failure, metabolic acidosis is the usual finding.

Alterations in Acid-Base Balance

An acid-base imbalance is produced when the ratio of 1:20 between acid and base content is altered (Table 13-14). A primary disease or process may alter one side of the ratio (e.g., CO_2 retention in pulmonary disease). The compensatory process attempts to maintain the other side of the ratio (e.g., increased renal bicarbonate reabsorption). When the compensatory mechanism fails, an acid-base imbalance results. The compensatory process may be inadequate because either the pathophysiologic process is overwhelming or there is insufficient time for the compensatory process to function.

Acid-base imbalances are classified as *respiratory* or *metabolic*. Respiratory imbalances affect carbonic acid concentrations; metabolic imbalances affect the base bicarbonate. Therefore acidosis can be caused by an increase in carbonic acid (respiratory acidosis) or a decrease in bicarbonate (metabolic acidosis). Alkalosis can be caused by a decrease in carbonic acid (respiratory alkalosis) or an increase in bicarbonate (metabolic alkalosis).

Respiratory Acidosis. Respiratory acidosis (carbonic acid excess) occurs whenever there is hypoventilation (Table 13-14). Carbon dioxide and, subsequently, carbonic acid accumulate in the blood. Carbonic acid dissociates, liberating H^+, and there is a decrease in pH. If carbon dioxide is not eliminated from the blood, acidosis results from the accumulation of carbonic acid (Fig. 13-16, *A*).

The kidneys conserve bicarbonate and secrete increased concentrations of hydrogen ion into the urine. In acute respiratory acidosis the renal compensatory mechanisms begin to operate within 24 hours. Therefore a normal serum bicarbonate level usually can be found until the kidneys have compensated for the imbalance.

Respiratory Alkalosis. Respiratory alkalosis (carbonic acid deficit) occurs with hyperventilation (Table 13-15). Anxiety, CNS disease, sepsis, and mechanical overventilation all increase ventilation and decrease the PCO_2 level. This leads to decreased carbonic acid and alkalosis (Fig. 13-16, *A*).

Compensated respiratory alkalosis is uncommon unless the patient has been maintained on a ventilator or has a CNS problem. A decreased bicarbonate level differentiates compensated respiratory alkalosis from acute or uncompensated respiratory alkalosis.

Metabolic Acidosis. Metabolic acidosis (base bicarbonate deficit) occurs when an acid other than carbonic acid accumulates in the body or when bicarbonate is lost from body fluids (Table 13-14 and Fig. 13-16, *B*). In both cases a bicarbonate deficit results. Acetoacetic acid accumulation in diabetic ketoacidosis and lactic acid accumulation with shock are examples of accumulation of acids. Severe diarrhea results in loss of bicarbonate. In renal disease the kidneys lose their ability to reabsorb bicarbonate and secrete hydrogen ions.

Table 13-14 Acid-Base Imbalances

Common Causes	Pathophysiology	Laboratory Findings
Respiratory Acidosis		
Chronic obstructive pulmonary disease Barbiturate or sedative overdose Chest wall abnormality (e.g., obesity) Pneumonia Atelectasis Respiratory muscle weakness (e.g., Guillain-Barré syndrome) Mechanical underventilation	CO_2 retention from hypoventilation Impaired respiratory efforts caused by airway obstruction, weakened respiratory muscles, or depressed respiratory center Compensatory response to HCO_3^- retention by kidney	Plasma pH ↓ PCO_2 ↑ HCO_3^- normal (uncompensated) HCO_3^- ↑ (compensated) Urine pH <6 (compensated)
Respiratory Alkalosis		
Hyperventilation (caused by hypoxia, high altitudes, anxiety, fear, pain, exercise, fever) Stimulated respiratory center caused by septicemia, encephalitis, brain injury, salicylate poisoning Mechanical overventilation	Increased CO_2 excretion from hyperventilation Compensatory response of HCO_3^- excretion by kidney	Plasma pH ↑ PCO_2 ↓ HCO_3^- normal (uncompensated) HCO_3^- ↓ (compensated) Urine pH >6 (compensated)
Metabolic Acidosis		
Diabetic ketoacidosis Lactic acidosis Starvation Severe diarrhea Renal tubular acidosis Renal failure Gastrointestinal fistulas Shock	Gain of fixed acid, inability to excrete acid, loss of base Compensatory response of CO_2 excretion by lungs	Plasma pH ↓ PCO_2 ↓ (compensated) HCO_3^- ↓ Urine pH <6 (compensated)
Metabolic Alkalosis		
Severe vomiting Excess gastric suctioning Diuretic therapy Potassium deficit Excess $NaHCO_3$ intake Excessive mineralocorticoids	Loss of strong acid or gain of base Compensatory response of CO_2 retention by lungs	Plasma pH ↑ PCO_2 ↑ (compensated) HCO_3^- ↑ Urine pH >6 (compensated)

The compensatory response is to increase CO_2 excretion by the lungs. The patient often develops Kussmaul breathing (deep, rapid breathing). In addition, the kidneys attempt to excrete additional acid.

Metabolic Alkalosis. Metabolic alkalosis (base bicarbonate excess) occurs when a loss of acid (prolonged vomiting or gastric suction) or a gain in bicarbonate (ingestion of baking soda) occurs (Table 13-14 and Fig. 13-16, *B*). The compensatory mechanism is a decreased respiratory rate to increase CO_2. Renal excretion of bicarbonate also occurs.

Clinical Manifestations

Clinical manifestations of acidosis and alkalosis are summarized in Tables 13-15 and 13-16. Because a normal pH is vital to all cellular reactions, the clinical manifestations of acid-base imbalances are generalized and nonspecific. The actual compensatory mechanisms also produce some clinical manifestations. For example, the deep, rapid respirations of a patient with metabolic acidosis are an example of respiratory compensation. In alkalosis, hypocalcemia may concurrently be found and accounts for many of the clinical manifestations.

Blood Gas Values. Blood gas values provide essential information for evaluation of acid-base problems.[11] These include pH, PCO_2, and HCO_3^-. Diagnosis of acid-base disturbances and identification of compensatory processes are done by correlating the pH with the PCO_2 and HCO_3^-. First, it is necessary to determine whether the pH is alkalotic (>7.45) or acidotic (<7.35) and then whether the PCO_2 level or HCO_3^- is the primary cause of the pH change. For example, acidosis is caused by high carbon dioxide levels or low bicarbonate levels. Next, determine whether the body is attempting to compensate for the pH change. For example, if the primary problem is respiratory acidosis (low pH with an elevated PCO_2), are the kidneys compensating by reabsorbing more bicarbonate? If compensatory mechanisms are functioning, the pH will return toward 7.40. The body will not overcompensate for pH changes.

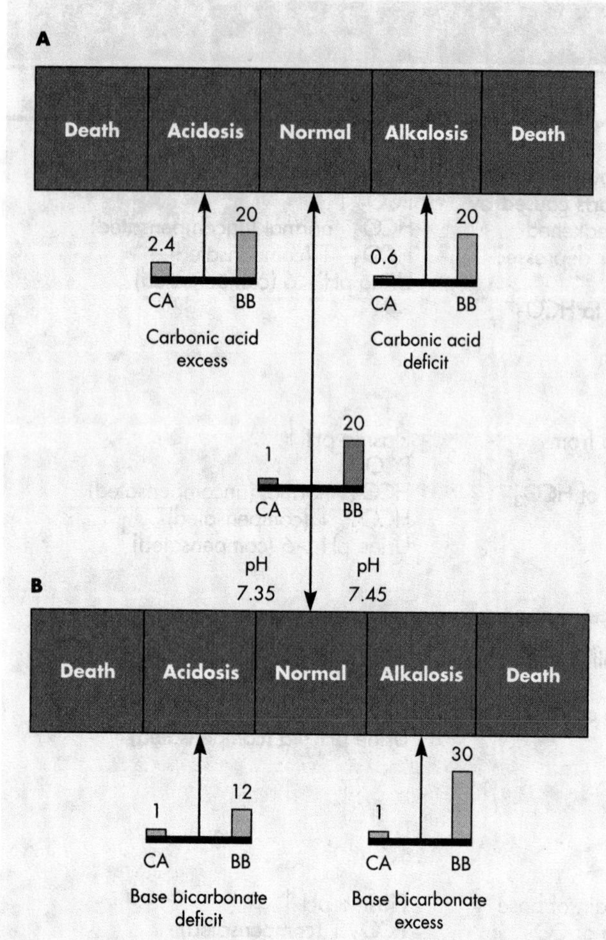

Fig. 13-16 Kinds of acid-base imbalances. ***A,*** Respiratory imbalances as a result of carbonic acid excess and carbonic acid deficit. ***B,*** Metabolic imbalances as a result of bicarbonate deficit and base bicarbonate excess.

Mixed acid-base problems are also possible. An example of a mixed acidosis appears in a patient in cardiopulmonary arrest. Hypoventilation elevates the carbon dioxide level, and anaerobic metabolism produces lactic acid. Circulating bicarbonate levels fall as the HCO_3^- buffers the lactic acid. The blood gases of this patient reflect an acidotic pH, an increased PCO_2, and a decreased HCO_3^-. An example of a mixed alkalosis is the case of a patient who is hyperventilating because of postoperative pain and is also losing acid secondary to nasogastric suctioning. (Refer to the laboratory findings section of Table 13-14 for the blood gas findings of the four major acid-base disturbances.)

Blood gas analysis will also show the PCO_2 and oxygen saturation. These values are used to identify hypoxemia. Either arterial or venous blood can be used for sampling as long as only one is consistently used for comparison. The arterial method is usually preferred. The values of blood gases differ slightly between arterial and venous samples (Table 13-17).

Table 13-15 Clinical Manifestations of Acidosis

Respiratory ($\uparrow PCO_2$)	Metabolic ($\downarrow HCO_3^-$)
Appearance	
Drowsiness Unconscious	Drowsiness Coma Dehydration
Behavior	
Disorientation Dizziness	Disorientation
Cardiovascular	
Decreased blood pressure Ventricular fibrillation Peripheral vasodilatation	Bradycardia Peripheral vasodilatation
Gastrointestinal	
No significant findings	Nausea, vomiting, diarrhea, abdominal pain
Neuromuscular	
Headache Muscular twitching Convulsions	Headache Muscular twitching
Respiratory	
Rapid, shallow breaths or hypoventilation with hypoxia	Deep, rapid respirations

ASSESSMENT OF FLUID, ELECTROLYTE, AND ACID-BASE IMBALANCES

Subjective Data

Important Health Information

Past health history. The patient should be questioned about any past health history of problems involving the kidneys, heart, GI system, or lungs that could affect the present fluid and electrolyte balance. Information about specific diseases such as diabetes mellitus, diabetes insipidus, ulcerative colitis, and Crohn's disease should be obtained from the patient.

Medications. An assessment of the patient's current and past use of medications is important. The ingredients in many drugs, especially over-the-counter drugs, are often overlooked as sources of sodium, potassium, calcium, magnesium, and other electrolytes. Many prescription drugs can cause fluid and electrolyte problems, including diuretics, corticosteroids, and electrolyte supplements.

Surgery or other treatment. The patient should be asked about past or present renal dialysis, kidney surgery, and bowel or kidney surgery resulting in a temporary or permanent external collecting system such as a colostomy or nephrostomy.

Functional Health Patterns

Health perception–health management pattern. If the patient is currently experiencing a problem related to fluid

Table 13-16 Clinical Manifestations of Alkalosis

Respiratory ($\downarrow PCO_2$)	Metabolic ($\uparrow HCO_3^-$)
Appearance	
Lethargy	Confusion Dizziness
Behavior	
Lightheadedness Confusion	Irritability Nervousness Confusion
Cardiovascular	
Tachycardia Dysrhythmias	Tachycardia Dysrhythmias
Gastrointestinal	
Nausea Vomiting Epigastric pain	Anorexia Nausea Vomiting
Neuromuscular	
Tetany Numbness Tingling of extremities Hyperreflexia	Tremors Hypertonic muscles Muscle cramps Tetany Tingling of fingers and toes Seizures
Respiratory	
Hyperventilation	Hypoventilation

and electrolyte balance, a careful description of the illness including onset, course, and treatment should be obtained.

Nutritional-metabolic pattern. The patient should be questioned regarding diet, especially whether he has been on a special diet such as a reducing, low-sodium, or fad diet. If the patient is on a special diet, such as low sodium or high potassium, his ability to comply with the dietary prescription should be determined.

Elimination pattern. Note should be made of the patient's usual bowel and bladder habits. Any deviations from the expected elimination pattern such as diarrhea, nocturia, or polyuria should be carefully documented.

Activity-exercise pattern. The patient's exercise pattern is important to determine because excessive perspiration secondary to exercise could result in a fluid and electrolyte problem. Also, the patient's exposure to extremely high temperatures as a result of leisure or work activity should be determined. The patient should be asked what practices are followed to replace fluid and electrolytes lost through excessive perspiration.

Cognitive-perceptual pattern. The patient should be queried about any changes in sensations such as numbness, tingling, fasciculations, or muscle weakness that could indicate a fluid and electrolyte problem. Additionally, both the patient and the family should be asked if any changes in mentation or alertness have been noted such as confusion, memory impairment, or lethargy.

Table 13-17 Normal Arterial and Venous Blood Gas Values

Parameter	Arterial	Venous
pH	7.35-7.45	7.35-7.45
PCO_2	35-45 mm Hg	40-45 mm Hg
Bicarbonate	20-30 mEq/L (mmol/L)	20-30 mEq/L (mmol/L)
PO_2*	80-100 mm Hg	40-50 mm Hg†
Oxygen saturation	96%-100%	60%-85%
Base excess	±2.0	±2.0

*Decreases above sea level and with increasing age.
†Oxygen tension is defined as the significant difference between the PO_2 concentrations of arterial and venous blood.

Objective Data

Physical Examination. There is no specific physical examination to assess fluid and electrolyte balance. Common abnormal assessment findings of major body systems offer clues to possible fluid and electrolyte imbalances (Table 13-18).

Laboratory Values. Normal serum electrolyte values are a good starting point for identifying fluid and electrolyte imbalance (see Table 13-4). However, they often provide only cursory information. Serum electrolyte values reflect the concentration of that electrolyte in the ECF. They do not necessarily provide information concerning the concentration of the electrolyte in the ICF. For example, the majority of the potassium in the body is found intracellularly. Changes in serum potassium values may be the result of a true deficit or excess of potassium or may reflect the movement of potassium into or out of the cell.

An abnormal serum sodium level may reflect a sodium problem or, more likely, a water problem. A reduced hematocrit value could indicate anemia, or it could be caused by fluid volume excess.

Therapeutic Management

In all cases of fluid, electrolyte, and acid-base imbalances the treatment is directed toward correction of the underlying cause. The specific diseases or disorders that cause these imbalances are discussed in various chapters throughout this text. IV fluid and electrolyte therapy are commonly used to treat many different fluid and electrolyte imbalances.

INTRAVENOUS FLUID AND ELECTROLYTE REPLACEMENT

Many patients need *maintenance* IV fluid therapy only while they cannot take oral fluids (e.g., during and after surgery). Other patients need *corrective* or *replacement* therapy for losses that have already occurred.[1] The amount and type of solution are determined by the normal daily maintenance requirements and by imbalances identified by laboratory results. The normal daily requirement for fluids and electrolytes is as follows:

Table 13-18 Common Assessment Abnormalities: Fluid and Electrolyte Imbalances

Finding	Possible Cause
Skin	
Poor skin turgor	Fluid volume deficit
Cold, clammy skin	Sodium deficit, shift of plasma to interstitial fluid
Pitting edema	Fluid volume excess
Flushed, dry skin	Sodium excess
Pulse	
Bounding pulse	Fluid volume excess, shift of interstitial fluid to plasma
Rapid, weak, thready pulse	Shift of plasma to interstitial fluid, sodium deficit, fluid volume deficit
Weak, irregular, rapid pulse	Severe potassium deficit
Weak, irregular, slow pulse	Severe potassium excess
Blood Pressure	
Hypotension	Fluid volume deficit, shift of plasma to interstitial fluid, sodium deficit
Hypertension	Fluid volume excess, shift of interstitial fluid to plasma
Respirations	
Deep, rapid breathing	Metabolic acidosis
Shallow, slow, irregular breathing	Metabolic alkalosis
Shortness of breath	Fluid volume excess
Moist crackles	Fluid volume excess, shift of interstitial fluid to plasma
Skeletal Muscle	
Cramping of exercised muscle	Calcium deficit
Carpal spasm (Trousseau's sign)	Calcium deficit
Flabby muscles	Potassium deficit
Positive Chvostek's sign	Calcium deficit
Behavior or Mental	
Picking at bedclothes	Potassium deficit, magnesium deficit
Indifference	Fluid volume deficit, sodium deficit
Apprehension	Shift of plasma to interstitial fluid
Extreme restlessness	Potassium excess, fluid volume deficit
Confusion and irritability	Potassium deficit, fluid volume excess

Electrolytes: Na^+—100 to 150 mEq; K^+—40 to 60 mEq
Glucose: 150 to 200 g (1 g equals approximately 4 kcal)
Fluid: 1500 ml/m^2 body surface (265 ml for a 70 kg adult with 1.76 m^2 body surface)

An example of normal daily maintenance IV therapy is presented in Table 13-19.

Solutions

Hypotonic. A hypotonic solution provides more water than electrolytes, diluting the ECF. Osmosis then produces a movement of water from the ECF to the ICF. After osmotic equilibrium has been achieved, the ICF and the ECF have the same osmolality, and both compartments have been expanded. Examples of hypotonic fluids are given in Table 13-20. Maintenance fluids are usually hypotonic solutions (e.g., 0.225% NaCl) because normal daily losses are hypotonic. Additional electrolytes (e.g., KCl) may be added to maintain those levels.

Although 5% dextrose in water is considered an isotonic solution, the dextrose is quickly metabolized, and the net result is the administration of free water (hypotonic). One liter of a 5% dextrose solution provides 50 g of dextrose or 170 calories. Although this amount of dextrose is not enough to meet caloric requirements, it helps to prevent ketosis associated with starvation. Pure water cannot be administered IV because it would cause hemolysis of red blood cells.

Isotonic. Administration of an isotonic solution expands only the ECF. There is no net loss or gain from the ICF. An isotonic solution is the ideal fluid replacement for a patient with an ECF volume deficit. Examples of isotonic solutions include lactated Ringer's solution and 0.9% NaCl. Lactated Ringer's solution contains sodium, potassium, chloride, calcium, and lactate (the precursor of bicarbonate) in about the same concentrations as those of the ECF.

Hypertonic. A hypertonic solution initially raises the osmolality of ECF and expands it. Examples are listed in Table 13-20. In addition, the higher osmotic pressure draws water out of the cells into the ECF. Hypertonic solutions (e.g., 3% NaCl) require frequent monitoring of blood pressure, lung sounds, and serum sodium levels and should be used with caution.

Although concentrated dextrose and water solutions (10% dextrose or greater) are hypertonic solutions, once the dextrose is metabolized, the net result is the administration of water. The free water provided by these solutions will ultimately expand both the ECF and ICF. The primary use of these solutions is in the provision of calories. Concentrated dextrose solutions may be combined with amino acid solutions, electrolytes, vitamins, and trace elements to provide total parenteral nutrition (TPN). Solutions containing 10% dextrose or less may be administered through a peripheral IV line. Solutions with greater concentrations of dextrose must be administered through a central line. (TPN is discussed in Chapter 37.)

Intravenous Additives. In addition to the basic solutions that provide water and a minimum amount of calories and electrolytes, there are additives to replace specific losses. These additives are mentioned previously during the discussion of the particular electrolyte deficiencies. KCl, calcium chloride, magnesium sulfate, and lactate are common additives to the basic (IV) solutions.

Recommendations for giving potassium vary, but, in general, no more than 10 mEq per hour is considered safe

Table 13-19 Normal Daily Maintenance Requirements for Fluids and Electrolytes

Maintenance IVs	Volume	NaCl	K^+	Glucose
5% dextrose and 0.45% normal saline with 20 mEq KCl	2000 ml	154 mEq	40 mEq	100 g
10% dextrose in water ($D_{10}W$)	1000 ml			100 g/L
	3000 ml	154 mEq	40 mEq	200 g

Table 13-20 Composition and Use of Commonly Prescribed Crystalloid Solutions

Solution	Tonicity	mOsm/L (mmol/L)	Glucose (g/L)	Indications and Considerations
Dextrose in Water				
5%	Isotonic	278	50	■ Provides free water necessary for renal excretion of solutes ■ Used to replace water losses and treat hypernatremia ■ Provides 170 calories/L ■ Does not provide any electrolytes
10%	Hypertonic	556	100	■ Provides free water only, no electrolytes ■ Provides 340 calories/L
Saline				
0.45%	Hypotonic	154	0	■ Provides free water in addition to Na^+ and Cl^- ■ Used to replace hypotonic fluid losses ■ Used as maintenance solution although it does not replace daily losses of other electrolytes ■ Provides no calories
0.9%	Isotonic	308	0	■ Used to expand intravascular volume and replace extracellular fluid losses ■ Only solution that may be administered with blood products ■ Contains Na^+ and Cl^- in excess of plasma levels ■ Does not provide free water, calories, other electrolytes ■ May cause intravascular overload or hyperchloremic acidosis
3.0%	Hypertonic	1026	0	■ Used to treat symptomatic hyponatremia ■ Must be administered slowly and with extreme caution because it may cause dangerous intravascular volume overload and pulmonary edema
Dextrose in Saline				
5% in 0.225%	Isotonic	355	50	■ Provides Na^+, Cl^-, and free water ■ Used to replace hypotonic losses and treat hypernatremia ■ Provides 170 calories/L
5% in 0.45%	Hypertonic	432	50	■ Same as 0.45% NaCl except provides 170 calories/L
5% in 0.9%	Hypertonic	586	50	■ Same as 0.9% NaCl except provides 170 calories/L
Multiple Electrolyte Solutions				
Ringer's Solution	Isotonic	309	0	■ Similar in composition to plasma except that it has excess Cl^-, no Mg^{2+}, and no HCO_3^- ■ Does not provide free water or calories ■ Used to expand the intravascular volume and replace extracellular fluid losses
Lactated Ringer's (Hartmann's) Solution	Isotonic	274	0	■ Similar in composition to normal plasma except does not contain Mg^{2+} ■ Used to treat losses from burns and lower gastrointestinal tract ■ May be used to treat mild metabolic acidosis but should not be used to treat lactic acidosis ■ Does not provide free water or calories

Modified from Horne MM, Swearingen PL: *Pocket guide to fluid, electrolyte, and acid-base balance*, ed 2, St Louis, 1993, Mosby.

CRITICAL THINKING EXERCISES

CASE STUDY

FLUID AND ELECTROLYTE IMBALANCE

Patient Profile

Robert S is a 54-year-old man admitted to the oncology unit with a primary diagnosis of carcinoma of the lung complicated by severe chronic obstructive pulmonary disease (COPD) and the recent development of SIADH.

Subjective Data

- Health has rapidly deteriorated during past 6 months
- Underweight with recent weight loss of 20 pounds (9.1 kg)
- Smoker for 35 years
- Difficulty expressing his problems
- Recently divorced from second wife

Objective Data

Physical Examination

- Blood pressure 130/88 mm Hg, pulse 110, respirations 32 and labored; appears confused and lethargic.

Diagnostic Studies

- Serum sodium 128 mEq/L (mmol/L)
- Serum osmolality 260 mOsm/kg (mmol/kg)
- Arterial blood gases pH 7.25
  PCO_2 90 mm Hg
  PO_2 54 mm Hg
  HCO_3^- 38 mEq/L (mmol/L)

Critical Thinking Questions

1. What is the probable cause of Robert's sodium imbalance? Which clinical manifestations may be related to sodium imbalance?
2. Given the patient's problems, what signs and symptoms should the nurse monitor?
3. Explain the reason for Robert's abnormal serum osmolality.
4. Discuss the role of ADH in the regulation of fluid balance.
5. Analyze the arterial blood gas results. What is the likely etiology of the acid-base imbalance? Is the body compensating for this disturbance?
6. Discuss the type and tonicity of fluid therapy most appropriate for Robert.
7. Based on the assessment data presented, write one or more nursing diagnoses. Are there any collaborative problems?

for routine administration. Potassium can be safely diluted as 40 mEq/L of solution with a maximum of 60 mEq/L.

Plasma Expanders. Plasma expanders stay in the vascular space and increase the oncotic pressure. Plasma expanders include colloids, dextran, and hetastarch. Colloids are protein solutions such as plasma, albumin, and commercial plasmas (e.g., Plasmanate). Dextran is a complex synthetic sugar. Because dextran is metabolized slowly, it remains in the vascular system for a prolonged period but not as long as the colloids. Hetastarch is a synthetic colloid that works similarly to dextran.[2]

If the patient has lost blood, whole blood or packed red blood cells are necessary to restore hemoglobin. Packed red blood cells have the advantage of giving the patient primarily red blood cells; the blood bank can use the plasma for blood components. Also, packed cells have a decreased plasma volume, which may be a significant consideration in the patient who has received plasma expanders in emergency treatment of blood loss. Whole blood with its additional fluid volume may cause circulatory overload.

REVIEW QUESTIONS

The number of the question corresponds to the same-numbered objective at the beginning of the chapter.

1. The majority of the body's fluid is contained in which fluid space?
   a. Intravascular
   b. Interstitial
   c. Intracellular
   d. Extracellular

2. Active transport of solutes from one fluid compartment to another requires
  a. energy.
  b. a favorable concentration gradient.
  c. a carrier molecule.
  d. a membrane permeable to the solute.

3. Changes in which of the following will cause movement of water into or out of the cells?
  a. ECF potassium
  b. ECF osmolality
  c. ICF calcium
  d. ICF hydrogen

4. Decreased production of ADH would be evidenced by
  a. hyperkalemia.
  b. decreased thirst.
  c. hyponatremia.
  d. polyuria.

5. Implementation of nursing care for the patient with hypernatremia might include
  a. administration of hypotonic intravenous fluids.
  b. increased water intake for patients on nasogastric suction.
  c. fluid restriction.
  d. administration of a cation exchange resin.

6. In respiratory acidosis, compensation would be accomplished by
  a. the lungs eliminating CO_2.
  b. the kidneys eliminating bicarbonate.
  c. the lungs retaining CO_2.
  d. the kidneys retaining bicarbonate.

7. Nasogastric suction might cause which acid-base imbalance?
  a. Metabolic alkalosis
  b. Respiratory acidosis
  c. Metabolic acidosis
  d. Respiratory alkalosis

8. Poor skin turgor, hypotension, and a rapid, thready pulse suggest which imbalance?
  a. Fluid volume excess
  b. Fluid volume deficit
  c. Sodium excess
  d. Potassium deficit

9. The ideal fluid replacement for the patient with an ECF fluid volume deficit is
  a. hypotonic.
  b. isotonic.
  c. hypertonic.
  d. a plasma expander.

REFERENCES

1. Horne MM, Heitz UE, Swearingen PL: *Fluid, electrolyte, and acid-base balance: a case study approach,* St Louis, 1991, Mosby.
2. Prielipp RC, Heyneker TJ, Prough DS: Fluid and divalent cation therapy in the critically ill patient, *Int Anesthesiol Clin* 31:21, 1993.
3. Rose BD: *Clinical physiology of acid-base and electrolyte disorders,* ed 4, New York, 1994, McGraw-Hill.
4. Horne MM, Swearingen PL: *Pocket guide to fluids, electrolytes and acid-base balance,* ed 2, St Louis, 1993, Mosby.
5. Cogan MG: *Fluid and electrolytes–physiology and pathophysiology,* Norwalk CT, 1991, Appleton & Lange.
6. Nussbaum SR: Pathophysiology and management of severe hypercalcemia, *Endocrin Metab Clin North Am* 22:343, 1993.
7. Hawthorne JL, Schneider SM, Workman ML: Common electrolyte imbalances associated with malignancy, *AACN Clinical Issues* 3:714, 1992.
8. Workman ML: Magnesium and phosphorus: the neglected electrolytes, *AACN Clinical Issues* 3:655, 1992.
9. Altura BM, Altura BT: Cardiovascular risk factors and magnesium: relationships to atherosclerosis, ischemic heart disease, and hypertension, *Magnes Trace Elem* 10:182, 1991-92.
10. Campbell RK, Nader J: Pharmacy update-magnesium deficiency and diabetes, *Diabetes Educator* 18:17, 1992.
11. Shapiro BA, Peruzzi WT, Templin R: *Clinical application of blood gases,* ed 5, St Louis, 1994, Mosby.

SECTION II BIBLIOGRAPHY

Books

Cogan MG: *Fluid and electrolytes: physiology and pathophysiology,* Norwalk, CT, 1991, Appleton and Lange.

DeVita VT, Helman S, Rosenberg SA, editors: *Cancer: principles and practice of oncology,* ed 4, Philadelphia, 1993, JB Lippincott.

Horne MM, Heitz UE, Swearingen PL: *Fluid, electrolyte, and acid-base balance: a case study approach,* St Louis, 1991, Mosby.

Horne MM, Swearingen PL: *Pocket guide to fluids, electrolytes and acid-base balance,* ed 2, St Louis, 1993, Mosby.

Maxwell MH, Kleeman CR, Narins RG: *Clinical disorders of fluid and electrolyte metabolism,* ed 5, New York, 1994, McGraw-Hill.

McCorkle R, editor: *Pocket companion for cancer nursing,* Philadelphia, 1994, WB Saunders.

Metheny NM: *Fluid and electrolyte balance: nursing considerations,* ed 2, Philadelphia, 1992, JB Lippincott.

Middleton E and others, editors: *Allergy: principles and practices,* ed 4, St Louis, 1993, Mosby.

Million RR, Cassisi NJ: *Management of head and neck cancer: a multidisciplinary approach,* ed 2, Philadelphia, 1994, JB Lippincott.

Roitt IM: *Essential immunology,* ed 8, Boston, 1994, Blackwell Scientific.

Rose BD: *Clinical physiology of acid-base and electrolyte disorders,* ed 4, New York, 1994, McGraw-Hill.

Rupprecht CE: Current topics in microbiology and immunology, New York, 1994, Springer Verlag.

Shapiro BA, Peruzzi WT, Templin R: *Clinical application of blood gases,* ed 5, St Louis, 1994, Mosby.

Vander AJ: *Renal physiology,* ed 4, New York, 1991, McGraw-Hill.

Weldy NJ: *Body fluids and electrolytes–a programmed presentation,* ed 6, St Louis, 1992, Mosby.

Journals

Altura BM, Altura BT: Cardiovascular risk factors and magnesium: relationships to atherosclerosis, ischemic heart disease and hypertension, *Magnes Trace Elem* 10:182, 1992.

*Arathuzik D: Effects of cognitive-behavioral strategies on pain in cancer patients, *Cancer Nurs* 17:207, 1994.

Arieff AI, Ayus JC: Pathogenesis of hyponatremic encephalopathy–current concepts, *Chest* 103:607, 1993.

Arsenian MA: Magnesium and cardiovascular disease, *Prog Cardiovasc Dis* 35:271, 1993.

Belani CP and others: Instruction in the techniques and concept of supportive care in oncology, *Support Care Cancer* 2:50, 1994.

Blaylock B: The aging immune system and common infections in elderly patients, *J Et Nurs* 20:63, 1993.

*Bottorff JL: The use and meaning of touch in caring for patients with cancer, *Oncol Nurs Forum* 20:1531, 1993.

Bourke E, Delaney V: Assessment of hypocalcemia and hypercalcemia, *Clin Lab Med* 13:157, 1993.

Bourke E, Yanagawa N: Assessment of hyperphosphatemia and hypophosphatemia, *Clin Lab Med* 13:183, 1993.

Bright MA: Public health initiatives in cancer prevention and control, *Semin Oncol Nurs* 9:139, 1993.

Burgess L: Facing the reality of head and neck cancer, *Nurs Stand* 8:30, 1994.

Burnard P: The content of AIDS counselling workshops for nursing students, *Nurse Educ Today* 13:369, 1993.

Campbell RK, Nader J: Pharmacy update–magnesium deficiency and diabetes, *Diabetes Educ* 18:17, 1992.

Carpenter JS, Brockopp DY: Evaluation of self-esteem of women with cancer receiving chemotherapy, *Oncol Nurs Forum* 21:751, 1994.

Cullen L: Interventions related to fluid and electrolyte balance, *Nurs Clin North Am* 27:569, 1992.

Curtiss CP: Trends and issues for cancer care in rural communities, *Nurs Clin North Am* 28:241, 1993.

Driggers DL, Nussbaum JS, Haddock KS: Role modeling: an education strategy to promote effective cancer pain management, *Oncol Nurs Forum* 20:959, 1993.

*Duncan IB, Batchelor C: Assessment of the effectiveness of body substance precautions as the infection control system of a large teaching hospital, *Am J Infect Control* 21:302, 1993.

Dwyer K, Barone JE, Rogers JF: Severe hypophosphatemia in postoperative patients, *Nutr Clin Prac* 7:279, 1992.

Eakes GG: Chronic sorrow: a response to living with cancer, *Oncol Nurs Forum* 20:1327, 1993.

*Ferrell-Torry AT, Glick OJ: The use of therapeutic massage as a nursing intervention to modify anxiety and the perception of cancer pain, *Cancer Nurs* 16:93, 1993.

Glaus A: Assessment of fatigue in cancer and non-cancer patients and in healthy individuals, *Support Care Cancer* 1:305, 1993.

Grassman D: Development of inpatient oncology educational and support programs, *Oncol Nurs Forum* 20:669, 1993.

Graydon JE and others: Bridging the gap between research and clinical practice: a collaborative approach, *Oncol Nurs Forum* 20:953, 1993.

Gurevich I: Body substance isolation, *Infect Control Hosp Epidemiol* 13:191, 1992.

Hagopian GA: Cognitive strategies used in adapting to a cancer diagnosis, *Oncol Nurs Forum* 20:759, 1993.

Hall TG, Schaiff RA: Update on the medical treatment of hypercalcemia of malignancy, *Clinical Pharmacology* 12:117, 1993.

Hanson EJ: An exploration of the taken-for-granted world of the cancer nurse in relation to stress and the person with cancer, *J Adv Nurs* 19:12, 1994.

Hawthorne JL, Schneider SM, Workman ML: Common electrolyte imbalances associated with malignancy, *AACN Clin Issues* 3:714, 1992.

Hodgson SF, Hurley DL: Acquired hypophosphatemia, *Endocrinol Metab Clin North Am* 22:297, 1993.

Holtzclaw BJ: Monitoring body temperature, *AACN Clin Issues Crit Care Nurs* 4:44, 1993.

*Houldin AD, McCorkle R, Lowery BJ: Relaxation training and psychoimmunological status of bereaved spouses. A pilot study, *Cancer Nurs* 16:47, 1993.

Imm A, Carlson RW: Fluid resuscitation in circulatory shock, *Crit Care Clin* 9:313, 1993.

Innerarity SA: Hyperkalemic emergencies, *Crit Care Nurs Q* 14:32, 1992.

Jackson BS: Hope and wound healing, *J Et Nurs* 20:73, 1993.

Johnson CC: Knowledge of immunology is essential to plan effective nursing for immunocompromised patients, *Intensive Crit Care Nurs* 10:121, 1994.

Kumasaka LM, Dungan JM: Nursing strategy for initial emotional response to cancer diagnosis, *Cancer Nurs* 16:296, 1993.

Kupin WL, Narvins RG: The hyperkalemia of renal failure: pathophysiology, diagnosis and therapy, *Contrib Nephrol* 102:1, 1992.

*Langius A, Bjorvell H, Lind MG: Oral- and pharyngeal-cancer patients' perceived symptoms and health, *Cancer Nurs* 16:214, 1993.

Lin EM and others: Improving ambulatory oncology nursing practice. An innovative educational approach, *Cancer Nurs* 16:53, 1993.

Ljutic D, Rumboldt Z: Should glucose be administered before, with, or after insulin, in the management of hyperkalemia? *Ren Fail* 15:73, 1993.

Lynch P and others: Implementing and evaluating a system of generic infection precatuions: body substance isolation, *Am J Infect Control* 18:1, 1990.

Mack E and others: Reaching poor populations with cancer prevention and early detection programs, *Cancer Pract* 1:35, 1993.

Mahon SM, Casperson DS: Nursing management of malignancy induced hypercalcemia, *JUN* 10:1367, 1992.

Mallon DF and others: Exposure to blood borne infections in health care workers, *Med J Aust* 157:592, 1992.

Meyer I: Sodium polystyrene sulfonate: a cation exchange resin used in treating hyperkalemia, *ANNA J* 20:93, 1993.

Miller SJ, Simpson J: Medication-nutrient interactions: hypophosphatemia associated with sucralfate in the intensive care unit, *Nutr Clin Pract* 6:199, 1991.

*Millward S, Barnett J, Thomlinson D: A clinical infection control audit programme: evaluation of an audit tool used by infection control nurses to monitor standards and assess effective staff training, *J Hosp Infect* 24:219, 1993.

Mocsny N: Toxoplasmic encephalitis in the AIDS patient, *Rehabil Nurs* 28:20, 1993.

Neumark DE: Providing information about advance directives to patients in ambulatory care and their families, *Oncol Nurs Forum* 21:771, 1994.

Nussbaum SR: Pathophysiology and management of severe hypercalcemia, *Endocrinol Metab Clin North Am* 22:343, 1993.

*Olsen SJ, Frank-Stromborg M: Cancer prevention and screening activities reported by African-American nurses, *Oncol Nurs Forum* 21:487, 1994.

*Post-White J, Carter M, Anglim MA: Cancer prevention and early detection: nursing students' knowledge, attitudes, personal practices, and teaching, *Oncol Nurs Forum* 20:743, 1993.

Prelipp RC, Heyneker TJ, Prough DS: Fluid and divalent cation therapy in the critically ill patient, *Int Anesthesiol Clin* 31:21, 1993.

Rhiner M and others: A structured nondrug intervention program for cancer pain, *Cancer Pract* 1:137, 1993.

Rice R: Principles of universal precautions/body substance isolation, *Home Healthc Nurse* 11:55, 1993.

Roup BJ: OSHA's new standard: exposure to blood borne pathogens, *AAOHN J* 41:136, 1993.

Rude RK: Magnesium metabolism and deficiency, *Endocrinol Metab Clin North Am* 22:377, 1993.

Secor VH: Mediators of coagulation and inflammation: relationship and clinical significance, *Crit Care Nurs Clin North Am*, 5:411, 1993.

*Sheehan DK and others: Level of cancer pain knowledge among baccalaureate student nurses, *J Pain Symptom Manage* 7:478, 1992.

Shell JA, Smith CK: Sexuality and the older person with cancer, *Oncol Nurs Forum* 21:553, 1994.

Simpson S: Methicillin resistant *Staphylococcus aureus* and its implications for nursing practice: a literature review, *Nurs Prac* 5:2, 1992.

*Sloman R and others: The use of relaxation for the promotion of comfort and pain relief in persons with advanced cancer, *Contemp Nurse* 3:6, 1994.

Underwood SM, Hoskins D: Increasing nursing involvement in cancer prevention and control among the economically disadvantaged: the nursing challenge, *Semin Oncol Nurs* 10:89, 1994.

Underwood SM and others: Obstacles to cancer care: focus on the economically disadvantaged, *Oncol Nurs Forum* 21:47, 1994.

Wilkinson S: Good communication in cancer nursing, *Nurs Stand* 7:35, 1992.

Winson G: Gastrointestinal problems in patients with AIDS, *Nurs Times* 90:36, 1994.

Woodward W, Thobaben M: Special home healthcare nursing challenges: patients with cancer, *Home Healthc Nurse* 12:33, 1994.

Yates P: Towards a reconceptualization of hope for patients with a diagnosis of cancer, *J Adv Nurs* 18:701, 1993.

---

*Nursing research-based articles.

Organizations

Action on Smoking and Health
2013 H Street, NW
Washington, DC 20006
202-659-4310

AIDS Clinical Trials Information Service
P. O. Box 6003
Rockville, MD 20849-6003
800-874-2572 (800-TRIALS-A)
800-243-7012 (TTY/TDD)
301-738-6616 (FAX)

AIDS Education and Training Centers
5600 Fishers Lane
Room 4C-03
Rockville, MD 20857
301-443-6364
301-443-8890 (FAX)

American Cancer Society
1599 Clifton Road NE
Atlanta, GA 30329
404-320-3333

American Association for Cancer Education (AACE)
Educational Research and Development
University of Alabama at Birmingham
Community Health Science Building, Room 401
933 South 19th Street
Birmingham, AL 35294
205-934-6641

American Association for Cancer Research (AACR)
Public Ledger Building, Suite 816
Sixth and Chestnut Streets
Philadelphia, PA 19106
215-440-9300

American Foundation for AIDS Research
733 Third Avenue, 12th floor
New York, NY 10017
212-682-7440
212-682-9812 (FAX)

American Society of Clinical Oncology (ASCO)
435 North Michigan Avenue, Suite 1717
Chicago, IL 60611
312-644-0828

Association for Practitioners in Infection Control
505 East Hawley Street
Mundelein, IL 60060

Association for Professionals in Infection Control and Epidemiology, Inc.
1016 16th Street NW
Washington, DC 20036
202-296-APIC

Association of Community Cancer Centers (ACCC)
11600 Nebel Street, Suite 201
Rockville, MD 20852
301-984-9496

Association of Nurses in AIDS Care
704 Stonyhill Road, Suite 106
Yardley, PA 19067
215-321-2371
FAX: 215-321-2370

Asthma and Allergy Foundation of America
1717 Massachusetts Avenue, Suite 305
Washington, DC 20036

Cancer Fax
NCI International Cancer Information Center
9030 Old Georgetown Road
Building 82, Room 219
Bethesda, MD 20892
301-402-5874 on fax machine handset
301-496-8880 for technical assistance
FAX # 301-402-0212

Cancer Federation, Inc.
21250 Box Spring Road
Morena Valley, CA 92388
714-682-7989

Cancer Information Service (CIS)
NIH Bldg. 31, Room 10A 24
Bethesda, MD 20892
1-800-4-CANCER
1-800-638-6070–Alaska
524-1234 - Hawaii; in Oahu, dial direct; call collect from neighboring islands

CDC National AIDS Clearinghouse
P.O. Box 6003
Rockville, MD 20849-6003
800-458-5231
800-243-7012 (TTY/TDD)
301-738-6616 (FAX)

CDC National AIDS Hotline
P.O. Box 13827
Research Triangle Park, NC 27709
800-342-AIDS
800-344-7432 (Spanish)
800-243-7889 (TTY/TDD)

Centers for Disease Control
1600 Clifton Road NE
Atlanta, GA 30333

Choice in Dying
250 West 57th Street
New York, NY 10107
212-246-6962

Concern for Dying
250 West 57th Street
New York, NY 10843

HIV Telephone Consultation Service from San Francisco General Hospital
800-933-3413

Institute of Allergy and Infectious Disease
9000 Rockville Pike
Bethesda, MD 20892

International Society of Nurses in Cancer Care
Mulberry House, The Royal Marsden Hospital
Fulham Road
London SW3 6JJ
071-252-8171, ext. 2123

Johanna's On Call to Mend Esteem
Cancer Rehabilitation Nurse Consultants
199 New Scotland Avenue
Albany, NY 12208
518-482-4178

National Association of People with AIDS
1413 K Street NW, 8th Floor
Washington, DC 20005
202-898-0414
202-898-0435 (FAX)
703-998-3144 (BBS)

National Hospice Organization
1901 North Moore Street, Suite 901
Arlington, VA 22209

Oncology Nursing Society
501 Holiday Drive
Pittsburgh, PA 15220
412-921-7373

AHCPR Guidelines

Guides developed and published by The Agency for Health Care Policy and Research (AHCPR). The Patient Guides are available in English and Spanish. The guidelines can be obtained by writing to: Center for Research Dissemination and Liaison, AHCPR Clearinghouse, P.O. Box 8547, Silver Spring, MD 20907, or by calling 1-800-358-9295. The Guidelines are as follows:

Management of cancer pain. Clinical Practice Guideline. AHCPR Pub. No. 92-0592.

Management of cancer pain: adults. Quick Reference Guide for Clinicians. AHCPR Pub. No. 92-0593.

Managing cancer pain. A Patient's Guide. AHCPR Pub. No. 92-0595.

Evaluation and management of early HIV infection. Clinical Practice Guideline. AHCPR Publ No. 92-0572.

Managing early HIV infection. Quick Reference Guide for Clinicians. AHCPR Publ No. 92-0573.

Understanding HIV. A Consumer Guide. AHCPR Pub. No. 92-0574.

HIV and your child. A Consumer Guide. AHCPR Pub. No. 92-0576.

THE SURGICAL EXPERIENCE

Section Three

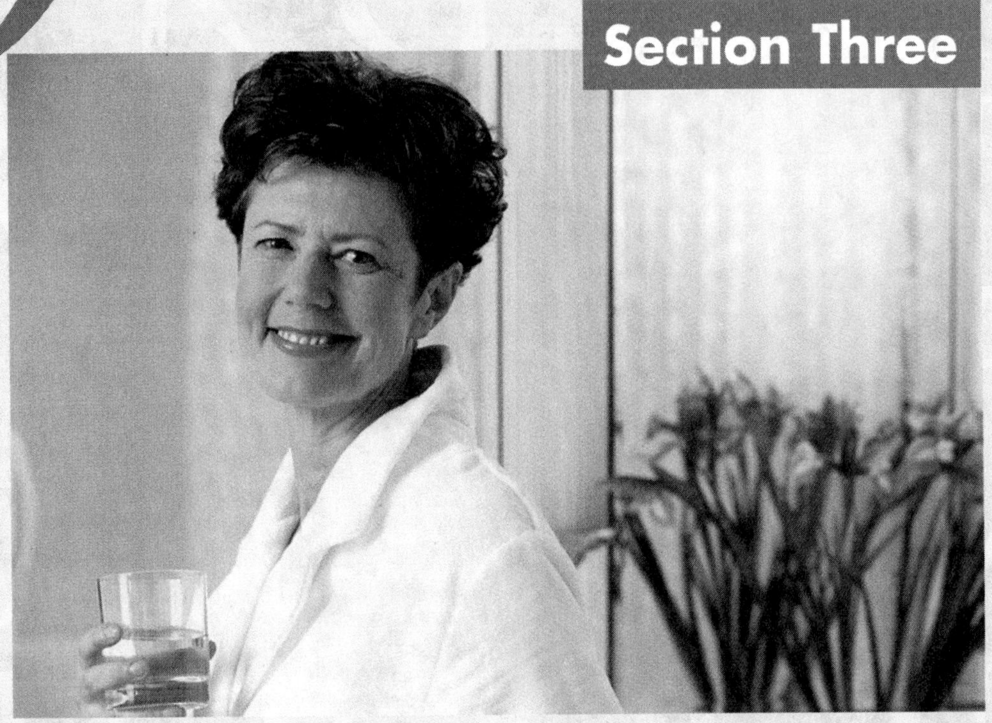

Chapter 14

NURSING ROLE IN MANAGEMENT
Preoperative Patient

Kim Litwack

Learning Objectives

1. Identify the usual purposes of surgery.
2. Describe the purpose and components of a preoperative assessment.
3. Interpret the significance of data related to the preoperative patient's health status and operative risk.
4. Explain the components and purpose of informed consent for surgery.
5. Describe the nursing role in the psychologic and educational preparation of the surgical patient.
6. Discuss the day of surgery preparation for the surgical patient.
7. Identify the purpose and types of preoperative medication.
8. Identify the special considerations of preoperative preparation for the older adult surgical patient.

Surgery can be defined as the art and science of treating diseases, injuries, and deformities by operation and instrumentation. The surgical procedure involves the interaction of the patient, the surgeon, and the nurse. Surgery may be performed for any of the following purposes:

1. *Diagnosis:* Lymph node biopsy or exploratory laparoscopy
2. *Cure:* Removal of a ruptured appendix or benign ovarian cyst
3. *Palliation:* Cutting a nerve root (rhizotomy) to remove symptoms of pain, or creating a colostomy to bypass an inoperable bowel obstruction
4. *Cosmetic improvement:* Repairing a burn scar or changing breast shape (mammoplasty)
5. *Prevention:* Removal of a mole before it becomes malignant or removal of the colon in familial polyposis to prevent cancer

Specific suffixes are commonly used in combination with identifying a body part or organ in naming surgical procedures (Table 14-1).

Surgery may be a carefully planned and anticipated event in a person's life (elective surgery). The need for surgery may sometimes arise with sudden and unanticipated urgency (emergency surgery). Both elective and emergency surgery may be performed in a variety of settings. The setting in which a surgical procedure may be safely and effectively performed is influenced by the extent of the surgery, the possible complications, and the general condition of the patient.

In the past the patient scheduled for a surgical procedure was admitted to the hospital the day before surgery to complete appropriate preoperative assessments and laboratory testing. Surgery was usually performed in a hospital operating room (OR) and involved a hospital stay of several days. Today, because of increased interest in cost containment and advances in technology, the majority of surgical patients are admitted to the hospital on the day of surgery (same day admission) or not admitted at all (outpatient).

An increasing number and type of surgical procedures are being performed as ambulatory procedures in emergency rooms, doctor's offices, freestanding surgical clinics, and outpatient surgery units in hospitals. Ambulatory surgical procedures can be performed with the use of a general or local anesthetic, usually take less than two hours, require less than a 3-hour stay in the postanesthesia care unit (PACU), and do not require an overnight hospital stay.

The popularity of ambulatory surgery has steadily increased during the last decade. In some cases this concept has been mandated by third-party payers—private insurance companies, government insurers (Medicare and Medicaid), and health management organizations. Ambulatory surgery is generally preferred by patients, physicians, and third-party payers for several reasons. Patients like the

---

Reviewed by Susan S. Fairchild, RN, MSN, CNOR, CS, Doctoral Candidate-EdD, Assistant Professor–Nursing, Barry University, Miami Shores, FL.

Table 14-1 Suffixes Describing Surgical Procedures

Suffix	Meaning	Example
-ectomy	Excision or removal of	Appendectomy
-lysis	Destruction of	Electrolysis
-orrhaphy	Repair or suture of	Herniorrhaphy
-oscopy	Looking into	Endoscopy
-ostomy	Creation of permanent opening into	Colostomy
-otomy	Cutting into or incision of	Tracheotomy
-plasty	Repair or reconstruction of	Mammoplasty

convenience, physicians prefer the flexibility in scheduling, and the cost is usually less for both the patient and the insurer. Ambulatory surgery generally involves fewer laboratory tests, fewer preoperative and postoperative medications, less psychologic stress (especially in young children and older adults), and less susceptibility to hospital-acquired infections.

Regardless of where the surgery is performed, the nurse plays a significant role in preparing the patient for surgery, maintaining surveillance of the patient during surgery, preventing complications, and facilitating recovery following surgery. To perform this role effectively, the nurse must have certain basic information. First, the nurse must establish the nature of the disorder requiring surgery and any coexisting disease processes. Second, the nurse must know the individual patient's response to a stressful situation. Third, the nurse must assess the results of appropriate diagnostic tests done preoperatively. Finally, the nurse must consider the bodily alterations and possible risks and complications associated with the surgical procedure.

The preoperative nursing measures included in this chapter are those that are applicable to the preparation of any surgical patient. Specific measures in preparation for particular surgical procedures (e.g., abdominal, thoracic, or orthopedic surgery) are covered in other chapters of this text.

PSYCHOSOCIAL REACTIONS TO SURGERY

Even when planned well in advance, surgery is a psychologic and a physiologic experience that elicits the stress response. The stress response is a desirable mechanism that enables the body to adapt and heal in the postoperative period. If stressors or the response to the stressors are excessive, the stress response can be magnified and recovery can be affected. The nurse who is aware of a patient's perceived or actual stressors can provide support and the needed information during the preoperative period so that stress will not become distress. (See Chapter 5 for a discussion of stress.)

Emotional reactions to impending surgery and hospitalization often intensify in the older adult. Hospitalization may represent to the patient a physical decline and loss of health, mobility, and independence. The older adult may view a hospital as a place to die or as a stepping-stone to nursing home placement. The nurse can be instrumental in allaying anxieties and fears and maintaining and restoring the self-esteem of the older adult during the surgical experience (see end of chapter for Gerontologic Considerations).

Common Fears

Fear of pain and discomfort is nearly universal. It includes concern about feeling pain during and after surgery. The nurse can reassure the patient that surgery will not begin before the anesthetic has taken effect and that adequate anesthesia is maintained throughout the procedure. The nurse can encourage the patient to talk with the anesthesia care provider (ACP) for clarification. The nurse can help the patient who fears postoperative pain by emphasizing the availability of drugs for pain relief.

Fear of the unknown is also extremely common. It is based on lack of information about what to expect during the surgical experience and on the uncertainty about the outcome of surgery. The dread of cancer, so prevalent in society, often contributes to this fear, both when the surgery is for diagnostic purposes and when the diagnosis is known. The patient may have totally unrealistic expectations of what surgery will be like. This may be a result of past experiences or the vicarious experiences provided by friends' stories and the mass media, especially television. The nurse can relieve the patient's fear of the unknown by providing accurate, specific information about what to expect. The surgeon should be informed if the patient requires any additional information or if the fear seems excessive.

Fear of mutilation or alteration of body image may be a factor, not only when radical surgery or amputation is to be performed, but also when less extensive surgery is required. The prospect of blood being shed provokes anxiety in some persons. The presence of even a small scar on the body is abhorrent to others. A person's body image and the perception of a threat to it are unique. The nurse must listen to and assess the patient's concern about this aspect of surgery with an open, nonjudgmental attitude.

Fear of death may be greater when patients know that they have a malignancy or are a poor surgical risk. However, it may be experienced by others who are contemplating even minor procedures. Surgery may be postponed if the patient is convinced that it will lead to death. Attitude and emotional state influence the surgical outcome. The nurse should inform the surgeon if a patient expresses fear related to survival.

Fear of anesthesia may include concern about an unpleasant induction or aftereffects, hazards or complications (such as brain damage or paralysis), or loss of control while under its influence. The nurse can reassure the patient that anesthesia does not have the effect of "truth serum." The patient also needs to know that it is not usual for persons to reveal their deepest secrets while under anesthesia. The anesthesiologist can provide detailed information about what the patient can expect to experience with the particular agents to be used.

Fear of disruption of life pattern may be present in varying degrees. It may range from fear of permanent disability to concern about not being able to play golf for a few weeks. Concerns about separation from family and about how spouse or children are managing are common. Financial concerns may be related either to an anticipated loss of income or to the costs of surgery.

PATIENT INTERVIEW

Screening before surgery usually begins with a patient interview. The interview allows for the development of a relationship between the patient and the nurse. The interview is often the patient's first contact with the surgical facility and will frequently set the tone of the patient's opinion of the entire experience. The prescreening interview may occur in advance of or on the day of surgery.

The primary purposes of the patient interview are to obtain patient information, to provide information about surgery and anesthesia, and to get the patient's consent for surgery. The interview is also a time to assess the patient's emotional state and readiness for surgery, to explore the patient's expectations about surgery and anesthesia, and to reinforce and clarify these expectations as indicated. The interview provides an opportunity for the patient and family to ask questions about surgery, anesthesia, and postoperative care.

The preoperative interview also allows for assessment of the patient's and family's emotional response to surgery (see research box on p. 356). The nurse who is aware of a patient's and family's perception of stressors can provide the support needed during the preoperative period so that stress will not become distress. Emotional reactions to surgery and anesthesia vary. The extent of a patient's and family's fears will be influenced by past surgical experiences, knowledge, hopes about the outcome of surgery, and personal coping mechanisms.

The nurse records preoperative data about the patient (Fig. 14-1) to be used as a basis for comparison during the intraoperative and postoperative periods, as well as to individualize postoperative care.

ASSESSMENT OF THE PREOPERATIVE PATIENT

Although nursing assessment and intervention are discussed separately, both are simultaneously done in practice. The overall goal of preoperative assessment is patient safety and includes the following specific assessments:

1. Determine the adequacy of the patient's health status to undergo the proposed surgery.
2. Identify and correct (if possible) any operative risk factors.
3. Determine whether surgery should be done as an inpatient, outpatient, or same-day admission.
4. Establish baseline data for comparison in the postoperative period.
5. Plan and institute preoperative care.
6. Select the anesthetic medication and technique best suited to the patient and type of surgery to be performed.

Subjective Data

Psychosocial Assessment. A psychosocial assessment of the preoperative patient should gather information about how the patient perceives the surgical experience (Table 14-2). This information can be gathered by the nurse during the admission nursing interview and throughout the ongoing nurse-patient relationship. The extremely anxious patient also needs additional consideration during the assessment process. The nurse must avoid introducing new concepts or terms that may increase the anxiety level and further impair thought processes and cognitive ability.

Past Health History. Initially, the nurse will explore the patient's understanding of the need for surgery and specific patient complaints that may have caused the patient to seek medical attention. For example, a patient scheduled for a total-knee replacement may indicate problems with increasing pain and mobility limitations.

Women should be asked about menstrual and obstetric history. This includes obtaining the date of the patient's last menstrual period. The purpose for obtaining this information is to avoid possible maternal and fetal exposure to anesthetics during the first trimester of pregnancy. This type of questioning may be embarrassing for a teenager in the presence of parents or guardians. The nurse may elect to ask these questions with parents or guardians out of the room.

Obtaining information about the patient's family health history is also important, including any adverse reactions to or problems with anesthesia. Anesthesiologists were first made aware of a phenomenon, later to be known as malignant hyperthermia, when a young man in Australia reported that 10 of his family members died while undergoing anesthesia. The genetic predisposition for malignant hyperthermia is now well documented. (For further information on malignant hyperthermia, see Chapter 15.)

A family history of cardiac and endocrine disease should be investigated. A family history of sudden cardiac death, myocardial infarction, and coronary artery disease should alert the nurse to the possibility of similar diseases in the patient. A family history of diabetes should also be investigated because of the familial predisposition to both insulin-dependent diabetes (IDDM) and non–insulin-dependent diabetes (NIDDM).

The last component of the patient history is the systems review. Specific questions should be asked to confirm the presence or absence of disease. Systems alterations may influence the choice of anesthetic agents and techniques, intraoperative monitoring priorities, and the type of care administered postoperatively. If the patient is being evaluated before the day of surgery, the review of systems, combined with patient history data, will suggest the need for preoperative laboratory tests. Many physiologic stressors may put the patient at risk for surgical complications, whether the surgery is an elective or an emergency proce-

(Text continued on p. 356.)

Rush-Presbyterian-St. Luke's Medical Center
Chicago, Illinois

Patient Data Base-Nursing Assessment
___ Same Day Admission ___ General Admission

REASON FOR THIS HOSPITAL ADMISSION: ____________

HOW DO YOU RATE YOUR HEALTH (PATIENT'S)? POOR ______ FAIR ______ GOOD ______ EXCELLENT ______
PLEASE EXPLAIN ____________

ALLERGIES (FOOD, MEDICATION, OTHER) & TYPE OF REACTION: ____________

MEDICATION HISTORY

PLEASE LIST ALL PRESCRIPTION AND NON-PRESCRIPTION MEDICATIONS WHICH YOU ARE CURRENTLY TAKING

NAME OF MEDICATION	DOSE OF MEDICATION	TIME OF DAY MEDICATION IS TAKEN	NAME OF MEDICATION	DOSE OF MEDICATION	TIME OF DAY MEDICATION IS TAKEN

DO YOU SMOKE? YES ______ NO ______ AMT ______ /DAY HAVE YOU SMOKED IN THE PAST? YES ______ NO ______
HOW MUCH ALCOHOL DO YOU DRINK? ____________
DO YOU TAKE ANY OTHER ANY DRUGS? YES ______ NO ______ TYPE OF DRUG: ____________

DISCHARGE PLANNING

MARITAL STATUS: MARRIED ______ SINGLE ______ DIVORCED ______ WIDOWED ______ CHILDREN: YES ______ # ______ NO ______
OCCUPATION: ____________ NUMBER OF YEARS ______
NAME AND PHONE NUMBER OF IMMEDIATE FAMILY MEMBER OR FRIEND: ____________
NONE: ______
LEVEL OF EDUCATION: GRADE SCHOOL ______ HIGH SCHOOL ______ COLLEGE ______
WHAT IS YOUR PRIMARY LANGUAGE? ____________

HAVE YOU USED HOME HEALTH CARE SERVICES? YES ______ NO ______ IF YES, WHICH AGENCY: ______
WHERE WILL YOU GO AFTER BEING DISCHARGED FROM THE HOSPITAL: HOME ______ REHAB. FACILITY ______
NURSING HOME ______ UNCERTAIN ______ OTHER ______
WHAT TYPE OF ASSISTANCE DO YOU THINK YOU MIGHT NEED AFTER LEAVING THE HOSPITAL? ______

UNSURE AT THIS TIME: ____________

Fig. 14-1 Adult surgical data base.

NUTRITION

WHAT IS YOUR NORMAL DIET?

GENERAL ___ SPECIAL ___

ARE YOU HAVING:	**YES**	**NO**
CHANGES IN APPETITE?	___	___
CHANGES IN THIRST?	___	___
INTOLERANCE TO FOOD?	___	___
IF YES, TO WHAT TYPES OF FOOD:		
PROBLEMS CHEWING OR SWALLOWING?	___	___
DO YOU HAVE LOOSE TEETH?	___	___

SLEEP PATTERN

	YES	**NO**
DO YOU HAVE DIFFICULTY SLEEPING?	___	___
DO YOU USE SLEEPING PILLS OR SPECIAL ROUTINES TO HELP YOU SLEEP?	___	___

PLEASE SPECIFY: ___

ACTIVITY

	YES	**NO**
DO YOU EXERCISE REGULARLY?	___	___
DO YOU HAVE SUFFICIENT ENERGY FOR ACTIVITIES?	___	___
HAVE YOU HAD AN INCREASE IN FALLS OR STUMBLING?	___	___

DESCRIBE: ___

ELIMINATION

DO YOU:	**YES**	**NO**
MOVE YOUR BOWELS DAILY?	___	___
IF NO, HOW OFTEN:		
HAVE CONSTIPATION?	___	___
HAVE DIARRHEA?	___	___
USE A LAXATIVE? (TYPE):	___	___
HAVE AN INCREASE IN URINARY FREQUENCY?	___	___
LOSE CONTROL OF BLADDER?	___	___
USE ANY URINARY/OSTOMY APPLIANCE? (TYPE):	___	___

PERCEPTUAL PATTERN

DO YOU HAVE PROBLEMS WITH:	**YES**	**NO**
SENSATION?	___	___
VISION?	___	___
HEARING?	___	___
PAIN?	___	___

DESCRIBE ANY PAIN YOU CURRENTLY HAVE. INCLUDE THINGS THAT CAUSE IT AND RELIEVE IT: ___

COPING / STRESS

HAVE YOU EVER EXPERIENCED:	**YES**	**NO**
MOOD SWINGS?	___	___
DEPRESSION?	___	___
ANXIETY?	___	___
DO YOU HAVE ANY QUESTIONS OR CONCERNS REGARDING SEXUAL ACTIVITY?	___	___
HAVE THERE BEEN ANY MAJOR CHANGES IN YOUR LIFE WITHIN THE PAST YEAR?	___	___
DO YOU HAVE FINANCIAL CONCERNS RELATED TO YOUR HEALTH CARE OR HOSPITALIZATION?	___	___

COMMENTS: ___

SPIRITUAL

	YES	**NO**
DO YOU HAVE ANY RELIGIOUS OR CULTURAL BELIEFS THAT WE SHOULD BE AWARE OF WHILE YOU ARE HOSPITALIZED?		

IF YES, EXPLAIN: ___

RELATIONSHIP PATTERNS

DO YOU LIVE: ALONE ___ WITH OTHERS ___

APARTMENT ___ HOUSE ___ OTHER ___

ARE THERE STAIRS? YES ___ # ___ NO ___

DO YOU HAVE SOMEONE AVAILABLE TO ASSIST YOU AFTER YOU GO HOME? YES ___ NO ___

PLEASE SPECIFY WHO: ___

ACTIVITIES OF DAILY LIVING

PLEASE CHECK (√) ANY AREAS WITH WHICH YOU NEED HELP:

EATING ___ BATHING ___ COMBING HAIR ___

GETTING DRESSED: UPPER ___ LOWER ___

MOVING TO/FROM: BED ___ WHEEL CHAIR ___ TOILET ___ TUB/SHOWER ___

CAN YOU MOVE ALONE WHILE: SITTING ___ STANDING ___ IN BED ___

DO YOU HAVE/USE:	**YES**	**NO**	BROUGHT TO HOSPITAL **YES**	**NO**
DENTURES: FULL/UPPER	___	___	___	___
FULL/LOWER	___	___	___	___
PARTIAL/UPPER	___	___	___	___
PARTIAL/LOWER	___	___	___	___
GLASSES:	___	___	___	___
CONTACT LENSES:	___	___	___	___
HEARING AID:	___	___	___	___
WALKER:	___	___	___	___
CRUTCHES:	___	___	___	___
CANE:	___	___	___	___
WHEEL CHAIR:	___	___	___	___
PROSTHETIC DEVICE:	___	___	___	___

PLEASE SPECIFY: ___

Fig. 14-1—cont'd Adult surgical data base.

PLEASE ANSWER THE FOLLOWING QUESTIONS ABOUT YOUR HEALTH HISTORY BY PLACING A CHECK(√) IN THE APPROPRIATE COLUMN. YOU MAY USE THE SPACE UNDER "COMMENTS" TO ADD ANY ADDITIONAL INFORMATION ABOUT YOUR HEALTH HISTORY.

DO YOU HAVE OR HAVE YOU EVER HAD:	**YES**	**NO**	**COMMENTS:**
ARTHRITIS OR JOINT PROBLEMS?	___	___	
ASTHMA, BRONCHITIS, PNEUMONIA OR BREATHING DIFFICULTIES?	___	___	
BLEEDING DISORDERS OR PROBLEMS WITH BLOOD CLOTS?	___	___	
CIRCULATION PROBLEMS?	___	___	
DIABETES?	___	___	
DIZZINESS OR FAINTING?	___	___	
LIVER PROBLEMS?	___	___	
HEART PROBLEMS?	___	___	
HIGH BLOOD PRESSURE?	___	___	
INFECTIOUS DISEASE:			
HEPATITIS?	___	___	
TUBERCULOSIS?	___	___	
AIDS?	___	___	
OTHER: ___			
KIDNEY, BLADDER OR PROSTATE PROBLEMS?	___	___	
RASHES, SORES OR REDDENED AREAS?	___	___	
IF YES, WHERE: ___			
SEIZURES?	___	___	
STOMACH PROBLEMS?	___	___	
STROKE?	___	___	
OTHER HEALTH PROBLEMS: ___			

HAVE ANY MEMBER(S) OF YOUR FAMILY (BLOOD RELATIONS) HAD ANY OF THE FOLLOWING PROBLEMS:

	YES	**NO**	**RELATIONSHIP**		**YES**	**NO**	**RELATIONSHIP**
HEART DISEASE?	___	___	___	DIABETES?	___	___	___
HIGH BLOOD PRESSURE?	___	___	___	CANCER?	___	___	___
STROKE?	___	___	___	PROBLEMS WITH ANESTHESIA?	___	___	___
OTHER HEALTH PROBLEMS?	___	___	___				

LIST ANY PREVIOUS SURGERIES YOU HAVE HAD:

SURGERY: DATE:

___

___

___

___

___

WHAT TYPE OF ANESTHESIA HAVE YOU HAD?

GENERAL ___ LOCAL ___ OTHER ___

PLEASE DESCRIBE ANY PROBLEMS YOU HAD WITH PREVIOUS ANESTHESIA OR SURGERY (SUCH AS NAUSEA, DIFFICULTY WAKING UP, ALLERGIC REACTIONS, ETC.):

___

___

FEMALE PATIENTS ONLY: WHAT WAS THE DATE OF YOUR LAST MENSTRUAL PERIOD? ___

DO YOU HAVE ANY REASON TO BELIEVE YOU MIGHT BE PREGNANT? YES ___ NO ___

PATIENT / FAMILY SIGNATURE: ___ DATE: ___

INTERVIEWER / REVIEWER: ___ DATE: ___

UNABLE TO OBTAIN SUBJECTIVE INFORMATION DUE TO: ___

Fig. 14-1—cont'd Adult surgical data base.

DAY OF ADMISSION

DATE: ______ TIME: ______ A.M./P.M. MODE OF ARRIVAL: W/C ____ CART ____ AMBULATORY ____

ACCOMPANIED BY: ______ PATIENT SEX: M ____ F ____ AGE: ____

DISPOSITION OF VALUABLES: HOSPITAL VAULT ____ SENT HOME ____ NONE ____

DISPOSITION OF BELONGINGS / PROSTHESIS: FAMILY ____ STORAGE ____ WITH PATIENT ____

SPECIFY TYPE OF BELONGINGS / PROSTHESIS: ______

COMPLETE THIS SECTION FOR ALL SAME DAY SURGICAL AND GENERAL ADMISSION PATIENTS:

GENERAL APPEARANCE:

PULSE: ______ RESP: ______ BP: ______ TEMP: ______ ALERT & ORIENTED x 3: ______

REG: ______ UNLABORED: ______ LYING: ______ WEIGHT: ______ HEIGHT: ______

IRREG: ______ BREATH SOUNDS: SITTING: ______

APICAL / RADIAL CLEAR & BILATERALLY: STANDING: ______

______ EQUAL: ______ RT. / LT. ARM ______

ADDITIONAL COMMENTS: ______

RN SIGNATURE ______ DATE: ______ TIME: ______

COMPLETE THIS SECTION FOR ALL GENERAL ADMISSION PATIENTS:

CIRCULATION/SKIN: Movement, circulation, & sensation intact in all extremities ____

Skin color: WNL ____ Other ______

Skin lesions: Yes ____ No ____ Location/size ______ Braden score: ______

Edema: Yes ____ No ____ Location/degree ______

ABDOMEN: Soft, nontender, nondistended ____ Other: ______

Bowel sounds: Normal ____ Other: ______ Date of last bowel movement: ______

Stoma/Ostomy/Tubes: ______

NEUROMUSCULAR: Gait: Steady ____ Unsteady ____ Muscle tone: Good ____ Fair ____ Poor ____

Joint swelling: Yes ____ No ____ Where ______

ADDITIONAL COMMENTS: ______

RN SIGNATURE ______ DATE: ______ TIME: ______

ORIENTATION TO UNIT:	YES	NO	PT. UNABLE		YES	NO	PT. UNABLE
Tour of room complete	____	____	____	Safety precautions explained	____	____	____
Visiting policies explained	____	____	____	Identification/allergy band on	____	____	____
Demonstrates use of call light	____	____	____				

RN SIGNATURE ______ DATE: ______ TIME: ______

Fig. 14-1—cont'd Adult surgical data base.

Table 14-2 Psychosocial Assessment of the Preoperative Patient

Situational Changes
- Determine support systems, including family, significant others, group and institutional structure, and religious and spiritual orientation.
- Define current degree of personal control, decision making, and independence.
- Consider the impact of surgery and hospitalization and the possible effects on lifestyle.

Concerns with The Unknown
- Identify specific areas of concern.
- Identify expectations of surgery, changes in current health status, and effects on daily living.

Concerns with Body Image
- Identify current roles or relationships and view of self.
- Determine perceived or potential changes in role or relationships and their impact on body image.

Past Experiences
- Review previous surgical experiences, hospitalizations, and treatments.
- Determine responses to those experiences (positive and negative).
- Identify current perceptions of surgical procedure in relation to the above and information from others (e.g., a neighbor's view of a personal surgical experience).

Knowledge Deficit
- Identify understanding of the surgical procedure, including preparation, care, interventions, activities, restrictions, and expected outcomes.
- Identify the accuracy of information the patient has received from others, including health team, family, friends, and neighbors.

RESEARCH

Implications for Nursing Practice

ANXIETY OF FAMILY MEMBERS OF SURGICAL PATIENTS

Citation Leske JS: Anxiety of elective surgical patients' family members. *AORN J* 57:1091-1103, 1993.

Purpose Determine anxiety levels of family members of patients undergoing elective surgery.

Methods Descriptive, correlational design was used to measure family members' (n = 50) STAI S-Anxiety levels, mean arterial pressures (MAP), heart rate (HR), and the relationship between selected characteristics (e.g., age and education of family member, length of surgical procedure). The study was done during the intraoperative waiting period.

Results and Conclusions The mean anxiety scores were one standard deviation higher than the norm for adults. Older family members had higher anxiety scores and increased MAP and HR. There was no difference between the anxiety scores of men and women. Family members with the lower levels of education had higher anxiety levels and increased MAP and HR. The length of the surgical procedure did not correlate significantly with anxiety scores. The anxiety scores remained high regardless of how long surgery lasted.

Implications for Nursing Practice Family members of patients having even simple, routine, elective procedures experience anxiety, particularly during the intraoperative period. Ironically, during this time period there is little communication between health care professionals and family members. Interventions that reduce the anxiety of family members need to be developed to enable family members to help the patient recover after surgery.

dure. A physiologic assessment of the preoperative patient is presented in Table 14-3.

Cardiovascular system. The purpose of evaluating a patient's cardiovascular function is to determine the presence of preexisting disease or functional problems (e.g., mitral valve prolapse) that may increase perioperative risk. It is important to inquire about any history of cardiac problems, including hypertension, angina, dysrhythmias, and myocardial infarction. The patient may respond or understand questions better if asked in lay terms about a history of high blood pressure, chest pain, palpitations, or heart attack. It is also important to inquire about any history of congestive heart failure and edema (e.g., swelling or fluid retention). The nurse should also inquire whether the patient has seen a cardiologist in the past, is using cardiac medications, or has ever undergone any cardiac surgical procedures, including catheterization, pacemaker insertion, or bypass surgery.[1]

Ideally, the patient who has had a myocardial infarction should wait at least 6 months for elective surgery to decrease the risk of reinfarction.[2,3] If the patient has a history of hypertension, medical approval by an internist is recommended.[4] If the patient has a history of congenital, rheumatic, or valvular heart disease, antibiotic prophylaxis before surgery may be used to decrease the risk of bacterial endocarditis.[5]

The patient with recognized dysrhythmias will be monitored electrocardiographically during and after surgery. The patient who receives digitalis therapy will have serum potassium levels carefully monitored to avoid the adverse and toxic effects of anesthetic agents. Dehydration may require preoperative correction with fluid therapy. Although a preoperative fluid balance assessment should be completed for all patients, it is especially critical for the older adult because the reduced adaptive capacity leaves a narrow margin of safety between overhydration and underhydration.

Respiratory system. It is important to inquire about any history of dyspnea (at rest or with exertion), coughing (dry or productive), hemoptysis, and asthma. If a patient has a history of asthma, the nurse should inquire about the patient's use of bronchodilators and the frequency and triggers of an asthma attack.

Table 14-3 Physiologic Assessment of the Preoperative Patient

Cardiovascular Status
- Identify acute or chronic problems; focus on the presence of angina, hypertension, congestive heart failure, and recent history of myocardial infarction.
- Assess baseline pulses: apical, radial, and pedal for rate and characteristics (compare one side to the other).
- Assess for the presence of edema (including dependent areas), noting location and severity.
- Assess neck veins for distention.

Respiratory Status
- Identify acute or chronic problems; note the presence of infection or chronic obstructive lung disease.
- Note the history of smoking, including the time interval since the last cigarette and the number of pack years. (Remember that although smoking should be discouraged preoperatively, it may be difficult for patients to stop during this time of anxiety.)
- Assess breath sounds for clarity; determine baseline respiratory rate, pattern, and the use of accessory muscles of respiration.

Integumentary and Musculoskeletal Status
- Assess mucous membranes for dryness and intactness.
- Determine skin status; note drying, bruising, or breaks in integrity of surface.
- Note any limitations in range of motion, weakness, or impairments to ambulation.

Nutritional Status
- Weigh patient.
- Determine recent weight loss through a diet history (e.g., a negative nitrogen balance may lead to postoperative complications of delayed or impaired wound healing, fluid imbalances, and infection).
- Assess food and fluid intake patterns (older adults frequently have a preexisting nutritional deficit).
- Identify any drug therapies that may affect electrolyte balance. Consider prescribed and over-the-counter medications (e.g., potassium-depleting diuretics, excessive use of laxatives or antacids).
- Assess the presence of dentures and bridges (loose dentures or teeth may be dislodged during intubation).

See related body system chapters for more specific assessments and related laboratory studies.

The patient should be asked about any recent or chronic upper respiratory infections. The presence of an upper airway infection normally results in the cancellation or postponement of elective surgery because the patient is at an increased risk of bronchospasm, laryngospasm, decreased oxygen saturation, and problems with secretions. The patient with a history of chronic obstructive pulmonary disease (COPD) and asthma is also at risk for postoperative pulmonary complications.[6,7]

The patient who smokes should be encouraged to abstain preoperatively but may find this difficult during a time of heightened anxiety. Any physical condition likely to influence or compromise respiratory function should also be noted. These include obesity and spinal, chest, and airway deformities. Depending on the patient's history and physical examination, baseline pulmonary function tests and arterial blood gases (ABGs) may be ordered preoperatively.

Central nervous system. Preoperative evaluation of neurologic functioning includes assessing the patient's ability to respond to questions, to follow commands, and to maintain orderly thought patterns. Appropriateness of response and thought must be evaluated. This is particularly important for the patient who is expected to prepare for surgery and to complete preoperative preparation on an outpatient basis. If deficits are noted, careful assessment should determine its extent and if the problem can be corrected before surgery. If the problem cannot be corrected, it is important to determine whether there are appropriate resources and support to assist the patient.

It is also important to inquire about any history of cerebrovascular accidents (strokes), transient ischemic attacks, spinal cord injury, and diseases of the nervous system, including cerebral palsy, myasthenia gravis, and other neuromuscular disorders.[8]

Renal system. Because many people in the United States and Canada are affected by renal disease, it is important to include questions about preexisting renal disease.[9] Renal dysfunction is associated with a number of alterations, including fluid and electrolyte imbalances, coagulopathies, increased risk for infection, and impaired wound healing. Another important consideration is the recognition that many medications are metabolized and excreted by the kidney. A decrease in renal function may contribute to an altered response to medications and unpredictable drug elimination.

Hepatic system. The liver is involved in glucose homeostasis, fat metabolism, protein synthesis, drug and hormone metabolism, and bilirubin formation and excretion.[10] The liver detoxifies many anesthetics and adjunctive drugs. Therefore, hepatic dysfunction will result in systemic effects. In addition, the patient with liver disease may have problems with glucose control, clotting abnormalities, and response to drug effects, all of which may increase perioperative risk.

Musculoskeletal system. It is important, particularly in the elderly, to inquire about a history of musculoskeletal problems.[11] If the patient has arthritis, all affected joints should be identified. Mobility restrictions may influence intraoperative and postoperative positioning and postoperative ambulation. If the neck is affected, intubation and airway management may be difficult. Any mobility aids such as a cane, walker, or crutches should be brought with the patient to the hospital on the day of surgery.

Nutritional status. Assessment of nutritional status includes recognition of two problems that can increase operative risk—obesity and nutritional deficiencies. Obesity makes access to the surgical site more difficult and thus prolongs the surgery.[12] It predisposes the patient to wound dehiscence, wound infection, and incisional herniation because adipose tissue impairs approximation of the wound edges and is less vascular than other tissues. The inhalation anesthetic is absorbed and stored by adipose tissue and then released postoperatively. Therefore the obese patient requires more anesthetic and recovers more slowly from its effects.

Nutritional deficiencies of protein and vitamins A, C, and B complex are particularly significant because each of these substances is essential for wound healing. The older adult is often at risk for malnutrition and fluid volume deficits associated with poor eating habits and a lack of dentition, as well as economic restrictions. Nutritional deficiencies impair the ability to recover from surgery. Surgery may be postponed until the patient gains or loses weight and deficiencies are corrected.

Endocrine system. Diabetes is a risk factor for both anesthesia and surgery. The diabetic patient is at risk for the development of hypoglycemia, ketosis, cardiovascular alterations, delayed wound healing, and infection.[13] It will be important to clarify with the patient's surgeon or anesthesia provider whether the patient should take the usual dose of insulin on the day of surgery. Some practitioners prefer the patient take only half of the usual dose; others ask that the patient take either the usual dose or take no insulin at all.

Infection. Although the presence of an acute infection often results in the cancellation of elective surgery, patients with active chronic infections such as acquired immunodeficiency syndrome (AIDS) and tuberculosis may still have surgery. When preparing the patient for surgery, it should be remembered that infection control precautions need to be taken with every patient.

Medications. The patient should be questioned about current medication use, including the use of over-the-counter medications. This is an important area to explore because these medications may interact with anesthetics, often increasing or decreasing potency and effectiveness. It is especially important to consider the effects of drugs used for heart disease, hypertension, immunosuppression, anticoagulation, and endocrine replacement.

In addition, knowledge about current medication usage can alert the nurse to obtain and evaluate laboratory tests. For example, if the patient is receiving warfarin (Coumadin) or aspirin, a coagulation profile should be obtained. A patient on diuretic therapy may need to have a potassium level obtained. If the patient is taking medications for dysrhythmias, a preoperative electrocardiogram (ECG) should be obtained.[14] Insulin or antidiabetic agents used in the management of the patient with diabetes may require dose or agent adjustments during the perioperative period because of increased body metabolism, stress, and anesthesia. Tranquilizers potentiate the effect of narcotics and barbiturates, which are agents used for anesthesia. Antihypertensive medication may predispose the patient to shock from the combined effect of the medication and the vasodilator effect of some anesthetic agents.

The nurse should also determine whether the patient is correctly taking currently prescribed medications. Is the patient taking the medication as ordered, or has the patient stopped taking the medication because of cost, side effects, or the feeling that ongoing therapy is no longer needed? Inquiry about medication use provides an ideal area for patient teaching and for referral of the patient to the physician who prescribed the medication.

When inquiring about medication use, it is important to ask about medication intolerance and drug allergies. *Medication intolerance* usually results in side effects that are uncomfortable or unpleasant for the patient but are not life threatening. These effects include nausea, constipation, diarrhea, and rash. A true *drug allergy* produces an anaphylactic or anaphylactoid reaction, causing cardiopulmonary compromise, including hypotension, tachycardia, bronchospasm, and possibly, pulmonary edema. By being aware of medication intolerance and drug allergies, it will be possible to avoid the use of these drugs, and ideally maintain patient comfort, safety, and stability. If a medication intolerance or drug allergy is noted, the patient's chart should be labeled accordingly, and an allergy wrist band should be put on the patient on the day of surgery.

It is also important to inquire about nondrug allergies, including allergies to foods, chemicals, and pollen. The patient with a history of allergic responsiveness has a greater potential for demonstrating hypersensitivity reactions to drugs administered during anesthesia.[15]

Although it may be difficult or embarrassing, the patient should be asked about possible drug use, abuse, and addiction. The categories of drugs most likely to be used and abused include tobacco, alcohol, opioids, marijuana, and cocaine. Questions should be asked matter-of-factly, and the patient should be encouraged to respond truthfully. Surprisingly, when patients become aware of the potential interactions of these drugs with anesthetic medications, most patients will respond honestly about their drug use. Specific to smoking, the patients should be encouraged to stop 6 weeks before surgery to decrease the risk of intraoperative and postoperative respiratory complications.[16] Alcohol will place the surgical patient at risk when used chronically (see Chapter 8). When liver function is affected, metabolism of anesthetic agents is prolonged, nutritional status is altered, and the potential for postoperative complications is increased.

Surgery and Other Treatments. The patient should be questioned about previous surgical procedures and anesthetics. These answers will provide information about the patient's exposure to anesthetics and about any postoperative complications that may have occurred. For example, the patient may report having had an allergic reaction to a medication or may have developed pneumonia after a previous surgery.

Table 14-4 Key Questions: Preoperative Patient

Health Perception–Health Management Pattern
- What has the doctor explained to you about your surgery?
- Have you had surgery before?*
- Have you or any family members ever experienced any problems with anesthesia?*
- Do you smoke?* If yes, how many packs daily? For how many years?
- Do you have any chronic illnesses?*
- Are you taking any medications?* Are you allergic to any medication?*
- What is your usual use of alcohol?

Nutritional-Metabolic Pattern
- What is your usual or present height and weight?
- Have you had a recent weight gain or loss?*
- Do you have any food preferences or dislikes?*
- Do you have any difficulty chewing or swallowing?*
- Do you take vitamins?*
- Do you have any problems healing?*

Elimination Pattern
- Do you experience any problems with constipation?*
- Do you experience any problems with urinary elimination?*

Activity-Exercise Pattern
- Do you have a history of high blood pressure or cardiac disease?*
- Do you have any history of dyspnea, coughing, hemoptysis, COPD, or asthma?*
- Do you presently have an upper respiratory infection?*
- Do you have any musculoskeletal problems that might affect positioning during surgery or activity level after surgery?*
- Do you have any limitation in mobility of your neck?*
- Do you require any special equipment for ambulation?*

Sleep-Rest Pattern
- Describe any problems you have with sleeping.
- Do you use sleeping pills?*

Cognitive-Perceptual Pattern
- Do you wear glasses, contact lenses, or hearing aid?*
- How would you describe your pain tolerance?
- What methods have you found effective for pain relief?

Self-Perception–Self-Concept Pattern
- How do you feel about having this surgery?
- Have you experienced any changes in the way you feel about yourself or your body?*

Role-Relationship Pattern
- Will this surgery create any problems in your usual roles or relationships?*
- Will you have the support you feel you need following discharge?

Sexuality-Reproductive Pattern
- Do you expect this surgery to have any impact on your usual sexual activity?*

Coping–Stress Tolerance Pattern
- How do you feel about this surgery?
- Do you feel you will be able to cope following this surgery?

Value-Belief Pattern
- Do you have a conflict between your planned surgery and your value or belief system?*

COPD, Chronic obstructive pulmonary disease.
*If yes, describe.

Functional Health Patterns. It is important to review each functional health pattern of the patient before surgery. Key questions to ask a preoperative patient are listed in Table 14-4.

Objective Data

Physical Examination. It is a requirement of the Joint Commission for the Accreditation of Healthcare Organizations (JCAHO) that all patients admitted to the OR have a documented physical examination in the chart. This examination may be done in advance of surgery or on the day of surgery. It may be performed by a nurse, surgeon, internist, or anesthesiologist.

In consideration of the patient interview and physical examination, the ACP will assign the patient a physical status rating. This rating is designed to be an indicator of perioperative risk and overall outcome. Table 14-5 defines the current physical status classification rating scale.

Laboratory Testing. Ideally, preoperative laboratory tests should be ordered on the basis of the individual patient history and physical examination. However, many facilities have a written protocol for preoperative laboratory tests. Commonly ordered preoperative laboratory tests can be found in Table 14-6. It is often the responsibility of the nurse sending the patient to surgery to ensure that laboratory data are on the chart. In some institutions it is the nurse who screens the data for abnormalities, informing the surgeon and ACP as appropriate.

NURSING MANAGEMENT

PREOPERATIVE PATIENT

Preoperative Teaching

If the patient is an inpatient, most of the patient and family teaching should be done the evening before surgery. If the patient is an outpatient, the teaching is frequently done on the day of the preoperative interview and reinforced on the morning of surgery. Some ambulatory surgical centers have the staff telephone the patients the evening before surgery to answer last minute questions and to reinforce teaching.

The positive values of preoperative teaching include an increased satisfaction with nursing care by the patient and nurse, as well as a reduction in fear and anxiety, postoperative vomiting, postoperative pain and the use of pain medications, the number of complications, the duration of hospitalization, and the recovery time following discharge. In

Table 14-5 Preoperative Rating of Patient's Physical Status

Rating	Examples
I. Healthy patient with no systemic disease	Patient with no significant past or present health history
II. Mild systemic disease without functional limitations	Patient with a history of asthma controlled with β-agonist inhaler
III. Severe systemic disease associated with definite functional limitations	Patient with history of chronic asthma controlled with β-agonist inhaler, oral theophylline, and inhaled steroids; not wheezing
IV. Severe systemic disease that is ongoing threat to life	Patient with a history of asthma, poorly controlled with theophylline and oral steroids; PaO_2 50 mmHg; wheezing; chest x-ray changes
V. Patient unlikely to survive for more than 24 hr with or without surgery	Patient in status asthmaticus, intubated, ventilated, IV steroids, IV aminophylline

IV, Intravenous.

addition, the patient has a right to know what to expect and how to participate effectively during the surgical experience.

Preoperative teaching includes information about preoperative routines, such as the approximate time of surgery and postoperative recovery, and the purpose and goals of postanesthesia care and routines. The patient may receive instruction about deep breathing, use of incentive spirometry, and use of patient-controlled analgesia pumps. The patient will also receive surgery-specific information. For example, a patient having a total joint replacement will be instructed about the use of an immobilizer and, possibly, about the use of an epidural catheter for postoperative pain control. A patient having open heart surgery will be told about the intensive care unit and its routines.

Preoperative teaching also includes information about any preoperative preparation required before surgery. These preparations may include the need for a preoperative shower or enema. The patients will also need to be instructed about preoperative food and fluid restrictions. The patient is usually instructed to have nothing by mouth (NPO), including food and fluids after midnight on the evening before surgery. This protocol may vary if the patient is having local anesthesia. It will be important to verify the NPO protocol of a specific institution when instructing patients. Restriction of fluids and food is designed to minimize the potential risk of aspiration upon induction of anesthesia and to decrease the risk of postoperative nausea and vomiting. The patient who has not followed this instruction may have surgery delayed or canceled.

In preparing the patient psychologically for surgery, the nurse must strike a balance between telling so little that the patient is unprepared and telling so much that the patient is overwhelmed. The nurse who observes carefully and listens sensitively to the patient can usually determine how much information is enough in each instance.

The nurse should be particularly aware of the effect of anxiety on learning and should allow time for repetition,

Table 14-6 Common Preoperative Laboratory Tests

Test	Area Assessed
Urinalysis	Renal status, hydration, urinary tract infection and disease
Chest x-ray	Pulmonary disorders, cardiac enlargement
Blood studies: RBC, Hb, Hct, WBC, WBC differential	Anemia, immune status, infection
Electrolytes	Metabolic status, renal function
ABGs, oximetry	Pulmonary and metabolic function
Prothrombin or partial thromboplastin time	Bleeding tendencies
Fasting blood sugar	Metabolic status, diabetes mellitus
Creatinine	Renal function
Blood urea nitrogen	Renal function
Electrocardiogram	Cardiac disease, electrolyte abnormalities
Pulmonary function studies	Pulmonary status
Type and cross-match	Blood availability for replacement (elective surgery patients may have own blood available)
Pregnancy	Reproductive status

ABGs, Arterial blood gases; *Hb,* hemoglobin; *Hct,* hematocrit; *RBC,* red blood cell count; *WBC,* white blood cell count.

NURSING CARE PLAN Preoperative Patient*

Planning: Outcome Criteria	Nursing Interventions and Rationales
➤ **NURSING DIAGNOSIS**	Anxiety *related to* lack of knowledge about preoperative routines, physical preparation for surgery, postoperative care, and potential body image change *as manifested by* signs of anxiety ranging from mild to high, such as verbal expression of concern, restlessness, irritability, agitation, and crying; repeated questioning about impending surgery
State anxiety relieved or maintained at tolerable level; have relaxed facial expression and body movements; express feeling less anxious; express an understanding of preoperative routine, surgery, and postoperative routine; have vital signs within normal limits; give informed consent.	For lack of knowledge about preoperative routines, encourage patient to verbalize concerns. Provide information as patient requests it *to give information in order to make informed choices.* Instruct patient about time of surgery, food or fluid restrictions, informed consent, physical preparation required, operating room environment, intravenous lines, other likely drains, anesthesia. Instruct patient about role and responsibility during the preoperative phase *to reduce anxiety.* For lack of knowledge about physical preparation for surgery, explain the purpose of the particular bowel or skin preparation ordered, if any, *to reduce anxiety related to these procedures.* For lack of knowledge about postoperative care, describe awakening in the recovery room. Explain why fluids may be restricted; explain the purpose of frequent vital signs assessment; teach how to turn, cough, and deep breathe; explain pain control and other comfort measures that may be used *to reduce anxiety and the incidence of postoperative complications and to increase patient cooperation.* For lack of knowledge about potential body image changes specifically related to the expected bodily changes associated with the respective surgery, assess patient's areas of concern—use of blood products, presence of scar, change in body structure or function; identify impact on roles—economic, occupational, emotional; identify support services; make referrals as needed; ensure privacy; use open communication, active listening, and nonjudgmental responses; observe verbal and nonverbal cues; notify physician if fear of death is overwhelming *as high stress levels can affect anesthesia and the postoperative course.*

*This general preoperative care plan is used in conjunction with a surgical care plan specific to the type of surgery being performed.

reinforcement, and verification of the patient's understanding. All teaching should be documented in the patient's medical record. A nursing care plan related to the problem of anxiety of the preoperative patient is presented above.

Preoperative Teaching for Outpatients. The outpatient and family should also receive instruction about day of surgery events, including patient registration, parking, what to wear, what to bring, and the need to have a responsible adult present for transportation home after surgery.

In addition, the patient should be told the time to arrive and the time of surgery. It is often one to two hours before the actual scheduled time of surgery to allow for completion of preoperative paperwork and preparation.

Legal Preparation for Surgery

Before nonemergency surgery can be legally performed, the patient must sign a voluntary and informed consent in the presence of a witness. This document protects the patient, surgeon, and the hospital and its employees (Fig. 14-2). Informed consent is an active, shared decision-making process between the provider and the recipient of care.

For consent to be valid, three conditions must be met.[17] First, there must be *adequate disclosure* of the diagnosis; the nature and purpose of the proposed treatment; the risks and consequences of the proposed treatment; the probability of a successful outcome; the availability, benefits, and risks of alternative treatments; and the prognosis if treatment is not instituted. Second, the patient must demonstrate *sufficient comprehension* of the information being provided. Because preoperative medications may cloud a patient's comprehension, the operative consent must be signed before any preoperative medication is given. Third, the recipient of care must *give consent voluntarily.* The patient must not be persuaded or coerced in any way to undergo the procedure.

Although the physician is ultimately responsible for obtaining the consent, the nurse may be responsible for obtaining and witnessing the patient's signature on the consent form. At this time the nurse can be a patient advocate,

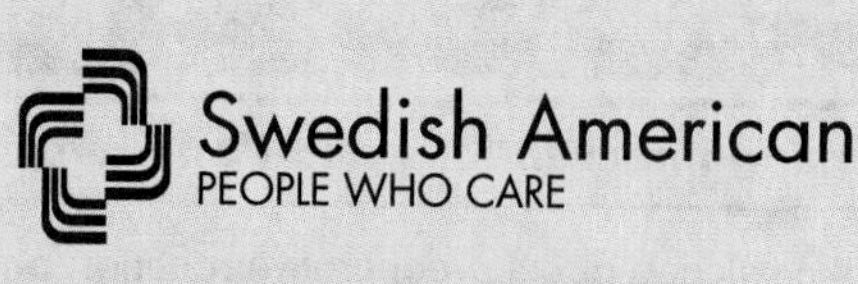

CONSENT TO OPERATION, ANESTHETICS, OBSTETRICAL PROCEDURES, AND OTHER MEDICAL SERVICES

Date ______________________ Time ______________ AM PM

1) I authorize the performance on ______________________ (Name of patient)
of the following operation ______________________
to be performed under the direction of Dr. ______________________

2) I consent to the performance of operations and procedures in addition to or different from those now contemplated whether or not arising from presently unforeseen conditions, which the above named doctor or associates or assistants may consider necessary or advisable in the course of the operation.

3) I consent to the administration of such anesthetics as may be considered necessary or advisable by the physician for this service with the exception of ______________________ (State "None," "Spinal Anesthesia," etc.)

4) I consent to the photographing or televising of the operation or procedures to be performed, including appropriate portions of my body for medical, scientific, or educational purposes, provided my identity is not revealed by the pictures or by descriptive texts accompanying them.

5) For the purpose of advancing medical education, I consent to the admittance of observers to the operating room.

6) I consent to the disposal by hospital authorities of any tissues or parts that may be removed.

7) I am aware that sterility may result from this operation. I know that a sterile person is not capable of becoming a parent.

8) The nature and purpose of the operation, possible alternative methods of treatment, the risks involved, and the possibility of complications have been fully explained to me. No guarantee or assurance has been given by anyone as to the results that may be obtained.

____
(Signature of Patient or Authorized Person to Consent for Patient)

____
(Witness)

*Note: Cross out any paragraphs above that do not apply.

Fig. 14-2 Operative consent form.

verifying that the patient (or family member) understands the consent form and its implications. The nurse has an important role as a patient advocate in ensuring that consent for surgery is truly voluntary and informed. The patient needs to be aware that permission may be withdrawn at any time, including after the permit has been signed.

If the patient is a minor, unconscious, or mentally incompetent to sign the permit, the written permission may be signed by a responsible family member. Local hospital policies should be checked for further clarification on this matter.

A true medical emergency may override the need to obtain consent. When immediate medical treatment is

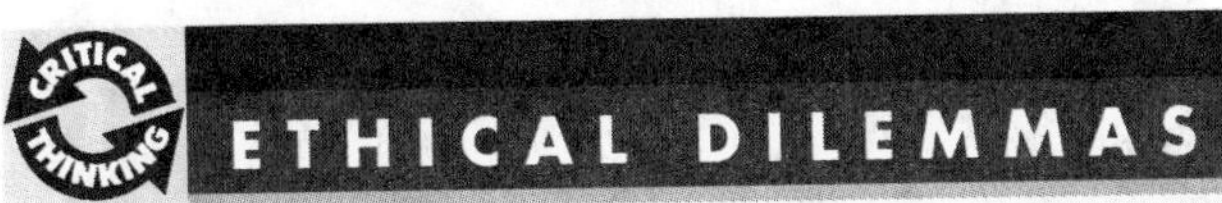

INFORMED CONSENT

Situation The nurse discusses a patient's impending surgery in the preoperative holding area. It becomes obvious that this competent adult patient was not fully informed of the alternatives to this surgery. The patient has signed the consent form but clearly was not fully informed about other options. What should the nurse do?

Discussion Informed consent requires that patients be fully informed about the need for surgery, the nature of the surgery, and the alternatives to surgery. If this patient was not fully counseled about alternatives, informed consent for this surgery could not have been given. No one should attempt to coerce a patient into signing a consent form or witness a form that has not been fully explained. The nurse needs to make sure that the patient discusses with the surgeon any and all questions and concerns about the surgery before any anesthetics are administered. The patient's rights to full disclosure are of greater importance than maintaining the surgical schedule.

ETHICAL AND LEGAL PRINCIPLES

- Elements of informed consent include competency of the patient to understand the information and make a decision; full disclosure of risks, benefits and alternatives; and voluntary (not coerced) consent.
- A patient's autonomy and bodily integrity are best upheld and protected by full disclosure of risks, benefits, and alternatives.
- Medical paternalism would maintain the position that (1) medical professionals know what is best for patients, (2) patients can never fully understand enough to give fully informed consent, and (3) the contract with the patient implies consent to appropriate treatment. It is unethical and illegal if this attitude denies a patient complete information on the grounds that full disclosure might be worse than withholding information or alternatives.

needed to preserve life or to prevent serious impairment to life and the individual patient is incapable of giving consent, the next of kin may give consent. If reaching the next of kin is not possible, the physician may institute treatment without written consent. A note will be written in the chart documenting the medical necessity of the procedure. Procedures for obtaining consent vary among states and institutions. The nurse should be aware of the state's nurse practice act and the institutional or agency policies that apply to an individual situation.

Advance Directives. With advances in technology and pharmacology, new limits have been reached in the artificial support of patients through artificial ventilation, hydration, and nutrition. Ethical issues of withholding care and withdrawing care challenge all health care providers. The issue of withholding care is distinctly different from withdrawing life-sustaining treatment once it has been initiated. Health care providers have several options available related to withdrawing care, which may vary somewhat from state to state. These options include the following:

1. Obtain a court order to withdraw treatment.
2. Wait for death.
3. Follow advance directives, including a living will and durable power of attorney.
4. Follow verbal refusal of the patient for life support.
5. Follow directives of a surrogate decision maker.

As these situations are often unexpected and occur suddenly, it is now required by law that before surgery inpatients be provided the opportunity to sign advance directives, including a living will and power of attorney. Many centers offer the forms to outpatients as well. A living will recognizes the right of a person to make a written declaration instructing his physician to withhold or withdraw death-delaying procedures in the event that the person becomes terminally ill and is unable to express his wishes. It may be signed by any patient 18 years of age and older in the presence of two witnesses. A durable power of attorney for health care recognizes the right of an individual to delegate control over treatment decisions to another person in the event that the individual becomes incompetent.[18] Figures 14-3 and 14-4 provide examples of these forms. It is often the nurse who is responsible for providing the forms to the patient, for answering questions, and for placing the signed forms in the chart.

Day of Surgery

Day of surgery preparation will vary a great deal depending on whether the patient is an inpatient or an outpatient. If the patient is an inpatient, it will be the responsibility of the hospital nurse to ensure that the patient is ready and appropriately prepared for surgery. If the patient is an outpatient, the patient or family member will share the responsibility for preoperative preparation. The nursing responsibility immediately before surgery includes final preparation of the patient, as well as checking to determine that all orders have been carried out and that records are complete and ready to accompany the patient to the OR.

The patient should be assisted as necessary in dressing for surgery. Most institutions require that a patient wear a hospital gown with no underclothes. Some surgery centers allow the patient to wear underwear, depending on the surgical procedure to be performed. It is recommended that the patient wear no cosmetics or nail polish, because observation of skin color will be important and equipment used to monitor oxygenation will be placed on the patient's fingertip (pulse oximeter). An identification band should be put on the patient and, if applicable, an allergy band. All patient valuables should be returned to a family member or locked up according to institutional protocol. If the patient prefers not to remove a wedding ring, the ring can be taped securely to the finger to prevent loss. All prostheses, including dentures, contact lenses, and glasses are generally removed to prevent loss or damage to them. Consideration should be given to the privacy and self-esteem needs of the patient.

DURABLE POWER OF ATTORNEY FOR HEALTH CARE

POWER OF ATTORNEY made this ______________ day of ______________ 19 ______

1. I, the undersigned, hereby appoint (insert name and address of agent) ______________________________

as agent to act for me and in my name to make any and all decisions for me concerning my personal care, medical treatment, hospitalization and health care and to require, withhold or withdraw any type of medical treatment or procedure, even though my death may ensue. My agent shall have the same access to my medical records that I have, including the right to disclose the contents to others. My agent shall also have full power to make disposition of any part or all of my body for medical purposes, authorize an autopsy and direct the disposition of my remains. (Neither the attending physician nor any other health care provider may act as your agent.)

2. The powers granted above shall be subject to the following rules or limitations (if none, leave blank):

____

____

(The subject of life-sustaining treatment is of particular importance. For your convenience in dealing with that subject, some general statements concerning the withholding or removal of life-sustaining treatment are set forth below. If you agree with one of these statements, you may initial that statement; but do not initial more than one.)

____ (I do not want my life prolonged nor do I want life-sustaining treatment to be provided or continued if my agent believes the burdens of the treatment outweigh the expected benefits. I want my agent to consider the relief of suffering, the expense involved and the quality as well as the possible extension of my life in making decisions concerning life-sustaining treatment.

____ (I want my life to be prolonged and I want life-sustaining treatment to be provided or continued unless I am in a coma which my attending physician believes to be irreversible, in accordance with reasonable medical standards at the time of reference. If and when I have suffered irreversible coma, I want life-sustaining treatment to be withheld or discontinued.

____ (I want my life to be prolonged to the greatest extent possible without regard to my condition, the chances I have for recovery or the cost of the procedures.

3. This power of attorney shall become effective on ______________________________
4. This power of attorney shall terminate on ______________________________
5. If any agent named by me shall die, become legally disabled, resign, refuse to act or be unavailable, I name the following (each to act alone and successively, in the order named) as successors to such agent:

____

____

6. If a guardian of my person is to be appointed, I nominate the following to serve as such guardian (If same as agent, leave blank):

____

7. I am fully informed as to all the contents of this form and understand the full import of this grant of power to my agent.

Signed ______________________________
Principal

The principal has had an opportunity to read the above form and has signed the form or acknowledged his or her signature or mark on the form in my presence.

______________________________ Residing at ______________________________
(Witness)

(You may, but are not required to, request your agent and successor agents to provide specimen signature below. If you include specimen signature in this Power of Attorney, you must complete the certification opposite the signatures of the agents.)

Specimen signatures of agent (and successors)	I certify that the signature of my agent (and successors) are correct.
______________ (agent)	______________ (principal)
______________ (successor agent)	______________ (principal)
______________ (successor agent)	______________ (principal)

Fig. 14-3 Durable power of attorney for health care form.

The patient should be encouraged to void before going into surgery. This should be done before the administration of any preoperative medication. Many preoperative medications have the potential to interfere with balance and judgment and could result in a patient fall. Urination before surgery prevents involuntary elimination under anesthesia, lessens the chance of accidental nicking of the bladder during surgery, and reduces the possibility of urinary retention during early postoperative recovery. When surgery is in the area of the bladder, as in gynecological procedures, an indwelling catheter may be inserted either preoperatively in the holding room or in the OR.

The use of a preoperative checklist (Fig. 14-5) will help to ensure that no detail has been omitted. The nurse should

LIVING WILL DECLARATION

This declaration is made this __________ day of ______________________ ,19 _____ (month, year). I, ____, being of sound mind, willfully and voluntarily make known my desires that my moment of death shall not be artificially postponed.

If at any time I should have an incurable and irreversible injury, disease, or illness judged to be a terminal condition by my attending physician who has personally examined me, and has determined that my death is imminent except for death delaying procedures. I direct that such procedures which would only prolong the dying process be withheld or withdrawn, and that I be permitted to die naturally with only the administration of medication, sustenance, or the performance of any medical procedure deemed necessary by my attending physician to provide me with comfort care.

In the absence of my ability to give directions regarding the use of such death delaying procedures, it is my intention that this declaration shall be honored by my family and physician as the final expression of my legal right to refuse medical or surgical treatment and accept the consequences from such refusal.

Signed ______________________________

City, County and State of Residence ____

The declarant is personally known to me and I believe him or her to be of sound mind. I did not sign the declarant's signature above for or at the direction of the declarant. At the date of this instrument I am not entitled to any portion of the estate of the declarant according to the laws of intestate succession or to the best of my knowledge and belief, under any will of declarant or other instrument taking effect at declarant's death, or directly financially responsible for declarant's medical care.

Witness ______________________________

Witness ______________________________

Fig. 14-4 Living will declaration.

determine that all preoperative orders and procedures have been completed and that the chart and documentation is complete before giving any preoperative medications. It is especially important to verify the presence of a signed operative consent, laboratory data, a history and physical examination report, a record of any consultations, baseline vital signs, and nurses' notes complete to that point.

Preoperative Medications

Preoperative medications are used for a variety of reasons, as summarized in Table 14-7. A patient may receive a single drug or combination of drugs (Table 14-8). Benzodiazepines and barbiturates are used for their sedative and amnestic properties. H_2-receptor antagonists are used to prevent the risks of aspiration. Anticholinergics are given to

St. Joseph Hospital, Inc.
Albuquerque, New Mexico
☐ St. Joseph Hospital
☐ St. Joseph West Mesa Hospital

ADDRESSOGRAPH

PREOPERATIVE CHECK LIST

Name of Procedure ______
Date of Surgery ______

	INITIALS O.R.	UNIT
1. Operative Permit signed and on chart: (initial if completed)		
2. History and Physical in chart: (initial if present)		
3. New Progress and Doctor's order sheet on chart: (initial if present)		
4. Consultation: ______ NA ______		
5. Laboratory results: Hct: ______ Hgb: ______ K+ ______		
6. Miscellaneous Pre-Op Lab studies: SMAC ______ Chest X-Ray ______ ECG ______ Type & Cross Match ______ # of units ______		
7. Allergies: ______ NKA ______ Front of chart labelled ______ NPO ______		
8. Prosthetic removed: Contact lenses ______ glasses ______ limb ______ eyes ______ hearing aid ______ dentures ______ removable bridgework ______ capped teeth present ______ location ______ etc. ______		
9. Old chart to O.R. with patient: ______ Not requested ______ No old chart ______		
10. Preoperative Medication given: ______ TIME: ______ None ordered ______		
11. Vital Signs: (time taken) ______ B.P. ______ P ______ R ______ T ______		
12. Skin prep on unit: ______ wash ______ scrub ______ shower ______		
13. Wearing hospital gown: ______ other: ______		
14. Hairpins and/or wig removed: ______ NA ______		
15. Make-up, false eyelashes and nail polish removed: ______ NA ______		
16. Disposition of valuables: (money, credit cards) To business office ______ family ______ none ______ To O.R. with patient: Rings (taped) ______ religious articles ______ NONE ______		
17. Antiembolism stockings/bandages: Applied ______ with patient ______ NA ______		
18. Urinary status: voided ______ catheterized ______ indwelling cath ______		
19. Medications to O.R. with patient: ______ none ______		
20. Addressograph on chart ______		
21. Chart and transport slip checked ______		
Chart signed off ______		

Signature and Title	initials

Signature and Title	initials

SJH #6010-110(5/84)

Fig. 14-5 Preoperative checklist.

reduce secretions. Narcotics may be given to decrease intraoperative anesthetic requirements and to decrease any pain associated with placement of IV catheters or other preoperative monitors. Antiemetics may be given to decrease nausea and vomiting.

Other medications that may be administered preoperatively include antibiotics, heparin, eye drops, and routine prescription medications. Antibiotics may be ordered for a patient with a history of congenital or valvular heart disease to prevent the development of bacterial endocarditis. They may also be ordered for the patient undergoing surgery where wound contamination is either a potential risk (e.g., gastrointestinal surgery) or where wound infection could have serious postoperative consequences (e.g., cardiac and

Table 14-7 Purposes of Preoperative Medication

Relieve apprehension and anxiety
Promote sedation and amnesia
Provide analgesia
Facilitate induction of anesthesia
Prevent nausea and vomiting
Prevent autonomic reflex response
Decrease anesthetic requirements
Decrease respiratory and gastrointestinal secretions

joint replacement surgery). Antibiotics are most commonly administered IV and may be started either preoperatively or in the OR.[19]

The use of low-dose subcutaneous heparin administered 6 to 12 hours preoperatively has been shown to reduce the rate of deep venous thrombosis and pulmonary embolism by 60%. As most patients are not admitted to the hospital preoperatively, it has also been shown that heparin therapy may be started up to 2 days after surgery with similar outcomes.[20]

Eye drops are commonly ordered and administered preoperatively for the patient undergoing cataract and other eye surgery. Many times the patient will require multiple sets of eye drops, administered at 5-minute intervals. It is important to administer these drugs as ordered and on time to adequately prepare the eye for surgery.

Administering preoperative medications would be easier if two lists of medications were developed; the first would list the medications that are always given on the day of surgery, and the second would list those that are never given on the day of surgery. It would facilitate patient teaching and eliminate confusion. Unfortunately, such lists do not exist. Most patients will be advised to take routine cardiac, antihypertensive, and asthma medications on the day of surgery. It is important to carefully check written preoperative orders and to clarify which medications should be taken on the day of surgery. In the case of insulin it is important to clarify the dose.

Premedications may be administered orally, IV, subcutaneously, or IM. Oral medications should be given 60 to 90 minutes before the patient arrives in the OR. Because patients are fluid restricted before surgery, it is important for the patient to swallow these medications with only a minimal amount of water. Intramuscular and subcutaneous injections should be given 30 to 60 minutes before arrival (minimally 20 minutes).[19] Intravenous medications are usually administered to the patient upon arrival to the preoperative holding area or OR. Once the medication is given, charting should be completed because the patient is now prepared for surgery and ready for transport to the OR. Premedication should be administered to the patient after all other preoperative preparation has been completed. The patient should be told that the medications will help with relaxation, and drowsiness may occur without loss of consciousness. If an anticholinergic is used, the patient needs to know that although the mouth will feel dry, no fluids should be taken.

Transportation to the Operating Room

If the patient is an inpatient, the OR staff sends transport personnel to the patient's room with a cart to transport the patient to surgery. The nurse assists the patient in transferring from the hospital bed to the OR cart, and the side rails of the cart are raised and secured. The nurse should ensure that the chart goes with the patient, as well as any ordered preoperative equipment, such as the patient's inhaler if the patient is an asthmatic or antiembolism devices. In many institutions the family may accompany the patient to the holding area.

Table 14-8 Frequently Used Preoperative Medications

Class	Purpose and Effects	Drug
Benzodiazepines	Reduce anxiety Induce sedation Induce amnesia	Midazolam Diazepam Lorazepam
Narcotics	Relieve discomfort during preoperative procedures	Morphine Meperidine Fentanyl
H_2-receptor antagonists	Increase gastric pH Decrease gastric volume	Cimetidine Famotidine Ranitidine
Antacid	Increase gastric pH	Sodium citrate
Antiemetics	Increase gastric emptying Decrease nausea and vomiting	Metoclopramide Droperidol
Anticholinergics	Decrease oral and respiratory secretions Prevent bradycardia Induce amnesia (scopolamine only)	Atropine Glycopyrrolate Scopolamine

If the patient is an outpatient, the patient may be transported to the OR by cart, wheelchair, or may even walk accompanied to the OR. In all cases it is important for the nurse to ensure patient safety in transport.

Because the patient is leaving the nursing unit or outpatient area for surgery, it will be important for the nurse to instruct the family where to wait for the patient during surgery. Many hospitals have a surgical waiting room where personnel communicate the status of the patient and the surgical schedule with the OR staff. It is in this waiting room that the surgeon can locate the family after surgery and where families can be notified that the surgery is complete.

While the patient is in surgery the hospital nurse can prepare the patient's room in consideration of the patient's needs after surgery. The bed is remade and, if necessary, disposable pads are placed for any anticipated drainage. Any additional necessary equipment including IV poles, oxygen equipment, suction equipment, and additional pillows for positioning should also be placed in the room. By having these items readily available and the room ready, patient transfer from the PACU or the OR will be smooth.

Gerontologic Considerations

Approximately 24% of all surgical procedures are performed on patients older than 65 years of age.[21] The most frequently performed procedures in the older adult are cataract extraction, prostatectomy, herniorraphy, cholecystectomy, and hip stabilization.[22]

The risks associated with anesthesia and surgery increase in the older patient. In general, the older the patient, the greater the risk of complications after surgery. The surgical risk in the older adult relates to normal physiologic aging changes that compromise organ function, reduce reserve capacity, and limit the body's ability to adapt to stress. This decreased ability to cope with stress, compounded by the additional burden of one or more chronic illnesses, anxiety, and the surgery itself, increases the risk of complications. The increased risks are not only a result of aging, but are caused by the increased prevalence of coexisting diseases and by a decline in basic organ system functioning, which is independent of disease processes. It is important to consider the physiologic status or condition of the patient in planning care and not simply the chronologic age.

When preparing the older adult for surgery, it is important to obtain a detailed history and complete physical examination. Often this patient will be referred to an internist for medical approval before surgery. Preoperative laboratory tests, including an ECG and a chest x-ray, will be important in planning the choice and technique of anesthesia. Inquiry about family support will also be important. With the increase in outpatient surgical procedures and shorter postoperative hospitalizations, family support is an important consideration in the continuity of care for the older patient.

The nurse must remember that the thought processes and cognitive abilities may be slowed or impaired in some older adults. In addition, vision and hearing may be diminished. Therefore the older patient may require increased time to complete preoperative testing, dress for surgery, understand preoperative instructions, and complete any needed preoperative preparation.

Adding to situational change and loss, the perceived threat or loss of health associated with surgery may be overwhelming to the older adult. This overwhelming loss, which can affect independence, lifestyle, and self-esteem, may result in ineffective coping. The nurse must be particularly alert when assessing and caring for the older adult surgical patient. An event that has little effect on a younger patient may be overwhelming to the older patient.

CRITICAL THINKING EXERCISES

CASE STUDY

PREOPERATIVE PATIENT

Patient Profile

Mrs. Frances D., an 82-year-old retired librarian, is admitted to the hospital with complaints of abdominal pain, alternating diarrhea and constipation, and blood in her stool.

Subjective Data

- Has history of hypertension for 40 years
- Takes hydrochlorthiazide
- Has history of diabetes mellitus, type II, since age of 60
- Takes NPH insulin every morning and regular insulin before meals
- Has surgical history that includes a C-section at age 30 and appendectomy at age 19
- Has not eaten for 2 days and has had decreasing oral intake for the past 2 weeks
- Reports a 10-pound weight loss
- Sleeps poorly at night and is drowsy during the day
- Lives alone and has no immediate family

Objective Data

Physical Examination

- Alert, well-oriented, slightly obese older woman with painful, palpable abdominal mass

Diagnostic Studies

- Ultrasound—abdominal mass in area of transverse colon
- Hematocrit—27%
- Stool for guaiac—positive

Therapeutic Management

Scheduled for explorotomy laparotomy, colon resection, and possible colostomy

Critical Thinking Questions

1. What factors may influence Mrs. D's response to hospitalization and surgery?
2. Given Mrs. D's history, what preoperative laboratory tests would you want to assess and why?
3. What potential perioperative complications might you expect for Mrs. D.?
4. What topics would you include in Mrs. D's preoperative teaching plan?
5. Based on the assessment data presented, write one or more appropriate nursing diagnoses. Are there any collaborative problems?

NURSING RESEARCH ISSUES

1. Can a patient interview effectively predict the need for specific preoperative laboratory tests as opposed to using a predetermined list of required preoperative laboratory tests?
2. Does the preoperative administration of antiemetics to specific patient groups reduce the incidence of nausea and vomiting in the postoperative period?
3. Does the nurse use preoperative patient interview data in planning preoperative instruction?
4. Is there a difference in the accuracy of preoperative assessment data collected by a patient-completed form as compared with a nurse-completed questionnaire?

REVIEW QUESTIONS

The number of the question corresponds to the same-numbered objective at the beginning of the chapter.

1. Which of these surgical procedures involves removal of a body organ?
  a. Herniorrhaphy
  b. Cholecystectomy
  c. Mammoplasty
  d. Colostomy

2. A patient reports having an allergy to penicillin. Which of the following questions would elicit the most useful information for the nurse?
  a. When did the reaction occur?
  b. What infection did you have that required penicillin?
  c. What type of allergic reaction did you have?
  d. Did you notify your physician of the allergy?

3. Which patient is at greatest risk for surgical and anesthetic complications?
  a. A 3-year-old boy scheduled for a hernia repair
  b. An 80-year-old scheduled for an exploratory laparotomy
  c. An 18-year-old scheduled for an emergency appendectomy
  d. A 42-year-old scheduled for a breast biopsy

4. Mr. Jensen, an alert 75-year-old man, is to undergo elective hip surgery. The operative permit must be signed in the presence of a witness by

a. Mr. Jensen.
b. Mr. and Mrs. Jensen.
c. either Mr. or Mrs. Jensen.
d. Mr. Jensen and the surgeon.

5. A nursing intervention to assist the patient in coping with fear of pain would be to

a. describe the degree of pain expected.
b. explain the availability of pain medication.
c. inform the patient of the frequency of pain medication.
d. divert the patient when talking about pain.

6. Which measure should be done last on the morning of surgery?

a. Administrating preanesthetic medication
b. Asking patient to void in the bathroom
c. Removing jewelry and locking up securely
d. Checking chart for signed consent form

7. Which of the following statements is correct?

a. A preoperative diazepam (Valium) tablet should be administered within 15 minutes of scheduled surgery.
b. An intramuscular injection of secobarbital should be administered 2 hours before the scheduled surgery.
c. Intravenous medications can only be administered by an anesthesiologist on the day of surgery.
d. Preoperative medications may help reduce anesthetic requirements.

8. A primary consideration in the instruction of the older preoperative patient is

a. using large-print material.
b. teaching early in the morning.
c. standing very close to aid communication.
d. recognizing that cognitive function may be decreased.

REFERENCES

1. Mangano D: Perioperative cardiac morbidity: concepts and controversies. *ASA Refresher Course Lectures* 44:131, 1993.
2. Barash P: The high-risk patient for non-cardiac surgery: preoperative evaluation. *ASA Refresher Course Lectures* 44:231, 1993.
3. Tarhan S: Myocardial infarction after general anesthesia, *JAMA* 220:1451, 1988.
4. Hulyalker A, Miller E: Evaluation of the hypertensive patient. In M Rogers and others, editors: *Principles and practice of anesthesiology,* St Louis, 1993, Mosby.
5. Mangano D: Perioperative cardiac risk evaluation, *ASA Refresher Course Lectures,* 115:1, 1989.
6. Hotchkiss A: Perioperative management of the patient with chronic obstructive pulmonary disease, *Int Anesthesiol Clin* 26:134, 1988.
7. Stein M, Cassara E: Preoperative pulmonary evaluation and therapy for surgical patients, *JAMA* 211:787, 1970.
8. Ross A, Tinker J: Evaluation of the adult patient with cardiac problems. In M Rogers and others, editors: *Principles and practice of anesthesiology,* St Louis, 1993, Mosby.
9. Miller C: Evaluation of the patient with renal disease. In M Rogers and others, editors: *Principles and practice of anesthesiology,* St Louis, 1993, Mosby.
10. Stoelting R, Diendorf S: *Anesthesia and co-existing disease,* ed 3, New York, 1993, Churchill-Livingstone.
11. Bourke D, Yates H: Evaluation of the patient with orthopedic disease. In M Rogers and others, editors: *Principles and practice of anesthesiology,* St Louis, 1993, Mosby.
12. Snyder D, Humphrey L: Evaluation of the obese patient. In M Rogers and others, editors: *Principles and practice of anesthesiology,* St Louis, 1993, Mosby.
13. Ross A, Tinker J: Preoperative evaluation of the healthy patient. In M Rogers and others, editors: *Principles and practice of anesthesiology,* St Louis, 1993, Mosby.
14. Roizen M: Routine preoperative evaluation. In RD Miller, editor: *Anesthesia,* ed 3, New York, 1990, Churchill-Livingstone.
15. Hirshman C: Anaphylaxis and anesthesia, *ASA Refresher Course Lectures* 233:1, 1989.
16. Litwack K: *Post anesthesia care nursing,* ed 2, St Louis, 1995, Mosby.
17. Silva M, Zeccolo P: Informed consent: the right to know and the right to choose, *Nurs Manage* 17:18, 1986.
18. Brown M, Burck J: Implementation of the patient self-determination act and health care surrogate act: legal and ethical guidelines, Chicago, 1992, Rush Presbyterian St. Luke's Medical Center.
19. Moyers J: Premedication. In M Rogers and others, editors: *Principles and practice of anesthesiology,* St Louis, 1993, Mosby.
20. Symreng T: Thrombosis prophylaxis. In M Rogers and others, editors: *Principles and practice of anesthesiology,* St Louis, 1993, Mosby.
21. McLeskey C: Anesthesia for the geriatric outpatient. In P Barash and others, editors: *Clinical anesthesia,* Philadelphia, 1991, Lippincott.
22. Callahan L: General considerations in planning anesthetic care for the geriatric patient, *Anes Today* 3:10, 1991.

Chapter 15

NURSING ROLE IN MANAGEMENT

Patient During Surgery

Patricia Robertson Hercules **Darlene Batson**

Learning Objectives

1. Describe the physical environment of the operating room and the holding area.
2. Describe the functions of the members of the surgical team.
3. Identify needs experienced by the patient undergoing surgical procedures.
4. Discuss the role of the perioperative nurse when managing the care of the patient undergoing surgery.
5. Describe basic principles of aseptic technique used in the operating room.
6. Differentiate between general and regional or local anesthesia, including advantages, disadvantages, and rationale for choice of the anesthetic technique.
7. Identify the basic techniques and drugs used to induce and maintain general anesthesia.
8. Discuss techniques for administering local and regional anesthetics.
9. Discuss the characteristics of adjunct agents used with general anesthesia.

Nursing care of the surgical patient requires an understanding of surgery and surgical interventions. This knowledge allows the nurse to monitor the patient's response to the stressors related to the surgical experience. Use of the nursing process during the operative phase of care is necessary as a framework for the delivery of care. The needs of the patient determine the type of nursing care delivered. These needs are based on the current health status of the patient and the type of surgical intervention anticipated.

Historically, surgical interventions have taken place in the traditional environment of the operating room (OR) suite. Today some surgical procedures are also performed in alternative surgical environments, including endoscopy units, cardiac catheterization laboratories, emergency rooms, radiology outpatient surgical centers, and physician offices.

For the purposes of this chapter, the traditional OR suite and role and function of the perioperative nurse will be used to discuss the management of the patient during the surgical experience.

Reviewed by Susan S. Fairchild, RN, MSN, CNOR, CS, Doctoral Candidate, Assistant Professor, Nursing, Barry University, Miami Shores, FL and James H. Mulchay, RN, BA, CRNA, Staff Anesthetist, Anesthesia Professional Association, Ft Lauderdale, FL.

PHYSICAL ENVIRONMENT

Operating Room

The traditional surgical environment is a unique acute-care setting removed from other hospital clinical units. It is controlled geographically, environmentally, and bacteriologically, and it is restricted in terms of the inflow and outflow of personnel (Fig. 15-1). It is preferable to have the physical location of the OR adjacent to the postanesthesia care unit (PACU) and the surgical intensive care unit. This allows for close collaboration for postanesthesia recovery and intensive care follow-up. Careful consideration of the design, location, and control of the physical environment assists with the prevention of infection and provides physical safety and comfort for the patient and the OR team.

Several methods are used to prevent the transmission of infection. Filters and controlled airflow in the ventilating systems provide dust control. Positive air pressure in the rooms prevents air from entering the OR from the halls and corridors. Dust-collecting surfaces such as open shelves, windows, and ledges are omitted. Materials that are resistant to the corroding effects of strong disinfectants are used. The functional design facilitates the practice of aseptic technique by the OR team.

Physical safety and comfort are aided by the use of OR furniture that is conductive, adjustable, easy to clean, and easy to move. All equipment is checked frequently to ensure electrical safety. Line isolation monitors are installed

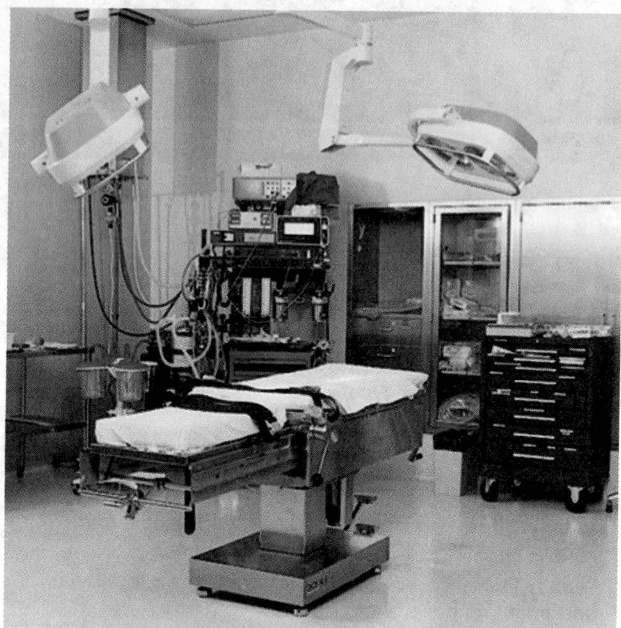

Fig. 15-1 Traditional operating room.

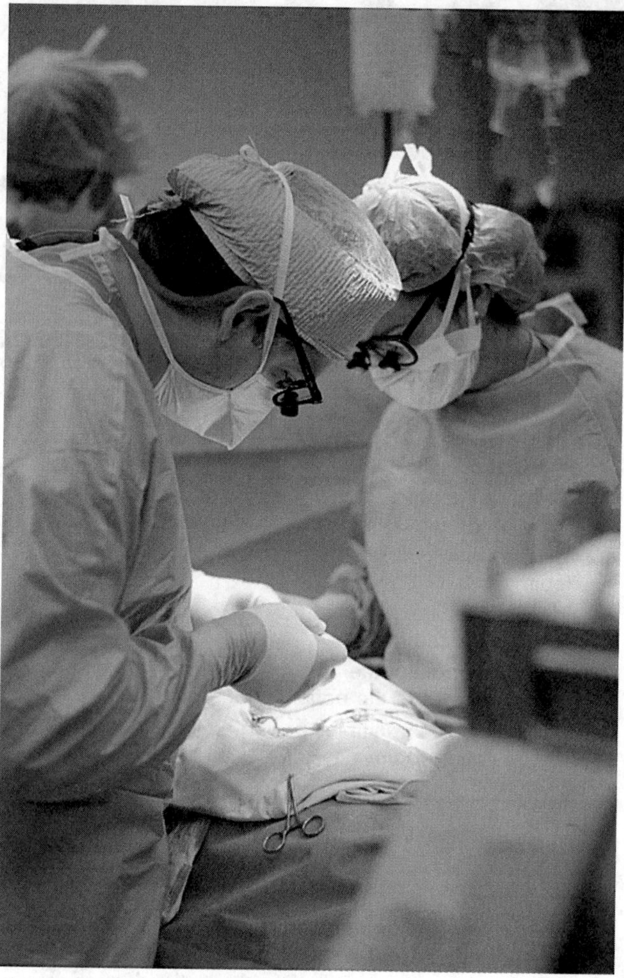

Fig. 15-2 The complexity of the operative procedure does not allow for the influx of extra personnel or visitors.

to assess proper function of all electrical equipment devices. The lighting is designed to provide a low- to high-intensity range for a precise view of the surgical site. A communication system provides a means for the delivery of routine and emergency messages.[1,2,3]

The temperature is controlled from 68° F to 75° F (20° C to 24° C), and the humidity is regulated at a minimum of 50% to facilitate patient comfort under the surgical drapes, team comfort during the procedure, and an environment that is unfavorable to bacterial incubation and growth.[1,3]

The privacy of the patient is achieved by restricting the influx of hospital personnel and visitors. Special permission must be obtained to enter the suite during the surgical procedure. The complexity of an ongoing operative procedure does not allow for the presence of extraneous personnel and visitors (Fig. 15-2).

Holding Area

The holding area, frequently called the preoperative holding area, is a special waiting area inside or outside the surgical suite. The size varies according to hospital design and can range from a centralized area to accommodate numerous patients to a small designated area immediately outside the actual room scheduled for the surgical procedure. In the holding area the perioperative nurse makes the final identification and assessment before the patient is transferred into the OR for surgery.[4,5] Many minor procedures can also be performed in the holding area, such as inserting intravenous (IV) catheters and arterial lines and removing casts.

In some settings another area for holding is identified as the admission, observation, and discharge (AOD) area. This area is designed to allow early morning admissions for outpatient surgery, same day admission, and inpatient holding before surgery. In this holding area the nurse can assess the patient for preoperative data, observe the patient both before and after surgery, and allow recovery for a sufficient length of time before discharge to either the home or an inpatient room. The AOD area significantly impacts the patient's stay throughout outpatient surgery and prevents unnecessary overnight stays in the inpatient setting.[4,5]

Some institutions permit the family or a friend to wait with the patient until it is time to be transferred to the OR. Separation from loved ones just before surgery can produce anxiety, and allowing them to stay with the patient alleviates stress.

THE SURGICAL TEAM

Registered Nurse

When the patient awaiting surgery arrives from home or is transported from the acute-care inpatient area to the holding area, the nurse is usually the first member of the surgical team encountered. Along with the final assessment and necessary tasks before the surgery, the nurse provides physical comfort measures and assists in reducing the patient's anxiety.

The perioperative nurse is a registered nurse who implements patient care based on the nursing process. Different

Table 15-1 Intraoperative Activities of the Perioperative Nurse

Circulating and Nonsterile Activities	Scrub and Sterile Activities
▪ Review anatomy, physiology, and surgical procedure. ▪ Assist with preparing the room. Practice aseptic technique. Monitor the activities of others. Ensure that needed items are available and sterile (if required). Check mechanical and electrical equipment and environmental factors. Arrange the furniture in workable order. ▪ Identify and assess the patient and coordinate the intraoperative nursing care. ▪ Check the chart and relate pertinent data. ▪ Admit the patient to the operating room suite. ▪ Assist with transferring the patient to the operating table. ▪ Participate in insertion and application of monitoring devices. ▪ Protect the patient during induction of anesthesia. ▪ Position the patient. ▪ Prepare the patient's skin for the surgical incision. ▪ Monitor the draping procedure and all activities requiring asepsis. ▪ Complete the intraoperative record. ▪ Record, label, and send tissue specimens and cultures to proper locations. ▪ Measure blood and fluid loss. ▪ Record amount of drugs and medications used during local anesthesia. ▪ Coordinate all activities in the room with team members and other health-related personnel and departments. ▪ Count sponges, needles, and instruments. ▪ Monitor practices of aseptic technique in self and others. ▪ Accompany the patient to the PACU. ▪ Report pertinent information to the PACU nurses.	▪ Review anatomy, physiology, and surgical procedure. ▪ Assist with preparation of the room. ▪ Scrub, gown, and glove self and other members of the surgical team. ▪ Prepare the instrument table and organize sterile equipment for functional use. ▪ Assist with the draping procedure. ▪ Pass instruments to the surgeon and assistants by anticipating their needs. ▪ Count sponges, needles, and instruments. ▪ Monitor practices of aseptic technique in self and others. ▪ Keep track of irrigation solutions used for calculation of blood loss. ▪ Report amounts of local anesthetic and epinephrine solutions used by anesthetist.

OR, Operating room; *PACU*, postanesthesia care unit.

functions may be assumed by the perioperative nurse that involve either *sterile* or *nonsterile* activities. If the nurse is not scrubbed, gowned, and gloved and remains in the unsterile field, the function of *circulating* is implemented. If the nurse follows the designated scrub procedure, is gowned and gloved in sterile attire, and remains in the sterile field, the function of *scrubbing* is implemented. Some specific intraoperative activities of each function are outlined in Table 15-1.

The perioperative nurse is not limited to task-oriented duties and actively implements nursing care throughout the patient's surgical experience. Examples of nursing activities that characterize each phase surrounding the surgical experience are presented in Table 15-2.

Licensed Practical Nurse and Surgical Technologist

In many institutions the scrubbed function is performed by a trained OR surgical technologist or a licensed practical nurse. The scrubbed, or assistive person assists the surgeon by passing instruments and implementing other technical functions during the surgical procedure. This role is supervised by and can also be assumed by a registered nurse.

Surgeon and Assistant

The surgeon is the physician who performs the surgical procedure. The surgeon may be the patient's primary physician or one who was selected by the patient's physician or the patient. The surgeon is primarily responsible for the following:

1. Preoperative patient history and physical assessment, including need for surgical intervention, choice of surgical procedure, and management of preoperative workup
2. Patient safety and management in the OR
3. Postoperative management of the patient

Table 15-2 Examples of Nursing Activities Surrounding the Surgical Experience

Before	During	After
Assessment ***Home, Clinic, and Holding Areas*** ▪ Initiate initial preoperative assessment ▪ Plan teaching methods appropriate to patient's needs ▪ Involve family in interview ***Surgical Unit*** ▪ Complete preoperative assessment ▪ Coordinate patient teaching with other nursing staff ▪ Develop a plan of care ***Surgical Suite*** ▪ Verify surgical suite ▪ Assess patient's level of consciousness ▪ Review chart ▪ Identify patient ***Planning*** ▪ Determine a plan of care	**Implementation** ***Maintenance of Safety*** ▪ Ensure that the sponge, needle, and instrument counts are correct ▪ Position the patient Functional alignment Exposure of surgical site Maintenance of position throughout procedure ▪ Apply grounding device to patient ▪ Provide physical support ***Monitoring of Physical Status*** ▪ Report changes in patient's pulse, respirations, temperature, and blood pressure ▪ Distinguish normal from abnormal cardiopulmonary data ***Monitoring of Psychologic Status*** ▪ Provide emotional support to patient ▪ Stand near or touch patient during procedures and induction ▪ Continue to assess patient's emotional status ▪ Communicate patient's emotional status to other appropriate members of the health care team ***Communication of Intraoperative Information*** ▪ State patient's name ▪ State type of surgery performed ▪ Provide contributing intraoperative factors (e.g., drain, catheters) ▪ State physical limitations ▪ State impairments resulting from surgery ▪ Report patient's preoperative level of consciousness ▪ Communicate necessary equipment needs	**Evaluation** ***Postanesthesia and Discharge Area*** ▪ Determine patient's immediate response to surgical intervention ***Surgical Unit*** ▪ Evaluate effectiveness of nursing care in the operating room ▪ Determine patient's level of satisfaction with care given during perioperative period ▪ Evaluate products used on patient in the operating room ▪ Determine patient's psychologic status ▪ Assist with discharge planning ***Home and Clinic*** ▪ Seek patient's perception of surgery in terms of the effects of anesthetic agents, impact on body image, immobilization ▪ Determine family's perceptions of surgery

The surgeon's assistant is usually a physician who functions in an assisting role during the surgical procedure. The assistant usually holds retractors to expose surgical areas and assists with hemostasis and suturing. In some instances, especially in educational settings, the assistant may perform some portions of the operative procedure under the direct supervision of the surgeon.

In some institutions the surgeon's assistant is a registered nurse or a nonphysician who functions in the role of the assistant under the direct supervision of the physician. Hospital policies define this role and physician responsibility when the assistant's position is filled by a nonphysician.

Anesthesia Care Provider

The term *anesthesia care provider* (ACP) may be defined as "one who administers anesthesia" and can refer to an anesthesiologist or a nurse anesthetist. An anesthesiologist is a medical doctor who has completed a residency in the field of anesthesia and is credentialed by the American Board of Anesthesiology. A nurse anesthetist is a registered nurse who has passed a national certification examination to become a certified registered nurse anesthetist (CRNA). Both the anesthesiologist and the CRNA are qualified to administer anesthetics to the patient and assume responsibility for the maintenance of physiologic homeostasis throughout the intraoperative period.

Anesthesia may be provided by the anesthesiologist or CRNA, working alone or in combination. The latter is often referred to as the *anesthesia team* approach. When working in the team approach, the anesthesiologist assumes the responsibility of supervision of the CRNA while the CRNA administers the anesthesia. When the CRNA is practicing

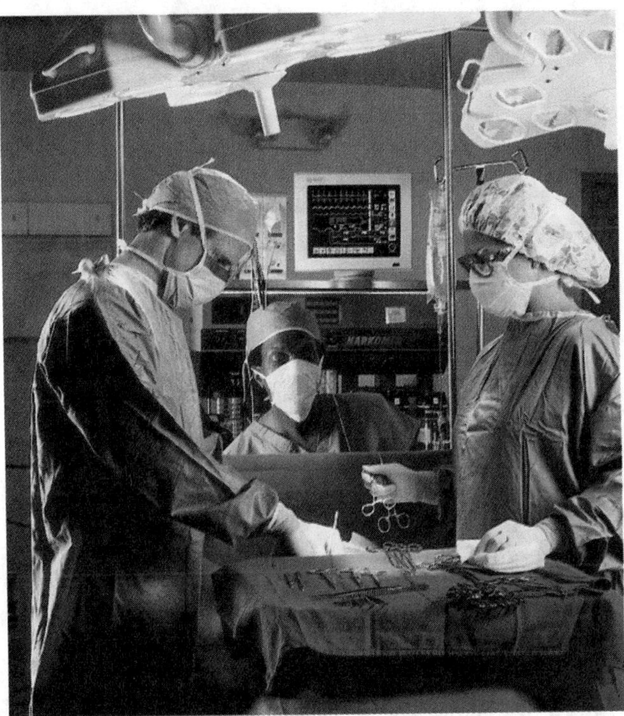

Fig. 15-3 Members of the surgical team collaborate about the care of the paient before, during, and after the surgical procedure.

alone, the surgeon assumes the responsibility for medical supervision. The ACP is also governed by state practice acts and the policies of the hospital where the provider is practicing.

The responsibilities generally accepted by the ACP are the following:

1. Assess the patient preoperatively to determine the safest anesthetic for the particular patient's needs and anticipated operative procedure.
2. Prescribe preoperative and adjunctive medications.
3. Administer the anesthetic during the surgical procedure, and inform the surgeon if difficulties arise during the patient's anesthetic course.
4. Administer fluids and electrolytes, medications, and blood products throughout the surgical procedure.
5. Supervise the postanesthesia recovery of the patient in the PACU, and document the patient's postanesthetic recovery in the first 24 hours.

In preparation for and carrying out the surgical procedure, members of the surgical team (circulating nurse, scrub assistant, surgeon, assistant, and ACP) collaborate to ensure that the patient is receiving the best possible care (Fig. 15-3).

NURSING MANAGEMENT

SURGICAL PATIENT

Before Surgery

The preoperative assessment of the surgical patient establishes baseline data for intraoperative and postanesthesia care. Assessment data that are provided by the patient and family in the holding area and data from the inpatient nursing units are important to ensure that a plan of care can be developed.

Psychosocial Assessment. The perioperative nurse who cares for the patient in the OR is knowledgeable about the ongoing activities that occur when a patient is transferred into the surgical suite. This knowledge allows for informative and reassuring explanations, especially to the anxious patient. General questions regarding surgery or anesthesia can usually be answered by the perioperative nurse. Examples of these questions include, "When will I go to sleep?" "Who will be in the room?" "When will my doctor arrive?" "How much of my body will be exposed and to whom?" "Will I be cold?" "When will I wake up?" Specific questions relating to details of the surgical procedure and anesthesia are referred to the surgeon or ACP.

It is especially important that the perioperative nurse has knowledge of the patient's spiritual and cultural habits and beliefs. Care must be taken that infringement on the patient's rights and privileges is not made without consent.

Physical Assessment. Physical assessment data that are specifically important to intraoperative nursing care include baseline data such as vital signs, height, weight, age, allergic reactions, condition and cleanliness of skin, skeletal and muscle impairments, perceptual difficulties, level of consciousness, and any sources of pain or discomfort. Vital signs are important as baseline data when drugs and anesthetics are administered. These data provide a means to evaluate the effects of intraoperative medications. Height and weight of the patient guide the nurse regarding the width and length of the operating table. Age can indicate the need for extra warmth because age can reflect the rate of basal metabolism. Some allergic reactions may be avoided with such simple measures as a change in "prepping" solutions or the type of tape used with dressings. The condition and cleanliness of the skin determine the amount and type of intraoperative skin preparation solutions and will alert the team to the potential for infection as a result of open or closed skin lesions. Knowledge of skeletal and muscle impairments helps to prevent injury during positioning. Perceptual difficulty, such as a vision or hearing impairment, will guide the nurse in adapting communication techniques to individual needs. An altered level of consciousness necessitates increased safety and protection techniques. Communicating identified sources of pain to other health team members prevents subjecting the patient to unnecessary discomfort.

Chart Assessment. Required chart data vary with hospital policy, patient condition, and specific surgical procedures. Examples of data that are routinely obtained during the preoperative assessment include the results of the following:

1. History and physical examination
2. Urinalysis
3. Complete blood cell count
4. Serum electrolyte values
5. Chest x-ray
6. Electrocardiogram
7. Diagnostic tests

A knowledge of these chart data will contribute to an understanding of past and present history, cardiopulmonary status, and potential for infection.

Admitting the Patient. Hospital policy designates the exact procedure that should be followed when admitting the patient to the holding area and OR suite. A general routine includes initial greeting, extension of human contact and warmth, and proper identification. The identification process includes asking the patient to state his name, the surgeon's name, and the operative procedure and location. In addition, the hospital identification numbers are compared with the patient's own identification band and chart. The patient is further identified by the surgeon before anesthesia induction. In some institutions identification may take place in the holding area and, in others, in the OR itself.

The admitting procedure is continued with reassessment of the patient and allowance of time for last-minute questions. The nurse continues to review the chart for the previously mentioned data and notes any abnormalities or changes. The patient is questioned concerning valuables, prostheses, and last intake of food and fluid. Validation is made that the correct preoperative medication was given, if ordered. A warm blanket, pillow, or position adjustment is provided if the patient is uncomfortable. Most hospitals require the patient's hair to be covered just before transfer.

During Surgery

Room Preparation. Before transferring the patient into the scheduled OR, the nurse spends significant time preparing the room to ensure privacy, safety, and prevention of infection. Surgical attire (specially designed pants or dresses, masks, protective eyewear, caps or hoods, and shoe covers) is worn by all persons entering the OR suite (Fig. 15-4). All electrical and mechanical equipment is checked for proper functioning. Aseptic technique is practiced as each surgical item is opened and placed systematically on the instrument table. Sponges, needles, and instruments are counted to ensure accurate retrieval at the close of the procedure.[4]

During this time and during the procedure the functions of the teams are delineated. While touching only those items in the sterile field, the scrub assistant scrubs hands and arms and dresses in sterile surgical gowns and gloves. The circulating nurse remains in the unsterile field and implements those activities that permit touching all unsterile items and the patient.

Transferring the Patient. Once the patient has been properly identified and the OR has been adequately prepared, the patient is transported into the room for the surgery. Each time a patient is transferred from one bed to another, the wheels of the stretcher should be locked, and a sufficient number of personnel should be available to lift, guide, and prevent accidental falling. Once the patient is on the operating table, safety straps should be snugly placed across the patient's thighs. At this time the monitor leads (e.g., electrocardiograph leads) are usually applied and an IV catheter is inserted if it was not in place when the patient arrived from the holding area.

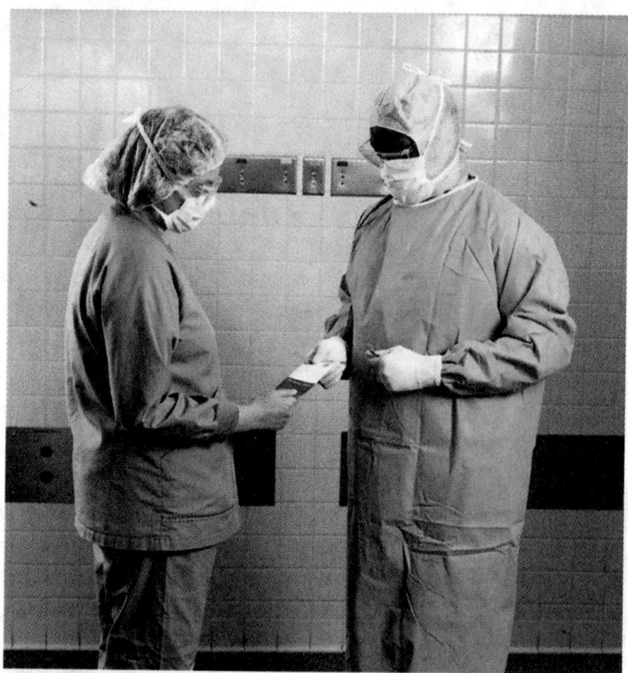

Fig. 15-4 Surgical attire is worn by all persons entering the operating room suite.

Scrubbing, Gowning, and Gloving. All sterile members of the surgical team (scrub assistant, surgeon, surgical technologist, and assistant) are required to cleanse their hands and arms by scrubbing with a brush and detergent before entering the sterile field. This is done to eliminate dirt and skin oil to decrease the microbial count as much as possible. The surgical scrub helps prevent the growth of microbes beneath the surgical glove and gown. The detergent used should be a broad-spectrum microbicidal agent. The procedure should involve a minimum of 5 minutes of mechanical friction with a specially designed sterile surgical brush. During the actual procedure of scrubbing, the team members' fingers and hands should be scrubbed first with progression to the arms and elbows. The hands should be held higher than the elbows at all times to prevent detergent suds and water from draining from the unclean (above elbows) to the clean and previously scrubbed areas (hands and fingers).[1,3,6]

Once the scrub procedure is completed, the team members enter the room to clothe themselves in the surgical gowns and gloves. Because the gowns and gloves are sterile, it is permissible for the scrubbed people to manipulate and organize all sterile items for use during the procedure.

Basic Aseptic Technique. To prevent infections, aseptic technique is practiced in the OR to prevent the entrance of microorganisms into the surgical wound. This is implemented through the creation and maintenance of a sterile field (Fig. 15-5). The center of the sterile field is the site of the surgical incision. Inanimate items in the sterile field include surgical items and equipment that have been sterilized by appropriate sterilization methods.

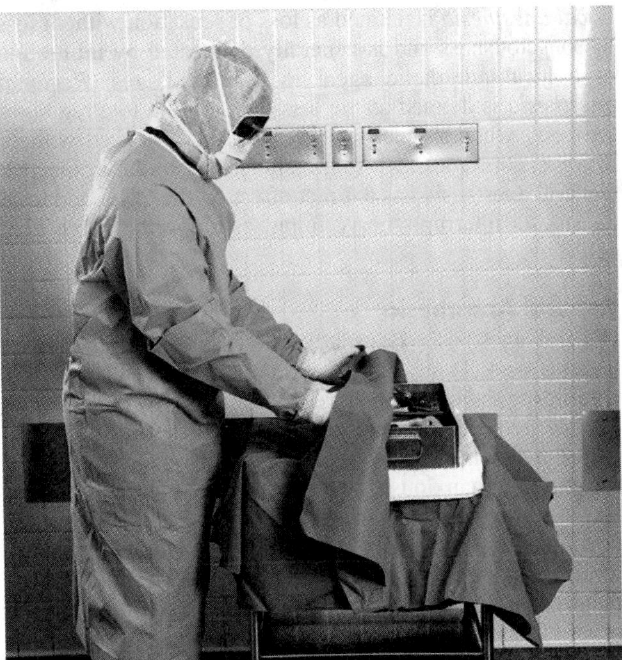

Fig. 15-5 A sterile field is created before surgery.

There are specific principles that the team members should understand to practice aseptic technique. Unless these principles are followed, the safety of the patient is compromised, and the potential for postoperative infection is increased. Table 15-3 presents basic principles of aseptic technique.[1,3,6]

In addition to following the principles of aseptic technique, the surgical team is responsible for following the guidelines established by the U.S. Occupational Safety and Health Administration (OSHA) to protect the patient and the team from exposure to bloodborne pathogens. These guidelines emphasize universal precautions, engineering and work practice controls, and the use of personal protective equipment such as gloves, gowns, aprons, caps, shoe covers, face shields, masks, and protective eye wear. This is especially important in the OR environment because of the high potential for exposure to bloodborne pathogens.[7,8]

Assisting the Anesthesia Team. While the perioperative nurse checks the OR to complete its preparation, the anesthesia team prepares the patient for the administration of the anesthetic. The nurse must understand the mechanism of anesthetic administration and the pharmacologic effects of the agents. The nurse should know the location of all emergency drugs and equipment in the OR area.

The circulating nonsterile perioperative nurse may be involved in placing monitoring devices to be used during the surgical procedure (e.g., urinary catheter, electrocardiogram [ECG] leads) and the electrical grounding pad. If the patient is to have a general anesthetic, the nurse remains at the patient's side to ensure safety and to assist the ACP. These responsibilities may include obtaining blood pressure measurements, starting an IV line, and protecting the patient from falling.

Table 15-3 Principles of Basic Aseptic Technique in the Operating Room

1. All materials that enter the sterile field must be sterile.
2. Sterilization is the only means by which an item can be considered sterile; if it comes in contact with an unsterile item, it becomes contaminated.
3. Contaminated items should be removed immediately from the sterile field.
4. Sterile team members must wear only sterile gowns; once dressed for the procedure, the team should recognize that all parts of the gown are considered unsterile except the front from chest to table level and the sleeves to 2 in above the elbow.
5. A wide margin of safety must be maintained between the sterile and unsterile field.
6. Team members' motions should be from sterile to sterile or from unsterile to unsterile.
7. Tables are considered sterile only at tabletop level, and items extending beneath this level are considered contaminated.
8. The edges of a sterile package are considered contaminated once the package has been opened.
9. Bacteria travel on airborne particles and will enter the sterile field with excessive air movements and currents.
10. Bacteria travel with moisture and liquids by capillary action from surface to surface.
11. Bacteria harbor on the patient's and the team members' hair, skin, and respiratory tracts.

Positioning the Patient. Positioning the patient usually follows induction of a general anesthetic. If an alternative anesthetic technique (e.g., epidural or local anesthesia) is used, the ACP will indicate when to begin the positioning of the patient. When positioning for the surgical procedure, care must be used to (1) provide correct skeletal alignment; (2) prevent undue pressure on nerves, bony prominences, eyes, and skin; (3) provide for adequate thoracic excursion; (4) prevent occlusion of arteries and veins; (5) avoid stretching and compression of nerve tissue; (6) provide modesty in exposure; and (7) recognize and respect individual needs such as previously assessed aches, pains, or deformities. It is a nursing responsibility to secure the extremities, provide adequate padding and support, and obtain sufficient physical or mechanical help to avoid unnecessary straining of self or patient.

Various positions in which the patient may be positioned include supine, prone, Trendelenburg, lateral, kidney, lithotomy, jackknife, and sitting. The supine is the most common position used. It is suited for surgery involving the abdomen, heart, and breast. Following anesthesia, the head is turned toward the extended arm. The prone position allows easy access for back surgeries (e.g., laminectomies). The lithotomy position is used for some pelvic organ surgery (e.g., vaginal hysterectomy). The sitting position is used for some craniotomies.[1]

Preparing the Surgical Site. The purpose of skin preparation, or "prepping," is to reduce the number of

Table 15-4 Expected Outcomes for the Surgical Patient

- Demonstration of knowledge of the physiologic and psychologic responses to surgical intervention
- Absence of infection
- Maintenance of skin integrity
- Freedom from injury related to positioning, extraneous objects, or chemical, physical, and electrical hazards
- Maintenance of fluid and electrolyte balance
- Satisfaction with pain relief
- Participation in the rehabilitative process

organisms available to migrate to the surgical wound. The task of prepping is usually the responsibility of the circulating nurse.

The skin is prepared by mechanically scrubbing or cleansing around the surgical site with antimicrobial agents identified as being nonallergic to the patient. In most cases the nurse removes excess hair from the area. The area is then scrubbed in a circular motion. The principle of scrubbing from the clean area (site of the incision) to the dirty area (periphery) is observed at all times. A liberal area is cleansed to allow for added protection and unexpected occurrences during the procedure.

After preparation of the skin, the sterile members of the surgical team drape the area. Only the site to be incised is left exposed.

After Surgery

Through constant observation of the surgical progress, the ACP anticipates the end of the surgical procedure and uses anesthetic agents so that their effects will be minimal at the conclusion. This also allows greater physiologic control of the patient during the transfer to the PCU.

The ACP and the surgeon or another member of the surgical team accompany the patient to the PCU. A report of the patient's status and the procedure is communicated. The OR nurse evaluates the patient's response to nursing care based on outcome criteria established when the plan of care was developed (Table 15-4).[2,9,10]

CLASSIFICATION OF ANESTHESIA

The anesthetic technique and agents are selected by the ACP in collaboration with the surgeon and the patient. Factors contributing to the decision include the patient's current health status and history, emotional stability, and factors relating to the operative procedure (e.g., length, position, site). The ACP validates this information during the preoperative assessment, makes the final decision, obtains anesthesia consent, and writes orders for the preoperative medication.

Anesthesia is classified according to the effect that it has on the patient's sensorium (central nervous system [CNS]) and pain perception. *General anesthesia* is defined as the loss of sensation with a loss of consciousness and reflexes. *Local anesthesia* is defined as loss of sensation without loss of consciousness and is generally delineated by infiltration of a local anesthetic agent in a limited area. *Regional anesthesia* is defined as the loss of sensation to a region of the body when a specific nerve branch is blocked without loss of consciousness (e.g., spinal or epidural blocks). General anesthesia has a direct effect on the CNS, and local anesthesia interrupts nerve impulses along the nerve fiber cells.

General Anesthesia

General anesthesia is usually the category of choice for patients who (1) are having surgical procedures that require significant skeletal muscle relaxation, last for long periods of time, require awkward positions because of the location of the incisional site, or require control of respiration; (2) are extremely anxious; (3) refuse or have contraindications for local or regional anesthetic techniques; and (4) are uncooperative secondary to emotional status, maturity, intoxication, head injury, or muscle disorders. General anesthetics may be administered by an IV, inhalation, or rectal route (Table 15-5).

Intravenous Induction Agents. Virtually all routine adult general anesthetics begin with an IV induction agent. These agents have a smooth and rapid action that patients find desirable, but a single dose lasts only a few minutes. These agents can be separated into barbiturates and nonbarbiturate hypnotics.

Barbiturates. Traditionally the IV agents used to induce general anesthesia have been the short-acting barbiturates. Of those available, the two most frequently used are thiopental sodium (Pentothal) and sodium methohexital (Brevital).

Induction with both agents is rapid. In higher doses these agents can cause cardiovascular depression, hypotension, tachycardia, and respiratory depression. Leakage of the barbiturates into the tissue surrounding the vein can cause severe pain and damage because of the alkalinity of the drugs. If they are injected into an artery, arterial spasms may occur.[11]

Rectal administration of short-acting barbiturates is used only occasionally today because acceptable pharmacologic alternatives are available. This type of anesthetic is most frequently administered to children to produce a sleep state before the use of other anesthetics.

Nonbarbiturate hypnotics. Etomidate (Amidate) and propofol (Diprivan) are nonbarbiturate hypnotic agents. Etomidate produces less cardiovascular or respiratory depression than propofol or barbiturates. This feature makes it an attractive alternative in potentially unstable patients. Cardiovascular and respiratory depression is dose-related with propofol. A side effect common to both agents is pain on injection. Etomidate also can cause myoclonia and postoperative nausea and vomiting. Propofol can be used as an induction agent and to maintain general anesthetic levels. Its extremely rapid elimination may favor its use in short (less than 2 hours) outpatient procedures in which shortened recovery time and early discharge are important. Propofol also causes less nausea and vomiting than many

Table 15-5 General Anesthesia Drugs and Methods

Intravenous Agents
Barbiturates
Thiopental sodium (Pentothal)
Sodium methohexital (Brevital)
Nonbarbiturate Hypnotic
Etomidate (Amidate)
Propofol (Diprivan)
Inhalation Agents
Volatile Liquids
Halothane (Fluothane)
Enflurane (Ethrane)
Isoflurane (Forane)
Desflurane (Suprane)
Gaseous Agents
Nitrous oxide
Anesthesia Adjuncts
Narcotics
Fentanyl (Sublimaze)
Sufentanil (Sufenta)
Alfentanil (Alfenta)
Morphine sulfate
Meperidine hydrochloride (Demerol)
Muscle Relaxants
Depolarizing agents
Succinylcholine (Anectine)
Nondepolarizing agents
Vecuronium (Norcuron)
Atracurium (Tracrium)
Pancuronium (Pavulon)
Tubocurarine (Curare)
Metocurine (Metubine)
Gallamine (Flaxedil)
Pipecuronium (Arduan)
Doxacurium (Nuromax)
Rocuronium (Zemuron)
Sedative-Hypnotics
Midazolam (Versed)
Diazepam (Valium)
Antiemetics
Droperidol (Inapsine)
Ondansetron (Zofran)
Metoclopramide (Reglan)
Prochlorperazine (Compazine)
Promethazine (Phenergan)
Dissociative Anesthetics
Ketamine (Ketalar)

other anesthetic agents.[11] Propofol must be used within 6 hours from the time it is open because it has been shown to support the rapid growth of microorganisms if contaminated within that time. The patient with a soybean allergy history should not be given propofol.

Inhalation Agents. The inhalation agents used for general anesthesia may be *volatile liquids* (liquid at room temperature) or *gases* (gas at room temperature). Volatile liquids are vaporized into a gaseous state together with a carrier gas such as oxygen.

Inhalation agents enter the body through the alveoli in the lungs. Ease of administration and excretion by ventilation, as well as control of depth through respiratory rate and depth, make them desirable agents. One undesirable characteristic is the irritating effect of inhalation agents on the respiratory tract. Complications that may arise are coughing, laryngospasm (muscular spasms of the larynx), bronchospasm, increased secretions, and, at deep levels of anesthesia, respiratory depression. In addition, some of the agents stimulate the vomiting center of the brain, potentially causing postoperative aspiration.

Inhalation agents are used to maintain the anesthetic state. They may be administered through a mask, laryngeal mask airway, endotracheal tube, or tracheostomy. Proper positioning of the endotracheal tube must be ensured. In an anesthesia setting, possible esophageal placement of the ET is checked by positive endtidal CO_2. (The monitor for CO_2 is in the anesthesia machine's circuit.) Auscultation of the chest should be done to detect endobronchial intubation (in which the tube is inserted too far and only one lung is ventilated). If either complication is detected immediately, the problem can be corrected quickly without catastrophic results.

The endotracheal tube with an inflated cuff permits mechanical ventilation, control of ventilation with an open airway, easy access to the tracheobronchial tree for suctioning, and less chance for regurgitation of stomach contents and aspiration of secretions. In emergency surgical procedures when the patient has ingested food or drink, the circulating nurse will frequently be responsible for applying pressure on the anterior neck over the cricoid cartilage (Sellick maneuver). This compresses the esophagus to prevent passive vomiting and aspiration of stomach contents before inflation of the protective cuff. The nurse must be certain that suction is readily available to the ACP at the time of induction and throughout the intraoperative period.

Complications of endotracheal intubation include those primarily associated with its insertion and removal. These include damage to teeth and lips, laryngospasm, laryngeal edema, postoperative sore throat, and hoarseness caused by injury or irritation of the vocal cords or surrounding tissues.[12]

After the endotracheal tube is removed, the nurse should be ready to assist with management of respiratory complications. Oxygen, suction apparatus, emergency drugs, and equipment for reinsertion of the endotracheal tube must be readily available.

Volatile liquids. Volatile liquid anesthetics include the halogenated agents consisting of halothane, enflurane, isoflurane, and desflurane. They are nonexplosive when used in their usual concentration. Although there are variations among the agents, all are bronchodilators, vasodilators, and muscle relaxants. Postoperative incidence of nausea and vomiting is low with the use of these drugs. Because these agents are eliminated rapidly and there is little remaining analgesia, the postanesthesia nurse should evaluate the patient for the early onset of pain.

Halothane (Fluothane) is a halogenated hydrocarbon that is nonexplosive and the least irritating of all agents to the respiratory tract. During its administration, cardiac depression and peripheral vasodilatation resulting in hypotension may occur. Although hepatic inflammation and damage have occurred after the use of halothane, it is theorized that these occurrences may be linked to a problem with its metabolism. Because halothane has a documented history of hepatotoxicity, its use has decreased dramatically because agents not similarly metabolized have become available. Use of this agent is still prevalent in inhalation inductions in children because its odor is nonirritating and more pleasant than other inhalation agents in current use.

Halothane sensitizes the myocardium to the presence of catecholamines, which increases the incidence of ventricular dysrhythmias. For this reason the nurse must inform the ACP that the surgeon will be injecting local solutions containing epinephrine before every injection and carefully record the dose used.

Enflurane (Ethrane) is a halogenated ether that is nonexplosive and rapid acting. It allows for ready management of cardiovascular status and produces minimal respiratory secretions. It is also a good muscle relaxant and provides for rapid postoperative recovery with minimal nausea and vomiting. Seizure activity has been seen during enflurane anesthesia at high concentrations. Recovery is rapid, and there is little residual analgesia.

Isoflurane (Forane) is an isomer of enflurane but with very different properties. It is even more rapid acting than enflurane. Its metabolism by the body is minimal, and it has not been found to be toxic to any organs of the body. Isoflurane also causes less cardiovascular depression than either halothane or enflurane and therefore may be better tolerated in some situations. Isoflurane may produce tachycardia, but this can be generally diminished by decreasing the concentration or adding other anesthesia adjuncts. Because the vapors are irritating to an awake patient, isoflurane is seldom used for induction.

Desflurane (Suprane) is the newest halogenated agent. It is nonexplosive and has the lowest metabolism, thus decreasing toxicity. It decreases systemic blood pressure but, like isoflurane, does not cause severe cardiac depression. In addition, tachycardia does not appear at light levels. This agent is also irritating to the airways and is not recommended for mask induction. Its low solubility allows more sensitive control of the depth in response to surgical stimuli and faster emergence from anesthesia than other halogenated agents.

Gaseous agents. Nitrous oxide is a gaseous agent that provides more analgesia than unconsciousness. It is the most commonly used diluent because of its favorable qualities. The use of nitrous oxide speeds the passage of volatile anesthetics into the patient. When it is administered in combination with other anesthetic agents, its potentiating effects allow smaller amounts of the accompanying drugs. Its primary harmful effect results from administration without a sufficient amount of oxygen, leading to varying degrees of hypoxia and respiratory depression. Its effects are readily reversible by its discontinuation. A major concern with the use of nitrous oxide is that significant cardiac depression can occur with its use. This may cause problems if the patient has significant cardiac disease or dysfunction. Nitrous oxide has also been shown to cause an increased incidence of nausea and vomiting because of its effects on the middle and inner ear. Nitrous oxide readily diffuses into existing air spaces in the body and can cause problems if the increase in pressure cannot be equalized.

Compressed air may be used with oxygen for the patient in whom nitrous oxide use would be precluded. These situations may include (1) severe cardiac disease, (2) history of nausea and vomiting with nitrous oxide use, (3) laser surgery of the airway, (4) inner ear and some eye surgeries, (5) procedures in which air embolism is a risk (e.g., craniotomies, laparoscopies), and (6) surgery involving compliant spaces (e.g., bowel obstruction, pneumothorax).

Adjuncts to General Anesthesia. As mentioned previously, general anesthesia is rarely limited to one agent. Drugs added to an anesthetic (other than IV induction agents or inhalation agents) are called *adjuncts*. These agents are added to the anesthetic for several reasons that include pain relief, amnesia, and muscle relaxation. Adjuncts include opiates, neuromuscular blocking agents (muscle relaxants), and sedative hypnotics. Because the goal of the ACP is optimal operating conditions and rapid awakening of a comfortable and pain-free patient, combinations of these adjuncts are chosen to accomplish this goal. Opiates decrease the concentrations of inhalation agents needed and allow for analgesia to continue into the postoperative period. Use of muscle relaxants also decreases the concentrations of the inhalation agents that would be required to ensure optimal muscular relaxation for surgery. Using low dose inhalation agents and narcotics may sometimes allow recall of events under anesthesia, but addition of a hypnotic agent aids in ensuring an amnestic state.

Opiates. Opiates are also called *narcotics*. The most common opiates in use in anesthesia today are fentanyl (Sublimaze), sufentanil (Sufenta), and alfentanil (Alfenta). These are all synthetic opiates. Sufentanil and alfentanil are analogs of fentanyl. These agents are all extremely potent but, at the same time, short acting. Sufentanil is the most potent of these opiates, and alfentanil is the least potent. Narcotics in high doses, combined with muscle relaxants, can serve in an anesthetic capacity, but recall has been observed. For this reason, hypnotic agents or subanesthetic doses of volatile agents are often added to this technique. Morphine sulfate and, occasionally, meperidine hydrochloride (Demerol) are used, but they tend to have more undesirable side effects. Both are mostly used for postoperative pain management.

The primary disadvantages of all opiates are respiratory depression evidenced by a decreased respiratory rate and nausea and vomiting. These effects should be closely evaluated in the postanesthesia period.

Neuromuscular blocking agents. Neuromuscular blocking agents (muscle relaxants) are a group of agents given to the patient to produce paralysis. These agents can produce deep muscle relaxation without relationship to the level of anesthesia, and they are potentiated by halogenated agents.

The degree of relaxation is important because adequate surgical exposure is essential for many procedures. The nurse should know that patient awareness occasionally occurs under deep relaxation-light anesthesia techniques. For this reason, vigilance to the appropriateness of audio stimulation in the room is constantly necessary.

The two categories of muscle relaxants, or neuromuscular blocking agents, are *depolarizing agents* and *nondepolarizing agents*. Depolarizing agents such as succinylcholine (Anectine) depolarize the motor end plate and prevent further depolarization. This yields paralysis until uptake, and metabolism of the agent occurs and allows nerve conduction to return to normal function, usually within 3 to 10 minutes. Nondepolarizing agents such as vecuronium (Norcuron), atracurium (Tracrium), tubocurarine (Curare), pancuronium (Pavulon), metocurine (Metubine), gallamine (Flaxedil), mivacurium (Mivacron), pipecuronium (Arduan), doxacurium (Nuromax), and rocuronium (Zemuron) interfere with nerve impulse transmission at the myoneural junction by competing at the motor end plate with acetylcholine. As with the depolarizing agents, the end result is paralysis with the effects lasting much longer than with the depolarizing agents.

Disadvantages involving the administration of muscle relaxants are of special concern to the postanesthesia nurse. The duration of their action may be longer than the surgical procedure, or reversal agents may not be effective in completely eliminating the residual effects. The patient should be carefully observed for airway patency and respiratory muscle movement. Lack of movement or poor return of reflexes and strength may indicate the need for an artificial airway and ventilator. If the patient is intubated, the endotracheal tube should not be removed without careful assessment of return of muscular strength and tidal volume. A patient's strength should be evaluated by a combination of the ability to lift the head off the bed and hold it up for a few seconds, tidal volumes, and negative inspiratory pressure.

Sedative-hypnotics. Sedative-hypnotics are agents that cause amnesia and sedation. Their use varies from induction of general anesthesia to sedation and sleep as supplementation of local and regional anesthesia. Their use for induction of general anesthesia involves the use of higher doses than would be used in an awake patient. These agents should be given in small incremental doses until the desired effect is reached. Such administration allows the nurse to closely observe the patient for the side effects of these agents, which are mainly respiratory depression, airway obstruction, apnea, and cardiovascular depression. Respiratory depression is the most frequent side effect, but it is generally not seen unless the agents are administered too rapidly, the dose is too high, or other potentiating compounds such as narcotics or other sedative hypnotics have been administered.

The most commonly used hypnotics are in the benzodiazapine class: diazepam (Valium) and midazolam (Versed). Because of its superior amnestic properties and shorter action, midazolam is presently the most frequently used hypnotic in anesthesia.

Antiemetics. Antiemetics are medications that reduce or eliminate the incidence of nausea and vomiting. One of the most commonly used agents for this purpose in anesthesia is droperidol (Inapsine). This agent has antiemetic properties at all doses and heavy sedation and tranquilization properties at higher doses. As with hypnotics, droperidol will potentiate the depressant effect of any other medication given to the patient. Ondansetron (Zofran), a drug previously used for treating nausea in chemotherapy, is now approved for use in anesthesia settings. It prevents nausea and vomiting by blocking serotonin peripherally, centrally, and in the small intestine. Metoclopramide (Reglan) may be given to cause the stomach contents to empty more rapidly into the small bowel, and it is commonly used postoperatively. Other antiemetics such as prochlorperazine (Compazine) or promethazine (Phenergan) are sometimes prescribed, but their use is usually in a postoperative setting.

Dissociative Anesthetics. Dissociative anesthetics interrupt associative brain pathways while blocking sensory pathways. The patient may appear catatonic but is actually asleep. The agent administered as a dissociative anesthetic is ketamine hydrochloride (Ketalar). It is particularly advantageous because this agent does not relax upper airway muscles and tissues. The probability of airway obstruction is minimal, but secretions and reflexes are increased, and aspiration is possible. Therefore ketamine should never be administered without resuscitative equipment immediately available. Because ketamine has minimal cardiac depressant effects and may even elevate blood pressure, it is a suitable agent in the patient who is a poor surgical risk.

Ketamine's principal disadvantage is the production of undesirable psychologic reactions that appear during emergence. The likelihood of these reactions is reduced by keeping the total dose of the drug as low as possible and by using benzodiazepines. The nurse should approach the patient slowly and quietly; a startling touch and loud sounds may elicit hallucinatory reactions. Ketamine may be administered IV or IM. Ketamine's flashback effect (recurrence of bad dreams) precludes its use in adults and adolescents, but it is still useful in the pediatric or geriatric patient in whom hallucinogenic incidence is much less. Intramuscular administration of ketamine is occasionally used in children who are uncooperative or need painful procedures. Ketamine produces a sleepy, cooperative state that is conducive to other anesthetic agents or techniques.

Local Anesthesia

Local anesthetics allow an operative procedure to be performed on a part of the body without loss of consciousness. All local anesthetics act by blocking the conduction of nerve impulses through altering nerve cell permeability to sodium, resulting in a decrease in the degree of membrane depolarization to prevent the development of a propagated action potential.[13]

Local anesthetics frequently administered are procaine hydrochloride, tetracaine hydrochloride (Pontocaine), dibucaine hydrochloride (Nupercaine), lidocaine hydrochloride (Xylocaine), mepivacaine hydrochloride (Carbocaine), and bupivacaine hydrochloride (Marcaine).

Advantages. Advantages of local anesthesia are numerous when the patient is assessed as suitable. A suitable recipient is the patient who is not allergic to the drug, who is having a surgical procedure that does not require an unconscious state or extreme muscular relaxation, and whose anxiety or apprehension is not excessive. Because loss of consciousness does not occur, the induction and recovery hazards of a general anesthetic do not exist. Minimum equipment is needed, and the cost is lower. Local anesthesia is especially beneficial for the person who has ingested liquids or solid food before surgery or who is having minor procedures performed on an outpatient basis.

Disadvantages. Disadvantages of local anesthesia include lack of patient cooperation because of awareness during the procedure, lack of feasibility of localizing some anatomic sites, and unanticipated rapid absorption of the agent into the bloodstream in unsuspected circumstances. Manifestations of overdose and rapid absorption include light-headedness, dizziness, ringing in ears, loss of consciousness, and seizure activity. In addition, cardiovascular toxicity may occur, including dysrhythmias and decreased cardiac output.

Methods of Administration. There are a variety of methods for administering local anesthetics (Table 15-6). *Topical application* is application of the agent directly to the skin, mucous membrane, or open surface. *Local infiltration* is injection of the agent into the tissues through which the surgical incision will pass. *Regional application* is injection of the agent at some location along the conductive nerve pathway to and from the region selected to be anesthetized; regional application is achieved away from the surgical field.

There are several types of regional anesthesia. The *nerve block* is the injection of a specific nerve at a given point, such as an intercostal, median, or axillary nerve block. The *intravenous regional block* with a tourniquet (Bier block) is the injection of a local anesthetic IV into an extremity after a tourniquet has been applied and the extremity exsanguinated. The tourniquet should always remain inflated a minimum of 30 minutes. The patient should be closely observed when the tourniquet is released because it is possible to have symptoms of local anesthetic overdose at that time. The *field block* is a type of infiltration anesthesia in which the anesthetic is injected around the area of the surgical procedure by a series of injections. The *central nerve block* is the type that anesthetizes the spinal cord nerves (motor and sensory) near its origin. The *spinal block* affects the nerves in the subarachnoid space, and the *epidural block* affects the nerve roots passing through the epidural space. The epidural block may use a thoracic or lumbar approach; a sacral approach is called a caudal.

Table 15-6 Methods for Administering Local Anesthetics

Topical Application

Local Infiltration

Regional Application—Conduction Block
- Nerve block
- Intravenous regional block—Bier block
- Field block
- Central nerve blocks
  - Spinal block
  - Epidural block
    - Lumbar-peridural block
    - Caudal-sacral block

Epidural and Spinal Anesthesia. Spinal anesthesia is achieved by the injection of a local anesthetic agent into the spinal fluid in the subarachnoid space. In epidural anesthesia the local anesthetic is injected into the epidural space between two vertebrae. Once injected, sensory and motor sympathetic routes of the nerve cell are anesthetized. Anesthesia spreads to the uppermost desired level as additional fibers are gradually affected.

Epidural or spinal analgesia is administered primarily for surgery of the lower abdomen and lower extremities. During the surgical procedure the patient can remain conscious or be sedated. Thoracic and lumbar epidurals are indicated to augment general anesthesia and offer postoperative pain relief for surgical sites innervated by nerves above the lumbar approach (e.g., thoracic surgery). The onset of spinal anesthesia is faster than that of epidural anesthesia because the drug is placed in closer proximity to the nerve, but the end result with either technique is equally profound. The patient must be closely observed for signs of sympathetic nervous system blockade, especially with spinal anesthesia. These include hypotension, bradycardia, and nausea and vomiting. If the block extends upward, the patient may experience inadequate respiratory excursion and apnea. The level of the sensory and sympathetic block is controlled by the site of injection, amount and strength of drug used, rapidity of injection, patient's height and weight, specific gravity of the solution, position of the patient at the time of injection, and position maintained on the operating table.

An advantage of epidural over spinal anesthesia is a decreased incidence of headache. The headache experienced after spinal anesthesia is thought to occur following leakage of spinal fluid at the site of injection. The incidence of headache is decreasing with the common use of smaller-gauge spinal needles (25 to 27 gauge). A headache following an epidural may occur when a 17 to 18-gauge needle is advanced too far, and the dura is punctured, resulting in the leakage of cerebrospinal fluid (CSF).

Additional Anesthesia Mechanisms

Controlled hypotension is a technique used to decrease the amount of expected blood loss by lowering the blood pressure during the administration of anesthetics. *Hypothermia* is the deliberate lowering of the body temperature to decrease body metabolism and thus reduce the need for oxygen. *Cryoanesthesia* involves cooling or freezing a localized area to block pain impulses of localized nerve impulses. *Hypnoanesthesia* uses hypnosis to produce an alteration in pain consciousness. *Acupuncture* achieves loss of sensation by the use of intense local stimulation with fine-gauge needles at meridian points throughout the body.

Gerontologic Considerations

Although anesthetic agents have become safer throughout the years, the older adult demonstrates varying and unique responses to the anesthetizing process. Several physiologic alterations may occur because of the aging process. The older adult shows decreased adaptive responses to heat and cold and altered drug metabolism. Although the patient may be able to maintain homeostasis, the older adult is progressively unable to restore it when disease, trauma, or drugs are present.

The older adult experiences a decrease in respiratory protective reflexes. These include decreased ability to cough, decreased thoracic compliance, and degeneration of lung parenchymal tissue. This series of alterations in pulmonary status may lead to a 30% increase in the work of ventilation by age 60. Organ function declines linearly after age 30 at the rate of 1% per year. These changes cause a decreased ability to readily eliminate pharmacologic agents; consequently, these changes have many implications for the surgical experience. Reactions to anesthetic agents need to be carefully monitored and their postoperative elimination assessed before the patient is left without close supervision.[14]

Circulatory function in the older adult is altered because of plaque formation and decreased elasticity in the vasculature. Cardiac function is often compromised, and compensatory responses to changes in blood pressure and volume are limited. Circulating blood volume is decreased, and hypertension is common. Circulatory parameters need to be closely monitored throughout surgery and during the postanesthesia period.

Renal perfusion in the older adult normally decreases; the result is a reduction in the ability to eliminate drugs that are excreted by the kidney. This increases the patient's susceptibility to renal failure. Renal function needs to be carefully assessed intraoperatively and in the postoperative phase of the patient's care. Liver metabolism of anesthetic agents is also decreased. In addition, anesthetic pharmacology in the elderly person is complex because anesthetics are being superimposed on multiple medications that the patient takes on a maintenance basis.

Many older adults experience a decrease in their ability to communicate and follow directions as a result of alterations in sight or hearing. This factor poses a special need for clear and concise communication in the OR, especially when preoperative sedation is superimposed on the existing sensory deficit. Skin elasticity in the older adult is decreased because of loss of collagen. As a result, the skin is sensitive to injury from tape, electrodes, warming and cooling blankets, and certain types of dressing. In addition, the older adult often has fragile bones and osteoarthritis. These factors reinforce the need for careful transferring, lifting, and positioning techniques.[15]

Catastrophic Events in the Operating Room

Unanticipated intraoperative events occasionally occur. Although some might be anticipated (e.g., cardiac arrest in an unstable patient, massive blood loss during trauma surgery, or loss of ability to ventilate a patient), others are unanticipated by the OR team. Two of these events are latex allergic reactions and malignant hyperthermia.

Latex Allergy Reaction. Latex allergy is a diagnosis that has only recently been recognized. Latex is used in gloves, catheters, intubation tubes, anesthesia masks, and many other devices. Reactions have ranged from urticaria to systemic anaphylaxis. During anesthesia the symptoms typically appear within 30 minutes but range from 10 minutes to 5 hours. The patient must be treated immediately, and a latex-free environment must be instituted. Latex allergy protocols should be set up in each institution. Identified risk groups include health care workers and others with frequent latex exposures, patients with some disease states (e.g., spina bifida), and those with documented reactions (e.g., itching, rash) to latex-containing objects such as balloons. Currently a latex allergy protocol is available through the American Association of Nurse Anesthetists (AANA).[16] Latex allergies are also discussed in Chapter 10.

Malignant Hyperthermia. Malignant hyperthermia is a rare, life-threatening disorder that may be triggered by drugs commonly used in anesthesia. It is an autosomal dominant trait with variable expression in affected individuals. The main defect is altered cellular calcium metabolism in muscle cells. Triggering agents include various anesthetic agents (most commonly succinylcholine and inhaled halogenated agents), emotional stress, and trauma.

Characteristics of malignant hyperthermia include generalized muscular rigidity, high fever, tachypnea, tachycardia, metabolic acidosis, dysrhythmias, hypoxia, and hypertension. Although the disorder can occur postoperatively, it usually occurs during induction or maintenance of anesthesia. Once triggered, the patient will die unless treated immediately and vigorously. The initial drug of choice is dantrolene sodium (Dantrium), commonly stored in a preassembled treatment pack. A treatment protocol is available from the Malignant Hyperthermia Association of the United States and is usually displayed in the OR.[17]

To prevent this problem, it is important to obtain a careful family history. The patient known or suspected to have this disorder can be anesthetized with minimal risks if appropriate precautions are taken.

REVIEW QUESTIONS

The number of the question corresponds to the same-numbered objective at the beginning of the chapter.

1. Which of the following characteristics of the operating room environment facilitates the prevention of infection in the surgical patient?
   a. Conductive furniture
   b. Filters in the ventilating system
   c. Explosion-proof electrical plugs
   d. Adjustable lighting
2. Select from the following the activity that is *not* a function of the registered nurse in the operating room.
   a. Administering local anesthetic
   b. Checking electrical equipment

c. Implementing the nursing process
d. Scrubbing for the surgical procedure

3. Which of the following is a need of the patient undergoing surgery?
a. Privacy
b. Comfort measures
c. Reduction of anxiety
d. All of the above

4. Preoperative assessment by the perioperative nurse is initiated in a variety of settings. Which setting is inappropriate for preoperative patient assessment?
a. Home or clinic setting
b. Clinical unit
c. Postanesthesia care unit
d. Preoperative holding areas

5. When scrubbing at the scrub sink, the surgical team members should
a. hold hands higher than the elbows.
b. scrub from elbows to hands.
c. scrub for a minimum of 10 minutes.
d. scrub without mechanical friction.

6. Mrs. Jones is scheduled for an abdominal hysterectomy. She is extremely anxious and has a tendency to hyperventilate when upset. Which type of anesthetic would be most appropriate for Mrs. Jones?
a. General anesthetic
b. Spinal block

7. Intravenous induction for general anesthesia is the method of choice for most patients because
a. they are nonexplosive agents.
b. induction is rapid and pleasant.
c. the patient is not intubated.
d. the odor of the agent is not offensive.

8. The injection of the local anesthetic into the tissues through which the surgical incision will pass is the technique of
a. topical application.
b. nerve block.
c. regional application.
d. local infiltration.

9. Which of the following is not a purpose of adjunct agents in general anesthesia?
a. Induce general anesthesia
b. Provide pain relief
c. Ensure muscle relaxation
d. Induce amnesia

REFERENCES

1. Atkinson LJ, Kohn ML: *Berry and Kohn's introduction to operating room techniques,* ed 7, New York, 1992, Mosby.
2. Groah L: *Operating room nursing,* ed 2, San Mateo, Calif., 1990, Appleton and Lange.
3. Meeker MH, Rothrock JC: *Alexander's care of the patient in surgery,* ed 9, St Louis, 1991, Mosby.
4. DeLong DL: Preoperative holding area, *AORN J* 55:563, 1992.
5. Longinow LT, Rzeszewski LB: The holding room, *AORN J* 57:914, 1993.
6. Association of Operating Room Nurses: Recommended practices for basic aseptic technique. In *AORN Standards of Practice,* Denver, 1993, Association of Operating Room Nurses.
7. Department of Labor, Occupational Safety and Health Administration, Federal Register, vol 56, no 235, part 1920, Dec 6, 1991.
8. Fairchild SS: *Perioperative nursing,* Boston, 1993, Jones and Bartlett.
9. Association of Operating Room Nurses: Patient outcome standards. In *AORN Standards and Recommended Practices,* Denver, 1993, Association of Operating Room Nurses.
10. Phippen ML, Wells MP: *Perioperative nursing practice,* Philadelphia, 1993, Saunders.
11. Siler JN, Fisher SM, Boon P: A comparative study of total intravenous anesthesia technique versus a standard anesthetic technique for outpatient surgical procedures, *Semin Anes* 11(Suppl 1):14, 1992.
12. Miller RD: *Anesthesia,* ed 3, New York, 1990, Churchill Livingstone.
13. Scott DB: *Techniques of regional anaesthesia,* Norwalk, CT 1989, Appleton and Lange/Mediglobe.
14. Blitt CD: *Monitoring in anesthesia and critical care medicine,* ed 2, New York, 1990, Churchill Livingstone.
15. Katz J, Benumot JL, Kadis LB: *Anesthesia and uncommon diseases,* ed 3, Philadelphia, 1990, Saunders.
16. American Association of Nurse Anesthetists: Latex allergy protocol, *AANA* 61:223, 1993.
17. Malignant Hyperthermia Association of the United States: Suggested therapy for malignant hyperthermia emergency. *MHaus Internationa,* Darien, CT.

Chapter 16

NURSING ROLE IN MANAGEMENT
Postoperative Patient

Kim Litwack

Learning Objectives

1. Identify the components of an initial postanesthesia assessment.
2. Identify the nursing responsibilities in admitting patients to the postanesthesia care unit (PACU).
3. Explain the etiology and nursing assessment and management of potential problems of patients in the PACU.
4. Describe the initial nursing assessment and management immediately after transfer from the PACU to the general care unit.
5. Explain the etiology and nursing assessment and management of potential problems during the postoperative period.
6. Identify the information needed by the postoperative patient in preparation for discharge.

The postoperative period begins immediately after surgery and continues until the patient is discharged from medical care. This chapter focuses on the common features of postoperative nursing care for the patient undergoing surgery. The problems and nursing care related to specific surgical procedures are discussed in the appropriate chapters of this text.

POSTOPERATIVE CARE IN THE POSTANESTHESIA CARE UNIT

The patient's immediate recovery period is supervised by a postanesthesia care nurse, an educated specialist working in a specially equipped environment. The postanesthesia care unit (PACU) is located adjacent to the operating room (OR) to minimize transportation of the patient immediately after surgery and to provide ready access to anesthesia and surgical personnel.

Postanesthesia Care Unit Admission

The initial admission of the patient to the PACU is a joint effort between the anesthesia care provider (ACP) and the PACU nurse. This collaborative effort fosters a smooth transfer of care. To ensure patient safety and continuity of care, the ACP gives a verbal report to the admitting PACU nurse. A complete report includes details of the surgical and anesthetic course, preoperative conditions warranting or influencing the surgical or anesthetic outcome, and PACU treatment plans. Table 16-1 summarizes the components of a complete anesthesia report.[1]

A priority in admitting a patient to the PACU is an assessment designed to:

1. Determine the patient's physiologic status at the time of admission to the PACU
2. Allow periodic reevaluation of the patient so that physiologic trends become apparent
3. Establish the patient's baseline parameters
4. Assess the ongoing status of the surgical site
5. Assess recovery from anesthesia, noting residual effects
6. Allow comparison of current patient status with discharge criteria[2]

A specific assessment priority is an evaluation of respiratory and circulatory adequacy.[3] Assessment will be made of the patient's airway patency and rate and quality of respirations. Breath sounds should be auscultated throughout all lung fields.

Oxygen therapy will be used if the patient has had general anesthesia or the ACP orders it. Oxygen therapy is given via nasal cannula or face mask. The use of oxygen aids the elimination of anesthetic gases and helps to meet the increased demand for oxygen needed in the immediate postoperative period. If the patient requires postoperative

---

Reviewed by Susan S. Fairchild, RN, MSN, CNOR, CS, Doctoral candidate-EdD, Assistant Professor–Nursing, Barry University, Miami Shores, FL.

Table 16-1 Postanesthesia Admission Report

General Information
- Patient name
- Age
- Anesthesia care provider
- Surgeon
- Surgical procedure

Intraoperative Management
- Anesthetic medications
- Other medications received preoperatively or intraoperatively
- Blood loss
- Fluid replacement totals, including blood transfusions
- Urine output

Intraoperative Course
- Unexpected anesthetic events or reactions
- Unexpected surgical events
- Vital signs and monitoring trends
- Results of intraoperative laboratory tests

Patient History
- Indication for surgery
- Medical history, medications, allergies

Postanesthesia Care Unit Plan
- Potential and expected problems (with plan for intervention)
- Suggested PACU course
- Acceptable parameters for laboratory test results
- PACU discharge plan

PACU, Postanesthesia care unit.

Table 16-2 Clinical Manifestations of Inadequate Oxygenation

Central Nervous System
- Restlessness
- Agitation
- Muscle twitching
- Seizures
- Coma

Cardiovascular System
- Hypertension
- Hypotension
- Tachycardia
- Bradycardia
- Dysrhythmias

Integumentary System
- Cyanosis
- Poor capillary refill
- Skin flushed and moist

Pulmonary System
- Increased to absent respiratory effort
- Use of accessory muscles
- Abnormal airway sounds
- Abnormal arterial blood gases

Renal System
- Urine output <0.5 ml/kg/hr

ventilation, a ventilator will be provided. Pulse oximetry monitoring will be initiated because it provides a noninvasive means of assessing the adequacy of oxygenation.

During this initial assessment, any signs of inadequate oxygenation and ventilation should be identified (Table 16-2). Any evidence of respiratory compromise requires prompt intervention. Commonly occurring respiratory problems for patients in the PACU are discussed on p. 389.

Electrocardiographic (ECG) monitoring will be initiated to determine cardiac rate and rhythm. Any deviation from preoperative findings should be noted and evaluated. Blood pressure should be measured and compared with baseline readings. Any invasive monitoring (e.g., arterial blood pressure monitoring) will be initiated. Body temperature and skin color and condition should also be assessed. Any evidence of inadequate circulatory status requires prompt intervention. Commonly occurring cardiovascular problems for patients in the PACU are discussed on p. 391.

The initial neurologic assessment will focus on level of consciousness; orientation; sensory and motor status; and size, equality, and reactivity of the pupils. The patient may be awake, drowsy but arousable, or asleep. Occasionally the patient may wake up agitated in what is referred to as *emergence delirium.* If the patient has had a regional anesthetic (e.g., spinal or epidural), sensory and motor blockade may still be present.

The assessment of the renal system focuses on intake and output and electrolyte status. Intraoperative fluid totals will be communicated as part of the anesthesia report. The PACU nurse will note the presence of all intravenous (IV) lines, irrigation solutions and infusions, and all output devices, including catheters and wound drains. Intravenous infusions will be regulated according to postoperative orders.

The PACU nurse will also assess the surgical site, noting the condition of any dressings and the type and amount of any drainage. Postoperative orders related to site care will be instituted. All data obtained in the admission assessment are documented on a PACU record, a form specific to postanesthesia and postsurgical care (Fig. 16-1).

Even the patient who has been told what to expect after surgery may be frightened or confused on awakening in the strange environment. Because hearing is the first sense to return in the unconscious patient, the nurse should explain all activities from the moment of admission to the PACU. Orientation includes explaining to the patient that the surgery is completed, that he is in the recovery room, the family or significant other has been notified, noting who is caring for the patient and what is being done, and what time it is.

After the initial assessment is completed, the PACU nurse will continue to apply the skills of ongoing assessment, diagnosis, and intervention. The patient's response to intervention is also noted. The goal of PACU care is to identify actual and potential patient problems that may occur as a result of anesthetic administration and surgical intervention and to intervene appropriately. The American

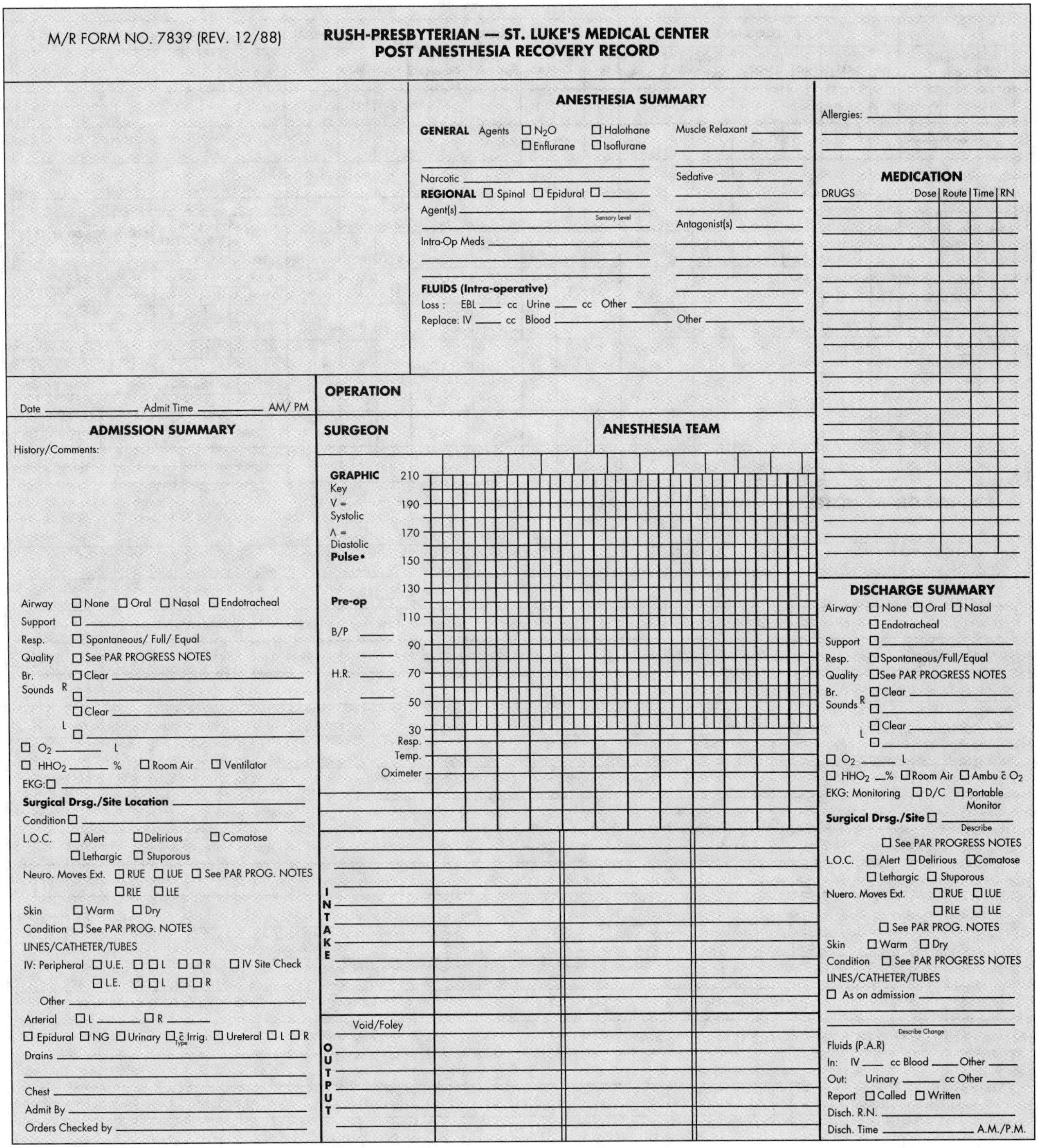

M/R FORM NO. 7839 (REV. 12/88)

RUSH-PRESBYTERIAN — ST. LUKE'S MEDICAL CENTER
POST ANESTHESIA RECOVERY RECORD

ANESTHESIA SUMMARY

GENERAL Agents ☐ N_2O ☐ Halothane ☐ Enflurane ☐ Isoflurane

Muscle Relaxant ______

Narcotic ______

Sedative ______

REGIONAL ☐ Spinal ☐ Epidural ☐ ______

Agent(s) ______ Sensory Level

Antagonist(s) ______

Intra-Op Meds ______

FLUIDS (Intra-operative)

Loss: EBL ____ cc Urine ____ cc Other ______

Replace: IV ____ cc Blood ______ Other ______

Allergies: ______

MEDICATION

DRUGS	Dose	Route	Time	RN

Date ______ Admit Time ______ AM/ PM

OPERATION

SURGEON

ANESTHESIA TEAM

ADMISSION SUMMARY

History/Comments:

Airway ☐ None ☐ Oral ☐ Nasal ☐ Endotracheal

Support ☐ ______

Resp. ☐ Spontaneous/ Full/ Equal

Quality ☐ See PAR PROGRESS NOTES

Br. Sounds R ☐ Clear ______ ☐ ______

L ☐ Clear ______ ☐ ______

☐ O_2 ____ L

☐ HHO_2 ____ % ☐ Room Air ☐ Ventilator

EKG: ☐ ______

Surgical Drsg./Site Location ______

Condition ☐ ______

L.O.C. ☐ Alert ☐ Delirious ☐ Comatose ☐ Lethargic ☐ Stuporous

Neuro. Moves Ext. ☐ RUE ☐ LUE ☐ See PAR PROG. NOTES ☐ RLE ☐ LLE

Skin ☐ Warm ☐ Dry

Condition ☐ See PAR PROG. NOTES

LINES/CATHETER/TUBES

IV: Peripheral ☐ U.E. ☐ ☐ L ☐ ☐ R ☐ IV Site Check

☐ L.E. ☐ ☐ L ☐ ☐ R

Other ______

Arterial ☐ L ______ ☐ R ______

☐ Epidural ☐ NG ☐ Urinary ☐ Type c̄ Irrig. ☐ Ureteral ☐ L ☐ R

Drains ______

Chest ______

Admit By ______

Orders Checked by ______

GRAPHIC Key V = Systolic Λ = Diastolic **Pulse•**

210, 190, 170, 150, 130, 110, 90, 70, 50, 30

Pre-op

B/P ______

H.R. ______

Resp.

Temp.

Oximeter

INTAKE

Void/Foley

OUTPUT

DISCHARGE SUMMARY

Airway ☐ None ☐ Oral ☐ Nasal ☐ Endotracheal

Support ☐ ______

Resp. ☐ Spontaneous/Full/Equal

Quality ☐ See PAR PROGRESS NOTES

Br. Sounds R ☐ Clear ______ ☐ ______

L ☐ Clear ______ ☐ ______

☐ O_2 ____ L

☐ HHO_2 ____% ☐ Room Air ☐ Ambu c̄ O_2

EKG: Monitoring ☐ D/C ☐ Portable Monitor

Surgical Drsg./Site ☐ ______ Describe

☐ See PAR PROGRESS NOTES

L.O.C. ☐ Alert ☐ Delirious ☐ Comatose ☐ Lethargic ☐ Stuporous

Nuero. Moves Ext. ☐ RUE ☐ LUE ☐ RLE ☐ LLE

☐ See PAR PROG. NOTES

Skin ☐ Warm ☐ Dry

Condition ☐ See PAR PROGRESS NOTES

LINES/CATHETER/TUBES

☐ As on admission ______

Describe Change

Fluids (P.A.R)

In: IV ____ cc Blood ____ Other ____

Out: Urinary ____ cc Other ____

Report ☐ Called ☐ Written

Disch. R.N. ______

Disch. Time ______ A.M./P.M.

Fig. 16-1 Postanesthesia care unit record.

		ARTERIAL GASES							ELECTROLYTES					Hg/Hct		INITIAL	SIGNATURE & TITLE
Time	Parameters O_2 or Vent.	pH	pCO_2	pO_2	HCO_3	Total CO_2	BE	O_2 Sat %	Na	K	Cl	Ca	Glucose	Hg	Hct		

TESTS/PROCEDURES		
TEST	TIME DONE/SENT	COMMENTS OR RESULTS
EKG		
MODEL S		
SMA_6		

X-RAY EXAMINATION	TIME DONE
☐ CXR	
☐ PELVIS	

P.A.R. PROGRESS NOTES

Fig. 16-1—cont'd Postanesthesia care unit record.

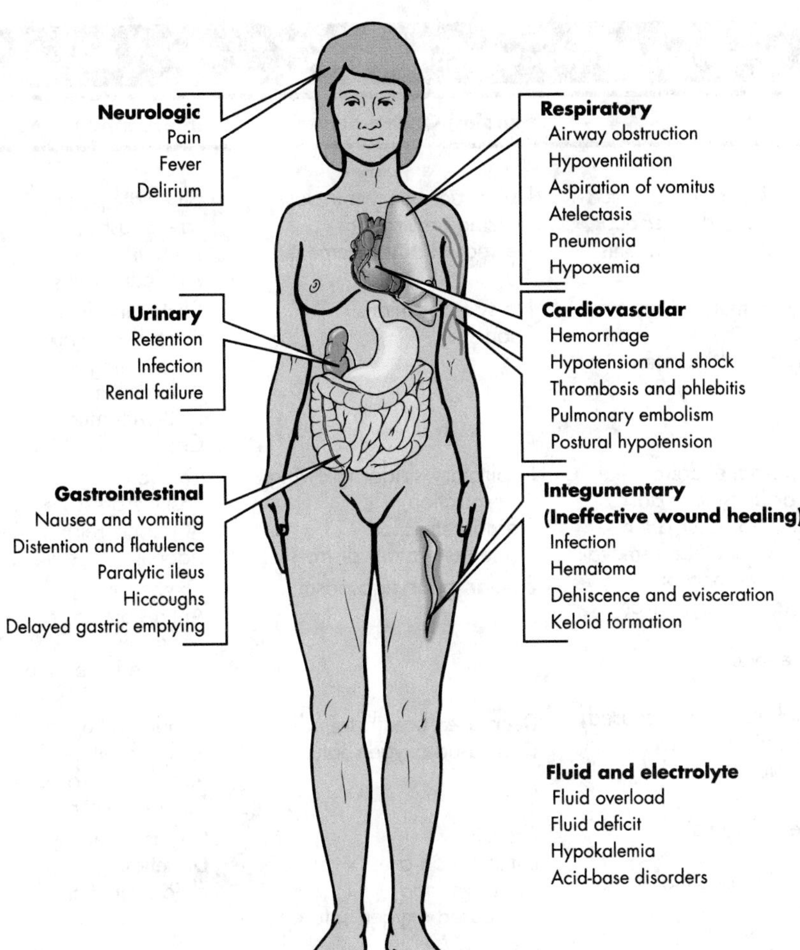

Fig. 16-2 Potential problems in the postoperative period.

Society of Postanesthesia Nursing (ASPAN) has defined Standards of Postanesthesia Nursing Practice (1995) to guide PACU care of adult, pediatric, and geriatric patients.[4]

Common postoperative problems include airway compromise (obstruction), respiratory insufficiency (hypoxemia and hypercarbia), cardiac compromise (hypotension, hypertension, and dysrhythmias), neurologic compromise (emergence delirium and delayed awakening), hypothermia, pain, and nausea and vomiting (Fig. 16-2). Each of these problems and appropriate nursing interventions are discussed.

Potential Alterations in Respiratory Function

Etiology. In the immediate postanesthetic period the most common causes of airway compromise include obstruction, hypoxemia, and hypoventilation (Table 16-3). Patients at particular risk include those who have had general anesthesia, are older, smoke heavily, have lung disease, or have undergone airway, thoracic, or abdominal surgery. However, respiratory complications may occur with any patient who has been anesthetized.

Airway obstruction is most commonly caused by blockage of the airway by the patient's tongue (Fig. 16-3). The base of the tongue falls backward against the soft palate and occludes the pharynx. It is most pronounced in the supine position and in the patient who is extremely somnolent after surgery. Other less common causes of airway obstruction include laryngospasm, retained secretions, and laryngeal edema.

Hypoxemia, specifically a PaO_2 of less than 60 mm Hg, is characterized by a variety of nonspecific clinical signs and symptoms, ranging from agitation to somnolence, hypertension to hypotension, and tachycardia to bradycardia. Pulse oximetry may indicate a low oxygen saturation (less than 90%). Arterial blood gas results will confirm hypoxemia if the PaO_2 is less than 60 mm Hg.

The most common cause of postoperative hypoxemia is atelectasis.[5] Atelectasis may be the result of bronchial obstruction caused by retained secretions or decreased respiratory excursion. Hypotension and low cardiac output states can also contribute to the development of atelectasis.[6] Other causes of hypoxemia that may occur in the PACU include pulmonary edema, pulmonary embolism, aspiration, and bronchospasm.

Hypoventilation, a common complication in the PACU, is characterized by a decreased respiratory rate, hypoxemia, and an increasing $PaCO_2$ (hypercapnia). Hypoventilation may occur as a result of depression of the central respiratory drive (secondary to anesthetic exposure or pain medi-

Table 16-3 Common Immediate Postoperative Respiratory Complications

Complications and Causes	Mechanisms	Nursing Observations	Intervention
Airway Obstruction			
Tongue falling back	Muscular flaccidity associated with decreased consciousness and muscle relaxants	Use of accessory muscles Snoring respirations Decreased air movement	Stimulate patient Jaw thrust Chin lift Artifical airway
Retained thick secretions	Secretion stimulation by anesthetic agents Dehydration of secretions	Noisy respirations Rhonchi	Suctioning Deep breathing and coughing IV hydration IPPB with mucolytic agent Chest physical therapy
Laryngospasm	Irritation from endotracheal tube or anesthetic gases Most likely to occur after endotracheal tube removal	Inspiratory stridor (crowing respiration) Sternal retraction Acute respiratory distress	Oxygen Positive pressure ventilation IV muscle relaxant Lidocaine or steroids
Laryngeal edema	Allergic drug reaction Mechanical irritation from intubation Fluid overload	Similar to laryngospasm	Oxygen Antihistamines or steroids Sedatives Possible intubation
Hypoxemia			
Atelectasis	Bronchial obstruction caused by secretions or decreased lung volumes	Decreased breath sounds Decreased oxygen saturation	Humidified oxygen Deep breathing Incentive spirometry Early mobilization
Pulmonary edema	Increase in hydrostatic pressure Decrease in interstitial pressure Increase in capillary permeability	Crackles Infiltrates on chest x-ray Fluid overload Decreased oxygen saturation	Oxygen therapy Diuretics Fluid restriction
Pulmonary embolism	Thrombus dislodged from periphery; lodged in pulmonary artery	Acute tachypnea Dyspnea Tachycardia Hypotension Decreased oxygen saturation	Oxygen therapy Cardiopulmonary support Heparin therapy
Aspiration	Inhalation of gastric contents	Bronchospasm Atelectasis Crackles Respiratory distress Decreased oxygen saturation	Oxygen therapy Cardiac support Antibiotics or steroids
Bronchospasm	Increase in smooth muscle tone with closure of small airways	Wheezing Dyspnea Tachypnea Decreased oxygen saturation	Oxygen therapy Bronchodilators
Hypoventilation			
Depression of central respiratory drive	Medullary depression from anesthetics, narcotics, sedatives	Shallow respirations Decreased respiratory rate or apnea Hypoxemia Increased $PaCO_2$	Stimulation Reversal or narcotics or benzodiazepines Mechanical ventilation
Poor respiratory muscle tone	Neuromuscular blockade Neuromuscular disease	As above	Reversal of paralysis Mechanical ventilation
Mechanical restriction	Tight casts, dressings, positioning, and obesity prevent lung expansion	As above	Elevate head of bed Repositioning Loosen dressings
Pain	Shallow breathing to prevent incisional pain	As above Complaints of pain Guarding behavior	Analgesic therapy in reduced dose

IPPB, Intermittent positive pressure breathing; *IV*, intravenous.

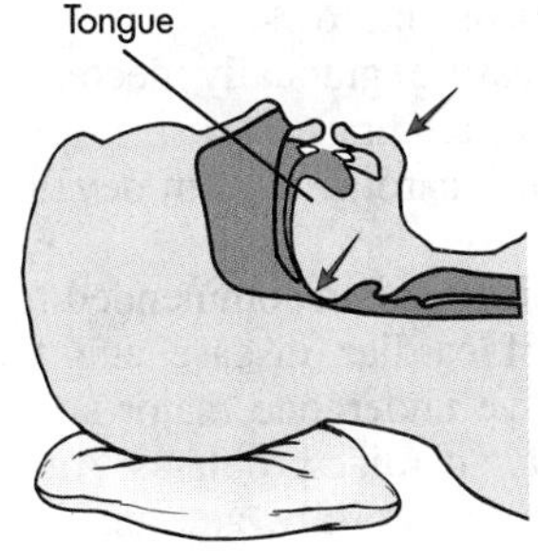

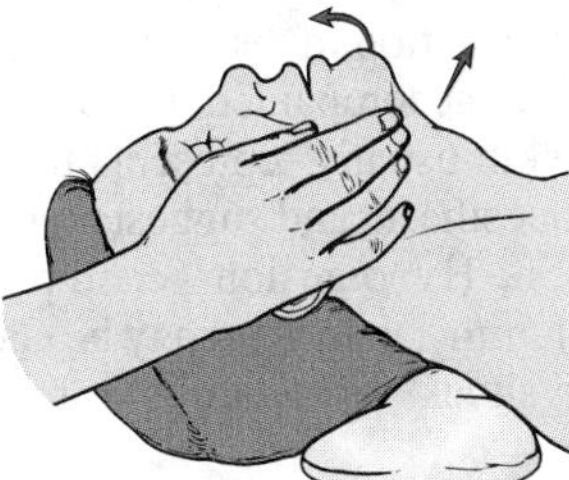

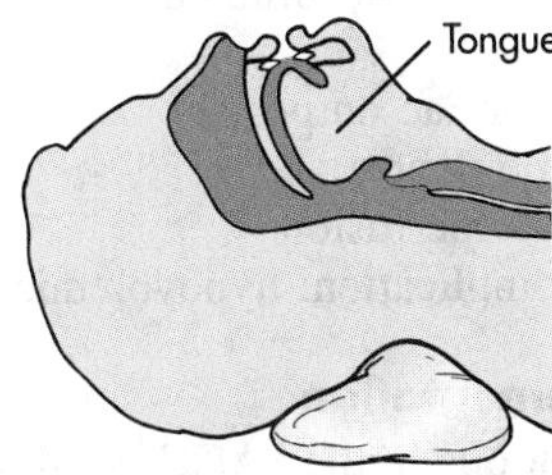

Fig. 16-3 Etiology and relief of airway obstruction as a result of occlusion by the patient's tongue.

cation), poor respiratory muscle tone (secondary to neuromuscular blockade or disease), or a combination of both.

NURSING MANAGEMENT

RESPIRATORY COMPLICATIONS

Nursing Assessment

For an adequate respiratory assessment, the nurse needs to evaluate airway patency, chest symmetry, and the depth, rate, and character of respirations. The nurse can place a cupped hand over the patient's nose and mouth to evaluate the forcefulness of exhaled air.

The chest wall should be observed for symmetry of movement with a hand placed lightly over the xiphoid process. It should also be determined whether abdominal or accessory muscles are being used for breathing. If the muscles are moving excessively, it may indicate respiratory distress.

Breath sounds should be auscultated anteriorly, laterally, and posteriorly. Decreased or absent breath sounds will be detected when airflow is diminished or obstructed. The presence of crackles or wheezes may indicate the need for suctioning of secretions.

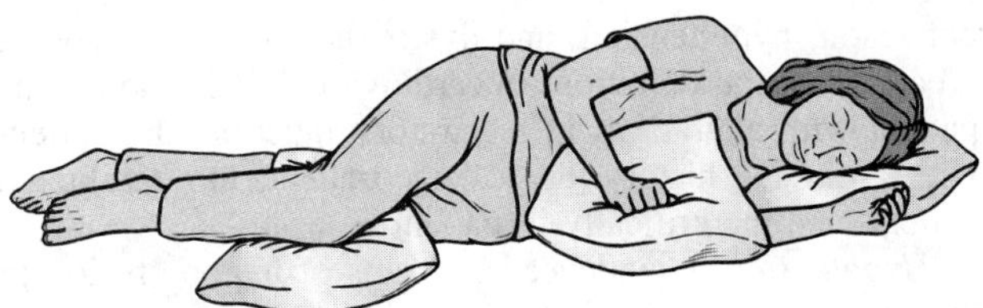

Fig. 16-4 Positioning of patient during recovery from general anesthesia.

The regular monitoring of vital signs permits the nurse to recognize early signs of respiratory distress. The presence of hypoxemia from any cause may be reflected by rapid breathing, gasping, apprehension, restlessness, and a rapid or thready pulse. Impaired ventilation may initially be detected by the observation of slowed breathing or diminished chest and abdominal movement during the respiratory cycle.

The characteristics of sputum or mucus should be noted and recorded. Mucus from the trachea and throat is colorless and thin in consistency. Sputum from the lungs and bronchi is thick with a slight yellow tinge.

Nursing Diagnoses

Nursing diagnoses and collaborative problems related to potential respiratory complications for the patient in the PACU include, but are not limited to, the following:

- Ineffective airway clearance
- Ineffective breathing pattern
- Impaired gas exchange
- Risk for aspiration
- Potential complication: hypoxemia

Nursing Implementation

In the PACU, nursing interventions are designed to both prevent and treat respiratory problems. Proper positioning of the patient to facilitate respirations and protect the airway is essential. Unless contraindicated by the surgical procedure, the unconscious or semiconscious patient is positioned in a lateral position (Fig. 16-4). Once conscious the patient is usually returned to a supine position with the head of the bed elevated. This position maximizes expansion of the thorax by decreasing the pressure of the abdomen on the diaphragm.

Deep breathing is encouraged to facilitate gas exchange and to promote the return to consciousness. The patient should be taught to take in slow, deep breaths, ideally through the nose, to hold the breath, and to then slowly exhale. A patient can perform this type of breathing independently or with the aid of an incentive spirometer. This type of breathing is also useful as a relaxation strategy when the patient is anxious or in pain. Other nursing interventions will be specific to the cause of the respiratory complication, as detailed in Table 16-3.

Potential Alterations in Cardiovascular Function

Etiology. In the immediate postanesthetic period the most common cardiovascular complications include hypotension, hypertension, and dysrhythmias. The person at greatest risk for alterations in cardiovascular function is the patient with alterations in respiratory function, the patient with a cardiac history, the elderly patient, the debilitated patient, and the critically-ill patient.

Hypotension is evidenced by signs of hypoperfusion to the vital organs, especially the brain, heart, and kidneys. Clinical signs of disorientation, loss of consciousness, chest pain, oliguria, and anuria reflect loss of physiologic compensation. Intervention must be timely to prevent the devastating complications of myocardial ischemia or infarction, cerebral ischemia, renal ischemia, and bowel infarction.[7]

The most common cause of hypotension in the PACU is unreplaced fluid and blood loss. As a result, treatment will be directed toward restoring circulating volume. If there is no response to fluid administration, then myocardial dysfunction should be considered to be the cause of hypotension.

Primary cardiac dysfunction, as may occur in the case of myocardial infarction, cardiac tamponade, or pulmonary embolism, results in an acute fall in cardiac output. Secondary myocardial dysfunction occurs as a result of the negative chronotrope (rate) and negative inotrope (force) effects of medications, such as beta blockers, digoxin, or narcotics.[6]

Other causes of hypotension include decreased low systemic vascular resistance, dysrhythmias, and measurement errors that may occur if a blood pressure cuff is incorrectly sized.

Hypertension is defined as a 20% to 30% increase above the resting blood pressure. Hypertension, a common finding in the PACU, is most frequently the result of sympathetic stimulation that may be the result of pain, bladder distention, or respiratory compromise. Hypertension may also be the result of hypothermia and preexisting hypertension, and it may be seen after vascular and cardiac surgery as a result of revascularization.

Dysrhythmias are most commonly the result of an identifiable cause as opposed to myocardial injury. The leading causes include hypokalemia, hypoxemia, hypercarbia, alterations in acid-base status, circulatory instability, and preexisting heart disease. Hypothermia, pain, surgical stress, and many anesthetic agents are also capable of causing dysrhythmias.[8]

NURSING MANAGEMENT

CARDIOVASCULAR COMPLICATIONS

Nursing Assessment

The most important aspect of the cardiovascular assessment is frequent monitoring of vital signs. They are usually monitored every 15 minutes, or more often until stabilized, and then at less frequent intervals. Postoperative vital signs should be compared with preoperative and intraoperative readings to determine when the signs are stabilizing at a normal level for the patient's situation. The ACP or surgeon should be notified if the following occur:

1. Systolic blood pressure is less than 90 mm Hg or greater than 160 mm Hg.
2. Pulse rate is less than 60 beats per minute (bpm) or greater than 120 bpm.
3. Pulse pressure narrows.
4. Blood pressure gradually decreases during several consecutive readings.
5. An irregular cardiac rhythm develops.

Cardiac monitoring is recommended for any patient who has a history of cardiac disease and for all older adult patients who have undergone major surgery, regardless of whether they have cardiac problems. An apical-radial pulse should be assessed carefully, and any irregularities should be reported.

Assessment of skin color, temperature, and moisture provides valuable information in detecting cardiovascular problems. Hypotension accompanied by a normal pulse and warm, dry, pink skin usually represents the residual vasodilating effects of anesthesia and suggests only a need for continued observation. Hypotension accompanied by a rapid pulse and cold, clammy, pale skin may be caused by impending hypovolemic shock and requires immediate treatment.

Nursing Diagnoses

Nursing diagnoses and collaborative problems related to potential cardiovascular complications for the patient in the PACU include, but are not limited to, the following:

- Decreased cardiac output
- Fluid volume deficit
- Altered tissue perfusion
- Potential complication: hypovolemic shock

Nursing Implementation

Nursing interventions in the PACU are designed to prevent and treat cardiovascular complications. Treatment of hypotension should always begin with oxygen therapy. Volume status should be assessed, and errors of blood pressure measurement should be ruled out. Primary cardiac dysfunction may require pharmacologic intervention. Secondary cardiac dysfunction may require discontinuation of causative medications. Peripheral vasodilatation may require vasoconstrictive agents to normalize systemic vascular resistance.

Treatment of hypertension will center on addressing the cause of sympathetic stimulation and eliminating the precipitating cause. Treatment may include the use of analgesics, assistance in voiding, and correction of respiratory problems. Rewarming will correct hypothermia-induced hypertension. If the patient has preexisting hypertension or has undergone cardiac or vascular surgery, pharmacologic intervention designed to reduce blood pressure will usually be required.

Because the majority of dysrhythmias seen in the PACU have identifiable causes, treatment is directed toward eliminating the cause. Correction of these physiologic alterations will, in most instances, correct the dysrhythmias. In the event of life-threatening dysrhythmias, protocols of advanced cardiac life support will be applied (see Chapter 33).

Potential Alterations in Neurologic Function

Etiology. Postoperatively, *emergence delirium* remains the neurologic alteration that causes the most concern to the practitioner. Emergence delirium is defined as a condition characterized by extreme alterations in arousal, orientation, perception, affect, and attention.[9] The patient is frequently combative. Common causes of emergence delirium include hypoxemia, adverse reactions to anesthetic medications, chemical dependency, metabolic alterations, pain, bladder distention, and hypothermia.[10]

Delayed awakening may also be a problem postoperatively. Fortunately, the most common cause of delayed awakening is prolonged drug action, particularly of narcotics, sedatives, and inhalational anesthetics, as opposed to neurologic injury.

NURSING MANAGEMENT

NEUROLOGIC ALTERATIONS

Nursing Assessment

The patient's level of consciousness, orientation, and ability to follow commands should be assessed. The size, reactivity, and equality of the pupils should be determined. The patient's sensory and motor status should also be assessed. If the neurologic status is altered, possible causes should be determined.

Nursing Diagnoses

Nursing diagnoses related to potential neurologic alterations in the patient in the PACU include, but are not limited to, the following:

- Sensory/perceptual alterations
- Risk for injury
- Altered thought processes
- Impaired verbal communications

Nursing Implementation

The most common cause of postoperative agitation is hypoxemia. As a result, attention must be addressed toward evaluation of respiratory function. Once hypoxemia has been ruled out as the cause of postoperative delirium and all potentially known causes have been addressed, sedation may prove beneficial in controlling the agitation and for providing for patient and staff safety. Emergence delirium is time limited and will resolve before the patient is discharged from the PACU. Because the most common cause of delayed awakening is prolonged drug action, usually delays in awakening spontaneously resolve with time. If necessary, benzodiazepines and narcotics may be pharmacologically reversed with antagonists.

Until the patient is awake and able to communicate effectively, it will be the responsibility of the PACU nurse to act as a patient advocate and to maintain patient safety at all times. This includes having the side rails up, securing IV lines and artificial airways, verifying the presence of identification and allergy bands, and monitoring physiologic status.

Hypothermia

Etiology. Hypothermia, defined as a body temperature of less than 96° F (35.5° C), occurs when heat loss exceeds heat production.[11] Hypothermia may be the result of *radiant heat loss* (loss of heat from a warm body to a cold OR), *convective heat loss* (loss of heat from the body to ambient air), *conductive heat loss* (loss of heat from a warm body to a cold OR table), or *evaporative loss* (loss of heat from exposed viscera to the air).[1,3]

Although all patients are at risk for hypothermia, the older, debilitated, or intoxicated patient is at an increased risk. Long surgical procedures and prolonged anesthetic administration also place the patient at an increased risk for hypothermia.[3]

Hypothermia has the potential to compromise physiologic stability and increase perioperative risk. Oxygen demand is increased and metabolic processes slow down, decreasing metabolism and elimination of anesthetic agents. Renal transport decreases, cardiac rate and rhythm disturbances may develop, and central nervous system (CNS) depression is accentuated. Systemic vascular resistance is increased as a result of peripheral vasoconstriction.[1]

NURSING MANAGEMENT

HYPOTHERMIA

Nursing Assessment

Vital signs, including temperature, should be determined. The color and temperature of the skin should also be assessed.

Nursing Diagnoses

The nursing diagnosis specific to the patient with hypothermia includes, but is not limited to, altered body temperature.

Nursing Implementation

Passive rewarming (i.e., shivering) raises basal heat metabolism. Active rewarming requires the application of external warming devices and may include warm blankets, heated aerosols, radiant warmers, forced air warmers, or heated water mattresses. When using any external warming device, body temperature should be monitored at 15-minute intervals, and care should be taken to prevent burns. In addition, oxygen therapy is used to treat the increased demand for oxygen.

Pain and Discomfort

Etiology. Despite the availability of analgesic medications and pain-relieving techniques, pain remains a common problem for the patient in the PACU and during the postoperative period. Pain may be the result of surgical manipulation, positioning, the presence of internal devices such as an endotracheal tube or catheter, or may occur as the patient begins to mobilize postoperatively. Other sources of physical and emotional discomfort include anxiety about the outcome of surgery, embarrassment from having removed dentures or other prostheses, shivering, and a full bladder.[1]

NURSING MANAGEMENT

PATIENT IN PAIN

Nursing Assessment

The patient should be observed for indications of pain (e.g., restlessness). In addition, the patient should be questioned about the degree and characteristics of the pain.

Nursing Diagnoses

Nursing diagnoses for the patient experiencing pain and discomfort include, but are not limited to, the following:

- Pain
- Anxiety

Nursing Implementation

Interventions for pain include pharmacologic and behavioral therapy. Intravenous narcotics provide the most rapid relief. More sustained relief may be obtained through the use of epidural catheters, patient-controlled analgesia, or regional anesthetic blockade. Comfort measures, including touch, reuniting the patient and family, and rewarming also contribute to patient comfort.

Pain management is most likely to be successful if the treatment plan is initiated with involvement of the patient, the ACP, and the PACU nurse (see research box). The goals should be to determine the most effective therapy, medication, and dose and to determine the best response to therapy. Once discharged from the PACU to an inpatient unit, the medical-surgical nurse will replace the PACU nurse as a member of the pain management team. For more information on nursing assessment and management of patients in pain, see Chapter 6.

Nausea and Vomiting

Etiology. Nausea and vomiting remain significant problems in the immediate postoperative period. These problems are responsible for unanticipated admission of day surgery patients, increased patient discomfort, delays in discharge, and patient dissatisfaction with the surgical experience.[12]

Numerous factors have been identified as contributing to the development of nausea and vomiting, including anesthetic agents and techniques, gender (female), weight (obesity), type of surgery (eye, testicular, and gynecologic), and a history of nausea and vomiting after surgery or motion sickness.[12]

NURSING MANAGEMENT

NAUSEA AND VOMITING

Nursing Assessment

The patient should be questioned about feelings of nausea. If vomiting occurs, it is important to determine the quantity, characteristics, and color of the vomitus.

Nursing Diagnoses

Nursing diagnoses specific to the patient experiencing nausea and vomiting include, but are not limited to, the following:

- Nausea and vomiting
- Risk for fluid volume deficit

Nursing Implementation

Intervention is primarily the use of antiemetic drugs. In the PACU, oral fluids should be given only as indicated and tolerated. Intravenous fluids will provide hydration until the patient is able to tolerate oral fluids. Care should also be taken to prevent aspiration if the patient vomits while still sleepy from anesthesia. Having suction equipment readily available at the bedside and turning the patient's head to the side will help to protect the patient from aspiration.

RESEARCH

Implications for Nursing Practice

PAIN IN POSTOPERATIVE PATIENTS

Citation Webb MR, Kennedy MG. Behavior responses and self-reported pain in postoperative patients, *J Post Anesth Nurs* 9:91-95, 1994.

Purpose Investigate the relationship of the patient's self-report of pain to the total score of a PACU Behavioral Pain Rating Scale (BPRS).

Methods Descriptive-correlational study used the BPRS, the patient's self-report of pain, and the hospital's patient-controlled analgesia (PCA) pain-rating scale to investigate pain measurement. Pain assessments (at five different time intervals) were collected from a convenience sample of 36 gynecologic patients during the first 6 postoperative hours.

Results and Conclusions Pain scores were highest in the immediate postoperative period and continued throughout 2 hours. The BPRS consistently showed a moderate-to-high relationship with the patient's self-report of pain, and the BPRS had a stronger relationship with the patient's self-reported pain than with the hospital's PCA pain scale.

Implications for Nursing Practice The assessment of pain is difficult. The nurse frequently relies on the subjective assessment of the patient's pain. The findings of this study provide data about the effectiveness of a brief pain assessment scale. Regardless of the clinical setting, the nurse needs to use efficient and valid tools to assess the patient's pain levels.

Surgical Care of the Patient in the PACU

In addition to meeting the postanesthesia needs of the patient in the PACU, the PACU nurse will also attend to the surgery-specific (e.g., abdominal, thoracic) needs of the patient. The nursing assessment and management of the patient having a specific surgical procedure are discussed in the appropriate chapters of this text.

Discharge from the PACU

The patient leaving the PACU may be discharged to an inpatient unit, intensive care unit, ambulatory care unit, or home. The choice of discharge site will be based on patient acuity, access to follow-up care, and the potential for postoperative complications.

The decision to discharge the patient from the PACU will be based on written discharge criteria. Discharge from an ambulatory care PACU will require that the patient meet

Table 16-4 Postanesthesia and Ambulatory Surgery Discharge Criteria

PACU Discharge Criteria
- Patient awake or baseline
- Vital signs stable
- No excess bleeding or drainage
- No respiratory depression
- Oxygen saturation >90%
- Report given

Ambulatory Surgery Discharge Criteria
- All PACU discharge criteria met
- No IV narcotics for last 30 min
- Minimal nausea and vomiting
- Voided if appropriate to surgical procedure or orders
- Able to ambulate if appropriate to patient's age and not contraindicated
- Responsible adult present to accompany patient
- Discharge instructions given and understood

IV, Intravenous; *PACU,* postanesthesia care unit.

additional criteria. Examples of discharge criteria are provided in Table 16-4.

CARE OF THE POSTOPERATIVE PATIENT ON THE CLINICAL UNIT

Before discharging the patient from the PACU, the PACU nurse will provide a verbal report about the patient to the receiving nurse. The report will summarize the operative and postanesthetic period.

The nurse who receives the patient on the clinical unit will assist PACU transport personnel in transferring the patient from the PACU cart onto the bed. Care must be taken to protect IV lines, wound drains, dressings, and traction devices. The use of a draw sheet and sufficient personnel will facilitate transfer.

Vital signs should be obtained, and patient status should be compared with the report provided by the PACU. Documentation of the transfer is then completed, followed by a more in-depth assessment (Table 16-5). Postoperative orders and appropriate nursing care are then initiated.

Although many of the potential problems that may occur in the PACU are time limited to the immediate postoperative period, there are a number of potential complications that may occur during the extended postoperative recovery period on the medical-surgical unit. Nursing assessment and management are based on awareness of the potential complications of surgery in general, as well as complications specific to the surgical procedure. A general nursing care plan for the postoperative patient is presented on p. 396.

Early ambulation is the most significant general nursing measure to prevent postoperative complications. Since it was first advocated nearly 40 years ago, the value of early ambulation has been obvious. The exercise associated with walking (1) increases muscle tone; (2) improves gastrointestinal (GI) and urinary tract function; (3) stimulates circulation, which prevents venous stasis and speeds wound healing; and (4) increases vital capacity and maintains normal respiratory function.[13] Ambulation is especially important for the older adult patient because hazards of immobility develop earlier, last longer, and may have more lasting effects in the older adult.[14]

Table 16-5 Nursing Assessment and Care of Patient on Admission to Clinical Unit

- Record time of patient's return to unit
- Take baseline vital signs
  Assess airway and breath sounds
- Assess neurologic status, including level of consciousness and movement of extremities
- Assess wound, dressing, drainage tubes
  Note type and amount of drainage
  Connect tubing to gravity or suction drainage
- Assess color and appearance of skin
- Assess urinary status
  Note time of voiding
  Note presence of catheter and total output
  Check for bladder distention or urge to void
  Note catheter patency
- Assess pain and discomfort
  Note last dose and type of pain control
  Note current pain intensity
- Position for airway maintenance, comfort, safety (bed in low position, side rails up)
- Check IV infusion
  Note type of solution
  Note amount of fluid remaining
  Note flow rate
  Check integrity of insertion site and size of catheter
- Attach call light within reach, and reorient patient to use of call light
- Ensure that emesis basin and tissues are available
- Determine emotional condition and support
  Check for presence of family member or significant other
- Check and carry out postoperative orders

IV, Intravenous.

Potential Alterations in Respiratory Function

Etiology. Atelectasis and pneumonia can occur in the postoperative surgical patient and are particularly common after abdominal and thoracic surgery.[15] *Atelectasis* (alveolar collapse) occurs when mucus blocks bronchioles or when the amount of alveolar surfactant (the substance that holds the alveoli open) is reduced (Fig. 16-5). As air becomes trapped beyond the plug and is eventually absorbed, the alveoli collapse. Atelectasis may affect a portion or an entire lobe of the lungs.

The postoperative development of mucous plugs and decreased surfactant production are directly related to hypoventilation, constant recumbent position, ineffective coughing, and smoking. Increased bronchial secretions occur

NURSING CARE PLAN Postoperative Patient*

Planning: Outcome Criteria	Nursing Interventions and Rationales
➤ **NURSING DIAGNOSIS**	Pain *related to* surgical incision and reflex muscle spasm *as manifested by* complaints of pain, tense and guarded body posture, facial grimacing, restlessness, irritability, moaning, diaphoresis, tachycardia, hypertension, or hypotension
Express satisfaction with pain relief; have no interference with postoperative recovery.	Assess pain for character, location, and effectiveness of relief measures *to plan appropriate interventions.* Position *to relieve pain.* Assure patient of efforts to reduce pain. Administer analgesics as ordered *to relieve pain by interrupting CNS pathways.* Assess effectiveness. Convey accepting attitude *so patient does not become defensive about pain.* Use nonpharmacologic pain relievers in addition to pharmacologic intervention such as distraction, massage, and imagery *to reduce need for drugs.*
➤ **NURSING DIAGNOSIS**	Nausea and vomiting *related to* distention, medication and anesthesia effects, and stimulation of vomiting center or chemoreceptor trigger zone *as manifested by* complaints of nausea, refusal to take fluids and solids, and observed or reported vomiting
Have reduced or no episodes of nausea and vomiting.	Assess precipitating factors and eliminate when possible (e.g., unpleasant smells, sights) *to prevent initiating episode of nausea or vomiting.* Control pain *to reduce or eliminate response.* Maintain patency of nasogastric tube if present *to prevent accumulation of gastric contents and subsequent vomiting.* Advance diet only as tolerated. Monitor effects of medications, especially narcotics *to determine if this is a possible source of the nausea.* Administer antiemetics as indicated. Assess bowel sounds *to determine presence, frequency, and characteristics.*
➤ **NURSING DIAGNOSIS**	Risk for infection *related to* surgical incision, inadequate nutrition and fluid intake, presence of environmental pathogens, invasive catheters, and immobility
Have no evidence of infection such as fever, pain or swelling at operative site, or purulent wound drainage.	Monitor for and report the following *to determine possible presence of infection:* elevated body temperature; red, swollen, warm area surrounding incision or indwelling catheters; elevated white blood cell count; elevated pulse and respiratory rate; purulent drainage from wound. Use strict aseptic technique in providing wound care, including hand washing and sterile dressing technique, *to prevent wound contamination.* Monitor daily caloric intake. Ensure a minimum of 2000 calories and 2500 ml fluid/day (greater if metabolic demands are increased) *to ensure adequate calories for tissue repair.* Weigh daily and notify physician if greater than 5% weight loss from baseline *to modify nutritional plan.* Minimize exposure to environmental pathogens by avoiding contact between patient and others with infection *to prevent cross contamination.* Maintain aseptic technique in care of invasive lines. Monitor patient daily *to detect any changes indicative of infection.* Report to physician. Help patient turn, cough, and breathe deeply q1-2hr while awake *to prevent respiratory infection.*
➤ **NURSING DIAGNOSIS**	Ineffective airway clearance *related to* ineffective cough and tenacious secretions *as manifested by* abnormal breath sounds, shallow respirations, nonproductive cough
Have clear breath sounds, effective cough.	Provide pain relief before asking the patient to cough and breathe deeply *to encourage cooperation and pain-free performance.* Provide a minimum of 2500 ml/day of fluids unless contraindicted *to liquefy secretions for easier removal.* Provide preoperative teaching of proper coughing and deep-breathing techniques *to increase probability of good postoperative technique.* Assist patient with turning, coughing, and deep breathing q1-2hr while awake *to aid in removal of secretions and prevent formation of mucous plug.* Monitor use of incentive spirometer *to maintain airway patency.* Discourage smoking. Suction if necessary *to remove secretions the patient is unable to remove unaided.* Monitor breath sounds and temperature *to detect early signs of infection.* Assist with early mobility *to increase respiratory excursion.*

continued

NURSING CARE PLAN Postoperative Patient*—cont'd

Planning: Outcome Criteria	Nursing Interventions and Rationales
➤ **NURSING DIAGNOSIS**	Anxiety *related to* lack of knowledge about follow-up care *as manifested by* frequent questioning about self-care at home, agitation concerning difficulty in performing any part of self-care at home, concern over absence of assistance at home
Express satisfaction with own knowledge and skill level or with plan made for home care.	Teach patient and family about signs and symptoms of infection to observe and report, nutritional needs of patient, activity restrictions, wound care, and medication requirements *to decrease anxiety and increase sense of control.* Ensure patient's or family member's skills in performing self-care before discharge, or arrange for referral for home care *to assure continuity of care using appropriate technique.* Allow sufficient practice in technical skills such as dressing change for patient and family member *to become confident.* Together with patient, identify aspects of self-care with which assistance may be needed *so appropriate referrals can be made.* Make appropriate referrals. Assist patient to plan follow-up care with surgeon *to avoid delay in appropriate follow-up treatment.*
➤ **NURSING DIAGNOSIS**	Constipation *related to* inadequate intake, decreased physical activity, and medications that decrease bowel activity *as manifested by* hard, formed stool, straining at stool, or defecation less than 3 times per week
Resume usual bowel pattern.	Assess bowel elimination *to determine need for intervention.* Maintain fluid intake of 2500 ml or more *to soften fecal mass.* Provide increased fiber in diet if appropriate *to increase fecal bulk and retention of fluid in fecal mass.* Increase activity as tolerated *to increase peristalsis.* Administer stool softeners as ordered *to soften fecal mass.*

COLLABORATIVE PROBLEMS

Nursing Goals	Nursing Interventions and Rationales
➤ **POTENTIAL COMPLICATION**	Hemorrhage *related to* ineffective vascular closure or alterations in coagulation
Monitor operative site for signs of hemorrhage, report deviations from acceptable parameters, and carry out appropriate medical and nursing interventions.	Observe surgical site and dressings regularly (q hr for 4 hr, then q4hr) *to detect signs of bleeding, including dependent sites.* Monitor vital signs regularly from q 15 min to q2-4hr as indicated *to detect signs of hypovolemia.* Report abnormalities such as decreasing blood pressure, rapid pulse and respirations, cool and clammy skin, pallor, and bright red blood on dressing. Monitor for changes in mental status such as restlessness and sense of impending doom *as indicators of inadequate cerebral perfusion.* Monitor hematocrit and hemoglobin levels as ordered *because decreases can indicate hemorrhage.* Monitor platelet levels as ordered *because decreases may indicate bleeding tendencies.* Monitor prothrombin and thrombin levels as ordered *because elevations may indicate bleeding tendencies.*
➤ **POTENTIAL COMPLICATION**	Thromboembolism *related to* dehydration, immobility, vascular manipulation, or injury
Monitor for signs of thromboembolism, report deviation from acceptable parameters, and carry out appropriate medical and nursing interventions.	Assess every shift *to detect signs of thromboembolism such as redness, swelling, pain; increased warmth along path of vein; positive Homans' sign; edema or pain in extremity; chest pain; hemoptysis; tachypnea; dyspnea; and restlessness.* Teach or perform range of motion to lower extremities and encourage early ambulation *to maintain muscle contractions and adequate vascular flow.* Avoid pressure under knees from bed or pillows *to avoid pressure on veins, constriction of circulation, or pooling and stasis of blood.* If ordered, apply antiembolism stockings and sequential compression device; remove every shift for 1 hr *to allow for skin assessment.* Maintain adequate hydration *to prevent hypovolemia and subsequent sludging of cells.*

continued

NURSING CARE PLAN Postoperative Patient*—cont'd

Nursing Goals	Nursing Interventions and Rationales
➤ **POTENTIAL COMPLICATION**	Urinary retention *related to* horizontal positioning, pain, fear, analgesic and anesthetic medications, or surgical procedure
Monitor for signs of urinary retention, report deviation from acceptable parameters, and carry out appropriate medical and nursing interventions.	Assess for bladder pain and distention, decreased or absent urinary output *to determine if a problem is present.* Monitor intake and output *to determine fluid balance.* Percuss bladder routinely for 48 hr postoperatively *to assess for distention.* Notify physician if no urine output within 6 hr after surgery. Position patient in as normal position as possible for voiding. Provide privacy. Use appropriate pain measures *to reduce anxiety so voiding will be easier.* Provide explanation and encouragement *to relieve patient's fears.* Monitor urinary effects of analgesic and anesthetic medications *because they could be a source of urinary retention.*
➤ **POTENTIAL COMPLICATION**	Paralytic ileus *related to* bowel manipulation, immobility, pain medication, and anesthetics
Monitor for signs of paralytic ileus, report deviation from acceptable parameters, and carry out appropriate medical and nursing interventions.	Assess every shift for abdominal distention, presence of flatus and stool, bowel sounds, or nausea and vomiting *to determine if paralytic ileus is present.* Maintain NPO status until peristalsis returns and ensure patency of nasogastric tube *to prevent vomiting.* Provide frequent oral hygiene for patient comfort.

CNS, Central nervous system; *NPO,* nothing by mouth.
*This is a general nursing care plan for the postoperative patient. It should be used in conjunction with a nursing care plan specific to the type of surgery being performed.

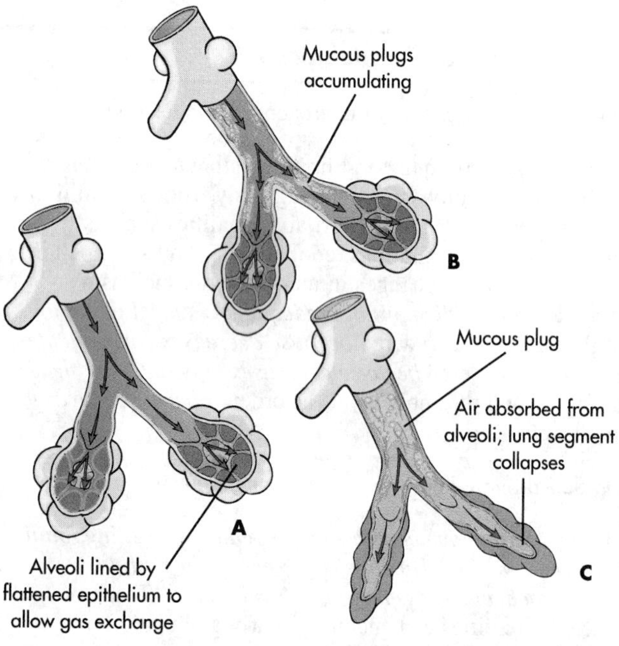

Fig. 16-5 Postoperative atelectasis. ***A,*** Normal bronchiole and alveoli. ***B,*** Mucous plugs in bronchiole. ***C,*** Collapse of alveoli resulting from atelectasis following absorption of air.

when the respiratory passages are irritated by heavy smoking, acute or chronic pulmonary infection or disease, and the drying of mucous membranes that occurs with intubation, inhalation anesthesia, and dehydration. Without intervention, atelectasis can progress to pneumonia when microorganisms grow in the stagnant mucus and an infection develops.

NURSING MANAGEMENT

RESPIRATORY FUNCTION

Nursing Assessment

Nursing assessment of the patient's respiratory rate, patterns, and breath sounds is essential to identify potential respiratory problems.

Nursing Diagnoses

Nursing diagnoses related to potential alterations in respiratory function for the postoperative patient include, but are not limited to, the following:

- Ineffective airway clearance
- Ineffective breathing patterns
- Ineffective gas exchange
- Potential complication: pneumonia
- Potential complication: atelectasis

Nursing Implementation

Deep-breathing and coughing techniques help the patient to prevent alveolar collapse and move respiratory secretions to larger airway passages for expectoration. The patient should be assisted to breathe deeply 10 times every hour. Diaphragmatic or abdominal breathing is accomplished by inhaling slowly and deeply through the nose, holding the breath for a few seconds, and then exhaling slowly and completely through the mouth. The patient's hands should be placed lightly over the lower ribs and upper abdomen. This allows the patient to feel the abdomen rise during inspiration and fall during expiration.

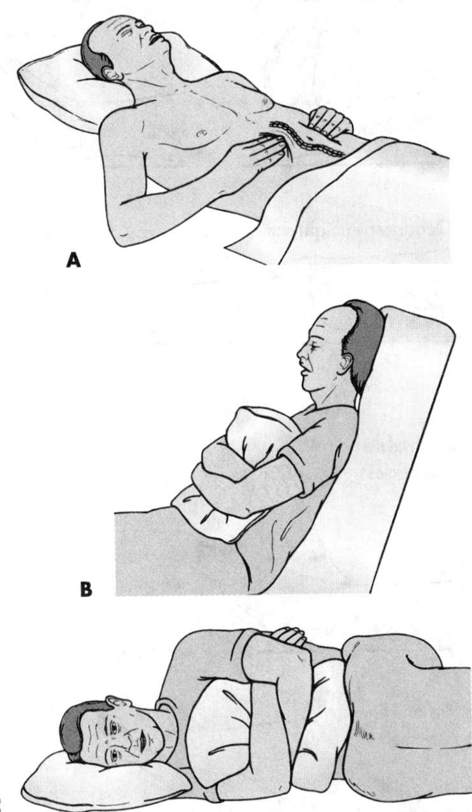

Fig. 16-6 Techniques for splinting a wound when patient is coughing.

Following four to six deep breaths, the patient should cough deeply from the lungs rather than the throat. If secretions are present in the respiratory passages, deep breathing often will move them up to stimulate the cough reflex without any voluntary effort by the patient, and they can then be expectorated.

Splinting the incision with a pillow or a rolled blanket provides support to weakened muscles and also aids in coughing and expectoration of secretions (Fig. 16-6). Incentive spirometry is increasingly used as an adjunct to traditional deep breathing and coughing techniques.[16]

The patient's position should be changed every 1 to 2 hours to allow full chest expansion and increase perfusion of both lungs. Ambulation, not just sitting in a chair, should be aggressively carried out as soon as physician approval is given. Adequate and regular analgesic medication should be provided because incisional pain often is the greatest deterrent to patient participation in effective ventilation and ambulation. The patient should also be reassured that these activities will not cause the incision to separate. Adequate hydration, either parenteral or oral, is essential to maintain the integrity of mucous membranes and to keep secretions thin and loose for easy expectoration.

Potential Alterations in Cardiovascular Function

Etiology. Postoperative fluid and electrolyte imbalances are contributing factors to alterations in cardiovascular function. They may develop as a result of a combination of the body's normal response to the stress of surgery, excessive fluid losses, and improper IV fluid replacement. The body's fluid status directly affects cardiac output. Fluid retention during the first 2 to 5 postoperative days is a result of the stress response (see Chapter 5). This body response serves to maintain both blood volume and blood pressure. Fluid retention results from the secretion and release of two hormones by the pituitary—adrenocorticotropic hormone (ACTH) and antidiuretic hormone (ADH). ACTH stimulates the adrenal cortex to secrete aldosterone and cortisol. These adrenocortical hormones promote sodium and water retention, which increases blood volume. ADH release leads to a decrease in urinary output, which ultimately increases blood volume.

Fluid overload may occur during this period of fluid retention when IV fluids are administered too rapidly, when chronic (e.g., cardiac or renal) disease exists, or when the patient is an older adult. Conversely, fluid deficit may be related to slow or inadequate fluid replacement, which leads to decreases in cardiac output and tissue perfusion. Untreated preoperative dehydration or intraoperative or postoperative losses from vomiting, bleeding, wound drainage, or suctioning may be contributing factors to fluid deficits.

Hypokalemia can be a consequence of urinary and GI tract losses, and it results when potassium is not replaced in IV fluids. The loss of potassium directly affects the contractility of the heart and thus may also contribute to decreased cardiac output and overall body tissue perfusion. Adequate replacement of potassium is usually 40 mEq per day. However, it should not be given until adequate renal function has been established. A urine output of at least 0.5 ml/kg per hour is generally considered indicative of adequate renal function.

Cardiovascular status is also affected by the state of tissue perfusion or blood flow. The stress response contributes to an increase in clotting tendencies in the postoperative patient by increasing platelet production and circulating levels of glucocorticoids. Blood clots may form in leg veins as a result of inactivity, body position, and pressure, all of which lead to venous stasis and decreased perfusion. Deep vein thrombosis, especially common in the older adult, obese individual, and immobilized patient, is a potentially life-threatening complication because it may lead to pulmonary embolism.[13] Superficial thrombophlebitis is an uncomfortable but less ominous complication that may develop in a leg vein as a result of venous stasis or in the arm veins as a result of irritation from IV catheters or solutions. If a piece of a clot becomes dislodged, it can cause a pulmonary infarction of a size proportionate to the vessel in which it lodges.

Syncope (fainting) is another factor that reflects the cardiovascular status. It may indicate decreased cardiac output, fluid deficits, or defects in cerebral tissue perfusion. Syncope frequently occurs as a result of postural hypotension when the patient ambulates. It is more common in the older adult or in the patient who has been immobile for long periods of time. Normally when the patient quickly moves to a standing position, the arterial pressoreceptors respond to the accompanying fall in blood pressure with sympathetic nervous stimulation, which produces vasoconstriction. This sympathetic nervous system response causes an increase in, and therefore maintains, blood pressure. These sympathetic and vasomotor functions may be diminished in the older adult and the immobile or postanesthetic patient. Consequently, syncope develops when the patient sits up rapidly or during ambulation.

NURSING MANAGEMENT

CARDIOVASCULAR FUNCTION

Nursing Assessment

Specific assessment of cardiovascular function includes the regular monitoring of the patient's blood pressure, heart rate, pulses, and skin temperature and color. Results should be compared with preoperative status and the immediate postoperative and intraoperative findings.

Nursing Diagnoses

Nursing diagnoses related to potential altered cardiovascular function in the postoperative patient include, but are not limited to, the following:

- Altered cardiac output: decreased
- Fluid volume deficit
- Fluid volume excess
- Altered tissue perfusion
- Activity intolerance
- Potential complication: thromboembolism

Nursing Implementation

An accurate intake and output record should be kept during the postoperative period, and laboratory findings (e.g., electrolytes, hematocrit) should be monitored. Nursing responsibilities relating to IV management are critical during this period. In particular the nurse should be alert for symptoms of too slow or too rapid a rate of fluid replacement. Assessment should also be made of the infusion site for discomfort and the hazards associated with the IV administration of potassium (see Chapter 13). Thirst is one of the most annoying discomforts with which the postoperative patient must contend. This may be related to the drying effects of anticholinergic drugs, anesthetic gases, and fluid deficits. Adequate and regular mouth care is helpful while the patient cannot ingest food or drink by mouth.

Leg exercises (Fig. 16-7) should be encouraged 10 to 12 times every 1 to 2 hours. The muscular contraction produced by these exercises and by ambulation facilitates venous return from the lower extremities. The ambulating patient should pick up the feet rather than shuffling them so that muscular contraction is maximized. When confined to bed, the patient should alternately flex and extend the legs. When the patient is sitting in a chair or lying in bed, there should be no pressure to impede venous flow through the popliteal space. Crossed legs, pillows behind the knees, and elevation of the knee gatch must be avoided.

Some surgeons routinely prescribe elastic stockings or mechanical aids such as sequential compressive devices to stimulate and enhance the massaging and milking actions that are transmitted to the veins when leg muscles contract.[17] The nurse must remember that these aids are useless if the legs are not exercised and may actually impair circulation if the legs remain inactive or if the devices are sized or applied improperly. When in use, elastic stockings must be removed and reapplied at least once every shift for skin care and inspection. The skin of the heels and posttibial areas is particularly susceptible to increased pressure and breakdown.

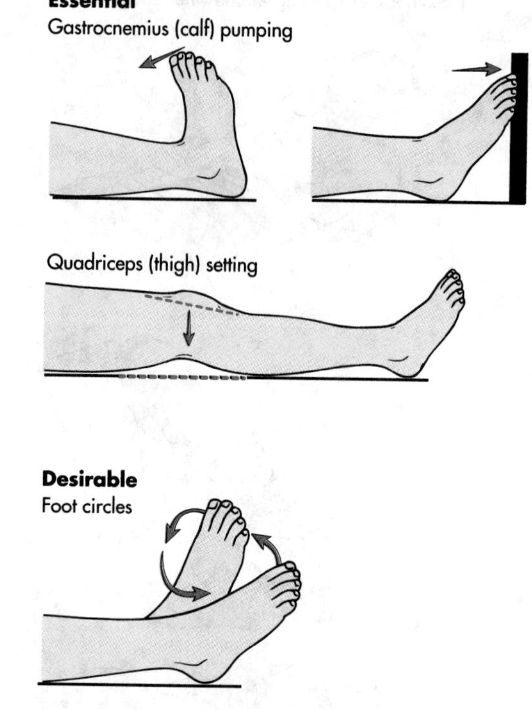

Fig. 16-7 Postoperative leg exercises.

The use of low-dose heparin therapy (5000 units subcutaneously every 8 to 12 hours) is a prophylactic measure for venous thrombosis and embolism. Low-dose heparin does not significantly increase the risk of bleeding during surgery or in the postoperative period. However, this prophylactic measure is not routine and remains controversial.[13,17]

The nurse may prevent syncope by making changes slowly in the patient's position. Progression to ambulation can be achieved by first raising the head of the patient's bed for 1 to 2 minutes and then by assisting the patient to stand beside the bed while monitoring the radial pulse for rate and quality. If no changes or complaints are noted, ambulation can be started. If faintness occurs, the nurse can help the patient sit on the edge of the bed while continuing to monitor the pulse. If changes occur or if the patient complains of feeling faint during ambulation, the nurse should provide assistance to a nearby chair or ease the patient to the floor. The patient should remain in either location until recovered and then be helped back to the bed. If faintness occurs, it is often frightening for the patient and for the unprepared nurse, but syncope poses no real physiologic danger, although injury can result from a fall.

Potential Alterations in Urinary Function

Etiology. Low urine output (800 to 1500 ml) in the first 24 hours may be expected, regardless of fluid intake. This low output is caused by increased aldosterone and ADH secretion resulting from the stress of surgery, fluid restriction before surgery, and loss of fluids caused by evaporation during surgery, drainage, and diaphoresis. By the second or third day, the patient will diurese after fluid has been mobilized, and the immediate stress reaction subsides.

Actual urinary retention can occur in the postoperative period for a variety of reasons. Anesthesia depresses the nervous system, including the micturition reflex arc and the higher centers that influence it. This allows the bladder to fill more completely than normal before the urge to void is felt. Anesthesia also impedes voluntary micturition. Anticholinergic and narcotic drugs may also interfere with the ability to initiate voiding or to empty the bladder completely.

Retention is more likely to occur after lower abdominal or pelvic surgery because spasm or guarding of the abdominal and pelvic muscles interferes with their normal function in micturition. Pain may alter perception and interfere with the patient's awareness of the less intense sensation arising as the bladder fills. Voiding ability is probably impaired to the greatest extent by immobility and the recumbent position in bed. Lack of skeletal muscle activity decreases smooth muscle (bladder detrusor) tone, and the supine position reduces the ability to relax the perineal muscles and external sphincter.

Oliguria, the diminished output of urine related to intake, is associated with acute renal failure and is a less common although more serious problem after surgery. It may result from renal ischemia caused by inadequate renal perfusion or altered cardiovascular function.

NURSING MANAGEMENT

URINARY FUNCTION

Nursing Assessment

The urine of the postoperative patient should be examined for both quantity and quality. The color, amount, consistency, and odor of the urine should be noted. Indwelling catheters should be assessed for patency, and urine output should be at least 0.5 ml/kg per hour. If a catheter is not present, the patient should be able to void approximately 200 ml of urine following surgery. Most people urinate within 6 to 8 hours after surgery. If no voiding occurs, the abdominal contour should be inspected and the bladder palpated and percussed for distention.

Nursing Diagnoses

Nursing diagnoses and collaborative problems related to potential altered urinary function in the postoperative patient include, but are not limited to, the following:

- Altered patterns of urinary elimination
- Potential complication: acute urinary retention

Nursing Implementation

The nurse may facilitate voiding by normal positioning of the patient—sitting for women and standing for men. Providing reassurance to the patient regarding the ability to void and the use of techniques such as running water, drinking water, or pouring warm water over the perineum may also be of assistance. Ambulation, preferably to the bathroom, and the use of a bedside commode are additional helpful measures to assist in voiding.

The surgeon often leaves an order to catheterize the patient in 8 to 12 hours if voiding has not occurred. Because of the possibility of infection associated with catheterization, the nurse should first try other measures to induce voiding and validate that the bladder is actually full. If the bladder becomes overdistended, it is traumatized and more susceptible to infection if catheterization becomes necessary. In assessing the need for catheterization, the nurse should consider fluid intake during and after surgery and determine bladder fullness (e.g., palpable fullness above the symphysis pubis, discomfort when pressure is applied over the bladder, or the presence of the urge to void). Straight catheterization is preferred because of the possibility of infection associated with an indwelling catheter.

Potential Alterations in Gastrointestinal Function

Etiology. Slowed GI function and altered patterns of food intake may lead to the development of several distressing postoperative symptoms that are most pronounced after abdominal surgery. Nausea and vomiting may be caused by the action of anesthetics or narcotics, delayed gastric emptying, slowed peristalsis resulting from the handling of the bowel during surgery, and resumption of oral intake too soon after surgery.

Abdominal distention is another common problem caused by decreased peristalsis as a result of handling of the intestine during surgery and limited dietary intake after surgery. Motility of the large intestine may be reduced for 3 to 5 days, although motility in the small intestine resumes within 24 hours. Swallowed air and GI secretions may accumulate in the colon, producing flatulence and gas pains.

Hiccoughs (singultus) are intermittent spasms of the diaphragm caused by irritation of the phrenic nerve, which innervates the diaphragm. Postoperative sources of direct irritation of the phrenic nerve may be gastric distention, intestinal obstruction, intraabdominal bleeding, and a subphrenic abscess. Indirect irritation of the phrenic nerve may be produced by acid-base and electrolyte imbalances. Reflex irritation may come from drinking hot or cold liquids or from the presence of a nasogastric tube. Hiccoughs usually last a short time and subside spontaneously; occasionally they may be persistent but are rarely debilitating.

NURSING MANAGEMENT

GASTROINTESTINAL FUNCTION

Nursing Assessment

The abdomen should be auscultated in all four quadrants to determine the presence, frequency, and characteristics of the bowel sounds. Bowel sounds are frequently absent or diminished in the immediate postoperative period when peristalsis is decreased.

Nursing Diagnoses

Nursing diagnoses and collaborative problems related to potential alterations in GI function in the postoperative patient may include, but are not limited to, the following:

- Nausea and vomiting
- Altered comfort: hiccoughs
- Altered nutrition: less than body requirements
- Potential complication: paralytic ileus

Nursing Implementation

Depending on the nature of the surgery, the patient may resume oral intake as soon as the gag reflex returns. Sometimes the patient is kept on nothing by mouth (NPO) status for several days until bowel sounds are heard. Although the patient is receiving nothing by mouth, IV infusions are given to maintain fluid and electrolyte balance. A nasogastric tube may be used to decompress the stomach to prevent nausea, vomiting, and abdominal distention. When oral intake is allowed after the return of bowel sounds, clear liquids are begun, and the IV infusion is continued, usually at a reduced rate. If oral intake is well tolerated by the patient, the IV is discontinued, and the diet is advanced until a regular diet is tolerated.

While the patient is on NPO status, regular mouth care is essential for comfort and stimulation of salivary glands. Nausea and vomiting may be prevented or relieved by the administration of an antiemetic drug given IV, intramuscularly, or by rectal suppository. In some instances a nasogastric tube is inserted when symptoms persist.

Abdominal distention may be prevented or minimized by early and frequent ambulation and by resumption of a normal diet, both of which stimulate intestinal peristalsis. The nurse should assess the patient regularly to detect the resumption of normal intestinal peristalsis as evidenced by the return of bowel sounds and the passage of flatus.

The patient may need to be encouraged to expel flatus and to be assured that expulsion is necessary and desirable. Gas pains, which tend to become pronounced on the second or third postoperative day, may be relieved by ambulation and frequent repositioning. Positioning the patient on the right side permits gas to rise along the transverse colon and facilitates its release. Bisacodyl (Dulcolax) suppositories may be ordered to stimulate peristalsis and expulsion of flatus.

The postoperative patient who is hiccoughing should first be assessed in an attempt to determine the cause. In many instances simple irrigation of the nasogastric tube to restore patency will solve the problem. Techniques such as holding the breath while drinking water, swallowing 1 or 2 teaspoons of sugar, and rebreathing carbon dioxide from a paper bag may help.

Potential Alterations of the Integument

Etiology. Surgery generally involves an incision through the skin and underlying tissues. An incision disrupts the protective skin barrier and needs wound healing, which is one of the major concerns of the postoperative period.

An adequate nutritional state is essential for wound healing. Amino acids are readily available for the healing process because of the catabolic effects of the stress response. The patient who was well nourished preoperatively can tolerate the postoperative delay in nutritional intake. However, the patient with preexisting nutritional deficits, such as with chronic diseases (e.g., diabetes, ulcerative colitis, alcoholism), are more prone to problems of wound healing. Wound healing is also a concern for the older adult and is affected by multiple factors.[18]

Wound infection may result from contamination of the wound from three major sources—exogenous flora present in the environment and on the skin, oral flora, and intestinal flora. The incidence of wound sepsis is higher in patients who are malnourished, immunosuppressed, or older, or who have had a prolonged hospital stay or a lengthy surgical procedure (lasting more than 3 hours). Infection may involve the entire incision and may extend downward through the deeper tissue layers. An abscess may form locally, or the infection may penetrate entire body cavities, as in peritonitis. Evidence of wound infection usually does not become apparent before the third to the fifth postoperative day. The signs include local manifestations of redness, swelling, and increasing pain and tenderness at the site. Systemic signs are fever and leukocytosis.

An accumulation of fluid in a wound may create pressure, impair circulation and wound healing, and predispose to infection. Because of these reasons the surgeon may place a drain in the incision or make a stab wound adjacent to the incision to allow for drainage. These drains may be made of soft rubber and drain into a dressing, or they may be firm catheters attached to a Hemovac or other source of gentle suction. Wound healing and complications are discussed in Chapter 9.

NURSING MANAGEMENT

SURGICAL WOUNDS

Nursing Assessment

Nursing assessment of the wound and dressing requires knowledge of the type of wound, drains inserted, and expected drainage related to the specific type of surgery. A small amount of serous drainage is common from any type of wound. If a drain is in place, a moderate to large amount of drainage may be expected. For example, an abdominal incision with accompanying Penrose drain is expected to have a moderate amount of serosanguineous drainage in the first 24 hours. In contrast, an inguinal herniorrhaphy should have only minimal serous drainage during the postoperative period.

In general, drainage is expected to change from sanguineous (red) to serosanguineous (pink) to serous (straw-colored) during a period of hours and days. Bloody drainage may be normal after certain types of surgery (e.g., chest surgery). However, it should not last more than a few hours and should spontaneously decrease in volume. A continuation of bleeding or an increase in drainage after it has once subsided often signals a problem. Wound infection may be accompanied by purulent drainage. *Wound dehiscence* (separation and disruption of previously joined wound edges) may be preceded by a sudden discharge of brown, pink, or clear drainage.

Nursing Diagnoses

Nursing diagnoses related to potential alterations in the integumentary system of the postoperative patient include, but are not limited to, the following:

- Impaired tissue integrity
- Risk for infection

Nursing Implementation

When drainage occurs on the dressing, it should be circled with a pen and marked with the date and time. The type, amount, color, consistency, and odor of drainage should be noted and recorded. Expected drainage from tubes is outlined in Table 16-6. The effect of position changes on drainage should also be assessed. The surgeon should be notified of any excessive or abnormal drainage and significant changes in vital signs.

The incision may be initially covered with a transparent, impermeable, adherent dressing immediately after surgery. If there are no drains or drainage after 24 to 48 hours, the incision may be opened to the air. Agency policy determines whether the nurse may change the initial operative dressing or simply reinforce it if the dressing is saturated.

When a dressing is changed, the number and type of drains present should be noted. Care should be taken to avoid dislodging drains during dressing removal. When the dressing is changed, the incision site should be examined carefully. The area around the sutures may be slightly reddened and swollen, which is an expected inflammatory response. However, the skin around the incision should be normal color and temperature. Abnormal findings include unusually warm skin around the incision, purple hard areas in the site (possibly from hemorrhage into the tissue), and other signs of infection. The nurse should wear gloves when removing a dressing. Sterile technique should be used when any new dressing is applied. If healing is by primary intention, little or no drainage is present, and no drains are in place. A single-layer dressing is sufficient. When drains are in place, when moderate to heavy drainage is occurring, or when healing occurs other than by primary intention, a multiple-layer dressing is needed. Wound care is discussed in Chapter 9.

Potential Alterations in Neurologic Function

Etiology. Pain and fever are two clinical manifestations mediated by the CNS that may present problems for the postoperative patient. The assessment and management of the patient in pain are discussed in Chapter 6.

Postoperative pain is produced by the interaction of a number of physiologic and psychologic factors. The skin and underlying tissues have been traumatized by the incision and retraction during surgery. In addition, there may be reflex muscle spasms around the incision. Anxiety and fear, sometimes related to the anticipation of pain, create tension and further increase muscle tone and spasm. The effort and movement associated with deep breathing, coughing, and changing position may aggravate pain by creating tension or pull on the incisional area.

When the internal viscera is cut, no pain is felt. However, pressure in the internal viscera elicits pain. Therefore deep visceral pain may signal the presence of a complication such as intestinal distention, bleeding, or abscess formation.

Postoperative pain is usually most severe within the first 48 hours and subsides thereafter. Variation is considerable, according to the procedure performed and the patient's individual pain tolerance or perception.

Table 16-6 Expected Drainage from Tubes and Catheters

Substance	Daily Amount	Color	Odor	Consistency
Indwelling Catheter				
Urine	500-700 ml, 1-2 days postoperative; 1500-2500 ml thereafter	Clear, yellow	Ammonia	Watery
Gastrostomy Tube				
Gastric contents	Up to 1500 ml/day	Pale, yellow-green Bloody following GI surgery	Sour	Watery
Nasogastric Tube				
Gastric contents	Up to 1500 ml	Pale yellow-green Bloody following GI surgery	Sour	Watery
Hemovac				
Wound drainage	Variable with procedure	Variable with procedure Usually serosanguineous	Same as wound dressing	Variable
T Tube				
Bile	500 ml	Bright yellow to dark green	Acid	Thick

GI, Gastrointestinal.

Temperature variation in the postoperative period provides valuable information about the patient's status. Hypothermia may be present in the immediate postoperative period while the patient is recovering from the effects of anesthesia and body heat loss during surgery. Fever may occur at any time during the postoperative period (Table 16-7). A mild elevation (up to 100.4° F [38° C]) during the first 48 hours usually reflects the surgical stress response. A moderate elevation (higher than 38° C) is caused more frequently by respiratory congestion or atelectasis and less frequently by dehydration. After the first 48 hours a moderate to marked elevation (higher than 99.9° F [37.7° C]) is usually caused by infection.

Wound infection, particularly from aerobic organisms, is often accompanied by a fever that spikes in the afternoon or evening and returns to near normal levels in the morning. The respiratory tract may be infected secondary to stasis of secretions in an atelectatic region. The urinary tract may be infected secondary to catheterization. Superficial thrombophlebitis may occur at the IV site or in the leg veins. The latter may produce a temperature elevation between 7 and 10 days after surgery.

Intermittent high fever accompanied by shaking chills and diaphoresis suggests septicemia. This may occur at any time during the postoperative period because microorganisms may have been introduced into the bloodstream during surgery, especially in GI or genitourinary (GU) procedures, or picked up later from the site of a wound or a urinary or vein infection.

NURSING MANAGEMENT

NEUROLOGIC FUNCTION

Nursing Assessment

The initial aspect of the neurologic assessment is a determination of the level of consciousness. The anesthetized

Table 16-7 Significance of Postoperative Temperature Changes

Time After Surgery	Temperature	Possible Causes
Up to 12 hr	Hypothermia to 94° F (34.5° C)	Effects of anesthesia Body heat loss in surgical exposure
First 24-48 hr	Elevation to 100.4° F (38° C) Above 100.4° F (38° C)	Inflammatory response to surgical stress Lung congestion, atelectasis Dehydration
Third day and later	Elevation above 100° F (37.7° C)	Wound infection Urinary infection Respiratory infection Phlebitis

patient resumes consciousness in a predictable pattern. By the time the patient returns to the clinical unit, he is usually awake or easily arousable. The nurse needs to be alert for possible deepening of anesthesia effects, especially when administering pain medication in the early postoperative period.

Pain assessment may be difficult in the early postoperative period. The patient may not be able to verbalize the presence or severity of pain. The nurse should observe for behavioral clues of pain such as a wrinkling face or brow, a clenched fist, moaning, diaphoresis, and an increased pulse rate.

Nursing Diagnoses

Nursing diagnoses related to potential alterations in neurologic function of the postoperative patient may include, but are not limited to, the following:

- Sensory/perceptual alterations
- Pain
- Risk for altered body temperature

Nursing Implementation

Postoperative pain relief is a nursing responsibility because the surgeon's orders for analgesic medication and other comfort measures are usually written on an as needed basis. During the first 48 hours or longer, narcotic analgesics (e.g., morphine) are required to relieve moderate-to-severe pain. After that time, nonnarcotic analgesics may be sufficient as pain intensity decreases.

Nurses must examine their own attitudes toward pain and suffering. Too often nurses undermedicate patients in an attempt to protect them from addiction, an imagined hazard that simply does not exist during the few days of extreme postoperative discomfort. Studies have shown that the nurse tends to give less pain medication to the older adult and female patients.[19,20]

During the first 24 to 48 hours, the patient should be medicated freely every 3 to 4 hours if necessary because (1) the greatest relief is obtained when an analgesic is administered as pain is beginning rather than when it has become more severe and (2) relative freedom from pain is essential to gain the patient's cooperation in activities of deep breathing, coughing, turning, and ambulating.[20] When the patient does request pain medication, it should be given promptly because time perception is altered by pain and minutes can seem like hours.

Analgesic administration should be timed to ensure that it is in effect during activities that may be painful for the patient, such as ambulating. Although narcotic analgesics are often essential for the postoperative patient's comfort, there are undesirable side effects. Side effects such as slowed intestinal peristalsis, nausea and vomiting, respiratory and cough depression, and hypotension are most common with the opiates.

Before administering any analgesic, the nurse should first assess the nature of the patient's pain, including location, quality, and intensity. If it is incisional pain, analgesic administration is appropriate. If it is remote chest or leg pain, medication may simply mask a complication that must be reported and documented. If it is gas pain, narcotic medication can aggravate it. The nurse should notify the physician and request a change in the order if the analgesic either fails to relieve the pain or makes the patient excessively lethargic or somnolent.

PCA and epidural analgesia are two alternative approaches for pain control. The goals of PCA are to provide immediate analgesia and to maintain a constant, steady blood level of the analgesic agent. PCA involves self-administration of predetermined doses of analgesia by the patient. The route of delivery may be IV, oral, or epidural.

Epidural analgesia is the infusion of pain-relieving medications through a catheter placed into the epidural space surrounding the spinal cord. The goal of epidural analgesia is delivery of medication directly to opiate receptors in the spinal cord. The administration may be intermittent or constant and is monitored by the nurse. The overall effectiveness and the technique of administration result in a constant circulating level and a total reduced dose of medication.

A number of other measures may be helpful in preventing or relieving postoperative pain. If abdominal surgery has been performed, the patient should be instructed to use the limbs rather than the abdominal muscles in turning and getting out of bed. Techniques of controlled breathing or relaxation may be used for pain relief. Both methods have a similar rationale, which includes anxiety reduction, attention distraction, muscle relaxation, and provision of a sense of control over the pain experience.[20] Transcutaneous electrical nerve stimulation (TENS) has also been effective in decreasing pain perception in postoperative patients.[21]

The nurse's role with respect to postoperative fever may be preventive, diagnostic, and therapeutic. Meticulous asepsis is a preventive measure that should be maintained with regard to the wound and IV site, and frequent observation for early signs of inflammation.

The patient's temperature is usually measured every 4 hours for the first 48 hours postoperatively and then less frequently if no problems develop. If fever develops, chest x-rays may be taken and, depending on the suspected cause, cultures of the wound, urine, or blood are obtained. If infection is the source of the fever, antibiotics are started intramuscularly (IM) or by IV piggyback as soon as cultures have been obtained. If the fever is extreme (105.8° F [41° C]), antipyretic drugs and body-cooling measures may be employed.

Potential Alterations in Psychologic Function

Etiology. Anxiety and depression may occur in the postoperative patient for many reasons (see Chapter 14). These states may be more pronounced in the patient who has had radical surgery (e.g., colostomy) or amputation or whose findings suggest a poor prognosis (e.g., inoperable tumor). A history of a neurotic or psychotic disorder should alert the nurse to the possibility of postoperative anxiety and depression. However, these responses may develop in any patient as part of the grief response to loss of a body organ or disturbance in body image and may be exacerbated by a lowered response to stress.

Confusion or delirium may arise from a variety of psychologic and physiologic sources, including fluid and electrolyte imbalance, hypoxemia, drug toxicity, sleep deprivation, and sensory alteration, deprivation, or overload. Delirium tremens caused by alcohol withdrawal may be responsible for as much as 25% of all postoperative delirium.[10] Delerium tremens is a reaction characterized by restlessness, insomnia and nightmares, tachycardia, apprehension, confusion and disorientation, irritability, and auditory or visual hallucinations, and it may be treated by the administration of alcohol, sedation, or patient restraint (see Chapter 8).

NURSING MANAGEMENT

PSYCHOLOGIC FUNCTION

Nursing Diagnoses

Nursing diagnoses related to potential alterations in psychologic function in the postoperative patient include, but are not limited to, the following:

- Anxiety
- Ineffective individual coping
- Body image disturbance

Nursing Implementation

The nurse attempts to prevent psychologic problems in the postoperative period by providing adequate support for the patient. Supportive measures include taking time to listen and talk with the patient, offering explanations and genuine reassurance, and encouraging the presence and assistance of significant others. The nurse must observe and evaluate the patient's behavior to distinguish a normal reaction to the stress situation from one that is becoming abnormal or excessive. The recognition of the alcohol withdrawal syndrome in a patient not previously known to be an alcoholic presents a particular challenge. Any unusual or disturbed behavior should be reported immediately so that diagnosis and treatment may be instituted.

Planning for Discharge and Follow-Up Care

Preparation for the patient's discharge is an ongoing process throughout the surgical experience that begins during the preoperative period. The informed patient is therefore prepared as events unfold and gradually assumes greater responsibility for self-care during the postoperative period. As the day of discharge approaches, the nurse should be certain that the patient has the following information:

1. Care of wound site and any dressings
2. Action and possible side effects of any medications; when and how to take them
3. Activities allowed and prohibited; when various physical activities can be resumed safely (e.g., driving a car, returning to work, sexual intercourse, leisure activities)
4. Dietary restrictions or modifications
5. Symptoms to be reported (e.g., development of incisional tenderness or increased drainage, discomfort in other parts of the body)
6. Where and when to return for follow-up care
7. Answers to any individual questions or concerns

CRITICAL THINKING EXERCISES

CASE STUDY

POSTOPERATIVE PATIENT

Patient Profile

Mr. Edward G., 74-year-old retired college professor, has just undergone a left hip pinning after a fall. The surgery, performed while the patient was under general anesthesia, was uneventful.

Subjective Data

- Has been in excellent health before fall
- Played tennis three times each week
- Walked 20 to 30 miles per week
- Always had problems sleeping
- Difficulty hearing, wears hearing aid
- Upset with injury and its impact on activity
- Has no relatives or friends to assist with care

Objective Data

Admitted to PACU with pillows between his legs, two peripheral IV catheters, a self-suction drain from the hip dressing, and an indwelling urinary catheter

Therapeutic Management

Postoperative orders include:

- Vital signs per PACU routine
- D5/.45 NS at 100 ml/hr
- PCA morphine 1 mg q 6 min (30 mg max in 4 hr) for pain
- Advance diet as tolerated
- Triflow spirometry every hour while awake

Critical Thinking Questions

1. What are the potential postanesthetic problems that the nurse might expect with Mr. G.?
2. What nursing interventions would be appropriate to prevent these complications from occurring?
3. What factors may predispose Mr. G. to the following problems: atelectasis, infection, nausea and vomiting?
4. How should it be determined when Mr. G. is sufficiently recovered from general anesthesia to be discharged to the clinical unit?
5. What potential postoperative problems might the nurse on the clinical unit expect?
6. Based on the assessment data presented, write one or more appropriate nursing diagnoses. Are there any collaborative problems?

NURSING RESEARCH ISSUES

1. Does early mobilization of specific patient groups prevent the development of postoperative respiratory complications?
2. What are the unique differences in discharging a patient to home as opposed to a clinical unit?
3. Does the use of written discharge criteria accurately predict patient readiness for discharge?
4. Is patient-controlled intravenous delivery of narcotics more effective in controlling postoperative pain than intramuscular injections of narcotics?
5. Does an early phone call from a nurse during the first week of postoperative discharge reduce the occurrence of hospital readmission and postoperative complications?

If the physician has not provided information about particular diet or activity prescriptions or restrictions, the nurse should either obtain this information or encourage the patient to do so. Attention to complete discharge instruction may prevent needless distress for the patient. Written instructions are important for reinforcing verbal information. The nurse should specifically document in the record the discharge instructions provided to the patient and family. For the patient, the postoperative phase of care continues and extends into the recuperative period. Assessment and evaluation of the patient after discharge may be accomplished by a follow-up call or by a visit from a home health nurse.

Ambulatory Surgery Discharge. The patient leaving an ambulatory surgery setting must be able to provide a degree of self-care and must be mobile and alert. Postoperative pain and nausea and vomiting must be controlled. Overall, the patient must be stable and near the level of preoperative functioning for discharge from the unit. On discharge, both specific and general instructions are given to the patient verbally and reinforced with written directions. The patient may not drive and must be accompanied by a responsible adult at the time of discharge. A follow-up evaluation of the patient's status is made by telephone, and any specific questions and concerns are addressed.

REVIEW QUESTIONS

The number of the question corresponds to the same-numbered objective at the beginning of the chapter.

1. As soon as the patient enters the PACU, the nurse routinely
   a. initiates range of motion to extremities.
   b. assesses level of consciousness.
   c. starts a unit of whole blood.
   d. removes the oropharyngeal airway.

2. Which of these nursing actions is *not* desirable during recovery from general anesthesia?
   a. Encouraging deep breathing and coughing
   b. Placing the patient in a supine position
   c. Suctioning to remove excess respiratory secretions
   d. Auscultating the patient's chest bilaterally

3. Which of the following patients is at greatest risk for postoperative nausea and vomiting?
   a. 45-year-old, 70 kg man following an arthroscopy under epidural anesthesia
   b. 81-year-old, 55 kg woman following a cystoscopy under local anesthesia
   c. 14-year-old, 40 kg boy following an orchiopexy under general anesthesia
   d. 23-year-old, 125 kg woman following a diagnostic laparoscopy under general anesthesia

4. Following admission to the clinical unit, which assessment data requires the most immediate attention?
   a. Temperature of 94.3° F (34.6° C)
   b. Blood pressure of 90/60 mm Hg
   c. Oxygen saturation of 85%
   d. Respiratory rate of 13/min

5. A urine output averaging 20 ml/hr for the first postoperative day
   a. is a normal expected finding.
   b. is normal if the patient had genitourinary surgery.
   c. requires an evaluation of the patient's fluid status.
   d. requires a return to the operating room.

6. Which of the following should the patient have in preparation for discharge?
   a. Rationale for abstinence from sexual intercourse for 4 to 6 weeks
   b. Need to call hospital clinical unit to report any abnormal signs or symptoms
   c. Time frame for when various physical activities can be resumed
   d. Referral to nutritional center for management of dietary restrictions

REFERENCES

1. Litwack K: *Post anesthesia care nursing,* ed 2, St Louis, 1995, Mosby.
2. Litwack K: Immediate postoperative care: a problem-oriented approach. In Vender J, Spiess B, editors: *Post anesthesia care,* Philadelphia, 1992, Saunders.
3. Litwack K: Post-anesthesia assessment: what medical-surgical nurses need to know, *MedSurg* 2:294, 1993.
4. American Society of Post Anesthesia Nurses: *Standards for perianesthesia nursing practice,* Richmond, 1992, The Society.
5. Feeley T: The postanesthesia care unit. In Miller R, editor: *Anesthesia,* ed 3, New York, 1990, Churchill-Livingstone.

*6. Litwack K, Saleh D, Schultz P: Postoperative pulmonary complications, *Crit Care Nurs Clin North Am* 3:77, 1991.

7. Mecca R: Postanesthesia recovery. In Barash P, Cullen B, Stoelting R, editors: *Clinical Anesthesia,* Philadelphia, 1989, Lippincott.

*8. Tremblay D and others: Arrhythmias in the PACU, *Crit Care Nurs Clin North Am* 3:95, 1991.

9. Merck, Sharpe, and Dohme Pharmaceuticals: *Merck manual,* ed 15, Rathway, 1987.
10. Lipov E: Emergence delirium in the PACU, *Crit Care Nurs Clin North Am* 3:145, 1991.

*11. Litwack K: Practical points in the management of hypothermia, *JOPAN* 3:339, 1988.

*12. Litwack K, Parnass S: Practical points in the management of nausea and vomiting, *J Postanesth Nurs* 3:275, 1988.

13. Moser K: Venous thromboembolism: state of the art, *Am Rev Respir Dis* 141:235, 1990.

*14. Jackson M: Elder care: implication of surgery in very elderly patients, *AORN J* 50: 859, 1989.

15. Howie J: How and when should I respond to postoperative fever?, *Am J Nurs* 89:984, 1989.
16. Spearing C: Incentive spirometry: inspiring your patient to breathe deeply, *Nursing* 17:50, 1987.
17. Fahey V: An indepth look at deep vein thrombosis, *Nursing* 19:86, 1989.
18. Wysocki A: Surgical wound healing, *AORN J* 49:502, 1989.
19. McCaffery M: *Pain assessment and intervention in clinical practice,* St Louis, 1993, Mosby.
20. Acute Pain Management Guideline Panel: *Clinical practice guideline: acute pain management: operative or medical procedures and trauma.* AHCPR Pub #92-0032, Rockville, MD, 1992, US Department of Health and Human Services.

*21. Hargraves A, Lander J: Use of transcutaneous electric nerve stimulation for postoperative pain, *Nurs Res* 38:159, 1989.

SECTION III BIBLIOGRAPHY

Books

Barash P, Cullen B, Stoelting R, editors: *Clinical anesthesia,* ed 2, Philadelphia, 1992, JB Lippincott.

Breslow M, Miller C, Rogers M: *Perioperative management,* St Louis, 1990, Mosby.

Burden N: *Ambulatory surgical nursing,* Philadelphia, 1993, WB Saunders.

Eliopoulos C: *A guide to the nursing of the aging,* ed 2, Baltimore, 1992, Williams & Wilkins.

Kersten L: *Comprehensive respiratory nursing: a decision-making approach, Philadelphia, 1989, WB Saunders.*

Meeker M, Rothrock J, editors: *Alexander's care of the patient in surgery,* ed 10, St Louis, 1995, Mosby.

Phippen M, Wells MP: *Perioperative nursing practice,* Philadelphia, 1994, WB Saunders.

Journals

Balcom C: The new code of ethics: implications for perioperative nurses, *Can Oper Room Nurs* 12:6, 1994.

Batson VD: Conscious sedation: implications for perioperative nursing practice, *Semin Perioper Nurs* 2:45, 1993.

Botti MA, Hunt JO: The routine of post anaesthetic observations, *Contemp Nurse* 3:52, 1994.

---

*Nursing research-based articles.

Clark KL: Nursing patient care rounds in the postanesthesia care unit setting, *J Post Anesth Nurs* 9:20, 1994.

Davis LA, O'Rourke NC: Pulmonary embolism: early recognition and management in the postanesthesia care unit, *J Post Anesth Nurs* 8:338, 1993.

DeWolf-Bosek M, Fitzpatrick J: A nursing perspective on advanced directives, *Medsurg Nurs* 1:33, 1993.

Dunscombe A, Riall CT: Celebrating 40 years of progress in perioperative nursing techniques, *AORN* 60:742,751, 1994.

Heitz L, Symreng T, Scamman FL: Effect of music therapy in the postanesthesia care unit: a nursing intervention, *J Post Anesth Nurs* 7:22, 1992.

Horstman P, Helmick L, Sions JA: Perioperative nursing model redesign, *Nurs Manage* 25:80A, 1994.

Kang SB and others: Postanesthesia nursing care for ambulatory surgery patients post-spinal anesthesia, *J Post Anesth Nurs* 9:101, 1994.

King CA: A perioperative nursing challenge: trauma in the OR, *Todays OR Nurse* 15:5, 1993 (editorial).

Kolodner D: Advanced medical directives after Cruzan, *Medsurg Nurs* 1:56, 1993.

Leino-Kilpi H, Vuorenheimo J: Perioperative nursing care quality. Patients' opinions, *AORN J* 57:1061, 1993.

*Leske JS: Anxiety of elective surgical patients' family members. Relationship between anxiety levels, family characteristics, *AORN J* 57:1091, 1993.

Litwack K, editor: Postanesthesia care nursing, *Nurs Clin North Am* 28:483, 1993.

Litwack K: Post-anesthesia assessment: what medical-surgical nurses need to know, *Medsurg Nurs* 2:294, 1993.

Litwack K, editor: Pain and postanesthesia management, *Crit Care Nurs Clin North Am* 3:1, 1991.

Lord EV: General anesthesia: what the perioperative nurse needs to know, *Semin Perioper Nurs* 2:4, 1993.

Reis JG: Colors of the spectrum. Perioperative nursing, *Nurs Spect* 4:16, 1994.

Rivellini D: Local and regional anesthesia. Nursing implications, *Nurs Clin North Am* 28:547, 1993 (review).

Shapiro G, editor: Postanesthesia care unit problems, *Anesth Clin North Am* 8:223, 1990.

Steelman VM, Bulechek GM, McCloskey JC: Toward a standardized language to describe perioperative nursing, *AORN J* 60:786, 1994.

Stuttard D: The effects of minimally invasive surgery on the future of perioperative nursing, *Can Oper Room Nurs* 12:5, 1994.

Summers S: Inadvertent hypothermia: clinical validation in postanesthesia patients, *Nurs Diagr* 3:54, 1992.

Thornhill AM: Perioperative nursing in a national health care system, *AORN J* 60:302, 1994.

Vogelsang J: Patients who develop postanesthesia shaking increase body temperature at the same rate as those who do not develop shaking, *J Post Anesth Nurs* 8:3, 1993 (see comments).

Vogelsang J: Patients talk about their postanesthesia shaking experiences, *J Post Anesth Nurs* 9:214, 1994.

---

*Nursing research-based articles.

Organizations

American Association of Nurse Anesthetists
222 South Prospect Avenue
Park Ridge, IL 60068-4001
708-692-7050
FAX: 708-692-6968

American Association of Operating Room Nurses
10170 East Mississippi Avenue
Denver, CO 80231

American Society of Post Anesthesia Nurses
11512 Allecingie Parkway
Richmond, VA 23235
804-379-5516

Association of Operating Room Nurses
2170 South Parker Road, Suite 300
Denver, CO 80231-5711
303-755-6300

Intravenous Nurses Society
2 Brighton Street
Belmont, MA 02178

PROBLEMS RELATED *to* ALTERED SENSORY INPUT

Section Four

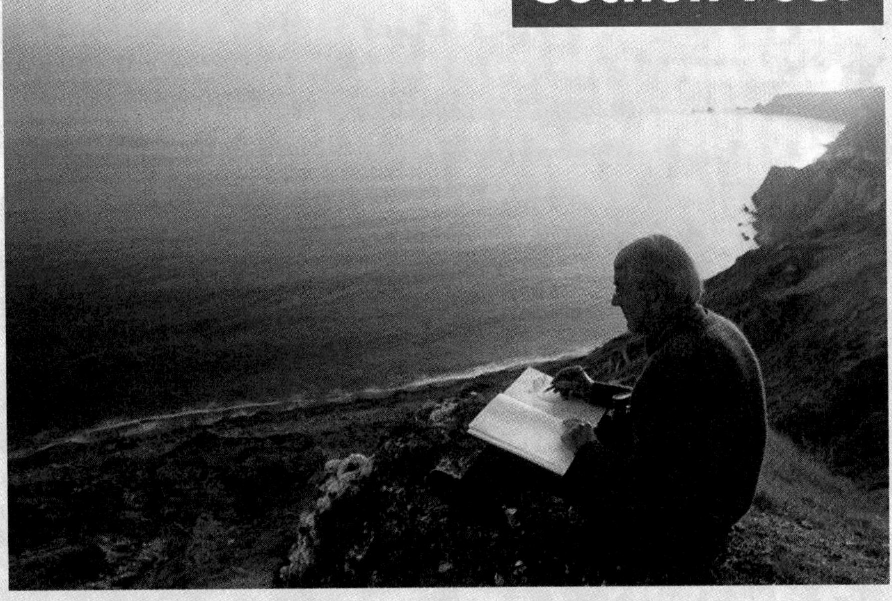

Chapter 17

NURSING ASSESSMENT

Vision and Hearing

Kate Goldblum **Idolia Cox Collier**

Learning Objectives

1. Describe the structures and functions of the visual and auditory systems.
2. Describe the physiologic processes involved in normal vision and hearing.
3. Identify significant subjective and objective assessment data related to the visual and auditory systems that should be obtained from the patient.
4. Describe the appropriate techniques used in the physical assessment of the visual and auditory systems.
5. Differentiate normal findings from common abnormal findings of a physical assessment of the visual and auditory systems.
6. Describe age-related changes in the visual and auditory systems, and describe differences in assessment findings.
7. Describe the purpose, significance of results, and nursing responsibilities related to diagnostic studies of the visual and auditory systems.

STRUCTURES AND FUNCTIONS OF THE VISUAL SYSTEM

The visual system consists of the internal and external structures of the eyeball, the refractive media, and the visual pathways. The internal structures are the iris, lens, ciliary body, choroid, and retina. The external structures are the eyebrows, eyelids, eyelashes, lacrimal system, conjunctiva, cornea, sclera, and extraocular muscles. The entire visual system is important for visual function. Light reflected from an object in the field of vision passes through the transparent structures of the eye and, in doing so, is *refracted* (bent) so that a clear image can fall on the retina. From the retina, the visual stimuli travel through the visual pathway to the occipital cortex where they are perceived as an image.

General Structure and Visual Function

Eyeball. The eyeball, or globe, is composed of three layers (Fig. 17-1). The tough outer layer is composed of the sclera and the transparent cornea. The middle layer consists of the uveal tract (iris, choroid, and ciliary body) and the innermost layer is the retina. The anterior chamber lies between the iris and the posterior surface of the cornea, whereas the posterior chamber lies between the anterior surface of the lens and the posterior surface of the iris. These chambers are filled with aqueous humor secreted by the ciliary body (Fig. 17-2). The anatomic space between the posterior lens surface and the retina is filled with the vitreous gel.

Refractive Media. For light to reach the retina, it must pass through a number of structures: the cornea, aqueous humor, lens, and vitreous. Each structure has a different density and plays a role in helping the image fall focused on the retina. The transparent cornea is the first structure through which light passes. It is responsible for the majority of light refraction necessary for clear vision.[1]

Aqueous humor, a clear watery fluid, fills the anterior and posterior chambers of the anterior cavity of the eye. Aqueous humor is produced by the ciliary process and passes through the pupil from the posterior chamber into the anterior chamber (Fig. 17-2). It drains through the trabecular meshwork located in the angle formed by the cornea and iris and into the canal of Schlemm. This circular canal conveys fluid into scleral veins, which enter the circulation of the body. The aqueous humor bathes and nourishes the lens and the endothelium of the cornea. Excess production or decreased outflow can elevate intraocular pressure above the normal 10 to 21 mm Hg, a condition known as *glaucoma.*

The lens is a biconvex structure located behind the iris and supported in place by small fibers called *zonules.* The primary function of the lens is to bend light rays, allowing the rays to fall onto the retina. The lens shape is modified by action of the ciliary zonules as part of *accommodation,* a process that allows the patient to focus on near objects, such as in reading. Because light rays pass through the lens,

Reviewed by Mary S. Merchant, RN, MSN, CCM, Outcome Manager, Medical University of South Carolina, Charleston, SC.

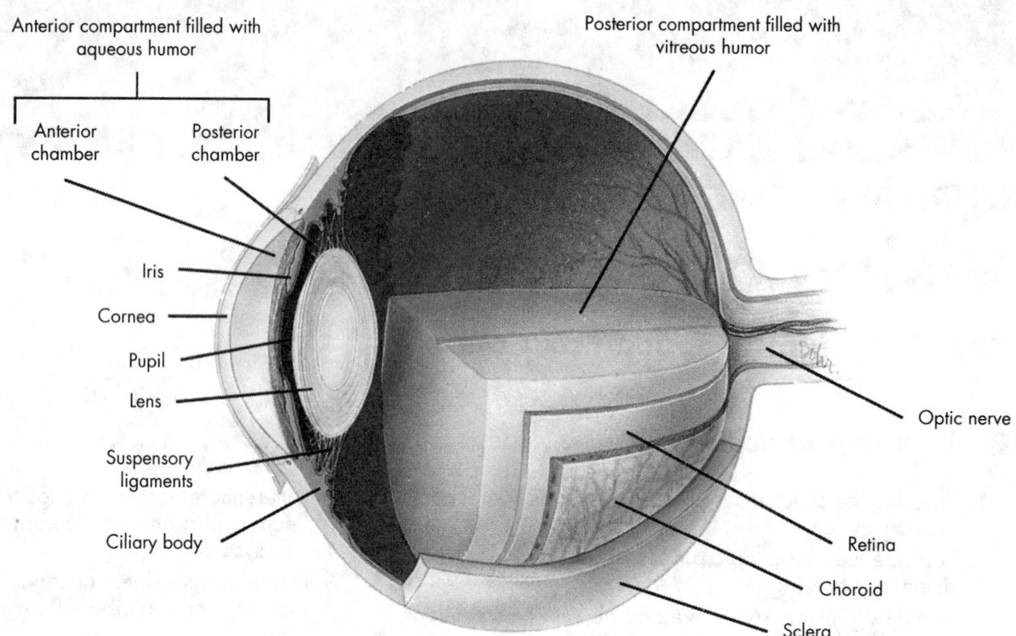

Fig. 17-1 The human eye.

the lens must remain clear. Anything altering the clarity of the lens affects light transmission.

Vitreous humor is located in the posterior cavity, the large area behind the lens and in front of the retina (Fig. 17-1). Light passing through the vitreous may be blocked by any nontransparent substance within the vitreous. The effect on vision varies, depending on the amount, type, and location of the substance blocking the light. For example, in the case of hemorrhage into the vitreous, little light will reach the retina, and vision will be severely compromised.

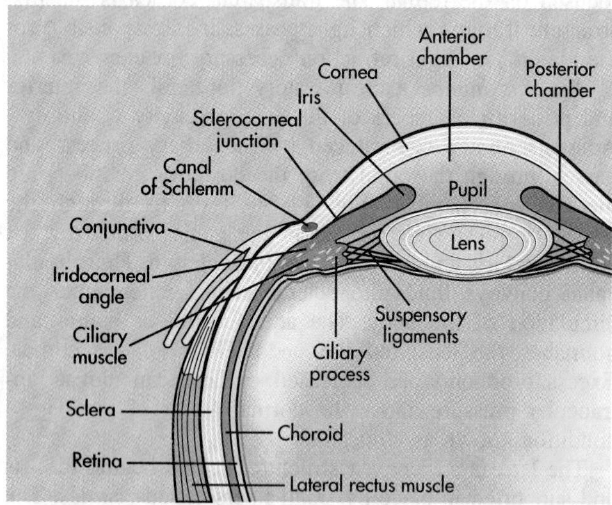

Fig. 17-2 Close-up view of ciliary body, zonules, lens, and anterior and posterior chambers. The aqueous humor flows from the ciliary process, over the anterior lens, and into the anterior chamber through the pupil, where it drains through the canal of Schlemm.

However, cellular debris that accumulates from normal cell metabolism will cause only a relatively small shadow on the retina (a "floater"). The vitreous becomes more liquid with aging.[2]

Refractive Errors. *Refraction* is the ability of the eye to bend light rays so that they fall on the retina. In the normal eye, parallel light rays are focused through the lens into a sharp image on the retina. This condition is termed *emmetropia* and means that light is focused exactly on the retina, not in front of it or behind it. When the light does not focus properly, it is called a *refractive error.*

The individual with *myopia* can see near objects clearly (nearsightedness), but objects in the distance are blurred. This condition occurs when an image is focused in front of the retina, either because the eye is too long, or because there is excessive refracting power (Fig. 17-3, *A*). A concave lens is used to correct the light refraction so that objects seen in the distance are focused clearly on the retina (Fig. 17-3, *B*).

The individual with *hyperopia* can see distant objects clearly (farsightedness), but close objects are blurred. This condition occurs when an image is focused behind the retina, either because the eye is too short, or because there is inadequate refracting power (Fig. 17-3, *C*). A convex lens is used to correct the refraction (Fig. 17-3, *D*).

Astigmatism is caused by an unevenness in the corneal or lenticular curvature, causing horizontal and vertical rays to be focused at two different points on the retina, which results in visual distortion. It can be myopic or hyperopic in nature in relation to where the image falls.

Presbyopia is a form of hyperopia, or farsightedness, that occurs as a normal process of aging, usually around age 40. As the lens ages and becomes less elastic, it loses refractive power, and the eye can no longer accommodate

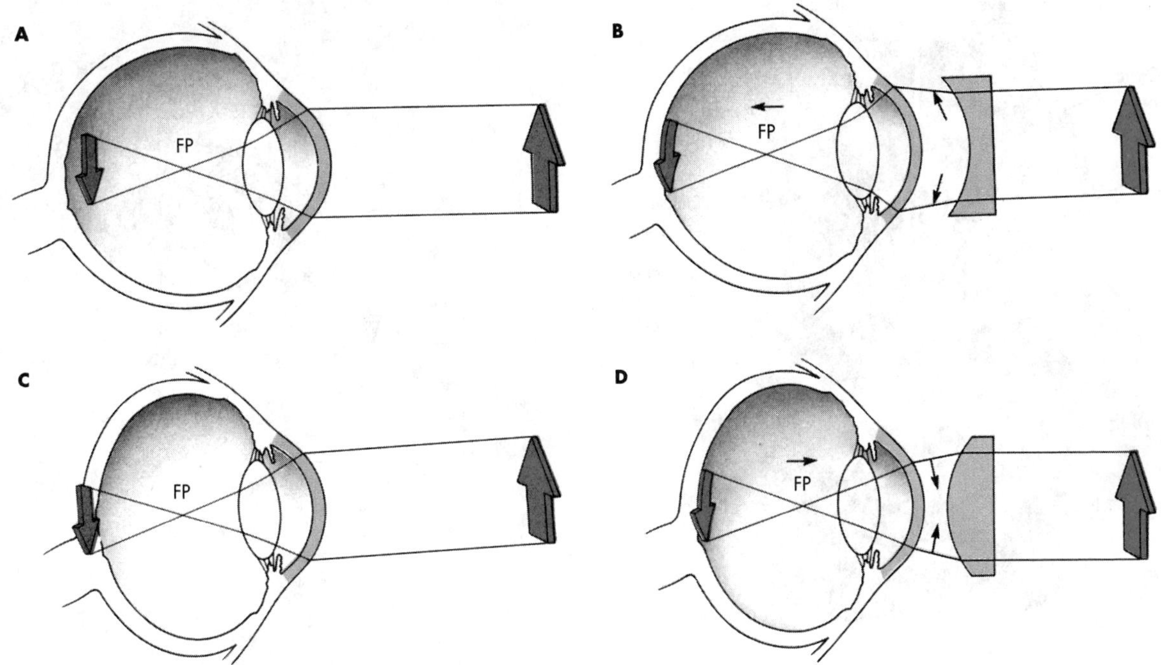

Fig. 17-3 Refraction disorders. ***A*** and ***B,*** Abnormal and corrected refraction observed in myopia and ***C*** and ***D,*** hyperopia. *FP,* Focal point.

for near vision. As with hyperopia, convex lenses are used to correct the light refraction so that the presbyopic individual can see clearly to read and accomplish other near-vision tasks.

Visual Pathways. Once the image travels through the refractive media, it is focused on the retina inverted and reversed left to right (Fig. 17-4). For example, if the visualized object is in the upper part of the left temporal visual field, it will be focused in the lower part of the nasal retina, upside down and as a mirror image. From the retina, the impulses travel through the optic nerve to the optic chiasm where the nasal fibers of each eye cross over to the other side. Fibers from the left field of both eyes form the left optic tract and travel to the left occipital cortex. The fibers from the right field of both eyes form the right optic tract and travel to the right occipital cortex. This arrangement of the nerve fibers in the visual pathways allows determination of the anatomic location of abnormalities in those nerve fibers by interpretation of the specific visual field defect (Fig. 17-4).

External Structures and Functions

Eyebrows, Eyelids, and Eyelashes. The eyebrows, eyelids, and eyelashes serve an important role in protecting the eye. They provide a physical barrier to dust and foreign particles (Fig. 17-5). The eye is further protected by the surrounding bony orbit and by fat pads located below and behind the globe, or eyeball.

The *upper* and *lower eyelids* join at the medial and lateral canthi, forming the *palpebral fissure,* which normally measures 10 to 12 mm.[3] The upper eyelid blinks spontaneously approximately 15 times a minute. Blinking distributes tears over the anterior surface of the eyeball and helps control the amount of light entering the visual pathway.

The *eyelids* open and close through the action of muscles innervated by cranial nerve VII (CN VII) or the facial nerve. Muscular action also helps hold the eyelids against the eyeball. The *tarsal plate,* a tough sheet of connective tissue within the lids, maintains the shape of the eyelids. When open the upper eyelid rests just below the *limbus* (the junction of the cornea and sclera). Sebaceous glands, located in the eyelids, help form the lipid layer of the tear film.

Conjunctiva. The conjunctiva is a transparent mucous membrane that covers the inner surfaces of the eyelids (the palpebral conjunctiva) and also extends over the sclera (bulbar conjunctiva), forming a "pocket" under each eyelid. This structure takes on the pink color of the underlying tissue. The bulbar conjunctiva terminates at the corneal-scleral limbus and contains tiny blood vessels, most visible in the periphery. Glands in the conjunctiva secrete mucus and tears.

Sclera. The sclera is composed of collagen fibers meshed together to form an opaque structure commonly referred to as the "white" of the eye. It comprises the posterior five-sixths of the external eye and encircles the globe to join the cornea at the limbus. The sclera forms a tough shell that helps protect the intraocular structures.

Cornea. The transparent and avascular cornea comprises the anterior one-sixth of the globe and allows light to enter the eye. The curved cornea refracts (bends) incoming

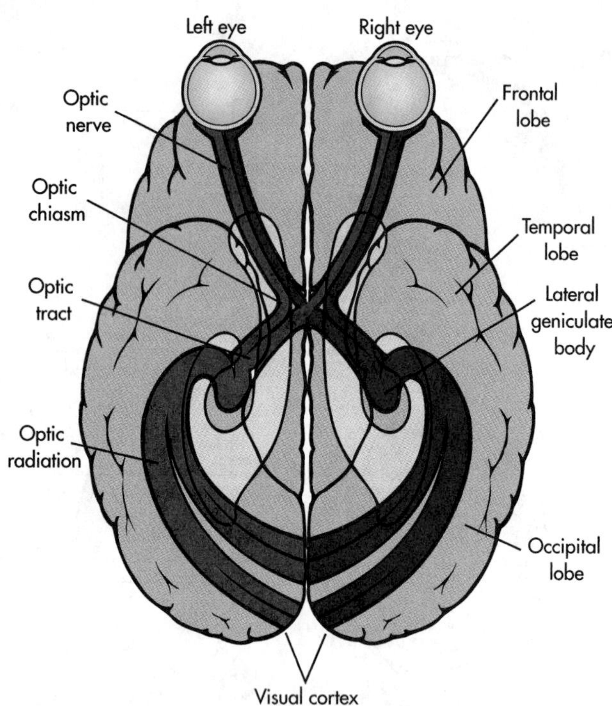

Fig. 17-4 The visual pathway. Fibers from the nasal portion of each retina cross over to the opposite side of the optic chiasma, terminating in the lateral geniculate body of the opposite side. Location of a lesion in the visual pathway determines the resulting visual defect.

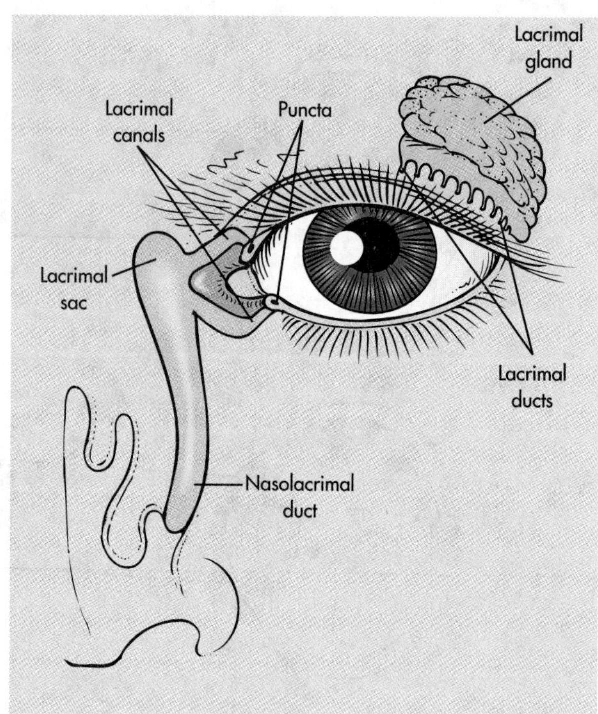

Fig. 17-5 External eye and lacrimal apparatus. Tears produced in the lacrimal gland pass over the surface of the eye and enter the lacrimal canal. From there the tears are carried through the nasolacrimal duct to the nasal cavity.

light rays to help focus them on the retina. It is one of the most highly-developed sensitive tissues in the body and is innervated by the trigeminal nerve (CN V).

The cornea consists of five layers: the epithelium, Bowman's layer, the stroma, Descemet's membrane, and the endothelium. The *epithelium* consists of a layer of cells that helps protect the eye by serving as a barrier to fluid loss and to the entry of pathogens. The *stroma* consists of collagen fibrils separated by the ground substance, which has a unique ability to hold water. The stroma is normally relatively water-free in order to maintain transparency. Any abnormality that disrupts the normal state of stromal hydration can result in stromal edema with a resulting loss of corneal clarity and a decrease in visual acuity. The corneal endothelium also consists of a single layer of cells, but unlike the cells of the epithelium, which regenerate if destroyed, the endothelial cells are limited in their regenerative ability. When these cells are damaged or destroyed, repair of an endothelial defect occurs primarily by the enlargement and spreading of the cells around the defect.

The avascular cornea obtains oxygen primarily through absorption from the tear film layer that bathes the epithelium. A small amount of oxygen is obtained from the aqueous humor through the endothelial layer, which is also responsible for transporting other nutrients into the corneal tissues.

Lacrimal Apparatus. The lacrimal system consists of the lacrimal gland and ducts, the lacrimal canals and puncta, the lacrimal sac, and the nasolacrimal duct. In addition to the lacrimal gland, other glands provide secretions to make up the mucous, aqueous, and lipid layers of the tear film that covers the anterior surface of the globe. The tear film moistens the eye and provides oxygen to the cornea. Lid and globe movements are both involved in spreading tears over the anterior surface of the eye. The tears are drained from the eye through the upper and lower puncta, then through the lacrimal sac, and finally through the nasolacrimal duct into the nose (Fig. 17-5).

Extraocular Muscles. Each eye is moved by three pairs of extraocular muscles: the superior and inferior rectus muscles, the medial and lateral rectus muscles, and the superior and inferior oblique muscles (Fig. 17-6). Neuromuscular coordination produces simultaneous movement of the eyes in the same direction (*conjugate movement*).

Internal Structures and Functions

Iris. The iris provides the color of the eye. This structure has a small round opening in its center, the *pupil*, which allows light to enter the eye. The pupil constricts via action of the iris sphincter muscle (innervated by CN III) and dilates via action of the iris dilator muscle (innervated by CN V) to control the amount of light that enters the eye. The constrictor muscle of the iris is stimulated by light falling on the retina and by accommodation. The autonomic nervous system also affects pupil size. Sympathetic stimulation results in contraction of the radial muscle and

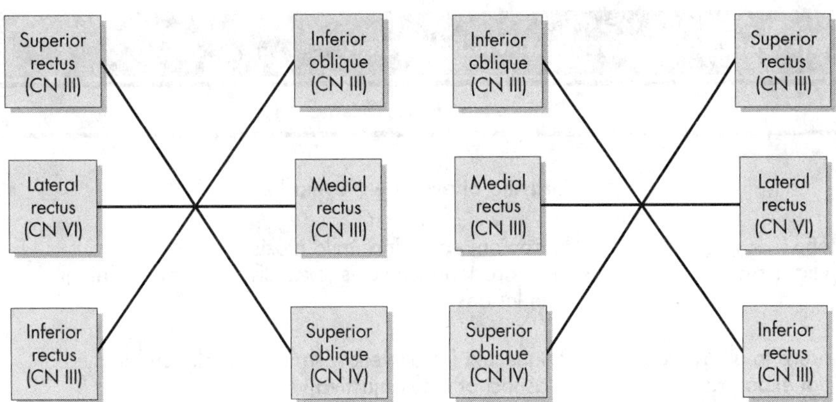

Fig. 17-6 Cardinal fields of gaze with corresponding muscles and nerves.

dilation of the pupil. Parasympathetic stimulation results in contraction of the circular muscle and constriction of the pupil.

Crystalline Lens. The crystalline lens is a biconvex, avascular, transparent structure located behind the iris. It is supported by the anterior and posterior *ciliary zonules*. The lens is composed of thick gelatinous material enclosed in a clear capsule. The primary function of the lens is to bend light rays so that they fall onto the retina. *Accommodation* occurs when the eye focuses on a near object and is facilitated by contraction of the ciliary body, which changes the shape of the lens.

Ciliary Body. The ciliary body consists of the ciliary muscles, which surround the lens and lie parallel to the sclera, the ciliary zonules, which attach to the lens capsule, and the ciliary processes, which constitute the terminal portion of the ciliary body. The ciliary processes lie behind the peripheral part of the iris and secrete aqueous humor.

Choroid. The choroid is a highly vascular structure that serves to nourish the ciliary body, the iris, and the outer portion of the retina. It lies inside and parallel to the sclera and extends from the area where the optic nerve enters the eye to the ciliary body (Fig. 17-1).

Retina. The retina is the innermost layer of the eye that extends and forms the optic nerve. Neurons make up the major portion of the retina. Therefore retinal cells are unable to regenerate if destroyed. The retina lines the inside of the eyeball, extending from the area of optic nerve to the ciliary body (Fig. 17-1). It is responsible for converting images into a form the brain can understand and process as vision. The retina is composed of two types of photoreceptor cells: rods and cones. *Rods* are stimulated in dim or darkened environments, and *cones* are receptive to colors in bright environments. There are approximately 130 million photoreceptors in each human retina, with rods outnumbering cones by approximately 13:1.[4] The center of the retina is the *fovea centralis,* a pinpoint depression composed only of densely-packed cones. This area of the retina provides the sharpest visual acuity. Surrounding the fovea is the *macula,* an area less than 1 square millimeter, which has a high concentration of cones and is relatively free of blood vessels.[5] Nourishment to the macula comes from two sources: the choroid and the underlying pigment epithelium, which is the deepest layer of the retina.

With the exception of the macula, the retina is nourished by retinal arterioles and veins. This blood supply enters the eye through the optic disc, located nasally from the macula. The optic disc is the area where the optic nerve (CN II) exits the eyeball. Within the disc is the *physiologic cup*, a depression that can be visualized through the pupil with an ophthalmoscope. The retinal veins and arteries can also be visualized in this way and can provide information about the vascular system in general.

Effects of Aging on the Visual System

Every structure of the visual system is subject to changes as the individual ages. Whereas many of these changes are relatively benign, others may result in severely compromised visual acuity in the older adult. The psychosocial impact of poor vision or blindness can be highly significant. Some common changes in the visual structures that occur with normal aging are outlined in Table 17-1.

ASSESSMENT OF THE VISUAL SYSTEM

Assessment of the visual system may be as simple as determining a patient's visual acuity or as complex as collecting complete subjective and objective data pertinent to the visual system. To do an appropriate ophthalmic evaluation, the nurse must determine which parts of the data collection are important for each particular patient.

Subjective Data

Important Health Information

Past health history. Information about the patient's past health history should include both ocular and nonocular history. In addition, the nurse should ask the patient specifically about systemic diseases, such as diabetes, hypertension, cancer, rheumatoid arthritis, syphilis and other sexually transmitted diseases (STDs), acquired immunodeficiency syndrome (AIDS), muscular dystrophy, myasthenia gravis, multiple sclerosis, inflammatory bowel disease, and hypothyroidism or hyperthyroidism because many of these diseases have ocular manifestations. It is particularly important to determine if the patient has any history of cardiac or pulmonary disease because β-adrenergic blocking agents are often used to treat glaucoma. These medications can slow heart rate, decrease blood pressure, and exacerbate asthma or emphysema.[6]

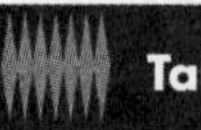

Table 17-1 Gerontologic Differences in Assessment: Visual System

Changes	Differences in Assessment Findings
Eyebrows and Eyelashes	
Loss of pigment in the hair	Graying of eyebrows, eyelashes
Eyelids	
Loss of orbital fat, decreased muscle tone	Entropion, ectropion, mild ptosis
Tissue atrophy, prolapse of fat into eyelid tissue	Blepharodermachalasis (excessive upper lid skin)
Sun damage to skin	Skin lesions
Conjunctiva	
Tissue damage related to chronic exposure to ultraviolet light or to other chronic environmental exposure	Pinguecula (small yellowish spot usually on the medial aspect of the conjuctiva)
Sclera	
Lipid deposition	Scleral color yellowish as opposed to bluish
Cornea	
Cholesterol deposits in peripheral cornea	Arcus senilis (milky or yellow ring encircling periphery of cornea)
Tissue damage related to chronic exposure	Pterygium (thickened, triangular bit of pale tissue that extends from the inner canthus of eye to the nasal border of the cornea)
Decrease in water content, atrophy of nerve fibers	Decreased corneal sensitivity
Epithelial changes	Loss of corneal luster
Accumulation of lipid deposits	Blurring of vision
Lacrimal Apparatus	
Decreased tear secretion	
Malposition of the eyelid resulting in tears overflowing the lid margins instead of draining through the puncta	Dryness, tearing, irritated eyes
Iris	
Increased rigidity of iris	Decreased pupil size
Dilator muscle atrophy or weakness	Slower recovery of pupil size after light stimulation
Loss of pigment	Change of iris color
Ciliary muscle becomes smaller, stiffer	Decrease in near vision and accommodation
Lens	
Biochemical changes in lens proteins, oxidative damage, chronic exposure to ultraviolet light	Cataracts
Increased rigidity of lens	Presbyopia
Opacities in the lens (may also be related to opacities in the cornea and vitreous)	Complaints of glare
Accumulation of yellow substances	Yellow color
Retina	
Retinal vascular changes related to arteriosclerosis and hypertension	Narrowed, pale, straighter arterioles; acute branching
Decrease in cones	Changes in color perception
Loss of photoreceptor cells, loss of retinal pigment, epithelial cells, and melanin	Decreased visual acuity
Age-related macular degeneration as a result of vascular changes	Loss of central vision
Vitreous	
Liquefaction and detachment of the vitreous	Increased complaints of "floaters"

A history of tests for visual acuity should be obtained, including the date of the last examination and change in lenses. The nurse should specifically ask about a history of strabismus, amblyopia, cataracts, retinal detachment, or glaucoma. Any trauma to the eye, its treatment, and sequelae should be noted.

The patient's nonocular history can be significant in assessing or treating the ophthalmic condition. Specifically, the nurse should ask the patient about previous surgeries or treatments related to the head, as well as about previous trauma to the head.

Medications. If the patient takes medication, the nurse should obtain a complete list, including over-the-counter (OTC) medicines, eye drops, and herbal or "natural" supplements or substances. Many patients do not think OTC drugs, eye drops, or herbal agents are "real" medica-

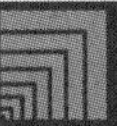

Table 17-2 Key Questions: Patient with a Visual Problem

Health Perception–Health Management Pattern
- Describe the change in your vision. Describe how this affects your daily life.
- Do you wear protective eyewear (sunglasses or safety goggles)?*
- Do you wear contact lenses? If so, how do you take care of them?
- If you use eye drops, how do you instill them?
- Do you have any allergies that cause eye symptoms?*
- Do you have a family history of cataracts or macular degeneration?*

Nutritional-Metabolic Pattern
- Do you take any nutritional supplements?*
- Does your visual problem affect your ability to obtain and prepare food?*

Elimination Pattern
- Do you have to strain to defecate?*

Activity-Exercise Pattern
- Are your activities limited in any way by your eye problem?*
- Do you participate in any leisure activities that have the potential for eye injury?*

Sleep-Rest Pattern
- Are your eyes affected by the amount of sleep you get?*

Cognitive-Perceptual Pattern
- Does your eye problem affect your ability to read?*
- Do you have any eye pain?* Do you have any eye itching, burning, or foreign body sensation?*

Self-Perception-Self-Concept Pattern
- How does your eye problem make you feel about yourself?

Role-Relationship Pattern
- Do you have any problems at work or home because of your eyes?*
- Have you made any changes in your social activities because of your eyes?*

Sexuality-Reproductive Pattern
- Has your eye problem caused a change in your sex life?*
- For women—Are you pregnant? Do you use birth control?*

Coping–Stress Tolerance Pattern
- Do you feel able to cope with your eye problem?*
- Are you able to acknowledge the effects of your eye problem on your life?*

Value-Belief Pattern
- Do you have any conflicts about the treatment of your eye problem?*

*If yes, describe.

tions and may not mention their use unless specifically questioned. However, many of these drugs have ocular effects. For example, many cold preparations contain a form of epinephrine that can dilate the pupil. The nurse should specifically ask whether the patient uses any prescription drugs such as corticosteroids, thyroid medications, or agents such as oral hypoglycemics and insulin to lower blood glucose levels. Cortisone preparations can contribute to the development of glaucoma or cataracts. It is especially important to indicate whether the patient is taking any β-adrenergic blocking medications, because these can be potentiated by the β-blocking agents used to treat glaucoma. The nurse should also note the use of any antihistamines or decongestants, because these drugs can cause ocular dryness.

Each drug the patient uses should correspond with a disease or disorder described in the patient's history. If a medication cannot be correlated with a disease or disorder, the nurse should ask the patient to explain why the drug is used. Finally, the nurse should determine whether the patient has allergies to medications or other substances.

Surgery and other treatments. Surgical procedures related to the eye or brain should be noted. Brain surgery and the subsequent swelling can cause pressure on the optic nerve or tract resulting in visual alterations. Any laser procedures to the eye should also be documented. The effect of any eye surgery or laser treatment on visual acuity is important information for the nurse to obtain.

Functional Health Patterns. The ophthalmic patient may seek health care for a specific problem or for regular ophthalmic care. When the patient needs routine ophthalmic care, the nurse will focus the assessment of functional patterns on issues related to health maintenance or promotion. When the patient has a recognized problem, the nurse will direct the assessment to identify those issues related to the patient's specific problem.

Ocular problems do not always affect the patient's visual acuity. For example, patients with blepharitis or diabetic retinopathy may not have any visual deficit. The nurse should be aware that many conditions can cause vision loss. The focus of the functional health pattern assessment is dependent on the presence or absence of vision loss and whether the loss is permanent or temporary. Table 17-2 lists suggested questions to obtain data relating to the functional health patterns.

Health perception–health management pattern. The patient's age is pertinent in considering cataracts, macular problems, degenerative lid disorders, glaucoma, and other ophthalmic conditions. Men are more likely than women to have color-blindness.[7] African-Americans and older individuals are at higher risk of damage to the optic nerve from glaucoma.[8]

The ophthalmic patient in a clinic or office setting is often seeking routine eye care or a change in the prescription of eye wear. However, there can be some underlying concern that the patient may not mention or even recognize.

Even the hospitalized or surgical patient may not completely understand why he is receiving care. The nurse should obtain this information by asking, "Why are you here today?"

The patient's visual health can affect activities at home or at work. It is important to know how the patient perceives the current health problem. As outlined in Table 17-2, the nurse can guide the patient in defining the current problem and how it affects the patient's normal activities. The nurse should also assess the patient's ability to accomplish all necessary self-care, especially any eye care related to the patient's ophthalmic problem.

The nurse needs to assess the patient's ocular health care activities. The patient may not recognize the importance of eye safety practices such as wearing protective eyewear during potentially hazardous activities or avoiding noxious fumes and other eye irritants. Information about the use of sunglasses in bright lights should be obtained. Prolonged exposure to ultraviolet (UV) light can affect the retina. Night driving habits and any problems encountered should be noted. Today, millions of people wear contact lenses, but many do not care for them properly.[9] The type of contact lenses used and the patient's wearing and care habits may provide information for teaching.

Information about allergies should be obtained. Allergies often cause eye symptoms such as itching, burning, watering, drainage, and blurred vision.

Many hereditary systemic diseases (e.g., sickle cell anemia) can significantly affect ocular health. In addition, many refractive errors and other eye problems are hereditary. For these reasons the nurse should obtain a careful family history of both ocular and nonocular diseases. Specifically, the nurse should ask if the patient has a family history of diseases such as arteriosclerosis, diabetes, thyroid disease, hypertension, arthritis, or cancer. The nurse should also determine whether the patient has a family history of ocular problems such as cataracts, tumors, glaucoma, refractive errors (especially myopia and hyperopia), or retinal degenerative conditions (e.g., macular degeneration, retinal detachment, retinitis pigmentosa).

Nutritional-metabolic pattern. The patient's intake of antioxidant vitamins and trace minerals can be important to ocular health. Adequate intake of vitamins C and E may be beneficial in preventing or delaying retinal damage, and zinc deficiency is linked to erythematous scales in the periorbital area.[10,11]

Elimination pattern. Straining to defecate (Valsalva maneuver) can raise the intraocular pressure. Although there is some evidence that elevating the intraocular pressure by normal activities is not detrimental to the surgical incision made during eye surgery, many surgeons do not want the patient straining. The nurse should assess the patient's usual pattern of elimination and determine whether there is the potential for constipation in the patient who has had ophthalmic surgical procedures.

Activity-exercise pattern. The patient's usual level of activity or exercise may be affected by reduced vision, by symptoms accompanying an ocular problem, or by activity restrictions following a surgical procedure. For example, a patient with *hyphema* (intraocular bleeding) may be on bed rest or have severely restricted activity. The diabetic patient with lower limb prostheses will have additional ambulation difficulties if diabetic retinopathy with vision loss is present.

The nurse should also inquire about leisure activities during which the patient may incur an ocular injury. For example, gardening, woodworking, and other craft activities can result in corneal or conjunctival foreign bodies or even penetrating injuries of the globe. Injuries to the globe or bony orbit can also occur after blows to the head or eye during sports activities such as racquetball, baseball, and tennis. Cross-country skiers may develop corneal fungal ulcers after an abrasion caused by low-hanging tree limbs. Other leisure activities such as needlepoint, fly tying, or bird-watching may have high-level visual demands and produce eye strain.

Sleep-rest pattern. In the otherwise healthy person, lack of sleep may cause ocular irritation, especially in the patient who wears contact lenses. Normal sleep patterns may be disrupted in the patient with painful eye problems such as corneal abrasions. The patient with alkali burns of the eye requires continuous irrigation of the ocular surface until the pH of the conjunctival sac returns to normal levels.[12] Normal sleep will be disrupted during this time.

Cognitive-perceptual pattern. The entire assessment of the ophthalmic patient focuses on the sense of sight, but it is important not to overlook other cognitive or perceptual problems. For example, the functional ability of a patient with a visual deficit will be further compromised if the patient also has hearing problems. The patient who cannot see to read has increased difficulty in following postoperative instructions if there is also trouble hearing or remembering verbal instructions. The patient who does not understand or read English may require written or verbal instructions and information in the native language.

Eye pain is always an important symptom to assess. Corneal abrasions, iritis, and acute glaucoma manifest with pain and are serious eye problems. Infections and foreign bodies can also cause less severe eye discomfort and are also potentially serious. If eye pain is present the patient should be questioned about treatment and response.

Self-perception–self-concept pattern. The loss of independence that can follow a partial or complete loss of vision, even if the condition is temporary, can have devastating effects on the patient's self-concept. The nurse should carefully evaluate the potential effect of vision loss on the patient's self-image. For instance, disabling glare from a cataract may prevent nighttime driving or even limit daytime driving resulting in a diminished self-image. In today's highly mobile society, loss of ability to drive can represent a significant loss of independence and self-esteem. The patient with severe ptosis or other disfiguring ophthalmic conditions may be embarrassed by his appearance and suffer from a poor self-image.

Role-relationship pattern. The patient's ability to maintain the necessary or desired roles and responsibilities in the home, work, and social environments can be negatively affected by ocular problems. For example, macular degeneration may decrease the patient's visual acuity to a level inadequate to function at work. Many occupations place workers in conditions in which eye injury may occur. For example, factory workers may be at risk from flying metal debris. Information should be obtained about eye-safety practices, such as the use of goggles or safety glasses. Workers can also be exposed to eye strain in the office from video display terminals, poor lighting, and glare.

The patient with diabetes may not be able to see well enough to self-administer insulin. This patient may resent the dependence on a family member who takes over this function. The patient with exophthalmos may be embarrassed by his appearance and avoid usual social activities. The nurse should sensitively inquire if the patient's preferred roles and responsibilities have been affected by the ocular problem.

Sexuality-reproductive pattern. The inactivity that may be associated with low vision, blindness, and certain eye problems and surgeries can negatively affect a patient's sexuality. The patient with severe vision loss may develop such a poor self-image that the ability to be sexually intimate is lost. The nurse can assure the patient that low vision or blindness does not affect a person's ability to be sexually expressive. For many sexually expressive acts, touch is more important than vision.

The female patient in her childbearing years should avoid medications, such as demecarium and isoflurophate, that may cause fetal abnormalities.[9] If a patient with low vision or blindness has a family, assistance with childrearing tasks may be necessary. The nurse should determine the need and availability of help if this situation is present.

Coping–stress tolerance pattern. The patient with temporary or permanent visual problems will experience emotional stress. The nurse should assess the patient's coping level, coping mechanisms, and availability of social and personal support systems.

The patient with permanent visual loss experiences the usual stages of grief after the loss. The nurse should assess the potential need for psychosocial counseling and eventual vocational rehabilitation.

Value-belief pattern. The nurse must be sensitive to the individual values and spiritual beliefs of each patient, because the patient makes decisions regarding ophthalmic care based on those values and beliefs. It can be difficult to understand why a patient refuses treatment that has potential benefit or wants treatment that may have limited potential benefit. The nurse should assess the patient's value-belief pattern that serves as the basis for making those decisions.

Objective Data

Physical Examination. Physical examination of the visual system includes inspecting the ocular structures and determining the status of their respective functions. Physiologic functional assessment includes determining the patient's visual acuity, determining the patient's ability to judge closeness and distance, assessing extraocular muscle function, evaluating the visual fields, observing pupil function, and measuring the intraocular pressure. Assessment of ocular structures should include examining the ocular adnexa, external eye, and internal structures. Some structures, such as the retina and blood vessels, must be visualized with the aid of various ophthalmic observation equipment, such as the biomicroscope and the ophthalmoscope.

Assessment of the visual system may include all of the following components, or it may be as brief as measuring the patient's visual acuity. The nurse will assess what is appropriate and necessary for the specific patient. All of the following assessments are in the nurse's scope of practice, but some require special training. Normal physical examination findings are outlined in Table 17-3. Age-related changes and differences in assessment findings are listed in Table 17-1. Ophthalmic assessment techniques are summarized in Table 17-4, and common assessment abnormalities are listed in Table 17-5.

Initial observation. The initial observation of the patient can provide information that will help the nurse focus the assessment. When first encountering the patient, the nurse may observe that the patient is dressed in clothing with unusual color combinations. This may indicate a color vision deficit. The nurse may also note an unusual head position. The patient with diplopia may hold the head in a skewed position in an attempt to relieve the problem. The patient with a corneal abrasion or photophobia will cover the eyes with the hands to try to block out room light. The nurse can make a crude estimate of depth perception by extending a hand for the patient to shake.

During the initial observation, the nurse should also observe the overall facial and ophthalmic appearance of the patient. The eyes should be symmetrical and normally placed on the face. The globes should not have a bulging or sunken appearance.

Assessing functional status

VISUAL ACUITY. The nurse should always record the patient's visual acuity for medical and legal reasons. The nurse must document the patient's visual acuity before the patient receives any care.

The patient sits or stands 20 feet (6 meters) from the Snellen chart with the usual correction (glasses or contact lenses) left in place unless they are used solely for reading. The nurse asks the patient to cover the left eye and read the smallest line that the patient can read comfortably. If the patient reads that line with two or fewer errors, the examiner instructs the patient to read the next lower line.

Table 17-3 Normal Physical Assessment Findings of the Visual System

Visual acuity 20/20; no diplopia. External eye structures intact without lesions or deformities. Conjunctiva clear; sclera white without redness. PERRLA. Lens clear. EOMs full; red reflex intact. Lacrimal apparatus nontender without drainage. Retinal vessels normal with no hemorrhages or spots.

EOMs, Extraccula movement; *PERRLA*, pupils equal round, reactive to light and accommodation.

Table 17-4 Ophthalmic Assessment Techniques

Technique	Description	Purpose
■ Visual acuity testing	Patient reads from Snellen chart at 20 ft (distance vision test) or Jaeger's chart at 14 in (near vision test); examiner notes smallest print patient can read on each chart.	To determine patient's distance and near visual acuity
■ Extraocular muscle function testing	Examiner has patient follow a light source or other fixation object through a complete field of gaze; in the cover-uncover test, examiner covers patient's eye and then uncovers it to see if eye has deviated under the cover.	To determine if patient's extraocular muscles are functioning in a normal manner, with no underaction or overaction
■ Confrontation visual field test	Patient faces examiner, covers one eye, fixates on examiner's face and counts number of fingers that the examiner brings into patient's field of vision.	To determine if patient has a full field of vision, without obvious scotomas
■ Pupil function testing	Examiner shines light into patient's pupil and observes pupillary response; each pupil is examined independently; examiner also checks for consensual and accommodative response.	To determine if patient has normal pupillary response
■ Tonometry	Applanation tonometer is gently touched to the anesthetized corneal surface; examiner looks through ocular of slit lamp microscope, adjusts pressure dial until mires are aligned and notes intraocular pressure reading.	To measure intraocular pressure (normal pressure is 10-21 mm Hg)
■ Slit lamp microscopy	Patient is seated with chin placed in chin rest; slit beam illuminates ocular structures; examiner looks through magnifying ocular to assess various structures.	To provide magnified view of the conjunctiva, sclera, cornea, anterior chamber, iris, lens, and vitreous
■ Ophthalmoscopy	Examiner holds ophthalmoscope close to patient's eye, shining light into back of eye and looking through aperture on ophthalmoscope; examiner adjusts dial to select one of the lenses in ophthalmoscope that produces the desired amount of magnification to inspect ocular fundus.	To provide magnified view of retina and optic nerve head
■ Color vision testing	Patient identifies numbers or paths formed by pattern of dots in series of color plates.	To determine patient's ability to distinguish colors
■ Stereopsis testing	From a series of plates, patient identifies geometric pattern or figure that appears closer to patient when viewed through special spectacles that provide a three dimensional view.	To determine patient's ability to see objects in three dimensions; to test depth perception
■ Keratometry	Examiner aligns the projection and notes the readings of corneal curvature.	To measure the corneal curvature; often done before fitting contact lenses, before doing refractive surgery, or after corneal transplantation

The nurse notes the smallest line the patient can read with two or fewer errors, and records the standard of 20 feet (6 meters) and then the distance in feet on the line of the Snellen chart the patient read successfully. The nurse records the visual acuities using the ophthalmic abbreviations for right eye (*OD*, or *oculus dexter*), left eye (*OS*, or *oculus sinister*), and both eyes (*OU*, or *oculus uterque*). For example, for the patient who reads to the 30-foot (9 meter) line with the right eye, the nurse records the acuity as 20/30 OD. A visual acuity of 20/30 means that from 20 feet (6 meters) away, the patient can read the same letters that the person with normal vision can read from 30 feet (9 meters) away. *Legal blindness* is defined as the best-corrected vision in the better eye of 20/200 or less.[6] The nurse then

Table 17-5 Common Assessment Abnormalities: Eye

Findings	Description	Possible Etiology and Significance
SUBJECTIVE DATA		
▪ Pain	Foreign body sensation	Superficial corneal erosion or abrasion; can result from contact lens wear or trauma; conjunctival or corneal foreign body; usually lessened with lid closure
	Severe, deep, throbbing	Anterior uveitis, acute glaucoma, infection; acute glaucoma also associated with nausea, vomiting
▪ Photophobia	Persistent abnormal intolerance to light	Inflammation or infection of cornea or anterior uveal tract (iris and ciliary body)
▪ Blurred vision	Gradual or sudden inability to see clearly	Refractive errors, corneal opacities, cataracts, retinal changes (detachment, macular degeneration), optic neuritis or atrophy, central retinal vein or artery thrombosis, refractive changes related to fluctuations in control of diabetic hyperglycemia
▪ Scotoma	Blind or partially blind area in the visual field	Disorders of the optic chiasm, glaucoma, central serous chorioretinopathy, age-related macular degeneration, injury, migraine headache
▪ Spots, floaters	Patient describes seeing spots, "spider webs," "curtain" or floaters within the field of vision	Most common cause is vitreous liquefication (benign phenomenon); other possible causes include hemorrhage into the vitreous humor, retinal holes or tears, impending retinal detachment, vitreous detachment, intraocular hemorrhage, chorioretinitis
▪ Dryness	Discomfort, sandy, gritty, irritation, or burning	Decreased tear formation or changes in tear composition because of aging or various systemic diseases
▪ Halo around lights	Presence of a halo around lights	Refractive changes, corneal edema as a result of a sudden rise in intraocular pressure in angle-closure glaucoma or secondary glaucoma
▪ Glare	Headache, ocular discomfort, reduced visual acuity	Related to corneal inflammation or to opacities in the cornea, lens, or vitreous that scatter the incoming light; can also result from light scatter around edges of an intraocular lens; worse at night when pupil dilated
▪ Diplopia	Double vision	Abnormalities of extraocular muscle action related to muscle or cranial nerve pathology
OBJECTIVE DATA		
Eyelids		
▪ Allergic reactions	Redness, excessive tearing, and itching of lid margins	Many possible allergens; associated eye trauma can occur from rubbing itchy eyelids
▪ Hordeolum (sty)	Small, superficial white nodule along lid margin	Infection of a sebaceous gland of eyelid; causative organism is usually bacterial (most commonly *Staphylococcus aureus*)
▪ Chalazion	Reddened, swollen area on eyelid; involves deeper tissues than hordeolum; can be inflamed and tender	Granuloma formed around a sebaceous gland; occurs as a foreign body reaction to sebum in the tissue; can develop from a hordeolum or from rupture of a sebaceous gland with resulting sebum in the tissue
▪ Blepharitis	Redness, swelling, and crusting along lid margins	Bacterial invasion of lid margins; often chronic
▪ Dacryocystitis	Redness, swelling, and tenderness of medial area of lower lid (in region of lacrimal sac)	Blockage of nasolacrimal duct and subsequent infection
▪ Xanthelasma	Raised, yellowish plaques on eyelids usually on nasal portion	Lipid disorders; may be a normal finding

continued

Table 17-5 Common Assessment Abnormalities: Eye—cont'd

Findings	Description	Possible Etiology and Significance
▪ Ptosis	Drooping of upper lid margin, unilateral or bilateral	Mechanical causes as a result of eyelid tumors or excess skin; myogenic causes attributable to conditions involving the levator muscle or myoneural junction, such as myasthenia gravis; neurogenic causes affecting third cranial nerve that innervates the levator muscle; or aponeurogenic causes resulting in dehiscence in central part of aponeurosis
▪ Entropion	Inward turning of upper or lower lid margin, unilateral or bilateral	Congenital causes resulting in developmental abnormalities; spastic entropion caused by increased orbicularis muscle tone; cicatricial type characterized by scarring and contraction of tarsus and conjunctiva; involutional entropion related to horizontal eyelid laxity; can cause irritation and tearing
▪ Ectropion	Outward turning of lower lid margin	Mechanical causes as a result of eyelid tumors, herniated orbital fat, or extravasation of fluid; cicatricial ectropion caused by contraction or loss of tissue, such as with thermal or chemical injury; paralytic ectropion occurs when orbicularis muscle function is disturbed as with Bell's palsy; involutional ectropion characterized primarily by laxity of lateral canthal tendon; often associated with tearing
▪ Lid lag	Slower or absent closing of one lid	Possible involvement of CN VII
▪ Blepharospasm	Increased blink rate; when severe spasms occur, inability to open eyelids	Inflammation; involvement of CNs V and VII; can occur as a response to bright lights
▪ Decreased blink	Decreased rate of eyelid closure	Decreased corneal sensation; possible involvement of CN VII; dry eye and corneal damage may result if blink rate significantly decreased
Conjunctiva		
▪ Conjunctivitis	Redness, swelling of conjunctiva; may be itchy	Bacterial or viral infection; may be allergic response or inflammatory response to chemical exposure
▪ Subconjunctival hemorrhage	Appearance of blood spot on sclera; may be small or can affect entire sclera	Conjunctival blood vessels rupture, leaking blood into the subconjunctival space; caused by coughing, sneezing, eye rubbing, or minor trauma; generally requires no treatment
▪ Pinguecula	Raised area (growth) on conjunctiva; horizontally oriented in medial area of bulbar conjunctiva	Degenerative lesion related to chronic ultraviolet light or other environmental exposure
Sclera		
▪ Jaundice	Yellowish color of entire sclera	Jaundice related to liver dysfunction; yellow color normal after diagnostic study requiring intravenous fluorescein injection
Cornea		
▪ Corneal abrasion	Localized painful disruption of the epithelial layer of cornea, can be visualized with fluorescein dye	Trauma, overwear or improper fit of contact lenses
▪ Corneal opacity	Whitish area of normally transparent cornea; may involve entire cornea	Scar tissue formation related to inflammation; infection, trauma; degree of visual acuity deficit depends on location and size of opacity
▪ Pterygium	Triangular, horizontally-oriented thickening of bulbar conjunctiva that extends past corneoscleral border onto cornea	Commonly thought to be an extension of a pinguecula; degenerative lesion related to chronic ultraviolet light or other environmental exposure; surgical removal necessary if progression to central cornea

continued

Table 17-5 Common Assessment Abnormalities: Eye—cont'd

Findings	Description	Possible Etiology and Significance
Globe		
▪ Exophthalmos	Protrusion of globe beyond its normal position within bony orbit; sclera often visible above iris when eyelids are open	Intraocular or periorbital tumors; thyroid eye disease; swelling or tumors of the frontal sinus; dry eye and corneal damage may occur as a result of inability to close eye normally
Pupils		
▪ Mydriasis	Pupil is larger than normal (dilated)	Emotional influences, trauma, acute glaucoma (fixed, mid-dilated), systemic or local drugs, head injury
▪ Miosis	Pupil is smaller than normal	Iritis, morphine and similar drugs, glaucoma treated with miotic agents
▪ Anisocoria	Pupils are unequal (constricted)	Central nervous system disorders; slight difference in pupil size is normal in a small percentage of the population
▪ Dyscoria	Pupil is irregularly shaped	Congenital causes (e.g., iris coloboma); acquired causes (e.g., trauma, iris-fixated intraocular lens implant, posterior synechiae, surgery on iris)
▪ Abnormal response to light or accommodation	Pupils respond asymmetrically or abnormally to light stimulus or accommodation	Central nervous system disorders, general anesthesia
Iris		
▪ Heterochromia	Irides are different colors	Congenital causes (Horner's syndrome); acquired causes (chronic iritis, metastatic carcinoma, diffuse iris nevus or melanoma)
▪ Iridokinesis	Iris appears to shake on movement of eye	Aphakia
Extraocular Muscles		
▪ Strabismus	Deviation of eye position in one or more directions	Overaction or underaction of one or more extraocular muscles; can be congenital or acquired; neuromuscular involvement; CN III, IV, or VI involved
Visual Field Defect		
▪ Peripheral	Partial or complete loss of peripheral vision	Glaucoma, complete or partial interruption of visual pathway; migraine headache
▪ Central	Loss of central vision	Macular disease
Lens		
▪ Cataract	Opacification of lens, pupil can appear cloudy or white when opacity is visible behind pupil opening	Aging, trauma, electrical shock, diabetes, chronic systemic steroid therapy, congenital
▪ Subluxation or dislocation	Edge of lens may be seen through pupil; "setting sun" sign	Trauma, systemic disease (e.g., Marfan's syndrome)

asks the patient to cover the right eye, and the process is repeated.

If the patient cannot read letters, the examiner can use an eye chart with pictures or numbers. A second option is an eye chart that presents the letter E in four different directions. The examiner asks the patient to point in the direction the E faces.

To evaluate visual acuity when the patient is unable to see the 20/400 letter, the nurse holds up a number of fingers 3 to 5 feet (0.9 to 1.5 meters) in front of the patient and asks the patient to count them. If the patient is unable to count the fingers, the nurse holds up a different number of fingers at successively closer distances up to 1 foot and again asks the patient to count them. The examiner tests the opposite eye in the same manner and records the acuities of each eye. If the patient could count the number of fingers at 2 feet (0.6 meters), the nurse records the acuity as *FC* or *CF* ("finger counting" or "counts fingers") at 2 feet (0.6 meters). If the patient cannot count fingers, the nurse asks the patient to indicate if moving the hand is seen in front of the face. This level of visual acuity is *HM* ("hand motion"). *LP* ("light projection") is the term for a patient's visual acuity if only light can be seen.

If the patient has a complaint of visual problems at near, and for all patients 40 years of age or older, the nurse tests the near visual acuity. The patient is instructed to hold a Jaeger chart 14 inches (35.6 cm) from the eyes. The nurse covers the patient's left eye with the occluder, asks the patient to read successively smaller lines of print from the chart and records the visual acuity that corresponds to the smallest line of print the patient can read comfortably. The procedure is repeated while covering the right eye. A near acuity of $Jaeger_1$ (J_1) indicates that the patient can read 4 point type at 14 inches (35.6 cm), and is considered normal. A near acuity of J_{10} indicates that the smallest print the patient can read at 14 inches (35.6 cm) is 14 point type and is moderately impaired. Normal newspaper print is 8 point type.

If the nurse must assess visual acuity without access to an eye chart, an accurate assessment is still possible. Examples of other stimuli acceptable for use include newsprint or the label on a container. The examiner records the acuity as "reads newspaper headline at _____ inches."

Extraocular Muscle Functions. The nurse observes the corneal light reflex to evaluate eye position. In a darkened room, the nurse asks the patient to look straight ahead while a penlight is shone directly on the cornea. The light reflection should be located in the center of both corneas as the patient faces the light source.

The *cover-uncover test* will also detect extraocular muscle imbalance. While the examiner covers one eye of the patient, the patient looks at an object in front of the patient (e.g., the examiner's nose). The examiner then uncovers the eye, observing for movement of the uncovered eye. If the uncovered eye moves to look at the object, it was deviated under the cover before the cover was removed. In other words, the covered eye is observed for movement to focus when uncovered. Both eyes are tested. In the alternating cover test, the nurse covers one eye and then the other (one eye is covered at all times), again observing for movement of the uncovered eye. Movement of either eye during the cover-uncover test or the alternating cover test indicates *strabismus* (inability of the eyes to focus together).

The nurse also tests the extraocular movements of the eyes. The nurse asks the patient to follow a fixation object, such as the examiner's index finger or a light, through the nine cardinal fields of gaze while keeping the head facing forward (Fig. 17-6). The eyes should follow equally with parallel and coordinated movements. While the patient looks at each field of gaze, the nurse observes for *nystagmus,* which is a rhythmic jerking motion of the eyes. It is a normal finding on far lateral gaze but not in other positions.

Visual Fields. Tests of the visual fields assess peripheral vision. A simple but gross method of determining visual fields is the *confrontation test.* The patient and nurse sit facing each other 2 to 3 feet (0.6 to 0.9 meters) apart. The patient and the examiner cover opposite eyes. For example, the nurse covers her left eye, while the patient covers his right eye. Covering eyes in this manner allows the nurse and the patient to have approximately the same field of vision. The examiner brings one, two, or three fingers into the field of vision, equidistant between the examiner and the patient. Without moving the eyes to the left or right, the patient reports the number of fingers extended as soon as he is able to do so. The fingers are brought in from six different peripheral areas. For example, the nurse will ask the patient to count fingers from the 2, 4, and 6 o'clock positions. Any difference from the examiner's field is noted. Use of the examiner's field as the standard is acceptable only if the examiner's field of vision is normal. The examiner tests each eye separately. Test results for the normal eye are described as "confrontation fields full." The nurse should note whether the patient used corrective lenses during the test. If the nurse detects a defect in the patient's visual field, its location is described in terms of direction (nasal or temporal) and position (superior or inferior). If the nurse suspects an abnormality, the patient should be referred to an ophthalmologist for visual field perimetry (see Table 17-6).

Pupil Function. Pupil function is determined by inspecting the pupils and their reactions to light. The pupils should be equal in size, round, and react briskly to light. In a small percentage of the population the pupils are unequal in size (*anisocoria*). The pupils should react to light directly (the pupil constricts when a light shines into the *same* eye) and consensually (the pupil constricts when a light shines into the *opposite* eye). The nurse should also check the accommodative response by having the patient fixate on an object held 2 to 3 feet (0.6-0.9 m) away and then bringing the object closer to the patient until the patient is fixating on the object at 6 to 8 inches (15 to 20 cm) away. The pupils should constrict when the patient tries to focus on the near object.

Intraocular Pressure. Intraocular pressure can be measured by using a Schiotz or air-puff tonometer, but the most accurate readings are obtained by applanation tonometry (Fig. 17-7). The surface of the anesthetized cornea is applanated by the tonometer, and the cornea is observed through the biomicroscope. The normal intraocular pressure ranges from 10 to 21 mm Hg.

Assessing structures. The structures that constitute the visual system are assessed primarily by inspection. The visual system is unique because the nurse can directly inspect not only the external structures but also many of the internal structures. The iris, lens, vitreous, retina, and optic nerve can all be visualized directly through the clear cornea and pupil opening.

This direct inspection requires the examiner to use special observation equipment such as the slit lamp biomicroscope and the ophthalmoscope. This equipment permits examination of the conjunctiva, sclera, cornea, anterior chamber, iris, lens, vitreous, and retina under magnification. With the *slit lamp microscope,* a narrow beam, or slit, of light is directed onto the eye to brightly illuminate a small section. The patient's chin is positioned in a chin rest to stabilize the head. The *ophthalmoscope* is a hand-held instrument with a light source and magnifying lenses that is

Table 17-6 Diagnostic Studies: Visual System

Study	Description and Purpose	Nursing Responsibilities*
■ Retinoscopy	Objective (though inexact) measure of refractive error; hand-held retinoscope directs focused light into the eye, refractive error distorts the light, distortion is neutralized to determine refractive error; useful for patient unable to cooperate during process of subjective refraction (e.g., preverbal or confused patients.)	Procedure is painless; may need to help patient hold head still. Pupil dilation will make it difficult to focus on near objects; dilation may last from 3-4 hr.
■ Refractometry	Subjective measure of refractive error; multiple lenses are mounted on rotating wheels; patient sits looking through apertures at Snellen acuity chart, lenses are changed; patient chooses lenses that make acuity sharpest; cycloplegic drugs used to paralyze accommodation during refraction process.	Same as Retinoscopy
■ Visual field perimetry	Detailed mapping of the visual field; study uses semicircular, bowl-like instrument that presents patient with a light stimulus in various parts of the bowl; specific pattern of visual field loss used to diagnose glaucoma and certain neurologic deficits.	Procedure is painless but may be fatiguing; elderly or debilitated patient may need rest periods; patient must fixate on center target for accurate testing.
■ Gonioscopy	Examination of anterior chamber angle where iris and cornea meet; special mirrored lens is applanated against patient's anesthetized cornea to provide a magnified view of the angle; status of angle is diagnostic of open-angle, narrow-angle, or angle-closure glaucoma.	Patient may feel uncomfortable with gonioscope lens on eye despite corneal anesthesia; gently irrigate goniogel (used to lubricate lens) from the eye after procedure so patient does not abrade anesthetized cornea while attempting to wipe gel away.
■ Ultrasonography	A-scan probe is applanated against patient's anesthetized cornea; used primarily for axial length measurement used in calculating power of intraocular lens implanted after cataract extraction; B-scan probe is applied to patient's closed lid; used more often than A-scan for diagnosis of ocular pathology such as intraocular foreign bodies or tumors, vitreous opacities, retinal detachments.	Procedure is painless (cornea is anesthetized for A-scan).
■ Indirect ophthalmoscopy	Indirect ophthalmoscope is worn on examiner's head; light is projected through a hand-held lens into patient's eye; stereoscopic view is larger and provides a better view of peripheral retina; always used when some retinal abnormality is suspected.	Light source is bright, patient may be uncomfortably photophobic, especially because pupil is dilated.

continued

held close to the patient's eye to visualize the posterior part of the eye. There is no pain or discomfort associated with these examinations.

As with other skills, using this equipment requires some special training and practice. However, special equipment provides the means for a thorough ophthalmic assessment that gives the nurse information not only about the ocular structures themselves but also about the patient's systemic condition.

Eyebrows, Eyelashes, and Eyelids. All structures should be present and symmetric, and without deformities, redness, or swelling. Eyelashes extend outward from the lid margins. The eyelids are positioned symmetrically with the upper and lower eyelids approximately at the corneal-scleral limbus and the lid margins against the globe. In normal closing, the upper and lower eyelid margins just touch. The lacrimal puncta should be open and positioned properly against the globe, with no swelling or redness around the lower puncta indicating lacrimal sac inflammation. If the sac is inflamed, pressure over the lacrimal sac may cause purulent material to ooze from the puncta. Inspecting the eyelids with the slit lamp microscope pro-

Table 17-6 Diagnostic Studies: Visual System—cont'd

Study	Description and Purpose	Nursing Responsibilities*
■ Fluorescein angiography	Fluorescein (a nonradioactive, noniodine dye) is intravenously injected into antecubital or other peripheral vein, followed by serial photographs (over a 10-min period) of the retina through dilated pupils; provides diagnostic information about flow of blood through pigment epithelial and retinal vessels; often used in diabetic patients to accurately locate areas of diabetic retinopathy before laser destruction of neovascularization.	If extravasation occurs, fluorescein is toxic to tissues; systemic allergic reactions are rare, but nurse should be familiar with emergency equipment and procedures; tell patient that dye can sometimes cause transient nausea or vomiting; yellow discoloration of urine and skin is normal and transient.
■ Electroretinography	Objective measurement of electrical response of the retina to a flash of light; uses contact lens electrode; study is helpful in diagnosing diffuse retinal damage, with or without ophthalmoscopic changes.	Explain procedure to patient; assure that patient is comfortably positioned.
■ Amsler grid test	Test is self-administered using a hand-held card printed with a grid of lines (similar to graph paper); patient fixates on center dot and records any abnormalities of the grid lines, such as wavy, missing or distorted areas; used to monitor macular problems.	Regular testing is necessary to identify any changes in macular function immediately.
■ Schirmer tear test	Study measures tear volume produced throughout fixed time period; one end of a strip of filter paper is placed in lower lid cul-de-sac; area of tear saturation is measured after 5 min; useful in diagnosing keratoconjunctivitis sicca.	Test may be done with closed or open eyes.
■ Tensilon test	Edrophonium chloride (Tensilon) injected; in patients with ptosis caused by myasthenia gravis, the drooping lid immediately lifts.	Tensilon effect is very short-lived; consequently, drug is useful only in diagnosis, not treatment.

*Patient education regarding the purpose and method of testing is a nursing responsibility for all diagnostic procedures.

vides a magnified view useful for the patient who may have minor inflammation or even lice along the lid margins.

Conjunctiva and Sclera. The nurse can easily examine the conjunctiva and sclera at the same time. The examiner evaluates the color, smoothness, and presence of lesions. To examine the palpebral conjunctiva, the examiner places a forefinger over the cheekbone and gently pulls down. This maneuver exposes the palpebral conjunctiva of the lower lid for the nurse to assess color (normally pale pink), texture (normally smooth), and the presence of lesions or foreign bodies. The bulbar conjunctiva covering the sclera is normally clear, with fine blood vessels visible. These blood vessels are more common in the periphery.

The sclera is normally white, but it may take on a yellowish hue in the older individual because of lipid deposition. A pale blue cast caused by scleral thinning can also be normal in the older adult and in the infant (who have naturally thinner scleras). The blue cast is actually the vascular choroid showing through. A slight yellow cast may also be found in some dark-pigmented persons, such as African-Americans and Native Americans. Again, the slit lamp microscope is useful in those situations when the nurse may want a closer view of these external structures.

Cornea. A light is shone obliquely on the cornea while the nurse observes the surface of the cornea for smoothness, clarity, and foreign bodies. The surface should be smooth and without irregularities. The cornea should be clear, transparent, and shiny. In an older patient, *arcus senilis,* which is a white ring at the limbus, is normal. The nurse can determine whether there are abrasions or defects in the corneal epithelium by using a fluorescein test strip. This is done by moistening the test strip with a drop of sterile saline solution, touching it to the lower conjunctival sac, and instructing the patient to blink several times to distribute the solution across the cornea. Any corneal abrasions or defects will stain a brilliant green.

The slit lamp microscope is particularly useful in examining the cornea. The slit beam focused on the cornea and viewed through the microscope provides more information about the thickness and clarity of the cornea than is possible by viewing it without magnification.

A normal corneal reflex is indicative of intact functioning of the trigeminal nerve (CN V). The nurse tests the corneal reflex only when there is strong suspicion of a defect. It is frequently performed in cases of known or suspected brain death. The nurse should not perform this

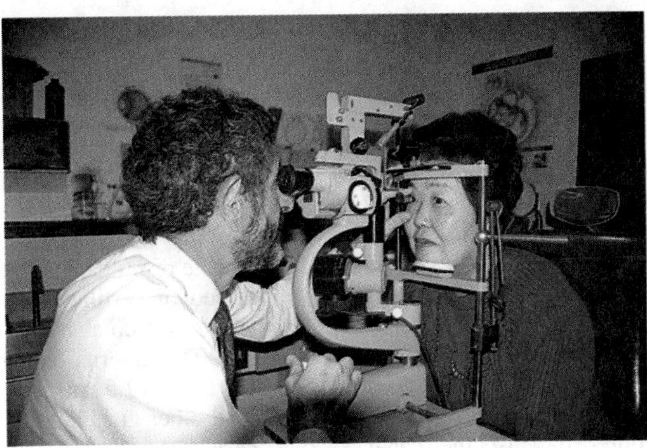

Fig. 17-7 Applanation tonometry.

test in the patient wearing contact lenses or in the patient who may have a corneal abrasion. A wisp of cotton is brought in laterally and lightly touched against the cornea. The patient with an intact corneal reflex will blink with both eyes when the cornea is touched and may tear profusely as a response to the irritation.

ANTERIOR CHAMBER. The nurse can use either a hand-held oblique light or the slit lamp microscope to inspect the anterior chamber. The iris should appear flat and not bulging toward the cornea. The area between the cornea and the iris should be clear with no blood or purulent material visible in the anterior chamber. Because blood and purulent material have a viscosity greater than aqueous humor, they will settle to the lower portion of the chamber, if present.

IRIS. Both irides should be of similar color and shape. However, a color difference between the irides occurs normally in a small portion of the population. The iris should be inspected with the upper lid raised. Any area of missing iris will be evident, because the absence of the colored iris tissue leaves what appears to be a dark, abnormally-shaped "pupil." Round or notched areas of missing iris tissue are often the result of cataract or glaucoma surgery. The nurse should determine the cause of these areas and document the findings.

LENS AND VITREOUS HUMOR. These internal structures are normally clear and should not be visible behind the pupil with the unaided eye. However, with the slit lamp microscope, the examiner can see small or early opacities in the lens or vitreous "floaters." The lens can become dislocated in the patients with Marfan's syndrome or as a result of trauma. This is readily seen with the microscope, and a dislocated lens may even be visible without it.

RETINA AND OPTIC NERVE. To assess these structures, the nurse uses an ophthalmoscope to magnify the ocular structures and bring them into crisp focus. Blood vessels in the vascular choroid are visible through the retinal tissues as is the optic disc (where the optic nerve enters the back of the eye). The ability to directly view arteries, veins, and the optic nerve in this manner is unique.

When using the ophthalmoscope, the nurse directs the beam of light obliquely into the patient's pupil. The red reflex should be visible. This reflex results from the light reflecting off the pink color of the retina. Any dense areas in the lens, such as a cataract, will decrease the red reflex. The reflex is followed inward until the fundus, or back of the eye, comes into view. Both arterioles and veins can be seen. Arterioles are smaller, thinner, and lighter red and reflect light better than veins. The nurse should examine the areas where arterioles and veins cross for nicking or narrowing. These changes are associated with diabetes and hypertension.

The examiner follows a blood vessel toward the optic nerve. The optic nerve or disc is examined for size, color, and abnormalities. The disc is creamy yellow with distinct margins. A slight blurring of the nasal margin is common.

A central depression in the disc, called the *physiologic cup,* may be seen. This area is the exit site for the optic nerve. The cup should be less than one-half the diameter of the disc. The nurse should document the presence of any unusual rings or crescents surrounding the disc.

There are normally no hemorrhages or exudates present in the fundus (retinal background). Careful inspection of the fundus can reveal the presence of retinal holes, tears, detachments, or lesions. Small hemorrhages can be associated with diabetes or hypertension and can appear in various shapes, such as dots or flames. Finally, the nurse examines the macula for shape and appearance. This area of high reflectivity is devoid of any blood vessels.

The nurse can obtain important information about the vascular system and the central nervous system (CNS) through direct visualization with an ophthalmoscope. Skilled use of this instrument requires practice, and it is not unusual for the nurse to be frustrated initially.

Special assessment techniques.

COLOR VISION. Testing the patient's ability to distinguish colors can be an important part of the overall assessment because some occupations may require accurate color discrimination. The Ishihara color test determines the patient's ability to distinguish a pattern of color in a series of color plates. In individuals of European ancestry, approximately 6% of males and 0.3% of females have a congenital color vision defect. The incidence of congenital color vision defects in individuals of non-European ancestry is lower.[7] Older adults have a loss of color discrimination at the blue end of the color spectrum and loss of sensitivity throughout the entire spectrum.

STEREOPSIS. Stereoscopic vision allows a patient to see objects in three dimensions. Any event that causes a patient to have monocular vision (e.g., enucleation, patching) results in the loss of stereoscopic vision. When stereopsis is not present, the individual's ability to judge distances is impaired. This disability can have serious consequences if the patient trips over a step when walking or follows too closely to another vehicle when driving. The nurse can test the patient's stereopsis by having them identify whether a series of objects is in front of or behind other objects when viewed through special spectacles.

CORNEAL CURVATURE. The curvature of the front surface of the cornea can be measured with a *keratometer.* This instrument projects a series of concentric circles of light onto the corneal surface. The examiner aligns the projection and notes the corneal curvature readings. Keratometry is used to assess the status of the corneal curvature after corneal transplantation, to determine the shape of the cornea when fitting contact lenses, and to evaluate astigmatism before corrective surgery. A newer technique to assess the corneal curvature converts multiple corneal video images into a color-coded corneal map.[11]

Diagnostic Studies. Diagnostic studies provide important information to the nurse in monitoring the patient's condition and planning appropriate interventions. These studies are considered objective data. Table 17-6 presents common diagnostic studies of the visual system.

DIAGNOSTIC STUDIES OF THE VISUAL SYSTEM

Diagnostic tests provide specific information about the structures and functions of the visual system. Although the physician and technician often do special diagnostic testing, the ophthalmic nurse can perform all types of testing. The nurse generalist does not usually perform these specialized tests. Almost all ophthalmic diagnostic testing is done with special equipment in the physician's office or outpatient clinic (Table 17-6). Similar tests are sometimes ordered for both ophthalmic and neurologic problems.

STRUCTURES AND FUNCTIONS OF THE AUDITORY SYSTEM

The auditory system is composed of the peripheral auditory system and the central auditory system. The *peripheral system* includes the structures of the ear itself: the external, middle, and inner ear (Fig. 17-8). This system is concerned with the reception and perception of sound. The inner ear functions in hearing and balance. The *central system* (the brain and its pathways) integrates and assigns meaning to what is heard.

External Ear

The external ear is composed of the auricle or pinna and the auditory canal. The *auricle* is composed of cartilage and connective tissue covered with epithelium, which also lines the external auditory canal (Fig. 17-8). The external auditory canal in the adult is approximately 1 inch (2.5 cm) long and has a slight S shape. Sebaceous and other glands in the outer half of the canal secrete *cerumen,* or wax. By waterproofing the ear canal, cerumen functions to protect the epithelium from maceration and dehydration.[14]

Hair is present in the outer half of the canal. This hair may be profuse and coarse, especially in the older male patient. The inner half of the ear canal is quite sensitive. The function of the external ear and canal is to collect and transmit sound waves to the tympanic membrane (eardrum). This shiny, translucent, pearl-gray membrane is composed of skin, connective tissue, and mucous membrane. It is obliquely positioned at the medial end of the canal.

Middle Ear

Mucous membrane lines the middle ear and is continuous from the nasal pharynx via the eustachian tube. The middle

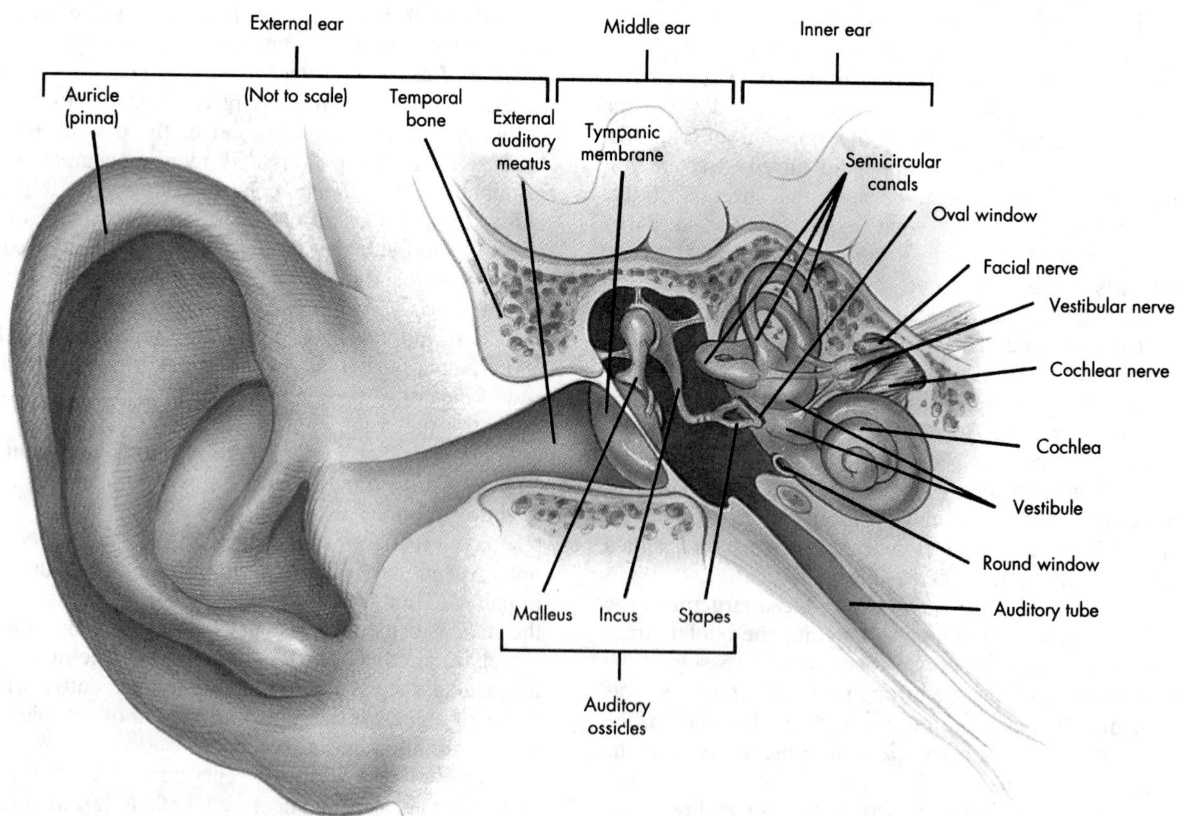

Fig. 17-8 External, middle, and inner ear.

ear cavity, which is located in the temporal bone, contains the *malleus, incus,* and *stapes* bones (collectively called the *ossicular chain*). The malleus articulates with the incus, which articulates with the head of the stapes. These articulations are freely movable synovial joints. The footplate of the stapes is positioned in the oval window and vibrates, causing the fluid in the inner ear to be set in motion. The round window covered with mucous membrane also opens into the inner ear and allows for dissipation of the fluid disturbances (round window reflex). The superior part of the middle ear is called the *epitympanum* or the attic, and also communicates with air cells within the mastoid bone. The air cells are lined with the same mucous membrane as the middle ear.

The *middle ear cavity* is filled with air, and equalization of atmospheric air pressure is accomplished by the eustachian tube. This tube is opened during yawning or swallowing. Blockage of the tube can occur with allergies, nasopharyngeal infections, and enlarged adenoids. Of clinical significance is the fact that the facial nerve (CN VII) traverses above the oval window of the middle ear. The thin, bony covering of the facial nerve (CN VII) can become eroded or traumatized by chronic ear infection, skull fracture, or trauma during ear surgery resulting in problems related to voluntary facial movements, eyelid closure, and taste discrimination.

The external and middle portions of the ear function to conduct and amplify sound waves from the environment. This portion of sound conduction is referred to as *air conduction*. Problems in these two parts of the ear may cause conductive hearing loss, resulting in an alteration in the patient's perception or sensitivity to sounds.

Inner Ear

The middle ear interfaces with the inner ear where the stapes meets the oval window. The *inner ear* is composed of the bony labyrinth and the membranous labyrinth and houses the end organ receptors for hearing and balance. The receptor organ for hearing is the *cochlea*, a coiled structure. It contains the *organ of Corti*, whose tiny hair cells respond to stimulation of selected portions of the basilar membrane according to pitch. This mechanical stimulus is converted into an electrochemical impulse and then transmitted by the acoustic portion of CN VIII to the brain.

Three *semicircular canals* and the utricle and saccule make up the organ of balance. These structures make up the membranous labyrinth, which is housed in a bony labyrinth. The membranous labyrinth is filled with endolymphatic fluid while the bony labyrinth is filled with perilymphatic fluid. The perilymphatic fluid cushions these two sensitive organs and communicates with the brain and the subarachnoid spaces of the brain. The nervous stimuli are communicated by the vestibular portion of CN VIII.

Pathology of the inner ear or along the nerve pathway from the inner ear to the brain can result in *sensorineural hearing loss*. This may result in an alteration of the patient's perception or sensitivity to high-pitched tones. These may be experienced as a decrease in intensity, muffling of the intensity (increased sensitivity to loud sounds), or decrease in ability to understand spoken words (distortion). Problems within the central auditory system from the cochlear nuclei to the cortex cause *central hearing loss*. This type of hearing loss causes difficulty in understanding the meaning of the words heard. (Types of hearing loss are discussed in Chapter 18.)

Transmission of Sound. Sound waves are conducted by air and picked up by the auricles and auditory canal. The taut tympanic membrane is struck by the sound waves, causing it to vibrate. The ossicles amplify sound waves received by the tympanic membrane and transmit the waves to the inner ear via the stapes by a lever action. The footplate of the stapes vibrates in the oval window to conduct sound waves to the inner ear.[15]

Once sound has been transmitted to the liquid medium of the inner ear, the disturbance is picked up by the tiny sensory hair cells of the cochlea, which initiate nerve impulses. These impulses are carried by nerve fibers to the main branch of the acoustic portion of CN VIII (acoustic) and then to the brain.

Effects of Aging on the Auditory System

Age-related changes of the auditory system can result in impaired hearing. *Presbycusis*, the decreased ability to hear high-frequency sounds, is caused by decreased efficiency of the cochlea as a result of loss of auditory neurons, decreased vascularity in the cochlea, and loss of hair cells in the organ of Corti. *Tinnitus*, or ringing in the ears, may accompany the hearing loss that results from the aging process. Exposure to loud noises earlier in life can result in increased hearing loss with age. Hearing loss, especially in the older adult, can have serious consequences on the life-style, leading to increased isolation, decreased socialization, and subsequent deterioration.[16] As the average life span increases, the number of people with progressive changes in the auditory system will also increase. Early identification of problems will ensure a more active and healthy patient population in their seventh and eighth decades (Table 17-7).

ASSESSMENT OF THE AUDITORY SYSTEM

Assessment of the auditory system includes assessment of the vestibular (balance) system because the two systems are so intimately related. It is often difficult to separate the symptomatology between the two systems. The nurse must help the patient to describe symptoms and problems in order to differentiate the source of the problems. Key questions to ask a patient with an auditory problem are listed in Table 17-8.

Initially the nurse should try to categorize symptoms related to dizziness and vertigo and separate them from symptoms related to hearing loss or tinnitus. The symptoms can be combined later in the assessment to help to make the diagnosis and plan for the patient.

Subjective Data

Important Health Information

Past health history. Many problems related to the ear are sequelae of childhood illnesses or result from problems of adjacent organs. Consequently a careful assessment of past health problems is important.

Table 17-7 Gerontologic Differences in Assessment: Auditory System

Changes	Differences in Assessment Findings
External Ear	
Increased production of and drier cerumen	Occlusion of canal with earwax; potential hearing loss
Increased hair growth	Visible hair
Middle Ear	
Atrophic changes of tympanic membrane	Conductive hearing loss
Inner Ear	
Hair cell degeneration, neuron degeneration in auditory nerve and central pathways, reduced blood supply to cochlea	Presbycusis, diminished sensitivity to high-pitched sounds, impaired speech reception, tinnitus
Less effective vestibular apparatus in semicircular canals	Alterations in balance and body orientation

The patient needs to be questioned about previous problems regarding the left and right ears, especially problems experienced during childhood. The frequency of acute middle ear infections (otitis media), perforations of the eardrum, drainage, complications, and history of mumps, measles, or scarlet fever should be recorded.

Congenital hearing loss can result from rubella or influenza in the first trimester of pregnancy. Therefore pregnant women and other young women of childbearing age are questioned regarding whether they were vaccinated against rubella or have ever had rubella. If the patient is uncertain about having had rubella, a serology test for measles antibody can be performed. A titer of 1:32 or more indicates immunity. The absence (or low levels) of rubella antibody titers indicates that the patient is susceptible to rubella infection.[17]

Problems such as dizziness, tinnitus, and hearing loss are recorded in the patient's words. Often it is difficult for the patient to describe the dizziness. However, it is important that the patient describe the dizziness in detail using his own words. This careful description could help to differentiate the cause.

Medications. Information about present or past medications that are *ototoxic* (cause damage to CN VIII) and can produce hearing loss, tinnitus, and disequilibrium should be obtained. The amount of aspirin used and the frequency of its use are important because tinnitus can result from high aspirin intake. Aminoglycosides, antibiotics, salicylates, antiprotozoal agents, chemotherapeutic drugs, diuretics, and non-steroidal antiinflammatory drugs (NSAIDs) are the most important drug groups that are potentially ototoxic.[18] Careful monitoring is essential. Many drugs produce inner ear damage that is reversible with cessation of treatment.

Surgery and other treatments. Information regarding previous hospitalizations for ear surgery as well as for tonsillectomy and adenoidectomy should be obtained. Hospitalization or treatment for head injury should also be documented because a head injury may result in decreased or lost hearing. Use and satisfaction with a hearing aid should be documented. The need for regular removal of impacted cerumen should be noted.

Functional Health Patterns. Hearing and balance problems can affect all aspects of a person's life. In order to assess the impact, based on a functional health pattern approach key questions can be asked (Table 17-8).

Health perception–health management pattern. The nurse should note the onset of hearing loss, whether sudden or gradual. It should be recorded who noted the onset, whether it be the patient, family, or significant others. Gradual hearing losses are most often noted by those who communicate with the patient. Sudden losses and those exacerbated by some other condition are most often reported by the patient.

Information about allergies is important because the eustachian tube can become edematous and prevent aeration of the middle ear. This occurs more frequently in children.

Information regarding family members with hearing loss and type of hearing loss is important. Some congenital disorders are hereditary. The age of onset of presbycusis also follows a familial pattern. Because prematurity can cause hearing problems, information about the patient's gestational age is also important. Premature infants may have been treated with an ototoxic drug. If knowledge of this event is important, it may be necessary to examine hospital records.

The patient should be questioned about practices that are used to preserve hearing. Use of protective ear covers is a good practice for persons in high-noise situations. If the patient is a swimmer, the frequency and duration of swimming and use of ear protection should be documented. Also, it is important to note the type of water in which the swimming takes place.

Nutritional-metabolic pattern. Both alcohol and sodium affect the amount of endolymph retained in the inner ear system. Patients with Meniere's disease generally notice some improvement with alcohol restriction and a low sodium diet. Improvements and exacerbations associated with food intake should be noted. The patient should also be questioned about any ear pain or discomfort associated with chewing or swallowing that might cause a reduction in the amount of food consumed. This problem is often associated with a problem in the middle ear.

Elimination pattern. Elimination patterns and their association with otologic problems are mainly of interest in the patient with perilymph fistula or the patient who is immediately postoperative. If the patient experiences fre-

Table 17-8 Key Questions: Patient with a Hearing or Balance Problem

Health Perception–Health Management Pattern

Hearing

Have you had a change in your hearing?* If yes, how does this change affect your daily life?

Do you use any devices to improve your hearing (e.g., hearing aid, special volume control, headphones for television or stereo)?*

How do you protect your hearing?

Do you have any allergies that result in ear problems?*

Balance

Is your walking affected by dizziness or vertigo?*

Does movement cause nausea or vomiting?*

Can you drive or walk alone? If no, elaborate.

Are there any times of the day when your symptoms are worse?*

Tinnitus

How long have you experienced ringing in your ears? Has it changed?*

When does it bother you the most?

What things have you tried that help?

Nutritional-Metabolic Pattern

Do you have any food allergies that affect your ears?*

Do you notice any differences in symptoms with changes in diet?*

Elimination Pattern

Does straining during a bowel movement cause you ear pain?*

Does your ear problem cause nausea that interferes with your food intake?*

Does chewing or swallowing cause you any ear discomfort?*

Activity-Exercise Pattern

Does you ear problem result in any change in your usual activity or exercise?*

Do you need help with certain activities (lifting, bending, climbing stairs, driving, speaking) because of symptoms?*

Do you have any limitations in activities of daily living because of your symptoms?*

Sleep-Rest Pattern

Is your sleep disturbed by symptoms of tinnitus or dizziness?*

Cognitive-Perceptual Pattern

Do you experience pain associated with your hearing or balance problem?* What relieves the pain? What makes it worse?

Is your ability to communicate and understand affected by your symptoms?*

Self-Perception–Self-Concept Pattern

Have these changes affected your self-esteem or feeling of independence?*

Role-Relationship Pattern

What effect has your ear problem had on your work, family, or social life?

Are you able to recognize the effects of your ear problem on your life?*

Do you consider your ear problem a stressor?*

Sexuality-Reproductive Pattern

Has your ear problem caused a change in your sex life?*

Coping–Stress Tolerance Pattern

What coping mechanisms do you use during time of exacerbation of symptoms?

Do you feel able to cope with your hearing or balance problem? If no, describe.

Value-Belief Pattern

Do you have a conflict between your planned treatment and your value-belief system?*

*If yes, describe.

quent constipation or straining with bowel or bladder elimination, this may interfere with healing of a perilymph fistula or its repair. The patient who is poststapedectomy especially needs to prevent the increased intracranial (and consequent inner ear) pressure associated with straining during bowel movements. Stool softeners are sometimes ordered postoperatively for the patient who reports chronic problems with constipation.

Activity-exercise pattern. Activity-exercise review is most important when assessing the patient with vestibular problems. The patient should be questioned specifically about activities that relieve or exacerbate symptoms of dizziness or bring on nausea or vomiting. The patient with chronic vertigo syndrome (benign paroxysmal positional nystagmus and vertigo, or BPPNV) notes that the symptoms improve throughout the day as adjustment to the visual and positional input from the environment occurs.

If dizziness is a problem, the patient should be questioned about the onset, duration, frequency, and precipitating factors of this symptom.

Patients with Meniere's syndrome demonstrate increasing inability to compensate for environmental input as the day progresses. Symptoms are experienced particularly in the evening. The nurse and the patient should identify a list of activities and exercises that affect dizziness and vertigo. The patient may undergo habituation exercises to help control the symptomatology. Habituation exercises involve the frequent repetition of an activity that causes symptoms until the body adjusts and the activity is no longer a problem.

Sleep-rest pattern. The patient with chronic tinnitus should be questioned about sleep problems. Tinnitus can disturb sleep and activities conducted in a quiet environment. If a sleep problem is associated with tinnitus, the patient should be asked if any masking devices or techniques are used or have been tried to drown out the more annoying tinnitus.

Cognitive-perceptual pattern. Pain is associated with some ear problems, particularly those involving the middle ear. If pain is present, the patient should be asked to recount the pain experience and the treatments used for relief. The effect on the pain level when the auricle is moved should be noted.

Hearing loss is associated with many middle and inner ear problems. The nurse or family may report the patient's decreased hearing, or the patient may express concern about perceived hearing loss. If decreased hearing is noted the patient and family should be questioned about the duration, severity, and circumstances associated with the decreased hearing.

Self-perception–self-concept pattern. The patient should be asked to describe how the ear problem has affected life and the feelings about themselves. Hearing loss and chronic vertigo are particularly problematic for the patient. Hearing loss can result in many embarrassing social situations that leave the patient with a diminished self-concept. The nurse should sensitively question the patient about the occurrence of such situations.

The patient with chronic vertigo may occasionally be accused of alcoholic intoxication. The patient should be asked if this has ever happened and how the situation was handled.

Role-relationship pattern. The patient should be questioned about the effect the ear problem has had on family life, work responsibilities, and social relationships. Hearing loss can result in strained family relations and misunderstandings. Failure to acknowledge the hearing loss and seek assistance can further compromise a family situation.

The patient should be questioned regarding employment or contact with environments that have excessive noise levels, such as work with jet engines and machinery, contact with the firing of firearms, and electromagnified music. The use of preventive devices worn in noisy environments is important to document.

Many jobs are contingent upon the ability to hear accurately and respond appropriately. If a hearing loss is present, the nurse should gather detailed information on the effect this has on the patient's job. The patient should be helped to realistically evaluate the job situation.

Hearing loss often leaves the patient feeling isolated and cut off from valued social relationships. The nurse should gather information about social activities such as playing cards, going to movies, and attending church from before and since the hearing loss occurred. Comparison of the frequency and enjoyment of the events can indicate if a problem is present.

The unpredictability of vertigo attacks can have devastating effects on all aspects of a patient's life. Ordinary activities such as driving, child care, housework, climbing stairs, and cooking all have an element of danger. The patient should be asked to describe the effect of the vertigo on the many roles and responsibilities of life. Compensatory practices to avoid the development of dangerous situations should also be noted.

Sexuality-reproductive pattern. It should be determined if ear problems related to hearing loss or deafness have interfered with the establishment of a satisfying sex life. Although intimacy does not depend on the ability to hear, it could interfere with establishing a relationship that could develop into a sexual relationship or maintaining a current relationship.

Coping–stress tolerance pattern. The patient should be asked to describe the usual coping style, tolerance for stress, stress-reducing behaviors, and available support. This information enables the nurse to determine if the patient's resources are adequate to meet the demands imposed by the ear problem. If the nurse concludes that the patient seems unable to manage the situation produced by the ear problem, outside intervention may be necessary. Denial is a common response to a hearing problem and should be assessed.

Value-belief pattern. The patient should be questioned about any conflicts produced by the problem or treatment related to values or beliefs. Every effort should be made to resolve the problem so the patient does not experience additional stress.

Objective Data

Physical Examination. The nurse can collect valuable objective data regarding the patient's ability to hear during the health-history interview. Clues such as posturing of the head and appropriateness of responses should be noted. Does the patient ask to have certain words repeated? Does the patient intently watch the examiner but miss comments when not looking at the examiner? Such observations are significant and should be recorded. This is also important because the patient is often not aware of hearing losses or does not admit to changes in hearing until moderate losses have occurred. A normal assessment of the ear is recorded as shown in Table 17-9. Age-related changes of the auditory system and differences in assessment findings are listed in Table 17-7.

External ear. The external ear is observed and palpated before inspection of the external canal and tympanum. The auricle, preauricular area, and mastoid area are inspected for equality of conformation of both ears, color of skin, nodules, swelling, redness, and lesions. The auricle and mastoid areas are then palpated for tenderness and nodules. Grasping the auricle may elicit pain, especially if inflammation of the external ear or canal is present.

External auditory canal and tympanum. Before inserting an otoscope, the nurse should inspect the canal opening for patency, palpate the tragus, and move the ear about to check for discomfort. After inspecting the canal opening for patency, an otoscopic examination is performed. A

Table 17-9 Normal Physical Assessment Findings of the Auditory System
Ears symmetric in location and shape. Auricles and tragus nontender, without lesions. Canal clear, tympanic membrane intact, landmarks and light reflex intact. Able to hear low whisper at 30 cm; Rinne test results AC > BC; Weber test results, no lateralization.

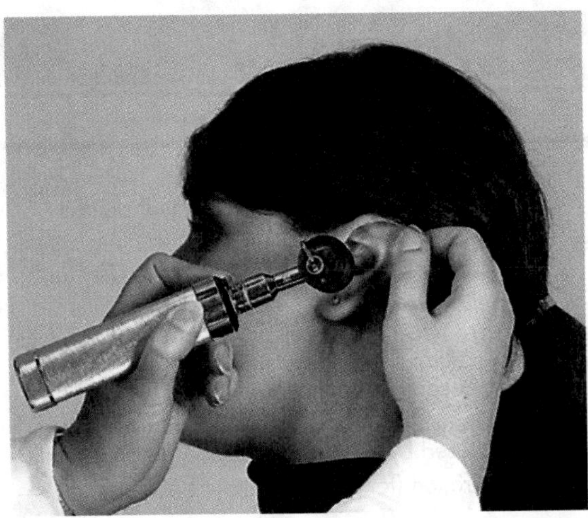

Fig. 17-9 Otoscopic examination of the adult ear. Auricle is pulled up and back. The hand holding the otoscope is braced against the face for stabilization.

speculum slightly smaller than the size of the ear canal is selected. The patient's head is tipped to the opposite shoulder. In the adult patient, the top of the auricle is grasped and gently pulled up and back to straighten the canal. The otoscope, held in the examiner's right hand and stabilized on the patient's head by the fingers, is inserted slowly (Fig. 17-9). The canal is observed for the color and amount of cerumen. If a large amount of cerumen is present, the tympanum may not be visible. The tympanum is observed for color, landmarks, contour, and intactness (Fig. 17-10).

The tympanic membrane separates the external ear from the middle ear. It is pearl-gray, white, or pink; shiny; and translucent. The anteroinferior quadrant is situated obliquely in the ear canal and is farthest from the examiner. The major landmarks are formed by the short process of the malleus superiorly, the handle or manubrium, and the

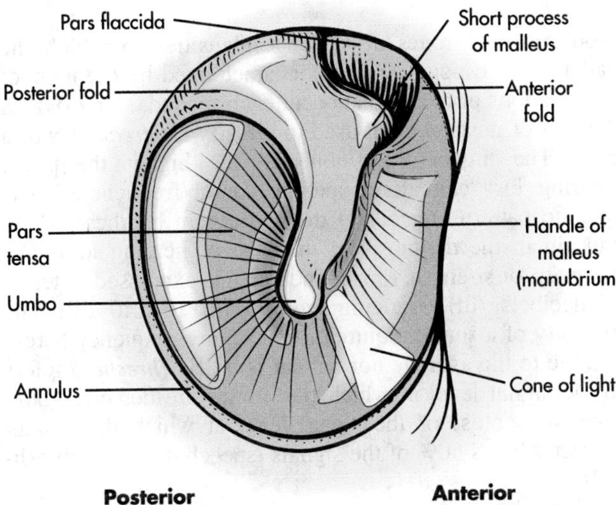

Fig. 17-10 Normal landmarks of the right tympanic membrane as seen through an otoscope.

umbo. From the innermost part of the tympanum a light reflex or cone of light is formed with the point directed toward the umbo. The circumference of the tympanum is surrounded by a dense, whitish, fibrous ring, or *annulus,* except in the superior area. The tympanum within the annulus is taut and is called the *pars tensa*. Superior to the short process of the malleus is the *pars flaccida,* or flaccid part of the tympanum. The malleolar folds are anterior and posterior to the short process of the malleus. Table 17-10 summarizes common assessment abnormalities of the auditory system. The middle and inner ear cannot be examined directly with the otoscope because of the tympanic membrane.

Diagnostic Studies. Diagnostic studies provide important information to the nurse in monitoring the patient's condition and planning appropriate interventions. These studies are considered to be objective data. Table 17-11 presents diagnostic studies common to the auditory system.

DIAGNOSTIC STUDIES OF THE AUDITORY SYSTEM

Tests for Hearing Acuity

Tests involving the whispered and spoken voice can provide gross screening information about the patient's ability to hear. Audiometric testing provides more specific information that can be used for diagnosis and treatment.

In the whispered test the examiner stands 12 to 24 inches (30 to 61 cm) to the side of the patient and, after exhaling, speaks using a low whisper. A louder whisper is used if the patient does not respond correctly. Spoken voice, increasing in loudness, is similarly used. The patient is asked to repeat numbers or words or answer questions. Each ear is tested. The ear not being tested is masked with the patient occluding the ear or with the examiner moving a finger rapidly, close to the ear canal.

In another test a ticking watch is placed 0.5 to 2 inches (1.3 to 5 cm) from the ear being tested, and the opposite ear is masked. The patient with normal hearing should be able to hear the ticking. However, with the advent of quartz movement watches, ticking watches are harder to find and the variation among watches makes this test a difficult one for assessing hearing acuity. The patient with sensorineural loss may not be able to hear the high-pitched tones of a ticking watch.

Tuning-Fork Tests. Tuning-fork tests aid in differentiating between conductive and sensorineural hearing loss. Tuning forks of 250, 500, and 1000 Hz are generally used for this examination. Both skill and experience are necessary to ensure accurate results. If a problem is suspected, further evaluation by pure-tone audiometry is essential. The most common tuning-fork tests are the Rinne and the Weber tests.

For the *Rinne test* the base of an activated tuning fork is held alternately on the mastoid bone and in a position that is 0.5 to 2 inches (1.3 to 5 cm) from the ear canal. The patient reports whether the sound is louder behind the ear (on the mastoid bone) or next to the ear canal. When the sound is no longer perceived behind the ear, the fork is shifted next to the ear canal until the patient indicates that the sound is no longer heard. The Rinne test is *positive* when the patient reports that air conduction is heard longer

Table 17-10 Common Assessment Abnormalities: Ear

Findings	Description	Possible Etiology and Significance
External Ear and Canal		
■ Sebaceous cyst behind ear	Usually within skin, possible presence of black dot (opening to sebaceous gland)	Removal or incision and drainage if painful
■ Tophi	Hard nodules in the helix or antihelix consisting of uric acid crystals	Associated with gout, metabolic disorder; further diagnosis needed
■ Impacted cerumen	Wax that has not normally been excreted from the ear; no visualization of eardrum	Decreased hearing possible, sensation of fullness in auditory canal, removal necessary before otoscopic examination
■ Discharge in canal	Infection of external ear, usually painful	Swimmer's ear, infection of external ear; possibly caused by ruptured eardrum and otitis media
■ Swelling of pinna, pain	Infection of glands of skin, hematoma caused by trauma	Aspiration (for hematoma)
■ Scaling or lesions	Change in usual appearance of skin	Seborrheic dermatitis, squamous cell carcinoma
■ Exostosis	Bony growth extending into canal causing narrowing of canal	Possible interference with visualization of tympanum, usually asymptomatic
Tympanum		
■ Retracted eardrum	Appearance of shorter, more horizontal malleus; absent or bent cone of light	Absorption of air from middle ear, blockage of eustachian tube, negative pressure in middle ear
■ Hairline fluid level, yellow-amber bubbles above fluid level	Caused by transudate of blood and serum, meniscus of fluid producing hairline appearance	Serous otitis media
■ Bulging red or blue eardrum, lack of landmarks	Fluid-filled middle ear, pus, blood	Acute otitis media, perforation possible
■ Early stage hyperemic vessels	Complaint of severe pain	Usually in children
■ Perforation of eardrum (central or marginal)	Previous perforations of the eardrum that have failed to heal (in adults); thin, transparent layer of epithelium surrounding eardrum	Chronic otitis media
■ Recruitment	Disproportionate loudness of sound from malfunction of inner ear	Hearing aid difficult to use

than bone conduction. This can indicate normal hearing or a sensorineural loss. If the patient hears the tuning fork better by bone conduction, the Rinne test is negative and indicates that a conductive hearing loss is present.

For the *Weber test* an activated tuning fork is placed on the midline of the skull, the forehead, or the teeth. The patient is asked to indicate where the sound is heard best. The normal response is perception of equal loudness bilaterally. If a patient has a conductive hearing loss in one ear, sound is heard louder (lateralizes) in that ear. If a sensorineural loss is present, sound is louder (lateralizes) in the good ear.

Results of tuning fork tests are subjective. The patient with inconsistent test results or questionable results should be referred for more objective audiometric evaluation.

Audiometry. Audiometry is useful as a screening test for hearing acuity and as a diagnostic test for determining the degree and type of hearing loss. The audiometer produces pure tones at varying intensities to which the patient can respond. Sound is characterized by the number of vibrations or cycles that occur each second. Hertz (Hz) is the unit of measurement used to classify the *frequency* of a tone. The higher the frequency, the higher the pitch. Hearing loss can affect specific sound frequencies. The specific pattern created on the audiogram by these losses can aid in the diagnosis of the type of hearing loss. The *intensity,* or strength, of a sound wave is expressed in terms of decibels (dB), ranging from 0 dB to 140 dB. The intensity of a sound required to make any frequency barely audible to the average normal ear is 0 dB. *Threshold* refers to the signal level at which pure tones are detected (pure tone thresholds) or the signal level at which the patient correctly hears 50% of the signals (speech detection thresholds).

Normal speech presented comfortably loud is approximately 40 to 65 dB; a soft whisper is 20 dB. Normally, a

Table 17-11 Diagnostic Studies: Auditory System

Study	Description and Purpose	Nursing Responsibility
Auditory		
Pure-tone audiometry	■ Sounds are presented through earphones in soundproof room. ■ Patient responds nonverbally when sound is heard. ■ Response is recorded on an audiogram. ■ Purpose is to determine hearing range of patient in terms of dB and Hz for diagnosing conductive and sensorineural hearing loss.	Nurse does not usually participate in examination.
Bone conduction	■ Vibrator is placed on mastoid process and hearing by bone conduction is recorded. Diagnoses conductive hearing loss.	
One-syllable word lists	■ Words are presented and recorded at comfortable level of hearing to determine percentage correct and word understanding.	
High-frequency pure tones of 12,000 to 15,000 Hz	■ Normally, patient can hear pure tone for 1 min. Those with pressure on CN VIII will not hear pure tones. Levels of intensity are increased, which patient cannot hear. ■ If patient could not hear tones before administration of ototoxic drug, decrease at this level during drug administration indicates cochlear damage and need to discontinue use of drug.	Nurse does not usually participate in examination.
Evoked response audiometry or audiometric brainstem response	■ Procedure is similar to electroencephalogram (See Table 53-9) ■ Electrodes are attached to patient in a darkened room. ■ Electrodes are placed typically at the vertex, mastoid process, or earlobes and forehead. A computer is used to isolate the auditory from other electrical activity of the brain. ■ Test is useful for uncooperative patient or patient who cannot volunteer useful information.	Explain procedure to patient. Do not leave patient alone in the darkened room.
Cortical (stimulus, pure tone, or broadband)	■ Test focuses on electrical activity at cerebral cortex level.	
Brainstem (stimulus, pure tone, or broadband)	■ Study measures electrical peaks along auditory pathway of inner ear to brain and gives possible diagnosis of acoustical neuromas, brainstem problems, or vascular accident.	
Vestibular		
Caloric test stimulus	■ Endolymph of the semicircular canals is stimulated irrigation of cold (20° C) or warm (36° C) solution into ear. ■ Patient is seated or in supine position. ■ Observation of type of nystagmus, nausea and vomiting, falling, vertigo produced is helpful in diagnosing disease of labyrinth. ■ Decreased function is indicated by decreased response and indicates disease of vestibular system. ■ Other ear is tested similarly and results are compared.	Observe patient for vomiting; assist if necessary. Ensure patient safety.
Electronystagmography	■ Electrodes are placed near patient's eyes and movement of eyes (nystagmus) is recorded on graph during specific eye movements and when ear is irrigated. ■ Study diagnoses diseases of vestibular system.	
Posturography	■ Balance test that can isolate one semicircular canal from others to determine site of lesion.	Inform patient that test is time-consuming and uncomfortable; test can be discontinued at any time at patient's request.

child and a young adult can hear frequencies from about 16 to 20,000 Hz, but hearing is most sensitive between 500–4000 Hz. This is similar to the frequencies contained in speech. A 40 to 45 dB loss in these frequencies causes moderate difficulty in hearing normal speech. A hearing aid is helpful because it amplifies sound. A patient with a loss primarily in the higher frequencies, such as 4000 through 8000 Hz, has difficulty distinguishing the high-pitched consonants. Words such as cat, hat, and fat may not be perceived accurately because the important information conveyed by the consonant is not heard. A hearing aid makes sound information louder but not clearer and so may not be helpful to the patient who has problems with *discrimination* of sounds or sound information because the consonants are still not heard sufficiently to make speech intelligible.

Screening audiometry. *Screening audiometry* is the testing of large numbers of persons with a fast, simple test to detect possible hearing problems. A pass-fail criterion is used to screen persons who will or will not be given additional diagnostic testing. Persons who fail the screening should be referred for threshold audiometry.

In screening audiometry, the audiometer is usually set at a hearing level of 10 to 20 dB. The patient wears earphones as the tester sweeps across the available signal frequencies. The patient is directed to raise a hand when a sound is heard. Responses to air-conducted tones are checked at each frequency setting.

Pure-tone audiometry. A *pure-tone audiometer* produces pure tones at varied frequencies and intensities. Threshold audiometry generally determines detection thresholds for seven frequencies from 250 to 8000 Hz. The intensity is plotted against the frequency on an audiogram (Fig. 17-11). The right ear is represented by a red circle and the left ear by a blue X on the audiogram.

In a quiet setting a tone loud enough to be clearly heard by the patient is presented. The threshold level for frequency is then determined. A person with thresholds at 25 dB or higher will demonstrate problems in everyday communication situations. Usually the lower limit used for acceptable hearing for children is 15 to 20 dB because a child's ability to develop adequate speech is dependent on sound information received. A 26 dB hearing loss is used as a guideline for further action. A hearing aid or surgery is rarely recommended for a hearing loss of less than 26 dB.[19]

Specialized Tests

An audiologist can perform many additional tests since the advent of newer audiometers and computers that record electrical activity from the middle ear, inner ear, and brain (Table 17-11). The most common test performed by the audiologist is pure-tone audiometry done under ideal testing conditions. A soundproof room is used for greater accuracy of results. The audiologist can also test bone conduction to aid in differentiating sensorineural from conductive hearing losses. The more specialized tests of the auditory system are most often performed in an outpatient setting by an audiologist. The nursing responsibilities involved include: (1) explaining the exam in general terms, (2) informing the patient if there are any dietary restrictions such as caffeine or other stimulants, and (3) advising the patient if sedation will be used.

Other more sophisticated tests are also available to determine the origin of certain hearing losses. These include evoked potential studies or auditory brain stem response, and electrocochleography. Computerized tomography (CT) and magnetic resonance imaging (MRI) scans are used to diagnose the site of a lesion, such as a tumor of the auditory nerve.

Test for Vestibular Function

Nystagmus, an abnormal rhythmic jerking motion of the eyes within the field of binocular vision, can be caused by disturbances in the endolymph fluid. The movement of the endolymph fluid stimulates receptor cells and causes nystagmus. Lesions in the CNS and drug toxicity can also cause nystagmus. In a test for nystagmus the patient looks straight ahead and then follows the examiner's finger to an extreme lateral gaze. Quick jerking movements along the way, except on extreme lateral gaze, are considered abnormal. Caloric testing and electronystagmography also test the function of the vestibular system.

The *caloric test* is done to determine the function of the vestibular system. The external ear is irrigated with cold or warm water, which causes disturbances in the endolymph. The patient's reaction is observed for type of eye movements. This observation may be made subjectively by examiner or objectively by placing electrodes around the eyes. A normal individual will exhibit nystagmus when water is instilled in the ear, with cold water producing a nystagmus directed opposite the side of instillation. Peripheral or brain lesions are suspected in the patient where no nystagmus is elicited by caloric testing. Drugs that may affect the test include alcohol, CNS depressants, and barbiturates. The patient's use of these drugs should be known to the physician before testing.

Posturography. In the past few years, more sophisticated tests of the balance system have been developed including platform posturography and rotational chair tests. These tests isolate one semicircular canal from the others to determine the site of a lesion causing vestibular disturbance. They can also provide hard data concerning the degree of disability caused by the disorder. These tests are time consuming and, in the vestibularly disabled patient, can cause great distress and discomfort, particularly nausea and vomiting. The patient needs pretest instructions regarding intake of substances that can affect test results. In addition, the patient requires reassurance that the test can be discontinued if stimulation to the vestibular systems cannot be tolerated.

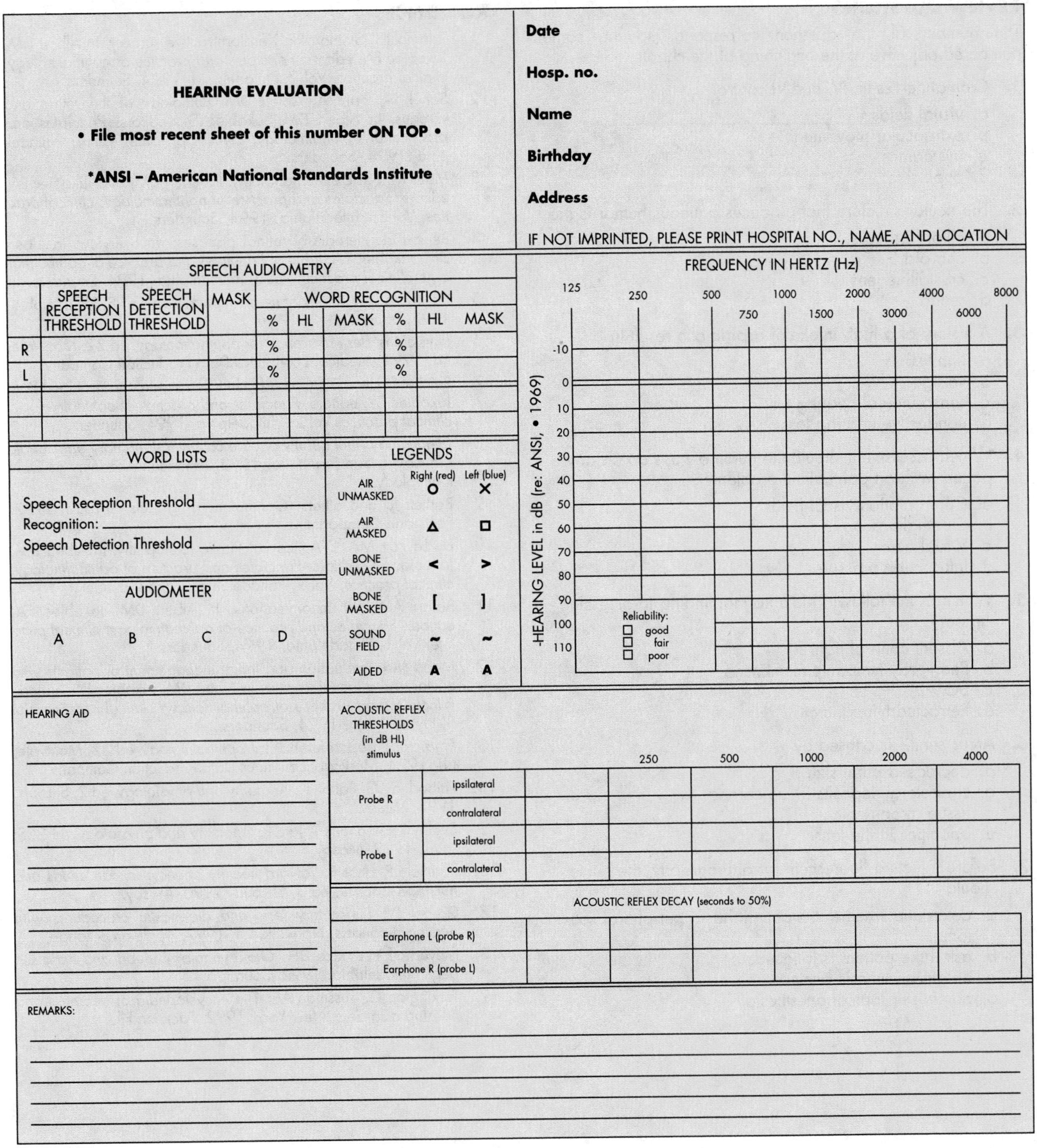

HEARING EVALUATION

• File most recent sheet of this number ON TOP •

***ANSI – American National Standards Institute**

Date

Hosp. no.

Name

Birthday

Address

IF NOT IMPRINTED, PLEASE PRINT HOSPITAL NO., NAME, AND LOCATION

SPEECH AUDIOMETRY

	SPEECH RECEPTION THRESHOLD	SPEECH DETECTION THRESHOLD	MASK	WORD RECOGNITION					
				%	HL	MASK	%	HL	MASK
R				%			%		
L				%			%		

WORD LISTS

Speech Reception Threshold ____

Recognition: ____

Speech Detection Threshold ____

AUDIOMETER

A B C D

LEGENDS

	Right (red)	Left (blue)
AIR UNMASKED	O	X
AIR MASKED	△	□
BONE UNMASKED	<	>
BONE MASKED	[	]
SOUND FIELD	~	~
AIDED	A	A

FREQUENCY IN HERTZ (Hz)

125 250 500 750 1000 1500 2000 3000 4000 6000 8000

-HEARING LEVEL in dB (re: ANSI, • 1969)

-10 0 10 20 30 40 50 60 70 80 90 100 110

Reliability:
□ good
□ fair
□ poor

HEARING AID

ACOUSTIC REFLEX THRESHOLDS (in dB HL) stimulus

		250	500	1000	2000	4000
Probe R	ipsilateral					
	contralateral					
Probe L	ipsilateral					
	contralateral					

ACOUSTIC REFLEX DECAY (seconds to 50%)

Earphone L (probe R)					
Earphone R (probe L)					

REMARKS:

Fig. 17-11 The patient's hearing level is plotted on the audiogram.

REVIEW QUESTIONS

The number of the question corresponds to the same-numbered objective at the beginning of the chapter.

1. Cranial nerves III, IV, and VI control
   a. visual fields.
   b. extraocular movement.
   c. nystagmus.
   d. pupil size.

2. The ocular structure that produces aqueous humor is the
   a. ciliary process.
   b. choroid.
   c. crystalline lens.
   d. retina.

3. A history of a high intake of aspirin can result in
   a. tinnitus.
   b. vertigo.
   c. sensorineural hearing loss.
   d. conductive hearing loss.

4. Which assessment should the nurse *always* do on any patient with an ophthalmic problem?
   a. Confrontation visual fields
   b. Ophthalmoscopy
   c. Visual acuity
   d. Intraocular pressure

5. Which of the following is a normal finding in assessing the ear?
   a. Absent cone of light
   b. Pearl-gray tympanic membrane
   c. BC > AC
   d. Retracted tympanum

6. Arcus senilis is caused by
   a. decreased pupil size.
   b. cholesterol deposits in the cornea.
   c. tissue atrophy.
   d. opacities in the lens.

7. Before injecting fluorescein for angiography, the nurse should
   a. determine whether the patient has a peripheral scotoma.
   b. ask if the patient is fatigued.
   c. obtain an emesis basin.
   d. administer topical anesthesia.

REFERENCES

1. Talamo JH, Steinert RF: Keratorefractive surgery. In Albert DM, Jakobiec FA, editors: *Principles and practice of ophthalmology: clinical practice,* Vol 1, Philadelphia, 1994, Saunders.
2. Sahel JA, Brini A, Albert DM: Pathology of the retina and vitreous. In Albert DM, Jakobiec FA, editors: *Principles and practice of ophthalmology: clinical practice,* Vol 4, Philadelphia, 1994, Saunders.
3. Maus M: Basic eyelid anatomy. In Albert DM, and Jakobiec FA, editors: *Principles and practice of ophthalmology: clinical practice,* Vol 3, Philadelphia, 1994, Saunders.
4. Berson EL: Hereditary retinal diseases: an overview. In Albert DM, Jakobiec FA, editors: *Principles and practice of ophthalmology: clinical practice,* Vol 2, Philadelphia, 1994, Saunders.
5. Guyton AC: *Textbook of medical physiology,* ed 8, Philadelphia, 1991, Saunders.
6. *Physicians' desk reference for ophthalmology,* ed 22, Montvale, NJ, 1994, Medical Economics Data Production Company.
7. Reichel E: Hereditary cone dysfunction syndromes. In Albert DM, Jakobiec FA, editors: *Principles and practice of ophthalmology: clinical practice,* Vol 2, Philadelphia, 1994, Saunders.
8. *Glaucoma panel quality of care committee: primary open-angle glaucoma,* San Francisco, 1992, American Academy of Ophthalmology.
9. Bartlett JD and others: *Ophthalmic drug facts,* St Louis, 1992, Facts and Comparisons.
10. De La Paz MA, D'Amico DJ: Photic retinopathy. In Albert DM, Jakobiec FA, editors: *Principles and practice of ophthalmology: clinical practice,* Vol 2, Philadelphia, 1994, Saunders.
11. Bajart AM: Lid inflammations. In Albert DM, Jakobiec FA, editors: *Principles and practice of ophthalmology: clinical practice,* Vol 1, Philadelphia, 1994, Saunders.
12. Mead MD: Evaluation and initial management of patients with ocular and adnexal trauma. In Albert DM, Jakobiec FA, editors: *Principles and practice of ophthalmology: clinical practice,* Vol 5, Philadelphia, 1994, Saunders.
13. *Physicians' desk reference for ophthalmology,* ed 22, Montvale, NJ, 1994, Medical Economics Data Production Company.
14. Thibodeau G, Patton K: *Anatomy and physiology,* ed 2, St Louis, 1993, Mosby.
15. Seeley R, Stephens T, Tate P: *Anatomy and physiology,* ed 2, St Louis, 1992, Mosby.
16. Ebersole P, Hess P: *Toward healthy agency: human needs and nursing response,* ed 3, St Louis, 1990, Mosby.
17. Corbet JV: *Laboratory tests and diagnostic procedures with nursing diagnosis,* Norwalk, CT, 1992, Appleton & Lange.
18. Meyerhoff WL, Rice DH: *Otolaryngology: head and neck surgery,* Philadelphia, 1992, Saunders.
19. Turkington C, Sussman AE: *The encyclopedia of deafness and hearing disorders,* New York, 1992, Facts on File.

Chapter 18

NURSING ROLE IN MANAGEMENT

Vision and Hearing Problems

Kate Goldblum **Idolia Cox Collier**

Learning Objectives

1. Describe the types of refractive errors and appropriate corrections.
2. Describe the etiology and management of extraocular disorders.
3. Explain the pathophysiology, clinical manifestations, and therapeutic and nursing management of the patient with selected intraocular disorders.
4. Describe the nursing measures that promote the health of the eyes and ears.
5. Explain the general preoperative and postoperative care of the patient undergoing surgery of the eye or ear.
6. Describe the action and uses of common pharmacologic agents used in treating problems of the eyes and ears.
7. Explain the pathophysiology, clinical manifestations, and therapeutic and nursing management of common ear problems.
8. Compare the causes, management, and rehabilitative potential of conductive and sensorineural hearing loss.
9. Explain the use, care, and patient education related to assistive devices for eye and ear problems.
10. Describe the common causes and assistive measures for uncorrectable visual impairment and deafness.
11. Describe the measures used to assist the patient in adapting psychologically to decreased vision and hearing.

VISUAL PROBLEMS

Health Promotion and Maintenance

The nurse's role as a health educator with individuals, groups, and communities is extremely important in preventing health problems that have the potential for visual impairment. In addition to health education, the nurse can promote visual health by early recognition of conditions or situations that carry a high risk of visual impairment. Following is information about those adult conditions and situations amenable to nursing interventions:

1. Glaucoma and diabetic retinopathy are significant causes of preventable visual impairment. Early recognition of these conditions is extremely important in promoting visual health. The nurse can advocate and provide assistance for screening programs. In addition, the nurse should provide health information regarding the importance of regular ophthalmic examinations, especially to the patient at high risk for these disorders. The nurse can provide this information to an individual patient, groups of patients, or the general community.

2. Ocular trauma can lead to blindness or severe visual impairment. Many injuries can be prevented by identifying and correcting situations that may lead to eye injuries such as (1) failure to properly use eye protection during potentially hazardous work, hobby, or sports activities; (2) improper handling or storing of chemicals, especially strong alkalis or acids; (3) inappropriate response to ocular injuries, particularly failure to institute prompt, continuous ocular irrigation after exposure to a potentially toxic substance; and (4) failure to properly use seat belts or infant and child vehicle restraint devices. The nurse should take an active role in educating the patient about these potentially harmful situations.

3. As contact lens wear becomes increasingly common and contact lens companies continue to market directly to consumers, many people have become casual about wearing and caring for their lenses. Although contact lenses are generally safe and effective, they can be a significant potential source of ocular problems when the patient does not use or care for lenses properly. The nurse should promote ocular health by teaching the patient correct wearing and cleaning techniques and recommending appropriate ophthalmic follow-up. Using incorrect solutions can be associated with severe ocular problems, and the nurse should stress using only approved contact lens solutions.

Reviewed by Mary S. Merchant, RN, MSN, CCM, Outcome Manager, Medical University of South Carolina, Charleston, SC.

CULTURAL & ETHNIC Considerations

HEARING AND VISUAL PROBLEMS

- Caucasians have a higher incidence of hearing impairment than African-Americans or Asian-Americans.
- Incidence and severity of glaucoma is increased among African-Americans when compared with Caucasians.
- Native Americans and African-Americans have a higher incidence of astigmatism than Caucasians.
- Native Americans have an increased incidence of otitis media when compared with Caucasians.

4. Women of childbearing age should be immunized against rubella, or German measles, to prevent congenital blindness in infants, which can result from rubella infection in the mother during the first trimester of pregnancy.[1] Persons who come in contact with this group of women, especially those who work in health care agencies, must be immunized as well.

5. Genetically transmitted syndromes and conditions often have ocular manifestations. The nurse working with the patient of childbearing age should be prepared to make referrals for genetic counseling when appropriate.

CORRECTABLE REFRACTIVE ERRORS

The most common visual problem is *refractive error.* This defect of the refracting media of the eye prevents light rays from converging into a single focus on the retina. Defects are due to irregularities of the corneal curvature, the focusing power of the lens, or the length of the eye. The major symptom is blurred vision. In some cases the patient may also complain of ocular discomfort, eyestrain, or headaches. The patient with refractive errors uses corrective lenses to improve the focus of light rays on the retina (Fig. 18-1).

Myopia (nearsightedness) is the most common refractive error with approximately 25% of Americans exhibiting this disorder. The prevalence of *hyperopia* (farsightedness) and *presbyopia* (farsightedness resulting from a decrease in the accommodative ability of the eye as a result of aging) is less common. However, approximately 80 million Americans wear some form of spectacle correction for refractive errors, approximately 25 million wear contact lenses, and several hundred thousand more have had keratorefractive surgery to correct refractive errors.[2] Table 18-1 summarizes the types of refractive errors and the appropriate corrections. Contrary to common belief, uncorrected refractive errors do not worsen the error, nor do they cause further pathology. However, refractive errors in young children should be corrected because children may develop *amblyopia* (reduced vision in the affected eye) if their refractive error is uncorrected.[2]

Myopia

Myopia causes light rays to be focused in front of the retina. Myopia may occur because of excessive light refraction by the cornea or lens or because of an abnormally long eye. Myopia may also occur because of lens swelling that occurs when blood glucose levels are elevated, as in uncontrolled diabetes. This myopia is transient and variable, fluctuating with the blood glucose level. During childhood, especially during adolescence when the child's growth rate increases, myopia may progress rapidly and require frequent changes in the patient's glasses. This excessive lengthening of the eye is often attributable to genetic factors.[3]

Hyperopia

Hyperopia (farsightedness) causes the light rays to focus behind the retina and requires the patient to use accommodation to focus the light rays on the retina for near and far objects. This type of refractive error occurs when the cornea or lens do not have adequate focusing power or when the eyeball is too short.

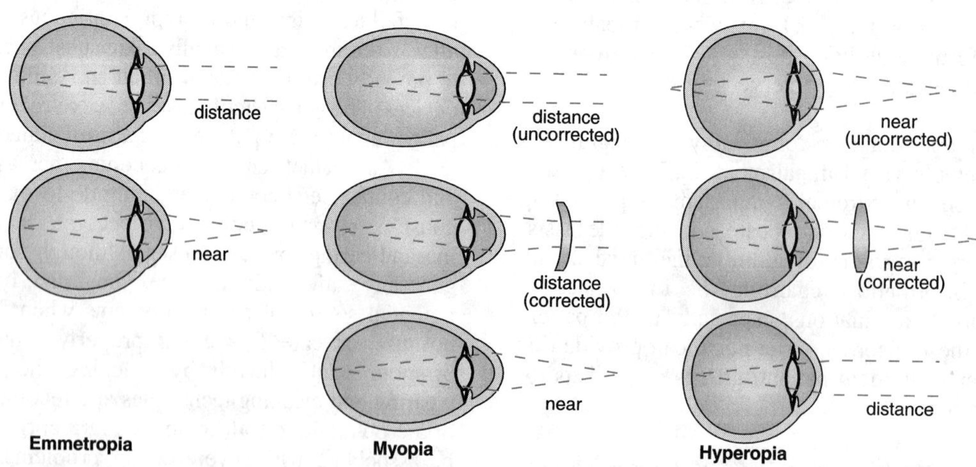

Fig. 18-1 Emmetropic, myopic, and hyperopic eyes with corrected and uncorrected vision.

Table 18-1 Correction of Refractive Errors

Description	Symptoms	Type of Spectacles	Type of Contact Lenses*
Emmetropia Normal vision; light focuses on retina without accommodation for distance vision and with accommodation for near vision	None; vision is normal	Not indicated	Not indicated; some emmetropic patients wear tinted lenses for cosmetic reasons
Myopia Nearsightedness; light focuses in front of retina because eyeball is too long or because cornea or lens have excessive refractive power; light focuses *on* retina with accommodation for near vision	Blurred distance vision; patient may squint in an attempt to improve focus	Concave (minus); lens bends light rays outward	Rigid or soft; daily wear or extended wear
Hyperopia Farsightedness; light focuses behind retina because eyeball is too short or because cornea or lens have inadequate refractive power; light focuses *on* retina for distance vision	Blurred near vision; ocular fatigue from accommodative effort	Convex (plus); lens bends light rays inward	Rigid or soft; daily wear or extended wear
Astigmatism Light focuses at no clear point on the retina because corneal surface is irregularly curved; can occur with any of the above refractive errors	Blurred vision; ocular fatigue	Cylinder; lens bends light rays in different directions to align in a focused point	Rigid or soft toric; daily wear or extended wear
Presbyopia Light does not focus on retina for near vision because the aging crystalline lens can no longer accommodate	Blurred near vision; patient may attempt to obtain clear vision by holding objects further from the eyes	Convex for near vision; can be reading glasses or bifocals with reading correction in lower part of lens	Bifocal rigid or soft; monovision (one eye corrected for distance, one for near)
Aphakia Crystalline lens is absent because of congenital defect, trauma, or surgery (cataract extraction); eye loses approximately 30% of its refractive power	No near vision; if one eye is involved, the retinal image is one third larger than in the normal eye	Thick, convex; almost never used after cataract extraction today because of visual distortion, discomfort from heavy glasses, poor appearance, and superiority of IOL as aphakic correction	Rigid, soft; daily wear or extended wear; not used after cataract extraction in most cases today because of difficulty in handling lenses, complications related to wear, and superiority of IOL as aphakic correction

IOL, Intraocular lens.
*See Table 18-2 for explanation of contact lens types.

Presbyopia

Presbyopia is the loss of accommodation because of age. As the eye ages, the crystalline lens becomes larger, firmer, and less elastic. These changes decrease the eye's accommodative ability. The accommodative ability continues to decline with each decade of life and, by approximately age 70, the accommodative power of the lens declines to zero.[4] When this occurs, the patient cannot focus on near objects without some form of visual aid.

Astigmatism

Astigmatism is caused by an unequal corneal curvature. This irregularity causes the incoming light rays to be bent unequally. Consequently, the light rays do not come to a single point of focus on the retina.

Aphakia

Aphakia is defined as the absence of the crystalline lens. The lens may be absent congenitally, or it may be removed during cataract surgery. A lens that is traumatically dislocated results in functional aphakia, although the lens remains in the eye. Because it accounts for approximately 30% of ocular refractive power, the absence of the lens results in a significant refractive error.[5] Without the focusing ability of the lens, images are projected behind the retina.

Nonsurgical Corrections

Glasses. Myopia, hyperopia, presbyopia, astigmatism, and aphakia can be modified by using the appropriate corrective lens (Table 18-1). Myopia requires a minus corrective lens (concave), whereas hyperopia, presbyopia, and aphakia all require a plus corrective lens (convex). Glasses for presbyopia are often called reading glasses because they are usually worn for close work only. The presbyopic correction may also be combined with a correction for another refractive error, such as myopia or astigmatism. In these combined glasses the presbyopic correction is in the lower portion of bifocal or trifocal glasses. A newer type of correction for presbyopia, the "no-line" bifocal, is actually a multifocal lens that allows the patient to see clearly at any distance.

Aphakic glasses are very thick, making them heavy and unattractive to wear. The high degree of correction also causes images to be magnified about 25%. The glasses can provide good central vision but distort peripheral vision. This magnification and visual distortion is often unacceptable to the aphakic patient. With the modern surgical procedures prevalent today, patients seldom wear aphakic glasses for correction because of the associated visual problems. Astigmatism can occur in conjunction with any of the other refractive errors.

Contact Lenses. Contact lenses are another way to correct refractive errors. Contact lenses generally provide better vision than glasses because the patient has more normal peripheral vision without the distortion and obstruction of the glasses and their frames. Aphakic contact lenses magnify objects only approximately 7% and are visually superior to aphakic glasses.[6] However, many older patients have difficulty handling and caring for contact lenses. Table 18-2 describes the various types of contact lenses and the advantages and disadvantages of each.

Lenses may be either rigid or flexible (soft lenses). Rigid contact lenses ride on the tear film layer of the cornea and are held in place by surface tension. Blinking causes the tear film to move under and over the contact lens providing oxygen for the cornea. If the oxygen supply to the cornea is decreased, it becomes swollen, visual acuity decreases, and the patient experiences severe discomfort.

Because soft contact lenses do not ride on the corneal tear film layer, the cornea cannot receive oxygen from the tear film. Instead, the cornea receives oxygen through the soft contact lens, which is permeable to oxygen. Rigid gas permeable contact lenses also allow oxygen to reach the cornea through the lens itself.

Altered or decreased tear formation can make wearing contact lenses difficult. Tear production can be disturbed by antihistamines, decongestants, diuretics, birth control pills, and the hormones produced by pregnancy. Allergic conjunctivitis can also affect contact lens wear.

In general the nurse needs to know whether the patient wears contact lenses, the frequency of medical supervision, pattern of wear (daily versus extended), and care practices. The patient must remove daily wear lenses each night. The patient with extended wear lenses may generally wear the lenses as long as 1 week before removing them for cleaning, sterilizing, and an overnight period without lens wear. The nurse must be able to identify whether contact lenses are present and should know how to remove them in an emergency situation. Shining a light obliquely on the eyeball can help the nurse visualize a contact lens. If the patient can sit upright, the nurse can remove a rigid contact lens as follows: (1) wash hands with nonoily soap, rinse thoroughly, and dry with a lint-free towel; (2) stand at the patient's side (right side to remove right lens, left side to remove left lens); (3) place index finger of one hand near the lateral canthus; (4) hold the other hand beneath the patient's eye to catch the lens as it falls from the eye; (5) instruct the patient to blink; (6) as the patient blinks, use the index finger at the lateral canthus to gently pull the upper and lower lid tissue outward and slightly upward. The lens will fall into the nurse's hand and should be stored in a case filled with the appropriate solution and labeled with the patient's name. If the patient cannot sit upright, or otherwise cooperate with the procedure, the nurse can remove a hard contact lens with a small suction cup designed for that purpose.

With the patient in any position, the nurse can remove a soft contact lens as follows: (1) wash hands with nonoily soap, rinse thoroughly, and dry with a lint-free towel; (2) stand at the patient's side (right side if right-handed, left side if left-handed); (3) place the middle finger of the dominant hand against the lower eyelid; (4) gently pull the lower eyelid down against the cheekbone; (5) with the thumb and index finger, slide the lens down off the cornea and onto the sclera; (6) bring the thumb and index finger together, gently pinching the lens off the eye. The nurse should store the lens in a case filled with normal saline solution and label the case with the patient's name.

Table 18-2 Types of Contact Lenses

Type	Description	Advantages	Disadvantages	Wearing Schedule
Rigid Lenses				
■ Standard	Rigid plastic; smaller than cornea	Can be tinted for easier visibility out of the eye; longer lasting; least expensive to purchase; corrects all types of refractive errors	Requires separate care solutions for cleaning, storing, wetting; new patients (or those resuming wear after a period of nonwear) must gradually increase wearing time; initially uncomfortable, requires adaptation to obtain adequate comfort level; daily wear only	Daily wear; sleeping in lenses (either inadvertantly or not) can cause corneal edema or severe pain from lack of oxygen
■ Gas permeable	Similar to standard rigid lenses, but plastic allows oxygen to pass through to cornea	Longer lasting than soft lenses; corrects all types of refractive errors; more comfortable initially than standard hard lenses; less adaptation time and fewer problems with corneal edema than standard hard lenses; flexible wearing schedule	Requires separate care solutions for cleaning, storing, wetting; more expensive to purchase	Daily wear or extended wear
Soft Lenses				
■ Standard	Soft, flexible plastic; covers entire cornea and a small rim of sclera	Fits snugly on eye, allowing less invasion of foreign particles under the lens; initially more comfortable and less adaptation time than rigid lenses; can be worn intermittently	Less durable and more expensive than rigid lenses (cost may be similar to gas permeable rigid lenses); more susceptible to surface protein deposition that causes discomfort and vision problems; requires cleaning, sterilizing, and enzymatic removal of protein deposits; cannot correct for higher degrees of astigmatism	Daily wear only; sleeping in these lenses causes similar problems as sleeping in standard rigid lenses

continued

The patient should know the signs and symptoms of contact lens problems that need to be managed by the eye care professional. The patient may remember these symptoms better if the nurse uses the mnemonic device ***RSVP*** for ***Redness, Sensitivity, Vision*** problems, and ***Pain.*** The nurse must stress the importance of removing contact lenses *immediately* if any of these problems occur.

Surgical Corrections

Keratorefractive Surgery and Photorefractive Keratectomy. Keratorefractive surgery (surgery to alter the corneal curvature) is a new method of refractive correction that remains controversial. This surgical category includes a variety of procedures including those in which the surgeon either (1) makes cuts in the cornea, (2) removes some corneal tissue, or (3) does a graft to replace or add corneal tissue. Myopia is the refractive error most commonly corrected by keratorefractive surgery because it can be corrected by *radial keratotomy*, a relatively noninvasive technique when compared with other more complicated procedures. In radial keratotomy the surgeon makes radial incisions in the patient's cornea, leaving an uncut optical zone in the center. Although 88% of eyes in one prospective study had uncorrected visual acuities greater than or equal to 20/40,[7] there remains a real risk of serious complications such as operative infection and corneal scarring that the patient must evaluate when considering this procedure.[2,8]

Table 18-2 Types of Contact Lenses—cont'd

Type	Description	Advantages	Disadvantages	Wearing Schedule
▪ High water content	Similar to standard soft lenses, but with a higher water content	Similar to standard soft lenses; allow more oxygen through lens so lens can be worn up to a week at a time without removal	Similar to standard soft lenses (with the exception that these can be extended wear); greater risk of complications related to contact lens wear than with daily wear lenses	Daily wear or extended wear
▪ Toric	Similar to other soft lenses; special design to correct astigmatism	Similar to other soft lenses; can be custom ordered to correct patient's individual type of astigmatism	Similar to other soft lenses; more expensive than other types of lenses; can be more difficult to fit than nontoric soft lenses	Daily wear or extended wear
▪ Disposable	Similar to other soft lenses but thinner	Similar to other soft lenses; frequent replacement decreases risk of complications related to contact lens wear	Similar to other soft lenses; cost may be greater (can be similar, depending on prevalent charges for replacement lenses)	Daily wear or extended wear; each lens can be worn as long as 2 wk before disposal
▪ Daily disposable	Similar to disposable	Similar to other soft lenses; daily disposal decreases risk of complications; good for patient who wears lenses only occasionally; no cleaning or disinfection necessary	Greater expense	Daily wear only; each lens is worn for 1 day and then discarded

Photorefractive keratectomy is another procedure that uses an excimer laser to reshape the corneal surface, primarily to correct myopia. There is some evidence that this will be more predictable than radial keratotomy, but today it is still an investigational procedure.[9]

Intraocular Lens Implantation. The most common reason for aphakia is surgical removal of the lens during cataract extraction. In the past, the aphakic patient had to use either aphakic spectacles or, more recently, contact lenses for aphakic correction. However, the most common method of correction today is the surgical implantation of an *intraocular lens* (IOL), usually at the time of the initial cataract extraction. The IOL is a small plastic lens that can be implanted either in the anterior or posterior chamber and provides very little optical distortion, especially compared with aphakic spectacles or even aphakic contact lenses. The type of IOL implanted depends on the cataract extraction technique and the surgeon's preference, but currently most IOLs are placed in the posterior chamber.

UNCORRECTABLE VISUAL IMPAIRMENT

The patient with correctable errors of vision is not functionally impaired. When no correction is possible, the patient's visual impairment may be moderate or profound.

Significance

Approximately 4.8 million people in the United States have severe visual impairment, which is defined as the inability to read newsprint even with glasses. Of those individuals, only 9% have no useful vision, and the remaining 91% are considered partially sighted. The partially sighted individual may have significant visual abilities. Although visual acuity less than 20/50 is often considered a visual impairment, some states require only 20/70 visual acuity to obtain a commercial driver's license.[10] It is important in working with the visually impaired patient to understand that a person classified as blind may have useful vision. Appropriate responses and interventions are dependent on the nurse's understanding of each patient's visual abilities.

Levels of Visual Impairment

The patient may be categorized by the level of visual loss.[11] *Total blindness* is defined as no light perception and no usable vision. *Functional blindness* is present when the patient has some light perception but no usable vision. The patient with total or functional blindness is considered legally blind and may use vision substitutes such as guide dogs and canes for ambulation and Braille for reading. Vision enhancement techniques are not helpful.

Table 18-3 Definition of Legal Blindness in the United States

- Central visual acuity for distance of 20/200 or worse in the better eye (with correction)
- Visual field no greater than 20° in its widest diameter or in the better eye

The *legally blind* individual meets the criteria developed by the federal government to determine eligibility for federal and state assistance and income tax benefits (Table 18-3). The legally blind individual has some usable vision. The *partially sighted* individual who is not legally blind has a corrected visual acuity greater than 20/200 in the better eye and greater than 20 degrees of visual field, but the visual acuity is 20/50 or worse in the better eye. The patient who is partially or legally blind can benefit greatly from vision enhancement techniques.

NURSING MANAGEMENT

SEVERE VISUAL IMPAIRMENT

Nursing Assessment

It is important to determine how long the patient has had a visual impairment because recent loss of vision has different implications for nursing care. The nurse should determine how the patient's visual impairment affects normal functioning. This may be done by questioning the patient about the level of difficulty encountered when doing certain tasks. For example, the nurse may ask how much difficulty the patient has when reading a newspaper, writing a check, moving from one room to the next, or viewing television. Other questions will help the nurse determine the personal meaning that the patient attaches to the visual impairment. The nurse can ask how the vision loss has affected specific aspects of the patient's life, whether the patient has lost a job, or what activities the patient does not engage in because of the visual impairment. The patient may attach many negative meanings to the impairment because of societal views of blindness. For example, the patient may view the impairments as punishment, or view himself as useless and burdensome. It is also important to determine the patient's primary coping strategies, emotional reactions, and the availability and strength of the patient's support systems.

Nursing Diagnoses

Specific nursing diagnoses depend upon the degree of visual impairment and how long it has been present. General nursing diagnoses for the visually impaired patient include, but are not limited to, the following:

- Sensory-perceptual alteration related to visual deficit
- Risk for injury related to visual impairment and inability to see potential dangers
- Self-care deficit related to visual impairment
- Fear related to inability to see potential danger or accurately interpret environment
- Grieving related to loss of functional vision
- Self-esteem disturbance related to loss of visual function and self-sufficiency
- Risk for impaired social interactions related to visual deficits
- Risk for diversional activity deficit related to inability to perform usual activities
- Risk for social isolation related to increased difficulty in sustaining previous relationships

Planning

The overall goals are that the patient with recently impaired vision, or the patient with unsuccessful adjustment to longstanding visual impairment, will (1) make a successful adjustment to the impairment, (2) verbalize feelings related to the loss, (3) identify personal strengths and external support systems, and (4) use appropriate coping strategies. If the patient has been functioning at an appropriate or acceptable level, the goal of the patient is to maintain the current level of function.

Nursing Implementation

Health Maintenance and Promotion. The nurse should encourage the partially sighted patient with preventable causes for further impairment to seek appropriate health care. For example, the patient with vision loss from diabetic retinopathy or glaucoma may prevent further visual impairment by complying with prescribed therapies and suggested ophthalmic evaluations.

Acute Intervention. The nurse provides emotional support and direct care to the patient with recent visual impairment. Active listening and grief work facilitation are important components of nursing care for the recently visually impaired patient. The nurse should allow the patient to express anger and grief and should help the patient identify fears and successful coping strategies. The family is intimately involved in the experiences that follow visual loss. With the patient's knowledge and permission, the nurse should include family members in discussions and encourage members to express their concerns.

Many are uncomfortable around the blind or partially sighted individual because people are not sure what behaviors are appropriate. The nurse is responsible for knowing what is appropriate so that the patient does not become uncomfortable in the nurse's presence. Sensitivity to the patient's feelings without being overly solicitous or stifling the patient's independence is vital in creating a therapeutic nursing presence. The nurse should always communicate in a normal conversational tone and manner with the patient, and the nurse should address the patient, not a family member or friend that may be with the patient. Common courtesy dictates introducing oneself and any other persons who approach the blind or partially sighted patient and saying goodbye upon leaving. Making eye contact with the partially sighted patient accomplishes several objectives. It ensures that the nurse speaks while facing the patient so the patient has no difficulty hearing the nurse. The nurse's head position validates that the nurse is attentive to the patient. Also, establishing eye contact ensures that the nurse will perceive the patient's facial or movement cues about reactions and responses.

The nurse should explain any activities or noises occurring in the patient's immediate surroundings. Orientation to the environment lessens the patient's anxiety or discomfort and facilitates independence. In orienting the partially sighted or blind patient to a new area, the nurse should identify one object as the focal point and describe the location of other objects in relation to it. For example the nurse may say, "The bed is straight ahead, approximately 10 steps. The chair is to the left, and the nightstand is to the right, near the head of the bed. The bathroom is to the left of the foot of the bed."

The nurse should assist the patient to each major object in the area, using the sighted-guide technique. When using this technique, the nurse stands slightly in front and to one side of the patient and offers an elbow for the patient to hold. The nurse serves as the sighted guide, walking slightly ahead of the patient with the patient holding the back of the nurse's arm (Fig. 18-2). When using this technique in any situation, the nurse should describe the environment to help orient the patient. For example the nurse may say, "We're going through an open doorway and approaching 2 steps down. There's an obstacle on the left." To assist the patient to sit, place one of his hands on the back of the chair.

When the partially sighted or blind patient places an object in a certain position, it should not be moved without the knowledge and consent of the patient. Objects on a table or food tray can be described in terms of the hours on a clock face. For example the nurse may say, "Your book is at the 12 o'clock position, and your magnifier is at the 3 o'clock position," or "The eggs are at the 9 o'clock position, bacon at the 3 o'clock position, and toast at the 12 o'clock position." If the nurse is uncertain about providing help, it is perfectly appropriate to ask the patient if assistance is needed and, if so, how to provide it.

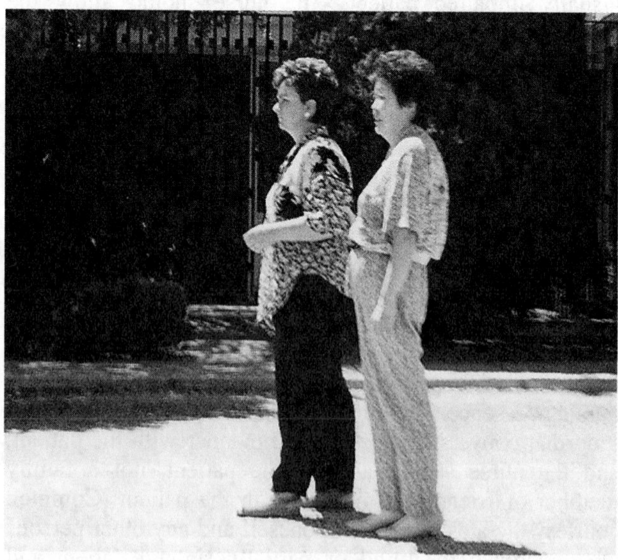

Fig. 18-2 Sighted-guide technique. The nurse serves as the sighted guide, walking slightly ahead of the patient with the patient holding the back of the nurse's arm.

Chronic and Home Management. Rehabilitation after partial or total loss of vision can foster independence, self-esteem, and productivity. The nurse should know what services and devices are available for the partially sighted or blind patient and be prepared to make appropriate referrals for those services and devices. For the legally blind patient, the primary resource for services is the state agency for rehabilitation of the blind.[12] A list of agencies that serves the partially sighted or blind patient is available from the American Foundation for the Blind, 15 West 16th Street, New York, NY 10011. Many of these agencies are listed in the bibliography section.

Braille or talking books for reading and a cane or guide dog for ambulation are examples of vision substitution techniques. These are usually most appropriate for the patient with no functional vision. For most patients who have some remaining vision, vision enhancement techniques can provide enough help for many patients to learn to ambulate, read printed material, and accomplish activities of daily living (ADLs).

Optical devices for vision enhancement. *Telescopic lenses* for near or far vision and *magnifiers* of various types can often enhance the patient's remaining vision enough to allow the performance of many previously impossible tasks and activities. Most of these devices require some training and practice for successful use. Closed circuit television can provide up to 60× magnification, allowing some patients to read, write, use computers, and do crafts. Although these systems are expensive and have limited portability, they are available in some public or university libraries.

Nonoptical methods for vision enhancement. *Approach magnification* is a simple but sometimes overlooked technique for enhancing the patient's residual vision. The nurse can recommend that the patient sit closer to the television or hold books closer to the eyes, which the patient may be reluctant to do unless encouraged. *Contrast enhancement* techniques include watching television in black and white, placing dark objects against a light background (e.g., a white plate on a black place mat), using a black felt-tip marker, and using contrasting colors (e.g., a red stripe at the edge of steps or curbs). *Increased lighting* can be provided by halogen lamps, direct sunlight, or gooseneck lamps that can be aimed directly at the reading material or other near objects. *Large type* is often helpful, especially in conjunction with other optical or nonoptical vision enhancements.

Gerontologic Considerations

The elderly patient is at an increased risk for vision loss because cataracts, glaucoma, diabetic retinopathy, macular degeneration, and other potential causes of visual impairment are more common in the older patient. The older patient may have other deficits such as cognitive impairment or limited mobility, which further impact the ability to function in usual ways. Societal devaluation of the elderly may compound the self-esteem or isolation issues associated with the older patient's visual impairment. Financial resources may meet normal needs but can be inadequate in meeting increased demands of vision services or devices.

TRAUMA

Although the eyes are well protected by the bony orbit and by fat pads, everyday activities can result in ocular trauma. Ocular injuries can involve the ocular adnexa, the superficial structures, or the deeper ocular structures. In the United States an estimated 1.3 million eye injuries occur each year. Of these injuries, 40,000 result in permanent visual impairment.[4] Table 18-4 outlines emergency management of the patient with an eye injury. Types of ocular trauma include blunt injuries, penetrating injuries, or chemical exposure injuries. Causes of ocular injuries include automobile accidents, accidental occurrences such as falls, sports and leisure activities, assaults, or work-related situations. The patient with major trauma and concurrent ocular trauma often has elevated blood alcohol levels.[13]

Trauma is often a preventable cause of visual impairment. The nurse's role in individual and community education is extremely important in reducing the incidence of ocular trauma.

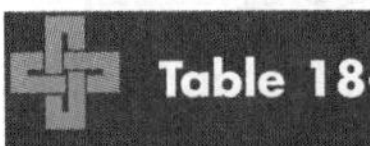

Table 18-4 Emergency Management: Eye Injury

Possible Etiologies

Foreign bodies (glass, metal, wood), blunt or penetrating trauma, chemical or thermal burns

Possible Assessment Findings

- Pain
- Photophobia
- Visible foreign body
- Redness, swelling, ecchymosis
- Tearing
- Absent eye movements
- Fluid drainage from eye: blood, CSF, aqueous humor
- Abnormal or decreased vision

Management

- Determine mechanism of injury.
- Assess patient for associated systemic injuries (airway, breathing, circulation).
- Begin ocular irrigation *immediately* in the case of chemical exposure; do not stop until emergency personnel arrive to continue irrigation; sterile, pH-balanced, physiologic solution is best, but, if unavailable, use any nontoxic liquid.
- Do not attempt to treat the injury (except as noted above for chemical exposure).
- Do not put medication or solutions in the eye.
- Do not put pressure on the eye.
- Cover the eye(s) with dry, sterile patches and a protective shield.
- Do not give the patient any food or fluids.

CSF, Cerebrospinal fluid.

EXTRAOCULAR DISORDERS

Inflammation and Infection

One of the most common conditions encountered by the ophthalmologist is inflammation or infection of the external eye. Many external irritants or microorganisms affect the lids and conjunctiva and can involve the avascular cornea. It is a nursing responsibility to teach the patient appropriate interventions related to the specific disorder.

Hordeolum. A hordeolum (commonly called a sty) is an infection of the sebaceous glands in the lid margin. The most common bacterial infective agent is *Staphylococcus aureus*.[14] A red, swollen, circumscribed, and acutely tender area develops rapidly. The nurse should instruct the patient to apply warm, moist compresses at least four times a day until the abscess drains. This may be the only treatment necessary. If there is a tendency for recurrence, the patient should perform lid scrubs daily. In addition, appropriate antibiotic ointments or drops may be indicated.

Chalazion. A chalazion is an inflammation of a sebaceous gland in the lids. It may evolve from a hordeolum or may occur as a primary inflammatory response to the material released into the lid tissue when a blocked gland ruptures. The chalazion appears as a swollen, nonpainful, reddened area, usually on the upper lid. Initial treatment is similar to that for a hordeolum. If warm, moist compresses are ineffective in causing spontaneous drainage, the ophthalmologist may surgically remove the chronic lesion (this is normally an office procedure), or the ophthalmologist may inject the chronic lesion with steroids.

Blepharitis. Blepharitis is a common chronic bilateral inflammation of the lid margins. The lids are red rimmed with many scales or crusts on the lid margins and lashes. The patient may primarily complain of itching but may also experience burning, irritation, and photophobia. Conjunctivitis may occur simultaneously.

If the blepharitis is caused by a staphylococcal infection, therapeutic management includes the use of an appropriate ophthalmic antibiotic ointment. Seborrheic blepharitis, related to seborrhea of the scalp and eyebrows, is treated with an antiseborrheic shampoo for the scalp and eyebrows. Often blepharitis is caused by both staphylococcal and seborrheal microorganisms, and the treatment must be more vigorous to avoid hordeolum, keratitis (inflammation of the cornea), and other eye infections. Conscientious hygienic practices involving skin and scalp need to be emphasized. Gentle cleansing of the lid margins with baby shampoo can effectively soften and remove crusting.

Conjunctivitis. Conjunctivitis is an infection or inflammation of the conjunctiva. Conjunctival infections may be caused by bacterial, viral, or chlamydial microorganisms. Conjunctival inflammation may result from exposure to allergens or chemical irritants (including cigarette smoke). The tarsal conjunctiva (lining the interior surface of the lids) may become inflamed as a result of a chronic foreign body in the eye, such as a contact lens or an ocular prosthesis.

Bacterial infections. Acute bacterial conjunctivitis (pinkeye) is a common infection. Although it occurs in every age group, epidemics commonly occur in children because of their poor hygienic habits. In adults and children the most common causative microorganism is *Staphylococcus aureus. Streptococcus pneumoniae* and *Haemophilus influenzae* are other common causative agents, but they are seen more often in children than adults. The patient with bacterial conjunctivitis may complain of irritation, tearing, redness, and a mucopurulent drainage. Although this typically occurs initially in one eye, it spreads rapidly to the unaffected eye. It is usually self-limiting, but treatment with antibiotic drops will shorten the course of the disorder. Careful handwashing and using individual or disposable towels will help prevent spreading the condition.

Viral infections. Conjunctival infections may be caused by many different viruses. The patient with *viral conjunctivitis* may complain of tearing, foreign body sensation, redness, and mild photophobia. Unless other ocular structures become involved, this condition is usually mild and self-limiting. However, it can be severe with increased discomfort, subconjunctival hemorrhaging, or formation of *symblepharon* (adhesions between the bulbar and palpebral conjunctiva). Adenovirus conjunctivitis may be contracted in contaminated swimming pools and through direct contact with an infected patient.[15] Good hygiene practices will decrease spread of the virus. Treatment is usually palliative. If the patient is severely symptomatic, topical steroids provide temporary relief but have no benefit in the final outcome. Antiviral drops are ineffective and therefore not indicated.

Chlamydial infections. Adult inclusion conjunctivitis (AIC) is caused by the oculogenital type of *Chlamydia trachomatis*. It is becoming more prevalent in the United States because of the increase in sexually transmitted chlamydial disease.[16] The patient complains of a mucopurulent ocular discharge, irritation, redness, and lid swelling. Systemic symptoms may be present as well. For unknown reasons, this type of chlamydial infection does not carry the long-term consequences of *trachoma* (a sight-threatening keratoconjunctivitis caused by a different type of the *Chlamydia trachomatis* bacteria). It also differs in that it is common in economically developed countries, whereas trachoma is rarely seen except in underdeveloped countries. The more benign nature of AIC may be related to lack of reexposure to the microorganism, the age of the patient at initial exposure, or a lower degree of pathogenicity of the oculogenital organism.[17]

Although topical treatment may be successful in the adult with chlamydial conjunctivitis, these patients have a high risk of concurrent chlamydial genital infection, as well as other sexually transmitted diseases. Consequently, all patients should be referred for further evaluation and systemic antibiotic therapy. The nurse's responsibility with the patient with chlamydial conjunctivitis includes education about the ocular condition, as well as the sexual implications of the condition.

Allergic conjunctivitis. Conjunctivitis caused by exposure to some allergen can be mild and transitory or severe enough to cause significant swelling, sometimes ballooning the conjunctiva beyond the eyelids. The defining symptom of allergic conjunctivitis is itching. The patient may also complain of burning, redness, and tearing. Acutely, the patient may also have white or clear exudate. If the condition is chronic, the exudate is thicker and becomes mucopurulent. In addition to pollens, the patient may develop allergic conjunctivitis in response to animal dander, ocular solutions and medications, or even contact lenses. The nurse should instruct the patient to avoid the allergen if it is known. Artificial tears can be effective in diluting the allergen and washing it from the eye. Effective topical medications include antihistamines, cromolyn, and steroids.

Keratitis. Keratitis is an inflammation or infection of the cornea that can be caused by a variety of microorganisms or by other factors. The condition may involve the conjunctiva and the cornea. When it involves both, the disorder is *keratoconjunctivitis*.

Bacterial infections. The intact cornea provides an effective defense against infection. However, when the epithelial layer is disrupted, the cornea can become infected by a variety of bacteria. The infected cornea can develop an ulcer with a mucopurulent exudate adherent to the ulcer. Topical antibiotics will generally be effective, but eradicating the infection may require subconjunctival antibiotic injection or, in severe cases, intravenous (IV) antibiotics. Risk factors include mechanical or chemical corneal epithelial damage, soft contact lens wear (particularly with extended wear), debilitation, nutritional deficiencies, immunosuppressed states, and contaminated products (e.g., lens care solutions and cases, topical medications, and cosmetics).[18]

Viral infections. Herpes simplex virus (HSV) keratitis is the most frequently occurring infectious cause of corneal blindness in the Western hemisphere.[15] It is a growing problem, especially with immunosuppressed patients. It may be caused by HSV-1 or HSV-2 (genital herpes), although HSV-2 ocular infection is much less common. The resulting corneal ulcer has a characteristic dendritic (tree-branching) appearance, and it is often, although not always, preceded by infection of the conjunctiva or eyelids. Pain and photophobia are common. Up to 40% of patients with herpetic keratitis will heal spontaneously. The spontaneous healing rate increases to 70% if the cornea is debrided to remove infected cells. Therapeutic management includes corneal debridement followed by topical therapy with idoxuridine drops or ointment (Stoxil, Herplex, IDU) for 2 to 3 weeks. Corticosteroids are contraindicated because they contribute to a longer course, possible deeper ulceration of the cornea, and systemic complications. If the ulcer is not responsive to idoxuridine within 1 to 2 weeks, vidarabine (Vira-A) or trifluorothymidine (Viroptic) may be used topically. Pharmacologic therapy may also include acyclovir (Zovirax). Recurrent dendritic keratitis may be a problem.

The varicella-zoster virus (VZV) causes both chickenpox and *herpes zoster ophthalmicus* (HZO). HZO may occur by reactivation of an endogenous infection that has persisted in latent form after an earlier attack of varicella or by direct or indirect contact with a patient with chickenpox or herpes zoster. It occurs most frequently in the older adult and in the immunosuppressed patient. Therapeutic management of acute HZO may include narcotic or nonnarcotic analgesics for the pain, topical corticosteroids to reduce the inflammatory process, antiviral agents such as acyclovir (Zovirax) to reduce viral replication, mydriatic agents to dilate the pupil and relieve pain, and topical antibiotics to combat secondary infection. The patient may apply warm compresses and povidone-iodine gel to the affected skin (gel should not be applied near the eye).

Epidemic keratoconjunctivitis (EKC) is the most serious ocular adenoviral disease. EKC is spread by direct contact, including sexual activity. In the medical setting, contaminated hands and instruments can be the source of spread. The patient may complain of tearing, redness, photophobia, and foreign body sensation. In most patients, the disease involves only one eye. Treatment is primarily palliative and includes ice packs and dark glasses. In severe cases, therapy can include mild topical steroids to temporarily relieve symptoms and topical antibiotic ointment to lubricate the cornea when membranes are present.[15] The nurse's most important role is to educate the patient and family members regarding good hygienic practices to avoid spreading the disease.

Chlamydial infections. Trachoma is a severe keratoconjunctivitis caused by a variety of the *Chlamydia trachomatis* organism. It is the most common ocular disease in the world, affecting 500 million persons and often leading to blindness from corneal scarring.[16] Trachoma is especially prevalent in the Middle East, Africa, India, Southeast Asia, and South America, but it affects only isolated groups in the Southwestern United States. Transmission of the disease is through contact with contaminated hands, bedding, linens, and eye-seeking flies. Treatment with topical and systemic antibiotics is effective but difficult to provide in the developing countries most afflicted with the disease. It is a preventable cause of blindness, requiring better sanitation and health delivery systems, as well as improved education.

Other causes of keratitis. Keratitis may also be caused by fungi (most commonly by the *Aspergillus, Candida,* and *Fusarium* species), especially in the case of ocular trauma in an outdoor setting where fungi are prevalent in the soil and moist organic matter. *Acanthamoeba* keratitis is caused by a parasite that is associated with contact lens wear, probably as a result of contaminated lens care solutions or cases. Homemade saline solution is particularly vulnerable to *Acanthamoeba* contamination. The nurse should instruct the patient who wears contact lenses about good lens care practices. Medical treatment of fungal and *Acanthamoeba* keratitis is difficult. Only one antifungal eye drop (natamycin) is approved by the Food and Drug Administration (FDA), and the *Acanthamoeba* organism is resistant to most drugs. If antimicrobial therapy fails, the patient may require a corneal transplant.

Exposure keratitis occurs when the patient cannot adequately close the eyelids. The patient with *exophthalmos* (protruding eyeball) from thyroid eye disease or masses posterior to the globe is susceptible to exposure keratitis.

NURSING MANAGEMENT

INFLAMMATION AND INFECTION OF THE EYES

Nursing Assessment

The nurse should assess ocular changes such as edema, redness, decreasing visual acuity, or discomfort, and document the findings in the patient's record. The nurse's assessment should also consider the psychosocial aspects of the patient's condition, especially when the patient has visual impairment associated with the condition.

Nursing Diagnoses

Nursing diagnoses specific to the patient with inflammation or infection of the external eye include, but are not limited to, the following:

- Pain related to irritation or infection of the external eye
- Anxiety related to uncertainty of cause of disease and outcome of treatment
- Sensory-perceptual alteration: visual related to diminished or absent vision

Planning

The overall goals are that the patient with inflammation or infection of the external eye will (1) maintain or improve visual acuity, (2) maintain an acceptable level of comfort and functioning during the course of the specific ocular problem, (3) avoid spread of infection, (4) promote appropriate health-seeking behaviors, and (5) comply with the prescribed therapy.

Nursing Implementation

Health Maintenance and Promotion. Careful asepsis and frequent, thorough hand washing are essential to prevent spreading organisms from one eye to the other, to other patients, to family members, and to the nurse. The nurse should dispose of any contaminated dressings in a proper waste container. The patient and family need information about avoiding sources of ocular irritation or infection and responding appropriately if an ocular problem occurs. The patient with infective disorders that may have a sexual mode of transmission or an associated sexually transmitted disease (STD) needs specific information about those disorders. The patient with contact lenses often does not comply with care regimens. The patient needs information about appropriate use and care of lenses and lens care products. The nurse should encourage the patient to follow the recommended regimens.

Acute Intervention. The nurse may apply warm or cool compresses if indicated for the patient's condition. Darkening the room and providing an appropriate analgesic are other comfort measures. If the patient's visual acuity is decreased, the nurse may need to modify the patient's environment or activities for safety.

The patient may require eye drops as frequently as every hour. If the patient receives two or more different drops, the nurse should stagger the eye drops to promote maximum absorption. For example, if two different eye drops are ordered hourly, the nurse should administer one drop on the hour and one drop on the half hour. This staggered schedule promotes maximum absorption.

The patient who needs frequent eye-drop administration may experience sleep deprivation. Common symptoms include short attention span, irritability, confusion, and disorientation. Grouping necessary activities together and allowing periods of rest, in addition to providing a quiet environment, may be beneficial. The sleep-deprived patient may recognize abnormal behavior and be concerned or embarrassed. The nurse should reassure the patient that this behavior change is a normal consequence of lack of sleep.

Chronic and Home Management. The patient's primary need in the home environment is for information about required care and how to accomplish that care. The nurse should provide the patient and family with information about proper hygiene techniques to prevent contamination or limit spread of infectious disorders. The patient and family also need information about proper techniques for medication administration. If the patient's vision is compromised, the nurse should provide suggestions for alternative ways to accomplish necessary daily activities and self-care. The patient who wears contact lenses and develops infections should discard all opened or used lens care products and cosmetics to decrease the risk of reinfection from contaminated products (a common problem and probable source of infection for many patients).

Gerontologic Considerations

The older patient may become confused or disoriented when visually compromised. The combination of decreased vision and confusion increases the risk of falls, which have potentially serious consequences for the older adult. Decreased vision may also compromise the older patient's abilities to function, increasing concerns about maintaining independence and affecting the self-image. Decreased manual dexterity may make the instillation of prescribed eye drops difficult for some older adults.

Dry Eye Disorders

Complaints of *dry eye* are caused by a variety of ocular disorders characterized by decreased tear secretion or increased tear film evaporation. *Keratoconjunctivitis sicca* is caused by lacrimal gland dysfunction from an autoimmune mechanism. If the patient with keratoconjunctivitis sicca has associated dry mouth, the patient has *primary Sjögren's syndrome*. If the patient has associated rheumatoid arthritis, scleroderma, or systemic lupus erythematosus, the patient has *secondary Sjögren's syndrome*. Meibomian gland dysfunction leads to a lipid deficiency in the tear film and subsequent increased rate of tear film evaporation. Increased palpebral fissure width (e.g., in thyroid eye disease) also results in increased tear film evaporation. The patient complains of a sandy-gritty sensation that typically worsens during the day and is better in the morning after eye closure with sleep. Treatment is directed at the underlying cause. With meibomian gland dysfunction, hot compresses and lid margin massage help express lipid into the tear film. With decreased tear secretion, the patient may use artificial tears or ointments but should avoid preserved products and use them sparingly because preservatives in the drops or overuse can cause further ocular irritation. In severe cases the ophthalmologist may temporarily or permanently surgically occlude the puncta, effectively providing the ocular surface with more available tears.

Strabismus

Strabismus is a condition in which the patient cannot consistently focus 2 eyes simultaneously on the same object. One eye may deviate in (*esotropia*), out (*exotropia*), up (*hypertropia*), or down (*hypotropia*). Strabismus in the adult may be caused by thyroid disease, neuromuscular problems of the eye muscles, entrapment of the extraocular muscles in orbital floor fractures, retinal detachment repair, or cerebral lesions. In the adult the primary complaint with strabismus is double vision.

Corneal Disorders

Corneal Scars and Opacities. The cornea is an optically transparent tissue that allows light rays to enter the eye and focus on the retina, thus producing a visual image. Any corneal wound causes the stroma to become abnormally hydrated and decreases the normal transparency. If a corneal defect does not heal in a normal, rapid fashion, persistent stromal edema may lead to corneal irregularity or scarring.[19] Corneal scars and the resulting opacities may occur as a complication of ulcerative keratitis, after ocular trauma from lacerations or chemical injuries, or as a complication of keratorefractive surgery. Opacities may also be congenital or associated with congenital glaucoma. Many of the corneal dystrophies disturb the normal transmission of light through the cornea as well. A rigid contact lens can be effective in correcting the irregular astigmatism that results from corneal scars. In other situations the treatment for corneal scars or opacities is *penetrating keratoplasty* (corneal transplant). In penetrating keratoplasty the ophthalmic surgeon removes the full thickness of the patient's cornea and replaces it with a donor cornea or "button" that is sutured into place. Although corneal problems leading to blindness are uncommon, a corneal transplant can restore vision that otherwise would be lost. Approximately 40,000 transplants are performed in the United States each year.

The time between the donor's death and the removal of the tissue should be as short as possible. Most surgeons prefer this interval to be 8 hours or less, but some eye banks provide donor eyes that have remained in the donor for as long as 18 hours.[20] The eye banks test donors for human immunodeficiency virus (HIV) and hepatitis A, B, and C. The tissue is preserved in a special nutritive solution, and it can be kept for a week or longer in the storage media. Improved methods of tissue procurement and preservation, refined surgical techniques, postoperative topical corticosteroids, and careful follow-up have decreased graft rejection. The nurse plays an important role in promoting tissue donation through education of the individual and the community, as well as by functioning in defined tissue-procurement procedures.

Keratoconus. Keratoconus is a bilateral degenerative disease that is familial but has no exclusive inheritance pattern. It can be associated with Down syndrome, atopic dermatitis, Marfan syndrome, aniridia (congenital absence of the iris), and retinitis pigmentosa (hereditary disease characterized by bilateral primary degeneration of the retina beginning in childhood and progressing to blindness by middle age).

The anterior cornea thins and protrudes forward, taking on a cone shape. Keratoconus appears during adolescence and slowly progresses between the ages of 20 and 60. The only symptom is blurred vision caused by the variable astigmatism associated with the altered corneal shape. The astigmatism may be corrected with glasses or rigid contact lenses. The cornea can perforate as central corneal thinning progresses. Penetrating keratoplasty is indicated before perforation in advanced cases.

INTRAOCULAR DISORDERS

Cataract

A *cataract* is an opacity within the crystalline lens. The patient may have a cataract in one or both eyes. If present in both eyes, one cataract may affect the patient's vision more than the other.

Significance. Cataracts are the third leading cause of preventable blindness and the most common cause of self-declared visual disability in the United States. Approximately 50% of Americans between the ages of 65 and 74 have some degree of cataract formation, and for those older than 75, the incidence increases to approximately 70%. Cataract removal is the most common surgical procedure for Americans older than 65, with U.S. surgeons performing approximately 1.25 million cataract extractions in 1988.[21] Congenital cataracts are relatively common, occurring in 1 of every 250 newborns (0.4%).[22]

Etiology and Pathophysiology. Although most cataracts are age-related (*senile cataracts*), they can be associated with other factors. These include blunt or penetrating trauma; congenital factors, such as maternal rubella; radiation or ultraviolet (UV) light exposure; certain drugs such as systemic corticosteroids or long-term topical steroids; and ocular inflammation. The patient with diabetes mellitus tends to develop cataracts at a younger age than does the patient in the nondiabetic population.

Cataract development is mediated by a number of factors. In senile cataract formation, it appears that altered metabolic processes within the lens cause an accumulation of water and alterations in the lens fiber structure. These changes affect lens transparency, causing vision changes.

Clinical Manifestations. The patient with cataracts may complain of a decrease in vision, abnormal color perception, and glare. Glare is due to light scatter caused by the lens opacities, and it may be significantly worse at night when the pupil dilates. The visual decline is gradual, but the rate of cataract development varies from patient to patient. Some patients may complain of a sudden loss of vision because they inadvertently cover their unaffected eye, and

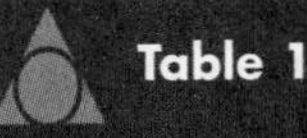

Table 18-5 Therapeutic Management: Cataract

Diagnostic
- Visual acuity measurement
- Ophthalmoscopy (direct and indirect)
- Slit lamp microscopy
- Glare testing, potential acuity testing in selected patients
- Keratometry and A-scan ultrasound (if surgery is planned)
- Other tests may be indicated to differentiate visual loss of cataract from visual loss of other causes (e.g., visual field perimetry)

Therapeutic

Nonsurgical management
- Change prescription of glasses
- Strong reading glasses or magnifiers
- Increased lighting
- Lifestyle adjustment
- Reassurance

Preoperative
- Mydriatic, cycloplegic agents
- Nonsteroidal antiinflammatory drugs
- Topical antibiotics
- Antianxiety medications

Surgery
- Removal of lens
  - Phacoemulsification
  - Extracapsular extraction
  - Intracapsular extraction (technique used much less frequently today)
- Correction of surgical aphakia
  - Intraocular lens implantation (most frequent type of correction)
  - Contact lens
  - Aphakic spectacles (rarely used)

Postoperative
- Topical antibiotic
- Topical steroid or other antiinflammatory agent
- Mild analgesia if necessary
- Eye shield and activity as preferred by patient's surgeon

the decreased acuity of the eye with cataracts becomes "suddenly" apparent. Secondary glaucoma can also occur if the enlarging lens causes increased intraocular pressure.

Diagnostic Studies. Diagnosis is based on decreased visual acuity or other complaints of visual dysfunction. The opacity is directly observable by ophthalmoscopic or slit lamp microscopic examination. As noted earlier, a totally opaque lens creates the appearance of a white pupil. Table 18-5 outlines other diagnostic studies that may be helpful in evaluating the visual impact of a cataract.

Therapeutic Management. The presence of a cataract does not necessarily indicate a need for surgery. For many patients the diagnosis is made long before they actually decide to have surgery. Other therapy may postpone or even negate the need for surgery.

Nonsurgical management. Currently, there is no available treatment to "cure" cataracts other than surgical removal. If the cataract is not removed, the patient's vision will continue to deteriorate. However, palliative measures alone may help the patient. Often, changing the patient's glasses prescription can improve the level of visual acuity, at least temporarily. Other visual aids, such as strong reading glasses or magnifiers of some type, may help the patient with close vision. Increasing the amount of light to read or accomplish other near vision tasks is another useful measure. The patient may be willing to adjust lifestyle to accommodate for visual decline. For example, if glare makes it difficult to drive at night, a patient may elect to drive only during daylight hours or to have a family member drive at night. Sometimes informing and reassuring the patient about the disease process makes the patient comfortable about choosing nonsurgical measures, at least temporarily.

Surgical management. When palliative measures no longer provide an acceptable level of visual function, the patient is an appropriate candidate for surgery. In some instances factors other than the patient's visual needs may influence the need for surgery. Lens-induced problems such as increased intraocular pressure may require lens removal. Opacities may prevent the ophthalmologist from obtaining a clear view of the retina in the patient with diabetic retinopathy or another sight-threatening pathology. In those cases the cataract may be removed to allow visualization of the retina and adequate management of the problem.

PREOPERATIVE PHASE. When the patient's decreasing vision interferes with functional activities, such as work, driving, reading, and ADLs, surgery becomes an acceptable option. The patient's occupational needs and lifestyle changes are also factors affecting the decision to have surgery. The patient should have a complete ophthalmic assessment. In addition, the surgeon will use axial length measurements obtained by ultrasonography and corneal curvature measurements obtained by keratometry to calculate the appropriate intraocular lens power. The patient's preoperative preparation should include an appropriate history and physical examination. Because almost all patients have local anesthesia, many physicians and surgical facilities do not require an extensive preoperative physical assessment. However, most cataract patients are older adults and may have several medical problems that should be evaluated and controlled before surgery. The surgeon may order preoperative antibiotic eye drops. The patient should not have food or fluids for approximately 6 to 8 hours before surgery.

Almost all cataract patients are admitted to a surgical facility on an outpatient basis. The patient is normally admitted several hours before surgery to allow adequate time for necessary preoperative procedures. The nurse will instill dilating drops (Table 18-6) and a nonsteroidal antiinflammatory eye drop to reduce inflammation and to help maintain pupil dilatation. The patient often receives preoperative antianxiety medication before the local anesthesia injection.

INTRAOPERATIVE PHASE. Cataract extraction is an intraocular procedure. In *intracapsular extraction* the entire lens is removed with the capsule intact. In *extracapsular extraction* the anterior capsule is opened, and the lens nucleus and cortex are removed, leaving the remaining capsular bag intact. Although some surgeons still perform intracapsular extraction (and it may be necessary in instances of trauma), the intracapsular technique has been largely replaced by extracapsular extraction as the procedure of choice in the United States.[21] In extracapsular extraction, the surgeon can remove the lens nucleus by "scooping" it out with a lens loop, or by *phacoemulsification,* in which the nucleus is fragmented by ultrasonic vibration and aspirated from inside the capsular bag (Fig. 18-3). In either case the remaining cortex is aspirated with an irrigation and aspiration instrument. The placement and type of incision varies among surgeons. Corneoscleral incisions require closure with sutures, while scleral tunnel incisions are self-sealing and require no closing suture. The incision required for phacoemulsification is considerably smaller than those required with intracapsular or standard extracapsular surgery.

Almost all patients now have an intraocular lens implanted at the time of cataract extraction surgery. Because most patients have an extracapsular procedure, the lens of choice is a posterior chamber lens that is implanted in the capsular bag behind the iris. At the end of the procedure, the patient receives injections of subconjunctival steroid and antibiotic medications. Then an antibiotic and steroid ointment is applied, and the patient's eye is covered with a patch and protective shield. The patch is usually worn overnight and removed during the first postoperative visit.

POSTOPERATIVE PHASE. Unless complications occur, the patient is usually ready to go home within a few hours after the surgery as soon as the effects of sedative agents have dissipated. Postoperative medications usually include antibiotic and steroid drops to prevent infection and decrease the postoperative inflammatory response. There is some evidence that postoperative activity restrictions and nighttime eye shielding are unnecessary.[23] However, many ophthalmologists still prefer that the patient avoid activities that increase the intraocular pressure, such as bending or stooping, coughing, or lifting. Opthalmologists may also recommend using an eye shield over the operative eye at night for protection.

The ophthalmologist will usually see the patient four to five times at increasing intervals throughout the 6 to 8 weeks following surgery. During each postoperative examination the surgeon will measure the patient's visual acuity, check anterior chamber depth, assess corneal clarity, and measure intraocular pressure. A flat anterior chamber may cause adhesions of the iris and cornea. The cornea may become hazy or cloudy from intraoperative trauma to the endothelium. Even on the first postoperative day the patient's uncorrected visual acuity in the operative eye may be good. However, it is not unusual or indicative of any problem if the patient's visual acuity is reduced immediately after surgery. The postoperative eye drops will be gradually reduced in frequency and finally discontinued when the eye has healed. When the eye is fully recovered, the patient will receive a final glasses prescription. Although the majority of the postoperative refractive error is corrected with the intraocular lens, the patient will still need glasses for near vision and for any residual refractive error.

Table 18-6 Common Topical Medications for Pupil Dilatation

Drug	Onset	Duration	Nursing Considerations
Mydriatics			
▪ α-adrenergic agonists that produce pupillary dilatation by contraction of iris dilator muscle; these have little cycloplegic action (paralysis of accommodation)			Patient with dark irides may need larger doses; photophobia common and patient needs dark glasses; produces transient stinging and burning; contraindicated in patient with narrow angle-glaucoma because angle-closure glaucoma may be produced; can produce significant cardiovascular effects; use punctal occlusion, especially in older and susceptible patients
▪ Phenylephrine HCl (NeoSynephrine, Mydfrin)	45-60 min	4-6 hr	May cause tachycardia and elevated blood pressure, especially in elderly patient; can cause a reflexive decrease in heart rate when blood pressure rises; use punctal occlusion to limit systemic absorption
▪ Hydroxyamphetamine hydrobromide (Paredrine)	45-60 min	4-6 hr	Used diagnostically to differentiate postganglionic, central, or preganglionic Horner's syndrome
Cycloplegics			
▪ Anticholinergic agents that produce paralysis of accommodation (cycloplegia) by blocking the effect of acetylcholine on the ciliary body muscles; produce pupillary dilatation (mydriasis) by blocking effect of acetylcholine on iris sphincter muscle			Patient with dark irides may need larger doses; photophobia common and patient needs dark glasses; produces transient stinging and burning; contraindicated in patient with narrow-angle glaucoma because angle-closure glaucoma may be produced; when used in inflammatory disorders such as uveitis or iritis desired effect is to place iris and ciliary body at rest, increasing patient comfort; may help prevent posterior synechiae (adhesion of iris to cornea or lens)
▪ Tropicamide (Mydriacyl, Tropicacyl)	20-40 min	4-6 hr	1% solution used in cycloplegic refraction; 0.5% solution used in fundus examination
▪ Cyclopentolate HCl (AK-Pentolate, Cyclogyl, Ocu-Pentolate, Pentolair)	30-75 min	6-24 hr	Has been associated with psychotic reactions and behavioral disturbances, usually in children (especially in stronger concentrations); used in cycloplegic refraction, fundus examination, and uveitis
▪ Homatropine hydrobromide (AK-Homatropine, Isopto Homatropine)	30-60 min	1-3 days	Used in cycloplegic refraction, uveitis; may be used for pupil dilatation to allow patient to see around a central lens opacity
▪ Scopolamine (Isopto Hyoscine)	20-60 min	3-7 days	Used in cycloplegic refraction, uveitis
▪ Atropine (Atropisol, Atropair, Bufopto, Atropine, Isopto Atropine, Ocu-Tropine)	30-180 min	6-12 days	Used in cycloplegic refraction, uveitis

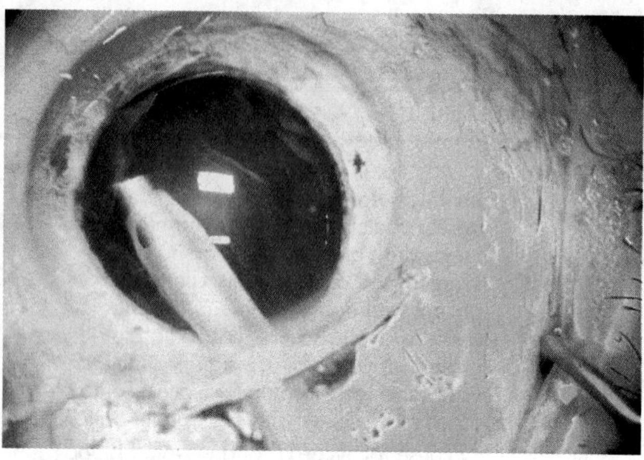

Fig. 18-3 Phacoemulsification of a cataractous lens through a self-sealing, scleral-tunnel incision. Note the circular opening in the anterior lens capsule.

RESEARCH

Implications for Nursing Practice

PRIMARY NURSING, DISCHARGE TEACHING, AND PATIENT SATISFACTION IN POSTCATARACT PATIENTS

Citation McGrory A, Assmann S: A study investigating primary nursing, discharge teaching, and patient satisfaction of ambulatory cataract patients. *Insight: the journal of the American society of ophthalmic registered nurses,* 19:8-13, 1994.

Purpose To investigate the impact of the primary nursing model of care on discharge teaching and satisfaction of cataract patients having surgery.

Method Experimental group (n = 36) received primary nursing with the same nurse providing care from the morning of surgery through discharge and postoperative phone call 24 to 48 hours later. The control group (n = 36) received care by different nurses during the preoperative and postoperative phases, and a third nurse made the postoperative phone call. Data were collected with instruments developed for the study related to knowledge level and patient satisfaction.

Results and Conclusions Knowledge levels were high, and there were no significant differences between the primary and control groups in total score or in subscores on self-care, normal side effects, or complications. Women had significantly higher scores than men. There was a high level of satisfaction with care, and almost all patients felt ready to go home when discharged.

Implications for Nursing Practice Primary nursing is not a critical factor in patient knowledge and satisfaction following cataract surgery. Well-prepared knowledgeable nurses, regardless of what method was used to deliver the patient teaching, provided equally significant knowledge and achieved comparable satisfaction following cataract surgery.

NURSING MANAGEMENT

CATARACTS

Nursing Assessment

The nurse should assess the patient's distance and near visual acuities. If the patient is going to have surgery, the nurse should especially note the visual acuity in the patient's unoperated eye. With this information the nurse can determine how visually compromised the patient may be while the operative eye is patched and healing. In addition, the nurse assesses the psychosocial impact of the patient's visual disability and the patient's level of knowledge regarding the disease process and therapeutic options. Postoperatively it is important to assess the patient's level of comfort and ability to follow the postoperative regimen. The nursing care plan on p. 455 outlines the nursing care for the patient following eye surgery.

Nursing Diagnoses

Nursing diagnoses specific to the patient with a cataract include, but are not limited to, the following:

- Decisional conflict related to lack of knowledge about the condition and treatment options
- Impaired self-care deficit related to visual deficit
- Anxiety related to lack of knowledge about the surgical and postoperative experience

Planning

Preoperatively the overall goals are that the patient with a cataract will (1) make informed decisions regarding therapeutic options and (2) experience minimal anxiety. Postoperatively the overall goals are that the patient with a cataract will (1) understand and comply with postoperative therapy, (2) maintain an acceptable level of physical and emotional comfort, and (3) remain free of infection or other complications.

Nursing Implementation

Health Maintenance and Promotion. There are no proven measures to prevent cataract development. However, it is probably prudent (and certainly does no harm) to suggest that the patient wear sunglasses, avoid extraneous or unnecessary radiation, and maintain appropriate intake of antioxidant vitamins through good nutrition. The nurse can also provide information about vision enhancement techniques for the patient who chooses not to have surgery.

Acute Intervention. Preoperatively the patient with cataracts needs accurate information about the disease process and the treatment options, especially because cataract surgery is considered an elective procedure. For the patient who wants or needs to see better than is possible with medical interventions only, cataract surgery may not seem elective. However, in most cases there is no harm in not having surgery except that the patient has some degree of visual disability. The nurse should be available to give the patient and the family information to help them make an informed decision about appropriate treatment.

NURSING CARE PLAN Patient After Eye Surgery

Planning: Outcome Criteria	Nursing Interventions and Rationales
➤ **NURSING DIAGNOSIS**	Anxiety *related to* actual or potential permanent visual impairment *as manifested by* irritability and restlessness, frequent questions about outcome
Verbalizes realistic understanding and acceptance of expected outcome; exhibits hopeful attitude regarding best possible outcome	Use active listening techniques, encouraging patient to communicate *to allow patient to vent feelings and to validate patient's emotional responses.* Give careful explanations of all treatments and activities *to allow patient to feel a measure of control in the situation.* Include patient's family in planning and teaching *to foster their support of the patient.*
➤ **NURSING DIAGNOSIS**	Risk for injury *related to* visual impairment or presence of eyepatch
Has no incidence of injury; verbalizes feelings of security about personal safety	Advise patient to use side rails *to provide orientation to sides of bed.* Alter patient's environment *to reduce possibility of injuries as a result of unfamiliarity with the environment.* Assist with ambulation and ADLs *to reduce opportunities for injuries and provide verbal cueing.* Teach patient and family about possible sources of injury in the home environment *to allow them to identify and correct potentially harmful situations.*
➤ **NURSING DIAGNOSIS**	Pain *related to* surgical manipulation of tissue *as manifested by* verbal expressions and nonverbal cues of pain and pressure in the affected eye
Expresses satisfaction with pain control	Apply warm or cold compresses using clean washcloth *to reduce edema of eyelid and conjunctiva and provide soothing sensation.* Administer and teach patient to use analgesic as ordered *to relieve pain.* Report and teach patient to report increasing or unremitting pain *to allow early recognition and treatment of possible complications.*
➤ **NURSING DIAGNOSIS**	Altered health maintenance *related to* lack of knowledge regarding postoperative regimen and signs and symptoms of possible complications *as manifested by* questions about postdischarge care and status or inability to perform necessary postoperative care activities
Knows postoperative regimen; demonstrates correct technique in performing eye care procedures	Provide written and verbal discharge instructions to patient and family regarding eye care, medications, activity restrictions, and follow-up care schedule *to ensure understanding and prevent complications.* Teach patient and family signs and symptoms of possible complications *to allow early recognition and treatment.* Provide opportunity for patient and family to perform return demonstration of necessary postoperative care activities *to ensure correct technique.*
➤ **NURSING DIAGNOSIS**	Risk for self-care deficit *related to* visual impairment and activity restrictions
Has care needs met with or without assistance	Assist patient with ADLs as needed or requested *to maintain health and self-esteem.* Help patient and family identify self-care deficits and alternative methods of accomplishing those activities and refer to community support agencies if necessary *to assure availability of necessary assistance after discharge.*

continued

For the patient who elects to have surgery, the nurse is able to provide information, support, and reassurance about the surgical and postoperative experience that can reduce or alleviate the patient's anxiety. The nurse should inform all patients that they will not have depth perception until their patch is removed (usually within 24 hours). This will necessitate special considerations to avoid possible falls or other injuries. The patient with a significant visual impairment in the unoperated eye will require more assistance while the operative eye is patched. Once the patch is removed (usually within 24 hours) most patients with visual impairment in the unoperated eye will have adequate vision for necessary activities because the implanted IOL provides immediate visual rehabilitation in the operated eye. Occasionally the patient may require 1 or 2 weeks for the visual acuity in the operated eye to reach an adequate level for most of the visual needs. This patient will also need some special assistance until the vision improves. The postoperative cataract patient usually experiences little or no pain. There may be some scratchiness in the operative eye. Mild analgesics are usually sufficient to relieve these problems. If pain increases the patient should notify the surgeon because this may indicate hemorrhage, infection, or increased IOP. The nurse should also instruct the patient to

NURSING CARE PLAN Patient After Eye Surgery—cont'd

Planning: Outcome Criteria	Nursing Interventions and Rationales
➤ NURSING DIAGNOSIS Risk for impaired home maintenance *related to* visual impairment and activity restrictions	
Expresses satisfaction with home situation; demonstrates ability to maintain home in personally satisfying condition with or without assistance	Help patient and family identify home maintenance activity deficits and alternative methods of accomplishing those activities and refer to community support agencies if necessary *to assure availability of assistance to maintain home.*
➤ NURSING DIAGNOSIS Risk for infection *related to* presence of surgical wound	
Remains free of infection; demonstrates proper hygiene techniques; performs eye care activities correctly	Teach patient and family proper hygiene and eye care techniques *to assure that medications, dressings, and surgical wound are not contaminated during necessary eye care.* Teach patient and family about signs and symptoms of infection and when and how to report those *to allow early recognition and treatment of possible infection.*

COLLABORATIVE PROBLEMS

Nursing Goals	Nursing Interventions and Rationales
➤ POTENTIAL COMPLICATION Increased intraocular pressure *related to* surgery or postoperative activities	
Monitor for signs of increased intraocular pressure, report deviations from acceptable parameters, and carry out appropriate medical and nursing interventions	Monitor for and teach patient and family to report presence of blurred or cloudy vision, halos around lights, severe and unrelieved eye pain, nausea and vomiting *to allow early recognition and treatment of possible increased intraocular pressure.* Instruct patient to comply with postoperative restrictions on bending, coughing, and Valsalva maneuver *to prevent increased intraocular pressure.* Reinforce need to comply with eye medication routine *to avoid increased intraocular pressure because of improper medication use.*

ADLs, Activities of daily living; *CNS,* central nervous system.

notify the surgeon if there is increased or purulent drainage, increased redness, or any decrease in visual acuity.

Chronic and Home Management. For the cataract patient who has not had surgery, the nurse can suggest ways in which the patient may modify activities or lifestyle to accommodate the visual deficit produced by the cataract. The nurse should also provide the patient with accurate information about appropriate long-term eye care.

The trend toward outpatient surgery has clearly affected the patient with cataracts. Typically the patient remains in the surgical facility for only few hours instead of a few days. This shift in practice patterns has dramatically affected how the nurse provides the patient with postoperative care and teaching. The patient and the family are now responsible for almost all postoperative care, and the nurse should give them written and verbal instructions before discharge. These instructions should include information about postoperative eye care, activity restrictions, medications, follow-up visit schedule, and signs and symptoms of possible complications. The patient's family should be included in the instruction, because some patients may have difficulty with self-care activities, especially if the vision in the unoperated eye is poor. The nurse should provide an opportunity for the patient and family to present return demonstrations of any necessary self-care activities.

Most patients will experience little visual impairment following surgery. This is because (1) IOL implants provide immediate visual rehabilitation, (2) many patients achieve a usable level of visual acuity within a few days following surgery, (3) patients remain patched for only 24 hours, and (4) many patients have good vision in their unoperated eye. A few patients may experience significant visual impairment postoperatively. These include patients who do not have an IOL implanted at the time of surgery, who require several weeks to achieve a usable level of visual acuity following surgery, or with poor vision in their unoperated eye. For those patients the time between surgery and receiving aphakic glasses or contacts can be a period of significant visual disability. The nurse can suggest ways in which the patient and the family can modify activities and the environment to maintain an adequate level of safe functioning. Suggestions may include getting assistance with steps, removing area rugs and other potential obstacles, preparing meals for freezing before surgery, or obtaining audio books for diversion until visual acuity improves.

Gerontologic Considerations

Most patients with cataracts are elderly. When the older patient is visually impaired, even temporarily, the patient may experience a loss of independence, lack of control over his life, and a significant change in self-perception. Societal devaluation of the older individual complicates these experiences. The older patient often needs emotional support and encouragement as well as specific suggestions to allow a maximum level of independent function. The nurse can assure the older patient that cataract surgery can be accomplished safely and comfortably with minimal sedation. The change to outpatient surgery for cataract extraction is particularly beneficial for the older patient who may become confused or disoriented during hospitalization.

Retinal Detachment

A *retinal detachment* is a separation of the sensory retina and the underlying pigment epithelium, with fluid accumulation between the two layers.

Significance. The incidence of nontraumatic retinal detachment is approximately 1 of every 10,000 individuals each year. This number increases when aphakic individuals are included because retinal detachment is more likely to occur in aphakic patients. Including traumatic retinal detachments increases the incidence only slightly. In the patient with no other risk factors who has had a retinal detachment in one eye, the risk of detachment in the second eye is approximately 10%. Almost all patients with untreated, symptomatic retinal detachment will become blind in the involved eye.[24]

Etiology and Pathophysiology. There are many causes of retinal detachment. The most common cause is a retinal break. *Retinal breaks* are an interruption in the full thickness of the retinal tissue, and can be classified as tears or holes. *Retinal holes* are atrophic retinal breaks that occur spontaneously. Retinal tears can occur as the vitreous shrinks during aging and pulls on the retina. The retina tears when the traction force exceeds the strength of the retina. Once there is a break in the retina, liquid vitreous can enter the subretinal space between the sensory layer and the retinal pigment epithelium layer, causing a *rhegmatogenous* retinal detachment. Less frequently, retinal detachment can occur when abnormal membranes mechanically pull on the retina. These are called *tractional* detachments. A third type of retinal detachment is the *secondary* or *exudative* detachment that occurs with conditions that allow fluid to accumulate in the subretinal space (e.g., choroidal tumors or intraocular inflammation). Risk factors for retinal detachment are listed in Table 18-7.

Clinical Manifestations. Patients with a detaching retina describe symptoms that include *photopsia* (light flashes), floaters, and a "cobweb," "hairnet," or ring in the field of vision. Once the retina has detached, the patient describes a painless loss of peripheral or central vision, "like a curtain" coming across the field of vision. The area of visual loss corresponds to the area of detachment. If the detachment is in the superior nasal retina, the visual field loss will be in the inferior temporal area. If the detachment is small or develops slowly in the periphery, the patient may not be aware of a visual problem.

Diagnostic Studies. Visual acuity measurements should be the first diagnostic procedure with any complaint of vision loss (see Table 18-8). The ophthalmologist or nurse can directly visualize the retinal detachment using direct and indirect ophthalmoscopy or slit lamp microscopy in conjunction with a special lens to view the far periphery of the retina. Ultrasound may be useful to identify a retinal detachment if the retina cannot be directly visualized (e.g., when the cornea, lens, or vitreous is hazy or opaque).

Therapeutic Management. The ophthalmologist will carefully evaluate the patient with retinal breaks to determine

Table 18-7 Risk Factors for Retinal Detachment

High Myopia
Premature, accelerated rate of vitreous detachment; increased incidence of lattice degeneration

Aphakia
Retinal tears that presumably occur because of surgical disturbance of the vitreous

Proliferative Diabetic Retinopathy
Vitreous remains attached to areas of neovascularization as normal process of vitreal contraction occurs

Retinal Lattice Degeneration
Retinal holes common in lattice degeneration; vitreous remains attached to areas of degeneration as the normal process of vitreal contraction occurs

Ocular Trauma
Retinal breaks after blunt or penetrating trauma allow fluid to accumulate in the subretinal space

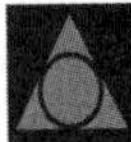

Table 18-8 Therapeutic Management: Retinal Detachment

Diagnostic
- Visual acuity measurement
- Ophthalmoscopy (direct and indirect)
- Slit lamp microscopy
- Ultrasound if cornea, lens, or vitreous are hazy or opaque

Therapeutic

Preoperative
- Mydriatic, cycloplegic
- Photocoagulation of retinal break that has not progressed to detachment

Surgery to seal retinal breaks and relieve traction on the retina
- Photocoagulation
- Cryoretinopexy
- Diathermy
- Scleral buckling procedure
- Draining of subretinal fluid
- Vitrectomy
- Intravitreal bubble

Postoperative
- Topical antibiotic
- Topical steroid
- Analgesia
- Mydriatics
- Positioning and activity as preferred by patient's surgeon

if prophylactic laser photocoagulation or cryopexy is necessary to avoid possible retinal detachment. Some retinal breaks are not likely to progress to detachment, and the ophthalmologist will simply watch the patient, giving precise information about the warning signs and symptoms of impending detachment and instructing the patient to seek immediate evaluation if any of those signs or symptoms are recognized. The general ophthalmologist will usually refer the patient with retinal detachments to a retinal specialist. Retinal detachment treatment has two objectives. The first is to seal any retinal breaks, and the second is to relieve inward traction on the retina. Several techniques are used to accomplish these objectives.

Photocoagulation, cryopexy, and diathermy. These techniques seal retinal breaks by creating an inflammatory reaction that causes a chorioretinal adhesion or scar. *Laser photocoagulation* involves using an intense, precisely focused light beam, such as the argon laser or a xenon light, to create an inflammatory reaction. The light is directed at the area of the retinal break. This produces a scar that seals the edges of the hole or tear and prevents fluid from collecting in the subretinal space, causing a detachment. The ophthalmologist may use photocoagulation alone if there is a single small tear with little or no detachment in the periphery and minimal subretinal fluid. For retinal breaks accompanied by significant detachment, the retinal surgeon may also use photocoagulation intraoperatively in conjunction with scleral buckling. Tears or holes without accompanying retinal detachment may be treated prophylactically with laser photocoagulation if the ophthalmologist judges them to be at high risk of progressing to retinal detachment. When used alone, laser therapy is an outpatient procedure that requires no anesthetic, and the patient usually experiences minimal adverse symptoms during or following the procedure.

Two other methods used to seal retinal breaks are *cryopexy* and *diathermy*. These procedures involve using extreme cold or heat to create the inflammatory reaction that produces the sealing scar. The ophthalmologist applies the cryoprobe or diathermy instrument to the external globe in the area over the tear. Cryotherapy is used more frequently today because there is less tissue reaction. It is usually done on an outpatient basis under local anesthesia. As with photocoagulation, cryotherapy may be used alone or during scleral buckling surgery. The patient may experience significant discomfort following cryopexy. The nurse should encourage the patient to take the prescribed pain medication following the procedure.

Scleral buckling. Scleral buckling is an extraocular surgical procedure that involves indenting the globe so the pigment epithelium, choroid, and sclera move toward the detached retina. This not only helps seal retinal breaks, but also helps relieve inward traction on the retina. The retinal surgeon sutures a silicone implant against the sclera causing the sclera to buckle inward. The surgeon may place an encircling band over the implant if there are multiple retinal breaks, if the surgeon cannot locate suspected breaks, or if there is widespread inward traction on the retina (Fig. 18-4). If present, subretinal fluid may be drained by inserting a small gauge needle to facilitate contact between the retina and the buckled sclera. Scleral buckling is usually accomplished under local anesthesia, and the patient may be discharged on the first postoperative day. Many surgeons now perform scleral buckling surgery as an outpatient procedure.

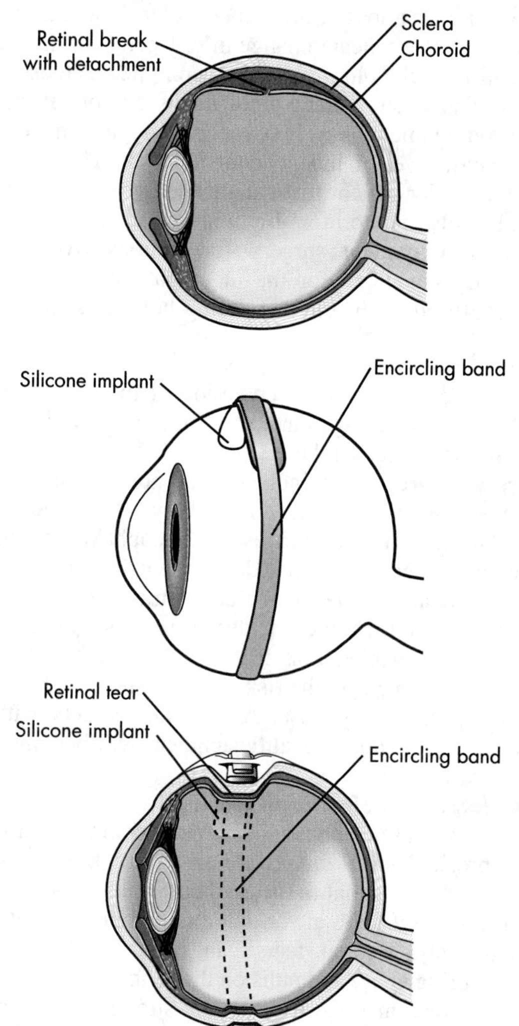

Fig. 18-4 Retinal break with detachment: surgical repair by scleral buckling technique.

Intraocular procedures. In addition to the extraocular procedures described, retinal surgeons may use one or more intraocular procedures in treating some retinal detachments. *Pneumatic retinopexy* is the intravitreal injection of special gases to form a temporary bubble in the vitreous that closes retinal breaks and provides apposition of the separated retinal layers. Because the intravitreal bubble is temporary, this technique is combined with cryopexy or scleral buckling. The patient with an intravitreal bubble must position the head so that the bubble is in contact with the retinal break. It may be necessary for the patient to maintain this position for up to 16 hours a day for 5 days.[25] Special liquids or oil may also be used to form an intravitreal bubble.

Vitrectomy (surgical removal of the vitreous) may be used to relieve traction on the retina, especially when the traction results from proliferative diabetic retinopathy. Vitrectomy may be combined with scleral buckling to provide a dual effect in relieving traction. In *proliferative vitreoretinopathy* (PVR), membranes develop in the vitreous cavity and on the retinal surface, exerting traction that causes folds in the retina. Vitrectomy may be combined with membrane peeling to relieve traction in those cases.

Postoperative considerations in scleral buckling and intraocular procedures. Reattachment is successful in 90% of retinal detachments. Visual prognosis varies, depending on the extent, length, and area of detachment. Postoperatively, the patient may be on bed rest and may require special positioning to maintain proper position of an intravitreal bubble. Length of hospitalization varies according to physician preference and third-party payer guidelines. The patient may use multiple topical medications, including antibiotics, antiinflammatory agents, or dilating agents. Activity recommendations vary according to physician preference, extent of the detachment, and the particular repair procedure.

NURSING MANAGEMENT

RETINAL DETACHMENT

Nursing Assessment

The nurse should elicit a careful description of the patient's visual symptoms and determine visual acuity. Confrontation visual fields may reveal a peripheral scotoma. If familiar with the techniques, the nurse may also visualize a detachment directly by ophthalmoscopy or slit lamp microscopy.

Nursing Diagnoses

Nursing diagnoses specific to the patient with retinal detachment include, but are not limited to, the following:

- Pain related to surgical correction and unusual positioning
- Fear related to possibility of permanent vision loss in affected eye
- Self-care deficit syndrome related to imposed activity restrictions and visual deficits.

Planning

The overall goals are that the patient with retinal detachment will (1) experience minimal anxiety throughout the event, and (2) maintain an acceptable level of comfort postoperatively.

Nursing Implementation

The nurse should teach the patient with a high risk of retinal detachment the signs and symptoms of retinal detachment. The nurse can also promote use of proper protective eyewear to help avoid retinal detachments related to trauma.

In most cases retinal detachment is an urgent situation, and the patient is confronted suddenly with the need for surgery. The patient needs emotional support, especially during the immediate preoperative period when preparations for surgery produce additional anxiety. When the patient experiences postoperative pain, the nurse should administer prescribed pain medications and teach the patient to take the medication as necessary after being discharged. The patient may go home within a few hours of surgery or may remain in the hospital for several days, depending on the surgeon and the type of repair. Discharge planning is important, and the nurse should begin this process as early as possible because the patient may not remain hospitalized long.

The type and amount of activity restriction following retinal detachment surgeries varies greatly. The nurse should verify the prescribed level of activity with each patient's surgeon and help the patient plan for any necessary assistance related to activity restrictions. The nurse should teach the patient the signs and symptoms of retinal detachment because the risk of retinal detachment in the other eye is approximately 10%.[24]

Age-Related Macular Degeneration

Age-related macular degeneration (AMD) is an entity that is not precisely defined. However, for the purposes of this discussion, AMD is defined as a retinal degenerative process involving the macula and resulting in varying degrees of central vision loss.

Significance. AMD is the leading cause of uncorrectable vision loss in adults over 52 years of age. The incidence of vision loss increases with age, with 2.2 percent of patients over 65 years of age blind in one or both eyes from AMD. With increasing numbers of elderly persons in the population, it is estimated that by 1995 AMD will result in unilateral or bilateral blindness in approximately 745,000 patients more than 65 years of age.[26]

Etiology and Pathophysiology. Little is known about the etiology of AMD. Although it is clearly related to retinal aging, there is no explanation for the fact that not all aged retinas develop AMD and vision loss. The pathophysiologic mechanism may be an abnormal accumulation of waste material in the retinal pigment epithelium.[27] Some evidence suggests that cigarette smokers have a significantly higher risk of developing one form of AMD.[28]

Clinical Manifestations. The hallmark sign of AMD is the appearance of *drusen* in the fundus. Drusen appear as yellowish exudates beneath the retinal pigment epithelium and represent localized or diffuse deposits of extracellular debris. The patient may complain of blurred vision, the presence of scotomas, or *metamorphopsia* (distortion of vision).

Diagnostic Studies. In addition to visual acuity measurement, the primary diagnostic procedure is ophthalmoscopy. The examiner looks for drusen and other fundus changes associated with AMD. The Amsler grid test (Table 17-7) may help define the involved area and provides a baseline for future comparison. Fundus photography and IV fluorescein angiography may be helpful in further defining the extent and type of degenerative disease.

Therapeutic Management. Therapy for AMD is problematic because laser treatment is only beneficial for some patients. Laser treatment may help reduce visual loss in the patient with choroidal neovascularization. Laser treatment seals any leakage in the neovascular area, at least preventing progression of visual loss. However, in most cases of AMD, laser treatment is not helpful. Zinc nutritional supplements are another possible treatment to slow or halt progression of visual loss. Unfortunately, this therapy is also of questionable value. When no treatment is possible, or when treatment fails, the patient with AMD can benefit from low-vision aids, such as magnifying lenses.

The extent of this problem continues to grow as the number of individuals more than 65 years of age increases. The permanent loss of central vision associated with AMD has significant psychosocial implications for nursing care. Nursing management of the patient with uncorrectable visual impairment is discussed in that section and is appropriate for the patient with AMD. It is especially important when caring for the patient to avoid giving them the impression that "nothing can be done" about their problem. While it is true that therapy will not recover lost vision (and is not even appropriate in most cases) much *can* be done to augment the remaining vision. Just knowing that the ophthalmologist and nurse have not abandoned any attempt to help them can give these patients a more positive outlook.

Diabetic Retinopathy

Diabetic retinopathy is a complication of diabetes mellitus that affects the retinal blood vessels. Eventually, most patients with diabetes mellitus will develop some abnormalities in the retinal vessels.

Significance. Diabetic retinopathy is the cause of the majority of new cases of legal blindness in working-age Americans. Less retinopathy is associated with the diabetic patient who has noninsulin-dependent diabetes mellitus (NIDDM, Type II). Of those with insulin-dependent diabetes mellitus (IDDM, Type I), approximately 25% will develop retinopathy within 5 years of diagnosis. The incidence of retinopathy increases over time, with 80% of patients with IDDM exhibiting retinopathy after 15 years. The most sight-jeopardizing form of retinopathy, proliferative diabetic retinopathy, occurs in about 25% of patients with IDDM after 15 years.[26]

Etiology and Pathophysiology. The retinal vascular changes in diabetes are probably caused initially by alterations in various biochemical processes. This results in weakening of the microvessel walls, microaneurysm formation, capillary dilatation, decreased capillary blood flow, and capillary atrophy. The retina becomes ischemic and releases substances that stimulate growth of new vessels that may bleed easily. Systemic conditions that may affect the course of development of diabetic retinopathy include hypertension, elevated lipids and triglycerides, kidney disease, elevated creatinine, and cardiovascular disease.

Clinical Manifestations. The earliest and most treatable stages of diabetic retinopathy often produce no visual symptoms. Because of this, the diabetic patient must have regular examinations by an ophthalmologist for early detection and appropriate treatment of the disorder. Retinal vascular changes visible in the retina of the patient with diabetes are classified as *nonproliferative diabetic retinopathy* (NPDR) or *proliferative diabetic retinopathy* (PDR). In NPDR microaneurysms, hemorrhages, and fatty deposits appear in the retina. In PDR new vessels form (neovascularization) on the surface of the retina and in the optic disc. These new vessels are often accompanied by fibroglial tissue growth. The areas of neovascularization may bleed into the vitreous. When this occurs, the patient may complain of a sudden, often severe loss of vision because the blood in the vitreous obscures vision. The neovascular areas also form a firm adhesion to the posterior vitreous face that can result in a tractional retinal detachment as the vitreous recedes.

Leakage may also cause *macular edema*, a swelling around the macular area. The macular edema may not produce any visual symptoms even if it is apparent on retinal examination. It is characterized as clinically significant if the patient has a decrease in visual acuity.

Diagnostic Studies. Careful ophthalmoscopic and slit lamp microscopic retinal examinations are the most important diagnostic tools to identify diabetic fundus changes and should be a regular part of care for the diabetic patient (Table 18-9). Fluorescein angiography demonstrates dye leakage from abnormal retinal and subretinal vessels and identifies retinal areas amenable to focal laser treatment. If the vitreous humor is opaque in advanced disease, ultrasonography may be useful to identify retinal detachment.

Therapeutic Management. Until recently little could be done to treat diabetic retinopathy. Since the 1970s three major research groups have contributed valuable information about appropriate and effective treatment for diabetic retinopathy. These groups include the Diabetic Retinopathy Study Research Group, the Diabetic Retinopathy Vitrectomy Study Research Group, and the Early Treatment Diabetic Retinopathy Study Research Group.[29] Current treatment recommendations include early laser photocoagulation of the retina. When there is vision loss from macular edema, *focal* laser treatment is appropriate.

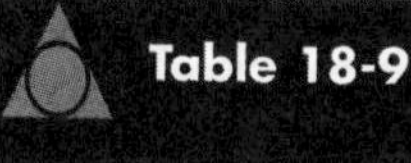

Table 18-9 Therapeutic Management: Diabetic Retinopathy

Diagnostic
- Visual acuity measurement
- Ophthalmoscopy (direct and indirect)
- Slit lamp microscopy
- Fluorescein angiography
- Ultrasonography if vitreous is hazy or opaque

Therapeutic
- Photocoagulation
- Vitrectomy
- Retinal detachment repair
- Proper management of other systemic conditions that may affect progression of diabetic retinopathy

Focal treatment is directed to a specific area of leakage identified by fluorescein angiography. *Panretinal photocoagulation* (PRP) is a scatter technique in which thousands of laser burns are placed in the retinal periphery. PRP is generally recommended when there is moderate to severe neovascularization.

Photocoagulation with the argon laser coagulates the microaneurysms and new growth of vessels in and on the retina and may require several treatments. Simply destroying the newly formed vessels does not eliminate the underlying hypoxic state that stimulates new vessel growth. PRP destroys the hypoxic retina, reducing its oxygen requirement and reducing the stimulus for new blood vessel growth.

Topical anesthetic is generally adequate for laser treatment. Pain is usually transient but occasionally requires retrobulbar anesthesia. The patient may experience some loss of peripheral or central vision, and the dark adaptation may be affected.

Photocoagulation is not possible when there is significant vitreous or retinal hemorrhage. In those cases *vitrectomy* is useful to surgically remove the vitreous and vitreal membranes. Vitrectomy is indicated when there is a vitreous hemorrhage that does not clear or when the hemorrhage is obscuring the retina in the patient who needs photocoagulation. It is also indicated when vision loss is caused by traction on the macula or when there is a combined traction-rhegmatogenous retinal detachment. Vitrectomy is an intraocular procedure, and possible complications include the risk of further vitreous hemorrhage, cataract formation, glaucoma, and endophthalmitis. Despite the risks, vitrectomy has been an important development in treating the ocular complications of diabetes. Since the 1970s, vitrectomy has offered the only hope for the patient with severe vision loss from vitreous hemorrhage or severe PDR complicated by vitreal involvement. Despite these clinical advances, diabetic retinopathy remains a disease that cannot be cured—only treated. Although it is not proven, proper management of certain systemic conditions may help control the progression of diabetic retinopathy.[30]

Glaucoma

Glaucoma is not one disease but rather a group of disorders characterized by increased intraocular pressure. Increased intraocular pressure ultimately damages the optic nerve, leading to visual field loss. Initially the patient has no signs or symptoms of the disease. The patient is unlikely to notice visual field loss until it is severe, especially if the loss occurs first in one eye. Glaucoma may occur congenitally, as a primary disease, or secondary to other ocular or systemic conditions. If not recognized and treated, glaucoma may cause blindness that could have been prevented in most patients.

Significance. Glaucoma is the second-leading cause of permanent blindness in the United States and the leading cause of blindness among African-Americans. At least 2 million persons have glaucoma, and of these, more than 50% are unaware that they have the disease. Another 5 to 10 million persons have elevated intraocular pressure, placing them at increased risk of developing the disease. The incidence among older Americans is even higher, with 1 in 50 Caucasians and 1 in 10 African-Americans exhibiting glaucoma.[31]

Etiology and Pathophysiology. Although vision loss from glaucoma results from damage to the optic nerve and retina, the mechanism that causes increased intraocular pressure involves the anterior part of the eye. The ciliary body secretes approximately 4 to 5 ml of aqueous humor a day. This bathes the lens with nutrients and then flows through the pupil into the anterior chamber, where it bathes the corneal endothelium. Aqueous humor exits the eye through the trabecular meshwork and the canal of Schlemm in the iridocorneal angle of the anterior chamber (see Fig. 17-2). Increased intraocular pressure results from a decrease in aqueous humor outflow, and in some cases may also be related to an increased production of aqueous humor. The outflow of aqueous humor can be decreased by several mechanisms.

In *primary open-angle glaucoma* (POAG), decreased aqueous outflow is most likely caused by increased resistance to outflow in the trabecular meshwork. The increased pressure affects the sensitive nerve tissue of the optic disc, causing ischemia. As ischemia of the optic nerve tissue occurs, the patient begins to lose peripheral vision. Glaucomatous optic nerve damage with the resulting visual field loss is more likely to occur in the patient with a family history of glaucoma, with increasing age, in the African-American patient, and in the patient with diabetes mellitus or cardiovascular disease.[32] Vision loss can progress toward blindness if the intraocular pressure is not controlled.

In *primary angle-closure glaucoma* (PACG), the iridocorneal angle closes, blocking aqueous outflow. PACG represents approximately 10% of the total number of glaucoma cases in the United States. It is caused by *pupillary block,* in which the lens blocks the pupillary opening, preventing the flow of aqueous humor into the anterior chamber where it would normally drain through the trabecular meshwork. The lens may also push the iris forward, causing the peripheral iris to cover the trabecular meshwork and blocking the outflow channels. This may occur with lens enlargement, which occurs naturally throughout life. In addition to this normal enlargement, the lens also moves slightly more anterior as the individual ages. These changes result in some degree of contact between the posterior iris and the anterior lens, blocking the pupil and causing the iris to bulge forward. Contact between the two structures is usually not complete and results in *relative pupillary block* (RPB). RPB glaucoma may develop slowly or occur intermittently.

Pupillary block may also occur as a result of pupil dilatation in the patient with anatomically narrow angles. Dilatation causes peripheral iris bulging with the same result of covering the trabecular meshwork and blocking the outflow channels. Although pupillary block glaucoma is rare, it occurs suddenly and constitutes an ocular emergency. An acute attack may be precipitated by situations during which the pupil remains in a middilated state long enough to cause an acute and significant rise in the intraocular pressure. This may occur because of drug-induced mydriasis, emotional excitement, or darkness. Drug-induced mydriasis may occur not only from topical ophthalmic preparations but also from many systemic medications (both prescription drugs and over-the-counter [OTC] drugs). The nurse should check drug documentation before administering medications to the patient with narrow-angle glaucoma and should instruct the patient *not* to take any mydriatic-producing medications.

In *secondary glaucoma,* increased intraocular pressure results from other ocular or systemic conditions that may block the outflow channels in some way. Secondary glaucoma may be associated with various inflammatory processes that produce cells that can block the outflow channels. Inflammatory processes may also damage the trabecular meshwork. Trauma, intraocular or periorbital neoplasms, iris neovascularization, and other ocular or systemic disorders may also be associated with secondary glaucoma.

Clinical Manifestations. POAG develops slowly and without symptoms. The patient with POAG reports no symptoms of pain or pressure. The patient usually does not notice the gradual visual field defects that develop until the peripheral vision has been severely compromised. Eventually the patient with untreated glaucoma has "tunnel vision" in which only a small center field can be seen, and all peripheral vision is absent.

Acute angle-closure glaucoma causes definite symptoms, including sudden, excruciating pain in or around the eye. This can be accompanied by nausea and vomiting. Visual symptoms include seeing colored halos around lights, blurred vision, and ocular redness. The acute pressure rise may also cause corneal edema, giving the cornea a steamy appearance.

Manifestations of subacute or chronic angle-closure glaucoma appear gradually. The patient who has had a previous, unrecognized episode of subacute angle-closure glaucoma may report a history of blurred vision, colored halos around lights, ocular redness, or eye or brow pain.

Diagnostic Studies. Intraocular pressure (IOP) is usually elevated in glaucoma. Normal IOP by applanation tonometry is 10 to 21 mm Hg. In the patient with elevated pressures, the ophthalmologist will usually repeat the measurements during a period of time and at various times of the day to verify the elevation. In open-angle glaucoma, IOP is usually between 22 and 32 mm Hg. In acute angle-closure glaucoma, IOP may be 50 mm Hg or higher.

In open-angle glaucoma, slit lamp microscopy reveals a normal angle. In angle-closure glaucoma, the examiner may note a markedly narrow or flat anterior chamber angle, an edematous cornea, a fixed and moderately dilated pupil, and ciliary injection. Gonioscopy (Table 17-7) allows better visualization of the anterior chamber angle.

Measures of peripheral and central vision provide other diagnostic information. Whereas central acuity may remain 20/20 even in the presence of severe peripheral visual field loss, visual field perimetry may reveal subtle changes in the peripheral retina early in the disease process, long before actual scotomas develop. When visual field defects begin to appear, the initial scotoma is a small, football-shaped defect that gradually progresses to a nasal and superior field defect in chronic open-angle glaucoma. In acute angle-closure glaucoma, central visual acuity will be reduced if the patient has corneal edema, and the visual fields may be markedly decreased.

As glaucoma progresses, *optic disk cupping* occurs. This is visible with direct or indirect ophthalmoscopy. The optic disc becomes wider, deeper, and paler (light gray or white). Optic disk cupping may be one of the first signs of chronic open-angle glaucoma. Optic disk photographs are useful for comparison over time to demonstrate an increase in the cup-to-disc ratio and progressive blanching (Fig. 18-5).

Therapeutic Management. The primary focus of glaucoma therapy is to keep the IOP low enough to prevent the patient from developing optic nerve damage. This damage is manifested by increasing visual field loss and progressive optic disk cupping. Specific therapies vary with the type of glaucoma. The diagnostic and therapeutic management of glaucoma is summarized in Table 18-10.

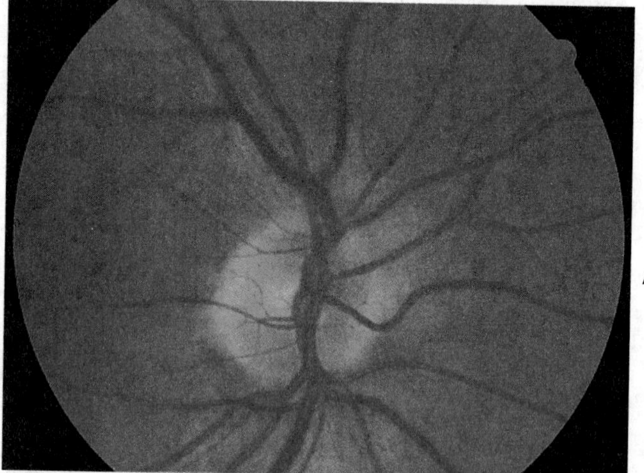

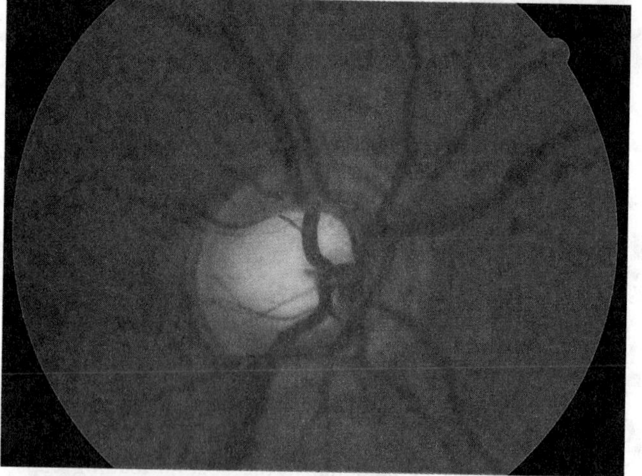

Fig. 18-5 ***A,*** In the normal eye, the optic cup is pink with little cupping. ***B,*** In the glaucomatous eye, the optic disk is bleached, and optic cupping is present. (Note the appearance of the retinal vessels, which travel over the edge of the optic cup and appear to dip into it.)

Chronic open-angle glaucoma. Initial treatment in chronic open-angle glaucoma is pharmacologic (Table 18-11). With all pharmacologic therapy, the patient must understand that continued treatment and supervision is necessary because the medications control but do not cure the disease.

Argon laser trabeculoplasty (ALT) is another therapeutic option to lower IOP that is indicated when pharmacologic control is not successful or when occasionally the patient either cannot or will not use the pharmacologic agents. ALT is an outpatient procedure that requires only topical anesthetic. The topical drops anesthetize the cornea before the gonioscopy lens is applied, allowing visualization of the treatment area. Approximately 50 laser "spots" are evenly spaced around the superior or inferior 180° of the trabecular meshwork. The laser stimulates scarring and contraction of the trabecular meshwork, opening the outflow channels. ALT reduces IOP approximately 75% of the time.[33] A second 180° area may be treated in a subsequent procedure. The patient uses topical steroids for approximately 3 to 5 days following surgery. The most common complication is an acute postoperative IOP rise. Because the decrease in pressure is gradual, the patient continues taking the preoperative glaucoma medication. The ophthalmologist examines the patient 1 week after the procedure and again 4 to 6 weeks following surgery.

A *filtering procedure,* such as trabeculectomy, may be indicated if medical management and laser therapy are not successful. In this procedure the surgeon makes conjunctival and scleral flaps, removes part of the iris and trabecular meshwork, and closes the scleral flap loosely. Aqueous humor may now "percolate" out through the area of missing iris where it is trapped under the repaired conjunctiva and absorbed into the systemic circulation. The success rate of filtering surgery is 75% to 85%. Mitomycin or 5-fluorouracil may increase the success rate by preventing scarring and subsequent closure of the opening created during surgery.

Cyclocryotherapy is another procedure that reduces IOP. The cryoprobe is touched to the sclera outside of the ciliary body. This freezes parts of the ciliary body, causing local destruction of the ciliary tissue and decreasing production of aqueous humor. The procedure may be repeated and can also be used in treating acute glaucoma.

A *Molteno implant* is another surgical option, usually reserved for the patient in whom filtration surgery has failed. It involves surgical placement of a small tube and reservoir to shunt aqueous humor from the anterior chamber to the implanted reservoir. Complications include ocular hypotony, wound leak, shunt tube obstruction, hyphema, excessive scar tissue formation, and cataract formation.

Acute angle-closure glaucoma. Acute angle-closure glaucoma is an ocular emergency that requires immediate intervention. Miotics and oral or IV hyperosmotic agents are usually successful in immediately lowering the IOP (Table 18-11). A laser peripheral iridotomy or surgical iridectomy is necessary for long-term treatment and prevention of subsequent episodes. These procedures allow the aqueous humor to flow through a newly created opening in the iris and into normal outflow channels. One of these procedures may be performed on the other eye as a precaution, because many patients have an acute attack in the other eye.

Secondary glaucoma. Secondary glaucoma is managed by treating the underlying problem and by using antiglaucoma drugs. If treatment fails, glaucoma can progress to absolute glaucoma, resulting in a hard, sightless, and usually painful eye requiring *enucleation* (surgical removal of the eye).

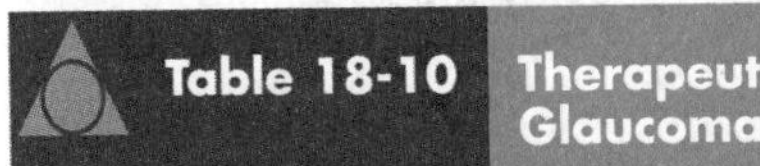

Table 18-10 Therapeutic Management: Glaucoma

Diagnostic
- Visual acuity measurement
- Tonometry
- Ophthalmoscopy (direct and indirect)
- Slit lamp microscopy
- Gonioscopy
- Visual field perimetry
- Fundus photography

Therapeutic

Chronic open-angle glaucoma
- Pharmacologic management
  - β-adrenergic receptor blocking agents
  - Adrenergic agents
  - Cholinergic agents (miotics)
  - Carbonic anhydrase inhibitors
- Surgical management
  - Argon laser trabeculoplasty
  - Trabeculectomy
  - Cyclocryotherapy destruction of ciliary body
  - Molteno implant

Acute angle-closure glaucoma
- Topical cholinergic agent
- Hyperosmotic agent
- Laser peripheral iridotomy
- Surgical iridectomy

NURSING MANAGEMENT

DIABETIC RETINOPATHY OR GLAUCOMA

Diabetes and glaucoma are chronic conditions that have long-term significant sight-threatening implications. Nursing interventions for the patient with these disorders have an underlying similarity because both disorders require chronic management, and both are causes of preventable visual impairment. Nursing management is focused on the chronicity of the diseases and on the fact that visual impairment is preventable in most cases with proper therapeutic management.

Nursing Assessment

Because glaucoma and diabetic retinopathy are chronic conditions requiring long-term management the nurse must carefully assess the patient's ability to understand and comply with the rationale and regimen of the prescribed therapy. In addition, the nurse should assess the patient's psychologic reaction to the diagnosis of a potentially sight-threatening chronic disorder. The nurse must include

Table 18-11 Medications Used for Treatment of Acute and Chronic Glaucoma

Drug	Action	Side Effects	Nursing Considerations
β-Adrenergic Receptor Blocking Agents			
Betaxolol (Betoptic)	β_1 cardioselective blocker; probably decreases aqueous humor production	Transient ocular discomfort; systemic reactions rarely reported but include bradycardia, heart block, pulmonary distress, headache, depression	Topical drops; minimal effect on pulmonary and cardiovascular parameters; contraindicated in patient with bradycardia, greater than first degree heart block, cardiogenic shock, or overt cardiac failure; systemic absorption can have additive effect with systemic β-blocking agents; teach patient to occlude puncta
Carteolol (Ocupress) Levobunolol (Betagan) Metipranolol (Optipranolol) Timolol maleate (Timoptic)	β_1 and β_2 noncardioselective blockers; probably decrease aqueous humor production	Transient ocular discomfort; blurred vision; photophobia; blepharoconjunctivitis; bradycardia; decreased blood pressure; bronchospasm; headache; depression	Topical drops; same as betaxolol; these noncardioselective β-blockers are also contraindicated in patients with asthma or severe COPD
Adrenergic Agonists			
Dipivefrin (Propine)	α- and β-adrenergic agonist; converted to epinephrine inside the eye; decreases aqueous humor production, enhances outflow facility	Ocular discomfort and redness; tachycardia; hypertension	Topical drops; contraindicated in patient with narrow-angle glaucoma; teach punctal occlusion to patient at risk of systemic reactions
Epinephrine (Epifrin; Eppy; Glaucon; Epitrate; Epinal; Eppy/N)	Same as dipivefrin	Same as dipivefrin, but can be more pronounced	Topical drops; same as dipivefrin
Apraclonidine (Iopidine)	α-adrenergic agonist; probably decreases aqueous humor production	Ocular redness; irregular heart rate	Topical drops; used to control or prevent acute postlaser IOP rise (used 1 hour before, and immediately after ALT and iridotomy, Nd:YAG laser capsulotomy); teach patient at risk of systemic reactions to occlude puncta
Cholinergic Agents (Miotics)			
Carbachol (Isopto Carbachol)	Parasympathomimetic; stimulates iris sphincter contraction, causing miosis and opening of trabecular meshwork, facilitating aqueous outflow; also partially inhibits cholinesterase	Transient ocular discomfort; headache; browache; blurred vision; decreased dark adaptation; syncope; salivation; dysrhythmias; vomiting; diarrhea; hypotension; rarely, retinal detachment in susceptible individual	Topical drops; caution patient about decreased visual acuity caused by miosis, particularly in dim light
Pilocarpine (Akarpine; Isopto Carpine; Pilocar; Pilopine; Piloptic; Pilostat)	Parasympathomimetic; stimulates iris sphincter contraction, causing miosis and opening of trabecular meshwork, facilitating aqueous humor outflow	Same as carbachol	Topical drops; same as carbachol

continued

Table 18-11 Medications Used for Treatment of Acute and Chronic Glaucoma—cont'd

Drug	Action	Side Effects	Nursing Considerations
Physostigmine (Eserine; Isopto Eserine)	Temporary cholinesterase inhibitor; enhances effect of endogenous acetylcholine on iris and ciliary muscle, causing miosis	Allergic conjunctivitis; browache; lid twitching; accommodative spasm	Topical ointment; rarely used
Echothiophate iodide (Phospholine Iodide)	Long-acting cholinesterase inhibitor; enhances effect of endogenous acetylcholine on iris and ciliary muscle, causing miosis	Retinal detachment; ocular discomfort and redness; activation of latent iritis or uveitis; iris cysts; conjunctival thickening with obstruction of nasolacrimal canals can occur with prolonged use; lens opacities; cardiac irregularities; paradoxical rise in IOP	Topical drops; rarely used
Demecarium bromide (Humorsol)	Same as echothiophate iodide	Same as echothiophate iodide; also headache; browache; blurred vision	Topical drops; rarely used
Isoflurophate (Floropryl)	Same as echothiophate iodide	Same as demecarium	Topical ointment; rarely used
Carbonic Anhydrase Inhibitors			
Acetazolamide (Diamox) Dichlorphenamide (Daranide) Methazolamide (Neptazane)	Decreases aqueous production	Paresthesias, especially "tingling" in extremities; hearing dysfunction or tinnitus; loss of appetite; taste alteration; GI disturbances; drowsiness; confusion	Oral nonbacteriostatic sulfonamides; anaphylaxis and other sulfa-type allergic reactions may occur in patient allergic to sulfa; diuretic effect can lower electrolyte levels; ask patient about aspirin use; drug should not be given to patient on high-dose aspirin therapy
Hyperosmolar Agents			
Glycerine liquid (Ophthalgan; Osmoglyn Oral)	Increases extracellular osmolarity so intracellular water moves to the extracellular and vascular spaces, reducing IOP	Nausea; vomiting; headache; confusion, disorientation; dysrhythmia, severe dehydration	Oral liquid; used in acute glaucoma attacks or preoperatively when decreased IOP is desired; assess patient for susceptibility to pulmonary edema and CHF before administering hyperosmolar agents
Isosorbide solution (Ismotic)	Same as glycerine	Nausea; vomiting; headache; confusion; disorientation; syncope; lethargy; irritability	Oral liquid; same as glycerine
Mannitol solution (Osmitrol)	Same as glycerine	Nausea; vomiting; diarrhea; thrombophlebitis; hypertension; hypotension; tachycardia	IV solution; same as glycerine

ALT, Argon laser trabeculoplasty; *CHF,* congestive heart failure; *COPD,* chronic obstructive pulmonary disease; *GI,* gastrointestinal, *IOP,* intraocular pressure; *IV,* intravenous.

the patient's family in the assessment process because the chronic nature of these disorders impacts the family in many ways. Some families may become the primary providers of necessary care, such as eye drop administration or insulin injections, if the patient is unwilling or unable to accomplish these self-care activities. The nurse also assesses visual acuity, visual field, IOP, and fundus changes when appropriate.

Nursing Diagnoses

Nursing diagnoses specific to the patient with glaucoma and diabetic retinopathy include, but are not limited to, the following:

- Risk for noncompliance related to the inconvenience and side effects of glaucoma medications
- Risk for injury related to visual acuity deficits
- Risk for self-care deficits related to visual acuity deficits
- Pain related to pathophysiologic process and surgical correction

Planning

The overall goals are that the patient with glaucoma or diabetic retinopathy will (1) have no progression of visual impairment, (2) understand the disease process and therapeutic rationales, (3) comply with all aspects of therapy (including medication administration and follow-up care), and (4) have no postoperative complications.

Nursing Implementation

Health Maintenance and Promotion. The nurse has an important role in educating the patient and family about the risk of glaucoma or diabetic retinopathy. In addition, the nurse should stress the importance of early detection and treatment in preventing visual impairment from those disorders. This knowledge should encourage the patient to seek appropriate ophthalmic health care. The nurse may fulfill this teaching role by educating individual patients and families, groups of patients, or entire communities, depending on the nurse's practice setting. The patient should know that the incidence of glaucoma increases with age and that a comprehensive ophthalmic examination is invaluable in identifying persons with glaucoma or those at risk of developing glaucoma. The current recommendation is for an ophthalmologic examination every 2 to 4 years for persons between the ages of 40 and 64, and every 1 to 2 years for persons age 65 or older. African-Americans in every age category should have examinations more often because of the increased incidence and more aggressive course of glaucoma in these individuals.[34] The patient with diabetic retinopathy should be aware of the benefit of early laser treatment for proliferative retinopathy and the importance of early detection.

Acute Intervention. Acute nursing interventions are directed primarily toward the patient with acute angle-closure glaucoma and the surgical patient. The patient with acute angle-closure glaucoma requires immediate medication to lower the IOP, which the nurse must administer in a timely and appropriate manner according to the ophthalmologist's prescription. This patient may also be uncomfortable, and appropriate nursing comfort interventions may include darkening the environment, applying cool compresses to the patient's forehead, and providing a quiet and private space for the patient. Most surgical procedures for glaucoma or diabetic retinopathy are outpatient procedures. Acutely, the patient needs postoperative instructions and may require nursing comfort measures to relieve discomfort related to the procedure.

Chronic and Home Management Because of the chronic natures of these disorders, the patient with glaucoma or diabetic retinopathy needs encouragement to follow the therapeutic regimen and follow-up recommendations prescribed by their ophthalmologist. The patient needs accurate information about the disease processes, the normal course of the conditions, and the treatment options, including the rationales underlying each option. In addition, the patient with glaucoma needs information about the purpose, frequency, and technique for administration of prescribed antiglaucoma agents. In addition to verbal instructions, all patients should receive written information that contains the same information. This should be sufficiently detailed to provide all the necessary information without being so extensive that the patient becomes overwhelmed. The patient with glaucoma may be encouraged to comply with the medication regimen if the nurse encourages consideration of the sight-saving nature of the drops. The nurse can further encourage compliance by helping the patient identify the most convenient and appropriate times for medication administration or advocating a change in therapy if the patient reports unacceptable side effects. The diabetic patient has many nursing care needs in addition to the ophthalmic considerations. These are discussed in Chapter 46.

Gerontologic Considerations

Many older patients with glaucoma have systemic illnesses or take systemic medications that may affect their glaucoma therapy. In particular, the patient using a β-blocking glaucoma agent may experience an additive effect if a systemic βG-blocking medication is also being taken. All β-blocking glaucoma agents are contraindicated in the patient with bradycardia, greater than first degree heart block, cardiogenic shock, and overt cardiac failure. The noncardioselective β-blocker glaucoma agents are also contraindicated in the patient with severe chronic obstructive pulmonary disease (COPD) or asthma. The hyperosmolar agents may precipitate congestive heart failure (CHF) or pulmonary edema in the susceptible patient. The older patient is more likely to be on aspirin therapy for rheumatoid arthritis, and the carbonic anhydrase inhibitors are contraindicated in the patient on high-dose aspirin therapy. The adrenergic agents can cause tachycardia or hypertension, which may have serious consequences in the older patient. The nurse should teach the older patient to occlude the puncta to limit the systemic absorption of glaucoma medications. Special considerations for the older patient with diabetes are discussed in Chapter 46.

Intraocular Inflammation and Infection

The term *uveitis* is used to describe inflammation of the uveal tract, the retina, the vitreous body, or the optic nerve. This inflammation may be caused by bacteria, viruses, fungi, or parasites. *Cytomegalovirus retinitis* (CMV retinitis), is an opportunistic infection that occurs in patients with acquired immunodeficiency syndrome (AIDS), and in other immunosuppressed patients. The etiology of sterile intraocular inflammation includes autoimmune disorders, AIDS, malignancies, or those associated with systemic diseases such as juvenile rheumatoid arthritis and inflammatory bowel disease. Pain and photophobia are common symptoms.

Endophthalmitis is an extensive intraocular inflammation of the vitreous cavity. Bacteria, viruses, fungi, or parasites can all induce this serious inflammatory response. The mechanism of infection may be *endogenous,* in which the infecting agent arrives at the eye through the bloodstream, or *exogenous,* in which the infecting agent is introduced through a surgical wound or a penetrating injury. Although rare, most cases of endophthalmitis are a devastating complication of intraocular surgery or penetrating ocular injury and can lead to irreversible blindness within hours or days. Manifestations include ocular pain, photophobia, decreased visual acuity, headaches, upper lid edema, reddened and swollen conjunctiva, and corneal edema.

When all the layers of the eye (vitreous, retina, choroid, and sclera) are involved in the inflammatory response, the patient has *panophthalmitis*. In the final stages of extensive cases, the scleral coat may undergo bacterial or inflammatory dissolution. Subsequent rupture of the globe spreads the infection into the orbit or eyelids.

Treatment of intraocular inflammation is dependent on the underlying cause. Intraocular infections require antimicrobial agents, which may be delivered topically, subconjunctivally, intravitreally, systemically, or in some combination. Sterile inflammatory responses require antiinflammatory agents such as steroids. The site and severity of the sterile inflammatory response determines whether topical, subconjunctival, or systemic steroids are necessary.

The patient with intraocular inflammation is usually uncomfortable and may be noticeably anxious and frightened. The patient may fear sudden and total loss of vision. In some cases this fear is realistic, and the nurse should provide accurate information and emotional support to the patient and the family. In severe cases enucleation may be necessary. When the patient has lost visual function or even the entire eye, the patient will grieve the loss. The nurse's role includes helping the patient through the grieving process.

Enucleation

Enucleation is the removal of the eye. The primary indication for enucleation is a blind, painful eye. This may result from absolute glaucoma, infection, or trauma. Enucleation may also be indicated in ocular malignancies, although many malignancies can be managed with cryotherapy, radiation, and chemotherapy. An extremely rare indication is *sympathetic ophthalmia*, in which the untraumatized eye develops an inflammatory response following the primary eye trauma. In this situation the traumatized eye is enucleated. The surgical procedure includes severing the extraocular muscles close to their insertion on the globe, inserting an implant to maintain the intraorbital anatomy, and suturing the ends of the extraocular muscles over the implant. The conjunctiva covers the joined muscles, and a clear conformer is placed over the conjunctiva until the permanent prosthesis is fitted. A pressure dressing helps prevent postoperative bleeding.

Postoperatively the nurse observes the patient for signs of complications including excessive bleeding or swelling, increased pain, displacement of the implant, or temperature elevation. Patient instruction should include instillation of topical ointments or drops and wound cleansing. The nurse should also instruct the patient in the method of inserting the conformer into the socket in case the conformer falls out. The patient is often devastated by the loss of an eye, even when enucleation occurs following a lengthy period of painful blindness. The nurse should recognize and validate the patient's emotional response and provide support to the patient and the family.

Approximately 6 weeks following surgery the wound is sufficiently healed for the permanent prosthesis. The prosthesis is fitted by an ocularist and designed to match the remaining eye. The patient should learn how to remove, cleanse, and insert the prosthesis. Special polishing is required periodically to remove dried protein secretions.

The nurse may need to remove the prosthesis when the patient is unable to do so. After thorough hand washing, the nurses pulls the patient's lower lid down and toward the cheekbone. The prosthesis will usually slip out (Fig. 18-6). A special small suction tip may be used if necessary. The prosthesis should be cleaned with a mild soap, rinsed well, and stored in a container lined with soft material to prevent damage. The patient's name should be clearly marked on the container. To reinsert the prosthesis, the nurse opens the upper lid by pressure on the upper bony orbit, places the top of the prosthesis under the upper lid, and pulls the lower lid

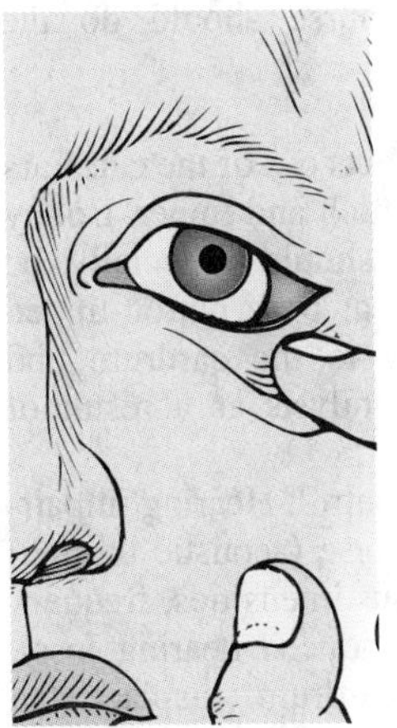
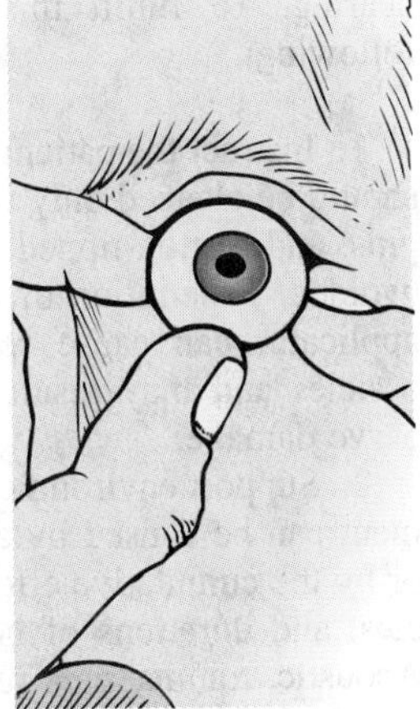

Fig. 18-6 Removal of ocular prosthesis.

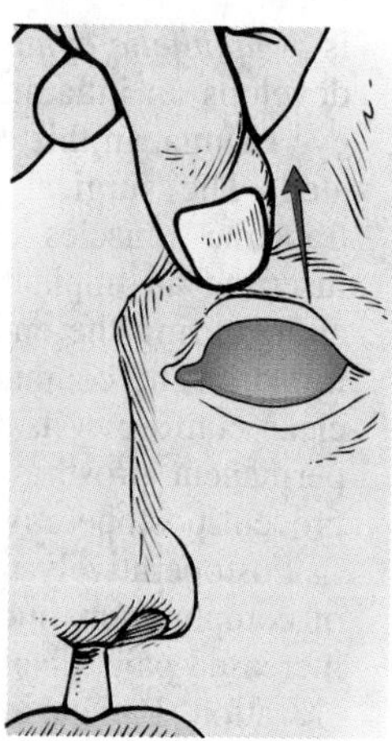
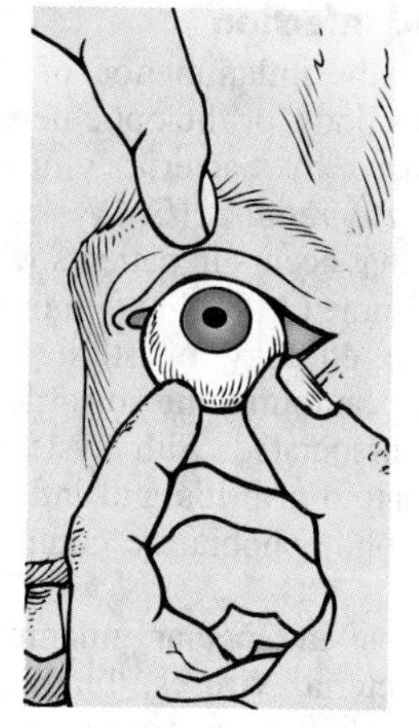
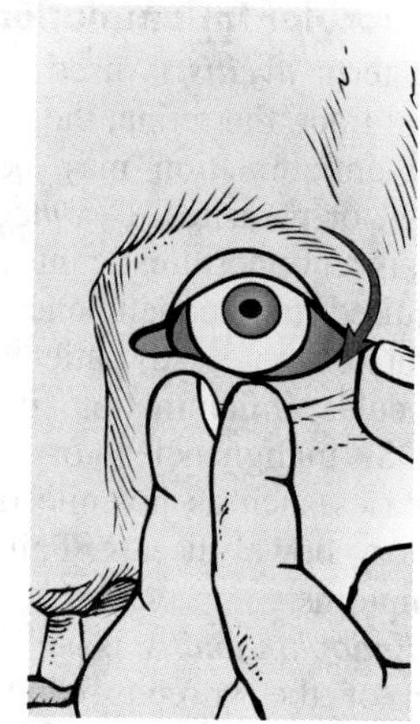

Fig. 18-7 Insertion of ocular prosthesis.

down. The lower edge of the prosthesis will slip under the lower lid with a little pressure on the prosthesis (Fig. 18-7).

Ocular Manifestations of Systemic Diseases

Many systemic diseases have significant ocular manifestations. Although it is not the purpose of this discussion to provide a full description of these disorders, it is important for the nurse to recognize that many systemic diseases have ocular symptoms. Conversely, ocular signs and symptoms may be the first finding or complaint in the patient with systemic diseases. One example is the patient with undiagnosed diabetes who seeks ophthalmic care for blurred vision. A careful health history and examination of the patient can reveal that the underlying cause of the blurred vision is lens swelling caused by uncontrolled hyperglycemia. Another example is the patient who seeks care for a conjunctival lesion. The ophthalmologist may be the first health care professional to make the diagnosis of AIDS based on the presence of a conjunctival Kaposi's sarcoma (KS). Table 18-12 lists some systemic diseases and the associated ophthalmic manifestations.

HEARING PROBLEMS

Health Promotion and Maintenance

The nurse has an important role in the preservation of hearing. To fulfill this role, the nurse should do the following:

1. Instruct the patient to keep objects out of the ear. Ears should be cleaned only with a washcloth and finger. Bobby pins and cotton-tipped applicators should especially be avoided. Penetration of the middle ear by a cotton-tipped applicator can cause serious injury to the eardrum and ossicles and may result in facial paralysis as a result of nerve damage.

2. Support environmental noise control. Hearing impairment can be caused by acute loud noise (acoustic trauma) or by the cumulative effects of various intensities, frequencies, and durations of noise (noise-induced hearing loss). Acoustic trauma can rupture the eardrum, displace the ossicles of the middle ear, and damage the organ of Corti in the inner ear. Noise-induced hearing loss is probably caused by high-intensity stimulation of the cochlear resulting in vasoconstriction and ischemia.

   Sensorineural hearing loss as a result of increased and prolonged environmental noise, such as amplified sound, is occurring in young adults at an increasing rate. Health teaching regarding avoidance of continued exposure to noise levels greater than 85 to 95 dB is essential. Table 18-13 describes the range of sounds audible to humans. Continued exposure to noise causes some persons to be more irritable and tense.

   The nurse should monitor noise levels in hospitals and at home to promote rest and recovery from illness. Interventions such as seeking different and less noisy equipment or a different time to use noisy equipment are possible solutions. In work environments known to have high noise levels (greater than 90 dB), ear protection should be worn. Occupational Safety and Health Administration (OSHA) standards require ear protection for workers in environments where the noise levels exceed 90 dB consistently. A variety of protectors is available that are worn over the ears or in the ears to prevent hearing loss. Periodic audiometric screening should be part of the health maintenance policies of industry. This provides baseline data on hearing to measure subsequent hearing loss.

   The nurse should participate in hearing conservation programs in work environments. A hearing conservation program has four main features: sound measurement, engineering and administrative controls, personal hearing protection, and audiometric monitoring of the population at risk.[37] Often a multidisciplinary team including an industrial hygienist, engineer, nurse, and audiometric technician is responsible for such a program.

   Ear protection should be worn during skeet shooting and other recreational pursuits with high noise levels. Young adults should be encouraged to keep amplified music to a reasonable level and limit their exposure time. Hearing loss caused by noise is not reversible.

3. Promote childhood and adult immunizations, including the measles, mumps, rubella (MMR) immunization. Various viruses can cause deafness as a result of fetal damage and malformations affecting the ear. Deafness will

Table 18-12 Ocular Manifestations of Systemic Diseases or Syndromes

Systemic Entity	Ocular Manifestations
▪ AIDS	Herpes zoster ophthalmicus, keratitis (bacterial and viral), CMV retinitis, endophthalmitis (bacterial and fungal), cotton-wool spots and microvasculopathy of the retina, KS of eyelids, conjunctiva
▪ Albinism	Decreased visual acuity, photophobia, nystagmus, strabismus
▪ Diabetes mellitus	Fluctuating refractive errors, diabetic retinopathy, macular edema, rubeosis irides, premature cataract development, increased incidence of glaucoma
▪ Down syndrome	Myopia, cataracts, nystagmus, strabismus, keratoconus, upward and outward slant of palpebral fissures
▪ Hypertension	Cotton-wool spots and hemorrhage of the retina, retinal lipid deposits
▪ Systemic lupus erythematosus	Dry eye, retinal changes, uveitis, scleritis
▪ Marfan's syndrome	Lens dislocation, high myopia, keratoconus, retinal detachment
▪ Rheumatoid arthritis	Dry eye, keratitis, scleritis
▪ Scleroderma	Dry eye, cotton-wool spots and hemorrhage of the retina, fibrotic eyelid changes
▪ Infections	
Botulism	Blurred vision, ptosis, diplopia, fixed, dilated pupil
Endocarditis	Subconjunctival or retinal petechiae
Tuberculosis	Conjunctivitis, keratitis, uveitis
Leprosy	Conjunctivitis, keratitis, uveitis, ptosis
Genital herpes	Herpes simplex keratitis
CMV infection	CMV retinitis
Measles	Conjunctivitis, keratitis, retinopathy
Congenital rubella	Cataracts, glaucoma
Histoplasmosis	Chorioretinal lesions, subretinal neovascularization
Toxoplasmosis	Necrotic retinal lesions, vitreal inflammation, retinochoroiditis
Lyme disease	Conjunctivitis, keratitis, episcleritis, panophthalmitis, retinal detachment, diplopia
Syphilis	Conjunctivitis, keratitis, uveitis, retinal detachment, macular edema, lens dislocation, glaucoma (congenital syphilis)
▪ Temporal arteritis	Vision loss, palsies of CN III, IV, and VI, nystagmus, ptosis
▪ Thyroid disease	Lid retraction, lid lag, exophthalmos, abnormal eye movement, increased IOP
▪ Vitamin deficiencies	
A	Night blindness, corneal ulceration
B	Optic neuropathy, corneal changes, retinal hemorrhage, nystagmus
C	Hemorrhage in anterior chamber, retina, conjunctiva
D	Exophthalmos

AIDS, Acquired immunodeficiency virus; *CMV*, cytomegalovirus; *CN*, cranial nerve; *IOP*, intraocular pressure; *KS*, Kaposi's sarcoma.

occur following exposure to rubella up to 16 weeks of gestation. Congenital defects following exposure to rubella after 20 weeks are rare.[35] Women who are susceptible to rubella can be vaccinated safely and effectively with a live attenuated rubella virus vaccine during the immediate puerperium.[36] This is an ideal time to vaccinate because there is no risk of inadvertently vaccinating a pregnant woman.

4. Monitor the patient's reaction to drugs that are known to cause ototoxicity. Ototoxic drugs are capable of damaging one or both branches of the auditory nerve (CN VIII) and the inner ear. Signs and symptoms of cochlear toxicity are tinnitus and sensorineural hearing loss. Damage in the vestibule and semicircular canals can result in vertigo, horizontal nystagmus, nausea and vomiting, and a spinning or rocking motion while sitting still. Risk factors associated with ototoxicity include the patient who is very young or very old, has a history of hearing loss, has renal or hepatic disease, uses two or more potentially ototoxic drugs, is dehydrated, has bacteremia, and has a history of previous exposure to loud noise or cranial irradiation.[38]

Drugs commonly associated with ototoxicity include aspirin, cinchona alkaloids (quinidine), loop diuretics, cisplatin, and aminoglycosides. The patient who is receiving these drugs should be assessed for development or exacerbation of signs and symptoms associated with ototoxicity. When these symptoms develop, immediate withdrawal of the offending drug may prevent further damage and may cause the symptoms to disappear. When withdrawal of the

Table 18-13 Range of Sounds Audible to Human Ear

Typical Decibel	Example
0	Lowest sound audible to the human ear
30	Quiet library, soft whisper
40	Living room, quiet office, bedroom away from traffic
50	Light traffic at a distance, refrigerator, gentle breeze
60	Air conditioner at 20 ft, conversation, sewing machine
70	Busy traffic, office tabulator, noisy restaurant. At this decibel level, noise may begin to affect hearing if exposure is constant.
Hazardous Zone	
80	Subway, heavy city traffic, alarm clock at two feet, factory noise. These noises are dangerous if exposure to them lasts for more than 8 hr.
90	Truck traffic, noisy home appliances, shop tools, lawn mower. As loudness increases, the "safe" time exposure decreases; damage can occur in less than 8 hr.
100	Chain saw, stereo headphones, pneumatic drill. Even 2 hr of exposure can be dangerous at this decibel level; with each 5 dB increase the safe time is cut in half.
120	Rock band concert in front of speakers, sandblasting, thunderclap. The danger is immediate; exposure at 120 dB can injure ears.
140	Gunshot blast, jet plane. *Any* length of exposure time is dangerous; noise at this level may cause actual pain in the ear.
180	Rocket launching pad. Without ear protection, noise at this level causes irreversible damage; hearing loss is inevitable.

From American Academy of Otolaryngology, 1983,

drug therapy is life-threatening, the patient should be advised of the possibility of permanent hearing loss.

5. Identify the patient who has a potential for hearing loss. Children who are chronic mouth breathers need referral. Enlarged adenoids can block the nasal passages, as well as the eustachian tube, preventing aeration of the middle ear. This also predisposes the child to serous otitis media. Children who have acute otitis media frequently need to be watched for signs of chronic otitis media. It is important that children complete the full course of antibiotics prescribed for the acute episode.

6. Be observant of symptoms that indicate hearing loss at all ages. These symptoms include asking others to speak up, answering questions inappropriately, not responding when not looking at the speaker, straining to hear, cupping hands around ear, showing irritability with others who do not speak up, and increasing sensitivity to slight increases in noise level. Often the patient is not aware of minimal hearing loss or may compensate by using these mannerisms. Children will often be inattentive, bored, or uncooperative when they have decreased hearing caused by a middle ear infection (conductive type of loss) or an inner ear problem (sensorineural loss). Hearing loss in the older adult is most often first noticed by family and friends and not the patient.

EXTERNAL EAR AND CANAL

Trauma

Trauma to the external ear can cause injury to the subcutaneous tissue that may result in a hematoma. If the hematoma is not aspirated, an inflammation of the membranes of the ear cartilage (perichondritis) can result. Antibiotics are given to prevent infection. Blows to the ear can also cause hearing loss if there is dislocation of the ossicles of the middle ear or if a perforation of the eardrum results. It is important to obtain a careful history of the accident and to assess the hearing of a patient who has had a blow to the ear or side of the head.

External Otitis

The skin of the external ear and canal is subject to the same problems as skin anywhere on the body. *External otitis* involves inflammation or infection of the epithelium of the auricle and ear canal. It is a more common finding in the summer. Swimming in contaminated waters is frequently implicated and is called *swimmer's ear*. Trauma caused by picking the ear or the use of sharp objects, such as hairpins, frequently causes the initial break in the skin.

Etiology. External otitis may be caused by infections, dermatitis, or both. Bacteria or fungi may be the cause. The bacteria most commonly cultured are *Pseudomonas aeruginosa, Proteus vulgaris, Escherichia coli,* and *Staphylococcus aureus*. The most common fungi are *Candida albicans* and *Aspergillus* organisms. Fungi are often the causative agents of external otitis, especially in warm, moist climates. The warm, dark environment of the ear canal provides a good medium for the growth of microorganisms.

Clinical Manifestations and Complications. Pain is one of the first signs of external otitis. It is caused by the stretching of the tight epithelium of the ear canal by the inflammatory process. Pain is especially noted on movement of the auricle or on application of pressure to the tragus (directly in front of the ear). Drainage from the ear may be serosanguineous or purulent. If it is the result of an infection caused by a *Pseudomonas* organism, the drainage will be green and have a musty smell. Temperature elevations occur when there is extensive involvement of the tissue. The swelling of the ear canal can block hearing and cause dizziness.

THERAPEUTIC AND NURSING MANAGEMENT

EXTERNAL OTITIS

Diagnosis is made by observation with the otoscope light using the largest speculum the ear will accommodate without causing the patient unnecessary discomfort. The eardrum may be normal if it can be seen. Culture and sensitivity

Table 18-14 Therapeutic Management: External Otitis

Diagnostic
- Otoscopic examination
- Culture and sensitivity

Therapeutic
- Analgesics (depending on severity)
- Warm compresses
- Cleansing of canal
- Ear wick
- Antibiotic otic drops
- Systemic antibiotics

studies of the drainage may be done. Aspirin or codeine will usually control the pain. After the ear canal is cleansed, a wick of cotton is placed in the canal to help deliver the antibiotic eardrops. Cotton wicks should be used with caution in patients, such as the very young and confused or psychotic patients, who may push them farther into the ear. Topical antibiotics include polymyxin B, colistin, neomycin, and chloromycetin. Nystatin is used for fungal infections. Corticosteroids may also be used unless the etiology of the problem is a fungal infection. Corticosteroids are contraindicated in fungal infections. If the surrounding tissue is involved, systemic antibiotics are prescribed. Warm, moist compresses or heat may be prescribed. Improvement should occur in 48 hours, but more time is required for complete resolution.

Careful handling and disposal of material saturated with drainage are important. Otic (ear) drops should be administered at room temperature because cold drops can elicit dizziness in the patient by stimulation of the semicircular canals. The tip of the dropper should not touch the auricle during administration to prevent contamination of the entire bottle of drops when the dropper is replaced in the bottle. The ear is positioned so that the drops can run down the canal. This position should be maintained for 2 minutes after eardrop administration to allow dispersion of drops. The diagnostic and therapeutic management of external otitis is shown in Table 18-14.

Cerumen and Foreign Bodies in the External Ear Canal

Impacted cerumen can cause discomfort and decreased hearing, which is often described as a hollow sensation. In the older person, the earwax becomes drier and harder and is not easily removed from the canal.[39] Water that enters the canal during a shower or swimming may cause swelling of the cerumen, resulting in complete blockage of the canal. Management involves irrigation of the canal with body-temperature solutions. Special syringes can be used and vary from the simple bulb syringe to special irrigating equipment used in the physician's office or clinic (Fig. 18-8). The patient is placed in a sitting position with an emesis basin under the ear. The auricle is pulled up and back, and the flow of solution is directed to the top of the

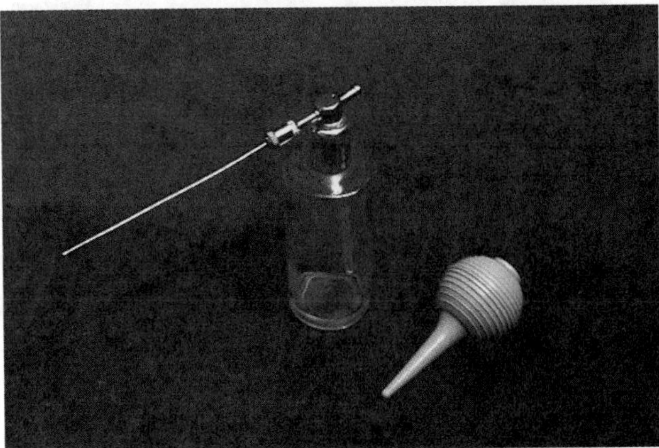

Fig. 18-8 Types of equipment used to irrigate the external ear canal. A bulb syringe (*right*) and an ear irrigation apparatus used in doctors' offices and clinics (*left*) are shown.

canal. It is important that the ear canal not be completely occluded with the syringe tip. If this irrigation does not remove the wax, a special cerumen spoon can be used. Mild lubricant drops may be used (sometimes overnight) to soften the earwax, and irrigation may then be effective in removing the impacted cerumen.

The list of objects removed from the ear is extensive and includes animate, inanimate, vegetable, and mineral objects. The major problem of foreign body removal is the isthmus of the canal. Attempts to remove the object occasionally result in pushing it beyond the isthmus. This trauma causes edema, which can trap the object and make removal difficult.

Animate objects must be killed before removal.[40] Olive oil, mineral oil, or ether can be used to kill or stupefy the insect. Irrigation can then be used to flush the insect out. If a wood tick has become attached to the tissue, it can be removed with ear forceps. Care should be taken to avoid crushing the wood tick, which leaves its head attached to the tissue.

Malignancy of the External Ear

Malignancies of the external ear (other than skin cancers) and canal are uncommon. The predominant signs include a chronic ulcer of the auricle and persistent drainage from the canal. This drainage is tinged with blood and does not diminish with treatment. Therapeutic management includes biopsy and other diagnostic studies to determine invasion of underlying tissue and bone. Treatment involves surgery. If the malignancy involves the ear canal and temporal bone, radical surgery of the middle and inner ear with resection of the facial nerve (CN VII), auditory nerve (CN VIII), and part of the temporal bone may be necessary.

The amount of resection is determined by the extent of disease. Basal cell carcinoma of the auricle accounts for approximately 1.5% of all basal cell carcinomas of the head and neck. It is usually attributed to sun exposure. These skin cancers can be simply excised surgically, or they may be serially excised using a special technique to microscopically examine the tissue to be sure that all residual cancer cells are resected. This procedure is known as Mohs' micrographic chemosurgery. These skin cancers are usually not life-threatening, and the cure rate after resection is greater than 95% in most cases.

MIDDLE EAR AND MASTOID

Acute Otitis Media

The most common problem of the middle ear is *acute otitis media,* usually a childhood disease associated with colds, sore throats, and blockage of the eustachian tube. The earlier the initial episode, the greater the risk of subsequent episodes. Predisposing factors include young age, congenital abnormalities, immune deficiencies, passive smoke inhalation, eustachian tube damage from viral infections, family history of otitis media, and allergic rhinitis. Although most patients have mixed infections, bacteria are the predominant etiologic agents. Pain, fever, malaise, headache, and reduced hearing are clinical manifestations of acute otitis media.

Therapeutic management involves the use of antibiotics to eradicate the causative organism. Surgical intervention is generally reserved for the patient who does not respond to medical treatment. A *myringotomy* involves an incision in the tympanum to release the increased pressure and exudate in the ear. Prompt treatment of an episode of acute otitis media generally prevents spontaneous perforation of the tympanic membrane. In the adult patient where allergy may be an accompanying factor, antihistamines may also be prescribed as part of the medication regimen. Otherwise, antihistamines have not proven effective.[42] Since the advent of treatment with antibiotics, the incidence of severe and prolonged infections of the middle ear and mastoid has been greatly reduced except in areas where health care is inadequate or people have limited access to health care.

Chronic Otitis Media and Mastoiditis

Significance and Etiology. Untreated or repeated attacks of acute otitis media may lead to the chronic condition. Chronic infection of the middle ear is more common in the person who experienced episodes of acute otitis media in early childhood. Organisms involved in chronic otitis media include *Staphylococcus aureus, Streptococcus, Proteus mirabilis, Pseudomonas aeruginosa,* and *E. coli.* Because the mucous membrane is continuous, both the middle ear and the air cells of the mastoid can be involved in the chronic infectious process.

Clinical Manifestations. *Chronic otitis media* is characterized by a purulent, foul-smelling discharge accompanied by hearing loss and occasionally by ear pain, nausea, and episodes of dizziness. The patient may complain of hearing loss that may be due to destruction of the ossicles, a tympanic membrane perforation, or the accumulation of fluid in the middle ear space. Occasionally a facial palsy or an attack of vertigo may alert the patient to this condition. Chronic otitis media is usually painless, but if pain is present, it indicates fluid under pressure.

Untreated conditions can result in an eardrum perforation and the formation of a cholesteatoma (a cystic mass found in the middle ear composed of epithelial cells and cholesterol). Enzymes produced by it may destroy the adjacent bones, including the ossicles. Unless removed surgically a cholesteatoma can cause extensive damage to the structures of the middle ear, can erode the bony protection of the facial nerve, may create a labyrinthine fistula, or even invade the dura, threatening the brain. In addition to cholesteatoma, other complications of chronic otitis media include sensorineural deafness, facial weakness, lateral sinus thrombosis, brain or subdural abscess, and meningitis.[43]

Diagnostic Studies. Otoscopic examination may reveal a marginal or central perforation of the eardrum (Fig. 18-9). A central perforation has tympanum remaining around all points of the circumference. Some eardrums may be healed but have an area that is more flaccid and thinner, indicative of a previous perforation. Culture and sensitivity tests are necessary to identify the organisms involved and the appropriate antibiotic to use. The audiogram may demonstrate no loss in hearing or a loss as great as 50 to 60 dB if the ossicles have been partially destroyed or disarticulated (separated). X-rays, polytomography, or a computerized tomography (CT) scan of the temporal bone may demonstrate bone destruction, absence of ossicles, or the presence of a mass, most likely a cholesteatoma.

Therapeutic Management. The aim of treatment is to rid the middle ear of infection (Table 18-15). Systemic antibiotic therapy based on the sensitivity study is initiated. In addition, the patient may need to undergo frequent evacuation of drainage and debris in an outpatient setting. Antibiotic eardrops and 2% acetic acid drops are also used to reduce infection. If there is a recurrence, the patient may need to be treated with parenteral antibiotics.

Often chronic tympanic membrane perforations will not heal in response to conservative treatment, and surgery is necessary. Surgery to restore the structure and function to the middle ear is called a *tympanoplasty* (Table 18-16). Diseased tissue is removed, and the ossicles are examined and evaluated in reconstructing the conductive mechanism. This may be done with the use of partial or total ossicular prostheses in combination with a fascia graft to repair the perforation of the tympanic membrane. The incision may be endaural (incision within the ear canal) or postauricular

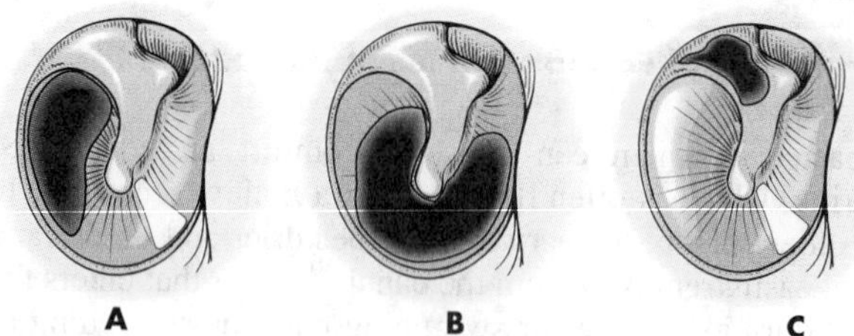

Fig. 18-9 Three common tympanic perforations. ***A,*** Small central perforation (hearing is usually good). ***B,*** Large central perforation around the handle of the malleus (hearing is usually poor). ***C,*** Marginal perforation of Shrapnell's membrane (hearing is usually good). Cholesteatomas commonly occur in patients with a marginal perforation and are always present with attic perforation.

(behind the auricle or ear) depending on the amount of involvement.

A *mastoidectomy* is often performed concurrently with tympanoplasty to remove diseased tissue and the source of infection. A modified mastoidectomy attempts to preserve functioning by removing as little structural tissue as possible. Removal of tissue stops at the middle ear structures that appear capable of functioning in the conduction of sound. A radical mastoidectomy, which involves complete removal of all middle ear structures, is required when disease is extensive or when complete exposure is necessary. No attempt is made to restore conductive hearing. The middle ear and mastoid become one large cavity. This surgery is rarely performed today, but it was not uncommon before antibiotics were available to treat ear infections. Patients seen today with a history of this type of surgery would have been children or young adults in the early 1940s or may have been raised in a culture or country without adequate medical treatment.

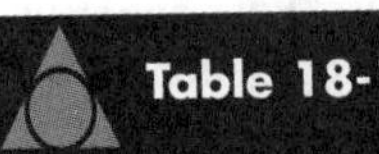

Table 18-15 Therapeutic Management: Chronic Otitis Media

Diagnostic
- Otoscopic examination
- Culture and sensitivity
- Mastoid x-ray

Therapeutic
- Ear irrigations
- Acetic acid (equal amounts of white vinegar and warm water)
- Otic drops, powders
- Systemic antibiotics
- Surgery
  - Tympanoplasty*
  - Mastoidectomy (modified)
- Analgesics
- Antiemetics

*See Table 18-16.

Table 18-16 Types of Tympanoplasty

Type	Description
I	Absorbable Gelfoam sponge placed in middle ear to support fascia or vein graft under the tympanic membrane
II	Fascia or perichondrium grafted over remnant of malleus to correct ossicular defect
III	Removal of necrosed ossicles except for stapes, with fascia or perichondrium graft placed over stapes
IV	Removal of necrosed ossicles except for footplate of the stapes, with fascia or perichondrium graft placed over footplate
V	Fenestration made into horizontal semicircular canal and then closed with fascia or perichondrium graft

NURSING MANAGEMENT

FOLLOWING TYMPANOPLASTY

Routine preoperative care is provided before tympanoplasty and includes teaching postoperative expectations. Postoperative concerns are the avoidance of complications such as disruption of the repair during the healing phase, facial nerve paralysis (rare), and increased pressure in the middle ear (see the nursing care plan on p. 474). The patient is instructed to avoid blowing the nose because this causes increased pressure in the eustachian tube and the middle ear cavity and could dislodge the graft to the tympanum. Coughing and sneezing can cause similar disruption and are to be avoided if possible. If the patient must cough or sneeze, leaving the mouth open will reduce the pressure increase. It is essential that the patient be helped when getting up the first time, because dizziness, loss of balance, and a resulting fall may occur.

A cotton ball dressing is used for an endaural incision. If a postauricular incision is used and a drain is in place, a mastoid dressing is used. A 4 inch by 4 inch dressing is cut to fit behind the ear, and fluffs are applied over the ear to prevent the outer circular head dressing from placing pressure on the auricle. It is necessary to monitor the tightness of the dressing (to prevent tissue necrosis) and the amount and type of drainage postoperatively.

Serous Otitis Media

Serous otitis media (effusion of the middle ear) is an accumulation of sterile fluid in the middle ear. The fluid may be thin, mucoid, or mucopurulent. The middle ear fluid can become thick and mucoid (called glue ear) and may be bloody. It may occur at any age but is more frequent in children. The fluid usually collects because of a malfunction of the eustachian tube, which commonly follows upper respiratory and chronic sinus infections, barotrauma (caused by pressure change), or otitis media. If the eustachian tube does not open and allow equalization of atmospheric pressure, negative pressure within the middle ear pulls (effuses) fluid from the tissues and capillaries. Allergic reaction of the mucosa and subsequent edema can also cause blockage of the eustachian tube and cause fluid within the ear. Overgrowth of nasopharyngeal lymphoid tissue and chronic sinusitis are also factors that may contribute to middle ear effusion.

Complaints include a feeling of fullness of the ear, pressure, and decreased hearing. The patient does not experience pain, fever, or discharge from the ear. Otoscopic examination may reveal a normal tympanic membrane or minimal dullness and retraction. Tympanometry and pneumotoscopy may demonstrate limited tympanic membrane motion.

Decongestants, antihistamines, and glucocorticoids, as well as antibiotics, have been used in the treatment of serous effusions. Exercises such as swallowing and gum chewing are used to open the eustachian tube. In addition, the patient may be taught Valsalva's maneuver (nose and mouth are closed off, forcing air into middle ear through the eustachian tube). If the effusion is not relieved in a few days or a week, a myringotomy is performed, usually under

NURSING CARE PLAN Patient After Middle Ear Surgery

Planning: Outcome Criteria	Nursing Interventions and Rationales
➤ **NURSING DIAGNOSIS**	Pain *related to* surgical incision and localized pressure and edema *as manifested by* verbalization of pain, isolation, withdrawal
Verbalize satisfaction with pain relief.	Assess degree of pain *to plan appropriate intervention.* Report excessive ear pain immediately. Administer analgesics as needed *to relieve pain by interrupting CNS pathways.* Assess and document effectiveness. Encourage patient to avoid sudden movements *that increase pain.* Do not position patient on operative side *to avoid accumulation of fluid and subsequent increase in pain.*
➤ **NURSING DIAGNOSIS**	Risk for injury *related to* decreased hearing acuity and dizziness
Identify factors that increase risk of injury; formulate plan to alter environment to reduce risk and experience no incidence of injury	Assess patient for decreased hearing, lack of awareness of environmental warning sounds, dizziness when upright *to determine injury potential*; determine patient's hearing level *to plan appropriate interventions.* Assist with assessing environment *to identify and alter injury risk factors.* Assess and monitor dizziness. Assist with ambulation as needed. Instruct patient to change positions slowly, keep eyes straight ahead, and move head and body as a unit *to prevent dizziness and the possibility of falling.* Structure environment to reduce visual input *that exacerbates dizziness.* Put patient in a quiet darkened room *to reduce stimulus for dizziness.* When transfering patient in a wheelchair, move slowly down hallways *to prevent dizziness.*
➤ **NURSING DIAGNOSIS**	Impaired verbal communication *related to* hearing loss *as manifested by* unawareness of being addressed, no tracking of sound, inappropriate response when addressed, verbalization of inability to hear part or all of spoken communication, inattentive, use of loud or soft speaking voice (depending on type of hearing problem)
Express satisfaction with communication pattern; use alternative method to communicate (if indicated)	Assess ability to receive verbal messages *to determine extent of problem and plan appropriate interventions.* Use techniques such as slowed speech and speaking directly into better or nonoperated ear *to increase ability to hear.* Attempt to determine whether a message has been received accurately *to evaluate effectiveness of interventions.*
➤ **NURSING DIAGNOSIS**	Social isolation *related to* inability to make meaningful contact with another secondary to hearing deficit *as manifested by* solitary lifestyle; few, if any, visitors or phone calls; verbalization of feelings of aloneness
Express satisfaction with amount and kind of social contacts	Assess patient preference for social activities *to individualize interventions.* Suggest names of groups with persons with similar disabilities *so common feelings and problems can be shared.*
➤ **NURSING DIAGNOSIS**	Altered health maintenance *related to* lack of knowledge of self-care and signs and symptoms of complications *as manifested by* frequent questioning related to self-care and complications, inability to answer or incorrect responses regarding self-care and possible complications
Have adequate knowledge base to take care of self and identify complications	Instruct patient not to blow nose or cough and to sneeze with mouth open *to prevent fluctuation of air pressure in middle ear.* Give written instructions *so patient has accurate reference for self-care.* Teach self-care and signs and symptoms of complications *to increase patient's sense of control.*

continued

NURSING CARE PLAN Patient After Middle Ear Surgery—cont'd

COLLABORATIVE PROBLEMS AND COMPLICATIONS

Nursing Goals	Nursing Interventions and Rationales
➤ **POTENTIAL COMPLICATION** Bleeding from operative site *related to* surgical incision	
Monitor for bleeding, report deviation from acceptable parameters, and carry out appropriate medical and nursing interventions	Assess, record, and report unusual bleeding or drainage from operative site. Elevate head of bed 30 degrees *to decrease intravascular pressure.*
➤ **POTENTIAL COMPLICATION** Facial nerve damage *related to* edema	
Monitor for bleeding, report deviation from acceptable parameters, and carry out appropriate medical and nursing interventions	Monitor to detect inability to perform activities controlled by facial nerve such as wrinkling eyebrows and nose, closing lids, smiling and baring teeth symmetrically *to detect problem.* Notify physician if problem observed *so early treatment can be initiated.*

local or topical anesthesia and an operating microscope. A ventilating tube is frequently used for the person who has recurrent serous otitis media or dysfunction of the eustachian tube. The patient who has a ventilating tube in the eardrum must be instructed not to swim or get water in the ear. Despite efforts to correct inadequate middle ear aeration, eustachian tube dysfunction may persist, causing collapse of the eardrum, conductive hearing loss, and formation of a cholesteatoma.

Otosclerosis

Otosclerosis, an autosomal dominant disease, is the fixation of the footplate of the stapes in the oval window by bony overgrowth. It is a common cause of conductive hearing loss in young adults, especially women, and may be accelerated during pregnancy. It is a common finding in children who have a rare disease known as osteogenesis imperfecta. Otosclerosis involves both ears but at different rates. Spongy bone develops from the bony labyrinth, causing immobilization of the footplate of the stapes, which reduces the transmission of vibrations to the inner ear fluids. Hearing loss is typically bilateral, although one ear frequently shows a greater hearing loss. The patient is often unaware of the problem until the loss becomes so severe that communication is difficult. Loss of hearing usually becomes increasingly severe. Otosclerosis is rare in African-Americans.

Otoscopic examination may reveal a pinkish-orange discoloration of the tympanum (Schwartz's sign) caused by the vascular and bony changes within the middle ear. The Rinne test, using the 512 Hz tuning fork, favors bone conduction. Bone conduction is equal to or greater than air conduction (BC > AC). This is a negative Rinne test. Weber's test lateralizes to the poor ear or to the ear with the greater conductive hearing loss. An audiogram demonstrates good hearing by bone conduction, but poor hearing is demonstrated by air conduction or an air-bone gap audiogram. Usually at least a difference of 20 dB to 25 dB between air-conduction and bone-conduction levels of hearing is seen.

Therapeutic Management. A *stapedectomy* is the surgical treatment for otosclerosis and is usually performed with the patient under local anesthesia. The poorer-hearing ear is repaired first, and the other ear is operated on at a later date. (The therapeutic management of otosclerosis is shown in Table 18-17.)

In stapedectomy an endaural incision is made using the operating microscope for visualization. Generally the stapes superstructure is removed, and a small hole is made in the footplate. A prosthesis made of wire, polyethylene, or some other synthetic material completes the ossicular chain. Sound is then conducted with the prosthesis. The tympanum is rolled back into place, and packing is placed in the external ear canal. A cotton ball dressing is placed in the

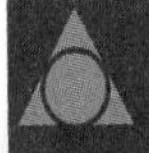

Table 18-17 Therapeutic Management: Otosclerosis

Diagnostic
- Otoscopic examination
- Rinne test (512 Hz tuning fork)
- Weber test
- Audiometry
- Tympanometry

Therapeutic
- Hearing aid
- Surgery (stapedectomy)
- Analgesics
- Antiemetics
- Antibiotics
- Antimotion drugs

outer portion of the ear canal. During surgery the patient will often report an immediate improvement in hearing in the operative ear. Because of the accumulation of blood and fluid in the middle ear, the hearing level decreases postoperatively but does return to near-normal levels. In 90% to 95% of patients, normal hearing is restored.[43]

A *perilymph fistula* (incomplete closure of the oval window) can occur with symptoms of widely fluctuating hearing levels, tinnitus, and dizziness. Approximately 6% of patients may develop a sensorineural hearing loss. An audiogram is repeated when the ear heals.

NURSING MANAGEMENT

OTOSCLEROSIS

Nursing management of the patient undergoing a stapedectomy and for the patient who has undergone a tympanoplasty is similar. (See the above nursing care plan). Postoperatively, the patient may experience dizziness, nausea, and vomiting because of stimulation of the labyrinth intraoperatively. Some patients will demonstrate nystagmus on lateral gaze because of disturbance of the perilymph. Care should be taken to decrease as much as possible sudden movements by the patient that may bring on or exacerbate episodes of dizziness. Actions (coughing, sneezing, lifting, bending, straining during bowel movements) that increase intracranial pressure should also be minimized.

INNER EAR PROBLEMS

Three symptoms that indicate disease of the inner ear are vertigo (whirling), sensorineural hearing loss, and tinnitus (ringing in the ear). Symptoms of vertigo arise from the vestibular labyrinth, whereas hearing loss and tinnitus arise from the auditory labyrinth. There is an overlap between manifestations of inner ear problems and CNS disorders.

Ménière's Disease

Ménière's disease (endolymphatic hydrops) is characterized by the triad of symptoms caused by inner ear disease: episodic vertigo, tinnitus, and fluctuating sensorineural hearing loss. It incapacitates the patient because of sudden, severe attacks of vertigo. Symptoms usually begin at approximately 40 years of age. In 85% of patients with Ménière's disease, only one ear is affected.

The cause of the disease is unknown, but it results in an excessive accumulation of endolymph in the membranous labyrinth. The volume of endolymph increases until the membranous labyrinth ruptures, mixing high-potassium endolymph with low-potassium perilymph. These changes lead to degeneration of the delicate vestibular and cochlear hair cells. Attacks of vertigo are sudden and often occur without warning. Attacks may be preceded by an aura consisting of a sense of fullness in the ear, increasing tinnitus, and a decrease in hearing. Before vertigo attacks the patient may report inner ear "fullness." The patient complains that the environment is whirling wildly and experiences the feeling of being pulled to the ground (often called "drop attacks"). Some patients report that they feel as if they are whirling in space. The duration may be hours or days, and attacks may occur several times a year. Autonomic symptoms include pallor, sweating, nausea, and vomiting.

The clinical course of the disease is highly variable. Low-pitched *tinnitus* may be present continuously in the affected ear or be intensified during an attack. Hearing loss fluctuates, but it decreases with each attack of vertigo.

THERAPEUTIC AND NURSING MANAGEMENT

MÉNIÈRE'S DISEASE

Therapeutic management of Ménière's disease (Table 18-18) includes diagnostic tests to rule out CNS disease. The audiogram demonstrates a hearing loss in the low tones. Vestibular tests indicate decreased function.

The glycerol test may suggest the diagnosis of Ménière's disease. An oral dose of glycerol is given, and hearing threshold and speech discrimination are tested 1 to 3 hours after administration. Improvement in hearing or speech discrimination supports a diagnosis of Ménière's disease. The improvement is attributed to the osmotic effect of glycerol that pulls fluid from the inner ear.

During the acute attack, atropine may be given to decrease the autonomic nervous system function. Diazepam (Valium) is often used instead of atropine. Acute vertigo is treated symptomatically with bed rest, sedation, and antiemetics or drugs for motion sickness administered orally,

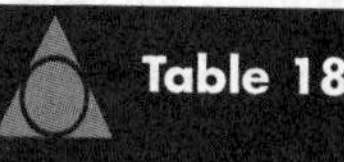

Table 18-18 Therapeutic Management: Ménière's Disease

Diagnostic
- History
- Audiometric studies, including speech discrimination, tone decay
- Vestibular tests, including caloric test, positional tests
- Electronystagmography
- Neurologic examination
- Glycerol test

Therapeutic

Acute (one or more)
- Sedative (Diazepam [Valium])
- Anticholinergic (atropine)
- Vasodilator (histamine)
- Antihistamine (diphenhydramine [Benadryl])

Chronic (one or more)
- Diuretics
- Antihistamines
- Vasodilators
- Neuroleptics
- Vitamins
- Diazepam (Valium)
- Low-salt diet
- Restriction of caffeine, nicotine, and alcohol intake

Conservative surgical intervention
- Endolymphatic shunt
- Vestibular nerve section

Destructive surgical intervention
- Labyrinthotomy
- Labyrinthectomy

rectally, or IV. The patient requires reassurance and counseling that the condition is not life-threatening. Management between attacks may include vasodilatation, diuretics, antihistamines, a low-sodium diet, and other interventions. Diazepam (Valium) and Antivert (Bonamine plus nicotinic acid) are commonly used to reduce the dizziness. Over a period of time, most patients respond to the prescribed medications but must learn to live with the unpredictability of the attacks. Approximately 80% of patients experience improvement with therapeutic management.[43] Conservation of hearing is a main concern for most patients.

Frequent and incapacitating attacks, reduced quality of life, and threatened employment are indications for surgical intervention. Surgical decompression of the endolymphatic sac is performed to reduce the pressure on the cochlear hair cells and to prevent further damage and sensorineural hearing loss. If relief is not achieved with endolymphatic shunt surgery and hearing remains good, vestibular nerve resection may be performed to alleviate vertigo and preserve hearing. When involvement is unilateral, surgical ablation of the labyrinth, resulting in loss of the vestibular and hearing cochlear function, is performed. Careful therapeutic management can decrease the possibility of progressive sensorineural loss in many patients.

Nursing interventions are planned to minimize vertigo and keep the patient safe. During the acute attack the patient is kept in a quiet, darkened room in a comfortable position. Because motion aggravates the whirling and roaring sensations, the patient is moved only for essential care. Fluorescent or flickering lights or watching television may exacerbate symptoms and are avoided when possible. An emesis basin should be available, because vomiting is common. To minimize the risk of falling the nurse should keep the siderails up when the patient is in bed. The bed should be kept in the low position. The patient should be instructed to call for assistance when getting out of bed. Medications and fluids are administered parenterally, and intake and output are monitored. When the attack subsides the patient is assisted with ambulation because unsteadiness may remain. Similar nursing care is provided after surgical ablation of the labyrinth. The patient will have severe tinnitus and vertigo, which decrease during a period of days or weeks as the brain adjusts to loss of vestibular input and postural stability is regained.

Presbycusis

Presbycusis is hearing loss associated with aging, which results in high pitched sounds becoming inaudible and hearing becoming increasingly restricted to low-frequency sounds. High-frequency sounds such as the consonants f, p, t, k, ch, sh, and st become increasingly difficult for the older adult to hear. Because consonants are the letters by which spoken words are recognized, the ability of the older adult with presbycusis to understand the spoken word is greatly affected. There may be a significant difference between what was said and what was heard, leading to confusion and embarrassment.

The cause of presbycusis is related to degenerative changes in the inner ear such as loss of hair cells, reduction of blood supply, diminution of endolymph production, decreased basilar membrane flexibility, and loss of neurons in the cochlear nuclei. Table 18-19 describes the classification of specific causes and associated hearing changes of presbycusis. Often, more than one type of presbycusis may be present in the same person. The prognosis for hearing depends on the cause of the presbycusis. Sound amplification with the appropriate device is often effective in improving the understanding of speech. In other situations an audiologic rehabilitation program can be valuable.

The older adult is often reluctant to use a hearing aid for amplification. In our society a hearing aid is often associated with aging. Most hearing aids and the necessary batteries are small in size, and neuromuscular changes such as stiff fingers, enlarged joints, and decreased sensory perception often make the care and handling of a hearing aid a difficult and frustrating experience for an older person.

Table 18-19 Classification of Presbycusis

Type	Cause	Hearing Change and Prognosis
▪ Sensory	Atrophy of organ of Corti; degeneration of hair cells	Loss of high-pitched sounds, little effect on speech understanding; good response to sound amplification
▪ Neural	Degenerative changes in cochlea and spiral ganglion	Loss of speech discrimination; amplification alone not sufficient
▪ Metabolic	Atrophy of blood vessels in wall of cochlea with interruption of essential nutrient supply	Uniform loss for all frequencies accompanied by recruitment*; good response to hearing aid
▪ Mechanical	Atrophic changes in structures involved with vibration of cochlear partition	Hearing loss increases from low to high frequencies; speech discrimination affected with higher frequency losses; helped by appropriate forms of amplification

*Abnormally rapid increase in loudness as sound intensity increases.

Labyrinthitis

Infection or inflammation of the inner ear may affect the cochlear or vestibular portion of the labyrinth or both areas. Infection can enter from the meninges, the middle ear, or the bloodstream. Symptoms of vertigo, tinnitus, and sensorineural hearing loss are a result of problems in the labyrinth. *Nystagmus*, an abnormal rhythmic, jerking movement of the eyes, accompanies the vertigo and has a horizontal beat. Nystagmus is caused by abnormal currents in the endolymph fluid, causing the eyes to have a rhythmic jerking movement with a quick and a slow component.

Suppurative labyrinthitis from infection causes severe vertigo similar to that of an attack of Ménière's disease. It lasts for days to weeks, progressing until vestibular function is destroyed. Complete destruction of the cochlear portion occurs, causing deafness. Loss of vestibular input causes extreme unsteadiness in the patient. The patient requires physical therapy to recondition the brain to interpret vestibular input. *Vestibular neuronitis* causes vertigo, nausea, vomiting, and nystagmus. A viral infection may be the cause. The patient recovers after a week or more. Tinnitus is not present, and hearing loss does not occur. Toxic labyrinthitis is caused by ototoxic drugs that may cause vertigo. However, most ototoxic drugs affect the cochlea, resulting in tinnitus and eventually, hearing loss.

Acoustic Neuroma

An *acoustic neuroma* is a benign tumor that occurs where the acoustic nerve (CN VIII) enters the internal auditory canal or the temporal bone from the brain. It is important that early diagnosis be made because the neuroma can compress the facial nerve and arteries within the internal auditory canal. Once the tumor has expanded and become an intracranial neoplasm, more extensive surgery is necessary, reducing the chances of preserving hearing and normal facial nerve function. It can expand into the cerebellopontine angle and involve other cranial nerves and the brain by compression.

Early symptoms are associated with eighth cranial nerve compression and destruction. They include unilateral, progressive, sensorineural hearing loss, unilateral tinnitus, and intermittent vertigo. One of the earliest symptoms of an acoustic neuroma is reduced touch sensation in the posterior ear canal. Diagnostic tests include neurologic, audiometric, and vestibular tests, and tomograms (CT scans) and magnetic resonance imaging (MRI).

Surgery to remove small tumors is performed through the middle cranial fossa or retrolabyrinthine approach that preserves hearing and vestibular function. A translabyrinthine approach is usually used for medium-sized tumors and when hearing is minimal. Although hearing is destroyed by this approach, advantages include good access to the tumor and preservation of the facial nerve. Posterior cranial fossa or translabyrinthine approaches are used for large tumors (larger than 3 cm). It is almost impossible to preserve residual hearing when the tumor is larger than 2 cm.

HEARING IMPAIRMENT AND DEAFNESS

Incidence

Communication disorders are the primary handicapping disability in the United States. Twenty million persons in the United States have impaired hearing in one or both ears. The majority of persons lost their hearing as adults. Hearing impairment is common among older adults. Nearly half of the persons who need assistance with hearing disorders are 65 years of age or older. Between 2% and 4% of children have a hearing loss, with 3 million school-age children affected.[44]

Etiology and Types of Hearing Loss

Conductive hearing loss occurs in the outer and middle ear and impairs the sound being conducted from the outer to the inner ear. It is caused by conditions interfering with air conduction, such as impacted cerumen, middle ear disease, and otosclerosis. Antibiotics, tubes in the eardrum, and surgery usually correct the problem. The audiogram demonstrates an air-bone gap of at least 15 dB.

An air-bone gap occurs when hearing sensitivity by bone conduction is significantly better than by air conduction. The patient may speak softly because she hears her voice, which is conducted by bone, as being loud. This patient hears better in a noisy environment. A hearing aid is helpful for a patient with a 40 to 50 dB loss or more, although the device often is not necessary because of the excellent results of treatment of the underlying problem.

Sensorineural hearing loss is caused by impairment of function of the inner ear or its central connections. Congenital and hereditary factors, noise trauma during a period of time, aging (presbycusis), Ménière's disease, and ototoxicity can cause sensorineural hearing loss. Systemic diseases, such as certain collagen diseases, diabetes, syphilis, and Paget's disease, can also cause sensorineural deafness. The two main problems associated with sensorineural loss are the ability to hear sound but not to understand speech and lack of understanding of the problem by others. The ability to hear high-pitched sounds diminishes with sensorineural hearing loss. Consonants are high-pitched sounds that give intelligibility to speech. Words become difficult to distinguish, and sound becomes muffled. An audiogram demonstrates a loss in dB levels of the 4000 Hz range, which can progress to the 2000 Hz range. A hearing aid may help the patient who has a 30 dB loss or more by reducing the strain of trying to hear, but the sounds will still be muffled. *Presbycusis*, degenerative change of the inner ear, is a major cause of sensorineural hearing loss, especially in the older adult. It is a progressive problem that results in many social and emotional problems for the affected older adult. The control of inner ear diseases such as Ménière's disease can prevent further hearing loss. If the sensorineural loss is caused by an ototoxic drug, further loss should not occur if the drug is discontinued.

Mixed hearing loss is caused by a combination of conductive and sensorineural losses. Careful evaluation is needed before corrective surgery for conductive loss is planned because the sensorineural component of the hearing loss will still remain.

Central hearing loss is caused by problems in the CNS from the auditory nucleus to the cortex. The patient is unable to understand or to put meaning to the incoming sound. *Functional hearing loss* may be caused by an emotional or psychologic factor. The patient does not seem to hear or respond to pure-tone subjective hearing tests, but no organic cause can be identified. A careful history is helpful because there is usually a reference to deafness within the family. Psychologic counseling may help. Referral to qualified hearing and speech services is indicated.

Hearing loss can also be classified by the decibel (dB) level or loss as recorded on the audiogram. Normal hearing is in the 0 to 25 dB range. A mild impairment is present at the 30 dB hearing level. A moderate impairment is in the 31 to 55 dB range. A moderate to severe impairment is in the 56 to 70 dB range. The severely impaired have a loss in the 70 to 90 dB range. The profoundly deaf have a loss greater than 90 dB. Many persons in this last group are the congenitally deaf.

Manifestations of Hearing Loss

If the hearing loss is congenital and profound, the great difficulty in learning speech and conceptual thinking is evident. Rehabilitation must be started early.

Deafness is often called the "unseen handicap" because it is not until conversation is initiated with a deaf adult that the difficulty in communication is realized. It is important that the health professional be aware of the need for thorough validation of the deaf person's understanding of health teaching. Descriptive visual aids can be helpful. Because of the difficulty in communication, deaf persons often seek relationships with other deaf persons. The person who develops hearing loss later in life varies in the amount of loss and the reactions to it.

Interference in communication and interaction with others can be the source of many problems for the patient and family. Often the patient refuses to admit or may be unaware of impaired hearing. Irritability is common because of the intentness with which the patient must listen to understand speech. The loss of clarity of speech in the patient with sensorineural hearing loss is most frustrating. The patient may hear what is said but not understand it. Withdrawal, suspicion, loss of self-esteem, and insecurity are commonly associated with advancing hearing loss.

Rehabilitation of the Patient with Impaired Hearing

Hearing Aids. It is important that the patient with a suspected hearing loss have a hearing assessment by a qualified audiologist including examination and audiometric testing. If a *hearing aid* is indicated, it should be fitted by an audiologist or a speech and hearing specialist. There are many types of aids available each with advantages and disadvantages: the body-worn aid, the eyeglasses style, the behind-the-ear style, the in-the-ear style (Fig. 18-10), and the implantable hearing aid. The conventional hearing aid amplifies sounds and sends them into the damaged ear. In the inner ear these louder sounds stimulate whatever hair cells remain functional. Hair cells transduce acoustic energy into the electrochemical signals that excite auditory nerve fibers. For the patient with bilateral hearing impairment, binaural hearing aids provide the best sound lateralization and speech discrimination. Patient acceptance of a hearing aid may present a real problem. The nurse needs to be prepared to give careful instruction on its use and maintenance and to assist the patient during the period of adjustment.

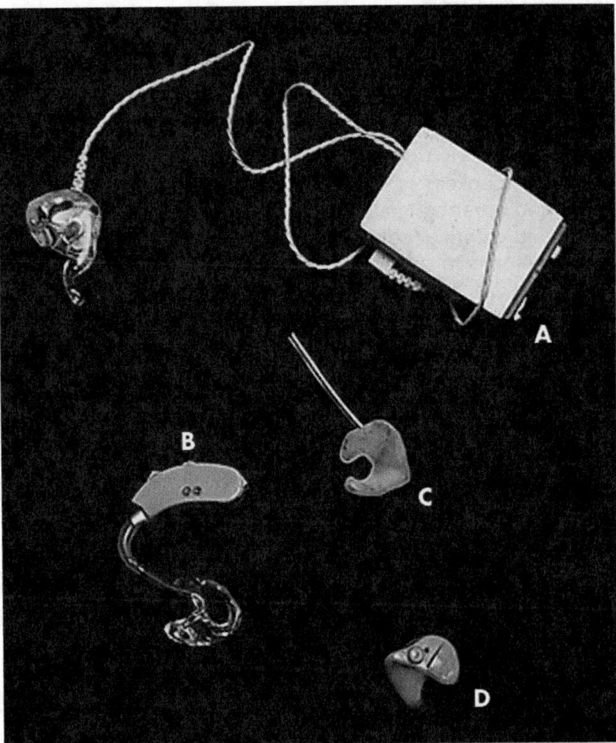

Fig. 18-10 Types of hearing aids. ***A,*** Older aid with a battery pack worn on the body and a wire connected to the ear mold. ***B,*** Behind-the-ear battery with ear mold. ***C,*** Small ear canal mold with battery. ***D,*** Newer, smaller mold worn in the ear canal.

Initially, use of the hearing aid should be restricted to quiet situations in the home. The patient needs to first adjust to voices (including the patient's own) and household sounds. The patient should also experiment by increasing and decreasing the volume as situations require. As adjustment to the increase in sounds and background noise occurs, the patient will be ready to try a different listening environment, such as a small party where several people will be talking simultaneously. Next the environment can be expanded to the outdoors. After adapting to controlled situations, the patient will be ready to encounter environments such as the shopping mall or grocery store. Adjustment to different environments occurs gradually during weeks to months, depending on the individual patient.

When the hearing aid is not being worn, it should be placed in a dry cool area where it will not be inadvertently damaged or lost. The battery should be disconnected or

Table 18-20 Communicating with the Patient with Impaired Hearing

Nonverbal Aids
Draw attention with hand movements.
Have speaker's face in good light.
Avoid covering mouth or face with hands.
Avoid chewing, eating, smoking while talking.
Maintain eye contact.
Avoid distracting environments.
Avoid careless expression that the patient may misinterpret.
Use touch.
Move close to better ear.
Avoid light behind speaker.
Verbal Aids
Speak normally and slowly.
Do not overexaggerate facial expression.
Do not overenunciate.
Use simple sentences.
Rephrase sentence; use different words.
Write name or difficult words.
Avoid shouting.
Speak in normal voice directly into better ear.

removed. Battery life averages 1 week, and patients should be advised to purchase only a month's supply at a time. Earmolds should be cleaned weekly or as needed. Toothpicks or pipe cleaners may be used to clear a clogged eartip.

Speech Reading. Speech reading, commonly called lip reading, can be helpful in increasing communication. It allows for approximately 40% understanding of the spoken word. The patient is able to use visual cues associated with speech, such as gestures and facial expression, to help clarify the spoken message. In speech reading, many words will look alike to the patient (e.g., rabbit and woman). If the patient wears glasses, the glasses should be used to facilitate speech reading. The nurse can help the patient by using and teaching verbal and nonverbal communication techniques as described in Table 18-20. If a hearing aid is used, it should be readily available to the patient.

Cochlear Implant. The cochlear implant is being used as a hearing device for the profoundly deaf. The system consists of a surgically embedded coil beneath the skin behind the ear and an electrode wire placed in the cochlea. The implanted parts interface with externally worn components. The system stimulates auditory nerve fibers by an electric current so signals reach the brainstem's auditory nuclei and ultimately, the auditory cortex. The implant is intended for use with the patient whose profound deafness is either congenital or acquired. The patient impaired by a hearing loss after language has been acquired benefits most from cochlear implants. The adult who was born deaf or became deaf before learning to speak is generally not considered a candidate for cochlear implants.[42]

The implant offers the profoundly deaf the ability to hear environmental sounds, such as telephones, doorbells, garbage disposals, footsteps, and fire alarms. Current multichannel implant technology provides a lot of information about speech.[44] Extensive training and rehabilitation are essential to receive maximum benefit from these implants. The positive aspects of a cochlear implant include providing sound to the person who heard none, improving lipreading, monitoring the loudness of the person's own speech, improving the sense of security, and decreasing feelings of isolation. With continued research the cochlear implant may offer the possibility of aural rehabilitation for a range of hearing problems.

Assisted Listening Devices. Numerous devices are now available to assist the hearing impaired person. Direct amplification devices, amplified telephone receivers, light systems that flash when activated by sound, an infrared septum for amplifying the sound of the television, and a combination FM receiver and hearing aid are all possible aids that can be explored by the nurse based on each patient's needs.

CRITICAL THINKING EXERCISES

CASE STUDY

CATARACT EXTRACTION

Patient Profile

Mr. O., a 62-year-old man, was admitted to the hospital for extraction of a cataract in his left eye.

Subjective Data

- Noticed a gradual decrease in visual acuity in his left eye
- Bothered by glare, especially when in bright lights

Objective Data

Physical Examination

- Has visual acuity of 20/80 OS and 20/40 OD with correction (bifocal lens)
- Has nuclear cataract OS and small cataract OD on bimicroscopic examination

Therapeutic Management

Preoperative Orders

- Atropine 1% gtts ṫ OS, h.s. and in AM
- Neosporin ophthalmic gtts ṫ OS, h.s. and in AM
- Phenylephrine 10% gtts ṫ OS; cyclopentolate 2% gtts ṫ OS; preoperatively q15 min × 3
- Diazepam (Valium) 10 mg PO with small amount of water on call to surgery
- NPO after midnight

The surgery was performed with the patient under local anesthesia. The lens was removed by extracapsular extraction. An IOL was inserted in the posterior chamber. Mr. O. returned to his room with an eye pad and a metal shield on the treated eye.

Critical Thinking Questions

1. Explain the etiology of Mr. O.'s symptoms.
2. Why were the preoperative eye medications given? What are the actions of each?
3. What are the advantages of the IOL used for Mr. O.?
4. What precautions need to be taken with the operative eye?
5. What will vision of the left eye be when the patch is removed?
6. What topics should the nurse include in the discharge teaching?
7. Based on the assessment data presented, write one or more appropriate nursing diagnoses. Are there any collaborative problems?

NURSING RESEARCH ISSUES

1. Are there any differences in patient outcomes and patient satisfaction when patient education is provided by the ophthalmic nurse as compared to an ophthalmic technician?
2. What factors are most important in increasing patient compliance with a glaucoma medication regimen?
3. Does the patient with a cataract experience a significant improvement in quality of life after cataract extraction?
4. What factors in the nursing care of the patient with significant visual impairment from age-related macular degeneration are indicators of improved patient outcomes?
5. What sleeping position provides the greatest comfort immediately following a tympanoplasty?
6. Compare the effectiveness of different types of sound protectors in high-noise environments.
7. Why do persons with hearing aids choose not to use them?

*A list of agencies that serve the blind can be obtained from the American Foundation for the Blind, 15 West 16th Street, New York, NY 10011. Many of these agencies are listed following the section bibilography.

REVIEW QUESTIONS

The number of the question corresponds to the same-numbered objective at the beginning of the chapter.

1. Presbyopia occurs in the older individual because
   a. the person may have poor nutritional status.
   b. it is associated with cataract development.
   c. the crystalline lens becomes inflexible.
   d. the retina degenerates.

2. The most important nursing intervention in the patient with epidemic keratoconjunctivitis is
   a. teaching the patient and family members good hygiene techniques.
   b. determining near visual acuity.
   c. accurately measuring IOP.
   d. teaching the patient about the disease process.

3. The patient with diabetic retinopathy should understand that
a. he will probably go blind.
b. the condition is untreatable.
c. ophthalmic examinations should be a regular part of his care.
d. diet and exercise will not affect the outcome.

4. Rubella can cause hearing problems if
a. exposure is before 16 weeks gestation.
b. exposure is after 20 weeks gestation.
c. the mother is vaccinated during the puerperium.
d. the mother had rubella before age 18.

5. In preparing the patient for retinal detachment surgery, the nurse should
a. begin explaining how to care for an ocular prosthesis.
b. teach the family how to recognize when the patient is hallucinating.
c. assess the patient's level of knowledge about retinal detachment and provide information appropriate to the situation.
d. assure the patient that he can expect 20/20 vision following surgery.

6. The nurse should instruct the patient with glaucoma that
a. he should see his family practitioner or internist every 2 months.
b. if he uses drops properly, he can expect full resolution of the glaucoma.
c. punctal occlusion will lessen systemic absorption of glaucoma eye drops.
d. his increased IOP is often painful.

7. All of the following are correct related to otosclerosis *except*
a. it is uncommon in African-Americans.
b. it is always unilateral.
c. the footplate of the stapes becomes fixed.
d. hearing loss progresses over time.

8. The patient who has a sensorineural hearing loss will
a. have difficulty understanding speech.
b. hear low-pitched sounds better.
c. not benefit from discontinuing ototoxic drugs.
d. not experience muffled sounds with a hearing aid.

9. The patient with extended wear contact lenses may
a. wear lenses up to 1 week without removal.
b. moisten the lenses with saliva if necessary.
c. continue lens wear if mild to moderate irritation or redness is experienced.
d. use any saline solution as long as it is hypertonic.

10. The person with a severe hearing loss may do all of the following *except*
a. not admit to having a problem.
b. avoid other hearing-impaired persons.
c. become irritable from the effort of trying to hear.
d. suffer a loss of self-esteem.

11. The patient with permanent visual impairment
a. may experience the same grieving process that other losses precipitate.
b. feels most comfortable with other visually impaired persons.
c. usually needs others to speak louder so he can communicate more effectively.
d. cannot generally make a successful emotional adjustment to his loss.

REFERENCES

1. Petersen RA, Hunter DG, Mudai S: Retinopathy of prematurity. In Albert DM, Jakobiec FA, editors: *Principles and practice of ophthalmology: clinical practice,* vol 4, Philadelphia, 1994, WB Saunders.
2. Refractive Errors Panel of the Quality of Care Committee: *Low to moderate refractive errors,* San Francisco, 1991, American Academy of Ophthalmology.
3. Pruett RC: Pathologic myopia. In Albert DM, Jakobiec FA, editors: *Principles and practice of ophthalmology: clinical practice,* vol 2, Philadelphia, 1994, WB Saunders.
4. Guyton AC: *Textbook of medical physiology,* ed 8, Philadelphia, 1991, WB Saunders.
5. Mead MD, Sieck EA, Steinert RF: Optical rehabilitation of aphakia. In Albert DM, Jakobiec FA, editors: *Principles and practice of ophthalmology: clinical practice,* vol 2, Philadelphia, 1994, WB Saunders.
6. Tortora CM, Hersh PS, Blaker JW: Optics of intraocular lenses. In Albert DM, Jakobiec FA, editors: *Principles and practice of ophthalmology: clinical practice,* Vol 5, Philadelphia, 1994, WB Saunders.
7. Deitz MR and others: Long-term (5–12 year) follow-up of metal-blade radial keratotomy procedures, *Arch Ophthalmol* 112:614, 1994.
8. Can surgery free you from glasses? *Consumer Reports,* 59:87, 1994.
9. Stark WJ and others: Clinical follow-up of 193-nm ArF excimer laser photokeratectomy, *Ophthalmology,* 99:805, 1992.
10. *Physicians' desk reference of ophthalmology,* Montvale, NJ, 1994, Medical Economics Data Production Company.
11. Kraut JA, McCabe CP: The problem of low vision: definition and common problems. In Albert DM, Jakobiec FA, editors: *Principles and practice of ophthalmology: clinical practice,* Vol. 5, Philadelphia, 1994, WB Saunders.
12. Brandt JT, Nason FE: Community resources for the ophthalmic practice. In Albert DM, Jakobiec FA, editors: *Principles and practice of ophthalmology: clinical practice,* Vol. 5, Philadelphia, 1994, WB Saunders.
13. Sastry SM and others: Ocular trauma among major trauma victims in a regional trauma center, *J Trauma,* 34:223, 1993.
14. Bajart AM: Lid inflammations. In Albert DM, Jakobiec FA, editors: *Principles and practice of ophthalmology: clinical practice,* Vol. 5, Philadelphia, 1994, WB Saunders.
15. Pavan-Langston D: Viral disease of the cornea and external eye. In Albert DM, Jakobiec FA, editors: *Principles and practice of ophthalmology: clinical practice,* Vol. 5, Philadelphia, 1994, WB Saunders.
16. Avery RK, Baker AS: Chlamydial disease. In Albert DM, Jakobiec FA, editors: *Principles and practice of ophthalmology: clinical practice,* Vol. 5, Philadelphia, 1994, WB Saunders.
17. Adamis AP, Schein OD: Chlamydia and acanthamoeba infections of the eye. In Albert DM, Jakobiec FA, editors: *Principles and practice of ophthalmology: clinical practice,* Vol. 5, Philadelphia, 1994, WB Saunders.
18. Foulks GN: Bacterial infections of the conjunctiva and cornea. In Albert DM, Jakobiec FA, editors: *Principles and practice of ophthalmology: clinical practice,* Vol. 5, Philadelphia, 1994, WB Saunders.
19. Talamo JH, Steinert RF: Keratorefractive surgery. In Albert DM, Jakobiec FA, editors: *Principles and practice of ophthalmology: clinical practice,* Vol. 5, Philadelphia, 1994, WB Saunders.

20. Boruchoff SA: Penetrating keratoplasty. In Albert DM, Jakobiec FA, editors: *Principles and practice of ophthalmology: clinical practice,* Vol. 5, Philadelphia, 1994, WB Saunders.
21. Anterior Segment Panel of the Quality of Care Committee: *Cataract in the otherwise healthy adult eye,* San Francisco, 1991, American Academy of Ophthalmology.
22. Streeten BW: Pathology of the lens. In Albert DM, Jakobiec FA, editors: *Principles and practice of ophthalmology: clinical practice,* Vol. 5, Philadelphia, 1994, WB Saunders.
23. Perkins RS, Olson RJ: A new look at postoperative instructions following cataract extraction, *Ophthalmic Surg,* 22:66, 1991.
24. Retina Panel of the Quality of Care Committee: *Preferred practice pattern: retinal detachment,* San Francisco, 1990, American Academy of Ophthalmology.
25. Haynie GD, D'Amico DJ: Scleral buckling surgery. In Albert DM, Jakobiec FA, editors: *Principles and practice of ophthalmology: clinical practice,* Vol. 5, Philadelphia, 1994, WB Saunders.
26. Retina Panel of the Quality of Care Committee: *Preferred practice pattern: macular degeneration,* San Francisco, 1990, American Academy of Ophthalmology.
27. Sahel JA, Brini A, Albert DM: Pathology of the retina and vitreous. In Albert DM, Jakobiec FA, editors: *Principles and practice of ophthalmology: clinical practice,* Vol. 5, Philadelphia, 1994, WB Saunders.
28. The Eye Disease Case Control Study Group: Risk factors for neovascular age-related macular degeneration, *Arch Ophthalmol* 110:1701, 1992.
29. Garcia CA, Ruiz RS: Ocular complications of diabetes, *Clin Symp* 44:2, 1992.
30. Aiello LM: Diagnosis, management, and treatment of nonproliferative diabetic retinopathy and macular edema. In Albert DM, Jakobiec FA, editors: *Principles and practice of ophthalmology: clinical practice,* Vol. 5, Philadelphia, 1994, WB Saunders.
31. Glaucoma Panel of the Quality of Care Committee: *Preferred practice pattern: primary open-angle glaucoma,* San Francisco, 1992, American Academy of Ophthalmology.
32. Thomas JV: Primary open-angle glaucoma. In Albert DM, Jakobiec FA, editors: *Principles and practice of ophthalmology: clinical practice,* Vol. 5, Philadelphia, 1994, WB Saunders.
33. Richter CU: Laser Therapy of open-angle glaucoma. In Albert DM, Jakobiec FA, editors: *Principles and practice of ophthalmology: clinical practice,* Vol. 5, Philadelphia, 1994, WB Saunders.
34. Retina Panel of the Quality of Care Committee: *Preferred practice pattern: comprehensive adult eye evaluation,* San Francisco, 1990, American Academy of Ophthalmology.
35. Fanaroff AA, Martin RJ: *Neonatal-perinatal medicine,* St Louis, 1992, Mosby.
36. Novy M: The normal puerperium. In DeCherney A, Pernoll M, editors, *Current obstetric and gynecologic diagnosis and treatment,* ed 8, Norwalk, Conn, 1994, Appleton and Lange.
37. Alberti PW: Occupational hearing loss. In Ballenger JJ, editor: *Diseases of the nose, throat, ear, head, and neck,* ed 14, Philadelphia, 1991, Lea and Febiger.
38. Haybach PJ: Tuning into ototoxicity, *Nurs,* 23:34, 1993.
39. Carnevali DL, Patrick M: *Nursing management for the elderly,* ed 3, Philadelphia, 1993, Lippincott.
40. Ballenger JJ: *Diseases of the nose, throat, ear, head, and neck,* ed 14, Philadelphia, 1991, Lea and Febiger.
41. Daly KA: Epidemiology of otitis media, *Otolaryngol Clin North Am,* 24:775, 1991.
42. Drake AF: Modern management of otitis media, *Hosp Med,* 29:116, 1993.
43. Silverstein H, Wolfson R, Rosenberg S: Diagnosis and management of hearing loss, *Clin Symp* 44:2, 1992.
44. Schuller DE, Schleuning AJ: *DeWeese and Saunders' Otolaryngology—head and neck surgery,* ed 8, St Louis, 1994, Mosby.
45. Telischi F, Hodges A, Balkany T: Cochlear implants for deafness, *Hosp Pract* 29:55, 1994.

Chapter 19

NURSING ASSESSMENT

Integumentary System

Eileen Enny Leach **Anne Marie Ruszkowski**

Learning Objectives

1. Describe the structures and functions of the integumentary system.
2. Describe age-related changes in the integumentary system and differences in assessment findings.
3. Describe the significant subjective and objective data related to the integumentary system that should be obtained from a patient.
4. Describe specific assessments to be made during the physical examination of the skin and appendages.
5. Explain the critical components for describing a lesion.
6. Describe the appropriate techniques used in the physical assessment of the integumentary system.
7. Explain the structural and assessment differences in black skin.
8. Differentiate normal from common abnormal findings of a physical assessment of the integumentary system.
9. Describe the purpose, significance of results, and nursing responsibilities of diagnostic studies related to the integumentary system.

The integumentary system is composed of the skin, hair, nails, and glands. The skin is further divided into three layers: epidermis, dermis, and subcutaneous tissues (Fig. 19-1).

STRUCTURES AND FUNCTIONS OF THE SKIN AND APPENDAGES

Structures

The epidermis is the outermost structure of the multiple layers of the skin. The dermis, the second layer, contains a framework of connective tissue. The subcutaneous tissue is composed of fat deposits in modified connective tissue and adipose tissue.

Epidermis. The epidermis, the avascular outermost layer of the skin, is thin—approximately 0.06 mm to 0.1 mm depending on the skin site. It is nourished by diffusion from blood vessels in the dermis, and waste products are removed in the same way. The two types of cells of the epidermis are melanocytes (5%) and keratinocytes (95%).

Melanocytes are scattered throughout the basal layer (stratum basale) of the epidermis. They produce melanin, a pigment that gives color to the skin and protects the body from injurious ultraviolet (UV) light ray damage. All races have approximately the same number of melanocytes. The wide range of skin colors is caused by the size and distribution of the melanosomes produced by the melanocytes. Sunlight and hormones stimulate melanin production.

Keratinocytes develop from cells in the basal layer of the epidermis. After division, one cell remains in the basal cell layer and is called a basal cell. The other keratinocyte moves to the skin surface (stratum corneum of the epidermis), where it flattens, dehydrates, and becomes keratinized.[1] The upward movement of keratinocytes from the basement membrane to the stratum corneum takes approximately 14 days. The sloughing of the stratum corneum takes an additional 14 to 30 days. If dead cells slough off too rapidly, the skin will appear thin, eroded, or atrophic. If new cells form faster than old cells shed, the skin becomes scaly and thickened. Deviations in this cycle account for many dermatologic problems. Keratinocytes produce a specialized protein, *keratin*, which is vital to the protective barrier function of the skin.

Dermis. The dermis (1 mm to 4 mm thick) is the layer beneath the epidermis and the principal mass of the skin. It is primarily made up of fibrils of collagen. In addition, there are blood vessels, nerves, lymphatic vessels, hair follicles, involuntary muscle fibers, and sebaceous and sweat glands found in the dermis. Collagen, water, and a gel-like ground substance serve to support the structures of the epidermis and dermis. Collagen is responsible for the mechanical strength of the skin.

The dermis is divided into two layers, the upper or *papillary* layer and the lower or *reticular* layer. The papil-

---

Reviewed by Sandra Somma, RN, BSN, Staff Nurse, Yale New Haven Hospital, New Haven, CT.

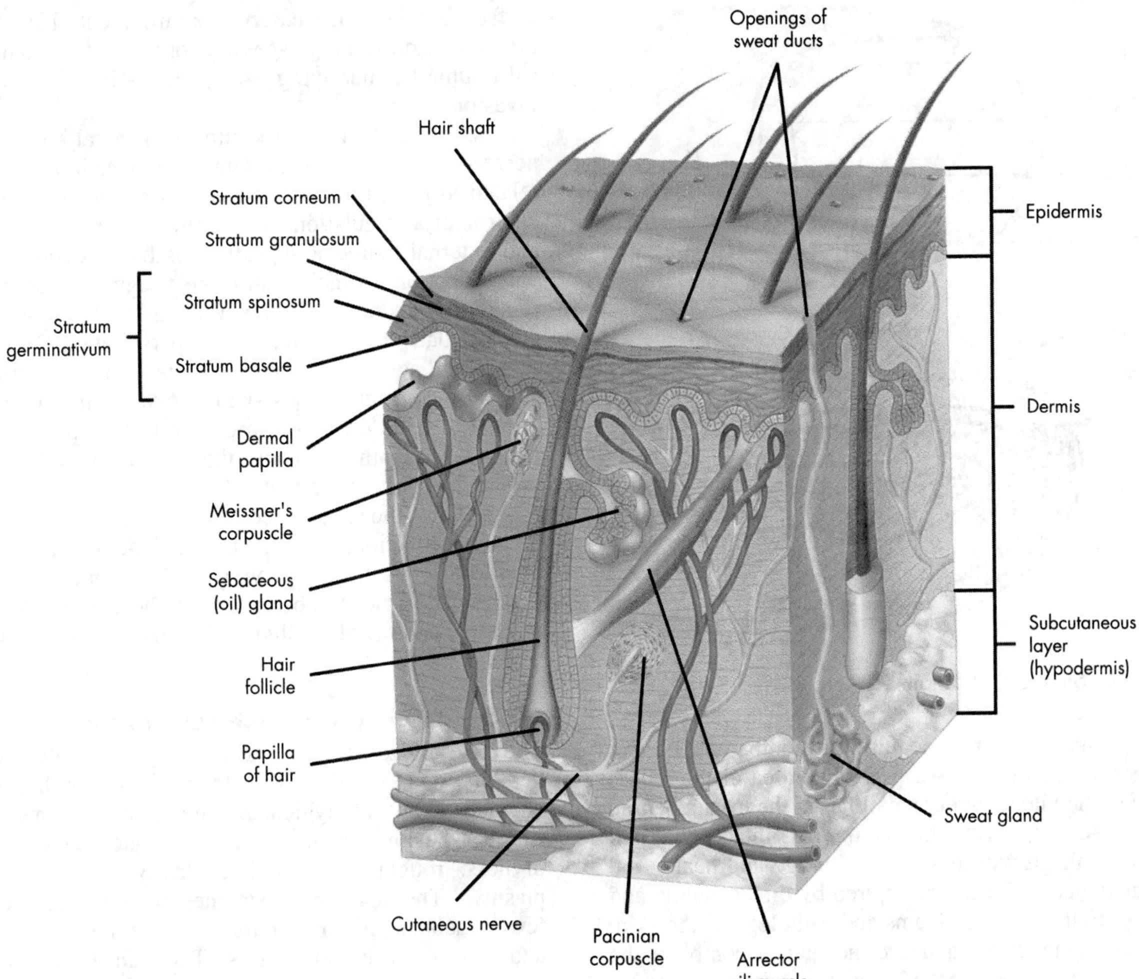

Fig. 19-1 Microscopic view of the skin in longitudinal section. The epidermis is shown raised at one corner to reveal the dermal papillae.

lary layer is arranged into parallel rows of microscopic structures called papillae, which produce the ridges of the skin that are individual footprints or fingerprints. The reticular layer is composed of white fibrous tissue that supports the blood vessels. The dermis gives the skin substance, provides support, and absorbs and reduces environmental stress and strain.

Subcutaneous Tissue. Subcutaneous tissue, although not actually part of the skin, is traditionally discussed with skin because it attaches the skin to underlying muscle and bone; in addition, blood vessels and nerves that supply the skin run through it.[2] It consists of loose connective tissue with collagen and elastin fibers. The anatomic distribution of subcutaneous tissue is a secondary sex characteristic and is also controlled by heredity, age, and eating habits. This layer supports, nourishes, insulates, and cushions the skin.

Epidermal Appendages. Appendages of the skin include the hair, nails, and glands (apocrine, eccrine, and sebaceous). These originate from the epidermal layer, although they are anatomically located in both the epidermis and the dermis. They receive nutrients, electrolytes, fluids, and innervation from the dermis. Hair and nails are specialized keratin that becomes dry and firm.

Hair covers the entire body except for the palms of the hand, the soles of the feet, and parts of the external reproductive organs. Its main function is protection of delicate structures. The color of the hair is a result of genetic factors and is determined by the amount of pigmentation in the hair shaft. Hair grows approximately 1 cm per month, 50 to 100 hairs are lost each day, and its rate of growth is not affected by cutting. The growth of hair occurs in several phases. Each hair goes through a resting (*telogen*), growth (*anagen*), and transitional (*catagen*) phase. Each hair grows independently of one another so not all hairs are in the same phase at the same time. Chemical, mechanical, or psychologic factors can convert all hair to the atrophy phase, resulting in baldness.

Nails grow from the nail matrix, which is usually hidden by skin at the base of the nail (Fig. 19-2). Nails grow at one third the rate of hair. Fingernails grow faster than toenails. A lost fingernail usually regenerates in 3½ to 6 months,

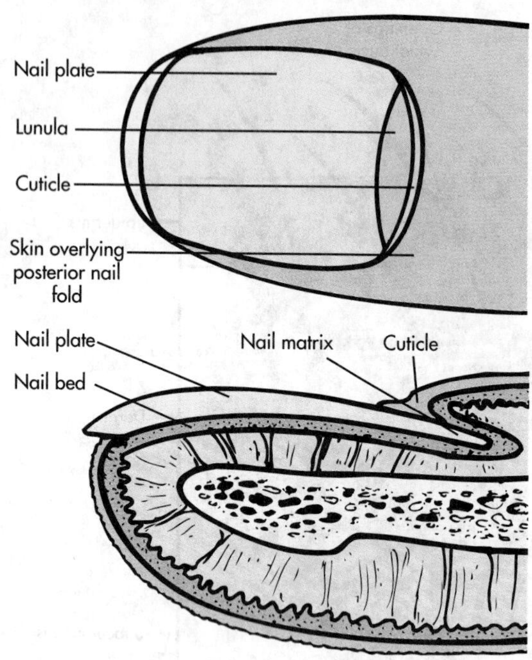

Fig. 19-2 Structure of a nail.

whereas a lost toenail may require 12 months or more for regeneration. The crescent-shaped white area of the nail is the *lunula.* The viable part of a nail lies in the matrix behind the lunula. As long as the matrix remains intact, new nail will grow. Nail growth may vary with age and health and hormonal status. Nails can be injured by direct trauma and are subject to the same problems and pathology as the skin.

Sebaceous, apocrine, and eccrine glands complete the epidermal or accessory appendages. The *sebaceous glands* secrete sebum, a complex lipid mixture that is emptied into the hair shaft. These glands depend on the male hormone androgen to initiate and continue production. Sebaceous glands are present on all areas of the skin except the palms and soles. They are most numerous and largest on the face, scalp, upper chest, and back. The amount of secretion is controlled by the endocrine system and varies with age, puberty, and pregnancy.

Apocrine gland secretion, which occurs primarily in the axillae, breast areolae, anogenital area, ear canals, and eye lids, serves no known function in human beings.[3] A milky substance is secreted that becomes odoriferous when altered by skin surface bacteria. The activity of these glands is mediated by adrenergic innervation.

Eccrine, or sweat, *glands* are present almost everywhere on the body, especially on the forehead, palms, and soles. There are approximately 3000 sweat glands per square inch of skin.[4] Sweat has the same composition as plasma but is less concentrated. The main function of sweat glands is to cool the body by evaporation, to excrete waste products through the pores of the skin, and to moisturize surface cells.

Functions of the Skin

The skin is the largest organ of the body. Its primary function is to protect the underlying tissue by acting as a surface barrier to the external environment. The skin also protects by preventing excessive loss of water and mechanical trauma to underlying tissue and by inhibiting bacterial invasion.

The skin is the major receptor for general sensation. The nerve endings in the skin supply information to the brain related to pain, touch, pressure, and temperature. The skin controls heat regulation by its ability to respond to internal and external temperature variations by vasoconstriction or vasodilatotion. Coincidental to heat regulation is the skin's function of excretion. Between 600 ml and 900 ml of water are lost daily through insensible perspiration. In addition, sebum and sweat are secreted by the skin and lubricate the skin surface. Endogenous synthesis of vitamin D, which is critical to bone metabolism, occurs in the epidermis. Vitamin D is synthesized by the action of UV light on previtamin D in epidermal cells.

The fat of the subcutaneous layer insulates the body. The aesthetic functions of the skin include the mirroring of emotions as well as displaying the individual identity of a person. The role of absorption at the cutaneous level is unknown and may be influenced by the integrity of the skin surface.

Effects of Aging on the Integumentary System

The rate of age-related skin changes is influenced by heredity and a personal history of sun, radiation, and chemical exposure, hygiene practices, nutrition, and general state of health. Changes that are related to age include dryness, roughness, wrinkling, laxity, and benign neoplasms.[5] The epidermis becomes flattened and contains fewer melanocytes. In addition, the dermis loses volume and has fewer blood vessels. The hair becomes depigmented and thinner. There is often a nailplate abnormality. Exposure to UV rays is the major contributor to the look of aging skin. Wrinkling of sun-exposed areas such as the face is worse than sun-shielded areas such as the buttocks. In addition, a decrease in the level of sex hormones and atrophy of the skin and epidermal appendages correlate with the look of aging.

A variety of neoplasms appear on the skin as part of the aging process. These benign growths include *seborrheic keratoses, cherry angiomas,* and *skin tags.* A common premalignant lesion is an *actinic keratosis,* which appears on areas of chronic sun exposure, especially in the person who has a fair complexion and light eyes. This individual is also at increased risk for cutaneous squamous cell epithelioma and basal cell carcinoma.

Poor nutrition contributes to aging of the skin through a decrease in protein, calories, and vitamins. With aging, collagen stiffens, elastic fibers degenerate, and the amount of subcutaneous tissue decreases. These changes, with the added effects of gravity, lead to wrinkling (Fig. 19-3). Blood vessels close to the skin give a ruddy appearance. With aging, sweating diminishes as eccrine glands become less active. The rate of hair and nail production decreases as a result of atrophy of the involved structures. Vitamin deficiencies can cause dry, thin hair that has a tendency to fall out. See Table 19-7 for age-related changes in the skin.

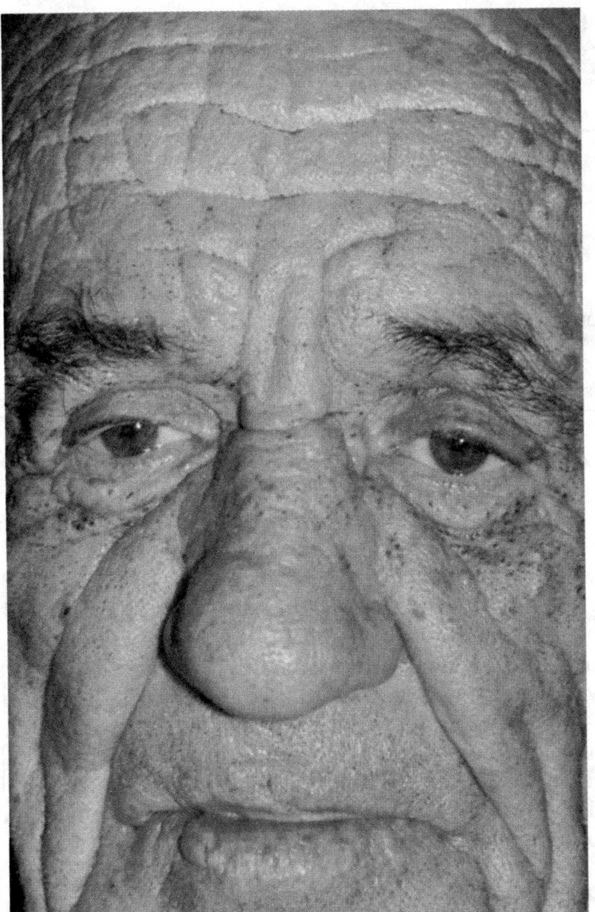

Fig. 19-3 Photoaging. Wrinkling becomes coarse and deep rather than fine, and the skin is thickened.

ASSESSMENT OF THE INTEGUMENTARY SYSTEM

Assessment of the skin begins at the initial contact with the patient and continues throughout the examination. Specific areas of the skin are examined during examination of other areas of the body unless the chief complaint is that of a dermatologic nature. A general statement about the skin should be recorded (Table 19-1), and specific problems should be noted under the appropriate system. The patient's skin type should be determined and recorded (Table 19-2). In addition, questions presented in Table 19-3 should also be asked when a skin problem is noted.

Table 19-1 Normal Physical Assessment of the Integumentary System

Skin even-toned and warm; good turgor; no petechiae, purpura, lesions, or excoriations. Nails pink, round, and mobile with 160° angle. Hair shiny and full; amount and distribution appropriate for age and sex; no flaking.

Subjective Data

Important Health Information

Past health history. Past health history will indicate previous trauma or surgery involving the skin. The nurse should determine if the patient has experienced any dermatologic manifestations of systemic problems such as jaundice (liver disease), delayed wound healing (diabetes mellitus), pruritus (Hodgkin's disease), and increased sweating (hyperthyroidism). Table 20-14 lists additional problems. Specific information related to food and drug allergies and skin reactions to insect bites and stings should be obtained. A history of excessive or unprotected exposure to UV light as well as radiation treatments should be noted.

Medications. The patient should be questioned about skin-related problems that occurred as a result of taking prescription or over-the-counter medications. A careful medication history is important, especially in relation to vitamins, steroids, hormones, antibiotics, and antimetabolites, because these medications often cause dermatologic side effects.

The nurse needs to document the use of prescription or over-the-counter medications used specifically to treat a primary skin problem such as acne or a secondary skin problem such as itching. If a preparation is used, the name, length of use, method of application, and effectiveness of the medication should be recorded.

Surgery and other treatments. It is important to determine if any surgical procedures, including cosmetic surgery, were performed on the skin. If a biopsy was done, the result should be recorded. Any treatments specific for a skin problem such as phototherapy or for a health problem such as radiation therapy should also be noted.

Functional Health Patterns

Health perception–health management pattern. The nurse should ask about the patient's health practices related to the integumentary system, such as usual habits related to daily hygiene and brand names of cosmetic products. The use, type, and sun protection factor (SPF) number of sun protection agents should be documented. Assessment of the use of personal care products (e.g., shampoos and moisturizing agents), including brand name, quantity, and frequency, should be made. A description of any current skin problem including onset, course, and treatment should be noted.

Information should be obtained about family history of any skin diseases, including congenital and familial diseases (e.g., alopecia, ichthyosis, and psoriasis) and systemic diseases with dermatologic manifestations (e.g., diabetes, blood dyscrasias, collagen-vascular diseases, and allergic disorders). In addition, a history of skin cancer, particularly melanoma, should be noted.

Nutritional-metabolic pattern. The nurse should ask the patient about any changes in the condition of skin, hair, nails, and mucous membranes and whether they are related to dietary changes. A diet history will reveal the adequacy of nutrients essential to healthy skin such as vitamins A, D, E, and C; dietary fat; and protein. Food allergies that cause cutaneous eruptions should be noted. Obese patients should be asked if they have areas of chafing or maceration where moisture accumulates in overlapping skin areas.

Table 19-2 Skin Types

Reaction to Sun	Characteristics	Population Example
I. Always sunburns easily, never tans	Fair skin; blue eyes; blond or red hair	Celtic, Northern European
II. Always sunburns easily, tans minimally	Fair skin; blue, green, or light brown eyes; blond, red, or light brown hair	Germanic, European
III. Sunburns moderately, tans gradually	Medium color skin; brown eyes; brown hair	Southern European
IV. Sunburns minimally, tans always	Light brown skin; dark eyes; dark hair	Mediterranean, Asian, Latin American
V. Rarely sunburns, tans profusely	Brown skin; dark brown eyes; dark hair	African, Native American, East Indian
VI. Never sunburns, tans deeply	Dark skin; black eyes; black hair	African

Elimination pattern. The patient should be questioned about conditions of the skin, which can indicate alterations in fluid balance such as dehydration, edema, and pruritus. If incontinence is a problem, the condition of the skin in the anal and perineal areas should be determined.

Activity-exercise pattern. Information should be obtained about environmental and occupational hazards, including exposure to known cutaneous carcinogens, photosensitizers, chemical and mechanical irritants, and allergens. The patient should be asked to report changes in skin that occur during exercise.

Sleep-rest pattern. The patient should be questioned about disturbances in sleep patterns caused by a skin condition. For example, pruritus can be very distressing and cause major alterations in sleep. Also, poor sleep and resulting tiredness is often reflected in a patient's face by dark circles under the eyes and a laxity to the facial skin. These observations should be noted by the nurse.

Cognitive-perceptual pattern. The nurse should ascertain the patient's perception of the sensations of heat, cold, and touch. Pain associated with a skin condition should be noted, especially when observed in intact skin. Joint pain related to the patient's skin condition should be recorded.

Self-perception–self-concept pattern. Assessment should be made of the feelings of loss, inadequacy, rejection, and prejudice in relation to the patient's skin condition. The patient should be observed for signs of loss of self-esteem and poor body image.

Role-relationship pattern. It is important to determine how the patient's skin condition affects relationships with family members, peers, and business associates. Assessment should be made of changes in lifestyle relative to the skin condition.

The patient should be questioned regarding the skin effect of environmental factors such as exposure to irritants, sun, and unusually cold or unhygienic conditions related to recreation or occupation. Skin rashes caused by allergies and irritants are among the most common occupational problems.

Sexuality-reproductive pattern. The nurse should tactfully question and assess the effect of the patient's skin condition on sexual activity. Note should also be made of the reproductive status of the female patient relative to possible therapeutic interventions. For example, isotretinoin (Accutane) is a teratogenic drug that causes abnormal fetal development and, consequently, should not be used by a woman who could become pregnant.

Coping–stress tolerance pattern. Assessment should be made of whether the patient observes that stress exacerbates the skin condition. The patient should be questioned as to what coping mechanisms are used to deal with this stress.

Value-belief pattern. The patient should be questioned about cultural or religious beliefs that could potentially influence the perception of self image. Assessment should also be made of values and beliefs that would influence or limit the choice of treatment options.

Objective Data

Physical Examination. Characteristics of *primary (basic) skin lesions* are shown in Fig. 19-4. *Secondary skin lesions* are shown in Fig. 19-5. General principles of the assessment of the skin are as follows:

1. Have a well-lit, private room of moderate temperature with exposure to daylight.
2. Ensure that the patient is completely undressed for an adequate skin examination.
3. Be systematic, and proceed from head to toe.
4. Compare symmetrical parts.
5. Perform a general inspection and then a lesion-specific examination.
6. Use the metric system for measurements.
7. Use appropriate terminology and nomenclature when reporting or recording.

Because dermatology is a descriptive discipline, it is most useful to be able to communicate using a common language. Photographs are useful to document findings.

Inspection. The skin is inspected for color, vascularity, and presence of lesions. The critical factor in assessment of *skin color* is change. A skin color that is normal for a particular patient can be a sign of a pathologic condition in another patient. The color of the skin depends on the amount of melanin (brown), carotene (yellow), oxyhemoglobin (red), and reduced hemoglobin (bluish-red) present at a particular time. The most reliable areas in which to

Table 19-3 Key Questions: Patient with an Integumentary Problem

Health Perception–Health Management Pattern
- Describe your routine daily hygiene.
- What products are you currently using?
- Describe your current skin condition, including onset, course, and treatment, if any.
- Do you have any pets?*

Nutritional-Metabolic Pattern
- Describe any changes in the condition of your skin, hair, nails, and mucous membranes.
- Are the conditions related to changes in your diet, including supplemental vitamins and minerals?*

Elimination Pattern
- Have you noticed changes in skin temperature, including excessive sweating or dryness?*

Activity-Exercise Pattern
- Do your hobbies or leisure activities involve the use of any chemicals that are potentially toxic to the skin?*
- What is your sun protection program?

Sleep-Rest Pattern
- Does your skin condition keep you awake or awaken you after you have fallen asleep?

Cognitive-Perceptual Pattern
- Do you have any unusual sensations of heat, cold, or touch?*
- Do you have any pain associated with your skin condition?*
- Do you have any joint pain?*

Self-Perception–Self-Concept Pattern
- How does your skin condition make you feel about yourself?

Role-Relationship Pattern
- Has your skin condition changed your relationships with others?*
- Have you changed your lifestyle because of your skin condition?*
- Are there any unusual chemical or occupational hazards at your current or previous work place or home?*

Sexuality-Reproductive Pattern
- Has your skin condition changed your intimate relationships with others?*
- Has your birth control method, if used, caused a skin problem?*

Coping–Stress Tolerance Pattern
- Are you aware of anything that changes your skin condition?*
- Do you feel that stress plays a role in your skin condition?*
- How do you handle stress?

Value-Belief Pattern
- Are there any cultural beliefs that influence your thinking or feelings about your skin condition?*
- Are there any treatment options that you would be opposed to using?*

*If yes, describe.

assess color are the areas of least pigmentation, such as the sclera, conjunctiva, nail beds, lips, and buccal mucosa. Activity, emotions, cigarette smoking, and edema as well as respiratory, cardiovascular, and hepatic problems can all directly affect the color of the skin.

The skin is examined for problems related to *vascularity,* such as areas of bruising, and vascular and purpuric lesions, such as angioma, petechiae, or purpura. Reaction to direct pressure should be noted. If a lesion blanches on direct pressure and then refills, the redness is due to dilated blood vessels. If the discoloration remains, it is the result of subcutaneous or intradermal bleeding.

If *lesions* are found on the skin, the type, color, size, distribution and grouping, location, and consistency should be recorded. Skin lesions are usually described by using words that describe the lesions' configuration (pattern in relation to other lesions, Table 19-4) and distribution (arrangement of lesions over an area of skin, Table 19-5).

Palpation. Palpation of the skin provides information about temperature, turgor and mobility, moisture, and texture. *Temperature* of the skin is best assessed by palpating the upper lip, palms, or forehead with the backs of the hands. The temperature of the skin increases when blood flow to the dermis is increased. There will be a localized temperature increase with burns and local inflammation. A generalized increase in temperature will result from fever. A decreased body temperature may occur when shock, chilling, or emotional trauma is present.

Turgor and *mobility* refer to the elasticity of the skin. There is a loss of turgor with dehydration and aging. The nurse assesses turgor by gently pinching an area of skin over the sternum. Skin with good turgor will immediately return to its original position.

Moisture of the skin is the dampness or dryness of the skin. Moisture increases in *intertriginous* (overlying surfaces) areas. The amount of moisture on the skin varies with the temperature of the environment, muscular activity, and body temperature. Skin generally becomes drier with increasing age. High humidity causes increased skin moistness.

Texture refers to the fineness or coarseness of the skin. Changes in texture can reflect local trauma or systemic disease. Increased thickness is often work related and should not be mistaken for a pathologic condition. Increased thickness can also be the result of repeated injury through rubbing or itching and may indicate an underlying problem.

Diagnostic Studies. Diagnostic studies provide important information to the nurse in monitoring the patient's condition and planning appropriate interventions. These studies are considered to be objective data. Table 19-6 contains diagnostic studies common to the integumentary system.

Assessment of Black Skin

The degree of color of the black-skinned person is genetically determined. The dark skin color results from the reflection of light as it strikes the underlying skin pigment. Increased activity of melanocytes results in large amounts

Macule
A circumscribed, flat discoloration, which may be brown, blue, red, or hypopigmented

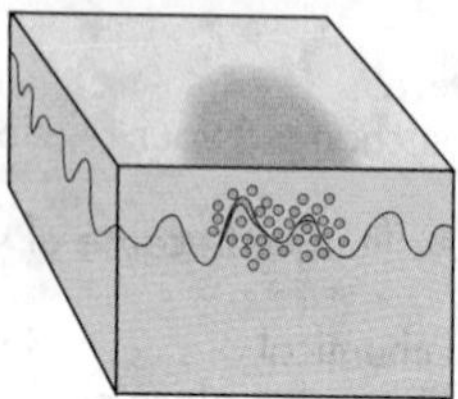

Vesicle
A circumscribed collection of free fluid up to 0.5 cm in diameter

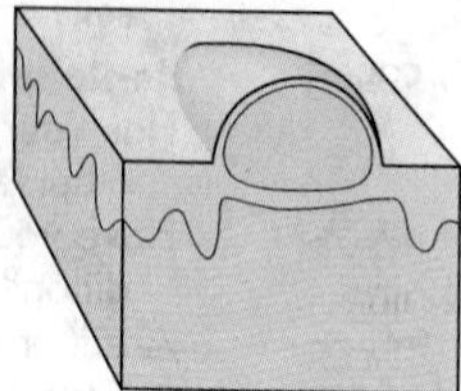

Plaque
A circumscribed, elevated, superficial, solid lesion more than 0.5 cm in diameter, often formed by the confluence of papules

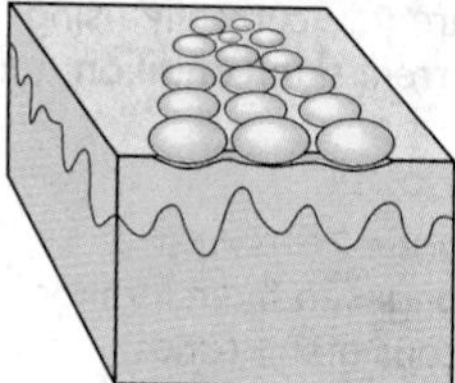

Nodule
A circumscribed, elevated, solid lesion more than 0.5 cm in diameter; a large nodule is referred to as a tumor

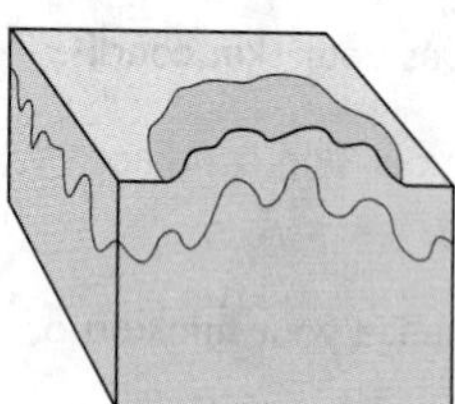

Papule
An elevated solid lesion up to 0.5 cm in diameter; color varies; papules may become confluent and form plaques

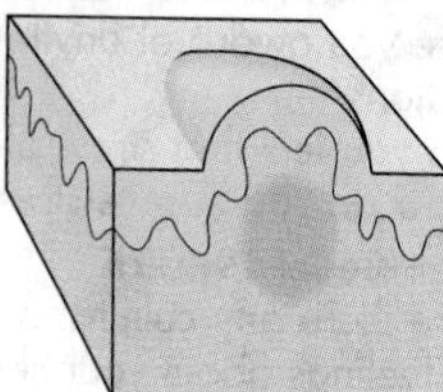

Pustule
A circumscribed collection of leukocytes and free fluid that varies in size

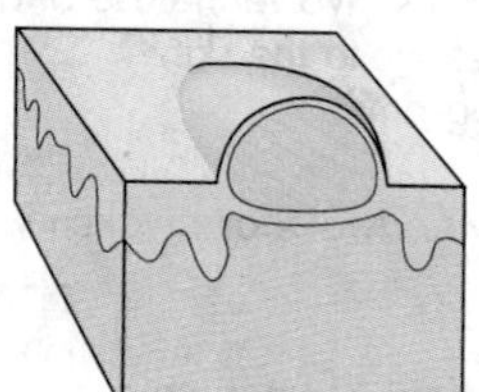

Wheal
A firm edematous plaque resulting from infiltration of the dermis with fluid; wheals are transient and may last only a few hours

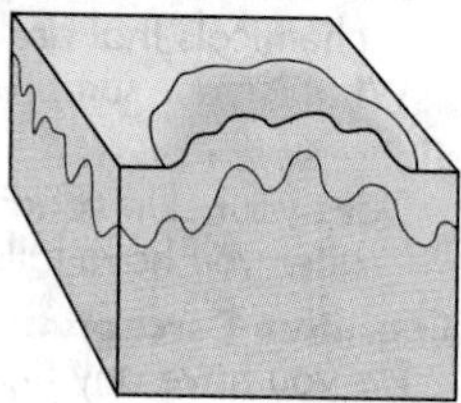

Fig. 19-4 Characteristics of primary skin lesions.

Scales
Excess dead epidermal cells that are produced by abnormal keratinization and shedding

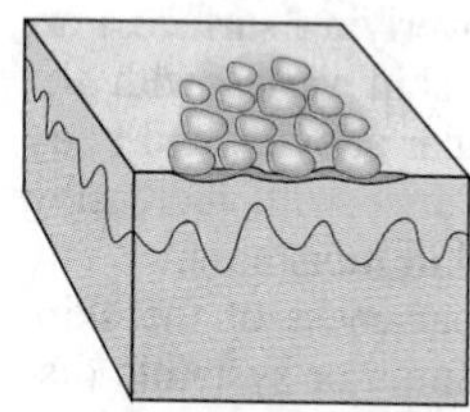

Scar
An abnormal formation of connective tissue implying dermal damage; after injury or surgery scars are initially thick and pink but become white and atrophic

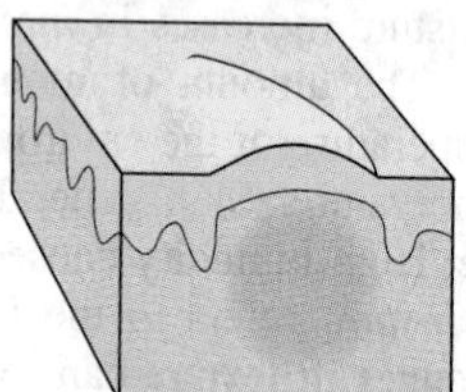

Erosions
A focal loss of epidermis; erosions do not penetrate below the dermoepidermal junction and therefore heal without scarring

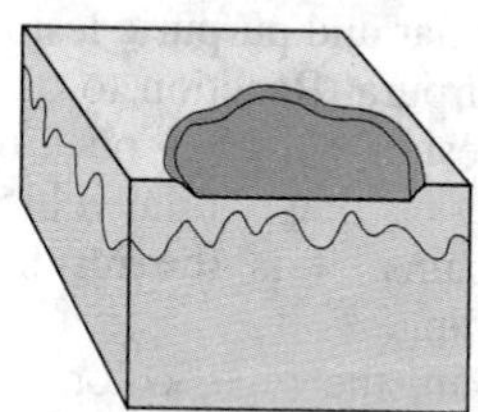

Ulcers
A focal loss of epidermis and dermis; ulcers heal with scarring

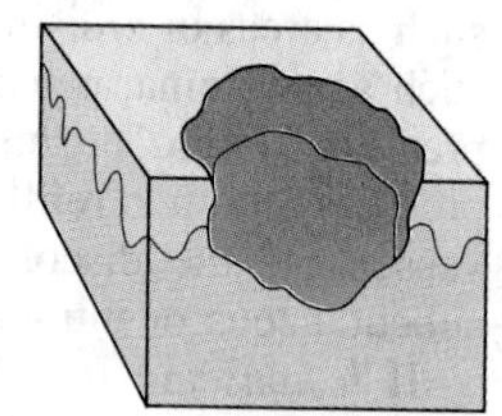

Fissure
A linear loss of epidermis and dermis with sharply defined, nearly vertical walls

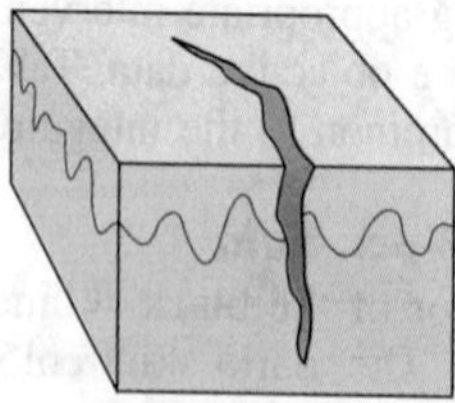

Atrophy
A depression in the skin resulting from thinning of the epidermis or dermis

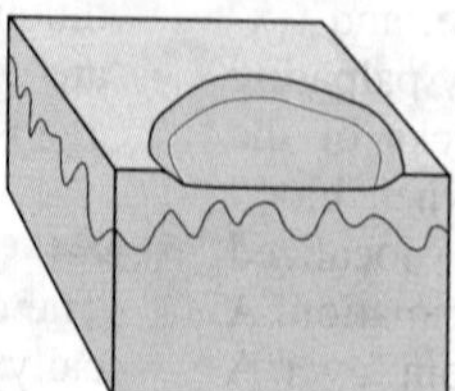

Crusts
A collection of dried serum and cellular debris; a scab

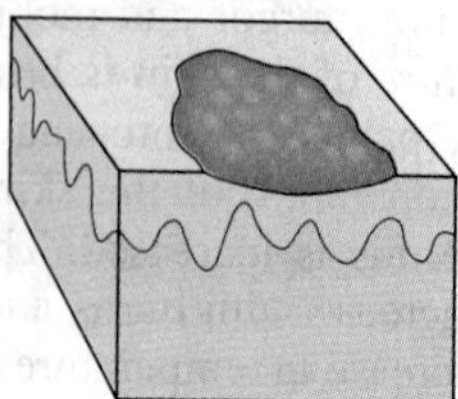

Fig. 19-5 Characteristics of secondary skin lesions.

Table 19-4 Configuration Terminology

Name	Appearance
Annular	Ring shaped
Gyrate	Ring-spiral shape
Iris lesions	Concentric rings or "bull's eyes"
Linear	In a line
Nummular, discoid	Coinlike
Polymorphous	Occurring in several forms
Punctuate	Marked by points or dots
Serpiginous	Snakelike

Table 19-5 Distribution Terminology

Term	Description
Asymmetric	Unilateral distribution
Confluent	Merging together
Diffuse	Wide distribution
Discrete	Separate from other lesions
Generalized	Diffuse distribution
Grouped	Cluster of lesions
Localized	Limited areas of involvement that are clearly defined
Satellite	Single lesion in close proximity to a large grouping
Solitary	A single lesion
Symmetric	Bilateral distribution
Zosteriform	Bandlike distribution along a dermatome area

of melanin production and accounts for the darker skin color. This increased melanin forms a natural sun shield for black skin and results in a decreased incidence of skin cancer in blacks.

The structures of black skin are no different than those of lighter skin, but they are more difficult to assess. Practice and comparison are necessary. Assessment of color is more easily made in areas where the epidermis is thin, such as the lips and mucous membranes.[6] Rashes are often difficult to observe and may need to be palpated.

Black skin is predisposed to certain skin conditions, including pseudofolliculitis, keloids, and mongolian spots. Because of the darkness of the skin of some individuals, color often cannot be used as an indicator of systemic conditions (e.g., flushed skin with fever).

Age-Related Assessment Differences

There are many changes in the skin of the aging person. Although many changes are not serious except for their cosmetic effect, others are more serious and need careful evaluation. Age-related changes in the integumentary system and differences in assessment findings are listed in Table 19-7. Common assessment abnormalities of the skin are described in Table 19-8.

DIAGNOSTIC STUDIES

The main diagnostic techniques related to skin problems are inspection of an individual lesion and a careful history related to the problem. If a definitive diagnosis cannot be made by these techniques, other tests may be indicated (Table 19-6).

Biopsy is the most common diagnostic test used in the evaluation of a skin lesion. A biopsy is indicated in all conditions in which malignancy is suspected or a specific diagnosis is questionable. Techniques include punch, incisional, excisional, and shave or subsection biopsies that can be both therapeutic and diagnostic. The method used depends on factors such as the site of the biopsy, cosmetic result desired, type of tissue to be removed (e.g., flat or elevated), and simplicity of technique.[7]

Other diagnostic procedures used include cultures for fungal, bacterial, and viral infections. *Immunofluorescence* is a special technique used on specimens and may be indicated in certain conditions such as bullous diseases and systemic lupus erythematosus. *Patch testing* and *photopatch testing* may be used in the evaluation of contact, photoallergic, and photodistributed dermatitis.

Table 19-6 Diagnostic Studies: Integumentary System

Study	Description and Purpose	Nursing Responsibility
Biopsy		
■ Punch	Special punch biopsy instrument of appropriate size is used. Instrument rotated to appropriate level to include dermis and some fat. Suturing may or may not be done.	Verify that consent form is signed (if needed). Assist with preparation of site, anesthesia, procedure, and hemostasis. Apply dressing, and give postprocedure instructions to patient. Properly identify specimen.
■ Excisional	Useful when good cosmetic results and entire removal is desired. Skin closed with subcutaneous and skin sutures.	Same as above
■ Incisional	Elliptical incision made in lesion too large to excise. Adequate specimen obtained without causing an extensive cosmetic defect.	Same as above
■ Shave (subsection)	Single-edged razor blade used to shave off lesions. Performed on superficial lesions. Provides full thickness specimen of stratum corneum.	Same as above
Microscopic Tests		
■ Potassium hydroxide	Hair, scales, or nails are examined for hyphae of fungal infection. Specimen is put on a glass slide, and 10% to 40% concentration of potassium hydroxide is added.	Instruct patient regarding purpose of test. Prepare slide.
■ Tzanck test (Wright's, Glesma's, and Papanicolaou stain)	Fluid and cells from vesicles or bullae are examined to diagnose herpes virus. Specimen is put on slide, stained, and examined microscopically for multinucleated giant cells.	Inform patient of purpose of test. Use sterile technique for collection of fluid.
■ Culture	The test will identify fungal, bacterial, and viral organisms. For fungi, scraping is performed if the fungus is systemic involving the skin. For bacteria, material is obtained from intact pustules, bullae, or abscesses. For viruses, bullae are scraped, and exudate is taken from center of lesion.	Instruct patient regarding purpose and specific procedure. Properly identify specimen. Follow instructions for storage of specimen if not sent to laboratory.
■ Mineral oil slides	To check for infestations, scrapings are placed on slide with mineral oil.	Instruct patient of purpose of test. Prepare slide.
■ Immunofluorescent studies	Some cutaneous diseases have specific, abnormal antibody proteins that can be identified by fluorescent studies. Both skin and serum can be examined.	Inform patient of purpose of test. Assist in obtaining specimen.
Miscellaneous		
■ Wood's light	Examination of skin with long-wave ultraviolet light causes specific substances to fluoresce (e.g., *Pseudomonas* organisms, erythrasma, fungal infections, vitiligo)	Explain purpose of examination. Inform patient it is not painful.
■ Diascopy	Examination of the skin using gentle pressure with a transparent object to check lesion vascularity.	Explain procedure to patient.
■ Patch test	Used to determine whether patient is allergic to any testing material. Small amount of potentially allergenic material applied under occlusion usually to skin or back.	Explain purpose and procedure to patient. Instruct patient to return in 48 hr for removal of allergens and evaluation. Inform patient if reevaluation is needed at 96 hr.

Table 19-7 Gerontologic Differences in Assessment: Integumentary System

Changes	Differences in Assessment Findings
Skin	
▪ Decreased subcutaneous fat, muscle laxity, degeneration of elastic fibers, collagen stiffening	Increased wrinkling, sagging breasts and abdomen, redundant flesh around eyes, slowness of skin to flatten when pinched together (tenting)
▪ Decreased extracellular water, surface lipids, and sebaceous gland activity	Dry, flaking skin with possible signs of excoriation caused by pruritus
▪ Less active apocrine and sebaceous gland activity	Dry skin with minimal to no perspiration
▪ Increased capillary fragility and permeability	Evidence of bruising
▪ Increased melanocytes in basal layer with pigment accumulation	Senile lentigines on face and back of hands
▪ Diminished blood supply	Decrease in rosy appearance of skin and mucous membranes; cool to touch; diminished awareness of pain, touch, temperature, and peripheral vibration
▪ Decrease in proliferative capacity	Diminished rate of wound healing
Hair	
▪ Decreased melanin and melanocytes	Graying hair
▪ Decreased oil	Dry, coarse hair; scaly scalp
▪ Decrease in density of hair follicles	Thinning and loss of hair; loss of hair in outer one half or one third of eyebrow
▪ Cumulative androgen effect; decreasing estrogen levels	Facial hirsutism; baldness
Nails	
▪ Decreased peripheral blood supply	Thick, brittle nails with diminished growth
▪ Increased keratin	Ridging
▪ Decreased circulation	Prolonged return of blood to nails on blanching

Table 19-8 Common Assessment Abnormalities: Skin

Finding	Description	Possible Etiology and Significance
Alopecia	Loss of hair (localized or general)	Heredity, friction, rubbing, traction, trauma, infection, inflammation, chemotherapy, pregnancy, stress, emotional shock, tinea capitis, immunologic factors
Angioma	Tumor consisting of blood or lymph vessels	Normal increase with aging, liver disease, pregnancy, varicose veins
Carotenemia (carotenosis)	Yellow discoloration of skin, no yellowing of sclerae, most noticeable on palms and soles	Vegetables containing carotene (e.g., carrots, squash), hypothyroidism
Comedo (blackheads and whiteheads)	Keratin, sebum, microorganism, and epithelial debris within a dilated follicular opening	Acne vulgaris
Cyanosis	Slightly bluish gray or dark purple discoloration of the skin and mucous membranes caused by presence of excessive amounts of reduced hemoglobin in capillaries	Cardiorespiratory problems; vasoconstriction, asphyxiation, anemia, leukemia, and malignancies
Cyst	Sac containing fluid or semisolid material	Obstruction of a duct or gland, parasitic infection
Depigmentation (vitiligo)	Congenital or acquired loss of melanin resulting in white, depigmented areas	Genetic, chemical and pharmacologic agents, nutritional and endocrine factors, burns and trauma, inflammation and infection
Ecchymosis	Large, bruiselike lesion caused by collection of extravascular blood in dermis and subcutaneous tissue	Trauma, bleeding disorders
Erythema	Redness occurring in patches of variable size and shape	Heat, certain drugs, alcohol, ultraviolet rays, any problem that causes dilatation of blood vessels to the skin
Excoriation	Superficial excavations of epidermis	Pruritus, trauma
Hematoma	Extravasation of blood of sufficient size to cause visible swelling	Trauma, bleeding disorders
Hirsutism	Male distribution of hair in women and children	Abnormality of gonads or adrenal glands, decrease in estrogen levels, familial trait
Intertrigo	Dermatitis of overlying surfaces of the skin	Moisture, obesity, *Monilia* infections
Jaundice	Yellow (in Caucasians) or yellowish-brown (in African-Americans) discoloration of the skin, best observed in the sclera secondary to increased bilirubin in the blood	Liver disease, red blood cells hemolysis; pancreatic cancer, common bile duct obstruction
Keloid	Hypertrophied scar beyond margin of incision or trauma	Predisposition more common in blacks
Lichenification	Thickening of the skin with accentuated skin markings	Repeated scratching, rubbing, and irritation
Mole (melanocytic nevus)	Benign overgrowth of melanocytes	Defects of development; excessive numbers and large, irregular moles often familial
Petechiae	Pinpoint, discrete deposit of blood less than 1 mm to 2 mm in the extravascular tissues and visible through the skin or mucous membrane	Inflammation, marked dilatation, blood vessel trauma, blood dyscrasias that result in bleeding tendencies (e.g., thrombocytopenia)
Telangiectasia	Visibly dilated, superficial, cutaneous small blood vessels, commonly found on face and thighs	Aging, acne, sun exposure, alcohol, liver failure, steroid medication, irradiation, certain systemic diseases, and skin tumors; normal variant
Tenting	Failure of skin to return immediately to normal position after gentle pinching	Aging, dehydration, cachexia
Varicosity	Increased prominence of superficial veins	Interruption of venous return (e.g., from tumor, incompetent valves, inflammation)

REVIEW QUESTIONS

The number of the question corresponds to the same-numbered objective at the beginning of the chapter.

1. The primary function of the skin is
a. absorption.
b. sensation.
c. protection.
d. excretion.

2. The most important factor in aging of skin relates to
a. nutrition.
b. sun exposure.
c. exercise.
d. use of makeup.

3. Environmental hazards to the skin include all of the following *except*
a. excessive UV light.
b. irritants.
c. allergens.
d. polypharmacy.

4. When examining a patient, the nurse should do all of the following *except*
a. keep the room well lit and at a moderate temperature.
b. allow the patient to remain dressed.
c. observe and describe specific lesions.
d. wear gloves when palpating a draining lesion.

5. When documenting the appearance of a lesion, the nurse should include all of the following *except*
a. type and color.
b. distribution and grouping.
c. location and size.
d. aggravating factors.

6. The most important assessment technique related to the skin is
a. inspection.
b. palpation.
c. percussion.
d. auscultation.

7. Black skin is predisposed to
a. atopic dermatitis.
b. keloids.
c. sunburn.
d. skin cancer.

8. The most common cause of an excoriation is
a. vasoconstriction.
b. scratching.
c. moisture.
d. hemolysis.

9. If a more definitive diagnosis of a lesion is needed, the most common diagnostic tool used is
a. Tzanck test.
b. Wood's light.
c. potassium hydroxide.
d. biopsy.

REFERENCES

1. Hill MJ: The skin: anatomy and physiology, *Dermatol Nurs* 2:13, 1990.
2. Seeley R, Stephens T, Tate P: *Anatomy and physiology,* ed 2, St Louis, 1992, Mosby.
3. Arnold HL, Odom RB, James WD, editors: *Andrews' diseases of the skin,* ed 8, Philadelphia, 1990, Saunders.
4. Thibodeau G, Patton K: *Anatomy and physiology,* ed 2, St Louis, 1993, Mosby.
5. Gilchrest BA: Aging of the skin, in Fitzpatrick TB and others: *Dermatology in general medicine,* ed 4, New York, 1993, McGraw-Hill.
6. Fitzpatrick T, Bernhard J: Clinical-pathologic correlations of skin leasions: approach to diagnosis, in Fitzpatrick TB and others: *Dermatology in general medicine,* ed 4, New York, 1993, McGraw-Hill.
7. Sauer G: *Manual of skin diseases,* ed 6, Philadelphia, 1991, Lippincott.

Chapter 20

NURSING ROLE IN MANAGEMENT
Integumentary Problems

Eileen Enny Leach **Anne Marie Ruszkowski**

Learning Objectives

1. Describe health promotion and maintenance practices related to the skin.
2. Explain the etiology, clinical manifestations, and therapeutic and nursing management of common acute dermatologic problems.
3. Describe the psychologic and physiologic effects of chronic dermatologic conditions.
4. Explain the etiology, clinical manifestations, and management of malignant dermatologic disorders.
5. Explain the etiology, clinical manifestations, and management of bacterial, viral, and fungal infections of the integumentary system.
6. Explain the etiology, clinical manifestations, and management of infestations and bites.
7. Explain the etiology, clinical manifestations, and management of dermatologic disorders related to allergies.
8. Explain the etiology, clinical manifestations, and management related to benign dermatologic disorders.
9. Describe the dermatologic manifestations of common systemic diseases.
10. Explain the indications and nursing management related to plastic surgery and skin grafts.
11. Explain the etiology, clinical manifestations, and management of pressure sores.

Problems of the skin often present difficult management challenges. Although clothing and cosmetics can disguise or cover some skin problems, many problems cannot be hidden so easily. The emotional impact of skin problems is often more serious than the problem itself. For instance, acne is little more than a nuisance in relation to systemic health. To the adolescent attempting to establish personal identity, however, acne can be a barrier to acceptance in a peer group and pleasant social outlets.

A dichotomy often exists between the actual seriousness of a skin problem and its emotional impact. The therapeutic and nursing management of integumentary problems is presented before specific problems are discussed. These general considerations common to many dermatologic problems also apply to many specific diseases.

THERAPEUTIC AND NURSING MANAGEMENT OF INTEGUMENTARY PROBLEMS

Health Promotion and Maintenance

Health promotion and maintenance practices related to problems of the skin often parallel practices appropriate for general good health. The skin reflects both physical and psychologic well-being. Specific health promotion and maintenance activities appropriate to good skin health include avoidance of environmental hazards, adequate rest and exercise, proper hygiene and nutrition, and cautious use of self-treatment.

Environmental Hazards

Sun. Many people are unaware that the effects of years of exposure to the sun are cumulative and damaging. The ultraviolet (UV) rays of the sun cause degenerative changes in the dermis that result in premature aging from loss of elasticity and thinning, wrinkling, and drying of the skin. Prolonged and repeated sun exposure is a major factor in precancerous and cancerous lesions. Actinic damage, actinic keratoses, basal cell epithelioma, squamous cell epithelioma, and malignant melanoma are dermatologic problems associated directly or indirectly with sun exposure.[1]

The nurse should be a strong advocate of moderation in sun exposure. Vitamin D_3 is produced in the skin and is necessary for vitamin D synthesis; however, only a few minutes of sun on small areas of the body meet this need. Specific wavelengths of the sun (Table 20-1) have different effects on the skin. Ultraviolet B (UVB) appears to be the major factor in the development of skin cancer, whereas ultraviolet A (UVA) augments the carcinogenic effects of UVB. Tanning is the body's defense against further sunburn and is caused by increased production of melanin. When sun exposure is excessive, the turnover time of the skin is shortened and results in peeling. The fair-skinned person,

Reviewed by Sandra Somma, RN, BSN, Staff Nurse, Yale New Haven Hospital, New Haven, CT.

Table 20-1 Wavelengths of the Sun and Effect on Skin

Wavelength	Nanometer Rating	Effect
Short (UVC)	Below 290	Does not reach earth; blocked by atmosphere.
Middle (UVB)	280-320	Causes sunburn and cumulative effect of sun damage.
Long (UVA)	320-400	Can produce elastic tissue damage and actinic skin damage; contributes to formation of skin cancer.

who has smaller amounts of the natural protection afforded by melanin, should be especially cautious about excessive sun exposure.

Sunscreens can filter UVA and UVB wavelengths. There are two types of sunscreen—chemical and physical. *Chemical sunscreens* are designed to absorb or filter UV light, resulting in diminished light penetration into the epidermis. *Physical sunscreens* are thick and opaque and reflect UV radiation. They block all UVA and UVB radiation and all visible light.

The Food and Drug Administration has rated popular sunscreen products according to their *sun protection factor* (SPF). This is a method of measuring the effectiveness of a sunscreen in filtering and absorbing UVB radiation. There is no similar rating of products to screen UVA. The patient should be taught to look for the term "broad spectrum" on the packaging indicating a wide range of absorbance, particularly for UVB wavelengths.

Para-aminobenzoic acid (PABA) has been removed from many sunscreen products because it stains clothing and can cause contact dermatitis. Although rare, allergic contact dermatitis and photoallergic contact dermatitis have been reported following the use of certain chemical sunscreens (PABA and others).[2]

Consumers need to select the sunscreen most appropriate for their needs. PABA and PABA esters, cinnamates, salicylates, and methyl anthranilate block UVB rays. Parsol blocks UVA rays and is added to some sunscreens. The benzophenones block both UVA and UVB rays[3] (Table 20-2). Waterproof sunscreens should be used by swimmers and by persons who perspire profusely. Directions accompanying specific products should be followed as application time before exposure varies according to the product.

The general recommendation is that everyone should use a sunscreen with a minimum SPF 15 daily.[4] Sunscreens with an SPF of 15 or more filter 92% of the UVB responsible for erythema and make sunburn unlikely in most individuals. Although sunscreens with an SPF as high as 50 are available, very little unbiased, published scientific data compare high SPF products to those of SPF 15.

Table 20-2 Sunscreen Ingredients and Ultraviolet Light Protection

Chemical Sunscreens	
Benzophenones	UVA and UVB
PABA and PABA esters	UVB
Cinnamates	UVB
Salicylates	UVB
Miscellaneous	
Methyl anthranilate	UVB
Parso 1789	UVA
Physical Sunscreens	
Titanium dioxide	UVA and UVB
Zinc oxide	UVA and UVB

UVA, ultraviolet A; *UVB*, ultraviolet B.

The nurse can also inform the patient about other means of protection from the damaging effects of the sun, such as wearing a large-brimmed hat and a long-sleeved shirt of a lightly woven fabric or carrying an umbrella. The patient needs to know that the rays of the sun are most dangerous between 10 AM and 2 PM standard time or 11 AM and 3 PM daylight saving time, regardless of the latitude. Even on overcast days a serious sunburn can occur, since up to 80% of UV rays can penetrate through the clouds. Other factors that increase the possibility of a sunburn include being at high altitudes, in snow (which reflects 85% of the sun's rays), or in or near water.[5] Patients should be warned of the dangers of tanning booths and sunlamps, which are predominantly UVA. No presently available sunscreen blocks all UVA.

Certain topical and systemic medications potentiate the sun's effect, even with brief exposure. Common photosensitizing medications are listed in Table 20-3. The chemicals in these medications absorb light and release energy that harms cells and tissues. The clinical picture of drug-induced photosensitivity is that of an exaggerated sunburn with swelling; erythema; papular, plaque-like lesions; and vesicles.[6] Skin that is at risk for photosensitivity reactions

CULTURAL & ETHNIC Considerations

INTEGUMENTARY PROBLEMS

- African-Americans and Native Americans have a low incidence of skin cancer.
- Caucasians, especially those living in sunny climates, have a high incidence of skin cancer.
- Skin assessment may be difficult in individuals with darker skin. The oral mucous membranes and conjunctiva are areas where pallor, cyanosis, and jaundice are more readily detected. The palms of the hands and soles of feet can also be used for assessment of the skin of darker individuals.

Table 20-3 Drugs that May Cause Photosensitivity

Antidysrhythmics	**Diuretics**
Amiodarone	Thiazides
Quinidine	Chlorothiazides
Antihistamines	**Psychotherapeutics**
Diphenhydramine	Chlorpromazine
Antiinfectives	Promazine
Sulfonamides	Thioridazine
Tetracyclines	**Psoralens**
Chloroquine	**Retinoids**
Griseofulvin	**Sulfonylureas**
Nalidixic acid	**Others**
Antineoplastics	Phenistatin
Dacarbazine	Coal tar
Fluorouracil	

can be protected by the use of sunscreen products. The nurse has a role in educating the patient who is taking these medications about their photosensitizing effect.

Irritants and allergens. The nurse needs to reinforce the need to avoid exposure to known irritants (e.g., ammonia, harsh detergents). In addition, allergens that have troubled the patient in the past or that are known to produce problems on exposure (e.g., poison ivy) should be avoided. Many irritants and allergens have a cumulative effect, producing more serious dermatoses on repeated exposure. Patch testing (application of allergens) is necessary to determine the most likely sensitizing agent and to establish a strategy of avoidance.

Prescribed and over-the-counter (OTC) medications used to treat a variety of conditions may cause dermatologic reactions. In fact, drugs are the most frequently identified cause of urticaria and should always be suspected when this condition occurs. The eruption may occur up to 10 days after exposure to the offending drug.[7]

Radiation. Although most radiology departments are extremely cautious in protecting themselves and their patients from the effects of excessive radiation, the nurse should help the patient make intelligent decisions about radiologic procedures. X-rays can be invaluable in both diagnosis and therapy, but indiscriminate use can cause serious side effects to the skin and to other body processes. In the past (30 years ago), cystic acne was treated with radiation. This information is important, since the patients who were thus treated have an increased incidence of basal cell carcinoma (BCC).

Rest and Sleep. Rest and sleep are important health-promotion considerations in relation to the skin. Although the exact effects of sleep are not known, it is thought to be restorative. Rest reduces the threshold of itching and the potential skin damage from the resultant scratching.

Exercise. Exercise increases circulation and dilates the blood vessels. In addition to the healthy glow produced by exercise, the psychologic effects can also improve one's appearance and mental outlook. However, the exerciser needs to avoid overexposure to heat, cold, and sun during outdoor exercise.

Hygiene. Hygienic practices should match the skin type, lifestyle, and culture of the patient. The person with oily skin will need to cleanse the skin with a drying agent more often than the person with dry skin. Dry skin might benefit from superfatted soaps and other measures to increase moisture, such as the application of moisturizers to the skin.

The normally acidic skin (pH 4.2 to 5.6) and perspiration protect against bacterial overgrowth. Most soaps are alkaline and cause a neutralization of the skin surface and loss of protection. Using more neutral soaps and avoiding hot water and vigorous rubbing can noticeably decrease local irritation and inflammation.

In general, the skin and hair should be washed often enough to remove excess oil and excretions and to prevent odor. An older person should avoid the use of harsh soaps and shampoos and should decrease the frequency of bathing because of the skin's increasing dryness. Moisturizers should be used after a bath or shower, while the skin is still damp, to seal in this moisture.

Nutritional Management. A well-balanced diet adequate in all food groups can produce healthy skin, hair, and nails. Certain elements are particularly essential to good skin health. These include the following:

1. *Vitamin A*—Essential for maintenance of normal cell structure, specifically in epithelial cells.
2. *Vitamin B complex*—Essential to complex metabolic functions. Deficiencies of niacin and pyridoxine manifest as dermatologic symptoms such as erythema, bullae, and seborrhea-like lesions.
3. *Vitamin C (ascorbic acid)*—Essential for connective tissue formation and normal wound healing. Absence causes damage to the dermis.
4. *Vitamin K*—Deficiency interferes with normal prothrombin synthesis in the liver and can lead to cutaneous purpura.
5. *Protein*—Adequate supply is necessary for cell synthesis.
6. *Unsaturated fatty acids*—Necessary to maintain the function and integrity of cellular and subcellular membranes in tissue metabolism, especially linoleic and arachidonic acids.

Obesity has an adverse effect on the skin. The increased subcutaneous fat deposits can lead to stretching and overheating. Overheating secondary to the greater insulation provided by fat causes an increase in sweating, which has an adverse effect on normal or inflamed skin. Obesity also has an influence on the development of type II diabetes and its concomitant skin complications (see Chapter 46).

Self-treatment. The nurse needs to increase the patient's awareness of the dangers of self-diagnosis and treatment. The wide variety of OTC skin preparations can indeed confuse the consumer. General instructions that the nurse can discuss with the patient stress the duration of the treatment and the need to follow package directions closely.

Skin problems are generally slow to produce symptoms and slow to resolve. If the package directions of an OTC drug says its use should not exceed 7 days, this warning should be heeded. If the directions say to apply twice daily, the urge to double the dose and hasten the cure must be avoided. If any systemic signs of inflammation or extension of the skin problem develop (e.g., an increased number of lesions or increased erythema or swelling), self-care should be stopped and the help of a professional should be enlisted.

General Measures to Treat Acute Dermatologic Problems

Diagnostic Studies. A careful patient history is of prime importance in the diagnosis of skin problems. The clinician must be skilled at detecting any evidence that could lead to the cause of an extraordinary number of skin problems. After a careful history and physical examination, individual lesions are inspected. On the basis of the history, physical examination, and appropriate diagnostic tests, medical, surgical, or combination therapy will be planned.

Therapeutic and Pharmacologic Management. Many treatment methods are used in dermatology. Some are disease-specific, whereas others work for unknown reasons. Advances in this field have brought relief to the person with a previously chronic, untreatable condition. Many of the specific therapeutic treatments require specialized equipment and are usually reserved for use by the dermatologist. Pharmacologic treatments are prescribed by many clinicians. The effectiveness of these treatments can often be related to the base (or vehicle) in which the medication is prepared. Table 20-4 summarizes the common agents used as bases for topical preparations and their therapeutic considerations.

Table 20-4 Common Bases for Topical Medications

Agent	Therapeutic Considerations
■ Powder	Promotion of dryness, increase in evaporation, absorbing of moisture possible, common base for antifungal preparations
■ Lotion	Suspension of insoluble powders in water; cooling and drying, with residual powder film after evaporation of water; useful in subacute pruritic eruptions
■ Cream	Emulsions of oil and water, most common base for topical medications, lubrication, and protection
■ Ointment	Oil with differing amounts of water added in suspension, lubrication and prevention of dehydration, petrolatum most common
■ Paste	Mixture of powder and ointment, used when drying effect necessary because moisture is absorbed

Phototherapy. Two types of UV light, or a combination of the two (UVA, UVB), are used to treat many dermatologic conditions. Ultraviolet wavelengths cause erythema, desquamation, and pigmentation and may cause a temporary suppression of basal cell mitosis followed by a rebound increase in cell turnover.

Psoralen plus UVA light (PUVA) is a form of phototherapy. The photosensitizing drug psoralen is given to the patient 90 minutes before exposure to UVA to enhance the effect of UV light in the UVA spectrum (Table 20-1). Usually a moisturizing agent or a tar preparation is applied to the affected area in a thin layer before exposure to UVB. Conditions that are responsive to effective wavelengths with or without drugs include atopic dermatitis, cutaneous T-cell lymphoma, pruritus, psoriasis, and vitiligo.

Ultraviolet light in the specific wavelengths can be produced artificially. Therapeutic doses of UVA and UVB can be measured and used to treat spectrum-specific diseases (Fig. 20-1). Frequent skin assessments must be performed on all patients receiving phototherapy. Inappropriate exposure to UV light can result in basal or squamous cell carcinoma (SCC), as well as severe erythema or burns to the skin. The patient should be cautioned about the potential hazards of using photosensitizing chemicals and further exposure to UV rays from sunlight or artificial UV light during the course of phototherapy. Protective eyewear that blocks 100% of UV light is prescribed for the patient receiving PUVA, since psoralen is absorbed by the lens of the eye. The eyewear is used to prevent cataract formation. The patient is instructed to use the eyewear for 24 hours after taking the medication when outdoors or near a bright window because UVA penetrates glass. The recent evidence of immunosuppressive effects of PUVA requires careful ongoing monitoring.

Radiation therapy. The use of radiation for the treatment of cutaneous malignancies varies greatly according to local practice and availability. Even if radiotherapy is

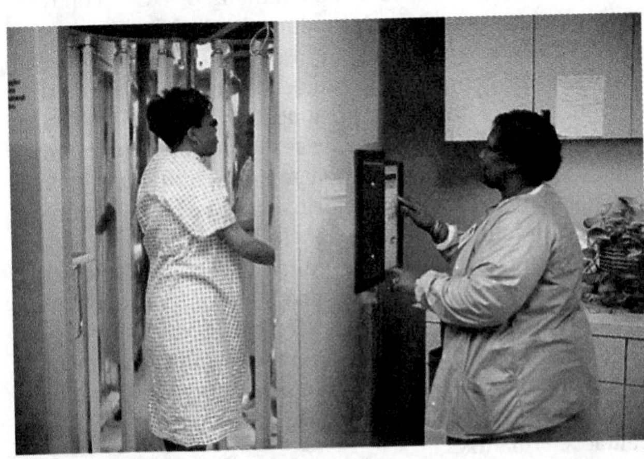

Fig. 20-1 Patient receiving phototherapy, a method for treating spectrum-specific diseases.

planned, a biopsy must first be performed to obtain a pathologic diagnosis.[8]

Radiation to malignant cutaneous lesions is a painless treatment that is similar in cost to surgery and produces minimal damage to surrounding tissue. It is a particularly effective treatment for the older adult or debilitated patient who cannot tolerate even a minor surgical procedure and for the nose, eyelids, and canthal areas, where preservation of the surrounding tissue is of prime consideration. Careful shielding is necessary to prevent ocular lens damage if the irradiated area is around the eyes.

Radiation therapy usually requires multiple visits and is most effective on lesions above the neck. However, it produces permanent alopecia of the irradiated areas. Adverse effects include telangiectasia, atrophy, hyperpigmentation, depigmentation, ulceration, chronic radiodermatitis, and squamous cell carcinoma. (Radiation therapy is discussed in Chapter 12).

Total-body skin irradiation (the body is bombarded with high-energy electrons) may be the treatment of choice or adjunctive therapy for cutaneous T-cell lymphoma. Treatment follows a lengthy course, and toxicity to internal organs must be avoided. The patient experiences transient loss of hair and radiation dermatitis with transient loss of sweat gland function. This treatment ages the skin about 20 years.

Laser technology. Laser technology is gaining in importance as an efficient surgical tool for many types of dermatologic procedures. Lasers are able to produce measurable, repeatable, consistent zones of tissue damage. They can cut, coagulate, and vaporize tissue to some degree. The wavelength determines the type of delivery system used and the intensity of the energy delivered.

The surgical use of laser energy requires a focusing device to produce a small, high-density spot of energy that can be carefully and controllably directed to the operative site. Written policies and procedures should cover laser safety and should be reviewed by all personnel working with laser equipment. Laser light does not accumulate in body cells and cannot cause cellular changes or damage. No monitoring or shielding devices are necessary. Dermatologic uses of laser surgery include coagulation of vascular lesions, removal of tatoos, and treatment of BCC, condylomas, plantar warts, keloids, and many other lesions.

Antibiotics. Antibiotics are used topically and systemically to treat dermatologic problems and are often used in combination with other treatments. Topical antibiotics should always be applied to clean skin. Occlusive dressings should not be used. Common topical antibiotics include bacitracin (used for gram-positive organisms), neomycin and gentamicin (used for Staphylococcus and most gram-negative organisms), and erythromycin (used for gram-positive cocci [staphylococci and streptococci] and gram-negative cocci and bacilli). Topical erythromycin and clindamycin (solutions or gels) are used in the treatment of acne vulgaris. Many of the more popular systemic antibiotics are not used topically because of the danger of allergic contact dermatitis.

If there are signs of systemic infection, a systemic antibiotic should be used. Systemic antibiotics are useful in the treatment of bacterial infections and acne vulgaris. The most frequently used antibiotics are synthetic penicillin, erythromycin, and tetracycline. These drugs are particularly useful for erysipelas; cellulitis; carbuncles; and severe, infected eczema. Cultures of the lesion can guide the choice of the antibiotic. The patient requires specific instructions on the proper technique of taking or applying the antibiotic. For instance, oral tetracycline must be taken on an empty stomach and never with a dairy product, which would interfere with absorption.

Corticosteroids. Corticosteroids are particularly effective in treating a wide variety of dermatologic conditions and can be used topically, intralesionally, or systemically. *Topical corticosteroids* are used for their local antiinflammatory action, as well as for their antipruritic effects. Attempts to diagnose a lesion should be made before a steroid preparation is applied because steroids will mask the clinical manifestations. Steroids are useful in the treatment of many dermatoses. Once a sufficient amount of medication is dispensed, limits should be set on the duration and frequency of application. With prolonged use the more potent steroid formulations can cause adrenal suppression, especially if occlusive dressings are used. High-potency corticosteroids may produce side effects, including atrophy of the skin resulting from impaired cell mitosis and collagen production from capillary fragility, striae, and susceptibility to bruising with prolonged use. In general, dermal and epidermal atrophy does not occur until a steroid has been used 2 to 3 weeks. If drug use is discontinued at the first sign of atrophy, recovery will usually occur in several weeks.[9] Rosacea eruptions, severe exacerbations of acne vulgaris, and dermatophyte infections may also occur. Rebound dermatitis is not uncommon when therapy is stopped.

Low-potency corticosteroids such as hydrocortisone act more slowly but can be used for a longer period without producing serious side effects. Low-potency corticosteroids are used on the face and intertriginous areas. The potency of a particular preparation is related to the concentration of the active drug in it. The ointment form represents the most efficient delivery system. Creams and ointments should be applied in thin layers and slowly massaged into the site 1 to 4 times a day as prescribed. The nurse must stress that only a small amount of medication is necessary—more is *not* better.

Intralesional corticosteroids are injected directly into or just beneath the lesion. This method provides a reservoir of medication whose effect will last several weeks to months. Intralesional injections are commonly used in the treatment of psoriasis, alopecia areata (patchy hair loss), cystic acne, hypertrophic scars, and keloids. A 2.5 to 10 mg/ml suspension of triamcinolone acetonide (Kenalog) is the most common dose range for intralesional injection. A small amount is injected into the site of each lesion.

Systemic corticosteroids can have remarkable results in the treatment of dermatologic conditions. However, they often have undesirable systemic effects (see Chapter 44). Steroids can be administered as short-term therapy for such acute conditions as contact dermatitis from poison ivy. Long-term steroid therapy for dermatologic conditions is reserved for chronic bullous diseases, severe systemic effects of collagen and immunologic responses, and as a last resort when other therapies have failed. The side effects of both topical and systemic long-term steroid therapy must always be considered when such therapy is used to treat chronic skin conditions.

Antihistamines. Antihistamines are used to treat conditions that exhibit urticaria; angioedema; pruritus associated with many dermatologic problems such as atopic dermatitis, psoriasis, and contact dermatitis; and other allergic cutaneous reactions. Antihistamines compete with histamine for the receptor site, thus preventing its pharmacologic response. Antihistamines have anticholinergic, antipruritic, and sedative effects. Several different antihistamines may have to be tried before the satisfactory therapeutic effect is achieved. A major side effect of some antihistamines is sedation. The patient should be warned about sedative effects, a particular problem when one is driving or operating heavy machinery. Because of their long half-life and their anticholinergic effects, antihistamines should be used with particular caution in the older adult.

Topical fluorouracil. Fluorouracil (5-FU), a topical cytotoxic agent with selective toxicity for sun-damaged cells, is available in three strengths (1%, 2%, and 5%). It is used for the treatment of premalignant skin disease, especially actinic keratosis. Since systemic absorption of the drug is minimal, systemic side effects are virtually nonexistent. When a diagnosis of skin cancer has been established, 5-FU is generally not used.[10]

Patient compliance is the major problem with the use of 5-FU. The medication produces painful, eroded areas over the damaged skin within 4 days. Treatment must continue with applications 1 to 2 times a day for 2 to 4 weeks. Healing may take up to 3 weeks after the medication is stopped (Fig. 20-2). Since fluorouracil is a photosensitizing drug, the patient must be instructed to avoid sunlight during treatment. The patient needs to be educated about the effect of the medication and should be warned that the skin will look worse before it looks better. Fluorouracil causes dermatitis, so the patients can plan social activities accordingly. After effective treatment, treated skin is smooth and free of actinic keratoses, although sometimes a second course is necessary.

Disease-specific drugs. Many dermatologic conditions are treated by specific drug preparations, which are outlined in tables throughout this chapter.

Surgical Interventions. Certain dermatologic conditions are best treated by surgical methods.

Electrodesiccation and electrocoagulation. Electrical energy can be converted to heat by the tip of an electrode. This results in tissue being destroyed by burning. The major uses of this type of therapy are point coagulation of bleeding vessels and destruction of small telangiectasias. *Electrodesiccation* usually involves more superficial destruction, and a monopolar electrode is used. *Electrocoagulation* has a deeper effect, with better hemostasis and an increased possibility of scarring. A dipolar electrode is used for electrocoagulation.

Curettage. Curettage is the removal of tissue by means of an instrument with a circular cutting edge attached to a handle. The tissue is scooped away. Although the curette is not usually strong enough to cut normal skin, it is useful for removing many types of small skin tumors, such as warts, molluscum contagiosum, seborrheic keratoses, and small basal and squamous cell cancers. The area to be curetted is anesthetized before the procedure. Hemostasis is obtained by use of one of several methods: electrocoagulation, ferric subsulfate (Monsel's solution), gelatin foam, aluminum

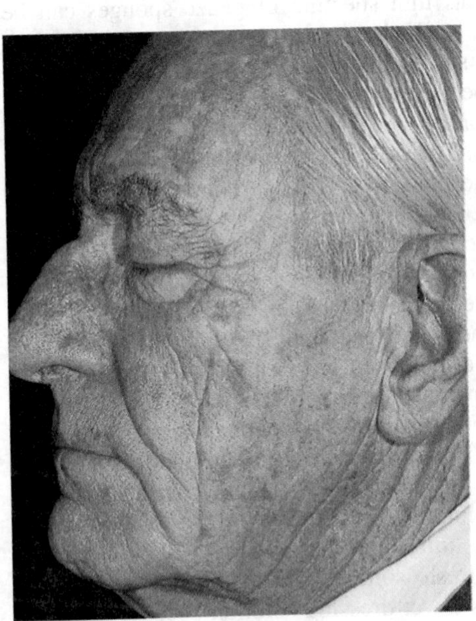

A

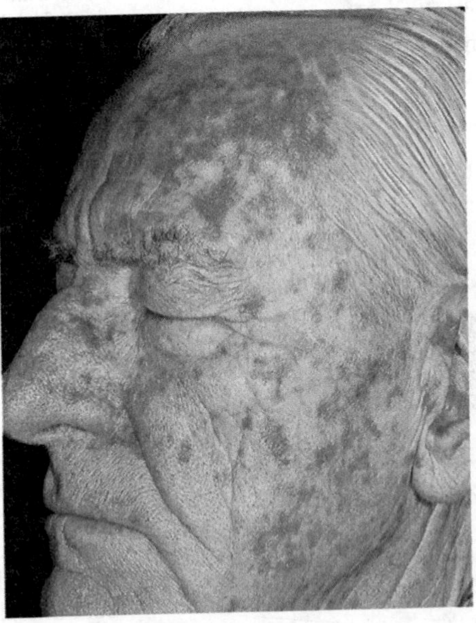

B

Fig. 20-2 Actinic Keratosis. ***A,*** Diffuse involvement of the forehead. Lesions are superficial. Lesions on the cheek were not clinically apparent. ***B,*** Treatment with topical 5-FU. Maximum intensity of inflammation was reached 3 weeks after starting treatment. The medication has inflamed the cheek lesions that were not clinically apparent before treatment.

chloride, or a gauze pressure dressing. A small scar may result. The specimen may be sent for biopsy.

Punch biopsy. Punch biopsy is a common dermatologic procedure used to obtain a tissue sample for histologic study or to remove small lesions. Its use is generally reserved for lesions of less than 0.5 cm. Before anesthesia is used, the biopsy area is outlined so that landmarks will not be obscured by the anesthetizing agent. The biopsy punch cores out a small cylinder of skin when its sharp edge is twirled between the fingers. The core of skin is snipped from the subcutaneous fat and appropriately preserved for examination (Fig. 20-3). Hemostasis is achieved by using the same methods as with curettage, but sites of 3 mm or larger are often closed with sutures. Other types of biopsies are discussed in Chapter 19 and displayed in Table 19-8.

Cryosurgery. Some skin lesions can be destroyed by freezing. Topical liquid nitrogen is the agent most commonly used for cryosurgery. Although the exact mechanism is not clearly understood, the use of liquid nitrogen causes death or destruction of the treated skin.

Liquid nitrogen is a cold, liquefied gas with a temperature of 20° F (4° C). For cells to be destroyed, the agent used must go to at least 320.8° F (196° C). Liquid nitrogen can explode if kept in an airtight container.

Liquid nitrogen can be applied topically (directly onto the benign or precancerous lesion) with a cotton swab or with the appropriate container (Cry-AC) for several freeze-and-thaw cycles. The patient is informed that a cold sensation will be felt. The lesion will first become swollen and red, and it may blister. Next, a scab will form and fall off in 1 to 3 weeks. The skin lesion will be sloughed along with the scab. Growth of new skin will follow. Cryosurgery is a useful treatment for common and genital warts, cutaneous tags, seborrheic keratoses, actinic keratoses, and many other less common skin conditions. Cryosurgery is inexpensive, rapid, and leaves minimal scarring. The major disadvantage of this treatment is lack of a tissue specimen.

Excision. Excision should be considered if the lesion involves the dermis. Complete closure of the excised area usually results in a good cosmetic result. To minimize scarring, a pressure dressing should be applied.

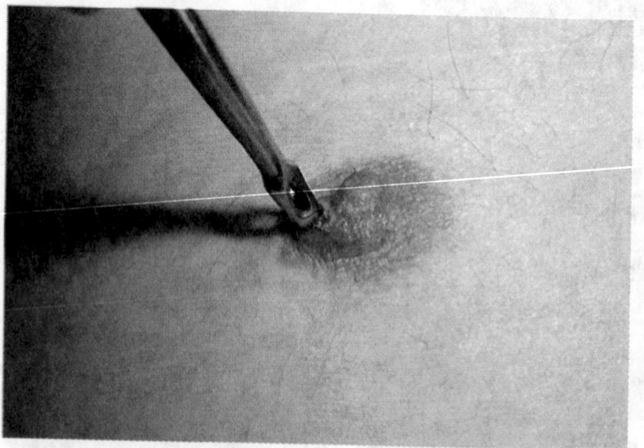

Fig. 20-3 Punch biopsy for pathology specimen.

Another type of excision is the *Mohs micrographic surgery,* a microscopically controlled excision of a cutaneous malignancy. This procedure sections the surgical specimen horizontally, so that 100% of the surgical margin can be examined. Any residual tumor not removed by the first surgical excision can be removed in serial excisions performed the same day. The benefit of this treatment is preservation of normal tissue, producing the smallest possible wound. Mohs micrographic surgery is an outpatient procedure.

NURSING MANAGEMENT

DERMATOLOGIC PROBLEMS

Acute Interventions

Dermatologic conditions are not commonly the primary reasons for hospitalization; however, the hospitalized patient may exhibit concurrent skin problems that warrant nursing intervention and patient education.

If the nursing care is in an acute-care setting, the nurse will both administer and teach the appropriate treatments. If the patient is in an outpatient setting, the nursing focus will be on patient education, with opportunities provided for demonstration and redemonstration. Subsequent visits provide the opportunity to evaluate patient understanding and treatment effectiveness.

Nursing interventions related to dermatologic conditions fall into broad categories. They are applicable to many skin problems in both inpatient and outpatient settings. The nursing care for a patient with chronic skin lesions is presented in the care plan on p. 504.

Wet Dressings. The use of wet dressings is a common dermatologic procedure used to dry exudative lesions, relieve itching, suppress inflammation, and debride a wound. In addition, wet dressings will increase penetration of topical medications, promote sleep by relieving discomfort, and enhance removal of scales, crusts, and exudate. Such materials as thin sheeting or gauze sponges can be used for dressings. Ingenuity is sometimes required when odd-shaped parts of the body must be covered.

The prescribed dressing is put into fresh solution, held until it is no longer dripping, and applied to the affected area (Fig. 20-4). The dressing should be left in place 15 to 30 minutes. The compress is then removed and replaced with a new one. This treatment may be used 2 to 4 times a day or continuously. If the skin appears macerated, the dressings should be discontinued for 2 to 3 hours. The patient should be protected from discomfort and chilling by protection of linens and bedclothes with pads or plastic.

Common solutions used for wet dressings are listed in Table 20-5. Tap water at room temperature is the most common solution. Potassium permanganate must be completely dissolved before use because the undissolved crystals may burn the skin. This solution must be freshly prepared to maintain its oxidative properties. Potassium permanganate solution that turns brown should be discarded and a fresh solution made. Boric acid is not recommended as a wet dressing solution because of potential systemic toxicity from percutaneous absorption, espe-

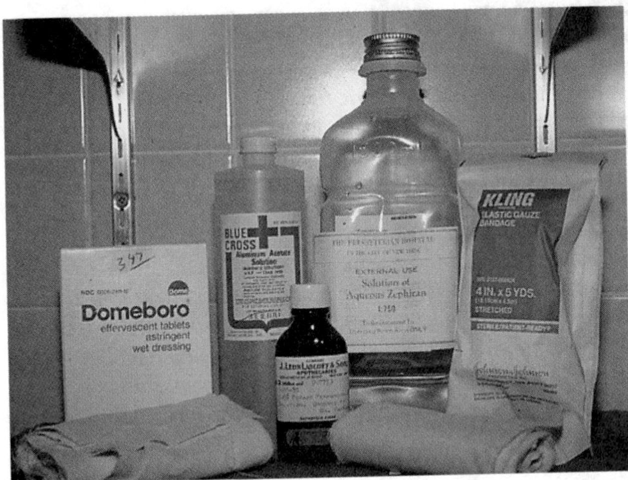

Fig. 20-4 Wet dressings, a common dermatologic procedure, use many different types of dressings and solutions.

cially on open skin. The best solution to use on the eyes is plain, cool water.

Wet dressings do not need to be sterile. They should be cool when an antiinflammatory effect is desired and tepid when the purpose is to debride an infected, crusted lesion. These treatments are excellent ways to remove the scabs left by the collection of debris at a wound site.

Baths. Baths are appropriate when large body areas need to be treated. They also have sedative and antipruritic effects. Some medications, such as oilated oatmeal, potassium permanganate, and sodium bicarbonate, can be added directly to the bathwater. One cup of the mixture can be added to 2 cups of water and then added to the bathwater. The bathtub should be half-full of water. Both the bathwater and the prescribed solution should be at a temperature that is comfortable for the patient. The patient can soak for 15 to 20 minutes 3 to 4 times a day, depending on the severity of the dermatitis and the patient's discomfort. It is important to stress to the patient that the skin not be towel-dried but gently patted to prevent increased irritation and inflammation. The addition of oils makes the bathtub extremely slippery and therefore should be avoided. If oils are used in the bathtub, the utmost caution must be used in transferring the patient to prevent accidents. To sustain the moisturizing effect, lubrication should be applied to the skin directly after the bath. This helps to retain the moisture in the hydrated cells.

Topical Medications. A thin layer of ointment, cream, or lotion should be applied to clean skin and spread evenly in a downward motion. An alternate method is to apply the medication directly onto the dressings. Pastes are designed to protect the affected area. They should be applied thickly with a tongue blade or a gloved hand. Draining lesions and lesions with greasy medication can be covered with a light dressing to prevent soiling clothes. The patient needs specific directions on the proper application of prescribed topical medications.

Control of Pruritus. Pruritus (itching) can be caused by almost any physical or chemical stimulus to the skin, such as drugs, insects, and dry skin. The itch sensation is carried by the same nonmyelinated nerve fibers as pain. If the epidermis is damaged or absent, the sensation will be felt as pain rather than itch.

The itch-scratch-itch cycle needs to be broken to prevent excoriation and eventual lichenification. Control of pruritus also is important because it is difficult to diagnose a lesion that is excoriated and inflamed.

Certain circumstances make itching worse. Anything that causes vasodilation, such as heat or rubbing, should be avoided. Dryness of the skin lowers the itch threshold and increases the itch sensation. Any internal or external factor that increases blood flow to an area increases itching.

Measures that the nurse can use or teach the patient to use to break the itch cycle should be attempted. A cool environment may cause vasoconstriction and decrease itching. The use of topical corticosteroids reduces inflammation

Table 20-5 Wet Dressing Solutions

Agent	Preparation	Use
Acetic acid	Vinegar is 5% acetic acid; make 1% solution by adding ½ cup of white vinegar to 1 pint of water	Bactericidal
Burow's solution (aluminum sulfate and calcium acetate)	One packet or tablet in 1 pint of water produces a modified 1:40 Burow's solution	Mildly antiseptic for acute inflammation
Magnesium sulfate (Epsom salt)	8 tsp to 1 L of water	Debridement, cleansing
Potassium permanganate	1 crushed 65 mg tablet to 250 ml of water	Antiseptic, disinfectant
Silver nitrate	1 tsp of 50% stock to 1 L of water	Antiseptic, disinfectant
Sodium bicarbonate	8 tsp to 1 L of water	Antipruritic
Sodium chloride	2 tsp to 1 L of water	Antipruritic, cleansing, debridement
Water	Tap water, does not need to be sterile	Debridement, cleansing

NURSING CARE PLAN Patient With Chronic Skin Lesions

Planning: Outcome Criteria	Nursing Interventions and Rationales
➤ **NURSING DIAGNOSIS**	Altered comfort: pruritus *related to* presence of skin lesions *as manifested by* itching, areas of excoriated skin, agitation, and anxiety over itching sensation
Express satisfactory control of pruritus.	Decrease environmental irritants (e.g., heat, scratchy coverings) *to reduce vasodilatation and sensory stimulation.* Use topical and systemic antiinflammatory medications *to reduce inflammation and cause vasoconstriction.* Provide a cool environment *to promote vasoconstriction.* Use cool, wet dressings, soaks, and baths *to cause vasoconstriction and promote comfort.* Administer antihistamines as necessary *to reduce feeling the need to scratch* Keep patient's nails trimmed short *to prevent skin excoriation from scratching.* Provide diversional activities *to distract patient from discomfort of pruritus.*
➤ **NURSING DIAGNOSIS**	Risk for infection *related to* open lesion, presence of environmental pathogens and exudate
Show no evidence of secondary infection such as redness, edema, or exudate.	Monitor for open, draining lesions; redness, swelling, and pain at lesion sites; lymphadenopathy and fever; indications of scratching *to detect presence of infection.* Teach patient measures to prevent scratching, such as tepid baths and a cool environment *to reduce itchy sensation and subsequent excoriation and creation of a portal of entry for infection.* Practice and teach careful hand washing and proper disposal of dressings and contaminated linens *to prevent secondary infections.* Inform patient of dangers of scratching.
➤ **NURSING DIAGNOSIS**	Altered comfort: dry skin *related to* inadequate fluid intake, too frequent cleansing, dryness from treatment medications *as manifested by* dry, flaking skin
Have moist, well-lubricated skin.	Use nonirritating moisturizing agents *to keep skin moist and reduce water loss.* Provide adequate fluid (2000 to 3000 ml/day) and fat intake *to keep skin well hydrated.* Avoid frequent bathing. Encourage use of superfatted soap *to prevent drying of skin and encourage moisture retention.* Apply skin lotion or cream immediately after bathing *to trap moisture from bathing in the skin.*
➤ **NURSING DIAGNOSIS**	Self-esteem disturbance *related to* presence of unsightly lesions *as manifested by* verbalization of self-disgust and despair over appearance of lesions, isolation, reluctance to look at lesions or participate in self-care
Express realistic hope for resolution of open lesions, maintain normal social relationships.	Discuss situation with patient in open, accepting manner *to assist patient to express feelings.* Do not show shock or disgust at the sight of lesions *to prevent further decrease in self-esteem.* Touch the patient, if appropriate to the situation, *as reluctance to touch the patient may be demoralizing.* Provide counseling, if indicated, *to assist patient in accepting the situation.*

continued

and causes vasoconstriction. Menthol, camphor, or phenol can be used to numb the itch receptors. Systemic antihistamines can be used if necessary to provide relief to a patient while the underlying cause of the pruritus is diagnosed and treated. The principal side effect of antihistamines is sedation. This may, in fact, be desirable, since pruritus is often worse at night and interferes with sleep.[11]

Wet dressings can be used effectively to relieve pruritus. Thin, old sheets are placed in warm water, wrung out, and placed over the pruritic area. After 10 to 15 minutes the dressing is removed, the skin patted dry, and a lubricant applied. This procedure can be repeated as necessary for comfort. Topical antipruritic medications should be applied as directed by the physician.

Prevention of Spread. Although most skin problems are not contagious, infection control precautions indicate the need for gloves. Procedures should be explained in order to avoid demoralizing an already sensitive patient. If in doubt, however, the nurse should wear gloves until a definite diagnosis has been established. The most common contagious lesions that should be easily recognized by nurses include impetigo, staphylococcus, pyoderma, primary chancre and secondary syphilis lesions, scabies, and pediculosis. Careful hand washing and safe disposal of soiled dressings are the best means of preventing spread of skin problems.

Prevention of Secondary Infections. Open lesions on the skin are susceptible to invasion by other organisms.

NURSING CARE PLAN Patient With Chronic Skin Lesions—cont'd

Planning: Outcome Criteria	Nursing Interventions and Rationales
➤ **NURSING DIAGNOSIS**	Altered health maintenance *related to* lack of knowledge of disease process, management plan, prevention of scarring, care of lesions, possible cosmetic surgery, and use of OTC medications *as manifested by* questions on self-care activities and possibilities for surgery to improve appearance, lack of understanding of disease process or management plan
Verbalize confidence in ability to care for self and explore surgical options, describe disease process and management plan, seek medical help (if self-medication is ineffective or condition worsens).	Answer questions completely *to foster knowledge base of pertinent issues.* Teach patient about disease process, management plan, care of lesions *to foster independence and boost confidence in ability to manage self-care.* Discuss possible cosmetic surgery options *so patient can make informed decisions.* Advise patient to carefully follow guidelines for OTC medications *to prevent misuse or worsening of condition.* Inform patient of signs that indicate a worsening of the condition, such as increase in number of lesions, increase in erythema and swelling, and fever *so medical assistance will be sought promptly.*
➤ **NURSING DIAGNOSIS**	Anxiety *related to* chronicity of problem and personal appearance *as manifested by* verbalization of anxiety and frustration over chronicity of problem and appearance of skin from scarring and lichenification, request for information on suitable cover-up techniques
Express hope regarding cessation of new lesions, improved appearance with use of cosmetics.	Encourage patient to continue medical regime *to enhance appearance and reduce awareness of lesions.* Counsel patient regarding healthy life practices. Advise patient on skilled use of cosmetics *to maximize improvement possibilities.* Involve family members for support.
➤ **NURSING DIAGNOSIS**	Social isolation *related to* decreased activities secondary to poor self-image, fear of rejection, and lack of knowledge related to cover-up techniques *as manifested by* lack of social activities, verbalization of dissatisfaction with social life
Express satisfaction with social life.	Encourage socialization in patient's interest areas *to reduce sense of isolation and worthlessness.* Arrange psychiatric referral, if indicated. Teach skillful use of cosmetics, cover-up agents, and clothing *to maximize personal appearance and encourage socialization.*

OTC, Over-the-counter.

Meticulous hygiene, hand washing, and dressing changes are important to prevent secondary infections. Also, the patient should be warned about scratching lesions, which can cause excoriations and create a portal of entry for pathogens. The patient's nails should be trimmed short to minimize trauma from scratching.

Specific Skin Care. The nurse is often in a position to advise the patient about skin care following simple dermatologic surgical procedures, such as skin biopsy, excision, and cryosurgery. Patient follow-up should be individualized. In general, instructions would include dressing changes, use of topical antibiotics, and the signs and symptoms of infection.

Oozing wounds are best treated with wet to dry dressings (for debridement) and an antibiotic ointment. The ointment will inhibit infection and keep the bandage from sticking. If the bandage gets wet, both ointment and bandage need to be reapplied.

Initially, a scab should be left alone to be a protective coating for the damaged skin under it. Scabs should be kept dry. They can be covered during the day for cosmetic purposes but should be exposed at night. If a scab gets wet, it should be dried gently. After awhile, the scab should be removed gently, after soaking, to encourage healing and remove a site for bacterial growth.

A wound with stitches is handled much like an oozing wound. The area should be covered with a pressure bandage, and an antibiotic ointment should be used. Stitches will generally be removed in 4 to 10 days, although facial stitches may be removed earlier to prevent scarring. Sometimes every other stitch will be removed after the third day. Incision lines require daily cleansing, usually with plain tap water. If necessary a topical antibiotic is applied and the wound is either covered with a dry sterile dressing or left open to air. The patient may experience some swelling and discomfort in the first 24 hours. Mild analgesics such as acetaminophen should control the discomfort. The patient needs to know the manifestations of inflammation such as redness, fever, or increased pain or swelling, and signs of infection, such as purulent drainage. Any of these manifestations should be reported to the health care provider.

Chronic and Home Management

Psychologic Effects of Chronic Dermatologic Problems. The emotional toll is indeed heavy for persons who suffer from chronic skin problems such as eczema, psoriasis, and atopic and seborrheic dermatitis. The sequelae of chronic skin problems could result in employment problems with subsequent financial implications, a frail and easily damaged body image, problems with sexuality, and increasing and progressive frustration. The usual lack of systemic overt illness coupled with the visibility of the skin lesions present real problems to the patient.

The nurse must continue to be optimistic and help the patient comply with the prescribed regimen. The patient must be allowed to verbalize the "why me?" question, even though there is no ready answer. Reinforcement of the prescribed hygiene and treatment measures is an important part of the nursing management.

Many lesions can be camouflaged with the skillful use of cosmetics. Individual sensitivity to product ingredients must always be considered in the selection of a cosmetic product. Oil-free, hypoallergenic cosmetics are available and could be beneficial to the allergic patient. Rehabilitative cosmetics are available to help camouflage and deemphasize such lesions as vitiligo or melasma (tan to brown patches on the face) or postoperative wound sites. These products are opaque, smudge resistant, and water resistant.

In addition to specific skin conditions that tend to chronicity, other factors affecting the outcome of long-term dermatologic problems include skin type, history of previous exacerbations, family history, complications, intolerance to therapy, environmental factors, lack of adherence to the prescribed regimen, endocrine factors, and psychologic factors. Lesions that follow a chronic pattern often are associated with lichenification and scarring.

Physiologic Effects of Chronic Dermatologic Problems. *Scarring* and *lichenification* are the result of chronic dermatologic problems. Scars occur when ulceration takes place and reflects the pattern of healing in the area. Scars are pink and vascular at first. As scars age they become avascular and white with increasing strength. Different parts of the body scar differently. Scars usually remain conspicuous except on the face and neck, where they heal fairly well because of a good blood supply.

The location of the scar is the determining factor with respect to cosmetic implications. Facial scars are the most damaging psychologically because they are so visible. Creative use of cosmetics can do much to mask the scarring of chronic skin conditions. The best treatment is prevention of scarring by controlling the problem in the acute phase.

Lichenification, another consequence of chronic skin problems, is the thickening of skin from proliferation of keratinocytes with accentuation of the normal markings of the skin. Lichenification is caused by scratching or rubbing of the skin and is often associated with atopic dermatoses and pruritic conditions. Although any area of the body may be affected, the hands and forearms are common sites. Treatment of the cause of the itching is the key to prevention of lichenification. Excoriations are often evident in the thickened skin as a result of the pruritus.

DERMATOLOGIC DISORDERS

Malignant Conditions

Malignant neoplasms of the skin exhibit the characteristics of all malignant conditions (see Chapter 12). However, skin malignancies generally grow slowly (Fig. 20-5). Adequate and early treatment can lead to a complete cure. The fact that skin lesions are very visible increases the likelihood of early detection and diagnosis.

The presence of a lesion that persists and does not heal is highly suspicious. Evidence from the patient's history related to skin type, history of sun exposure, an outdoor versus indoor occupation, history of genetic diseases characterized by intolerance to sunlight (e.g., albinism), exposure to tar and systemic arsenicals, in addition to the persistent lesion are indications for a biopsy of the lesion.

General Risk Factors. Two different patterns of sun exposure are associated with skin cancer. In the first pattern, solar exposure alone causes skin cancer in a manner modulated by individual differences in sensitivity and in total exposure. In the second type, intense intermit-

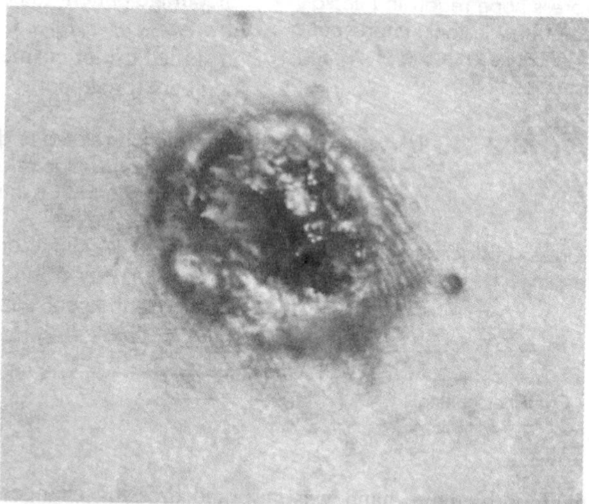

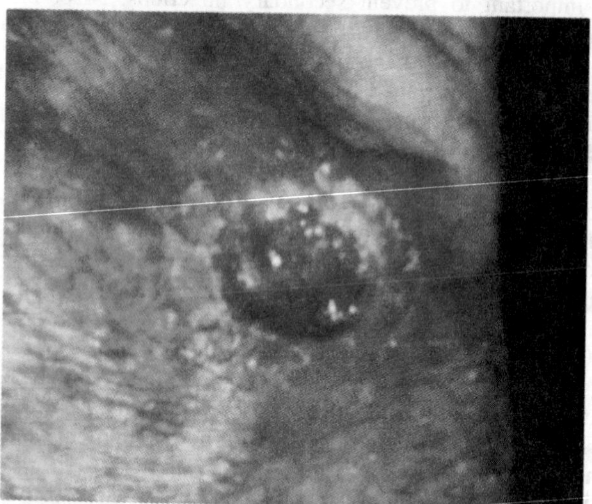

Fig. 20-5 Basal cell carcinoma. Note the typical pearly border.

tent exposure and the presence of precursors and lesions are risk factors. In fact, three severe sunburns early in life are enough to increase a person's subsequent risk of cutaneous melanoma.[12]

The incidence of skin cancer increases with age in persons who have accumulated substantial sun exposure. Dark-skinned persons are less susceptible to skin cancers because of the naturally occurring increase in melanin, the most effective sunscreen. The incidence of skin cancer increases with proximity to the equator (latitude) and high altitude because of the increased intensity of UVB exposure. Depletion of the stratosphere ozone layer has also been implicated in the recent increase of skin cancer. For instance, it is estimated that every 1% reduction in atmospheric ozone will result in a 2% increase in UVB radiation and in a 3% to 6% increase in the incidence of squamous cell carcinoma.[13]

Nonmelanoma Skin Cancers. Nonmelanoma skin cancer is the most common form of neoplasm in countries with large numbers of Caucasian inhabitants and high exposure to UV light. In the United States there are more than half a million new cases yearly. The most common sites for development of nonmelanoma skin cancer include the face, head, neck, back of the hands, and arms.[10] A biopsy should be performed to confirm the diagnosis before specific treatment is started.

Although the number of deaths attributable to nonmelanoma skin cancer is small, the tumors have an inherent potential for severe local destruction, permanent disfigurement, and disability. The most common etiologic factor, chronic sun exposure, should be consciously avoided by the use of sunscreens and protective clothing.

Actinic keratoses. Actinic keratoses is a premalignant form of SCC. Actinic keratoses are hyperkeratotic papules and plaques that occur on sun-exposed areas. The lesions present as skin-colored macules and papules with dry, rough adherent scales. Although many forms of treatment are used, the use of 5-FU over the affected area for 14 to 21 days is popular. This drug has no effect on healthy skin and other lesions.

Basal cell carcinoma. Basal cell carcinoma is a malignancy arising from epidermal basal cells. The noduloulcerative BCC, the most common type, and superficial BCC have distinct clinical manifestations (see Table 20-6). Multiple treatment modalities are used depending on the tumor location and histologic subtype, history of recurrence, and patient characteristics. Treatment modalities include electrodesiccation and curettage, excision, cryosurgery, radiation therapy, Mohs surgery, topical chemotherapy, and intralesional interferon.[14]

Squamous cell carcinoma. Squamous cell carcinoma is a malignant neoplasm of keratinizing epidermal cells. It frequently occurs on skin previously damaged by burns, scars, and irradiation. Unlike BCC, SCC has the potential to metastasize. Clinical manifestations are described in Table 20-6. Treatment consists of surgical excision, radiation, and Mohs surgery. Cryosurgery and electrodesiccation and curettage have been used successfully in small primary tumors. There is a high cure rate with early detection and treatment.

Cutaneous T-cell lymphoma. Cutaneous T-cell lymphoma, another type of skin cancer, consists of malignant T-cells. This type of skin cancer presents in different forms: from a small area of involvement with little or no spread, to a wide area of involvement resulting in disfigurement, pain, spread to internal organs, and death. In its early stages, the plaques may be confused with eczema or psoriasis. As the disease progresses, cutaneous tumors and lymph node involvement may appear. Immunotherapy combined with PUVA chemotherapy, and extracorporeal photephoresis (ECP) are treatments currently being used to treat T-cell lymphoma.[15]

Extracorporeal photopheresis involves removing plasma and white cells, including lymphocytes, from the body, irradiating them with UVA in the presence of a photoactive drug, and subsequently reinfusing them. The reinfusion of damaged clonal cells is thought to cause a reaction comparable to that of a vaccine. Use of ECP is reserved for the lymphoma patient who has an immune system capable of responding to modified malignant cells reintroduced after ECP. A general immunosuppression is not induced by ECP.

Dysplastic nevus syndrome. An abnormal mole pattern called *dysplastic nevus syndrome* (DNS) indicates an increased risk of melanoma. There are two subtypes of DNS, *familial* and *sporadic.* The earliest clinically detectable abnormality associated with this syndrome is an increase in the number of morphologically normal-looking nevi from the age of 2 to 6 years. Another proliferation occurs around adolescence, and new nevi appear throughout life.[7] Obtaining a detailed family history related to melanoma and DNS is an important epidemiologic responsibility of the clinician.

Malignant Melanoma. Malignant melanoma, a tumor of the skin originating from melanocytes, is the most serious skin cancer and the eighth most common cancer in the United States. Melanoma has the ability to metastasize to any organ including the brain and heart.[7] A family's tendency to sunburn easily and a positive family history of skin cancer are significant risk factors for the development of malignant melanoma. Figure 20-6 presents the *ABCDs* of melanoma detection. The incidence of melanoma has doubled every 10 years in the last 30 years. Risk factors that may contribute to this increase include UV radiation; lack of skin pigmentation; genetic, hormonal, and immunologic factors; and societal and lifestyle changes that lead to greater skin exposure.[12] Cutaneous melanoma is nearly 100% curable by excision if diagnosed when the malignant cells are restricted to the epidermis. If melanoma spreads to regional lymph nodes, the patient has a 50% five-year survival rate. If metastasis occurs, treatment is largely palliative.

There are four types of cutaneous melanomas. The most important prognostic factor is the stage at the time of presentation. Superficial (radial) growth is a period when three types of lesions—superficial spreading, lentigo maligna, and acral lentigines—increase in size but do not penetrate deeply. The fourth type, nodular melanoma, has no recognizable radial growth phase and usually presents as a deeply invasive lesion, fully capable of early metastasis.

Table 20-6 Malignant Conditions of the Skin

Etiology and Pathophysiology	Clinical Manifestations	Treatment and Prognosis
Actinic Keratoses ▪ Actinic (sun) damage (precursor of squamous cell carcinoma)	Flat or slightly elevated, dry, hyperkeratotic scaly papule; possibly flat, rough, or verrucous; adherent scale, which returns when removed; often multiple; rough scale on red base; often on erythematous sun-exposed areas; increase in number with age	Curettage, electrosurgery, cryosurgery, chemical caustics, topical application of 5-fluorouracil over entire area for 14-21 days; no effect on healthy skin and other lesions; recurrence possible even with adequate treatment; untreated lesions possibly leading to squamous cell carcinoma (1% incidence)
Dysplastic Nevus Syndrome ▪ Morphologically between common acquired nevi and melanoma; histogenetic precursor of cutaneous malignant melanoma	Often larger than 5 mm; irregular border, possibly notched; variegated color mixture of tan, brown, black, red, and pink with single mole; presence of at least one flat portion, often at edge of mole; frequently multiple; uncommon before puberty; most common site on back, but possible in uncommon mole sites such as scalp or buttocks	Marker of increased risk for melanoma; careful monitoring of persons suspected of familial tendency to melanoma or dysplastic nevus syndrome necessary to increase likelihood of early diagnosis of melanoma; indication for excisional biopsy for suspicious lesions
Basal Cell Carcinoma ▪ Change in basal cell; no maturation or normal keratinization; continuing division of basal cells and formation of enlarging mass; related to excessive sun exposure, genetic skin type, arsenicals, x-ray irradiation, scars, and some types of nevi; basal cells possibly pigmented but absent in nevi	***Nodular and ulcerative*** Small, slowly enlarging papule; borders semitranslucent or "pearly," with overlying telangiectasia; erosion, ulceration, and depression of center; normal skin markings lost ***Superficial*** Erythematous, sharply defined, barely elevated multinodular plaques with varying scaling and crusting; similar to eczema but not pruritic	Excisional surgery, chemosurgery, electrosurgery, cryosurgery; 95% cure rate; slow-growing tumor that invades local tissue; metastasis rare
Squamous Cell Carcinoma ▪ Frequent occurrence on previously damaged skin (e.g., from sun, irradiation, scar); malignant tumor of squamous (prickle) cell of epidermis; invasion of dermis, surrounding skin; metastasis possible	***Early*** Firm nodules with indistinct borders with scaling and ulceration; opaque ***Late*** Covering of lesion with scale or horn from keratinization; most common on sun-exposed areas such as face and hands	Surgical removal, cryosurgery, radiation therapy, chemosurgery, Mohs procedure or microscopically controlled excision, electrodesiccation, and curettage; untreated lesion possibly metastasizes to regional lymph nodes; high cure rate with early detection and treatment
Cutaneous T-Cell Lymphoma ▪ Origination in skin; chronic, slowly progressing disease with grave prognosis; possible etiologies of environmental toxins and chemical exposure	Prevalent in twice as many men as women in United States; classic presentation involving three stages—patch, plaque, and tumor; history of persistent macular eruption followed by gradual appearance of indurated plaques	Topical nitrogen mustard, radiation therapy, systemic chemotherapy, PUVA, and extracorporeal photopheresis; 5-yr life expectancy with only skin manifestations and no treatment; greatly decreased survival rate with generalized erythroderma with exfoliation and abnormal cells in bloodstream

continued

Table 20-6 Malignant Conditions of the Skin—cont'd

Etiology and Pathophysiology	Clinical Manifestations	Treatment and Prognosis
Malignant Melanoma		
▪ Neoplastic growth of melanocytes anywhere on skin, eyes, or mucous membranes; classification according to major histologic mode of spread; potential invasion and widespread metastases	Irregular color, irregular surface, irregular border; variegated color including red, white, blue, black, gray, brown; flat or elevated, eroded or ulcerated; often under 1 cm in size; most common sites in males and females on back; in females in chest and lower legs	Wide excision, full-thickness surgical removal; correlation of survival rate with depth of invasion; poor prognosis unless diagnosis and treatment early; spreading by local extension, regional lymphatic vessels, and bloodstream; adjuvant therapy after surgery possibly necessary if lesions greater than 1.5 mm in depth
Kaposi's Sarcoma		
▪ Multicentric neoplasms that occur with increasing frequency in HIV-infected individuals. Occurs predominantly in homosexual men. Multiple vascular nodules appearing in the skin, mucous membranes, and viscera. Severity ranges from minor to fulminant with extensive cutaneous and visceral involvement	Wide range of presentation. Initially, small reddish, purple nodules on skin; lesions range in size from a few mm to several cm, can cause lymphedema and disfigurement particularly when confluent; systemic involvement has symptoms associated with organ (e.g., lungs and shortness of breath)	Diagnosis based upon biopsy of suspicious lesion. Treatment dependent on severity of lesions and patient's immune status; attempt to avoid treatments to further suppress immune system; possible treatments include localized radiation, intralesional vinblastine, combination chemotherapy and cryotherapy

HIV, Human immunodeficiency virus; *PUVA,* psoralen ultraviolet A.

The initial treatment of malignant melanoma is a wide surgical excision with a margin of normal skin. Subsequent treatment modalities such as regional node dissection, chemotherapy, nonspecific immunotherapy, chemoimmunotherapy, and radiation may be planned depending on the staging of the disease.

Infections

Bacterial Infections. The skin is covered with numerous microorganisms, especially bacteria. *Staphylococcus epidermidis* and diphtheroids are the most common bacteria present on the skin. The skin provides an ideal environment for bacterial growth, with abundant supplies of warmth, nutrients, and water.

Bacterial infection (*pyoderma*) occurs when the balance between the host and the microorganisms is altered. This can occur as a primary infection following a break in the skin, as a secondary infection to already damaged skin, or as a sign of a systemic disease (Table 20-7).

Healthy persons can develop bacterial skin infections. Predisposing factors such as moisture, obesity, skin disease, systemic corticosteroids and antibiotics, chronic disease, and diabetes mellitus all increase the likelihood of infection. Good hygienic practices and general good health inhibit

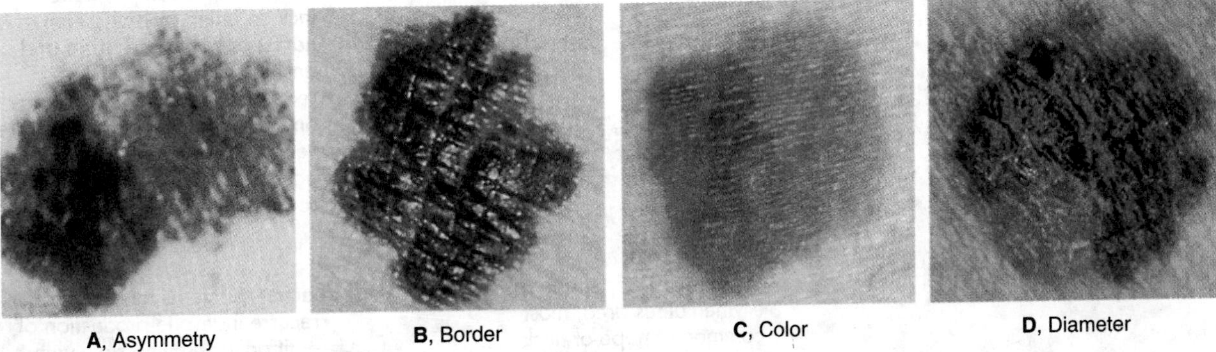

Fig. 20-6 The *ABCDs* of melanoma. ***A,*** Asymmetry (one half unlike the other). ***B,*** Border (irregular-scalloped or poorly circumscribed border). ***C,*** Color varied from one area to another; shades of tan and brown; black; sometimes white, red, or blue; change in shape, size, or color of mole. ***D,*** Diameter larger than 6 mm as a rule (diameter of a pencil eraser)

Table 20-7 Common Bacterial Infections of the Skin

Etiology and Pathophysiology	Clinical Manifestations	Treatment and Prognosis
Impetigo ■ Group A β-hemolytic streptococci, staphylococci, or combination of both; associated with poor hygiene and low socioeconomic status; primary or secondary infection; contagious	Vesiculopustular lesions that develop thick, honey-colored crust surrounded by erythema; pruritic; most common on face	***Systemic antibiotics*** 400,000 units oral penicillin qid × 10 days, 600,000 units of benzathine penicillin IM in single injection, or 250 mg erythromycin qid × 10 days ***Local treatment*** Warm saline or aluminum acetate soaks followed by soap-and water removal of crusts; topical antibiotic cream; with no treatment, glomerulonephritis possible when streptococcal strain nephritogenic; meticulous hygiene essential
Folliculitis ■ Usually staphylococci; present in areas subjected to friction, moisture, oil, or grease	Small pustule at hair follicle opening with minimal erythema; development of crusting; most common on scalp, beard, extremities in men; tender to touch	Soap (e.g., Hibiclens) and water cleansing; topical antibiotics (e.g., Bactroban); warm compresses of water or aluminum acetate solution; healing usually without scarring; if lesions extensive and deep, possible scarring and loss of involved hair follicles
Furuncle ■ Deep infection with staphylococci around hair follicle, often associated with severe acne or seborrheic dermatitis	Tender erythematous area around hair follicle; draining of pus and core of necrotic debris on rupture; most common on face, back of neck, axillae, breasts, buttocks, perineum, thighs; painful	Incision and drainage, occasionally antibiotics, meticulous care of involved skin, frequent application of warm, moist compresses
Furunculosis ■ Increased incidence in patients who are obese, chronically ill, or regularly exposed to grease or oils or who have diabetes mellitus	Lesions as above; malaise, regional adenopathy, elevated temperature	Warm compresses; systemic antibiotic after culture and sensitivity study of drainage (usually semi-synthetic, penicillinase-resistant, oral penicillin such as cloxacillin and oxacillin); measures to reduce surface staphylococci include antimicrobial cream to nares, armpits, and groin and antiseptic to entire skin; often recurrent with scarring; incision and drainage of soft lesions; prevention or correction of predisposing factors; meticulous personal hygiene
Carbuncle ■ Multiple, interconnecting furuncles	Many pustules appearing in erythematous area, most common at nape of neck	Treatment same as furuncles; often recurrent despite production of antibodies; healing slow with scar formation

continued

Table 20-7 Common Bacterial Infections of the Skin—cont'd

Etiology and Pathophysiology	Clinical Manifestations	Treatment and Prognosis
Cellulitis		
▪ Inflammation of subcutaneous tissues; possibly secondary complication or primary infection; often following break in skin; *S. aureus* and streptococci usual causative agents; deep inflammation of subcutaneous tissue from enzymes produced by bacteria	Hot, tender, erythematous, and edematous area with diffuse borders; malaise and fever	Moist heat, immobilization and elevation, systemic antibiotic therapy, hospitalization if severe; progression to gangrene possible if untreated
Erysipelas		
▪ Superficial cellulitis primarily involving the dermis; group A β-hemolytic streptococci	Red, hot, sharply demarcated plaque that is indurated and painful; bacteremia possible; most common on face and extremities; toxic signs, such as fever, elevated white blood cell count, headache, malaise	Systemic antibiotics—usually penicillin; hospitalization often required

IM, Intramuscular.

bacterial infections. If an infection is present, the resulting drainage is infectious. Meticulous skin hygiene is necessary to prevent spread of the infection.

Trauma is a common predisposing factor to skin infection. Table 20-8 outlines the emergency management of a patient with a skin wound.

Viral Infections. Viral infections of the skin are as difficult to treat as are those anywhere in the body. A virus requires living cells to survive. When a cell is infected by a virus, a lesion can result (Fig. 20-7). Lesions can also result from an inflammatory response to the viral infection (Table 20-9). Herpes simplex, herpes zoster, and warts are the most common viral infections affecting the skin.

Fungal Infections. Because of the large number of identified fungi, it is almost impossible to avoid exposure to some pathologic varieties. Many fungi have valuable functions as in food preparation (e.g., molds, cheese) and drug synthesis (e.g., penicillin). However, some fungi can cause serious infections. Common fungal infections of the skin are presented in Table 20-10.

Microscopic examination of the scraping of suspicious lesions in 10% to 20% potassium hydroxide is an easy, inexpensive diagnostic measure to determine the presence of fungus. The appearance of hyphae (threadlike structures) is indicative of a fungal infection (Fig. 20-8).

Infestations and Insect Bites

The possibilities for exposure to insect bites and infestations are almost limitless (Table 20-11). In many instances, an allergy to the venom plays a major role in the reaction. In other cases, the clinical manifestations are the results of a reaction to the eggs, feces, or body parts of the invading organism (Fig. 20-9). Certain persons will react with a severe hypersensitivity (anaphylaxis), which can be life threatening.

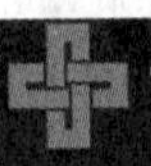

Table 20-8 Emergency Management: Skin Wound

Possible Etiology

Forceful contact with penetrating or blunt object resulting in contusions, avulsions, lacerations, abrasions

Possible Assessment Findings

Redness, swelling
Bleeding
Pain
Surrounding nerve and vascular impairment
Discoloration of skin
Fear and anxiety

Management

- Monitor airway if wound involves face, neck, head, or chest.
- Assess for bleeding areas; control with pressure dressing.
- Rule out other injuries.
- Check wound for impaled objects, pieces of glass, or debris.
- Do not attempt to remove any penetrating object. Stabilize for removal in controlled environment.
- Cleanse wound with isotonic solution.
- For an avulsed wound, fold the skin flap back into normal position and then control bleeding.
- Apply bulky sterile dressing to area and immobilize injured part.
- Determine need for tetanus toxoid (see Table 62-6).

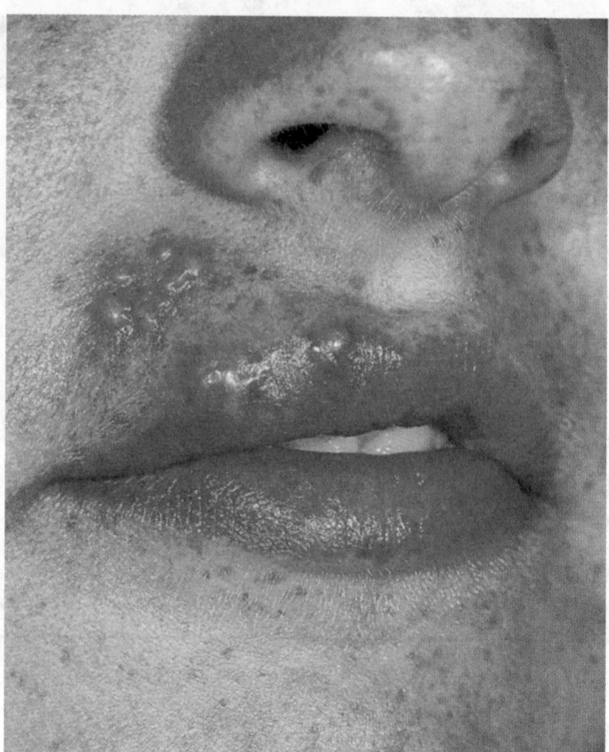

Fig. 20-7 Herpesvirus on the lips. Typical presentation with tense vesicles appearing on the lips and extending onto the skin.

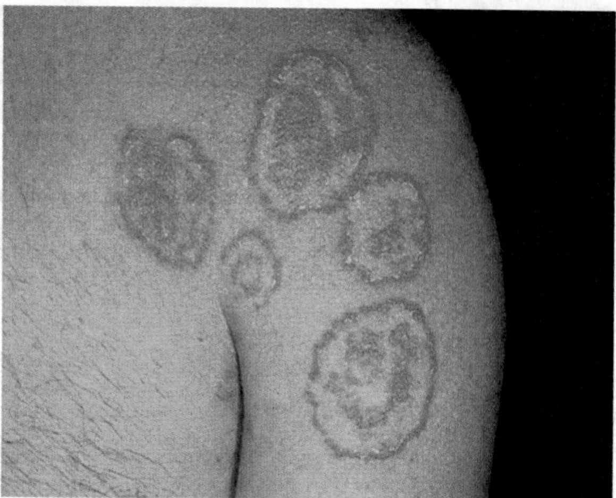

Fig. 20-8 Tinea corporis. A classic presentation with an advancing red scaly border. The reason for the designation "ring worm" is obvious.

Prevention of insect bites by avoidance or by the use of repellents is somewhat effective. Meticulous hygiene related to personal articles, clothing, bedding, examination and care of pets, and careful selection of sexual partners can reduce the incidence of infestations. A rash on exposed body parts only is highly suggestive of an insect bite. Routine inspection is necessary if there is a risk of tick bites and Lyme disease.

Allergic Dermatologic Problems

Dermatologic problems associated with allergies and hypersensitivity reactions present a real challenge to the clinician (Table 20-12). The pathophysiology related to allergic and contact dermatitis is discussed in Chapter 10. A careful family history and discussion of exposure to possible offending agents will provide valuable data. Patch testing involves the application of allergens to the patient's skin (usually on the back). After 48 hours the test sites are examined for erythema, vesicles, or both. Patch testing is used to determine possible causative agents. This information is valuable to the patient. The best treatment of allergic dermatitis is avoidance. The extreme pruritus of contact dermatitis and its potential for chronicity make it a frustrating problem for the patient, the nurse, and the dermatologist.

Benign Dermatologic Problems

Although the list of benign dermatoses is extensive, some of the most commonly seen and distressing problems are summarized in Table 20-13.

DERMATOLOGIC MANIFESTATIONS OF SYSTEMIC DISEASES

Dermatologic manifestations of systemic disease may be either specific or nonspecific. Specific conditions display the same pathophysiologic process in relation to the skin as the internal disease process. Nonspecific conditions do not resemble the internal problem but are helpful in establishing a diagnosis. The skilled clinician should always consider the possibility that a particular dermatosis is a clue to an internal, less obvious problem.

Certain life changes have recognized associated dermatoses. At puberty, male- or female-pattern hair growth will be evident as a secondary sex characteristic. Increased apocrine gland activity can lead to body odor. The increased sebaceous gland activity stimulated by androgens can result in seborrhea and acne.

Pregnancy is characterized by physiologic skin changes, including hyperpigmentation and increased perspiration. *Menopause* is often accompanied by hot flashes, increased perspiration, facial hair growth, and varying degrees of scalp hair loss. Skin problems related to aging include dryness, wrinkling, hyperpigmentation, and actinic changes. Dermatologic manifestations of systemic diseases are presented in Table 20-14.

PLASTIC SURGERY

Elective Cosmetic Surgery

The possible cosmetic changes that can be made surgically are almost limitless. Cosmetic surgery includes such techniques as breast enlargement; breast reduction; chemical, mechanical, and surgical face-lift; eyelid lift; hair transplant; nose corrections; removal of double chin; correction of receding or prominent chin; abdomen or thigh lift; buttocks reduction; correction of elephant ears; and liposuction of many body areas.

The reasons for the surgery are as varied as are the techniques. The most common reason that people suffer the discomfort and financial expense (most cosmetic surgeries

Table 20-9 Common Viral Infections of the Skin

Etiology and Pathophysiology	Clinical Manifestations	Treatment and Prognosis
Herpes Simplex Virus Type 1 Generally oral infections; virus remaining in nerve root ganglion and possibly returning to skin to produce recurrence when exacerbated by sunlight, trauma, menses, stress, and systemic infection; contagious to those not previously infected; increase in severity with age, transmission by respiratory droplets or virus-containing fluid, such as saliva or cervical secretions; no protection against subsequent infection in other areas with episodes of infection in one area	***First episode*** Symptoms occurring 3-7 days or more after contact; painful local reaction; grouped vesicles on erythematous base; systemic symptoms, such as fever and malaise possible or asymptomatic presentation possible ***Recurrent*** Small; recurrence in similar spot; characteristic grouped vesicles on erythematous base	Symptomatic medication; soothing, moist compresses; petrolatum to lesions; scarring not usual result; antiviral agents such as acyclovir (Zovirax)
Herpes Simplex Virus Type 2 Generally genital infections; recurrence more frequent than oral-labial infections	Same as for herpes simplex virus Type 1	Same as for herpes simplex virus Type 1
Herpes Zoster Activation of the varicella-zoster virus; frequent occurrence in immunosuppressed patients; potentially contagious to anyone who has not had varicella or who is immunosuppressed	Linear patches along dermatome of grouped vesicles on erythematous base; usually unilateral and on trunk; burning, pain, and neuralgia preceding outbreak; mild to severe pain during outbreak	Symptomatic; wet compresses, white petrolatum to lesions; analgesia; mild sedation at bedtime; systemic corticosteroids to shorten course and decrease likelihood of postherpetic neuralgia (controversial); usual healing without complications but scarring possible; postherpetic neuralgia possible
Verruca Vulgaris Caused by human papillomavirus; spontaneous disappearance in 1-2 yr possible; mildly contagious by autoinoculation; specific response dependent on body part affected	Circumscribed, hypertrophic, flesh-colored papule limited to epidermis; painful on lateral compression	Multiple treatments, including surgery—scoop removal with scissors and curette; liquid nitrogen therapy; blistering agents—cantharidin; keratolytic agents—salicylic acid; CO_2 laser therapy, treatment can result in scarring
Plantar Warts Caused by human papillomavirus	Wart on bottom surface of foot, growing inward because of pressure of walking or standing; painful when pressure applied; interrupted skin markings; cone-shaped with black dots (thrombosed vessels) when pared	Usual treatment is frequent paring followed by application of patches of impregnated chemicals to continue to decrease regrowth; over-aggressive destruction possibly resulting in painful, hypertrophic scar

Table 20-10 Commun Fungal Infections of the Skin and Mucous Membranes

Etiology and Pathophysiology	Clinical Manifestations	Treatment and Prognosis
Candidiasis Caused by yeastlike fungus of *Candida albicans;* also known as moniliasis; 50% of adults symptom-free carriers; presenting in warm, moist areas such as crural area, oral mucosa, and submammary folds; HIV infection, chemotherapy, radiation, and organ transplantation related to depression of cell-mediated immunity that allow yeast to become pathogenic; production of symptoms by imbalance between host and normal inhabitant of gastrointestinal tract, mouth, and vagina	***Mouth*** White, cheeselike patches leaving erosions when removed ***Vagina*** Vaginitis, with red, edematous, painful vaginal wall, white patches; vaginal discharge; pruritus; pain on urination and intercourse ***Skin*** Diffuse papular erythematous rash with pinpoint satellite lesions around edges of affected area	Microscopic examination and culture; nystatin or other specific medication as vaginal suppository or oral lozenge; abstinence or use of condom; eradication of infection with appropriate medication; skin hygiene to keep it clean and dry; mycostatin powder effective on skin lesions; avoidance of lubricants
Tinea Corporis Various dermatophytes, commonly referred to as ringworm	Typical annular appearance, well-defined margins with fine cigarette paper scale; erythematous	Cool compresses; topical antifungals for isolated patches; creams or solutions
Tinea Cruris Various dermatophytes, commonly referred to as jock itch	Well-defined border in groin area	Topical antifungal cream or solution
Tinea Unguium Various dermatophytes	Only few nails on one hand affected; nails on toes possibly affected; fungal scale close to outer margin of lesion; brittle, thickened, broken nails with white or yellow discoloration	Topical antifungal cream or solution; griseofulvin moderately successful on fingernails; poor response on toenails; debridement of toenails to normal contour if problematic
Tinea Pedis Various dermatophytes, commonly referred to as athlete's foot	Interdigital scaling and maceration; erythema and blistering; pruritus; painful	Topical antifungal cream or solution

HIV, Human immunodeficiency virus.

are not covered by insurance) of cosmetic surgery is to improve their body image. People project their personal image of themselves. If they feel better about themselves as a result of cosmetic surgery, they will often act more confident and self-assured. Social position and economic considerations may be part of the decision. Persons who support a youth-oriented society often feel uncomfortable doing business with someone who appears to be aging. Also, increased longevity provides a larger population to whom cosmetic surgery is especially appealing.

Regardless of the reason the patient elects to have cosmetic surgery, the nurse should maintain a supportive, nonjudgmental attitude. If the patient wishes to change a body feature perceived as unattractive and makes a personal decision to undergo cosmetic surgery, the nurse should support this decision.

Chemical Face-Lift or Peel. A chemical face peel uses a cauterant to the skin to cause a controlled burn. This results in superficial destruction of the upper layers of the skin and a tightening of the deep layers. The most common indications for a chemical peel include pigmentation problems, skin damage resulting from radiation, freckles, superficial acne scarring, and actinic and seborrheic keratoses.

A solution (buffered phenol, trichloroacetic acid, or other exfoliation acids) is applied to the skin with care taken to avoid the eyes. Posttreatment care is prescribed specifically by the physician. It may include refraining from activities, talking, and chewing, and applying compresses and topical ointments. There may be moderate swelling and crusting for 1 week. Within 7 to 8 days new skin will appear, and healing will be complete by 10 days. Redness will persist for 6 to 8 weeks, and a pink tone will be apparent for several months. Once healing is complete, the skin will have a more youthful appearance because of a new superficial layer of skin.

Because there is a reduction of melanin as a result of this procedure, the patient must be instructed to absolutely avoid the sun for 6 months to prevent unsightly hyperpigmentation. Chemical peeling is accepted as a treatment for wrinkles and certain types of hyperpigmentation.

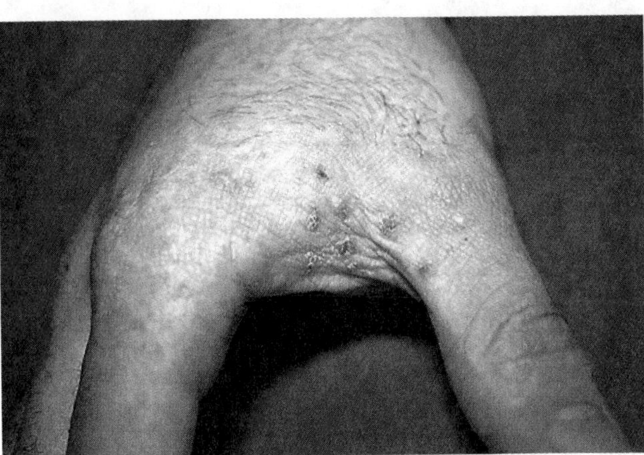

Fig. 20-9 Scabies on a hand.

Topical Tretinoin. Topical application of tretinoin (Retin A) provides some reversal of photodamaged skin. Fine and coarse wrinkling improves. There is a reduction in the number of lentigines (age spots) and in the color of freckles. Actinic keratoses decrease in number. Deep wrinkles and expression lines are usually not affected by tretinoin. The main adverse effect is a cutaneous reaction characterized by erythema, swelling, and scaling, which generally improves when treated with emollients or when application of tretinoin is stopped or decreased to every other day.[16]

The response to tretinoin appears to be dose related. The usual dose is 0.025%, 0.05%, or 0.1% in a cream or gel base. Gradual introduction to tretinoin begins with application every other day, aiming for nightly application as tolerated. Treatment is not usually stopped when inflammation occurs unless the inflammation is severe. Maximum response occurs after 8 to 12 months of treatment. Thereafter application 3 to 4 times a week should maintain improvement. A sunscreen must be used in combination with tretinoin to prevent further sun damage and to protect against the greater photosensitivity that the patient experiences during tretinoin therapy.

Dermabrasion. Dermabrasion is the removal of the epidermis and a portion of the superficial layer of the dermis with preservation of sufficient epidermal adnexa to allow for spontaneous reepithelialization of the abraded surface. Dermabrasion is used to treat acne scars, hypertrophic scars, and sun-damaged and wrinkled skin and to correct pigmentary abnormalities, usually on the face. There has been marked improvement in the tools used for this procedure.

In general, the instructions to the patient who has dermabrasion are focused on prevention of drying. Emollients or antibiotic ointments and wet soaks are included in the instructions and are to be applied at varying times on particular postoperative days. The patient is instructed to use a heavy layer of emollient when not using wet soaks. Instructions for postoperative wound care vary widely among practitioners. Specific care needs to be well understood by the patient. Sunscreens (SPF 30) should be used when the patient is outdoors. The most common complications include hyperpigmentation, hypopigmentation, keloids, herpes simplex, milia, persistent erythema, telangiectasia, and infection.

Face-lift. A face-lift (rhytidectomy) is the lifting and repositioning of the lower two thirds of the face and neck to improve appearance (see Fig. 20-10 on p. 519). Indications for this procedure include the following:

1. Redundant soft tissue resulting from dermatitis (e.g., smallpox or acne scarring)
2. Asymmetric redundancy of soft tissues (e.g., facial palsy)
3. Redundant soft tissue resulting from trauma
4. Preauricular lesions
5. Redundant soft tissues resulting from solar elastosis (sagging of the skin from sun damage), changes in body weight, and the effects of gravity
6. Restoration of body image

The surgical approach and lines of incisions vary according to the nature of the deformity and the position of the hairline. Prevention of hematoma formation is the most important postoperative consideration. A pressure dressing is usually used the first 24 to 48 hours to reduce the possibility of hematoma formation. Complications can occur if the person smokes or is involved in vigorous exercise. Once the dressing is removed, there is little pain. The sutures are removed sometime from the fifth to the tenth postoperative day. Antibiotics are used at the discretion of the surgeon, since infection is not a common problem.

Liposuction. Liposuction is a technique for removing subcutaneous fat to improve facial and body contours. Although not a substitute for diet and exercise, it can be successful in removing areas of fat from virtually any body area that is resistant to other techniques.

Although relatively free of complications, possible contraindications for liposuction include use of anticoagulants, history of inflammatory disease, uncontrolled hypertension, diabetes mellitus, and poor cardiovascular status. Persons under 40 years of age with good skin elasticity are the best candidates. However, patients ranging in age from 16 to 70 years can be treated successfully.[7]

The procedure is usually performed on an outpatient basis with the aid of local anesthesia. One or more sessions may be necessary, depending on the size of the area to be treated. A blunt-tipped cannula is inserted through a one half inch incision and pushed into the fat to break it loose from the fibrous stroma. Multiple repeated thrusts disrupt the fat and create tunnels (see Fig. 20-11 on p. 522). The loosened fat is removed with a very powerful suction and the area is taped. Firm bandaging helps to contour the skin and reduce the chance of postoperative bleeding and fluid accumulation. It may take several months for the final results to be evident.

NURSING MANAGEMENT

COSMETIC SURGERY

Many cosmetic surgical procedures are performed in well-equipped day surgery units or in plastic surgeons' office surgery suites. There are several nursing interventions

Table 20-11 Common Infestations and Insect Bites

Name	Etiology and Pathophysiology	Clinical Manifestations	Treatment and Prognosis
▪ Bees and wasps	Hymenoptera	Intense, burning, local pain; swelling and itching; severe hypersensitivity possibly leading to anaphylaxis	Cool compresses; local application of antipruritic lotion; antihistamines if indicated; usually uneventful recovery
▪ Bedbugs	Cimicidae; feeding periodic, usually at night; present in furniture, walls during day	Wheal surrounded by vivid flare; firm urticaria transforming into persistent lesion; severe pruritis; often grouped in threes appearing on noncovered parts of body	Bedbug controlled by chlorocyclohexane; lesions usually requiring no treatment; severe itching possibly requiring use of antihistamines or topical steroids
▪ Pediculosis Head lice Body lice Pubic lice	*Pediculus humanus* var. *capitis* *Pediculus humanus* var. *corporis;* *Phthirius pubis;* obligate parasites that suck blood, leave excrement and eggs on skin, live in seams of clothing (if body lice) and in hair as nits; reaction results from delayed hypersensitivity to saliva and feces acting on antigen; transmission of pubic lice often by sexual contact	Minute, red, noninflammatory; points flush with skin; progression to papular wheallike lesions; pruritis; secondary excoriation, especially parallel linear excoriations in intrascapular region; firmly attached to hair shaft in head and body lice	γ-Benzene hexachloride or pyrethrins to treat various parts of body; application as directed; contact screening with bed partners, playmates, shared head gear
▪ Scabies	*Sarcoptes scabiei;* penetration of stratum corneum; depositing of eggs; allergic reaction due to presence of eggs, feces, mite parts; transmission by direct physical contact, only occasionally by shared personal items	Severe itching, especially at night, usually not on face; presence of burrows, especially in interdigital webs, flexor surface of wrists, and anterior axillary folds; redness, swelling, vesiculation	10% crotamiton, γ-benzene hexachloride, benzyl benzoate 12-25%; complete eradication possible; recurrence possible; treatment of sexual partner in positively diagnosed scabies; antibiotics if dermatitis and secondary infections present
▪ Ticks	*Borrelia burgdorferi;* spirochete transmitted by ticks in certain areas at any time during 2-yr life cycle, most commonly during nymphal stage; endemic areas that include Northeast, Mid-Atlantic states, parts of Midwest and West	Spreading, ringlike rash 3-4 wk after bite; commonly in groin, buttocks, axillae, trunk, and upper arms and legs; warm, itchy, or painful rash; flulike symptoms; cardiac, arthritic, and neurologic manifestations possible; unreliable laboratory test; no acquired immunity	Oral antibiotics, such as doxycycline, tetracycline; intravenous antibiotics for arthritic, neurologic, and cardiac symptoms; rest and healthy diet

appropriate for the patient who has cosmetic surgery, regardless of where the surgery is done.

Preoperative Management

A major consideration relates to informed consent and realistic expectations of what cosmetic surgery can accomplish. Although this information is usually provided by the surgeon, the nurse can and should reinforce this information and answer questions and concerns. For instance, a face-lift has little or no effect on deep wrinkling of the forehead and temples, deep nasolabial grooves, or vertical lip wrinkles. Before-and-after–treatment photographs of similar cases are often useful in helping the patient to set realistic expectations.

The patient also needs to understand the time frame for healing. Complete results may not be evident until 1 year after the procedure. The oozing, crusting phase of the abrasive procedures must be explained so the patient can plan to take time off from work if this seems necessary. The final results of the cosmetic procedures are affected by age,

Table 20-12 Common Allergic Conditions of the Skin

Etiology and Pathophysiology	Clinical Manifestations	Treatment and Prognosis
Contact Dermatitis		
Manifestation of delayed hypersensitivity, absorbed agent acting as antigen, sensitization after several exposures, appearance of lesions 2-7 days after contact with allergen	Red, hivelike papules and plaques; sharply circumscribed with occasional vesicles; exposed areas more common; usually pruritic; relation of area of dermatitis to causative agent (e.g., metal allergy and dermatitis on ring finger)	Topical corticosteroids, antihistamines; skin lubrication; elimination of contact allergen; avoidance of irritating affected area; systemic steroids if sensitivity severe
Urticaria		
Usually allergic phenomena; presence of edema in upper dermis resulting from a local increase in permeability of capillaries, usually from histamine	Spontaneously occurring and rounded elevations, varying size, usually multiple	Removal of source; antihistamine therapy
Drug Reaction		
Any drug that acts as antigen and causes hypersensitivity reaction possible cause, certain drugs more prone to reactions (e.g., penicillin) mediated by circulating antibodies	Rash of any morphology; often red, macular and papular, semiconfluent, generalized rash with abrupt onset; appearance as late as 14 days after cessation of drug; possibly pruritic	Withdrawal of drug if possible; antihistamines, local or systemic corticosteroids possibly necessary
Atopic Dermatitis		
Exact cause unknown, often beginning in infancy and decreasing in incidence with age, association with allergic conditions, elevation of IgE levels common, genetically determined, often family history, decreased itch threshold, stress and increased water contact (e.g., frequent hand washing, thumb sucking), other possible agents	Scaly, red to red-brown, circumscribed lesions; accentuation of skin markings; pruritic; symmetric eruptions common in antecubital and popliteal space in adults	Topical corticosteroids, phototherapy, coal tar therapy, intralesional steroids, lubrication of dry skin, systemic steroids if severe, reduction of stress, antibiotics for secondary infection

IgE, Immunoglobin E.

general state of health, and skin type. If a health problem is present, efforts should be made to correct or control the problem before the procedure is performed.

Postoperative Management

Most cosmetic procedures are not very painful. Mild analgesics are usually sufficient to keep the patient comfortable.

Even though infection is not a common problem after cosmetic surgery, the nurse needs to assess the surgical sites for signs of infection. The patient should be aware of signs of infection and told to report any such signs and symptoms immediately so that appropriate antibiotic intervention can be started.

If the surgery involves alteration in the circulation to the skin, such as the undermining done in a face-lift, a careful monitoring of adequate circulation is necessary. Warm, pink skin that blanches on pressure indicates that adequate circulation is present in the surgical area.

Skin Grafts

Uses. Skin grafts may be necessary to protect underlying structures or to reconstruct areas for cosmetic or functional purposes. Ideally, wounds heal by primary intention. However, large, surgically created wounds, trauma, and chronic wounds can cause extensive tissue destruction, making primary intention healing impossible. In these cases, skin grafting may be necessary. Improved surgical techniques make it possible to graft skin, bone, cartilage, fat, fascia, muscles, and nerves. For cosmetically pleasing results, the color, thickness, texture, and hair-bearing nature of skin used for grafting must be chosen to match the recipient site. (Skin grafting is discussed in Chapter 21.)

Table 20-13 Common Benign Conditions of the Skin

Etiology and Pathophysiology	Clinical Manifestations	Treatment and Prognosis
Acne		
Inflammatory disorder of sebaceous glands; more common in teenagers but possible development in adulthood; persistence into adulthood possible; secondary result of iodides, bromides, corticosteroids, androgen-dominant birth control pills	Noninflammatory lesions, including comedones (blackheads) and closed comedones (whiteheads); inflammatory lesions, including papules and pustules; most common on face, neck, and upper back	Mechanical removal of multiple lesions with comedo extractor after comedo opened with fine needle or blade; topical application of benzoyl peroxide as antibacterial and peeling agent; use of peeling and irritating agents such as retinoic acid; long-term antibiotic therapy—topical or systemic; phototherapy; aim of treatment to suppress new lesions; spontaneous remission possible; often improvement with exposure to sun Use of isotretenoin (Accutane) for severe cystic acne to possibly provide lasting remission; contraindicated in pregnant women or women intending to become pregnant while on drug; monitoring of liver function tests, cholesterol, and triglycerides essential
Moles		
Grouping of normal cells derived from melanocyte-like precursor cells; hereditary determination possible	Hyperpigmented areas that vary in form and color; flat, slightly elevated, haloid, verrucoid, polypoid, dome-shaped, sessile, or papillomatous; preservation of normal skin markings; hair growth possible	No treatment necessary except for cosmetic reasons; skin biopsy for diagnostic decisions
Psoriasis		
Chronic dermatitis, which involves excessively rapid turnover of epidermal cells; family predisposition	Sharply demarcated scaling plaques of the scalp, elbows, and knees; palms, soles, and fingernails possibly affected; localized or general, intermittent or continuous	Aim of retarding growth of epidermal cells; difficult to medicate; usually topical corticosteroids, tar, anthralin; intralesional injection of corticosteroids for chronic plaques; sunlight; ultraviolet light, alone or with topical or systemic potentiation; no cure; control possible; antimetabolities (especially methotrexate) for difficult cases
Seborrheic Keratoses		
Benign, genetically determined growths; found in increasing number with age; no association with sun exposure	Irregularly round or oval, flat-topped papules or plaques; surface often warty; appearance of being stuck on; increase in pigmentation with age of lesion; usually multiple and possibly itchy	Removal by curettage or cryosurgery for cosmetic reasons or to eliminate source of irritation; minimal scarring
Skin Tags		
Common after midlife; appearance on neck, axillae, and upper trunk	Small, skin-colored, soft, pedunculated papules	No treatment unless for cosmetic reasons or because of repeated trauma; surgical removal possible (if requested); usually just "clipping off" without anesthesia
Lipoma		
Benign tumor of adipose tissue, often encapsulated, most common in 40- to 60-year-old age group	Rubbery, compressible, round mass of adipose tissue; single or multiple; variable in size, possibly extremely large; most common on trunk, back of neck, and forearms	Usually no treatment, biopsy to differentiate from liposarcoma, excision usual treatment (when indicated)

continued

Table 20-13 Common Benign Conditions of the Skin—cont'd

Etiology and Pathophysiology	Clinical Manifestations	Treatment and Prognosis
Vitiligo		
Unknown cause; genetically influenced, most noticeable in dark-skinned persons and those with summer tan; complete absence of melanocytes; noncontagious	Focal amelanosis (complete loss of pigment); macular; variation in size and location; usually symmetric and permanent	Attempts at repigmentation with sunlight and psoralens; depigmentation of pigmented skin with extensive disease (>50% of body involved); cosmetics and stains for camouflage and to deemphasize vitiliginous areas
Lentigo		
Increased number of normal melanocytes in basal layer of epidermis; senile lentigos ("liver spots") related to aging and sun exposure	Hyperpigmented, brown to black, flat lesion; usually on sun-exposed areas	Treatment only for cosmetic purposes, liquid nitrogen; possible recurrence in 1-2 yr

Types. The two types of skin grafts are free grafts and skin flaps. *Free grafts* are further classified according to the method of providing a blood supply to the grafted skin. One method is to transfer the graft (epidermis and part or all of the dermis) to the recipient site from the donor site. If the graft is an autograft (from the patient's own body) or an isograft (from an identical twin), it will revascularize and become fixed to the new site. Chapter 21 discusses full and split skin grafts in detail. Another method of free skin grafting is reconstructive microsurgery. With the use of an operating microscope, circulation is immediately established in the free flap by anastomosis of the blood vessels from the skin flap to the vessels in the recipient site.

Skin flaps involve moving a section of skin and subcutaneous tissue from one part of the body to another without terminating the vascular attachment. The vascular attachment is called a *pedicle.* Skin flaps are used to cover wounds with a poor vascular bed, to add padding, and to cover wounds over cartilage and bone. There may be a need for intermediate flap placement if the recipient site is far removed from the donor site. For instance, a skin flap from the thigh to the head would require an intermediate graft.

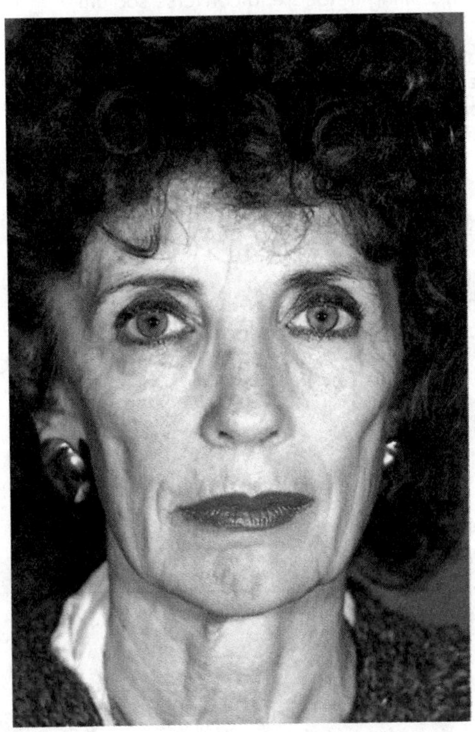

A

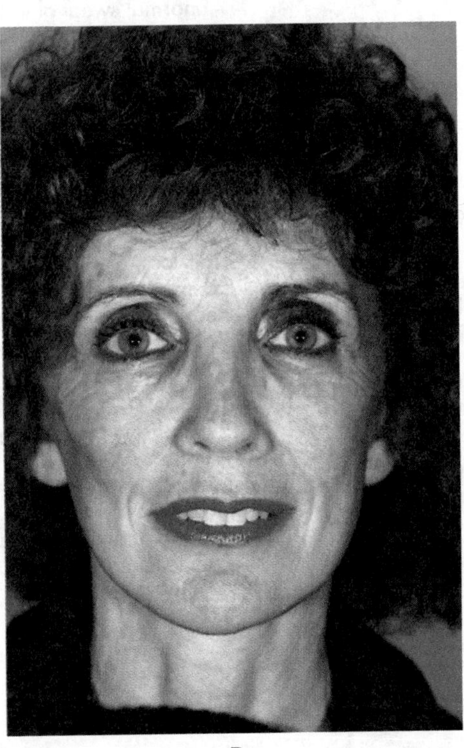

B

Fig. 20-10 ***A,*** Before face-lift. ***B,*** After face-lift.

Table 20-14 Dermatologic Manifestations of Systemic Problems*

Systemic Problem	Dermatologic Manifestations
Endocrine	
Hyperthyroidism	Increased sweating, warm skin with persistent flush, thin nails, vitiligo and alopecia, fine, soft hair
Hypothyroidism	Cold, dry, pale to yellow skin; slighly hyperkeratotic epidermis with follicular plugging; generalized nonpitting edema; dry, coarse, brittle hair; brittle, slow-growing nails
Glucocorticoid excess (Cushing's syndrome), induced endogenously or exogenously	Atrophy; striae; epidermal thinning; telangiectasia; acne, decreased subcutaneous fat over extremities; thin, loose dermis; impaired wound healing; increased vascular fragility; mild hirsutism; excessive collection of fat over clavicles, back of neck, abdomen, and face; increased incidence of pyodermas
Addison's disease	Loss of body hair (especially axillary), generalized hyperpigmentation (especially in folds)
Androgen excess	Enlarged facial pores, male sex characteristics, acne, acceleration of coarse hair growth
Androgen deficiency—postpuberty	Development of sparse hair; marked reduction in sebum production
Hypoparathyroidism	Opaque, brittle nails with transverse ridges; coarse, sparse hair with patchy alopecia; eczematous and exfoliative dermatitis; hyperkeratotic and maculopapular eruptions
Hyperpituitarism (acromegaly)	Coarsened skin, deepened lines; increased oiliness and sweating; acne; increased number of nevi, hyperpigmentation; hypertrichosis
Hypopituitarism (Froëlich's syndrome)	Smooth skin; scant hair growth; obesity; small, thin fingernails
Diabetes mellitus	Increased xanthomas and carotene, shin spots, necrobiosis lipoidica diabeticorum, delayed wound healing
Gastrointestinal	
Ulcerative colitis, Crohn's disease	Pyoderma gangrenosum, mouth ulcers
Liver disease and biliary tract obstruction	Jaundice, itching, pigmentary abnormalities, alterations in nails and hair, spider angiomas, telangiectasia
Deficiency of essential fatty acids	Scaly skin
Malabsorption syndrome	Acquired ichthyosis
Cystic fibrosis	Abnormal sweat gland function resulting in failure to converse sodium
Musculoskeletal and Connective Tissue	
Systemic lupus erythematosus	Maculopapular semiconfluent rash (butterfly rash)
Scleroderma	Leathery hardening and stiffness of skin
Dermatomyositis	Edema; purplish-red upper eyelids; butterfly rash; scaly, macular erythema over knuckles; linear telangiectasia of posterior nail fold
Metabolic	
Lipidoses	Xanthomas
Vitamin A deficiency	Generalized dry hyperkeratoses (pyrynoderma)
Hypervitaminosis A	Hair loss, dry skin
Vitamin B_1 (thiamine) deficiency	Edema, redness of soles of feet
Vitamin B_2 (riboflavin) deficiency	Red fissuers at corner of mouth, glossitis
Nicotinic acid (niacin) deficiency	Pellagra; redness of exposed areas of hand or foot; face or neck; infected dermatitis
Immune	
Drug sensitivity	Rash of any morphology
Serum sickness	Pruritus
Cancer of breast, stomach, lung, uterus, kidney, ovary, colon, bladder	Metastasis to skin
Hodgkin's disease	Pruritus and nonspecific erythemas
Lymphomas	Papules, nodules, plaques, pruritus

continued

Table 20-14 Dermatologic Manifestations of Systemic Problems*—cont'd

Systemic Problem	Dermatologic Manifestations
Cardiovascular	
Arteriosclerosis	Decreased oxygenation leading to gangrene
Rheumatic heart disease	Petechiae, urticaria, rheumatoid nodules, erythema nodosum and multiforme
Periarteritis nodosa	Periarteritis nodules
Thromboangiitis obliterans (Buerger's disease)	Superficial migrating thrombophlebitis, pallor or cyanosis, gangrene, ulceration
Respiratory	
Inadequate oxygenation secondary to respiratory disease	Cyanosis
Hematologic	
Anemia	Pallor, hyperpigmentation, pale mucous membranes, hair loss, nail dystrophy
Clotting disorders	Purpura, petechiae, ecchymosis
Renal	
Chronic renal failure	Dry skin, pruritis, uremic frost, pallor, dry skin, bruises
Reproductive	
Primary syphilis	Chancre
Secondary syphilis	Generalized skin lesions
Late benign syphilis	Gummas
Paget's disease	Eczematous patch of nipple and areola
Neurologic	
Syringomyelia, chronic sensory polyneuropathies, spinal cord trauma	Trophic changes in skin due to sensory denervation, pressure ulcers, anesthesia, paresthesias

*Refer to the systemic disease for specific information.

The flap is advanced to the recipient site when circulation is well established at the intermediate site. The type of flap and the route of transfer are individually determined according to the needs of the patient and the nature of the defect to be repaired.

Soft tissue expansion is a technique of providing skin for resurfacing a defect, such as a burn scar, or for removing a disfiguring mark, such as a tattoo. A subcutaneous tissue expander of an appropriate size and shape is placed under the skin, usually as an outpatient procedure. Weekly expansion with saline solution can be done in a health care setting or by the patient at home. This expansion procedure is repeated until the skin reaches the size needed for the repair. This may take from several weeks to 3 to 4 months. Once sufficient skin is available, the old incision is opened, the expander is removed, and the soft tissue is ready to be used as an advancement flap. The tissue expander next to a defect retains the primary tissue characteristics such as color and texture.

NURSING MANAGEMENT

SKIN GRAFTS

After a skin graft, several areas need to be assessed. The most critical assessment is related to the vascular supply to the grafted site. If the area is not covered by a dressing, it should be regularly assessed for color, warmth, capillary refill, and turgor. If the grafted area has a dressing, it is usually left in place until removed by the surgeon. Systemic signs of infection, such as fever and pain, must be monitored.

Although pain is not usually a major problem, the nurse should provide pain relief when necessary. Conversation, diversion, massage, and medication should be used to maintain patient comfort. The immobility enforced by certain grafting procedures presents the expected potential complications of pneumonia, pulmonary emboli, and pressure ulcers. Aggressive measures by the nurse should be instituted to prevent such complications.

Skin grafting may involve long periods of hospitalization, with the constant threat of graft death. Because this is a particularly difficult time emotionally for the patient, the nurse needs to be supportive and understanding. Expectations of the results of the graft must be realistic if the patient is not to suffer depression. The family and friends of the patient need consideration and explanation of procedures and restrictions imposed by the grafting procedures.

PRESSURE ULCERS

Etiology and Pathophysiology

A pressure ulcer is a lesion caused by unrelieved pressure or from tissue layers sliding over other tissue layers (shearing). The result is damage to underlying tissues. More than 95% of all pressure ulcers occur over a bony prominence, primarily the pelvic girdle.[17] Pressure ulcers are graded or staged according to their degree of tissue damage (Table 20-15).[18]

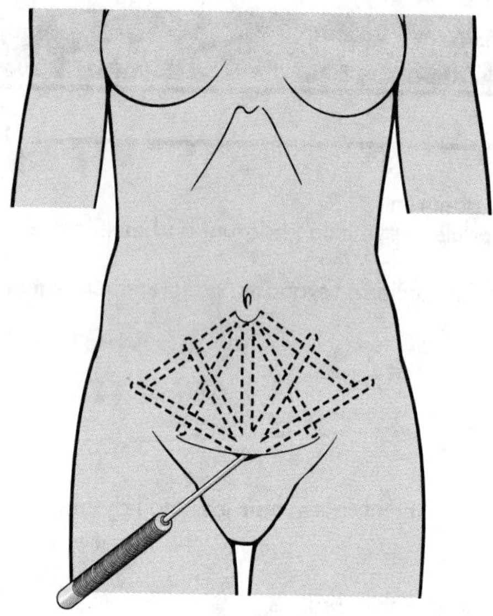

Fig. 20-11 Liposuction. Site of incision and tunneling pattern for abdominal liposuction procedure.

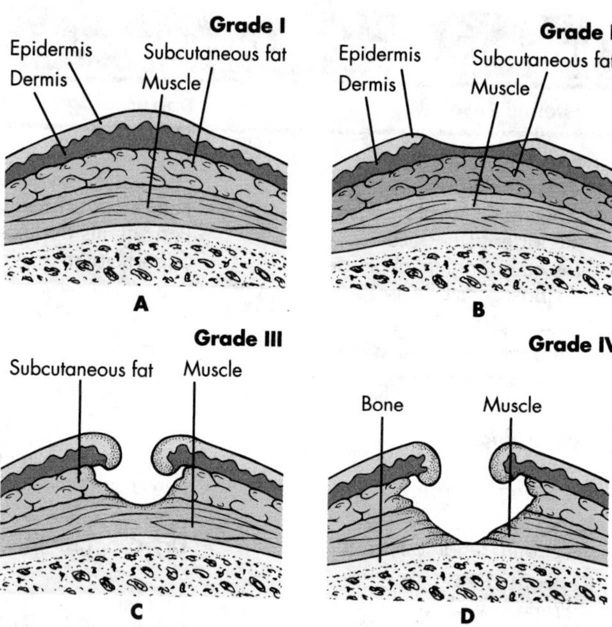

Fig. 20-12 Staging of pressure sores. ***A,*** Stage I. Erythema not resolving within 30 minutes of pressure relief. Epidermis remains intact. Reversible with intervention. ***B,*** Stage II. Partial-thickness loss of skin layers involving epidermis and possibly penetrating into but not through dermis. May manifest as blistering with erythema or induration; wound base is moist and pink, painful, and free of necrotic tissue. ***C,*** Stage III. Full-thickness tissue loss extending through dermis to involve subcutaneous tissue. Manifests as shallow crater unless covered by eschar (If wound involves necrotic tissue, staging cannot be confirmed until wound base is visible.) May include necrotic tissue; undermining, sinus tract formation; exudate; and infection. Wound base is usually not painful. ***D,*** Stage IV. Deep tissue destruction extending through subcutaneous tissue to fascia and possibly involving muscle layers, joint, and bone. Manifests as a deep crater. May include necrotic tissue; undermining, sinus tract formation; exudate; and infection. Wound base is usually not painful.

In addition to pressure and shearing force, other factors that predispose to the development of pressure ulcers include impaired circulation, anemia, contractures, mental deterioration, physical dependence, immobility, incontinence, old age, hyperglycemia, and poor nutrition.

Clinical Manifestations

The clinical manifestations of pressure ulcers depend on the stage of the ulcer. Figure 20-12 describes the four stages of pressure ulcer development. Identification of Stage I pressure ulcers may be difficult in patients with dark skin. Also, when eschar is present, accurate staging of the pressure ulcer is not possible until the eschar has sloughed or the wound has been débrided.[19] If the pressure ulcer becomes infected, the patient may display systemic signs of infection, such as leukocytosis and fever. In addition, the pressure ulcer may increase in size, odor, and drainage, have necrotic tissue, and be indurated, warm, and painful. The most common complication of a pressure ulcer is recurrence.[20]

Table 20-15 Classifying Pressure Ulcers

The National Pressure Ulcer Advisory Panel recommends the following staging system for classifying pressure ulcers according to their depth:

Stage I
Nonblanchable erythema of intact skin

Stage II
Partial-thickness skin loss involving dermis or epidermis, with superficial abrasion, blister, or shallow crater

Stage III
Full-thickness skin loss involving damage or necrosis of subcutaneous tissue; damage may extend down to, but not through, fascia

Stage IV
Full-thickness skin loss with extensive destruction, tissue necrosis, or damage to muscle, bone, or supporting structures

From Bergstrom N: *Pressure sores in adults: prediction and prevention,* Rockville, Md, 1992, US Dept Health and Human Services.

THERAPEUTIC AND NURSING MANAGEMENT

PRESSURE ULCERS

The current trend is to keep a pressure sore slightly moist, rather than dry, to enhance reepithelialization. In addition to the nurse, other members of the health team, such as the plastic surgeon, the nutritionist, the physical therapist, and the occupational therapist can provide valuable input into complex treatment necessary to prevent and treat pressure ulcers.

Both conservative and surgical management strategies are used in the treatment of pressure ulcers, depending on their stage and condition. Therapeutic and nursing management will be discussed together, since the activities are interrelated.

Nursing Assessment

Subjective and objective data that should be obtained from a person with a pressure ulcer are presented in Table 20-16.

Nursing Diagnoses

Nursing diagnoses are determined when the problem and etiologic factors are supported by clinical data. Nursing diagnoses related to pressure ulcers may include, but are not limited to, those presented in the nursing care plan on p. 524.

Planning

The overall goals are that the patient with a pressure ulcer will (1) have no upgrading of the ulcer stage, (2) reduce or eliminate the factors that predispose to pressure ulcers, (3) not develop an infection in the pressure ulcer, and (4) have no recurrence.

Nursing Implementation

Health Maintenance and Promotion. A primary nursing responsibility is the identification of the patient at risk for the development of pressure ulcers. Factors that put a patient at risk for the development of pressure ulcers include impaired circulation, postoperative state, obesity, malnutrition, moisture, elevated body temperature, anemia, contractures, mental deterioration, physical dependence, immobility, incontinence, and old age. Systemic illnesses such as diabetes, collagen disease, vascular diseases, leprosy, and neurologic disorders that affect sensation result in greater risk of ulcer formation. Both obesity and emaciation put patients at increased risk.

Prevention remains the best treatment for pressure ulcers. Pressure-reduction devices, such as alternating pressure mattresses, egg-crate–like mattresses, wheelchair cushions, padded commode seats, foam boots, and lift sheets are useful in preventing pressure and shearing force. However, they are not adequate substitutes for frequent repositioning.

Table 20-16 Nursing Assessment: Pressure Ulcer

Subjective Data

Important health information

Past health history: Stroke, spinal cord injury; prolonged bed rest or immobility; circulatory impairment; altered level of consciousness; advanced age; diabetes; anemia; trauma

Medications: Use of narcotics, hypnotics, muscle paralyzers, corticosteroids

Surgery or other treatments: Recent surgery

Functional health patterns

Nutritional-metabolic: Obesity, emaciation; fluid intake; typical dietary intake

Elimination: Incontinence

Activity-exercise: Usual daily activities

Cognitive-perceptual: Pain in pressure ulcer area; altered sensation in pressure ulcer area

Objective Data

General

Fever

Integumentary

Diaphoresis, edema, and redness, especially over bony areas such as sacrum, hips, elbows, heels, knees, ankles, shoulders, and ear rims; hydration status, staging*

Possible findings

Leukocytosis, positive cultures for microorganisms from pressure ulcer

*See Fig. 20-12.

RESEARCH

Implications for Nursing Practice

INTRAOPERATIVE PRESSURE SORE PREVENTION

Citation Hoshowsky VM, Schramm CA: Intraoperative pressure sore prevention: an analysis of bedding materials, *Research in Nursing and Health* 17:333, 1994.

Purpose To evaluate patient characteristics, surgical experience variables, and operating room (OR) table surfaces as determinants in pressure sore development.

Methods Descriptive study using 505 surgical patients. Preoperatively, patients were assessed using an adapted Hemphill's Guidelines for Assessment of Pressure Sore Potential, and heels and knees were inspected for absence or presence of skin breakdown. Various mattress and overlay combinations were used in the OR under the heel and knee section. Postoperatively, patients' heels and knees were again visually inspected.

Results and Conclusions None of the 505 patients developed pressure sores of severity Stages II through IV in the immediate postoperative period. Stage I pressure sores occurred in 85 patients (16.8%). Factors predictive of pressure sore formation include time on the OR table longer than 2.5 hours, presence of vascular disease, age over 40 years, and a preoperative Hemphill scale rating of 4 or more. Also, the foam and gel mattress and the viscoelastic overlay were significantly better for preventing skin changes than was the standard foam mattress.

Implications for Nursing Practice Identification of predictive factors for pressure sore formation assists the OR nurse in identifying a subset of patients who need special attention and handling during the intraoperative period. Patients who are in this subset would benefit from the use of preventive bedding material identified in this study. Information about the best type of pressure sore preventive bedding could be used by the OR nurse manager in making purchasing decisions based on usual patient populations.

NURSING CARE PLAN Patient With a Pressure Ulcer

Planning: Outcome Criteria	*Nursing Interventions and Rationales*
➤ **NURSING DIAGNOSIS**	Impaired skin integrity *related to* pressure and inadequate circulation *as manifested by* evidence of pressure sore from grade I to grade III; complaints of pain or discomfort in affected area; presence of risk factors such as immobility, old age, debilitation, diminished mental status, poor nutrition, pronounced bony prominences, incontinence, altered cutaneous sensation
Have intact skin.	Assess causative factors such as activity, mobility, presence or absence of sensory deficits, nutrition and hydration status, circulation and oxygenation, skin moisture status *to reduce or eliminate factors that contribute to development or extension of the pressure ulcer.* Assess and document wound in relation to location, size of granulation tissue visible or epithelialization, necrotic tissue, local or systemic infection, presence and character of exudate, including volume, color, consistency, and odor *to provide baseline data for determining improvement or worsening of pressure ulcer.* Classify wound *to direct treatment.* Use pressure relief device if indicated. Institute position change schedule *to avoid prolonged pressure in one area.* Keep head of bed at or below 30-degree angle and flat when not contraindicated *to avoid sacral and buttock pressure from gravity.* Use assistive devices (e.g., trapeze, turning sheets, lifts) to aid patient movement. Protect patient's skin from excess moisture *to prevent maceration.* Institute 2000 to 3000 calories/day (more if increased metabolic demands), 2000 ml/day of fluid *to provide calories, protein, and fluids necessary for tissue repair.* Initiate prescribed treatment based on stage of the pressure ulcer. Monitor progress of wound on a regular basis *to determine effectiveness of treatment plan.* Educate patient and family about cause, prevention, and treatment of pressure ulcer *to prevent recurrence.* Refer for definitive treatment if indicated.

COLLABORATIVE PROBLEMS

Nursing Goals	*Nursing Interventions and Rationales*
➤ **POTENTIAL COMPLICATION**	Stage IV pressure ulcer *related to* extension of pressure ulcer
Monitor for signs of worsening of pressure ulcer to stage IV or presence of stage IV pressure ulcer, report deviations from acceptable parameters, and carry out appropriate medical and surgical interventions.	Assess for signs of stage IV pressure ulcer *such as penetration of muscle, bone, or supporting tissues.* Reduce factors that contribute to the extension of pressure ulcer *such as malnutrition, unrelieved pressure, shear forces, and moisture.* Carry out interventions appropriate to treatment being used.

Modified from *Standards of care: dermal wounds: pressure sores,* Irvine, CA, 1992. International Association for Enterostomal Therapy

Acute Intervention. Once a pressure ulcer has developed, the nurse should initiate interventions based on the grade, size, and presence of infection. Careful documentation should be made of the size of the pressure ulcer. A plastic ruler or lesion-measuring card can be used to note the ulcer's maximum length and width in centimeters. To find the depth of the ulcer, it should be gently probed with a sterile cotton-tipped applicator. The length of the portion of the applicator that probed the ulcer can then be measured. If possible, pictures of the pressure ulcer should be taken initially and at regular intervals during the course of treatment.

A *stage I pressure ulcer* will usually heal completely once the pressure on the affected area is relieved. The affected area should not be massaged because it may increase tissue trauma. The involved area can be covered with a transparent dressing, which is an adhesive, sterile dressing that is impermeable to water and bacteria but permeable to moisture vapor and oxygen. This dressing can be left in place for the 1 to 2 weeks that it takes for the area to heal.

A *stage II pressure ulcer* is reversible if detected early. After irrigation with the prescribed solution, a transparent dressing with a pouch to collect exudate can be applied. The dressing should be reapplied if the edges become loose. This ulcer takes 2 to 4 months to heal.

A *stage III pressure ulcer* is usually irrigated daily, and a transparent dressing with a pouch or a hydrocolloid dressing is applied. (This type of dressing is discussed in Chapter 9.) A hydrocolloid dressing interacts with exudate to form a hydrated gel over the wound. The gel protects the new tissue from being damaged. These dressings are relatively impermeable to oxygen. Both the transparent and the hydrocolloid dressings are contraindicated for an infected

CRITICAL THINKING EXERCISES

CASE STUDY

BASAL CELL CARCINOMA

Patient Profile

John Martin, 67, is a fair-skinned, balding, retired construction worker who comes to the dermatology clinic for evaluation.

Subjective Data

- Has a six-month history of papule on the right side of his nose.
- States that scab forms, falls off, and reforms.
- Worries that lesion could be cancer and require extensive, disfiguring surgery

Objective Data

Physical Examination

- Has 1 cm x 2 cm lesion with semitranslucent border with absence of normal skin markings
- Telangiectasia overlies lesion

Diagnostic Studies

- Biopsy results: basal cell epithelioma

Critical Thinking Questions

1. What risk factors in this patient support the diagnosis?
2. What are the usual clinical characteristics of a basal cell carcinoma?
3. What is the usual diagnostic protocol for a basal cell epithelioma?
4. What treatment options are available for a basal cell epithelioma?
5. What would you tell Mr. Martin about the potential for metastasis of this lesion?
6. Based on the assessment data presented, write one or more appropriate nursing diagnoses. Are there any collaborative problems?

NURSING RESEARCH ISSUES

1. How does facial scarring secondary to a chronic skin condition affect the body image of a patient?
2. What nursing measures are most effective in relieving the pruritus associated with a dermatologic problem?
3. Compare preoperative expectations of the patient undergoing cosmetic surgery with postoperative satisfaction.
4. What are the most common reasons for patient noncompliance in the use of sunscreens?

pressure ulcer or one with exposed muscles, tendons, or bones (grade IV).

A *stage IV pressure ulcer* is treated by debridement, intravenous fluids, and antibiotics. The ulcers may take months or even years to heal (Fig. 20-13). A wet-to-dry gauze dressing is applied daily after irrigation of the wound with a prescribed solution. Enzymes may be used to liquefy necrotic tissue. With the use of a sterile technique, the affected area should have a saline-soaked gauze dressing gently packed into the wound. Once the wound is clean, surgical debridement may be necessary. Reconstruction of the pressure ulcer site by such measures as split-thickness grafts, free skin flap procedures, and myocutaneous flaps may be necessary.[21]

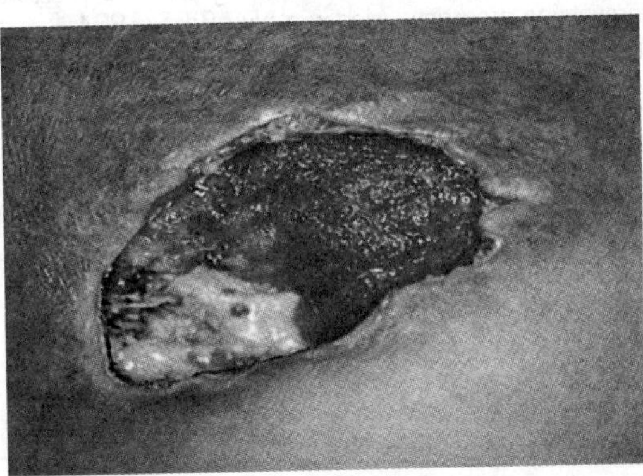

Fig. 20-13 Stage IV pressure ulcer.

The maintenance of adequate nutrition is an important nursing responsibility for the patient with a pressure ulcer. Often the patient is debilitated and has a poor appetite secondary to inactivity. The caloric intake needed to correct and maintain a nutritional balance may be as high as 4200 calories a day. Oral feedings should be high in calories and proteins and should be supplemented with vitamins. Nasogastric feedings can be used to supplement the oral feedings. If necessary, parenteral nutrition consisting of amino acid and glucose solutions is used when oral and nasogastric feedings are inadequate. The nursing care plan presents care for the patient with a pressure ulcer.

Chronic and Home Management. Since recurrence of pressure ulcers is common, the education of both the patient and the care provider in prevention techniques is extremely important. The care provider needs to know the etiology of pressure ulcers, prevention techniques, early signs, nutritional support, and care techniques for active pressure ulcers. Since the patient with a pressure ulcer often requires extensive care for other health problems, it is important that the nurse support the caregiver through the added responsibility of pressure ulcer treatment.

REVIEW QUESTIONS

The number of the question corresponds to the same-numbered objective at the beginning of the chapter.

1. Photodamage prevention can be accomplished by all of the following *except*
   a. use of sunscreens and sun blocks.
   b. avoidance of sun exposure between 10 AM and 2 PM.
   c. using protective clothing.
   d. only tanning at a tanning salon.

2. The most common medication used for the treatment of contact dermatitis is
   a. topical corticosteroids.
   b. antibiotics.
   c. keratolytics.
   d. antipruritics.

3. Chronic pruritus can lead to
   a. basal cell carcinoma.
   b. photodamage.
   c. skin tags.
   d. lichenification.

4. The most common etiologic factor related to skin cancer is
   a. chronic sun exposure.
   b. excessive cleaning.
   c. prolonged irritation.
   d. inadequate vitamin C intake.

5. The pathogen involved in impetigo is
   a. *Escherichia coli.*
   b. *Pseudomonas aeruginosa.*
   c. *Proteus.*
   d. group A β-hemolytic *streptococci.*

6. Scabies is spread by
   a. systemic involvement.
   b. contaminated articles.
   c. direct physical contact.
   d. airborne transfer.

7. A common site for the lesions associated with atopic dermatitis is the
   a. palmar surface of the feet.
   b. antecubital space.
   c. temporal area.
   d. buttocks.

8. A common benign skin problem associated with aging is
   a. psoriasis.
   b. skin tags.
   c. vitiligo.
   d. lipomas.

9. Skin manifestation of chronic liver disease would include all of the following *except*
   a. increased pruritus.
   b. jaundice.
   c. changes in color.
   d. atrophy.

10. Important patient instruction after a chemical peel or dermabrasion include all of the following *except*
   a. how to apply ointment.
   b. use of a drying soap.
   c. use of sunscreens.
   d. how to keep the treated area moist.

11. Which stage of pressure ulcer might require surgical debridement?
   a. Stage I.
   b. Stage II.
   c. Stage III.
   d. Stage IV.

REFERENCES

1. Frankel DH: Mohs micrographic surgery for nonmelanoma skin cancer, *Hosp Pract* 25:16, 1990.
2. Bargoil S, Erdman L: Safe tan: an oxymoron, *Cancer Nurs* 16:140, 1993.
3. Rumsfield J: Sunscreens: what you and your patients should know, *Dermatol Nurs* 2:142, 1990.
4. Nicol N, Fenske N: Photodamage: cause, clinical manifestations and prevention, *Dermatol Nurs* 5:4, 1993.
5. DeLeo VA: *Photosensitivity,* New York, 1992, Igaku-Shoin.
6. Morrow G: *Drug-induced photosensitivity,* Yale New Haven Hospital Pharmacy Bulletin for Nurses 13:2, 1992.
7. Habif TF: *Clinical dermatology: a color guide to diagnosis and therapy,* ed 3, St Louis, 1995, Mosby.
8. Mackie RM: *Skin cancer,* Chicago, 1989, Year-Book Medical Publishers.
9. Stoughton RB, Cornell R: Corticosteroid. In Fitzpatrick T and others: *Dermatology in general medicine,* ed 4, New York, 1993, McGraw-Hill.
10. Shupack JL, Stiller MJ, Webster GF: Cytotoxic agents and dermatologic therapy. In Fitzpatrick TB and others: *Dermatology in general medicine,* vol. II, New York, 1993, McGraw-Hill.
11. Greco P, Ende J: An office-based approach to the patient with pruritus, *Hosp Prac,* 27:121, 1992.
12. Hoffman S and others: Melanoma: clinical characteristics, *Hosp Prac,* 29:37, 1994.
13. Frankel D: Squamous cell carcinoma of the skin, *Hosp Prac,* 28:99, 1992.
14. Washington CV: Skin cancer. In Isselbacher K and others, editors: *Harrison's principles of internal medicine,* ed 13 New York, 1994, McGraw-Hill.
15. Gollnick H, Osianowski M, Orfanos C: A new treatment for a dangerous cancer, *Skin Canc Found J,* 12:49, 1994.
16. Gilchrest B: Skin aging and photoaging, *Dermatol Nurs* 2:79, 1990.
17. Murray M, Blaylock B: Maintaining effective pressure ulcer prevention programs, *MedSurg Nurs* 3:85, 1994.
18. Bergstrom N: *Pressure sores in adults: prediction and prevention,* Rockville, Md, 1992, US Dept. Health and Human Services.
19. Pressure ulcers in adults: prediction and prevention, Clinical Practice Guideline Number 3, USDHHS, AHCPR Pub. no. 92-0047, Rockville, Md, 1992.
20. Goodman T, Thomas C, Rappaport N: Skin ulcers: overview, nursing implications, *AORN J* 52:24, 1990.
21. Schmidling R, Gordon S, Davenport B: Treating pressure ulcers with a myocutaneous flap, *Nurs* 22:56, 1992.

Chapter 21

NURSING ROLE IN MANAGEMENT
Burn Patient

Kathleen C. Solotkin   Cindy J. Knipe

Learning Objectives

1. Describe the causes and prevention of burn injuries.
2. Describe the burn injury classification system.
3. Differentiate between the involved structures and the clinical appearance of partial- and full-thickness burns.
4. Identify the parameters used to determine the severity of burns.
5. Describe the pathophysiologic changes, clinical manifestations, and therapeutic and nursing management of each burn phase.
6. Explain fluid and electrolyte shifts during the emergent and acute burn phases.
7. Differentiate among the nutritional needs of the burn patient during the three burn phases.
8. Explain the physiologic and psychosocial aspects of burn rehabilitation.
9. Describe the therapeutic and nursing management of the emotional needs of the burn patient and family.
10. Describe the special needs of the nursing staff caring for the burn patient and the possible ways to meet those needs.
11. Discuss the issues involved and rationale of preparing the burn patient to return home.
12. Describe the interventions the nurse may use in the management of pain in the burn patient.

SIGNIFICANCE

An estimated 2.5 million Americans seek medical care each year for burns. Approximately 100,000 are hospitalized, and 70,000 require intensive care services. An estimated 12,000 of these people die annually as a direct result of their burns. Children (especially preschool-aged children) and older adults account for more than two thirds of all burn fatalities.[1]

The major cause of fires in the home is carelessness with cigarettes. Other causes of burns include hot water from water heaters set above 140° F (60° C), cooking accidents, space heaters, combustibles such as gasoline and charcoal lighter fluid, steam from radiators, and chemicals.

Health Promotion and Maintenance

Most burn injuries can be prevented. The nurse as a citizen and health care provider is in a good position to conduct home safety assessments and to educate people about burn injuries before accidents occur. Home safety measures include the use of smoke alarms and fire extinguishers. Families should have fire drills, and each family member should know where to go and what to do in case of a fire. Local fire departments can inform the public of regional fire codes as well as perform home safety checks.

Knowledge of potential sources for burn injury allows problem solving for burn prevention (Tables 21-1 and 21-2). Teaching people proper use of appliances (e.g., space heaters), electrical cords, wiring, outlets, outdoor grills, and hot water heaters can prevent burn injury. The nurse can be instrumental in teaching home care of minor burns to the public. The industrial nurse should teach burn prevention in the work setting.

PATHOPHYSIOLOGY

Burn wounds occur when there is contact between tissue and an energy source, such as heat, chemicals, electrical current, or radiation. The resulting local effects are influenced by the intensity of the energy, the duration of exposure, and the type of tissue injured. Immediately after the injury there is an increase in blood flow to the area surrounding the wound. This is followed by the release of various vasoactive substances from the burned tissue, which results in increased capillary permeability. Fluid then shifts from the intravascular compartment to the interstitial space, producing edema and hypovolemia.[2]

Reviewed by Judy Knighton, BScN, MScN, Patient Unit Manager and Clinical Nurse Specialist—Burns, Ross Tilley Burn Centre at The Wellesley Hospital, Toronto, Ontario, Canada.

Table 21-1 Common Places and Causes of Burn Injury

Occupational Hazards	
Steam pipes	Electricity from power lines
Chemicals	Combustible fuels
Hot metals	
Tar	
Home and Recreational Hazards	
Hot water heaters set higher than 140° F (60° C)	Improper use of outdoor grills
Multiple extension cords per outlet	Improper use of flammables (e.g., starter fluid, gasoline, kerosene)
Frayed or defective wiring	Hot grease or liquids from cooking
Pressure cookers	Excessive exposure to sunlight
Microwaved food	Electrical storms
Radiators	
Open space heaters	
Carelessness with cigarettes or matches	

Table 21-2 Causes of Thermal Burn Injury

Cause	Examples
Flame	Clothing ignited with fire
Flash	Flame burn associated with explosion (combustible fuels)
Scald	Hot bath water Spilled hot beverages Hot grease or liquids from cooking Steam burns (pressure cookers, microwaved food, automobile radiators)
Contact	Hot metal (outdoor grill) Hot, sticky tar

TYPES OF BURN INJURY

Various types of burn may be seen alone or in combination with others. Initial management of any burn should focus first on protection of the caregiver (especially important in chemical and electrical injuries), followed by limb and lifesaving interventions. In many situations, actual wound care is not addressed during the initial resuscitation.

Thermal Injury

The most common type of burn is thermal injury, which can be caused by flame, flash, scald, or contact with hot objects (Table 21-2 and Fig. 21-1).[3]

Chemical Injury

Chemical injuries are the result of tissue injury and destruction from necrotizing substances. With chemical injuries, it is important to remove the person from the burning agent, or vice versa. The latter is accomplished by lavaging the affected area with copious amounts of water. Any clothing containing the chemical should be removed, otherwise the burning process will continue as long as the chemical is in contact with the skin.

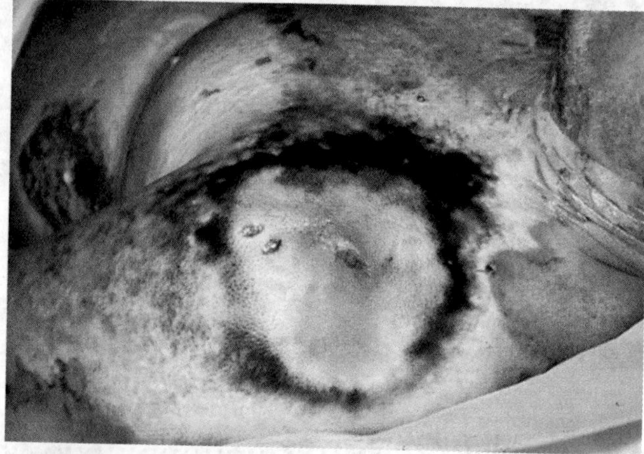

A

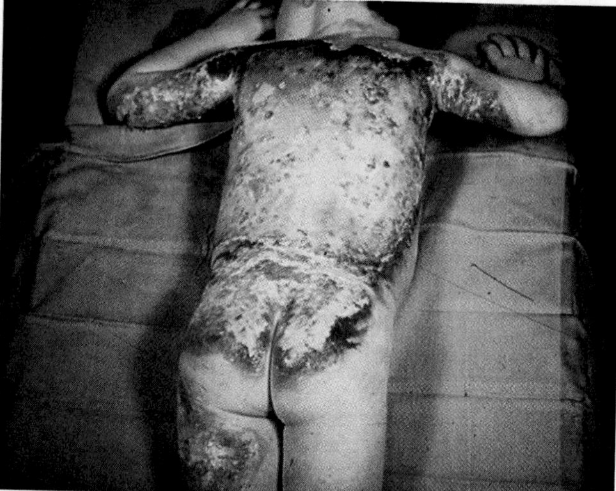

B

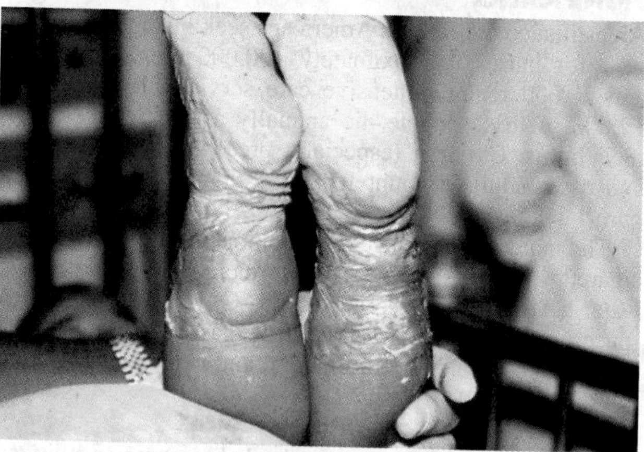

C

Fig. 21-1 Types of burn injury. ***A,*** Patient with full-thickness thermal burn of the shoulder. ***B,*** Full-thickness burns to back. ***C,*** Partial-thickness burns secondary to immersion in hot water.

Chemicals can produce respiratory and systemic symptoms as well as skin or eye injuries. When chlorine is inhaled, toxic gas produces respiratory distress. Byproducts of burning substances (e.g., carbon) are toxic to the sensitive respiratory mucosa. Tissue destruction may continue for up to 72 hours after a chemical injury.

Chemical burns are most commonly caused by acids. However, alkali burns also occur, and they are more difficult to manage than acid burns. Alkaline substances are not neutralized by tissue fluids as readily as acid substances. Alkalies adhere to tissue, causing protein hydrolysis and liquefaction. This damage continues even when the alkali is neutralized. Examples of alkalies that cause burn injury are cleaning agents, drain cleaners, and lyes.

Smoke and Inhalation Injury

Smoke and inhalation of hot air or noxious chemicals can cause damage to the tissues of the respiratory tract. Breathing hot air may cause damage to the respiratory mucosa, although it seldom happens because the vocal cords and glottis close as a protective mechanism. Gases are cooled to body temperature before they reach the lung parenchyma. Smoke inhalation injuries are an important determinant of mortality in fire victims. Inhalation injuries are present in 20% to 30% of the patients admitted to burn centers and 60% to 70% of patients who die in burn centers.[4]

There are three types of smoke and inhalation injuries:

1. *Carbon monoxide poisoning.* Carbon monoxide (CO) poisoning and asphyxiation account for the majority of deaths at the fire scene. CO is produced by the incomplete combustion of burning materials. It is subsequently inhaled and displaces oxygen (O_2) on the hemoglobin molecule, causing hypoxia and ultimately death when levels are high. Often the victims of fires, especially those who have been trapped in a closed space, will have elevated carboxyhemoglobin levels. If CO intoxication is suspected, the patient should be quickly treated with 100% humidified O_2 and the carboxyhemoglobin level should be measured when feasible.[5]
2. *Inhalation injury above the glottis.* This injury may be caused by the inhalation of hot air, steam, or smoke. Mucosal burns of the oropharynx and larynx are manifested by redness, blistering, and edema. Mechanical obstruction can occur quickly, presenting a true medical emergency. Often a reliable clue that this injury is likely is the presence of facial burns, singed hair, hoarseness, and painful swallowing.
3. *Inhalation injury below the glottis.* A general principle to remember is that inhalation injury above the glottis is thermally produced, and below the glottis it is usually chemically produced. The tissue injury to the lower respiratory tract is related to the length of exposure to smoke or toxic fumes. Symptoms may not appear until 12 to 24 hours after the burn, and then they may manifest as acute respiratory distress syndrome.[6]

These patients must be observed closely for signs of respiratory distress or compromise and must be treated quickly and efficiently if they are to survive. Respiratory tract complications from burn injury are discussed in detail later in this chapter.

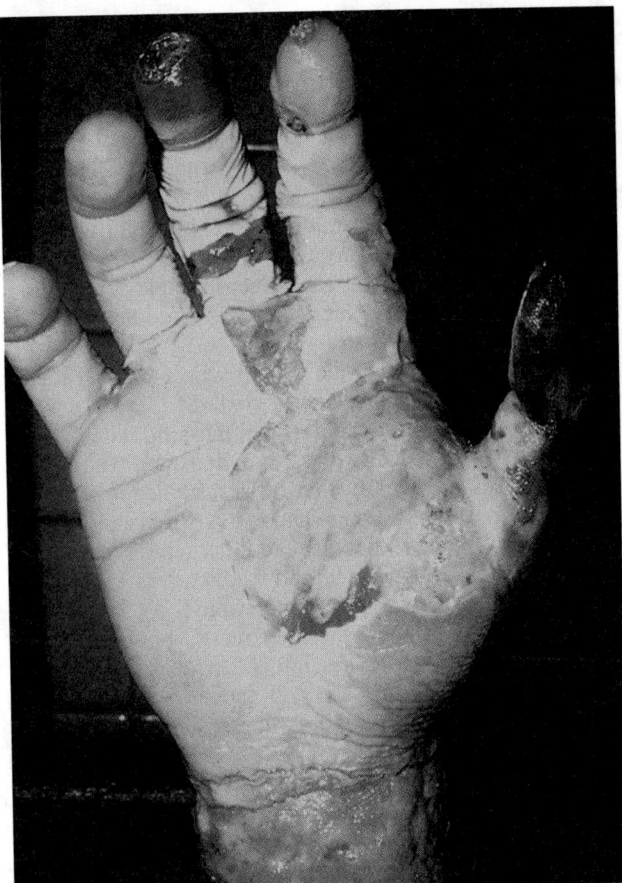

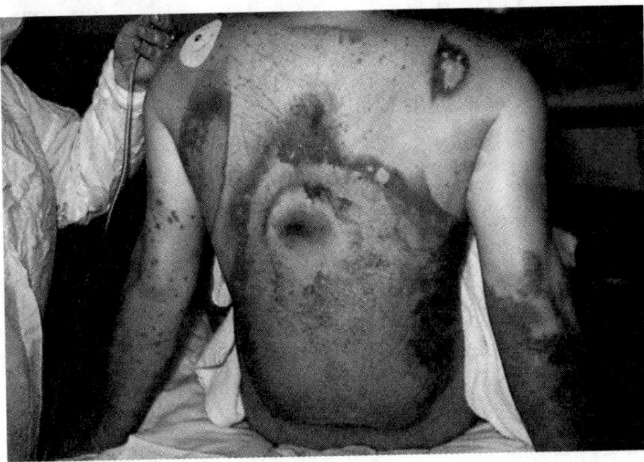

Fig. 21-2 Electrical injury produces heat coagulation of blood supply and contact area as electric current passes through the skin. ***A,*** Hand. ***B,*** Back.

Electrical Injury

Electrical injury results from coagulation necrosis that is caused by intense heat generated from an electric current (Fig. 21- 2). It can also result from direct damage to nerves and vessels causing tissue anoxia and death. The severity of the electrical injury depends on the amount of voltage, tissue resistance, current pathways, and surface area in contact with the current and on the length of time the current flow was sustained. Tissue densities offer various amounts of resistance to electric current. For example, fat and bone offer the most resistance, whereas nerves and blood vessels offer the least resistance. Current that passes through vital organs (e.g., brain, heart, kidneys) will produce more profound damage than current that passes through other tissue. In addition, electrical sparks may have ignited the patient's clothing, causing a combination of thermal and electrical injury.

Nursing assessment of the patient with electrical injury should be thorough. Often the wounds of electric current entry and exit are all that are visible, masking the possibility of extensive, underlying tissue damage. Noting the patient's position when the injury was sustained in conjunction with identifying the entry and exit wounds can help the nurse assess which underlying organ structures may have been affected. Contact with electric current can cause tetanic muscle contractions strong enough to fracture the long bones and vertebrae. Another reason to suspect long bone or spinal fractures is a fall. Most electrical injuries occur when the victim is elevated above the ground (e.g., during the work of a utility pole lineperson) and comes in contact with a current source. For this reason all patients with electrical burns should be treated for a potential cervical spine injury. This includes cervical spine immobilization during transport and subsequent spinal x-rays to rule out any injury.

Electrical injury puts the patient at risk for cardiac arrest or dysrhythmias, severe metabolic acidosis, and myoglobinuria, which can lead to acute renal tubular necrosis. The electrical shock event can cause immediate cardiac standstill or fibrillation. If this occurs, cardiopulmonary resuscitation (CPR) should be initiated immediately. Delayed cardiac dysrhythmias or arrest may also occur without warning during the first 24 to 48 hours after injury; therefore the patient should be monitored continuously. Because of extensive tissue destruction and cell rupture, severe metabolic acidosis develops within minutes after the injury, even in the absence of cardiac arrest. Arterial blood gas (ABG) analysis should be performed to assess the acid-base balance. Sodium bicarbonate may be administered in amounts sufficient to maintain the serum pH at near-normal levels.

Myoglobin is released from muscle tissue into the circulation whenever massive muscle damage occurs. It is then transported to the kidneys where it can mechanically block the renal tubules because of its large size. This process can result in acute tubular necrosis (ATN) and eventual acute renal failure if not appropriately treated (see Chapter 44). Treatment consists of infusing Ringer's lactate solution at a rate to maintain urine output at 75 to 100 ml per hour until urine samples indicate that the myoglobin has been flushed from the circulatory system. In addition, an osmotic diuretic (e.g., mannitol) may be given to maintain urine output. (Cold thermal injury, or frostbite, is discussed in Chapter 62.)

CLASSIFICATION OF BURN INJURY

The treatment of burns is related to the severity of the injury. Severity is determined by (1) depth of burn, (2) extent of burn calculated in percent of total body surface area (TBSA), (3) location of burn, (4) age of victim, (5) concomitant injury, and (6) past health history indicating risk factors for recovery.

Depth

Burn injury involves the destruction of the integumentary system. The skin is divided into three layers, which include the epidermis, dermis, and subcutaneous tissue (Fig. 21-3). The *epidermis*, or nonvascular outer layer of the skin, is approximately as thick as a sheet of paper. It is composed of many layers of nonliving epithelial cells that provide a protective barrier to the skin, hold in fluids and electrolytes, regulate heat, and keep harmful agents in the external environment from injuring or invading the body. The *dermis*, which lies below the epidermis, is approximately 30 to 45 times thicker than the epidermis. The dermis contains connective tissues with blood vessels and highly specialized structures consisting of hair follicles, nerve endings, sweat glands, and sebaceous glands. Under the dermis lies the *subcutaneous tissue*, which contains major vascular networks, fat, nerves, and lymphatics. The subcutaneous tissue acts as a shock absorber and heat insulator for the underlying structures, which include the muscles, tendons, bones, and internal organs.

In the past, burns were defined by degrees: first-degree, second-degree, and third-degree burns. The American Burn Association now advocates a more explicit definition categorizing the burn according to depth of skin destruction: partial-thickness and full-thickness burns. Table 21-3 reflects the comparison of the depth of injury.

Extent

Two commonly used guides for determining the extent of a burn wound are the Lund-Browder chart (Fig. 21-4, *A*) and the Rule of Nines (Fig. 21-4, *B*). (Only partial-thickness and full-thickness burns are included in calculating TBSA.) The Lund-Browder chart is considered more accurate because the patient's age in proportion to relative body-area size is taken into account. The Rule of Nines, which is easy to remember, is considered adequate for initial assessment. For irregular- or odd-shaped burns, the palmar surface of the patient's hand is considered to be approximately 1% of the TBSA. The extent of a burn is often revised after edema has subsided and demarcation of zones of injury has occurred.

Location

The location of the burn wound has a direct relationship to the severity of the burn injury. Burns of the face and neck and circumferential burns of the chest may inhibit respiratory function by virtue of mechanical obstruction secondary to edema or eschar formation. These injuries may also indicate the possibility of inhalation injury and respiratory mucosal damage.

Burns of the hands, feet, joints, and eyes are of concern because they make self-care impossible and jeopardize later

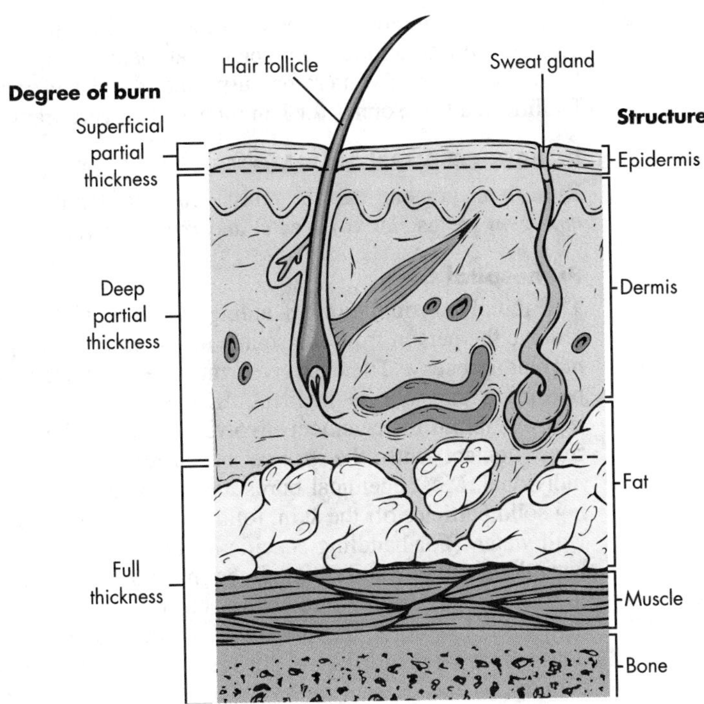

Fig. 21-3 Cross section of skin indicating the degree of burn and structures involved.

function. Hands and feet are difficult to manage medically because of superficial vascular and nerve-supply systems.

The ears and nose, composed mainly of cartilage, are susceptible to infection because of poor blood supply to the cartilage. Burns of the buttocks or genitalia are susceptible to infection and may be the source of emotional conflict because of the pain involved and possible disfigurement. Circumferential burns of the extremities can cause circulatory compromise distal to the burn with subsequent neurologic impairment of the affected extremity.

Age

Because of an immature immune system and generally poor host defense mechanisms, an infant is less able to cope with burn injuries. The older adult heals more slowly and has more difficulty with rehabilitation than a child or younger

Table 21-3 Classification of Burn Injury Depth

Classification	Clinical Appearance	Cause	Structure*
Partial-thickness skin destruction			
▪ Superficial (First-degree)	Erythema, blanching on pressure, pain and mild swelling, no vesicles or blisters (although after 24 hr skin may blister and peel)	Superficial sunburn Quick heat flash	Only superficial devitalization with hyperemia is present. Tactile and pain sensation intact.
▪ Deep (Second-degree)	Fluid-filled vesicles that are red, shiny, wet (if vesicles have ruptured); severe pain caused by nerve injury; mild-to-moderate edema	Flame Flash Scald Contact burns	Epidermis and dermis involved to varying depth. Some skin elements, from which epithelial regeneration can occur, remain viable.
Full-thickness skin destruction ▪ (Third- and fourth-degree)	Dry, waxy white, leathery, or hard skin; visible thrombosed vessels; insensitivity to pain and pressure because of nerve destruction; possible involvement of muscles, tendons, and bones	Flame Scald Chemical Tar Electric current	All skin elements and nerve endings destroyed. Coagulation necrosis present.

*See Fig. 21-3.

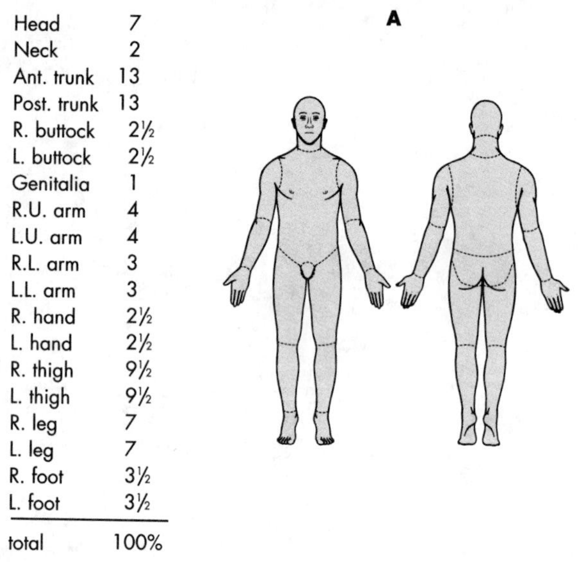

B

Head & neck	9%
Arms	9%
Ant. trunk	18%
Post. trunk	18%
Legs	18%
Perineum	1%
total	100%

Fig. 21-4 ***A,*** Lund-Browder chart. By convention, areas of partial-thickness injury are colored in blue and areas of full-thickness injury in red. Superficial partial-thickness burns are not calculated. ***B,*** Rule of Nines chart.

adult. Infection of the burn wound and pneumonia are common complications in the older patient.

Risk Factors

Any patient with preexisting cardiovascular, pulmonary, or renal disease has a poorer prognosis for recovery because of the tremendous demands placed on the body by a burn injury. The patient with diabetes mellitus or peripheral vascular disease is at high risk for gangrene and poor healing, especially with foot and leg burns. General physical debilitation from any chronic disease, including alcoholism, drug abuse, and malnutrition, renders the patient less physiologically competent to deal with a burn injury. In addition, the patient who concurrently sustained fractures, head injuries, or other trauma, has a poorer prognosis for recovery from the burn injury.

Major Versus Minor Burns

The American Burn Association classifies burns into major, moderate uncomplicated, and minor injuries by depth, extent, location, and risk factors (Table 21-4). The American Burn Association recommends that major burn injuries be treated at burn centers or burn units that have optimal facilities and personnel for handling such severe trauma.

PHASES OF BURN MANAGEMENT

Burn management can be classified into three phases: *emergent* (resuscitative), *acute*, and *rehabilitative*.

Prehospital Care

The initial consideration in aiding the burn victim is to remove the person from the source of the burn and stop the burning process. The caregiver must be protected from becoming part of the incident. In the case of electrical injuries, initial management involves removing the patient from contact with the source of current by a trained individual. Most chemical burns are best treated by brushing solid particles off the skin, followed by thorough lavage with water. (For handling specific agents, please refer to a hazardous materials text). Small thermal burns (10% or less of TBSA) may be covered with a clean, cool, tap water-dampened towel for the patient's comfort and protection until definitive medical care is instituted. It is believed that cooling of the injured area (if small) within 1 minute minimizes the depth of injury. Tap water is acceptable for flushing. Time should not be wasted trying to find sterile water or saline solution.

If the thermal burn is large, primary considerations are focused on the "ABCs": *Airway*: check for patency, soot around nares, or singed nasal hair; *Breathing*: check for adequacy of ventilation; and *Circulation*: check for presence and regularity of pulses.[7] If the burn is large, it is not advisable to immerse the burned body part in cool water because doing so would lead to extensive heat and electrolyte loss. The burn should never be packed in ice. As much clothing as possible should be removed. The patient should be wrapped in a dry, clean sheet or blanket to prevent further contamination of the wound and to provide warmth.

The burn patient may also have sustained other injuries that take priority over the burn wound.[8] It is important for the individual involved in the prehospital phase of burn care to adequately communicate the circumstances of the injury to the receiving hospital. This is especially important when the injury involved entrapment in a closed space, hazardous chemicals, or possible trauma.

Prehospital care of the patient with various types of burns is presented in tables that describe chemical burns (Table 21-5), inhalation injury (Table 21-6), electrical burns (Table 21-7), and thermal burns (Table 21-8).

Emergent Phase

Definition. The *emergent* (resuscitative) *phase* is the period of time required to resolve the immediate problems resulting from burn injury. This phase may last from burn onset to 5 or more days, but it usually lasts 24 to 48 hours. This phase begins with fluid loss and edema formation and continues until fluid mobilization and diuresis begin.

Pathophysiologic Changes

Fluid and electrolyte shifts. The greatest initial threat to a major burn victim is hypovolemic shock. It is caused by a

Table 21-4 American Burn Association Adult Burn Classification

Magnitude of Burn Injury	Partial Thickness* (Second-Degree)	Full Thickness* (Third-Degree)	Other Factors
Minor	<15%	<2%	Does not involve special care areas (eyes, ears, face, hands, feet, perineum); excludes electrical injury, inhalation injury, complicated injury (fractures), all poor-risk patients (extremes of age, concomitant disease)
Moderate uncomplicated	15-25%	<10%	Excludes electrical injury, inhalation injury, complicated injury, all poor-risk patients; does not involve special care areas
Major	>25%	>10%	Includes all burns involving hands, face, eyes, ears, feet, or perineum; includes inhalation injury, electrical injury, complicated burn injury, and all poor-risk patients

*Figures indicate percentage of total body surface area involved.

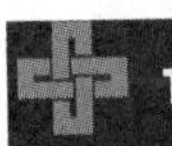

Table 21-5 Emergency Management: Chemical Burns

Possible Etiologies

Exposure to strong acids, alkali, corrosive materials, or organophosphates

Possible Assessment Findings

Burning, degeneration of exposed tissues
Discoloration of injured exposed skin
Localized pain
Edema of surrounding tissue
Respiratory distress if chemical inhaled
Paralysis, decreased muscle coordination (if organophosphate)

Management

- Wear appropriate protective garb.
- Remove the chemical from contact with patient's body.
- Flush chemical from wound and surrounding area with saline solution or water. Brush off lime and other powders.
- Remove clothing including shoes, watches, jewelry, and contact lenses (if face exposed).
- Blot, *do not rub,* skin dry with clean towels.
- Cover all burned areas with dry, sterile dressing or clean, dry sheet.
- Monitor airway if airway exposed to chemicals.
- Attempt to determine type of chemical exposure.

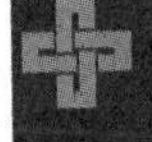

Table 21-6 Emergency Management: Inhalation Injury

Possible Etiologies

Exposure of respiratory tract to intense heat, flames, inhalation of noxious chemicals, smoke, CO gas

Possible Assessment Findings

Rapid, shallow respirations
Increasing hoarseness
Coughing
Singed nasal or facial hair
Sooty, smoky breath
Productive cough that is black, gray, or bloody
Irritation of upper airways or burning pain in throat or chest
Difficulty swallowing
Restlessness, anxiety

Management

- Remove patient from toxic environment.
- Establish and maintain airway. Anticipate need for intubation if respiratory distress.
- Administer high flow O_2 (100%) by nonrebreather mask.
- Be prepared to intubate if respiratory distress occurs.
- Remove patient's clothing.
- Establish IV line with large-gauge needle.
- Monitor vital signs including level of consciousness and O_2 saturation.
- Place patient in high Fowler's position unless spinal injury suspected.
- Assess for facial and neck burns or other signs of trauma.
- Prepare for emergency endotracheal intubation if indicated.

IV, Intravenous.

massive shift of fluids out of blood vessels as a result of increased capillary permeability. As the capillary walls become more permeable, water, sodium, and later plasma proteins (especially albumin) move into the interstitial spaces and other surrounding tissue (Fig. 21-5). The colloidal osmotic pressure decreases with progressive loss of protein from the vascular space. This results in more fluid shifting out of the vascular space into the interstitial spaces. (Fluid accumulation in the interstitium is called *second spacing.*) Fluid also moves to areas that normally have minimal to no fluid, a phenomenon called *third spacing.* Examples of third spacing in burn injury are exudate and blister formation.

Table 21-7 Emergency Management: Electrical Burns

Possible Etiologies
Exposure to electric current (e.g., lightning, electric wires, utility wires)

Possible Assessment Findings
Leathery, white charred skin
Burn odor
Impaired touch sensation
Minimal or absent pain
Dysrhythmias
Depth of wound difficult to visualize; assume injury greater than seen
Entrance and exit wounds

Management
- Remove patient from contact with current source by trained personnel.
- Avoid contact with electric current during rescue.
- Assess for patent airway, breathing, and circulation.
- Initiate CPR if necessary.
- Establish and maintain airway.
- Maintain cervical spine precautions.
- Administer high flow O_2 (100%) by nonrebreather mask.
- Establish IV line with large-gauge needle.
- Remove patient's clothing.
- Assess burn areas, especially entrance and exit sites.
- Check pulses distal to burns.
- Monitor HR and rhythm.
- Cover burn sites with dry sterile dressing.
- Assess for any other injuries (e.g., fractures).
- Monitor vital signs including level of consciousness.

CPR, Cardiopulmonary resuscitation; *HR,* heart rate; *IV,* intravenous.

The net result of the fluid shift is intravascular volume depletion. Edema, decreased blood pressure (BP), increased pulse, and other manifestations of hypovolemic shock are clinically detectable signs (see Chapter 7). If not corrected, these events can lead to irreversible shock and death.

Another source of fluid loss is insensible loss by evaporation from large, denuded body surfaces. The normal insensible loss of 30 to 50 ml per hour may increase to as much as 200 to 400 ml per hour in the severely burned patient.

The circulatory status is also impaired because of hemolysis of red blood cells (RBCs). The RBCs are hemolyzed by a circulating factor released at the time of the burn as well as by the direct insult of the burn injury. Thrombosis in the capillaries of burned tissue causes an additional loss of circulating RBCs. An elevated hematocrit is commonly caused by hemoconcentration. After fluid balance has been restored, lowered hematocrit levels are found secondary to dilution, and an anemic state is more readily detectable.

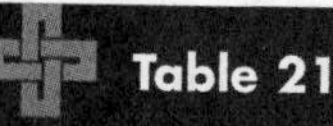

Table 21-8 Emergency Management: Thermal Burns

Possible Etiologies
Contact with hot liquids or solids, flash flame, open flame, steam or UV rays

Possible Assessment Findings

Partial-thickness (superficial) burns
Redness
Pain
Moderate to severe tenderness
Minimal edema
Blanching with pressure

Partial-thickness (deep) burns
Moist blebs, blisters
Mottled white, pink to cherry red
Hypersensitive to touch or air
Moderate to severe pain
Blanching with pressure

Full-thickness burns
Shock (e.g., tachycardia, hypotension)
Dry, leathery eschar
White, waxy, dark brown, or charred appearance
Strong burn odor
Impaired sensation when touched
Absence of pain with severe pain in surrounding tissues
Lack of blanching with pressure

Management
- Remove patient from environment; stop the burning process.
- Establish and maintain airway; inspect the face and neck for singed nasal hair, hoarseness of voice, stridor, soot in the sputum. Anticipate need for intubation.
- Administer high flow humidified O_2 (100%) by nonrebreather mask.
- Establish IV line with large-gauge needle.
- Administer fluid (see text).
- Monitor vital signs including level of consciousness and O_2 saturation.
- Remove clothing and jewelry.
- Examine and treat for other associated injuries (e.g., fractured ribs, pneumothorax).
- Determine depth, extent, and severity of burn.
- Anticipate need for analgesia and tetanus prophylaxis.
- Cover large burns with dry, sterile dressing.
- Apply cool compresses or immerse in cool water for minor injuries only (less than 10% TBSA burn).
- Transport as soon as possible to a burn center.

IV, Intravenous; *TBSA,* total body surface area; *UV,* ultraviolet.

Sodium and potassium are involved in electrolyte shifts. Sodium rapidly shifts to the interstitial spaces and remains there until edema formation ceases (Fig. 21-6). A potassium shift develops initially because injured cells and hemolyzed RBCs release potassium into the extracellular spaces.

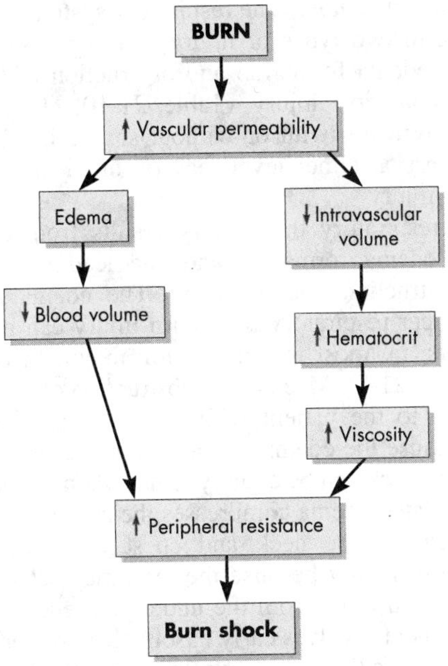

BURN

↑ Vascular permeability

Edema

↓ Intravascular volume

↓ Blood volume

↑ Hematocrit

↑ Viscosity

↑ Peripheral resistance

Burn shock

Fig. 21-5 At the time of major burn injury, the capillaries increase in permeability. All fluid components of the blood begin to leak into the interstitium, causing edema and a decreased blood volume. The red blood cells and white blood cells do not leak. Therefore the hematocrit increases and the blood becomes viscous. The combination of decreased blood volume and increased viscosity produces increased peripheral resistance. Burn shock, a type of hypovolemic shock, rapidly ensues and continues for about 24 hours.

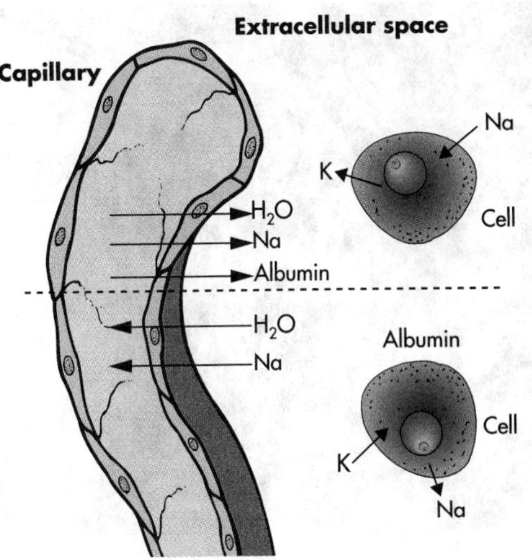

Fig. 21-6 The effects of burn shock during the first 24 hours are shown (*above the dotted line*). As the capillary seal is lost, the interstitial edema fluid is formed. The cellular integrity is also altered, with sodium moving into the cell in abnormal amounts and potassium leaving the cell. The shifts after the first 24 hours are shown (*below the dotted line*). The water and sodium move back into the circulating volume through the capillary. The albumin remains in the interstitium. Potassium is transported into the cell and sodium is transported out as the cellular integrity returns.

Toward the end of the emergent phase, if fluid replacement is adequate, capillary membrane permeability will be restored. Fluid loss and edema formation cease. Interstitial fluid gradually returns to the vascular space (Fig. 21-6). Clinically, diuresis is noted with low urine specific gravities. Serum potassium levels may be markedly elevated initially as fluid mobilization brings potassium from the interstitium to the vascular space. Hypokalemia may occur later as a result of the loss of potassium from diuresis and potassium movement back into cells. Serum sodium levels increase as sodium returns to the vascular space. Normal serum sodium values occur later with loss of sodium in urine.

Inflammation and Healing. Burn injury causes coagulation necrosis whereby tissues and vessels are damaged or destroyed. Polymorphonuclear leukocytes and monocytes accumulate at the site of injury. Fibroblasts and newly formed collagen fibrils appear and begin wound repair within the first 6 to 12 hours after injury. (The inflammatory response is discussed in Chapter 9.)

Immunologic Changes. Burn injury causes widespread impairment of the immune system.[9] The skin barrier to invading organisms is destroyed, circulating levels of immunoglobulins are decreased, and many changes in white blood cells (WBCs), both quantitative and qualitative, occur. Depression of neutrophil chemotactic, phagocytic, and bactericidal activity is found after burn injury. Burn size-related alterations of lymphocyte populations include decreased T-helper cells and increased T-suppressor cells. In addition, decreased levels of interleukin-1 (produced by macrophages) and interleukin-2 (produced by lymphocytes) are also found in some patients with burn injury. All of these changes in the immune system can make the burn patient more susceptible to infection.

Clinical Manifestations. The burn patient may be in shock from pain and hypovolemia. Areas of full-thickness and deep partial-thickness burns are frequently anesthetic because the nerve endings are destroyed. Superficial partial-thickness burns are painful. Blisters filled with fluid and protein may occur in partial-thickness burns. The patient may experience an intense thirst because of the relative fluid loss. The fluid is not actually lost from the body as much as it is sequestered in the interstitial spaces and third spaces. It is hard to visualize severe dehydration in someone who is so obviously edematous. The patient will have minimal urine output and will have signs of adynamic ileus as a result of the body's response to massive trauma and potassium shifts. Shivering may occur as a result of chilling that is caused by heat loss, anxiety, or pain.

The patient may be disoriented and have difficulty recalling the sequence of events that preceded the burn injury. Unconsciousness in a burn patient is usually not a result of the burn. The most common reason is hypoxia associated with smoke inhalation. Other possibilities include head trauma and an overdose of sedative or pain medication.

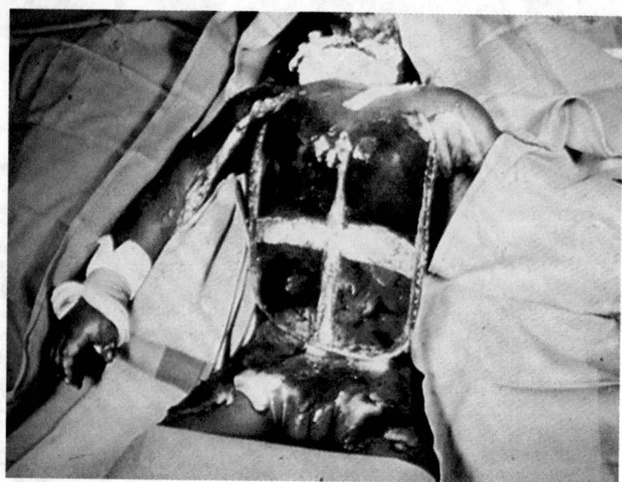

Fig. 21-7 Escharotomy of the chest and abdomen.

Complications. The three major organ systems most susceptible to complications during the emergent phase of burn injury are the cardiovascular, respiratory, and renal systems.

Cardiovascular system. Cardiovascular system complications include dysrhythmias and hypovolemic shock, which may progress to irreversible shock.[10] Circulation to the extremities can be severely impaired by circumferential burns and subsequent edema formation. These processes occlude the blood supply causing ischemia, necrosis, and eventually gangrene. *Escharotomies* (incisions through the eschar) are frequently performed to restore circulation to compromised extremities (Fig. 21-7).

Initially there is an increase in blood viscosity with burn injuries because of the fluid loss that occurs in the emergent period. Microcirculation is impaired because of the damage to skin structures that contain small capillary systems. These two events result in a phenomenon called *sludging*. Sludging can be corrected by adequate fluid replacement, which is calculated with one of the burn resuscitation formulas (Table 21-9).

Respiratory system. The respiratory system is especially vulnerable to two types of injury: (1) upper airway burns that cause edema formation and obstruction of the airway and (2) inhalation injury (Table 21-10). Upper airway distress may occur with or without smoke inhalation, and airway injury at either level may occur in the absence of cutaneous injury.

Upper respiratory tract injury results from direct heat injury or edema formation and can lead to mechanical airway obstruction and asphyxia. The edema associated with an upper respiratory tract burn injury can be massive and occurs in most patients with major thermal burn injuries (Fig. 21-8). Mechanical obstruction of the airway is not limited to the patient with flame burns of the upper airway because the edema that accompanies scald burns to the face and neck can be equally lethal when the pressure of the accumulated edema compresses the airway externally.[11] Flame burns to the neck and chest may contribute to respiratory difficulty because the inelastic eschar becomes tight and constricting from the underlying edema.

Management involves early nasotracheal or endotracheal intubation before the airway is actually compromised. Early intubation eliminates the necessity for emergency tracheostomy after respiratory problems have become apparent. In general the patient with major injuries involving burns to the face and neck requires intubation within 1 to 2 hours after burn injury. (Nasotracheal and endotracheal intubations are discussed in Chapter 23.) After intubation, the patient may be placed on ventilatory assistance, and the delivered oxygen concentration is determined by assessing ABG values. Extubation may be indicated when the edema resolves, usually 3 to 6 days after burn injury, unless severe inhalation injury is involved. Escharotomies may be needed to relieve respiratory distress secondary to circumferential, full-thickness burns of the neck and trunk.

Inhalation injury refers to a direct insult at the alveolar level secondary to the inhalation of chemical fumes or smoke. The result is interstitial edema that prevents the diffusion of oxygen from the alveoli into the circulatory system. The patient with smoke inhalation frequently exhibits *no* physical manifestations of injury during the first

Table 21-9 Formulas for Estimating Fluid Replacement of an Adult Burn Patient

	First 24 Hours		Second 24 Hours
Formula	**Crystalloids**	**Colloids**	**Glucose in Water**
Brooke (modified)	Lactated Ringer's solution: 2.0 ml/kg/% burn; ½ given during first 8 hr; ½ given during next 16 hr	0.3 to 0.5 ml/kg/% burn	Amount to replace estimated evaporative losses
Parkland (Baxter)	Lactated Ringer's solution: 4 ml/kg/% burn; ½ given first 8 hr; ¼ given each next 8 hr	20-60% of calculated plasma volume	Amount to replace estimated evaporative losses

Table 21-10 Clinical Manifestations of Respiratory Injury Associated with Burns

Upper Respiratory Tract Injury
Edema, hoarseness, difficulty swallowing, copious secretions, stridor, substernal and intercostal retractions, total airway obstruction

Inhalation Injury
Initial absence of manifestations possible; high degree of suspicion if patient was trapped in fire and has facial burns, singed nasal or facial hair; dyspnea, carbonaceous sputum, wheezing, hoarseness, altered mental status

24 hours after sustaining a major burn. The only diagnostic indicator may be a history of prolonged exposure to smoke or fumes; therefore the nurse must be especially sensitive to signs of respiratory distress such as increased agitation or change in the rate or character of respirations. Sputum that contains carbon may be present. Generally there is no correlation between the extent of TBSA burn and severity of inhalation injury because inhalation injury is a factor of time exposure plus the type and density of the material inhaled. The initial chest x-ray may appear normal, and the ABG values may be within the normal range.

Within 6 to 12 hours after injury in which smoke inhalation is probable, the patient should have a fiberoptic bronchoscopy to assess the lower respiratory tract. Significant findings include the appearance of carbonaceous material, mucosal edema, vesicles, erythema, hemorrhage, and ulceration. A radioactive xenon^{133} ventilation-perfusion scan may be used to assess the ventilatory removal of gases that are normally expelled. The patient with inhalation injury has delayed clearance of gas. The results of the scan may also demonstrate areas containing no gas or areas in which the gas remains for many minutes. A disadvantage of this test is that the patient must be transported to the special radiology unit of the hospital.

Impaired gas exchange related to CO poisoning often accompanies smoke inhalation. Inhalation of CO can produce significant hypoxemia. CO, produced by incomplete combustion of carbon-containing materials, has an affinity for hemoglobin 200 times that of oxygen. Carboxyhemoglobin concentration should be measured as soon as the patient reaches the hospital. The presence of increased concentrations of carboxyhemoglobin suggests that the patient has inhaled a significant amount of smoke. The characteristic cherry-red skin and mucous membranes associated with CO poisoning may not be present in the patient with burn shock because of the decrease in blood flow to the skin.

Treatment of inhalation injury includes administration of humidified air and 100% oxygen as required. The patient should be placed in a high Fowler's position (unless contraindicated by a possible spinal injury), encouraged to cough and deep breathe every hour, repositioned every 1 to 2 hours, given chest physiotherapy, and suctioned as necessary. If respiratory failure is impending, nasotracheal or endotracheal intubation should be performed and the patient should be supported with mechanical ventilation. Positive end-expiratory pressure (PEEP) may be used to prevent collapse of the alveoli and progressive respiratory failure (see Chapter 26). Bronchodilators may be administered intravenously to treat severe bronchospasm. CO poisoning is treated by administering 100% O_2 until the carboxyhemoglobin levels return to normal. Hyperbaric O_2 therapy may also be useful in accelerating the excretion of CO.[12]

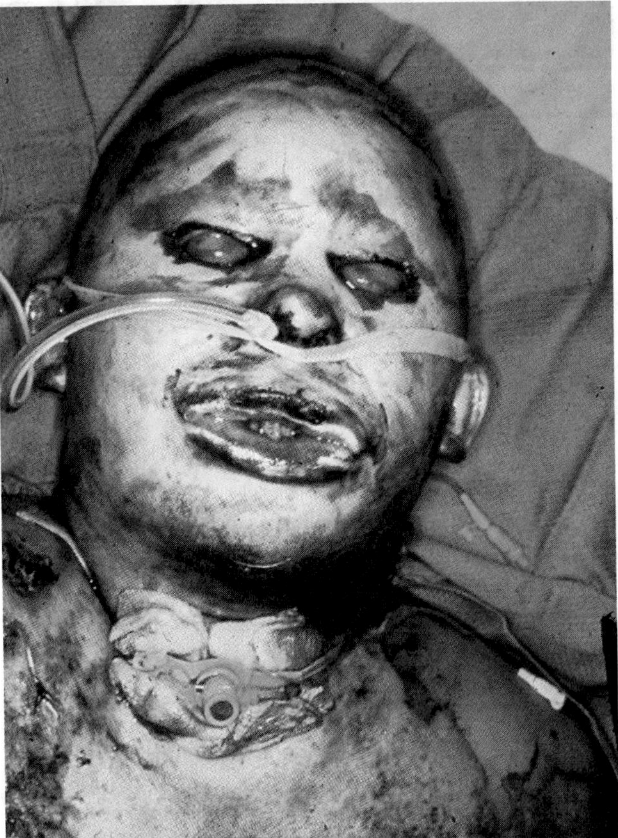

Fig. 21-8 Patient with massive upper airway edema requiring a tracheostomy to prevent airway obstruction.

The patient with preexisting pulmonary problems (e.g., chronic obstructive pulmonary disease) is more likely to sustain respiratory infection. Pneumonia is a common complication of major burns (especially in the older adult) because of debilitation, abundant microbial flora, and the relative immobility of the patient. If fluid replacement is vigorous, the patient can succumb to pulmonary edema.

Renal system. The most common renal complication of a burn in the emergent phase is ATN. Because of the

Table 21-11 Therapeutic Management: Burn Patient

Emergent Phase	Acute Phase	Rehabilitation Phase
Fluid therapy Assess fluid needs.* Begin IV fluid replacement. Insert indwelling catheter. Monitor urine output. Wound care Start hydrotherapy or cleansing. Debride as necessary. Assess extent and depth of burns. Initiate topical antibiotic therapy. Administer tetanus toxoid or tetanus antitoxin.	Fluid therapy Replace fluids, depending on individual patient needs. Administer RBCs (if necessary). Wound care Assess wound daily. Observe for complications. Continue hydrotherapy. Continue debridement (if necessary). Early excision and grafting Provide homografts. Provide autografts. Care for donor site.	Counsel and teach patient and family. Encourage and assist patient in resuming self-care. Begin physical therapy for maintenance and rehabilitation of motion. Correct contractures and scarring (surgery, physical therapy, or splinting). Discuss possible cosmetic or reconstructive surgery.

IV, Intravenous; *RBCs*, red blood cells.
*See Table 21-12.

hypovolemic state, blood flow to the kidneys is decreased, causing renal ischemia. If this continues, acute renal failure may develop.

With full-thickness and electrical burns, myoglobin (from muscle cell breakdown) and hemoglobin (from RBC breakdown) are released into the bloodstream and occlude renal tubules. Adequate fluid replacement and diuretics can counteract myoglobin and hemoglobin obstruction of the tubules.

Therapeutic Management. From the onset of the burn event until the patient is stabilized, medical therapy predominantly consists of airway management, fluid therapy, and wound care (Table 21-11). As soon as the patient arrives at a health care facility, at least one (and usually two) large bore intravenous (IV) replacement line is secured, preferably by percutaneous puncture. If this is not feasible, a jugular or subclavian line is inserted through unburned or even burned tissue. A cutdown is a final measure but is rarely used because of the high incidence of infection and sepsis. It is critical to establish IV access that can accommodate large volumes of fluid.

Fluid therapy. IV fluid therapy is usually instituted in the patient with burns greater than 20% of TBSA. The type of fluid replacement is determined by size and depth of burn, age of the patient, and individual considerations such as dehydration in the preburn state or preexisting chronic illness. Each burn center has a preference for a replacement regime, which is used almost exclusively. Fluid replacement is accomplished with either crystalloid solutions (physiologic saline, lactated Ringer's, or 5% dextrose and saline) or colloids (albumin, dextran, or other commercially prepared solutions).

Of the many formulas that are used for fluid replacement, the Brooke formula and the Parkland (Baxter) formula are the most commonly employed (Table 21-9). All formulas are estimates. The Parkland formula has been widely used because it is easy to calculate and monitor and

Table 21-12 Fluid Resuscitation with the Parkland (Baxter) Formula*

Formula
4 ml lactated Ringer's solution
per
kg body weight
per
% TBSA burn
= total fluid requirement for first 24 hr after burn

Application
½ of total in first 8 hr
¼ of total in second 8 hr
¼ of total in third 8 hr

Example
For a 70 kg patient with a 50% TBSA burn:
4 ml × 70 kg × 50% TBSA burn = 14,000 ml
= 14 L in 24 hr
½ of total in first 8 hr = 7000 ml (875 ml/hr)
¼ of total in second 8 hr = 3500 ml (436 ml/hr)
¼ of total in third 8 hr = 3500 ml (436 ml/hr)

TBSA, Total body surface area.
*Formulas are guidelines. Fluid is administered at a rate to produce 30 to 50 ml of urine output per hour.

it provides a reliable method of fluid replacement for most patients.

As noted in Table 21-12, the Parkland formula gives fluid in the following manner: 4 ml lactated Ringer's solution per kilogram of body weight per percent TBSA burned. This quantity is calculated for the first 24 hours, with one half of the total quantity given in the first 8 hours after injury because it is during that period that fluid loss is greatest. (*Note*: This 24 hours is not calculated from time of arrival to hospital but from the time of injury.) One quarter of the total quantity is then given in the second 8-hour

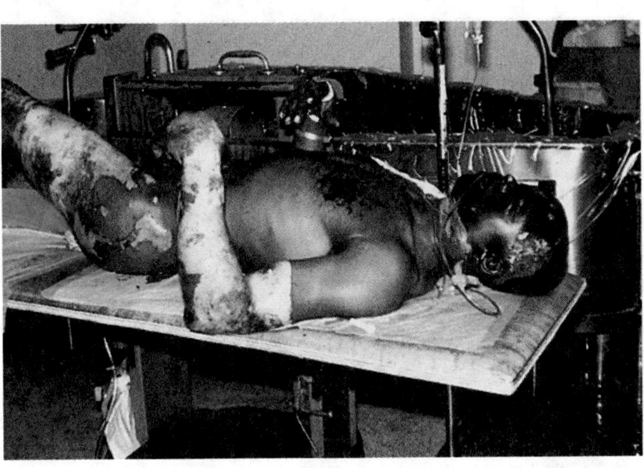

Fig. 21-9 Patient is being bathed in a tank. Bathing presents an opportunity for physical therapy as well as wound care.

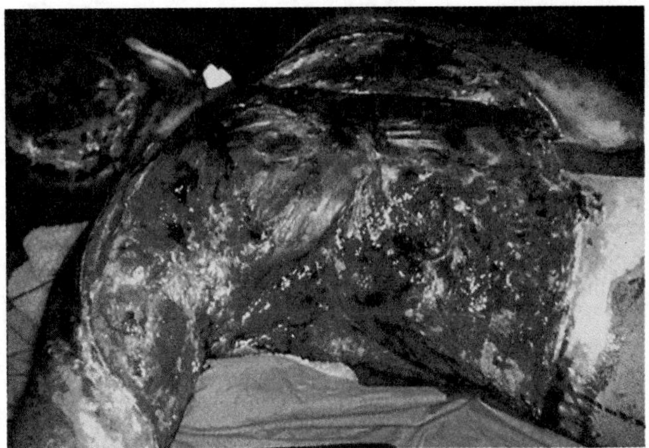

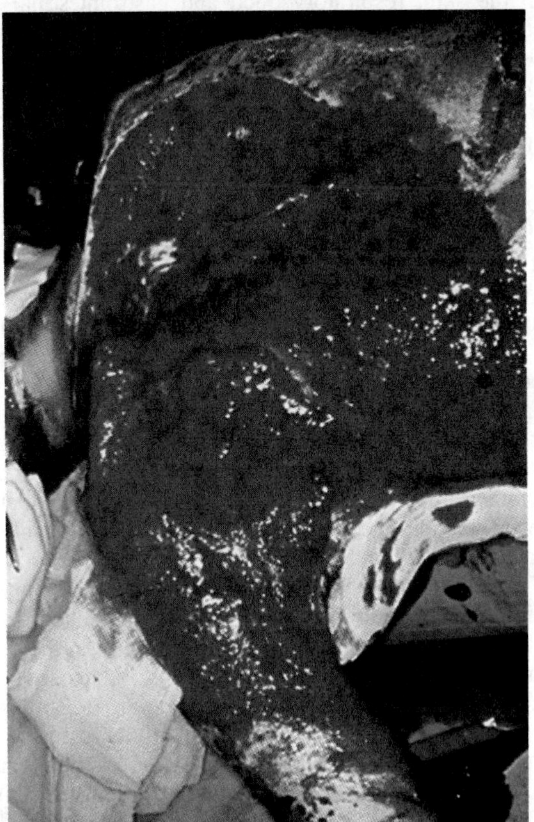

Fig. 21-10 Operative debridement of full-thickness burns secondary to an electrical injury. ***A,*** Before debridement. ***B,*** After debridement.

period, and the final quarter is given in the last 8-hour period (Table 21-12).

The second 24 hours of fluid replacement consists of ensuring adequate dextrose in water replacement to maintain a serum sodium level below 140 mEq/L (140 mmol/L). Colloidal solutions (e.g., Plasmanate, albumin) are also routinely given. The amount is calculated with a formula and the patient's body weight, which predicts the replacement volume. Colloidal solutions are not usually given until the second 24 hours, when capillary permeability begins to return to normal, because premature infusion of colloid solutions could result in leakage out of the vascular space as a result of increased capillary permeability. After this time, the plasma remains in the vascular space and expands the circulating volume.

Assessment of the adequacy of fluid replacement is best made by use of more than one parameter, and urinary output is the most commonly used. Assessment parameters include the following:

1. Urine output: 30 to 50 ml/hr in an adult
2. Cardiopulmonary factors: BP* (systolic ≥90 to 100 mm Hg), pulse rate (≤100), respiration (16 to 20 breaths per minute)
3. Sensorium: alert and oriented to time, place, and person

Wound care. Wound care should be delayed until a patent airway, adequate circulation, and adequate fluid replacement have been established. Goals of wound care are to (1) cleanse and debride the area of necrotic tissue and debris that would promote bacterial growth, (2) minimize further destruction to viable skin, and (3) promote patient comfort.

Cleansing and debridement can be done in a tank (Fig. 21-9), shower, or bed. Debridement may need to be done in the operating room (OR) (Fig. 21-10). During these procedures, loose, necrotic skin is removed. Large blisters may be opened to eliminate media for bacterial growth. All burned areas with hair (except eyebrows) should be shaved, including the head and perineum. Thereafter, daily shaving is required to minimize pathogen accumulation. Care should be

*BP is most appropriately measured by an arterial line. Peripheral measurement is often invalid because of early vasoconstriction and edema.

taken to accomplish this procedure as quickly and deftly as possible. Immersion in a tank for longer than 20 to 30 minutes can cause electrolyte loss from open burned areas. Prolonged immersion can lead to chilling after the bath and cross-contamination of wounds from one area of the body to another. Because of these factors, some institutions do not submerge the patient. The water does not need to be sterile, and tap water not exceeding 104° F (40° C) is acceptable. Because pathogenic organisms are present on the burn wound, a surgical detergent, disinfectant, or cleansing agent may be used. The patient may be bathed two times daily to limit the amount of bacterial growth.

Infection is the most serious threat to further tissue injury and possible sepsis. The source of infection in burn wounds is the patient's own residual flora, predominately from the skin, respiratory tract, and gastrointestinal (GI) tract. The prevention of cross-contamination from one patient to another is a priority for nursing care. Two methods of wound treatment used to control infection are the *open method* and the *closed method.*[13] In the open method the patient's burn is covered with a topical antibiotic and has no dressing. The closed method uses sterile gauze dressings impregnated with or laid over a topical antibiotic. These dressings are changed two to three times every 24 hours.

When the patient's wounds are exposed, the staff must wear hats, masks, gowns, and gloves. When removing dressings and washing the wound, the nurse should use nonsterile disposable gloves. Sterile gloves are used when applying ointments and sterile dressings. In addition, the room must be kept warm (approximately 85° F [29.4° C]). All attire is changed before the nurse treats another patient. Careful hand washing is also required to prevent cross-contamination. After the patient has been treated in the tub, the tank and agitators are disinfected with a chemical preparation.

Coverage is the primary goal for burn wounds. Survival is directly related to prevention of wound contamination. Because there is rarely enough unburned skin in the major burn patient for immediate skin grafting, other temporary wound closure methods are used. Allograft or homograft skin (usually from cadavers) is commonly used for wound closure (Table 21-13). However, rejection occurs because the host's immune system acts against the foreign substance.

Other measures. Routine lab tests are performed initially and serially to monitor electrolyte balance. Blood for measurement of ABGs may be drawn to determine adequacy of ventilation and perfusion. Physical therapy is begun immediately, sometimes in the tank. Early range-of-motion (ROM) exercises are necessary to facilitate mobilization of the extravasated fluid back to the vascular bed. Exercise of body parts also maintains function and reassures the patient that movement is still possible.

Pharmacologic Management. Tetanus toxoid is given routinely to all burn patients because of the likelihood of anaerobic burn-wound contamination. In the absence of active immunization within 10 years before the burn injury, tetanus immunoglobulin should be administered.

Analgesics are ordered to promote patient comfort. Early in the postburn period, IV pain medications should be given because (1) GI function is slowed or impaired because of shock or paralytic ileus, and (2) intramuscular (IM) injections will not be absorbed adequately in burned or edematous areas, causing pooling of medications in the tissues. When fluid mobilization begins, the patient could be inadvertently overdosed from the interstitial accumulation of previous IM medications.

Common narcotics used for pain control are listed in Table 21-14. The need for analgesia should be evaluated early rela-

Table 21-13 Sources of Grafts

Source	Graft Name	Coverage
Porcine skin	Heterograft or xenograft (different species)	Temporary (3 days to 2 wk)
Cadaveric skin	Homograft or allograft (same species)	Temporary (3 days to 2 wk)
Patient's own skin	Autograft	Permanent
Patient's own skin and cell culture	Cultured epithelial autograft	Permanent

Table 21-14 Drugs Commonly Used in Burn Treatment

Types and Names of Drugs	Purpose
Nutritional Support	
Vitamins A, C, E, and multivitamins	Promotes wound healing
Minerals: zinc, folate, iron (ferrous sulfate, ferrous gluconate)	Promotes cellular integrity and hemoglobin formation
Analgesia and Sedative	
Morphine	Diminishes pain perception
Meperidine (Demerol)	Diminishes pain perception
Methadone	Relieves pain, elevates mood
Haloperidol (Haldol)	Produces antipsychotic and sedative effects, promotes sleep
Midazolam (Versed)	Has short-acting amnestic properties
Gastrointestinal Support	
Cimetidine (Tagamet)	Decreases incidence of Curling's ulcer
Nystatin (Mycostatin)	Prevents overgrowth of *Candida albicans* in oral mucosa
Mylanta, Maalox	Neutralizes stomach acid

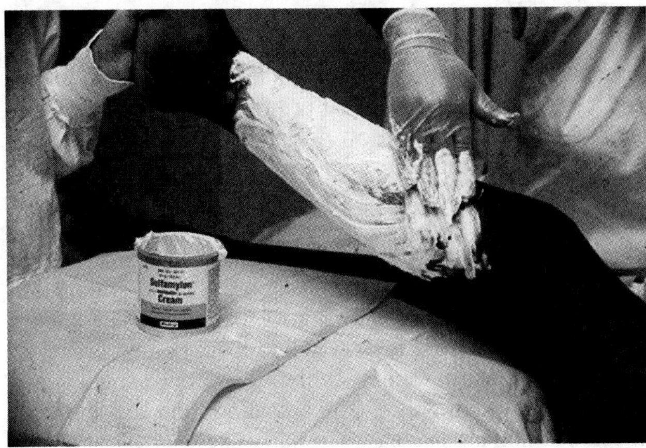

Fig. 21-11 Patient being treated with mafenide (Sulfamylon).

tive to the burn injury. The drug of choice for pain control is morphine, but meperidine and methadone may also be used. These drugs provide adequate pain control and a sedative effect. The patient may be in great pain with large burns (especially those that are predominantly partial-thickness). Withholding pain medication in the emergent and acute phases of burn recuperation is not only inhumane but also unethical.

After the wound is cleansed, topical antibacterial agents are applied and may be covered with a light dressing or left open to air (Fig. 21-11). Systemic antibiotics are not usually used in controlling burn wound flora, especially after 48 hours, because there is little or no blood supply to the burn eschar, and consequently, there is little delivery of the antibiotic to the wound. Some burn centers prophylactically administer IV penicillin for the first 3 to 4 days to reduce the proliferation of gram-positive organisms. Topical burn agents penetrate the eschar, thereby inhibiting bacterial invasion of the wound (Table 21-15). Silver sulfadiazine is commonly used because it is effective, and unlike mafenide (Sulfamylon), it is painless. Systemic sepsis remains a leading cause of death in the patient with major burns because resistant organisms develop with exposure of bacteria to topical agents over time. Most burn centers use one topical agent almost exclusively and change to another at the first sign of microorganism resistance. Systemic antibiotic therapy is initiated when the clinical diagnosis of invasive burn wound sepsis is made or when some other source of sepsis is identified (e.g., pneumonia).

A variety of drugs may be administered to the burn patient (Table 21-15). Frequently, superinfections develop in the patient's mucous membranes (mouth and genitalia) as a result of antibiotic therapy and low resistance in the host. The offending organism is usually *Candida albicans*. This is treated with nystatin (Mycostatin) mouthwash. When a normal diet is resumed, yogurt or Lactobacillus (Lactinex) may be given by mouth to reintroduce the normal intestinal flora that have been destroyed by antibiotic therapy. Supplemental vitamins and iron may be given as early as the emergent phase. However, the need for these supplements usually does not occur until the acute phase.

Nutritional Management. Fluid replacement takes priority over nutritional needs in the initial emergent phase. The patient with large burns frequently develops paralytic ileus within a few hours as a result of the body's response to major trauma. A nasogastric tube is inserted and connected to low intermittent suction for decompression. When bowel sounds return at 48 to 72 hours after injury, alimentation can be initiated beginning with clear liquids and progressing to a diet high in protein and calories.

A hypermetabolic response proportional to the size of the wound is observed. Resting metabolic expenditure may be increased by 50% to 100% above normal for major burns. Core temperature is elevated. Plasma catecholamines, which stimulate heat production, and substrate mobilization are increased. Massive catabolism is characterized by protein mobilization and increased gluconeogenesis. Caloric needs are often in the 5000 kcal per day range. Failure to supply ad-

Table 21-15 Topical Antibiotic Therapy Used in Burn Wound Therapy

Drug	Indications for Use	Advantages	Disadvantages
Silver sulfadiazine (Silvadene)	Gram-positive and gram-negative organisms, *Candida albicans*	Wide-spectrum antibacterial action; no limit to motion because of light or no dressing; fast, painless, easy to apply	Possible depression of granulocyte formation; possible allergic reaction to sulfa component in susceptible patients
Mafenide acetate (Sulfamylon)	Gram-positive and gram-negative organisms, most anaerobes	Wide-spectrum antibacterial action; most effective of all topical antibiotics; penetration of eschar better than other agents; open treatment of burn wound possible; good treatment for electrical burns	Pain on application for 15-30 min; acid-base derangements because it is a carbonic anhydrase inhibitor; allergic reaction to sulfa component in susceptible patients

equate calories and protein actually leads to malnutrition. The patient is not freely given water to drink. Rather, calorie-containing liquids are given because of the great need for calories and the potential for water intoxication.

Major advances have been made in the area of liquid nutritional supplementation (see Chapter 37). A thin latex feeding tube can be advanced by fluoroscopic guidance into the duodenum, bypassing the stomach. This allows for quicker absorption of nutrients and a decrease in the nausea and vomiting associated with high-volume tube feedings into the stomach. This patient can be maintained on a more continuous feeding schedule, which does not have to be interrupted by surgical interventions. Because the liquid goes past the pyloric sphincter, the patient does not have to remain without food or water for extended periods before surgery, as is required when the tube is in the stomach.

NURSING MANAGEMENT

EMERGENT PHASE

In the emergent phase, patient survival depends on quick and thorough assessment and intervention. It may be the nurse who makes the initial assessment of depth, degree, and percent of burn and who coordinates the actions of the burn team. The nurse assesses the adequacy of fluid replacement, provides wound care, and offers support to the patient and family. (See the nursing care plan on p. 543.)

Care of special areas is initiated by the nurse. The face is vascular and subject to a greater amount of edema. The face is treated by the open method because facial dressings cause disorientation and confusion. Eye care for corneal burns or edema is done with slightly warmed physiologic saline rinses as often as every hour. Periorbital edema can prevent opening of the eyes. This can be frightening to the patient; the nurse must assure the patient that the swelling is not permanent and that vision will soon be restored. Instillation of methylcellulose drops or artificial tears into the eyes for moisture provides additional comfort and prevents corneal abrasions.

Hands and arms should be extended and elevated on pillows or in slings to minimize edema. Ears should be kept free of pressure because of their poor vascularization and predisposition to infection. The patient with ear burns is not allowed to use pillows because of the danger of the burned ear sticking to the pillow case, thereby causing bleeding, pain, or infection of the ear cartilage. The patient with neck burns is not allowed to use pillows in order to prevent wound contraction.

The perineum must be kept clean and as dry as possible. In addition to providing hourly urine outputs, an indwelling catheter prevents urine contamination of the perineal area. Frequent perineal and catheter care is essential.

Acute Phase

The acute phase begins with the mobilization of extracellular fluid and subsequent diuresis. The acute phase is concluded when the burned area is completely covered or when the wounds are healed. This may take weeks or many months.

Pathophysiologic Changes. Burn injury involves pathophysiologic changes in many body systems. Diuresis from fluid mobilization occurs, and the patient is no longer grossly edematous. Areas that are full- or partial-thickness burns are more evident. Bowel sounds return. The patient is now aware of the enormity of body changes and the presence of pain. Healing begins when WBCs have surrounded the burn wound and phagocytosis begins. Necrotic tissue begins to slough. Fibroblasts lay down matrices of the collagen precursors that eventually form granulation tissue. Kept free from infection, a partial-thickness burn wound will heal from the edges and from below; however, full-thickness burn wounds, unless extremely small, must be covered by skin grafts. Often, healing time and length of hospitalization are decreased by early excision and grafting.

Clinical Manifestations. Full-thickness wounds will be dry and waxy white to dark brown and will have little to no sensation because nerve endings have been destroyed. Partial-thickness wounds are pink to cherry red and wet and shiny with serous exudate. These wounds may or may not have intact blisters and are painful when touched or exposed to air. With time, the margins of full-thickness eschar will begin to separate, allowing for debridement of the wound. Usually full-thickness wounds will require surgical debridement and skin grafting to speed the healing process.

Partial-thickness wounds will also form eschar but will not be as thick, so they will begin separating sooner and healing more quickly. Once partial-thickness eschar is removed, epithelialization begins at the wound margins and appears as red or pink scar tissue. The epithelial buds eventually close in the wound, and the wound heals spontaneously without surgical intervention. This is expected to occur in 10 to 14 days.

Laboratory Values. Because the body is attempting to reestablish fluid and electrolyte homeostasis in the initial acute phase, it is important to follow serum values closely.

Sodium. *Hyponatremia* can occur with silver nitrate topical antibiotic therapy as a result of sodium loss through the eschar. If hydrotherapy is too lengthy (usually longer than 20 to 30 minutes), the hypotonicity of the bath water pulls sodium from the open burn areas. Other causes of hyponatremia include excessive GI drainage, diarrhea, and excessive water intake. Symptoms of hyponatremia include weakness, dizziness, muscle cramps, fatigue, headache, tachycardia, and confusion. The burn patient may also develop a dilutional hyponatremia called *water intoxication*. To avoid this condition, the patient should drink fluids other than water, such as juices or soft drinks.

Hypernatremia may be seen after successful fluid replacement if copious amounts of hypertonic solutions were required. Other causes of hypernatremia include improper tube feeding therapy or improper fluid administration. Manifestations of hypernatremia include thirst; dried, furry tongue; lethargy; confusion; and, possibly, convulsions.

Potassium. *Hyperkalemia* is noted if the patient has renal failure, adrenocortical insufficiency, or massive deep muscle injury with large amounts of potassium released from damaged cells. Cardiac dysrhythmias and ventricular failure can occur with excessive elevations (potassium level

NURSING CARE PLAN Burn Patient

Planning: Outcome Criteria	Nursing Interventions and Rationales: Emergent Phase	Acute Phase	Rehabilitative Phase
➤ **NURSING DIAGNOSIS**	Risk for fluid volume deficit *related to* evaporative loss, plasma loss, and shift of fluid into interstitium secondary to burn injury		
Have output >30-50 ml/hr, stable vital signs, clear sensorium, sodium and potassium levels within acceptable range, systolic BP > 90 mm Hg.	Assess every 1-2 hours: pulses, BP, circulation, and sensation to all extremities; mental status; intake and output; pulmonary function *to determine status of major body systems.* Establish large-bore IV access *for initial fluid resuscitation.* Monitor weight daily *to evaluate nutritional status and determine caloric needs.* Monitor serial laboratory tests *to determine adequacy of fluid replacement.* Give fluids according to patient needs.	Use emergent phase interventions as necessary. Monitor electrolyte levels regularly. Provide oral fluids if patient is able to drink *to increase fluid intake and patient comfort.*	No intervention is required.
➤ **NURSING DIAGNOSIS**	Pain *related to* burn injury, treatments, and shearing injuries *as manifested by* demonstration of discomfort and pain		
Verbalize satisfaction with level of pain control. Demonstrate tolerable level of pain.	Administer IV analgesia as needed *to keep pain at a tolerable level.* Keep patient warm *to promote comfort and prevent energy use caused by shivering.* Elevate burned arms on pillows. Administer medication for pain 30 min before interventions *to relax patient and make planned intervention more tolerable.* Evaluate effectiveness of medication. Provide emotional support. Reposition patient carefully using lifting sheet as necessary *to avoid further damage to skin and minimize pain.*	Plan adequate rest periods *to facilitate coping abilities and to foster healing.* Administer medication before interventions. Plan diversional activities *to distract patient from present situation.*	Be aware that patient's pain is replaced by itchiness. Keep skin lubricated with water-based moisturizers *to prevent drying and increase in itching.* Teach patient to watch for injuries to new skin.

continued

NURSING CARE PLAN Burn Patient—cont'd

Planning: Outcome Criteria	Nursing Interventions and Rationales: Emergent Phase	Acute Phase	Rehabilitative Phase
➤ NURSING DIAGNOSIS Total self-care deficit *related to* pain, immobility, and perceived helplessness *as manifested by* inability or unwillingness to participate in self-care			
Exhibit optimal performance of self-care.	Assess patient's ability to perform self-care activities *to plan appropriate interventions.* Assist or intervene as appropriate. Assist patient in remaining in emotional control *to reduce feelings of helplessness.*	Increase patient's self-care activities as appropriate. Ensure that patient participates in planning care as able *to increase sense of control and to be certain that patient preferences are considered.*	Assess and arrange for needed adaptations in living arrangements and lifestyle *to accommodate optimal self-care.*
➤ NURSING DIAGNOSIS Impaired physical mobility *related to* joint contractures secondary to pain and immobility *as manifested by* difficulty in performing active ROM, pain on movement; assumption of position of comfort that may be dysfunctional; reluctance to ambulate and participate in self-care; fear of activities that involve joint movement			
Have maximum potential ROM of all extremities, absence of contractures.	Initiate and encourage passive and active ROM during hydrotherapy and during waking hours *to prevent or minimize contractures and muscle atrophy.* Maintain neck, arms, legs in extension positions. Keep hands in functional position. Help patient to ambulate as tolerated.	Increase mobility and activity as tolerated *to reduce the possibility of mobility problems.* Teach ways to avoid contractures. Have patient assume as much self-care as possible *to exercise extremities and reduce feelings of helplessness.* Use anticipatory guidance and teaching *to alleviate anxiety.*	Plan daily program with patient and appropriate resources *to provide continuing activity program as needed.*
➤ NURSING DIAGNOSIS Altered nutrition: less than body requirements *related to* increased caloric demands and inability to ingest increased requirements *as manifested by* weight loss, low serum albumin level, inability or unwillingness to ingest food			
Maintain a positive nitrogen balance, have weight loss not >10% of preburn body weight.	Chart caloric intake *to monitor adequacy of diet.* Maintain patient NPO with nasogastric tube to low intermittent suction *to allow for decompression of the stomach secondary to ileus.* Assess return of bowel sounds *to determine when oral intake can be resumed.* Initiate and monitor hyperalimentation and IV fluid replacement. Institute progressive diet *to meet nutritional needs if bowel sounds are present.*	Continue to monitor peristalsis. Offer high-protein, high-carbohydrate diet *to meet increased nutritional needs and prevent malnutrition.* Assess patient food preferences and offer favored food when patient is able to eat. Encourage family to bring food from home when appropriate. Titrate tube feedings to patient tolerance *to prevent diarrhea.*	Continue to meet nutritional needs. Once skin coverage is achieved, reduce calories *to prevent excess weight gain (if necessary).*

continued

NURSING CARE PLAN Burn Patient—cont'd

Planning: Outcome Criteria	Nursing Interventions and Rationales: Emergent Phase	Acute Phase	Rehabilitative Phase
➤ **NURSING DIAGNOSIS** Risk for infection *related to* impaired skin integrity, endogenous flora, and suppressed immune response			
Have wound free of debris and loose necrotic tissue, minimum infection, rapid infection control.	Use good hand-washing technique. Use sterile technique during topical antibiotic application and dressing changes *to prevent contaminating burn area.* Ensure that hydrotherapy and debridement last for no longer than 30 min per session *to reduce loss of electrolytes, chilling and cross-contamination.* Shave appropriate areas *to remove possibility of contamination.* Evacuate blisters and remove devitalized tissue *to eliminate medium for bacterial growth.* Cleanse area around eyes with normal saline solution (if burned). Apply topical antibiotic or sterile dressings as indicated; start systemic antibiotics IV (if indicated) *to decrease probability of infection.* Give tetanus vaccine if necessary. Observe wound daily for separation of eschar; check wound margins for cellulitis *so treatment can be initiated early.* Monitor VS and temperature.	Monitor burn wound margins *to detect signs of infection* such as purulent drainage, edema, redness. Note any change in behavior or sensorium *as a possible precursor to sepsis.* Perform hydrotherapy and debridement carefully. Monitor body temperature, WBC counts, and urine output *to detect signs of sepsis.* Monitor donor sites *to detect possible infection.*	Instruct patient and family about signs and symptoms of infection *so early treatment can be initiated.* Teach family how to perform dressing changes *to ensure proper technique and increase their sense of control.*

continued

>7 mEq/L [7 mmol/L]). Muscle weakness and electrocardiographic changes are observed clinically (see Chapter 13).

Hypokalemia is observed with silver nitrate therapy and lengthy hydrotherapy. Other causes of this deficit include vomiting, diarrhea, prolonged GI suction, and prolonged IV therapy without potassium supplementation. Constant potassium losses occur through the burn wound.

Complications

Infection. The course of recovery from major burn injury is seldom smooth. The body's first line of defense, the skin, has been destroyed by burn injury. Pathogens often proliferate before phagocytosis has begun. The media for pathogenic growth are favorable. If bacterial density at the junction of the eschar with underlying viable tissue rises to greater than 10^5/g, the patient has a wound infection. In the presence of an infection, localized inflammation, induration, and suppuration will be seen at the burn wound margins. Partial-thickness burns can convert to full-thickness burns in the presence of infection. A histologic examination of a burn-wound biopsy is the most reliable means of differentiating colonization of nonviable tissue from invasive infection of viable tissue.

NURSING CARE PLAN Burn Patient—cont'd

Planning: Outcome Criteria	Nursing Interventions and Rationales: Emergent Phase	Acute Phase	Rehabilitative Phase
➤ NURSING DIAGNOSIS Anxiety *related to* pain, separation from family, guilt associated with injury, lack of knowledge about treatment and outcome, financial needs, and appearance *as manifested by* questions about treatment and prognosis, withdrawn or overtly angry behavior, expression of concerns about scarring			
Verbalize reduction of anxiety, have body language indicating rest and comfort; verbalize change in self-image.	Administer and evaluate effectiveness of medication for pain before interventions. Encourage family visits and participation in care *to increase feelings of support.* Be open to patient's expressions of feelings about burn event *so patient has opportunity to vent feelings and discuss situation freely.* Provide information or explanation as assessment indicates *because a well-informed patient is able to make better decisions about care.* Describe burn process, signs and symptoms to patient and family on admission. Explain therapeutic interventions, precautionary measures, gowning, hand washing, and visiting policy on admission *to elicit cooperation and decrease anxiety.*	Assist patient and family in setting realistic expectations of near and distant future *as anticipatory guidance decreases anxiety and inaccurate perceptions.*	Provide avenues for patient and family to maintain contact with hospital personnel after discharge *to promote continuity of care and minimize anxiety.* Consider referral to support group. Plan counselling if needed.
➤ NURSING DIAGNOSIS Grieving (family, individual) *related to* change in body image, actual or perceived impact of injury on lifestyle, role relationships, and occupation *as manifested by* crying, withdrawal, unwillingness to look at self or participate in self-care, expression of concern about impact of injury on lifestyle			
Verbalize realistic goals regarding future lifestyle, accept altered body image.	Reassure patient and family that swelling will subside in 2-4 days *so patient realizes that it is not permanent.*	Plan for family interaction *to foster feeling of support and reduce sense of isolation.* Assist patient to progress through stages of grief and acceptance at own pace *because people differ widely in their grief timetable.* Be realistic and positive during interventions. Set goals within limitations *so patient can feel a sense of accomplishment when a goal is achieved and progress can be documented.*	Assess need for and provide means of professional counselling (psychologic and vocational) if appropriate *to reduce impact of the burn event on the patient's life.* Reassure patient that appearance of burn wounds will continue to improve even after healing has taken place.

BP, Blood pressure; *IV,* intravenous; *NPO,* nothing by mouth; *ROM,* range of motion; *VS,* vital signs; *WBCs,* white blood cells.

Wound infection may progress to transient bacteremia from wound manipulation (e.g., after debridement and hydrotherapy). The patient may develop an invasive infection or sepsis. Manifestations of sepsis include an elevated temperature, increased pulse and respiratory rate, decreased BP, and decreased urine output. There may be mild confusion, chills, malaise, and loss of appetite. The WBC count will usually be between 10,000 (10×10^9/L) and 20,000/μl (20×10^9/L). There are functional defects in the WBCs, and the patient remains immunosuppressed for a period after the burn injury. The causative organisms of sepsis are usually gram-negative bacteria (e.g., *Pseudomonas, Proteus* organisms), putting the patient at further risk for septic shock.

When sepsis is suspected, cultures should be obtained immediately from all possible sources: urine, oropharynx, IV site, and wound. However, treatment should not be delayed pending results of the culture and sensitivity studies. Therapy will begin with antibiotics appropriate for the usual residual flora of the particular burn center. The topical antibiotic that is used may be continued or may be changed to another agent. At this stage, the patient's condition is critical, requiring close monitoring of vital signs.

Cardiovascular and respiratory systems. The same cardiovascular and respiratory system complications may be present in the acute phase as in the emergent phase.

Neurologic system. Neurologically, the patient usually has no physically based problems unless severe hypoxia from respiratory injuries or complications from electrical injuries occur. However, a poorly understood phenomenon is likely to be seen. The patient can become extremely disoriented, may withdraw or become combative, and has hallucinations and frequent nightmarelike episodes. Delirium is more acute at night and occurs more often in the older patient. This is a transient state lasting from a day or two to several weeks. Various causes have been considered, including electrolyte imbalance, massive stress, cerebral edema, sepsis, and intensive care unit (ICU) psychosis syndrome.

Musculoskeletal system. The musculoskeletal system takes center stage for complications during the acute phase. As the burns begin to heal and scar tissue forms, the skin is less supple and pliant. ROM may be limited, and contractures can occur. Rigorous physical therapy is imperative to maintain optimal joint function. A good time for exercise is during and after hydrotherapy when the skin is softer. Passive and active ROM should be performed on all joints. The patient with neck burns should sleep without pillows or with the head hanging slightly over the top of the mattress to encourage hyperextension. Splints should be used to keep joints in functional positions.

Gastrointestinal system. The GI system also exhibits complications. Adynamic ileus results from sepsis. However, diarrhea is more commonly present than ileus and can be caused by the use of supplemental feedings or antibiotics. Constipation can occur as a side effect of narcotic analgesics and decreased mobility. *Curling's ulcer*, a type of gastroduodenal ulcer characterized by diffuse superficial lesions including mucosal erosion, is caused by a generalized stress response resulting in decreased production of mucus and increased gastric acid secretion. The best treatment for Curling's ulcer is the prophylactic use of antacids and cimetidine (Tagamet), which prevents histamine stimulation of hydrochloride (HCL) secretion. Many major burn patients also have occult blood in their stools during the acute phase.

Endocrine system. *Stress diabetes* may be seen transiently because of stress-mediated cortisol and catecholamine release resulting in increased mobilization of glycogen stores and subsequent conversion to glucose. There is also an increase in insulin production and release. However, insulin's effectiveness is decreased, leading to an elevated blood glucose level. Later, hyperglycemia can be caused by the supranormal caloric intake necessary to meet the metabolic requirements. When this occurs, the treatment is supplemental insulin, not decreased feeding. Serum glucose is checked frequently and an appropriate amount of insulin is given if hyperglycemia is present. Glucometers may also be used to assess blood glucose; serum glucose samples are more accurate than glucometers. As the patient's metabolic demands are met and less stress is placed on the entire system, this stress-induced condition is reversed.

Therapeutic Management. The four predominant therapeutic interventions in the acute phase are fluid replacement, wound care, early excision and grafting, and ROM exercises.

Fluid replacement. Fluid replacement continues from the emergent phase into the acute phase on the basis of patient needs. IV therapy is provided to replace fluid losses, administer medications, and administer transfusions. The type of fluid replacement depends on the patient's specific needs. Common types of replacement are normal saline solution, Ringer's lactate solution, and various concentrations of glucose in saline solution or water. Packed RBCs, fresh frozen plasma, and Plasmanate are also commonly given at this time.

Wound care. Wound care consists of daily observation, assessment, and debridement. Wound care is usually done by nursing staff and involves active debridement of the wound with forceps and scissors. If the eschar is thick and hard as in full-thickness burns, a grid escharotomy may be necessary. This procedure involves cross-hatching the eschar. This is painless for the patient because nerve endings have been damaged by the burning process. The grid eschar allows more of the burn surface to be "an edge," thus promoting eschar separation from viable tissue. A grid eschar has been less commonly performed in recent years because the preferred treatment is early excision of the eschar.

Excision and grafting. Current therapeutic management of burn wounds involves early removal of the necrotic tissue followed by application of split-thickness autograft skin. This therapy has changed the management and mortality of the burn patient in the past 10 years. In the past, major burn patients had low rates of survival because healing and wound coverage took so long that the patient usually succumbed first to infection or malnutrition. Now, mortality rates can be greatly reduced and morbidity can be decreased by early intervention. Candidates for early excision and grafting are those with stable cardiovascular systems after initial fluid resuscitation.

During the procedure of excision and grafting, eschar is removed down to subcutaneous tissue or fascia, depending on the degree of injury. The graft must be placed on clean, viable tissue to achieve good adherence. Hemostasis is achieved by pressure and application of topical thrombin or epinephrine, after which the wound is covered with autograft skin (Table 21-13). With early excision, function is restored and scar tissue formation is minimized. Because the dead tissue is planed off until viable tissue is reached, extensive bleeding is expected to occur, which may pose a problem when grafting is performed. Clots between the graft and the wound keep the graft from adhering to the wound. One method of managing the clotting problem is to excise the wound on one day and to graft it on the next day. The excised wounds are soaked every 4 hours with an antibiotic solution between the surgeries. This will also ensure that the wound has been excised to viable tissue, because it can be visualized with a clear field to check the depth.

Donor skin is taken from the patient for grafting by means of a dermatome, which removes a thin layer (split-thickness) of skin from an unburned site (Fig. 21-12). The donor skin can be meshed to allow for greater wound coverage, or it may be applied as a sheet graft for a better cosmetic result in grafting of face, neck, and hands.

Cultured epithelial autografts. In the patient with large body surface area burns, limited unburned skin may be available as a donor site for grafting, and available skin may also be unsuitable for harvesting. In the past few years, cultured epithelial autograft (CEA) has become available to burn centers in the United States, Canada, South America, and Europe. CEA is grown from biopsies obtained from the patient's own skin. The initial step in this process involves taking one to two small (2 to 3 cm long by 1 cm wide) biopsy specimens from unburned skin (usually the groin or axilla). This procedure is performed as soon as possible after the patient has been identified as a candidate for this type of grafting, and it can usually be done at the bedside while the patient is under local anesthesia. The specimen is sent to a commercial laboratory where the skin biopsy specimens are disaggregated into single cells and are subsequently cultivated in a culture medium that contains epidermal growth factor. During the following 18 to 25 days the originally cultivated keratinocytes expand up to 10,000 times until they form confluent sheets that can be used as skin grafts. The cultured grafts are returned to the burn center where they are grafted on the patient's excised burn wounds.

CEA grafts generate permanent skin coverage as they originate from the patient's own cells. CEA is applied surgically utilizing the same procedure as with split-thickness autograft. CEA grafts generally form a seamless, smooth replacement skin tissue (Fig. 21-13) and have played an important role in the survival of the patient with major burns with limited skin for donor harvesting. In 24 days, enough CEA can be generated to cover the entire body surface.[14]

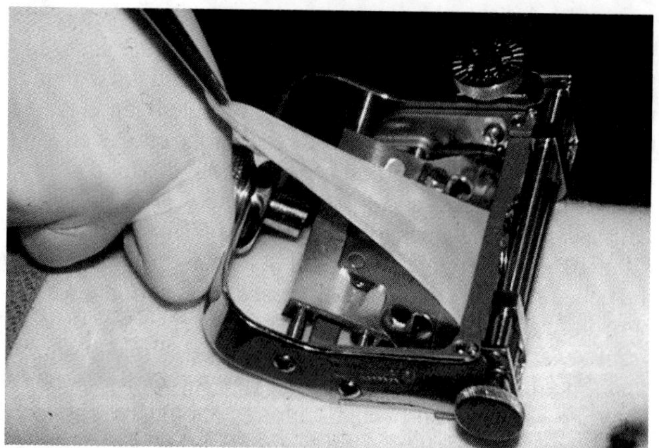
A

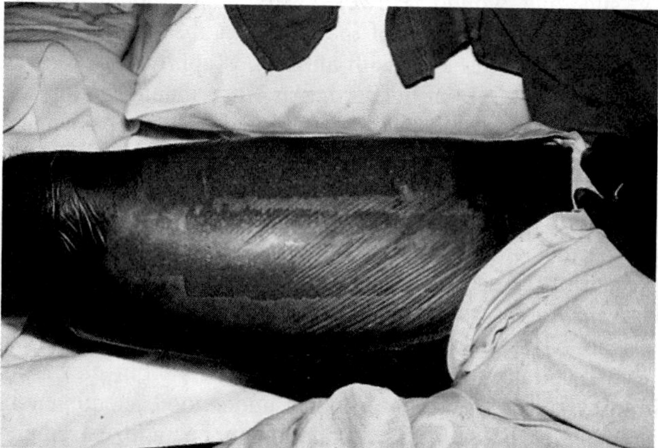
B

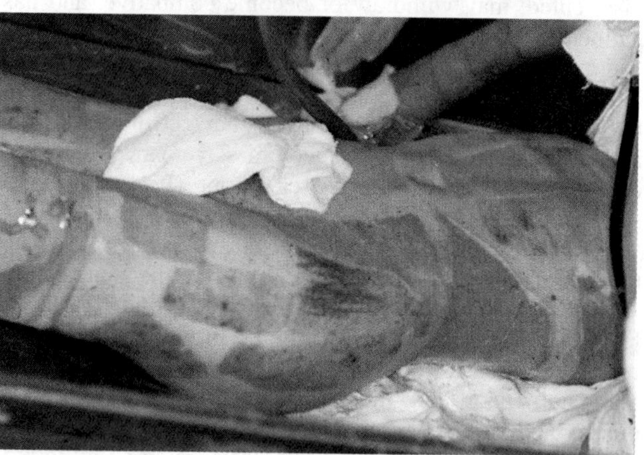
C

Fig. 21-12 ***A,*** The surgeon harvests skin from a patient's thigh using a dermatome. ***B,*** Appearance of donor site after harvesting split thickness skin graft. Donor site is covered with a transparent occlusive dressing. ***C,*** Healed donor site.

Nutritional Management. The goals of nutritional management of the burn patient during the acute phase are to minimize energy demands and provide adequate calories to promote healing.

The burn patient is in a hypermetabolic and highly catabolic state as a result of the burn injury. Decreasing catecholamine release by minimizing pain, fear, anxiety,

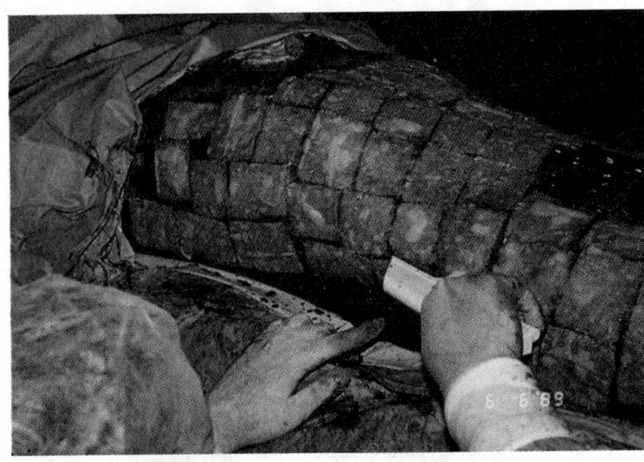

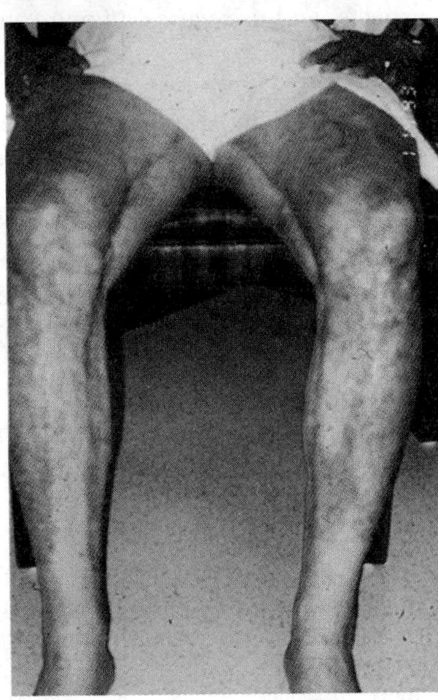

Fig. 21-13 Patient with cultured epithelial autograft. ***A,*** Intraoperative application of cultured epithelial autograft. ***B,*** Appearance of healed cultured epithelial autograft.

and cold can maximize patient comfort and conserve energy. Infection also consumes a great deal of energy.

Daily caloric intake is crucial. Estimated caloric needs for 24 hours for the adult with burns of greater than 20% TBSA can be calculated by the following formula:

(25 kcal × kg of body weight) + (40 kcal × % TBSA burn)

Caloric needs are often 5000 kcal a day. By the end of the first week after burn injury, the patient's caloric and nutritional requirements should be met. The patient should be encourged to eat high-protein, high-carbohydrate foods to meet increased caloric needs. Ideally the patient should not lose more than 10% of preburn weight. Caloric requirements should be recalculated at least biweekly to prevent overfeeding and subsequent weight gain.

Optimally the patient should take a normal diet by mouth as soon as bowel function returns. If this is not possible, a feeding tube can be placed and a complete liquid diet administered. Diet supplements can be given by mouth or IV in the form of total parenteral nutrition (see Chapter 37).

If family members wish to bring in the patient's favorite foods, this should be encouraged. Appetite is usually diminished, and constant encouragement may be necessary to achieve adequate intake.

NURSING MANAGEMENT

ACUTE PHASE

During this phase, wound care consumes most of the nursing care hours. Yet this should not negate the importance of supportive care, comfort and hygiene measures, and physical therapy.

Pain Assessment and Management

One of the most critical functions a nurse performs during this phase is pain assessment and management. It becomes difficult in burn nursing to separate empathy from sympathy and to act appropriately when the patient is so vulnerable and ill. Almost every intervention that is performed for the patient causes pain. The patient may experience rare moments of relative comfort, but the patient knows that these moments will not last. The nurse must understand the physiologic as well as the psychologic bases of pain (see Chapter 6). Allowing the patient to ventilate feelings of anger, hostility, and frustration serves to assist the patient in expression of the pain.

There are several interventions that the nurse may try to help the patient deal with pain.[15] These interventions can also help the nurse cope with interventions that cause pain. First, it is helpful to get an order for a dosage range of a narcotic (e.g., morphine sulfate 5 to 10 mg IV every 1 to 3 hours for pain). When the order is written this way, it allows the nurse some freedom to try medicating the patient according to responses to the medication. That is, the nurse may find that giving morphine 5 mg every hour works better than giving 10 mg every 3 hours. This method should include the patient's input if alert and also gives the patient some control over the pain. If the patient is unable to participate, the nurse will have to assess response to medication by physiologic parameters (i.e., heart rate, BP, and respiratory rate).

The second intervention is the use of several drugs in combination. This includes the use of morphine with haloperidol (Haldol), diazepam (Valium), or midazolam (Versed). The effect of midazolam is short-term memory loss, so if it is given 15 to 20 minutes before a dressing change, the patient will not recall the event. Midazolam lasts about 30 to 60 minutes after it is administered. Buprenorphine (Buprenex) is another drug that has come into use recently. The mechanism of action is not entirely understood, but it is proposed that it exerts its analgesic effect via high-affinity binding to opiate receptors in the central nervous system (CNS). It is a narcotic antagonist so it cannot be used in combination with other narcotic analgesics. Buprenorphine may work well for the patient who does not obtain relief even with high doses of narcotics.

A third method of managing pain is an alternative manner in which the nurse and patient work together to find a way to cope with pain. It involves the use of relaxation tapes, visualization, guided imagery, biofeedback, and meditation. These techniques are used as adjuncts to traditional narcotic treatment of pain. They are not meant to be used exclusively to control pain in the burn patient.

The nurse works with the patient to identify the best strategy to manage the pain using one or more of these techniques. Visualization and guided imagery can be helpful to the nurse as well as the patient. These two techniques can take several forms but the easiest method is for the nurse to ask questions about a favorite hobby or recent vacation destinations. The nurse can then explore these areas further by asking questions that make the patient visualize and describe a favorite hobby or most recent vacation. When using this method, both the nurse and the patient have to think of other things besides the task at hand (e.g., a dressing change) to keep the conversation flowing. It is up to the nurse to maintain the exchange. Relaxation tapes can also be helpful, especially when played at night to help the patient fall asleep. The use of these techniques involves a close nurse-patient relationship and can leave both with a sense of accomplishment.

The most important point to remember about pain management is that the more control that the patient has in managing pain, the more successful it will be. There has been a recent trend toward the use of patient-controlled analgesic (PCA) pumps. An IV solution is made up to contain a certain dose of a narcotic per milliliter (e.g., morphine 2 mg/ml). The patient has a control that can be operated to deliver a preset dose of the IV narcotic. The machine is locked into this dose, so there is no possibility of the patient getting more than what is prescribed. Results of this method are promising and may be a way in which burn centers can help to manage pain in their patients. (PCA is discussed in Chapters 6 and 16.)

Wound Care

Debridement, dressing changes, topical antibiotic therapy, graft care, and donor site care are done 2 to 3 times daily. Appropriate coverage of the graft (if it is not kept open to air) should include fine-mesh gauze in closest proximity to the graft before other dressings are applied. Xeroform dressing, a fine mesh, absorbent gauze impregnated with 3% bismuth tribromophenate, may be used over grafted areas. It has a petrolatum base that keeps the gauze from adhering to graft sites, and it also has mild antibacterial properties.

Sheet skin grafts must be free of serous collections or blebs. Blebs prevent the graft from interfacing and growing to the wound itself. Evacuation of blebs is done by aspiration with a tuberculin syringe or by pricking or cutting the peripheral margin of the bleb and rolling (with a sterile swab) the fluid from the center of the bleb to the exit site. The bleb should never be rolled to the edge of the graft. This only serves to separate adherent graft from the wound.

Donor site care methods have been controversial throughout the years. While the majority of burn centers continue to utilize heat lamp treatments with a xeroform-covered donor site to facilitate drying, many new methods are being evaluated across the country. The average healing time for a donor site is 10 to 14 days. Several of the newer methods potentially can decrease this healing time, which would facilitate earlier reharvesting of skin at the site. One new method of treatment is to cover the xeroform donor site with bacitracin ointment 24 hours postoperatively. This is then covered with a bulky dressing that is changed twice daily, allowing for a moist environment with some topical antibiotic coverage.

Some centers are using a transparent dressing that adheres to the periphery of the donor site. This permits an occlusive, yet visible wound. Pigskin, Silvadene, and calcium alginate dressings are also being used with varying degrees of success. Each donor site dressing has specific nursing care aspects, and use varies among centers.

Emotional Support

Because the nurse has the most prolonged contact with the patient and family, it is natural for the nurse to be seen as an important source of emotional support. The nurse must assist the patient in maintaining personal worth and reestablishing a satisfactory body image. The nurse must have an almost unlimited supply of patience and understanding. Often the health care worker is the target for anger and hostility from the patient who has no other focus or method of expressing these feelings.

Working with the family can be a challenge for the nurse. Family members need to see the importance of reestablishment of a patient's independence. Family members will be confused by all the changes they see in the various burn phases. It is helpful for the family to view the burned areas frequently so that they can see the progress of healing. The nurse should involve the family as team members during the patient's hospitalization.

The stress of the burn injury occasionally precipitates a psychiatric crisis. Treatment by a psychiatrist who can prescribe psychotropic drugs is indicated when this occurs. Early psychiatric intervention is also crucial if the patient has been previously treated for a psychiatric disorder or if the burn injury was the result of a suicide attempt.

The diagnosis of posttraumatic stress disorder is being made with increasing frequency in the burn patient. It is felt that early intervention by appropriate professionals is associated with improved outcomes. (See research box on p. 551.)

Rehabilitation Phase

The *rehabilitation phase* is defined as beginning when the patient's burn wound is covered with skin or healed and the patient is capable of assuming some self-care activity. This can occur as early as 2 weeks to as long as 2 or 3 months after the burn injury. Goals for this period are to assist the patient in resuming a functional role in society and to accomplish functional and cosmetic reconstruction.

Pathophysiologic Changes and Clinical Manifestations. The burn wound heals either by primary intention or by grafting. Layers of epithelialization begin rebuilding the tissue structure destroyed by the burn injury. Collagen fibers present in the new scar tissue help healing

RESEARCH

Implications for Nursing Practice

HOPE IN PATIENT WITH CRITICAL BURN INJURIES

Citation Anderson FD, Maloney JP, Redland AR: Study of hope in patients with critical burn injuries, *J Burn Care Rehab* 14:207-214, 1993.

Purpose To determine factors that affect feelings of hope in patients with critical burn injuries

Methods This qualitative study involved a convenience sample of nine male patients with burn injuries ranging from 23-70% of total body surface area. Audiotaped, semistructured interviews using open-ended questions were conducted. Content analysis technique was used to determine the nursing behaviors that influenced the patients' level of hope. In this study, hope was viewed as a dynamic process with past, present, and future dimensions.

Results and Conclusions The majority of factors that patients identified as affecting their levels of hope evolved from the present dimension. The factors that affected each patient's level of hope were contingent upon where the patient was in the psychologic recovery process that occurs after burn injury. The effectiveness of nursing actions is contingent upon consideration of where the patient is in this recovery process.

Implications for Nursing Practice The caregiver needs to assess feelings about the amount of hope that is appropriate for any given patient. A thorough nursing assessment that is relevant to the patient's hope structure should be made. Outcome criteria for the evaluation of the therapeutic support of hope should be developed on an individual basis.

and add strength to weakened areas. After healing, the new skin appears flat and pink. In approximately 4 to 6 weeks the area becomes raised and hyperemic. If adequate ROM is not instituted, the new tissue will shorten, causing contracture. Mature healing is reached in 6 months to 1 year when suppleness has returned and the pink or red color has faded to a slightly lighter hue than the surrounding unburned tissue. It takes longer for more heavily pigmented skin to regain its dark color because many of the melanocytes are destroyed. Often skin never regains its original color.

Scarring has two components: discoloration and contour. The discoloration of scars fades with time. However, scar tissue tends to develop altered contours; that is, it is no longer flat or slightly raised but becomes elevated and enlarged above the original burn injury area. Pressure can help to keep a scar flat. Gentle capillary pressure is maintained on the healed burn with pressure garments. These garments are worn up to 24 hours a day for as long as 1 year after burn injury. They may be removed for short periods while bathing.

The patient will experience discomfort from itching where healing is occurring. Nivea or similar lotions and diphenhydramine (Benadryl) serve to ease the itching. As "old" epithelium is replaced by new cells, flaking will occur. The newly formed skin is extremely sensitive to trauma. Blisters are likely to form from slight pressure or friction. Additionally, these newly healed areas can be hypersensitive or hyposensitive to cold, heat, and touch. Grafted areas are more likely to be hyposensitive until peripheral nerve regeneration occurs. Healed burn areas must be protected from direct sunlight for 1 year to prevent hyperpigmentation and sunburn injury.

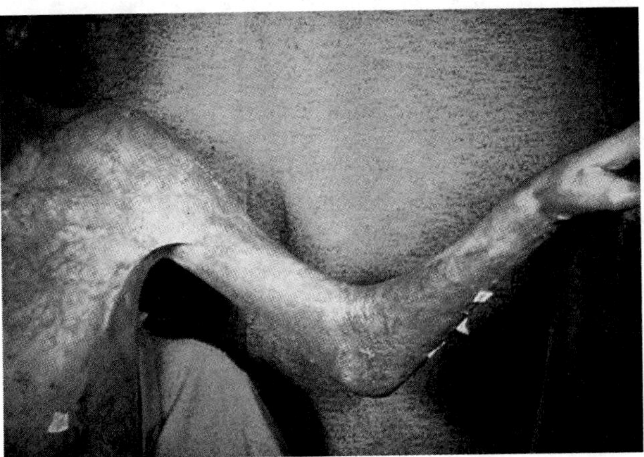

Fig. 21-14 Contracture of axilla.

Complications. The most common complications of burn injury are skin and joint contractures and hypertrophic scarring (Fig. 21-14). Because of pain, the patient will prefer to assume a flexed position for comfort. This position predisposes the wounds to contracture formation. Positioning, splinting, and exercise should be instituted on admission to minimize this complication. These procedures should be continued until the skin matures.

Areas that are most susceptible to contracture formation include the anterior and lateral neck areas, axillae, antecubital fossae, fingers, groin areas, popliteal fossae, and ankles. These areas encompass major joints. Not only does the skin over these areas develop contractures, but the underlying tissues such as the ligaments and tendons also have a tendency to shorten in the healing process. Therapy is aimed at extension of body parts because the flexors are stronger than the extensors. Legs should be wrapped before ambulation after grafting and donor site healing. This pressure prevents blister formation and promotes venous return. Once the skin is completely healed, pressure garments can replace leg wraps to grafted areas.

THERAPEUTIC AND NURSING MANAGEMENT

REHABILITATION PHASE

Members of the health care team share responsibility for assisting the patient to return to optimal function during the rehabilitation phase. Because of the severe psychologic impact of burn injury, health care providers must be sensitive and attuned to the patient's feelings. They must assist the patient to adjust emotionally by encouraging them to ventilate their fears regarding loss of function, deformity, disfigurement, and financial burdens. Care should also be taken to address individual spiritual and ethnic needs. Having expressed these fears, the patient can then be assisted in a realistic appraisal of the particular situations, emphasizing what they *can* do, not what they *cannot* do. An individual's self-esteem is usually adversely affected by a burn injury. In some an overwhelming fear may be the loss of relationships because of perceived or actual physical disfigurement. In a society that values physical beauty, alterations in body image commonly result in psychologic distress. Allowing appropriate independence and encouraging the patient to assist in the care of others with burn trauma will involve the patient in activities that may help to restore self-esteem. Counseling continues after the patient goes home. The patient needs reassurance that the feelings during this period of adjustment are normal and that frustration is to be expected as they attempt to resume the normal lifestyles.

During the rehabilitation phase, both patient and family are actively learning how to care for the healing wounds. Because the patient may go home with unhealed open areas, instruction will be needed in dressing changes and wound care. An emollient cream (e.g., Nivea) should be used routinely on healed areas to keep the skin supple and to decrease itching and flaking. The patient and family will need anticipatory guidance to know what to expect physiologically as well as psychologically during recovery.

Cosmetic or reconstructive surgery is often needed for major burns. It is important that the patient understand the need for or possibility of reconstructive surgery before leaving the hospital.

The role of exercise and appropriate physical therapy cannot be overemphasized. The progression of physical therapy from hydrotherapy to passive ROM, active ROM, stretching, ambulation, and ultimate restoration of function is a lengthy and painful process that lasts for at least 1 year after burn injury. Constant encouragement and reassurance are necessary to maintain a patient's morale. The patient soon regards physical therapy as an integral part of treatment.

Nutritional Management

By this time in the patient's recovery, the negative nitrogen balance should have been corrected. However, it is still important to maintain a high-calorie, high-protein diet. The problem with anorexia decreases at this time. As the oral intake increases, tube feedings are gradually tapered and discontinued. The patient with a functional problem associated with eating (especially burn injury to the hands) may need assistance from occupational therapy to obtain devices to correct or lessen the problem. Often all that is necessary is padding the handle of a fork or spoon with several layers of gauze so that a better grip is established.

Toward the end of hospitalization, the patient occasionally needs assistance from a dietitian. Because they have been encouraged to eat during the lengthy wound healing period, some patients may have difficulty controlling their appetite and avoiding unwanted weight gain as healing approaches completion.

Gerontologic Considerations

The older patient presents many challenges for the burn team. Normal aging puts the patient at risk for injury because of the possibility of an unsteady gait, failing eye sight, and diminished hearing. Once injured the older adult has more complications in the emergent and acute phases of burn resuscitation because of preexisting medical conditions that may be present. For example, an older patient with diabetes, congestive heart failure, and chronic obstructive pulmonary disease will have morbidity and mortality rates exceeding a healthy younger patient. In the older patient, pneumonia is a frequent complication, wounds take longer to heal, and surgical procedures are less well tolerated. Because of all of these problems, strategies to prevent burn injuries are especially important in this population.

EMOTIONAL NEEDS OF THE PATIENT AND FAMILY

Because of the suddenness and severity of burn trauma, the patient and family are plunged into physical and emotional crises.[16] The health care provider must be prepared to assess psychoemotional cues and provide appropriate intervention throughout the course of recovery.

The patient may experience thoughts and feelings that are frightening and disturbing, such as guilt about the burn accident, reliving the experience, fear of death, and concern about future therapy and the concomitant pain. Families may share any or all of these feelings. At times, family members will feel helpless when trying to assist their loved ones. During this period of adjustment, the nurse should provide time for the patient and the families to be alone. Family members may also be encouraged to assist with position changes and eating.

For the nurse to adequately deal with the enormous range of emotional responses that the burn patient may exhibit, it is important to have an understanding of the circumstances of the burn, past family interactions, and past coping experiences with stressful stimuli. At any time the various emotional responses of fear, anxiety, anger, guilt, and depression may be experienced (Table 21-16).

A common emotional response is *regression*. The patient will revert to behavior that helped in coping with stressful situations in the past. Frank psychosis can also be observed. Unless the patient had a psychiatric condition before the burn injury, this psychosis is usually transient. Major emotional tasks confront the patient and the families. As more and more independence is expected from the patients, new fears must be confronted: "Can I do it?" "Am I a desirable partner, parent?" Open communication must exist in the patient's environment during this phase of recovery.

Therapeutic intervention for the patient at this point does not necessarily require the involvement of a psychiatrist. Nurses, physicians, social workers, or anyone else who has a rapport with the patient and a good understanding of personal feelings in such situations can be therapeutic. The patient can best convey some of these negative but normal emotions to a health care provider with whom the patient can communicate. Acknowledgment that the feelings are real and valid can do much to help the patient. The nurse

Table 21-16 Emotional Responses of Burn Patients

Emotion	Possible Verbal Expression
Fear	Will I die? What will happen next? Will I be disfigured? Will my spouse or friend still love me?
Anxiety	I feel out of control. What's happening to me? When will it end?
Anger	Why did this happen to me? Those nurses enjoy hurting me.
Guilt	If only I'd been more careful. I was punished because I was bad.
Depression	It's no use going on like this. I don't care what happens to me. I wish people would leave me alone.

should not belittle or scorn a patient's regression but should be firm and consistent in assisting the patient to cope.

The difficult issue of *sexuality* must be met with honesty. Physical appearance will be altered in the patient who has sustained a major burn. Acceptance of this alteration is difficult at first for the patient and family. The nature of skin injury in itself causes modifications in processing sexual stimuli. Touch is an important part of sexuality. Immature scar tissue may make the sensation of touch unpleasant or may dull it. This is usually transient, but the patient and family need to know that it is normal and receive anticipatory guidance from health care personnel to avoid undue emotional strain.

Family and patient support groups may be beneficial in meeting the patient's and family's emotional needs. Speaking with others who have experienced burn trauma can be beneficial, both in terms of reaffirming that the patient is feeling normal and in allowing for the sharing of helpful advice.

SPECIAL NEEDS OF THE NURSING STAFF

A logical extension of the emotional trauma experienced by the patient includes the emotional trauma for the nurse.[17] The nurse must deal with the patient who, at times, is unpleasant and hostile and with the fact that burn therapy is almost always painful. The nurse will sometimes see many hours of patient care suddenly destroyed by sepsis and death. Because of long hospitalizations and intense contact, the relationships between the caregiver and the care receiver can result in strong bonds that can be healthy and healing or destructive and draining. The burn patient can develop demanding or punitive attitudes, which may cause the nurse to be reluctant to provide care. The nurse and patient can also develop warm, trusting, mutually satisfying relationships not only during hospitalization but also during long-term rehabilitation. Sometimes the bond can be so strong that the patient has difficulty separating from the hospital and staff. The frequency and intensity of family contact can also be rewarding as well as draining to the nurse. Newcomers to burn nursing often find it difficult to cope with not only the deformities caused by burn injury but also the odor, the unpleasant sight of the wound, and the reality of the pain that accompanies the burn.

However, many nurses believe that the care they provide makes a critical difference in helping patients to survive and cope with the severe injury. It is this belief that keeps nurses caring for burn patients and their families.

Support services for the burn nurse in the form of group meetings led by a psychiatrist, psychologist, psychiatric clinical nurse specialist, or social worker can be helpful. Such meetings help the nursing staff to cope with difficult feelings that may be experienced when caring for the burn patient. The nurse may need the opportunity to ventilate feelings of anger and hostility to an impartial listener. This therapeutic communication process may make the difference between the nurse who can deliver effective nursing care and the nurse who provides mere custodial patient care.

INNOVATIONS IN BURN RESEARCH

The burn nurse can be an active participant in research on many levels. Because the field of burn care is rapidly changing, there must be a continued awareness of new literature and treatments and a willingness to call into question practices that do not have scientific support. Multidisciplinary research is abundant in the areas of initial management, fluid resuscitation, inhalation injury, antibiotic therapy, nutrition, and pain management. Some other common areas of research involving the burn nurse and the burn patient are centered around injury prevention and nursing interventions that are the most effective means of preparing patients, families, and community nurses for posthospitalization care.[18] Grafting materials and techniques are under constant study in an attempt to find the best substitute for skin that was lost.

CRITICAL THINKING EXERCISES

CASE STUDY

SEVERE BURN PATIENT

Patient Profile

Sylvia, a 24-year-old woman, was brought to the emergency department with extensive full-thickness burns to nearly her entire body. Her gas stove exploded while she was manually lighting a burner.

Subjective Data

- Complains of feeling very cold
- Cannot remember the accident
- Is hoarse and has difficulty talking
- Expresses a great deal of fear

Objective Data

Physical Examination

- Is awake and oriented but in obvious distress
- Has dark brown, leathery burns involving entire body except feet and ankles
- Has hair and eyebrows that are singed
- Is unable to palpate peripheral pulses; apical pulse-140

Critical Thinking Questions

1. What are the first priorities in the prehospital environment? How should her airway be managed?
2. Why would Sylvia be considered at high risk for an inhalation injury?
3. What intervention should the nurse anticipate in a patient with full thickness circumferential burns to the chest and extremities?
4. Describe the rationale for Sylvia's lack of pain and her complaints of being cold. What medications might be considered to promote her comfort?
5. What fluid and electrolyte disturbances would be expected in the first 48 hours of Sylvia's hospitalization? Explain the physiologic bases for these changes.
6. What measures should be taken to support Sylvia's family?
7. Based on the assessment data presented, write one or more appropriate nursing diagnoses. Are there any collaborative problems?

NURSING RESEARCH ISSUES

1. What nursing interventions are most effective in preparing patients, families, and community nurses for the early discharge and posthospitalization phases of burn care?
2. What nursing interventions are most effective in the management of burn pain in the acute phase of recovery?
3. What nutritional supplements are best tolerated in the emergent and acute phases of burn recovery?

REVIEW QUESTIONS

The number of the question corresponds to the same-numbered objective at the beginning of the chapter.

1. Extent of electrical injury can be difficult to assess because
  a. victims are often in shock.
  b. the entry and exit wounds are deep.
  c. internal damage is not readily apparent.
  d. electrical injury is usually smaller than thermal injury.

2. Which of the following is least likely to result in a full-thickness burn injury?
  a. Scald injury
  b. Sunburn
  c. Chemical burn
  d. Electrical injury

3. A partial-thickness burn has which of the following characteristics?
  a. Red, shiny, wet appearance
  b. Generalized erythema with no vesicles
  c. Exposed fascia
  d. Dry, waxy appearance

4. The extent of burns is assessed by
  a. looking at which body parts are involved.
  b. determining preexisting risk factors.
  c. using guides to indicate burn location relative to total body surface.
  d. estimating what is a full-thickness as opposed to what is partial-thickness burn.

5. Silver sulfadiazine is an effective topical antibiotic because it
  a. is rapidly absorbed by blood.
  b. is effective against bacterial growth and has few side effects.
  c. is a carbonic anhydrase inhibitor.
  d. maintains adequate pH of the newly forming skin buds.

6. Which of the following events occurs during the early emergent phase?
  a. Large proteins adhere to vascular walls
  b. Potassium moves into the cell
  c. Sodium and water are sequestered in interstitial fluid
  d. RBCs hemolyze from large volumes of rapidly administered fluid

7. To maintain a positive nitrogen balance in a major burn, the patient must

a. eat at least 500 calories three times a day.
b. eat rice and whole wheat for the chemical effect on nitrogen balance.
c. increase normal adult caloric intake by approximately three times.
d. eat a high-protein, low-carbohydrate diet.

8. A burn patient is said to be in the rehabilitative phase when

a. the burn wound is healed or closed.
b. physical therapy is no longer needed.
c. scars have faded and skin looks normal.
d. the patient can return to work.

9. It is important for the burn patient and family to

a. see the burn wound three times a day.
b. talk frequently with the nurse about the patient's progress.
c. allow the nurse to do total care for the patient to prevent infection.
d. avoid discussion of the patient's progress to minimize false hope.

10. The burn nurse needs

a. special psychologic training.
b. to be sensitive to the needs of the patient and family.
c. much physical strength because of the patient's debilitation.
d. to hide all personal feelings from the patient and family.

11. Discharge planning begins

a. after the emergent phase.
b. after grafting.
c. at least 1 week before discharge.
d. on admission.

12. Pain management of the burn patient involves

a. giving set dosage of medications at scheduled times.
b. sympathizing with the patient.
c. using traditional and alternative methods of pain control.
d. having the nurse maintain control of the patient's medication.

REFERENCES

1. Advanced Burn Life Support Curriculum, Lincoln, NE, 1993.
2. Lightfoot H, Vukich L: Burn, electrical, and lightning injuries. In Lee G, editor: *Flight nursing: principles and practice,* St Louis, 1991, Mosby.
3. Dyer C, Roberts D: Thermal trauma, *Nurs Clin North Am* 25:85, 1990.
4. Wilding PA: Care of respiratory burns—hard work can bring spectacular results, *Prof Nurse* 5:412, 1990.
5. Advanced Trauma Life Support Curriculum, American College of Surgeons Committee on Trauma, Chicago, 1993.
6. Marvin J: Thermal injuries. In Cardona V and others, editors: *Trauma nursing: from resuscitation through rehabilitation,* Philadelphia, 1994, Saunders.
7. Robertson C, Fenton O: ABC of major trauma: management of severe burns, *Br Med J* 301:282, 1990.
8. Smith G, Savinski-Bozinko G: Giving emergency care for burns, *Nursing* 19:55, 1989.
9. Robins EV: Immunosuppression of the burned patient, *Crit Care Nurs Clin North Am* 1:767, 1989.
10. Robins EV: Burn shock, *Crit Care Nurs Clin North Am* 2:299, 1990.
11. Jarlsberg CR: Action stat! Neck and chest burns, *Nursing* 20:33, 1990.
12. Lazear SE: Tissue integrity: burns. In Neff JA, Kidd PS, editors: *Trauma nursing: the art and science,* St Louis, 1993, Mosby.
13. Bayley EW: Wound healing in the patient with burns, *Nurs Clin North Am* 25:205, 1990.
14. Siwy BK, Compton CC: Cultured epidermis: Indiana University Medical Center's experience, *J Burn Care Rehabil* 13:130, 1992.

*15. van der Does W: Pain and anxiety ratings during burn care, *Nurs Times* 86:53, 1990.

16. Roberts D, Appleton V: Psychosocial care of burn-injured patients, *Plast Surg Nurs* 9:62, 1989.

*17. Lewis KF and others: Survey of perceived stressors and coping strategies among burn unit nurses, *Burns* 16:109, 1990.

*18. Bayley EW and others: Research priorities for burn nursing: rehabilitation, discharge planning and follow-up care, *J Burn Care Rehabil* 13:471, 1992.

SECTION IV BIBLIOGRAPHY

Books

Albert DM, Jakobiec FA: *Principles and practice of ophthalmology: basic sciences,* Philadelphia, 1994, WB Saunders.

Arnold HL, Odom RB, James WD, editors: *Andrews' diseases of the skin,* ed 8, Philadelphia, 1990, WB Saunders.

Coleman WP and others: *Cosmetic skin surgery: principles and techniques,* St Louis 1990, Mosby.

Cummings CW and others: *Otolaryngology—head and neck surgery,* ed 2, St Louis, 1992, Mosby.

Davson H: *Physiology of the eye,* ed 5, New York, 1990, Pergamon Press.

DeWeese DD and others: *Otolaryngology—head and neck surgery,* ed 8, St Louis, 1994, Mosby.

Dolecek R and others, editors: *Endocrinology of thermal burns: pathophysiologic mechanisms and clinical interpretation,* Philadelphia, 1990, Lea & Febiger.

Geefand SA: *Hearing: an introduction to psychological and physiological acoustics,* ed 2, New York, 1990, Marcel Dekker.

Glasscock III ME, Jackson CG, Josey AF: *Handbook of audiology,* St Louis, 1990, Mosby.

Gold D, Weingeist TA, editors: *The eye in systemic disease,* Philadelphia, 1990, JB Lippincott.

Habif TP: *Clinical dermatology: a color guide to diagnosis and therapy,* ed 2, St Louis, 1990, Mosby.

Hart W, editor: *Adler's physiology of the eye: clinical application,* ed 9, St Louis, 1992, Mosby.

Jaffe N: *Cataract surgery and its complications,* ed 5, St Louis, 1990, Mosby.

Jordan RE, editor: *Immunologic diseases of the skin,* Norwalk, CT, 1991, Appleton & Lange.

Jurkiewicz MJ and others: *Plastic and reconstructive surgery: principles and practices,* St Louis, 1990, Mosby.

Laibson PR: *The year book of ophthalmology,* St Louis, 1993, Mosby.

Leibovic KN, ed: *Science of vision,* New York, 1990, Springer-Verlag.

Lever WF, Schaumburg G: *Histopathology of the skin,* ed 7, Philadelphia, 1990, JB Lippincott.

---

*Nursing research-based articles.

Moschella SL, Hurley H: *Dermatology,* ed 3, Philadelphia, 1992, WB Saunders.

Newell F: *Ophthalmology: principles and concepts,* ed 7, St Louis, 1992, Mosby.

Ophthalmic drug facts, St Louis, 1992, Facts and Comparisons, Inc.

Journals

Alderman C: Psoriasis: whose skin is it anyway, *Nurs Stand* 4:26, 1990.

Allen AW: Retinal surgery, *Ophthalmol Clin North Am* 7:1, 1994.

Bayley EW: Wound healing in the patient with burns, *Nurs Clin North Am* 25:205, 1990.

Brechtelsbauer DA: Adult hearing loss, *Prim Care* 17:249, 1990.

*Cobb N, Maxwell G, Silverstein P: Patient perception of quality of life after burn injury: results of an eleven-year survey, *J Burn Care Rehabil* 11:330, 1990.

DeWitt S: Nursing assessment of the skin and dermatologic lesions, *Nurs Clin North Am* 25:235, 1990.

Dolinger RD: Pressure sores and optimum skin care, *J Palliat Care* 6:50, 1990.

Edmonds SE: Resources for the visually impaired, *J Ophthalmic Nurs Technol* 9:14, 1990.

Fishbaugh J: Lessons on dilation, *Insight* 19:30, 1994.

Gallagher CM: The young adult with recent vision loss: a pilot case study, *Insight* 16:8, 1991.

Gilchrist V: Assessment and education of the diabetic with vision loss, *Insight* 18:9, 1993.

Hardy MA: A pilot study of the diagnosis and treatment of impaired skin integrity: dry skin in older persons, *Nurs Diagn* 1:57, 1990.

Hill MJ: The skin: anatomy and physiology, *Dermatol Nurs* 2:13, 1990.

Hinchcliffe S: Benign and malignant skin conditions: *Nursing* 4:28, 1990.

Hinchcliffe S: Skin lesions 2: a study involving pigmented areas, *Nursing* 4:30, 1990.

Hotter AN: Wound healing and immunocompromise, *Nurs Clin North Am* 25:193, 1990.

*Hubler J, Detrick D: Endophthalmitis: an investigational process, *Insight* 19:18, 1994.

Hunt L: Nutrients and the eye, *Insight* 19:25, 1994.

Jones PL, Millman A: Wound healing and the aged patient, *Nurs Clin North Am* 25:263, 1990.

Kee CC: Sensory impairment: factor x in providing nursing care to the older adult, *J Community Health Nurs* 7:45, 1990.

Knight DB, Scott H: Contracture and pressure necrosis, *Ostomy Wound Manage* 26:60, 1990.

McConnell EA: Clinical do's and don'ts: placing your patient in the lateral position, *Nursing* 20:65, 1990.

*McGrory A, Assmann S: A study investigating primary nursing, discharge teaching, and patient satisfaction of ambulatory cataract patients, *Insight* 19:8, 1994.

Payne RL, Martin ML: The epidemiology and management of skin tears in older adults, *Ostomy Wound Manage* 26:26, 1990.

Schremp PS, editor: Ophthalmic nursing, *Nurs Clin North Am* 27:703, 1992.

Smalley PJ: Lasers in otolaryngology, *Nurs Clin North Am* 25:645, 1990.

*Smith SC, Folk JC, Losch ME: Effects of collaborative education on patient satisfaction and knowledge, *Insight* 17:20, 1992.

*Steinberg EP and others: The VF-14: an index of functional impairment in patients with cataracts, *Arch Ophthalmol* 112:630, 1994.

Tenpas DM: Multidisciplinary team approach to skin care, *Ostomy Wound Manage* 26:50, 1990.

VanEtten NK, Sexton P, Smith R: Development and implementation of a skin care program, *Ostomy Wound Manage* 27:40, 1990.

Ward RS and others: Prosthetic use in patients with burns and associated limb amputations, *J Burn Care Rehabil* 11:361, 1990.

*Nursing research-based articles.

Organizations

American Academy of Facial, Plastic and Reconstructive Surgery
1110 Vermont Avenue, NW
Washington, DC 20005

American Association of Tissue Banks (AATB)
1350 Beverly Road, Suite 220-A
McLean VA 22101

American Burn Association
c/o Cleon W. Goodwin, M.D., Secretary
New York Hospital-Cornell Medical Center
525 East 68th Street, Room L706
New York, NY 10021

American Council of the Blind
1010 Vermont Avenue NW, Suite 1100
Washington, DC 20005

American Diabetes Association National Service Center
1660 Duke Street
Alexandria, VA 22314

The American Foundation for the Blind
15 West 16th Street
New York, NY 10011

American Printing House for the Blind
P.O. Box 6085
1839 Frankfort Avenue
Louisville, KY 40206

American Society of Ophthalmic Registered Nurses, Inc.
P.O. Box 193030
San Francisco, CA 94119
415-561-8513

American Society of Plastic and Reconstructive Surgical Nurses, Inc.
East Holly Avenue
Box 56
Pitman, NJ 08071-0056
609-256-2340

American Speech-Language-Hearing Association
10801 Rockville Pike
Rockville, MD 20852

American Trauma Society
8903 Presidential Parkway, Suite 512
Upper Marlboro, MD 20772

Associated Services for the Blind
919 Walnut Street
Philadelphia, PA 19107

Association for Education and Rehabilitation of the Blind and Visually Impaired
206 North Washington Street, Suite 320
Alexandria, VA 22314

Association for Macular Diseases
210 East 64th Street
New York, NY 10021

Blind Outdoor Leisure Development
St. Mary's Church
533 East Main Street
Aspen CO 81611

Canadian Association of Burn Nurses
c/o Judy Knighton
The Wellesley Hospital
160 Wellesley Street E
Toronto, Ontario, Canada M4Y 1J3

Center for Independent Living
817 Broadway, 11th Floor
New York, NY 10003

Dermatology Nurses Association
East Holly Avenue, Box 56
Pitman, NJ 08071-0056
609-256-2330

Fight for Sight
160 East 56th Street, Eighth floor
New York, NY 10022

Foundation for Glaucoma Research
490 Post Street, Suite 830
San Francisco, CA 94102

Guide Dogs for the Blind, Inc.
P.O. Box 1200
San Raphael, CA 94915

IBM National Support Center for Persons with Disabilities
P.O. Box 2150
Atlanta, GA 30301-2150

International Association of Laryngectomees
c/o American Cancer Society
1599 Clifton Road, NE
Atlanta, GA 30329

International Society for Burn Injuries
2005 Franklin Street #660
Denver, CO 80205

Library of Congress National Library Service for the Blind and Physically Handicapped
1291 Taylor Street, NW
Washington, DC 20543

National Association for the Deaf
814 Thayer Avenue
Silver Spring, MD 20910

National Association for the Visually Handicapped
22 West 21st Street
New York, NY 10010

National Eye Institute/National Institutes of Health
Bldg 31, Room 6A32
9000 Rockville Pike
Bethesda, MD 20892

National Federation for the Blind
1800 Johnson Street
Baltimore, MD 21230

National Fire Protection Association (NFPA)
Batterymarch Park
Quincy, MA 02269

National Institute for Burn Medicine
909 East Ann Street
Ann Arbor, MI 48104

National Institutes of Health/National Eye Institute
US Department of Health and Human Services
9000 Rockville Pike
Bethesda, MD 10892

National Psoriasis Foundation
6443 Southwest Beaverton Highway, Suite 210
Portland, OR 97221

National Safe Kids Campaign
111 Michigan Avenue NW
Washington, DC 20010-2970

National Society to Prevent Blindness, Inc.
500 East Remington Road
Schaumberg, IL 60173

Office of Disease Prevention and Health Promotion (ODPHP)
National Health Information Center
P.O. Box 1133
Washington, DC 20013-1133

Phoenix Society (Burn Rehabilitation)
11 Rust Hill Road
Levittstown, PA 19056

Recording for the Blind, Inc.
20 Roszel Road
Princeton, NJ 08540

Talking Books: National Library Service for the Blind and Visually Handicapped
Library of Congress
Washington, DC 20540

The Seeing Eye
P.O. Box 375
Morristown, NJ 07960-0375

AHCPR Guidelines

Guides developed and published by The Agency for Health Care Policy and Research (AHCPR). The Patient Guides are available in English and Spanish. The guidelines can be obtained by writing to: Center for Research Dissemination and Liaison, AHCPR Clearinghouse, P.O. Box 8547, Silver Spring, MD 20907, or by calling 1-800-358-9295. The Guidelines are as follows:

Cataract in adults. A Patient's Guide. AHCPR Pub. No. 92-0544.

Cataract in adults: management of functional impairment. Clinical Practice Guideline. AHCPR Pub. No. 92-0542.

Guideline Overview: Otitis media with effusion in young children. AHCPR Pub. No. 94-0620.

Management of cataract in adults. Clinical Practice Guideline. Quick Reference Guide for Clinicians. AHCPR Pub. No. 92-0543.

Parent Guide: Middle ear fluid in young children. AHCPR Pub. No. 94-0624.

Pressure ulcer treatment. Guideline overview. AHCPR Pub. No. 95-0650.

Pressure ulcer treatment. Quick Reference Guide for Clinicians. AHCPR Pub. No. 95-0653.

Pressure ulcers in adults: prediction and prevention. Clinical Practice Guideline. AHCPR Pub. No. 92-0047.

Pressure ulcers in adults: prediction and prevention. Quick Reference Guide for Clinicians. AHCPR Pub. No. 92-0050.

Preventing pressure ulcers. A Patient's Guide. AHCPR Pub. No. 92-0048.

Quick Reference Guide for Clinicians. Managing Otitis media with effusion in young children. AHCPR Pub. No. 94-0623.

Treating pressure sore. Consumer Guide. AHCPR Pub. No. 95-0654.

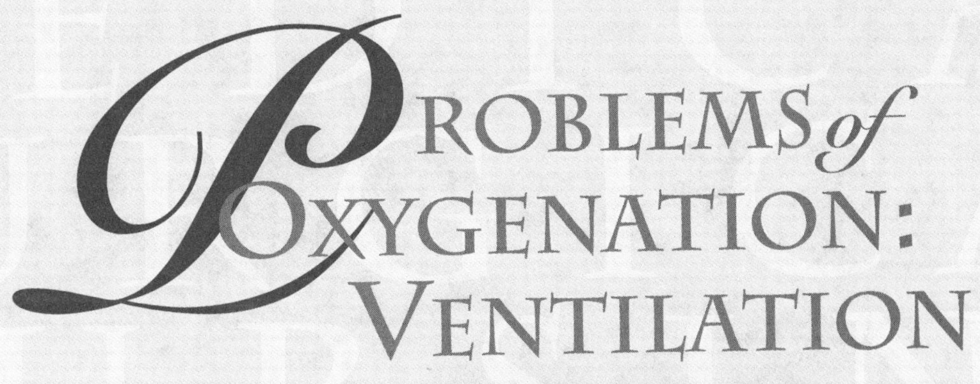

Problems of Oxygenation: Ventilation

Section Five

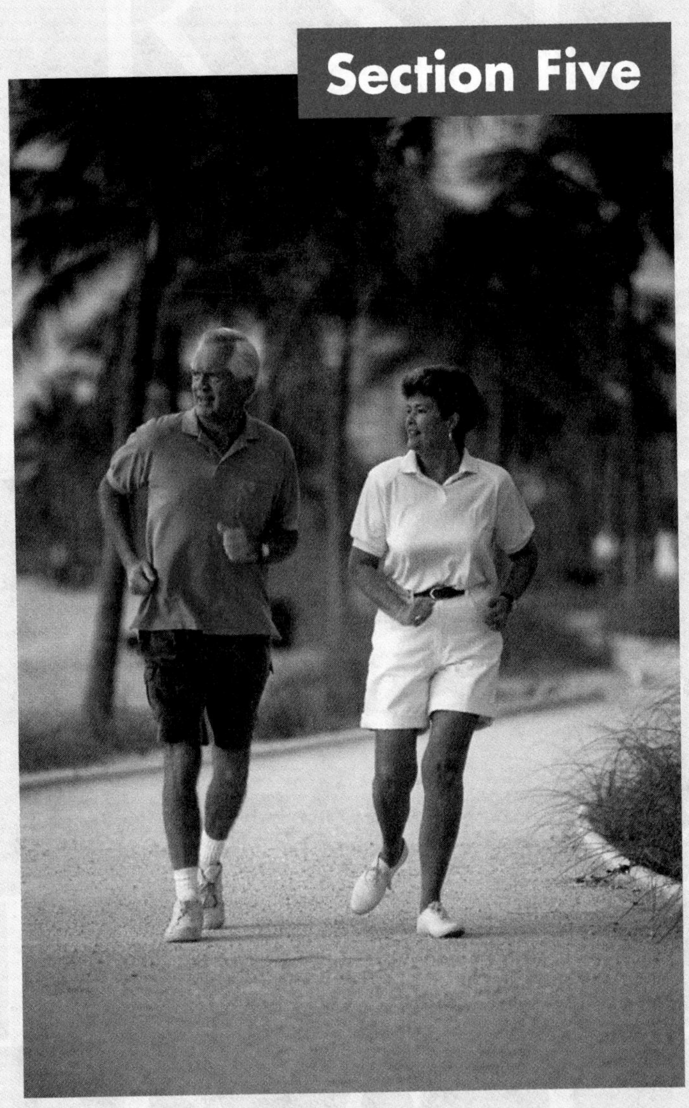

MEDICA
SURGICA
NURSIN
MEDICA
SURGICA
NURSIN
MEDICA
SURGICA
NURSIN
MEDICA
SURGICA

Chapter 22

NURSING ASSESSMENT

Respiratory System

Leslie A. Hoffman **Jan D. Manzetti**

Learning Objectives

1. Describe the structures and functions of the upper respiratory tract, the lower respiratory tract, and the chest wall.
2. Describe the process that initiates and controls inspiration and expiration.
3. Describe the process of gaseous diffusion within the lungs.
4. Identify the functions of the respiratory defense mechanisms.
5. Describe the significance of arterial blood gas values and the oxyhemoglobin dissociation curve in relation to respiratory function.
6. Identify the signs and symptoms of inadequate oxygenation and the implications of these findings.
7. Describe age-related changes in the respiratory system and differences in assessment findings.
8. Identify the significant subjective and objective assessment data that should be obtained from a patient.
9. Describe the techniques used in physical assessment of the respiratory system.
10. Differentiate normal from common abnormal findings on physical assessment of the respiratory system.
11. Describe the purpose, nursing responsibilities, and significance of the results related to diagnostic studies of the respiratory system.

This chapter includes an overview of the structure and function of the respiratory system, physiology of respiration, respiratory defense mechanisms, and age-related changes in respiratory function. In addition, this chapter describes the processes used to identify changes in functional health patterns, physical examination findings, and diagnostic tests commonly associated with the patient with respiratory system dysfunction.

STRUCTURES AND FUNCTIONS

The primary purpose of the respiratory system is gas exchange, which involves the transfer of oxygen and carbon dioxide between the atmosphere and the blood. The respiratory system is divided into two parts, the *upper respiratory tract* and the *lower respiratory tract* (Fig. 22-1). The upper respiratory tract includes the nose, pharynx, adenoids, tonsils, epiglottis, larynx, and trachea. The lower respiratory tract consists of the bronchi, bronchioles, alveolar ducts, and alveoli. With the exception of the right and left main stem bronchi, all lower airway structures are contained within the lungs. The right lung is divided into three lobes (upper, middle, and lower) and the left lung into two lobes (upper and lower) (Fig. 22-2). The structures of the chest wall (ribs, pleura, muscles of respiration) are also essential to respiration.

Upper Respiratory Tract

The *nose* is made of bone and cartilage. Internally, the nose is divided into two passages, or nares, by the septum. The interior of the nose is shaped into rolling projections called *turbinates* that increase the surface area for warming and moistening air. The internal nose opens directly into the *sinuses*. The nasal cavity connects with the pharynx, a tubular passageway that is subdivided from above downward into three parts: the *nasopharynx*, the *oropharynx*, and the *laryngopharynx*.

The nose, like the rest of the respiratory tract, is lined with *mucous membrane*. As air enters the nose, it is warmed, moistened, and filtered by very small hairs. These actions serve a protective function. Inhaled particles that are larger than 10 microns (e.g., dust, bacteria) are trapped by nasal hairs or impact on mucous membranes, thereby preventing them from reaching the lower airways. By the time air enters the alveoli, it should be 100% saturated with water vapor. Most of this humidification occurs in the nose. When humidifying air, the body loses approximately 250 ml of water a day, a process called *insensible loss*.[1-5]

Reviewed by Donna Wilson, RN, RRT, MSN, Pulmonary Clinical Nurse Specialist, Memorial Sloan Kettering Cancer Center, New York, NY.

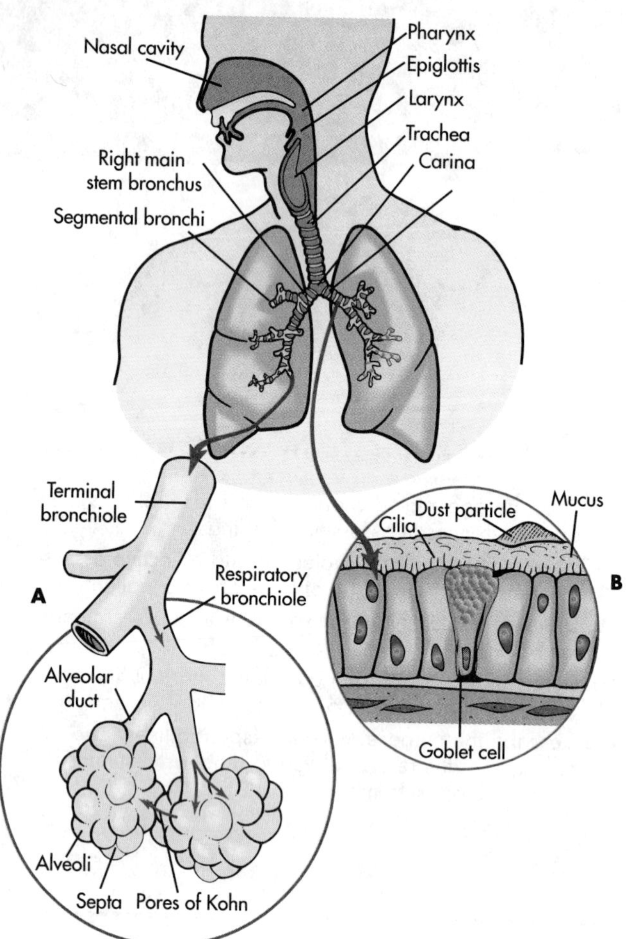

Fig. 22-1 Structures of the respiratory tract. ***A,*** Pulmonary functional unit. ***B,*** Ciliated mucous membrane.

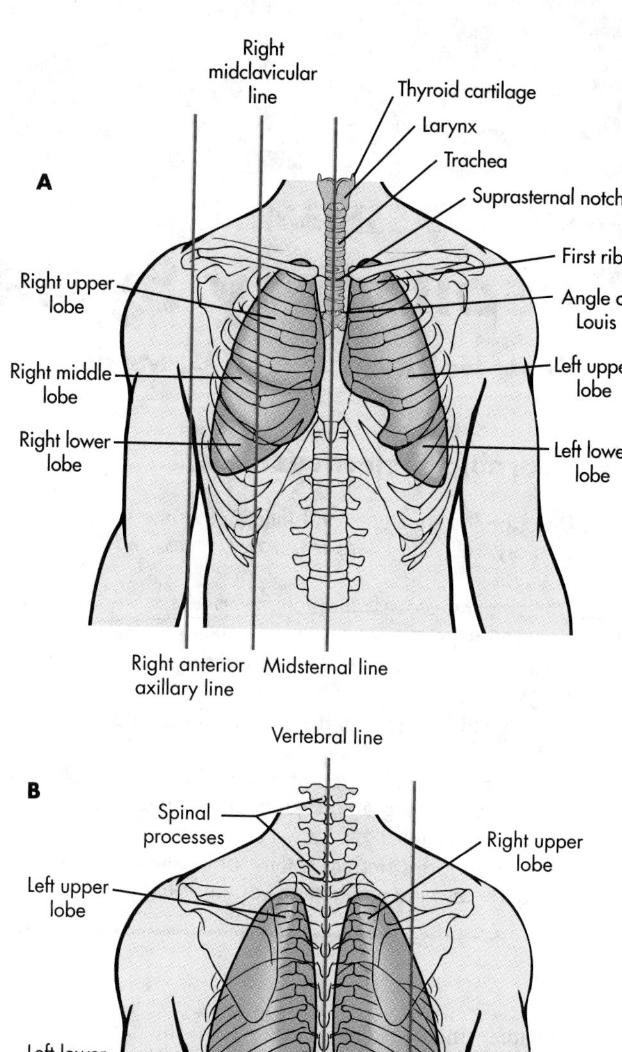

Fig. 22-2 Landmarks and structures of chest wall. ***A,*** Anterior view. ***B,*** Posterior view.

The olfactory nerve endings (receptors for the sense of smell) are located in the roof of the nose. The *adenoids* and *tonsils*, which are small masses of lymphatic tissue, are found in the nasopharynx and the oropharynx, respectively. Air can enter the oropharynx through the nose or the mouth. However, the mouth breather loses the filtering and humidifying functions of the nose.

The *epiglottis* is a small flap of tissue at the base of the tongue. During swallowing, the epiglottis covers the larynx, preventing solids and liquids from entering the lungs. If the epiglottis does not perform this protective function, food or liquids could be aspirated into the lungs. The patient with a tracheostomy is prone to aspiration because the presence of the tracheostomy tube interferes with normal function of the epiglottis (see Chapter 23). Liquids are more likely to be aspirated than are solids.[1,6]

After passing through the oropharynx, air moves through the laryngopharynx and the larynx, where the *vocal cords* are located, and then down into the trachea. The *trachea* is a cylindric tube about 5 inches (10 to 12 cm) long and 1 inch (1.5 to 2.5 cm) in diameter.[1] It is supported by U-shaped cartilages, which keep the trachea from collapsing. On the posterior surface, the cartilages of the trachea are bridged by connective tissue and smooth muscle. This design allows the esophagus to expand when a bolus of food is swallowed. The trachea bifurcates into the right and left main stem bronchi at a point called the *carina*. The carina is located at the level of the manubriosternal junction. The manubriosternal junction is sometimes called the *angle of Louis*. The carina is very sensitive, and touching it, as might occur during insertion of a suction catheter, elicits vigorous coughing.[1-5]

Lower Respiratory Tract

Once air passes the carina, it is in the lower respiratory tract. The main stem bronchi, pulmonary vessels, and nerves enter the lungs through a slit called the *hilus*. The right main stem bronchus is shorter, wider, and straighter than the left main stem bronchus. For this reason, aspiration is more likely in the right lung than in the left lung.

The main stem bronchi subdivide several times to form the lobar, segmental, and subsegmental bronchi. Further divisions form the bronchioles. The most distant bronchioles are called the *respiratory bronchioles*. Beyond these lie the *alveolar ducts* and *alveolar sacs*. The bronchioles are encircled by smooth muscles that constrict and dilate in response to various stimuli. The terms *bronchoconstriction* and *bronchodilatation* are used to refer to a decrease or increase in the diameter of the airways caused by contraction of these muscles. The different appearance of the airways in emphysema, chronic bronchitis, and asthma is illustrated in Fig. 22-3.

No exchange of oxygen or carbon dioxide takes place until air enters the respiratory bronchioles. The area of the respiratory tract from the nose to the respiratory bronchioles serves only as a conducting pathway and is therefore termed the *anatomic dead space* (V_D) or *conducting zone*. This space must be filled with every breath, but the air that fills it is not available for gas exchange. In adults, a normal tidal volume (V_T), or volume of air exchanged with each breath, is about 500 ml. Of each 500 ml inhaled, about 150 ml remains in the V_D.[1-5]

After moving through the conducting zone, air reaches the respiratory bronchioles and *alveoli* (Fig. 22-4). Alveoli are small sacs that form the functional unit of the lungs. The alveoli are interconnected by *pores of Kohn*, which allow movement of air from alveolus to alveolus (see Fig. 22-1). Bacteria can also move through these pores, resulting in an extension of respiratory infection to previously noninfected areas. The 300 million alveoli in the adult have a total volume of about 2500 ml and a surface area for gas exchange that is about the size of a tennis court. The alveoli are separated from the capillaries by the *interstitial layer* or *space* (Fig. 22-5). The alveolar-capillary membrane is very thin (less than 1/5000 of an inch or 1 μm) and is the site of gaseous exchange. In conditions such as pulmonary edema, excess fluid fills the interstitial space and alveoli, markedly impairing gas exchange.[1-5]

Surfactant. The lung can be conceptualized as a collection of 300 million bubbles (alveoli), each 0.3 mm in diameter.[1] Such a structure is inherently unstable and, as a consequence, the alveoli have a natural tendency to collapse. The alveolar surface is composed of two kinds of cells, Type I and Type II. Type I cells provide structure and Type II cells secrete *surfactant* (see Fig. 22-5). Surfactant lowers surface tension in the alveoli, thereby reducing the amount of pressure needed to inflate the alveoli and decreasing the tendency of the alveoli to collapse.[2] Normally, each person takes a slightly larger breath, termed a *sigh*, after every five to six breaths. This sigh stretches the alveoli and causes surfactant to be secreted by Type II cells.

Normal lung function depends on the continuous production and secretion of surfactant. When insufficient surfactant is present, the alveoli collapse. The term *atelectasis*

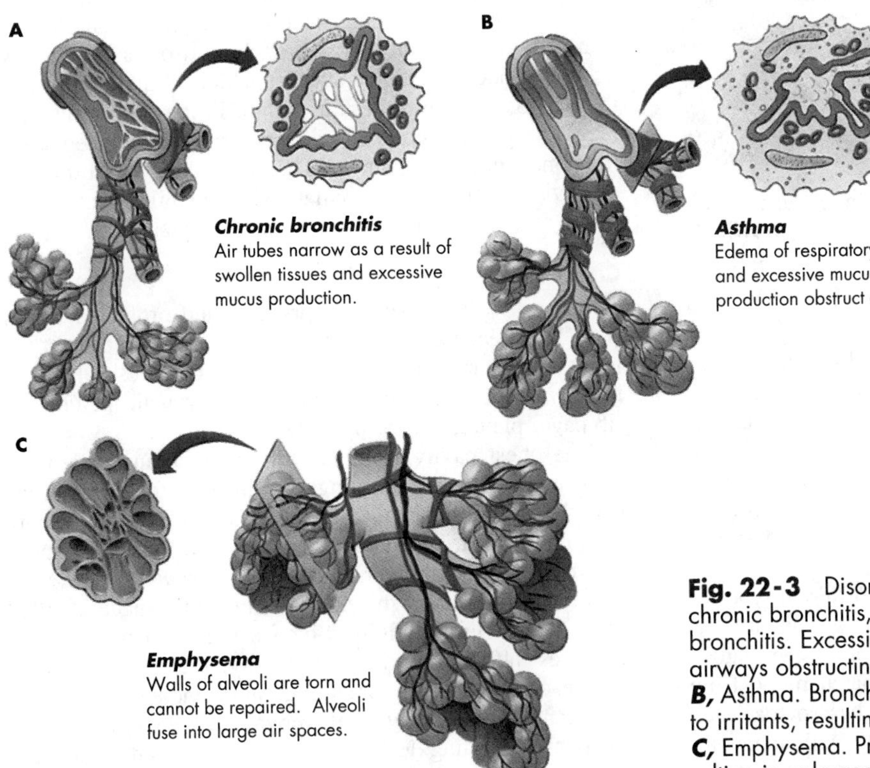

Fig. 22-3 Disorders of the airways in patients with chronic bronchitis, asthma, and emphysema. ***A,*** Chronic bronchitis. Excessive amounts of mucus accumulate in the airways obstructing airflow and impairing ciliary function. ***B,*** Asthma. Bronchial smooth muscle constricts in response to irritants, resulting in airflow obstruction and wheezing. ***C,*** Emphysema. Proteolytic enzymes destroy lung tissue resulting in enlarged air sacs and impaired gas exchange.

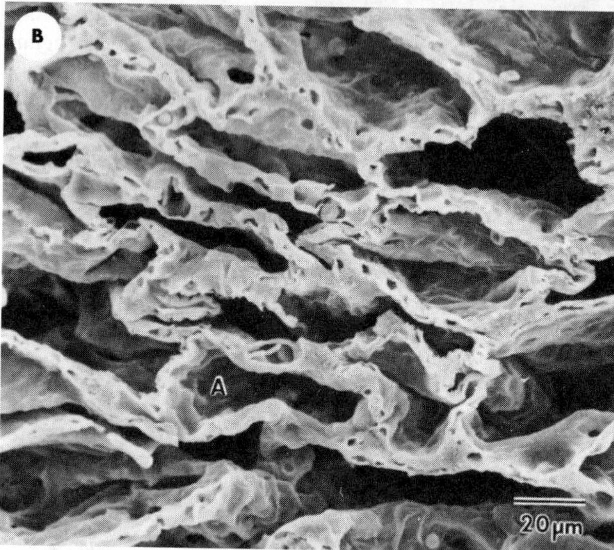

Fig. 22-4 Scanning electron micrograph of lung parenchyma. ***A,*** Alveoli *(A)* and alveolar capillary *(arrow).* ***B,*** Effects of atelectasis. Alveoli *(A)* are partially or totally collapsed.

refers to collapsed, airless alveoli (see Fig. 22-4). The postoperative patient is at risk for atelectasis because of the tendency to resist taking deeper, sigh breaths because of pain (see Chapter 16). In acute respiratory distress syndrome (ARDS), fluid enters the alveoli as a result of damage to the alveolar-capillary membrane, resulting in inactivation or destruction of surfactant and widespread atelectasis (see Chapter 26).

Blood Supply. The lungs have two different types of circulation, pulmonary and bronchial. The pulmonary circulation provides the lungs with blood for gas exchange. The *pulmonary artery* receives deoxygenated blood from the right ventricle of the heart and branches so that each *pulmonary capillary* is directly connected with many alveoli. Oxygen and carbon dioxide exchange occurs at this

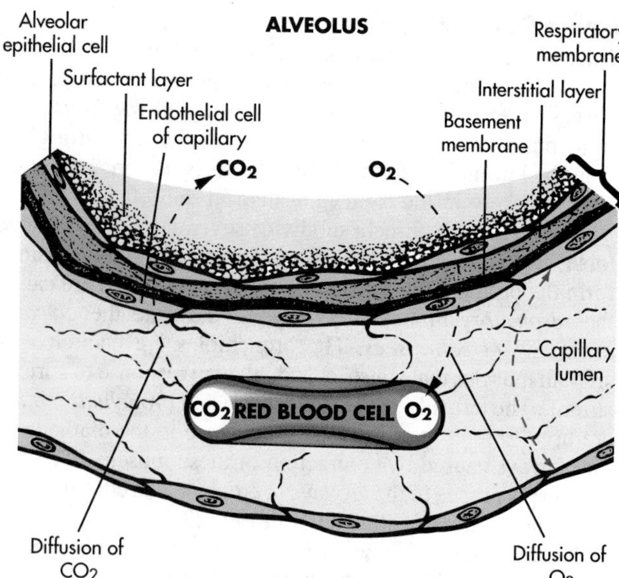

Fig. 22-5 A small portion of the respiratory membrane greatly magnified. An extremely thin interstitial layer of tissue separates the endothelial cell and basement membrane on the capillary side from the epithelial cell and surfactant layer on the alveolar side of the respiratory membrane. The total thickness of the respiratory membrane is less than 1/5000 of an inch.

point. The *pulmonary veins* return oxygenated blood to the left atrium of the heart.

The *bronchial circulation* starts with the bronchial arteries, which arise from the thoracic aorta. Bronchial circulation provides oxygen to the bronchi and other pulmonary tissues. Blood returns from the bronchial circulation through the azygos vein into the left atrium. In the lung transplant recipient, the bronchial circulation is not reconnected when the donor lung is implanted. Therefore, the donor bronchus depends on collateral circulation for viability until local tissue revascularization occurs[7] (see Chapter 24).

Chest Wall

The *chest wall* is shaped, supported, and protected by 24 ribs (12 on each side). The ribs and the sternum protect the lungs and heart from injury and are sometimes called the *thoracic cage.* The structures of the chest wall include the rib cage, pleura, and respiratory muscles.

The chest cavity is lined with a membrane called the *parietal pleura* and the lungs are lined with a membrane called the *visceral pleura.* The parietal and visceral pleura are joined and form a closed, double-walled sac. The space between the pleural layers, termed the *intrapleural space,* is a potential space. In the normal adult, this space is filled with a thin film of fluid, which serves two purposes: it provides lubrication, allowing the layers of pleura to slide over each other during breathing; and it increases cohesion between the pleural layers, thereby facilitating expansion of the pleura and lung during inspiration. Fluid is drained from the pleural space by the lymphatic circulation.

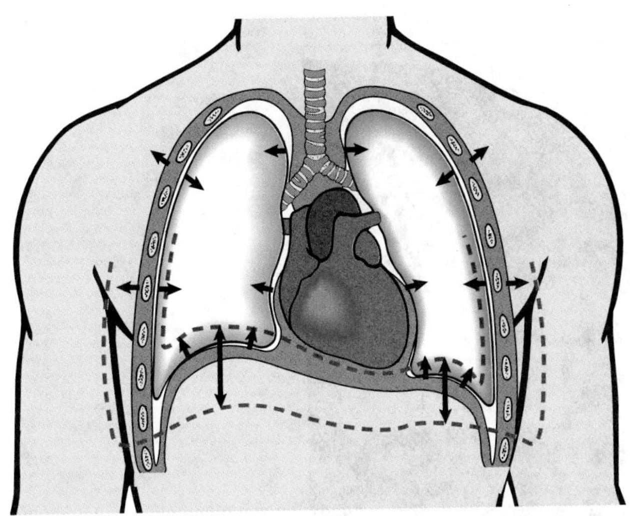

Fig. 22-6 Frontal section of chest showing movement of the lungs and chest wall during inspiration and expiration. During inspiration, the inspiratory muscles contract and the chest expands. Alveolar pressure becomes subatmospheric with respect to pressure at the airway opening and air flows into the lungs. During expiration, the inspiratory muscles relax. Recoil of the lung causes alveolar pressure to exceed pressure at the airway opening and air to flow out of the lungs. *Single arrows* show excursion of the lungs and chest wall. *Double arrows* show movement of the lung bases.

Normally, the pleural space contains 20 to 25 ml of fluid. Several pathologic conditions may cause the accumulation of greater amounts of fluid, termed a *pleural effusion.* Pleural fluid may accumulate because malignant cells block lymphatic drainage or because there is an imbalance between intravascular and oncotic fluid pressures, such as occurs in congestive heart failure. Bacterial infection that extends to the pleura may also cause fluid accumulation. The term *empyema* is used to designate presence of purulent pleural fluid. Pleuritic pain is a symptom of conditions involving the pleura. Pleuritic pain is caused when the parietal pleura is involved, as the visceral pleura does not contain pain receptors.

The *diaphragm* is the major muscle of respiration. During inspiration, the diaphragm contracts, pushing the abdominal contents downward. At the same time, the external intercostal muscles and parasternal muscles contract, increasing the lateral and anteroposterior dimension of the chest.[1] This causes the size of the thoracic cavity to increase (Fig. 22-6). As a consequence, *intrathoracic pressure* decreases, causing air to enter the lungs.

The diaphragm is innervated by the right and left *phrenic nerves,* which arise from the spinal cord between C3 and C5, the third and fifth cervical vertebrae. If the phrenic nerve is injured, diaphragm function will be impaired. Causes of phrenic nerve injury include blunt, penetrating, or surgical trauma. Injury to the phrenic nerve results in *hemidiaphragm paralysis* with paralysis on the side of the injury.[1] Spinal cord injuries at or above the level of C5 typically result in total diaphragm paralysis. The patient with such an injury cannot breathe a normal V_T without assistance of a mechanical ventilator, since only a V_T of 50 to 100 ml (normal 500 ml) can be achieved. If the spinal cord injury is at the level of C6 or below, the patient typically retains sufficient phrenic and diaphragmatic function to breathe without a mechanical ventilator.

Physiology of Respiration

Ventilation. Ventilation involves *inspiration* (movement of air into the lungs) and *expiration* (movement of air out of the lungs). Air moves in and out of the lungs because intrathoracic pressure changes in relation to pressure at the airway opening. Contraction of the diaphragm and intercostal and scalene muscles increases chest dimensions, thereby decreasing intrathoracic pressure. Gas flows from an area of higher pressure (atmospheric) to one of lower pressure (intrathoracic) (see Fig. 22-6). Some conditions (e.g., phrenic nerve paralysis, rib fractures, neuromuscular disease) may limit diaphragm or chest wall movement and cause the patient to breathe with smaller V_Ts. As a result, the lungs do not fully inflate, and gas exchange is impaired. Interventions used to reverse this problem include mechanical ventilation, phrenic nerve stimulation, and nerve blocks to relieve pain from rib fractures.

In contrast to inspiration, expiration is passive. The elastic recoil of the chest wall and lungs allows the chest to passively return to its normal position. Intrathoracic pressure rises, causing air to move out of the lungs. Some conditions cause respiration to become an active process. For example, this may occur during an asthmatic exacerbation or when a patient with emphysema has severe dyspnea (see Chapter 25). During active or "labored" respirations, the scalene muscles and sternocleidomastoid muscles assist with expiration.

Elastic Recoil and Compliance. Elastic recoil is the tendency for the lungs to recoil after being stretched or expanded. The elasticity of lung tissue is due to the elastin fibers found in the alveolar walls and surrounding the bronchioles and capillaries.

Compliance (distensibility) is a measure of the elasticity of the lungs and thorax. When *compliance* is decreased, the lungs are more difficult to inflate. Examples include conditions that increase fluid in the lungs (e.g., pulmonary edema and ARDS); conditions that make lung tissue less elastic (e.g., pulmonary fibrosis or sarcoidosis); and conditions that restrict lung movement (e.g., pleural effusion). Compliance is increased as a result of aging and when there is destruction of alveolar walls and loss of tissue elasticity, as in emphysema.

Diffusion. Oxygen and carbon dioxide move back and forth across the alveolar capillary membrane by *diffusion.* The overall direction of movement is from the area of higher concentration to the area of lower concentration. Thus, oxygen moves from alveolar gas (atmospheric air) into the arterial blood and carbon dioxide from the arterial blood into the alveolar gas. Diffusion continues until equilibrium is reached (see Fig. 22-5).[2]

The ability of the lungs to oxygenate arterial blood adequately is determined by examination of the *arterial*

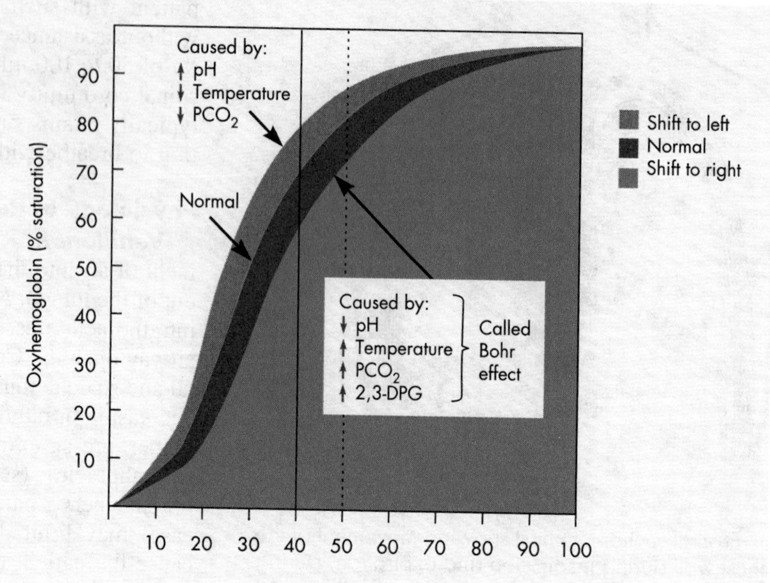

Fig. 22-7 Oxygen-hemoglobin dissociation curve. The effects of acidity and temperature changes are shown.

oxygen tension (PaO_2) and *arterial oxygen saturation* (SaO_2). Oxygen is carried in the blood in two forms, dissolved oxygen and oxygen in chemical combination with hemoglobin. The PaO_2 represents the amount of oxygen dissolved in the plasma and is expressed in millimeters of mercury (mm Hg). The SaO_2 is the amount of oxygen bound to hemoglobin in comparison with the amount of oxygen the hemoglobin can carry. The SaO_2 is expressed as a percentage. For example, if the SaO_2 is 90%, then 90% of the hemoglobin attachments for oxygen have oxygen bound to them.

Oxygen-Hemoglobin Dissociation Curve. The affinity of hemoglobin for oxygen is described by the *oxygen-hemoglobin dissociation curve* (Fig. 22-7). Oxygen delivery to the tissues depends on the amount of oxygen transported to the tissues and the ease with which hemoglobin gives up oxygen once it reaches the tissues. In the upper flat portion of the curve, fairly large changes in the PaO_2 cause a small change in hemoglobin saturation. For this reason, if the PaO_2 drops from 100 to 60 mm Hg, the saturation of hemoglobin changes only 7% (from the normal 97% to 90%). Thus, the hemoglobin remains 90% saturated despite a 40 mm Hg drop in the PaO_2. This portion of the curve also explains the reason the patient is considered adequately oxygenated when the PaO_2 is greater than 60 mm Hg. Increasing the value above this level causes little change in hemoglobin saturation, and if high concentrations of oxygen can be avoided, there is less risk of oxygen toxicity. *Oxygen toxicity* refers to alveolar injury caused by high oxygen concentrations, that is, greater than 40% to 60%.[8]

The lower portion of the oxyhemoglobin-dissociation curve indicates a different type of phenomenon. As the hemoglobin becomes further desaturated, larger amounts of oxygen are released for tissue use. This is an important method of maintaining the pressure gradient between the blood and the tissues. It also ensures an adequate oxygen supply to peripheral tissues, even if oxygen delivery is compromised.[8]

Many factors alter the affinity of hemoglobin for oxygen. When the oxygen dissociation curve *shifts to the left*, blood picks up oxygen more readily in the lungs but delivers oxygen less readily to the tissues. This is seen in alkalosis, hypothermia, and with a decrease in arterial carbon dioxide tension ($PaCO_2$) (see Fig. 22-7). The patient with a condition that causes a leftward shift of the curve, such as the hypothermia that follows open heart surgery, may be given higher concentrations of oxygen until the body temperature normalizes. This helps to compensate for decreased oxygen unloading in the tissues. When the curve *shifts to the right*, the opposite occurs. Blood picks up oxygen less rapidly in the lungs but delivers oxygen more readily to the tissues. This is seen in acidosis, hyperthermia, and when the $PaCO_2$ is increased.[8,9]

Two methods are used to assess the efficiency of gas transfer in the lung: analysis of arterial blood gases (ABGs) and oximetry. These measures are usually adequate if the patient is stable and not critically ill. The critically ill patient often has a condition that impairs tissue oxygen delivery. In this patient, venous oxygen tension and venous oxygen saturation may also be assessed (see Chapter 26).

Arterial Blood Gases. ABGs are measured to determine oxygenation status and acid-base balance. ABG analysis includes measurement of the PaO_2, $PaCO_2$, acidity (pH), and bicarbonate (HCO_3) in arterial blood. The SaO_2 is also calculated during this analysis.[8-10]

Table 22-1 Normal Arterial and Venous Blood Gas Values*

Laboratory Value	Arterial Blood Gases: Sea Level BP 760 mm Hg	Arterial Blood Gases: 1 Mile Above Sea Level (5280 ft) BP 629 mm Hg	Mixed Venous Blood Gases	
pH	7.35-7.45	7.35-7.45	pH	7.34-7.37
PaO_2	80-100 mm Hg	65-75 mm Hg	PvO_2	38-42 mm Hg
SaO_2	>95%†	>95%†	SvO_2	60-80%†
$PaCO_2$	35-45 mm Hg	35-45 mm Hg	$PvCO_2$	44-46 mm Hg
HCO_3	22-26 mEq/L	22-26 mEq/L	HCO_3	24-30 mEq/L

BP, Barometric pressure; PvO_2, partial pressure of oxygen in venous blood; SvO_2, venous oxygen saturation.
*Assumes patient is ≤60 years of age and breathing room air.
†The same normal values apply when SpO_2 and SvO_2 are obtained by oximetry.

Blood for ABG analysis can be obtained by *arterial puncture* or from an *arterial catheter* that is typically placed in the radial or femoral artery. Both techniques are invasive and allow only intermittent analysis. *Continuous intraarterial blood gas monitoring* is also possible via a fiberoptic sensor or oxygen electrode inserted into an arterial catheter.[11] An arterial catheter and continuous blood gas monitoring permit ABG sampling without repeated punctures.

Normal values for ABGs are given in Table 22-1. The normal PaO_2 decreases with advancing age.[8] The normal PaO_2 also varies in relation to the distance above sea level. At higher altitudes, the barometric pressure is lower, resulting in a lower inspired oxygen pressure (PiO_2) and a lower PaO_2 (Table 22-1). Most airplanes are pressurized to approximate an altitude of 8000 feet above sea level. A normal person can expect a 16 to 32 mm Hg fall in PaO_2 at this altitude.[12] The patient who is already receiving oxygen therapy or the patient with a PaO_2 less than 72 mm Hg while breathing room air needs careful evaluation before air travel. Supplemental oxygen or a change in liter flow may be required during the flight. If oxygen is required, the airline should be contacted several weeks in advance to determine the procedures regarding air travel with oxygen.[12,13]

Mixed Venous Blood Gases. For the patient with a normal or near normal cardiac status, an assessment of PaO_2 or SaO_2 is usually sufficient to determine adequate oxygenation. This is often *not* true for the patient with impaired cardiac output or hemodynamic instability. Such a patient may have inadequate tissue oxygen delivery or abnormal oxygen consumption. The amount of oxygen delivered to the tissues and the amount of oxygen consumed can be determined by analyzing the *mixed venous* oxygen tension (PvO_2) and *venous oxygen saturation* (SvO_2).

A catheter positioned in the pulmonary artery, termed a *pulmonary artery* (PA) *catheter*, is used for mixed venous sampling (see Chapter 61). Blood drawn from a PA catheter is termed a *mixed venous* sample because it consists of venous blood that has returned to the heart from all tissue beds and "mixed" in the right ventricle. Normal mixed venous values are given in Table 22-1.

When tissue oxygen delivery is inadequate or when inadequate oxygen is transported to the tissues by the hemoglobin, PvO_2 falls. When PvO_2 falls to 27 mm Hg, the limits of compensation are such that any further fall will most likely result in cellular death. This is considered preterminal unless reversal is fairly rapid. Monitoring of mixed venous values can provide important information about the ability to meet tissue oxygen demands.

Oximetry. ABG values provide accurate information about oxygenation and acid-base balance. However, they are invasive, require laboratory analysis, and expose the patient to the risk of bleeding from an arterial puncture. Arterial oxygen saturation can be monitored continuously and noninvasively (i.e., without a blood sample) using *pulse oximetry*. The technique involves attaching a probe to the ear, finger, toe, or bridge of the nose (Fig. 22-8).

A pulse oximeter emits two wavelengths of light, one red and one infrared, which pass from a light emitting diode

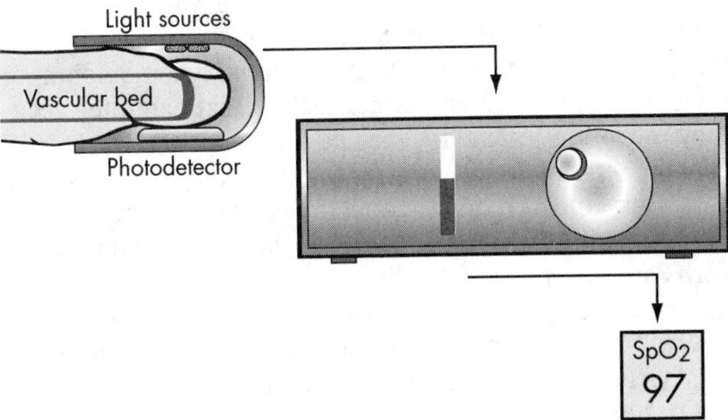

Fig. 22-8 A pulse oximeter passes light from a light-emitting diode through a vascular bed to a photodetector. The oximeter compares the amount of light emitted and absorbed and calculates the SpO_2. The oximeter displays SpO_2 as a digital reading.

Table 22-2 Critical Values for PaO_2 and SpO_2*

PaO_2 (%)	SpO_2 (%)	Considerations
≥70	≥94	Adequate unless patient is hemodynamically unstable or has oxygen-unloading problem. With a low cardiac output, dysrhythmias, a leftward shift of the oxyhemoglobin dissociation curve, or carbon monoxide inhalation, higher values may be desired. Benefits of a higher blood oxygen value need to be balanced against the risk of oxygen toxicity.
60	90	Adequate in almost all patients. Values are at steep part of oxygen-hemoglobin dissociation curve. Provides adequate oxygenation but with less margin of error than above.
55	88	Adequate for patients with chronic hypoxemia if no cardiac problems occur. These values are also used as criteria for prescription of continuous oxygen therapy.
40	75	Inadequate but may be acceptable on a short-term basis if the patient also has carbon dioxide retention. In this situation, respirations may be stimulated by a low PaO_2. Thus the PaO_2 cannot be raised rapidly. The nurse may use oxygen therapy by mask at a low concentration (24–28%) to gradually increase the PaO_2. Monitoring for dysrhythmias is necessary.
<40	<75	Inadequate. Tissue hypoxia and cardiac dysrhythmias can be expected.

*The same critical values apply for SpO_2 and SaO_2.

(positioned on one side of the probe) to a photodetector (positioned on the opposite side). Well-oxygenated blood absorbs light differently than deoxygenated blood does. The oximeter determines the amount of light absorbed by the vascular bed and uses this information to calculate the saturation. Since arterial oxygen saturation can be determined from ABGs or by oximetry, *SpO_2* is used to indicate the value obtained by pulse oximetry. SpO_2 and heart rate are displayed on the monitor as a digital reading. The normal SpO_2 is greater than 95%.[14]

Pulse oximetry is particularly valuable in intensive care units (ICUs), during exercise testing, and when determining oxygen flow rates for the patient on long-term oxygen therapy. Changes in SpO_2 can be quickly detected and modifications made in the plan of care (Table 22-2).[15] Pulse oximetry does not provide any information about ventilation status (pH, $PaCO_2$). Thus, use of pulse oximetry does not eliminate the need for ABGs.[14,15]

Values obtained by pulse oximetry become less accurate if the SpO_2 is less than 70%. At this level, the oximeter may display a value that is ±3% of the actual value, for example, if the SpO_2 is 70%, the actual value can range from 67% to 73%. Pulse oximetry is also inaccurate if there are hemoglobin variants, such as carboxyhemoglobin or methemoglobin, present. Other factors that can alter accuracy of pulse oximetry include motion, low perfusion, anemia, bright fluorescent lights, intravascular dyes, and dark skin color. If there is doubt about the accuracy of the SpO_2 reading, an ABG analysis should be obtained to verify accuracy.

The technique of oximetry can also be used to monitor SvO_2.[16,17] With SvO_2 monitoring, the light-emitting probe is placed in one lumen of the PA catheter. A decrease in SvO_2 suggests that less oxygen is being delivered to the tissues or that more oxygen is being consumed. Changes in SvO_2 provide an early warning of a change in cardiac output and tissue oxygen delivery. The clinician can immediately assess the effect of treatment or routine interventions such as positioning or suctioning (Fig. 22-9). Normal SvO_2 is 60% to 80%.

Oxygen Delivery. Information from ABGs or oximetry is used to assess adequacy of oxygenation. Several questions need to be asked to determine if oxygenation is adequate:

1. What is the patient's SpO_2 or PaO_2 compared to expected normal values? (Normal values are given in Table 22-1.)
2. What is the degree of hypoxemia and trend? Has there been a rapid decline in SpO_2 or PaO_2? A sudden drop in blood oxygen level can be life threatening. A gradual decline is tolerated with fewer symptoms. Critical values for SpO_2 and PaO_2 are given in Table 22-2.
3. Are there signs or symptoms of inadequate oxygenation? Changes in respiratory, cardiovascular, central nervous system, and renal function are seen when tissue oxygen delivery is inadequate (Table 22-3). Because the brain is very sensitive to a decrease in tissue oxygen delivery, the very first evidence of hypoxemia may be apprehension, restlessness, or irritability. If these signs or symptoms are observed, a change in the management plan is needed.

Control of Respiration

The respiratory center is composed of cell clusters in the medulla. These cells respond to chemical and mechanical signals from the body. Impulses are sent from the medulla to the respiratory muscles through the spinal cord and phrenic nerves. Respiration is controlled by chemoreceptors and mechanical sensors.

Chemoreceptors. A chemoreceptor is a receptor that responds to a change in the chemical composition ($PaCO_2$ and pH) of the fluid around it. Central chemoreceptors are located in the medulla and respond to changes in the hydrogen ion (H^+) concentration. An increase in the H^+ concentration (acidosis) causes the medulla to increase the respiratory rate and V_T. A decrease in H^+ concentration

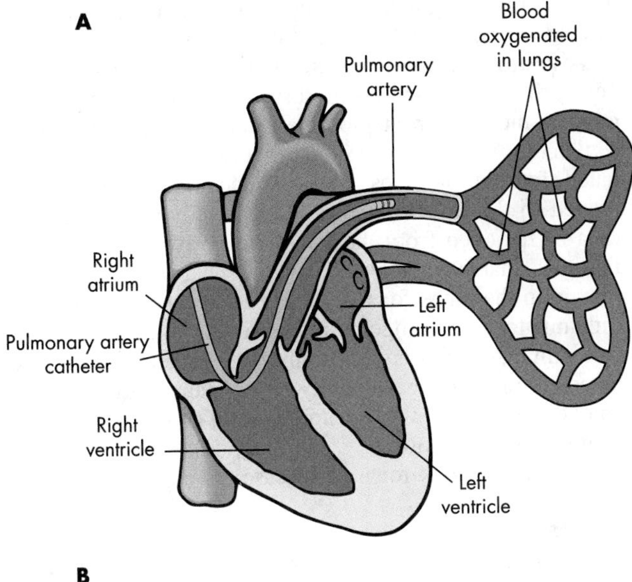

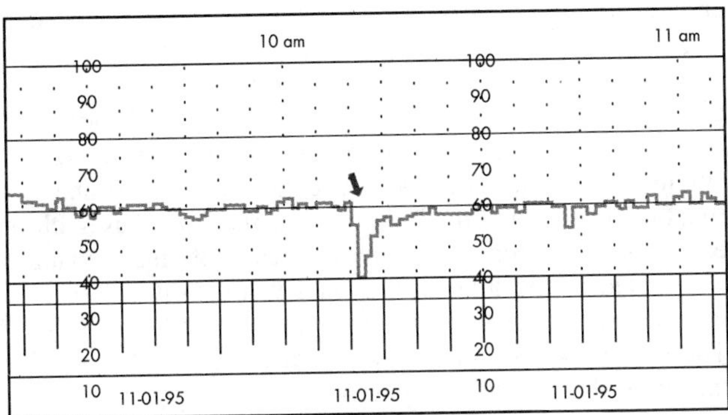

Fig. 22-9 Technology used to monitor SvO_2. ***A,*** Catheter placed in the pulmonary artery contains a fiberoptic probe. Light emitted from this probe is reflected from red blood cells. The oximeter compares the amount of light emitted and absorbed from this and calculates SvO_2. ***B,*** SvO_2 tracing. The SvO_2 decreased from 60% to 40% during endotracheal suctioning (*arrow*). Although the fall was greater than 10%, recovery was rapid.

(alkalosis) has the opposite effect. Changes in $PaCO_2$ regulate ventilation primarily by their effect on the pH of the cerebrospinal fluid. When the $PaCO_2$ level is increased, more CO_2 is available to combine with H_2O and form carbonic acid (H_2CO_3). This lowers the cerebrospinal fluid pH and stimulates an increase in respiratory rate. The opposite process occurs with a decrease in $PaCO_2$ level.

Peripheral chemoreceptors are located in the carotid bodies at the bifurcation of the common carotid arteries and in the aortic bodies above and below the aortic arch. The peripheral chemoreceptors respond to decreases in PaO_2 and pH and to increases in $PaCO_2$. These changes also cause stimulation of the respiratory center.

In a healthy person an increase in $PaCO_2$ or a decrease in pH causes an immediate increase in the respiratory rate.

Table 22-3 Signs and Symptoms of Inadequate Oxygenation

Signs and Symptoms	Onset
Respiratory	
Tachypnea	Early
Dyspnea on exertion	Early
Dyspnea at rest	Late
Use of accessory muscles	Late
Retraction of interspaces on inspiration	Late
Pause for breath between sentences, words	Late
Cardiovascular	
Tachycardia	Early
Mild hypertension	Early
Dysrhythmias (e.g., premature ventricular contractions)	Early or late
Hypotension	Late
Cyanosis	Late
Cool, clammy skin	Late
Central Nervous System	
Unexplained apprehension	Early
Unexplained restlessness or irritability	Early
Unexplained confusion or lethargy	Early or late
Combativeness	Late
Coma	Late
Other	
Diaphoresis	Early or late
Decreased urinary output	Early or late
Unexplained fatigue	Early or late

The process is very precise. The $PaCO_2$ does not vary more than about 3 mm Hg if lung function is normal. Conditions such as chronic obstructive pulmonary disease (COPD) alter lung function and may result in chronically elevated $PaCO_2$ levels (see Chapter 25).

Mechanical Receptors. Mechanical receptors are located in the lungs, upper airways, chest wall, and diaphragm. They are stimulated by a variety of physiologic factors, such as irritants, muscle stretching, and alveolar wall distortion. Signals from the stretch receptors aid in the control of respiration. As the lungs inflate, pulmonary stretch receptors activate the inspiratory center to inhibit further lung expansion. This is called the *Hering-Breuer reflex* and it prevents overdistention of the lungs. Impulses from the mechanical sensors are sent through the vagus nerve to the brain. Juxtacapillary (J) receptors are believed to cause the rapid respiration (tachypnea) seen in pulmonary edema. These receptors are stimulated by fluid entering the pulmonary interstitial space.

Respiratory Defense Mechanisms

Respiratory defense mechanisms are very efficient in protecting the lungs from inhaled particles, microorganisms, and toxic gases. The defense mechanisms include filtration of air, the mucociliary clearance system, the cough reflex, reflex bronchoconstriction, and alveolar macrophages.

Filtration of Air. Nasal hairs filter the inspired air. In addition, the abrupt changes in direction of airflow that occur as air moves through the nasopharynx and larynx increase air turbulence. This causes particles and bacteria to come in contact on the mucosa lining these structures. Most large particles (greater than 5 μm in diameter) are removed in this manner.

The velocity of airflow slows greatly after it passes the larynx, facilitating the deposition of smaller particles (1 to 5 μm in size). They settle out like sand in a river, a process referred to as *sedimentation*. Particles less than 1 μm in size are too small to settle in this manner and are deposited in the alveoli. Particle size is very important. Particles greater than 5 μm in size are less dangerous because they are removed in the nasopharynx or bronchi and do not reach the alveoli.

Mucociliary Clearance System. Below the larynx, movement of mucus is accomplished by the *mucociliary clearance system*. This term is used to indicate the interrelationship between the secretion of mucus and the ciliary activity. Mucus is continually secreted at a rate of about 100 ml per day by goblet cells and submucosal glands. It forms a mucous blanket that contains the impacted particles and debris from distal lung areas (see Fig. 22-1). The small amount of mucus normally secreted is swallowed without being noticed. Secretory immunoglobulin A (IgA) in the mucus contributes to protection against bacteria and viruses.

Cilia cover the airways from the level of the trachea to the respiratory bronchioles (see Fig. 22-1). Each ciliated cell contains approximately 200 cilia, which beat rhythmically about 1000 times per minute in the large airways, moving mucus toward the mouth. The ciliary beat is slower further down the tracheobronchial tree. As a consequence, particles that penetrate more deeply into the airways are removed less rapidly. Ciliary action is impaired by dehydration, smoking, inhalation of high oxygen concentrations, infection, and ingestion of drugs such as atropine, alcohol, and anesthetics. Patients with chronic bronchitis often have repeated upper respiratory infections. Cilia are often destroyed during these infections, resulting in impaired secretion clearance, a chronic productive cough, and frequent respiratory infections.

Cough Reflex. The cough is a protective reflex action that clears the airway by a high-pressure, high-velocity flow of air. It is a backup for mucociliary clearance, especially when this clearance mechanism is overwhelmed or ineffective. Coughing is only effective in removing secretions above the subsegmental level. Secretions below this level need to be moved upward by the mucociliary mechanism or by interventions such as postural drainage before they can be removed by coughing.

Reflex Bronchoconstriction. Another defense mechanism is reflex bronchoconstriction. In response to the inhalation of large amounts of irritating substances (e.g., dusts, aerosols), the bronchi constrict in an effort to prevent entry of the irritants. A person with hyperactive airways, such as a person with asthma, experiences bronchoconstriction after inhalation of cold air, perfume, or other strong odors.

Alveolar Macrophages. Ciliated cells are not found below the level of the respiratory bronchioles. The primary defense mechanism at the alveolar level is *alveolar macrophages*. Alveolar macrophages rapidly phagocytize inhaled foreign particles such as bacteria. The debris is moved to the level of the bronchioles for removal by the cilia or removed from the lungs by the lymphatic system. Particles that cannot be adequately phagocytized tend to remain in the lungs for indefinite periods and can stimulate inflammatory or fibrogenic responses. Coal dust and silica can stimulate a fibrous reaction (see Chapter 24). Because alveolar macrophage activity is impaired by cigarette smoke, the smoker who is employed in an occupation with heavy dust exposure (e.g., mining, foundries), is at an especially high risk for lung disease.

Effects of Aging

Age-related changes in the respiratory system can be divided into alterations in structure, defense mechanisms, and respiratory control.[18] See Table 22-4 for age-related changes and assessment implications.

Structural alterations include a decrease in elastic recoil of the lung and a decrease in chest wall compliance. The anteroposterior diameter of the thoracic cage increases. Within the lung, there is a decrease in the number of functional alveoli. Small airways in the lung bases close earlier in expiration. As a consequence, more inspired air is distributed to the lung apices, and ventilation is less well matched to perfusion, causing a lowering of the PaO_2.[18] The PaO_2 associated with a given age can be calculated by means of the following equation:[18]

$$PaO_2 \text{ (mm Hg)} = 103.5 - (0.42 \times \text{age [yr]})$$

For example, the normal PaO_2 for a patient 80 years of age is $103.5 - (0.42 \times 80) = 70$ mm Hg, as compared to a PaO_2 of 93 mm Hg for a 25-year-old person.

Respiratory defense mechanisms are less effective because of a decline in cell-mediated immunity and formation of antibodies. The alveolar macrophages are less effective at phagocytosis. An elderly patient has a less forceful cough and fewer and less functional cilia. Formation of secretory IgA, an important mechanism in neutralizing the effect of viruses, is diminished.[18]

Respiratory control is altered, resulting in a more gradual response to changes in blood oxygen or carbon dioxide level. The PaO_2 drops to a lower level and the $PaCO_2$ rises to a higher level before the respiratory rate changes.

There is much variability in the extent of these changes in persons of the same age. The elderly patient who has a significant smoking history, is obese, and is diagnosed with a chronic illness is at greatest risk of adverse outcomes.

ASSESSMENT OF THE RESPIRATORY SYSTEM

Correct diagnosis depends on an accurate health history and a thorough physical examination. A respiratory assessment can be done as part of a comprehensive physical examina-

Table 22-4 Gerontologic Differences in Assessment: Respiratory System

Changes	Differences in Assessment Findings
Structure	
↓ elastic recoil ↓ chest wall compliance ↑ anteroposterior diameter ↓ functioning alveoli	Barrel chest appearance; ↓ chest wall movement; ↓ respiratory excursion; ↓ vital capacity; ↑ functional residual capacity; diminished breath sounds particularly at lung bases; ↓ PaO_2 and SaO_2; normal pH and $PaCO_2$
Defense Mechanisms	
↓ cell-mediated immunity ↓ specific antibodies ↓ cilia function ↓ cough force ↓ alveolar macrophage function	↓ cough effectiveness; ↓ secretion clearance; ↑ risk of upper respiratory infection, influenza, or pneumonia. Respiratory infections may be more severe and last longer.
Respiratory Control	
↓ response to hypoxemia ↓ response to hypercapnia	Greater ↓ in PaO_2 and ↑ in $PaCO_2$ before respiratory rate changes. Significant hypoxemia or hypercapnia may develop from relatively small incidents. Retained secretions, excessive sedation, or positioning that impairs chest expansion may substantially alter PaO_2.

tion, or as an examination in itself. Judgment must be used in determining whether all or part of the history and physical examination will be completed based on problems presented by the patient and the degree of respiratory distress. If respiratory distress is severe, only pertinent information should be obtained and a thorough assessment should be deferred until the patient's condition stabilizes.

Subjective Data

Important Health Information

Past health history. The nurse should determine the frequency of upper respiratory problems (e.g., colds, sore throats, sinus problems, or allergies) and if weather changes affect these problems. The patient with allergies should be questioned about possible precipitating factors such as medications, pollen, smoke, or pet exposure. Characteristics of the allergic reaction, such as runny nose, wheezing, scratchy throat, or tightness in the chest, and severity, should be documented. The frequency of asthma exacerbations and cause, if known, should also be determined.

A history of lower respiratory problems such as asthma, COPD, pneumonia, and tuberculosis should also be elicited. Respiratory symptoms are often manifestations of problems that involve other body systems. Therefore the patient should be asked if there is a history of other health problems in addition to those involving the respiratory system. For example, the patient with cardiac dysfunction may experience dyspnea as a consequence of congestive heart failure. The patient with human immunodeficiency virus (HIV) infection may experience frequent respiratory infections because immune function is compromised.

Medications. The patient should be questioned carefully about prescription and over-the-counter drugs used to manage respiratory problems, such as antihistamines, bronchodilators, corticosteroids, cough suppressants, and antibiotics. Information about the reason for taking the medication, its name, the dose and frequency, length of time taken, its effect, and any side effects should be obtained.

It should also be noted if the patient is using oxygen to ease a breathing problem. If so, the amount, method of administration, and effectiveness of the therapy should be documented. Safety practices related to using oxygen should also be assessed.

Surgery or other treatments. The nurse should determine if the patient has been hospitalized for a respiratory problem. If so, the dates, therapy (including surgery), and current status of the problem should be recorded.

The nurse needs to ask about the use of respiratory treatments such as nebulizer, humidifier, postural drainage, and percussion. The frequency of these treatments and the results obtained are important for the nurse to know.

Functional Health Patterns. Key questions to ask a patient with a respiratory problem are presented in Table 22-5.

Health perception–health management pattern. The patient should be asked if there has been a perceived change in health status within the last several days, months, or years. In COPD, lung function declines slowly over many years. The patient may not notice this decline because activity is altered to accommodate reduced exercise tolerance. If an upper respiratory infection is superimposed on a chronic problem, dyspnea and decreased exercise tolerance may occur very quickly.

The nurse should describe the course of the patient's illness including when it began, the type of symptoms, and factors that alleviate or aggravate these symptoms. The most common signs and symptoms of respiratory disease are runny nose, sore throat, cough, sputum production, hemoptysis, wheezing, breathlessness, and chest pain. Because of the chronic nature of respiratory problems, the patient may relate a change in symptoms rather than the onset of new symptoms when describing the present illness.

Table 22-5 Key Questions: Patient with a Respiratory Problem

Health Perception–Health Management Pattern
- Describe your daily activities. Has there been a change in activities you can perform in the last several days? months? years? If changed, was this because of your health?
- How do your breathing problems affect your self-care abilities?
- Have you ever smoked? Do you smoke now? If yes, how many cigarettes each day and for how long? Did you stop or cut back on your smoking because of your health?*
- Have you had a Pneumovax vaccination? When was your last flu shot?
- What types of alcoholic beverages do you drink? How often?
- Do you ever use drugs to get high?* How often?
- What equipment helps you manage your respiratory problems? How often do you use it? Does it help? Cause problems?

Nutritional-Metabolic Pattern
- Have you recently lost weight because of difficulty eating secondary to a respiratory problem? How much? Voluntarily?
- Do any particular foods affect your sputum production or breathing?*

Elimination Pattern
- Does your respiratory problem make it difficult for you to get to the toilet?*
- Are you inactive because of dyspnea to the point where it causes constipation?

Activity-Exercise Pattern
- Are you ever short of breath during exercise?* At rest?*
- Do you get too short of breath to do the things you want to do?*
- Is your home one-story? Two stories? How many steps from the street to your door?
- Are you able to maintain your typical activity pattern? If not, explain.

Sleep-Rest Pattern
- Do breathing problems cause you to awaken during the night?*
- Can you lie flat at night? If not, how many pillows do you use? Do you need to sleep upright in a chair?

Cognitive-Perceptual Pattern
- Do you have any pain associated with breathing?*
- Do you ever feel restless, irritable, or confused without a reason?*
- Do you have difficulty remembering things?*

Self-Perception–Self-Concept Pattern
- Describe how your respiratory problems have changed your life.
- Do you ever go out without using your oxygen? When and why?

Role-Relationship Pattern
- Has your respiratory problem caused any difficulties in your work, family, or social relationships?*

Sexuality-Reproductive Pattern
- Has your respiratory problem caused a change in your sexual activity?*
- Do you want to discuss ways to decrease dyspnea during sexual activity?

Coping–Stress Tolerance Pattern
- How often do you leave your home?
- Would you want to join a support group? Pulmonary rehabilitation program?
- Does stress have an effect on your breathing?*
- What effect does your respiratory problem have on your emotions?

Value-Belief Pattern
- How often do you miss taking your medications? Why?
- Do you think the things you have been told to do for your respiratory problems really help? If not, why?

*If yes, describe.

Such changes should be carefully documented because they often suggest the cause of the illness. For example, a change in the volume, tenacity (thickness), or color of sputum suggests onset of a lower respiratory tract infection.

The patient should be questioned about a family history of respiratory problems that may be genetic, such as cystic fibrosis or emphysema resulting from alpha$_1$ antitrypsin deficiency. A history of family exposure to tuberculosis bacilli should be noted.

The nurse should ask where the patient has lived and traveled. Risk factors for tuberculosis include prior residence in Asia, Africa, or Latin America. Risk factors for fungal infections of the lung include living or travel in the Southwest (coccidioidomycosis) and the Mississippi River Valley (histoplasmosis).

The nurse should also ask about current and past smoking habits and quantify exposure in pack-years. This is done by multiplying the number of packs smoked per day by the number of years smoked. For example, a person who smoked 1½ packs per day for 10 years has a 15 pack-year history. The risk of lung cancer rises in direct proportion to the number of cigarettes smoked. Smoking increases the risk of COPD and exacerbates symptoms of asthma and chronic bronchitis.

The nurse should ask if the patient received immunization for pneumococcal pneumonia (Pneumovax) and influenza (flu). Influenza vaccine should be administered yearly in the fall. Repeat vaccination with Pneumovax is not advised unless the patient is at high risk for fatal pneumococcal disease (asplenic patient) or likely to experience a rapid decline in antibody levels (transplant recipient).[19]

The patient should be asked about the use of equipment to manage respiratory symptoms (e.g., home oxygen therapy equipment, metered dose inhaler [MDI] or nebulizer for medication administration, a positive airway pressure device for relief of sleep apnea). The patient should be questioned about the type of equipment used, frequency of use, its effect, and any side effects. The patient should be asked to demonstrate use of the MDI. Many patients do not know how to correctly use MDI devices (see Chapter 25).[21] The elderly are more likely to experience problems learning correct MDI inhalation technique.[22]

Nutritional-metabolic pattern. Weight loss is a symptom of many respiratory diseases. The nurse should determine if weight loss was intentional and, if not, if food intake is altered by anorexia (from medications), fatigue (from hypoxemia, increased work of breathing), early satiety (from lung hyperinflation), or social isolation. Anorexia and weight loss are common symptoms in patients with COPD, acquired immunodeficiency syndrome (AIDS), lung cancer, and tuberculosis. Fluid intake should also be noted. Dehydration can result in thickened mucus, which can cause airway obstruction.

Weight gain indicates possible fluid retention from cardiovascular dysfunction. Excessive weight interferes with normal ventilation and may cause sleep apnea (see Chapter 23).

Elimination pattern. Healthy elimination habits depend on the ability to reach a toilet when necessary. Activity intolerance secondary to dyspnea could result in urinary incontinence. Dyspnea can also be the cause of limited mobility which, in turn, can cause constipation. The patient with dyspnea should be questioned about both of these possibilities.

Activity-exercise pattern. The nurse should determine if the patient's activity is limited by dyspnea at rest or during exercise. The nurse should also note whether the patient's housing (e.g., number of steps, levels) poses a problem that increases social isolation.

The nurse should also inquire if the patient is able to carry out activities of daily living without dyspnea or other respiratory symptoms. If unable, the amount and type of care needed should be documented. Immobility and sedentary habits can be risk factors for hypoventilation leading to atelectasis or pneumonia.

Sleep-rest pattern. The nurse should ask if the patient can sleep throughout the night. The patient with asthma or COPD may awaken at night with chest tightness, wheezing, or coughing. This suggests a need for a longer-acting bronchodilator or other medication change. The patient with cardiovascular disease (e.g., congestive heart failure) may sleep with the head elevated on several pillows. The patient with sleep apnea may complain of snoring, insomnia, and daytime drowsiness. The occurrence of night sweats should be documented because this event can be a manifestation of tuberculosis.

Cognitive-perceptual pattern. Because hypoxia can cause neurologic symptoms, the nurse should ask about apprehension, restlessness, and irritability, which can indicate inadequate cerebral oxygenation (see Table 22-3). Hypoxemia interferes with the ability to learn and retain information.[23] For this reason, teaching may be more effective if another person is present during the teaching session to provide reinforcement at a later date.

The patient's ability to cooperate with the treatment plan should be assessed. Cognitive impairment may cause noncompliance or resistance to therapy. Failure to participate in needed therapy can result in exacerbation of respiratory problems.

The nurse should inquire about any discomfort or pain with breathing. A complaint of chest pain needs to be explored carefully to rule out cardiac involvement. Respiratory system problems such as pleurisy, fractured ribs, and costochondritis cause chest pain. Pleuritic pain is described as a sharp, stabbing pain associated with movement or deep breathing. Fractured ribs cause localized sharp pain associated with breathing. The pain of costochondritis is along the borders of the sternum and is associated with breathing.

Self-perception–self-concept pattern. Dyspnea limits activity, impairs ability to fulfill normal developmental role functions, and often alters self-esteem. Concern about a highly visible nasal cannula may cause the patient to resist using oxygen in public. The nurse should ask how the patient views body image in relation to that of others. Referral to a support group or pulmonary rehabilitation program may be beneficial in developing a support system and coping strategies.[24]

Role-relationship pattern. Acute or chronic respiratory problems can seriously affect performance in work or other related activities. The nurse needs to ask about the impact of activity, medications, oxygen, and special routines (e.g., pulmonary hygiene for cystic fibrosis) on the patient's family, job, and social life.

Progression of chronic respiratory problems that severely limit activity may have a negative impact on the patient's roles and responsibilities at home or on the job. The patient should be asked if any problems in these areas are present.

The nurse should document the nature of the patient's work and the frequency and intensity of exposure to fumes, toxins, asbestos, coal, or silica. Patient-specific allergens such as dust or fumes, which could be present in the work environment, should be investigated. Hobbies such as woodworking (sawdust) or pottery (silica) and exposure to animals (allergies) may also cause respiratory problems.

Sexuality-reproductive pattern. Most patients can continue to have good sexual relationships despite marked physical limitations. In a tactful manner, the nurse needs to determine whether breathing difficulties have caused alterations in sexual activity. If so, teaching can be provided about positions which decrease dyspnea during sexual activity and alternate strategies for sexual fulfillment.[25]

Coping–stress tolerance pattern. Dyspnea causes anxiety and anxiety exacerbates dyspnea. The result is a vicious cycle—the patient avoids activities that cause dyspnea, becoming more deconditioned and more dyspneic. The outcome is often physical and social isolation. The nurse should ask how often the patient leaves home and interacts with others. Referral to a support group or pulmonary rehabilitation program may be beneficial.[24]

The chronic nature of many respiratory problems such as COPD and asthma can cause prolonged stress. Inquiry should be made into the patient's coping strategies to manage this protracted stress.

Value-belief pattern. The nurse should determine the patient's adherence to the management regimen. If suboptimal, reasons for lack of adherence should be explored, including culturally-specific beliefs, failure to note benefit, or other reasons.

Objective Data

Physical Examination. Vital signs, including temperature, pulse, respirations, and blood pressure, are important data to collect before examination of the respiratory system.

Nose. The nose is inspected for inflammation, deformities, and symmetry. The nurse tilts the patient's head backward and pushes the tip of the nose upward gently. With a nasal speculum and a good light, the interior of the nose is inspected. The mucous membrane should be pink and moist, with no evidence of edema (bogginess), exudate, or bleeding. The nasal septum should be observed for deviation, perforations, and bleeding. Some nasal deviation is normal in an adult. The turbinates should be observed for *polyps*, which are abnormal, fingerlike projections of swollen nasal mucosa. Polyps may result from long-term irritation of the mucosa, as from allergies.

Mouth and pharynx. Using a good light source, the nurse inspects the interior of the mouth for color, lesions, masses, gum retraction, bleeding, and poor dentition. The tongue is inspected for symmetry and presence of lesions. The nurse observes the pharynx by pressing a tongue blade against the middle of the back of the tongue. The pharynx should be smooth and moist, with no evidence of exudate, ulcerations, or swelling. The color, symmetry, and any enlargement of the tonsils are noted. The nurse stimulates the gag reflex by placing a tongue blade on the back of the pharynx. A normal response (gagging) indicates that the ninth and tenth cranial nerves are intact and that the airway is protected.

Neck. The nurse inspects the neck for symmetry and presence of tender or swollen areas. The lymph nodes are palpated while the patient is sitting erect with the neck slightly flexed. Progression is front to back from the nodes around the ears, to the nodes at the base of the skull, and then to those located under the angles of the mandible to the midline. The patient may have small, mobile, nontender nodes *(shotty nodes)*, which are not a sign of a pathologic condition. Tender, hard, or fixed nodes are indicative of disease. The location and characteristics of any nodes that are palpated are described.

Thorax and lungs. Imaginary lines can be pictured on the chest to help in identifying abnormalities (see Fig. 22-2). Abnormalities can be described in relation to their location to these lines (e.g., 2 cm from the right midclavicular line).

Chest examination is best performed in a well-lighted, warm room with measures taken to ensure the patient's privacy. Depending on the clinician's preference, either the anterior or the posterior chest may be examined first.

INSPECTION. The patient's anterior side of the chest should be exposed. If able, the patient should sit upright or lean on the bedside table. First, the nurse observes the patient's appearance and notes any evidence of respiratory distress, such as tachypnea, inability to lie flat, or use of accessory muscles. Next, the nurse determines the shape and symmetry of the chest. Chest movement should be equal on both sides and anteroposterior (AP) diameter ⅓ to ½ the side-to-side diameter. An increase in AP diameter (e.g., *barrel chest*) may be a normal aging change or result from lung hyperinflation. The nurse observes for abnormalities in the sternum (e.g., *pectus carinatum*, a prominent protrusion of the sternum, and *pectus excavatum*, an indentation of the lower sternum above the xiphoid process).[26,27]

Next the respiratory rate, depth, and rhythm should be observed. The normal rate is 12 to 20 breaths per minute; in the elderly, it is 16 to 25 breaths per minute. Inspiration (I) should take half as long as expiration (E) (e.g., I:E = 1:2). The nurse should observe for abnormal breathing patterns, such as *Kussmaul's* (rapid, deep breathing), *Cheyne-Stokes* (a rhythmic increase and decrease in rate separated by periods of apnea), or *Biot's* respirations (irregular breathing with apnea every 4 to 5 cycles).

Skin color provides clues to respiratory status. *Cyanosis* is best observed in a dark-skinned patient in the conjunctivae, lips, palms, and soles of the feet. Causes of cyanosis include hypoxemia or decreased cardiac output. The fingers should be inspected for evidence of *clubbing* (an increase in the angle between the base of the nail and the fingernail to 180 degrees or more, usually accompanied by an increase in the depth, bulk, and sponginess of the end of the finger).[28,29]

When the nurse is inspecting the posterior part of the chest, the patient should be asked to lean forward with arms folded. This position moves the scapula away from the spine, so there is more exposure of the area to be examined. The same sequence of observations that were done on the anterior part of the chest is performed on the posterior part. In addition, any spinal curvature is noted. Spinal curvatures that affect breathing include *kyphosis*, *scoliosis*, and *kyphoscoliosis*.

PALPATION. The nurse determines tracheal position by gently placing the index fingers on either side of the trachea just above the suprasternal notch and gently pressing backward. Normal tracheal position is midline; deviation to the left or right is abnormal. Tracheal deviation occurs with pneumothorax (toward the collapsed lung), pneumonectomy (toward the surgical side), and lobar atelectasis (toward the collapsed lobe).

The nurse determines symmetry of chest expansion and extent of movement at the level of the diaphragm. The nurse places the hands over the lower anterior chest wall along the costal margin and moves them inward until the thumbs meet at midline. The patient is asked to breathe deeply, and the nurse observes the movement of the thumbs away from each other. Normal expansion is 1 inch (2.5 cm). On the posterior side of the chest, the nurse places the hands at the level of the tenth rib and moves the thumbs until they meet over the spine (Fig. 22-10).

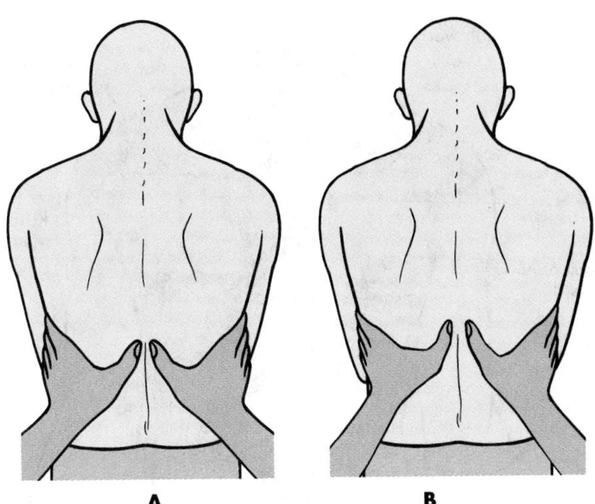

Fig. 22-10 Estimation of thoracic expansion. ***A,*** Exhalation. ***B,*** Maximal inhalation.

Normal chest movement is equal. Unequal expansion occurs when air entry is limited by conditions involving the lung (e.g., atelectasis, pneumothorax), the chest wall (e.g., incisional pain), or the pleura (e.g., pleural effusion). Equal but diminished expansion occurs in conditions that produce a hyperinflated or barrel chest or in neuromuscular disease (e.g., amyotrophic lateral sclerosis, spinal cord lesions). Movement may be absent or unequal over a pleural effusion, atelectasis, or pneumothorax.

Tactile fremitus is vibration of the chest wall produced by vocalization. To elicit this, the nurse places the palms of the hands against the patient's chest and asks the patient to repeat a phrase such as "ninety-nine." The nurse moves the hands from side to side and from top to bottom on the patient's chest (Fig. 22-11). All areas of the chest should be palpated and vibrations compared from similar areas. Tactile fremitus is most intense in the first and second interspace lateral to the sternum and between the scapulae because these areas are closest to the major bronchi. Fremitus is less intense farther away from these areas.[28,29]

Increase, decrease, or absence of fremitus should be noted. Increased fremitus occurs when the lung becomes filled with fluid or more dense. This is noted in pneumonia, lung tumors, and above a pleural effusion (the lung is compressed upward). Fremitus is decreased if the hand is farther from the lung (e.g., pleural effusion) or the lung is hyperinflated (e.g., barrel chest). Absent fremitus may be noted with pneumothorax or atelectasis. The anterior of the chest is more difficult to palpate for fremitus because of the presence of large muscles and breast tissue.

Rhonchal fremitus is a palpable vibration caused by air traveling past thick mucus. It can be felt with the hand on the chest and may change or clear with coughing.

PERCUSSION. Percussion is done to assess density or aeration of the lungs. Percussion sounds are described in Table 22-6. (The technique for percussion is described in Chapter 4.)

The anterior of the chest is usually percussed with the patient in a semisitting or supine position. Starting below the clavicles, the nurse percusses downward, interspace by interspace (see Fig. 22-11). The area over lung tissue should be resonant, with the exception of the area of cardiac dullness (Fig. 22-12). For percussion of the posterior of the chest, the patient should sit leaning forward with arms folded. The posterior of the chest should be resonant over lung tissue to the level of the diaphragm (Fig. 22-13).

AUSCULTATION. During chest auscultation, the patient is instructed to breathe slowly and deeply through the mouth. The nurse should proceed from the lung apices to the bases, comparing opposite areas of the chest (see Fig. 22-11). The stethoscope should be placed over lung tissue, not over

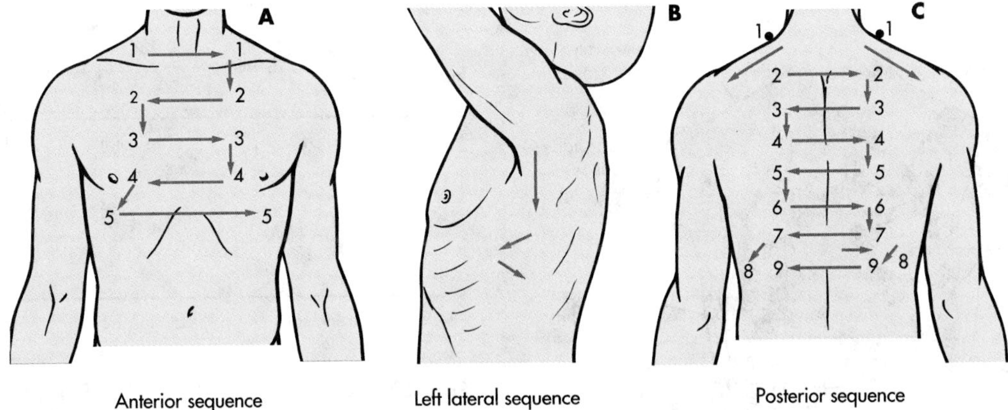

Fig. 22-11 Sequence for examination of the chest. ***A,*** Anterior sequence. ***B,*** Lateral sequence. ***C,*** Posterior sequence. For palpation, place the palms of the hands in the position designated as "1" on the right and left sides of the chest. Compare the intensity of vibrations. Continue for all positions in each sequence. For percussion, tap the chest at each designated position, moving downward from side-to-side, while comparing percussion notes. For auscultation, place the stethoscope at each position. Listen to at least one inspiratory and expiratory cycle.

Table 22-6 Percussion Sounds

Sound	Description
▪ Resonance	Low-pitched sound heard over normal lungs
▪ Hyperresonance	Loud, lower-pitched sound than normal resonance heard over hyperinflated lungs, such as in chronic obstructive lung disease and acute asthma
▪ Tympany	Drumlike, loud, empty quality heard over gas-filled stomach or intestine, or pneumothorax
▪ Dull	Medium-intensity pitch and duration heard over areas of "mixed" solid and lung tissue, such as over the top area of the liver, partially consolidated lung tissue (pneumonia), or fluid-filled pleural space
▪ Flat	Soft, high-pitched sound of short duration heard over very dense tissue where air is not present

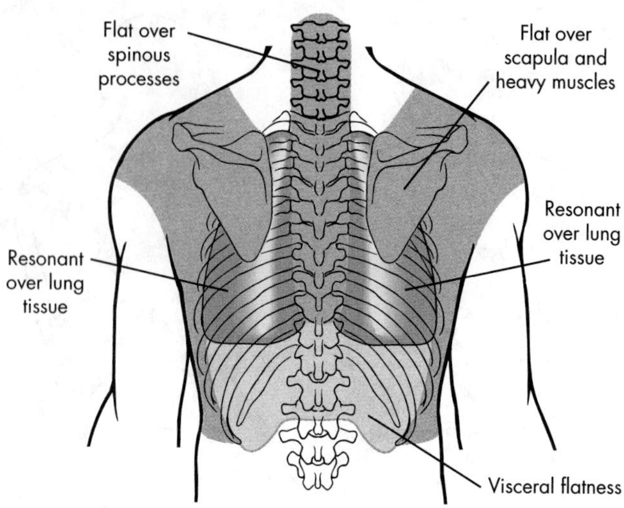

Fig. 22-13 Diagram of percussion areas and sounds in the posterior side of the chest. Percussion proceeds from the lung apices to the lung bases, comparing sounds in opposite areas of the chest.

bony prominences. At each placement of the stethoscope, the nurse should listen to at least one cycle of inspiration and expiration. Note the pitch (e.g., high, low), duration of sound, and adventitious or abnormal sounds. Normal and adventitious sounds are more easily understood by visualization of a diagrammatic model (Fig. 22-14).

There are three normal breath sounds: vesicular, bronchovesicular, and bronchial. *Vesicular sounds* are relatively soft, low-pitched, gentle, rustling sounds. They are heard over all lung areas except the major bronchi. *Bronchovesicular sounds* have a medium pitch and intensity and are heard anteriorly over the main stem bronchi on either side of the sternum and posteriorly between the scapulae. Inspiration is equal to expiration. *Bronchial sounds* are louder and higher-pitched and resemble air blowing through a hollow pipe. There is a gap between inspiration and expiration, reflecting the short pause between these respiratory cycles. Bronchial sounds are heard over the manubrium.[26,27]

The term *abnormal breath sounds* is used to describe bronchial or bronchovesicular sounds heard in the peripheral lung fields. *Adventitious sounds* include *crackles, rhon-*

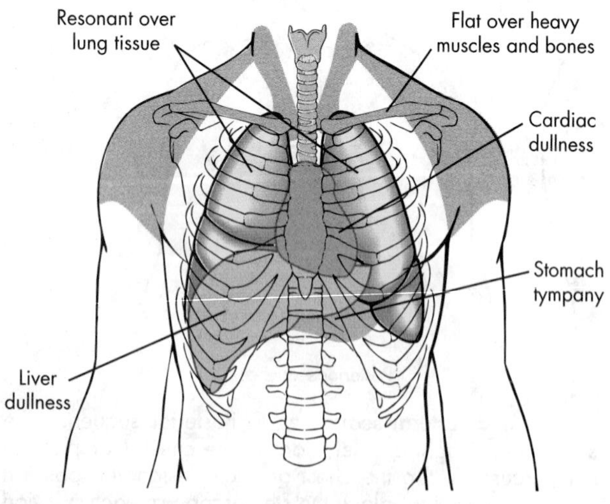

Fig. 22-12 Diagram of percussion areas and sounds in the anterior side of the chest.

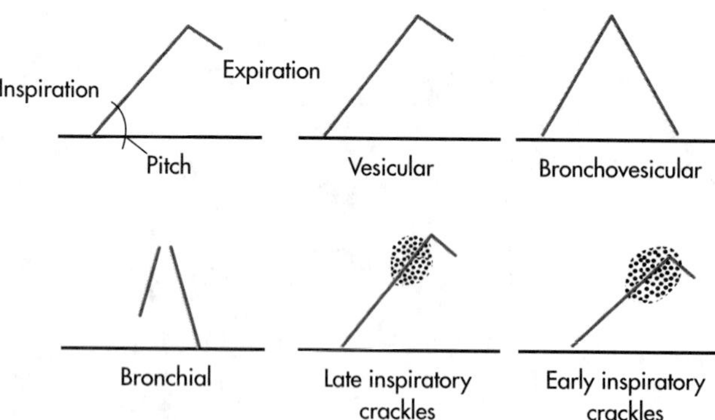

Fig. 22-14 Diagrammatic model of breath sounds. Inspiration is shown by the upstroke and expiration by the downstroke. Vesicular sounds have a 3:1 ratio, with inspiration longer than expiration. Bronchovesicular sounds have a 1:1 ratio, with inspiration and expiration equal, and bronchial sounds have a 2:3 ratio, with a gap between inspiration and expiration. Fine and coarse crackles are typically heard at points marked by the showers of dots.

Table 22-7 Common Assessment Abnormalities: Thorax and Lungs

Finding	Description	Possible Etiology and Significance*
Inspection		
▪ Pursed lip breathing	Exhalation through mouth with lips pursed together to slow exhalation.	COPD, asthma. Suggests ↑ breathlessness. Strategy taught to slow expiration, ↓ dyspnea.
▪ Tripod position; inability to lie flat	Leaning forward with arms and elbows supported on overbed table.	COPD, asthma in exacerbation, pulmonary edema. Indicates moderate to severe respiratory distress.
▪ Accessory muscle use; intercostal retractions	Neck and shoulder muscles used to assist breathing. Muscles between ribs pull in during inspiration.	COPD, asthma in exacerbation, secretion retention. Indicates severe respiratory distress, hypoxemia.
▪ Splinting	Voluntary ↓ in tidal volume to ↓ pain on chest expansion.	Thoracic or abdominal incision. Chest trauma, pleurisy.
▪ ↑ AP diameter	AP chest diameter equal to lateral. Slope of ribs more horizontal (90°) to spine.	COPD, asthma, cystic fibrosis. Lung hyperinflation. Advanced age.
▪ Tachypnea	Rate >20 breaths/min; >25 breaths/min in elderly.	Fever, anxiety, hypoxemia. Magnitude of ↑ above normal rate reflects increased work of breathing.
▪ Kussmaul's respirations	Regular, rapid, and deep respirations.	Metabolic acidosis. ↑ in rate aids body in ↑ CO_2 excretion.
▪ Cyanosis	Bluish color of skin best seen in ear lobes, under the eyelids, or nail beds.	↓ oxygen transfer in lungs, ↓ cardiac output. Nonspecific, unreliable indicator.
▪ Clubbing of fingers	↑ in depth, bulk, sponginess of distal digit of finger.	Chronic hypoxemia. Cystic fibrosis, lung cancer.
Palpation		
▪ Tracheal deviation	Leftward or rightward movement of trachea from normal midline position.	Nonspecific indicator of change in position of mediastinal structures. Medical emergency if caused by tension pneumothorax.
▪ Altered tactile fremitus	Increase or decrease in vibrations.	↑ in pneumonia, pulmonary edema; ↓ in pleural effusion, atelectatic area, lung hyperinflation; absent in pneumothorax, large atelectasis.
▪ Altered chest movement	Unequal or equal but diminished movement of two sides of chest with inspiration.	Unequal movement caused by atelectasis, pneumothorax, pleural effusion, splinting; equal but diminished movement caused by barrel chest, restrictive disease, neuromuscular disease.
Percussion		
▪ Hyperresonance	Loud, lower-pitched sound over areas that normally produce a resonant sound.	Lung hyperinflation (COPD), lung collapse (pneumothorax), air trapping (asthma).
▪ Dullness	Medium-pitched sound over areas that normally produce a resonant sound.	↑ density (pneumonia, large atelectasis), ↑ fluid pleural space (pleural effusion).

continued

chi, *wheezes*, and *pleural friction rubs*. Table 22-7 describes these sounds and gives possible etiologies.

A record of the normal physical assessment of the respiratory system is shown in Table 22-8. Chest examination findings in common pulmonary problems are presented in Table 22-9. Common assessment abnormalities are presented in Table 22-7. Age-related changes in the respiratory system and assessment findings are presented in Table 22-4.

Diagnostic Studies. Diagnostic studies provide important information to the nurse in monitoring the patient's condition and planning appropriate interventions. These studies are considered to be objective data. Diagnostic studies of the respiratory system are presented in Table 22-10.

DIAGNOSTIC STUDIES

Blood Studies

Common blood studies used to assess the respiratory system are the hemoglobin (Hb), hematocrit (Hct), and ABG determinations (see Tables 22-1 and 22-2). Table

Table 22-7 Common Assessment Abnormalities: Thorax and Lungs—cont'd

Finding	Description	Possible Etiology and Significance*
Auscultation		
▪ Fine crackles	Series of short, explosive, high-pitched sounds heard just before the end of inspiration; result of rapid equalization of gas pressure when collapsed alveoli or terminal bronchioles suddenly snap open; similar sound to that made by rolling hair between fingers just behind ear	Interstitial fibrosis (asbestosis), interstitial edema (early pulmonary edema), alveolar filling (pneumonia), loss of lung volume (atelectasis)
▪ Coarse crackles	Series of short, low-pitched sounds caused by air passing through airway intermittently occluded by mucus, unstable bronchial wall, or fold of mucosa; evident on inspiration and, at times, expiration; similar sound to blowing through straw under water; increase in bubbling quality with more fluid	Congestive heart failure, pulmonary edema, pneumonia with severe congestion, COPD
▪ Rhonchi	Continuous rumbling, snoring, or rattling sounds from obstruction of large airways with secretions; most prominent on expiration; change often evident after coughing or suctioning	COPD, cystic fibrosis, pneumonia
▪ Wheezes	Continuous high-pitched squeaking sound caused by rapid vibration of bronchial walls; first evident on expiration but possibly evident on inspiration as obstruction of airway increases; possibly audible without stethoscope	Bronchospasm (caused by asthma), airway obstruction (caused by foreign body, tumor), COPD
▪ Stridor	Continuous musical sound of constant pitch; result of partial obstruction of larynx or trachea	Croup, epiglottitis, vocal cord edema after extubation, foreign body
▪ Absent breath sounds	No sound evident over entire lung or area of lung	Pleural effusion, mainstem bronchi obstruction, large atelectasis
▪ Pleural friction rub	Creaking or grating sound from roughened, inflamed surfaces of the pleura rubbing together; evident during inspiration and expiration and no change with coughing; usually uncomfortable, especially on deep inspiration	Pleurisy, pneumonia, pulmonary infarct
▪ Bronchophony, whispered pectoriloquy	Spoken or whispered syllable more distinct than normal on auscultation	Pneumonia
▪ Egophony	Spoken "e" similar to "a" on auscultation because of altered transmission of voice sounds	Pneumonia, pleural effusion

AP, Anteroposterior; *COPD,* chronic obstructive pulmonary disease.
*Limited to common etiologic factors. (Further discussion of conditions listed may be found in Chapters 23 through 26.)

22-10 describes nursing responsibilities associated with these tests.

Oximetry

Oximetry is used to noninvasively monitor SpO_2 and SvO_2 (see Tables 22-1 and 22-2). Nursing care associated with oximetry is discussed in Table 22-10.

Sputum Studies

Sputum samples can be obtained by expectoration or bronchoscopy, a technique in which a flexible scope is inserted into the airways. The specimens may be examined for culture and sensitivity to identify an infecting organism (e.g., *Mycobacterium, Pneumocystis carinii*) or to confirm a diagnosis (e.g., malignant cells). Nursing responsibilities

Table 22-8 Normal Physical Assessment of the Respiratory System

- Nose is symmetric with no deformities. Nasal mucosa is pink and moist with no edema, exudate, or blood. Nasal septum is straight, without perforations. No polyps are evident.
- Oral mucosa is light pink and moist, with no exudate or ulcerations.
- Tonsils are present and not inflamed or enlarged.
- Pharynx is smooth, moist, and pink.
- Neck is symmetric and trachea is in the midline. No nodes are palpable.
- Chest has a normal configuration, with no evidence of injury. Respirations are normal, at the rate of 14/min. Excursion is equal bilaterally, with no increase in tactile fremitus. Percussion is resonant throughout. Breath sounds are resonant throughout, without crackles, rhonchi, or wheezes. No axillary nodes are palpable.

for specimen collection are given in Table 22-10. Regardless of whether specimens are ordered, it is important to observe the sputum for color, blood, volume, and viscosity.

Skin Tests

Skin tests may be performed to test for allergic reactions or exposure to tuberculous bacilli or fungi. Skin tests involve the intradermal injection of an antigen. A positive result indicates the patient has been exposed to the antigen. It does not indicate that disease is currently present. A negative result indicates there has been no exposure or there is depression of cell-mediated immunity such as occurs in HIV infection.

Nursing responsibilities are similar for all skin tests. First, to prevent a false-negative reaction, the nurse should be certain that the injection is intradermal and not subcutaneous. After the injection, the sites should be circled and the patient instructed not to remove the marks. When charting administration of the antigen, the nurse should draw a diagram of the forearm and hand and label the injection sites. The diagram is especially helpful when more than one test is administered.

Table 22-9 Chest Examination Findings in Common Pulmonary Problems

Problem	Inspection	Palpation	Percussion	Auscultation
▪ Chronic bronchitis	Barrel chest; cyanosis	↓ movement ↑ fremitus	Hyperresonant or dull if consolidation	Crackles; rhonchi; wheezes
▪ Emphysema	Barrel chest; tripod position; use of accessory muscles	↓ movement	Hyperresonant or dull if consolidation	Crackles; rhonchi; diminished if no exacerbation
▪ Asthma: In exacerbation	Prolonged expiration; tripod position; pursed lips	↓ movement ↓ fremitus if hyperinflation	Hyperresonance	Wheezes; ↓ breath sounds (silent chest) ominous sign if no improvement (severely diminished air movement)
Not in exacerbation	Normal	Normal	Normal	Normal
▪ Pneumonia	Tachypnea; use of accessory muscles; duskiness or cyanosis	Unequal movement if lobar involvement; ↑ fremitus over affected area	Dull over affected areas	Early: Bronchial sounds lower in chest Later: Crackles; rhonchi
▪ Atelectasis	No change unless involves entire segment, lobe	If small, no change. If large, ↓ movement; ↑ fremitus	Dull over affected areas	Crackles (may disappear with deep breaths); absent sounds if large
▪ Pulmonary edema	Tachypnea; labored respirations; cyanosis	↓ or normal movement	Dull or normal depending on amount of fluid	Fine or coarse crackles
▪ Pleural effusion	Tachypnea; use of accessory muscles	↓ movement; ↑ fremitus above effusion; absent fremitus over effusion	Dull	Diminished or absent over effusion; egophony over effusion
▪ Pulmonary fibrosis	Tachypnea	↓ movement	Normal	Crackles

Table 22-10 Diagnostic Studies: Respiratory System

Study	Description and Purpose	Nursing Responsibility
Blood Studies		
▪ Hemoglobin	This test reflects amount of hemoglobin available for combination with oxygen. Venous blood is used. *Normal level* for adult male is 13-16 g/dl; *normal level* for adult female is 12-14 g/dl.	Explain procedure and its purpose.
▪ Hematocrit	This test reflects ratio of red blood cells to plasma. Increased hematocrit (polycythemia) found in chronic hypoxemia. Venous blood is used. *Normal* for adult man is 42-50%; *normal* for adult woman is 40-48%.	Explain procedure and its purpose.
▪ ABGs	Arterial blood is obtained through puncture of radial or femoral artery or through arterial catheter. ABGs are performed to assess acid-base balance, need for oxygen therapy, change in oxygen therapy, or change in ventilator settings.* Continuous ABG monitoring is also possible via a sensor or electrode inserted into the arterial catheter.	Indicate whether patient is using oxygen (percentage, L/min). Avoid change in oxygen therapy or interventions (e.g., suctioning, position change) for 20 min before obtaining sample. Cleanse skin with alcohol swab and assist with positioning (e.g., palm up, wrist slightly hyperextended if radial artery is used). Collect blood into heparinized syringe. To ensure accurate results, expel all air bubbles, and place sample in ice, unless it will be analyzed in less than 1 min. Apply pressure to artery for 5 min after specimen is obtained to prevent hematoma formation at the arterial puncture site.
▪ Oximetry	This test monitors SaO_2 or SvO_2. Device attaches to the earlobe, finger, or nose for SpO_2 monitoring or is contained in a pulmonary artery catheter for SvO_2 monitoring. Oximetry is used for continuous monitoring in ICUs, inpatient and outpatient settings, and exercise testing.†	Apply monitoring probe to finger, earlobe, or bridge of nose. When interpreting SpO_2 and SvO_2 values, first assess patient status and presence of factors that can alter accuracy of pulse oximeter reading. For SpO_2, these include motion, low perfusion, bright lights, use of intravascular dyes, dark skin color. For SvO_2, these include change in O_2 delivery or O_2 consumption. For SpO_2, notify physician of ±4% change from baseline or ↓ to <90%. For SvO_2, notify physician of ±10% change from baseline or ↓ <60%. Institute changes or modify plan of care as needed if values are not within expected range.
Sputum Studies		
▪ Culture and sensitivity	Single sputum specimen is collected in a sterile container. Purpose is to diagnose bacterial infection, select antibiotic, and evaluate treatment.	Instruct patient on how to produce a good specimen (see Gram stain). If patient cannot produce specimen, bronchoscopy may be used (see Fig. 22-16).
▪ Gram stain	Staining of sputum permits classification of bacteria into gram-negative and gram-positive types. Results guide therapy until culture and sensitivity results are obtained.	Instruct patient to expectorate sputum into the container after coughing deeply. Obtain sputum (mucoidlike), not saliva. Obtain specimen in early morning because secretions collect during night. If unsuccessful, try increasing oral fluid intake unless fluids are restricted. Collect sputum in sterile container (sputum trap) during suctioning or by aspirating secretions from the trachea. Send specimen to laboratory promptly.
▪ Acid-fast smear and culture	This test is performed to collect sputum for acid-fast bacilli (tuberculosis). A series of 3 early morning specimens is used.	Instruct patient on how to produce a good specimen (see Gram stain). Cover specimen and send to laboratory for analysis.

continued

Table 22-10 Diagnostic Studies: Respiratory System—cont'd

Study	Description and Purpose	Nursing Responsibility
▪ Cytology	Single sputum specimen is collected in special container with fixative solution. Purpose is to determine presence of abnormal cells that may indicate malignant condition.	Send specimen to laboratory promptly. Instruct patient on how to produce a good specimen (see Gram stain). If patient cannot produce specimen, bronchoscopy may be used (see Fig. 22-16).
Radiology		
▪ Chest x-ray	This test is used to screen, diagnose, and evaluate change. Most common views are posteroanterior and lateral.	Instruct patient to undress to waist, put on gown, and remove any metal between neck and waist.
▪ Computed tomography (CT)	This test is performed for diagnosis of lesions difficult to assess by conventional x-ray studies, such as those in the hilum, mediastinum, and pleura. Images obtained show body structures in cross section (see Fig. 22-15).	Same as for chest x-ray.
▪ Magnetic resonance imaging (MRI)	This test is used for diagnosis of lesions difficult to assess by CT scan (e.g., lung apex near the spine).	Same as for chest x-ray. Instruct the patient to remove all metal (e.g., jewelry, watch) before test.
▪ Ventilation-perfusion ($\dot{V}/\dot{Q}$)	This test used to identify areas of the lung not receiving airflow (ventilation) or blood flow (perfusion). It involves injection of radioisotope and inhalation of small amount of radioactive gas (xenon). A gamma-detecting device is used to record radioactivity. Ventilation without perfusion suggests pulmonary embolus.	Same as for chest x-ray. Also check for dye allergy. No precautions needed afterward because the gas and isotope transmit radioactivity for only a brief interval.
▪ Pulmonary angiogram	This study is used to visualize pulmonary vasculature and locate obstruction or pathologic conditions such as pulmonary embolus. A radiopaque dye is injected, usually through a catheter, into the pulmonary artery or right side of the heart.	Same as for chest x-ray. Know that dye injection may cause flushing, warm sensation, and coughing. Check pressure dressing site after procedure. Monitor blood pressure, pulse rate, and circulation distal to injection site. Report and record significant changes.
▪ Positron emission tomography (PET)	This test is used to distinguish benign and malignant lung nodules. It involves IV injection of a radioisotope with short half-life.	Same as for chest x-ray study. No precautions needed afterward because isotope only transmits radioactivity for brief interval.
Endoscopic Examinations		
▪ Bronchoscopy	This study is typically performed in outpatient procedure room. Flexible fiberoptic scope is used for diagnosis, biopsy, specimen collection, or assessment of changes. It may also be done to suction mucous plugs or to remove foreign objects.	Instruct patient to be on NPO status for 6-12 hr. Obtain signed permit. Give diazepam if ordered by physician before procedure to aid relaxation. After procedure, keep patient NPO until gag reflex returns and monitor for laryngeal edema. If biopsy was done, monitor for hemorrhage and pneumothorax.
▪ Mediastinoscopy	This test is used for inspection and biopsy of lymph nodes in mediastinal area.	Prepare patient for surgical intervention. Obtain signed permit. Afterward, monitor as for bronchoscopy.
Biopsy		
▪ Lung biopsy	Specimens may be obtained by transbronchial or open-lung biopsy. This test is used to obtain specimens for laboratory analysis.	Same as bronchoscopy if procedure done with bronchoscope, and same as thoracotomy if open-lung biopsy done. Obtain signed permit.

continued

Table 22-10 Diagnostic Studies: Respiratory System—cont'd

Study	Description and Purpose	Nursing Responsibility
Other		
▪ Thoracentesis	This test is used to obtain specimen of pleural fluid for diagnosis, to remove pleural fluid, or to instill medication. The physician inserts a large-bore needle through the chest wall into pleural space. Chest x-ray is always obtained after procedure to check for pneumothorax.	Explain procedure to patient and obtain signed permit before procedure. Position patient upright, instruct not to talk or cough, and assist physician during procedure. Apply dressing after procedure. Observe for signs of inadequate oxygenation after procedure. If large volume of fluid is removed, monitor for decrease in shortness of breath. Send labeled specimens to laboratory.
▪ Pulmonary function test	This test is used to evaluate lung function. It involves use of a spirometer to diagram air movement as patient performs prescribed respiratory maneuvers.‡	Avoid scheduling immediately after mealtime. Explain procedure to patient. Provide rest after the procedure.

ABGs; Arterial blood gases; *ICUs,* intensive care units; *IV,* intravenous; *NPO,* nothing by mouth.
*For normal values, see Tables 22-1 and 22-2.
†For normal values see Tables 22-12 and 22-13.
‡See Figs. 22-8 and 22-9.

When reading test results, the nurse should use a good light. If induration is present, a marking pen should be brought in from the periphery on all four sides of the induration. As the pen touches the raised area, a mark should be made. The nurse then determines the diameter of the induration in millimeters. Reddened, flat areas are not measured.[28-31] See Table 22-11 for a description of reactions that indicate a positive tuberculosis skin test.

Radiographic Studies

Chest X-ray. A chest x-ray is the most commonly used test for respiratory diagnosis. It is also used to assess progression of disease and response to treatment. The most common views used are the posteroanterior (PA) and lateral. (See Table 22-10 for nursing responsibilities related to chest x-rays.)

Computed Tomography. A computed tomography (CT) scan may be used to examine cross sections of the entire body. CT scans are used to evaluate areas that are difficult to assess by conventional x-ray, such as the mediastinum, hilum, and pleura. With the addition of a contrast enhanced medium-or high-resolution technique, all structures of the thorax can be inspected for evidence of disease (Fig. 22-15).[32]

Magnetic Resonance Imaging. While in a strong magnetic field, the alignment of spinning nuclei can be changed with a superimposed radiofrequency and the rate at which they return to alignment with the field can be measured. Magnetic resonance imaging (MRI) uses this technique to produce images of body structures. MRI has limited indications. It is most useful when evaluating images near the lung apex or spine, and for distinguishing vascular from nonvascular structures.[32]

Ventilation-Perfusion Scan. A ventilation-perfusion ($\dot{V}/\dot{P}$) scan is used primarily to check for the presence of a pulmonary embolus. There is no specific preparation or aftercare. An intravenous (IV) radioisotope is given for the perfusion portion of the test, and the pulmonary vasculature is outlined and photographed. For the ventilation portion, the patient inhales a radioactive gas, which outlines the alveoli, and another photograph is taken. Normal scans show homogeneous radioactivity. Diminished or absent radioactivity suggests lack of perfusion or airflow.

Pulmonary Angiography. Pulmonary angiography is used to confirm the diagnosis of an embolus if findings of the lung scan are inconclusive. A series of x-rays is taken after radiopaque dye is injected into the pulmonary artery. This test also detects congenital and acquired lesions of the pulmonary vessels.

Positron Emission Tomography. Positron emission tomography (PET) scans involve the use of radionuclides with short half-lives. PET scans are used to distinguish benign and malignant solitary pulmonary nodules. Because malignant lung cells have an increased uptake of glucose, the PET scan, which uses an IV glucose preparation, can demonstrate increased uptake of glucose in malignant lung cells.

Endoscopic Examinations

Bronchoscopy. Bronchoscopy is a procedure in which the bronchi are visualized through a fiberoptic tube. Bronchoscopy may be used to obtain biopsy specimens, assess changes resulting from treatment, and remove mucous plugs or foreign bodies. Small amounts (30 ml) of sterile saline may be injected through the scope and withdrawn and examined for cells, a technique termed *bronchoalveolar lavage* (BAL). BAL is used to diagnose *Pneumocystis carinii* pneumonia (Fig. 22-16).

Bronchoscopy can be performed in an outpatient procedure room or surgical suite, with the patient lying down or seated. After the nasal pharynx and oral pharynx are anesthetized with local anesthetic, the bronchoscope is

Table 22-11 Interpreting Skin Reactions to Tuberculosis Testing

Size of Induration	Consider Positive in the Following Groups
5 mm or greater	▪ Recent close contact with person diagnosed with infectious TB. ▪ Chest x-ray with fibrotic lesions likely to be healed TB. ▪ Known or suspected HIV infection.
10 mm or greater	▪ Other medical risk factors known to substantially ↑ risk of TB once infection has occurred (e.g., diabetes mellitus, immunosuppressive therapy, end-stage renal disease, cancer of oropharynx or upper GI tract). ▪ Foreign-born from high prevalence countries (e.g., Southeast Asia, Africa, Latin America). ▪ Medically underserved groups, homeless. ▪ Residents of long-term care facilities, prisons. ▪ IV drug users.
15 mm or greater	▪ All other persons.
False negative reactions may occur in persons who were infected with TB many years ago and persons with an active current infection.	Causes include: ▪ immunosuppression, overwhelming TB infection. ▪ testing too soon after exposure to TB (up to 10 wk may be required to develop immune response). ▪ aging (may result in delayed-type hypersensitivity). ▪ long time since TB infection. Sensitivity to tuberculin may wane over the years, resulting in a negative reaction. However, the tuberculin test may stimulate (*boost*) ability to react to tuberculin, causing a positive reaction to future tests.
10-25% of persons with TB have a negative reaction if tested with tuberculin.	*Two-step testing* is therefore recommended for individuals likely to be tested often, (i.e., health care providers and individuals who may have delayed hypersensitivity). Interpret as follows: ▪ 1st test positive, consider the person infected. ▪ 1st test negative, repeat 1-3 weeks later. ▪ 2nd test positive, consider active or prior infection (depending on risk factors) and care for accordingly. ▪ 2nd test negative, consider uninfected. Interpret future positive test as a new infection.

GI, gastrointestinal; *HIV*, human immunodeficiency virus; *IV*, intravenous; *TB*, tuberculosis.

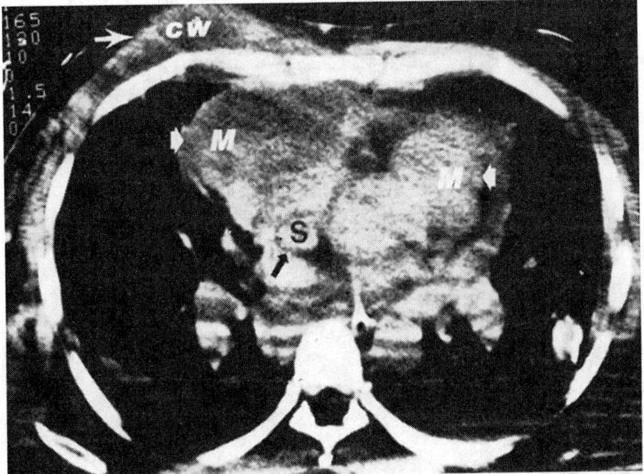

Fig. 22-15 Computed tomographic (CT) scan of the chest. *Arrows* indicate a large mediastinal mass (*M*) invading the lung, chest wall (*CW*), and superior vena cava (*S*).

coated with lidocaine (Xylocaine) and inserted, usually through the nose, and threaded down into the airways. Bronchoscopy can be done on mechanically ventilated patients. The scope is inserted through the endotracheal tube. The nursing care for this procedure is described in Table 22-10.

Mediastinoscopy. For mediastinoscopy, a scope is inserted through a small incision in the suprasternal notch and advanced into the mediastinum to inspect and biopsy lymph nodes. The test is used to diagnose carcinoma, granulomatous infections, and sarcoidosis. The procedure is performed in the operating room and the patient is given a general anesthetic.

Lung Biopsy

Lung biopsy may be done transbronchially or as an open-lung biopsy. The purpose is to obtain tissue, cells, or secretions for evaluation. *Transbronchial lung biopsy* involves passing a forceps or needle through the bronchoscope. A specimen is obtained with forceps or aspirated through a needle (Fig. 22-17). Specimens can be cultured or examined for malignant cells. A combination of transbronchial lung biopsy and BAL is used to differentiate infection and rejection in lung transplant recipients. Nursing care is the same as for fiberoptic bronchoscopy. *Open-lung biopsy*

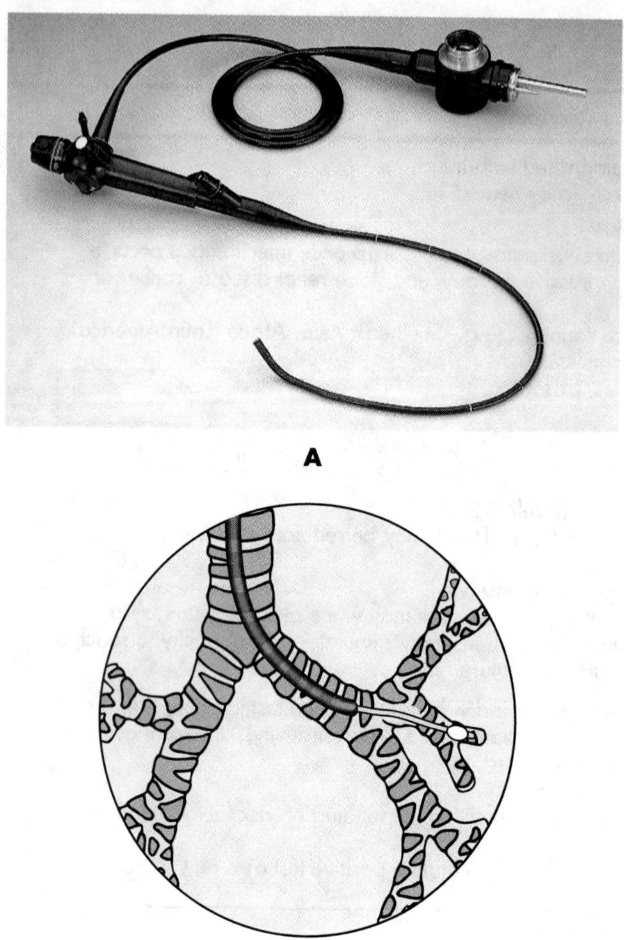

A

B

Fig. 22-16 Fiberoptic bronchoscope. ***A,*** The transbronchoscopic balloon-tipped catheter and the flexible fiberoptic bronchoscope. ***B,*** The catheter is introduced into a small airway and the balloon inflated with 1.5 to 2 ml air to occlude the airway. Bronchial alveolar lavage (BAL) is performed by injecting and withdrawing 30 ml aliquots of sterile saline solution, gently aspirating after each instillation. Specimens are sent to the laboratory for analysis.

is used when pulmonary disease cannot be diagnosed by other procedures. The patient is anesthetized, the chest is opened with a thoracotomy incision, and a biopsy specimen obtained. Nursing care for the procedure is the same as for any patient who has a thoracotomy (see Chapter 24).

Thoracentesis

Thoracentesis is the insertion of a needle through the chest wall into the pleural space to obtain specimens for diagnostic evaluation, remove pleural fluid, and instill medication into the pleural space (Fig. 22-18). The patient is positioned sitting upright with elbows on an overbed table. Feet and legs should be well supported. The skin is cleansed and a local anesthetic (Xylocaine) instilled subcutaneously. A chest tube may be inserted to permit further drainage of fluid. (Nursing care is described in Table 22-10.)

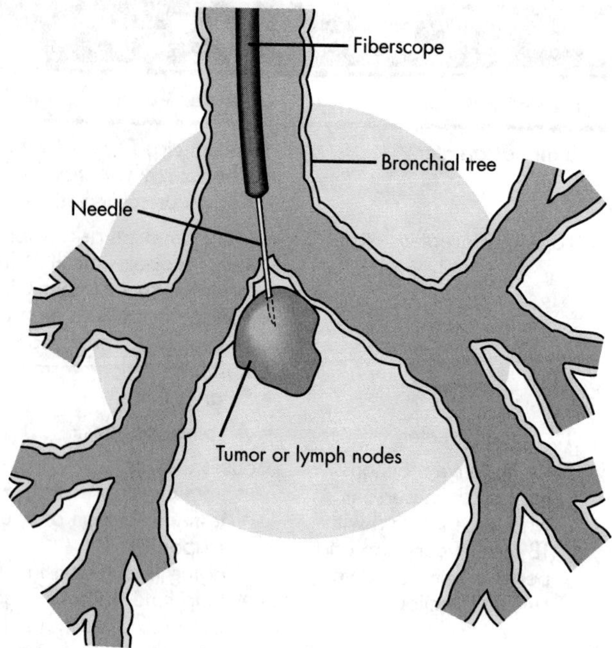

Fig. 22-17 Transbronchial needle biopsy. The diagram shows a transbronchial biopsy needle penetrating the bronchial wall and entering a mass of subcarinal lymph nodes or tumor.

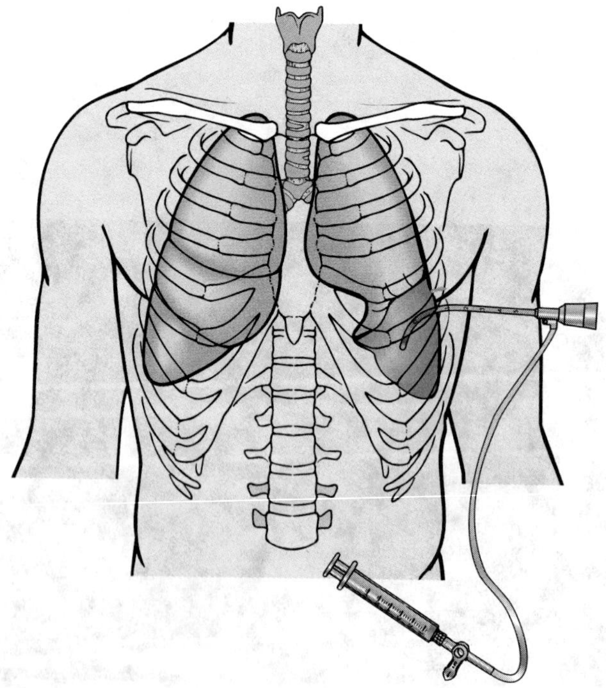

Fig. 22-18 Thoracentesis. The needle has penetrated the fluid-filled pleural space to remove fluid.

Table 22-12 Lung Volumes and Capacities

Parameter	Definition	Normal Values
Volumes		
▪ Tidal volume (V_T)	Volume of air inhaled and exhaled with each breath; only a small proportion of total capacity of lungs	0.5 L
▪ Expiratory reserve volume (ERV)	Additional air that can be forcefully exhaled after normal exhalation is complete	1.0 L
▪ Residual volume (RV)	Amount of air remaining in lungs after forced expiration; air available in lungs for gas exchange between breaths	1.5 L
▪ Inspiratory reserve volume (IRV)	Maximum volume of air that can be inhaled forcefully after normal inhalation	3.0 L
Capacities		
▪ Total lung capacity (TLC)	Maximum volume of air that lungs can contain (TLC = IRV + V_T + ERV + RV)	6.0 L
▪ Functional residual capacity (FRC)	Volume of air remaining in lungs at end of normal exhalation (FRC = ERV + RV); increase or decrease possible with lung disease	2.5 L
▪ Vital capacity (VC)	Maximum volume of air that can be exhaled after maximum inspiration (VC = IRV + V_T + ERV); higher VC for men (generally)	4.5 L
▪ Inspiratory capacity (IC)	Maximum volume of air that can be inhaled after normal expiration (IC = V_T + IRV)	3.5 L

Pulmonary Function Tests

Pulmonary function tests (PFTs) measure lung volumes and airflow. The results of PFTs are used to diagnose pulmonary disease, monitor disease progression, evaluate disability, and evaluate response to bronchodilators. PFTs are performed with the use of a spirometer. The patient's age, sex, height, and weight are first obtained. This information is entered into the PFT computer and used to calculate the predicted value for each test. The patient inserts a mouthpiece, takes as deep a breath as possible, and exhales as hard, fast, and long as possible. Verbal coaching is given to ensure that the patient continues blowing out until exhalation is complete. The computer determines the actual value, predicted (normal) value, and percentage of the predicted value for each test. A normal value is 80% to 120% of the predicted value. Normal values for PFTs are shown in Tables 22-12 and 22-13 and Fig. 22-19.

Pulmonary function parameters can also be used to determine the need for mechanical ventilation or the readiness to be weaned from ventilatory support. Measurements of vital capacity, maximum inspiratory pressure (MIP), and minute ventilation are used to make this determination (see Table 22-12 and Chapter 26).

Exercise Testing

Exercise testing is used in diagnosis, in determining exercise capacity, and for disability evaluation. A complete exercise test involves walking on a treadmill while expired oxygen and carbon dioxide, respiratory rate, heart rate, and rhythm are monitored. A modified test (desaturation test)

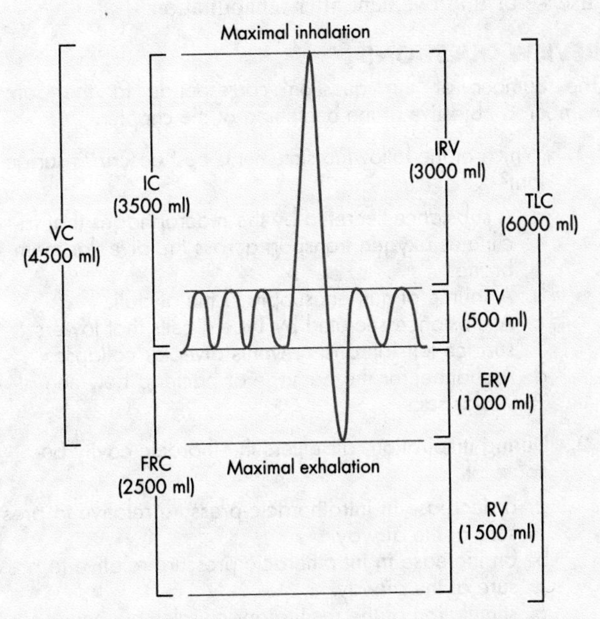

Fig. 22-19 Relationship of lung volumes and capacities.

Table 22-13 Common Measures of Pulmonary Function

Measure	Description	Normal Value*
▪ Forced vital capacity (FVC)	Amount of air that can be quickly and forcefully exhaled after maximum inspiration	Over 80% of predicted
▪ Forced expiratory volume in first second of expiration (FEV_1)	Amount of air exhaled in first second of FVC; valuable clue to severity of airway obstruction	Over 80% of predicted
▪ FEV_1/FVC	Dividing of value for FEV_1 by value for FVC; useful in differentiating obstructive and restrictive pulmonary dysfunction	Over 80% of predicted
▪ Forced midexpiratory flow rate ($FEF_{25-75\%}$)	Measurement of airflow rate in middle half of forced expiration; early indicator of disease of small airways	Over 80% of predicted
▪ Maximal voluntary ventilation (MVV)	Deep breathing as rapidly as possible for specified period; test for airflow, muscle strength, coordination, airway resistance; important factor in exercise tolerance	About 170 L/min
▪ Peak expiratory flow rate (PEFR)	Maximum airflow rate during forced expiration; aid in monitoring bronchoconstriction in asthma	Up to 600 L/min
▪ Maximum inspiratory pressure(MIP)	Amount of negative pressure generated on inspiration; indication of ability to breathe deeply and cough	−25 cm H_2O minimum

*Normal values vary with height, weight, age, and sex of patient.

may also be used. In this case, only SpO_2 is monitored. A desaturation test can also be used to determine the oxygen flow needed to maintain the SpO_2 at a safe level during exercise in patients who use home oxygen therapy.

A *timed walk* can also be used to measure exercise capacity. The patient is instructed to walk as far as possible during a timed period (6 or 12 minutes), stopping when short of breath, and continuing when able. The distance walked is measured and used to monitor progression of disease or improvement after rehabilitation.

REVIEW QUESTIONS

The number of the question corresponds to the same-numbered objective at the beginning of the chapter.

1. Which of the following statements best describes surfactant?
   a. A substance secreted by the macrophages that facilitates oxygen transport across the alveolar membrane.
   b. A source of nutrient supply to the alveoli.
   c. A substance secreted by Type II cells that lowers surface tension and prevents alveolar collapse.
   d. A channel for the passage of bacteria between alveolar sacs.

2. During inspiration, air enters the thoracic cavity because of
   a. a decrease in intrathoracic pressure relative to pressure at the airway.
   b. an increase in intrathoracic pressure relative to pressure at the airway.
   c. stimulation of the respiratory muscles by the chemoreceptors.
   d. an increase in carbon dioxide and decrease in oxygen in the blood.

3. The ability of the lungs to adequately oxygenate the arterial blood is determined by examination of the
   a. arterial carbon dioxide tension.
   b. venous carbon dioxide tension.
   c. carboxyhemoglobin level.
   d. arterial oxygen tension.

4. The most important respiratory defense mechanism distal to the respiratory bronchioles is the
   a. alveolar macrophage.
   b. reflex bronchoconstriction.
   c. mucociliary clearance mechanism.
   d. impaction of particles.

5. A rightward shift of the oxygen-hemoglobin dissociation curve
   a. interferes with release of oxygen at the tissue level.
   b. causes oxygen to have a greater affinity for hemoglobin.
   c. facilitates release of oxygen at the tissue level.
   d. is caused by metabolic alkalosis.

6. Signs and symptoms of inadequate oxygenation include all of the following *except*
   a. tachypnea, dyspnea on exertion.
   b. tachycardia, mild hypertension.
   c. unexplained apprehension, restlessness, irritability.
   d. increased peripheral perfusion, increased urine output.

7. Changes associated with the aging process include all of the following *except*
   a. a decrease in chest wall compliance.
   b. a decrease in pulmonary artery blood flow.
   c. a decrease in cell-mediated immunity.
   d. a decreased response to hypoxemia and hypercapnia.

8. When assessing activity-exercise patterns related to respiratory health, the nurse inquires about

a. willingness to wear oxygen in public.
b. ability to sleep through the entire night.
c. dyspnea during rest or exercise.
d. recent weight loss or weight gain.

9. When percussing the chest, the nurse should compare sounds heard

a. at the lung base and apex.
b. on the anterior and posterior chest.
c. on the left and right anterior and posterior chest in the same areas.
d. over the scapulae and manubrium.

10. Adventitious breath sounds include all of the following *except*

a. bronchovesicular sounds.
b. crackles.
c. wheezing.
d. rhonchi.

11. Examination of sputum specimens is used in the diagnosis of all the following *except*

a. tuberculosis.
b. pneumonia.
c. emphysema.
d. cancer of the lung.

REFERENCES

1. Corbridge T, Irvin CG. Pathophysiology of chronic obstructive pulmonary disease with emphasis on physiologic and pathologic correlations. In Casaburi R, Petty TL, editors: *Principles and practice of pulmonary rehabilitation,* Philadelphia, 1993, Saunders.
2. Dettemeier PA: *Pulmonary nursing care,* St Louis, 1992, Mosby.
3. Kersten LD: *Comprehensive respiratory nursing: a decision-making approach,* Philadelphia, 1989, Saunders.
4. Stone KS: Respiratory physiology. In Clochesy JM and others, editors: *Critical care nursing,* Philadelphia, 1993, Saunders.
5. Vander AJ, Sherman JH, Luciano DS: *Human physiology: the mechanisms of body function,* ed 5, New York, 1990, McGraw-Hill.
6. Elpern EH and others: Pulmonary aspiration in mechanically ventilated patients with tracheostomies, *Chest* 105:563, 1994.
7. Patterson GA: Double lung transplantation, *Clin Chest Med* 11:227, 1990.
8. Malley WJ: *Clinical blood gases: application and noninvasive alternatives,* Philadelphia, 1990, Saunders.
9. Mims BC: Interpreting ABGs, *RN* 54:42, 1991.
10. Anderson S: ABGs: six easy steps to interpreting blood gases, *Am J Nurs* 90:42, 1990.
11. Dellinger RP, Zimmerman JL: Continuous intra-arterial blood gas monitoring. In Vincent JL, editor: *Yearbook of intensive care and emergency medicine,* Berlin, 1992, Springer-Verlag.
12. Cooper CB. Long-term oxygen therapy. In Casaburi R, Petty TL, editors: *Principles and practice of pulmonary rehabilitation,* Philadelphia, 1993, Saunders.
13. Gong H: Air travel and oxygen therapy in cardiopulmonary patients, *Chest* 101: 1104, 1992.
14. Szaflarski NL: Use of pulse oximetry in critically ill adults, *Heart Lung* 18:444, 1989.
15. Grossbach I: Studies in pulse oximetry monitoring, *Crit Care Nurse* 13: 63, 1993.
16. Hayden RA: Trend-spotting with an SvO_2 monitor, *Am J Nurs* 93:26, 1993.
17. Copel LC and Stolarik A: Continuous SvO_2 monitoring: a research review, *DCCN* 10:202, 1991.
18. Britt TL: Elderly patients. In Clochesy JM and others, editors: *Critical care nursing,* Philadelphia, 1993, Saunders.
19. Gardner P, Schaffner W: Immunization of adults, *New Engl J Med* 328:1252, 1993.
20. Timby BK: Pneumocystosis in patients with acquired immunodeficiency syndrome, *Crit Care Nurse* 12:64, 1992.
21. National Asthma Education Program: *Guidelines for the diagnosis and management of asthma,* Bethesda, MD, Dept of Health and Human Services, 1991, DHHS publication 91-3042.
22. Chapman KR, Love L, Brubaker H: A comparison of breath-activated and conventional metered-dose inhaler inhalation techniques in elderly subjects, *Chest* 104:1332, 1993.
23. Incalzi RA and others: Chronic obstructive pulmonary disease: an original model of cognitive decline, *Am Rev Respir Dis* 148:418, 1993.
24. Vale F, Reardon JZ, ZuWallack RL: The long-term benefits of outpatient pulmonary rehabilitation on exercise endurance and quality of life, *Chest* 103:42, 1993.
25. Hoffman LA, Berg J, Rogers RM: Daily living with COPD, *Postgrad Med,* 86:153, 1989.
26. Freedberg PD, Hoffman LA, Cagno JA: *Physical examination of the chest* (40 minute videocassette), Philadelphia, 1988, Saunders.
27. Steismeyer JK: A four-step approach to pulmonary assessment, *Am J Nurs* 93:22, 1993.
28. Avey MA: TB skin testing: how to do it right, *Am J Nurs* 93:42, 1993.
29. Boutotte J: TB the second time around, *Nursing* 13:42, 1993.
30. O'Brien LM, Bartlett KA: TB plus HIV, *Am J Nurs* 92:28, 1992.
31. Summartojo E: When tuberculosis treatment fails: a social behavioral account of patient adherence, *Am Rev Respir Dis* 147:1311, 1993.
32. Weinberger SE: Recent advances in pulmonary medicine, *New Engl J Med* 328:1389, 1993.

Chapter 23

NURSING ROLE IN MANAGEMENT

Upper Respiratory Problems

Adele A. Large   Leslie A. Hoffman

Learning Objectives

1. Describe the clinical manifestations and nursing management of problems of the nose.
2. Describe the clinical manifestations and nursing management of problems of the paranasal sinuses.
3. Describe the clinical manifestations and nursing management of inflammatory problems of the pharynx and larynx.
4. Discuss the nursing management of the patient who requires endotracheal intubation or a tracheostomy.
5. Identify the steps involved in suctioning an airway and performing tracheostomy care.
6. Describe the risk factors and warning symptoms associated with oral cancer and cancer of the larynx.
7. Discuss the nursing management of the patient with a laryngectomy.
8. Describe the methods used in voice restoration for the patient with temporary or permanent loss of speech.

The structures that make up the upper respiratory tract are the nose, paranasal sinuses, pharynx, larynx, and trachea. As a person breathes these structures are subjected to repeated exposure to microorganisms, fumes, gases, and carcinogens. For this reason, disorders involving the upper respiratory tract are common.

STRUCTURAL AND TRAUMATIC DISORDERS OF THE NOSE

Deviated Septum

Deviated septum most commonly occurs as a result of nasal trauma or congenital disproportion, in which the cartilaginous septum is too large for the area. The main symptom of a deviated nasal septum is obstruction of nasal breathing. On inspection, the septum is bent to one side with the air passage reduced. Minor septal deviations cause no symptoms. Major deviations may cause cosmetic deformity, epistaxis, or sinusitis.[1] *Epistaxis* results from nasal crusting because of an alteration in air flow. *Sinusitis* results from obstruction of mucus drainage into the nose. Discomfort from nasal obstruction is variable and is not always related to the amount of nasal blockage.[1]

A *nasal septoplasty* may be performed to surgically correct the deformity when major symptoms or discomfort occur. The deviated septum is reconstructed, aligned, and straightened, and complications are rare. Health promotion is aimed at the prevention of precipitating factors, such as accidental falls sustained in childhood.

Nasal Fracture

Nasal fracture is most often caused by trauma sustained as a result of an injury. Complications of the fracture include airway obstruction and cosmetic deformity. Nasal fractures are classified as unilateral, bilateral, or complex. A *unilateral fracture* typically produces little or no displacement. *Bilateral fractures,* the most common fractures, give the nose a flattened look. Powerful frontal blows cause *complex fractures,* which may also shatter frontal bones. Diagnosis of nasal fracture is based on the health history, direct observation of internal and external nasal structures, and x-ray findings.

On inspection, the patient's nose may be deviated to one side or depressed, with epistaxis evident and a positive history of trauma. The nurse should note the presence of edema or hematoma and the patient's ability to breathe through each side of the nose. The nose is inspected internally for septal deviation, hemorrhage, and leakage of cerebrospinal fluid. If clear drainage is observed, a specimen may be sent to the laboratory to determine if it is cerebrospinal fluid (CSF). Injury of sufficient force to fracture nasal bones causes considerable swelling of soft tissues. With extensive swelling, it may be difficult or impossible to verify the extent of deformity until reexamination several days after the injury when edema is subsiding.

Reviewed by Donna J. Wilson, RN, MSN, RRT, Pulmonary Clinical Nurse Specialist, Memorial Sloan Kettering Cancer Center, New York, NY.

Ice may be gently applied to the face and nose to reduce edema and bleeding. When a fracture is confirmed, the goal of therapeutic management is to realign the fracture by open or closed reduction. This will reestablish the cosmetic appearance and proper function of the nose and provide an adequate airway.

The goals of nursing management are to reduce edema, prevent complications, educate the patient, and provide emotional support. If the injury is severe, surgical intervention such as open reduction (septoplasty or rhinoplasty) may be required.

Rhinoplasty

Rhinoplasty is surgical reconstruction of the nose. It is performed for cosmetic reasons or to improve airway function when trauma or developmental deformities result in nasal obstruction. Assessment of expectations is a critical aspect of the patient's preparation for rhinoplasty. Body image is multidimensional and includes perception of the body as a physical, psychologic, and social entity. For this reason any actual or perceived alteration, such as a deformed or enlarged nose, can affect one's self-esteem and interactions with others. The patient's expectations concerning surgical results should be assessed with regard to the expected change. Photographs made to life-size measurements can be used to simulate the appearance after the reconstruction. These photographs may help the patient decide whether to undergo rhinoplasty. Expected results of surgery should be explained frankly and truthfully to avoid disappointment.

Procedure. Rhinoplasty is performed with the use of regional anesthesia. The entire nose is anesthetized by injection of lidocaine at points that block involved nerve pathways, preventing pain transmission. The patient is given preoperative sedation and additional sedation in the operating room (OR) just before the lidocaine injection. Tissue may be added or removed, and the nose may be lengthened or shortened. Plastic implants may be used to reshape the nose. Postoperatively, Steri-Strips are placed to hold the skin against the septal cartilage. Packing is inserted to apply pressure and to prevent bleeding or septal hematoma formation. A plastic splint is molded to the new shape of the nose. The packing is typically removed the day after surgery, and the splint is removed in 3 to 5 days.

NURSING MANAGEMENT

RHINOPLASTY

To reduce the risk of bleeding, the patient should be instructed to refrain from taking aspirin-containing drugs for 2 weeks before surgery. Nursing diagnoses specific to the patient undergoing a rhinoplasty include, but are not limited to, those presented in the nursing care plan on p. 590. Nursing interventions during the immediate postoperative period include assessment of respiratory status and observation of the surgical site for hemorrhage and edema. Health teaching is important because time in the hospital is limited. The outcome of rhinoplasty is most often satisfactory and pleasing to the patient.

Epistaxis

Epistaxis (nosebleed) occurs as a result of bleeding from a rich network of veins located in the anterior nasal septum (i.e., Kiesselbach's plexus or posterior nasal septum). Anterior bleeding usually stops spontaneously or can be self-treated, but posterior bleeding may require medical care.[1] Causes of epistaxis include trauma to the nose, nasogastric tube insertion, nasal intubation, cocaine use, nasal crusting, and nasal picking. Conditions that prolong bleeding time or alter platelet counts may predispose the patient to epistaxis. Bleeding time may also be prolonged if the patient takes aspirin or nonsteroidal antiinflammatory drugs (NSAIDs). Conditions such as hypertension may increase the risk of epistaxis if blood pressure is elevated.

Therapeutic Management. Simple first aid measures may be effective in stopping epistaxis. It is important to (1) keep the patient quiet; (2) place the patient in a sitting position, leaning forward, or if that is not possible, in a reclining position with head and shoulders elevated; (3) apply direct pressure by pinching the entire soft lower portion of the nose for 10 to 15 minutes; (4) apply ice compresses to the nose, and have the patient suck on ice; (5) partially insert a small gauze pad into the bleeding nostril, and apply digital pressure if bleeding continues; and (6) obtain medical assistance if bleeding does not stop.[2]

If first aid is not effective, management involves localization of the bleeding site and application of a vasoconstrictive agent or cauterization of the problem vessel.[2] In addition, the nose may be packed. Anterior packing may consist of ribbon gauze impregnated with antibiotic ointment that is wedged firmly in the desired location and remains in place for 48 to 72 hours. If posterior packing is required, inflatable balloons may be used as the nasal pack or gauze may be inserted (Fig. 23-1).[3] Strings attached to the packing are brought to the outside and taped to the cheek for ease of removal. Packing is painful because sufficient pressure must be applied to stop the bleeding.[2]

NURSING MANAGEMENT

EPISTAXIS

If bleeding can be controlled with the use of a vasoconstrictive agent, cauterization, or anterior packing, the patient can be discharged after being taught about home care. The patient should be instructed to avoid vigorous nose blowing, strenuous activity, lifting, and straining for 4 to 6 weeks. The patient should be taught to sneeze with the mouth open and to avoid the use of aspirin-containing products or NSAIDs, if possible. The patient should receive a medication for pain and an antibiotic to prevent infection.

The patient with posterior packing requires hospitalization. After packing, some patients experience a decrease in PaO_2 and an increase in $PaCO_2$. Because these changes may be life-threatening in the older patient, admission to an intensive care unit (ICU) may be necessary.[2] The nurse should monitor respiratory rate and rhythm, oxygen saturation using pulse oximetry (SpO_2), and observe for signs of

NURSING CARE PLAN Patient with a Rhinoplasty

Planning: Outcome Criteria	Nursing Interventions and Rationales
➤ **NURSING DIAGNOSIS**	Altered health maintenance *related to* lack of knowledge of postoperative course, pain management, and prevention of complications *as manifested by* questioning about care, anxiety
Correctly verbalize information about expected routine and self-care.	Explain surgical procedure, expected postoperative course, and required self-care *to decrease anxiety and increase patient cooperation.* Answer questions as needed.
➤ **NURSING DIAGNOSIS**	Ineffective breathing pattern *related to* presence of packing and nasal edema *as manifested by* abnormal respiratory rate, rhythm, or depth; mucosal swelling, ecchymosis
Have normal respiratory rate, rhythm, and depth. Have minimal to no swelling or bruising.	Instruct patient to not blow nose, to sneeze with mouth open, and to avoid coughing *to avoid dislodging packing.* Instruct patient to maintain semi-Fowler's position and minimize facial movement for 48 hr *to prevent increase in facial edema.* Apply 4 by 4-in pads dipped in ice water to incisional area for 24 hr *to minimize pain and swelling.*
➤ **NURSING DIAGNOSIS**	Pain *related to* incisional edema or inadequate comfort measures *as manifested by* report of pain, facial expression indicative of pain, dry mucous membranes
Have minimal or no pain; satisfaction with pain control; moist, intact mucous membranes.	Describe to patient the amount of pain to expect *to decrease anxiety and foster cooperation.* Instruct patient in correct analgesic schedule. Teach patient to apply iced 4 by 4-in pads for 24 hr *to reduce edema and pain by vasoconstriction.* Teach patient to avoid use of aspirin-containing analgesics *to decrease possibility of bleeding.* Teach patient gentle cleaning techniques, such as use of cotton swabs and water-soluble jelly or hydrogen peroxide when packing has been removed *to promote cleanliness and comfort and to decrease infection.*
➤ **NURSING DIAGNOSIS**	Body-image disturbance *related to* postoperative edema and changed facial appearance *as manifested by* verbalization of concern about appearance, anxiety
Report feeling less anxious and more optimistic about positive surgical outcome.	Inform patient that most facial edema subsides gradually in 1 mo *to decrease anxiety.* (It may take as long as 8 mo for all edema to subside). Help patient to remain realistic regarding surgical results *to avoid disappointment.*

COLLABORATIVE PROBLEMS

Nursing Goals	Nursing Interventions and Rationales
➤ **POTENTIAL COMPLICATION**	Nasal hemorrhage *related to* inadequate hemostasis and high vascularity of operative site
Monitor for signs of bleeding, report deviation from acceptable parameters, and carry out appropriate medical and nursing interventions.	Teach patient to report continued drainage of serosanguineous fluid from operative site after 24 hr, and to avoid taking aspirin or aspirin-containing drugs because *aspirin products increase the potential for bleeding.* Report to physician any fresh bleeding or displacement of the packing *so early treatment of hemorrhage is initiated.*

aspiration and infection. Nasal packing may predispose to toxic shock syndrome because it promotes production of an endotoxin produced by certain strains of *Staphylococcus aureus* that may be present in the nasal cavity.[1] Mouth care should be provided, and a call bell should be placed within reach. Nasal dryness can be decreased by breathing humidified oxygen. A nasal sling (a folded 2 by 2 inch gauze pad) should be taped over the nares to absorb drainage. Posterior packs are usually removed after 4 to 5 days. Before removal the packing may be saturated with hydrogen peroxide. After removal, the nares may be gently cleaned and lubricated with petroleum jelly.

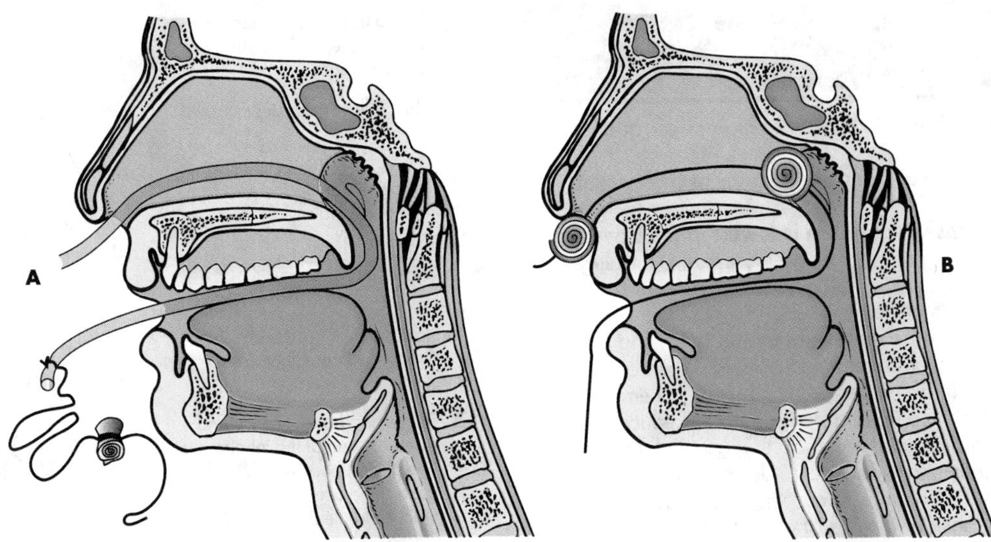

Fig. 23-1 Method for placing posterior nasal pack. ***A,*** Catheter is passed through the bleeding side of the nose and pulled out through the mouth with a hemostat. Strings are tied to the catheter and the pack is pulled up behind the soft palate and into the nasopharynx. ***B,*** Nasal pack in position in the posterior nasopharynx. Dental roll at the nose helps to maintain correct position.

INFLAMMATION AND INFECTION OF THE NOSE AND PARANASAL SINUSES

Allergic Rhinitis

Allergic rhinitis (hay fever) is the reaction of the nasal mucosa to a specific antigen (allergen). Attacks of *seasonal rhinitis* usually occur in the spring and fall and are caused by allergy to pollens from trees, flowers, or grasses. The typical attack lasts for several weeks (most commonly during the hay fever season), disappears, and recurs at the same time the following year. *Perennial rhinitis* is present intermittently or constantly. Symptoms are usually caused by specific environmental triggers such as pet dander, dust mites, molds, odors, or particular foods. Because symptoms of perennial rhinitis resemble those of the common cold, the patient may believe the condition is a continuous or repeated "cold."

Allergic rhinitis is caused by an immunoglobulin E (IgE)-mediated reaction. The first step involves sensitized mast cells with allergen-specific IgE coming into contact with the inciting allergen. Next, the mast cell degranulates, releasing mediators (such as histamine, leukotrienes, thromboxanes, and prostaglandins) that trigger the acute phase of the allergic reaction. These mediators act on the respiratory mucosa to produce symptoms of sneezing, itching, and rhinorrhea. In addition, these mediators cause relaxation of smooth muscle in blood vessels, increased capillary permeability, and nasal congestion.[3] (The allergic reaction is discussed in Chapter 10.)

Clinical Manifestations. Manifestations of allergic rhinitis are nasal congestion (caused by edema); sneezing; watery, itchy eyes and nose; altered sense of smell; and thin watery nasal discharge.[4] The nasal turbinates appear pale, boggy, and swollen. The turbinates may fill the air space and press against the nasal septum. The posterior ends of the turbinates can become so enlarged that they obstruct sinus aeration or drainage and result in sinusitis.

With chronic exposure to allergens, the patient's responses include increased congestion, pressure, and postnasal drip. The patient may complain of cough, hoarseness, or the recurrent need to clear the throat. Congestion may be sufficient to cause snoring. Nasal polyps may be present if the allergy has persisted for a long time.

Therapeutic Management. Several steps are used in managing allergic rhinitis. The most important step involves identifying triggers of allergic reactions by monitoring when symptoms occur and instituting measures to minimize exposure to these triggers (Table 23-1). Drug therapy may involve the use of antihistamines, decongestants, nasally inhaled cromolyn, or nasally inhaled steroids (Fig. 23-2). An antihistamine or decongestant is typically used first. If this therapy is not effective, intranasal administration of steroids or a cromolyn spray may be used (Table 23-2). Immunotherapy involves controlled exposure to small amounts of a known antigen through weekly injections with the goal to decrease sensitivity.[3,4] Therapy is initiated when a specific allergen has been identified, triggers cannot be avoided, and medications are not well tolerated or are ineffective in symptom management.[3]

NURSING MANAGEMENT

ALLERGIC RHINITIS

The patient should be instructed to keep a diary of times when the allergic reaction occurred and the activities that precipitated the reaction. Steps can then be taken to avoid these triggers (Table 23-1). The patient receiving drug therapy needs careful instructions about proper use (Table 23-2). The patient who is using classic antihistamines should

Table 23-1 How to Reduce Symptoms of Allergic Rhinitis

1. **Stay indoors if pollen levels are high or air quality is poor.**
2. **Avoid trips to woodlands in seasons of high pollen production.**
3. **Plan vacations when pollen is lowest in the travel area.** The best time to visit the Northeast is late July or early August. Avoid the West Coast in August. Europe has little or no ragweed.
4. **Eliminate dust mite reservoirs by the following actions:** Cover mattresses and pillows. Wash bedding weekly in hot water (135° F [60° C]). Remove carpets. Minimize upholstered furniture. Reduce indoor humidity to less than 50%. Avoid tightly sealed homes and workplaces. Use air conditioners in warm humid months. If carpets cannot be removed, consider the use of an acaricide (e.g. chemical that controls mite growth or mite allergens). Examples are (1) benzyl benzoate, a powder that is sprinkled on carpets and reduces mite counts if used regularly and (2) tannic acid, an agent that denatures mite and cat allergen. Both are recommended only if carpets cannot be removed.
5. **Keep closets and basements well-aired and dry.** Keep closet and linen drawers open. Do not let damp or wet clothing lie in hampers.
6. **Avoid scented soaps and perfumes.** Substitute nonallergenic products.
7. **Minimize animal exposure if it triggers allergy symptoms.** Keep pets out of the bedroom. Wash the pet weekly. If symptoms persist, consider removing pet from the home.

Modified from *How a Nasal Inhaler Works to Control Your Allergy.* Rhone-Poulenc Rorer Pharmaceuticals, Inc. and Mabry RL: A step-care approach to the treatment of upper respiratory allergy, *Otolaryngol Head Neck Surg* 107:828, 1992.

Before using the inhaler, gently blow your nose, making sure your nostrils are clear.

Then follow these steps:

1. Remove the protective cap from the nasal inhaler.
2. Shake the canister well.
3. Hold the inhaler between the thumb and forefinger.
4. Tilt the head back slightly and insert the end of the inhaler into one nostril, pointing it slightly toward the outside nostril wall. Hold the other nostril closed with one finger.
5. Press down on the canister to release one dose and, at the same time, inhale gently.
6. Hold your breath for a few seconds, then breathe out slowly through the mouth.
7. Withdraw the inhaler from the nostril and repeat the process for the other nostril. If more than one puff is prescribed per nostril, repeat steps 4-6.
8. Replace the protective cap on the inhaler.

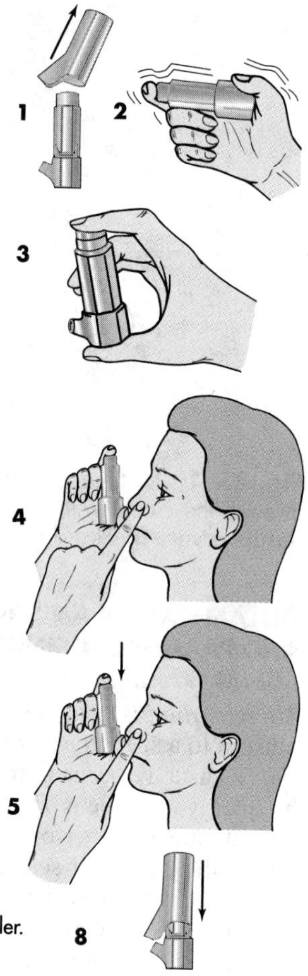

Fig. 23-2 Method for using an intranasal inhaler.

be warned about sedative side effects. Nonsedating antihistamines eliminate or reduce drowsiness but are more costly. If nasal decongestant sprays are prescribed, the patient should be warned about the dangers of long-term use. These sprays cause constriction of nasal vessels but have no effect on the allergic response. The patient who uses such sprays more than 3 days may experience *rhinitis medicamentosa* (rebound nasal congestion). Nasal vessels constrict and then dilate, causing chronic nasal obstruction. This outcome may cause use of more of the drug with less effect.[3,4] Intranasal cromolyn or steroid sprays are effective for seasonal and perennial rhinitis. The best relief is often obtained by combining an intranasal corticosteroid spray and a nonsedating antihistamine.[4-6]

Acute Viral Rhinitis

Acute viral rhinitis (common cold or acute coryza) is caused by viruses that invade the upper respiratory tract. It is the most prevalent infectious disease and is spread by airborne droplet sprays emitted by the infected person while breathing, talking, sneezing, and coughing, or by direct hand contact. Colds occur frequently because of multiple infections with many antigenically unrelated viruses.

Frequency increases in the winter months, when people stay indoors and overcrowding is more common. Other factors, such as chilling, fatigue, physical and emotional stress, and the patient's compromised immune status may increase susceptibility.

The patient with acute viral rhinitis typically first experiences tickling, irritation, sneezing, or dryness of the nose or nasopharynx, followed by copious nasal secretions, some nasal obstruction, watery eyes, elevated temperature, general malaise, and headache. After the early profuse secretions, the nose becomes more obstructed, and the discharge is thicker and more purulent. The general symptoms improve and the nasal passages reopen and normal breathing is established within a few days.[7]

Therapeutic Management. Rest, fluids, proper diet, antipyretics, and analgesics are recommended. Complications include pharyngitis, sinusitis, otitis media, tonsillitis,

Table 23-2 Drug Therapy for Allergic Rhinitis and Sinusitis

Preparation*	Mechanism of Action	Side Effects	Nursing Actions
Antihistamines			
Classic			
■ Diphenhydramine (Benadryl) ■ Clemastine (Tavist) ■ Chlorpheniramine (Chlor-Trimeton) ■ Brompheniramine (Dimetane) ■ Phenothiazine (Phenergan)	Bind with H_1 receptors on target cells, blocking histamine binding. Relieve acute symptoms of allergic response (itching, sneezing, excessive secretions, mild congestion).	Cross blood-brain barrier, bind to H_1 receptors in brain. Cause sedative and hypnotic effects. Have anticholinergic effects and may cause palpitations, tachycardia, blurred vision, constipation, or urinary retention.	Warn patient that operating machinery and driving may be dangerous because of sedative effect. Teach patient to report palpitations, change in heart rate, blurred vision, change in bowel, bladder habits. Instruct patient to avoid using alcohol with antihistamines because of additive depressant effect.
Nonsedating			
■ Acrivastine (Prolert) ■ Astemizole (Hismanal) ■ Terfenadine (Seldane) ■ Loratidine (Claritin)	Bind with H_1 receptors, blocking histamine binding. Inhibit release of mediators by preventing mast cell degranulation.	Limited affinity for brain H_1 receptors. Little sedation, few effects on psychomotor, vision, bladder functions.	Teach patient to expect few, if any, side effects. Rapid onset of action, and no drug tolerance with prolonged use. More expensive than classic antihistamines.
Decongestants			
Oral			
■ Pseudoephedrine (Sudafed) ■ Phenylpropanolamine (Dura-Vent)	Stimulate adrenergic receptors on blood vessels, promoting vasoconstriction and reducing nasal edema and rhinorrhea. Efficacy and side effects relate to α and β adrenergic receptor stimulation.	CNS stimulation, causing insomnia, excitation, headache, irritability, increased blood and ocular pressure, dysuria, palpitations, tachycardia.	Advise patient of adverse reactions. Advise that some preparations are contraindicated for patients with cardiovascular disease, hypertension, diabetes, glaucoma, prostate hyperplasia, hepatic disease, and renal disease.
Topical (nasal)			
■ Oxymetazoline (Dristan) ■ Phenylephrine (Neo-Synephrine)	Same as oral decongestants.	Same as oral decongestants, plus rhinitis medicamentosa (rebound nasal congestion).	Teach patient that these drugs should not be used for more than 3 days or more than 3 to 4 times a day. Longer use increases risk of rhinitis medicamentosa.

continued

and chest infections. Unless symptoms of these complications are present, antibiotic therapy is not indicated. Antibiotics have no effect on viruses and, if taken injudiciously, may produce resistant organisms.

NURSING MANAGEMENT

ACUTE VIRAL RHINITIS

During the cold season, the patient with a chronic illness or a compromised immune status should be advised to avoid crowded, close situations, and other persons who have obvious cold symptoms. The nurse should recommend that the patient get adequate rest. If the patient cannot avoid such contacts, frequent hand washing may prevent contamination through direct spread.

Nursing diagnoses specific to the patient with an upper respiratory infection include, but are not limited to, those presented in the nursing care plan on p. 595. Interventions are directed toward relieving annoying symptoms and instructing the patient in prevention of secondary bacterial

Table 23-2 Drug Therapy for Allergic Rhinitis and Sinusitis—cont'd

Preparation*	Mechanism of Action	Side Effects	Nursing Actions
Corticosteroids *Intranasal spray*			
▪ Beclomethasone (Vancenase-AQ) ▪ Flunisolide (Nasalide) ▪ Triamcinolone (Nasacort)	Antiinflammatory effect. Precise mechanism of action in nose is unknown. Systemic effects may occur with greater-than-recommended doses.	Mild transient nasal burning and stinging. In rare instances, localized fungal infection with *Candida albicans*.	Teach patient correct use (Fig. 23-2). Instruct patient to use on regular basis and not prn. Reinforce that spray acts to decrease inflammation and effect is not immediate, as with decongestant sprays. Discontinue use if nasal infection develops.
Antiinflammatory Agents *Intranasal spray*			
▪ Cromolyn spray (Nasalcrom) ▪ Nedocromil spray	Inhibits inflammatory response and degranulation of sensitized mast cells after exposure to specific allergens.	Minimal side effects. Occasional burning or nasal irritation.	Teach patient correct use (Fig. 23-2). Reinforce that spray prevents symptoms and should be used prophylactically, such as 10-15 min before exposure to allergen (gardening, hiking, pet contact) and before pollen season. Use should continue until exposure ends.

CNS, Central nervous system; H_1, hystamine type 1.
*Partial listing of available medications.

invasion. The patient should be encouraged to drink increased amounts of fluids to liquefy secretions. Antihistamine or decongestant therapy reduces postnasal drip and significantly decreases the severity of cough, nasal obstruction, and nasal discharge.

The patient should also be taught to recognize the symptoms of secondary bacterial infection, such as a temperature higher than 100.4° F (38° C), exudate on the tonsils, tender swollen glands, and a sore, red throat. In the patient with pulmonary disease, signs of infection include a change in consistency, volume, or color of sputum. Because infection can progress rapidly, the patient with chronic respiratory disease may be taught to inspect the sputum and to begin a 10- to 14-day course of antibiotics if any changes occur. The patient with pulmonary disease who has not been taught when to begin antibiotics should make contact with the physician if a change in the characteristics of the sputum is noticed.

Influenza

Influenza (flu) epidemics occur every year in the United States and, in years of low activity, are associated with approximately 10,000 deaths. In more severe years, as many as 40,000 deaths have occurred.[8,9] Most of these deaths, approximately 80% to 90%, occurred in persons more than 65 years of age, particularly those with cardiac or pulmonary disease. Influenza is preventable, yet only 20% to 30% of persons at high risk for complications receive prophylactic vaccination (Table 23-3).[8]

Influenza virus has a remarkable ability to change over time, which accounts for its ability to cause widespread illness. Minor changes develop each winter. If the change is minor, most patients will have some previous immunity. Major changes occur every 10 to 30 years. Few patients have immunity to major changes and pandemics may occur. Influenza virus occurs in 3 strains—A, B, and C. Subtypes are named by the strain, site of isolation, and year such as A/Beijing/95.[8]

Clinical Manifestations. The onset of flu is typically abrupt with systemic symptoms of headache, fever, chills, and myalgia accompanied by a cough and sore throat. Milder symptoms, similar to the common cold, may also occur. Physical findings are usually minimal with normal assessment on chest auscultation. Dyspnea and diffuse crackles are signs of pulmonary complications. In uncomplicated cases, symptoms usually subside within 7 days.[10] Some patients, particularly older patients, may experience weakness or lassitude that persists for weeks. The convalescent phase may be marked by hyperreactive airways and a chronic cough. Important factors in making a diagnosis are the patient's health history, clinical findings, and knowledge of other cases of influenza in the community.

NURSING CARE PLAN Patient with Upper Respiratory Infection

Planning: Outcome Criteria	Nursing Interventions and Rationales
➤ NURSING DIAGNOSIS	Altered respiratory function *related to* mucosal edema *as manifested by* cough, increased nasal and respiratory secretions, inability to tolerate breathing of cold air
Have decreased or absent cough, normal secretion production.	Humidify air as needed *to assist in moisturizing respiratory mucosa.* Encourage intake of fluids *to assist in liquefying secretions.* Administer antihistamine-decongestant prn *to reduce postnasal drip and cough.* Administer throat lozenges or antitussive prn *to provide throat and cough relief.* Instruct patient to place a scarf or mask over the nose and mouth when breathing cold air *to prevent drying and irritation of oral and respiratory mucosa.*
➤ NURSING DIAGNOSIS	Risk for ineffective thermoregulation *related to* infection
Have temperature ≤ to 100.4° F (38° C), absence of chills and diaphoresis, adequate state of hydration.	Assess for temperature >100.4° F (38° C) and diaphoresis *so early intervention can be initiated.* Check temperature *to provide ongoing assessment of temperature and response to treatment.* Give antipyretic medications prn *to reduce temperature.* Use cooling sponge bath prn *to assist in temperature reduction by heat dissipation.* Keep patient dry and lightly covered *to avoid chilling and a subsequent rise in temperature secondary to muscle contraction.* Encourage increased fluid intake *to replace fluid lost through perspiration and to assure adequate circulating volume to promote adequate renal function.* Monitor intake and output.
➤ NURSING DIAGNOSIS	Activity intolerance *related to* physical discomfort, fatigue, and inadequate comfort measures *as manifested by* complaints of aches, pains; sense of weakness
Have absence of aches, pain, fatigue.	Encourage bed rest or reduction of physical activity *to conserve energy.* Give analgesics (such as aspirin or acetaminophen) prn *to promote comfort.*

COLLABORATIVE PROBLEMS

Nursing Goals	Nursing Interventions and Rationales
➤ POTENTIAL COMPLICATION	Viral/bacterial pneumonitis *related to* secondary infection
Monitor for signs of pneumonitis, report positive signs, and carry out appropriate medical and nursing interventions.	Instruct patient about proper diet, rest, and activity *to avoid progression of illness.* Teach patient to report symptoms that do not resolve, such as increase in fever, dyspnea, or secretion production or change in volume, color, or consistency of secretions; tender glands; and tonsil exudate *to promote early detection of any complications.* Administer antibiotics as prescribed if bacterial infection develops.

The most common complication of influenza is pneumonia. *Primary viral influenzal pneumonia* is the least common, but potentially most serious complication. The patient develops symptoms of influenza that become more severe, rather than resolving, and may be fatal. Respiratory distress is often sufficient to require mechanical ventilation. The patient with secondary bacterial pneumonia experiences gradual improvement of symptoms for 2 to 3 days and then develops cough and purulent sputum. The elderly patient and the patient with cardiac and pulmonary disease are most at risk. Treatment with antibiotics is usually effective if started early. Mixed viral and bacterial pneumonia, the most common complication, involves symptoms of both types of pneumonia.[10]

THERAPEUTIC AND NURSING MANAGEMENT

INFLUENZA

The patient with influenza usually requires only symptomatic therapy. The elderly patient and the patient who has a chronic illness may require hospitalization. Antibiotics are not indicated unless secondary bacterial infection occurs. The primary goals in nursing management are supportive measures directed toward relief of symptoms and prevention of secondary infection.

Influenza immunization is the most effective measure for preventing or minimizing influenza symptoms.[11] To be effective, the vaccine must be given in the fall before exposure to the flu virus occurs. The nurse should advocate that the patient at increased risk for influenza-related com-

Table 23-3 Indications for Influenza Immunization

Groups at Increased Risk
- Persons ≥65 years old
- Residents of nursing or chronic care facilities
- Adults and children of any age with chronic pulmonary or cardiovascular disorders
- Adults and children who have regular medical follow-ups or who have been hospitalized during the preceding year because of chronic metabolic diseases, renal dysfunction, hemoglobinopathies, or immunosuppression
- Children receiving long-term aspirin therapy and who are therefore at risk of developing Reye's syndrome after influenza

Groups That Can Transmit Influenza to High-Risk Persons
- Hospital and outpatient health care workers who are in contact with high-risk patients
- Nursing home and chronic-care facility employees who have patient contact
- Providers of home care to high-risk persons
- Household members of high-risk persons

Other Groups
- Any person wishing to reduce chances of acquiring influenza
- Pregnant women at increased risk for influenza complications
- Persons infected with HIV
- Foreign travelers to the tropics at any time of year or to the Southern Hemisphere from April through September.

Modified from *Influenza News'93,* American Lung Association.
HIV, Human immunodeficiency virus.

plications receive the vaccination during routine office visits or, if hospitalized, at the time of discharge (Table 23-3). High priority should also be given to groups that can transmit influenza to high-risk persons, such as health care workers. By being vaccinated, the nurse can decrease the risk of transmitting influenza to those who have less ability to cope with the effects of this illness.

Many adults are reluctant to be vaccinated. Current vaccines are highly purified, and reactions are extremely uncommon. Soreness at the injection site is usually the only side effect in the person who receives the vaccine. The only contraindication to vaccination is hypersensitivity to eggs, since the vaccine is produced in eggs.

Amantadine (Symmetrel) may prevent influenza or decrease severity of symptoms if given before or within 48 hours of exposure. The drug is presumed to act by inhibiting virus shedding and must be taken daily for the duration of the outbreak. The high-risk patient who is exposed to persons with influenza or who has influenza (with no prior vaccination) may benefit from taking amantadine.[10]

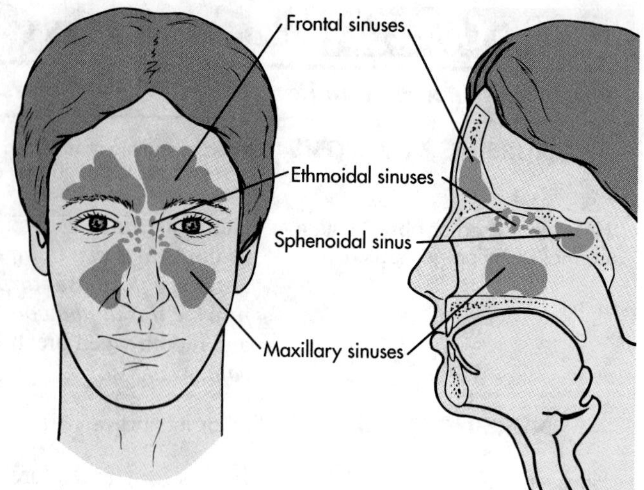

Fig. 23-3 Location of the sinuses.

Sinusitis

Sinusitis is classified as acute, subacute, or chronic, depending on the duration of symptoms. *Acute sinusitis* is an inflammation of one or more of the sinus cavities and lasts up to 3 weeks (Fig. 23-3). The most common cause is upper respiratory tract infection (URI), which results in obstruction of sinus drainage and bacterial invasion. The term *chronic sinusitis* is used when symptoms persist for more than 3 months. Sinus infections that persist for longer than 3 weeks but less than 3 months are termed *subacute sinusitis.*[12,13]

Clinical Manifestations. *Acute sinusitis* causes significant pain over the affected sinus, purulent nasal drainage, nasal obstruction and congestion, fever, and malaise. The patient looks and feels sick. If the patient leans forward, increased pain is experienced. Assessment involves inspection of the nasal mucosa and palpation of the sinus points for pain. Findings that indicate acute sinusitis include a hyperemic and edematous mucosa, enlarged turbinates, and tenderness over the involved sinuses. Pain is caused by the accumulation of pus and absorption of air behind a blocked ostium. In some instances, location of the pain marks the site of infection. The patient may also experience recurrent headaches that change in intensity with position or when secretions drain.

Chronic sinusitis is difficult to diagnose because symptoms may be nonspecific. The patient is rarely febrile. Although there may be facial pain, nasal congestion, and increased drainage, severe pain and purulent drainage are often absent. Symptoms may mimic those seen with allergies. X-rays of the sinuses or a sinus computed tomography (CT) scan may be performed to confirm the diagnosis. CT scans may show the sinuses to be opaque (filled with fluid), partially opaque (filled with air and fluid), or the mucous membrane to be thickened (Fig 23-4). Nasal endoscopy may be used to examine the sinuses and obtain drainage for culture. This test involves insertion of a rigid or flexible scope that allows extensive examination of the nasal cavity.[13]

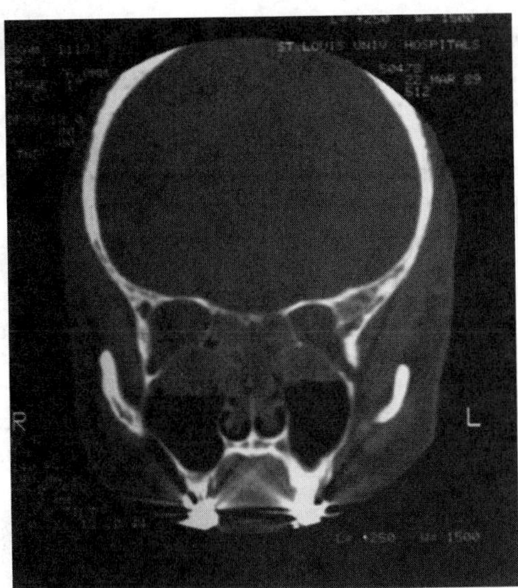

Fig. 23-4 Computed tomography (CT) scan of the sinuses. Bilateral air fluid levels are indicated by the dark (fluid) and light (air) contrast in the area of the maxillary sinuses.

THERAPEUTIC AND NURSING MANAGEMENT

SINUSITIS

Therapy for acute sinusitis includes topical and oral decongestants, mucolytics, and antibiotics (Table 23-2). Steam inhalations or saline administered by nasal spray may be used to assist in liquefying secretions. If no improvement occurs within 2 to 3 days, the antibiotic is changed to a broader spectrum drug. Duration of therapy is usually 10 to 14 days. Mixed bacterial flora are typically present in chronic sinusitis, and infections are difficult to eliminate. Broad-spectrum antibiotics are used for 3 to 6 weeks. The nurse should teach the patient to continue therapy for at least 1 week after symptoms are gone. Classic antihistamines increase mucous viscosity and promote continued symptoms, therefore their use should be avoided. Nonsedating antihistamines do not cause this problem.

The patient with persistent or recurrent sinus complaints not alleviated by medical therapy may require nasal endoscopic surgery to relieve anatomic sinus blockage caused by mucosal or turbinate hypertrophy or septal deviation. This is an outpatient procedure performed while the patient is under local or general anesthesia. Discomfort is minimal and more than 80% of those who have the procedure report substantial symptomatic improvement. The patient can return to work in 5 days but should limit strenuous activity for 3 to 4 weeks.[13,14] Nursing diagnoses specific to the patient with acute sinusitis include, but are not limited to, those presented in the following nursing care plan.

OBSTRUCTION OF THE NOSE AND PARANASAL SINUSES

Polyps

Nasal polyps are benign projections of edematous mucous membrane that form slowly in response to repeated inflammation of the sinus or nasal mucosa. Once nasal polyps are present, they enlarge, partly by growing and partly by swelling from increased edema, until they protrude into the airway or occlude the nose. Polyps may be multiple or bilateral, and they can exceed the size of a grape. The patient may be anxious about the polyps and fear that they are malignant.

Clinical manifestations are nasal obstruction, nasal discharge (usually clear mucus), and speech distortion. Nasal polyps can be removed with endoscopic or laser surgery, but recurrence is common.

Foreign Bodies

A variety of *foreign bodies* may lodge in the upper respiratory tract. Inorganic foreign bodies such as buttons and beads may cause no symptoms, lie undetected, and be accidentally discovered on routine examination. Organic foreign bodies such as wood, cotton, and paper produce a local inflammatory reaction and nasal discharge, which may become purulent and foul smelling. Foreign bodies should be removed from the nose through the route of entry. Sneezing with the opposite nostril closed may be effective. Irrigation of the nose or pushing the object backward should not be done, because either could cause aspiration and airway obstruction. If the object cannot be removed by sneezing or blowing the nose, the patient should see a physician.

PROBLEMS RELATED TO THE PHARYNX

Acute Pharyngitis

Acute pharyngitis can be caused by a bacterial, viral, or fungal infection. Acute follicular pharyngitis ("strep throat") results from *Streptococcal* bacterial invasion. Gonorrhea and herpes simplex virus (HSV) may cause pharyngitis as a result of transmission during orogenital contact. Acquired immunodeficiency syndrome (AIDS) must be considered as a potential diagnosis in any patient who has symptoms of pharyngitis, tonsillitis, and cervical lymphadenopathy. AIDS is characterized by a profound defect in cell-mediated immunity that leads to opportunistic infections. (Management of the patient with AIDS is discussed in Chapter 11.)

Clinical Manifestations. Symptoms of acute pharyngitis may range in severity from complaints of a "scratchy throat" to pain so severe that swallowing is difficult. White, irregular patches suggest infection with *Candida albicans,* commonly seen in the patient who is immunosuppressed or who has AIDS. In viral infections, the throat may appear mildly red with some congestion of blood vessels. In strep throat, the throat is typically an intense red-purple with patchy yellow exudate and hypertrophy of lymphoid tissue. In diphtheria, a gray-white false membrane, termed a *pseudomembrane,* is seen covering the oropharynx, nasopharynx, and laryngopharynx and sometimes extends to the trachea. Appearance is not always diagnostic. Cultures are done to establish the cause and direct appropriate management. Even with severe infection, cultures may be negative.

NURSING CARE PLAN Patient with Acute or Chronic Sinusitis

Planning: Outcome Criteria	Nursing Interventions and Rationales
➤ NURSING DIAGNOSIS	Pain *related to* sinus obstruction, inflammation or infection, and inadequate comfort measures *as manifested by* pain over involved sinuses or infected nasal discharge
Have no pain when pressure applied over involved sinus, drainage of secretions; use correct technique when using nasal inhalers; have normal temperature.	Encourage increased fluid intake (8 to 10 glasses of water daily) to liquefy secretions and use of steam inhalations (15-min vaporization of boiled water), saline nasal sprays, or bedside humidifier to promote secretion drainage. Instruct patient to maintain semi-Fowler's position (head of bed elevated 30 degrees) to promote sinus drainage. Administer analgesics prn to relieve sinus pain and decongestants to relieve swelling and improve breathing. Teach patient proper use of medications to ensure maximum benefit. Discourage smoking because smoking is an irritant to nasal passages. Administer antibiotics as indicated to treat infection.
➤ NURSING DIAGNOSIS	Altered nutrition: less than body requirements *related to* decreased appetite and altered taste sensation *as manifested by* inadequate food intake, less than recommended daily allowance
Have usual appetite; maintain normal body weight.	Encourage frequent oral hygiene *to enhance taste of food and remove foul-tasting drainage.* Provide nutritious, attractive foods *to stimulate appetite.*
➤ NURSING DIAGNOSIS	Altered health maintenance *related to* lack of knowledge of self-care, pain management, and prevention of chronic sinusitis *as manifested by* anxiety, questioning about care, continued purulent nasal discharge, sinus pain and cough
Have no nasal discharge, cough or sinus pressure; give an accurate description of self-care requirements related to hydration, infection control, and pain management.	Instruct patient on use of pain, mucolytic, decongestant, and antibiotic medications, local hydration techniques, and nutrition and hydration issues *to increase the patient's knowledge of self care.* Answer questions completely about self-care responsibilities *to promote health through knowledgeable self-care.* Instruct patient to follow interventions for acute sinusitis *to provide for early treatment and avoid chronic condition.* Teach patient to avoid factors that predispose to exacerbations, such as swimming and diving. If allergy is cause, follow instructions regarding environmental control, drug therapy, and immunotherapy *to reduce the sinus inflammation and prevent sinus infection.*
➤ NURSING DIAGNOSIS	Risk for infection *related to* impaired mucosal integrity
Have no inflammation; have normal temperature and white blood cell count.	Check temperature periodically. Report a temperature of >100.4° F (38° C), *which may indicate infection.* Instruct patient to take medications as prescribed and report continued symptoms or a change in symptoms to health care provider *because these symptoms may indicate need for change in antibiotic regimen.* Report any signs of infection to physician.

THERAPEUTIC AND NURSING MANAGEMENT

ACUTE PHARYNGITIS

The goals of nursing management are infection control, symptomatic relief, and prevention of secondary complications. Because cultures can be negative even when infection is present, the patient suspected of having strep throat is often treated with antibiotics. *Candida* infections are treated with nystatin, an antifungal antibiotic. The preparation should be held in the mouth as long as possible before it is swallowed, and treatment should continue until symptoms are gone. The patient should be encouraged to increase fluid intake and to take cool, bland liquids and gelatin that will not irritate the pharynx. Citrus juices should be avoided because they irritate the mucous membrane.

Peritonsillar Abscess

Peritonsillar abscess typically occurs as a complication of acute pharyngitis or acute tonsillitis if bacterial infection results in invasion of one or both tonsils. The tonsils may enlarge sufficiently to threaten airway patency. The patient will experience a high fever, leukocytosis, and chills. Treatment consists of intravenous (IV) antibiotic therapy. Early detection and treatment may clear the infection and prevent abscess development. If an abscess develops, incision and drainage are required. An emergency tonsillectomy may be performed or an elective tonsillectomy may be scheduled after the infection has subsided.

Sleep Apnea Syndrome

Sleep apnea syndrome is a condition characterized by repetitive cessation of airflow during sleep. Airflow obstruction occurs when the tongue and the soft palate fall backward and partially or completely obstruct the pharynx (Fig. 23-5). The obstruction may last from 15 seconds to as long as 90 seconds. During the apneic period, the patient experiences severe hypoxemia (decreased PaO_2) and hypercapnia (increased $PaCO_2$). These changes are ventilatory stimulants and cause the patient to partially awaken. The patient has a generalized startle response, snorts and gasps, which causes the tongue and soft palate to move forward and the airway to open. Apnea and arousal cycles occur repeatedly, as many as 200 to 400 times during 6 to 8 hours of sleep.[15]

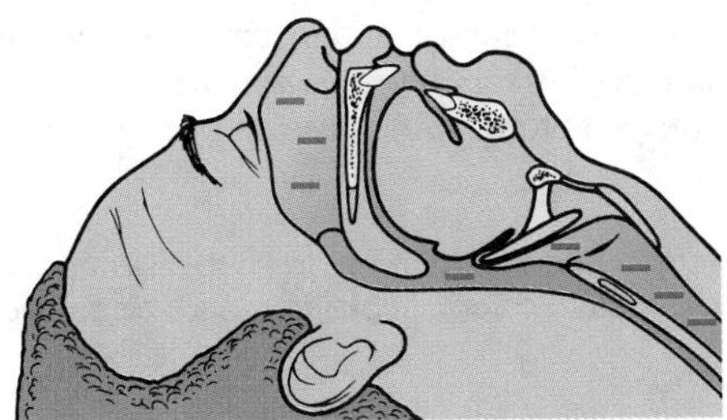

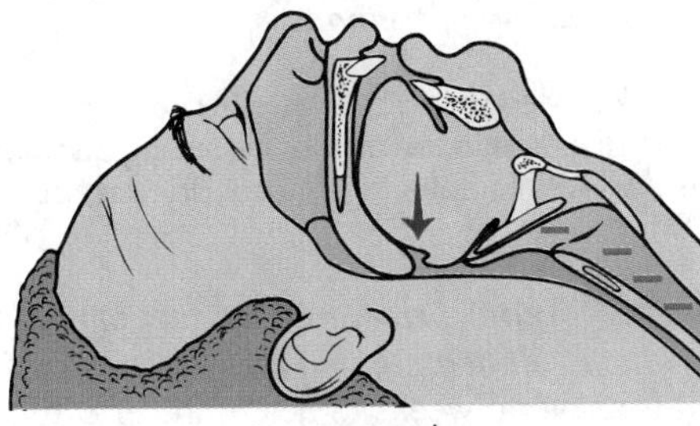

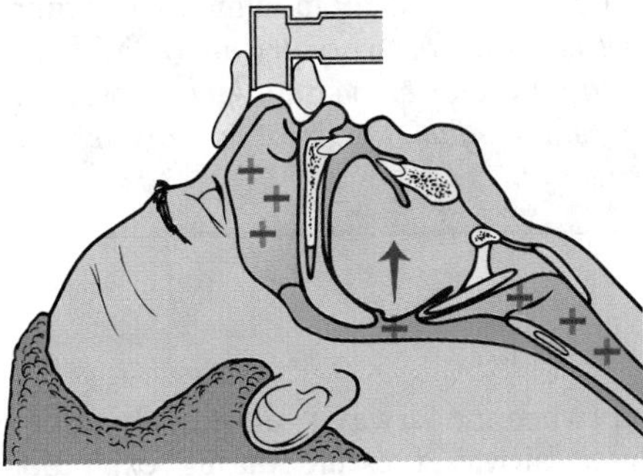

Fig. 23-5 How sleep apnea occurs. ***A,*** The patient predisposed to obstructive sleep apnea (OSA) has a small pharyngeal airway. ***B,*** During sleep, the pharyngeal muscles relax, allowing the airway to close. Lack of airflow results in repeated apneic episodes. ***C,*** With nasal continuous positive airway pressure (CPAP), positive pressure splints the airway open, preventing airflow obstruction.

The cause of sleep apnea is not definitely known. However, three factors appear to be involved: (1) an anatomically small pharyngeal airway, (2) altered neural control of the respiratory muscles, and (3) hormonal imbalance. Sleep apnea occurs in 2% to 5% of otherwise healthy men. The disorder is 7 to 10 times more common in men than women.[15-17]

Clinical Manifestations and Diagnostic Studies. Clinical manifestations of sleep apnea include frequent awakening at night, insomnia, and excessive daytime sleepiness. The patient's bed partner may complain about loud snoring. The snoring may be so loud that both persons cannot sleep in the same room. Other symptoms include morning headaches (from hypercapnia), personality changes, and irritability. Symptoms of sleep apnea alter many aspects of the patient's lifestyle. Chronic sleep loss predisposes a person to diminished ability to concentrate, impaired memory, failure to accomplish daily tasks, and interpersonal difficulties. The male patient may experience impotence. Vehicular accidents may be more common in the patient with sleep apnea. Family life and the patient's ability to maintain employment are also often compromised. As a result, the patient may experience severe depression.[15,16] The patient should be assessed to determine psychologic adjustment, and appropriate referral should be made if problems are identified.

Diagnosis of sleep apnea is made during an overnight sleep study with the use of polysomnography. The patient's chest and abdominal movement, oral airflow, nasal airflow, SaO_2, ocular movement, and heart rate and rhythm are monitored, and time in each sleep stage is determined. A diagnosis of sleep apnea requires documentation of 5 or more apneic episodes each hour or 30 or more apneic episodes each night.[15]

Therapeutic and Nursing Management of Sleep Apnea. Mild sleep apnea may respond to simple measures. The patient should be instructed to avoid sedatives and alcoholic beverages for 3 to 4 hours before sleep. If a supine position makes the apnea worse, the patient can be kept from using this position by placing a golf ball or other object in a pouch in the back of the pajama shirt. Referral to a weight loss program may be beneficial if the patient is obese, because excessive weight exacerbates symptoms. The patient may find a support group beneficial. The patient can share concerns and feelings with others who have the same problems and discuss strategies for resolving these problems.

If simple measures are not effective, nasal continuous positive airway pressure (CPAP) may be used (Fig 23-6). With nasal CPAP, the patient applies a nasal mask to the face that is attached to a high flow blower. The blower is adjusted to maintain sufficient positive pressure (5 to 15 cm H_2O) in the airway during inspiration and expiration to prevent airway collapse. Although nasal CPAP is effective, compliance with this therapy is poor even when symptoms of sleep apnea are relieved.[18,19] Nursing management is important in assisting the patient to develop a regimen that promotes comfort and adherence with this therapy. As a result of the continuous airflow, the patient may experience

NURSING CARE PLAN Patient with Sleep Apnea

Planning: Outcome Criteria	Nursing Interventions and Rationales
➤ **NURSING DIAGNOSIS**	Sleep pattern disturbance *related to* inability to sleep normally because of airflow obstruction during sleep *as manifested by* snoring; restlessness during sleep; morning headache; reports of falling asleep while eating, carrying on a conversation, driving
Recognize relationship between sleep and breathing problem; seek treatment; avoid driving until symptoms resolve.	Assist patient to recognize that breathing problems may be cause of symptoms *to foster seeking help to resolve problem.* Assess severity of symptoms *to determine their effect on the patient's life and urgency for treatment.* Teach patient and spouse that problems are result of airflow obstruction and should respond to treatment *to encourage compliance with CPAP therapy.* Teach need to avoid driving until management is effective *because daytime sleepiness may result in falling asleep while driving.*
➤ **NURSING DIAGNOSIS**	Self-esteem disturbance *related to* changes in body image, role performance, and personal identity *as manifested by* withdrawal from social contacts, change in usual pattern of responsibility
Attend support groups such as Alert, Well, and Keeping Energetic (AWAKE); express positive feelings about self.	Assess patient's ability to understand and cope with symptoms experienced *to determine effectiveness of coping.* Inform patient and spouse about support groups *to share concerns and feelings with other patients with sleep apnea and to discuss strategies to deal with the problem.* Assess patient for symptoms of depression because *this is a common occurrence in sleep apnea.*
➤ **NURSING DIAGNOSIS**	Altered nutrition: greater than body requirements *related to* increased appetite and inadequate exercise *as manifested by* inability to regulate caloric intake to reduce or maintain normal weight
Initiate a weight-loss program; achieve weight goal.	Assist patient to recognize that obesity may be contributing to present illness *because this is a common predisposing factor.* Educate patient about weight-loss methods *to provide encouragement by knowledge of a variety of methods.*
➤ **NURSING DIAGNOSIS**	Altered health maintenance *related to* lack of knowledge regarding self-care or perception that benefits of treatment do not outweigh the disadvantages *as manifested by* questioning about care; noncompliance with use of nasal CPAP; complaints of nasal dryness, burning, congestion; presence of epistaxis, conjunctivitis
State purpose and demonstrate proper use of mask; adhere to plan of care; have resolution of conjunctivitis, and epistaxis; have correct fit of mask.	Teach patient how to apply CPAP device *to insure correct use.* Instruct patient that device will create a positive pressure, *which will help to hold airway open during sleep.* Teach that therapy must be used for several weeks to determine effectiveness *to prevent discouragement.* Teach patient that conjunctivitis and epistaxis result from dry air blowing into eyes and nose. Instruct patient to use room humidifier or humidifier incorporated in airway circuit *because treatments are very drying to nasal mucosa.* For traveling, humidifier can be replaced by use of chin strap. A corticosteroid or saline nasal spray may also be used *to reduce inflammation of or moisturize nasal mucosa.* Check mask *to determine correct fit.*

CPAP, Continuous positive airway pressure.

nasal dryness, burning, or congestion that may be relieved by use of a room humidifier or a humidifier incorporated into the airway circuit.[19] When the patient is traveling, the humidifier can be replaced by a chin strap. Intranasal steroid or saline nasal sprays may also help minimize dryness and congestion. Another problem is discomfort from the high pressure, especially if airway pressures exceed 12 cm H_2O. A device that provides bilevel positive pressure airway pressure (BiPAP) may help to resolve this problem. BiPAP delivers a higher airway pressure during inspiration (when the airway is most likely to be occluded) and a lower airway pressure during expiration (patient exhales against less resistance).

Sleep apnea may also be managed surgically with a *tracheostomy* or *uvulopalatopharyngoplasty* (UVPP). UVPP involves excision of the tissues of the soft palate, uvula, and posterior lateral pharyngeal wall with the goal of removing the obstructing tissue. UVPP typically relieves snoring but may not alter sleep apnea symptoms. Tracheostomy relieves symptoms of sleep apnea because the airway opening is

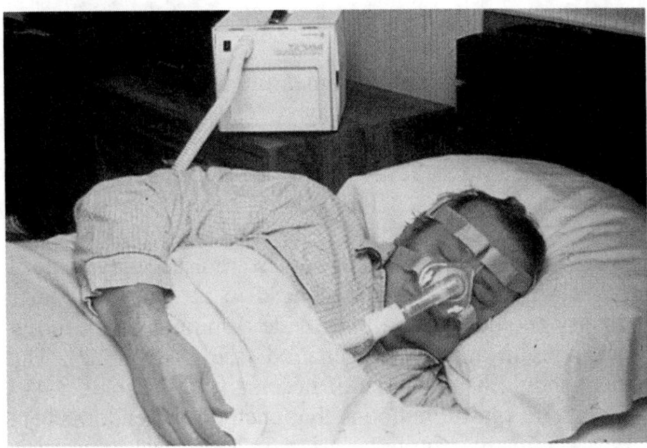

Fig. 23-6 Management of sleep apnea often involves sleeping with a nasal mask in place. The pressure supplied by air coming from the compressor opens the oropharynx and nasopharynx.

below the site of airflow obstruction. However, the patient may not wish to have a permanent tracheostomy, and this option is not used unless all other therapies are unsuccessful or unacceptable. Nursing diagnoses specific to the patient with sleep apnea include, but are not limited to, those presented in the following nursing care plan.

PROBLEMS RELATED TO THE TRACHEA AND LARYNX

Airway Obstruction

Airway obstruction may be complete or partial. Complete airway obstruction is a medical emergency. Partial airway obstruction may occur as a result of aspiration of food or a foreign body. In addition, partial airway obstruction may result from laryngeal edema following extubation, laryngeal or tracheal stenosis, and neurologic depression. Symptoms include stridor, use of accessory muscles, suprasternal and intercostal retractions, wheezing, restlessness, tachycardia, and cyanosis. Prompt assessment and treatment are essential because partial obstruction may quickly progress to complete obstruction. Interventions to maintain a patent airway include use of the obstructed airway (Heimlich) maneuver, cricothyroidotomy, endotracheal intubation, and tracheostomy. The patient may have few symptoms if the obstruction is minor. Unexplained or recurrent symptoms indicate the need for additional tests, such as a chest x-ray, pulmonary function tests, and bronchoscopy.

Endotracheal Intubation

Endotracheal intubation is the insertion and placement of a tube into the trachea through the nose (nasal intubation) or mouth (oral intubation) (Fig. 23-7). Indications for endotracheal intubation are to (1) prevent or relieve upper airway obstruction, (2) prevent aspiration, (3) facilitate secretion removal, and (4) provide a closed system for positive pressure ventilation.[20] The patient who requires endotracheal intubation is often in acute respiratory distress and has an altered level of consciousness.

If *oral intubation* is selected, the patient is placed in a supine position with the head extended, the neck fully flexed, and the jaw pulled forward. The endotracheal tube is passed through the mouth and vocal cords and into the trachea with the aid of a laryngoscope or bronchoscope. If *nasal intubation* is performed, insertion is performed by manipulating the tube through the nose, nasopharynx, and vocal cords. An oral endotracheal tube is easier to insert and easier to suction. Problems with oral intubation include easy dislodgement, poor toleration, and difficulty with oral hygiene. Nasal tubes are more easily secured, and may be better tolerated by the patient. However, their use is associated with serious complications, including sinusitis, otitis media, and epistaxis after removal.[20]

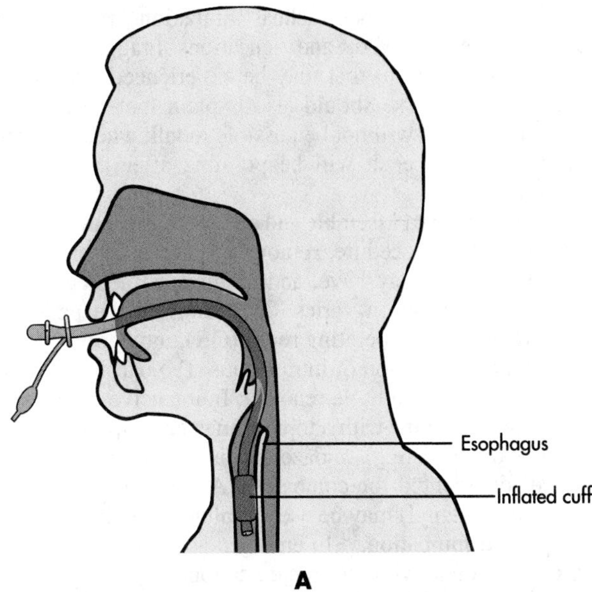

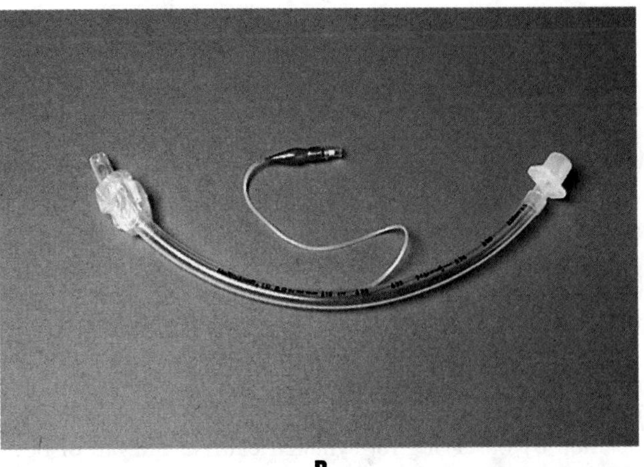

Fig. 23-7 Endotracheal tube. ***A,*** Tube in position in airway with cuff inflated and ***B,*** before placement.

NURSING MANAGEMENT

ENDOTRACHEAL INTUBATION

Before intubation, the nurse should ensure that the patient is properly oxygenated. If the patient is conscious, the nurse should explain why endotracheal intubation is necessary, the procedure involved, and sensations (gagging and a feeling of suffocation) that may be experienced during the procedure. The nurse should also explain that because of the inflated cuff, it will not be possible to talk when the tube is in place but speech will be possible after the tube is removed.

The nurse should assemble and check the equipment to be used during the procedure, remove any dentures or partial plates the patient may have, and administer medication as ordered. Premedication varies, depending on the patient's health status. In the operating room (OR), intubation is preceded by administration of intravenous (IV) barbiturates (to induce sleep) and a muscle relaxant. In intensive care units, premedication begins with a topical anesthetic spray. A hypnotic and amnestic (e.g., midazolam) is used if the patient is agitated, disoriented, or combative. A narcotic with rapid onset (e.g., fentanyl) may be used to blunt the pain of laryngoscopy and intubation.[20] In emergency situations, intubation may be done without premedication.

After intubation, nursing responsibilities include (1) assessing correct tube placement, (2) inflating the cuff, (3) assessing oxygenation status and acid-base balance and reporting untoward changes, (4) suctioning to remove secretions, (5) providing mouth care, (6) alternating placement of oral tubes to prevent pressure necrosis, (7) preventing accidental disconnection from the ventilator or extubation, and (8) preventing cuff overinflation.

Airway Management. After placement, the cuff is inflated and the tube secured. When inserted, the endotracheal tube may inadvertently enter the esophagus instead of the trachea. If inserted too far the tube may be in the right mainstem bronchus, rather than just above the carina (the site where the trachea branches into the right and left bronchi). The nurse should immediately verify correct tube position by observing for symmetrical rise and fall of both sides of the chest and auscultation of bilateral breath sounds. A device that detects exhaled CO_2 and indicates this by color change may also be used. A color change from purple to yellow indicates CO_2 in the exhaled air, confirming entry into the lungs.[21] If correct tube position is not verified, the physician should *immediately* reposition the tube because this is an emergency. No oxygen will be delivered to the lungs or the entire tidal volume will be delivered to one lung, placing the patient at risk for *pneumothorax.*[20]

Two approaches may be used to secure the endotracheal tube: adhesive tape or a tube holder. If adhesive tape is used, the tube will be taped securely to the face. If a tube holder is used, the straps will be placed around the patient's head and a device (e.g., plastic, Velcro strip) positioned to hold the tube in place. The Secure-Easy endotracheal tube holder has been shown to allow less movement and to cause less facial skin breakdown than adhesive tape or other types of tube holders.[22,23]

After the tube is secured, a chest x-ray is taken to confirm correct placement. The tip of the endotracheal tube should be 2 to 3 cm above the carina.[24] The number of centimeters the tube extends beyond the teeth or gums should be recorded on the patient's chart. Correct placement should be verified at least once each shift by one of the following: (1) presence of bilateral breath sounds, (2) same tube protrusion as prior measurement, or (3) tip 2 to 3 cm above carina on chest x-ray.

The endotracheal tube is connected to humidified oxygen by means of a T tube or to a mechanical ventilator. Arterial blood gases (ABGs) should be assessed 10 to 20 minutes after intubation to determine oxygenation status and acid-base balance. These values are used to evaluate if mechanical ventilator settings need to be changed. Pulse oximetry should be used to provide continuous monitoring of changes in arterial oxygenation (see Chapter 22). The patient should be suctioned if necessary[25,26] (Table 23-4).

Cuffs are plastic balloons that encircle the endotracheal tube. A cuff is required during endotracheal intubation because the tube passes through the epiglottis, splinting it open (see Fig. 23-7). The patient cannot protect the airway from aspiration. The cuff is inflated by injecting air into the fine-bore tubing leading to the cuff. The cuff should be inflated with the least amount of air that will allow delivery of an adequate tidal volume and prevent aspiration.

The nurse should record cuff pressure after intubation and once every shift to confirm that the cuff is properly inflated. Normal capillary perfusion is 30 mm Hg. To insure adequate tracheal perfusion, cuff pressure should not exceed 20 mm Hg or 25 cm H_2O. Overinflation predisposes to tracheal necrosis because excessive pressure obstructs blood flow through tracheal capillaries. The steps in cuff inflation are: (1) inflate the cuff to *minimal occluding volume* (MOV) by adding air until no leak is heard at peak inspiratory pressure (end of ventilator inspiration) when a stethoscope is placed over the trachea (Fig. 23-8); (2) for the spontaneously breathing patient, inflate until no sound is heard after a deep breath or after inhalation with a manual resuscitation bag (MRB); (3) verify cuff pressure is within the accepted range with a manometer; and (4) record the value in the chart. (See Table 23-5 for nursing management of artificial airways and monitoring of cuff pressure.)

Meticulous care is required to prevent skin excoriation or pressure sores as a result of pressure from the tube, tube-holder, or adhesive tape. To prevent these complications, the adhesive tape may be removed once a day and the tube moved to the other side of the mouth. If a tube holder is used the straps can be loosened, the area under the straps massaged, and the straps reapplied. Mouth care and shaving can be done at this time. This procedure must be performed by two nurses. One nurse holds the tube and the second performs the care. Because tube position may change during repositioning or when the straps are adjusted, the presence of bilateral breath sounds should always be confirmed after completion of the procedure. Some clinicians do not advocate routine repositioning of endotracheal tubes because of the risk of tube movement or extubation.

Mouth care should be provided at least once every 8 hours. The presence of an oral endotracheal tube stimulates oral secretions. If not removed, secretions can dry and crust in the mouth and provide a medium for bacterial growth. Frequent mouth care is refreshing to the patient and should be a part of the daily care routine.

Table 23-4 Procedure for Suctioning an Endotracheal Tube or Tracheostomy

1. Assess need for suctioning every 2 hr. Indications include coarse crackles or rhonchi over large airways, moist cough, increase in peak inspiratory pressure on mechanical ventilator, restlessness or agitation if accompanied by decrease in PaO_2. Do not suction routinely.
2. If suctioning is indicated, explain procedure to patient.
3. Collect necessary sterile equipment, such as suction catheter, gloves, water, cup, drape (usually in disposable set). If closed suction is used, the catheter is enclosed in a plastic sleeve and reused for 24 hr. No additional equipment is needed.[23]
4. Check suction source and regulator. Adjust pressure until dial reads −120 to −150 mm Hg with tubing occluded.
5. Wash hands. Put on goggles and gloves.
6. Provide preoxygenation by adjusting ventilator to deliver 100% O_2 or use reservoir-equipped MRB connected to 100% oxygen at 15 L/min. MRB is more likely to cause an increase in MAP.[24]
7. Use sterile technique to open package, fill cup with water, put on gloves, and connect catheter to suction. Designate one hand as contaminated for disconnecting, bagging, and operating the suction control. Suction water through the catheter to test system.
8. Assess SaO_2, heart rate, and rhythm to provide baseline for detecting change during suctioning.
9. Preoxygenate with 3 to 4 breaths of 100% O_2 by ventilator or MRB.
10. Gently insert catheter until obstruction is met. *Do not* apply suction during insertion.
11. Withdraw the catheter 1 to 2 cm and apply suction intermittently while withdrawing catheter in a rotating manner. If secretion volume is large, apply suction continuously.
12. *Limit suction time to 10 seconds.* Discontinue suctioning if heart rate decreases from baseline by 20 bpm, increases from baseline by 40 bpm, a dysrhythmia occurs, or SaO_2 decreases to less than 90%.
13. After each suction pass, oxygenate with 3 to 4 breaths by ventilator or MRB.
14. Rinse catheter with sterile water.
15. Limit insertions of suction catheter to three passes.
16. Oxygenate with 3 to 4 breaths by ventilator or MRB after last suction pass.
17. Return ventilator oxygen concentration to prior setting.
18. Rinse catheter and suction the oropharynx or use mouth suction.
19. Dispose of catheter by wrapping it around fingers of gloved hand and pulling glove over catheter. Discard equipment in proper waste container.
20. Auscultate to assess changes in lung sounds. Record time, amount, and character of secretions and response to suctioning.

bpm, Beats per minute; *MAP,* mean arterial pressure; *MRB,* manual resuscitation bag.

Communicating with the intubated patient can be a frustrating experience. In order to communicate more effectively, the nurse should have available a variety of methods. A *magic slate* or pad and pencil should be provided if the patient can use his hands. Additional options for communication include an alphabet board, flash cards, photo boards, lip reading, and hand signals.[27]

Extubation. Extubation (tube removal) should be performed as soon as possible. The health care team should assess the patient's status each day to determine whether (1) the underlying condition has improved so that intubation is no longer required, (2) spontaneous respiration can be maintained without the ventilator, and (3) the patient can cough, clear secretions, and protect the airway. (See Chapter 61 for additional criteria predicting ability to wean from mechanical ventilation).

If assessment indicates that weaning criteria have been met, extubation can be planned. Extubation should be attempted only by trained persons and persons trained in reintubation should be present. The nurse selects a time when the patient is rested, explains the procedure, and places the patient in a sitting position. The endotracheal tube and the area above the cuff (oropharynx) are suctioned. The tape or tube holder is loosened, the cuff deflated, and while the patient takes deep breath, the tube is removed at peak inspiration. Once the tube is removed, the patient is encouraged to cough to clear secretions. The mouth is suctioned and humidified oxygen is administered through a face mask. The patient is observed for signs of laryngospasm (e.g., stridor, dyspnea) and respiratory distress (e.g., restlessness, irritability, tachycardia, tachypnea). A pulse oximeter should be used to monitor SaO_2. If the patient cannot tolerate extubation, immediate reintubation may be necessary.

Tracheostomy

A *tracheotomy* is a surgical incision into the trachea for the purpose of establishing an airway. A *tracheostomy* is the tracheal stoma or opening that results from tracheotomy (Fig. 23-9). Correct placement of the tube requires careful dissection. For this reason a tracheotomy is not performed as an emergency unless required to relieve upper airway obstruction. A tracheotomy can be performed in the ICU with the patient under local anesthesia, but it is performed most frequently in the OR.

Indications for tracheostomy are to (1) bypass an upper airway obstruction, (2) facilitate removal of secretions, (3) facilitate weaning from a respirator by reducing anatomic

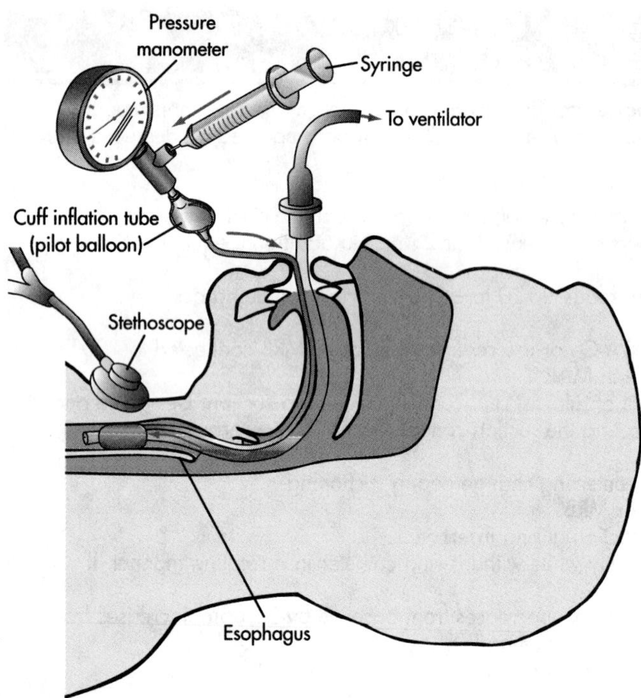

Fig. 23-8 Technique to inflate a cuff and check cuff pressure. The cuff is inflated until no leak is heard at peak inspiratory pressure (end of ventilator inspiration). A stethoscope is then placed over the trachea or, for spontaneously breathing patients, after a deep breath or inhalation with a manual resuscitation bag. A manometer is used to verify that cuff pressure is within the accepted range. (See Table 23-5 and the nursing care plan on p. 608 for related nursing management.)

dead space and lowering airway resistance, (4) permit long-term mechanical ventilation, and (5) improve patient comfort. Patient comfort may be increased because no tube is present in the mouth. The patient can eat and speak if the tracheostomy cuff can be deflated or a speaking tube is used. Because the tube is more secure, patient mobility is increased.[28-30] Most clinicians believe a tracheostomy should be performed after 7 to 10 days of mechanical ventilation if extubation is not possible, or earlier, if it appears likely that an extended period of mechanical ventilation will be required.[28-30]

NURSING MANAGEMENT

TRACHEOSTOMY

Before the tracheotomy, the nurse should explain to the patient and the family the purpose of the procedure and inform them that the patient will not be able to speak if an inflated cuff is used. The patient and the family should be told that normal speech will be possible as soon as the cuff can be deflated.

A variety of tubes are available to meet the individual needs of the patient (Fig. 23-9 and Table 23-5). All tracheostomy tubes contain an outer cannula and a faceplate or flange, which rests on the neck between the clavicles. In addition, all tubes have an obturator that is positioned in the

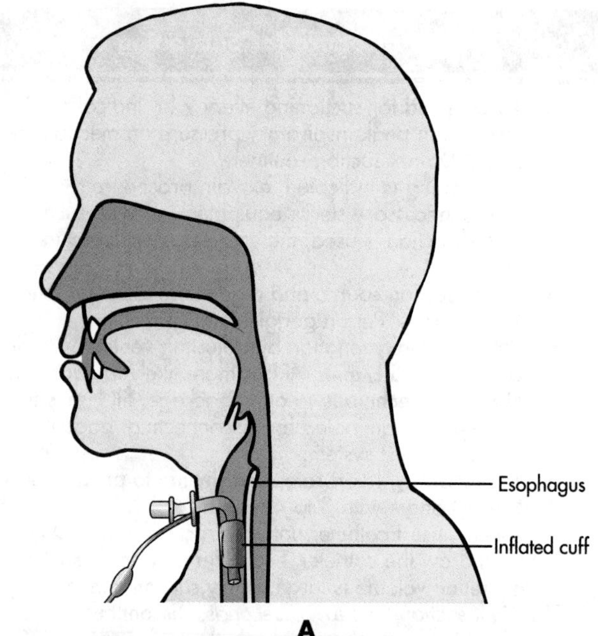

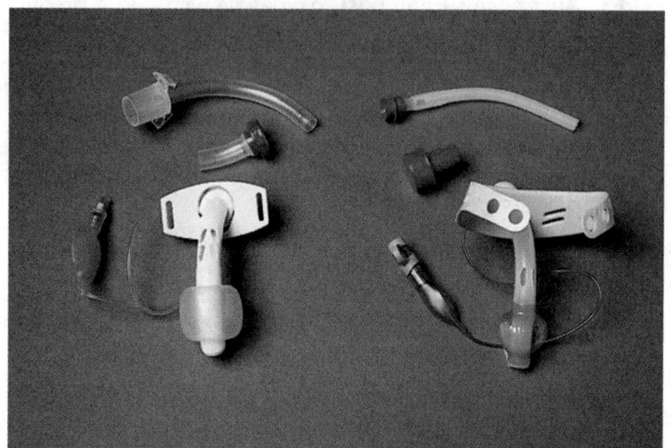

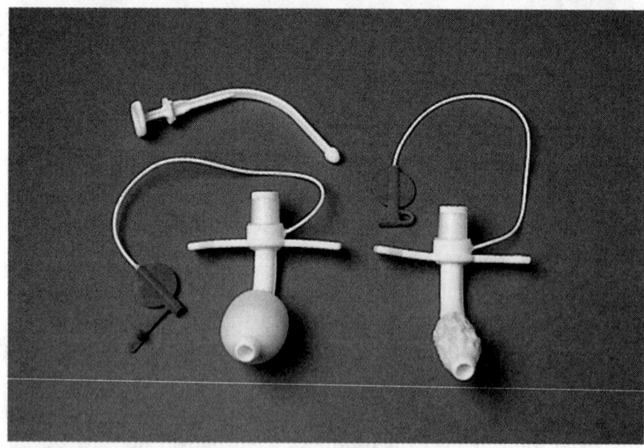

Fig. 23-9 Types of tracheostomy tubes. ***A,*** Tracheostomy tube inserted in airway with inflated cuff. ***B,*** Shiley and Portex fenestrated tracheostomy tube with cuff, inner cannula, decannulation plug, and pilot balloon. ***C,*** Bivona (Fome) tracheostomy tube with foam cuff and obturator (one cuff is deflated on tracheostomy tube). (See Table 23-5 and the nursing care plan for related nursing management.)

Table 23-5 Artificial Airways: Characteristics and Nursing Management

Tube	Characteristics	Nursing Management
Disposable oral or nasal endotracheal tube pilot balloon (see Fig. 23-7).	When properly inflated, low-pressure, high-volume cuff distributes cuff pressure over large area, minimizing pressure on tracheal wall.	■ Inflate the cuff to MOV by slowly injecting air into the cuff until no leak is heard at peak inspiratory pressure (end of ventilator inspiration), when a stethoscope is placed over the trachea (Fig. 23-8). If the patient is breathing spontaneously, inflate cuff until no sound is heard after deep breath or during inhalation with MRB. Verify pressure is within accepted range with a manometer. Record value in chart. ■ Monitor and record cuff pressure q8hr using above technique. Cuff pressure should be $\leq$20 mm Hg or $\leq$25 cm H_2O to allow adequate tracheal capillary perfusion. If needed, remove or add air to the pilot tubing using a syringe and stopcock. Afterward, verify cuff pressure is within accepted range with manometer. ■ Report inability to keep the cuff inflated or need to use progressively larger volumes of air to keep cuff inflated. Potential causes include tracheal dilatation at the cuff site or a crack or slow leak in the housing of the one-way inflation valve. If the leak is caused by tracheal dilatation, the physician may intubate the patient with a larger tube. Cracks in the inflation valve may be temporarily managed by clamping the small bore tubing with a hemostat. The tube should be changed within 24 hr.
Fenestrated tracheostomy tube (Shiley, Portex) with cuff, inner cannula, and decannulation plug (see Figs. 23-9*B*, 23-12*A*).	When inner cannula is removed, cuff deflated, and plug inserted, air flows around tube and through fenestration in outer cannula, up over vocal cords. Patient can then speak.	■ Assess risk of aspiration before removing inner cannula. Deflate cuff. Have patient swallow a small amount of clear liquid or 30 ml of water that contains a few drops of blue food coloring. Note coughing. Suction trachea to check for the presence of colored secretions. If no aspiration is noted, a fenestrated tube may be used. ■ Never insert plug in tracheostomy tube until cuff is deflated and inner cannula remove. Prior insertion will prevent patient from breathing (no air inflow) and may precipitate a cardiac arrest. ■ Assess for signs of respiratory distress when a fenestrated cannula is first used. If this occurs, the cap should be removed, the inner cannula replace, and the cuff reinflated. ■ Monitor cuff pressure q8hr as noted above.

continued

inner cannula when the tube is inserted into the airway. After insertion the obturator is immediately removed so that air can flow through the tube.[31] The obturator should be kept at the patient's bedside. In the case of accidental decannulation the obturator is required for placement of the tracheostomy tube.

Some tracheostomy tubes have two cannulas—an outer cannula, which remains in place, and an inner cannula, which can be removed for cleaning (Fig. 23-9 and Table 23-6). The cleaning procedure removes mucus that has accumulated on the inside of the tube. If humidification is adequate, this accumulation of mucus should not occur and a tube without an inner cannula can be used.

Both cuffed and uncuffed tracheostomy tubes are available. A tracheostomy tube with an inflated cuff should always be used if the patient is at risk of aspiration or needs mechanical ventilation. Procedures for care of a cuffed tracheostomy tube are the same as for a cuffed endotracheal tube. When the patient can protect the lower airway from aspiration and does not require mechanical ventilation, a cuffless tracheostomy tube can be used.

Care should be taken to not dislodge the tracheostomy tube during the first few days when the stoma is not mature or healed. Because tube replacement can be difficult, several precautions are required: (1) a replacement tube of equal or smaller size is kept at the bedside, readily available for emergency reinsertion; (2) the first tube change is performed by a physician usually no sooner than 7 days after the tracheotomy and (3) tracheostomy tapes are not changed for at least 24 hours after the insertion procedure (Fig. 23-10).

Retention sutures are often placed in the tracheal cartilage when the tracheostomy is performed. The free ends should be taped to the skin in a place and manner that leaves them accessible if the tube is dislodged. If dislodged, the nurse should immediately attempt to replace the tube. The retention sutures are grasped and the opening is spread. The obturator is inserted in the replacement tube, a water-soluble lubricant is applied to the tip, and the tube is inserted in the

Table 23-5 Artificial Airways: Characteristics and Nursing Management—cont'd

Tube	Characteristics	Nursing Management
Speaking tracheostomy tube (Portex, National) with cuff, two external tubings (see Figs. 23-9*B* and 23-12*B*).	Has two tubings, one leading to cuff and second to opening above the cuff. When port is connected to air source, air flows out of opening up over the vocal cords, allowing speech with cuff inflated.	▪ Once tube is inserted, wait 2 days before use so that the stoma can close around the tube to prevent leaks. ▪ When patient desires to speak, connect port to compressed air (or oxygen). Be certain to identify correct tubing. If gas enters the cuff, it will overinflate and rupture, requiring an emergency tube change. Use lowest flow (typically 4-6 L/min), which results in speech. High flows dehydrate mucosa. ▪ Cover port adaptor. This will cause the air to flow upward. Instruct the patient to speak in short sentences because voice becomes a whisper with long sentences. ▪ Disconnect flow when patient does not want to speak to prevent mucosal dehydration. ▪ If desired, use system to monitor aspiration risk. Give the patient ice chips with 5-6 drops of blue food coloring with cuff inflated. Suction via port. If dye is suctioned, patient has aspirated. Volume of aspirate can be judged by collecting secretions in sputum trap. ▪ Monitor cuff pressure q8hr as noted above.
Tracheostomy tube (Bivona Fome-Cuf) *foam-filled cuff* (see Fig. 23-9*C*).	Cuff filled with silicone foam. Before insertion, cuff is deflated. After insertion, cuff is allowed to fill passively with air. Pilot tubing is not capped, and no cuff pressure monitoring is required.	▪ When inserting tube, withdraw all air using a 60 ml syringe, then cap pilot balloon tubing to prevent air entry. After tube is inserted, remove cap from pilot tubing allowing cuff to reinflate. ▪ Do not inject air into tubing or cap tubing while it is in patient. Air will flow in and out in response to pressure changes (head turning). Place tag on tubing alerting staff not to cap or inflate cuff. ▪ Once each shift assess ability to easily deflate cuff. Difficulty deflating cuff indicates need for tube change. Tube can be used for up to 1 mo in the patient on home mechanical ventilation. This is a good choice for the patient who requires inflated cuff at home because teaching about cuff pressure is simplified.
Tracheostomy button (Olympic) with spacers, outer cannula, plug (see Fig. 23-14).	Maintains stoma patency and ability to talk with plug in place. Plug removal allows suctioning and easy re-intubation if needed.	▪ Do not insert button before assessing aspiration risk (see above). ▪ Measure stoma size and add spacers as needed. Insert lubricated button in stoma. Insert plug in button. This causes the petals at the back of the button to flare and hold button in stoma. ▪ After insertion, rotate button 180° to make certain not adhering to tracheal tissue. ▪ Instruct patient to clean stoma daily with hydrogen peroxide and remove and clean button at least twice a week. If button is not removed, tissue may granulate around petals, predisposing to bleeding.

MOV, Minimal occluding volume; *MRB*, manual resuscitation bag.

stoma at a 45-degree angle to the neck. If insertion is successful, the obturator is removed immediately so that air can flow through the tube.

If the tube cannot be replaced, the level of respiratory distress is assessed. Minor dyspnea may be alleviated by use of semi-Fowler's position until assistance arrives. Severe dyspnea may progress to respiratory arrest. If this situation occurs, the stoma should be covered with a sterile dressing, and the patient should be ventilated with bag-mask ventilation until help arrives. The patient who has had a laryngectomy needs to be ventilated with stoma ventilation, because there is no communication between the tracheal and upper airways.

After the first tube change, the tube should be changed approximately once a month. When a tracheostomy has been in place for several months, the tract will be well formed. The patient can then be taught to change the tube and suction the tracheostomy at home (Fig. 23-11). Teaching will vary, depending on the illness of the patient and the device selected. Nursing diagnoses specific to the patient with a tracheostomy include, but are not limited to, those presented in the nursing care plan on p. 608.

Swallowing Dysfunction. The patient who cannot protect the airway from aspiration requires an inflated cuff. However, an inflated cuff may promote swallowing dysfunction because the cuff interferes with the normal func-

Table 23-6 Tracheostomy Care

1. Explain procedure to patient.
2. Collect necessary sterile equipment such as suction catheter, gloves, water, basin, drape, tracheostomy ties, tube brush or pipe cleaners (usually in a disposable set), 4 × 4s, hydrogen peroxide (3%), and tracheostomy dressing (optional).
3. Position patient in semi-Fowler's position.
4. Assemble needed materials on bedside table next to patient.
5. Suction and oxygenate patient (see Table 23-4).
6. Wash hands. Put on goggles and gloves.
7. Unlock and remove inner cannula.*
8. If disposable inner cannula is used, replace with new cannula. If nondisposable cannula is used:
   - Immerse inner cannula in 3% hydrogen peroxide and clean inside and outside of cannula using tube brush or pipe cleaners.
   - Drain hydrogen peroxide from cannula. Immerse cannula in sterile water. Remove from sterile water and shake dry.
   - Insert inner cannula into outer cannula with the curved part downward and lock in place.
9. Remove dried secretions from stoma using 4 × 4 in pad soaked in hydrogen peroxide. Rinse with sterile water and another 4 × 4 pad. Gently pat dry area around the stoma.
10. Change tracheostomy ties (Fig. 23-10).† To prevent accidental tube removal, secure the tracheostomy tube by gently applying pressure to flange of the tube.
11. As an alternative, the patient may prefer tracheostomy ties made of velcro, which are easier to adjust. Plastic intravenous tubing may also be preferred because it is easily cleaned and dries without the need to replace the ties.
12. Unless excessive amounts of exudate are present, avoid using a tracheostomy dressing. If drainage is excessive, place dressing around tube (see Fig. 23-10). Change the dressing frequently. Wet dressings promote infection and stoma irritation.

*Many tracheostomy tubes do not have inner cannulas. Care for these tubes includes all steps except those for inner cannula care.
†Do not change tracheostomy ties for 24 hours after the tracheotomy procedure.

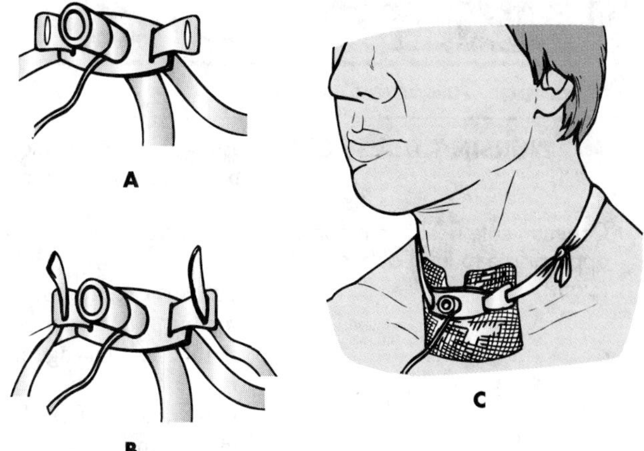

Fig. 23-10 Changing tracheostomy ties. ***A,*** A slit is cut about 1 inch (2.5 cm) from the end. The slit end is put into the opening of the cannula. ***B,*** A loop is made with the other end of the tape. ***C,*** The tapes are tied together with a double knot on the side of the neck.

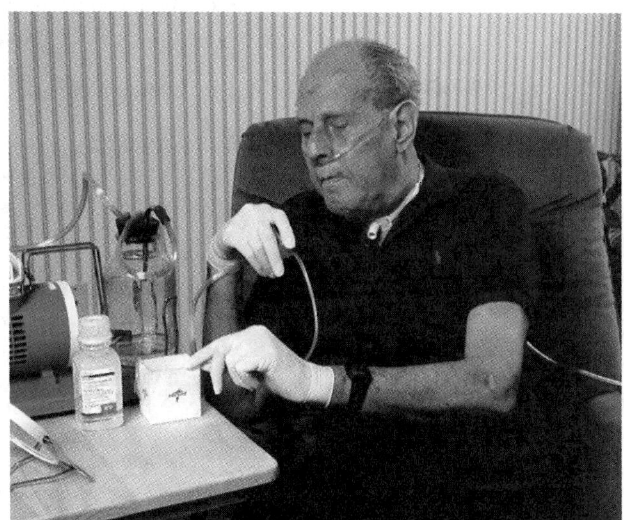

Fig. 23-11 Suctioning the tracheostomy at home. Patient is rinsing catheter after suctioning own tracheostomy.

tion of muscles used to swallow. For this reason, it is important to evaluate the risk for aspiration with the cuff deflated. The patient may be able to swallow without aspirating when the cuff is deflated but not when it is inflated. The cuff may then be left deflated or a cuffless tube substituted.

To evaluate aspiration risk, the cuff is deflated and the patient is instructed to swallow a small amount of clear liquid or 30 ml of water that has blue food coloring added. Any coughing is noted. Next, the trachea is suctioned to check for the presence of blue-colored secretions. If there is no indication of aspiration, the patient is judged to have competent epiglottic function without risk for aspiration.

Speech with a Tracheostomy Tube. A number of techniques can be used to promote speech in the patient with a tracheostomy. The spontaneously breathing patient may be able to talk during expiration by simply deflating the cuff and occluding the tube. If the patient is on mechanical ventilation, speech may be possible by allowing a constant airleak around the cuff (*minimal leak technique*). In addition, tracheostomy tubes and valves have been designed to facilitate speech with a tracheostomy. The nurse can be an advocate in promoting use of these specialized devices. Their use can provide great psychologic benefit and facilitate self-care for the patient with a tracheostomy.

NURSING CARE PLAN Patient with a Tracheostomy

Planning: Outcome Criteria	Nursing Interventions and Rationales
➤ **NURSING DIAGNOSIS**	Impaired verbal communication *related to* use of artificial airway and cuff *as manifested by* anxiety, inability to communicate or signs of frustration
Communicate needs in manner appropriate to level of consciousness.	Assess patient's level of consciousness *to determine approach and plan of care.* If patient is alert, provide call bell within easy reach, magic slate, pad and pencil, artificial larynx, or communication board with illustrations of requests *as alternative means of communication.* Reassure patient that speech will return when cuff can be deflated (if laryngectomy has not been performed) *to allay fear that situation is permanent.* Read lips for cues. Provide for continuity of care *to decrease frustration associated with multiple caregivers.* Suggest use of tubes (fenestrated, speaking tracheostomy tube, valve) *to permit speech.*
➤ **NURSING DIAGNOSIS**	Ineffective airway clearance *related to* difficulty expectorating sputum *as manifested by* adventitious sounds on auscultation, tenacious secretions, increase in restlessness, change in mentation, ineffective or absent cough
Maintain patent airway; secretions expectorated without need to suction airway, chest clear to auscultation.	Assess for respiratory distress *to determine need for interventions.* Assist patient to semi-Fowler's position (if tolerated) *to allow for more forceful cough and to relieve dyspnea.* Suction airway. Monitor humidification system *to ensure provision of adequate humidity* if secretions are tenacious. Teach patient to inhale 4 or 5 times through nose, breathe out through airway, and then cough, if not on ventilator *to facilitate expectoration.* Encourage oral fluids (if tolerated) *to liquefy secretions.*
➤ **NURSING DIAGNOSIS**	Risk for infection *related to* bypass of airway defense mechanisms and impaired skin integrity
Have normal WBC count and temperature, white secretions, no erythema or purulent secretions.	Monitor for elevated white blood cell (WBC) count and temperature, change in color of secretions, purulent secretions *to detect signs of infection.* Use strict aseptic technique for suctioning tracheostomy during hospitalization *to reduce occurrence of infection.* Wash hands before touching equipment. Change oxygen-delivery equipment q48hr *to prevent contaminated tubing from being a source of infection.* Empty condensate into waste receptacle (not into humidifier or nebulizer) *to keep from contaminating water that will come in contact with patient.* Keep stoma clean and dry with frequent tracheostomy care. Report to physician any elevation in temperature or WBC count, change in secretion color, and purulent drainage from stoma *because these events may indicate presence of an infection and need for treatment.*
➤ **NURSING DIAGNOSIS**	Altered nutrition: less than body requirements *related to* decreased oral intake, altered taste sensation, and swallowing difficulty *as manifested by* inadequate caloric intake and weight loss
Have usual appetite, maintenance of normal body weight.	Provide ongoing caloric count *to assess adequacy of diet.* Monitor weight *to provide information for evaluation.* Provide food and beverages that patient prefers *to increase likelihood of consumption.* Perform mouth care q8hr *to promote patient comfort and appetite.*
➤ **NURSING DIAGNOSIS**	Impaired swallowing *related to* tracheostomy tube *as manifested by* inability to swallow without difficulty with cuff inflated
Have normal swallowing function with cuff deflated or with cuff inflated (if former not tolerated).	Assess swallow and gag reflexes by deflating cuff, asking patient to swallow small amount of clear liquid or 30 ml water colored with blue food coloring *to determine presence of aspiration.* Note coughing *as indicator of aspiration.* Suction trachea and check for colored secretions. (If none present, patient may tolerate eating with cuff deflated.)

continued

NURSING CARE PLAN Patient with a Tracheostomy—cont'd

Planning: Outcome Criteria	*Nursing Interventions and Rationales*
➤ **NURSING DIAGNOSIS**	Ineffective management of therapeutic regimen *related to* lack of knowledge about care of tracheostomy at home *as manifested by* questioning about care (patient and family), agitation, and restlessness when planning for discharge
Demonstrate techniques by patient and family for suctioning, care of equipment and tracheostomy care; verbalize expected outcomes and time to contact health care professionals (if problems arise) by patient and significant other.	Assess ability of patient and family to provide care at home, including airway care, ability to respond appropriately to emergencies *to determine if home care is feasible*. Teach clean suction technique, good hand washing, home preparation of sterile saline solution, use of one catheter for 24 hr, methods of cleaning and reusing catheters, clean technique for tracheostomy care *so patient can properly care for self at home*. Make referral for visiting nurse or home care *to provide ongoing assistance and support*. Provide opportunities for patient to discuss care and concerns about caring for tracheostomy at home *to alleviate anxiety*.

COLLABORATIVE PROBLEMS

Nursing Goals	*Nursing Interventions and Rationales*
➤ **POTENTIAL COMPLICATION**	Hypoxemia *related to* misplaced or improperly functioning tube
Monitor for signs of hypoxemia, report deviations from acceptable parameters, and carry out appropriate medical and nursing interventions.	Assess patient for restlessness, agitation, confusion, tachycardia, bradycardia, dysrhythmias; SaO_2 less than 90%; accidental expulsion of tube from airway *to determine if tube is placed properly*. Elevate head of bed if tolerated. Auscultate chest *to determine need for suctioning*. If course crackles, rhonchi are present, suction airway. Check tube position and function. If tube is misplaced from airway, grasp the retention sutures and spread opening. Lubricate tube and insert with obturator in place at 45° angle to neck. If successful, remove obturator immediately. If tube cannot be reinserted, assess the level of respiratory distress *to determine whether patient can breathe without tube for a short interval*. Notify the physician. If distress is severe, ventilate with bag-mask or bag-stoma (laryngectomy) until assistance arrives *to ensure adequate ventilation*.

A *speaking tracheostomy tube* has two tubings. One connects to the cuff and is used for cuff inflation. The second connects to an opening just above the cuff (Fig. 23-12). When the second tubing is connected to a low-flow (4 to 6 L/min) air source, sufficient air moves up over the vocal cords to permit speech. The patient can then speak, although the cuff is inflated.

A *fenestrated tube* is typically used by the patient who can swallow without risk of aspiration but requires suctioning for secretion removal. It may also be used by the patient who requires mechanical ventilation for fewer than 24 hours a day (Figs. 23-9 and 23-12). The tube has openings on the surface of the outer cannula that permit air from the lungs to flow over the vocal cords. When a fenestrated tube is used, the patient can breathe spontaneously through the larynx, speak, and cough up secretions. However, the tracheostomy tube remains in place. Suctioning can still be done. The tube can also be connected to a mechanical ventilator.

Before this device is used, the patient's ability to swallow without aspiration is determined (see Table 23-5 and the nursing care plan). If there is no aspiration, the inner cannula is removed and the cuff deflated before the cap is placed in the tube (see Fig. 23-12). It is important to perform the steps in order because severe respiratory distress may result if the tube is capped before the inner cannula is removed and the cuff is deflated. The nurse should frequently assess the patient for signs of respiratory distress when a fenestrated cannula is first used. If the patient is not able to tolerate the procedure, the cap should be removed, the inner cannula replaced, and the cuff reinflated.

When *speaking tracheostomy valves* are used, the cuff is deflated and the valve is placed over the tracheostomy tube (Fig. 23-13). The speaking valve contains a thin plastic diaphragm that opens on inspiration and closes on expiration. During inspiration, air flows in through the valve. During expiration, the diaphragm moves against the plastic cover and air flows upward over the vocal cords. The cuff must be deflated to allow exhalation. Ability to tolerate cuff deflation without aspiration or respiratory distress must also be evaluated in patients using this device.[31]

A *tracheostomy button* is a short outer tube that extends from the skin to the anterior tracheal wall (Fig. 23-14). No

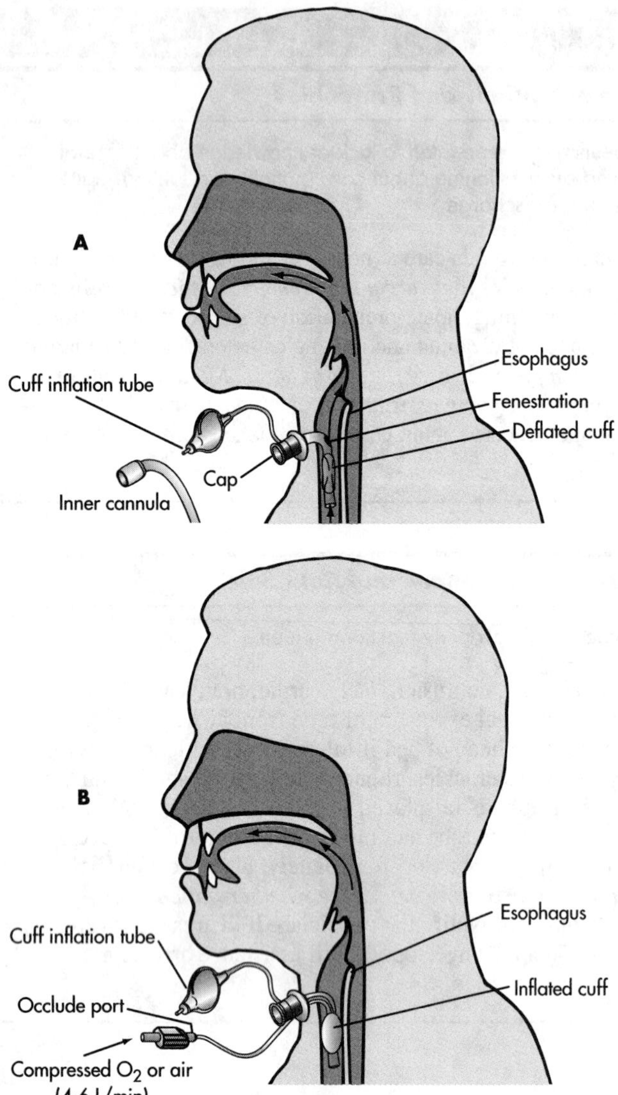

Fig. 23-12 Speaking tracheostomy tubes. ***A,*** Fenestrated tracheostomy tube with cuff deflated, inner cannula removed, and tracheostomy tube capped to allow air to pass over the vocal cords. ***B,*** Speaking tracheostomy tube. One tubing is used for cuff inflation. The second tubing is connected to a source of compressed air or oxygen. When the port on the second tubing is occluded, air flows up over the vocal cords, allowing speech with an inflated cuff. (See Table 23-5 and the nursing care plan for related nursing management.)

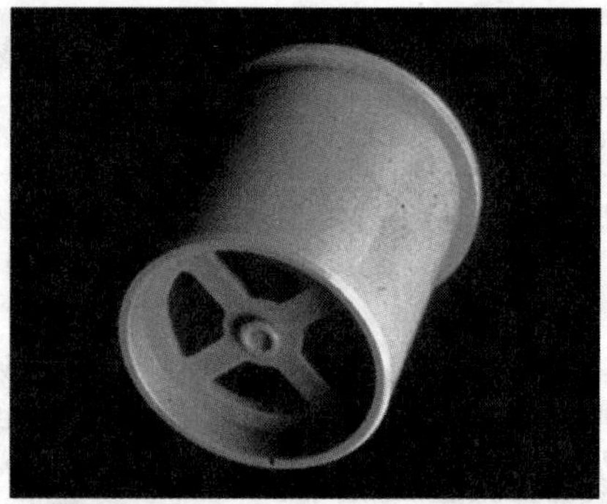

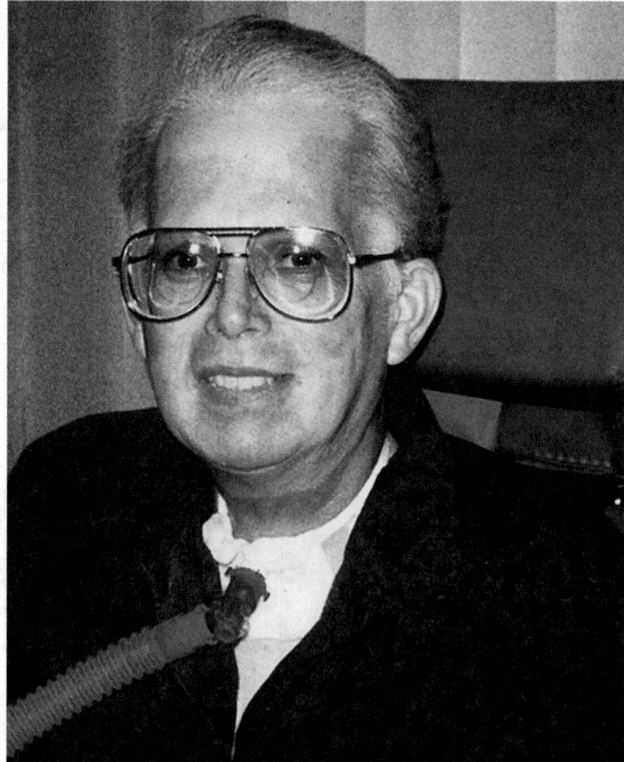

Fig. 23-13 Passy-Muir speaking tracheostomy valve. The valve is placed over the tracheostomy opening after cuff deflation. The device is used for the patient who requires an inflated cuff for mechanical ventilation or sleep apnea management at night but who can breathe spontaneously without problems with the cuff deflated during the day.

tube is present in the airway. The button is used for short periods (e.g., several weeks) to evaluate ability to tolerate tube removal.[29] The button can be plugged, permitting normal speech and coughing. If suctioning is needed, the plug can be quickly removed. If the button is not tolerated, it can be removed and the tracheostomy tube reinserted.

Decannulation. When the patient can expectorate secretions and maintain adequate gas exchange without mechanical ventilation, the tracheostomy tube can be removed. The stoma is covered with a dressing and tape. Epithelial tissue begins to form in 24 to 48 hours, and the opening will close in several days. Surgical intervention is not required.

Laryngeal Polyps

Laryngeal polyps may develop on the vocal cords from vocal abuse (e.g., excessive talking, singing) or irritation (e.g., cigarette smoking). The most common symptom is hoarseness. Large polyps may cause dyspnea and stridor. Polyps may be treated conservatively with voice rest. Surgical removal may be indicated for benign polyps because they are sometimes later found to be malignant.

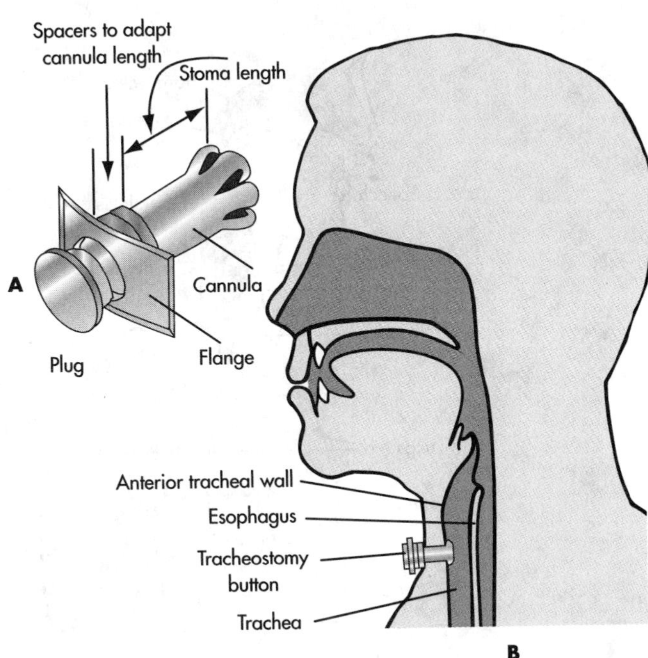

Fig. 23-14 Olympic tracheostomy button. ***A,*** Parts of the tracheostomy button. The button consists of a cannula, spacers that adapt the button to the length of the stoma, and a plug that fits into the cannula. The plug is removed for suctioning. ***B,*** Tracheostomy button inserted into the stoma. The button extends from the stoma opening to the anterior tracheal wall.

Cancer of the Head and Neck

In 1992 there were an estimated 42,800 new cases of cancer involving the head and neck and 11,600 deaths from this type of cancer. Approximately 4 times as many men as women have head and neck cancer. The usual time of diagnosis is after the age of 50. Although this cancer represents only approximately 5% of cancer cases, disability is great because of the potential loss of voice, disfigurement, and social consequences. Although specific causes of head and neck cancer are not known, there are some well-known risk factors. The patient will most likely have smoked or used other forms of tobacco. Heavy alcohol intake appears to have a potentiating effect. There is also evidence that chronic infection with Epstein-Barr or papilloma virus increases the risk of head and neck cancer.[32,33]

Clinical Manifestations. The nurse is in a key position to detect early signs of head and neck cancer. Early detection is critical. If the cancer is localized, survival is improved and the need for extensive surgery is reduced. Symptoms are often not reported, however, because the patient does not know the significance or fears the consequences.

Early signs and symptoms of upper airway cancers vary with the location of the tumor. Cancer of the oral cavity may cause pain that is aggravated by movement of the affected structure or acidic foods, ulcers that do not heal, or change in fit of dentures. Cancers of the oropharynx, hypopharynx, and supraglottic larynx rarely produce early symptoms and are usually diagnosed in later stages. The patient may complain of persistent unilateral sore throat or otalgia (ear pain). Hoarseness may be a symptom of early laryngeal cancer. If hoarseness lasts longer than 2 weeks, a medical evaluation is indicated. Some patients experience what may feel like a lump in the throat or a change in voice quality. Late stages of head and neck cancers have easily detectable signs and symptoms including pain, dysphagia, decreased mobility of the tongue, airway obstruction, and cranial neuropathies.[32,33]

The nurse should thoroughly examine the oral cavity including the area under the tongue and dentures. The floor of the mouth and tongue and the lymph nodes in the neck should be bimanually palpated. There may be thickening of the normally soft and pliable oral mucosa. *Leukoplakia* (white patch) or *erythroplakia* (red patch) may be seen and should be noted for later biopsy. Both leukoplakia and *carcinoma in situ* (localized to a defined area) may precede invasive carcinoma by many years.[32,33]

Diagnostic Studies. If lesions are suspected, the upper airways may be examined using an indirect laryngoscopy that involves using a laryngeal mirror to visualize the laryngeal area and determine mobility of the larynx and vocal cords. Presence of a tumor restricts tissue mobility. A flexible nasopharyngoscope may also be used. A CT scan or magnetic resonance imaging (MRI) may be performed to detect the extent of local and regional spread. Neoplastic tissue is identifiable because it contains tissue of greater density or because it distorts, displaces, or destroys normal anatomical structures. Typically, multiple biopsy specimens are also obtained to determine the extent of the disease.

Therapeutic Management. On the basis of the information obtained, a decision will be made about the stage of the disease by means of the tumor, nodes, metastasis (TNM) system. This system identifies the stage of disease (Stage I to Stage IV) and guides principles of treatment. Approximately one third of patients have highly confined lesions that are Stage I or II. Such a patient can undergo surgery or radiation therapy with the goal of cure. This goal is achieved in 80% of patients with Stage I disease and in 60% of patients with Stage II disease. In Stage III or IV disease, fewer than 30% of patients are cured.[32]

Choice of treatment is based on such factors as extent of disease, cosmetic considerations, patient desires, and urgency of treatment. More advanced disease is managed with combinations of surgery and radiation therapy or surgery and chemotherapy. Clinical trials have shown that induction chemotherapy (that is, chemotherapy given before surgery) may allow less extensive surgery and reduce the incidence of metastasis. However, survival is not improved. Even if initial therapy is curative, the patient will most probably experience a second primary cancer. Strategies to prevent a second primary cancer involve chemoprevention, or giving drugs such as retinoids to suppress or prevent development of invasive cancer. Several studies indicate that this strategy reduces the occurrence of secondary cancers. Radiation therapy and surgical interventions are the only curative modalities for cancer of the head and neck.[32,33]

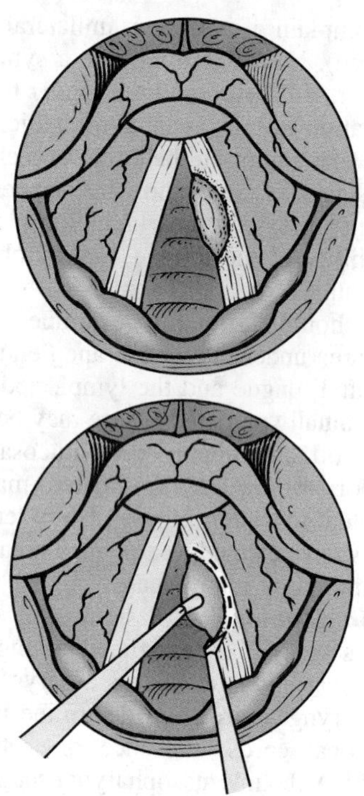

Fig. 23-15 Excision of laryngeal cancer. This cancer of the right vocal cord meets criteria for resection by transoral cordectomy. The cord is fully mobile and the lesion can be fully exposed. It does not approach or cross the anterior commissure.

Early vocal cord lesions are typically managed by radiation therapy. This therapy is usually successful in eliminating the tumor and preserving the quality of the voice. If treatment is not successful, several surgical interventions may be performed. A *cordectomy* may be performed with a laser for superficial tumors involving 1 cord. The cordectomy is a smaller version of a hemilaryngectomy (Fig. 23-15). A *hemilaryngectomy* is open laryngeal surgery to remove 1 or 1½ vocal cords and requires a tracheostomy. A *supraglottic laryngectomy,* or a partial laryngectomy, involves removing the false vocal cords and epiglottis. Although these procedures allow the voice to be preserved, it usually remains hoarse.

Advanced lesions are managed by a *total laryngectomy* in which the entire larynx and preepiglottic region are removed and a permanent tracheostomy is performed. Airflow patterns before and after total laryngectomy are shown in Fig. 23-16. *Radical neck dissection* frequently accompanies total laryngectomy. Depending on the extent of involvement, extensive dissection and reconstruction may be performed. The patient may refuse surgical intervention or may be judged to be at too high a risk for the procedure. Radiation therapy may be used as the sole treatment in this circumstance. Chemotherapy and radiation therapy may be used in the patient with advanced lesions to preserve the larynx to avoid a total laryngectomy.

Brachytherapy, a concentrated form of radiation therapy, involves placement of a radioactive source directly into or near the tumor. The goal is to deliver high doses of radiation

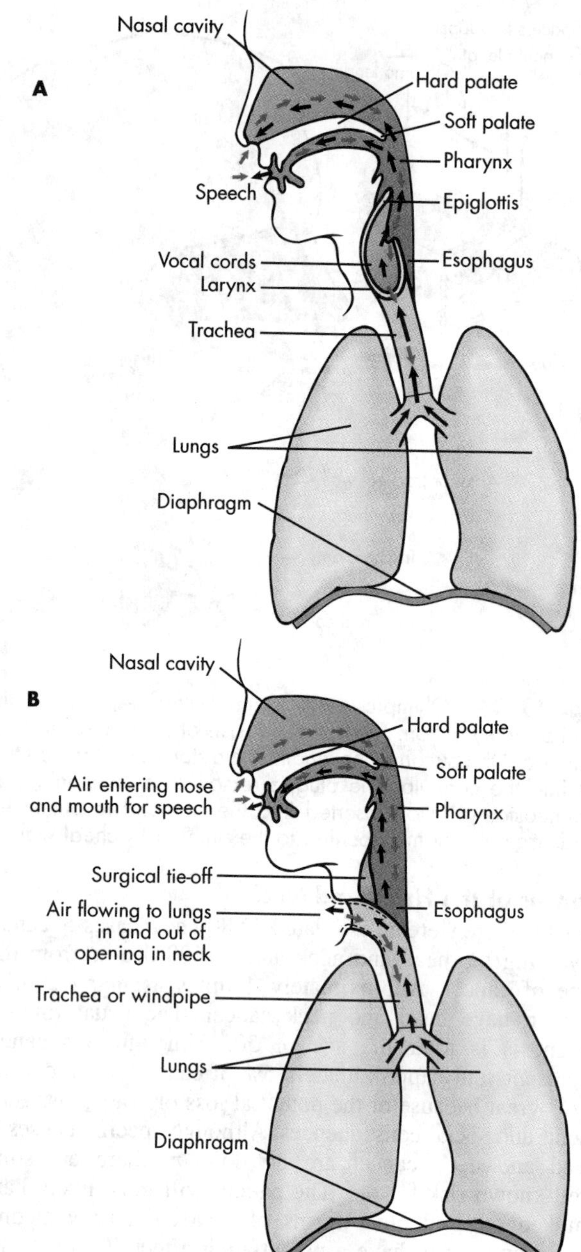

Fig. 23-16 ***A,*** Normal airflow in and out of the lungs. ***B,*** Airflow in and out of the lungs after total laryngectomy. The patient who uses esophageal speech traps air in the esophagus and releases it to create sound.

to the target area and to limit exposure of surrounding tissues. Thin hollow plastic needles are inserted into the tumor area. A radioactive source, iridium seeds, is placed in the needles. The seeds emit continuous radiation. Brachytherapy can be used alone or combined with external radiation or surgical intervention.[32]

Nutritional Management. The patient with extensive head and neck surgery will likely return from the OR with a nasogastric tube in place. Initially the tube is used for gastric decompression and then later for tube feedings. It is the responsibility of the nurse to assess correct placement and function of the tube (see Chapter 37). Gastric distention may lead to vomiting, aspiration, stress on the suture line, or wound contamination. The patient who undergoes extensive surgical procedures may require tube feedings to maintain nutrition until healing is sufficient to permit oral intake.

Changes in swallowing after surgery can be anticipated. The type and degree of difficulty will vary, depending on type of surgical procedure. When a supraglottic laryngectomy is performed, the surgeon excises the upper portion of the larynx, including the epiglottis and false vocal cords. The patient can speak because the true vocal cords remain intact. However, new swallowing techniques must be learned to compensate for removal of the epiglottis. To swallow, the patient performs a Valsalva maneuver (forced exhalation against a closed glottis). The Valsalva maneuver exaggerates the normal swallowing process and tightly closes the vocal cords, facilitating food passage into the stomach.

Table 23-7 Nursing Assessment: Cancer of the Head and Neck

Subjective Data

Important health information

Past health history: Heavy tobacco use (cigarettes, pipes, cigars, smokeless tobacco), chronic and heavy alcohol use, exposure to fumes, pollution, or radiation

Medications: Use of OTC medication for sore throat

Functional health patterns

Health perception–health management: Family history of head and neck cancers

Nutritional-metabolic: Mouth ulcer that does not heal, change in fit of dentures, swallowing difficulty, weight loss, change in appetite

Activity-excercise: Sensation of lump in throat, cough, hemoptysis, hoarseness, change in voice quality, chronic laryngitis

Cognitive-perceptual: Sore throat, pain on swallowing, referred ear pain

Objective Data

Gastrointestinal

White or red patches inside mouth, ulceration of mucosa, asymmetric tongue, exudate in mouth or pharynx, thickening of mucosa

Respiratory

Hoarseness, palpable neck mass and lymph nodes (tender, hard, fixed), tracheal deviation; stridor (late sign)

Possible findings

Mass on direct or indirect laryngoscopy; tumor on soft tissue x-ray, CT scan, or MRI; positive biopsy

CT, Computed tomography; *MRI,* magnetic resonance imaging; *OTC,* over-the-counter.

NURSING MANAGEMENT

CANCER OF THE HEAD AND NECK

Nursing Assessment

Subjective and objective data that should be obtained from a person with head and neck cancer are presented in Table 23-7.

Nursing Diagnoses

Nursing diagnoses are determined when the problem and the etiologic factors are supported by clinical data. Nursing diagnoses for the patient with head and neck cancer include, but are not limited to, those presented in the nursing care plan on p. 614.

Planning

The overall goals are that the patient with head or neck cancer will have (1) a patent airway, (2) no spread of cancer, (3) no complications related to therapy, (4) adequate nutritional intake, (5) minimal to no pain, (6) appropriate communication methods, and (7) acceptable body image.

Nursing Implementation

Health Maintenance and Promotion. Development of head and neck cancer is closely related to personal habits, primarily cigarette smoking. The cigarette smoker has an increased risk of lung cancer as well as head and neck cancer. Alcohol has been implicated as a potentiating factor for some head and neck cancers. Head and neck cancer may also be associated with the use of chewing tobacco. Snuff dipping, or the placement and retention of tobacco in the cheek, is a common practice in some areas of the United States. The long-term snuff user is at increased risk of oral cancer. The nurse should include information about these risk factors in health teaching. If cancer has been diagnosed, smoking cessation is still important. The patient with head and neck cancer who continues to smoke during radiation therapy has lower rates of response and survival than the patient who does not smoke during radiation therapy.[34]

Acute Intervention. The patient and the family must be taught about the type of therapy to be performed and care required. This should include (1) changes as a result of radiation therapy or surgical intervention, (2) duration of change, (3) change in the voice and ability to eat, (4) alternate methods of speech, (5) self-help groups and community resources, and (6) emotional adjustments to be anticipated. It is vital to include the patient and significant other in all aspects of teaching and care.[1]

Assessment of the patient's concerns is integral to the plan of care. The patient and family need to deal with the psychologic impact of the diagnosis of cancer and possible need for altered methods of communication. The care plan should include assessment of the patient's support system. The patient may not have someone to provide assistance after discharge, may not be employed, or may be employed in a job that cannot be continued. A social worker should be consulted if problems are identified.

Radiation therapy. The nurse can suggest interventions to reduce side effects of radiation therapy.[1] Dry mouth, the most frequent and annoying problem, typically begins within a few weeks of treatment. The patient's salivadecreases in volume and becomes thick. The change may be temporary or permanent. The volume of secretions can be increased with the use of sugarless gum, candy, and artifi-

NURSING CARE PLAN Patient Having Radical Neck Surgery or a Permanent Laryngectomy

Planning: Outcome Criteria	Nursing Interventions and Rationales
➤ NURSING DIAGNOSIS	Anxiety *related to* lack of knowledge regarding surgical procedure, postoperative course, pain management, and prevention of complications *as manifested by* questioning about impending surgery, agitation, and restlessness
Have a decrease in anxiety about surgery and a calm appearance; verbalize confidence regarding surgical procedure.	Assess knowledge desired by patient to allay fears and answer questions. Facilitate discussion of expected alterations in physical appearance; encourage sharing feelings and concerns to begin adjustment and acceptance. Give information about what to expect after surgery (e.g., pain management, tracheostomy, nasogastric tube, drainage tubes) to reduce patient's sense of helplessness and increase sense of control. Establish means of communication preoperatively so patient will have means of communication postoperatively.
➤ NURSING DIAGNOSIS	Ineffective airway clearance *related to* difficulty expectorating sputum and presence of tracheostomy *as manifested by* ineffective or absent cough; rhonchi or coarse crackles on auscultation; abnormal rate, pattern of breathing
Have secretions cleared with coughing, lungs clear on auscultation, normal respiratory rate and pattern.	Auscultate chest and monitor respiratory rate pattern q4hr for 24 hr and monitor SaO_2 or ABGs to determine adequacy of respirations. Encourage deep breathing and coughing and suction prn to clear secretions. Administer supplemental humidification as prescribed to liquefy secretions.
➤ NURSING DIAGNOSIS	Altered tissue perfusion *related to* tissue edema and disruption of vascular and lymphatic drainage *as manifested by* swollen and tense skin, and serous drainage from wound drainage tubes
Have decrease in tissue edema; serous drainage with decreased volume; no swelling, tenseness, or warmth in area over skin flaps; stable vital signs.	Maintain head of bed at 30 to 40 degrees to decrease tissue edema. Monitor HR, BP, Hb, Hct to detect excessive bleeding. Monitor patency of drainage tubes, amount, color of drainage to determine if drainage is excessive. Assess skin flap integrity q4hr (for warmth, swelling, color) to determine if flap is viable. Clean incision as prescribed to prevent infection.
➤ NURSING DIAGNOSIS	Altered nutrition: less than body requirements *related to* inability to ingest food secondary to pain, edema at surgical site, dysphagia, and presence of a nasogastric tube *as manifested by* absence of oral intake
Resume normal oral intake, swallow without coughing or aspirating; maintain or gain weight (if appropriate).	Provide frequent oral hygiene to promote comfort, improve appetite, remove drainage, and prevent infection. Deliver tube feedings as ordered to provide adequate nutrients while wound heals. Allow several days for wound healing. When oral feedings begin, give clear liquids and advance as tolerated to allow patient time to adjust to initiation of oral intake.
➤ NURSING DIAGNOSIS	Impaired verbal communication *related to* removal of vocal cords *as manifested by* inability or unwillingness to use voice rehabilitation methods
Be able to communicate clearly using method of choice.	Anticipate needs to reduce frustration of not having needs met because of unfamiliarity with alternate communication method. Answer call bell immediately. Communicate to staff that patient cannot speak. Instruct in alternate methods of communication (e.g., magic slate, communication board). Refer patient to speech therapist to learn use of voice prosthesis, electrolarynx, or esophageal speech.
➤ NURSING DIAGNOSIS	Body-image disturbance *related to* altered facial appearance *as manifested by* unwillingness to participate in self-care, view self in mirror, or visit with others
Participate in self-care; be willing to view self in mirror and visit with others.	Assess preoperative body image to determine importance of physical appearance to patient. Assess patient's readiness to view and touch reconstructed area to plan resumption of self-care. Assist and encourage patient to do so. Encourage support from family members. Refer to a support group to obtain information and support from firsthand experience. Encourage patient to verbalize feelings about body image and to participate in self-care to foster acceptance of altered physical appearance. Prepare visitors to prevent shocked response as this could be very demoralizing to patient.

continued

NURSING CARE PLAN Radical Neck Surgery/Permanent Laryngectomy—cont'd

Planning: Outcome Criteria	Nursing Interventions and Rationales
➤ **NURSING DIAGNOSIS** Pain *related to* surgical procedure *as manifested by* report of discomfort, facial mask of pain	
Verbalize that pain is controlled, to patient's satisfaction; express comfort.	Assess patient's manifestations of pain such as facial expression, reluctance to cough or move to *plan appropriate interventions.* Administer pain medication as prescribed and assess effectiveness. Monitor edema at incision site *because edema causes pressure on nerves and increased pain.* Logroll head and chest *to prevent strain on sutures.* Teach self-support of head and neck by interlocking hands behind head to provide support when moving to sitting position *to prevent strain on sutures.*
➤ **NURSING DIAGNOSIS** Ineffective management of therapeutic regimen *related to* lack of knowledge about home care after discharge *as manifested by* verbalized concern about ability to manage self-care at home	
Verbalize techniques and rationale for self-care; demonstrate techniques to be used in carrying out self-care; know when to contact health care professionals for problem solving.	Assess ability of patient to learn information *to avoid premature instruction.* Provide written instructions for patient and significant other *because an accurate reference reduces error.* Teach patient to perform suction in front of mirror and provide positive reinforcement *to ensure correct performance of technique.* Teach cleansing of tracheostomy or laryngectomy tube, voice prosthesis. Supervise care until patient and family are comfortable with techniques. Teach patient to cover stoma before performing such activities as shaving and applying makeup *to avoid inhalation of foreign materials.* Teach patient to report changes such as stoma narrowing, difficulty in swallowing, and lump in throat *to detect possible recurrence of tumor or tracheal stenosis.* Make referral for home health care visit *to evaluate self-care.*

ABGs, Arterial blood gases; *BP,* blood pressure; *Hb,* hemoglobin; *Hct,* hematocrit; *HR,* heart rate.

cial saliva. Good oral hygiene is performed with normal saline and a small amount of hydrogen peroxide. Increased fluid intake may help relieve symptoms. Additional side effects of radiation therapy include taste changes and stomatitis. Stomatitis is most common if the oral cavity is in the field of therapy. Irritation, ulceration, and pain are common complaints. Rinses of half-strength hydrogen peroxide or baking soda and water can be used to clean and soothe irritated tissues. Commercial mouthwashes and hot or spicy foods should be avoided because they are irritating. If the problem is severe, a mixture of equal parts of antacid, diphenhydramine (Benadryl), and topical lidocaine can be used.

Skin over the radiated area often becomes reddened and sensitive to touch. All exposure to the sun should be avoided to reduce discomfort. Corticosteroid sprays may be used to provide symptomatic relief.

Good nutrition is important during radiation therapy because calories and protein are needed for tissue repair. Antiemetics or analgesics may be given before meals to reduce nausea and mouth pain. Bland foods may be better tolerated. Caloric intake may be increased by adding dry milk to foods during preparation, selecting foods high in calories, and using oral supplements. If adequate intake cannot be maintained, nasogastric feedings may be used.

Preoperative teaching. Teaching must include information about expected changes in speech after surgical intervention. The nurse or speech pathologist should demonstrate alternate means of communicating other than speaking. The patient may find relief from anxiety by learning more about what to anticipate after the surgical intervention or may only want limited information. Most teaching will then need to be done after the surgery.

Postoperative management. After surgical intervention has been performed, airway management is the primary concern. The patient will be placed in a semi-Fowler's position to decrease edema and place less tension on the suture lines. Vital signs should be monitored frequently because of the risk of hemorrhage. Immediately after surgery, the patient with a laryngectomy requires frequent suctioning because secretions or saliva cannot be swallowed.

Secretions also typically change in consistency over time. The patient may initially have copious secretions that diminish and thicken as time goes on. If the patient develops mucous plugs or thick secretion, a 2 to 3 ml bolus of normal saline should be instilled into the airway to loosen secretions enough for the patient to clear the airway either through coughing or suctioning (see the nursing care plan for the patient with a tracheostomy, p. 608). With teaching, the patient can learn to use the bolus technique at home if necessary. The patient may also benefit from the use of a humidifier.

Pressure dressings, packing, or drainage tubes (Hemovac, Jackson Pratt) may be used for wound management, depending on the type of surgical procedure. If skin flaps are employed, dressings are typically not used. This allows better visualization of the incision and avoids excessive pressure on tissue. Patency of drainage tubes should be monitored every 4 hours for 24 hours to ensure that they are properly removing serous drainage. If the tubing becomes obstructed, fluid will accumulate under the skin flap and predispose to impaired wound healing and infection. After drainage tubes are removed, the area should be closely monitored to detect any swelling. If fluid continues to accumulate, aspiration may be necessary.

Voice rehabilitation. A speech therapist or speech pathologist should meet with the patient to discuss voice restoration. The International Association of Laryngectomees, an association of laryngectomy patients, focuses on assisting patients to reestablish speech. Local groups, called "Lost Cord Clubs," identify members who can visit the patient, preferably preoperatively.

Several options are available to restore speech. These include use of a voice prosthesis, an electrolarynx, and esophageal speech. The most commonly used voice prosthesis is the Blom-Singer prosthesis (Fig. 23-17). This soft plastic device is inserted into a fistula made between the esophagus and the trachea. The puncture may be created at the time of surgery or afterward, depending on the preference of the surgeon. The prosthesis allows air from the lungs to enter the esophagus but prevents aspiration. To speak, the patient blocks the stoma with the finger. Air moves from the lungs, through the prosthesis, into the esophagus, and out the mouth. Speech is produced the same as before surgery by moving the tongue and lips to form sound into words. A valve is also available for use with this prosthesis. When the valve is in place, the stoma does not need to be closed to speak. The patient using this prosthesis should be instructed to avoid eating foods (e.g. cheese, pasta, beans) that may clog the device. The prosthesis needs to be cleaned and should be replaced with a new one when it becomes blocked with mucus.[35]

The *electrolarynx* is a hand-held, battery-powered device that creates speech with the use of sound waves. One device, the Cooper-Rand, uses a plastic tube placed in the corner of the roof of the mouth to create vibrations. To create the most normal sound when using this device, the patient should (1) avoid trying to use the tongue to hold the tube in place; (2) compress the tone generator for short intervals and speak in phrases, rather than full sentences; (3) speak using large movements of the lips, tongue, and jaw, rather than keeping the mouth partially closed; (4) talk face-to-face with the listener; and (5) practice because development of skill takes time. Another type of artificial larynx is placed against the neck rather than in the mouth (Fig. 23-18). With experience the patient can learn to move the lips in ways that create normal-sounding speech. With both devices, voice pitch is low, and the sound resembles that of a robot or machine.

Esophageal speech is a method of swallowing air, trapping it in the esophagus, and releasing it to create sound. The air causes vibration of the pharyngoesophageal segment and sound (which initially is similar to a belch). With practice, 50% of patients will develop some speech skills, but only 10% will develop fluent speech.

Stoma care. Before discharge, the patient should be instructed in the care of the laryngectomy stoma.[35] The area around the stoma should be washed daily with a moist cloth. If a laryngectomy tube is in place, the tube will need to be removed daily and cleaned in the same manner as a tracheostomy tube (Table 23-6). A scarf, a loose shirt, or a crocheted stoma shield can be used to shield the stoma. The

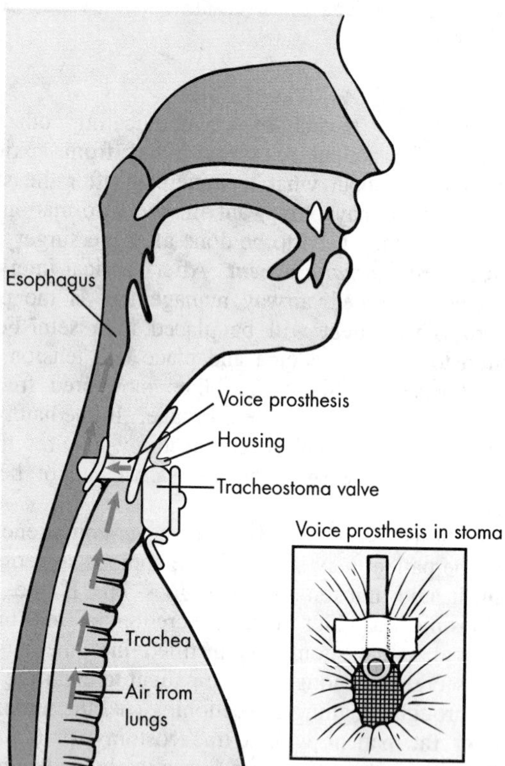

Fig. 23-17 Blom-Singer voice prosthesis and tracheostoma valve. With this prosthesis and valve, the patient with a laryngectomy can speak normally. The insert shows laryngectomy stoma and voice prosthesis with tracheostoma valve removed.

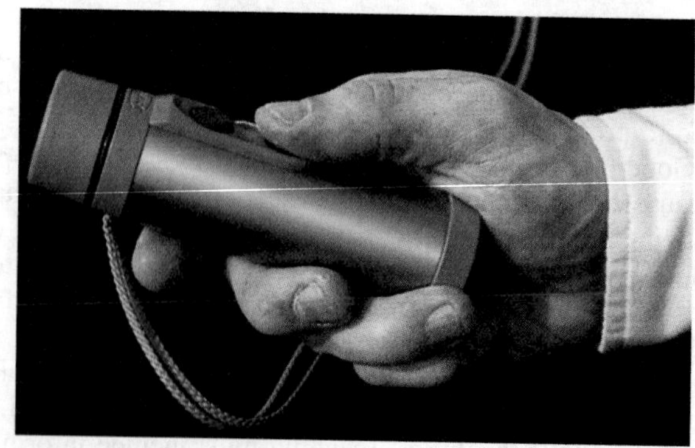

Fig. 23-18 Artificial larynx. Battery-powered electronic artificial larynx for patient who has total laryngectomy.

patient should cover the stoma when coughing, because mucus may be expectorated. Also, the stoma should be covered during any activity (such as shaving, applying makeup) that might lead to inhalation of foreign materials. Because water can easily enter the stoma, the patient should wear a plastic collar when taking a shower. Swimming is contraindicated. Initially, humidification will be supplied by oxygen mist through the tracheostomy adaptor. Later, a bedside humidifier can be substituted. A high oral fluid intake must be maintained, especially in dry weather. The patient should be told the importance of wearing a Medic-Alert bracelet or other identification that alerts others in an emergency situation of the use of neck breathing (Fig. 23-19).

Since the patient no longer breathes through the nose, the ability to smell smoke and food may be lost. Advise the patient to install smoke detectors in the home. It is important for food to be colorful, attractively prepared, and nutritious, because taste may also be diminished.

Chronic and Home Management. The patient can resume exercise, recreation, and sexual activity when able. Most patients can return to work 1 to 2 months after laryngectomy. However, as many as 50% never return to full-time employment. The changes that follow laryngectomy are upsetting. Loss of speech, loss of the ability to taste and smell, inability to produce audible sounds (including laughing and weeping), and the presence of a permanent tracheal stoma that produces undesirable mucus are often overwhelming to the patient. Although changes in body image resulting from the surgical procedure are discussed before surgery, the patient may not be prepared for the reality of the changes. If the patient has a significant other, the reaction of this person to the patient's altered appearance is important. Acceptance by another person can promote an improved self-image. Encouraging the patient to participate in self-care activities is another important part of rehabilitation.

Despite the use of surgical interventions and radiation therapy, the cure rate is disappointingly low for advanced head and neck cancer. Reasons include a high death rate from causes unrelated to cancer (e.g., cirrhosis, chronic obstructive lung disease, malnutrition, cardiovascular disease), development of a second primary tumor, and failure to control the disease. Metastatic cancer of the larynx is often painful, leaving the affected person in a severely debilitated state. If pain is a problem, a pain control regimen should be identified to provide comfort and referral should be made to a hospice, if indicated.

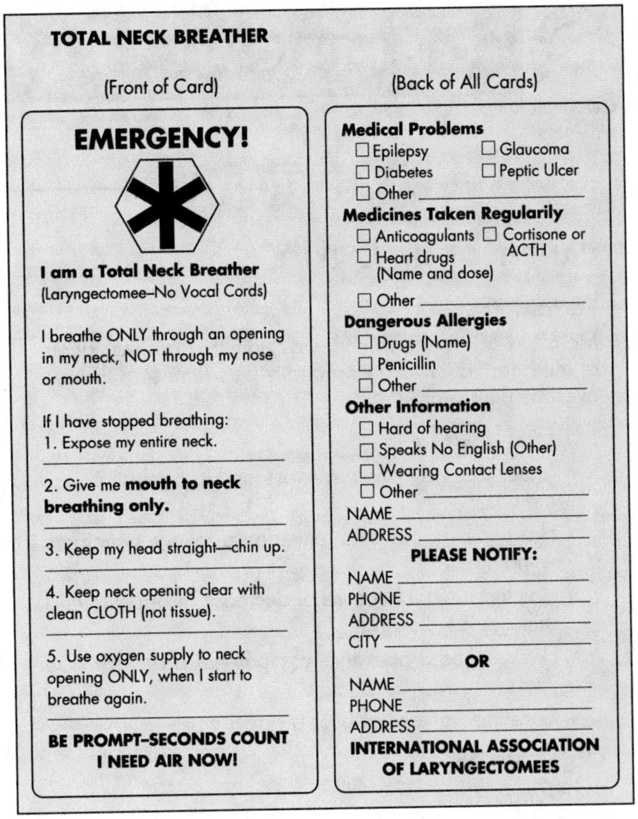

TOTAL NECK BREATHER

(Front of Card)

EMERGENCY!

I am a Total Neck Breather
(Laryngectomee–No Vocal Cords)

I breathe ONLY through an opening in my neck, NOT through my nose or mouth.

If I have stopped breathing:
1. Expose my entire neck.
2. Give me **mouth to neck breathing only.**
3. Keep my head straight—chin up.
4. Keep neck opening clear with clean CLOTH (not tissue).
5. Use oxygen supply to neck opening ONLY, when I start to breathe again.

BE PROMPT–SECONDS COUNT
I NEED AIR NOW!

(Back of All Cards)

Medical Problems
☐ Epilepsy ☐ Glaucoma
☐ Diabetes ☐ Peptic Ulcer
☐ Other ____

Medicines Taken Regularly
☐ Anticoagulants ☐ Cortisone or ACTH
☐ Heart drugs (Name and dose)
☐ Other ____

Dangerous Allergies
☐ Drugs (Name)
☐ Penicillin
☐ Other ____

Other Information
☐ Hard of hearing
☐ Speaks No English (Other)
☐ Wearing Contact Lenses
☐ Other ____
NAME ____
ADDRESS ____

PLEASE NOTIFY:
NAME ____
PHONE ____
ADDRESS ____
CITY ____

OR
NAME ____
PHONE ____
ADDRESS ____

INTERNATIONAL ASSOCIATION OF LARYNGECTOMEES

Fig. 23-19 Emergency identification of a neck breather.

CRITICAL THINKING EXERCISES

CASE STUDY

CANCER OF THE LARYNX

Patient Profile

Mr. C., a 60-year-old man, was admitted for evaluation of mild pain on swallowing and a persistent sore throat over the past year.

Subjective Data

- States that his symptoms worsened in the last 2 months
- Has used various cold remedies to relieve symptoms without relief
- Has lost weight because of decrease in appetite and difficulty swallowing
- Has smoked 3 packages of cigarettes a day for 40 years
- Consumes 6 cans of beer a day

Objective Data

Laryngoscopy

- Enlarged cervical nodes

CT scan

- Subglottic lesion with lymph node involvement

Therapeutic Management

- Total laryngectomy with tracheostomy with inflated cuff
- Nasogastric tube

Critical Thinking Questions

1. What information in the assessment suggests that Mr. C. might be at risk for cancer of the larynx?
2. What diagnostic tests are typically performed to evaluate the extent of this problem?
3. What teaching should the nurse plan for Mr. C. before and after laryngectomy?
4. Discuss methods used to restore the voice after laryngectomy. How do these methods differ in regard to the techniques used to produce speech after removal of the vocal cords?
5. What teaching is required to assist this patient to assume self-care after his surgery? What precautions should the patient take because of his stoma?
6. Based on the assessment data presented, write one or more nursing diagnoses. Are there any collaborative problems?

NURSING RESEARCH ISSUES

1. In what ways does sleep apnea affect patient's quality of life?
2. After a laryngectomy what methods of voice restoration provide the most satisfaction for the patient?
3. What are the most effective ways for a patient with a tracheostomy to communicate?
4. What is the quality of life of patients following a radical neck dissection?
5. What factors are most likely to promote compliance with CPAP therapy?

REVIEW QUESTIONS

These questions correspond to the same-numbered objectives at the beginning of the chapter.

1. Mr. J. was seen in clinic for an episode of epistaxis that was controlled by placement of anterior nasal packing. Which of the following should *not* be included in teaching before discharge?

a. Avoid vigorous nose blowing and strenuous activity.
b. Sneeze with the mouth open.
c. Use aspirin or aspirin-containing compounds for pain relief.
d. Take antibiotic at prescribed intervals.

2. Ms. S. is diagnosed with allergic rhinitis. She reports severe nasal congestion, sneezing, and watery, itchy eyes and nose most of the year. Which of the following should *not* be included in her teaching?

a. Keep diary of times the allergic reaction occurs and what precipitates it.
b. Limit the duration of use of nasal decongestant spray to 10 days.
c. Try to remove triggers of allergic symptoms from the home.
d. Never use an intranasal corticosteroid spray and nonsedating antihistamine at the same time.

3. Ms. P. asks for instruction about proper use of an intranasal corticosteroid spray prescribed for her sinusitis. When teaching, the nurse should include all of the following *except*

a. reinforce that spray acts to decrease risk of infection from the sinusitis.
b. instruct her to use the inhaler on a regular basis and not prn.
c. instruct her to discontinue use if a nasal infection develops.
d. reinforce that spray should be directed toward the outside nostril wall when inhaling.

4. All of the following groups should receive yearly influenza vaccination *except*

a. persons with an allergic reaction to egg protein.
b. residents of nursing homes.
c. adults with chronic pulmonary or cardiovascular problems.
d. health care professionals in contact with high-risk patients.

5. Mr. C. is diagnosed with sleep apnea. He would like to avoid using a nasal CPAP device, if possible. Which of the following strategies would *not* be appropriate in helping him achieve this goal?

a. Referral to a weight loss program, if he is obese.
b. Placing golf balls in a pocket sewn in the back of his pajamas.
c. Avoiding alcohol or sedatives for 3 to 4 hours before sleep.
d. Keeping a diary of events that trigger his sleep apnea.

6. To prevent excessive pressure on tracheal capillaries, pressure in the cuff on an endotracheal tube or tracheostomy should be

a. <30 mm Hg or <35 cm H_2O.
b. <20 mm Hg or <25 cm H_2O.
c. sufficient to fill the pilot balloon until it is tense.
d. monitored every 2 to 3 days.

7. Mr. P. is intubated with an endotracheal tube as a result of acute respiratory failure secondary to pneumococcal pneumonia. You would suction him

a. routinely every 2 hours.
b. when rhonchi or coarse crackles are heard on auscultation.
c. when his cuff is deflated.
d. after completion of the nasogastric feeding.

8. Which of the following is *not* an early symptom of cancer of the head and neck?

a. Pain when eating acidic foods.
b. Mouth ulcers that do not heal.
c. Change in fit of dentures.
d. Decreased mobility of the tongue.

9. Nursing management of the patient immediately after a total laryngectomy includes all of the following *except*

a. changing the surgical dressing.
b. ensuring that the nasogastric tube is patent.
c. placing the patient in semi-Fowler's position.
d. monitoring function of the drainage tubes.

10. When using a voice prosthesis, the patient

a. swallows air using a Valsalva maneuver.
b. places a vibrating device in the mouth or on the neck.
c. blocks the stoma entrance with the finger, causing air to travel up over the vocal cords.
d. places a speaking valve over the laryngectomy stoma.

REFERENCES

1. Sigler BA, Schuring LT: *Ear, nose, and throat disorders,* St Louis, 1993, Mosby.
2. Josephson GD, Godley FA, Stierna P: Practical management of epistaxis, *Med Clin North Am* 75:1311, 1991.
3. Mabry RL: A step-care approach to the treatment of upper respiratory allergy, *Otolaryngol Head Neck Surg* 107:828, 1992.
4. O'Hollaren MT, Bardana EJ: Successfully managing chronic rhinitis, *J Resp Dis* 11:565, 1990.
5. Findlay S and others: Efficacy of once-a-day intranasal administration of triamcinolone acetonide in patients with seasonal allergic rhinitis, *Ann Allergy* 68:228, 1992.
6. Nurse's guide to OTC allergy products, *Nurs* 23:67, 1993.
7. Colman BH: *Hall & Colman's diseases of the nose, throat, ear, and head and neck: a handbook for students and practitioners,* New York, 1992, Churchill Livingstone.
8. Beckett WS, Fiebach NH: Influenza and pneumococcal vaccines: 1993-1994 update, *J Resp Dis* 114:1068, 1993.
9. Gardner P, Schaffner W: Immunization of adults, *N Engl J Med* 328:1252, 1993.
10. Dolin R: Influenza. In Isselbacher KJ and others: *Harrison's principles of internal medicine,* ed 13, New York, 1994, McGraw-Hill.
11. American Lung Association: Influenza news '93, Recommendations of the advisory committee on immunization practices, Centers for Disease Control, 1993.
12. Williams JW, Simel DL: Does this patient have sinusitis? *JAMA* 270:1242, 1993.
13. Bolger WE, Kennedy DW: Current perspectives on sinusitis in adults, *J Resp Dis* 13:421, 1992.
14. Hoffman SR and others: Symptom relief after endoscopic sinus surgery: an outcomes-based study, *Ear Nose Throat J* 72:413, 1993.
15. Smolley LA: How to help patients with obstructive sleep apnea, *J Resp Dis* 11:723, 1990.
16. Dement WC, Mitler MM: It's time to wake up to the importance of sleep disorders, *JAMA* 269:1548, 1993.
17. Young T and others: The occurrence of sleep-disordered breathing among middle-aged adults, *N Engl J Med* 328:1230, 1993.
18. Reeves-Hoche MK, Meck R, Zwillich C: Nasal CPAP: an objective evaluation of patient compliance, *Am J Resp Crit Care Med* 149:149, 1994.
19. Strumpf DA and others: Alternative methods of humidification during use of nasal CPAP, *Resp Care* 35:217, 1990.
20. Hall JB, Schmidt GA, Wood LDH: *Principles of critical care companion hand book,* New York, 1993, McGraw Hill.
21. Pagan P: How to use a disposable end-tidal CO_2 detector, *Nurs* 24:50, 1994.
22. Kaplow R, Bookbinder M: A comparison of four endotracheal tube holders, *Heart Lung* 23:59, 1994.
23. Tasota F and others: Evaluation of two methods used to stabilize oral endotracheal tubes, *Heart Lung* 16:140, 1987.

24. Harshbarger SA and others: Effects of a closed tracheal suction system on ventilatory and cardiovascular parameters, *Amer J Crit Care* 1992:57, 1992.
25. Mancinelli-Beck J, Beck SL: Preventing hypoxemia and hemodynamic compromise related to endotracheal suctioning, *Amer J Crit Care* 1992:62, 1992.
26. Dettenmeier PA: *Pulmonary nursing care,* St Louis, 1992, Mosby.
27. Williams ML: An algorithm for selecting a communication technique with intubated patients, *Dimens Crit Care Nurs* 11:222, 1992.
28. Heffner JE: Timing of tracheotomy in mechanically ventilated patients, *Am Rev Respir Dis* 147:768, 1993.
29. Hoffman LA: Timing of tracheostomy, *Respir Care* 39:378, 1994.
30. Lewis RJ: Tracheostomies: indications, timing and complications, *Clin Chest Med* 13:137, 1992.
31. Weilitz PB, Dettenmeier PA: Test your knowledge of tracheostomy tubes, *Amer J Nurs* 94:46, 1994.
32. Vokes EE and others: Head and neck cancer, *N Engl J Med* 328:184, 1993.
33. Hanson DG: Detecting and identifying upper airway cancers–early, *J Resp Dis* 13:78, 1992.
34. Browman GP and others: Influence of cigarette smoking on the efficacy of radiation therapy in head and neck cancer, *N Engl J Med* 328:159, 1993.
35. Lochart JS, Bryce J: Restoring speech with tracheoesophageal puncture, *Nurs* 23:59, 1993.

Chapter 24

NURSING ROLE IN MANAGEMENT

Lower Respiratory Problems

Joyce Tremper Mitchell

Learning Objectives

1. Describe the pathophysiology, types, clinical manifestations, and therapeutic and pharmacologic management of pneumonia.
2. Explain the nursing role in management of the patient with pneumonia.
3. Describe the pathogenesis, classification, clinical manifestations, complications, diagnostic abnormalities, and therapeutic, pharmacologic, and nursing management of tuberculosis.
4. Identify the causes, clinical manifestations, and therapeutic and nursing management of pulmonary fungal infections.
5. Explain the pathophysiology, clinical manifestations, and therapeutic and nursing management of bronchiectasis and lung abscess.
6. Identify the indications for oxygen therapy, methods of delivery, and complications of oxygen administration.
7. Identify the causative factors, clinical features, and management of occupational lung diseases.
8. Describe the causes, risk factors, pathogenesis, clinical manifestations, and therapeutic and nursing management of lung cancer.
9. Describe the risks associated with cigarette smoking, various methods of smoking cessation, and the role of the nurse in assisting the patient to stop smoking.
10. Identify the mechanisms involved and the clinical manifestations of pneumothorax, fractured ribs, and flail chest.
11. Describe the purpose, methods, and nursing responsibilities related to chest tubes.
12. Explain the types of chest surgery and appropriate preoperative and postoperative care.
13. Compare and contrast extrapulmonary and intrapulmonary restrictive lung disorders in terms of causes, clinical manifestations, and management.
14. Describe the pathophysiology, clinical manifestations, and management of pulmonary hypertension and cor pulmonale.
15. Discuss the use of lung transplantation as a treatment for pulmonary disorders.

There is a wide variety of problems that affect the lower respiratory system. Lung diseases that are characterized primarily by an obstructive disorder, such as asthma, emphysema, chronic bronchitis, and cystic fibrosis, are discussed in Chapter 25. All other lower respiratory problems are discussed in this chapter.

PULMONARY INFECTIONS

Pulmonary infections annually rank among the top ten causes of death in the United States. Bacterial pneumonia remains the leading infectious cause of death in spite of the availability of antimicrobial agents.[1] Tuberculosis, although potentially curable and preventable, is still a significant public health problem in the United States, Canada, and the rest of the world.

Acute Bronchitis

Acute bronchitis is a common pulmonary infection that occurs most frequently in the patient with chronic obstructive pulmonary disease (COPD), but it also occurs in other patients, usually as a sequela to an upper respiratory tract infection. The patient's symptoms include fever, cough, tachypnea, purulent sputum, and occasionally, pleuritic chest pain. When the patient's chest is auscultated, diffuse rhonchi and crackles may be heard. Chest x-ray differentiates acute bronchitis from pneumonia, because there is usually no evidence of consolidation or infiltrates with bronchitis. The origin of most cases of acute bronchitis is viral, but bacterial causes (*Streptococcus pneumoniae* or *Haemophilus influenzae*) are also common.

Reviewed by Mary Beth Egloff-Parr, RN, MSN, CCRN, Pulmonary Clinical Nurse Specialist, Sharp Memorial Hospital, San Diego, CA.

Acute bronchitis does not require hospitalization unless the patient shows symptoms of dehydration. Treatment is generally with a broad-spectrum antibiotic (e.g., ampicillin, tetracycline, or erythromycin) for 7 to 10 days. The patient with COPD who has symptoms of acute bronchitis is usually treated empirically with broad-spectrum antibiotics, and modifications in therapy are made if they prove ineffective. Often the patient with COPD is taught to recognize symptoms of acute bronchitis and to begin a course of antibiotics when symptoms occur. Many clinicians believe that a more severe infection often results if the patient delays taking antibiotics until after an examination by a physician. This delay may cause serious consequences for the patient with severe chronic lung disease.

When educating the patient on the use of antibiotics, it is important to stress that the full course of the drug must be taken to minimize the development of resistant organisms. In addition, timing of drug dosing related to food intake and avoidance of certain foods taken concurrently with certain medications (e.g., milk and antacids with tetracycline) should be discussed with the patient.

Pneumonia

Significance. *Pneumonia*, or *pneumonitis*, is an acute inflammation of the lung parenchyma. Until 1936 pneumonia was the leading cause of death in the United States. Then sulfa drugs and penicillin were discovered and used to treat pneumonia. However, in spite of antibiotics, pneumonia is still common, and some types of the disease have a high mortality rate. Approximately 1% of the American population will have pneumonia at some time in their lives. Pneumonia is the sixth leading cause of death in the United States.[1]

Pathophysiology

Normal defense mechanisms. Normally, the airway distal to the larynx is sterile because of protective defense mechanisms. These mechanisms include (see Chapter 22):

1. Filtration and humidification of air
2. Warming of inspired air
3. Epiglottis closure over the trachea
4. Cough reflex
5. Mucociliary escalator mechanism
6. Secretion of immunoglobulin A
7. Alveolar macrophages

Factors predisposing to pneumonia. Pneumonia is more likely to result when defense mechanisms become incompetent or are overwhelmed by the virulence or quantity of infectious agents. Decreased consciousness depresses the cough and epiglottal reflexes, which may allow aspiration of oropharyngeal contents into the lungs. Tracheal intubation interferes with the normal cough reflex and the mucociliary escalator mechanism. It also bypasses the upper airways in which filtration and humidification of air normally take place. The mucociliary escalator mechanism is impaired by air pollution, cigarette smoking, viral upper respiratory tract infections (URIs), and normal changes of aging. In cases of malnutrition the formation and function of lymphocytes and polymorphonuclear leukocytes are altered. Certain diseases such as leukemia, alcoholism, and diabetes mellitus are associated with an increased frequency of gram-negative bacilli in the oropharynx.[2] (Gram-negative bacilli are not normal flora.) Altered oropharyngeal flora can also occur secondary to antibiotic therapy given for an infection elsewhere in the body. The factors predisposing to pneumonia are shown in Table 24-1.

Table 24-1 Factors Predisposing to Pneumonia

Smoking
Air pollution
Altered consciousness: alcoholism, head injury, seizures, anesthesia, drug overdose
Tracheal intubation (endotracheal intubation, tracheostomy)
Upper respiratory tract infection
Chronic diseases: chronic lung disease, diabetes mellitus, heart disease, uremia, cancer
Immunosuppression ▪ Drugs (corticosteroids, cancer chemotherapy, immunosuppressive therapy after organ transplant) ▪ HIV
Malnutrition
Inhalation or aspiration of noxious substances
Debilitating illness
Bed rest and prolonged immobility
Altered oropharyngeal flora

HIV, Human immunodeficiency virus.

Acquisition of organisms. Organisms that cause pneumonia reach the lung by three methods:

1. Aspiration from the nasopharynx or oropharynx. Many of the organisms that cause pneumonia are normal inhabitants of the pharynx in healthy adults.
2. Inhalation of microbes present in the air. Examples include *Mycoplasma pneumoniae* and fungal pneumonias.
3. Hematogenous spread from a primary infection elsewhere in the body.

Types of Pneumonia. Pneumonia can be caused by bacteria, viruses, Mycoplasma organisms, fungi, protozoa (e.g., *Pneumocystis carinii*), chemicals, dust, gases, and a variety of other organisms and materials (Table 24-2). Pneumonia is usually classified according to the causative organism. Sometimes pneumonia is classified on the basis of areas and type of lung involvement (Fig. 24-1).

Gram-positive bacterial pneumonias. Gram-positive bacteria (*S. pneumoniae, Staphylococcus aureus*, and group A β-hemolytic streptococci) account for most bacterial pneumonias acquired in the community. Recently *S. aureus* has become an increasingly common cause of nosocomial pneumonia. The most common type of pneumonia is pneumococcal pneumonia caused by *S. pneumoniae*.

Table 24-2 Comparison of Types of Pneumonia

Causative Agent	Characteristics	Clinical Manifestations and Complications
Gram-Positive Bacterial Pneumonias		
▪ Pneumococcal pneumonia *(Streptococcus pneumoniae)*	URI usually preceding, usual involvement of 1 or more lobes, incubation period of 1-3 days, peak incidence in winter and spring, damage to host by overwhelming growth of organism, necrosis of lung tissue (unusual), chest x-ray shows lobar infiltration,* nasopharyngeal carriers, frequent finding of herpes labialis in association with pneumonia, risk factors of chronic heart or lung disease, diabetes mellitus, cirrhosis	Abrupt onset, elevated temperature, tachypnea, chills and rigor, productive cough (often bloody, rusty, or green), nausea, vomiting, malaise, myalgia, weakness, pleuritic chest pain, atelectasis, lung abscess (rare), pleural effusions (25-50%), empyema, metastatic infection (meninges, joints, heart valves), bacteremia (25%)
▪ Staphylococcal pneumonia *(Staphylococcus aureus)*	Acquisition via hematogenous route or via aspiration into lungs; nasopharyngeal carriers (35-50% of population); necrotizing infection causing destruction of lung tissue; chest x-ray shows bronchopneumonia;* risk factors of chronic lung disease, leukemia, other debilitating diseases; influenza infection (10-14 days earlier) often preceding; drug abusers, diabetics, patients on long-term hemodialysis at risk as carriers; occurrence more frequent in hospitalized patients than in persons in community; prolonged antibiotic therapy usually necessary; high mortality rate in chronically debilitated patients, newborns	Abrupt onset, chills, high fever, productive cough with sputum (often bloody and purulent), tachypnea, progressive dyspnea, pleuritic chest pain, empyema, pleural effusions, lung abscess
▪ Streptococcal pneumonia *(Streptococcus pyogenes)*	Occurrence in military populations after influenza epidemics and sporadically in community, often associated with strep throat, occurrence most frequent in winter, transmission to lung by inhalation or aspiration, destruction of lung tissue, chest x-ray shows bronchopneumonia	Fever (usually >102.2° F [39° C]), chills, cough, pharyngitis, hemoptysis, pleuritic chest pain, dyspnea, myalgia, empyema (common), pleural effusions, bacteremia, mediastinitis, pneumothorax, bronchiectasis
▪ Anthrax pneumonia *(Bacillus anthracis)*	Association with agricultural or industrial exposure (e.g., individuals working with animal hair or contaminated animal hides or bones), transmission to lung via inhalation, formation of spores, ingestion and transport of spores to hilar lymph nodes (site of multiplication of bacteria) by alveolar macrophages, hemorrhagic pneumonitis possible	Early manifestations: insidious onset (2-4 days), mild fever, myalgia, malaise, fatigue, nonproductive cough Later manifestations: dyspnea, profuse diaphoresis, cyanosis
Gram-Negative Bacterial Pneumonias		
▪ Friedländer's pneumonia *(Klebsiella pneumoniae)*	Most common gram-negative pneumonia acquired outside hospital; alcoholics, diabetics, persons with chronic lung disease, and postoperative patients at risk; transmission to lungs via aspiration of oropharyngeal organisms; chest x-ray shows lobar consolidation;* rapid progession to lung abscess possible; high mortality and morbidity rates	Sudden onset, fever, cough, purulent sputum, hemoptysis, malaise, pleuritic chest pain, extensive lung necrosis, lung abscess, empyema, pericarditis, meningitis

continued

Table 24-2 Comparison of Types of Pneumonia—cont'd

Causative Agent	Characteristics	Clinical Manifestations and Complications
Gram-Negative Bacterial Pneumonias—cont'd		
▪ Pseudomonas pneumonia (*Pseudomonas aeruginosa*)	Most common gram-negative hospital-acquired pneumonia; predisposition from endotracheal intubation, intermittent positive-pressure breathing treatments, suctioning, respiratory therapy equipment; high mortality rate in critically ill patients; chest x-ray shows nodular bronchopneumonia;* persons with chronic lung disease, debilitating diseases, tracheostomies, cancer, and kidney transplants or those taking immunosuppressive drugs or broad-spectrum antibiotics at risk; high mortality rate (50-90%)	High fever, cough, copious sputum, hypoxia, cyanosis, lung abscess
▪ Influenza pneumonia (*Haemophilus influenzae*)	Increase in incidence; transmission to lung by endogenous aspiration; chest x-ray shows bronchopneumonia in multiple lobes or lobar consolidation; alcoholics and persons with chronic lung disease, recent viral infections, and immune deficiencies at risk; high mortality rate, especially in older adult patients	Usually gradual onset, sometimes abrupt; fever; chills; cough; purulent sputum; hemoptysis; sore throat; dyspnea; nausea and vomiting; pleuritic chest pain; pleural effusions; lung abscess (common); empyema (common)
▪ Legionnaires' disease (*Legionella pneumophila*)	Occurrence in outbreaks or sporadic, transmission to lung from airborne organisms, proliferation of organisms in water reservoirs (e.g., air-conditioning cooling towers), cigarette smokers and persons with serious underlying diseases (e.g., chronic lung or heart conditions) at increased risk, erythromycin effective	Myalgia (initially), headache (initially), fever, chills, nonproductive cough, pleuritic chest pain, nausea and vomiting, diarrhea, mental confusion, respiratory failure (major complication), healing with fibrosis common
Anaerobic Bacterial Pneumonias		
▪ Anaerobic streptococci ▪ Fusobacteria ▪ *Bacteroides* species	Transmission to lung usually by aspiration of oropharyngeal secretions but occasionally via blood from GI or GU tract or wound infections; three or four anaerobes usually causing infections; persons with poor dental hygiene, periodontal disease, and history of altered consciousness at risk; chest x-ray often shows lung abscess, empyema, necrotizing pneumonia	Similar to pneumococcal pneumonia, except for insidious onset; foul-smelling sputum; necrotizing pneumonitis (aspiration induced); lung abscess; empyema
Mycoplasma Pneumonia		
▪ Mycoplasma pneumonia (*Mycoplasma pneumoniae*)†	Transmission from person to person by respiratory droplets; incubation period of 9-21 days; involvement of epithelial lining of respiratory system; common in children, military populations, college-age groups; increase in cold agglutinin titer in serum or complement fixation with negative bacterial culture; chest x-ray shows interstitial pneumonia, often bilaterally*	Gradual onset; URI, including fever (low-grade), nasal congestion, pharyngitis; lower respiratory tract involvement (e.g., bronchitis, bronchiolitis); headache; malaise; cough (initially usually nonproductive); maculopapular rashes

continued

Table 24-2 Comparison of Types of Pneumonia—cont'd

Causative Agent	Characteristics	Clinical Manifestations and Complications
Viral Pneumonias ■ Influenza viruses ■ Adenovirus ■ Parainfluenza viruses ■ Respiratory syncytial virus	Influenza A most common in civilian adults; responsible for about one half of all pneumonias; peak incidence in winter; transmission from person to person by respiratory droplets; usually self-limiting; symptomatic treatment; adverse effect on many respiratory defense mechanisms, predisposing patients to secondary bacterial pneumonia; chest x-ray shows interstitial pneumonia*	Fever, chills, headache, myalgia, anorexia, sneezing, nasal congestion, cough (initially nonproductive)
Protozoan Pneumonia ■ Interstitial plasma cell pneumonia (*Pneumocystis carinii*)	Opportunistic infection; persons with immunosuppression (e.g., recipients of organ transplants, patients with HIV infection, and those with hematologic malignancies) at highest risk; presentation similar to other atypical pneumonias	Cough (usually nonproductive), fever, night sweats, dyspnea (may be only with exertion)

GI, Gastrointestinal; *GU*, genitourinary; *HIV*, human immunodeficiency virus; *URI*, upper respiratory tract infection.
*See Fig. 24-1.
†Organism has characteristics of both bacteria and viruses.

Gram-negative bacterial pneumonias. There has been an increasing incidence of aerobic gram-negative bacterial pneumonias. They account for 20% of community-acquired pneumonias and 40% to 60% of hospital-acquired pneumonias.[3] Organisms that cause gram-negative pneumonias include *Klebsiella, Pseudomonas, Haemophilus, Serratia, Escherichia coli*, and *Proteus*. Most of these organisms enter the lung after aspiration of particles from the patient's own pharynx. Immunosuppressive therapy, general debility, endotracheal intubation, and prolonged antibiotic therapy may be predisposing factors. Respiratory therapy equipment that is not cleaned regularly is a potential source of infection.

Anaerobic bacterial pneumonias. Most anaerobic pneumonias are caused by aspiration of oropharyngeal secretions. Infections usually involve multiple organisms, and aerobic organisms are also found in many cases of anaerobic pneumonia.

Mycoplasma pneumonia. The transmission of mycoplasma pneumonia is from person to person by respiratory droplets. Intrafamily or intragroup (e.g., the military) spread is common. It is the most common community-acquired pneumonia in young adults. Mycoplasma pneumonia is usually treated with antibiotics (e.g., tetracycline).

Viral pneumonias. Viruses are the most common cause of pneumonia in infants and children. In adults viruses account for a small number of lower respiratory tract infections.

The initial manifestations of viral pneumonia are highly variable but are usually similar to those of influenza and include fever, myalgia, headache, rhinorrhea, and dry cough. On chest x-ray there is usually an interstitial pattern of lung involvement. The x-ray may demonstrate extensive pulmonary involvement, although there are minimal physical findings on examination. These types of pneumonias are typically mild and self-limiting and result in no permanent lung damage in previously healthy individuals. Treatment is usually for relief of symptoms because antibiotics are not effective. The most common pulmonary complication of influenza is secondary bacterial pneumonia.[3]

Primary influenza viral pneumonia syndrome, although rare, is severe and may be fatal. It occurs primarily in the patient who is an older adult, is debilitated, or has chronic lung or heart disease. The alveoli fill with fibrin, fluid, red blood cells (RBCs), and macrophages. These individuals have severe hypoxemia, tachycardia, and tachypnea. The mortality rate is high in spite of ventilatory support. If the individual survives, pulmonary fibrosis is a common complication.

Viral pneumonia is also found in association with systemic viral diseases such as measles, varicella-zoster (VZV), and herpes simplex (HSV). Varicella pneumonia is more common in adults with chicken pox than in children.

Two antiviral drugs, amantadine and rimantadine, are approved for parenteral use in treatment of viral respiratory infections, and they have been shown to have therapeutic benefit in uncomplicated cases of influenza infections in adults.[4] Vaccines against adenovirus and influenza are currently available. Because adenovirus pneumonia is not common in the general population, the use of adenovirus vaccine has been limited to high-risk groups, such as military recruits. Influenza vaccine is considered a mainstay of prevention and is recommended annually for use in the individual considered to be at risk of serious influenza.

Amantadine has also been used as a chemoprophylactic agent against influenza A virus infections. It acts by pre-

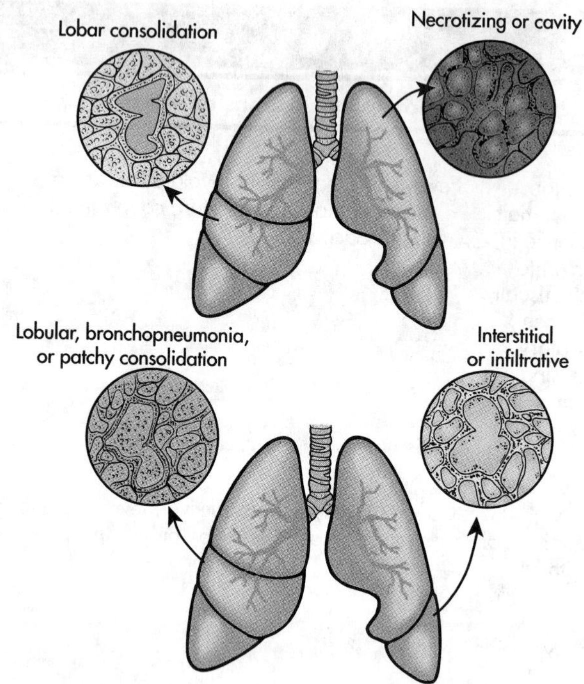

Fig. 24-1 Types of pneumonia. *Lobar*: Entire lobe is consolidated. Exudate chiefly intraalveolar *(inset)*. *Pneumococcus* and *Klebsiella* are common infecting organisms. *Necrotizing*: Granuloma may undergo caseous necrosis and form a cavity. Fungi and tubercle bacillus are common infecting organisms. *Lobular*: Patchy distribution displayed. Fibrinous exudate is chiefly in bronchioles. *Staphylococcus* and *Streptococcus* are common infecting organisms. *Interstitial*: Perivascular exudate and edema found between the alveoli, caused by viral or mycoplasma infection.

venting the penetration of the virus into the host cell. It is used primarily in outbreaks of the virus and in the high-risk individual. Amantadine needs to be given daily throughout the period of influenza exposure. Side effects are uncommon and consist primarily of reversible minor central nervous system (CNS) effects.

Fungal pneumonia. Fungi may also be a cause of pneumonia (see section on Pulmonary Fungal Infections).

Aspiration pneumonia. Aspiration pneumonia is frequently called *necrotizing pneumonia* because of the pathologic changes in the lungs. It usually follows aspiration of material in the mouth into the trachea and subsequently the lungs. The aspirated material, either food, water, or vomitus, is the triggering mechanism for the pathology of this type of pneumonia.

If the aspirated material is an inert substance (e.g., barium or nonacid stomach contents), the initial manifestation is usually caused by obstruction of airways. When the aspirated materials contain gastric acid, there is chemical injury to the lung parenchyma with infection as a secondary event usually 48 to 72 hours later. The infecting organism is usually one of the normal oropharyngeal flora, and the clinical manifestations proceed as those of a classic pneumococcal or streptococcal pneumonia. Multiple organisms, including both aerobes and anaerobes, are isolated from the sputum of the patient with aspiration pneumonia.

The person who has aspiration pneumonia usually has a history of loss of consciousness (e.g., as a result of seizure, anesthesia, head injury, alcohol intake). With loss of consciousness the gag and cough reflexes are depressed, and aspiration is more likely to occur. The dependent portions of the lung are most often affected, primarily the superior segments of the lower lobes, which are dependent in the supine position.

Pneumonia in the compromised host. Certain patients with an altered immune response are highly susceptible to respiratory infections. Individuals considered at high risk include those who have severe protein-calorie malnutrition, immune deficiencies, transplants, and patients who are being treated with radiation therapy, chemotherapy drugs, and corticosteroids (especially for a prolonged period). The individual has a variety of altered conditions, including altered B- and T-lymphocyte function, depressed bone marrow function, and decreased levels or function of neutrophils and macrophages. In addition to the causative agents (especially gram-negative bacteria), other agents that cause pneumonia in the immunosuppressed patient are *Pneumocystis carinii,* cytomegalovirus (CMV), and fungi.

Pneumocystis carinii, a protozoan organism, rarely causes pneumonia in the healthy individual. In this type of pneumonia the chest x-ray usually shows a diffuse bilateral alveolar pattern of infiltration. In widespread disease the lungs are massively consolidated. Clinical manifestations are insidious and include fever, tachypnea, tachycardia, dyspnea, nonproductive cough, and hypoxemia. Pulmonary physical findings are minimal in proportion to the serious nature of the disease. Treatment consists of a 14-day course of trimethoprim-sulfamethoxazole (Bactrim) as the primary agent and pentamidine isethionate. The mortality rate for an initial episode of *P. carinii* pneumonia (PCP) is approximately 40%. With a second infection the mortality rate rises to 75%.[5] If left untreated, the mortality rate is 100%. In populations at high risk for development of *P. carinii* pneumonitis (e.g., patients with hematologic malignancies or acquired immunodeficiency virus [AIDS]), secondary prophylaxis with trimethoprim-sulfamethoxazole may be advocated. Aerosols of pentamadine isethionate have shown promising results as a treatment option for PCP and as a prophylactic measure.[6] In addition, the patient may be given drug treatment for the primary disease, such as zidovudine (Retrovir). (See Chapter 11).

CMV, also called *cytomegalic inclusion virus,* is a common cause of viral pneumonia in the immunocompromised patient, particularly in a transplant recipient. CMV, a type of herpes virus, gives rise to latent infections and reactivation with shedding of infectious virus. This type of interstitial pneumonia can be a mild disease or it can be fulminant and produce pulmonary insufficiency and death. Often, CMV coexists with other opportunistic bacterial, fungal, or protozoan agents in causing pneumonia. There is no definitive therapy available for this type of pneumonia.[4]

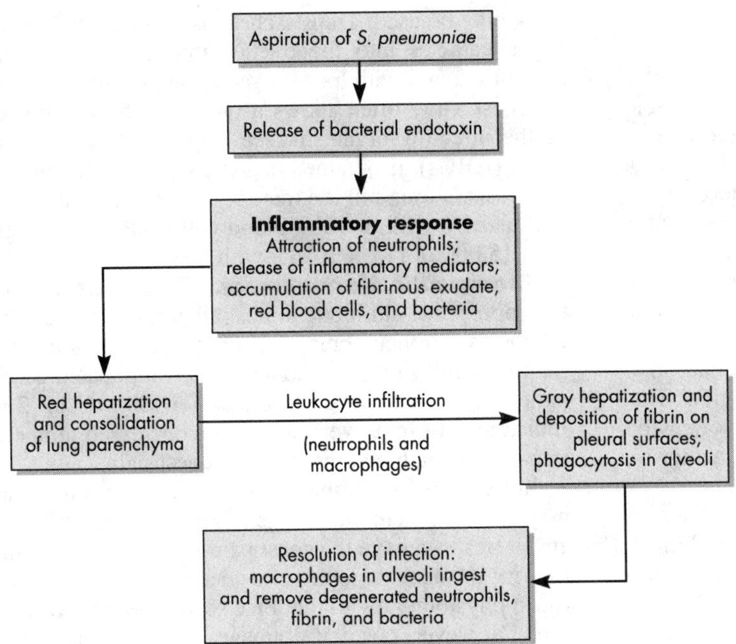

Fig. 24-2 Pathophysiologic course of pneumococcal pneumonia.

Pneumococcal Pneumonia

Pathophysiology. Pneumococcal pneumonia is the most common cause of bacterial pneumonia. There are four characteristic stages of the disease process:

1. *Congestion.* After the pneumococcus organisms reach the alveoli via droplets or saliva, there is an outpouring of fluid into the alveoli. The organisms multiply in the serous fluid, and the infection is spread. The pneumococci damage the host by their overwhelming growth and interference with lung function.
2. *Red hepatization.* There is massive dilatation of the capillaries, and alveoli are filled with organisms, neutrophils, RBCs, and fibrin (Fig. 24-2). The lung appears red and granular, or liver-like, which is why the process is called *hepatization.*
3. *Gray hepatization.* Blood flow decreases, and leukocytes and fibrin consolidate in the affected part of the lung.
4. *Resolution.* Complete resolution and healing occur if there are no complications. The exudate becomes lysed and is processed by the macrophages. The normal lung tissue is restored, and the person's gas-exchange ability returns to normal.

Clinical manifestations. Typically an URI precedes a case of pneumococcal pneumonia. The incubation period is 1 to 14 days. Manifestations include an acute onset of fever; chills; productive cough with greenish, bloody, or rusty sputum; and pleuritic chest pain. Nausea and vomiting are also observed, and systemic manifestations such as malaise, myalgia, and weakness are common. Tachycardia, tachypnea, and chest splinting are commonly found. Findings on physical examination of the chest may include dullness to percussion, diminished or bronchial breath sounds in the affected part of the lung, crackles, and a pleural friction rub. The patient's skin may have a dusky appearance because of hypoxemia. If the lower lobes are involved, the patient may experience mild to severe abdominal pain.

Complications. Pneumococcal pneumonia generally runs an uncomplicated course. The associated mortality rate is approximately 10% when there is associated bacteremia, leukopenia, or multiple (2 to 3) lobes involved. However, in patients more than 65 years of age with bacteremia or involvement of more than three lobes the mortality is 60%.[3] Complications that do develop are more frequently found in individuals with underlying chronic diseases. Complications may include the following:

1. *Pleurisy* (inflammation of the pleura) is a relatively common accompanying problem of pneumonia. Pain develops when the parietal and visceral pleurae rub together.
2. *Pleural effusion* occurs in many patients. Usually, the effusion is sterile and is reabsorbed in 1 to 2 weeks. Occasionally, it requires aspiration by means of thoracentesis.
3. *Atelectasis* (collapsed, airless alveoli) of one or part of one lobe may occur. These areas usually clear with effective coughing and deep breathing or vigorous tracheal suctioning.
4. *Delayed resolution* results from persistent infection and is seen on x-ray as residual consolidation. Usually, the physical findings return to normal within 2 to 4 weeks. Delayed resolution occurs most frequently in the patient who is older, malnourished, alcoholic, or has COPD.
5. *Lung abscess* is *not* a common complication of pneumococcal pneumonia. It is seen more frequently with

other types of pneumonia, such as staphylococcal and gram-negative pneumonias (see section on Lung Abscess).

6. *Empyema* (accumulation of purulent exudate in the pleural cavity) is relatively infrequent but requires antibiotic therapy and drainage of the exudate by a chest tube or open surgical drainage.

7. *Pericarditis* results from spread of the infecting organism from an infected pleura or via a hematogenous route to the pericardium (the fibroserous sac around the heart).

8. *Arthritis* results from systemic spread of the organism. The affected joints are swollen, red, and painful, and a purulent exudate can be aspirated.

9. *Meningitis* caused by pneumococcus is second only to meningococcus as a cause of purulent meningitis. The patient with pneumococcal pneumonia who is disoriented, confused, or somnolent should have a lumbar puncture to evaluate the possibility of pneumococcal meningitis.

10. *Endocarditis* can develop when the organisms attack the endocardium and the valves of the heart. The clinical manifestations are similar to those of acute bacterial endocarditis (see Chapter 34).

Diagnostic Studies for Pneumonia. The common diagnostic measures for pneumonia are presented in Table 24-3. Immediate identification of the organism is critical in order to institute appropriate antimicrobial therapy. Blood and sputum cultures may take 24 to 72 hours. Therefore a Gram stain of the sputum provides the information on which the initial therapy is based. Usually, the predominant organism can be identified on a Gram stain. If the patient cannot voluntarily produce a sputum specimen, procedures such as transtracheal aspiration and fiberoptic bronchoscopy may be used. Transtracheal aspiration involves inserting a catheter into the trachea through the cricothyroid membrane and withdrawing secretions for testing.

Chest x-ray often shows a typical pattern characteristic of the infecting organism (see Table 24-2). Arterial blood gases (ABGs), if obtained, usually reveal hypoxemia. Leukocytosis is found in the majority of patients with pneumonia, usually with a white blood cell (WBC) count greater than 15,000/μl (15 × 10^9/L) with a shift to the left.

Therapeutic Management. Prompt treatment with the appropriate antibiotic almost always cures bacterial and mycoplasma pneumonia. Currently, there is no effective treatment for viral pneumonia. In uncomplicated cases, the patient responds to drug therapy within 1 to 2 days. Indications of improvement include decreased temperature, improved breathing, and reduced chest pain.

In addition to antibiotic therapy, supportive measures may be used, including oxygen therapy to treat hypoxemia, analgesics to relieve the chest pain, and antipyretics such as aspirin or acetaminophen to decrease the temperature. Chest physiotherapy to mobilize secretions has been widely used. However, postural drainage and percussion probably offer no benefit to the patient who has uncomplicated pneumonia without chronic lung disease. During the acute febrile phase, the patient's activity should be restricted, and rest should be encouraged and planned.

Most individuals with mild to moderate illness who have no other underlying disease process can be treated on an outpatient basis. If there is a serious underlying disease or if the pneumonia is accompanied by severe dyspnea, hypoxemia, or other complications, the patient should be hospitalized.

Pneumococcal vaccine. Pneumococcal vaccine has been available since 1983, and its use is indicated primarily for the individual considered at high risk who (1) has chronic illnesses such as lung and heart disease and diabetes mellitus, (2) is recovering from a severe illness, (3) is 65 years of age or older, or (4) is in a nursing home or other long-term care facility.

The vaccine is not recommended for pregnant women, children less than 2 years of age, or those with febrile disease. Usually, 0.5 ml is given subcutaneously. The current recommendation is that it is good for the person's lifetime. However, in the immunosuppressed individual at high risk for development of fatal pneumococcal infection (e.g., asplenic patient; patient with nephrotic syndrome, renal failure, or AIDS; or transplant recipient), it is felt that revaccination should be considered every 5 to 6 years. Revaccination should be considered every 3 to 5 years for children with nephrotic syndrome, asplenia, or sickle cell anemia who would be 10 years of age or older at the time of revaccination.[7]

Pharmacologic Management of Pneumonia. The introduction of sulfonamides in the 1930s and penicillin in the 1940s revolutionized the treatment of pneumonia. Today penicillin is still the drug of choice for a great number of bacterial pneumonias. The main problems with the use of antibiotics in pneumonia are the development of resistant strains of organisms and the patient's hypersensitivity or allergic reaction to certain antibiotics. Table 24-4 outlines

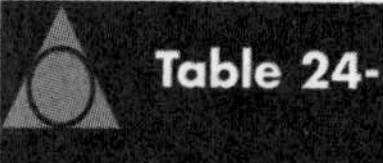

Table 24-3 Therapeutic Management: Bacterial Pneumonia

Diagnostic
- History and physical examination
- Gram stain of sputum
- Sputum culture and sensitivity test (transtracheal aspiration or bronchoscopy with aspiration if unable to obtain via cough or induced production of sputum)
- Chest x-ray
- ABGs (if indicated)
- Complete blood count
- Blood cultures

Therapeutic
- Appropriate antibiotic therapy*
- Increased fluid intake (at least 3 L q24hr)
- Limited activity or bed rest
- Antipyretics
- Analgesics
- Oxygen therapy (if indicated)
- Aerosol therapy

ABGs, Arterial blood gases.
*See Table 24-4.

Table 24-4 Antibiotic Drug Therapy Used for Pneumonia

Drug	Common Side Effects	Comments
Penicillins		
■ Penicillin G (Bicillin), penicillin G with procaine, penicillin V, ampicillin, amoxicillin, carbenicillin (Geopen), methicillin, nafcillin, oxacillin, cloxacillin, dicloxacillin, piperacillin (Pipracil), azlocillin (Axlin), ticarcillin (Ticar), bacampicillin (Spectrobid), amoxicillin and potassium clavulanate (Augmentin)	Low incidence of side effects, hypersensitivity reactions (15%), neurotoxicity (from procaine penicillin), hepatotoxicity, neutropenia, interstitial nephritis (especially from methicillin)	Frequently drug of choice in treatment of bacterial and anaerobic pneumonias, broad-spectrum activity, monitoring for superinfection necessary
Cephalosporins		
■ Cephalothin (Keflin),* cephapirin (Cefadyl),* cefazolin (Ancef, Kefsol),* cephradine (Anspor),* cephalexin (Keflex), cefotaxime (Claforan),‡ moxalactam (Moxam),‡ cefoperazone (Cefobid),‡ cefamandole (Mandol),† cefaclor (Ceclor),† cefotetan disodium (Cefotan),‡ cefoxitin sodium (Mefoxin)†	GI disturbances, phlebitis (from IV administration), nephrotoxicity, hypersensitivity reactions (2-5%)	Primary therapy in *Klebsiella* pneumonia along with an aminoglycoside; useful for therapy when mixed infection present; broad-spectrum activity; use when patient has known hypersensitivity to penicillins; rapid absorption from gastrointestinal tract
Aminoglycosides		
■ Kanamycin (Kantrex), gentamicin (Garamycin), tobramycin (Nebcin), amikacin (Amikin), neomycin (Neobiotic)	Nephrotoxicity, ototoxicity, hypersensitivity reactions, neuromuscular blockade	Particularly effective against gram-negative bacilli, poor absorption after oral administration, monitoring of blood urea nitrogen and serum creatinine necessary, assessment of hearing before and during therapy necessary
Miscellaneous Drugs		
■ Erythromycin	GI disturbances, infrequent hypersensitivity reactions, reversible hepatotoxicity, phlebitis (with IV administration)	Primary therapy for Legionnaires' disease, drug of choice for treatment of mycoplasma pneumonia
■ Tetracycline	GI, photosensitivity, hypersensitivity	Primarily effective against gram-positive bacilli, alteration of GI absorption with antacid or milk ingestion
■ Clindamycin	GI disturbances, hypersensitivity reactions	Particularly effective against anaerobic bacteria, also effective against gram-positive bacteria
■ Chloramphenicol	Bone marrow suppression, optic neuritis	Broad-spectrum antibiotic, not for treatment of minor infections
■ Vancomycin	Nephrotoxicity, ototoxicity, phlebitis	IV administration necessary, infrequent use for pulmonary infections, effective against gram-positive organisms
■ Lincomycin	GI disturbances, hypersensitivity reactions	Not a first choice drug but useful for patients allergic to penicillin
■ Aztreonam (Azactam)	GI, CNS disturbances	Bactericidal against gram-negative aerobic pathogens
■ Ciprofloxacin (Cipro)	GI, CNS disturbances	Broad-spectrum activity

CNS, Central nervous system; *GI*, gastrointestinal; *IV*, intravenous;
*First generation.
†Second generation.
‡Third generation; increased activity against gram-negative and resistant organisms and less activity against gram-positive organisms than first-generation agents.

the major antimicrobial agents used in the treatment of pneumonia and respiratory infections. It is extremely important to accurately identify the infecting organism so that the appropriate drug therapy can be instituted. Initial antimicrobial therapy is based in large part on the results of the Gram stain smear analysis. More definitive information may be obtained later from the sputum culture and sensitivity test, and the antibiotic can be changed if indicated.

In acute cases, antibiotics are usually given parenterally for the first few days and then administered orally. In mild cases, oral administration is adequate for the duration of the illness. It is extremely important that the patient continue taking the antibiotics for the prescribed period (usually at least 10 days) to prevent a relapse of pneumonia and the development of resistant strains of the organism. Before antibiotics are given, it is necessary to obtain the patient's health history regarding possible drug allergies.

Nutritional Management of Pneumonia. Fluid intake of at least 3 liters a day is important in the supportive treatment of pneumonia. If oral intake cannot be maintained, IV administration of fluids and electrolytes may be necessary for the acutely ill patient. A blenderized or processed liquid diet may be tolerated better than solid food by the patient in the acute phase of pneumonia. An intake of at least 1500 calories a day should be maintained to provide energy for the increased metabolic processes in the patient. Small, frequent meals are tolerated better by the dyspneic patient.

Table 24-5 Nursing Assessment: Pneumonia

Subjective Data
Important health information
Past health history: Lung cancer, COPD, cigarette smoking, alcoholism, diabetes, chronic debilitating disease, AIDS, exposure to chemical toxins, dust, or allergen
Medications: Use of antibiotics, corticosteroids, chemotherapy, or any other immunosuppressants
Surgeries and other treatment: Recent abdominal or thoracic surgery, splenectomy, any surgery with general anesthesia
Functional health patterns
Health perception–health management: Recent URI, fatigue, malaise
Nutritional-metabolic: Anorexia, nausea, vomiting; fever, chills
Activity-exercise: Prolonged bed rest or immobility, weakness, dyspnea, cough (productive or dry)
Cognitive-perceptual: Pain with breathing, chest pain, headache, myalgia

Objective Data
General
Restlessness or lethargy; splinting of affected area
Integumentary
Diaphoresis or dry skin with poor turgor; pallor, flushing, or circumoral and nail-bed cyanosis
Respiratory
Tachypnea; pharyngitis; asymmetric chest movements or retraction; decreased excursion; nasal flaring; use of accessory muscles (neck, abdomen); grunting; crackles, rhonchi, bronchial or absent breath sounds, pleural friction rub on auscultation; dull over consolidated areas, tactile fremitus; pink, rusty, purulent, green, yellow, or white sputum (amount may be scant to copious) on percussion
Cardiovascular
Tachycardia
Neurologic
Changes in mental status; confusion to delirium
Possible findings
Leukocytosis; abnormal ABGs with decreased or normal PaO_2, decreased $PaCO_2$, and increased pH initially, and later decreased PaO_2, increased $PaCO_2$, and decreased pH; positive sputum gram stain and culture; nonsegmental consolidation with air bronchograms and patchy or diffuseinfiltrates on chest x-ray

ABGs, Arterial blood gases; *AIDS,* acquired immunodeficiency syndrome, *COPD,* chronic obstructive pulmonary disease; *URI,* upper respiratory tract infection.

NURSING MANAGEMENT

PNEUMONIA

Nursing Assessment

Subjective and objective data that should be obtained from an individual with pneumonia are presented in Table 24-5.

Nursing Diagnoses

Nursing diagnoses are determined when the problem and etiologic factors are supported by clinical data. Nursing diagnoses related to pneumonia may include, but are not limited to, those presented in the nursing care plan for the patient with pneumonia on p. 631.

Planning

The overall goals are that the patient with pneumonia will have (1) clear breath sounds, (2) normal breathing patterns, (3) normal chest x-ray, and (4) no complications related to pneumonia.

Nursing Implementation

Health Promotion and Maintenance. There are many nursing interventions to help prevent the occurrence as well as the morbidity associated with pneumonia. Teaching the individual to practice good health habits, such as proper diet and hygiene, adequate rest, and regular exercise, can maintain the natural resistance to infecting organisms. If possible, exposure to URIs should be avoided. If a URI occurs, it should be treated promptly with supportive measures (e.g., rest, fluids, antipyretics). If symptoms persist for more than 3 or 4 days, the person should obtain medical care. The individual at high risk for pneumonia (e.g., the chronically ill and older adult) should be encouraged to obtain both influenza and pneumococcal vaccines.

In the hospital, the nursing role involves identifying the patient at risk (Table 24-1) and taking measures to prevent the development of pneumonia. The patient with altered consciousness should be placed in positions (e.g., side-lying, upright) that will prevent aspiration. The patient

NURSING CARE PLAN Patient With Pneumonia

Planning: Outcome Criteria	Nursing Interventions and Rationales
➤ NURSING DIAGNOSIS	Ineffective breathing pattern *related to* pneumonia, anxiety, and pain *as manifested by* rapid respirations, dyspnea, tachypnea, nasal flaring, altered chest excursion, inability to lie down
Have respiratory rate of 12-18 breaths/min; express feeling of comfort.	Assess degree of pain and anxiety *to provide guidelines for intervention.* Take vital signs and auscultate lungs q2-4hr *to provide ongoing data on patient's response to therapy.* Monitor ABGs if ordered *to assess oxygenation status.* Administer oxygen as indicated *to maintain optimal oxygen level and increase patient comfort.* Assess effectiveness of O_2 therapy. Decrease anxiety (e.g., with relaxation techniques, diversion) and provide a quiet, restful environment *to encourage rest and to prevent a relapse.* Position patient in semi-Fowler's or other comfortable position for breathing (may use reclining chairs) *to maximize lung expansion.*
➤ NURSING DIAGNOSIS	Ineffective airway clearance *related to* pain, positioning, fatigue, and thick secretions *as manifested by* ineffective cough or thick, tenacious sputum; abnormal breath sounds; dyspnea
Have clear breath sounds, effective cough with expectoration of sputum, normal chest x-ray or evidence of resolution.	Assist patient to cough by splinting chest, and teach patient how to cough effectively (inhale slowly through nose, exhale, and cough) *to clear airways by bringing secretions to the mouth.* Provide receptacle and tissues *for disposal of sputum.* Provide means of oral hygiene after production of sputum *as a comfort measure and to remove pathogens from the mouth.* Give expectorants *to increase bronchial fluid production and promote expectoration* and cough suppressants *to relieve nonproductive cough* as ordered. Provide humidification of inhaled air *to maintain moisture of nasal and oral mucosa.* Maintain fluid intake of 3 L daily *to liquefy secretions.* Use chest physiotherapy, if indicated, *to mobilize secretions.* Observe characteristics of sputum and report any significant changes (e.g., from mucoid to grossly purulent) *to insure early identification and treatment of infection.*
➤ NURSING DIAGNOSIS	Pain *related to* pleuritis and ineffective pain management or comfort measures *as manifested by* pleuritic chest pain, pleural friction rub, shallow respirations, decreased breath sounds
Have decreased or absent pain, full lung excursion; express satisfaction with pain control.	Assess pain level and location *to provide information on need for analgesia and other types of pain relief.* Administer analgesics as ordered *to relieve pain by interrupting CNS pathways.* Position patient comfortably such as in semi-Fowler's position *to maximize ventilation.* Premedicate with analgesics before uncomfortable therapies are given *to promote cooperation and patient comfort.* Assist with intercostal nerve block if necessary *to treat pleuritic pain unresponsive to analgesics.* Observe for possible complications (e.g., pleural effusion, empyema) if pain persists *so appropriate treatment can be initiated.* Perform nonpharmacologic pain interventions such as back rubs, distraction, and relaxation techniques *to relieve pain and reduce the need for analgesia.*
➤ NURSING DIAGNOSIS	Risk for transmission of infection *related to* lack of knowledge of preventive measures
Practice infection prevention measures.	Teach patient to cover nose and mouth during sneeze or cough and to use tissues when coughing and expectorating sputum *to reduce factors that contribute to the spread of infection.* Place used tissues in wax-lined paper bag, and dispose of properly *to reduce possibility of spread of pathogens to others.* Wash hands thoroughly after contact with infected patient *to reduce the risk of cross-contamination.* Teach patient to practice these techniques at home as well as in the hospital *to promote health and reduce spread of infection.* Do not put infectious patient in same room with patient at high risk for pneumonia (e.g., patient who is recovering from surgery, has chronic lung disease, is immunosuppressed, or is an older adult) *to reduce risk of nosocomial infection.*

continued

NURSING CARE PLAN Patient With Pneumonia—cont'd

Planning: Outcome Criteria	Nursing Interventions and Rationales
➤ **NURSING DIAGNOSIS**	Risk for health maintenance deficit *related to* lack of knowledge regarding treatment regimen after discharge
Follow regimen, including medications, fluid therapy, activity schedule.	Assess ability to continue self-care at home *to identify patient's knowledge about self-care and ability to manage self-care.* Encourage patient to continue on full course of antibiotic therapy *to prevent relapse of pneumonia and development of resistant strains of the organism.* Instruct patient on importance of rest and limited activity *to maintain progress toward recovery and prevent relapse.* Encourage patient to obtain adequate rest, nutrition, and fresh air *to assist healing process.* If indicated, encourage patient to stop or decrease cigarette smoking *to improve mucociliary clearance mechanism.* Teach patient to continue coughing and deep breathing exercises *to remove secretions and improve ventilation.* Teach patient importance of follow-up care and need to seek medical attention for symptoms related to respiratory infections *to prevent relapse.* Encourage patient who has chronic illness (e.g., heart, lung, diabetes mellitus), is recovering from severe illness, is ≥65 yr, or is in nursing home or other long-term care facility, to obtain vaccinations (pneumococcal and influenza) *because this person is at risk for pneumonia.*
➤ **NURSING DIAGNOSIS**	Altered nutrition: less than body requirements *related to* increased metabolism, fatigue, anorexia, nausea, and vomiting *as manifested by* weight loss
Maintain normal body weight, adequate strength to perform ADLs.	Assist with meals *to conserve energy.* Determine patient's food preferences and provide when possible *to promote ingestion of adequate nutrients.* Provide means of oral hygiene before meals *to remove foul tastes related to sputum or medications.* Provide frequent, small meals *to prevent pressure on diaphragm and minimize energy expense.* Monitor environment *to reduce negative stimuli.* Monitor patient's weight and caloric intake *to assess need to adjust diet.*
➤ **NURSING DIAGNOSIS**	Altered comfort *related to* fever *as manifested by* diaphoresis, chills, flushing, thirst, headache, malaise
Have normal body temperature; express increased comfort as fever subsides.	Administer antibiotics as prescribed *to treat infection.* Observe for side effects and toxicity associated with antibiotic therapy *because hypersensitivity or allergic reaction may occur with antibiotics.* Administer antipyretics as ordered *to reduce fever and increase patient's comfort.* Take temperature q2-4hr. Observe for continuing or recurring fever and report finding to physician *because this may indicate worsening of illness.* Provide fluid intake (at least 3 L/day) *to replace fluid loss caused by fever and diaphoresis.* Provide frequent clothing and linen changes if diaphoresis occurs *to keep patient comfortable and dry and prevent chilling.* Provide cooling measures (reduced clothing and bedlinens, tepid baths, hypothermia blanket) to lower metabolic rate and reduce oxygen consumption.
➤ **NURSING DIAGNOSIS**	Activity intolerance *related to* fatigue, treatment regime, interrupted sleep and wake cycle, hypoxia, and weakness *as manifested by* fatigue, unwillingness or inability to exert self, dyspnea, increased pulse and respiration, dizziness on exertion
Verbalize feeling of being rested; cooperate with required activities.	Provide bed rest and limit physical activity *to conserve oxygen.* Assess response to activity *to evaluate patient's hypoxemia* and plan changes accordingly. Limit visitors and long conversations. Plan nursing care in blocks *to ensure periods of uninterrupted rest.* Maintain a pleasant, calm environment. Place needed items (e.g., tissues, call bell) within easy reach *to conserve energy while facilitating independence.*

COLLABORATIVE PROBLEMS

Nursing Goals	Nursing Interventions and Rationales
➤ **POTENTIAL COMPLICATION**	Hypoxemia *related to* impaired gas exchange in lungs
Monitor for signs of hypoxemia, report deviations from acceptable parameters; carry out appropriate medical and nursing interventions.	Administer oxygen and antibiotics as ordered *to treat hypoxemia and infection.* Monitor vital signs as indicated. Assess and monitor mental status (restlessness, anxiety, confusion, combative reactions), and respiratory status (cyanosis and changes in respiratory rate). Report changes from baseline values *to provide early treatment.*

ABGs, Arterial blood gases; *ADLs,* activities of daily living; *CNS,* central nervous system.

ETHICAL DILEMMAS

GUARDIANSHIP

Situation A 32-year-old man, institutionalized almost all of his life for profound developmental disabilities, is hospitalized for his fourth aspiration-related pneumonia in the last year. His physician believes that a feeding tube would solve the problem of aspiration and wants the family to agree to the procedure. The family believes his life span should not be extended by artificial means and refuses consent for the procedure. The hospital is considering seeking a court-appointed guardian because the family is not acting in the best interest of the patient.

Discussion Disagreeing with the physician is not necessarily grounds for the family to be considered inappropriate guardians. In cases of profound developmental disabilities, it is difficult to distinguish who has the patient's *best interests* at heart: the family, the institution paid to attend to the patient, specialists who focus on a specific medical condition, or disability advocates. This patient presents a medical condition that could probably be alleviated by the surgical placement of a feeding tube. However, there has yet to be a discussion about how the patient will adapt to the tube, what pleasures of taste he would lose, or how this would affect his ongoing care. Seeking a guardian hearing before these considerations would be premature.

ETHICAL AND LEGAL PRINCIPLES

- The state's position in favor of treating incompetent patients in order to preserve their life can be in direct opposition to the longheld assumption that parents have the right to make decisions for their incompetent adult children.
- Substituted judgment, basing the decision on what the patient would have decided, is not possible in cases of the never-competent patient. However, best interest judgment can be based on the experience of the patient and extrapolation of the value, meaning, and pleasure the patient receives from life.
- Usually any person can petition the court for protection of an incompetent person. Courts are reluctant to intervene if the parents are functioning in a reasonable fashion. The law should be the last resort for treatment decisions.

should be turned and repositioned at least every 2 hours to facilitate adequate lung expansion and to discourage pooling of secretions.

The patient who has a feeding tube generally requires attention to the positioning of the tube to prevent aspiration (see Chapter 37). Although the distal end of the feeding tube is small, an interruption in the integrity of the lower esophageal sphincter of the stomach still exists, which can allow reflux of gastric and intestinal contents.

The patient who has difficulty swallowing (e.g., stroke patient) needs assistance in eating, drinking, and taking medication to prevent aspiration. The patient who has recently had surgery and others who are immobile need assistance with turning, coughing, and deep-breathing measures at frequent intervals (see Chapter 16). The nurse must be careful to avoid overmedication with narcotics or sedatives, which can cause a depressed cough reflex and accumulation of fluid in the lungs. The gag reflex should be present in the individual who has had local anesthesia to the throat before the administration of fluids or food.

Strict medical asepsis and adherence to infection control guidelines should be practiced by the nurse to reduce the incidence of nosocomial infections. The patient with an infection should not be placed in the same room with a patient who is recovering from surgery or a patient with chronic lung disease. Respiratory therapy equipment should be properly cleaned and changed, and disposable equipment should be used as much as possible. Strict sterile aseptic technique should be used when suctioning a patient.

Acute Intervention. Although many patients with pneumonia are treated on an outpatient basis, the nursing care plan for a patient with pneumonia is applicable to both these individuals and inhospital patients. It is important for the nurse to remember that pneumonia is an acute, infectious disease. Although most cases of pneumonia are potentially completely curable, complications can result. The nurse must be aware of these complications and their manifestations.

Chronic and Home Management. The patient needs to be reassured that complete recovery from pneumonia is possible. It is extremely important to emphasize the need to take all of the prescribed medication and to return for follow-up medical care and evaluation. Adequate rest is needed to maintain progress toward recovery and to prevent a relapse. The patient needs to be told that it may be weeks before the usual vigor and sense of well-being are felt. A prolonged period of convalescence may be necessary for the older adult or chronically ill patient.

The patient considered to be at high risk for pneumonia should be told about available vaccines and should discuss them with the health care provider. Deep-breathing and coughing exercises should be practiced for 6 to 8 weeks after the patient is discharged from the hospital.

Tuberculosis

Tuberculosis (TB) is a bacterial infectious disease transmitted by *Mycobacterium tuberculosis*. It usually involves the lungs, but it also occurs in the kidneys, bones, lymph nodes, and meninges and can be disseminated throughout the body.

Significance. With the introduction of chemotherapy in the late 1940s and early 1950s, there was a dramatic decrease in the prevalence of TB. Today 10 to 15 million people are infected with or harbor the tubercle bacillus. The majority of these individuals have healed or dormant TB. There have been approximately 26,000 cases a year of new active TB. Approximately 10% of these cases represented relapses.[8] These statistics indicate that TB, in spite of being potentially curable and preventable, is still a major public health problem in the United States. The major factors that have contributed to the resurgence of TB have been (1) the

Clinical Pathway for Simple Pneumonia

Landmark Medical Center — Diagnostic Related Group 90 — Prescribed Length of Stay 4.9 Days (1995)
Date of this draft: ________ — Caremap® form Data base/kardex Section1 Admission—day 3

Casetype description: Simple pneumonia and/or pleurisy, age > 17 without complications.

Admission date: ____ Time: ____ AM/PM
Physician: ________
Primary nurse: ________
Consult: ________ Date: ____
Consult: ________ Date: ____
Allergies: ________

Precautions: ________
Restrictions: ________

Code status
DNR: ___ Full code: ___ Chemical code: ___
Limited (✔) chart: ________

Advance directive
Type: ________
Location: ________

Discharge plan
Home: independent ____ with services ____
Nursing home: return ____ placement ____
Rehab: ____ Other: ____

Support systems
Contact: ________
Relation: ________
Telephone: day ____ night ____
Religion: ____ Anointed: ____

Caremap® authors
L. Puppi, MD.
T. Verma, MD.
I. Girard, Microbiology
L. Gagne, Radiology
N. Bradley, RN.C., BSN, ANM. 1E
D. Chenot, RN.
J. Pomfret, RN. ED.
R. Ferry, RN., VNS.
P. Bibeault, RN. BSN., NM CCU.
T. Johnson, RD. Nutrition Services
R. Wagner, R.Ph., Clinical Pharmacist
A. Jacobs, RN.C., CareMap® Project Manager
D. Douglas, MSN., RN., CNA, Assistant Vice President Patient

Medical/surgical history:

Date																
Interventions-	**Day 1 ED/ Direct admission**	**D**	**E**	**N**	**Day 1 Nursing unit**	**D**	**E**	**N**	**Day 2**	**D**	**E**	**N**	**Day 3**	**D**	**E**	**N**
Consults/ assessments **if patient placed in ICU/CCU on admission—evaluate daily for transfer out of unit**	ER MD assessment RN assessment ***Special Considerations:** Onset of symptoms Alcohol/smoking history Environmental exposure TB history/exposure to birds Family/colleague illness Underlying disease Recent dental work I & O +/−Notify primary MD +/−Quantify hemoptysis				RN admission assessment *(Note method of breathing, use of accessory muscles, etc.) VS per unit standard *(Include lung sounds) I & O +/− Need for influenza vaccination				VS per unit standard *(with lung sounds) I & O Nutrition screening				VS per unit standard *(with lung sounds) I & O			

continued

CLINICAL PATHWAY FOR SIMPLE PNEUMONIA—cont'd

Date															
Interventions-	**Day 1 ED/ Direct admission**	**D**	**E**	**N**	**Day 1 Nursing unit**	**D**	**E**	**N**	**Day 2**	**D**	**E**	**N**	**Day 3**	**D**	**E**	**N**
Specimens/Tests	CBC stat Chemical profile and lytes ABGs Blood culture Sputum gram stain with C & S (respiratory therapist to induce if necessary) CXR PA and LAT (if patient able) +/−ECG				Serology ■ Legionella ■ Mycoplasma ■ Chlamydia ■ Immune deficiency ■ Mumps panel ■ IFA/IgG/IgM				Review culture Results +/− ABGs/pulse oximetry +/− CXR +/− Sinus films +/− Additional testing as indicated				+/− Additional testing as indicated. +/− CXR (if follow-up film not already done)			
Treatments	+/− Chest patient				Respiratory therapy per MD order				Respiratory therapy per MD order				Respiratory therapy per MD order			
Medications	O_2 after ABGs—per patient criteria IV IV antibiotic Acetaminophen +/−Mucoevacuant agent +/−Other analgesia with pleuritic pain				*Review patient's own meds O_2 per criteria IV IV antibiotic Acetaminophen +/− Other analgesia +/− Mucoevacuant agent				O_2 per criteria IV Reassess antibiotic +/− Continue antibiotic (pending culture results) Acetaminophen/other analgesia +/− Patient's own meds				DC/renew O_2 IV/INT IV antibiotic Acetaminophen/analgesia +/− Patient's own meds			
Nutrition*	Push fluids (if no nausea/vomiting)				Appropriate diet Push fluids				Appropriate diet Push fluids +/− Diet supplements				Appropriate diet Push fluids +/− Diet supplements			
Activity/safety	HOB elevated 30°-60° +/− BRP with help				HOB elevated 30°-60° Activity as Tolerated with CBR DVT prophylaxis +/− Fall prevention program				Activity as Tolerated +/− DVT prophylaxis +/− Fall prevention program				Activity as Tolerated +/− DVT prophylaxis +/− Fall prevention program			
Teaching *Include family	Paced Breathing Re: need for sputum specimen Orient to surroundings				Orient to unit +/− Incentive spirometry instructions				Proper disposal of contaminated tissues +/− Reinforce incentive spirometry				Discuss infection control principles			
Discharge planning Patient care review	+/− Notify nursing home of admission				Review home environment				Address indentified needs				Patient care review to follow			
Signature Log																

continued

Clinical Pathway for Simple Pneumonia—cont'd

Date

Problem/Focus	Day 1 ED	D	E	N	Day 1 Unit	D	E	N	Day 2	D	E	N	Day 3	D	E	N
Ineffective airway clearance and impaired gas exchange r/t: ▪ **Nonproductive cough** ▪ **Tachypnea/ tachycardia** ▪ **Stasis of secretions r/t poor cough effort, fatigue, pleuritic pain** ▪ **Potential aspiration**	Respirations slowed Less tachycardia Oxygenation improved				Respirations slowed Less tachycardia Continuing improvement in oxygenation				Respirations slowed Less tachycardia Less tachypneic Lung sounds clearing Improved cough mechanism				Depth and rate of respirations near baseline Improved activity/ exercise tolerance			
Pain/discomfort r/t: ▪ **Fever/chills/ rigors** ▪ **Sore throat** ▪ **GI symptoms (N-V-D)** ▪ **Pleuritic pain** ▪ **Coughing**	Patient verbalizes "feeling better" after initial treatment				Patient verbalizes acceptable comfort level with treatment and medication				Comfortable as evidenced by ability to rest Responding to treatment as evidenced by decreasing fever/N-V-D controlled				Comfortable as evidenced by ability to rest			
Lack of knowledge ▪ **Type of pneumonia** ▪ **Medical treatment** ▪ **Infection control principles**	Verbalizes basic understanding of treatment plan				Verbalizes basic understanding of treatment plan and unit regime				Demonstrates appropriate coughing technique after teaching				Demonstrates effective coughing techniques Appropriate disposal of contaminated tissues			
Anxiety r/t: ▪ **Increased shortness of breath** ▪ **Treatments and tests** ▪ **Unfamiliar environment**	Verbalizes less anxious after treatment and initial teaching				Demonstrates improved coping ability by participating in care and teaching				Improved coping as evidenced by increased participation in care and teaching				Able to identify remaining feelings of anxiety			

Partial Care Map Day 1 to Day 3 for Simple Pneumonia. Developed by Landmark Medical Center, Woonsocket, RI. Licensed by The Center for Case Management, Inc., South Natick, MA.

ABGs, Arterial blood gases; *BRP,* bathroom privileges; *C&S,* culture and sensitivity; *CBC,* complete blood count; *CBR,* complete bed rest; *CCU,* coronary case unit; *CXR,* chest x-ray; *DC,* discontinue; *DNR,* do not resuscitate; *DVT,* deep vein thrombosis; *ED,* emergency department; *GI,* gastrointestinal; *HOB,* head of bed; *I&O,* intake and output; *ICU,* intensive care unit; *INT,* intermittent; *LAT,* lateral; *NVD,* nausea, vomiting, diarrhea; *PA,* posterior-anterior; *r/t,* related to; *TB,* tuberculosis; *VS,* vital signs.

*Document Outcome Achievement on Problem/Focus form. A focused progress note is required on all unmet outcomes.

CULTURAL & ETHNIC Considerations

TUBERCULOSIS

- TB in the United States and Canada tends to be a disease of the older population, urban poor, minority groups, and patient with AIDS.
- At all ages the incidence of TB among non-Caucasians is at least twice that of Caucasians.
- Ethnic groups that have a high incidence of TB include foreign-born people from Asia, Africa, and Latin America. Native Americans, Alaskan Natives, African-Americans, and Asian-Americans are also ethnic groups with a high incidence of TB.
- Southeastern Asian, Haitian, and Hispanic immigrants have incidence rates of TB similar to those of the countries from which they came.

emergence of multidrug-resistant strains of *M. tuberculosis* and (2) epidemic proportions of TB among patients with HIV infections.

Multidrug-resistant strains of TB have developed because TB patients' compliance to drug therapy was not monitored and therefore faltered, leading to treatment failure and development of resistant strains. Patients were lost to follow-up treatment or placed on drug regimens to which their infections were no longer susceptible. In general there was decreased vigilance in treating patients diagnosed with TB.

Individuals at risk for TB include homeless persons, residents of inner-city neighborhoods, foreign-born persons (especially from Haiti and Southeastern Asia), older adults, those in institutions (nursing homes, prisons), and the socioeconomically disadvantaged and medically underserved of all races. Immunosuppression from any etiology (e.g., HIV infection, malignancy) increases the risk of TB infection. The incidence of TB is high in a few areas of the United States where there is a large population of Native Americans, such as Arizona and New Mexico, and in counties near the Mexican border.

The tubercle bacillus may remain dormant for many years and then reactivate and produce clinical TB. Infection with *M. tuberculosis* involves a lifelong relationship between humans and the tubercle bacillus because the dormant organisms may remain alive in the host for life. The infected host has been referred to as a "walking time bomb" in whom TB may develop and because the host may serve as a source of infection for others.

Pathophysiology. *M. tuberculosis*, a gram-positive, acid-fast bacillus, is usually spread via airborne droplets, which are produced when the infected individual coughs, sneezes, or speaks. Once released into a room, the organisms are dispersed and can be inhaled. Brief exposure to a few tubercle bacilli rarely causes an infection. Rather, it is more commonly spread to the individual who has had repeated close contact with an infected person. TB is not highly infectious, and transmission usually requires close, frequent, or prolonged exposure. The disease cannot be spread by hands, books, glasses, dishes, or other fomites.

When the bacilli are inhaled, they pass down the bronchial system and implant themselves on the respiratory bronchioles or alveoli. The lower parts of the lungs are usually the site of initial bacterial implantation. After implantation, the bacilli multiply with no initial resistance from the host. The organisms are engulfed by phagocytes (initially neutrophils and later macrophages) and may continue to multiply within the phagocytes.

While a cellular immune response is being activated, the bacilli can be spread through the lymphatic channels to regional lymph nodes and via the thoracic duct to the circulating blood. Thus organisms may be spread throughout the body before sufficient activation of the cell-mediated immune response is available to bring the infection under control. The organisms find favorable environments for growth primarily in the upper lobes of the lungs, kidneys, epiphyseal lines of the bone, and cerebral cortex.

Eventually the acquired cellular immunity limits further multiplication and spread of the infection. A characteristic tissue reaction called an *epithelioid cell granuloma* results after the cellular immune system is activated. This granuloma (also called an *epithelioid cell tubercle*) is a result of fusion of the infiltrating macrophages. The granuloma is surrounded by lymphocytes. This reaction usually takes 10 to 20 days.

The central portion of the lesion (called a *Ghon tubercle*) undergoes necrosis characterized by a cheesy appearance and hence is named *caseous necrosis*. The lesion may also undergo liquefactive necrosis in which the liquid sloughs into connecting bronchi and produces a cavity. Tubercular material may enter the tracheobronchial system, allowing airborne transmission of infectious particles.

Healing of the primary lesion usually takes place by resolution, fibrosis, and calcification. The granulation tissue surrounding the lesion may become more fibrous and form a collagenous scar around the tubercle. A *Ghon complex* is formed, consisting of the Ghon tubercle and regional lymph nodes. Calcified Ghon complexes may be seen on chest x-ray.

When a tuberculous lesion regresses and heals, the infection enters a latent period in which it may persist without producing a clinical illness. The infection may remain dormant for life, or it may develop into clinical disease if the persisting organisms begin to multiply rapidly.

If the initial immune response is not adequate, control of the organisms is not maintained, and clinical disease results. Certain individuals are at a higher risk for clinical disease, including those who are immunosuppressed for any reason (e.g., patients with AIDS, those receiving cancer chemotherapy or long-term prednisone therapy), or have diabetes mellitus.

Approximately 5% of individuals are incapable of containing the initial infective process. An additional 5% of those who do produce an effective immune response later lose this capability; dormant bacilli then begin to multiply, and the disease is reactivated. The reasons for reactivation are not well understood, but they are related to decreased resistance found in older adults, individuals with concomitant diseases, and those who receive immunosuppressive therapy.

Classification. In 1974 the American Thoracic Association and American Lung Association adopted a classification system that covers the entire population. This classification system has since been revised (Table 24-6).

Clinical Manifestations. In the early stages of TB the person is usually free of symptoms. Many cases are found incidentally when routine chest x-rays are taken, especially in older adults.

Systemic manifestations may initially consist of fatigue, malaise, anorexia, weight loss, low-grade fevers (especially in the late afternoon), and night sweats. These manifestations are related to the lymphokine production that is stimulated by the immune response to the tubercle bacilli. The weight loss may not be excessive until late in the disease and is often attributed to overwork or other factors. Irregular menses may also be present in premenopausal women.

A characteristic pulmonary manifestation is a cough that becomes frequent and produces mucoid or mucopurulent sputum. Chest pain characterized as dull or tight may also be present. Hemoptysis is not a common finding and is usually associated with more advanced cases. Sometimes TB has more acute, sudden manifestations; the patient has high fever, chills, generalized flulike symptoms, pleuritic pain, and a productive cough.

The HIV-infected patient with TB often has atypical physical examinations and chest x-ray findings. Classical signs such as fever, cough, and weight loss may be attributed to PCP or other HIV-associated opportunistic diseases. Clinical manifestations of respiratory problems need to be carefully investigated to determine the cause.

Complications

Miliary TB. If a necrotic Ghon complex erodes through a blood vessel, large numbers of organisms invade the bloodstream and spread to all body organs. This is called *miliary* or *hematogenous TB*. The patient may be either acutely ill with fever, dyspnea, and cyanosis or chronically ill with systemic manifestations of weight loss, fever, and GI disturbance. Hepatomegaly, splenomegaly, and generalized lymphadenopathy may be present.

Pleural effusion. A pleural effusion is caused by the release of caseous material into the pleural space. The bacteria-containing material triggers an inflammatory reaction and a pleural exudate of protein-rich fluid. A form of pleurisy called *dry pleurisy* may result from a superficial tuberculous lesion involving the pleura. It appears as localized pleuritic pain on deep inspiration.

Tuberculous pneumonia. Acute pneumonia may result when large amounts of tubercle bacilli are discharged from the liquefied necrotic lesion into the lung or lymph nodes. The clinical manifestations are similar to those of bacterial pneumonia, including chills, fever, productive cough, pleuritic pain, and leukocytosis.

Other organ involvement. Although the lungs are the primary site of TB, other body organs may also be involved. The meninges may become infected. Bone and joint tissue may be involved in the infectious disease process. The kidneys, adrenal glands, lymph nodes, and both female and male genital tracts may also be infected.

Diagnostic Studies

Tuberculin skin testing. The body's immune response can be demonstrated by hypersensitivity to a tuberculin skin test. A positive reaction occurs 3 to 10 weeks after the initial infection, corresponding to the time needed to mount an immune response.

Purified protein derivative (PPD) of tuberculin is used primarily to detect the delayed hypersensitivity response. (The procedure for performing the tuberculin skin test is described in Chapter 22.) Once acquired, sensitivity to tuberculin tends to persist throughout life. A positive reaction indicates the presence of a tuberculous infection, but it does not show whether the infection is dormant or active, causing a clinical illness.

Because the response to TB skin testing may be decreased in the immunosuppressed patient, induration reactions less than 10 mm may be considered positive. See Table 22-11 for the guidelines in interpreting TB skin tests.

Chest x-ray. Although the findings on chest x-ray examination are important, it is not possible to make a diagnosis of TB solely on the basis of this examination. This is because other diseases can mimic the appearance of TB. The abnormality most commonly found in TB is multinodular

Table 24-6 Classification of Tuberculosis (TB)

Class 0
No TB exposure, not infected (no history of exposure, negative tuberculin skin test)

Class 1
TB exposure, no evidence of infection (history of exposure, negative tuberculin skin test)

Class 2
TB infection without disease (significant reaction to tuberculin skin test, negative bacteriologic studies, no x-ray findings compatible with tuberculosis, no clinical evidence of tuberculosis)

Class 3
TB infection with clinically active disease (positive bacteriologic studies or both a significant reaction to tuberculin skin test and clinical or x-ray evidence of current disease)

Class 4
No current disease (history of previous episode of TB or abnormal, stable roentgenographic findings in a person with a significant reaction to tuberculin skin test; negative bacteriologic studies if done; no clinical or x-ray evidence of current disease)

Class 5
TB suspect (diagnosis pending); person should not be in this classification for more than 3 mo

Modified from American Thoracic Society: *Diagnostic standards and classification of tuberculosis*, New York, 1990, *American Review of Respiratory Disease* 142:725, 1990.

lymph node involvement with cavitation in the upper lobes of the lungs. This is often referred to as the *parenchymal lymph node complex*. Calcification of the lung lesions generally occurs within several years of the infection.

Bacteriologic studies. The demonstration of tubercle bacilli bacteriologically is essential for establishing a diagnosis. Microscopic examination of stained sputum smears for acid-fast bacilli is usually the first bacteriologic evidence of the presence of tubercle bacilli. This is a quick, easy examination that provides the physician with valuable information. A major disadvantage is that more than 10,000 bacteria per milliliter of specimen are required to produce a positive smear. In addition to sputum, material for examination can be obtained from gastric washings, cerebrospinal fluid (CSF), or pus from an abscess.

The most accurate means of diagnosis is a culture technique. The major disadvantage of this method is that it takes 2 weeks or more for the mycobacterium to grow. The advantage is that it can detect small quantities (as few as 10 bacteria per milliliter of specimen).

Therapeutic Management. The treatment of TB rarely requires inhospital treatment. Most patients are treated on an outpatient basis (Table 24-7), and many can continue to work and maintain their lifestyles with few changes. Hospitalization may be used for diagnostic evaluation, for the severely ill or debilitated, and for those who experience adverse drug reactions or treatment failures.

The mainstay of TB treatment is pharmacologic. Drug therapy is used to treat an individual with clinical disease as well as to prevent disease in an infected person.

Pharmacologic Management

Active disease. In view of the growing prevalence of multidrug-resistant TB, the patient with active TB should be managed aggressively. Treatment of TB usually consists of a combination of at least three drugs. In areas known to have high incidence of drug resistance, initial therapy is with three or more drugs. The reason for combination therapy is to increase the therapeutic effectiveness and decrease the development of resistant strains of *M. tuberculosis*. It has been shown that single-drug therapy can result in rapid development of resistant strains.

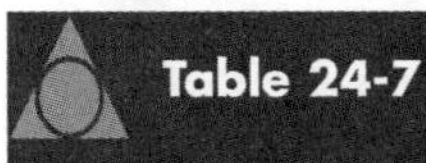

Table 24-7 Therapeutic Management: Tuberculosis

Diagnostic
- Health history and physical examination
- Tuberculin skin test
- Chest x-ray
- Bacteriologic studies
  - Sputum smear
  - Sputum culture

Therapeutic
- Long-term treatment with antimicrobial drugs*
- Follow-up bacteriologic studies

*See Table 24-8.

The four primary drugs used are isoniazid, rifampin, streptomycin, and ethambutol (Table 24-8). A new combination drug, Rifamate, consists of 150 mg of isoniazid and 300 mg of rifampin. Other drugs are primarily used for treatment of resistant strains or if the patient develops toxicity to the primary drugs. Many "second-line" drugs carry a greater risk of toxicity and require closer monitoring.

A problem with antituberculous therapy is the length of time medication must be taken. In the past, 18 to 24 months was the usual period of time required for individuals to adhere to the medical regimen. Shorter courses of therapy (6 to 9 months) have been shown to be effective. Although there are variations, the protocol for initial treatment consists of using isoniazid, rifampin, and ethambutol for 2 months, followed by 4 months of isoniazid and rifampin. An additional 3 months of therapy is given if cultures are negative (Table 24-9).

Treatment in areas where drug resistance is known to be a problem consists of initial addition of drugs not in the resistance pattern for that area. Drug regimens should be adapted to the resistance pattern evident from sputum. At least 2 drugs are administered to which the individual's bacilli are sensitive.[9] In follow-up care for patients on long-term therapy, it is important to monitor the effectiveness of drugs and the development of toxic side effects. Usually sputum specimens are initially obtained weekly and then monthly to assess the effectiveness of the medication. The regimen is considered to be effective if the patient converts to a negative sputum status.

Although TB tends to have a rapidly progressive course in the patient coinfected with HIV, it responds well to standard medication. The coinfected patient should receive antituberculosis treatment for at least 6 months beyond the conversion of sputum cultures to negative status.

An important reason for follow-up care in the patient with TB is to ensure adherence to the treatment regimen. Noncompliance is a major factor in the emergence of multidrug resistance and treatment failures. Many individuals do not adhere to the treatment program in spite of understanding the disease process and the value of treatment. As a result, directly observed therapy (DOT) is recommended as part of most treatment regimens. The patient needs to have follow-up visits for 12 months after completion of therapy to check for the development of resistant strains.

Prophylactic treatment. Pharmacologic management can be used to prevent a TB infection from developing into a clinical disease. Isoniazid prophylaxis is recommended for all adult tuberculin reactors with additional risk factors for active TB. The indications for preventive therapy (chemoprophylaxis) are presented in Table 24-10. Close contacts of individuals with infectious clinical TB should be examined with tuberculin skin tests. Close contacts who are less than 4 years of age should be given treatment even if the tuberculin skin test is negative.

Some individuals carry dormant TB infections that may develop into active disease in some situations. Examples include positive reactors who (1) demonstrate some degree

Table 24-8 Drug Therapy Used in Tuberculosis

Drug	Mechanisms of Action	Side Effects	Comments
First-Line Drugs			
▪ Isoniazid (INH)	Interferes with DNA metabolism of tubercle bacillus	Peripheral neuritis, hepatotoxicity, hypersensitivity (skin rash, arthralgia, fever), optic neuritis, vitamin B_6 neuritis	Metabolism primarily by liver and excretion by kidneys, pyridoxine (vitamin B_6) administration during high-dose therapy as prophylactic measure, use as single prophylactic agent for active TB in individuals whose PPD converts to positive, ability to cross blood-brain barrier
▪ Rifampin	Has broad-spectrum effects, inhibits RNA polymerase of tubercle bacillus	Hepatitis, febrile reaction, GI disturbance, peripheral neuropathy, hypersensitivity	Most common use with isoniazid, low incidence of side effects, suppression of effect of birth control pills, possible orange urine
▪ Ethambutol (Myambutol)	Inhibits RNA synthesis and is bacteriostatic for the tubercle bacillus	Skin rash, GI disturbance, malaise, peripheral neuritis, optic neuritis	Side effects uncommon and reversible with discontinuation of drug, most common use as substitute drug when toxicity occurs with isoniazid or rifampin
▪ Streptomycin	Inhibits protein synthesis and is bactericidal	Ototoxicity (eighth cranial nerve), nephrotoxicity, hypersensitivity	Cautious use in older adults, those with renal disease, and pregnant women
Second-Line Drugs			
▪ Ethionamide	Inhibits protein synthesis	GI disturbance, hepatotoxicity, hypersensitivity	Valuable retreatment of resistant organisms Contraindication in pregnancy
▪ Capreomycin	Inhibits protein synthesis and is bactericidal	Ototoxicity, nephrotoxicity	Cautious use in older adults
▪ Kanamycin	Interferes with protein synthesis	Ototoxicity, nephrotoxicity	Use in selected cases for retreatment of resistant strains
▪ Pyrazinamide	Bactericidal effect (exact mechanism is unknown)	Fever, skin rash, hyperuricemia, jaundice (rare)	High rate of effectiveness when used with streptomycin or capreomycin
▪ Para-aminosalicylic acid (PAS)	Interferes with metabolism of tubercle bacillus	GI disturbance (frequent), hypersensitivity, hepatotoxicity	Interference with absorption of rifampin, infrequent use
▪ Cycloserine	Inhibits cell-wall synthesis	Personality changes, psychosis, rash	Contraindication in individuals with a history of psychosis, use in retreatment of resistant strains

DNA, Deoxyribonucleic acid; *GI,* gastrointestinal; *PPD,* purified protein derivative; *RNA,* ribonucleic acid; *TB,* tuberculosis.

of immunosuppression (e.g., person who is on prolonged steroid therapy or has HIV infection), (2) have a malignant condition such as Hodgkin's disease, or (3) have diabetes mellitus. The individual with any of these characteristics will benefit from prophylactic treatment for TB.

The drug generally used in prophylactic chemotherapy is isoniazid. It is effective and inexpensive and can be administered orally. Isoniazid is usually administered once daily for 6 months in an uncomplicated case or for 12 months for the individual with abnormal chest x-rays or who is HIV positive.

Bacille Calmette-Guérin vaccine. Bacille Calmette-Guérin (BCG) is a live attenuated vaccine that has limited usefulness in the United States because of the low rate of TB infection. It is recommended for the person who has a negative tuberculin skin test but who is repeatedly exposed

Table 24-9 Regimen Options for the Initial Treatment of Tuberculosis among Children and Adults

TB without HIV Infection	
Option 1	Daily isoniazid, rifampin, and pyrazinamide for 8 wk followed by 16 wk of isoniazid and rifampin daily or 2-3 times/wk* in areas where the isoniazid resistance rate is not documented to be <4%. Ethambutol or streptomycin should be added to the initial regimen until susceptibility to isoniazid and rifampin demonstrated. Continue treatment for at least 6 mo and 3 mo beyond culture conversion. Consult a TB medical expert if patient is symptomatic or smear or culture positive after 3 mo.
Option 2	Isoniazid, rifampin, pyrazinamide, and streptomycin or ethambutol for 2 wk followed by 2 times/wk administration of the same drugs for 6 wk (by DOT), subsequently, with 2 times/wk administration the isoniazid and rifampin for 16 wk (by DOT). Consult a TB medical expert if the patient is symptomatic or smear or culture positive after 3 mo.
Option 3	Treat by DOT, 3 times/wk with isoniazid, rifampin, pyrazinamide and ethambutol or streptomycin for 6 mo. Consult a TB medical expert if patient is symptomatic or smear or culture positive after 3 mo.
TB with HIV Infection	
	Option 1, 2, or 3 can be used, but treatment regimens should continue for a total of 9 mo and at least 6 mo beyond culture conversion.

Modified from Centers for Disease Control: Initial therapy for tuberculosis in the era of multidrug resistance, *MMWR* 42 (RR-7):1, 1993.
DOT, Directly observed therapy; *HIV,* human immunodeficiency virus; *TB,* tuberculosis.
*All regimens administered 2 times/week or 3 times/week should be monitored by DOT for the duration of therapy.

Table 24-10 Indications for Preventive TB Therapy

- Newly infected patient
- Person with known or suspected HIV infection and positive skin test
- Exposure of household members and other close associates to newly diagnosed patient
- Significant tuberculin skin test reactors with abnormal chest x-ray study
- Significant tuberculin skin test reactors in special clinical situations (person takes corticosteroids; has diabetes mellitus, silicosis, gastrectomy, or end stage renal disease)
- Other significant tuberculin skin test converters (≥10mm increase within a 2-yr period for those less than 35 yr old; ≥15mm increase for those greater than 35 yr old; all children less than 2 yr old with a >10 mm skin test)
- Other significant tuberculin skin test reactors in person less than 35 yr old (persons born outside of United States from high-prevalence countries; medically underserved low-income populations including high risk racial or ethnic populations, such as African-Americans, Hispanic, and Native Americans; residents of facilities for long-term care)

Modified from American Thoracic Society: Control of tuberculosis in the United States, *American Review of Respiratory Disease* 146:1623, 1992.

to pulmonary tuberculosis (e.g., person assigned to work in countries with a high-prevalence rate). It is also used for young children in countries with a high rate of TB. The vaccine does not reduce the chance of natural infection but may decrease the seriousness of clinical TB if it does occur.

NURSING MANAGEMENT

TUBERCULOSIS

Nursing Assessment

It is important to determine whether the patient was ever exposed to a person with TB. The patient should be assessed for productive cough, night sweats, afternoon temperature elevation, weight loss, pleuritic chest pain, and crackles over the apices of the lungs. If the patient has a productive cough, an early morning sputum specimen will be required for an acid-fast bacillus (AFB) smear to detect the presence of mycobacteria.

Nursing Diagnoses

Nursing diagnoses that are specific to the patient with TB include, but are not limited to, the following:

- Ineffective breathing pattern related to decreased lung capacity
- Altered nutrition: less than body requirements related to chronic poor appetite, fatigue, and productive cough
- Risk for noncompliance related to lack of knowledge of disease process, lack of motivation, and long-term nature of treatment
- Altered health maintenance related to lack of knowledge about the disease process and therapeutic regimen
- Activity intolerance related to fatigue, decreased nutritional status, and chronic febrile episodes

Planning

The overall goals are that the patient with TB will (1) comply with therapeutic regime, (2) have no recurrence of disease, (3) have normal pulmonary function, and (4) take appropriate measures to prevent the spread of the disease.

Nursing Implementation

Health Promotion and Maintenance. The ultimate goal related to TB in the United States is eradication. The public health nurse and clinical nurse have especially important responsibilities. Selective screening programs in known high-risk groups are of value in detecting individuals with TB. The person with a positive tuberculin skin test should have a chest x-ray to assess for the presence of TB. Another important measure is to identify the contacts of the individual who has TB. These contacts should be assessed for the possibility of infection and the need for chemoprophylactic treatment.

When an individual has respiratory symptoms such as cough, dyspnea, or productive sputum, especially if accompanied by a history of night sweats and/or unexplained weight loss, the nurse should assess for the presence of TB. Even if the suspected respiratory problem is something else, such as emphysema, pneumonia, or lung cancer, it is possible that the patient may also have TB.

Acute Intervention. Acute in-hospital care is seldom required for the patient with TB. If hospitalization is needed, it is usually for a brief period. Respiratory isolation (in a negative pressure room with at least six completed air exchanges each hour) is indicated until the patient has been on adequate drug therapy for at least 2 weeks and has shown a clinical response to therapy. It is recommended that isolation be maintained on the patient with drug resistant TB until smears are negative on 3 consecutive days.[10] The patient who is unlikely to transmit tubercle bacilli (i.e., patient without a cough) does not necessarily need to be placed in respiratory isolation. Masks are of limited value unless they are made of fabric designed to filter out droplet nuclei. High-efficiency particulate air (HEPA) masks may be indicated because they can remove almost 100% of particles greater than 3 μm in diameter.[10] Any mask used needs to be molded to fit tightly around the nose and mouth.

The patient should be taught to cover the nose and mouth with paper tissue every time he coughs, sneezes, or produces sputum. The tissues should be thrown into a paper bag and disposed of with the trash, burned, or flushed down the toilet. Masks are necessary only during face-to-face contacts. It is preferable that the patient wears the mask. The patient should also be taught careful hand-washing techniques after handling sputum and soiled tissues.

Special precautions should be taken during high-risk procedures such as sputum induction, bronchoscopy, endoscopy, or pentamidine aerosol treatment. These procedures should only be conducted in negative pressure rooms, and masks (preferably HEPA filter masks) should be worn.

Most treatment failures occur because the patient neglects to take the medication, discontinues it prematurely, or takes it irregularly. It is important for the nurse to develop a therapeutic, consistent relationship with each patient. The nurse needs to understand the patient's lifestyle and to provide flexibility in planning a program that facilitates the patient's participation in and completion of therapy. The nurse should educate the patient so that the need for dedication to the prescribed regimen is fully understood by the patient. Ongoing reassurance helps the patient understand that faithfulness can mean cure. If the patient cannot or will not adhere to a self-administered medication regimen, medication may have to be given by a responsible person on a daily or intermittent basis. Notification of the public health department is essential if drug compliance is questionable so that follow-up of close contacts can be accomplished. In many cases the public health nurse will be responsible for DOT.

Some patients may feel that there is a social stigma attached to TB. These feelings need to be discussed, and the patient needs to be reassured that an individual with TB can be cured if the prescribed regimen is followed. Many people still remember when TB patients were sent away to TB sanitariums and isolated from society. The health care worker's attitude toward individuals with TB should be no different from the attitude toward those with pneumonia. Both diseases are infectious and potentially curable. The American Lung Association provides excellent literature

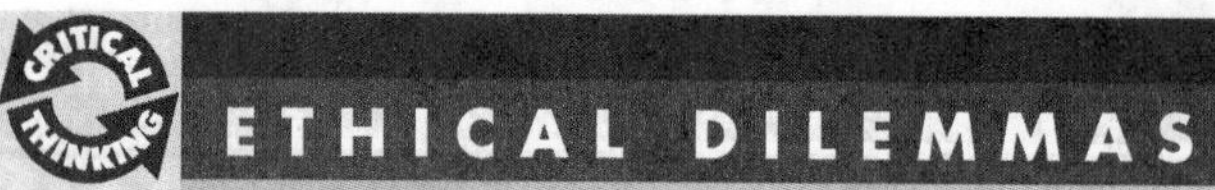

PATIENT COMPLIANCE

Situation The health clinic for the homeless discovers that a patient with TB has not been complying with taking his medication. He tells the nurse that it is hard for him to get to the clinic to obtain the medication, much less to keep on a schedule. The nurse is concerned not only about this patient, but also about the risks for the other people at the shelter, in the park, and at the meal sites.

Discussion TB is a public health concern as well as this individual's problem. Homelessness does not lend itself toward good compliance with medical treatment unless the patient is highly motivated and able to cope with daily living issues as well as the medical condition. If the TB is not treated appropriately, the patient may not only infect others, but the disease may develop a resistance to the medication, possibly leading to an even more resistant strain of the TB bacillus. There are two patients in this case, this particular patient and the public. In order to effectively help this person with his treatment program, social services need to be involved. It might be possible to place him in a halfway house or group home until his treatment is completed. In any case if he is unable or unwilling to cooperate, the public health officials need to be involved so that the public is protected.

ETHICAL AND LEGAL PRINCIPLES

- Patient autonomy may be overridden by concerns about protecting the health of the public.
- Compliance with a medical treatment plan helps to assure the goals of treatment. If a patient cannot comply, the medical goals of treatment are compromised.
- The interests of public health may be included in state statutes allowing medical personnel to detain and treat a patient with infectious diseases.

for teaching about the disease as well as providing emotional support to the patient and family.

Chronic and Home Management. Many patients lack the incentive to comply with their drug regimen. The most cost effective way of ensuring that the patient actually takes the medication is through DOT. A spouse, grown child, or other relative living with the patient may be asked to supervise drug taking. Sometimes coworkers or public health nurses are needed.

When the chemotherapy regimen has been completed, most individuals can be considered adequately treated. Follow-up care may be indicated during the subsequent 12 months, including bacteriologic studies and chest x-ray. Because approximately 5% of individuals experience relapses, the patient should be taught to recognize the symptoms that indicate recurrence of TB. If these symptoms occur, immediate medical attention should be sought.

The patient needs to be instructed about certain factors that could reactivate TB, such as immunosuppressive therapy, malignancy, and prolonged debilitating illness. If the patient experiences any of these events, the health care provider needs to be told so that reactivation of TB can be closely monitored. In some situations it may be necessary to put the patient on anti-TB chemotherapy.

Atypical Mycobacteria. Pulmonary disease that closely resembles TB may be caused by atypical acid-fast mycobacteria. This type of pulmonary disease is indistinguishable from TB clinically and radiologically but can be differentiated by bacteriologic culture. These organisms are not believed to be airborne and thus are not transmitted by droplet nuclei.

Atypical mycobacteria that affect the lung include *M. kansasii*, *M. scrofulaceum*, *M. intracellularis*, and *M. xenopi*. These bacteria (especially *M. avium-intracellulare* and *M. scrofulaceum*) may also invade the cervical lymph nodes, causing lymphadenitis. This type of pulmonary disease typically occurs in white men with a history of COPD or silicosis. *M. avium-intracellulare* is a common cause of opportunistic infections in the patient with HIV infection.

Treatment depends on identification of the causative agent and determination of drug sensitivity. Many of the drugs used in treating TB are employed in combating infections from atypical mycobacteria.

Pulmonary Fungal Infections

Pulmonary fungal infections are increasing in incidence. They are found most frequently in seriously ill patients being treated with corticosteroids, antineoplastic and immunosuppressive drugs, or multiple antibiotics; they are also found in patients with AIDS.[11] Types of fungal infections are presented in Table 24-11. These infections are not transmitted from person to person, and the patient does not have to be placed in isolation. The clinical manifestations are similar to those of bacterial pneumonia. Skin and serology tests are available to assist in identifying the infecting organism. However, identification of the organism in a sputum specimen or in other body fluids is the best diagnostic indicator.

Therapeutic Management. Amphotericin B is the drug most widely used in treating serious systemic fungal infections. It must be given IV to achieve adequate blood and tissue levels because it is poorly absorbed from the GI tract. Amphotericin B is considered a toxic drug with many possible side effects, including hypersensitivity reactions, fever, chills, malaise, nausea and vomiting, thrombophlebitis at the injection site, and abnormal renal function. Many of the side effects during infusion can be avoided by using aspirin or diphenhydramine (Benadryl) 1 hour before the infusion. Additionally, the infusion is best tolerated if given in less than 1 hour. Inclusion of a small amount of hydrocortisone hemisuccinate in the infusion helps to decrease the irritation of the veins, which is important because infusions are given two to three times weekly. Monitoring of renal function is essential while a person is receiving this drug. Renal changes are at least partially reversible. Amphotericin infusions are incompatible with most other drugs. Amphotericin is frequently administered every other day after an initial period of several weeks of daily therapy. Total treatment with the drug may range from 4 to 10 weeks.

Oral imidazole compounds with antifungal activity such as ketoconazole or fluconazole have been successful in the treatment of coccidioidomycosis, especially in diseases that affect skin and soft tissue. Their effectiveness in treatment of more severe coccidioidal infections has been shown and allows an alternative to the use of Amphotericin B in many cases.[12] The action of the imidazoles is primarily to control the fungal infection and localize it rather than to cure it. Effectiveness of therapy can be monitored with fungal serology titers.

5-Fluorocytosine has also been used in selected types of pulmonary fungal infections. It is given orally and becomes widely distributed in the body. Adverse reactions include abdominal discomfort, diarrhea, hepatotoxicity, and bone marrow suppression.

Bronchiectasis

Pathophysiology. *Bronchiectasis* is a disorder characterized by permanent, abnormal dilatation of one or more large bronchi. The pathophysiologic change that results in dilatation is destruction of the elastic and muscular structures of the bronchial wall. There are two pathologic types of bronchiectasis: saccular and cylindrical (Fig. 24-3). *Saccular bronchiectasis* occurs mainly in large bronchi and is characterized by cavity-like dilatations. The affected bronchi end in large sacs. *Cylindrical bronchiectasis* involves medium-sized bronchi that are mildly to moderately dilated. A subtype of cylindrical, *fusiform bronchiectasis*, tends to involve more "pouching" of the bronchi as opposed to dilatation seen with cylindrical bronchiectasis.

Almost all forms of bronchiectasis are associated with bacterial infections. Infections cause the bronchial walls to weaken, and pockets of infection begin to form. When the walls of the bronchial system are injured, the mucociliary mechanism is damaged, allowing bacteria and mucus to accumulate within the pockets. The infection becomes worse and results in bronchiectasis.

Table 24-11 Fungal Infections of the Lung

Organism	Characteristics
Histoplasmosis *Histoplasma capsulatum*	Indigenous to soil of North American river valleys, inhalation of mycelia into lungs, infected individual often free of symptoms, generally self-limiting, chronic disease similar to TB
Coccidioidomycosis *Coccidioides immitis*	Indigenous to semiarid regions of Southwestern United States, inhalation of arthrospores into lungs, suppurative and granulomatous reaction in lungs, symptomatic infection in one third of individuals
Blastomycosis *Blastomyces dermatitidis*	Indigenous to Southeastern and Midwestern United States, inhalation of fungus into lungs, progression of disease often insidious, possible involvement of skin
Cryptococcosis *Crytococcus neoformans*	True yeast, indigenous worldwide in soil and pigeon excreta, inhalation of fungus into lungs, possible meningitis
Aspergillosis *Aspergillus niger* or *Aspergillus fumigatus*	True mold inhabiting mouth, widely distributed, invasion of lung tissue resulting in possible necrotizing pneumonia: in individual with asthma, allergic bronchopulmonary aspergillosis may require corticosteroid therapy
Candidiasis *Candida albicans*	Leading cause of mycotic infections in hospitalized and immunocompromised hosts, ubiquitous and frequent colonization of upper respiratory and GI tracts, infections often following broad-spectrum antibiotic therapy (systemic or inhaled), possible development of localized pulmonary infiltrate to widespread bilateral consolidation with hypoxemia
Actinomycosis *Actinomyces israeli*	Not a true fungus, pseudohyphae present; anaerobic, gram-positive, higher bacteria with branching hyphae; presence of necrotizing pneumonia after aspiration; pneumonitis, commonly in lower lobes with abscess or empyema formation
Nocardiosis *Nocardia asteroides*	Not a true fungus; aerobic, higher bacteria with branching hyphae; soil saprophyte widely distributed in nature; acquisition of infection from nature; rarely present in sputum without accompanying disease

GI, Gastrointestinal; *TB*, tuberculosis.

A recent classification of bronchiectasis divides it into designations of *localized* or *generalized* based upon the underlying cause.[13] *Localized bronchiectasis* results from necrotizing or lobar pneumonia whose bronchiectatic sequelae are limited to one area of the lung or from focal airway obstructions. Obstructive processes of any kind can predispose an individual to bronchiectasis. Examples include lung tumors, tumor masses in the chest cavity, aspirated foreign objects, and thick, tenacious secretions such as those found in chronic bronchitis. The obstruction causes the bronchi and bronchioles to distend and balloon out below the level of obstruction. This provides a good place for organisms to proliferate.

The most common cause of *generalized bronchiectasis* is multifocal necrotizing bacterial infection, but other conditions such as congenital factors, recurrent gastric aspiration, and toxic inhalations can predispose persons to the development of bronchiectasis. Congenital factors include altered bronchial structures such as cysts and cul-de-sacs, which lead to pooling of secretion. A defect in cilia, causing them to be immobile, is also associated with the development of bronchiectasis. In cystic fibrosis, there is retention and thickening of mucus that may plug the airways. A variety of immunodeficiency diseases are associated with recurrent bacterial pneumonias. Some inhalation exposures, particularly to irritant gases such as oxides of sulfur and nitrogen, have been noted as causes of bronchiectasis.

The disease process is often believed to start in childhood as an acquired disorder, beginning with respiratory complications secondary to influenza, measles, or whooping cough. Recurring lower respiratory tract infections are another pattern of disease in childhood that may predispose an individual to bronchiectasis. This pattern is typically seen in the individual who has cystic fibrosis, asthma, α-1 antitrypsin deficiency, or immunodeficiency diseases.

Clinical Manifestations. The primary manifestations of bronchiectasis vary considerably, depending on the extent and location of the disease process. They include chronic cough with production of mucopurulent sputum, hemoptysis, and recurrent pneumonia. The cough is paroxysmal and is often stimulated with position changes. Other manifestations include exertional dyspnea, fatigue, weight loss, anorexia, and fetid breath. Sinusitis frequently accompanies diffuse bronchiectasis. The manifestations of ad-

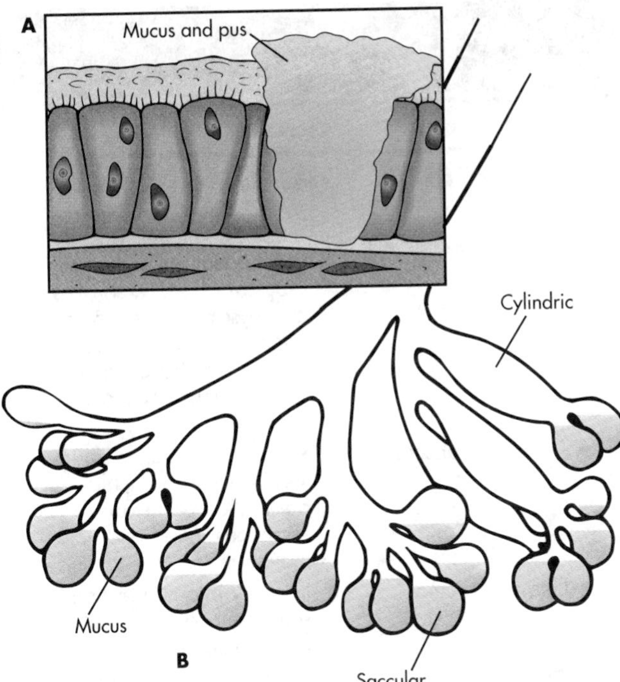

Fig. 24-3 Pathologic changes in bronchiectasis. ***A,*** Longitudinal section of bronchial wall where chronic infection has caused damage. ***B,*** Collection of purulent material in dilated bronchioles, leading to persistent infection.

vanced, widespread bronchiectasis are generalized wheezing, digital clubbing, and cor pulmonale.

Diagnostic Studies. An individual with a chronic productive cough with copious sputum (which may be blood streaked) should be suspected of having bronchiectasis. Characteristic findings in the health history, such as childhood diseases complicated by respiratory infections or chronic bronchitis, are significant. Chest x-rays are usually done and may show streaky infiltrates. Bronchography involves instilling liquid radiopaque material into the bronchial system via a catheter or bronchoscope, and in the past it was useful in evaluating individuals with moderate to severe cases of bronchiectasis. With the availability of computed tomography (CT) scanning, bronchography has become all but obsolete.[13] Bronchoscopy may be useful in identifying the source of secretions or sites of hemoptysis in the individual with a chronic productive cough.

Collecting sputum to evaluate its quantity, characteristics, and microbial content may provide additional information regarding the severity of impairment and the presence of active infection. Pulmonary function studies may be abnormal in advanced bronchiectasis, showing a decrease in vital capacity, expiratory flow, and maximum voluntary ventilation and an increase in ventilation-perfusion mismatching with resultant hypoxemia. A complete blood count may be normal or show evidence of anemia and leukocytosis.

Therapeutic Management. Bronchiectasis is difficult to treat. Antibiotics are the major form of treatment and should be given on the basis of sputum culture results. Other forms of drug therapy may include bronchodilators, mucolytic agents, and expectorants. Maintaining good hydration is important to liquefy secretions. Postural drainage is vital to facilitate expectoration of sputum. (Postural drainage is discussed in Chapter 25.) The individual should reduce exposure to excessive air pollutants and irritants, avoid cigarette smoking, and obtain pneumococcal and influenza vaccinations.

Surgical resection of parts of the lungs, although not used as often as previously, may be done if more conservative treatment is not effective. Surgical resection of an affected lobe or segment may be indicated for the patient with repeated bouts of pneumonia, hemoptysis, and disabling complications. Surgery is not advisable when there is diffuse or widespread involvement.

NURSING MANAGEMENT

BRONCHIECTASIS

Health Maintenance and Promotion

The incidence of bronchiectasis has shown a decline in recent years. This is partially because of the administration of measles and pertussis vaccines, which decreases the incidence of bronchiectasis caused by these diseases. Early detection and treatment of lower respiratory tract infections prevent them from developing into complications such as bronchiectasis. Any obstructing lesion or foreign body should be removed promptly. Other measures to decrease the occurrence or progression of bronchiectasis include avoiding cigarette smoking and decreasing exposure to pollution. Children with persistent coughs should receive evaluations to determine the source of the problem.

Acute and Chronic Interventions

An important nursing goal is to promote drainage and removal of bronchial mucus. The patient should be taught effective deep-breathing exercises and effective ways to cough (see Table 25-12). Postural drainage should be done on affected parts of the lung (see Fig. 25-12). Some individuals require elevation of the foot of the bed by 4 to 6 inches to facilitate drainage. Pillows may be used in the hospital and at home to help the patient assume postural drainage positions. Administration of the prescribed antibiotics, bronchodilators, or expectorants is important. The patient needs to understand the importance of taking the prescribed regimen of drugs to obtain maximum effectiveness. The patient should be aware of possible side or adverse effects that must be reported to the physician.

Rest is important to prevent overexertion. Bed rest may be indicated during the acute phase of the illness. Chilling and excess fatigue should be avoided.

Good nutrition is important and may be difficult to maintain because the patient is often anorexic. Oral hygiene to cleanse the mouth and remove dried sputum crusts may improve the patient's appetite. Offering foods that are appealing may also increase the desire to eat. Adequate hydration to help liquefy secretions and thus make it easier to remove them is extremely important. Unless there are contraindications such as concomitant congestive heart failure or renal disease, the patient should be instructed to drink at least 3 L of fluid daily. To accomplish this, the patient should be advised to increase fluid consumption from the baseline by increasing intake by one glass per day until the goal is reached. Generally the patient should be counseled to use low-sodium fluids to avoid systemic fluid retention.

Direct hydration of the respiratory system may also prove beneficial in the expectoration of secretions. Usually a bland aerosol with normal saline solution delivered by a jet-type nebulizer is used. The patient with bronchiectasis should avoid ultrasonic nebulizers because they often induce bronchospasm. At home a steamy shower can prove effective; expensive equipment that requires frequent cleaning is usually unnecessary. It is important that the patient medicate with an inhaled bronchodilator 10 to 15 minutes before using a bland aerosol to prevent bronchoconstriction.

The patient and family should be taught to recognize significant manifestations to be reported to the health care provider. These manifestations include increased sputum production, grossly bloody sputum, increasing dyspnea, fever, chills, and chest pain.

Lung Abscess

Pathophysiology. *Lung abscess* is a pus-containing lesion of the lung parenchyma that gives rise to a cavity. The cavity is formed by necrosis of the lung tissue. In many cases the causes and pathogenesis of lung abscess are similar to those of pneumonia. The most common etiologic factor of a lung abscess is aspiration of material into the lungs (Table 24-12). In addition to producing infection, the organisms involved cause necrosis of the lung tissue. Examples include enteric gram-negative organisms (e.g., *Klebsiella*), *S. aureus*, and anaerobic bacilli. Lung abscess can also result from hematogenously spread lung infarct secondary to pulmonary embolus, malignant growth, TB, and various parasitic and fungal diseases of the lung.

The areas of the lung most commonly affected are the apical segments of the lower lobes and the posterior segments of the upper lobes. Fibrous tissue usually forms around the abscess in an attempt to wall it off. The abscess may erode into the bronchial system, causing the production of foul-smelling sputum. It may grow toward the pleura and cause pleuritic pain. Multiple small abscesses can occur within the lung.

Clinical Manifestations and Complications. The onset of a lung abscess is usually insidious, especially if anaerobic organisms are the primary cause. A more acute onset occurs with aerobic organisms. The most common manifestation is cough producing purulent sputum (often dark brown) that is foul smelling and foul tasting. Hemoptysis is common, especially at the time that an abscess ruptures into a bronchus. Other common manifestations are fever, chills, prostration, pleuritic pain, dyspnea, cough, and weight loss. The history may reveal a predisposing condition such as alcoholism, pneumonia, or oral infection.

Physical examination of the lungs indicates dullness to percussion and decreased breath sounds on auscultation

Table 24-12 Common Causes of Lung Abscess

Type of Abscess	Cause
▪ Aspiration abscess	Alcoholism, postanesthesia, oversedation, coma (e.g., diabetes, seizures, gastroesophageal reflux disease, drug overdose, cerebrovascular accident), oral infection, food or foreign body, laryngeal palsy, carcinoma of esophagus ("spill-over" aspiration)
▪ Malignant abscess	Necrotic bronchial carcinoma, secondary to bronchial obstruction and stasis of secretions, head and neck malignancies
▪ Pulmonary embolus	Pulmonary infarct infection, septic emboli, fragments from bacterial endarteritis
▪ Infection	Pneumonia, pyogenic bacteria (notably *S. aureus*), defective ciliary action, ineffective expectoration, infected cysts, necrotic lesions, subdiaphragmatic infections (usually liver), open chest wounds

From Kinney M and others: *AACN's clinical reference for critical-care nursing*, ed 3, St Louis, 1993, Mosby.

over the segment of lung involved. There may be transmission of bronchial breath sounds to the periphery if the communicating bronchus becomes patent and drainage of the segment begins. Crackles may also be present in the later stages as the abscess drains. Oral examination often reveals dental caries, gingivitis, and periodontal infection.

Complications that can occur include chronic pulmonary abscess, hemorrhage from abscess erosion into blood vessels, brain abscess as a result of the spread of infection, bronchopleural fistula, and empyema from abscess perforation into the pleural cavity.

Diagnostic Studies. A chest x-ray taken before drainage of the abscess will reveal a circumscribed area of infiltration. After the abscess is drained, a chest x-ray will show an area of consolidation with a wall around a lucent zone. Sputum culture and Gram stain are necessary to identify the infecting organism. Bronchoscopy may be used in cases of abscess in which drainage is delayed or in which there are factors that suggest an underlying malignancy. Leukocytosis is usually present.

Therapeutic Management. Antibiotics given for a prolonged period (up to 6 weeks) are usually the primary method of treatment. Penicillin has historically been the drug of choice because of the frequent presence of anaerobic organisms. However, recent studies suggesting the presence of β-lactamase production by the anaerobic bacteria involved in abscesses of the lung indicate that drugs such as clindamycin or metronidazole in combination with penicillin should be used as primary therapy. Clindamycin is definitely the drug of choice for infections involving putrid abscesses with large cavities or for the patient who has severe systemic toxicity.[14] Chest physiotherapy and postural drainage are sometimes used to drain abscesses located in the lower or posterior portions of the lung. Surgery is rarely indicated but occasionally may be necessary when reinfection of a large cavitary lesion occurs or to establish a diagnosis when there is evidence of an underlying neoplasm or chronic associated disease. The use of bronchoscopy for drainage of an abscess is controversial. Some clinicians believe that this procedure may spread the infection to other parts of the lung. If used, bronchoscopy should not be performed until after 24 to 48 hours of antimicrobial therapy.

NURSING MANAGEMENT

LUNG ABSCESS

Drainage of the abscess and treatment of the infection are the primary goals. The patient should be taught how to cough effectively. Chest physiotherapy will help to loosen secretions. Postural drainage according to the lung area involved will aid the removal of secretions (see Fig. 25-12). Frequent (every 2 to 3 hours) mouth care is needed to relieve the putrid odor and taste from the foul-smelling sputum. Diluted hydrogen peroxide and mouthwash are often effective.

Because of the need for prolonged antibiotic therapy, the patient must be aware of the importance of continuing the medication for the prescribed period. The patient needs to know about untoward side effects to be reported to the health care provider. Sometimes the patient is asked to return periodically during the course of antibiotic therapy for repeat cultures and sensitivity tests to ensure that the infecting organism is not becoming resistant to the antibiotic. When antibiotic therapy is completed, the patient is reevaluated.

Rest, good nutrition, and adequate fluid intake are all supportive measures to facilitate recovery. If dentition is poor and dental hygiene is not adequate, the patient should be encouraged to obtain dental care.

OXYGEN THERAPY

Oxygen (O_2) therapy is frequently used in the treatment of respiratory problems. Oxygen is a colorless, odorless, tasteless gas that constitutes 20.95% of the atmosphere. Used clinically it is considered a drug. Administering supplemental O_2 raises the partial pressure of O_2 (PO_2) in inspired air.

Indications

Oxygen is usually administered to treat hypoxemia caused by (1) *respiratory disorders* such as COPD, cor pulmonale, pneumonia, atelectasis, lung cancer, and pulmonary emboli; (2) *cardiovascular disorders* such as myocardial infarction, dysrhythmias, angina pectoris, and cardiogenic shock; and (3) *CNS disorders* such as overdose of narcotics, head injury, and disordered sleep (sleep apnea).

Methods

The goal of O_2 administration is to supply the patient with adequate O_2 to maximize the O_2-carrying ability of the blood. There are various methods of O_2 administration (Table 24-13 and Figs. 24-4 and 24-5). The method selected depends on factors such as the fraction of inspired O_2 (FIO_2) and humidification required, patient cooperation, and comfort.

Oxygen delivery systems are classified as low- or high-flow systems based upon whether the system provides the entire inspired atmosphere to a patient in a fixed oxygen concentration. Most methods of O_2 administration are *low-flow devices* that deliver O_2 in concentrations that vary with the person's respiratory pattern. In contrast the Venturi mask is a *high-flow device* that delivers fixed concentrations of O_2 independent of the patient's respiratory pattern. With the Venturi mask, O_2 is delivered to a small jet (Venturi device) in the center of a wide-based cone (Fig. 24-4). Air is *entrained* (pulled through) openings in the cone as O_2 flows through the small jet. The mask has large vents through which exhaled air can escape. The degree of restriction or narrowness of the jet determines the amount of entrainment and dilution of pure O_2 with room air and thus the concentration of O_2. Mechanical ventilators are another example of a high flow O_2 delivery system.

Humidification and Nebulizers

Oxygen obtained from cylinders or wall systems is dry. Dry oxygen has an irritating effect on mucous membranes and dries secretions. Therefore it is important that O_2 be humidified when administered, either by humidification or nebulization. A common device used for humidification when the patient has a catheter, cannula, or low-flow mask is a *bubble humidifier*. It is a small plastic jar filled with sterile distilled water that is attached to the O_2 source by means of a flowmeter. O_2 passes into the jar, bubbles through the water, and then goes through tubing to the patient's catheter, cannula, or mask. The purpose of the bubble humidifier is to restore the humidity conditions of room air. However, the need for bubble humidifiers at flow rates between 1 and 4 L per minute is controversial when humidity in the environment is adequate.

Another means of administering humidified O_2 is via a *nebulizer*. It delivers particulate water mist (aerosols) with a high degree of humidity. The humidity can be raised by heating the water, which increases the ability of the gas to hold moisture. Heated (98.6° F [37° C]) and humidified (100%) gas is required when the upper airway is bypassed. When nebulizers are used, large-size tubing should be employed to connect the device to a face mask or T bar. If small-size tubing is used, condensation can occlude the flow of O_2.

Complications

Combustion. Oxygen supports combustion and increases the rate of burning. This is why it is important that

Table 24-13 Methods of Oxygen Administration

Advantages	Disadvantages	Nursing Interventions
Low Flow Delivery Devices		
Nasal cannula		
Cannula may be used by a restless patient. It is a safe and simple method that is relatively comfortable and acceptable. It is useful for a patient requiring low O_2 concentrations (e.g., those with chronic CO_2 retention). It allows patient to move about in bed. Patient can eat, talk, or cough while wearing device.	Cannula is difficult to maintain in position and can be easily dislodged. Patient must be alert and cooperative to keep cannula in proper place. High-flow rates (>5 L/min) dry nasal membranes and may cause pain in frontal sinuses.	Nasal cannula should be stabilized when caring for a restless patient. A flow rate of 2 L/min gives an O_2 concentration of approximately 28%. Amount of O_2 inhaled depends on room air and patient's breathing pattern. Most patients with COPD can tolerate 2 L/min via cannula.
Simple face mask		
O_2 can be given quickly for short periods. O_2 concentrations of 35-50% can be achieved with flow rates of 6-12 L/min. Mask provides adequate humidification of inspired air.	Lack of patient tolerance results in inadequate therapy. Mask may be uncomfortable because tight seal must be maintained between face and mask. Mask may produce pressure necrosis of the skin and confines heat radiating from the face about nose and mouth. It must be removed to eat or drink.	Wash and dry under mask q2hr. Mask needs to fit snugly. Nasal cannula may be provided while patient is eating. Watch for pressure necrosis at the top of ears from elastic straps. (Gauze or other padding may be used to alleviate this problem.) Method requires at least 5 L/min flow to prevent accumulation of expired air in the mask.
Nasal catheter		
Catheter allows continuous uninterrupted O_2 therapy. Patient receives O_2 even if a mouth breather. Catheter does not interfere with patient care. It is rarely used.	Catheter must be inserted into nasopharynx through a nostril and can produce excoriation of the nares. High-flow rates (>6 L/min) can cause drying of nasal membranes. Inadvertent gas flow distends the stomach. Cannula does not permit a high degree of humidification and must be taped to patient's face.	Catheter should be changed q8hr, alternate the nostrils. Distance that catheter is to be inserted is measured from distance between tip of nose and earlobe. A flow rate of 5-6 L/min gives an O_2 concentration of approximately 30%. Method is best used for short-term therapy.
Partial rebreathing mask		
Mask is lightweight and easy to use. Reservoir bag conserves O_2. Concentrations of 40-60% can be achieved using flow rates of 6-10 L/min.	Mask cannot be used with a high degree of humidity.	Method is useful when blood O_2 concentrations must be raised. It is not recommended for patient with COPD and should never be used with a nebulizer. Bag should not be allowed to deflate during inspiration.
Non-breathing mask		
High concentrations of O_2 can be delivered accurately. O_2 flows into bag and mask during inhalation. Valve prevents expired air from flowing back into bag. Concentrations of 60-90% can be achieved.	Mask cannot be used with a high degree of humidity.	Mask should fit snugly. Flow rate must be sufficient to keep bag from collapsing during inspiration.

continued

smoking be prohibited in the area in which O_2 is being used. A "No Smoking" sign should be prominently displayed on the patient's door. The patient should also be cautioned against smoking cigarettes with O_2 prongs or a catheter in place.

Carbon Dioxide Narcosis. In some cases of respiratory distress, increasing the O_2 flow rate may be quite harmful. Normally, carbon dioxide (CO_2) accumulation is a major stimulant of the respiratory center. However, the individual with a long-standing history of COPD or who is heavily sedated may have a tendency to hypoventilate and to retain CO_2. Gradually, the respiratory center loses its sensitivity to the elevated CO_2 level. For these individuals the major stimulant of respiration becomes hypoxemia.

Table 24-13 Methods of Oxygen Administration—cont'd

Advantages	Disadvantages	Nursing Interventions
Oxygen-conserving cannula Cannula has a built-in reservoir that increases O_2 concentration delivered and allows patient to use lower flow, usually 30-50%, which increases comfort and lowers cost. It is reportedly more comfortable than standard cannulas.	Cannula cannot be cleaned: manufacturer recommends changing cannula every week. It is more expensive than standard cannulas and requires evaluation with ABGs and oximetry to determine correct flow for patient. Cannula is highly visible.	Method is generally indicated for patient requiring long-term O_2 therapy at home versus during hospitalization. It may be "moustache" or "pendant" type.
Transtracheal catheter[†] Catheter is less visible. Flow requirement may be reduced 60-80%, which greatly increases amount of time available from portable source of O_2. Less nasal irritation occurs.	Patient and family must learn care for tracheostoma and how to replace catheter. Procedure is invasive. Procedure and replacement adds costs to O_2 therapy.	Method may not be appropriate for patient with excessive mucus production from "clogging."
Face tent Tent is ideal for providing moderate- to high-density aerosol. O_2 concentration administered varies with O_2 flow rate.	Face tent is less reliable than face mask for maintaining high inspiration of O_2 concentration.	Open plastic mask fits under chin. Temperature of aerosol needs to be checked to maintain at or near body temperature. It is rarely used.
Tracheostomy collar Collar can deliver high humidity and O_2 via tracheostomy.	Condensed fluid in tubing may drain into tracheostomy. Secretions collect inside collar and around tracheostomy. O_2 concentration is lost into atmosphere because collar does not fit tightly.	Collar attaches to neck with elastic strap and should be removed and cleaned at least q4hr to prevent aspiration of fluid and infection.
Tracheostomy T bar Tight fit allows better O_2 and humidity delivery than tracheostomy collar.	Condensed fluid in tubing may drain into tracheostomy.	T bar needs to be removed for suctioning. Mörch swivel may be used to eliminate the need for removal. It should be emptied as necessary.
Tent or incubator Tent or incubator has ability to control temperature and humidity.	Tent or incubator has limited usefulness. It is difficult to maintain adequate concentrations of O_2. Method isolates patient from environment.	Tent should be flushed with O_2 every time it is opened. Nurse should assess for leaks around canopy.
High Flow Delivery Devices		
Venturi mask* Mask can deliver precise, high-flow rates of O_2. Lightweight plastic, cone-shaped device is fitted to face. Masks are available for delivery of 24%, 28%, 31%, 35%, 40%, and 50% O_2. Adaptors can be applied to increase humidification.	Mask is uncomfortable and must be removed when patient eats. Patient can talk but voice may be muffled. Other disadvantages are the same as those discussed for the simple face mask.	Entrainment device on mask must be changed to deliver higher concentrations of O_2. Method is especially helpful for administering low, constant O_2 concentrations to patients with COPD. Air entrainment ports must not be occluded.

ABGs, Arterial blood gases; *COPD,* chronic obstructive pulmonary disease.
*See Fig. 24-4.
†See Fig. 24-7.

When O_2 is administered in high concentrations, the hypoxic stimulus is eliminated and the rate and depth of ventilation will decrease. The patient will subsequently develop hypercapnia and eventually CO_2 narcosis.

It is critical to start O_2 at low flow rates until arterial blood gases (ABGs) can be obtained. ABGs are used as a guide to determine what FIO_2 level is sufficient and can be tolerated. The patient's mental status and vital signs should be assessed before starting O_2 therapy and frequently thereafter.

Oxygen Toxicity. Pulmonary O_2 toxicity may result from prolonged exposure to a high PaO_2. The development of O_2 toxicity is determined by patient tolerance, exposure time, and effective dose. It is believed that high concentrations of O_2 may inactivate pulmonary surfactant and lead to the development of the acute respiratory distress syndrome

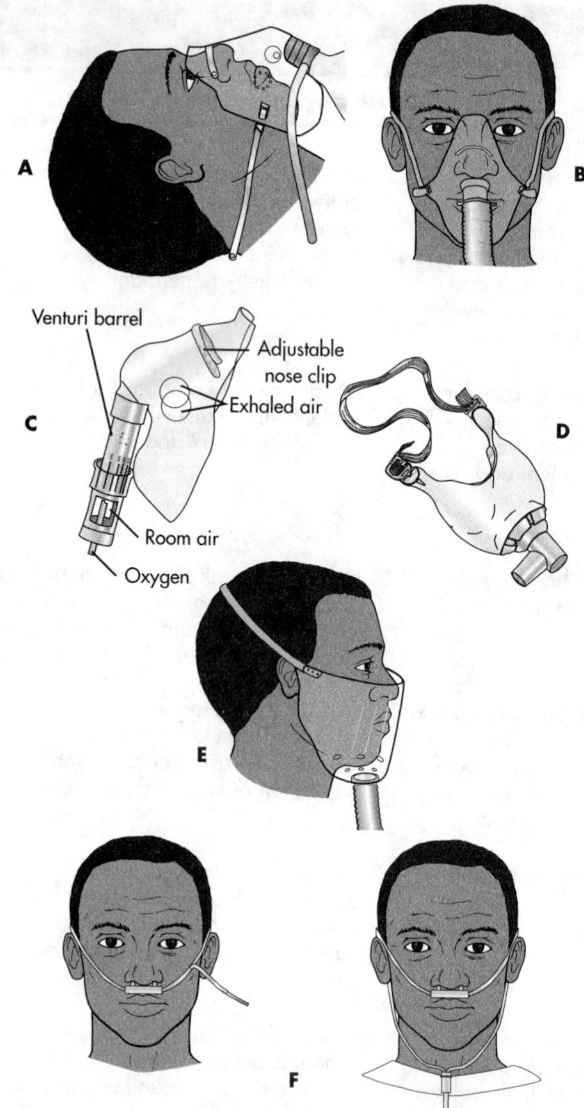

Fig. 24-4 Methods of oxygen administration. Shown are: ***A***, Non-rebreathing mask. ***B***, Aerosol mask. ***C***, Venturi mask. ***D***, Tracheostomy mask. ***E***, Face tent. ***F***, Standard nasal cannulas.

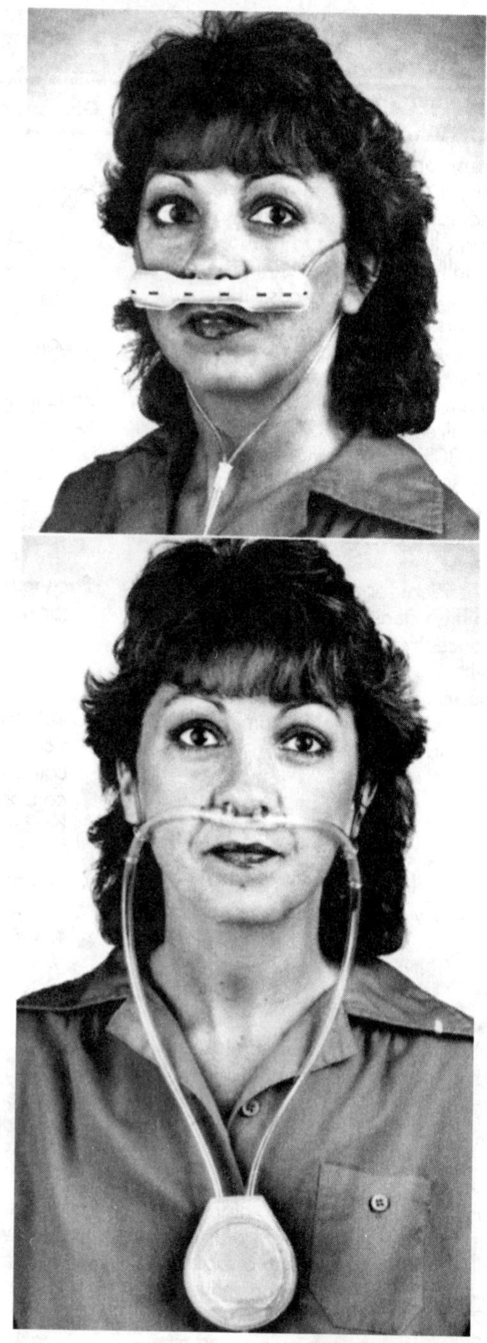

Fig. 24-5 Oxygen-conserving cannulas. Moustache-type oxygen-conserving cannula and pendant-type oxygen-conserving cannula.

(ARDS). The lungs from individuals who die after prolonged administration of 100% O_2 show some or all of the following abnormalities on autopsy:[15]

1. Lungs are heavy, "beefy," and edematous.
2. Hyaline membranes cover many alveoli, alveolar ducts, and respiratory bronchioles.
3. Many alveoli are filled with hemorrhagic exudate.
4. Alveolar septa are markedly increased.

Early manifestations of O_2 toxicity are reduced vital capacity, cough, substernal chest pain, nausea and vomiting, paresthesia, nasal stuffiness, sore throat, and malaise. The later stages of O_2 toxicity affect the alveolar-capillary gas exchange unit, causing edema and production of copious sputum. The end stage of O_2 toxicity is progressive fibrosis of the lungs.

Prevention of O_2 toxicity is very important for the patient who is receiving O_2. The amount of O_2 administered should be just enough to maintain the PaO_2 within a normal or acceptable range for the patient. ABGs should be monitored frequently to evaluate the effectiveness of therapy as well as to guide the tapering of supplemental O_2. A safe limit of O_2 concentrations has not yet been estab-

NURSING CARE PLAN Patient Receiving Oxygen

Planning: Outcome Criteria	*Nursing Interventions and Rationales*
➤ NURSING DIAGNOSIS	Risk for impaired skin integrity *related to* the O_2 administration device and humidity
Have no skin breakdown from breathing device.	Ensure that strap is not too tight *to prevent excessive pressure.* Remove O_2 device every shift and wash and dry skin *to stimulate and clean the area and prevent skin maceration.* Pad any pressure points *to reduce pressure from the equipment.* Observe tops of ears for skin breakdown of pressure points *because this is a common area of pressure ulcer formation.*
➤ NURSING DIAGNOSIS	Altered oral and nasal mucous membranes *related to* O_2 therapy *as manifested by* drying, redness, cracking of nasal mucosa, possibly bleeding
Have no evidence or complaints of mucosal discomfort.	Assess oral and nasal mucosa every shift *to detect signs of mucosal irritation.* Use water-based jelly on lips and nasal mucosa *to provide lubrication.* (Oil-based lubricants are contraindicated.) Do not obstruct cannula outlets with jelly. Provide frequent oral hygiene *to maintain patient comfort and reduce opportunity for infection.* Provide humidification via humidifier or nebulizing device *to maintain moisture of nasotracheal mucosa.*
➤ NURSING DIAGNOSIS	Risk for infection *related to* presence of environmental pathogens and bacterial contamination of equipment
Have no evidence of respiratory infection.	Remove mask or collar and cleanse with water q4-8hr *to remove potentially infectious material.* Clean skin carefully *to reduce pathogens on the skin.* Change disposable equipment frequently *to prevent infection.* Remove secretions that are coughed out; empty container *to prevent exposure to pathogenic material.*
➤ NURSING DIAGNOSIS	Risk for injury related to fire hazard secondary to O_2-enriched environment
Have no incidence of fire caused by O_2 equipment.	Post "No Smoking" warning sign prominently *to remind everyone of fire hazard.* Do not use electric razors, portable radios, open flames, wool blankets, or mineral oils *because each of these has potential to cause fire with oxygen present.* Do not allow smoking in room *because it can cause a fire.* Teach patient about precautions related to home O_2 therapy *to eliminate the risk of fire at home.*

COLLABORATIVE PROBLEMS

Nursing Goals	*Nursing Interventions and Rationales*
➤ POTENTIAL COMPLICATION	CO_2 narcosis in patient with COPD *related to* excessive oxygen administration in a person with hypercapnia
Monitor for CO_2 narcosis as evidenced by a rising $PaCO_2$ or decreased level of consciousness, report deviations from acceptable parameters, and carry out appropriate medical and nursing interventions.	Identify patient at risk for CO_2 narcosis such as those with a history of COPD and CO_2 above normal (>45 mm Hg) with or without abnormal pH *so problem can be identified early.* Administer O_2 only at ordered level *because increasing the O_2 flow rate will remove the hypoxemic drive in people with COPD and hypercapnia.* Monitor results of ABGs *to evaluate the effectiveness of therapy as well as to guide the tapering of supplemental oxygen.* Assess baseline level of consciousness, respiratory rate, and pulse rate *to have comparative values for future assessments* and monitor frequently *to evaluate response to therapy.* Teach patient and family not to increase O_2 flow rate unless directed to do so by a physician or nurse *to prevent problems related to removing the patient's hypoxic drive.*
➤ POTENTIAL COMPLICATION	O_2 toxicity *related to* enriched O_2 environment
Administer minimal O_2 therapy to maintain PaO_2 at adequate level.	Administer O_2 at the lowest level that produces acceptable ABGs *because of the potential for O_2 toxicity.* Monitor ABGs frequently *to determine what FIO_2 level is sufficient.* Monitor patient for manifestations of O_2 toxicity (substernal discomfort, cough, nasal congestion, sore throat, confusion). Do not attempt to use FIO_2 more than 50% for >24 hr unless specifically indicated *because of the potential for oxygen toxicity above this level.*

ABGs, Arterial blood gases; *COPD,* chronic obstructive pulmonary disease.

lished. All levels above 50% and used for longer than 24 hours should be considered potentially toxic. Levels of 40% and below may be regarded as relatively nontoxic and may not result in development of significant O_2 toxicity if the exposure period is short.

Absorption Atelectasis. Normally nitrogen, which constitutes 79% of the air we breathe, is not absorbed into the bloodstream, and it prevents alveolar collapse. When high concentrations of O_2 are given, nitrogen is washed out of the alveoli and replaced with O_2. If airway obstruction occurs, the O_2 is absorbed into the bloodstream and the alveoli collapse. This process is called absorption atelectasis.

Infection. Infection can be a major hazard of O_2 administration. Heated nebulizers present the highest risk. The constant use of humidity supports bacterial growth with the most common infecting organism being *Pseudomonas aeruginosa*. Disposable equipment that operates as a closed system should be used and changed every 48 hours to prevent infection. There should be a hospital policy stating the required frequency of equipment changes based upon the type of equipment used at that particular institution. Both equipment and respiratory secretions should be gram stained and cultured frequently. (Nursing care of the patient who is receiving O_2 therapy is presented in the nursing care plan on p. 651.)

Chronic Oxygen Therapy at Home

Improved prognosis has been noted in patients with COPD who receive nocturnal or continuous O_2 to treat hypoxemia. The longer that the continuous daily use of O_2 is maintained, the greater the improvement.[16] This improved prognosis results from preventing progression of the disease and subsequent cor pulmonale, thus decreasing the development of fatal dysrhythmias. Data that suggest effectiveness of chronic supplemental O_2 have been gathered only on patients with underlying COPD. However, most clinicians believe that these data apply to other chronic hypoxemic pulmonary disorders.

The potential benefit of long-term O_2 therapy should be evaluated when the patient's condition has stabilized. There should be an accurate, current diagnosis and an optimal medical regimen prescribed by a physician knowledgeable in the treatment of respiratory disease. Short-term home O_2 therapy (1 to 30 days) may be indicated for the patient in whom hypoxemia persists after discharge from the hospital. For example, the patient with underlying COPD who develops a serious respiratory infection may continue to have clearing of the infection after completion of antibiotic therapy and discharge from the hospital. This patient may demonstrate continued hypoxemia for 4 to 6 weeks after discharge.

If a patient has a PaO_2 of less than 55 mm Hg (at sea level), it is generally considered that potential benefit can be gained from long-term O_2 therapy. The patient who demonstrates PaO_2 greater than 55 mm Hg but who also has evidence of hypoxia and organ dysfunction, such as secondary pulmonary hypertension, secondary erythrocytosis, impaired mental status, and CNS dysfunction, are also considered candidates for chronic O_2 therapy.[17] Medicare guidelines for reimbursement of the cost of home oxygen therapy follow these criteria. However, a PaO_2 of less than 59 mm Hg and an O_2 saturation of less than 89% are used as points of reference to determine necessity for chronic supplemental oxygen unless there is additional documentation by a physician regarding the presence of severe hypoxemic end organ dysfunction.

The need for O_2 during exercise may be demonstrated by showing significant desaturation with exertion and an increased tolerance for exercise when using supplemental O_2. The necessity for O_2 therapy during sleep to control sleep-induced hypoxemia is not well delineated. Significant nocturnal desaturation with associated sleep disturbance, cardiac dysrhythmias, or pulmonary hypertension should be demonstrated. Preferably these effects should be abolished by the use of O_2.

Technology for evaluation and monitoring patients for O_2 therapy includes arterial puncture for ABGs, placement of an indwelling arterial line for continuous monitoring, and pulse oximetry. Another method, transcutaneous monitoring, has been developed and is useful in neonatal intensive care unit (ICU) settings, but its reliability in adults is variable and thus not beneficial.[18] (Chapter 26 discusses methods to monitor oxygenation status of patients.)

ABGs provide the information necessary to evaluate acid-base and oxygenation status of a patient. However, technical errors that can decrease their validity are possible (e.g., too much heparin, failure to properly ice the sample, or improper calibration of the ABG equipment). Pulse oximetry should be used to avoid excessive invasive techniques during evaluation studies. An oximeter is a machine that measures light transmission through a thin layer of tissue (e.g., ear lobe, finger) and reports O_2 saturation of the arterial blood, giving a constant digital display.[19] It can be used to monitor saturation continuously during sleep, changes in position, and exertion to determine an individualized prescription for O_2 use. In addition, oximetry is useful in determination of O_2 requirements during hospitalization and during the weaning process from ventilatory support. (Pulse oximetry is discussed in Chapters 22 and 26.)

Periodic reevaluations are necessary for the patient who is using chronic supplemental O_2. Generally the recommendation is that the patient should be reevaluated every 6 months during the first year of therapy and annually after that, as long as the patient remains stable. This frequency of reevaluation is used by Medicare and other third party payors for reimbursement determinations.

Nasal cannulas, either regular or the O_2-conserving type (Table 24-13), are usually used to deliver O_2 from a central source in the home. The source may be a liquid O_2 storage system, compressed O_2 in tanks, or an O_2 concentrator or extractor, depending on the patient's home environment, activity level, and proximity to an O_2 supply company (Table 24-14). The patient can use extension tubing (up to 50 feet) without adversely affecting the O_2 flow delivery to increase mobility in the home, provided that the flowmeter is the back pressure-compensated type. Small portable systems may be provided for the patient who remains active outside the home (Fig. 24-6).

Table 24-14 Home Oxygen Delivery Systems

System	Advantages	Disadvantages	Comments
■ Liquid oxygen (reservoir/ portable unit)	Portable unit can be refilled by patient from reservoir. Portable unit holds 6-8 hr supply at 2 L/min; reservoir will last approximately 7-10 days at 2 L/min continuously.	Liquid system slightly more expensive, depending on location; not available everywhere; generally limited to urban areas.	As liquid warms to gas, some is vented from the system. In summer, evaporation is accelerated and may decrease reservoir duration to <1 wk.
■ Compressed tank O_2 (H or J tank/E or A cylinder for portable)	Good availability in most areas. Portability possible with cart. Aluminum E or A cylinders available that are markedly lighter than steel and easier to maneuver.	Duration of H or J tank at 2 L/min flow about 50 hr; storage of 4-5 large cylinders in the home necessary to have 1-wk to 10-day supply; portable cylinder on cart is cumbersome and heavy. Duration of E cylinder at 2 L/min approximately 4-5 hr; A cylinder at 2 L/min will last approximately 8-10 hr.	Some smaller tanks (D or M) may be used; these can be refilled from large cylinders and weigh about 10 lb. Tank can be carried on shoulder strap or placed on portable cart.
■ Concentrator or extractor (E or A cylinder for portable)	On wheels, movable from room to room; weekly delivery of supply not necessary, because unit delivers oxygen continuously; compact, excellent system for rural or homebound patient.	Older models can be noisy; increase in electricity bill by $20-$30 a month (not reimbursable by insurance); >3 L flow resulting in significant decrease in concentration.	Concentrator should be kept in room other than bedroom; extension tubing should be used if noise disturbs sleep.
■ Demand delivery system	Simple to use; delivery rate changes with respiratory rate, (i.e., the faster the patient's rate, the higher the rate of delivery).	Mechanically complex; only safe use with portable system when patient is awake (unless there is an alarm to detect disconnection of patient. Oxygenation possibly less efficient with exertion.	System may be a separate unit that can be used with liquid or cylinder, or can be "built in" to portable liquid oxygen unit.

Reservoir cannulas operate on the principle of storing O_2 in a small reservoir during exhalation. The O_2 is then delivered to the patient during the subsequent inhalation, almost like a bolus effect. The reservoir cannulas can reduce flow requirements by approximately 50%. Newer reservoir cannulas are available, and they may be less visible than the original moustache type. One is the pendant type (Fig. 24-5), and another fits onto the frame of eyeglasses.

Recent technologic advances in the delivery of chronic O_2 therapy include transtracheal O_2 delivery and intermittent-demand O_2 delivery systems. The greatest stimulus for these advances has been the increasingly high cost of home O_2 therapy. However, other benefits in addition to less waste of O_2 and therefore lower cost include the potential for less nasal irritation, prolonged availability of portable O_2 stores, and in the case of transtracheal O_2, less visibility of the O_2 delivery device.[20]

Transtracheal O_2 delivery requires a surgical procedure to insert the small O_2 catheter into the patient's trachea (Fig. 24-7). Nursing care involves teaching the patient and family how to care for the tracheostoma including how to clean and change the transtracheal catheter. Delivery of supplemental O_2 transtracheally reduces the flow requirement by 30% to 50%.[20]

Intermittent-demand delivery systems are mechanically complex devices. They deliver "pulses" of O_2 to the patient, usually during inspiration, and thus eliminate wasted flow during exhalation as is experienced during continuous flow. There are intermittent-demand units that

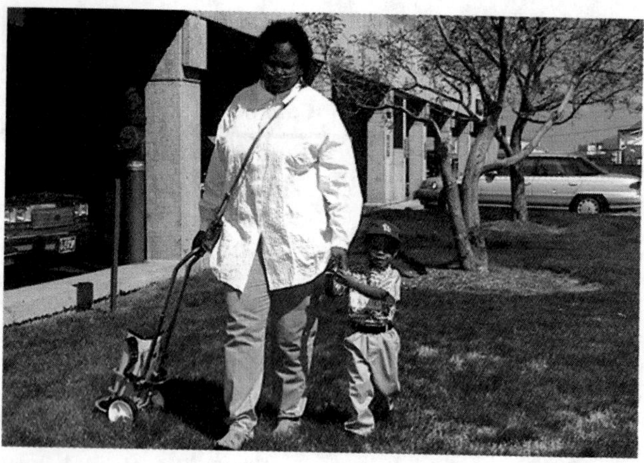

Fig. 24-6 Portable liquid oxygen system.

operate independently of a particular system as well as units that are built into the delivery device itself.

Home O_2 systems are usually rented from a company that sends a respiratory therapist or pulmonary nurse specialist to the patient's home. The therapist teaches the patient how to use the O_2 system, how to care for it, and how to recognize when the supply is running low and needs to be reordered.

The patient who uses home O_2 should be encouraged to remain active and to travel normally. If travel is by automobile, arrangements can be made for O_2 to be available at the destination point. O_2 supply companies can often assist in these arrangements. If a patient wishes to travel by airplane, the airlines require notification of the need for O_2 during the flight when reservations are made. Because the cabins are pressurized to an elevation of 7000 or 8000 feet, the patient who uses supplemental O_2 should have O_2 provided during flight. The plane's O_2 system must be used. The patient may not use the O_2 systems during flight because they are not properly pressurized. Most airlines will allow portable reservoirs (liquid or tank) to be carried in the baggage compartment for use at the point of destination as long as they are empty and the valves are left open. Some patients may need to avoid prolonged exposure to high elevations during travel unless they are instructed by their physician regarding adjustments in their O_2 flow to attempt to compensate for altitude.

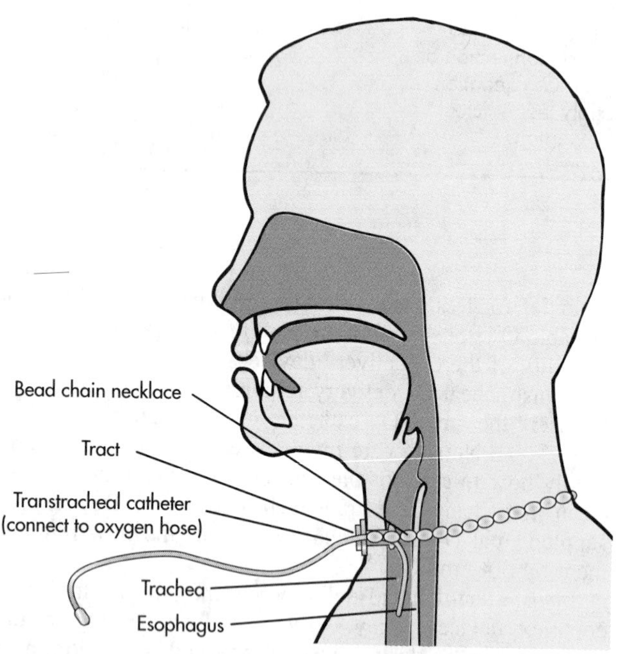

Fig. 24-7 Transtracheal catheter for oxygen administration.

OCCUPATIONAL LUNG DISEASES

Occupational lung diseases result from inhaled dust or chemicals.[21] The duration of exposure and the amount of inhalant have a major influence on whether the exposed individual will have lung damage. Another factor is the susceptibility of the host.

Pneumoconiosis is a general term for lung diseases caused by inhalation and retention of dust particles. The literal meaning of pneumoconiosis is "dust in the lungs." Examples of this condition are silicosis, asbestosis, and berylliosis. The classic response to the inhaled substance is diffuse parenchymal infiltration with phagocytic cells. This eventually results in *diffuse pulmonary fibrosis* (excess connective tissue). Fibrosis is the result of tissue repair after inflammation. Pneumoconiosis and other occupational lung diseases are presented in Table 24-15.

Chemical pneumonitis results from exposures to toxic chemical fumes. Acutely there is diffuse parenchymal injury characterized as pulmonary edema. Chronically the clinical picture is that of bronchiolitis obliterans, which is usually associated with a normal chest radiograph or shows hyperinflation. An example is silo filler's disease.

Hypersensitivity pneumonitis or extrinsic allergic alveolitis is the response seen when antigens are inhaled to which an individual is allergic. Examples include bird fancier's lung and farmer's lung.

Lung cancer is associated with exposure to a substantial number of chemicals including arsenic (used in oil refining, copper smelting, pesticides, tanning, and mining), nickel, petroleum products, and radiation. It is estimated that approximately 12% of lung cancer deaths are related to occupational exposures.[22]

Clinical Manifestations

Acute symptoms of pulmonary edema may be seen following early exposures to chemical fumes. However, symptoms of many occupational lung diseases may not occur until at least 10 to 15 years after the initial exposure to the inhaled irritant. Dyspnea and cough are often the earliest manifestations. Chest pain and productive cough and sputum production usually occur later. Complications that often result are pneumonia, chronic bronchitis, emphysema, and lung cancer. Cor pulmonale is a late complication, especially in conditions characterized by diffuse pulmonary

Table 24-15 Occupational Lung Diseases

Disease	Agents/Industries	Description	Complications
▪ Asbestosis	Asbestos fibers present in insulation, construction material (roof tiling, cement products), shipyards, textiles (for fireproofing), automobile clutch and brake linings	Disease appears 15-35 yr after first exposure, Interstitial fibrosis develops. Pleural plaques, which are calcified lesions, develop on pleura. Dyspnea, basal crackles, and decreased vital capacity are early manifestations.	Bronchogenic carcinoma,especially in cigarette smokers; mesothelioma (rare type of cancer affecting pleura and peritoneal membrane)
▪ Berylliosis	Beryllium dust present in aircraft manufacturing, metallurgy, rocket fuels	Noncaseating granulomas form. Acute pneumonitis occurs after heavy exposure. Interstitial fibrosis can also occur.	Progress of disease possible after removal of stimulating inhalant
▪ Bird fancier's, breeder's, or handler's lung	Bird droppings or feathers	Hypersensitivity pneumonitis is present.	Progressive fibrosis of lung
▪ Byssinosis	Cotton, flax, and hemp dust (textile industry)	Airway obstruction is caused by contraction of smooth muscles. Chronic disease results from severe airway obstruction and decreased elastic recoil.	Progression of chronic disease after cessation of dust exposure
▪ Coal worker's pneumoconiosis (black lung)	Coal dust	Incidence is high (20-30%) in coal workers. Deposits of carbon dust cause lesions to develop along respiratory bronchioles. Bronchioles dilate because of loss of wall structure. Chronic airway obstruction and bronchitis develop. Dyspnea and cough are common early symptoms.	Progressive, massive lung fibrosis; increased risk of chronic bronchitis and emphysema with smoking
▪ Farmer's lung	Inhalation of airborne material from moldy hay or similar matter	Hypersensitivity pneumonitis occurs. *Acute* form is similar to pneumonia, with manifestations of chills, fever, and malaise. *Chronic*, insidious form is type of pulmonary fibrosis.	Progressive fibrosis of lung
▪ Siderosis	Iron oxide present in welding materials, foundries, iron ore mining	Dust deposits are found in lung.	
▪ Silicosis	Silica dust present in quartz rock in mining of gold, copper, tin, coal, lead; also present in sandblasting, foundries, quarries, pottery making, masonry	In *chronic* disease, dust is engulfed by macrophages and may be destroyed, resulting in fibrotic nodules. *Acute* disease results from intense exposure in short time period. Within 5 yr, it progresses to severe disability from lung fibrosis.	Increased susceptibility to tuberculosis; progressive, massive fibrosis; high incidence of chronic bronchitis
▪ Silo filler's disease	Nitrogen oxides from fermentation of vegetation in freshly filled silo	Chemical pneumonitis occurs.	Progressive bronchiolitis obliterans

fibrosis. Manifestations of these complications can be the reason the patient seeks health care.

Pulmonary function studies often show reduced vital capacity. A chest x-ray will often reveal lung involvement specific to the primary problem. High resolution CT scans have been shown to be useful in detecting early parenchymal involvement.

Occupational asthma refers to the development of symptoms of shortness of breath, wheezing, cough, and chest tightness as a result of exposure to fumes or dust that trigger an allergic response. The obstruction may initially be reversible or intermittent, but continued exposure results in permanent obstructive changes. The best-known causative agent in occupational asthma is toluene diisocyanate (TDI), which is used in the production of rigid polyurethane foam.[23]

Therapeutic Management

The best approach to management is to try to prevent or decrease occupational risks. Well-designed, effective ventilation systems can reduce exposure to irritants. Wearing masks is appropriate in some occupations. Periodic inspections and monitoring of workplaces by agencies such as the Occupational Safety and Health Agency (OSHA) and the National Institute for Occupational Safety and Health (NIOSH) reinforce the obligations of employers to provide a safe work environment.

Cigarette smoking adds increased insult to the lungs, and the person at risk for occupational lung disease should not smoke. Additionally, recent evidence implicates secondhand smoke as an important source of occupational exposure with increased risk for development of lung cancer.[24] This has led to regulations requiring a smoke-free workspace for all employees.

Early diagnosis is essential if the disease process is to be halted. The best treatment is to decrease or stop exposure to the harmful agent. Some places of employment at which there is a known risk of lung disease may require periodic chest x-rays and pulmonary function studies for exposed employees. These measures can detect pulmonary changes before symptoms develop.

There is no specific treatment for most occupational lung diseases. Treatment is directed toward providing symptomatic relief. If there are coexisting problems, such as pneumonia, chronic bronchitis, emphysema, or asthma, they are treated.

LOWER RESPIRATORY TRACT MALIGNANCIES

Lung Cancer

Significance. Primary lung cancer is the leading cause of death in men and women who have malignant disease in the United States. Until recently, many more cases of lung cancer were found in men than in women. That situation is changing, probably because cigarette smoking has become socially acceptable for women since the 1930s and 1940s. The male to female ratio for lung cancer is about 1.4:1, only slightly greater for men.[25] Beginning in 1986, deaths from lung cancer in women exceeded deaths from all other cancers and are expected to continue to increase.[26]

CULTURAL & ETHNIC Considerations

LUNG CANCER

- Lung cancer occurs more frequently and has a higher mortality rate among non-Caucasians.
- Lung cancer is the most common newly diagnosed cancer among African-Americans.
- Prevalence of cigarette smoking is higher among African-Americans and Hispanics than Caucasians.

The mortality rate from lung cancer has increased during the past 50 years. In the past decade the death rate has escalated sharply for both men and women. In 1994 there were 153,000 deaths from lung cancer with 94,000 of these men. The overall 5-year survival rate is 13%, which is the poorest prognosis for any cancer other than cancers of the pancreas, liver, and esophagus.

Lung cancer most commonly occurs in individuals more than 50 years of age who have a long history of cigarette smoking. The disease is found most frequently in persons 40 to 75 years of age.

Causes and Risk Factors. Cigarette smoking as a chronic respiratory irritant is by far the major risk factor in the development of lung cancer. Smoking is responsible for approximately 80% to 90% of all lung cancers.[25] About one of every ten heavy smokers eventually develops lung cancer. Cigarette smoking causes a change in the bronchial epithelium, which usually returns to normal when smoking is discontinued. The risk of lung cancer is gradually lowered when smoking ceases and continues to decline with time.[23] It is estimated that it takes approximately 15 years for the risk for lung cancer of a former smoker to equal that of a nonsmoker.

The risk of developing lung cancer is directly related to total exposure to cigarette smoke measured by total number of cigarettes smoked in a lifetime, depth of inhalation, and tar and nicotine content of the cigarettes smoked. The report of the Surgeon General presented data that showed that side stream smoke is qualitatively similar to main stream smoke and concluded that involuntary (secondhand) smoking poses a risk for the development of lung cancer in nonsmokers.[24] One study reports that nonsmoking wives of smokers have a 34% higher rate of lung cancer than nonsmoking wives of nonsmokers.[27] Heredity may play a role in both the tendency to smoke and the predisposition to develop lung cancer. Because only a few persons (1 of 10) at high risk actually develop lung cancer, there is probably a difference in the host's ability to deal with the repeated insult of smoking.

Those who smoke pipes and cigars have also been shown to have an increased risk of developing lung cancer, which is slightly higher than that of nonsmokers. Cigar smokers are at higher rate for lung cancer than are pipe smokers. However, heavy smoking of small cigars and inhalation of smoke from small cigars have been shown to

RESEARCH

IMPLICATIONS FOR NURSING PRACTICE

SMOKING CESSATON

Citation Hill HA and others: A longitudinal analysis of predictors of quitting smoking among participants in a self-help intervention trial, *Addic Behav* 19:159-173, 1994.

Purpose To determine predictors of abstinence from smoking.

Methods Descriptive longitudinal study involving adult smokers (n = 2021) belonging to a health maintenance organization who were offered free "do-it-yourself" assistance in quitting smoking. Subjects were randomized into four groups including three intervention groups receiving various quitting aids, and a control group who was given a resource guide describing available self-help material. Self-reported smoking status was assessed at 8, 16, and 24 months following enrollment.

Results and Conclusions Quit status for all subjects at 8, 16, and 24 months indicated quit rates of 16%, 18%, and 20%, respectively. Seventeen items emerged as significant predictors of the ability to quit smoking. These included support from significant others, confidence in one's ability to become a nonsmoker, having set a quit date, having previously quit for more than 90 days, being married, and perceiving weight control as a serious problem. Factors negatively associated with success in quitting included higher nicotine dependence, greater tension, and presence of smoking-related medical conditions.

Implications for Nursing Practice This study indicates that emphasis should be put on psychosocial or motivational factors and quitting activities as important factors in predicting long-term abstinence. High self-efficacy and benefits of social support are important positive influences in quitting smoking. The nurse can assist the patient in quitting smoking by helping the patient gain confidence in the ability to quit and soliciting support from significant others.

correlate with the rates of lung cancer observed in cigarette smokers.

Another major risk factor for lung cancer is inhaled carcinogens. These include asbestos, nickel, iron and iron oxides, uranium, polycyclic aromatic hydrocarbons, chromates, arsenic, and air pollution. Exposure to these substances is common for employees of industries involved in mining, smelting, or chemical or petroleum manufacturing.[22] The cigarette smoker who is also exposed to one or more of these chemicals or to high amounts of air pollution is at significantly higher risk for lung cancer.

Lung cancer does occur in individuals who have never smoked or worked with carcinogens. The reasons for this are not known but heredity may play a part. The host's response to environmental insults is important in determining who develops lung cancer.

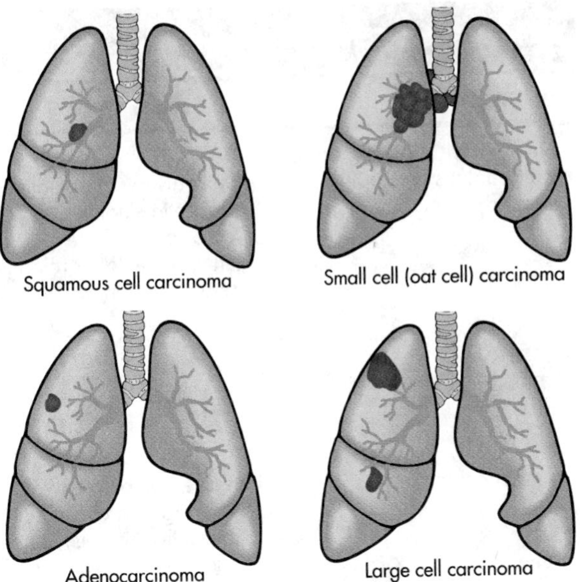

Fig. 24-8 Predominant sites of types of lung cancer.

Another possible risk factor is preexisting pulmonary diseases such as TB, pulmonary fibrosis, bronchiectasis, and COPD. Chronic inflammatory conditions often precede cancer. The incidence of lung cancer correlates with the degree of urbanization and population density. One reason for this may be increased exposure to irritants and pollutants.

Pathophysiology. The pathogenesis of primary lung cancer is not well understood. More than 90% of cancers originate from the epithelium of the bronchus (bronchogenic). They grow slowly, and it takes 8 to 10 years for a tumor to reach 1 cm in size, which is the smallest detectable lesion on an x-ray. Lung cancers occur primarily in the segmental bronchi or beyond and have a preference for the upper lobes of the lungs (Fig. 24-8). Pathologic changes in the bronchial system show nonspecific inflammatory changes with hypersecretion of mucus, desquamation of cells, reactive hyperplasia of the basal cells, and metaplasia of normal respiratory epithelium to stratified squamous cells.

Primary lung cancers are often categorized into histologic types (Table 24-16). They metastasize primarily by direct extension and via the blood circulation and the lymph system. The common sites for metastatic growth are the liver, brain, bones, scalene lymph nodes, and adrenal glands.

Paraneoplastic syndrome. Certain lung cancers cause the paraneoplastic syndrome, which is characterized by various manifestations caused by certain substances (e.g., hormones, enzymes, antigens) produced by the tumor cells. Small cell carcinomas are most commonly associated with the paraneoplastic syndrome. The systemic manifestations are the following:

1. *Hormonal* (Table 24-17)
2. *Dermatologic*, including dermatomyositis and acanthosis nigricans

Table 24-16 Comparison of the Types of Primary Lung Cancer

Cell Type	Risk Factors	Characteristics	Response to Therapy
Nonsmall Cell Lung Cancer			
▪ Squamous cell (epidermoid) carcinoma	Almost always associated with cigarette smoking, is associated with exposure to environmental carcinogens (e.g., uranium, asbestos)	Accounts for 30-35% of lung cancers; is more common in men; arises from the bronchial epithelium, produces earlier symptoms because of bronchial obstructive characteristics; does not have a strong tendency to metastasize, metastasizes locally by direct extension, causes cavitating pulmonary lesions	Surgical resection is often attempted, life expectancy is better than for undifferentiated (anaplastic) carcinoma
▪ Adenocarcinoma	Has been associated with lung scarring and chronic interstitial fibrosis, is not related to cigarette smoking	Accounts for approximately 50% of lung cancers, is more common in women; often has no clinical manifestations until widespread metastasis is present, metastasizes via bloodstream, is most commonly located in peripheral portions of lungs*	Surgical resection is often attempted, cancer does not respond well to chemotherapy
▪ Large cell undifferentiated	High correlation with cigarette smoking and exposure to environmental carcinogens	Accounts for 5-10% of lung cancers, commonly causes cavitation, is highly metastatic via lymphatics and blood, commonly peripheral rather than central	Surgery is not usually attempted because of high rate of metastases, tumor may be radiosensitive but often recurs
Small Cell Lung Cancer			
▪ Small cell anaplastic undifferentiated (includes oat cell)	Associated with cigarette smoking, exposure to environmental carcinogens	Accounts for 15-25% of lung cancers, is most malignant form, tends to spread early via lymphatics and bloodstream, is frequently associated with endocrine disturbances, predominantly central and can cause bronchial obstruction and pneumonia	Cancer has poorest prognosis; however, recent chemotherapy gains have been substantial: 70% response rate with chemotherapy; radiation is used as adjuvant therapy, as well as palliative measure; average median survival is <1 yr

*See Fig. 24-8.

3. *Neuromuscular*, including peripheral neuropathy, cortical cerebellar degeneration, and a syndrome similar to myasthenia gravis
4. *Vascular* and *hematologic*, including thrombocytopenic purpura, anemia, leukemia-like reaction, thrombophlebitis, and nonbacterial endocarditis
5. *Connective tissue*, including nonspecific arthralgias, hypertrophic pulmonary osteoarthropathy, and digital clubbing.

Clinical Manifestations. The clinical manifestations of lung cancer are usually nonspecific and appear late in the disease process. Manifestations depend on the type of primary lung cancer. Often there is extensive metastasis before symptoms become apparent. Persistent pneumonitis that is a result of obstructed bronchi may be one of the earliest manifestations, causing fever, chills, and cough.

One of the most significant symptoms, and often the one reported first, is a persistent cough that may be productive

Table 24-17 Ectopic Hormone Syndromes of Lung Cancer

Syndrome	Ectopic Hormone	Most Common Cell Type
Cushing's syndrome	Adrenocorticotropic hormone	Oat cell (small cell)
Syndrome of inappropriate antidiuretic hormone	Antidiuretic hormone	Oat cell (small cell)
Hypercalcemia	Parathyroid hormone	Squamous cell
Gynecomastia	Follicle-stimulating hormone	Large cell
Carcinoid syndrome	5-hydroxyindoleacetic acid (5-HIAA) from serotonin breakdown.	Oat cell (small cell)
		Bronchial adenoma (adenocarcinoma)

of sputum. Blood-tinged sputum may be produced because of bleeding caused by malignancy, but hemoptysis is not a common early presenting symptom. Chest pain may be present and localized or unilateral, ranging from mild to severe. Dyspnea and an auscultatory wheeze may be present if there is bronchial obstruction.

Later manifestations may include nonspecific systemic symptoms such as anorexia, fatigue, weight loss, and nausea and vomiting. Hoarseness may be present as a result of involvement of the recurrent laryngeal nerve. Unilateral paralysis of the diaphragm, dysphagia, and superior vena cava obstruction may occur because of intrathoracic spread of the malignancy. There may be palpable lymph nodes in the neck or axilla. Mediastinal involvement may lead to pericardial effusion, cardiac tamponade, and dysrhythmias.

Diagnostic Studies. Chest x-rays are widely used in the diagnosis of lung cancer. Anyone who has had a cough or a change in a cough for more than 2 to 3 weeks should be evaluated by chest x-ray examination. The findings may show the presence of the tumor or abnormalities related to the obstructive features of the tumor such as atelectasis and pneumonitis. The x-ray can also show evidence of metastasis to the ribs or vertebrae and the presence of pleural effusion. Lung tomograms may be used to locate the tumor and to estimate the extent of involvement of nearby structures.

CT scans are also used in the diagnosis of lung cancer. With CT scans, the location and extent of masses in the chest can be identified as well as any mediastinal involvement or lymph node enlargement. Magnetic resonance imaging (MRI) is a radiographic technique that may be used in combination with or instead of CT scans. The most recent advance in imaging techniques, the positron-emission tomography (PET), promises to be a useful diagnostic tool in early detection of cancers as well as in staging and monitoring the effects of treatment. PET allows measurement of differential metabolic activity in normal and diseased tissues.[28]

A definitive diagnosis of lung cancer is made by identifying malignant cells. Sputum specimens are usually obtained for cytologic studies and may identify tumors that involve the bronchial wall. An early-morning specimen that has been obtained by having the patient cough deeply provides the most accurate results. However, malignant cells may not be obtained even in the presence of a lung cancer.[29]

The use of the fiberoptic bronchoscope is important in the diagnosis of lung cancer, particularly when the lesions are endobronchial or are in close proximity to an airway. It provides direct visualization and allows biopsy specimens to be obtained. A biopsy is usually the best method for establishing the presence of a malignant tumor.

Mediastinoscopy involves the insertion of a scope via a small anterior chest incision into the mediastinum. This is done to examine for metastasis in the anterior mediastinum or hilum or in the chest extrapleurally. It is also used to determine the stage of the lung cancer, which is important in determining the treatment plan.

Other diagnostic studies include radionuclide scans of the liver, spleen, bone, or brain and scalene lymph node biopsy to determine metastatic spread. Pulmonary angiography and lung scans may be performed to assess overall pulmonary status. Fine-needle aspiration (FNA) may be used to obtain a tissue sample to determine tumor histology. FNA is most useful in cases involving a peripheral lesion near the chest wall, and it is usually attempted in an effort to avoid a thoracotomy. If a thoracentesis is performed to relieve a pleural effusion, the fluid should be analyzed for malignant cells. (Table 24-18 summarizes the diagnostic management of lung cancer.)

Staging. Staging of nonsmall cell lung cancer (NSCLC) is performed according to the American Joint Committee's TNM staging system in a manner similar to that for other tumors (Table 24-19). Assessment criteria are *T*, which denotes tumor size, location, and degree of invasion; *N*, which indicates regional lymph node involvement; and *M*, which represents the presence or absence of distant metastases. Depending on the TNM designation, the tumor is then staged, which assists in estimating prognosis and appropriate therapy.

Staging of small cell lung cancer (SCLC) has not been useful because the cancer has usually metastasized by the time a diagnosis is made. Instead, SCLC is determined to be *limited* (confined to one hemothorax and to regional lymph nodes) or *extensive* according to a staging system for SCLC developed by the Veterans Affairs Lung Cancer Study Group.[30]

Therapeutic Management

Surgical resection. Surgical resection is usually the only hope for cure in lung cancer. Unfortunately, detection is often so late that the tumor is no longer localized and is

Table 24-18 Therapeutic Management: Lung Cancer

Diagnostic
Health history and physical examination
Chest x-ray
Sputum for cytologic study
Bronchoscopy
Spirometry (preoperative)
Mediastinoscopy
Scalene node biopsy
Pulmonary angiography
Lung scan
CT scan
FNA
MRI
Therapeutic
Surgery
Radiation therapy
Chemotherapy
Immunotherapy
Phototherapy (Nd-YAG Laser)

CT, Computed tomography; *FNA,* fine-needle aspiration; *MRI,* magnetic resonance imaging.

not amenable to resection. Resectability of the tumor is a major consideration in planning the surgical intervention. Oat cell (small cell) carcinomas usually have widespread metastasis at the time of diagnosis. Therefore surgery is usually contraindicated. In contrast, squamous cell carcinomas are more likely to be treated with surgery because they remain localized, or if they metastasize they primarily do so by local spread.

When the tumor is considered operable with a potential for cure, the patient's cardiopulmonary status must be evaluated to determine the ability to withstand surgery. This is done by clinical studies of pulmonary function, ABGs, and others, as indicated by the individual's status. Contraindications for thoracotomy include hypercapnia, pulmonary hypertension, cor pulmonale, and markedly reduced lung function. Coexisting conditions such as cardiac, renal, and liver disease are also contraindications for surgery.

A tumor may be potentially resectable but if it is located in a critical area, such as the trachea or too close to the heart, it may be considered inoperable. The type of surgery performed is usually a *lobectomy* (removal of one or more lobes of the lung) and less often a *pneumonectomy* (removal of one entire lung).

Radiation therapy. Radiation therapy is used as a curative approach in the individual who has a resectable tumor but who is considered a poor surgical risk. Adenocarcinomas are the most radioresistant type of cancer cell. Although small-cell carcinomas are radiosensitive, radiation (even when used in combination with chemotherapy) does not significantly improve the mortality rate because of the early metastases of this type of cancer.

Radiation therapy is also done as a palliative procedure to reduce distressing symptoms such as cough, hemoptysis, bronchial obstruction, and superior vena cava syndrome. It can be used to treat pain that is caused by metastatic bone lesions or cerebral metastasis. Radiation used as a preoperative or postoperative adjuvant measure has not been found to significantly increase survival in the patient with lung cancer.[31]

Chemotherapy. Chemotherapy may be used in the treatment of nonresectable tumors or as adjuvant therapy to surgery in NSCLC with distant metastases. Multidrug regimens (i.e., protocols including combination chemotherapy) using cyclophosphamide, methotrexate, methyl CCNU, and vincristine have increased the survival rate in patients with oat cell carcinomas. Most persons with SCLC enjoy partial or complete responses to combination chemotherapy. However, the patient needs to be aware that a cure or long-term survival is rarely a reality.

Chemotherapy has not shown any significant results when used for treatment of squamous cell carcinoma and adenocarcinoma. Symptomatic improvement and tumor regression will usually last for only a period of months.

Biologic response modifiers. Biologic response modifiers (BRM) as adjuvant therapy have been used in individuals with cancer including malignant lung tumors. (BRM are discussed in Chapter 12.)

Laser surgery. Laser surgery, with the use of the Nd-YAG laser via a fiberoptic bronchoscope, makes it possible to remove obstructing bronchial lesions as large as 2 cm in depth.[32] It is a complicated procedure that often requires general anesthesia to control the patient's cough reflex. Relief of the symptoms from airway obstruction as a result of thermal necrosis and shrinkage of the tumor can be dramatic. However, it is not a curative therapy for cancer.

NURSING MANAGEMENT
LUNG CANCER

Nursing Assessment

It is important to determine the understanding of the patient and the family concerning the diagnostic tests (those completed as well as those planned), the diagnosis or potential diagnosis, the treatment options, and the prognosis. At the same time the nurse can assess the level of anxiety experienced by the patient and the support provided and needed by the patient's significant others. Subjective and objective data that should be obtained from a patient with lung cancer are presented in Table 24-20.

Nursing Diagnoses

Nursing diagnoses specific to the patient with lung cancer include, but are not limited to, the following:

- Ineffective airway clearance secondary to increased tracheobronchial secretions
- Anxiety related to lack of knowledge of diagnosis or unknown prognosis and treatments
- Pain from pressure of tumor on surrounding structures and erosion of tissues
- Altered nutrition: less than body requirements related to increased metabolic demands, increased secretions, weakness, and anorexia

Table 24-19 Lung Cancer TNM Classifications

Tumor Definitions

T_x Tumor proved by cytologic studies but not visualized by radiograph or bronchoscope
T_0 No evidence of tumor
T_{is} Carcinoma in situ
T_1 Tumor 3 cm or less in greatest dimension, surrounded by lung or visceral pleura, without invasion proximal to lobar bronchus
T_2 Tumor greater than 3 cm in diameter or invading visceral pleura or with atelectasis or obstructive pneumonitis extending to the hilum; proximal extent of tumor at least 2 cm from carina
T_3 Tumor with direct extension into chest wall, diaphragm, mediastinal pleura, or pericardium without involvement of mediastinal viscera; tumor within 2 cm of carina but not involving carina
T_4 Tumor invading mediastinal viscera or carina or with malignant pleural effusion

Nodal Involvement

N_0 No nodal metastasis
N_1 Metastasis to peribronchial or ipsilateral hilar lymph nodes
N_2 Metastasis to ipsilateral mediastinal or subcarinal lymph nodes
N_3 Metastasis to contralateral mediastinal or hilar lymph nodes or any scalene or supraclavicular node

Distant Metastases

M_0 No known metastasis
M_1 Presence of distant metastasis

Stage Grouping

Stage	T	N	M
Occult Carcinoma	T_x	N_0	M_0
Stage 0	T_{is}	Carcinoma in situ	M_0
Stage I	T_1	N_0	M_0
	T_2	N_0	M_0
Stage II	T_1	N_1	M_0
	T_2	N_1	M_0
Stage IIIA	T_3	N_0	M_0
	T_3	N_1	M_0
	$T_{1\text{-}3}$	N_2	M_0
Stage IIIB	Any T	N_3	M_0
	T_4	Any N	M_0
Stage IV	Any T	Any N	M_1

TNM, Tumor node metastases.

- Altered health maintenance related to lack of knowledge about the disease process and therapeutic regimen
- Ineffective breathing pattern related to decreased lung capacity

Planning

The overall goals are that the patient with lung cancer will have (1) effective breathing patterns, (2) adequate airway clearance, (3) adequate oxygenation of tissues, (4) minimal to no pain, and (5) realistic attitude toward treatment and prognosis.

Nursing Implementation

Health Promotion and Maintenance. The best way to halt the epidemic of lung cancer is for people to stop smoking. In agreement with this primary prevention goal the U.S. Surgeon General has set forth the objective of achieving a smokeless society by the year 2000.[33] Important nursing activities to assist in the progress toward this goal include promoting smoking cessation programs and actively supporting education and policy changes deterring social, economic, and political patterns that have, in the past, encouraged smoking. Some recent important changes that have occurred as the result of nonsmokers' assertions that sidestream smoke is a health hazard are laws requiring designation of nonsmoking areas in most public places or prohibiting it altogether and a ban on smoking on most domestic airline flights. Other actions aimed at controlling tobacco use include restrictions on tobacco advertising on television and warning label requirements for cigarette packaging. These are examples of beginning steps toward the goal of a smokeless society. Other strategies may be to ban cigarettes and other tobacco products or to tax them heavily to prevent many people, such as adolescents, from taking up the habit or continuing it. Despite the small advances being made, strong political influences by tobacco-producing states remain. For example, low taxes still exist on the sale of cigarettes.

For the individual who does have a tobacco habit, efforts should be made to assist the smoker to stop smoking. Nicotine's addictive properties make quitting a difficult task and requires much support. Research into smoking behaviors and successful strategies to promote smoking cessation is ongoing. However, many factors are recognized as being important in the initiation and continuation of smoking, such as peer pressure, rebelliousness, curiosity, self-image, environmental cues, and psychologic needs. Programs designed to assist the individual to stop smoking use strategies such as education, environmental control, social support, and slow nicotine withdrawal with varying degrees of success. Other methods offered in smoking cessation programs may involve hypnosis, behavioral interventions, nicotine weaning (with products such as nicotine polacrilex gum or transdermal patches), and aversion therapy. The most successful programs combine a behavior modification approach with pharmacologic intervention to decrease nicotine dependence.[34] Group support programs, individual therapy, and self-help options are also available.

Most smokers have tried to quit smoking several times, and relatively few are successful. The nurse needs to be aware of resources in the community to assist the individual who is interested in quitting. Local chapters of the American Lung Association and the American Cancer Society have information on available programs.

An important part of concentrated efforts to prevent smoking-related health problems is recognizing what influences people, particularly children and adolescents, to begin smoking. Programs developed to help children explore the external influences (e.g., peer pressure) that may cause one to start smoking and that help them identify alternative behaviors make it less likely for these children to start smoking. An emphasis on the health hazards of smoking, as well as on those of other addictive behaviors, should be part of the total curriculum beginning in elementary schools.

The nurse who smokes is in a difficult position to help the patient change smoking habits. The nurse as a role model can do much to facilitate or harm educational attempts with persons in the community as well as in the hospital. Therefore if the nurse smokes, the nurse must try to stop before serving as a role model for the patient. A smoker turned nonsmoker may be in a good position to suggest strategies for success.

Screening chest x-rays every 6 to 12 months may be of value for the individual considered at high risk for lung cancer. This consideration applies to persons employed in uranium mining, asbestos-related industries, iron foundries, and other industries with known respiratory carcinogens, as well as to those who are heavy cigarette smokers.

When a nurse is obtaining a health history from a patient (even a patient with nonrespiratory problems), it is important to get information related to respiratory carcinogens. The patient should be asked about occupational exposure to asbestos, uranium, arsenic, nickel, iron and iron oxides, and excessive exposure to air pollution. In addition, a detailed history of cigarette smoking should be obtained. This information should be used to evaluate the patient's risk of developing lung cancer and also to teach the patient about early recognition of symptoms. Anyone with a history of exposure to respiratory carcinogens who has pneumonitis that persists for longer than 2 weeks in spite of antibiotic therapy should be evaluated for the possibility of lung cancer.

The individual with a chronic cough or a change in the character of a cough should be encouraged to obtain care. In addition, the person with chronic or recurring respiratory infections should be carefully evaluated, especially if the person smokes cigarettes.

Acute Intervention. Care of the patient with lung cancer will initially involve support and reassurance during the diagnostic evaluation. (Specific nursing measures related to the diagnostic studies are outlined in Chapter 22.)

Another major responsibility of the nurse is to help the patient and the family deal with the diagnosis of lung

Table 24-20 Nursing Assessment: Lung Cancer

Subjective Data

Important health information

Past health history: Smoking history (number of cigarettes smoked per day, years of smoking, amount of tar and nicotine in cigarettes); exposure to second-hand smoke; airborne carcinogens (e.g., asbestos, uranium, chromates, hydrocarbons, arsenic) or other pollutants; urban living environment; chronic lung disease, including TB, COPD, bronchiectasis

Medications: Use of cough medicines or other respiratory medications

Functional health patterns

Health perception–health management: Frequent respiratory infections; family history of lung cancer

Nutritional-metabolic: Anorexia, nausea, vomiting, dysphagia (late); weight loss; jaundice (liver metastasis); fever, chills

Activity-exercise: Persistent cough (productive or nonproductive); dyspnea, hemoptysis (late symptom)

Cognitive-perceptual: Chest pain or tightness, shoulder and arm pain, headache, bone pain (late symptom)

Objective Data

General

Neck and axillary lymphadenopathy, paraneoplastic syndromes (syndrome of inappropriate ADH; ACTH secretion; hypercalcemia; vascular, neuromuscular, dermatologic, and connective tissue disorders)

Respiratory

Wheezing, hoarseness, stridor, unilateral diaphragm paralysis, pleural effusions (late signs)

Cardiovascular

Edema of neck and face (superior vena cava syndrome), finger clubbing, pericardial effusion, cardiac tamponade, dysrhythmias (late signs)

Neurologic

Unsteady gait (brain metastasis)

Musculoskeletal

Pathologic fractures, muscle wasting (late)

Possible findings

Low serum sodium and hypercalcemia (paraneoplastic syndrome); observance of lesion on chest x-ray, CT scan, or lung scan; positive sputum or bronchial washings for cytologic studies; positive fiberoptic bronchoscopy and biopsy findings

ACTH, Adrenocorticotropic hormone; *ADH,* antidiuretic hormone; *COPD,* chronic obstructive pulmonary disease; *CT,* computed tomography; *TB,* tuberculosis.

cancer. The patient may feel guilty about cigarette smoking having caused the cancer and need to discuss this feeling with someone who has a nonjudgmental attitude. Questions regarding each patient's condition should be answered honestly. Additional counseling from a social worker, psychologist, or member of the clergy may be needed.

Specific care of the patient will depend on the treatment plan. Postoperative care for the patient having surgery is discussed later in this chapter. Care of the patient undergoing radiation therapy and chemotherapy is discussed in Chapter 12. The nurse has a major role in providing patient comfort, teaching methods to reduce pain, and assessing indications for hospitalization (see Chapter 12).

Chronic and Home Management. The patient who has had a surgical resection with intent to cure should be followed up carefully for manifestations of metastasis. The patient and family should be told to contact the physician if symptoms such as hemoptysis, dysphagia, chest pain, and hoarseness develop.

For many individuals who have lung cancer, little can be done to significantly prolong their lives. Radiation therapy and chemotherapy can be used to provide palliative relief from distressing symptoms. Constant pain becomes a major problem. (Measures used to relieve pain are discussed in Chapter 6. Care of the patient with cancer is discussed in Chapter 12.)

Other Types of Lung Tumors

Other types of primary lung tumors include sarcomas, lymphomas, and bronchial adenomas. Bronchial adenomas are small tumors that arise from the lower trachea or major bronchi and are considered malignant because they are locally invasive and frequently metastasize. Clinical manifestations of bronchial adenomas include hemoptysis, persistent cough, localized obstructive wheezing, and purulent bronchitis. There may be secondary bronchiectasis in long-standing cases. Bronchial adenomas frequently cause endocrine paraneoplastic manifestations. They can usually be treated successfully with surgical resection.

The lungs are a common site for secondary metastases and are more often affected by metastatic growth than by primary lung tumors. The pulmonary capillaries, with their extensive network, are ideal sites for tumor emboli. In addition, the lungs have an extensive lymphatic network. The primary malignancies that spread to the lungs often originate in the gastrointestinal (GI) or genitourinary (GU) tracts and in the breast. General symptoms of lung metastases are chest pain and nonproductive cough.

Benign tumors of the lung are generally classified as *mesenchymal*. Their occurrence is rare, and they have the potential to become malignant. The most common mesenchymal tumors are chondromas, which arise in the bronchial cartilage, and leiomyomas, which are myomas of smooth, nonstriated muscle fibers.

Hamartomas of the lung are mixtures of fibrous tissue, fat, and blood vessels. They are congenital malformations of the connective tissue of the bronchiolar walls.

CHEST TRAUMA AND THORACIC INJURIES

Traumatic injuries fall into two major categories: (1) blunt trauma and (2) penetrating trauma. *Blunt trauma* occurs when the body is struck by a blunt object such as a steering wheel. The external injury may appear minor, but the impact may cause severe, life-threatening internal injuries such as a ruptured spleen. *Contrecoup trauma*, a type of blunt trauma, is caused by the impact of parts of the body against other objects. This type of injury differs from blunt trauma primarily in the velocity of the impact. Internal organs are rapidly forced back and forth within the bony structures that surround them so that internal injury is sustained not only on the side of the impact but also on the opposite side where the organ or organs hit bony structures. If the velocity of impact is great enough, organs and blood vessels can literally be torn from their points of origin. Many head injuries are caused by contrecoup trauma.

Penetrating trauma occurs when a foreign body impales or passes through the body tissues (e.g., gunshot wounds, stabbings). Table 24-21 describes selective traumatic inju-

Table 24-21 Common Traumatic Chest Injuries and Mechanisms of Injury

Mechanism of Injury	Common Related Injury
Blunt Trauma	
Blunt steering-wheel injury to chest	Rib fractures, flail chest, pneumothorax, hemopneumothorax, cardiac contusion, pulmonary contusion, cardiac tamponade, great vessel tears
Shoulder-harness seat belt injury	Fractured clavicle, dislocated shoulder, rib fractures, pulmonary contusion, pericardial contusion, cardiac tamponade
Crush injury (e.g., heavy equipment, crushing thorax)	Pneumothorax and hemopneumothorax, flail chest, great vessel tears and rupture, decreased blood return to heart with decreased cardiac output
Penetrating Trauma	
Gunshot or stab wound to chest	Open pneumothorax, tension pneumothorax, hemopneumothorax, cardiac tamponade, esophageal damage, tracheal tear, great vessel tears

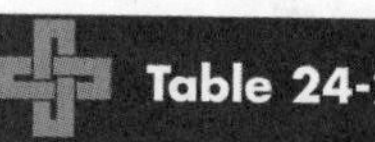

Table 24-22 Emergency Management: Chest Injury

Possible Etiologies

Blunt (e.g., fall, motor vehicle accident, struck by an object) or penetrating trauma (e.g., knife, gunshot wound)

Possible Assessment Findings

Obvious trauma to chest wall (e.g., bruising, open wound)
Chest pain
Dyspnea, shortness of breath, difficulty in breathing
Cough (with or without hemoptysis)
Asymmetric chest movement
Cyanosis of mouth, face, nail beds, mucous membranes
Rapid, weak pulse
Decreased blood pressure
Deviation of trachea
Distended neck veins
Audible air escaping from chest
Subcutaneous emphysema
Decreased breath sounds on side of injury
Muffled heart sounds

Management

- Establish and maintain airway. Anticipate need for intubation if respiratory distress evident.
- Administer high flow humidified O_2 using nonrebreather mask.
- Establish IV access with two large gauge catheters.
- Remove clothing to assess injury sites.
- Monitor vital signs, level of consciousness, oxygen saturation, urinary output.
- Assess for tension pneumothorax and, if present, do a needle thoracostomy.
- Dress sucking chest wound with nonporous dressing taped on three sides.
- *Do not* remove impaled objects; stabilize them with bulky dressings.
- Assess for other injuries such as bleeding and treat appropriately.
- Put patient in a semi-Fowler's position or lay patient on the injured side if breathing is easier.

ries as they relate to the categories of trauma and the mechanism of injury. Emergency care of the patient with a chest injury is presented in Table 24-22.

Thoracic injuries range from simple rib fractures to life-threatening tears of the aorta, vena cava, and other major vessels. The most common thoracic emergencies and their management are described in Table 24-23.

Pneumothorax

A *pneumothorax* is a complete or partial collapse of a lung as a result of an accumulation of air in the intrapleural space. This condition should be suspected after any blunt trauma to the chest wall. Pneumothorax may be closed or open. Pneumothorax associated with trauma may be accompanied by hemothorax, a condition called *hemopneumothorax*.

Closed Pneumothorax. Closed pneumothorax has no associated external wound. The most common form is a *spontaneous pneumothorax*, which is caused by rupture of small blebs on the visceral pleural space. The cause of the blebs is unknown. This condition occurs most commonly in male cigarette smokers between 20 and 40 years of age. There is a tendency for this condition to recur.

Other causes of closed pneumothorax include the following:

1. Injury to the lungs from mechanical ventilation
2. Injury to the lungs from insertion of a subclavian catheter
3. Perforation of the esophagus
4. Injury to the lungs from broken ribs
5. Ruptured blebs or bullae in a patient with COPD

Open Pneumothorax. Open pneumothorax occurs when air enters the pleural space through an opening in the chest wall (Fig. 24-9, *B*). Examples include stab or gunshot wounds and surgical thoracotomies. A penetrating chest wound is often referred to as a *sucking chest wound.*

An open pneumothorax should be covered with a vented dressing. (A vented dressing is one secured on three sides with the fourth side left untaped.) This allows air to escape from the vent and decreases the likelihood of tension pneumothorax developing. If the object that caused the open chest wound is still in place, it should not be removed until a physician is present.

Tension Pneumothorax. Tension pneumothorax may result from either an open or a closed pneumothorax. In an open chest wound, a flap may act as a one-way valve; thus, air can enter on inspiration but cannot escape. Intrathoracic pressure increases, the lung collapses, and the mediastinum shifts toward the unaffected side, which is subsequently compressed. As the intrathoracic pressure increases, cardiac output is altered because there is decreased venous return and compression of the great vessels. Tension pneumothorax is a medical emergency because both the respiratory and circulatory systems are affected. Nurses and paramedics are now being trained to insert large-bore needles and chest tubes into the chest wall to release the trapped air. Tension pneumothorax may also occur when chest tubes are clamped or become blocked in a patient after insertion for treatment of pneumothorax. Unclamping the tube or relief of the obstruction will remedy this situation.

Hemothorax. Hemothorax is an accumulation of blood in the intrapleural space. It is frequently found in association with open pneumothorax and is then called a *hemopneumothorax.* Causes of hemothorax include chest trauma, lung malignancy, complication of anticoagulant therapy, pulmonary embolus, and tearing of pleural adhesions.

Clinical Manifestations. The patient with a pneumothorax has respiratory distress including shallow, rapid respirations, dyspnea, and air hunger. Chest pain and a cough with or without hemoptysis may be present. On

Table 24-23 Clinical Manifestations and Emergency Management of Thoracic Injuries

Injury	Definition	Clinical Manifestation	Emergency Management
▪ Pneumothorax	Collection of air between chest wall and lung	Dyspnea, pain, decreased movement of involved chest wall, diminished breath sounds on injured side	Insertion of large-bore needle with attached one-way valve to release air from pleural cavity, chest tube insertion to underwater seal or one-way valve, application of vented dressing
▪ Hemothorax	Collection of blood between chest wall and lung, usually occurring with pneumothorax	Same as pneumothorax	Insertion of chest tube and aspiration of pleural cavity, treatment of hypovolemic shock if present
▪ Tension pneumothorax	Collection of air between chest wall and lung; no escape of air during expiration; rapid increase of air in pleural cavity, causing shifting of intrathoracic organs and increased intrathoracic pressure	Cyanosis, air hunger, violent agitation, trachea deviated to side opposite injury, subcutaneous emphysema	Insertion of chest tube or large-bore needle to relieve air pressure in thorax and treat hypoxia
▪ Flail chest	Fracture of two or more adjacent ribs in two or more places, causing loss of stability of chest wall; possibly occurring with pneumothorax, hemothorax, and tension pneumothorax	Paradoxical movement of chest wall and respiratory distress	Humidified O_2 therapy, reexpansion of the lung, IV fluids (some situations requiring intubation and mechanical ventilation), intercostal nerve blocks to relieve pain, judicious use of systemic analgesics, rapid administration of IV fluids
▪ Cardiac tamponade	Rapid collection of blood in pericardial sac from laceration of blood vessels, pericardium's inelasticity preventing heart from pumping blood	Muffled and distant heart sounds, failing or absent blood pressure or pulses, steadily increasing central venous pressure; distention of neck veins possible	Cardiopulmonary resuscitation if no pulses present, immediate aspiration of blood from pericardium with needle and syringe by physician, surgery to repair torn vessel

IV, Intravenous.

auscultation there are no breath sounds over the affected area, and hyperresonance may be heard. A chest x-ray shows the presence of pneumothorax.

If a tension pneumothorax develops, severe respiratory distress, tachycardia, and cyanosis occur. The trachea and point of maximal impulse (PMI) shift to the unaffected side.

Therapeutic Management. If the amount of air or fluid accumulated in the intrapleural space is minimal, no treatment is needed because it will gradually be absorbed. If the amount of air or fluid is minimal, the pleural space can be aspirated with a large-bore needle. Needle aspiration is often a lifesaving measure. The most definitive and common form of treatment of pneumothorax and hemothorax is to insert a chest tube and connect it to water-seal drainage.

Repeated spontaneous pneumothorax may need to be treated surgically by a partial pleurectomy or by application of an irritating agent such as tetracycline to the pleural surfaces via a pleural catheter to promote adherence of the pleurae to one another, which is a procedure called *pleurodesis* or *sclerosing*. Tetracycline is the most common agent used in pleurodesis although quinacrine solution has been used and has been shown to be effective. Pleurodesis is a painful procedure. The patient should be prepared to expect the discomfort, and analgesics should be administered before the instillation of the sclerosing agent.[35]

Fractured Ribs

Rib fractures are the most common type of chest injury resulting from trauma. Ribs 4 through 9 are most com-

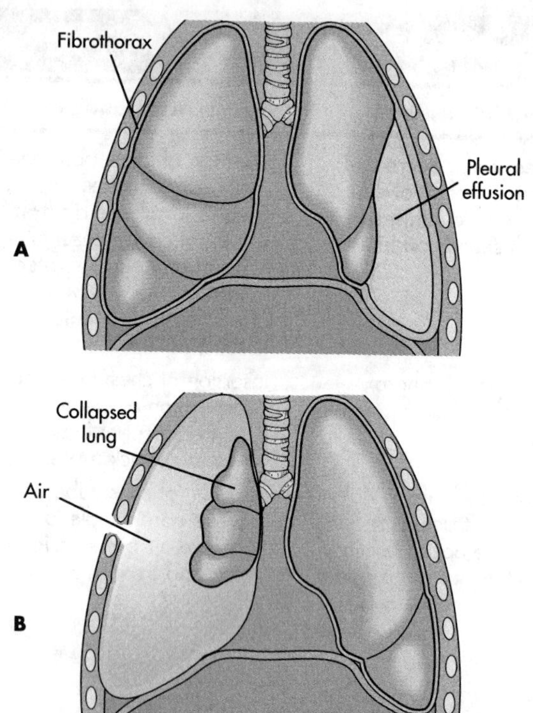

Fig. 24-9 Disorders of the pleura. ***A***, Fibrothorax resulting from an organization of inflammatory exudate and pleural effusion. ***B***, Collapse of lung resulting from an open pneumothorax.

monly fractured because they are least protected by chest muscles. If the fractured rib is splintered or displaced, it may damage the pleura and lungs.

Clinical manifestations of fractured ribs include pain (especially on inspiration) at the site of injury. The individual splints the affected area and takes shallow breaths to try to decrease the pain. Because the individual is reluctant to take deep breaths and cough, atelectasis may develop because of decreased ventilation.

The main goal in treatment is to decrease pain so that the patient can breathe adequately to promote good chest expansion. Intercostal nerve blocks with local anesthesia are most frequently used to provide pain relief. The nerves of the affected ribs and the two intercostal nerves above and below the injured rib are also blocked. The effect of the anesthesia lasts for a period of hours to days. It needs to be repeated as necessary to provide pain relief. Strapping the chest with tape or using a binder is not common practice. Most physicians believe that these measures should be avoided because they reduce lung expansion and predispose the individual to atelectasis. Narcotic drug therapy must be individualized and used with caution because these drugs can depress respirations.

Flail Chest

Flail chest results from multiple rib fractures, causing instability of the chest wall (Fig. 24-10). The chest wall cannot provide the bony structure necessary to maintain bellows action and ventilation. The affected (flail) area will move paradoxically to the intact portion of the chest during respiration. During inspiration the affected portion is sucked in, and during expiration it bulges out. This paradoxical chest movement prevents adequate ventilation of the lung in the injured area. This defect itself does not cause hypoxia. The major difficulty in flail chest is that the underlying lung has been injured. Associated pain and this lung injury, giving rise to loss of compliance, will contribute to the alteration in breathing patterns and lead to hypoxia.

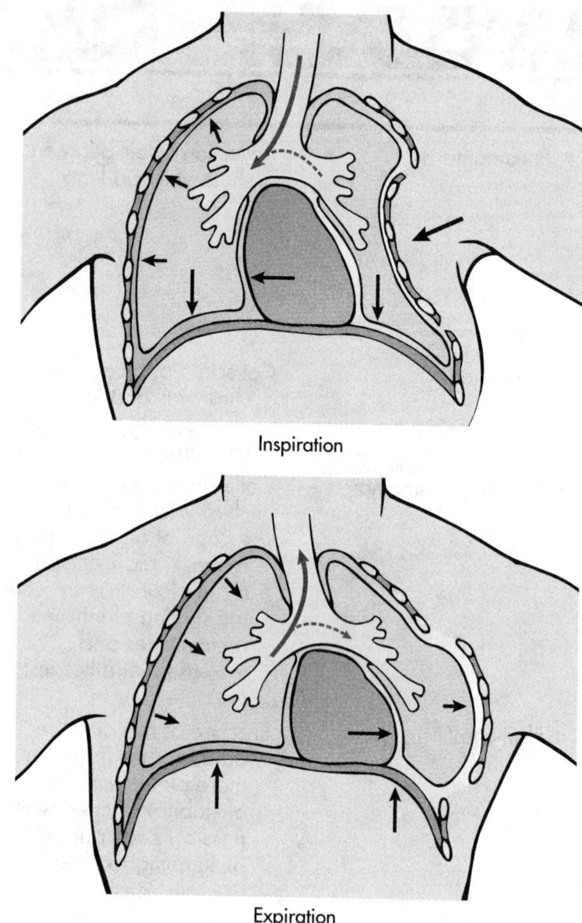

Fig. 24-10 Flail chest produces paradoxical respiration. On inspiration the flail section sinks in with the mediastinal shift to the uninjured side. On expiration the flail section bulges outward with the mediastinal shift to the injured side.

A flail chest is usually apparent on visual examination of the unconscious patient. The patient manifests rapid, shallow respirations, cyanosis, and tachycardia. A flail chest may not be initially apparent in the conscious patient as a result of splinting of the chest wall. The patient moves air poorly, and movement of the thorax is asymmetrical and uncoordinated. Palpation of abnormal respiratory movements, crepitus of the rib, chest x-ray, and ABGs assist in the diagnosis.

Initial therapy consists of adequate ventilation, humidified O_2, and careful administration of crystalloid IV solutions. The definitive therapy is to reexpand the lung and ensure adequate oxygenation. Although many patients can be managed without the use of mechanical ventilation, a short period of intubation and ventilation may be necessary until the diagnosis of the lung injury is complete.

Positive end-expiratory pressure (PEEP) used with mechanical ventilation to improve oxygenation will maintain positive pressure in the lungs throughout the respiratory cycle (mechanical ventilation is discussed in Chapter 61). The lung parenchyma and fractured ribs will heal with time.

Chest Tubes and Pleural Drainage

Under normal conditions, intrapleural pressure is below atmospheric pressure (approximately 4 to 5 cm H_2O below atmospheric pressure during expiration and approximately 8 to 10 cm H_2O below atmospheric pressure during inspiration). (Intrapleural pressure and the intrapleural space are described in Chapter 22.) If intrapleural pressure becomes equal to atmospheric pressure, the lungs will collapse (pneumothorax). Air can enter the intrapleural space by a variety of mechanisms including traumatic chest injury (e.g., gunshot wound, fractured rib), thoracotomy, and spontaneous pneumothorax. Excess fluid accumulation can occur in the pleural space as a result of impaired lymphatic drainage (e.g., from malignancy) or changes in the colloid osmotic pressure (e.g., congestive heart failure). Empyema is purulent pleural fluid, which may be associated with lung abscesses or pneumonia.

Small accumulations of air or fluid in the pleural space may not require removal by thoracentesis or chest-tube insertion. Instead it may be reabsorbed throughout a period of time. The purposes of chest tubes and pleural drainage are to remove the air and fluid and to restore normal intrapleural pressure so that the lungs can reexpand.

Chest Tube Insertion. A physician can insert a chest tube in the emergency department (ED), at the patient's bedside, or in the operating room (OR), depending on the situation. In the OR the chest tube is inserted via the thoracotomy incision. In the ED or at the bedside the patient is placed in a sitting position or is lying down with the affected side elevated. The area is prepared with antiseptic solution, and the site is infiltrated with a local anesthetic agent. After a small incision is made, one or two chest tubes are inserted into the pleural space. One catheter is placed anteriorly through the second intercostal space to remove air (Fig. 24-11). The other is placed posteriorly through the eighth or ninth intercostal space to drain fluid and blood. The tubes are sutured to the chest wall, and the puncture wound is covered with an airtight dressing. During insertion, the tubes are kept clamped. After the tubes are in place in the pleural space, they are connected to drainage tubing and pleural drainage. Each tube may be connected to a separate drainage system and suction. More commonly, a Y connector is used to attach both chest tubes to the same drainage system.

Pleural Drainage. Most pleural drainage systems have three basic compartments, each with its own separate function. The three compartments were bottles in early drainage systems and were known as the *three-bottle system* (Fig. 24-12).

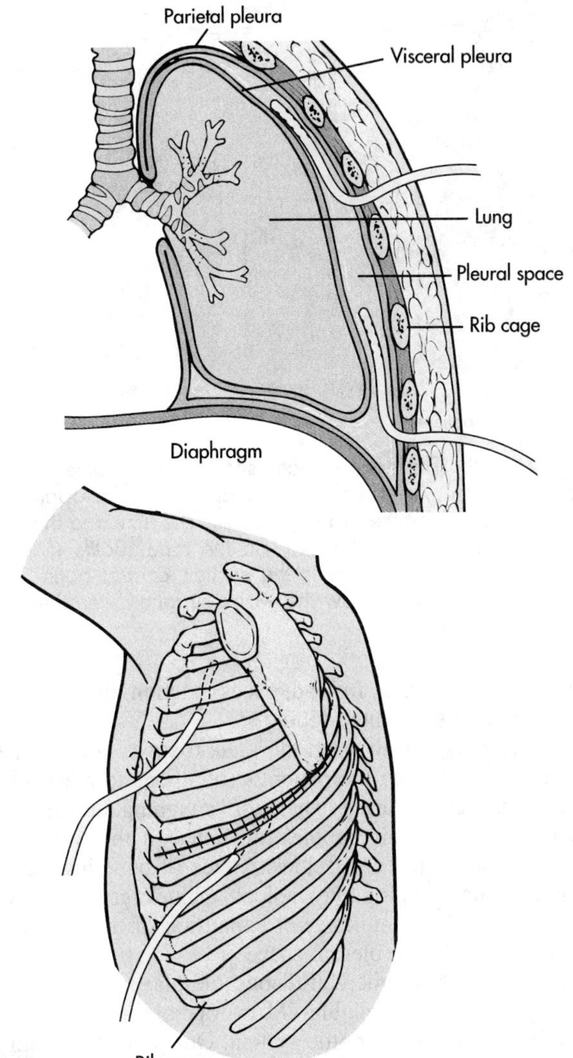

Fig. 24-11 Placement of chest tubes.

The first compartment, or *collection chamber*, receives fluid and air from the chest cavity. The air in the chamber is vented to the second compartment called the *water-seal chamber*, which acts as a one-way valve. Air enters from the collection chamber via a connector that enters under water in the second compartment. The air bubbles up through the water, and no air can reenter the collection chamber because of the water seal.

A third compartment, which is used to apply controlled suction to the system, is called the *suction control chamber*. The suction control bottle uses a tubing partially submerged in a column of water, which is also vented to the atmosphere (Fig. 24-12). Suction is applied to the bottle through a separate opening. The amount of suction applied is regulated by the depth of the tubing in the water, not by the amount of suction applied to the system. An increase in suction does not result in an increase in negative pressure

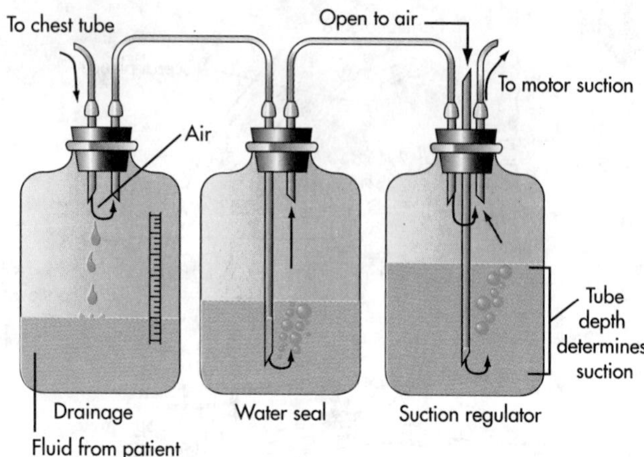

Fig. 24-12 Three-bottle water-seal suction. *Bottle I* is the drainage bottle. A vertical piece of tape should be applied to the outer surface of the drainage bottle. The time and the fluid level should be marked hourly on the tape. *Bottle II* is the water-seal bottle. *Bottle III* is the suction control bottle. The length of glass tube below the water surface determines the amount of suction.

applied to the system. Instead, excess suction merely draws in air through the vented tubing.

The removal of air from the pleural space is facilitated during periods when the patient's intrathoracic pressure is increased, such as during exhalation, coughing, or sneezing. As a result, more air bubbles are noted in the water-seal chamber during these activities. A lack of bubbling during exhalation or coughing may indicate a blockage in the chest tube (e.g., kinking, clotting) or expansion of the lung with no further air in the pleural space.

A variety of commercial disposable plastic chest drainage systems are available. Most operate on the same principles as the three-bottle system. One popular system is the Pleur-evac shown in Fig. 24-13. (Note the correspondence of the chambers to the bottles shown in the three-bottle system in Fig. 24-12.)

These units can be used only for collection or for both collection and water seal. The manufacturer's suggestions for use are included with the equipment. The plastic units allow the patient mobility and decrease the risk of breaking or spilling the drainage system.

Heimlich valves. Another device that may be used to evacuate air from the pleural space is the Heimlich valve. This valve is a collapsible rubber tube that is attached to the external end of the chest tube. The valve opens whenever the pressure is greater than atmospheric pressure and closes when the reverse occurs. The Heimlich valve functions like a water seal and is usually used for emergency transport or in special home care situations.[36]

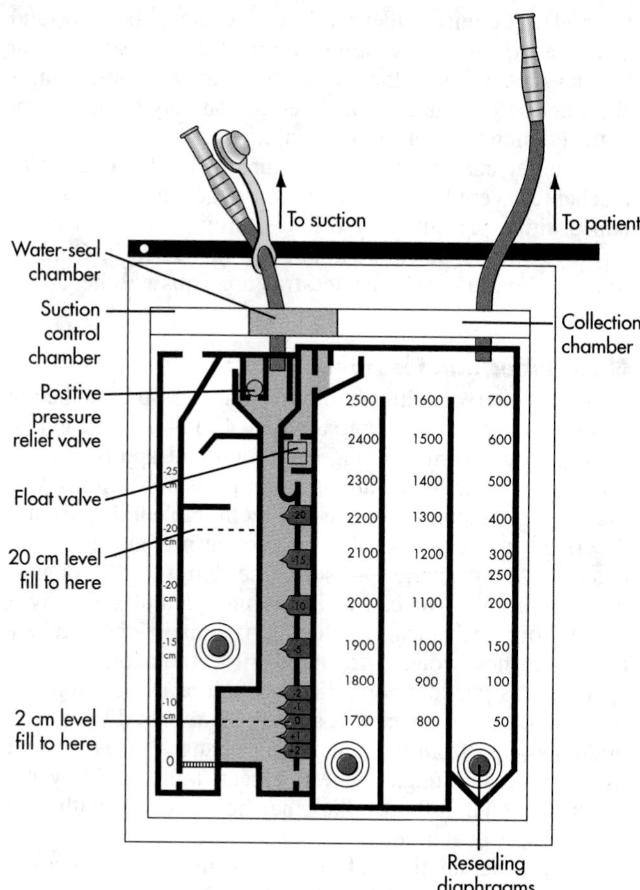

Fig. 24-13 Pleur-evac disposable chest suction system.

NURSING MANAGEMENT

CHEST TUBES

Some general guidelines for nursing care of the patient with chest tubes and water-seal drainage systems include the following:

1. Keep all tubing as straight as possible and coiled loosely. Do not let the patient lie on it.
2. Keep all connections between chest tubes, drainage tubing, and the drainage collector tight. Taping at connections and at the top of the bottle helps prevent air leaks.
3. Keep the water seal and suction control chamber at the appropriate water levels by adding sterile water as needed because water loss by evaporation may occur.
4. Place a piece of tape on the outside of the drainage bottle. The time of measurement and the fluid level should be marked according to the prescribed orders. Marking intervals may range from once per hour to every 8 hours. Any change in the quantity or characteristics of drainage (e.g., clear yellow to bloody) should be reported to the physician and recorded.
5. Observe for air bubbles in the water-seal chamber and fluctuations in the glass tube or chest tubes. Air should be bubbling out from the glass tube. If no fluctuations are observed (rising with inspiration and falling with expiration in the spontaneously breathing patient; the opposite occurs during positive-pressure mechanical ventilation), the drainage system is blocked or the lungs are reexpanded. If bubbling increases, there may be an air leak.
6. Check for bubbling in the water seal. Normally, this is intermittent. When bubbling is continuous and constant, the nurse may determine the source of the air leak by momen-

NURSING CARE PLAN Patient After Thoracotomy

Planning: Outcome Criteria	Nursing Interventions and Rationales
➤ **NURSING DIAGNOSIS**	Ineffective airway clearance *related to* inability to cough secondary to pain from surgical procedure and positioning *as manifested by* rhonchi, wheezes, complaints of pain, inability to cough or deep breathe, temperature elevation, atelectasis on chest x-ray
Have lungs clear to auscultation; be able to clear secretions.	Place patient in semi-Fowler's position *to improve cardiac output and to maximize lung excursion.* Assist patient to turn, deep breathe, and cough q1-2hr initially *to help move or drain the lungs of accumulated secretions.* Splint chest incision *to facilitate breathing exercises and coughing.* Plan coughing exercises after pain relief is obtained *to achieve maximum lung inflation and to open closed airways.* Auscultate lungs before and after deep-breathing and coughing regimes *to evaluate effectiveness of intervention.* Perform postural drainage, percussion, and vibration over nonoperative site *so gravity will aid in moving secretions from lungs.* Humidify air *to liquefy secretions for easier expectoration.* Perform suctioning if necessary *to assist in removing secretions from airway.* Observe the color and characteristics of sputum *to obtain information about possible infection or dehydration.*
➤ **NURSING DIAGNOSIS**	Impaired gas exchange *related to* air and fluid collections in pleural space *as manifested by* chest tube or tubes with drainage, decreased breath sounds on surgical side, abnormal ABGs
Have full expansion of lungs, normal breath sounds bilaterally, normal ABGs.	Monitor chest drainage system (see text) *to assure adequate ventilation and to detect hemorrhage.*
➤ **NURSING DIAGNOSIS**	Ineffective breathing pattern *related to* pain, position, and possible complication on affected side *as manifested by* shortness of breath, shallow respirations, use of accessory muscles
Have respiratory rate 12-18 breaths/min; ease of respiration.	Administer O_2 via nasal prongs or mask (if ordered). Assess respiratory rate q1-2hr *to evaluate patient's response to therapy.* Auscultate lungs q2-3hr *to evaluate the quality and depth of patient's respirations and the need for tracheal aspiration.* Monitor the results of ABGs *to have a quantitative measure of patient's response.* Observe for manifestations of complications such as pneumothorax or hemothorax with symptoms of acute shortness of breath, shallow rapid respirations, dyspnea, cough, and air hunger. Assist patient with deep breathing *to provide encouragement and improve results.* Position patient for comfort and ease of breathing *to increase compliance with respiratory treatments.* Encourage use of incentive spirometer q2-3hr *to provide visual feedback to the patient on effectiveness of respirations.*
➤ **NURSING DIAGNOSIS**	Anxiety *related to* feelings of dyspnea and pain *as manifested by* anxious facial expression, inability to cooperate with instructions to breathe slowly
Express relief from anxiety; be able to manage level of anxiety.	Stay with patient during procedures *to provide encouragement and explanations.* Evaluate chest tubes *to validate proper functioning.* Provide feedback about effective breathing *to provide encouragement and reduce anxiety.* Administer pain medication as ordered *because pain increases anxiety and decreases compliance with necessary treatments.* Monitor the effectiveness *to determine if satisfactory pain relief was obtained.* Use nonpharmacologic measures such as distraction and relaxation techniques *to augment therapeutic effects of analgesia and reduce need for analgesia.*

ABGs, Arterial blood gases.

tarily clamping the tubing at successively distal points away from the patient until the bubbling ceases. Retaping tubing connections or replacing the drainage apparatus may be necessary to prevent the air leak.

7. Monitor the patient's clinical status. Vital signs should be taken frequently, lungs auscultated, and the chest wall observed for any abnormal chest movements.

8. Never elevate the drainage system to the level of the patient's chest because this will cause fluid to drain back into the lungs. Secure the bottles to the metal drainage stand or racks. The drainage bottles should not be emptied unless they are in danger of overflowing.

9. Encourage the patient to cough and breathe deeply periodically to facilitate lung expansion.

10. Check the position of the bottle. If the bottle is overturned and the water seal is disrupted, return the bottle to an upright position and encourage the patient to take a few deep breaths, followed by forced exhalations and cough maneuvers.

Milking and stripping of chest tubes may briefly increase the amount of negative pressure applied to the pleural space. The increased negative pressure should enhance the evacuation of fluid in chest tubes and prevent the development of clots and obstruction from the stagnation of fluids. Although further study is still needed to evaluate the effects of routine stripping of pleural and mediastinal tubes on the lung and mediastinal tissue, present practice advocates the use of these procedures when there is bloody drainage or when the fluid in the collection bottle tends to clot. When chest tubes are used for air collection alone, stripping and milking is not usually performed.[37] Each clinical situation should be evaluated individually, and unit protocol and physician preferences should be ascertained before initiation of stripping and milking. The nurse should keep in mind that these procedures can cause the patient to experience pain and that dislodgement of the tube may occur if the tube is not stabilized above the area that is being stripped.

Clamping of chest tubes is no longer advocated as routine clinical practice unless they become disconnected.[38] The danger of a rapid accumulation of air in the pleural space causing tension pneumothorax is far greater than that of a small amount of atmospheric air entering the pleural space. Chest tubes may be *momentarily* clamped to change the drainage apparatus or to check for air leaks.[39] Continuous clamping may be ordered by the physician before discontinuing the use of the chest tube once it has been determined that normal pleural pressures have been reestablished and the lung has been reexpanded. If a chest tube becomes disconnected the most important intervention is reestablishment of the water-seal system immediately and attachment of a new drainage system as soon as possible. In some hospitals when disconnection occurs, the chest tube is immersed in sterile water (about 2 cm) until the system can be reestablished. It is important for the nurse to know the unit protocol, individual clinical situation (whether an air leak exists), and physician preference before resorting to prolonged chest tube clamping.

Chest Tube Removal. The patient with chest tubes may have daily chest x-rays to follow the course of lung reexpansion. The chest tubes are removed when the lungs are reexpanded and fluid drainage has ceased. Sometimes the amount of suction is decreased or the tubes are clamped off for a period of time before they are removed. If the tubing is clamped, the patient must be observed closely for signs and symptoms of tension pneumothorax. The tube is removed by cutting the sutures, applying a sterile petroleum jelly gauze dressing, having the patient take a deep breath, exhaling, and bearing down (Valsalva maneuver), and then removing the tube. Sometimes pain medication is given before chest tube removal. The site is covered with an airtight dressing, the pleura seals itself off, and the wound is healed in several days. The wound should be observed for drainage and should be reinforced if necessary. The patient should be observed for any manifestations of respiratory distress, which may signify a recurrent or new pneumothorax.

CHEST SURGERY

Chest surgery is performed for a variety of reasons, some of which are unrelated to primary lung problems. For example, a thoracotomy is performed for heart and esophageal surgery. The types of chest surgery are compared in Table 24-24.

Preoperative Care

Before chest surgery, baseline data are obtained on the respiratory and cardiovascular systems. Diagnostic studies usually performed are pulmonary function studies, chest x-rays, lung scans, electrocardiograph (ECG), ABGs, blood urea nitrogen (BUN), serum creatinine, blood glucose, serum electrolytes, and complete blood count. Additional studies of cardiac function such as cardiac catheterization may be done for the patient who is to undergo a pneumonectomy. A careful physical assessment of the lungs, including percussion and auscultation, should be done. This will allow the nurse to compare preoperative and postoperative findings.

The patient should be encouraged to stop smoking before surgery to decrease secretions and increase O_2 saturation. In the anxious period before surgery this is not an easy thing for the habitual smoker to do. Postural drainage may be indicated to help drain the lungs of accumulated secretions. This is especially indicated for the patient with a lung abscess or bronchiectasis.

Preoperative teaching should include exercises for effective deep breathing and coughing or incentive spirometry. If the patient practices these techniques before surgery, the techniques will be easier to perform postoperatively. The patient should be told that adequate medication will be given to reduce the pain, and the patient is helped to splint the incision with a pillow to facilitate deep breathing and coughing.

For most types of chest surgery, chest tubes are inserted and connected to water-sealed drainage systems. The purpose of these tubes should be explained to the patient. In addition, O_2 is frequently given the first day after surgery.

Table 24-24 Chest Surgeries

Type	Description	Indication	Comments
▪ Lobectomy	Removal of one lobe of lung	Lung cancer, bronchiectasis, TB, emphysematous bullae, benign lung tumors, fungal infections	Most common lung surgery, postoperative insertion of two chest tubes, expansion of remaining lung tissue to fill up space
▪ Pneumonectomy	Removal of entire lung	Lung cancer (most common), extensive TB, bronchiectasis, lung abscess	Done only when lobectomy or segmental resection will not remove all diseased lung, no drainage tubes (generally), fluid gradually filling space where lung has been removed, turning of patient with unaffected side dependent contraindicated, position of patient on back or operative side with head elevated
▪ Segmental resection	Removal of one or more lung segments	Bronchiectasis, TB	Technically difficult, done to remove lung segment, insertion of chest tubes, expansion of remaining lung tissue to fill space
▪ Wedge resection	Removal of small, localized lesion that occupies only part of a segment	Lung biopsy, excision of small nodules	Need for chest tubes postoperatively
▪ Decortication	Removal or stripping of thick, fibrous membrane from visceral pleura	Empyema	Use of chest tubes and drainage postoperatively
▪ Exploratory thoracotomy	Incision into thorax to look for injured or bleeding tissues	Chest trauma	Use of chest tubes and drainage postoperatively
▪ Thoracotomy not involving lungs*	Incision into thorax for surgery on other organs	Hiatal hernia repair, open heart surgery, esophageal surgery, tracheal resection, aortic aneurysm repair	—
▪ Thoracoplasty	Removal of ribs without entering pleura	Reduction of size of chest cavity	Historical importance in treating TB, possible use to decrease lung size in area of chronic empyema, use before resectional surgery (rarely)
▪ Endoscopic thoracotomy or video fluoroscopy	One to four 1-in incisions through which a special fiberoptic camera is introduced as well as other instruments and suction	Patient without prior thoracotomy; peripheral or mediastinal lesions; lung function must be sufficient to undergo conventional thoracotomy	Possible complications include heavy bleeding, diaphragmatic perforation, air emboli, tension pneumothorax; chest tube is inserted through one of the incisions; incisions may be sutured or closed with adhesive wound approximating strips

TB, Tuberculosis.
*For comments on thoracotomy not involving the lungs, see discussion of individual diseases in text.

Range-of-motion exercises on the surgical side similar to those for the mastectomy patient should be taught (see Chapter 49).

The thought of losing part of a vital organ is frequently frightening. The patient should be reassured that the lungs have a large degree of functional reserve. Even after the removal of one lung there is enough lung tissue to maintain adequate oxygenation. However, the patient should be instructed to include adequate rest periods to allow compensation for the decreased diffusion capacity that occurs.

The nurse should be available to deal with the questions asked by the patient and the family. Questions should be answered honestly. The nurse should try to facilitate the expression of concerns, feelings, and questions. (General preoperative care and teaching are discussed in Chapter 14.)

Surgical Interventions

Thoracotomy surgery is considered major surgery because the incision is large, cutting into bone, muscle, and cartilage. The two types of thoracic incisions are *median sternotomy*, performed by splitting the sternum, and *lateral thoracotomy*. The median sternotomy is primarily used for surgery involving the heart. The two types of lateral thoracotomy are posterolateral and anterolateral. The posterolateral thoracotomy is used for most surgeries involving the lung. The incision is made from the anterior axillary line below the nipple level posteriorly at the fourth, fifth, or sixth intercostal space. It is rarely necessary to remove the ribs. Strong mechanical retractors are used to gain access to the lung. The anterolateral incision is made in the fourth or fifth intercostal space from the sternal border to the midaxillary line. This procedure is commonly used for surgery or trauma victims, mediastinal operations, and wedge resections of the upper and middle lobes of the lung.

The extensiveness of the thoracotomy incision often results in severe pain for the patient after surgery. Because muscles have been severed, the patient is reluctant to move the shoulder and arm on the surgical side. Chest tubes are placed in the pleural space except in pneumonectomy surgery. In a pneumonectomy the space from which the lung was removed gradually fills with serosanguineous fluid.

Endoscopic thoracotomy or *video thoracoscopy* is a new procedure, which in many cases can avoid the impact of a full thoracotomy. The procedure involves three to four 1-inch incisions made on the chest that allows a special fiberoptic camera and instruments to be inserted and manipulated. The candidate for this type of procedure should not have a prior history of conventional thoracic surgery because the probability of adhesion formation would make access more difficult. The patient whose lesions are in the lung periphery or the mediastinum is a better candidate because of better accessibility. The patient considered for endoscopic thoracotomy should have sufficient pulmonary function preoperatively to allow the surgeon to perform conventional thoracotomy if complications occur (e.g., heavy bleeding). Other complications that may occur are diaphragmatic perforation, air emboli, persistent pleural air leaks, and tension pneumothorax.[40]

There are many benefits of endoscopic thoracotomy when compared with a conventional thoracotomy procedure. These include less adhesion formation, minimal blood loss, less time under anesthesia, no ICU confinement in most cases, shorter hospitalization and faster recovery, less pain, and no need for postoperative rehabilitation therapy because of minimal disruption of thoracic structures.[41]

Chest tubes are placed at the end of the procedure through one of the incisions. The incisions are closed with sutures or a wound approximating adhesive bandage. Nursing assessment and care postoperatively include monitoring respiratory status and lung reexpansion with the chest tubes and checking the incisions for drainage or dehiscence. A return to prior activities should be encouraged as quickly as possible.[41]

Postoperative Care

Specific measures related to the care after a thoracotomy are presented in the nursing care plan on p. 669. The specific follow-up care depends on the type of surgical procedure. General postoperative care is discussed in Chapter 16.

RESTRICTIVE RESPIRATORY DISORDERS

Restrictive respiratory disorders are characterized by decreased compliance of the lungs or chest wall or both. This is in contrast to obstructive disorders, which are characterized by increased resistance to airflow. Pulmonary function tests are the best means to use in differentiating between restrictive and obstructive respiratory disorders (Table 24-25). Restrictive disorders are characterized by reduced vital capacity (VC) and reduced total lung capacity (TLC), with a normal or reduced functional residual capacity (FRC) and

Table 24-25 Relationship of Lung Volumes to Type of Ventilatory Impairment

Interpretation	FVC	FEV_1	FEV_1/FVC	RV	TLC
Normal	Normal	Normal	Normal	Normal	Normal
Airway obstruction	Normal or low	Low	Low	High	High
Lung restriction	Low	Normal or low	Normal or high	Normal or low	Low
Obstruction and restriction	Low	Low	Low	Variable	Variable

FEV_1, Forced expiratory volume in 1 second; *FVC*, functional vital capacity; *RV*, residual volume; *TLC*, total lung capacity.

residual volume (RV). Obstructive disorders are characterized by normal or decreased VC, increased TLC, reduced ratio of forced air expiration volume in the first second of expiration (FEV_1) to functional vital capacity (FVC), increased FRC, and increased RV. Mixed obstructive and restrictive disorders are often manifested. For example, a patient may have both chronic bronchitis (an obstructive problem) and pulmonary fibrosis (a restrictive problem).

Restrictive problems are generally categorized into extrapulmonary and intrapulmonary disorders. Extrapulmonary causes of restrictive lung disease include disorders involving the CNS, neuromuscular system, and chest wall (Table 24-26). In these disorders the lung tissue is normal. Intrapulmonary causes of restrictive lung disease involve the pleura or the lung tissue (Table 24-27).

Pleural Effusion

Types. Pleural effusion is a collection of fluid in the pleural space (Fig. 24-9, *A*). It is not a disease but rather a sign of a serious disease. It is frequently classified as *transudative* or *exudative* according to whether the protein content of the effusion is low or high, respectively. A transudate occurs primarily in noninflammatory conditions and is an accumulation of protein-poor, cell-poor fluid. Transudative pleural effusions (also called *hydrothorax*) are caused by (1) increased hydrostatic pressure found in congestive heart failure (CHF) or (2) decreased oncotic pressure (from hypoalbuminemia) found in chronic liver or renal disease. In these situations, fluid movement is facilitated out of the capillaries and into the pleural space.

An exudate is an accumulation of fluid and cells in an area of inflammation. An exudative pleural effusion results from increased capillary permeability characteristic of the inflammatory reaction. This type of effusion occurs secondary to pulmonary inflammations or malignancies.

The type of pleural effusion can be determined by a sample of pleural fluid obtained via thoracentesis (a procedure done to remove fluid from the pleural space). Exudates have a specific gravity above 1.015 and a high protein content, and the fluid is clear or pale yellow. Transudates have a lower specific gravity and low to no protein content. The fluid is dark yellow or amber. The fluid can also be analyzed for red and white blood cells, malignant cells, bacteria, glucose, pH, and lactic dehydrogenase.

An *empyema* is a pleural effusion that contains pus. It is caused by conditions such as pneumonia, TB, and lung abscess. A complication of empyema is *fibrothorax*, in which there is fibrous fusion of the visceral and parietal pleurae (Fig. 24-9, *A*).

Clinical Manifestations. Common clinical manifestations of pleural effusion are progressive dyspnea and decreased movement of the chest wall on the affected side. There may be pleuritic pain from the underlying disease. Physical examination of the chest will indicate dullness to percussion and absent or decreased breath sounds over the affected area. The chest x-ray will indicate an abnormality if the effusion is greater than 250 ml. Manifestations of empyema include the manifestations of pleural effusion as well as fever, night sweats, cough, and weight loss. A thoracentesis reveals an exudate containing thick, purulent material.

Thoracentesis. If the cause of the pleural effusion is not known, a diagnostic thoracentesis is needed to obtain pleural fluid for analysis (see Fig. 22-18). If the degree of pleural effusion is severe enough to impair breathing, a therapeutic thoracentesis is done to remove fluid.

A thoracentesis is performed by having the patient sit on the edge of a bed and lean forward over a bedside table. The puncture site is determined by chest x-ray and percussion of the chest is used to assess the maximum degree of dullness. The skin is cleaned with an antiseptic solution and anesthetized locally. The physician inserts the thoracentesis needle into the intercostal space. Fluid can be aspirated with a syringe, or tubing can be connected to allow fluid to drain into a sterile collecting bottle. After the fluid is removed, the needle is withdrawn, and a bandage is applied over the insertion site.

Usually only 1000 to 1200 ml of pleural fluid are removed at one time to prevent mediastinal shift and compromised venous return. A follow-up chest x-ray should be done to detect a possible pneumothorax that could have been induced by perforation of the pleura. During and after the procedure the patient should be observed for any manifestations of respiratory distress.

Therapeutic Management. The main goal of management of pleural effusions is to treat the underlying cause. For example, adequate treatment of CHF with diuretics and sodium restriction will result in decreased pleural effusions. The treatment of pleural effusions secondary to malignant disease represents a more difficult problem. These types of pleural effusions are frequently recurrent and accumulate quickly after thoracentesis. Infusions of cancer chemotherapeutic agents directly into the pleural space are used to decrease the number of recurrent effusions.

Treatment of empyema is directed at drainage of the pleural space via thoracentesis or a closed thoracotomy tube. Appropriate antibiotic therapy is also needed to eradicate the causative organism. If a fibrothorax results from the empyema and causes severe pulmonary restriction, a decortication surgical procedure is done in which the pleural membranes are separated.

Pleurisy

Pleurisy (also called *pleuritis*) is an inflammation of the pleura. The most common causes are pneumonia, TB, chest trauma, pulmonary infarctions, and neoplasms. The inflammation usually subsides with adequate treatment of the primary disease. Pleurisy can be classified as *fibrinous* (dry), with fibrinous deposits on the pleural surface, or *serofibrinous* (wet), with increased production of pleural fluid that may result in pleural effusion.

The pain of pleurisy is typically abrupt and sharp in onset and is aggravated by inspiration. The patient's breathing is shallow and rapid to avoid unnecessary movement of the pleura and chest wall. A pleural friction rub may occur, which is the sound over areas where inflamed visceral and parietal pleura rub over one another during inspiration. This

Table 24-26 Extrapulmonary Causes of Restrictive Lung Disease

Disease or Alteration	Description	Comments
Central Nervous System		
■ Head injury, CNS lesion (e.g., tumor, cerebrovascular accident)	Injury to or impingement on respiratory center, causing hypoventilation or hyperventilation; relationship of manifestations to increased intracranial pressure (see Chapter 54)	Management is directed toward treating the underlying cause, maintaining the airway, using mechanical ventilation for supportive care, and assessing for manifestations of increased intracranial pressure.
■ Narcotic and barbiturate use	Depression of respiratory center, respiratory rate of <12 breaths/min	Respiratory depression is caused by drug overdose or inadvertent administration of drugs to a person with respiratory difficulty. These drugs should not be administered to a person with a respiratory rate of <12 breaths/min.
Neuromuscular System		
■ Guillain-Barré syndrome	Acute inflammation of peripheral nerves and ganglia; paralysis of intercostal nerves leading to diaphragmatic breathing; paralysis of vagal preganglionic and postganglionic fibers leading to reduced ability of bronchioles to constrict, dilate, and respond to irritants	Patient often has to be put on mechanical ventilation for supportive care (see Chapter 57).
■ Amyotrophic lateral sclerosis	Progressive degenerative disorder of the motor neurons in the spinal cord, brain stem, and motor cortex; respiratory system involvement as a result of interruption of nerve transmission to respiratory muscles, especially diaphragm	See Chapter 57 for clinical manifestations and management.
■ Myasthenia gravis	Defect in neuromuscular junction, respiratory system involvement as a result of interruption of nerve transmission to respiratory muscles	See Chapter 57 for clinical manifestations and management.
■ Muscular dystrophy	Hereditary disease; eventual involvement of all skeletal muscles; paralysis of respiratory muscles, including intercostals, diaphragm, and accessory muscles	Pulmonary problems develop late in disease process.
Chest Wall		
■ Chest-wall trauma (e.g., flail chest, fractured rib)	Rib fracture causing inspiratory pain; voluntary splinting of chest, resulting in shallow, rapid breathing; impaired ventilatory ability caused by paradoxical breathing (see text)	—
■ Pickwickian syndrome (extreme obesity)	Excess adipose tissue interfering with chest-wall and diaphragmatic excursion, somnolence from hypoxemia and CO_2 retention, polycythemia from chronic hypoxia	Weight loss generally causes reversal of symptoms. Prevention and prompt treatment of respiratory infections are important. Condition is worsened in supine position.
■ Kyphoscoliosis	Posterior and lateral angulation of the spine; restriction of ventilation as a result of alteration in thoracic excursion; increase in work of breathing; pattern of rapid, shallow breathing; reduction of lung volume; compression of alveoli and blood vessels	Only small number of persons with condition develop severe respiratory problems.

CNS, Central nervous system.

Table 24-27 Intrapulmonary Causes of Restrictive Lung Disease

Disease or Alteration	Description
Pleural Disorders	
▪ Pleural effusion	Accumulation of fluid in pleural space secondary to altered hydrostatic or oncotic pressure, fluid collection >250 ml, showing up on chest x-ray
▪ Pleurisy	Inflammation of pleura, classification as fibrinous (dry) or serofibrinous (wet), wet pleurisy accompanied by an increase in pleural fluid and possibly resulting in pleural effusion
▪ Pneumothorax	Accumulation of air in pleural space with accompanying lung collapse
Parenchymal Disorders	
▪ Atelectasis	Condition of lung characterized by collapsed, airless alveoli; possibly acute (e.g., in postoperative patient) or chronic (e.g., in patient with malignant tumor)
▪ Pneumonia	Acute inflammation of lung tissue caused by bacteria, viruses, fungi, chemicals, dusts, and other factors
▪ Pulmonary fibrosis	Excessive connective tissue in the lungs resulting from healing and tissue repair after inflammation, possible localized fibrosis (e.g., from lung abscess, TB, pneumonia) or diffuse (e.g., from pneumoconiosis, sarcoidosis, cystic fibrosis, Hamman-Rich syndrome), progressive dyspnea on exertion as a result of decreased compliance of lungs and increased work of breathing. Diffuse pulmonary fibrosis is progressively disabling and frequently fatal.
▪ ARDS*	Atelectasis, pulmonary edema, congestion, and hyaline membrane lining the alveolar wall; result of variety of conditions, including shock lung, O_2 toxicity, gram-negative sepsis, cardiopulmonary bypass, and aspiration pneumonia.

ARDS, Acute respiratory distress syndrome; TB, tuberculosis.
*See Chapter 26 for clinical manifestations and management.

sound is usually loudest at peak inspiration but can be heard during exhalation as well.[42]

Treatment of pleurisy is aimed at treating the underlying disease and providing pain relief. Taking analgesics as well as lying on or splinting the affected side may provide some relief. The patient should be taught to splint the rib cage when coughing. Intercostal nerve blocks may be done if the pain is severe.

Atelectasis

Atelectasis is a condition of the lungs characterized by collapsed, airless alveoli. The most common cause of atelectasis is airway obstruction that is as a result of retained exudates and secretions. This is frequently observed in the postoperative patient. Normally the pores of Kohn provide for collateral passage of air from one alveolus to another. Deep inspiration is necessary to open the pores effectively. For this reason, coughing and deep-breathing exercises are important in preventing atelectasis in the high-risk patient (e.g., postoperative, immobilized patient). Pulmonary fibrosis can occur as a complication of chronic atelectasis. (The prevention and treatment of atelectasis are discussed in Chapter 16.)

Pulmonary Fibrosis

A common cause of diffuse pulmonary fibrosis is occupational inhalation of organic and inorganic substances. Other causes of diffuse pulmonary fibrosis include the Hamman-Rich syndrome (an unusual form of interstitial pneumonia) and sarcoidosis. Sarcoidosis is the presence of granulomatous lesions and proliferation of lymph tissue, which can involve any body organ including the lungs. The disease is most common in African-Americans between the ages of 20 and 35. The clinical course of the disease varies from self-limiting to progressive, widespread granulomatous inflammation and fibrosis. Marked pulmonary fibrosis can be present with severe restrictive lung disease. Cor pulmonale can develop in the advanced stages. There is no specific treatment for sarcoidosis. Often the disease is self- limiting, and the patient gets well without treatment. Corticosteroids have been used to relieve symptoms and suppress the acute inflammation.

VASCULAR LUNG DISORDERS

Pulmonary Edema

Pulmonary edema is an abnormal accumulation of fluid in the alveoli and interstitial spaces of the lungs. It is a complication of various heart and lung diseases (Table 24-28). It is considered a medical emergency and may be life threatening.

Normally, there is a balance between the hydrostatic and oncotic pressures in the pulmonary capillaries. If the hydrostatic pressure increases or the colloid oncotic pressure decreases, the net effect will be fluid leaving the pulmonary capillaries and entering the interstitial space. This stage is referred to as *interstitial edema.* At this stage the lymphatics can usually drain away the excess fluid. If fluid continues to leak from the pulmonary capillaries it will enter the alveoli. This stage is referred to as *alveolar edema.* Pulmonary edema interferes with gas exchange by

Table 24-28 Causes of Pulmonary Edema

Congestive heart failure
Overhydration with intravenous fluids
Hypoalbuminemia: nephrotic syndrome, hepatic disease, nutritional disorders
Altered capillary permeability of lungs: inhaled toxins, inflammation (e.g., pneumonia), severe hypoxia, near drowning
Mechanical ventilation
Lymph malignancies
Respiratory distress syndrome (e.g., O_2 toxicity)
Unknown causes: neurogenic condition, narcotic overdose, high altitude

causing an alteration in the diffusing pathway between the alveoli and the pulmonary capillaries.

The most common cause of pulmonary edema is left-sided CHF. (The clinical manifestations and management of pulmonary edema are described in Chapter 32.) Chronic forms of pulmonary edema are not common. This condition can be asymptomatic for a long period of time while structural changes such as pulmonary fibrosis result. An early manifestation of this condition may be paroxysmal nocturnal dyspnea as a result of increased hydrostatic pressure in the lungs in the recumbent position.

Pulmonary Embolism

Pulmonary embolism is the most frequently encountered pulmonary illness in a general hospital and is responsible for more than 50,000 deaths annually in the United States.[43] A pulmonary embolism is caused by thrombotic occlusion of the pulmonary arterial system. The most common source of the thrombus is the deep veins of the legs. The thrombus breaks loose and travels as an embolus until it lodges in the pulmonary vasculature.

The result of the thromboembolic occlusion is complete or partial occlusion of the pulmonary arterial blood flow to parts of the lung. Thus the lung is ventilated but not perfused. As the pressure increases in the pulmonary vasculature, pulmonary hypertension may result. (Pulmonary embolism is described in detail in Chapter 35.)

Pulmonary Hypertension

Pathophysiology. Normally the pulmonary circulation is characterized by low resistance and low pressure. Cardiac output can increase significantly with no increase in the pressure in the pulmonary vasculature. In pulmonary hypertension the pulmonary pressure is elevated because of an increase in pulmonary vascular resistance to blood flow through small arteries and arterioles. A 60% to 70% reduction in the vascular bed is required before pulmonary hypertension develops. The increase in vascular resistance may be anatomic or vasomotor related in origin. The reasons for an anatomic increase in vascular resistance include (1) loss of capillaries as a result of alveolar wall damage, as found in COPD, (2) stiffening of the pulmonary vasculature, as found in pulmonary fibrosis, and (3) obstruction of blood flow, as found with pulmonary emboli.

Vasomotor increase in pulmonary vascular resistance is found in conditions characterized by alveolar hypoxia and hypercapnia. These conditions cause localized vasoconstriction and shunting of blood away from poorly ventilated alveoli. Alveolar hypoxia and hypercapnia can be caused by a wide variety of conditions, including the pickwickian syndrome, kyphoscoliosis, neuromuscular diseases, and other conditions characterized by alveolar hypoventilation with normal lungs.

It is possible to have a combination of anatomic restriction and vasomotor constriction. This is found in the patient with long-standing chronic bronchitis who has chronic hypoxia in addition to loss of lung tissue.

Pulmonary hypertension is almost always caused by pulmonary or cardiac disorders. However, *primary pulmonary hypertension* is not associated with either pulmonary or cardiac disease. The person with this disorder is typically a woman between the ages of 20 and 40.[44] The basic cause of the problem is unknown. No definitive therapy is available, and the course is often continual downhill progression often occurring within several years of onset of symptoms.

Clinical Manifestations. The most common manifestations of pulmonary hypertension are dyspnea and weakness. These symptoms initially occur only when there is an increased cardiac output (e.g., during exercise or with fever) or during hypoxia (e.g., with pulmonary infection). Eventually the condition occurs even during rest. Pulmonary hypertension increases the work load of the right ventricle and causes right ventricular hypertrophy, a condition called *cor pulmonale*.

Cor Pulmonale

Cor pulmonale is characterized by hypertrophy of the right ventricle secondary to a respiratory disorder. Pulmonary hypertension is usually a preexisting condition in the individual with cor pulmonale. Cor pulmonale may be present with or without overt cardiac failure. The most common cause of acute cor pulmonale is a massive pulmonary embolism. However, cor pulmonale is usually chronic, resulting from alveolar hypoxia in COPD. Almost any disorder that affects the respiratory system can cause cor pulmonale. The etiology and pathogenesis of pulmonary hypertension and cor pulmonale are outlined in Fig. 24-14.

Clinical Manifestations. Clinical manifestations of cor pulmonale include dyspnea, cough, retrosternal or substernal pain, and fatigue. Chronic hypoxia leads to polycythemia and increased total blood volume and viscosity of the blood. Compensatory mechanisms that are secondary to hypoxemia can aggravate the pulmonary hypertension. Episodes of cor pulmonale in a person with underlying chronic respiratory problems are frequently triggered by an acute respiratory tract infection.

If heart failure accompanies cor pulmonale, additional manifestations such as peripheral edema; weight gain; distended neck veins; full, bounding pulse; and enlarged liver will also be found. (CHF is discussed in Chapter 32.)

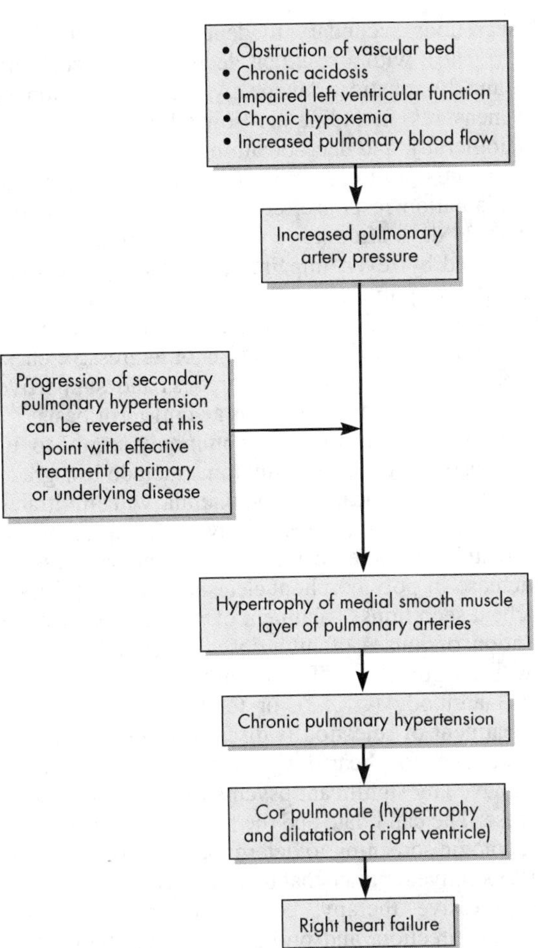

Fig. 24-14 Pathogenesis of pulmonary hypertension and cor pulmonale.

A chest x-ray will show an enlarged right ventricle and pulmonary artery.

Therapeutic Management. The primary management of cor pulmonale is directed at treating the underlying pulmonary problem that precipitated the heart problem (Table 24-29). Low-flow O_2 therapy is used to correct the hypoxemia and reduce vasoconstriction in chronic states of respiratory disorders. In acute states (e.g., those caused by pulmonary emboli), higher concentrations of O_2 may be required. If fluid and electrolyte and acid-base imbalances are present, they need to be corrected. Diuretics and a low-sodium diet will help to decrease the plasma volume and the load on the heart. Bronchodilator therapy is indicated if the underlying respiratory problem is because of an obstructive disorder. Antibiotic therapy is indicated if the cor pulmonale was precipitated by an infection. The use of digitalis may be necessary to treat the accompanying heart failure. If digitalis is used, smaller doses than usual are recommended because hypoxemia predisposes the patient to digitalis toxicity. Antidysrhythmic drugs are given if indicated. Phlebotomies may be needed in the patient with hematocrits more than 60 g/dl (600 g/L) to reduce the hematocrit and blood volume.

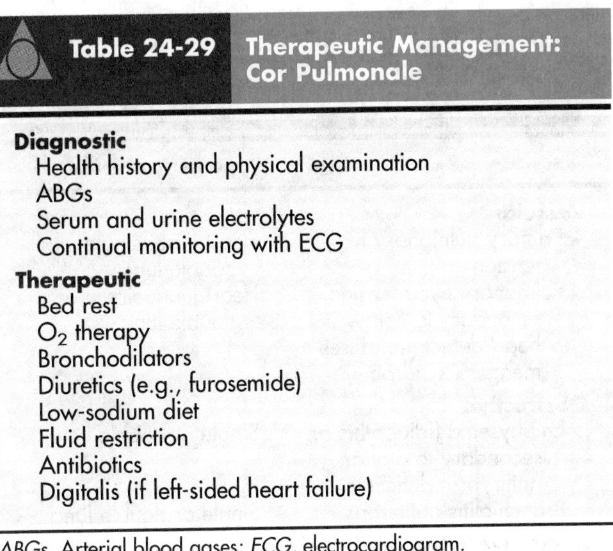

Table 24-29 Therapeutic Management: Cor Pulmonale

Diagnostic
- Health history and physical examination
- ABGs
- Serum and urine electrolytes
- Continual monitoring with ECG

Therapeutic
- Bed rest
- O_2 therapy
- Bronchodilators
- Diuretics (e.g., furosemide)
- Low-sodium diet
- Fluid restriction
- Antibiotics
- Digitalis (if left-sided heart failure)

ABGs, Arterial blood gases; *ECG,* electrocardiogram.

Chronic management of cor pulmonale resulting from COPD is similar to that described for COPD (see Chapter 25). Continuous low-flow O_2 during sleep, exercise, and small, frequent meals may allow the patient to feel better and be more active. Vasodilator therapy has been evaluated as a possible treatment for pulmonary hypertension and has been shown to produce sustained hemodynamic and symptomatic improvement in approximately two thirds of patients. However, the efficacy of long-term vasodilator therapy in the treatment of pulmonary hypertension has not been impressive.[44] Anticoagulation has also been used with success. New approaches include the use of high-dose calcium channel blockers and continuous IV infusion of prostacyclin.[45] When medical treatment fails, heart-lung or lung transplantation has become an option for some patients.

LUNG TRANSPLANTATION

In 1968 the first heart-lung transplant was performed in the United States. In the 1980s successful transplantation of the lungs was performed. Since then the area of lung transplantation has continued to rapidly evolve. Improved selection criteria, technical advances, and better methods of immunosuppression have resulted in improved survival rates (75% 1- and 2-year survival rate for most heart-lung recipients; 78% 1-year and 74% 2-year survival rates for single lung transplant recipients).[46]

Selection criteria have changed dramatically, and there are variances dependent on the type of lung transplantation advocated. Not only is transplantation an option for the patient with primary pulmonary hypertension but also for the patient with chronic pulmonary diseases, including cystic fibrosis.[47] Table 24-30 illustrates the variety of pulmonary disorders potentially treatable with some type of lung transplantation. Heart-lung transplants are recom-

Table 24-30 Pulmonary Diseases Treatable with Lung or Heart-Lung Transplantation

Disorder	Type of Transplant
Vascular	
Primary pulmonary hypertension	Heart-lung, single or double lung
Pulmonary hypertension secondary to congenital heart defect (i.e., Eisenmenger's syndrome).	Heart-lung, single or double lung
Obstructive	
Emphysema (idiopathic or secondary to $alpha_1$ antitrypsin deficiency)	Single or double lung
Bronchiolitis obliterans	Single or double lung
Ineffective/Obstructive	
Cystic fibrosis	Double lung, heart-lung
Bronchiectasis	Double-lung, heart-lung
Fibrotic	
Idiopathic pulmonary fibrosis	Single lung
Secondary pulmonary fibrosis	Single lung

From Onofrio JM, Emory B: Selection of patients for lung transplantation, *Med Clin North Am* 76:1207, 1992.

mended for the patients with pulmonary hypertension or with irreversible cardiac disease. However, there is evidence that single lung transplantation can markedly correct pulmonary hypertension and resultant cor pulmonale.

Immunosuppressive therapy usually includes cyclosporine, azathioprine, and prednisone. These drugs are discussed in Chapter 44. New approaches with agents such as FK506, RS-61443, Rapamycin, and monoclonal antibodies promise to improve survival and hopefully further reduce posttransplant rejection.[48]

Contraindications for lung transplantation are divided into absolute and relative categories. Absolute contraindications include "physiologic" (not chronologic) age greater than 60 years, a person who currently smokes cigarettes, a patient with malignancy or a recent history of malignancy or other end-stage dysfunction secondary to systemic disease, such as systemic lupus erythematosus or sclerodema. Relative contraindications are patients who are ventilator-dependent, have recent use of steroid therapy, or those with a history of previous cardiothoracic surgery (because of possible adhesions).[48]

Early pulmonary postoperative complications of heart-lung transplantation include respiratory dysfunction, the "implantation response," and infection. Initially, patients experience a shallow breathing pattern and difficulty in clearing secretions secondary to denervation of the lung below the trachea, with a resultant decrease in mucociliary clearance and lymphatic drainage. Aggressive pulmonary clearance measures, including aerosolized bronchodilators, chest physiotherapy, and deep-breathing and coughing techniques, are mandatory to minimize potential complications.

The implantation response, commonly encountered between 4 and 24 days after surgery, is a reversible phenomenon manifested by fever, impaired gas exchange, tachypnea, and diffuse pulmonary infiltrates. The causes are believed to be denervation, lymphatic disruption, ischemia, and surgical trauma. Treatment consists of aggressive chest physiotherapy, administration of diuretics, and supportive mechanical ventilation as needed on a short-term basis.[49]

Rejection of lung transplants is commonly seen 7 to 10 days after transplantation, and symptoms include low grade fever, tachypnea, dyspnea, and hypoxemia with infiltrates and pleural effusion on chest x-ray.[48] Other signs of rejection include an increase in pulmonary artery pressure and an increase in polymorphonuclear neutrophils (PMNs) in the tracheal secretions. Treatment of rejection consists of administration of pulses of high-dose IV methylprednisolone as well as polyclonal T-cell antibody (ATG), monoclonal CD3 antibody (OKT3), or total lymphoid irradiation.[48] (Treatment of rejection is discussed in Chapter 44.)

The candidate for heart-lung or lung transplantation should not have any significant psychiatric disorders or systemic disease. The candidate and the family undergoes thorough psychologic screening to determine the ability to cope with a postoperative regimen that requires strict adherence to immunosuppressive therapy, continuous monitoring for early signs of infection, and prompt reporting of manifestations of infection for medical evaluation. Additionally, they must have the financial ability, either through medical insurance or private funds, to afford the procedure, postoperative immunosuppressive drugs, and medical follow-up care.

Bronchoalveolar lavage may be used as well as technetium 99m lung scans to show decreased arterial flow to the transplanted lung and detect rejection earlier than demonstrable by radiographic evidence. Infection in the transplant recipient is the most significant cause of morbidity and death. The immunosuppression necessary to prevent rejection makes the recipient susceptible to many pathogens, including bacterial, fungal, viral, nocardial, and protozoal organisms. Infections are primarily pulmonary and are usually either nosocomial or opportunistic in nature. A late complication of lung transplantation procedures is obliterative bronchiolitis that involves fibrotic plugging of the terminal bronchioles. It is manifested by decreases in pulmonary functions and is the target for further research to understand its etiology as well as treatment. As heart-lung and lung transplantation continues to evolve, hope for a prolonged life with improved quality may be realistic for some individuals with end-stage heart and lung disease.

CRITICAL THINKING EXERCISES

CASE STUDY

TUBERCULOSIS

Patient Profile

Mr. G., a 56-year-old Hispanic male, was admitted to the hospital with symptoms of right-sided chest pain and coughing up blood.

Subjective Data

- Has been homeless and living on the street for the past 6 months
- Has had increasingly severe pain in the right side during the past 2 weeks
- Describes the pain as "like a knife stabbing him" and is almost unable to breathe when it hits
- Thinks he has lost weight because he needs a rope to hold up pants
- Describes frequent episodes of awakening in the night soaking wet

Objective Data

Physical Examination

- Thin, disheveled man appearing older than stated age.
- Chest auscultation revealed diffuse rhonchi.

Diagnostic Studies

- Serum albumin 2.8 g/dl (28 g/L)
- WBC 20,000/μl (20×10^9/L)
- Induced sputum specimen gray with red streaking
- Stain of sputum revealed many acid-fast bacilli

Chest X-ray

- Diffuse alveolar infiltrates in lower right lobe accompanied by small pleural effusion

Critical Thinking Questions

1. What types of infectious disease precautions should be taken related to his hospitalization?
2. What clinical manifestations of TB did Mr. G. exhibit? Explain their pathophysiologic bases.
3. With a new diagnosis of TB, what drugs will probably be given to Mr. G.?
4. What will the nurse need to consider in planning discharge arrangements for Mr. G.?
5. Based on the assessment data presented, write one or more appropriate nursing diagnoses. Are there any collaborative problems?

NURSING RESEARCH ISSUES

1. What are effective measures that a nurse can institute to increase patient compliance with long-term antituberculosis medication?
2. Compare the effectiveness of various smoking cessation methods (e.g., hypnosis, aversion therapy, nicotine weaning).
3. What position should a patient assume following lung surgery for comfort and maximum oxygenation?
4. Does an aggressive nurse-managed community program related to TB therapy increase patient compliance with therapy?
5. Is there a significant improvement in the quality of life of the patient following lung transplantation?

REVIEW QUESTIONS

The number of the question corresponds to the same-numbered objective at the beginning of the chapter.

1. Which of the following statements characterize pneumococcal pneumonia?

a. Generally causes an interstitial type of pneumonia
b. Usually self-limiting and treated symptomatically
c. Characterized by productive cough with rust-colored sputum
d. Most common complication is pneumothorax

2. Which of the following would not be considered an appropriate nursing intervention for the patient with pneumonia?

a. Performing postural drainage every 2 to 3 hours
b. Teaching the patient proper disposal of soiled tissues
c. Allowing the patient to sleep in the semi-Fowler's position
d. Administering analgesics for chest pain

3. Clinical manifestations of TB include
a. chest pain and morning sweats.
b. productive cough and high-grade fevers.
c. night sweats and cough.
d. hemoptysis and rust-colored sputum.

4. All of the following are types of fungal infections *except*
a. histoplasmosis.
b. coccidioidomycosis.
c. aspergillosis.
d. mycoplasmosis.

5. Bronchiectasis is characterized by
a. bronchoconstriction and mucosal edema.
b. hypersensitivity of small bronchioles.
c. chronic dilatation of the bronchi.
d. rupture of bronchi secondary to fibrosis.

6. The major advantage of a Venturi mask is that it can
a. deliver a precise concentration of O_2.
b. provide continuous 100% humidity.
c. be used while a patient eats and sleeps.
d. deliver as much as 80% O_2.

7. A common pathophysiologic characteristic of many types of pneumoconiosis is
a. diffuse airway obstruction.
b. diffuse pulmonary fibrosis.
c. benign tumor growth.
d. liquefactive necrosis.

8. The type of lung cancer generally associated with the best prognosis because it is potentially surgically resectable is
a. squamous cell carcinoma.
b. small cell carcinoma.
c. adenocarcinoma.
d. undifferentiated large cell carcinoma.

9. Which of the following would probably *not* be considered a risk associated with the development of lung cancer?
a. Living in rural environment
b. Heredity
c. Cigar smoking
d. Preexisting pulmonary disease

10. A common cause of flail chest is
a. multiple rib fractures.
b. spontaneous pneumothorax.
c. kyphoscoliosis.
d. atelectasis.

11. The purpose of closed chest-tube drainage is to
a. prevent the escape of air from the pleural space.
b. produce additional negative alveolar pressure.
c. equalize the pressure in the chest cavity.
d. remove air and fluid from the pleural space.

12. Nursing measures that should be instituted after a thoracotomy include all the following *except*
a. range-of-motion exercises on the affected upper extremity.
b. keeping the patient off the unaffected side after a pneumonectomy.
c. monitoring chest-tube drainage and functioning.
d. using a shoulder sling to immobilize the affected upper extremity.

13. The Guillain-Barré syndrome causes respiratory problems primarily by
a. depressing the CNS.
b. paralyzing the diaphragm secondary to trauma.
c. interrupting nerve transmission to respiratory muscles.
d. deforming chest-wall muscles.

14. Which of the following descriptions best characterizes cor pulmonale?
a. Right ventricular hypertrophy secondary to increased pulmonary vascular resistance
b. Right ventricular hypertrophy secondary to congenital heart disease
c. Pulmonary congestion secondary to left ventricular failure
d. Excess serous fluid collection in the alveoli secondary to heart failure

15. For which of the following conditions is lung transplantation not indicated?
a. End-stage COPD
b. Primary pulmonary hypertension
c. Cystic fibrosis
d. Adenocarcinoma of the lung

REFERENCES

1. Boring CC and others: Cancer statistics, 1994, *CA Cancer J Clin* 44:7, 1994.
2. Johnson CC, Finegold SM: Pyogenic bacterial pneumonia, lung abscess, and empyema. In Murray JF, Nadel JA, editors: *Textbook of respiratory medicine,* ed 2, Philadelphia, 1994, Saunders.
3. Blinkhorn RJ: Community-acquired pneumonia. In Baum GL, Wolinsky E, editors: *Textbook of pulmonary diseases,* ed 5, New York, 1994, Little, Brown.
4. Hayden FG, Gwaltney JM: Viral infections. In Murray JF, Nadel JA, editors: *Textbook of respiratory medicine,* ed 2, Philadelphia, 1994, Saunders.
5. Timby BK: Pneumocystosis in patients with acquired immunodeficiency syndrome, *Crit Care Nurse* 12:64, 1992.
6. Petersen C, Mills J: Parasitic infections. In Murray JF, Nadel JA: *Textbook of respiratory medicine,* ed 2, Philadelphia, 1994, Saunders.
7. Update: tuberculosis elimination–United States, *MMWR* 39:153, 1990.
8. Boutotte J: T.B. the second time around, *Nursing* 23:42, 1993.
9. Elpern EH, Girzadas AM: Tuberculosis update: new challenges of an old disease, *Medsurg Nurs* 2:176, 1993.
10. Adler JJ: Hospital-acquired tuberculosis: addressing the challenge, *Hosp Prac* 28:109, 1993.
11. Farazan S: Fungal infections of the lung. In Farazan S: *A concise handbook of respiratory disease,* ed 3, East Norwalk, CT, 1992, Appleton and Lange.
12. Galgiani JN: Coccidiodomycosis, *West J Med* 159:153, 1993.
13. Murray JF: New presentations of bronchiectasis, *Hosp Prac* 26:55, 1991.
14. Bartlett JG: Antibiotics in lung abscess, *Semin Respir Infect* 6:103, 1991.

15. Massaro D: Oxygen: toxicity and tolerance, *Hosp Pract* 24:95, 1986.
16. Crockett AJ and others: The effects of home oxygen therapy on hospital admission rates in chronic obstructive airways disease, *Monaldi Archives for Chest Disease* 48:445, 1993.
17. Tarpy SP, Farber HW: Chronic lung disease: when to prescribe home oxygen, *Geriatrics* 49:27, 1994.
18. O'Donohue WJ: Technical and therapeutic advances in home oxygen therapy, *Monaldi Archives for Chest Disease* 48:458, 1993.
19. Klaas MA, Cheng EY: Early response to pulse oximetry alarms with telemetry, *J Clin Monit* 10:178, 1994.
20. Kampelmacher MJ and others: Long-term oxygen therapy, *Neth J Med* 44:141, 1994.
21. Epler GR: Clinical overview of occupational lung disease, *Radiol Clin North Am* 30:1121, 1992.
22. McLoud TC: Occupational lung disease, *Radiol Clin North Am* 29:931, 1991.
23. Hendrick DJ: Management of occupational asthma, *Eur Resp J* 7:961, 1994.
24. Report of the Surgeon General: The health consequences of involuntary smoking, *US Department of Health and Human Services.*
25. Cresanta JL: Epidemidogy of cancer in the United States, *Prim Care* 19:419, 1992.
26. Elpern EH: Lung cancer. In Groenwald SL: *Cancer nursing: principles and practice,* ed 3, Boston, 1990, Jones and Bartlett.
27. Phillips AJ: The relationship between smoking and health—a review of the evidence, *Can J Public Health* 85:77, 1994.
28. Gupta NC, Frick MP: Clinical applications of positron emission tomography in cancer, *CA Cancer Clin* 43:235, 1993.
29. Flehinger BJ, Melamed MR: Current status of screening for lung cancer, *Chest Surgery Clinics of North America* 4:1, 1994.
30. Glover J, Miaskowski C: Small cell lung cancer: pathophysiologic mechanisms and nursing implications, *Oncol Nurs Forum* 21:87, 1994.
31. Hazuka MB, Bunn PA: Controversies in the non-surgical treatment of Stage III non-small cell lung cancer, *Am Rev Respir Dis* 145:967, 1992.
32. Maran JN, Gray MA: Pulmonary laser therapy, *Am J Nurs* 88:828, 1988.
33. Kviz FJ and others: Age and readiness to quit smoking, *Prev Med* 23:211, 1994.
34. Wong JG: How to help your patients quit smoking: strategies that work, *Postgrad Med* 94:197, 1993.
35. Light RW: Malignant pleural effusions. In *Pleural diseases,* ed 2, Philadelphia, 1990, Lea and Febiger.
36. Spouge AR, Thomas HA: Tension pneumothorax after reversal of a Heimlich valve, *Am J Roentgenol* 158:763, 1992.
37. Gross SB: Current challenges, concepts, and controversies in chest tube management, *Clin Issues Crit Care Nurs* 4:260, 1993.
38. Erickson RS: Mastering the ins and outs of chest drainage, part 2, *Nursing* 19:46, 1989.
39. Managing chest drainage problems, *Nursing* 23:32J, 1993.
40. Tampinco-Golos IC: Endoscopic thoracotomy, *Nursing* 23:62, 1993.
41. Nicholson C, Coleman CA, Mack M: Are you ready for video thoracoscopy? *Am J Nurs* 93:54, 1993.
42. Snider GL: History and physical examination. In Baum GL, Wolinsky E: *Textbook of pulmonary diseases,* ed 5, New York, 1994, Little, Brown.
43. Moser K: Pulmonary embolism. In Baum GL, Wolinsky E: *Textbook of pulmonary diseases,* ed 5, New York, 1994, Little, Brown.
44. Tahir MZ: Long-term survival in primary pulmonary hypertension, *Hosp Prac* 27:219, 1992.
45. Rubin W: Primary pulmonary hypertension. Practical therapeutic recommendations, *Drugs* 43:37, 1992.
46. Calhoon JH; Grover FL, Gibbons, WJ: Single lung transplantation alternative indications and techniques, *J Thorac Cardiovasc Surg* 101:816, 1991.
47. Orofrio JM, Emory B: Selection of patients for lung transplantation, *Med Clin North Am* 76:1207, 1992.
48. McCarthy PM, and others: Lung and heart lung transplantation: the state of the art, *Cleve Clin J Med* 59:307, 1992.
49. Kirk AJ, Colquhoun IW, Dark JH: Lung preservation: a review of current practice and future directions, *Ann Thorac Surg* 56:990, 1993.

Chapter 25

NURSING ROLE IN MANAGEMENT

Obstructive Pulmonary Diseases

Pamela Becker Weilitz   Trisch Van Sciver

Learning Objectives

1. Describe the etiology, pathophysiology, clinical manifestations, and therapeutic and pharmacologic management of asthma.
2. Describe the nursing role in management of the patient with asthma.
3. Differentiate among the etiology, pathophysiology, clinical manifestations, complications, and therapeutic and pharmacologic management of chronic bronchitis and emphysema.
4. Describe the effects of cigarette smoking on the lungs.
5. Explain the respiratory therapy and nursing management of the patient with chronic bronchitis and emphysema.
6. Describe the pathophysiology, clinical manifestations, and therapeutic and nursing management of the patient with cystic fibrosis.

Chronic obstructive pulmonary disease (COPD) is a descriptive term for diseases characterized by increased resistance to airflow as a result of airway obstruction or airway narrowing. Airway obstruction may be the result of accumulated secretions, edema, and swelling of the inner lumen; bronchospasm; or destruction of lung tissue. Emphysema and chronic bronchitis are the most common forms of COPD. Asthma, a reactive airway disease, is also a chronic obstructive lung disease. The patient with asthma has variations in airflow over time, whereas the limitation in expiratory airflow in the patient with emphysema or chronic bronchitis is generally more constant. The patient with a diagnosis of COPD may have distinguishing features of two or all three of these diseases. Cystic fibrosis, another form of COPD, is a genetic disorder that produces airway obstruction because of changes in glandular secretions.

ASTHMA

Asthma is a lung disease characterized by airway obstruction, inflammation, and increased responsiveness to a variety of stimuli. The airway obstruction may resolve spontaneously or with treatment, and in some patients, it may not resolve completely. The hyperresponsiveness of the airways is variable, producing spontaneous fluctuations in the severity of obstruction. The clinical course of asthma is unpredictable, ranging from paroxysms of dyspnea, wheezing, and cough, which may be mild and difficult to detect, to severe and unremitting symptoms such as in status asthmaticus.

Significance

Asthma affects an estimated 12 million persons in the United States. The prevalence of asthma has increased more than 60% in the last 10 years.[1] The morbidity rate associated with asthma is dramatic. It affects school attendance, occupational choices, physical activity, and many other aspects of life. The mortality rate related to asthma has more than doubled since 1978. African-Americans are twice as likely to die from asthma as Caucasians. Between the ages of 15 and 44 years, the asthma death rate for African-Americans is at least five times higher than for Caucasians. The high mortality rates related to asthma may be related to an inaccurate assessment of disease severity, increase of allergens in the environment, delay in seeking help, inadequate medical treatment, limited access to health care, and noncompliance with prescribed therapy.[2,3]

Pathophysiology

The most common etiologic factor of asthma is nonspecific *hyperirritability* or *hyperresponsiveness* of the tracheobronchial tree. The airway hyperresponsiveness seen in asthma is caused by bronchoconstriction in response to physical, chemical, and pharmacologic agents. Asthma has been traditionally considered a disease characterized by bronchospasm; however, the pathophysiologic changes associated

Reviewed by Janet Crimslik, RN, MSN, CS, Pulmonary Clinical Nurse Specialist, Department of Health and Hospitals, Boston City Hospital, Boston, MA.

RESEARCH

IMPLICATIONS FOR NURSING PRACTICE

IMPACT OF ASTHMA ON PATIENTS

Citation Janson-Bjerklie S, Ferketich S, Benner P: Predicting the outcomes of living with asthma, *Res Nurs Health* 16:241-250, 1993.

Purpose To explore the impact of person and disease predictors on psychosocial and morbidity outcomes in adults with chronic asthma.

Methods Descriptive study using 95 asthmatic adults who were followed for 60 days. Standardized questionnaires were used to measure panic-fear, uncertainty, appraisal of social support and life change, coping, and anticipating self-care strategies. Asthma was rated as mild, moderate, or severe. Qualitative interviews were used to elicit descriptions of coping with episodes of asthma during the study period.

Results and Conclusions Amount of distress during an asthma attack, perceived danger from asthma, and appraisal of social support were predictors of emergency room visits. Self-care, perceived life stress, nocturnal symptoms, and amount of distress during an asthma episode were predictors of depression. The patient using self-care strategies to prevent asthma attacks felt less depressed. Financial status and the absence of nocturnal symptoms predicted life satisfaction.

Implications for Nursing Practice Control of nocturnal symptoms and restoration of normal sleep patterns may be an essential first step in asthma management. Psychosocial variables influence symptom perception, treatment, and emotional responses to illness episodes. Depression is associated with increased asthma morbidity and mortality. The nurse needs to become involved in identifying the asthma patient at greatest risk and to plan interventions to decrease the morbidity and mortality associated with asthma.

with asthma are the result of inflammatory responses in the airways.

The *early-phase response* in asthma is characterized by bronchospasm, which induces the inflammatory sequelae of the late-phase response (Fig. 25-1). The early-phase response is triggered when an allergen or irritant cross-links IgE receptors on mast cells found beneath the basement membrane of the bronchial wall (Fig. 25-2). The mast cells become activated with subsequent release of granules (Table 9-8) and disruption of the phospholipid cell membrane. Both processes result in the release of histamine, bradykinin, leukotrienes, prostaglandins, platelet-activating factor, and chemotactic factors. A similar process can occur in a susceptible patient after exercise. These mediators cause an intense inflammatory reaction associated with the classic immediate reaction of asthma, which consists of bronchial smooth muscle constriction, increased vasodilatation and permeability, and epithelial damage. Clinically the

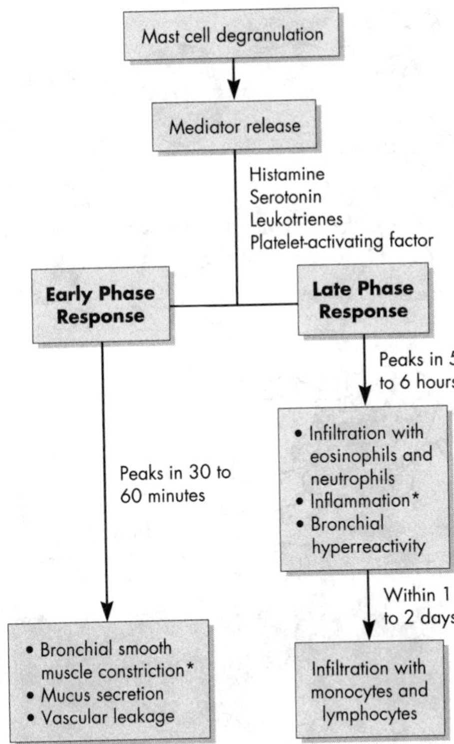

Fig. 25-1 Early and late phase responses of asthma. Items with an *asterisk* are primary processes.

effects are bronchospasm, increased mucus secretion, edema formation, and increased amounts of tenacious sputum (Figs. 25-1 and 25-3). This immediate response peaks within 30 to 60 minutes of exposure to the trigger (e.g., allergen, irritant) and subsides in another 30 to 90 minutes. Clinically the patient has wheezing, chest tightness, and dyspnea.

The *late-phase response* in asthma peaks 5 to 6 hours after exposure and may last for several hours or days. It is characterized primarily by inflammation. Eosinophils and neutrophils infiltrate the airways. These cells can subsequently release mediators that cause mast cells to release histamine and other mediators that eventually set up a self-sustaining cycle. In addition, lymphocytes and monocytes influx into the area.

These series of reactions, which make up the late-phase response, heighten airway reactivity that in turn worsens the symptoms of future asthma attacks. The person becomes hyperresponsive to specific allergens and nonspecific stimuli such as air pollution, cold air, and dust. Identifying the original trigger may be difficult at this point, and less stimulation is required to produce a reaction. The airway hyperreactivity may be related to the exposure of sensory nerves as a result of epithelial injury caused by the repeated late-phase responses. Increased airway resistance leads to air trapping in the alveoli and hyperinflation of the lungs.

Approximately 50% of adults with an early-phase response to an allergen will also have a late-phase response. In the case of nonallergenic irritants the frequency is 30%

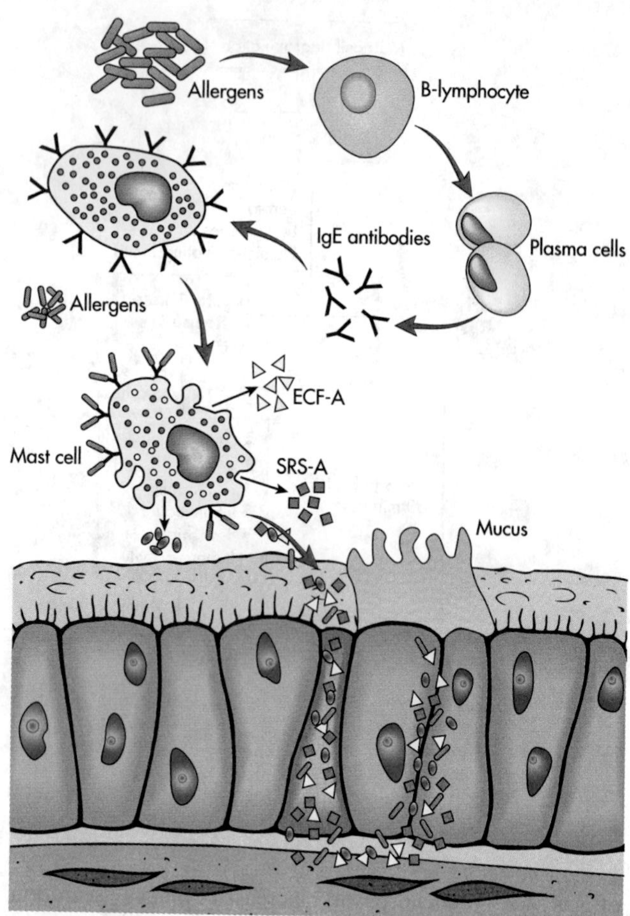

Fig. 25-2 The early phase response in asthma is triggered when an allergen or irritant cross-links IgE receptors on mast cells, which are then activated to release histamine and other inflammatory mediators.

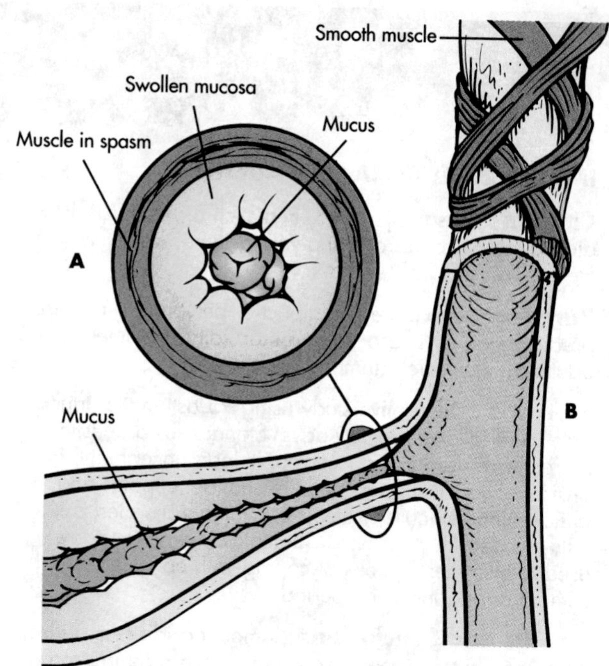

Fig. 25-3 Factors causing expiratory obstruction in asthma. ***A,*** Cross section of a bronchiole occluded by muscle spasm, swollen mucosa, and mucus in the lumen. ***B,*** Longitudinal section of a bronchiole.

to 40%. The underlying epithelial damage and airway hyperreactivity may persist for several weeks or more after resolution of the airway obstruction.[4]

The prominent pathophysiologic features of asthma are a reduction in airway diameter and an increase in airway resistance related to mucosal inflammation, constriction of bronchial smooth muscles, and excess production of mucus (Fig. 25-4). Accompanying these changes are bronchial muscle hypertrophy, basement membrane thickening, mucous gland hypertrophy, thick and tenacious sputum, hyperinflation and air trapping in the alveoli, increased work of breathing, alterations in respiratory muscle function, abnormal distribution of both ventilation and perfusion, and altered arterial blood gases (ABGs). Although asthma is considered a disease of the airways, eventually all aspects of pulmonary function are compromised during an asthma attack.

In addition to the inflammatory aspects of asthma, alterations in the neural control of the airways have been postulated. It is possible, however, that these defects are secondary to the inflammatory process. The autonomic

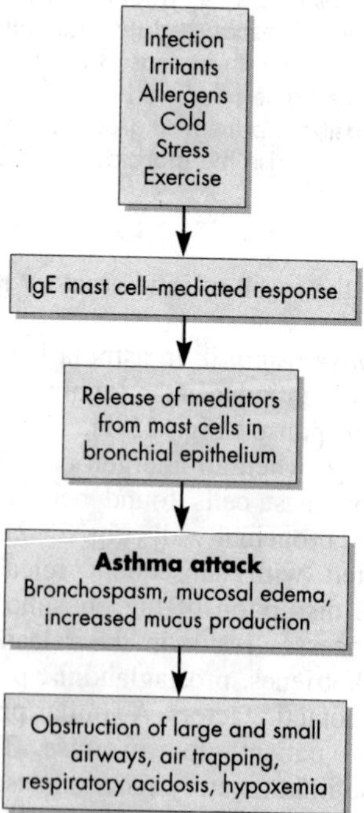

Fig. 25-4 Pathophysiology of asthma.

nervous system, consisting of the parasympathetic and sympathetic systems, innervates the bronchi. Bronchial muscle tone is regulated by the parasympathetic nervous system via the vagus nerve. Afferent and efferent impulses are conducted through the vagus nerve to the medulla and back to the lungs. When airway nerve endings are stimulated by mechanical or chemical stimuli (e.g., air pollution, cold air, dust, allergens), increased release of acetylcholine causes bronchoconstriction.

Both α- and β-adrenergic receptors of the sympathetic nervous system are located in the bronchi. When the α receptors are stimulated, bronchoconstriction occurs. When the β receptors (β_2 receptors are primarily located in the bronchi) are stimulated, bronchodilatation occurs. Epinephrine and β_2-adrenergic drugs act primarily on β receptors.

Triggers of Asthma Attacks (Table 25-1)

Allergens. In some persons with asthma, an exaggerated IgE response to certain allergens (e.g., dust, pollen, grasses, animal danders) occurs. These allergens attach to IgE receptors on mast cells (Fig. 25-2). The IgE-mast cell complexes remain for a long time so that a second exposure to the allergen triggers mast cell degranulation even years after the initial exposure to the antigen. (Allergic reactions are discussed in Chapter 10.)

Respiratory infections. Respiratory infections (especially viral infections) are one of the most common precipitating factors of an acute asthma attack. Bacterial respiratory infections, with the exception of sinusitis, do not play a major role in exacerbations of asthma. Infections cause inflammatory changes in the tracheobronchial system and alter the mucociliary mechanism. Therefore they increase the hyperresponsiveness of the bronchial system. Increased airway responsiveness can last from 2 to 8 weeks after the infection in both normal and asthmatic persons. A respiratory infection may trigger airway inflammation and cause asthma that subsides in 2 to 3 weeks, or it may trigger asthma that continues for several months and then subsides spontaneously or after medical intervention. The patient should avoid people with colds or flu, get yearly influenza vaccinations, and avoid taking over-the-counter (OTC) cold remedies unless approved by the health care provider.

Exercise. Asthma that is induced or exacerbated during physical exertion is called exercise-induced asthma (EIA). Provocation of bronchospasm by exercise is probably operative to some extent in every person with asthma, and in some it may be the only trigger mechanism that will produce symptoms. Typically, EIA occurs after several minutes of vigorous exercise (e.g., jogging, aerobics, walking briskly, climbing stairs) and is characterized by bronchospasm, shortness of breath, and wheezing. β_2-agonists, cromolyn (Intal), and nedocromil (Tilade) have successfully maintained bronchodilatation during exercise when they were inhaled immediately before exercise. The patient should perform a brief warm-up of stretching for 2 to 3 minutes before exercise. When exercising in cold or dry climate conditions, breathing through a scarf or mask may decrease the likelihood of symptoms.

Drugs and food additives. Sensitivity to drugs may occur in some asthmatic persons. In some asthmatics who ingest aspirin or nonsteroidal antiinflammatory drugs (NSAIDs) (e.g., indomethacin), wheezing will develop in approximately 2 hours. Some patients are sensitive to salicylates, which are found in many foods, beverages, and flavorings. β-blockers (e.g., propanolol [Inderal]) may trigger asthma because they inhibit adrenergic stimulation of the bronchioles and thus prevent bronchodilatation. Other agents that may precipitate asthma in the susceptible patient are tartrazine (yellow dye No. 5 found in many foods), vitamins, and sodium metabisulfate (a food preservative commonly found in fruits, beer, and wine and used extensively in salad bars to protect vegetables from oxidation).

These agents are thought to interfere with prostaglandin metabolic pathways, leading to enhanced production of leukotrienes, some of which are potent bronchoconstrictors. The onset of a typical reaction occurs 15 minutes to 3 hours after ingestion and is marked by profuse rhinorrhea, often accompanied by macular erythema or nausea, vomiting, intestinal cramps, and diarrhea. Acute asthma begins after the nasal symptoms appear. Pretreatment with steroids or cromolyn does not prevent the reaction. Epinephrine and theophylline, given shortly after the onset, usually control symptoms.

Although sensitivity to salicylates persists for many years, the nature and severity of the reaction can change over time. Dietary restrictions of tartrazine (if applicable) and avoidance of aspirin and NSAIDs are required.

Emotional stress. Another factor often discussed in relationship to the etiology of asthma is psychologic or emo-

Table 25-1 Triggers of Acute Asthma Attacks

▪ Allergen inhalation Animal danders House dust mite Pollens Molds ▪ Air pollutants Exhaust fumes Perfumes Oxidants Sulfur dioxides Cigarette smoke Aerosol sprays ▪ Viral upper respiratory infection ▪ Paranasal sinusitis ▪ Exercise and cold, dry air ▪ Drugs Aspirin Nonsteroidal antiinflammatory drugs β-adrenergic blockers	▪ Occupational exposure Metal salts Wood and vegetable dusts Industrial chemicals and plastics Pharmaceutical agents ▪ Food additives Sulfites (bisulfites and metabisulfites) Tartrazine ▪ Menses ▪ Gastroesophageal reflux ▪ Emotional stress

tional stimuli. Asthma is not a psychosomatic disease; however, psychologic factors can interact with the asthmatic response to worsen or ameliorate the disease process. An asthma attack caused by any trigger can produce panic and anxiety, which are not unexpected emotions during this experience. The extent to which psychologic factors contribute to the induction and continuation of any given acute exacerbation is unknown, but it probably varies from patient to patient and in the same patient from episode to episode.

Clinical Manifestations

Asthma is characterized by an unpredictable and variable course. An attack of asthma may have an abrupt onset or may be more gradual. Attacks often occur at night and may last for a few minutes to several hours. Between attacks the patient may be asymptomatic with normal pulmonary function. In some persons, however, compromised pulmonary function may result in a state of continuous asthma and chronic debilitation.

The characteristic clinical manifestations of asthma are wheezing, cough, dyspnea, and chest tightness after exposure to a precipitating factor or trigger. Expiration may be prolonged. Instead of a normal inspiratory-expiratory ratio of 1:2, it may be prolonged to 1:3 or 1:4. Normally the bronchioles constrict during expiration; however, because of the bronchospasm, edema, and mucus in the bronchioles, the airways become narrower than usual. Thus it takes longer for the air to move out of the bronchioles. This produces the characteristic wheezing, air trapping, and hyperinflation.

Wheezing is an unreliable sign to gauge the severity of an attack. Many patients with minor attacks wheeze loudly, whereas others with severe attacks do not wheeze. The patient with severe asthmatic attacks may have no audible wheezing because of the marked reduction in airflow. For wheezing to occur, the patient must be able to move enough air to produce the sound. Wheezing usually occurs first on exhalation. As asthma progresses the patient may wheeze during inspiration and expiration. Severely diminished breath sounds are an ominous sign, indicating severe obstruction and impending respiratory failure.

The cough may be nonproductive. Mobilizing secretions may be difficult, indicating production of thick, tenacious, white, gelatinous mucus and widespread bronchiolar mucus plugging. In some patients with asthma, cough is the only symptom. The bronchospasm may not be severe enough to cause airflow obstruction, but it can increase bronchial tone and cause irritation and stimulation of the cough receptors.

The person with asthma has difficulty moving air in and out of the lungs, which creates a feeling of suffocation. Therefore during an acute attack, the person with asthma sits upright or slightly bent forward, using the accessory muscles of respiration to try to get enough air. The more difficult the breathing becomes, the more anxious the patient feels.

Examination of the patient during an acute attack usually reveals signs of hypoxemia, which may include restlessness, increased anxiety, inappropriate behavior, increased pulse and blood pressure, and pulsus paradoxus greater than 12 mm Hg. The respiratory rate is significantly increased (usually greater than 30 breaths per minute) with the use of accessory muscles. Percussion of the lungs indicates hyperresonance, and auscultation indicates the presence of inspiratory or expiratory wheezing. Diminished or absent breath sounds may indicate a significant decrease in air movement resulting from exhaustion and an inability to generate enough muscle force to ventilate.

Classification of Asthma

Asthma can be classified as mild, moderate, or severe. *Mild asthma* is defined as cough or chest tightness one to two times a week without limitation in physical activity between episodes. The patient is treated as needed and can achieve peak expiratory flow rates (PEFRs) of 80% or greater than predicted. Spirometry shows minimal to no evidence of airway obstruction with normal expiratory flow volumes and lung volumes.

The patient with *moderate asthma* experiences cough, wheezing, or chest tightness on most days that results in a mild to moderate reduction in physical activity. Cough and wheezing are often present between exacerbations. Nocturnal symptoms can occur as often as two to three times a week, and significant exacerbations can occur one to two times a year. The patient with moderate asthma has PEFRs that show 20% variability between morning and evening measurements. This patient is usually only able to achieve PEFRs of 60% to 80% of predicted. Spirometry reveals airway obstruction with decreased expiratory flow at low volumes. Lung volumes may be increased because of hyperinflation.

The patient with *severe asthma* has significant daily symptoms that result in major limitations in their activities of daily living (ADLs) and exercise tolerance. There are frequent, severe exacerbations. The patient with severe asthma is almost nightly awakened by the asthma and complains of chest tightness when awakening in the morning. The patient may be hospitalized a few times a year for respiratory insufficiency or respiratory failure with intubation and mechanical ventilation. PEFRs are less than 60% of predicted with a 30% variability between the morning and the evening. Spirometry reveals marked evidence of obstruction, with decreased expiratory flow volumes that may not normalize between exacerbations. Total lung volumes are increased because of chronic hyperinflation.

Complications

Severe acute asthma can result in complications such as rib fractures, pneumothorax, pneumomediastinum, atelectasis, pneumonia, and status asthmaticus.

Status Asthmaticus. Status asthmaticus is a severe, life-threatening complication of asthma that may be refractory to the usual treatment. An axiom describes status asthmaticus: "The longer it lasts, the worse it gets, and the worse it gets, the longer it lasts." Acute asthmatic attacks account for nearly 1 million emergency department (ED) visits a year in the United States, with hundreds of thousands of hospital admissions each year.[1] Of the persons with asthma admitted to the hospital, approximately 10% require intensive care unit (ICU) monitoring or ventilatory assistance for status asthmaticus.[5]

Causes of status asthmaticus include viral illnesses, ingestion of aspirin or other NSAIDs, emotional stress, increases in environmental pollutants or other allergen exposure, abrupt discontinuation of drug therapy (especially corticosteroids and theophylline), abuse of aerosol medication, and ingestion of β-adrenergic blocking agents.[6] The patient usually reports a history of poorly controlled asthma progressing over days or weeks.

The clinical manifestations of status asthmaticus result from increased airway resistance as a consequence of edema, mucus plugging, and bronchospasm with subsequent air trapping and hyperinflation. The patient has clinical manifestations similar to those of asthma, but they are more severe and more prolonged. Extreme anxiety, fear of suffocation, severely increased work of breathing, and diaphoresis are common. Absence of diaphoresis may indicate significant dehydration. Sternocleidomastoid, intercostal, and supraclavicular muscle retractions reflect increased work of breathing. If obtainable, the PEFR is usually less than 100 to 150 L per minute.

Although wheezing is often audible without a stethoscope, auscultation may not always be reliable because the airflow obstruction may be so severe in some patients that audible wheezing or other abnormal lung sounds may not be produced because of insufficient airflow. The chest appears fixed in a hyperinflated position and is often described as "tight," indicating severely decreased movement of air through the constricted bronchial airways.

Forced exhalation with the use of the abdominal musculature can result in increased intrathoracic pressure transmitted to the great vessels and heart. Neck vein distention and a pulsus paradoxus of 40 mm Hg or higher may result. (Pulsus paradoxus is described in Chapter 34.) Hypertension, sinus tachycardia, and ventricular dysrhythmias may occur. These three conditions are related to hypoxemia, catecholamines from an endogenous response to hypoxia, and underlying coronary artery disease in the older adult population. Electrocardiogram (ECG) results may show sinus tachycardia or signs of strain on the right side of the heart secondary to pulmonary vasoconstriction, which may be seen as P-pulmonale and a right axis deviation.

Hypoxemia with hypocapnia usually occurs initially as the patient attempts to hyperventilate and maintain adequate oxygenation and ventilation. As the severity of the attack increases, the work of breathing increases, making it more difficult for the patient to overcome the increased resistance to breathing. The patient becomes fatigued, causing more carbon dioxide (CO_2) retention. ABGs deteriorate to normocapnia (normal arterial CO_2 pressure) and then ultimately to hypercapnia and hypoxemia (Table 25-2). A moderate elevation in $PaCO_2$ may be tolerated without intubation and mechanical ventilation if the patient remains alert and cooperative and continues to improve during the first 2 to 3 hours of treatment.

Complications of status asthmaticus include pneumothorax, pneumomediastinum, acute cor pulmonale with right ventricular failure, and severe respiratory muscle fatigue leading to respiratory arrest. Repeated attacks of status asthmaticus can lead to irreversible emphysema. Death from status asthmaticus is usually the result of respiratory arrest or cardiac failure.

Diagnostic Studies

Wheezing and respiratory distress characterize a variety of disorders, including asthma, chronic bronchitis, emphy-

Table 25-2 Arterial Blood Gas Results Correlated with Clinical Manifestations During an Acute Asthmatic Attack

Time Frame	pH	$PaCO_2$	PaO_2	Physiologic Event	Clinical Manifestations
Early in attack	↑	↓	↓	Alveolar hyperventilation→ hypocarbia Hypoxemia secondary to ventilation-perfusion mismatch Adequate alveolar ventilation CO_2 not being eliminated as well	Use of all accessory muscles of ventilation to overcome increased airway resistance Increased heart rate, diaphoresis, chest tightness, cough, wheezing
Progressive attack	N	N	↓	Decrease in effective alveolar ventilation Hypercarbia indicating that ventilation is no longer adequate	Tiring of patient and difficulty with increased work of breathing
Prolonged attack, status asthmaticus	↓	↑	↓	Alveolar hypoventilation → respiratory acidosis Worsening hypoxemia as result of hypoventilation and ventilation-perfusion mismatch	Exhaustion, diminished breath sounds, intubation and mechanical ventilation necessary

sema, cystic fibrosis, pulmonary edema, upper airway and bronchial obstruction, tracheobronchitis, bronchiolitis, aspiration, and pulmonary embolism. Certain diagnostic studies must be performed to determine whether these symptoms are caused primarily by asthma (Table 25-3). The severity of the clinical manifestations of asthma determines the appropriate diagnostic studies.

In the patient who is not in distress, a detailed history may indicate previous attacks of a similar nature, often precipitated by a known cause. Seasonal attacks may indicate pollen triggers. Attacks that occur at night may be caused by sleeping with a cat, sleep apnea, gastroesophageal reflux, or mattress dust mites. It is important to determine whether the patient can sleep through the night or participate in an aerobic exercise program. This information helps to identify asthma triggers.

Pulmonary function tests are usually within normal limits between attacks if the patient has no other underlying pulmonary disease. Pulmonary function tests are frequently used to diagnose asthma and are important for an objective measurement of airflow obstruction. The patient with asthma usually has a decrease in forced expiratory volume in one second (FEV_1), PEFR, FEV to forced vital capacity (FVC) ratio (FEV_1/FVC), and forced expiratory flow rate measured during the middle of a FVC ($FEF_{25-75\%}$), with the degree of obstruction depending on the values obtained. (The normal values for pulmonary function tests are discussed in Chapter 22.)

These parameters decrease from their baseline levels during an exacerbation and in some patients may be within normal limits during a remission. Confirmation of the diagnosis can be made by inducing bronchospasm with bronchial provocation testing with known quantities of bronchial irritants such as histamine, methacholine, and cold air. An increase of 15% or more in the FEV_1 in response to a bronchodilator when the patient is not experiencing an exacerbation is another diagnostic indicator of asthma.

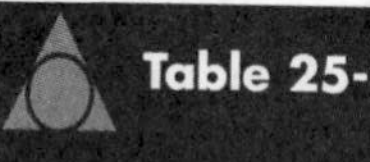

Table 25-3 Therapeutic Management: Asthma

Diagnostic
- Health history and physical examination
- Pulmonary function studies including response to bronchodilator therapy
- Chest x-ray
- Measurement of ABGs or oximetry
- Allergy skin testing (if indicated)
- Sputum specimen for Gram stain and culture (if indicated)
- Blood level of eosinophils and IgE

Therapeutic

Prevention and maintenance
- Elimination of causative factors or triggers (if known)
- Desensitization (immunotherapy) (if indicated)
- β_2-adrenergic drugs (inhaled or oral)
- Theophylline compound (oral) (if indicated)
- Corticosteroids (inhaled or oral)
- Cromolyn sodium (inhaled)
- Nedocromil (Tilade) (inhaled)
- Assessment of home and work environment
- Progressive plan of exercise

Acute asthma
- Inhaled β_2-adrenergic drugs
- Nasal or mask O_2
- IV aminophylline (if indicated)
- IV or oral corticosteroids
- Inhaled or nebulized anticholinergic agents
- Fluid intake of 3 L/day

Status asthmaticus
- Inhaled β_2-adrenergic drugs or anticholinergic agents
- IV aminophylline (if indicated)
- O_2 by mask or nasal prongs
- IV corticosteroids
- IV fluids
- IV magnesium (if indicated)
- Intubation and assisted ventilation (if indicated)

ABGs, Arterial blood gases; *IV*, intravenous.

Eosinophils in the sputum and serum eosinophilia (greater than or equal to 5% of the total white blood cell [WBC] count) and elevated serum IgE levels are highly suggestive of asthma in a symptomatic patient. A chest x-ray in an asymptomatic patient with asthma is usually normal. During an acute attack the chest x-ray shows hyperinflation. In a mild asthma attack, ABGs (if obtained) would indicate respiratory alkalosis with an arterial oxygen pressure (PaO_2) near normal. Hypercapnia and respiratory and metabolic acidosis indicate severe disease. In mild asthma pulse oximetry monitoring is sufficient to determine oxygenation status.

Allergy skin testing may be of some value to determine sensitivity to specific antigens. However, a positive skin test does not necessarily mean that the allergen (antigen) is causing the asthma attack. On the other hand, a negative allergy test does not mean that the asthma is not allergy related. A radioallergosorbent test (RAST) is sometimes used to identify allergic causes in certain patients who show negative skin tests and in those who should not be tested (e.g., patients with severe eczema).

If the patient has wheezing and acute distress, it is not feasible to obtain a detailed health history (although a family member may supply some pertinent information). During an acute attack of asthma, bedside spirometry (specifically FEV_1 or FVC, but usually PEFR) may be used to monitor pulmonary function test results. Serial spirometric parameters, oximetry, and measurement of ABGs help provide information about the severity of the attack and the response to therapy. ABG changes during the stages of an asthmatic attack are listed in Table 25-2. A complete blood cell count (CBC) and serum electrolytes are also obtained to help direct the course of therapy.

A sputum specimen for Gram stain and culture may be obtained to rule out the presence of bacterial infection, especially if the patient has purulent sputum, a history of upper respiratory tract infection (URI), a fever, or an elevated WBC count. A chest x-ray obtained during an acute attack may show findings resembling emphysema with the presence of hyperinflation. Occasionally the chest x-ray reveals complications of asthma such as mucoid impaction, atelectasis, and pneumomediastinum.

Therapeutic Management

The initial treatment of asthma is to alleviate bronchoconstriction with bronchodilator therapy (Table 25-3). In the past, theophylline was the first-line drug for asthma, but it has now been replaced by other bronchodilators and anti-inflammatory agents. Currently β_2-adrenergic agonists are the most effective bronchodilators in use.

Prevention and Maintenance of Chronic Asthma. The patient who has persistent airflow obstruction and frequent attacks of asthma should be taught to avoid triggers of acute attacks and to premedicate before exercising. The choice of drug therapy depends on the severity of symptoms. The patient with mild to moderate asthma or EIA should use inhaled β_2-adrenergic agents or cromolyn (Intal) before exercising or when anticipating exposure to allergens known to cause asthma. Inhaled steroids and nedocromil (Tilade) are used in mild to moderate asthma when symptoms warrant. For moderate to severe asthma, inhaled corticosteroids, oral sustained-release theophylline drugs, inhaled cromolyn, and inhaled ipratropium (Atrovent) can be used to alleviate symptoms. Some persons require continuous oral corticosteroids, which should be maintained at as low a dosage as possible and administered on alternate days (if possible) to reduce systemic side effects. Methotrexate and troleandomycin (TAO) have been used experimentally in the patient with chronic steroid-dependent asthma or COPD who has required high doses of oral prednisone. Methotrexate and TAO are used in combination with methylprednisolone (Medrol) to decrease the required dose of this drug by prolonging its half-life.

Acute Asthma. A patient frequently comes to the ED or a physician's office in acute respiratory distress. The choice of treatment of acute asthma depends on the severity of the attack and response to initial therapy. Severity can be measured objectively by measuring FEV_1 or PEFR. Assessing the degree or amount of change from the patient's personal best PEFR (if known) can help to determine the severity of the attack. Oxygen (O_2) therapy should be started immediately, and its administration should be monitored by pulse oximetry and in more severe cases by measurement of ABGs. Initial therapy should include inhaled β_2-adrenergic-agonist drugs administered by metered-dose inhaler (MDI) using spacer devices or nebulizer. Generally aerosolized medications by nebulizer therapy are given every 20 minutes to 4 hours as necessary.

Although the value of administering aminophylline in the treatment of acute asthma has been questioned, intravenous (IV) aminophylline should be considered if the asthma attack is severe or there is minimal or no response to inhaled β_2-agonists. Corticosteroids are indicated if the initial response is insufficient (e.g., no response within 30 to 60 minutes), if the patient has had several recent asthma attacks, or if the patient is receiving steroid therapy. The choice of oral or IV administration of corticosteroids depends on the severity of the attack. Nebulized ipratropium or glycopyrrolate (Robinul), both of which are anticholinergics, may be administered every 4 to 6 hours if the patient does not respond. Therapy should be continued until the patient is breathing comfortably, wheezing has disappeared, and pulmonary function study results are near baseline values.

Status Asthmaticus. Management of the patient with status asthmaticus aims at correcting hypoxemia and improving ventilation. Most of the therapeutic measures are the same as acute asthma. It may be necessary, however, to increase the frequency and dose of inhaled bronchodilators. When an MDI is used, the typical dose is two to six puffs every 5 to 20 minutes, depending on the medication selected (Table 25-4). Therapy with inhaled agents is usually initiated despite prior home use, because drug delivery at home may have been submaximal and higher doses given under supervision may be beneficial. Frequent continuous nebulization of β-adrenergic agonists may be required.

Continuous monitoring of the patient is critical. Obtaining even a PEFR during a severe asthma attack is usually not possible. IV aminophylline administration may be added to the treatment regimen if the patient does not respond to β-adrenergic agonists. IV corticosteroids are administered, although their peak effect is not apparent for 6 to 12 hours. IV methylprednisolone is administered every 4 to 6 hours. Anticholinergic drugs such as ipratropium (Atrovent) or nebulized glycopyrrolate also may be added to the treatment regimen if severe obstruction persists. The usual dose of ipratropium is two to four puffs every 4 to 6 hours. Magnesium, which acts by relaxing the bronchial smooth muscle, has been used in certain situations to treat status asthmaticus.

Supplemental O_2 is given by Venturi mask or nasal prongs (typically 2 L/min) to achieve a PaO_2 of at least 60 mm Hg or an O_2 saturation of greater than or equal to 90%. An arterial catheter may be inserted to facilitate frequent ABG monitoring. Because the patient's insensible loss of fluids is increased and the metabolic rate is increased, IV fluids are given to provide optimal hydration. Sodium bicarbonate administration is usually limited to treatment of severe metabolic or respiratory acidosis (pH less than 7.29), because effective bronchodilatation by adrenergic agents is not possible if the patient has extreme acidosis. Bronchoscopy, although rarely performed during an acute attack, may be necessary to remove thick mucous plugs.

Occasionally, asthma attacks are so severe that the patient requires mechanical ventilation if there is no response to treatment. Indications for mechanical ventilation are persistence or progressive CO_2 retention and respiratory acidosis, clinical deterioration indicated by fatigue and hypersomnolence, and cardiopulmonary arrest. In status asthmaticus the goals of initiating mechanical ventilation are to achieve a PaO_2 greater than or equal to 60 mm Hg, O_2 saturation greater than or equal to 90%, and a normal pH. Heliox therapy, which is a mixture of oxygen and helium, is sometimes used during mechanical ventilation to decrease airway resistance and improve ventilation.

Louder wheezing may actually occur in the airways that are responding to the therapy as airflow in the airways increases. As improvement continues and airflow increases,

CLINICAL PATHWAY FOR ASTHMA

UNITY HOSPITAL
Emergency Department
Anticipated Recovery Path

Chief Complaint: **Asthma**

Expected Length of Stay 30 Minutes–3 Hours

Admitted per:______

Date:______ Time:______

LMP:______ WT:______

Urgent______

Emergent______

Scheduled______

Allergies ______

Present Medications ______

Chronic Illness ______

Nursing Interventions: Any deviation from normal must be documented on the nursing progress record.

15 minutes	1 hour	2 hours	3 hours
Time:____ Presenting history and precipitating events Time:____ Assessments per standard: A. T, P, R, BP B. Alert ☐ Yes ☐ No C. Orient: time, person, place, situation ☐ Yes ☐ No D. Skin: color____ warm____ dry____ E. Normal home treatment:____ Quantity used:____ F. Quality of respiratory effort (circle) regular; full; labored; shallow; rapid. G. Accessory muscles used: ☐ Yes ☐ No H. Lung sounds:____ I. Recent URI ☐ Yes ☐ No Sputum produced ☐ Yes ☐ No Describe:	Time:____ Document response to any nursing intervention: Time:____ P, R, BP	Time:____ Document response to any nursing intervention: Time:____ P, R, BP	Time: P, R, BP____ Disposition: Time: Admit: Report called to: By whom: Discharge time: A. Reinforce asthma pamphlet ☐ Yes ☐ No B. Reinforce inhaler use ☐ Yes ☐ No C. Reinforce steroid use ☐ Yes ☐ No D. Reinforce ↑ fluids, rest ☐ Yes ☐ No Verbalized understanding ☐ Yes ☐ No RN Signature

continued

breath sounds increase and wheezing decreases. As the patient begins to respond to therapy and symptoms begin to subside, it is important to remember that despite the disappearance of most of the bronchospasm, the edema and cellular infiltration of the airway mucosa and the viscous mucous plugs may take several days to improve. Thus intensive therapy must be continued even after clinical improvement has occurred. IV steroids are usually tapered rapidly, and the patient is placed on oral steroids, which are tapered over several weeks. Inhaled steroids are usually added when the oral steroid dose is tapered. IV aminophylline (if used), frequent airway care with aerosolized medications, and chest physiotherapy (if indicated) are continued for several days after clinical improvement is noted. The patient's cough often becomes productive of mucous

(Text continued on p. 695.)

Clinical Pathway for Asthma—cont'd

	15 minutes	1 hour	2 hours	3 hours
Activity	Position of comfort: Describe: ______ ______	↑ activity as tolerated ____ ______ SOB with exertion ☐ Yes ☐ No Return of symptoms ☐ Yes ☐ No Tolerate lowered HOB s̄ SOB ☐ Yes ☐ No		Activity______ ______ ______ ______
IV	IV ordered solution ☐ Yes ☐ No			
Medications	A. Stable, age appropriate: initiate asthma protocol: ______ B. Unstable, or not fulfilling criteria: order per MD. Anticipate: O_2 ______ Albuterol neb ☐ Yes ☐ No Time neb: ______ Initiated by: ______ Theophylline, steroids, epinephrine	Albuterol neb ☐ Yes ☐ No Time neb: ______ Initiated by: ______ Theophylline, steroids, epinephrine	Albuterol neb ☐ Yes ☐ No Time neb: ______ Initiated by: ______ Theophylline, steroids, epinephrine	**Expected outcomes:** 1. RR appropriate for age. 2. Pulse oximeter >97% on room air (variations based on patient's chronic condition) 3. Patient verbalizes proper use of inhaler and quantity to be used. 4. Patient verbalizes signs and symptoms of increasing respiratory distress and a plan of action. 5. Appropriate disposition made. 6. Peak flow: >350 for adult
Treatments	A. Pulse oximetry: ______ Room air/O_2 ______ B. Peak flow: before neb: ______ after neb: ______	A. Pulse oximetry: ______ Room air/O_2 ______ B. Peak flow: before neb: ______ after neb: ______	A. Pulse oximetry: ______ Room air/O_2 ______ B. Peak flow: before neb: ______ after neb: ______	
Lab	CBC, theophylline level, anticipate ABGs. Time drawn: ______		Lab results on chart within 1 hour of being drawn: ____ ______ Time back: ______	
Radiology				
Consult				
Discharge planning	Anticipate needs for ancillary services: SS, PHN, ______		Appropriate referrals made: ☐ Yes ☐ No	
Teaching		Assess knowledge of: Asthma triggers ☐ Yes ☐ No Use of inhaler ☐ Yes ☐ No Danger signs ☐ Yes ☐ No Previous need for steroids ☐ Yes ☐ No		
Support Psycho/Social	A. Explain projected course of treatment and time frame ☐ Yes ☐ No B. Answer questions of patient and family ____ ______			

Anticipated Recovery Paths are originated from a CareMap® tool. CareMap® tools provide guidance in the case management process for a specified case type. Using CareMap® tools in actual practice requires consideration of individual patient needs. Developed by HealthSpan, Unity Hospital, Coon Rapids, MN. Licensed by Center for Case Management, South Natick, MN.

ABGs, Arterial blood gases; *BP,* blood pressure; *CBC,* complete blood count; *HOB,* head of bed; *IV,* intravenous; *LMP,* last menstrual period; *LOS,* length of stay; *neb,* nebulization; *P,* pulse; *PHN,* Public Health Nurse; *R,* respirations; *RR,* respiratory rate; *SOB,* shortness of breath; *SS,* Social Services; *T,* temperature; *URI,* upper respiratory infection; *WT,* weight.

Table 25-4 Drugs Used in the Treatment of Asthma and COPD

Drug	Route of Administration	Mechanisms of Action	Side Effects	Comments
***β*-Adrenergic Agonist**				
Metaproterenol (Alupent, Metaprel)	Nebulizer, oral tablets, elixir, MDI	Stimulates β-adrenergic receptors, producing bronchodilatation. Increases mucociliary clearance.	Tachycardia, BP changes, nervousness, palpitations, muscle tremors, nausea, vomiting, vertigo, insomnia, dry mouth, headache, hypokalemia.	Should not be used in patient with angina or other cardiac disorders. Has fairly rapid onset of action (5-10 min). Duration of action is 3-4 hr. Oral lasts up to 8 hr.
Albuterol (Proventil, Ventolin)	Nebulizer, MDI, oral tablets, rotahaler	Selectively stimulates β_2 receptors, producing bronchodilatation.	Same as above but cardiac effects are less.	Has slow onset of action (15 min). Duration of action is 4-8 hr, extended-release lasts 8-12 hr.
Pirbuterol (Maxair)	MDI	Same as above.	Same as metaproterenol but cardiac effects are less.	
Isoetharine (Bronkometer, Bronkosol)	Nebulizer, MDI	Same as above.	Same as above.	Pink appearance of sputum may result. Has fast onset of action (5 min) but short duration of 2-3 hr.
Terbutaline (Bicanyl, Brethine, Brethaire)	Oral tablets, nebulizer,* subcutaneous, MDI	Same as above.	Same as above.	Has slow onset of action (except nebulized and subcutaneous route). Duration of action is 4-6 hr.
Bitolterol (Tornalate)	MDI	Same as above.	Same as above.	Duration of action is 4-8 hr.
Epinephrine (Adrenalin)	Subcutaneous, MDI, nebulizer	Stimulates α, β_1, and β_2 receptors. Stimulates β_2 receptors, producing bronchodilatation.	Headache, dizziness, palpitations, tremors, restlessness, hypertension, dysrhythmias, tachycardia	Used primarily to treat severe bronchial asthma attacks. Should not be used in patient with dysrhythmias or hypertension. Instruct patient regarding self-administration of inhalants.
Isoproterenol (Isuprel)	MDI, subcutaneous, nebulizer, IV (rarely used)	Stimulates β_1 and β_2 receptors. Primarily affects β_2 receptors. Acts quickly.	Tachycardia, headache, nausea, palpitations, tremor, insomnia, dysrhythmias	Instruct patient regarding self-administration of inhalants. Abuse can lead to excessive cardiac side effects. Duration of action is 1-2 hr. Used primarily today for pulmonary function testing.
Antiinflammatory Agents				
Corticosteroids				
Hydrocortisone (Solu-Cortef)	IV	Have antiinflammatory and immunosuppressive effects. Decrease edema in bronchial airways. Act synergistically with β_2-agonists. Decrease mucus secretion. Effective in late-phase reaction of asthma.	Cushingoid appearance, skin changes (acne, striae, bruising), osteoporosis, increased appetite, obesity; peptic ulcer, hypertension, hypokalemia, cataracts, menstrual irregularities, muscle weakness, immunosuppression, catabolism, dysphonia, growth retardation	Alternate-day therapy minimizes side effects. Oral dose should be taken in morning with food or milk. When given in high doses, patient must be observed for epigastric distress. H_2 blockers (ranitidine, cimetidine) and antacids may help minimize GI effects. The patient taking long-term steroids may be given vitamin D and calcium to prevent osteoporosis. Should never be abruptly discontinued but tapered gradually over time to prevent adrenal insufficiency. If during tapering patient has recurrence of symptoms, physician should be notified. May be used concomitantly with bronchodilator.
Methylprednisolone (Medrol)	Oral			
(Solu-Medrol)	IV			
Prednisone	Oral			

continued

Table 25-4 Drugs Used in the Treatment of Asthma and COPD—cont'd

Drug	Route of Administration	Mechanisms of Action	Side Effects	Comments
Beclomethasone (Vanceril, Beclovent)	MDI, nasal spray, ophthalmic solution	Same as above. Acts locally in respiratory tract with relatively little systemic absorption.	Oral thrush infections, hoarseness, irritated throat, dry mouth, cough, few systemic effects	Not recommended for acute asthma attack. Rinse mouth with water or mouthwash after use to prevent oral fungal infections. Use of space device with MDI may decrease incidence of thrush. Use after MDI bronchodilator. MDI steroids may be discontinued during acute asthma attack. Nasal spray and eye drops are used for allergic rhinitis.
Triamcinolone acetonide (Azmacort)	MDI	Same as above.	Same as above.	Same as above. Advantage is that it has a built-in spacer device.
Flunisolide (AeroBid, AeroBid-M)	MDI	Same as above.	Same as above.	Aerobid-M contains menthol.
Mast cell stabilizer				
Cromolyn sodium (Aarane, Intal)	Nebulizer, spin inhaler, MDI, nasal spray, ophthalmic solution	Inhibits release of histamine and SRS-A by acting directly on mast cell. May act by interference with calcium ion influx across cell membrane. Exact mechanism unknown.	Irritation of throat, relatively nontoxic effects, bronchospasm	Used for asthma (e.g., before exercise) prophylactically if allergen is causative agent. Instruct patient in correct use of inhaler. May follow treatment with glass of water to reduce pharyngeal irritation. May take 4-6 wk before clinical response occurs. Nasal spray used for allergic rhinitis.
Nedocromil (Tilade)	MDI	Similar to cromolyn but with broad-spectrum effects.	Same as above. Transient unpleasant taste, rhinitis	
Anticholinergics				
Atropine, ipratropium (Atrovent) Glycopyrrolate (Robinul)	Nebulizer, MDI	Blocks action of acetylcholine, resulting in bronchodilatation.	Drying of oral mucosa, cough, flushing of skin, bad taste, fewer systemic effects with glycopyrrolate	Atropine is contraindicated in patient with glaucoma and bladder neck obstruction. Ipratropium bromide can be used in patients with glaucoma and bladder neck obstruction. Half-life of ipratropium is 3-4 hr. Its duration is longer than that of atropine. Atropine's duration of action is longer than that of β_2-agonists. These drugs can be used alone or in conjunction with β-agonists in nebulizers. Alternating schedules of β-adrenergic agonists and atropine administration may be helpful in some patients. Temporary blurred vision will occur if sprayed in eyes.

continued

Table 25-4 Drugs Used in the Treatment of Asthma and COPD—cont'd

Drug	Route of Administration	Mechanisms of Action	Side Effects	Comments
Methylxanthine Derivatives				
Slow-acting agents: Slo-Phyllin, Aminophylline, Theolair, Choledyl, Somophyllin *IV agent:* Aminophylline *Sustained-release agents:* Aminodur, Dura-tabs, Choledyl SA, Constant-T, Theo-Dur, Theolair-SR, Elixophyllin, Slo-Bid Gyrocaps, Theo-Dur Sprinkles *24-hr agents:* Theo-24, Uniphyl	Oral tablets, IV, elixir, rectal suppositories (rarely used)	Major effects are relaxation of bronchial smooth muscles and improved contractility of fatigued diaphragm. Other effects are mild diuresis, increased gastric acid secretion, stimulation of mucociliary clearance, stimulation of CNS and respiration, pulmonary vasodilatation, improved exercise tolerance.	Tachycardia, BP changes, dysrhythmias, anorexia, nausea, vomiting, nervousness, irritability, headache, muscle twitching, flushing, epigastric pain, diarrhea, insomnia, palpitations	Wide variety of response to drug metabolism exists. Half-life is decreased by smoking and is increased by heart failure and liver disease. Cimetidine, ciprofloxacin, erythromycin, and several other drugs may rapidly increase theophylline levels. Gastrointestinal side effects may be alleviated by taking drug with food or antacids. Patient should be instructed to lie down if dizziness is experienced. Patient must be encouraged to take drugs even when feeling well. Extra doses should not be taken when symptoms are present unless prescribed by physician. Side effects should be reported but medication not stopped unless symptoms are severe. Sustained-release tablets should be taken whole and not chewed or crushed. If patient has difficulty swallowing, bead-filled preparations may be used, and they can be emptied onto food but should not be chewed.
Mucolytics				
Acetylcysteine (Mucomyst) (10% and 20%)	Nebulizer	Enzyme breaks down mucoproteins. Decreases viscosity of mucus and enhances mobilization of secretions.	Bronchospasm, hemoptysis, nausea, vomiting	After administration of mucolytics, secretions may become profuse. Use of mucolytic agents may not be necessary if patient is kept well hydrated and humidified. Usually combined with bronchodilator when administered.
Iodinated glycerol (Organidin)	Oral tablets, elixir	Increases output of thin respiratory tract secretions. Liquefies mucus.	GI irritation, rash, thyroid gland enlargement	Same as above, except agent is not usually combined with bronchodilator.

BP, Blood pressure; *CNS,* central nervous system; *GI,* gastrointestinal; *IV,* intravenous; *MDI,* metered-dose inhaler; *SRS-A,* slow-reacting substance of anaphylaxis.
*Not currently approved by FDA for nebulization.

plugs and breath sounds improve. If the patient is asked to perform a forced expiratory maneuver, a faint wheeze may still be heard. Finally, the patient can be switched to oral bronchodilators and can use a β_2- adrenergic MDI before discharge.

Pharmacologic Management

Bronchodilators. Three classes of bronchodilator drugs currently used in asthma therapy are β-adrenergic agonists, methylxanthine derivatives, and anticholinergics (see Table 25-4).

β-Adrenergic agonist drugs. β-Agonists are by far the most effective bronchodilators currently available for asthma.[7] They relax the smooth muscle of the airways from the trachea to the terminal bronchioles and play a role in increasing mucociliary clearance. Activation of β-adrenergic receptors on airway smooth muscle leads to activation of adenylate cyclase and to an increase in intracellular cyclic adenosine monophosphate (cAMP) and subsequent bronchodilatation.

Inhaled β_2-agonists such as metaproterenol (Alupent), albuterol (Proventil, Ventolin), terbutaline (Brethaire), bitolterol (Tornalate), and pirbuterol (Maxair) have an onset of action within minutes and are effective for 4 to 8 hours. All but metaproterenol are β_2 specific. Inhaled β-agonists are indicated for the short-term relief of bronchoconstriction and are the treatment of choice for acute exacerbations of asthma. β-agonists are also useful in preventing bronchospasm precipitated by exercise and other stimuli because they prevent mediator release from mast cells and block acetycholine release from cholinergic nerves. They do not inhibit either the late-phase response or the subsequent bronchial hyperresponsiveness. If used frequently, inhaled β_2-agonists may produce tremors, anxiety, tachycardia, palpitations, and nausea.

Longer-acting inhaled β_2 agonists include salmeterol (Serevent). Salbuterol (Salbuvent) is a long-acting (8 to 12 hour) β-agonist MDI that has been available in Europe and will soon be available in the United States. There is no indication for the administration of nonselective β-adrenergic agonists (e.g., isoproterenol), which are associated with a high incidence of cardiovascular side effects (e.g., tachycardia, palpitations) because of their stimulation of β_1-adrenergic receptors. Patient education should stress that these drugs are used only every 12 hours and are not used as reserve therapy to obtain quick relief from bronchospasm like the shorter-acting β-agonists.

Orally administered β-agonists are less useful because of the increased incidence of side effects. The most common side effects are tremor, tachycardia, and palpitations. However, these drugs may be useful for nocturnal asthma or severe asthma. Excessive use of β-agonists may cause hypokalemia. Therefore their use should be monitored carefully in patients on long-term diuretic or corticosteroid therapy.

Methylxanthine derivatives. Methylxanthine derivative (theophylline) preparations are less effective bronchodilators than inhaled β-agonists.[8] The trend is now toward introducing theophylline as an additional bronchodilator later in the therapeutic regimen. Theophylline may have a synergistic effect with β-agonists. It is not effective as an inhalant and must be given orally or IV as aminophylline. Sustained-release theophylline preparations are preferable for maintenance therapy.

Although the exact mechanism of action is unknown, the main therapeutic action of methylxanthine derivatives is bronchodilatation, which is useful in the early-phase response. Only minimal bronchodilatation occurs at therapeutic theophylline concentrations.

Theophylline alleviates the early phase of asthma attacks and the bronchoconstrictive portion of the late-phase asthmatic response; however, it has no effect on bronchial hyperresponsiveness. Long-acting theophylline products administered at bedtime may be used to treat the patient with nocturnal asthma. The main problem with theophylline is the relatively high incidence of side effects, which include nausea, headache, gastrointestinal (GI) distress, tachycardia, cardiac dysrhythmias, and seizures.

Theophylline administration requires monitoring of its serum concentrations for safe and effective use. Many foods, drugs, and pathophysiologic conditions can alter the metabolism of theophylline. The end result can be subtherapeutic or toxic concentrations with previously appropriate doses. Drugs that inhibit the metabolism of theophylline include cimetidine, erythromycin, ciprofloxacin, diltiazem, verapamil, and allopurinol.

Anticholinergic drugs. Airway diameter is predominantly controlled by the parasympathetic division of the autonomic nervous system. The effects of acetylcholine on the airways are increased mucus secretion and smooth muscle contraction, resulting in bronchoconstriction. Anticholinergic agents (e.g., ipratropium) inhibit only the component of bronchoconstriction related to the parasympathetic nervous system. Thus these drugs are less effective than β-agonists and are usually used in combination with other bronchodilators. Anticholinergic agents produce most of their bronchodilatation in larger airways in contrast to β_2-agonists that act primarily in smaller airways.

The onset of action of anticholinergics is slower than β-agonists, peaking at 1 hour and lasting longer, usually up to 8 hours. Systemic side effects of inhaled anticholinergics are uncommon because they are poorly absorbed. For some asthma and COPD patients less responsive to β_2-agonists, ipratropium is effective either alone or in combination with β_2-agonists.

Antiinflammatory Drugs. Because chronic inflammation is a primary component of asthma, corticosteroids, which suppress the inflammatory response, are important therapeutic agents. These drugs do not have an immediate bronchodilatory effect and are used to potentiate the action of the bronchodilators.[8]

Corticosteroids. Although corticosteroids are remarkably effective in suppressing the inflammation induced by asthma, they are still greatly underused.[8] Steroids do not block the classic immediate response to irritants, allergens, or exercise but they do block the late-phase response and subsequent bronchial hyperresponsiveness. The onset of action of corticosteroids occurs approximately 3 to 6 hours after oral administration. They act by inhibiting the release of mediators from macrophages and eosinophils, reducing the microvascular leakage in the airways, inhibiting the influx of inflammatory cells into the reactive site, and decreasing peripheral blood eosinophilia.

Inhaled steroids must be administered for at least 4 to 5 days before a therapeutic effect can be seen. Steroids given by inhalation (e.g., beclomethasone, flunisolide, triamcinolone) are active topically and can control the disease without systemic side effects. When administered in the aerosol form as MDIs, little systemic absorption occurs, thus eliminating the side effects that result from adrenal suppression seen with oral or IV glucocorticoids.

Oropharyngeal candidiasis, hoarseness, and dry cough are local adverse effects caused by inhalation of corticosteroids. These problems can be reduced or prevented by using a spacer with the MDI and by rinsing the mouth with water after each use. Short courses of orally administered steroids are indicated for acute exacerbations of asthma. Side effects associated with short-term therapy include insomnia, heartburn, mood swings, blurry vision, headache, increased appetite, and weight gain. Maintenance doses of oral corticosteroids may be necessary to control asthma in a minority of patients with severe chronic asthma when long-term therapy is required. A single dose in the morning to coincide with endogenous cortisol production and alternate-day dosing is associated with fewer side effects. Side effects of long-term corticosteroid therapy are discussed in Chapter 47.

Cromolyn sodium. Cromolyn sodium is often classified as a mast cell stabilizer; however, its exact mechanism of action is unknown. It inhibits the immediate response from exercise and allergens and prevents the late-phase response. Long-term administration can reduce bronchial hyperreactivity and prevent the increased bronchial hyperreactivity associated with pollens in susceptible asthmatics. It is the antiinflammatory drug of choice in children, but it can also be used successfully in adults for seasonal asthma. It is particularly effective in exercise-induced asthma. Patient education should emphasize the rationale for use and the correct method of administration of cromolyn.

Nedocromil sodium (Tilade) is a new bronchial antiinflammatory agent that has a broad spectrum of effects. It is similar to cromolyn because it inhibits both the immediate and late phases of asthmatic response as well as reduces bronchial hyperreactivity. It can be used as a pretreatment therapy before exposure to environmental irritants, cold air, allergens, or exercise. It is most effective in mild to moderate asthma where frequent bronchodilator therapy is required. The usual dosage is two puffs four times a day, but twice a day dosages are sometimes used. The most common side effects are a transient, mild, unpleasant taste and rhinitis.

Leukotreine Antagonists or Inhibitors. Leukotriene antagonists, or synthesis inhibitors, a new class of drugs, are currently being investigated for the treatment of asthma. Leukotrienes are potent bronchoconstrictors, and some also cause airway edema and inflammation, thus contributing to the symptoms of asthma. Exactly where these drugs will fit into asthma management remains to be seen. So far some of these drugs have shown promise in helping to decrease the needed doses of oral steroids and controlling symptoms in patients with severe recalcitrant asthma.

Patient Teaching Related to Drug Therapy. Information about medications should include the name, dosage, method of administration, and schedule taking into consideration meal times and other ADLs, purpose, side effects, appropriate action if side effects occur, consequences of improper use, and the importance of refilling the prescription before the medication runs out. A sample medication instruction sheet for the patient is presented in Fig. 25-5.

One of the major factors in asthma management is the correct administration of medications. The majority of asthma medications are administered only or preferably by inhalation. Inhalation of drugs is often preferred to oral administration because a lower dose is needed and systemic side effects are reduced. In addition, the onset of action of bronchodilators is faster. Inhalation devices include nebulizers and MDIs (Fig. 25-6). Nebulizers, which generally deliver a larger dose of medication, are usually used for severe asthma. MDIs are usually effective, but some persons, particularly older adults, may have problems with the coordination needed to activate the MDI and inhale the medication. Poor coordination can be solved by the use of spacer devices (Aerochamber, Inspireease) (Fig. 25-7) or the use of a breath-activated MDI (Maxair Autoinhaler). If the patient is still unable to receive adequate medication, a nebulizer may be used.

The patient should be given instructions on the use of MDIs (Fig. 25-6). Recent studies indicate that 24% to 67% of patients using MDI are performing the technique incorrectly. Because at best only 10% to 15% of the inhaled medication reaches the lung, correct use of MDI technique is imperative. Problems commonly observed with MDI use are presented in Table 25-5. It is helpful to observe the patient from the side and evaluate each step in the MDI process. Even experienced asthmatic inhaler users frequently make errors in technique. Videos (available from pharmaceutical companies) on correct inhaler technique can be helpful.

The inhaler should be cleaned by removing the dust cap and rinsing it in warm water (Fig. 25-6). The amount of medication left in the canister can be determined by the method described in Fig. 25-6.

The patient who needs to use several MDIs are often unclear about the order in which to take the medications. As a general rule, β_2-agonists should be used first to open the airway. Corticosteroid inhalers should be used last because they require mouth rinsing after use to prevent oral candidiasis. Numbering the inhalers in order of use and marking the number of puffs in large, indelible markers on the inhaler has proved valuable for some patients.

One of the major problems with metered-dose drugs is the potential for overuse (i.e., using them much more frequently than prescribed rather than seeking needed medical care), especially β-agonist MDIs. As a patient develops additional asthmatic symptoms, the β-agonist MDI will be

Medication Instructions for Pulmonary Patients

Name: ____________________

Your diagnosis is: ☐ Chronic Obstructive Pulmonary Disease (COPD) ☐ Chronic Bronchitis ☐ Emphysema ☐ Asthma ☐ ____________________

Your medications are checked and the dosage is written.

☐ OXYGEN at ________ liters per minute for ________ hours a day.

☐ Oxygen is prescribed to decrease the strain on your heart and to keep oxygen in your blood (PaO_2) normal.

☐ BRONCHODILATOR MEDICINES

These medications relax the muscles around your air tubes (bronchial tubes) and keep your air tubes open (dilated) so that you can breathe easier.

Important: Bronchodilator medications may have other effects that you'll notice. These include upset stomach,heartburn, and palpitations and feeling jittery or nervous and muscle tremors. Taking the pills with food or an antacid can help. If these side effects are bothersome, please let us know. Also, it is important not to overuse your bronchodilator inhaler or nebulizer treatment. Only use it every 2-3 hours for shortness of breath. If you find that you need it more often, contact us.

☐ PILLS

☐ Theodur ________ milligram (mg) tablets, take ________ tablets every ________ hours.
☐ Brethine/bricanyl (Terbutaline) ________ mg tablets, take ________ tablets every ________ hours.
☐ Alupent (Metaproterenol) ________ mg tablets, take ________ tablets every ________ hours.
☐ Ventolin (Albuterol) ________ mg tablets, take ________ tablets every ________ hours.

☐ INHALERS

☐ Alupent (Metaproterenol) – White
☐ Ventolin (Albuterol) – Blue
☐ Proventil (Albuterol) – Yellow
☐ Brethair (Terbutaline) – Yellow and white
☐ Maxair (Pirbuterol) – Blue and white
☐ Serevent (Salmeterol) – Turquoise

Use ___ puff(s) of your inhaler:
☐ 4 times a day (e.g. with meals and at bedtime) and every 2-3 hours as needed for increased shortness of breath
____

☐ Atrovent (Ipratropium)–Green and white
A bronchodilator with a different mode of action than those above, it is frequently used in combination with above inhalers. Use ___ puff(s) of Atrovent 4 times a day.
____

☐ Rotohaler (Ventolin or Proventil)

☐ Use ___ capsule(s) 4 times a day (e.g. with meals and at bedtime) and every 2-3 hours as needed for shortness of breath.

NEBULIZER TREATMENTS
☐ Alupent (Metaproterenol) use ______ cc in ______ cc of saline, take ______ times a day, and every 2-3 hours as needed for shortness of breath.
☐ Ventolin/Proventil (Albuterol) use ______ cc in ______ cc of saline, take ______ times a day, and every 2-3 hours as needed for shortness of breath.
☐ Atrovent (Ipratropium) use ______ cc ______ times a day. Do not dilute further with saline.
____

continued

Fig. 25-5 Medication instructions for pulmonary patients.

used repeatedly. β-agonists help by relieving bronchospasm; they do not treat the inflammatory response. Therefore the patient must receive explicit instructions in the correct therapeutic use of these drugs.

Poor compliance with asthma therapy is a major problem in the long-term management of chronic asthma. The patient will use β-agonist inhalers because they provide immediate relief of symptoms. However, the patient often does not take prophylactic therapy (inhaled steroids or cromolyn) regularly because no immediate benefit is seen. It is important to explain to the patient the importance and purpose of taking inhaled steroid therapy regularly and to emphasize that maximal improvement may take weeks.

Nonprescription Combination Drugs. Several nonprescription combination products are available as over-the-counter (OTC) drugs. They are usually combinations of a bronchodilator, expectorant, and sedative (Table 25-6). These agents are advertised as drugs to relieve bronchospasm. In general they should be avoided by the person with obstructive lung disease. Many persons consider these drugs safe because they can be obtained without a prescription. Some of the dangers of these drugs are as follows:[9]

1. Epinephrine, found in Primatene spray, acts only for a short time, and rebound bronchospasm may occur. When taken with propranolol and other β-adrenergic blockers, it

☐ CORTICOSTEROIDS (Steroids)

These medications are all relatives of the hormone cortisol, which is normally produced by your body. They help to dilate the bronchial tubes, decrease the swelling of the bronchial tube lining, and decrease lung inflammation. All steroids must be taken on a regular schedule because they do not give immediate effects; rather, they prevent wheezing, so they are *not* to be used as you "need" them, but regularly to prevent symptoms. They must never be discontinued suddenly, and they should be taken only as directed by your physician.

☐ Prednisone _____ milligram (mg) tablets, take _____ tablets every morning _____ tablets every other morning as listed in the following schedule:

____

____

____

Note: Always take your prednisone in the morning (if it is only once a day) and with milk or food.

☐ STEROID INHALERS

☐ Vanceril (Beclomethasone) – Pink ☐ Beclovent (Beclomethasone) – Brown

☐ Azmacort (Triamcinolone acetonide) – White ☐ Aerobid (Flunisolide) – Purple and gray

Take _____ puffs _____ times a day (1-2 minutes) after you take your bronchodilator inhaler or nebulizer treatment. Eat food or rinse your mouth with water after using.

☐ Intal (Cromolyn sodium) ☐ Tilade (Nedocromil)

This is a medication that is used to prevent asthma (wheezing). Since it only works to prevent asthma, it must be taken regularly. Take _____ puffs of Intal Inhaler _____ times a day.
Take _____ mg liquid medication in your nebulizer _____ times a day. Cromolyn may be taken about 1-2 minutes after your bronchodilator inhaler of nebulizer treatment.

☐ OTHER MEDICATIONS

☐ Diuretics (water pills): ______________________________

☐ Antibiotics (fight infection): Please complete your entire prescription of antibiotics: ______________________________

☐ Antihypertensives (lower blood pressure and decrease the work of your heart): ______________________________

☐ Potassium supplements (replace potassium that is lost with certain diuretics and with prednisone): ______________________________

☐ Stomach medications (decrease stomach acid secretion or relieve heartburn): ______________________________

☐ Other medications: ______________________________

Fig. 25-5—cont'd Medication instructions for pulmonary patients.

can lead to a rise in BP.[9] An increase in cardiac dysrhythmias may be seen in the patient who combines epinephrine and digitalis.

2. Theophylline, taken with other xanthines including caffeine, has an additive effect. Side effects include central nervous system (CNS) and cardiovascular effects, vomiting, nausea, and anorexia.[9]

3. A combination of ephedrine (found in many OTC decongestants) and theophylline causes synergistic stimulation of the central nervous and cardiovascular systems.[9] Side effects include nervousness, heart palpitations and dysrhythmias, tremors, and insomnia.

4. Phenobarbital interferes with the action of steroids and is contraindicated in the asthmatic patient receiving steroid therapy.

5. Freon, a gas used as a propellant in some MDIs, can cause bronchospasm and possibly cardiac dysrhythmias.

An important teaching responsibility of the health professional is to warn the patient about the dangers associated with nonprescription combination drugs. These drugs are especially dangerous to a patient with underlying cardiac problems. The patient who insists on or persists in taking one of these medications should be cautioned to read and follow the accompanying directions on the label. Another way of discouraging the use of these drugs is to carefully monitor and reevaluate the effectiveness of the prescribed drug therapy. The drug regimen may have to be adjusted to help the patient obtain maximum relief from bronchospasm. An attitude of understanding and caring will often

Correct Use of a Metered-Dose Inhaler

Using a metered-dose inhaler (MDI) is a good way to take asthma medicines. There are few side effects because the medicine goes right to the lungs and not to other parts of the body. It takes only 5 to 10 minutes for the medicine to have an effect compared to liquid asthma medicines, which can take 1 to 3 hours. Inhalers can be used by all asthma patients age 5 and older. A spacer or holding chamber attached to the inhaler can help make taking the medicine easier. These devices are helpful to people having trouble using an inhaler.

The inhaler must be cleaned often to prevent buildup that will clog it and reduce how well it works.

- The guidelines that follow will help you use the inhaler the right way.
- Ask your doctor or nurse to show you how to use the inhaler.

Using the Inhaler

1. Remove the cap and hold the inhaler upright.
2. Shake the inhaler.
3. Tilt your head back slightly and breathe out.
4. Use the inhaler in any one of these ways.
   (A is the best way, but C is okay if you are having trouble with A or B).
   A. Open mouth with inhaler 1 to 2 inches away
   B. Use spacer
   C. In the mouth

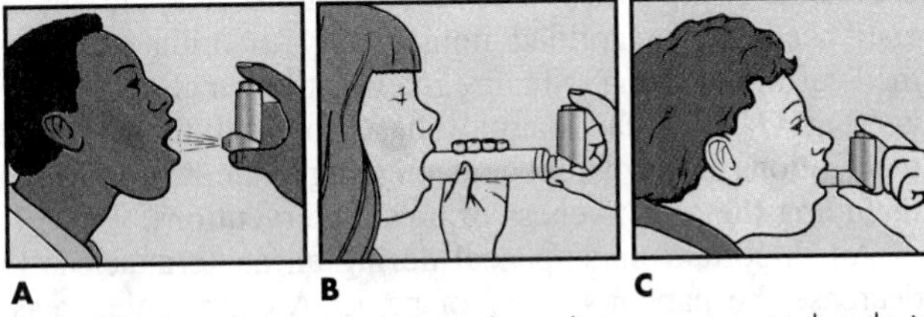

5. Press down on the inhaler to release the medicine as you start to breathe in slowly.
6. Breathe in *slowly* for 3 to 5 seconds.
7. Hold your breath for 10 seconds to allow the medicine to reach deeply into your lungs.
8. Repeat puffs as prescribed. Waiting 1 minute between puffs may permit the second puff to go deeper into the lungs.

Note: Dry powder capsules are used differently. To use a dry powder inhaler, close your mouth tightly around the mouthpiece and inhale very fast.

Cleaning

1. Once a day clean the inhaler and cap by rinsing it in warm running water. Let it dry before you use it again. Have another inhaler to use while it is drying.
2. Twice a week wash the plastic mouthpiece with mild dishwashing soap and warm water. Rinse and dry well before putting it back.

Checking How Much Medicine Is Left in the Canister

1. If the canister is new, it is full.
2. An easy way to check the amount of medicine left in your metered dose inhaler is to place the canister in a container of water and observe the position it takes in the water.

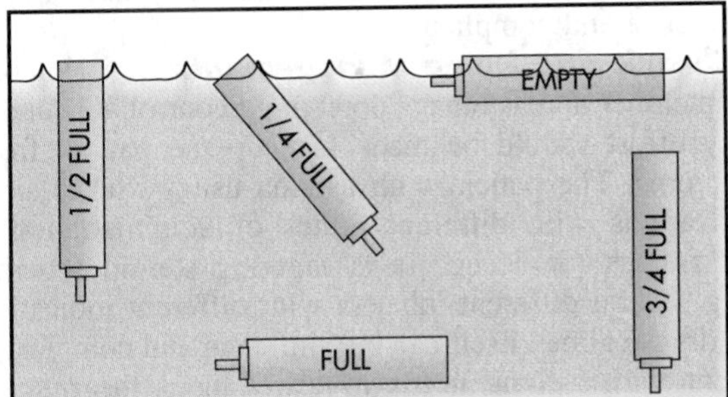

Fig. 25-6 Correct use of a metered-dose inhaler.

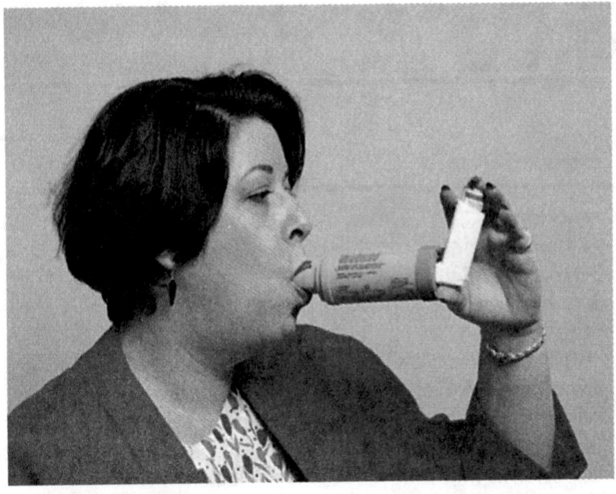

Fig. 25-7 Example of an AeroChamber spacer used with a metered-dose inhaler.

reassure the patient that the health care worker is concerned. This may prevent the patient from attempting to find relief at the local drugstore.

NURSING MANAGEMENT

ASTHMA

Nursing Assessment

If a patient can speak and is not in acute distress, a detailed health history, including identification of any precipitating factors and what has helped to alleviate attacks in the past, can be taken. Subjective and objective data that should be obtained from a patient with asthma are presented in Table 25-7.

Nursing Diagnoses

Nursing diagnoses are determined when the problem and etiologic factors are supported by clinical data. Nursing diagnoses related to asthma may include, but are not limited to, those presented in the nursing care plan on p. 702.

Table 25-5 Problems Encountered with Metered-Dose Inhaler Use

1. Failing to coordinate activation with inspiration
2. Activating MDI in the mouth while breathing through nose
3. Inspiring too rapidly
4. Not holding the breath for 10 sec (or as close to 10 sec as possible)
5. Holding MDI upside down or sideways
6. Inhaling more than 1 puff with each inspiration
7. Not shaking MDI before use
8. Not waiting a sufficient amount of time between each puff (1 min is recommended)
9. Not tilting head back and opening mouth, causing medication to bounce off teeth, tongue, or palate
10. Not having adequate strength to activate MDI

MDI, Metered-dose inhaler.

Table 25-6 Nonprescription Combination Asthma Drugs

Drug Product	Ingredients		
	Sympathomimetic	Xanthine	Other
Amodrine	Ephedrine	Aminophylline	Phenobarbital
Asthma Nefrin inhalant	Epinephrine	—	Chlorobutanol
Bronkaid tablets	Ephedrine	Theophylline	Guaifenesin
Bronkaid mist	Epinephrine	—	Ascorbic acid, alcohol
Bronkotabs	Ephedrine	Theophylline	Guaifenesin, phenobarbital
Primatene M tablets	Ephedrine	Theophylline	Pyrilamine
Primatene P tablets	Ephedrine	Theophylline	Phenobarbital
Primatene Mist	Epinephrine	—	Ascorbic acid, alcohol
Tedral	Ephedrine	Theophylline	Phenobarbital
Vaponefrin inhalant	Epinephrine	—	Chlorobutanol
Verquad	Ephedrine	Theophylline	Guaifenesin, phenobarbital

Planning

The overall goals are that the patient with asthma will have (1) normal breath sounds, (2) normal or baseline pulmonary function, (3) increased energy, (4) decreased incidence of asthma attacks, and (5) adequate knowledge to participate in and carry out management.

Nursing Implementation

Health Promotion and Maintenance. The nursing role in preventing asthma attacks or decreasing their severity focuses primarily on teaching the patient and family. The patient should be taught to avoid known personal triggers for asthma (e.g., cigarette smoke, pet dander) and irritants (e.g., cold air, aspirin, foods, cats, indoor air pollution). If cold air cannot be avoided, dressing properly with scarves or using a mask helps reduce the risk of an asthma attack. Aspirin and NSAIDs (e.g., indomethacin) should be avoided if they are known to precipitate an attack. Many OTC drugs contain aspirin, and the patient should be instructed to read the labels carefully. β-adrenergic blocking agents (e.g., propranolol) are contraindicated because they inhibit brochodilatation. Desensitization (immunotherapy) may be partially effective in decreasing the patient's sensitivity to known allergens (see Chapter 10).

Prompt diagnosis and treatment of upper respiratory tract infections (URI) may prevent an exacerbation of asthma. If occupational irritants are involved as etiologic factors, the patient may need to consider changing jobs. The patient should be encouraged to maintain a fluid intake of 2 to 3 L per day, good nutrition, and adequate rest. If exercise is planned, administering a β-agonist or cromolyn 10 to 15 minutes before the activity should prevent bronchospasm.

Acute Intervention. During an acute attack of asthma, it is important to monitor the patient's respiratory and cardiovascular systems. This includes auscultating lung sounds; taking the pulse rate, respiratory rate, and BP; and monitoring ABGs, pulse oximetry, and PEFR rates. The patient's work of breathing (i.e., use of accessory muscles, degree of fatigue) and response to therapy also should be evaluated. If the patient's condition deteriorates, the physician needs to be notified immediately to initiate prompt medical intervention. Nursing interventions include administering O_2, bronchodilators, chest physical therapy, and medications (as ordered) and ongoing patient monitoring including the effectiveness of these interventions.

An important nursing goal during an acute attack is to decrease the patient's sense of panic. A calm, quiet, reassuring attitude may help the patient relax. The patient should be positioned comfortably (usually sitting) to maximize chest expansion. Staying with the patient and being available provide additional comfort. Encouraging slow breathing using pursed lips for prolonged exhalation can be helpful.

When the acute attack subsides, the nurse should provide rest and a quiet, calm environment for the patient. When the patient has recovered from exhaustion, the nurse should attempt to obtain information about the patient's health history and pattern of asthma. If family members are present, they may be able to provide information about the patient's health history. A thorough physical assessment should be completed (Table 25-7). This information is important in planning an individualized nursing care plan for the patient. Well-thought-out written plans involving the patient and significant others increase the patient's knowledge and control of the situation and may help improve confidence and compliance.

Chronic and Home Management. It is important to remember that asthma is potentially controllable and that every effort should be made to keep the patient free of symptoms. The patient with asthma usually takes several medications with different routes of administration and time frames for dosage (e.g., tapering steroid schedules, using several different inhalers with different indications). The drug regimen itself can be confusing and complex. The patient with asthma needs to learn about the numerous medications and to develop self-management strategies. The patient and the health professional need to monitor the patient's responsiveness to medication. It is easy to undermedicate or overmedicate a patient with asthma unless

Table 25-7 Nursing Assessment: Asthma

Subjective Data

Important health information

Past health history: Allergic rhinitis; exposure to pollen, danders, feathers, mold, dust, inhaled irritants, weather changes, exercise, smoke, sinus infection, gastroesophageal reflux

Medications: Use and discontinuance of steroids, bronchodilators, cromolyn sodium; medications that may precipitate an attack such as aspirin, NSAIDs, β-blockers, cholinergics, antibiotics

Functional health patterns

Health perception–health management: Recent URI or sinus infection, family history of allergies or asthma, fatigue

Activity-exercise: Decreased exercise tolerance; dyspnea, cough, sputum production (amount, character, color), chest tightness, feelings of suffocation, air hunger

Sleep-rest: Interrupted sleep, insomnia

Coping–stress tolerance: Fear, anxiety, emotional distress

Objective Data

General

Anxiety, restlessness or exhaustion, confusion, appearance, body position

Integumentary

Diaphoresis, cyanosis (circumoral, nailbed)

Respiratory

Wheezing, crackles, diminished or absent breath sounds, and rhonchi on auscultation; sputum (thick, white, tenacious), increased work of breathing with use of accessory muscles; intercostal and supraclavicular retractions; tachypnea with hyperventilation; prolonged expiration

Cardiovascular

Tachycardia, pulsus paradoxus, jugular venous distention, hypertension or hypotension, premature ventricular contractions

Possible findings

Abnormal ABGs during attacks, decreased O_2 saturation, elevated serum IgE, positive skin tests for allergens, chest x-ray demonstrating hyperinflation with attacks, abnormal pulmonary function tests showing decreased flow rates, FVC, FEV_1, PEFR, and FEV_1/FVC ratio that improve between attacks and with bronchodilators

ABGs, Arterial blood gases; *FEV_1,* forced expiratory volume at 1 second; *FVC,* forced vital capacity; *NSAIDs,* nonsteroidal antiinflammatory drugs; *PEFR,* peak expiratory flow rate; *URI,* upper respiratory tract infection.

careful monitoring is ongoing. Some patients may benefit from keeping a diary to record medication use, the presence of wheezing or coughing, PEFR, the drug's side effects, and the activity level. This information will be valuable in helping the health care provider adjust the medication. The patient needs to understand the importance of continuing the medication even when symptoms are not present. If worsening bronchospasm or severe side effects of the drugs occur, the patient needs to seek medical attention.

The patient should be taught to maintain a fluid intake of 2 to 3 L per day. Good nutrition and avoidance of overeating are other important measures. Physical exercise (e.g., swimming, walking, stationary cycling) within the patient's limit of tolerance is also beneficial. If dyspnea occurs on exertion, it can be prevented with the use of a β-adrenergic MDI. Adequate rest and uninterrupted (from asthma symptoms) sleep are important.

The patient needs to be instructed to recognize triggers of an acute exacerbation so that it will be possible to medicate early, continue medication according to individually predetermined protocols until symptoms improve, or seek emergency care at a predetermined place. Many patients with asthma have peak flowmeters at home to monitor their PEFRs. A decrease in the PEFR may indicate a need for adjustment in the medication and may help prevent a severe exacerbation. It may be appropriate to notify the physician if the predetermined PEFR, as set by the physician, decreases significantly. It is most helpful for the physician or nurse to write a detailed individual asthma management plan about what to do with medications once early warning signs of an acute exacerbation occur.

It is also helpful for the patient to develop a plan with a significant other that defines what can be done to help the patient during an asthmatic attack. The significant other needs to know where the patient's inhalers, oral medications, and emergency phone numbers are located. The significant other can also be instructed on how to decrease the patient's anxiety if an asthma attack occurs.

Counseling may be indicated to help the patient and the family resolve personal, family, social, and occupational problems that have resulted from asthma. Relaxation therapies (e.g., yoga, meditation, relaxation techniques, and breathing techniques) may be of value in helping a patient relax respiratory muscles and decrease the respiratory rate. A healthy emotional outlook can also be important in preventing future asthma attacks. One resource that can be used when teaching the patient about asthma is the American Lung Association, which has educational materials about asthma, including the *Asthma Handbook.*

EMPHYSEMA AND CHRONIC BRONCHITIS

The clinical use of the terms COPD and *chronic obstructive lung disease* (COLD) is common. COPD may be defined "as the process characterized by the presence of chronic bronchitis and/or emphysema that may lead to the development of obstructed airways; the airway obstruction may be partially reversible and is often accompanied by airway hyperreactivity."[10] Although the preferred terms are *emphysema* or *chronic bronchitis,* there is usually some overlap between them.

Significance

More than 23 million persons in the United States have emphysema and chronic bronchitis.[11] COPD is the fifth leading cause of death in the United States,[11] and it accounts for almost 4% of all the deaths in the United States.[12] The death

NURSING CARE PLAN Patient with Asthma

Planning: Outcome Criteria	Nursing Interventions and Rationales
➤ NURSING DIAGNOSIS	Ineffective breathing pattern *related to* increased airway resistance caused by bronchospasm, mucosal edema, and mucus production *as manifested by* dyspnea, wheezing, rapid respiratory rate, use of accessory muscles
Have absence of wheezing and chest tightness, return of appropriate breath sounds indicating better airflow, respiratory rate of 12-24/min; ABGs, oximetry, PEFR, and pulmonary function tests within normal limits or returned to baseline.	Provide comfortable position (e.g., bed rest in high Fowler's position or recliner chair) *to maximize chest expansion and promote prolonged expiratory phase to reduce trapped air.* Administer bronchodilators as ordered *to treat bronchospasm.* Administer O_2 as ordered *to increase oxygen saturation.* Auscultate breath sounds *to monitor effectiveness of treatment and patient status.* Monitor ABGs and pulse oximetry *to monitor oxygen saturation,* PaO_2*, and* $PaCO_2$. Assess BP, HR, respiratory rate, and level of consciousness *to determine change in status and effectiveness of interventions.* Premedicate with bronchodilators before doing deep-breathing and coughing exercises or chest physiotherapy *to open airways for more efficient movement of sputum toward mouth.* Evaluate effectiveness of nebulizer treatments by noting degree of respiratory distress, secretion clearance, PEFR, and oximetry *to assess need for increase or decrease in frequency of treatments.* Teach patient to breathe deeply through the nose and exhale two to three times as long as inspiration through pursed lips *to remove trapped air and increase* PaO_2. Assess and document breathing pattern including respiratory rate, depth, relationship of inspiration to exhalation, use of accessory muscles, presence of chest discomfort *to provide ongoing parameters to measure effects of treatment.* Assist with pulmonary function tests if ordered.
➤ NURSING DIAGNOSIS	Ineffective airway clearance *related to* bronchospasm, ineffective cough, excessive mucus production, tenacious secretions, and fatigue *as manifested by* ineffective cough, inability to raise secretions, adventitious breath sounds
Have breath sounds indicating good air movement, effective and productive cough of clear or white secretions.	Monitor and control environment for possible allergens (e.g., dust, smoke, flowers) *to reduce exacerbating asthma attack.* Auscultate lungs *to provide baseline and ongoing data.* Assess patient's ability to cough effectively *to determine need for intervention.* Teach effective coughing techniques *so patient can clear airways by propelling secretions toward mouth for expectoration.* If patient is unable to cough and expectorate secretions, evaluate possible causes (e.g., respiratory muscle fatigue, thick secretions, severe bronchospasm, decreased level of consciousness) *so that appropriate intervention can be initiated.* As ordered, assist in and evaluate administration of bronchodilator drugs, mucolytic drugs (iodinated glycerol, guaifenesin), steroid therapy, chest physiotherapy *to improve respiratory status.* Observe and note character and quantity of coughed or suctioned sputum and secretions *to determine presence of infection.* If ordered, send sputum for Gram stain and culture and sensitivity.
➤ NURSING DIAGNOSIS	Activity intolerance *related to* fatigue secondary to increased work of breathing and inadequate oxygenation *as manifested by* inability or unwillingness to ambulate, increase in pulse and respirations on exertion
Feel rested, have increased energy to do self-care activities.	Evaluate fatigue in relationship to work of breathing (signs of hypercapnia, hypoxemia). Use portable O_2 or extension tubing hooked to O_2 *so patient can move about freely as tolerated.* Plan 1- to 2-hr rest periods. Provide total care for patient at onset with progressive self-care as tolerated *to decrease energy utilization during acute phase.* Use gentle massage or heating pad *to alleviate muscle fatigue and chest and abdominal discomfort.* Provide small amounts of liquid, progressing to soft diet *to reduce energy required for ingestion and digestion.* Promote plan of ambulation *to increase exercise tolerance.*

continued

NURSING CARE PLAN Patient with Asthma—cont'd

Planning: Outcome Criteria	Nursing Interventions and Rationales
➤ **NURSING DIAGNOSIS**	Sleep pattern disturbance *related to* dyspnea, anxiety, frequent assessments and treatments, and side effects of some medications *as manifested by* dyspnea, inability to sleep or able to sleep only for short intervals, inability to fall asleep, not rested on awakening, dissatisfaction with sleep
Sleep several hours at a time, feel rested on awakening, verbalize satisfaction with sleep pattern.	Administer O_2 as ordered *to reduce hypoxia and subsequent anxiety.* Plan nursing care *so that uninterrupted periods of sleep are possible.* If possible, administer medications that increase HR several hours before bedtime *to minimize effect on sleep.* Observe for signs and symptoms of sleep apnea syndrome such as frequent awakening at night, insomnia, and excessive daytime sleepiness *so appropriate interventions can be initiated.*
➤ **NURSING DIAGNOSIS**	Anxiety *related to* difficulty breathing, perceived or actual loss of control, and fear of suffocation *as manifested by* anxiety over condition, restlessness, elevated vital signs
Have calm feeling, less anxiety over asthma.	Interact with patient in a calm, unhurried, supportive manner. Give simple, concise explanations and demonstrating and repeating (as necessary) *to increase understanding and foster cooperation.* Encourage and demonstrate slow, deep breathing with pursed lip breathing *to assist patient in improving respiratory status.* Do *not* sedate unless a light sedative is ordered. If sedated, monitor for respiratory depression. Stay with the patient *to provide reassurance and reduce anxiety.* Anticipate patient's needs. Provide anticipatory guidance for patient to prevent excaberations. Promptly treat any exacerbations of an attack *to prevent development of status asthmaticus.* Place patient in room near nurses station *to provide reassurance that help is nearby and to allow for frequent observation.* Teach relaxation techniques *to reduce anxiety.* Explain that some medications (e.g., β_2-agonists, corticosteroids, theophylline) may further increase anxiety and irritability.
➤ **NURSING DIAGNOSIS**	Risk for respiratory infection *related to* decreased pulmonary function, ineffective airway clearance, and possible steroid therapy
Have no sputum or clear to white sputum, normal temperature, clear chest x-ray.	Assess for manifestations of a respiratory infection such as elevated temperature, pulse, and respiration; productive cough; change in color, consistency or amount of sputum, adventitious breath sounds. If sputum is mucopurulent, obtain sputum Gram stain and culture and sensitivity *to determine infecting organism.* Administer antibiotic as ordered *to treat the infection.* Monitor temperature q4hr and as needed, sputum character and quantity *to assess for signs of infection.* Monitor for localized decrease in breath sounds, decreased PaO_2, inability to raise secretions *to determine a worsening of condition.* Provide deep-breathing and coughing exercises (if needed) *to improve breathing and raise secretions.* Monitor all respiratory treatments that are administered *to evaluate effectiveness.*

continued

rate from emphysema and chronic bronchitis, at more than 18,000 deaths a year, has risen by 22% in the last decade. The mortality rate 10 years after diagnosis is more than 50%. Caucasian men account for more than one third of the deaths.[12] Most patients with COPD are men who are usually older than 45 years of age. The number of women with COPD is on the rise because of the increased number of women smoking cigarettes.[11]

Etiology

Chronic irritation of the lungs is the primary etiologic mechanism in COPD. There are three major irritants: cigarette smoke, infection, and inhaled irritants. The development of COPD is extremely variable and depends on the inherent host susceptibility and on the nature and severity of exposure to the irritant. The host susceptibility factors that cause some people to develop pathologic lung changes and others to remain symptom free are unclear and still under investigation. One known host susceptibility is alpha$_1$-antitrypsin (AAT) deficiency (see Fig. 25-8).

Cigarette Smoking. Cigarette smoking is the most common cause of COPD in the United States. Clinically significant airway obstruction develops in 15% of smokers, and 80% to 90% of COPD deaths in the United States are

NURSING CARE PLAN Patient with Asthma—cont'd

Planning: Outcome Criteria	Nursing Interventions and Rationales
➤ **NURSING DIAGNOSIS**	Risk for fluid volume deficit *related to* inadequate intake secondary to fatigue, excessive loss resulting from tachypnea, and diaphoresis
Have moist mucous membranes and thin, easily expectorated sputum.	Assess for manifestations of fluid volume deficit such as thick sputum, dry mucous membranes and skin, decreased urinary output *to determine extent of problem.* Administer IV fluids as ordered. Encourage oral fluids to 3000 ml/day *to ensure adequate fluid intake.* Provide for oral hygiene *to remove foul-tasting expectorant.* Monitor intake and output and body weight *to use as indicators of fluid adequacy.* May use humidified O_2 equipment *to liquefy secretions for easier expectoration.* Assess viscosity and ease of expectorating sputum *because dry, difficult-to-expectorate sputum indicates dehydration.* Monitor vital signs *because increasing pulse and decreasing BP may indicate fluid volume deficit.*
➤ **NURSING DIAGNOSIS**	Ineffective management of therapeutic regimen *related to* lack of knowledge about management of bronchospasm, medications, use of nebulizer or metered-dose inhaler, role of proper rest and activity, adequate hydration, signs and symptoms of respiratory infection, and factors that may precipitate an asthma attack *as manifested by* frequent questioning about all aspects of long-term management
Have minimal or no symptoms of bronchospasm, respiratory rate of 12-20/min, knowledge of home management program and importance of adequate fluid intake, sleep, knowledge of patient's asthma triggers and appropriate actions for avoidance, pretreatment, and management of asthma.	Administer bronchodilators as prescribed *to reduce bronchospasm.* Increase activity as tolerated. Assess patient's response to bronchodilators, hydration, and increased activity *to evaluate effectiveness of plan.* Assess patient's understanding and develop a teaching plan for home care including proper balance of rest and activity; names, actions, side effects, frequency, and dose of prescribed medications; use of nebulizer, inhaler, and peak flowmeter; use of inhaled bronchodilator before strenuous activity to prevent attack; and avoidance of allergens and irritants *to increase patient's sense of control and decrease anxiety.* Explain effect of dehydration on sputum production and consequent effect on bronchospasm. Assist in planning patient's self-administered fluid intake *to ensure adequacy and prevent dehydration.* Explain factors that may contribute to infections and assist in planning preventive measures and explain method to evaluate color, character, and amount of sputum on regular basis *to ensure early recognition of infection.* Review physician's orders related to infection and acute attack (take medications as ordered or seek medical attention). Assist in identifying factors that precipitate attacks *to develop plans to prevent them.* Stress importance of taking medications regularly as ordered. Teach patient to seek medical attention if medicine does not relieve attack or if dyspnea occurs at night. Teach patient technique of breathing in through nose and out through pursed lips, two to three times *to prevent bronchiolar collapse and maintain open airways.* Inform patient about American Lung Association and its services and literature such as *Living with Asthma to provide support group for ongoing help.*

ABGs, Arterial blood gases; *BP,* blood pressure; *HR,* heart rate; *IV,* intravenous; *PEFR,* peak expiratory flow rate.

related to cigarette smoking.[11] For most Americans who die of lung diseases related to cigarette smoking, death is preceded by a long period of debilitating morbidity characterized by frequent hospitalizations and loss of many years of productivity. In addition to being linked with emphysema, chronic bronchitis, and lung cancer, cigarette smoking has also been implicated as a factor in cancers of the mouth, pharynx, larynx, esophagus, pancreas, kidney, stomach, cervix, and bladder. Approximately 172,000 deaths were attributed to lung cancer in 1994. Cigarette smoking is responsible for approximately 87% of deaths from lung cancer.[13]

When cigarettes are smoked, approximately 4000 chemicals and gases are inhaled into the lungs. Many carcinogens have been isolated from cigarette smoke; 3,4-benzpyrene is the most dangerous. At least 43 other components have been identified as carcinogens, cocarcinogens, tumor promoters, tumor initiators, and mutagens. Nicotine is probably not a carcinogen, but it has other deleterious effects. It acts by stimulating the sympathetic nervous system, resulting in increased HR, increased peripheral vasoconstriction, increased BP, and increased cardiac work load. These effects of nicotine compound the problems in a person with coronary artery disease (CAD).

Table 25-8 Effects of Tobacco Smoke on the Respiratory System

Area of Defect	Acute Effects	Long-Term Effects
Respiratory mucosa		
Nasopharyngeal	↓ Sense of smell	Cancer
Tongue	↓ Sense of taste	Cancer
Vocal cords	Hoarseness	Chronic cough, cancer
Bronchus and bronchioles	Bronchospasm, cough	Chronic bronchitis, asthma, cancer
Cilia	Paralysis, sputum accumulation, cough	Chronic bronchitis, cancer
Mucous glands	↑ Secretions, ↑ cough	Hyperplasia and hypertrophy of glands, chronic bronchitis
Alveolar macrophages	↓ Function	Increased incidence of infection
Elastin and collagen fibers	↑ Destruction by proteases, ↓ function of antiproteases (alpha$_1$-antitrypsin), ↓ synthesis and repair of elastin	Emphysema

Cigarette smoke has several direct effects on the respiratory tract (Table 25-8). The irritating effect of the smoke causes hyperplasia of cells, including goblet cells, which subsequently results in increased production of mucus. Hyperplasia reduces airway diameter and increases the difficulty in clearing secretions. Smoking reduces the ciliary activity and may cause actual loss of ciliated cells. Smoking also produces abnormal dilatation of the distal air space with destruction of alveolar walls. Many cells develop large, atypical nuclei, which is considered a precancerous condition.

After only 1 year of smoking, changes in small airway function can develop. In the early stages these changes are mostly inflammatory with mucosal edema and an influx of inflammatory cells. In later stages, however, peribronchiolar fibrosis is present. These inflammatory changes in small airways can be reversed with smoking cessation, at least in the younger person.

Carbon monoxide (CO), a component of tobacco smoke, is present in similar concentrations in automobile exhaust. CO has a high affinity for hemoglobin and combines with it more readily than does O_2, thereby reducing the smoker's O_2-carrying capacity. The smoker inhales a lower percentage of O_2 than normal, resulting in less O_2 available at the alveolar level. The heart's need for O_2 is increased because of the sympathetic stimulatory effect of nicotine. Because the blood's O_2-carrying capacity is reduced, the heart must pump more rapidly to adequately supply tissues with O_2. CO also seems to impair psychomotor performance and judgment and may cause psychologic stress.

Exposed nonsmokers are affected by involuntary exposure to smoke (*passive smoking*). Effects in children are an increased incidence of respiratory illnesses and decreased lung growth. In adults, involuntary smoke exposure is associated with decreased pulmonary function, increased risk for lung cancer, and increased mortality from ischemic heart disease.[13]

Smoking rates in the United States among adults have decreased from more than 40% in 1965 to 25.5% in 1990.[13] This decrease in smoking can be related to the widespread publicity of the harmful effects of smoking and the vocal response of nonsmokers who are concerned about the effects of passive smoking. By 1989 nearly half of all living adults who had ever smoked had quit. Unfortunately, the decline in prevalence has lagged among women, teenagers, young adults, and the less educated.

A major theory regarding the relationship between cigarette smoking and emphysema is that cigarette smoke may cause an imbalance between proteolytic enzymes that digest lung connective tissue and protease inhibitors, one of which is AAT. Other evidence indicates that oxidants in tobacco smoke can inactivate AAT. In the presence of cigarette smoke, neutrophils and macrophages in the lung release proteases that destroy lung tissue. Other chemicals in cigarettes may interfere with normal repair and synthesis of lung elastic fibers.

Infection. Recurring respiratory tract infections are a major contributing factor to the aggravation and progression of COPD. Recurring infections impair normal defense mechanisms, making the bronchioles and alveoli more susceptible to injury. In addition, the person with COPD is more prone to respiratory infections, which subsequently intensify the pathologic destruction of lung tissue and the progression of COPD. The most common causative organisms are *Haemophilus influenzae, Streptococcus pneumoniae*, and *Moraxella catarrhalis*. Retained secretions provide a good medium for their proliferation.

Inhaled Irritants. The incidence of COPD is higher in urban than in rural areas. This difference may be partially explained by the air pollution and occupational irritants (e.g., coal dust, potash) to which persons are exposed. Inhaled irritants cause a nonspecific inflammatory response. More macrophages and neutrophils are found in the lungs. Proteases released from these cells can destroy alveoli, and this process has been implicated in the pathogenesis of COPD.

Exposure to occupational gases and dusts can cause lung fibrosis and focal areas of emphysema. Exposure to air pollution and occupational irritants worsens the dyspnea of COPD by causing bronchospasm and mucosal edema.

Heredity. A form of familial primary emphysema is related to a deficiency of AAT that normally has an inhibitory effect on proteolytic enzymes. The level of AAT is controlled by a pair of autosomal codominant genes. Low levels of AAT are related to homozygosity for the deficiency gene (ZZ), intermediate levels to heterozygosity (MZ), and normal values to homozygosity for the normal gene (MM). The incidence of ZZ homozygous individuals ranges from 1 out of 3500 persons to 1 out of 1670 persons, and 5% to 10% of persons are heterozygous.[14] In the homozygous group, onset of symptoms often occurs by the age of 40, and the disease is found as frequently in women as in men. The people with this type of emphysema are primarily of Northern European origin.

Emphysema results when lysis of lung tissues by proteolytic enzymes from neutrophils and macrophages occurs because of the AAT deficiency. Normally AAT inhibits the action of these enzymes. Therefore lower levels of AAT result in insufficient inactivation and subsequent destruction of lung tissue. Smoking greatly exacerbates the disease process in these patients. IV or nebulizer-administered AAT (Prolastin) augmentation therapy has recently been approved for persons with AAT deficiency. The infusions are administered weekly.[15] Its effectiveness in slowing the progression of the disease continues to be evaluated.

Aging. Some degree of emphysema is common in the lungs of the older person, even a nonsmoker. Aging results in changes in the lung structure, the thoracic cage, and the respiratory muscles. Clinically significant emphysema, however, is usually not caused by aging alone.

As people age there is gradual loss of the elastic recoil of the lung.[16] The lungs become more rounded and smaller. The number of functional alveoli decrease as a result of the loss of the alveolar supporting structures and loss of the intraalveolar septum. These changes are similar to those seen in the patient with emphysema.[17] Thinner alveolar walls contribute to loss of alveolar septal tissue and alveolar capillaries. With fewer capillaries available for gas exchange, arterial oxygen levels decrease. The PaO_2 falls at a rate of 4 mm Hg for each decade of life, beginning after 20 years of age. The surface area available for gas exchange decreases from 80 m^2 at 20 years of age to 65 to 70 m^2 by 70 years of age.

Thoracic cage changes result from osteoporosis and calcification of the costal cartilages. The thoracic cage becomes stiff and rigid, and the ribs are less mobile. The shape of the rib cage gradually changes because of the increased functional residual capacity (FRC), causing it to expand and become rounded.[16] These changes result in a decreased compliance of the chest wall and an increase in the work of breathing.

The respiratory muscles, and all other muscles, weaken with aging. Breathing in the older adult is less efficient because the chest wall is stiffer and there is decreased muscle strength. It is common for the older adult to use the accessory muscles of respiration.

Pathophysiology

It is common clinically to find a combination of emphysema and chronic bronchitis in the same person, often with one condition predominating (Fig. 25-8).

Emphysema. Emphysema is a condition of the lungs characterized by abnormal, permanent enlargement of the air spaces distal to the terminal bronchioles, accompanied by destruction of their walls, and without obvious fibrosis. Structural changes include (1) hyperinflation of alveoli; (2) destruction of alveolar walls; (3) destruction of alveolar capillary walls; (4) narrowed, tortuous, small airways; and (5) loss of lung elasticity.

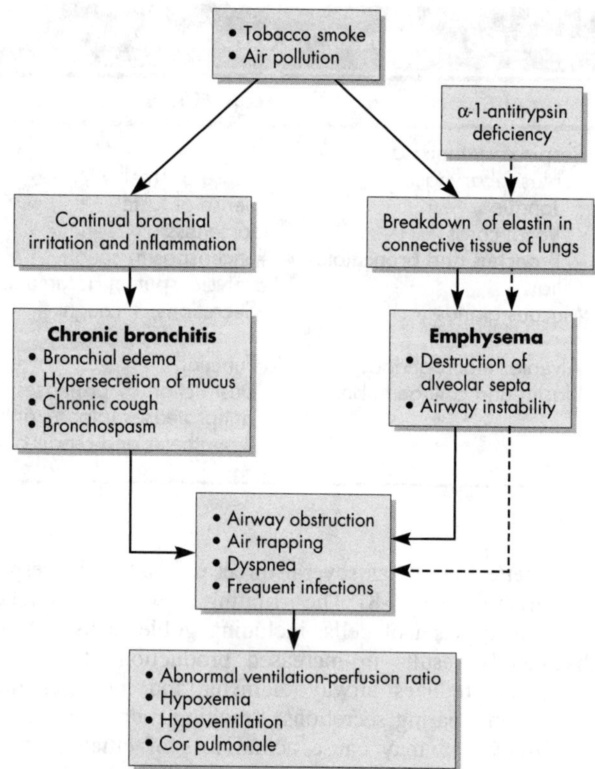

Fig. 25-8 Pathophysiology of chronic bronchitis and emphysema. *Dashed arrows,* role of α_1-antitrypsin deficiency, if present.

There are two major types of emphysema, *centrilobular* and *panlobular* (Fig. 25-9). In centrilobar emphysema the primary area of involvement is the central part of the lobule. Respiratory bronchioles enlarge, the walls are destroyed, and the bronchioles become confluent. Chronic bronchitis is often associated with centrilobular emphysema, which is more common than panlobular emphysema.

In contrast, panlobular emphysema involves distention and destruction of the whole lobule. Respiratory bronchioles, alveolar ducts and sacs, and alveoli are all affected. There is progressive loss of lung tissue and a decreased alveolar-capillary surface area. Severe panlobular emphysema is usually found in persons with AAT deficiency. In some patients with emphysema, bullae (large cystic areas) develop. When emphysema is severe, it is difficult to distinguish the two types, which may coexist in the same lung.

The pathophysiologic mechanisms involved in emphysema are not totally understood. Small bronchioles become obstructed as a result of mucus, smooth muscle spasm, the inflammatory process, and collapse of bronchiolar walls. Recurrent infectious processes lead to increased production and stimulation of neutrophils and macrophages. These cells release proteolytic enzymes that can destroy alveolar

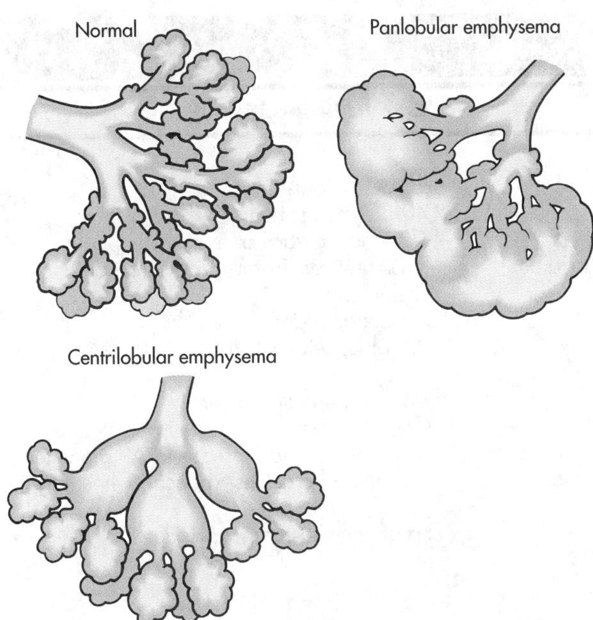

Fig. 25-9 Morphologic types of emphysema. In panlobular emphysema the entire primary lobule is involved, with destruction and distention distal to the respiratory bronchioles. In centrilobular emphysema, destruction is central, involving primarily the respiratory bronchioles.

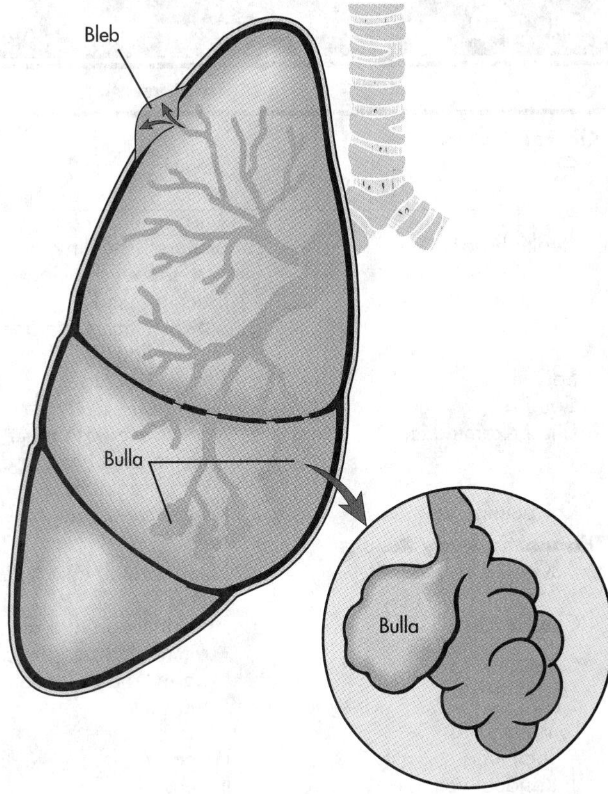

Fig. 25-10 Pulmonary blebs and bullae.

tissue. This process results in more inflammation, more edema, and exudate formation.

In a healthy person there is a balance between elastases and proteases and antiproteases; in smokers the numbers of polymorphonuclear neutrophils and macrophages are increased. Release of their elastases and proteases may overwhelm the normal antiprotease defense. In addition, smoking inactivates AAT. In AAT-related emphysema, AAT activity is greatly diminished and may be overwhelmed by normal protease activity.

In emphysema, elastin and collagen, the supporting structures of the lung, are destroyed. As a result there is no pull or traction on the walls of the bronchioles. Like air being blown into a paper bag, air goes into the lungs easily but is unable to come out on its own and remains in the lung. Thus the bronchioles tend to collapse (especially on expiration) and air is trapped in the distal alveoli, resulting in hyperinflation and overdistention of the alveoli. This trapped air in the lungs gives the patient the typical barrel-chested appearance. In emphysema the lungs can be inflated easily but can deflate only partially. As more alveoli are destroyed and alveoli coalesce, larger air spaces called *blebs* (in the visceral pleura) and *bullae* (in the lung parenchyma) may develop (Fig. 25-10).

Because of the loss of alveolar walls and the capillaries surrounding them, the amount of surface area that is available for diffusion of O_2 in the blood decreases. The patient with emphysema compensates for this problem by increasing the respiratory rate to increase alveolar ventilation. Typically the patient with pure emphysema does not have difficulty with hypoxemia at rest until late in the disease. However, hypoxemia may develop during exercise, and the patient may benefit from supplemental O_2. Hypercapnia and respiratory acidosis do not develop until late in the disease process.

Chronic Bronchitis. Chronic bronchitis is excessive production of mucus in the bronchi accompanied by a recurrent cough that persists for at least 3 months of the year during at least 2 successive years. Pathologic changes in the lung consist of (1) hyperplasia of mucous-secreting glands in the trachea and bronchi, (2) increase in goblet cells, (3) disappearance of cilia, (4) chronic inflammatory changes and narrowing of small airways, and (5) altered function of alveolar macrophages, leading to increased bronchial infections. Frequently the airways are colonized with organisms. Infections can occur when the organisms increase. Excess amounts of mucus are found in the airways and sometimes may occlude small bronchioles. Eventually, scarring of the bronchial walls may occur. In contrast to emphysema, the alveolar structure and capillaries are normal.

Chronic inflammation is the primary pathologic mechanism involved in causing the changes characteristic of chronic bronchitis. The inflammatory response causes vasodilatation, congestion, and mucosal edema. The mucous glands are stimulated to become hyperplastic. This hyperplasia, inflammatory swelling, and excess, thick mucus cause narrowing of the airway lumen and result in diminished airflow. Greater resistance to airflow increases the work of breathing. Hypoxemia and hypercarbia develop more frequently in chronic bronchitis than in emphysema because of the tendency for hypoventilation as well as

Table 25-9 Comparison of Emphysema and Chronic Bronchitis*

	Emphysema	Chronic Bronchitis
Clinical Features		
Age	30-40 yr (onset) 60-70 yr (disabling)	20-30 yr (onset) 40-50 yr (disabling)
Body build	Thin	Tendency toward obesity
Health history	Generally healthy, occasional insidious dyspnea, smoking	Recurrent respiratory tract infections, smoking
Weight loss	Often marked	Absent or slight
Dyspnea	Slowly progressive and eventually disabling	Variable, relatively late
Sputum	Scanty, mucoid	Copious, mucopurulent
Cough	Negligible	Considerable
Chest examination	Marked increase in AP diameter, quiet or diminished breath sounds, limited diaphragmatic excursion	Slight to marked increase in AP diameter, scattered crackles, rhonchi, wheezing
Cor pulmonale	Rare except terminally	Frequent with many episodes
Diagnostic Study Results		
ABGs	Near normal, mild ↓ PaO_2, normal or ↓ $PaCO_2$	↓ PaO_2, ↑ $PaCO_2$
Chest x-ray	Hyperinflation, flat diaphragm, attenuated peripheral vessels, small or normal heart, widened intercostal margins	Cardiac enlargement, normal or flattened diaphragm, evidence of chronic inflammation, congested lung fields
Lung volumes		
Total lung capacity	Increased	Normal or slightly increased
Residual volume	Increased	Increased
Vital capacity	Decreased	Decreased
FEV_1	Decreased	Decreased
FEV_1/FVC	Decreased (<70%)	Decreased (<70%)
Hematocrit and hemoglobin	Normal until late in disease	Increased
Pathology	Panlobular emphysema	Centrilobular emphysema

ABGs, Arterial blood gases; *AP*, anteroposterior; *FEV_1*, forced expiratory volume in 1 second; *FVC*, forced vital capacity.
*Most persons with COPD have features of both pulmonary emphysema and chronic bronchitis.

ventilation-perfusion mismatch (i.e., a disproportionate relationship between ventilation and perfusion). Because the constricted bronchioles are clogged with mucus, there is a physical barrier to ventilation. In addition, there is a diminished respiratory drive, with a tendency to hypoventilate and retain CO_2. As a result, many areas of the lung are not ventilated, and O_2 diffusion cannot occur. Frequently the patient with chronic bronchitis requires O_2 both at rest and during exercise as the disease progresses. Peribronchial fibrosis may also result from the healing process secondary to inflammatory changes.

Coughing is stimulated by retained mucus that cannot adequately be removed as a result of decreased cilia and lessened mucociliary activity. The cough is often ineffective to remove secretions adequately because the person cannot inspire deeply enough to cause air to flow distal to retained secretions. Frequently, bronchospasm develops in the patient with chronic bronchitis. Bronchospasm is usually more common in the patient with a history of cigarette smoking or asthma. The bronchospasm adds to the already increased airway resistance, resulting in further increased work of breathing and impaired gas exchange.[18]

Clinical Manifestations

The clinical manifestations of COPD vary from those of pure emphysema to those of pure chronic bronchitis. Most patients with COPD have features of both (Table 25-9).

Emphysema. An early symptom of emphysema is dyspnea, which becomes progressively more severe. The patient will first complain of dyspnea on exertion that progresses to interfering with ADL to dyspnea at rest. Minimal coughing is present, with no sputum or small amounts of mucoid sputum. As more alveoli become overdistended, increasing amounts of air are trapped. This causes a flattened diaphragm and an increased anteroposterior (AP) diameter of the chest, forming the typical barrel chest. Effective abdominal breathing is decreased because of the flattened diaphragm from the overdistended lungs. The person becomes more of a chest breather, relying on the intercostal and accessory muscles. This type of breathing, however, is not that effective because the ribs become fixed in an inspiratory position.

Hypoxemia (especially during exercise) may be present, but hypercapnia does not develop until late in the disease. The person is characteristically thin and underweight, but

Table 25-10 Correlation of FEV_1 with Probable Clinical Manifestations

Approximate FEV_1 (ml)	Probable Clinical Manifestation
1500	Shortness of breath just beginning to be noticed
1000	Shortness of breath with activity
500	Shortness of breath at rest

FEV_1, Forced expiratory volume in 1 second.

the exact cause for this is not well understood. One possibility is that the patient is in a hypermetabolic state with increased energy requirements that are partly due to the increased work of breathing. Even when the patient has adequate calorie intake, weight loss is still experienced. The patient with emphysema has protein-calorie malnutrition with loss of lean muscle mass and subcutaneous fat. (Malnutrition is discussed in Chapter 37.)

Later in the course of the disease, secondary chronic bronchitis may develop. In advanced stages, finger clubbing may be present in both emphysema and chronic bronchitis. Other characteristics are presented in Table 25-10.

Chronic Bronchitis. The earliest symptom in chronic bronchitis is usually a frequent, productive cough during most winter months. It is often exacerbated by respiratory irritants and cold, damp air. Bronchospasm can occur at the end of paroxysms of coughing. Frequent respiratory infections are another common manifestation. Somewhat later, dyspnea on exertion may develop. A history of cigarette smoking for many years is almost always present. Unfortunately, a patient often attributes chronic cough to smoking rather than lung disease, thus delaying initiation of treatment.

Hypoxemia and hypercapnia result from hypoventilation caused by increased airway resistance. The bluish-red color of the skin results from polycythemia and cyanosis. Polycythemia develops as a result of increased production of red blood cells (RBCs) secondary to the body's attempt to compensate for chronic hypoxemia. Hemoglobin concentrations may reach 20 g/dl (200 g/L) or more. Cyanosis develops when there is at least 5 g/dl (50 g/L) or more of circulating unoxygenated hemoglobin.

A person with chronic bronchitis is usually of normal weight or heavyset, with a robust appearance. Emphysema of the centrilobular type frequently develops.

Complications

Cor pulmonale. Cor pulmonale is hypertrophy of the right side of the heart, with or without heart failure, resulting from pulmonary hypertension. In COPD, pulmonary hypertension is caused primarily by constriction of the pulmonary vessels in response to alveolar hypoxia, with acidosis further potentiating the vasoconstriction (Fig. 25-11). Chronic alveolar hypoxia also causes arteriolar muscle hypertrophy. Chronic hypoxia also stimulates erythropoiesis, which causes polycythemia and increases the viscosity of the blood.

Normally the right ventricle and pulmonary circulatory system are low-pressure systems compared with the left ventricle and systemic circulation. When pulmonary hypertension develops, the pressures on the right side of the heart must increase to push blood into the lungs. Eventually, right-sided heart failure develops.

The clinical manifestations of cor pulmonale are related to dilatation and failure of the right ventricle with subsequent intravascular volume expansion and systemic venous congestion. Heart sound changes include accentuation of the pulmonic component of the second heart sound, right-sided ventricular diastolic S_3 gallop, and early systolic ejection click along the left sternal border. ECG changes include increased P-wave amplitude (P-pulmonale) in leads II, III, and aVF; a tendency for right axis deviation; and incomplete right bundle branch block. Overt manifestations of right-sided heart failure may develop, which include distended neck veins (jugular venous distention), hepatomegaly with right upper quadrant tenderness, ascites, epigastric distress, peripheral edema, and weight gain.

Therapeutic management of cor pulmonale is continuous low-flow O_2. Long-term O_2 therapy can reverse the progression of pulmonary hypertension in the patient with COPD.[19] Although use of digitalis is not indicated for right-sided heart failure, it is used when a left-sided heart failure is present. Dietary salt restriction is sometimes recommended, especially if overt congestive heart failure (CHF) is present. Although diuretics are generally used, they are prescribed with caution because of their tendency to deplete potassium and chloride and reduce intravascular volume and cardiac output. (Cor pulmonale is discussed further in Chapter 24.)

Acute Respiratory Failure. The most common event leading to acute respiratory failure in COPD is acute respiratory tract infection (usually viral) or acute bronchitis. An exacerbation of cor pulmonale occurring either alone or simultaneously with other etiologic causes of acute respiratory failure may lead to acute respiratory failure. Discontinuing bronchodilator or steroid medication may also precipitate respiratory failure. The use of β-blocker medications (e.g., propranolol [Inderal]) may also exacerbate acute respiratory failure in the patient with an asthmatic component to the COPD.

The indiscriminate use of sedatives and narcotics, especially in the preoperative or postoperative patient who retains CO_2, may suppress ventilatory drive and lead to ventilatory failure. Hypercapnia (elevated CO_2) presents a serious problem when O_2 therapy is being given. Because of the persistent elevation of CO_2, the respiratory center no longer responds to increases in CO_2 by stimulating breathing. Therefore hypoxemia becomes the primary respiratory stimulant. If too much O_2 is administered, the hypoxic drive is abolished and breathing slows or stops. The person with COPD who retains CO_2 should be treated with low flow rates of O_2 with careful monitoring of ABGs. Surgery or severe, painful illness involving the chest or abdominal organs may lead to splinting and ineffective ventilation and respiratory failure. Careful preoperative screening, which includes pulmonary function tests and ABG monitoring, is important in the patient with a heavy smoking history and COPD to prevent postoperative pulmonary complications.[20] (Respiratory failure is defined and discussed in Chapter 26.)

Peptic Ulcer and Gastroesophageal Reflux. The incidence of peptic ulcer disease is increased in the person

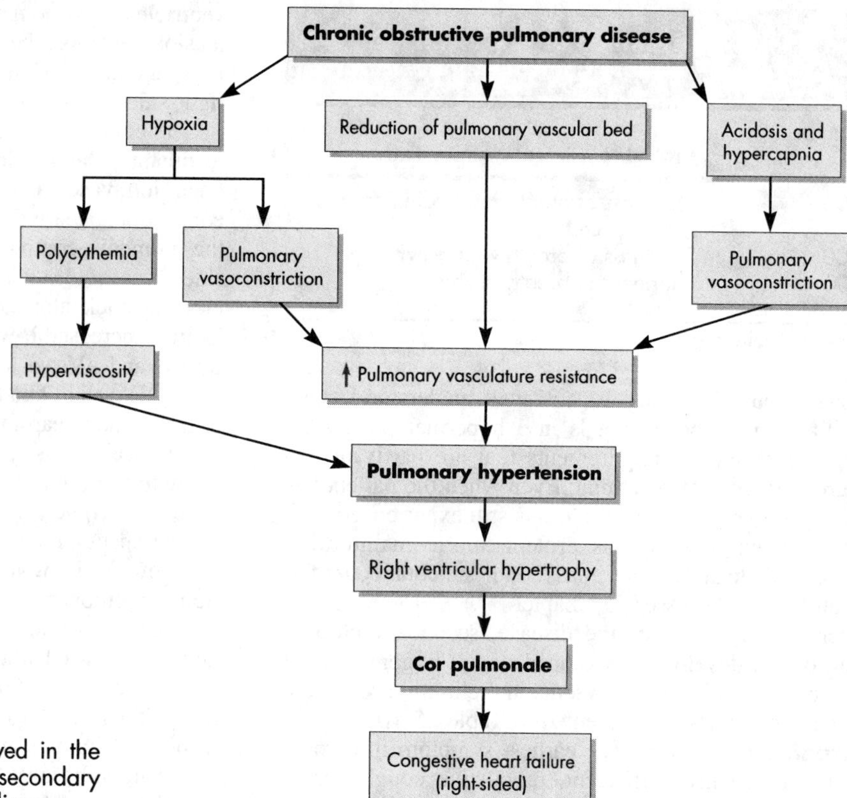

Fig. 25-11 Mechanisms involved in the pathophysiology of cor pulmonale secondary to chronic obstructive pulmonary disease.

with COPD. The reason for this occurrence is not known. It may be because of side effects from the long-term use of bronchodilator or steroid drugs. Another factor may be the stressful nature of the disease. It is important to test gastric aspirates and feces for occult blood.

Gastroesophageal reflux, which may or may not be associated with a hiatal hernia, occurs frequently in the patient with COPD and may aggravate respiratory symptoms. The reflux and accompanying heartburn may be aggravated or even precipitated by theophylline or β-adrenergic drugs. As a result of esophageal irritation or aspiration into the tracheobronchial tree, reflux airway constriction and obstruction may occur. (Treatment of hiatal hernia and gastroesophageal reflux is discussed in Chapter 38.)

Pneumonia. Pneumonia is a frequent complication of COPD. The most common causative agents are *S. pneumoniae, H. influenzae*, and viruses. The most common manifestation is purulent sputum. Systemic manifestations such as fever, chills, and leukocytosis may not be present. (Treatment of pneumonia is discussed in Chapter 24.)

Diagnostic Studies

An important goal of the diagnostic workup is to determine the major disease component of COPD and the severity of progression. These factors enable the health care provider to design an individualized treatment plan. Chest x-rays taken early in the disease may not show abnormalities. Later in the disease the findings presented in Table 25-9 may be present.

Pulmonary function studies are useful in diagnosing and assessing the severity of COPD. The most significant findings are related to increased resistance to expiratory airflow. Typical findings are as follows:

1. Reduced FEV_1
2. Reduced forced expiratory flow $(FEF)_{25\text{-}75\%}$
3. Reduced maximum voluntary ventilation (MVV)
4. Reduced vital capacity (VC)
5. Reduced FEV_1/FVC ratio
6. Reduced diffusing capacity for carbon monoxide
7. Increased residual volume (RV)
8. Increased total lung capacity (TLC)
9. Increased FRC

When the FEV_1/FVC ratio is less than 70%, it suggests the presence of obstructive lung disease. The value of FEV_1 in milliliters can provide a rough guideline to determine the severity of the patient's lung disease and the degree of disease progression. When compared with previous values, it can also provide a fair estimate of the level of expected activity tolerance for the patient (Table 25-10).

ABGs are usually monitored. In the later stages of COPD, typical findings are low PaO_2, elevated $PaCO_2$, decreased pH, and increased bicarbonate levels. In the early stages there may be a normal or only slightly decreased PaO_2 and a normal $PaCO_2$.

An exercise test to determine O_2 saturation in the blood with pulse oximetry or an arterial line with ABGs may be performed to evaluate whether desaturation occurs with exercise. An ECG may be normal or show signs indicative of right ventricular failure (e.g., low voltage, right axis deviation, P-pulmonale). An echocardiogram or gated pool

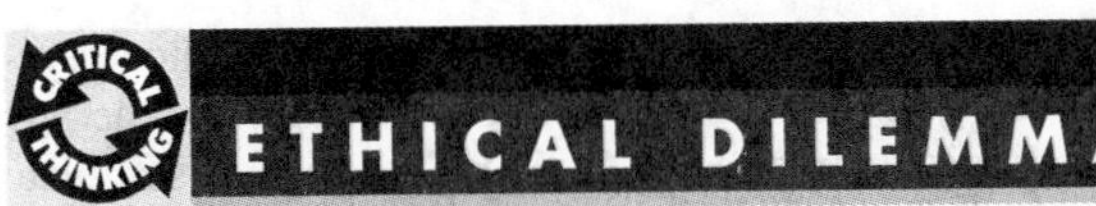

ETHICAL DILEMMAS

LIVING WILL

Situation A 79-year-old man with emphysema is admitted to the hospital with respiratory failure. His living will was executed 5 years ago, and a copy was given to his wife and physician at that time. The wife brings the document to the intensive care unit and tells the nurse that the hospital must stop treating her husband and allow him to die as he requested. However, the oldest son is threatening the hospital with a lawsuit if its staff does not provide full care to his father.

Discussion A legally executed living will is binding in most states. If the patient is not mentally competent or physically able to explain his wishes regarding continuation of medical treatment, then this advance directive is designed to speak for him. The son has no legal right to object to this directive if the document was duly executed by the patient when he was competent. Under the Patient Self-Determination Act (PSDA), the hospital would have asked the patient about his advance directives at the time of admission if he had been competent. His physician is obligated to follow the patient's directives if (1) the physician agrees that the patient is terminally ill and another physician concurs with that diagnosis and (2) it does not conflict with the physician's beliefs. If this physician is unable to follow the directives, the physician must transfer the care of this patient to another physician who will honor them. Professional counseling should be sought for the son and the wife because they face the patient's impending death.

ETHICAL AND LEGAL PRINCIPLES

- The Patient Self-Determination Act was enacted in 1990. All health care facilities and agencies that receive Medicaid or Medicare reimbursements are covered under the act. It requires that upon admission, information be given to the patient regarding the rights to make medical decisions for themselves and to execute advance directives (Living Wills and Durable Powers of Attorney for Health Care Decisions).
- Living Wills are a patient's advance directives regarding terminal illness or condition, and, in some states, persistent vegetative state. They specifically request that certain life-sustaining treatments be withheld or withdrawn and may also indicate the refusal of such maintenance medical care as artificial hydration and nutrition. Not all states have these statutes, and the laws vary in definition and content.
- A legally executed Living Will is the expression of a patient's wishes and should hold the same weight as the verbal expression of a currently competent patient. In this case the son's wishes do not outweigh his father's wishes.

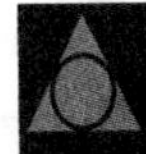

Table 25-11 Therapeutic Management: Chronic Obstructive Pulmonary Disease

Diagnostic
Health history and physical examination
Chest x-ray
Pulmonary function tests
Sputum specimen for Gram stain and culture (if indicated)
ABG monitoring
ECG
Exercise testing with oximetry or ABG monitoring
Echocardiogram or cardiac nuclear scans
Therapeutic
Treatment of respiratory infections
Bronchodilator therapy
β-adrenergic agonists
Anticholinergic agents (ipratropium)
Long-acting theophylline preparations
Corticosteroids
PEFR monitoring (if indicated)
Chest physiotherapy and postural drainage (if indicated)
Breathing exercises and retraining
Hydration of 3 L/day (if not contraindicated)
Cessation of cigarette smoking
Appropriate rest periods
Patient and family education
Influenza immunization yearly
Pneumovax immunization
Low flow rate O_2 (if indicated)
Progressive plan of exercise
Pulmonary rehabilitation program

ABGs, Arterial blood gases; *ECG,* electrocardiogram; *PEFR,* peak expiratory flow rate.

nuclear blood studies (see Chapter 29) can be used to evaluate right-sided as well as left ventricular function.

Therapeutic Management

In general, COPD is an irreversible process. The reversible components are airway size and secretions. Certain patients with COPD have emphysema that may be described as fixed airway disease; that is, there is no reversibility. The primary goals of therapeutic management are to (1) improve ventilation, (2) promote secretion removal, (3) prevent complications and progression of symptoms, and (4) promote patient comfort and participation in care[21] (Table 25-11). The majority of these patients are treated as outpatients. They are hospitalized for acute exacerbations and complications such as respiratory failure, pneumonia, and CHF.

Cessation of cigarette smoking in the early stages is probably the most significant factor in slowing the progression of the disease. After discontinuation of smoking, the accelerated decline in pulmonary function slows and returns to the more normal level of nonsmokers. Thus the sooner the smoker stops, the less pulmonary function is lost and the sooner the symptoms decrease, particularly cough and sputum production. The health care provider has a responsibility to inform each smoking patient about the effects of smoking, offer suggestions and guidelines on how to quit, and refer them to a smoking cessation program. The use of nicotine gum, nicotine transdermal patches, or clonidine patches may be helpful in minimizing the effects of nicotine withdrawal. These adjunctive therapies should be combined with other modalities such as support groups, education materials, and behavior modification programs. Hypnosis and acupuncture have also been helpful. Regardless of the methods used to stop smoking, the most important factor is that the person is committed to stopping.

Other environmental or occupational irritants should be evaluated for their possible negative effect, and ways to control or avoid them should be determined. For example, aerosol hair sprays and smoke-filled rooms should be avoided. The patient with COPD should have a vaccination with influenza virus vaccine yearly and with pneumococcal vaccine once in a lifetime.[18] Pneumococcal revaccination is recommended every 5 to 6 years for the patient who has depressed immune function. The patient with COPD is extremely susceptible to pulmonary infections. Respiratory infections should be treated as soon as possible. Often the best indication of the presence of a respiratory infection is the increasing quantity, viscosity, or purulence of sputum. Some patients are given a 7- to 10-day supply of antibiotics and are instructed to begin taking them at the first signs of change in sputum. The most common antibiotics given are ampicillin, amoxicillin, amoxicillin with clavulanate (Augmentin), tetracycline, erythromycin, and trimethoprim-sulfamethoxazole.

Bronchodilator drug therapy is often helpful in relieving symptoms. Although patients with COPD do not respond as dramatically as those with asthma to bronchodilator therapy, a reduction in dyspnea and an increase in FEV_1 are usually achieved. Most physicians believe that bronchodilator therapy is best given as maintenance therapy rather than as a treatment for acute symptoms. However, the routine use of bronchodilator therapy in all patients with COPD is controversial, especially in people with pure emphysema.

β-adrenergic agonists are routinely used as bronchodilators in the treatment of COPD. The preferred route of administration is by MDI or nebulizer. Anticholinergic agents, especially ipratropium by inhaler, are even more effective bronchodilators than β-agonists in the patient with emphysematous COPD. Because they are poorly absorbed systemically, inhaled anticholinergics have almost no side effects. These drugs are best taken on a regular basis. The use of long-acting theophylline in the treatment of COPD is controversial. Although it has some action as a mild bronchodilator in the patient with partial reversibility of airflow obstruction, its main value may be to improve contractility of the diaphragm and decrease diaphragmatic fatigue. Theophylline, a respiratory stimulant, may also be useful in a patient who hypoventilates.

The use of corticosteroid therapy in COPD also is controversial. The persons most likely to benefit from these drugs has a history of childhood asthma, has bronchospasm, has a relatively short duration of disease, or has frequent exacerbations that do not respond to therapy with β-agonists and theophylline.

Mucolytic expectorants (e.g., guaifenesin, iodinated glycerol, glycerol guiacolate) may be effective as adjuvant therapy in treating mucus-complicated COPD. These agents stimulate the bronchial glands to secrete more fluid. Initial use may result in increased coughing, sputum production, and shortness of breath as mucus is moved from the airways.

Home oxygen therapy is the only intervention in the patient with COPD that has been shown to increase life span. It may increase the life span of hypoxemic COPD patients by 6 to 7 years.[20] Home O_2 therapy is used in the patient who has significant hypoxemia. For medical reimbursement, Medicare guidelines require that the patient who receives home oxygen therapy have a PaO_2 of less than or equal to 55 mm Hg or a SaO_2 less than or equal to 88%. Medicare guidelines for the patient with a PaO_2 between 56 and 59 mm Hg or an SaO_2 of 89% include a secondary diagnosis of edema, CHF, or pulmonary hypertension, with a right axis with P waves greater than 2.5 mm in leads II, III, and aVF or polycythemia with a hematocrit greater than 56%. O_2 may be prescribed for continuous use, only at night, or with exercise. Long-term administration of O_2 is probably the most effective therapy for the prevention and treatment of cor pulmonale. (O_2 therapy is discussed in Chapter 24.)

Surgical Therapy for COPD. There are currently two types of lung volume reduction surgery available for patients with emphysematous-bullous COPD. One type is thorascopic bullectomy in which a thoracoscope is inserted into the pleura at affected sites and bullae can be treated by laser or stapled. Another type is reduction pneumoplasty, which requires a median sternotomy to remove bullae. The exact mechanism for improvement in lung function and clinical status is not known. Little is known about the complications and long-term results. It is theorized that by removing bullae, thus reducing the chest size, the respiratory muscles are at a more efficient length and work better. Removing bullae also allows for decompression of "normal" lung sections.

Respiratory Care

Respiratory care is usually a collaborative effort involving respiratory therapists and nurses. Respiratory care includes breathing retraining, effective cough techniques, chest physiotherapy, and aerosol-nebulization therapy.

The patient with COPD develops an increased respiratory rate with a prolonged expiration to compensate for dyspnea. In addition, the accessory muscles of breathing in the neck and upper part of the chest are used excessively to promote chest wall movement. These muscles are not designed for long-term use and as a result the patient experiences increased fatigue. Breathing exercises can assist the patient during rest and activity (e.g., lifting, walking, stair climbing). The main types of breathing exercises are (1) pursed-lip breathing and (2) diaphragmatic breathing.

The purpose of using *pursed-lip breathing* is to prolong exhalation and thereby prevent bronchiolar collapse and air trapping. The patient is taught to inhale slowly through the nose and then to exhale slowly through pursed lips, almost as if whistling. Exhalation should be at least twice as long as inhalation. It is helpful to have the nurse demonstrate the breathing exercises so the patient can imitate the action. The following techniques can be used to teach pursed-lip breathing:

1. Blow through a straw in a glass of water with the intent of forming small bubbles.
2. Blow at a lit candle enough to bend the flame without blowing it out.
3. Steadily blow a table-tennis ball across a table.

Diaphragmatic (abdominal) breathing focuses on using the diaphragm instead of the accessory muscles to achieve maximum inhalation and to slow the respiratory rate. The patient should be made aware of the difference between chest breathing and abdominal breathing. This can be achieved by having the patient lie down or assume a semi-Fowler's position and by placing one hand on the chest and the other on the abdomen. The patient should observe which hand moves during inspiration. The abdomen should protrude on inhalation with diaphragmatic breathing and contract on exhalation as the diaphragm pushes the air out of the lungs. The nurse should emphasize the value of diaphragmatic movement in increasing lung expansion.

To practice diaphragmatic breathing, the patient should keep the hand on the abdomen and concentrate on filling up the abdomen by inhaling slowly through the nose. Another technique is to wrap a towel gently around the abdomen and to pull it tight during exhalation. The patient then attempts to stretch the towel with slow inhalation by diaphragmatic breathing. On exhalation the patient uses pursed-lip breathing and draws the towel tighter to promote effective expiration.

Another technique to assist in diaphragmatic breathing is to place a small pillow, magazine, or book on the abdomen. This approach provides tactile stimulation and visual feedback. If the object rises on inspiration, the patient is given positive feedback that diaphragmatic breathing is taking place.

Pursed-lip breathing and diaphragmatic breathing should be practiced together for eight to 10 repetitions three or four times a day. These techniques give the patient more control over breathing, especially during exercise and periods of dyspnea.

In the setting of extreme acute dyspnea when the patient is hospitalized for infection or heart failure, it is more important to focus on helping the patient slow the respiratory rate by using the principles of pursed-lip breathing. Diaphragmatic (abdominal) breathing requires more energy and thus should be taught only when the patient has achieved a stable rehabilitative state such as before discharge or in a home care rehabilitation program.

Effective Coughing. Many patients with COPD have developed ineffective coughing patterns that do not adequately clear their airways of sputum. In addition, they fear they may develop spastic coughing, resulting in dyspnea. Guidelines for effective coughing are presented in Table 25-12. Huff coughing is an effective technique that the patient can be easily taught. The main goals of effective coughing are to conserve energy, reduce fatigue, and facilitate removal of secretions.

Table 25-12 Guidelines for Effective Coughing

1. Patient assumes a sitting position with head slightly flexed, shoulders relaxed, knees flexed, and forearms supported by pillow, and if possible, with feet on the floor.
2. Patient then drops head and bends forward while using slow, pursed-lip breathing to exhale.
3. Sitting up again, patient uses diaphragmatic breathing to inhale slowly and deeply.
4. Patient repeats steps 2 and 3 three to four times to facilitate mobilization of secretions.
5. Before initiating a cough, patient should take a deep abdominal breath, bend slightly forward, and then huff cough (cough three to four times on exhalation). Patient may need to support or splint thorax or abdomen to achieve a maximum cough.

Chest Physiotherapy. Chest physiotherapy (CPT) is indicated in the patient with (1) excessive bronchial secretions who has difficulty clearing secretions with expectorated sputum production greater than 25 to 30 ml a day, (2) evidence or suggestion of retained secretions in the presence of an artificial airway, or (3) lobar atelectasis caused by or suspected of being caused by mucus plugging.[22]

Chest physiotherapy consists of percussion, vibration, and postural drainage (Table 25-13). Percussion and vibration are manual or mechanical techniques used to augment postural drainage. Postural drainage uses the principle of gravity to assist in bronchial drainage. Percussion and vibration are used after the patient has assumed a postural drainage position to assist in loosening the mobilized secretions. Percussion, vibration, and postural drainage may assist in bringing secretions into larger, more central airways. Effective coughing is then necessary to help raise these secretions. After each drainage position change, the patient should be given time to cough and deep breathe. These techniques are individualized based on the patient's pulmonary condition and response to the initial treatment. Sometimes it takes several hours after CPT for secretions to be expectorated. It is important to evaluate CPT for both its effectiveness and relief of the patient's symptoms. CPT should be performed by an individual who has been properly trained. Complications associated with improperly performed CPT include fractured ribs, bruising, and discomfort to the patient. CPT may not be beneficial and may be stressful for some patients. Some patients may develop hypoxemia and bronchospasms with CPT.

Postural drainage. The lungs are divided into five lobes, with three on the right side and two on the left side. There are 18 segments in the lungs, which can be drained by 18 positions. Figure 25-12 shows the modified postural drainage positions most often used in clinical practice. The purpose of various positions in postural drainage is to drain each segment toward the larger airways. The postural drainage positions are determined by the areas of involved lung, which are assessed by chest x-rays, percussion, palpation, and auscultation. Aerosolized bronchodilators

Table 25-13 Steps in Chest Physiotherapy

1. Perform procedure 1 hr before meals or 1-3 hr after meals.
2. Administer bronchodilator (if nebulized or MDI is ordered) approximately 15 min before procedure.
3. Collect needed equipment such as tissues, emesis basin, paper bag, and pillows.
4. Help patient assume correct position for postural drainage based on findings from x-ray, auscultation, palpation, and percussion of chest. Position should be maintained for 5-15 min to mobilize secretions via gravity.
5. Observe patient during treatment to assess tolerance. Particularly observe breathing and color changes, especially duskiness in face.
6. Have patient take several deep abdominal breaths.
7. Percuss appropriate area for 1-2 min.
8. Vibrate the same area while the patient exhales 4-5 deep breaths.
9. Assist patient to cough while assuming same position. Splinting with towel or hands may be necessary to aid in effective coughing. Patient may have to assume sitting position to generate enough airflow to expel secretions. (Coughing productively may be a long waiting process that may occur 30 min after procedure.) Suction may be necessary if coughing is not effective.
10. Repeat percussion, vibration, and coughing until patient no longer expectorates mucus.
11. Repeat same procedure in all necessary positions.
12. After procedure, help patient assume a comfortable position, assist with oral hygiene, and discard used tissues.
13. Evaluate and chart effectiveness of treatment by amount of sputum produced and the results of auscultation. Also chart patient tolerance.

MDI, Metered-dose inhaler.

and hydration therapy is frequently administered before postural drainage. The chosen postural drainage position is maintained for 5 to 15 minutes. The degree of slope can be obtained with pillows, blocks, books, or a tilt board.

The frequency and choice of postural drainage positions depend on the location of retained secretions and patient tolerance to dependent positions. A common order is two to four times a day. In acute situations, postural drainage may be performed as frequently as every 1 to 2 hours. The procedure should be planned to occur and be completed at least 1 hour before meals and 3 hours after meals.

If a patient has difficulty in assuming various positions, adaptations will need to be made by reducing the angle or length of time of the procedure. A side-lying position can be used for the patient who cannot tolerate a head-down position. Some positions for postural drainage (e.g., Trendelenburg) should not be performed on the patient with chest trauma, hemoptysis, heart disease, or head injury, and in other situations where the patient's condition is not stable.

Percussion. Percussion is performed in the appropriate postural drainage position with the hands in a cuplike position (Fig. 25-13). The hands are cupped, and the fingers and thumbs are closed. The cupped hand should create an air pocket between the patient's chest and the hand. Both hands are cupped and used in an alternating rhythmic fashion. Percussion is accomplished with flexion and extension of the wrists. If it is performed correctly, a hollow sound should be heard. The air-cushion impact facilitates the movement of thick mucus. A thin towel should be placed over the area to be percussed, or the patient may choose to wear a T-shirt or hospital gown. Percussion should not be performed over the kidneys, sternum, spinal cord, or any tender or painful area. Other contraindications to percussion include hemoptysis, carcinoma, and induced bronchospasm.

Vibration. Vibration is accomplished by tensing the hand and arm muscles repeatedly and pressing mildly with the flat of the hand on the affected area while the patient slowly exhales a deep breath. The vibrations facilitate movement of secretions to larger airways. Mild vibration is tolerated better than percussion and can be used in situations where percussion may be contraindicated. Commercial vibrators are available for hospital and home use.

Aerosol-Nebulization Therapy. Devices that deliver a suspension of fine particles of liquid in a gas are commonly used to deliver medications to the COPD patient. Nebulizers are usually powered by a compressed air or O_2 generator. At home the patient may have an air-powered compressor; in the hospital, wall O_2 or compressed air is used to power the nebulizer.

Aerosolized medication orders must include the medication, dose, diluent, and whether it is to be nebulized with O_2 or compressed air. If O_2 is inadvertently used, a patient could become apneic if hypoxia was the primary respiratory stimulant. Medication is nebulized or reduced to a fine spray, and depending on several factors, including droplet size, it can be inhaled into the patient's tracheobronchial tree. The advantage to aerosol-nebulization therapy is a rapid-acting form of administration with few systemic effects. Medications that are routinely nebulized include albuterol, metaproterenol, isoetharine, isoproterenol, ipratropium, terbutaline, glycopyrrolate, acetylcysteine, and cromolyn. Other medications that can be administered by nebulization include antibiotics (gentamicin, tobramycin) and pentamidine.

The patient is placed in an upright position that allows for most efficient breathing to ensure adequate penetration and deposition of the aerosolized medication. The patient must breathe slowly and deeply through the mouth and hold inspiration for 2 to 3 seconds. Deep diaphragmatic breathing helps to ensure deposition of the medication. The patient is instructed to do normal tidal breathing in between these larger forced vital capacity breaths to prevent alveolar hypoventilation and dizziness. After the treatment the patient should be instructed to cough effectively. Postural drainage and CPT are ideally administered after bronchodilator medications are given.

A disadvantage of nebulizer equipment use is the possibility that the nebulizer unit will be a source of respiratory

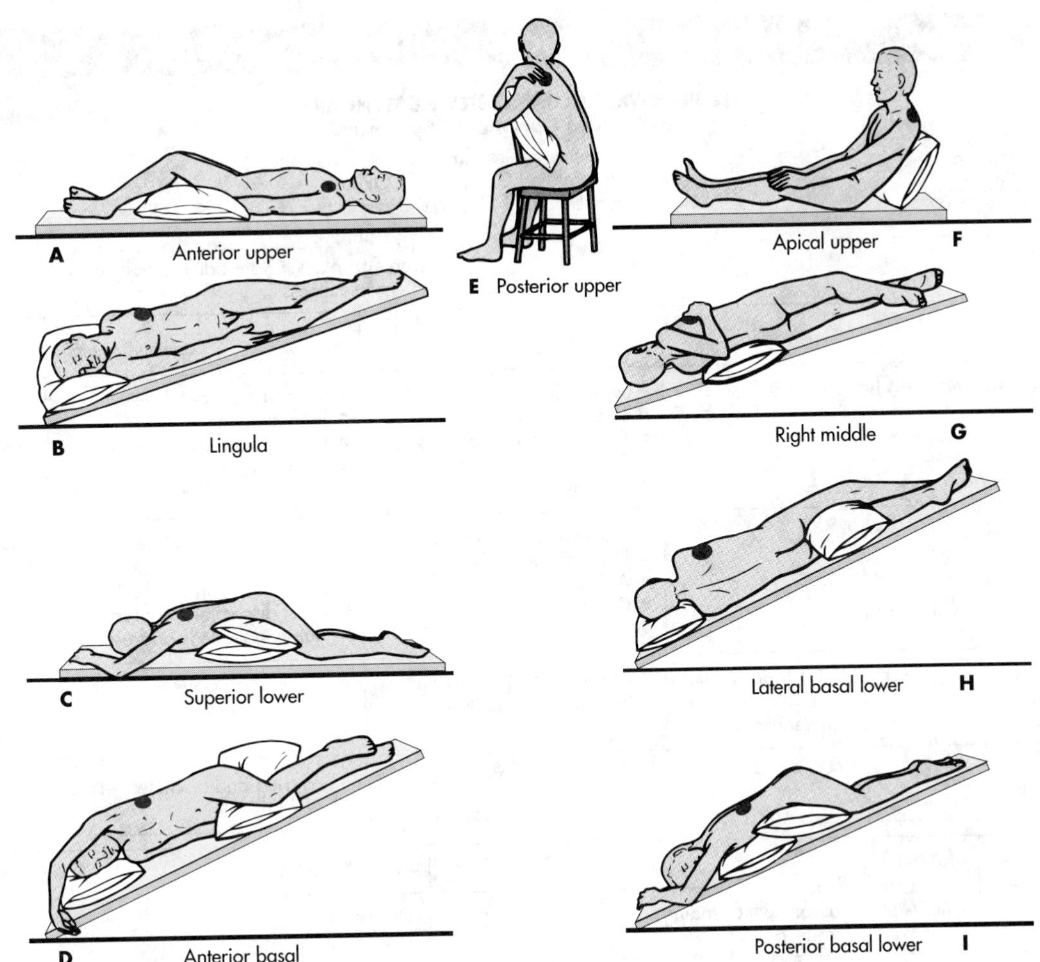

Fig. 25-12 Representative positions for postural drainage. *Shaded area* in each drawing indicates the segment of the lung in which drainage is promoted.

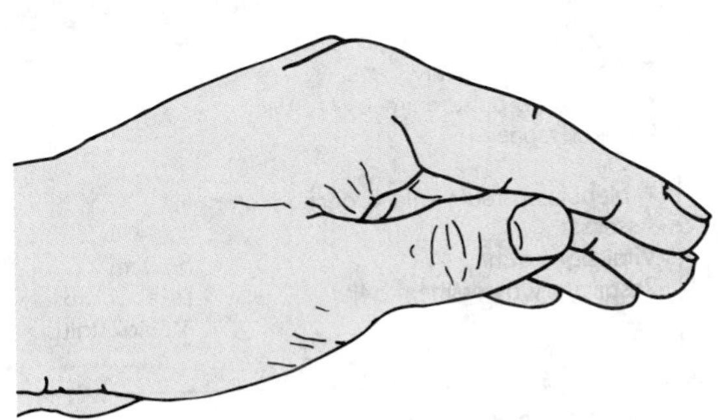

Fig. 25-13 Cupped-hand position for percussion. The hand should be cupped as though scooping up water.

infection. Because home nebulization is used for the patient with COPD, it is important for the health professional in the hospital and home care setting to review cleaning procedures for home respiratory equipment with the patient. A frequently used, effective home-cleaning method is to wash the nebulizer daily in soap and water, rinse it with water, and soak it for 20 to 30 minutes in a 1:1 white vinegar-water solution followed by a water rinse and air drying. Commercial respiratory cleaning agents may also be used if directions are followed carefully. Cleaning the nebulizer in the top shelf of an automatic dishwasher saves time, and the hot water destroys most organisms.

Peak Flow Meters. The patient with COPD can be taught how to correctly use a peak flow meter to monitor the clinical condition. The patient with severe disease may produce peak flow readings of less than 50 L per minute. Patients with mild to moderate disease may have PEFR that are clinically more useful. As with asthma, it is helpful to quantify the degree of clinical symptoms and response to therapy.

Intermittent Positive-Pressure Breathing. Intermittent positive-pressure breathing (IPPB) is the use of a pressure-limited ventilator to deliver a gas volume with humidity or aerosol medication. The machine applies positive pressure, forcing a prescribed volume of air into the lungs. IPPB can transiently decrease the work of breathing and improve ventilation. Although this modality of treatment is rarely used in COPD, it can be used for the patient with severe end-stage respiratory muscle failure to improve ventilation. IPPB may be used for atelectasis unresponsive to incentive spirometry.

Clinical Pathway for Chronic Obstructive Pulmonary Disease

NORTHWEST COMMUNITY HEALTHCARE
Coordinated Caremap™ Summary
Timeframe (minutes, hours, days, weeks, visits)
Diagnostic Related Group 88—COPD
National Length of Stay: 6.0 Days

Code status:________________
NWCH: 6.0 days

Physician:________________
Demographics: Older adult (usually over 65) with chronic illness

Area of treatment	Timeframe	Clinical focus	Expected outcomes
Emergency department	2-4 hr	■ Open airway (breathing) ■ Chest discomfort ■ Fluid intake and balance ■ Rule out infection ■ Anxiety	■ Improved oxygen levels in blood ■ Breathing easier ■ Lung sounds show improved air movement ■ Anxiety addressed ■ Underlying infection addressed
Hospital	6 days	■ Diet and nutritional needs ■ Physical condition ■ Airway ■ Chest discomfort	■ Improvement in oxygen levels in blood ■ Ease of breathing improved ■ COPD teaching protocol followed ■ Chest discomfort reduced ■ Nutritional needs addressed
Physician's Office	First visit 7-14 days after discharge with regular checkups thereafter	■ Chronic airway problems ■ Recent illness resolved	■ Return to previous level of functioning

This plan has been reviewed and discussed with me.

Patient's Name ________________ Signature ________________

Categories of care	Area: ER — Time: 2-4 hr	Area: Hospital — Time: Day 1
Consults	MESA physician on call/attending Respiratory care tech	Dietitian prn Discharge Planner prn
Tests/Specimens	Chest x-ray, ABGs/Pulse oximetry, CBC, electrolytes, ECG, UA (Cultures)	
Treatments/therapy ■ Respiratory Status	<u>Respiratory status addressed</u> Date ______ Initials ______ ■ Decreasing anxiety ■ Less dyspnea ■ Improved ABGs ■ O_2 ■ Nebulizer treatments/bronchodilator ■ Pursed lip breathing **Assess:** Vital signs q1hr and prn Respiratory assessment q1hr and prn Level of anxiety Mental status Sputum	<u>Improving respiratory status from ER</u> Date ______ Initials ______ ■ Decreasing anxiety ■ Improving pulse oximetry/ABGs ■ Less dyspnea ■ O_2 ■ Nebulizer treatments/bronchodilator **Assess:** Vital signs q4hr Respiratory assessment q4hr Sputum Level of anxiety Mental status
Fluid balance	<u>Hydration status addressed</u> Date ______ Initials ______ ■ IVs per MD order ■ I & O **Assess:** Breath sounds Skin turgor Presence of peripheral edema Mucous membranes dry/moist	<u>Stabilizing hydration status balanced I & O</u> Date ______ Initials ______ ■ Daily weight ■ IVs per MD order ■ I & O **Assess:** Breath sounds Presence of peripheral edema Skin turgor Mucous membranes dry/moist

continued

Clinical Pathway for Chronic Obstructive Pulmonary Disease—cont'd

Categories of care	Area: ER Time: 2-4 hr	Area: Hospital Time: Day 1
Diet	As tolerated	Nutritional needs addressed Date Initials ■ O_2 cannula for meals if on face mask ■ Obtain order for dietitian to see for nutritional assessment if indicated ■ Good oral hygiene **Assess:** Nutritional status Albumin Weight
Medications	Medications per MD's order	Demonstrates proper use of MDI if ordered Date ____ Initials ____ ■ Refer to patient teaching protocol
Activity	Expresses acceptable breathing comfort level Date ____ Initials ____ ■ Head of bed up ■ Overbed table with pillow to lean on ■ Keep head in good alignment with patient airway **Assess:** Decreased dyspnea with positioning Able to expectorate secretions	■ OOB as tolerated ■ Up in chair tid **Assess:** Current physical condition Ability to complete ADLs Current baseline activity level Patient response to activity ■ Increased SOB ■ Increased anxiety
Miscellaneous	Patient/SO verbalizes understanding need for admission Date ____ Initials ____ ■ Type of unit ■ Admitting process	Become familiar with proper breathing techniques during ADLs/activities Date ____ Initials ____ ■ Pursed-lip breathing (refer to teaching protocol)
Discharge planning		■ Refer to discharge plan if indicated **Assess:** Current living arrangements Discharge planning needs Level of independence Use of O_2/home
		Initials [ ] D [ ] E [ ] N

Partial critical pathway for COPD. The complete plan is for a 6-day hospitalization. Developed by Northwest Community Hospital, Arlington Heights, IL. Licensed by the Center for Case Management, South Natick, MA.
ABGs, Arterial blood gases; *ADLs,* activities of daily living; *CBC,* complete blood count; *COPD,* chronic obstructive pulmonary disease; *ER,* emergency room; *I & O,* intake and output; *IV,* intravenous; *MDI,* metered-dose inhaler; *NWCH,* Northwest Community Hospital; *OOB,* out of bed; *SO,* significant other; *SOB,* shortness of breath.

Nutritional Management

The patient with COPD should try to keep body weight for height in standard range. Weight loss and malnutrition are commonly seen in the patient with severe emphysema. The cause of this weight loss is unknown, but it is thought to be caused by increased energy expenditure or inadequate caloric intake. Eating becomes an effort, especially in the later stages of COPD. It is difficult for some patients to hold their breath while swallowing; therefore inadequate amounts of food are eaten. Other proposed reasons for malnutrition include loss of appetite related to a decreased sense of taste and smell and gastrointestinal disturbances.

To decrease dyspnea and conserve energy, the patient should rest at least 30 minutes before eating and should select foods that can be prepared in advance. Exercises and treatments should be avoided at least 1 hour before and after eating. The exertion involved in the preparation and eating of food is often fatiguing. The use of a microwave oven may help to conserve patient energy in food preparation. Many patients with COPD have feelings of bloating and early satiety when eating. This sensation can be attributed to swallowing air while eating, side effects of medication (especially corticosteroids and theophylline), and the abnormal position of the diaphragm relative to the stomach in association with hyperinflation. A full stomach puts pressure on the diaphragm and decreases lung movement. Liquid, blenderized, or commercial diets may be helpful. Foods that require a great deal of chewing should be avoided or served in another manner (e.g., grated, pureed). Cold foods may give less of a sense of fullness than hot foods.

The patient with emphysema has a greater than normal nutritional requirement for protein and calories. A high-calorie, high-protein diet is recommended and can be divided into five to six small meals a day. High-protein, high-calorie nutritional supplements can be offered between meals. Ice cream added to these supplements can help to increase calories. (Nutritional supplements are discussed in Chapter 37). A high carbohydrate diet may need to be avoided in the patient who retains CO_2 because carbohydrates metabolize into CO_2 and increase the CO_2 load of the patient. In most cases just getting the patients to eat adequate amounts of any foods can be difficult. Gas-forming foods should be avoided. If the patient has O_2 prescribed, use of supplemental O_2 by nasal prongs while eating may also be beneficial. Fluid intake should be at least 3 L a day unless contraindicated for other medical conditions, such as heart failure. Fluids should be taken between meals (rather than with them) to prevent excess stomach distention and to decrease pressure on the diaphragm. Sodium restriction may be indicated if there is accompanying heart failure.

Loss of appetite and nausea may also occur as a result of increased production of mucus and as an effect of some of the prescribed medications. If anorexia is a problem, various strategies can be used, including having the patient eat high-calorie food first; having favorite foods available; and adding butter, mayonnaise, or sauces to supply additional calories. Taking medicines with milk or meals and performing bronchial drainage procedures approximately 1 hour before meals may help. The patient who is overweight, more commonly seen in chronic bronchitis, needs to be placed on a low-fat diet to assist in weight reduction.

NURSING MANAGEMENT

EMPHYSEMA AND CHRONIC BRONCHITIS

Nursing Assessment

Subjective and objective data that should be obtained from a person with emphysema or chronic bronchitis are presented in Table 25-14.

Nursing Diagnoses

Nursing diagnoses are determined when the problem and etiologic factors are supported by clinical data. The nursing diagnoses related to emphysema and chronic bronchitis may include, but are not limited to, those presented in the nursing care plan on p. 720.

Planning

The overall goals are that the patient with COPD will have (1) return of baseline respiratory function, (2) ability to perform ADL, (3) relief from dyspnea, (4) no complications related to COPD, and (5) knowledge and ability to implement a long-term treatment regimen.

Nursing Implementation

Health Promotion and Maintenance. The incidence of COPD would decrease if more people would choose not to start smoking or would stop smoking. Avoiding or controlling exposure to occupational and environmental pollutants and irritants is another preventive measure to maintain healthy lungs. (These factors are discussed in the section on nursing management of lung cancer in Chapter 24.)

Early detection of small-airway disease is important. The person who has smoked for only a few years may have early evidence of obstructive airways. These changes often cannot be detected from pulmonary function studies until extensive damage is present. It is extremely important for the person to stop smoking and avoid inhaling irritants while the disease is still reversible. Failure to follow this advice will inevitably lead to irreversible COPD.

As health care professionals, nurses who smoke should reevaluate the smoking behavior and its relationship to their health. It is also important for nurses to counsel patients and peers regarding the harmful effects of smoking and to encourage them to quit. Referring patients and peers to self-help groups in the community may be especially valuable. These groups are sponsored by organizations such as the American Lung Association, American Cancer Society, and American Heart Association. These groups also have literature available that provides helpful guidelines, encouragement, and support. Nurses need to participate actively in developing policies establishing smoke-free working environments for themselves and others, controlling smoking in public places, requiring self-extinguishing cigarettes to prevent fire deaths and injuries, prohibiting advertising and tobacco promotions, and mandating health warning labels on cigarette packages.

Early diagnosis and treatment of respiratory tract infections are other ways to decrease the incidence of COPD. Avoiding exposure to large crowds in the peak periods for influenza may be necessary, especially for the older adult and the person with a history of respiratory problems. Influenza and pneumococcal pneumonia vaccines are recommended for the patient with COPD.

Families with a history of AAT deficiency need to be aware of the genetic nature of the disease. Genetic counseling may be appropriate for the patient who is planning to have children.

Acute Intervention. The patient with COPD will require acute intervention for complications such as pneumonia, cor pulmonale, and acute respiratory failure. (The nursing care for these conditions is discussed in Chapters 24 and 26.) Once the crisis in these situations has been resolved, the nurse can assess the degree and severity of the underlying respiratory problem. (The section on assessment in Chapter 22 provides a beginning basis to use in obtaining information from the patient.) The information obtained will help to plan the nursing care.

Chronic and Home Management. By far the most important aspect in the long-term care of the patient with COPD is education (Table 25-15). Because COPD is a chronic, debilitating disease, the patient will benefit by being able to exert some control over the disease. Because each COPD patient has different learning expectations,

Table 25-14 Nursing Assessment: Patient with Emphysema or Bronchitis

Subjective Data

Important health information

Past health history: Smoking (including passive smoking, pack years); long-term exposure to chemical pollutants, respiratory irritants, occupational fumes, dust, previous hospitalizations

Medications: Use of O_2, bronchodilators, steroids, antibiotics, anticholinergics, OTC drugs

Functional health patterns

Health perception–health management: Recurrent respiratory tract infections, family history of respiratory disease, fatigue

Nutritional-metabolic: Anorexia, weight loss or gain

Activity-exercise: Inability to perform ADLs; palpitations, swelling of feet; dyspnea (progressive), especially on exertion; recurrent cough; sputum production (color, odor, viscosity, amount); orthopnea

Sleep-rest: Insomnia; sitting up position for sleeping, paroxysmal nocturnal dyspnea

Cognitive-perceptual: Chest and abdominal soreness, headache

Objective Data

General

Debilitation, anxiety, restlessness, position assumed

Integumentary

Cyanosis (bronchitis), pallor or ruddy color, poor skin turgor, clubbing, easy bruising

Respiratory

Respiratory distress; rapid, shallow breathing; inability to speak; prolonged expiratory phase; pursed-lip breathing; wheezing; rhonchi, crackles, diminished or bronchial breath sounds; decreased chest excursion and diaphragm movement; use of accessory muscles; hyperresonant or dull chest sounds on percussion

Cardiovascular

Tachycardia, dysrhythmias (especially multifocal atrial tachycardia), edema of lower extremities, pulsus paradoxus, JVD, distant heart tones, right-sided S_3

Musculoskeletal

Muscle atrophy, increased anteroposterior diameter (barrel-chest)

Possible findings

Abnormal ABGs, polycythemia, pulmonary function tests showing expiratory airflow obstruction (e.g., low FEV_1, low FEV_1/VC, large RV, low PEFR compared to baseline decreased expiratory flow rate), chest x-ray showing flattened diaphragm and hyperinflation or infiltrates, ECG showing dysrhythmias

ABGs, Arterial blood gases; *ADLs,* activities of daily living; *ECG,* electrocardiogram; *FEV_1,* forced expiratory volume in 1 second; *JVD,* jugular venous distention; *OTC,* over-the-counter; *PEFR,* peak expiratory flow rate; *RV,* residual volume; *VC,* vital capacity.

motivations and needs, teaching must be adapted individually. Therefore it is important to assess the patient's level of knowledge, motivations, and goals before beginning to teach or develop a teaching plan. The nurse should help the patient understand that it is possible to plan treatment aimed at preserving lung function and slowing the progression of the disease. Patient and family participation in the treatment plan is essential. Respiratory care, as well as other related approaches, will be ongoing.

The health professional usually finds that it is not realistic to teach everything at one time. For example, if the patient has been hospitalized recently for acute respiratory failure resulting from a respiratory infection, the focus of teaching may be on helping the patient identify the signs and symptoms of a respiratory infection (e.g., fever, increased dyspnea, purulent sputum, increased use of inhalers or nebulizer treatments without relief) and writing a plan with input from the patient that may be used if these symptoms recur. The plan may include the following: notify the physician, increase fluid intake, increase nebulizer treatments (e.g., from twice a day to four times a day) with the physician's order, begin taking prescribed antibiotics, monitor for decrease or increase in symptoms, and notify the physician of the effects of these interventions.

Pulmonary rehabilitation. Pulmonary rehabilitation should be considered for the patients with symptomatic COPD. According to the American Thoracic Society, the objectives of pulmonary rehabilitation are to (1) control and alleviate as much as possible the symptoms and pathophysiologic complications of respiratory impairment and (2) teach the patient how to achieve optimal capability for carrying out ADL. The overall goal is to increase the quality of life. The components of pulmonary rehabilitation include physical therapy (e.g., bronchial hygiene, exercise conditioning, breathing retraining, energy conservation), nutrition, and education and other topics such as smoking cessation, environmental factors, health promotion, psychologic counseling, and vocational rehabilitation. Although much of this intervention should be routinely included in the comprehensive approach to the patient with COPD, the referral of the patient to a structured pulmonary rehabilitation program should also be considered for the patient with moderate to severe COPD.

Activity considerations. Energy conservation is another important component in COPD rehabilitation. This patient is typically an upper thoracic and neck breather who uses accessory muscles rather than the diaphragm. Thus the patient has difficulty performing upper-extremity activities, particularly those activities that require arm elevation above the head.[23] Exercise training of the upper extremities may improve function and reduce dyspnea. Frequently the patient has already adapted alternative energy-saving practices for ADL. Alternative methods of hair care, shaving, showering, and reaching may need to be explored. An occupational therapist may help with ideas in these areas. Assuming a tripod posture (elbows supported on a table,

(Text continued on p. 724.)

NURSING CARE PLAN Patient with Chronic Obstructive Pulmonary Disease

Planning: Outcome Criteria	Nursing Interventions and Rationales
➤ NURSING DIAGNOSIS	Ineffective airway clearance *related to* expiratory airflow obstruction, ineffective cough, environmental irritants leading to hypersecretion and decreased mucociliary transport, decreased airway humidity, and infection in airways *as manifested by* difficulty in expectorating sputum, presence of abnormal breaths sounds, ineffective or absent cough, no audible breath sounds
Expectorate sputum without difficulty, have normal breath sounds for patient and effective coughing.	Evaluate cough pattern and encourage cough. Facilitate deep breathing by elevating head or sitting patient up *to maximize ventilation and prolong expiratory phase, which reduces trapped air.* Position *to facilitate cough and prevent aspiration.* Ensure hydration (oral intake approximately 2-3 L/day, humidified ambient air) *to liquefy secretions for easier expectoration.* Provide CPT (positioning, percussion, and vibration) when indicated *to use effect of gravity in removing secretions.* Coordinate inhaled bronchodilator administration *to facilitate clearance of retained secretions.* Minimize exposure to environmental irritants and pathogenic organisms *to prevent secondary infection.* Promote smoking cessation *to reduce the effect of smoke on the lungs (e.g., increase in mucus production and a decrease in ciliary action) and to slow progression of the disease.* Teach alternative cough techniques (e.g., quad, huff), signs and symptoms of infection, and airway clearance techniques *to prepare patient for self-care at home.*
➤ NURSING DIAGNOSIS	Ineffective breathing pattern *related to* obstruction of airflow, increased work of breathing, respiratory muscle fatigue or failure, and anxiety *as manifested by* respiratory rate <11 or >24 breaths/min, abnormal inspiratory-expiratory ratio, irregular breathing rhythm (e.g., use of accessory muscles of breathing inappropriate to level of activity), discoordinated abdominal-thoracic muscle motion
Report decrease in dyspnea; have respiratory rate, rhythm, depth, and timing within normal limits; use accessory muscles appropriate to activity level.	Evaluate breathing patterns *to provide baseline data and determine appropriate intervention.* Position patient *to maximize respiratory effort* (i.e., sitting with stabilization of shoulders). Administer O_2 if appropriate at low flow *to avoid depressing respiratory drive.* Initiate techniques *to conserve energy.* Provide relaxation training (e.g., biofeedback, progressive muscle relaxation, imagery). Use airway clearance techniques *to facilitate breathing by raising mucus.* Teach and demonstrate pursed-lip and abdominal breathing *to maximize ventilation and minimize air trapping.*
➤ NURSING DIAGNOSIS	Impaired gas exchange: hypercapnia *related to* alveolar hypoventilation *as manifested by* headache on awakening, $PaCO_2$ >45 mm Hg and abnormal for patient's baseline
Have $PaCO_2$ of 35-45 mm Hg or usual compensated baseline value, demonstrate correct techniques to normalize $PaCO_2$ (e.g., secretion clearance and bronchodilator therapies), improved mental status.	Provide frequent stimulation (e.g., talking, turning, positioning) *to keep patient moving and to mobilize secretions.* Teach pursed-lip breathing *to prolong expiratory phase and slow rate.* Avoid use of respiratory depressants *to ensure adequate alveolar ventilation.* Administer and teach appropriate use of bronchodilator *to treat bronchospasm and narrowing of bronchi.* Teach potential hazard of excessive levels of inspired O_2 to patient with blunted CO_2 drive *because excess O_2 will depress respiratory drive.* Teach signs, symptoms, and consequences of hypercapnia (e.g., confusion, somnolence, headache, irritability, decrease in mental acuity, increase in respiration, facial flush, diaphoresis) *so problem can be recognized early and treatment initiated.* Teach avoidance of CNS depressants, *which further depress respirations.*

continued

NURSING CARE PLAN Patient with Chronic Obstructive Pulmonary Disease—cont'd

Planning: Outcome Criteria	Nursing Interventions and Rationales
➤ **NURSING DIAGNOSIS**	Impaired gas exchange: hypoxemia *related to* alveolar hypoventilation, intrapulmonary shunting, low ventilation-perfusion ratio, diffusion impairment, decreased ambient O_2, and decreased barometric pressure (high altitude) *as manifested by* PaO_2 <60 mm Hg or SaO_2 <90% at rest
Have return of PaO_2 to normal range for patient, increased independence in ADLs, improved mental status.	Administer O_2 if appropriate *to increase O_2 saturation without depressing respiratory drive.* Teach and monitor proper placement of supplementary O_2 devices (e.g., nasal cannula) *to maximize delivery of O_2.* Select O_2 supply systems and devices (e.g., nasal cannulas, mask) that are appropriate to patient ADLs (e.g., rest, sleep, exercise) *to minimize impact on preferred lifestyle.* Avoid unnecessary activity and provide assistance with ADLs *to minimize hypoxemia secondary to activity.* Teach and encourage deep breathing and pursed-lip breathing *to clear airways by propelling secretions towards mouth and to minimize air trapping.* Implement airway clearance techniques, if appropriate. Teach patient and family early signs and symptoms of impaired gas exchange (e.g., increased respiratory rate, irritability, anxiety, restlessness, dyspnea) *so interventions can be initiated promptly.* Administer and teach appropriate use of bronchodilator. Counsel patient about management of hypoxemia associated with air travel or increased altitude. Advise avoidance of respiratory depressants.
➤ **NURSING DIAGNOSIS**	Dyspnea *related to* increased airway resistance (bronchospasm and retained secretions), psychologic stress provoking and worsening dyspnea (anxiety, depression, fear), noxious environmental stimuli, and air trapping *as manifested by* unpleasant breathing sensation (shortness of breath, breathlessness), gasping, truncated speech patterns, abnormal use of accessory muscles at rest
Have diminished sensation of unpleasant breathing, less anxiety.	Administer and teach effective use of drugs and equipment (e.g., bronchodilators, diuretics, antibiotics, analgesics, mood elevators) *to achieve optimal benefits of drugs with minimal adverse side effects.* Schedule rest and activity *to provide adequate rest while maintaining adequate activity.* Provide relaxation training (e.g., biofeedback, imagery, progressive muscle relaxation). Provide psychomotor distraction techniques *to desensitize dyspnea (e.g., progressive exercise with coaching).* Assist patient to assume position of comfort (e.g., tripod position, elevated backrest, supported upper extremities to correct shoulder girdle) *to maximize respiratory excursion.* Remove or limit noxious environmental stimuli *to prevent source of irritation.* Teach, encourage, and demonstrate pursed-lip breathing *to prolong expiratory phase and reduce CO_2 retention.*
➤ **NURSING DIAGNOSIS**	Self-care deficit *related to* lowered energy level, hypoxemia, and depression *as manifested by* dependency, fatigue, weakness, muscle wasting, shortness of breath on exertion or rest, inadequate intake, poor personal hygiene
Accomplish ADLs by self or with partial or total assistance; have decrease in shortness of breath on exertion.	Assess type of self-care deficits *to have baseline data for planning care.* Teach measures such as lifting on exhalation, using assistive devices for work activities, transferring techniques, pacing activities, and planning periods of rest *to conserve energy.* Refer for occupational therapy when appropriate *for expert analysis of energy conserving aids and activities.* Administer O_2, if appropriate. Teach appropriate physical conditioning exercises *to increase strength and endurance.* Investigate need for personal assistance in home and refer to agencies that provide necessary assistance *to ensure that basic needs are met.*

continued

NURSING CARE PLAN Patient with Chronic Obstructive Pulmonary Disease—cont'd

Planning: Outcome Criteria	Nursing Interventions and Rationales
➤ NURSING DIAGNOSIS	Altered nutrition: less than body requirements *related to* poor appetite, lowered energy level, shortness of breath, gastric distention, sputum production, and depression *as manifested by* weight loss >10% of ideal body weight, serum albumin level below normal laboratory values, weight loss, weakness, muscle wasting, dehydration, decreased muscle tone, poor skin integrity, lack of interest in food
Maintain body weight within normal range for height and age.	Assess dietary preferences and dental status *to plan appropriate diet.* Monitor daily caloric intake *to determine adequacy of intake relative to weight.* Identify foods that require little work to prepare or eat *to keep energy expense related to food at a minimum.* Plan periods of rest after food intake *to compensate for blood flow diversion to the GI tract for digestion.* Provide menu suggestions for high-protein, high-calorie foods. Provide high-protein, high-calorie liquid supplements if necessary *to provide adequate calories and protein to prevent weight loss and muscle wasting.* Teach patient to avoid gas-producing foods *to prevent bloating and interference with respiratory excursion.* Provide O_2 supplement during meals as required and prescribed. Refer to agency for financial or nutritional assistance as necessary (e.g., Meals-on-Wheels, food stamps) *to ensure nutritional adequacy after discharge.* Be aware that patient may benefit from six small meals throughout the day, *because this reduces bloating.*
➤ NURSING DIAGNOSIS	Fluid volume excess *related to* fluid retention secondary to cor pulmonale or steroid use *as manifested by* peripheral or sacral edema; increased dyspnea; abnormal breath sounds (crackles, wheezes); weight gain >3 lb in 1 wk or 2 lb on consecutive days; JVD; taut, shiny skin; pedal edema
Have no evidence of fluid retention, baseline weight for patient.	Auscultate chest and heart *to detect abnormal sounds.* Continually assess change in activity level; JVD; edema and amount of pitting; serum electrolytes, Hb and Hct levels *because these provide cues to fluid retention.* Monitor input, output, and daily weights *to assess for fluid retention.* Teach positions *to enhance venous return.* Teach patient to weigh self daily and report weight gain >3 lb/wk or 2 lb on consecutive days without evidence of other cause *for early detection of fluid retention.* Elevate head of bed if patient is dyspneic *to decrease pulmonary congestion, decrease venous return, and lower the diaphragm.* Teach patient to report increase in dyspnea *to ensure early treatment and prevent anxiety.* Administer O_2, if appropriate. Provide bed or chair rest during acute phase. Monitor and teach effectiveness of drug therapy (e.g., diuretics) *to ensure safe and correct use.* Restrict sodium intake, if prescribed, *to reduce fluid retention.*
➤ NURSING DIAGNOSIS	Sleep pattern disturbance *related to* anxiety, depression, hypoxemia and hypercapnia, and shortness of breath *as manifested by* insomnia, lethargy, fatigue, restlessness, irritability; decreased level of ADLs; morning headaches; decreased PaO_2 with or without increased $PaCO_2$; orthopnea, paroxysmal nocturnal dyspnea
Verbalize feeling of being rested, have improvement in sleep pattern.	Identify usual sleep habits *to provide baseline data.* Assist patient to identify sources of discomfort and wakefulness. Observe for signs and symptoms of sleep apnea syndrome. Identify patient-specific methods of relaxation, and teach patient relaxation methods *to foster sleep.* Encourage exercise and activity during daylight hours *as this will improve sleep at night.* Instruct patient on position for easier breathing. Instruct patient to eat small evening meals *to reduce amount of oxygen to digestive system and prevent nocturnal dyspnea.* Administer O_2, if appropriate, *to increase PaO_2.* Encourage verbalization of feelings *to provide outlet for feelings.* Assist patient to identify source of help during night *to reduce feelings of anxiety and isolation.* Instruct patient in maintaining an environment conducive to rest (e.g., clothing, temperature, position, noise level). Teach potential dangers in use of respiratory depressants, *which further depress respirations and increase $PaCO_2$.* Teach avoidance of alcoholic beverages, caffeine products, or other stimulants before bedtime *to reduce interference with sleep.* Teach signs and symptoms of early hypoxemia and hypercapnia *so that early intervention can be initiated.* Administer sedatives as prescribed *to prevent excess anxiety.*

continued

NURSING CARE PLAN Patient with Chronic Obstructive Pulmonary Disease—cont'd

Planning: Outcome Criteria	*Nursing Interventions and Rationales*
➤ **NURSING DIAGNOSIS**	Sexual dysfunction *related to* physiologic alterations, hypoxemia, shortness of breath, effect of medications, and psychologic factors *as manifested by* decrease in desire for or interest in sex; decrease in social interactions with actual or potential sexual partners; avoidance of discussion of subject; inappropriate verbal or physical sexual behaviors; decrease in sexual activity; report of impotence; divorce or breakup of relationships; decrease in interest in appearance; increase in passivity; increase in feelings of hopelessness
Verbalize satisfaction with sexual functioning.	Determine basis for dysfunction (physical or psychologic) *to plan appropriate interventions*. Teach use of O_2 during and use of β-agonist MDI 10 min before sexual activities, if appropriate, *to reduce dyspnea secondary to hypoxemia*. Provide opportunity for patient and significant other to discuss feelings regarding problem *to foster sharing and mutual problem solving*. Help partner to understand change *so guilt and blame do not enter relationship*. Teach effects of medication and recommend modification, if necessary. Encourage patient and partner to explore other means of sexual expression and planning of sexual activity in terms of energy levels during the day *so that means of sexual expression is maintained*. Counsel patient and partner on sexual positions *to conserve energy*. Refer for counseling, if indicated.
➤ **NURSING DIAGNOSIS**	Risk for disturbance in self-concept, body image, self-esteem, role performance *related to* changes in body appearances, function, personal and societal role, and increased physical and psychologic dependence
Maintain social contacts; express positive feelings about self.	Assess patient for carelessness in dress and grooming; expression of depression or anxiety; difficulty in decision making; withdrawal from social situations, family interactions, and work-related responsibilities; ineffectual social interactions; verbal and nonverbal expression of decrease in self-worth; increase in dependent behaviors *to determine whether there is a self-concept problem*. Determine basis for disturbance in self-concept *to plan appropriate interventions*. Help patient identify and optimize physical and psychologic strengths. Help patient maintain social interactions by participation in family and social activities *to increase sources of pleasure and maintain self-esteem*. Help family or significant others to understand patient's limitations and need for acceptance *so they will continue to provide support to the patient*. Help family understand patient's need for independence and feeling of significant worth *to prevent family from treating patient as an invalid*. Refer for psychologic intervention or to support groups as needed.
➤ **NURSING DIAGNOSIS**	Risk for infection *related to* decreased pulmonary function, possible steroid therapy, ineffective airway clearance, and lack of knowledge regarding signs and symptoms of infection and preventive measures
Demonstrate behaviors designed to minimize risk of infection; seek medical attention for appropriate interventions; have no infection.	Assess for change in color, quantity, odor, and viscosity of sputum; difficulty in mobilizing secretions; foul oral odor; increase in cough; increase in dyspnea; fever; chills; diaphoresis; increase in respiratory rate; abnormal breath sounds (gurgles, wheezing); hypoxemia or hypercapnia; excessive fatigue *to determine whether an infection is present*. Teach patient to use good handwashing techniques and avoid contact (whenever possible) with persons with respiratory infections *to minimize source of infection*. Encourage patient to obtain vaccines for influenza and pneumococcal pneumonia *to decrease occurrence or severity of influenza or pneumonia*. Teach proper care and cleaning of home respiratory equipment *to eliminate these sources of infection*. Instruct patient to seek medical attention for manifestations of early infection *so that treatment can be started promptly*. Teach patient to initiate plan of care previously discussed with physician when infections occur (e.g., increase fluid intake, begin antibiotics, increase or begin steroids) *so that appropriate self-care is initiated promptly*.

ADLs, Activities of daily living; *CNS*, central nervous system; *CPT*, chest physiotherapy; *GI*, gastrointestinal; *Hb*, hemoglobin; *Hct*, hematocrit; *JVD*, jugular venous distention; *MDI*, metered-dose inhaler.

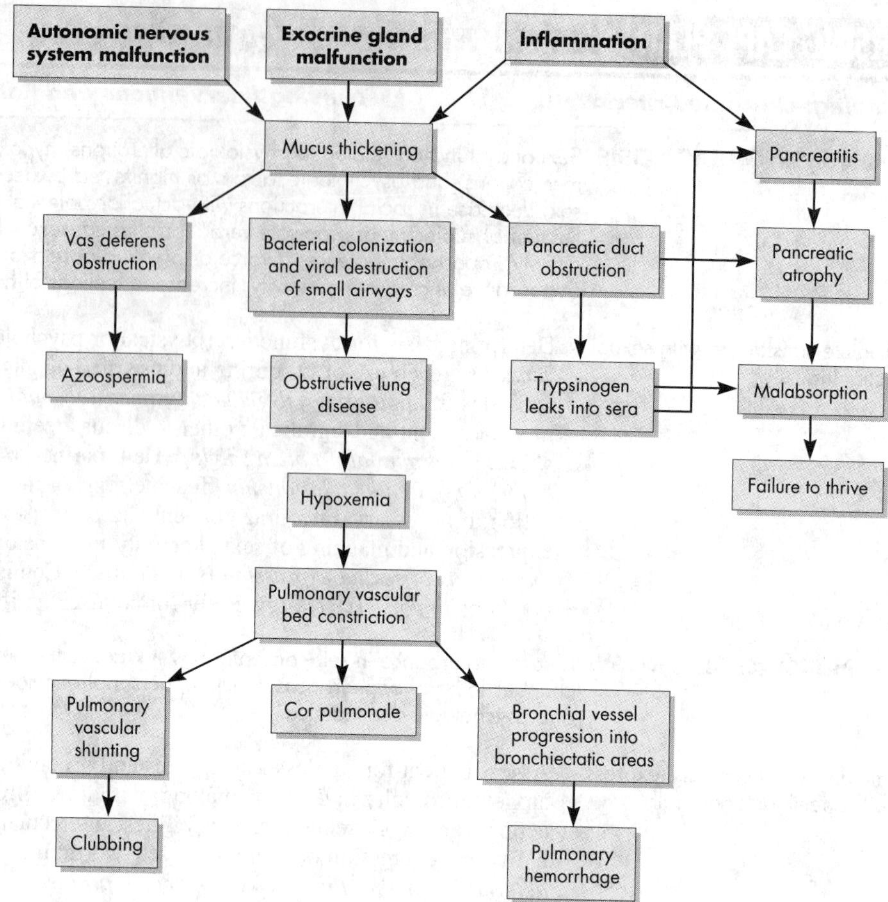

Fig. 25-14 Progression of cystic fibrosis.

Table 25-15 Components of a Teaching Plan for the Patient with Obstructive Pulmonary Disease

- Basic understanding of lung function and pathophysiology
- Basic understanding of drug, O_2, respiratory, and other therapies
- Knowledge of the signs and symptoms of respiratory infection, heart failure, and bronchospasm; what to do if these occur
- Knowledge of good nutrition
- Knowledge of the importance of exercise
- Knowledge of energy conservation techniques
- Demonstration of abdominal breathing and pursed-lip breathing
- Demonstration of peak flow monitoring and chest physiotherapy including vibration, percussion, and postural drainage, when indicated
- Steps for healthy psychologic coping

chest in fixed position) and a mirror placed on the table during use of an electric razor or hair dryer conserves much more energy than when the patient stands in front of a mirror to shave or blow-dry hair. The patient should be encouraged to make a schedule and plan daily and weekly activities so as to leave plenty of time for rest periods. The patient should also try to sit as much as possible when performing activities. Another energy-saving tip is to exhale when pushing, pulling, or exerting effort during an activity.

Walking is by far the best physical exercise for the COPD patient. Coordinated walking with slow, pursed-lip breathing without breath holding is a difficult task that requires conscious effort and frequent reinforcement. During coordinated walking and breathing, the patient is taught to breathe through the nose while taking one step, then to breathe out through pursed lips while taking two to four steps (the number depends on the patient's tolerance). Walking should occur at a slow pace with rest periods when necessary so the patient can sit or lean against an object such as a tree or post. The patient may need to ambulate using O_2. Once the patient is able to successfully perform coordinated walking with pursed-lip breathing, diaphragmatic breathing may also be incorporated if the patient has practiced and mastered this technique at rest. The nurse should walk with the patient, giving verbal reminders when necessary regarding breathing (inhalation and exhalation) and steps. Walking with the patient helps to decrease anxiety and to maintain a slow pace; it also enables the nurse to observe the patient's actions and physiologic responses to the activity. Many patients with moderate or severe COPD are anxious and fearful of walking or performing exercise. These patients and their families require much support while they build the confidence they need to walk or to perform daily exercises.

The patient should be encouraged to walk 15 to 20 minutes a day with gradual increases. Severely disabled patients can begin at a slow pace by walking for 2 to 5 minutes three times a day and slowly building up to 20 minutes a day, if possible. Adequate rest periods should be allowed. Some patients benefit from using their β-agonist MDI approximately 10 minutes before exercise. Parameters that may be monitored in the patient with mild COPD are resting pulse and pulse rate after walking. Pulse rate after walking should not exceed 75% to 80% of the maximum heart rate (maximum heart rate is age in years subtracted from 220). In the patient with other than mild COPD and without significant heart disease, it is usually dyspnea and the limitation in breathing rather than increased HR that limits the exercise. Thus it is better to use the patient's perceived sense of dyspnea as an indication of exercise tolerance.

The patient should be told that shortness of breath will probably increase during exercise (as it does for a healthy individual) but that the activity is not being overdone if this increased shortness of breath returns to baseline within 5 minutes after the cessation of exercise. The patient should be told to wait 5 minutes after completion of exercise before using their β-agonist MDI to allow a chance to recover. During this time, slow, pursed-lip breathing should be used. If it takes longer than 5 minutes to return to the baseline, the patient most likely has overdone it and needs to proceed at a slower pace during the next exercise period. The patient may benefit from keeping a diary or log of the exercise program. The diary can help provide a realistic evaluation of the patient's progress. In addition, the diary can help motivate the patient and add to the patient's sense of accomplishment. Stationary cycling can also be used either alone or with walking. Cycles are particularly valuable when weather prevents walking outside.

Sexual activity. Modifying but not abstaining from sexual activity can also contribute to a healthy psychologic well-being. Using an inhaled bronchodilator before sexual activity can help ventilation. The patient with COPD will also use less energy if these quidelines are followed: (1) plan sexual activity during the part of the day when breathing is best, (2) use slow pursed-lip breathing, (3) refrain from sexual activity after eating or other strenuous activity, (4) do not assume a dominant position, and (5) do not prolong foreplay. These aspects of sexual activity require open communication between partners regarding their needs and expectations.

Sleep. Adequate sleep is extremely important. Getting adequate amounts of sleep can be difficult for the COPD patient. Medications may cause irritability and insomnia. Many patients with COPD have postnasal drip or nasal congestion that may cause coughing and wheezing at night. Nasal saline sprays before sleep and in the morning may help. The physician may also prescribe a nasal decongestant or nasal steroid inhaler that may be used at bedtime. Long-acting theophylline preparations frequently aid in promoting sleep by decreasing bronchospasm and airway obstruction. If the patient is a restless sleeper, snores, stops breathing while asleep, and has a tendency to fall asleep during the day, sleep apnea may be present (see Chapter 23).

Home oxygen therapy. Long-term use of O_2 therapy has improved the quality of life for many patients with COPD. The use of controlled, low-flow O_2 at home can improve the patient's exercise tolerance and appetite and alleviate pulmonary hypertension. (Increased pulmonary vascular resistance is associated with alveolar hypoxia.) If pulmonary hypertension is reduced, the risk of cor pulmonale decreases. In addition, chronic hypoxia is partially corrected, and secondary polycythemia is less likely to develop. One of the major benefits of O_2 use at home is that the patient has a sense of well-being and gains more freedom in the choice of activities. Oxygen may be prescribed for continuous use, nocturnal use, and use during exercise and ambulation. Because hypoxemia worsens during sleep in some patients with COPD, nocturnal supplemental O_2 is indicated. (O_2 therapy is discussed in Chapter 24.)

Psychosocial considerations. Healthy psychologic coping is often the most difficult task to accomplish. People with COPD frequently have to deal with many lifestyle changes that may involve decreased ability to care for themselves, decreased energy for social activities, and loss of a job.

When a patient with COPD is first diagnosed or when a patient has complications that require hospitalization, the nurse should expect a variety of emotional responses from the person ranging from denial and guilt to depression. Guilt may result from the knowledge that the disease was caused largely by cigarette smoking. Depression may be experienced as the severity and chronicity of the disease are realized. Denial may result if the disease is not yet severe enough to cause much physical limitation. The nurse needs to convey a sense of understanding and caring to the patient.

Emotions frequently encountered include anxiety, depression, social isolation, denial, and dependence. Expression of these emotions becomes complicated because of the relationship of emotional expression to breathing. For example, anxiety normally produces an increase in respiratory rate, and depression usually goes along with inactivity, which in the COPD patient can translate into decreased exercise tolerance, increased dyspnea, increased dependence, and ultimately, worsening of depression.[20] A vicious cycle of emotional entrapment can occur. Learning new ways to express emotions with the use of relaxation techniques involving breathing can be helpful. Slowing the pace with frequent rest periods, open and honest communication with supportive significant others, and avoidance of anxiety-producing situations (if necessary) may need to be learned.

CULTURAL & ETHNIC Considerations

OBSTRUCTIVE PULMONARY DISEASES

- African-Americans have a higher mortality rate from asthma than Caucasians.
- Caucasians have the highest incidence of cystic fibrosis.
- Cystic fibrosis is uncommon among African-Americans and Asian-Americans.

The patient with COPD may benefit from several relaxation techniques. One is the use of a progressive relaxation technique in which the patient listens either to a tape or to the patient's own or another voice and gradually begins to tighten and relax muscle groups. Relaxation may begin in the head and neck area and end in the legs. Self-hypnosis, biofeedback, meditation, and massage (self-massage or massage from others) are other alternative relaxation therapies. Support groups at local American Lung Associations, hospitals, and clinics can also be helpful.

The patient frequently asks whether moving to a warmer or drier climate will help. In general, such a move is not significantly beneficial. Moving to places with an elevation of 4000 feet or more should be discouraged because of the lower partial pressure of O_2 found in the air at higher elevations. A disadvantage of moving may be that a person leaves an occupation, friends, and familiar environment, which could be psychologically stressful. Any advantage gained from a different climate may be outweighed by the psychologic effects of the move.

CYSTIC FIBROSIS

Cystic fibrosis (CF) is an autosomal recessive, multisystem disease characterized by altered function of the exocrine glands involving primarily the lungs, pancreas, and sweat glands. Abnormally thick, abundant secretions from mucous glands can lead to a chronic, diffuse, obstructive pulmonary disorder in almost all patients. Exocrine pancreatic insufficiency is associated with about 85% to 90% of cases of CF. Sweat glands excrete increased amounts of sodium and chloride.

Significance

Cystic fibrosis affects approximately 30,000 persons in the United States. The disease occurs primarily in Caucasians, with a frequency of 1 in 2500 births among Caucasians and 1 in 17,000 births among African-Americans. Both sexes are equally affected. Approximately 4% to 5% of the general population are carriers of the gene transmitting CF. Approximately 20% of these are young adults.[24] The first signs and symptoms typically occur in children, but some patients are not diagnosed until they are adults.

CF was once exclusively a pediatric disease; however, because of improved and aggressive treatment, the median survival of patients with CF has increased from less than 2 years in 1950 to almost 25 years of age currently. More than 25% reach adulthood, and many survive into their thirties and forties.[24] Each person has an individual spectrum of the disease and time course of deterioration.

Pathophysiology

CF is an autosomal recessive disease resulting from mutations in a gene located on chromosome 7. The most common mutation in the CF gene is known as the CF transmembrane regulator (CFTR). The primary defect in CF is abnormally regulated chloride channel activity. This defect alters ionic transport of sodium and chloride across epithelial surfaces. The high concentrations of sodium and chloride in the sweat of the patient with CF results from decreased chloride reabsorption in the sweat duct. The basic pathophysiologic mechanism is obstruction of exocrine gland ducts with thick, viscous secretions that adhere to the lumen of the ducts (Fig. 25-14). The glands distal to the duct eventually undergo fibrosis.

In the respiratory system, both upper and lower respiratory tracts can be affected. Upper respiratory tract manifestations may be present and include nasal polyposis. The hallmark of respiratory involvement in CF is its effect on the airways. The disease progresses from being a disease of the small airways (chronic bronchiolitis) to an entity that eventually involves the larger airways and finally causes destruction of lung parenchyma. Thick secretions obstruct bronchioles and lead to air trapping and hyperinflation of the lungs. The stasis of mucus provides an excellent growth medium for bacteria. The most common organisms cultured from the sputum of a patient with CF are *S. aureus, H. influenzae*, and *Pseudomonas aeruginosa*.

Lung disorders that can result include pneumonia, bronchiolitis, bronchitis, bronchiectasis, atelectasis, and emphysema. There is progressive loss of lung tissue from inflammation and scarring, and the resultant chronic hypoxia leads to pulmonary hypertension and cor pulmonale. Blebs and large cysts in the lung are also severe manifestations of lung destruction. Other pulmonary complications include hemoptysis, which can sometimes be fatal, and pneumothorax.

Initially, CF is an obstructive lung disease caused by the overall obstruction of the airways with mucus. Later, CF also progresses to a restrictive lung disease because of the fibrosis, lung destruction, and thoracic wall changes. Death usually results from extensive respiratory infection. Cor pulmonale is a common late complication caused by extensive loss of lung tissue and chronic hypoxia.

Pancreatic insufficiency is caused primarily by mucus plugging the pancreatic duct and its branches, which results in fibrosis of the acinar glands of the pancreas. The exocrine function of the pancreas is altered and may stop completely. Pancreatic enzymes such as trypsinogen, lipase, and amylase do not reach the intestine to digest ingested nutrients. There is malabsorption of fat, protein, and fat-soluble vitamins (e.g., Vitamins A, D, E, K). Fat malabsorption results in steatorrhea, and protein malabsorption results in failure to grow and gain weight. In advanced pancreatic insufficiency, diabetes mellitus may occur if the islets of Langerhans become fibrotic.

The sweat glands of the CF patient secrete normal volumes of sweat but are unable to absorb sodium chloride from sweat as it moves through the sweat duct. Therefore they excrete four times the normal amount of sodium and chloride in sweat. This abnormality does not seem to affect the general health of the person, but it is useful as a diagnostic indicator.

The liver may become involved. Biliary cirrhosis may not be recognized until late in the disease. Hepatobiliary disease is common in the older patient. Chronic cholestasis, inflammation, fibrosis, and portal hypertension can occur. Intestinal obstructions can also occur. Once resolved, they recur in almost one half of patients.

The function of the reproductive system is altered. This finding is important because more persons with CF are living to adulthood. The male adult is usually sterile (although not impotent) as a result of structural changes in the vas deferens, seminal vesicles, and epididymis. The female adult usually has delayed menarche. During exacerbations, menstrual irregularities and secondary amenorrhea are fairly common for the woman. She may be unable to become pregnant because of the increased viscosity of the cervical mucus. Women with CF do become pregnant, but the fertility rate is lower than in healthy women. The baby is heterozygous (and hence a carrier) for CF if the father is not a carrier. If the father is a carrier, there is a 50% chance that the baby will have CF.

Clinical Manifestations

The clinical manifestations of CF vary depending on the severity of the disease. An initial finding of meconium ileus in the newborn infant is present in 10% of persons with CF. Early manifestations in childhood are failure to grow, clubbing, persistent cough with mucus production, tachypnea, and large, frequent bowel movements. A large, protuberant abdomen may develop with an emaciated appearance of the extremities. Other respiratory problems that may be indicative of CF are recurring lung infections such as bronchiolitis, bronchitis, and pneumonia.

The severity and progression of the disease vary from person to person. In the last decade, it has been shown that with early diagnosis and immediate institution of intensive care, the prognosis can be significantly improved.

Complications

Pneumothorax is common (greater than 10% of patients) in patients with cystic fibrosis. The presence of small amounts of blood in sputum is common in the CF patient with lung infection. Massive hemoptysis is life threatening. With advanced lung disease, digital clubbing becomes evident in almost all patients with CF. Respiratory failure and cor pulmonale are late complications of CF.

Diagnostic Studies

The main diagnostic test for CF is the sweat chloride test with the pilocarpine iontophoresis method. Pilocarpine carried by a small electric current is used to stimulate sweat production. The sweat is collected on filter paper or gauze and then analyzed for sodium and chloride concentrations. The test takes approximately 40 minutes. Values greater than 65 mEq/L for both sodium and chloride are suggestive of CF, especially in a person who has other clinical features of the disease. The degree of sodium and chloride elevation does not necessarily correlate with the severity of the disease. Fetal diagnosis can now be made by analyzing gene markers from the chorionic villus tissue. Other diagnostic studies include chest x-ray, pulmonary function tests, fecal analysis for fat, and duodenoscopy for quantitative determination of enzymes.

DNA analysis is not used in the primary diagnosis because of the large number of CF mutations. It is likely, however, that DNA analysis will be performed increasingly in the CF patient to corroborate the diagnosis.

Therapeutic Management

The major objectives of therapy in CF are to promote clearance of secretions, control infection in the lungs, and provide adequate nutrition. Ultimately, gene therapy may be the treatment of choice.

Management of pulmonary problems in CF aims at relieving airway obstruction and controlling infection. Drainage of thick bronchial mucus is assisted by aerosol and nebulization treatments of medications used to liquefy mucus and to facilitate coughing. The abnormal viscoelastic properties of CF secretions are primarily caused by mucus glycoproteins and DNA from degenerated neutrophils. Agents that degrade the high concentrations of DNA in CF sputum (e.g., Pulmozyme [human recombinant DNAase]) decrease sputum viscosity and increase airflow during short-term administration. Bronchodilators (e.g., β_2 agonists, theophylline) may be used. They have a short-term effect and no long-term benefit. CPT (e.g., postural drainage, vibration, and percussion) has been the mainstay of treatment for some time.

Aerobic exercise seems to be effective in clearing the airways. Important needs to consider when planning an aerobic exercise program for the patient with CF are (1) frequent rest periods interspersed throughout the exercise regimen, (2) meeting increased nutritional demands of exercise, (3) observing for manifestations of hyperthermia, and (4) drinking large amounts of fluid and replacing salt losses.

More than 95% of CF patients die of complications resulting from lung infection. Antimicrobial treatment is initiated for the treatment of infection. The use of antibiotics should be carefully guided by sputum culture results. Early intervention with antibiotics is useful, and long courses of antibiotics are the usual treatment. Prolonged high-dose therapy may be necessary because many drugs are abnormally metabolized and rapidly excreted in the patient with CF. Pharmacokinetic and kidney function studies therefore should be monitored closely. Oral agents commonly used are trimethoprim-sulfamethoxazole, tetracycline, chloramphenicol, cephalosporins, antistaphylococcal penicillins, and new oral quinolones, especially ciprofloxacin. Although oral and aerosolized antimicrobial therapy is usually adequate 20% to 80% of the time, some patients require a 2- to 4-week course of IV antimicrobial therapy. If home facilities are adequate, the CF patient and the family may choose to continue parenteral therapy at home. The usual treatment for acute infectious exacerbations is aminoglycosides, penicillin, or third-generation cephalosporins. Aerosolized bronchodilators and antiinflammatory agents (e.g., cromolyn) are used in selected patients, particularly before chest physical therapy (see Table 25-4). The patient with cor pulmonale or hypoxemia may require home O_2 therapy (O_2 therapy is discussed in Chapter 24). Sclerosing of the pleural space or partial pleural stripping and pleural abrasion performed surgically are usually indicated for recurrent episodes of pneumothorax.

CF has become a leading indication for either heart-lung or lung transplantation. (Lung transplants are discussed in Chapter 24.) Lung transplantations for the patient with CF have resulted in significant improvement of pulmonary function, with no recurrence of lung disease.

The management of pancreatic insufficiency includes pancreatic enzyme replacement (e.g., lipase, pancrease, Cotazym-S, and Creon) administered before each meal and snack. A high-calorie, high-protein diet and multivitamins are recommended. Fat restriction usually is not necessary. Fat-soluble vitamins (vitamins A, D, E, and K) need to be supplemented. Use of caloric supplements improves nutritional status. Added dietary salt is indicated whenever sweating is excessive, such as during hot weather, in the presence of fever, or from intense physical activity.

Table 25-16 Nursing Assessment: Patient with Cystic Fibrosis

Subjective Data

Important health information

Past health history: Allergic rhinitis, excessive sputum production

Medications: Use and discontinuance of steroids, bronchodilators, antibiotics, oxygen

Functional health patterns

Health perception–health management: Recurrent respiratory and sinus infections, family history of CF, fatigue

Nutritional-metabolic: Dietary intolerances, intestinal gas, voracious appetite

Activity-exercise: Decreased exercise tolerance; dyspnea, cough, excessive mucus or sputum production

Cognitive-perceptual: Abdominal pain

Objective Data

General

Anxiety, restlessness, salty breath, failure to thrive

Integumentary

Cyanosis (circumoral, nailbed), salty skin

Respiratory

Persistent runny nose, diminished breath sounds, sputum (thick, white, tenacious), increased work of breathing, use of accessory muscles of respiration, barrel chest

Gastrointestinal

Protuberant abdomen; abdominal distention; foul, fatty stools

Cardiovascular

Tachycardia, digital clubbing

Possible finding

Abnormal ABGs and pulmonary function tests; abnormal sweat chloride test, chest x-ray, fecal fat

ABGs, Arterial blood gases; CF, cystic fibrosis.

NURSING MANAGEMENT

CYSTIC FIBROSIS

Nursing Assessment

Subjective and objective data that should be obtained from the patient with cystic fibrosis are presented in Table 25-16.

Nursing Diagnoses

Nursing diagnoses related to CF may include, but are not limited to:

- Ineffective airway clearance related to abundant, thick bronchial mucus, weakness, and fatigue
- Ineffective breathing pattern related to bronchoconstriction, anxiety, airway obstruction
- Impaired gas exchange related to recurring lung infections
- Altered nutrition related to dietary intolerances, intestinal gas, and altered pancreatic enzyme production
- Altered growth and development related to physical, emotional, and social effects of a serious chronic illness

Planning

The overall goals are that the patient with CF will have (1) adequate airway clearance, (2) reduced risk factors associated with respiratory infections, (3) ability to perform ADL, (4) no complications related to CF, and (5) active participation in planning and implementing a therapeutic regimen.

Nursing Implementation

Health Promotion and Prevention. The nurse and other health professionals can assist young adults to gain independence by helping them assume responsibility for their care and for their vocational or school goals. A major problem that needs to be discussed is sexuality. Delayed or irregular menstruation is not uncommon. There may be delayed development of secondary sex characteristics such as breasts in girls or prolonged short stature in boys. The person may use the illness to avoid certain events or relationships. On the other hand, the healthy person hesitates to make friends with someone who is sick. Other crises and life transitions that must be dealt with in the young adult include building confidence and self-respect on the basis of achievements, persevering with employment goals, developing motivation to achieve, learning to cope with the treatment program, and adjusting to the need for dependence if health fails.

The issue of marrying and having children is difficult. Many men with CF are sterile. Women with the disease may have difficulty becoming pregnant. In addition, any children produced will either be a carrier of CF or have the disease. Another concern is the shortened life span of the parent with CF, and the parent's ability to care for the child

CRITICAL THINKING EXERCISES

CASE STUDY

ASTHMA

Patient Profile

Mrs. S, 30, comes to the ED with severe wheezing, dyspnea, and anxiety. She was in the ED only 6 hours ago with an acute asthma attack.

Subjective Data

- Treated in the ED previously with nebulized albuterol and responded quickly
- Can only speak one- to three-word sentences
- Is allergic to cigarette smoke
- Began to experience increased shortness of breath and tightness in her chest when she returned home
- Used albuterol MDI repeatedly at home without relief

Objective Data

Physical Examination

- Uses accessory muscles to breathe
- Has audible wheezing
- Respiratory rate 34/min
- Auscultation reveals no air movement in lower lobes
- HR: 126 bpm

Diagnostic Studies

ABGs: PaO_2 80 mm Hg
$PaCO_2$ 35 mm Hg
pH 7.46

PEFR: 150 L/min (personal best: 400 L/min)

Critical Thinking Questions

1. Why did Mrs. S. return to the ED? Explain the pathophysiology of this exacerbation of asthma.
2. What are the nursing care priorities for Mrs. S.?
3. What are the complications the nurse must be ready for based on her assessment?
4. What should be included in her discharge plan of care?
5. Based on the assessment data presented, write one or more nursing diagnoses. Are there any collaborative problems?

NURSING RESEARCH ISSUES

1. What effect does a planned exercise program have on respiratory function in the patient with COPD?
2. Can the use of relaxation techniques reduce dyspnea in the patient with asthma or COPD?
3. What types of breathing retraining techniques result in the greatest improvement in oxygenation?
4. What are the most common patient care problems with an adult who has CF?
5. What are the most effective nursing care measures to promote airway clearance?
6. What are the most effective measures to improve upper arm strength and endurance and reduce dyspnea in the patient with COPD?

must be taken into consideration. Genetic counseling may be an appropriate suggestion for the couple considering having children.

Acute Intervention. Acute intervention for the patient with CF includes relief of bronchoconstriction, airway obstruction, and airflow limitation. Interventions include aggressive CPT, antibiotics, oxygen therapy, and corticosteroids in severe disease. Good nutrition is important to support the immune system.

Chronic and Home Management. CPT is the mainstay of intervention for ineffective airway clearance in this population (see p. 713). Home management of cystic fibrosis includes an aggressive plan of postural drainage with percussion and vibration, aerosol-nebulization therapy, and breathing retraining. The patient is taught controlled coughing techniques, deep breathing exercises, and progressive exercise conditioning such as a bicycling program or arm ergometry.

The family and the person with CF have a great financial and emotional burden. The cost of drugs, special equipment, and continual care is often a great financial hardship. As CF patients are living to childbearing age, family planning and genetic counseling are important. The burden of living with a chronic disease at a young age can be emotionally overwhelming. Community resources are often available to help the family. In addition, the Cystic Fibrosis Foundation can be of assistance.

Regardless of how well the person is coping with living with the disease, a normal life span is not possible. As the person continues toward and into adulthood, the nurse and other skilled health professionals need to be available to help the patient and family cope with complications resulting from the disease and to prepare for dying.

REVIEW QUESTIONS

The number of the question corresponds to the same-numbered objective at the beginning of the chapter.

1. Asthma is best characterized as
   a. an obstructive disease with loss of alveolar walls.
   b. an inflammatory disease.
   c. a steady progression of bronchoconstriction.
   d. a chronic obstructive disorder characterized by mucus production.

2. The teaching plan for the asthmatic patient includes all of the following *except*
   a. preventing or limiting exposure of the patient to allergens.
   b. isolating the patient to prevent respiratory infections.
   c. correct use of MDI.
   d. deep-breathing and coughing exercises to clear the airway.

3. A plan of care for the patient with COPD would include all of the following *except*
   a. annual influenza vaccine.
   b. chronic steroid therapy.
   c. reduction of risk factors for infection.
   d. alterations in ADLs.

4. Which of the following effects does cigarette smoking have on the respiratory system?
   a. Hyperplasia of goblet cells and increased production of mucus
   b. Increased proliferation of ciliated cells
   c. Hypertrophy of the alveolar membrane
   d. Destruction of all alveolar macrophages

5. One of the most important things a nurse can teach a patient with emphysema is to
   a. obtain adequate rest in the supine position.
   b. move to a hot, dry climate.
   c. know the early signs of infection.
   d. perform CPT.

6. Diagnostic studies that would probably be abnormal in a person with CF are
   a. pancreatic enzymes and hormones.
   b. pulmonary function study and sweat test.
   c. sweat test and vitamin B tolerance test.
   d. insulin tolerance and blood sugars.

REFERENCES

1. National Institute of Health: *Guidelines for the diagnosis and management of asthma,* MD, 1991, Publication No. 91-3042, US Department of Health and Human Services.
2. *ALA memo, update details XIII,* New York, 1990, American Lung Association.
3. Allen and Hansburys Respiratory Institute: Asthma not adequately treated in United States, *Air Currents* 4:1, 1993.
4. Bone RC: Bronchial asthma: diagnostic and treatment issues. *Hosp Pract* 28:45, 1993.
5. Weiss KB and others: Changing patterns of asthma mortality: identifying target populations at high risk, *JAMA* 264:1683, 1990.
6. Bjerklie SJ: Status asthmaticus, *Am J Nurs* 90:52, 1990.
7. Barnes PJ: A new approach to the treatment of asthma, *New Engl J Med* 321:1517, 1989.
8. Kelly HW: Long-term management of asthma, *J Pharm Prac* 5:167, 1992.
9. Rodman M: Over-the-counter interactions: asthma medications, *RN* 56:40, 1993.
10. Snider GL: Chronic obstructive pulmonary disease: risk factors, pathophysiology and pathogenesis, *Annu Rev Med* 40:411, 1989.
11. Jess LW: Chronic bronchitis and emphysema airing the differences, *Nursing* 22:34, 1992.
12. Feinleib M and others: Trends in COPD morbidity and mortality in the United States, *Am Rev Respir Dis* 140:S9, 1989.
13. Cancer facts and figures—1994, American Cancer Society.
14. Buist AS: Alpha-1-antitrypsin deficiency in lung and liver disease, *Hosp Pract* 24:51, 1989.
15. American Thoracic Society: Guidelines for the approach to the patient with severe hereditary alpha-1-antitrypsin deficiency, *Am Rev Respir Dis* 140:1491, 1989.
16. Gail DB, Lenfant C: The aging respiratory system. In Evans JG, Williams TF, editors: *Oxford textbook of geriatric medicine,* New York, 1992, Oxford Univ Press.
17. Pierson DJ: Effects of aging on the respiratory system. In Pierson DJ, Kacmarek RM, editors: *Foundations of respiratory care,* New York, 1992, Churchill Livingstone.
18. Petty TL, Raff MJ: Controlling bronchitis flare-ups in COPD, *Patient Care* 25:81, 1991.
19. Petty TL: Home oxygen—a revolution in the care of advanced COPD, *Med Clin North Am* 74:715, 1990.

*20. Weaver TE, Narsavage GL: Physiological and psychological variables related to functional status in chronic obstructive pulmonary disease, *Nurs Res* 41:286, 1992.

21. Ferguson GT, Cherniack RM: Management of chronic obstructive pulmonary disease, *New Engl J Med* 328:1017, 1993.
22. American Association of Respiratory Care: AARC clinical practice guidelines, *Respir Care* 36:1418, 1991.

*23. Breslin EH: Dyspnea-limited response in chronic obstructive pulmonary disease: reduced unsupported arm activities, *Rehabil Nurs* 17:12, 1992.

24. Davis PB: Cystic fibrosis: new perceptions, new strategies, *Hosp Pract* 27:79, 1992.

*Nursing research-based articles.

Chapter 26

NURSING ROLE IN MANAGEMENT

Respiratory Failure

Trisch Van Sciver

Learning Objectives

1. Describe the types, mechanisms, etiology, and clinical manifestations of acute respiratory failure.
2. Describe the therapeutic and nursing management of the patient in acute respiratory failure.
3. Describe the etiology, pathophysiology, and clinical manifestations of acute respiratory distress syndrome.
4. Explain the therapeutic and nursing management of the patient with acute respiratory distress syndrome.

ACUTE RESPIRATORY FAILURE

Acute respiratory failure is present when alveolar ventilation is inadequate to meet the body's needs. The lungs can no longer adequately oxygenate the blood. Although no universal definition exists, the most common definition of acute respiratory failure is an arterial oxygen pressure (PaO_2) of less than 50 mm Hg and/or an arterial carbon dioxide pressure ($PaCO_2$) of more than 50 mm Hg measured at rest on room air at sea level. Other manifestations of acute respiratory failure are acute dyspnea, significant respiratory acidemia (pH $<$7.3), or both. In most patients at least two of these criteria are present.

Acute respiratory failure in a patient with chronic restrictive or obstructive lung disease cannot be defined according to the criteria used for the patient with normal lungs. The patient with chronic pulmonary diseases is able to tolerate and compensate for a significant degree of hypoxemia and/or hypercapnia. Commonly, the stable, ambulatory patient with chronic pulmonary disease maintains PaO_2 levels of 60 mm Hg or lower and/or $PaCO_2$ levels of 50 mm Hg or higher with a normal pH. In chronic lung disease, acute respiratory failure can be defined as alveolar ventilation inadequate to oxygenate the blood sufficiently, as evidenced by an acute decrease in PaO_2 and/or increase in $PaCO_2$ from the patient's baseline parameters, accompanied by an acid pH.

Risk Factors

The critically ill patient is at risk for respiratory distress and/or acute respiratory failure. This patient already has sustained significant injury to one or more body systems. Because there are so many functional systemic interrelationships in the body, disequilibrium in one body system frequently leads to disequilibrium in other systems.

The patient who has undergone recent abdominal or thoracic surgery is at risk for respiratory failure as a result of splinting of the incision, abdominal distention, restrictive bandages, tubes, and reduced ventilation because of pain. The extremely obese patient also may be at an increased risk of respiratory failure because of the restriction of ventilation. The comatose patient or patient with decreased level of consciousness and depression of the respiratory center (e.g., after anesthesia, narcotic use, head injury, or cerebral vascular accident [CVA]) is prone to aspiration pneumonia and respiratory failure. The patient who has sustained a thoracic or spinal cord injury is predisposed to ineffective ventilation. Because of a loss of normal respiratory or protective mechanisms and decreased ventilatory reserve, the patient who has lung disease or who smokes heavily is at risk for acute respiratory failure, especially when an infection develops or surgery is needed. The immunosuppressed patient is also prone to acute respiratory failure for similar reasons. Finally, the older adult is also at risk for acute respiratory failure because of the reduction in ventilatory capacity that accompanies aging, especially when other risk factors are present.

Prevention and Early Detection

Measures to help prevent respiratory failure include preoperative screening and evaluation of all high-risk patients. Pulmonary function tests should be performed and arterial blood gas (ABG) levels assessed preoperatively in the high-risk patient to determine the operative risk and to establish baseline parameters for postoperative care. Measures to optimize ventilation such as bronchodilators, incen-

Reviewed by Janet Crimlisk, MS, CS, RN, Pulmonary Clinical Nurse Specialist, Department of Health and Hospitals, Boston City Hospital, Boston, MA.

GLOSSARY OF ABBREVIATIONS

ABGs	Arterial blood gases
D (A–a) O_2	Alveolar to arterial O_2 difference
FIO_2	Fraction of inspired O_2
PaO_2	Partial pressure of oxygen in arterial blood
P_AO_2	Partial pressure of oxygen in alveoli
$PaCO_2$	Partial pressure of carbon dioxide in arterial blood
P_ACO_2	Partial pressure of carbon dioxide in alveoli
$P\bar{v}O_2$	Partial pressure of oxygen in mixed venous blood
PEFR	Peak expiratory flow rate (maximum airflow during a forced expiration)
$\dot{Q}_S/\dot{Q}_T$	Shunt fraction (relationship of unoxygenated blood to total blood volume)
SaO_2	Oxygen saturation in blood as measured by arterial blood gas analysis
SpO_2	Oxygen saturation in blood as measured by pulse oximetry
$S\bar{v}O_2$	Mixed venous oxygen saturation
$\dot{V}/\dot{Q}$	Ventilation-perfusion ratio (relationship of ventilation to perfusion in the lungs)
V_D	Anatomic dead space
V_E	Minute ventilation – product of V_T × respiratory rate
V_T	Tidal volume

tive spirometry, and coughing and deep-breathing techniques are important to prepare the patient for surgery. Preoperative teaching is essential, especially for the patient having thoracic or abdominal surgery, because of the higher incidence of postoperative complications for this patient. Cessation of smoking, even 24 hours before surgery, improves mucociliary function, mucus clearance, and oxygenation as a result of decreased carbon monoxide (CO) levels. Early postoperative ambulation and sitting in an upright position beginning on the first postoperative day for at least several times each day are important.

Frequent monitoring of the respiratory status of the critically ill patient is imperative. ABG analysis is often an initial part of the work-up during admission to the intensive care unit (ICU). Astute observation and measurement of the patient's respiratory status assist in early detection of respiratory problems. These measurements include the respiratory rate, pattern, and depth; frequent assessment of breath sounds; vital signs and level of consciousness; pulse oximetry; peak expiratory flow rates (PEFR) (if indicated); and/or ABGs. Subjective patient evaluation is also important. Early recognition of the clinical symptoms of respiratory distress and immediate implementation of corrective measures may prevent further deterioration and failure of the patient's respiratory mechanisms.

Pathophysiology

Respiratory failure can be divided into two categories. *Type I,* or *hypoxemic respiratory failure,* occurs when there is a low PaO_2 and a normal or low $PaCO_2$. *Type II,* or *hypercapnic respiratory failure,* occurs when there is a low PaO_2 with an elevated $PaCO_2$.

Table 26-1 Classification and Mechanisms of Acute Respiratory Failure

Type I (Hypoxemic) Respiratory Failure
- Ventilation-perfusion mismatch
- Shunting
- Diffusion abnormalities
- Alveolar hypoventilation

Type II (Hypercapnic) Respiratory Failure
- Alveolar hypoventilation
- Ventilation-perfusion mismatch

Table 26-2 Causes of Type I (Hypoxemic) Respiratory Failure*

Pneumonia	Collagen diseases of lung
Asthma	Sarcoidosis
Chronic and acute bronchitis	Asbestosis
Emphysema	Acute respiratory distress syndrome
Pulmonary embolus	Sepsis
Cystic fibrosis	Interstitial lung disease
Pulmonary edema	

*This list is not inclusive.

Mechanisms of Type I (Hypoxemic) Respiratory Failure. *Severe hypoxemia,* or *low O_2 tension,* in the arterial blood (PaO_2 <50 to 60 mm Hg), can contribute to the development of hypoxia or lack of tissue O_2 and acute respiratory failure. Arterial O_2 levels are not solely responsible for effective tissue oxygenation. The hemoglobin (Hb) level, Hb O_2-carrying capacity, cardiac output, and distribution of blood flow to the tissues are all involved in the delivery of O_2 to the tissues and thus determine the state of tissue oxygenation.

Mechanisms that may cause hypoxemia and subsequent acute hypoxemic respiratory failure are (1) ventilation-perfusion ($\dot{V}/\dot{Q}$) mismatch, (2) shunts, (3) diffusion abnormalities, and (4) alveolar hypoventilation (Table 26-1). Type I respiratory failure typically involves a disease process in the lung itself. Clinical causes of type I respiratory failure are listed in Table 26-2. A common cause is acute lung injury or acute respiratory distress syndrome (ARDS).

Ventilation-perfusion mismatch. Altered ($\dot{V}/\dot{Q}$) relationships in the lungs, or $\dot{V}/\dot{Q}$ mismatch, is the most common

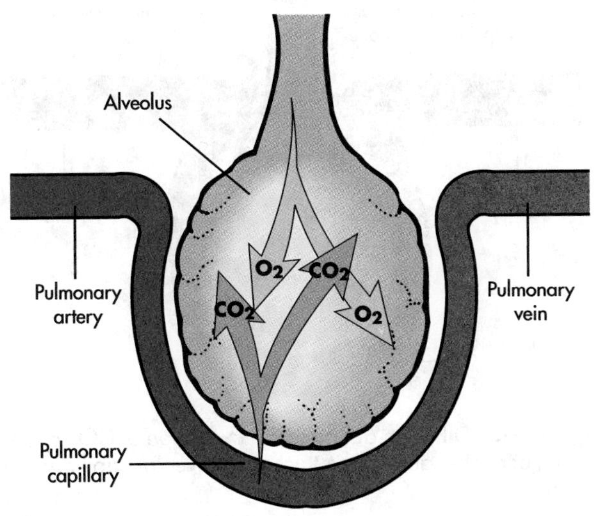

Fig. 26-1 Normal gas exchange unit in the lung.

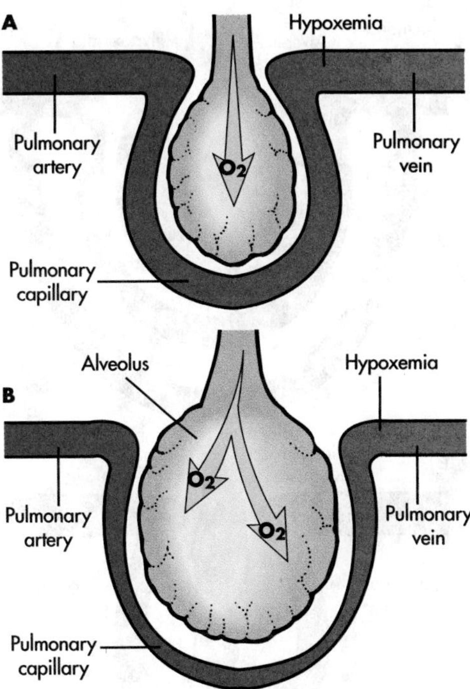

Fig. 26-2 Gas exchange unit illustrating $\dot{V}/\dot{Q}$ mismatch. ***A,*** $\dot{V}/\dot{Q}$ mismatch with decreased ventilation and normal perfusion. Note the limited ventilation. ***B,*** $\dot{V}/\dot{Q}$ mismatch with normal ventilation and decreased perfusion. Note the narrowing of the blood vessel.

cause of hypoxemia. The $\dot{V}/\dot{Q}$ relationship means that where there is ventilation in the lung, there must be matching blood perfusion to that area for efficient gas exchange to occur (Fig. 26-1). In the normal lung the overall $\dot{V}/\dot{Q}$ ratio is 0.8. Normal resting alveolar ventilation is approximately 4 L per minute and cardiac output is approximately 5 L per minute in an adult with a resultant $\dot{V}/\dot{Q}$ of 4:5, or 0.8. An alteration or mismatch occurs if there is blood flow to areas of decreased or absent ventilation, or if there is ventilation to areas of decreased or absent blood flow (Fig. 26-2). Changes in thoracic resistance and compliance also can affect $\dot{V}/\dot{Q}$ ratio in the lungs.

Examples of processes that cause $\dot{V}/\dot{Q}$ mismatch are pneumonia, atelectasis, chronic and acute bronchitis, severe emphysema, asthma, and pulmonary embolism. In pulmonary embolism, ventilation is sustained in an area that is not perfused. In some processes, there is sustained perfusion of poorly ventilated zones of the lung.

Shunts. Shunting is also a cause of hypoxemia (Fig. 26-3). A shunt occurs when blood enters the arterial system from the venous system without being exposed to ventilated areas of the lung. Essentially, the blood is shunted from the right to the left side of the heart without participating in gas exchange. Blood that has a PaO_2 similar to venous blood is then mixed with arterial blood as it enters the left atrium of the heart.

A shunt can be viewed as an extreme $\dot{V}/\dot{Q}$ imbalance. The most common shunts are extrapulmonary and include those that occur in congenital heart disease through atrial or septal defects or a patent ductus arteriosus. These represent an anatomic shunt of blood from the right to the left side of the heart, bypassing gas exchange in the lung. Shunting can occur in situations in which the blood perfuses large areas of nonventilated or underventilated alveoli (as in consolidated pneumonia) or the blood bypasses alveoli (as in pulmonary emboli).

Intrapulmonary anatomic shunts are associated with arteriovenous fistulas in congenital defects. Anatomic-like or intrapulmonary shunts develop when there is obstruction to the flow of gas to lobes or segments of the lung, as in pneumonia with consolidation.

The classic difference between $\dot{V}/\dot{Q}$ mismatch and anatomic-like shunts is demonstrated by having the patient breathe 100% O_2 for 15 to 20 minutes. The patient with $\dot{V}/\dot{Q}$ mismatch will increase the PaO_2 to more than 400 mm Hg, whereas the patient with a shunt cannot increase the PaO_2 despite receiving high concentrations of O_2. In $\dot{V}/\dot{Q}$ mismatch, the increased fraction of inspired O_2 (FIO_2) delivered to poorly or intermittently ventilated areas provides enough O_2 to correct the ventilation problem, increasing the PaO_2 and saturating the Hb. In a patient with shunting, however, the increased FIO_2 does not correct the oxygenation problem because mixed venous blood continues to flow through the shunted area. The poorly oxygenated blood from the shunt area mixes with blood that has perfused normal alveoli and lowers the PaO_2 of the blood, resulting in a minimal or no increase in PaO_2.

Diffusion abnormalities. Diffusion abnormalities are also a cause of hypoxemia. These abnormalities indicate an impairment in the equilibration between the O_2 pressure in the alveoli (P_AO_2) and in the pulmonary capillaries (Fig. 26-4). Diffusion does not occur normally for the following reasons:

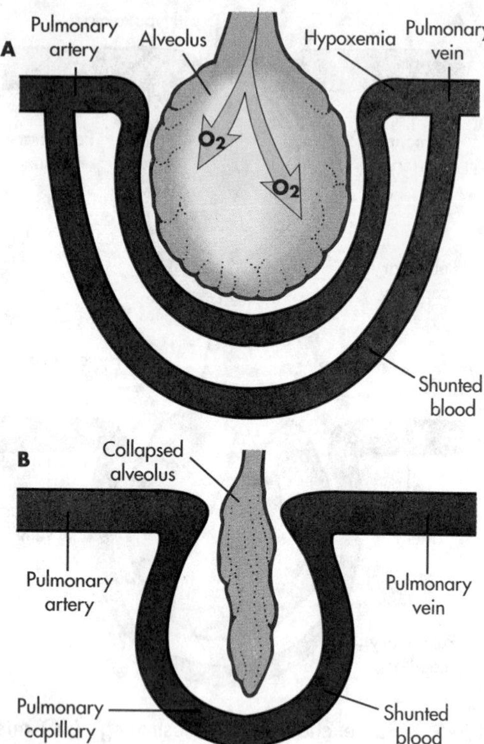

Fig. 26-3 Two types of shunts. ***A,*** Anatomic shunt. The vessel that receives no ventilation has shunted blood mixing with oxygenated blood. ***B,*** Anatomic-like shunt. Perfusion continues in the absence of ventilation, and blood cannot be oxygenated.

1. The contact time for the red blood cells (RBCs) at the capillary membrane is decreased (e.g., intense physical exercise increases blood flow and thus decreases contact time).
2. Pulmonary capillary blood is reduced as a result of obstruction or destruction of vessels (e.g., large bullae cause vascular obstruction in severe emphysema).
3. The blood-gas membrane is thickened (e.g., in fibrosis, pulmonary edema).

A combination of these effects also may occur. Hypoxemia caused by diffusion impairment can be corrected by the administration of 100% O_2. The rate of movement of O_2 across the alveolar-capillary membrane is proportional to the difference in pressures between the alveolar gas and capillary blood. As FIO_2 in the alveoli increases, PAO_2 increases and O_2 transfer across the alveolar-capillary membrane occurs.

Severe diffusion problems must be present to cause a clinical decrease in the PAO_2. Hypercapnia usually is not present because CO_2 diffuses 20 times more easily than O_2 across the respiratory membrane. Diseases in which a diffusion abnormality may contribute to hypoxemia include diffuse interstitial fibrosis, collagen-vascular disease of the lung (e.g., scleroderma, systemic lupus erythematosus), asbestosis, sarcoidosis, interstitial pneumonia, and cardiogenic pulmonary edema). Patients usually have concurrent $\dot{V}/\dot{Q}$ abnormalities or shunt problems.

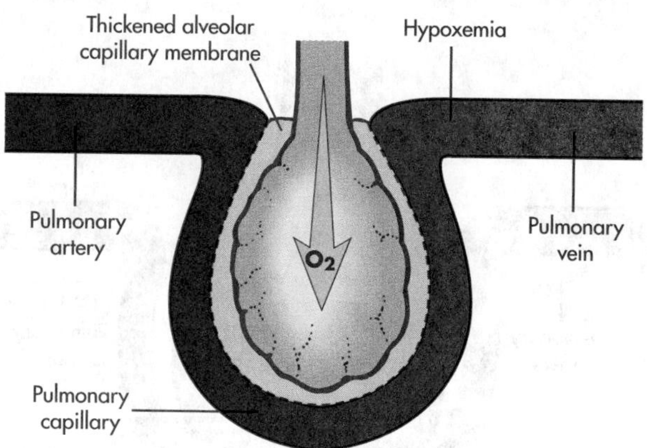

Fig. 26-4 Diffusion abnormality. Exchange of CO_2 and O_2 cannot occur because of the thickened alveolar-capillary membrane.

Alveolar hypoventilation. Alveolar hypoventilation ($PaCO_2$ >50 mm Hg) is a generalized decrease in ventilation of the lungs with a buildup of CO_2 in the blood. Hypoventilation is commonly the result of diseases outside of the lungs (e.g., sleep apnea, neuromuscular diseases). Although alveolar hypoventilation is primarily a mechanism of type II respiratory failure, it is mentioned here because it can cause hypoxemia.

Interrelationship of mechanisms. Hypoxemic respiratory failure frequently is caused by a combination of $\dot{V}/\dot{Q}$ mismatch, shunting, diffusion abnormalities, and hypoventilation. The patient with acute respiratory failure secondary to acute pneumonia has a $\dot{V}/\dot{Q}$ imbalance because the inflammation, edema, and hypersecretion of exudate within the bronchioles and terminal respiratory units obstruct airways and impair ventilation in the alveoli. Hypoventilation can result from pain from pleuritic inflammation and subsequent shallow breathing. Interstitial edema caused by secretion and fluid accumulation can cause diffusion abnormalities. Consolidation of lung lobules as a result of secretion accumulation and alveolar collapse can cause shuntlike effects.

Pathophysiologic Effects of Hypoxemia. *Hypoxia* (decreased oxygenation of the tissues) occurs when the amount of O_2 in the blood is not adequate to support aerobic metabolism. Aerobic metabolism provides the energy for cellular activities in which O_2 is used. CO_2 is the waste product of aerobic metabolism. When O_2 insufficiency persists, the cells must shift from aerobic to anaerobic metabolism. Anaerobic metabolism uses more fuel and produces less energy and is less efficient than aerobic metabolism. The waste product of anaerobic metabolism, lactic acid, is more difficult than CO_2 to remove from the body because it has to be buffered with sodium bicarbonate. When the body does not have adequate amounts of sodium bicarbonate to buffer the lactic acid produced by anaerobic metabolism, metabolic acidosis and cell death occur.

Hypoxemia and metabolic acidosis have adverse effects on the vital organs, especially the heart and central nervous system (CNS). Permanent brain damage may occur because of the depressant effect on the brain. The heart tries to compensate for the decreased O_2 level in the blood by increasing heart rate and cardiac output. As oxygenation decreases and acidosis increases, however, the heart muscle is unable to function and a slowing and eventual cessation of cardiac activity occurs, resulting in systemic shock. Renal function is also impaired, and sodium retention, proteinuria, edema formation, tubular necrosis, and uremia may occur. Gastrointestinal (GI) system alterations include abnormal liver function, abdominal pain, and bowel infarction.

Mechanisms of Type II (Hypercapnic) Respiratory Failure. Mechanisms that cause type II (hypercapnic) respiratory failure are alveolar hypoventilation and ventilation-perfusion mismatch (see Table 26-1). Clinical causes of Type II respiratory failure are listed in Table 26-3.

Alveolar hypoventilation. Alveolar ventilation is the volume of gas per breath that is available for gas exchange in functioning alveoli. When an adult takes a normal breath (tidal volume or V_T) of 500 ml, approximately 150 ml of this gas never reaches the alveoli to be involved in gas exchange. This 150 ml is called the *anatomic dead space* (V_D) and is about one-third of V_T or approximately equal in number to a person's weight in pounds (a 150-pound person has approximately 150 ml of V_D). The remaining 350 ml is the gas available for alveolar ventilation per breath.

Adequate alveolar ventilation is necessary to exchange O_2 for CO_2 in the alveoli. The $PaCO_2$ is directly related to the amount of CO_2 produced metabolically and inversely related to the effective alveolar ventilation. Therefore increased $PaCO_2$ indicates decreased alveolar ventilation (hypoventilation) and decreased $PaCO_2$ indicates increased alveolar ventilation (hyperventilation). For the $PaCO_2$ to remain constant, alveolar ventilation must increase or decrease in proportion to the CO_2 produced metabolically.

Alveolar hypoventilation occurs when effective ventilation of the alveoli is no longer adequate for the body's metabolic rate. Less O_2 is supplied and less CO_2 is removed. Consequently, alveolar and arterial CO_2 levels increase and O_2 levels decrease. Alveolar hypoventilation is commonly caused by diseases outside the lungs, and often the lungs are normal.

Ventilation-perfusion mismatch. In addition to causing a decreased PaO_2, an elevated $PaCO_2$ may develop in $\dot{V}/\dot{Q}$ mismatch. This may occur in a patient who has an increased work of breathing, most likely secondary to a large increase in airway resistance. Increased airway resistance is likened to breathing through a narrow tube. This condition occurs in severe bronchospasm, although fluid and secretions in the airways could produce similar results. Because the patient does not have the energy or ability to overcome this increased resistance, ventilation decreases and $PaCO_2$ increases.

PATHOPHYSIOLOGIC EFFECTS OF HYPERCAPNIA. The main physiologic feature of hypoventilation is *hypercapnia* (elevated $PaCO_2$ greater than 50 mm Hg). This occurs because ventilation is inadequate to remove the CO_2 produced by cellular metabolism. A subsequent physiologic effect of increased $PaCO_2$ is a decrease in PaO_2. As the level of CO_2 increases in the blood ($PaCO_2$), the level of CO_2 in the alveoli also increases. Less space is left in the alveoli for O_2. This results in a decrease in PaO_2 that is proportional to the rise in $PaCO_2$.

Another physiologic effect of hypercapnia is increased $PaCO_2$ is decreased pH. Respiratory acidosis results as CO_2 accumulates in the plasma ($CO_2 + H_2O \rightleftarrows H_2CO_3 \rightleftarrows H^+ + HCO_3^-$). A significant increase in plasma bicarbonate does not occur in acute hypercapnia because it takes the kidney 48 to 72 hours to retain enough bicarbonate to compensate for the acidemia. In contrast, in chronic hypercapnia the plasma bicarbonate is elevated and thus arterial pH is within the normal range. In chronic hypercapnia, metabolic alkalosis compensates for the respiratory acidosis.

Another physiologic effect of hypercapnia is the *chloride shift.* A low serum chloride level occurs in acute respiratory failure. The mechanism for this is as follows: As bicarbonate ions (HCO_3^-) move from the cells to the plasma to buffer the H_2CO_3, the chloride ions move into the cell to maintain electroneutrality. As the CO_2 accumulates, and with it hydrogen ions (H^+), the serum becomes more acidic. H^+ enters the cells and potassium ions (K^+) move out of cells to the plasma in an attempt to achieve electroneutrality. Initially, serum K^+ may be increased, but as the acidemia becomes prolonged or more pronounced, total body K^+ (both intracellular and extracellular) is depleted as the excess extracellular K^+ is excreted by the kidneys. Thus the patient can demonstrate both hypokalemia and hypochloremia as a result of respiratory failure.

Hypoxemia alone can cause vasoconstriction of the pulmonary circulation, resulting in pulmonary hypertension and shunting of blood away from the alveoli. Respiratory acidemia seems to potentiate this effect. Therefore as CO_2

Table 26-3 Causes of Type II (Hypercapnic) Respiratory Failure*

- Sedative and narcotic overdosage
- Postoperative anesthetic depression
- Excessive O_2 tensions (especially in the presence of chronic hypercapnia)
- Sleep apnea
- Neuromuscular diseases
  - Guillain-Barré syndrome
  - Myasthenia gravis
  - Bulbar poliomyelitis
  - Multiple sclerosis
  - Amyotrophic lateral sclerosis
- Spinal cord trauma
- Muscular dystrophy
- Severe chronic obstructive pulmonary disease
- Severe asthma
- Bronchiectasis
- Severe kyphoscoliosis
- Cystic fibrosis
- Chest trauma
- Upper airway obstruction

*This list is not inclusive.

Table 26-4 Clinical Manifestations of Acute Respiratory Failure

	Hypoxemia	Hypercapnia
Manifestations	Restlessness, agitation, disorientation, confusion, delirium, loss of consciousness, dyspnea	Headache, somnolence, dizziness, coma
Findings	Cardiac dysrhythmias; tachycardia; hypertension; tachypnea; cyanosis (may not be present until hypoxemia is severe); pale, cool, clammy skin	Hypertension; tachycardia; asterixis; warm, flushed skin; diaphoresis; bounding pulse; papilledema; decreased deep tendon reflexes

rises, with the subsequent development of acidosis, the elevation of the pulmonary artery pressure increases relative to the level of hypoxemia.

Clinical Manifestations

Clinical manifestations of respiratory failure are related either to the increase in $PaCO_2$ and/or to the decrease in PaO_2 (Table 26-4). The onset of symptoms is related to the rate of buildup of CO_2, the decrease of O_2, and the ability of the patient's compensatory mechanisms to overcome these changes. When the patient's compensatory mechanisms fail to facilitate removal of CO_2 and conserve O_2, symptoms of tissue hypoxia and/or hypercapnia in the vital organs appear. The patient may have rapid, shallow respirations because the lungs contain fluid and are noncompliant and stiff. The patient may increase the respiratory rate in an effort to blow off accumulated CO_2. As CO_2 continues to increase, a slower respiratory rate may indicate that the patient is no longer able to eliminate accumulated CO_2.

Acceptable ABG values may be present, but the patient may be working extremely hard to attain them. Accessory muscles may be used during inspiration and expiration. During normal tidal breathing, the diaphragm moves about 3 to 5 cm. With forced inspiration or expiration, however, diaphragmatic excursion may be as much as 10 cm. Accessory muscles of inspiration include the scalene muscles, which elevate the first two ribs, and the sternocleidomastoids, which raise the sternum. Small muscles of the neck, head, and face play a minor role as accessory inspiratory muscles. Normally, expiration is passive. When expiration becomes active during distress or increased exercise, the abdominal muscles and internal intercostals are used. Intercostal and supraclavicular retractions are indications that these muscles are being used to aid in ventilation.

The patient with advanced chronic obstructive pulmonary disease (COPD) and inspiratory muscle fatigue may exhibit asynchronous respirations. Normally, the thorax and abdomen move synchronously outward on inspiration and inward on exhalation. During asynchronous breathing an outward movement of the abdomen occurs during exhalation and an inward movement occurs during inspiration. Asynchronous breathing probably results from inefficient diaphragm position and maximal use of accessory muscles of respiration.

The length of inspiration compared with that of expiration (I/E ratio), which is normally 1:1.5, may be decreased (e.g., 1:5). The expiratory time is usually prolonged in airway obstruction. The pattern of respiratory response to activity may be altered. The patient may use few accessory muscles at rest, but may activate more muscle groups with increased activity.

The position that the patient assumes is also a clue to the effort associated with breathing. The patient may prefer to sit straight up or lean forward, resting on the elbows, or to lie partially on one side or the other depending on the location of the pulmonary disease. Asymmetric chest expansion may occur from splinting an incision or trauma site, pleural effusion, pneumothorax, or a paralyzed hemidiaphragm. Pursed-lip or open-mouth breathing may be used. The patient who is working hard to breathe may become extremely diaphoretic and may be able to speak only two or three words at a time between breaths.

Because of the increased work of breathing, wide swings in intrathoracic pressure may occur during inspiration and expiration. Thus the nurse may be able to detect a pulsus paradoxus of greater than 10 mm Hg during inspiration. (The physiology of pulsus paradoxus is described in Chapter 34.) The degree of paradox can aid in assessing the degree of respiratory distress. A paradox of as much as 50 mm Hg can be present in severe respiratory distress. Improvement in paradox usually correlates with clinical improvement. However, in severe respiratory distress an exhausted patient is not able to generate enough respiratory effort to produce intrathoracic pressure changes of the magnitude necessary for a paradox to occur.

In mild hypoxemia at sea level (PaO_2 <80 mm Hg) the sympathetic nervous system is stimulated, producing an increased heart rate and cardiac output. Peripheral vasoconstriction also occurs to shunt blood to vital organs and to increase blood pressure (BP). The skin may become pale, cool, and clammy. In pure hypercapnic ventilatory failure, vasodilatation occurs. Thus the patient may have warm, flushed skin and a bounding pulse.

Clinical manifestations of hypoxemia related to the cardiovascular system include tachycardia, mild hypertension (partly from the release of catecholamines), increased cardiac output, cardiac dysrhythmias, and potentially deleterious effects on cardiac function with subsequent heart failure. These manifestations are especially evident in the presence of coronary artery disease and pulmonary hypertension (secondary to alveolar hypoxia) and are further aggravated by respiratory acidosis (if present). With severe, prolonged hypoxemia, bradycardia and hypotension may result.

CNS alterations may occur as a result of the combination of hypoxemia, increased $PaCO_2$, and acidemia. The patient may complain of a headache because increased $PaCO_2$ causes vasodilatation of cerebral blood vessels and increased cerebral blood flow. Cerebrospinal pressure may be elevated and the patient may exhibit drowsiness, confusion, papilledema, slurred speech, restlessness, fluctuations of mood, tremors, convulsions, coma, decreased deep tendon reflexes, and *asterixis* (flapping tremor). Tachycardia and hypertension also may be present.

Cyanosis may occur as the level of PaO_2 decreases; however, this is a very late sign of hypoxemia. Cyanosis occurs when there is at least 5 g/dl (50 g/L) of reduced or unoxygenated Hb in capillary blood. The skin of the lips, ear lobes, nailbeds, and oral mucous membranes in adults often are assessed for peripheral cyanosis. Alterations in local capillary blood flow are responsible for peripheral cyanosis. Central cyanosis is usually observed in the tongue and sublingual region. In dark-skinned individuals the tongue is the best site to observe for cyanosis.[1]

Cyanosis may not occur in the anemic patient despite decreased PaO_2 because Hb is decreased. In contrast, a patient with polycythemia may appear cyanotic even though the O_2 content is normal (e.g., "blue bloater" COPD patient with chronic bronchitis). Cyanosis by itself is not a reliable indicator of oxygenation status; it must be evaluated together with other clinical parameters.

The patient with COPD may be able to tolerate a significant degree of hypoxemia and hypercapnia. Clinical signs of hypercapnia (e.g., tachycardia, papilledema, decreased deep tendon reflexes, confusion) may be apparent if the CO_2 retention is of rapid onset. If chronic hypercapnia has been a feature of the patient's disease, these clinical signs are often absent or subtle. Only when the condition progresses to lethargy and coma may the diagnosis of respiratory failure be clinically obvious. For this reason it is important to closely observe the patient with COPD for subtle changes in respiratory pattern and mental status.

Diagnostic Studies

Evaluation of Oxygenation (Table 26-5)

Arterial blood gases. The most specific diagnostic study used to determine respiratory failure is ABGs. If the patient is critically ill, an indwelling catheter may be inserted into an artery for monitoring pressures. This arterial line can be used to obtain frequent arterial blood gases.

The PaO_2 and O_2 saturations are useful in assessing oxygenation. The desirable range for PaO_2 is usually 60 to 80 mm Hg in the critically ill patient; this range usually provides an arterial saturation of at least 90%. For a review of ABG interpretations see Table 22-1. These levels are monitored as indicated by the patient's respiratory status to detect changes, trends, and response to therapy. Pulse oximetry is frequently used for monitoring of oxygenation status, but in respiratory failure, ABGs are necessary to obtain both oxygenation (PaO_2) and ventilation ($PaCO_2$) status.

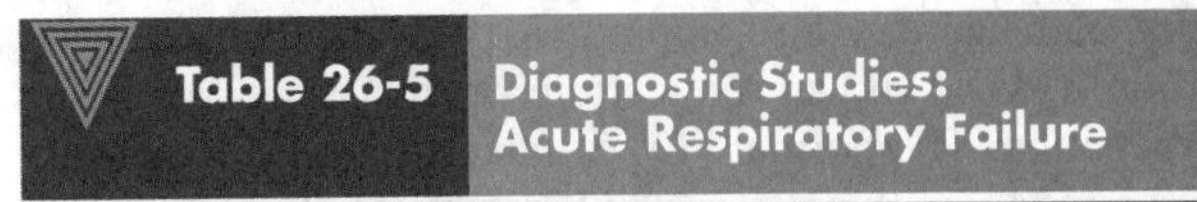
Table 26-5 Diagnostic Studies: Acute Respiratory Failure

Evaluation of Oxygenation
- Arterial blood gas analysis (PaO_2, O_2 saturation)
- Pulse oximetry (SpO_2)
- Mixed venous oxygen ($P\bar{v}O_2$)
- Shunt equation ($\dot{Q}_S/\dot{Q}_T$)
- Alveolar-arterial oxygen difference $D(A\text{-}a)O_2$
- Arterial-alveolar ratio (a/A gradient or PaO_2/PAO_2 ratio)
- Hypoxemia score (PaO_2/FIO_2 ratio)

Evaluation of Ventilation
- Arterial blood gas analysis ($PaCO_2$)
- Capnography ($PetCO_2$)
- Tidal volume (V_T)
- Forced vital capacity (FVC)
- Minute ventilation or volume (V_E)
- Negative inspiratory force (NIF) or maximum inspiratory pressure (MIP)
- Physiologic dead space (V_D/V_T ratio)

Pulse oximetry. Pulse oximetry is used frequently to monitor O_2 saturation. (Oxygen saturation obtained by pulse oximetry may be abbreviated as SpO_2.) The pulse oximeter works by electronically measuring the optical density of light absorbed by the arterial blood. The oxisensor is placed on the finger, toe, nose, or ear. A beam of light passes through the tissue and measures oxyhemoglobin as a percentage of total hemoglobin. The SpO_2 and heart rate are displayed on the monitor. Accurate oxygen saturation measurement depends on accurate probe fit and adequate tissue perfusion. Falsely low oximetry readings may occur with decreased cardiac output, low BP, peripheral vasoconstriction, dark nail polish, deeply pigmented skin, high bilirubin levels, and motion artifact. Falsely high values occur in CO poisoning and dyshemoglobinemias. Backscatter from high intensity ambient light (sunlight, surgical lamps) and electrical interference also can cause inaccuracies.[2] To assure accurate SpO_2 readings, the patient's pulse can be checked and compared to the oximeter's reading.

The pulse oximeter is relatively accurate at arterial O_2 saturation (SaO_2) levels of 80% to 100%. Below the 80% level it is less accurate, but is still clinically useful. When the PaO_2 is approximately 60 mm Hg, the Hb is 90% saturated with O_2 (SaO_2). The relationship between PaO_2 and oxygen saturation is discussed in Chapter 22.

Pulse oximetry is not helpful in evaluating ventilatory status. To evaluate ventilatory status, it is more reliable to observe for clinical signs of hypoventilation and increased work of breathing such as decreased V_T and minute ventilation; change in respiratory rate, pattern, mental status; and behavior changes such as confusion, lethargy, and stupor.

Mixed venous oxygen tension. Blood from the pulmonary artery port (mixed venous blood) of the pulmonary artery catheter can be sampled. Mixed venous blood O_2 tension (PvO_2) is an indication of the state of tissue oxygenation. The normal PO_2 of mixed venous blood is 35 to 40 mm Hg, with an average O_2 saturation (SvO_2) of 75% (acceptable range of 60% to 80%). An increase in PvO_2 to more than 60 mm Hg indicates that the tissues are not extracting and using O_2, or are not being perfused (e.g., in cyanide poisoning). A decrease in PvO_2 (to less than 35 mm Hg) indicates that the tissues are using more O_2 than they would normally.

It is possible to directly monitor the SvO_2 of mixed venous blood with a special fiberoptic flow-directed thermodilution pulmonary artery catheter. Continuous SvO_2 monitoring can decrease the need for frequent ABG determinations. Clinically, a decreased PaO_2 and SvO_2 is evident in severe hypoxemia caused by decreased PaO_2, decreased O_2-carrying capacity of Hb, or decreased cardiac output.

Shunt equation. In clinical situations involving significant hypoxemia, the degree of physiologic (also called venous admixture) shunt can be calculated or estimated. Physiologic shunt is the amount of blood unoxygenated or shunted ($\dot{Q}s$) in relation to the total volume of blood ($\dot{Q}T$). In a healthy person 2% to 5% of the cardiac output returns to the left heart unoxygenated by way of the bronchial and thesbian veins; this is known as a normal anatomic shunt. When 20% to 29% of the cardiac output is shunted, this indicates significant intrapulmonary disease and can be life threatening in a patient with limited cardiovascular or CNS function. A shunt of more than 30% is potentially life threatening and usually requires aggressive management that includes mechanical ventilation. Clinical states that produce shunts include ARDS, pulmonary edema, pneumonia, and atelectasis. Monitoring of $\dot{Q}_S/\dot{Q}_T$ (shunt fraction) is helpful in evaluating responses to therapies such as diuretics, antibiotics, and positive end expiratory pressure (PEEP) therapy. The degree of shunt can be measured using data from the pulmonary artery catheter.

Alveolar-arterial oxygen difference. The alveolar to arterial oxygen difference $D(A\text{–}a)O_2$ is used as an indication of gas exchange efficiency. This measurement assesses the oxygen difference between the alveolus (A) and the artery (a). The normal gradient between PAO_2 and PaO_2 is 10 mm Hg when breathing room air. This difference increases with age. As FIO_2 increases, $D(A\text{-}a)O_2$ also increases until it is approximately 100 mm Hg when the patient with normal lungs is breathing 100% oxygen. Values vary with changes in FIO_2 and lung function. The alveolar-arteriolar oxygen difference is also referred to as the A-a gradient and written as $P(A\text{-}a)O_2$.

Hypoxemia score. The hypoxemia score is defined as the ratio of PaO_2 divided by FIO_2 and is a reflection of the severity of the disease. It ranges from less than 100 (severe problem) to more than 300 (minimal to no problem).

Evaluation of Ventilation (see Table 26-5)

Arterial blood gases. $PaCO_2$ is the partial pressure of CO_2 in the arterial blood measured by ABG analysis. It is the primary indicator of effectiveness of alveolar ventilation. When $PaCO_2$ rises, it indicates decreased, ineffective ventilation, or hypoventilation. A decrease in $PaCO_2$ indicates hyperventilation. $PaCO_2$ values greater than 50 mm Hg indicate hypoventilation. For a detailed discussion of ABGs see Chapter 22.

Capnography. Capnography is a noninvasive method to assess adequacy of ventilation. It is used for intubated patients on mechanical ventilation. A sampling tube leading to a capnograph withdraws gas from the patient's airway. The partial pressure of CO_2 is measured during the entire respiratory cycle and can be displayed digitally and as a wave form (capnogram) on an oscilloscope. The capnograph provides a measure of the end-tidal partial pressure of carbon dioxide ($PetCO_2$) which is a reliable estimate of $PaCO_2$ in normal lungs. Capnography has significant limitations when used to monitor a patient with severe respiratory failure and during weaning from mechanical ventilation. Thus measurements need to be correlated closely with $PaCO_2$. Capnography has been used to detect inadvertent esophageal intubation.

Tidal volume. VT is the volume of air passively exhaled during a normal breathing cycle. Normal predicted VT is about 7 ml/kg of ideal body weight. VT less than 300 ml or greater than 700 ml in the spontaneously breathing adult patient is abnormal and requires further evaluation. Conditions that cause VT to decrease include atelectasis, pneumonia, chest trauma, congestive heart failure (CHF), pulmonary edema, and chronic and acute lung diseases.

Forced vital capacity. Forced vital capacity (FVC) is the maximal volume of air that can be forcibly exhaled from the lungs after a maximal inhalation. Normal values for a healthy adult range from 60 to 80 ml/kg of ideal body weight. A healthy adult requires a minimum FVC of 15 ml/kg to ensure effective cough and adequate ventilation to prevent atelectasis.

Minute ventilation or volume. Minute ventilation or volume (VE) is the product of VT and respiratory rate. This represents the total volume of gas inspired or exhaled by the patient in 1 minute. The average VE for a normal healthy adult is 4 to 8 L per minute. This is an important calculation in estimating work of breathing.

Maximum inspiratory pressure or negative inspiratory force. Maximum inspiratory pressure (MIP) or negative inspiratory force (NIF) is the maximum inspiratory pressure that the patient is capable of generating against a closed airway. The determinants of NIF are respiratory muscle strength, patient effort, ventilatory drive, and lung volume. An advantage of this measurement as compared with FVC is that it can be performed on the patient who is unresponsive or comatose. When the patient exhales, at end exhalation the airway is occluded. During this time the patient is making maximal efforts to breathe and this effort is recorded on the manometer. Normal NIF is in excess of −80 cm H_2O. However, a patient who can generate −20 cm H_2O within 20 seconds can be assumed to have a vital capacity of 15 ml/kg or greater.[3] This measure is useful in assessing respiratory muscle strength before weaning from mechanical ventilation and in neuromuscular dysfunction causing respiratory muscle weakness.

Physiologic dead space. Dead space volume is that inspired volume of air that does not come in contact with pulmonary capillary blood for oxygenation. The normal dead space in a healthy adult is approximately 30% of the V_T or the equivalent of V_D. V_D is made up of the conducting airways and is normally about 2 ml/kg of ideal body weight. Physiologic dead space is V_D plus alveolar dead space (alveolar dead space is alveoli that are ventilated but not perfused).

Miscellaneous Diagnostic Studies. Other routine studies performed are chest x-ray, complete blood cell count (CBC), serum electrolytes, urinalysis, and electrocardiogram (ECG). Cultures of the sputum and blood are obtained as necessary to determine sources of possible infection. If pulmonary embolus is suspected, a ($\dot{V}/\dot{Q}$) lung scan or pulmonary angiography may be performed. Pulmonary function tests may be performed to determine respiratory function.

In severe respiratory failure, measurement of cardiac output and mixed venous blood gases by a thermodilution pulmonary artery catheter (see Chapter 61) is important in determining the amount of blood flow to tissues and the response to treatment. Pulmonary artery, pulmonary capillary wedge, and left atrial pressures are monitored to determine whether the accumulation of fluid in the lungs is the result of cardiac or pulmonary problems. These parameters also are monitored to determine the response of the lungs and heart to hypoxemia and the patient's response to therapy. (Hemodynamic monitoring is discussed in detail in Chapter 61.)

THERAPEUTIC AND NURSING MANAGEMENT

ACUTE RESPIRATORY FAILURE

Nursing Assessment

Subjective and objective data that should be obtained from a person with acute respiratory failure are presented in Table 26-6.

Table 26-6 Nursing Assessment: Acute Respiratory Failure

Subjective Data

Important health information

Past health history: Smoking (pack years), previous hospitalizations related to lung disease, chronic lung disease

Medications: Use of O_2, inhalers, home nebulizers, OTC medications

Surgery and other treatments: Previous intubation and mechanical ventilation

Functional health patterns

Health perception–health management: Fatigue

Nutritional-metabolic: Bloatedness, decreased appetite, heartburn, weight gain or loss; chills, diaphoresis

Activity-exercise: Dyspnea (at rest, with activity), wheezing, cough (productive or nonproductive)

Sleep-rest: Changes in sleep patterns

Cognitive-perceptual: Headaches, chest pain or tightness

Objective Data

General

Appearance (indications of anxiety, fear), state of alertness, speech pattern, position assumed, muscle wasting, diaphoresis

Respiratory

Accessory muscle use; breathing pattern (during rest and activity) including rate, rhythm, I/E ratio; chest symmetry or asymmetry; retractions; tactile fremitus, crepitus, or deviated trachea on palpation; resonant, hyperesonant, or dull percussion note; absent, diminished, or adventitious breath sounds; inspiratory stridor; pleural friction rub; bronchial or bronchovesicular sounds heard in other than normal location; surgical scars (thoracotomy)

Cardiovascular

Peripheral edema (lower extremities, sacrum, periorbital), jugular venous distention, true central cyanosis (tongue), tachycardia, dysrhythmias, extra heart sounds (S_3, S_4)

Gastrointestinal

Ascites, epigastric tenderness, hepatojugular reflex distention, tympany

Diagnostic findings

$\downarrow$ pH, $\uparrow\downarrow$ $PaCO_2$, $\downarrow$ PaO_2, $\downarrow$ O_2 Sat, $\downarrow$ PEFR, $\downarrow$ V_T, $\downarrow$ FVC, $\downarrow$ V_E, $\downarrow$ NIF; abnormal $D(A\text{-}a)O_2$, a/A ratio, PaO_2/FIO_2 ratio, $\dot{Q}_S/\dot{Q}_T$, $P\bar{v}O_2$, V_D/V_T ratio; altered values of serum electrolytes, Hb, hematocrit; abnormal findings on chest x-ray film, pulmonary artery and pulmonary capillary wedge pressures

OTC, Over-the-counter.

Nursing Diagnoses

Nursing diagnoses are determined when the problem and etiologic factors are supported by clinical data. Nursing diagnoses related to acute respiratory failure may include, but are not limited to, those in the nursing care plan on p. 740.

Planning

The overall goals are that the patient with respiratory failure will have (1) ABG values within patient's baseline, (2) baseline breath sounds, and (3) absence of dyspnea or dyspnea at patient's baseline.

Nursing Implementation

Management of acute respiratory failure depends on the underlying disease process (Table 26-7); however, several aspects of management are common to many types of respiratory failure. Therapeutic management and nursing management of acute respiratory failure are strongly interdependent and are presented together.

Maintenance of Adequate Oxygenation

Oxygen administration. If hypoxemia is secondary to hypoventilation, provision and maintenance of adequate ventilation usually will overcome the problem of gas exchange. Hypoxemia secondary to $\dot{V}/\dot{Q}$ mismatch usually responds favorably to the lowest concentration of O_2 (administered by mask or cannula) necessary to maintain a PaO_2 of at least 55 to 60 mm Hg. Hypoxemia secondary to shunting is usually refractory (refractory hypoxemia) to the administration of high concentrations of O_2 by mask and ultimately requires mechanical ventilation. The patient with

NURSING CARE PLAN Patient with Acute Respiratory Failure

Planning: Outcome Criteria	Nursing Interventions and Rationales
➤ **NURSING DIAGNOSIS**	Ineffective airway clearance *related to* accumulation of secretion, exudate, sputum in airways, decreased level of consciousness, presence of an artificial airway, thoracic and/or abdominal neuromuscular dysfunction, pain, and expiratory airflow obstruction *as manifested by* difficulty in expectorating sputum, presence of abnormal breath sounds (e.g., rhonchi, crackles), ineffective or absent cough
Have no abnormal breath sounds (e.g., rhonchi, crackles), or normal baseline breath sounds for patient with chronic respiratory disease, presence of effective cough, easy expectoration of sputum, ability to perform airway clearance procedures.	Evaluate patient's ability to cough *to determine effectiveness and need for assistance in removing secretions.* Humidify inspired air if upper airway is bypassed or O_2 is being used at >3 L/min *to prevent drying of mucosa.* Perform tracheobronchial suctioning if coughing is ineffective, or if artificial airway is present *to remove retained secretions and improve oxygenation.* Consider minitracheostomy if patient meets criteria. Perform chest physiotherapy *to enhance removal of secretions.* Splint chest or abdominal incision with pillow or hand *to reduce pain and allow deeper, more effective breathing and coughing.* Turn q2hr *to prevent stasis of secretions and promote optimal ventilation.* Stabilize artificial airway *to prevent accidental extubation.* Ensure adequate fluid intake of 2-3 L/24 hr as indicated *to liquefy secretions and prevent dehydration.* Administer prescribed bronchodilator and mucolytic medications *to promote better air flow and secretion removal*
➤ **NURSING DIAGNOSIS**	Ineffective breathing pattern *related to* neuromuscular impairment, pain, musculoskeletal impairment, anxiety, CNS depression, respiratory muscle fatigue or failure, increased work of breathing, expiratory obstruction to airflow, and weaning attempt *as manifested by* respiratory rate <11 or >24 breaths/min, alteration of I/E ratio, irregular breathing rhythm (e.g., use of accessory muscles of breathing inappropriate to level of activity), need for mechanical ventilation
Have respiratory rate, depth, timing within normal limits for patient; have respiratory rhythm within normal limits for age; have synchronous thoracoabdominal movement; use of accessory muscles appropriate to level of activity.	Provide comfort measures (e.g., positioning, analgesics) *to reduce anxiety and allow for maximum patient cooperation with respiratory procedures.* Provide mechanical support (e.g., IPPB, NIPPV, mechanical ventilation) if indicated *to prevent or treat acute respiratory failure and maintain adequate oxygenation and ventilation.* Evaluate potential to wean from mechanical ventilation *to determine patients' ability to adjust to lowered levels of mechanical ventilator support.*
➤ **NURSING DIAGNOSIS**	Risk for fluid volume excess *related to* increases in peripheral or pulmonary fluid secondary to cor pulmonale, heart failure, or acute respiratory distress
Have a reduction in weight toward normal range, return of PaO_2 to patient's normal range, absence of abnormal breath sounds, decreased sensation of dyspnea, decrease in or absence of signs of peripheral edema, decreased pulmonary artery or pulmonary capillary wedge pressure.	Assess for manifestations of fluid volume excess such as PaO_2 <60 mm Hg; increasing dyspnea; abnormal breath sounds (crackles); weight gain >2-3 lb on consecutive days; jugular venous distention; taut, shiny skin; peripheral or sacral edema *to identify if problem is present.* Monitor fluid status by intake and output, daily weights, jugular venous distention, and pulmonary artery or pulmonary capillary wedge pressures (when appropriate) *as the accumulation of lung water can aggravate and prevent alveolar ventilation.* Assist with ventilatory support measures (e.g., mechanical ventilation) when appropriate *to prevent tissue hypoxia.* Restrict fluid intake and administer diuretics (if prescribed) *to prevent heart failure secondary to fluid overload.*

continued

NURSING CARE PLAN Patient with Acute Respiratory Failure—cont'd

Planning: Outcome Criteria	*Nursing Interventions and Rationales*
➤ **NURSING DIAGNOSIS**	Altered nutrition: less than body requirements *related to* poor appetite, lowered energy level, shortness of breath, presence of sputum, presence of artificial airway, and increased caloric requirements *as manifested by* >10% below ideal body weight, serum albumin level below normal laboratory values, weight loss, weakness, muscle wasting, dehydration, decreased muscle tone, poor skin integrity, presence of artificial airway or mechanical ventilation
Be within 10% of ideal body weight, have serum albumin level within normal laboratory values, have stabilized or increasing weight not as a result of fluid retention.	Provide high-protein, high-calorie, enteral or parenteral nutrition as prescribed *to meet increased nutritional requirements resulting from fever, anxiety, pain, and increased work of breathing.* Monitor serum albumin or transferrin levels *to determine adequacy of protein and iron and potential for anemia and muscle wasting.* Take measures *to prevent aspiration* (e.g., positioning, small-bore feeding tube). Monitor fluid status (intake and output, weight) *to avoid fluid overload and subsequent heart failure.* With parenteral nutrition, monitor for signs of CO_2 increase during weaning as result of carbohydrate loads *as carbohydrates may increase CO_2 levels in patients with hypercapnia.*
➤ **NURSING DIAGNOSIS**	Anxiety *related to* dyspnea, intubation, severity of illness, loss of personal control, and uncertain outcome *as manifested by* increased pulse, respiratory rate, and BP; agitation, restlessness; verbalization of anxiety over health situation.
Have decreased anxiety, relaxed demeanor, increased sense of personal control, verbalization of hopeful attitude about outcome.	Perform interventions in calm, assured manner *to decrease patient's anxiety and foster hope about the outcome.* Reassure patient of competence of caregivers *to encourage patient to relax and allow caregivers to deliver needed care.* Answer questions simply and honestly *to provide patient with needed information for decision making.* Teach and demonstrate to patient slow pursed-lip breathing; explain sensations patient may experience during procedures (e.g., suctioning); explain equipment, procedures, and treatments in familiar terms so patient can purposefully select coping strategies *to reduce anxiety and fear.*
➤ **NURSING DIAGNOSIS**	Dyspnea *related to* increased airway resistance, air trapping or hyperinflation, decreased lung compliance, and decreased chest wall compliance*

COLLABORATIVE PROBLEMS

Nursing Goals	*Nursing Interventions and Rationales*
➤ **POTENTIAL COMPLICATION**	Hypoxemia *related to* alveolar hypoventilation, intrapulmonary shunting, $\dot{V}/\dot{Q}$ mismatch, diffusion impairment
Manage and minimize complications of hypoxemia; monitor patient's PaO_2 and O_2 Sat for deviation from baseline.	Assess patient for PaO_2 <60 mm Hg or SaO_2 <90% at rest (for acute patients on room air at sea level), PaO_2<60 mm Hg or SaO_2 <88% during exercise (for chronic patients on room air at sea level), tachycardia, ↑ BP, dyspnea on exertion, restlessness, fatigue, true central cyanosis, and change in mentation. Position patient (e.g., elevate head of bed 45 degrees, use tripod position) *to promote optimal gas exchanges.* Assist with ventilatory support measures (e.g., mechanical ventilation, NIPPV), *to improve patient's respiratory status.* Monitor oximetry and ABGs *to evaluate gas exchange in lungs.* Ensure adequate hydration *to liquefy secretions.* Monitor cardiac and ECG for dysrhythmias *as hypoxemia may precipitate cardiac dysrhythmias.*
➤ **POTENTIAL COMPLICATION**	Hypercapnia *related to* alveolar hypoventilation and $\dot{V}/\dot{Q}$ mismatch
Manage and minimize complications of hypercapnia; monitor patient's $PaCO_2$ and blood pH for deviations from baseline; $PaCO_2$ <40 mm Hg or patient's baseline value, pH 7.35 to 7.45.	Assess for $PaCO_2$ >50 mm Hg with pH <7.35, headache on awakening, and somnolence *to determine presence of hypercapnia.* Administer drugs prescribed *to reverse respiratory depression (e.g., Narcan).* Withhold sedative drugs unless discussed with physician *as they can further depress respiration.* Monitor forced vital capacity in patients with neuromuscular weakness *to evaluate as a potential cause of CO_2 retention.* Monitor ventilatory parameters such as MIP ≥−20 cm H_2O, vital capacity ≤10-15 ml/kg, respiratory rate >35 breaths/min, increasing lethargy or drowsiness *to detect changes that suggest possible increase in $PaCO_2$.* Assist with ventilatory support measures (e.g., mechanical ventilation, NIPPV), if needed. Monitor level of consciousness.

ABGs, Arterial blood gases; *BP,* blood pressure; *CNS,* central nervous system; *ECG,* electrocardiogram; *I/E,* inspiratory-expiratory; *IPPB,* intermittent positive pressure breathing; *MIP,* maximum inspiratory pressure; *NIPPV,* noninvasive positive pressure ventilation.
*See the nursing care plan for the patient with chronic obstructive pulmonary disease in Chapter 25.

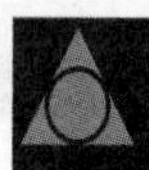

Table 26-7 Therapeutic Management: Acute Respiratory Failure

Maintenance of Adequate Oxygenation
- O_2 administration to keep PaO_2 >60 mm Hg
- Maintenance of adequate Hb concentration
- Maintenance of adequate cardiac output
- Prevention and assessment of tissue hypoxia
- Measures to decrease stress and anxiety and promote comfort

Improvement of Alveolar Ventilation
- Maintenance of patent airway
  - Effective coughing
  - Suctioning
  - Positioning
- Measures to assist in liquefaction and movement of secretions
  - Humidification
  - Adequate hydration
  - Chest physiotherapy (if indicated)
  - Aerosols and ultrasonic nebulization
- Relief of bronchospasm
  - Bronchodilators
  - Aerosolized bronchodilators
  - Corticosteroids (when indicated)
- Reduction of pulmonary congestion
  - Diuretics
- Ventilatory assistance
  - Continuous positive pressure breathing (CPPB)
  - Noninvasive positive pressure ventilation (NIPPV)

Treatment of Underlying Cause of Failure

Continuous Monitoring and Evaluation of Treatment

chronic pulmonary disease requiring O_2 should receive controlled O_2 through a nasal cannula (1 to 3 L/min) or Venturi mask. The Venturi mask is a high flow O_2 system that provides an exact concentration of O_2. In contrast, low flow through a nasal cannula delivers O_2 concentrations that vary with the patient's minute ventilation. Both low-flow O_2 and the Venturi mask generally correct severe arterial hypoxemia in chronically ill patients without unduly suppressing respiration by reducing the hypoxic drive. (Other methods of O_2 administration are discussed in Chapter 24.)

Maintenance of hemoglobin concentration and cardiac output. To ensure adequate O_2 delivery to the tissues, keeping the patient's PaO_2 equal to 60 mm Hg or greater will provide adequate O_2 saturation. When the PaO_2 is 60 mm Hg or greater, the Hb is 90% saturated (see Fig. 22-7). An adequate Hb concentration of 9 to 10 g/dl (90 to 100 g/L) or greater and maintenance of an adequate cardiac output are also important in ensuring adequate O_2 delivery.

BP should be maintained at the most beneficial level for each patient. Usually, a systolic BP of at least 90 mm Hg is adequate to maintain perfusion to the vital organs. A urine output of 0.5 ml/kg per hour or more is an indication of adequate renal perfusion. If the systolic BP is at least 90 mm Hg, changes in mental status may be attributed to the levels of O_2 and CO_2 in the blood rather than to decreased perfusion to the brain. Cardiac output may be measured using a pulmonary artery catheter. If cardiac output is decreased, medications (e.g., sympathomimetics) or fluids may be administered.

Prevention and assessment of tissue hypoxia. Close observation for clinical manifestations of vital organ hypoxia is needed, including frequent assessment of the patient's mental and neurologic status for clouding of sensorium, poor concentration, restlessness, stupor, lethargy, somnolence, tremors, slurred speech, depressed tendon reflexes, and asterixis. Cardiovascular status assessment includes direct or indirect BP monitoring; monitoring of cardiac output, pulmonary artery and wedge pressures and cardiac rate and rhythm; and assessment for symptoms of right-sided and left-sided heart failure. The older patient and the patient with coronary artery disease are especially susceptible to the effects of decreased tissue O_2 on the myocardium.

Fluid and electrolyte levels should be assessed carefully. Serial evaluations of serum electrolytes are made to determine excesses or deficiencies. Incremental replacement of potassium may be indicated if the patient is hypokalemic. Continuous or serial monitoring of oxygenation status is essential.

Measures to decrease stress and promote comfort. The patient should be maintained in an atmosphere as quiet and relaxed as possible. Rising levels of stress and anxiety can further increase O_2 demands. The respiratory rate also can be increased. A patient often feels powerless, with a loss of personal control as dyspnea increases and the need for invasive supportive treatment increases. Four key types of loss of control that the patient may experience have been defined.[4] These include physiologic loss of control when breathing problems can no longer be controlled, cognitive loss of control when thoughts become frightening and anxiety-producing, environmental loss of control when one feels helpless to control the equipment or situation, and decisional loss of control when one feels others are making all the decisions.

Several nursing strategies can help the patient restore some degree of personal control over all of these areas. In a patient with COPD, increasing dyspnea results in decreased time for exhalation, increased air trapping, and an enhanced sense of breathlessness. Teaching slow-pursed lip breathing techniques can help the patient feel some sense of control over breathing. Fear of suffocation or death is not uncommon. Thus the patient must be supported both emotionally and physically at this time. Providing reassurance, spending time with the patient, and ensuring that help can be received immediately (e.g., by making a call light readily available) may help to decrease the patient's anxiety level. Anxiety also may be reduced through the use of progressive relaxation, guided imagery, and meditation. Frequently, a family member or friend will have a soothing effect on the patient. It is important to evaluate the effect of visitors on the patient's anxiety level. It is also important to let the patient choose who, when, and how long to visit if this is possible.

A patient in respiratory distress (especially in the presence of chronic lung disease) often prefers to be in an open area without curtains or with a door or window open. Activity should be kept to a minimum within reason. Positioning the patient for comfort and for the most efficient ventilation is important. The patient should be asked what position seems best to ease breathing. Frequent rest periods need to be provided, and efficient scheduling (pacing) of care, treatments, assessments, and diagnostic studies are important to help with conserving the patient's energy.

The patient with pronounced acute hypercapnia is often sleepy. In this case it is important to keep the patient awake and breathing at regular intervals because sleeping will result in further hypoventilation. Patting the patient on the back, keeping the lights on, and giving frequent reminders to breathe can help. Interpreting facial expressions and body language, using questions that require short yes-and-no answers or head nodding, or using a word board for communication will help to limit the amount of energy the patient expends for communication.

It is helpful to explain to the patient the possible sensations that may be encountered with each new experience (e.g., suctioning, drawing ABGs) so that coping strategies can be purposefully selected. Using common names for equipment such as "TV screen" for the monitor and explaining equipment, procedures, and treatments in familiar terms can help reduce anxiety and the feeling of potential threat.

Measures to increase physical comfort are also important. A cool cloth placed on the forehead to remove perspiration and to refresh the face is usually appreciated. Sips of cool water or ice chips (if tolerated) also can be offered. Mouth care is especially important for the patient who is a mouth breather because of the drying effects of inspired air on the mucous membranes. Removing a perspiration-soaked gown, lightly sponging the patient's upper torso, and helping the patient into a dry gown will often suffice for a daily bath.

Improvement of Alveolar Ventilation. In respiratory failure the work of breathing is increased and often the CO_2 production is excessive in relation to the amount of alveolar ventilation that is occurring. Reduction of both CO_2 production and the work of breathing, with subsequent improvement in alveolar ventilation, can be accomplished by instituting therapeutic measures to relieve airway obstruction or pulmonary congestion. If these intensive measures fail, mechanical ventilation may be required to assist or control the ventilation.

Maintenance of a patent airway. Maintenance of a patent airway is essential. Obstruction of the airway caused by the accumulation of secretions or bronchospasm occurs frequently. If secretions are obstructing the airway, the patient should be encouraged to cough. Effective coughing requires a deep inhalation, effective glottic closure, and high expiratory flows (see Table 25-12). These abilities need to be evaluated to determine whether the cough is effective.

The patient with neuromuscular weakness may have a flow limitation as a result of decreased volume and an inability to produce adequately high pleural pressures. Augmented coughing may be helpful in this patient or in an exhausted patient. Augmented coughing is performed by placing the flat palm of the hand or hands on the thorax (rib springing) in the area where the presence of secretions has been detected by auscultation or on the abdominal musculature below the xiphoid process. As the patient ends the deep inspiration and begins expiration, the hands should be moved forcefully downward, facilitating chest compression or increased abdominal pressure. This measure helps to produce muscle movement, increases pleural pressure and expiratory flows, and augments or assists the cough. Coughing at the end of expiration is helpful in the patient with severe airway obstruction because it can cause compression of the more distal or peripheral airways and may help "milk" or move secretions into the proximal airways. Frequently, having the patient breathe as deeply as possible (if able) may stimulate the cough. "Huff" coughing with the glottis open may be used for the patient who has problems with glottic closure, such as one who has endotracheal or tracheal tubes in place.

Positioning the patient either by elevating the head of the bed to at least 45 degrees (if tolerated) or by using a reclining chair bed may maximize thoracic expansion. A patient with only one functioning lung should be positioned with the unaffected lung in the dependent position. This positioning is important in preventing hypoxemia because the "down" lung gets more perfusion. If the diseased lung was down, more $\dot{V}/\dot{Q}$ mismatch would occur. Consequently, recording and noting the patient's position and FIO_2 level when drawing ABGs are important in evaluating the results. The patient should be lying on the side if there is any possibility that the tongue will obstruct the airway or that aspiration may occur. An oral or nasal airway should be kept at the bedside for use if necessary.

If the patient's cough is ineffective in removing secretions, nasopharyngeal or nasotracheal suctioning is indicated. Minitracheostomy (mini-trach) has been used in some centers to facilitate suctioning a patient who has an ineffective cough, respiratory muscle weakness, or postoperative incisional pain that limits secretion removal and cough, or difficulty performing "blind" endotracheal suctioning (suctioning without an endotracheal tube in place). The mini-trach is a 4 mm indwelling plastic cuffless cannula inserted through the cricothyroid membrane. It can be used to instill sterile saline to elicit cough and for suctioning with #10 French catheters. Contraindications for this procedure include absence of a gag reflex, history of aspiration, and the need for long-term ventilation.[5]

Adequate oxygenation and monitoring of the patient are essential during suctioning procedures. Although rarely indicated, bronchoscopy may be used to remove secretions, especially if they are extremely thick and tenacious.

Measures to liquefy and mobilize secretions. If bronchial secretions are thick, viscous, and difficult to raise, efforts to thin them should be made. Adequate hydration is necessary to keep secretions thin and easy to remove.

Aerosols of sterile normal saline solutions administered by a nebulizer may be used to liquefy secretions. The patient's response to aerosol therapy must be assessed. Aerosol therapy may induce bronchospasm, severe bouts of coughing, and decreased PaO_2. Nebulized acetylcysteine (e.g., Mucomyst) or other mucolytic agents have been used to thin secretions. These agents usually are mixed together with a bronchodilator; however, the value of these agents is questionable. They may be irritating, cause erythematous changes, and may induce bronchospasm.

Chest physiotherapy in certain situations (e.g., sputum production greater than 30 ml/day) can be an effective means of improving the removal of retained secretions (see Fig. 25-12). If tolerated, postural drainage, percussion, and vibration performed manually or by a mechanical vibrator to the affected lung segments may assist in moving secretions to larger airways where they can be removed by effective coughing or suctioning. If suctioning or other measures to mobilize secretions are ineffective, it may become necessary to insert an endotracheal or tracheostomy tube to facilitate suctioning of secretions. Mucolytic agents (e.g., guaifenesin, iodinated glycerol) may be helpful if the patient can swallow.

Relief of bronchospasm. Relief of bronchospasm (if present) will aid in maximal bronchodilatation and increase effective alveolar ventilation. An intravenous (IV) loading dose of aminophylline may be administered in an acute attack of bronchospasm. Severe bronchospasm may be treated with IV infusions of isoproterenol (Isuprel) or terbutaline (Brethaire) as a final effort to prevent intubation and mechanical ventilation. Aerosolized β-agonist bronchodilators such as metaproterenol (Alupent) or albuterol (Ventolin; Proventil) (see Table 25-4) also may be administered at regular intervals depending on the patient's response. These bronchodilators can be administered by a hand-held nebulizer or by a metered-dose inhaler. Nebulized glycopyrolate (Robinul) or ipratropium (Atrovent) together with a β-agonist bronchodilator may be administered in COPD exacerbations.

The patient's response to β-adrenergic bronchodilators should be monitored and charted. Bronchodilator administration sometimes results in an initial worsening of arterial hypoxemia. This change is due to redistribution of the inspired gas away from areas that continue to be perfused to areas with decreased perfusion. Administration of an O_2-enriched gas mixture simultaneously with the bronchodilator may help to alleviate the subsequent hypoxemia. (Side effects and nursing management related to bronchodilators are discussed in Chapter 25 and Table 25-4).

Corticosteroids frequently are used in conjunction with bronchodilating agents when bronchospasm and inflammation are present. The dose of steroids depends on the severity of bronchospasm and the patient's clinical status (see Chapter 25).

Reduction of pulmonary congestion. Pulmonary congestion precipitating acute respiratory failure can occur as a result of right-sided or left-sided heart failure or leakage of fluid into the pulmonary interstitial space because of a defective capillary-alveolar membrane as in pulmonary edema (either cardiac or noncardiac in etiology). The accumulation of fluid in the lung can further aggravate and inhibit alveolar ventilation. Therefore it is important for the nurse to monitor for signs and symptoms of heart failure and to be able to interpret the pressures obtained by the pulmonary artery catheter.

Diuretics may be used to treat pulmonary congestion. Digitalization is not usually recommended unless left ventricular failure or atrial fibrillation is present. If digitalis is used, ABGs, ECG, and serum electrolytes are monitored closely, because digitalis in the presence of hypoxemia, hypokalemia, and acidemia can increase cardiac irritability. Close monitoring of edema, daily weights, and intake and output is imperative.

Ventilatory assistance. If intensive measures fail to improve alveolar ventilation and the patient continues to deteriorate clinically, mechanical ventilation may be instituted to assist or control ventilation. (See Table 61-11 for guidelines for determining the need for mechanical ventilation.) Clinical observation of the patient is important in making a decision to institute mechanical ventilation.

A patient with chronic lung disease needs to be evaluated on the basis of limited pulmonary function because the patient's baseline values often meet the criteria for mechanical ventilation. Patient assessment includes monitoring clinical manifestations of respiratory disease and the response to therapy. For example, a patient with an acute exacerbation of asthma usually demonstrates significant hypocapnia and respiratory alkalemia with hypoxemia in the early stages rather than hypercapnia and respiratory acidemia with hypoxemia. In this patient a rise in $PaCO_2$, especially into the normal range, is an ominous sign because it signifies exhaustion and impending respiratory failure. Ventilatory support is imperative.

Noninvasive positive pressure ventilation (NIPPV) is used as a treatment for selected patients with acute or chronic respiratory failure. NIPPV can be used without endotracheal intubation; instead a nasal or face mask is applied and a volume of air is delivered to the patient at preset inspiratory or expiratory pressures. Bilevel positive airway pressure (BIPAP) indicates that different positive pressure levels are set for inspiration and expiration. Continuous positive airway pressure (CPAP) indicates that there is a constant or continuous positive pressure on the airway during inspiration and expiration.

The main goal of NIPPV is to improve ventilation. The advantages of NIPPV are to improve patient comfort; reduce the need for sedation; avoid the complications of endotracheal intubation, including upper airway trauma, sinusitis, otitis, and nosocomial pneumonia; and maintain airway defenses, speech, and swallowing. Limitations include the need for the patient to be alert and to be able to cooperate, lack of direct access to the airway, which could promote mucous plugging or atelectasis in the patient with copious secretions, facial skin ulcers caused by mask pressure, or aerophagia.[6]

NIPPV is most useful in treating chronic respiratory failure resulting from restrictive thoracic disease (kyphoscoliosis; neuromuscular diseases such as multiple sclerosis and muscular dystrophies). NIPPV, however, has been used for the patient with COPD in acute respiratory failure with limited success. NIPPV is also useful in the patient who refuses invasive mechanical ventilation but still desires treatment, as well as for the patient requesting limited palliative ventilatory support in terminal illnesses.[7] NIPPV is not appropriate for the patient who has absent respirations, excessive secretions, decreased level of consciousness, high oxygen requirements, facial trauma, or hemodynamic instability. The use of NIPPV in the acute care setting could possibly result in a greater time commitment for nursing staff than traditional mechanical ventilation.

Treatment of the Underlying Cause of Respiratory Failure. In a patient with absolute hypoventilation, the primary problem usually can be diagnosed rapidly, and appropriate therapy initiated. When the problem is drug overdose, dialysis or other methods to promote excretion of the drug are used. Bronchoscopy or lung biopsy may need to be performed to obtain specimens for determining the underlying respiratory disease. Specific treatment measures are available for the patient with myasthenia gravis, whereas the patient with Guillain-Barré syndrome often requires long-term ventilatory support until the disease process runs its course. Infection is often the primary cause of acute respiratory failure in the immunosuppressed patient. Appropriate cultures must be obtained and antibiotic therapy begun as soon as possible.

Continuous Monitoring of the Effects of Treatment. A flowchart that shows the patient's ABG measurements and results of other laboratory and clinical studies, including vital signs, pulmonary artery and wedge pressures, weights, intake and output, medications and dosage, electrolytes, CBC, and respiratory parameters, is extremely helpful. Accurate, clear documentation of objective and subjective assessments on the patient's flowchart is an important aspect of care. Management of the patient should be evaluated regularly, and the therapeutic regimen should be altered as indicated by the patient's response.

ACUTE RESPIRATORY DISTRESS SYNDROME

ARDS is a sudden, progressive disorder consisting of pulmonary edema of noncardiac origin, severe dyspnea, hypoxemia refractory to supplemental O_2, reduced lung compliance, and diffuse pulmonary infiltrates. ARDS previously was thought of as a syndrome limited to the lungs. ARDS, however, is either a cause or a consequence of the systemic inflammatory response syndrome (SIRS), which occurs in the host as a response to a severe insult. SIRS is characterized by widespread inflammation or clinical responses to inflammation occurring in a patient with a variety of insults. When SIRS is the result of infection, the term *sepsis* is used. Clinical manifestations of SIRS include (1) a temperature greater than 100.4° F (38° C), (2) heart rate greater than 90 beats per minute, (3) tachypnea (>20 respirations/minute or $PaCO_2$ <32 mm Hg), (4) white blood cell count less than 4000/µl or greater than 12,000/µl, and (5) more than 10% neutrophils in band forms.[8] (SIRS is discussed in Chapter 61.)

ARDS itself may initiate SIRS, or it may be one of the earliest manifestations of the multiple organ dysfunction syndrome (MODS), which develops as a consequence of

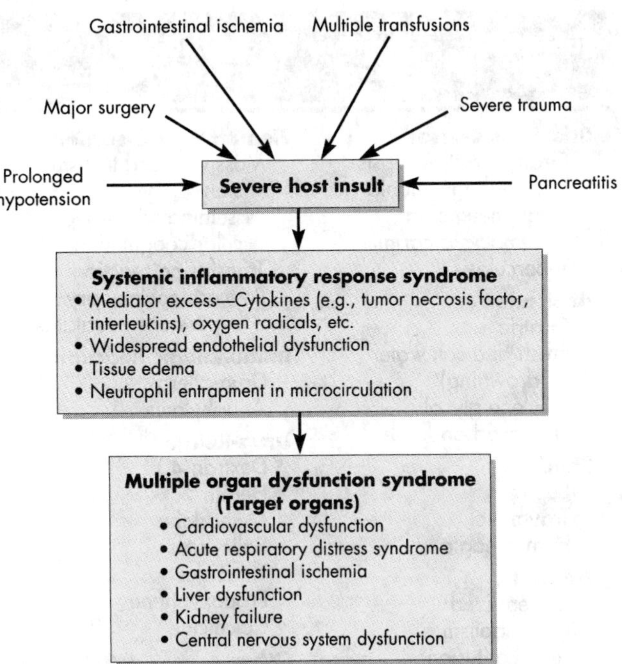

Fig. 26-5 Relationship of systemic inflammatory response syndrome, multiple organ dysfunction syndrome, and acute respiratory distress syndrome.

SIRS. MODS results from progressive failure of several interdependent organ systems following a significant insult, such as trauma, burns, infection, aspiration, multiple blood transfusions, pulmonary contusions, or pancreatitis.[9] Figure 26-5 presents the events surrounding SIRS, MODS, and ARDS. (MODS is discussed in Chapter 61.)

Risk factors for development of SIRS and MODS include inadequate or delayed resuscitation, persistent infection or inflammation, hemorrhagic shock, multiple trauma with massive tissue injury, age of 65 years or older, alcohol abuse, bowel infarction, malnutrition, diabetes, corticosteroids, cancer, presence of a large hematoma, and surgical misfortunes.[9] Many clinical disorders cause either direct lung injury (e.g., pneumonia, gastric aspiration) or indirect lung injury caused by mediators produced by the SIRS (e.g., sepsis, multiple trauma, pancreatitis, burns).

Clinical disorders associated with the development of ARDS are listed in Table 26-8. Septic shock is the major risk factor for ARDS. The patient who has gram-negative septic shock and ARDS has a mortality rate of 70% to 90%.[10]

The incidence of ARDS in the United States is estimated at more than 150,000 cases a year, often striking previously healthy people. The mortality rate from ARDS of approximately 50% to 76% is usually due to MODS.[11]

Pathophysiology

The initial insult to the lungs in ARDS occurs in the patient who has a variety of disorders (see Table 26-8). Because ARDS does not develop in every patient with these types of clinical disorders, it is assumed that there is a disturbance in

Table 26-8 Conditions Predisposing to Acute Respiratory Distress Syndrome

Infectious Causes	**Hematologic Disorders**
Gram-negative sepsis	Massive blood transfusion
Bacterial pneumonia	Disseminated intravascular coagulation
Viral pneumonia	Transfusion reaction
Pneumocystis carinii	Postcardiopulmonary bypass or resuscitation
Tuberculosis	**Immunologic Reactions**
Aspiration	Drug allergy
Gastric	Anaphylaxis
Fresh and salt water (drowning)	**Drug-Related**
Ethylene glycol	Dextran 40
Hydrocarbon fluids	Heroin
Shock	Methadone
Septic	Salicylates
Traumatic	Thiazides
Hemorrhagic	Propoxyphene
Trauma	Colchicine
Generalized	**Other**
Fat embolism	Radiation pneumonitis
Lung contusion	Amniotic fluid emboli
Multiple major fractures	Increased intracranial pressure
Head injury	High altitude
Burns	Fluid overload
Metabolic Disorders	Eclampsia
Pancreatitis	Goodpasture's syndrome
Uremia	Drug overdose
Diabetic ketoacidosis	Bowel infarction
Inhaled Toxic Agents	Dead fetus
O_2	
Smoke	
Toxic gases	

Table 26-9 Mediators of Acute Lung Injury

- Complement component C5a
- Neutrophil products, including proteases and O_2 radicals
- Monocyte and macrophage products, including tumor necrosis factors, interleukin-1, and granulocyte colony-stimulating factor
- Arachidonic acid metabolites, including prostaglandins and leukotrienes
- Coagulation products, including kallikreins, kinins, fibrin degradation products, and plasminogen-activating factor
- Histamine
- Serotonin
- Endotoxin
- Elastase
- Collagenase

normal protective mechanisms. Despite the heterogeneity of the disorders that cause ARDS, the common abnormal finding is diffuse alveolar-capillary membrane damage with subsequent leakage of fluid from the vascular space into the interstitium and alveoli.

An exact cause for the damage to the alveolar-capillary membrane is not known; however, many cellular and humoral mediators are thought to be involved (Table 26-9 and Fig. 26-6). (These mediators are discussed in Chapters 9 and 10.) Release of these inflammatory mediators results in structural damage to the lungs, increased vascular permeability, development of microemboli of platelets and fibrin within the pulmonary vasculature, vasoconstriction leading to increased vascular resistance, and bronchoconstriction.

The pathophysiologic changes in ARDS are divided into three phases: (1) injury or exudative, (2) reparative or proliferative, and (3) fibrotic.

Injury or Exudative Phase. The injury or exudative phase occurs approximately 1 to 7 days (usually 24 to 48 hours) after the initial direct lung injury or host insult. An influx of neutrophils, which adhere to the pulmonary microcirculation, causes damage to the vascular endothelium. The end result is alveolar capillary and endothelial cell injury, increasing the permeability of the vessels. Because of this disruption in the normal alveolar-capillary membrane in ARDS, alveolar fluid accumulates (proteinaceous pulmonary edema) (Fig. 26-7).

Normally, the force tending to push fluid out of the capillary is the capillary hydrostatic pressure (also known in the lungs as *pulmonary capillary wedge pressure*). The force tending to pull fluid into the capillaries is the colloidal osmotic pressure in the blood. The net balance of these forces results in a normal continuous filtration of fluid from the pulmonary capillaries into the interstitial space. Alveolar type I cells that line the alveolar wall make the alveolus virtually impermeable to fluid and solute flow from the interstitium. As fluid in the interstitium accumulates, equilibrium is maintained by flow of fluid into peribronchial and perivascular spaces and thus into the lymphatics. With excessive fluid accumulation, however, lymph channels become compressed by the fluid and the fluid moves from the interstitium into the alveolus, ultimately producing alveolar or pulmonary edema.

The earliest phase of pulmonary edema is characterized by engorgement of the peribronchial and perivascular interstitial spaces and is known as *interstitial edema.* When fluid crosses the alveolar epithelium into the alveolar spaces, the alveoli fill with fluid. Because the alveoli are unventilated, blood passing through them cannot be oxygenated.

In ARDS, alveolar type I and type II cells (which produce surfactant) are damaged. The result is further fluid and protein accumulation, which inactivates surfactant. Surfactant normally lowers the surface tension of the alveolar lining fluid and maintains alveolar stability by preventing alveolar collapse, increasing lung compliance, and decreasing the work of breathing. As a consequence of the damage to the alveolar type II cells and inactivation of existing surfactant, the alveoli become increasingly unstable and tend to collapse unless filled with interstitial fluid. This change in the alveoli results in atelectasis and causes further compromise of the gas exchange in the lungs.

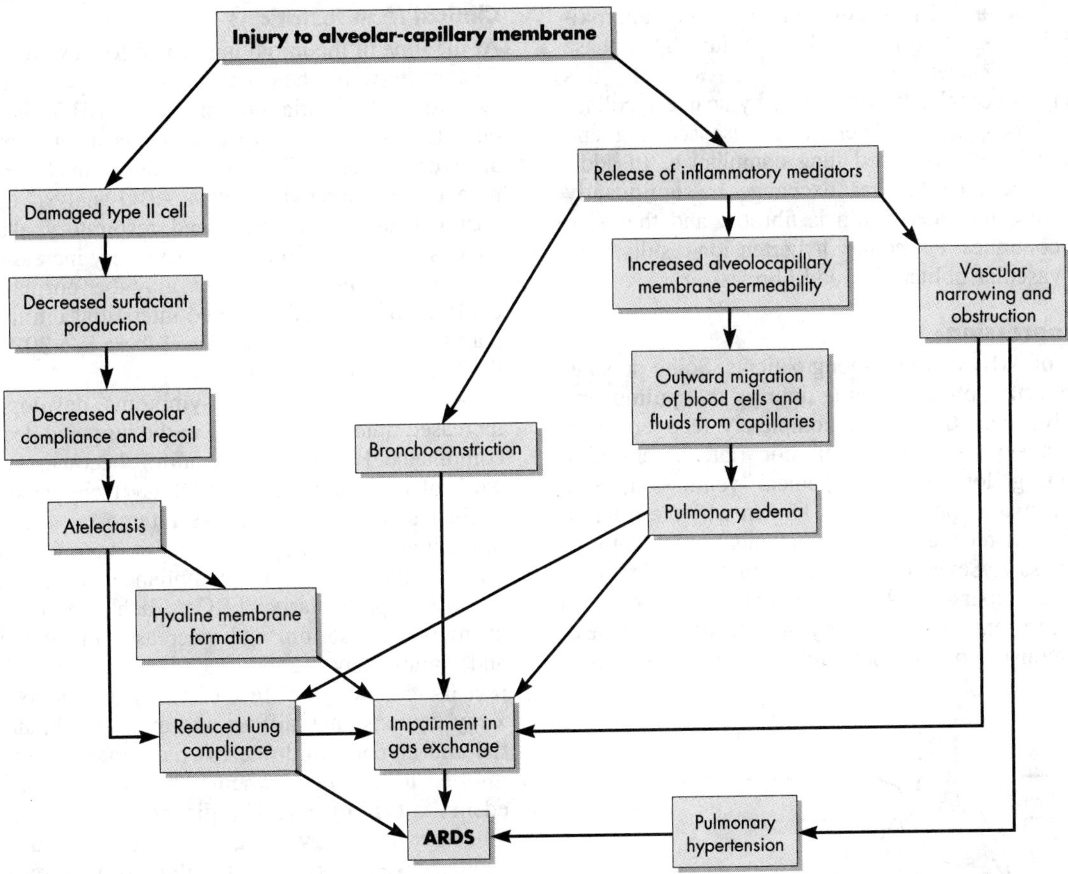

Fig. 26-6 Pathophysiology of acute respiratory distress syndrome (ARDS).

Also during this stage, hyaline begins to line the alveolar membrane. These hyaline membranes are thought to result from the exudation of high-molecular-weight substances (particularly fibrinogen) in the edema fluid. Hyaline membranes contribute to the development of fibrosis and atelectasis, leading to a decrease in gas exchange capability and lung compliance.

The essential disturbances that characterize the injury or exudative phase of ARDS are interstitial and alveolar edema (noncardiogenic pulmonary edema) and atelectasis. Severe $\dot{V}/\dot{Q}$ mismatch and shunting of blood occur as blood flows through alveoli that are collapsed or filled with fluid. Diffusion limitations and impairment may occur because of thickening of alveolar-capillary interfaces. Hypoxia and subsequent severe hypoxemia that is refractory to increasing concentrations of O_2 (refractory hypoxemia) develop.

The lungs become stiff and less compliant because of the loss of surfactant, interstitial edema, and alveolar collapse. Large inspiratory pressures must be generated by the respiratory muscles to inflate the noncompliant lungs. Changes in airway resistance also increase respiratory work. The work of breathing is greatly increased and the functional residual capacity (FRC) is decreased as a result of alveolar collapse, alveolar filling, and interstitial thickening.

Both hypoxemia and the stimulation of juxtacapillary receptors in the stiff lung parenchyma (J reflex) cause an increase in respiratory frequency and decreased V_T. This change results in alveolar hyperventilation, which causes increased removal of CO_2. The alveolar hyperventilation and a reflexive increase in cardiac output attempt to compensate for the severe hypoxemia. As alveoli collapse and fill with fluid, however, increased shunting of blood occurs, and alveolar hypoventilation and symptoms of decreased cardiac output and decreased tissue perfusion develop.

Reparative or Proliferative Phase. The reparative or proliferative phase begins 1 to 2 weeks after the initial lung injury. During this phase, there is an influx of granulocytes, monocytes, and lymphocytes and fibroblast proliferation as part of the inflammatory response. The injured lung has an immense regenerative capacity after acute lung injury.

The proliferative phase is complete when the diseased lung becomes characterized by dense, fibrous tissue. Increased pulmonary vascular resistance and pulmonary hypertension may occur in this stage secondary to fibroblasts and inflammatory cells, obliterating the pulmonary vasculature. Lung compliance continues to decrease as a result of interstitial fibrosis. Hypoxemia worsens because of the thickened alveolar membrane, causing diffusion defects and shunting. If the reparative phase persists, widespread fibrosis results; if the proliferative phase is arrested, the lesions resolve.

Fibrotic Phase. The fibrotic phase occurs approximately 2 to 3 weeks after the initial lung injury. This phase is also called the *chronic* or *late phase* of ARDS. By this time the lung is completely remodeled by sparsely collagenous and fibrous tissues. There is diffuse scarring and fibrosis, resulting in decreased lung compliance. In addition, the surface area for gas exchange is significantly reduced because the interstitium is fibrotic, and therefore hypoxemia continues. Pulmonary hypertension results from pulmonary vascular obliteration and fibrosis.

Clinical Progression

Progression of ARDS varies among patients. Some persons survive the acute phase of lung injury; the pulmonary edema resolves and the patient completely recovers in a few days. Others go on to the fibrotic (late or chronic) stage, requiring long-term mechanical ventilation, and chance of survival is poor. It is not known why the injured lungs repair and recover in some patients, and in others ARDS progresses. Several factors seem to be important in determining the course of ARDS, including the nature of the initial injury, extent and severity of coexisting diseases, and the pulmonary complications related to intensive care.

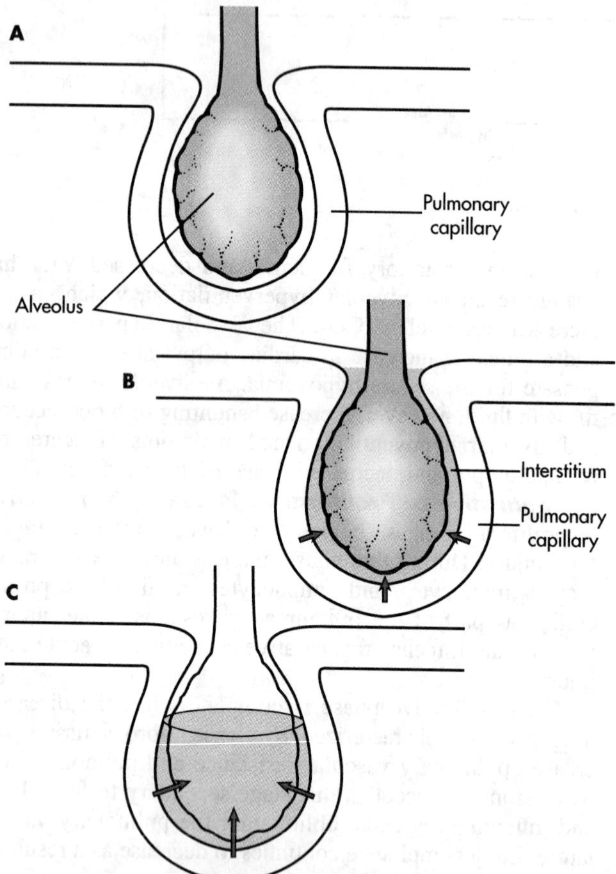

Fig. 26-7 Stages of edema formation in acute respiratory distress syndrome. ***A,*** Normal alveolus and pulmonary capillary. ***B,*** Interstitial edema occurs with increased flow of fluid into the interstitial space. ***C,*** Alveolar edema occurs when the fluid crosses the blood-gas barrier.

Clinical Manifestations

At the time of the initial injury and for several hours to 1 to 2 days afterward, the patient may not experience respiratory symptoms. The initial presentation of ARDS is often insidious. The patient may exhibit dyspnea, tachypnea, cough, and restlessness. Chest auscultation may be normal or reveal fine, scattered crackles. ABG analysis usually demonstrates mild hypoxemia and respiratory alkalosis. The alkalosis results from the compensatory increase in alveolar ventilation. The chest x-ray may be normal or exhibit evidence of minimal scattered interstitial infiltrates. Edema may not show on the x-ray until there is a 30% increase in fluid content in the lung.[12]

As ARDS progresses, symptoms develop related to increased fluid accumulation in the lung and decreased lung compliance. Respiratory discomfort becomes evident as the work of breathing increases. Noisy tachypneic and hyperpneic respirations, as well as intercostal and suprasternal retractions, may be present. Pulmonary function tests in ARDS reveal decreased compliance and decreased lung volumes, particularly FRC. Tachycardia, diaphoresis, changes in sensorium with decreased mentation, cyanosis, and pallor may be present. Chest auscultation usually reveals scattered to diffuse crackles and rhonchi. The chest x-ray demonstrates diffuse and extensive bilateral interstitial and alveolar infiltrates. A pulmonary artery catheter is inserted to determine whether the cause of the pulmonary edema is cardiogenic. The diagnosis of ARDS or noncardiogenic pulmonary edema is confirmed if the pulmonary capillary wedge pressure is within normal limits. Typically, pulmonary artery pressures increase.

Progressive arterial hypoxemia, despite increased FIO_2 by mask, cannula, or endotracheal tube, is a *hallmark* of ARDS (Table 26-10). This development is referred to as *refractory hypoxemia*. The $D(A\text{-}a)O_2$ (the alveolar-arterial oxygen difference), or the difference between PAO_2 and PaO_2, can be as high as 200 to 500 mm Hg (normal <15 to 25 mm Hg). A calculated $\dot{Q}_S/\dot{Q}_T$ more than 30% of the cardiac output and an a/A ratio of less than 0.3 are other diagnostic signs. ABG values may demonstrate a normal $PaCO_2$ despite severe dyspnea and hypoxemia. An elevated $PaCO_2$ signifies that the patient is no longer able to compensate in response to hypoxemia and other stimuli.

As ARDS progresses it is associated with profound respiratory distress requiring endotracheal intubation and assisted ventilation. Bronchial breath sounds are frequently

Table 26-10 Diagnostic Findings in Acute Respiratory Distress Syndrome

Hypoxemia Severe refractory hypoxemia (a/A ratio of <0.3)

Chest x-ray Diffuse bilateral interstitial and alveolar infiltrates

Pulmonary capillary wedge pressure <18 cm H_2O (excluding left ventricular failure)

Decreased lung compliance High ventilatory pressures

associated with this stage. The chest x-ray is often termed "white out" or "white lung," because consolidation and coalescing infiltrates pervade the lungs, leaving few recognizable air spaces. Pleural effusions also may be present.[13] Severe hypoxemia, hypercapnia, and metabolic acidosis, with symptoms of target organ or tissue hypoxia, may ensue if prompt therapy is not instituted.

Complications

Complications (Table 26-11) may develop as a result of ARDS itself or treatment. The major cause of death in ARDS is MODS, often accompanied by sepsis. The organs most commonly involved are the kidneys, liver, and heart; the systems most often involved are the CNS, hematologic, and GI systems.

Nosocomial pneumonia is a frequent complication of acute respiratory failure, occurring in 20% of mechanically ventilated patients and in as many as 68% of patients with ARDS.[13] Risk factors predisposing to nosocomial infections include impaired host defenses, contaminated support equipment or invasive monitoring devices, and colonization of the respiratory tract. In addition, organisms can be transmitted by a health care provider in contact with the patient. Gastric colonization aspiration or reflux, with subsequent tracheal appearance of gastric organisms, has been found in patients on H_2 blockers (e.g., cimetidine [Tagamet]) or antacids. Frequent monitoring of sputum smears and cultures and the quality, quantity, and consistency of sputum should be assessed. The presence of fever warrants a work-up to determine the source of infection. Serial chest x-rays and blood cell counts with a WBC differential must be closely monitored.

Table 26-11 Complications Associated with Acute Respiratory Distress Syndrome

Infection	**Renal Complications**
Nosocomial pneumonia	**Cardiac Complications**
Catheter-related infection	Decreased cardiac output
Sepsis (bacteremia)	Dysrhythmias
Respiratory Complications	**Hematologic Complications**
Pulmonary emboli	Anemia
Pulmonary barotrauma (e.g., pneumothorax, pneumomediastinum, subcutaneous emphysema)	Thrombocytopenia
	Disseminated intravascular coagulation
O_2 toxicity	**CNS Complications**
Pulmonary fibrosis	**Endotracheal Intubation Complications**
Gastrointestinal Complications	Laryngeal ulceration
Stress ulceration and hemorrhage	Tracheal ulceration
Ileus	Tracheal malacia
Pneumoperitoneum	Tracheal stenosis

CNS, Central nervous system.

The diagnosis of pneumonia is difficult, especially in a patient with diffuse infiltrates already present. The distinction between tracheobronchial colonization and pneumonia is not readily apparent. New techniques and technologies have improved diagnostic sensitivity. These include quantitative cultures obtained from the use of a protected specimen brush that bypasses the upper airway or bronchoalveolar lavage (BAL) with bronchoscopy.[14]

Observing and changing vascular cannula sites as necessary may prevent sepsis. All stopcocks should be capped or covered and old blood flushed from them to prevent bacterial contamination and growth.

Barotrauma or volutrauma in a mechanically ventilated patient (caused by rupture of overdistended alveoli) results in the presence of alveolar air in locations where it is not usually found. Clinical manifestations of this air collection or barotrauma are pulmonary interstitial emphysema, pneumothorax, subcutaneous emphysema, pneumoperitoneum, pneumomediastinum, and tension pneumothorax. Risk factors for barotrauma include high ventilator tidal volumes and high inflation and inspiratory airway pressures secondary to low lung compliance and PEEP. High levels of intrinsic or auto PEEP may predispose to barotrauma as well. The mean airway pressure appears to be a major determinant of barotrauma. A growing body of evidence, however, suggests that lung volume or lung overdistention is a more important variable as a determinant of barotrauma.

Patient symptoms of barotrauma may include agitation, worsening hypoxemia, and hypotension. Cardiovascular collapse may indicate a tension pneumothorax. It is important to monitor peak and mean airway pressures and also to feel for subcutaneous emphysema as evidenced by crepitation in the patient's neck, face, chest, axillae, and abdomen. X-ray evaluation is necessary to make the diagnosis of barotrauma. Pneumothorax is treated as discussed in Chapter 24. Other manifestations of barotrauma are closely monitored and lower inflation pressures are maintained.

Stress ulcers, occurring most frequently in the fundus of the stomach, develop in a majority of critically ill patients with acute respiratory failure. Bleeding from these ulcers occurs more frequently in ARDS than in other causes of acute respiratory failure. Bleeding occurs in 30% of ventilated patients compared to only 3% of nonventilated patients.[14] Management strategies include correction of predisposing conditions such as hypotension, shock, and acidosis. Prophylactic management includes either monotherapy or combination therapy with antacids, histamine-receptor blockers (e.g., cimetidine or ranitidine), sucralfate, and enteral nutrition. Close assessment of the patient for signs of active and occult bleeding is important. Emesis, nasogastric drainage, and stools should be tested for the presence of blood. The hematocrit levels should be monitored.

Disseminated intravascular coagulation (DIC) may occur with ARDS. (The pathophysiology of DIC is discussed in Chapter 28.) Frequent monitoring of platelet counts, fibrinogen level, and partial thromboplastin and prothrombin times is helpful in the early detection of DIC. Observation and assessment of bleeding from venipuncture sites and mucous membranes and during endotracheal suction are important. The patient also should be observed for the presence of bruises and petechiae.

Renal failure and abnormalities of sodium and water balance can occur because of the effects of hypoxemia, hypercapnia, and acidosis on renal function. Other causes of renal failure include hypotension, shock, and nephrotoxic drugs such as aminoglycosides and radiographic contrast medium. The mortality rate is near 80% for the patient with acute respiratory failure who develops renal failure.[14] The urinary system also can be a source of sepsis. Fluid excess secondary to increased antidiuretic hormone occurs in approximately 50% of patients with acute respiratory failure. Renal function should be regularly assessed by monitoring blood urea nitrogen, serum creatinine levels, daily weights, and intake and output.

THERAPEUTIC AND NURSING MANAGEMENT

ACUTE RESPIRATORY DISTRESS SYNDROME

Nursing Assessment

Because ARDS causes acute respiratory failure, the subjective and objective data that should be obtained from a person with ARDS are the same as that for acute respiratory failure (see Table 26-6).

Nursing Diagnoses

Nursing diagnoses are determined when the problem and etiologic factors are supported by clinical data. Nursing diagnoses related to ARDS may include, but are not limited to, those described for acute respiratory failure and are presented in the nursing care plan on p. 740.

Planning

The overall goals are that the patient with ARDS will have (1) a PaO_2 within limits of normal for age, (2) SaO_2 greater than 90%, (3) patent airway, and (4) clear lungs on auscultation.

Nursing Implementation

Preventive measures for ARDS include those for acute respiratory failure. Astute observation of the respiratory status of a patient at increased risk is especially important. Judicious fluid administration and monitoring of the fluid status by intake and output records, weights, clinical manifestations of increased fluid in the lung (e.g., crackles, deteriorating ABGs, increased work of breathing), and body fluid accumulation (e.g., jugular venous distention; sacral, periorbital, or peripheral edema; hepatomegaly; splenomegaly) are important. Expeditious treatment of the initial disorder (e.g., prompt treatment with antibiotics or surgery to remove the source of infection in sepsis and maintenance of BP and renal blood flow in shock) is necessary and may prevent further deterioration of the patient and the development of ARDS and subsequent MODS.

At the time of the initial lung injury and for as long as 12 to 48 hours thereafter, the patient may be free of respiratory symptoms or signs of distress. Usually, abnormal findings on physical examination are indications that ARDS has progressed beyond the initial stages. Prompt recognition of clinical manifestations and treatment may help to prevent the development of ARDS.

Table 26-12 Principles of Therapeutic Management of ARDS

- Identify and treat underlying condition
- Establish an airway (usually endotracheal tube)
- Institute mechanical ventilation
  - Volume-cycled ventilator
  - PEEP
- Maintain oxygenation
  - O_2 administration
  - Packed RBCs
- Increase cardiac output and maintain blood pressure
  - Dolbutamine
  - Dopamine
- Monitor oxygenation and cardiac output
  - Arterial line
  - Pulmonary artery catheter
  - Oximetry
- Maintain fluid balance
  - Colloids, crystalloids
  - Diuretics
- Treat infections

ARDS, Acute respiratory distress syndrome; *PEEP*, positive end expiratory pressure; *RBCs*, red blood cells.

Management of ARDS includes many of the therapeutic and nursing regimens used in acute respiratory failure. Measures to improve alveolar ventilation and maintain adequate PaO_2 in the management of acute respiratory failure also apply to ARDS. Many therapeutic and nursing therapies, however, are unique to ARDS (Table 26-12).

Treatment of the Underlying Disorder. Sepsis is often an initiating mechanism of ARDS. Prompt culture of exudates, secretions, and blood and surgical débridement (if indicated) of an infected area are necessary. Antibiotic therapy should be instituted as soon as possible.

If severe arterial hypotension and shock are the initiating factors, restoration of adequate BP is essential. Frequently, overzealous administration of fluids in the attempt to restore BP leads to circulatory overload and pulmonary edema. Other conditions contributing to ARDS are presented in Table 26-8.

Maintenance of Adequate Oxygenation. O_2 administration through a face mask or nasal cannula (prongs) is usually inadequate to treat the refractory hypoxemia of ARDS. The rule of thumb for O_2 administration is to give the patient the lowest concentration of O_2 in inspired air that suffices to maintain a PaO_2 of approximately 60 mm Hg. When the FIO_2 concentration exceeds 0.5 for more than a few days, O_2 toxicity is virtually inevitable.

Endotracheal intubation with subsequent mechanical ventilation is almost always required. Lower tidal volumes and higher respiratory rates may help to decrease peak airway pressures, thus decreasing the risk of barotrauma. The respiratory rate of the ventilator is set to keep the pH at

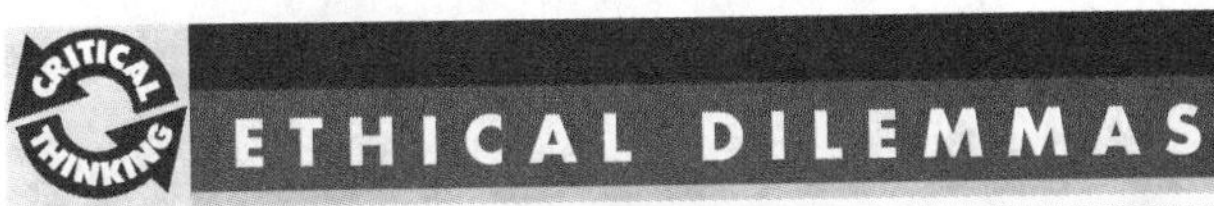

ENTITLEMENT TO TREATMENT

Situation A 35-year-old European tourist had a hang-gliding accident while touring the United States. He is taken to the emergency department of the regional trauma center for treatment of internal injuries, loss of blood, and severe pelvic fractures. He has become septic with a rare organism, is now in renal failure, and has acute respiratory distress syndrome. Despite a 5% to 6% chance of survival, his wife and parents want all possible measures to be taken.

Discussion He is not a U.S. resident or citizen, was intentionally involved in a (potentially) dangerous activity, and has no insurance coverage. According to federal law a patient may not be refused admission to an emergency department for acute care. His family believes that his condition entitles him to treatment. His overall prognosis is grim, but his individual conditions can be treated with modern technology and expensive antibiotics. There is still a question about the futility of continuing his treatment. The hospital may be left with an enormous uncompensated bill for this patient, whether or not he survives. Many hospitals suffer the same dilemma with U.S. residents and citizens who are unable to pay for their treatment.

ETHICAL AND LEGAL PRINCIPLES

- Under the Emergency Medical Treatment and Labor Act (also known as COBRA Act), hospitals receiving federal money under Medicare must provide emergency screening and treatment to stabilize a patient before transfer to another facility.
- The Hill-Burton Act requires states to provide sufficient hospitals and necessary services for those unable to pay.
- Medically futile treatment need not be offered by the hospital. If the family or patient demands obviously futile treatment, the medical team should seek clarification of the goals of such treatment (i.e., recovery, survival, continuing biologic existence, nonabandonment of the patient.) There is no legal right to require medical treatment in cases where the treatment goals cannot be met.

7.35 to 7.45 and to prevent alkalosis, which may impair O_2 unloading at the tissue level, depress cardiac output, and initiate dysrhythmias.

When adequate oxygenation is not achieved by conventional mechanical ventilation and when the PaO_2 remains less than 60 mm Hg with an FIO_2 of more than 0.5 to 0.6, the use of PEEP is indicated. PEEP is a ventilatory maneuver that applies positive pressure to the airway and lungs at the end of exhalation. Expiration normally occurs when the pressure in the chest becomes equal to atmospheric pressure or zero. When positive pressure is applied to the lung at the end of expiration, the lung is kept partially expanded and the alveoli are prevented from totally collapsing. The mechanism of action of PEEP is related to its ability to recruit or open up collapsed alveoli and increase the FRC. It also acts in this way to decrease shunting and improve oxygenation and lung compliance. O_2 delivery and $\dot{Q}_s/\dot{Q}_T$ may be monitored to help determine appropriate levels of PEEP.

Pressure control ventilation, inverse ratio ventilation, high frequency ventilation, and permissive hypercapnia (low tidal volumes that allow $PaCO_2$ to increase slowly, maintaining normal pH and low airway pressures) are all ventilatory techniques that have been used in ARDS. For a discussion of mechanical ventilation, see Chapter 61.

Extracorporeal membrane oxygenation (ECMO) and extracorporeal CO_2 removal ($ECCO_2R$) pass blood across a gas-exchanging membrane outside the body and then return oxygenated blood back to the body. $ECCO_2R$ with low frequency positive pressure ventilation allows the lung to heal while the lung is not functional.[15]

Maintenance of Cardiac Output and Hemoglobin Concentration. Continuous hemodynamic monitoring of the patient with ARDS who is receiving ventilator and PEEP therapy is required. An arterial line should be inserted to obtain continuous recording of BP and to make it easier to obtain frequent ABG measurements. (Specific nursing measures for the patient with an indwelling arterial cannula are discussed in Chapter 61.)

Cardiac output can be assessed by the thermodilution port of the pulmonary artery catheter. Mixed venous O_2 samples also can be obtained from the distal part of the catheter. Calculation of the arterial venous oxygen $(A - V)O_2$ difference can be performed by determining PvO_2. The $(A - V)O_2$ is the difference in the O_2 content of arterial and mixed venous blood. This value gives an indication of cardiac output if thermodilution is not available. The normal $(A - V)O_2$ difference is 4.5 volume % to 6 volume %, and an $(A - V)O_2$ difference of more than 6 volume % suggests impaired O_2 delivery. It is important to be able to assess cardiac output accurately by using one of these methods to determine the effects of PEEP and other therapies on the patient's cardiopulmonary status.

If cardiac output falls, it may be necessary to administer fluids or colloid solutions or to lower PEEP. Use of inotropic drugs such as dolbutamine (Dolbutrex) or dopamine (Intropin) also may be necessary.

The hemoglobin is usually kept at levels of more than 9 to 10 g/dl (90 to 100g/L) with an adequate saturation of more than 90% (when PaO_2 is more than 50 to 60 mm Hg). Packed RBCs may be administered to increase the O_2-carrying capacity of the blood.

Maintenance of Fluid Balance. Maintenance of fluid balance is precarious in the patient with ARDS. Leaky capillaries increase fluid in the lungs and cause pulmonary edema. However, the patient may be volume depleted and prone to hypotension and decreased cardiac output from mechanical ventilation and PEEP.

Generally, diuretics are used to treat the patient. The pulmonary capillary wedge pressure (which indicates the fluid status of the left side of the heart) is kept as low as possible without impairing cardiac output. The patient is

CRITICAL THINKING EXERCISES

CASE STUDY

ACUTE RESPIRATORY DISTRESS SYNDROME

Patient Profile

Mr. J. is a 65-year-old man who was admitted to the surgical intensive care unit after surgery for multiple gunshot wounds in the abdomen. He had extensive abdominal surgery during which he received a combination of 8 units of packed red blood cells and whole blood. He has a pulmonary artery catheter in place.

Subjective Data

- Complains of shortness of breath

Objective Data

Physical Examination

- BP 100/60
- Pulse 120 bpm
- Respirations 30/min

Diagnostic Studies

- Chest x-ray: Diffuse alveolar infiltrates
  Pulmonary capillary wedge pressure 7-10 mm Hg

Arterial Blood Gases (on 0.4 FIO_2)

- pH 7.1
- PaO_2 65 mm Hg
- $PaCO_2$ 50 mm Hg
- O_2 saturation 85%
- Has not responded to increasing concentrations of O_2

Therapeutic Management

- Endotracheal intubation
- Mechanical ventilation

Critical Thinking Questions

1. Briefly discuss the pathophysiology of ARDS as it relates to the systemic inflammatory response syndrome and multiple organ dysfunction syndrome.
2. How is ARDS different from cardiogenic pulmonary edema?
3. What are possible causes of ARDS in Mr. J.?
4. Why does the patient with ARDS not increase PaO_2 in response to higher FIO_2 ?
5. Based on the assessment data presented, write one or more appropriate nursing diagnoses. Are there any collaborative problems?

usually placed on mild fluid restriction, and diuretics are used as necessary. The patient is maintained with strict intake and output and daily weights. Electrolytes and fluid status are monitored.

Future Trends in Pharmacologic Therapy

During the last ten years pharmacologic agents to treat ARDS have been researched extensively. Monoclonal antibodies are being studied for their effects in binding endotoxin and interleukins, thus limiting or preventing mediator-induced damage to the alveolar capillary endothelium. Prostaglandin E_1 (PGE_1), a vasodilator, is being studied for its use in decreasing systemic and pulmonary vascular resistance. Inhaled nitric oxide (NO) is another vasodilator currently being studied for its effects on decreasing pulmonary artery pressure and improving oxygenation. Surfactant, a lipid-protein complex produced by alveolar type II cells, which decreases surface tension and maintains lung compliance, is also being used in ARDS. Surfactant replacement therapy has been effective in respiratory distress syndrome in infants. The use of corticosteroids in the acute phase of ARDS has not proven beneficial in multicentered trials. The use of steroids in the chronic phases of ARDS, however, may be indicated if the patient is not responding to conventional treatment.

REVIEW QUESTIONS

The number of the question corresponds to the same-numbered objective at the beginning of the chapter.

1. Which of the following is *not* a cause of type I hypoxemic respiratory failure?

a. $\dot{V}/\dot{Q}$ mismatch
b. Shunting
c. Diffusion abnormalities
d. Alveolar hyperventilation

2. Which of the following may enhance ventilation in the patient with expiratory wheezing and prolonged exhalation?

a. Bronchodilator administration (IV, aerosol)
b. Ultrasonic nebulization with normal saline solution
c. Aerosolized acetylcysteine (Mucomyst)
d. Administration of a large volume of IV fluids

3. The most common early clinical manifestations of ARDS that the nurse may observe are

a. cyanosis and apprehension.
b. dyspnea and tachypnea.
c. respiratory distress and frothy sputum.
d. hypotension and tachycardia.

4. Which of the following is true concerning fluid management in the stable ARDS patient?

a. Pulmonary capillary wedge pressure is maintained at high levels.
b. Pulmonary capillary wedge pressure is kept as low as possible without impairing cardiac output.
c. Diuretics and fluid restriction are rarely used.
d. Frequent and vigorous administration of salt-poor albumin is used.

REFERENCES

1. Carpenter K: A comprehensive review of cyanosis, *Crit Care Nurse* 13:66, 1993.
2. Grossbach I: Case studies in pulse oximetry monitoring, *Crit Care Nurse* 13:63, 1993.
3. Shapiro BA and others: *Clinical applications of respiratory care,* ed 4, St Louis, 1991, Mosby.
4. White BS and Roberts SL: Powerlessness and the pulmonary alveolar edema patient, *Dimens Crit Care Nurs* 12:127, 1993.
5. Callaghan and others: Minitracheostomy: an alternative to "blind" endotrachael suctioning, *Dimens Crit Care Nurs* 13:38, 1994.
6. Meyer T, Hill N: Noninvasive positive pressure ventilation to treat respiratory failure, *Ann Intern Med* 120:760, 1994.
7. Freichels T: Palliative ventilatory support: use of noninvasive positive pressure ventilation in terminal respiratory insufficiency, *Am J Crit Care* 3:6, 1994.
8. Bone RC and others: Definitions for sepsis and organ failure and guidelines for the use of innovative therapies in sepsis, *Chest* 101:1644, 1992.
9. Beal C: Multiple organ failure syndrome in the 1990s, *JAMA* 271:226, 1994.
10. Thijs LG: Septic shock: etiology, clinical manifestations, pathophysiology, and treatment. In Bone R, editor: *Pulmonary and critical care medicine,* vol 2, St Louis, 1993-1994, Mosby.
11. Suchyta MR and others: The adult respiratory distress syndrome—a report of survival and modifying factors, *Chest* 101:1074, 1992.
12. George R and others: *Chest medicine: essentials of pulmonary and critical care medicine,* ed 2, New York, 1990, Williams & Wilkins.
13. Bone R: The acute respiratory distress syndrome (ARDS). In Bone R, editor: *Pulmonary and critical care medicine,* vol 2, St Louis, 1993-1994, Mosby.
14. Pingleton S: Management of complications of acute respiratory failure. In Bone R, editor: *Pulmonary and critical care medicine,* vol 2, St Louis, 1993-1994, Mosby.
15. Atkins PJ, Egloff ME, Wilms DC: Respiratory consequences of multisystem crisis: the adult respiratory distress syndrome, *Crit Care Nurs Q* 16:27, 1994.

SECTION V BIBLIOGRAPHY

Books

Bordow RA, Moser KM: *Manual of clinical problems in pulmonary medicine,* Boston, 1991, Little, Brown.

Dettenmeier PA: *Pulmonary nursing care,* St Louis, 1992, Mosby.

Eubanks DH, Bone RC: *Comprehensive respiratory care, A learning system,* St Louis, 1990, Mosby.

Fishman A, editor: *Pulmonary diseases and disorders,* ed 3, New York, 1992, McGraw-Hill.

Harrington G: *The asthma self-care book,* New York, 1991, Harper Collins.

Hogshead N, Couzans G: *Asthma and exercise,* New York, 1991, Henry Holt.

Karetzky M, Cunha BA, Brandsetter RD: *The pneumonias,* New York, 1993, Springer-Verlag.

Khan MG: *Cardiac and pulmonary management,* London, 1993, Lea & Febiger.

McPherson SP: *Respiratory therapy equipment,* ed 4, St Louis, 1990, Mosby.

Schlossberg D: *Tuberculosis,* ed 3, New York, 1994, Springer-Verlag.

Moser K and others, editors: *Shortness of breath, a guide to better living and breathing,* ed 4, St Louis, 1991, Mosby.

Traver GA, Mitchell JT, Flodquist-Priestley: *Respiratory care. A clinical approach,* Gaithersburg, MD, 1991, Aspen.

Weilitz PB: *Pocket guide to respiratory care,* St Louis, 1991, Mosby.

West JB: *Pulmonary pathophysiology: the essentials,* ed 4, Philadelphia, 1992, Williams & Wilkins.

West JB: *Respiratory physiology: the essentials,* ed 4, Baltimore, 1990, Williams & Wilkins.

Wilkins RL, Sheldon RL, Krider SJ: *Clinical assessment in respiratory care,* ed 2, St Louis, 1990, Mosby.

Journals

Anderson B: Inability to sustain spontaneous ventilation, *Nurs Diagn* 3:164, 1992.

Atkins PJ, Egloff ME, Willms DC: Respiratory consequences of multisystem crisis: the adult respiratory distress syndrome, *Crit Care Nurs Q* 16:27, 1994.

Barnes G, Betts AV: Asthma explained, *Nurs Stand* 6:9, 1992.

*Bjerklie S, Ferketich S, Benner P: Predicting the outcomes of living with asthma, *Res Nurs Health* 16: 241, 1993.

*Blackler P, Sinclair D: Audit of inhaled asthma therapy, *Nurs Stand* 7:28, 1993.

Bouley GH, Froman R, Shah H: The experience of dyspnea during weaning, *Heart Lung* 21:471, 1992.

*Breslin EH and others: Standardization of a device to measure unsupported arm exercise endurance in chronic obstructive pulmonary disease, *Nurs Res* 41:292, 1992.

*Breslin EH, Roy C, Robinson CR: Physiological nursing research in dyspnea: a paradigm shift and a metaparadigm exemplar, *Scholar Inq Nurs Pract* 6:81, 1992.

Brockopp DY and others: Nursing knowledge: acute postoperative pain management in the elderly, *J Gerontol Nurs* 19:31, 1993.

Brown RL, Wessel J, Warner BW: Nutrition considerations in the neonatal extracorporeal life support patient, *Nutr Clin Pract* 9:22, 1994.

*Bruera E, Schoeller T, MacEachern T: Symptomatic benefit of supplemental oxygen in hypoxemic patients with terminal cancer: the use of the N of 1 randomized controlled trial, *J Pain Symptom Manage* 7:365, 1992.

Busse W: Asthma in the 1990s, *Postgrad Med* 92:177, 1992.

Carpenter KD: A comprehensive review of cyanosis, *Crit Care Nurse* 13:66, 1993.

Chapman KR: Diagnostic dilemmas in obstructive airway disease, *Hosp Pract* 28:71, 1993.

*Dirkes S, Dickinson S, Valentine J: Acute respiratory failure and ECMO, *Crit Care Nurse* 12:39, 1992.

Elpern EH, Girzadas AM: Tuberculosis update: new challenges of an old disease, *MEDSURG Nurs* 2:176, 1993.

Etches RC: Respiratory depression associated with patient-controlled analgesia: a review of eight cases, *Can J Anaesth* 41:125, 1994.

*Nursing research-based articles.

*Ferrell-Torry AT, Glick OJ: The use of therapeutic massage as a nursing intervention to modify anxiety and the perception of cancer pain, *Cancer Nurs* 16:93, 1993.

*Fiorentini A: Potential hazards of tracheobronchial suctioning, *Intensive Crit Care Nurs* 8:217, 1992.

*Fleming BM, Coombs DW: A survey of complications documented in a quality-control analysis of patient-controlled analgesia in the postoperative patient, *J Pain Symptom Manage* 7:463, 1992.

*Folden SL: Definitions of health and health goals of participants in a community-based pulmonary rehabilitation program, *Public Health Nurs* 10:31, 1993.

Franklin RA: Smoking, *Nurs Clin North Am* 27:631, 1992.

*Gift AG, Austin DJ: The effects of a program of systemic movement on COPD patients, *Rehabil Nurs* 17:6, 1992.

*Gift AG, Moore T, Soeken K: Relaxation to reduce dyspnea and anxiety in COPD patients, *Nurs Res* 41:242, 1992.

*Grant JP: Nutrition care of patients with acute and chronic respiratory failure, *Nutr Clin Pract* 9:11, 1994.

*Hanania NA and others: Medical personnel's knowledge of and ability to use inhaling devices. Metered-dose inhalers, spacing chambers, and breath-activated dry powder inhalers, *Chest* 105:111, 1994.

Hayden RA: What keeps oxygenation on track? *Am J Nurs* 92:32, 1992.

Hess D, Kacmarek RM: Techniques and devices for monitoring oxygenation, *Respir Care* 38:646, 1993.

Hough A: Making sense of sputum retention, *Nurs Times* 88:33, 1992.

Hudson LD: Pharmacologic approaches to respiratory failure, *Respir Care* 38:754, 1993.

Hunter FC, Mitchell S: Managing ARDS, *RN* 56:52, 1993.

*Innes MH: Management of an inadequately ventilated patient, *Br J Nurs* 1:780, 1992.

*Innes MH: Managing upper airway obstruction, *Br J Nurs* 1:732, 1992.

*Janson-Bjerklie S and others: Clinical markers of asthma severity and risk: importance of subjective as well as objective factors, *Heart Lung* 21:265, 1992.

*Janson-Bjerklie S, Ferketich S, Benner P: Predicting the outcomes of living with asthma, *Res Nurs Health* 16:241, 1993.

Jordon K: Chest trauma. How to detect and react to, *Nursing* 20:34, 1990.

*Kayser FH: Changes in the spectrum of organisms causing respiratory tract infections: a review, *Postgrad Med J* 68(suppl 3):17, 1992.

Kearney ML: Adult respiratory distress syndrome following thoracic trauma, *Crit Care Nurs Clin North Am* 5:723, 1993.

Kendrick AH, Smith EC: Respiratory measurements. 2: Interpreting simple measurements of lung function, *Prof Nurse* 7:748, 1992.

*Kerr ME, Brucia J: Hyperventilation in the head-injured patient: an effective treatment modality? *Heart Lung* 22:516, 1993.

*Knebel AR: When weaning from mechanical ventilation fails, *Am J Crit Care* 1:19, 1992.

Lowry PW, Tompkins LS: Nosocomial legionellosis: a review of pulmonary and extrapulmonary syndromes, *Am J Infect Control* 21:21, 1993.

Malseed RT, Wilson BA: Isoniazid and rifampin therapy for tuberculosis: what patients need to know, *MEDSURG Nurs* 2:236, 1993.

*Narsavage GL, Weaver TE: Physiologic status, coping, and hardiness as predictors of outcomes in chronic obstructive pulmonary disease, *Nurs Res* 43:90, 1994.

Pasero CL, McCaffrey M: Avoiding opioid-induced respiratory depression, *Am J Nurs* 94(4):24, 1994.

*Rosenberg T, Manfreda J, Hershfield ES: Two-step tuberculin testing in staff and residents of a nursing home, *Am Rev Respir Dis* 148:1537, 1993.

*Rutten-Van Molken MPMH, VanDooreslaer EKA, Rutten FFH: Economic appraisal of asthma and COPD care: a literature review 1980-1991, *Soc Sci Med* 35:161, 1992.

Salerno M, Huss K, Huss RW: Allergen avoidance in the treatment of dust-mite allergy and asthma, *Nurse Pract* 17:53, 1992.

*Sarna L and others: Nutritional intake, weight change, symptom distress, and functional status over time in adults with lung cancer, *Oncol Nurs Forum* 20:481, 1993.

Sharp JA: Which peak flow meter? *Nurs Times* 89:61, 1993.

*Sheehan DK and others: Level of cancer pain knowledge among baccalaureate student nurses, *J Pain Symptom Manage* 7:478, 1992.

*Spessert CK, Weilitz PB, Goodenberger DM: A protocol for initiation of nasal positive pressure ventilation, *Am J Crit Care* 2:54, 1993.

Stiesmeyer JK: A four-step approach to pulmonary assessment, *Am J Nurs* 93:22, 1993.

*Tettersell MJ: Asthma patient's knowledge in relation to compliance with drug therapy, *J Adv Nurs* 18:103, 1993.

*Tittle MB, Moody L, Becker MP: Severity of illness and resource allocation in DNR patients in ICU, *Nurs Econ* 10:210, 1992.

*Weilitz PB: Weaning a patient from mechanical ventilation, *Crit Care Nurse* 13:33, 1993.

*Wigal JK, Creer TL, Kotses H: The COPD self-efficacy scale, *Chest* 99:1193, 1991.

Young NA, Gorzeman J: Managing pneumothorax and hemothorax, *Nursing* 21:56, 1991.

Yu VL: Legionnaire's disease: New understanding of community-acquired pneumonia, *Hosp Pract* 28:63, 1993.

Resources

A Newsletter for People with Asthma
123 Monticello Avenue
Annapolis, MD 21401

Alert, Well and Keeping Energetic (AWAKE), a health awareness group for patients with sleep disordered breathing. For information, write
AWAKE Network
P.O. Box 534
Bethel Park, PA 15102

Breathing Disorders: Your complete exercise guide.
Neil F. Gordan, Human Kinetics Pub.
P.O. Box 5076
Champaign, IL 61825-5076
800-747-4457

Explicit and detailed exercise guidelines for people with asthma, chronic bronchitis, and emphysema, 1993.

Breathing Disorder During Sleep, a patient-teaching booklet provided by the US Department of Health and Human Services, NIH. Publication NO. 93-2966.

Consumer Update on Asthma—Nancy Sander: 9-page layman's version of the guidelines for the Diagnosis and Management of Asthma. Issued by National Asthma Education program
P.O. Box 30105
Bethesda, MD 20824-0105

Healthlines—bimonthly newsletter for teenagers with asthma. Published by Renee Theodorakis who has founded a support group for young people called "Support for Asthmatic Youth." Call 516-625-5735 or write 1080 Glencove Avenue, Glen Head, NY 11545 for more information.

Lung Line Patients who have a question about lung disease can call 1-800-222-LUNG, a toll-free information service staffed by reg-

*Nursing research-based articles.

istered nurses with special education in respiratory care. Offered by National Jewish Center for Immunology and Respiratory Medicine, Denver, CO, Monday through Friday, 10:30 AM to 7 PM (EST). In Denver, the number is 398-1477.

Newsletter for people with asthma (free):
Allen & Hanburys Respiratory Institute
P.O. Box 1409
West Caldwell, NJ 07007-1409

Newsletter for people with asthma (free):
Schering Corporation
Proventil Advisor
P.O. Box 263
Rutherford, NJ 07070-9841

NHLBI, Asthma Reading and Resource List (60 pages, over 115 items, and indexed). Available from the National Asthma Education program
NHLBI Information Center
P.O. Box 30105
Bethesda, MD 20824-0105
301-951-3260
Single copies are free

Shower Shields can be purchased from C.L. Sheldon
P.O. Box 128
Watertown MA, 01272 (Sheldon Shower and Shampoo Shield)
or

Lost Chord Club of Southern California
c/o Richard Winter
10755 Hortense Avenue
Toluca Lake, CA 91602

Emergency identification tags can be purchased from Medic-Alert Foundation, Turlock, CA 95381-1009 or by calling (209) 634-4917. This organization provides a wallet card and identification tags.

Organizations

American Lung Association, National Headquarters
1740 Broadway
New York, NY 10019
212-315-8700

American Speech-Language-Hearing Association
10801 Rockville Pike
Rockville, MD 20852

Asthma and Allergy Foundation of America
1717 Massachusetts Avenue NW, Suite 305
Washington, DC 20036
202-265-0265

Asthma Care Association of America
P.O. Box 568
Spring Valley Road
Ossining, NY 10562
914-762-2110

Canadian Lung Association
75 Alberta, Suite 908
Ottawa, Ontario K1P 5E7
613-237-1208

Cancer Information Line and Antismoking Helpline
800-4-CANCER
800-638-6070 - Alaska
800-524-1234 - Hawaii; in Oahu, dial direct

Cystic Fibrosis Foundation
6931 Arlington Road, #200
Bethesda, MD 20814

International Association of Laryngectomees
c/o American Cancer Society
1599 Clifton Road NE
Atlanta, GA 30329

International Association of Laryngotomies (IAL)
777 Third Avenue
New York, NY 10017

Respiratory Nursing Society
5700 Old Orchard Road, 1st floor
Skokie, IL 60077-1057
708-966-8673
708-966-9418

Society of Otorhinolaryngology and Head/Neck Nurses
116 Canal Street, Suite A
New Smyrna Beach, FL 32168
904-428-1695
FAX: 904-423-7566

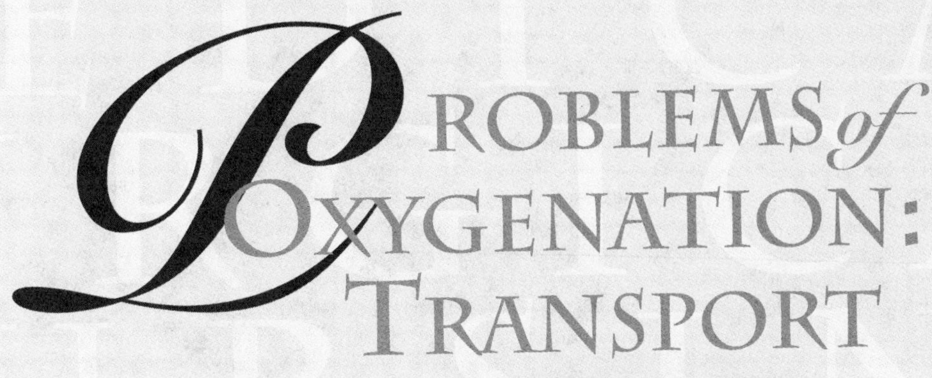

Problems of Oxygenation: Transport

Section Six

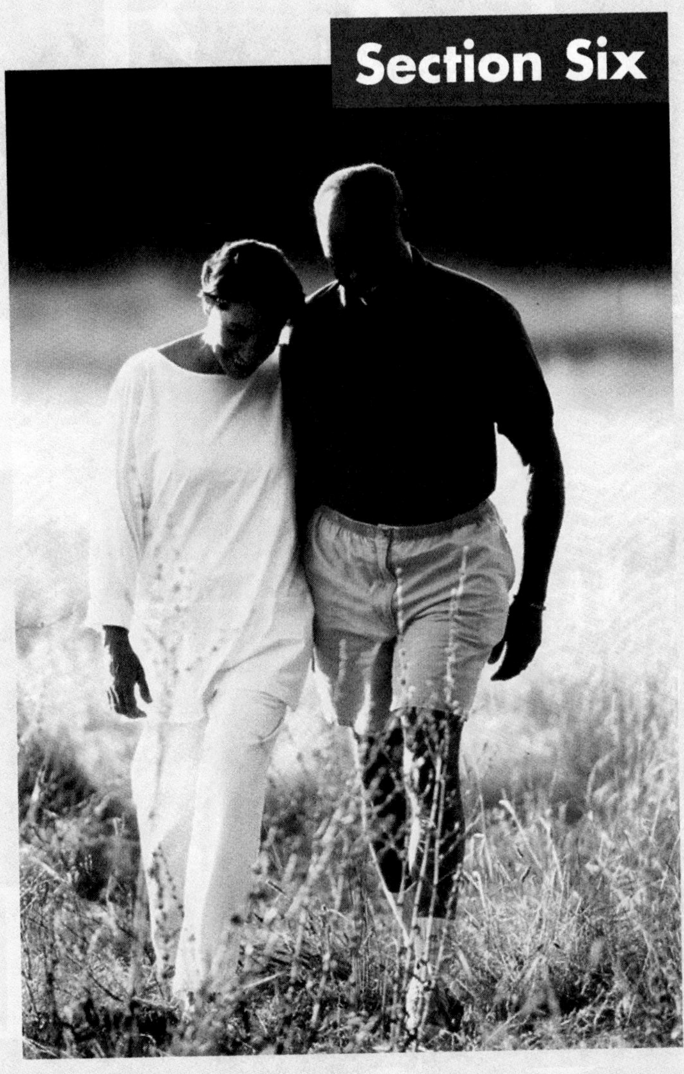

MEDICA
SURGICA
NURSIN
MEDICA
SURGICA
NURSIN
MEDICA
SURGICA
NURSIN
MEDICA
SURGICA

Chapter 27

NURSING ASSESSMENT
Hematologic System

Marie Whedon **Lynne Daly** **Bonnie Jennings**

Learning Objectives

1. Describe the structures and functions of the hematologic system.
2. Differentiate among the different types of blood cells and their functions.
3. Explain the process of hemostasis.
4. Describe the age-related changes in the hematologic system and differences in hematologic parameters.
5. Identify the significant subjective and objective assessment data related to the hematologic system that should be obtained from a patient.
6. Describe the appropriate techniques used in the physical assessment of the hematologic system.
7. Differentiate normal from common abnormal findings of a physical assessment of the hematologic system.
8. Describe the purpose, significance of results, and nursing responsibilities related to diagnostic studies of the hematologic system.

Hematology is the study of blood and blood-forming tissues. This includes the blood cells, the bone marrow, the spleen, and the lymph system. A basic knowledge of hematology is useful in clinical settings to evaluate the patient's ability to transport oxygen and carbon dioxide, coagulate blood, and combat infections. Another important homeostatic function of the blood cells is removing old and dead cells. This function is accomplished by the *mononuclear phagocyte system* (MPS). The MPS, formerly known as the reticuloendothelial system, is composed of monocytes and macrophages. The role of the MPS in phagocytosis and the immune response is described in Chapters 9 and 10.

STRUCTURES AND FUNCTIONS OF THE HEMATOLOGIC SYSTEM

Bone Marrow

Bone marrow is the soft material that fills the central core of bones. It is the blood-forming tissue that produces the three major cell components of the blood: *erythrocytes* (red blood cells [RBCs]), *leukocytes* (white blood cells [WBCs]), and *platelets.* The blood components develop from a common stem cell, but as they mature and differentiate several distinct cell types evolve (Fig. 27-1). An understanding of the function of particular blood cell types enhances the nurse's ability to interpret laboratory data.

Reviewed by Kathleen Dietz-Lovett, MA, MS, RN, Clinical Nurse Specialist, Oncology, Marstons Mills, MA.

In the fetus, most of the bone marrow actively produces blood cells. However, in the adult, active production of marrow is generally limited to the ends of long bones, vertebrae, flat cranial bones, sternum, ribs, scapulae, clavicles, pelvis, and sacrum.

Blood Cells

Erythrocytes. *Erythropoiesis,* which is the production of erythrocytes, or RBCs, is largely regulated by cellular oxygen requirements and general metabolic activity. The process of erythropoiesis is stimulated by hypoxia and controlled hormonally by *erythropoietin,* a hormone synthesized and released by the kidney. Erythropoietin stimulates the bone marrow to increase erythrocyte production. Erythropoiesis is also influenced by the availability of nutrients, with iron, vitamin B_{12}, and folic acid being the essential nutrients for erythropoiesis.[1]

Several distinct cell types evolve during erythrocyte maturation (Fig. 27-1). The *reticulocyte* is an immature erythrocyte. The reticulocyte count measures the rate at which new RBCs appear in the circulation. Reticulocytes are capable of maturing to mature erythrocytes within 48 hours of release into circulation. Therefore assessing the number of reticulocytes is a useful means of evaluating the adequacy of erythrocyte production. The functions of erythrocytes include transport of gases (both oxygen and carbon dioxide) and assistance in maintaining the acid-base balance through the buffering capability of hemoglobin.

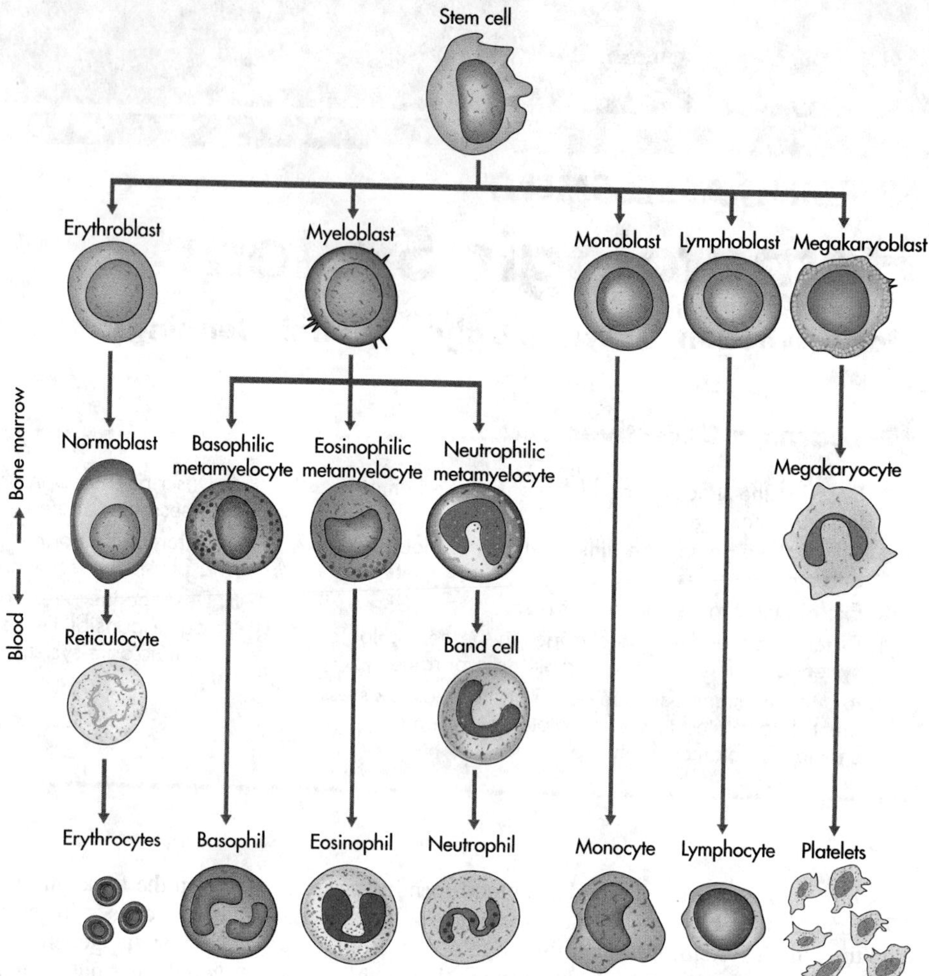

Fig. 27-1 Development of blood cells.

Hemoglobin, the major component of erythrocytes, gives them their characteristic red color when combined with oxygen. Iron and protein form the molecular structure of hemoglobin. The function of hemoglobin is to transport oxygen. Therefore, although adequate oxygen may be inspired into the lungs, it may not reach the tissues unless there is an adequate amount of hemoglobin to carry it. Consequently the significance of any type of anemia is its effect on tissue oxygenation.

Hemolysis (destruction of erythrocytes) by macrophages removes abnormal, defective, damaged, and old RBCs from circulation. Hemolysis occurs in the bone marrow, liver, and spleen, and it increases bilirubin production. The normal life span of an erythrocyte is 120 days.

Leukocytes. Leukocytes, the white cells of the blood, also develop in a series of cell types that vary in maturity (Fig. 27-1). The three general classes of mature circulating leukocytes are *granulocytes, monocytes,* and *lymphocytes.* The main function of the granulocytes and monocytes is *phagocytosis* of bacteria and foreign particles that invade the body. Phagocytosis is a process by which cells ingest or engulf any unwanted organism and then digest and kill it. The main function of lymphocytes is related to the immune response (see Chapter 10).

Granulocytes. Granulocytes, which contain granules in their cytoplasm, consist of *neutrophils, eosinophils,* and *basophils.* They are also known as *polymorphonuclear leukocytes* (PMNs).

The maturation cycle of neutrophils is shown in Fig. 27-1. Following the metamyelocyte stage, the neutrophil matures into a band or stab, followed by a mature PMN. The band or stab stage is similar to the metamyelocyte except that the nucleus has become horseshoe-shaped. Although band cells are sometimes found in the peripheral circulation of normal persons and are capable of phagocytosis, the mature neutrophil is much more effective at phagocytosis. The nucleus of the neutrophil is segmented into two to five lobes connected by thin chromatin strands, hence the nickname "segs" for these mature neutrophils.

Neutrophils have strong phagocytic activity. They are the primary phagocytic cells involved in acute inflammatory responses. *Eosinophils* have a similar but reduced ability for phagocytosis. One of their primary functions is to engulf antigen-antibody complexes formed during an allergic response. They also are able to defend against parasitic infections. *Basophils* have a limited role in phagocytosis. Their granules in the cytoplasm contain heparin, serotonin, and histamine. If a basophil is stimulated by an antigen or by tissue injury, it will respond by releasing its granules. This is part of the response seen in allergic and inflammatory reactions.

Monocytes. Monocytes are produced in the bone marrow and circulate briefly in the blood. They are large, slow-moving, potent phagocytic cells that can ingest small or large masses of matter, such as bacteria, dead cells, tissue debris, and old or defective RBCs. Monocytes are the second type of WBCs to arrive at the scene of an injury (neutrophils are the first). When monocytes leave the blood and enter and remain in the tissues, they differentiate into specialized phagocytes called *macrophages.*

In tissues, resident macrophages are given special names (e.g., Kupffer cells in the liver, osteoclasts in the bone, and alveolar macrophages in the lung). They protect the body from pathogens at these entry points and are more phagocytic than monocytes. Macrophages also interact with lymphocytes to facilitate the humoral and cellular immune responses.

Lymphocytes. Lymphocytes are produced in the bone marrow and form the basis of the cellular and humoral immune responses. Two lymphocyte subtypes are B cells and T cells. B cells mediate the humoral immune response. When B cells are stimulated by antigens, they are activated to form specialized antibody factories, called plasma cells. Plasma cells produce antibodies, also known as *immunoglobulins,* that mediate humoral immunity.

T-cell precursors originate in the bone marrow and then migrate to the thymus gland for further differentiation. The T cells mediate cellular immunity, and they are involved in the cellular immune response against intracellular viruses, tuberculosis, contact irritants (e.g., poison ivy), cancer, parasites, fungi, and transplant antigens that provoke rejection of organs. Various subtypes of T cells have been identified. Among these are the T-helper cells and the T-suppressor cells. Human immunodeficiency viral (HIV) infections cause decreases and alterations of T-helper cells, leaving the individual vulnerable to the previously mentioned pathogens as well as malignancies. (The details of lymphocyte function are presented in Chapter 10.)

Platelets. Platelets, or *thrombocytes,* are derived from megakaryocytes (see Fig. 27-1). The primary function of platelets is to aid in blood clotting. Platelet performance depends on both quantitative and qualitative features.[2] Platelets must be available in sufficient numbers (quantitatively sufficient) and must be structurally sound to work properly (qualitatively adequate). Platelets are also involved in homeostasis by maintaining capillary integrity by working as "plugs" to close any openings in the capillary wall. At the site of any damage, platelet activation is initiated. Increasing numbers of platelets accumulate to form a platelet plug. Platelets are also important in the process of clot shrinkage and retraction.

Spleen

Another component of the hematologic system is the spleen, which is located in the upper left quadrant of the abdomen.The functions of the spleen can be classified into four general groups:

1. *Hematopoietic function.* The spleen produces RBCs during fetal development.
2. *Filter function.* The splenic structure provides an ideal filter mechanism. For example, the spleen removes old and defective erythrocytes from the circulation by the MPS. Another example of filtering involves the reuse of iron. The spleen is able to catabolize hemoglobin released by hemolysis and return the iron component of the hemoglobin to the bone marrow for reuse.
3. *Immune function.* The spleen contains a rich supply of lymphocytes and monocytes.
4. *Storage function.* Approximately 30% of the platelet mass is stored in the spleen.

Lymph System

The *lymph system,* consisting of lymphatic capillaries, ducts, and lymph nodes, carries fluid from the interstitial spaces to the blood. It is by means of the lymph that proteins, fat from the gastrointestinal (GI) tract, and certain hormones are able to return to the blood. The lymph system also returns excess interstitial fluid to the blood, which is important in preventing the development of edema.

Lymph fluid is pale yellow interstitial fluid that has diffused through lymphatic capillary walls. It circulates through a special vasculature, much as blood moves through blood vessels. The formation of lymph fluid increases when interstitial fluid pressure rises, thereby forcing more fluid into the lymph system. When too much interstitial pressure develops or when something interferes with the reabsorption of lymph, *lymphedema* develops. The lymphedema that may occur as a complication of a radical mastectomy is often caused by the obstruction of lymph flow resulting from the removal of nodes.

The lymphatic capillaries are thin-walled, endothelium-lined vessels that have an irregular diameter. They are somewhat larger than blood capillaries and do not contain valves. Lymphatic capillaries unite to form lymphatic vessels that carry all lymph to either the right lymphatic duct or the thoracic duct. These large lymphatic ducts drain into subclavian veins in the neck.

The lymph nodes are also a part of the lymphatic system. Structurally the nodes are small, round to bean-shaped organs of varying sizes. A primary function of lymph nodes is filtration of bacteria and foreign particles carried by lymph. Lymph nodes are distributed throughout the body along lymph vessels. They are situated both superficially and deep. The superficial nodes can be palpated, but the deep nodes must be visualized radiographically.

Liver

The liver functions as a filter but also produces all the procoagulants that are essential to hemostasis and blood coagulation. (Other functions of the liver are described in Chapter 41).

Normal Clotting Mechanisms

Hemostasis is a normal homeostatic process of blood clotting and blood lysing.[3] Blood clotting minimizes blood loss when various body structures are injured. Three components contribute to normal clotting: *vascular response, platelet response,* and *plasma clotting factors.*

Vascular Response. When a blood vessel is injured, an immediate local vasoconstrictive response occurs. Vasoconstriction reduces the leakage of blood from the vessel not only by restricting the vessel size but also by pressing the endothelial surfaces together. The latter reaction enhances vessel wall stickiness and maintains closure of the vessel even after the vasoconstriction subsides. Vascular spasm may last for 20 to 30 minutes, thus allowing time for the platelet response and plasma clotting factors to be activated.

Platelet Response. Platelets are activated when they are exposed to interstitial collagen from an injured blood vessel. Platelets stick to one another and form clumps. The stickiness is known as *adhesiveness,* and the formation of clumps is called *aggregation* or *agglutination.* When a blood vessel is injured, the circulating platelets are exposed to the collagen from the inner lining of the vessel. This interaction causes the platelets to release substances such as platelet factor 3 (PF3), serotonin, and epinephrine, which facilitate coagulation. At the same time, platelets release adenosine diphosphate (ADP), which increases platelet adhesiveness and aggregation, thereby enhancing the formation of a platelet plug.

In addition to their independent contribution to clotting, platelets also facilitate the reactions of the plasma clotting factors. As Fig. 27-2 shows, platelet lipoproteins stimulate necessary conversions in the clotting process.

Plasma Clotting Factors. The plasma clotting factors are labeled with both names and Roman numerals (Table 27-1). Plasma proteins circulate in inactive forms until stimulated to initiate clotting through one of two pathways, *intrinsic* or *extrinsic.* The intrinsic pathway is activated by collagen exposure from endothelial injury when the blood vessel is damaged. The extrinsic pathway is initiated when tissue thromboplastin is released extravascularly from injured tissues.

Regardless of whether clotting is initiated by substances internal or external to the blood vessel, coagulation ultimately follows the same final common pathway of the clotting cascade. *Thrombin,* in the common pathway, is the most powerful enzyme in the coagulation process (Fig. 27-2). It converts fibrinogen to fibrin, which is an essential component of a blood clot.

Anticoagulants. Just as some blood elements foster coagulation (procoagulants), others interfere with clotting (anticoagulants). This countermechanism to blood clotting serves to keep blood in its fluid state. Anticoagulation may be achieved by two means, antithrombins and fibrinolysis. As the name implies, *antithrombins* keep blood fluid by antagonizing thrombin, a powerful coagulant. Endogenous heparin is an example of an anticoagulant.

The second means of maintaining blood in its fluid form is *fibrinolysis.* The fibrinolytic system is initiated when plasminogen is activated to plasmin (Fig. 27-3). Thrombin is one of the substances that can activate the conversion of plasminogen to plasmin, thereby propagating fibrinolysis. The plasmin attacks either fibrin or fibrinogen by splitting the molecules into smaller elements known as fibrin split products (FSPs) or fibrin degradation products (FDPs). (More information about FSPs can be found in Table 27-6 and in the discussion of disseminated intravascular coagulation in Chapter 28.)

If fibrinolysis is excessive, the patient will be predisposed to bleeding. In such a situation, bleeding results from the destruction of fibrin in platelet plugs or from the effects of increased FSPs, which include impaired platelet aggregation, reduced prothrombin, and an inability to stabilize fibrin.

Effects of Aging on the Hematologic System

Physiologic aging is a gradual process that involves cell loss and organ atrophy. After age 30, marrow cellularity (stem cells) decreases from approximately 80% to approximately 50% at age 65. After age 65, cellularity decreases to 30%.[4] Although the remaining stem cells maintain their functional capacity to divide, there are fewer because they are gradually replaced by nonfunctional fat cells. In the bone marrow, decreased cellularity and decreased marrow reserves leave the older adult more vulnerable to problems with clotting, oxygen transport, and fighting infection. This will result in a diminished ability of an older adult to compensate for an acute or chronic illness.[4]

Hemoglobin levels begin to decrease in both men and women after middle age, with the lowest levels seen in the oldest patients. Approximately 12% to 20% of older patients are anemic. Although iron deficiency is usually responsible for the low hemoglobin levels, the cause of anemia in many older patients has no known etiology. Iron absorption is not impaired in the older patient, but nutritional intake of iron-rich foods is decreased and the use of iron supplements may be decreased. It is essential to assess for indications of disease processes such as GI bleeding before concluding decreased hemoglobin levels are caused solely by aging. The osmotic fragility of RBCs is increased in the older person, and this may account for the increased mean corpuscular volume (MCV) and the decreased mean corpuscular hemoglobin concentration (MCHC) of RBCs of the older person.

The total WBC count and differential are generally not affected by aging.[5] Leukocyte function is also well preserved. However, during an infection, the older adult may only have a minimal elevation in the total white blood cell count. These laboratory findings suggest a diminished marrow granulocyte reserve in older adults. Platelets are unaffected by the aging process. The effects of aging on hematologic studies are presented in Table 27-2. (Immune changes related to aging are presented in Chapter 10.)

ASSESSMENT OF THE HEMATOLOGIC SYSTEM

Much of the evaluation of the hematologic system is based on a thorough health history. Consequently, the nurse must be knowledgeable about what to include in the health history so that questions may be phrased in a manner eliciting the most information related to the hematologic

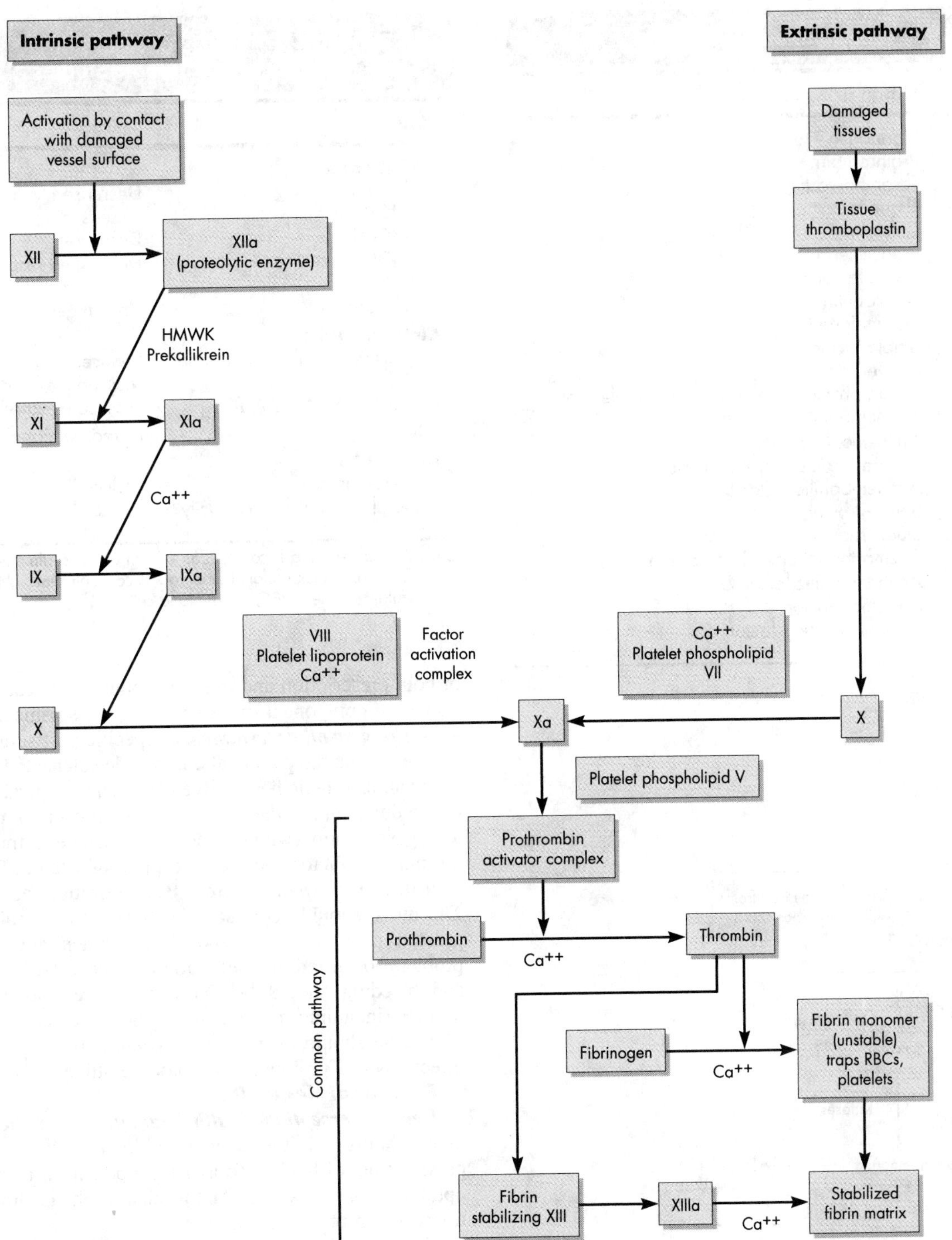

Fig. 27-2 Coagulation mechanism showing steps in the intrinsic pathway and extrinsic pathway. *RBCs,* Red blood cells.

problem. Key questions to ask a patient with a hematologic problem are presented in Table 27-3.

Subjective Data

Important Health Information

Past health history. It is important to learn whether the patient has had prior hematologic problems. A previous laboratory determination of anemia must be explored, as should diagnoses of mononucleosis, malabsorption, liver disorders (e.g., hepatitis, cirrhosis), and spleen disorders. Diseases of the blood, such as leukemia, should be documented.

Medications. Many drugs may interfere with normal hematologic function (Table 27-4). Antineoplastic agents used to treat malignant disorders may cause depression of the bone marrow (see Chapter 12). A complete drug history

Table 27-1 Coagulation Factors

Factor	Name or Synonym
I	Fibrinogen
II	Prothrombin
III	Thromboplastin Tissue factor
IV	Calcium
V	Proaccelerin Labile factor Ac globulin
VI	Not assigned
VII	Stable factor Convertin Serum prothrombin conversion accelerator
VIII	Antihemophilic globulin Antihemophilic factor
IX	Plasma thromboplastin component Antihemophilic factor B
X	Stuart-Prower factor Stuart factor
XI	Plasma thromboplastin antecedent Antihemophilic factor C
XII	Hageman factor
XIII	Fibrin-stabilizing factor

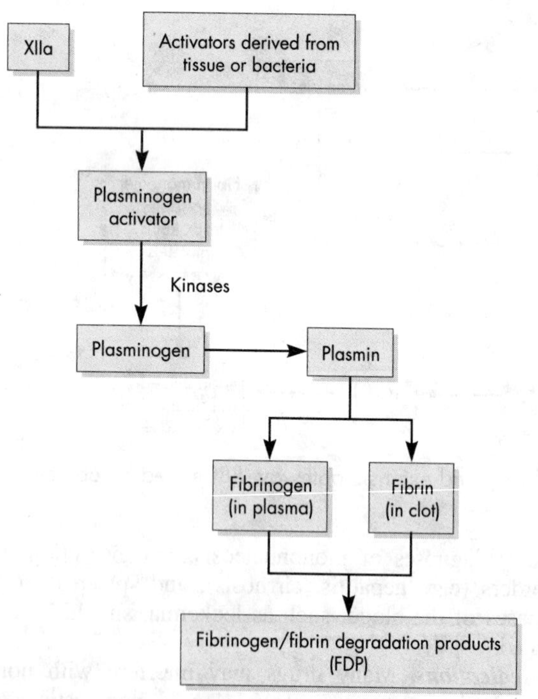

Fig. 27-3 Fibrinolytic system.

Table 27-2 Effects of Aging on Hematologic Studies

Study	Changes
CBC studies	
Hb	Decreased
MCV	Increased
MCHC	Decreased
WBC count	Diminished response to infection
Platelets	Unchanged
Clotting studies	
Partial thromboplastin time	Reduced
Fibrinogen	May be elevated
Factors V, VII, VIII, IX	May be elevated
ESR	Increased significantly
Iron studies	
Serum iron	Reduced
Total iron-binding capacity	Reduced

CBC, Complete blood count; *ESR,* erythrocyte sedimentation rate; *MCHC,* mean corpuscular hemoglobin concentration; *MCV,* mean corpuscular volume; *WBC,* white blood cell.

of both prescription and over-the-counter medications is an important component of a hematologic assessment.

Surgery or other treatments. Specific past surgical procedures to ask the patient about include splenectomy, tumor removal, prosthetic heart valve placement, surgical excision of the duodenum (where iron absorption occurs), partial or total gastrectomy (which removes parietal cells, thus reducing intrinsic factor and the absorption of vitamin B_{12}), and ileal resection (where vitamin B_{12} absorption takes place). The nurse should also ascertain how wound healing progressed postoperatively and if and when any bleeding problems occurred in relation to the surgery. Wound healing and bleeding should be discussed as responses to past injuries (including minor trauma) and to dental extractions. The nurse should also ask the patient about any recurring infections and problems with blood clotting.

Functional Health Patterns

Health perception–health management pattern. The nurse should ask the patient to describe the usual and present state of health. To assist the patient in maintaining optimal health, it is important to identify the health perceptions, health practices, and preventive practices.

Complete biographic data are needed including age, sex, race, and ethnic background. There is a known genetic influence in certain hematologic conditions as well as in other blood diseases that follow familial patterns. For example, sickle cell disease occurs primarily in African-Americans, and pernicious anemia occurs most commonly in persons of Northern European descent.

When a family health history is taken, the following health problems should be explored: jaundice, anemia, malignancies, RBC dyscrasias such as sickle cell disease, and bleeding disorders (e.g., hemophilia). The number of

Table 27-3 Key Questions: Patient with a Hematologic Problem

Health Perception–Health Management Pattern
- Do you have any difficulty performing daily activities because of a lack of energy?*
- Do you smoke or drink alcohol?*
- Have you ever received a blood transfusion?*
- Is there any family history of anemia, cancer, bleeding, or clotting problems?*
- List the medications you are taking.

Nutritional-Metabolic Pattern
- Do you have any difficulties with eating, chewing, or swallowing?*
- How has your appetite been?
- Do you take any vitamins, nutritional supplements, or iron?*
- Is nausea and vomiting a problem for you?*
- Have you had any unusual bleeding or bruising?*
- Have there been recent changes in the condition of your skin?*
- Have you experienced night sweats or cold intolerance?*
- Have you noticed any swelling in your armpits, neck, or groin?*

Elimination Pattern
- Have you had black or tarry stools?*
- Have you noticed any blood in your urine?*
- Have you had any decrease in urinary output?*
- Do you ever have diarrhea?*

Activity-Exercise Pattern
- Have you experienced excessive fatigue recently?*
- Do you have any shortness of breath at rest? With activity?*
- Do you have any limitations in joint motion?*
- Do you have a problem with unsteady gait?*
- After activity do you ever notice bleeding or bruising?*

Sleep-Rest Pattern
- Do you feel fatigued? Are you more fatigued than usual?*
- Do you feel rested upon awakening? If no, explain.

Cognitive-Perceptual Pattern
- Have you experienced any numbness or tingling?*
- Have you had any problems with your vision, hearing, or taste?*
- Have you noticed any changes in your mental functions?*
- Do you have any pain such as bone, joint, or abdominal pain, or abdominal fullness?*
- Do you have pain when moving your joints?*
- Have your muscles been sore or achy recently?*

Self-Perception–Self-Concept Pattern
- Does your health problem make you feel differently about yourself?*
- Do you have any physical changes that cause you distress?*

Role-Relationship Pattern
- Does your occupation bring you into contact with hazardous substances?*
- Has your present illness caused a change in your roles and relationships?*

Sexuality-Reproductive Pattern
- Woman: When was your last menses? Did you consider your cycle normal? How long does your bleeding usually last? Have you had any increase in cramping or clotting?*
- Men: Do you experience impotence?*
- Has your hematologic problem caused any sexual problems that concern you?*

Coping–Stress Tolerance Pattern
- Do you have a support system to assist you when needed?
- What coping strategies do you use during exacerbation of symptoms?

Value-Belief Pattern
- How do you feel about blood transfusions?
- Do you have any conflicts between your planned therapy and your value-belief system?*

*If yes, describe.

previous blood transfusions and possible complications during administration should be determined. Known allergies and allergic reactions, including anaphylaxis, should be documented.

Risk factors such as alcohol and cigarette use that might disrupt the hematologic system must be assessed. Alcohol use must be tactfully explored. Alcohol is a caustic agent to GI mucosa, and damage to the GI tract secondary to alcohol can cause local bleeding. Hematemesis (bright red, brown, or black vomitus) can be a symptom of this problem and should be investigated. Chronic alcohol abusers frequently have vitamin deficiencies. Alcohol also exerts a damaging effect on the liver, where several clotting factors are produced. Consequently, bleeding problems can develop and should be anticipated in cases of known alcohol abuse.

Nutritional-metabolic pattern. During the patient interview and assessment, the nurse will obtain the patient's weight and determine if the patient has experienced any recent changes associated with anorexia, nausea, vomiting, or oral discomfort. A dietary history may provide clues about the cause of erythrocyte deficiencies. Iron, vitamin B_{12}, and folic acid are necessary for the development of RBCs. Iron and folic acid deficiencies are associated with inadequate intake of foods such as liver, meat, eggs, whole-grain and enriched breads and cereals, potatoes, leafy green vegetables, dried fruits, legumes, and citrus fruits. Folic acid deficiencies may be offset by a diet including foods that are also high in iron.

Any changes in the skin's texture or color should be explored. The patient should be asked about any bleeding of gum tissue. Any petechiae or ecchymotic areas on the skin should be noted. If present, the frequency, size, and cause should be documented. Petechiae pinpoint an accumulation of blood in the skin or mucous membranes. Small vessels leak under pressure, and the platelet numbers are insufficient to stop the bleeding. Petechiae are more likely to occur where clothing constricts the circulation.

Table 27-4 Drugs Affecting Hematologic Function and Laboratory Values

Drug	Clinical Use	Hematologic Effect
Aminosalicylic acid (Pamisyl, PAS)	Antituberculin	Leukocytosis secondary to hypersensitivity
Amphotericin B (Fungizone)	Antifungal	Anemia
Acetylsalicylic acid (aspirin) and aspirin-containing compounds (e.g., Empirin, Percodan)	Analgesic, antipyretic, antiinflammatory	Reduced platelet aggregation, prolonged bleeding time
Azathioprine (Imuran)	Immunosuppression	Anemia, leukopenia
Carbamazepine (Tegretol)	Anticonvulsant	Anemia, leukopenia, thrombocytopenia
Chloramphenicol (Chloromycetin)	Antibiotic	Anemia, neutropenia, thrombocytopenia
Chlorothiazide (Diuril)	Diuretic	Thrombocytopenia (occasional)
Oral contraceptives and diethylstilbestrol	Birth control, menopausal symptoms, functional uterine bleeding, cancer of prostate	Increase in factors II, V, VII, VIII, IX, X; increase in fibrinogen; increase in thrombin; decrease in prothrombin and partial thromboplastin times; increase in coagulation and thromboemboli formation (overall)
Diphenylhydantoin (Dilantin)	Anticonvulsant, antidysrhythmic	Anemia
Epinephrine (Adrenalin)	Sympathomimetic	Leukocytosis
Glucocorticoids (ACTH, prednisone)	Antiinflammatory	Lymphopenia, neutrophilia
Isoniazid (INH)	Antituberculin	Neutropenia
Methyldopa (Aldomet)	Antihypertensive	Hemolytic anemia
Phenacetin (APC, Empirin compound)	Analgesic, antipyretic	Anemia
Phenylbutazone (Butazolidin)	Antiinflammatory	Anemia, leukopenia, neutropenia, thrombocytopenia
Procainamide hydrochloride (Pronestyl)	Antidysrhythmic	Agranulocytosis
Quinidine sulfate	Antidysrhythmic	Agranulocytosis, anemia, thrombocytopenia
Trimethoprim-sulfamethoxazole (Bactrim, Septra)	Antibacterial	Anemia, leukopenia, neutropenia, thrombocytopenia
Antineoplastic agents	Immunosuppression, malignancies	Anemia, leukopenia, thrombocytopenia
Nonsteroidal antiinflammatory drugs	Antiinflammatory, analgesic, antipyretic	Inhibition of platelet aggregation

The patient should also be questioned about any swelling in the neck, armpits, or groin. A careful description of the swelling should be made and should include size, texture, movability, and tenderness. Primary lymph tumors are usually not painful. A nontender swollen lymph node may be a sign of Hodgkin's disease or non-Hodgkin's lymphoma.

Any incidents of fever need to be explored thoroughly. It should be determined if the patient currently has a fever, recurring fevers, chills, or night sweats.

Elimination pattern. The patient should be asked if blood has been noted in the urine or stool or if black, tarry stools have occurred. Also, any decrease in urinary output or diarrhea should be documented.

Activity-exercise pattern. Because fatigue is a prominent symptom in many hematologic disorders, the patient should be asked about feelings of tiredness. Weakness and complaints of heavy extremities should also be determined. Symptoms of apathy, malaise, dyspnea, or palpitations should be documented. Any change in the patient's ability to perform activities of daily living (ADLs) should be noted.

Sleep-rest pattern. The patient's feeling of being rested after a night's sleep should be determined. Fatigue secondary to a hematologic problem often will not be resolved following sleep.

Cognitive-perceptual pattern. Pain may also be caused by a hematologic problem and should be assessed. Arthralgia (joint pain) may indicate an autoimmune disorder or may be caused by gout secondary to increased uric acid production as a result of a hematologic malignancy or hemolytic anemia. Aching bones may result from pressure of expanding bone marrow. *Hemarthrosis* (blood in a joint) occurs in the patient with bleeding disorders and can be painful.

Paresthesias, numbness, and tingling may be related to a hematologic disorder and should be noted. Any changes in vision, hearing, taste, or mental status should also be carefully assessed.

Self-perception–self-concept pattern. The effect of the health problem on the patient's perception of self and personal abilities should be determined. The effect of certain problems, such as bruising, petechiae, and lymph node swelling, on the patient's personal appearance should also be assessed.

Role-relationship pattern. The patient should be questioned about any past or present occupational or household exposures to radiation or chemicals. If such exposure has occurred, the type, amount, and duration of the exposure should be determined.

It is known that a person who has been exposed to radiation, as a treatment modality or by accident, has a higher incidence of certain hematologic problems. The same is true of a person who has been exposed to chemicals (e.g., benzene, lead, naphthalene, and phenylbutazone). The patient should also be questioned about a history in the military. Many Vietnam veterans were exposed to dioxin-containing defoliant (Agent Orange), which has been linked with leukemia and lymphoma. The nurse also needs to assess the impact of the present illness on the patient's usual roles and responsibilities.

Sexuality-reproductive pattern. A careful menstrual history should be obtained from women including the age at which menarche and menopause began, duration and amount of bleeding, incidence of clotting and cramping, and any associated problems. Any intrapartum or postpartum bleeding problems should also be documented. Men should be asked if they have any problems related to impotence because this is not uncommon in men with hematologic problems.

Coping–stress tolerance pattern. The patient with a hematologic problem often needs assistance with ADLs. The patient should be asked if adequate support is available to meet daily needs. The patient's usual methods of handling stress should also be determined. In the patient with platelet disorders, the potential for hemorrhage can be so frightening that usual life patterns may be drastically curtailed affecting the person's quality of life. The nurse needs to explore the accuracy of the patient's understanding of the problem.

Value-belief pattern. Often the person with hematologic problems needs a blood transfusion or other treatment involving body tissue. The nurse should determine if these types of treatments are problematic for the patient. In addition, the nurse should determine if the planned therapy causes any conflicts with the patient's value-belief system. The nurse should be cognizant of cultural differences related to blood and blood transfusions.

Objective Data

Physical Examination. A complete physical examination is necessary to accurately examine all systems that affect or are affected by the hematologic system (see Chapter 4). For example, a decreasing level of consciousness may be caused by an intracranial hemorrhage, and this indicates the need for a neurologic examination. Increasing abdominal girth may be related to an enlarged spleen or abdominal bleeding. This finding warrants the need for a complete GI examination. The nurse must be aware that signs and symptoms can be caused by hematologic problems, even though these are not the obvious cause (Table 27-5).

Lymph nodes are distributed throughout the body. The superficial nodes can be evaluated by light palpation (Fig. 27-4). Deep nodes are detected radiographically. Lymph nodes should be assessed symmetrically with regard to location, size (in centimeters), degree of fixation (e.g., movable, fixed), tenderness, and texture.

The examiner should lightly palpate lymph nodes over the appropriate areas.[6] The pads of the index and third fingers are most often used when assessing the lymph nodes. The examiner should gently roll the skin over the area and concentrate on feeling for possible lymph node enlargement. When not specifically examined for their status, lymph nodes are usually palpated during the examination of the region where the nodes are located. For example, the axillary lymph nodes are examined at the completion of a breast examination.

It is important to develop a sequence when examining the lymph nodes. The lymph nodes of the head and neck drain areas of the mouth, throat, abdomen, breast, thorax, and arms. A convenient sequence for examination is preauricular, posterior auricular, occipital, tonsillar, submaxillary, submental, superficial cervical, posterior cervical chain, deep cervical chain, and supraclavicular (Fig. 27-4).

The axillary lymph nodes drain lymph from the chest wall, breasts, arms, and hands. The pectoral, subscapular, and lateral groups of nodes are palpated next. The epitrochlear nodes, located in the antecubital fossa between the biceps and triceps muscles, are then examined. These nodes drain specific areas of the forearm and hand. The inguinal lymph nodes, which drain the lower extremities, are palpated last.

Lymph nodes are generally not palpable unless there is residual enlargement from a previous or current infection.[6] It may be normal to find small (0.5 to 1.0 cm), mobile, discrete, firm, nontender nodes, known as *shotty nodes.* Tender nodes are usually a result of inflammation, whereas hard or fixed nodes suggest malignancy.

Additional hematologic data can also be acquired from other body systems. It is important to include careful inspection of the skin (see Chapter 19) and palpation of the liver and spleen (see Chapter 36) in a hematologic assessment. The most direct means of evaluating the hematologic system is through laboratory analysis and other diagnostic studies.

DIAGNOSTIC STUDIES

The nurse should recognize the need to thoroughly explain any diagnostic procedures to the patient. It is common for a patient to be anxious when faced with illness. Therefore instructions must be simple, clear, and repeated when necessary to decrease anxiety and ensure the patient's compliance with preparatory protocols. Whether studies are performed on an outpatient or an inpatient basis, written instructions regarding the procedures facilitate compliance. If a diverse ethnic population is served, it is helpful to have instructions translated into the patients' dominant language.

The repeated acquisition of blood specimens may be distressing for the patient. Some patients and staff members become concerned that the amount of blood withdrawn for tests could lead to adverse effects. Although multiple blood studies may be uncomfortable, it is only in rare situations that diagnostic blood withdrawal predisposes the patient to significant volume loss.

Table 27-5 Common Assessment Abnormalities: Hematologic System

Finding	Possible Etiology and Significance
Skin	
Pallor of skin or nail beds	Decrease in quantity of hemoglobin (anemia)
Flushing	Increase in hemoglobin (polycythemia)
Jaundice	Accumulation of bile pigment caused by rapid or excessive hemolysis
Purpura, petechiae, ecchymoses, hematoma	Hemostatic deficiency of platelets or clotting factors resulting in hemorrhage into the skin
Excoriation and pruritus	Scratching from intense pruritus secondary to disorders such as Hodgkin's disease
Leg ulcers	Common in sickle cell disease, especially prominent on the malleoli on the ankles
Brownish discoloration	Hemosiderin and melanin from the breakdown of erythrocytes
Cyanosis	Increase in amounts of reduced hemoglobin (secondary polycythemia)
Telangiectasis	Hyperemic spot caused by capillary or small artery dilatation; small angioma with a tendency to hemorrhage
Angioma	A benign tumor consisting primarily of blood or lymph vessels
Spider nevus	Branched growth of dilated capillaries resembling a spider; associated with liver disease, elevated estrogen levels as in pregnancy
Eyes	
Jaundiced sclera	Accumulation of bile pigment because of rapid or excessive hemolysis
Conjunctival pallor	Reduction in quantity of hemoglobin (anemia)
Retinal hemorrhages	More frequent in concurrent states of thrombocytopenia and anemia than with thrombocytopenia alone
Mouth	
Pallor	Reduction in quantity of hemoglobin (anemia)
Gingival and mucosal ulceration	Neutropenia
Gingival infiltration (swelling, reddening, bleeding)	Leukemia caused by impeded movement of granulocytes and monocytes through gingiva-tooth attachment into mucous membrane or by inability of impaired leukocytes to combat oral infections
Gingival or mucosal bleeding	Hemorrhagic diseases, thrombocytopenia
Smooth tongue texture	Pernicious and iron deficiency anemia
Lymph Nodes	
Lymphadenopathy, tenderness	Normal response to infection in infants and children; cancerous invasion causative factor in adults; enlargement caused by infection, foreign infiltrates, or metabolic disturbances, especially with lipids
Chest	
Widened mediastinum	Enlarged lymph nodes
Generalized sternal tenderness	Leukemia resulting from increased bone marrow cellularity, causing increase in pressure and bone erosion
Localized sternal tenderness	Multiple myeloma as a result of stretching of periosteum
Tachycardia	Compensatory mechanism in anemia to increase cardiac output
Widened pulse pressure	Compensatory mechanism in anemia to increase cardiac output by increasing stroke volume
Murmurs	Usually systolic murmur in anemia caused by increased quantity and speed of low-viscosity blood going through pulmonic valve
Bruits (especially carotid bruits)	Anemia caused by increased flow of low-viscosity blood swirling through blood vessels
Abdomen	
Hepatomegaly	Leukemia
Splenomegaly	Leukemia, lymphomas, mononucleosis
Splenic bruits and rubs	Splenic infarction
Nervous System	
Pain and touch, position and vibratory sensation, tendon reflexes	Impaired nervous system function because of vitamin B_{12} deficiency or compression of nerves by masses
Back and Extremities	
Back pain	Acute hemolytic reaction from flank pain because of renal involvement with hemolysis; multiple myeloma from enlarged tumors that stretch periosteum or weaken supportive tissue, causing ligament strain and muscle spasm
Arthralgia	Leukemia as a result of aching in bones that contain marrow, sickle cell disease from hemarthrosis
Bone pain	Bone invasion by leukemia cells, bone demineralization resulting from various hematopoietic malignancies enhancing possibility of pathologic fractures

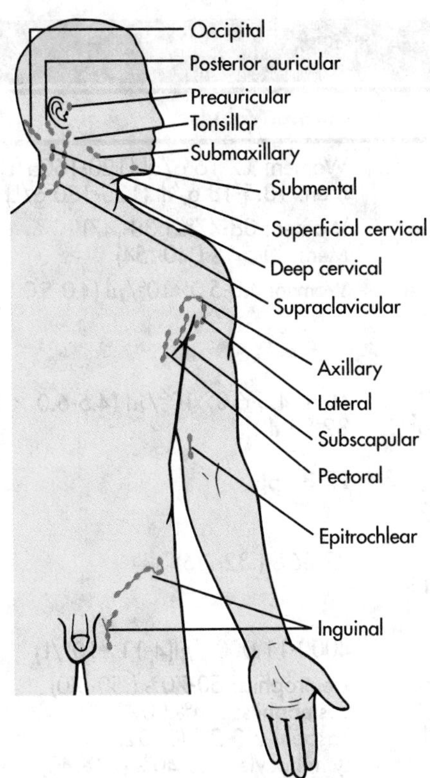

Fig. 27-4 Palpable superficial lymph nodes.

Finally the nurse must capitalize on all appropriate opportunities to use independent nursing assessment and clinical judgment. For example, when there is a suspicion of bleeding, it is important to perform guaiac tests of the stool, nasogastric secretions, or emesis and a Hematest of the urine.

Laboratory Studies

Complete Blood Count. The complete blood count (CBC) involves several laboratory tests (Table 27-6), each of which serves to assess the three major blood cells formed in the bone marrow. Although the status of each cell type is important, the entire system may be disrupted by diseases as well as by treatment of diseases. When the entire CBC is suppressed, a condition known as *pancytopenia* exists. In such cases the patient needs care directed toward the management of anemia, infection, and hemorrhage (see Chapter 28). The effects of aging on hematologic studies are presented in Table 27-2.

Red blood cells. Normal values of some RBC tests are reported separately for men and for women because normal values are based on body mass and men usually have a larger body mass than women.

The *hemoglobin* (Hb) value is reduced in cases of anemia, hemorrhage, and states of hemodilution, such as those that occur when the fluid volume is excessive. Increases in hemoglobin are found in polycythemia or in states of hemoconcentration, which can develop from volume depletion.

The *hematocrit* (Hct) value is determined by spinning blood in a centrifuge, which causes erythrocytes and plasma to separate. The erythrocytes, being the heavier elements, settle to the bottom. Reductions and elevations of hematocrit value are seen in the same conditions that raise and lower the hemoglobin value. The hematocrit value generally equals three times the hemoglobin value.

The *total RBC count* is reported as RBC $\times$ $10^6/\mu l$. However, total RBC count is not always reliable in determining the adequacy of RBC function. Consequently, other data, such as hemoglobin, hematocrit, and RBC indices, must also be evaluated. The RBC count is altered by the same conditions that raise and lower the hemoglobin and hematocrit values.

RBC indices are special indicators that reflect RBC volume, color, and hemoglobin saturation. These parameters may provide insight into the cause of anemia. (The significance of these parameters is discussed further in Chapter 28.)

White blood cells. The *white blood cell differential* is of considerable significance because it is possible for the total WBC count to remain essentially normal despite a marked change in one type of leukocyte. For example, a patient may have a normal WBC count of 8800/μl while the differential count may show a relative proportion of lymphocytes to be 10%. This is an abnormal finding that warrants further investigation.

An important concept related to neutrophil counts is the shift to the left. When infections are severe, more granulocytes are released from the bone marrow as a compensatory mechanism. To meet the increased demand, many young, immature PMNs or bands are released into circulation. The usual laboratory procedure is to report the WBCs in order of maturity (see Fig. 27-1), with the less mature forms on the left side of the written report. Consequently the existence of many immature cells is referred to as a *shift to the left.*

Platelet count. Bleeding may occur when platelet counts are depressed, which is a condition known as *thrombocytopenia.* If platelets are functioning properly, most hematologists believe that a patient can undergo necessary surgery with platelet counts as low as 50,000/μl (normal count is 150,000 to 400,000/μl). Once platelet counts drop to between 20,000 and 30,000/μl, spontaneous hemorrhage is probable. When platelets are depressed to 10,000/μl, the possibility of intracerebral hemorrhage is significantly increased. Clotting studies are presented in Table 27-7.

Erythrocyte Sedimentation Rate. Erythrocyte sedimentation rate (ESR, or sed rate) measures the sedimentation or settling of RBCs and is used as a nonspecific measure of many diseases, especially inflammatory conditions. Increased ESRs are common during acute and chronic inflammatory reactions when cell destruction is increased. They are also found in persons with malignancy, myocardial infarction, and end-stage renal disease. Although the ESR is a nonspecific test, it is often used as a routine screening procedure.

Blood Typing and Rh Factor. Blood group antigens (A and B) are found on RBC membranes and form the basis

Table 27-6 Complete Blood Count Studies

Study	Description and Purpose	Normal Values
Hb	Measurement of gas-carrying capacity of RBC	Women: 12-16 g/dl (120-160g/L) Men: 13.5-18 g/dl (135-180 g/L)
Hct	Comparison of volume of RBC to volume of plasma as percent of total blood volume	Women: 38-47% (.38-.47) Men: 40-54% (.40-.54)
Total RBC count	Count of number of circulating RBCs	Women: 4.0-5.0×$10^6/\mu l$ (4.0-5.0 × 10^{12}/L) Men: 4.5-6.0×$10^6/\mu l$ (4.5-6.0 × 10^{12}/L)
Red cell indices		
$MCV = \frac{Hct \times 10}{RBC \times 10^6}$	Determination of relative size of RBC; low MCV reflection of microcytosis, high MCV reflection of macrocytosis	82-98 fl
$MCH = \frac{Hb \times 10}{RBC \times 10^6}$	Measurement of average weight of Hb/RBC; low MCH indication of microcytosis or hypochromia, high MCHC indication of macrocytosis	27-33 pg
$MCHC = \frac{Hb}{Hct} \times 100$	Evaluation of RBC saturation with Hb; low MCHC indication of hypochromia, high MCHC evident in spherocytosis	32-36% (.32-.36)
WBC count	Measurement of total number of leukocytes	4000-11,000 /μl(4-11×10^9/L)
WBC differential	Determination of whether each kind of WBC is present in proper proportion, determination of absolute value by multiplying percentage of cell type by total WBC count and dividing by 100	Neutrophils: 50-70% (.50-.70) Eosinophils: 2-4% (.02-.04) Basophils: 0-2% (0-.02) Lymphocytes: 20-40% (.20-.40) Monocytes: 4-8% (.04-.08)
Platelet count	Measurement of number of platelets available to maintain platelet clotting functions (not measurement of quality of platelet function)	150,000-400,000 /μl (150-400 × 10^9/L)

Hb, Hemoglobin; *Hct*, hematocrit; *MCH*, mean corpuscular hemoglobin; *MCHC*, mean corpuscular hemoglobin concentration; *MCV*, mean corpuscular volume; *RBC*, red blood cell; *WBC*, white blood cell.

Table 27-7 Clotting Studies

Study	Description and Purpose	Normal Values
Prothrombin time	Assessment of extrinsic coagulation by measurement of factors I, II, V, VII, X	12-15 sec
Activated partial thromboplastin time	Assessment of intrinsic coagulation by measuring factors I, II, V, VIII, IX, X, XI, XII; longer with use of heparin	30-45 sec
Bleeding time	Measurement of time small skin incision bleeds; reflection of ability of small blood vessels to constrict	1-6 min
Thrombin time	Reflection of adequacy of thrombin; prolonged thrombin time indication that coagulation is inadequate secondary to decreased thrombin activity	8-12 sec
Fibrinogen	Reflection of level of fibrinogen; increase in fibrinogen possible indication of enhancement of fibrin formation, making patient hypercoagulable; decrease in fibrinogen indication that patient possibly predisposed to bleeding	200-400 mg/dl (2.0-4.0 g/L)
Fibrin split products	Reflection of degree of fibrinolysis; reflection of excessive fibrinolysis and predisposition to bleed (if present); possible indication of disseminated intravascular coagulation	<10 mg/L
Protamine sulfate tests	Reflection of presence of fibrin monomer (portion of fibrin remaining after elements that polymerize and stabilize clot detach); positive test indication of predisposition to bleed and possible presence of disseminated intravascular coagulation	Negative

Table 27-8 ABO Blood Group Names and Compatibilities*

Blood Group	Red Blood Cell Agglutinogen(s)	Serum Agglutinin(s)	Compatible Donor Blood Groups	Incompatible Donor Blood Groups
A	A	Anti-B	A and O	B and AB
B	B	Anti-A	B and O	A and AB
AB	A and B	Neither	A, B, AB, and O	None
O	Neither (universal donor)	Anti-A and anti-B	O	A, B, and AB

*ABO blood groups are named for the antigen found on the RBCs. Compatibility is based on the antibodies present in the serum.

Table 27-9 Miscellaneous Laboratory Blood Studies

Study	Description and Purpose	Normal Values
ESR	Measurement of RBCs that settle to bottom of test tube in 1 hr; certain blood elements, especially protein, possibly affecting results	Women: 1-20 mm in 1 hr Men: 1-15 mm in 1 hr
Reticulocyte count	Measurement of immature RBCs; reflection of bone marrow activity in producing RBCs	0.5-1.5% of RBC count (0.005-0.015 of RBC count)
Bilirubin	Measurement of degree of RBC hemolysis or liver's inability to excrete normal quantities of bilirubin; increase in indirect bilirubin with hemolytic problems	Total: 0.2-1.3 mg/dl (3.4-22 μmol/L) Direct: 0.1-0.3 mg/dl (1.7-5.1 μmol/L) Indirect: 0.1-1.0 mg/dl (1.7-17 μmol/L)
Iron		
Serum iron	Reflection of amount of iron combined with proteins in serum; accurate indication of status of iron storage and use	50-150 μg/dl (9.0-26.9 μmol/L)
Total iron-binding capacity	Measurement of percentage of saturation of transferrin, a protein that binds iron; evaluation of amount of extra iron that can be carried	250-410 μg/dl (45-73 μmol/L)
Coombs' test	Differentiation among types of hemolytic anemias; detection of immune antibodies	
Direct	Detection of antibodies that are attached to RBCs	Negative
Indirect	Detection of antibodies in serum	Negative

ESR, Erythrocyte sedimentation rate; *RBCs,* red blood cells.

for the ABO blood typing system. The presence or absence of one or both of the two inherited antigens is the basis for the four blood groups: A, B, AB, and O. Blood group A has A antigens, group B has B antigens, group AB has both antigens, and group O has neither A nor B antigens. Each person has antibodies in the serum called *anti-A* and *anti-B* that react with A or B antigens. These antibodies are found when the corresponding antigen is absent from the RBC surface. For example, B antibodies are found in persons with blood group A (Table 27-8).

Blood reactions based on ABO incompatibilities result from intravascular hemolysis of the RBCs. Erythrocytes agglutinate when a serum antibody is present to react with the antigens on the RBC membrane. For example, agglutination would occur in the blood of a person with Type A blood when blood is transfused from a person with B antigens (i.e., Type B or AB) into the person with Type A blood. The anti-B antibodies in the Type A blood would react with the B antigens, thus initiating the process that results in RBC hemolysis.

The Rh system is based on a third antigen, D, which is also found on the RBC membrane. Rh-positive persons have the D antigen, whereas Rh-negative persons do not. Approximately 85% of persons are Rh positive and 15% are Rh negative.[7] As a result of transfusion therapy or during childbirth, an Rh-negative person may be exposed to Rh-positive blood. Such exposure results in formation of an antibody, anti-D, which acts against Rh antigens. (Rh-positive persons normally have no anti-D.) The person is then sensitized to Rh-positive blood, and a second exposure to Rh-positive blood will cause a severe hemolytic reaction. A Coombs' test can be used to evaluate the person's Rh status (Table 27-9).

Lymphangiography

Lymphangiography is radiologic visualization of the lymph system after the injection of dye. The purpose of this procedure is to assess deep lymph nodes. It is particularly useful in detecting lymph node involvement in malignant conditions. This test may be used in conjunction with other tests like computerized tomography (CT) scans or gallium scans to fully identify lymph nodes involved with cancer. Allergies to shellfish and iodine, and previous reactions to dyes should be ascertained before doing a lymphangiogram.

The procedure begins with the intracutaneous injection of a blue dye into the webs of the toes. (It is less commonly done through the hands.) The dye is absorbed by the lymph vessels, making them visible through the skin on the dorsum of the foot. Once visible the dorsum of each foot is injected with a local anesthetic agent, and a small superficial incision is made over the lymph vessels. The lymph vessel is then cannulated with a small needle. Once the needle is inserted it is important that the patient not move the feet to avoid the possibility of dislodging the needle. When the lymph vessels are cannulated, a radiopaque oil is injected slowly by means of an automated pump. The usual dose of oil for an adult is 7 ml in each foot administered for a duration of 45 to 60 minutes. Fluoroscopy may be used during the injection to watch the filling of the lymph vessels. Immediately after the dye has been injected several x-rays will be taken from various angles. A second set of x-rays will be taken the next day when the lymph channels are emptied. The incisions on the feet are sutured closed when the procedure is complete.

The lymph nodes can also be seen by means of isotopic (technetium 99m) lymphangiography. Compared with radiographic lymphangiography, isotopic lymphangiography is less invasive and does not require dye injection. However, the isotope's short life prevents serial studies.

Nursing responsibilities related to lymphangiography and other common studies of the hematologic system are presented in Table 27-10.

Biopsies

Biopsy procedures specific to hematologic assessment are bone marrow examination and lymph node biopsy. In general, these procedures are done when a diagnosis cannot be established from a peripheral blood smear or when more information about the possible hematologic problem is needed.

Bone Marrow Examination. Bone marrow examination is important in the evaluation of many hematologic disorders. It involves the aspiration or biopsy of bone marrow with a syringe and needle. The aspirate is made into smears that are useful for cytologic diagnosis.

The site of bone marrow aspiration is determined by the age of the patient and the skill of the physician or specially credentialed nurse. In adults, the sites most easily aspirated are the anterior and posterior iliac crests. The tibia may provide an additional site in young children. Although hazards of bone marrow aspiration are minimal, there is a possibility of penetrating the bone and damaging underlying structures.

The skin over the puncture site is cleansed with a bactericidal agent. The skin, subcutaneous tissue, and periosteum are infiltrated with a local anesthetic agent. In addition, systemic analgesics or tranquilizers are often administered before the procedure to minimize pain and decrease anxiety. The patient may be uncomfortable when the periosteum is infiltrated. Once the area is anesthetized, the special marrow needle is inserted through the cortex of the bone. The stylet of the needle is then removed, the hub is attached to a 10 ml syringe, and 0.2 to 0.5 ml of the fluid marrow is aspirated. The aspiration is experienced by the patient as a suction pain, which may be quite uncomfortable although it lasts for only a few seconds.

After the marrow aspiration, the needle is removed. Pressure is applied over the aspiration site to ensure hemostasis. If the patient is thrombocytopenic, pressure may be required for 5 to 10 minutes or longer.

If a bone biopsy is required, the preparatory procedure remains the same, but a different needle is used. The needle has a cutting blade that allows a specimen of the bone to be removed. When either a marrow aspirate or a biopsy specimen is acquired, a glass slide is carefully prepared with a thin film of the marrow.

Lymph Node Biopsy. Lymph node biopsy involves obtaining lymph tissue for histologic examination to determine the diagnosis and therapy. This may be accomplished by either an open biopsy or a closed (needle) biopsy. In the open biopsy procedure, an incision is made, and the lymph node and surrounding tissue are dissected whenever possible. Care must be taken because neoplastic cells can be disseminated during the biopsy procedure if the scalpel passes through tissues containing cancerous cells. An open biopsy is performed in the operating room using either local or general anesthesia.

A closed (needle) biopsy may also be performed to analyze lymph tissue. This bedside or outpatient technique is performed by a skilled physician. Sterile technique is essential throughout the procedure. Nursing personnel must recognize the possibility of insidious bleeding, and direct pressure should be applied to the area after the biopsy procedure to achieve hemostasis. Frequent observations of the site for bleeding, and monitoring of vital signs should be done, especially if the platelet count is low. The sterile dressing should be changed as ordered, and the wound should be inspected for healing and infection. It is important to recognize that if a needle biopsy is negative, it may signify only that the cancer cells were not a part of the tissue in the biopsy specimen. However, a positive finding is sufficient evidence for confirming a diagnosis.

Table 27-10 Diagnostic Studies: Hematologic System

Study	Description and Purpose	Nursing Responsibility
Urine Studies		
Bence Jones protein	An electrophoretic measurement is used to detect the presence of the Bence Jones protein, which is found in most cases of multiple myeloma. Negative finding indicates that patient is normal.	Acquire random urine specimen.
Radioisotope Studies		
Liver/spleen scan	Radioactive isotope is injected intravenously. Images from the radioactive emissions are used to evaluate the structure of the spleen and liver. Patient is not a source of radioactivity.	No specific nursing responsibilities
Bone scan	Same procedure as for the spleen scan except used for the purpose of evaluating the structure of the bones.	No specific nursing responsibilities
Isotopic lymphangiography	Radionuclide study is used to assess lymph nodes and lymph system. Technetium 99m is used. Technique is less invasive than radiographic lymphangiography.	No specific nursing responsibilities
Radiologic Studies		
Lymphangiography	Purpose is to evaluate deep lymph nodes. Radiopaque oil-based dye is infused slowly into the lymph vessels via small needles in the dorsum of each foot. Radiographs are taken immediately and on next day.	Inform the patient about what to anticipate. Obtain consent form. Assess for iodine sensitivity. Give preoperative sedation, if indicated. Instruct patient that urine will be blue from the dye excretion for 1-2 days. Inform patient that transient fever, general malaise, and diffuse muscle aches may be experienced for 12-24 hr. Watch for signs of oil embolus to lungs (hacking cough, dyspnea, pleuritic pain, and hemoptysis).
Computed tomography	Noninvasive radiologic examination using computer-assisted x-ray evaluates the spleen, liver, or lymph nodes.	No specific nursing responsibilities
Magnetic resonance imaging	Noninvasive procedure produces sensitive images of soft tissue without using contrast dyes. No ionizing radiation is required. Technique is used to evaluate spleen, liver, and lymph nodes.	Instruct patient to remove all metal objects and ask about any history of surgical insertion of staples, plates, or other metal appliances. Inform patient of need to lie still in small chamber.
Biopsies		
Bone marrow	Technique involves removal of bone marrow through a locally anesthetized site to evaluate the status of the blood-forming tissue. It is used to diagnose multiple myeloma, all types of leukemia, and some lymphomas. It is also done to assess efficacy of leukemic therapy.*	Explain procedure to patient. Obtain signed consent form. Consider preprocedure analgesic administration to enhance patient comfort and cooperation. Apply pressure dressing after procedure. Assess biopsy site for bleeding.
Lymph node biopsy	Purpose is to obtain lymph tissue for histologic examination to determine diagnosis and therapy.	Explain procedure to patient. Obtain signed consent form. Use sterile technique in dressing changes after procedure. Carefully evaluate wound for healing. Assess patient for complications, especially bleeding and edema.
Open	Test is performed in operating room with direct visualization of the area.	
Closed (needle)	Test is performed at bedside or in office.	
Blood Studies[†]		

*See Chapter 28.
[†]See Tables 27-4, 27-6, and 27-8.

REVIEW QUESTIONS

The number of the question corresponds to the same-numbered objective at the beginning of the chapter.

1. An important function of the spleen in the adult is
   a. RBC production.
   b. monocyte production.
   c. removal of defective or senescent erythrocytes.
   d. platelet production.

2. Which of the following are both types of granulocytes?
   a. Basophils and neutrophils
   b. Monocytes and eosinophils
   c. Thrombocytes and lymphocytes
   d. Erythrocytes and eosinophils

3. Which of the following substances are necessary for converting prothrombin to thrombin?
   a. Fibrinogen and factor IX
   b. Thromboplastin and calcium
   c. Platelet factor III and factor V
   d. Fibrin-stabilizing factor and sodium

4. All of the following changes in the hematologic system are associated with normal aging *except*
   a. decreased hemoglobin.
   b. decreased bone marrow cellularity.
   c. decreased WBC count.
   d. no change in platelet counts.

5. Which of the following information obtained from the health history has a significant relationship to the hematologic system?
   a. Multiple pregnancies
   b. Early menopause
   c. Jaundice
   d. Bladder surgery

6. Which of the following statements accurately describes the technique to palpate lymph nodes?
   a. Gentle, firm pressure should be applied to deep lymph nodes.
   b. Normally superficial lymph nodes are not palpable.
   c. The index and third fingers should lightly palpate superficial lymph nodes.
   d. The tips of the second, third, and fourth fingers should apply firm pressure for palpation.

7. Which of the following is considered a normal finding of the lymph node examination?
   a. Shotty nodes
   b. Firm, tender nodes
   c. Hard, fixed nodes
   d. Mobile, hard nodes

8. Immediately following a bone marrow biopsy and aspiration the nurse should instruct the patient to
   a. lie still with a sterile pressure dressing intact.
   b. cleanse the site immediately with povidone iodine.
   c. lie with knees slightly bent and head elevated.
   d. expect to receive a blood transfusion .

REFERENCES

1. Spivak JL: The application of recombinant erythropoietin in anemic patients with cancer, *Semin Oncol* 19:25, 1992.
2. George JN, Shattil SJ: The clinical importance of acquired abnormalities of platelet function, *N Engl J Med* 324:27, 1991.
3. Jandl JH: *Blood: pathophysiology,* Boston, 1991, Blackwell Scientific.
4. Williams WJ, editor: *Hematology in the aged,* New York, 1990, McGraw-Hill.
5. Mezey MD, Rauckhorst LH, Stokes SA: Assessment of the cardiac, vascular, respiratory, and hematopoietic systems. In *Health assessment of the older individual,* ed 2, New York, 1993, Springer.
6. Mudge-Grout CL: *Immunologic Disorders,* St Louis, 1992, Mosby.
7. Belcher AE: *Blood disorders,* St Louis, 1993, Mosby.

Chapter 28

NURSING ROLE IN MANAGEMENT

Hematologic Problems

Marie Bakitas Whedon

Learning Objectives

1. Describe the general clinical manifestations and complications of anemia.
2. Differentiate between the etiologic and morphologic classifications of anemia.
3. Describe the etiologies, specific clinical manifestations, diagnostic findings, and therapeutic, pharmacologic, and nursing management of anemia caused by decreased erythrocyte production: iron-deficiency, megaloblastic, and aplastic anemias and anemia of chronic disease.
4. Explain the nursing management of anemia secondary to blood loss.
5. Describe the pathophysiology, clinical manifestations, and therapeutic and nursing management of anemia caused by increased erythrocyte destruction, including sickle cell disease and acquired hemolytic anemias.
6. Describe the pathophysiology and therapeutic and nursing management of polycythemia.
7. Explain the pathophysiology, clinical manifestations, and therapeutic and nursing management of various types of thrombocytopenia.
8. Describe the types, clinical manifestations, diagnostic findings, and therapeutic and nursing management of hemophilia and von Willebrand disease.
9. Explain the pathophysiology, diagnostic findings, and therapeutic and nursing management of disseminated intravascular coagulation.
10. Describe the etiology, clinical manifestations, and therapeutic and nursing management of neutropenia.
11. Describe the pathophysiology, clinical manifestations, and therapeutic and nursing management of myelodysplastic syndromes.
12. Compare and contrast the major types of leukemia regarding age at onset and distinguishing clinical and laboratory findings.
13. Explain the therapeutic and nursing management of acute and chronic leukemias.
14. Compare Hodgkin's and non-Hodgkin's lymphomas in terms of clinical manifestations, staging, and therapeutic and nursing management.
15. Describe the pathophysiology, clinical manifestations, and therapeutic and nursing management of multiple myeloma.
16. Describe the role of the spleen in hematologic disorders and related therapeutic management.
17. Describe the nursing management of the patient receiving transfusions of blood and blood components.

ANEMIA

Definition and Classification

Anemia is a reduction below normal in the number of erythrocytes, the quantity of hemoglobin, and the volume of packed red cells (hematocrit) caused by rapid blood loss, impaired production of erythrocytes, or increased destruction of erythrocytes. Because red blood cells (RBCs) transport oxygen (O_2), erythrocyte disorders can lead to tissue hypoxia. This hypoxia accounts for many of the clinical manifestations of anemia. Anemia is not a specific disease; it is a manifestation of a pathologic process. Anemia is identified and classified by laboratory evaluation. Once anemia is identified, further investigation must be done to determine its cause.[1]

Anemia can result from primary hematologic problems or can develop as a secondary consequence of defects in other body systems. The many kinds of anemia can be grouped according to either a *morphologic* or an *etiologic* classification. Morphologic classification is based on descriptive, objective laboratory information about erythrocyte size and color. (The terms used in this classification system are explained in Chapter 27.) Etiologic classification is related to the clinical conditions causing the anemia, such as decreased erythrocyte production, blood loss, or increased erythrocyte destruction (Table 28-1). Although the

Reviewed by Kathy Dietz-Lovett, Oncology CNS, Marstons Mills, MA. Acknowledgment for manuscript review to Solveig Erickson, MD, Department of Hematology-Oncology, Dartmouth Hitchcock Medical Center, Lebanon, NH, and Carol Femia, RN, BS, graduate student, Master's program, Massachusetts General Institute of Health Professions.

Table 28-1 Etiologic Classification of Anemia

Decreased Erythrocyte Production
- Decreased hemoglobin synthesis
  - Iron deficiency
  - Thalassemias (decreased globin synthesis)
  - Sideroblastic anemia (decreased porphyrin)
- Defective DNA synthesis
  - Vitamin B_{12} deficiency
  - Folic acid deficiency
- Decreased number of erythrocyte precursors
  - Aplastic anemia
  - Anemia of leukemia and myelodysplasia
  - Chronic diseases or disorders

Blood Loss
- Acute
  - Trauma
  - Blood vessel rupture
- Chronic
  - Gastritis
  - Menstrual flow
  - Hemorrhoids

Increased Erythrocyte Destruction*
- Intrinsic
  - Abnormal hemoglobin (HbS—sickle cell anemia)
  - Enzyme deficiency (G6PD)
  - Membrane abnormalities (paroxysmal nocturnal hemoglobinuria)
- Extrinsic
  - Physical trauma (prosthetic heart valves, extracorporeal circulation)
  - Antibodies (isoimmune and autoimmune)
  - Infectious agents and toxins (malaria)

DNA, Deoxyribonucleic acid; *G6PD*, glucose-6-phosphate dehydrogenase; *HbS*, hemoglobin S.
*Hemolytic anemias.

morphologic system is the most accurate means of classifying anemias, it is easier to discuss patient care by focusing on the etiologic problem. Table 28-2 relates morphologic classifications to various etiologies.

Mechanisms to Compensate for Hypoxia

Regardless of the source of anemia, a decrease in erythrocytes reduces the blood's O_2-carrying capacity, which leads to tissue hypoxia. The physiologic effects of anemia are caused by tissue hypoxia and activation of compensatory mechanisms that attempt to meet cellular O_2 needs. The four major compensatory responses to anemia include the following:

1. A shift of the oxygen-hemoglobin dissociation curve to the right, thereby facilitating removal of more O_2 by the tissues at the same partial pressure of O_2 (Fig. 28-1)
2. Redistribution of blood from tissues that have a low O_2 requirement (e.g., skin) to tissues that have higher O_2 needs (e.g., brain, muscle, myocardium)
3. Increased cardiac output (CO) achieved by increased heart rate (HR) or increased stroke volume (SV) to meet O_2 demands of the tissues

Table 28-2 Relationship of Morphologic Classification and Etiologies of Anemia

Morphology	Etiology
Normocytic, normochromic	Acute blood loss, hemolysis, chronic renal disease, chronic disease, cancers, sideroblastic anemia, refractory anemia, diseases of endocrine dysfunction, aplastic anemia, pregnancy
Macrocytic, normochromic	Vitamin B_{12} deficiency, folic acid deficiency, liver disease (including effects of alcohol abuse), postsplenectomy
Microcytic, hypochromic	Iron-deficiency anemia, thalassemia, lead poisoning

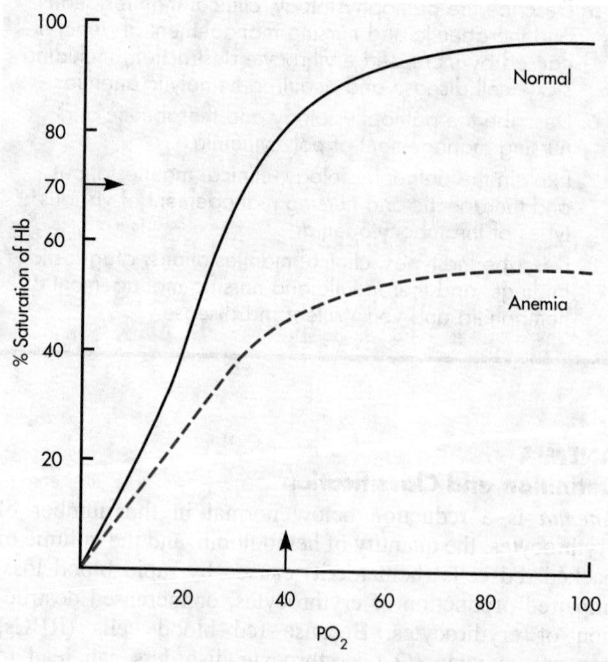

Fig. 28-1 Oxygen-hemoglobin dissociation curve. The oxygen-hemoglobin curve of a normal person (*solid line*) with hemoglobin (Hb) of 15 g/dl compared to that of a person with anemia (*dashed line*) with hemoglobin of 6 g/dl. The shift to the right seen with the anemic person is a compensatory mechanism. While the O_2 transport capability of hemoglobin is decreased with the shift to the right, hemoglobin release of O_2 to the tissues is facilitated; that is, hemoglobin gives up O_2 more readily when the curve shifts to the right.

Table 28-3 Clinical Manifestations of Anemia

Body System	Severity of Anemia		
	Mild (Hb 10-14 g/dl [100-140 g/L])	Moderate (Hb 6-10 g/dl [60-100 g/L])	Severe (Hb <6 g/dl [<60 g/L])
Integument	None	None	Pallor, jaundice,* pruritus*
Eyes	None	None	Icteric conjunctiva and sclera,* retinal hemorrhage, blurred vision
Mouth	None	None	Glossitis, smooth tongue
Cardiovascular	Palpitations	Increased palpitations	Tachycardia, increased pulse pressure, systolic murmurs, intermittent claudication, angina, CHF, MI
Pulmonary	Exertional dyspnea	Dyspnea	Tachypnea, orthopnea, dyspnea at rest
Neurologic	None	None	Headache, vertigo, irritability, depression, impaired thought processes
Gastrointestinal	None	None	Anorexia, hepatomegaly, splenomegaly
Musculoskeletal	None	None	Bone pain
General	None	Fatigue	Sensitivity to cold, weight loss, lethargy

CHF, congestive heart failure; *Hb,* hemoglobin; *MI,* myocardial infarction.
*Caused by hemolysis.

4. Increased rate of RBC production (within 4 to 5 days) after erythropoietin synthesis (by the kidneys) has increased in response to tissue hypoxia

Clinical Manifestations

The clinical manifestations of anemia are primarily caused by the body's response to tissue hypoxia. The intensity of the manifestations varies depending on the severity of the anemia and the presence of coexisting diseases. The severity of anemia can be determined by the hemoglobin (Hb) levels. *Mild* states of anemia (Hb 10 to 14 g/dl [100 to 140 g/L]) may exist without causing symptoms. If symptoms develop, they are usually caused by an underlying disease or a compensatory response to heavy exercise. These symptoms include palpitations, dyspnea, and diaphoresis. In cases of *moderate* anemia (Hb 6 to 10 g/dl [60 to 100 g/L]), the cardiopulmonary symptoms may be increased and may be associated with rest as well as activity. The patient with *severe* anemia (Hb less than 6 g/dl [60 g/L]) displays many clinical manifestations involving multiple body systems (Table 28-3).

Integumentary Changes. Integumentary changes include pallor, jaundice, and pruritus. The pallor results from reduced amounts of hemoglobin and reduced blood flow to the skin. Jaundice occurs when there is an increased concentration of serum bilirubin, which increases when hemolysis of RBCs occurs. Pruritus occurs because of increased serum and skin bile salt concentrations. In addition to the skin, the sclera of the eyes and mucous membranes should be evaluated for jaundice because they reflect the integumentary changes more accurately, especially in a dark-skinned individual.

Cardiopulmonary Manifestations. Cardiopulmonary manifestations of severe anemia result from additional attempts by the heart and lungs to provide adequate amounts of oxygen to the tissues. CO is maintained by increasing the pulse rate. The low viscosity of the blood contributes to the development of systolic murmurs and bruits. In extreme cases or when concomitant heart disease is present, angina pectoris and high output failure may occur if myocardial O_2 needs cannot be met. Myocardial infarction (MI) may also occur. Congestive heart failure (CHF), cardiomegaly, pulmonary and systemic congestion, ascites, and peripheral edema may develop if the heart is overworked for an extended period of time.

NURSING MANAGEMENT

ANEMIA

This section will discuss general nursing management of anemia. Specific care related to various types of anemia is discussed later in this chapter.

Nursing Assessment

Subjective and objective data that should be obtained from an individual with anemia are presented in Table 28-4.

Nursing Diagnoses

Nursing diagnoses specific to the patient with anemia include, but are not limited to, those presented in the nursing care plan for the patient with anemia on p. 779.

Table 28-4 Nursing Assessment: Anemia

Subjective Data

Important health information

Past health history: Recent blood loss or trauma; chronic liver, endocrine, or renal disease (including dialysis); GI disease (malabsorption syndrome, ulcers, gastritis, or hemorrhoids); inflammatory disorders; exposure to radiation or chemical toxins (arsenic, lead, benzenes, copper)

Medications: Use of vitamin and iron supplements; aspirin, anticoagulants, oral contraceptives, phenobarbital, penicillins, NSAIDs, phenacetin, quinine, quinidine, phenytoin (Dilantin), methyldopa (Aldomet), sulfonamides

Surgery and other treatments: Recent surgery, small bowel resection, gastrectomy, prosthetic heart valves

Functional health patterns

Health perception–health management: Family history of anemia; malaise

Nutritional-metabolic: Nausea, vomiting, anorexia, weight loss; dysphagia, dyspepsia, heartburn, pica; night sweats, cold intolerance

Elimination: Hematuria, decreased urinary output; diarrhea, constipation, flatulence, tarry stools

Activity-exercise: Muscle weakness and decreased strength; dyspnea, orthopnea, cough, hemoptysis; palpitations

Cognitive-perceptual: Headache; abdominal, chest, and bone pain; painful tongue; paresthesias of feet and hands; disturbances in vision, taste, or hearing; vertigo

Sexuality-reproductive: Menorrhagia, metrorrhagia; recent or current pregnancy

Objective Data

General

Lethargy, apathy, general lymphadenopathy, fever

Integumentary

Pale skin and mucous membranes; blue or pale white sclera; poor skin turgor; brittle, spoon-shaped fingernails; jaundice; petechiae; ecchymoses; nose or gingival bleeding; poor healing; dry, brittle, thinning hair

Respiratory

Tachypnea

Cardiovascular

Tachycardia, systolic murmur, intermittent claudication, ankle edema, dysrhythmias, postural hypotension

Gastrointestinal

Hepatosplenomegaly; glossitis; beefy, red tongue; stomatitis; abdominal distention

Neurologic

Confusion, impaired judgment, irritability, ataxia, unsteady gait, paralysis

Possible findings

↓Hb; ↓ Hct; ↓ serum iron, ferritin, folate, or vitamin B_{12}; heme(guaiac) positive stools

GI, Gastrointestinal; *Hb,* hemoglobin; *Hct,* hematocrit; *NSAIDs,* nonsteroidal antiinflammatory drugs.

Planning

The overall goals are that the patient with anemia will (1) be able to participate in activities of daily living (ADLs), (2) experience no fatigue with activity, (3) have a nutritional intake containing essential nutrients for erythropoiesis, and (4) understand and comply with the therapeutic regimen.

Nursing Implementation

The numerous causes of anemia necessitate different nursing interventions specific to the needs of the patient. Nevertheless, there are certain general components of care for all patients with anemia. These are presented in the nursing care plan for the patient with anemia on p. 779.

Dietary and lifestyle changes (described with specific types of anemia) can reverse some anemias so that the patient can return to the former state of health. Acute interventions include blood transfusions, pharmacologic management (e.g., erythropoietin, vitamin replacements), and oxygen therapy. However, correcting the etiology of the anemia is ultimately the goal of therapy. Chronic management of anemias most often requires dietary and lifestyle changes. Long-term transfusion therapy or erythropoeitin injections may occasionally be required.

Gerontologic Considerations

Anemia is common in older adults. Women more than 60 years of age have a prevalence as high as women in childbearing years.[2] Nutritional deficiencies account for the majority of anemia seen in older adults. Physical debilitation and depression among older adults can interfere with their ability to maintain adequate nutrition[3] (Table 28-5). Many signs and symptoms of anemia are unrecognized in the older adult or are mistakenly attributed to aging. These symptoms include confusion, ataxia, fatigue, worsening angina, and CHF. Multiple comorbid conditions in older adults increase the likelihood of occurrence of many types of anemia. However, these same conditions and the bias about what constitutes "normal aging" also contribute to the difficulty in diagnosing reversible causes. For example, an easily reversible iron deficiency anemia presenting as ataxia may go unrecognized and untreated in an older patient. The nurse can play a major role in providing appropriate health assessment and related interventions for the older adult.

ANEMIA CAUSED BY DECREASED ERYTHROCYTE PRODUCTION

Normally RBC production is in equilibrium with RBC destruction and loss. This balance ensures that an adequate number of erythrocytes are available at all times. RBCs must be replenished on a regular basis because they are viable for only 120 days. Three significant alterations in erythropoiesis may occur that decrease RBC production: (1) decreased hemoglobin synthesis may lead to iron-deficiency anemia, thalassemia, and sideroblastic anemia; (2) defective DNA synthesis in RBCs may lead to megaloblastic anemias (e.g., vitamin B_{12} deficiency, folic acid deficiency); and (3) diminished availability of erythrocyte precursors may result in aplastic anemia and anemia of chronic disease (Table 28-1).

Iron-Deficiency Anemia

Iron-deficiency anemia, one of the most common chronic hematologic disorders, is found in 10% to 30% of the population in the United States. Regardless of economics or

NURSING CARE PLAN Patient with Anemia

Planning: Outcome Criteria	*Nursing Interventions and Rationales*
➤ **NURSING DIAGNOSIS**	Activity intolerance *related to* decreased hemoglobin and imbalance between oxygen supply and demand *as manifested by* difficulty in tolerating increased activity (e.g., increased BP, pulse, respiration), statement of feeling fatigued with minimal exertion
Feel rested; participate in ADLs (e.g., bathing, dressing, grooming, feeding) to greatest extent possible; have vital signs within acceptable range.	Plan care to alternate periods of rest and activity *to provide activity without tiring the patient.* Strive for a 1:3 rest to activity ratio; assist patient with ADLs as needed. Place objects within patient's reach *to reduce physiologic demands brought on by exertion.* Limit visitors, phone calls, noise, and interruptions by hospital staff *to reduce demands placed on patient.* Monitor vital signs *to evaluate activity tolerance.* Monitor Hct and Hb *as a guide to planning activities.*
➤ **NURSING DIAGNOSIS**	Altered nutrition: less than body requirements *related to* disease, treatment, and lack of knowledge of adequate nutrition *as manifested by* weight loss, low serum albumin, decreased iron levels, vitamin deficiencies, weight below normal for height, weakness, poor color and skin turgor, inadequate dietary intake
Consume well-balanced, high-caloric diet and adequate intake of nutrients necessary for RBC production; maintain weight, then gradually increase within range of ideal.	Teach basics of good nutrition, especially importance of including nutrients needed for RBC production *to increase intake of essential nutrients needed for hematopoiesis.* With input from patient, establish range of optimal weight outcomes and dietary plan *to involve patient and increase compliance.* Teach and monitor use of a food diary *to increase patient's awareness of actual intake as compared to necessary intake.* Encourage oral hygiene before and after meals *to enhance taste.* Give antacids or other agents before meals as ordered *to reduce gastric distress.*
➤ **NURSING DIAGNOSIS**	Self-care deficit: partial to total *related to* weakness and fatigue *as manifested by* inability to accomplish part or all of ADLs
Plans for accomplishment of ADLs by patient or with assistance.	Assess patient's ability to perform ADLs *to determine the need for interventions.* Assist patient with self-care as needed *to ensure needs are met.* Pace activities and intersperse periods of rest *to prevent hypoxemia and fatigue.* Plan help if needed at discharge *so activities of daily living can be accomplished at home.*
➤ **NURSING DIAGNOSIS**	Impaired physical mobility *related to* fatigue and weakness *as manifested by* inability to ambulate independently, reluctance to self-mobilize
Maintain joint functioning; increase mobility as is realistic for state of health.	Assess patient's ability to ambulate *to determine degree of hypoxia.* Determine appropriate activity levels given the patient's degree of disability *to maximize patient's mobility while ensuring safety.* Promote active or passive range of motion as indicated *to maintain strength and function of all joints.*

continued

geography, iron-deficiency anemia is most common in infants, children, women who are premenopausal or pregnant, and older adults.

Iron is present in all RBCs as heme in hemoglobin and in a stored form. The heme in hemoglobin accounts for two thirds of the body's iron. The other one third of iron is stored as ferritin and hemosiderin in macrophages in the bone marrow, spleen, and liver. Normally, 1 mg of iron is lost daily through the gastrointestinal (GI) tract, sweat, and urine. When the stored iron is not replaced, hemoglobin production is reduced.

Etiology. Iron deficiency may develop from inadequate dietary intake, malabsorption, blood loss, or hemolysis. Iron is obtained from dietary intake. Approximately 1 mg of every 10 to 20 mg of iron ingested is absorbed in the duodenum. Therefore only approximately 5% to 10% of ingested iron is absorbed. This amount of dietary iron is adequate to meet the needs of men and older women, but it may be inadequate for those individuals who have higher iron needs (e.g., children, pregnant women). Table 28-5 lists nutrients needed for erythropoiesis.

Malabsorption of iron may occur after certain types of GI surgery and in malabsorption syndromes. Iron absorption primarily occurs in the duodenum. Surgical procedures such as Billroth I or II often involve the removal of or bypass of the duodenum (see Chapter 40). Malabsorption syndromes commonly involve disease of the upper small intestine, where iron is normally absorbed. The absorption of iron is impeded in malabsorption states because the disease has altered or destroyed the absorptive surface.

NURSING CARE PLAN Patient with Anemia—cont'd

Planning: Outcome Criteria	Nursing Interventions and Rationales
➤ **NURSING DIAGNOSIS**	Anxiety *related to* inability to care for self and lack of knowledge of cause of weakness and prognosis *as manifested by* frequent questioning about reason for weakness and outcome of disease; restlessness, apathy; concern about ability for self-care
Adapt to condition; cooperate with plan of care; express confidence that needs will be met.	Teach patient about causes of weakness and course of disease *to promote realistic expectations and decrease anxiety about weakness.* Include family in teaching *to promote understanding and cooperation with treatment plan.* Answer questions accurately and honestly. Assess need for assistance *to help patient make realistic plans related to future care.*
➤ **NURSING DIAGNOSIS**	Altered health maintenance *related to* lack of knowledge about lifestyle adjustments, appropriate nutrition, and medication regimen *as manifested by* questioning about lifestyle adjustments, diet, medication prescriptions
Demonstrate knowledge about lifestyle changes, nutrition, and medication regimens.	Review and teach patient about lifestyle changes and nutrition and medication information *to promote compliance.* Teach about and monitor response to supplemental drugs that aid in RBC production *because it is difficult to correct severe anemia by diet alone.* Suggest follow-up resources to help patient maintain gains and adjustments throughout recovery.
➤ **NURSING DIAGNOSIS**	Risk of injury: falls *related to* weakness and dizziness
Adjust mobility to minimize risk for fall; experience no injuries from falling.	Monitor for risk factors for falls such as unsteady gait, dizziness when changing positions or ambulating. Teach patient to change position slowly *to prevent dizziness caused by cerebral hypoxia.* Discourage patient from ambulating alone *to avoid injury.* Assess vital signs before ambulating *to identify low BP and need to modify ambulation plan.* Assess home environment *to minimize risks for falling at home.*

COLLABORATIVE PROBLEMS

Nursing Goals	Nursing Interventions and Rationales
➤ **POTENTIAL COMPLICATION**	Hypoxemia *related to* decreased Hb
Monitor for signs of hypoxemia, report deviations from acceptable parameters and carry out appropriate medical and nursing interventions.	Assess for manifestations of hypoxemia such as dyspnea, decrease in O_2 saturation, increase in $PaCO_2$, cyanosis *to initiate early intervention.* Administer O_2 as ordered *to saturate all available Hb.* Transfuse with blood products as ordered *to increase Hb.* Change patient's position slowly; evaluate dizziness *as sign of cerebral hypoxia.* Monitor Hb *to determine severity of anemia and response to treatment.*

ADLs, Activities of daily living; *BP,* blood pressure; *Hb,* hemoglobin; *Hct,* hematocrit; *RBC,* red blood cell.

Blood loss is a major cause of iron deficiency in adults. Two milliliters of whole blood contain 1 mg of iron. The major sources of chronic blood loss are from the GI and genitourinary (GU) systems. GI bleeding is often not apparent and therefore may exist for a considerable time before the problem is identified. Loss of 50 to 75 ml of blood from the upper GI tract is required to cause stools to appear as *melena.* The black color of melena results from the iron in the RBCs. Common causes of GI blood loss in the adult are peptic ulcer, gastritis, esophagitis, diverticuli, hemorrhoids, and neoplasia. GU blood loss occurs primarily from menstrual bleeding. The average monthly menstrual blood loss is about 45 ml and causes the loss of about 22 mg of iron. Postmenopausal bleeding is rarely significant but also can contribute to anemia in a susceptible older woman.

Pregnancy contributes to iron deficiency because of the diversion of iron to the fetus for erythropoiesis, blood loss at delivery, and lactation. In addition to anemia of chronic renal failure, dialysis treatment may induce iron-deficiency anemia because of the blood lost in the dialysis equipment and frequent blood sampling.

Clinical Manifestations. In the early course of iron-deficiency anemia, the patient may be free of symptoms. As

Table 28-5 Nutritional Management: Nutrients Needed for Erythropoiesis

Nutrient	Role in Erythropoiesis	Food Sources
Vitamin B_{12}	RBC maturation	Red meats, especially liver
Folic acid	RBC maturation	Green leafy vegetables, liver, meat, fish, legumes, whole grains
Iron	Hemoglobin synthesis	Liver and muscle meats, eggs, dried fruits, legumes, dark green leafy vegetables, whole-grain and enriched bread and cereals, potatoes
Vitamin B_6	Hemoglobin synthesis	Meats (especially pork and liver), wheat germ, legumes, potatoes, cornmeal, bananas
Amino acids	Synthesis of nucleoproteins	Eggs, meat, milk and milk products (cheese, ice cream), poultry, fish, legumes, nuts
Vitamin C	Conversion of folic acid to its active forms, aids in iron absorption	Citrus fruits, leafy green vegetables, strawberries, cantaloupe

the disease becomes chronic, any of the general manifestations of anemia may develop (Table 28-3). In addition, specific clinical symptoms may occur related to iron-deficiency anemia. Pallor is the most common finding, and *glossitis* (inflammation of the tongue) is the second most common; another finding is *cheilitis* (inflammation of the lips). In addition, the patient may report headache, paresthesias, and a burning sensation of the tongue, all of which are caused by lack of iron in the tissues.

Diagnostic Studies. Laboratory abnormalities characteristic of iron-deficiency anemia are presented in Table 28-6. Other diagnostic studies are done to determine the cause of the iron deficiency. For example, endoscopy and colonoscopy may be used to detect GI bleeding.

Therapeutic and Pharmacologic Management. The main goal of the therapeutic management of iron-deficiency anemia is to treat the underlying disease that is causing reduced intake (e.g., malnutrition, alcoholism) or absorption of iron. In addition, efforts are directed toward replacing iron (Table 28-7). This may be done through increasing the intake of iron. The patient should be taught which foods are good sources of iron (Table 28-5). If nutrition is already adequate, increasing iron intake by dietary means may not be reasonable because it is difficult for nutritional intake to exceed 7 mg of iron per 1000 kcal without the use of dietary supplements (e.g., an 8-oz steak supplies 8 mg of iron). Consequently, oral or, occasionally, parenteral iron supplements are used. If the iron deficiency is from significant acute blood loss, transfusion of packed RBCs may be required.

Oral iron should be used whenever possible because it is inexpensive and convenient. Many iron preparations are available. Four factors that should be considered in the administration of iron are the following:

1. The dosage should provide 150 to 200 mg elemental iron daily. This can be ingested in three or four daily doses, with each tablet or capsule of the iron preparation containing between 50 and 100 mg of iron (e.g., a 325-mg tablet of ferrous sulfate contains 50 mg of elemental iron).
2. Iron is best absorbed in an acidic environment. For this reason and to avoid binding the iron with food, iron should be taken about an hour before meals, when the duodenal mucosa is most acidic. Taking iron with vitamin C (ascorbic acid) or orange juice, which contains ascorbic acid, also enhances iron absorption. Gastric side effects, however, may necessitate ingesting iron with meals. Enteric-coated iron may be ineffective because the iron may not be released in an area in the intestine that facilitates absorption.
3. Undiluted liquid iron may stain the patient's teeth; therefore it should be diluted and ingested through a straw.
4. Mild GI side effects of iron administration may occur, including pyrosis (heartburn), constipation, and diarrhea. If side effects develop, the dose and type of iron supplement may be adjusted. For example, many individuals who need supplemental iron cannot tolerate ferrous sulfate because of the effects of the sulfate base. However, ferrous gluconate may be an acceptable substitute. All patients should know that the use of iron preparations will cause their stools to become black because excess iron is excreted by the GI tract. Constipation is common, and the patient should be told about this side effect because constipation may be a reason for decreased patient compliance.

In some situations, it may be necessary to administer iron parenterally. Parenteral use of iron is indicated for malabsorption, intolerance of oral iron, a need for iron beyond oral limits, and poor patient compliance in taking the oral preparations of iron. Parenteral iron can be given intramuscularly (IM) or intravenously (IV).

Because IM iron solutions may stain the skin, separate needles should be used for withdrawing the solution and for injecting the medication. Approximately 0.5 ml of air should be left in the syringe to clear the iron completely from the syringe. Iron should be given deep IM in the upper outer quadrant of the buttocks, with a 2-inch to 3-inch needle with a 19 to 20 gauge. Preferably, no more than 2 ml of iron is given in a single injection. A Z-track technique should be used for injection to prevent leakage of the iron solution to the subcutaneous (SC) tissue. The site should not be massaged after the injection is given.

Table 28-6 Laboratory Study Findings in Anemias

	Iron Deficiency	Thalassemia Major	Vitamin B_{12} Deficiency	Folic Acid Deficiency	Aplastic Anemia	Chronic Disease	Acute Blood Loss	Chronic Blood Loss	Sickle Cell Anemia	Hemolytic Anemia
Hb/Hct	↓	↓	↓	↓	↓	↓	↓	↓	↓	↓
MCV	↓	N	↑	↑	N	N	N	↓	N	N
MCH	↓	N	N or slight ↓	N or slight ↓	N	N	N	↓	N	N
MCHC	↓	N	↑	↑	N	N	N	↓	N	N
Reticulocytes	N or ↓	↑	↓	N	↓	N	N	N or ↑	↑	↑
Serum iron	↓	↑	N	N	±N	↓	N	↓	N to ↑	↑
TIBC	↑	↑	N	N	±N	↓	N	↓	N to ↓	↓
Bilirubin	N to ↓	↑	N	N	N	±N	N	N to ↓	↑	N to ↑
Platelets	N or ↑	—	↓	—	↓	↑	—	↑	↑	—
Other findings	—	—	↓vitamin B_{12}, positive Schilling test, achlorhydria	↓ folate	↓ WBC	—	—	—	See Table 28-11	—

Hb, Hemoglobin; *Hct,* hematocrit; *MCH,* mean corpuscular hemoglobin; *MCHC,* mean corpuscular hemoglobin concentration; *MCV,* mean corpuscular volume; *N,* normal; *TIBC,* total iron-binding capacity; *WBC,* white blood cell.

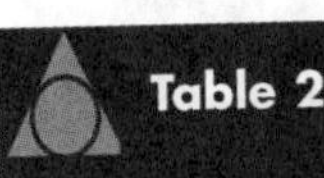

Table 28-7 Therapeutic Management: Iron-Deficiency Anemia

Diagnostic
History and physical examination
Hct and Hb levels
RBC count, including morphology
Reticulocyte count
Serum iron
Serum ferritin
Total iron-binding capacity
Fecal examination for occult blood
Therapeutic
Identification and treatment of underlying cause
Administration of ferrous sulfate or ferrous gluconate
Administration of iron dextran IM or IV
Diet rich in foods containing iron
Nutritional education
Transfusion of packed RBCs (symptomatic patient only)

Hb, Hemoglobin; *Hct*, hematocrit; *IM*, intramuscular; *IV*, intravenous; *RBCs*, red blood cells.

NURSING MANAGEMENT

IRON-DEFICIENCY ANEMIA

It is important to recognize groups of individuals who are at an increased risk for the development of iron-deficiency anemia. These include infants, teenage girls, premenopausal and pregnant women, persons from low socioeconomic backgrounds, older adults, and individuals experiencing blood loss. Diet teaching, with an emphasis on foods high in iron, is important for these groups. Supplemental iron is especially important for the pregnant woman. Appropriate nursing measures are presented in the nursing care plan for the patient with anemia on p. 779.

If anemia is present, it is important to discuss with the patient the need for diagnostic studies to identify the cause. The Hb level and RBC count should be reassessed to evaluate the response to therapy. Compliance with dietary and drug therapy needs to be emphasized. To replenish the body's iron stores, the patient should take iron therapy for 2 to 3 months after the Hb level returns to normal. An older adult patient may require lifelong iron supplementation. If the Hb level remains low, the patient must be reevaluated for the cause of anemia.

Thalassemia

Another cause of decreased erythrocyte production is known as *thalassemia.* As in iron deficiency, it is a disease of inadequate production of normal hemoglobin. Hemolysis also occurs in thalassemia, but insufficient production of normal hemoglobin is the predominant problem. In contrast to iron-deficiency anemia, in which heme synthesis is the problem, thalassemia involves a problem with the globin protein. Therefore the basic defect of thalassemia is abnormal hemoglobin synthesis.

Etiology. Thalassemias are a group of autosomal recessive genetic disorders commonly found in members of ethnic groups whose origins are near the Mediterranean Sea. An individual with thalassemia may have a heterozygous or homozygous form of the disease. A person who is heterozygous has one thalassemic gene and one normal gene and is said to have *thalassemia minor* or *thalassemic trait,* which is a mild form of the disease. A homozygous person has two thalassemic genes, causing a severe condition known as *thalassemia major.*

Clinical Manifestations. The patient with thalassemia minor is frequently asymptomatic because the patient adjusts to the gradually acquired chronic state of anemia. Occasionally, splenomegaly may develop in this patient, and mild jaundice may occur if malformed erythrocytes are rapidly hemolyzed. The person who has thalassemia major is pale and displays other general symptoms of anemia (see Table 28-3). In addition, the person has pronounced splenomegaly and hepatomegaly. Jaundice from RBC hemolysis is prominent. Chronic bone marrow hyperplasia leads to expansion of the marrow space. This may cause thickening of the cranium and maxillary cavity, leading to an appearance resembling Down syndrome. Thalassemia major is a life-threatening disease in which growth, both physical and mental, is often retarded.

Therapeutic Management. The laboratory abnormalities of thalassemia major are summarized in Table 28-6. Thalassemia minor requires no treatment because the body adapts to the reduction of normal hemoglobin. Thalassemia major is usually treated with blood transfusions and chelation therapy (therapy to reduce the iron overloading that sometimes occurs with chronic transfusion therapy). Medication and diet therapy are not effective in treating thalassemia. Transfusions are administered to keep the Hb level at approximately 10 g/dl (100 g/L). This level is low enough to foster the patient's own erythropoiesis without enlarging the spleen. Because RBCs are sequestered in the enlarged spleen, thalassemia may be treated by splenectomy. However, even with therapeutic management, the person with thalassemia major will gradually progress to a fatal outcome from effects of chronic iron overload (from the RBC transfusions) on the heart.[4] A rare patient has also been treated with HLA-compatible bone marrow transplantation. In this approach an attempt is made to change the defective marrow stem cells to ones that are capable of normal erythropoeisis.

Megaloblastic Anemias

Megaloblastic anemias are disorders caused by impaired DNA synthesis and characterized by the presence of large RBCs. When DNA synthesis is impaired, defective RBC maturation results. The RBCs are large (macrocytic) and abnormal and are referred to as *megaloblasts.* Macrocytic RBCs are easily destroyed because of their fragile membranes. Although the overwhelming majority of megaloblastic anemias result from vitamin B_{12} and folate deficiencies, this type of red cell deformity can also occur from suppression of DNA synthesis by drugs, from inborn errors of vitamin B_{12} and folic acid metabolism, and from erythroleukemia (an erythropoietic malignancy) (Table 28-8). Common forms of megaloblastic anemia are vitamin B_{12} deficiency (e.g., pernicious anemia) and folic acid deficiency.

Table 28-8 Classification of Megaloblastic Anemias

Vitamin B_{12} Deficiency
- Dietary deficiency
- Deficiency of gastric intrinsic factor
  - Pernicious anemia
  - Gastrectomy
- Intestinal malabsorption
- Increased requirement

Folic Acid Deficiency
- Dietary deficiency
- Impaired absorption
- Increased requirement

Drug-Induced Suppression of DNA Synthesis
- Folate antagonists
- Metabolic inhibitors
- Alkylating agents
- Nitrous oxide

Inborn Errors
- Hereditary orotic aciduria
- Defective folate metabolism
- Lesch-Nyhan syndrome
- Defective transport of vitamin B_{12}

Erythroleukemia

DNA, Deoxyribonucleic acid.

CULTURAL & ETHNIC *Considerations*

HEMATOLOGIC PROBLEMS

- Sickle cell disease has a high incidence among African-Americans.
- Thalassemia has a high incidence among African-Americans and people of Mediterranean origin.
- Tay-Sachs disease has the highest incidence in families of Eastern European Jewish origin, especially the Ashkenazic Jews.
- Pernicious anemia has a high incidence in Scandinavians and African-Americans.

Vitamin B_{12} Deficiency. Normally, a protein known as *intrinsic factor* (IF) is secreted by the parietal cells of the gastric mucosa. IF is required for vitamin B_{12} (extrinsic factor) absorption. Therefore if intrinsic factor is not secreted, vitamin B_{12} cannot be absorbed. (Vitamin B_{12} is normally absorbed in the distal ileum.) In pernicious anemia, gastric secretion of intrinsic factor is defective. Although once fatal, pernicious anemia is now treatable. The term *pernicious anemia* has been used inappropriately to describe any vitamin B_{12} deficiency. However, pernicious anemia is only one cause of vitamin B_{12} deficiency, and the term should be used only to describe the situations in which the gastric mucosa is clearly not secreting IF (Table 28-8).

Etiology. Pernicious anemia is a disease of insidious onset that generally begins in middle age or later (usually after age 40). In this condition, IF secretion fails because of gastric mucosal atrophy. Pernicious anemia is an autoimmune disease; the gastric atrophy of pernicious anemia probably results from destruction of the parietal cells.

Pernicious anemia occurs frequently in persons of Northern European ancestry, particularly Scandinavians, and African-Americans. In African-Americans, the disease tends to begin early, occurs with high frequency in women, and is often severe.

Vitamin B_{12} deficiency can occur in a patient who has a total gastrectomy or small bowel resection involving the ileum. Vitamin B_{12} deficiency results from the loss of IF-secreting gastric mucosal surface or impaired absorption of vitamin B_{12} in the distal ileum.

Clinical manifestations. General symptoms of anemia related to vitamin B_{12} deficiency develop because of tissue hypoxia (Table 28-3). GI manifestations include a sore tongue, anorexia, nausea, vomiting, and abdominal pain. Typical neuromuscular manifestations include weakness, paresthesias of the feet and hands, reduced vibratory and position senses, ataxia, muscle weakness, and impaired thought processes ranging from confusion to dementia. Because vitamin B_{12} deficiency–related anemia has an insidious onset, it may take several months for these manifestations to develop.

Diagnostic studies. Laboratory data reflective of vitamin B_{12} deficiency anemia is presented in Table 28-6. The erythrocytes appear large (macrocytic) and have abnormal shapes. This structure contributes to erythrocyte destruction because the cell membrane is fragile. Additional studies may need to be performed. Serum vitamin B_{12} levels will be reduced. A gastric analysis is done to ascertain the cause of the vitamin B_{12} deficiency. A nasogastric tube is inserted, pentagastrin is injected to stimulate gastric juice secretion, and the gastric juice is aspirated via the nasogastric tube for a period of time. If analysis of the gastric juice reveals *achlorhydria* (the absence of free hydrochloric acid in a pH never lower than 3.5), depressed parietal cell function can be determined.

Another means of assessing parietal cell function is by a Schilling test. After radioactive vitamin B_{12} is administered to the patient, the amount of vitamin B_{12} excreted in the urine is measured. An individual who cannot absorb vitamin B_{12} excretes only a small amount of this radioactive form. The same procedure may be followed with the addition of IF parenterally. Absorption of vitamin B_{12} when IF is added is diagnostic of pernicious anemia.

Therapeutic and pharmacologic management. Regardless of how much vitamin B_{12} is ingested, the patient is not able to absorb it if IF is lacking or there is impaired absorption in the ileum, so dietary management is not a reasonable approach for vitamin B_{12} replacement. However, the patient should be instructed on adequate dietary intake to maintain good nutrition (Table 28-6). The treatment of vitamin B_{12} deficiency is based on replacing vitamin B_{12}. Without vitamin B_{12} administration, these individuals will die in 1 to 3 years. As long as supplemental vitamin B_{12} is used, the anemia can be controlled. Hematologic manifestations can be completely reversed. However, most long-standing (>3 months) neuromuscular complications will not be reversed by this therapy.

Parenteral administration of vitamin B_{12} (cyanocobalamin or hydroxycobalamin) is the treatment of choice. The efficacy of vitamin B_{12} injections in altering the otherwise fatal course cannot be overemphasized. The dosage and frequency of vitamin B_{12} administration may vary. A typical treatment schedule consists of 1000 μg cobalamin IM daily for 2 weeks, then weekly until the Hct is normal, then monthly for life.

NURSING MANAGEMENT

PERNICIOUS ANEMIA

Because of the familial predisposition involved, patients who have a positive family history of pernicious anemia should be evaluated for symptoms. Although disease development cannot be prevented, early detection and treatment can lead to reversal of symptoms.

The nursing measures presented in the nursing care plan for the patient with anemia are appropriate for the patient with vitamin B_{12} deficiency anemia. In addition to these measures, the nurse should ensure that injuries are not sustained because of the diminished sensations to heat and pain resulting from the neurologic impairment. The patient must be protected from burns and trauma. If heat therapy is required, the patient's skin must be evaluated at frequent intervals to detect redness. Irritation from nasogastric tubes and restrictive clothing may not be perceived by the patient because of reduced pain sensations.

Ongoing care is primarily related to ensuring good patient compliance in returning for monthly vitamin B_{12} injections. There must also be careful follow-up to assess for neurologic difficulties that were not fully corrected by adequate vitamin B_{12} replacement therapy. Because the potential for gastric carcinoma is increased in pernicious anemia, the patient should have frequent and careful evaluation for this problem.

Folic Acid Deficiency. Folic acid deficiency also causes megaloblastic anemia. Folic acid is required for DNA synthesis leading to RBC formation and maturation. Four common causes of folic acid deficiency are the following:

1. Poor nutrition, especially a lack of leafy green vegetables, liver, citrus fruits, yeast, dried beans, nuts, and grains
2. Malabsorption syndromes, particularly small bowel disorders
3. Drugs that impede the absorption and use of folic acid (e.g., methotrexate, oral contraceptives) and anticonvulsants (e.g., phenobarbital, diphenylhydantoin)
4. Alcohol abuse and anorexia

The clinical manifestations of folic acid deficiency are similar to those of vitamin B_{12} deficiency. The disease develops insidiously, and the patient's symptoms may be attributed to other coexisting problems such as cirrhosis or esophageal varices. GI disturbances include dyspepsia and a smooth, beefy red tongue. The absence of neurologic problems is an important diagnostic finding. This lack of neurologic involvement differentiates folic acid deficiency from vitamin B_{12} deficiency.

The diagnostic findings for folic acid deficiency are presented in Table 28-6. In addition, the serum folate level is low (normal is 3 to 25 ng/ml [7 to 57 nmol/L]), the serum vitamin B_{12} level is normal, and the gastric analysis is positive for hydrochloric acid.

Folic acid deficiency is treated by replacement therapy. The usual dose is 1 mg per day by mouth. In malabsorption states, up to 5 mg per day may be required. The duration of treatment depends on the reason for the deficiency. The patient should be encouraged to eat foods containing large amounts of folic acid (see Table 28-5).

Anemia of Chronic Disease

Hypoproliferative anemias (decreased erythrocyte precursors) may develop in several chronic conditions. One specific cause is end-stage renal disease. There is a relationship between the degree of anemia and the severity of uremia. Although several mechanisms may be involved in the development of anemia with renal disease, the primary factor is decreased erythropoietin, a hormone made in the kidneys that is necessary for erythropoiesis. With impaired renal function, decreased levels of erythropoietin are produced (see Chapter 44).

Other chronic, inflammatory, or malignant diseases can lead to the *anemia of chronic disease.* Chronic liver disease may also contribute to the development of anemia. Anemia may result from the folic acid deficiencies caused by inadequate nutrition in abusers of alcohol or from blood loss caused by chronic gastritis. The use of alcohol itself may reduce erythropoiesis. Anemia may also result from splenomegaly, which is commonly found in advanced stages of cirrhosis (see Chapter 41).

Chronic inflammation and malignant tumors are other conditions in which anemia may be present. The mechanisms involved include increased RBC destruction accompanied by a failure to augment erythropoiesis to compensate for the rise in destruction. Chemotherapy with heavy metals (e.g., cisplatin, carboplatin) for malignant diseases is a common cause of anemia in neoplastic disease.[5] Anemia related to human immunodeficiency virus (HIV) and its treatment with AZT are other causes of anemia.

Chronic endocrine diseases may also lead to anemia. Hypopituitary and hypothyroid states both lead to reduced tissue metabolism; therefore tissue oxygen needs are diminished, leading to a reduced production of erythropoietin by the kidneys. Adrenal hypofunction caused by either adrenalectomy or Addison's disease also results in anemia.

Anemia of chronic disease must first be recognized and differentiated from anemias of other etiologies. Findings of elevated serum ferritin and increased iron stores will distinguish it from iron deficiency anemia. Effective treatment for anemia of chronic disease begins with specific therapy of the underlying etiology. The anemia of chronic disease is not responsive to iron, folic acid, or vitamin B_{12}. Because the anemia is rarely severe, blood transfusions are rarely indicated. Anemia related to end-stage renal disease does respond to erythropoietin therapy (see Chapter 44).

Aplastic Anemia

One of the most severe forms of anemia related to reduced erythrocyte production is a group of disorders termed *aplastic* or *hypoplastic* anemias. These anemias are life-threatening stem cell disorders characterized by hypoplastic, fatty bone marrow that result in pancytopenia. Aplastic anemia is somewhat of a misnomer because in most cases all marrow elements—erythrocytes, leukocytes, and platelets—are quantitatively decreased, although they are qualitatively normal.[6]

Etiology. The incidence of aplastic anemia is low, affecting approximately 4 persons per 1 million. There are various etiologic classifications for aplastic anemia, but they can be divided into two major groups: congenital or acquired (Table 28-9).

1. Congenital origin caused by chromosomal alterations (approximately 30% of the aplastic anemias that appear in childhood are inherited).
2. Acquired as a result of exposure to ionizing radiation, chemical agents (e.g., benzene, insecticides, arsenic, alcohol), viral and bacterial infections (e.g., hepatitis, parvovirus, miliary tuberculosis), and prescribed medications (e.g., alkylating agents, analgesics, anticonvulsants, antimetabolites, antimicrobials, gold). The causes of 70% of acquired cases of aplastic anemia are idiopathic.[6]

Clinical Manifestations. Aplastic anemia usually develops insidiously. Clinically the patient may have symptoms caused by suppression of any or all bone marrow elements. General manifestations of anemia such as fatigue and dyspnea, as well as cardiovascular and cerebral responses, may be seen (Table 28-3). The patient with granulocytopenia is susceptible to infection and generally has a fever. Thrombocytopenia is manifested by a predisposition to bleed (e.g., petechiae, ecchymoses, epistaxis).

Diagnostic Studies. The diagnosis is confirmed by laboratory studies. Because all marrow elements are affected, hemoglobin, white blood cell (WBC), and platelet values are often decreased in aplastic anemia (Table 28-6). However, the RBC indices are normal. The condition is therefore classified as a normocytic, normochromic anemia. The reticulocyte count is low. Bleeding time is prolonged.

Aplastic anemia can be further evaluated by assessing various iron studies. The serum iron and total iron-binding capacity (TIBC) are elevated as initial signs of erythroid suppression. Bone marrow examination may be done for any anemic state. However, the findings are especially important in aplastic anemia because the marrow is hypocellular, with increased yellow marrow (fat content), a finding referred to as a *dry tap.*

Table 28-9 Causes of Aplastic Anemia

Congenital	
Fanconi syndrome	
Familial aplastic anemia	
Acquired	
Radiation	Viral and bacterial infections
Chemical agents and toxins	Pregnancy
Drugs	Idiopathic

THERAPEUTIC AND NURSING MANAGEMENT

APLASTIC ANEMIA

Management of aplastic anemia is based on identifying and removing the causative agent (when possible) and providing supportive care until the pancytopenia reverses. Nursing interventions appropriate for the patient with pancytopenia from aplastic anemia are presented in the nursing care plans for the patient with anemia (p. 779), thrombocytopenia (p. 798), and neutropenia (p. 809). Nursing actions are directed at preventing complications from infection and hemorrhage.

The prognosis of untreated aplastic anemia is poor (approximately 75% fatal). However, advances in medical management, including bone marrow transplantation and immunosuppressive therapy with antithymocyte globulin (ATG) and cyclosporine, have improved outcomes significantly.[6] ATG is a horse serum containing polyclonal antibodies against human T cells. The rationale for this therapy is that aplastic anemia is an immune-mediated disease. (ATG and cyclosporine are discussed in Chapter 44.)

The treatment of choice for adults less than 45 years of age who have a human leukocyte antigen (HLA)–matched sibling donor is allogeneic bone marrow transplantation. The best results occur in a younger patient who has not had previous transfusions.[7] Prior transfusions increase the risk of graft rejection.

For the older adult or the patient without HLA-matched siblings, the treatment of choice is immunosuppression with ATG or cyclosporine. Response to this therapy may be only partial, but transfusions usually can be avoided.

ANEMIA CAUSED BY BLOOD LOSS

Anemia resulting from blood loss may be caused by either acute or chronic problems.

Acute Blood Loss

Acute blood loss occurs as a result of sudden hemorrhage. Causes of acute blood loss include trauma, complications of surgery, and diseases that disrupt vascular integrity. There are two clinical concerns in such situations. First, there is a sudden reduction in the total blood volume that can lead to hypovolemic shock. Second, if the acute loss is more gradual, the body maintains its blood volume by slowly increasing the plasma volume. Consequently, the circulating fluid volume is preserved, but the number of erythrocytes available to carry O_2 is significantly diminished.

Table 28-10 Clinical Manifestations of Acute Blood Loss

Volume Lost (%)	Clinical Manifestations
10	None
20	No detectable signs or symptoms at rest, tachycardia with exercise and slight postural hypotension
30	Normal supine blood pressure and pulse at rest, postural hypotension and tachycardia with exercise
40	Blood pressure, central venous pressure, and cardiac output below normal at rest; rapid, thready pulse and cold, clammy skin
50	Shock and potential death

Clinical Manifestations. The clinical manifestations of anemia from acute blood loss are caused by the body's attempts to maintain an adequate blood volume and meet O_2 requirements. Table 28-10 summarizes the clinical manifestations of patients with varying degrees of blood volume loss. It is essential to understand that clinical symptoms are valuable indicators of the degree of blood loss because laboratory data may not accurately reflect the severity of hemorrhage for 2 to 3 days.

The nurse should be alert to the patient's expression (verbal or nonverbal) of pain. Internal hemorrhage may cause pain because of tissue distention, organ displacement, and nerve compression. Pain may be localized or referred. In the case of retroperitoneal bleeding, the patient may not experience abdominal pain. Instead, the patient may have numbness and pain in a lower extremity secondary to compression of the lateral cutaneous nerve, which is located in the region of the first to third lumbar vertebrae. The major complication of acute blood loss is shock (see Chapter 7).

Diagnostic Studies. When blood volume loss is sudden, the body reacts by vasoconstriction. Because plasma volume has not yet had a chance to increase, the loss of RBC mass is not reflected in laboratory data, and the results may seem normal or high for 2 to 3 days. However, once the plasma is replaced by endogenous and exogenous means, the RBC mass is less concentrated. At this time, erythrocytes, Hb, and Hct levels are usually low and reflect the blood loss.

Therapeutic Management. Therapeutic management is initially concerned with (1) replacing blood volume to prevent shock and (2) identifying the source of the hemorrhage and stopping the blood loss. IV fluids used in emergencies include dextran, Hetastarch, albumin, or crystalloid electrolyte solutions such as lactated Ringer's. The amount of infusion varies with the solution used. (Management of shock is discussed in Chapter 7.)

Once volume replacement is established, attention can be directed to correcting RBC loss. The body needs 2 to 5 days to manufacture more RBCs in response to increased erythropoietin. Consequently, blood transfusions (packed RBCs) may be needed if the blood loss is significant.

The patient may also need supplemental iron because the iron supply affects the marrow production of erythrocytes. When anemia exists after acute blood loss, dietary sources of iron will probably not be adequate to maintain iron pools. For every 2 ml of blood lost, 1 mg of iron is also lost. Therefore oral or parenteral iron preparations are administered.

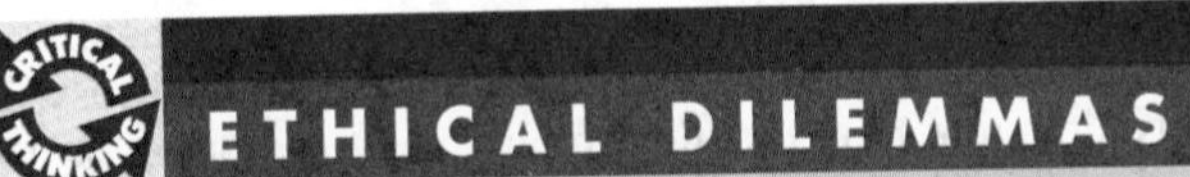

RELIGIOUS ISSUES

Situation An elderly woman is transferred from a nursing home because of gastrointestinal bleeding from an unknown cause. Some of her family members tell the nurse that she is a Jehovah's Witness and must not receive blood products. If she does not have exploratory surgery and transfusions, the physicians believe that she will die.

Discussion A competent adult has the right to make medical decisions based on religious beliefs. If the patient is not able to communicate her wishes and has no advance directives, a determination must be made about her religious beliefs before treatment decisions are made. Appropriate methods to make this determination would be consulting with the local church officials, inquiring about a wallet card identifying her religious affiliation and beliefs, and discussing her religious beliefs and involvement with the family. Jehovah's Witnesses believe that if they receive blood products, there are eternal consequences. If there is doubt about the patient's involvement in this church or commitment to the tenets of this article of faith, potentially lifesaving surgery and transfusion would be acceptable.

ETHICAL AND LEGAL PRINCIPLES

- The competent adult patient has the right to refuse medical treatment whether or not the refusal is based on religious beliefs.
- If a patient is not competent and has no advance directives, health care providers must protect the patient by determining whether it is the *patient's* belief that is the basis for refusing treatment.
- In two cases involving Jehovah's Witnesses in the 1960s, judges' decisions were based on the competency of the patient. A competent patient's wish to refuse treatment was upheld; an incompetent patient's wishes were not clear, and the transfusion was ordered.

NURSING MANAGEMENT

ACUTE BLOOD LOSS

In the case of trauma, it may be impossible to prevent the situation leading to the blood loss. For the postoperative patient, careful evaluation of blood loss from various drainage tubes and dressings facilitates early assessment of the source of bleeding and related appropriate treatment.

The nursing care plan for the patient with anemia is relevant to the anemia resulting from acute blood loss. In this situation, blood product replacement (described at the end of this chapter) is almost certainly necessary.

Once the source of hemorrhage is identified, blood loss is controlled, and fluid and blood volume are replaced, the anemia should begin to correct itself. There should be no need for long-term treatment of this type of anemia.

Chronic Blood Loss

The sources of *chronic blood loss* are similar to those of iron-deficiency anemia (e.g., bleeding ulcer, hemorrhoids, menstrual and postmenopausal blood loss). The effects of chronic blood loss are usually related to the depletion of iron stores and are usually considered as iron-deficiency anemia. Management of chronic blood loss anemia involves identifying the source and stopping the bleeding. Supplemental iron may be required. The nursing measures presented in the nursing care plan for the patient with anemia (p. 779) are relevant to anemia of chronic blood loss.

ANEMIA CAUSED BY INCREASED ERYTHROCYTE DESTRUCTION

The third major cause of anemia is the destruction, or *hemolysis,* of RBCs at a rate that exceeds production. Hemolysis can occur because of problems intrinsic or extrinsic to the RBCs. *Intrinsic hemolytic anemias* result from defects in the RBCs themselves caused by abnormal hemoglobin (e.g., sickle cells), enzyme deficiencies that alter glycolysis (glucose-6-phosphate dehydrogenase [G6PD] deficiency), or RBC membrane abnormalities. Intrinsic hemolytic anemias are usually hereditary. More common are the *extrinsic hemolytic anemias,* which are acquired. The patient's RBCs are normal, but damage is caused by external factors such as trapping of cells within the sinuses of the liver or spleen, antibody-mediated destruction, toxins, or mechanical injury (e.g., prosthetic heart valves).

The two sites of hemolysis are classified as *intravascular* or *extravascular.* Intravascular destruction occurs within the circulation; extravascular hemolysis takes place in the macrophages of the spleen, liver, and bone marrow. The spleen is the primary site of the destruction of RBCs that are old, defective, or moderately damaged. Figure 28-2 indicates the sequence of events involved in extravascular hemolysis.

The patient with hemolytic anemia manifests the general symptoms of anemia (see Table 28-3) and clinical manifestations specific to this type of anemia. Jaundice is likely because the increased destruction of RBCs causes an elevation in bilirubin levels. The spleen and liver may enlarge because of their hyperactivity, which is related to macrophage phagocytosis of the defective erythrocytes.

In all causes of hemolysis a major focus of treatment is to maintain renal function. When an RBC is hemolyzed, the hemoglobin molecule is released and filtered by the kidneys. The hemoglobin molecule can obstruct the renal tubule and lead to acute tubular necrosis (see Chapter 44).

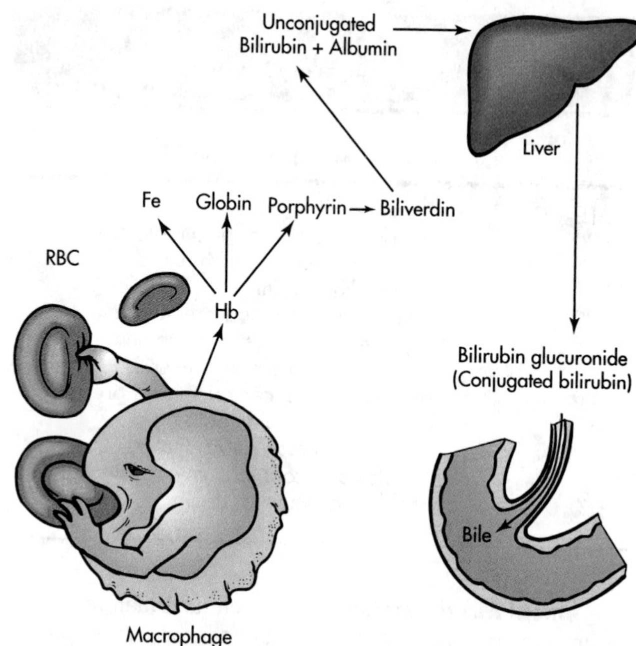

Fig. 28-2 Sequence of events in extravascular hemolysis. *Hb,* Hemoglobin; *RBC,* red blood cell.

Sickle Cell Disease

Sickle cell disease is a genetic disorder characterized by production of abnormal Hb, anemia, and acute and chronic tissue damage from vascular blockage by trapped abnormal RBCs. The most common type of sickle cell disease is sickle cell anemia, which produces abnormal Hb (hemoglobin S [HbS]) instead of normal Hb (hemoglobin A [HbA]). The disease affects more than 50,000 Americans and is predominant in African-Americans, occurring in an estimated prevalence of 1 in 375 live births. It can also affect people of Mediterranean, Caribbean, South and Central American, Arabian, or East Indian ancestry. It is an incurable type of anemia that is often fatal by middle age.[8]

Etiology. Sickle cell anemia is an autosomal recessive genetic disorder in which the person is homozygous for HbS. Some persons may have *sickle cell trait,* a mild condition that may be asymptomatic. A person with sickle cell trait is heterozygous, with approximately one fourth of the hemoglobin in the abnormal S form and three fourths in the normal A form (Fig. 28-3). If two parents have sickle cell trait, there is a 25% chance with each pregnancy that the child will have sickle cell anemia. The mutation that causes HbS to develop involves one amino acid. One valine amino acid is substituted for a glutamic acid. This substitution leads to an abnormal linking reaction that causes the development of deformed crescent-shaped cells when O_2 tension is lowered (Fig. 28-4).

Pathophysiology. When hypoxia occurs in a patient with sickle cell disease, the HbS assumes various crescent or sickle shapes. Erythrostasis develops when sickled red cells are trapped in small blood vessels. The erythrostasis causes further O_2 deprivation, which potentiates more

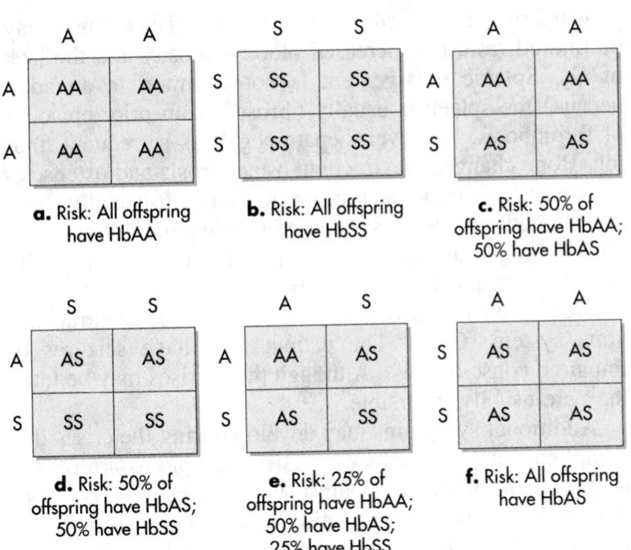

Fig. 28-3 Inheritance patterns of sickle cell disease. The boxes represent the possible genetic make-up of children from parents with various genotypes.

sickling. The increased concentration of sickle cells makes the circulation more sluggish, thus exerting a profound effect on all major organs. The abnormal shape of the hemoglobin is recognized by the body, and the cell is hemolyzed. Initially the sickling is reversible on reoxygenation but eventually becomes irreversible, with cells being hemolyzed. *Sickle cell crises* (exacerbations of sickling) develop only if a patient becomes extremely hypoxic.

Clinical Manifestations. Infants do not manifest symptoms until 10 to 12 weeks of age, at which time most of the fetal hemoglobin (HbF) has been replaced by HbS. Children manifest a general impairment of growth and development and a failure to thrive. Puberty is delayed, but considerable growth occurs in late adolescence.

Most patients with sickle cell anemia are in reasonably good health most of the time. This state of relative well-being is periodically interrupted by crisis, which may have sudden onset and occasionally fatal outcome. The painful crisis is caused by an increased rate of sickling. On deoxygenation, the RBC containing HbS changes from a biconcave disc to an elongated, crescent or sickle cell. These sickling cells clog the small capillaries. The resulting hemostasis promotes a self-perpetuating cycle of local hypoxia, deoxygenation of more erythrocytes, and more sickling. As blood vessels become occluded, thrombosis

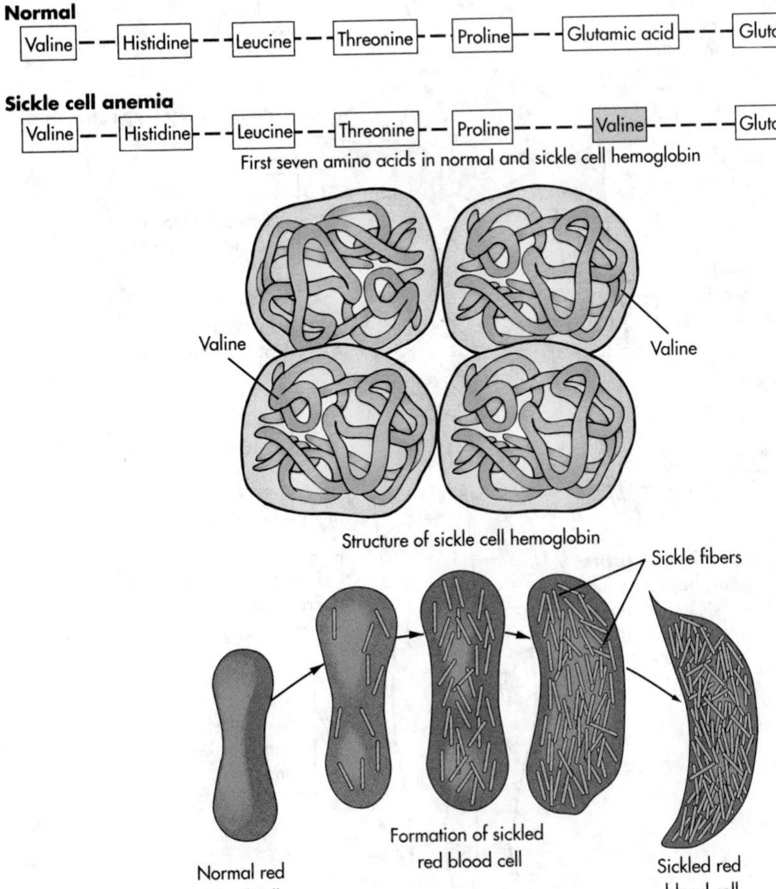

Fig. 28-4 Sickle cell hemoglobin is produced by a recessive allele of the gene encoding the β chain of hemoglobin. It represents a single amino acid change from glutamic acid to valine at the sixth position in the chain. In the folded β-chain molecule the sixth position contacts the α chain, and the amino acid change causes the hemoglobins to aggregate into long chains, altering the shape of the cell.

occurs. This can ultimately lead to necrosis of the infarcted tissue from lack of O_2.

Precipitating factors include conditions that cause hypoxia or deoxygenation of the RBCs, such as viral or bacterial infections, high altitudes, emotional or physical stress, surgery, and blood loss. Crises can also be precipitated by elevated blood viscosity, which may result from dehydration caused by vomiting, diarrhea, or diaphoresis. Sometimes the crisis occurs spontaneously, with no apparent precipitating event. The frequency of sickle cell crisis varies. Crises may occur frequently and then may not recur for months or years. The attack may last for 4 to 6 days.

These attacks may appear suddenly and affect various parts of the body, especially the chest, abdomen, bones, and joints (Fig. 28-5). Organs that have a high need for O_2 are most immediately affected and form the basis for many of the complications of sickle cell disease. The heart may become ischemic and enlarged, leading to electrocardiographic changes. Pulmonary infarctions may cause chest pain and ultimately lead to cor pulmonale. The kidneys may be injured from the increased blood viscosity and the lack of O_2. Splenic enlargement is not common in an adult because the spleen is usually fibrosed from prior episodes of thrombosis. However, hepatomegaly is a frequent finding. Bone changes may include osteoporosis and osteosclerosis after infarction. Aching in the joints, especially those of the hands and feet, is a common complaint. Chronic leg ulcers can result from the hypoxia and are especially prevalent around the ankles.

Sickle cell crises occasionally involve the central nervous system (CNS). The patient may have seizures or impaired consciousness. Although these crises may be fatal, they are usually reversible.

Additional symptoms may develop during the crises that complicate sickle cell anemia. These symptoms are related to pain and aplasia. The pain may occur spontaneously or may be precipitated by infection and cold intolerance. The pain usually begins in the extremities and lasts for 4 to 6

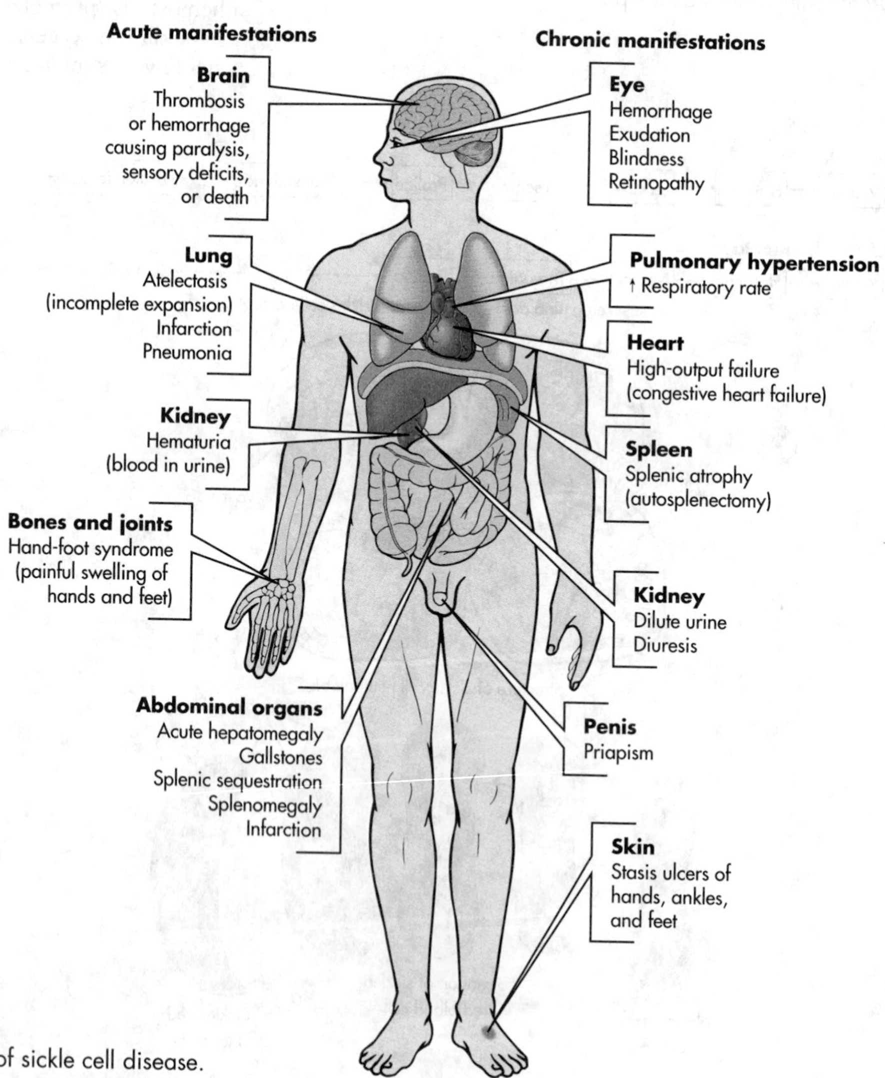

Fig. 28-5 Clinical manifestations of sickle cell disease.

days. Aplastic crises occur when a stressor significantly decreases erythropoiesis. The anemia is therefore exacerbated as hemolysis continues.

Shock is also a possible development in sickle cell crisis. Capillary hypoxia may result in changes in membrane permeability, leading to plasma loss, hemoconcentration, and further circulatory stagnation, causing a reduction of the circulating fluid volume.

The patient with sickle cell disease is particularly prone to infection. One reason for this is the failure of the spleen to phagocytize foreign substances because of impairment of splenic function. Pneumonia is the most common infection and often is of pneumococcal origin. Infections need to be treated vigorously with antibiotics.[8]

Diagnostic Studies. Screening tests to identify sickle cell disease or trait are available (Table 28-11). A person with sickle cell anemia has a severe form of hemolytic anemia. The Hb level usually ranges from 5 to 11 g/dl (50 to 110 g/L). The mean RBC survival time is 10 to 15 days. As a result of the accelerated RBC breakdown, the patient has characteristic clinical findings of hemolysis (jaundice, elevated serum bilirubin levels) and abnormal laboratory test results (Table 28-6). Skeletal x-rays will demonstrate bone and joint deformities and flattening. Magnetic resonance imaging may be used to diagnose a cerebrovascular accident caused by blocked cerebral vessels from sickled cells.

Therapeutic Management. Therapeutic care for a patient with sickle cell anemia is essentially supportive. There is no specific treatment for the disease. Therapy is usually directed toward alleviating the symptoms from complications of the disease. For example, chronic leg ulcers may be treated with bed rest, antibiotics, warm saline soaks, mechanical or enzyme débridement, and dressings.

Sickle cell crises may require hospitalization. O_2 may be administered to alter hypoxia and control sickling. Rest is instituted to reduce metabolic requirements, and fluids and electrolytes are administered to reduce blood viscosity and maintain renal function. Analgesics are used to treat pain. Transfusion therapy is indicated when an aplastic crisis occurs.

Because these patients have an increased need for folic acid, it is important for them to obtain daily supplements. Blood transfusions should be used judiciously to treat a crisis. They have little if any role in the treatment between crises. In general, iron therapy is not indicated.

Hydroxyurea therapy significantly increases HbF levels and reduces hemolysis. Its therapeutic effects are currently being investigated. Additional investigation is focusing on stimulating the production of HbF by other agents such as butyrate and erythropoietin. Bone marrow transplantation is also being investigated as a treatment for sickle cell anemia.

NURSING MANAGEMENT

SICKLE CELL ANEMIA

Because of the hereditary nature of sickle cell disease, genetic counseling is the only form of prevention. For genetic counseling to be effective, screening must be done to detect someone who has sickle cell trait.

The basic care for the patient with sickle cell anemia is discussed in the nursing care plan for the patient with anemia. Long-term care for the patient is also of great importance. Long-term management is based mostly on patient education. The patient and family must understand the basis of the disease and the reasons for supportive care. (Sources of patient education are available.[8]) The patient must be taught ways to avoid crises, which include taking steps to reduce the chance of developing hypoxia, such as avoiding high altitudes, and seeking medical attention quickly to counteract problems such as upper respiratory tract infections. Education on pain control is also needed because the pain during a crisis may be severe and often requires considerable analgesia.

Glucose-6-Phosphate Dehydrogenase Deficiency

Glucose-6-phosphate dehydrogenase (G6PD) is an RBC enzyme that acts as the initial catalyst in glycolysis. *G6PD deficiency* is a sex-linked disorder and directly affects the erythrocyte's ability to resist oxidative damage. Consequently, when G6PD is reduced, there is a decrease in glucose use by the RBCs. If erythrocytes are exposed to

Table 28-11 Laboratory Assessment of Sickle Cell Trait and Sickle Cell Anemia

Study	Description	Sickle Cell Trait	Sickle Cell Anemia
Peripheral smear	Small amount of peripheral blood specimen is smeared on a slide.	Normal	Partially or completely sickled cells
Sickle cell preparation	Blood specimen reaction is observed in hypoxic setting.	Sickle cells	Sickle cells
Sickledex	Blood is mixed with a solution that deoxygenates HbS; this becomes insoluble and causes turbidity. Development of cloudiness is positive for presence of HbS.	Positive	Positive
Hemoglobin electrophoresis	Blood specimen is exposed to electric field and types of hemoglobin are separated.	HbS and HbA	HbS

oxidative foods and drugs, the metabolic needs of RBCs increase. However, the G6PD deficiency interferes with glucose metabolism and leads to damage of older RBCs, which are then destroyed by hemolysis.

G6PD deficiency is relatively common, especially in African-Americans and in persons of Mediterranean heritage. Hemolytic episodes are triggered by viral and bacterial infections. Drugs and toxins also cause hemolysis in persons deficient in G6PD. Drugs that may cause oxidative problems include antimalarial drugs, sulfonamides, nitrofurantoins, analgesics (e.g., phenacetin), and chloramphenicol.

Managing the hemolysis seen in G6PD deficiency is relatively easy. Because only older RBCs are destroyed by the oxidative agent, the younger cells survive. The cause of the hemolytic reaction must be removed. During the period of acute hemolysis, the patient will require rest, adequate hydration, and assessment of kidney function. Attention should be focused on preventing the hemolytic disorders by treating infections promptly and screening African-American patients for G6PD deficiency before giving an oxidant drug.

Acquired Hemolytic Anemia

Extrinsic causes of hemolysis can be separated into three categories: (1) physical factors, (2) immune reactions, and (3) infectious agents and toxins. Physical destruction of RBCs results from the exertion of extreme force on the cells. Traumatic events causing disruption of the RBC membrane include hemodialysis, extracorporeal circulation used in heart-lung bypass, and prosthetic heart valves. In addition, the force needed to push blood through abnormal vessels, such as those that have been burned or affected by angiopathic disease (e.g., diabetes mellitus), may also physically damage RBCs.

Antibodies may destroy RBCs by the mechanisms involved in antigen-antibody reactions. The reactions may be of an *isoimmune* or *autoimmune* type. Isoimmune reactions occur when antibodies develop against antigens from another person of the same species. Blood transfusion reactions typify this response, especially when donor cells are hemolyzed by the recipient's antibodies because of an ABO mismatch. Another isoimmune reaction is known as *hemolytic disease of the newborn* (HDN). In the past this disorder was referred to as *erythroblastosis fetalis.* In this situation, maternal antibodies that have been previously sensitized either through previous pregnancy or transfusion destroy the RBCs of the fetus, resulting in a hemolytic anemia.

Autoimmune reactions result when individuals develop antibodies against their own erythrocytes. Autoimmune hemolytic reactions may be idiopathic, developing with no prior hemolytic history as a result of the immunoglobulin IgG covering the red cells, or secondary to other autoimmune diseases (e.g., systemic lupus erythematosus), leukemia, lymphoma, or drugs (penicillin, indomethacin, phenylbutazone, phenacetin, quinidine, quinine, and methyldopa).

The third category of acquired hemolytic disorders is caused by infectious agents and toxins. Infectious agents can foster hemolysis in four ways: (1) by invading the RBC and destroying its contents (e.g., parasites such as in malaria); (2) by releasing hemolytic substances (e.g., *Clostridium perfringens*); (3) by generating an antigen-antibody reaction; and (4) by contributing to splenomegaly as a means of increasing the removal of damaged erythrocytes from the circulation.

Various agents may be toxic to RBCs and cause hemolysis. These hemolytic toxins involve chemicals such as oxidative drugs, arsenic, lead, copper, and snake venom.

Laboratory findings in hemolytic anemia are presented in Table 28-6. Treatment and management of acquired hemolytic anemias involve general supportive care until the causative agent can be eliminated or at least rendered less injurious to the erythrocytes. Supportive care may include administering corticosteroids and blood products or removing the spleen.

POLYCYTHEMIA

Polycythemia is the production and presence of increased numbers of RBCs. The increase in erythrocytes can be so great that blood circulation is impaired as a result of the increased blood viscosity (hyperviscosity) and volume (hypervolemia).

Etiology

The two types of polycythemia are *primary polycythemia,* or *polycythemia vera,* and *secondary polycythemia* (Fig. 28-6). Their etiologies and pathogenesis differ, although their complications and clinical manifestations are similar. Polycythemia vera is a neoplastic disease arising from a chromosomal mutation in a single pluripotent stem cell. Therefore not only are erythrocytes involved but also granulocytes and platelets, leading to increased production of each of these blood cells. The disease develops insidiously and follows a chronic, vacillating course. It usually develops in patients more than 50 years of age. With this myeloproliferative disorder the patient has enhanced blood viscosity and blood volume and congestion of organs and tissues with blood.

Secondary polycythemia is caused by hypoxia rather than a defect in the evolution of the RBC. Hypoxia stimulates erythropoietin production in the kidney, which in turn stimulates erythrocyte production. The need for O_2 may be due to high altitude, pulmonary disease, cardiovascular disease, alveolar hypoventilation, defective O_2 transport, or tissue hypoxia. Consequently, secondary polycythemia is a physiologic response in which the body tries to compensate for a problem rather than a pathologic response. (Secondary polycythemia is discussed in Chapter 25.)

Clinical Manifestations and Complications

Circulatory manifestations of polycythemia vera are because of the hypertension caused by hypervolemia and hyperviscosity. They are often the first symptoms and include subjective complaints of headache, vertigo, dizziness, tinnitus, and visual disturbances. In addition, the patient may experience angina, CHF, intermittent claudication, and thrombophlebitis, which may be complicated by embolization. These manifestations are caused by blood

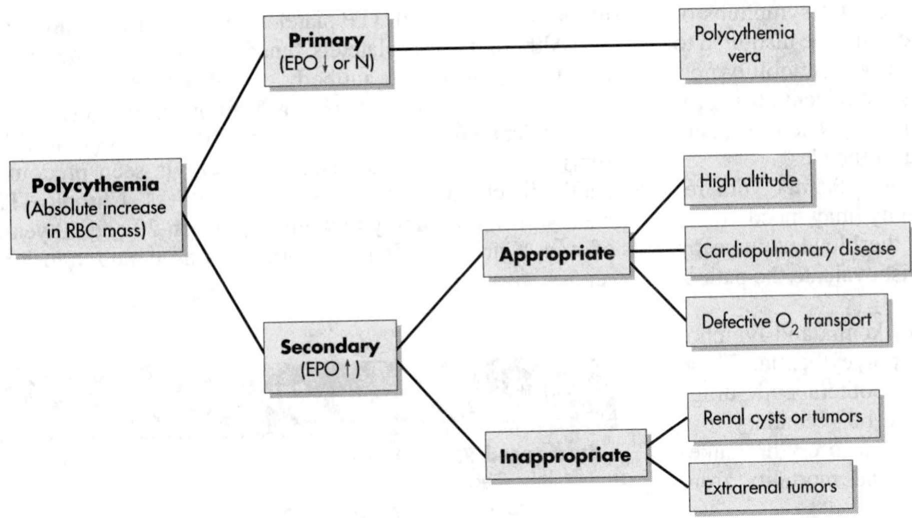

Fig. 28-6 Differentiating between primary and secondary polycythemia. *EPO*, erythropoietin; *N*, normal; *RBC*, red blood cell.

vessel distention, impaired blood flow, circulatory stasis, thrombosis, and tissue hypoxia caused by the hypervolemia and hyperviscosity. The most common serious complication is cerebrovascular accident. Generalized pruritus may be a striking symptom and is related to histamine release from an increased number of basophils and mast cells.

Hemorrhagic phenomena caused by either vessel rupture from overdistention or inadequate platelet function may result in petechiae, ecchymoses, epistaxis, or GI bleeding. Hemorrhage can be acute and catastrophic.

Hepatomegaly and splenomegaly from organ engorgement may contribute to patient complaints of satiety and fullness. The patient may also experience pain from peptic ulcer caused by either increased gastric secretions or liver and spleen engorgement. *Plethora* (ruddy complexion) may also be present.

Hyperuricemia is caused by the increase in cell destruction that accompanies the excessive cell production. Uric acid is one of the products of cell destruction. As cell destruction increases, uric acid production also increases, thus leading to hyperuricemia. This problem may cause a secondary form of gout.

Diagnostic Studies

The following laboratory manifestations are seen in a patient with polycythemia vera: (1) elevated hemoglobin and RBC count; (2) elevated WBC count with basophilia; (3) elevated platelets (thrombocytosis) and platelet dysfunction; and (4) elevated leukocyte alkaline phosphatase, uric acid, and vitamin B_{12} levels.

Bone marrow examination in polycythemia vera shows hypercellularity of RBCs, WBCs, and platelets. Splenomegaly is found in 90% of patients with primary polycythemia but does not accompany secondary polycythemia.

Therapeutic Management

Once the diagnosis of polycythemia vera is made, treatment is directed toward reducing blood volume and viscosity and bone marrow activity. Phlebotomy may be done to diminish blood volume until the desired Hct level is achieved. The aim of phlebotomy is to reduce and keep the Hct less than 45% to 48%. Generally, at the time of diagnosis 300 to 500 ml of blood may be removed every other day until the Hct is reduced to normal levels. An individual managed with repeated phlebotomies eventually becomes deficient in iron, although this effect is rarely symptomatic. Iron supplementation should be avoided. Hydration therapy is used to reduce the blood's viscosity. Myelosuppressive agents such as busulfan (Myleran), hydroxyurea (Hydrea), melphalan (Alkeran), and radioactive phosphorus may be given to inhibit bone marrow activity. Allopurinol may reduce the number of acute gouty attacks. Antiplatelet agents, such as aspirin and dipyridamole, used to prevent thrombotic complications are controversial because of increased irritation of the gastric mucosa resulting in GI symptoms, including bleeding.

NURSING MANAGEMENT

POLYCYTHEMIA VERA

Primary *polycythemia vera* is not preventable. However, because secondary polycythemia is generated by any source of hypoxia, problems may be prevented by maintaining adequate oxygenation. Therefore controlling chronic pulmonary disease and avoiding high altitudes may be important.

When acute exacerbations of polycythemia vera develop, the nurse has several responsibilities. Depending on the institution's policies, the nurse may either assist with or perform the phlebotomy. Fluid intake and output must be judiciously evaluated during hydration therapy to avoid fluid overload (which further complicates the circulatory congestion) and underhydration (which can cause the blood to become even more viscous). If myelosuppressive agents are used, the nurse must administer the drugs as ordered, observe the patient, and teach the patient about medication side effects.

Assessment of the patient's nutritional status in collaboration with the dietitian may be necessary to offset the inadequate food intake that can result from GI symptoms of fullness, pain, and dyspepsia. Activities must be instituted to decrease thrombus formation. The relative immobility normally imposed by hospitalization puts the patient at risk for thrombus formation. Active or passive leg exercises, and ambulation when possible, should be initiated.

Because of its chronic nature, polycythemia vera requires ongoing evaluation. Phlebotomy may need to be done every 2 to 3 months, reducing the blood volume by about 500 ml each time. The nurse must evaluate the patient for the development of complications.

Although the incidence is small, leukemia and lymphomas develop in some patients with polycythemia. These occurrences may be caused by the chemotherapeutic drugs used to treat the disease, or they may be secondary to a disorder in the stem cells that progresses to erythroleukemia. The major cause of morbidity and mortality from polycythemia vera is thrombosis.

PROBLEMS OF HEMOSTASIS

The hemostatic process involves the vascular endothelium, platelets, and coagulation factors, which normally function in concert to arrest hemorrhage and repair vascular injury. (These mechanisms are described in Chapter 27). Disruption in any of these components may result in bleeding or thrombotic disorders.

Three major disorders of hemostasis discussed in this section are (1) thrombocytopenia (low platelet count), (2) hemophilia and von Willebrand disease (inherited disorders of specific clotting factors), and (3) disseminated intravascular coagulation.

Thrombocytopenia

Etiology. Thrombocytopenia is a reduction of platelets below the normal range of 150,000 to 400,000/μl (150 to 400×10^9/L). Acute, severe, or prolonged decreases from this normal range can result in abnormal hemostasis that manifests as prolonged bleeding from minor trauma to spontaneous bleeding without injury.[4]

Platelet disorders can be inherited (e.g., Wiskott-Aldrich syndrome), but the vast majority are acquired. Acquired disorders can occur because of decreased platelet production or increased platelet destruction (Table 28-12). Many of these abnormalities of platelet number occur following ingestion of some foods and medications (Table 28-13). Aspirin doses as low as 60 mg (a baby aspirin) can alter the function of circulating platelets. Normal function is restored with the generation of newly formed platelets. However, abnormalities caused by food and medications (with the exception of aspirin) are rarely significant causes of serious bleeding in a healthy person.[9] It is important for the nurse to be aware of the numerous conditions that may affect platelet production and destruction.

Immune thrombocytopenic purpura. The most common acquired thrombocytopenia is a syndrome of abnormal destruction of circulating platelets known as *immune thrombocytopenic purpura* (ITP). It was originally termed *idiopathic* thrombocytopenic purpura because its cause was unknown; however, it is now believed that ITP is an autoimmune disease. In ITP platelets are coated with antibodies. Although these platelets function normally, when they reach the spleen, the antibody-coated platelets are recognized as foreign and are destroyed by macrophages.

Platelets normally survive 8 to 10 days, but in ITP, survival is only 1 to 3 days. Acute ITP is seen predominantly in children following a viral illness. Chronic ITP occurs most commonly in women between 20 and 40 years of age. Chronic ITP has a gradual onset, and transient remissions occur.

Table 28-12 Causes of Thrombocytopenia

Decreased Platelet Production
- Inherited
  - Fanconi syndrome (pancytopenia)
  - Hereditary thrombocytopenia
- Acquired
  - Aplastic anemia
  - Hematologic malignant disorders
  - Myelosuppressive drugs
  - Chronic alcoholism
  - Exposure to ionizing radiation
  - Viral infections
  - Deficiencies of vitamin B_{12}, folic acid

Increased Platelet Destruction
- Nonimmune
  - Thrombotic thrombocytopenic purpura
  - Pregnancy
  - Infection
  - Drug induced
  - Severe burns
- Immune
  - Immune thrombocytopenic purpura
  - Human immunodeficiency virus infection
  - Drug induced
- Splenomegaly

Table 28-13 Drugs, Spices, and Vitamins That Can Cause Abnormalities of Platelet Function

Suppression of Platelet Production
- Thiazide diuretics, alcohol, estrogen, chemotherapeutic drugs

Abnormal Platelet Aggregation
- Nonsteroidal antiinflammatory drugs: ibuprofen (Advil, Motrin, Aleve), indomethacin (Indocin), naproxen (Naprosyn)
- Antibiotics: penicillins, cephalosporins
- Analgesics: aspirin and aspirin-containing drugs (see Table 28-16)
- Spices: ginger, cumin, tumeric, cloves, garlic
- Vitamins: vitamin C, vitamin E

Thrombotic thrombocytopenia purpura. Thrombotic thrombocytopenia purpura (TTP) is an uncommon syndrome characterized by microangiopathic hemolytic anemia, thrombocytopenia, neurologic abnormalities, fever (in the absence of infection), and renal abnormalities. The disease is associated with enhanced agglutination of platelets, which form microthrombi that deposit in arterioles and capillaries. The cause of the platelet agglutination is unknown. TTP is seen primarily in adults between 20 and 50 years of age, with a slight female predominance. The syndrome is occasionally precipitated by the use of estrogen or by pregnancy. TTP is a medical emergency because bleeding and clotting occur simultaneously.

Clinical Manifestations. Despite different etiologies, clinical manifestations of thrombocytopenia are similar. Thrombocytopenia is most commonly manifested by the appearance of small, flat, pinpoint red or reddish brown microhemorrhages known as *petechiae.* When the platelet count is low, RBCs may leak out of the blood vessels to cause petechiae. When petechiae are numerous, the resulting reddish skin bruise is known as *purpura.* Larger purplish lesions caused by hemorrhage are called *ecchymoses* (Fig. 28-7). Ecchymoses may be flat or raised; pain and tenderness sometimes are present.

Prolonged bleeding after routine procedures such as venipuncture or IM injection may also indicate thrombocytopenia. Because the bleeding may be internal, the nurse must also be aware of manifestations that reflect this type of blood loss, including weakness, fainting, dizziness, tachycardia, abdominal pain, and hypotension.

The major complication of thrombocytopenia is hemorrhage. The hemorrhage may be insidious or acute and internal or external. It may occur in any area of the body, including joints, retina, and brain. Cerebral hemorrhage may be fatal in persons with ITP. Insidious hemorrhage may first be detected by discovering the anemia that accompanies blood loss.

Diagnostic Studies. The platelet count is decreased in cases of thrombocytopenia. Any reduction below 150,000/μl (150×10^9/L) may be termed *thrombocytopenia.* However, prolonged bleeding from trauma or injury does not usually occur until platelet counts are less than 50,000/μl (50×10^9/L). When the count drops below 20,000/μl (20×10^9/L), spontaneous, life-threatening hemorrhages (e.g., intracranial bleeding) can occur. Platelet transfusions are generally not recommended until the count is below 20,000/μl (20×10^9/L) unless the patient is actively bleeding.

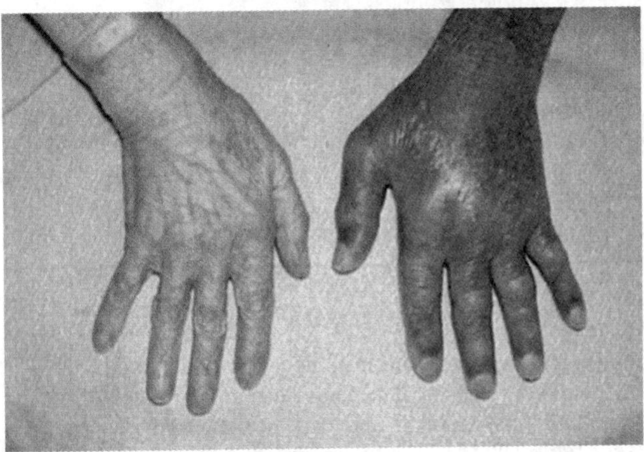

Fig. 28-7 Example of ecchymoses.

The bleeding time is a test of primary hemostasis and will be prolonged in any disorder of platelet function. Laboratory tests that assess secondary hemostasis or coagulation, such as the prothrombin time (PT) and partial thromboplastin time (PTT), can be normal even in severe thrombocytopenia. When destruction of circulating platelets is the etiology, bone marrow analysis shows megakaryocytes (precursors of platelets) to be normal or increased, even though circulating platelets are reduced. Additionally, special blood analyses using flow cytometry and other techniques can detect antiplatelet antibodies as the source of destruction. Bone marrow examination is done to rule out production problems as the cause of thrombocytopenia (e.g., leukemia, aplastic anemia, and other myeloproliferative disorders).

Anemia is present in proportion to the amount of blood lost. Therefore it is important to monitor Hb and Hct values and to observe the patient for cardiopulmonary distress and other manifestations of anemia. When thrombocytopenia occurs with anemia characterized by altered RBC morphology, including spherocytes, fragmented cells (schistocytes), and pronounced reticulocytosis, a diagnosis of TTP should be suspected. These findings are partially as a result of intravascular fibrin deposition causing a "slicing" of red cells. In TTP, thrombocytopenia may be severe, but coagulation studies are normal.

Therapeutic Management. Therapeutic management of thrombocytopenia differs based on the etiology of the thrombocytopenia as a destruction or production problem. Discussion of management strategies for these different etiologies follows.

Immune thrombocytopenic purpura. Multiple therapies are used to manage the patient with ITP (Table 28-14). Corticosteroids are used to treat ITP because of their ability to suppress the phagocytic response of splenic macrophages. This alters the spleen's recognition of platelets and increases the platelets' life spans. In addition, corticosteroids depress autoimmune antibody formation. Initial treatment is with prednisone, which reduces the binding of antibody to the platelet surface. Corticosteroids also reduce capillary fragility and bleeding time. The mechanism of action for this response is poorly understood.

Treatment may also include high doses of IV immunoglobulin in the patient who is unresponsive to corticosteroids or splenectomy. The immunoglobulin works by competing with the antiplatelet antibodies for macrophage receptors. IV immunoglobulin effectively raises the platelet count, but the beneficial effects are temporary.

Danazol, an androgen, has been used with success in some patients. Immunosuppressive therapy used in refractory cases includes vincristine, vinblastine, azathioprine, and cyclophosphamide.

Table 28-14 Therapeutic Management: Thrombocytopenia

Diagnostic
- History and physical examination
- Platelet count
- Bleeding time
- Bone marrow aspiration and biopsy
- Hematocrit and hemoglobin levels

Therapeutic
- Immune thrombocytopenic purpura
  - Corticosteroids
  - Platelet transfusions
  - Intravenous immunoglobulin
  - Danazol
  - Immunosuppressives (cyclophosphamide, azathioprine)
  - Splenectomy
- Thrombotic thrombocytopenic purpura
  - Plasma infusion
  - Plasmapheresis and plasma exchange
  - High-dose prednisone
  - Splenectomy
- Decreased production problem
  - Identification and treatment of cause
  - Corticosteroids
  - Platelet transfusions
  - Thrombopoietin (investigational)

Splenectomy is indicated if the patient does not respond to prednisone initially or requires unacceptably high doses to maintain an adequate platelet count. Approximately 80% of patients benefit from splenectomy, resulting in a complete or partial remission. The effectiveness of splenectomy is based on four factors. First, the spleen contains an abundance of the macrophages that sequester and destroy platelets. Second, structural features of the spleen enhance antibody-coated platelets and macrophage interaction. Third, some antibody synthesis occurs in the spleen; thus antiplatelet antibodies decrease after splenectomy. Fourth, the spleen normally sequesters approximately one third of the platelets, so its removal increases the number in circulation.

Platelet transfusions may be used to increase platelet counts in cases of life-threatening hemorrhage. Platelets should not be administered prophylactically because of the possibility of antibody formation. ABO compatibility is not a necessary prerequisite for platelet transfusions. However, after multiple platelet transfusions, a patient may develop anti-HLA antibodies to the transfused platelets. Therefore by using lymphocyte typing to match HLA types of the donor and the recipient, multiple platelet transfusions can be given with fewer complications. In addition, the patient may be premedicated with an antihistamine (e.g., diphenhydramine) and hydrocortisone to decrease the possibility of reacting to platelet transfusions. Sometimes meperidine (Demerol) is used for symptomatic treatment of platelet transfusion reactions in combination with an antihistamine and corticosteroids. The mechanism of action of meperidine in controlling this reaction is not well understood, but it is believed to reset the temperature-regulating center in the hypothalamus. Aspirin and aspirin-containing compounds (see Table 28-15) should be avoided in the patient with thrombocytopenia.

Table 28-15 Products Containing Aspirin and Aspirin-like Compounds

Nonprescription	Prescription
Alka-Seltzer Antacid/Pain Reliever Effervescent Tablets	Darvon Compound-65
Alka-Seltzer Plus Cold Medicine Tablets	Disalcid Capsules/Tablets
Anacin Caplets/Tablets	Easprin Tablets
Anacin Maximum Strength Tablets	Empirin with Codeine Tablets
Arthritis Pain Formula Tablets	Equagesic Tablets
Arthritis Strength Bufferin Tablets	Fiorinal Capsules/Tablets
Ascriptin Caplets/Tablets	Fiorinal with Codeine Capsules/Tablets
Ascriptin A/D Caplets	Lortab ASA Tablets
Aspergum	Magsal Tablets
Bayer Aspirin Caplets/Tablets	Mono-Gesic Tablets
Bayer Children's Chewable Tablets	Norgesic and Norgesic Forte Tablets
Bayer Plus Tablets	Percodan and Percodan-Demi Tablets
Maximum Bayer Caplets/Tablets	Robaxisal Tablets
8-Hour Bayer Extended-Release Tablets	Salflex Tablets
BC Powder	Soma Compound Tablets
BC Cold Powder	Soma Compound with Codeine Tablets
Buffaprin Caplets/Tablets	Synalgos-DC Capsules
Bufferin Arthritis Strength Caplets	Talwin Compound Tablets
Bufferin Caplets/Tablets	Trilisate Tablets/Liquid
Cama Arthritis Pain Reliever Tablets	
Doan's Pills Caplets	
Ecotrin Caplets/Tablets	
Empirin Tablets	
Excedrin Extra-Strength Caplets/Tablets	
Midol Caplets	
Mobigesic Analgesic Tablets	
Norwich Tablets	
P-A-C Analgesic Tablets	
Sine-Off Tablets, Aspirin Formula	
St. Joseph Adult Chewable Aspirin	
Therapy Bayer Caplets	
Trigesic	
Ursinus Inlay-Tabs	
Vanquish Analgesic Caplets	

Thrombotic thrombocytopenic purpura. TTP is treated with emergency plasma infusion or plasmapheresis. The mechanism for the therapeutic response is not fully understood. Treatment should be continued daily until the patient is in complete remission. Splenectomy, corticosteroids, and dextran (antiplatelet agent) have also been used with success.

Acquired thrombocytopenia from decreased platelet production. The therapeutic management of acquired thrombocytopenia is based on identifying the cause and treating the disease or removing the causative agent. If the precipitating factor is unknown and being investigated, the patient may receive corticosteroids to enhance capillary integrity. Platelet transfusions are given if life-threatening hemorrhage develops. Splenectomy is not used because the spleen is not contributing to the thrombocytopenia.

Often, acquired thrombocytopenia is caused by another underlying condition (e.g., aplastic anemia or leukemia) or therapy used to treat another problem. For example, in acute leukemia all blood cell types may be depressed. Additionally, the patient may receive chemotherapeutic drugs that cause bone marrow suppression. If the patient can be adequately supported throughout the course of chemotherapy-induced thrombocytopenia, the disease-related thrombocytopenia will also resolve.

Thrombopoeitin, similar to erythropoeitin, is a specific hematopoeitic growth hormone that can stimulate the bone marrow to produce platelets. Currently thrombopoietin is in the investigational stages.[10]

NURSING MANAGEMENT

THROMBOCYTOPENIA

Nursing Assessment

Subjective and objective data that should be obtained from a patient with thrombocytopenia are presented in Table 28-16.

Table 28-16 Nursing Assessment: Thrombocytopenia

Subjective Data

Important health information

Past health history: Recent hemorrhage, excessive bleeding, or viral illness; cancer (especially leukemia or lymphoma); aplastic anemia; systemic lupus erythematosus; alcoholism; cirrhosis; chronic renal failure; exposure to radiation or toxic chemicals

Medications: Use of thiazide diuretics, furosemide (Lasix), aspirin, acetaminophen, estrogens, gold salts, nonsteroidal antiinflammatory drugs, phenylbutazone, penicillins, cephalothin, streptomycin, sulfonamides, quinidine, quinine, phenobarbital, methyldopa, phenytoin (Dilantin), diabinese, meprobamate, chemotherapy drugs

Functional health patterns

Health perception–health management: Fatigue, malaise

Nutritional-metabolic: Bleeding gingiva; coffee-ground or bloody vomitus; easy bruising

Elimination: Hematuria, blood in stools

Activity-exercise: Weakness, fainting; epistaxis, hemoptysis; dyspnea

Cognitive-perceptual: Pain and tenderness in bleeding areas (e.g., abdomen, head, extremities)

Sexuality-reproductive: Menorrhagia, metrorrhagia

Objective Data

General

Fever, lethargy

Integumentary

Petechiae, ecchymoses, purpura

Cardiovascular

Tachycardia, hypotension (significant bleeding)

Gastrointestinal

Blood-filled bullae in mouth, splenomegaly, abdominal distention, positive stools for occult blood (guaiac)

Neurologic

Slurred speech, decreased level of consciousness (CNS bleeding)

Possible findings

Platelet count $<150,000/\mu l$ ($150 \times 10^9/L$), prolonged bleeding time

Nursing Diagnoses

Nursing diagnoses related to a patient with thrombocytopenia include, but are not limited to, those presented in the following nursing care plan.

Planning

The overall goals are that the patient with thrombocytopenia will (1) have no gross or occult bleeding, (2) maintain vascular integrity, and (3) manage home care to prevent any complications related to an increased risk for bleeding.

Nursing Interventions

Health Promotion and Maintenance. It is important for the nurse to discourage excessive use of over-the-counter (OTC) medications known to be possible causes of acquired thrombocytopenia. Many medications contain aspirin as an ingredient (Table 28-15). Aspirin reduces platelet adhesiveness, thus potentially contributing to thrombocytopenia.

It is also important for the nurse to encourage persons to have a complete medical evaluation if manifestations of bleeding tendencies (e.g., prolonged epistaxis, petechiae) develop. In addition, the nurse must observe for early signs of thrombocytopenia in the patient receiving cancer chemotherapy drugs.

Acute Intervention. The goal during acute episodes of thrombocytopenia is to prevent or control hemorrhage (see the nursing care plan for the patient with thrombocytopenia on p. 798). In the patient with thrombocytopenia, bleeding is usually from superficial sites; deep bleeding (into muscles, joints, abdomen) usually occurs only when clotting factors are diminished. It is important to emphasize that a seemingly minor nosebleed may lead to hemorrhage in a patient with severe thrombocytopenia. Bleeding from the posterior nasopharynx may be difficult to detect because the blood may be swallowed. If an IM or SC injection is unavoidable, the use of a small-gauge needle and applica-

NURSING CARE PLAN Patient with Thrombocytopenia

Planning: Outcome Criteria	Nursing Interventions and Rationales
➤ **NURSING DIAGNOSIS**	Risk for altered cardiopulmonary, cerebral, or renal tissue perfusion *related to* acute or chronic blood loss *as manifested by* prolonged bleeding from venipuncture site or injection site, epistaxis, gingival bleeding, GI and genitourinary bleeding, ecchymoses, petechiae, bleeding within CNS.
Have pulse, respirations, BP within acceptable range of patient's normal; no evidence of gross or occult bleeding, including absence of CNS bleeding; receive required blood products with appropriate intervention if transfusion reaction occurs; adequate urine output (>0.5 ml/kg/hr).	Evaluate mucous membranes and skin each shift or more often *to detect presence of epistaxis, petechiae, ecchymoses, hematomas.* Test excretions regularly for occult blood and observe for blood in emesis, sputum, feces, urine, nasogastric secretions, wound secretions *to detect potential presence of hemorrhage.* Assess complete blood count and platelet count daily or more often if warranted *to monitor for hemorrhage.* Estimate blood loss *to determine need for transfusion.* Assess for retinal hemorrhage (visual impairment). Do not administer aspirin or aspirin-containing products *because of their effects on platelet adhesiveness.* Teach patient to avoid OTC medications that contain aspirin (Table 28-15). Use ice, packing, or direct pressure *to control active bleeding.* Teach patient to avoid Valsalva maneuver (e.g., straining at stool); administer stool softeners as ordered; avoid rectal temperatures, suppositories, and enemas; teach patient to cough, sneeze, and blow nose gently; administer medications to suppress vomiting and coughing *to avoid activities that could cause hemorrhage.* Evaluate mental status for alterations (e.g., headaches, vertigo, irritability, confusion) *to identify CNS bleeding.* Administer platelets or other blood components as ordered *to treat bleeding or replace blood loss from hemorrhage.* Understand various purposes of transfusion therapy, differentiate various types of blood products, administer and monitor blood products properly, intervene with transfusion reactions *to ensure safe administration of appropriate blood products.*
➤ **NURSING DIAGNOSIS**	Risk for altered oral mucous membranes *related to* treatment, disease, or blood-filled bullae.
Have pink, moist, lesion-free oral mucosa, tongue, and lips; no irritation or injury to mucous membrane; adequate nutritional intake	Assess oral mucosa daily for presence of blood-filled bullae in mouth; bleeding; tender gingivae and lips *to provide data for planning interventions.* Remove dentures daily and examine oral cavity *to assess underlying gums and mouth for bullae or bleeding areas.* Provide oral hygiene with minimal friction: use soft-bristle toothbrush, cotton swabs, mild mouthwash, or irrigating syringe *to gently cleanse mouth without trauma.* Evaluate integrity of nares, especially if nasogastric tube, endotracheal tube, or nasal O_2 is in use *to determine need for prophylactic or treatment interventions.*
➤ **NURSING DIAGNOSIS**	Risk for impaired tissue integrity *related to* interventions and tissue sensitivity to trauma.
Maintain tissue integrity; have no evidence of petechiae, ecchymoses, purpura, hematoma.	Assess for risk factors such as multiple skin punctures and signs such as bruising after even minor pressure or trauma *to enable early detection and intervention.* Initiate IV therapy judiciously; consider use of long-term venous access devices *to reduce number of venipunctures.* Avoid IM and SC injections; if used, apply local pressure with dry, sterile 2 × 2-in gauze for 5-10 min after needle is removed *to prevent bleeding into tissue surrounding puncture site.* Use electric razor for shaving *to reduce potential for skin nicks.* Reduce frequency of cuff blood pressures and alternate extremities used for readings; pad rails and other firm surfaces, especially if patient is combative or at risk for seizures; be gentle when turning patient or changing dressings *to reduce tissue trauma and subsequent bleeding into tissue.* Administer prophylactic platelet transfusions before necessary invasive procedures (if ordered) *to minimize risk of hemorrhage.*

continued

NURSING CARE PLAN Patient with Thrombocytopenia—cont'd

Planning: Outcome Criteria	Nursing Interventions and Rationales
➤ **NURSING DIAGNOSIS**	Ineffective management of therapeutic regimen *related to* lack of knowledge of disease process, activity, nutrition, and medication *as manifested by* frequent questioning about disease management; anxiety, restlessness; inability to answer or incorrect answering of disease-related questions.
Verbalize or demonstrate by patient or family required knowledge and skills to manage home care.	Assess learning needs related to disease management *to plan appropriate interventions.* Teach patient about disease process, medication, and activity and dietary recommendations *to decrease anxiety and prevent complications.* Discuss complications and signs that should be reported, such as trauma prevention, need for high fluid intake, medication management, and need for periods of rest and exercise *so patient will be knowledgeable and able to manage own care or direct others in care.* Provide opportunities for patient to verbalize concerns *because discussing these with a supportive other decreases anxiety.* Foster care decisions and planning by patient *to increase patient's sense of control and self-esteem.*

BP, Blood pressure; *CBC,* complete blood count; *CNS,* central nervous system; *GI,* gastrointestinal; *IM,* intramuscular; *IV,* intravenous; *OTC,* over-the-counter; *SC,* subcutaneous.

tion of direct pressure for at least 5 to 10 minutes after injection is indicated.

In a woman with thrombocytopenia, menstrual blood loss may exceed the usual amount and duration. Counting sanitary napkins used during menses is another important intervention to detect excess blood loss. Fifty milliliters of blood will completely soak a sanitary napkin. Suppression of menses with hormonal agents may be indicated during predictable periods of thrombocytopenia to reduce blood loss from menses (e.g., during chemotherapy and bone marrow transplantation).

The proper administration of platelet transfusions is an important nursing responsibility. Platelet concentrates, derived from fresh whole blood, can increase the platelet level effectively. One unit of platelets, a yellow liquid that is usually 30 to 50 ml in volume, can be derived by centrifuging 500 ml of whole blood. Platelet concentrates from multiple units of blood (usually from six to eight different donors) can be pooled together for a single administration. The degree of increase or increment from a pooled platelet product varies widely and is usually measured by performing a platelet count within 1 hour following the transfusion.

Platelet transfusions can also be prepared by pheresing single donors. This may be indicated when HLA-matched platelets are needed, especially for patients requiring multiple platelet transfusions. In this procedure, blood is removed from the donor, the platelets are removed, and the rest of the blood is reinfused into the donor. This procedure takes several hours and results in 200 to 400 ml of platelets and plasma.

Once acquired from a donor, platelets can be stored at room temperature for 1 to 5 days. Gentle agitation of the bag is useful to prevent the platelets from adhering to the plastic. The actual transfusion procedure (described later in this chapter) may vary among institutions but may involve the use of specialized leukocyte reduction filters. In a severely immunocompromised patient these products are also radiated to further ensure WBC removal and prevent the complication of graft-versus-host disease (see Chapter 10).

Chronic and Home Management. The patient with ITP who is receiving corticosteroids should be monitored frequently for the response to therapy. If the ITP is reversed by splenectomy, there is usually no recurrence. The person with acquired thrombocytopenia must be taught to avoid causative agents when possible (see Table 28-13). If the causative agents cannot be avoided (e.g., chemotherapy), the patient should learn to avoid injury or trauma during these periods and to detect the clinical signs and symptoms of bleeding caused by thrombocytopenia. The patient with either ITP or acquired thrombocytopenia should have planned periodic medical evaluations to assess the patient's status and to intercede in situations in which exacerbations and bleeding are likely to occur.

Hemophilia and von Willebrand Disease

Hemophilia is a hereditary bleeding disorder caused by defective or deficient coagulation factors. The two major forms of hemophilia, which can occur in mild to severe forms, are *hemophilia A* (classic hemophilia, factor VIII deficiency) and *hemophilia B* (Christmas disease, factor IX deficiency). *von Willebrand disease* is a related disorder involving a congenitally acquired deficiency of the von Willebrand coagulation protein. Factor VIII is synthesized in the liver and circulates complexed to von Willebrand protein (vWF).

Hemophilia A is the most common form of hemophilia; it makes up approximately 80% of all cases. The incidence of hemophilia A is approximately 1 in 10,000 men; hemophilia B is seen in 1 in 100,000 men. von Willebrand disease is considered the most common congenital bleeding disorder in humans, with estimates as high as 1 in 100. However, because this disease can also exist in mild to severe forms, life-threatening hemorrhage in afflicted pa-

Table 28-17 Comparison of Hemophilic States

Disorder	Deficiency	Inheritance Pattern
Hemophilia A	Factor VIII	Recessive sex-linked (transmitted by female carriers, displayed almost exclusively in men)
Hemophilia B	Factor IX	Recessive sex-linked (transmitted by female carriers, displayed almost exclusively in men)
von Willebrand disease	vWf and platelet dysfunction	Autosomal dominant, seen in both sexes Recessive (in severe forms of the disease)

vWF, von Willebrand factor.

tients is rare (1 in 1 million).[11] The deficiency and inheritance patterns of these three forms of inherited coagulapathies are compared in Table 28-17.

Clinical Manifestations and Complications. Clinical manifestations and complications related to hemophilia include (1) slow, persistent, prolonged bleeding from minor trauma and small cuts; (2) delayed bleeding after minor injuries (the delay may be several hours or days); (3) uncontrollable hemorrhage after dental extractions or irritation of the gingiva with a hard-bristle toothbrush (Fig. 28-8); (4) epistaxis, especially after a blow to the face; (5) GI bleeding from ulcers and gastritis; (6) hematuria from GU trauma and splenic rupture resulting from falls or abdominal trauma; (7) ecchymoses and subcutaneous hematomas (common); (8) neurologic signs, such as pain, anesthesia, and paralysis, which may develop from nerve compression caused by hematoma formation; and (9) *hemarthrosis* (bleeding into the joints) (Fig. 28-9), which may lead to joint deformity severe enough to cause unresolvable crippling (most commonly in the knees, elbows, shoulders, hips, and ankles).

These manifestations are especially important when seen in children because the disease may not yet be diagnosed. In adults, these developments may be the first sign of a newly diagnosed mild form of the disease that escaped detection through a childhood free of major injuries, dental procedures, or surgeries. However, these manifestations can also suggest that the hemophilia is poorly controlled. All clinical manifestations relate to bleeding, and any bleeding episode in persons with hemophilia may result in death from hemorrhage.

Hemophilia had been considered primarily a disease of childhood because of early death from complications. At the beginning of the century the median life expectancy was 11 years. By the 1970s advances in its treatment enabled persons with hemophilia to have a median life expectancy of 68 years. Unfortunately, the AIDS epidemic has reduced this figure to 49 years.[12] Many persons with hemophilia became seropositive for human immunodeficiency virus (HIV) infection, which was transmitted via cryoprecipitates and factor concentrates. Before 1986 donated blood and blood products were not tested for HIV

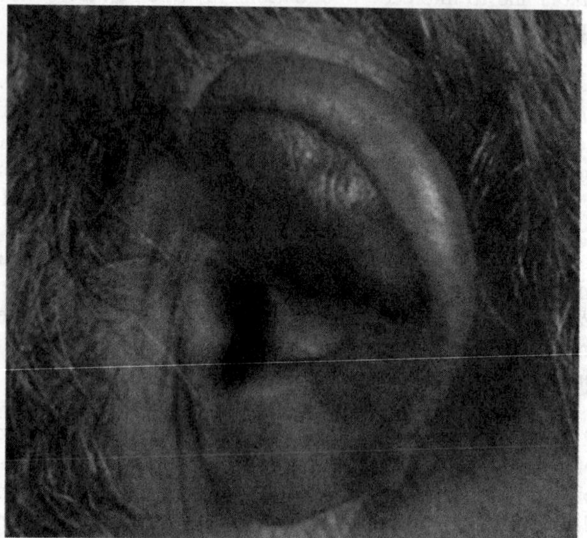

Fig. 28-8 Hematoma that developed in a person with hemophilia after trauma to the ear.

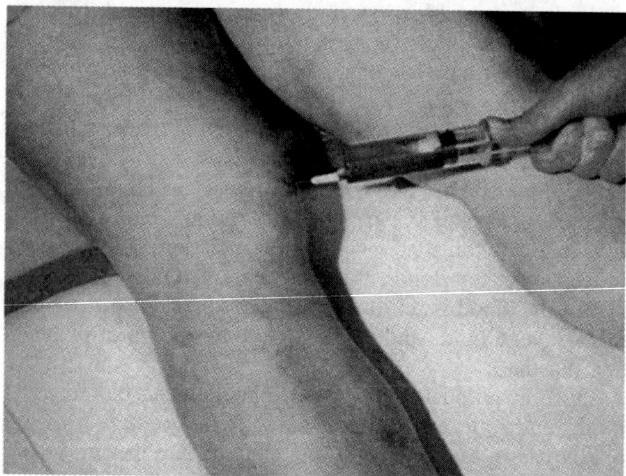

Fig. 28-9 Acute hemarthrosis of right knee in a patient with severe hemophilia. Blood is being aspirated with a needle and syringe.

Table 28-18 Laboratory Results in Hemophilia

Test	Comments
Prothrombin time	No involvement of extrinsic system
Thrombin time	No impairment of thrombin-fibrinogen reaction
Platelet count	Adequate platelet production
Partial thromboplastin time	Prolonged because of deficiency in any intrinsic clotting system factor
Bleeding time	Prolonged in von Willebrand disease because of structurally defective platelets, normal in hemophilia A and B because platelets not affected
Factor assays	Reduction of factor VIII in hemophilia A, vWF in von Willebrand disease, reduction of factor IX in hemophilia B

Table 28-19 Concentrate Factors Used in Treating Hemophilia

Factor VIII	
Plasma-derived products	***Recombinant products****
Monoclate	Recombinate
Hemofil	Kogenate
Profilate	
Koate	
Humate	
Factor IX	
Plasma-derived products	
Alpha-Nine	Bebulin
Mononine	Autoplex
Konyne	FEIBA
Profilnine	Hyate

*Produced by hamster cell lines transfected with a gene for factor VIII.

antibody. Routine testing is now used, all factor concentrates are prepared from plasma obtained from HIV-seronegative donors, and the product is heat-treated to further reduce the likelihood of transmission of both HIV and hepatitis B and C viruses.[13] The development of hepatitis C in hemophilia patients was also common for many years because of lack of an available test to detect it and the use of pooled blood products. Hepatitis C antibody screening is now routinely done on all donated blood and blood products.

Diagnostic Studies. Laboratory studies are used to determine the type of hemophilia present. Any factor deficiency within the intrinsic system (factors VIII, vWF, IX, XI, or XII) will yield the laboratory results presented in Table 28-18.

Therapeutic and Pharmacologic Management. The goals of therapeutic management are to prevent and treat bleeding. The therapeutic regimens for persons with hemophilia or von Willebrand disease focus on maintaining adequate blood levels of the deficient clotting factors. This goal is achieved by assessing clinical manifestations, determining blood levels of the involved factors, and administering the necessary factors.

Replacement of deficient clotting factors is the primary means of supporting a patient with hemophilia. In addition to treating acute crises, replacement therapy may be given before surgery and dental care as a prophylactic measure. The standard therapeutic products are described in Table 28-19. Fresh frozen plasma, once commonly used for replacement therapy, is rarely used today. Cryoprecipitate, which primarily contains factor VIII and fibrinogen, is prepared from plasma, frozen rapidly, and kept frozen until used. Before administration, the cryoprecipitate is thawed slowly.

Most patients with hemophilia A use factor VIII concentrate, which is prepared from multiple donors and supplied as a lyophilized powder. A number of processes have increased the safety of factor VIII therapy. First, heat-treating the concentrate in solution or after lyophilization inactivates HIV. Second, treating the concentrate with chemicals, including solvent-detergent mixtures, can specifically inactivate lipid-envelope viruses. Highly purified factor VIII can be produced by adsorbing and eluding factor VIII from monoclonal antibody columns. The discovery of the factor VIII gene in 1984 and recombinant DNA techniques have allowed for the production of factor VIII by recombinant DNA technology (see Chapter 10). This product appears to be equivalent to its plasma-derived counterpart; because donors are not involved, it should prevent infectious complications.[12]

Factor IX deficiency is treated with factor IX concentrate, which is available as a lyophilized concentrate and contains prothrombin and factors VII and X. Monoclonally purified or recombinant factor IX preparations are undergoing clinical trials.

For mild hemophilia or certain subtypes of von Willebrand disease, desmopressin acetate (also known as DDAVP), a synthetic analog of vasopressin, may be used to stimulate an increase in factor VIII and von Willebrand factor. This drug acts on endothelial cells to cause the release of von Willebrand factor, which subsequently binds with factor VIII, thus increasing their concentration. Beneficial effects (e.g., decreased bleeding time) of DDAVP, when administered IV, are seen within 30 minutes and can last for more than 12 hours. Because the effect of DDAVP is relatively short-lived, the patient needs to be closely monitored and repeated doses may be necessary. It is an appropriate therapy for procedures such as dental extractions or care. An intranasal form has been developed and may be indicated for home therapy for some patients with mild to moderate forms of the disease.[12]

Complications of treatment of hemophilia include development of inhibitors to factors VIII or IX, transfusion-transmitted infectious disorders, allergic reactions (more commonly seen with the use of cryoprecipitate), and thrombotic complications with the use of factor IX because it contains activated coagulation factors. Because of the improved viral-depleting processes and donor screening practices, the risk of HIV and hepatitis transmission is greatly reduced from the pre-1986 incidence.

The most common difficulties with acute therapeutic management are starting factor replacement therapy too late and stopping it too soon. Generally, minor bleeding episodes should be treated for at least 72 hours. Surgery and traumatic injuries may dictate support for 10 to 14 days. Because of the short half-life of the factors, regular intermittent or continuous infusions have been used to manage bleeding episodes or expected traumatic procedures. Chronically, development of inhibitors to the factor products has occurred and requires individualized expert patient management.

NURSING MANAGEMENT

HEMOPHILIA

Nursing Implementation

Health Promotion and Maintenance. Because of the hereditary nature of hemophilia, referral for genetic counseling is essential when considering preventive measures. This is especially important because persons with hemophilia are living longer and reaching an age when reproduction is possible.

Acute Intervention. Nursing interventions are related primarily to controlling bleeding and include the following:

1. Stop the topical bleeding as quickly as possible by applying direct pressure or ice, packing the area with Gelfoam or fibrin foam, and applying topical hemostatic agents such as thrombin.
2. Administer the specific coagulation factor concentrate ordered to raise the patient's level of the deficient coagulation factor.
3. When joint bleeding occurs, it is important to totally rest the involved joint, in addition to administering antihemophilic factors to help prevent crippling deformities from hemarthrosis. The joint may be packed in ice. Analgesics are given to reduce severe pain. However, aspirin should *never* be used. As soon as bleeding ceases, it is important to encourage mobilization of the affected area through range-of-motion (ROM) exercises and physical therapy. Actual weight bearing is avoided until all swelling has resolved and muscle strength has returned.
4. Manage any life-threatening complication that may develop as a result of hemorrhage. Examples include nursing interventions to prevent or treat airway obstruction from hemorrhage into the neck and pharynx, as well as early assessment and treatment of intracranial bleeding.

Chronic and Home Management. Home management is a primary consideration for the patient with hemophilia because the disease follows a progressive, chronic course. The quality and the length of life may be significantly affected by the patient's knowledge of the illness and how to live with it. The patient and family can be referred to the local chapter of the National Hemophilia Society to encourage associations with other individuals who are dealing with the problems of hemophilia. The nurse must provide ongoing assessment of the patient's adaptation to the illness. Psychosocial support and assistance should be readily available as needed.

Most of the long-term care measures are related to patient education. The patient with hemophilia must be taught to recognize disease-related problems and to learn which problems can be resolved at home and which require hospitalization. Immediate medical attention is required for severe pain or swelling of a muscle or joint that restricts movement or inhibits sleep and for a head injury, a swelling in the neck or mouth, abdominal pain, hematuria, melena, and skin wounds in need of suturing.

Daily oral hygiene must be performed without causing trauma. Understanding how to prevent injuries is another consideration. This is no easy task; there are many potential sources of trauma. The patient can learn to participate in noncontact sports (e.g., golf) and wear gloves when doing household chores to prevent cuts or abrasions from knives,

---

RESEARCH

Implications for Nursing Practice

SPIRITUAL CARE FOR PATIENTS

Citation Clark C, Heidenreich T: Spiritual care for the critically ill, *Am J Crit Care* 4:77-81, 1995.

Purpose To identify factors that contribute to providing spiritual care for patients in intensive care units.

Methods Descriptive research design was used for this replication study conducted on a convenience sample of 63 patients in the intensive care unit of a large military hospital. A trained interviewer asked each participant three open-ended questions regarding (1) events that created hope or a sense of well-being, (2) events that created negative feeling that influenced recovery, and (3) factors that would have helped the patient's sense of well-being. The interviews took place 1 to 2 days after discharge from the intensive care unit. Content analysis was used to determine predominant patterns.

Results and Conclusions Three themes were identified as integral to the spiritual well-being of critical care patients: care providers, family/friends, and religion/faith. Nursing interventions identified for the three themes include establishing trusting relationships, providing in-depth spiritual assessment, conveying technical competence, and acting as facilitator among family, clergy, and other providers.

Implications for Nursing Practice Spiritual well-being is the center of a healthy lifestyle and enables holistic integration of one's inner resources. Helping patients maintain spiritual well-being is a complex process for caregivers. Key nursing interventions derived from this study include listening to patients' concerns and maintaining and conveying technical competence.

hammers, and other tools. The patient should wear a Medic-Alert tag to ensure that health care providers know about the hemophilia in case of an accident.

The patient needs information about routine follow-up care, and the compliance with scheduled visits must be assessed. A reliable person can be taught to self-administer some of the factor replacement therapies at home. With the exception of intranasal DDAVP this will require providing instructions regarding venipuncture and infusion techniques.

Disseminated Intravascular Coagulation

Disseminated intravascular coagulation (DIC) is a serious bleeding disorder resulting from abnormally initiated and accelerated clotting. Subsequent decreases in clotting factors and platelets ensue, which may lead to uncontrollable hemorrhage. The term *DIC* can be misleading because it suggests that blood is clotting. However, the paradox of this condition is characterized by the profuse bleeding that results from the depletion of platelets and clotting factors. DIC is always caused by an underlying disease. The underlying disease must be treated for the DIC to resolve.

Etiology. DIC is not a disease; it is an abnormal response of the normal clotting cascade stimulated by another disease process or disorder. The diseases and disorders known to predispose a patient to DIC are listed in Table 28-20. DIC can occur as an acute, catastrophic condition, or it may exist at a subacute or chronic level. Each condition may have one or multiple triggering mechanisms to start the cascade. For example, tumors and traumatized or necrotic tissue release tissue factor into circulation. Endotoxin from gram-negative bacteria activates several steps in the coagulation cascade.

Initially in DIC, the normal coagulation mechanisms are enhanced. Abundant intravascular thrombin, the most powerful coagulant, is produced (Fig. 28-10). It catalyzes the conversion of fibrinogen to fibrin and enhances platelet aggregation. There is widespread fibrin and platelet deposition in capillaries and arterioles, resulting in thrombosis. Excessive clotting activates the fibrinolytic system, which in turn lyses the newly formed clots, creating fibrin-split (fibrin-degradation) products. These products have anticoagulant properties and inhibit normal blood clotting. Ultimately with fibrin-split products accumulating and clotting factors being depleted, the blood loses its ability to clot. Therefore a stable clot cannot be formed at injury sites. This situation predisposes the patient to hemorrhage.

Chronic DIC is most commonly seen in patients with long-standing illnesses such as malignant disorders or autoimmune diseases. The incidence of DIC associated with malignancy ranges from 10% to 75%, depending on the malignancy studied.[14] Occasionally these patients have subclinical disease manifested only by laboratory abnormalities. However, the clinical spectrum ranges from easy bruising to hemorrhage and from hypercoagulability to thrombosis.

Clinical Manifestations. There is no well-defined sequence of events in acute DIC. Bleeding in a person with no previous history or obvious cause should be questioned because it may be one of the first manifestations of acute DIC. Other nonspecific manifestations can include weakness, malaise, and fever.

There are both bleeding and thrombotic manifestations in DIC. *Bleeding manifestations* of DIC are multifactorial (Fig. 28-10) and result from consumption and depletion of platelets and coagulation factors, as well as clot lysis and formation of fibrin-split products that have anticoagulant properties. Bleeding manifestations include integumentary problems, such as pallor, petechiae, oozing blood, venipuncture site bleeding, hematomas, and occult hemorrhage; respiratory problems, such as tachypnea, hemoptysis, and orthopnea; cardiovascular problems, such as tachycardia and hypotension; GI changes, such as abdominal distention and bloody stools; urinary problems, such as hematuria; neurologic changes, such as vision changes, dizziness, headache, changes in mental status, and irritability; and musculoskeletal changes, such as bone and joint pain.

Table 28-20 Predisposing Conditions to Development of Disseminated Intravascular Coagulation

Acute DIC
- Shock
  - Hemorrhagic
  - Cardiogenic
  - Anaphylactic
- Septicemia
- Hemolytic processes
  - Transfusion of mismatched blood
  - Acute hemolysis from infection or immunologic disorders
- Obstetric conditions
  - Abruptio placenta
  - Amniotic fluid embolism
  - Septic abortion
- Tissue damage
  - Extensive burns and trauma
  - Heat stroke
  - Severe head injury
  - Transplant rejections
  - Postoperative damage, especially after extracorporeal membrane oxygenation
  - Fat and pulmonary emboli
  - Snakebites
  - Glomerulonephritis
  - Acute anoxia (e.g., after cardiac arrest)
  - Prosthetic devices

Subacute DIC
- Malignant disease
  - Acute leukemias
  - Metastatic cancer
- Obstetric
  - Retained dead fetus

Chronic DIC
- Liver disease
- Systemic lupus erythematosus
- Localized malignancy

DIC, Disseminated intravascular coagulation.

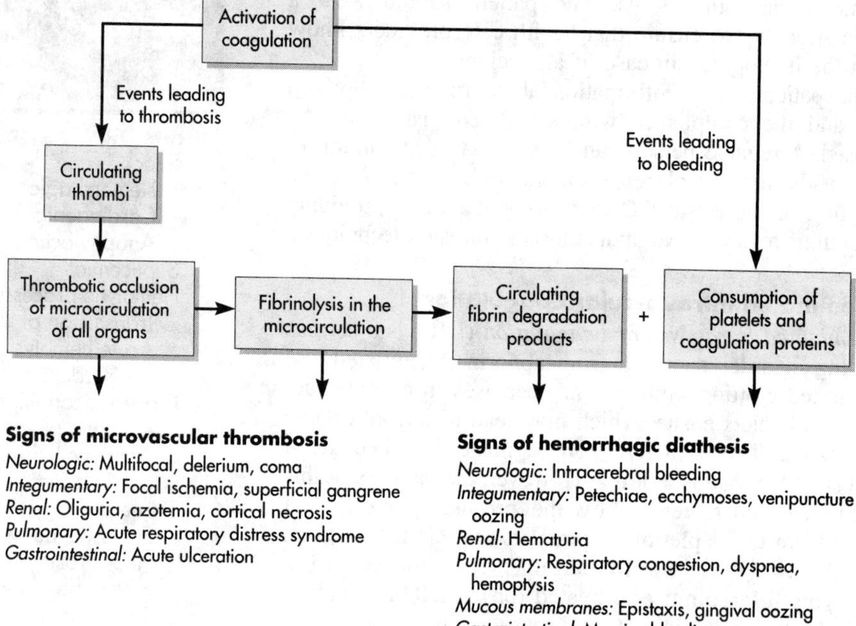

Fig. 28-10 The sequence of events that occurs during disseminated intravascular coagulation (DIC), leading to the clinical appearance of thrombotic and hemorrhagic phenomena.

Thrombotic manifestations are a result of fibrin or platelet deposition in the microvasculature (Fig. 28-10) and include integumentary changes, such as acral cyanosis, ischemic tissue necrosis (e.g., gangrene), and hemorrhagic necrosis; respiratory changes, such as tachypnea, dyspnea, pulmonary emboli, and acute respiratory distress syndrome; cardiovascular changes, such as ECG changes and venous distention; GI changes, such as abdominal pain and paralytic ileus; and urinary changes, such as oliguria.

Diagnostic Studies. Tests used to diagnose acute DIC and their findings are listed in Table 28-21. As more clots are made in the body, more breakdown products from fibrinogen and fibrin are also formed. These are called *fibrin-split products* (FSPs) or *fibrin-degradation products* (FDPs), and they work in three ways to interfere with blood coagulation. First, they coat the platelets and interfere with platelet function. Second, they interfere with thrombin and thereby disrupt coagulation. Third, the FSPs attach to fibrinogen, which interferes with the polymerization process necessary to form a stable clot. A much more specific test that is replacing measurement of FSP is the D-Dimer assay. D-Dimer, a specific polymer resulting from the breakdown of fibrin (and not fibrinogen), is a much more specific marker of the degree of fibrinolysis. In general, tests that measure *raw materials* needed for coagulation (e.g., platelets and fibrinogen) are reduced, and values that measure *times to clot* are prolonged. Fragmented erythrocytes (schistocytes), indicative of partial occlusion of small vessels by fibrin thrombi, may be found on blood smears.

Therapeutic Management. It is important to diagnose DIC quickly, institute therapy that will resolve the underlying causative disease or problem, and provide supportive care for the manifestations resulting from the pathology of DIC itself. The treatment of DIC remains controversial and under investigation as researchers attempt to determine the most suitable means of managing this dangerous syndrome. Consequently it is imperative that the nurse maintain an ongoing awareness of current modes of therapy. Regardless of the etiology, treating the primary disease process is essential to the resolution of DIC.

Depending on its severity, a variety of different methods are used to provide supportive and symptomatic management of DIC (Fig. 28-11). First, if chronic DIC is diagnosed

Table 28-21 Laboratory Abnormalities of Acute Disseminated Intravascular Coagulation

Test	Finding (Incidence)
Screening Tests	
Prothrombin time	Prolonged (75%) Normal or shortened (25%)
Partial thromboplastin time	Prolonged (50-60%)
Activated partial thromboplastin time	Prolonged
Thrombin time	Prolonged
Fibrinogen	Reduced
Platelets	Reduced to below 100,000/μl (100 × 10^9/L) to 5000/μl (5 × 10^9/L) in some
Special Tests	
Fibrin-split products (FSP)*	Elevated (75-100%)
Factor assays (for factors V, VII, VIII, X, XIII)	Reduced
D-Dimers (cross-linked fibrin fragments)	Elevated (more reliable than FSP)
Antithrombin III	Reduced (90%)

*Fibrin-degradation products (FDP).

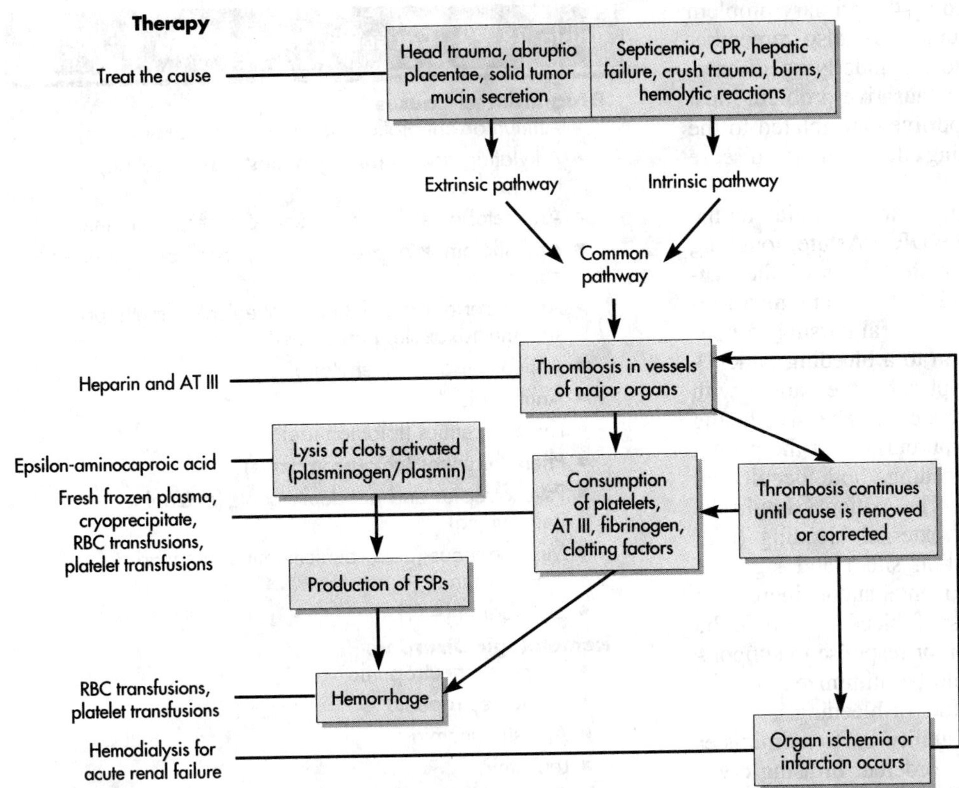

Fig. 28-11 Intended sites of action for therapies in disseminated intravascular coagulation. *CPR*, cardiopulmonary resuscitation; *FSP*, fibrin-split products; *RBC*, red blood cell.

in a patient who is not bleeding, no therapy for DIC is necessary. Treatment of the underlying disease may be sufficient to reverse the DIC (e.g., antineoplastic therapy when DIC is caused by malignancy). Second, when the patient with DIC is bleeding, therapy is directed toward providing support with necessary blood products while treating the primary disorder. The blood products are administered on the basis of specific component deficiencies. Platelets are given to correct thrombocytopenia, cryoprecipitate replaces factor VIII and fibrinogen, and fresh frozen plasma (FFP) replaces all clotting factors except platelets and provides a source of antithrombin.

A patient with manifestations of thrombosis is often treated by anticoagulation with either unfractionated (low or high dose) or low-molecular-weight heparin. The use of heparin in the treatment of DIC remains controversial. Antithrombin III (AT III), a cofactor of heparin that becomes depleted during DIC, has been used alone or in conjunction with heparin when levels of this factor are low. Hirudin, a thrombin inhibitor and neutralizer, is also being studied as a blocker of the abnormal coagulation process.[14] Another treatment that has been used is epsilon aminocaproic acid (EACA, Amicar) because of its ability to inhibit fibrinolysis. The use of EACA is controversial because it can enhance thrombosis. Generally it is used only as adjunctive therapy to heparin. Blood product support with platelets, cryoprecipitate, and FFP is usually reserved for a patient with life-threatening hemorrhage. The concern is that one is adding "fuel to the fire" of already activated coagulation. However, it may be the only method to avoid fatal hemorrhage in some patients. Therapy will stabilize a patient, prevent exsanguination or massive thrombosis, and permit institution of definitive therapy to treat the underlying cause.

Chronic DIC does not respond to oral anticoagulants, but it can be controlled with long-term, low-dose SC or IV heparin. Some patients with indolent tumors and severe, chronic DIC may need continuous infusion of heparin with portable pumps.

NURSING MANAGEMENT
DISSEMINATED INTRAMUSCULAR COAGULATION

Nursing Diagnoses

Nursing diagnoses for DIC include, but are not limited to, the following:

- Altered cerebral, cardiopulmonary, renal, GI, and peripheral tissue perfusion related to bleeding and sluggish or diminished blood flow secondary to thrombosis
- Pain related to bleeding into tissues and diagnostic procedures
- Risk for decreased CO related to fluid volume deficit and hypotension
- Anxiety related to fear of the unknown, disease process, diagnostic procedures, and therapy

Nursing Implementation

Nurses must be alert to the possible development of DIC and especially to the precipitating factors listed in Table 28-20. This may be difficult because the nurse is focusing on the complex care often required by the primary problem that precipitated the DIC. The nurse must also remember that because DIC is secondary to an underlying disease, appropriate care for managing the causative problem must be provided while providing supportive care related to the manifestations of DIC. Correcting the primary disease (when possible) will help resolve the DIC.

Appropriate nursing interventions are essential to the survival of a patient with acute DIC. Astute, ongoing assessment; active attention to manifestations of the syndrome; and institution of appropriate treatment measures are challenging and sometimes paradoxical nursing responsibilities (i.e., administering heparin to a bleeding patient). Table 28-16 and the nursing care plan for the patient with thrombocytopenia (p. 798) provide a comprehensive listing of assessments and interventions appropriate for the patient with DIC. Early detection of bleeding, both occult and overt, must be a primary goal. The patient should be thoroughly assessed for signs of external bleeding (e.g., petechiae, oozing at IV or injection sites) and signs of internal bleeding (e.g., changes in mental status, increasing abdominal girth, pain). Any sites of bleeding should be carefully monitored for progression or response to supportive therapies. Tissue damage should be minimized and the patient protected from additional foci of bleeding.

An additional nursing responsibility is to administer blood products properly if they are ordered. Infusing cryoprecipitate or FFP is similar to giving any other blood product (see Table 28-36). Cryoprecipitate comes in bags of 10 to 20 ml each. When it is used to treat DIC, multiple bags of cryoprecipitate may be required to support the patient. A unit of FFP that contains 200 to 280 ml takes about 20 minutes to thaw.

NEUTROPENIA

Leukopenia refers to a decrease in the total WBC count (granulocytes, monocytes, and lymphocytes). *Granulocytopenia* is a deficiency of the subset of WBCs called granulocytes, which include neutrophils, eosinophils, and basophils. The neutrophilic granulocytes, which play a major role in phagocytizing pathogenic microbes, are closely monitored in clinical practice as an indicator of a patient's risk for infection. A reduction in the neutrophil subset of granulocytes is called *neutropenia.* (Some clinicians use the terms *granulocytopenia* and *neutropenia* interchangably because the largest constituency of the granulocyte family is the neutrophils.) The absolute neutrophil count is determined by multiplying the total WBC count by the percentage of neutrophils. For example, a person with a total WBC of 9800/μl (9.8×10^9/L) and a neutrophil percentage of 72% would have a total of neutrophil count of 7056/μl (7.1×10^9/L). Neutropenia is defined as a neutrophil count of less than 1000 to 1500/μL (1 to 1.5 $\times 10^9$/L).[15] However, in considering the clinical significance of neutropenia it is important to know the rapidity of the decrease in the neutrophil count (gradual or rapid), degree of neutropenia, and duration. The faster the drop, the more profound the marrow suppression and the greater the likelihood of developing infection.

Table 28-22 Causes of Neutropenia

Drug-Induced Causes
- Antitumor antibiotics (daunorubicin, doxorubicin)
- Alkylating agents (nitrogen mustards, busulfan, chlorambucil)
- Antimetabolites (methotrexate, 6-mercaptopurine)
- Antiinflammatory drugs (aminopyrine, phenylbutazone)
- Antibacterial drugs (chloramphenicol, trimethoprim-sulfamethoxazole, penicillins)*
- Anticonvulsants (phenytoin)*
- Antithyroids*
- Hypoglycemics (tolbutamide)*
- Phenothiazines (chlorpromazine)*
- Psychotropics and antidepressants (clozapine, imipramine)
- Miscellaneous (gold, penicillamine, mepacrine, amodiaquine)
- Zidovudine (AZT)

Hematologic Disorders
- Idiopathic neutropenia
- Cyclic neutropenia
- Aplastic anemia
- Leukemia

Autoimmune Disorders
- Systemic lupus erythematosus
- Felty's syndrome
- Rheumatoid arthritis

Infections
- Viral (e.g., hepatitis, influenza, HIV, measles)
- Fulminant bacterial infection (e.g., typhoid fever, miliary tuberculosis)

Miscellaneous
- Severe sepsis
- Bone marrow infiltration (e.g., carcinoma, tuberculosis, lymphoma)
- Hypersplenism (e.g., portal hypertension, Felty's syndrome, storage diseases e.g., Gaucher's disease)
- Nutritional deficiencies (Vitamin B_{12}, folic acid)

HIV, Human immunodeficiency virus.
*Infrequent causes of neutropenia.

Neutropenia is not a disease; it is a syndrome that occurs with a variety of conditions or diseases (Table 28-22). It can also be an expected effect, side effect, or unintentional effect of taking certain medications. The most common cause of neutropenia is iatrogenic, resulting from widespread use of cytotoxic and immunosuppressive therapy used in the treatment of malignancies and autoimmune diseases. A brief overview of the clinical, diagnostic, and therapeutic implications of neutropenia is provided as a foundation for considering the effect of neutropenia in other diseases of WBCs that follow in this chapter.

Clinical Manifestations

The patient with neutropenia is predisposed to infection with nonpathogenic organisms that normally constitute normal body flora, as well as opportunistic pathogens. When the WBC count is depressed or immature WBCs are present, normal phagocytic mechanisms are impaired. Because of the diminished phagocytic response, the classic signs of inflammation—redness, heat, and swelling—may not occur. WBCs are the major component of pus; therefore, in the patient with neutropenia, pus formation (e.g., as a visible skin lesion or as pulmonary infiltrates on a chest x-ray) is also absent. Therefore the presence of fever is of great significance in recognizing the presence of infection in a neutropenic patient.[16]

When fever occurs in a neutropenic patient, it is generally assumed to be caused by infection and requires immediate attention because the immunocompromised, neutropenic patient lacks normal protective mechanisms. This can lead to a rapid and sometimes fatal progression of minor infections to sepsis. The mucous membranes of the throat and mouth, the perianal area, and the pulmonary system are common entry points for pathogenic organisms in susceptible hosts. Clinical manifestations related to infection at these sites include complaints of sore throat and dysphagia, appearance of ulcerative lesions of the pharyngeal and buccal mucosa, diarrhea, rectal tenderness, vaginal itching or discharge, shortness of breath, or nonproductive cough. These seemingly minor complaints can progress to fever, chills, sepsis, and septic shock if not recognized and treated in early stages.

Systemic infections caused by bacterial, fungal, and viral organisms are common in patients with neutropenia. The patient's own flora (normally nonpathogenic) have been identified as contributing significantly to life-threatening infections such as pneumonia. Organisms that are known to be common sources of infection include gram-positive *Staphylococcus aureus* and gram-negative organisms such as *Escherichia coli, Pseudomonas aeruginosa,* and *Klebsiella pneumoniae. Pneumocystis carinii* is an especially serious cause of pneumonia. Fungi that are involved include *Candida* (usually *C. albicans*) and *Aspergillus.* Viral infections caused by reactivation of herpes simplex and zoster are common following prolonged periods of neutropenia.[17]

Diagnostic Studies

The primary diagnostic tests for assessing neutropenia are the peripheral WBC count and bone marrow aspiration and biopsy (Table 28-23). A total WBC count of less than 5000/μl (5 × 10^9/L) reflects leukopenia. However, only a differential count can confirm the presence of neutropenia (neutrophil count <1000 to 1500/μl [1 to 1.5 × 10^9/L]). If the differential WBC count reflects an absolute neutropenia of 500 to 1000/μl (0.5 to 1.0 × 10^9/L), the patient is at moderate risk for a bacterial infection; an absolute neutropenia of less than 500/μl (0.5 × 10^9/L) places the patient at severe risk.

A peripheral blood smear is used to assess for immature forms of WBCs. The Hct level, reticulocyte count, and platelet count are done to evaluate general bone marrow function. Bone marrow aspirations and biopsies are done to examine cellularity and cell morphology. Additional studies may be done as indicated to assess spleen and liver function.

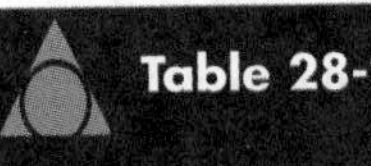

Table 28-23 Therapeutic Management: Neutropenia

Diagnostic
- History and physical examination
- WBC count with differential count
- WBC morphology
- Hct and Hb values
- Reticulocyte and platelet count
- Bone marrow aspiration or biopsy
- Cultures of nose, throat, sputum, urine, stool, obvious lesions, blood (as indicated)
- Chest x-ray

Therapeutic
- Identification and removal of cause of neutropenia (if possible)
- Identification of site of infection (if present) and causative organism
- Antibiotic therapy
- Hematopoietic growth factors (G-CSF, GM-CSF)
- Protective (reverse) isolation
- High-efficiency particulate air filtration
- Laminar airflow isolation

G-CSF, Granulocyte colony-stimulating factor; *GM-CSF,* granulocyte-macrophage colony-stimulating factor; *Hb,* hemoglobin; *Hct,* hematocrit; *WBC,* white blood cell.

Therapeutic Management

The factors involved in therapeutic management of neutropenia include (1) determining the cause of the neutropenia; (2) identifying the offending organisms if infection has developed; (3) instituting prophylactic, empiric, or therapeutic antibiotic therapy; (4) administering hematopoeitic growth factors (e.g., granulocyte colony-stimulating factor [G-CSF] and granulocyte-macrophage colony-stimulating factor [GM-CSF]); and (5) instituting protective isolation practices, such as strict hand washing, visitor restrictions, private room, high-efficiency particulate air (HEPA) filtration, or laminar airflow (LAF) environment (Table 28-23).

Occasionally the cause of the neutropenia can be easily removed (e.g., by termination of phenothiazines). However, neutropenia can also be a side effect that must be tolerated as a necessary step in therapy (e.g., chemotherapy or radiation therapy). In some situations the neutropenia resolves when the primary disease is treated (e.g., tuberculosis).

One aspect of vigilant monitoring of the neutropenic patient is constantly evaluating for signs and symptoms of infection. Early identification of a potentially infective organism depends on acquiring cultures from various sites. Serial blood cultures (at least two) and cultures of sputum, throat, lesions, wounds, urine, and feces are essential in the surveillance of the patient. It may also be necessary to do a tracheal aspiration, bronchoscopy with bronchial brushings, or lung biopsy to diagnose the cause of pneumonic infiltrates. Despite these many tests, the causative organism is usually identified only in approximately one third of patients.[16]

When a febrile episode occurs in a neutropenic patient, antibiotic therapy must be initiated immediately. The life-threatening nature of infection in a neutropenic host necessitates the institution of broad-spectrum antibiotics before the determination of a specific causative organism by culture. Administration of antibiotics is usually by the IV route because of the rapidly lethal effects of infection. However, some oral antibiotics are highly effective and routinely used for prophylaxis against infection in some neutropenic patients. Antibiotics are often used in combinations because of their synergistic effects. Combinations of antibiotics are also used in the event that multiple organisms are responsible for the infectious symptoms. Usually an aminoglycoside is used with an antipseudomonal penicillin or cephalosporin. Regardless of the combination, the nurse must observe for side effects of antimicrobial agents. Side effects common to aminoglycosides include nephrotoxicity and ototoxicity; side effects common to cephalosporins include rashes, fever, and pruritus.

G-CSF (filgrastim [Neupogen]) and GM-CSF (Sargramostim [Leukine, Prokine]) can be used to treat a neutropenic patient. These factors are especially beneficial in enhancing granulocyte recovery after chemotherapy and shorten the period of vulnerability to fatal infections. These CSFs also have the potential benefit of enhancing the phagocytic and cytotoxic activities of neutrophils.

An important consideration in the care of a neutropenic patient is the determination of the best means to protect the patient whose own defenses against infection are compromised. The principles to keep in mind to accomplish this goal are (1) the patient's normal flora is the most common source of microbial colonization and infection; (2) transmission of organisms from humans most commonly occurs by direct contact with the hands; (3) air, food, water, and equipment provide additional opportunities for infection transmission; and (4) health care providers with transmittable illnesses and other patients with infections can also be sources of infection transmission under certain conditions.[18,19]

Strict hand washing by all persons coming in contact with the compromised patient is the major method to prevent transmission of harmful pathogens. The Center for Disease Control and Prevention (CDC) advocates hand washing before, during, and after care. This seemingly routine technique has a significant effect in reducing infection. It must be emphasized and enforced despite its seeming simplicity.

The CDC also encourages separating immunocompromised patients from those who are infected or who have conditions that increase the probability of transmitting infections (e.g., poor hygiene caused by lack of understanding or cognitive dysfunction). Private rooms are useful whenever possible. HEPA filtration is an air-handling method with a high flow filtering system that can reduce or eliminate the number of aerosolized pathogens in the environment. Although it is expensive to install, it is often used for a patient with severe prolonged neutropenia. Care routines in an HEPA environment are essentially the same as care in any other private room.[16,19]

LAF rooms are controversial, are extremely expensive, require complex care routines, and are warranted for only the most severely immunocompromised patients.[16,19] Their purpose is to create a "sterile" environment to prevent infection transmission in the patient whose treatment caused severe, prolonged neutropenia (e.g., certain patients with leukemia who are receiving chemotherapy or waiting for bone marrow recovery). These rooms can provide a virtually sterile environment by filtering the air through extremely efficient air filters and using a blower system that provides a laminar flow of air free from convection and conduction currents. Sterile garments, water, and food also contribute to maintaining environmental sterility. Although LAF rooms can reduce the incidence of hospital-acquired infections in severely neutropenic persons, long-term survival has not been increased in most of these patients. Furthermore, unless the patient's own flora, a major source of infection, are reduced to a minimum through the use of prophylactic topical and oral antibiotics, this environment has no advantage over a HEPA-filtered room. There are also psychologic effects to a patient isolated in an LAF room.

NURSING MANAGEMENT

NEUTROPENIA

The nursing measures presented in the nursing care plan on p. 809 are important in the treatment of the patient with neutropenia. The value of effective nursing care in reducing the development of infection or limiting its extent cannot be overemphasized. Regular assessment and early detection of infectious sources is a key role for the nurse in reducing morbidity and mortality from infection.

MYELODYSPLASTIC SYNDROMES

Myelodysplastic syndromes (MDS) are a group of hematologic disorders characterized by a change in the quantity and quality of bone marrow elements. Other terms used to describe this hematologic disorder include preleukemia, hematopoietic dysplasia, refractory anemia with excessive myeloblasts, subacute myeloid leukemia, oligoblastic leukemia, and smoldering leukemia.[20]

Etiology

The etiology of MDS is unknown. Its manifestations result from neoplastic transformation of the pluripotent hematopoietic stem cell within the bone marrow. MDS is referred to as a clonal disorder because some bone marrow stem cells continue to function normally while others (a specific clone) do not. Occasionally one type of MDS transforms into another. In approximately 30% of cases, MDS will progress to acute myelogenous leukemia. Typically, life-threatening anemia, thrombocytopenia, and neutropenia will occur during the advanced stage of MDS.

The abnormal clone of the stem cells is usually found in the bone marrow but eventually may be found in circula-

NURSING CARE PLAN Patient with Neutropenia

Planning: Outcome Criteria	Nursing Interventions and Rationales
➤ **NURSING DIAGNOSIS**	Risk for infection *related to* decreased neutrophils and altered response to microbial invasion and presence of environmental pathogens.
Be free from signs and symptoms of infection; have minimal exposure to environmental pathogens.	Monitor for fever without evidence of redness, heat, swelling; absolute neutrophil count <1000/μl *to identify signs of and potential for infection.* Evaluate for presence of chills and malaise and determine temperature q4hr; report elevations >100.4° F (38° C) to physician *so appropriate interventions (e.g., IV antibiotics) can be initiated promptly.* Administer acetaminophen *as an antipyretic after evaluating fever if ordered by physician.* Avoid using aspirin if patient is thrombocytopenic *to avoid adverse effect on hemostasis and increasing risk for hemorrhage.* Be aware of chills, complaints of being cold when environment is warm, sore throat, persistent cough, chest pain, burning on urination, rectal pain, confusion *because these may be local and systemic signs of infection.* Use proper skin preparation techniques for initiating and maintaining IVs, caring for venous access devices, or obtaining blood culture specimens *to reduce the risk of introducing infection through the skin.* Evaluate fluid status during febrile episodes *to maintain adequate hydration and patient comfort.* Assess intake and ouput to include fluid lost through perspiration *to be as accurate as possible.* Assess skin turgor and mucous membranes *to evaluate state of hydration.* Institute antibiotic therapy as ordered. Dilute IV medication adequately and infuse at appropriate rate *to diminish vein irritation.* Establish administration schedule *to maximize pharmacologic effects and minimize side effects of drugs.* Assess for superinfections *that may develop with extended use of antibiotics.* Recognize need for prompt initiation of antimicrobial therapy *because of the rapidly lethal effects of infection.* Institute good hand washing technique with antiseptic solution for all persons in contact with patient; place patient in private room; limit or screen visitors and hospital staff members with colds or potentially communicable illnesses *to prevent the transmission of harmful pathogens to patient.* Routinely culture common sources of contamination (e.g., bathtubs or shower heads, respiratory therapy equipment) *to determine possible environmental sources of harmful pathogens.* Avoid invasive procedures to the greatest extent possible (e.g., venipunctures, urinary catheters, enemas, rectal suppositories). Teach patient necessary personal hygiene techniques (e.g., hand washing, pulmonary hygiene) *to decrease the colonization of organisms at these sites because this can lead to infection from these various sources.* Provide meticulous perianal care *to prevent perirectal abscess.* Administer hematopoietic growth factors as ordered (e.g., G-CSF, GM-CSF) *to raise patient's WBC count and reduce infection risk during periods of neutropenia.*
➤ **NURSING DIAGNOSIS**	Risk for altered oral mucous membranes *related to* treatment, disease, nausea, vomiting, or anorexia.
Have pink, moist, lesion-free oral mucosa, tongue, lips; no inflammation, lesions, crusts, or hardened debris; no evidence of infection; no discomfort with talking or swallowing.	Assess oral mucosa daily *to determine presence of oral or pharyngeal ulcerations, stomatitis, oral infections.* Remove dentures daily *to assess condition of underlying gums* and evaluate fit *to avoid loose dentures causing a lesion.* Distinguish infectious from noninfectious stomatitis *so appropriate treatment can be initiated.* Administer a topical or systemic antifungal (as ordered) for candidiasis. Encourage patient to use mouthwash q2hr such as baking soda, normal saline solution, diphenhydramine (Benadryl) elixir, Maalox, xylocaine *for comfort.* Use soft-bristle toothbrushes, toothettes, or an irrigating syringe *to cleanse mouth and prevent trauma.* Avoid lemon and glycerine swabs and hydrogen peroxide *because these are drying to oral mucosa.* Apply topical anesthetic such as viscous lidocaine (Xylocaine) *to minimize discomfort* and an oral antiseptic such as chlorhexidine *to minimize colonization of harmful pathogens.* Apply water-soluble lubricants and moisturizers to lips *to keep lips moist and minimize cracking.*

G-CSF, Granulocyte colony-stimulating factor; *GM-CSF,* granulocyte-macrophage colony-stimulating factor; *IV,* intravenous; *WBC,* white blood cell.

tion. In contrast to acute myelogenous leukemia (AML), in which the leukemic cells show little normal maturation, the clonal cells in MDS always display some degree of maturity. Disease progression is slower than in AML. However, eventually the bone marrow is replaced partly or wholly by the abnormal cells.

Clinical Manifestations. Most cases of MDS are discovered as a result of testing for complications of anemia, thrombocytopenia, or neutropenia. However, there are other cases in which there are no symptoms and diagnosis results from a routine complete blood count (CBC).

Infection and bleeding are common and result from either inadequate numbers of circulating cells or from poorly functioning cells. Neutropenia usually precedes infection. Some patients may have normal numbers of granulocytes but become infected as a result of the ineffective functioning of these circulating granulocytes.

Diagnostic Studies. Bone marrow aspiration and biopsies are essential for both the diagnosis and the classification of the specific types of myelodysplasia. In MDS the bone marrow is normocellular, hypocellular, or hypercellular in the presence of peripheral cytopenias. MDS is staged according to clinical and laboratory findings. The relationship between the number of circulating blast cells and the number of blast cells in the bone marrow serves as the main indicator of prognosis in this disease.

Therapeutic Management

Supportive treatment of MDS is based on the premise that the aggressiveness of treatment should match the aggressiveness of the disease. Supportive treatment consists of simple hematologic monitoring (serial bone marrow and peripheral blood examinations), antibiotic therapy, or transfusions with blood products. Side effects and toxicities from supportive treatment include anemia, thrombocytopenia, and blood transfusion reactions.

Androgens and corticosteroids have been used in patients with bone marrow failure with little effect. Treatment with androgens has not improved bone marrow function and has not affected survival. Further immunosuppression associated with corticosteroid treatment may outweigh the benefits. Side effects of corticosteroid therapy include moon faces, fragile skin, and increased risk of infection.

Differentiation-inducing agents have been investigated in an attempt to correct the defective maturation of the hematopoietic stem cells clone in the marrow. Some agents have been shown to transform nonfunctional immature blasts and promyelocytes into functional mature granulocytes.[20] These agents include retinoic acid (Tretinoin) and cytosine arabinoside. Response rates have ranged from no response to improvement in survival in some patients. Side effects and toxicities from retinoic acid include dry skin, dry lips, myalgias, lethargy, and hypercalcemia. Bone marrow transplantation, biologic response modifiers, and colony-stimulating factors have also been used in an attempt to correct bone marrow dysfunction of MDS. However, because of the aggressiveness of these treatments, they are not often tolerated by older patients.

NURSING MANAGEMENT

MYELODYSPLASTIC SYNDROME

Nursing care of a patient with MDS is similar to that of a patient with manifestations of anemia (see the nursing care plan for the patient with anemia), thrombocytopenia (see the nursing care plan for the patient with thrombocytopenia), and neutropenia (see the nursing care plan for the patient with neutropenia). The nurse needs to educate the patient about the risks of infection, bleeding, and fatigue.

LEUKEMIA

Leukemia is the general term used to describe a group of malignant disorders affecting the blood and blood-forming tissues of the bone marrow, lymph system, and spleen. Leukemia occurs in all age groups. It results in an accumulation of dysfunctional cells because of a loss of regulation in cell division. It follows a progressive course that is eventually fatal if untreated. An estimated 28,600 new cases were diagnosed in 1994.[21] Table 28-24 summarizes the relative incidences of the different subtypes and their hallmark features. Although often thought of as a disease of children, the number of adults affected with leukemia is 10 times that of children.

Etiology

Regardless of the specific type of leukemia, there is generally no single causative agent in the development of leukemia. Most leukemias result from a combination of factors, including genetic and environmental influences.[22] Chromosomal changes, first recognized in chronic myelogenous leukemia (which involves Philadelphia chromosome), have led to discoveries of how normal genes, once transformed, can result in abnormal genes (oncogenes) capable of causing many types of cancers, including leukemias (see Chapter 12). Chemical agents (e.g., benzene), chemotherapeutic agents (e.g., alkylating agents), viruses, radiation, and immunologic deficiencies have all been associated with the development of leukemia in susceptible hosts. There is an increased incidence of leukemia in radiologists, persons who lived near nuclear bomb test sites or nuclear reactor accidents (e.g., Chernobyl), survivors of the bombing of Nagasaki and Hiroshima, and persons previously treated with radiotherapy or chemotherapy. Although RNA retroviruses cause a number of leukemias in animals, a viral cause for a human leukemia has been established only for some patients with adult T-cell leukemia, which is caused by the human T-cell leukemia virus type I (HTLV-1). This form of leukemia is endemic in southwestern Japan and parts of the Caribbean and central Africa.

Pathophysiology

Acute leukemia is characterized by the clonal proliferation of immature hematopoietic cells. The leukemia arises following malignant transformation of a single hematopoietic progenitor, followed by cellular replication and expansion of the transformed clone. The most prominent characteristic

Table 28-24 Types of Leukemia

Type/Incidence*	Age of Onset	Clinical Manifestations	Diagnostic Findings
Acute myelogenous leukemia—23%	Increase in incidence with advancing age, peak incidence between 60-70 yr of age	Fatigue and weakness, headache, mouth sores, minimal hepatosplenomegaly and lymphadenopathy, anemia, bleeding, fever, infection, sternal tenderness	Low RBC count, Hb, Hct; low platelet count; low to high WBC count with myeloblasts; greatly hypercellular bone marrow with myeloblasts
Acute lymphocytic leukemia—14%	Before 14 yr of age, peak incidence between 2-9 yr of age and in older adults	Fever; pallor; bleeding; anorexia; fatigue and weakness; bone, joint, and abdominal pain; generalized lymphadenopathy; infections; weight loss; hepatospleno-megaly; headache; mouth sores; neurologic manifestations; including CNS involvement, increased intracranial pressure, secondary to meningeal infiltration	Low RBC count, Hb, Hct; low platelet count; low, normal, or high WBC count; transverse lines of rarefaction at ends of metaphysis of long bones on x-ray; hypercellular bone marrow with lymphoblasts; lymphoblasts also possible in cerebral spinal fluid
Chronic myelogenous leukemia—17%	25-60 yr of age, peak incidence around 45 yr of age	No symptoms early in disease, fatigue and weakness, fever, sternal tenderness, weight loss, joint pain, bone pain, massive splenomegaly, increase in sweating	Low RBC count, Hb, Hct; high platelet count early, lower count later; increase in polymorphonuclear neutrophils, normal number of lymphocytes, and normal or low number of monocytes in WBC differential; low leukocyte alkaline phosphatase; presence of Philadelphia chromosome in 90% of patients
Chronic lymphocytic leukemia—29%	50-70 yr of age, rare below 30 yr of age, predominance in men	No symptoms usually, detection of disease often during examination for unrelated condition, chronic fatigue, anorexia, splenomegaly and lymphadenopathy, hepatomegaly	Mild anemia and thrombocytopenia with disease progression; increase in peripheral lymphocytes; increase in presence of lymphocytes in bone marrow

CNS, Central nervous system; *Hb*, hemoglobin; *Hct*, hematrocrit, RBC, red blood cell; *WBC*, white blood cell.
*This is the incidence based on all types of leukemia; the number does not add up to 100% because approximately 17% are unclassifiable.

of the neoplastic cell in acute leukemia is a defect in maturation beyond the myeloblast or promyelocyte level in acute myelogenous leukemia and the lymphoblast level in acute lymphocytic leukemia.

Chronic lymphocytic leukemia (CLL) is a neoplasm of activated B lymphocytes. The CLL cells, which morphologically resemble mature, small lymphocytes of the peripheral blood, accumulate in the bone marrow, blood, lymph nodes, and spleen in large numbers.

Chronic myelogenous leukemia (CML) is a clonal stem cell disorder characterized by greatly increased myelopoiesis and the presence of the Philadelphia chromosome. Although no specific etiologic agent has been identified, an increased incidence of CML was observed in survivors of the atomic bomb in Japan. The incidence of CML in these individuals was dose related.

Clinical Manifestations

The clinical manifestations of leukemia are varied (see Table 28-24). Essentially they relate to problems caused by bone marrow failure and the formation of masses composed of leukemic infiltrates. Bone marrow failure results from (1) inadequate production of normal marrow elements and (2) bone marrow crowding by abnormal cells, leading to marrow suppression. The patient is predisposed to anemia, thrombocytopenia, and decreased number and function of WBCs.

As leukemia progresses, fewer normal blood cells are produced. Abnormal WBCs continue to accumulate because

Table 28-25 The French-American-British (FAB) Classification of Acute Myelogenous Leukemias

Classification	Category	Abbreviation	Percent of Cases
AML M1	Myeloblastic leukemia	AML	19%
AML M2	Myeloblastic leukemia with maturation	AML	29%
AML M3	Promyelocytic leukemia	APL	9%
AML M4	Myelomonocytic leukemia	AMML	19%
AML M5	Monocytic leukemia	AMoL	15%
AML M6	Erythroleukemia	AEL	4%
AML M7	Megakaryoblastic leukemia	AMegL	4%
AML M0	Undifferentiated leukemia		1%

they do not go through the normal cell life cycle to death. The increased numbers of WBCs can lead to infiltration and damage to the bone marrow, lymph nodes, spleen, and other organs, including the CNS. Leukemic infiltration leads to problems such as splenomegaly, hepatomegaly, lymphadenopathy, bone pain, meningeal irritation, and oral lesions. Solid masses resulting from collections of leukemic cells, called *chloromas,* can also occur.

Diagnostic Studies and Classification

The goal of diagnostic studies is to define the subclass or specific type of leukemia so that the appropriate treatment and prognosis can be determined. Peripheral blood evaluation and bone marrow examination are the primary methods of diagnosing and classifying the subtypes of leukemia. (See Tables 28-25 and 28-26 for these classifications.) Morphologic, histochemical, immunologic, and cytogenetic methods are all used to identify cell subtypes and stage of development of leukemic cell populations. Further studies such as lumbar puncture and CT scan can determine the presence of leukemic cells outside of the blood and bone marrow.

The two major categories of leukemia are acute and chronic. In the past, these designations had significant prognostic implications related to the duration of the illness. However, current therapeutic measures have increased the survival of patients with certain forms of acute leukemia beyond that of patients with certain forms of chronic leukemia. Although the terms *acute* and *chronic* are still used, they refer primarily to cell maturity and the nature of the disease onset. In acute leukemia, the bone marrow is infiltrated with young, undifferentiated, immature cells, often referred to as *blasts.* The disease has a rapid onset and requires immediate and aggressive intervention. The bone marrow in an individual with chronic leukemia consists primarily of differentiated mature WBCs, and the disease onset is more gradual.

Table 28-26 French-American-British (FAB) Classification of Acute Lymphocytic Leukemia

L1	Common childhood leukemia
L2	Adult acute lymphocytic leukemia
L3	Rare subtype, blasts resembling those in Burkitt's lymphoma

Additional classification of leukemia is done by identifying the type of leukocyte involved, whether of myelogenous origin (granulocyte, monocyte, erythrocyte, megakaryocyte) or of lymphocytic origin. By combining the acute and chronic categories with the cell type involved, specific types of leukemia can be identified. Four major types of leukemia are acute lymphocytic leukemia (ALL), acute myelogenous leukemia (AML) (also called acute nonlymphoblastic leukemia [ANLL]), chronic myelogenous (granulocytic) leukemia (CML), and chronic lymphocytic leukemia (CLL). Other defining features of these leukemic subtypes are presented in Table 28-24.

Leukemias are classified using the French-American-British (FAB) classification system. The FAB system divides acute myelogenous leukemia into seven subtypes (Table 28-25) according to the direction of differentiation along one or more cell lines and the degree of cellular maturation. Three types of acute lymphocytic leukemia (Table 28-26) are distinguished by certain cytologic features and the degree of heterogeneity of the leukemic cell population. The traditional AML (ANLL) and ALL labels are used in conjunction with the FAB nomenclature. Additional work is being done using monoclonal antibodies, molecular cell markers, and genetic probes to more accurately distinguish among the many types of leukemic WBCs and their precursors to facilitate diagnosis and classification of leukemia.

Acute Myelogenous Leukemia. AML is also referred to as ANLL, as previously mentioned. Although only one fourth of all leukemias are of this subtype, it makes up approximately 85% of the acute leukemias in adults. Its onset is often abrupt and dramatic. A patient may have serious infections and abnormal bleeding.

AML is characterized by uncontrolled proliferation of myeloblasts, the precursors of granulocytes. There is hyperplasia of the bone marrow and spleen. The clinical manifestations are usually related to replacement of normal hematopoietic cells in the marrow by leukemic cells and, to a lesser extent, to infiltration of other organs (Table 28-25).

Some AML subtypes are accompanied by additional specific clinical manifestations. For example, the patient with the M5 subtype, acute *monocytic leukemia,* has weakness and fatigue progressing to exhaustion, anorexia, pallor, chills, and fever, as well as findings of gingival hyperplasia or inflammation, bleeding, and infection. M3, promyeloctyic leukemia, is often accompanied by bleeding caused by procoagulant cells initiating DIC. M6 is a rare form of leukemia that affects RBCs, known as *erythroleukemia* or *DiGugliemo's syndrome.* It is considered a WBC disorder because ultimately the disease progresses to affect granulocytes.

Acute Lymphocytic Leukemia. ALL is most common in children and accounts for 15% of acute leukemia in adults. In ALL, immature lymphocytes proliferate in the bone marrow. Fever is present in the majority of patients at the time of diagnosis. Symptoms may appear abruptly with bleeding or fever, or they may be insidious with progressive weakness, fatigue, and bleeding tendencies. CNS manifestations are especially common in ALL and represent a serious problem. Leukemic meningitis caused by arachnoid infiltration occurs in many patients with ALL.

Chronic Myelogenous Leukemia. CML is also referred to as *chronic granulocytic leukemia* (CGL). CML is caused by excessive development of neoplastic granulocytes in the bone marrow. The excess neoplastic granulocytes move into the peripheral blood in massive numbers and ultimately infiltrate the liver and spleen. Immature and mature granulocytes are found in the bone marrow and peripheral blood, but mature cells are dominant peripherally.

The chromosomal abnormality found in 90% of individuals with CML is an exchange of genetic information between chromosome pairs 9 and 22 and is called the *Philadelphia chromosome.* This alteration is directly attributed to the disease process.[22] Complications of CML are related to a blast crisis in which chronic leukemia transforms to acute disease (infiltration of more immature cells). In a blastic crisis increased numbers of myeloblasts are found in both the bone marrow and blood. The chronic phase of CML can persist for 2 to 4 years and can usually be well controlled with treatment. Currently the only curative therapy for CML is bone marrow transplantation with an HLA-matched donor.[7] Without treatment the chronic phase of the disease will ultimately progress to a more symptomatic *accelerated phase,* ending in a brief blastic phase in which the disease resembles its acute counterpart. Once CML transforms to an accelerated or blastic phase, it is often refractory to therapy and the patient may live for only a few months.

Chronic Lymphocytic Leukemia. CLL is characterized by the production and accumulation of functionally inactive but long-lived, mature-appearing lymphocytes. The type of lymphocyte involved is usually the B cell. The lymphocytes infiltrate the bone marrow, spleen, and liver. Lymph node enlargement throughout the body is commonly present. There is an increased incidence of infection. CLL tends to cluster in families. Complications from CLL are uncommon initially but may develop as the disease advances. Pressure on nerves from enlarged lymph nodes can cause pain and even paralysis. Mediastinal node enlargement can lead to pulmonary symptoms. Because CLL is a disease of older adults, treatment decisions must be made by considering the progression of the disease and the side effects of treatment. Many individuals in the early stages of CLL require no treatment. As the disease progresses, various treatments can be used to control symptoms.

Hairy Cell Leukemia. Hairy cell leukemia accounts for approximately 2% of all adult leukemias. It is a chronic disease of lymphoproliferation predominantly involving B lymphocytes that infiltrate the bone marrow and spleen. Cells have a "hairy" appearance under the microscope. The spleen sequesters increasing numbers of normal hematopoietic cells, making splenomegaly a common finding. Hairy cell leukemia is usually seen in male patients over 40 years of age. A patient with hairy cell leukemia usually has symptoms from splenomegaly, pancytopenia, infection caused by impaired host defense, or vasculitis. Many asymptomatic patients are detected on routine CBC. α-Interferon, deoxycoformycin (Pentostatin), and 2 chlorodeoxyadenosine (2 CDA) are effective agents in the treatment of this type of leukemia. Virtually all patients treated with α-interferon respond to therapy. Cladribine (Leustatin) can also be used in the treatment of hairy cell leukemia. This drug is given in a single continuous IV infusion for 7 days. Complete remissions are rare, but retreatment of recurrent disease is often successful.

Unclassified Leukemias. Occasionally the subtype of leukemia cannot be identified. The malignant leukemic cells may have lymphoid, myeloid, or mixed characteristics. Often these patients do not respond to treatment. Typically a patient with undifferentiated leukemia has a poorer prognosis. Response to treatment will help to identify if a correct diagnosis has been made.

Therapeutic and Pharmacologic Management

Once a diagnosis of leukemia has been made, therapeutic management includes remission induction with chemotherapeutic drugs and, sometimes, radiation therapy. Other considerations include regular examination of patients on an ongoing basis to evaluate their progress and supportive interventions to prevent complications of the disease and the therapy (e.g., hemorrhage, infection). The nurse needs to understand the principles of cancer chemotherapy, including cellular kinetics, the use of multiple drugs rather than single agents, and the cell cycle. (See the section on chemotherapy in Chapter 12.)

Attaining remission is the initial goal of treatment for leukemia. Although not all forms of leukemia are considered curable at this time, attaining an initial remission or disease control is currently a realistic option for the majority of patients. In complete remission there is no evidence of overt disease on physical examination, and the bone marrow and peripheral blood appear normal. A lesser state of control is known as partial remission. Partial remission is characterized by no overt clinical disease and a normal peripheral blood smear, but there is still evidence of disease in the bone marrow. The survival period after diagnosis is increasing as a result of attaining and maintaining remissions. Each time there is a relapse, the succeeding remis-

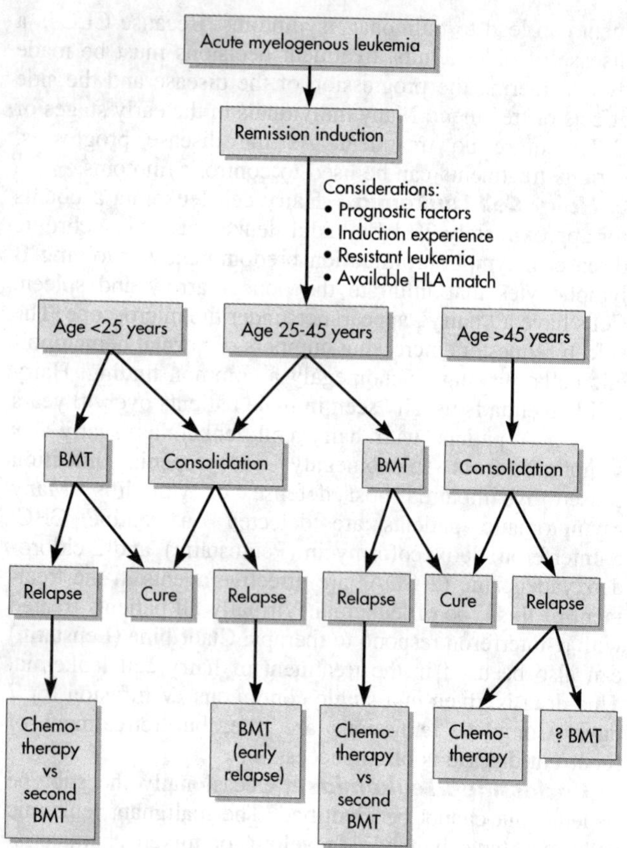

Fig. 28-12 Treatment considerations and options for a patient with acute myelogenous leukemia. *BMT,* Bone marrow transplant.

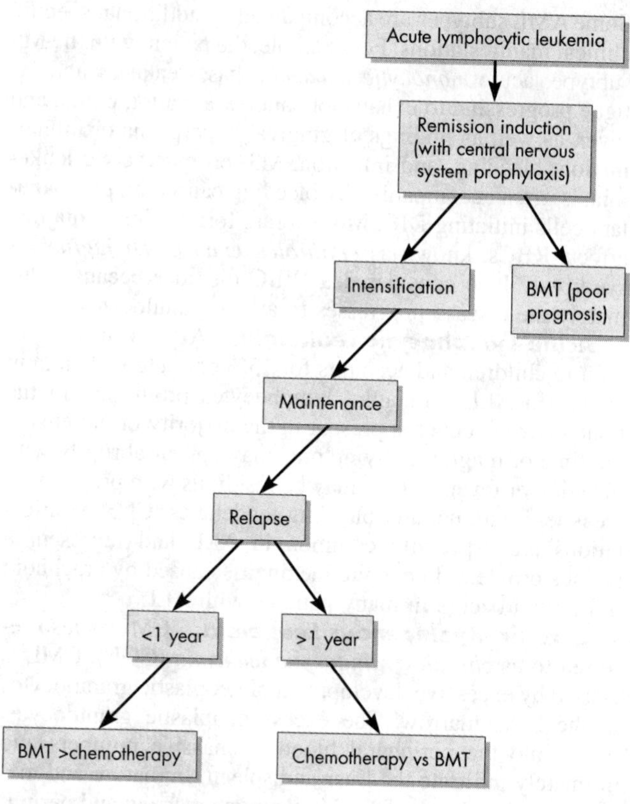

Fig. 28-13 Treatment considerations and options for a patient with acute lymphocytic leukemia. *BMT,* Bone marrow transplant.

sion may be more difficult to achieve and shorter in duration (See Figs. 28-12 and 28-13). With each subsequent therapy a patient needs to consider the likelihood of attaining remission versus experiencing potentially life-threatening side effects.

The chemotherapeutic treatment of acute leukemia is divided into stages. The first stage, *induction therapy,* is the attempt to induce or bring about a remission. Induction is aggressive treatment that seeks to destroy leukemic cells in the tissues, peripheral blood, and bone marrow. During induction therapy a patient may become devastatingly ill and predisposed to complications because the bone marrow is severely depressed by the drugs. Throughout induction, therapeutic and nursing interventions focused on anemia, thrombocytopenia, and neutropenia may significantly affect the patient's survival. Common chemotherapy for induction of acute myelogenous leukemia includes cytosine arabinoside, an antimetabolite, given for 7 days, and 3 days of anthracycline therapy (including daunorubicin, doxorubicin, idarubicin, amsacrine, or mitoxantrone). This "7 + 3" protocol is considered a standard therapy at the present time and results in a 65% to 80% remission induction rate.[20]

Terms used to describe postremission chemotherapy include intensification, consolidation, and maintenance. *Intensification,* or high-dose therapy, may be given immediately after induction therapy for several months. This therapy may use the same drugs as those used in induction but at higher dosages. Other drugs that target the cell in a different way than those used for induction may also be added. *Consolidation therapy* is started after a remission is achieved. It may consist of one or two additional courses of the same drugs used during induction or involve high-dose therapy (intensive consolidation). The purpose of consolidation therapy is to eliminate remaining leukemic cells.

Maintenance therapy is treatment with lower doses of the same drugs used in induction or other drugs given every 3 to 4 weeks for a prolonged period, usually years. Usually there are few complications and this therapy is well tolerated. The goal is to maintain the remission once it is achieved, thereby keeping the body free of leukemic cells. The patient with lymphocytic leukemia can undergo maintenance therapy for a number of years. However, in acute myelogenous types of leukemia, it is rarely effective and therefore rarely administered.[20]

In addition to chemotherapy, corticosteroids and radiation therapy can also have a role in the complex therapeutic plans for the patient with leukemia. Total body radiation may be used to prepare a patient for bone marrow transplantation, or it may be restricted to certain areas (fields) such as the liver and spleen or other organs affected by infiltrates. In acute lymphocytic leukemia, prophylactic intrathecal methotrexate is given to decrease the chance of CNS involvement, which is common in this particular type of leukemia. When CNS leukemia does occur, cranial radiation is given. The use of biologic response modifiers in the treatment of leukemia is being investigated (see Chapter 12).

Chemotherapy Regimens. The chemotherapeutic agents used to treat leukemia vary. The choice of drugs and the sequence of therapy depend on the preference of the oncologist and on current research findings. Table 28-27 lists chemotherapeutic agents used to treat leukemia. Table 28-28 gives examples of treatment regimens used in various types of leukemia.

Combination chemotherapy is the mainstay of treatment for leukemia. The three purposes for using multiple drugs are to (1) decrease drug resistance, (2) minimize the toxicity of high doses of single agents by using multiple drugs with varying toxicities, and (3) interrupt cell growth at multiple points in the cell cycle.

Acronyms made from the letters of the drugs used in combination chemotherapy may be used to identify the regimen. For example, *COAP* stands for cyclophosphamide, Oncovin, arabinoside, and prednisone. This combination of drugs is used to treat acute leukemia.

Bone Marrow Transplantation. Bone marrow transplantation (BMT) is another form of therapy used for patients with different forms of leukemia, including ALL, AML, and CML. This treatment modality is also used for other hematologic malignancies, such as Hodgkin's disease, non-Hodgkin's lymphoma, solid tumors (e.g., breast cancer), and some nonmalignant disorders, including aplastic anemia and

Table 28-27 Chemotherapeutic Agents Used to Treat Leukemia

Drug Classification	Drug Name
Alkylating agents	Busulfan (Myleran) Chlorambucil (Leukeran) Cyclophosphamide (Cytoxan)
Antitumor antibiotics	Daunorubicin (Cerubidine) Doxorubicin (Adriamycin) Mitoxantrone (Novantrone) Idarubicin (Idamycin)
Antimetabolites	Cytarabine/cytosine arabinoside (Cytosar/Ara-C) 6-mercaptopurine (Purinethol), Methotrexate (Folex, Mexate) 6-thioguanine (6-TG) Fludarabine (Fludara)
Corticosteroid	Prednisone
Nitrosoureas	Carmustine (BCNU)
Plant alkaloid	Vincristine (Oncovin) Vinblastine (Velban)
Miscellaneous	L-Asparaginase (Elspar) Hydroxyurea (Hydrea) Etoposide (VP-16)

Table 28-28 Treatments Used in Leukemia

Drug Therapy	Other Therapy
Acute Myelogenous Leukemia	
Daunorubicin, cytosine arabinoside, doxorubicin, idarubicin, 6-thioguanine, mitoxantrone, combination chemotherapy of antitumor antibiotic and cytosine arabinoside or antitumor antibiotic and cytosine arabinoside and thioguanine	Bone marrow transplant
Acute Lymphocytic Leukemia	
Daunorubicin, doxorubicin, vincristine, prednisone, L-asparaginase, cyclophosphamide, methotrexate, 6-mercaptopurine, cytosine arabinoside, combination chemotherapy of cyclophosphamide and vincristine and prednisone and antitumor antibiotic and L-asparaginase, combination chemotherapy of daunorubicin and cytosine arabinoside and 6-mercaptopurine and vincristine and prednisone	Cranial radiation therapy, intratheca methotrexate
Chronic Myelogenous Leukemia	
Busulfan (Myleran); hydroxyurea (Hydrea); combination chemotherapy including any of the following: cytosine arabinoside, thioguanine, daunorubicin, methotrexate, prednisone, vincristine, L-asparaginase, carmustine, 6-mercaptopurine	Radiation (total body or spleen), bone marrow transplant, interferon, leukapheresis
Chronic Lymphocytic Leukemia	
Chorambucil (Leukeran), cyclophosphamide (Cytoxan), prednisone (CVP protocol (cyclophosphamide, vincristine, and prednisone), fludarabine	Radiation (total body, lymph nodes, or spleen), splenectomy, colony-stimulating factors, interferon

congenital immunodeficiencies. In leukemia, the goal of BMT is to totally eliminate leukemic cells from the body using combinations of chemotherapy and total body irradiation. This treatment also eradicates the patient's bone marrow stem cells, which are then replaced with those of an HLA-matched sibling or volunteer donor (allogeneic), an identical twin (syngeneic), or with the patient's own marrow (autologous) that was removed (harvested) before the intensive therapy.[7, 23-25]

Bone marrow stem cells are aspirated from the pelvis, usually from the iliac crest, but they can also be obtained from the sternum or ribs. A newer method of obtaining bone marrow stem cells is through an apheresis procedure that separates them from circulating blood.[25] These peripheral blood stem cells have essentially the same capacity to repopulate the marrow and create a new hematopoeitic system. An advantage of collecting stem cells by this method is that it avoids the need for an operating room procedure under general anesthesia, which is usually done when performing a traditional bone marrow harvest.

Autologous bone marrow, harvested from the patient during remission either from the bone or by peripheral pheresis, is sometimes treated (purged) to remove residual leukemic cells. Several immunologic and chemical agents have been used for this purpose. The bone marrow is then cryopreserved (frozen) and stored until it is used for transplantation.

Regardless of the harvesting method, the specially prepared marrow is infused IV into the recipient following intensive chemotherapy and radiation therapy. The marrow stem cells reconstitute, or *rescue,* the recipient's hematopoeitic system. Usually 2 to 4 weeks are required for the transplanted marrow to start producing hematopoeitic blood cells. This period has been reduced when peripheral blood stem cells have been used. Presumably these cells contain more mature cells than marrow-derived stem cells. During this pancytopenic period it is critical for the patient to be in a protective isolation environment receiving supportive care. RBC and platelet transfusions may be necessary to maintain circulating blood cells during this time.

The primary complications of patients with allogeneic BMT are graft-versus-host disease (GVHD), relapse of leukemia (especially ALL), and infection (especially interstitial pneumonia). GVHD is mediated by competent T cells infused with the donor marrow that mount an attack against the recipient's immune system (see Chapter 10). Relapse of the underlying disease is also a difficult problem to solve because of the inability for even intensive therapy to eliminate every leukemic cell. The intent of BMT is cure. Because it is a highly toxic therapy, the patient must weigh the significant risks of treatment-related death or treatment failure (relapse) with the hope of cure.[26,27]

NURSING MANAGEMENT

LEUKEMIA

Nursing Assessment

Subjective and objective data that should be obtained from a patient with leukemia are presented in Table 28-29.

Table 28-29 Nursing Assessment: Leukemia

Subjective Data

Important health information

Past health history: Exposure to chemical toxins (e.g., benzene, arsenic), radiation, or viruses (Epstein-Barr, HTLV-1); chromosome abnormalities (e.g., in patients with Down syndrome, Klinefelter's syndrome, Fanconi's syndrome), organ transplantation; frequent infections; bleeding tendencies

Medications: Use of phenylbutazone, chloramphenicol, chemotherapy

Surgery and other treatments: Radiation exposure, prior radiation and chemotherapy for cancer

Functional health patterns

Health perception–health management: Family history of leukemia; fatigue, malaise

Nutritional-metabolic: Mouth sores, weight loss; chills, fever, night sweats; nausea, vomiting, anorexia, dysphagia, early satiety; easy bruising

Elimination: Hematuria, decreased urine output; diarrhea, dark stools

Activity-exercise: Progressive weakness; dyspnea, epistaxis, cough

Cognitive-perceptual: Headache; bone tenderness; muscle cramps; sore throat; bone, joint, abdominal pain; paresthesias, numbness, tingling, visual disturbances

Sexuality-reproductive: Prolonged menses, menorrhagia, impotence

Objective Data

General

Generalized lymphadenopathy, lethargy

Integumentary

Pallor or jaundice; petechiae, ecchymoses, purpura, reddish brown to purple cutaneous infiltrates, purple skin tumors, macules, and papules

Cardiovascular

Tachycardia, systolic murmurs

Neurologic

Seizures, disorientation, confusion, decreased coordination, cranial nerve palsies, papilledema

Musculoskeletal

Muscle wasting

Possible laboratory findings

Low, normal, or high WBC count with shift to the left (↑ blast cells); anemia, decreased hematocrit and hemoglobin, thrombocytopenia, Philadelphia chromosome; hypercellular bone marrow aspirate or biopsy with myeloblasts, lymphoblasts, greatly reduced normal cells

Respiratory

Abnormal lung sounds (e.g., rhonchi, crackles)

Gastrointestinal

Gingival bleeding and hyperplasia; oral herpes and *Candida* infections; perirectal irritation and infection; splenomegaly, hepatomegaly

WBC, White blood cell.

Nursing Diagnoses

Nursing diagnoses related to leukemia include those appropriate for anemia, thrombocytopenia, and neutropenia (see the appropriate nursing care plans in this chapter).

Planning

The overall goals are that the patient with leukemia will (1) understand and cooperate with the treatment plan, (2) experience minimal side effects and complications associated with both the disease and its treatment, and (3) feel hopeful and supported during the periods of remission and relapse.

Nursing Implementation

Acute Intervention. The nursing role during acute phases of leukemia is extremely challenging because the patient has many physical and psychosocial needs. As with other forms of cancer, the diagnosis of leukemia can evoke great fear and be equated with death. It may be viewed as a hopeless, horrible disease with many painful and undesirable consequences. The diagnosis of leukemia elicits many emotional responses based on the realization that life is finite. The nurse has a special responsibility in helping the patient and family deal with these feelings. The nurse must help the patient realize that although the future may be uncertain, one can have a meaningful quality of life while in remission or with disease control. The family also needs help in adjusting to the stress of this abrupt onset of serious illness (e.g., dependence, withdrawal, changes in role responsibilities, and alterations in body image) and the losses imposed by the sick role. The diagnosis of leukemia often brings with it the need to make difficult decisions at a time of profound stress for the patient and family.

The nurse is an important advocate in helping the patient and family understand the complexities of treatment decisions and expected side effects and toxicities. A patient empowered by knowledge of the disease and treatment can have a more positive outlook and improved quality of life. A patient may require isolation or may need to temporarily relocate to an appropriate treatment center. These situations can lead a patient to feel deserted and isolated at the time when the most support is needed. The nurse has contact with a patient 24 hours a day, and can help reverse feelings of abandonment and loneliness by balancing the demanding technical needs with a humanistic, caring approach. Therefore a nurse faces a special challenge in learning how to meet the intense psychosocial needs of a patient with leukemia while continuing to offer the complex physical care that is usually required. Consulting with other health professionals (e.g., psychiatric clinical specialists, oncology clinical specialists, social workers) may help the nurse develop the skills required to meet the many needs of a patient with leukemia.

From a physical care perspective, the nurse is challenged to make astute assessments and plan care to help the patient survive the severe side effects of chemotherapy. The life-threatening results of bone marrow suppression (anemia, thrombocytopenia, neutropenia) require aggressive nursing interventions (see the appropriate nursing care plans). Additional complications of chemotherapy may affect the patient's GI tract, nutritional status, skin and mucosa, cardiopulmonary status, liver, kidneys, and neurologic system. (Nursing interventions to reduce discomfort related to these problems are discussed in Chapter 12.)

The nurse must be knowledgeable about all drugs being administered. This includes the mechanism of action, purpose, routes of administration, usual doses, potential side effects, safe-handling considerations, and toxic effects of the drugs. In addition, the nurse must know how to assess laboratory data reflecting the effects of the drugs. Patient survival and comfort during aggressive chemotherapy are significantly affected by the quality of nursing care.

Chronic and Home Management. Ongoing care for the patient with leukemia is necessary to monitor for signs and symptoms of disease control or relapse. For a patient requiring long-term or maintenance chemotherapy the fatigue of long-term chronic disease management can become arduous and discouraging. Therefore a patient and the significant other must be educated to understand the importance of the continued diligence in disease management and the need for follow-up care. At a minimum the patient and significant other must be taught about the drugs and when to seek medical attention.

The goals of rehabilitation for long-term survivors of childhood and adult leukemia are to manage the physical, psychologic, social, and spiritual consequences and delayed effects from the disease and its treatment. Assistance may be needed to reestablish the various relationships that are a part of the patient's life. Friends and family may not know how to interact with the patient. The patient and family must learn to regain attitudes of health and life while facing the real fear of relapse of disease. Involving the patient in survivor networks, support groups, or services such as CanSurmount and Make Today Count may help the patient adapt to living after a life-threatening illness. Exploring resources in the community (e.g., American Cancer Society, Leukemia Society, Meals-on-Wheels, wheelchair taxis) may reduce the financial burden and the feelings of dependence. Spiritual support may give the patient inner strength and peace.

It is expected that the patient will need support in adapting to any physical limitations or changes imposed by the illness. Vigilant follow-up care by providers who are aware of the unique needs of a cancer survivor is of the utmost importance for early recognition and treatment of long-term or delayed physical, psychologic, and social effects. The nurse may involve other health care providers in meeting the patient's needs. However, often these needs will require the initiation of a referral or consultation. For example, physical therapy personnel may be asked to develop an exercise program to prevent posttreatment deficits caused by drug-induced peripheral neuropathy. These needs can also include other concerns such as growth and development concerns for childhood survivors, vocational retraining, and reproductive concerns for a patient of childbearing age.[26] The long-term recovery following treatment for leukemia affects the quality of the patient's life.

LYMPHOMAS

Lymphomas are malignant neoplasms originating in the bone marrow and lymphatic structures resulting in the proliferation of lymphocytes. The cause for the currently rising incidence is not entirely understood, although AIDS-related lymphoma is certainly a factor. Lymphomas are the fifth most common type of cancer in the United States.[18] Two major types of lymphoma—Hodgkin's disease and non-Hodgkin's lymphoma (NHL)—are discussed in this chapter. A comparison of these two types of lymphoma is presented in Table 28-30.

Hodgkin's Disease

Hodgkin's disease, which makes up 15% of all lymphomas, is a malignant condition characterized by proliferation of abnormal giant, multinucleated cells, called *Reed-Sternberg cells,* which are located in lymph nodes. Although it was the first of the diseases known as lymphomas to be identified by Thomas Hodgkin in 1832, the actual origin of the malignant Reed-Sternberg cell remains elusive. The disease has a bimodal age-specific incidence, occurring most frequently in persons from 15 to 35 years of age and above 50 years of age. In adults, it is twice as prevalent in men as in women.

Etiology. Although the cause of Hodgkin's disease remains unknown, several key factors are thought to play a role in its development. The main interacting factors include infection with Epstein Barr virus (EBV), genetic predispositions, and exposures to occupational toxins.

Normally, the lymph nodes are composed of connective tissues that surround a fine mesh of reticular fibers and cells. In Hodgkin's disease the normal structure of lymph nodes is destroyed by hyperplasia of monocytes and macrophages. The main diagnostic feature of Hodgkin's disease is the presence of Reed-Sternberg cells in lymph node biopsy specimens. The disease is believed to arise in a single location (it originates in lymph nodes in 90% of patients) and then spreads along adjacent lymphatics. It eventually infiltrates other organs, especially the lungs, spleen, and liver. In approximately two thirds of patients the cervical lymph nodes are the first to be affected. When the disease begins above the diaphragm, it remains confined to lymph nodes for a variable period of time. Disease originating below the diaphragm frequently spreads to extralymphoid sites such as the liver.

Table 28-30 Comparison of Hodgkin's Disease and Non-Hodgkin's Lymphoma

	Hodgkin's	Non-Hodgkin's
Cellular origin	Unknown	B lymphocytes (90%) T lymphocytes (10%)
Spread at presentation	Localized to regional	Disseminated
B symptoms	Common	Uncommon
Histopathologic classification	Singular	Many different classifications (see Table 28-33)
Curability	>75%	30-40%

Clinical Manifestations. The onset of symptoms in Hodgkin's disease is usually insidious. The initial development is most often enlargement of cervical, axillary, or inguinal lymph nodes. This lymphadenopathy affects discrete nodes that remain movable and nontender. The enlarged nodes are not painful unless pressure is exerted on adjacent nerves.

The patient may notice weight loss, fatigue, weakness, fever, chills, tachycardia, or night sweats. A group of initial findings including fever, night sweats, and weight loss (referred to as *B symptoms*) correlate with a worse prognosis. After the ingestion of even small amounts of alcohol, individuals with Hodgkin's disease may complain of a rapid onset of pain at the site of disease. The cause for the alcohol-induced pain is unknown. Generalized pruritus without skin lesions may develop. Cough, dyspnea, stridor, and dysphagia may all reflect mediastinal node involvement.

In more advanced disease there is hepatomegaly and splenomegaly. Anemia results from increased destruction and decreased production of erythrocytes. Other physical signs vary depending on where the disease has spread. For example, intrathoracic involvement may lead to superior vena cava syndrome, enlarged retroperitoneal nodes may cause palpable abdominal masses or interfere with renal function, jaundice may occur from liver involvement, and spinal cord compression leading to paraplegia may occur with extradural involvement. Bone pain occurs as a result of osteoblastic bone lesions.

Diagnostic and Staging Studies. Peripheral blood analysis, lymph node biopsy, bone marrow examination, and radiologic evaluation are important means of evaluating Hodgkin's disease. Peripheral blood analysis often reveals a microcytic hypochromic anemia, neutrophilic leukocytosis (15,000 to 28,000/μl [15 to 28 $\times$ 10^9/L]), which may be associated with lymphopenia, and an increased platelet count. Leukopenia and thrombocytopenia may develop, but they are usually a consequence of treatment, advanced disease, or superimposed hypersplenism. Other blood studies may show hypoferremia caused by excessive iron uptake by the liver and spleen, elevated leukocyte alkaline phosphatase from liver and bone involvement, hypercalcemia from bone involvement, and hypoalbuminemia.

Excisional lymph node biopsy offers a definitive means of diagnosis. If removed, an enlarged peripheral lymph node can be examined histologically for the presence of the diagnostic Reed-Sternberg cells.

Bone marrow biopsy is performed as an important aspect of staging. In Hodgkin's disease there may be indications of granulocytic and megakaryocytic hyperplasia, but these findings are not unique to Hodgkin's disease. Reed-Sternberg cells may also be found in the bone marrow of patients with advanced disease.

Radiologic evaluation can help to define all sites of the disease. Chest x-rays, radioisotope studies, and computed tomography (CT) scans may show mediastinal lymphadenopathy, renal displacement caused by retroperitoneal node enlargement, abdominal lymph node enlargement, and liver, spleen, bone, and brain infiltration. Some clinicians also use lymphangiography, a radiographic dye study that uses blue dye injected into the lymphatic system to assess the lymph nodes and lymph vessels. This test can also visualize the sometimes difficult to see retroperitoneal structures.

Diagnostic studies are conducted to assess the stage of Hodgkin's disease. However, there also is a need to demonstrate the actual extent of disease involvement. In the past, a surgical procedure (called a *staging* laparotomy including splenectomy) was performed to visualize the actual extent of disease involvement. Technologic advances such as CT scanning have augmented the array of techniques available for noninvasive evaluation. Although controversial, many institutions continue to use surgical staging to ensure accurate identification of all sites of disease involvement.

Therapeutic and Pharmacologic Management. Using all of the information from the various tests, a stage of disease is determined (Fig. 28-14). Treatment decisions are made based on the stage of disease. Staging involves determining the extent and involvement of the disease. This is important because Hodgkin's disease may be localized or diffuse. Treatment depends on the nature of the disease. The nomenclature used in staging involves an A or B classification, depending on whether symptoms are present when the disease is found, and a Roman numeral (I to IV) that reflects the location and extent of the disease.

Once the stage of Hodgkin's disease is established, therapeutic management focuses on selecting a treatment plan (Table 28-31). Treatment for Hodgkin's disease has improved considerably and is aimed at cure. The least amount of treatment is used to achieve cure yet minimize the short-term and long-term complications. Radiation therapy given to affected areas over 4 to 6 weeks can cure 95% of patients with stage I or stage II disease. Combination chemotherapy is used in some early stages in patients believed to have resistant disease or at high risk for relapse. Stage IIIA disease is treated with both radiotherapy and chemotherapy. The role of radiation as a supplement to chemotherapy in stages III and IV varies depending on sites of disease. Advances in treatment now enable some stage IIIB and stage IV diseases to be cured with high-dose chemotherapy and bone marrow or peripheral stem cell transplantation.

Intensive chemotherapy with or without the use of bone marrow transplantation and hematopoeitic growth factors is the treatment of choice for advanced Hodgkin's disease (stages IIIB and IV). Combination chemotherapy works well because, as in leukemia, drugs are used that have an additive antitumor effect without increasing side effects. As with leukemia, therapy must be aggressive; therefore potentially life-threatening problems are encountered in an attempt to achieve a remission.[28]

Two chemotherapy regimens called *MOPP* and *ABVD* have been used alone and in combination to induce remissions in 80% of patients. The acronyms are described in Table 28-32. About 60% to 70% of these patients will be cured.

Maintenance chemotherapy does not contribute to increased survival once a complete remission is achieved. Occasionally, single drugs may be administered palliatively to patients who cannot tolerate intensive combination therapy. A serious consequence of the treatment for Hodgkin's disease is the later development of secondary malignancies (see Chapter 12).

NURSING MANAGEMENT

HODGKIN'S DISEASE

The nursing care for Hodgkin's disease is largely based on managing pancytopenia and other side effects of therapy. Because the survival of patients with Hodgkin's disease

Table 28-31 Guidelines for Treatment of Hodgkin's Disease

Stage	Recommended Therapy
I, II (A or B)	Radiation
I, II (A or B, with mediastinal mass >⅓ diameter of the chest)	Combination chemotherapy followed by radiation to involved field
$IIIA_1$ (minimal abdominal disease)	Radiation
$IIIA_2$ (extensive abdominal disease)	Combination chemotherapy with radiation to involved sites
IIIB	Combination chemotherapy
IV (A or B)	Combination chemotherapy

Table 28-32 Two Chemotherapeutic Regimens for Hodgkin's Disease

Drug	Schedule
MOPP	
Nitrogen **M**ustard	Days 1 and 8
Vincristine (**O**ncovin)	Days 1 and 8
Procarbazine	Days 1-14
Prednisone (cycles 1 and 4 only)	Days 1-14
ABVD	
Doxorubicin (**A**driamycin)	Days 1 and 15
Bleomycin	Days 1 and 15
Vinblastine	Days 1 and 15
Dacarbazine (DTIC)	Days 1 and 15

Repeat cycle every 28 days for a minimum of six cycles. Complete remission must be documented before discontinuing therapy. Therapy may continue for two cycles after remission.

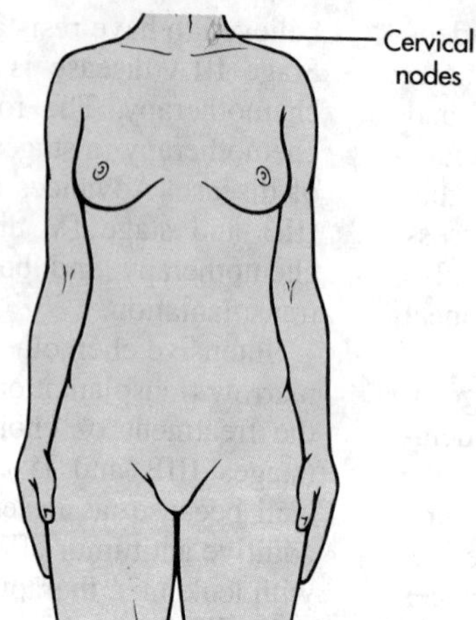

Stage I
Involvement of a single lymph node or a single extranodal site

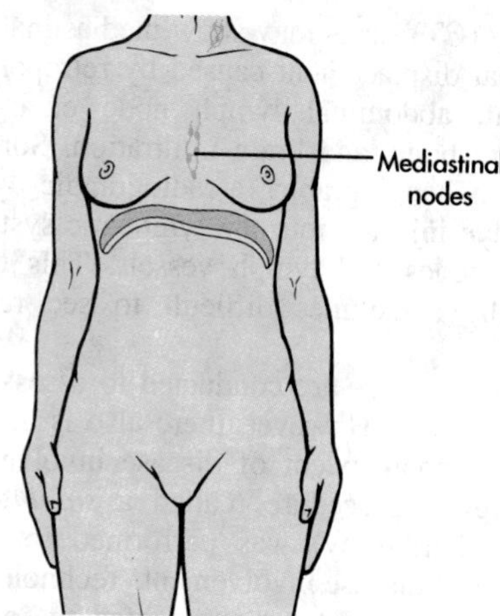

Stage II
Involvement of two or more lymph node regions on the same side of the diaphragm or localized involvement of an extranodal site and one or more lymph node regions of the same side of diaphragm

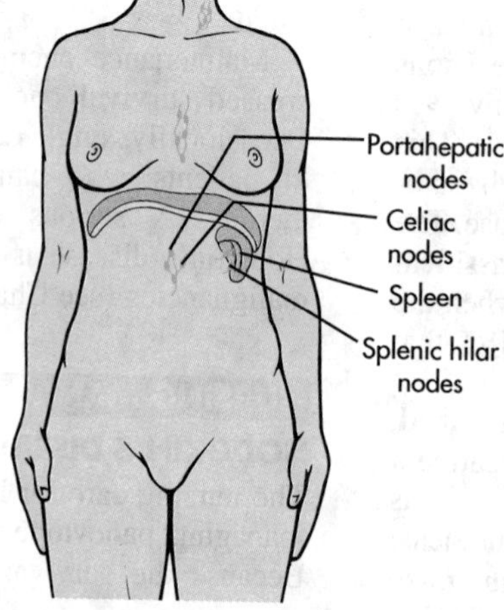

Stage III
Involvement of lymph node regions on both sides of the diaphragm. May include a single extranodal site, the spleen or both; now subdivided into lymphatic involvement of the upper abdomen in the spleen (splenic, celiac, and portal nodes) (*Stage* III_1) and the lower abdominal nodes in the periaortic, mesenteric, and iliac regions (*Stage* III_2)

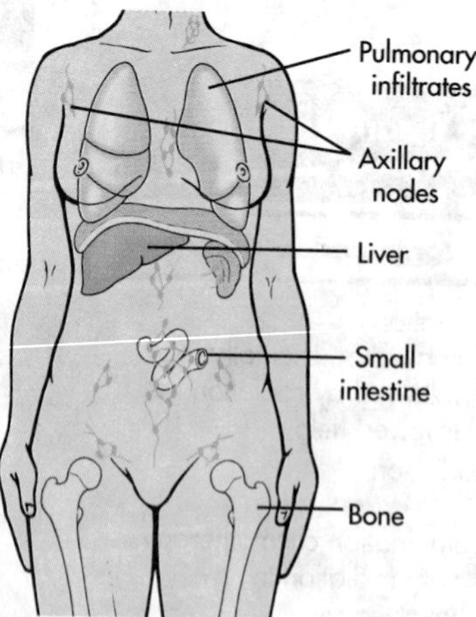

Stage IV
Diffuse or disseminated disease of one or more extralymphatic organs or tissues with or without associated lymph node involvement; the extranodal site is identified as *H*, hepatic; *L*, lung; *P*, pleura; *M*, marrow; *D*, dermal; *O*, osseous

Fig. 28-14 Staging system for Hodgkin's disease and non-Hodgkin's lymphoma.

depends on their response to treatment, supporting the patient through the immunosuppressive state is extremely important.

The patient undergoing radiotherapy will need special nursing consideration. The skin in the radiation field requires special attention. Also, the nurse must understand the concepts related to administration of radiotherapy (see Chapter 12).

Psychosocial considerations are just as important as they are with leukemia. Although the prognosis for Hodgkin's disease is better than that for many forms of cancer or leukemia, patients must still be helped to deal with all of the physical, psychologic, social, and spiritual consquences of their disease. Evaluation of patients for long-term effects of therapy are important because delayed consequences of disease and treatment may not be apparent for many years.[29] (Secondary malignancies and delayed effects are discussed in Chapter 12.)

Non-Hodgkin's Lymphoma

Non-Hodgkin's lymphomas (NHL) are a heterogeneous group of malignant neoplasms of the immune system affecting all ages. They are classified according to different cellular and lymph node characteristics (Table 28-33). As more information about the cell types is discovered, evolving schemas have been used to describe different subtypes. A variety of clinical presentations and courses are recognized, from indolent to rapidly progressive disease. Common names for different types of NHL include *Burkitt's lymphoma, reticulum cell sarcoma,* and *lymphosarcoma.* There is no hallmark feature in NHLs that parallels the Reed-Sternberg cell of Hodgkin's disease. However, all NHLs involve lymphocytes arrested in various stages of development.[30]

NHLs can originate outside the lymph nodes, the method of spread can be unpredictable, and the majority of patients have widely disseminated disease at the time of diagnosis. The primary clinical manifestation is painless lymph node enlargement. Because the disease is usually disseminated when it is diagnosed, other symptoms will be present depending on where the disease has spread (e.g., hepatomegaly with liver involvement).

Patients with high-grade lymphomas may have lymphadenopathy and constitutional ("B") symptoms such as fever, night sweats, and weight loss. The peripheral blood is usually normal, but some lymphomas may occur in a "leukemic" phase.

Diagnostic studies used for NHL resemble those used for Hodgkin's disease. Lymph node biopsy establishes the cell type and pattern. Staging, as described for Hodgkin's disease, is used to guide therapy (Fig. 28-14). The prognosis for NHL is generally not as good as that for Hodgkin's disease.

Treatment for NHL involves radiotherapy and chemotherapy (Table 28-34). Ironically, more aggressive lymphomas are more responsive to treatment and more likely to be cured. In contrast, indolent lymphomas have a naturally long course but are difficult to effectively treat. Radiotherapy alone may be effective for treatment of stage I disease, but combination radiation therapy and chemotherapy are used for other stages. Initial chemotherapy uses alkylating agents such as cyclophosphamide and chlorambucil. However, numerous combinations have been used to try to overcome the resistant nature of this disease. The most common chemotherapeutic regimen is CHOP (cyclophosphamide, doxorubicin [Adriamycin], vincristine [Oncovin], prednisone). Other combination therapies include cyclophosphamide, vincristine, prednisone (CVP) and cyclophosphamide, vincristine [Oncovin], procarbazine, and prednisone (COPP). Furthermore, high-dose therapy with

Table 28-33 Classification of Non-Hodgkin's Lymphomas

Low Grade
- Small lymphocytic
- Follicular, small cleaved cell
- Follicular, mixed small cleaved and large cell

Intermediate Grade
- Follicular, large cell
- Diffuse, small cleaved cell
- Diffuse, mixed; small and large
- Diffuse, large cell

High Grade
- Large cell, immunoblastic
- Lymphoblastic
- Small noncleaved cell

Table 28-34 Guidelines for Treatment of Non-Hodgkin's Lymphoma

	Recommended Therapy	
Grade	**Stage I, II_1***	**Stages II_2,† III, IV**
Low	Localized irradiation	Observation until disease progression, then palliative irradiation or single-agent or combination chemotherapy
Intermediate	Combination chemotherapy with localized radiation	Combination chemotherapy
High	Combination chemotherapy (high dose) with localized radiation	Combination chemotherapy (high dose)

*Stage II_1 = nonbulky disease.
†Stage II_2 = bulky disease >10 cm or ⅓ diameter of chest.

peripheral blood stem cell or bone marrow transplantation is also commonly employed. Biologic response modifiers (BRMs), such as α-interferon, interleukin-2, and tumor necrosis factor, are also being investigated for treatment of NHL. (BRMs are discussed in Chapter 12.)

MALIGNANCIES OF PLASMA CELLS

Multiple Myeloma

Multiple myeloma, or plasma cell myeloma, is a condition in which neoplastic plasma cells infiltrate the bone marrow and destroy bone. A patient usually lives for approximately 2 years after diagnosis if untreated. The incidence of multiple myeloma is approximately 2 to 3 per 100,000 people, which is similar to that of Hodgkin's disease or chronic lymphocytic leukemia. The disease is twice as common in men as in women and usually develops after 40 years of age, with a peak incidence around 55 years of age.

Pathophysiology. There are many hypotheses regarding the etiology of multiple myeloma (e.g., chronic inflammation, chronic hypersensitivity reactions, viral influences), but no actual cause has been identified. The disease process involves excessive production of plasma cells. Plasma cells are activated B cells, which produce immunoglobulins that normally serve to protect the body (see Chapter 10). However, in multiple myeloma the malignant plasma cells infiltrate the bone marrow and produce abnormal and excessive amounts of immunogloblulin (usually IgG, IgA, IgD, or IgE). This abnormal immunoglobulin is known as a *myeloma protein.* Furthermore, plasma cell production of excessive and abnormal amounts of cytokines (IL-4, IL-5, IL-6) also plays an important role in the pathologic process of bone destruction. As myeloma protein increases, normal plasma cells are reduced, which further compromises the body's normal immune response. Ultimately, the plasma cells destroy bone and invade the lymph nodes, liver, spleen, and kidneys.

Clinical Manifestations. Multiple myeloma develops slowly and insidiously. The patient often does not manifest symptoms until the disease is advanced, at which time skeletal pain is the major manifestation. Pain in the pelvis, spine, and ribs is particularly common. Diffuse osteoporosis develops as the myeloma protein destroys more bone. Osteolytic lesions are seen in the skull, vertebrae, and ribs. Vertebral destruction can lead to collapse of vertebrae with ensuing compression of the spinal cord, requiring emergency measures to prevent paraplegia (e.g., radiation, surgery, chemotherapy). Loss of bone integrity can lead to the development of pathologic fractures. Bony degeneration also causes calcium to be lost from bones, eventually causing hypercalcemia.

Hypercalcemia may cause renal, GI, or neurologic changes such as polyuria, anorexia, and confusion. In addition, cell destruction contributes to the development of hyperuricemia, which, along with the high protein levels caused by the presence of the myeloma protein, can result in renal failure from renal tubular obstruction and interstitial nephritis from the uric acid precipitates. The patient may display symptoms of anemia, thrombocytopenia, and granulocytopenia, all of which are related to the replacement of normal bone marrow elements with plasma cells.

Diagnostic Studies. Evaluating multiple myeloma involves laboratory, radiologic, and bone marrow examination. High serum protein may be present as evidenced by an "M" spike on serum electrophoresis. Pancytopenia, hyperuricemia, hypercalcemia, and elevated creatinine may also be found. In addition, an abnormal globulin known as *Bence Jones protein* is found in the urine of a patient with multiple myeloma.

Radiologic studies, including bone scans, are done to establish the degree of bone involvement. The studies document the presence of diffuse bony lesions, demineralization, and osteoporosis in affected areas of the skeleton.

Bone marrow analysis shows significantly increased numbers of plasma cells in the bone marrow. Other components of the marrow, particularly megakaryocytes, may be normal.

Therapeutic Management. The therapeutic approach involves managing both the disease and its symptoms because with treatment the chronic phase of multiple myeloma may last for more than 10 years. Ambulation and adequate hydration are used to treat hypercalcemia, hyperuricemia, and dehydration. Weight bearing helps the bones reabsorb some calcium, and fluids dilute calcium and prevent protein precipitates from causing renal tubular obstruction. Control of pain is another goal of therapeutic management. Analgesics, orthopedic supports, and localized radiation help to reduce the skeletal pain.

Chemotherapy is used to reduce the number of plasma cells. The agents most frequently used are the alkylating drugs, including melphalan (Alkeran), cyclophosphamide (Cytoxan), chlorambucil (Leukeran), and carmustine (BCNU). Corticosteroids may be added because they exert an antitumor effect in some patients. The VAD regimen (vincristine, doxorubicin [Adriamycin], and dexamethasone) can be used for patients who do not respond to alkylating agents. Radiotherapy is another important component of treatment, primarily because of its palliative effect on localized lesions. Bone marrow transplantation is being investigated in the treatment of multiple myeloma.

Drugs may be used to treat complications of multiple myeloma. For example, allopurinol (Zyloprim) may be given to reduce hyperuricemia, and IV furosemide promotes renal excretion of calcium. Calcitonin and pamidronate (Aredia) may be used to treat moderate to severe hypercalcemia.

NURSING MANAGEMENT

MULTIPLE MYELOMA

The focus of care for the neuromuscular system has to do with the bony involvement and sequelae from bone breakdown. Maintaining adequate hydration is a primary nursing consideration to minimize problems from hypercalcemia. Fluids are administered to attain a urinary output of 1.5 to 2 L per day. This may require an intake of 3 to 4 L. In addition, weight bearing helps bones to reabsorb some of the calcium, and corticosteroids may augment the excretion of calcium. Once chemotherapy is initiated, the uric acid levels rise because of the increased cell destruction. Hyperuricemia must be resolved by ensuring adequate hydration and using allopurinol.

Because of the potential for pathologic fractures, the nurse must be careful when moving and ambulating the patient. A slight twist or strain in the wrong area (e.g., a weak area in the patient's bones) may be sufficient to cause a fracture.

Pain management requires innovative and knowledgeable nursing interventions. If radiotherapy is used to diminish pain from localized myeloma lesions, appropriate skin care techniques must be used. Mild analgesics, such as NSAIDs, acetaminophen, or acetaminophen with codeine, may be more effective than potent analgesics in diminishing bone pain. Braces, especially for the spine, may also help control pain. As in any pain management situation, the nurse is responsible for assessing the patient and for implementing necessary nursing measures to reduce and hopefully alleviate the pain (see Chapter 6).

The patient's psychosocial needs require sensitive, skilled management. As with leukemia, it is important to help the patient and significant others adapt to changes fostered by chronic sickness, to deal with reality rather than create fantasies, and to adjust to the losses related to the disease process. The symptoms of multiple myeloma remit and exacerbate. Consequently acute care is needed at various times during the course of the illness. The final, acute phase is unresponsive to treatment and usually short in duration. The way in which patients and families deal with confronting death may be affected by the manner in which they learned to accept and live with the chronic nature of the disease.

DISORDERS OF THE SPLEEN

The spleen performs many functions (see Chapter 27) and is affected by many illnesses. There are many different causes of splenomegaly (Table 28-35). The term *hypersplenism* refers to the occurrence of splenomegaly and peripheral cytopenias (anemia, leukopenia, thrombocytopenia). The degree of splenic enlargement varies with the disease. For example, massive splenic enlargement occurs with chronic myelocytic leukemia, hairy cell leukemia, and thalassemia major. Mild splenic enlargement occurs with congestive heart failure and systemic lupus erythematosus.

When the spleen enlarges, its normal filtering and sequestering capacity increases. Consequently there is often a reduction in the number of circulating blood cells. A slight to moderate enlargement of the spleen is usually asymptomatic and found during a routine examination of the abdomen. Even massive splenomegaly can be well tolerated, but the patient may complain of abdominal discomfort and early satiety. Other techniques to assess the size of the spleen include ^{99}Tc-colloid liver-spleen scan, CT scan, and ultrasound scan.

Occasionally laparotomy and splenectomy are indicated in the evaluation or treatment of splenomegaly. Splenectomy can have a dramatic effect in increasing peripheral RBC, WBC, and platelet counts. Another major indication for splenectomy is splenic rupture. The spleen may rupture from trauma, inadvertent tearing during other surgical procedures, and diseases such as mononucleosis.

Table 28-35 Causes of Splenomegaly

- Hereditary hemolytic anemias
  - Sickle cell disease
  - Thalassemia
- Autoimmune cytopenias
  - Acquired hemolytic anemia
  - Immune thrombocytopenia
- Infections and inflammations
  - Bacterial endocarditis
  - Infectious mononucleosis
  - Systemic lupus erythematosus
  - Sarcoidosis
  - Human immunodeficiency virus infection
  - Viral hepatitis
- Infiltrative diseases
  - Acute and chronic leukemia
  - Lymphomas
  - Polycythemia vera
- Congestion
  - Cirrhosis of the liver
  - Congestive heart failure

Nursing responsibilities for the patient with spleen disorders vary depending on the nature of the problem. Splenomegaly may be painful and may require analgesic administration; care in moving, turning, and positioning; and evaluation of lung expansion because spleen enlargement may impair diaphragmatic excursion. If anemia, thrombocytopenia, or leukopenia develops from splenic enlargement, nursing measures must be instituted to support the patient and prevent life-threatening complications. If splenectomy is performed, the nurse must provide the meticulous care warranted after any surgery. In addition, there must be special observation for hemorrhage, which could lead to shock, fever, and abdominal distention.

After splenectomy, immunologic deficiencies may develop. IgM levels are reduced, and IgG and IgA values remain within normal limits. Postsplenectomy patients are especially vulnerable to infection. A younger patient is at significantly greater risk than an older patient, but the risk is present for all ages. This patient is highly susceptible to infection from encapsulated organisms such as pneumococcus. This complication is prevented by immunization with polyvalent pneumococcal vaccine (e.g., Pneumovax).

BLOOD COMPONENT THERAPY

Blood component therapy is frequently used in managing hematologic diseases. Many therapeutic and surgical procedures depend on blood product support. However, blood component therapy only temporarily supports the patient until the underlying problem is resolved. Because transfusions are not free from hazards, they should be used only if necessary. Nurses must be careful to avoid developing a complacent attitude about this common but potentially dangerous therapy.

Traditionally, the term *blood transfusion* meant the administration of whole blood. Blood transfusion now has a broader meaning because of the ability to administer specific components of blood such as platelets, RBCs, or plasma (Table 28-36).

Table 28-36 Blood Products*

Description	Special Considerations	Indications for Use
Packed RBC		
Packed RBCs are prepared from whole blood by sedimentation or centrifugation. One unit contains 250-350 ml.	Use of RBCs for treatment allows remaining components of blood (e.g., platelets, albumin, plasma) to be used for other purposes. There is less danger of fluid overload. Packed RBCs are preferred RBC source because they are more component specific.	Severe or symptomatic anemia, acute blood loss.
Frozen RBC		
Frozen RBCs are prepared from RBCs using glycerol for protection and frozen. They can be stored for 3 yr at −188.6° F (−87° C).	They must be used within 24 hr of thawing. Successive washings with saline solution remove majority of WBCs and plasma proteins.	Autotransfusion, patient with previous febrile reactions to transfusions. Infrequently used because filters remove most WBCs.
Platelets		
Platelets are prepared from fresh whole blood within 4 hr after collection. One unit contains 30-60 ml of platelet concentrate.	Multiple units of platelets can be obtained from one donor by plateletpheresis. They can be kept at room temperature for 1-5 days depending on type of collection and storage bag used. Bag should be agitated periodically. Expected increase is 10,000/μl/U. Failure to have a rise may be due to fever, sepsis, splenomegaly, or DIC.	Bleeding caused by thrombocytopenia, platelet levels <10,000-20,000/μl (10-20×10^9/L)
Fresh-Frozen Plasma		
Liquid portion of whole blood is separated from cells and frozen. One unit contains 200-250 ml. Plasma is rich in clotting factors but contains no platelets. It may be stored for 1 yr. It must be used within 2 hr after thawing.	Use of plasma in treating hypovolemic shock is being replaced by pure preparations such as albumin plasma expanders.	Bleeding caused by deficiency in clotting factors (e.g., DIC, hemorrhage, massive transfusion)
Albumin		
Albumin is prepared from plasma. It can be stored for 5 yr. It is available in 5% or 25% solution.	Albumin 25 g/100 ml is osmotically equal to 500 ml of plasma. Hyperosmolar solution acts by moving water from extravascular to intravascular space.	Hypovolemic shock, hypoalbuminemia
Cryoprecipitates and Commercial Concentrates		
Cryoprecipitate is prepared from fresh frozen plasma, with 10-20 ml/bag. It can be stored for 1 yr. Once thawed, must be used.	See Table 28-20.	Replacement of clotting factors, especially factor VIII and fibrinogen.

DIC, Disseminated intravascular coagulation; *Hct*, hematocrit; *RBCs*, red blood cells; *WBCs*, white blood cells.
*Component therapy has replaced the use of whole blood, which accounts for less than 10% of all transfusions.

Administration Procedure

Blood components can be administered safely through a 19- or larger gauge needle into a free-flowing IV line. Larger size needles (e.g., 19 gauge) may be preferred if rapid transfusions are given. Smaller-size needles can be used for platelets, albumin, and cryoprecipitates. The blood administration tubing with a filter should have a stopcock or other means to develop a closed system, with blood open to one port and isotonic saline solution infusing through the other. Dextrose solutions or lactated Ringer's should not be used because they induce RBC hemolysis. No other additives (including medications) should be given via the same tubing as the blood unless the tubing is cleared with saline solution.

When the blood or blood components have been obtained from the blood bank, positive identification of the donor blood and recipient must be made. Improper product-to-patient identification causes 90% of transfusion reactions, thus placing a great responsibility on nursing personnel to carry out the identification procedure appropriately. The nurse should follow the policy and procedures at the place of employment. The blood bank is responsible for typing and crossmatching the donor's blood with the recipient's blood.

The blood should be administered as soon as it is brought to the patient. It should not be refrigerated on the nursing unit. If the blood is not used right away, it should be returned to the blood bank.

During the first 15 minutes of blood infusion, the nurse should stay with the patient. If there are any untoward reactions, they are most likely to occur at this time. The rate of infusion during this period should be no more than 2 ml/min. Blood should not be infused quickly unless an emergency exists. Rapid infusion of cold blood may cause the patient to become chilled. If rapid replacement of large amounts of blood is necessary, a blood-warming device should be used.

After the first 15 minutes, the rate of infusion is governed by the clinical condition of the patient and the product being infused. Most patients not in danger of fluid overload can tolerate the infusion of one unit of packed cells over 2 hours. The transfusion should not take more than 4 hours to administer. Blood remaining after 4 hours should not be infused because of the length of time it has been removed from refrigeration.

Blood Transfusion Reactions

If a transfusion reaction occurs, the following steps should be taken: (1) stop the transfusion; (2) maintain a patent IV line with saline solution; (3) notify the blood bank and the physician immediately; (4) recheck identifying tags and numbers; (5) monitor vital signs and urine output; (6) treat symptoms per physician order; (7) save the blood bag and tubing and send them to the blood bank for examination; (8) complete transfusion reaction reports; (9) collect required blood and urine specimens at intervals stipulated by hospital policy to evaluate for hemolysis; and (10) document on transfusion reaction form and patient chart. The blood bank and laboratory are responsible for identifying the type of reaction.

The complications of transfusion therapy may be significant and necessitate judicious evaluation of the patient. Blood transfusion reactions can be classified as acute or delayed (Tables 28-37 and 28-38).

Acute Reactions

Acute hemolytic reactions. The most common cause of hemolytic reactions is transfusion of ABO-incompatible blood (see Table 27-8). This is an example of a type II cytotoxic hypersensitivity reaction (see Chapter 10). Severe hemolytic reactions are rare. Most mistakes are caused by mislabeling specimens and administering blood to the wrong individual.

When an acute hemolytic reaction occurs, antibodies in the recipient's serum react with antigens on the donor's RBCs. This results in agglutination of cells, which can obstruct capillaries and block blood flow. Hemolysis of the RBCs releases free hemoglobin into the plasma. The hemoglobin is filtered by the kidney and may be found in the urine (hemoglobinuria). Hemoglobin may obstruct the renal tubules, leading to acute renal failure (see Chapter 44).

The clinical manifestations of an acute hemolytic reaction may be mild or severe and usually develop within the first 15 minutes of transfusion. Free hemoglobin in blood and urine specimens obtained at the onset of the reaction will provide evidence of an acute hemolytic reaction. Delayed transfusion reactions may occur 2 to 14 days after the administration of blood. (The clinical manifestations and nursing management for the patient with a hemolytic reaction are presented in Table 28-37.)

Febrile reactions. Febrile reactions are most commonly caused by leukocyte incompatibility. Many individuals who receive five or more transfusions develop circulating antibodies to WBCs. Febrile reactions can often be prevented by using filters to leukocyte deplete RBCs and platelets. Leukocyte-poor blood products (filtered, washed, or frozen) can also be used to prevent febrile reactions.

Mild allergic reactions. Allergic reactions result from the recipient's sensitivity to plasma proteins of the donor's blood. These reactions are more common in an individual with a history of allergies. Antihistamines may be used to prevent allergic reactions. Epinephrine or corticosteroids may be used to treat a severe reaction.

Circulatory overload. An individual with cardiac or renal insufficiency is at risk for developing circulatory overload. This is especially true if a large quantity of blood is infused in a short period of time. When blood is needed, it should be infused as slowly as possible, and the patient can be monitored with central venous pressure readings. Central venous pressure readings above 15 cm H_2O usually indicate circulatory overload. If a pulmonary artery catheter is in place, pulmonary capillary wedge pressure readings above 18 mm Hg indicate elevated left atrial pressure and impending heart failure.

Sepsis. Blood products can become infected from improper handling and storage. Bacterial contamination of blood products can result in bacteremia, sepsis, or septic shock. However, with careful handling, bacterial contamination and growth rarely occur.

Massive blood transfusion reaction. An acute complication of transfusing large volumes of blood products is

Table 28-37 Acute Transfusion Reactions

Reaction	Cause	Clinical Manifestations	Management	Prevention
Acute hemolytic	Infusion of ABO-incompatible whole blood, RBCs or components containing 10 ml or more of RBCs. Antibodies in the recipient's plasma attach to antigens on transfused red blood cells causing RBC destruction.	Chills, fever, low back pain, flushing, tachycardia, tachypnea, hypotension, vascular collapse, hemoglobinuria, acute jaundice, dark urine, bleeding, acute renal failure, shock, cardiac arrest, death	Treat shock if present. Draw blood samples for serologic testing slowly to avoid hemolysis from the procedure. Send urine specimen to the laboratory. Maintain BP with IV colloid solutions. Give diuretics as prescribed to maintain urine flow. Insert indwelling urinary catheter or measure voided amounts to monitor hourly urine output. Dialysis may be required if renal failure occurs. Do not transfuse additional RBC-containing components until blood bank has provided newly crossmatched units.	Meticulously verify and document patient identification from sample collection to component infusion.
Febrile, nonhemolytic (most common)	Sensitization to donor WBCs, platelets, or plasma proteins.	Sudden chills and fever (rise in temperature of $>1°$ C), headache, flushing, anxiety, muscle pain.	Give antipyretics as prescribed—avoid aspirin in thrombocytopenic patients. *Do not restart transfusion* unless physican orders	Consider leukocyte-poor blood products (filtered, washed, or frozen).
Mild allergic	Sensitivity to foreign plasma proteins.	Flushing, itching, urticaria (hives).	Give antihistamine as directed. If symptoms are mild and transient, transfusion may be restarted slowly. Do not restart transfusion if fever or pulmonary symptoms develop.	Treat prophylactically with antihistamines.
Anaphylactic and severe allergic	Sensitivity to donor plasma proteins. Infusion of IgA proteins to IgA-deficient recipient who has developed IgA antibody.	Anxiety, urticaria, wheezing, progressing to cyanosis, shock, and possible cardiac arrest	Initiate CPR, if indicated. Have epinephrine ready for injection (0.4 ml of a 1:1000 solution SC or 0.1 ml of 1:1000 solution diluted to 10 ml with saline for IV use). *Do not restart transfusion.*	Transfuse extensively washed RBC products, from which all plasma has been removed. Use blood from IgA-deficient donor.
Circulatory overload	Fluid administered faster than the circulation can accommodate.	Cough, dyspnea, pulmonary congestion, headache, hypertension, tachycardia, distended neck veins.	Place patient upright with feet in dependent position. Administer prescribed diuretics, oxygen, morphine. Phlebotomy may be indicated.	Adjust transfusion volume and flow rate based on patient size and clinical status. Have blood bank divide unit into smaller aliquots for better spacing of fluid input.
Sepsis	Transfusion of bacterially infected blood components.	Rapid onset of chills, high fever, vomiting, diarrhea, marked hypotension, or shock	Obtain culture of patient's blood and send bag with remaining blood and tubing to blood bank for further study. Treat septicemia as directed—antibiotics, IV fluids, vasopressors.	Collect, process, store, and transfuse blood products according to blood banking standards and infuse within 4 hr of starting time.

Modified from Transfusion Therapy Guidelines for Nurses, National Blood Resources Education Program, US Department Health and Human Services.
BP, Blood pressure; *CPR*, cardiopulmonary resuscitation; *IV*, intravenous; *RBCs*, red blood cells; *SC*, subcutaneous; *WBCs*, white blood cells.

Table 28-38 Delayed Transfusion Reactions

Reaction	Clinical Manifestations
Delayed hemolytic	Fever, mild jaundice, decreased hematocrit. Occurs as early as 3 days or as late as several months, but usually 7-14 days posttransfusion as the result of destruction of transfused red blood cells by alloantibodies not detected during crossmatch. Generally, no acute treatment is required, but hemolysis may be severe enough to warrant further transfusions.
Hepatitis B	Elevated liver enzymes (AST and ALT), anorexia, malaise, nausea and vomiting, fever, dark urine, jaundice. Usually resolves spontaneously within 4-6 wk. Chronic carrier state can develop and can result in permanent liver damage. Treat symptomatically. (See Chapter 41.)
Hepatitis C	Similar to hepatitis B, but symptoms are usually less severe. Chronic liver disease and cirrhosis may develop. Before introduction of anti-HCV test, accounted for 90-95% of all posttransfusion hepatitis. Treat symptomatically. (See Chapter 41.)
Human immunodeficiency virus (HIV)	Can be asymptomatic for up to several years or may develop flulike symptoms within 2-4 wk. Later signs and symptoms include weight loss, diarrhea, fever, lymphadenopathy, thrush, pneumocystis pneumonia. Current estimated risk of HIV infection from a single blood transfusion ranges from 1:30,000 to 1:300,000, reflecting geographic variance. (See Chapter 11.)
Iron overload	Excess iron is deposited in the heart, liver, pancreas, and joints, causing dysfunction. Congestive heart failure, dysrhythmias, impaired thyroid and gonadal function, diabetes, arthritis, cirrhosis. Commonly occurs in patients receiving >100 units for chronic anemia over a period of time. Treat symptomatically. Deferoxamine (Desferal), which chelates and removes accumulated iron via the kidneys, may be administered IV or SC.
Graft-versus-host disease	Fever, rash, diarrhea, hepatitis. Result of replication of donor lymphocytes (graft) in the transfusion recipient (host). No effective therapy available. To prevent, irradiate blood products intended for immunocompromised patients. Some believe that irradiated blood products are indicated for first degree family members' donations also. (See Chapter 10.)
Other	Other infectious diseases and agents may be transmitted via transfusion, including cytomegalovirus, HTLV-I, and those causing malaria.

Modified from Transfusion Therapy Guidelines for Nurses, National Blood Resources Education Program, US Department Health and Human Services.
ALT, Alanine aminotransferase; *AST,* aspartate aminotransferase; *IV,* intravenous; *SC,* subcutaneous.

massive blood transfusion reaction. Massive blood transfusion reactions can occur when replacement of RBCs or blood exceeds the total blood volume within 24 hours. In this situation, an imbalance of normal blood elements can result because clotting factors, albumin, and platelets are not found in RBC transfusions.

Additional problems such as hypothermia, citrate toxicity, hypocalcemia, and hyperkalemia may occur when massive blood transfusions are given. Hypothermia with cardiac dysrhythmias can result from rapid infusion of large quantities of cold blood. Blood-warming equipment can prevent this problem. Citrate toxicity and hypocalcemia can occur from the use of large quantities of blood products, which usually have citrate as part of the storage solution; calcium binds to the citrate. Citrate toxicity is likely to develop when blood is transfused at a rate of 1 unit in 10 minutes (or 8 to 10 units of RBC within a few hours). Symptoms such as muscle tremors and ECG changes may be observed with hypocalcemia but can be prevented or reversed by the infusion of 10% calcium gluconate (10 ml with every liter of citrated blood).[31] Hyperkalemia results when potassium leaks from red cells in stored blood. Mild to severe signs and symptoms can occur, including nausea, muscle weakness, diarrhea, paresthesias, flaccid paralysis of the cardiac or respiratory muscles, and cardiac arrest. Electrolyte monitoring is an important aspect of care when massive transfusions are necessary.

Delayed Transfusion Reactions. Delayed transfusion reactions include delayed hemolytic reactions (discussed previously), infections, iron overload, and GVHD (Table 28-38).

Infection. Infectious agents transmitted by blood transfusion include hepatitis B and C viruses, HIV, human herpesvirus type 6 (HSV-6), EBV, human T-cell leukemia (HTLV-1), cytomegalovirus (CMV), and malaria. Hepatitis is the most common viral infection transmitted, although its incidence has been decreasing. Hepatitis B virus can be detected in the blood by the presence of hepatitis B surface antigen (HBsAg). It is now becoming more apparent that hepatitis non-A, non-B viruses are responsible for a large number of cases of hepatitis (see Chapter 41). A new test for hepatitis C (the most common type of non-A, non-B hepatitis) antibodies in donor blood is used to exclude the use of any donated blood testing positive for hepatitis C. Therefore the risk of transmission of hepatitis C is reduced.

In the past, HIV was transmitted by contaminated blood and blood products. This posed a serious problem for an individual who received infected transfusions. Patients with hemophilia who received antihemophiliac factors, which had been prepared from pooled plasma of a large number of donors of which some donors were infected, have a high rate of HIV infection from transfusion sources. Presently, the use of recombinant antihemophilic factors (see Table 28-19), donor education, donor screening, and

CRITICAL THINKING EXERCISES

CASE STUDY

LEUKEMIA

Patient Profile

J., a 35-year-old man, went to the emergency department because of severe bruising following a fall while hiking.

Subjective Data

- Complains of oral pain and white patches covering his tongue.
- Has had a 2-month history of fatigue, malaise, and flu symptoms.
- Has taken numerous prescribed antibiotics and increased rest and sleep in the past 2 months without relief of symptoms.

Objective Data

Physical Examination

- Has bruises and ecchymoses from fall.
- Gingiva has petechiae and patchy white spots.
- Temperature 102.2° F (39° C)
- Has splenomegaly.

Laboratory Results

- Hct 30%
- WBC 120,000/μl (120×10^9/L)
- Platelet count 25,000/μl (25×10^9/L)

Bone Marrow Biopsy

- Multiple myeloblasts (>50%)

Critical Thinking Questions

1. What components of the laboratory test results suggest acute leukemia?
2. How is acute myelogenous leukemia treated?
3. What is the prognosis for J.?
4. What are the main priorities for patient teaching with a newly diagnosed young adult with leukemia?
5. Based on the assessment data presented, write one or more nursing diagnoses. Are there any collaborative problems?

NURSING RESEARCH ISSUES

1. What nursing interventions can assist the patient to manage fatigue from anemia?
2. How effective are different types of isolation procedures in the prevention of infection in an immunocompromised patient?
3. What is the quality of life for a patient following bone marrow transplantation?
4. What is the impact on the family when one of its members is receiving chemotherapy for leukemia?
5. What are the most effective ways to train a nurse to administer blood and blood products?
6. How does hemophilia affect the lifestyle of an affected individual?

HIV-antibody testing have greatly reduced the transmission of HIV by blood transfusion or factor replacement therapy.

Autotransfusion

Autotransfusion, or autologous transfusion, consists of removing whole blood from a person and transfusing that blood into the same person. The problems of incompatibility, allergic reactions, and transmission of disease can be avoided. There are various reasons and methods of autotransfusion. These include the following:

1. *Autologous donation* or *elective phlebotomy* (*predeposit transfusion*): A person donates blood before a planned surgical procedure. The blood can be frozen and stored for up to 3 years. Usually the blood is stored without being frozen and is given to the person within a few weeks of donation. This technique is especially beneficial to the patient with a rare blood type or for any patient that might be expected to require limited blood product support during a major surgical procedure (e.g., elective joint surgery).
2. *Autotransfusion:* A newer method for replacing blood volume involves safely and aseptically collecting, filtering, and returning the patient's own blood lost during a major surgical procedure or from a traumatic injury. This system was originally developed in response to patients' concerns about the safety of blood from blood products. However, today it provides an important way to safely replace volume and stabilize bleeding patients.[32] Collection devices can be attached to drains following chest or orthopedic procedures. Sometimes the collection device is a component of the drainage system. Some systems allow blood to be automatically and continuously reinfused; others require collection for a period of time (usually no longer than 2 to 4 hours) and then are reinfused. Drainage after the first 24 hours or drainage that is suspected to contain pathogens should not be reinfused. Anticoagulants may or may not be added before reinfusion. Development of clots after blood is filtered through the collection system can sometimes prevent reinfusion of the blood. Sometimes blood that has been collected has become depleted of its normal coagulation factors; therefore monitoring coagulation studies in the patient receiving an autotransfusion is important.

REVIEW QUESTIONS

The number of the question corresponds to the same-numbered objective at the beginning of the chapter.

1. Cardiopulmonary effects in severely anemic patients include
   a. cardiomegaly and pulmonary fibrosis.
   b. cyanosis and pulmonary edema.
   c. dyspnea and tachycardia.
   d. ventricular dysrythmias and wheezing.

2. A microcytic, normochromic anemia may be caused by
   a. iron deficiency anemia.
   b. folic acid deficiency.
   c. vitamin B_{12} deficiency.
   d. sickle cell anemia.

3. Nursing intervention for a patient with the anemia of chronic disease includes
   a. teaching self-injection of erythropoietin.
   b. monitoring RBC size.
   c. dietary teaching.
   d. monitoring urine intake and output.

4. Chronic blood loss anemia mimics
   a. sickle cell anemia.
   b. anemia of chronic disease.
   c. iron deficiency anemia.
   d. megaloblastic anemia.

5. The nursing management of a patient in sickle cell crisis includes
   a. aggressive analgesic and oxygen therapy.
   b. platelet administration and monitoring of CBC.
   c. blood transfusions and iron replacement.
   d. bed rest and heparin therapy.

6. The hypervolemia and hyperviscosity of polycythemia can lead to which complication?
   a. Pulmonary edema
   b. DIC
   c. Thrombosis
   d. Cardiomyopathy

7. When providing care for a patient with thrombocytopenia, the nurse must avoid administering aspirin or aspirin-containing products because they
   a. disguise fever.
   b. destroy RBCs.
   c. increase intracranial pressure.
   d. interfere with platelet aggregration.

8. von Willebrand factor is associated with which other coagulation protein?
   a. Factor VIII
   b. Factor VII
   c. Factor VI
   d. Thrombin

9. Disseminated intravascular coagulation is
   a. a hereditary disorder that may lead to diffuse hemorrhage.
   b. an acquired disorder that may lead to diffuse hemorrhage.
   c. a hereditary disorder that may lead to localized hemorrhage.
   d. an acquired disorder that may lead to localized hemorrhage.

10. Which of the following nursing actions are appropriate when caring for a hospitalized patient with severe neutropenia and infection?
   a. Strict hand washing, antibiotic administration, frequent temperature assessment
   b. Oral care, red blood cell administration, daily electrolyte monitoring
   c. Perirectal care, platelet administration, radiation therapy
   d. Monitoring lung sounds, electrocardiogram, and invasive blood pressures

11. Myelodysplastic syndromes can be characterized as
   a. rapidly fatal disorders of hematopoiesis.
   b. indolent, serious hematopoeitic disorders that can exist for years.
   c. a syndrome caused by exposure to ionizing radiation.
   d. a blood disorder that is eventually reversible.

12. Which of the following types of leukemia is most likely characterized by the description "common but rarely fatal in older adults"?
   a. Acute lymphocytic leukemia
   b. Acute myelocytic leukemia
   c. Chronic lymphocytic leukemia
   d. Chronic granulocytic leukemia

13. Multiple drugs are used in predetermined combinations to treat leukemia and lymphoma because
   a. the chance that one drug will be effective is increased.
   b. they are more effective without having overlapping side effects.
   c. they can interrupt cell growth at multiple points in the cell cycle.
   d. there are fewer toxic effects and side effects.

14. One major differences between Hodgkin's disease and non-Hodgkin's lymphoma is
   a. Hodgkin's disease occurs only in young adults.
   b. non-Hodgkin's lymphoma is treated only with radiation therapy.
   c. Hodgkin's disease is considered curable.
   d. non-Hodgkin's lymphoma requires a staging laparotomy.

15. A patient with multiple myeloma becomes confused and lethargic. Which diagnostic finding could explain these clinical manifestations?
   a. Hypercalcemia
   b. CNS myeloma
   c. Hyperkalemia
   d. Hyperuricemia

16. Expected changes in hematologic laboratory values after a splenectomy include
   a. increased platelet count.
   b. RBC abnormalities.
   c. decreased hemoglobin.
   d. leukopenia.

17. Leukocyte reduction filters for red cells and platelets can decrease which of the following complications of transfusions?
   a. Chills and back pain
   b. Transmission of cytomegalovirus and alloimmunization
   c. Fluid overload and pulmonary edema
   d. Leukostasis and neutrophilia

REFERENCES

1. Berne RM, Levy MN: *Physiology,* ed 3, St Louis, 1993, Mosby.
2. Beard JL, Ashraf R, Smiciklas-Wright H: Iron nutrition in the elderly. In Watson RR, editor: *Handbook of nutrition in the elderly,* ed 2, Boca Raton, FL, 1994, CRC Press.
3. Lipschitz DA: Anemia. In Hazzard WR and others, editors: *Principles of geriatric medicine and gerontology,* ed 3, New York, 1994, McGraw-Hill.
4. Jandl JH: *Blood: pathophysiology,* Boston, 1991, Blackwell Scientific.
5. Nissenblatt MJ: *Managing cancer-related anemia,* NJ, 1994, Ortho Biotech (monograph).
6. Billett HH: Aplastic anemia: the role of immunosuppression, *Hosp Pract* 27:35, 1992.
7. Whedon MB: Allogeneic bone marrow transplantation: clinical indications, process, outcomes. In Whedon MB, editor: *Bone marrow transplantation: principles, practice, and nursing insights,* Boston, 1991, Jones & Bartlett.
8. Sickle Cell Disease Guideline Panel: Sickle cell disease: screening, diagnosis, management, and counseling in newborns and infants. Clinical Practice Guideline No. 6, AHCPR Pub No 93-0562, Rockville, MD, 1993, Agency for Health Care Policy and Research, Public Health Service, US Department of Health and Human Services.
9. George JN, Shattil SJ: The clinical importance of acquired abnormalities of platelet function, *N Engl J Med* 324:27, 1991.
10. Schick BP: Hope for treatment of thrombocytopenia, *N Engl J Med* 331:875, 1994.
11. Vosburgh E: Rational intervention in von Willebrand's disease, *Hosp Pract* 28:31, 1993.
12. Hoyer LW: Hemophilia A, *N Engl J Med* 330:38, 1994.
13. The National Hemophilia Foundation, Medical and Scientific Advisory Council: *Recommendations concerning HIV infection, AIDS, and hepatitis in the treatment of hemophilia,* Medical Bulletin #206, July 9, 1994, Hemophilia Information Exchange.
14. Wheeler A, Rubenstein EB: Current management of disseminated intravascular coagulation, *Oncology* 8:69, 1994.
15. Van Der Meer JWM: Defects in host defense mechanisms. In Rubin RR, Young LS, editors: *Clinical approach to infection in the compromised host,* ed 3, New York, 1994, Plenum Medical.
16. Wade JC: Epidemiology and prevention of infection in the compromised host. In Rubin RR, Young LS, editors: *Clinical approach to infection in the compromised host,* ed 3, New York, 1994, Plenum Medical.
17. Caudell KA, Whedon MB: Hematopoietic complications. In Whedon MB, editor: *Bone marrow transplantation: principles, practice, and nursing insights,* Boston, 1991, Jones & Bartlett.
18. Rowe JM, Lazarus HM: Are protected environments necessary for recipients of bone marrow transplants? In response, *Ann Intern Med* 121:76, 1994.
19. Mooney BR, Reeves SA, Larson E: Infection control and bone marrow transplantation, *Am J Infect Control* 21:131, 1993.
20. Wujcik D: Leukemia. In Groenwald SL and others, editors: *Cancer nursing principles and practice,* ed 3, Boston, 1993, Jones & Bartlett.
21. *Cancer facts and figures,* 1994, American Cancer Society.
22. Whedon MB, Elshamy M: Biology of leukemia. In Wujcik D, editor: *Nursing issues in adult acute leukemia,* New York, 1993, PRR.
23. Vose JM, Armitage JO: Bone marrow transplantation for Hodgkin's disease and lymphoma, *Annu Rev Med* 44:255, 1993.
24. Vose JM, Armitage JO, Kessinger A: High-dose chemotherapy and autologous transplant with peripheral-blood stem cells, *Oncology* 7:23, 1993.
25. Whedon MB: Autologous bone marrow transplantation: clinical indications, process, outcomes. In Whedon MB, editor: *Bone marrow transplantation: principles, practice, and nursing insights,* Boston, 1991, Jones & Bartlett.

*26. Whedon MB, Damianos F: Nursing care issues in patients undergoing autologous bone marrow transplantation, *Oncology* 7:78, 1993.

*27. Whedon MB, Ferrell BR: Quality of life in adult bone marrow transplant patients: beyond the first year, *Semin Oncol Nurs* 10:42, 1994.

28. McFadden ME: Malignant lymphomas. In Groenwald SL and others, editors: *Cancer nursing principles and practice,* ed 3, Boston, 1993, Jones & Bartlett.

*29. Yellen SB, Cella DF, Bonomi A: Quality of life in people with Hodgkin's disease, *Oncology* 7:41, 1993.

30. Longo DL and others: Lymphocytic lymphomas. In Devita VT, Hellman S, Rosenberg SA, editors: *Cancer: principles and practice of oncology,* Philadelphia, 1993, Lippincott.
31. Gloe D: Common reactions to transfusions, *Heart Lung* 20:506, 1991.
32. Gobel BH: Bleeding disorders. In Groenwald SL and others, editors: *Cancer nursing principles and practice,* ed 3, Boston, 1993, Jones & Bartlett.

SECTION VI BIBLIOGRAPHY

Books

Beutler E: *Williams hematology,* ed 5, New York, 1994, McGraw-Hill.

Handin RI, Lux SE, Stossel TP: *Blood: principles and practice of hematology,* Philadelphia, 1995, JB Lippincott.

Mazza JF, editor: *Manual of clinical hematology,* ed 2, Boston, Little, Brown.

Rodak BF, editor: *Diagnostic hematology,* Philadelphia, 1995, WB Saunders.

Turgeon ML, editor: *Clinical hematology. Theory and procedures,* ed 2, Boston, 1993, Little, Brown.

Wiernik PH: *Neoplastic diseases of the blood,* ed 2, New York, 1991, Churchill Livingstone.

Journals

*Bertero C, Ek AC: Quality of life of adults with acute leukaemia, *J Adv Nurs* 18:1346, 1993.

Binkley LS, Whittaker A: Erythropoietin use in the critical care setting, *AACN Clin Issues Crit Care Nurs* 3:640, 1992.

Cherry-Peppers G, Davis V, Atkinson JC: Sickle-cell anemia: a case report and literature review, *Clin Preventive Dentistry* 14:5, 1992.

de Misa RF, Megido M: Autoimmune hemolytic anemia and cutaneous T cell lymphoma: review of the literature, *Acta Haematol* 89:168, 1993.

DeBacker A and others: Totally implantable central venous access devices in pediatric oncology—our experience in 46 patients, *Eur J Pediatr Surg* 3:101, 1993.

Doheny MO and others: Caring for the orthopaedic patient with sickle cell disease, *Orthop Nurs* 11:41, 1992.

Ellenberger BJ, Haas L, Cundiff L: Thrombotic thrombocytopenia purpura: nursing during the acute phase, *DCCN* 12:58, 1993.

Fasola G and others: Infections in patients with acute nonlymphocytic leukemia nursed with central or peripheral venous access, *Tumori* 79:112, 1993.

Fiske DN, McCoy HE, Kitchens CS: Zinc-induced sideroblastic anemia: report of a case, review of the literature, and description of the hematologic syndrome, *Am J Hematol* 46:147, 1994.

Frassoldati A and others: Hairy cell leukemia: a clinical review based on 725 cases of the Italian Cooperative Group (ICG

*Nursing research-based articles.

HCL). Italian Cooperative Group for Hairy Cell Leukemia, *Leuk Lymphoma* 13:307, 1994.

Harris MG, Bean CA: Changing the role of the nurse in the hematology-oncology outpatient setting, *Oncol Nurs Forum* 18:43, 1991.

Heron D: Leukaemia and bone marrow transplant nursing. Talking about a revolution, *Nurs Stand* 7:52, 1992.

Hiromoto BM, Dungan J: Contract learning for self-care activities. A protocol study among chemotherapy outpatients, *Cancer Nurs* 14:148, 1991.

Kantarjian HM: Adult acute lymphocytic leukemia: critical review of current knowledge, *Am J Med* 97:176, 1994.

Kelly C and others: A change in flushing protocols of contral venous catheters, *Oncol Nurs Forum* 19:599, 1992.

Kenny SA: Effect of two oral care protocols on the incidence of stomatitis in hematology patients, *Cancer Nurs* 13:345, 1990.

Kurtz A: Disseminated intravascular coagulation with leukemia patients, *Cancer Nurs* 16:456, 1993.

Litwach K: Bleeding and coagulation in the PACU, *Crit Care Nurs Clin North Am* 3:121, 1991.

Lovett RB, Wagner L, McMillan S: Validity and reliability of a pediatric hematology oncology patient acuity tool, *J Pediatr Oncol Nurs* 8:122, 1991.

Paschall FE: Thrombotic thrombocytopenic purpura: the challenges of a complex disease process, *AACN Clin Issues Crit Care Nurs* 4:655, 1993.

Rogers BB: Taxol: a promising new drug of the '90s, *Oncol Nurs Forum* 20:1483, 1993.

Schwarzinger I and others: Hypergranular acute lymphoblastic leukemia (ALL). Report of a case and review of the literature, *Ann Hematol* 67:301, 1993.

Shibata K and others: Essential thrombocythemia terminating in acute leukemia with minimal myeloid differentiation—a brief review of recent literature, *Acta Haematol* 91:84, 1994.

Sirchia G and others: Quality control of red cell filtration at the patient's bedside, *Transfusion* 34:26, 1994.

Skov T and others: Leukaemia and reproductive outcome among nurses handling antineoplastic drugs, *Br J Indust Med* 49:855, 1992.

Stalfelt AM, Wadman B: Assessing quality of life in leukemia: presentation of an instrument for assessing quality of life in patients with blood malignancies, *Qual Assur Health Care* 5:201, 1993.

Timmerman PR: Intravenous immunoglobulin in oncology nursing practice, *Oncol Nurs Forum* 20:69, 1993.

Tugal O and others: Recurrent benign intracranial hypertension due to iron deficiency anemia. Case report and review of the literature, *Am J Pediatr Hematol Oncol* 16:266, 1994 (review).

Yeager KA, Miaskowski C: Advances in understanding the mechanisms and management of acute myelogenous leukemia, *Oncol Nurs Forum* 21:541, 1994.

Organizations

National Association for Sickle Cell Disease
3345 Wilshire Blvd., Suite 1106
Los Angeles, CA 90010-1880
800-421-8453

National Hemophilia Foundation
110 Green Street, Room 303
New York, NY 10012
212-219-8180

Leukemia Society of America
600 Third Avenue
New York, NY 10017
212-573-8484

Sickle Cell Disease Foundation of Greater New York
1 West 125th Street, Room 206
New York, NY 10027

AHCPR Guidelines

Guides developed and published by The Agency for Health Care Policy and Research (AHCPR). The Patient Guides are available in English and Spanish. The guidelines can be obtained by writing to: Center for Research Dissemination and Liaison, AHCPR Clearinghouse, P.O. Box 8547, Silver Spring, MD 20907, or by calling 1-800-358-9295. The Guidelines are as follows:

Sickle cell disease: screening, diagnosis, management, and counseling in newborns and infants. AHCPR Pub. No. 92-0562.

Sickle cell disease: comprehensive screening and management in newborns and infants. AHCPR Pub. No. 92-0563.

Sickle cell disease in newborns and infants: A Guide for Parents. AHCPR Pub. No. 92-0564.

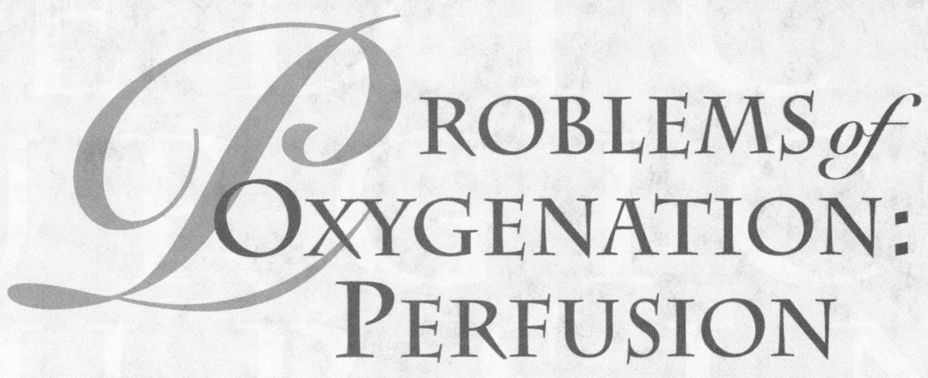

Problems of Oxygenation: Perfusion

Section Seven

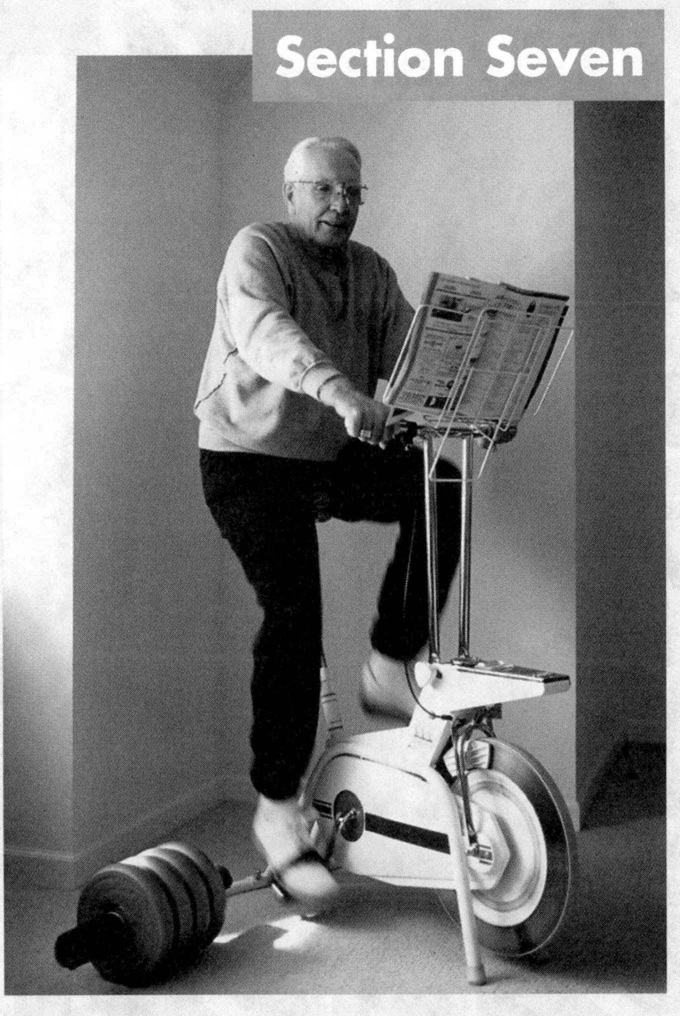

Chapter 29

NURSING ASSESSMENT

Cardiovascular System

Lori D. Finlay

Learning Objectives

1. Describe the anatomic location and function of the following cardiac structures: pericardial layers, atria, ventricles, semilunar valves, and atrioventricular valves.
2. Describe coronary circulation and the areas of heart muscle supplied by each blood vessel.
3. Explain the normal sequence of events involved in the conduction pathway of the heart.
4. Describe the structure and function of arteries, capillaries, and veins.
5. Define blood pressure and the mechanisms involved in its regulation.
6. Identify the significant subjective and objective assessment data related to the cardiovascular system that should be obtained from a patient.
7. Describe the appropriate techniques used in the physical assessment of the cardiovascular system.
8. Differentiate normal from common abnormal findings of a physical assessment of the cardiovascular system.
9. Describe the age-related changes of the cardiovascular system and differences in assessment findings.
10. Describe the purpose, significance of results, and nursing responsibilities of invasive and noninvasive diagnostic studies of the cardiovascular system.
11. Identify waveforms of a normal electrocardiogram and components of the normal sinus rhythm.

STRUCTURES AND FUNCTIONS OF THE CARDIOVASCULAR SYSTEM

Heart

Structure. The heart is a four-chambered muscular organ approximately the size of a fist. It is the pump of the cardiovascular system. The heart lies within the thorax between the lungs in the mediastinal space. Its beating is often palpable at the fifth intercostal space approximately 2 inches left of the midline (Fig. 29-1). This pulsation, arising at the apex of the heart, is known as the *point of maximum impulse* (PMI).

The heart wall is composed of three layers. The *endocardium* is the thin inner lining, the *myocardium* is the middle muscular layer, and the *epicardium* is the outer serous membrane. The *pericardium (pericardial sac)* surrounds the heart, enclosing it the way a glove encloses a fist. This sac consists of a visceral (inner) layer and a parietal (outer) layer. The visceral layer is in contact with the epicardium. Between the visceral and parietal layers is the *pericardial space.* A small amount of fluid in this space acts as a lubricant and reduces the friction caused by the movement of the layers with each contraction.

The heart's four chambers are separated by a septum, with two chambers on the right side and two chambers on the left side. The upper chambers on each side are the *atria,* and the lower chambers are the *ventricles.* The atrial myocardium is thinner than that of the ventricles. The left ventricular wall is much thicker than the right ventricular wall. Its added thickness provides the force for the left ventricle to pump blood into the systemic circulation. The smaller right ventricle pumps against a lower pressure into the lungs.

Blood Flow through the Heart

Cardiac valves. The right atrium receives venous blood from the inferior and superior venae cavae and the coronary sinus. The blood then passes through the *tricuspid valve* into the right ventricle. With each contraction, the right ventricle pumps blood into the pulmonary artery. At the entrance to the pulmonary artery is the *pulmonic valve.*

Blood from the lungs flows into the left atrium by way of the pulmonary veins. It then passes through the *mitral valve* and into the left ventricle. As the heart contracts, blood is ejected through the aortic valve into the aorta and thus enters the systemic circulation (Fig. 29-2).

Reviewed by Katie Drake Speer, RN, MSN, Assistant Professor, Tuskegee University School of Nursing and Allied Health, Tuskegee Institute, AL.

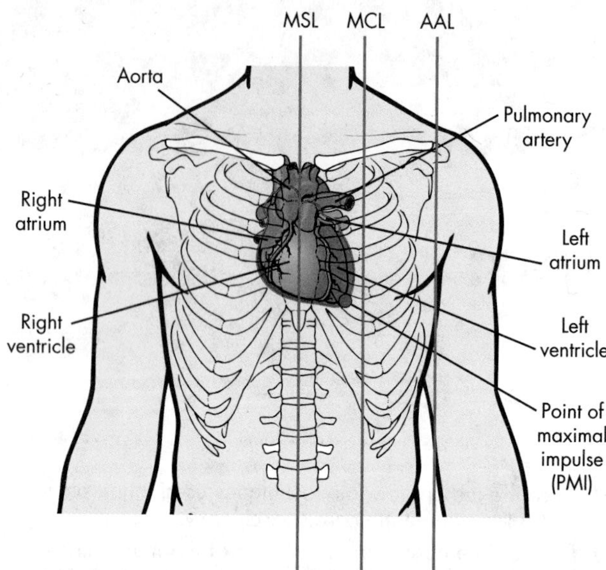

Fig. 29-1 Orientation of the heart within the thorax. Red lines indicate the midsternal line (MSL), midclavicular line (MCL), and anterior axillary line (AAL).

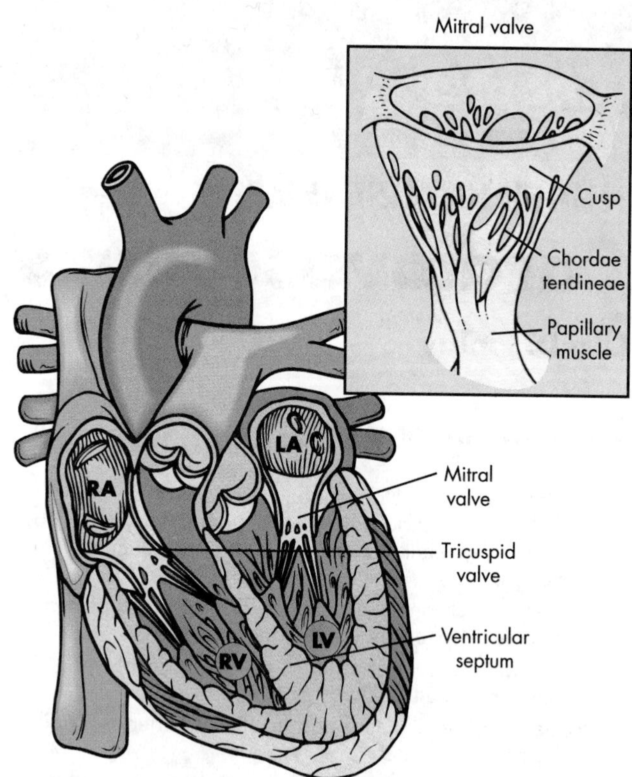

Fig. 29-3 Anatomic structures of the atrioventricular (AV) valves. *LA,* Left atrium; *LV,* left ventricle; *RA,* right atrium; *RV,* right ventricle.

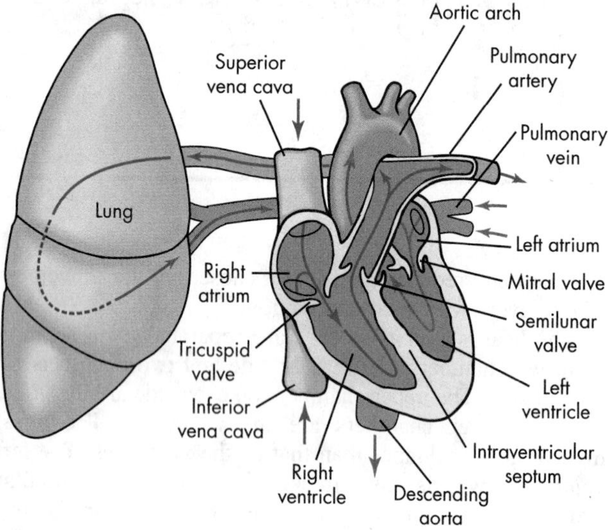

Fig. 29-2 Schematic representation of blood flow through the heart. *Arrows* indicate direction of flow.

The four valves of the heart serve to keep blood flowing in one direction. The atrioventricular (AV) valves (tricuspid and mitral) prevent backflow of blood into the atria at the start of each contraction of the ventricles. The cusps of the valves are attached to thin strands of fibrous tissue called *chordae tendineae* (Fig. 29-3). These strands are anchored in papillary muscles projecting from the walls of the ventricles. During ventricular contraction the support of the valves by the chordae tendineae prevents the eversion of the valves into the atria. The pulmonic and aortic valves prevent blood from regurgitating into the ventricles at the end of each ventricular contraction. These valves, also known as *semilunar valves,* have three cusps.

Blood Supply to the Myocardium. The myocardium has its own coronary circulation that allows for constant delivery of oxygenated blood so contraction can continue. Immediately above the cusps of the aortic valve are the sinuses of Valsalva, with openings to the right and left coronary arteries. Blood flow into the coronary arteries occurs primarily during diastole. The branches of the coronary arteries carry blood to different areas of the myocardium (Fig. 29-4). The right coronary artery and its branches usually supply the right atrium, the right ventricle, and a portion of the posterior wall of the left ventricle. The left coronary artery and its branches (left anterior descending artery and left circumflex artery) supply the left atrium and the massive walls of the left ventricle. In 90% of all persons, the *AV node,* part of the cardiac conduction system, receives its blood supply from the right coronary artery. For this reason, obstruction of this artery often causes serious defects in cardiac conduction.

If blood flow through any part of the coronary arterial system is interrupted, an imbalance between oxygen supply and demand occurs. *Ischemia* is a consequence of this imbalance. Ischemia, which is a reversible cellular injury, produces tissue hypoxia, a decreased energy supply, and a buildup of toxic metabolic wastes.[1] The overall effect of this ischemia on the heart depends on the size of the area

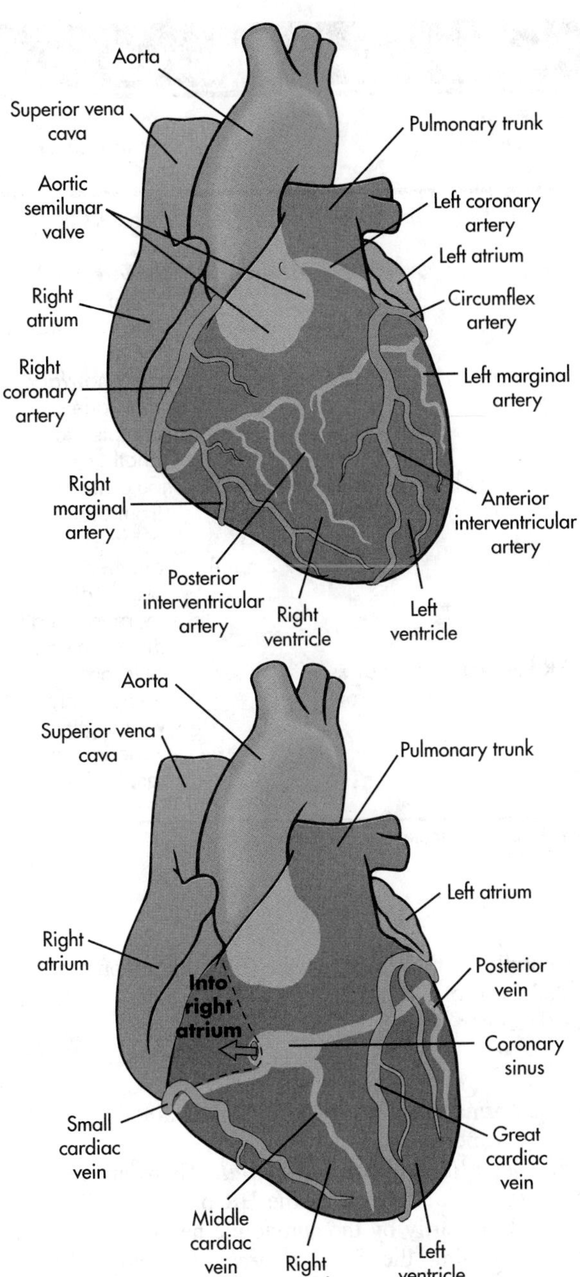

Fig. 29-4 Coronary arteries and veins.

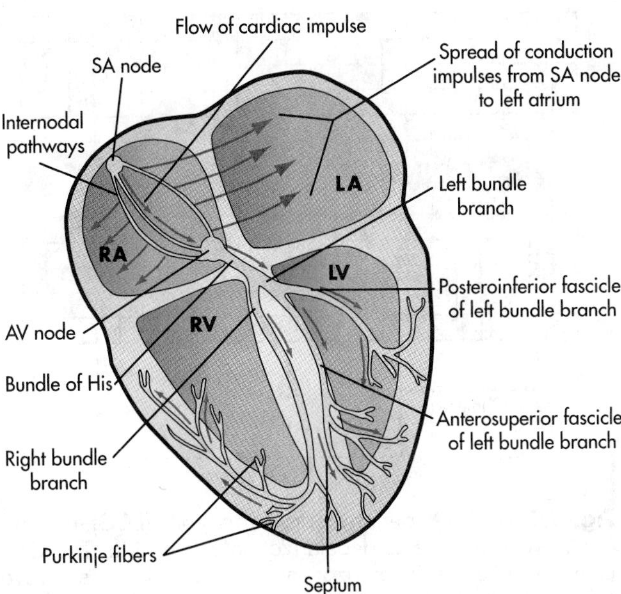

Fig. 29-5 Conduction system of the heart. *LA,* Left atrium; *LV,* left ventricle; *RA,* right atrium; *RV,* right ventricle; *SA,* sinoatrial.

deprived of oxygen (O_2). If blood flow is reduced gradually, alternate routes may develop in enough time to nourish the endangered myocardium. These alternate routes are called *collateral circulation* and may be compared with a detour for a road blocked with traffic.

The divisions of coronary veins parallel the coronary arteries. Most of the blood from the coronary system drains into the coronary sinus, which empties into the right atrium near the entrance to the inferior vena cava (Fig. 29-4).

Conduction System. In the heart wall are pathways of special myocardial tissue for the wave of excitation that triggers each contraction of the heart muscle. This wave, or *action potential,* is the consequence of a sudden change in the membrane potential of node cells that occurs because of the rapid influx of sodium ions into the cells and the outflux of potassium ions. This shift in electrolytes reduces the polarized condition that exists when node cells are at rest (i.e., electrically negative inside, positive outside), and the cell membranes become *depolarized.* The action potential created at that instant moves in concentric waves throughout the atria. This wave of conduction starts at the *sinoatrial* (SA) *node,* a tiny knob of tissue in the wall of the right atrium, near the entrance of the superior vena cava (Fig. 29-5). The normal heartbeat begins as an action potential generated in the SA node. Therefore the SA node is called the *pacemaker* of the heart. Each impulse generated at the SA node travels swiftly through the muscle fibers of both atria.

The mechanical contraction of the heart muscle follows the depolarization of the cells. Contraction occurs when the actin and myosin filaments of the contractile units of the heart come together. Calcium, which flows into the cell after depolarization, initiates this contraction. Because the muscle fibers are in contact with one another, the walls of the atria contract almost as one unit.

The action potential travels through the atria to the AV node, located in the right atrium near the ventricle. The action potential pauses briefly in the AV node, which allows contraction and emptying of the atria to proceed before contraction of the ventricles begins. The excitation then moves through the *bundle of His* and along the interventricular septum by way of the *left* and *right bundle branches.* The left bundle branch has two fascicles, an anterior and a posterior. From there the action potential

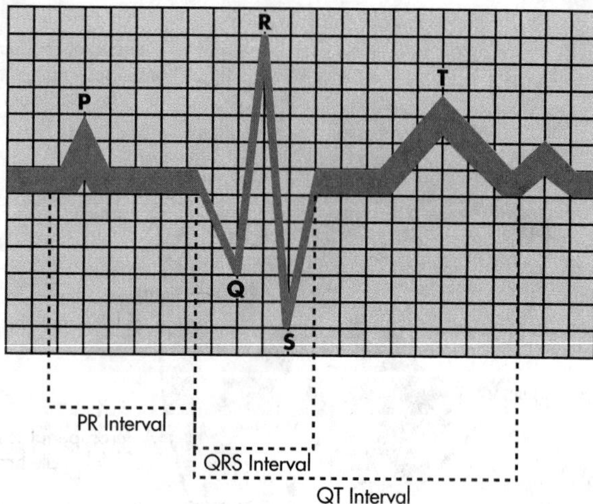

Fig. 29-6 The normal electrocardiogram (ECG) pattern. The P wave represents depolarization of the atria. The QRS complex indicates depolarization of the ventricles. The T wave represents repolarization of the ventricles. The PR interval is a measure of the time required for the impulse to spread from the sinoatrial node to the ventricles.

Table 29-1 Electrocardiogram Waves

Normal Waveforms and Intervals	Normal Timing	Normal Sinus Rhythm*
P	0.06-0.12 sec	Precedes QRS-T waves
QRS	0.06-0.10 sec	Follows each P wave
T	0.16 sec	Follows each QRS wave
PR interval	0.12-0.20 sec	Should not vary from one complex to another
QT interval	Varies with pulse rate (0.31-0.38 sec at heart rate of 72 bpm)	Should not vary from one complex to another Should not be more than half the RR interval
RR interval	Varies with pulse rate	Should be equidistant, with slight variations on respiration

bpm, Beats per minute.
*At 60-100 bpm.

diffuses widely through the walls of both ventricles by means of *Purkinje fibers.* The conduction system allows coordinated contraction of the heart chambers.

The cardiac cycle starts with depolarization of the SA node. Its climax is ejection of blood into the pulmonary and systemic circulations. It ends with *repolarization* when the contractile fiber cells and the conduction pathway cells regain their resting polarized condition. Cardiac muscle cells have a compensatory mechanism that makes them unresponsive or *refractory* to restimulation during the action potential. During systole there is an *absolute refractory period* during which cardiac muscle does not respond to any stimuli. After this period, cardiac muscle gradually recovers its excitability and a *relative refractory period* occurs by early diastole.

Electrocardiogram. The action potential of the heart can be detected on the body surface and is recorded as an electrocardiogram (ECG). The letters *P, QRS,* and *T* are used to identify the separate waveforms (Fig. 29-6). The first wave, P, begins with the firing of the SA node and represents depolarization of the fibers of the atria. The QRS wave represents depolarization from the AV node throughout the ventricles. There is a delay of impulse transmission through the AV node that accounts for the time sequence between the end of the P wave and the beginning of the QRS wave. The last component of the cardiac cycle, the T wave, represents repolarization of the ventricles.

Intervals between these waves reflect the length of time it takes for the impulse to travel from one area of the heart to the other. These time intervals can be measured (Table 29-1), and deviations from these time references often indicate pathology.

Cardiac Output. Cardiac output (CO) is the amount of blood pumped by each ventricle in 1 minute. It is calculated by multiplying the *stroke volume* (SV) (the amount of blood ejected from one ventricle with one heartbeat) by the *heart rate* (HR) per minute:

$$CO = SV \times HR$$

For the normal adult at rest, CO is maintained in the range of 4 to 8 L per minute.[2]

Factors affecting cardiac output. There are numerous factors that can affect either the HR or the SV. The HR is regulated primarily by the autonomic nervous system. The factors affecting the SV are *preload, contractility,* and *afterload.*[3]

Starling's law states that the more fibers are stretched, the greater their force of contraction. The volume of blood in the ventricles at the end of diastole, before the next contraction, is called *preload.* Preload determines the amount of stretch placed on myocardial fibers. The greater the amount of stretch placed on myocardial fibers, the greater the force of the next contraction; thus SV is increased. Nitrate drugs (e.g., nitroglycerin, isosorbide [Isordil]) are commonly used to decrease preload because they primarily dilate veins. Thus, venous return, which indirectly determines the SV, is decreased.

Contractility, another factor affecting SV, can be increased by norepinephrine released by the sympathetic nervous system, as well as by epinephrine, whether produced endogenously by the body or administered as a drug.

Increasing contractility raises the SV by increasing ventricular emptying. Digitalis is one of the medications commonly used to increase contractility of heart muscle.

Afterload is the peripheral resistance against which the left ventricle must pump. Afterload is affected by the size of the ventricles, wall tension, and arterial pressure. An increase in afterload usually means an increase in the work of the heart. If the arterial pressure is elevated, the ventricles will meet increased resistance to ejection of blood. Eventually this can result in ventricular hypertrophy (enlargement of the cardiac muscle tissue without an increase in the size of cavities). Thus increased afterload results from increased arterial pressure. Certain classes of drugs, such as arterial vasodilators (e.g., hydralazine [Apresoline]) and angiotensin-converting enzyme (ACE) inhibitor agents (e.g., captopril [Capoten]), decrease afterload, thus increasing SV and CO. Such drugs are used in the treatment of conditions in which afterload is increased (e.g., congestive heart failure, hypertension).

Cardiac Reserve. Considering the numerous factors affecting CO, the fact that the cardiovascular system is able to adjust to the body's demands is a marvel. For example, the demand for increased output occurs with hypovolemia, exercise, and stress. The ability to respond to these demands and increase CO threefold or fourfold is referred to as *cardiac reserve.*

The increase in CO results from an increase in HR or SV. The HR can increase to as high as 180 beats per minute (bpm) for short periods without deleterious effects. The SV can be increased by increasing either preload or contractility.

Vascular System

Blood Vessels. The three major types of blood vessels in the vascular system are the *arteries, veins,* and *capillaries.* Arteries travel away from the heart and, except for the pulmonary artery, carry oxygenated blood. Veins travel toward the heart and, except for the pulmonary veins, carry deoxygenated blood. Small arteries are called *arterioles,* and small veins are called *venules.* Blood circulates from the heart into arteries, arterioles, capillaries, venules, veins, and back to the heart.

Arteries and arterioles. The arterial system differs from the venous system by the amount and type of tissue that makes up arterial walls (Fig. 29-7). The large arteries have thick walls that are composed mainly of elastic tissue. This elastic property creates a low-resistance reservoir for blood as well as a recoil that propels blood forward into the circulation. Large arteries also contain some smooth muscle. Examples of large arteries are the aorta and the pulmonary artery.

Arterioles have relatively little elastic tissue but a lot of smooth muscle. They respond readily to autonomic nervous control by dilating or constricting. The amount of blood flow to each organ and various tissues is directly related to the degree of constriction of the arteriole lumen. Arterioles serve as the major control of arterial blood pressure and distribution of blood flow.

Capillaries. The thin capillary wall is made up of endothelial cells, with no elastic or muscle tissue present

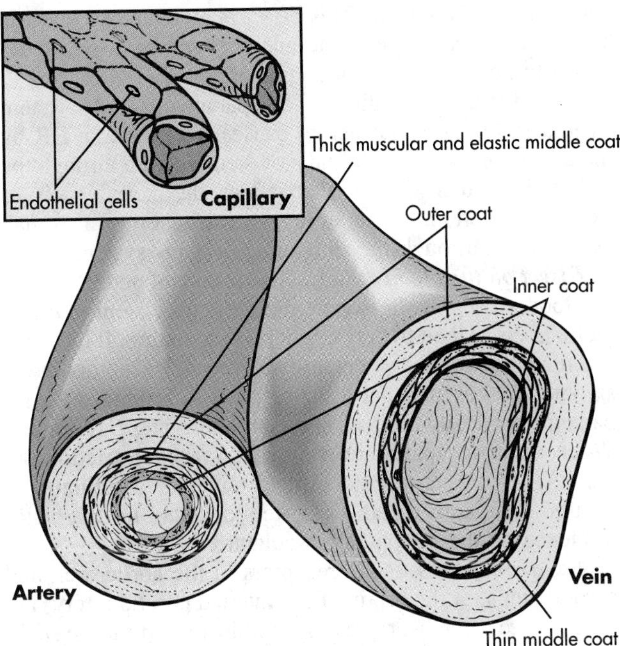

Fig. 29-7 Comparative thickness of layers of the artery, vein, and capillary.

(Fig. 29-7). There are an estimated 25,000 miles of capillaries in an adult.[2] The exchange of cellular nutrients and metabolic end products takes place through these many thin-walled vessels.

Veins and venules. Veins are large-diameter, thin-walled vessels that return blood to the right atrium (Fig. 29-7). The larger veins contain semilunar valves at intervals to maintain the blood flow toward the heart and to prevent backward flow. The amount of blood in the venous system is affected by a number of factors, including arterial flow, compression of veins by skeletal muscles, alterations in thoracic and abdominal pressures, and right atrial pressure.

The largest veins are the *superior vena cava,* which returns blood to the heart from the head, neck, and arms, and the *inferior vena cava,* which returns blood to the heart from the lower part of the body. These large-diameter vessels are affected by the pressure in the right side of the heart. Elevated right atrial pressure can cause distended neck veins or liver engorgement as a result of resistance to blood flow.

Venules are relatively small tubules made up of a small amount of muscle and connective tissue. Venules collect blood from various capillary beds and channel it to the larger veins.

Regulation of the Cardiovascular System

Autonomic Nervous System. The autonomic nervous system consists of the *sympathetic system* and the *parasympathetic system.*

Effect on the heart. Stimulation of the sympathetic nervous system increases the HR, the speed of impulse conduction through the AV node, and the force of atrial and ventricular contractions. This effect is mediated by specific sites in the heart called β-adrenergic *receptors,* which respond to norepinephrine and epinephrine.

In contrast, stimulation of the parasympathetic system (mediated by the vagus nerve) causes a decrease in HR by the action on the SA node and slows conduction through the AV node. Other factors that affect the heart, such as exercise, emotion, temperature, and medications, also may be mediated through the autonomic nervous system.

Effect on the blood vessels. The source of neural control of blood vessels is the autonomic nervous system. Sympathetic fibers extend to the peripheral vasculature. It has been postulated that vessels contain two types of receptors in the smooth muscle and that these respond differently to sympathetic nerve stimulation. These are the α and β receptors. When the α receptors are stimulated, vasoconstriction occurs. When the β receptors are stimulated, vasodilatation occurs. The parasympathetic system does not have a major influence on the peripheral vasculature.

Baroreceptors. Baroreceptors in the aortic arch and carotid sinus (at the origin of the internal carotid artery) are sensitive to stretch or pressure within the arterial system. Stimulation of these receptors sends information to the vasomotor center in the brain stem. This results in inhibition of the sympathetic nervous system and enhancement of the parasympathetic influence, causing a decreased HR and peripheral vasodilatation.

Decreased arterial pressure causes the opposite effect. Baroreceptors control only temporary changes, such as changes in position.

Chemoreceptors. Chemoreceptors are located in the aortic arch and carotid body. They are capable of initiating changes in HR and arterial pressure in response to chemical stimulation. They are stimulated by decreased arterial O_2 pressure (PO_2), increased arterial carbon dioxide pressure (PCO_2), and decreased plasma pH. When the chemoreceptor reflexes are stimulated, they subsequently stimulate the vasomotor center to increase cardiac activity.

Blood Pressure

The arterial blood pressure (BP) is a measure of the pressure exerted by blood against the walls of the arterial system. The *systolic* pressure is the peak pressure exerted against the arteries when the heart contracts. The *diastolic* pressure is the residual pressure of the arterial system during cardiac relaxation. BP is usually expressed as the ratio of systolic to diastolic pressure.

The two main factors influencing BP are CO and systemic vascular resistance (SVR):

$$BP = CO \times SVR$$

SVR is the force opposing the movement of blood. This force is created primarily in small arteries and arterioles.

Measurement of Arterial Blood Pressure. BP can be measured by invasive and noninvasive techniques. The invasive technique consists of catheter insertion into an artery. The catheter is attached to a recording device, and the pressure is measured directly (see Chapter 61).

However, the easiest technique is the noninvasive, indirect measurement of BP with a sphygmomanometer and a stethoscope. The sphygmomanometer consists of an inflatable cuff and a pressure gauge. The BP is measured externally by listening for sounds, called *Korotkoff sounds,* produced over an artery when it is constricted. The brachial artery is the usual site for taking BP.

The balloon cuff is inflated to a pressure in excess of the systolic pressure. This causes blood flow in the artery to cease. As the pressure in the cuff is lowered, Korotkoff sounds are heard. Korotkoff sounds are divided into five phases. The *first phase* is a tapping sound caused by the spurt of blood into the constricted artery as the pressure in the cuff is gradually deflated. This sound is considered the *systolic measurement.* The *second phase* begins with a murmur, usually 10 to 15 mm Hg below the systolic tap. The *third phase* begins 14 to 20 mm Hg below the second phase and begins when the murmur changes again to a crisper, more intense tapping sound. This sound is higher pitched, with no discernible murmur. The *fourth phase* begins when this tapping sound becomes muffled and less intense. This sound represents the diastolic pressure, or lowest pressure before the next ventricular beat. The *fifth phase* occurs when the sound disappears.[4] Controversy exists as to whether the fourth phase or the fifth phase is the accurate indicator of diastolic pressure. Thus, for greatest accuracy, the diastolic pressure should be recorded as both the muffled sound and the disappearance of sound (e.g., 120/84/80).[4]

Occasionally the sounds will be heard all the way to zero. In this case the BP should be recorded as 120/80/0. In actual practice, BP is often recorded as two numbers. The first number indicates the appearance of sound, and the second number represents the cessation of sound.

In addition to the manual technique, another noninvasive way to measure BP indirectly is to use an automatic cycling device. These automated BP monitors have been found to correlate closely with the results obtained by auscultating BP.

Ambulatory BP monitoring may be used to diagnose hypertension more accurately in some patients (see Chapter 30). The monitor consists of a BP cuff and a microprocessing unit that fits into a pouch and hangs from the shoulder or attaches to a belt. Most units weigh less than a pound and are battery operated. This method records a patient's BP at preset intervals during routine activities. At the end of the monitoring period (usually 24 hours), the data that are recorded and stored in the microprocessing unit are transferred to a printer for interpretation.

Pulse Pressure and Mean Arterial Pressure. Pulse pressure is the difference between the systolic and diastolic pressures. It is normally about one third of the systolic pressure. If the BP is 120/80, the pulse pressure is 40. An increased pulse pressure may occur in exercise or in arteriosclerosis of the larger arteries. A decreased pulse pressure may be found in cardiac failure or hypovolemia.

Another measurement related to BP is *mean arterial pressure* (MAP). It is not the average of the diastolic and systolic pressures because the duration of diastole exceeds that of systole at normal HRs. MAP is calculated by adding the diastolic pressure to one third of the pulse pressure:

$$MAP = \text{diastolic pressure} + \tfrac{1}{3}\ \text{pulse pressure}$$

A person with a BP of 120/60/0 has a MAP of 80.

Effects of Aging on the Cardiovascular System

There is some controversy related to the effects of aging on the cardiovascular system. This is partly because of the presence of atherosclerosis in many older adults, which makes it difficult to separate physiologic from pathologic alterations. Age-related changes are presented in Table 29-6.

The most important cellular changes in the cardiac structure are related to collagen and elastin. With increased age, the amount of collagen in the heart increases and elastin decreases. These changes affect the contractile and distensible properties of the myocardium. The deposition of lipofuscin (brown lipid) is the most specific cellular age-related change. However, it does not appear to have any effect on myocardial function.

In addition to collagen degeneration, heart valves also undergo lipid accumulation and calcification. The aortic valve is usually more involved than the mitral valve.

The resting HR is not markedly affected by aging. However, one of the major age-associated alterations in the cardiovascular response to exercise is a striking decrease in the cardiac response (e.g., decreased SV, CO, and HR).

The number of pacemaker cells in the SA node decreases with age. By age 75, a person may have only 10% of the normal number of pacemaker cells.[5] This increases the likelihood of sinus node dysfunction with sustained sinus bradycardia. Fibrosis and increased microcalcification of the conduction system, as well as an almost 50% reduction of bundle of His fibers, may also precipitate chronic heart block. A normal ECG of an aging patient may show small, inconspicuous increases in PR, QRS, and QT intervals. There is also a decrease in the amplitude of QRS complex (probably a result of left ventricular thickening).

The number and function of β-adrenergic receptors in the heart decrease with age. Therefore, the older adult is less sensitive to β-adrenergic agonist drugs.

With aging, the amount of elastin in arterial walls decreases, apparently as a result of destruction. The elastin and collagen alterations cause a thickened intimal layer and fibrosed medial layer in the coronary arteries, resulting in rigidity associated with coronary artery disease.[5] This imitation of atherosclerosis has caused some of the confusion associated with cardiovascular aging. There is an increase in pulse pressure in the older adult because of an increase in systolic pressure and a lower rate of increase in the diastolic pressure. These changes are related to loss of vascular distensibility and elastic recoil. Despite the changes associated with aging, the heart is able to function adequately under normal circumstances, and hypertension should not be considered a normal consequence of aging.[5]

ASSESSMENT OF THE CARDIOVASCULAR SYSTEM

Subjective Data

A careful health history and physical examination should aid the nurse in differentiating symptoms that reflect a cardiovascular problem from problems of other body systems. For instance, it is important to determine if weight gain is because of overeating or a manifestation of fluid retention. Is shortness of breath caused by congestive heart failure (CHF) or chronic obstructive pulmonary disease (COPD)? Common chief cues that should alert the nurse to the possibility of underlying cardiovascular problems need to be explored and documented (Table 29-2).

Important Health Information

Past health history. Many illnesses affect the cardiovascular system directly or indirectly. The patient should be questioned about a history of chest pain, shortness of breath, alcoholism or excessive drinking, anemia, rheumatic fever, streptococcal sore throat, congenital heart disease, stroke, syncope, hypertension, thrombophlebitis, intermittent claudication, varicosities, and edema.

Medications. An assessment of the patient's current and past use of medication should be made. This includes both over-the-counter (OTC) drugs and prescription drugs. For example, aspirin, which prolongs the blood-clotting time, is contained in many drugs used to alleviate cold symptoms.

A medication assessment should list the name of the drug and the patient's understanding of its purpose and side effects. Specific categories of drugs frequently used in the patient with cardiovascular problems include antihypertensives, anticoagulants, diuretics, glycosides, and nitrates. Drugs that may adversely affect the cardiovascular system also should be assessed. Some of these, and examples of their effect on the cardiovascular system, are as follows:

Table 29-2 Cues to Cardiovascular Problems

Symptom	Description
Fatigue	No energy, need more rest than usual, normal activities result in tiring
Fluid retention	Weight gain, bloated feeling; swelling; tightening of clothing; shoes no longer fitting comfortably; marks or indentations left from constricting garments
Irregular heartbeat	Sensation of heart in throat or skipped beats, racing heart; dizziness
Dyspnea	Air hunger, especially after exertion; pillows or upright chair necessary for sleep
Pain	Indigestion, burning, numbness, tightness, or pressure in midchest; epigastric or substernal pain, radiating to shoulder, neck, arms
Tenderness in calf of leg	Inability to bear weight; swelling of the involved extremity; inflamed, warm skin over vein
	Distended, discolored, tortuous veins in calves of legs; ache in lower extremities after standing for short periods

Tricyclic antidepressants	Dysrhythmias
Phenothiazines	Dysrhythmias and hypotension
Oral contraceptives	Thrombophlebitis
Doxorubicin (Adriamycin)	Cardiomyopathy
Lithium	Dysrhythmias
Corticosteroids	Sodium and fluid retention
Theophylline preparations	Tachycardia and dysrhythmias
Recreational or abused drugs	Tachycardia and dysrhythmias

Surgery or other treatments. The patient should also be asked about specific treatments, past surgeries, or hospital admissions related to cardiovascular problems. Any hospitalizations for diagnostic workups or cardiovascular symptoms should be explored. It should be noted whether an ECG or a chest x-ray was taken for baseline data.

Functional Health Patterns. The strong correlation between components of a patient's lifestyle and cardiovascular health supports the need to review each functional health pattern. Key questions to ask a person with a cardiovascular problem are listed in Table 29-3.

Health perception–health management pattern. The nurse should ask the patient about the presence of cardiovascular risk factors. Major risk factors include elevated serum lipids, hypertension, and cigarette smoking. Obesity, a sedentary or stressful lifestyle, and diabetes mellitus should also be investigated as minor risk factors.

If the patient smokes, the number of pack years of smoking (number of packs smoked per day multiplied by the number of years the patient has smoked) should be estimated. The patient's attitude about smoking, as well as

Table 29-3 Key Questions: Patient with a Cardiovascular Problem

Health Perception–Health Management Pattern
- Have you noticed an increase in cardiovascular symptoms such as chest pain or dyspnea?*
- Do you practice any preventive measures to decrease cardiac risk factors?*
- Do you foresee any potential self-care problems because of your cardiovascular problem?*

Nutritional-Metabolic Pattern
- Describe your usual daily dietary intake including fat, sodium, and fluid.
- What is your present weight? What was your weight one year ago? If different, explain.
- Does eating cause fatigue or shortness of breath?*

Elimination Pattern
- Do your feet or ankles ever swell?*
- Have you ever taken medication to help you get rid of excess fluid?*

Activity-Exercise Pattern
- Are your activities or exercise limited because of your cardiovascular problem?*
- Are your activities of daily living restricted because of your cardiovascular problem?*
- Do you experience any discomfort or side effects as a result of exercise or activity?*

Sleep-Rest Pattern
- How many pillows do you sleep on at night?
- How many times a night do you awaken to urinate?
- Do you ever wake up suddenly and feel as if you cannot catch your breath?*

Cognitive-Perceptual Pattern
- Have you noticed any changes in your memory or level of awareness?*
- Do you ever experience dizziness?*
- Do you find it difficult to verbally express yourself?*
- Do you experience any pain (e.g., chest pain, leg pain with activity) as a result of your cardiovascular problem?*

Self-Perception–Self-Concept Pattern
- Have your perceptions of yourself changed since you were diagnosed with a cardiovascular disease?
- How has your cardiovascular disease affected your life and your self-esteem?

Role-Relationship Pattern
- Describe how this illness has affected the roles that you play in your daily life.
- Describe how this illness has affected your relationships.
- How have your significant others been affected by your disease?

Sexuality-Reproductive Pattern
- Has your sexual behavior changed?*
- Do you experience any cardiac-related symptoms during intercourse?*
- Do any of your medications affect your ability to participate in sexual activities?*

Coping–Stress Tolerance Pattern
- Do you practice any stress reduction techniques?*
- Describe your normal coping mechanisms for stress.
- Who or where would you turn to during a time of stress? Are these people or services helping you now?*
- Do you feel capable of handling your present health situation? Explain.
- Do you experience any cardiovascular symptoms such as chest pain or palpitations during times of stress?*

Values-Belief Pattern
- What influence has your value-belief system had during your illness?
- Do you feel any conflicts between your value-belief system and your planned therapy?*
- Describe any cultural or religious beliefs that may influence the treatment of your cardiovascular problem.

*If yes, describe.

attempts to stop, should be documented. Alcohol use should also be recorded. This information should include type of beverage, amount, frequency, and any changes in the reaction to it. The use of habit-forming drugs, including recreational drugs, also should be noted. Finally, of importance for teaching and discharge planning, is knowledge of the patient's perception of how this illness may impact the future level of wellness and ability for self-care.

A question about the patient's allergies is appropriate. The nurse should determine whether a drug reaction or allergic reaction was ever experienced. If the patient has been treated for allergies, understanding of this therapy should be ascertained. The patient should also be asked whether an anaphylactic reaction has ever been experienced.

Confirmed illnesses of blood relatives can highlight any hereditary or familial tendencies toward coronary artery disease, peripheral vascular disease, hypertension, bleeding, cardiac disorders, diabetes mellitus, atherosclerosis, and stroke. In addition, disorders affecting the vascular system, such as intermittent claudication and varicosities, may be familial. Finally, a family health history of noncardiac conditions such as asthma, renal disease, and obesity should be assessed because they can affect the cardiovascular system.

Nutritional-metabolic pattern. Being underweight or overweight may indicate potential cardiovascular problems. Thus it is important to assess the patient's weight history in relation to height and build. A typical day's diet should be examined for its adequacy in relation to the patient's lifestyle. The amount of salt, saturated fats, and triglycerides in the patient's diet should be determined. In addition to actual food habits, which are influenced greatly by ethnicity, the patient's attitudes and plans in relation to diet should be investigated. Food intake and exercise patterns should be complementary.

Elimination pattern. Skin color, temperature, and turgor may provide excellent information about circulatory problems. Atherosclerosis may produce cool, cyanotic extremities, and edema may indicate heart failure. The patient on diuretics may report increased urinary elimination. Problems with constipation should be documented as straining at stool (Valsalva maneuver) should be avoided in a patient with cardiovascular problems.

Cardiovascular problems may impair the patient's ability to get to a toilet as quickly as necessary. The patient should be questioned about this if incontinence or constipation are problematic.

Activity-exercise pattern. The benefit of exercise to cardiovascular health is indisputable, with sustained aerobic exercise being most beneficial. The nurse should carefully inquire about the types of exercise done, the duration and frequency of each, and the occurrence of any unwanted effects. The length of time the exercise program has been practiced should be recorded, along with participation in individual or group sports. Any symptoms indicative of cardiovascular problems such as lightheadedness, chest pain, shortness of breath, or claudication during exercise should be noted.

The patient should also be questioned about any limitations in activities of daily living (ADL) as a result of a cardiovascular problem. Such problems are often associated with fatigue and depression, which are common symptoms of cardiac disease. The nurse should also gather information about the patient's leisure and recreational activities. Any decrease in previous abilities should be noted.

Sleep-rest pattern. Although there are many possible causes, cardiovascular problems are often the cause for interrupted sleep. Paroxysmal nocturnal dyspnea (attacks of shortness of breath especially at night that awaken the patient) are associated with advanced heart failure. Many patients with heart failure may need to sleep with their head elevated on pillows. The nurse should note the number of pillows needed for comfort.

Cognitive-perceptual pattern. It is important that the nurse ask both the patient and significant others about cognitive-perceptual problems. Any pain associated with the cardiovascular system such as chest pain and claudication should be reported. Cardiovascular problems such as dysrhythmias, hypertension, and stroke may cause problems with vertigo, language, and memory.

Self-perception–self-concept pattern. If a cardiovascular event has been of acute origin, the patient's self-perception is often affected. Invasive diagnostic and palliative procedures often lead to body image concerns for the patient. When the cardiovascular disease is chronic in nature, the patient may not be able to identify the cause but can often describe the inability to "keep up" previous levels of activity or accomplishments. This too may affect the patient's self-esteem. Hence, it is essential to inquire about the effects of the illness on the patient.

Role-relationship pattern. The patient's sex, race, and age are all related to cardiovascular health and are therefore important basic information. In addition, discussing the patient's marital status, role in the household, number of children and their ages, living environment, and significant others assist the nurse in identifying strengths and support systems in the patient's life. The nurse must assess the patient's level of satisfaction or dissatisfaction in each assigned role, which may alert the clinician to possible areas of stress or conflict.

Sexuality-reproductive pattern. The patient should be asked about the effect of the cardiovascular problem on the sexual patterns and satisfaction. It is common for the patient to have a fear of sudden death during sexual intercourse, causing a major alteration in sexual behavior. Fatigue or shortness of breath may also curtail sexual activity.

Many medications used to treat cardiovascular problems, particularly those used to treat hypertension, can result in impotence (Table 30-7). This side effect may result in noncompliance with medical treatment. Counseling of both the patient and partner may be indicated.

Coping–stress tolerance pattern. The patient should be asked to identify areas that cause stress or anxiety. Potentially stressful areas include marital relationships, family, occupation, church, friends, finances, and housing. Although many persons enjoy certain activities, these activities can be stressful at the same time that they are rewarding. The usual methods of coping with stress should be investigated. Behaviors such as explosive, rapid speech and emotions such as anger and hostility have been associated with a risk of cardiac disease.[6] The patient and the family should be asked about the frequency of these types of behavior.

Adjustment to cardiovascular disease has been linked to the degree of social support.[7] Thus information about support systems such as family, extended family and friends, psychologists, religious groups or others, may provide excellent resources for developing a plan of care.

Values-belief pattern. Individual values and beliefs, impacted greatly by culture, may play a significant role in the level of conflict a patient faces when dealing with a diagnosis of cardiovascular disease. Some patients may attribute their illness to punishment by "their God," while others may feel a "higher power" may assist them. Knowledge of a patient's values and beliefs will give the nurse and allied professionals excellent information to intervene during periods of crisis. It is also important to determine if the proposed plan of care causes any conflict with the patient's value system.

Objective Data

Physical Examination

Blood pressure. After the patient's general appearance has been observed, vital signs, including BP, heart and respiratory rate, and temperature, are taken. The BP should be measured while the patient is sitting, lying, and standing. An appropriate cuff size should be used for accurate readings. Normally there is a reduction of up to 15 mm Hg in the systolic blood pressure and 3 to 5 mm Hg in the diastolic blood pressure in the standing position. BP measurements should be taken in both arms. These readings may vary from 5 to 15 mm Hg. A greater variance indicates pathology. BP in the lower extremities is expected to be 10 mm Hg higher than in the upper extremities.

Peripheral vascular system

INSPECTION. Inspection of the skin color, hair distribution, and venous blood flow provides information about arterial blood flow and venous return. The extremities should be inspected for conditions such as edema, thrombophlebitis, varicose veins, and lesions such as stasis ulcers. Edema in the extremities can be caused by gravity, interruption of venous return, or elevation of right atrial pressure.

A measure used for assessing arterial flow to the extremities is the *capillary filling time.* The patient's nail beds are squeezed to produce blanching and observed for the return of color. With normal arterial capillary perfusion, the color will return within 3 seconds.

The large veins in the neck (*internal* and *external jugular*) should be inspected while the patient is gradually elevated to an upright position. Distention and prominent pulsations of these neck veins can be caused by right atrial pressure elevation.

PALPATION. Palpation of the pulses in the neck and extremities also provides information on arterial blood flow. The pulses should be palpated to assess the volume and

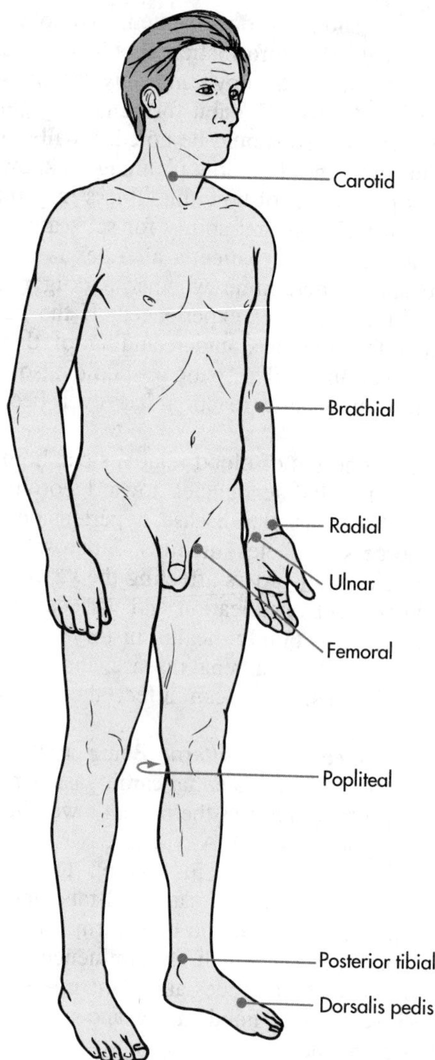

Fig. 29-8 Common sites for palpating arteries.

pressure within each vessel. Characteristics of the arteries on the right and left sides of the body should be compared. It is important to palpate each carotid pulse separately to avoid vagal stimulation and subsequent dysrhythmias.

When palpating the arteries identified in Figure 29-8, the assessor should note the pressure of the pulse wave or how far the vessel wall distends when the pulse occurs. This judgment of the pulsation volume is recorded as *normal, bounding, thready,* or *absent.* A scale may be used to document pulse volume or amplitude:[8]

0—Absent
1+ —Weak, thready
2+ —Normal
3+ —Full, bounding

The *rigidity* (hardness) of the vessel should also be noted. The normal pulse will feel like a tap, whereas a vessel wall that is narrowed or bulging will vibrate. A term for a palpable vibration is *thrill.*

Table 29-4 Common Assessment Abnormalities: Cardiovascular System

Findings	Description	Possible Etiology and Significance
Pulse		
Pulse volume		
Bounding	Sharp, brisk, rapidly rising pulse	Bradycardia, anemia, aortic valve incompetence
Thready	Weak, slowly rising pulse	Blood loss, mitral valve stenosis
Absent	Lack of pulse	Atherosclerosis, thrombus, trauma
Thrill	Vibration of vessel or chest wall	Aneurysm, aortic regurgitation
Rigidity	Stiffness or inflexibility of vessel wall	Hardening or thickening of wall, atherosclerosis
Bruit	Humming heard through stethoscope placed over vessel	Narrowing of vessel, atherosclerosis, or aneurysm
Tachycardia	Heart rate greater than 100 bpm	Exercise, anxiety, shock, need for increased cardiac output
Bradycardia	Heart rate less than 60 bpm	Rest, SA node (pacemaker) damage, athletic conditioning, side effect of drugs (e.g., β-blocker medications)
Dysrhythmia	Irregular heart rate, skipped heartbeats	Damage to cardiac conduction pathway, ischemia, side effect of drugs
Venous Abnormalities		
Distended neck veins	Vertical distance between intersection of angle of Louis and level of jugular distention greater than 3 cm with patient sitting at 45° angle	Elevated right atrial pressure
Pitting edema of lower extremities or sacral area	Visible finger indentation after application of firm pressure	Interruption of venous return to heart, fluid in tissues
Thrombophlebitis	Inflammation of vein associated with red, warm, tender, hard vein; edema, pain, tenderness of extremity	Venous stasis, damage to endothelial layer of vein, hypercoagulability of blood
Positive Homans' sign	Presence of calf pain during sharp dorsiflexion of foot	Thrombophlebitis
Skin		
Unusually warm hands or feet	Warmer than normal	Possible thyrotoxicosis and severe anemia
Cold hands or feet	Cold to touch, external covering necessary for comfort	Intermittent claudication, peripheral arterial obstruction, low cardiac output
Central cyanosis	Bluish or purplish tinge in central areas such as tongue, conjunctivae, inner surface of lips	Incomplete O_2 saturation of arterial blood due to pulmonary or cardiac disorders (e.g., congenital defects)
Peripheral cyanosis	Bluish or purplish tinge in extremities or in nose and ears	Reduced blood flow because of heart failure, vasoconstriction, cold environment
Color changes in extremities with postural change	Pallor, cyanosis, mottling of skin after limb elevation; glossy skin	Chronic decreased arterial perfusion
Stasis ulcers	Darkly pigmented, edematous areas of skin; open or oozing fluid	Poor venous return, varicose veins, incompetent venous valves
Extremities		
Clubbing of nail beds	Obliteration of normal angle between base of nail and skin	Endocarditis, congenital defects, prolonged O_2 deficiency
Splinter hemorrhages	Small red to black streaks under fingernails	Infective endocarditis (infection of endocardium, usually in area of cardiac valves)
Abnormal capillary filling time	Blanching of nail bed for more than 3 sec after release of pressure	Reduced arterial capillary perfusion, anemia
Varicose veins	Visible dilated, tortuous vessels in lower extremities	Incompetent valves in vein
Asymmetry in limb circumference	Measurable swelling of involved limb	Thrombophlebitis, varicose veins

continued

Table 29-4 Common Assessment Abnormalities: Cardiovascular System—cont'd

Findings	Description	Possible Etiology and Significance
Cardiac Auscultatory Abnormalities		
Third heart sound (S_3)	Extra heart sound, low pitched, ending in early diastole, similar to sound of a gallop	Left ventricular failure; mitral valve regurgitation, volume overload, hypertension (possible)
Fourth heart sound (S_4)	Extra heart sound, low pitched, ending in late diastole, similar to sound of a gallop	Forceful atrial contraction from resistance to ventricular filling (e.g., in left ventricular hypertrophy, pulmonary stenosis, hypertension, coronary artery disease, aortic stenosis)
Cardiac murmurs	Turbulent sounds occurring between normal heart sounds; characterization by loudness, pitch, shape, quality, duration, timing	Cardiac valve disorder, abnormal blood flow patterns

bpm, Beats per minute; *SA,* sinoatrial.

AUSCULTATION. An artery that has a narrowed or bulging wall may also create an abnormal buzzing or humming called a *bruit.* It can be heard through a stethoscope placed over the vessel. Auscultation of major arteries such as the abdominal aorta, carotids, and femoral should be part of the initial cardiovascular assessment. Abnormalities of the vascular system are described in Table 29-4.

Thorax

INSPECTION AND PALPATION. An overall inspection of the bony structures of the thorax, including the sternoclavicular joints, the manubrium, and the upper part of the sternum, is the initial step in the examination. Pulsations of the aortic arch or the innominate arteries may be observed or palpated in this area in some normal persons. Thrills caused by abnormalities of these vessels may also be detected.

The next step in examining the thorax is to inspect the areas where the cardiac valves project their sounds by identifying the *intercostal spaces* (ICSs). The raised notch, *angle of Louis,* that is created where the manubrium and the body of the sternum are joined is readily palpable in the midline of the sternum. The angle of Louis is at the level of the second rib and can therefore be used to count ICSs and locate specific auscultatory areas.

The following auscultatory areas can be located (Fig. 29-9): the *aortic area* in the second ICS to the right of the sternum, the *pulmonic area* in the second ICS to the left of the sternum, the *tricuspid area* in the fifth left ICS close to the sternum, and the *mitral area* in the left midclavicular line at the level of the fifth ICS. A fifth auscultatory area is *Erb's point,* located at the third left ICS near the sternum.

Normally, no pulsations are felt in these areas unless the patient has a thin chest wall. Valvular disorder may be suspected if abnormal pulsations or thrills are felt. Next, the epigastric area, which lies on either side of the midline just below the xyphoid process, is inspected and palpated. The pulsation of the abdominal aorta may be visible and can normally be palpated here. Next, the precordium, which is located between the apex and the sternum, is inspected for heaves. *Heaves* are sustained lifts of the chest wall in the precordial area that can be seen or palpated. They may be caused by left ventricular enlargement. Normally no pulsations are seen or felt here.

The mitral valve area is inspected for the PMI while the patient is recumbent. This pulsation or ventricular thrust normally has a short duration and lies within the midclavicular line in the fifth ICS (apex). If the PMI is not visible, the area should be palpated by placing the palm of the right hand in the apical area and feeling for the thrust. If the PMI is palpable, its position is recorded in relation to the midclavicular line and ICSs. When the PMI is left of the midclavicular line, the heart may be enlarged.

PERCUSSION. The borders of the right and left sides of the heart can be estimated by percussion. The nurse stands to the right of the recumbent patient and percusses along the curve of the rib in the fourth and fifth ICSs, starting at the midaxillary line. The percussion note over the heart is dull in comparison with the resonance over the lung and is recorded in relation to the midclavicular line.

AUSCULTATION. The movement of the cardiac valves creates some turbulence in the blood flow. The vibration of the blood causes normal heart sounds (Fig. 29-10). These sounds can be heard through a stethoscope placed on the chest wall. The first heart sound (S_1), which is associated with the closure of the tricuspid and mitral (AV) valves, has a soft *lub* sound. The second heart sound (S_2), which is associated with the closure of the aortic and pulmonic (semilunar) valves, has a sharp *dub* sound. S_1 signals the beginning of systole, the period of ventricular contraction. S_2 signals the beginning of diastole, the period of ventricular relaxation (Fig. 29-11). The nurse should listen to the auscultatory areas in sequence with both the diaphragm and bell of the stethoscope.

The first and second heart sounds are heard best with the diaphragm of the stethoscope because they are high-pitched. Extra heart sounds (S_3 or S_4), if present, are heard best with the bell of the stethoscope because they are low pitched. It is important to explain that the nurse will be listening to the

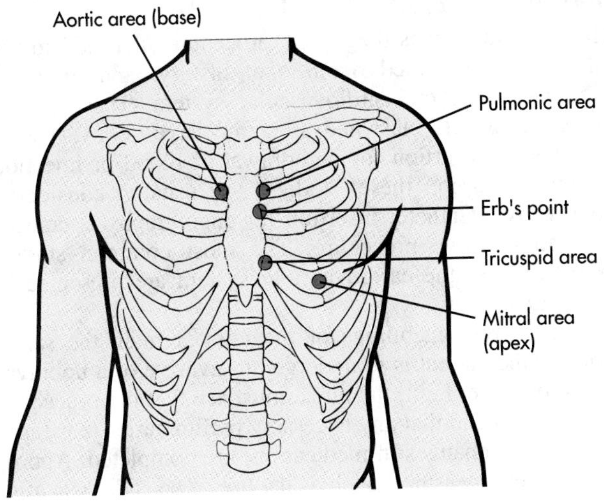

Fig. 29-9 Cardiac auscultatory areas.

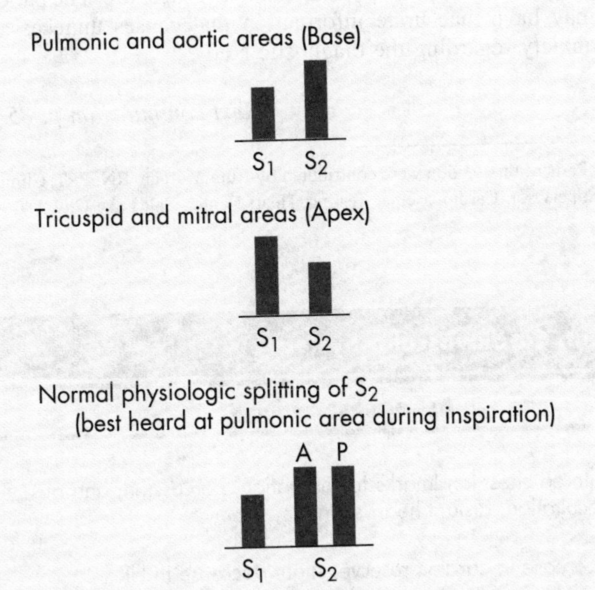

Fig. 29-10 Heart sounds. *A*, Aortic; *P*, Pulmonic.

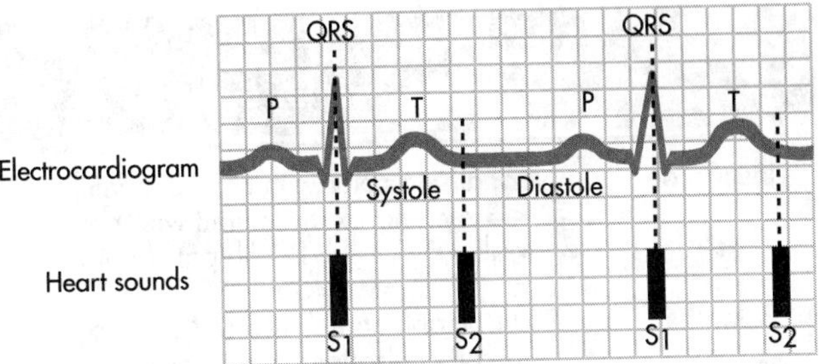

Fig. 29-11 Relationship of electrocardiogram, cardiac cycle, and heart sounds.

patient's heart in several different positions such as leaning forward while sitting and in the left lateral decubitus position. Leaning forward while sitting accentuates sounds from the second ICSs (aortic and pulmonic areas). The left lateral decubitus position accentuates sounds produced at the mitral area.

Initially the nurse listens at the apical area with the diaphragm of the stethoscope while simultaneously palpating the radial pulse. If fewer radial than apical pulses are counted, a *pulse deficit* is present. A patient with a pulse deficit should have the apical and radial pulse taken often to monitor this abnormality. A judgment about the rhythm (regular or irregular) is also made when listening at the apex.

Palpating the carotid artery while auscultating is also important because it allows differentiation of S_1 from S_2 and systole from diastole. Because S_1 (lub) occurs almost simultaneously with ventricular ejection, it is heard when the carotid pulse is felt. When listening at the other valvular areas, the nurse should always concentrate on the periods of systole and diastole as well as on the first and second heart sounds.

Normally no sound is heard between S_1 and S_2 during the periods of systole and diastole. Sounds that are heard during these periods probably represent abnormalities and should be described. An exception to this is a normal splitting of S_2, which is best heard at the pulmonic area during inspiration. Splitting of this heart sound can be abnormal if it is heard during expiration or if it is constant (fixed) during the respiratory cycle.

Murmurs are sounds produced by turbulent blood flow through the heart or the walls of large arteries. Most murmurs are the result of cardiac abnormalities, but some occur in normal cardiac structures. Murmurs are graded on a six-point scale of loudness and recorded as a Roman numeral ratio; the numerator is the intensity of the murmur and the denominator is always VI, which indicates that the six-point scale is being used. Number *I* indicates a soft, faint murmur; number *VI* indicates a murmur that can be heard without a stethoscope.[8]

If an abnormal sound is heard, it should be documented. This description should include the timing (during systole or diastole), location (the site on the chest where it is heard the loudest), pitch (heard best with the diaphragm or the bell of the stethoscope), position (heard best when patient is recumbent, sitting and leaning forward, or in the left lateral decubitus position), characteristic (harsh, musical, soft, short, long), and any other abnormal findings (irregular cardiac rhythms or palpable chest wall heaves) associated with the sound.

The abnormal sounds occurring during systole and diastole are classified as either murmurs or extra sounds. The most common abnormal sounds and abnormal assessment findings are described in Table 29-4. A method of recording data from the cardiovascular assessment is presented in

Table 29-5 Normal Physical Assessment of the Cardiovascular System

Inspection	Normal skin color with capillary refill <3 sec; thorax symmetric with no visible PMI; no JVD with patient at 45° angle
Palpation	PMI palpable in fifth ICS at MCL; no forceful pulsations, thrills, or heaves; slight palpable pulsations of abdominal aorta in epigastric area; carotid and extremity pulses 2+ and equal bilaterally; no evidence of impaired arterial flow or venous return in lower extremities
Percussion	Unable to distinguish right sided heart border
Auscultation	S_1 and S_2 heard; HR 72 and regular; no murmurs or extra heart sounds

HR, Heart rate; *ICS,* intercostal space; *JVD,* jugular venous distention; *MCL,* midclavicular line; *PMI,* point of maximum impulse.

Table 29-5. Table 29-6 lists the cardiovascular assessment changes associated with aging.

Diagnostic Studies. Diagnostic studies provide important information to the nurse in monitoring the patient's condition and planning appropriate interventions. These studies are considered to be objective data. Diagnostic studies of the cardiovascular system are presented in Table 29-7.

DIAGNOSTIC STUDIES*

There are numerous diagnostic procedures that add to the information obtained from the history and physical examination of the cardiovascular system. These procedures are usually classified as noninvasive or invasive. If only needle insertion for withdrawal of blood or injection of dye is used, these studies are usually considered noninvasive. Catheter insertion for angiography is considered an invasive procedure. The most common studies used to assess the cardiovascular system are presented in Table 29-7.

Certain responsibilities of the nurse remain the same, whether the patient is to undergo an invasive or a noninvasive procedure. First, the nurse must see that the procedure is scheduled and that any necessary preliminaries (e.g., special diets or changes in medication) are completed. Appropriate safety measures, such as the use of bedside rails after administration of preprocedure medications or identification of patient allergies, should be instituted. Comfort measures, such as oral care before the procedure, are important. The nurse must also check to see that the patient's permission for the procedure has been obtained if it is required. It is important that the patient understand the procedure. The patient may have inaccurate information that causes unnecessary anxiety regarding the diagnostic study.

(Text continued on p. 853).

*Parts of this section were contributed by Ruth Morgan, RN, PRT, Clinical Supervisor, Cardiovascular Testing, Heart Center, Salt Lake City, UT.

Table 29-6 Gerontologic Differences in Assessment: Cardiovascular System

Changes	Differences in Assessment Findings
Chest Wall	
Senile kyphosis	Altered chest landmarks for palpation, percussion, and auscultation; distant heart sounds
Heart	
Myocardial hypertrophy, increase in collagen and scarring, decrease in elasticity	Decrease in cardiac reserve, slight decrease in HR
Downward displacement	Difficulty in isolating apical pulse
Decrease in CO, HR, SV in response to exercise or stress	Slowed, decreased response to stress; slowed recovery from activity
Cellular aging changes and fibrosis of conduction system	Decrease in amplitude of QRS complex and lengthening of PR, QRS, and QT intervals; left axis deviation; irregular cardiac rhythms
Valvular rigidity from calcification, sclerosis, or fibrosis, impeding complete closure of valves	Systolic murmur (aortic or mitral) possible without being indication of cardiovascular pathology
Blood Vessels	
Arterial stiffening caused by loss of elastin in arterial walls, thickening of intima of arteries and progressive fibrosis of media	Elevation in systolic and possibly diastolic BP (e.g., 160/90); possible widened pulse pressures; more pronounced arterial pulses; pedal pulses often not detectable; color and temperature changes in extremities; loss of hair on lower legs
Increase in tortuosity and varicosities of veins	Ulcerated, inflamed, painful, or cordlike varicosities

BP, Blood pressure; *CO,* cardiac output; *HR,* heart rate; *SV,* stroke volume.

Table 29-7 Diagnostic Studies: Cardiovascular System

Study	Description and Purpose	Nursing Responsibility
Noninvasive		
Chest x-ray	Patient is placed in two upright positions to examine lung fields and size of heart. The two common positions are anterior-posterior and left lateral. Normal heart size and contour for individual's age, sex, and size noted.	Inquire about frequency of recent x-rays and possibility of pregnancy. Provide lead shielding to areas not being viewed. Remove any jewelry or metal objects that may obstruct view of heart and lungs.
ECG	Small electrodes placed on surface of chest and extremities allowing ECG machine to pick up electrical conduction patterns from different angles as they pass through heart. Technique can detect rhythm of heart, site of pacemaker, position of heart, size of atrium and ventricles, and presence of injury.	Inform patient that no discomfort is involved. Instruct patient to hold still to alleviate movement or muscle tremors.
Ambulatory ECG Monitoring		
Holter monitoring	Recording of ECG rhythm for 24-48 hr and then correlating rhythm changes with symptoms. Normal patient activity encouraged to simulate conditions that produce symptoms. Five electrodes placed on chest and recorder is used to store information until it is recalled, printed, and analyzed for any rhythm disturbance. It can be performed on an inpatient or outpatient basis.	Preparation of skin and application of electrodes and leads. Explain importance of keeping accurate diary of activities and symptoms. Tell patient that no bath or shower can be taken during monitoring.
Transtelephonic event recorders	Allows more freedom in wearing and recording than regular Holter monitor. Records rhythm disturbances that are not frequent enough to be recorded in one 24-hr period. Some units have electrodes attached to chest and have a loop of memory that captures the onset and end of an event. Other types placed directly on patient's wrist, chest, or fingers and have no loop of memory, but record patient's ECG in real time. Recordings are transmitted over the phone to a receiving unit and then printed out for review. Tracings can then be erased and unit can be reused.	Instruction in use of equipment for recording and transmitting of transient events. Careful instruction of skin preparation for lead placement or steady skin contact for units not requiring electrodes. This will ensure reception of optimal ECG tracings for analysis.
Exercise treadmill test	Various protocols used to evaluate effect of exercise tolerance on myocardial function. A common protocol uses 3 min stages at set speeds and elevation of treadmill belt. Continual monitoring of vital signs and ECG rhythms or ischemic changes important in the diagnosis of left ventricular function and coronary artery disease.	Instruct patient to wear comfortable clothes and shoes that can be used for walking and running. Instruct patient about procedure and application of lead placement. Monitor vital signs and obtain 12-lead ECG before, during each stage of exercise, and after exercise until all vital signs and ECG changes have returned to normal.
Echocardiogram M-Mode Two-dimensional Cardiac doppler Color flow imaging	Small transducer that emits and receives ultrasound waves placed in four positions on chest above heart. Transducer records sound waves that are bounced off heart. Also records direction and flow of blood through heart and transforms it to audio and graphic information that measures valvular abnormalities, congenital cardiac defects, and cardiac function.	Place patient in a supine position on left side facing equipment. Instruct family and patient about procedure and sensations (pressure and mechanical movement from head of transducer). No contraindications to procedure exist.

continued

Table 29-7 Diagnostic Studies: Cardiovascular System—cont'd

Study	Description and Purpose	Nursing Responsibility
Stress echocardiogram	Combination of exercise treadmill test and echocardiogram. Resting images of heart taken with ultrasound and then patient exercises to peak heart rate. Postexercise images taken immediately after exercise (within one minute of stopping exercise). Differences in left ventricular wall motion and thickening before and after exercise are evaluated.	Instruct and prepare patient for exercise treadmill. Inform patient that ultrasound is not harmful and the importance of speed in returning to exam table for imaging after exercise. Contraindications include any patient unable to reach peak exercise.
Dobutamine echocardiogram	Used as substitute for exercise stress test in individual unable to walk on treadmill. Dobutamine (a positive inotropic agent) infused IV and dosage increased in 5-min intervals while echocardiogram performed to detect wall motion abnormalities at each stage.	Start IV infusion. Administer dobutamine. Monitor vital signs before, during, and after test until baseline achieved. Monitor patient for signs and symptoms of distress during procedure.
Transesophageal echocardiogram	Use of a long tube or probe that has an ultrasound transducer in the tip. As patient swallows transducer end, the physician controls angle and depth from other end. As it passes down the esophagus, it sends back clear images of heart size, wall motion, valvular abnormalities, and possible source of thrombi without interference from lungs or chest ribs. Sometimes a contrast media injected intravenously for evaluating direction of blood flow if an atrial or ventricular septal defect suspected. Doppler ultrasound and color flow imaging can also be used concurrently.	Instruct patient to be NPO for at least 6 hr before test. A tranquilizer will be given and throat locally anesthetized, so if done as an outpatient, a designated driver is needed. Monitor vital signs and oxygen saturation levels and perform suctioning continually during procedure. Explain to patient proper procedure for easy passage of transducer. Assist patient to relax.
Nuclear cardiology	Study involves IV injection of radioactive isotopes. Radioactive uptake is counted over heart by scintillation camera. It supplies information about myocardial contractility, myocardial perfusion, and acute cell injury.	Explain procedure to patient. Establish IV line for injection of isotopes. Explain that radioactive isotopes used are small, diagnostic amounts and will lose most radioactivity in a few hours. Inform patient that he will be lying down on back with arms extended over head for a period of about 20-30 min.
Thallium imaging	Thallium 201 injected IV and used to evaluate blood flow in different parts of heart. Cold spots correlate with areas of infarction. For stress testing, IV thallium given 1 min before patient reaches maximum HR on bicycle or treadmill. Patient then required to continue exercise for 1 min to circulate radioactive isotope. Actual scanning must be done within 5-10 min postexercise. A second resting scan is performed 2-4 hr later and compared to postexercise.	Explain procedure to patient. Instruct patient to only eat a light meal between scans.
Dipyridamole thallium scan	As with a thallium exercise test, dipyridamole (Persantine) is also injected. Dipyridamole acts as powerful vasodilator and will increase blood flow to well-perfused coronary arteries. Scanning procedure same as with thallium scan.	Explain procedure to patient. Instruct patient not to ingest caffeine products or aminophylline 12 hr before procedure.

continued

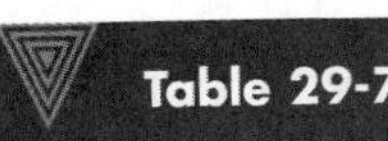

Table 29-7 Diagnostic Studies: Cardiovascular System—cont'd

Study	Description and Purpose	Nursing Responsibility
Technetium pyrophosphate scanning	Technetium 99m pyrophosphate injected IV and taken up in area of MI, producing hot spots. Maximum results produced when performed 1-6 days after suspected MI. Waiting period after injection is 1½-2 hr. Scan usually done in nuclear medicine department. It can be done in critical care unit in some hospitals.	Explain procedure to patient.
Blood pool imaging	Technetium 99m pertechnetate injected IV. Single injection allows sequential evaluation of heart for several hours. Study indicated for patient with recent MI or CHF, especially if not recovering well. It can be used to measure effectiveness of various cardiac medications and can be done at patient's bedside.	Explain procedure to patient. Inform patient that procedure involves little or no risk.
Positron emission tomography	Uses two radionuclides. Nitrogen-13-ammonia injected IV first and scanned to evaluate myocardial perfusion. A second radioactive isotope, fluoro-18-deoxyglucose then injected and scanned to show myocardial metabolic function. In normal heart, both scans will match, but in an ischemic or damaged heart, they will differ. Patient may or may not be stressed. A baseline resting scan usually obtained for comparison.	Instruct patient on procedure. Explain that he will be scanned by a machine and will need to stay still for a period. Patient's glucose level must be between 60 and 140 mg/dl (3.3-7.8 μmol/L) for accurate glucose metabolic activity. If exercise is included as part of testing, patient will need to be NPO and refrain from tobacco and caffeine before test.
Magnetic resonance imaging	Noninvasive imaging technique obtains information about cardiac tissue integrity, aneurysms, ejection fractions, CO, and patency of proximal coronary arteries. It does not involve ionizing radiation and is extremely safe procedure. It provides images in multiple planes with uniformly good resolution. It has limited use in critical care patient because of access and equipment problems. It cannot be used in person with any implanted metallic devices.	Explain procedure to patient. Inform patient that small diameter of the cylinder, along with loud noise of the procedure, may cause panic or anxiety. Antianxiety medications and music may be recommended.
Serum Enzymes	CK enzymes present in heart, skeletal muscle, and brain. Within 4-6 hr of MI, CK is elevated. It returns to normal within 48-72 hr. *Normal:* <160 U/ml (2.67 μkat/L) (male) <130 U/ml (2.17 μkat/L) (female)	Avoid CK elevation created by IM injections that damage muscle cells.
CK-MB fraction	Immunochemical process using monoclonal antibodies that measures this cardiospecific isoenzyme within 10-30 min. Concentrations >7.5 ng/ml highly indicative of MI.	Serial sampling should be done in conjunction with ECG.
AST (SGOT)	Within 6-8 hr after MI, AST rises. It peaks within 24-48 hr and returns to *normal* in 4-8 days. It is not specific to cardiac muscle damage. *Normal:* 7-40 U/ml (0.12-0.67 μkat/L)	Because AST can be elevated by other disorders such as liver damage, thorough history is important.
Myoglobin	Low molecular protein that is 99-100% sensitive for myocardial injury. Serum concentrations rise as early as 1 hr after MI and peak in 4-12 hr. *Normal:* 250-450 ng/ml	Cleared from the circulation rapidly and therefore must be measured within first 18 hr of onset of chest pain.

continued

Table 29-7 Diagnostic Studies: Cardiovascular System—cont'd

Study	Description and Purpose	Nursing Responsibility
LDH	LDH has five different isoenzymes. Pattern of elevation similar to that of AST after MI except that LDH remains elevated for 5-7 days. *Normal:* 50-150 U/L (.83-2.5 μkat/L)	When drawing blood, make certain it is not hemolyzed because will falsely raise LDH level.
LDH_1 and LDH_2	LDH isoenzyme subgroups are contained in heart muscle. Test determines LDH_1/LDH_2 ratio. If $LDH_1/LDH_2 > 1$, it is indicative of MI.	
Serum Lipids		
Cholesterol	Cholesterol is a blood lipid. Elevated cholesterol considered a risk factor for atherosclerotic heart disease. Level can be measured at any time of day in nonfasting state. *Normal level:* 140-200 mg/dl (3.62-5.17 mmol/L) (varies with age and sex)	Explain procedure to patient. Cholesterol levels can be obtained in nonfasting state but for triglyceride levels and lipoproteins, fasting state for at least 12 hr (except for water) necessary and no alcohol intake allowed for 24 hr before testing.
Triglycerides	Triglycerides are mixtures of fatty acids. Elevations associated with cardiovascular disease. *Normal:* 40-190 mg/dl (.45-2.15 mmol/L) (varies with age)	
Lipoproteins	Electrophoresis done to separate lipoproteins into HDL, LDL, and VLDL, and chylomicrons. There are marked day-to-day fluctuations in serum lipid levels. More than one determination is needed for accurate diagnosis and treatment. *Normal:* Desirable LDL is <130 mg/dl (3.4 mmol/L) (varies with age)	
Drug levels	Blood tests done to determine therapeutic and toxic levels of drugs in body.	Ensure appropriate timing of test with medication schedule.
Digoxin	Therapeutic level is 1-2 ng/ml; toxic level is >3 ng/ml.	
Quinidine	Therapeutic level is 2.5-5 μg/ml; toxic level is >5 μg/ml.	
Propranolol (Inderal)	Therapeutic level is 20-85 ng/ml; toxic level is >150 ng/ml.	
Invasive		
Cardiac catheterization	Study involves insertion of catheter into heart. Information can be obtained about O_2 saturation and pressure readings within chambers. Dye can be injected to assist in examining structure and motion of heart. Procedure is done by insertion of catheter into a vein (for right side of heart) or an artery (for left side of heart) (see text).	Before procedure, obtain written permission. Withhold food and fluids for 6-18 hr before procedure. Give sedative, if ordered. Inform patient about use of local anesthesia, insertion of catheter, and feeling of warmth and fluttering sensation of heart as catheter is passed. Note that patient may be instructed to cough or take a deep breath when catheter is inserted and that patient is monitored by ECG throughout procedure. After procedure, assess circulation to extremity used for catheter insertion. Check peripheral pulses, color, and sensation of extremity every 15 min for 1 hr and then with decreasing frequency. Observe injection site for swelling and bleeding. Place sandbag over arterial site, if indicated. Monitor vital signs. Assess for abnormal HR, dysrhythmias, and signs of pulmonary emboli (respiratory difficulty).

continued

Table 29-7 Diagnostic Studies: Cardiovascular System—cont'd

Study	Description and Purpose	Nursing Responsibility
Coronary angiography	Study involves injection of radiopaque dye directly into coronary arteries by same procedure as for cardiac catheterization. It is used to evaluate patency of coronary arteries and collateral circulation.	Same as for cardiac catheterization.
Electrophysiology study	Invasive study used to record intracardiac electrical activity using catheters (with multiple electrodes) inserted via the femoral vein into right side of heart. Catheter electrodes record the electrical activity in different cardiac structures. In addition, dysrhythmias can be induced.	Obtain written consent. Antidysrhythmic medications may need to be discontinued several days before study. Keep patient NPO 6-8 hr before test. Give premedication to promote relaxation and throughout procedure if ordered. Place patient on cardiac monitor after procedure.
Hemodynamic monitoring	Hemodynamic monitoring of arterial BPs, pulmonary artery pressures, pulmonary capillary wedge pressures, and CO discussed in Chapter 61.	
Peripheral arteriography and venography*	Study involves injection of radiopaque dye into either arteries or veins. Serial x-rays taken to detect and visualize any atherosclerotic plaques, occlusions, aneurysms, or traumatic injury.	Carefully explain procedure to patient. Give mild sedative, if ordered. Check extremity with puncture site for pulsation, warmth, color, and motion after procedure. Inspect insertion site for bleeding or swelling. Observe patient for allergic reactions to dye.
Digital subtraction angiography	This type of arteriography involves IV injection of contrast media. Catheter is threaded into superior vena cava. When contrast media circulate through arteries, computerized subtraction technique "subtracts" structures that block clear view of arteries. Most portions of cardiovascular system (except coronary arteries) can be studied by this technique. It can be performed on an outpatient basis and has fewer complications than arteriography. Fluoroscopy used to help position catheter.	Keep patient NPO 2 hr before test. Inform patient that slight feeling of warmth may be experienced as contrast medium is injected and that ECG monitoring is done throughout procedure. Explain to patient that test takes about 1 hr.

AST, Aspartate aminotransferase; *BP,* blood pressure; *CHF,* congestive heart failure; *CK,* creatine kinase; *CO,* cardiac output; *ECG,* electrocardigram; *HDL,* high-density lipoproteins; *HR,* heart rate; *IM,* intramuscular; *IV,* intravenous; *LDH,* lactic dehydrogenase; *LDL,* low-density lipoproteins; *MI,* myocardial infarction; *NPO,* nothing by mouth; *SGOT,* serum glutamic-oxaloacetic transaminase; *VLDL,* very low-density lipoproteins.
*Additional peripheral vascular diagnostic studies are found in Table 35-8.

Noninvasive Studies

Chest X-Ray. A radiographic picture can depict cardiac contours, heart size and configuration, and anatomic changes in individual chambers (Fig. 29-12). The radiographic image records any displacement or enlargement of the heart, and it is more accurate than percussion in determining the size of the heart. In addition to cardiac abnormalities, the presence of extra fluid around the heart may be detected by these radiographic images.

Electrocardiogram. The basic P, QRS, and T waveforms (Table 29-1) are used to assess cardiac function. Deviations from the normal sinus rhythm can indicate abnormalities in heart function.

There are numerous types of electrographic monitoring including *resting, exercise* or *stress testing,* and *continuous ambulatory monitoring.* A resting ECG helps to identify primary conduction abnormalities, cardiac dysrhythmias, cardiac hypertrophy, pericarditis, myocardial ischemia, site and extent of myocardial infarction (MI), pacemaker performance, and effectiveness of drug therapy. It is used to monitor recovery from an MI.

In an exercise or stress ECG, the person pedals a stationary bicycle or walks on a treadmill while ECG and BP measurements are taken to evaluate the heart's response to physical stress. This test is valuable in assessing asymptomatic cardiac disease and helping to define limits for exercise programs.

Continuous ambulatory ECG can provide more diagnostic information than a standard resting ECG, which records less than 1 minute of the heart's activity. In this test, a portable Holter monitor is attached to the patient, and the ECG is recorded during a 24- to 48-hour period while the person performs usual activities. The person records these activities in a log book so cardiac responses to level of activity can be studied.

ECG leads. Recording of an ECG involves the use of five electrodes. An electrode is placed on each of the four limbs. The right-leg electrode is used as an inactive ground

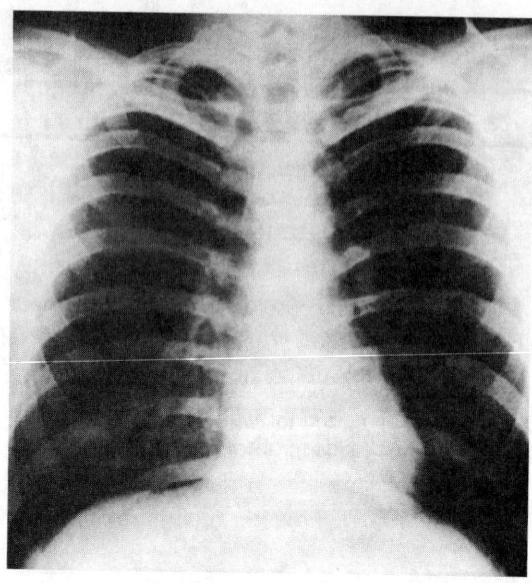

Fig. 29-12 Chest x-ray showing outline of the heart.

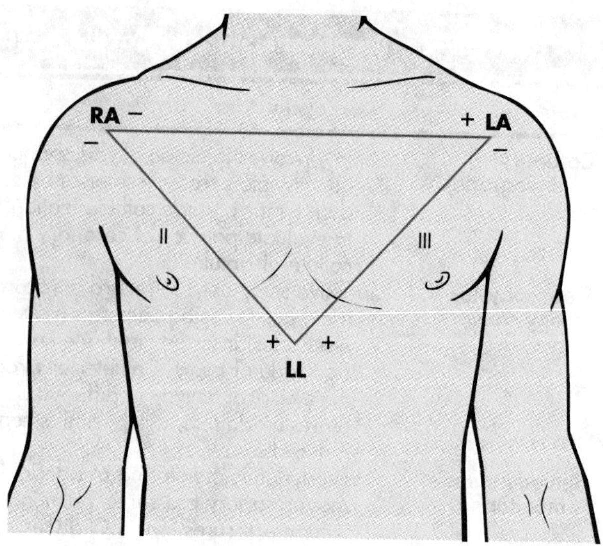

Fig. 29-13 Conventional polarity of the three standard leads is indicated by + and –.

electrode. The fifth electrode is used for various placements on the precordium.

Electrical impulses generated by the heart are picked up by the electrodes, magnified by an amplifier, and recorded. The recording is done by machines that produce a direct tracing by a stylus on paper. The paper contains a graphic background that permits rapid interpretation of the waveforms.

Each combination of electrodes used in standard electrocardiography is called a *lead.* Each lead gives a continuous recording of changes in potential (or voltage) during the cardiac cycle between any two of the electrodes or between one electrode and a combination of others.

Like a camera taking a picture from different angles, ECG leads take pictures of the myocardium. In a standard 12-lead ECG, five electrodes attached to the arms, legs, and chest measure current, or take pictures, from 12 different views or leads. The three limb leads are I, II, and III (Fig. 29-13). Lead I records the direction of electric current and voltage detected between the right- and left-arm electrodes. Lead II is a right-arm and left-leg combination. Lead III records the electrical activity using the left-arm and left-leg electrodes. The unipolar augmented limb leads (aVR, aVF and aVL) measure electrical potential between one augmented limb lead and the electrical midpoint of the remaining two leads. The fifth electrode is placed in various locations, starting at the right sternal border in the fourth ICS (V_1) and moving across the chest (V_1 through V_6), as indicated in Fig. 29-14. These are known as *chest* or *V* leads.

Unfortunately, the 12-lead ECG has limitations, with some areas of the myocardium left completely invisible to "the camera's vision." Because of lead placement, invisible areas of the myocardium include the right ventricle and the posterior wall of the left ventricle. If a more definitive diagnosis is needed for a posterior wall or right ventricular infarct, then an 18-lead ECG must be obtained. Similar to the 12-lead ECG, the additional six leads of the 18-lead ECG are obtained by moving the fifth electrode across the *right* side of the chest (Fig. 29-15).

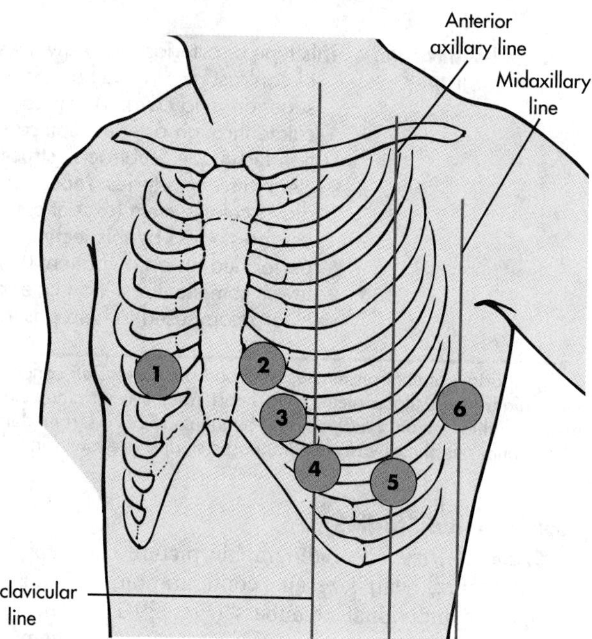

Fig. 29-14 Placement of chest leads for a 12-lead electrocardiogram.

Ambulatory Electrocardiogram Monitoring. Two types of ambulatory ECG monitoring devices include continuous (e.g., Holter monitoring) and noncontinuous (e.g., transtelephonic event recorders).

Holter monitoring. In Holter monitoring a recorder is worn by the patient for 24 to 48 hours, and the resulting

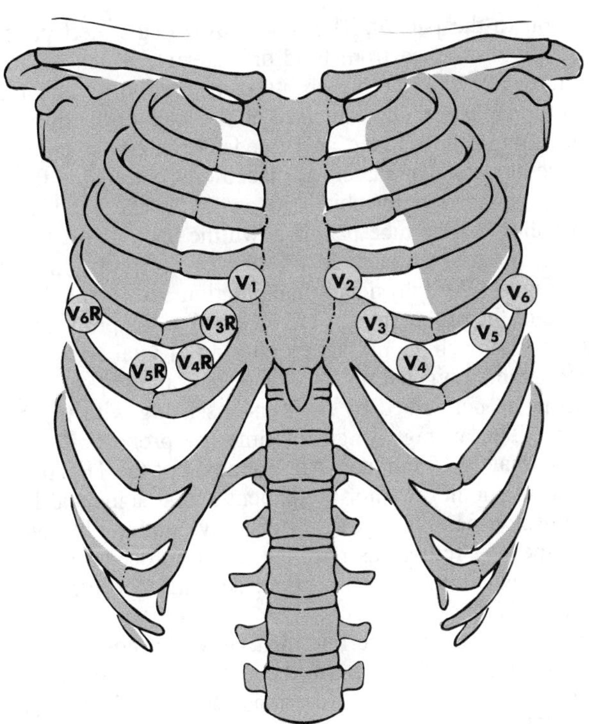

Fig. 29-15 Left precordial chest leads and right chest leads V_3R, V_4R, V_5R, V_6R.

ECG information is then stored until it is played back for printing and evaluation. Two types of recorders are used for this diagnostic technique. The first type is a conventional recorder that is battery operated and records data on magnetic tape cassettes. After the recordings are complete, they are played back, analyzed, and printed out by a specialized computer system for editing by trained personnel. The second type of recorder uses a microcomputer that analyzes the data on line and stores this for processing and immediate information without input from personnel. Both units must be worn with five electrodes attached to the chest to give either a two-channel or three-channel view of the ECG. Holter monitoring gives the patient freedom to perform those activities that are associated with the cardiovascular symptoms while documenting any ECG changes associated with these activities.

Transtelephonic event recorders. This type of ambulatory monitoring differs from Holter monitoring by allowing flexibility of use and catching those events that are not frequent enough to be recorded in a 24 to 48 hour period. These devices are also battery operated and carried by the patient. The size of these units ranges from a small transistor radio to a 3 inch by 1 inch rectangle that allows the patient freedom of movement and ease of recording events. While some of the units have electrodes that need to be attached to the chest area, others have metal conducting surfaces that will also pick up ECG tracings when moistened and placed on the chest, wrist, or finger. Once events are stored in memory, the patient can transmit the tracings over the phone to a receiving unit that prints out the ECG tracing for analysis. The tracings on the event recorder can then be erased, and the unit can be used again until documentation of symptoms or rhythm disturbances has been completed. A disadvantage of this type of monitoring is that if the event occurs for only a short duration, the symptoms may be over before the patient puts on the device.

Exercise Treadmill Testing. This test is set up in protocols that define the length of each step as well as the speed and elevation of the treadmill belt. The placement of electrodes is similar to a regular 12-lead placement for the chest leads V1 through V6. However, the limb-lead placement is altered to reduce the amount of muscle interference on the ECG while exercising. Limb leads are placed on upper and lower chest walls to alleviate muscle interference during exercise. Resting blood pressures and ECGs are performed in the supine position, while standing, and after hyperventilation to provide a baseline for comparison of any changes during exercise. These are performed because hyperventilation and a change in position can often change the appearance of the ECG.

As the patient exercises, the blood pressure, ECG, and often the oxygen saturation level are measured and monitored to make certain that the test is performed safely. The patient exercises to either peak HR (calculated by subtracting the person's age from 220) or to peak exercise tolerance at which time the test is terminated and the treadmill is slowed while the patient continues walking. (The test can also be terminated for moderate to severe chest discomfort, or significant ST segment depression indicating ischemic changes associated with coronary artery disease.) After the treadmill belt is stopped, the patient lies down to rest. The ECG is monitored postexercise for rhythm disturbances or, if ECG changes did occur with exercise, for return to baseline.

There are certain instances where regular treadmill tests are not indicated for diagnosing coronary artery disease (CAD). These include situations where existing left bundle branch blocks, predominantly paced rhythms, and ECG changes caused by medications (e.g., digoxin) are present. Other factors that influence the results of the test are electrolyte imbalances, severe hypertension, or the inability to reach maximum HR. Other treadmill procedures like thallium perfusion scans or exercise echocardiograms may be more accurate in these situations. If the patient is unable to exercise, dobutamine echocardiograms may be used. Dobutamine will stimulate the HR to mimic the ECG response to exercise.

Echocardiogram. The echocardiogram (ultrasound cardiogram) uses ultrasound waves (high-frequency sound waves) to record the movement of the structures of the heart. In the normal heart, ultrasonic sound waves directed at the heart are reflected back in typical configurations (Fig. 29-16). The echocardiogram provides information about abnormalities of (1) valvular structure and motion, (2) cardiac chamber size and contents, (3) ventricular muscle and septal motion and thickness, (4) the pericardial sac, and (5) the ascending aorta.

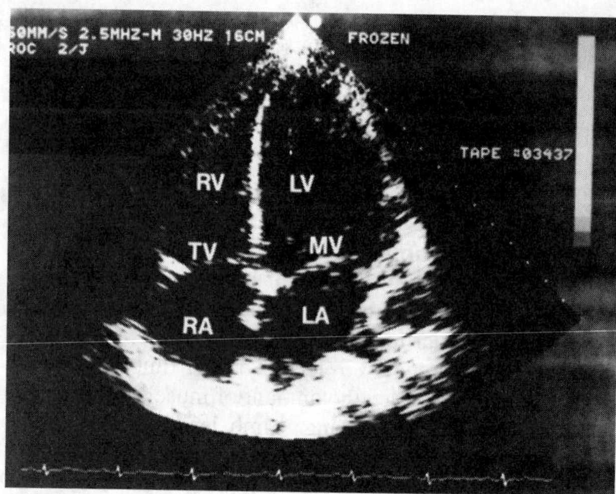

Fig. 29-16 Apical four-chamber two-dimensional echocardiographic view in a normal patient. *LA,* Left atrium; *RA,* right atrium; *TV,* tricuspid valve; *LV,* left ventricle; *RV,* right ventricle; *MV,* mitral valve.

Two commonly used types are the *M-mode* (motion-mode) and the *two-dimensional* (2-D, real-time, cross-sectional) echocardiogram. In the M-mode, a single ultrasound beam is directed toward the heart, recording the motion of the intracardiac structures, as well as detecting wall thickness and chamber size. The 2-D echocardiogram sweeps the ultrasound beam through an arc, producing a cross-sectional view in real time, and shows correct spatial relationships among the structures. Abnormalities in myocardial wall motion can be detected by a 2-D echocardiogram before the electrical changes are noted on an ECG. Thus 2-D echocardiography has been shown to be an adjunctive tool in the diagnosis of an acute myocardial infarction when the patient has a positive clinical history but a nondiagnostic ECG.[9]

Transesophageal echocardiography (TEE), a form of M-mode echocardiography, is used when a traditional approach is nondiagnostic. The TEE uses a modified, flexible endoscope probe with an ultrasound transducer in the tip for imaging of the heart and great vessels. This probe is attached to the regular ultrasound machine so that M-mode, 2-D images, pulsed doppler, and color flow imaging can be used. The TEE provides information on left ventricular function and wall motion. In addition, it can evaluate valvular prosthetic dysfunction, bacterial endocarditis, congenital heart disease, aortic dissection, and aortic aneurysm.[10]

This technique can be used in more than one setting. It has proven helpful in intraoperative procedures because it does not interfere with the operative field and provides continuous monitoring of heart function. Knowledge regarding the adequacy of valve repair, valve replacement, and septal closures can be obtained before removal of cardiopulmonary bypass.

Outpatient TEE procedures are becoming more popular with the advantage of equipment availability and cost reduction to the patient. The procedure for the alert patient requires abstinence from food or water for at least 6 to 8 hours to alleviate the possibility of aspiration. Oropharyngeal topical anesthetics are used on the back of the throat to reduce gag reflexes, and an IV sedative is administered to reduce anxiety. The patient is placed on the left side facing the equipment with the chin bent toward the chest and is told to swallow as the tube passes down the back of the throat. This helps to facilitate the passage of the probe into the esophagus. With physician manipulation and angulation of the tip of the probe, images are obtained as the probe passes into the stomach. Continual monitoring of vital signs, heart rhythm, and oxygenation status and suctioning of secretions need to be performed by the nurse assisting with the procedure. The average length of time the probe is down is approximately 15 minutes. After removal of the TEE probe, the nurse should monitor the patient's vital signs and level of consciousness. The patient must have nothing by mouth until the gag reflex has returned. If the procedure is performed on an outpatient basis, a designated driver is required.

The risks of TEE are minimal. However, complications may include perforation of the esophagus, hemorrhage, dysrhythmias, vasovagal reactions, and transient hypoxemia. TEE is contraindicated if the patient has a history of esophageal disorders, dysphagia, or radiation therapy to the chest wall.

An additional measurement used in conjunction with the echocardiogram is the *cardiac doppler.* Like the echocardiogram, it is based on the doppler effect, which refers to a change in frequency of sound, light, or other waves caused by the motion of the source. The classic example is the change in the pitch of a train whistle as it moves past a stationary observer. The cardiac doppler adds quantitative and qualitative information on valvular abnormalities, congenital cardiac defects, and cardiac function. The characteristics of the measured blood flow can be evaluated by means of the audio and graphic display of the spectral analysis that is seen along with the echocardiographic imaging.[11]

One of the newest developments in cardiac ultrasound is doppler color flow imaging (CFI) or color doppler echocardiography. This technology is a combination of doppler flow information and 2-D echo imaging. The different colors seen on the echo image provide information about both direction and velocity of blood flow. Thus this technology has provided the best anatomically and physiologically correct picture of blood flow through the beating heart. Detection of pathologic conditions, such as valvular leaks and congenital defects (septal defects), can be diagnosed with much greater ease.[11]

Stress echocardiography, a combination of treadmill test and ultrasound images, evaluates segmental wall motion abnormalities.[12] By using a digital computer system to produce images before and after exercise, wall motion and segmental function can be clearly seen. Baseline echo images are taken, and the patient is exercised to either maximum HR or peak exercise tolerance. The treadmill is then terminated abruptly, and the patient lies down again in the imaging position on the left side. Postexercise images are stored for comparison with resting images.

To ensure accuracy of results, this test must be done immediately after exercise because within 1 minute after exercise the heart begins returning to normal function. This test adds only 10 to 15 minutes to a routine treadmill test and is a relatively low-cost, noninvasive procedure compared with the traditional cardiac radionuclide diagnostic examinations. There can be false-positive tests caused by severe hypertension or left bundle branch block with diffuse wall motion abnormalities at rest. False-negative tests may be caused by a delay in obtaining postexercise images and inability of the patient to reach peak maximal exercise.

Stress echocardiogram is particularly beneficial when (1) routine treadmill tests are nondiagnostic and further evaluation is needed, (2) factors make ECG uninterpretable for ischemic changes (e.g., in the presence of left bundle branch block, pacemakers, left ventricular hypertrophy, or medication changes), and (3) in women who often have an increased incidence of false-positive treadmill tests.

Nuclear Cardiology. Radioactive tracer studies are being used with increasing frequency to diagnose cardiovascular problems. Small amounts of radioactive isotopes are injected IV, and recordings are made of the radioactivity emitted over a specific area of the body. The total radiation exposure is minimal. The circulation of this tagged material can be used to detect coronary artery blood flow, intracardiac shunts, motion of ventricles, and size of the heart chambers. This procedure is also used in evaluating the site and extent of myocardial ischemia or infarction. The most commonly used nuclear imaging tests include thallium imaging, technetium pyrophosphate scanning, and blood pool imaging.[13]

Thallium imaging. Thallium imaging (also called *myocardial perfusion imaging*) involves the injection of thallium-201, an analogue of potassium. After IV injection, it accumulates in various regions of the myocardium in direct proportion to myocardial blood flow. Then it is subsequently taken up by healthy, viable myocardial cells. In the presence of severe coronary artery narrowing and decreased blood flow to an area, the accumulation of thallium in that area is decreased. This is referred to as a *perfusion defect.* Areas that do not take up thallium are often referred to as *cold spots* on the scan. Perfusion defects usually correlate with the degree of the myocardial ischemia or infarction.

Perfusion imaging with thallium is also used with exercise testing to determine whether the coronary blood flow changes with increased activity. Stress exercising imaging may show an abnormality even when a resting image is normal. This procedure is indicated to diagnose coronary artery disease, determine the prognosis in already diagnosed coronary disease, assess the physiologic significance of a known coronary lesion, and assess the effectiveness of various therapeutic modalities such as bypass surgery or angioplasty.[13]

If a patient is unable to tolerate exercise for a thallium stress test, then dipyridamole-thallium testing is an appropriate alternative. In this test an IV infusion of dipyridamole (Persantine) is given to dilate the coronary arteries and therefore simulate the effect of exercise. After the dipyridamole takes effect, the thallium is injected and the procedure proceeds. The patient is required to lie flat for 40 minutes while the pictures are taken.[13] Several hours later, repeat studies must be done. The patient must have nothing by mouth until the thallium imaging is complete. All caffeine and theophylline products must be held 12 hours before the study.

Technetium pyrophosphate scanning. This technique involves injection of the radionuclide technetium 99m pyrophosphate. In contrast to thallium, this radioisotope accumulates in ischemic or damaged myocardial tissue, thus forming a *hot spot* on the scan. This test can be used to detect and define the location and size of an acute MI, but it does not indicate old areas of infarction. It is most reliable when performed between 24 and 72 hours after the onset of symptoms. The patient with unstable angina pectoris may undergo these studies to differentiate chest pain from an acute MI. It is also valuable in diagnosing an acute MI when ECG or cardiac enzymes tests are inconclusive.

Blood pool imaging. Blood pool imaging (also called *radionuclide angiocardiography*) involves the IV injection of technetium 99m pertechnetate. It differs from the previous two tests in that the isotope stays in the bloodstream and is not picked up by myocardial tissue. In first-pass imaging the radioactivity is followed through the circulatory system with a scintillation camera. The size, shape, and sequence of filling of the various chambers of the heart can be studied. This allows for evaluation of right and left ventricular function, wall motion of both ventricles, and calculation of the ejection fraction (portion of isotope ejected during each heartbeat).

After the first-pass imaging, images of the blood pool of the heart throughout the cardiac cycle (*gated cardiac blood pool studies*) can be done. The radioisotope is tagged in vivo or in vitro to RBCs, and a scan of the heart then simultaneously reveals all the cardiac chambers and great blood vessels. The patient's ECG provides a gate, or physiologic marker, of when end diastole and end systole occur within the cardiac cycle. Multiple-gated acquisition scanning (MUGA), or blood pool imaging, can be used to record 16 to 32 points of a single cardiac cycle, yielding sequential images that can be studied like motion picture films. These studies can also be combined with exercise to evaluate cardiac reserve and function.

Positron emission tomography. Positron emission tomography (PET) is similar to thallium imaging, but it goes one step further in the evaluation of CAD by showing myocardial tissue viability. The patient is given nitroglycerin-13-ammonia, the first of two IV injections of radioisotope tracer to evaluate myocardial perfusion. Before this scan the patient may or may not exercise physically or exercise can be simulated with the use of drugs. A second IV injection or radioactive tracer is given, fluoro-18-deoxyglucose, to demonstrate myocardial metabolic function. This is determined by the level of glucose taken up by the cells. The two scans are then compared. In the normal heart, the scans will match in perfusion and metabolic function, but in the ischemic heart, the results will show a decrease in perfusion with an increase in the glucose metabolism.[14] This is because oxygen-deprived cells metabolize glucose more readily than normal tissue. Therefore the patient's blood glucose level must be normal for the metabolic function to be correct.

PET's ability to distinguish between viable and nonviable myocardial tissue allows for the identification of the appropriate candidates for bypass surgery or angioplasty. It is the most accurate of all diagnostic tests in the evaluation of CAD in both the symptomatic and asymptomatic patient. PET is not yet commonly used in most institutions because of the high cost of equipment and the short half-life of the isotopes needed for the study.

Indium-111 antimyosin antibody imaging. Antimyosin imaging is a new technique that involves the use of an antibody to myosin. This antibody, produced by recombinant deoxyribonucleic acid (DNA) technology, is specific for human cardiac myosin. Whereas other diagnostic techniques cannot always distinguish the stages of tissue damage and differentiate between acute and prior infarction, this antibody when labeled with radioisotope indium-111 can specifically detect necrotic myocardium. This technique has proven to be beneficial in the diagnosis of acute myocardial infarction (MI) when the results of ECG analysis or enzyme studies are inconclusive.[15]

Gloves must be worn when handling body fluids from these patients for at least 3 days after the injection. Like other radioactive procedures, exposure is contraindicated during pregnancy.

Antimyosin antibody imaging holds promise for diagnosis of a known or suspected acute MI. This procedure also has the potential to be used for detection of other conditions such as cardiac transplant rejection and myocarditis. In addition, because of the ability to identify areas of ischemia, this procedure may permit physicians to practice more aggressive management strategies for the patient at high risk.

Magnetic Resonance Imaging. Although not widely used because of equipment size and access, magnetic resonance imaging (MRI) allows detection and localization of MI areas. Some studies have shown that an MRI is comparable to other established imaging modalities in assessing infarct size and location.[16] Further research is needed to determine if this imaging technique will become more commonly used in diagnosing cardiac problems.

Blood Tests. There are numerous blood studies that contribute information about the cardiovascular system. For example, studies of the blood itself reflect the O_2 carrying capacity (RBC count and hemoglobin) and coagulation properties (clotting times). (See Chapter 27 for hematology studies.)

Enzymes. When cells are injured, they release their enzymes into the circulation. The enzymes characteristic of cardiac injury are creatine kinase (CK), lactic dehydrogenase (LDH), and serum aspartate aminotransferase (AST), formerly called serum glutamic-oxaloacetic transaminase (SGOT). Because these enzymes are found in a variety of body tissues, they can be elevated as a result of injury to the muscles, liver, and other organs. For example, an elevation of LDH can indicate heart, liver, skeletal muscle, lung, or kidney damage. For this reason, *isoenzymes,* multiple forms of an enzyme that have the same function, can be identified by electrophoresis and are organ specific. Their determination is a better indicator of cardiac injury than assessment of the total enzymes.

There are five isoenzymes of LDH, with LDH_1 and LDH_2 primarily found in the heart, RBCs, and kidneys; LDH_3 found in the lungs; and LDH_4 and LDH_5 found in the liver and skeletal muscle. Usually LDH_1 and LDH_2 levels rise 8 to 12 hours after an acute MI. An elevated LDH level in which LDH_1 levels exceed LDH_2 levels (the reversal of their normal pattern) is a reliable indication of acute MI.

AST is present in the heart, liver, skeletal muscles, kidneys, pancreas, and RBCs. Although a high correlation exists between an MI and elevated AST levels, no heart-specific isoenzymes exist to assist in identifying the specific organ damaged. Therefore testing for AST in assessment of myocardial injury is often considered superfluous.

CK is present in heart muscle, skeletal muscle, and brain tissue. CK-MM is found primarily in skeletal muscle, and the CK-BB is found in the brain and nervous tissue. CK-MB elevation is specific for myocardial tissue injury, and a rise may be detected within 2 to 4 hours after an MI.[17] CK-MB has been the "gold standard" in measuring the extent of myocardial damage. However, the traditional methodology (electrophoresis) to perform this test may take 1 to 2 hours, thereby decreasing the crucial "time-to-treatment" for the patient with acute chest pain. A rapid quantitative immunochemical determination of CK-MB using monoclonal antibody technology has now been developed and can confirm the diagnosis of acute MI within 10 minutes. In addition to the use of this assay, the nurse may perform a bedside test using reagent strips to determine CK-MB levels.[18]

Myoglobin and myosin light chains are two other markers of acute MI that are providing new techniques for diagnosis.[19] Myoglobin elevation is a sensitive indicator of myocardial injury, and serum elevations occur within 1 hour of injury. Although not currently in widespread use, these tests should prove to be beneficial in the early identification of myocardial infarction and may prevent inappropriate discharge from the emergency department.[19]

Blood lipids. Blood lipids consist of triglycerides, cholesterol, and phospholipids. They circulate in the blood bound to protein. Thus they are often referred to as *lipoproteins.*

Triglycerides are the main storage form of lipids and constitute approximately 95% of fatty tissue. *Cholesterol,* a structural component of cell membranes and plasma lipoproteins, is a precursor of glucocorticoids, sex hormones, and bile salts. In addition to being absorbed from food in the GI tract, cholesterol can also be synthesized in the liver. *Phospholipids* contain glycerol, fatty acids, phosphates, and a nitrogenous compound. Although formed in most cells, phospholipids usually enter the circulation as lipoproteins synthesized by the liver. *Apoproteins* are water-soluble proteins that combine with most lipids to form lipoproteins.

Different classes of lipoproteins contain varying amounts of the naturally occurring lipids. Electrophoresis is done to separate lipoproteins into the following groups:

1. *Chylomicrons:* Primarily exogenous triglycerides from dietary fat
2. *Very low-density lipoproteins* (VLDL): Primarily endogenous triglycerides with moderate amounts of phospholipids and cholesterol
3. *Low-density lipoproteins* (LDL): Mostly cholesterol with moderate amounts of phospholipids
4. *High-density lipoproteins* (HDL): About one-half protein and one-half phospholipids and cholesterol

An elevation in LDL has a strong and direct association with CAD; increased HDL has been inversely associated with the risk of CAD. High levels of HDL serve a protective role by mobilizing cholesterol from tissues. Although the association between elevated serum cholesterol levels and CAD exists, determination of total cholesterol level is not sufficient for the assessment of coronary risk. It is important to determine whether elevated cholesterol levels are related to increased LDL or HDL.

Two important considerations in the measurement of blood lipid levels are that the patient has to be fasting (12 to 14 hours) for useful information to be obtained and that there can be marked fluctuations from day to day in the same person. Therefore several measurements should be made before a definite diagnosis is made and dietary or drug therapy is implemented.

Recent evidence indicates that levels of plasma apolipoprotein A-1 (the major HDL protein) and apolipoprotein B (the major LDL protein) are better predictors of CAD than HDL or LDL. Therefore measurements of these lipoproteins may replace cholesterol-lipoprotein determinations in assessing the risk of CAD. (Blood lipids and their relationship to coronary artery disease are discussed in Chapter 31.)

Invasive Studies

Cardiac Catheterization. Cardiac catheterization is a definitive means of obtaining information about cardiac disorders. This procedure can be used to measure intracardiac pressures and O_2 levels in various parts of the heart, as well as CO. With injection of dye and x-ray visualization, the chambers of the heart can be outlined.

Cardiac catheterization is performed by insertion of a radiopaque catheter into the right or left side of the heart. For the right side of the heart, a catheter is inserted through an arm vein (basilic or cephalic) or a leg vein (femoral). The catheter is advanced into the vena cava, the right atrium, and the right ventricle. The catheter is further inserted into the pulmonary artery, where it can be wedged or lodged in position. This position is called the *pulmonary capillary wedge* position and can be used to measure pressures reflecting the function of the left side of the heart.

The left-sided approach is performed by insertion of a catheter into the brachial artery or the femoral artery. The catheter is passed in a retrograde manner up the aorta, across the aortic valve, and into the left ventricle.

Blood is taken from various chambers and analyzed for its O_2 content. Pressures in the various chambers are recorded. With the use of dye injections, the structures of the heart can be visualized, and the size of the chambers can be determined.

Complications of cardiac catheterization include looping, kinking, or breaking off of the catheter; blood loss; allergic reaction to the dye; infection, thrombus formation; air or blood embolism; dysrhythmias; MI; cerebrovascular accident; puncture of the ventricles, cardiac septum, lung tissue; and rarely, death.

The nurse has preprocedure and postprocedure responsibilities for the patient undergoing cardiac catheterization. The patient should be told how long the catheterization procedure will take (2 to 3 hours) and where it will take place. Most hospitals have a cardiac catheterization laboratory specifically designed for the procedure. (See Table 29-7 for the nursing responsibilities related to cardiac catheterization.)

Coronary Angiography. Coronary angiography (arteriography) is often done in conjunction with a cardiac catheterization. The left-sided catheter approach is modified so that the catheters are inserted up the aorta and into the openings of the coronary arteries. Dye is injected and x-rays are taken. The patient should be informed that a flush may be felt when the dye is injected. This procedure is useful in identifying any lesions, obstructions, or collateral circulation of the coronary arteries.

Coronary angiography is used to obtain information about the presence and severity of CAD. This is needed to confirm the diagnosis and to determine the therapy. The nursing responsibilities for this procedure are similar to those for a patient with a cardiac catheterization.

Electrophysiology Study. Electrophysiology study (EPS) is the direct study and manipulation of the electrical activity of the heart using electrodes placed inside the cardiac chambers. It provides information on sinus node function, atrioventricular conduction, and tachydysrhythmias. The individual who is considered for EPS includes someone with a history of syncope or cardiac electrical problems not diagnosed by noninvasive diagnostic studies.

Catheters are inserted via the femoral vein into the right side of the heart. These catheters are placed at specific anatomic sites within the heart to record electrical activity. Dysrhythmias can be triggered and treated with medication or defibrillation. EPS can provide valuable diagnostic information that can be used to guide management of the patient with significant dysrhythmias.

Blood Flow and Pressure Measurements

Peripheral vessel blood flow. Peripheral vessel blood flow can be assessed by injection of radiopaque material (arteriography and venography). With these tests, arterial occlusions and venous abnormalities can be located. (Additional studies of peripheral blood vessels are discussed in Chapter 35.)

Hemodynamic monitoring. Hemodynamic bedside monitoring of pressures of the cardiovascular system are frequently used to assess cardiovascular status. Invasive hemodynamic monitoring using intraarterial and pulmonary artery catheters can be used to monitor arterial BP, intracardiac pressures, and CO (see Chapter 61). *Central venous pressure* (CVP) monitoring is indicated when a patient has a significant alteration in fluid volume. The CVP reflects the pressure in the right atrium and is a measurement of preload. The CVP can be used as a guide in fluid volume replacement in hypovolemia and to assess the effect of diuretic administration in fluid overload.

CVP can be measured with a pulmonary artery catheter (see Chapter 61) or a central venous line threaded through the jugular or subclavian vein into the superior vena cava. Two different methods to take CVP measurements include a mercury (mm Hg) system or a water (cm H_2O) manometer system. The end of the catheter is connected to a three-way stopcock, a fluid system, and a water manometer or to a pressure transducer. The normal CVP is 2 to 9 mm Hg (3 to 12 cm H_2O).

For an accurate reading, the base of the manometer should be at the level of the right atrium. The pressure readings directly reflect the right ventricular filling and diastolic pressure. The CVP reading is influenced by the function of the left side of the heart, pressures in the pulmonary vessels, venous return to the heart, and the position of the patient when the reading is taken. The last factor must be kept in mind to obtain an accurate reading. The CVP reading is used less frequently since the introduction of pulmonary artery catheters.

REVIEW QUESTIONS

The number of the question corresponds to the same-numbered objective at the beginning of the chapter.

1. A semilunar valve is located between the
a. vena cava and right atrium.
b. right atrium and right ventricle.
c. right ventricle and pulmonary artery.
d. left atrium and left ventricle.

2. If a person had an MI of the anterior wall of the left ventricle, which of the following arteries is most likely occluded?
a. Left circumflex artery
b. Left anterior descending artery
c. Right marginal artery
d. Right anterior descending artery

3. Which of the following structures is *not* involved in the conduction pathway of the heart?
a. Sinuses of Valsalva
b. Purkinje fibers
c. Bundle branches
d. Bundle of His

4. At the level of which of the following blood vessels does diffusion of nutrients and metabolites occur?
a. Venules
b. Arterioles
c. Arteries
d. Capillaries

5. Chemoreceptors in the arch of the aorta and carotid body are stimulated by
a. decreased PCO_2.
b. increased pH.
c. decreased PO_2.
d. increased arterial pressure.

6. The purpose of testing for capillary filling time is to assess
a. arterial flow to the extremities.
b. venous circulation to the hands.
c. lymphatic obstruction of venous return.
d. thrombus formation in veins.

7. The auscultatory area in the left midclavicular line at the level of the fifth ICS is the
a. tricuspid area.
b. mitral area.
c. aortic area.
d. pulmonic area.

8. Palpable precordial thrills may be caused by
a. heart murmurs.
b. pulmonary edema.
c. gallop rhythms.
d. right ventricular hypertrophy.

9. Which of the following is not a cardiovascular change associated with aging?
a. Increased collagen in cardiac structures
b. Decreased resting HR
c. Decreased number of pacemaker cells
d. Calcification of cardiac valves

10. Which of the following is an important nursing responsibility for a patient having an invasive cardiovascular diagnostic study?
a. Tell patient that general anesthesia will be given.
b. Instruct patient to do a surgical scrub of the insertion site.
c. Check the peripheral pulses and percutaneous site.
d. Instruct patient about radioactive isotope injection.

11. A P wave on an ECG represents an impulse arising at the
a. AV node and spreading to the bundle of His.
b. AV node and depolarizing the atria.
c. SA node and repolarizing the atria.
d. SA node and depolarizing the atria.

REFERENCES

1. West CM: Ischemia. In Carrierii-Kohlman VK, Lindsey AM, West CM, editors: *Pathophysiological phenomena in nursing: human response to illness*, ed 2, Philadelphia, 1993, Saunders.
2. Eagan JS, Stewart SL, Vitello-Cicciu JM. *Quick reference to cardiac critical care nursing*, Gaithersburg, MD, 1991, Aspen Publ.
3. Clochesy JM and others: Cardiovascular anatomy and physiology. In Clochesy JM and others, editors: *Critical care nursing*, Philadelphia, 1993, Saunders.
4. Guzzetta CE, Dossey BM: *Cardiovascular nursing: holistic practice*, St Louis, 1992, Mosby.
5. Gawlinski A, Jensen GA: The complications of cardiovascular aging, *Am J Nurs* 11:26, 1991.
6. Friedman M: Type A behavior: its diagnosis, cardiovascular relation and the effect of its modification on recurrence of coronary artery disease, *Am J Cardiol* 64:12C, 1989.
7. Riegel B: Social support and psychological adjustment to chronic coronary heart disease: operationalization of Johnson's behavioral system model, *Adv Nurs Sci* 11:74, 1989.

8. Canobbio MM: *Cardiovascular disorders,* St Louis, 1990, Mosby.
9. Sabia P and others: Value of regional wall motion abnormality in the emergency room diagnosis of acute myocardial infarction, *Circulation* 84:185, 1991.
10. Beattie S, Meinhardt S: Transesophageal echocardiography: advanced technology for the cardiac patient, *Crit Care Nurse* 12:42, 1992.
11. Obeid A: Introduction to color doppler. In Obeid A, editor: *Echocardiography in clinical practice,* Philadelphia, 1992, Lippincott.
12. Obeid A: *Echocardiography in clinical practice,* Philadelphia, 1992, Lippincott.
13. Hochrein MA, Sohl L: Heart smart: a guide to cardiac tests, *Am J Nurs* 92:22, 1992.
14. Weikart CJ: New eye into the heart, *RN* 56:36, 1993.
15. Cimini DM: Indium-111 antimyosin antibody imaging: a promising new technique in the diagnosis of MI, *Crit Care Nurse* 12:44, 1992.
16. Krauss XH and others: Magnetic resonance imaging of myocardial infarction: correlation with enzymatic angiographic and radionuclide findings, *Am Heart J* 122:1274, 1991.
17. Gibler WB and others: Acute myocardial infarction in chest pain patient with nondiagnostic ECGs: serial CK-MB sampling in the emergency department, *Emerg Med* 21:504, 1992.
18. Downie AC and others: Bedside measurement of creatine kinase to get thrombolysis on the coronary care unit, *Lancet* 341:452, 1993.
19. Tucker JF and others: *Value of serial myoglobin values in the early diagnosis of acute myocardial infarction.* Abstracts of the 1992 Scientific Assembly, American College of Emergency Physicians, September, 1992.

Chapter 30

NURSING ROLE IN MANAGEMENT

Hypertension

Dee J. Trottier

Learning Objectives

1. Describe the mechanisms involved in the regulation of normal blood pressure.
2. Identify the risk factors associated with essential hypertension.
3. Describe the clinical manifestations and complications of hypertension.
4. Describe strategies for the primary prevention of essential hypertension.
5. Describe the therapeutic, pharmacologic, and dietary management of hypertension.
6. Discuss the management of the older adult patient with hypertension.
7. Describe the nursing management of the patient with hypertension, emphasizing patient education.
8. Describe the differences between clinical manifestations and management of hypertensive emergencies and hypertensive urgencies.

NORMAL REGULATION OF BLOOD PRESSURE

Blood pressure is primarily a function of cardiac output and systemic vascular resistance. The relationship is summarized by the following equation:

$$\text{Arterial blood pressure} = \text{Cardiac output} \times \text{Systemic vascular resistance}$$

Cardiac output (CO) is defined as the *stroke volume* (amount of blood pumped out of the left ventricle per beat [approximately 70 ml]) multiplied by the heart rate (HR) for 1 minute. CO is the major determinant of systolic blood pressure (SBP). *Systemic vascular resistance* (SVR) refers primarily to the vasomotor tone of the blood vessels in the peripheral vascular system. SVR is the force opposing the movement of blood. This force is created primarily in the small arteries and arterioles. A small change in the diameter of the arterioles creates a major change in the SVR. The venules can hold large amounts of the blood volume. If SVR is increased, a greater amount of pressure is needed to force the blood around the circulatory pathways and the work load of the heart is increased. SVR primarily affects the diastolic blood pressure (DBP).

The mechanisms that regulate blood pressure (BP) can affect either CO or SVR, or both. Regulation of BP is a complex process involving the nervous, renal, cardiovascular, and endocrine systems (Fig. 30-1). BP is regulated by both short-term (seconds to hours) and long-term (days to weeks) mechanisms. Short-term mechanisms are neural processes including baroreceptors and the autonomic nervous system. Long-term processes are hormonal and renal mechanisms that regulate arterial resistance and blood volume.

Nervous System

Sympathetic Nervous System. The nervous system, which reacts within seconds to minutes after a decrease in CO, increases arterial pressure primarily by activation of the sympathetic nervous system. When BP falls below normal levels, norepinephrine is released from sympathetic nerve endings, and both epinephrine and norepinephrine are secreted from the adrenal medulla. Sympathetic stimulation accelerates the HR and increases the force of myocardial contraction, which results in increased CO and sustains perfusion to vital organs, primarily the brain and heart. Sympathetic nervous system stimulation also causes the peripheral vasculature to constrict, leading to an increase in SVR. Sympathetic control is the most important factor related to increasing SVR.

Sympathetic nervous system receptors are classified as α_1, α_2, β_1, and β_2 receptors. β_1 Receptors in the heart respond to sympathetic stimulation with increased HR, increased force of contraction, and increased speed of conduction. α_1 Receptors are located primarily in the peripheral vasculature and cause vasoconstriction when

Reviewed by Patricia Lidbetter Bradley, RN, MEd, MSN, Nursing Faculty, John Abbott College, Ste. Anne De Bellevue, Quebec, Canada.

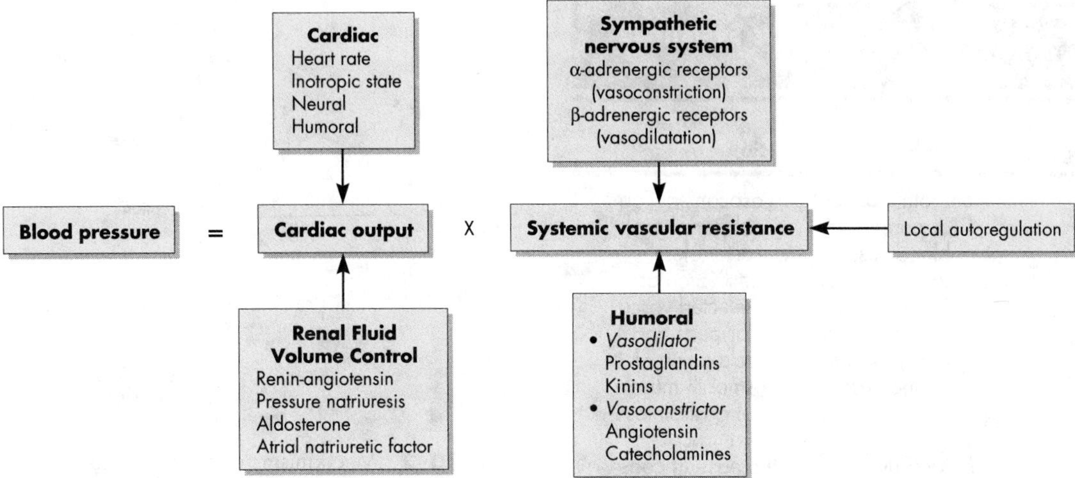

Fig. 30-1 Factors influencing blood pressure.

stimulated. The smooth muscles of the blood vessels have both α and β_2 receptors (Table 30-1).

The sympathetic vasomotor center is located in the medulla of the brain. During exercise the motor area of the cortex is stimulated, activating the vasomotor center and therefore the sympathetic nervous system through neuronal connections. This causes an appropriate increase in BP to accommodate the increased oxygen demand of the exercising muscles. During postural changes from lying to standing, there is a transient decrease in BP. The vasomotor center is stimulated and activates the sympathetic nervous system, causing peripheral vasoconstriction and increased venous return to the heart. If this response did not occur, there would be inadequate blood flow to the brain, resulting in dizziness. BP may be reduced by stimulation of the parasympathetic system, which decreases the HR (via the vagus nerve) and thereby decreases CO.

Baroreceptors. Baroreceptors (pressoreceptors) are specialized nerve receptors located in the carotid arteries and arch of the aorta. They are sensitive to stretching and, when stimulated by an increase in BP, send inhibitory impulses to the sympathetic vasomotor center in the brain stem. In addition, the vagus nerve is stimulated, resulting in dilatation of peripheral arterioles, a reduced HR, and decreased contractility of the heart.

A fall in BP leads to activation of the sympathetic nervous system. The result is constriction of the peripheral arterioles, increased HR, and increased contractility of the heart. The baroreceptors control only temporary changes in BP. In the presence of long-standing hypertension, the baroreceptors become adjusted to elevated levels of BP and recognize this level as "normal."

Renal System

The kidneys contribute to BP regulation by controlling sodium excretion and extracellular fluid (ECF) volume (see Chapter 42). Sodium retention results in water retention, which causes an increased ECF volume. This increases the venous return to the heart, increasing the stroke volume, which elevates the BP through an increase in CO.

The renin-angiotensin–aldosterone system also plays an important role in BP regulation. In response to sympathetic stimulation or decreased blood flow through the kidneys, renin is secreted from the juxtaglomerular apparatus in the kidney. Renin is an enzyme that activates angiotensinogen to angiotensin I; this is converted into angiotensin II, which can increase BP by two different mechanisms (see Fig. 42-6). First, it is a potent vasoconstrictor and increases vascular resistance, resulting in an immediate increase in BP. Second, angiotensin II increases BP indirectly by stimulating the adrenal cortex to secrete aldosterone, which causes sodium retention by the kidneys resulting in increased blood volume and increased CO (Fig. 30-2).

Prostaglandins (PGE_2 and PGI_2) secreted by the renal medulla have a vasodilator effect on the systemic circulation. This results in decreased systemic vascular resistance and lowering of BP. (Prostaglandins are discussed in Chapter 9.)

Endocrine System

Stimulation of the sympathetic nervous system results in release of epinephrine and norepinephrine by the adrenal medulla. These hormones raise the BP by causing vasoconstriction, which increases SVR. They also increase CO by increasing HR and myocardial contractility.

The adrenal cortex is stimulated by angiotensin II to release aldosterone. (Release of aldosterone is also regulated by other factors, such as low sodium levels; see Chapters 42 and 45.) Aldosterone stimulates the kidneys to retain sodium and therefore water. This increases BP by increasing CO (see Fig. 30-2).

An increased blood sodium level stimulates the release of antidiuretic hormone (ADH) by the posterior pituitary gland. ADH increases the ECF volume by stimulating the kidneys to retain water. The resulting increase in blood volume can cause an elevation in BP.

Table 30-1 Sympathetic Nervous System Receptors

Receptor	Location	Action When Stimulated
α_1	Smooth muscles of peripheral blood vessels	Vasoconstriction of peripheral arterioles
α_2	Smooth muscles of peripheral blood vessels and gastrointestinal tract	Constriction of selected vascular beds and relaxation of smooth muscle of gastrointestinal tract
β_1	Myocardium	Increase in contractility (positive inotropic effect)
β_2		Increase in heart rate (positive chronotropic effect)
		Increase in conduction through atria and ventricles (positive dromotropic effect)
	Smooth muscles of peripheral blood vessels and lungs	Mild vasodilatation of peripheral arterioles
		Bronchodilatation
Dopaminergic receptors	Primarily renal and mesenteric blood vessels	Vasodilatation

In the healthy person, these regulatory mechanisms function in response to the demands of the body. When hypertension develops, one or more of the BP-regulating mechanisms are defective. Therapeutic and nursing management is directed toward normalizing BP and preventing target organ damage.

HYPERTENSION

Definition

Hypertension is sustained elevation of BP. The diagnosis of hypertension is confirmed in the adult when the average of two or more resting BP measurements on at least two different visits reveals a SBP of 140 mm Hg or greater or a DBP of 90 mm Hg or greater.[1]

Significance

The status of hypertension control has improved considerably over the past 20 years. Large-scale education programs provided by various organizations have increased awareness of hypertension. The percentage of patients with hypertension on medication who have their BP controlled has also improved substantially. At the same time, cardiovascular mortality has decreased among all adult population groups in the United States. Because high BP is one of the major risk factors for coronary heart disease and the most important risk factor for cerebrovascular diseases, it is inferred that progress in detection, treatment, and control of hypertension has contributed greatly to the decline in the mortality rates of these diseases.[1]

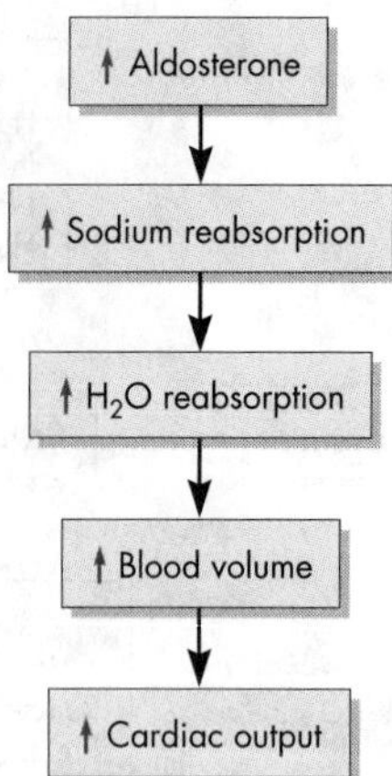

Fig. 30-2 Mechanisms of action of aldosterone.

Hypertension often causes no symptoms to motivate a person to seek treatment. When symptoms do occur, they are often nonspecific and are ignored or attributed to some other cause.

In the United States, 50 million people either have elevated BP (SBP of 140 mm Hg or greater or DBP of 90 mm Hg or greater) or are taking antihypertensive medication.[1] The incidence of hypertension increases with age and is higher in African-Americans than in Caucasians. In addition, African-Americans have a higher mortality rate at every level of BP elevation than do Caucasians. In both races, the prevalence is higher in less educated than more educated people. Hypertension is more prevalent in men than in women until the age of 55. After age 55, it is more prevalent in women.[1]

Classification

Table 30-2 defines the BP classification for people 18 years of age and older. Hypertension used to be classified as *mild, moderate,* or *severe,* but this system failed to convey the seriousness of the problem in the *mild* and *moderate* categories. Hypertension is now classified according to stages (1-4) with the addition of a *high normal* category. The person with BP in the high normal category is at higher risk for the development of definite hypertension, and should be monitored more frequently than the person with lower BP.[1] The etiology of hypertension can be classified as either *primary* (essential) or *secondary.*

PRIMARY (ESSENTIAL) HYPERTENSION

Essential hypertension accounts for 90% of all cases of hypertension, with the onset usually between the ages of 30

Table 30-2 Classification of Blood Pressure for Adults Age 18 Years and Older*

Category	Systolic (mm Hg)	Diastolic (mm Hg)
Normal†	<130	<85
High normal	130-139	85-89
Hypertension‡		
Stage 1 (Mild)	140-159	90-99
Stage 2 (Moderate)	160-179	100-109
Stage 3 (Severe)	180-209	110-119
Stage 4 (Very severe)	≥210	≥120

From US Department of Health and Human Services: The fifth report of the Joint National Committee on Detection, Evaluation, and Treatment of High Blood Pressure (JNC-V), Washington, DC, 1993, National Institutes of Health.

* Not taking antihypertensive drugs and not acutely ill. When systolic and diastolic pressures fall into different categories, the higher category should be selected to classify the individual's blood pressure status. For instance, 160/92 mm Hg should be classified as stage 2, and 180/120 mm Hg should be classified as stage 4. Isolated systolic hypertension (ISH) is defined as SBP ≥140 mm Hg and DBP <90 mm Hg and staged appropriately (e.g., 170/85 mm Hg is defined as stage 2 ISH).

† Optimal blood pressure with respect to cardiovascular risk is SBP <120 mm Hg and DBP <80 mm Hg. However, unusually low readings should be evaluated for clinical significance.

‡ Based on the average of two or more readings taken at each of two or more visits following an initial screening.

Note: In addition to classifying stages of hypertension based on average blood pressure levels, the clinician should specify presence or absence of target-organ disease and additional risk factors. For example, a patient with diabetes and a blood pressure of 142/94 mm Hg plus left ventricular hypertrophy should be classified as stage 1 hypertension with target-organ disease (left ventricular hypertrophy) and with another major risk factor (diabetes). This specificity is important for risk classification and management.

and 50 years. Although the exact cause of essential hypertension is unknown, several contributing factors, including greater than ideal body weight, sedentary lifestyle, increased sodium intake, and excessive alcohol intake, have been identified.

Pathophysiology and Risk Factors

For arterial pressure to rise, there must be an increase in either CO or SVR. Increased CO is sometimes found in the early and borderline hypertensive person. Later in the course of the disease, SVR rises and the CO returns to normal. If SVR is increased, a greater amount of pressure is required to pump blood throughout the body. The hemodynamic hallmark of hypertension is persistently increased systemic vascular resistance. This persistent elevation in SVR may come about in various ways. There is evidence that changes in the structure of the blood vessel walls occur with persistent stimulation by various pressor substances. These blood vessels increase their contractility, thereby sustaining the higher BP.[2]

There is probably no single cause of essential hypertension. It is multifactorial in origin, and only some of the factors have been identified. However, risk factors have been identified that are known to be related to the development of essential hypertension or contribute to the disease. These are presented in Table 30-3.

Heredity. The level of BP is strongly familial, although it is not known exactly what is inherited that leads to high BP. Studies of families and twins have shown poor correlation of BP for those who share only an environment. The correlation strengthens progressively as genetic similarity increases. Estimates of the genetic component of hypertension range from 25% to 61%.[2] It is hypothesized that some alteration in renal function may be implicated in the development of hypertension, and that this may be inherited. Studies in renal transplant patients who developed renal failure secondary to hypertension became normotensive after renal transplantation.[2]

Excess Sodium Intake. Excessive salt intake is considered responsible for initiation of hypertension in some people. Studies on populations with a low sodium intake (usually primitive hunter-gatherer societies) show little or no hypertension and no progressive increase in BP with age as is found in industrialized societies. In addition, when people from these societies adopt modern lifestyles, the prevalence of hypertension increases. When sodium is restricted in some hypertensive people, their BP falls. A high sodium intake may activate a number of pressor mechanisms and cause water retention. Although almost everyone in Western countries consumes a high sodium diet, only about 20% will develop hypertension. This indicates that some degree of sodium sensitivity must be present for high sodium intake to trigger the development of hypertension.[2]

Altered Renin-Angiotensin Mechanism. In some people with essential hypertension, excess quantities of renin are secreted by the kidney. This results in the conversion of angiotensinogen to angiotensin (see Fig. 42-6). Angiotensin causes direct arteriolar constriction and a secondary increase in aldosterone. This is followed by retention of sodium and water with resultant hypertension. In most patients with essential hypertension, the plasma renin level is normal, but in 10% to 17% of patients, the plasma level has been found to be elevated. These patients are said to have *high-renin essential hypertension.*

Stress and Increased Sympathetic Nervous System Activity. It has long been recognized that arterial pressure is influenced by factors such as anger, fear, and pain. Physiologic responses to stress, which are normally protective, may persist to a pathologic degree, resulting in increased sympathetic nervous system activity. Increased sympathetic stimulation results in increased vasoconstriction and an increased HR. Renin release is also stimulated. This results in activation of the angiotensin mechanism and increased aldosterone secretion, both leading to elevated BP. Studies have shown that people exposed to high levels of repeated psychologic stress develop hypertension to a greater extent than those who do not experience as much stress. As stress is a part of everyday life it may be that those who develop hypertension respond differently to stress.[2]

Table 30-3 Risk Factors in Essential Hypertension

Risk Factor	Description
▪ Age	Blood pressure (BP) rises progressively with increasing age. Elevated BP is present in approximately 50% of people over 65 years of age.
▪ Sex	More prevalent in men in young adulthood and early middle age. After age 55, more prevalent in women.
▪ Race	The incidence of hypertension is twice as great in African-Americans as in Caucasians.
▪ Family history	Level of BP is strongly familial. Risk of hypertension increases for those with a close relative having hypertension.
▪ Obesity	Weight gain is associated with increased frequency of hypertension. The risk is greatest with central abdominal obesity.
▪ Cigarette smoking	Smoking greatly increases the risk of cardiovascular disease. Hypertensive persons who smoke are at even greater risk for cardiovascular problems.
▪ Excess dietary sodium	High sodium intake can contribute to hypertension in some patients and can decrease the efficacy of certain antihypertensive medications.
▪ Elevated serum lipids	Elevated levels of cholesterol and triglycerides are primary risk factors in atherosclerosis. Hyperlipidemia is more common in hypertensive persons.
▪ Alcohol	Excessive alcohol intake is strongly associated with hypertension. Hypertensive patients should limit their daily intake to 1 oz of alcohol.
▪ Sedentary lifestyle	A regular exercise program can help control weight and may decrease BP.
▪ Diabetes	Hypertension is more common in patients with diabetes mellitus. When hypertension and diabetes coexist, complications are more severe.
▪ Socioeconomic status	Hypertension is more prevalent in lower socioeconomic groups and among the less educated.
▪ Stress	People exposed to repeated stress may develop hypertension more frequently than others. People who become hypertensive may respond differently to stress than others.

SECONDARY HYPERTENSION

Secondary hypertension is elevated BP with a specific cause that often can be corrected by surgery or medication. This type of hypertension accounts for less than 5% of hypertension in adults. If an adult over age 50 suddenly develops hypertension, especially if it is severe, a secondary cause should be suspected.[4] Causes of secondary hypertension include the following:

1. Coarctation or congenital narrowing of the aorta
2. Renal disease such as renal artery stenosis and parenchymal disease (see Chapter 43)
3. Endocrine disorders such as pheochromocytoma, Cushing's syndrome, and hyperaldosteronism (see Chapter 47)
4. Neurologic disorders such as brain tumors, quadriplegia, and head injury
5. Sleep apnea
6. Medications such as sympathetic stimulants, monoamine oxidase (MAO) inhibitors taken with tyramine-containing foods, estrogen replacement therapy, oral contraceptive pills, and nonsteroidal antiinflammatory drugs (NSAIDs)
7. Pregnancy-induced hypertension

Gerontologic Considerations

More than 50% of the U.S. population 65 years of age and older have elevated SBP or DBP, increasing the risk of cardiovascular disease and stroke.[5] The following age-related physical changes play a role in the pathophysiology of hypertension in the older adult:

1. Loss of tissue elasticity
2. Increased collagen content and stiffness of the myocardium
3. Increased peripheral vascular resistance
4. Decreased β-adrenergic sensitivity
5. Blunting of baroreceptor reflexes
6. Decreased renal function
7. Decreased renin response to sodium and water depletion

In the older adult taking antihypertensive medication, absorption of some drugs may be altered as a result of decreased splanchnic blood flow or gastrointestinal (GI) activity. Metabolism and excretion of drugs may also be prolonged.[5]

Careful technique is important in assessing BP in the elderly. In some older people, there is a wide gap between the first Korotkoff sound and subsequent beats. This is called the auscultatory gap. Failure to inflate the cuff enough may result in seriously underestimating the SBP. This problem can be avoided by palpating the radial artery while inflating the cuff to a level above the disappearance of the pulse.

Isolated Systolic Hypertension

Isolated systolic hypertension (ISH) is defined as a sustained elevation in SBP equal to or greater than 160 mm Hg

CULTURAL & ETHNIC
Considerations

HYPERTENSION

- African-Americans, Puerto Ricans, Cubans, and Mexican-Americans have a higher incidence of hypertension than do Caucasians.
- African-Americans have the highest incidence of hypertension.
- African-American women have a particularly high incidence of hypertension.
- African-Americans have a higher mortality rate related to hypertension than Caucasians.
- African-Americans and Caucasians living in the southeastern United States have a higher incidence of hypertension than similar ethnic groups living in other parts of the United States.

with a DBP less than 90 mm Hg. (A one-time isolated reading of increased SBP is not classified as ISH.) SBP in the range of 140 to 159 mm Hg with DBP less than 90 mm Hg constitutes borderline ISH.[1] Although ISH does occur in the young, it is much more common in the elderly and more prevalent in women and African-Americans.[6] Older adults often have ISH caused by loss of elasticity in large arteries from atherosclerosis.[7]

In the past, ISH was not treated because of the belief that excessive lowering of the DBP would occur, leading to greater problems. Side effects of medication were also a concern. The results of several studies have shown that it is both safe and beneficial to treat ISH in the elderly, and that to do so decreases the incidence of stroke and cardiovascular morbidity and mortality.[8, 9]

As with diastolic hypertension, treatment begins with lifestyle modifications, particularly if the BP is not severely elevated. If measures such as sodium and alcohol restriction, weight reduction for the overweight, and regular aerobic exercise are not sufficient to lower the SBP below 160 mm Hg, drug therapy is indicated.

Because of varying degrees of impaired baroreceptor reflex mechanisms, postural or orthostatic hypotension occurs often in older adults, especially in those with ISH. Postural hypotension in this age group is often associated with volume depletion or chronic disease states, such as decreased renal and hepatic function or electrolyte imbalance.[10] Antihypertensive drugs should be started at low doses and increased cautiously. BP should be measured in the standing and sitting positions at every visit.[6]

Pseudohypertension

Pseudohypertension or false hypertension can occur with sclerosis of the large arteries. As a result, a cuff pressure greater than the intraarterial pressure is needed to shut off the blood flow through the brachial artery. Pseudohypertension can result in a sphygmomanometer reading as much as 10 to 50 mm Hg higher than the actual arterial pressure. To detect this condition, Osler's maneuver is used. This maneuver is performed by inflating the BP cuff to a level above the SBP and then palpating the radial artery. If a pulseless radial artery is palpable even though the sphygomomanometer cuff is inflated to pressures high enough to occlude the brachial artery, pseudohypertension is a possibility. Pseudohypertension is fairly common in the elderly, and its incidence increases with age.[1]

The patient with pseudohypertension does not demonstrate the target organ damage that occurs with true hypertension, as the intraarterial BP is much lower than that recorded using a sphygmomanometer. The only way to accurately measure BP in this patient is by the use of an intraarterial catheter. Pseudohypertension does not need treatment, and there is no practical way to monitor BP in this patient.

CLINICAL MANIFESTATIONS

Hypertension is often called the "silent killer" because it is frequently asymptomatic, especially if the hypertension is mild or moderate. However, a patient with severe hypertension may experience a variety of symptoms. When symptoms develop, they may be secondary to effects on blood vessels in the various organs and tissues or to the increased work load of the heart. The most common symptom is headache in the occipital region that is worse in the morning on arising. In the supine position, CSF pressure increases secondary to increased BP, resulting in headache. When the person stands upright, the CSF pressure gradually decreases, and the headache disappears. Other possible manifestations of hypertension are fatigability, dizziness, palpitations, angina, and dyspnea. Blurring of vision and epistaxis (nosebleed) may occur as a result of vascular complications secondary to hypertension.

COMPLICATIONS

The most common complications of hypertension are target organ damage (Table 30-4) occurring in the heart (hypertensive heart disease), brain (cerebrovascular disease), peripheral vasculature (peripheral vascular disease), kidney (nephrosclerosis), and eyes (retinal damage).

Hypertensive Heart Disease

Coronary Artery Disease. Hypertension is a major risk factor for coronary artery disease and heart failure. The hypertensive patient is more susceptible to silent ischemia, unrecognized myocardial infarction (MI), and sudden cardiac death.[2] Elevated BP causes the entire inner lining of the arteriole to become thickened as a reaction to the high pressure. This characteristic change results from hyperplasia of connective tissues in the intima of the arteriole. These arteriolar changes account for a high incidence of coronary artery disease and the resulting problems of angina and MI.

Congestive Heart Failure. Congestive heart failure (CHF) occurs when the heart can no longer pump effectively against the increasing resistance. The greater resistance to blood flow increases the cardiac work load. To generate greater pressure, the myocardium of the left ventricle ini-

Table 30-4 Manifestations of Target-Organ Disease

Organ System	Manifestations
Cardiac	Clinical, electrocardiographic, or radiologic evidence of coronary artery disease Left ventricular hypertrophy or "strain" by electrocardiography or left ventricular hypertrophy by echocardiography Left ventricular dysfunction or cardiac failure
Cerebrovascular	Transient ischemic attack or stroke
Peripheral vascular	Absence of one or more major pulses in the extremities (except for dorsalis pedis) with or without intermittent claudication; aneurysm
Renal	Serum creatinine ≥1.5 mg/dl (130 μmol/L Proteinuria (1+ or greater) Microalbuminuria
Retinopathy	Hemorrhages or exudates, with or without papilledema

From US Department of Health and Human Services: The fifth report of the Joint National Committee on Detection, Evaluation, and Treatment of High Blood Pressure (JNC-V), Washington, DC, 1993, National Institutes of Health.

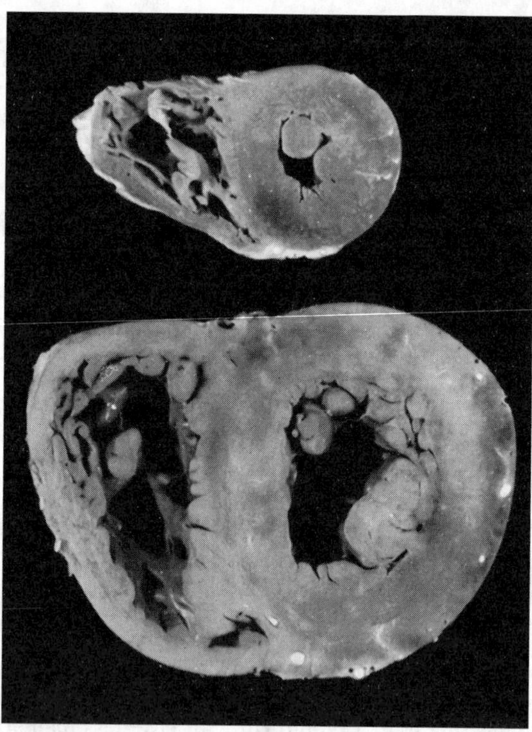

Fig. 30-3 Massively enlarged heart caused by hypertrophy of both ventricles. The normal heart weights 325 g. The heart with biventricular hypertrophy weighs 1100 g. The patient had suffered from severe systemic hypertension.

tially hypertrophies. When the hypertrophied ventricle can no longer function effectively, the left ventricle dilates (Fig. 30-3). Heart failure can result from excess dilatation (see Chapter 32). The patient may complain of shortness of breath on exertion and of paroxysmal nocturnal dyspnea. A chest x-ray will show an enlarged heart, and an electrocardiogram (ECG) will show electrical changes indicative of left ventricular hypertrophy.

Cerebrovascular Disease

Hypertension is the leading cause of stroke in the United States. As a result of hypertension, the blood vessels become more rigid because of thickening of vessel walls and replacement of smooth muscle tissue with fibrous tissue. The vessel is weakened by this process and tends to rupture more easily. Because of these abnormal processes, changes in cerebral circulation include the following:

1. Narrowing of the lumen of cerebral arterioles
2. Microaneurysms of small cerebral arteries
3. Progressive atherosclerotic changes
4. Increase in intracranial pressure

As a result of these changes, the patient may experience transient ischemic attacks (TIA) or a cerebrovascular accident (CVA) as a result of thrombosis of cerebral vessels, emboli from the heart, or intracerebral hemorrhage. Approximately 75% of strokes are caused by cerebral infarction, either from arterial thrombosis or embolism, another 15% to 20% are the result of hemorrhage, and a further 5% are the result of unknown causes.[2]

Hypertensive encephalopathy may occur after a marked rise in BP if the cerebral blood flow is not decreased by autoregulation. With the increase in BP, the cerebral vessels dilate and cerebral edema develops and produces a rise in intracranial pressure. The increased intracranial pressure may be sufficient to decrease or halt blood flow to the brain.

Peripheral Vascular Disease

As it does with other vessels, hypertension speeds up the process of atherosclerosis in the peripheral blood vessels leading to the development of aortic aneurysm, aortic dissection, and peripheral vascular disease (see Chapter 35). Intermittent claudication (ischemic muscle pain precipitated by activity and relieved with rest) is a classic symptom of peripheral vascular disease.

Nephrosclerosis

Hypertension is one of the leading risk factors for end-stage renal disease, especially in African-Americans. Some degree of renal dysfunction is usually present in the hypertensive patient, even one with a minimally elevated BP.[2] This disorder is the direct result of ischemia caused by the narrowed lumen of the intrarenal blood vessels. Gradual closure of the arteries and arterioles leads to destruction of

Table 30-5 Keith-Wagener Classification of Retinal Changes

Grade I	Vascular spasm and arteriolar narrowing in terminal branches of vessels
Grade II	Definite arteriovenous nicking (arterioles cross vein and compress it)
Grade III	Flame-shaped hemorrhages and fluffy cotton-wool exudates
Grade IV	Any of the above and papilledema (swelling of optic disk)

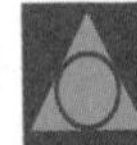

Table 30-6 Therapeutic Management: Hypertension

Diagnostic
- History and physical examination
- Routine urinalysis
- Serum electrolytes and uric acid levels
- BUN and serum creatinine levels
- Blood glucose (fasting, if possible) levels
- Complete blood count
- Serum lipid profile, cholesterol and triglycerides levels
- Chest x-ray
- ECG

Therapeutic
- Periodic monitoring of BP
  - Every 4-6 mo once BP is stabilized
- Diet
  - Restriction of sodium
  - Reduction of weight (if indicated)
  - Restriction of cholesterol and saturated fats
- Exercise program
- Cessation of smoking
- Modification of alcohol intake
- Antihypertensive drugs*

BP, Blood pressure; *BUN,* blood urea nitrogen; *ECG,* electrocardiogram.
*See Table 30-7.

the glomeruli, atrophy of the tubules, and eventual death of nephrons. These changes may eventually lead to renal failure. Common laboratory abnormalities are microalbuminuria, proteinuria, elevated blood urea nitrogen (BUN) and serum creatinine levels, and microscopic hematuria. The earliest symptom of renal dysfunction is usually nocturia.

Retinal Damage

An ophthalmoscope is used to visualize the blood vessels of the eye. The appearance of the retina provides important information about the severity and prognosis of the hypertensive process. The retina is the only place in the body where the blood vessels can be directly visualized. Therefore, retinal damage provides an indication of vessel damage in the heart, brain, and kidney. Manifestations of retinal damage include blurring of vision, retinal hemorrhage, and loss of vision.

Retinal changes are graded according to the severity of damage. The Keith-Wagener classification of retinal changes is presented in Table 30-5. Grade IV findings of papilledema are characteristic of malignant hypertension (discussed later in this chapter).

DIAGNOSTIC STUDIES

BP measurements should be taken in both arms when initially evaluating a patient's BP. If there is a difference between arms, the arm with the higher reading should be used for all subsequent measurements. This is because atherosclerotic narrowing of the subclavian artery may cause a falsely low reading on the side in which the narrowing occurs. The average of at least two BP measurements (taken 2 to 5 minutes apart while the patient is sitting) should be used to determine if the patient should return for subsequent evaluation.[1]

There is some controversy as to how extensive a diagnostic workup should be performed on a person with hypertension. Because most hypertension is classified as essential hypertension, testing for secondary causes is not routinely done. If the patient's age, history, physical examination findings, or severity of hypertension point to a secondary cause, further diagnostic tests may be indicated.

Table 30-6 lists basic laboratory studies that are performed in a person with sustained hypertension. Routine urinalysis, BUN, and serum creatinine levels are used to screen for renal involvement. Measurement of serum electrolytes, especially potassium levels, is important to detect hyperaldosteronism. Blood glucose levels are important because they can assist in identifying endocrine causes of hypertension, such as diabetes mellitus and Cushing's syndrome. Urinary catecholamine levels are used to diagnose pheochromocytoma. Serum cholesterol and triglyceride levels provide information about additional risk factors that predispose to atherogenesis. Uric acid levels are determined to establish a baseline, since the levels often rise with diuretic therapy. A chest x-ray provides baseline information regarding heart size, as well as aortic dilatation and rib notching, which occur in coarctation of the aorta. An ECG provides baseline information regarding the cardiac status.

Ambulatory Blood Pressure Monitoring

Some patients have elevated BP readings in a doctor's office and normal readings when BP is measured elsewhere. This phenomenon is referred to as "white coat" hypertension. When white coat hypertension is suspected, or when the BP is only slightly elevated, the doctor may use 24-hour ambulatory BP monitoring to help decide on appropriate treatment. The equipment includes a BP cuff and a small microprocessing unit that fits into a pouch worn on a shoulder strap or belt. The machine measures BP at preset intervals over the 24-hour period and can give the physician a better idea of the true status of the BP. The test is fairly expensive and not recommended for routine use but can be helpful in selected cases. If done, the test should be scheduled on a patient's regular work day as the results tend to be more indicative of the patient's usual BP.[11]

THERAPEUTIC MANAGEMENT

The goal in treating a hypertensive patient is to prevent the morbidity and mortality associated with high BP and to control BP by the least intrusive means possible[1] (see Table 30-6). Lifestyle modifications are indicated for the person with either borderline or sustained hypertension. These modification measures include dietary management, smoking cessation, regular exercise, and limitation of alcohol intake. (Management of risk factors is discussed in Chapter 31 and Table 31-4.) If the BP remains equal to or greater than 140/90 mm Hg after 3 to 6 months of lifestyle changes, drug therapy is indicated (Fig. 30-4). Some primary care providers choose to withhold drug therapy if the DBP is between 90 and 94 mm Hg. In this case, frequent monitoring of BP is indicated to promptly detect any further elevation. Other factors that may be considered in the decision to initiate drug therapy are the presence of target organ damage and the presence of other complications or risk factors.[1]

Follow-up monitoring of the BP is very important. The frequency of initial monitoring varies with the level of BP. After the BP has stabilized, it should be monitored every 4 to 6 months to ensure control and to assess for target organ damage.

Lifestyle Modifications

Dietary Changes. Dietary management of hypertension consists of sodium restriction, caloric restriction if the patient is overweight, and restriction of cholesterol and fat. The role of dietary potassium, calcium, and magnesium supplementation remains controversial.

Sodium restriction. Epidemiologic observations and clinical trials have shown an association between sodium intake and BP. Short-term studies have shown an average decrease of 4.9 mm Hg in SBP and 2.6 mm Hg in DBP with moderate reduction in sodium intake.[1]

The Joint National Committee recommends restricting sodium intake to less than 2.3 g (less than 6 g of salt [NaCl]) per day. This involves not adding salt in the preparation of foods or at meals and avoiding foods known to be high in sodium (see Table 32-11).

This level of sodium restriction may be enough to control hypertension in the patient with stage 1 hypertension. If drug therapy is needed, a lower dose may be effective if the patient also restricts sodium intake.[1]

Caloric and fat restriction. Obesity has a high correlation with hypertension. Abdominal obesity carries a higher risk than does excess weight carried in the hips and thighs. Weight reduction has a significant effect on lowering BP in many persons, and the effect is seen with even moderate weight loss. When a person decreases caloric intake, sodium and fat intake is also usually reduced. Therefore additional

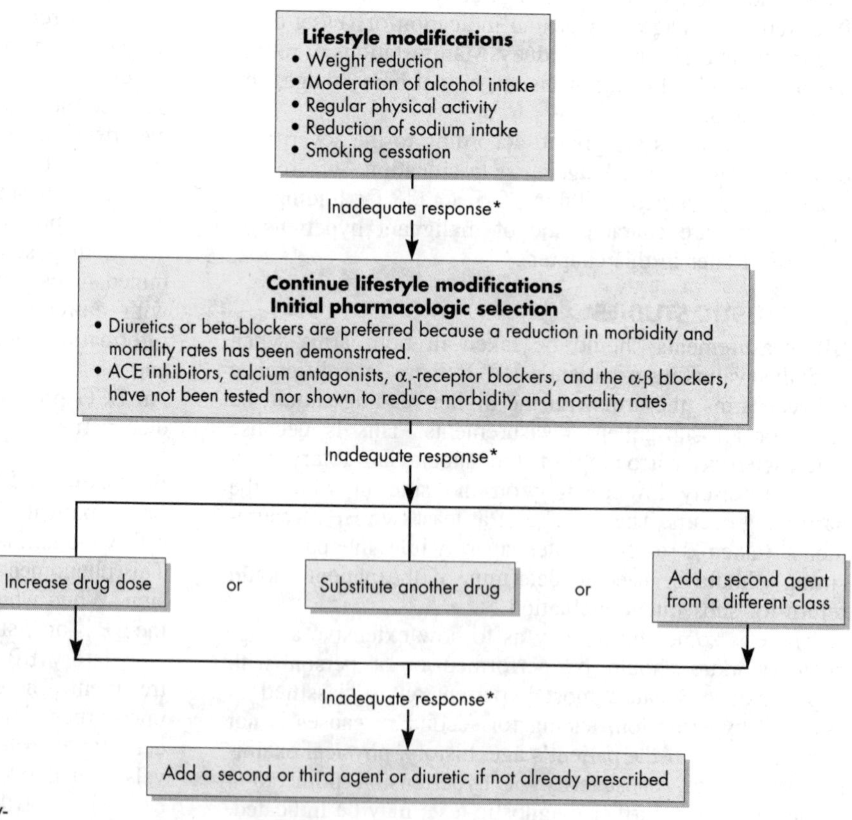

Fig. 30-4 Treatment algorithm for hypertension. *ACE*, Angiotensin-converting enzyme.

benefits are achieved with a weight-reduction diet. Lipid restriction should include limiting the intake of cholesterol as well as dietary fat. This practice may retard the progress of atherosclerosis (see Chapter 31).

Modification in Alcohol Consumption. Alcohol consumption is strongly associated with hypertension and available studies suggest that the consumption of three or more alcoholic drinks daily is a definite risk factor. The exact mechanism by which this occurs is unclear. It is possible that alcohol contributes to hypertension by its effects on renin or catecholamines or possibly a direct effect on vascular smooth muscle. Whatever the exact mechanism by which alcohol intake contributes to hypertension, it is estimated that from 5% to 11% of cases of hypertension can be attributed to excessive alcohol intake.[2] The patient should be advised to limit alcohol intake to 1 oz per day (the amount of alcohol in 2 oz of 100 proof whiskey, 8 oz of wine, or 24 oz of beer).[1]

Regular Exercise. Regular aerobic exercise such as walking, jogging, and swimming can help control BP, promote relaxation, and decrease or control body weight. Regular exercise of this type can reduce SBP in the hypertensive patient by approximately 10 mm Hg.[1] For a sedentary patient, moderate activity such as 30 to 45 minutes of brisk walking three to five times per week is recommended. The patient should be advised to increase exercise levels gradually. The patient with heart disease or other serious health problems needs a thorough examination, possibly including a stress test, before beginning an exercise program.[1]

Avoidance of Cigarette Smoking. Although cigarette smoking does not contribute to the development of hypertension, it is a major risk factor for cardiovascular disease, and avoidance of tobacco is essential. Everyone, especially a hypertensive patient, should be strongly advised not to smoke. The patient who continues to smoke may not receive the maximum effect of antihypertensive therapy.[1]

Stress Management. Although stress can raise BP on a short-term basis and has been implicated in the development of hypertension, controversy exists as to the benefit of stress management in the prevention and treatment of hypertension. Some studies of relaxation techniques and biofeedback have shown short- and long-term BP lowering effects. Consequently, some physicians recommend stress management techniques as routine management of hypertension.[12] Other studies have found little effect of stress management in the treatment of hypertension.[13, 14] The Joint National Committee does not recommend the use of relaxation techniques as definitive therapy or for the prevention of hypertension.[1]

Pharmacologic Management

The general goals of pharmacologic management of hypertension are to reduce and maintain the DBP at less than 90 mm Hg and to keep uncomfortable or disabling side effects of medications to a minimum (Table 30-7). The drugs currently available for treating hypertension have two main actions: reduction of SVR and decreased volume of circulating blood. The drugs used in the treatment of hypertension include diuretics, adrenergic (sympathetic)-inhibiting agents, vasodilators, angiotensin-converting enzyme (ACE) inhibiting agents, and calcium channel blockers (antagonists) (see Fig. 30-5 on p. 876).

Although the precise action of diuretics in the reduction of BP is unclear, it is known that they decrease sodium in the arteriolar walls, promote water excretion, reduce plasma volume, and reduce the vascular response to catecholamines. Adrenergic-inhibiting agents act by diminishing the sympathetic reflexes that increase BP. Vasodilators decrease the BP by dilating the arterioles. ACE inhibitors decrease BP by blocking the renin-angiotensin-aldosterone system, decreasing fluid volume, and decreasing SVR. Calcium channel blockers cause vasodilatation of peripheral arterioles by blocking the movement of extracellular calcium into cells (see Chapter 31).

The recommendation for treatment of stage 1 or 2 hypertension in the patient who remains uncontrolled after 3 to 6 months of lifestyle modification is monotherapy with either a diuretic or beta blocker. These are recommended as first-line drugs by the Joint National Committee as a result of studies that have shown decreased cardiovascular morbidity and mortality rates associated with their use.[1] Calcium channel blockers, ACE inhibitors, alpha-adrenergic blockers, and the combined alpha-beta adrenergic blockers are also effective in lowering BP and may be used as first-line drugs. The selection of a first-line drug is influenced by cost and the presence of other medical conditions. It is recommended that the drug be started at a low dose for several weeks. If, after 1 to 3 months, the BP is not controlled, the dose of the first-line drug can be increased, a second drug from a different class can be substituted, or a second drug from a different class can be added. If the addition of the second drug controls the BP, the doctor may try withdrawing the first drug. Many times, the patient with stage 1 or 2 hypertension can be controlled with only one drug.[1]

Before proceeding with the addition or substitution of medication, consideration should be given to possible reasons for the lack of response to drug therapy (see Table 30-8 on p. 877).

For stage 3 or 4 hypertension, the regimen is essentially the same, but the interval between medication changes may be shortened, and therapy may need to be started with more than one drug. The addition of a third or fourth drug, including the centrally acting alpha-adrenergic-blockers, peripheral-acting adrenergic antagonists, or direct vasodilators, may be necessary. These drugs are not suitable as initial monotherapy as they have a greater potential for side effects.[1]

After 1 year of good BP control, step-down therapy may be tried. The number of medications and their dosages are gradually decreased to the lowest amount that controls the BP. Regular follow-up is needed to detect any elevation of BP.[1]

Side effects and adverse effects of antihypertensive drugs may be so severe or undesirable that the patient does not comply with therapy. Table 30-7 describes the major

(Text continued on p. 876.)

Table 30-7 Antihypertensive Drug Therapy*

Agent	Mechanisms of Action	Side Effects and Adverse Effects	Nursing Considerations
Diuretics			
Thiazides and related diuretics			
Bendroflumethiazide (Naturetin) Benzthiazide (Aguatag, Exna) Chlorothiazide (Diuril) Chlorthalidone (Hygroton) Cyclothiazide (Anhydron) Hydrochlorothiazide (Esidrix, HydroDiuril, Oretic) Hydroflumethiazide (Saluron) Indapamide (Lozol) Metolazone (Zaroxolyn) Methyclothiazide (Enduron) Polythiazide (Renese) Quinethazone (Hydromox) Trichlormethiazide (Metahydrin, Nagua)	Act on ascending loop of Henle and distal tubule; prevent reabsorption of sodium and chloride; reduce ECF and CO, causing initial effect; reduce SVR, causing long-term effect; usually lower BP moderately within 3-4 days; higher than normal doses rarely add to effect on BP and can worsen adverse effects	Electrolyte imbalances, including hypercalcemia, hypochloremia, hypokalemia, hypomagnesemia, hyponatremia; orthostatic hypotension; hypercholesteremia; hyperglycemia; hypertriglyceridemia; hyperuricemia; GI manifestations, including anorexia, vomiting, diarrhea, pancreatitis; central nervous system effects, including dizziness, vertigo, headache; hematologic effects, including leukopenia, agranulocytosis, thrombocytopenia; hypersensitivity effects, including photosensitivity, purpura, rash; sexual dysfunction; weakness	Monitor for hypokalemia and alkalosis. Be aware that thiazides potentiate cardiotoxicity of digitalis by producing hypokalemia and that NSAIDs can decrease diuretic and antihypertensive effects of thiazide diuretics. Advise patient to supplement diet with potassium-rich foods. If potassium solution supplement needed, advise patient to drink it with fruit juice or water to minimize unpleasant taste.
Loop diuretics			
Bumetanide (Bumex) Ethacrynic acid (Edecrin) Furosemide (Lasix)	Act on ascending loop of Henle to prevent reabsorption of chloride and sodium; are more potent than thiazide diuretics; have shorter duration of action than thiazide diuretics and may be less effective for treatment of hypertension; furosemide reserved for patient with fluid retention that cannot be controlled with thiazides or for patient with impaired renal function	Same as thiazides, including fluid and electrolyte depletion and, in severe cases, cardiovascular collapse; also reversible hearing loss, metabolic alkalosis, GI upset (most common with ethacrynic acid)	Monitor for hypokalemia and alkalosis. Measure fluid intake and output and weigh patient daily. Be aware that effect of drug increases with dosage.
Potassium-sparing diuretics			
Amiloride (Midamor) Spironolactone (Aldactone) Triamterene (Dyrenium)	Used mainly with thiazide diuretics to prevent or correct hypokalemia; block sodium-potassium exchange mechanism in the distal portion of tubule; prevent sodium from being reabsorbed and retain potassium; triamterene and amiloride act on distal tubule to block potassium secretion independently of aldosterone; spironolactone blocks effect of aldosterone on kidney tubule	Renal insufficiency, hyperkalemia, GI disturbances, skin eruptions, hirsutism, headache, urticaria, drug fever, photosensitivity, gynecomastia in men, inability to achieve or maintain erection, menstrual irregularities, ataxia with spironolactone, and blood dyscrasias with triamterene	Monitor for hyperkalemia, especially in patients with renal impairment or diabetes, in older adult, and patient receiving other drugs that can lower aldosterone secretion, such as captopril and NSAIDs. Do not use potassium supplements.

continued

Table 30-7 Antihypertensive Drug Therapy*—cont'd

Agent	Mechanisms of Action	Side Effects and Adverse Effects	Nursing Considerations
Adrenergic Inhibitors			
β-Adrenergic blockers			
Acebutolol (Sectral) Atenolol (Tenormin) Betaxolol (Kerlone) Bisoprolol (Zebeta) Carteolol (Cartrol) Metoprolol (Lopressor) Nadolol (Corgard) Penbutolol (Levatol) Pindolol (Visken) Propranolol (Inderal) Timolol (Blocadren)	Reduce BP by decreasing CO, sympathetic stimulation, and renin secretion by kidney; reduce SVR (with long-term use)	Bronchospasm, heart failure, bradycardia, arterioventricular conduction block, impaired peripheral circulation, nightmares, depression, weakness, GI disturbances, insomnia, decreased exercise tolerance, sexual dysfunction masking hypoglycemic symptoms	Assess patient for manifestations of heart failure and heart block. Check pulse regularly. Be aware that drugs are contraindicated with a history of CHF, COPD, heart block, asthma, or diabetes mellitus and that sudden withdrawal can be hazardous in the patient with heart disease.
Centrally acting α blockers			
Clonidine (Catapres)†	Inhibits impulse through sympathetic nerve pathways; causes central α-receptor stimulation, decreasing sympathetic tone peripherally; results in dilatation of arterioles and veins; does not inhibit reflex responses as completely as drugs that act peripherally	Dry mouth, sedation, impotence, constipation, allergic reaction, dizziness, headache, fatigue, anxiety, severe rebound hypertension (if drug abruptly discontinued)	Suggest chewing gum or hard candy to relieve dry mouth. Be aware that alcohol and sedatives increase central nervous system depression. Use for hypertensive urgencies.
Guanabenz (Wytensin)	Same as clonidine	Same as clonidine	Same as clonidine
Guanfacine hydrochloride (Tenex)	Same as clonidine	Same as clonidine	Same as clonidine
Methyldopa (Aldomet)	Same as clonidine	Sedation, fatigue, orthostatic hypotension, decreased libido, impotence, dry mouth, hemolytic anemia, hepatotoxicity, GI disturbances, sodium and water retention, psychic depression	Instruct patient about daytime sedation and avoidance of hazardous activities. Be aware that activities requiring mental work may be an indication not to use drug. Give IV for hypertensive emergencies.
Peripheral-acting adrenergic antagonists			
Guanethidine (Ismelin)	Prevents release of norepinephrine, resulting in peripheral vasodilatation; usually lowers CO and reduces SBP more than DBP; produces greatest effects in standing position	Marked orthostatic hypotension, diarrhea, cramps, bradycardia, retrograde ejaculation, sodium and water retention; cumulative effects (over several weeks)	Because of adverse effects, drug is reserved for severe hypertension unresponsive to other drugs. It is not recommended for person with cerebral vascular insufficiency or coronary artery disease or in older adult because of orthostatic hypotension. The hypotensive effect is delayed for 2-3 days and lasts 7-10 days after withdrawal. Severe postural hypotension is aggravated by anything that stimulates vasodilatation (e.g., hot environment, alcohol, or hot shower). Use diuretic.
Guanadrel sulfate (Hylorel)	Same as guanethidine, except with shorter duration of action	Same as guanethidine	Same as guanethidine

continued

Table 30-7 Antihypertensive Drug Therapy*—cont'd

Agent	Mechanisms of Action	Side Effects and Adverse Effects	Nursing Considerations
Reserpine (Serpasil)	Acts both peripherally and centrally to deplete norepinephrine stores; results in peripheral vasodilatation	Nasal congestion, drowsiness, GI distress, mental depression, bizarre dreams, bradycardia, syncope, impotence	Be aware that history of depression is a contraindication. Monitor for depression and personality changes. Advise patient to eliminate barbiturates, alcohol, and narcotics.
α-Adrenergic blockers			
Phentolamine (Regitine)	Blocks α-adrenergic receptors, resulting in peripheral vascular dilatation	Acute prolonged hypotension, cardiac dysrhythmias, tachycardia, weakness, flushing	Use for pheochromocytoma.
Doxazosin (Cardura) Prazosin (Minipress) Terazosin (Hytrin)	Blocks peripheral vascular α-adrenergic receptors, resulting in dilatation of arterioles and veins	Profound orthostatic hypotension with syncope (1-3 hr after first dose), disappearing with continued use; headache; drowsiness; paresthesias; blurred vision; impotence; frequent urination; fluid retention	Prevent hypotension and syncope by giving small initial dose at bedtime and advising patient not to get up for 3 hr. Use cautiously in older adult because of orthostatic hypotension.
Combined α- and β-adrenergic blockers			
Labetalol (Normodyne, Trandate)	Has nonselective action, resulting in α-adrenergic blocking properties	Orthostatic hypotension, sexual dysfunction (more than other β-adrenergic blocking drugs); bronchospasm, peripheral vascular insufficiency	Same as β-blockers. Give IV for hypertensive emergencies.
Vasodilators			
Diazoxide (Hyperstat)	Has direct action (used only in hypertensive emergencies)	Sodium and water retention, hyperglycemia, hypotension, skin rash, fever, dysrhythmias, nausea, vomiting, chest pain, hyperuricemia	Inject via IV push within 30 sec. Administer diuretic because of sodium retention. Use cautiously in patient with diabetes or cerebrovascular insufficiency.
Hydralazine (Apresoline)	Acts primarily on smooth muscle of arterioles to cause vasodilatation and reduce SVR; usually decreases DBP and SBP proportionally and causes little orthostatic hypotension; acts more on arterioles than veins and is less potent than minoxidil	Tachycardia, fluid retention, nasal congestion, flushing, headache, palpitation, GI symptoms, hepatitis, CHF, angina exacerbation, lupuslike syndrome.	Be aware that headaches sometimes occur when drug is started or when dosage is increased. Discontinue drug if lupus-like syndrome occurs. Give drug IM or IV for hypertensive emergencies.
Minoxidil (Loniten)	Produces arterial vasodilatation with no venous effect	Reflex tachycardia, marked sodium and water retention (often not controllable with large doses of furosemide), CHF, weakness, hirsutism, aggravation of angina	Be aware that major disadvantage is reflex-increased sympathetic activity. Use only for treatment of severe hypertension resistant to other therapy. Use for hypertensive urgencies.

continued

Table 30-7 Antihypertensive Drug Therapy*—cont'd

Agent	Mechanisms of Action	Side Effects and Adverse Effects	Nursing Considerations
Nitroglycerin (Tridil)	Acts primarily as venous vasodilator; is effective in hypertensive emergencies, especially in patients with myocardial ischemia	Hypotension, headache	Closely monitor BP. Observe for drug tolerance, which may occur with repeated and prolonged use.
Sodium nitroprusside (Nipride)	Has direct action (used in hypertensive emergencies); is administered by continuous IV infusion with immediate effect	Hypotension, nausea, sweating, headache, restlessness, confusion, twitching, thiocyanate toxicity	Carefully titrate dosage to patient's response. Use intraarterial monitoring system. Be aware that drug is light sensitive and stable for 24 hr. Monitor thiocyanate levels.
Ganglionic Blockers			
Trimethaphan (Arfonad)	Blocks neural transmission at autonomic ganglia (used in hypertensive emergencies); is drug of choice for treatment of aortic dissection	Dry mouth, urinary retention, constipation, orthostatic hypotension, weakness, dilated pupils	Administer IV for rapid onset of action. Carefully titrate drug. Continually monitor BP after administration.
Angiotensin-Converting Enzyme Inhibitors			
Benazepril (Lotensin) Captopril (Capoten) Cilazapril (Inhibace) Enalapril (Vasotec) Fosinopril (Monopril) Lisinopril (Prinivil, Zestril) Perindopril (Aceon) Ramipril (Altace) Quinapril (Accupril)	Inhibit ACE, lowering SVR; is effective for essential hypertension and renovascular hypertension and in severe refractory hypertension; may be more effective than some three-drug regimens	Loss of taste (leading to severe anorexia), cough, fatal bone marrow depression, transient maculopapular rash, hyperkalemia, membranous-glomerulopathy, nephrotic syndrome, tachycardia, orthostatic hypotension	Use aspirin substitute because aspirin can decrease drug's effectiveness. Be aware that diuretics may not be required for effective therapy, but combination of diuretic and captopril is more effective than either drug alone. Use captopril for hypertensive urgencies
Enalaprilat (Vasotec IV)	Used when oral therapy is impractical	Given as IV infusion over at least 5 min	ACE inhibitors can cause fetal and neonatal morbidity and mortality when given to pregnant women.
Calcium Antagonists			
Amlodipine (Norvasc) Diltiazem (Cardizem) Felodipine (Plendil) Isradipine (Dynacirc) Nicardipine (Cardene) Nifedipine (Procardia) Verapamil (Isoptin) Verapamil SR (long-acting)	Cause vasodilatation of peripheral arterioles by blocking movement of extracellular calcium into cells, resulting in decreased SVR	Nausea, headache, hypotension, peripheral edema; reflex increase in HR (with nifedipine); reflex decrease in HR (with diltiazem); minimal change in HR (with verapamil); constipation (with verapamil and diltiazem)	Use with caution in patient with CHF; contraindicated with second- and third-degree heart block. Give nifedipine sublingually or have patient chew drug for hypertensive urgencies. Be aware that the higher the BP, the more significant the decrease in BP is once drug therapy is initiated.

ACE, Angiotensin-converting enzyme; *BP*, blood pressure; *CHF*, congestive heart failure; *CO*, cardiac output; *COPD*, chronic obstructive pulmonary disease; *DBP*, diastolic blood pressure; *ECF*, extracellular fluid; *GI*, gastrointestinal; *HR*, heart rate; *IM*, intramuscular; *IV*, intravenous; *NSAIDs*, nonsteroidal antiinflammatory drugs; *SBP*, systolic blood pressure; *SVR*, systemic vascular resistance.

*All drugs are normally given orally unless otherwise indicated.

†Available as a patch.

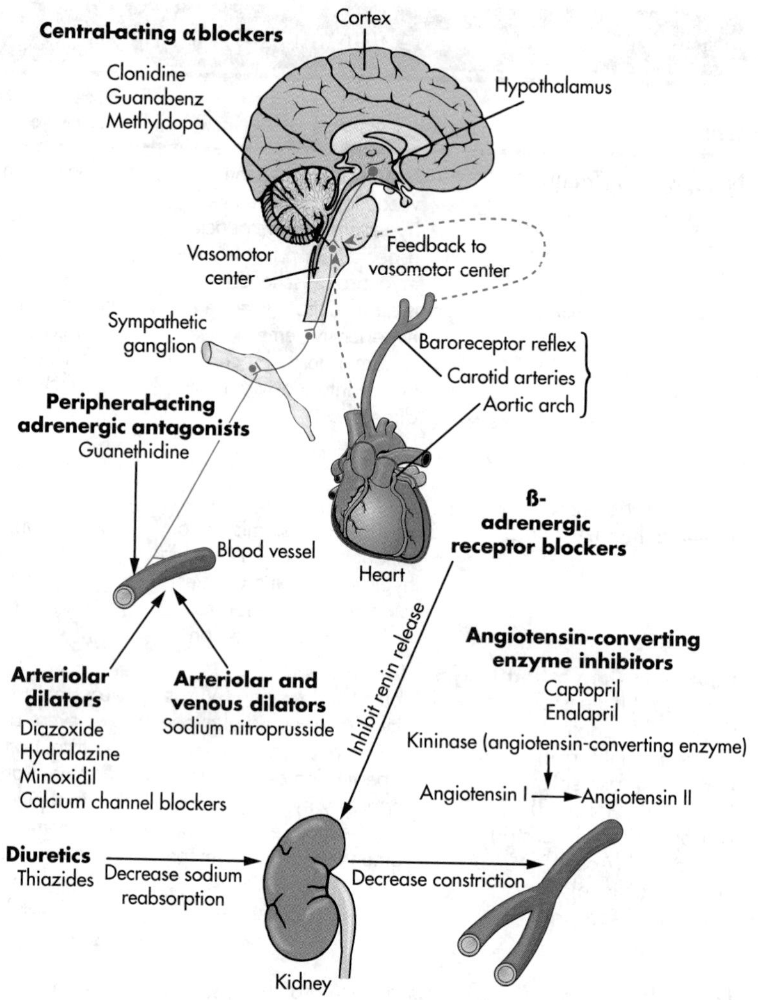

Fig. 30-5 Site and method of action of various antihypertensive drugs.

side effects of each drug. Hyperuricemia, hyperglycemia, and hypokalemia are common side effects with both thiazide and loop diuretics. Hyperkalemia can be a serious side effect of the potassium-sparing diuretics and ACE inhibitors. Impotence may occur with many of the diuretics. Orthostatic hypotension and sexual dysfunction are two undesirable effects of adrenergic-inhibiting agents. Tachycardia and orthostatic hypotension are potential adverse effects of both vasodilators and ACE inhibitors.

NURSING MANAGEMENT

HYPERTENSION

Nursing Assessment

Subjective and objective data that should be obtained from a patient with hypertension are presented in Table 30-9.

Nursing Diagnoses

Nursing diagnoses are determined when the problem and the etiologic factors are supported by the clinical data. Nursing diagnoses related to a patient with an elevated BP may include, but are not limited to, those presented in Table 30-10.

Planning

The overall goals are that the patient with hypertension will have (1) a decrease in BP, (2) no target organ damage, and (3) minimal or no unpleasant side effects of therapy.

Nursing Implementation

Health Maintenance and Promotion

Individual patient evaluation. The majority of cases of hypertension are identified through routine screening procedures such as insurance, preemployment, and military physical examinations. The nurse in these settings, as well as in most other practice settings, is in an ideal position to assess for the presence of hypertension, identify the risk factors for hypertension and coronary artery disease, and educate the patient regarding this disease. In addition to BP determination, a complete health assessment should include such factors as age, sex, race, diet history (including sodium and alcohol intake), weight patterns, and family history of heart disease, stroke, renal disease, and diabetes mellitus. Medications taken, both prescribed and over-the-counter, should be noted. The patient should be asked about any previous documentation of high BP and the results of treatment (if any).

Table 30-8 Causes for Lack of Responsiveness to Therapy

Nonadherence to Therapy
- Cost of medication
- Instructions not clear and/or not given to the patient in writing
- Inadequate or no patient education
- Lack of involvement of the patient in the treatment plan
- Side effects of medication
- Organic brain syndrome (e.g., memory deficit)
- Inconvenient dosing

Drug-related Causes
- Doses too low
- Inappropriate combinations (e.g., two centrally acting adrenergic inhibitors)
- Rapid inactivation (e.g., hydralazine)
- Drug interactions
  - Nonsteroidal antiinflammatory drugs
  - Oral contraceptives
  - Sympathomimetics
  - Antidepressants
  - Adrenal steroids
  - Nasal decongestants
  - Licorice-containing substances (e.g., chewing tobacco)
  - Cocaine
  - Cyclosporine
  - Erythropoietin

Associated Conditions
- Increasing obesity
- Alcohol intake more than 1 oz/day

Secondary Hypertension
- Renal insufficiency
- Renovascular hypertension
- Pheochromocytoma
- Primary aldosteronism

Volume Overload
- Inadequate diuretic therapy
- Excess sodium intake
- Fluid retention from reduction of blood pressure
- Progressive renal damage

Pseudohypertension

From US Department of Health and Human Services: The fifth report of the Joint National Committee on Detection, Evaluation, and Treatment of High Blood Pressure (JNC-V), Washington, DC, 1993, National Institutes of Health.

Initially, the BP is taken two or three times, at least 2 minutes apart, with the average pressure recorded as the value for that visit. Waiting for at least 2 minutes between readings allows the venous blood to drain from the arm and prevents inaccurate readings. The BP is initially measured with the patient in either the supine or the sitting position after at least 5 minutes of rest. BP should also be measured in the standing position. Usually the SBP decreases on standing, whereas the DBP increases.

BP measurements should be done under standardized conditions and with accurate equipment (Table 30-11). BP measurements of both arms should be performed initially to detect any differences between arms. Atherosclerotic narrowing of the subclavian artery can cause a falsely low reading on the side where the narrowing occurs. Therefore, the arm with the higher reading should be used for all subsequent BP measurements. The patient's arm is uncovered and placed at the level of the heart. The cuff should be inflated until no pulse is felt in the brachial artery located in the antecubital fossa of the arm being used. The cuff is then inflated an additional 10 to 20 mm Hg to ensure vascular occlusion. In an obese person, a cuff larger than the normal 12 to 14 cm cuff should be used to obtain accurate readings. The pressure is released at 2 mm Hg per second. Releasing any slower or faster may create inaccurate readings. Both SBP and DBP should be recorded, with the DBP recorded as the disappearance of sound.

Screening programs. The nurse involved in a screening program should be aware of general guidelines for BP detection and evaluation (Table 30-12). At the time of the

Table 30-9 Nursing Assessment: Hypertension

Subjective Data

Important health information

Past health history: History of cardiovascular, cerebrovascular, renal, or thyroid disease or diabetes mellitus; coarctation of aorta; pituitary disorders; smoking and alcohol use

Medications: Use of any prescription or over-the-counter medications; previous use of antihypertensive drug therapy

Functional health patterns

Health perception–health management: Family history of hypertension or cardiovascular disease, fatigue, epistaxis

Nutritional-metabolic: Salt and fat intake, weight gain or loss

Elimination: Nocturia

Activity-exercise: Dyspnea on exertion, palpitations on exertion

Cognitive-perceptual: Occipital headaches (especially in the morning), dizziness; blurred vision, paresthesias

Coping–stress tolerance: Stressful life events

Objective Data

Cardiovascular

BP consistently above 140 mm Hg systolic and 90 mm Hg diastolic, peripheral edema, retinal vessel changes, abnormal heart sounds, diminished or absent peripheral arterial pulses, bruits

Musculoskeletal

Muscle cramps

Possible findings

Abnormal serum electrolytes (especially potassium); elevated BUN, creatinine, glucose, cholesterol, and triglyceride levels; abnormal urinalysis; abnormal chest x-ray showing cardiomegaly, aortic dilatation, or rib notching; abnormal ECG demonstrating left ventricular hypertrophy

BP, Blood pressure; *BUN*, blood urea nitrogen; *ECG*, electrocardiogram.

Table 30-10 Nursing Diagnoses and Collaborative Problems Associated with Hypertension

Nursing Diagnoses

Altered health maintenance related to lack of knowledge of pathology, complications, and management of hypertension

Anxiety related to complexity of management regimen, possible complications, and lifestyle changes associated with hypertension

Altered sexuality related to effects of antihypertensive medication

Ineffective management of therapeutic regimen (specify) related to unpleasant side effects of medication, subsiding of symptoms, return of blood pressure to normal while on medication, lack of motivation, high cost of some medications, inconvenient schedule for taking medications, and lack of trusting relationship with health care provider

Body image disturbance related to diagnosis of hypertension

Collaborative Problems

Potential complication: Adverse effects from antihypertensive therapy

Potential complication: Hypertensive crisis

Potential complication: Cerebral vascular accident

Table 30-11 Appropriate Technique for Measuring Blood Pressure

1. Patient should be seated with the arm bared, supported, and positioned at heart level. The patient should not have smoked or ingested caffeine within 30 min before measurement.
2. Blood pressure should be taken in both arms initially.
3. Measurement should not begin until patient has had 5 min of quiet rest.
4. The appropriate cuff size must be used to ensure an accurate measurement. The rubber bladder should nearly (at least 80%) or completely encircle the arm. Several sizes of cuffs (e.g., child, adult, and large adult) should be available.
5. Measurements should be taken with a mercury sphygmomanometer, a recently calibrated aneroid manometer, or a calibrated electronic device.
6. Both systolic and diastolic pressures should be recorded. The disappearance of sound should be used for the diastolic reading.
7. Two or more readings (taken at least 2 min apart) should be averaged. If the first two readings differ by more than 5 mm Hg, additional readings should be obtained.
8. The patient should be informed of the reading and advised of the need for periodic remeasurement.

From US Department of Health and Human Services: The fifth report of the Joint National Committee on Detection, Evaluation, and Treatment of High Blood Pressure (JNC-V), Washington DC, 1993, National Institutes of Health.

BP measurement, each patient should be informed in writing of the numeric value of the reading and, if necessary, why further evaluation is important. Effort and resources should be focused on controlling BP in the person already identified as having hypertension; identifying and controlling BP in high-risk groups such as African-Americans, obese persons, and blood relatives of people with hypertension; and screening those with limited access to the health care system.[1]

Risk factors. Patient education regarding risk factors is appropriate for individual and mass screening programs. Populations at increased risk of developing hypertension are African-Americans, people with high-normal BP, those with a family history of hypertension, and people with one or more of the lifestyle factors mentioned previously.[3] Risk factors can easily be identified and modification discussed with the patient. (Health-promoting behaviors for risk factors related to coronary artery disease are discussed in Table 31-4.)

Acute Intervention. The majority of patients with hypertension are managed on an outpatient basis. The patient with a severely elevated BP, especially with significant target organ damage, may be hospitalized. The purpose of hospitalization is to lower the BP, determine the underlying cause of the hypertension, prevent or limit target organ damage, and treat the cause if it is secondary hypertension. The primary goal of the nurse at this stage of intervention is to assist in reducing BP and to begin patient education.

For the patient with severe hypertension, the nurse needs to monitor the BP every 1 to 2 hours and then with decreasing frequency as the pressure stabilizes. Antihypertensive drug therapy at this time may be given parenterally. This requires very frequent (every 2 to 5 minutes) BP checks, which can be done with an automated BP monitoring machine or an arterial catheter. Careful monitoring of vital signs provides information regarding the effectiveness of these drugs and the patient's response to therapy.

Regular, ongoing assessment is essential to evaluate the patient with severe hypertension. Frequent neurologic checks, including level of consciousness, pupillary size and reaction, movement of extremities, and reactions to stimuli, help to detect any changes in the patient's condition. Cardiac, pulmonary, and renal systems should be monitored for decompensation caused by the severe elevation in BP (e.g., pulmonary edema, CHF, angina, and renal failure).

If the patient has headaches, the nurse should assess when the headaches occur and what precipitating factors are present. In addition to lowering the BP, nursing interventions for headache include the modification of any environmental or emotional factors that may be contributing to the headache. Appropriate interventions include encouraging the patient to verbalize fears, answering questions concerning the hypertension, and eliminating excess noise in the patient's environment.

Table 30-12 Recommendations for Follow-Up Based on Initial Set of Blood Pressure Measurements for Adults Age 18 and Older

Initial Screening Blood Pressure (mm Hg)*		Recommendations
Systolic	Diastolic	Follow-up recommended*†
<130	<85	Recheck in 2 yr
130-139	85-89	Recheck in 1 yr‡
140-159	90-99	Confirm within 2 mo
160-179	100-109	Evaluate or refer to source of care within 1 mo
180-209	110-119	Evaluate or refer to source of care within 1 wk
≥210	≥120	Evaluate or refer to source of care immediately

From US Department of Health and Human Services: The fifth report of the Joint National Committee on Detection, Evaluation, and Treatment of High Blood Pressure (JNC-V), Washington, DC, 1992, National Institutes of Health.
* If the systolic and diastolic categories are different, follow recommendation for the shorter time follow-up (e.g., 160/85 mm Hg should be evaluated or referred to source of care within 1 mo).
† The scheduling of follow-up should be modified by reliable information about past blood pressure measurements, other cardiovascular risk factors, or target-organ disease.
‡ Consider providing advice about lifestyle modifications.

The patient with fatigue and anxiety should be provided with a schedule that alternates long rest periods with periods of light activity. It is important to plan for emotional as well as physical rest.

Chronic and Home Management. The primary nursing responsibilities for long-term management of the patient with hypertension are to assist in reducing BP and to begin or continue patient education (Table 30-13). Patient education includes the following:

1. Diet therapy
2. Drug therapy
3. Exercise
4. Home monitoring of BP (if appropriate)
5. Smoking cessation (if applicable)

Diet therapy. The patient and family, especially the member who prepares the meals, usually need to be educated about sodium-restricted diets. They need to be instructed on reading labels of over-the-counter drugs as well as packaged foods to identify hidden sources of sodium. It is helpful to review the patient's normal diet and to identify foods high in sodium. Analysis of a 3-day diet history will help to identify foods high in sodium in the patient's usual diet. (Weight-reduction diets are discussed in Chapter 37, and diets low in cholesterol and saturated fats are discussed in Chapter 31.)

Drug therapy. Side effects of antihypertensive drug therapy are common. (See the research box on p. 881.) The number or severity of side effects may be related to the dosage, and in certain cases it is necessary to change the drug or decrease the dosage. Side effects may be caused by an initial response to a drug and may decrease with long-term use of the drug. With some drugs, side effects can be alleviated by arranging a convenient schedule. For example, dry mouth and frequent voiding are common side effects of diuretics. Chewing sugarless gum or candy may relieve the dry mouth. When frequent urination interrupts sleep, diuretics work best taken early in the morning rather than at night. Side effects of vasodilators and adrenergic inhibitors decrease if the drugs are given in the evening. With some drugs, side effects can be decreased if the drugs are given with meals.

A common side effect of several of these drugs is orthostatic hypotension. This condition is caused by an alteration of the autonomic nervous system's mechanisms for regulating pressure, which are required for positional changes. Consequently, the patient may feel dizzy, weak, and faint when assuming an upright position after sitting or lying down. Specific measures to control or decrease orthostatic hypotension are presented in Table 30-13.

Sexual dysfunction may occur with many of the antihypertensive drugs (see Table 30-7) and can be a major reason that a male patient does not adhere to his treatment regimen. Rather than discussing a personal sexual problem with a health professional, the patient often finds it easier to discontinue using the drug. Often the nurse must approach the patient on this sensitive subject and encourage discussion of any sexual dysfunction that may be experienced. The sexual problems may be easier for the patient to discuss and handle once it has been explained that the drug may be the source of the problem and the side effects can be decreased or eliminated by changing to another antihypertensive drug.

Exercise. The patient needs assistance in developing a graduated exercise program. An aerobic exercise program based on the patient's current exercise activities can be planned. It is important to monitor the patient's long-term adherence to an exercise program.

Home monitoring. The patient should be assessed individually about the feasibility of being taught, or having a family member taught, to take BP readings at home. Often, home BP measurement gives a more valid indication of the BP because the patient is more relaxed. It is important to emphasize to the patient that a single reading is not as important as a series of readings over a period of time. The patient should be instructed to take BP readings weekly (unless otherwise instructed) once the BP has stabilized. A log of the BP measurements should be maintained by the patient and brought to office visits.

Home BP readings may help to achieve patient compliance by reinforcing the need to remain on therapy. A patient may become excessively concerned with the BP readings when using home monitoring. Generally, however, this practice should reassure the patient that the treatment is effective.

Patient noncompliance. A major problem in the long-term management of the patient with hypertension is poor compliance with the prescribed treatment regimen. The

Table 30-13 Teaching Plan for the Patient with Hypertension

When presenting information to the patient, the nurse should do the following:

1. Provide the numeric value of the patient's blood pressure (BP) and explain that it exceeds normal limits.
2. Inform patient that hypertension is usually asymptomatic and symptoms do not reliably indicate BP levels.
3. Explain that hypertension means elevated BP and does not relate to a "hyper" personality.
4. Explain that long-term follow-up and therapy are necessary.
5. Explain that therapy will not cure hypertension, but should control it.
6. Tell patient that controlled hypertension is usually compatible with an excellent prognosis and a normal lifestyle.
7. Explain the potential dangers of uncontrolled hypertension.
8. Be specific about the names, actions, dosages, and side effects of prescribed medications.
9. Tell patient to plan regular and convenient times for taking medications.
10. Tell patient not to discontinue drugs abruptly because withdrawal may cause a severe hypertensive reaction.
11. Tell patient not to double a dose when one has been missed.
12. Inform patient that if BP increases, not to take an increased medication dosage before consulting with the health care provider.
13. Tell patient not to take a medication belonging to someone else.
14. Inform patient that side effects of medication often diminish with time.
15. Tell patient to consult with the health care provider about changing drugs or dosages if impotence or other sexual problems develop.
16. Tell patient to supplement diet with foods high in potassium (e.g., citrus fruits and green leafy vegetables) if taking potassium-losing diuretics.
17. Tell patient to avoid hot baths, excessive amounts of alcohol, and strenuous exercise within 3 hr of taking medications that promote vasodilatation.
18. Explain that to decrease orthostatic hypotension, the patient should arise slowly from bed, sit on side of bed for a few minutes, stand slowly, not stand still for prolonged periods of time, do leg exercises to increase venous return, sleep with head of bed raised or on pillows, and lie or sit down when dizziness occurs.

reasons are many and include inadequate patient instruction, unpleasant side effects of drugs, relief of symptoms so that the patient feels "cured," return of BP to normal range while on medication, lack of motivation, high cost of drugs, and lack of a trusting relationship between the patient and the health care provider. In addition to using BP determinations as an indicator of compliance, the nurse should also assess the patient's diet, exercise program, and lifestyle.

Individual assessment to determine the reasons the patient is not complying with the treatment regimen and development of an individual plan with the patient's assistance are essential. The plan needs to be compatible with the patient's personality, habits, and lifestyle. Active patient participation increases the likelihood of adherence to the treatment plan. Measures such as involving the patient in scheduling medication convenient to a daily routine, helping the patient link pill-taking with another daily activity, and involving family members (if necessary) help increase patient compliance. Substituting combination tablets for multiple drugs once the BP is stabilized may also facilitate compliance, since the patient has to take fewer drugs each day and the cost is less. It is important to help the patient and the family understand that hypertension is a chronic condition that cannot be cured but can be controlled with drug therapy, diet therapy, an exercise program, periodic evaluation, and other relevant lifestyle changes.

HYPERTENSIVE CRISIS

Hypertensive crisis is a severe and abrupt elevation in BP and is potentially life threatening. A hypertensive crisis is not as common today as in the past.[15] However, when it does occur, prompt recognition and management is essential to decrease the threat to organ function and life. Hypertensive crisis related to cocaine or crack use is becoming a much more frequent problem. Other drugs such as amphetamines, phencyclidine (PCP), and lysergic acid diethylamide (LSD) may also precipitate hypertensive crisis that may be complicated by drug-induced seizures, stroke, MI, or encephalopathy.[16] In a patient with no history of hypertension, there is frequently a secondary cause.[17] Some causes of hypertensive crisis are presented in Table 30-14.

Hypertensive crisis is classified by the degree of organ damage and the rapidity with which the BP must be lowered. *Hypertensive emergency,* which develops over hours to days, is a situation in which a patient's BP is severely elevated with evidence of acute target organ damage, especially damage to the central nervous system. Possible complications include hypertensive encephalopathy, intracranial hemorrhage, acute left ventricular failure with pulmonary edema, renal failure, and dissecting aortic aneurysm. *Hypertensive urgency,* which develops over days to weeks, is a situation in which a patient's BP is severely elevated but there is no evidence of target organ damage. Hypertensive urgencies are usually caused by an exacerbation of previously existing hypertension.

Clinical Manifestations

A hypertensive emergency is often manifested as hypertensive encephalopathy, a syndrome in which a sudden rise in

Table 30-14 Causes of Hypertensive Crisis

Exacerbation of chronic hypertension
Renovascular hypertension
Preeclampsia, eclampsia
Pheochromocytoma
Drugs (cocaine, amphetamines, oral contraceptive pills)
Monoamine oxidase inhibitors taken with tyramine containing foods
Rebound hypertension (from abrupt withdrawal of clonidine or beta blockers)
Necrotizing vasculitis
Head injury
Acute aortic dissection

arterial pressure is associated with headache, nausea, vomiting, convulsions, confusion, stupor, and coma. Other common manifestations are blurred vision and transient blindness. The manifestations of encephalopathy are probably the results of cerebral edema and spasms of cerebral vessels.

Renal insufficiency ranging from minor impairment to complete renal shutdown may occur. Rapid cardiac decompensation with developing pulmonary edema is also possible.

Patient assessment is extremely important, especially monitoring for signs of neurologic dysfunction, retinal damage, CHF, pulmonary edema, and renal failure. The neurologic manifestations are often similar to the presentation of a CVA. However, a hypertensive crisis does not show focal or lateralizing signs often seen with a CVA.

Therapeutic Management

BP measurement alone is a poor indicator of the seriousness of the patient's condition and is not the major factor in deciding the treatment for a hypertensive crisis. The association between elevated BP and signs of new or progressive end-organ damage (e.g., cerebrovascular, cardiac, retinal, or renal damage) determines the seriousness of the situation. Initially, the treatment goal is a 25% decrease in mean arterial pressure (MAP) with a maximum DBP of 100 mm Hg. Lowering the BP too far or too fast may decrease cerebral perfusion and could precipitate a stroke. A patient who has aortic dissection needs to have the SBP lowered to 100 to 120 mm Hg as quickly as possible.[15]

When treating hypertensive emergencies, the MAP is often used instead of systolic and diastolic readings to guide and evaluate therapy. MAP is calculated as DBP + ⅓ pulse pressure (SBP − DBP):

$$\text{MAP} = \text{DBP} + \tfrac{1}{3}\ \text{pulse pressure (SBP} - \text{DBP)}$$

True hypertensive emergencies require hospitalization, parenteral administration of antihypertensive drugs, and intensive-care monitoring. However, oral agents may be administered in addition to the parenteral drugs to help make an earlier transition to long-term therapy. The intravenous (IV) drugs used for hypertensive emergencies are vasodilators such as sodium nitroprusside, nitroglycerin, diazoxide, and hydralazine; and adrenergic inhibitors such as phentolamine, labetalol, methyldopa; and the ACE inhibitor enalaprilat (Vasotec IV). Sodium nitroprusside is the most effective parenteral drug for the treatment of hypertensive emergencies.[17] The mechanisms of action and the adverse effects of these drugs are presented in Table 30-7.

The drugs are administered IV and have a rapid (within seconds to minutes) onset of action. The patient's BP and pulse should be taken every 2 to 3 minutes during the initial administration of these drugs. The use of an intraarterial line (see Chapter 61) or an automated BP monitoring machine (e.g., Dynamap) to monitor the BP is ideal. The rate of drug administration is titrated according to the level of BP. It is important to prevent hypotension and its effects in a person whose body has adjusted to hypertension. An excessive reduction in BP may cause stroke, MI, or visual changes. Continual ECG monitoring is frequently done to observe for cardiac dysrhythmias. Extreme caution is

RESEARCH

IMPLICATIONS FOR NURSING PRACTICE

SIDE EFFECTS OF ANTIHYPERTENSIVE MEDICATIONS

Citation Potempa K and others: Blood pressure and mood responses in hypertensive patients on antihypertensive medications, *J Am Acad Nurse Practitioners* 5:211-218, 1993.

Purpose To determine the effect of three antihypertensive medications (i.e., pindolol, propranolol, and hydrochlorothiazide) on changes in blood pressure and psychologic mood variables in hypertensive individuals.

Methods A randomized 3 × 2 factorial repeated measures experimental design was used with three randomly assigned drug treatment groups and two 4-week long treatment phases, an untreated and a drug-treated phase. Essential hypertensive subjects (n = 41) were monitored weekly for weight, blood pressure, heart rate, and psychologic mood measures including the Profile of Mood States (POMS) and the Beck Depression Inventory (BDI).

Results and Conclusions Pindolol, propranolol, and hydrochlorothiazide were equally effective in reducing systolic and diastolic blood pressure. However, pindolol and hydrochlorothiazide did not affect the resting heart rate. Hydrochlorothiazide was associated with a trend toward several negative mood changes in African-American subjects. Depression scores were significantly increased in African-American subjects taking hydrochlorothiazide.

Implications for Nursing Practice The nurse needs to be aware of the effects of antihypertensive medication on both physiologic and psychologic variables. Adequate assessment of these responses in the patient needs to be determined during treatment.

CRITICAL THINKING EXERCISES

CASE STUDY

ESSENTIAL HYPERTENSION

Patient Profile

Mr. R. is a 45-year-old African-American man with no previous history of hypertension. At a screening clinic, his BP was found to be 180/120 mm Hg.

Subjective Data

- Father died of stroke at age 60
- Mother is alive but has hypertension
- States that he feels fine and is not a "hyper" person
- Smokes one pack of cigarettes daily
- Drinks a 6-pack of beer on Friday and Saturday nights
- Believes that BP medication messes up his love life

Objective Data

Physical Examination

- Grade I/IV Keith Wagener retinopathy

Diagnostic Studies

- ECG—left ventricular hypertrophy
- Urinalysis—Protein 30 mg/dl (.3 gm/L)
- Serum creatinine level—1.6 mg/dl (141 μmol/L)

Therapeutic Management

- Low sodium diet
- Hydrochlorothiazide 25 mg/day

Critical Thinking Questions

1. What risk factors for hypertension are present?
2. What evidence of target organ damage is present?
3. What misconceptions about hypertension need to be corrected?
4. What areas would you focus on in teaching this patient about his illness?
5. Based on the assessment data presented, write one or more appropriate nursing diagnoses. Are there any collaborative problems?

NURSING RESEARCH ISSUES

1. Does a person believe that if the personal risk factors for hypertension are reduced, chances of developing hypertension will be reduced?
2. What are the perceptions and attitudes of the nurse toward the efficacy of hypertension screening?
3. Do the perceptions of daily stress in the hypertensive patient differ from the perceptions of daily stress in the nonhypertensive patient?
4. Do the patient and family members who are taught BP measurement by videotaped instruction measure BP as accurately as those who are taught by personal instruction?
5. Does home monitoring of BP increase the patient's compliance with antihypertensive therapy?

needed in treating the patient with coronary artery disease or cerebral vascular insufficiency. Hourly urinary output should be measured to assess renal perfusion.

Hypertensive urgencies usually do not require emergency IV medications but can be managed with oral agents. The patient with a hypertensive urgency may not need hospitalization, but requires frequent follow-up.[17] The oral drugs used for hypertensive urgencies, described in Table 30-7, are captopril, clonidine, and nifedipine. Sublingual or oral nifedipine is widely used for hypertensive urgencies, and has been shown to lower the BP within 10 to 15 minutes, with the maximal reduction in BP occurring within 30 minutes to 1 hour. Biting a nifedipine capsule and swallowing its contents with water, rather than taking the drug sublingually, is recommended in a hypertensive urgency. This method of administration provides for rapid therapeutic plasma levels of nifedipine, since absorption from the oral cavity is slow and incomplete. However, the disadvantage of oral medications such as nifedipine is the inability to regulate the dosage moment to moment, as can be done with IV medications.

Once the hypertensive crisis is resolved, it is important to determine the cause. The patient will need appropriate management and extensive education to avoid future crisis.

REVIEW QUESTIONS

The number of the question corresponds to the same-numbered objective at the beginning of the chapter.

1. Which of the following statements about BP regulation is incorrect?

a. Increased SVR causes an increased work load on the heart.

b. Baroreceptors are located in the peripheral blood vessels and are sensitive to stretch.

c. Sympathetic nervous system stimulation causes increased CO and SVR.

d. The kidneys contribute to BP regulation by controlling sodium excretion and ECF volume.

2. Which of the following risk factors does not contribute to the development of hypertension?

a. Cigarette smoking
b. Obesity
c. Sodium intake
d. Alcohol

3. Examples of target organ damage include both

a. renal dysfunction and left ventricular hypertrophy.
b. retinopathy and diabetes.
c. hypercholesterolemia and renal dysfunction.
d. headache and dizziness.

4. Which of the following is not considered a high risk population to be targeted in the primary prevention of hypertension?

a. Obese persons
b. African-American women
c. Smokers
d. Children of hypertensive parents

5. Which of the following is true about management of hypertension?

a. All patients with elevated BP require medication.
b. Lifestyle modifications are indicated for all persons with elevated BP.
c. It is not necessary to limit salt in the diet if taking a diuretic.
d. Obese persons must achieve a normal weight in order to lower BP.

6. Which of the following is not true about management of hypertension in the older adult?

a. Decreased regulatory controls in the older adult may cause variability in BP.
b. Absorption of some drugs may be decreased and excretion prolonged.
c. The older adult should be started on lower doses of medication than the younger adult.
d. Pseudohypertension must be followed closely in case it becomes true hypertension.

7. In teaching a hypertensive patient about medication, the nurse should know which of the following classes of drug is not appropriate as initial monotherapy?

a. ACE inhibitors
b. β-blockers
c. Vasodilators
d. Calcium channel blockers

8. Which of the following is not true regarding hypertensive emergencies and urgencies?

a. The level of BP determines whether a situation is an emergency or an urgency.
b. Oral drugs may be used in both hypertensive emergencies and urgencies.
c. Measurement of BP by an intraarterial catheter is often necessary in hypertensive emergencies.
d. Treatment of hypertensive urgencies does not always require hospitalization.

REFERENCES

1. Fifth report of the Joint National Committee on Detection, Evaluation and Treatment of High Blood Pressure (JNC-V), *Arch Intern Med* 153:154, 1993.
2. Kaplan NM: Primary hypertension: pathogenesis. In Fisher MG, editor: *Clinical hypertension*, ed 5, Baltimore, 1990, Williams and Wilkins.
3. National High Blood Pressure Education Program Working Group Report on Primary Prevention of Hypertension, *Arch Intern Med* 153:186, 1993.
4. Moorthy AV, Kochar MS: Nephrology and hypertension. In Kochar MS, editor: *Concise textbook of medicine*, ed 2, New York, 1990, Elsevier.
5. Weinberger MH: Hypertension in the elderly, *Hosp Pract* 27:103, 1992.
6. Mann SF: Systolic hypertension in the elderly: pathophysiology and management, *Arch Intern Med* 152:1977, 1992.
7. Berger DS, Li J: Concurrent compliance reduction and increased peripheral resistance in the manifestation of isolated systolic hypertension, *Am J Cardiol* 65:67, 1990.
8. SHEP Cooperative Research Group: Prevention of stroke by antihypertensive drug treatment in older persons with isolated systolic hypertension, *JAMA* 265:3255, 1991.
9. Dahlof B and others: Morbidity and mortality in the Swedish Trial in old patients with hypertension (STOP-hypertension), *Lancet* 338:1281, 1991.
10. Kochar MS: Hypertension in elderly patients: the special concerns in this growing population, *Postgrad Med* 91: 393, 1992.
11. Trottier DJ, Kochar MS: Around the clock blood pressure monitoring: how to get good results, *Nursing* 92:67, 1992.
12. Johnston DW: Stress management in the treatment of mild primary hypertension, *Hypertension* 17:III-63, 1991.
13. Montfrans G and others: Relaxation therapy and continuous ambulatory blood pressure in mild hypertension: a controlled study, *Br Med J* 300:1368, 1990.
14. The Trials of Hypertension Prevention Collaborative Research Group: The effects of nonpharmacologic interventions on blood pressure of persons with high normal levels: results of the trials of hypertension prevention, phase 1, *JAMA* 267:1213, 1992.
15. Moore RK and others: Alcohol consumption and blood pressure in the 1982 Maryland hypertension survey, *Am J Hyperten* 3:1, 1990.
16. Calhoun DA, Oparil SD: Treatment of hypertensive crisis, *N Engl J Med* 323:1177, 1990.
17. McKinney TD: Management of hypertensive crisis, *Hosp Pract* 27:133, 1992.

Chapter 31

NURSING ROLE IN MANAGEMENT

Coronary Artery Disease

Linda Griego **Mary Ann House-Fancher**

Learning Objectives

1. Describe the etiology and pathophysiology of coronary artery disease.
2. Explain the nursing role in health promotion and maintenance related to risk factors for coronary artery disease.
3. Describe the precipitating factors, types, clinical manifestations, and therapeutic and pharmacologic management of stable and unstable angina pectoris.
4. Explain the nursing role in the management of the patient with stable and unstable angina pectoris.
5. Describe the pathophysiology of myocardial infarction from the onset of injury through the healing process.
6. Describe the clinical manifestations, complications, diagnostic study abnormalities, and therapeutic management of myocardial infarction.
7. Describe the nursing role in the rehabilitative management of the patient following myocardial infarction.
8. Identify the emotional and behavioral reactions to myocardial infarction.
9. Describe the precipitating factors, types, clinical presentation, and therapeutic, pharmacologic, and surgical management of sudden cardiac death.

CORONARY ARTERY DISEASE

Coronary artery disease (CAD) is a type of blood vessel disorder that is included in the general category of atherosclerosis. *Atherosclerosis* is derived from two Greek words: *athere,* meaning "fatty mush," and *skleros,* meaning "hard." This word combination indicates that atherosclerosis begins as soft deposits of fat that harden with age. Atherosclerosis is often referred to as "hardening of the arteries." Although this condition can occur in any artery in the body, the atheromas (fatty deposits) have a preference for the coronary arteries. Arteriosclerotic heart disease (ASHD), cardiovascular heart disease (CVHD), ischemic heart disease (IHD), coronary heart disease (CHD), and CAD are synonymous terms used to describe this disease process. Other terms used to describe the disease mechanisms involved in CAD are *plaque formation, atheromatous deposits,* and *coronary occlusions.*

Significance

Cardiovascular diseases are the major cause of death in the United States (Fig. 31-1). The American Heart Association (AHA) reports that almost 490,000 persons die each year of heart attacks. Although this has decreased by 26.7% between 1980 and 1990, heart attacks or myocardial infarctions (MIs), are still the leading cause of all cardiovascular disease deaths and deaths in general. An estimated 70,020,000 persons have one or more forms of heart disease.[1] The estimated prevalence of CAD by age is presented in Fig. 31-2.

Etiology and Pathophysiology

Atherosclerosis is the major cause of CAD. It is characterized by a focal deposit of cholesterol and lipids, primarily within the intimal wall of the artery. The genesis of plaque formation is the result of complex interactions between the components of the blood and the elements forming the vascular wall.[1] The concept of endothelial injury is central to current theories of atherogenesis. Table 31-1 summarizes theories of atherogenesis, with endothelial injury being the leading theory for the cause of atherosclerotic disease.

Intact normal endothelium is nonreactive to platelets and leukocytes as well as coagulation, fibrinolytic, and complement factors. However, the endothelial lining can be altered as a result of chemical injuries, such as hyperlipidemia (nondenuding), or high-shear stress, such as hypertension (denuding). With either type of endothelial alteration, platelets are activated, and they release a growth factor that stimulates smooth muscle proliferation. The smooth muscle cell proliferation entraps lipids, which are calcified over time and form an irritant to the endothelium upon which

Reviewed by Juli Shea, RN, CCRN, MSN, Clinical Nurse Specialist–Critical Care, Oconee Memorial Hospital, Starr, SC.

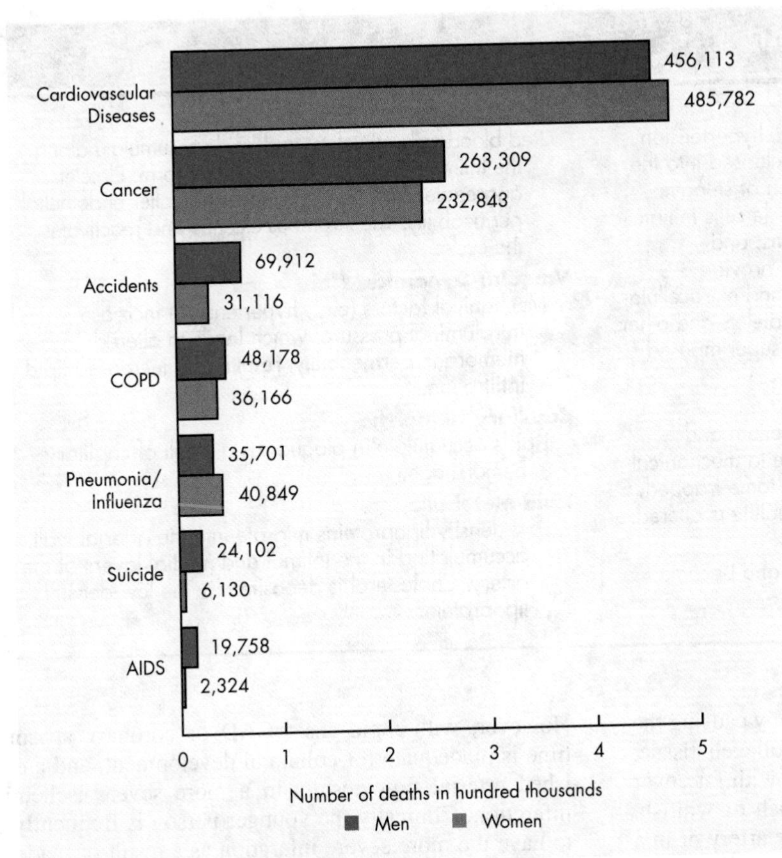

Fig. 31-1 Leading causes of death, men and women. *AIDS,* Acquired immunodeficiency syndrome; *COPD,* chronic obstructive pulmonary disease.

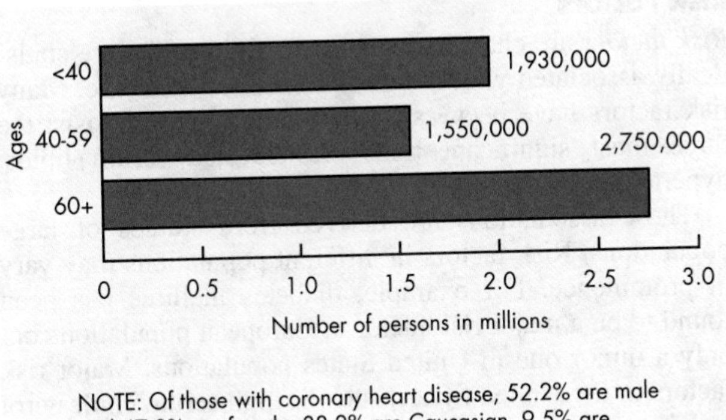

Fig. 31-2 Estimated prevalence of coronary heart disease.

platelets adhere and aggregate. Thrombin is generated, and fibrin formation and thrombi occur (Fig. 31-3). Endothelial replication is normally slow in adults, but in the presence of hypertension and hyperlipidemia, increased cell turnover leads to transient repeated denuding of the endothelium.

Development Stages. CAD takes many years to develop. When it becomes symptomatic, the disease process is usually well advanced. The stages of development in atherosclerosis are (1) fatty streak, (2) raised fibrous plaque resulting from smooth muscle cell proliferation, and (3) complicated lesion (Fig. 31-4).

Fatty streak. Fatty streaks, the earliest lesions of atherosclerosis, are characterized by lipid-filled smooth muscle cells. As streaks of fat develop within the smooth muscle cells, a yellow tinge appears. Fatty streaks are usually observed in the coronary arteries by age 15 and involve an increasing amount of surface area as the patient ages. It is generally believed that they are reversible.

Raised fibrous plaque. The raised fibrous plaque stage is the beginning of progressive changes in the arterial wall. These changes appear in the coronary arteries by the age of 30 and increase with age. The arterial wall changes are initiated by chronic endothelial injury that results from many factors, including elevated blood pressure (BP), high blood cholesterol, heredity, carbon monoxide produced by smoking, immune reactions, and possibly toxic substances within the blood. Normally the endothelium repairs itself immediately, but in the person with CAD the endothelium is *not* rapidly replaced, allowing low-density lipoproteins and growth factor from platelets to stimulate smooth muscle proliferation and thickening of the arterial wall. Once endothelial injury has occurred, lipoproteins (the carrier substances within the bloodstream) transport cholesterol and other lipids into the arterial intima (Fig. 31-4). Lipids may cause smooth muscle damage as well as contribute to plaque thickening and instability. As these lipids and other substances pass through the vessels, they

Table 31-1 Theories of Atherogenesis

Endothelial Injury
Endothelium is "injured" by hyperlipidemia, hypertension, or other chemical irritants. Factors are released into the subendothelium and induce the migration of smooth muscle cells into the intima. Smooth muscle cells initiate synthesis of collagen, elastic fiber proteins, and proteoglycans (a substance that tends to provide a nonthrombogenic surface). Intracellular and extracellular lipids begin to accumulate, as well as platelets and other clotting factors, and a lesion-associated superimposed thrombus is formed.

Lipid Infiltration
Lipids from the circulation enter the endothelium and accumulate in smooth muscle in response to mechanical or inflammatory trauma. Lipoproteins become trapped, and damage occurs. Endothelial permeability is altered.

Aging
Atherosclerotic changes occur in everyone and become more evident as aging progresses.

Thrombogenic
Red blood cells, platelets, and lipids accumulate along the intima of arteries. Microthrombi form. Platelets aggregate, releasing substances that alter endothelial permeability. The thrombus extends and reactivates the cycle.

Vascular Dynamics
Mechanical factors (e.g., hypertension) increase intraluminal pressure, which leads to altered membrane permeability, resulting in increased lipid infiltration.

Capillary Hemorrhage
Lipids accumulate in plaques as a result of capillary hemorrhage.

Lipid Metabolic
Low-density lipoproteins migrate into the arterial wall, accumulating in the intimal and medial layers of the artery. Cholesterol is deposited by the low-density lipoproteins.

adhere to the roughened, damaged wall, thereby causing the lesion buildup or structural abnormality. Collagen tissue, elastic fibers, and smooth muscle cells filled with fat cover the lesion. The fibrous plaque appears grayish or whitish. These plaques can form on one portion of the artery or in a circular fashion involving the entire lumen. The borders can be smooth or irregular with rough, jagged edges.[2]

Platelets also play a part in the hypertrophy of smooth muscle cells. Once the artery's inner wall has become damaged, platelets may accumulate in large numbers, leading to a thrombus. The thrombus may adhere to the wall of the artery, leading to narrowing or total occlusion of the artery.

Complicated lesion. The final stage in the development of the atherosclerotic lesion is the most dangerous. The plaque consists of a core of lipid materials (mainly cholesterol) within an area of dead tissue. With the incorporation of lipids, thrombi, damaged tissue, and some accumulation of calcium, the growing lesion becomes complex. As the lesion continues to grow and become complex, necrotic tissue that is dark and hardened appears within the arteries, causing rigidity and hardening. This complicated lesion may totally or partially occlude the artery.

Collateral Circulation. Normally some arterial branching, called *collateral circulation,* exists within the coronary circulation. The growth of collateral circulation is attributed to two factors: (1) the inherited predisposition to develop angioblastic properties and (2) the presence of chronic ischemia. When an atherosclerotic plaque occludes the normal flow of blood through a coronary artery and ischemia is chronic, increased collateral circulation develops (Fig. 31-5). When occlusion of the coronary arteries occurs slowly over a long period, there is a greater chance of adequate collateral circulation developing, and the myocardium may still receive an adequate amount of oxygen. However, with rapid-onset CAD or coronary spasm, the time is inadequate for collateral development, and a diminished arterial flow results in a more severe ischemia or infarction. Clinically the younger person is frequently seen to have the more severe infarction as a result of inadequate collateral formation.

Risk Factors

Risk factors are characteristics or conditions that are statistically associated with a high incidence of a disease. Many risk factors have been associated with atherosclerosis; the three most significant risks are elevated serum lipids, hypertension, and cigarette smoking.[3]

These associations are derived from studies of large populations. Risk factors in different populations may vary in prominence. For example, diabetes mellitus has been found to be a major risk factor in European populations but only a minor one in United States populations. Major risk factors in the United States, such as high serum cholesterol and hypertension, are less prevalent in Japanese, Puerto Rican, and Hawaiian populations.

Risk factors can be categorized as unmodifiable and modifiable (Table 31-2). *Unmodifiable* risk factors are age, gender, race, and genetic inheritance. *Modifiable* risk factors include elevated serum lipids, hypertension, smoking, obesity, sedentary lifestyle, and stress in daily living. Although control of diabetes is recommended, it has not been proven to decrease the incidence of CAD in the United States.

Data on risk factors have been obtained in several major studies. In the Framingham study (one of the most widely known), 5209 men and women were observed for 20 years.[3] Over time, it was noted that elevated serum cholesterol (>240 mg/dl), elevated systolic BP (>160 mm Hg), and cigarette smoking (one or more packs a day) were

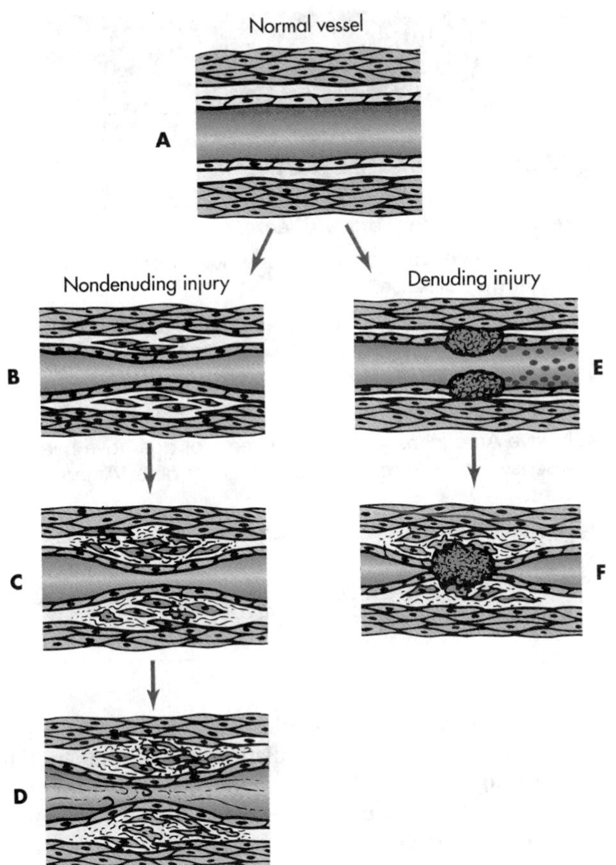

Fig. 31-3 Response to endothelial injury. ***A,*** Normal vessel, endothelium intact. ***B,*** Nondenuding injury (e.g., hyperlipidemia) with smooth muscle proliferation. ***C,*** Addition of collagen and fibroelastic tissues that narrow lumen. ***D,*** Narrowed lumen with calcification and irregular blood flow. ***E,*** Denuding injury with platelet adherence and aggregation or frank clot formation. ***F,*** Eventual thrombosis leading to infarction.

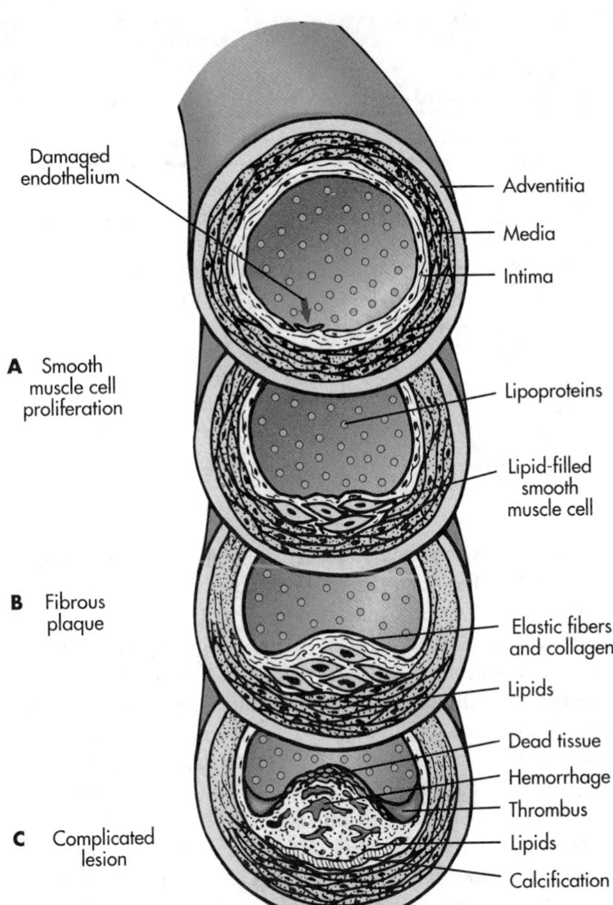

Fig. 31-4 The stages of development in the progression of atherosclerosis include ***A,*** smooth muscle cell proliferation, which creates ***B,*** a raised fibrous plaque and ***C,*** a complicated lesion.

positively correlated with an increased incidence of CAD. The younger the subject at the time of induction to the study, the more predictive were the values. Other implicated risk factors and indicators included diabetes mellitus, sedentary lifestyle, electrocardiographic (ECG) abnormalities, and reduced lung vital capacity.

Unmodifiable Risk Factors

Age, gender, and race. The incidence of MI is highest for the Caucasion, middle-aged man. After the age of 60, the incidence in men and women equalizes, although there is early evidence suggesting that more women are being seen with CAD earlier because of increased stress, increased cigarette smoking, presence of hypertension, and use of birth control pills. African-American males, although more prone to hypertension, are at less risk of CAD than Caucasians of the same age. Conversely, African-American females are at higher risk for CAD than Caucasian females.[1] MIs in the Asian population in the United States are less frequent than in Caucasians, but the rates are higher than in the countries of origin.

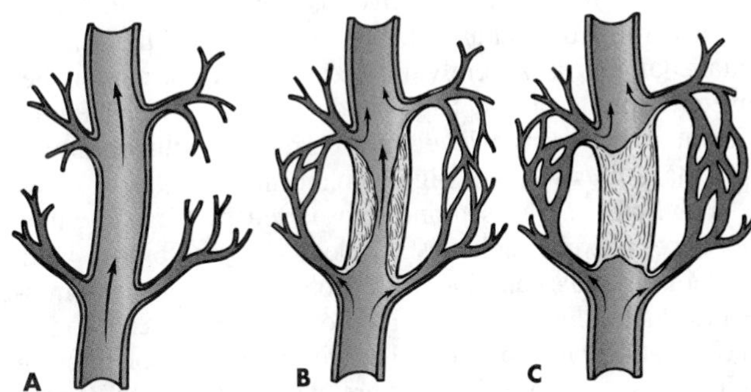

Fig. 31-5 Vessel occlusion with collateral circulation. ***A,*** Open, functioning coronary artery. ***B,*** Partial coronary artery closure with collateral circulation being established. ***C,*** Total coronary artery occlusion with collateral circulation bypassing the occlusion to supply the myocardium.

Table 31-2 Risk Factors in Coronary Artery Disease

Unmodifiable	Modifiable
Age Gender (men > women until 60 yrs of age) Race (African-Americans < Caucasians) Genetic predisposition and family history of heart disease	Major Elevated serum lipids Hypertension Cigarette smoking Physical inactivity Minor Obesity (>30% overweight) Diabetes mellitus* Stressful lifestyle

*May be hereditary.

CULTURAL & ETHNIC Considerations

CORONARY ARTERY DISEASE

- Caucasian, middle-aged males have the highest incidence of coronary artery disease.
- African-Americans have an early age of onset of coronary artery disease.
- African-American women have a higher incidence of coronary artery disease than Caucasian women.
- African-Americans have more severe coronary artery disease than Caucasians.
- Native Americans less than 35 years of age have heart disease mortality rates twice as high as other Americans.
- Hispanics have lower death rates from heart disease than non-Hispanics.
- Major modifiable cardiovascular risk factors for Native Americans are obesity and diabetes.

Family history and heredity. Genetic predisposition is an important factor in the occurrence of CAD, although the exact mechanism of inheritance is not fully understood. Some congenital defects in coronary artery walls predispose the person to the formation of plaques. Familial hyperlipoproteinemia, an autosomal dominant trait, has been strongly associated with CAD at early ages. In most cases of angina or MI, the patient can name a close family member who has died either suddenly of an unknown cause or of a documented heart attack.

Modifiable Major Risk Factors. The AHA has classified the modifiable risk factors as major and minor (contributing) risk factors. Major risk factors are those that medical research has shown to be definitely associated with a significant increase in the risk of the development of CAD. Minor risk factors are those associated with increased risk of CAD, but their significance and prevalence have not been precisely determined.[1]

Elevated serum lipids. An elevated serum lipid level is one of the four most firmly established risk factors for CAD.[1] The various types of serum lipids are presented in Fig. 31-6. More specifically, the risk of CAD is associated with a serum cholesterol level of more than 200 mg/dl (5.2 mmol/L) or a fasting triglyceride level of more than 150 mg/dl (1.7 mmol/L). The liver is capable of producing cholesterol from saturated fats, even when the dietary intake of fats is severely limited. A high correlation between cholesterol and triglyceride levels has been found. Elevated triglyceride levels are correlated with obesity, a sedentary lifestyle, and high alcohol intake.

For lipids to be used and transported by the body, they need to become soluble in blood by combining with proteins. Lipids combine with protein to form macromolecules called *lipoproteins*. Lipoproteins are vehicles for fat mobilization and transport. The different types of lipoprotein vary in composition and are classified as high-density lipoproteins (HDLs), low-density lipoproteins (LDLs), and very low-density lipoproteins (VLDLs) (see Fig. 31-6).

HDLs contain more protein by weight and less lipid than any other lipoprotein. HDLs carry lipids away from arteries and to the liver for metabolism (Fig. 31-7). Therefore high serum HDL levels are desirable. This process of HDL transport prevents lipid accumulation within the arterial walls. The higher the HDL levels in the blood, the lower the risk of CAD. HDL levels are generally higher in women than in men and are increased by physical activity and estrogen. The person who has had an MI has lower concentrations of HDL than matched controls. In general, HDL levels are high in children and women, decrease with age, and are low in persons with CAD. Current research on drug and dietary therapy is concentrating on ways to elevate HDL levels.

HDLs are broken down into HDL_2 and HDL_3. HDL_2 seems to protect the arteries from developing atherosclerosis. Exercise significantly raises HDL_2, which helps to clear out the fat load from the blood plasma. Premenopausal women have HDL levels approximately three times greater than men. After menopause, their HDL_2 levels quickly approximate those of men.

LDLs contain more cholesterol than any of the other lipoproteins and have an affinity for arterial walls.[4] Elevated LDL levels correlate most closely with an increased incidence of atherosclerosis. Therefore low serum LDL levels are desirable.

VLDLs contain most of the triglycerides. The direct correlation of VLDLs with heart disease is uncertain. High VLDL concentrations may increase the risk of premature atherosclerosis when associated with other factors such as diabetes, hypertension, and cigarette smoking.

Hypertension. The second major risk factor in CAD is hypertension, which is defined as a BP greater than or equal to 140/90 mm Hg. In the Framingham study, a threefold increase in the incidence of CAD was reported for middle-aged men with arterial pressures exceeding 160/95 mm Hg compared with those with BP of 140/90 mm Hg or less.[3] The cause of hypertension in 90% of those affected is

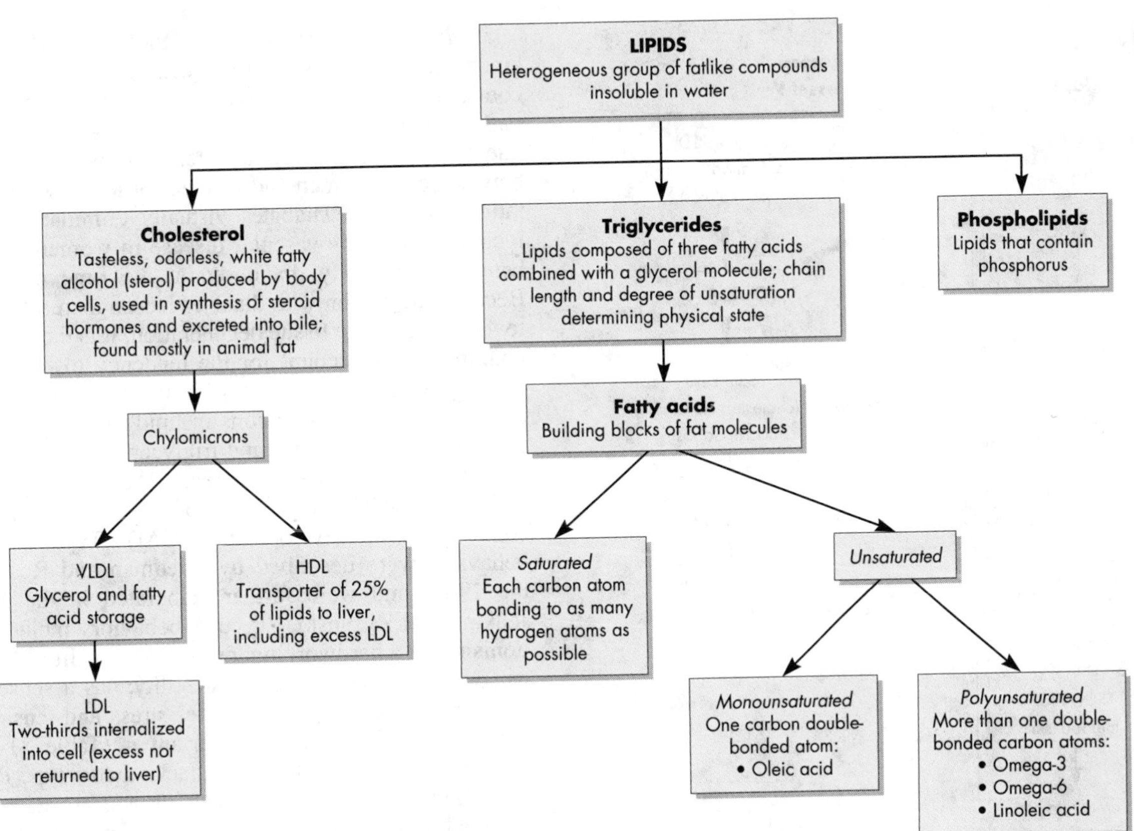

Fig. 31-6 Types of serum lipids. *HDL,* High-density lipoprotein; *LDL,* low-density lipoprotein; *VLDL,* very low-density lipoprotein.

unknown, but it is usually controllable with diet or medication.

The stress of a constantly elevated BP increases the rate of atherosclerotic development. This is related to the shearing stress, causing denuding injury of the endothelial lining. Atherosclerosis, in turn, causes narrowed, thickened arterial walls and decreases the distensibility and elasticity of vessels. More force is required to pump blood through diseased arterial vasculature, and this increased force is reflected in a higher BP. This increased work load is also manifested by left ventricular hypertrophy and a loss of efficiency with each contraction. Salt intake is positively correlated with elevated BP because of fluid retention, adding volume and increasing systemic vascular resistance (SVR) to the cardiac work load.

Smoking. The third major risk factor in CAD is cigarette smoking. Pipe and cigar smokers have not been found to have an increased risk of CAD. The risk of developing CAD is two to six times higher in cigarette smokers than in nonsmokers. There is some evidence that chronic exposure to environmental tobacco smoke also increases the risk of CAD.[5] Risk is proportional to the number of cigarettes smoked. Changing to lower nicotine or filtered cigarettes does not affect risk. Cessation of smoking has been shown to reduce the risk to nonsmoker levels with time.

Nicotine in cigarette smoke causes catecholamine (epinephrine, norepinephrine) release. These hormones cause an increased heart rate (HR), peripheral vasoconstriction, and increased BP. These changes increase the cardiac work load, necessitating greater myocardial oxygen consumption.

Carbon monoxide, a by-product of combustion, affects the oxygen-carrying capacity of hemoglobin by reducing the sites available for oxygen transport. Thus the effects of an increased cardiac work load, combined with the oxygen-depleting effect of carbon monoxide from smoking, significantly decrease the oxygen available to the myocardium. There is also some indication that carbon monoxide may be a chemical irritant as well, thus causing nondenuding injury to the endothelium.

Physical inactivity. Physical inactivity is the fourth major modifiable risk factor. Physical inactivity implies a lack of adequate physical exercise on a regular basis. Some practitioners define regular physical exercise as exercise that occurs at least three times a week for at least 30 minutes, causing perspiration and an increase in the HR by 30 to 50 beats per minute (bpm).

The mechanism by which physical inactivity predisposes to CAD is still unknown. It is thought that physically active people have increased HDL levels and that exercise enhances fibrinolytic activity, thus reducing the risk of clot formation. It is also believed that exercise encourages the development of collateral circulation.

Exercise training for those who are physically inactive is thought to decrease the risk of CAD through more efficient

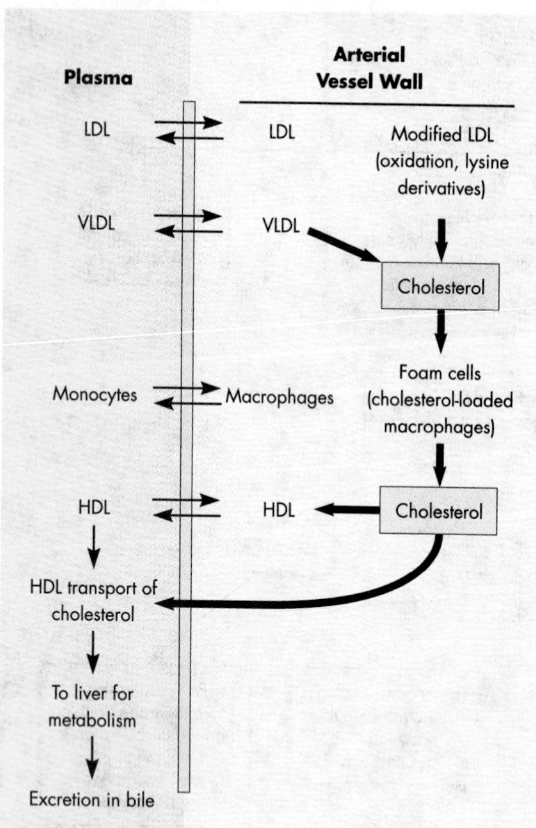

Fig. 31-7 Specific types of plasma lipoproteins (*LDL* and *VLDL*) deliver cholesterol to cells of the blood vessel wall, mostly to macrophages that become cholesterol foam cells. These are predominant early features of atherosclerotic lesions. *HDL* is an important cholesterol-transporting carrier, delivering cholesterol to the liver to be excreted in the bile.

lipid metabolism, increased HDL_2 production, and more efficient oxygen extraction from the working muscle groups, thereby decreasing the cardiac work load. It may be observed that physically active persons are seldom obese, thus eliminating two risk factors in CAD.[6]

Modifiable Minor Risk Factors

Obesity. The mortality from CAD is statistically higher in obese (defined as a weight 30% or more than that considered standard for a person's height and body build) persons than in persons of normal weight. The increased risk is proportional to the degree of obesity. However, obesity in the absence of other high-risk factors probably subjects a person to only a modest increase in risk. Obese persons are thought to produce increased levels of LDL, which are strongly implicated in atherosclerosis. Obesity is often associated with hypertension, which is three times more likely to develop in an obese person than in a person with normal weight. Obesity does not lead to hypertension, but hypertension is present in 60% of obese patients. As obesity increases, the heart size grows, causing increased myocardial oxygen consumption. In addition, there is an increase in Type II diabetes in the obese individual.

Diabetes mellitus. The incidence of CAD is greater among persons who have diabetes, even those with well-controlled blood sugars, than the general population. The patient with diabetes manifests CAD not only more frequently but also at an earlier age. There is no age difference between diabetic men and women for the onset of manifestations of CAD. Diabetes virtually eliminates the lower incidence of cardiovascular disease in women. Latent diabetes is frequently diagnosed at the time of infarction. Because the person with diabetes has an increased tendency toward connective tissue degeneration, it is thought that this condition may account for the tendency toward atheroma development seen in the diabetic population. Diabetic patients also have alterations in lipid metabolism and tend to have high cholesterol and triglyceride levels.[1]

Stress and behavior patterns. The Framingham study provided evidence that certain behaviors and lifestyles are conducive to the development of CAD.[3] Type A and type B behaviors were described by Friedman and Rosenman in the 1960s and were further elaborated in the 1970s by Jenkins and Zyzanski.[7] Type A behaviors include perfectionism and a hardworking, driving personality. The Type A person suppresses anger and hostility, has a sense of time urgency, is impatient, and creates stress and tension, often when a situation does not warrant it (Table 31-3). This person is more prone to heart attacks than a type B person, who is more easygoing, takes upsets in stride, knows personal limitations, takes time to relax, is not an overachiever, and is able to keep priorities in perspective. Although not all characteristics are present in one person all the time, people *tend* to be either type A or type B.

In the Framingham study, type A women manifested twice the incidence of CAD and three times the incidence of angina seen in type B women. Among type A men, there was a twofold risk of angina, MI, and CAD compared with type B men.[3]

Sympathetic stimulation and its effect on the heart is generally considered to be the physiologic mechanism by which stress predisposes to the development of CAD. Sympathetic stimulation causes an increased release of epinephrine and norepinephrine. This stimulation influences the heart by increasing the HR and intensifying the force of myocardial contraction, Therefore the demand for oxygen consumption greatly increases.

Health Promotion and Maintenance. The appropriate management of risk factors in CAD may prevent, modify, or retard the progression of the disease. In the United States during the past 20 to 30 years there has been a gradual and persistent decline in coronary deaths. The decline can be attributed to the efforts of consumers to become generally healthier and individual initiatives to alter hazardous lifestyles. Emphasis on prevention and early treatment of heart disease must be ongoing.

Identification of high-risk persons. In both the acute-care setting and the community, the nurse needs to identify the person at high risk for CAD. Screening for high risk involves obtaining personal and family health histories. The patient is questioned about a family history of heart disease in parents, grandparents, or siblings. The presence of any cardiovascular symptoms should be noted. Environmental

Table 31-3 Type A Personality Characteristics

Perfectionistic
Competitive
Aggressive
Constantly time-oriented
Has hurry sickness
Never says "no"
Compulsive
Impatient
Always tense
Unduly irritable
Obsessed with number of sales made, articles written, patients seen, forms completed
Holds in feelings
Never has leisure time
Rarely takes a relaxing vacation or day off

Modified from Friedman M, Roseman RH: *Type A behavior and your heart,* Greenwich, CT, 1974, Fawcett.

factors, such as eating habits, type of diet, and level of exercise, are assessed to elicit lifestyle patterns. A psychosocial history is included to determine smoking habits, alcohol ingestion, type A behaviors, recent life-stressing events, sleeping habits, and the presence of anxiety or depression. The place of work and the type of work can provide important information on the kind of activity performed; exposure to pollutants, allergens, or noxious chemicals; and the degree of emotional stress associated with employment.

The nurse needs to identify the patient's attitudes and beliefs about health and illness. This information can give some indication of how disease and lifestyle changes may affect the patient and can reveal possible misconceptions about heart disease. Knowledge of the patient's educational background is frequently helpful in deciding at what level to begin teaching. If the patient is taking medications, it is important to know what they are, when they are taken, and what the patient's attitude is regarding the taking of medications.

Management of high-risk persons. Once a high-risk person is identified, preventive measures can be taken. Risk factors such as age, gender, and genetic inheritance cannot be modified. However, the person with any of these risk factors can modify the risk of CAD by controlling or changing the additive effects of modifiable risk factors. For example, a young man with a family history of heart disease can decrease the risk of an MI by maintaining an ideal weight, getting adequate physical exercise, reducing intake of saturated fats, and not smoking.

The person who has modifiable risk factors needs to be encouraged and motivated to make changes in lifestyle to reduce the risk of heart disease. The nurse can play a major role in teaching health-promoting behaviors to the person at risk for CAD (Table 31-4). For highly motivated persons, knowing how to reduce this risk may be the only information needed to get them to make changes.

For the person who is less motivated to assume responsibility for health, the idea of risk factor reduction may be so remote that the person is unable to bring the threat of CAD into the real world. Especially in the absence of symptoms, few persons desire to make lifestyle changes. The nurse should first assist this person in clarifying personal values. Then by explaining the risk factors and having the person identify the personal vulnerability to various risks, the nurse may help the person to recognize the susceptibility to CAD. The nurse may also help the person to set realistic goals and allow the person to choose which risk factor to change first. Some persons will prove reluctant to change until they begin to manifest overt symptoms or actually suffer an infarction. Others, having suffered a heart attack, may find the idea of changing lifelong habits totally unacceptable. The nurse must be able to identify such attitudes and respect them as human rights.

Physical fitness. The last two decades have seen a surge of interest in attaining and maintaining health. Physical fitness has become a field of major importance. Communities are developing exercise programs for persons of all ages and with all health needs, ranging from aerobic exercise classes to cardiac walking-jogging programs. Local YMCAs often sponsor exercise classes, jogging courses, bicycling courses, and related offerings. Many shopping malls open their doors in the early morning to allow people to walk indoors. The AHA takes pride in its annual "Run for Your Life" race as well as other events dramatizing the need for physical activity to promote health. Many large corporations provide gymnasiums where their employees can exercise. For many people, running may be inadvisable; these people should be encouraged to pursue walking, swimming, or whatever exercise will accommodate their individual physical abilities.

Health education in schools. The recent awareness of the body and physical health is also seen in school systems. The school nurse has an important role in teaching good health practices. Besides teaching physical fitness topics, the school nurse can inform students on how the body functions and responds to daily living. Lifestyle habits can be positively influenced at early ages to decrease the need for drastic changes later in life that confront the students' parents. The school nurse must take advantage of the social climate that promotes health and health practices and find innovative ways to present these values to a receptive, youthful audience before the habits of that audience become inflexible. Health awareness programs have been initiated as early as preschool to try to establish health patterns for life. Follow-up on the effectiveness of early childhood health education will not yield data on cardiac risk for many years to come, yet the energy and effort to change lifestyle patterns cannot be left until adulthood when habits are set. The nurse can provide valuable consultation to schools and the educational process at all levels.

Nutritional Management. The patient with elevated serum cholesterol and triglyceride levels should first achieve a normal weight.[8,9] Then the patient should be maintained on a diet that emphasizes a decreased intake of saturated fat and cholesterol such as the step 1 diet recom-

Table 31-4 Management of Risk Factors in Coronary Artery Disease

Risk Factor	Health-Promoting Behaviors	Risk Factor	Health-Promoting Behaviors
▪ Hypertension	Have regular BP checkups. Take prescribed medications for BP control. Reduce salt intake. Stop smoking. Control or reduce weight. Exercise regularly.	▪ Elevated serum lipids	Reduce animal (saturated) fat intake. Reduce total fat intake. Adjust total caloric intake to achieve and maintain ideal body weight. Engage in regular exercise program. Increase amount of complex carbohydrates and vegetable proteins in diet.
▪ Smoking	Enroll in structured program to stop smoking if support system is needed. Change daily routines associated with smoking to reduce desire to smoke. Substitute other activities for smoking. Ask family members to support efforts to stop smoking.	▪ Physical inactivity	Develop and maintain routine for physical activity that is done at least three times a week. Increase activities to a fitness level.
▪ Obesity	Change eating patterns and habits. Reduce caloric intake. Exercise regularly to increase caloric expenditure. Avoid fad and crash diets, which are not effective in the long run. Avoid large, heavy meals.	▪ Stressful lifestyle	Increase awareness of behaviors that are detrimental to health. Alter patterns that are conducive to stress and rushing (e.g., get up 30 min earlier so breakfast is not eaten on way to work; take 20 min/day to meditate). Set realistic goals for self. Reassess priorities in light of health needs. Learn to cope with unavoidable stress. Avoid excessive and prolonged stress. Plan time for adequate rest and sleep.
▪ Diabetes mellitus*	Follow the recommended diet. Reduce weight and control diet. Monitor blood glucose levels regularly.		

BP, blood pressure.
*See Chapter 46 for additional health-promoting behaviors.

mended by the AHA.[9,10] Red meats, eggs, and milk products are major sources of saturated fat and cholesterol. If the serum triglyceride level is elevated, alcohol intake and simple sugars should be reduced or eliminated. If within 6 months there is no trend toward lower blood cholesterol, the patient should be placed on the step 2 diet of the AHA, which further restricts intake of saturated fats and cholesterol.[9,10] (Table 31-5)

The average reduction in total cholesterol levels with diet is 10% to 15%.[11] The highly motivated individual who adheres stringently to a low-fat diet may reduce total cholesterol more dramatically. Ornish has demonstrated regression in coronary atherosclerosis by lifestyle changes including a diet of less than 10 gm of fat a day.[12] Other investigators have also demonstrated regression in coronary atherosclerotic plaques with the combination of low-fat diet and pharmacologic management.[13,14] These studies demonstrated the importance of lowering cholesterol in the individual at risk for CAD.

Pharmacolgic Management. The person with serum cholesterol levels of more than 200 mg/dl (5.2 mmol/L) is at high risk for CAD and should be treated. Treatment usually begins with diet restriction, decreased dietary fat content, lower cholesterol intake, and exercise instruction. Serum cholesterol levels are reassessed after 6 months of diet therapy. If they remain elevated, drug therapy may be started (Table 31-6). Various pharmacologic agents are available to treat hyperlipidemia[14-16] (Table 31-7).

Drugs that increase lipoprotein removal. The major route of elimination of cholesterol is via conversion to bile acids in the liver. Two bile acid-sequestering agents are currently available. These resins primarily lower LDL cholesterol and also cause an increase in HDL. The resins are nonabsorbable compounds that interfere with the enterohepatic circulation of bile acids. There is increased conversion of cholesterol to bile acids and decreased hepatic cholesterol content.

The two resins that are available are cholestyramine (Questran) and colestipol (Colestid). A preparation of cholestyramine (Colybar) containing 4 gm of cholestyramine in a bar form has become available. Administration of these drugs can be associated with complaints related to palatability and with a variety of upper and lower gastrointestinal (GI) complaints, including constipation, abdominal pain, belching, heartburn, and nausea. The resins have been known to interfere with absorption of other drugs, such as warfarin, thiazides, thyroid hormones, and β-adrenergic blockers. Separating the time of administration of the resins from that of other drugs may decrease this side effect.

Drugs that restrict lipoprotein production. *Nicotinic acid* (niacin) is a B vitamin that has been used in conjunction with diet therapy. Nicotinic acid is highly effective in lowering cholesterol and triglyceride levels by interfering with their synthesis. Side effects of this drug may include severe flushing, pruritus, and GI distress.

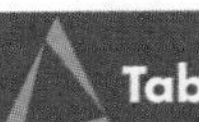

Table 31-5 Nutritional Management: Coronary Artery Disease

Comparison of Step 1 Low-Fat Diet and Step 2 Low-Fat Diet

Principles of Step 1 Diet

Visible fat (e.g., butter, cream, margarine, salad dressing, cooking oil) is restricted to 1 tsp/meal. Unsaturated vegetable oils should be used.

Only lean meats, skim milk or 1% milk, and no more than three egg yolks per week are used.

Food high in fat content (e.g., avocados, fat, meat, olives, nuts) are avoided.

Cooking methods such as steaming, baking, broiling, grilling, or stir-frying in small amounts of fat are recommended.

Principles of Step 2 Diet

Only leanest cuts of meats allowed.

Organ meats and shrimp are restricted because they are high in cholesterol although low in total fat.

Only one egg yolk per week is used because egg yolk is high in cholesterol. Egg white or egg substitutes may be used as desired.

Vegetable oils are used in cooking and food preparation. Coconut and palm oils are not allowed because of their high content of saturated fats. Choose margarine that contains 2 gm or less of saturated fat per tablespoon.

Skim milk is highly recommended. Low-fat yogurt and low-fat cheeses may be used. Low-fat ice milk, frozen yogurt, or sherbet may be used.

Sample Menus

	Step 1			Step 2		
Breakfast 1 fruit 1 starch 3 eggs/wk 1 fat 1 skim milk	½ cup orange juice ¾ cup dry cereal 1 poached egg 1 slice toast with 1 tsp butter or margarine 1 cup skim milk Coffee with sugar	1 banana ½ cup oatmeal 1 flour tortilla 1 cup skim milk Coffee with 1 tsp cream	¼ cantaloupe ½ cup corn meal mush 1 scrambled egg 1 slice toast with 1 tsp butter or margarine 1 cup skim milk Coffee with sugar	½ cup orange juice ¾ cup dry cereal Low-cholesterol egg 1 slice toast with 1 tsp special vegetable oil margarine 1 cup skim milk Coffee with sugar	1 banana ½ cup oatmeal 1 corn tortilla with 1 tsp special vegetable oil margarine 1 cup skim milk Coffee with sugar	¼ cantaloupe ½ cup corn meal mush 1 slice toast with 1 tsp special vegetable oil margarine 1 cup skim milk Coffee with sugar
Lunch 2 meat 2 starch 1 vegetable 1 starch 1 fat 1 dessert	2 oz baked chicken Mashed potato Tossed salad with vinegar, lemon juice Bread with 1 tsp margarine or butter Angel food cake Iced tea with sugar and lemon	3 oz lean hamburger Hamburger bun Lettuce, tomato, pickle, 1 tsp mustard Sherbet Carbonated beverage	2 oz baked fish Baked potato Zucchini Bread with 1 tsp butter or margarine Gelatin dessert Lemonade	3 oz baked chicken (skinless) Mashed potato with 1 tsp special vegetable oil margarine Tossed salad with vinegar, vegetable oil Angel food cake Iced tea with sugar and lemon	¾ cup dry cottage cheese with peach slices Saltine crackers Cucumber and tomato slices 1 tsp special vegetable oil Sherbet Carbonated beverage	4 oz baked fish Fried potatoes (cooked with allowed oils) Zucchini Cornbread (made with allowed oils) Gelatin dessert Lemonade

(continued)

Table 31-5 Nutritional Management: Coronary Artery Disease—cont'd

	Step 1			Step 2		
Dinner 2 meat 2 starch 1 vegetable 1 fat 1 fruit 1 skim milk	2 oz lean roast beef Rice Green beans Dinner roll with 1 tsp butter or margarine Canned peach 1 cup skim milk	Green chili stew (made with 2 oz lean beef cubes, potato slices, tomato, chili) 1 flour tortilla Pudding (made from skim milk and egg whites) Fruit punch	2 oz lean pork chop Corn on the cob Okra Bread with 1 tsp margarine or butter Watermelon slice Buttermilk	2 oz lean roast beef Rice with 1 tsp special vegetable oil margarine Green beans Dinner roll with 1 tsp special vegetable oil margarine Canned peach 1 cup skim milk	2 oz green chili stew (made with lean beef cubes, potato slices, tomato, chili) 1 corn tortilla with 1 tsp special vegetable oil margarine Pudding (made from skim milk and egg whites) Fruit punch	3 oz breaded lean pork chop Corn on the cob with 1 tsp special vegetable oil margarine Okra Biscuit (made with allowed oils) Watermelon slice Buttermilk

Clofibrate (Atromid) is effective primarily in lowering serum triglyceride levels and has some cholesterol-lowering activity as well. It appears to act by decreasing the synthesis of lipids. Side effects include malaise, nausea, diarrhea, and occasional increases in liver enzymes.

Gemfibrozil (Lopid) is primarily effective in lowering VLDL levels and triglycerides, and it also increases HDL cholesterol. Although most patients tolerate the drug well, complaints may include GI irritability.

Lovastatin (Mevacor) is a competitive inhibitor of the biosynthesis of cholesterol. Most patients may be successfully treated with either 20 mg or 40 mg a day. Side effects include rash, GI symptoms, insomnia, elevated liver enzymes, opacities of eye lenses, and rhabdomyolysis. A baseline eye examination may be required before administration of this drug is started. Liver enzymes may increase and then decrease to normal within 6 months following the initiation of treatment.

Drug therapy for hyperlipidemia is likely to be prolonged, perhaps continuing for a lifetime. It is essential that diet modification be used to minimize the need for drug therapy. The patient must fully understand the rationale and goals of treatment as well as the safety and side effects of drugs.[16]

CLINICAL MANIFESTATIONS OF CAD

There are three major clinical manifestations of CAD: angina pectoris, acute MI, and sudden cardiac death.

Angina Pectoris

Angina pectoris is literally translated as pain (angina) in the chest (pectoris). Myocardial ischemia is expressed symptomatically as angina. More specifically, angina pectoris is transient chest pain caused by myocardial ischemia. It usually lasts for only a few minutes (3 to 5 minutes) and commonly subsides when the precipitating factor (usually

Table 31-6 Treatment Decisions for High Blood Cholesterol Based on Low-Density Lipoprotein Cholesterol Levels

Patient Category	Initiation Level	LDL Goal
Dietary Therapy		
Without CAD and with fewer than two risk factors	≥160 mg/dl (4.1 mmol/L)	≤160 mg/dl (4.1 mmol/L)
Without CAD and with two or more risk factors	≥130 mg/dl (3.4 mmol/L)	≤130 mg/dl (3.4 mmol/L)
With CAD	>100 mg/dl (2.6 mmol/L)	≤100 mg/dl (2.6 mmol/L)
Drug Treatment		
Without CAD and with fewer than two risk factors	≥190 mg/dl (4.9 mmol/L)	≤130 mg/dl (4.1 mmol/L)
Without CAD and with two or more risk factors	≥160 mg/dl (4.1 mmol/L)	≤130 mg/dl (3.4 mmol/L)
With CAD	≥130 mg/dl (3.4 mmol/L)	≤100 mg/dl (2.6 mmol/L)

From Summary of the Second Report of the National Cholesterol Education Program (NCEP) Expert Panel on Detection, Evaluation, and Treatment of High Cholesterol in Adults (Adult Treatment Panel II), *JAMA* 269:3015, 1993.
CAD, Coronary artery disease; *LDL*, low-density lipoprotein.

Table 31-7 Drugs Used to Treat Hyperlipoproteinemia

Name	Mechanisms of Action	Side Effects	Nursing Considerations
Cholestyramine (Questran, Colybar)	Bile acid–binding resin, increases production of LDL receptors in liver Increases synthesis of cholesterol for use by liver as bile acids	Unpleasant gritty quality to taste GI disturbances (e.g., nausea, dyspepsia, constipation) Skin rash	Be aware that drug is effective and safe for long-term use, that side effects diminish with time, and that drug interferes with absorption of digoxin, thiazides, β blockers, fat-soluble vitamins, folic acid.
Colestipol (Colestid)	Same as cholestyramine	Same as cholestyramine	Same as cholestyramine.
Nicotinic acid (niacin, Nicobid, Niac, Nicospan)	Inhibits synthesis and secretion of VLDL and LDL from liver Increases HDL levels	Hot flashes and pruritus in upper torso and face GI disturbances (e.g., nausea and vomiting, dyspepsia, diarrhea)	Be aware that most side effects subside with time and that decreased liver function and dysrhythmias may occur with high doses. Have patient take aspirin ½ hr before drug to prevent flushing and take drug with meal.
Clofibrate (Atromid)	Promotes lipolysis of VLDL and reduces hepatic VLDL synthesis Reduces triglyceride levels	Nausea, diarrhea, weight gain Elevated liver enzymes	Monitor liver function tests.
Gemfibrozil (Lopid)	Reduces hepatic VLDL synthesis and inhibits VLDL secretion Reduces triglyceride levels	Mild GI disturbances (e.g., nausea and diarrhea)	Be aware that drug is generally well tolerated.
Lovastatin (Mevacor)	Increases liver rate of LDL removal from plasma Decreases liver synthesis of LDL	Rash, mild GI disturbances, insomnia, elevated liver enzymes, lens opacities, rhabdomyolysis	Be aware that drug is well tolerated with few side effects. Monitor patient with liver function tests and eye examinations.
Probucol (Lorelco)	Inhibits oxidation and tissue deposition of LDL Promotes clearance of LDLs Decreases cholesterol synthesis	Nausea, diarrhea, flatulence, abdominal pain, prolonged QT interval	Monitor ECG at intervals. Be aware that taking drug with meals may decrease side effects.

ECG, Electrocardiogram; *GI,* gastrointestinal; *HDL,* high-density lipoprotein; *LDL,* low-density lipoprotein; *VLDL,* very low-density lipoprotein.

exertion) is relieved. Typical exertional angina should not persist longer than 20 minutes after rest and administration of nitroglycerin.

Pathophysiology. Myocardial ischemia develops when the demand for myocardial oxygen exceeds the ability of the coronary arteries to supply it (see Table 31-8 on p. 899). The primary reason for insufficient flow is narrowing of coronary arteries by atherosclerosis. Although skeletal muscle extracts only 20% of available oxygen and maintains a reserve, the myocardium (at rest) extracts 60% to 85% of the available oxygen. If myocardial oxygen needs are not met from this near-maximum extraction, coronary blood flow is increased through vasodilatation and increased rate of flow.

In the person with CAD, the coronary arteries are unable to dilate to meet increased metabolic needs because they are already chronically dilated beyond the obstructed area. For ischemia as a result of atherosclerosis to occur, the artery is usually 75% or more stenosed. In addition, the diseased heart has difficulty increasing the rate of flow. This creates an oxygen deficit. In addition to atherosclerotic stenosis, oxygen deficit is caused by coronary artery spasm and coronary thrombosis. In coronary artery spasm the constriction is transient and reversible and causes either subtotal or total narrowing of the coronary artery. The coronary artery spasm is usually associated with an underlying atherosclerotic plaque, although spasms do occur in arteries without significant stenosis. The duration of the spasm determines whether the myocardium will sustain ischemia (not resulting in cell death) or actual infarction (resulting in cell death).

CLINICAL PATHWAY FOR ANGINA

Anticipated Recovery Plan

*As indicated by physician
Red check indicates MD order
PROFILE:
Case Type ANGINA
Diagnostic Related Group 140
Length of Stay 2 Days
Secondary Diagnosis________
Admission Date________
Surgery Date________

Physician________
Consults________
RN Initiated/reviewed with patient/family

Name________ Age________
Rm# ________

Allergies (in Red)	**Social History**	**Health History**	**Family/Emergency Phone/Religion**
Code Status / **Special Needs:** Visual ___ Hearing ___ Communication ___			

Staff Alert: (use pencil) Stat ECG with chest pain Date done____ Wt/Freq ____ Living will: Y/N In chart: Y/N	**Call if:** (use pencil)	**Daily labs:** (use pencil)	**Therapy:** OT/PT/RT (use pencil)

Collaborative focus areas (add additional areas to individualize)	**Initial patient/family outcomes**	**Intermediate patient/family outcomes**	**Discharge patient/family outcomes**	**Complete and initial**		
Pain related to imbalance of myocardial O_2 supply and demand	Patient/significant other state they will call nurse immediately if chest pain reoccurs.	Patient improved as evidenced by normal heart rate and rhythm, lack of discomfort with absence of controlled dysrhythmias.	**Record discharge date**	DATE Met before D/C	Met at D/C YES	NO
			1. Patient tolerates activity without chest pain or shortness of breath.			
Knowledge deficit re: disease/treatments	Patient/significant other verbalize anxieties, asking questions.	Patient/significant other verbalize understanding of disease process and continue to ask appropriate questions.	2. Heart rate/rhythm within baseline for patient.			
			3. BP within baseline for patient.			
			4. CAD/angina teaching completed (tracking only).			
			5. Patient/significant other verbalize understanding of diet, meals, activity.			
			6. No med changes 24 hr prior to discharge (for tracking only).			
			7. ECHO done (for tracking only).			
			8. EET ordered (for tracking only).			

continued

Clinical Pathway for Angina—cont'd

	Day Admission ______ Date ______	Day 1 ______ Date ______	Day 2 ______ Date ______
Nursing assessment	Compile/assess data. Assess pain and document effectiveness of pain meds. Notify MD of any chest discomfort Lung sounds q4hr Spot check oximeter q ______ Telemetry Assess activity tolerance q shift	Assess pain and document effectiveness of pain meds. Notify MD of any chest discomfort Lung sounds q shift Spot check oximeter q shift Telemetry Assess activity tolerance q shift	Assess pain and document effectiveness of pain meds. Notify MD of any chest discomfort Lung sounds q shift Spot check oximeter q shift DC telemetry Assess activity tolerance q shift
Treatments	O_2 prn chest pain	O_2 prn chest pain	O_2 prn chest pain
IV/Lines medications (see medication record)	Heplock	Heplock	DC Heplock
Activity/safety	BR with BRP Siderails × ______	Level 6 if pain-free and enzymes negative Siderails × ______	Level 6 Siderails × ______
Diet	NAS	NAS	NAS

continued

Other factors responsible for a discrepancy between myocardial oxygen needs and oxygen supply include low BP, low blood volume, drugs causing vasoconstriction, valvular disorders, stenosis of the coronary ostia (either congenital or secondary to syphilis), and aortic stenosis. Excessive catecholamine stimulation (e.g., from cocaine intoxication or overdose, chronic congestive heart failure), anemia, oxygen-hemoglobin disorders, and chronic lung disease may also contribute to myocardial ischemia.

The left ventricle (LV) is most susceptible to ischemia and injury because of its higher myocardial oxygen demand, larger mass, higher wall tension, and higher systemic pressures. Ischemia causes transient LV dysfunction resulting in an increased LV diastolic pressure. Ischemia also causes elevated pulmonary capillary wedge pressure (PCWP) and elevated right-sided heart pressure. These three factors eventually increase the oxygen deficit of the myocardium. Dysrhythmias may occur in the presence of myocardial ischemia because of cellular irritability. Dysrhythmias decrease the efficiency of the cardiac pump and thereby increase the need for myocardial oxygen while decreasing the available supply.

Research indicates that up to 90% of ischemia is asymptomatic.[17] This type of ischemia is referred to as *silent ischemia.* This creates an iceberg phenomenon, in which the angina is merely the tip of the iceberg. Ischemia with pain (angina) or without pain has the same prognosis. Diabetes mellitus and hypertension are associated with an increased prevalence of silent ischemia. This phenomenon occurs in patients with and without diabetes mellitus-related neuropathy. It is imperative to remember that when ischemia is present, whether it is asymptomatic or manifests as angina, the myocardium is at risk.

On the cellular level, the myocardium becomes cyanotic within the first 10 seconds of coronary occlusion, and ECG changes appear. With total occlusion of the coronary arteries, contractility ceases after several minutes, depriving the myocardial cells of glucose for aerobic metabolism. Anaerobic metabolism begins and lactic acid accumulates. Myocardial nerve fibers are irritated by the increased lactic acid and transmit a pain message to the cardiac nerves and upper thoracic posterior roots (the reason for referred cardiac pain to the left shoulder and arm). Under ischemic conditions, cardiac cells are viable for approximately 20 minutes. With restoration of blood flow, aerobic metabolism resumes and contractility is restored. Cellular repair also begins.

Clinical Pathway for Angina—cont'd

TEACHING SHEET
PATIENT EDUCATION—ANGINA

Date		Process/response Learner___ S/O___	Comments/initials (Readiness, special circumstances)	INIT.
	I. Anatomy a. Chambers b. Coronary arteries c. Blood flow			
	II. Restrictions a. Exercise before meals, or 1-2 hr after meals b. Rest periods c. Extreme temperatures d. Breath-holding isometrics			
	III. Risk factors a. Age b. Sex c. Family History d. Diabetes e. Cholesterol f. HTN g. Smoking h. Lack of exercise j. Obesity			
	IV. NTG (sublingual) a. Dark glass b. Date bottle/discard after 6 mo c. Sublingual ×3, q5min d. Side effects (biting, stinging, headache, faintness) e. Emergency call for no relief, "911"			
	V. Medications (list) a. Action b. Dosage c. Side effects d. Radial pulse demonstration e. Radial pulse return demonstration			
	VI. Cardiac tapes viewed (list) _Angina: A Message from your Heart _Taking Control (of Blood Pressure) _Other________ _Grocery Store Tour _Quitting Smoking			
	VII. Cardiac pamphlets given (list) _Healthy Heart Information _NTG Information Card _Other _Understanding Angina _Healthy Heart Nutrition			
	VIII. Referrals/Information a. Dietary 1. Diet type 2. Weight reduction Yes__ No__ b. Referral for exercise program/cardiac rehabilitation Yes__ No__ c. Stop Smoking in 5 Days d. Stress booklet			
	IX. Warning signs a. Chest discomfort b. Shortness of breath c. Nausea or vomiting d. Diaphoresis e. Cool, clammy skin f. Weakness, fainting			
	X. Mended Hearts visit			

Process/response key
G = Given information
V = Verbalizes understanding
D = Demonstration given
R = Return demonstration
I = Independent
RP = Reinforcement of previous instruction

Signature: ____________________

Developed by HealthSpan, Unity Hospital, Coon Rapids, MN. Licensed by Center for Case Management, South Natick, MN.
BP, Blood pressure; *BR*, bed rest; *BRP*, bathroom privileges; *CAD*, coronary artery disease; *D/C*, discharge; *DRG*, diagnostic related group; *EET*, exercise treadmill test; *HTN*, hypertension; *NAS*, no added salt; *OT*, occupational therapy; *NTG*, nitroglycerin; *PT*, physical therapy; *RT*, respiratory therapy; *SO*, significant other.

Table 31-8 Factors Determining Myocardial Oxygen Needs

Decreased Oxygen Supply	Increased Oxygen Demand or Consumption
↓ Hematocrit ↓ Hemoglobin-binding capacity ↓ Coronary blood flow ↑ Diastolic pressure ↑ Coronary vascular resistance Coronary spasm ↓ Blood Volume	↑ HR ↑ Contractility ↑ Left ventricular wall tension ↑ Systolic BP ↑ Ventricular volume ↑ Myocardial wall thickness

BP, Blood pressure; *HR,* heart rate.

Precipitating factors. Extracardiac factors may precipitate myocardial ischemia and anginal pain. These include the following:[18]

1. *Physical exertion,* which increases the HR. Increasing the HR decreases the time the heart spends in diastole, which is the time of greatest coronary blood flow. Walking outdoors is the most common form of exertion that produces an attack. Isometric exertion of the arms, as in raking leaves, painting, or lifting heavy objects, also causes exertional angina.
2. *Strong emotions,* which stimulate the sympathetic nervous system and increase the work of the heart. This results in an increase in HR, BP, and myocardial contractility.
3. *Consumption of a heavy meal* (especially if the person exerts afterward), which can increase the work of the heart. During the digestive process, blood is diverted to the GI system, causing a low flow rate in the coronary arteries.
4. *Temperature extremes,* either hot or cold, which increase the work load of the heart (blood vessels constrict in response to a cold stimulus; blood vessels dilate and blood pools in the skin in response to a hot stimulus). Cold weather also causes increased metabolism to maintain internal temperature regulation.
5. *Cigarette smoking,* which causes vasoconstriction and an increased HR because of nicotine's stimulation of catecholamine release. It also diminishes available oxygen by increasing the level of carbon monoxide.
6. *Sexual activity,* which increases the cardiac work load and sympathetic stimulation. In a person with severe CAD, the resulting extra work load of the heart may precipitate angina.
7. *Stimulants,* such as cocaine or caffeine, which cause increased HR and subsequent myocardial oxygen demand. Stimulation of catecholamine release is the precipitating factor.
8. *Circadian rhythm patterns* have been related to the occurrence of stable angina, Prinzmetal's angina, MI, and sudden cardiac death. These manifestations of CAD tend to occur in the early morning after awakening.

Types of Angina

Stable angina. Stable angina (classic) refers to chest pain occurring intermittently over a long period with the same pattern of onset, duration, and intensity of symptoms. Stable angina is usually exercise induced. Pain at rest is unusual. An ECG usually reveals ST segment depression, indicating subendocardial ischemia. The discomfort may be mild or severe and disabling, but it is usually infrequent. Stable angina can be controlled with medications on an outpatient basis. Because stable angina is often predictable, medications can be timed to provide peak effects during the time of day when angina is likely to occur. For example, if angina occurs when rising, the patient can take medication as soon as awakening and wait ½ to 1 hour before engaging in activity.

Unstable angina. Unstable angina (progressive, crescendo, or preinfarction angina) is different from stable angina. Unlike stable angina, it is unpredictable. The patient with stable angina may develop unstable angina, or unstable angina may be the first clinical manifestation of CAD. The patient with previously diagnosed stable angina will describe a significant change in the pattern of angina. It will be occurring with increasing frequency, easily provoked by minimal or no exercise, during sleep, or even at total rest. The patient without previously diagnosed angina will describe anginal pain that has progressed rapidly in the last few weeks to days that often culminates in rest pain.[19-21] Recent findings associate unstable angina with deterioration of a once stable atherosclerotic plaque. In the majority of cases, the once stable plaque has ruptured, exposing the intima to blood and stimulating platelet aggregation and local vasoconstriction with thrombus formation.[20,21] This unstable lesion is at increased risk of complete thrombosis of the lumen with progression to MI. This is why these patients require immediate hospitalization with ECG monitoring and bed rest. The unstable lesion can progress to an MI, or it can return to a stable lesion (Fig. 31-8). Aspirin and systemic anticoagulation are the treatments of choice for unstable angina. Because it is also believed that unstable angina may have a spasm component, calcium channel blockers are also frequently used.

Prinzmetal's angina. Prinzmetal's angina (variant angina) often occurs at rest, usually in response to spasm of a major coronary artery. It is a rare form of angina. The spasm may occur in the absence of atherosclerotic disease, as well as with documented disease. Prinzmetal's angina is not usually precipitated by increased physical demand. Coronary spasm can be described as a strong contraction of smooth muscle in the coronary artery caused by an increase in intracellular calcium ions. Factors that may precipitate coronary artery spasm include increased myocardial oxygen demand and increased levels of a variety of substances

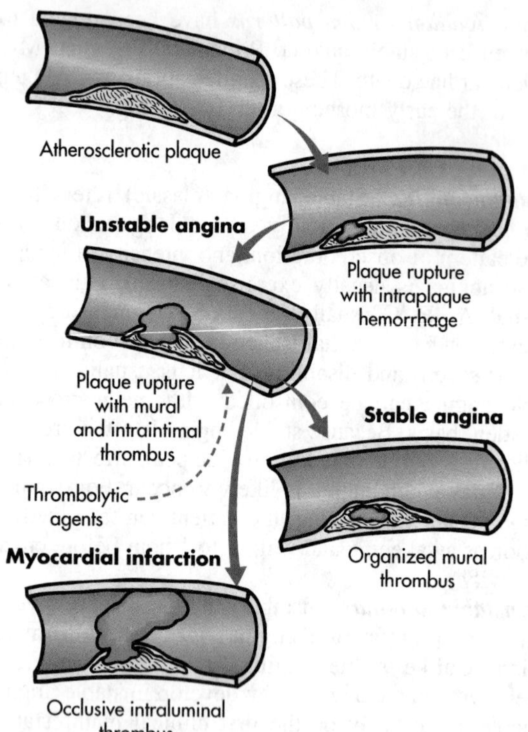

Fig. 31-8 Coronary thrombogenesis secondary to atherosclerotic plaque progression.

(e.g., histamine, angiotensin, epinephrine, norepinephrine, prostaglandins). When spasm occurs, the patient experiences pain and marked, transient ST segment elevation. The pain may occur during rapid eye movement (REM) sleep when myocardial oxygen consumption increases; it may be relieved by some form of exercise or it may disappear spontaneously. Cyclical, short bursts of pain at a usual time each day may also occur with this type of angina.

Nocturnal angina and angina decubitus. Nocturnal angina occurs only at night but not necessarily when the person is in the recumbent position or during sleep. *Angina decubitus* is chest pain that occurs only while the person is lying down and is usually relieved by standing or sitting.

Clinical Manifestations. The most common initial symptom of a patient with angina is chest pain or discomfort (Table 31-9). The exact cause of the pain is unknown, but neurogenic pain at the site of ischemia is most likely. On direct questioning, some patients may deny feeling pain but will refer to a vague sensation, a strange feeling, pressure, or ache in the chest. It is an unpleasant feeling, often described as a constrictive, squeezing, heavy, choking, or suffocating sensation. Many persons complain of severe indigestion or burning. Although most of the discomfort experienced by persons with angina appears substernally, the sensation may occur in the neck or radiate to various locations including the jaw, shoulders, and down the arms (Fig. 31-9). Often people will complain of pain between the shoulder blades and dismiss it as not being heart pain. Depending on the severity of the anginal attack, the person may remain motionless or may clench a fist over the sternal area. The person experiencing angina often refers to a feeling of anxiety and impending doom. Associated symptoms may include shortness of breath, cold sweat, weakness, or paresthesias of the arm(s). Relief of classic angina pectoris is usually obtained with rest or cessation of activity. Prinzmetal's angina differs from stable or unstable angina in that it is longer in duration and may wake people from sleep.

Complications. Dysrhythmias, such as premature contractions or fibrillations, may occur in a person with angina. The cells deprived of oxygen and nutrients may become irritable and develop into sites for ectopic pacemaker cells. Decreased myocardial contractility also occurs in the person experiencing angina.

Because some anginal pains may be vague, the patient may not perceive the discomfort as important and dismiss its occurrence. When chest pain is reported to a health care provider, the diagnosis of angina may not be the first consideration because many problems can mimic midthoracic discomfort. Exertional discomfort in any of the areas shown in Fig. 31-9 should be evaluated to rule out angina.

Diagnostic Studies. When a patient has a history indicating CAD, the physician may take several courses of action (Table 31-10). After a detailed health history and physical examination, a chest x-ray is usually taken to look for cardiac enlargement, cardiac calcifications, and pulmonary congestion. Laboratory tests may be done to ascertain serum lipid and cardiac enzyme values. Serum lipid levels are assessed to screen for positive risk factors, and enzyme levels are checked to rule out the occurrence of an infarction. An ECG is obtained and compared to an earlier tracing when possible.

Frequently, treadmill exercise testing is done for the patient with stable angina to examine ST segment changes during exercise as an indirect assessment of coronary artery perfusion. (Unstable angina is a contraindication for use of the treadmill.) Severely abnormal ECGs on exercise testing, indicating gross disease processes, may show the need for angiography. Unfortunately, the ECG stress test is not always conclusive for CAD. A false-positive reaction may be found (especially in women), and a false-negative reaction may be seen if the patient is exercised submaximally or if only one coronary artery is involved. Ambulatory 24-48 ECG monitoring with patient-recorded activity may be effective in identifying silent ischemia. It is also helpful in differentiating Prinzmetal's angina because the incidence of spasm occurs more commonly in early hours (5 to 6 AM).

Nuclear imaging is being widely used as a noninvasive measurement of myocardial perfusion. Thallium 201 is the isotope of choice to detect ischemia, and technetium 99m pyrophosphate is used to detect the "hot spots" of actual infarcted tissue. Thallium stress tests are also frequently performed. The patient is injected with thallium and pro-

Tale 31-9 Comparison of the Pain of Angina Pectoris and Myocardial Infarction

Angina	Myocardial Infarction
Precipitating Factors	
Stress, either physiologic (exertion) or psychologic Digestion of a heavy meal Valsalva maneuver during micturition or defecation Extremes of weather Hot baths or showers Sexual excitation	Exertion or at rest Physical or emotional stress Often no precipitating factors or any factor associated with angina
Location	
Midanterior chest Substernal Abdominal with radiation to neck, back, arms, fingers Diffuse, not easily located	Midanterior chest Substernal Subscapular, midscapular Diffuse Radiation to neck and jaw or down left arm or both arms to fingers
Description	
Deep sensation of tightness or a squeezing feeling Mild to moderate in severity or pressure Similar attacks each time Twinges or dullness in thoracic area	Severe pressure, squeezing, or heaviness with a crushing, oppressive quality Report of such severe pain that patient would rather die than experience pain again Residual "soreness" for several days following MI
Onset and Duration	
Gradual or sudden onset Usual duration of 15 min or less (usually no more than 30 min) Relief from nitroglycerin	Sudden onset Duration of 30 min to 2 hr No relief from rest or nitroglycerin
Associated Clinical Manifestations	
Apprehension Dyspnea Diaphoresis Nausea Desire to void Belching	Apprehension Nausea and vomiting Dyspnea Diaphoresis Extreme fatigue Dizziness or faintness (after abatement of pain)

MI, Myocardial infarction.

ceeds with exercise on a treadmill, with scanning done at peak exercise and 2 to 4 hours after exercise. For the patient unable to exercise, a dipyridamole thallium test may be done. The patient is injected with both dipyridamole and thallium and then scanned. Dipyridamole will cause apparent vasodilation in healthy arteries and thallium will "light up" the areas of the heart that are well perfused. Regions of the heart that are not well perfused will show up on the scan as a "cold spot." A repeat scan is done 2 to 4 hours later to see if the cold spots have reversed after the dipyridamole has worn off.

Positron emission tomography (PET), a noninvasive technique, is also useful in identifying and quantifying ischemia and infarction (see Chapter 29 and Table 29-7).

The physician may propose coronary angiography. This study allows visualization of the coronary arteries for obstruction and helps to determine the treatment and prognosis. The patient with unstable angina should undergo coronary angiography to evaluate the extent of the disease and to determine the most appropriate therapeutic modality. Coronary angiography is the only way to confirm the diagnosis of Prinzmetal's angina. This is often possible only with the intracoronary injection of ergonovine maleate to provoke a spasm.

Other new techniques for diagnosing coronary artery stenosis include the use of echocardiography with exercise. Stress echocardiograms may be used when a patient has an abnormal baseline ECG. The patient has a baseline echocardiogram before exercise stress testing and then proceeds with the treadmill exercise test. Immediately after the conclusion of the test, another echocardiogram is performed to detect any new regional abnormal wall motion. This increases the sensitivity of the treadmill test.

Another technique using an echocardiogram can be used for the patient who is unable to exercise. In this patient, a dobutamine stress echocardiogram can be performed. Echocardiography is done during a stepwise infusion of dobutamine, which causes a progressive increase in HR just

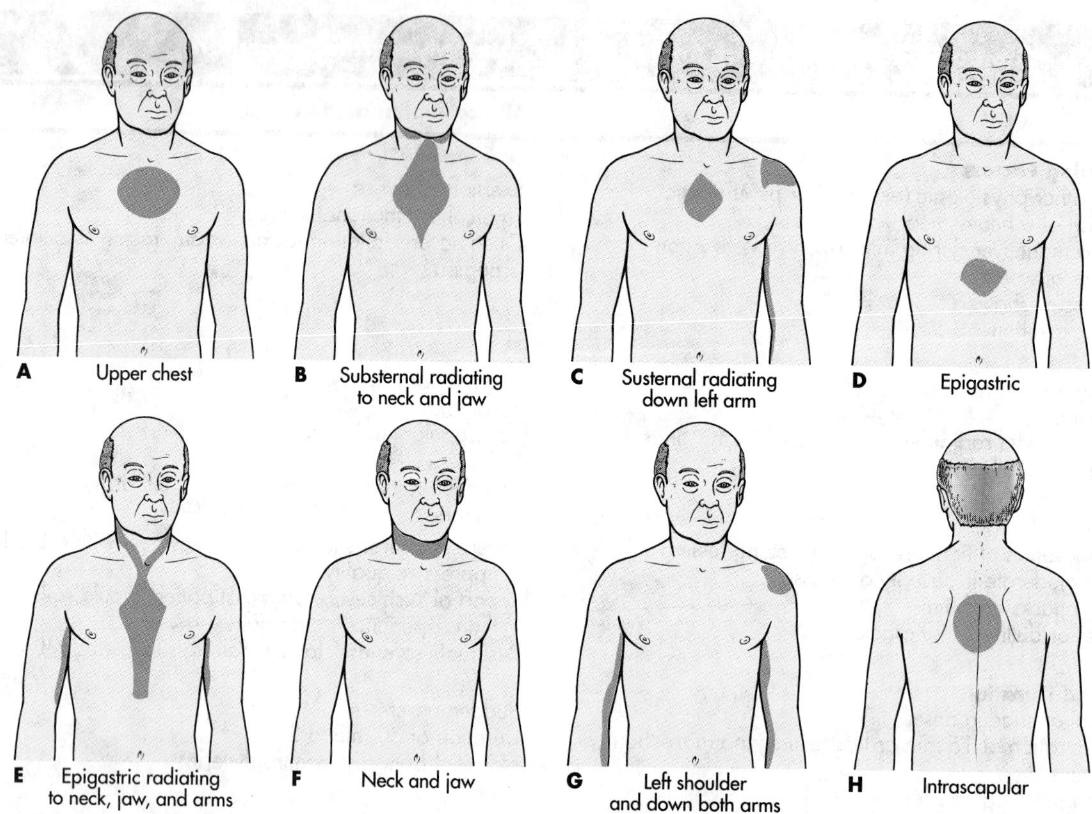

Fig. 31-9 Location of chest pain during angina or MI. ***A,*** Upper chest. ***B,*** Substernal, radiating to neck and jaw. ***C,*** Substernal, radiating down left arm. ***D,*** Epigastric. ***E,*** Epigastric, radiating to neck, jaw, and arms. ***F,*** Neck and jaw. ***G,*** Left shoulder and down both arms. ***H,*** Intrascapular.

as occurs with exercise; that is, the heart is being exercised chemically. Again, abnormality of the regional wall motion is determined. The test is stopped if a wall motion abnormality or angina develops, or the patient reaches the target HR or the peak dobutamine dose of 30 μg/kg per minute.

Therapeutic Management. The most common initial therapeutic intervention for angina is the use of nitrate therapy to enhance coronary blood flow (Table 31-10). Emergency care of the patient with chest pain is presented in Table 31-11. The treatment of CAD may include *percutaneous transluminal coronary angioplasty* (PTCA), *stent placement, atherectomy,* and *laser angioplasty.*

Percutaneous transluminal coronary angioplasty. A common intervention is PTCA.[22] In a catheterization laboratory a catheter equipped with an inflatable balloon tip is inserted into the appropriate coronary artery. When the lesion is located, the catheter is passed through and just past the lesion, the balloon is inflated, and the atherosclerotic plaque is compressed, resulting in vessel dilatation.

The advantages of PTCA are that (1) it provides an alternative to surgical intervention; (2) it is performed with local anesthesia; (3) it eliminates the recovery from thoracotomy required for bypass surgery and its complications; (4) the patient is ambulatory 24 hours after the procedure; (5) the length of hospital stay is approximately 1 to 3 days compared with the 5 to 7 day stay of someone having open

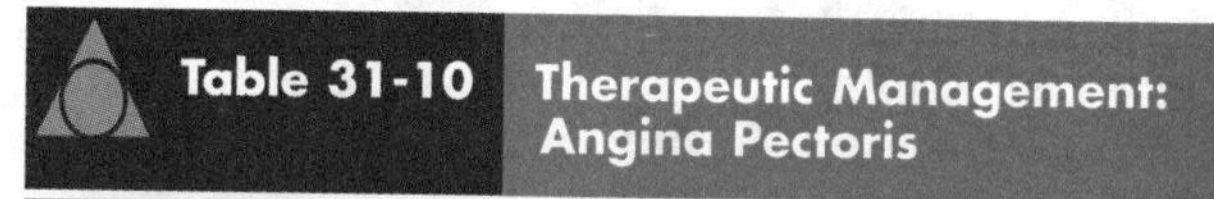
Table 31-10 Therapeutic Management: Angina Pectoris

Diagnostic
- History and physical examination
- Chest x-ray
- ECG
- Serum enzyme levels (CK, AST, LDH)
- Serum lipid levels
- Exercise stress tests
- Nuclear imaging studies
- Angiography studies
- Echocardiography

Therapeutic

Acute angina attacks
- Nitroglycerin (sublingual)

Chronic anginal prophylaxis
- Antithrombotic therapy (e.g., aspirin, dipyridamole)
- Nitroglycerin ointment (e.g., Nitrol)
- Transdermal controlled-release nitrates
- Long-acting nitrates (e.g., Isordil, Sorbitrate)
- β-Adrenergic blocking agents
- Calcium-channel blocking agents

AST, Aspartate aminotransferase; *CK, creatine kinase; ECG,* electrocardiogram; *LDH,* lactic dehydrogenase.

Table 31-11 Emergency Management: Chest Pain

Possible Etiologies
Chest trauma, angina, MI, dysrhythmia, pleurisy, pneumonia, pneumothorax, pericarditis, pulmonary edema, pulmonary emboli, stress, strenuous exercise, drugs, shock, aortic aneurysms, hiatal hernia, gastroesophageal reflux

Possible Assessment Findings
Pain located in chest, neck, arm, or shoulder
Cold, clammy skin
Diaphoresis
Nausea and vomiting
Abdominal pain
Heartburn
Dyspnea
Weakness
Anxiety: feeling of impending doom
Tachycardia, irregular HR, palpitations
Decreased BP
Fainting, loss of consciousness

Management
- Establish and maintain airway.
- Anticipate need for intubation if respiratory distress evident.
- Administer O_2 by nasal cannula if not in respiratory distress; otherwise use high flow O_2 (100%) by nonrebreather mask.
- Start 2 IV lines with large-gauge needles.
- Remove clothing; comfort and reassure patient.
- Monitor cardiac rate and rhythm.
- Monitor vital signs including level of consciousness.
- Do a 12-lead ECG.
- Be prepared to perform cardiopulmonary resuscitation, defibrillation, external pacing, or cardioversion.
- Assess severity and location of pain; medicate for pain as ordered.
- Obtain past health history including cardiac history.
- Assess for indications and contraindications for thrombolytic therapy.
- Prepare to initiate thrombolytic therapy if indicated.

BP, Blood pressure; *ECG,* electrocardiogram; *HR,* heart rate; *IV,* intravenous; *MI,* myocardial infarction.

heart surgery with a coronary artery bypass graft (CABG), thus reducing hospital costs; and (6) there is rapid return to work (approximately 1 week after PTCA) instead of a 2- to 8-week convalescence after CABG.

Many advancements have been made in PTCA during the last decade. Guidewires and catheters with greater flexibility have been developed enabling cardiologists to maneuver the catheters to distal and proximal lesions. Today PTCA is more frequently performed than CABG. Reduction of lesion size by greater than 20% occurs in 91%

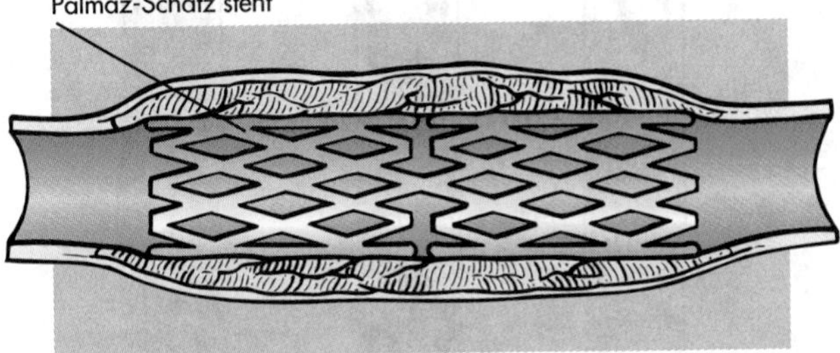

Fig. 31-10 Palmaz-Schatz stent, an articulated stainless steel mesh deployed by balloon inflation.

of patients.[22] New techniques have been developed to provide blood flow to the distal myocardium during balloon inflation increasing the safety of the procedure. Dilatation may also be done for stenotic grafts from a previous CABG, although these vessels usually require repeated dilatation.

The most serious complication of PTCA is dissection of the dilated artery where the intimal lesion is pushed farther up or down the intimal lining instead of being compressed. If the damage is extensive, the coronary artery could rupture, causing cardiac tamponade, ischemia and infarction, a fall in cardiac output (CO), and possible death. There is also danger from infarction should the lesion be calcified and a portion of the plaque dislodge and occlude the vessel distal to the catheter. The chance of coronary spasm from the mechanical irritation of the catheter is present, as well as chemical irritation from the contrast dye injection used to visualize the artery and catheter and balloon. Abrupt closure is another complication that can occur in the first 24 hours after PTCA. Factors related to abrupt closure include a diffuse, complicated lesion, severe stenosis (> 90%), presence of thrombus before dilatation, and lesions in vessels supplying collateral circulation.[22] The risk of restenosis after PTCA is approximately 30% in the first 3 to 6 months.[22] Restenosis occurs more commonly in smokers, diabetics, and patients with hypercholesteremia.

Stent placement. Stents are used to treat abrupt or threatened abrupt closure following PTCA. Stents are expandable meshlike structures designed to maintain vessel patency by compressing the arterial walls and resisting vasoconstriction[23,24] (Fig. 31-10). Stents are carefully placed over the angioplasty site to hold the vessel open. Because stents are thrombogenic, the patient must be kept on anticoagulation for at least 3 months. The primary complications from stent placement are hemorrhage and vascular injury. Less common complications are stent thrombosis, acute MI, emergency CABG, stent embolization, and coronary spasm.[24] The possibility of dysrhythmias is always present.

Atherectomy. Atherectomy is another technique used to treat CAD. With atherectomy the plaque is shaved off using a type of rotational blade (Fig. 31-11). Atherectomy decreases the incidence of abrupt closure as compared to PTCA. However, it is limited to use in proximal and middle portions of a vessel. It is superior to PTCA in lesions

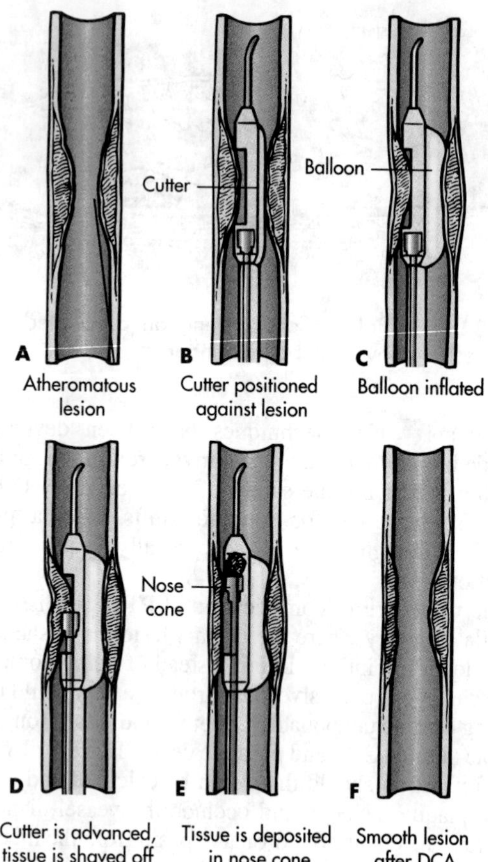

Fig. 31-11 Directional coronary atherectomy (DCA). ***A,*** Atheromatous lesion. ***B,*** DCA cutter is introduced over a guidewire into the coronary artery and positioned with the window against lesion. ***C,*** Balloon is inflated to maintain cutting position against the lesion. ***D,*** As the rotating cutter is advanced across lesion, atheromatous tissue is shaved off. ***E,*** Tissue is deposited in the nose cone. ***F,*** Smooth lesion after DCA.

located in branches or attachment sites of a bypass graft, but carries the same risk for thrombosis and restenosis rate as conventional PTCA.[23-25]

Laser angioplasty. In laser angioplasty a catheter is introduced through a peripheral artery into the diseased coronary artery. A small laser on the tip of the catheter vaporizes the plaqued areas of the artery, thereby facilitating blood flow. A disadvantage of this procedure is that the technique needs refinement so that the proper laser strength for a given thickness of atherosclerotic plaque will be known. Current research is perfecting this technique to move it from experimentation to therapeutic practice. The laser may also be used in the future to make a small opening in completely occlusive lesions, making them more amenable to angioplasty.[26]

Coronary artery bypass surgery. Generally, CABG is recommended if the patient has (1) significant left main coronary artery obstruction, (2) triple-vessel disease, or (3) two-vessel disease unresponsive to medical therapy. Bypass surgery is usually recommended for the person with unstable angina who demonstrates a poor response to therapy, requiring repeat angioplasty. The success of such treatment varies (see Chapter 32).

Pharmacologic Management

Antiplatelet aggregation therapy. Antiplatelet aggregation therapy is the first line of pharmacologic intervention in the treatment of angina. Aspirin is the drug of choice. Recent studies indicate that up to a 50% reduction in unstable angina progression to MI occurs with the use of aspirin.[18,20,21] As little as one baby aspirin daily may be effective in inhibiting platelet aggregation. Dipyridamole (Persantine) is also used as an antiplatelet-aggregation agent. The dose of dipyridamole varies but ranges from 25 to 75 mg orally three times a day.

Nitrates. Nitrates, which are commonly classified as vasodilators, are the next step in the treatment of angina. Nitrates produce their principal effects by the following:

1. Dilating peripheral blood vessels: This results in decreased SVR, venous pooling, and decreased venous blood return to the heart. Therefore myocardial oxygen requirements are lessened because of the reduced cardiac work load.
2. Dilating coronary arteries and collateral vessels: This may increase blood flow to the ischemic areas of the heart. However, when the coronary arteries are severely atherosclerotic, coronary dilatation is difficult to achieve.

NITROGLYCERIN. Nitroglycerin given sublingually (SL) will usually relieve pain in approximately 3 minutes and has a duration of approximately 20 to 45 minutes. The usual recommended dose is one tablet taken sublingually, which can be followed at 5-minute intervals with two more doses. If nitroglycerin tablets have been necessary and relief from anginal pain has not been obtained after 3 tablets and 15 minutes, the patient should be instructed to seek medical attention.

Nitroglycerin can be used prophylactically before undertaking an activity that the patient knows may precipitate an anginal attack. In these instances the patient can take a tablet 5 to 10 minutes before beginning the activity. Any changes in the usual pattern of pain, especially increasing frequency or nocturnal angina, should be reported to the physician.

Nitroglycerin tablets are marketed in light-resistant bottles closed with metal caps. Because they tend to lose potency, the patient should be advised to purchase a new supply every 6 to 9 months.

NITROGLYCERIN OINTMENT. Nitroglycerin (Nitrol and Nitropaste) is a 2% nitroglycerin topical ointment dosed by the inch. It is placed on the skin where it is absorbed, producing anginal prophylaxis for 3 to 6 hours. It has been found to be especially useful for nocturnal and unstable angina because it acts for a longer period of time than SL nitroglycerin. Its disadvantages include its messiness and its rapid absorption, necessitating repeated application.[27]

TRANSDERMAL CONTROLLED-RELEASE NITRATES. Currently there are two types of systems available for transdermal drug administration: reservoir and matrix. Transderm-Nitro is the reservoir type, in which the drug migrates to the absorption site through a rate-controlled permeable membrane. Nitro-Dur and Nitro-Disc are the matrix type, in which the drug is slowly dispersed through a polymer matrix to the skin absorption site. Both reservoir and matrix delivery systems offer the advantages of steady plasma levels within the therapeutic range during 24 hours, thus making only one application a day necessary. The reservoir system has the disadvantage of dose dumping if the reservoir seal is punctured or broken. An advantage of the matrix system is that there can be no dose dumping. Both systems achieve plasma steady states by 2 hours.

LONG-ACTING NITRATES. Long-acting nitrates such as isosorbide dinitrate (Isordil, Sorbitrate) are longer acting than SL nitroglycerin and, when used in adequate doses, are effective in reducing the incidence of anginal attacks. Their mechanisms of action and side effects are similar to those of nitroglycerin. The effects of oral isosorbide dinitrate may last for as long as 8 hours.

Because of the vasodilating properties of nitrates, the predominant side effect of nitrate drugs is headache from the dilatation of cerebral blood vessels. Sometimes the body can build up a tolerance to the drug so that the headaches abate but the principal antianginal effect is still present. However, the body has a tendency to develop a tolerance to the effects of nitrates.[28-29] A strategy found effective to combat this tolerance is providing a nitrate-free period within each 24-hour period. This nitrate-free period should be at night unless the patient experiences nocturnal angina. Other complications of the vasodilator drugs are orthostatic hypotension (nitrate syncope) and an aggravation of cerebral vascular insufficiency.

INTRAVENOUS NITROGLYCERIN. Intravenous (IV) nitroglycerin (Nitrol IV, Nitrostat IV, Nitro-Bid IV, Tridil) has been used in treating the hospitalized patient with unstable angina. It has an immediate onset of action and can be titrated to prevent, treat, and stop acute attacks of angina. The goal of therapy should aim at stopping anginal pain and reducing systolic BP by 15% or mean arterial pressure (MAP) by 10%.[20] IV nitroglycerin has also been used in treatment of MI. The rationale for use in MI has been to increase the collateral blood flow to the ischemic area and reduce myocardial oxygen demand because of decreasing preload and afterload. Tolerance is also a side effect of IV nitrate therapy. An effective strategy for this phenomenon is titrating down the dose at night during sleep and titrating the dose up during the day.

β-Adrenergic blocking agents. β-blocking agents available for the prophylaxis of angina are propranolol (Inderal), metoprolol (Lopressor), nadolol (Corgard), atenolol (Tenormin), oxyprendol (Trasicor), pindolol (Visken), and timolol (Blocadren). These drugs produce a direct decrease in myocardial contractility, HR, SVR, and BP, all of which reduce the myocardial oxygen demand. Side effects of the β-blockers may include bradycardia, hypotension, wheezing, and GI complaints. Many patients also complain of weight gain, depression, and sexual dysfunction. The β-blockers should not be discontinued abruptly without medical supervision.

Calcium-channel blocking agents. Calcium-channel blocking agents such as nifedipine (Procardia), verapamil (Calan, Isoptin), diltiazem (Cardizem), and nicardipine (Cardene) are the next step in the management of angina. Most of these agents have sustained-release versions for longer action with the hope of increased patient adherence. The three primary effects of calcium channel blockers are (1) systemic vasodilatation with decreased SVR, (2) decreased myocardial contractility, and (3) coronary vasodilatation. Each drug manifests these effects to a different degree. Calcium channel blockers have a depressant effect on the sinoatrial (SA) node rate of discharge, and the conduction velocity through the atrioventricular (AV) node is decreased, thus slowing the HR.

Cardiac muscle and vascular smooth muscle cells are more dependent on extracellular calcium than skeletal muscles and are therefore more sensitive to calcium channel-blocking agents. The effect of calcium channel blockers on smooth muscle of both coronary and systemic arteries is to cause relaxation and relative vasodilatation, thus increasing blood flow. Verapamil and diltiazem have antidysrhythmic properties (see Chapter 33). Myocardial perfusion is enhanced with calcium channel blockers by increased coronary blood flow through vasodilatation and reduction in myocardial oxygen demand mediated through a decrease in HR and afterload. Calcium channel-blocking agents have also been effective in controlling angina from either "fixed" atherosclerotic lesions or vasospasm. Verapamil, nifedipine, and diltiazem have also been shown to consistently decrease systemic BP in the hypertensive patient (see Table 30-7).

Calcium channel blockers potentiate the action of digoxin by increasing serum digoxin levels during the early part (first week) of therapy. Therefore serum digoxin levels should be closely monitored upon institution of this therapy, and the patient should be taught the signs and symptoms of digoxin toxicity.

NURSING MANAGEMENT

ANGINA

Nursing Assessment

Subjective and objective data that should be obtained from a patient with angina are presented in Table 31-12.

Nursing Diagnoses

Nursing diagnoses specific to the patient with angina include, but are not limited to, the following:

- Pain (chest pain or discomfort) related to ischemic myocardium
- Anxiety related to diagnosis and awareness of being a victim of heart disease, pain and limited activity tolerance, uncertainties about the future, diagnostic tests, and pending surgery
- Decreased CO related to myocardial ischemia affecting contractility
- Activity intolerance related to myocardial ischemia

Planning

The overall goals are that the patient with angina (1) will experience pain relief, (2) have reduced anxiety, (3) have

Table 31-12 Nursing Assessment: Angina Pectoris

Subjective Data
Important Health Information
Past health history: Previous history of MI, angina, aortic stenosis, or cardiomyopathy; hypertension, diabetes, anemia, lung disease; smoking
Medications: Use of nitrates, calcium-channel blockers, β-adrenergic blockers, antihypertensive drugs, illicit drugs
Functional Health Patterns
Health perception–health management: Family history of heart disease
Nutritional-metabolic: Indigestion, heartburn, nausea, belching; fat and sodium intake
Activity-exercise: Palpitations, dyspnea, dizziness
Cognitive-perceptual: Substernal chest pain or pressure (squeezing, constricting, aching, sharp, tingling) lasting <20 min; referral to arms (especially left), jaw, neck, shoulders, back; relief with rest or nitroglycerin

Objective Data
General
Anxiety
Integumentary
Diaphoresis, pallor
Cardiovascular
Tachycardia, pulsus alterans, dysrhythmias (especially ventricular), ventricular gallop, atrial gallop
Possible findings
Negative cardiac enzymes, elevated serum lipids; positive exercise stress test and thallium scans; demonstration of ST and T wave abnormalities on ECG; positive coronary angiography

ECG, Electrocardiogram; *MI,* myocardial infarction.

adequate knowledge of the problem and prescribed treatment, and (4) modify risk factors.

Nursing Implementation

Acute Intervention. Some of the main nursing objectives for the patient with angina are pain assessment, evaluation of treatment, and reinforcement of appropriate therapy. Because chest pain can be caused by many factors other than ischemia (e.g., pericarditis, valvular disease, pulmonary artery stenosis, MI, congestive cardiomyopathy), it is important to have a clear understanding of the patient's chest pain. The questions a nurse asks may elicit a history of anginal pain. The nurse should determine whether breathing in or out or changing positions makes the patient's chest pain better or worse. Anginal pain does not vary with body position or respirations. In contrast, the pain of pericarditis does. It should be ascertained whether the pain is deep or superficial, mild or intense. Cardiac pain is usually described as deep and intense, but occasionally it may be characterized as a dull ache. Few persons can successfully ignore cardiac pain.

The patient should be asked whether the pain is diffuse or well localized. Cardiac pain is usually diffuse. The patient may rub the entire chest to explain where the pain is occurring. The nurse should instruct the patient to quantify each pain experience by rating the pain on a scale from 1 to 10, with 10 being excruciating pain and 1 being barely noticeable pain. By doing this, the nurse can assess the effectiveness of treatment during a pain experience as well as discriminate between subsequent pain experiences.

If a nurse is present during an anginal attack, the following measures should be instituted: (1) administration of oxygen, (2) determination of vital signs, (3) 12-lead ECG, (4) prompt pain relief with a nitrate or a narcotic analgesic, (5) physical assessment of the chest, and (6) comfortable positioning of the patient. The patient will most likely appear distressed and have pale, cool, clammy skin. The BP and pulse rate will probably be elevated and an atrial gallop (S_4) sound may be heard. If a ventricular gallop (S_3) is heard, it may indicate LV decompensation. A murmur may be heard during an anginal attack secondary to ischemia of a papillary muscle. The murmur is likely to be transient and abates with the cessation of symptoms. Supportive and realistic assurance as well as a calm, soothing manner helps to reduce the patient's anxiety.

The patient needs to be instructed in the proper use of sublingual nitroglycerin. It should be easily accessible to the patient at all times. For protection from degradation, it should be kept in a tightly closed dark glass bottle. The patient should be instructed to place a nitroglycerin tablet beneath the tongue and allow it to dissolve. This should cause a fizzing or slightly warm feeling locally. The patient should be warned that HR may increase and a pounding headache, dizziness, or flushing may occur. The patient should be cautioned against quickly rising to a standing position because postural hypotension may occur after nitroglycerin ingestion. If the pain has not been relieved after 5 minutes, the patient should be told to take another nitroglycerin tablet. This procedure may be repeated for pain relief every 5 minutes, not to exceed the ingestion of three tablets. If pain persists after three doses, the patient should seek immediate medical attention.

Chronic and Home Management. The patient needs to be reassured that a long, productive life is possible, even with angina. Prevention of angina is preferable to its treatment, and this is where instruction is important. The patient needs to be educated regarding CAD and angina, precipitating factors, risk factors, and medications.

Patient teaching can be handled in a variety of ways. One-to-one contact between the nurse and the patient is often the most effective procedure. The time spent in providing daily care is often an ideal teaching period. Teaching tools, such as pamphlets, films at the bedside, a heart model, and especially written information, are necessary components of patient and family education.

The patient needs to be assisted in identifying factors that precipitate angina (see Table 31-9). The patient should be given instruction on how to avoid or control precipitating factors. For example, the patient should be cautioned to avoid exposures to extremes of weather and taught not to eat large, heavy meals. If a heavy meal is ingested, adequate rest should be planned for 1 to 2 hours after eating because blood is shunted to the GI tract to aid digestion.

The patient needs to be assisted in identifying personal risk factors in CAD. Once these risk factors are known, various methods of decreasing them should be discussed (see Table 31-4).

Educating the patient and the family about diets that are low in sodium and reduced in saturated fats may be appropriate. Maintaining ideal body weight is most important in controlling angina because weight above this level increases the myocardial work load and may cause pain. Eating large meals also contributes to angina, and the patient may need to eat several small meals in place of three moderate to large meals each day.

Adhering to a regular, individualized exercise program that conditions the heart rather than overstressing the myocardium is most important. The nurse should consult with a physician or a physical therapist in instructing the patient regarding an exercise program.

It is important to educate the patient and the family in the use of nitroglycerin. Nitroglycerin tablets or ointments may be used prophylactically before an emotionally stressful situation, sexual intercourse, or physical exertion (e.g., climbing a long flight of stairs).

Counseling should be provided to assess the psychologic adjustment of the patient and the family to the diagnosis of CAD and the resulting angina pectoris. Many patients feel a threat to their identity and self-esteem and are unable to fill their roles in society. These emotions are normal and real.

Myocardial Infarction

An MI occurs when ischemic intracellular changes become irreversible and necrosis results. Angina as a result of ischemia causes reversible cellular injury, and infarction is the result of sustained ischemia, causing irreversible cellular death (Fig. 31-12).

Prehospital mortality in patients with acute MI is approximately 30% to 50%. Mortality among patients who reach the hospital is approximately 5%. Most of these deaths occur within the first 3 to 4 days.[30]

Pathophysiology. Cardiac cells can withstand ischemic conditions for approximately 20 minutes before cellular death (necrosis) begins. Contractile function of the heart stops in the areas of myocardial necrosis. The degree of altered function depends on the area of the heart involved and the size of the infarct. Most infarcts involve the LV. A transmural MI occurs when the entire thickness of the myocardium in a region is involved (Fig. 31-13). A subendocardial MI (nontransmural) exists when the damage has not penetrated through the entire thickness of the myocardial wall.

Infarctions are described by the area of occurrence as anterior, inferior, lateral, or posterior wall infarctions (Fig. 31-14). Common combinations of areas are the anterolateral or anteroseptal MI. An inferior MI is also called a diaphragmatic MI (DMI).

The location and area of the infarct correlate with the part of the coronary circulation involved. For example, inferior wall infarctions are usually the result of right coronary artery lesions. Anterior wall infarctions are usually caused by lesions in the left anterior descending artery.

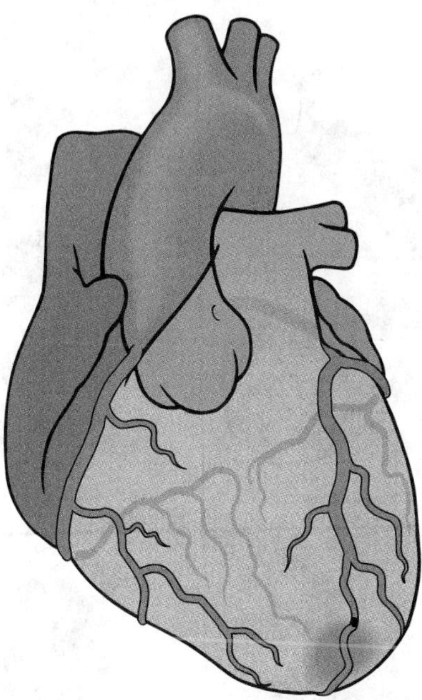

Fig. 31-12 Occlusion of coronary artery, resulting in a myocardial infarction.

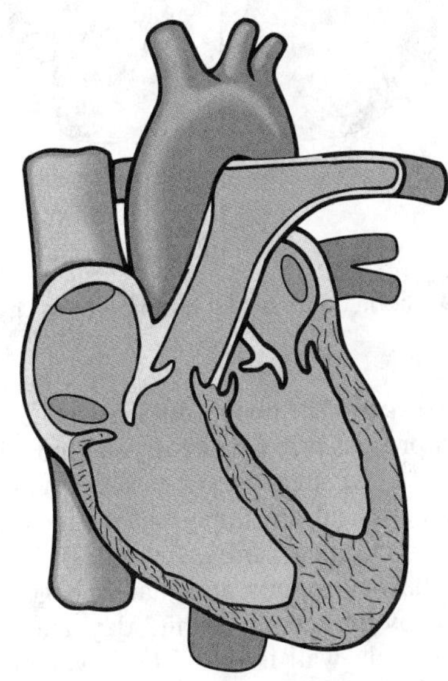

Fig. 31-13 Transmural myocardial infarction involving the thickness of the total wall.

Lesions in the left circumflex artery usually cause posterior or inferior MIs.

The degree of preestablished collateral circulation also determines the severity of infarction. In an individual with a history of heart disease, adequate collateral channels may have been established that provide the area surrounding the infarction site with a blood supply and oxygen. This is one explanation why the younger person who has a severe MI is often more likely to have a more serious impairment than an older person with the same degree of occlusion.

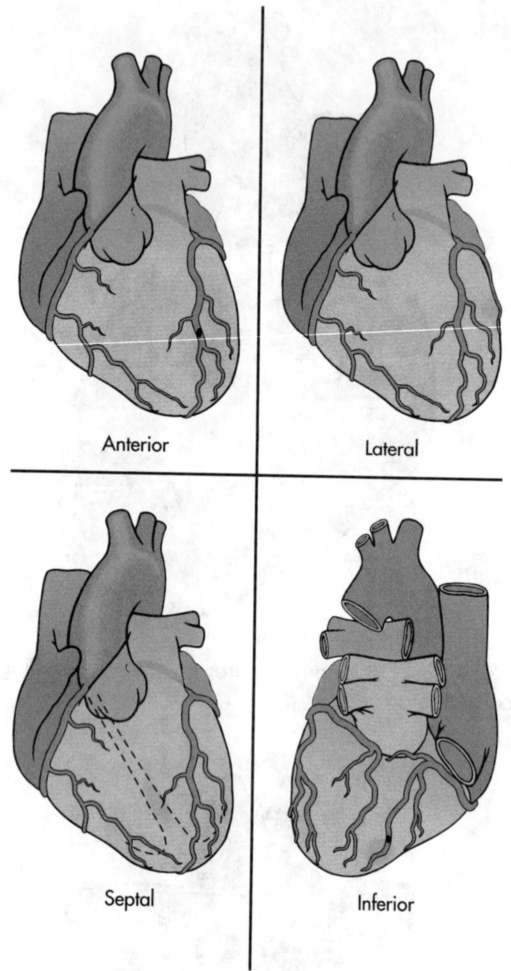

Fig. 31-14 Four common locations where myocardial infarction occurs.

Healing process. The body's response to cell death is the inflammatory process (see Chapter 9). Within 24 hours, leukocytes infiltrate the area. Enzymes are released from the dead cardiac cells and are important diagnostic indicators (see following section on Cardiac Enzymes). The proteolytic enzymes of the neutrophils and macrophages remove all necrotic tissue by the second or third day. During this time, the necrotic muscle wall is thin. The development of collateral circulation improves areas of poor perfusion and may limit the zones of injury and infarction. Once infarction takes place, catecholamine-mediated lipolysis and glycogenolysis occur. These processes allow the increased plasma glucose and free fatty acids to be used by the oxygen-depleted myocardium for anaerobic metabolism. For this reason, serum glucose levels are frequently elevated after MI and may be the reason for a pseudodiabetic state.

The necrotic zone is identifiable by ECG changes within 4 to 10 days and by technetium scanning 24 to 72 hours after the onset of symptoms. At this point, the phagocytes (neutrophils and monocytes) have cleared the necrotic debris from the injured area, and the collagen matrix that will eventually form scar tissue is laid down.

At 10 to 14 days after MI, the beginning scar tissue is still weak. The myocardium is considered to be especially vulnerable to increased stress because of the unstable state of the healing heart wall. (It is also at this time that the patient's activity level may be increasing so special caution and assessment is necessary.) By 6 weeks after MI, scar tissue has replaced necrotic tissue. At this time, the injured area is said to be healed. The scarred area is often less compliant than the surrounding fibers. This condition may be manifested by uncoordinated wall motion, ventricular dysfunction, or pump failure.

These changes in the infarcted muscle also cause changes in the unaffected myocardium as well. In an attempt to compensate for the infarcted muscle, the normal myocardium will hypertrophy and dilate. This process is called ventricular remodeling.[31,32] Remodeling of normal myocardium can lead to the development of late heart failure, especially in the individual with atherosclerosis of other coronary arteries.

Clinical Manifestations

Pain. Severe, immobilizing chest pain not relieved by rest or nitrate administration is the hallmark of an MI (see Table 31-9). The pain is caused by the inadequate oxygen supply to the myocardium. Persistent and unlike any other pain, it is usually described as a heaviness, tightness, or constriction. Common locations are substernal or retrosternal, radiating to the neck, jaw, and arms or to the back. It may occur while the patient is active or at rest, asleep or awake, and commonly occurs in the early morning hours. It usually lasts for 20 minutes or more and is described as more severe than anginal pain. The pain may be located atypically in the epigastric area. The patient may have taken antacids without relief. Some patients may not experience pain but may have "discomfort," weakness, or shortness of breath.

Nausea and vomiting. The patient may be nauseated and vomit. Nausea and vomiting can result from reflex stimulation of the vomiting center by the severe pain (see Chapter 39). These symptoms can also result from vasovagal reflexes from the area of the infarcted myocardium.

Sympathetic stimulation. During the initial phases of MI, increased catecholamines (norepinephrine and epinephrine) are released. The increased sympathetic nervous system stimulation results in diaphoresis and vasoconstriction of peripheral blood vessels. On physical examination, the patient's skin will be ashen, clammy, and cool. This condition is often referred to as a "cold sweat."

Fever. The temperature may increase within the first 24 hours up to 100.4° F (38° C) and occasionally to 102.2° F (39° C). The temperature elevation may last for as long as 1 week. This increase in temperature is a systemic manifestation of the inflammatory process caused by the infarcted myocardium.

Cardiovascular manifestations. The BP and pulse rate may be elevated initially. Later the BP may drop because of decreased CO. Urine output may be decreased. Crackles may be noted in the lungs, persisting for several hours to several days. Hepatic engorgement and peripheral edema may indicate overt cardiac failure. Jugular veins may be distended and may have obvious pulsations, indicating early right ventricular dysfunction and pulmonary congestion.

Cardiac examination may reveal abnormal precordial movements suggestive of ventricular aneurysm. Heart sounds may seem distant, but close auscultation may reveal splitting of heart sounds, indicating LV dysfunction. Other abnormal sounds suggesting ventricular dysfunction are S_3 and S_4. In addition, the presence of murmurs may indicate valve incompetency. A loud holosystolic apical presence of murmurs may indicate valve incompetency. A loud holosystolic apical murmur may occur as a result of papillary muscle rupture.

Complications

Dysrhythmias. The most common complications after an MI are dysrhythmias, present in 80% of MI patients. Dysrhythmias are caused by any condition that affects the myocardial cell's sensitivity to nerve impulses, such as ischemia, electrolyte imbalances, and sympathetic nervous system stimulation. The intrinsic rhythm of the heartbeat is disrupted, causing either a fast HR (tachycardia), a slow HR (bradycardia), or an irregular beat, all of which adversely affect the ischemic myocardium.

Life-threatening dysrhythmias occur most often with anterior wall infarction, pump failure, and shock. Complete heart block is seen in massive infarction. Ventricular fibrillation, a common cause of sudden death, is a lethal dysrhythmia that most often occurs within the first 4 hours after the onset of pain. Premature ventricular contractions (PVCs) may precede ventricular tachycardia and fibrillation. Ventricular dysrhythmias need immediate treatment. (See Chapter 33 for a detailed description of dysrhythmias and their management.)

Congestive heart failure. Congestive heart failure (CHF) is a complication that occurs when the pumping power of the heart has diminished. In the patient with an acute MI it is common to see some degree of LV dysfunction in the first 24 hours. Depending on the severity and extent of the injury, CHF occurs initially with subtle signs such as slight dyspnea, restlessness, agitation, or slight tachycardia. Jugular vein distention from right-sided heart failure, crackles heard in the lungs, distention of upper lobe veins on an upright chest x-ray, and the presence of an S_3 or S_4 heart sound may indicate the onset of heart failure. (The treatment of acute CHF is discussed in Chapter 32.)

Cardiogenic shock. Cardiogenic shock occurs when inadequate oxygen and nutrients are supplied to the tissues because of LV failure. It occurs when there is dysfunction of much of the LV because of infarction. Cardiogenic shock occurs in 10% to 15% of patients hospitalized with acute MI and has a high mortality rate. (Cardiogenic shock is discussed in Chapter 7).

Papillary muscle dysfunction. Papillary muscle dysfunction may occur if the infarcted area includes or is adjacent to these structures. Papillary muscle dysfunction causes mitral regurgitation, which increases the volume of blood in the left atrium. This condition aggravates an already compromised left ventricle. It is detected by a systolic murmur at the cardiac apex radiating toward the axilla. Papillary muscle rupture is a severe complication

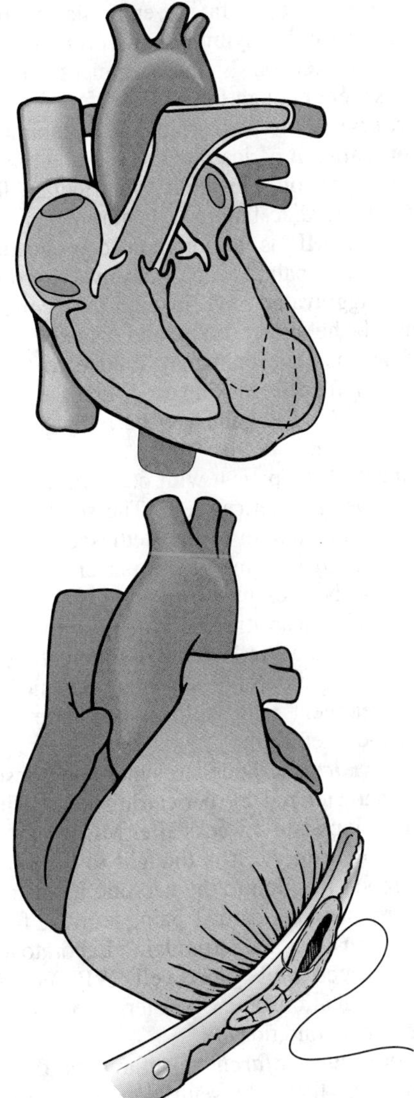

Fig. 31-15 Ventricular aneurysm and surgical repair.

causing massive mitral regurgitation, which results in dyspnea, gross pulmonary edema, and decreased CO. Treatment consists of rapid afterload reduction with nitroprusside or intraaortic balloon pumping and immediate open heart surgery with mitral valve replacement.

Ventricular aneurysm. Ventricular aneurysm results when the infarcted myocardial wall becomes thinned and bulges out during contraction (Fig. 31-15). In the acute stage after MI this is called an *ischemic bulge*. If the aneurysm still exists after scar tissue is laid down, it is called a *ventricular aneurysm*. Ventricular aneurysms are identified by palpation of ectopic impulses; bulges seen on x-ray, echocardiogram, or fluoroscopy; or persistent, long-term ST segment changes on an ECG. Ventricular angiography can definitively diagnose ventricular aneurysm.

The patient with a ventricular aneurysm may experience intractable CHF, dysrhythmias, and angina. Besides ventricular rupture, which is fatal, ventricular aneurysms harbor thrombi, cause dysrhythmias, and promote LV dysfunction. Surgical excision is the treatment for ventricular aneurysms severe enough to cause dysfunction.

Pericarditis. Acute pericarditis, an inflammation of the visceral or parietal pericardium, or both, may result in cardiac compression, lowered ventricular filling and emptying, and cardiac failure.[33] It may occur 2 to 3 days after an acute MI as a common complication of the infarction. Chest pain, which may vary from mild to severe, is aggravated by inspiration, coughing, and movement of the upper body and usually accompanies acute pericarditis. The pain may radiate to the back and down to the left arm, making it difficult to differentiate from an acute MI. The pain may be relieved by sitting in a forward position.

Assessment of the patient with pericarditis may reveal a friction rub over the pericardium. The sound may be best heard with the diaphragm of the stethoscope at the mid to lower sternal border. It may be persistent or intermittent. Fever may also be present.

Diagnosis of pericarditis can be made with serial 12-lead ECGs. ECG changes reflect the inflammation and may produce characteristic ST-T segment elevations that are persistent. Treatment may include pain relief by aspirin, steroids, or indomethacin.

Dressler syndrome. Dressler syndrome (post-MI syndrome) is characterized by pericarditis with effusion and fever that develops 1 to 4 weeks after MI. It may also occur after open heart surgery. It is thought to be caused by an antigen-antibody reaction to the necrotic myocardium. The patient experiences pericardial pain, fever, a friction rub, left pleural effusion, and arthralgia. Laboratory findings include an elevated white blood cell (WBC) count and an elevated sedimentation rate. Short-term corticosteroids are used to treat this condition.

Right ventricular infarction. Infarctions that primarily cause damage to the right ventricle (RV) are often seen with large inferior, inferolateral, or inferoposterior MIs. These RV infarctions can cause severe compromise of perfusion to the pulmonary system resulting in decreased filling of the LV. The patient will manifest symptoms of venous congestion such as distended jugular veins often with Kussmaul's sign (bulging of jugular veins on inspiration), hepatic congestion, and peripheral edema. Because the RV is unable to adequately pump blood through the pulmonary system and fill the LV, reduced LV filling will result in decreased contractility of the LV, hypotension, drop in CO, and tachycardia. ST elevation of right-sided chest leads (V_3 R and V_4 R) can be seen in the first few hours of an MI causing RV infarct. Treatment is aimed at increasing filling pressure of the LV by infusion of fluids carefully managed with pressure measurements using a pulmonary artery catheter and the use of inotropic agents to increase contractility of the RV.[34]

Pulmonary embolism. Pulmonary embolism may be seen in the patient with acute MI who has had bouts of CHF or dysrhythmias or has been extremely immobile because of prolonged bed rest. The source of the thrombus may be the roughened endocardium or leg veins. Early detection of emboli is accomplished by observing for pallor or cyanosis, heart failure unresponsive to treatment, and an unexplained pleural effusion. Acute massive pulmonary embolism causes sudden, severe dyspnea and is usually fatal. (Pulmonary emboli are discussed in more detail in Chapter 35.)

Diagnostic Studies. Three noninvasive diagnostic parameters are used to determine whether a person has sustained an acute MI: (1) the patient's history of pain, risk factors, and health history; (2) 12-lead ECG consistent with acute MI (ST-T wave elevations of greater than 1 mm or more in two contiguous leads); and (3) measurement of serial myocardial serum enzymes.

Clinical presentation. The patient's clinical presentation is important. However, many patients do not have the classic unrelenting chest pain characteristic of acute MI. The patient may complain of a feeling of weakness, severe indigestion, shortness of breath, or chest discomfort. Risk factor analysis may indicate the patient's propensity for an acute event. Any patient's presentation that is suggestive of an acute MI should be treated as quickly as possible to rule out an infarction.

ECG findings. Serial ECGs are approximately 80% specific for diagnosing an acute MI and represent a leading diagnostic criterion. Areas of ischemia or infarction may be noted on the ECG. Changes in rate and rhythm of the heart may also be diagnostic for abnormalities. Because the acute infarction is a dynamic process that occurs with time, the ECG may reveal the time sequence of ischemia, injury, infarction, and resolution of the infarction (Table 31-13).

The 12-lead ECG may be normal when the patient comes to the emergency department with a complaint of pain typical of ischemic chest pain, but within a few hours it may have changed to show the infarction process. These changes take place when cellular damage has occurred,

Table 31-13 Electrocardiogram Changes with Myocardial Infarction*

Phase I	Phase II	Phase III	Phase IV
Abnormal Q waves Elevated ST segment Inverted T waves	Gradual return of ST segment to baseline	Return of T waves to normal or near-normal configuration	Remnant Q wave

*Inferior wall infarction shows ST elevation, T inversion, and pathophysiologic Q wave in leads II, III, and aVF; inferolateral and posterolateral wall infarction shows reduced R and T inversion, with or without ST elevation in V_5, V_6, and aVL; posterior wall infarction shows mirror image of normal ECG; anterior wall infarction shows typical infarction pattern in leads I, aVL, V_2-V_6.

interrupting the normal electrical depolarization. Figure 31-16 correlates the anatomy with areas of infarction and with changes that occur on the 12-lead ECG. Changes that are present in the leads that examine infarcted areas of the heart are called indicative changes (i.e., they are indicative of infarction). Changes in the leads opposite infarcted areas are called reciprocal changes.

In general the area of infarction correlates more closely with side effects and complications than with mortality rates. With inferior wall damage, AV blocks are commonly seen because the right coronary artery perfuses the SA and AV node tissue in 80% to 90% of people. CHF, LV aneurysms, cardiogenic shock, and complete heart block are more frequently seen with anterior MI because the front surface of the LV and part of the septum are damaged. An inferior wall MI may also cause CHF, dysrhythmias, and cardiogenic shock.

Cardiac enzymes. An important diagnostic criterion for acute MI is laboratory assessment of serial cardiac serum enzymes. The cardiac enzymes are creatine kinase (CK), lactic dehydrogenase (LDH), and aspartate aminotransferase (AST). When cardiac cells die, their cellular enzymes are released into circulation. The increase in serum enzymes that occurs after cellular death can demonstrate whether cardiac damage is present and the approximate extent of the damage. (Figure 31-17 indicates the peak level and duration of these enzymes in the presence of MI.) Other causes of increased serum enzymes may make the differential diagnosis more difficult. These include pulmonary embolism, intramuscular damage, seizure activity, cardiopulmonary resuscitation, and other muscle-damaging events.

CK levels begin to rise approximately 6 hours after an acute MI and return to normal within 2 to 3 days. The CK enzymes may be fractionated into bands, including the MB band. The MB band is specific to the myocardial cell and may more specifically quantify myocardial damage. Depending on the individual laboratory, MB bands greater than 3% indicate MI.

Although the traditional cardiac enzymes are excellent diagnostic indicators of an acute MI, they are not immediately available to the physician or nurse because the laboratory needs time to analyze the results. Now there are noninvasive markers for the immediate diagnosis of an acute MI. They include CK, CK-MM and MB isoenzymes, myoglobin, and RP-30 isonitrile scanning. These markers aid in the rapid diagnosis of acute MI. All of these tests are not yet available in every clinical facility. (Enzyme studies are discussed in Chapter 29.)

Other measures. For the assessment of cardiac size and pulmonary congestion, an initial chest x-ray is helpful but not diagnostic of the acute MI. The appearance of distended upper lobe veins may indicate early LV dysfunction. The WBC count may rise to 12,000 to 14,000/μl (12 to 14 $\times$ 10^9/L) or higher. Increases in fasting blood glucose levels to 300 mg/dl (16.7 mmol/L) may also occur secondary to the body's stress response to injury.

Radionuclide imaging has become increasingly important in establishing the diagnosis of MI. Nuclear imaging is considered an extremely sensitive indicator of myocardial damage. Myocardial nuclear scans, done by injecting IV radioactive isotopes, can help establish the diagnosis of acute MI when other data are inconclusive. After an IV injection of thallium, the amount of thallium present in each myocardial region is determined by two factors: the amount of coronary blood flow to that region and the degree of viable myocardium. Ischemia or infarcted myocardial regions receiving little or no coronary blood flow accumulate little or no thallium. Such regions appear as cold spots on

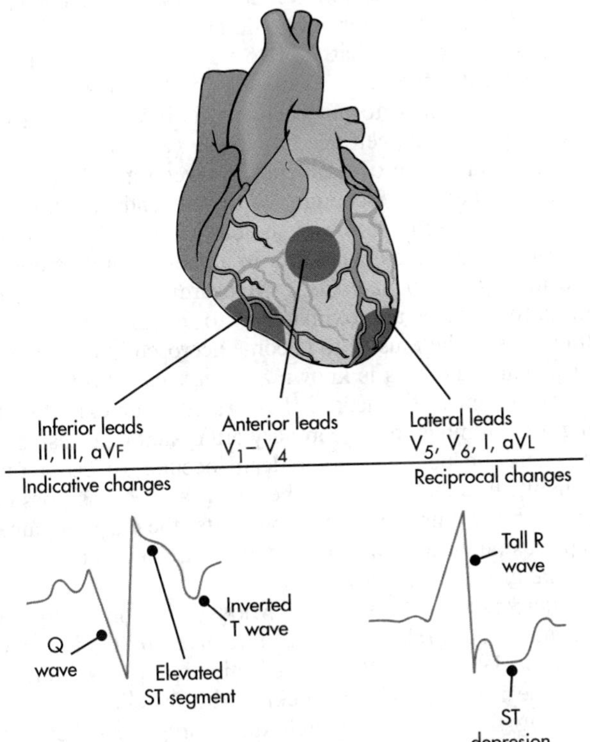

Fig. 31-16 Indicative changes occur in leads that examine the area of infarction. Reciprocal changes occur in leads opposite the area of infarction.

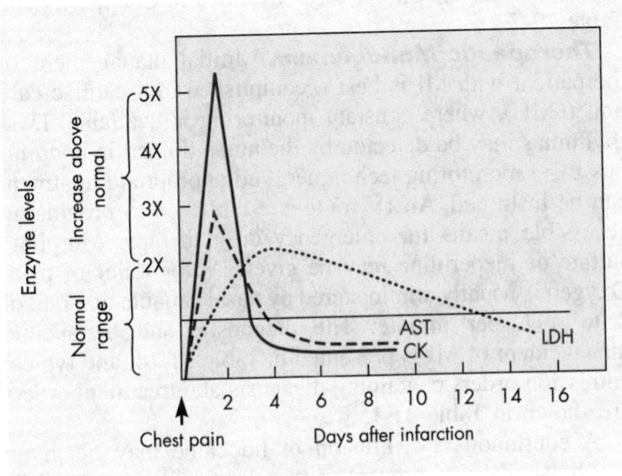

Fig. 31-17 Heart muscle enzyme levels in the blood after myocardial infarction. *AST,* Aspartate aminotransferase; *CK,* creatine kinase; *LDH,* lactic dehydrogenase.

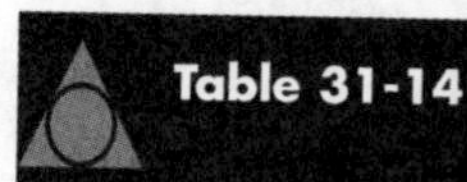

Table 31-14 Therapeutic Management: Myocardial Infarction

Diagnostic
- History and physical examination
- Serum enzyme levels (e.g., CK, AST, LDH)
- 12-lead ECG
- Chest x-ray
- CBC, thyroid profile
- Nuclear imaging studies
- Echocardiogram

Therapeutic
- IV therapy
- Continual ECG monitoring
- Morphine sulfate IV 2-4 mg/hr as needed (meperidine if patient is allergic to morphine)
- Oxygen therapy
- Monitoring of vital signs every 1-4 hr
- Lidocaine IV drip infusion (if ordered)
- Bed rest with progressive activity
- Recording of intake and output
- Thrombolytic therapy (as indicated)
- Anticoagulant therapy (e.g., heparin IV)
- Antithrombotic therapy (e.g., ASA)
- Nitroglycerin IV

ASA, Acetylsalicylic acid; *AST,* aspartate aminotransferase; *CBC,* complete blood count; *CK,* creatine kinase; *ECG,* electrocardiogram; *IV,* intravenous; *LDH,* lactic dehydrogenase.

the scan and thus indicate an area of ischemia or infarct. However, this technique does not differentiate old from new infarcts.

Technetium pyrophosphate scanning can localize areas of acute necrosis. When IV is given to the patient, technetium complexes with calcium in necrotic myocardial tissue. An area of infarct is visualized as a zone of increased radionuclide uptake and thus derives the name *hot spot.* Optimum time for imaging after an acute MI is 24 to 48 hours, but the scan may remain positive for as long as 10 days. (Nuclear imaging is also described in Chapter 29 and Table 29-7.)

Therapeutic Management. Initial management of the patient with MI is best accomplished in a cardiac care unit (CCU), where constant monitoring is available. Dysrhythmias may be detected by the nurse trained in continuous ECG monitoring techniques, and appropriate treatment can be instituted. An IV route is established to provide an accessible means for emergency drug therapy. Morphine sulfate or meperidine may be given IV for relief of pain. Oxygen is usually administered by nasal cannula at a rate of 2 to 4 L per minute. The diagnostic and therapeutic management of MI is presented in Table 31-14, and typical admission orders containing diagnosis and treatment orders are shown in Table 31-15.

A continuous IV infusion of lidocaine may be given prophylactically to prevent ventricular fibrillation, which is the greatest threat to life after MI. In many persons, episodes of fibrillation are preceded by premature ventricular contractions. The incidence of ventricular fibrillation has decreased to approximately 1% to 2%. Thus the use of prophylactic lidocaine is an area of much controversy. If the patient is past the first 4 to 6 hours, which is when ventricular fibrillation is greatest, or if the patient does not display premature ventricular contractions, prophylactic lidocaine may not be prescribed.

Vital signs are taken frequently during the first few hours after admission and are monitored closely thereafter. Bed rest and limitation of activity are usual initially, with a gradual increase in activity.

A pulmonary artery (PA) catheter and intraarterial line may be used to accurately monitor intracardiac, pulmonary artery, and systolic arterial pressures in complicated MI so that the most effective mode of treatment in the acute phase can be determined. In the presence of severe LV dysfunction, an intraaortic balloon pump (IABP) may be used to assist ventricular ejection and promote coronary artery perfusion. (Pulmonary artery catheters and IABP are discussed in Chapter 61).

Thrombolytic therapy. Thrombolytic therapy is the standard of practice in the treatment of acute MI. The goal in the treatment of acute MI is to salvage as much myocardial muscle as possible. Historically, treatment of acute MI had been directed at the patient's symptoms only (i.e., dysrhythmia and CHF), and nothing was done for the acute process of infarction. This treatment modality decreased mortality from 30% to approximately 15% in the 1970s. With the advent of thrombolytic therapy, treatment has progressed to actually stopping the infarction process instead of just treating symptoms. In the 1990s mortality rates have decreased to 2.5% to 5% with thrombolytic treatment.[35,36]

It is now known that 80% to 90% of all acute MIs are secondary to thrombus formation.[35,36] Perfusion to the myocardium distal to the occlusion is halted causing progressive ischemia, cell death, necrosis, and acute MI.

The acute MI process therefore takes time. The earliest tissue to become ischemic is the subendocardium (the innermost layer of tissue in the cardiac muscle). Necrosis spreads toward the epicardium in a phenomenon known as the *wave front of necrosis.*[36] Myocardial cells do not die instantly. It takes approximately 4 to 6 hours for the entire thickness of the muscle to become necrosed in the majority of patients, and this is known as a *transmural infarction.*

Treatment of the acute MI is geared to quickly dissolving the thrombus in the coronary artery and reperfusing the myocardium before cellular death occurs. To be of most benefit, thrombolytics must be given as soon as possible, preferably within that first 6 hours after the onset of pain. If reperfusion occurs within that time, a 25% reduction in mortality has been shown.[35]

INDICATIONS AND CONTRAINDICATIONS. The commonly used thrombolytics (Table 31-16) can be given by the intracoronary or IV route. IV thrombolytic therapy is preferred because it can be given quickly, with excellent results in opening the artery. Although these drugs have different mechanisms of action and different pharmacokinetics, they all produce an open artery by lysis of the thrombus in the coronary artery.

Table 31-15 Cardiac Care Unit Admission Orders

Admission
Continuous monitor, rhythm strips, and dysrhythmia analysis
Vital signs q2hr for first 8 hr, then q4hr from 6 AM to midnight or as needed
Intake and output hourly
IV infusion of 500 ml 5% dextrose and water to keep vein open
Diet: Determined by condition of patient *clear liquids and advance as tolerated*
Daily weight ✓
(Must be checked if wish to have done)
Oxygen 3 L/min by cannula or 5-8 L/min by mask
Absolute bed rest with bathroom privileges for 24 hr

CPR*
Defibrillation with 200 joules for ventricular fibrillation
Type of resuscitation:
DNR ____ EPS (treatment of dysrhythmias and defibrillation only—no CPR to be done) ____ Full ACLS ✓

Dysrhythmias
Lidocaine 75-100 mg bolus, then IV drip (500 ml 5% dextrose in water with 2 g lidocaine) of 2-4 mg/min for PVCs more than 6/min, R-on-T, multifocal or sequential PVCs at a rate >110
Atropine 0.5-1.0 mg IV for ventricular rate <50 with BP <90 and/or symptoms of poor cerebral perfusion

Medication
Pain
Severe *Morphine Sulfate 2-4 mg. IV every 5 min. until relief*
Mild *Acetaminophen 600 mg PO every 3-4 hr.*
Hypnotic *Restoril 5 mg po hs MR x 1*
Laxative *MOM 30 cc q hs prn* Stool softener *Colace 100 mg PO bid*
Antiemetic —
Antithrombotic *ASA i po q am*
Anticoagulant *(5% dextrose in water) Heparin 25,000 U/500 ml to run at 1000 U/hr; titrate to maintain PTT 1 1/2 - 2X baseline per unit protocol*

Laboratory
Cardiac profile on admittance and q8hr x 3
ECG Dates *4/5, 4/6, 4/7*
Serum K+ every other day while in CCU, PTT every am while on heparin
Routine lab UA, CBC, serum electrolytes, PTT
Other *Chest x-ray on admittance (if not done in ED)*

ACLS, Advanced cardiac life support; *ASA*, Acetylsalicylic acid; *BP*, blood pressure; *CBC*, complete blood count; *CPR*, cardiopulmonary resuscitation; *CCU*, cardiac care unit; *DNR*, do not resuscitate; *ECG*, electrocardiogram; *EPS*, electrophysiology study; *ED*, emergency department; *IV*, intravenous; *PO*, by mouth; *PRN*, as required; *PTT*, partial thromboplastin time; *PVC*, premature ventricular contraction; *UA*, urinary analysis.
*By certified personnel only.

Table 31-16 Thrombolytic Agents Used to Treat Myocardial Infarctions

Streptokinase
Urokinase
Tissue plasminogen activator (t-PA)
Anisoylated plasminogen-streptokinase activator complex (APSAC, Eminase)

Because all the thrombolytics produce lysis of the pathologic clot, they may also lyse homeostatic clots (such as in the stomach or over a postoperative site). Therefore patient selection is important because persons receiving thrombolytic therapy may have a minor or major bleeding episode as a consequence of therapy. Not all patients who have an acute MI are candidates for thrombolytic therapy (Table 31-17). Inclusion criteria to receive an IV thrombolytic agent are (1) chest pain typical of acute MI less than or equal to 6 hours in duration (some centers extend the time limit to 12 hours), (2) chest pain for more than 6 hours if intermittent with ongoing ischemia, and (3) 12-lead ECG findings consistent with acute MI, irrespective of location.[36]

Procedure. Once the patient has been assessed in the emergency department (ED) for risk factors of possible side effects of the therapy and is considered a candidate, IV thrombolysis can begin. An agent is selected according to the patient's profile and the physician's preference. Each hospital has a protocol to follow for administration of thrombolytic agents. However, there are several common factors. Blood is drawn, three lines for IV therapy are started, and all other invasive procedures are done before the thrombolytic agent is given, reducing the possibility of bleeding in the patient.

The time therapy begins is noted, and the patient is monitored frequently during the dose and maintenance

Table 31-17 Contraindications for Thrombolytic Therapy

Absolute Contraindications
- History of hemorrhagic stroke
- Uncontrolled hypertension
  - Systolic BP >200
  - Diastolic BP >120
- Recent surgery or trauma (within 2 wk)
- Active internal bleeding
- Known bleeding disorder
- Suspected aortic dissection

Relative Contraindications
- History of stroke
- Acute, poorly controlled hypertension (BP >180/110)
- Malignancy
- Recent, prolonged, traumatic CPR
- Acute pericarditis
- Pregnancy
- Active peptic ulcer
- Diabetic hemorrhagic retinopathy
- Atrial fibrillation

BP, Blood pressure; *CPR,* cardiopulmonary resuscitation.

protocol. ECG, vital signs, and heart and lung assessments are completed as often as every 5 minutes to evaluate the patient's response to therapy. When reperfusion occurs (i.e., the coronary artery that was occluded is patent, and blood flow is reestablished to the myocardium), several clinical markers may occur. These include chest pain resolution; return of ST segment to baseline on the ECG; the presence of reperfusion dysrhythmias; and marked, rapid rise of the CK enzyme within 3 hours of therapy, peaking within 12 hours.[37]

The nurse must closely monitor the patient for signs of reperfusion dysrhythmias including increase in premature ventricular contractions, ventricular tachycardia, ventricular fibrillation, and accelerated idioventricular rhythm. Sometimes bradycardia, AV blocks, and asystole can occur, depending on the location of the infarction. Unfortunately, these clinical markers do not always occur when the artery opens. If they do occur, the nurse should document their presence and have another ECG done.

Another major concern with therapy is reocclusion of the artery. In this situation the patient seems to have a reperfused artery and is stable. However, because the area around the thrombus is unstable, another clot may form or spasm of the artery may occur. Because of this possibility, most physicians begin heparin therapy. An IV bolus is given, followed by a heparin drip to maintain the patient's partial thromboplastin time (PTT) at one to two times normal. This prevents another clot from forming in the coronary artery. Despite this therapy, in approximately 12% to 15% of the patients in whom reperfusion occurs, another clot will develop. If another clot develops, the patient has similar complaints of chest pain, ECG changes, and hemodynamic compromise. The physician is notified and further action is taken to determine the cause of the reocclusion. The patient may go to the cardiac catheterization laboratory for further invasive diagnostic procedures or PTCA. Sometimes the patient will again receive thrombolytic therapy.

The major complication with thrombolytic therapy is bleeding. The patient is receiving an agent that causes clot dissolution and this may cause the patient to go into a lytic state. Minor bleeding is expected in this person. Prevention of bleeding is essential, and proper patient selection and screening are imperative. Ongoing nursing assessment is also essential. If minor bleeding does occur (such as surface bleeding from IV sites or gingival bleeding), it can be controlled and thrombolytic therapy should not be stopped. If, however, there is a major bleeding episode, such as massive GI or genitourinary (GU) bleeding, the physician should be notified and the thrombolytic therapy should be stopped. The nurse must pay particular attention to signs and symptoms of bleeding such as a drop in BP, an increase in HR, positive guaiac from the NG aspirate or stool, hematuria, a sudden change in the patient's level of consciousness, and oozing of blood from IV or catheter sites.

Cardiac catheterization. Although the treatment for acute MI is to lyse the thrombus and reperfuse the myocardium, some patients may not be candidates for thrombolytic therapy or may have a complicated course necessitating an emergent cardiac catheterization. The patient with acute MI may have a catheterization early in the treatment phase to locate the exact lesion (or lesions) and to assess the severity, the presence of collateral circulation, and LV function.

With actual visualization of the coronary artery system and LV function, the physician can prescribe a treatment modality most beneficial to the patient. Direct intracoronary thrombolytic therapy may be tried, PTCA may be performed, IABP insertion may be done, or the determination that CABG should be done can be made.

Percutaneous transluminal coronary angioplasty. PTCA may be performed emergently, especially in the patient exhibiting signs of cardiogenic shock or in the patient in which thrombolytic therapy was unsuccessful. PTCA is a nonoperative alternative to surgery for the patient who has coronary artery narrowing. Transluminal dilatation can increase the diameter of the artery with the use of percutaneous, fluoroscopically guided catheters to relieve stenotic or occlusive lesions.

The technique is similar to cardiac catheterization. A double-lumen polyvinyl balloon catheter is guided into the coronary artery to the site of the occlusion. The balloon is inflated at the site of stenosis, thereby directly increasing the diameter of the artery. After PTCA, regional coronary blood flow is increased and myocardial metabolism is restored. PTCA is therefore indicated for the relief of myocardial ischemia in the patient with noncalcified, occlusive, compressible coronary artery lesions. Emergent PTCA following MI has a slightly higher rate of abrupt closure than elective PTCA.[36] (Elective PTCA is described earlier in this chapter.)

Coronary artery bypass graft surgery. Coronary artery bypass graft (CABG) surgery may be a treatment choice in a select group of patients with acute MI (see Chapter 32).

Pharmacologic Management

IV nitroglycerin. IV nitroglycerin may be used in the initial therapeutic treatment of the patient with an acute MI.

CLINICAL PATHWAY FOR UNCOMPLICATED MYOCARDIAL INFARCTION

Diagnostic Related Group 122 Length of Stay 6.8 Days

Admit Date: ________ Discharge Date: ________

Pathway	Day 1		Day 2	Days 3-4	Days 5-6
Clinical Path Implemented (initial):					
Diagnostic Studies	■ Chem 7,12 CBC ■ Mg ■ Chest x-ray ■ PT/PTT q __ hr ■ Stool occult blood	■ Cardiac enzymes q8hr × 2 after initial labs ■ Pulse oximetry now ■ Consider ABGs ■ ECG	■ Echocardiogram ■ Consider cardiac enzymes 24 hr after initial series	Consider: ■ Cardiac enzymes ■ Holter monitor	■ Consider modified exercise treadmill testing and discharge if negative ■ If positive, consider cardiac catheterization ■ Consider signal average ECG (if low EF or significant ventricular ectopy on Holter)
Treatments	■ Consider thrombolytic therapy, complete questionnaire, identify eligibility ■ Oxygen ____ L/min ■ Cardiac monitoring ■ Pulse oximetry prn ■ If chest pain: ECG, SL NTG, call physician				
IV/Meds	■ IV heplock ■ IV fluids ____ @ ____ ■ NTG drip ____ ■ Heparin ■ Morphine IVP ■ Antidysrhythmics ■ Beta blockers IV/PO	■ SL NTG ____ ■ ASA ____ ■ Implement thrombolytic protocol ■ Stool softener	■ See med sheet	■ Consider weaning IV NTG	■ Consider discontinuing heparin
Consults	■ Cardiology		■ Consider cardiac rehab evaluation		
Nursing	■ ECG strips q shift prn (rhythm, ST segment analysis) ■ Monitor chest pain for site, duration, quality, radiation, relief using 1-5 pain scale, notify MD if increasing chest pain or ST elevations or changes in cardiac rhythm ■ Physical assessment q4hr prn X 24 hr, then q shift ■ Monitor lab values ■ I + O, admission wt. ■ No IM injections ■ VS q4hr prn ■ Provide emotional support and assistance to reduce patient/family anxiety				
Diet	■ Clear liquids until stable, then 2 g Na, low cholesterol, no caffeine				
Activity and Safety	■ Active and passive ROM ■ BR with bedside commode ■ Institute cardiac step levels ■ Routine safety measures		■ Cardiac step level ____ ■ Rest periods after meals	■ Cardiac step level ____	■ Cardiac step level ____
Teaching Patient and Family	■ Orient to unit ■ Explain diet, meds, activity ■ Call nurse with chest pain, rate on 1-5 scale ■ Explain all tests and procedures ■ Explain relationship among disease process, resulting symptoms, and therapy prescribed		■ Explain cardiac step levels ■ Teach taking of own pulse ■ Cardiac teaching ■ Films		
Discharge Planning	■ Initial assessment		■ Facilitate physician/RN/family conference ■ Assess need for follow-up care ■ Review Advance Directives by date of discharge ■ To consider: elective cardiac catheterization as outpatient		

continued

Clinical Pathway for Uncomplicated Myocardial Infarction—cont'd

Expected Outcomes: Uncomplicated MI

Problem List	Day 1	Day 2	Days 3-4	Days 5-6
Meets Expected Outcome (initial):				
Chest pain: Acute MI; validation of chest pain, discomfort, dyspnea	■ Verbalizes pain or discomfort on a 1-5 pt scale with 5 = worst pain imaginable and 0 = pain free ■ Verbalizes dyspnea	■ Pain managed ■ Non-verbal indicators such as grimacing will be absent	■ Pain free ■ Dyspnea resolving	■ Pain free at discharge ■ Denies dyspnea at rest or with activities
Activity intolerance: Imbalance of O_2 supply and demand 2° to decreased CO, dyspnea on exertion	■ Identifies activities that precipitate chest pain ■ Modifies activity as tolerated	■ Tolerates bedside commode/chair without chest pain ■ Participates in ADLs without chest pain ■ Progressive ROM prn	■ Tolerates level of activity ■ Maintains: RR <24/min, NSR or HR <110 or within 20 bpm of resting HR	■ Discharged at anticipated activity tolerance: BP change of <20 mm Hg and pain free ■ Identifies risks of immobility
Knowledge deficit: MI and implications for lifestyle changes; states concerns re: chest pain and disease process	■ States why admitted to hospital ■ States importance of notifying RN of chest pain	■ Demonstrates readiness to learn ■ Asks questions, reads MI packet, etc.	■ Demonstrates understanding of what an MI and angina are ■ Lists risk factors ■ Verbalizes understanding of diet ■ Selects appropriate items on menu ■ Takes own pulse	■ Verbalizes activity restrictions and rationale ■ Verbalizes understanding of discharge instructions. Will have completed MI teaching ■ Has plan to reaccess the EMS ■ Has discussed potential for OP cardiac catheterization with physician
Anxiety: Real or perceived threat of death, change in health status and unfamiliar environ. Verbalizes fear, is restless; hyperventilates; is withdrawn, angry	■ Verbalizes fears and concerns re: hospitalization ■ Asks questions	■ Shows appropriate coping mechanisms ■ Identifies support systems	■ Is coping ■ Exercises control by making decisions about care	■ Verbalizes resources and support systems available to assist on discharge
Alteration in cardiac output: BP <90 mm Hg systolic HR >100 bpm RR >20 min UO <30 ml/hr	■ BP stabilizing ■ UO >30 ml/hr	■ VS stable, hemodynamic parameters stabilized with or without intervention ■ UO >30 ml/hr ■ Lungs clear	■ BP maintained without IV fluid or vasoactive therapy	■ BP stabilized
Potential for bleeding: Risk of hemorrhage 2° to thrombolytics and heparin; bruising	■ Verbalizes understanding of reason to notify RN of any bleeding or bruising	■ No increased incidence of bruising, bleeding, or hematomas	■ No increased incidence of bruising, bleeding, or hematomas	■ States risk factors of anticoagulant therapy and when to notify physician

Other parts of this Clinical Pathway include Patient Pathways, Patient Education Documentation Record, and Physician's Orders. Developed by Nanticoke Memorial Hospital, Seaford, DE. Used with permission of and licensed by The Center for Case Management, Inc., South Natick, MA.
ADLs, Activities of daily living; *ASA,* acetylsalicylic acid; *BP,* blood pressure; *BR,* bed rest; *CBC,* complete blood count; *CO,* cardiac output; *ECG,* electrocardiogram; *EF,* ejection fraction; *EMS,* Emergency Medical System; *HR,* heart rate; *IM,* intramuscular; *I+O,* intake and output; *IV,* intravenous; *IVP,* intravenous pyelogram; *MI,* myocardial infarction; *NTG,* nitroglycerin; *OP,* outpatient; *PO,* oral; *prn,* as needed; *PT,* prothrombin time; *PTT,* partial thromboplastin time; *ROM,* range of motion; *RR,* respiratory rate; *SL,* sublingual; *UO,* urinary output; *VS,* vital signs.

Nitroglycerin given IV may reduce pain and decrease preload and afterload while increasing the myocardial oxygen supply. Its action may also increase collateral circulation to the ischemic areas of the myocardium. The dose of nitroglycerin is titrated to a dose that decreases the patient's pain while maintaining an adequate BP. The major side effect of IV nitroglycerin is headache or hypotension accompanied by diaphoresis, nausea, vomiting, and occasionally rate dysrhythmias.

Antidysrhythmic drugs. Dysrhythmias are the most common complications after an MI. (The drugs used in the treatment of dysrhythmias are discussed in Chapter 33.)

Morphine. Morphine sulfate is given for acute cardiac pain relief because it reduces anxiety and decreases the cardiac work load by lowering myocardial oxygen consumption, reducing contractility, lowering BP, and slowing the HR. Morphine is given IV because (1) after infarction there may be poor peripheral perfusion, which may cause pooling of medication, rendering the medication ineffective until the circulation is restored and at which time a drug overdose may occur, (2) serum enzymes are affected by an intramuscular (IM) injection, and (3) bleeding may occur at the site of the injection if the patient has received thrombolytic therapy or is on heparin.

Meperidine (Demerol) may be given, but it is used less frequently than morphine. Both drugs can depress respirations, which may cause hypoxia, a condition to be avoided in myocardial ischemia and infarction.

Positive inotropic drugs. Positive inotropic drugs that increase the heart's contractility may be used in the patient with acute MI. However, caution should be used. This group of drugs increases the heart's demand for oxygen (increased myocardial oxygen consumption [MVO_2]) at a time when therapy is used to decrease the demand and increase the heart's supply of oxygen (increased flow). Digitalis, amrinone (Inocor), and dobutamine (Dobutrex) are examples of drugs that increase the heart's pumping action (contractility). Their use is indicated when LV failure is present. Nursing interventions during the use of inotropic therapy should include frequent vital signs and heart and lung assessment for evidence of further LV failure or ischemia.

β-Blockers. The use of β-adrenergic blockers early in the acute phase of the MI and during a one-year follow-up regimen can decrease morbidity. The patient who uses β-blockers in the treatment of an acute MI and for 1 year following the infarction has a decreased chance of reinfarction and increased survival.[35,36]

Drug choice and dose depend on the physician. Nursing interventions during the use of β-blockers in acute MI should include frequent vital signs and heart and lung assessment. Bradycardia, heart block, and hypotension may result.

Calcium channel blockers. Calcium channel blockers may also be used in the treatment of acute MI, but have not been shown to be beneficial in reducing morbidity and mortality. They may be used in the treatment of MI where the patient also underwent PTCA to restore perfusion. In this setting, calcium channel blockers may be used to prevent coronary spasm.

Angiotensin-converting enzyme inhibitors. ACE inhibitors may be used following large transmural MIs. The use of ACE inhibitors in patients with large transmural MIs beginning approximately on the third day can help prevent ventricular remodeling and prevent or slow the progression of late heart failure. (See Chapter 30 for a discussion on ACE inhibitors.)

Stool softeners. After an MI the patient is predisposed to constipation as a result of bed rest and narcotic administration. Stool softeners such as dioctyl sodium sulfosuccinate (Colace) are given to facilitate and promote the comfort of bowel evacuation. This prevents straining and the resultant vagal stimulation from the Valsalva maneuver. (The Valsalva maneuver is explained in Chapter 40.) Vagal stimulation produces bradycardia and can provoke dysrhythmias. Another real danger of straining is that when the action is stopped, venous return to the heart is suddenly increased. This may result in overloading of a weakened heart.

Nutritional Management. Diet is restricted in saturated fats and cholesterol and is sometimes low in sodium to prevent fluid retention. The patient may have a clear liquid diet the first day when there may still be nausea.

NURSING MANAGEMENT

MYOCARDIAL INFARCTION

Nursing Assessment

Subjective and objective data that should be obtained from a patient with an MI are presented in Table 31-18.

Nursing Diagnoses

Nursing diagnoses specific to a patient with an MI include, but are not limited to, those presented in the nursing care plan on p. 919.

Planning

The overall goals are that the patient with a myocardial infarction (1) will experience relief of pain, (2) have no progression of MI, (3) receive immediate and appropriate treatment, (4) cope effectively with associated anxiety, (5) cooperate with rehabilitation plan, and (6) alter high-risk behaviors.

Nursing Implementation

Acute Intervention. Acute nursing interventions for the patient with MI are best done in a specialized care unit such as a CCU. Since the advent of CCUs in the early 1960s, medical and nursing care has improved dramatically, and countless lives have been saved.

Acute nursing intervention includes the initial CCU stay (2 to 3 days) and the rest of hospitalization (5 to 7 days). Priorities for nursing interventions in the initial phase of recovery after MI include pain assessment and relief, physiologic monitoring, promotion of rest and comfort, alleviation of stress and anxiety, and understanding of the patient's emotional and behavioral reactions. Proper management of these priorities decreases the oxygen needs of a compromised myocardium. In addition, the nurse needs to

Table 31-18 Nursing Assessment: Myocardial Infarction

Subjective Data
Important Health Information
Past health history: Previous angina or MI, hypertension, diabetes, smoking (pack years)
Medications: Use of nitrates, calcium blockers, antihypertensive medications, illicit drugs
Functional Health Patterns
Health perception–health management: Family history of heart disease
Nutritional-metabolic: Nausea, vomiting, indigestion, heartburn
Activity-exercise: Profound weakness, dyspnea, palpitations, syncope
Cognitive-perceptual: Severe substernal or precordial pain, described as heavy or crushing, lasting more than 30 min and not relieved by rest or nitrates; radiation to neck, back, or arms possible
Coping–stress tolerance: Feeling of impending doom, recurrent or persistent stress

Objective Data
General
Fever, anxiety, restlessness
Integumentary
Cold, clammy skin
Respiratory
Tachypnea, rales
Cardiovascular
Tachycardia or bradycardia; dysrhythmias (especially ventricular); elevated BP (initially); S_4, possible S_3; murmur and rub and diminished heart tones
Urinary
Decreased urinary output
Possible findings
Positive serum cardiac enzymes, leukocytosis; normal chest x-ray or signs of pulmonary congestion, cardiomegaly; positive radionuclide scan, coronary arteriography

BP, Blood pressure; *MI,* myocardial infarction.

institute measures to avoid the hazards of immobility while encouraging rest.

Pain. Morphine should be given as needed to eliminate or reduce chest pain. The nurse should instruct the patient to rate the pain on a scale of 1 to 10 to assist in the assessment and treatment of pain. Because a patient does not always verbalize pain, the nurse must be attuned to other manifestations of pain, such as restlessness, elevated pulse rate or BP, clutching of the bedclothes, or other nonverbal cues. Nitroglycerin IV, if given, should be titrated. Once pain is relieved, the nurse may have to deal with denial in a patient who interprets the absence of pain as an absence of cardiac damage. After the pain medication has been administered, the efficacy of the drug and the patient's response should be assessed and documented.

Monitoring. A patient has continuous ECG monitoring while in the CCU and usually after transfer to a step-down or general unit. The nurse should be trained in ECG interpretation so that dysrhythmias causing further deterioration of the cardiovascular status can be identified and treated. During the initial period after MI, ventricular fibrillation is the most common lethal dysrhythmia. In many patients, this dysrhythmia is preceded by PVCs or ventricular tachycardia (VT).

In addition to frequent vital signs, intake and output should be evaluated at least once a shift, and physical assessment should be carried out to detect deviations from the patient's baseline parameters. Included is the assessment of lung sounds and heart sounds and inspection for evidence of fluid retention (e.g., distended neck veins, hepatic engorgement, presacral or anterior tibial edema). Because a patient is frequently on strict bed rest initially, dorsiflexion of the feet (Homans' sign) to elicit deep calf pain should also be done to evaluate the presence of deep-vein thrombosis.

Assessment of the patient's oxygenation status is helpful, especially if the patient is receiving oxygen. Also, the nares should be checked for irritation or dryness, which can cause considerable discomfort if the nasal route is used for oxygen administration.

Rest and comfort. With a severe insult to the myocardium, as in the case of infarction, it is important for the nurse to promote rest and comfort. Bed rest may be ordered for the first 2 to 3 days in a severe MI. A patient with an uncomplicated MI may rest in a chair.

When sleeping or resting, the body requires less work from the heart than it does when active. It is important to plan nursing and therapeutic actions to ensure adequate rest periods free from interruption. Comfort measures that can promote rest are smooth bedclothes, frequent oral care, adequate warmth, dim lighting, a quiet atmosphere, and assurance that personnel are nearby and responsive to the patient's needs.

It is important that the patient understand the reasons why activity is limited. However, in spite of this limitation the patient is not completely restricted. Gradually the cardiac work load is increased through more demanding physical tasks so that the patient can achieve a discharge activity level adequate for home care. Phases of rehabilitation are outlined in Table 31-19.

Anxiety. Anxiety is present in all patients in various degrees. The nurse's role is to identify the source of anxiety and assist the patient in reducing it. If the patient is afraid of being alone, a family member should be allowed to sit quietly by the bedside or to check in with the patient frequently. If a source of anxiety is fear of the unknown, the nurse should explore these concerns with the patient and help with appropriate reality testing.

If anxiety is because of lack of information, the nurse should provide teaching appropriate to the patient's stated need and level. This does not mean that the nurse initiates the cardiac education protocol. Instead the nurse answers the patient's questions with clear, simple explanations sufficient to reduce the patient's anxiety.

It is important to start teaching at the patient's level rather than to present a prepackaged protocol. Usually, the patient is not yet ready to hear about the pathogenesis of

NURSING CARE PLAN Patient with Myocardial Infarction

Planning: Outcome Criteria	*Nursing Interventions and Rationales*
➤ **NURSING DIAGNOSIS**	Acute pain *related to* lactic acid production from myocardial ischemia and altered myocardial oxygen supply *as manifested* by severe chest pain, tightness or constriction, radiation of pain to neck, arms, or back
Express satisfaction with level of comfort.	Administer oxygen through nasal cannula *to increase oxygenation of myocardial tissue and prevent further tissue ischemia.* Administer morphine sulfate IV as needed to *decrease anxiety, aleviate pain, and decrease the cardiac work load by lowering myocardial oxygen consumption, reducing contractility, lowering BP, and slowing the HR.* Monitor vital signs q1-2hr *to provide on-going assessment of patient's response to treatment.* Assess mental status frequently because *confusion can indicate cerebral hypoxemia.* Continue to evaluate patient's level of comfort *as an evaluation of myocardial ischemia and response to treatment.* Explain the importance of reporting and rating any pain *so that it can be evaluated and treated.* Administer antianginal agents as ordered *to increase blood flow to myocardium, decrease work load, and reduce pain.*
➤ **NURSING DIAGNOSIS**	Altered cardiac tissue perfusion *related to* myocardial damage, ineffective CO, and potential pulmonary congestion *as manifested by* decrease in BP and urine output, crackles in lungs, hepatic engorgement and peripheral edema, splitting of heart sounds, presence of S_3 and S_4
Have BP and pulse within normal limits for individual, respiratory rate of 12-18/min.	Minimize cardiac workload during healing *to decrease the oxygen needs of the myocardium.* Explain necessity of bed rest and decreased activity *to promote patient cooperation.* Allow rest periods between concentrated nursing care times *to reduce fatigue and O_2 requirements of myocardium.* Provide long, uninterrupted rest periods *to promote cardiac rest and promote healing.* Monitor oxygen administration to *ensure adequacy of O_2* supply to the myocardium. Assess comfort level (try to keep patient free of pain) *because pain is an indication of myocardial ischemia and can produce anxiety, which increases O_2 needs.* Assess urine output *to determine adequacy of renal blood flow.* Assess vital signs q1-2hr *to evaluate patient's response to treatment.* Auscultate heart and lung sounds q2-3hr *to detect deviations from baseline parameters.* Provide low-fat, low-sodium diet.
➤ **NURSING DIAGNOSIS**	Impaired gas exchange *related to* ineffective breathing pattern and decreased systemic tissue perfusion secondary to decreased CO as manifested by confusion, somnolence, cyanosis, restlessness, irritability
Have improved blood gases, improved cerebral function (i.e., return of usual mental status), no evidence of cyanosis.	Treat pain *to reduce anxiety and decrease cardiac work.* Elevate head of bed *to allow gravity to lower the diaphragm and decrease the work of breathing and reduce venous return.* Relieve anxiety *because anxiety causes a release of catecholamines, which increase the cardiac work load.* Monitor effects of medications *to evaluate patient's response to treatment.* Hold morphine and notify physician if respiratory rate less than 10-12/min *because morphine is a respiratory depressant.* Maintain oxygen therapy as ordered *to increase oxygen supply to the myocardium.* Monitor blood gases and oximetry *to evaluate patient's oxygen saturation;* report abnormalities.
➤ **NURSING DIAGNOSIS**	Anxiety *related to* present status and unknown future, possible lifestyle changes, pain, and perceived threat of death *as manifested by* restfulness, agitation; verbalization of concern about many health-related aspects such as lifestyle changes and prognosis
Have physical and emotional comfort, sense of well-being.	Monitor anxiety level because *anxiety increases the need for O_2.* Assess stressors in patient's life *to identify possible sources of anxiety.* Determine patient's past coping mechanisms and effectiveness *to encourage use or assist in modifying if needed.* If patient needs information, provide it simply and clearly *so it can be understood.* Administer anti-anxiety agent as needed *to aid in reducing anxiety by depressing subcortical levels of CNS and limbic system.* Assess support systems and incorporate into plan of care if effective *because family may be most effective in reducing patient's stress.*

continued

NURSING CARE PLAN Patient with Myocardial Infarction—cont'd

Planning: Outcome Criteria	*Nursing Interventions and Rationales*
➤ **NURSING DIAGNOSIS**	Activity intolerance *related to* fatigue secondary to decreased CO and poor lung and tissue perfusion *as manifested by* fatigue with minimal activity, inability to care for self without dyspnea, and increase in pulse rate
Have minimal expenditure of energy in the first few days after MI.	Assess level of fatigue, weakness, and potential for activity progression *to provide baseline data for developing a care plan.* Meet patient's needs quickly and efficiently *to conserve energy and prevent anxiety.* Encourage patient to maintain bed rest until instructed otherwise *to reduce cardiac work load.* Have articles patient may want or need within easy reach *to minimize activity, conserve energy, and foster independence.* Monitor BP, pulse, respiration, and color *to monitor patient's response to activity and to adjust as necessary.* Administer O_2 prn during activity *to increase O_2 availability for cardiac and other organ perfusion.* Plan activity progression within limitations *to increase activity tolerance without rapidly increasing cardiac workload.*
➤ **NURSING DIAGNOSIS**	Self-esteem disturbance *related to* lack of control, illness event, and perceived or actual role changes *as manifested by* expression of feelings of helplessness and low self-esteem, minimal participation in self-care
Visualize recovery from MI as time-limited curtailment of normal activities; understand importance of limiting activity at this time; have realistic idea of future activities.	Allow patient as much autonomy as possible by giving necessary information *that will provide feeling of control.* Allow patient to assist in planning care *to reinforce value as a person and to maintain independence.* Inform patient of what to expect in hospital *to respect the right for information, decrease anxiety, and promote autonomy.*
➤ **NURSING DIAGNOSIS**	Constipation *related to* immobility, change in diet, possible fluid restriction, and medications *as manifested by* difficulty passing stool, dry and hard stool
Have normal bowel evacuation pattern.	Administer stool softeners as ordered *to facilitate and promote the comfort of bowel evacuation and to prevent straining and the resultant vagal stimulation from the Valsalva maneuver.* Provide bedside commode *because it is a more natural position than a bedpan and has been found to reduce the Valsalva maneuver.* Instruct patients to avoid straining *to prevent the Valsava maneuver.* Provide foods high in fiber *to add bulk to the stool.* If patient is unsuccessful, obtain laxative order from physician *to facilitate easier bowel evacuation.* Increase activity and ambulation as tolerated *to increase peristalsis and bowel motility.*
➤ **NURSING DIAGNOSIS**	Sleep pattern disturbance *related to* complex treatment regimen, pain, anxiety, stressful environment, and frequent interruptions *as manifested by* report of feeling tired on awakening, frequent napping, fitful sleep with frequent interruptions
Feel rested; have minimum interruptions during sleep.	Monitor flow of people into patient's room *to reduce noise and confusion and prevent sensory overload.* Plan nursing care to provide optimal rest *to encourage myocardial healing.* Provide calm, restful environment *to reduce stimuli and promote sleep.* Attempt to maintain patient's sleep-wake cycle *because lack of sleep impedes healing and may produce confusion.* If patient's condition is stable, do not awaken for vital signs *so that patient may have an uninterrupted sleep cycle.*

continued

NURSING CARE PLAN Patient with Myocardial Infarction—cont'd

Planning: Outcome Criteria	Nursing Interventions and Rationales
➤ **NURSING DIAGNOSIS**	Ineffective management of therapeutic regimen *related to* lack of knowledge of disease process, rehabilitation, home activities, diet, and medications *as manifested by* frequent questioning about illness, management, and aftercare
Describe causes of heart attack, appropriate response for future symptoms, recommended lifestyle changes, immediate plan of care, appropriate expectations after discharge, and activity and diet guidelines.	Teach at patient's level of understanding *to ensure that the information is understood* and *to increase likelihood of behavior change.* Provide guidelines with rationale for recommended actions to be taken *so patient has a clear understanding of why he is being asked to change specific behaviors.* Make recommendations to patient in a realistic manner *so that patient can see self carrying them out.* Include family when information is given, especially regarding homecoming, *to get the cooperation of the patient's most significant support system.* Be specific when giving discharge instructions; write them down for patient to take home *to be available for reference.*
➤ **NURSING DIAGNOSIS**	Grieving *related to* actual or perceived losses secondary to cardiac condition *as manifested by* possible losses, such as occupation, role, status, and previous lifestyle; denial of need to alter lifestyle
Begin to resolve grief over losses and changes; make positive plans for future.	Assess potential losses and changes that patient will need to make *to evaluate patient's perception of losses and changes and alter if unrealistic or unncessary.* Encourage discussion of ways to alter lifestyle to patient's satisfaction *to minimize impact of changes.* Assure patient of self-worth *to strengthen self-image.* Assist patient to plan realistic lifestyle adjustments *to increase the probability of compliance and avoid unnecessary changes.*

BP, Blood pressure; *CNS,* central nervous system; *CO,* cardiac output; *HR,* heart rate; *IV,* intravenous; *MI,* myocardial infarction.

Table 31-19 Phases of Rehabilitation

***Phase I**—Time when patient is in the CCU:* Activity level depends on severity of MI; patient may rest in bed or chair; attention focuses on management of pain, anxiety, dysrhythmias, and cardiogenic shock

***Phase II**—Time from transfer from the CCU to discharge from hospital:* Resumption of activities begins to the point of self-care at the time of discharge; information giving and teaching are appropriate at this time

***Phase III**—Time of convalescence at home:* Patient and family examine and possibly restructure lifestyles and roles; exercise program begins, commonly a walking program, which progresses daily during first week and then weekly; patient undergoes exercise treadmill test at about 8 wk to determine work load of recovering myocardium

***Phase IV**—Time of recovery and maintenance:* Involvement with the community rehabilitation program for physical training and fitness continues

CCU, Cardiac care unit; *MI,* myocardial infarction.

heart disease. The earliest questions usually relate to how the disease affects perceived control and independence. These questions usually include the following:

When will I leave the CCU?
When can I be out of bed?
When will I be discharged?
When can I return to work?
How much change will I have to make in my life?
Will this happen again?

The nurse should advise that a more complete teaching program begins once the patient is feeling stronger. Frequently the patient may not be able to consciously examine the most pervasive concern of all MI victims: Am I going to die? Even if a patient denies this concern, it is helpful for the nurse to initiate conversation by remarking that fear of dying is a common concern reported by most patients who have suffered an MI. This gives the patient "permission" to talk about an uncomfortable and fearful topic.

Emotional and behavioral reactions. The emotional and behavioral reactions of a patient are varied and frequently follow a predictable response pattern (Table 31-20). The role of the nurse in intervention is to understand what the patient is currently experiencing, to assist the patient in testing reality, and to support the use of constructive coping styles. Denial may be a positive coping style in the early phase of recovery from MI.

The nurse has an obligation to maximize and enhance the patient's support systems. This entails assessing the support structure of the patient and family and allowing it to function. Often the patient is separated from the most significant support system at the time of hospitalization. The nurse's role can include talking with the family, informing them of the patient's progress, allowing the patient and the family to interact as necessary, and supporting the family members who will be able to provide the necessary support to the

Table 31-20 Emotional and Behavioral Responses to Acute Myocardial Infarction

Denial
- May have history of ignoring symptoms related to heart disease
- Minimizes severity of medical condition
- Ignores activity restrictions
- Avoids discussing MI or its significance

Anger
- Is commonly expressed as "why did this happen to me?"
- May be directed at family, staff, or medical regimen

Anxiety and fear
- Fears death and long-term disability
- Overtly manifests apprehension, restlessness, insomnia, tachycardia
- Less overtly manifests increased verbalization, projection of feelings to others, hypochondriasis
- Fears activity, recurrent heart attacks, and sudden death

Dependency
- Is totally reliant on staff
- Is unwilling to perform tasks or activities unless approved by physician
- Wants to be monitored by ECG at all times
- Is hesitant to leave CCU or hospital

Depression
- Experiences mourning period concerning loss of health, altered body function, and changes in lifestyle
- Realizes seriousness of situation
- Begins to worry about future implications of health problem
- Shows manifestations of withdrawal, crying, anorexia, apathy
- May be more evident after discharge

Realistic acceptance
- Focuses on optimum rehabilitation
- Plans changes compatible with altered cardiac function

CCU, Cardiac care unit; *ECG*, electrocardiogram; *MI*, myocardial infarction.

patient. Open visitation is helpful in decreasing anxiety and increasing support for the patient with an MI.

Chronic and Home Management. *Rehabilitation* may be defined as the process of helping the patient adjust to a disability by teaching integration of all resources and concentrating more on existing abilities than on permanent disabilities. Cardiac rehabilitation is the restoration of a person to an optimal state of function in six areas: physiologic, psychologic, mental, spiritual, economic, and vocational. Many persons recover from an MI physically, yet they may never attain psychologic well-being because of misconceptions about the illness or a need to practice illness behaviors. Returning to work and resuming all activities have long been outcome measures of cardiac rehabilitation and are important in terms of the cost effectiveness of cardiac care and rehabilitation. A sample rehabilitation program is presented in Table 31-21.

In considering rehabilitation, the nurse and patient must recognize that CAD is a chronic disease. It will not be cured, nor will it disappear by itself. Therefore basic changes in lifestyle must be made to promote recovery and health. These changes must frequently be made at a time when a person is middle-aged and is already dealing with aging and all its associated stresses. The patient must also realize that recovery takes time. Resumption of physical activity after MI is slow and gradual. However, with appropriate and adequate supportive care, recovery is more likely to occur. (See the research box on p. 924.)

Patient education. Once the acute stage of MI has passed, the patient is transferred to a progressive care, or regular hospital unit. The goals of nursing care are ongoing. In addition, an important nursing goal is patient and family education. This teaching begins with the CCU nurse and progresses through the staff nurse to the community health nurse. The purpose of education is to give the patient and family the tools they need to make informed decisions about attainment of health. For teaching to be meaningful, the patient must be aware of the need to learn. Careful assessment of the patient's learning needs helps the nurse to set goals and objectives that are realistic.

The timing of the teaching is important. When patients or families are in crisis (either physiologic or psychologic), they may not have learning needs. It is important to remember that early questions should be answered initially in simple, brief terms, without detailed elaboration and that the answers to these questions require repetition and follow-up (elaboration). When the shock and disbelief accompanying a crisis subside, the patient and family are better able to focus on new information.

In addition to teaching the patient and the family what they wish to know, there are several types of information that are considered necessary in achieving health. A teaching plan for the patient with MI should include the following:

1. Anatomy and physiology of the heart and vessels
2. Cause and effect of atherosclerosis
3. Definition of terms (e.g., CAD, angina, MI, sudden death, CHF)
4. Signs and symptoms of angina and MI and reasons they occur
5. Healing after infarction
6. Identification of risk factors
7. Rationale for tests and treatments, including ECG, blood tests, and angiography and monitoring, rest, diet, and medications
8. Appropriate expectations about recovery and rehabilitation (anticipatory guidance)
9. Measures to take to promote recovery and health
10. Importance of the gradual, progressive resumption of activity

Some nurses have found that an algorithm sheet that lists these categories and who taught the information is helpful in documenting information given to the patient and family.

Table 31-21 In-Patient Rehabilitation: Seven-Step Myocardial Infarction Program (Revised 1992: Grady Memorial Hospital/Emory University School of Medicine)

Step	Date	Supervised Exercise	CCU/Ward Activity	Educational Activity
			Cardiac Care Unit (CCU)	
1	—	Active and passive ROM all extremities, in bed Teach patient ankle plantar and dorsiflexion—repeat hourly when awake	Partial self-care Feed self Dangle legs on side of bed Use bedside commode Sit in chair 15 min, 1-2 times/day	Orientation to CCU Personal emergencies, social service aid as needed Bedside teaching (CCU staff)
2	—	Active ROM all extremities, sitting on side of bed	Sit in chair 15-30 min, 2-3 times/day Complete self-care in bed	Orientation to rehabilitation team and program Smoking cessation Educational literature if requested Planning transfer from CCU
			Ward	
3	—	Warm-up exercises, 2 METs: Stretching Calisthenics Walk 50 ft and back at slow pace	Sit in chair ad lib To ward class in wheelchair Walk in room	Normal cardiac anatomy and function Development of atherosclerosis What happens when MI occurs
4	—	ROM and calisthenics, 2.5 METs Walk length of hall (75 ft) and back, average pace Teach pulse counting	OOB as tolerated Walk to bathroom Walk to ward class, with supervision	Coronary risk factors and their control
5	—	ROM and calisthenics, 3 METs Check pulse counting Practice walking few stairsteps Walk 300 ft bid	Walk to waiting room or telephone Walk in ward corridor prn	Diet Energy conservation Work simplification techniques (as needed)
6	—	Continue above activities Walk down flight of steps (return by elevator) Walk 500 ft bid Instruct on home exercise	Tepid shower or tub bath, with supervision To cardiac clinic teaching room, with supervision Predischarge exercise test (as appropriate)	Heart attack management: Medications Exercise Surgery Response to symptoms Family, community adjustments on return home
7	—	Continue above activities Walk up flight of steps Walk 500 ft bid Continue home exercise instruction; present information regarding outpatient exercise program	Continue all previous ward activities	Discharge planning Medications, diet, activity Return appointments Scheduled tests Return to work Community resources Educational literature Medication cards

Source: Reprinted with permission of Grady Memorial Hospital, Emory University School of Medicine.
Modified from Wegner N: Rehabilitation of the patient with coronary heart disease. In Schlant RC, Alexander RW: *Hurst's The Heart*, ed 8, 1994, New York, McGraw-Hill Book Co.
MET, metabolic equivalent; *MI*, myocardial infarction; *OOB*, out of bed; *OT*, occupational therapy, *ROM*, Range-of-motion.

RESEARCH

Implications for Nursing Practice

QUALITY OF LIFE IN PATIENTS TREATED FOR MI

Citation Papadantonaki A, Stotts NA, Paul SM: Comparison of quality of life before and after coronary artery bypass and percutaneous transluminal angioplasty, *Heart Lung* 23:45-52, 1994.

Purpose To compare quality of life, mood state, and physical functioning before and after revascularization in patients who have undergone CABG and PTCA

Methods Quasiexperiment using patients who had undergone elective CABG (n=44) and PTCA (n=32) with a mean age of 57.9 years of age. Quality of life, mood state, and physical functioning were measured before revascularization and 3 weeks after hospital discharge.

Results and Conclusions Patients who had undergone CABG and PTCA were similar in quality of life, mood state, and physical functioning before revascularization. Quality of life did not change from baseline in either group. Mood state and physical functioning improved for both CABG and PTCA groups after the procedure, but there was significantly greater improvement in the PTCA group.

Implications for Nursing Practice When evaluating the effectiveness of medical or surgical interventions, it is important to obtain both subjective and objective measurements. Knowing patients' perception about their quality of life, mood state, and physical functioning may assist nurses in planning care during hospitalization as well as after discharge.

When medical terminology is used, its meaning should be explained in lay terms. For example, it can be explained that the heart, a four-chambered pump, is a muscle that needs oxygen like all other muscles, and when vessels become narrowed by atherosclerosis, the process is similar to a buildup of mineral deposits inside water pipes, which causes less water to flow through at a higher pressure. It is a good idea for the nurse to have a model of the heart or to use a pad and pencil to sketch what is being explained. Literature written for a nonmedical audience is available through the American Heart Association.

Anticipatory guidance involves preparing the patient and the family for what to expect in the course of recovery and rehabilitation. By learning what to expect during treatment and recovery, the patient gains a sense of control over life. This sense of perceived control allows the patient to consciously consider stressors and thus possibly to promote recovery. The idea of perceived control is operationalized as the process by which the patient exercises choice and makes decisions by cutting back. Cutting back is one way of minimizing the psychophysiologic losses after MI (or any other life-changing event). The patient considers what must be cut back (changed), weighs this against what should be cut back, and finally determines what will be cut back. For example, a middle-aged man who smokes two packs of cigarettes a day, is 20 pounds overweight, and gets no physical exercise has a seemingly overwhelming task. He may decide that he *can* live with a weight-reduction diet and will get more exercise (although perhaps not daily) but that it is not possible for him to quit smoking. He reasons that because he is modifying two of the three risk factors, he will be safe if he cuts back on smoking. Ideally the smoking risk factors should be a priority for this patient, but if information regarding risks and effects of smoking is not accepted, the nurse must respect the patient's need for control.

Physical exercise. Exercise is an integral part of the rehabilitation program. It is necessary for optimal physiologic functioning and psychologic well-being. It has a direct, positive effect on maximal oxygen uptake, increasing CO, decreasing blood lipids, decreasing BP, increasing blood flow through the coronary arteries, increasing muscle mass and flexibility, improving the psychologic state, and assisting in weight loss and control. A regular schedule of moderate exercise, even after many years of sedentary living, is beneficial.

One method used to identify levels of physical activities is through metabolic equivalent (MET) units: 1 MET is the amount of oxygen needed by the body at rest—3.5 ml of oxygen per kilogram per minute or 1.4 calories/kg of body weight per minute. The MET is used to determine the energy costs of various exercises (Table 31-22).

In the hospital, the activity level is gradually increased so that by the time of discharge the patient can tolerate moderate-energy activities of 3 to 5 METs. Many patients with an uncomplicated MI are in the hospital only approximately 7 days. By day 4 or 5, the patient can stand in the room and perhaps even ambulate in the hallway. Many physicians order low-level treadmill tests before discharge to assess readiness for discharge, accurate HR for an exercise prescription, and potential for reinfarction. If tests are positive (i.e., ischemia at a low level of energy expenditure), the patient is evaluated for cardiac catheterization before discharge and possible bypass grafting. If the test is negative, a catheterization may be suggested for 1 month after discharge. Because of the short hospitalization, it is critical to give the patient specific guidelines for activity and exercise so that overexertion will not occur. It is helpful to stress that when the patient "listens to what the body is saying"—the most important facet of recovery—uncomplicated recovery should proceed.

Teaching the patient to check the pulse rate is a nursing responsibility. The patient should be taught the parameters within which to exercise. The patient should be told the maximum HR that should be present at any point. If the HR exceeds this level or does not return to the rate of the resting pulse, within a few minutes the patient should stop. The patient should be instructed to stop exercising if pain or dyspnea occurs.

In a normal, healthy person the minimum threshold for improving cardiorespiratory fitness is 60% of the age-pre-

Table 31-22 Energy Expenditure in Metabolic Equivalents

Activity	Calories Burned
Low-Energy Activities (less than 3 METs or less than 3 cal/min)	
Activities in hospital	
Resting supine	1.0
Sitting	1.2
Eating	1.4
Conversing	1.4
Washing hands, face	2.5
Activities outside hospital	
Sewing by hand	1.4
Sweeping floor	1.7
Painting, sitting	2.5
Driving car	2.8
Assembling radio	2.7
Sewing by machine	2.9
Moderate-Energy Activities (3-6 METs or 3-5 cal/min)	
Activities in hospital	
Sitting on bedside commode	3.6
Walking at 2.5 mph	3.6
Showering	4.2
Using bedpan	4.7
Walking at 3.75 mph	5.6
Activities outside hospital	
Bricklaying	4.0
Tractor plowing	4.2
Ironing, standing	4.2
Mopping	4.2
Bowling	4.4
Cycling at 5.5 mph on level ground	4.5
Golfing	5.0
Dancing	5.5
High-Energy Activities (6-8 METs or 6-8 cal/min)	
Ambulating with braces and crutches	8.0
Performing carpentry	6.8
Mowing lawn by hand	7.7
Playing singles tennis	7.1
Riding on trotting horse	8.0
Walking at 5 mph	6.5
Ascending stairs	7.0
Very High-Energy Activities (8-10 METs or 8-10 cal/min)	
Skiing	9.9
Jogging at 5 mph	8.0
Shoveling snow	8.5
Ascending stairs with a 17 lb load	9.0
Extremely High-Energy Activities (more than 10 METs or more than 11 cal/min)	
Playing handball	
Cycling at 13 mph	
Ascending stairs with a 22 lb load	

dicted maximum HR (which is calculated by subtracting the person's age from 220). The ideal training target HR is 80% of maximum HR. The patient who has been physically inactive and is just beginning an exercise program should do so under supervision whenever possible. The more important factor is the patient's response to exercise in terms of symptoms rather than absolute HR. This is a point that cannot be overstressed in teaching of the MI patient. In addition, a cardiac patient on medications (especially β blockers) may not be able to increase HR to any degree and should have a treadmill test to determine an individual target HR.

The basics for cardiac conditioning within the cardiac population include the following:

1. *Type of exercise*: Exercise should be regular, rhythmic, and repetitive, using large muscles to build up endurance (e.g., walking, cycling, swimming, rowing).
2. *Intensity*: Exercise intensity should be determined by the patient's HR. If a treadmill test has not been performed, the person recovering from MI should not exceed 20 bpm over the resting pulse rate.
3. *Duration*: Exercise can be from 20 to 30 minutes. It is important to begin slowly at personal tolerance (perhaps only 5 to 10 minutes) and build up to 30 minutes.
4. *Frequency*: The patient should exercise three times a week. If done at low duration (5 to 10 minutes), exercise can be done daily but is best done on nonconsecutive days.

In addition, it is helpful to teach the patient about "warm up" and "cool down" with exercise. Mild stretching for 3 to 5 minutes before the exercise activity and 5 minutes after the activity is sufficient. Activity should not be started or stopped abruptly.

The basic categories of exercise are static (*isometric*) and dynamic (*isotonic*). Most daily activities are a mixture of the two. Static exercise involves the development of tension during muscular contraction but produces little or no change in muscle length or joint movement. Lifting, carrying, and pushing heavy objects are primarily isometric activities. Since the HR and BP increase rapidly during isometric work, exercise programs involving isometric exercises should be limited.

Isotonic exercises involve changes in muscle length and joint movement with rhythmic contractions at relatively low muscular tension. Walking, jogging, swimming, bicycling, and jumping rope are examples of activities that are predominantly isotonic. Isotonic exercise can put a safe, steady load on the heart and lungs and may also improve the circulation in many organs.

Resumption of sexual activity. It is important to include sexual counseling for cardiac patients and their partners. This often-neglected area of discussion may be difficult for both patients and health care providers to approach. However, the cardiac patient's concern about resumption of sexual activity after MI often produces more stress than the physiologic act itself. It is reported that most cardiac patients, especially women, do not resume sexual activity after MI.[38] The majority of these patients changed their sexual behavior, not because of physical problems, but because they were concerned about sexual inadequacy, death during coitus, and impotence. The misconceptions held by these persons could have been clarified with specific counseling by a concerned and knowledgeable health care provider.

Before the nurse provides guidelines on resumption of sexual activity, it is important to know the physiologic status of the patient, the physiologic effects of sexual activity, and the psychologic effects of having a heart attack. Sexual activity for middle-aged men with their usual partners is no more strenuous than climbing two flights of stairs.

Most nurses are unsure of how and when to begin counseling about resumption of sex. It is helpful to consider sex as a physical activity and to discuss or explore feelings in this area when other physical activities are discussed. One helpful approach is: "Many people who have had a heart attack wonder when they will be able to resume sexual activity. Has this been of concern to you?" or "If this has been of concern to you, this information should be helpful." This type of nonthreatening statement brings up the topic, allows the patient to explore personal feelings, and gives the patient an opportunity to raise questions with the nurse or another health care provider. Common guidelines are presented in Table 31-23.

The patient needs to know that the inability to perform sexually after MI is common and that impotence usually disappears after several attempts. The nurse should reinforce the idea that patience and understanding usually solve the problem. The patient may assume the position of choice.

Table 31-23 Guidelines for Resumption of Sexual Activity After Myocardial Infarction

- Planning of resumption of sexual activity should correspond to sexual activity before the heart attack.
- Physical training (exercise) seems to improve the physiologic response to coitus; therefore daily exercise during recovery should be encouraged.
- Consumption of food and alcohol should be reduced before intercourse is anticipated (e.g., waiting 3-4 hr after ingesting a large meal before engaging in sexual activity).
- Familiar surroundings and a familiar partner reduce anxiety.
- Masturbation may be a useful sexual outlet and may reassure the patient that sexual activity is still possible.
- Temperature should be comfortable, not extreme. Hot or cold showers should be avoided just before and just after intercourse.
- Foreplay is desirable because it allows a gradual increase in heart rate before orgasm.
- Positions during intercourse are a matter of individual choice.
- Orogenital sex places no undue strain on the heart. This form of sexual expression depends entirely on the individuals involved.
- A relaxed atmosphere free of fatigue is optimal.
- Prophylactic use of nitrates is effective in decreasing angina during sexual activity.
- Anal intercourse may cause undue cardiac stress because of the possibility of inducing a vasovagal response.

It is not uncommon for a patient who experiences chest pain on physical exertion to have some angina during sexual stimulation or intercourse. The patient should be instructed to take nitroglycerin prophylactically. It is also helpful to have the patient avoid sex soon after a heavy meal or after excessive ingestion of alcohol, when extremely tired or stressed, or with unfamiliar partners. Anal intercourse is to be avoided because of the likelihood of eliciting a vasovagal response.

The patient should be counseled that resumption of sex depends on personal desires and on the physician's assessment of the extent of recovery. It is usually recommended that a patient refrain from sex until 4 to 8 weeks after MI. Some physicians believe that the patient should decide when ready to resume sex. Others say that a patient must be able to climb two flights of stairs briskly without dyspnea or angina before sexual activity can be resumed. There are medical practitioners whose experience leads them to believe that when the patient and the partner are ready emotionally, they are most likely ready physiologically.

Reading material on resumption of sexual activity may be presented to the patient to facilitate discussion. The nurse should return to clarify and explain as necessary. Calmly and matter-of-factly introducing the subject of resumption of sexual activity during teaching about physical activity has positive effects of eliciting questions and concerns that might not have otherwise surfaced. For example, the nurse might begin, "Sexual activity is like other forms of activity and should be gradually resumed after MI. If your ability to perform sexually is concerning you, the energy expenditure has been found to be no more than walking briskly or climbing two flights of stairs." This forms a factual basis for the patient to begin to seek information and explore personal feelings about resuming sex.

Sudden Cardiac Death

Sudden cardiac death is the unexpected collapse and cardiopulmonary arrest of a person within minutes to 1 hour after the onset of acute symptoms. It occurs secondary to natural (not accidental or traumatic) causes.[1] The afflicted person may or may not have a documented prior history of cardiovascular disease.

Significance. Sudden cardiac death accounts for approximately 250,000 deaths a year in the United States.[1] Sharma and Wyeth found that of 1070 persons who experienced sudden cardiac death, 325 survived the initial cardiopulmonary arrest.[39] Only 120 of these sudden cardiac death survivors were discharged from the hospital without neurologic impairment. Long-term follow-up of this survivor group revealed that only 44% were still alive after 6 years and that the vast majority of deaths in the survivor group were caused by recurrent sudden cardiac death. Other studies indicate that of those persons who survive sudden cardiac death, those that have cardiac arrest in the absence of acute MI are at high risk for recurrent sudden cardiac death.[1,40]

Etiology. In most instances, sudden cardiac death occurs as a primary manifestation of CAD, and victims usually have multivessel coronary atherosclerosis. However, many of these persons have no known history of cardiovascular disease. Less commonly, sudden cardiac death may occur as a result of a primary LV outflow obstruction. These obstructions may be secondary to such diseases as aortic stenosis, hypertrophic cardiomyopathy, and coarctation of the aorta.

Persons who experience sudden cardiac death as a result of CAD fall into two groups: those who had an acute MI, and those who did not have an acute MI. The latter group accounts for the majority of cases of sudden cardiac death.[1] In this instance, victims usually have no warning signs or no known precedent symptoms. Typically, death is a result of dysrhythmias, usually VT, ventricular fibrillation, or both. The patient is at risk of recurrence of sudden death, probably because of continued electrical instability of the myocardium that caused the initial event to occur.

The second, smaller group of patients includes those who have had acute MI and have suffered sudden cardiac death. In these cases the patients usually do have prodromal symptoms, such as chest pain and dyspnea, and they have less chance of recurrent sudden cardiac death than those who have not had MI.

Risk Factors. Persons at increased risk of sudden cardiac death include those with the following risk factors:

1. Male gender
2. Family history of premature atherosclerosis
3. Cigarette smoking
4. Diabetes
5. Hypercholesterolemia
6. Hypertension
7. Cardiomegaly

Therapeutic Management. Survivors of sudden cardiac death generally require a diagnostic workup to determine whether they have had an acute MI. Thus serial cardiac isoenzymes and ECGs must be obtained, and the patient must be treated accordingly. (See section on Therapeutic Management of MI.) In addition, because most persons with sudden cardiac death have CAD secondary to multivessel coronary atherosclerosis, cardiac catheterization is indicated to determine the possible location and extent of coronary artery occlusion. Percutaneous transluminal coronary angioplasty or CABG bypass graft surgery may be indicated (see Chapter 32).

Most sudden cardiac death patients have a lethal dysrhythmia that is associated with a high incidence of recurrence. Thus it is useful to know when those persons are most likely to have a recurrence and what pharmacologic regimen is the most effective treatment. Around-the-clock Holter monitoring and exercise stress testing may help elicit this information. An *electrophysiology study* (EPS) is most useful in aiding in this determination. This examination is performed under fluoroscopy; pacing electrodes are placed in selected intracardiac areas, and stimuli are selectively used to attempt to evoke dysrhythmias. The patient's response to various antidysrhythmic medications can be determined and monitored in a controlled environment.

Most commonly, a patient who has experienced sudden cardiac death can be treated with antidysrhythmic medications such as procainamide, quinidine, and amiodarone. However, some selected patients are refractory to pharmacologic therapy and may require the surgical implantation of a ventricular defibrillator (see Chapter 33).

The nurse caring for a survivor of sudden cardiac death needs to be attuned to the patient's psychosocial adaptation to this sudden "brush with death." Many of these patients develop a "time bomb" mentality. They fear the recurrence of cardiopulmonary arrest and may become anxious, angry, and depressed. Their families are likely to experience the same feelings. Wives of male survivors of sudden cardiac death often experience a great deal of anxiety and fear of recurrence. They often feel responsible for the prevention of another event.[41] The grief response varies among persons and families. The nurse should be attuned to the specific needs of the patient and the family and educate them accordingly while providing appropriate emotional support.

Gerontologic Considerations: Coronary Artery Disease

The incidence of cardiac disease is greatly increased in older adults and is the leading cause of death in older persons. Angina can be disabling in this population, and affected persons must place increased reliance on health care services to remain independent.[42]

The nurse caring for the older adult with CAD must be aware of the physiologic changes that occur in the cardiovascular system. Structural changes in the myocardium include increased collagen and fat deposition, myofibrillar degeneration, and endocardial thickening resulting in abnormalities in diastolic filling of the ventricles.[42,43] Calcification of the heart valves and degeneration of the conduction system can also occur. The majority of pacemakers are placed in persons more than 65 years of age. Also, resting HR decreases with age, and maximum HR with exercise decreases with age.

In the older adult, loss of elastic fibers and increased collagen in the arterial media diminish elasticity and distensibility of arteries.[42,43] These changes cause an increased systolic BP and SVR, which can result in accelerated atherosclerosis. These combined changes lead to a decrease in cardiac output (CO) by 1% a year. This is probably secondary to decreased contractility of the myocardium and increased afterload caused by the increase in SVR. In addition, decreased arterial wall elasticity blunts the responsiveness to baroreceptors in the aortic arch.[42,44] Circulating norepinephrine levels also increase with age. However, receptors may be less responsive to catecholamines.

The nurse must be aware of the changes in an older adult and must keep in mind the effect that nursing care may have on these patients. Because older adults have decreased responsiveness to catecholamines, their response to stress may be blunted; HR may not rise as quickly in response to pain or to declining CO. They often have atypical symptoms when experiencing an acute MI. Sudden shortness of breath may be more common than classic substernal chest pain.[45] Associated diaphoresis may not be a predominant manifestation of an MI. The sudden occurrence of symptoms such as profound weakness and dyspnea should be investigated.

Many of the antianginal agents that cause postural hypotension and decrease preload may not be well tolerated in the older patient secondary to the decreased responsiveness of the baroreceptors and impaired diastolic filling of the ventricles.[43-48] The patient who has been on bed rest should sit for 3 to 5 minutes before ambulating. Also, antianginal agents that can slow HR must be used with caution in the patient who may have degeneration of the conduction system. The patient may be at increased risk of drug toxicity because of declining hepatic and renal function.

The older patient should be included in a cardiac rehabilitation program. Activity performance, endurance, and ability to tolerate stress can be improved in the older adult with physical training. Positive psychologic benefits can be derived from a planned exercise program and can include increased self-esteem, heightened emotional well-being, and improved body image.[45-47]

When planning an exercise program for the older adult, the nurse should remember the following: (1) longer warm-up periods are needed, (2) longer periods of low-level activity or longer rest periods between sessions are advisable, and (3) heat intolerance may be caused by decreased ability to sweat efficiently. The patient should be taught to avoid exercising in extremes of temperature and to maintain a moderate pace. Target HR for an older adult is 60% to 75% of the maximum HR. The older adult should exercise a minimum of 30 to 40 minutes three or four times a week.

It is unknown if aggressive treatment of hypertension and hyperlipidemia will slow the progression of CAD in the older adult. However, cessation of cigarette smoking helps to decrease the risk of an MI at any age. Encouraging the older patient to adopt a healthy lifestyle may increase quality of life and may also reduce the risks of CAD.

Older adults have a greater incidence of unstable angina as well as more complications from an acute MI than younger patients.[42,44] Complications commonly found in an older patient with an acute MI include an increased incidence of atrial fibrillation, atrial flutter, complete heart block, CHF, myocardial rupture, and cardiogenic shock.[44] Given this greater risk, aggressive management with thrombolytic therapy of the older patient with an acute MI is recommended.[43,49]

β-Blocker therapy has also been shown to greatly benefit the older population, but side effects such as CHF and heart block are more common.[43] PTCA is another aggressive treatment used for controlling CAD in the older patient. However, in patients more than 70 years of age there is a significantly increased incidence of complications with this procedure.[50]

Elective CABG is generally well-tolerated in the older patient. However, the incidence of postoperative complications is high including dysrhythmias, stroke, and infection. The nurse caring for older adults must be aware that, although the benefits of treatment may outweigh risks in this population, complications are higher than in younger individuals. The nurse must be alert to early signs and symptoms of complications and aggressively try to prevent and treat them. Nursing research has shown that despite increased early postoperative complications, once these individuals are home their time of recovery is similar to patients younger than age 70.[51]

Women and Coronary Artery Disease

Traditionally CAD has been viewed as an affliction of middle-aged men, when in fact CAD is the number one killer of American women. Approximately 247,000 deaths occur from heart attacks in women per year.[52-54] Only recently has there been research focusing on the manifestations and course of CAD in women. Women tend to manifest CAD 10 years later in life than men and most women have symptoms of angina rather than MI.[52,53] The exercise treadmill test has a low sensitivity and specificity in women, and 30 to 40% of women will have false positive results.[54] This may be because women have lower hematocrits, higher pulmonary and systolic BP responses to exercise, and ST segment sagging from circulating estrogen. Thallium treadmill tests are more accurate than exercise treadmill tests in the detection of CAD in women.

Women also have a much higher mortality rate within 1 year following MI than men.[52] Women are also more likely to have reinfarction within 1 year.[53,54] This increased mortality was thought to be as a result of women developing CAD at a later age in life when they are more likely to have other illnesses such as diabetes, hypertension, and heart failure. However, even when these comorbidities have been taken into consideration, women still have a higher mortality following MI than men.

Women who have CABG surgery have a higher mortality rate and more complications postbypass than men. This is because women have smaller arteries, are older, and are referred more frequently for CABG with severe or unstable angina requiring urgent or emergent surgery.[53,54] Long-term survival rates are similar for men and women following CABG, but women report less relief from angina, poorer health, and more symptoms than men. Women also have higher rates of coronary dissection and hospital mortality than men following PTCA, but men have a higher incidence of restenosis.[55] However, women have decreased incidence of sudden cardiac death compared with men.

Although risk factors of CAD for men and women are similar, the significance of these risk factors may be different. Diabetes has been found to be a more important risk factor for women than men. Women with diabetes are at a greater risk for mortality from CAD than men with diabetes.[56] Studies have shown that estrogen replacement in postmenopausal women reduces their risk for CAD by 50%. Furthermore, estrogen replacement lowers LDL and raises HDL cholesterol in these women. Smoking, a major risk factor for both men and women, may also carry specific problems for women. Evidence has been found that smoking has been linked to a decrease in estrogen levels and hence early menopause. Wenger has identified cigarette smoking as the most powerful contributor to CAD in women younger than age 50.[53] Hypertension is a high risk factor for CAD in women. Even a 10 mm Hg increase in systolic BP in women is associated with a 20% to 30%

elevation in risk of CAD and stroke.[57] More studies are needed to evaluate the significance of risk factors and interventions to modify risk factors specifically in women.

Implications for Nursing. Because CAD in women more often manifests with angina and women have a poorer prognosis following acute MI, aggressive education about the reduction of risk factors and counseling about lifestyle modification should be implemented upon diagnosis of disease in an attempt to prevent an acute MI.[54] The nurse needs to recognize that women have significant post-MI and post-CABG morbidity and mortality. They need to be assessed for the presence of other diseases such as diabetes and hypertension that can impact their recovery. The nurse should closely assess for early complications following MI, PTCA, and CABG.

Because women generally develop CAD at a later age than men, they often are widowed or have older children who live far from them. The nurse needs to assess the patient's social support systems and refer to agencies that can assist in recovery where indicated. Cardiac rehabilitation programs are just as beneficial for women as men. Specific instruction needs to be given for activities that can be performed following recovery from MI or CABG. Because women often do not perceive housework as strenuous, they begin household chores early after hospital discharge. When they are unable to perform these chores, they may express feelings of guilt.[54]

CRITICAL THINKING EXERCISES

CASE STUDY

MYOCARDIAL INFARCTION

Patient Profile

M.T., a 46-year-old successful businessman, was rushed to the hospital by a rescue squad after experiencing crushing substernal pain radiating down his left arm. He also complained of dizziness and nausea.

Subjective Data

- Has a history of angina pectoris and hypertension
- Is overweight but recently lost 10 pounds
- Bowls occasionally
- Has three teenage children who are causing problems
- Recently experienced death of best friend and business partner who died from cancer

Objective Data

Physical Examination

- Diaphoretic, short of breath

Diagnostic Studies

- Cholesterol is 350 mg/dl (9.1 mmol/L).
- CK is 730 units/L (12.17 μkat/L).
- ECG shows premature ventricular contractions
- Tachycardia
- Inferolateral wall MI

Therapeutic Management

- Streptokinase 1.5 million units IVPB over 40 to 60 min
- Oxygen 2 L/min
- ASA 1 PO qd
- Bed rest
- Vital signs every hour
- Morphine 2-4 mg IV q 30 min prn for chest pain

Critical Thinking Questions

1. Which coronary artery was most likely occluded in M.T.'s coronary circulation?
2. Explain the pathogenesis of CAD. What risk factors may contribute to its development? What risk factors were present in M.T.'s life?
3. What is angina pectoris? How does angina differ from MI?
4. List the clinical manifestations that M.T. exhibited and explain their pathophysiologic bases.
5. Explain the significance of the results of the laboratory tests and ECG findings.
6. For each treatment measure M.T. received, explain the physiologic reason for its use.
7. Based on the assessment data presented, write one or more appropriate nursing diagnoses. Are there any collaborative problems?

NURSING RESEARCH ISSUES

1. Are patients with CABG more likely to make lifestyle changes than patients who are treated with PTCA?
2. Do the activities that precipitate angina differ between those who are older than 65 years as compared with younger people?
3. Is there a gender bias in the treatment of patients with CAD?
4. Does estrogen replacement delay the onset of symptomatic CAD in women?
5. Is a nurse-monitored rehabilitation program more effective than a self-monitored program?

REVIEW QUESTIONS

The number of the question corresponds to the same-numbered objective at the beginning of the chapter.

1. Which of the following changes occurs in the development of CAD?
- a. Formation of fibrous tissue around coronary artery orifices
- b. Accumulation of lipid and fibrous tissue within the coronary arteries
- c. Diffuse involvement of plaque formation in coronary veins
- d. Chronic vasoconstriction of coronary arteries leading to permanent vasospasm

2. Which of the following measures is not appropriate to include in a teaching plan to decrease risk factors for CAD?
- a. Modification of a stressful lifestyle
- b. Weight reduction and decreased dietary intake of saturated fats
- c. Reduction and control of hypertension
- d. Weight lifting to increase CO

3. Which of the following does not describe the pain associated with angina pectoris?
- a. Pain that is not relieved by nitroglycerin or rest
- b. Substernal chest pain precipitated by activity
- c. Crushing, heavy pain lasting 15 to 20 minutes
- d. Substernal pain radiating down the arm

4. Which of the following should be included in a teaching plan for a patient with angina?
- a. Prophylactic use of nitroglycerin
- b. Behavior modification to prevent recurrent MI
- c. Symptoms of digitalis toxicity
- d. Knowledge of foods that are high in potassium

5. Healing following MI is well established
- a. within 3 weeks after the infarction.
- b. when chest pain and dyspnea are not present.
- c. approximately 6 to 8 weeks after the infarction.
- d. at 4 to 6 days after the infarction.

6. The most common complication in the first week after MI is
- a. ventricular rupture.
- b. Dressler's syndrome.
- c. cardiogenic shock.
- d. dysrhythmias.

7. A patient 5 days after MI is restless and apprehensive. The nurse can help by
- a. structuring the environment and routine so that the patient can rest.
- b. encouraging the family to provide for patient's physical care and emotional support.
- c. allowing the patient to participate in planning and carrying out activities.
- d. providing all care by doing everything for the patient.

8. Three days after MI, a patient states that he does not understand what the alarm is about because his problem is just bad indigestion. His reaction is an example of
- a. anger.
- b. projection.
- c. depression.
- d. denial.

9. A post-MI patient being prepared for discharge should be instructed to
- a. take it easy until healing is complete.
- b. stay at home and avoid exposure to the environment.
- c. begin a graduated, progressive exercise program.
- d. do isometric exercises in a relaxed environment.

10. Sudden cardiac death is a primary manifestation of
- a. mitral valve disease.
- b. CHF.
- c. CAD.
- d. cardiomyopathy condition.

REFERENCES

1. American Heart Association: *1993 Heart and Stroke Facts Statistics,* 1992.
2. Lambert CR: Pathophysiology of stable angina pectoris. Angina pectoris mechanisms, diagnosis, and therapy, *Cardiol Clin* 9:1, 1991.
3. Kannel WB: CHD risk factors: a Framingham study update, *Hosp Pract* 25:119, 1990.
4. Dietschy JM: LDL cholesterol: its regulation and manipulation, *Hosp Pract* 25: 67, 1990.
5. Kannell WB: Update on the role of cigarette smoking in coronary artery disease, *Am Heart J* 101:319, 1989.
6. Fletcher GF: The value of exercise in preventing coronary atherosclerotic heart disease, *Heart Disease Stroke* 2:183, 1993.
7. Jenkins CD and others: Prediction of clinical coronary heart disease by a test for coronary prone behavior pattern, *N Engl J Med* 290:1271, 1974.
8. Stoy DB: Controlling cholesterol with diet, *Am J Nurs* 89:1625, 1989.
9. American Heart Association: *Nurses' cholesterol education handbook,* 1990.
10. American Heart Association: *Dietary treatment of high blood pressure and high blood cholesterol: a manual for patients,* 1990.
11. Carleton RA and others: Report of the expert panel on population strategies for blood cholesterol reduction, *Circulation* 83:2154, 1990.
12. Ornish D: Can lifestyle changes reverse coronary atherosclerosis? *Lancet* 336:129, 1990.
13. Brown BG and others: Regression of coronary artery disease as a result of intensive lipid-lowering therapy in men with high levels of apolipoprotein B, *N Engl J Med* 323:1289, 1990.
14. Kane JP and others: Regression of coronary atherosclerosis during treatment of familial hypercholesterolemia with combined drug regimens, *JAMA* 264:3007, 1990.
15. Stoy DB: Controlling cholesterol with drugs, *Am J Nurs* 89:1628, 1989.
16. Scheel M: Cholesterol, lipoproteins, lipid profiles: a challenge in patient education, *Focus Crit Care* 17:203, 1990.

17. Chuyun D, Ford CF, Yursha-Johnston M: Silent myocardial ischemia, *Focus Crit Care* 18:295, 1991.
18. Proudfit WL: Chest pain: angina pectoris and related states, *Heart Disease Stroke* 1:5, 1992.
19. Shuh PK: Pathophysiology of unstable angina. *Cardiol Clin* 9:11, 1991.
20. Gottlieb SO, Flaherty JT: Medical therapy of unstable angina pectoris. *Cardiol Clin* 9:89, 1991.
21. Matrisciano L: Unstable angina: an overview, *Crit Care Nurse* 12:30, 1992.
22. Faxon DP: Percutaneous angioplasty in stable and unstable angina. *Cardiol Clin* 9:99, 1991.
23. Gist HC, Mesrobian HD, Ziskind AA: New interventional techniques for coronary revascularization, *Heart Disease Stroke* 2:198, 1993.
24. Halfman-Franey M and others: Using stents in the coronary circulation: nursing perspectives, *Focus Crit Care* 18:132, 1991.
25. Holcomb SS: Atherectomy, *Nursing* 23:45, 1993.
26. Hall LT: Cardiovascular lasers: a look into the future, *Am J Nurs* 90:27, 1990.
27. McConnell EA: Applying nitroglycerin ointment correctly, *Nursing* 20:70, 1990.
28. Thandani U: Medical therapy in stable angina pectoris. *Cardiol Clin* 9:73, 1991.
29. Kalman JM: Nitrate tolerance: a new look at an old problem, *Focus Crit Care* 17:407, 1990.
30. Pasternak RC, Braunwald E: Acute myocardial infarction. In Isselbacher KJ and others, editors: *Harrison's principles of internal medicine,* ed 13, New York, 1994, McGraw-Hill.
31. Cuddy TE, Pfeffer MA: Indications and value of the use of captopril after myocardial infarction, *Heart Disease Stroke* 2:393, 1993.
32. Braunwald E, Pfeffer MA: Ventricular enlargement and remodeling following acute myocardial infarction: mechanisms and management, *Am J Cardiol* 68:1D, 1991.
33. Rodgers ML: Pericarditis, *Nursing* 20:52, 1990.
34. Norton M and others: Right ventricular infarction vs. left ventricular infarction: review of pathophysiology, medical treatment, and nursing care, *MedSurg Nursing* 2:203, 1993.
35. Antman EM, Braunwald E: Acute MI management in the 1990s, *Hosp Pract* 25:65, 1990.
36. ACC/AHA Task Force: Guidelines for the early management of patients with acute myocardial infarction, *J Am Coll Cardiol* 16:249, 1990.
37. Kleven MR: The critical care nurse's role in the noninvasive assessment of myocardial reperfusion. In Clochesy JM, Ward CR, editors: *AACN clinical issues in critical care nursing,* Philadelphia, 1990, Lippincott.
38. McCann ME: Sexual healing after heart attack, *Am J Nurs* 89:1133, 1989.
39. Sharma B, Wyeth R: Six-year survival of patients with and without painless myocardial ischemia and out of hospital ventricular fibrillation, *Am J Cardiol* 61:10F, 1988.
40. Moss AJ: Prevention of sudden cardiac death, *Hosp Prac* 27:165, 1992.
*41. Simons LH, Cunningham S, Catanzaro M: Emotional responses and experiences of wives of men who survive a sudden cardiac death event, *Cardiovas Nurs* 28:17, 1992.
42. Vetter NJ, Ford D: Angina among elderly people and its relationship with disability, *Age Ageing* 19:159, 1990.
43. Forman DE, Gutierrez-Bernal JL, Wei JY: Management of acute myocardial infarction in the very elderly, *Am J Med* 93:315, 1992.
44. Lewis JF, Maron BJ: Cardiovascular consequences of the aging process. *Geriatric cardiology, Cardiovasc Clin* 22:25, 1992.
45. Holm K, Penckofer S: Coronary heart disease: requisite knowledge for developing prevention strategies for the aging adult, *Prog Cardiovasc Nurs* 5:118, 1990.
46. Mark MD and others: Prognosis of coronary heart disease in the elderly patient: the CASS experience. In Coodley FL, editor: *Geriatric heart disease,* Littleton, MA, 1985, PSG Publishing.
47. Kannel WB: Epidemiology of cardiovascular disease in the elderly: an assessment of risk factors. *Geriatric cardiology, Cardiovasc Clin* 22:9, 1992.
48. Takemoto KA and others: Abnormalities of diastolic filling of the left ventricle associated with aging are less pronounced in exercise-trained individuals, *Am Heart J* 124:143, 1993.
49. House MA: Thrombolytic therapy for acute myocardial infarction: the elderly population, *AACN Clin Issues* 3:106, 1992.
50. McGrath MA and others: PTCA in elderly patients: hospital events, *Am J Crit Care* 2:171, 1992.
*51. Artinian NT, Duggan C, Miller P: Age differences in patient recovery patterns following coronary artery bypass surgery, *Am J Crit Care* 2:453, 1993.
52. American Heart Association: Silent epidemic: the truth about women and heart disease.
53. Wenger N: Coronary heart disease in women: A 'new' problem, *Hosp Prac* 27:59, 1992.
54. Wingate S: Women and coronary heart disease: implications for the critical care setting, *Focus Crit Care* 18:212, 1991.
55. Keresztes PA, Dan AJ: Estrogen and cardiovascular disease, *Cardiovasc Nurs* 28:1, 1992.
56. Holm K, Penckofer S: Cardiovascular risk factors in women, *J Myocard Ischemia* 4:25, 1992.
57. Hanson MJS: Modifiable risk factors for coronary heart disease in women, *Am J Crit Care* 3:177, 1994.

---

*Nursing research-based articles.

Chapter 32

NURSING ROLE IN MANAGEMENT

Congestive Heart Failure and Cardiac Surgery

Mary Ann House-Fancher   Linda Griego

Learning Objectives

1. Compare the pathophysiology of systolic and diastolic ventricular failure.
2. Discuss the compensatory mechanisms involved in congestive heart failure.
3. Describe the therapeutic, pharmacologic, nutritional, and nursing management of the patient with chronic congestive heart failure.
4. Describe the therapeutic and nursing management of the patient with acute congestive heart failure and pulmonary edema.
5. Compare the different types of cardiomyopathy regarding pathophysiology, clinical manifestations, and therapeutic and nursing management.
6. Describe the indications for cardiac transplantation and the nursing management of cardiac transplant recipients.
7. Describe the preoperative and postoperative management of the patient who has cardiac surgery.
8. Discuss the use of the ventricular assist device in ventricular failure and the related nursing care of the patient and family.

CONGESTIVE HEART FAILURE

Congestive heart failure (CHF) is a cardiovascular condition in which the heart is unable to pump an adequate amount of blood to meet the metabolic needs of the body's tissues. CHF is not a disease; it is a syndrome caused by a variety of pathophysiologic processes (Table 32-1). CHF is characterized by left ventricular dysfunction, reduced exercise tolerance, diminished quality of life, and shortened life expectancy.

Significance

CHF is associated with numerous types of heart disease, particularly with long-standing hypertension and coronary artery disease (CAD). Each year approximately 700,000 people in the United States die of heart disease, more than half of which are attributable to end-stage CHF.[1] Currently 2.3 to 3 million people in the United States have CHF. The American Heart Association (AHA) estimates that 400,000 to 500,000 new cases of CHF occur each year.[2]

The incidence of CHF dramatically increases with age—new cases of CHF double with each decade of life.[3] In patients more than 65 years of age, CHF is the most common hospital discharge diagnosis.[4] With the continuing increase in the proportion of older adults in the population and as mortality from CAD decreases, the prevalence of CHF is expected to rise.

In spite of the declining mortality from cardiovascular disease and cerebrovascular accidents in the United States and Canada, CHF continues to be a major cause of morbidity and mortality. CHF is associated with a high mortality rate. In the Framingham study, the 6-year mortality rates after the initial episodes of CHF were 82% for men and 67% for women.[4] These rates are four to eight times higher than those of the general population of the same age. The rate of sudden cardiac death in a patient with CHF is approximately five times higher than the rate for the general population.

Death rates from CHF are higher for men, African-Americans, and older individuals.[5] Mortality caused by CHF has been increasing during the last two decades.[6] There has recently been a decline in case-fatality rates, especially among older adults.[7] Results of large clinical trials have indicated that vasodilators and angiotensin-converting enzyme (ACE) inhibitors may decrease mortality in a patient with symptoms of CHF.[8]

The patient with CHF has an impaired quality of life, restrictions in functional capacity, and numerous symptoms.[5,6] Currently, CHF continues to have a poor prognosis and is likely to remain a major clinical and health care problem.

Reviewed by Roberta Ronayne, RN, BScN(ed), MSc(A), Assistant Professor, University of Ottawa, School of Nursing, Ottawa, Canada.

Table 32-1 Common Causes of Congestive Heart Failure

Chronic	Acute
Coronary artery disease	Acute myocardial infarction
Hypertensive heart disease	Dysrhythmias
Rheumatic heart disease	Pulmonary emboli
Congenital heart disease	Thyrotoxicosis
Cor pulmonale	Hypertensive crises
Cardiomyopathy	Rupture of papillary muscle
Anemia	Ventricular septal defect
Bacterial endocarditis	

Pathophysiology

Risk Factors. Although overt CAD and advancing age are the principle risk factors of CHF, there are also other factors, including hypertension, diabetes, cigarette smoking, obesity, high cholesterol levels, and proteinuria.[4] Hypertension is a major contributing factor, increasing the risk of CHF approximately threefold. The risk of CHF increases progressively with the severity of hypertension, and systolic and diastolic values equally predict risk. Diabetes predisposes an individual to CHF regardless of the presence of concomitant CAD or hypertension. Diabetes is more likely to predispose to CHF in women than in men.[5]

The presence of these risk factors should alert health care providers to the possibility of the development of CHF. A patient may remain asymptomatic while exhibiting clinical signs that reflect deteriorating myocardial functioning. These signs include rapid resting heart rate (HR), decreased vital capacity, an enlarged heart, electrocardiographic abnormalities, and, in particular, evidence of left ventricular hypertrophy.[5] The health care provider should include these parameters in assessing the patient with possible CHF.

Etiology. CHF may be caused by any interference with the normal mechanisms regulating cardiac output (CO). CO depends on (1) preload, (2) afterload, (3) myocardial contractility, (4) HR, and (5) metabolic state of the individual. Any alteration in these factors can lead to decreased ventricular function and the resultant manifestations of CHF. The major causes of CHF may be divided into two subgroups: (1) underlying cardiac diseases (Table 32-1) and (2) precipitating factors (Table 32-2). Underlying cardiac diseases that cause CHF may be congenital or acquired. Precipitating factors often increase the workload of the ventricles, causing a decompensated condition that leads to decreased myocardial function. Precipitating factors are generally more amenable to treatment than cardiac diseases. Prompt recognition and treatment of these precipitating factors can often result in successful patient outcomes.[1]

Pathology of Ventricular Failure. Ventricular failure can be described as (1) a defect in systolic function that results in impaired ventricular emptying or (2) a defect in diastolic function that causes an impairment in ventricular filling. It is now recognized that patients with heart failure actually comprise three distinct groups: (1) those with failure of systolic ejection, (2) those with abnormal resistance to diastolic filling, and (3) those with mixed systolic and diastolic dysfunction.[9]

Systolic failure. Systolic failure is the most common cause of CHF. It is a defect in the ability of the cardiac myofibrils to shorten, which decreases the muscles' ability to contract (pump). This causes the left ventricle to lose its ability to generate enough pressure to eject blood forward through the high-pressure aorta. Inability to move blood forward through the aorta results in (1) a decreased left ventricular ejection fraction (LVEF), (2) an acute increase in left ventricular end-diastolic pressure (LVEDP), (3) an increase in pulmonary capillary wedge pressure (PCWP), and (4) an increase in fluid accumulation in the pulmonary vascular bed (pulmonary congestion). Systolic failure is caused by impaired contractile function (e.g., myocardial infarction), increased afterload (e.g., hypertension), or mechanical abnormalities (e.g., valvular heart disease). Therefore systolic failure is characterized by low forward blood flow.

Diastolic failure. In contrast, diastolic failure is not a disorder of contractility, but of relaxation and ventricular filling. In fact, there is normal or hyperdynamic systolic function. Diastolic failure is characterized by high filling pressures and the resultant venous engorgement in both the pulmonary and systemic systems. The diagnosis of diastolic failure is made on the basis of the presence of pulmonary congestion and pulmonary hypertension in the setting of a normal ejection fraction.

Diastolic failure is usually the result of left ventricular hypertrophy from chronic systemic hypertension, aortic stenosis, or infiltrative and hypertrophic cardiomyopathy. Diastolic failure is commonly seen in older adults as a result of myocardial fibrosis and the hypertension so frequently seen in this population.[10]

Mixed systolic and diastolic failure. Systolic and diastolic failure of mixed origin is seen in disease states such as dilated cardiomyopathy (DCM), in which poor systolic function (weakened muscle function) is further compromised by dilated left ventricular walls that are unable to relax. This patient often has extremely poor ejection fractions, high pulmonary pressures, and biventricular failure (both ventricles may be dilated and have poor filling and emptying capacity).

The patient with ventricular failure of any type has low systemic arterial blood pressure, low CO, and poor renal perfusion. Poor exercise tolerance and ventricular dysrhythmias are also common.[11] When pulmonary congestion and edema are present, the diagnosis of CHF may be made. Whether a patient arrives at this point acutely from a myocardial infarction (MI) or chronically from worsening cardiomyopathy or hypertension, the body's response to this low CO is to mobilize its compensatory mechanisms to maintain CO and blood pressure (BP).

Compensatory Mechanisms. CHF can have an abrupt onset, as with acute MI, or it can be an insidious process resulting from slow, progressive changes. The overloaded heart resorts to certain compensatory mecha-

Table 32-2 Precipitating Causes of Congestive Heart Failure

Cause	Mechanism
Anemia	Decreases O_2-carrying capacity of the blood, stimulating ↑ in CO to meet tissue demands
Infection	Increases O_2 demand of tissues, stimulating ↑ CO
Thyrotoxicosis	Changes the tissue metabolic rate, accelerating HR and work load of the heart
Hypothyroidism	Indirectly predisposes to ↑ atherosclerosis; severe hypothyroidism decreases myocardial contractility
Dysrhythmias	May decrease CO and increase work load and O_2 requirements of the myocardial tissue
Bacterial endocarditis	Infection: increases metabolic demands and O_2 requirements Valvular dysfunction: causes stenosis and regurgitation
Pulmonary embolism	Increases pulmonary pressure and exerts a pressure load on the RV, leading to RV hypertrophy and failure
Pulmonary disease	Increases pulmonary pressure and exerts a pressure load on the RV, leading to RV hypertrophy and failure
Paget's disease	Increases work load of the heart by ↑ the vascular bed in skeletal muscle
Nutritional deficiencies	May decrease cardiac function by ↓ myocardial muscle mass and contractility
Hypervolemia	Increases preload and causes volume load on the RV

CO, Cardiac output; *HR,* heart rate; *RV,* right ventricle.

nisms to try to maintain adequate CO. The main compensatory mechanisms include (1) ventricular dilatation, (2) ventricular hypertrophy, (3) increased sympathetic nervous system stimulation, and (4) hormonal response.

Dilatation. Dilatation is an enlargement of the chambers of the heart. It occurs when pressure in the heart chambers (usually the left ventricle) is elevated over time. The muscle fibers of the heart stretch and thereby increase their contractile force. Initially this increased contraction leads to increased CO and maintenance of arterial blood pressure and perfusion. However, this increased contractility produces greater wall tension, and more myocardial oxygen is required for contraction. Therefore dilatation is a mechanism developed to cope with increasing blood volume. Eventually it becomes inadequate because the elastic elements of the muscle fibers are overstrained. Dilatation can progress to mitral valve incompetence and regurgitation, which further increase the cardiac work load.

Hypertrophy. In chronic CHF, hypertrophy is an increase in the muscle mass and the cardiac wall thickness from overwork and strain. It occurs slowly because it takes time for muscle tissue to develop. Hypertrophy generally follows persistent or chronic dilatation and thus further increases the contractile power of the muscle fibers. This will lead to an increase in CO and maintain tissue perfusion. As myocardial mass increases, the need for additional blood and oxygen increases. The oxygen requirement of the myocardium is referred to as MVO_2 demand. This additional demand cannot always be met in the patient with underlying heart disease.

Sympathetic nervous system activation. Sympathetic nervous system stimulation is often the first mechanism triggered in low CO states. However, it is the least effective compensatory mechanism. Because there is inadequate stroke volume and CO, there is increased sympathetic nervous system activation, resulting in the increased release of epinephrine and norepinephrine. This results in an increased heart rate, myocardial contractility, and peripheral vascular constriction. This increase of HR and contractility improves CO initially. However, over time these factors act in a detrimental fashion by increasing MVO_2 and increasing the workload of the already failing heart. The vasoconstriction causes an immediate increase in preload, which may increase CO initially. However, an increase in venous return to the heart, which is already volume overloaded, actually worsens ventricular performance. Peripheral vasoconstriction also causes an increase in afterload.

Hormonal response. As the CO falls, blood flow to the kidneys decreases, causing decreased glomerular blood flow. This is interpreted by the juxtaglomerular apparatus in the kidneys as decreased volume. In response the kidneys release renin, which converts angiotensinogen to angiotensin (see Chapter 42 and Fig. 42-6). Angiotensin causes (1) the adrenal cortex to release aldosterone, which causes sodium retention, and (2) increased vasoconstriction, which increases the arterial pressure.

The posterior pituitary senses the increased osmotic pressure from increased sodium retention and decreased blood volume, and it secretes antidiuretic hormone (ADH). ADH increases water reabsorption in the renal tubules, causing water retention and therefore increased blood volume.

The cycle previously detailed is a repeating cycle creating a downward spiral of the patient's condition. Blood volume is added to a system that is already overloaded and vasoconstriction increases afterload, causing an increased work load on the heart.

Cardiac compensation occurs when compensatory mechanisms succeed in maintaining adequate CO for tissue perfusion. Cardiac decompensation occurs when these mechanisms can no longer maintain adequate CO and clinical signs and symptoms appear as a consequence of inadequate tissue perfusion. Without treatment, this state is fatal. Even with treatment, the prognosis is poor.

Types of Congestive Heart Failure

CHF is usually manifested by biventricular failure, although one ventricle may precede the other in dysfunction.[9] Normally the pumping actions of the left and right sides of the heart complement each other, producing a continuous flow of blood. However, as a result of pathologic conditions, one side may fail while the other side continues to function normally for a period of time. Because of the prolonged strain, the functioning side of the heart will eventually fail, resulting in biventricular failure.

The most common form of initial heart failure is left-sided failure. CHF occurs in a retrograde fashion, progressing from the left ventricle (LV) to the pulmonary system to the right ventricle (RV) (Fig. 32-1). LV failure will usually lead to and be the main cause of right-sided failure. Right-sided failure can occur without preceding LV failure as a result of right ventricular MI or cor pulmonale (see Fig. 24-14). CHF will eventually develop in the majority of persons with moderate to severe cardiac disease.

Left-Sided Failure. Left-sided failure results from LV dysfunction, which causes blood to back up through the left atrium and into the pulmonary veins. The increased pulmonary pressure causes fluid extravasation from the pulmonary capillary bed into the interstitium and then the alveoli, which is manifested as pulmonary congestion and edema. The most common causes of left-sided failure are diseases of the coronary arteries, hypertension, cardiomyopathy, and rheumatic heart disease.

When a MI occurs, myocardial tissue is damaged and, with time, replaced by scar tissue. The ischemic tissue and the scar tissue are less elastic and have less contractility than undamaged myocardium. The loss of myocardial mass increases the work load on the remaining functional tissue. If the functioning myocardium cannot compensate for this

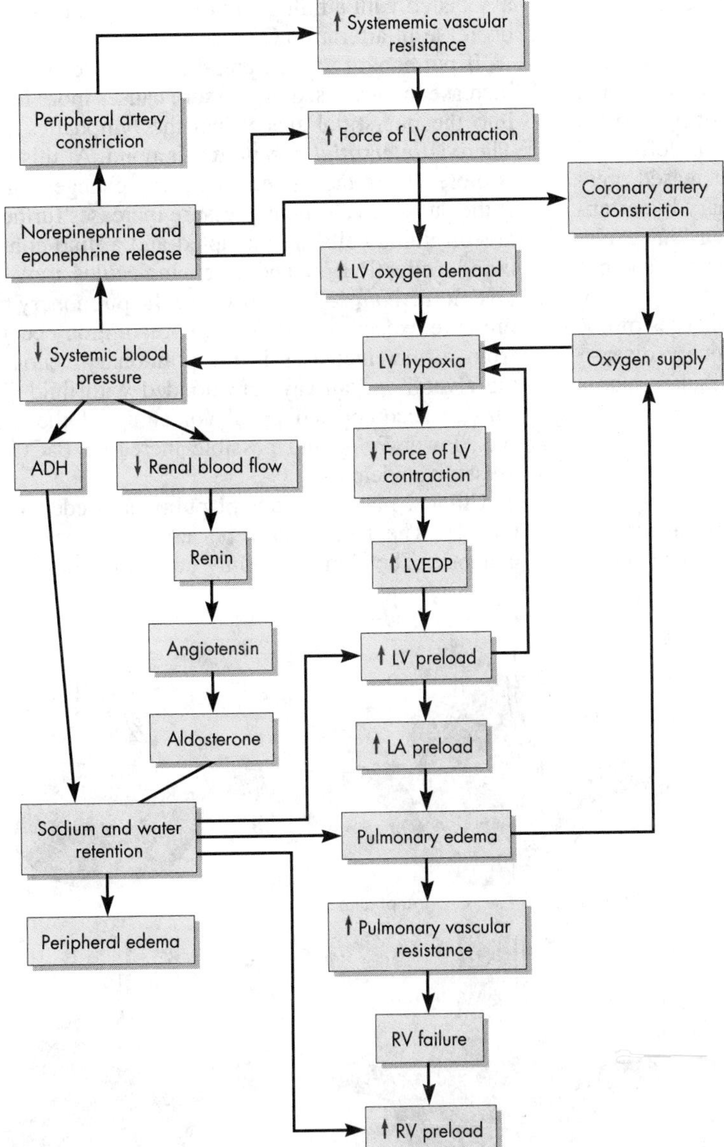

Fig. 32-1 Left heart failure (congestive heart failure) from elevated systemic vascular resistance. Left heart failure leads to right heart failure. Systemic vascular resistance and preload are exacerbated by renal and adrenal mechanisms. *ADH,* Antidiuretic hormone; *LA,* left atrial; *LV,* left ventricular; *LVEDP,* left ventricular end-diastolic pressure; *RV,* right ventricle.

loss, the volume of blood ejected from the ventricle is decreased and heart failure results. This failure may have a rapid onset (acute CHF) or a more insidious onset (chronic CHF).

When hypertension is present, the heart must pump blood against a high arterial pressure. Eventually this can lead to LV hypertrophy. Hypertrophic muscle has poor contractility and will result in failure with time. Cardiomyopathy (CMP) (discussed later in this chapter) is the third leading cause of CHF. There are different types of CMP, but the end result is loss of the LV's ability to maintain adequate CO, resulting in CHF. Rheumatic heart disease, stenosis, or insufficiency of the mitral or aortic valve increase the hemodynamic work load on the heart. (Rheumatic heart disease is discussed in Chapter 34.) With time, this results in failure of the LV and/or RV, requiring an increased amount of pressure that must be generated by the LV. In addition, the valve often fails to close completely and blood is regurgitated into the LV.

Right-Sided Failure. Right-sided failure from a diseased RV causes backward flow to the right atrium and venous circulation. Venous congestion in the systemic circulation results in peripheral edema, hepatomegaly, splenomegaly, congestion of the gastrointestinal (GI) tract, and jugular venous distention. The primary cause of right-sided failure is left-sided failure. In this situation, left-sided failure results in pulmonary congestion and increased pressure in the blood vessels of the lung (pulmonary hypertension). Eventually, chronic pulmonary hypertension results in right-sided hypertrophy and failure. Cor pulmonale (right ventricular dilatation and hypertrophy caused by pulmonary pathology) can also cause right-sided failure. Causes of cor pulmonale include chronic obstructive pulmonary disease (COPD) and pulmonary emboli. Right ventricular infarction may also cause RV failure.

Clinical Manifestations of Acute Congestive Heart Failure

Regardless of etiology, acute heart failure typically manifests as *pulmonary edema,* a term used to refer to an acute, life-threatening situation in which the lung alveoli become filled with serous or serosanguineous fluid (Fig. 32-2). The most common factor in the onset of pulmonary edema is LV failure caused by CAD. (Other etiologic factors are listed in Table 24-28.)

Although the mechanisms of the conditions resulting in pulmonary edema are not fully understood, pulmonary edema is most likely to result when an acute event occurs affecting the heart, such as an acute large MI. Pulmonary edema may also occur when compensatory mechanisms fail to effectively handle additional stress on the heart.

In most cases of left-sided heart failure, there is an increase in the pulmonary venous pressure caused by decreased efficiency of the LV. This results in engorgement of the pulmonary vascular system. As a result, the lungs become less compliant, and there is increased resistance in the small airways. In addition, the lymphatic system increases its flow to help maintain a constant volume of the pulmonary extravascular fluid. This early stage is clinically associated with a mild increase in the respiratory rate and a decrease in arterial PaO_2.

If pulmonary venous pressure continues to increase, the increase in intravascular pressure causes more fluid to move into the interstitial space than the lymphatics can handle. There is *interstitial edema* at this point. At this stage, there is more severe tachypnea, and x-ray changes can be noted. If the pulmonary venous pressure increases further, the tight alveoli lining cells are disrupted and a fluid containing red blood cells (RBCs) and large molecules moves into the alveoli (*alveolar edema*) because the pulmonary hydrostatic pressure exceeds normal. As the disruption becomes worse from further increases in the pulmonary venous pressure, the alveoli and airways are flooded with fluid (Fig. 32-2). This is accompanied by a worsening of the blood gases (i.e., lower PaO_2 and possible increased $PaCO_2$ and progressive acidemia).

Clinical manifestations of pulmonary edema are unmistakable. The patient may be agitated, pale, and possibly cyanotic. The skin is clammy and cold from vasoconstric-

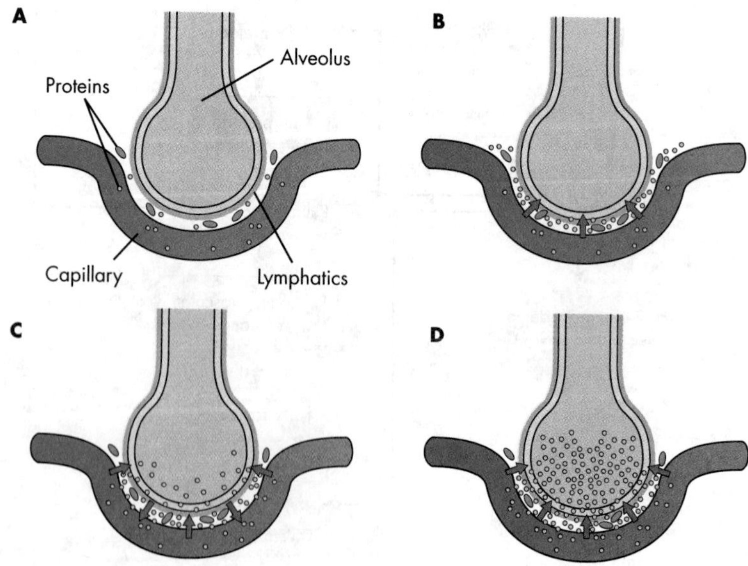

Fig. 32-2 As pulmonary edema progresses, it inhibits oxygen and carbon dioxide exchange at the alveolar capillary interface. ***A,*** Normal relationship. ***B,*** Increased pulmonary capillary hydrostatic pressure causes fluid to move from the vascular space into the pulmonary interstitial space. ***C,*** Lymphatic flow increases in an attempt to pull fluid back into the vascular or lymphatic space. ***D,*** Failure of lymphatic flow and worsening of left heart failure result in further movement of fluid into the interstitial space and into the alveoli.

tion caused by stimulation of the sympathetic nervous system. The patient has severe dyspnea, as evidenced by the obvious use of accessory muscles of respiration, a respiratory rate greater than 30 a minute, and orthopnea. There may be wheezing and coughing with the production of frothy, blood-tinged sputum. Auscultation of the lungs may reveal bubbling rales, wheezes, and rhonchi throughout the lungs. The patient's HR is rapid, and BP may be elevated or decreased depending on the severity of the edema.

Clinical Manifestations of Chronic Congestive Heart Failure

The clinical manifestations of chronic CHF depend on the patient's age, the underlying type and extent of heart disease, and which ventricle is failing to pump effectively. Table 32-3 lists the manifestations of LV and RV failure. The patient with chronic CHF will probably have manifestations of biventricular failure.

Fatigue. Fatigue is one of the earliest symptoms of chronic CHF. The patient notices fatigue after activities that normally are not tiring. The fatigue is caused by decreased CO, impaired circulation, and decreased oxygenation of the tissues. It is sometimes described as "sick fatigue" because of the decreased amounts of blood reaching the musculoskeletal system.

Dyspnea. Dyspnea is a common sign of chronic CHF. It is caused by increased pulmonary pressures secondary to interstitial and alveolar edema. This results in poor gas exchange because of fluid in the alveoli. The shortness of breath makes the patient conscious of air hunger that prompts rapid, shallow respirations. Dyspnea can occur with mild exertion or at rest. *Orthopnea* is shortness of breath that occurs when the patient is in a recumbent position.

Paroxysmal nocturnal dyspnea (PND) occurs when the patient is asleep. It is probably caused by the reabsorption of fluid from dependent body areas when the patient is recumbent. The patient awakens in a panic, has feelings of suffocation, and has a strong desire to seek respiratory relief by sitting up. Careful questioning of patients often reveals adaptive behavior such as sleeping with two or more pillows to aid breathing. A dry, hacking cough may be the first clinical symptom for the patient with CHF. Because there are increased pulmonary pressures and fluid accumulation in the lung tissues, the patient may have a persistent, dry cough, unrelieved with position or over-the-counter cough suppressants.

Tachycardia. Because CO is diminished, there is an increased sympathetic nervous system stimulation to compensate for low output. If the stroke volume decreases, the HR increases to maintain the CO. Tachycardia may be the first clinical sign of CHF.

Edema. Edema is a common sign of CHF. It may occur in the legs (peripheral edema), liver (hepatomegaly), abdominal cavity (ascites), lungs (pulmonary edema and pleural effusion), and other parts of the body. If the patient is in bed, sacral edema will most likely develop. Pressing the edematous skin with the finger may leave a transient indentation (*pitting edema*). The development of dependent edema or a sudden weight gain of 2 kg or more is often indicative of exacerbated CHF.

Nocturia. A person with chronic CHF will have decreased CO, impaired renal perfusion, and decreased urinary output during the day. However, when the person lies down at night, fluid movement from interstitial spaces back into the circulatory system is enhanced. This causes increased renal blood flow and diuresis. The patient may

Table 32-3 Clinical Manifestations of Heart Failure

Right-Sided Heart Failure	Left-Sided Heart Failure
Signs	**Signs**
RV heaves	LV heaves
Murmurs	Cheyne-Stokes respirations
Peripheral edema	Pulsus alternans (alternating pulses: strong, weak)
Weight gain	Increased HR
Edema of dependent body parts (sacrum, anterior tibias, pedal edema)	PMI displaced inferiorly and posteriorly (LV hypertrophy)
Ascites	↓ PaO_2, slight ↑ $PaCO_2$ (poor oxygen exchange)
Anasarca (massive generalized body edema)	Crackles (pulmonary edema)
Jugular venous distention	S_3 and S_4 heart sounds
Hepatomegaly (liver engorgement)	
Right-sided pleural effusion	
Symptoms	**Symptoms**
Fatigue	Fatigue
Dependent edema	Dyspnea (shallow respirations up to 32-40/min)
Right upper quadrant pain	Orthopnea (paroxysmal nocturnal dyspnea)
Anorexia and GI bloating	Dry, hacking cough
Nausea	Pulmonary edema
	Nocturia

GI, Gastrointestinal; *HR*, heart rate; *LV*, left ventricle; *PMI*, point of maximal impulse; *RV*, right ventricle.

complain of having to void six or seven times during the night.

Skin Changes. Because tissue capillary oxygen extraction is increased in a person with chronic CHF, the skin may appear dusky. It is also cool and may be cool to the touch from diaphoresis. Often the lower extremities are shiny and swollen, with diminished or absent hair growth. Chronic swelling may result in pigment changes causing the skin to appear brown in areas covering the ankles and lower legs. The peripheral vasoconstriction that occurs to shunt blood to vital organs is a minor compensatory mechanism in chronic CHF.

Behavioral Changes. Cerebral circulation may be impaired with chronic CHF, especially in the presence of more widespread atherosclerosis. The patient or family may report unusual behavior, including restlessness, confusion, and decreased attention span or memory.

Chest Pain. In the presence of atherosclerosis, CHF can precipitate chest pain because of decreased coronary perfusion from decreased CO and increased myocardial work. Anginal-type pain may accompany either acute or chronic CHF.

Weight Changes. Many factors contribute to weight changes. Initially there may be a progressive weight gain from fluid retention. The patient with CHF has an increased metabolic rate. At the same time, decreased oxygen and nutrients are transported to the tissues. Often the patient is too sick to eat. Abdominal fullness from ascites and hepatomegaly frequently causes anorexia and nausea. In many cases the muscle and fat loss is masked by the patient's edematous condition. The actual weight loss may not be apparent until after the edema subsides.

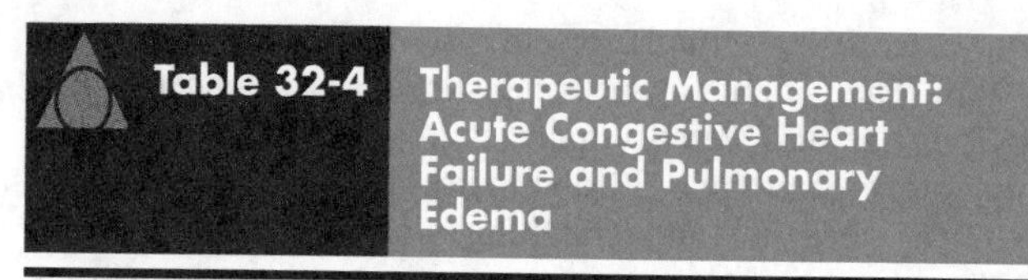

Table 32-4 Therapeutic Management: Acute Congestive Heart Failure and Pulmonary Edema

Diagnostic
- Health history and physical examination
- ABGs, serum chemistries, liver profile
- Chest x-ray
- Insertion of pulmonary artery catheter and peripheral arterial line
- Twelve-lead ECG and monitor
- Echocardiogram
- Nuclear imaging studies

Therapeutic
- Maintenance of patient in high Fowler's position
- Oxygen by mask or nasal catheter
- Morphine IV
- Diuretics IV (furosemide or bumetanide)
- Nitroglycerin IV
- Nitroprusside IV
- Inotropic therapy (see Table 32-7)
- BP, HR, RR, PCWP, urinary output at least q1hr
- Daily weights
- Possible cardioversion
- Endotracheal intubation and mechanical ventilation
- Treatment of underlying cause

ABGs, Arterial blood gases; *BP,* blood pressure; *ECG,* electrocardiogram; *HR,* heart rate; *IV,* intravenous; *PCWP,* pulmonary capillary wedge pressure; *RR,* respiratory rate.

Complications of Congestive Heart Failure

Pleural Effusion. Pleural effusion results from increasing pressure in the pleural capillaries. A transudation of fluid occurs from these capillaries into the pleural space. The pleural effusion usually develops in the right lower lobe initially. (Pleural effusion is discussed in Chapter 24.)

Left Ventricular Thrombus. With acute or chronic CHF, the enlarged LV and poor CO combine to increase the chance of thrombus formation in the LV. Many physicians initially administer anticoagulants to decrease the development of thrombus formation in patients with chronic CHF and in some patients with acute CHF. Once a thrombus has formed, it may also decrease LV contractility, decrease CO, and further worsen the patient's perfusion. The development of emboli from the thrombus is also a possibility.

Hepatomegaly. CHF can lead to severe hepatomegaly. The liver lobules become congested with venous blood. The hepatic congestion leads to impaired liver function. Eventually liver cells die, fibrosis occurs, and cirrhosis can develop (see Chapter 41).

Diagnostic Studies

The primary goal in diagnosis is to determine the underlying etiology of heart failure. Diagnostic measures to assess the cause and degree of heart failure include physical examination, chest x-ray, electrocardiogram (ECG), hemodynamic assessment, echocardiogram, and cardiac catheterization. Diagnostic studies used for the patient with acute CHF are presented in Table 32-4 and those for the patient with chronic CHF are presented in Table 32-5.

The chest x-ray is an important diagnostic measure for assessing and monitoring heart failure. Early abnormalities in CHF, such as prominent, congested upper lobe pulmonary veins, can be seen on x-ray studies. Later changes, such as interstitial pulmonary edema and pulmonary effusion, can also be seen. The degree of cardiac enlargement is also readily observed and is more accurate than percussing for cardiac enlargement.

An ECG is of value in confirming cardiac changes in chronic heart failure. Atrial enlargement is seen by P-wave changes in the early phases of CHF. LV hypertrophy can also be detected by high voltage, especially in V_5 and V_6 leads, and deep S waves in V_1 and V_2 leads. ECG can also be used to detect cardiac dysrhythmias and changes caused by myocardial ischemia or MI. Exercise-stress testing and nuclear imaging studies (see Chapter 29) may provide more valuable information than an ECG taken with the patient at rest.

Echocardiography can be used to measure the size of the cardiac chambers and to assess ventricular and valvular function. Cardiac catheterization and angiocardiography are useful in detecting underlying heart disease. Hemodynamic monitoring via a pulmonary artery catheter (right-sided heart catheterization) provides a means of directly assessing

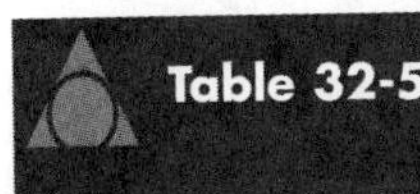

Table 32-5 Therapeutic Management: Chronic Congestive Heart Failure

Diagnostic
- Health history and physical examination
- Determination of underlying cause
- Serum chemistries, renal profile, liver profile
- Chest x-ray
- ECG
- Exercise-stress testing
- Nuclear imaging studies
- Echocardiogram
- Hemodynamic monitoring
- Cardiac catheterization

Therapeutic
- Treatment of underlying cause
- Oxygen therapy at 2-6 L/min
- Rest
- Digitalis preparations
- Diuretics*
- Vasodilator drugs
  - ACE-inhibitors
  - Nitrates
- Inotropic therapy
  - Amrinone (Inocor)
  - Milrinone (Primacor)
  - Dopamine (Intropin)
  - Dobutamine (Dobutrex)
- Antidysrhythmic agents
- Daily weights
- Sodium-restricted diet

ACE, Angiotensin-converting enzyme; *ECG*, electrocardiogram.
*See Table 32-9.

cardiac function. Determination of preload, afterload, contractility, CO, cardiac index, systemic vascular resistance, and work index can be made and treatment protocols devised for maximizing CO in the individual patient.

The New York Heart Association has developed functional guidelines for classifying people with CHF. The classification is based on the person's tolerance to physical activity (Table 32-6).

THERAPEUTIC AND NURSING MANAGEMENT

ACUTE CONGESTIVE HEART FAILURE AND PULMONARY EDEMA

The goal of therapy is to improve left ventricular function by decreasing intravascular volume, decreasing venous return, decreasing afterload, improving gas exchange and oxygenation, increasing CO, and reducing anxiety. Table 32-4 lists the major components of the therapeutic approach. Many of the measures may be done simultaneously.

Decreasing Intravascular Volume

Decreasing intravascular volume with the use of diuretics improves LV function by reducing venous return to the failing LV. A loop diuretic (e.g., furosemide, bumetanide) is the drug of choice for decreasing volume because it may be

Table 32-6 New York Heart Association Functional Classification of Persons with Congestive Heart Failure

Class 1
No limitation on physical activity; ordinary physical activity not resulting in symptoms

Class 2
Slight limitation on physical activity; no symptoms at rest, but symptoms possible with ordinary physical activity

Class 3
More severe limitations; patient usually comfortable at rest; clinical manifestations with unusual physical activities

Class 4
Inability to carry on any physical activity without producing symptoms; symptoms possible at rest

administered quickly by IV push and its action within the kidney occurs rapidly.

By decreasing venous return to the LV and thereby reducing preload, the overfilled LV contracts more efficiently and CO improves. This measure increases LV function, decreases pulmonary vascular pressures, and improves gas exchange.

IV nitroglycerin (NTG) is a vasodilator used in the treatment of acute and chronic CHF. NTG reduces circulating volume by decreasing preload and also increases coronary artery circulation by dilating the coronary arteries. Therefore NTG reduces preload, slightly reduces afterload (in high doses), and increases myocardial oxygen supply.

Decreasing Venous Return

Decreasing venous return reduces the amount of volume returned to the LV during diastole. This can be accomplished by placing the patient in a high Fowler's position with the feet horizontal in the bed or dangling at the bedside. This position helps decrease venous return because of the pooling of blood in the extremities. This position also increases the thoracic capacity, allowing for improved ventilation.

Decreasing Afterload

Afterload is the amount of wall tension the LV must develop during systole to eject blood into the aorta; that is, it is the amount of work the LV has to produce to eject blood to the systemic circulation. Systemic vascular resistance (SVR) is a determinant of afterload, as is LV filling. If afterload is reduced, the CO of LV improves and thereby decreases pulmonary congestion.

IV nitroprusside (Nipride) is a potent vasodilator that reduces preload and afterload. Because of its potent effects on the vascular system, it is the drug of choice for the patient with pulmonary edema. By reducing both preload and afterload (by arteriolar and venous dilatation), myocardial contraction improves, increasing CO and reducing pulmonary congestion. Complications of IV nitroprusside include hypotension, which may require the use of dobutamine IV to maintain a mean arterial BP greater than or equal to 60 mm Hg and thiocyanate toxicity that can develop after 48 hours of use. Morphine is also a drug that reduces preload and afterload. It dilates both the pulmonary and systemic blood vessels, a goal in decreasing pulmonary pressures and improving the exchange of gases.

Improving Gas Exchange and Oxygenation

Gas exchange may be improved by several measures. IV morphine decreases oxygen demands, which may be raised as a result of anxiety and subsequent increased musculoskeletal and respiratory activity. Administration of oxygen helps increase the percentage of oxygen in inspired air. (Oxygen therapy is discussed in Chapter 24.) In addition, an arterial line may be used to assess arterial pressure and to provide a site for withdrawal of specimens for blood gases. In severe pulmonary edema the patient may need to be intubated and placed on a mechanical ventilator.

Improving Cardiac Function

Digitalis improves LV function by its positive inotropic action. Digitalis increases contractility but also increases myocardial oxygen consumption. Newer inotropic drugs (e.g., dobutamine, amrinone) that increase myocardial contractility without increasing oxygen consumption are more effective. Dobutamine and amrinone also cause increased peripheral vasodilatation. Whatever increase in MVO_2 is induced by these agents is counteracted by subsequent vasodilatation. However, these drugs are potent vasoactive substances requiring close observation and monitoring of the patient.

Hemodynamic monitoring may become necessary if rapid resolution of symptoms does not occur with diuretics, morphine, and NTG or if the patient becomes hypotensive. Once a pulmonary artery catheter is in position, accurate measurement of PCWP may be made and effective therapy accomplished to maximize CO. A PCWP of 14 to 18 mm Hg will generally achieve the goal of increasing CO. BP control can also be maintained with other drugs if needed (see Chapter 30).

Reducing Anxiety

Reduction of anxiety is facilitated by the sedative action of morphine administered IV. When morphine is used, the patient must be watched closely for respiratory depression. In addition, a calm approach in providing care helps reduce anxiety.

Once the patient is more stable, determination of the cause of pulmonary edema is important. Diagnosis of systolic or diastolic failure will then determine further management protocols. Aggressive pharmacologic therapy may continue with IV forms of inotropic drugs, vasodilators, and ACE inhibitors. Nursing care focuses on continual physical assessment, hemodynamic monitoring, and monitoring the patient's response to treatment.

Therapeutic Management of Chronic Congestive Heart Failure (see Table 32-5)

One of the most important goals in the treatment of CHF is to treat the underlying cause. If dysrhythmias have precipitated the failure, they should be treated accordingly (see Chapter 33). If the underlying cause is hypertension, antihypertensives should be used in treatment (see Chapter 30). Valvular defects can be treated with surgery. If the cardiac dysfunction is a result of ischemic heart disease, specific interventions such as thrombolytic therapy and percutaneous transluminal coronary angiography (PTCA) or coronary artery bypass surgery may be warranted.

In a person with CHF, oxygen saturation of the blood is reduced because the blood is not adequately oxygenated in the lungs. Administration of oxygen improves saturation and assists greatly in meeting tissue oxygen needs. Thus oxygen therapy helps relieve dyspnea and fatigue. Optimally either arterial blood gases (ABGs) or pulse oximetry is used to monitor the effectiveness of oxygen therapy (see Chapter 24).

Physical and emotional rest allows the patient to conserve energy and decreases the need for additional oxygen. The degree of rest recommended depends on the severity of heart failure. A patient with severe CHF must be on bed rest with limited activity. A patient with mild CHF can be ambulatory with a restriction of strenuous activity. The patient should be instructed to participate in group activities with adequate recovery periods in between.

Pharmacologic Management of Chronic Congestive Heart Failure

General therapeutic objectives for pharmacologic management of CHF include (1) the identification of the type of CHF and underlying causes, (2) the correction of sodium and water retention and volume overload, (3) the reduction of cardiac work load, (4) the improvement of myocardial contractility, and (5) the control of precipitating and complicating factors.[12] Because CHF is a complex syndrome, it is unlikely that any single pharmacologic agent would be successful alone. A combination of drugs that meet the preceding objectives has been most successful in treating the patient with CHF.

Historically, LV systolic failure has been managed with positive inotropic agents (e.g., digitalis) to increase myocardial contractility and diuretic therapy to enhance sodium and water excretion, thereby controlling volume. LV volume overload (increased preload and afterload) exerts a major role in the development of LV dysfunction and has led to the addition of vasodilators in the treatment plan.[13,14]

Positive Inotropic Agents. The use of positive inotropic agents in the patient with CHF is directed at improving cardiac contractility to increase CO, decrease LV diastolic pressure, and decrease systemic vascular resistance. The types of positive inotropic agents are listed in Table 32-7.

Digitalis preparations. Digitalis preparations (cardiac glycosides) have been the mainstay in the treatment of CHF and have been used for more than 200 years. Currently,

Table 32-7 Positive Inotropic Agents Used To Treat Congestive Heart Failure

Sodium-potassium-ATPase inhibitors
Digitalis (Lanoxin)
β-Adrenergic agonists
Dopamine (Intropin)
Dobutamine (Dobutrex)
Phosphodiesterase inhibitors
Aminrone (Inocor)
Milrinone (Primacor)

digitalis is the only oral inotropic agent approved by the Food and Drug Administration (FDA) for use in the treatment of CHF. However, the use of digitalis preparations has recently become controversial, and they are now being used more judiciously. They are particularly useful in the treatment of heart failure accompanied by atrial flutter, fibrillation, and a rapid ventricular rate. Digitalis preparations increase the force or strength of cardiac contraction (inotropic action). They also decrease the conduction speed within the myocardium and slow the HR (chronotropic action). This action allows for more complete emptying of the ventricles, thus diminishing the volume remaining in the ventricles during diastole. CO increases because of an increased stroke volume (SV) from improved contractility.

With digitalis preparations, a digitalizing dose much higher than the maintenance dose is given to achieve adequate blood levels rapidly. The maintenance dosage varies from person to person.

The range between therapeutic and toxic effects is narrow and can be affected by other drugs (e.g., verapamil, aminoglycosides, anticholinergics) or concurrent disease processes (e.g., diabetic ketoacidosis, electrolyte imbalances). Monitoring the blood levels of digoxin is critical. The normal serum therapeutic range for digoxin is 1 to 2 ng/ml.

An individual receiving digitalis preparations is subject to digitalis toxicity (Table 32-8). Some of the earliest symptoms of toxicity are anorexia, nausea, and vomiting. Dysrhythmias are a common indication of digitalis toxicity. Although almost any dysrhythmia can occur, the types most frequently found are premature beats, atrial fibrillation, and first-degree heart block.

Hypokalemia is one of the most common causes of digitalis toxicity resulting in dysrhythmias because low serum potassium levels enhance ectopic pacemaker activity. Monitoring the serum potassium levels of patients receiving both digitalis preparations and potassium-losing diuretics (e.g., thiazides, loop diuretics) is essential. Other electrolyte imbalances, such as hypercalcemia and hypomagnesemia, can also precipitate toxicity.

Diseases of the kidney and liver increase the susceptibility to digitalis toxicity because most of the preparations are metabolized and eliminated by these organs. An older adult is especially prone to digitalis toxicity because digitalis accumulation occurs sooner with decreased liver and kidney function and slowed body metabolism, which occur with aging.

Table 32-8 Manifestations of Digitalis Toxicity

Cardiovascular System
Bradycardia; tachycardia; pulse deficit; dysrhythmias, including premature ventricular contractions, first-degree atrioventricular blocks, atrial fibrillation
Gastrointestinal System
Anorexia, nausea, vomiting, diarrhea, abdominal pain
Neurologic System
Headache, drowsiness, confusion, insomnia, muscle weakness
Visual System
Double vision, blurred vision, colored vision (usually green or yellow), visual halos

The usual treatment of toxicity consists of withholding the drug until the symptoms subside. In the case of life-threatening toxicity, digoxin immune Fab (ovine [Digibind]) is an antidote that can be given. The treatment of life-threatening dysrhythmias is instituted as needed (see Chapter 33).

β-Adrenergic agents. β-Adrenergic agonists include dopamine (Intropin), dobutamine (Dobutrex), epinephrine, and norepinephrine (Levophed). Stimulation of β-receptors results in an increase in cAMP within the myocardial cells and an increase in contractility. The β-adrenergic agents are typically used as a short-term treatment of acute exacerbations of CHF in the intensive care unit (ICU). Their role in long-term therapy of CHF is controversial. Potential problems related to long-term treatment with β-agonists include tolerance, increased ventricular irritability, and increased MVO_2.

Phosphodiesterase inhibitors. Inhibition of phosphodiesterase increases cyclic adenosine monophosphate (cAMP), which enhances calcium entry into the cell and improves myocardial contractility. Phosphodiesterase inhibitors are also potent vasodilators. They increase CO and reduce arterial pressure (decreased afterload). These drugs are not currently available in oral form; therefore they are limited to short-term use in the critical care setting.[15]

Aminrone (Inocor) strengthens myocardial contraction, increases CO, promotes peripheral vasodilatation, and decreases SVR, thus augmenting performance of the LV. Adverse reactions include dysrhythmias, thrombocytopenia, and GI effects. Because of aminrone's strong vasodilatory effect, hypotension may occur.

Milrinone (Primacor) is a newer phosphodiesterase inhibitor and appears to be more potent than aminrone (Inocor), better tolerated, and with fewer side effects (especially thrombocytopenia). Although milrinone has a direct positive inotropic effect, the improvement in cardiac function is probably a result of a combination of beneficial changes in preload and afterload, as well as inotropic effects.[15]

In summary, inotropic agents are clearly beneficial when used in the short term. However, controversy exists about their long-term role in the treatment of CHF. Although inotropic agents improve hemodynamic function and exercise tolerance, other effects may be harmful. Considerations to be weighed in the treatment of CHF patients include the potential to increase MVO_2, which can induce myocardial ischemia, exacerbate or stimulate dysrhythmias, and cause more rapid deterioration of muscle function.

Diuretics. Diuretics are used in heart failure to mobilize edematous fluid, reduce pulmonary venous pressure, and reduce preload (Table 32-9). If excess extracellular fluid is excreted, blood volume returning to the heart can be reduced and cardiac function improved.

Diuretics act on the kidney by promoting excretion of sodium and water. Many varieties of diuretics are available, and some have specific indications for use. Thiazide diuretics are usually the first choice in chronic CHF because of their convenience, safety, low cost, and effectiveness. They are particularly useful in treating edema secondary to CHF and in controlling hypertension. The thiazides inhibit sodium reabsorption in the distal tubule, thus promoting excretion of sodium and water.

Three potent diuretics, all classified as loop diuretics, are furosemide (Lasix), ethacrynic acid (Edecrin), and bumetanide (Bumex). These drugs act on the ascending loop of Henle to promote sodium, chloride, and water excretion. Furosemide is more commonly used in acute CHF and pulmonary edema because it is slightly more predictable in its response. Bumetanide is a short-acting diuretic with a rapid onset and a half-life of 1 to 1.5 hours. It is used when furosemide has not produced diuresis or when a patient is allergic to furosemide. Problems in using bumetadine include reduction in serum potassium levels, ototoxicity, and possible allergic reaction in the patient who is sensitive to sulfa-type drugs.

Spironolactone (Aldactone) and triamterene (Dyrenium) are potassium-sparing diuretics that promote sodium and water excretion but block potassium excretion. A combination of diuretics may be administered for maximum potential (see Table 32-9).

Because there are numerous effective diuretic agents available, the choice is usually based on whether the CHF is chronic or acute, on the degree or severity of symptoms, or on special needs caused by renal insufficiency or electrolyte abnormalities.

Vasodilator Drugs. Vasodilator drugs are the only class of drugs clearly shown to improve survival in overt heart failure. The goals of vasodilator therapy in the treatment of CHF include (1) increasing venous capacity, (2) improving ejection fraction through improved ventricular contraction, (3) slowing the process of ventricular

Table 32-9 Diuretic Therapy Used in Congestive Heart Failure*

Drugs	Mechanism of Action	Side Effects and Adverse Effects
Thiazides		
Chlorothiazide (Diuril) Hydrochlorothiazide (HydroDiuril, Oretic, Esidrix) Chlorthelidone (Hygroton) Indapamide (Lozol) Metolazone (Zaroxolyn)	Increase in sodium, chloride, and water excretion by inhibiting reabsorption of sodium and chloride in the distal tubule; excretion of potassium in conjunction with sodium	Hypokalemia, increased uric acid, hypercalcemia, hyperglycemia, dermatologic reactions
Loop Diuretics		
Furosemide (Lasix) Ethacrynic acid (Edecrin) Bumetanide (Bumex)	Potent diuretics that increase urine output by preventing sodium, chloride, and water reabsorption in the loop of Henle and distal tubule	Hypokalemia, hyperglycemia, hyperuricemia
Potassium-sparing Agents		
Spironolactone (Aldactone)	Inhibition of action of aldosterone in distal tubule; increased sodium excretion and potassium retention	Hyperkalemia, gynecomastia, amenorrhea, GI disturbances
Triamterene (Dyrenium)	Unknown mechanism of action; action on distal tubule to cause sodium excretion and potassium retention	Hyperkalemia, nausea and vomiting, leg cramps
Combination Agents		
Aldactazide (spironolactone and hydrochlorothiazide)	More potent diuretic effect than single agents alone	GI disturbances, dizziness, dry mouth, avoidance of hypokalemia possible
Dyazide (triamterene and hydrochlorothiazide)	Potassium-sparing effects	Same as above

GI, Gastrointestinal.
*For more information on diuretic therapy, see Table 30-7.

dysfunction, (4) decreasing heart size, and (5) avoiding stimulation of the neurohormonal responses initiated by the compensatory mechanisms of CHF.[16]

The beneficial effects of vasodilators in patients with severe CHF were first identified using sodium nitroprusside, which promotes both venous and arterial dilatation. Dramatic increases in CO and decreases in LV filling pressures were demonstrated following infusions, even in the patient whose LV failure was premorbid. Currently, vasodilators frequently are so beneficial in improving forward flow that mean systolic BP is not significantly reduced.[17] Vasodilators have been shown to produce favorable early hemodynamic effects, increased exercise tolerance, improved LV function, and beneficial effects on survival rates. Vasodilators include drugs that act primarily on the venous capacitance vessels, those that act primarily on the arteries, and some that possess a balanced effect.

Sodium nitroprusside. Nitroprusside is the most commonly used IV vasodilator in the management of acute CHF and pulmonary edema (see earlier in this chapter).

Nitrates. Nitrates cause vasodilatation by acting directly on the smooth muscle of the vessel wall. Their effects primarily involve increasing venous capacitance, dilating the pulmonary vasculature, and improving arterial compliance. Therefore the major hemodynamic effect of nitrates is to decrease preload. Nitrates are of particular benefit in the management of myocardial ischemia related to CHF because they promote vasodilatation of the coronary arteries.

Nitrates may activate reflex stimulation of the neurohormonal response and stimulate renin-angiotensin secretion. For these reasons, in the context of CHF, the action of nitrates may be enhanced by the administration of ACE inhibitors.[17] One specific deterrent to the use of nitrates in CHF is nitrate tolerance. This loss of pharmacologic activity may be caused by the activation of endogenous neurohormonal mechanisms. Frequent dosing with drug-free periods may help reduce this effect.

ACE inhibitors. ACE inhibitors have become the vasodilator of choice in the patient with mild to severe CHF. The conversion of angiotensin I to the potent vasodilator angiotensin II requires the presence of ACE. ACE inhibitors such as captopril (Capoten), enalapril (Vasotec), and lisinopril (Prinivil, Zestril) exert their effects through blocking ACE, resulting in decreased levels of angiotensin II. Plasma aldosterone levels are also reduced.[11]

Because CO is dependent on afterload in chronic CHF, the reduction in SVR seen with the use of ACE inhibitors produces a significant increase in CO. Furthermore, with the use of ACE inhibitors, although BP may be decreased, tissue perfusion is maintained or is increased as a result of improvement of CO and redistribution of regional blood flow. Other hemodynamic changes include a reduction in (1) pulmonary artery pressure, (2) right arterial pressure, and (3) left ventricular filling pressure.[14]

Activation of the sympathetic nervous system is augmented by the renin-angiotensin system, so treatment of CHF with an ACE inhibitor reduces norepinephrine levels and the effects of this potent catecholamine. Beneficial consequences of this decrease in sympathetic activity include (1) a reduction in ventricular wall stress (decreased afterload and work load of the LV), (2) decrease in ventricular dysrhythmias, and (3) increased vagal tone (decreased HR).[14]

Most vasodilators, with the exception of ACE inhibitors, activate the neurohormonal system. ACE inhibitors, especially captopril and enalapril, result in substantial hemodynamic and clinical improvement in the patient with heart failure. In addition, the use of ACE inhibitors is recommended not only in the patient with symptoms, but also in the patient with early LV dysfunction without overt symptoms.[14]

The differences between the three major ACE inhibitors—captopril, enalapril, and lisinopril—are related to onset and duration of action. Side effects may include symptomatic hypotension, chronic cough, and renal insufficiency (in high doses). Aging and baseline renal insufficiency slow the metabolism of ACE inhibitors and may therefore lead to increased serum drug levels.[11] It is recommended that these drugs be started at the lowest dose and that BP and renal function be monitored at regular intervals. Overall, ACE inhibitors are well tolerated by patients.[16]

Nutritional Management of Chronic Congestive Heart Failure

Diet education and weight management are critical to the patient's control of chronic CHF. The nurse or dietitian should obtain a detailed diet history, determining not only what foods the patient eats and when but also the sociocultural value of food. The nurse can use this data base to assist the patient in solving problems and developing an individual diet plan. The patient should be taught what foods are low and high in sodium and ways to enhance food flavors without the use of salt (e.g., substituting lemon juice and various spices).

The edema of chronic CHF is often treated by dietary restriction of sodium. The degree of sodium restriction depends on the severity of the heart failure and the effectiveness of diuretic therapy. Diets that are severely restricted in sodium are rarely prescribed because they are unpalatable and patient compliance is low.

The normal daily dietary intake of sodium ranges from 3 to 7 g. A commonly prescribed diet for a patient with mild CHF is a 2 g sodium diet (Table 32-10). All foods high in sodium should be eliminated (Table 32-11). For more severe CHF, sodium intake is restricted to 500 to 1000 mg. On this diet, milk, cheese, bread, cereals, canned soups, and some canned vegetables must be eliminated.

Fluid restrictions are not commonly prescribed for the patient with mild to moderate CHF. Diuretic therapy and digitalis preparations act as effective diuretics to promote fluid excretion. However, in moderate to severe CHF, fluid restrictions are usually implemented.

The patient and family need to be told which foods are high in sodium (see Table 32-11). Salt substitutes frequently contain potassium, and their use should be approved by the physician. The patient must be instructed on how to read labels to look for sodium as an ingredient.

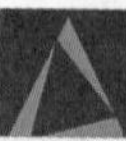

Table 32-10 Nutritional Management: Low-Sodium Diets

General Principles

Do not add salt or seasonings containing sodium when preparing foods.
Do not use salt at the table.
Avoid high-sodium foods.*
Limit milk products to 2 cups daily.

Sample Menu Plans for 2 g Sodium Diet*

Breakfast		
1 cup low-fat or skim milk ¾ cup puffed wheat Sugar Toast 1 tsp. margarine Scrambled egg substitute Coffee	½ cup low-fat or skim milk ½ cup cream of wheat Sugar Tortilla Coffee	½ cup low-fat or skim milk ½ cup grits Boiled egg 1 tsp butter 1 biscuit made with low-sodium baking powder Coffee
Lunch		
½ cup chicken salad sandwich with 1 tsp mayonnaise Fresh fruit 1 cup low-fat or skim milk Iced tea	½ cup pinto beans ½ cup chili with meat Tossed salad with oil and vinegar Tortilla ½ cup gelatin dessert Coffee	2 oz baked fish Carrots Roll and 1 tsp butter Canned fruit Coffee
Dinner		
3 oz roast beef 1 baked potato 2 tsp sour cream 1 tsp margarine ½ cup green beans 1 dinner roll ½ cup sherbet Coffee	3 oz broiled fish ½ cup fried potatoes ½ cup zucchini or corn 1 cup chocolate pudding Bread and 1 tsp margarine Coffee	3 oz baked chicken ½ cup boiled potatoes ½ cup greens cooked without salt pork 1 cup ice cream Sugar cookies Coffee

Modifications for Other Low-Sodium Diets

500 mg sodium diet
Restrict milk products to 1 cup daily.
Limit meat to 4 oz daily.
Use salt-free butter, bread, vegetables, and starches.

1000 mg sodium diet
Restrict milk products to 1 cup daily.
Use salt-free butter and vegetables.

4 g sodium diet
Allow cooking with small amounts of salt.
Allow 3 cups milk products daily.

*See Table 32-11.

When weight reduction is indicated to decrease the cardiac work load, the nurse and dietitian can assist the patient and family in menu planning. Instructing patients to weigh themselves daily is important for monitoring fluid retention, as well as weight reduction. Patients should be instructed to weigh themselves at the same time each day, preferably before breakfast, while wearing the same type of clothing. This helps ensure valid comparisons from day to day and helps identify early signs of fluid retention.

NURSING MANAGEMENT

CHRONIC CONGESTIVE HEART FAILURE

Nursing Assessment

Subjective and objective data that should be obtained from a patient with CHF include those presented in Table 32-12.

Nursing Diagnoses

Nursing diagnoses are determined when the problem and etiologic factors are supported by clinical data. Nursing diagnoses specific to the patient with CHF include, but are not limited to, those presented in the nursing care plan on p. 946.

Planning

The overall goals are that the patient with CHF will have (1) decreased peripheral edema, (2) decreased shortness of breath, (3) increased exercise tolerance, (4) compliance with medications prescribed, and (5) no complications related to CHF.

Nursing Implementation

Health Promotion and Maintenance. An important measure used to prevent heart failure is the treatment or

Table 32-11 High-Sodium Foods

Beverages	Mineral water, club soda, Dutch-processed cocoa
Breads	Saltines, baking powder biscuits, muffins, Bisquick, pretzels, salted snack crackers and chips; quick breads such as cornbread, nut bread; pancakes, waffles (including mixes)
Cereals	Instant cooked cereal, processed bran cereal, commercial granola
Dairy	Commercial buttermilk, regular cheese
Desserts	Commercial baked products, baked products and puddings made from mixes
Fats	Bacon fat, salted nuts or seeds, commercial dips (e.g., containing sour cream), regular salad dressings, mayonnaise
Juices	Tomato juice, V-8 juice, Clamato, Bloody Mary mixes
Meat	Smoked or cured products: bacon, ham, sausage, salt pork, hot dogs, lunch meat, corned or chipped beef, organ meats, shellfish, sardines, herring, anchovies, caviar, kosher meats, canned tuna fish and salmon, mackerel
Potato or substitute	Salted potato chips, salted french fries, instant potatoes, rice, noodle mixes
Seasonings	Salt, excessive amounts of baking powder, baking soda; celery, onion, and garlic salt and other seasoned salt and peppers; meat tenderizers, AćCent, MSG, worcestershire, soy sauce, mustard, catsup, horseradish, chili sauce, tomato sauce, barbeque sauce, steak sauce
Soup	Commercial soups, bouillon cubes, powdered dehydrated soups
Vegetables	Sauerkraut, tomato juice, V-8 juice, vegetables in creamed or seasoned sauces, frozen vegetables processed with salt or sodium
Miscellaneous	Olives; pickles; salted popcorn; commercially prepared, frozen, or canned entrees (e.g., pot pies, TV dinners); Mexican, Italian, Oriental dishes as ordinarily prepared

Table 32-12 Nursing Assessment: Congestive Heart Failure

Subjective Data

Important health information

Past health history: CAD (including recent MI), hypertension, cardiomyopathy, valvular or congenital heart disease, thyroid or lung disease, rapid or irregular heartbeat

Medications: Use of and compliance with any cardiac medications; use of diuretics, estrogens, corticosteroids, phenylbutazone, NSAIDs

Functional health patterns

Health perception–health management: Fatigue

Nutritional-metabolic: Nausea, vomiting, anorexia; sodium intake; weight gain

Elimination: Nocturia, decreased daytime urinary output

Activity-exercise: Dyspnea, orthopnea, cough; palpitations; dizziness, syncope

Sleep-rest: Number of pillows used for sleeping; paroxysmal nocturnal dyspnea

Cognitive-perceptual: Behavioral changes; chest pain or heaviness

Objective Data

Integumentary

Cool, diaphoretic skin; cyanosis or pallor, edema

Respiratory

Tachypnea, crackles, rhonchi, wheezes; frothy, blood-tinged sputum

Cardiovascular

Tachycardia, S_3, S_4, distended neck veins; peripheral edema (right-sided heart failure)

Gastrointestinal

Abdominal distention, hepatosplenomegaly, ascites, RUQ pain, discomfort, guaiac-positive stools

Neurologic

Restlessness, confusion, decreased attention or memory

Possible findings

Altered serum electrolytes (especially Na^+ and K^+), elevated BUN, creatinine, or liver function tests; chest x-ray demonstrating cardiomegaly, pulmonary congestion, and interstitial pulmonary edema; echocardiogram showing increased chamber size and decreased wall motion

ECG: atrial and ventricular enlargement

Hemodynamic findings: ↑ PAP, ↑ PCWP, ↓ CO, ↓ CI, ↓ O_2 saturation, ↑ SVR

BUN, Blood urea nitrogen; *CAD,* coronary artery disease; *CI,* cardiac index; *CO,* cardiac output; *ECG,* electrocardiogram; *MI,* myocardial infarction *NSAIDs:* nonsteroidal antiinflamatory drugs; *PAP,* pulmonary artery pressure; *PCWP,* pulmonary capillary wedge pressure; *RUQ,* right upper quadrant; *SVR,* systemic vascular resistance.

control of the underlying heart disease.[18] For example, in rheumatic valvular disease, valve replacement should be planned before lung congestion develops. Prophylactic antibiotics should be given to people with a known history of rheumatic heart disease when they undergo surgery or procedures involving instrumentation (e.g., cystoscopy, tooth extraction, and tooth cleaning).

NURSING CARE PLAN Patient with Congestive Heart Failure

Planning: Outcome Criteria	Nursing Interventions and Rationales
➤ **NURSING DIAGNOSIS**	Activity intolerance *related to* fatigue secondary to cardiac insufficiency, pulmonary congestion, and inadequate nutrition *as manifested by* dyspnea, shortness of breath, weakness, fatigue, increase or decrease in pulse on exertion, anorexia
Tolerate activity; have needs met to satisfaction.	Have patient rest in bed or chair when tired *to reduce cardiac work.* Provide emotional and physical rest *to reduce oxygen consumption and to relieve dyspnea and fatigue.* If patient is in bed, teach leg exercises *to prevent phlebothrombosis.* Assess patient daily for dyspnea, fatigue, and pulse rate *to determine level of activity that can be performed.* Provide frequent small feedings instead of three large meals a day *because increased CO is needed for digestion.* Teach patient about expenditure of energy on various activities *to promote self-monitoring of appropriate activities.*
➤ **NURSING DIAGNOSIS**	Sleep pattern disturbance *related to* nocturnal dyspnea, inability to assume favored sleep position, and nocturia *as manifested by* inability to sleep through night
Feel rested after sleep.	Explain etiology of nocturnal dyspnea *to reduce fear caused by waking up in acute dyspneic state.* Explore with patient alternative positions of comfort such as sleeping with two or more pillows *to relieve dyspnea.* Have patient take diuretics early in the day *to decrease urination during the night.*
➤ **NURSING DIAGNOSIS**	Fluid volume excess *related to* pump failure *as manifested by* edema, dyspnea on exertion, shortness of breath
Have reduced or absence of edema.	Evaluate degree of peripheral edema and measure abdominal girth daily *to provide data on patient's response to treatment.* Administer digitalis agents *to improve CO by improving contractility* and diuretics *to mobilize edematous fluid.* Assess intake and output q8hr *to monitor fluid balance.* Weigh patient daily *to monitor fluid retention and weight reduction.* Observe manifestations of hypokalemia because *hypokalemia sensitizes the myocardium to digitalis.* Provide sodium-restricted diet as ordered *to minimize further fluid retention.*
➤ **NURSING DIAGNOSIS**	Risk for impaired skin integrity *related to* edema or immobility
Have no breakdown of skin at edematous areas.	Monitor signs of edema, such as taut, shiny skin, sacral edema in bedfast patient, pitting edema, or dependent edema *to identify location and severity of edema.* Handle edematous skin gently *because tissue is painful and fragile.* Pad bony prominences *to reduce pressure and subsequent skin breakdown.* Assess edematous areas every shift for skin breakdown *because these areas have increased susceptibility to breakdown.* Perform passive ROM to extremities q4hr *to facilitate venous return of the fluid.* Turn and reposition q2hr *to prevent skin breakdown.*
➤ **NURSING DIAGNOSIS**	Impaired gas exchange *related to* increased preload, mechanical failure, or immobility *as manifested by* increased respiratory rate, shortness of breath, dyspnea on exertion
Have respiratory rate of 12-18/min.	Elevate head of bed to Fowler's position *to improve ventilation by decreasing venous return to the heart and increasing thoracic expansion.* Support patient's arms with pillows *to move arms off and away from chest to facilitate breathing.* Use footboard *to give patient a surface to press feet against to improve circulation through muscle contraction.* Administer oxygen by nasal cannula *to improve oxygen saturation, assist in meeting tissue oxygen needs, relieve dyspnea and fatigue.* Auscultate for lung and heart sounds q4hr *to evaluate patient's response to treatments.* Use pulse oximetry *to monitor oxygenation status.*

continued

NURSING CARE PLAN Patient with Congestive Heart Failure—cont'd

Planning: Outcome Criteria	*Nursing Interventions and Rationales*
➤ **NURSING DIAGNOSIS**	Anxiety *related to* dyspnea or perceived threat of death *as manifested by* restlessness, irritability, expression of feelings of life threat
Express feeling less apprehensive about condition and prognosis.	Assess facial expression and behavior for feeling of apprehension *to allow for early identification and treatment of anxiety.* Allow patient to ask questions *to relieve some anxiety by having accurate information.* Answer call light promptly and explain all procedures *to promote sense of security.* Demonstrate calm behavior with patient *to increase confidence in caregiver and relieve anxiety.* Use measures to decrease dyspnea (e.g., rest, elevation of head of bed) *to reduce anxiety and improve breathing.*
➤ **NURSING DIAGNOSIS**	Ineffective individual coping *related to* alterations in lifestyle, possible inability to use past coping methods, or perceived loss of control *as manifested by* use of ineffective coping behaviors such as shouting, blaming, anger, withdrawal, social isolation, increased dependency
Express satisfaction with self-participation in care; use positive coping strategies.	Teach patient about disease process and altered physiologic function *because increased understanding strengthens most patients' ability to cope.* Encourage patient to adopt lifestyle compatible with degree of heart impairment *to prevent worsening of heart failure or becoming a "cardiac cripple."* Assist patient and family in planning necessary changes *to facilitate long-term management.* Encourage the patient who seems discouraged or hopeless to plan and participate in own plan of care *to instill hope.* Question patient regarding concerns *to demonstrate attention to patient's priorities.* Support positive coping strategies *to build on patient's strengths.* Suggest alternate strategies *to replace ineffective ones.*
➤ **NURSING DIAGNOSIS**	Self-care deficit (total) *related to* dyspnea and fatigue *as manifested by* inability to perform part or all of ADLs
Achieve ADLs with assistance as necessary from health care provider.	Assist patient with all ADLs as needed *to meet patient needs and to relieve anxiety.* Assure patient of your willingness to assist with personal care *to allay fears of insecurity and embarrassment.* Advise family of patient's fluctuating abilities regarding self-care activities *to reduce family frustration regarding varying needs of patient.*
➤ **NURSING DIAGNOSIS**	Ineffective management of therapeutic regimen *related to* lack of knowledge regarding signs and symptoms of CHF, proper diet, and medications *as manifested by* lack of adherence to low-sodium diet and questioning of disease, diet, and medications
Express confidence regarding knowledge of disease process and dietary and medication regimen.	Teach patient manifestations to report, including shortness of breath at rest; swelling of ankles, feet, or abdomen; loss of appetite, nausea, or vomiting; weight gain of 1 to 2 kg in a 2-day period; frequent urination; persistent cough; changes in HR ± 20 bpm difference from usual *so patient will know signs and symptoms of worsening CHF.* Instruct patient on dietary restrictions (e.g., low-sodium diet, possible weight reduction) and medication regimen *to ensure adequate nutritional intake and that correct medications are taken.*

ADLs, Activities of daily living; *bpm,* beats per minute; *CHF,* congestive heart failure; *CO,* cardiac output; *HR,* heart rate; *ROM,* range-of-motion.

Another important preventive measure concerns early and continued treatment of hypertension. Hyperlipidemic states in persons with CAD should be managed with diet, exercise, and medication. The use of antidysrhythmic agents or pacemakers is indicated for people with serious dysrhythmias or conduction disturbances. When a patient is diagnosed with CHF, preventive care should focus on slowing the progression of the disease. Knowledge of the importance of following the medication, diet, and exercise regimens is paramount. The in-hospital nurse may request home care for the patient and family to provide for follow-up of care and to monitor the patient's response to treatment. Early detection of signs and symptoms of worsening failure may help modify care and prevent an acute episode requiring further hospitalization.

Acute Intervention. Many persons with CHF do not experience an acute episode. If they do, they are usually initially managed in a critical care unit and later transferred to a general unit when their condition has stabilized. The nursing care plan for the patient with CHF applies to the patient with stabilized acute or chronic CHF.

Chronic and Home Management. CHF is a chronic illness for most persons. Important nursing responsibilities are (1) educating the patient about the physiologic changes that have occurred and (2) assisting the patient to adapt to both the physiologic and psychologic changes. It must be emphasized to the patient that it is possible to live productively with this health problem. Home health care is a vital factor in preventing future hospitalization for this patient. Home nursing care will follow-up with ongoing clinical assessments, monitoring vital signs, and response to therapies. Managing these patients out of the hospital is a priority of care.

Patients with CHF are usually required to take medication for the rest of their lives. This often becomes difficult because a patient may be asymptomatic when CHF is under control. It must be stressed that the disease is chronic and that medication must be continued to keep the heart failure under control. The patient must understand the importance of maintaining adequate drug levels, as well as the danger of omitting or making up missed doses. In some situations, it is helpful to work out a system that helps the patient to remember to take the medication.

The patient should evaluate the action of the prescribed medication. The patient should be taught to recognize the manifestations of digitalis toxicity (see Table 32-8). The patient should also be taught how to take the pulse rate and to know under what circumstances drugs, especially digitalis preparations, should be withheld and a physician consulted. The pulse rate should always be taken for a full minute. A pulse rate lower than 50 to 60 beats per minute (bpm) may be a contraindication to taking a digitalis preparation unless specified otherwise by the physician. A slow pulse rate may indicate a need to alter the digitalis therapy. However, in the absence of primary heart block or the development of ventricular ectopy, a pulse rate of 60 bpm or less is not a contraindication to taking digitalis. A pulse rate of 50 bpm (especially in a patient who is also taking β-blocking drugs) may be acceptable.

The patient should also be taught the symptoms of hypokalemia if diuretics that cause potassium excretion are being taken. (Manifestations of hypokalemia are discussed in Chapter 13.) Hypokalemia sensitizes the myocardium to digitalis. Consequently, toxicity may develop from an ordinary dose of digitalis. Frequently the patient who is taking thiazide or loop diuretics is given supplemental potassium.

The nurse, physical therapist, or occupational therapist can instruct the patient in energy-saving and energy-efficient behaviors after an evaluation of daily activities has been done. For example, once the nurse understands the patient's daily routine, suggestions can be made for simplification of work or modification of an activity. Frequently the patient needs a prescription for rest after an activity. Many hard-driving persons need that "permission" to not feel "lazy." Sometimes an activity that the patient enjoys may need to be eliminated. In such situations the patient should be helped to explore alternative activities that cause less physical and cardiac stress. The physical environment may require modification in situations in which there is an increased cardiac work load demand (e.g., frequent climbing of stairs, inaccessibility to shopping areas). The nurse can help the patient identify areas where outside assistance can be obtained.

The nurse is also responsible for encouraging a patient who is discouraged and for motivating a patient who feels that the situation is unmanageable. This may require that the nurse assist the patient and family in making lifestyle changes that they can accept and follow. Often the nurse can begin this process by establishing small, achievable goals with the patient. Continuous support by the family and health care providers is important. If the patient does not adhere to the prescribed regimen, it is important to determine the reasons. After this evaluation process, it may be necessary to plan an alternative therapeutic regimen that is more compatible with the patient's lifestyle.

CARDIOMYOPATHY

CMP is a term used to describe a group of heart muscle diseases of unknown cause that primarily affect the structural or functional ability of the myocardium. This primary dysfunction is not associated with CAD, hypertension, valvular disease, vascular disease, or pulmonary disease. The etiology of cardiomyopathy is unknown.[19] Diagnosis of CMP is made by the patient's clinical manifestations and noninvasive and invasive cardiac procedures to rule out other causes of dysfunction. This patient is a particular challenge to the nurse and often has unique management and care needs.

CMPs can be classified as primary or secondary. Primary CMPs are those conditions in which the etiology of the heart disease is unknown. The heart muscle in this instance is the only portion of the heart involved, and other cardiac structures are unaffected. In secondary CMP the cause of the myocardial disease is known and is secondary to another disease process. Common causes of secondary CMP are ischemia, viral infections, alcohol intake, drug abuse, and pregnancy (Table 32-13).

The World Health Organization has classified CMP conditions into three general types: dilated (congestive), hypertrophic, and restrictive (Fig. 32-3).[19,20] Each of these types has its own pathogenesis, clinical presentation, and treatment protocols. All these types of CMP can lead to cardiomegaly and CHF (see Table 32-14 on p. 951).

Dilated Cardiomyopathy

Pathophysiology. *Dilated (congestive) cardiomyopathy* is the most common type of CMP, accounting for greater than 90% of all cases, and is characterized by cardiomegaly with ventricular dilatation, impairment of systolic function, atrial enlargement, and stasis of blood in the LV. Cardiomegaly is the result of primarily ventricular dilatation. Impaired systolic function results in decreased SV and reduced CO. In dilated CMP, a 15% to 20% decrease in ejection fraction is common.[21] Clinical sequence of this impaired systolic function closely resembles the situation in CHF. Because the ejection fraction falls and there is a lower CO, stasis of blood

Table 32-13 Causes of Secondary Cardiomyopathy

Dilated	Hypertrophic	Restrictive
Ischemic Valvular Infectious Pregnancy Metabolic Hypertension Cardiotoxic Alcohol Adriamycin Cobalt Cocaine	Genetic Hypertension Obstructive valvular disease Thyroid disease Glycogen storage disease Friedreich's ataxia Infants of diabetics	Amyloid Endomycardial fibrosis Löffler's disease Sarcoidosis Neoplastic tumor Ventricular thrombus

occurs. What makes this disorder unique from chronic CHF is that the walls of the ventricle do not become hypertrophic. This is thought to be caused by the rapid destruction of cells, leaving the ventricles with little time to develop extra muscle.[20] Deterioration is rapid after the development of symptoms, and as many as 20% to 50% of patients are expected to die within 1 year.

No specific cause has been identified, although dilated CMP often follows an infectious myocarditis. Thyrotoxicosis, diabetes mellitus, toxins (especially alcohol and cocaine), chemotherapeutic agents, nutritional deficiencies, pregnancy, and drugs causing a hypersensitivity reaction have all been associated with the development of dilated CMP. Regardless of the initial cause, it results in a diffuse inflammation and rapid degeneration of myocardial fibers that decrease contractile function.

Clinical Manifestations. The signs and symptoms of dilated CMP develop insidiously. The patient may have signs and symptoms of CHF. These symptoms can include a change in exercise tolerance, fatigue, dry cough, dyspnea, paroxysmal noctural dyspnea, orthopnea, palpitations, and anorexia. Signs can include S_3, S_4, tachycardia, pulmonary crackles, edema, weak peripheral pulses, pallor, hepatomegaly, and jugular venous distention. The patient may also have dysrhythmias or systemic embolization.

Diagnostic Studies. The diagnosis of dilated CMP is made on the basis of the patient's history and by ruling out other conditions that cause CHF. The chest x-ray shows cardiomegaly. Signs of pulmonary venous hypertension may be present, as well as pleural effusion. The ECG may reveal tachycardia and dysrhythmias. Conduction disturbances may also be present because of the stretching of the ventricular septum. Echocardiography is useful in distinguishing dilated CMP from other structural abnormalities. The size of the ventricular chamber can be assessed, the thickness of the heart muscle can be measured, and the valves can be evaluated.

Cardiac catheterization and coronary angiography are used in evaluating the manifestations of dilated CMP. The coronary arteries are usually normal, PCWP is elevated, and left atrial and LV end-diastolic pressures are elevated. Left ventriculogram may reveal abnormal wall motion caused by the dilatation, a thin wall, and dilated ventricles. Endomyocardial biopsy may be done at the time of the right heart catheterization. This rarely provides information significant for treatment, but it may rule out other diagnoses.

THERAPEUTIC AND NURSING MANAGEMENT

DILATED CARDIOMYOPATHY

Interventions focus on controlling CHF by enhancing myocardial contractility and decreasing afterload, similar to the treatment of chronic CHF (Table 32-15). Thus treatment is more palliative than curative. Digitalis is used in the presence of atrial fibrillation, diuretics are used to decrease preload, and vasodilators such as the ACE inhibitors are used to reduce afterload. Pharmacologic treatment, nutritional interventions, and cardiac rehabilitation may help alleviate symptoms of CHF and improve CO. A patient with secondary dilated CMP must be treated for the underlying disease process. For example, the patient with alcohol-induced dilated CMP must abstain from all alcohol intake.

Unfortunately, dilated CMP does not respond well to therapy. Intermittent dobutamine infusions, or "pulse inotropic therapy," is a therapy used in the treatment of dilated cardiomyopathy. The patient is admitted to the hospital for a 72-hour infusion of dobutamine. (Sometimes these infusions are done for an 8-hour period as an outpatient treatment.) After infusion, many patients experience an improvement in symptoms that lasts several weeks after therapy. Other therapy includes administration of antidysrhythmic agents and anticoagulation agents to prevent systemic embolization from mural thrombi that can form in the dilated ventricles. Because the cause of dilated CMP remains unclear, intervention is often unsatisfactory in producing a cure.

The patient with terminal end-stage cardiomyopathy may require cardiac transplantation. Currently approximately 50% of heart transplants are performed for treatment of cardiomyopathic conditions. Cardiac transplant recipients have a good prognosis for survival. However, donor hearts are difficult to obtain, and the surgical procedure is expensive. Many patients with dilated CMP die while awaiting heart transplantation.

Patients with dilated cardiomyopathy are very ill people with a grave prognosis who need expert nursing care. Nursing care should focus on monitoring the response to medications, monitoring for dysrhythmias, and preventing or rapidly detecting systemic emboli. The nurse should also educate the patient about the disease process and assist the patient in spacing daily activities to allow for periods of rest. This patient is in great need of emotional support. Information regarding candidacy for heart transplantation and the grave prognosis must be given honestly and empathically. A survivor of sudden cardiac death must be allowed to talk about the experience and express fears in an

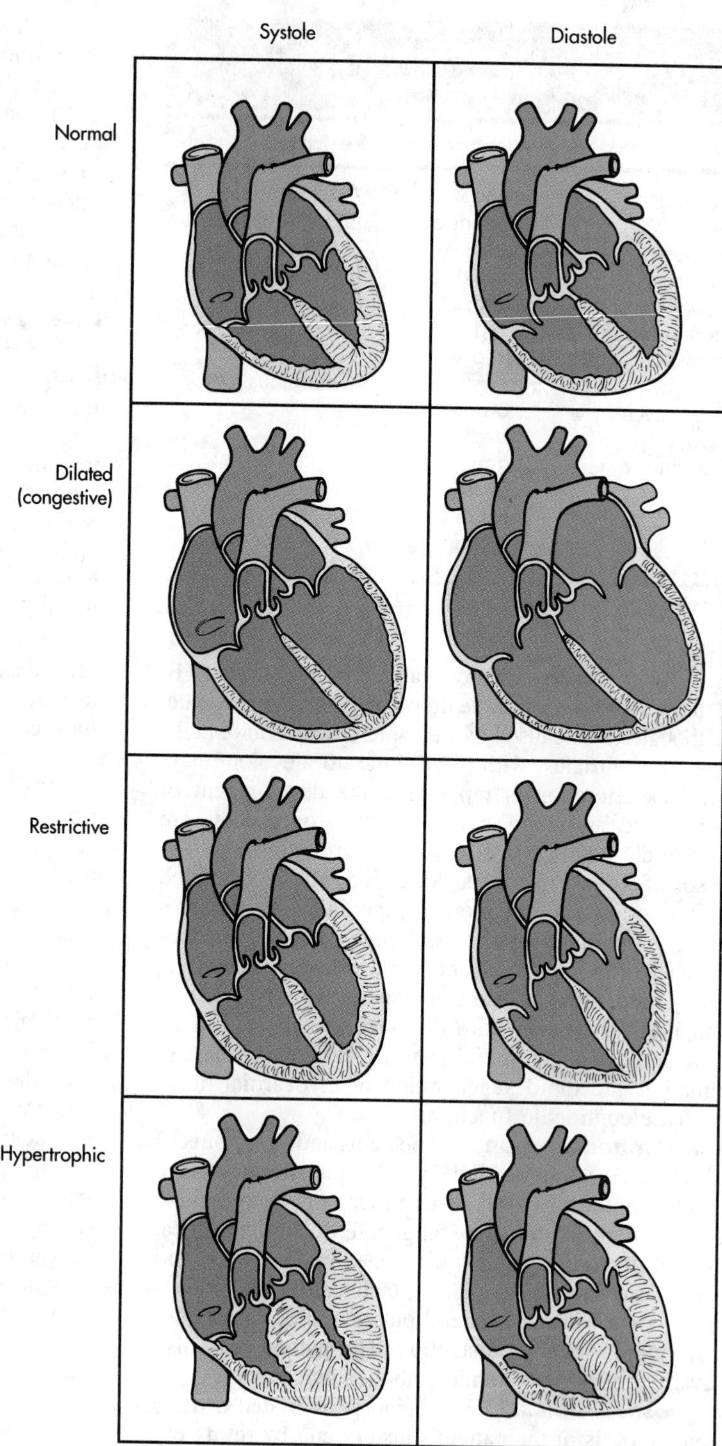

Fig. 32-3 Types of cardiomyopathies.

open atmosphere. The patient's family must learn cardiopulmonary resuscitation (CPR) and how to access emergency care in their neighborhood. The nurse should include family members and other support systems when planning a patient's care.

Home health care nursing can provide this patient and the family with the continuous assessments and therapeutic interventions that are required to maximize and maintain the functional status. Observing for signs and symptoms of worsening failure, dysrhythmias, and embolic formation are paramount in this patient, as well as monitoring drug responsiveness. Because the goal of therapy is to keep the patient functional and out of the hospital, home health nursing is an excellent resource for accomplishing these goals.

Table 32-14 Characteristics of Cardiomyopathies

Dilated	Hypertrophic	Restrictive
Etiology		
Idiopathic condition, alcoholism, pregnancy, myocarditis, nutritional deficiency (vitamin B_1), exposure to toxins and drugs, genetic disease	Inherited disorder (autosomal dominant), possible chronic hypertension	Amyloidosis, postradiation, post-open heart surgery, diabetes
Major Manifestations		
Fatigue, weakness, palpitations, dyspnea, dry cough	Exertional dyspnea, fatigue, angina, syncope, palpitations	Dyspnea, fatigue, palpitations
Cardiomegaly		
Moderate to marked	Mild	Mild to moderate
Contractility		
Decreased	Increased or decreased	Normal or decreased
Valvular Incompetence		
Atrioventricular valves, particularly mitral	Mitral valve	Mitral valve
Dysrhythmias		
Sinoatrial tachycardia, atrial and ventricular dysrhythmias	Tachydysrhythmias	Atrial and ventricular dysrhythmias
Cardiac Output		
Decreased	Decreased	Normal or decreased
Stroke Volume		
Decreased	Normal or increased	Decreased
Ejection Fraction		
Decreased	Increased	Normal or decreased
Outflow Tract Obstruction		
None	Increased	None

Hypertrophic Cardiomyopathy

Pathophysiology. *Hypertrophic cardiomyopathy* (HCM) produces asymmetric myocardial hypertrophy (Fig. 32-4) without ventricular dilatation. It seems to have an autosomal dominant genetic basis. HCM occurs less commonly than dilated CMP and is more common in men than in women.[21] It is usually diagnosed in young adulthood and is often seen in active, athletic individuals. Another name for this disorder is *idiopathic hypertrophic subaortic stenosis* (IHSS).

The four main characteristics of HCM are (1) massive ventricular hypertrophy; (2) rapid, forceful contraction of the LV; (3) impaired relaxation; and (4) obstruction to aortic outflow (not present in all patients). Ventricular hypertrophy is associated with a thickened intraventricular septum and ventricular wall. The end result is impaired ventricular filling as the ventricle becomes noncompliant and unable to relax. The primary defect of HCM is diastolic dysfunction. Impaired ventricular relaxation inhibits adequate filling of the ventricles during diastole. Decreased ventricular filling and obstruction to outflow can result in decreased CO, especially during exertion, when increased CO is needed (see Table 32-14).

Clinical Manifestations. Patient manifestations include exertional dyspnea, fatigue, angina, and syncope. The most common symptom is dyspnea, which is caused by an

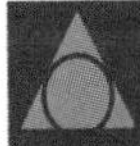

Table 32-15 Therapeutic Management: Cardiomyopathies

Diagnostic
- Health history and physical examination
- ECG
- Chest x-ray
- Echocardiogram
- Nuclear imaging studies
- Cardiac catheterization
- Endocardial biopsy

Therapeutic
- Treatment of underlying cause
- Digitalis (except in hypertrophic CMP in normal sinus rhythm)
- Diuretics
- ACE inhibitors
- Bed rest (if indicated)
- Anticoagulants (if indicated)
- Antidysrhythmics (if indicated)
- β-Adrenergic blocking agents (for hypertrophic CMP)
- Intermittent infusions of dobutamine (investigational)
- Heart transplant
- Surgical correction

ACE, Angiotensin-converting enzyme; *CMP*, cardiomyopathy; *ECG*, electrocardiogram.

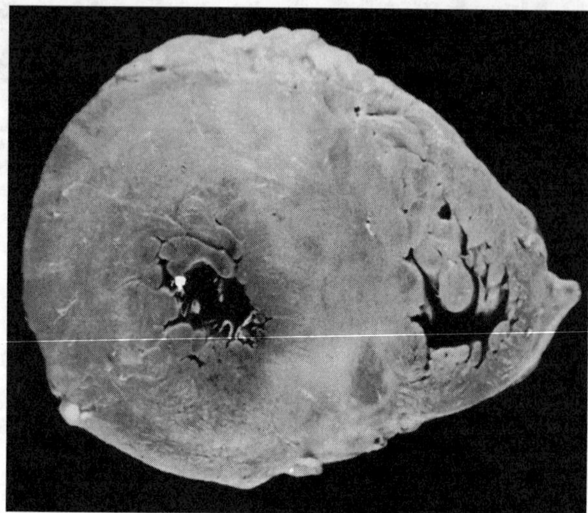

Fig. 32-4 Hypertrophic cardiomyopathy. Cross section through the ventricles is viewed from the base with the anterior surface at the bottom. Notice that the cavity of the left ventricle is unusually small, that the wall of the left ventricle is circumferentially thickened, and that the interventricular septum, especially anteriorly, is disproportionately thickened even more than the free wall (asymmetric septal hypertrophy). This individual was a 59-year-old woman who had hypertrophic cardiomyopathy complicated by mitral regurgitation and congestive heart failure; she died of ventricular fibrillation. Her heart weighed 500 g.

elevated left ventricular diastolic pressure. Fatigue is because of the resultant decrease in CO and in exercise-induced flow obstruction. Angina can occur and is most often caused by the increased LV muscle mass or compression of the small coronary arteries by the hypercontractile ventricular myocardium. This patient may also have syncope, especially during exertion. Syncope in this population is most often caused by an increase in obstruction to aortic outflow during increased activity, resulting in decreased CO and cerebral circulation. Syncope can also be caused by dysrhythmias. Palpitations are common in the patient and are most often caused by dysrhythmias. Common dysrhythmias include supraventricular tachycardia, atrial fibrillation, ventricular tachycardia, and ventricular fibrillation. Any of these dysrhythmias may lead to loss of consciousness or sudden cardiac death of the patient, which is the most common cause of death in this population.

Diagnostic Studies. The chest x-ray is usually normal except in a patient with severe disease causing an increased cardiac silhouette. Increased voltage and duration of the QRS complex are the most common abnormalities on the ECG. These findings usually indicate ventricular hypertrophy. Ventricular dysrhythmias are also frequently seen, with ventricular tachycardia the most common.

The echocardiogram is the primary diagnostic tool revealing the classic feature of HCM, which is LV hypertrophy. The echocardiogram may also demonstrate wall motion abnormalities and diastolic dysfunction. Cardiac catheterization may also be helpful in the diagnosis of HCM. Catheterization will document a pressure gradient if present and will also reveal depressed diastolic left ventricular compliance.

THERAPEUTIC AND NURSING MANAGEMENT

HYPERTROPHIC CARDIOMYOPATHY

Goals of intervention are to improve ventricular filling by reducing ventricular contractility and relieving LV outflow obstruction. These can be accomplished with the use of β-blockers or calcium channel blockers. Digitalis preparations are contraindicated in the patient unless they are used to treat atrial fibrillation. CHF may also be present in varying degrees but is usually not present until later stages. Antidysrhythmics are also used to control dysrhythmias; however, their use has not been proven to prevent sudden death in this group. An alternative treatment for ventricular dysrhythmias may be an implantable defibrillator (see Chapter 33). It has been found that ventricular or atrioventricular pacing can be beneficial for patients with HCM and outflow obstruction. By pacing the ventricles from the apex of the right ventricle septal depolarization occurs first, allowing the septum to move away from the left ventricular wall and reducing the degree of obstruction of the outflow tract.

Some patients may be candidates for surgical treatment of their hypertrophied septum. The indications for surgery include severe symptoms refractory to therapy with marked obstruction to aortic outflow. The surgery is called a *ventriculomyotomy* and *myectomy*. It involves incision of the hypertrophied septal muscle and resection of some of the hypertrophied muscle. Most patients have good symptomatic improvement after surgery and improved exercise tolerance.

The degree of impairment from HCM can range from mild to severe. Some patients have an abnormal ECG and know the disease is in their family but have no symptoms.

Nursing interventions focus on relieving symptoms, observing for and preventing complications, and providing emotional and psychologic support. Education should focus on teaching patients to adjust lifestyle to avoid strenuous activity and dehydration. Any activity or procedure that causes an increase in SVR (thus increasing the obstruction to forward flow) is dangerous for this group of patients and should be avoided. The patient should be taught to space activities and allow for rest periods.

Restrictive Cardiomyopathy

Pathophysiology. *Restrictive cardiomyopathy* is the rarest of the cardiomyopathic conditions. It is a disease of the heart muscle that impairs diastolic volume and stretch. Systolic function remains unaffected.

Although the specific etiology of restrictive CMP is unknown, a number of pathologic processes may be involved in its development. Myocardial fibrosis, hypertrophy, and infiltration produce stiffness of the ventricular wall. Secondary causes of restrictive CMP include amyloidosis, endocardial fibrosis, glycogen deposition, hemochromatosis, sarcoidosis, fibrosis of different etiology, and radiation to the thorax.

The principal characteristic of restrictive CMP is cardiac muscle stiffness. It is characterized by loss of ventricular compliance. The ventricles are resistant to filling and therefore demand high diastolic filling pressures to maintain CO. Systolic function is normal or near normal.

Clinical Manifestations. Angina, syncope, fatigue, and dyspnea on exertion are common signs. The most common symptom is that of exercise intolerance because the myocardium cannot increase CO by producing a tachycardia without further compromising the ventricular filling.

Signs and symptoms include those similar to CHF. The patient may have signs of both left-sided and right-sided heart failure, including dyspnea, peripheral edema, ascites, and hepatic dysfunction. Kussmaul's sign (bulging of the internal jugular neck veins on inspiration) may also be present.

Diagnostic Studies. The chest x-ray may be normal, or it may show cardiomegaly. Pleural effusions and pulmonary congestion may be evident in the patient with progression to CHF. The ECG may reveal a tachycardia at rest. The most common dysrhythmias are atrial fibrillation and complex ventricular dysrhythmias. Echocardiogram may reveal the thickened ventricular wall of restrictive CMP, small ventricular cavities, and a dilated atria. Endomyocardial biopsy, computed tomography (CT) scan, and nuclear imaging may be helpful in a definitive diagnosis.

THERAPEUTIC AND NURSING MANAGEMENT

RESTRICTIVE CARDIOMYOPATHY

Currently no specific treatment for restrictive CMP exists. Interventions are aimed at improving diastolic filling and the underlying disease process. Treatment includes conventional therapy for CHF and dysrhythmias. Heart transplant may also be a consideration. Nursing care is similar to the care of a patient with CHF. As in the treatment of patients with HCM, the patient should be taught to avoid situations that impair ventricular filling, such as strenuous activity, dehydration, and increases in SVR.

Crack Heart

Illicit or recreational drug abuse is a growing concern in the United States. The use of cocaine, as well as alcohol and heroin, has dramatically increased. With the advent of crack cocaine, the smokable form of cocaine, the incidence of fatal outcomes has also increased. Diagnosis such as acute MI in a 22-year-old person who uses cocaine is not uncommon. CMP caused by alcohol or cocaine use is seen with more frequency than ever before.

One significant problem is the increase in CMPs in young, previously healthy persons who have used cocaine.[22] The cocaine causes intense vasoconstriction of the coronary arteries and peripheral vasoconstriction, resulting in hypertension. This can result in increased MVO_2 and decreased oxygen supply to the myocardium and can cause ischemia and infarction. This may lead to an acute MI or ischemic CMP. High levels of catecholamines are seen in the person who uses cocaine, and this can also lead to cell damage in the myocardium. The CMP produced is difficult to treat. Interventions deal mainly with the CHF that ensues. The patient has a poor prognosis and is not usually considered a candidate for heart transplantation.

CARDIAC SURGERY

It has been estimated that more than 700,000 adult open heart procedures are performed annually in the United States.[23] Since the introduction of cardiopulmonary bypass in 1953 and the open heart surgery technique of Favalaro in 1967, modifications and technical improvements in the operating room and in perioperative patient care have abounded. Coronary artery bypass graft (CABG) procedures, heart valve repair and replacement, and heart transplantation have become routine surgical procedures. Cardiac surgery today provides pain relief, improvement of CHF, improvement in lifestyle, and improved survival for the patient undergoing open heart surgical treatment.

The nurse who cares for this patient has been challenged to keep pace with rapid technologic advances in patient care, as well as caring for a patient who 10 to 20 years ago would not have been a surgical candidate. Patients today are older, have worse LV function (patients with ejection fractions below 35%), have progressive disease, have had previous sternotomies, have other systemic diseases that increase the risk of operation (e.g., diabetes, severe hypertension, renal disease), and require emergency operations secondary to failed angioplasty or acute MI. These subgroups of patients require specialized nursing care (Fig. 32-5).

Myocardial Revascularization

Myocardial revascularization, or CABG, is the main surgical treatment for CAD (Fig. 32-6). Indications for surgery have changed during the last decade, especially with the advent of percutaneous transluminal coronary angioplasty (PTCA) (Table 32-16). The patient with CAD who has failed medical management or who has advanced disease is considered a candidate for surgical revascularization. A growing body of research indicates that surgical treatment,

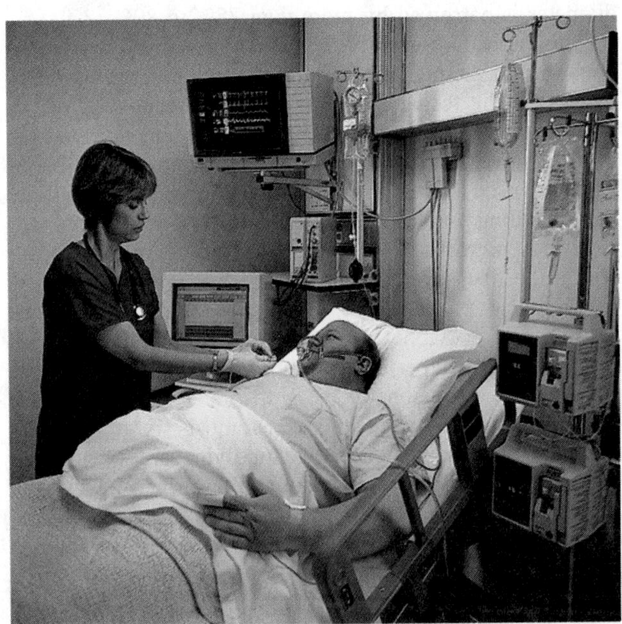

Fig. 32-5 Nurse in intensive care unit.

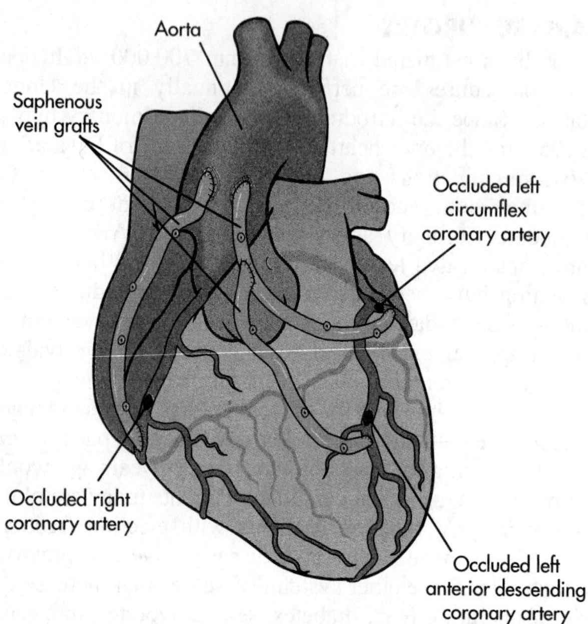

Fig. 32-6 Saphenous aortocoronary artery bypass or revascularization involves taking a piece of saphenous vein from the leg and creating a conduit for blood from the aorta to the area below the blockage in the coronary artery. A triple bypass is illustrated.

when compared with medical therapy, reduces angina, decreases overall costs, and improves patient survival.[24,25]

Surgical Procedure. The CABG operation consists of the construction of new conduits (vessels to transport blood) between the aorta, or other major arteries, beyond the obstructed coronary artery (or arteries). This procedure provides blood flow beyond the stenosis so that the myocardium distal to the obstruction continues to receive blood flow. The coronary artery is considered stenotic if its diameter is narrowed by more than 75% to 80%.

This procedure usually involves a graft from the saphenous vein or the internal mammary artery for aortocoronary bypass. In the former procedure, the saphenous vein from one of the legs of the patient is removed and reversed (so that the valves will not obstruct the blood flow). Saphenous veins are used as free grafts and anastomosed proximally to the ascending aorta and distally to one (or more) coronary artery. Approximately 10% of vessel occlusions occur within the first several weeks after surgery and are caused by technical problems or thrombosis at the distal graft anastomosis.[25] Saphenous veins used as grafts develop diffuse intimal hyperplasia, which contributes to ultimate stenosis and occlusions of the graft. Patency rates of these grafts are lower when the anastomosis is to a small coronary artery and to arteries supplying areas with scar tissue (infarction areas). The use of aspirin (325 mg PO daily) improves vein graft patency and is used postoperatively in the patient. Overall vein graft patency is estimated at 5 to 10 years.

The use of the internal mammary artery (IMA) as a conduit was introduced in 1968. Patency rates of the IMA are 85% to 95% at 10 years.[25] Because the patency rate of the IMA is higher than that of saphenous veins, the IMA may prove to be a better conduit for improving long-term prognosis.

Table 32-16 Indications for Cardiac Surgery
Aneurysm of sinus of Valsalva
Aortic stenosis and regurgitation
Atherosclerotic coronary artery disease
Constrictive pericarditis
Congenital heart defects
Dissecting aortic aneurysm
Mitral stenosis and regurgitation
Myocardial trauma or rupture
Tricuspid insufficiency or stenosis
Ventricular aneurysm
Ventricular septal defect
Ventricular dysrhythmias

Use of the left IMA, which is left attached to its origin from the left subclavian artery, is mobilized from the chest wall and anastomosed to the coronary artery distal to the stenosis. The right IMA may also be used in a similar fashion. The use of the left IMA and saphenous vein conduits together for patients with three-, four-, five-, or six-vessel bypass procedures is common.

If a patient has had previous CABG using saphenous vein grafts or IMA and at the time of reoperation has no conduits to harvest, the gastroepiploic artery or inferior epigastric artery may be used. These arteries are excellent conduits. However, use of these arteries creates the additional need for a laparotomy. This increases the length of surgery, and wound complications at the harvest site are not uncommon, especially in an obese or diabetic patient. Other arterial graft conduits, such as the splenic and radial arteries, have been used, but with slightly less successful patency rates than the IMA. Arm veins are more difficult to dissect and harvest, are thin and delicate, and may have been traumatized by previous intravenous injections. Because of the number of patients requiring reoperation, the use of alternative arteries and veins will become increasingly more common.

Postoperative Considerations. Revascularization surgery has an overall mortality rate of approximately 1% to 2%, with an 85% rate of functional improvement (85% of patients have their anginal pain completely eliminated).[25] CABG remains a palliative treatment for CAD and not a cure. It provides the patient with improved outcomes, quality of life, and survival.

Cardiovascular disease is the primary cause of morbidity and mortality for people more than 65 years of age. The number of older adults who are candidates for CABG has increased, and they have become a subpopulation of patients who have specialized needs before and after surgery. The mortality rate for patients more than 65 years of age has been reported to be as high as 22%, as opposed to 1% for those less than age 65.[26]

The results of coronary revascularization are less favorable for women than men. CAD is the leading cause of death among women. The severity of the clinical variables in women, including a more severe angina and poorer CHF score (despite a better ejection fraction) and the smaller mean diameter of the coronary vessels, are all considered possible causes of their increased risk of CABG. The mortality rate of women undergoing CABG is often double that of men the same age.

Nursing care for this patient involves caring for two surgical sites: the chest and the leg. The care of the leg wound is similar to the postoperative care after the stripping of varicose veins (see Chapter 35). The management of the chest wound, which involves a thoracotomy, is similar to that of other chest surgeries. (The nursing management of the patient with a thoracotomy is presented in the appropriate nursing care plan in Chapter 24.)

Valvular Surgeries

Successful replacement of diseased cardiac valves with valvular prostheses became a reality more than 30 years ago with the development of the Hacher and Starr caged ball prosthesis.[27] Since then, rapid technologic advances have occurred, and today there are a variety of protheses available for patients.

Heart valve prostheses can be broadly grouped into *mechanical valve* and *biologic (tissue) valve* categories (see Table 34-20). Both types of prostheses are associated with different valve-related complications, and the clinical superiority of one over the other has not been established. Before deciding which valve to use, factors in valve design, technical considerations, and long-term anticoagulation therapy should be considered.

Mechanical Valves. Currently available mechanical valves are long lasting and characterized by excellent durability. The durability of valves today usually exceeds the life expectancy of the patient requiring valvular replacement. Commonly used mechanical valves include the tilting disk valve and bileaflet valves, such as the St. Jude Medical, Björk-Shiley, and Medtronic-Hall valve.

Biologic Valves. Biologic valves are characterized by a low incidence of thromboembolism and valve thrombosis, and thus do not require long-term anticoagulation. The main concern with biologic valves is their unproven long-term durability and the potential risks, including reoperation, associated with tissue degeneration and failure. Biologic cardiac valve substitutes currently available include the porcine aortic valve, the bovine pericardial valve, and the aortic allograft (human cardiac) valves (also known as a homograft). The type of valve used depends on individual patient needs such as cardiac anatomic structure, age, past health history, contraindications to anticoagulation use, and lifestyle.

Both mitral valve disease and aortic valve disease may require valvular replacement when therapeutic management is no longer effective in the presence of increasing heart failure. Almost all cardiac valvular surgeries require cardiopulmonary bypass. A closed mitral commissurotomy is the only possible exception. It involves incising the fused leaflets of the mitral valves if there is no significant calcification of the valve. (Chapter 34 describes the causes, therapeutic management, and surgical intervention of valvular diseases.)

Ventricular Surgeries

Ventricular Septal Defects. Occasionally an adult may be diagnosed as having a ventricular septal defect (VSD) that is congenital in nature but had not been diagnosed early in life or progressed in size to cause oxygenation and exercise tolerance problems. A VSD repair involves a primary closure (suturing) or a patch (pericardial patch, or grafted with a Gortex or Dacron patch).

Ventricular septal rupture occasionally occurs as a complication of acute MI. Because this defect has a high mortality rate with medical treatment alone, surgical repair is indicated and may be performed on an emergency basis. The septal defect may be sutured or patched depending on the size of the rupture.

Ventricular Aneurysmectomy. Ventricular aneurysms located on the anterolateral or apical part of the LV may also be excised. These noncontracting areas interfere significantly with adequate cardiac contraction and CO. They are often a site for the development of mural thrombi within the ventricle. The ventricle is opened and allowed to collapse so that the thinned scar tissue is cut away and any thrombotic material removed before the ventricle is closed (see Fig. 31-15).

Septal Myotomy and Myectomy. Surgical intervention for HCM is indicated when the patient is symptomatic on optimal medical therapy and left ventricular outflow tract obstruction (LVOTO) is present. The goals of surgical therapy are to decrease LVOTO and improve quality of life. The most common operative procedure is left ventricular septal myotomy and myectomy. In this procedure, a portion of the hypertrophied septum is removed. A mitral valve replacement may be necessary to eliminate mitral insufficiency and decrease LVOTO. The outcomes for these patients are favorable. Postoperative complications include dysrhythmias such as heart block or tachydysrythmias. Another complication is VSD from septal perforation. During surgery a transesophageal echocardiogram is performed to detect a possible VSD before anastomosing the surgical incision.

Cardiomyoplasty

Cardiomyoplasty, a surgical method of augmenting cardiac function, usually involves the use of skeletal muscle such as the latissimus dorsi. The muscle is wrapped around the heart or the aorta, or it may be fashioned into a separate pumping chamber. The muscle is then stimulated with specialized burst pacing, which results in contraction and provides circulatory support. If clinical trials continue to produce favorable results, this procedure may become an important bridge to transplant. With the scarcity of donor hearts, the implications for skeletal muscle wrapping as a long-term alternative to transplant are promising.

Cardiac Transplantation

The first heart transplant was performed in 1967. Since that time, heart transplantation has developed into a viable option for the patient with terminal cardiac disease. Patients with CMP account for more than 50% of the cardiac transplant recipients. Dilated CMP is the most common type of CMP requiring transplantation. Inoperable CAD is the second most common indication for transplantation, accounting for 40% of candidates (Table 32-17).

Once an individual meets the criteria for cardiac transplantation, the goal of the evaluation process is to identify patients who would most benefit from a new heart. In addition to the physical examination, psychologic assessment of candidates is valuable. A complete history of coping abilities, family support system, and motivation to follow through with the transplant and the rigorous transplantation regimen is essential. The complexity of the transplant process may be overwhelming to a patient with inadequate support systems and a poor understanding of the lifestyle changes required after transplant.

Once potential recipients are placed on the transplant list, they may wait at home and receive ongoing medical care if their medical condition is stable. If their condition is not stable, they may require hospitalization for more intensive therapy. Unfortunately, the overall waiting period for a transplant is long, and many patients die while waiting for a transplant.

The decision to accept a donor heart is based on careful donor evaluation, size matching, blood type, and prediction of postoperative graft performance. Organ procurement coordinators must be familiar with the standard clinical criteria for brain death: absent cerebral function, apnea, absent brain stem function, and known causes of coma.

Donor and recipient matching is based on age, weight, and blood type. Most donor hearts are obtained at sites distant from the institution performing the transplant. The maximum acceptable ischemic time for cardiac transplant is 4 to 6 hours.

Table 32-17 Indications and Contraindications for Cardiac Transplantation

Indications
- Less than 62-65 yr of age*
- End-stage heart disease refractory to medical therapy
- Functional class III or IV status (NYHA)
- Vigorous and healthy individual (except for end-stage cardiac disease) who would benefit from procedure
- Compliance with medical regimens
- Demonstrated emotional stability, supportive family and friends
- Financial resources available

Contraindications†
- Systemic disease
- Active infection
- Pneumonia
- Recent or unresolved pulmonary infarction
- Severe pulmonary hypertension unrelieved with medication
- Cerebrovascular or peripheral vascular disease
- Moderate to severe azotemia or hepatic abnormalities
- Obesity
- History of drug or alcohol abuse or mental illness

NYHA, New York Heart Association.
*Age criteria may vary at different institutions.
†Contraindications may vary at different cardiac transplant centers.

In pairing donor and recipient, there must be ABO blood group compatibility, negative lymphocyte crossmatch, and avoidance of transplantation from a cytomegalovirus (CMV)-positive donor to a CMV-negative recipient. Human leukocyte antigen (HLA) matching (as discussed in Chapters 10 and 44) is not usually done in cardiac transplantation. This is because of the limited number of donors, time constraints (less than 4 to 6 hours required from removal from donor to surgical implantation), and lack of proven value of HLA matching on survival.

The recipient is prepared for surgery, and cardiopulmonary bypass is used. The usual surgical procedure involves removing the recipient's heart, except for the posterior right and left atrial walls and their venous connections. The recipient's heart is then replaced with the donor heart, which has been trimmed to match. Care is taken to preserve the integrity of the donor sinoatrial (SA) node so that a sinus rhythm may be achieved postoperatively.

Immunosuppressive therapy usually begins while the recipient is in the operating room and includes azathioprine (Imuran), corticosteroids, and cyclosporine, an antifungal immunosuppressant. (The mechanisms of action and side effects of these immunosuppressants are discussed in Chapter 44.) Cyclosporine was first used in heart transplantation in 1980. Currently it is usually used with corticosteroids for maintenance immunosuppression. Its use has resulted not only in reduced rejection, but also in slowing the rejection process so that early treatment can be instituted. As a result, rejection episodes have been less dangerous, and patient survival and rehabilitation have improved. Another immunosuppressant is OKT3, a monoclonal antibody specifically designed to react with T cells.[28] It is primarily used to treat acute rejection episodes. (OKT3 is discussed in Chapter 44.) OKT3 and antithymocytic globulin may also be used early as prophylactic agents after transplantation.

The postoperative care is similar to that of other open heart surgeries (see next section). Endomyocardial biopsies via the right internal jugular vein are performed at repeated intervals to detect rejection. In addition, peripheral blood T-lymphocyte monitoring is done to assess the recipient's immune status. With the use of cyclosporine, the usual parameters of rejection, such as change in ECG voltage, are less valid, and monitoring requires more frequent endomyocardial biopsies to detect rejection. Because cyclosporine may cause renal insufficiency, assessment of renal function using serum creatinine levels, BUN levels, and urine output must be performed.

The current report of the registry of the International Society for Heart and Lung Transplantation indicates that survival rates have improved. The 1-year survival rate was 72.8% from 1981 to 1985 as compared with a 1-year survival rate of 80% from 1986 to 1990. A greater increase in 5-year survival rates is also noted (70% as compared with 58%).

Because the patient is immunosuppressed, nursing management should involve prevention of infection, which is the leading cause of death in this population. Many deaths from infection occur during augmented immunosuppressive therapy for acute rejection episodes. Nursing care involves a great deal of emotional support and teaching of both the patient and the family, because transplantation is a last resort. In addition, often the patient is a long distance from home and significant others.

Advances in surgical technique and postoperative care have improved early survival rates after cardiac transplantation. Attention is directed toward improvements in immunosuppression and management of long-term complications. Nursing management continues to focus on promoting patient adaptation to the transplant process, monitoring, managing lifestyle changes, and ongoing education of the patient and family. Ongoing data collection and research continues in regard to quality of life, functional level, and rehabilitation of the cardiac transplant recipient.

Postoperative Complications

The possible complications resulting from cardiac surgery are summarized in Table 32-18.

Low Cardiac Output. The most common complication in the early postoperative period is low CO syndrome.

Table 32-18 Complications of Cardiac Surgery

Early Postoperative Period
Low CO syndrome caused by hypovolemia, acidosis, acute MI, CHF, drugs such as propranolol, mediastinal tamponade, pulmonary embolism, or incomplete or faulty surgical repair
Acute MI, especially with aortocoronary bypass surgery
Cardiac dysrhythmias
Hemorrhage
Pulmonary embolism, especially with saphenous vein aortocoronary bypass
Fever
Depression
Wound infection
Electrolyte disturbances
Systemic arterial hypertension
Cerebral infarcts caused by air or thrombus emboli
Confusion, agitation, and disorientation
Disseminated intravascular coagulation
Acute respiratory distress syndrome
Renal failure
Late Postoperative Period
Wound infection
Hepatitis
Pancreatitis (early or late)
Postpericardiotomy syndrome
Systemic arterial emboli and infective endocarditis, with valvular surgeries
Occlusion of graft

CHF, Congestive heart failure; *CO,* cardiac output; *MI,* myocardial infarction.

Regardless of the surgical procedure, most patients after open heart surgery are in a controlled state of shock caused by fluid shifts and varying vascular tone. Low CO may be caused by relative hypovolemia secondary to blood loss and vascular dilatation, or it may be caused by poor left ventricular function. It is evidenced by hypotension, oliguria, and cool extremities. If it is because of hypovolemia, the central venous pressure (CVP), left atrial pressure (LAP), and PCWP will be low.

The treatment for hypovolemia includes intravascular volume augmentation, calcium administration, and close observation for blood loss. Volume can be replaced by lactated Ringer's solution, colloids, or blood replacement in the form of packed RBCs (see Chapter 28). Blood is often transfused according to the measured loss in the chest tube drainage to prevent hypovolemia. Sometimes patients can be autotransfused, using a special chest tube drainage set to reinfuse blood into the patient. If the patient cannot be stabilized with transfusions, the patient may need to be returned to surgery. Careful recording of all intake and output (e.g., IV fluids, chest drainage, GI drainage, blood, urine, and medications) is essential to monitor fluid balance.

If the low output is secondary to poor LV function, there may be a high LAP, low BP, decreased urine output, and high CVP and PCWP. Pharmacologic intervention is needed and may include diuretics, inotropic agents, or vasopressor agents.

Cardiac Tamponade. Mediastinal or cardiac tamponade may be a cause of low output syndrome. Cardiac tamponade is pressure on the heart caused by the accumulation of fluid, such as blood, in the pericardium. Clinical manifestations include a decrease in chest tube drainage, decrease in the precordial pulsation, quiet heart sounds, and increased size of the heart on percussion. A chest x-ray shows an enlarged heart and a widened mediastinum. The ECG may show a decrease in the amplitude of the waves. The PCWP, LAP, and CVP are increased. Pulsus paradoxus, an abnormal (more than 10 mm Hg) fall in systolic BP on inspiration, may be present. It can be determined by taking the BP with a cuff. As the cuff is deflated, it is stopped at the first Korotkoff sound while the patient is breathing normally. If the Korotkoff sound is heard during both inspiration and expiration, no pulsus paradoxus exists. However, if the sound is heard only on expiration, the cuff is deflated slowly until the first Korotkoff sound is heard on both inspiration and expiration. If the difference in pressure between inspiration and expiration is greater than 10 mm Hg, the patient has significant pulsus paradoxus.

After open heart surgery the patient already has a mediastinal tube in place. Therefore the treatment for cardiac tamponade is one of the following:

1. Disconnect other chest tubes and clean out the mediastinal tube with a catheter.
2. Remove the tube, break up the clot by inserting a gloved finger into the stoma, and then reinsert a new chest tube.
3. Return the patient to the operating room, where bleeding can be further assessed and treated.

The other treatment for cardiac tamponade in the patient who does not have mediastinal tubes in place is pericardiocentesis. This procedure involves the insertion of a needle into the pericardium to remove fluid (see Fig. 34-6).

Dysrhythmias. Dysrhythmias are common postoperatively. A common cause of dysrhythmias is serum potassium imbalance (i.e., hyperkalemia or hypokalemia), necessitating frequent evaluation of serum potassium levels. Frequent PVCs and ventricular tachycardia may be seen early in the postoperative period. Potassium replacement is essential in the care of this patient. The nurse must also look to other causes of ventricular dysrhythmias, such as catheter placement, pH, and ischemia, that need to be evaluated and treated if necessary. Atrial flutter or fibrillation may occur as early as a few hours postoperatively, in the first 36 hours after aortocoronary bypass, or approximately 6 or 7 days postoperatively. Atrial dysrhythmias are treated prophylactically with drugs such as digoxin or metoprolol (Lopressor). (See Chapter 33 for treatment of dysrhythmias.) Atrial dysrhythmias are common with mitral and aortic valve replacements. The patient who has aortic valve replacement for aortic stenosis is at high risk for dysrhythmias. If PVCs are noted postoperatively, they are treated quickly with lidocaine. Pacing wires are inserted during surgery so that tachydysrhythmias can be paced in an overdrive method or bradydysrhythmias can be paced at a rate that will maximize CO.

Emboli. Pulmonary embolism occurs most often after the third postoperative day. It is common in the patient with saphenous aortocoronary bypass surgery. Because the clinical manifestations of pulmonary emboli are not always overt, the nurse should report to the physician any patient who has transient weakness, dyspnea, or faintness. Lung scans are often used in the diagnosis. Anticoagulation is the usual method of treatment. (The prevention and treatment of pulmonary emboli are discussed in Chapter 35.)

Arterial embolism may occur after aortic or mitral valve surgery. The patient is frequently placed on long-term anticoagulant therapy. The patient must be observed for evidence of a cerebral embolism, such as a sudden change in level of consciousness, slurring of speech, or one-sided weakness. Extremities should be assessed for evidence of embolization, including pain, pulselessness, pallor, paresthesia, and paralysis.

Fever. Fever is a common complication of cardiac surgery. Causes of a fever include atelectasis, urinary tract infection, pneumonia, thrombophlebitis, drug reaction, transfusion reaction, and wound infection. An elevated temperature increases the work load of the heart because it increases metabolism. The nurse is involved in preventing potential problems that cause fever and assisting in collecting information to assess the cause. The patient's body temperature is taken at least every 4 hours. Treatment is directed toward treating the cause and reducing the fever.

Another possible cause of fever is endocarditis. It rarely occurs in the first weeks postoperatively, probably because of the widespread use of prophylactic antibiotics. However, it can occur early with valvular replacements. (Endocarditis is discussed in Chapter 34.)

Intraoperative Myocardial Infarction. Of primary importance in all cardiovascular surgery, especially in bypass grafts, is the preservation of myocardial tissue. The incidence of intraoperative and perioperative MI may be as high as 25%. Several methods of preserving myocardial tissue during surgery have been developed, primarily cold cardioplegia. Immediately after the aorta is cross-clamped, a cold solution high in potassium is infused around the heart and into the aortic root. This process is repeated whenever the myocardial temperature rises to approximately 66°F (19°C). This technique lowers the myocardial oxygen consumption and the metabolic rate to prevent ischemia.

During the immediate postoperative period, serial ECGs are taken and cardiac enzymes are assessed to detect intraoperative infarction. It is sometimes difficult to assess if an intraoperative MI has occurred; enzymes may be elevated because of the surgical procedure itself, and an ECG may be difficult to evaluate (as with complete left bundle branch block). Preoperative and postoperative radionuclide scanning gives the best evaluation of coronary perfusion but is difficult to obtain in the immediate postoperative period. Nursing and medical interventions are aimed at preserving myocardial function at all times postoperatively. Monitoring SvO_2 and O_2 saturation gives the nurse a great deal of information about CO and O_2 utilization in this group of patients. If an infarct has occurred, the prognosis is worsened and the hospital stay is lengthened.

THERAPEUTIC AND NURSING MANAGEMENT

CARDIAC SURGERY

Preoperative Management

The preoperative period may vary from a few hours to a month or more depending on the patient's physical condition. Some conditions, such as a stab wound to the heart, require immediate surgical intervention. With other conditions, such as heart failure associated with mitral stenosis or regurgitation, the patient must be stabilized and prepared for surgery. It is desirable that the patient's cardiac and physical condition be stabilized before surgery. For example, dysrhythmias should be controlled, CHF treated, BP and CO maximized, and anginal pain relieved.

Extensive diagnostic studies are usually done before cardiac surgery. Most patients have a cardiac catheterization to measure changes in pressure and blood gases in cardiac chambers and across valves. This is performed to look for structural abnormalities or to confirm the diagnosis and to assess LV function. Coronary arteriography is also done to observe the coronary perfusion of the myocardium. Other diagnostic studies include echocardiograms, stress testing, nuclear imaging, ABGs, and Doppler studies to evaluate peripheral perfusion.

In addition, baseline data are obtained just before surgery. These include a chest x-ray, ECG, coagulation studies (e.g., clotting time, prothrombin time, fibrinogen, and platelets), complete blood count (CBC), urinalysis, serum electrolytes, BUN and serum creatinine levels, and cardiac enzymes. Some patients also have thyroid studies, liver function studies, and alkaline phosphate determinations.

Pulmonary function studies may be performed on patients with pulmonary disease or a history of smoking. ABGs may be done preoperatively as a baseline for postoperative care. The patient also has the blood typed and crossmatched.

Blood transfusions have become a major concern to many patients and their families. Preoperative teaching should include information regarding autotransfusion and autologous blood donation. If the surgery is planned, a patient may donate 1 unit of blood a week up to 3 units (3 weeks) and have fresh blood at the time of surgery (no freezing is required). A patient may also have the family donate blood (directed donor blood, which, when cross-typed, is given to the patient). Surgical procedures have improved with the use of blood cell savers and subsequent autotransfusion of blood from the surgical field, to the point where many patients require no blood after surgery. The patient may return home with lower hemoglobin and hematocrit levels but is treated successfully with iron replacement therapy and nutritional support.

Other baseline data obtained shortly before surgery include an accurate body weight to aid in fluid management and vital signs, including temperature because an elevated temperature is an indication for postponement of surgery.

To improve the respiratory status, the patient who smokes must stop smoking at least 1 week and preferably 1 month or more before surgery. This helps decrease the amount of bronchial secretions and thus reduces the postoperative risk of atelectasis and pneumonia. However, it may be difficult for many patients to stop smoking because of their anxiety about the surgery.

It may be necessary to modify the patient's medications to prevent adverse reactions. Digoxin may be discontinued 24 to 36 hours before surgery. This is usually done because digitalis toxicity may occur in the early postoperative period. (Digitalis preparations are usually not stopped in a patient with atrial fibrillation with a rapid ventricular response.) Propranolol (Inderal) may be tapered 24 hours to 2 weeks before surgery if the patient tolerates weaning (i.e., has no anginal or hypertensive episodes). However, a patient who requires propranolol may be given positive inotropic agents in the early postoperative period to counteract the effects of propranolol. If possible, aspirin or coumadin should be stopped 7 days before surgery. This may require the patient to be admitted preoperatively and be started on IV heparin for anticoagulation. Although tapering or stopping these drugs may appear to be beneficial, many patients who undergo emergency surgeries do not discontinue these medications and do well postoperatively.

If the patient has compensated heart failure, diuretics may be discontinued 24 to 48 hours before surgery. This will help reduce potassium loss and hypovolemia. The patient receiving long-acting insulins will be switched to regular insulin on a sliding-scale basis during the perioperative period. They remain on the sliding scale into the postoperative period when they start their cardiac diet. Other drugs that may need modification include corticosteroids, antihypertensives, and phenothiazines. The nurse should check with the physician concerning changes in any drug that is questionable.

To prevent incisional infections, the patient should be instructed to shower several times using a bacteriostatic soap (e.g., Betadine, hexachlorophene). In addition, the patient is usually started on parenteral antibiotics within 12 hours of surgery. The physician discusses at length with the patient and significant others the nature of the surgery, including the procedures, expected outcomes, possible complications, and postsurgical care.

Nursing management complements the various aspects of therapeutic management. Extensive preoperative teaching is a major responsibility of the nurse. It deals with general postoperative concerns (see Chapter 16), in addition to the specialized concerns related to cardiovascular surgery. A high level of anxiety is common because of the patient's perception of the central role of the heart in maintaining life. The purpose of teaching is to help reduce anxiety. The teaching may be more helpful to patients if the sensations that may be experienced are described in addition to the procedures to be performed. Table 32-19 outlines the topics that should be included. The patient should be encouraged to ask questions and discuss concerns. It is essential that the nurse report significant concerns to the physician so that a coordinated approach can be developed to deal with the patient's anxiety.

Family members should also be involved in the preoperative teaching. This will help to alleviate their anxiety so that they can support the patient more effectively during this period. It is important that the family know about the various tubes, lines, monitoring devices, and postoperative routines to be aware that these are normal procedures and that they are not an indication of trouble. The family may also be able to help provide comfort for the patient and identify unique needs of the patient, such as routines and habits. Many patients do not come to the hospital until the morning of surgery. In this situation, preoperative teaching should occur before this time, as an outpatient or in the physician's office.

Intraoperative Management

Many cardiovascular surgeries are being performed with the patient on a heart-lung machine or cardiopulmonary bypass. This allows the surgeon to work on the heart that has been put into asystole or a slowly contracting state. The heart-lung machine serves as a pump to circulate and oxygenate blood. The machine receives blood from catheters in the venae cavae or right atrium, oxygenates it, and returns the blood to the patient through a catheter in the aorta. This is usually done in conjunction with hypothermia (approximately 77 to 82°F [25 to 28°C] for bypass and valvular surgeries). The time on the heart-lung machine is closely monitored and kept to a minimum because the longer the patient is on it, the more complications may develop. In addition, careful anesthesia and precise monitoring of the cardiac rhythm, vital signs, blood gases, electrolytes, and coagulation status are components of the procedure.

At the end of the procedure, depending on the patient's condition (ventricular function) when coming off bypass, the surgeon may place monitoring lines for hemodynamic

Table 32-19 Preoperative Teaching List for Cardiovascular Surgery

Operating room	Provide trip to operating room to see area and meet staff (if desired) Provide trip to waiting room for family Inform patient that conversations and events from the operating room experience may be remembered
CCU or ICU	Provide trip to see area and meet staff (if desired)
Early postoperative period in CCU or ICU	Explain that patient may lose track of time and place and may have hallucinations (visual, auditory, taste) Explain ECG monitoring leads Discuss location and purpose of tubes and when they will be removed Discuss endotracheal tube; because patient cannot talk, devise method of calling a nurse Explain nasogastric tube Explain that arterial lines and monitors are used for pressure measurements Explain that venous lines and monitors are used for fluid or medication administration Explain that bloody red drainage will occur from the chest tubes and that a pulling sensation is felt when the tubes are removed Explain that retention catheter is used for input and output and ease of urine elimination Inform patient that thirst may be felt Discuss noise level, sounds, alarms
Postoperative routine	Explain mechanical ventilation Explain suctioning Explain the importance of coughing, deep breathing, and turning Discuss frequent monitoring of vital signs and continuous cardiac monitoring
Pain medications	Explain that patient can ask for pain medication to be comfortable Inform patient that the body will be achy and sore for the first week postoperatively
Nebulizer treatment	Provide demonstration of incentive spirometer
Post-CCU or post-ICU routines	Provide overview of discharge regimens
General care unit	Discuss emotional reaction Explain that depression is common and should be short-lived Explain discharge plans, home health care

CCU, Coronary care unit; *ECG*, electrocardiogram; *ICU*, intensive care unit; *IPPB*, intermittent positive-pressure breathing.

monitoring and management postoperatively. These may include pulmonary artery catheter, arterial line, a LAP line, and atrial and ventricular pacing wires. An intraaortic balloon pump may also need to be inserted in the operating room in cases of poor ventricular function.

Postoperative Management

Complications that may occur as a result of cardiac surgery are outlined in Table 32-18. Much of the postoperative management is directed toward the prevention or early detection of these complications. Postoperative assessment is outlined in Table 32-20. The physician and nurses work closely during this time with much overlapping of functions, depending on the policies of the institution.

On completion of cardiac surgery, the patient is transferred immediately to a coronary care unit (CCU) or ICU. (Some hospitals have separate heart recovery rooms because the CCU and the operating room are not always in close proximity.) The nursing staff should have been notified of the patient's estimated time of arrival and status so that all the equipment is ready to provide care.

On arrival the patient should already be lying on the postoperative bed. The patient should have been transferred directly from the surgical table to the postoperative bed to save time and energy. Usually a team of two nurses admits the patient on arrival to the unit. This is a crucial time for the patient because complications may occur early and during transport. When the patient arrives, the nurse team will connect the monitoring devices (e.g., ECG, arterial lines, O_2 saturation monitor) and suction equipment (e.g., chest tubes, NG tubes) so that the patient's hemodynamic parameters can be assessed immediately. The endotracheal tube is checked, and the patient is attached immediately to a preset mechanical ventilator. As soon as the equipment is properly connected and calibrated, the nurse should immediately assess the patient's neurologic, respiratory, and cardiac status to determine the level of anesthesia and the ventilation and perfusion status. Reports from the anesthesiologist and surgeon are often given during this initial assessment period. Baseline laboratory data are collected, including ABGs, serum electrolytes, CBC, clotting profile, lactate level, and cardiac enzymes. A chest x-ray is also taken immediately upon arrival to the ICU.

The nurse also collects baseline data on the cardiovascular status by checking the arterial blood pressure, PAP, PCWP, LAP (if a line was inserted during surgery), heart

Table 32-20 Postoperative Assessment

Nervous System
- Pupil size and reaction
- Orientation and level of consciousness
- Motor functioning

Respiratory System
- Placement of endotracheal tube
- Settings on mechanical ventilator
- Character of respirations
- Breath sounds and secretions
- Arterial blood gases

Cardiovascular and Hematologic Systems
- Cardiac rhythm
- Peripheral pulses
- Blood pressure
- Venous or pulmonary artery pressures
- Temperature
- Fluid status
- Chest tubes
- Coagulation status
- Cardiac output

Renal System
- Urinary output
- Urine character, color, specific gravity
- Electrolytes

Gastrointestinal System
- Nasogastric secretions
- Bowel sounds

Integumentary System
- Skin breakdown
- Incisional healing and drainage

Pain
- Quality or intensity
- Location

sounds, cardiac rhythm, and peripheral pulses and O_2 saturations. If the patient has an Oximetrix pulmonary artery catheter, venous O_2 saturation (SvO_2) can be monitored continuously. The patient's monitoring devices (e.g., pulmonary artery catheter, left atrial line, Oximetrix SvO_2 monitoring) depend on the patient's preoperative condition, the intraoperative procedures and findings, the surgeon's preference, and the unit's protocol. Many patients return from surgery with only a CVP line; others may require a pulmonary artery catheter, an LAP line, and a pacing wire and may be on the intraarterial balloon pump (IABP). These variations are of primary importance in preparing for the patient and in planning for care.

Once the initial assessment is made, the patient is placed on frequent vital signs (e.g., BP and HR continuously and then every 15 minutes for the first 4 hours, then every 30 minutes for 4 hours, and later every hour). After the patient has had the initial assessment, CO, cardiac index, and SVR measurements may be done to assess LV function. Other indicators may be measured at least every hour, such as urinary output, PCWP or PAP, temperature, breath sounds, and other respiratory parameters. In addition, the wave patterns for the arterial pressure, pulmonary artery (PA) catheter, LAP, O_2 saturation, SvO_2, and ECG are constantly monitored for significant changes. Peripheral pulses and warmth of extremities also need to be chcked every 1 to 2 hours.

Care of the patient's chest tubes is indicated by the surgeon's preference and the unit's protocol. Chest tubes must be kept patent so that blood from the mediastinum and pericardium can drain adequately. Plugging or clotting in the chest tube may obstruct the drainage and severely compromise the patient. Chest tube drainage (amount and character) is also assessed and recorded frequently (every 15 minutes for the first few hours postoperatively). (The nursing care of the patient with chest tubes is presented in Chapter 24.)

The patient also needs care to prevent problems associated with immobility. This includes turning from side to side. If the patient has an LAP line, surgeon preference will dictate the patient's mobility status. The head of the bed may be elevated 30 degrees when vital signs are stable. The patient may have antiembolic stockings in place. While on the ventilator, the patient needs to be suctioned (see Chapter 61). When the endotracheal tube is removed, the patient should cough and deep breathe. The patient can also sit in a chair, usually by the end of the first day postoperatively. Progressive ambulation is then encouraged.

Most tubes and lines are removed within 3 days of surgery. Because rest periods are important, care must be planned to allow for uninterrupted sleep, especially during the early period of intensive care. Pain medications are also important because they allow the patient to be active and to participate in coughing and deep-breathing exercises (see the following research box). The patient and the family need many explanations and much support. They should be allowed to spend as much time together as the patient's condition allows.

After a short period in the ICU, the patient is moved to a step-down area if further ECG monitoring or care is necessary; if the patient's condition is stable, the patient may be moved to a general surgical unit. After transfer, the patient's activity levels are gradually increased and nutritional patterns are resumed. Medication regimens are adjusted. Wound care is initiated according to physician preference or unit protocol. The patient is prepared for discharge, and referrals are made to appropriate community resources. Home regimens, including wound care, activity, and medications, are discussed, and the patient should be given written instructions. Wound care, diet, and activity levels should be discussed in specific terms with the patient and the family. Evaluation should be made of their level of knowledge and of the need for further teaching before discharge. Return appointments to the surgeon and referring physician are made before discharge so that the patient and family are aware of all follow-up procedures.

MECHANICAL ASSIST DEVICES

Decades of research have led to more effective means with which to care for the patient with end-stage heart disease. An exciting innovation in this area has been the development of ventricular assist devices (VADs) (Fig. 32-7). Pulsatile im-

RESEARCH

Implications for Nursing Practice

PAIN IN CARDIOVASCULAR SURGERY PATIENTS

Citation Puntillo K, Weiss SJ: Pain: its mediators and associated morbidity in critically ill cardiovascular surgical patients, *Nurs Res* 43:31-36, 1994.

Purpose To compare the effects of age, gender, personality adjustment, and analgesic administration on the magnitude of pain experienced in cardiac and abdominal vascular surgical patients.

Methods Descriptive study using 74 cardiac and abdominal vascular surgical patients during their first 3 postoperative days. Pain intensity was measured using a numerical rating scale and the McGill Pain Questionnaire. Personality adjustment was measured by the California Q-set. Analgesia data were obtained from the patients' charts.

Results and Conclusions Pain intensity in the cardiac surgical patients was moderate and did not diminish over the 3-day postoperative study period. Although these patients received small amounts of pain medication, it was the primary consistent mediator of pain magnitude after surgery. Patients with abdominal vascular surgery had a greater magnitude of pain sensation than cardiac patients. Women who had cardiac surgery reported a greater magnitude of pain sensation than men. Patients with greater pain intensity had a significantly greater incidence of atelectasis.

Implications for Nursing Practice Although a small amount of pain medication stabilized the pain experience, it was not sufficient to minimize the intensity of the patients' pain. This study also suggests that atelectasis is more likely to develop in those patients whose postoperative analgesia is less than optimal. The nurse who provides a patient with adequate analgesia may support the patient's abilities to deep breathe, cough, and ambulate and therefore minimize atelectasis development.

plantable ventricular assist systems began in 1984 with Novacor and in 1986 with Thermedics. These devices provide long-term support of CO and circulatory assist of the patient. Clinical trails on implanted VADs are likely to continue with total artificial heart studies to proceed into the next century.[29,30]

Mechanical circulating assist devices can be used as a bridge to transplant or as a temporary support to those with potential for regaining normal heart function. There are four general classifications of circulatory support system: (1) series mechanical ventricular assistance (e.g., IABP, cardiopulmonary bypass, axial flow pump); (2) parallel mechanical ventricular assistance; (3) mechanical replacement (total artificial heart); and (4) cardiomyoplasty.

Initially, failure to wean from cardiopulmonary bypass after surgery was the primary indicator for VAD support.

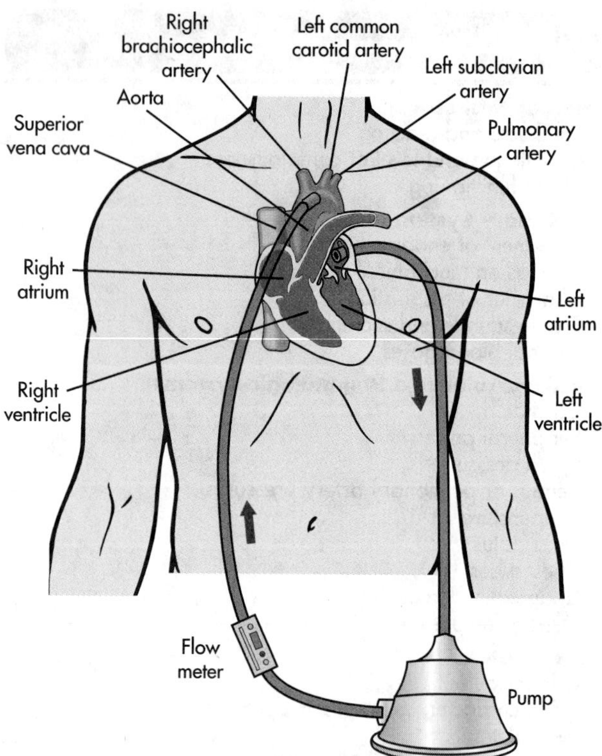

Fig. 32-7 Left ventricular assist device.

However, the role of VAD has expanded to include the patient with ventricular failure caused by MI and the patient awaiting cardiac transplantation. A VAD is a temporary device with the capability to partially or totally support circulation until the heart recovers or a donor heart can be obtained. Cannula sites depend on the type of device used. For support of the right side of the heart, the right atrium and pulmonary artery are cannulated. The LV apex can be cannulated for LV devices. Cannulation may occur at the bedside with femoral percutaneous technique or femoral cutdown. Direct cannulation of the atria and great vessels occurs in the operating room through a sternotomy.

Patient selection is critical. Three groups are recognized as potential candidates: (1) postcardiotomy patients; (2) those awaiting cardiac transplantation; and (3) patients with acute MI in cardiogenic shock. Exclusion criteria include (1) irreversible renal failure; (2) severe peripheral vascular disease; (3) symptomatic cerebrovascular disease; (4) cancer with metastasis; (5) severe hepatic disease; (6) coagulopathy or blood dyscrasia; (7) severe bacterial infection; (8) severe pulmonary disease; and (9) older than 65.[28] Device selection depends on the institution and physician approval to use investigational or FDA-approved devices.

Nursing care of the patient with a VAD is similar to that of the patient with IABP. Nursing care concerns include bleeding, cardiac tamponade, ventricular failure, infection, dysrhythmias, renal failure, nutritional support, activity versus immobilization, and psychologic support for the patient and family. Device-related complications include hemolysis and thromboembolism.

CRITICAL THINKING EXERCISES

CASE STUDY

CONGESTIVE HEART FAILURE

Patient Profile

Mrs. E., a 62-year-old Hispanic woman, was admitted to the medical unit with complaints of increasing dyspnea on exertion.

Subjective Data

- Had a severe MI at 58 years of age
- Has experienced increasing dyspnea of exertion during the last 2 years
- Had a respiratory tract infection, frequent cough, and edema in legs 2 weeks ago
- Cannot walk two blocks without getting short of breath
- Has to sleep with head elevated on three pillows
- Does not always remember to take digoxin and furosemide

Objective Data

Physical Examination

- Elderly woman in respiratory distress
- Diastolic heart murmur
- Moist crackles in both lungs
- Cyanotic lips and extremities

Diagnostic Studies

- Chest x-ray results: cardiomegaly with right and left ventricular hypertrophy; fluid in lower lobes of lungs

Therapeutic Management

- Digoxin 0.25 mg every day
- Lasix 40 mg bid
- 2 gm sodium diet
- Oxygen 6 L/min
- Daily weights

Critical Thinking Questions

1. Explain the pathophysiology of Mrs. E.'s heart disease.
2. What clinical manifestations of heart failure did Mrs. E. exhibit?
3. What is the significance of the findings of the chest x-ray?
4. Explain the rationale for each of the medical orders prescribed for Mrs. E.
5. What are appropriate nursing interventions for Mrs. E.?
6. What teaching measures should be instituted to prevent recurrence of an acute episode of heart failure?
7. Based on the assessment data presented, write one or more appropriate nursing diagnoses. Are there any collaborative problems?

NURSING RESEARCH ISSUES

1. What nursing measures are most effective in relieving shortness of breath in a patient with CHF?
2. What are effective ways of promoting optimum sleep-rest patterns in a patient with end-stage CHF?
3. What preoperative teaching methods are most effective in assisting the patient to prepare for a second open heart surgical procedure?
4. What are the psychoemotional needs of a spouse of an open heart surgical patient preoperatively and 2 months postoperatively?
5. How does quality of life change with time in a patient on a long-term ventricular assist device?

When the ventricle improves or transplantation occurs, the patient is taken to the operating room, where the VAD is removed. Cannula sites are packed and wounds are closed. Usual wound care is followed after the patient is returned to the ICU. Ideally this patient population recovers either through ventricular improvement or transplantation. However, many patients die. Nursing care should include the family as much as possible. Social workers and clergy should also be notified to help with family and friends.

The results of mechanical circulatory assist device use, at this relatively early phase in the development of these devices, have been encouraging. With the development of new mechanical pumps that will act as biologic donor hearts and as cardiac replacements, nursing care will be a challenge.

REVIEW QUESTIONS

1. Which of the following is not a manifestation of systolic ventricular failure?

a. Decreased ejection fraction
b. Increased PCWP
c. Increased fluid accumulation in the lungs
d. Decreased afterload

2. All of the following are compensatory mechanisms involved in CHF *except*

a. ventricular hypertrophy.
b. decreased sympathetic nervous system activation.
c. ventricular dilatation.
d. increased aldosterone secretion.

3. The goals of therapy for CHF include all of the following *except*

a. improve LV function.
b. decrease intravascular volume.
c. increase venous return.
d. treat the underlying cause.

4. In the management of a patient with acute pulmonary edema, which medication will reduce anxiety and improve oxygenation?

a. Morphine
b. Aminophylline
c. Amrinone
d. Dobutamine

5. Dilated cardiomyopathy is associated with

a. cardiomegaly with ventricular dilatation.
b. genetic basis.
c. atrial atrophy.
d. ventricular hyperplasia.

6. Which of the following does not accurately describe cardiac transplanation?

a. The most common complications are rejection and infection.
b. HLA-tissue typing is not important to decrease rejection episodes.
c. Endomyocardial biopsies are an important method to monitor possible rejection.
d. Surgical procedure involves removing all of recipient's own heart.

7. Common postoperative complications following cardiac surgery that the nurse needs to be aware of include all of the following *except*

a. hypovolemia.
b. fever.
c. hepatitis.
d. dysrhythmias.

8. The indications for the use of VADs include all of the following *except* the patient

a. is unconscious and unresponsive.
b. is awaiting cardiac transplantation.
c. has cardiogenic shock caused by an acute MI.
d. is unable to be weaned from cardiopulmonary bypass after open heart procedure.

REFERENCES

1. Committee to Evaluate the Artificial Heart Program; National Heart, Lung, and Blood Institute: *The artificial heart,* Washington, DC, 1991, National Academy Press.
2. American Heart Association: *1993 heart and stroke facts,* Dallas, 1992, National Center of the American Heart Association.
3. Funk M: Epidemiology of congestive heart failure, *Crit Care Nurs Clin North Am* 5:569, 1993.
4. Assey M: Heart disease in the elderly, *Heart Disease Stroke* 2:330, 1993.
5. Kannel WB, Plehn JF, and Cupples LA: Cardiac failure and sudden death in the Framingham study, *Am Heart J* 115:869, 1988.
6. National Heart, Lung, and Blood Institute: *Morbidity and mortality: chart book on cardiovascular, lung, and blood diseases,* Bethesda, MD, 1992, US Department of Health and Human Services.
7. Ghali JK, Cooper R, Ford E: Trends in hospitalization rates for heart failure in the United States, 1973-1986, *Arch Intern Med* 150:769, 1990.
8. Pitt B, Cohn JN, Franis GS: The effect of treatment on survival in congestive heart failure, *Clin Cardiol* 15:323, 1992.
9. Braunwald E, Grossman W: Clinical aspects of heart failure. In Braunwald E, editor: *Heart disease,* ed 4, Philadelphia, 1992, WB Saunders.
10. Conti RC: Ventricular diastolic dysfunction: clinical relevance, *Clin Cardiol* 15:399, 1992.
11. Cody RJ: Pharmacology of angiotensin-converting enzyme inhibitors as a guide to their use in congestive heart failure, *Am J Cardiol* 66:7D, 1990.
12. Muir AL, Nolan J: Modulation of venous tone in heart failure, *Am Heart J* 121:1948, 1991.
13. Kikin ML: Vasodilator therapy and survival in chronic congestive heart failure, *J Am Coll Cardiol* 19:1360, 1992.
14. Moser DK: Pharmacological management of heart failure: neurohormonal agents, *Crit Care Nurs Clin North Am* 5:599, 1993.
15. Nolan J and others: Acute effects of intravenous phosphodiesterase inhibition in chronic heart failure: simultaneous pre- and afterload reduction with a single agent, *Int J Cardiol* 35:3443, 1992.
16. Pratt NG: Neurohormonal response to ventricular failure: pharmacologic management, *J Cardiovasc Nurs* 8:49, 1993.
17. Cohn JN: Future directions in vasodilator therapy for heart failure, *Am Heart J* 121:969, 1991.
18. Cohn JN: The prevention of heart failure: a new agenda, *N Engl J Med* 327:725, 1992.
19. Purcell JA: Advances in the treatment of dilated cardiomyopathy. *AACN Clinical Issues in Critical Care Nursing,* 1:31, 1990.
20. Purcell JA, Holder CK: Cardiomyopathy, understanding the problem, *Am J Nurs* 89:59, 1989.
21. White-Williams C: Cardiomyopathy. In Kinney MR and others, editors: *Comprehensive cardiac care,* ed 7, Philadelphia, 1992, Mosby.
22. Bergstrom DL, Keller C: Drug-induced myocardial ischemia and acute myocardial infarction, *Crit Care Nurs Clin North Am* 4:273, 1992.
23. *1993 heart and stroke facts,* Dallas, 1993, The American Heart Association.
24. Lembo N, King S: Randomized trials of percutaneous transluminal coronary angioplasty, coronary artery bypass grafting or medical therapy in patients with coronary artery disease, *Coron Artery Dis* 1:449, 1990.
25. Kirklin JW and others: Guidelines and indications for coronary artery bypass graft surgery, ACC/AHA Task Force Report, *J Am Coll Cardiol* 17:543, 1991.
26. Horvath K and others: Favorable results of coronary artery bypass grafting in patients older than 75 years, *J Thorac Cardiovasc Surg* 99:92, 1990.
27. Starr A, Edwards MC: Mitral replacement: clinical experience with a ball-valve prosthesis, *Ann Surg* 154:726, 1961.
28. Vargo R, Dimengo JM: Surgical alternative for patients with heart failure, *AACN Clin Issues Crit Care Nurs* 4:244, 1993.
29. Quaal S: *Cardiac mechanical assistance beyond balloon pumping,* St Louis, 1993, Mosby.
30. Shively M, Verderber A, Fitzsimmons L: Caring for patients with ventricular assist devices, *J Cardiovasc Nurs* 8:91, 1994.

Chapter 33

NURSING ROLE IN MANAGEMENT

Dysrhythmias

Carolyn I. Johns

Learning Objectives

1. Identify the clinical characteristics and electrocardiographic patterns of common dysrhythmias.
2. Describe the therapeutic and nursing management of common dysrhythmias.
3. Differentiate between defibrillation and cardioversion, identifying indications for use and physiologic effects.
4. Describe the management of patients with temporary and permanent pacemakers.
5. Describe the management of a patient with an implantable cardioverter-defibrillator or a pacing cardioverter-defibrillator.
6. Explain the management of a patient undergoing electrophysiologic testing and radiofrequency catheter ablation therapy.
7. Explain the essential elements of Basic Cardiac Life Support.
8. Explain the essential elements of Advanced Cardiac Life Support.

DYSRHYTHMIA IDENTIFICATION AND TREATMENT

The ability to recognize *dysrhythmias,* which are abnormal cardiac rhythms, is an essential skill for the nurse. Prompt assessment of an abnormal cardiac rhythm and the patient's response to the rhythm is critical. This chapter describes basic principles of common dysrhythmias. For more information on dysrhythmias, the reader should refer to detailed texts on electrocardiographic (ECG) interpretation.[1-4] (The normal function of the electrical system of the heart is discussed in Chapter 29.) Therapeutic and nursing management of dysrhythmias, described in this chapter, includes drug therapy, pacemaker therapy, and principles of basic and advanced cardiac life support.

Conduction System: A Brief Review

There are four properties of cardiac tissue enabling the conduction system to initiate an electrical impulse, which is transmitted through the cardiac tissue stimulating muscle contraction (Table 33-1). The conduction system of the heart consists of specialized neuromuscular tissue located throughout the heart (see Fig. 29-5). Initiation of a normal cardiac impulse is begun in the *sinoatrial* (SA) *node* in the upper right atrium and is transmitted over the atrial myocardium via Bachmann's bundle and internodal pathways to the *atrioventricular* (AV) *node.* From the AV node, the impulse spreads through the bundle of His and down the left and right bundle branches, emerging in the Purkinje's fibers, which distribute the impulse to the ventricles.

Conduction to the point just before the impulse leaves the Purkinje's fibers takes place within the time of the PR interval of the ECG. When the impulse emerges from the Purkinje's fibers, ventricular depolarization occurs, producing mechanical contraction of the ventricles and the QRS complex on the ECG. The electrical activity of the heart is illustrated in Fig. 29-6.

Nervous Control of the Heart

The autonomic nervous system plays an important role in the rate of impulse formation, the speed of conduction, and

Table 33-1 Properties of Cardiac Tissue

Automaticity	Ability to initiate an impulse spontaneously and continuously
Contractility	Ability to respond mechanically to an impulse
Conductivity	Ability to transmit an impulse along a membrane in an orderly manner
Excitability	Ability to be electrically stimulated

Reviewed by Sandi Martin, RN, BSN, CCRN, Nurse Manager, Medical and Coronary Intensive Care, University of Utah Hospital, Salt Lake City, UT.

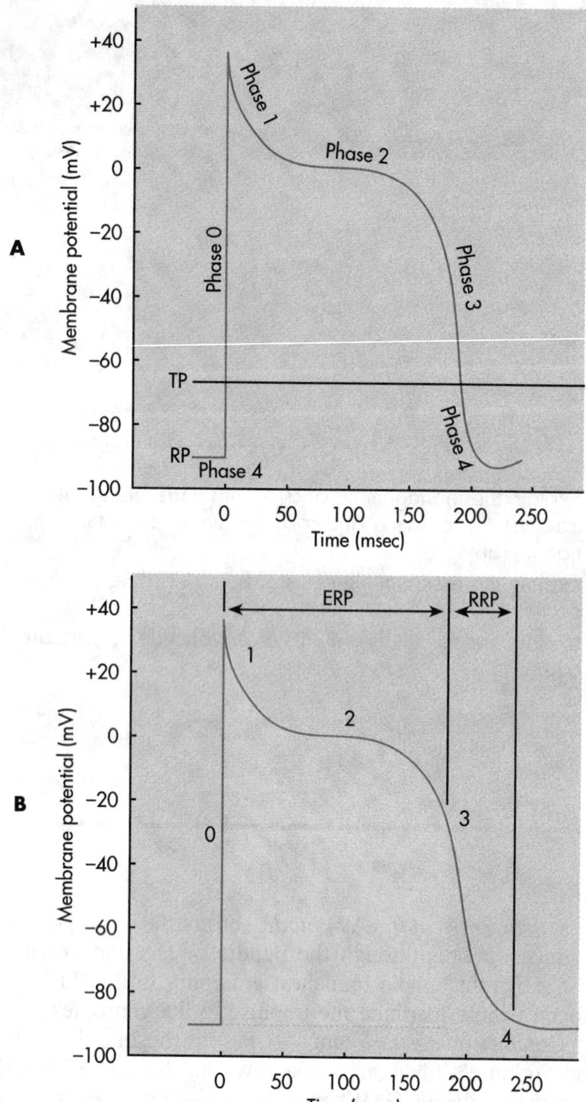

Fig. 33-1 ***A,*** Phases of the cardiac action potential. The electrical potential, measured in *mV,* is indicated along the vertical axis of the graph. Time, measured in milliseconds (*msec*), is indicated along the horizontal axis. The action potential consists of three to five phases, labeled as phase *0* through phase *4.* Each phase represents a particular electrical event or combination of electrical events. The events, the duration of the events and action potential, and the transmembrane potential vary with the type of cardiac cell being measured. ***B,*** Two parts of the refractory period. The effective refractory period (ERP) extends from phase 0 to approximately −60 mV in phase 3. The remainder of the action potential is the relative refractory period (RRP). *RP,* Resting potential; *TP,* threshold potential.

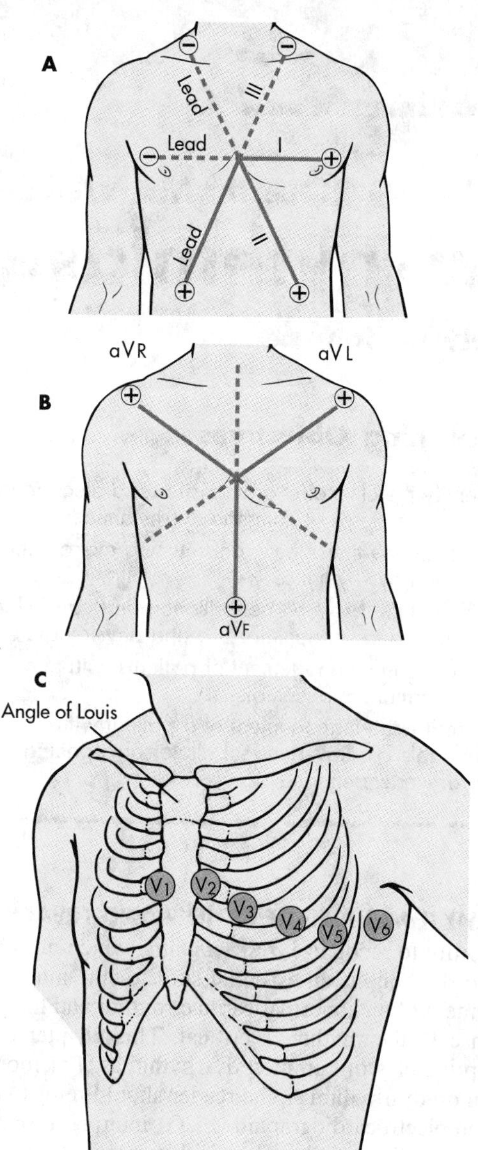

Fig. 33-2 ***A,*** Limb leads I, II, and III. Leads are located on the extremities. Illustrated are the angles from which these leads view the heart. ***B,*** Lead placement for augmented limb leads aVR , aVL , and aVF . These unipolar leads use the calculated center of the heart as their negative electrode. ***C,*** Lead placement for the chest electrodes: V_1 , fourth intercostal space at the right sternal border; V_2 , fourth intercostal space at the left sternal border; V_3, equidistant between V_2 and V_4 ; V_4 , fifth intercostal space at the left midclavicular line; V_5 , anterior axillary line and same horizontal level as V_4 ; V_6 , midaxillary line and same horizontal level as V_4.

the strength of cardiac contraction. The specific components of the autonomic nervous system that affect the heart are the right and left vagus nerve fibers of the parasympathetic fibers and the sympathetic nerves.

Stimulation of the vagus nerve causes a decreased rate of firing of the SA node, slowed impulse conduction of the AV node, and decreased force of cardiac muscle contraction. Stimulation of the sympathetic nerves that supply the heart has essentially the opposite effect on the heart.

Electrocardiogram Monitoring

The ECG is a graphic tracing of the electrical impulses produced in the heart. The deflections on the ECG are produced by the movement of charged ions across the

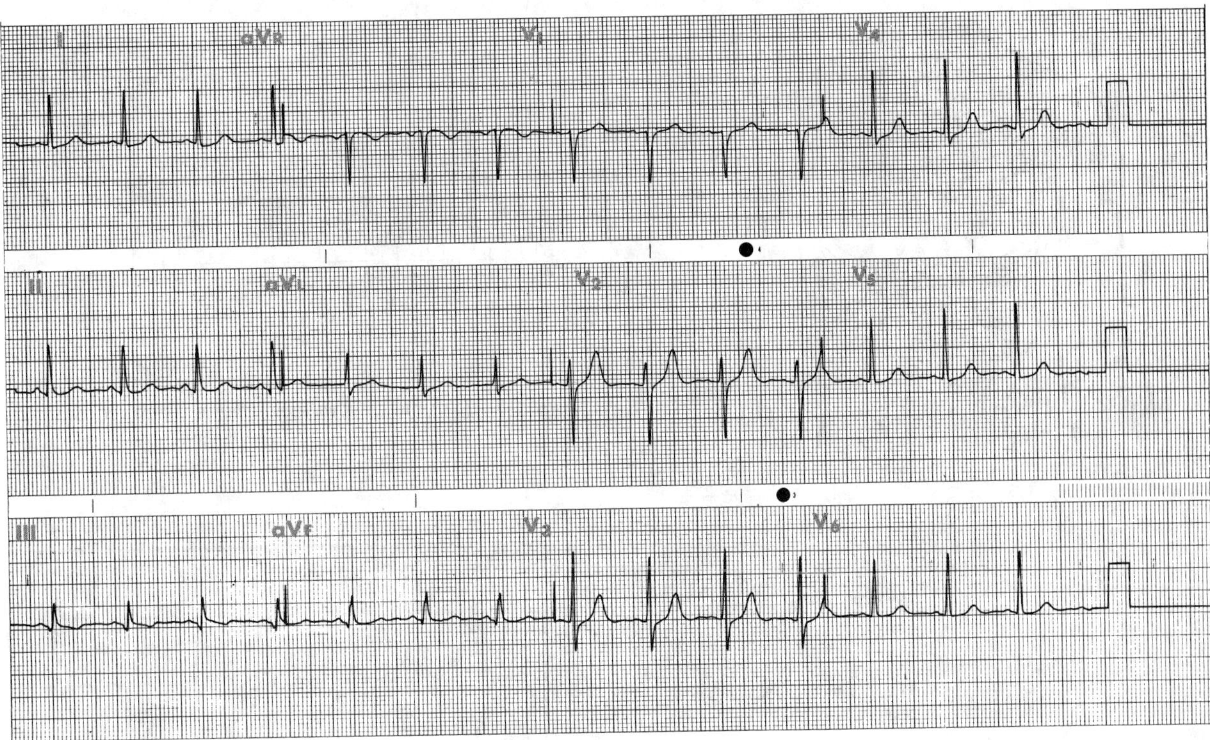

Fig. 33-3 Twelve-lead electrocardiogram showing a normal sinus rhythm.

membranes of myocardial cells, representing depolarization and repolarization.

The membrane of a cardiac cell is semipermeable, allowing it to maintain a high concentration of potassium and a low concentration of sodium inside the cell. A high concentration of sodium and a low concentration of potassium are maintained outside the cell. The inside of the cell when at rest, or in the *polarized* state, is negative compared with the outside. When a cell or groups of cells are stimulated, each cell membrane changes its permeability and allows sodium to migrate rapidly into the cell, making the cell positive compared with the outside (*depolarization*). A slower movement of ions across the membrane restores the cell to the polarized state, which is called *repolarization.* In Fig. 33-1, the phases are as follows: phase 4 is a polarized state; phase 0 is the upstroke of rapid depolarization; and phase 1, 2, and 3 represent repolarization. When antidysrhythmic drugs are used in a clinical setting, a nurse's understanding of the ionic shifts in the cardiac cell and the action potential mechanism is important. Antidysrhythmic drugs have a direct effect on the action potential.

Conventionally there are 12 recording leads in the ECG. Six of the 12 ECG leads measure electrical forces in the frontal plane (leads I, II, III, aVR, aVL, and aVF) (Fig. 33-2), and the remaining six leads (V_1 through V_6) measure the electrical forces in the horizontal plane (precordial lead sites). The 12-lead ECG may show changes that are indicative of structural changes or damage such as ischemia, infarction, enlarged cardiac chambers, electrolyte imbalance, or drug toxicity.[2] Obtaining 12 views of the heart that show cardiac rhythm is also helpful in the assessment of dysrhythmias. An example of a normal 12-lead ECG appears in Fig. 33-3.

When a patient's ECG is being continuously monitored, one or two single ECG leads are used. The most common leads used are lead II and lead MCL_1, which corresponds to V_1 in the standard 12-lead ECG (Fig. 33-4). These leads most clearly demonstrate the P wave and QRS complexes.

The ECG can be visualized continuously on a monitor oscilloscope. A recording of the ECG "strip" is done on ECG paper attached to the monitor. This provides documentation of the patient's rhythms and a means for thoroughly assessing and documenting dysrhythmias.

It is essential to know how to measure time and voltage on the ECG paper to correctly interpret an ECG. ECG paper consists of large (heavy lines) and small (light lines) squares (Fig. 33-5). Each large square incorporates 25 smaller squares (five horizontal and five vertical). Each small square represents 0.04 second horizontally and 0.1 mV vertically. This means that the large square equals 0.20 second and that 300 large squares equal 1.0 minute. Vertically, one large square is equal to 0.5 mV. These squares are used to calculate the heart rate (HR) and intervals between different ECG complexes.

A variety of ways can be used to calculate the HR from an ECG. Probably the most accurate way is to count the number of QRS complexes in a 1-minute time

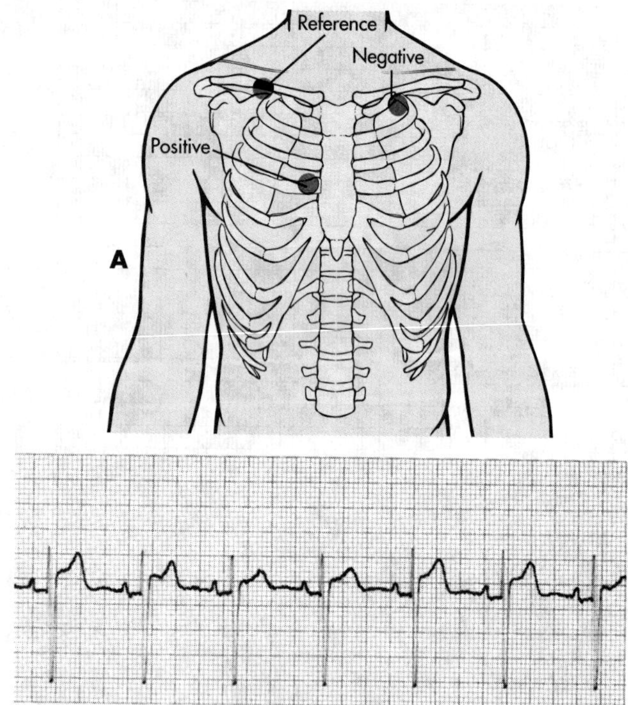

Fig. 33-4 ***A,*** Lead placement for MCL_1. ***B,*** Typical electrocardiogram tracing in lead MCL_1.

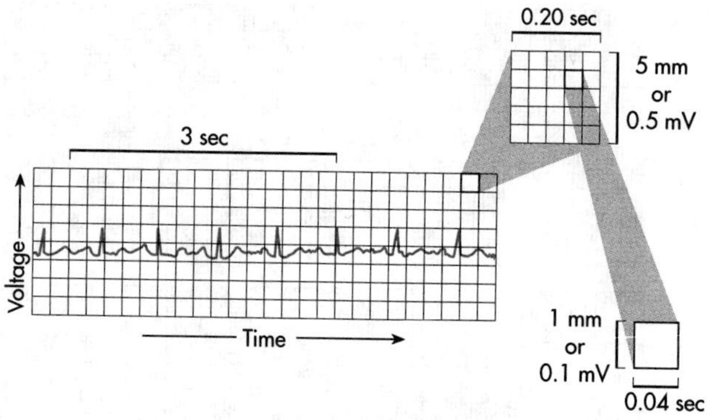

Fig. 33-5 Time and voltage on the electrocardiogram.

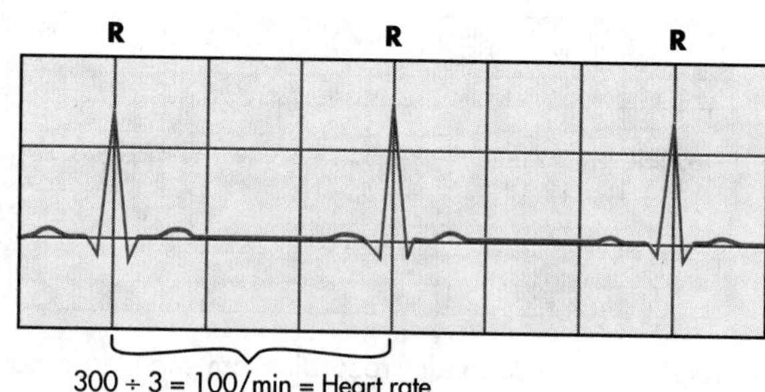

Fig. 33-6 When the rhythm is regular, heart rate can be determined at a glance.

interval; however, this method is cumbersome and time consuming. If the rhythm is regular, a simpler process can be used. Every 3 seconds a marker appears on the ECG paper. The nurse can count the number of QRS complexes in a 6-second interval and multiply that number by 10. This will yield the number of complexes or beats per minute (bpm).

Another rapid method for calculating the HR when a regular rhythm is present is to count the number of small squares between two QRS complexes (R-R interval). An R wave is the first upward deflection of the QRS complex. The nurse divides 1500 by the number of small squares to get the precise HR. This method is accurate only if the rhythm is regular.

The nurse can also count the number of large squares between two R waves and divide into 300 (Fig. 33-6). This method is also only accurate if the rhythm is regular.

An additional way to measure distances on the ECG grid is to use calipers. Calipers are used for fine measurements, especially for those components of a specific wave. Many times a P or R wave will not fall directly on a light or heavy line. The fine points of the calipers can be placed exactly on the components to be measured and then moved to another part of the grid for time measurement, which is accurate to 0.04 second.

ECG leads are attached to the patient's chest wall via an electrode pad fixed with electrical conductive paste. For best contact, hair on the chest wall should be shaved and skin should be prepared with acetone to remove excess oil and debris. In the case of a diaphoretic patient, benzoin may be applied to the skin before electrode placement. If leads and electrodes are not firmly placed, or if there is muscle activity or electrical interference from an outside source, an artifact may be seen on the monitor. An *artifact* is a distortion of the baseline and waveforms seen on the ECG (Fig. 33-7). Accurate interpretation of cardiac rhythm is difficult when artifact is present.

Telemetry Monitoring

Telemetry monitoring is the observation of a patient's HR and rhythm that is used for the diagnosis of dysrhythmias.[5] There are two types of systems used for detecting dysrhythmias by telemetry. The first type, a centralized monitoring system, requires a nurse or telemetry technician to constantly be observing all patients' rhythms at a central location. The second and most updated system of telemetry monitoring does not require constant nurse or technician surveillance. These systems have the capability of detecting and storing data on the type and frequency of dysrhythmias. Sophisticated alarm systems provide different levels of detection of dysrhythmias depending on the severity of the dysrhythmia. If used properly, these systems free the nurse from constant observation of monitors, while providing high-level dysrhythmia detection.[5]

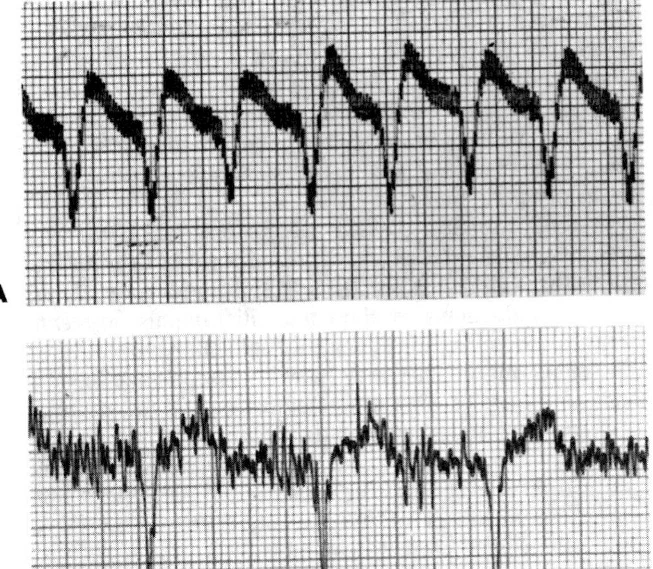

Fig. 33-7 ***A,*** Artifact—60-cycle interference. ***B,*** Artifact—muscular movement.

Assessment of Cardiac Rhythm

When assessing the cardiac rhythm the nurse must make an accurate interpretation of a dysrhythmia and immediately proceed to evaluate the consequences of that dysrhythmia for the individual patient. Assessment of the patient's hemodynamic response to a dysrhythmia provides guidance in therapeutic intervention. If possible, a determination of the cause of the dysrhythmia should be made. Tachycardias may cause a decrease in cardiac output (CO) and possible hypotension. Certain dysrhythmias may precipitate more life-threatening dysrhythmias.[6] The patient, not just the dysrhythmia, must be treated.

Normal sinus rhythm refers to the normal conduction pattern of the cardiac cycle, which originates in the SA node (Fig. 33-8). Figure 33-9 shows the normal electrical pattern of the cardiac cycle. Table 33-2 provides a description of ECG intervals and the significance of disturbances. The P wave represents the depolarization of the atrium (passage of an electrical impulse through the atrial muscle), resulting in atrial contraction. The QRS complex represents depolarization of the ventricles, resulting in ventricular contraction. The T wave represents repolarization of the ventricles, or the time at which the ventricles return to the prestimulated state. The PR interval represents the period during which the impulse spreads through the atria, AV node, bundle of His, and Purkinje fibers. The QRS interval represents the time it takes for depolarization of both ventricles. The QT interval represents the time it takes for complete depolarization and repolarization of the ventricles.

Electrophysiologic Mechanisms of Dysrhythmias

Disorders of impulse formation can initiate dysrhythmias. The heart has specialized cells found in the sinus node, parts of the atria, the AV node, and the His-Purkinje system, which are able to discharge spontaneously. This is called *automaticity.* Normally the main pacemaker of the heart is the sinus node, which spontaneously discharges at 60 to 100 times per minute (Table 33-3). A pacemaker from another site may be discharged in two ways. If the SA node discharges more slowly than a secondary or latent pacemaker, the electrical discharges from the secondary pacemaker may passively *escape* and discharge automatically at their intrinsic rates. These secondary pacemakers may originate from the AV node or the His-Purkinje system at rates of 40 to 60 times per minute and 30 to 40 times per minute, respectively. A second means by which latent pacemakers can originate occurs when the discharge rate is accelerated abnormally and other "pacemakers" take control of the sinus node. A premature beat or a series of premature beats can then occur from *ectopic foci* (abnormal cardiac impulse) in the atria, ventricles, or AV junction.

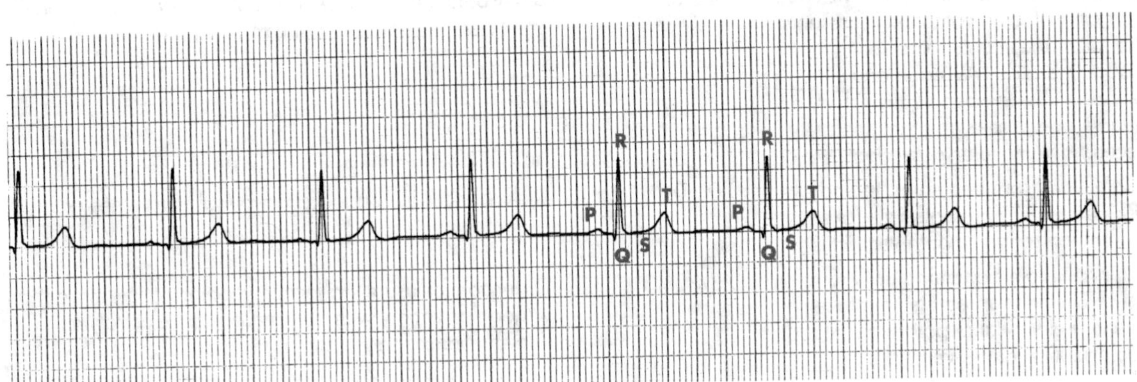

Fig. 33-8 Normal sinus rhythm in lead II.

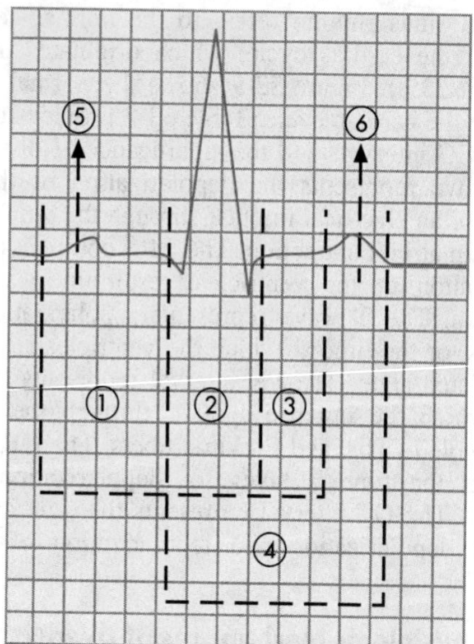

Fig. 33-9 The electrocardiogram complex as seen in a normal sinus rhythm. *1*, PR interval (normal is 0.12-0.20 sec); *2*, QRS complex (normal is 0.06-0.10 sec); *3*, ST segment (normal is 0.12 sec); *4*, QT interval (normal is 0.34-0.43 sec); *5*, P wave (normal is 0.06-0.12 sec); *6*, T wave (normal is 0.16 sec).

The impulse initiated by a pacemaker focus must be conducted to the entire heart chamber. The property of myocardial tissue that enables it to be depolarized by a stimulus is called *excitability.* This is an important part of the propagation of the impulse from one fiber to another. The level of excitability is determined by the length of time after depolarization during which the tissues can be restimulated. The recovery period after stimulation is called the *refractory phase* or *period.* The *absolute refractory phase* or *period* occurs when excitability is zero and heart tissue cannot be stimulated. The *relative refractory period* occurs slightly later in the cycle, and excitability improves. In states of full excitability, the heart is completely recovered. Figure 33-10 shows the relationship between the refractory period and the ECG.

If conduction is depressed and if some areas of the heart are blocked, the unblocked areas are activated earlier than the blocked areas. When the block is unidirectional, this uneven conduction may allow the initial impulse to *reenter* areas that were previously not excitable but have recovered. The reentering impulse may be able to depolarize the atria and ventricles, causing a premature beat. If the *reentrant excitation* continues, tachycardia occurs.

Dysrhythmias occur as the result of various abnormalities and disease states.[7] The cause of a dysrhythmia influences the treatment of the patient. Common causes of dysrhythmias are presented in Table 33-4.

Dysrhythmias occurring in out-of-hospital settings present problems of management. Determination of the rhythm by cardiac monitoring is a high priority. Emergency care of the patient with a dysrhythmia is outlined in Table 33-5. If indicated, the emergency medical system (EMS) is activated after the patient has been assessed.

Evaluation of Dysrhythmias

In addition to continuous ECG monitoring during hospitalization, several other methods are used to evaluate cardiac dysrhythmias and the effectiveness of antidysrhythmic drug therapy. An electrophysiology test (an invasive method) and Holter monitoring, exercise treadmill testing, and signal-averaged ECG (all noninvasive methods) can be performed on both an inpatient and an outpatient basis.

Table 33-2 Definition and Significance of Electrocardiogram Intervals*

Description	Duration (sec)	Significance of Disturbance
PR interval: From beginning of P wave to beginning of QRS complex; represents time taken for impulse to spread through the atria, AV node and bundle of His, the bundle branches, and Purkinje fibers, to a point immediately preceding ventricular activation	0.12-0.20	Disturbance in conduction usually in AV node, bundle of His, or bundle branches but can be in atria as well
QRS interval: From beginning to end of QRS complex; represents time taken for depolarization of both ventricles	0.06-0.10	Disturbance in conduction in bundle branches or in ventricles
QT interval: From beginning of QRS to end of T wave; represents time taken for entire electrical depolarization and repolarization of the ventricles	0.34-0.43	Disturbances usually affecting repolarization more than depolarization such as drug effects, electrolyte disturbances, and rate changes

*HR influences the duration of these intervals, especially those of the PR and QT intervals.

Table 33-3 Rates of the Conduction System

SA node	60-100 times/min
AV junction	40-60 times/min
Purkinje fibers	20-40 times/min

AV, Atrioventricular; *SA,* sinoatrial.

Table 33-4 Common Causes of Dysrhythmias

Drug effects or toxicity	Coffee, tea, tobacco
Myocardial cell degeneration	Electrolyte imbalances
Hypertrophy of cardiac muscle	Cellular hypoxia
Emotional crisis	Edema
Connective tissue disorders	Acid-base imbalances
Alcohol	Myocardial ischemia
	Degeneration of the conduction system

Electrophysiologic (EPS) testing is performed to identify different mechanisms of tachydysrhythmias as well as heart blocks, bradydysrhythmias, and dysrhythmic causes of syncope.[8] It can also be used to identify locations of accessory pathways and to determine the effectiveness of antidysrhythmic drugs. It involves introducing several electrode catheters transvenously to the right side of the heart with fluoroscopic guidance. Electrical stimulation to various areas of the atrium and ventricle is performed, and the inducibility of dysrhythmias is determined. This is a fairly unpleasant experience for most patients because ventricular tachycardia or ventricular fibrillation is often induced, and cardioversion and defibrillation are performed to convert the rhythm. Types of "near death" experiences have been reported by some patients. Emotional support by the nurse to the patient who has experienced this is important. Nursing care before and after the procedure is similar to that for cardiac catheterization. (EPS testing is also discussed in Chapter 29.)

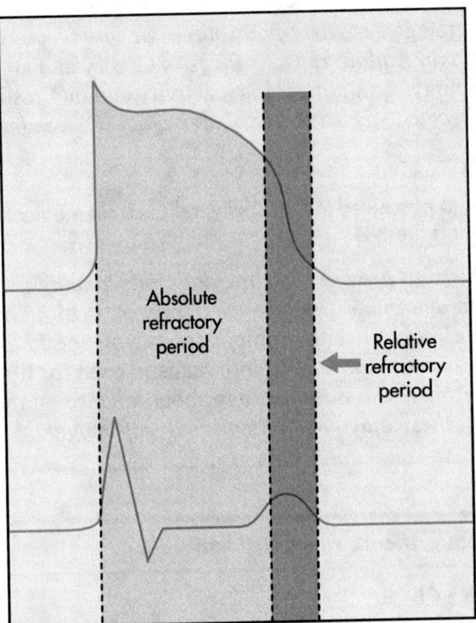

Fig. 33-10 Absolute and relative refractory periods correlated with the cardiac muscle's action potential and with an ECG tracing.

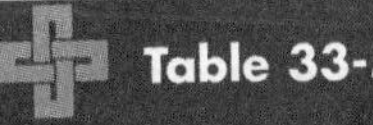

Table 33-5 Emergency Management: Dysrhythmia

Possible Etiologies

Poisoning, myocardial infarction, CHF, pulmonary disorders, drowning, electrolyte imbalances, shock, stress, drugs, electric shock, conduction defects

Possible Assessment Findings

Irregular HR and rhythm, palpitations
Chest, neck, shoulder, or arm pain
Dizziness, syncope
Dyspnea
Extreme restlessness
Decreased level of consciousness
Feeling of impending doom
Numbness, tingling of arms
Weakness and fatigue
Cold, clammy skin
Diaphoresis
Pallor
Nausea and vomiting

Management

- Establish and maintain airway. Anticipate need for intubation if respiratory distress evident.
- Administer O_2 via nasal cannula.
- Establish IV line with large-gauge needle.
- Apply cardiac electrodes and monitor patient's cardiac rhythm. Calculate HR. Determine regularity of rhythm.
- If cardiac rhythm is abnormal, report to physician and await drug orders.
- Be prepared to initiate CPR and defibrillation.
- Monitor vital signs including level of consciousness.
- Reassure patient. Provide calm environment.

CHF, Congestive heart failure; *CPR,* cardiopulmonary resuscitation; *HR,* heart rate; *IV,* intravenous.

NURSING CARE PLAN Patient with Dysrhythmias

Planning: Outcome Criteria	Nursing Interventions and Rationales
➤ **NURSING DIAGNOSIS**	Decreased CO *related to* dysrhythmias *as manifested by* sudden drop in BP, atrial or ventricular rate >100/min or <40/min, decreased mentation, chest pain, dyspnea, oliguria
Maintain mean arterial pressure >70 mm Hg, cardiac index >2 L/min, urine output >30 ml/hr; have cardiac rate and rhythm within normal limits; have normal mentation.	Assess ECG continuously for rhythm, rate, PR, QRS, and QT intervals to *monitor cardiac status.* Monitor vital signs. Assess and document excessive fatigue, activity intolerance, dyspnea, orthopnea, palpitations, chest pain, lightheadedness, dizziness and nausea as *subjective evidence of hemodynamic status.* Assess and document pulse rate and regularity, BP status, respiratory status (crackles, rhonchi, wheezing), heart sounds (murmurs, gallops), edema of extremities and sacrum, skin (diaphoretic, cool) as *objective evidence of hemodynamic status.* Use IV drugs, CPR, etc. per unit protocol *to treat dysrhythmias and sustain adequate CO.* Maintain at least one patent IV site *as vascular access for IV medications.* Provide supplemental oxygen as required *to maintain adequate tissue saturation.* Monitor serum electrolytes including potassium and magnesium *because high or low levels may exacerbate dysrhythmias.*
➤ **NURSING DIAGNOSIS**	Activity intolerance *related to* inadequate CO and medication effects *as manifested by* vertigo or syncope on position change, dyspnea on exertion, standing BP decreases >20 mm Hg, HR increases >20/min with positional change, ischemic pain
Maintain optimal activity level; have minimal changes in vital signs with return to baseline within 5 min of activity; experience no ischemic pain on activity; express increased comfort with activity.	Determine prehospital activity status *to provide baseline data for comparison with present activity status.* Assess respiratory and cardiac status before activity *to determine advisability of planned activity and provide baseline data for comparison with postactivity status.* Observe and document response to activity *to evaluate patient progress and plan future activity.* Encourage patient to assist in decision making about timing and level of activity *to foster self-care and sense of control.* Assess for medication side effects that affect activity (e.g., fatigue, dizziness, decreased myocardial contractility, exacerbation of dysrhythmias) *so medication or activity can be adjusted appropriately.*
➤ **NURSING DIAGNOSIS**	Fear *related to* development of life-threatening cardiac situation *as manifested by* refusal to move or participate in care, need for constant attention, asking many or no questions, intense focus on cardiac monitoring, poor attention span
Express understanding of treatment plan; have realistic expectations of outcome; participate in treatment plan; express increased psychologic and physiologic comfort; identify coping strategies.	Assess patient's coping ability and strategies *to identify resources or problems.* Encourage talking about feelings *so patient can explore reasons for fear.* Clarify and answer questions about cardiovascular pathology, symptomatology, activity and diet restrictions, medications, and procedures *because accurate knowledge often reduces fear.*
➤ **NURSING DIAGNOSIS**	Risk for body-image disturbance *related to* perceived vulnerability, reliance on medication and pacemaker, and necessity for adjusting lifestyle
Have accurate understanding of health problem and treatment plan; accept lifestyle adjustments.	Assess understanding of health problem *to provide baseline data for planning patient education.* Assess past body image *to determine significance of present health problem on patient's self-perception.* Discuss effect of health problem on body image *to assist clarification of feelings and accuracy of perception.* Explore realistic need for lifestyle changes *to prevent unnecessary adjustments.* Assess feelings about reliance on medication or pacemaker *to determine effect these may have on patient's self-image.*

COLLABORATIVE PROBLEMS

Nursing Goal	Nursing Interventions and Rationales
➤ **POTENTIAL COMPLICATION**	Cardiac arrest *related to* inadequate CO
Monitor for signs of significant cardiac dysrhythmias, report deviations from acceptable parameters; carry out appropriate medical and nursing interventions.	Assess for and recognize immediately cardiac dysrhythmias that can result in cardiac arrest. Initiate ACLS procedures according to unit protocol.

ACLS, Advanced Cardiac Life Support; *BP,* blood pressure; *CO,* cardiac output; *CPR,* cardiopulmunary resuscitation; *IV,* intravenous.

Table 33-6 Characteristics of Common Dysrhythmias

Pattern	Rate and Rhythm	P Wave	PR Interval	QRS Complex
NSR	60-100 bpm and regular	Normal	Normal	Normal
Sinus bradycardia	<60 bpm and regular	Normal	Normal	Normal
Sinus tachycardia	>100 bpm and regular	Normal	Normal	Normal
PAC	Usually 60-100 bpm and irregular	Abnormal shape	Normal or variable	Normal (usually)
PSVT	100-300 bpm and regular	Abnormal shape, may be hidden	Variable	Normal (usually)
Atrial flutter	*Atrial:* 250-350 bpm and regular *Ventricular:* >100 bpm and irregular	Sawtooth	Variable	Normal (usually)
Atrial fibrillation	*Atrial:* 350-600 bpm and irregular *Ventricular:* >100 bpm and irregular or possibly any rate	Chaotic	Not measurable	Normal (usually)
Junctional rhythms	40-140 bpm and regular	Abnormal (may be hidden)	Variable	Normal (usually)
First-degree heart block	Normal and regular	Normal	>0.20 sec	Normal
Second-degree heart block				
Type I (Mobitz I, Wenckebach)	*Atrial:* Normal and regular *Ventricular:* Slower and irregular	Normal	Progressively lengthened	Normal QRS width, with pattern of one nonconducted QRS
Type II (Mobitz II)	*Atrial:* Usually normal and regular or irregular *Ventricular:* Slower and regular or irregular	P wave occurs in multiples	Normal or prolonged	Widened QRS, preceded by two or more P waves
Third-degree heart block	Ventricular rate 20-40 bpm and regular	Normal, but no connection with QRS complex	Variable	Normal or widened, no connection with P waves
PVC	60-100 bpm and irregular	Not usually present	Not measurable	Wide and distorted
Ventricular tachycardia	100-250 bpm and regular or irregular	Not usually present	Not measurable	Wide and distorted
Ventricular fibrillation	Not measurable and irregular	Absent	Not measurable	Not measurable

bpm, Beats per minute; *NSR,* normal sinus rhythm; *PAC,* premature atrial contraction; *PSVT,* paroxysmal supraventricular tachycardia; *PVC,* premature ventricular contraction.

The Holter monitor is a device that records the ECG while the patient is ambulatory.[7] The device can record heart rhythm for 24 to 48 hours while the patient performs daily activities. The patient maintains a diary in which activities and any symptoms are recorded. Events in the diary can later be correlated with any dysrhythmias observed on the recording. The monitor is generally a useful device for detecting significant dysrhythmias and evaluating drug efficacy during a patient's normal activities. It can also be used for detecting ischemia by analyzing ST segments. A limitation of the device is that the patient who has frequent ventricular dysrhythmias, some of which may be lethal, may not have these dysrhythmias during the monitored time. Many physicians believe that EPS testing is more reliable for the determination of malignant dysrhythmias.

The signal-averaged ECG (SAECG) is a high-resolution electrocardiogram used to identify the patient at risk for developing complex ventricular dysrhythmias. A computerized program and ECG machine are used for the test. The identification of electrical activity called late *potentials* on the SAECG strongly suggests that the patient is at risk for developing serious ventricular dysrhythmias.[9]

Exercise treadmill testing is used for evaluation of cardiac rhythm response to exercise. Exercise-induced dysrhythmias can be reproduced and analyzed, and drug therapy can be evaluated. These tests are performed with routine treadmill testing protocols.

Types of Dysrhythmias

When assessing a cardiac rhythm, a systematic approach must be used. The recommended approach is to note the rate, rhythm, P wave, QRS complex, relationship of P wave to QRS complex, PR interval, QRS interval, and QT interval. Questions to consider are: Are premature ventricular complexes present? Are escape beats present? What is the dominant rhythm? What is the clinical significance of the dysrhythmia? What is the treatment for the particular dysrhythmia? Examples of the ECG tracings of common dysrhythmias are presented in Figs. 33-11 through 33-20. Descriptive characteristics of common dysrhythmias are presented in Table 33-6.

Sinus Bradycardia. In sinus bradycardia, the conduction pathway is the same as that in sinus rhythm, but the sinus node discharges at a rate of less than 60 beats per minute (bpm) (See Fig. 33-11, *A*).

Clinical associations. Sinus bradycardia is a normal sinus rhythm in aerobically trained athletes and in other individuals during sleep. It occurs in response to carotid sinus massage, the Valsalva maneuver, hypothermia, increased intraocular pressure, increased vagal tone, and administration of parasympathomimetic drugs. Disease states associated with sinus bradycardia are hypothyroidism, increased intracranial pressure, obstructive jaundice, and inferior wall myocardial infarction (MI).

Electrocardiogram characteristics. In sinus bradycardia, **HR** is less than 60 bpm, and **rhythm** is regular. The **P wave** precedes each QRS complex and has a normal contour and a fixed interval. The **PR interval** is normal, and the **QRS complex** has a normal contour and normal length.

Significance. The clinical significance of sinus bradycardia depends on how the patient tolerates it hemodynamically. Hypotension with decreased CO may occur in some circumstances. An acute MI may predispose the heart to escape dysrhythmias and premature beats.

Treatment. Treatment consists of administration of atropine, an anticholinergic drug, for the patient with symptoms. Pacemaker therapy may be required.

Sinus Tachycardia. The conduction pathway is the same in sinus tachycardia as that in normal sinus rhythm. The discharge rate from the sinus node is increased as a result of vagal inhibition or sympathetic stimulation. The sinus rate is greater than 100 bpm (Fig. 33-11, *B*).

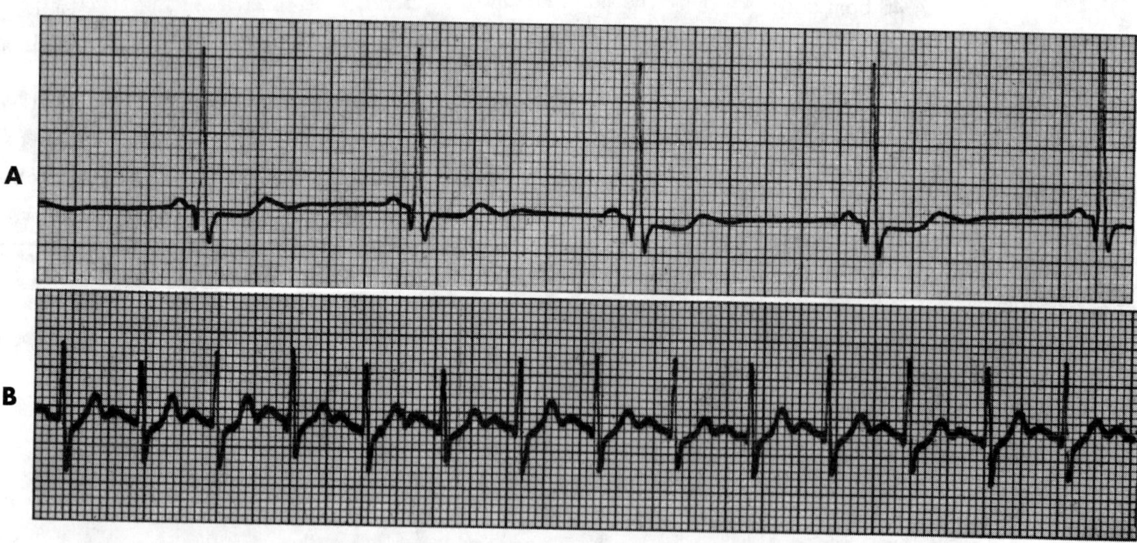

Fig. 33-11 ***A,*** Sinus bradycardia of 50 bpm. ***B,*** Sinus tachycardia of 140 bpm.

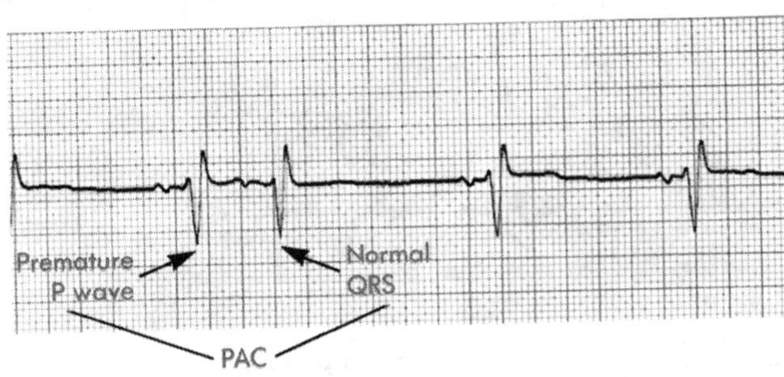

Fig. 33-12 Normally conducted premature atrial contraction (PAC). The early P wave is indicated by the *arrow*, and the QRS complex that follows is of normal shape and duration.

Clinical associations. Sinus tachycardia is associated with physiologic stressors such as exercise, fever, pain, hypotension, hypovolemia, anxiety, anemia, hypoxia, hypoglycemia, myocardial ischemia, congestive heart failure (CHF), and thyrotoxicosis. It can also be an effect of drugs such as epinephrine, norepinephrine, caffeine, atropine, theophylline, nifedipine, or hydralazine.

Electrocardiogram characteristics. In sinus tachycardia, **HR** is greater than 100 bpm, and **rhythm** is regular. The **P wave** is normal, precedes each QRS complex, and has a normal contour and fixed interval. The **PR interval** is normal, and the **QRS complex** has a normal contour.

Significance. The clinical significance of sinus tachycardia depends on the patient's tolerance of the increased HR. The patient may have symptoms of dizziness, and hypotension may occur. Increased myocardial oxygen consumption is associated with increased HR. Angina or an increase in infarct size may accompany persistent sinus tachycardia in the patient with an acute MI.

Treatment. Treatment is determined by underlying causes. In certain settings, β-blocker therapy (e.g., propranolol) is used to reduce HR and decrease myocardial oxygen consumption.

Premature Atrial Contraction. A premature atrial contraction (PAC) is a contraction originating from an ectopic focus in the atrium in a location other than the sinus node. It originates in the left or right atrium and travels across the atria by an abnormal pathway, creating a distorted P wave (Fig. 33-12). At the AV node, it is stopped (nonconducted PAC), delayed (lengthened PR interval), or conducted normally. It moves through the AV node, and in most cases it is conducted normally through the ventricles.

Clinical associations. In a normal heart, a PAC can result from emotional stress or the use of caffeine, tobacco, or alcohol. A PAC can also result from disease states such as infection, inflammation, hyperthyroidism, chronic obstructive pulmonary disease (COPD), heart disease (including atherosclerotic heart disease), valvular disease, and other diseases. A PAC can also be caused by enlarged atria.

Electrocardiogram characteristics. **HR** varies with the underlying rate and frequency of the PAC, and **rhythm** is irregular. The **P wave** has a different contour from that of a normal P wave. It may be notched or have negative deflection, or it may be hidden in the preceding T wave. The **PR interval** may be shorter or longer than a normal PR interval originating from the sinus node, but it is within normal limits. The **QRS complex** is usually normal. If the QRS interval is 0.10 second or longer, abnormal conduction through the ventricles is present.

Significance. A PAC may be a prelude to supraventricular tachycardias.

Treatment. Treatment depends on the patient's symptoms. Withdrawal of sources of stimulation such as caffeine may be warranted. Drugs such as digoxin, quinidine, procainamide, flecainide, and β-blockers can be used.

Paroxysmal Supraventricular Tachycardia. Paroxysmal supraventricular tachycardia (PSVT) is a dysrhythmia originating in an ectopic focus anywhere above the bifurcation of the bundle of His (Fig. 33-13). Identification of the ectopic focus is sometimes difficult with a 12-lead ECG. It occurs with the reentrant phenomenon (reexcitation of the atria when there is a one-way block). A run of repeated premature beats is initiated and is usually heralded by a PAC. *Paroxysmal* refers to an abrupt onset and termination. Termination is sometimes followed by a brief period of asystole. Some degree of AV block may be present. PSVT occurring via an accessory pathway is designated as *orthodromic* or *antidromic* tachycardia. *Orthodromic* refers to anterograde, or forward conduction through the AV node and retrograde, or backward conduction, through the accessory pathway. *Antidromic* refers to the opposite: anterograde conduction through the accessory pathway and retrograde conduction through the AV node.[7]

Clinical associations. In the normal heart, PSVT is associated with overexertion, emotional stress, changes of po-

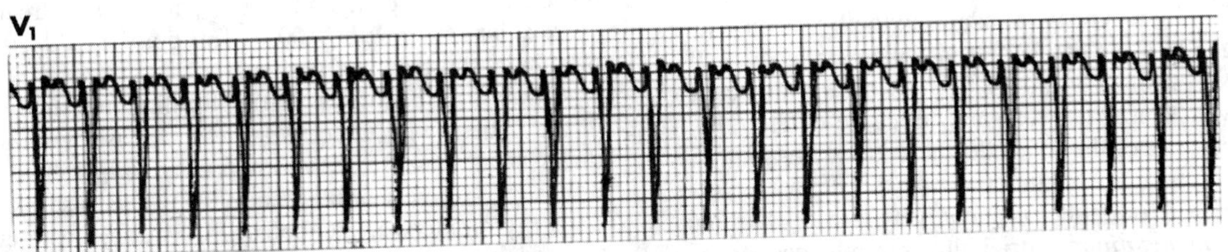

Fig. 33-13 A-V nodal reentrant paroxysmal supraventricular tachycardia with P wave at the end of the QRS complex.

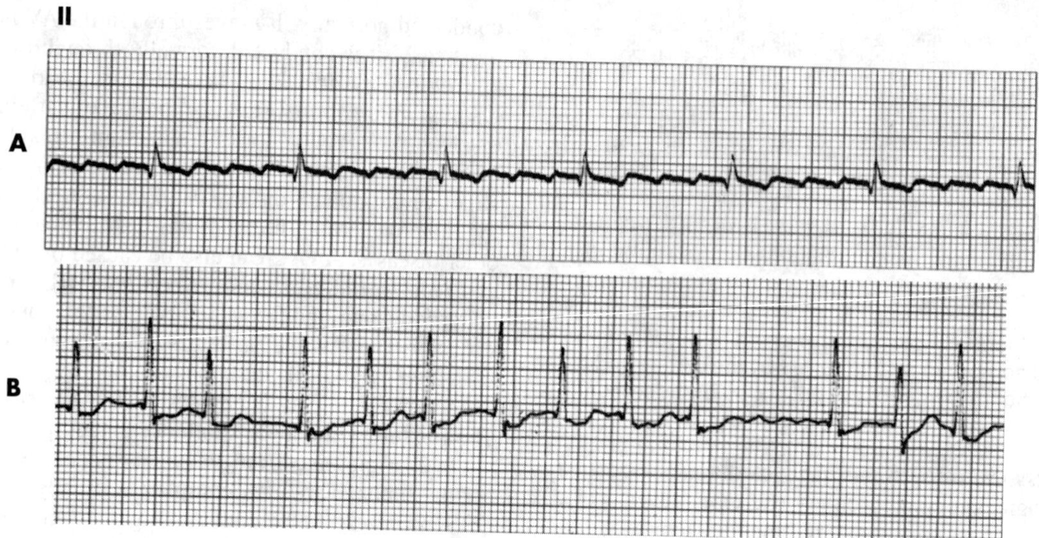

Fig. 33-14 ***A,*** Atrial flutter with a 4:1 conduction. ***B,*** Atrial fibrillation. Note the jagged, irregular baseline between the QRS complexes.

sition, deep inspiration, and stimulants such as caffeine and tobacco. In a disease state, PSVT is associated with rheumatic heart disease, Wolff-Parkinson-White (WPW) syndrome (conduction via accessory pathways), digitalis intoxication, coronary artery disease (CAD), or cor pulmonale.

Electrocardiogram characteristics. In PSVT, **HR** is 100 to 300 bpm, and **rhythm** is regular. The **P wave** is often hidden in the preceding T wave and has an abnormal contour. The **PR interval** may be prolonged, shortened, or normal, and the **QRS complex** may have a normal or abnormal contour.

Significance. The clinical significance of PSVT depends on symptoms and HR. A prolonged episode and HR greater than 180 bpm may precipitate a decreased CO with hypotension and myocardial ischemia.

Treatment. Treatment includes vagal stimulation and pharmacologic therapy. Vagal stimulation induced by carotid massage or the Valsalva maneuver may be used to treat PSVT. The drug of choice is adenosine, a drug with a short half-life (10 seconds) that successfully converts PSVT to sinus rhythm in a high percentage of patients.[7,10] Verapamil, diltiazem, digitalis, and propranolol can also be used. However, digitalis and calcium channel blockers can cause hemodynamic collapse in WPW syndrome. Persistent, recurring PSVT in WPW may ultimately be treated with radiofrequency catheter ablation of the accessory pathway.

Atrial Flutter. Atrial flutter is an atrial tachydysrhythmia identified by recurring, regular, sawtooth-shaped flutter waves (Fig. 33-14, *A*) and is best visualized in leads II, III, aVF, and V_1 on the 12-lead ECG. It is usually associated with a slower ventricular response. Because of the refractory characteristic of the AV node, there is usually some AV block in a fixed ratio of flutter waves to QRS complexes (e.g., 2:1, 3:1). Atrial flutter is a relatively rare dysrhythmia.

Clinical associations. Atrial flutter rarely occurs in a normal heart. In disease states, it is associated with CAD, hypertension, mitral valve disorders, pulmonary embolus, cor pulmonale, cardiomyopathy, hyperthyroidism, and the use of drugs such as digitalis, quinidine, and epinephrine.

Electrocardiogram characteristics. **Atrial rate** is 250 to 350 bpm. The **ventricular rate** varies according to the conduction ratio. In 2:1 conduction, the ventricular rate is typically found to be approximately 150 bpm. **Atrial rhythm** is regular, and **ventricular rhythm** is usually regular. The **P wave** is represented by sawtooth waves or F waves, the **PR interval** is variable, and the **QRS complex** is normal in contour.

Significance. High ventricular rates associated with atrial flutter can decrease CO and cause serious consequences such as heart failure, especially in the patient with underlying heart disease.

Treatment. The primary goal in treatment of atrial flutter is to slow the ventricular response by increasing AV block. Electrical cardioversion may be used to convert the atrial flutter to sinus rhythm in an emergency situation.[11] Drugs used include verapamil, digoxin, quinidine, procainamide, and β-blockers, as well as other antidysrhythmics.

Atrial Fibrillation. Atrial fibrillation is characterized by a total disorganization of atrial electrical activity without effective atrial contraction (Fig. 33-14, *B*). The ECG demonstrates baseline fibrillatory waves or undulations of variable contour at a rate of 300 to 600 per minute. Ventricular response is irregular, and if the patient is untreated, the ventricular rate will be 100 to 160 bpm. The dysrhythmia may be chronic or intermittent.

Clinical associations. Atrial fibrillation usually occurs in the patient with underlying heart disease, such as rheumatic heart disease, cardiomyopathy, hypertensive heart disease, CHF, pericarditis, and CAD. It is also associated with thyrotoxicosis, alcoholism, infection, gastroenteritis, and stress.

Electrocardiogram characteristics. During atrial fibrillation, **atrial rate** may be as high as 350 to 600 bpm.

Ventricular rate can vary from as low as 50 bpm to as high as 180 bpm. **Atrial rhythm** is chaotic, and **ventricular rhythm** is usually irregular. Ventricular rhythm may be regular if there is complete AV block (*ventricular escape rhythm*). The **P wave** shows fibrillatory waves, but no definite P wave can be observed. The **PR interval** is not measurable, and the **QRS complex** usually has a normal contour.

Significance. Atrial fibrillation can often result in a decrease in CO because of ineffective atrial contractions and a rapid ventricular response. Thrombi may form in the atria as a result of ineffective atrial contraction. Embolization to the arterial system may occur as a complication with subsequent development of a stroke.

Treatment. The goal of treatment is a decrease in ventricular response. In emergency situations, cardioversion may be used to convert atrial fibrillation to normal sinus rhythm. Medications used for pharmaceutical cardioversion or a decrease in ventricular response include digoxin, verapamil, diltiazem, quinidine, β-blockers, flecainide, propafenone, and sotalol.[12,13]

Junctional Dysrhythmia. Junctional rhythm refers to a dysrhythmia that originates in the area of the AV node. The impulse may move in a retrograde fashion that produces an abnormal P wave occurring just before or after the QRS complex or that is hidden in the QRS complex. The impulse usually moves normally through the ventricles. Junctional premature beats may occur, and they are treated in a manner similar to that for PACs. Other junctional dysrhythmias include *junctional escape rhythm* (Fig. 33-15), *accelerated junctional rhythm,* and *junctional tachycardia.* These dysrhythmias are treated according to the patient's tolerance of the rhythm and the circumstances.

Clinical associations. Junctional escape rhythm is often associated with the aerobically trained individual who has sinus bradycardia. It may occur with acute MI, especially inferior MI, and disease of the sinus node. Accelerated junctional rhythm and junctional tachycardia are observed with acute inferior MI, digitalis toxicity, and acute rheumatic fever and during open heart surgery.

Electrocardiogram characteristics. In junctional escape rhythm, **HR** is 40 to 60 bpm, in accelerated junctional rhythm it is 60 to 100 bpm, and in junctional tachycardia it is 100 to 140 bpm. **Rhythm** is regular. The **P wave** is abnormal in contour and inverted, or it may be hidden in the QRS complex. The **PR interval** is less than 0.12 second when the P wave precedes the QRS complex. The **QRS complex** is usually normal.

Significance. Junctional escape rhythm serves as a safety mechanism occurring when the primary pacemaker has not been activated. Escape rhythms such as this should not be suppressed. Accelerated junctional rhythm and junctional tachycardia indicate a problem with the sinus node. If these rhythms are rapid, they may result in a reduction of CO and possible heart failure.

Treatment. Treatment varies according to the type of junctional dysrhythmia. If a patient has symptoms with an escape junctional rhythm, atropine can be used. In accelerated junctional rhythm and junctional tachycardia caused by digoxin toxicity, the digoxin is withheld. In the absence of digitalis toxicity, propranolol, phenytoin, or verapamil may be used.

First-Degree AV Block. First-degree AV block is a type of AV block in which every impulse is conducted to the ventricles but the duration of AV conduction is prolonged (Fig. 33-16). This is manifested by a PR interval greater than 0.20 second. After the impulse moves through the AV node, it is usually conducted normally through the ventricles.

Clinical associations. First-degree AV block is associated with MI, chronic ischemic heart disease, rheumatic fever, hyperthyroidism, vagal stimulation, and drugs such as digitalis, β-blockers, flecainide, encainide, and IV verapamil.

Electrocardiogram characteristics. In first-degree AV block, **HR** is normal, and **rhythm** is regular. The **P wave** is normal, the **PR interval** is prolonged for more than 0.20 second, and the **QRS complex** usually has a normal contour.

Significance. First-degree AV block may be a precursor of higher degrees of AV block.

Treatment. There is no treatment for first-degree AV block.

Second-Degree AV Block, Type I. Type I AV block (Mobitz I, Wenckebach phenomenon) includes a gradual lengthening of the PR interval, which occurs because of the AV conduction time that is prolonged until an atrial impulse is nonconducted and a QRS complex is dropped (Fig. 33-16). Once a ventricular beat is dropped, the cycle repeats itself with progressive lengthening of the PR intervals until another QRS complex is dropped. The rhythm appears on the ECG in a pattern of grouped beats. The duration of the QRS complex is normal or prolonged. Type I AV block most commonly occurs in the AV node, but it can also occur in the His-Purkinje system.

Clinical associations. Type I AV block may result from use of drugs such as digoxin or β-blockers. It may also be

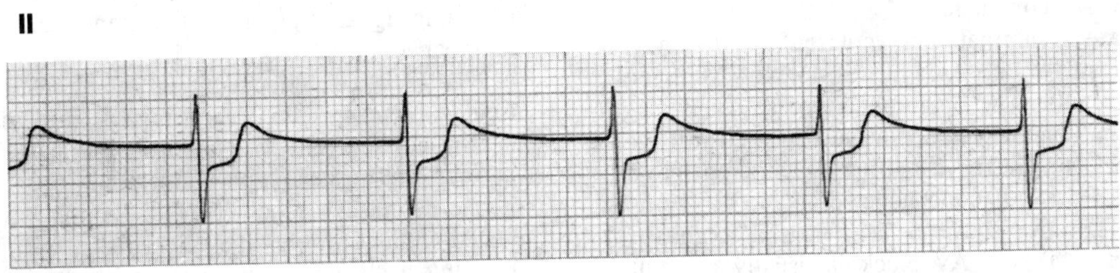

Fig. 33-15 Junctional rhythm of 57 beats per minute.

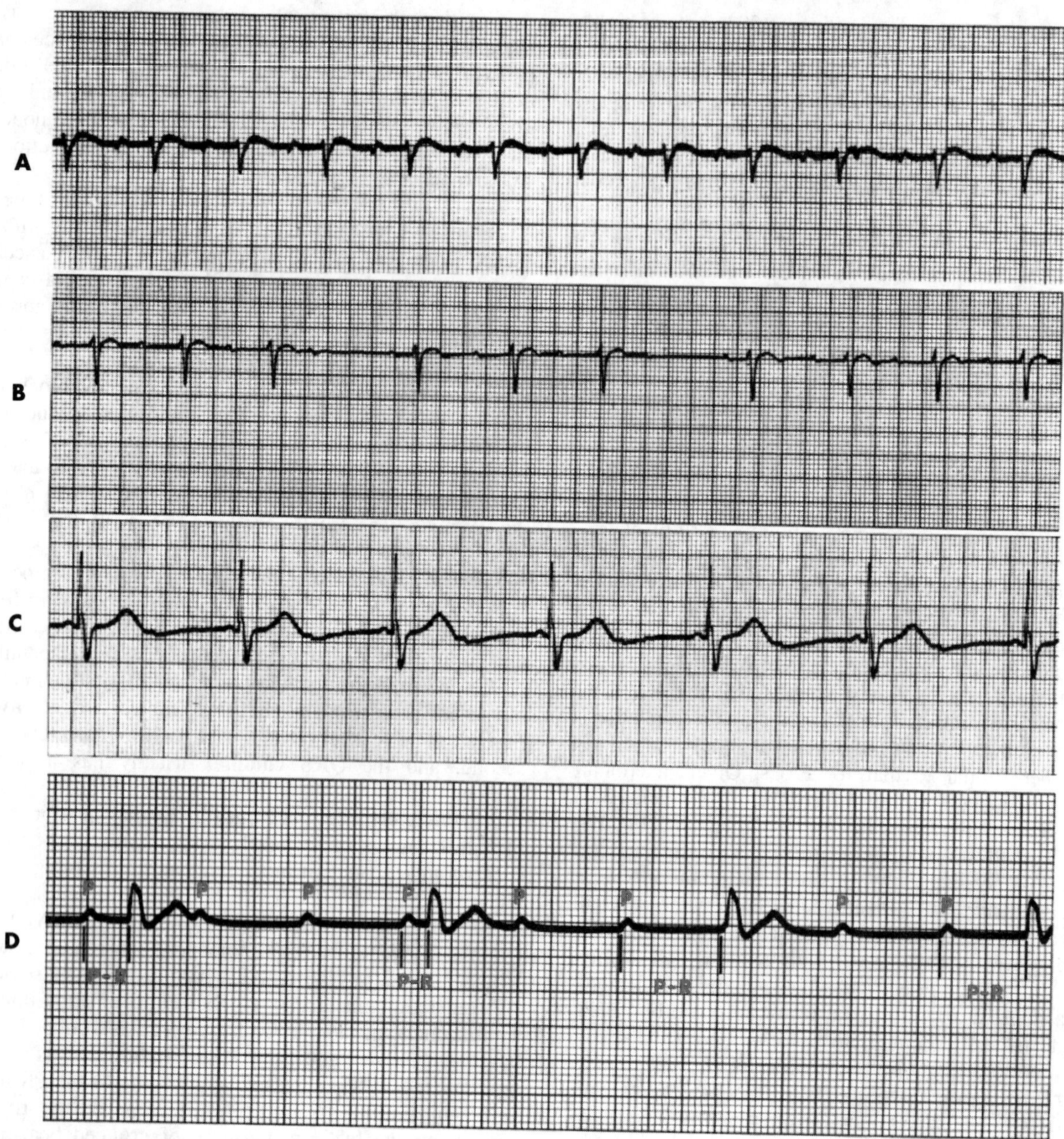

Fig. 33-16 Heart block. ***A,*** First-degree heart block. Note the delayed PR interval. ***B,*** Second-degree heart block, type I (Mobitz I, Wenckebach). ***C,*** Second-degree heart block, type II (Mobitz II). ***D,*** Complete heart block (third degree). The irregular PR intervals indicate the presence of a complete heart block.

associated with ischemic cardiac disease and other diseases that can slow AV conduction.

Atrial rate is normal, but **ventricular rate** may be slower as a result of dropped QRS complexes. **Ventricular rhythm** is irregular. The **PR interval** progressively lengthens before the nonconducted P wave occurs. The **P wave** has a normal contour. The **PR interval** lengthens progressively until a P wave is nonconducted and a QRS complex is dropped. The **QRS complex** has a normal contour.

Significance. Type I AV block is usually a result of myocardial ischemia in an inferior MI. It is almost always transient and is usually well tolerated. However, it may be a warning signal of an impending significant AV conduction disturbance.

Treatment. If the patient is symptomatic, atropine is used to increase HR, or a temporary pacemaker may be needed, especially if the patient has an acute MI.

Second-Degree Heart Block, Type II. In type II second-degree AV block (Mobitz II) a P wave is nonconducted without progressive antecedent PR lengthening, and this almost always occurs when a bundle branch block is present (Fig. 33-16). On conducted beats, the PR interval is constant. Second-degree heart block is a more serious type of block in which a certain number of impulses from the sinus node are not conducted to the ventricles. This occurs in ratios of 2:1, 3:1, and so on when there are two P waves to one QRS complex, three P waves to one QRS complex, and so on. It may occur with varying ratios. Type II AV block almost always occurs in the His-Purkinje system.

Clinical associations. Type II AV block is associated with rheumatic and atherosclerotic heart disease, acute anterior MI, digitalis toxicity, Lenègre's disease, and Lev's disease.

Electrocardiogram characteristics. **Atrial rate** is usually normal. **Ventricular rate** depends on the intrinsic rate and the degree of AV block. **Sinus rhythm** is regular, but **ventricular rhythm** may be irregular. The **P wave** has a normal contour. The **PR interval** may be normal or prolonged but remains fixed on conducted beats. The **QRS complex** widens to more than 0.12 second because of bundle branch block.

Significance. Type II AV block often progresses to third-degree AV block and is associated with a poor prognosis. The reduced HR may result in decreased CO with subsequent hypotension and myocardial ischemia. Type II AV block is an indication for therapy with a permanent pacemaker.

Treatment. Temporary treatment before the insertion of a permanent pacemaker involves the use of a temporary pacemaker. Drugs such as atropine, epinephrine, or dopamine can be tried as temporary measures to increase HR until pacemaker therapy is available.

Third-Degree AV Heart Block. Third-degree AV heart block, which is complete heart block, constitutes one form of AV dissociation in which no impulses from the atria are conducted to the ventricles (see Fig. 33-16). The atria are stimulated and contract independently of the ventricles. The ventricular rhythm is an escape rhythm, and the focus may be above or below the bifurcation of the His bundle.

Clinical associations. Third-degree heart block is associated with fibrosis or calcification of the cardiac conduction system, CAD, myocarditis, cardiomyopathy, open heart surgery, Lev's disease, Lenègre's disease, and some systemic diseases such as amyloidosis and scleroderma.

Electrocardiogram characteristics. The **atrial rate** is usually a sinus rate of 60 to 100 bpm. The **ventricular rate** depends on the site of the block. If it is in the AV node, the rate is 40 to 60 bpm, and if it is in the Purkinje system, it is 20 to 40 bpm. **Atrial** and **ventricular rhythms** are regular but asynchronous. The **P wave** has a normal contour. The **PR interval** is variable, and there is no time relationship between the P wave and the QRS complex. The **QRS complex** is normal if escape rhythm is initiated in the bundle of His or above. It is widened if escape rhythm is initiated below the bundle of His.

Significance. Third-degree AV block almost always results in reduced CO with subsequent ischemia and heart failure. Syncope from an AV block such as this may result from severe bradycardia or even periods of asystole.

Treatment. A temporary pacemaker may be inserted or an external pacemaker applied on an emergency basis in a patient with acute MI. The use of drugs such as atropine, epinephrine, and dopamine are temporary treatments to increase HR and support BP before pacemaker insertion.

Premature Ventricular Contractions. A premature ventricular contraction (PVC) is a contraction originating in an ectopic focus in the ventricles. It is the premature occurrence of a QRS complex, which is wide and distorted in shape, compared to a QRS complex initiated from the supraventricular tissue (Fig. 33-17). The QRS complex is usually wider than 0.12 second, and the T wave is generally large and opposite in direction to the major deflection of the QRS complex. Retrograde conduction may occur, and the P wave may be seen following the ectopic beat. PVCs that are initiated from different foci appear different in contour from each other and are called *multifocal PVCs.* When every other beat is a PVC, it is called *ventricular bigeminy.* When every third beat is a PVC, it is called *ventricular trigeminy.* Two consecutive PVCs are called *couplets.* Three consecutive PVCs are called *triplets. Ventricular tachycardia* occurs when there are three or more consecutive PVCs. When a PVC falls on the T wave of a preceding beat, the *R on T phenomenon* occurs and is considered to be dangerous because it may precipitate ventricular tachycardia or ventricular fibrillation.

Clinical associations. PVCs are associated with stimulants such as caffeine, alcohol, aminophylline, epinephrine, isoproterenol, and digoxin. They are also associated with hypokalemia, hypoxia, fever, exercise, and emotional stress. Disease states associated with PVCs include MI, mitral valve prolapse (MVP), CHF, and CAD.

Electrocardiogram characteristics. HR varies according to intrinsic rate and number of PVCs. **Rhythm** is irregular because of premature beats. A **retrograde P wave** is possible; the **P wave** is rarely visible and is usually lost in the QRS complex of PVC. The **PR interval** is not measurable. The **QRS complex** is wide and distorted in shape, more than 0.10 second.

Significance. PVCs are usually a benign finding in the patient with a normal heart. In heart disease, depending on frequency, PVCs may reduce the CO and precipitate angina and heart failure. PVCs in ischemic heart disease or acute MI represent ventricular irritability. They may also occur as *reperfusion dysrhythmias* after lysis of a coronary artery clot with thrombolytic therapy in acute MI, or following plaque reduction from a percutaneous coronary angioplasty (PTCA).

Treatment. Indications for treatment in an appropriate clinical setting include (1) six or more PVCs occurring per minute, (2) ventricular couplets and triplets, (3) multifocal PVCs, and (4) R on T phenomenon. If treatment is not initiated, ventricular tachycardia or ventricular fibrillation may occur. For treating PVCs, lidocaine is the drug of choice, with an initial IV bolus of 1 to 1.5 mg/kg followed by a second bolus of 0.5 to 1.5 mg/kg and continuous lidocaine infusion of 2 to 4 mg/min. Procainamide is the second drug of choice if lidocaine is ineffective.[11]

Ventricular Tachycardia. The ECG diagnosis of ventricular tachycardia is made when a run of three or more PVCs occurs. The QRS complex is distorted in appearance, with a duration exceeding 0.12 second and with the ST-T

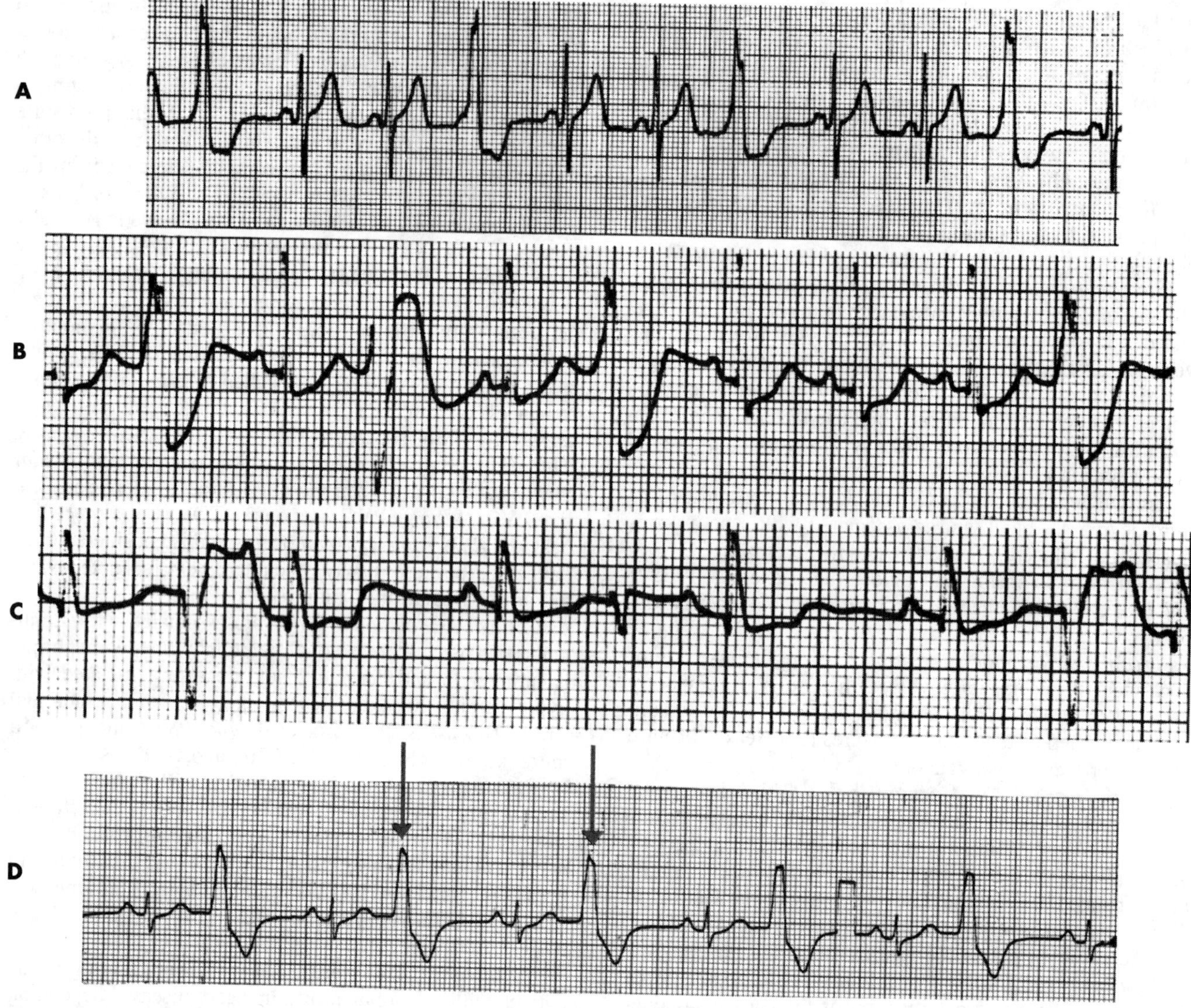

Fig. 33-17 Premature ventricular contractions (PVCs). ***A,*** Ventricular trigeminy. ***B,*** Multifocal PVC. ***C,*** Fusion (interpolated) PVCs. ***D,*** Ventricular bigeminy.

direction pointing opposite to the major QRS deflection (Fig. 33-18). It occurs when an ectopic focus or foci fire repetitively and the ventricle takes control as the pacemaker. The ventricular rate is 110 to 250 bpm, and the R-R interval may be irregular or regular. AV dissociation may be present, with P waves occurring independently of the QRS complex. The atria may also be depolarized by the ventricles in a retrograde fashion.

Ventricular tachycardia may be *sustained* (lasting longer than 30 seconds) or *nonsustained* (lasting 30 seconds or less). *Torsades de pointes* (Fig. 33-19) or polymorphic ventricular tachycardia is a type of ventricular tachycardia characterized by a QRS contour that gradually changes its polarity over a series of beats. It usually occurs when QT prolongation is present.

The appearance of ventricular tachycardia is an ominous sign because it usually indicates the presence of cardiac disease. It is considered to be a life-threatening dysrhythmia because of decreased CO and the possibility of deterioration of ventricular tachycardia to ventricular fibrillation, which is a lethal dysrhythmia.

Clinical associations. Ventricular tachycardia is associated with acute MI, CAD, significant electrolyte imbalances (e.g., potassium), cardiomyopathy, MVP, long QT syndrome, and coronary reperfusion after thrombolytic therapy. The dysrhythmia has also been observed in the patient who has no evidence of cardiac disease.

Electrocardiogram characteristics. **Ventricular rate** is 110 to 250 bpm. **Rhythm** may be regular or irregular. The **P wave** may be noted to "march through" the ventricular rhythm in AV dissociation, or it may occur after the QRS complex in a regular pattern of retrograde conduction. The **PR interval** is not measurable. The **QRS interval** is prolonged for more than than 0.10 second, and the QRS complex contour is distorted.

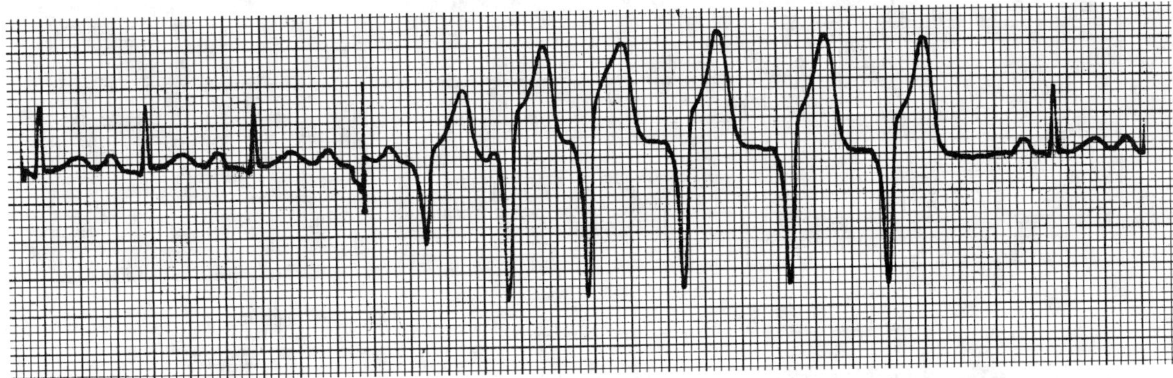

Fig. 33-18 Ventricular tachycardia.

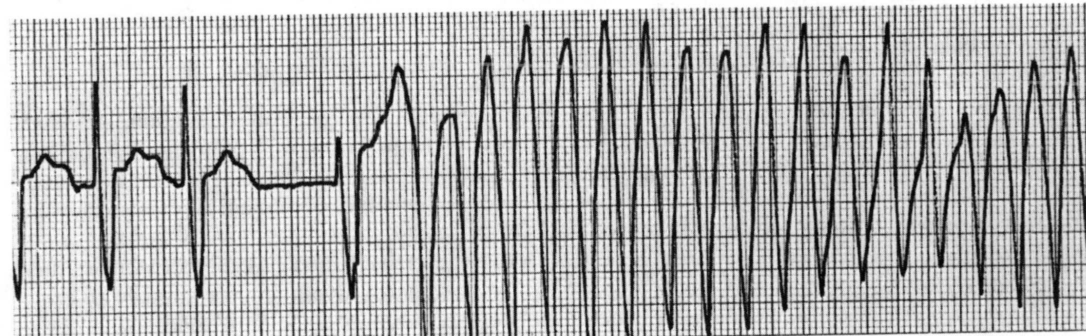

Fig. 33-19 Torsades de pointes.

Significance. Ventricular tachycardia may cause a severe decrease in CO as a result of decreased ventricular diastolic filling times and loss of atrial contraction. The result may be pulmonary edema, shock, and insufficient blood flow to the brain. The dysrhythmia must be treated quickly, even if it occurs only briefly and stops abruptly. Episodes may recur if prophylactic treatment is not begun.[11] Ventricular fibrillation may also develop.

Treatment. If the patient is hemodynamically stable, treatment consists of administration of a lidocaine bolus of 1 to 1.5 mg/kg/min with subsequent boluses of 0.5 to 1.5 mg/kg/min up to 3 mg/kg body weight. If this abolishes the tachycardia, a continuous lidocaine infusion of 2 to 4 mg/min should be started. If lidocaine is ineffective, IV procainamide may be tried. It may be given in an infusion of 20 mg/min until the dysrhythmia is suppressed, hypotension occurs, the QRS complex is widened by 50% of its original width, or a total of 17 mg/kg of the drug has been injected. If this treatment is successful, a continuous procainamide infusion of 2 to 4 mg/min should be started. A third drug of choice is bretylium, given IV at a dose of 5 mg/kg for several minutes and increased to 10 mg/kg at 15 to 30 minutes (not to exceed 30 to 35 mg/kg). A continuous infusion of bretylium (1 to 2 mg/min) may be started.[11]

The acute treatment of torsade de pointes can be quite different than that of more common ventricular tachycardias.[14,15] Magnesium sulfate infusion is the therapy of choice.[11,16,17] Other therapies indicated for torsade de pointes include isoproterenol or lidocaine infusions. Overdrive pacing is also used to suppress this dysrhythmia.[11]

If a patient is unconscious or hemodynamically unstable, immediate cardioversion, starting initially with 50 joules, is the recommended treatment. A defibrillator is used in the synchronized mode for cardioversion. The machine is timed to discharge on an R wave in order to effectively convert the ventricular tachycardia to a sinus rhythm. If a patient is awake before cardioversion, a sedative may be given before delivery of the electrical discharge.

Ventricular Fibrillation. Ventricular fibrillation is a severe derangement of the heart rhythm characterized on the ECG by irregular undulations of varying contour and amplitude (Fig. 33-20). This represents the firing of multiple ectopic foci in the ventricle. Mechanically the ventricle is simply "quivering," and no effective contraction or CO occurs.

Clinical associations. Ventricular fibrillation occurs in acute MI and myocardial ischemia and in chronic diseases such as CAD and cardiomyopathy. It may occur during cardiac pacing or cardiac catheterization procedures as a result of catheter stimulation of the ventricle. It may also occur with coronary reperfusion after thrombolytic therapy. Other clinical associations are accidental electrical shock, hyperkalemia, and hypoxemia.

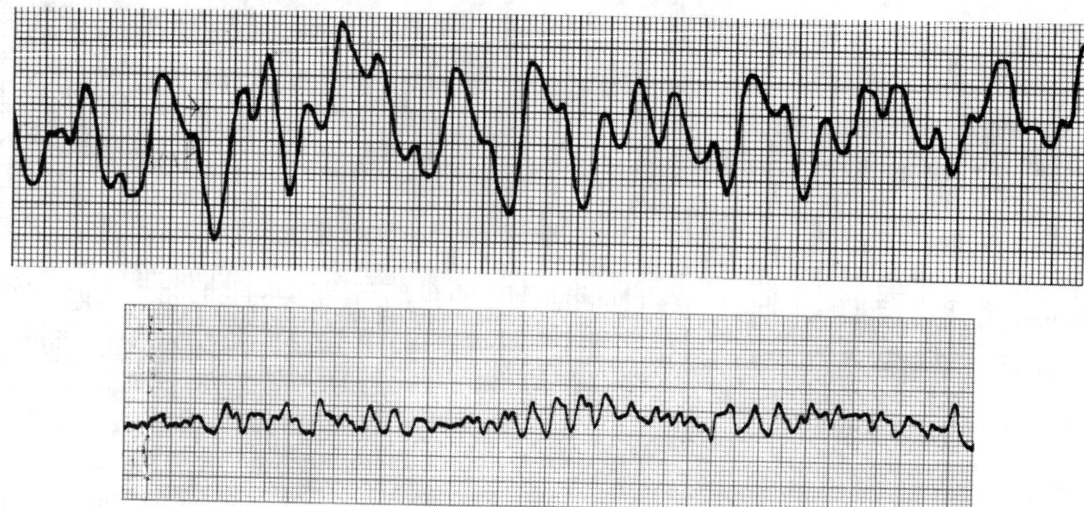

Fig. 33-20 Ventricular fibrillation.

Electrocardiogram characteristics. **HR** is not measurable. **Rhythm** is irregular and chaotic. The **P wave** is not visible, and the **PR interval** and the **QRS interval** are not measurable.

Significance. Ventricular fibrillation results in unconsciousness, absence of pulse, apnea, and seizures. If left untreated, the patient with this condition will die.

Treatment. Treatment consists of immediate initiation of CPR and initiation of advanced cardiac life support (ACLS) measures with use of defibrillation and definitive drug therapy. If a defibrillator is immediately available, there should be no delay in using it.

Asystole. Asystole represents the total absence of ventricular electrical activity. Occasionally, P waves can be seen. No ventricular contraction occurs because depolarization does not occur. This is a lethal dysrhythmia that requires immediate treatment. Ventricular fibrillation may masquerade as asystole; thus the rhythm should be assessed in more than one lead. The prognosis of a patient with asystole is poor.

Clinical associations. Asystole is usually a result of advanced cardiac disease, a severe cardiac conduction system disturbance, or end-stage CHF.

Significance. Generally the patient with asystole has end-stage cardiac function or has a prolonged arrest and cannot be resuscitated.

Treatment. Treatment consists of CPR with initiation of ACLS measures, which include intubation and IV therapy with epinephrine and atropine.[11]

Pulseless Electrical Activity. Pulseless electrical activity (PEA), a new term replacing *electromechanical dissociation,* describes a situation in which electrical activity can be observed on the ECG, but there is no mechanical activity of the ventricles and the patient has no pulse. Prognosis is poor unless the underlying cause can be identified and corrected. The most common correctable causes of PEA are hypovolemia, cardiac tamponade, tension pneumothorax, hypoxemia, hypothermia, and acidosis. Other less correctable causes of PEA include massive myocardial damage from infarction, prolonged ischemia during resuscitation, and pulmonary embolism. Treatment begins with CPR followed by intubation and IV therapy with epinephrine. Treatment is directed toward correction of the underlying cause.[11]

Prodysrhythmia. Antidysrhythmic drugs may cause life-threatening dysrhythmias similar to those for which they are administered. This concept is known as *prodysrhythmia.* The patient who has severe left ventricular dysfunction is the most susceptible to a prodysrhythmia. Class IA and IC drugs (Tables 33-7 and 33-8) as well as digoxin can cause a prodysrhythmic response. The first several days of drug therapy is the vulnerable period for developing prodysrhythmias. For this reason, the initiation of most oral antidysrhythmic drug regimens using these classes of drugs should be done in a monitored hospital setting.[16]

Antidysrhythmic Drugs

An increasing number of antidysrhythmic drugs have become available.[12-20] Table 33-7 categorizes major drug classifications by primary effects on the cardiac intracellular action potential. Table 33-8 includes pertinent data pertaining to the most commonly used drugs in each class.

Defibrillation

Defibrillation is the most effective method of terminating ventricular fibrillation. It is most effective when the myocardial cells are not anoxic or acidotic. Therefore defibrillation should ideally be performed within 15 to 20 seconds of the onset of the dysrhythmia. Defibrillation is accomplished by the passage of a direct current (DC) electrical shock through the heart that is sufficient to depolarize the cells of the myocardium. The intent is that subsequent repolarization of myocardial cells will allow the SA node to resume the role of pacemaker.[11] The output of a defibrillator is quantified in *joules* or *watts per second.* The recommended energy for initial shock in defibrillation is 200 joules with a second shock of 200 to 300 joules as needed

Table 33-7 Major Classifications of Antidysrhythmic Drugs

Classification
Classification I: Drugs That Depress Upstroke of Action Potential
Prolong repolarization
Quinidine
Procainamide
Disopyramide
Moricizine*
Accelerate repolarization
Lidocaine
Tocainide
Mexilitine
Have little or no effect on repolarization
Flecainide
Propafenone
Moricizine*
Classification II: β-Blockers
Propranolol
Nadolol
Timolol
Atenolol
Acebutolol
Esmolol
Metoprolol
Sotalol†
Labetalol
Classification III: Drugs That Prolong Repolarization
Bretylium
Amiodarone
Sotalol†
Classification IV: Calcium Channel Blockers
Diltiazem
Verapamil
Potassium Channel Opener
Adenosine

*Moricizine has both Class IA and IC properties.
†Sotalol has both Class II and Class III properties.

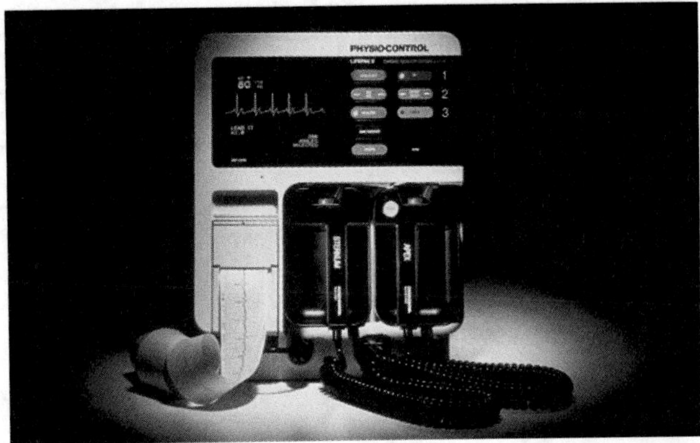

Fig. 33-21 Life-Pak II: Contains a monitor, defibrillator, and transcutaneous pacemaker.

and a third shock of 360 joules if defibrillation is unsuccessful. High doses of electricity during defibrillation have been found to cause myocardial damage; thus the lowest effective electrical output is the one with which to start.

A defibrillator is one part of standard emergency equipment available (Fig. 33-21). There are many different models of defibrillators. The nurse should be familiar with the operation of the type of defibrillator that is used in the emergency unit. Proficiency verification in use of the defibrillator is recommended annually for nursing staff members who use it.

The following steps are to be taken for defibrillation: (1) CPR should be in progress if the defibrillator is not immediately available; (2) the defibrillator should be turned on, and the proper energy level should be selected; and (3) someone should verify that the synchronizer switch is turned off. Conductive materials in the form of saline pads, electrode gel, or defibrillator gel pads are applied to the chest where defibrillator paddles will be placed. This decreases electrical impedance and helps to prevent burns. The paddles are charged by a button on the defibrillator or a button on the paddles themselves. The paddles are placed on the chest wall (Fig. 33-22); one is placed to the right of the sternum just below the clavicle, and the other is placed to the left of the precordium. The operator applies 20 to 25 pounds of pressure to the paddles. The operator calls "all clear" to ensure that personnel are not touching the patient or the bed at the time of discharge. The defibrillator is then discharged by depressing buttons on both paddles simultaneously.

Electrical cardioversion is the therapy of choice for hemodynamically unstable ventricular or supraventricular tachydysrhythmias. A synchronized circuit in the defibrillator is used to deliver a countershock that is programmed to occur during the QRS complex of the ECG.

The procedure for cardioversion is the same as for defibrillation with the following exceptions: If synchronized cardioversion is done on a nonemergency basis when the patient is awake and hemodynamically stable, the patient may be sedated with diazepam or midazolam before the procedure. Strict attention to maintenance of a patent airway is important in this situation. When a patient with supraventricular tachycardia or ventricular tachycardia is hemodynamically unstable, cardioversion is performed as quickly as possible.

Implantable Cardioverter-Defibrillator. In the past several years the implantable cardioverter-defibrillator (ICD) or automatic implantable cardioverter-defibrillator (AICD) has been developed as an acceptable treatment for the patient who has malignant ventricular dysrhythmias.[21-24] The patient who qualifies for this device has been shown by EPS to be prone to lethal tachydysrhythmias in spite of drug therapy. This new modality appears to significantly decrease cardiac mortality rates and has added a new dimension to the management of lethal dysrhythmias and the prevention of sudden cardiac death.

The ICD consists of a lithium battery-powered pulse generator housed in a titanium case weighing approxi-

Table 33-8 Antidysrhythmic Drugs

Drug	Indications	Major Pharmacologic Effects
Classification IA		
Quinidine	Symptomatic PVCs, ventricular tachycardia, atrial fibrillation, atrial flutter, PSVT	Decreases phase 0 of rapid depolarization of action potential (rapid sodium channel); slows phase 4 depolarization in Purkinje's fibers; inhibits conduction along fast limb of AV nodal or bypass tract reentrant dysrhythmias
Procainamide (Pronestyl, Procan)	Ventricular and supraventricular dysrhythmias	Similar effects as quinidine but does not prolong QT interval
Disopyramide (Norpace)	Ventricular and supraventricular dysrhythmias	Similar effects as quinidine and procainamide but with significant anticholinergic or atropine-like effects
Moricizine (Ethmozine)	Ventricular dysrhythmias	Reduces the fast, inward current carried by sodium ions. Shortens phase 2 and 3 repolarization, resulting in a decreased action potential duration and effective refractory period
Classification IB		
Tocainide (Tonocard)	Ventricular dysrhythmias	Primary amine analog of lidocaine; has similar effects as lidocaine; inhibits fast sodium current while shortening action potential duration (i.e., shortening of QT interval)
Mexilitine (Mexitil)	Ventricular dysrhythmias	Has similar effects as lidocaine; depresses inward sodium current, with a decrease in rate of rise of action potential; does not prolong QT interval
Lidocaine (Xylocaine)*		
Classification IC		
Flecainide (Tambocor)	Recurrent ventricular dysrhythmias, supraventricular dysrhythmias (effective in WPW syndrome)	Inhibits fast sodium current (Class I agent) and powerfully inhibits His-Purkinje conduction; prolongs PR and QRS intervals, causing prolongation of QT; inhibits AV nodal pathway in some AV nodal reentrant dysrhythmias
Moricizine (Ethmozine)†		
Propafenone (Rhythmol)	Ventricular dysrhythmias	Reduces upstroke velocity (phase 0) of the action potential. Reduces the fast, inward current of sodium ions in Purkinje's fibers, and less so in myocardial fibers. Prolongs AV conduction

continued

mately ½ pound. Lead wires are placed from the generator either on the epicardial surface or transvenously to the endocardium. There are monitoring leads and defibrillating leads (Fig. 33-23). The generator box is implanted subcutaneously in the abdomen. The ICD sensing system monitors the HR and rhythm and identifies ventricular tachycardia or ventricular fibrillation. Approximately 25 seconds after the sensing system detects a lethal dysrhythmia, the defibrillating mechanism delivers a 25-joule shock to the patient's heart muscle. If the first shock is unsuccessful, the generator recycles and can continue up to 4 to 7 shocks.[24]

The newest ICD implantation procedure involves a transvenous approach.[21] The previous approaches required thoracotomy or sternotomy, which carry an increased sur-

Adverse Effects	Nursing Considerations
Limiting side effects in at least 30% of patients, including nausea, diarrhea, headache, dizziness, tinnitus, fever, rash, thrombocytopenia, hemolytic anemia, anaphylaxis, and prolongation of QT interval with possible development of ventricular dysrhythmias including torsades de pointes (i.e., polymorphic ventricular tachycardia), representing prodysrhythmic effect (i.e., worsening of initial rhythm)	Assess carefully for side effects. Ensure continuous ECG monitoring at drug initiation. Reduce digoxin dose when quinidine therapy is started because quinidine increases blood digoxin levels.
GI intolerance, rash, agranulocytosis, drug-induced lupus syndrome, torsades de pointes, bundle branch block, AV block	Be aware that long-term therapy is not recommended because of risk of development of lupus-like syndrome and that procainamide does not affect digoxin levels.
Negative inotropic effects that may worsen heart failure; anticholinergic effects, including dry mouth, urinary hesitancy or retention, constipation; QRS and QT prolongation, producing torsades de pointes and other dysrhythmias	Be aware that the presence of heart failure is absolute contraindication to use of drug.
Most serious is prodysrhythmic effect. Others are nausea, conduction defects (sinus pauses, junctional rhythm, AV block), CHF, dizziness, anxiety, drug fever, urinary retention, blurred vision, GI upset, rash	Monitor heart rhythm carefully after initiation of therapy. Can cause sinus arrest in patient with underlying sinus node dysfunction. Be aware of the high risk of prodysrhythmia with this drug.
Neurologic effects, including dizziness, tremor, paresthesias; GI effects, including nausea, vomiting, diarrhea; severe effects, including leukopenia, thrombocytopenia, pulmonary fibrosis	Be aware that tocainide does not have negative inotropic effects and can be used safely in CHF.
Neurologic effects, including tremor, dysarthria, dizziness, paresthesias, diplopia, nystagmus, confusion, anxiety; GI effects, including nausea and vomiting	Be aware that mexilitine has a narrow therapeutic-toxic margin. Closely observe patient for side effects. Be aware that drug is important antidysrhythmic for patient with CHF and that it does not have negative inotropic properties.
Prodysrhythmic effect (aggravation of ventricular dysrhythmias in 5-12% of patients), decreased myocardial contractility (possibly exacerbating heart failure), dizziness, blurred vision, tremor, constipation, pruritus	Ensure continuous ECG monitoring after initiation of therapy. Frequently measure PR and QRS intervals. Be alert to any increase in ventricular dysrhythmias. Observe patient for any worsening of symptoms of CHF.
Dizziness, nausea and vomiting, unusual taste, constipation, angina, fatigue, dyspnea, headache, blurred vision, CHF, prodysrhythmias, first degree AV block, widened QRS, bradycardias, and atrial fibrillation	Assess carefully for side effects. Monitor HR during initiation of drug therapy. Digoxin and propranolol levels increase with concomitant administration of propafenone

continued

gical risk. The transvenous approach, with ICD electrodes placed transvenously rather than on the epicardium, decreases morbidity and medical costs related to surgical complications.

In addition to defibrillation capabilities, the newest ICDs, or "third generation" ICDs, are equipped with antitachycardia and antibradycardia pacemakers. These sophisticated devices use dysrhythmia algorithms that detect dysrhythmias and determine the appropriate programmed response. These devices initiate overdrive pacing of supraventricular and ventricular tachycardias, sparing the patient painful shocks from the defibrillator device. They also provide backup pacing for bradydysrhythmias occurring after defibrillation discharges.[22,23]

Table 33-8 Antidysrhythmic Drugs—cont'd

Drug	Indications	Major Pharmacologic Effects
Classification II		
***β*-Blockers**		
Nonselective		
Propranolol (Inderal) Nadolol (Corgard) Timolol (Blocadren) Pindolol (Visken)	Inappropriate sinus tachycardia, PSVT provoked by emotion or exercise, dysrhythmias of pheochromocytoma, exercise-induced ventricular dysrhythmias, dysrhythmias of MVP, acute myocardial ischemia and infarction	Induces β-adrenergic blockade; inhibits increases in HR, AV nodal conduction, myocardial contractility; shows cardioselective effect in some (i.e., predominant effect on β_1 receptors in heart, less effect on β_2 receptors in bronchial tree and peripheral vasculature)
Cardioselective		
Metoprolol (Lopressor) Atenolol (Tenormin) Acebutalol (Bectral)		
Esmolol (Brevibloc) Sotalol (Betapace)‡	For rapid, short-term control of ventricular rate in patient with atrial fibrillation or atrial flutter. Not intended for use in chronic settings	Ultra short-acting β-adrenergic blocking agent with a half-life of 9 minutes and β_1 cardioselectivity
Classification III		
Amiodarone (Cordarone)	Recurrent atrial fibrillation, supraventricular tachydysrhythmias associated with WPW syndrome, recurrent ventricular tachycardia, recurrent ventricular fibrillation	Prolongs action potential duration without significantly effective depolarization; increases refractory period of atrium, AV node, and ventricle; increases refractory period and slows conduction in accessory pathways in WPW syndrome; prolongs QT interval
Bretylium (Bretylol, Bretylate)* Sotalol (Betapace)	Ventricular dysrhythmias, atrial dysrhythmias	Class II: β-adrenergic antagonist Class III: Prolongs action potential duration
Classification IV		
Diltiazem,* verapamil*		
Potassium Channel Opener		
Adenosine (Adenocard)	Conversion to sinus rhythm of PSVT including those associated with accessory bypass tracts	Slows conduction time through the AV node and can interrupt the reentry pathways through the AV node

continued

The postoperative recovery period after implantation of an ICD is usually a prolonged hospitalization with careful observation for appropriate ICD response to dysrhythmias. The implantation procedure itself carries a low risk, and possible complications that the nurse should be aware of are similar to those for permanent pacemaker implantation (discussed later in chapter). Occasionally an ICD is implanted during open heart surgery, which results in a different risk and complication profile.

Education of the patient who is receiving an ICD is of extreme importance. The patient experiences a variety of emotions including fear of body image change, fear of recurrent dysrhythmias, expectation of pain with ICD discharge (described as a feeling of a blow to the chest), and anxiety about going home. Table 33-9 describes the discharge instructions for the patient with an ICD and the family.

Adverse Effects	Nursing Considerations
Decreased myocardial contractility with possible development of CHF, sinus bradycardia, asystole, AV block, bronchospasm, fatigue, impotence, insomnia, nightmares, hypoglycemia in patient with diabetes mellitus	Inform patient that abrupt discontinuation of β-blocking drugs can cause "rebound" syndrome.
Symptomatic hypotension, diaphoresis, dizziness, bradycardia, chest pain, syncope, pulmonary edema, heart block	Do not abruptly discontinue this drug (or any β-blocker). Withdrawal effects in patient with CAD may include severe angina and reflex tachycardia. May be more effective when used in conjunction with digoxin
Nausea, anorexia, insomnia, weakness, fatigue, microdeposits in cornea, thyroid dysfunction, pulmonary toxicity, hepatic toxicity, bluish discoloration of skin, exacerbation of ventricular dysrhythmias with torsades de pointes, worsening SA node dysfunction and abnormal AV node conduction; long half-life (possibly several weeks); weeks of therapy necessary for development of therapeutic level	Inform patient of potential toxicity. Ensure regular follow-up care to determine the best dosage and to check for toxicity with chest x-ray, pulmonary examinations, thyroid tests, and retinal examinations. Emphasize potential for bluish discoloration of skin. Educate patient about protecting from sun exposure with skin barriers of clothing and lotions. Caution patient about concomitant use with digoxin or coumadin.
Fatigue, decreased libido, exacerbation of heart failure, depression, exacerbation of peripheral vascular disease, bronchospasm; prodysrhythmias such as torsade de pointes, sustained VT or VF	Monitor patient with defibrillator readily available. Patient should be monitored and accompanied by nurse en route to tests and procedures. Assess closely for signs of CHF. Routinely monitor and assess ECG q shift for prolongation of QT interval. Monitor serum electrolytes, especially potassium. Teach diabetics that sotalol is similar to other β-blocker drugs and may mask symptoms of hypoglycemia.
Facial flushing, dyspnea, chest pressure, nausea, and lightheadedness are the most frequently reported. Because of the brief half-life (10 sec) of adenosine, side effects are generally brief and self-limiting	Important to inject adenosine rapidly, over 1-2 sec, in order for it to be effective. It should be injected directly into a vein or at the port closest to the IV site, followed by a rapid saline flush

AV, Atrioventricular; *CAD,* coronary artery disease; *CHF,* congestive heart failure; *ECG,* electrocardiogram; *GI,* gastrointestinal; *HR,* heart rate; *IV,* intravenous; *MVP,* mitral valve prolapse; *SA,* sinoatria; *PSVT,* paroxysmal supraventricular tachycardia; *PVC,* premature ventricular contraction; *VF,* ventricular fibrillation; *VT,* ventricular tachycardia; *WPW,* Wolff-Parkinson-White.

*See Table 33-17.

†See Classification IA.

‡See Classification III.

Pacemakers

The artificial cardiac pacemaker is an electronic device used in place of the SA node, the natural cardiac pacemaker of the heart. Implantable pacemakers were first developed in the 1950s. The artificial cardiac pacemaker is an electrical circuit in which the battery provides electricity that travels through a conducting wire to the myocardium, and the myocardium stimulates the heart to beat (i.e., it "captures" the heart).

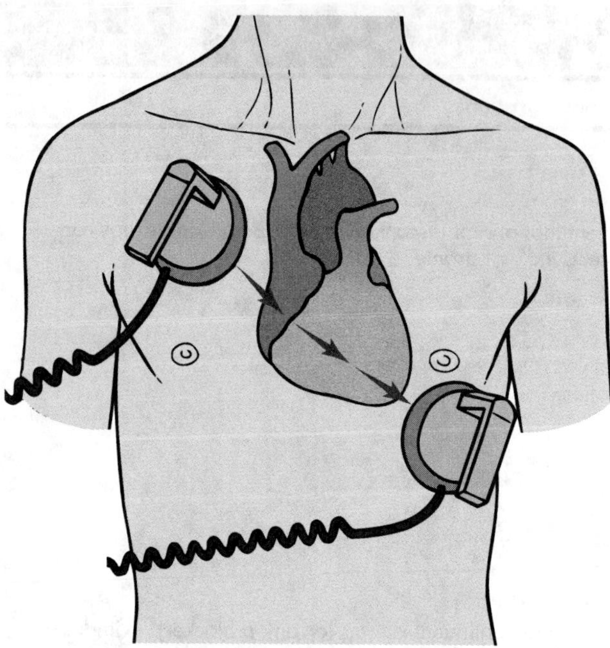

Fig. 33-22 Paddle placement and current flow in defibrillation.

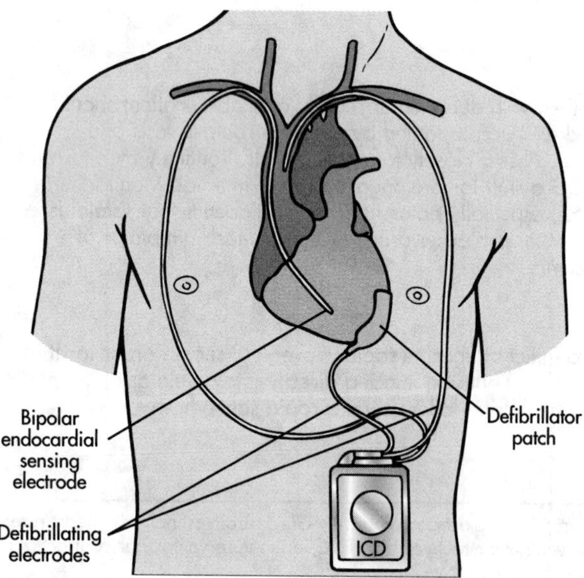

Fig. 33-23 The implantable cardioverter-defibrillator (ICD) pulse generator is placed in a subcutaneous pocket in the abdomen. Bipolar endocardial sensing electrode is placed in the right-ventricular apex. Defibrillating electrodes are positioned in the superior vena cava (spring lead) and over the apex of the heart (mesh patch covered with silicone and rubber).

Recent advances in technology have been applied extensively to pacemakers. This has resulted in sophisticated, noninvasive, programmable single- and dual-chambered pacemakers with specialized circuits that weigh only 40 to 50 g. Pacemakers have been developed that are more physiologically accurate, pacing both the atrium and the ventricle, as well as increasing HR when appropriate.[25-27]

Permanent pacemakers are those that are implanted totally within the body (Fig. 33-24), and *temporary pacemakers* are those with the power source outside the body (Fig. 33-25). The permanent pacemaker power source is implanted subcutaneously in the chest (Fig. 33-24, *B*) or abdomen and is attached to pacer electrodes, which are threaded transvenously to the right ventricle or the right atrium. Indications for insertion of permanent pacemaker are listed in Table 33-10.

Temporary pacemakers are usually used with a lead or wire threaded transvenously to the right ventricle and with a wire attached to a power source externally (Fig. 33-26). They are inserted in cardiac care units in emergency situations. Indications for temporary pacing are listed in Table 33-11.

The Intersociety Commission for Heart Disease (ICHD), the British Pacing and Electrophysiology Group (BPEG), and the North American Society of Pacing and Electro-

Table 33-9 Discharge Instructions for Patient and Family after ICD Implantation

1. When the ICD fires:
   - The patient should lie down.
   - One person should stay with the patient while another contacts the physician.
   - Someone should call an ambulance if patient loses consciousness. CPR should be delayed until device fires unsuccessfully 4-7 times or fails to fire after 30 sec.
   - If someone is touching the patient when the ICD fires, that person may feel a slight but harmless shock.
   - If alone, the patient should call an ambulance immediately and then lie down.
2. The ICD battery must be checked every 2 mo.
3. A "Medic-Alert" bracelet should be worn at all times.
4. An information card about the ICD should be easily accessible in the patient's wallet.
5. The manual for the patient provided by the ICD manufacturer should be read.
6. Family members should learn CPR.
7. The nurse should assist patient with the development of positive coping strategies to reduce stress.
8. Avoid electromagnetic and vibratory forces that may turn off the device.

CPR, Cardiopulmonary resuscitation; *ICD*, implantable cardioverter-defibrillator.

A

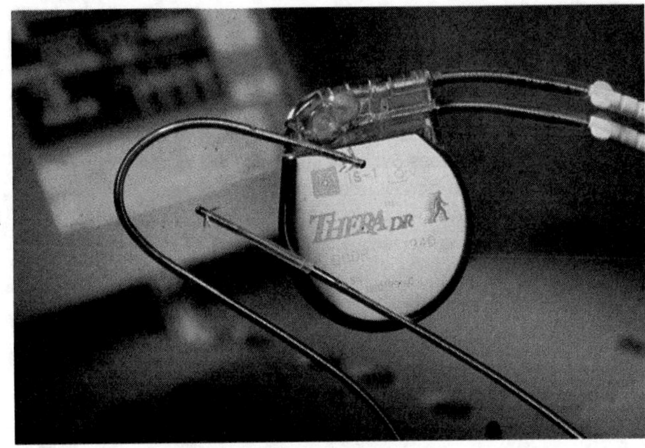

B

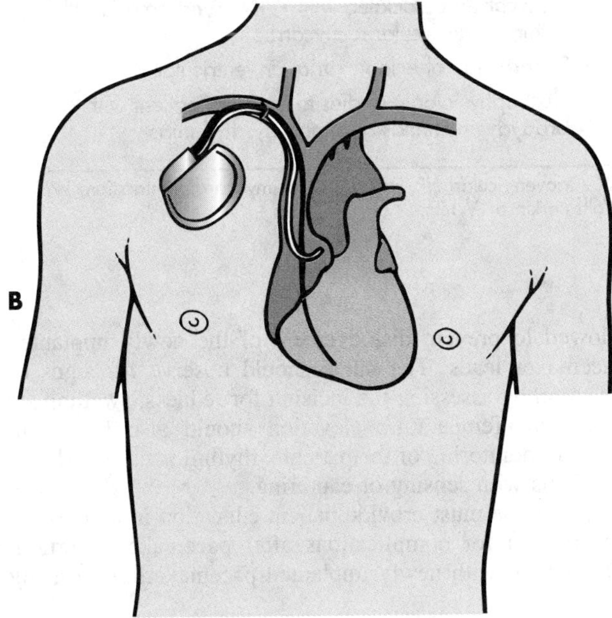

Fig. 33-24 ***A,*** Synergyst II, a new dual-chamber, rate-responsive pacemaker from Medtronic, Inc., is designed to detect body movement and automatically increase or decrease paced heart rates based on the level of physical activity. ***B,*** Cardiac leads in both the atrium and ventricle enable a dual-chamber pacemaker to sense and pace in both heart chambers.

physiology (NASPE) joined in the development of a five-position code that serves as abbreviations for permanent pacing devices (Table 33-12). The first-position code denotes the chamber or chambers paced. The second refers to the chamber or chambers sensed. The third refers to the mode of pacemaker response to the sensed event. The fourth position denotes programmability options and rate-modulation capabilities, and the fifth position indicates antitachycardia capabilities.[25]

Pacemaker malfunction is manifested by a failure to sense or a failure to capture. *Failure to sense* occurs when the pacemaker fails to recognize spontaneous atrial or ventricular activity, and it fires inappropriately (Fig. 33-27). Failure to sense may be caused by pacer lead fracture, battery failure, or displacement of electrode. *Failure to capture* occurs when the electrical charge to the myocardium is insufficient to produce atrial or ventricular contraction (Fig. 33-28). Failure to capture may be caused by pacer lead fracture, battery failure, electrode displacement, or fibrosis at the electrode tip.

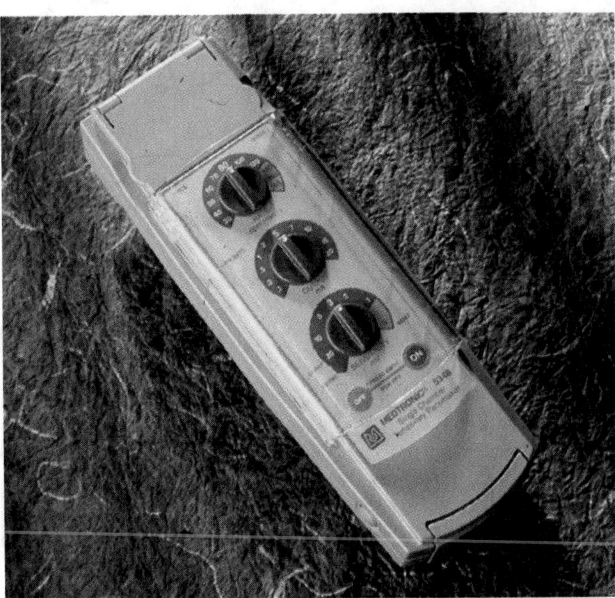

Fig. 33-25 Temporary external demand pacemaker.

Complications of invasive temporary or permanent pacemaker insertion include infection and hematoma formation at the site of insertion of the pacemaker power source, pneumothorax, failure to sense or capture with possible bradycardia and significant symptoms, perforation of the atrial or ventricular septum by the pacing wire, and appearance of "end-of-life" battery parameters on testing the pacemaker. A decrease in CO may also be seen when a ventricular demand-ventricular inhibited mode pacer is

Table 33-10 Indications for Permanent Pacemaker Therapy

Sinus node dysfunction
Third-degree AV block
Fibrosis or sclerotic changes of cardiac conduction system
Sick sinus syndrome
Mobitz II second-degree AV block
Hypersensitive carotid sinus syndrome
Chronic atrial fibrillation with slow ventricular response
Tachydysrhythmias
Bifascicular block

AV, Atrioventricular.

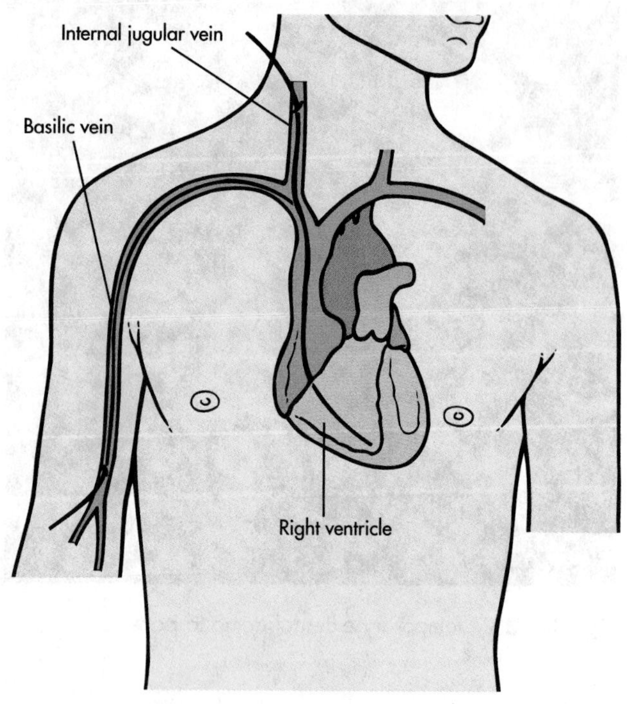

Fig. 33-26 Temporary pacemaker catheter insertion.

Table 33-11 Indications for Temporary Pacing

- Maintenance of adequate HR and rhythm during special circumstances such as surgery and postoperative recovery, cardiac catheterization or coronary angioplasty, during drug therapy that may cause bradycardia, and before implantation of a permanent pacemaker
- As prophylaxis after open heart surgery
- Acute anterior MI with second-degree or third-degree AV block or bundle branch block
- Acute inferior MI with symptomatic bradycardia and AV block
- Termination of AV nodal reentry or reciprocating tachycardia associated with WPW syndrome, atrial flutter, or ventricular tachycardia
- Suppression of ectopic atrial or ventricular rhythm
- Electrophysiologic studies to evaluate patient with bradydysrhythmias and tachydysrhythmias

AV, Atrioventricular; *HR,* heart rate; *MI,* myocardial infarction; *WPW,* Wolff-Parkinson-White.

inserted because of loss of atrial contractions (atrial "kick"). Measures taken to prevent and assess complications include prophylactic IV antibiotic therapy before and after insertion, assessment of chest x-ray after insertion to check lead placement and to rule out the presence of a pneumothorax, careful observation of insertion site, and continuous ECG monitoring of patient's rhythm. After pacemaker insertion, the patient is maintained on bed rest for 24 hours, and minimal arm and shoulder activity is allowed to prevent dislodgement of the newly implanted pacemaker leads. The nurse should observe for signs of infection by assessing the incision for redness, swelling, or discharge. Temperature elevation should also be noted. Careful monitoring of the patient's rhythm is used to detect problems with sensing or capturing.

The nurse must provide patient education in addition to observation for complications after pacemaker insertion. The patient with newly implanted pacemakers have many

Table 33-12 Pacemaker Terminology and Nomenclature

I. Chamber Paced	II. Chamber Sensed	III. Mode of Response	IV. Programmability	V. Tachydysrhythmia Functions
V, Ventricle	V, Ventricle	I, Inhibited	P, Programmable rate and output	B, Burst
A, Atrium	A, Atrium	T, Triggered	M, Multiprogrammability	N, Normal rate competition
D, Atrium and ventricle	D, Atrium and ventricle	D, Atrial triggered and ventricular inhibited	C, Programmable with telemetry	S, Scanning
O, None	O, None	O, None	O, None	E, External

Pacemaker Nomenclature*

VVI	Ventricular demand/ventricular inhibited
AAI	Atrial demand/atrial inhibited
DVI	AV sequential/ventricular inhibited
VAT	Atrial synchronous/P wave triggered
VDD	Atrial synchronous/ventricular inhibited
DDD	Universal/fully automatic

*First initial refers to chamber or chambers *paced;* second initial refers to chamber or chambers *sensed;* third initial refers to pacemaker's *response.*

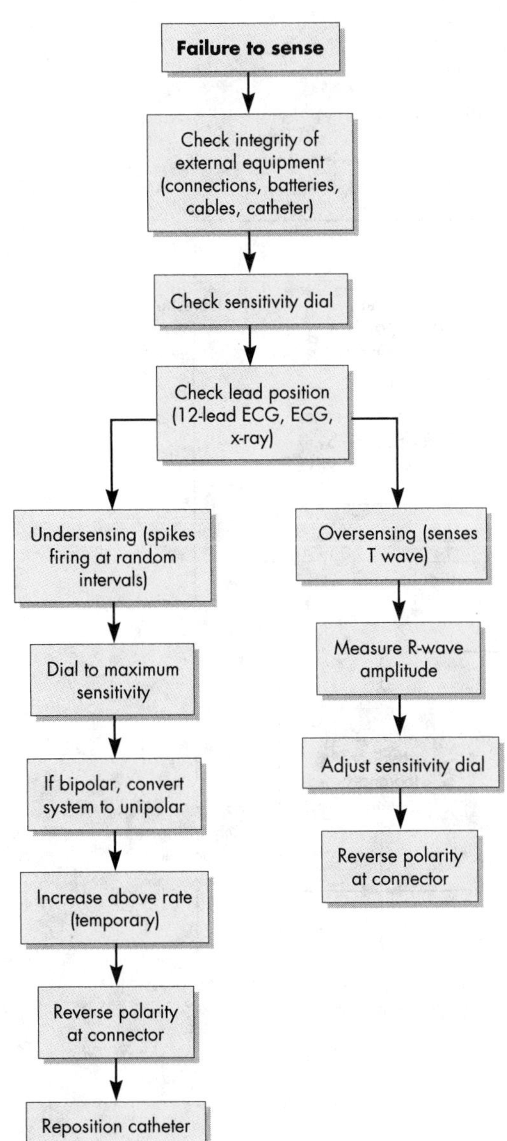

Fig. 33-27 Failure to sense.

questions about activity restrictions and fears concerning body image and becoming a "cardiac cripple" after the procedure. The goal of pacemaker therapy should be to enhance physiologic functioning and the quality of life.[25] This should be emphasized to the patient, and the nurse should give concrete advice on activity restrictions. Basic information for the patient with a pacemaker is outlined in Table 33-13.

Pacemaker function can be checked by magnet placement during ECG assessment in the pacemaker clinic, or it can be done from the home using telephone transmitter devices. The patient is sometimes given devices to place on the fingers or directly over the pacemaker battery generator with an attachment to the telephone. In this way, the heart rhythm can be transmitted to the pacemaker clinic.

External Pacemaker. The external pacemaker or transcutaneous pacemaker (TCP) has recently been reintroduced as a means of providing adequate HR and rhythm to the patient in an emergency situation (Fig. 33-29). Placement of the external pacemaker is a noninvasive procedure that should be used only temporarily until a transvenous pacemaker can be inserted or until more definitive therapy is available. The use of a TCP has become a cornerstone of therapy for asystole and bradycardia in the ACLS algorithms.[11]

The external pacemaker was used in the 1950s but lost favor in 1959 when internal pacemakers became available. Early external pacemakers were painful to use and required high voltage to maintain an acceptable cardiac rhythm. Modern external pacemakers have been modified to allow cardiac stimulation at lower voltage levels. The external pacemaker consists of a power source and a rate- and voltage-control device that is attached to two large electrode pads. One pad is positioned on the anterior part of the chest, usually on the V_2 or V_5 lead position, and the other pad is placed on the back between the spine and the left scapula at the level of the heart.[11]

Before initiating external pacemaker therapy, it is important to tell the patient what to expect. The uncomfortable muscle contractions that the pacemaker creates when the current passes through the chest wall should be explained. The patient should be reassured that the therapy is temporary and that every effort will be made to adjust the voltage settings of the pacemaker to improve comfort level.[23] Mild analgesia may also be given.

Catheter Ablation Therapy

Catheter ablation therapy is a revolutionary development in the area of antidysrhythmic therapy. In 1981 transcatheter ablation of the AV node was introduced as a treatment for supraventricular dysrhythmias. Radiofrequency energy (produced by high-frequency alternating current) has been most recently used to "burn" or ablate areas of the conduction system as definitive treatment of tachydysrhythmias.[28-30]

The procedure is done following EPS that is used to map the source of the dysrhythmia. An electrode-tipped ablation catheter is used to "burn" or ablate accessory pathways or ectopic sites in the atria, AV node, and ventricles. Catheter ablation is considered the nonpharmacologic treatment of choice for AV nodal reentrant tachycardia, reentrant tachycardia related to accessory bypass tracts, and to control the ventricular response of certain tachydysrhythmias. In some cases of uncontrolled ventricular response in atrial fibrillation or flutter, which is unresponsive to medical therapy, complete ablation of the AV node or bundle of His is performed.

The ablation procedure is a highly successful therapy with a low complication rate. Care of the patient following ablation therapy is similar to that of a patient undergoing cardiac catheterization (see Chapter 29).

CARDIOPULMONARY RESUSCITATION

Every nurse and physician should be skilled in CPR because *cardiac arrest,* the sudden cessation of breathing and adequate circulation of blood by the heart, may occur at

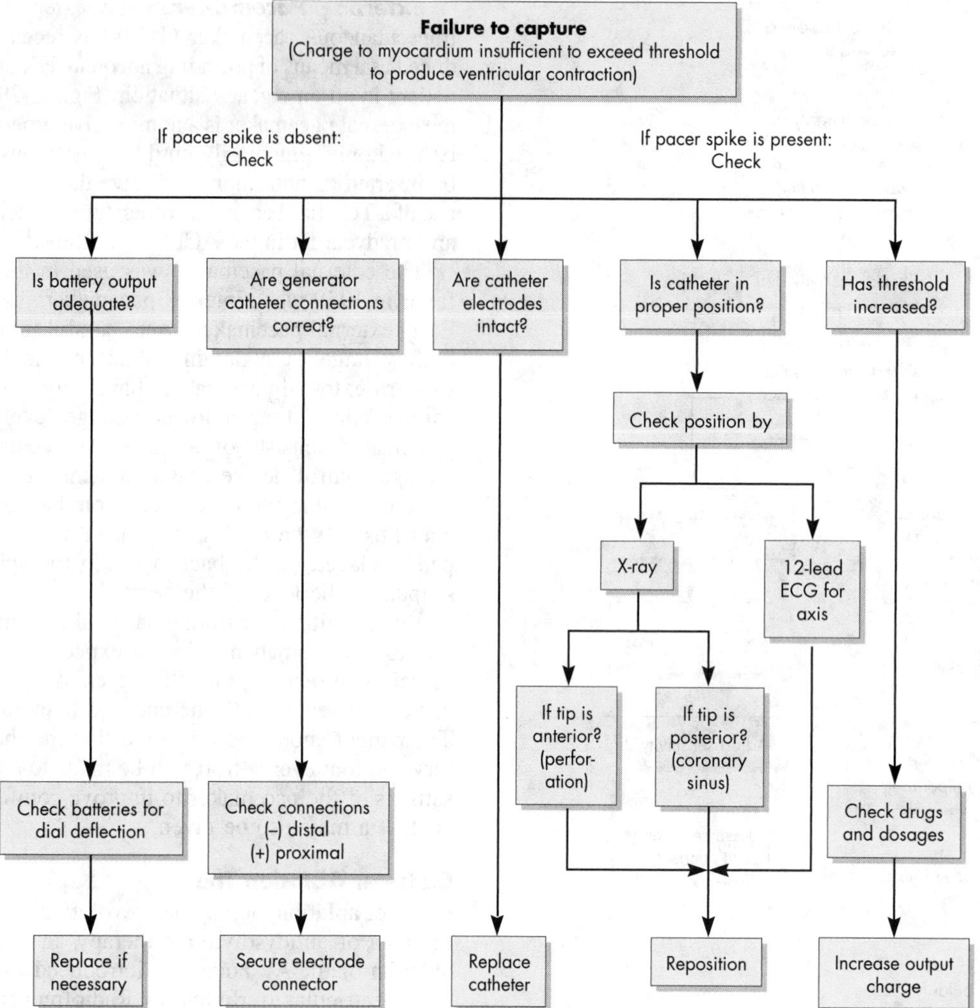

Fig. 33-28 Failure to capture.

any time or in any setting. CPR is the process of externally supporting the circulation and respiration of a person who has a cardiac arrest. Resuscitation measures are divided into two components, basic cardiac life support (BCLS) and ACLS. The American Heart Association establishes the standards for CPR and is actively involved in teaching BCLS and ACLS to health professionals. The American Heart Association recommends that nurses and physicians working with patients be certified in BCLS and ACLS. Certification involves attending formal classes and passing cognitive and motor skill tests.

CPR alone is not enough to save lives in most cardiac arrests. It is a vital link in the chain of survival that supports the victim until more advanced help is available. The chain of survival is composed of the following sequence: early activation of the EMS system, early CPR, early defibrillation, and early advanced care.[31]

Basic Cardiac Life Support

BCLS involves the external support of circulation and ventilation for a patient with cardiac or respiratory arrest through CPR.[31,32] Artificial respiration (mouth-to-mouth, mouth-to-mask, mouth-to-nose, mouth-to-stoma) and external chest compression substitute for spontaneous breathing and circulation. The major objective of performing CPR is to provide oxygen to the brain, heart, and other vital organs until appropriate therapeutic management and resuscitation efforts involving advanced life support methods can be initiated or until resuscitation efforts are ordered to be stopped.

Rapid intervention is the key to success and is critical in preventing biologic death or the death of brain cells. CPR must be initiated within 4 to 6 minutes of cardiac or pulmonary arrest. Brain cells begin to die (*brain death*) within 6 minutes of anoxia. It is critical that oxygenated blood be circulated during CPR. Unfortunately, even when CPR is performed with perfect technique, only 25% to 30% of the normal CO is achieved. National standards for knowledge and technique must be met for personnel to be certified to deliver CPR. Assessment of the victim must be stressed in teaching CPR. Each of the broad areas—**A**irway, **B**reathing, and **C**irculation (the ABCs of CPR)—should be reviewed.

Table 33-13 Educational Information for the Patient with a Pacemaker

- Maintain follow-up care with a physician because it is important to check the pacemaker site and to begin regular pacemaker function checks with magnet and ECG evaluation.
- Watch for signs of infection at incision site (e.g., redness, swelling, drainage).
- Keep incision dry for 1 wk after discharge.
- For activity restriction, avoid direct blows to generator site. (Avoid contact sports such as football or use of rifle.)
- Avoid close proximity to high-output electrical generators or to large magnets such as a MRI scanner. These devices can reprogram the pacemaker.
- Microwave ovens are perfectly safe to use and do not threaten pacemaker function.
- Travel without restrictions is allowed. The metal case of a small implanted pacemaker rarely sets off an airport security alarm.
- Learn how to take pulse rate.
- Carry pacemaker information card at all times, preferably in an easily accessible place such as a wallet or purse.

ECG, Electrocardiogram; *MRI*, magnetic resonance imaging.

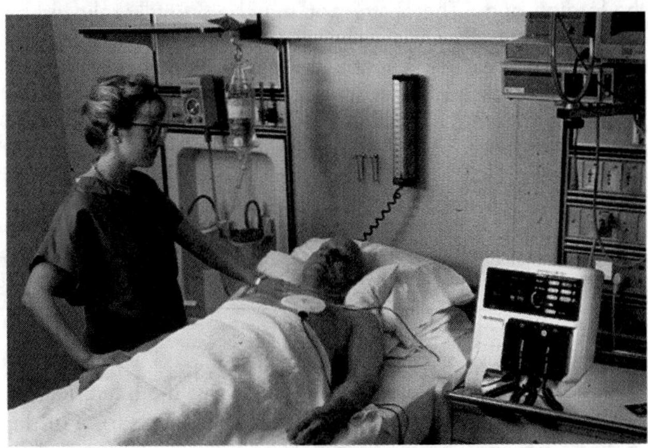

Fig. 33-29 Transcutaneous pacemaker.

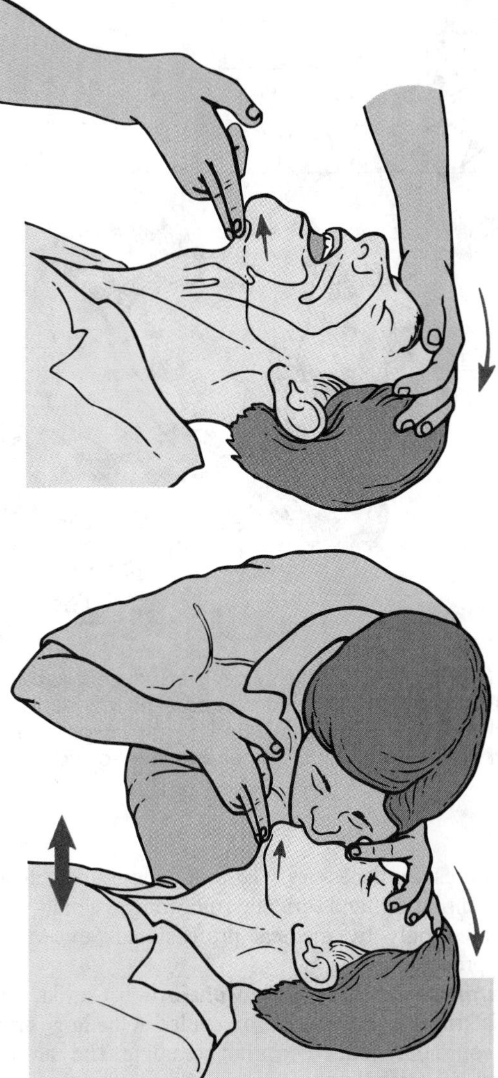

Fig. 33-30 The head-tilt/chin-lift maneuver is used to open the victim's airway to give mouth-to-mouth resuscitation. This procedure is carried out by placing one hand on the victim's forehead and applying firm, backward pressure with the palm to tilt the head back. The chin is lifted and brought forward with the fingers of the other hand.

Airway and Breathing. The first steps in administering BCLS are to confirm the absence of breathing and to establish a patent airway. Figure 33-30 demonstrates opening the airway and performing mouth-to-mouth ventilation. An adult's airway is opened by hyperextending the head. The *head-tilt/chin-lift manuever* is used and involves tilting the head back with one hand and lifting the chin forward with the fingers of the other hand. If no respirations are detected, the rescuer attempts to ventilate the victim with mouth-to-mouth resuscitation. Breaths are given with the victim's nostrils pinched and the rescuer's mouth placed around the victim's mouth to make a tight seal. Two slow breaths are given by the rescuer (1½ to 2 seconds per breath). The volume of air of each ventilation should be approximately 800 ml, which can be determined by noting a rise of 1 to 2 inches in the victim's chest. When the victim has a tracheostomy, ventilation should be given through the stoma.[11,31,32]

If air flow is obstructed, the rescuer should reposition the head and repeat the attempt to provide ventilation. If the victim cannot be ventilated after repositioning the head, the rescuer should proceed with maneuvers to remove foreign bodies that may be obstructing the airway (Table 33-14).

In those rare instances when airway obstruction is not relieved by methods described in Table 33-14, additional

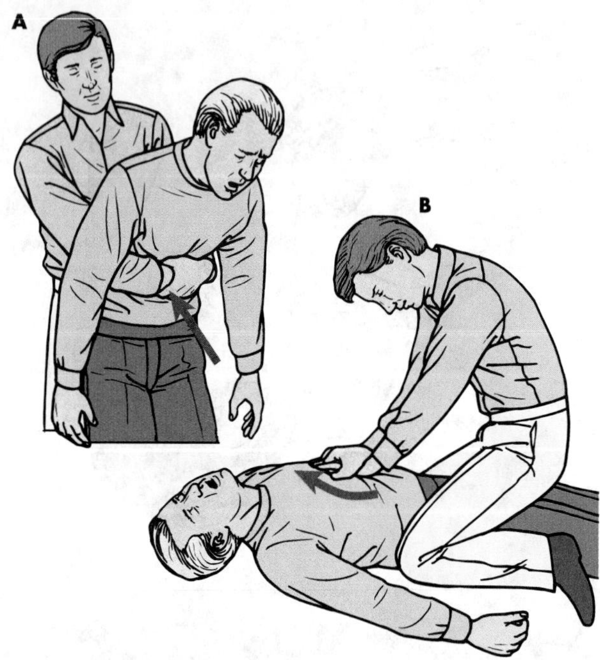

Fig. 33-31 ***A,*** Heimlich maneuver administered to a conscious (standing) victim of foreign body airway obstruction. ***B,*** Heimlich maneuver administered to an unconscious (lying) victim of foreign body airway obstruction—astride position.

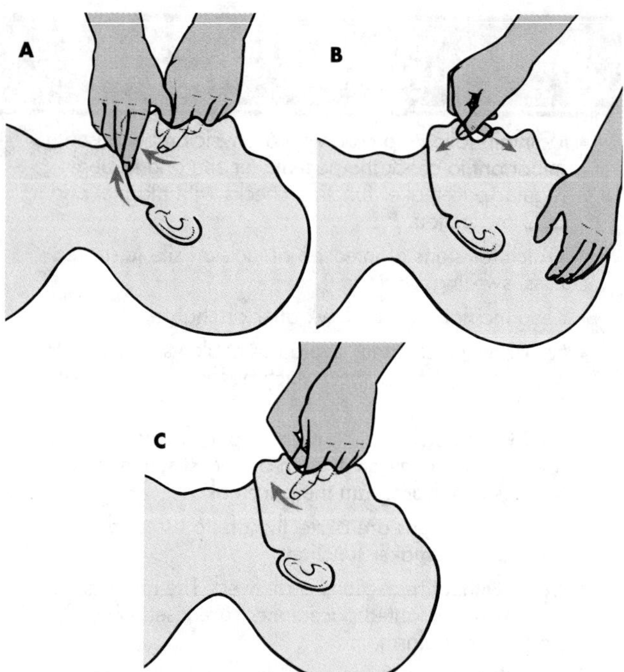

Fig. 33-32 ***A,*** Finger sweep maneuver administered to an unconscious victim of foreign body airway obstruction. With the victim's head up, the rescuer opens the victim's mouth by grasping both the tongue and the lower jaw between the thumb and fingers and lifting (tongue-jaw lift). This action draws the tongue from the back of the throat and away from the foreign body. The obstruction may be partially relieved by this maneuver. ***B,*** Crossed-finger technique for opening the airway. If the rescuer is unable to open the mouth with tongue-jaw lift, the crossed-finger technique may be used. The rescuer opens the mouth by crossing the index finger and thumb and pushing the teeth apart. ***C,*** The index finger of the rescuer's available hand is inserted along the inside of the cheek and deeply into the throat to the base of the tongue. A hooking motion is used to dislodge the foreign body and maneuver it into the mouth for removal.

procedures are necessary. These include transtracheal catheter ventilation and cricothyroidotomy, which must be attempted only by medical professionals experienced in these procedures.[11]

External Cardiac Compressions. Cardiac arrest is characterized by the absence of a pulse in the large arteries of an unconscious victim who is not breathing. The carotid artery is used to determine the absence of a pulse. After an airway has been established and two ventilations have been delivered, the rescuer checks the pulse. While maintaining the head-tilt position with one hand on the forehead, the rescuer locates the victim's trachea with two or three fingers of the other hand. The rescuer then slides these fingers into the groove between the trachea and the muscles of the side of the neck where the carotid pulse can be felt. The technique is more easily performed on the side nearest the rescuer. If no pulse is palpated, chest compressions should be initiated.[31]

The proper technique for administering chest compressions is shown in Fig. 33-33. External chest compression technique consists of serial, rhythmic applications of pressure on the lower half of the sternum. The victim must be in the horizontal supine position when the compressions are performed. The victim must be lying on a flat, hard surface, such as a CPR board (specially manufactured for use in CPR), a head board from a cardiac care unit bed, or if necessary, the floor. The rescuer should be positioned close to the side of the victim's chest.

The following guidelines have been established for proper hand placement[31] (see Fig. 33-33, *A*):

1. With the middle and index fingers of the hand nearest the victim's legs, the rescuer locates the lower margin of the victim's rib cage on the side next to the rescuer.
2. The fingers are moved up the rib cage to the notch where the ribs meet the sternum.
3. The middle finger is placed on this notch, and the index finger is placed next to it on the lower end of the sternum. (This allows proper placement above the xiphoid process and prevents possible laceration of the liver by the xiphoid process during compressions.)
4. The heel of the hand nearest the victim's head is placed on the lower half of the sternum, close to the index finger of the other hand. The long axis of the heel of the rescuer's hand should be placed on the long axis of the sternum.
5. The first hand is removed from the notch and placed on top of the hand on the sternum so that both hands are parallel to each other.

Table 33-14 Management of Foreign Body Airway Obstruction

Action	Helpful Hints
Conscious Adult	
1. Determine if victim is able to speak or cough.	Rescuer can ask "Are you choking?" Victim may be using the universal distress signal of choking: clutching the neck between thumb and index finger
2. Abdominal thrust: perform the Heimlich maneuver until the foreign body is expelled or the victim becomes unconscious (See Fig. 33-31).	Stand behind victim and wrap arms around victim's waist. Press fist into abdomen with quick inward and upward thrusts.
3. Chest thrust: for victims who are in advanced pregnancy or who are obese.	Chest thrusts: stand behind victim and place arms under victim's armpits to encircle the chest. Press with quick backward thrusts.
Victim Is or Becomes Unconscious	
1. Activate EMS.	Call 911.
2. Check for foreign body obstruction.	Sweep deeply into mouth with hooked finger to remove foreign body.
3. Attempt rescue breathing.	Open airway. Try to give two breaths. If needed, reposition the head and try again (See Fig. 33-32).
4. If airway is obstructed, perform Heimlich maneuver.	Kneel astride the victim's thighs. Place the heel of one hand on the victim's abdomen, in the midline slightly above the navel and well below the tip of the xyphoid. Place the second hand on top of the first. Press into the abdomen with quick upward thrusts.
5. Repeat sequence until successful.	Alternate these maneuvers in rapid sequence: finger sweep, rescue breathing attempt, and abdominal thrusts.

Modified from *Basic Life Support Heart Saver Guide: a student handbook for CPR and first aid for choking,* Dallas, 1993, American Heart Association.
EMS, Emergency medical services.

6. The fingers are extended or interlaced and must be kept off the chest.

The following guidelines have been established for proper compression technique (See Fig. 33-33):[31]

1. The elbows are locked into position, the arms are straightened, and the shoulders are positioned directly over the hands so that the thrust for each chest compression is straight down on the sternum.
2. The sternum must be depressed 1.5 to 2 inches (3.8 to 5.0 cm) for the normal-sized adult. The heart is compressed between the sternum and spine.
3. The external chest compression pressure is released to allow blood to flow into the heart. The time allowed for release of compression should be equal to the time required for compression.
4. The hands should not be lifted from the chest or the position changed in any way so that correct hand position is maintained.

Rescue breathing and chest compressions are combined for an effective resuscitation effort of the victim of cardiopulmonary arrest. When there is one rescuer, the rate of compression should be 80 to 100 compressions per minute with a compression-ventilation ratio of 15 compressions to 2 ventilations (Table 33-15). The compression rate for two-rescuer CPR is 80 to 100 per minute, with a compression-ventilation ratio of 5:1 (Table 33-16).

The victim's condition must be assessed during CPR to determine the effectiveness of compressions and to deter-

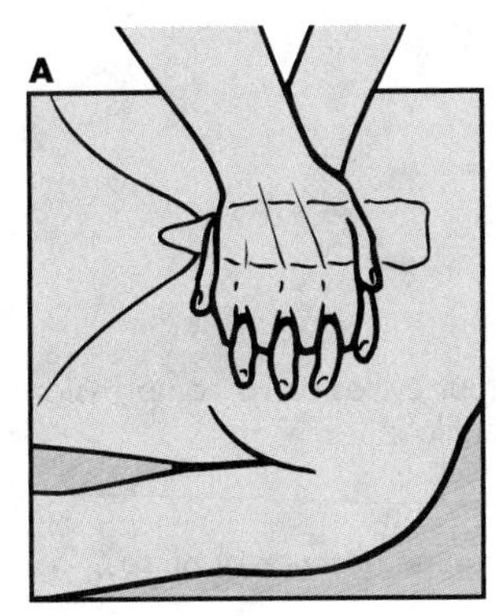

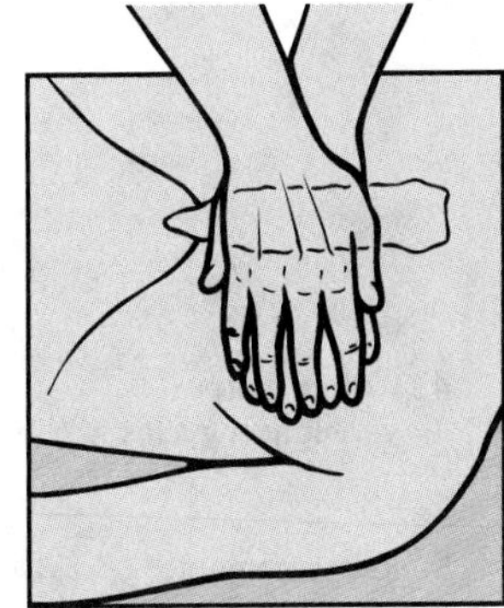
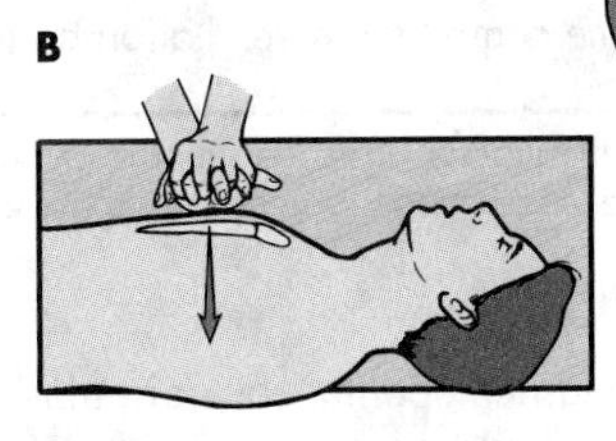

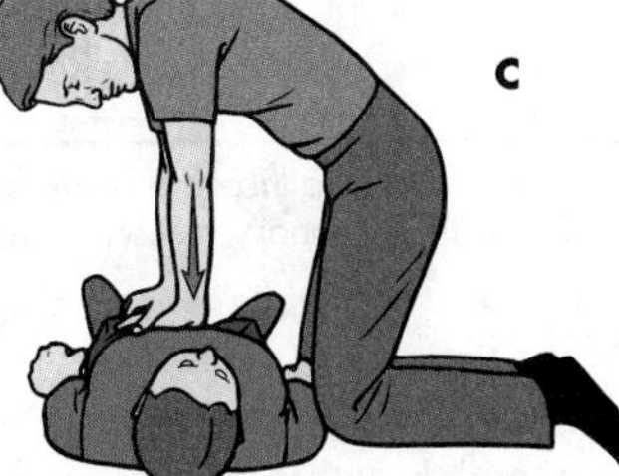

Fig. 33-33 Cardiopulmonary resuscitation (CPR). ***A,*** Position of the hands during application of external cardiac massage. ***B,*** When pressure is applied, the lower portion of the sternum is displaced posteriorly with the palm of the hand. ***C,*** To apply maximum downward pressure, the resuscitator leans forward so that both arms are at right angles to the patient's sternum and the elbows are locked.

Table 33-15 Adult One-Rescuer CPR

Step	Objective	Critical Performance
1. Airway	Assessment: Determine unresponsiveness.	Tap or gently shake shoulder. Shout "Are you OK?"
	Call for help.	Call out "Help!"
	Position the victim.	Turn on back as unit, if necessary, supporting head and neck (4-10 sec).
	Open the airway.	Use head-tilt/chin-lift maneuver.
2. Breathing	Assessment: Determine cessation of breathing.	Maintain open airway. With ear over mouth, observe chest: look, listen, feel for breathing (3-5 sec).
	Ventilate twice.	Maintain open airway. Seal mouth and nose properly. Ventilate two times at 1-1.5 sec/inflation. Observe chest rise (adequate ventilation volume). Allow deflation between breaths.
3. Circulation	Assessment: Determine absence of pulse.	Feel for carotid pulse on near side of victim (5-10 sec). Maintain head-tilt with other hand.
	Activate EMS system.	If someone responded to call for help, send person to activate EMS system. Total time, step 1—Activate EMS system: 15-35 sec.
	Begin chest compressions.	Kneel by victim's shoulders. Make landmark check before hands are placed. Maintain proper hand position throughout. Keep shoulders over victim's sternum. Maintain equal compression and relaxation. Compress 1.5-2 in. Keep hands on sternum during upstroke. Wait for complete chest relaxation on upstroke. Say any helpful mnemonic (e.g., one-and-two-and-three-and . . .). Remember that compression rate is 80-100/min (15/9-11sec).
4. Compression-ventilation cycles	Do four cycles of 15 compressions and two ventilations.	Maintain proper compression-ventilation ratio of 15 compressions to two ventilations per cycle. Observe chest rise: 1-1.5 sec/inflation; four cycles/52-73 sec.
5. Reassessment	Determine absence of pulse.	Feel for carotid pulse (5 sec). If there is no pulse, go to step 6.
6. Continuation of CPR	Ventilate twice.	Ventilate two times. Observe chest rise: 1-1.5 sec/inflation.
	Resume compression-ventilation cycles.	Feel for carotid pulse every few min.

Modified from *Healthcare provider's manual for basic life support,* Dallas, 1993, American Heart Association.
CPR, Cardiopulmonary resuscitation; *EMS,* emergency medical services.

mine whether the victim has resumed spontaneous circulation and breathing. The pulse should be checked by the ventilating rescuer during the compressions to assess the effectiveness of compressions in two-rescuer CPR. Chest compressions are stopped for 5 seconds at the end of the first minute and every few minutes thereafter to determine whether the victim has resumed spontaneous breathing and circulation. The goal of CPR is the return of spontaneous breathing and circulation, but it is rarely achieved without more definitive therapy with ACLS.

Advanced Cardiac Life Support

ACLS involves a systematic approach to treatment of cardiac emergencies with knowledge and skills necessary to provide early treatment. ACLS includes (1) basic life support (BLS); (2) the use of adjunctive equipment and special techniques for establishing and maintaining effective ventilation and circulation; (3) ECG monitoring and dysrhythmia recognition; (4) establishment and maintenance of IV access; (5) therapies for emergency treatment of patient with cardiac or respiratory arrest (including stabilization in the postarrest

Table 33-16 Adult Two-Rescuer CPR

Step	Objective	Critical Performance
1. Airway	*One rescuer (ventilator):*	
	Assessment: Determine unresponsiveness.	Tap or gently shake shoulder. Shout "Are you OK?"
	Position the victim.	Turn on back if necessary (4-10 sec).
	Open the airway.	Use a proper technique to open airway.
2. Breathing	Assessment: Determine cessation of breathing.	Look, listen, and feel for breath (3-5 sec).
	Ventilate twice.	Observe chest rise: 1-1.5 sec/inflation.
3. Circulation	Assessment: Determine absence of pulse.	Feel for carotid pulse (5-10 sec).
	State assessment results.	Say "No pulse."
	Other rescuer (compressor):	When another rescuer comes, first rescuer asks if EMS has been activated.
	Get into position for compressions.	Put hands, shoulders in correct position.
	Locate landmark notch.	Check landmark.
4. Compression-ventilation cycles	*Compressor:* Begin chest compressions.	Correct ratio compressions-ventilations is 5:1. Compression rate is 80-100/min (5 compressions/3-4 sec). Say any helpful mnemonic. Stop compressing for each ventilation.
	Ventilator: Ventilate after every fifth compression and check compression effectiveness.	Ventilate once (1-1.5 sec/inflation). Check pulse occasionally to assess compressions.
	(Minimum of 10 cycles)	(Time for 10 cycles: 40-53 sec)
5. Calling for switch	*Compressor:* Call for switch when tired.	Give clear signal to change roles. Compressor completes fifth compression. Ventilator completes ventilation after fifth compression.
6. Switching	Simultaneously switch:	
	Ventilator: Move to chest.	Become compressor. Get into position for compressions. Locate landmark notch.
	Compressor: Move to head.	Become ventilator. Check carotid pulse (5 sec). Say "No pulse." Ventilate once (1-1.5 sec/inflation).
7. Continuation of CPR	Resume compression-ventilation cycles.	Repeat step 4.

Modified from *Healthcare provider's manual for basic life support,* Dallas, 1993, American Heart Association.

phase); and (6) treatment of patient with suspected acute MI.[11]

The principle of early defibrillation has been emphasized in national emergency medical care organizations. With the invention of the automated external defibrillator (AED), which is simple to use and available throughout communities, more trained rescuers are available to provide early defibrillation.[33] The importance of early, effective BLS and defibrillation before entrance into the ACLS system cannot be overemphasized.

Drugs used in ACLS include oxygen therapy, IV fluids, morphine sulfate, drugs used for the control of HR and rhythm, and those used to improve CO and BP. Table 33-17 describes drugs used in cardiac emergencies.

Medical professionals trained in ACLS are taught treatment algorithms that are guidelines for definitive treatment of specific cardiac emergencies. The algorithm can be adjusted to fit the needs of a particular patient or situation. Emphasis is placed on maintaining the basics of airway, breathing, and circulation (ABC), and making judgments for effective treatment based on overall patient assessment.[11,18]

Nursing Role During a Code

There is potential for a "code" or cardiopulmonary arrest situation in all hospital settings. The nurse should be well prepared to participate in resuscitation of a patient. The nurse must be familiar with code protocols, emergency equipment in the crash cart, and keep current with BCLS and ACLS skills.[34,35]

It is important for the nurse to be familiar with the crash cart location and contents on the hospital unit. Most crash carts contain all necessary emergency supplies. Ideally, all crash carts in an individual hospital are organized in the same fashion.

Table 33-17 Drugs Commonly Used in Cardiac Emergencies

Drug	Indications	Major Pharmacologic Effect	Adverse Effects	Nursing Considerations
Oxygen	Hypoxia, acute MI, cardiopulmonary arrest	Used by all body cells for aerobic metabolism; improves tissue oxygenation	Oxygen toxicity	In emergency situations, administer oxygen.
Sodium bicarbonate	Metabolic and respiratory acidosis	Corrects metabolic acidosis by the following formula: $HCO_3^- + H^+ \leftrightarrow H_2CO_3 \leftrightarrow CO_2 + H_2O \leftrightarrow H_2CO_3$	Metabolic alkalosis, hypernatremia, water overload, possible worsening of intracellular acidosis	Be aware that drug is used only after more definitive maneuvers have proved unsuccessful. Do not mix it with any other agent.
Epinephrine (Adrenalin)	Asystole, pulseless electrical activity, bronchospasm, anaphylaxis	Stimulates α- and β-receptor sites, resulting in ↑ HR, ↑ myocardial contractile force, ↑ systemic vascular resistance, ↑ arterial blood pressure, ↑ myocardial oxygen consumption, ↑ coronary and cerebral blood flow, ↓ blood flow to kidneys and skin	Transient anxiety, palpitations, headache, tissue necrosis from local injections, increased blood glucose, increased oxygen consumption of heart, hypertension	Correct acidosis before IV administration of epinephrine. Do not mix with alkaline solutions.
Atropine	Symptomatic sinus bradycardia, asystole	↑ Discharge rate of the SA node (vagolytic action), ↓ refractory period and ↑ speed of conduction through AV node	Blurred vision, dry mouth, pupil dilatation, difficulty in voiding, increased bronchial secretions, PVCs, VT, or VF (especially in acute MI patient)	Give with morphine to counteract vagomimetic effect. Use with extreme caution in patient with myocardial ischemia because it may exacerbate ischemia.
Lidocaine (Xylocaine)	PVCs, VT, VF	↓ Automaticity of Purkinje's fibers, ↑ threshold for VF, ↓ conduction velocity and refractory period of Purkinje's fibers, prolonged conduction and refractoriness in ischemic tissue	Lethargy, confusion, slurred speech, tingling lips and tongue, disorientation, hypotension convulsions, SA arrest, heart block, bradycardia	Use with caution in patient with slow HR or heart block. Continuously monitor ECG of patient receiving this drug. Be aware that drug has slower detoxification in patient with liver dysfunction or reduced CO and in patient >70 yr of age.
Morphine	Pain with acute MI or acute pulmonary edema	Causes analgesic and sedative effects, ↑ venous pooling, ↓ left ventricular end diastolic pressure, ↓ myocardial oxygen consumption, ↓ left ventricular afterload, ↑ myocardial contractility, ↑ ventricular excitability	Respiratory depression, hypotension, confusion	Administer with caution. Be aware that morphine is a respiratory depressant. Reverse excessive narcosis with IV naloxone.
Calcium chloride	Lack of clear data demonstrating a beneficial effect of calcium salt administration during CPR	↑ Myocardial contractility, ↑ ventricular excitability	Moderate decrease in BP, hypercalcemia, local necrosis if extravasation occurs, bradycardia after rapid administration	Do not mix with sodium bicarbonate. Give slowly if heart is beating (can cause severe bradycardia or sinus arrest). Use cautiously with digitalized patient (can enhance toxicity).
Procainamide (Pronestyl)	PVCs, VT, supraventricular tachycardia	↑ Refractory period in atrium, ↓ excitability in atria and ventricles, ↓ automaticity of pacemaker cells, ↑ threshold to fibrillation, ↑ conduction time	GI distress, anorexia, nausea, vomiting, diarrhea; CNS depression and hallucinations; systemic lupus-like syndrome (arthralgia, fever, skin rash); hypotension, convulsions, AV block, PVCs, VF, agranulocytosis	Do not give to patient with complete heart block. When giving IV, monitor ECG and BP of patient. Stop drug if QRS complex widens or if PR or ST intervals become prolonged.

continued

Table 33-17 Drugs Commonly Used in Cardiac Emergencies—cont'd

Drug	Indications	Major Pharmacologic Effect	Adverse Effects	Nursing Considerations
Bretylium (Bretylol)	Resistant VT or VF not responsive to lidocaine, procainamide, defibrillation	Transiently increases BP and dysrhythmias followed by a decrease in BP and dysrhythmias as a result of sympatholytic action, ↑ myocardial contractility, ↑ VF threshold, ↑ refractory period of Purkinje's fibers and ventricular muscle	Postural hypotension, nausea and vomiting, increased sensitivity to catecholamines, aggravation of existing angina pectoris, parotid pain	Watch patient closely for hypersensitivity reaction if they are receiving catecholamine drugs concurrently. In patient with renal failure, watch closely for toxicity.
Verapamil (Calan, Isoptin)	Supraventricular tachycardia	Blocks slow inward current caused by changes in calcium and sodium, causes slow conduction and prolonged refractoriness in AV node	Hypotension in patient with reduced ventricular function, possible hypotension and AV block in those receiving concomitant IV β-blocker	Use with extreme caution in patient with sick sinus syndrome or AV block in absence of pacemaker.
Diltiazem (Cardizem)	Atrial fibrillation, atrial flutter, paroxysmal supraventricular tachycardia	Inhibits the influx of calcium ions during depolarization of cardiac cells. Slows AV nodal conduction time	Headache, CHF, AV block, dizziness, edema, bradycardia, constipation, nausea, palpitations, and hypotension	May produce a negative inotropic effect with heart failure resulting. Careful assessment of patient (especially those with CAD) for shortness of breath, rales, S_3 gallop, and other signs of CHF is important.
Magnesium sulfate	Recurrent and refractory VT and VF. Treatment of choice for torsade de pointes	Mechanism of action not entirely clear. It may be a calcium antagonist and block slow calcium channels. In the setting of hypomagnesemia, intracellular potassium may decrease, leading to increased cellular excitability. Magnesium replacement, instead of potassium, may resolve the problem	Sweating, depressed deep tendon reflexes, flushing, hypotension, heart block, circulatory collapse	Continue to monitor serum electrolytes including Mg^{++} and K^{+}. Monitor ECG rate, rhythm, QRS, and QT intervals. Nurse needs to recognize polymorphic VT (torsade de pointes) and be ready to treat with IV magnesium.
Dopamine (Intropin)	Cardiac decompensation, as with CHF or cardiogenic shock; open heart surgery; hypotension	Stimulates dopaminergic, β_2-adrenergic, and α-adrenergic receptors in a dose-dependent fashion: low doses (1-2 μg/kg/min) produce vasodilatation of renal, mesenteric, and cerebral arteries; medium doses (2-10 μg/kg/min) increase CO and modestly increase SVR and preload; high doses (>10 μg/kg/min) cause marked vasoconstriction	Tachycardia, ectopic dysrhythmias, nausea and vomiting, angina, dyspnea, headache, hypotension, palpitations, vasoconstriction, PVCs	Prevent extravasation by infusing into large vein. Do not mix with alkaline substance. Titrate dose to desired hemodynamic or renal response. Slow rate if an increased diastolic pressure results in a decreased pulse pressure. Continuously monitor ECG and BP.
Dobutamine (Dobutrex)	Cardiac decompensation, especially with CHF and cardiogenic shock	Stimulates β_1-receptor sites, ↑ myocardial contractility but not HR, slightly stimulates α- and β_2-vascular receptors (does not dilate renal and mesenteric arteries and does not have vasoconstrictive activity at higher doses)	Marked elevation in HR (30 bpm or more), marked elevation in BP (50 mm Hg), ventricular ectopy, nausea, headache, chest pain, palpitations, shortness of breath	Continuously monitor ECG, blood pressure, PCWP, and CO. Do not mix dobutamine with alkaline substance.

continued

Table 33-17 Drugs Commonly Used in Cardiac Emergencies—cont'd

Drug	Indications	Major Pharmacologic Effect	Adverse Effects	Nursing Considerations
Isoproterenol (Isuprel)	Temporary control of atropine-resistant bradycardia	Stimulates β-receptor sites (β_1 and β_2), ↑ myocardial contractility, ↑ HR, ↑ myocardial oxygen consumption, ↓ SVR, ↓ diastolic pressure (may reduce MAP), relaxes smooth muscle in bronchioles and GI tract	Sinus tachycardia; PVCs; VT; VF; hypotension in presence of hypovolemia, headache, flushing of skin, angina, nausea, tremor, dizziness, weakness, and sweating	Be aware that isoproterenol is contraindicated in the presence of digitalis-induced tachycardias. Use cautiously in presence of hypokalemia (↑ dysrhythmias). If ventricular irritability occurs, decrease IV infusion rate. Titrate IV dose to achieve HR of 60 bpm.
Digitalis (Ouabain, digoxin, digitoxin)	Atrial flutter, atrial fibrillation, paroxysmal supraventricular tachycardia, CHF	↑ Myocardial contractility, ↑ rate at which force is developed, ↑ refractory period of AV node, ↑ left ventricular end diastolic volume and pressure, ↑ ventricular automaticity, ↓ atrial automaticity	Cardiac effects of PVCs, junctional rhythms, AV block, VT, VF, PACs	Always assess pulse before giving the drug because many dysrhythmias are caused by digitalis. Monitor ECG when using IV administration. Be aware that reduced renal function, hypercalcemia, and hypokalemia predispose patient to digitalis toxicity. When giving drug with quinidine, decrease dose because quinidine reduces renal clearance of digoxin.
Amrinone (Inocor)	Severe CHF refractory to diuretics, vasodilators, and conventional inotropic agents	Inhibits phosphodiesterase, has inotropic and vasodilator effects, ↑ CO, ↓ SVR	Myocardial ischemia, thrombocytopenia, nausea and vomiting, myalgia, fever, hepatic dysfunction	Continuously monitor central hemodynamics. Be aware that drug contains metabisulfite, which is contraindicated in patients allergic to bisulfites.
Norepinephrine (Levophed)	Hypotension when total SVR is low	Acts as α- and β-adrenergic receptor agonist, ↑ myocardial contractility and ↑ peripheral vasoconstriction	Increased myocardial oxygen consumption, dysrhythmias	Continuously monitor hemodynamics and ECG. Be aware that ischemic necrosis and sloughing of tissues can occur with extravasations and that drug is contraindicated when hypotension is caused by hypovolemia.
Nitroprusside (Nipride)	Hypertensive emergency, acute left ventricular failure	Vasodilates arterioles and venules; causes increased CO in patient with elevated left ventricular filling pressure (increased CO caused more by decreased afterload than decreased preload); causes decreased ventricular filling pressure, mean PAP, SVR, and MAP	Acute effects, including hypotension, tachycardia, increased intracranial pressure; long-term effects, including fatigue, nausea, anorexia, disorientation, psychotic behavior, muscle spasm	Continuously infuse drug because its effect takes 3-5 min. Slow infusion rate if there is excessive increase in HR or lowering of blood pressure. When used for low-output states, monitor ECG, intraarterial pressure, PCWP, and CO. Be aware that the solution must be protected from light to prevent deterioration.

continued

Table 33-17 Drugs Commonly Used in Cardiac Emergencies—cont'd

Drug	Indications	Major Pharmacologic Effect	Adverse Effects	Nursing Considerations
Nitroglycerin	Angina pectoris, acute MI, left ventricular failure	Relaxes vascular smooth muscle; dilates venous smooth muscle in angina pectoris and MI, inhibiting venous return with reduced ventricular volume, ventricular pressure, and wall stress; dilates large coronary arteries, antagonizes vasospasm, and increases coronary collateral blood flow to ischemic myocardium, reduces left ventricular filling pressure and SVR in CHF	Headache, hypotension, bradycardia	Monitor hemodynamics if drug is given IV for CHF. Administer sublingual nitroglycerin while patient is sitting or lying down. Treat hypotension with fluid administration.
β-Blockers Propranolol (Inderal) Metoprolol (Lopressor)	Acute MI, angina pectoris, hypertension, atrial fibrillation, atrial flutter, PSVT, refractory VT or VF	Acts as β-adrenergic receptor blocking agent, ↓ HR and myocardial contractility, ↓ myocardial oxygen consumption, depresses automaticity of pacemakers and suppresses ectopic beats, prolongs AV conduction time and refractory period	Bradycardia, hypotension, heart block, fatigue, dizziness, blood sugar disturbances, insomnia, GI distress	Do not use in presence of bradycardia, heart block, and bronchospasm.
Furosemide (Lasix)	Emergency treatment of pulmonary congestion associated with left ventricular dysfunction, chronic heart failure	Inhibits reabsorption of sodium and chloride in the ascending loop of Henle; has direct venodilating effect that reduces venous return and central venous pressure	Dehydration; hypotension; sodium, potassium, and magnesium depletion; hyperosmolality; metabolic alkalosis; loss of hearing	Inject drug IV slowly for 1-2 min.

AV, Atrioventricular; *BP,* blood pressure; *CAD,* coronary artery disease; *CHF,* congestive heart failure; *CNS,* central nervous system; *CO,* cardiac output; *CPR,* cardiopulmonary resuscitation; *ECG,* electrocardiogram; *GI,* gastrointestinal; *HR,* heart rate; *IV,* intravenous; *MAP,* mean arterial pressure; *MI,* myocardial infarction; *PAC,* premature atrial contraction; *PAP,* pulmonary artery pressure; *PCWP,* pulmonary capillary wedge pressure; *PSVT,* paroxysmal supraventricular tachycardia; *PVC,* premature ventricular contraction; *SA,* sinoatrial; *SVR,* systemic vascular resistance; *VF,* ventricular fibrillation; *VT,* ventricular tachycardia.

*Diltiazem + Adenosine.

†See Table 33-8.

CRITICAL THINKING EXERCISES

CASE STUDY

DYSRHYTHMIA

Patient Profile

J.M., a 68-year-old retired postal worker, is admitted to the cardiac care unit following cardiac arrest. After defibrillation is performed by paramedics, J.M. is awake and lethargic but responding appropriately.

Subjective Data

- Has had two MIs and a history of CHF
- Has shortness of breath, even in a sitting position

Objective Data

Physical Examination

- Appears anxious
- BP 92/60 Pulse 98/min Respirations 28/min
- Lungs: bilateral coarse crackles
- Heart: S3 gallop at apex

Diagnostic Studies

- ECG: Frequent PVC
- Echocardiogram: severe left ventricular dysfunction with ejection fraction of 20%
- Serum potassium 2.9 mEq/L (2.9 mmol/L)

Therapeutic Management

Lidocaine infusion 2 mg/minute
Scheduled for EPS testing

Critical Thinking Questions

1. Why is J.M. at risk for sudden cardiac death (ventricular fibrillation)?
2. Explain the rationale for using lidocaine after ventricular fibrillation.
3. What methods may be used to assess the effectiveness of the antidysrhythmic drugs?
4. Would J.M. be a candidate for an ICD?
5. If J.M. had ventricular fibrillation again while on a lidocaine infusion, what other IV medications would be tried?
6. Explain the significance of the serum potassium value.
7. Based on the assessment data provided, write one or more appropriate nursing diagnoses. Are there any collaborative problems?

REVIEW QUESTIONS

1. Sinus bradycardia may require medical or pacemaker therapy for which of the following situations?
   a. Asymptomatic, aerobically-trained male with normal BP
   b. Patient with inferior MI with BP of 70/50
   c. Patient with hypothyroidism and BP of 120/80
   d. Patient on β-blocker therapy with BP of 120/80

2. Recommended treatment for second-degree AV block (Mobitz type I, Wenckebach phenomenon) with stable BP and no symptoms includes
   a. immediate insertion of temporary pacemaker.
   b. epinephrine 1 mg IV push.
   c. isoproterenol IV continuous drip.
   d. careful observation for symptoms of hypotension.

3. Defibrillation is indicated for
   a. third-degree AV block.
   b. ventricular fibrillation.
   c. ventricular tachycardia.
   d. atrial flutter.

4. Indications for permanent pacemaker therapy include all of the following *except*
   a. third-degree AV block.
   b. chronic atrial fibrillation with slow ventricular response.
   c. sick sinus syndrome.
   d. asymptomatic sinus bradycardia.

5. Which of the following is *not* an expected patient reaction to the recommendation for placement of an ICD?
   a. Denial
   b. Immediate acceptance
   c. Fear of change in body image
   d. Fear of recurrent sudden death

6. Important teaching for the patient who will be undergoing electrophysiologic monitoring includes all of the following except explaining that
   a. a catheter will be placed in a peripheral vein.
   b. dysrhythmias may be stimulated by the procedure.
   c. the patient will be asleep during the procedure.
   d. EPS testing can be used to map the source of dysrhythmias.

7. Which is the proper sequence for care of the obstructed airway victim who becomes unconscious?

a. Abdominal thrusts; finger sweep into mouth; call for second rescuer; attempt rescue breathing
b. Attempt rescue breathing; abdominal thrusts if still obstructed; finger sweep into mouth; call 911
c. Call 911; finger sweep into mouth; attempt rescue breathing; abdominal thrusts if still obstructed
d. Finger sweep into mouth; attempt rescue breathing; call 911; abdominal thrust if still obstructed

8. In addition to BLS, ACLS includes all of the following *except*

a. the use of drug therapy.
b. the use of adjunctive equipment.
c. ECG monitoring.
d. emergency surgical procedures.

REFERENCES

1. Marriott HJL, Conover MB: *Advanced concepts in arrhythmias*, ed 2, St Louis, 1989, Mosby.
2. Goldberger AL, Goldberger E: *Clinical electrocardiography: a simplified approach*, ed 5, St Louis, 1994, Mosby.
3. Thelan AL and others: *Textbook of critical care nursing: diagnosis and management*, ed 2, St Louis, 1994, Mosby.
4. Conover MB: *Understanding electrocardiography, arrhythmias, and the 12-lead ECG*, ed 6, St Louis, 1992, Mosby.
5. Sabol J and others: An innovative approach to telemetry monitoring, *Medsurg Nurs* 2:99, 1993.
6. Andreoli KG and others: *Comprehensive cardiac care*, ed 7, St Louis, 1991, Mosby.
7. Melio FR, Mallon WK, Newton E: Successful conversion of unstable supraventricular tachycardia to sinus rhythm with adenosine, *Ann Emerg Med* 22:709, 1993.
8. Mason JW: A comparison of electrophysiologic testing with holter monitoring to predict antiarrhythmic-drug efficacy for ventricular tachyarrhythmias, *N Engl J Med* 329:445, 1993.
9. Breithardt G and others: Standards for analysis of ventricular late potentials using high-resolution or signal-averaged electrocardiography, *Circulation* 83:1481, 1991.
10. McIntosh-Yellin NL, Drew BJ, Scheinman MM: Safety and efficacy of central intravenous bolus administration of adenosine for termination of supraventricular tachycardia, *J Am Coll Cardiol* 22:741, 1993.
11. Emergency Cardiac Care Committee and Subcommittees: American Heart Association: guidelines for cardiopulmonary resuscitation and emergency cardiac care, II: adult Basic Life Support, III: adult Advanced Cardiac Life Support, *JAMA* 268:2172, 1992.
12. Pritchett EL and others: Comparison of mortality in patients treated with propafenone to those treated with a variety of antiarrhythmic drugs for supraventricular arrhythmias, *Am J Cardiol* 72:108, 1993.
13. Shettigar UR, Toole GJ, Appunn DO: Combined use of esmolol and digoxin in the acute treatment of atrial fibrillation or flutter, *Am Heart J* 126:368, 1993.
14. Roden DM: Usefulness of sotalol for life-threatening ventricular arrhythmias, *Am J Cardiol* 72:51A, 1993.
15. Mason JW: A comparison of seven antiarrhythmic drugs in patients with ventricular tachyarrhythmias, *N Engl J Med* 329:452, 1993.
16. Lefor N, Cardello FP, Felicetta JV: Recognizing and treating torsades de pointes, *Crit Care Nurse* 12:23, 1992.
17. Owens MW, Daniel JN: IV magnesium sulfate in the treatment of ventricular tachycardia and acute myocardial infarction, *Crit Care Nurse* 13:83, 1993.
18. Herrmann DJ, Raehl CL: Optimizing resuscitation outcomes within pharmacologic therapy, *Crit Care Nurs Clin North Am* 5:247, 1993.
19. Woosley R, Sale M: QT interval: a measure of drug action, *Am J Cardiol* 72:36B, 1993.
20. Dunnington CS: Sotalol hydrochloride (Betapace): a new antiarrhythmic drug, *Am J Crit Care* 2:397, 1993.
21. Bardy GH and others: Implantable transvenous cardioverter-defibrillators, *Circulation* 87:1152, 1993.
22. Wietholt D and others: Clinical experience with antitachycardia pacing and improved detection algorithms in a new implantable cardioverter-defibrillator, *J Am Coll Cardiol* 21:885, 1993.
23. Porterfield JG and others: Experience with three different third-generation cardioverter-defibrillators in patients with coronary artery disease or cardiomyopathy, *Am J Cardiol* 72:301, 1993.
24. Schaffer YG, Chicca C, Fisher C: Caring for a patient with an AICD, *Nursing* 22:48, 1992.
25. Futterman LG, Lemberg L: Pacemaker update: 1992 Part I: general remarks and electrocardiographic assessment of pacemaker function, *Am J Crit Care* 1:118, 1992.
26. Futterman LG, Lemberg L: Pacemaker update Part II: Atrioventricular synchronous and rate-modulated pacemakers, *Am J Crit Care* 2:96, 1993.
27. Futterman LG, Lemberg L: Pacemaker update Part IV: Antitachycardia devices, *Am J Crit Care* 2:253, 1993.
28. Sheinman MM: Catheter ablation, *Circulation* 83:1489, 1991.
29. Futterman LG, Lemberg L: Radiofrequency catheter ablation for supraventricular tachycardias: Part I, *Am J Crit Care* 2:500, 1993.
30. Futterman LG, Lemberg L: Radiofrequency catheter ablation for supraventricular tachycardias: Part II, *Am J Crit Care* 3:77, 1994.
31. *Healthcare provider's manual for basic life support,* Dallas, 1992, American Heart Association.
32. Willens J: BCLS forecast, *Nursing* 21:53, 1991.
33. Barbiere CC, Liberatore K: Automated external defibrillators: an update of additions to the ACLS algorithms, *Crit Care Nurse* 12:17, 1992.
34. Willens J: Strengthen your life-support skills, *Nursing* 23:53, 1993.
35. Ellstrom K, Bella LD: Understanding your role during a CODE, *Nursing* 20:37, 1990.

Chapter 34

NURSING ROLE IN MANAGEMENT

Inflammatory and Valvular Heart Disease

Nancy Stoetzner Kupper **Ellen Stoetzner Duke**

Learning Objectives

1. Describe the etiology, pathophysiology, and clinical manifestations of infective endocarditis and pericarditis.
2. Discuss the therapeutic, pharmacologic, and nursing management of infective endocarditis and pericarditis.
3. Explain the importance of prophylactic antibiotic therapy in infective endocarditis.
4. Explain the etiology, clinical manifestations, and management of myocarditis.
5. Describe the etiology, pathophysiology, and clinical manifestations of rheumatic fever and rheumatic heart disease.
6. Discuss the therapeutic and nursing management of the patient with rheumatic fever and rheumatic heart disease.
7. Identify the etiologies of congenital and acquired valvular heart diseases.
8. Discuss the pathophysiology, clinical manifestations, and diagnostic studies for the various types of valvular heart problems.
9. Describe the therapeutic and nursing management of valvular heart disease.
10. Describe surgical interventions used in management of the patient with valvular heart problems.

INFLAMMATORY DISORDERS OF THE HEART

Infective Endocarditis

Infective endocarditis, previously known as bacterial endocarditis, is an infection of the endocardial surface with microorganisms present in the lesion.[1] The endocardium, the inner layer of the heart (Fig. 34-1), is contiguous with the valves of the heart. Therefore inflammation from infective endocarditis frequently affects the cardiac valves. Although bacteria are the most common cause of infective endocarditis, endocarditis can be caused by a variety of microorganisms.

Before the era of antibiotics, infective endocarditis was almost always fatal. The advent of penicillin therapy changed the prognosis dramatically, and mortality rates decreased appreciably. For example, the mortality rate of infective endocarditis from *Streptococcus viridans* is now less than 10%. In spite of the relatively uncommon nature of the disease, an estimated 5000 to 8000 new cases of endocarditis are diagnosed in the United States each year.[2] Infective endocarditis continues to pose a significant clinical challenge.

Reviewed by Linda Schakenbach, RN, MSN, CS, CCRN, Clinical Nurse Specialist, Surgical Nursing, Fairfax Hospital, Annandale, VA.

Classification. Two forms of infective endocarditis, *subacute* and *acute,* have been described. The subacute form has a longer clinical course of more insidious onset with less toxicity, and the causative organism is usually of low virulence (most often *Streptococcus viridans*). In contrast, the acute form has a shorter clinical course with a more rapid onset, increased toxicity, and a more pathogenic causative organism (usually *Staphylococcus aureus*).[1] Although this classification system has been used historically and may be conceptually useful, clinicians prefer to classify infective endocarditis based on the etiologic agent.

Etiology and Pathophysiology. The term *bacterial endocarditis* has been replaced by *infective endocarditis* because causative organisms include fungi, chlamydiae, rickettsiae, and bacteria (Table 34-1). Streptococci and staphylococci account for the majority of the cases.

Infective endocarditis occurs when turbulence within the heart allows the causative organism to infect previously damaged valves or other endothelial surfaces. The damage may occur in individuals with underlying cardiac conditions (Table 34-2). A variety of invasive procedures (e.g., surgical interventions, intravenous [IV] injection, and diagnostic procedures) can allow large numbers of organisms to enter the bloodstream and trigger the infectious process (Tables 34-2 and 34-5).

Table 34-1 Etiologic Organisms Associated with Infective Endocarditis

Streptococci
- α-Hemolytic streptococci
- Enterococci
- *Streptococcus bovis*
- *Streptococcus pneumoniae*

Staphylococci
- *Staphylococcus aureus*
- *Staphylococcus epidermidis*

Gram-negative Bacteria
- *Escherichia coli*
- *Klebsiella*
- *Pseudomonas*

Polymicrobic Endocarditis
- *Staphylococcus agalactiae* and methicillin susceptible *S. aureus*
- *Pseudomonas aeruginosa*, α-hemolytic streptococci, and *Micrococcus*

Haemophilus, Actinobacillus, Cardiobacterium, Eikenella, and Kingella

Modified from Durack DT: Amenable Infections: endocarditis, *Hosp Pract* (Suppl) 28:7, 1993.

Table 34-2 Predisposing Conditions to the Development of Infective Endocarditis

Cardiac Conditions
- Rheumatic heart disease
- Bifid aortic valves
- Mitral valve prolapse with murmur
- Cyanotic congenital heart disease
- Prosthetic valves
- Degenerative valvular lesions
- Prior endocarditis
- Marfan's syndrome
- Idiopathic hypertrophic subaortic stenosis (Asymmetric septal hypertrophy)

Noncardiac Diseases
- Nosocomial bacteremia
- Intravenous illicit drug use

Procedure-Associated Risks
- Intravascular devices (leading to nosocomial bacteremia)
- Procedures listed in Table 34-5

An increased frequency of endocarditis is seen in older adults, in patients after prosthetic valve replacement, and in IV drug abusers. Left-sided endocarditis is more common in patients with bacterial infections and underlying heart disease. The primary cause of right-sided (tricuspid) lesions is intravenous drug abuse, especially cocaine abuse.[3] Staphylococcal infections frequently occur in this patient population although gram-negative bacilli, yeasts, or fungi may be the infecting organisms.

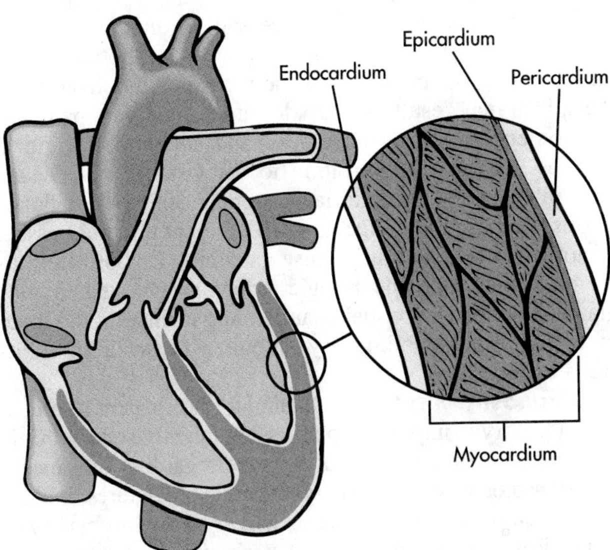

Fig. 34-1 Layers of the heart.

Vegetations, the primary lesions of infective endocarditis, consist of fibrin, leukocytes, platelets, and microbes that adhere to the valve surface or endocardium (Fig. 34-2). The loss of portions of these friable vegetations into the circulation results in embolization. Systemic embolization occurs from left-sided heart vegetations, progressing to organ (particularly the kidneys, spleen, and brain) and limb infarction. Right-sided heart lesions embolize to the lungs.

The infection may spread locally to cause damage to the valves or to their supporting structures. The resulting valvular incompetence and eventual invasion of the myocardium in the infectious disease results in congestive heart failure (CHF), generalized myocardial dysfunction, and sepsis (Fig. 34-3).

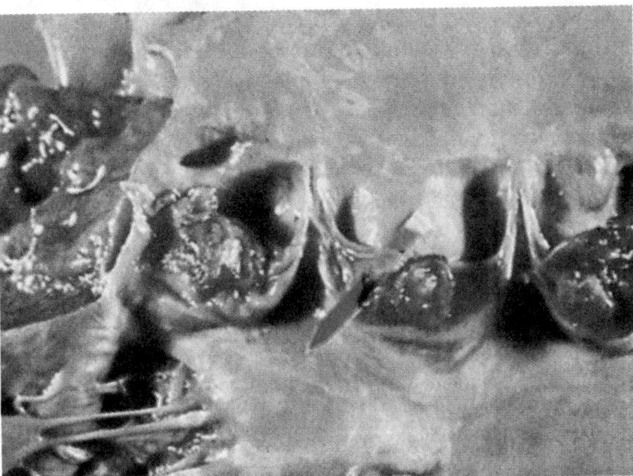

Fig. 34-2 Bacterial endocarditis of the mitral valve (caused by *Streptococcus viridans*).

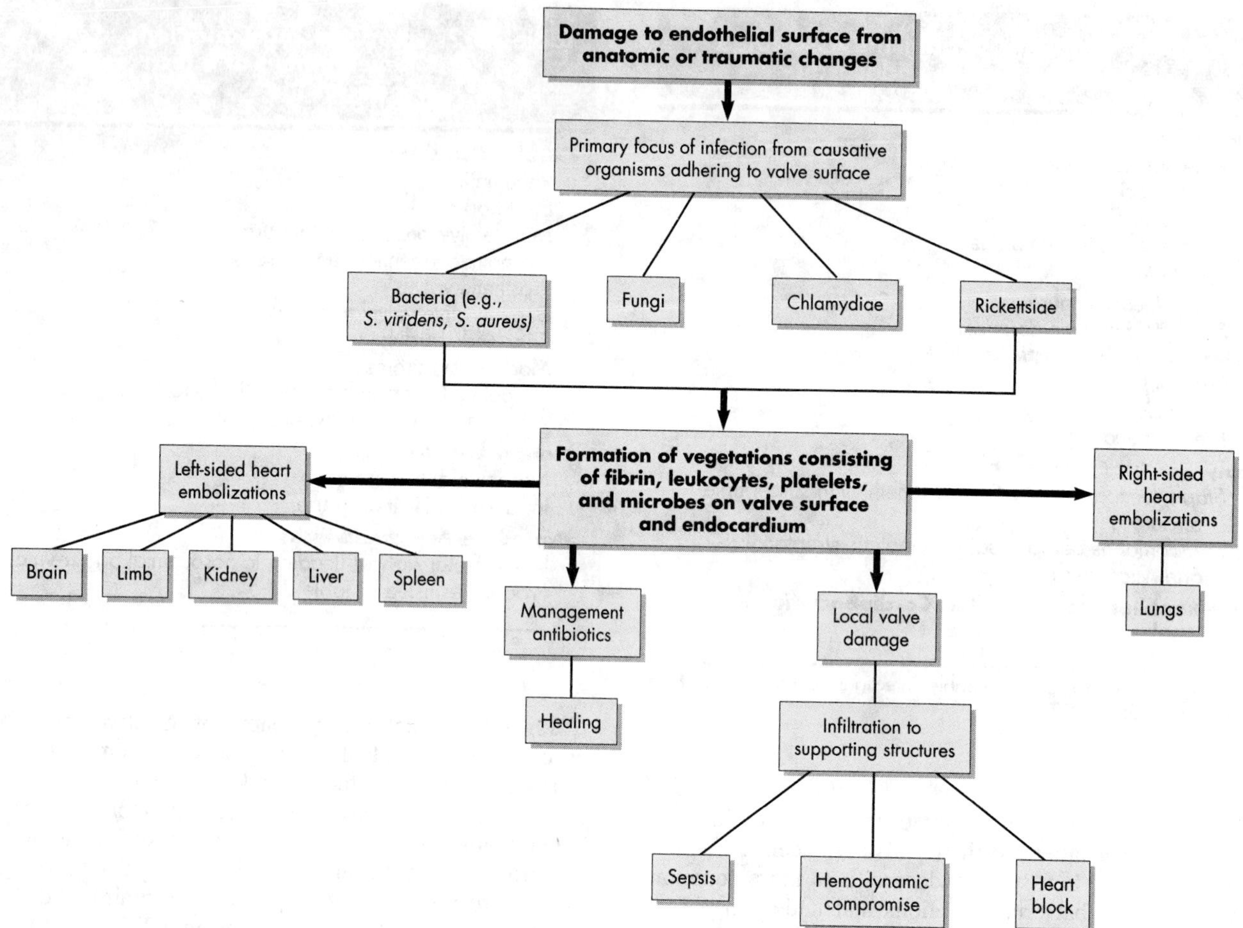

Fig. 34-3 Sequence of events in infective endocarditis.

Clinical Manifestations. The findings in infective endocarditis are nonspecific and can involve multiple organ systems. Fever occurs in more than 90% of patients with endocarditis. Other nonspecific manifestations that may accompany fever include chills, weakness, malaise, fatigue, and anorexia. Arthralgias, myalgias, back pain, abdominal discomfort, weight loss, headache, and clubbing of fingers may occur in subacute forms of endocarditis.

Vascular manifestations of infective endocarditis include *splinter hemorrhages* (black longitudinal streaks) that may occur in the nailbeds. Petechiae may occur as a result of fragmentation and microembolization of vegetative lesions and are common in the conjunctivae, the lips, the buccal mucosa, the palate, and over the ankles, the feet, and the antecubital and popliteal areas. *Osler's nodes* (painful, tender, red or purple, pea-size lesions) may be found on the fingertips or toes. *Janeway's lesions* (flat, painless, small, red spots) may be found on the palms and soles. Funduscopic examination may reveal hemorrhagic retinal lesions called *Roth's spots.*

The onset of a new murmur is frequently noted with infective endocarditis, with the aortic and mitral valves most commonly affected. The mitral murmur of endocarditis is generally a mid-to-late systolic regurgitant type. The aortic murmur may be early diastolic. Murmurs are often absent in tricuspid endocarditis because right-sided heart pressures are too low to hear. CHF occurs in up to 80% of patients with aortic valve endocarditis and in approximately 50% of patients with mitral valve endocarditis.[1]

Clinical manifestations secondary to embolization in various body organs may also be present. Embolization to the spleen may result in sharp, left upper quadrant pain and splenomegaly. Local tenderness and abdominal rigidity may be present. Embolization to the kidneys may cause pain in the flank, hematuria, azotemia, and glomerulonephritis. Emboli may lodge in small peripheral blood vessels of arms and legs and may cause gangrene. Embolization to the brain may cause neurologic problems such as hemiplegia, ataxia, aphasia, visual changes, and change in the level of consciousness. Pulmonary emboli may occur in right-sided endocarditis.

Diagnostic Studies. Obtaining the patient's recent health history is important in assessing infective endocarditis (Table 34-3). Inquiry should be made regarding any recent dental, urologic, surgical, or gynecologic procedures, including normal or abnormal obstetric delivery. Previous history of heart disease, recent cardiac catheterization, and skin, respiratory, or urinary tract infections should be documented.

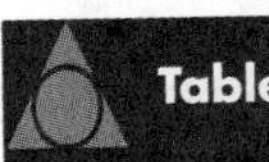

Table 34-3 Therapeutic Management: Infective Endocarditis

Diagnostic
- History and physical examination
- Blood culture and sensitivity
- WBC count with differential
- Rheumatoid factor
- Urinalysis
- Chest x-ray
- ECG
- Echocardiography
- Cardiac catheterization

Therapeutic
- Appropriate antibiotic therapy
- Antipyretics
- Rest
- Repetition of blood cultures and sensitivity tests
- Surgical valve repair or replacement (for severe valvular damage)

ECG, Electrocardiogram; *WBC*, white blood cell.

Table 34-4 Antibiotic Prophylaxis to Prevent Endocarditis in Cardiac Conditions (American Heart Association Guidelines)*

High-Risk Conditions
- Prosthetic heart valve (including biosynthetic valve)
- History of endocarditis
- Surgically constructed systemic-pulmonary shunts

Moderate-Risk Conditions
- Organic heart murmur
- Mitral valve prolapse with valvular regurgitation

Low-Risk Conditions (no prophylaxis)
- "Functional," "physiologic," or "innocent" heart murmur
- Mitral valve prolapse without valvular regurgitation
- History of rheumatic fever without heart murmur

Modified from Wahl MJ: Myths of dental-induced endocarditis, *Arch Intern Med* 154:141, 1994.
*Table lists common conditions, but is not inclusive.

Laboratory data, especially blood cultures, should also be assessed. Positive blood cultures are found in 90% to 95% of patients with infective endocarditis. Three sets of blood cultures (a set consists of one aerobic and one anaerobic culture from one site) should be performed over a 24-hour period. Negative cultures should be kept for 3 weeks if the clinical diagnosis remains endocarditis, because of the possibility of a slow-growing, fastidious, causative organism. The three sets of blood cultures may be obtained at 10-minute intervals if immediate antibiotic therapy is deemed necessary. Blood-culture bottles containing a resin to bind the antibiotic should be used if the patient is already receiving antibiotics. Culture-negative endocarditis may occur in those patients who have had previous antibiotic therapy, in patients with causative organisms that cannot be grown from blood using routine media (e.g., *Mycobacterium tuberculosis*), or in patients with right-sided infection of the heart.

A mild leukocytosis with average white blood cell (WBC) counts ranging from 10,000 to 11,000/μl (10-11 × 10^9/L) and erythrocyte sedimentation rates (ESR) greater than 30 mm per hour are often detectable. Microscopic hematuria and a positive rheumatoid factor may also be present in some patients with endocarditis.

Blood cultures are the primary diagnostic tool for the evaluation of infective endocarditis. Echocardiography is also useful in the diagnostic work-up for a patient with infective endocarditis when the blood cultures are negative, or for the patient who is a surgical candidate and has an active infection. Transesophageal echocardiograms and digital imaging using two-dimensional echocardiograms can correctly identify vegetations on valves. The use of echocardiography with prosthetic heart valves is not always useful because of resolution difficulties around the prosthetic device.

A chest x-ray examination is done to detect the presence of CHF. An electrocardiogram may reveal changes during endocarditis because the cardiac valves lie in proximity to cardiac conductive tissue, especially the atrioventricular (AV) node. Cardiac catheterization may be used when surgical intervention is being considered for patients with infective endocarditis.

Prophylactic Treatment. Cardiac lesions, prosthetic valves, acquired valvular disease, mitral valve prolapse, prior endocarditis, and noncardiac diseases are the principal risk factors for infective endocarditis.[2] Procedure-associated risks, including intravenous injection of recreational drugs and specific dental, medical, or surgical procedures must also be considered.[2,4] Antibiotic prophylaxis is recommended for patients with specific cardiac conditions before they undergo certain dental or surgical procedures (Table 34-4). Procedures that require endocarditis prophylaxis are summarized in Table 34-5. Specific antibiotic regimens are recommended for dental, respiratory tract, gastrointestinal (GI), and genitourinary (GU) procedures.[5] Antibiotic prophylaxis should also be instituted in high-risk patients who (1) are to undergo removal or drainage of infected tissue, (2) have indwelling cardiac pacemakers, (3) undergo renal dialysis, and (4) have ventriculoatrial shunts for management of hydrocephalus.[5-8]

Therapeutic Management. Accurate identification of the infecting organism is the key to successful treatment. The appropriate antibiotic (usually given intravenously) is chosen on the basis of sensitivity studies. Complete eradication of the organism generally takes weeks to achieve, and relapses are common. Traditionally this has meant a prolonged hospitalization for most patients with infective endocarditis. Currently, with the use of newer, more versatile antibiotics and in light of economic concerns, treatment of patients with infective endocarditis on an outpatient basis is becoming more common.[3] Table 34-6 outlines specific regimens for outpatient therapy of patients with endocardi-

Table 34-5 Procedures That Require Endocarditis Antibiotic Prophylaxis*

Oropharyngeal
- All dental procedures likely to produce gingival or mucosal bleeding (not simple adjustment of orthodontic appliances or shedding of deciduous teeth), including professional cleaning
- Tonsillectomy or adenoidectomy

Respiratory
- Surgical procedures or biopsy involving respiratory mucosa
- Bronchoscopy, especially with a rigid bronchoscope

Gastrointestinal
- Gallbladder surgery
- Colonic surgery
- Esophageal dilatation
- Sclerotherapy of esophageal varices
- Colonoscopy

Genitourinary
- Cystoscopy
- Prostatic surgery
- Urethral catheterization (in presence of infection)
- Urinary tract surgery (in presence of infection)
- Vaginal hysterectomy
- Vaginal delivery in presence of infection

Cardiac
- Placement of prosthetic heart valves
- Surgically constructed systemic pulmonary shunts

Other
- Incision and drainage of infected tissue
- Surgery involving infected soft tissue

Modified from Dajani AS and others: Prevention of bacterial endocarditis: recommendations by the American Heart Association, *JAMA* 264:2919, 1990.
*This table has selected procedures and is not all inclusive.

tis. Some patients require changes in antibiotics because of allergic reactions or other drug-related side effects.

The patient's antibiotic serum levels should be monitored periodically. Subsequent blood cultures may be performed to evaluate the effectiveness of antibiotic therapy. Blood cultures that remain positive indicate inadequate or inappropriate antibiotic administration, aortic root or myocardial abscess, or the wrong diagnosis (e.g., an infection elsewhere). Fever may persist for several days after treatment has been started and is treated with aspirin, acetominophen, fluids, and rest. Complete bed rest is usually not indicated unless the temperature remains elevated or there are signs of heart failure.

The results of pharmacologic management alone are generally poor in patients with fungal endocarditis and prosthetic valve endocarditis. Early valve replacement followed by prolonged pharmacologic management is recommended in these situations. Valve replacement has become an important adjunct procedure in the management of endocarditis, with use in greater than 25% of cases.

NURSING MANAGEMENT

INFECTIVE ENDOCARDITIS

Nursing Assessment

Subjective and objective data that should be obtained from a patient with infective endocarditis are presented in Table 34-7. Heart sounds should be assessed together with vital signs to detect a change in the character of the cardiac murmur and the presence of extradiastolic sounds. Arthralgia is common and may involve multiple joints and may be accompanied by myalgias. The patient should be assessed for joint tenderness, decreased range of motion (ROM), and muscle tenderness. The oral mucosa, conjunctivae, upper chest, and lower extremities should be examined for petechiae. A general systems assessment should be com-

Table 34-6 Treatment of Infective Endocarditis with Antibiotic Outpatient Therapy

Etiologic Agent or Clinical Situation	Antibiotic Regimen Options
Streptococcal endocarditis	IV/IM ceftriaxone*; IV/IM ceftriaxone* plus IV/IM gentamicin†; IV/IM ceftriaxone* followed by oral amoxicillin
Enterococcal endocarditis without renal failure	IV ampicillin plus IV/IM gentamicint†
Enterococcal endocarditis with renal failure	IV vancomycin‡
Staphylococcal endocarditis	IV nafcillin; IV vancomycin†
Right-sided staphylococcal endocarditis in IV drug abusers	IV nafcillin plus tobramycin

Modified from Durack DT: Amenable Infections: endocarditis *Hosp Pract Sympos* (Suppl) 28:9, 1993.
IM, Intramuscular; *IV*, intravenous.
*Endocarditis is not an FDA-approved indication for ceftriaxone therapy
†Serum concentrations should be monitored
‡Establish dose according to renal function and serum drug levels

Table 34-7 Nursing Assessment: Infective Endocarditis

Subjective Data

Important health information

Past health history: Valvular, congenital, or syphilitic cardiac disease (including valve repair or replacement); previous endocarditis, childbirth, staphylococcal or streptococcal infections

Medications: IV drug abuse, alcohol abuse, immunosuppressive therapy

Surgery and other treatments: Obstetric or gynecologic procedures; invasive techniques, including catheterization, cystoscopy, IV therapy; any dental or surgical procedure

Functional health patterns

Health perception–health management: Fatigue, malaise

Nutritional-metabolic: Weight gain or loss; anorexia; chills, diaphoresis

Elimination: Bloody urine

Activity-exercise: Arthralgias, myalgias; exercise intolerance, generalized weakness; cough, dyspnea on exertion, orthopnea; palpitations

Sleep-rest: Night sweats

Cognitive-perceptual: Chest pain, headache

Objective Data

General

Fever

Integumentary

Osler's nodes on extremities; splinter hemorrhages under nailbeds; Janeway's lesions on palms and soles; petechiae of skin, mucous membranes, or conjunctivae; purpura

Respiratory

Tachypnea, crackles

Hematologic

Anemia

Cardiovascular

Dysrhythmias, tachycardia, new or enhanced murmurs, S_3, S_4, retinal hemorrhages, peripheral edema

Possible findings

Leukocytosis, elevated ESR and cardiac enzymes; positive blood cultures; echocardiogram showing chamber enlargement, valvular dysfunction, and vegetations; chest x-ray showing cardiomegaly and pulmonary infiltrates; ECG demonstrating ischemia and conduction defects

ECG, Electrocardiogram; *ESR,* erythrocyte sedimentation rate; *IV,* intravenous.

pleted to facilitate recognition of hemodynamic and embolic complications.

Nursing Diagnoses

Nursing diagnoses are determined when the problem and the etiologic factors are supported by clinical data. Nursing diagnoses related to infective endocarditis may include, but are not limited to, those presented in the nursing care plan on p. 1010.

Planning

The overall goals are that the patient with infective endocarditis will (1) have normal cardiac function, (2) have no residual cardiac damage, (3) perform ADLs without fatigue, and (4) understand the therapeutic regimen to prevent recurrence of endocarditis.

Nursing Implementation

Health Maintenance and Promotion. The incidence of infective endocarditis can be decreased by identifying individuals who are at risk for the development of endocarditis. Assessment of the patient's history and an understanding of the disease process are crucial for planning and implementing appropriate health maintenance strategies.

Education is crucial for the patient's understanding of and adherence to the planned treatment regimen. The patient should understand the need to avoid persons with infection, especially upper respiratory, and to report cold, flu, and cough symptoms. The importance of avoiding excessive fatigue and the need to plan rest periods before and after activity should be carefully explained to the patient. Good oral hygiene, including daily care and regular dental visits, is also important. The patient must inform all healthcare providers performing dental, medical, or surgical procedures of the history of heart disease. The patient should understand the significance of the prescribed prophylactic antibiotic therapy before any invasive procedure. Education of the patient who is at risk or has had infective endocarditis helps reduce the incidence and recurrence of the disease.

Acute Intervention. A patient with infective endocarditis has many problems that require astute nursing management. (A nursing care plan for the patient with infective endocarditis is presented in the following nursing care plan.) Infective endocarditis generally requires treatment with antibiotics for 4 to 6 weeks. The patient usually requires in-hospital stabilization, and then may be treated with outpatient parenteral antibiotic therapy (OPAT). Some patients may not be candidates for OPAT and require a more prolonged hospitalization period.

Physical assessment findings are nonspecific (see Table 34-7) but can help confirm the diagnosis and aid the treatment plans. Fever, chronic or intermittent, is a common early sign. Frequent assessment of body temperature is important because persistent, prolonged temperature elevations may mean that the drug therapy is ineffective.

The patient needs adequate periods of physical and emotional rest. Bed rest may be necessary when fever is present or when there are complications (e.g., heart damage). Otherwise the patient may ambulate and perform moderate activity.

Laboratory data should be monitored to determine the effectiveness of the long-term, high-dose antibiotic therapy received by the patient. IV lines should be monitored for patency and antibiotics should be given when scheduled. The patient should be monitored continuously for undesirable reactions to drugs. To prevent problems because of immobility, the patient should wear elastic compression

NURSING CARE PLAN Patient with Infective Endocarditis

Planning: Outcome Criteria	Nursing Interventions and Rationales
➤ **NURSING DIAGNOSIS**	Altered comfort: Fever *related to* infection of cardiac tissue *as manifested by* temperature elevation, diaphoresis, chills, headache, malaise, tachycardia, and tachypnea
Have normal temperature 97.7°-99.7° F (36.5° -37.5° C); normal pulse (60-100 bpm); normal respiration (12-20 breaths/min); absence of chills, diaphoresis, headache.	Monitor temperature *to determine effectiveness of therapy.* Administer antipyretics or sedatives as ordered *to reduce fever and assist in sleep.* Reduce physical activity *to decrease cardiac work load.* Administer fluids (oral or parenteral) as ordered and tolerated *to replace insensible fluid loss and to maintain adequate blood volume.* Administer antibiotics *to treat the causative agent.* Monitor blood cultures and WBC count *to evaluate patient's response to treatment.* Wash patient with tepid water *to reduce fever and provide comfort.* Cover patient with light blankets *to prevent shivering and subsequent additional temperature elevation from increased muscular activity.*
➤ **NURSING DIAGNOSIS**	Decreased cardiac output *related to* valvular insufficiency and fluid overload *as manifested by* heart murmur, S_3, tachycardia, capillary refill time >3 sec, diminished peripheral pulses, adventitious breath sounds, decreased urine output, restlessness, confusion
Have sufficient cardiac output to maintain mean arterial BP ≥60 mm Hg and urine output greater than 0.5 ml/kg/hr.	Auscultate heart sounds, rate, and rhythm *to detect a change in the character of the cardiac murmur and the presence of extradiastolic sounds.* Monitor for new onset of murmurs *which could indicate infective endocarditis.* Assess capillary refill, skin color, and temperature *as indicators of effectiveness of peripheral circulation.* Assess for jugular venous distension *as indicator of fluid overload.* Assess for peripheral and sacral edema *as indicators of ineffective circulation or fluid overload.* Assess breath sounds *to identify pulmonary involvement, congestion, and fluid overload.* Provide O_2 therapy *to increase O_2 to the myocardium and to promote comfort by relieving hypoxemia.* Administer diuretics, inotropic therapy, and other medications as ordered *to promote diuresis and strengthen myocardial contractility.* Plan rest periods *to reduce cardiac work.* Assess urine output *to monitor renal function and evaluate fluid status.* Assess for changes in level of consciousness *to rule out embolization to the brain.* Assess BP *to evaluate the patient's response to treatment.*
➤ **NURSING DIAGNOSIS**	Activity intolerance *related to* generalized weakness and alteration in O_2 transport secondary to valvular dysfunction *as manifested by* fatigue, malaise, weakness, dyspnea, shortness of breath, pallor, cyanosis, confusion, vertigo, increased pulse, increase or decrease in RR and BP
Complete activities of daily living with no fatigue to minimal fatigue or physiologic distress; maintain activity as tolerated.	Monitor vital signs during activity *to evaluate cardiac response.* Monitor for signs of activity intolerance (e.g., tachycardia, hypertension, diaphoresis, shortness of breath) *to plan or alter activities.* Reduce activity if systolic BP goes down 10 mm Hg *as this may indicate impaired ability of the heart to respond appropriately to increased activity.* Teach patient to check pulse rate. Instruct patient to reduce activity if pulse increases >20 bpm and not to increase activity if resting pulse >100 bpm *since these signs indicate excessive cardiac effort.* Assist with activities as needed *to ensure that patient's basic needs are met.* Plan rest periods between activities *to reduce cardiac work load.* Use footboard or overhead trapeze *to encourage activity while on bedrest.*
➤ **NURSING DIAGNOSIS**	Anxiety *related to* critical illness and prolonged hospitalization *as manifested by* insomnia; restlessness; apprehension; withdrawal; helplessness; irritability; elevated pulse rate, BP, RR
Express reduction in anxiety; increase in psychologic and physiologic comfort; demonstrate usual sleep cycles.	Observe for verbal and physiologic signs of anxiety *to diagnose anxiety and initiate a plan of care.* Allow time for verbalization of fears related to illness *since discussing fears openly is helpful in allaying anxiety.* Encourage patient to discuss feelings and concerns about illness and hospitalization *to assess depth of feelings and accuracy of knowledge for planning interventions.* Explain how all procedures and activities relate to patient's treatment plan *to give patient information that may reduce anxiety.* Avoid unnecessary procedures during normal sleep hours *as sleep deprivation increases anxiety.* Assess and provide usual sleep aids *to enhance sleep since adequate sleep is helpful in preventing anxiety.* Teach patient relaxation techniques such as imagery and muscle relaxation *to directly reduce anxiety by eliciting the relaxation response.*

continued

NURSING CARE PLAN Patient with Infective Endocarditis—cont'd

Planning: Outcome Criteria	Nursing Interventions and Rationales
➤ **NURSING DIAGNOSIS**	Altered health maintenance *related to* lack of knowledge about disease and treatment process *as manifested by* nonperformance of desired prescribed health behaviors, verbalization of misconceptions about desired or prescribed health behaviors, requests for information
Verbalize increased understanding of disease process and self-care management.	Assess patient's knowledge about disease and treatment process *to identify teaching needs.* Establish what further information the patient needs. Allow time for questions *to increase patient's confidence in ability to manage self-care.* Discuss symptoms of recurrent infection (e.g., fatigue, malaise, chills, elevated temperature, anorexia) *so physician can be notified and treatment can be initiated promptly.* Explain need to avoid persons with infections. Encourage early treatment of common infections such as cold and flu *to reduce the risk of recurrent infective endocarditis.* Explain need to report endocarditis history to the physician performing invasive procedures such as dental or gingival therapy, diagnostic tests, or medical and surgical procedures *so prophylactic antibiotic therapy can be initiated to prevent the possibility of infection.* Explain the need for good oral hygiene *to remove oral bacteria.* Discuss names of prescribed medications, dosages, times of administration, purpose, and side effects *to promote safe medication therapy.*
➤ **NURSING DIAGNOSIS**	Diversional activity deficit *related to* restricted mobility and long-term hospitalization *as manifested by* restlessness and fidgeting; immobile, flat facial expression; unpleasant thoughts or feelings
Engage in identified diversional activities within prescribed limitation; verbalize relief from boredom.	Discuss the need for diversional activities with patient *to raise awareness and mutually plan to meet these needs.* Explore with patient potential diversional activities such as reading, puzzles, watching television, doing handicrafts. Encourage visitors and suggest family and friends send cards and letters *to maintain contact with patient.* Encourage family members to supply materials for the patient *since items of interest to the patient may not be available in the hospital.*
➤ **NURSING DIAGNOSIS**	Altered nutrition: less than body requirements *related to* anorexia *as manifested by* reported or recorded inadequate food intake, metabolic need greater than intake, muscle weakness, mental irritability, confusion
Increase amount and type of nutrient ingested; maintain weight.	Assess food preferences *so preferred foods will be available.* Weigh patient daily, use same scales and at the same time of day *to provide accurate evaluation of weight over time.* Assess for negative nitrogen balance *to correct protein intake and prevent excessive muscle wasting.* Provide caloric intake as ordered to meet body requirements *since inflammatory process raises caloric needs of patient.*

COLLABORATIVE PROBLEMS

Nursing Goals	Nursing Interventions and Rationales
➤ **POTENTIAL COMPLICATION**	Emboli *related to* dislodging of vegetations
Monitor for emboli to all systems, report deviations from expected parameters, and carry out medical and nursing interventions.	Assess breath sounds and RR, rhythm, volume, and use of accessory muscles *since pulmonary emboli may produce decreased breath sounds, increased RR, dyspnea, and use of accessory muscles.* Measure intake and output. Monitor color of urine and specific gravity *to evaluate renal function for decreased output and hematuria.* Assess for abdominal pain *since splenic emboli result in abdominal pain and splenomegaly.* Assess neurologic vital signs as needed *to detect signs of brain emboli.* Check temperature and pulse in extremities *since emboli may lodge in small peripheral blood vessels and cause gangrene.* Observe skin, eyes, mucous membranes for petechiae *which occur as a result of fragmentation and microembolization of vegetative lesions.* Check fingernails for splinter hemorrhages; fingers, toes, palms, and soles of feet for nodes; and skin surface for lesions *as these signs are indicative of emboli to the respective areas.* Observe for swelling, redness, calf tenderness *to identify possible signs of thrombophlebitis.* Apply elastic compression gradient stockings *to provide venous support to legs.* Teach patient leg exercises *to promote venous return and decrease the occurrence of thrombophlebitis.*

bpm, Beats per minute; *BP,* blood pressure; *RR,* respiratory rate; S_3, third heart sound; *WBC,* white blood cell.

gradient stockings, perform ROM exercises, and turn, cough, and deep breathe every 2 hours.

The patient may experience anxiety and fear associated with the illness. The nurse must recognize this problem and implement strategies to help reduce the patient's fears and anxieties.

Chronic and Home Management. Patients who receive OPAT will require vigilant home nursing care. Patients with active endocarditis are at risk for life-threatening complications, such as cerebral emboli and pulmonary edema. The adequacy of the home environment in terms of in-home companions and hospital access must be determined for successful management. After therapy is completed in either the home or the hospital setting, management will focus on educating the patient about the nature of the disease and on reducing the risk of reinfection. The patient should be instructed about symptoms that may indicate recurrent infection, such as fever, fatigue, malaise, and chills. If any of these symptoms occur, the patient should be aware of the importance of notifying the physician. The patient needs to be instructed about the need for prophylactic antibiotic therapy before any invasive procedure is performed (see Table 34-5). The nurse must explain to the patient the relationship of follow-up care, good nutrition, and early treatment of common infections (e.g., colds) to maintain good health.

Acute Pericarditis

Pericarditis is a syndrome caused by inflammation of the pericardial sac (the pericardium), which may occur on an acute basis.[12] The pericardium is composed of the inner serous membrane (*visceral pericardium*) that closely adheres to the epicardial surface of the heart and the outer fibrous (*parietal*) layer (see Fig. 34-1). The *pericardial space* is the cavity between these two layers, and in the normal state it contains less than 50 ml of serous fluid. Although the pericardium may be congenitally absent or surgically removed, it serves a useful anchoring function, provides lubrication to decrease friction during systolic and diastolic heart movements, and assists in preventing excessive dilatation of the heart during diastole.

Etiology and Pathophysiology. The common causes of acute pericarditis are listed in Table 34-8. Acute pericarditis in the adult patient is most often idiopathic, with a variety of suspected viral causes. The coxsackievirus B group is the most commonly identified virus and tends to elicit pleuropericarditis in adults (Bornholm disease) and myopericarditis in children. In addition to idiopathic or viral pericarditis, other causes of this syndrome include uremia, bacterial infection, acute myocardial infarction (MI), tuberculosis, neoplasm, and trauma.[9] Pericarditis in the acute MI patient may be described as two distinct syndromes.[10] Acute pericarditis immediately follows myocardial damage within the initial 48 to 72 hour period. Dressler's syndrome (late pericarditis) appears 2 to 4 weeks after infarction.

An inflammatory response is the characteristic pathologic finding in acute pericarditis. There is an influx of neutrophils, increased pericardial vascularity, and eventually fibrin deposition on the visceral pericardium (Fig. 34-4).

Table 34-8 Etiologies of Pericarditis

Infectious
- Viral causes, including coxsackievirus B, coxsackievirus A, echovirus, adenovirus, mumps, Epstein-Barr, varicella zoster, hepatitis B
- Bacterial causes, including pneumococci, staphylococci, streptococci, septicemia from gram-negative organisms
- Tuberculosis
- Fungal causes, including histoplasma, *Candida* species
- Infections such as toxoplasmosis, Lyme disease

Noninfectious
- Uremia
- Acute myocardial infarction
- Neoplasms, such as lung cancer, breast cancer, leukemia, Hodgkin's disease, lymphoma
- Trauma after thoracic surgery, pacemaker insertion, cardiac diagnostic procedures
- Radiation
- Dissecting aortic aneurysm
- Myxedema

Hypersensitive or Autoimmune
- Delayed postmyocardial-pericardial injury
- Postmyocardial infarction (Dressler's) syndrome
- Postpericardiotomy syndrome
- Rheumatic fever
- Drug reactions (e.g., from procainamide, hydralazine)
- Rheumatologic diseases, including rheumatoid arthritis, systemic lupus erythematosus, scleroderma, ankylosing spondylitis

Clinical Manifestations. Characteristic clinical manifestations found in acute pericarditis include chest pain, dyspnea, and a pericardial friction rub. The intense, pleuritic chest pain is generally sharpest over the left precordium or retrosternally but may radiate to the trapezius ridge and neck (mimicking angina), or sometimes to the epigastrium or abdomen (mimicking abdominal or other noncardiac pathologic conditions). The pain is aggravated by lying supine, deep breathing, coughing, swallowing, and moving the trunk and is eased by sitting up and leaning forward. The dyspnea accompanying acute pericarditis is related to the patient's need to breathe in rapid, shallow breaths to avoid chest pain and may be aggravated by fever and anxiety.

The hallmark finding in acute pericarditis is the *pericardial friction rub.* The rub is a scratching, grating, high-pitched sound believed to arise from friction between the roughened pericardial and epicardial surfaces.[10] It is best heard with the stethoscope diaphragm firmly placed at the lower left sternal border of the chest. The pericardial friction rub does not radiate widely or vary in timing from the heart beat, but may require frequent auscultation to identify because it may be elusive and transient. Timing the pericardial friction rub with the pulse (and not respirations) will help to distinguish it from pleural rub.

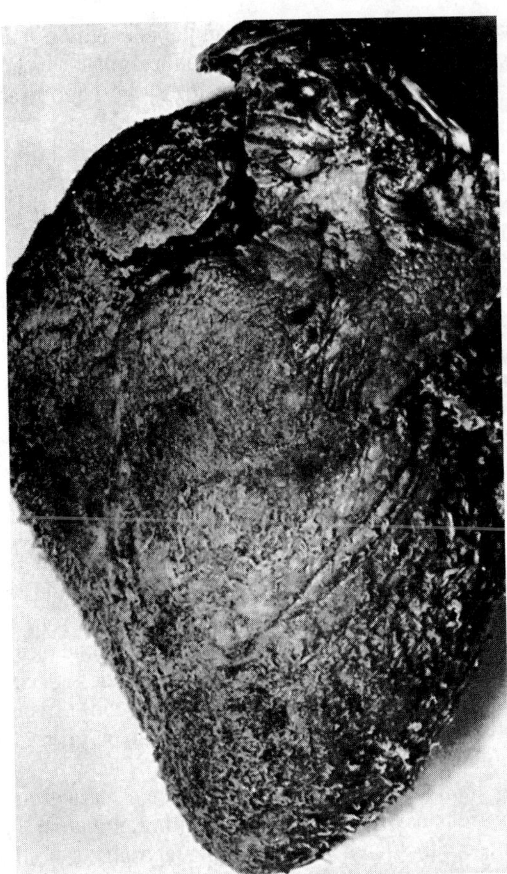

Fig. 34-4 Acute fibrinous pericarditis. There is a shaggy coat of fibrin covering the surface of the heart.

Complications. Two major complications that may result from acute pericarditis are *pericardial effusion* and *cardiac tamponade.* Pericardial effusion is generally a rapid accumulation of excess pericardial fluid that occurs in chest trauma. However, a slowly developing effusion may result, as in tuberculous pericarditis. Large effusions may compress adjoining structures. Pulmonary tissue compression can cause cough, dyspnea, and tachypnea. Phrenic nerve compression can induce hiccups, and compression of the recurrent laryngeal nerve may result in hoarseness. Heart sounds are generally distant and muffled, although blood pressure (BP) is usually maintained by compensatory changes.

Cardiac tamponade develops as the pericardial effusion increases in size. Compensatory mechanisms ultimately fail to adjust to the decreased cardiac output. The patient with pericardial tamponade is often confused, agitated, and restless and has tachycardia and tachypnea with a low-output state (Table 34-9). The neck veins are usually markedly distended because of jugular venous pressure elevation, and a significant *pulsus paradoxus* is present. Pulsus paradoxus, an inspiratory drop in systolic BP greater than 10 mm Hg, results because the normal inspiratory decline in systolic BP of less than 10 mm Hg is exaggerated in cardiac tamponade. The technique for measurement of pulsus paradoxus is outlined in Table 34-10.

Table 34-9 Clinical Manifestations of Cardiac Tamponade

- Decrease in systolic BP
- Narrowing pulse pressure
- Pulsus paradoxus (>10 mm Hg)
- Increase in venous pressure, distension of neck veins
- Tachycardia
- Tachypnea
- Possible friction rub
- Muffled heart sounds
- Low-voltage ECG
- Rapid enlargement of cardiac silhouette on chest x-ray
- Peripheral cyanosis
- Anxiety
- Chest pain

BP, Blood pressure; *ECG,* electrocardiogram.

Table 34-10 Measurement of Pulsus Paradoxus

1. Make determination during quiet breathing with stable rhythm.
2. Establish systolic pressure.
3. Inflate BP cuff until no sounds are heard with stethoscope.
4. Deflate cuff slowly until systolic sounds are heard on expiration and note the pressure.
5. Deflate cuff until systolic sounds are heard throughout the respiratory cycle and note the pressure.
6. Determine the difference between (4) and (5). This will equal the amount of paradox:

Sounds heard in expiration at	110 mm Hg
Sounds heard throughout cycle at	82 mm Hg
Amount of paradox	28 mm Hg

The difference is usually less than 10 mm Hg. If the difference is greater than 10 mm Hg, cardiac tamponade may be present.

BP, Blood pressure.

Diagnostic Studies (Table 34-11). ECG changes in acute pericarditis are key diagnostic clues and evolve over a period of hours to days or weeks. Four stages of ECG changes have been described: (1) initial diffuse ST segment elevations that concave upward and are present in all leads except aVR and V_1; (2) return of ST segments to baseline with T wave flattening several days later; (3) T wave inversion without the appearance of significant Q waves seen in acute MI; and (4) reversion of T wave changes to normal that may occur weeks or months later.[10] PR segment depression may also be present in the early stages of ST segment changes. The changes are believed to be caused by superficial myocardial inflammation or epicardial injury. Dysrhythmias can accompany these ECG

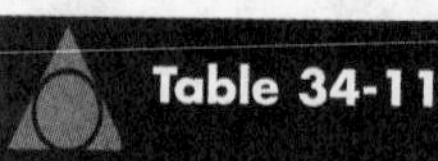

Table 34-11 Therapeutic Management: Acute Pericarditis

Diagnostic
- History and physical examination
- Auscultation of chest
- ECG
- Chest x-ray
- Echocardiography
- Pericardiocentesis
- Pericardial biopsy
- CT scan
- Nuclear scan of heart

Therapeutic
- Treatment of underlying disease
- Bed rest
- Aspirin
- Nonsteroidal antiinflammatory agents
- Corticosteroids
- Pericardiocentesis (for large pericardial effusion or tamponade)

CT, Computed tomography; *ECG,* electrocardiogram.

changes but are generally rare occurrences. When encountered, they are usually atrial dysrhythmias in patients who also have myocardial or valvular pathologic conditions.

The chest x-ray findings are generally normal or nonspecific in acute pericarditis unless the patient has a large pericardial effusion (Fig. 34-5). Echocardiographic findings are much more useful in determining the presence of a pericardial effusion or cardiac tamponade. Additional diagnostic studies such as gallium radionuclide heart scans may be performed, although their sensitivity in diagnosing pericarditis has not yet been determined.

Laboratory testing focuses on the possible etiology of the pericarditis. For example, elevated blood urea nitrogen (BUN) levels and serum creatinine levels may indicate uremic pericarditis, or a positive tuberculin skin test may suggest tuberculous pericarditis. The fluid obtained during pericardiocentesis (Fig. 34-6) or the tissue from a pericardial biopsy may also be studied to determine the cause of the pericarditis.

Therapeutic Management. Management of acute pericarditis is directed toward identification and treatment of the underlying problem (see Table 34-11). Antibiotics should be used to treat bacterial pericarditis. Corticosteroids are generally reserved for patients with pericarditis secondary to systemic lupus erythematosus, patients already taking corticosteroids for a rheumatologic or other immune system condition, or patients who do not respond to nonsteroidal antiinflammatory drugs. When necessary, prednisone is usually given according to a tapering dosage schedule (see Chapter 47). Discriminate and careful administration of corticosteroids is advised because of their numerous side effects, such as peptic ulcer disease, sodium retention, hyperglycemia, hypokalemia, and Cushing's syndrome (see Chapter 47).

The pain and inflammation of acute pericarditis are usually treated with nonsteroidal antiinflammatory agents. High-dose salicylates (300 to 900 mg orally four times a day) or indomethacin (25 to 50 mg orally four times a day) are commonly used.

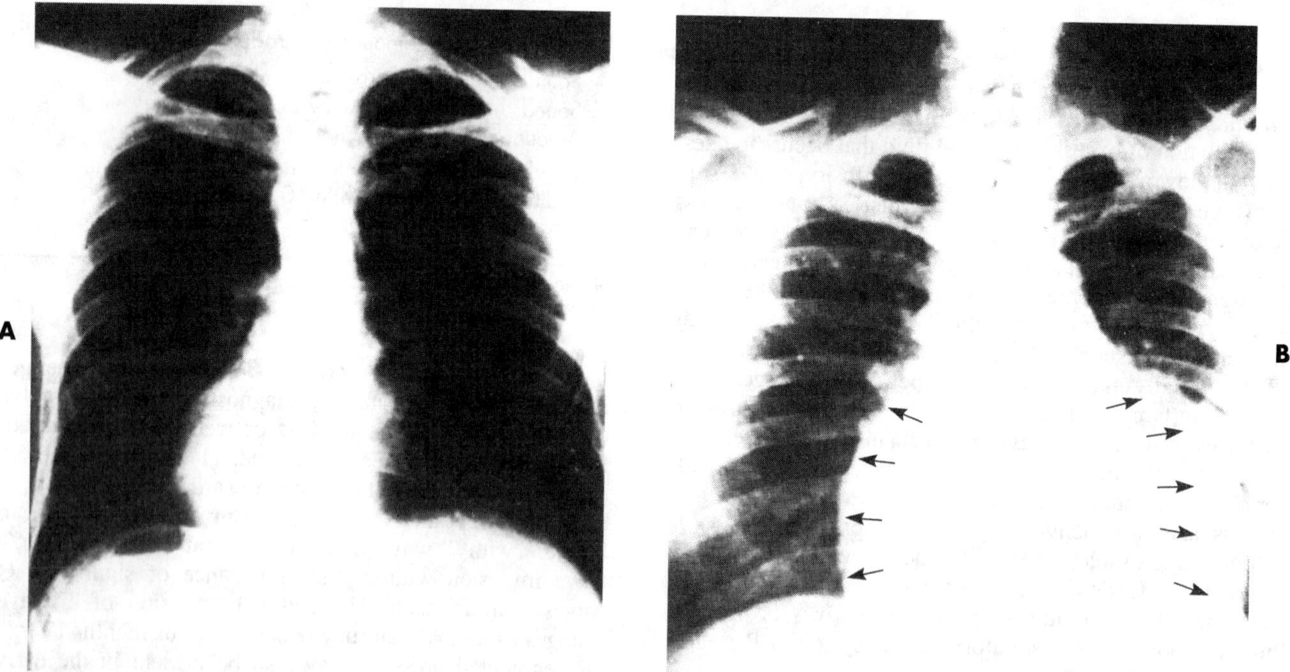

Fig. 34-5 ***A,*** X-ray of a normal chest. ***B,*** Pericardial effusion is present and the cardiac silhouette is enlarged with a globular shape (*arrows*).

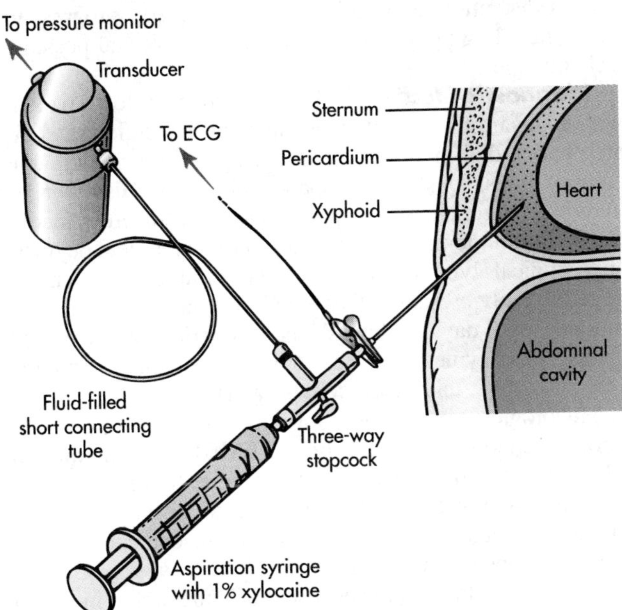

Fig. 34-6 Pericardiocentesis performed under sterile conditions in conjunction with electrocardiogram (ECG) and hemodynamic measurements.

Pericardiocentesis (Fig. 34-6) is usually performed when acute cardiac tamponade has reduced the patient's systolic BP 30 mm Hg or more from baseline. Hemodynamic support for the patient being prepared for the pericardiocentesis may include administration of volume expanders and inotropic agents. The procedure is usually performed in the cardiac care unit or cardiac catheterization laboratory under sterile conditions and in conjunction with ECG, echocardiogram, and hemodynamic measurements. A 16- to 18-gauge needle is inserted into the pericardial space to remove fluid for analysis and to relieve cardiac pressure. Complications from pericardiocentesis include dysrhythmias, pneumomediastinum, pneumothorax, myocardial laceration, cardiac tamponade, and coronary artery laceration.

NURSING MANAGEMENT

ACUTE PERICARDITIS

The management of the patient's pain and anxiety during acute pericarditis are primary nursing considerations. Assessment of the amount, quality, and location of the pain is important, particularly in distinguishing the pain of acute MI (or reinfarction) from the pain of pericarditis. Careful nursing observations should be made regarding ischemic chest pain, which is generally located retrosternal in the left shoulder and arm with a pressurelike, burning quality and is unaffected by posture. In contrast, pericarditic pain is usually located in the precordium, left trapezius ridge and has a sharp, pleuritic quality that changes with respirations. Relief from this pain is often obtained by leaning forward, and the pain is worsened by recumbency. The ECG also aids in distinguishing these types of pain because acute MI usually involves localized ST segment changes, as compared to the ST segment changes present in all leads except aVR and V_1 during acute pericarditis.

Pain relief measures include maintaining the patient on bed rest with the head of the bed elevated to 45 degrees and providing a padded overbed table for the patient. Antiinflammatory medications help to alleviate the patient's pain. However, because of the potential for GI problems with the use of high doses of these medications, nursing interventions should be directed toward management of this potential problem. Specific interventions include the administration of these drugs with food or milk, generally 30 minutes before or 2 hours after meals and instruction of the patient to avoid any alcoholic beverages while taking the medications.

Anxiety-reducing measures for the patient with acute pericarditis include providing simple, complete explanations of all procedures performed. These explanations are particularly important for the patient whose diagnosis of acute pericarditis is being established and for the patient who has already experienced an acute MI and has pericarditis (Dressler's syndrome).

The real potential for decreased cardiac output (CO) also exists for the patient with acute pericarditis because of the possibility of cardiac tamponade. Monitoring for the signs and symptoms of tamponade (see Table 34-9) along with preparations for possible pericardiocentesis are important nursing responsibilities.

Chronic Constrictive Pericarditis

Etiology and Pathophysiology. *Constrictive pericarditis* usually begins with an initial episode of acute pericarditis (often secondary to neoplasia, radiation, previous surgery, or idiopathic causes) and is characterized by fibrin deposition with a clinically undetected pericardial effusion. Organization and resorption of the effusion slowly follows with progression toward the chronic stage of fibrous scarring, thickening of the pericardium from calcium deposition, and eventual obliteration of the pericardial space. The fibrotic, thickened, and adherent pericardium encases the heart, thereby impairing the ability of the atria and ventricles to stretch adequately during diastolic filling.

Clinical Manifestations. Manifestations of chronic constrictive pericarditis occur over an extended time period and mimic those of CHF and cor pulmonale. They include dyspnea on exertion, lower extremity edema, ascites, fatigue, anorexia, and weight loss. The most prominent finding at the physical examination is elevated jugular venous pressure. Unlike cardiac tamponade, the presence of significant pulsus paradoxus is uncommon. Auscultatory findings include a *pericardial knock,* which is a loud early diastolic sound often heard along the left sternal border.

Diagnostic Studies. ECG changes may be nonspecific in chronic constrictive pericarditis but usually consist of low QRS voltage, generalized T wave inversion or flattening, and either P mitrale or atrial fibrillation. The cardiac silhouette on the chest x-ray may be normal or enlarged depending on the degree of pericardial thickening and the presence of a coexisting pericardial effusion. Echocardiographic findings may reveal a thickened pericardium, but without the presence of a large pericardial effusion. Distinctions between the myocardium and epicardium are difficult to ascertain.

Cardiac catheterization pressure tracings are more specific diagnostic tools in constrictive pericarditis. Abnormalities include elevation of the right and left atrial pressures with equilibration of these pressures during diastole. Other valuable diagnostic tools used to evaluate this condition are computed tomography (CT) and magnetic resonance imaging (MRI).

THERAPEUTIC AND NURSING MANAGEMENT

CHRONIC CONSTRICTIVE PERICARDITIS

Unless the patient is free of symptoms or the condition is inoperable, the treatment of choice for chronic constrictive pericarditis is a *pericardiectomy.* The pericardiectomy usually involves complete resection of the pericardium through a median sternotomy with the use of cardiopulmonary bypass. The postoperative prognosis is improved when the surgery is performed before the development of severe clinical disability. Postoperative nursing care after a pericardiectomy is similar to that of other open heart surgical procedures (see Chapter 32).

Myocarditis

Etiology and Pathophysiology. *Myocarditis,* a focal or diffuse inflammation of the myocardium, has been associated with a variety of etiologic agents, including viruses, bacteria, rickettsiae, fungi, parasites, radiation, and pharmacologic and chemical factors.[11] Viruses are the most common etiologic agent in the United States and Canada, with a predominance of RNA viruses (coxsackievirus A and B, echovirus, influenza A and B, and mumps virus).[11] Certain medical conditions such as metabolic disorders and collagen-vascular diseases (e.g., systemic lupus erythematosus) may also precipitate myocarditis. Myocarditis may also occur when no causative agent or factor can be identified. Myocarditis is frequently associated with acute pericarditis, particularly when it is caused by coxsackievirus B strains or echoviruses.

The pathophysiologic mechanisms of myocarditis are poorly understood because there is usually a period of several weeks after the initial infection before the development of manifestations of myocarditis. Immunologic mechanisms may play a role in the development of myocarditis. The majority of infections are benign, self-limiting, and subclinical, although viral myocarditis in infants and pregnant women may be virulent.

Clinical Manifestations. The clinical features for patients with myocarditis are variable, ranging from a benign course without any overt manifestations to severe heart involvement or sudden death. Fever, fatigue, malaise, myalgias, pharyngitis, dyspnea, lymphadenopathy, and GI complaints are early systemic manifestations of the viral illness.

Early cardiac manifestations appear 7 to 10 days after viral infection and include pericardial chest pain with an associated friction rub because pericarditis often accompanies myocarditis. Cardiac symptoms (S_3, crackles, jugular venous distention, and peripheral edema), may progress to CHF, including pericardial effusion, syncope, and possibly ischemic pain.

Diagnostic Studies. The ECG changes for a patient with myocarditis are often nonspecific and reflect associated pericardial involvement including diffuse ST segment abnormalities. Dysrhythmias and conduction disturbances may be present. Laboratory findings are also often inconclusive, with the presence of mild to moderate leukocytosis and atypical lymphocytes, elevated viral titers (virus is generally only present in tissue and fluid samples during the initial 8 to 10 days of illness), increased ESR, and elevated levels of enzymes such as the transaminases, creatine phosphokinase, and lactic dehydrogenase.

Histologic confirmation of myocarditis is possible through endomyocardial biopsy (EMB), a technique in which several small pieces of myocardial tissue are percutaneously removed from the right ventricle with a special instrument called a *bioptome* and microscopically examined. A biopsy done during the initial 6 weeks of acute illness is most diagnostic because this is the period in which lymphocytic infiltration and myocyte damage indicative of myocarditis are present. Special myocardial imaging techniques may also be used in the diagnostic evaluation of myocarditis.

Therapeutic Management. The specific treatment for myocarditis has yet to be established and usually consists of managing associated cardiac decompensation. Digoxin is often used to treat ventricular failure because it improves myocardial contractility and reduces ventricular rate. Digoxin should be used cautiously in patients with myocarditis, because of the increased sensitivity of the heart to the adverse effects of this drug and the potential toxicity with minimal doses. Oxygen therapy, bed rest, restricted activity, and maintenance of standby emergency equipment are general supportive measures used for management of myocarditis.

Immunosuppression with agents such as prednisone, azathioprine, and cyclosporine has been used in a limited number of patients with myocarditis to reduce myocardial inflammation and to prevent irreversible myocardial damage.[15] Administration of immunosuppressive agents is recommended only during the postinfectious stage of the disease, approximately 10 days after the onset of initial symptoms. If used early in the course of viral myocarditis, these drugs can actually increase tissue necrosis.[11] The use of corticosteroids for the treatment of myocarditis remains controversial because of the associated serious side effects and the lack of clear documentation of their efficacy.

NURSING MANAGEMENT

MYOCARDITIS

The potential for decreased CO is an ongoing nursing diagnosis in the care of the patient with myocarditis. Interventions focus on assessment for the signs and symptoms of CHF and institution of measures to decrease cardiac work load (e.g., use of semi-Fowler's position, spacing of activity and rest periods, and provisions for a quiet environment).

Prescribed medications that increase the heart's contractility and decrease the preload, afterload, or both are administered. Careful monitoring and evaluation of the patient taking these medications are necessary.

The patient may be anxious about the diagnosis of myocarditis, recovery from myocarditis, and therapy. Nursing measures include assessing the level of anxiety, instituting measures to decrease anxiety, and keeping the patient and family informed about therapeutic measures.

The patient who receives immunosuppressive therapy has additional problems of alterations in the immune response with the potential for infection and complications related to the therapy. Guidelines for care include monitoring for complications and providing the patient with a clean, safe environment by following proper infection control procedures.

The majority of individuals with myocarditis recover spontaneously. Occasionally, acute myocarditis progresses to chronic dilated cardiomyopathy (see Chapter 32).

Rheumatic Fever and Heart Disease

Rheumatic fever is an inflammatory disease of the heart potentially involving all layers (endocardium, myocardium, and pericardium). The resulting damage to the heart from rheumatic fever is called *rheumatic heart disease,* a chronic condition characterized by scarring and deformity of the heart valves.

Significance. Acute rheumatic fever (ARF) is a complication of up to 3% of sporadic upper respiratory infections caused by group A β-hemolytic streptococci.[12] Initial and recurrent episodes of ARF are most common from ages 6 through 15. Most recurrences occur within 2 years of the initial episode.[12] Recurrent attacks of rheumatic fever are twice as common between the ages of 11 and 22 as they are after the age of 22. The frequency of recurrence of rheumatic fever after streptococcal infection is greater in those patients with rheumatic heart disease than in those who have not had cardiac injury during previous attacks.[13] Attacks do occur in adulthood and are probably more common than previously believed. However, the sequelae of rheumatic heart disease are found primarily in young adults.

A spectacular decline in the incidence of rheumatic fever was observed in the 1960s and 1970s. By the 1980s rheumatic fever had almost disappeared in developed countries such as the United States. However, it remained frequent and severe in most of the Third World countries. Antibiotics, especially penicillin, are responsible for the decline in rheumatic fever. Antibiotics given within 9 days of the appearance of streptococcal sore throat, before the immune system completely responds, can prevent rheumatic complications.[14] A decrease in the prevalence of bacterial strains with the natural ability to trigger rheumatic complications has also contributed to the decline.

Since 1985, however, a startling reappearance of ARF in the United States and Canada has occurred. Outbreaks of the disease have occurred unexpectedly in white, middle-class families, many of whom lived in suburban or rural neighborhoods in Salt Lake City, Columbus, Akron, and Pittsburgh.[15] In searching for the cause of the reappearance, researchers have focused their efforts on isolating strains of group A streptococci. Researchers have isolated highly virulent mucoid strains of the same M protein serotypes that were prevalent in epidemic rheumatic fever more than 30 years ago. Another finding under consideration is the role of hyaluronate (a principal constituent of the group A streptococcal capsule) in the pathogenesis of the disease. Streptococcal hyaluronate, previously thought to be nonantigenic, induces the production of antibodies in animals. It is theorized that the body may have an allergic response to the streptococcus, or the host has an autoimmune response in which antibodies to the streptococci attack host tissue.[15] In the majority of new patients, a sore throat was never noted or reported. The infection that set off the immune system was so mild that the patient did not seek medical care. These reemergent strains of streptococci are capable of causing rheumatic fever, while producing such mild sore throats that no treatment is sought until it is too late to prevent complications.

Etiology. Rheumatic fever almost always occurs as a delayed sequela (usually after 2 to 3 weeks) of a group A β-hemolytic streptococcal infection of the upper respiratory system, usually a pharyngeal infection. Streptococcal infections of the skin are not associated with ARF, and some strains of group A β-hemolytic streptococci do not cause rheumatic fever. Although all attacks of rheumatic fever follow a streptococcal infection, only a few streptococcal infections are followed by rheumatic fever.

In addition to the infecting organisms, socioeconomic factors, familial factors, and the presence of an altered immune response have a predisposing role in the development of rheumatic fever. The incidence of rheumatic fever is higher in low socioeconomic groups and remains a major public health problem in the poorer countries of the Third World.[16] Crowded living conditions may be the major factor contributing to this finding. Neglect, inadequate treatment, poor nutrition, and a lowered state of health may be other reasons why lower socioeconomic groups in the United States and Canada and persons in Third World countries are more commonly affected. Rheumatic fever is more likely to develop in people living in urban areas than in rural communities. There also seems to be a familial tendency toward rheumatic fever, which may be genetically determined, possibly leading to an altered immune response.

Pathophysiology. The correlation of streptococcal pharyngitis with rheumatic fever is conclusive, but the pathogenic mechanisms by which the streptococcal infection causes inflammation of the heart and other tissues are not well defined. The organism is not demonstrable in the lesions when rheumatic fever appears several days or weeks after the acute streptococcal infection. Normally, antibodies are produced in response to infections with streptococcal organisms. Episodes of primary and recurrent ARF have been associated with a greater antibody response than those found with uncomplicated streptococcal sore throats.

Manifestations of ARF appear to be related (in susceptible individuals) to an abnormal immunologic response to an upper respiratory infection with group A β-hemolytic streptococci. ARF probably affects the heart, joints, central nervous system (CNS), and skin because of an abnormal humoral and cell-mediated immune response to group A hemolytic streptococcal cell membrane antigens. It is possible that these antigens cross-react with other tissues and bind to receptors on heart, muscle, joint, and brain cells triggering immune and inflammatory responses.[17] However, the direct relationship of this cross-reactive phenomenon to pathology is unproven, and streptococcus-induced autoimmunity as a mechanism to explain the rheumatic process remains a popular but unestablished pathogenetic concept.

Cardiac lesions and valvular deformities. About 40% of ARF episodes are marked by carditis, and all layers of the heart (endocardium, myocardium, and pericardium) may be involved. This generalized involvement gives rise to the term *rheumatic pancarditis.*

Rheumatic endocarditis is found primarily in the valves, with swelling and erosion of the valve leaflets. Vegetations form from deposits of fibrin and blood cells in areas of erosion. The lesions initially create fibrous thickening of the valve leaflets, fusion of commissures and chordae tendineae, and fibrosis of the papillary muscle. Valve leaflets may fuse and become thickened or even calcified, resulting in stenosis. Reduction in the mobility of valve leaflets may occur with failure of the leaflets to appose, resulting in regurgitation. The mitral and aortic valves are most commonly affected; less commonly involved are the tricuspid valve and, rarely, the pulmonic valve.

Myocardial involvement is characterized by *Aschoff's bodies,* which are nodules formed by a reaction to inflammation with accompanying swelling and fragmentation of collagen fibers. As Aschoff's bodies age, they become more fibrous, and scar tissue is formed in the myocardium. In addition to Aschoff's bodies, a diffuse cellular infiltrate is present in interstitial tissues. This interstitial myocarditis may be more important than nodular Aschoff's bodies in producing heart failure.

Rheumatic pericarditis affects both layers of the pericardium, which become thickened and covered with a fibrinous exudate, and a serosanguineous pericardial fluid may be present. When healing occurs, fibrosis and adhesions develop that partially or completely obliterate the pericardial sac, but constrictive pericarditis does not occur.

These pathophysiologic changes in the heart may occur as a result of an initial attack of rheumatic fever. However, recurrent infections may cause further structural damage.

Extracardiac lesions. The lesions of rheumatic fever are systemic, especially involving the connective tissue. The joints (polyarthritis), skin (subcutaneous nodules), CNS (chorea), and lungs (fibrinous pleurisy and rheumatic pneumonitis) can be involved in rheumatic fever.

Clinical Manifestations. The diagnosis of ARF is suggested by a clustering of signs and symptoms as well as from laboratory findings. When not observed in its most severe form, the disease may be difficult to differentiate from many illnesses with similar clinical manifestations. Criteria were established by T. D. Jones in 1944, revised by the American Heart Association in 1965, and updated in 1992 to provide a logical basis for diagnosis (Table 34-12).

The presence of two major criteria or one major and two minor criteria indicates a high probability of ARF. Either combination must have evidence of an existing streptococcal infection.

Major criteria. Carditis is the most important manifestation of ARF (see Table 34-12), with three signs including (1) an organic heart murmur or murmurs not usually present, usually from mitral or aortic regurgitation, or mitral stenosis; (2) cardiac enlargement and CHF occurring secondary to myocarditis; and (3) pericarditis resulting in distant heart sounds, chest pain, a pericardial friction rub or signs of effusion. Large effusions are rare but can lead to cardiac tamponade.

Polyarthritis, which is not a cause of permanent disability, is the most common finding in rheumatic fever. The inflammatory process affects the synovial membranes of the joints causing swelling, heat, redness, tenderness, and limitation of motion. The arthritis is migratory, affecting one joint and then moving to another. The larger joints are most frequently affected, particularly the knees, ankles, elbows, and wrists. The pain may prevent the patient from being able to walk.

Chorea (*Sydenham's chorea*) is the major CNS manifestation. It is characterized by weakness, ataxia, and choreic movement that is spontaneous, rapid, and purposeless, which tends to intensify with voluntary activity. Females under 18 years of age are primarily affected.

Erythema marginatum lesions are a less common feature of ARF. The bright-pink maplike macular lesions occur mainly on the trunk or inner aspects of the upper arm and thigh but never on the face. The rash is nonpruritic and nonpainful and is neither indurated nor raised. It is usually transitory (lasting for a few hours), may recur intermittently for months, and is exacerbated by heat (e.g., a warm bath).

Subcutaneous nodules are firm, small, hard, painless swellings found most commonly over bony prominences (e.g., knees, elbows, spine, scapulae). They frequently are not noticed by the person because the skin overlying the nodules moves freely and is not inflamed.

The presence of the major criteria of ARF vary among children and adults. In contrast to children, polyarthritis is

Table 34-12 Modified Jones Criteria for Acute Rheumatic Fever

Major Criteria	Minor Criteria
Carditis	Fever
Polyarthritis	Previous occurrence of rheumatic fever or rheumatic heart disease
Chorea	Arthralgia
Erythema marginatum	Prolonged PR interval
Subcutaneous nodules	Laboratory findings*

From American Heart Association: Jones criteria (revised) for guidance in the diagnosis of rheumatic fever, Dallas, 1992, American Heart Association.
*See Table 34-13.

the dominant clinical feature in adults, whereas carditis and subsequent valvular lesions are less prominent. In adults, two other major criteria, chorea and subcutaneous nodules, are usually not seen, and erythema marginatum occurs infrequently.

Minor criteria. Minor clinical manifestations (see Table 34-12) are frequently present and are helpful in recognizing the disease. These criteria are too nonspecific to make a definitive diagnosis because they frequently occur in other diseases. The minor criteria are used as supplemental data to confirm the presence of rheumatic fever. Laboratory test abnormalities in rheumatic fever are presented in Table 34-13.

Complications. The course of rheumatic fever cannot be predicted at the onset of the disease, but generalizations can be made. Within 6 weeks, 75% of the symptoms associated with ARF attacks abate, and 90% abate within 3 months. Less than 5% of the symptoms last for more than 6 months.[17] Once all evidence of rheumatic inflammation has abated, rheumatic fever does not recur in the absence of a new streptococcal infection. If the initial episode is not associated with carditis, there is little likelihood of subsequent cardiac damage if repeated attacks do occur.

A complication that can result from ARF is chronic rheumatic carditis. It results from changes in valvular structure that may occur months to years after an episode of ARF. Rheumatic endocarditis can result in fibrous tissue growth in valve leaflets and chordae tendineae with scarring and contractures. The mitral valve is most frequently involved. Other valves that may be affected are the aortic and tricuspid valves.

Diagnostic Studies. No single diagnostic test exists for rheumatic fever, but the results of combinations of laboratory studies suggest the presence of the disease (see Table 34-13). Throat cultures are usually negative at the onset of the disease because of the relatively long latent period of 10 days to several weeks after the precipitating infection. The most specific diagnostic test to confirm a recent group A streptococcal infection is measurement of the antistreptolysin O (ASO) titer. The ESR and measurement of C-reactive protein (CRP) are nonspecific tests indicative of a systemic inflammatory response.

An echocardiogram may show valvular insufficiency and pericardial fluid or thickening. A chest x-ray may show an enlarged heart if CHF is present. The most consistent electrocardiographic change is delayed AV conduction as evidenced in prolongation of the P-R interval. Other ECG changes are frequent but nondiagnostic.

Therapeutic Management. No specific treatment will cure rheumatic fever. Treatment consists of drug therapy and supportive measures (Table 34-14). Antibiotic therapy does not modify the course of the acute disease or the development of carditis. Penicillin eliminates residual group A β-hemolytic streptococci remaining in the tonsils and pharynx and prevents the spread of organisms to close contacts. Salicylates and corticosteroids are the two antiinflammatory agents most widely used in the management of ARF. Both are effective in controlling the fever and joint manifestations. Salicylates are used when arthritis is the main manifestation and corticosteroids if severe carditis is present.

Prolonged periods of bed rest have previously been recommended, but now the patient without carditis may be ambulatory as soon as acute symptoms have subsided and may return to normal activity when the antiinflammatory therapy has been discontinued. When carditis is present, ambulation is postponed until CHF has been controlled with treatment. Full activities should not be resumed until antiinflammatory therapy has been discontinued.

Table 34-13 Laboratory Test Abnormalities in Acute Rheumatic Fever

Antistreptolysin O titer	>250 IU/ml
Erythrocyte sedimentation rate	>15 mm/hr in men, >20 mm/hr in women
C-reactive protein	Positive
Throat culture	Positive for streptococci (usually negative)
WBC count	Elevated
Red blood cell parameters (Hct, Hb, RBCs)	Mild to moderate degree of normocytic, normochromic anemia

Hb, Hemoglobin; *Hct*, hematocrit; *RBC*, red blood cell; *WBC*, white blood cell.

NURSING MANAGEMENT

RHEUMATIC FEVER AND HEART DISEASE

Nursing Assessment

Subjective and objective data that should be obtained from a patient with rheumatic fever and heart disease are presented

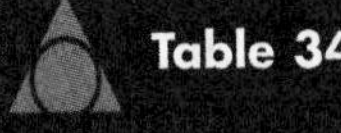

Table 34-14 Therapeutic Management: Rheumatic Fever

Diagnostic
- History and physical examination
- ASO titer
- Throat culture
- ESR
- C-reactive protein
- WBC count
- Chest x-ray
- Echocardiography
- ECG

Therapeutic
- Bed rest (modified)
- Benzathine penicillin (1.2 million units IM) or procaine penicillin (600,000 units IM) qd for 10 days
- Acetylsalicylic acid
- Corticosteroids

ASO, Antistreptolysin O; *ECG*, electrocardiogram; *ESR*, erythrocyte sedimentation rate; *IM*, intramuscular; *WBC*, white blood cell.

Table 34-15 Nursing Assessment: Rheumatic Fever

Subjective Data
Important health information
Past health history: Previous β-hemolytic streptococcal infection, previous rheumatic fever or rheumatic heart disease
Functional health patterns
Heath perception–health management: Malaise, fatigue
Nutritional-metabolic: Weight loss, anorexia
Activity-exercise: Generalized weakness; palpitations
Cognitive-perceptual: Chest pain, abdominal pain; joint pain and tenderness (especially large joints)

Objective Data
General
Low grade fever
Musculoskeletal
Signs of polyarthritis including swelling, heat, redness, limitation of motion (especially of knees, ankles, elbows, shoulders, and wrists)
Integumentary
Subcutaneous nodules and erythema marginatum
Cardiovascular
Tachycardia, pericardial friction rub, gallop rhythm, diastolic and systolic murmurs, peripheral edema
Neurologic
Chorea (involuntary, purposeless, rapid motions; facial grimaces)
Possible findings
Cardiomegaly on chest x-ray; prolonged PR interval; delayed AV conduction on ECG; valve abnormalities, chamber dilatation, and pericardial effusion on echocardiogram; laboratory abnormalities (see Table 34-13)

AV, Atrioventricular; *ECG,* electrocardiogram.

in Table 34-15. Rheumatic fever is five times more likely to occur in a person with a previous history of rheumatic fever than in the general population. A higher incidence of ARF occurs in lower socioeconomic groups and in crowded living conditions. This may be related to poor treatment of streptococcal infections.

The skin of the patient should be assessed for subcutaneous nodules and erythema marginatum. The procedure involves palpation for subcutaneous nodules over all bony surfaces and along extensor tendons of the hands and feet. The nodules range in size from 1 to 4 cm and are hard, painless, and freely movable. Erythema marginatum can occur on the trunk and inner aspects of the upper arm and thigh. The erythematous maplike macules do not itch and are not raised. The possible presence of these bright pink macules should be assessed in good light because the rash is difficult to observe.

Nursing Diagnoses

Nursing diagnoses are determined when the problem and etiologic factors are supported by clinical data. Nursing diagnoses related to rheumatic fever and heart disease may include, but are not limited to, those presented in the nursing care plan on rheumatic heart disease on p. 1021.

Planning

The overall goals are that the patient with rheumatic fever will (1) have no residual cardiac disease, (2) resume daily activities without joint pain, and (3) verbalize the ability to manage the disease.

Nursing Implementation

Health Promotion and Maintenance. Rheumatic fever is one of the few cardiovascular diseases that is preventable. Prevention is frequently classified as primary and secondary. *Primary prevention* involves early detection and immediate treatment of group A β-hemolytic streptococcal pharyngitis. Adequate treatment of streptococcal pharyngitis prevents initial attacks of rheumatic fever. Treatment consists of a single intramuscular (IM) injection of 0.6 to 1.2 million units of benzathine penicillin G or 10 days of oral penicillin G. If the patient is allergic to penicillin, clindamycin, vancomycin, or gentamicin may be substituted. Oral therapy requires faithful adherence to the full 10-day course of treatment. The nurse's role is to educate people in the community to seek medical attention for symptoms of streptococcal pharyngitis and to emphasize the need for adequate treatment of a streptococcal sore throat.

Secondary prevention focuses on the use of prophylactic antibiotics to prevent recurrent rheumatic fever. A person who has had rheumatic fever is more susceptible to a second attack after a streptococcal infection. The best prevention is monthly injections of benzathine penicillin G.[13] Alternative treatment is administration of oral penicillin, sulfonamide, erythromycin, or gentamicin one or two times a day. Prophylactic treatment should continue for life in individuals who had rheumatic carditis as children. Rheumatic fever without carditis after the age of 18 may need only 5 years of prophylactic antibiotic therapy, or may continue indefinitely in patients with frequent exposure to group A streptococcus.

Acute Intervention. The primary goals of managing a patient with ARF are to control and eradicate the infecting organism, prevent cardiac complications, relieve joint pain, fever, and other symptoms, and support the patient psychologically and emotionally. The nurse should administer antibiotics as ordered to treat the streptococcal infection and teach the patient that oral antibiotic therapy requires faithful adherence to the full 10-day course of therapy. Precautions with respiratory secretions should be maintained for 24 hours after initiation of antibiotic therapy. Tepid sponge baths should be given to relieve fever, and antipyretics should be administered as prescribed. Oral fluids should be encouraged if the patient is able to swallow; IV fluids should be administered as prescribed.

Promotion of optimal rest is essential to reduce the cardiac work load and to diminish the metabolic needs of the body. After the acute symptoms have subsided, the

NURSING CARE PLAN Patient with Rheumatic Fever and Heart Disease

Planning: Outcome Criteria	*Nursing Interventions and Rationales*
➤ **NURSING DIAGNOSIS**	Activity intolerance *related to* arthralgia *as manifested by* joint pain; related to congestive heart failure *as manifested by* malaise, fatigue, weakness, dyspnea, shortness of breath, confusion, vertigo, increased pulse, increase or decrease in respiratory rate and blood pressure (BP)
Perform activities of daily living with minimal or no fatigue or physiologic distress.	Assess patient's response to activity *to determine extent of problem and plan appropriate interventions.* Monitor heart rate and rhythm, BP, and respiratory rate before, during, and after activity *to determine degree of cardiac and pulmonary function.* Maintain bed rest during febrile periods *to promote resolution of inflammatory process and reduce cardiac work load.* Plan rest periods between activities *to balance demands that activity places on heart and to promote healing process.* Teach progressive exercise program after antiinflammatory therapy is discontinued, noting patient responses to activity *so that activity is increased to patient's ability.* Treat arthralgia with rest and medication for pain *to promote healing and enable limited activity.*
➤ **NURSING DIAGNOSIS**	Risk for injury *related to* chorea
Have no injuries as a result of uncontrolled body activity.	Monitor for weakness, ataxia, and choreic movement that is spontaneous, rapid, and purposeless which tends to intensify with voluntary activity *to initiate appropriate interventions for injury prevention.* Eliminate or minimize identified hazards in the environment *to reduce risk of injury.* Educate patient's family regarding need to safeguard home environment if appropriate *to reduce risk of injury at home.*
➤ **NURSING DIAGNOSIS**	Ineffective management of therapeutic regimen *related to* lack of knowledge concerning the need for long-term prophylactic antibiotic therapy and possible disease sequelae, lack of compliance, lack of resources *as manifested by* complications of rheumatic heart disease
Comply with treatment regimen; express confidence in managing disease; describe signs and symptoms of valvular heart disease.	Assess patient's knowledge, confidence, and resources for self-care *to initiate appropriate interventions.* Teach patient about the disease process, possible sequelae, and continued need for prophylactic antibiotics *to increase patient's control of disease and reduce the possibility of recurrence.* Provide patient with information on whom to contact when questions arise *so that long-term care is promoted.* Inform patient about the risk of exposure to streptococcal infections from such high-risk groups as children and military personnel *to reduce possibility of recurrence.* Teach patient the signs of valvular heart disease such as excessive fatigue, dizziness, palpitations, or dyspnea on exertion *as this is the most serious complication of rheumatic fever.* Provide educational resources to patient and family *to increase compliance with therapy.*

COLLABORATIVE PROBLEMS

Nursing Goals	*Nursing Interventions and Rationales*
➤ **POTENTIAL COMPLICATION**	Decreased cardiac output *related to* carditis and possible valvular defects
Monitor for signs of decreased cardiac output, report deviations from acceptable parameters, and carry out appropriate medical and nursing interventions.	Assess and monitor cardiac function regularly *to enable prompt intervention if abnormalities occur.* Promote optimal rest *to reduce cardiac work load and diminish the metabolic needs of the body.* Provide for rest in a quiet environment. Give explanations of treatment, listening to patient's concerns *as emotional stress increases work load of heart.* Administer medications as indicated *to treat fluid retention and improve cardiac contractility.* Monitor and replace electrolytes as necessary *since electrolyte imbalance can negatively affect cardiac function.*

patient without carditis should ambulate. The patient may resume normal activity after the antiinflammatory therapy is discontinued. If the patient has carditis with CHF, bed rest restrictions should be applied. Again, full activity should not be allowed until antiinflammatory therapy is discontinued. Nonstrenuous activities should be encouraged once recovery has begun.

Relief of joint pain is an important nursing goal. Painful joints should be positioned for comfort and proper alignment. Removal of covers from painful joints can be done with a bed cradle. Heat may be applied, and salicylates may be administered to relieve joint pain.

Psychologic and emotional care can be more important than physical care, especially because children and young adults are the primary patients, and the heart is often viewed as the center of life. Any alteration in cardiac function may be perceived as a threat to the person's body image.

Chronic and Home Management. Secondary prevention aims at preventing the recurrence of rheumatic fever. The patient with a previous history of rheumatic fever should be taught about the disease process, possible sequelae, and the continual need for prophylactic antibiotics. The patient must be made aware of the high risk of recurrence if a streptococcal infection develops and should be informed about the risk of exposure to streptococcal infections from contact with school-age children, individuals in military service, and people in healthcare positions. Ongoing patient education should encourage good nutrition and hygienic practices and reinforce the importance of receiving adequate rest.

The patient should be instructed in the use of prophylactic antibiotic therapy. The dosage of antibiotics used in maintenance prophylaxis of rheumatic fever is not adequate to prevent infective endocarditis when invasive procedures are performed. Additional prophylaxis is necessary if a patient with known rheumatic heart disease has dental or surgical procedures involving the upper respiratory, GI, or GU tract. The nurse must explain the difference between these two prophylactic programs.

The patient should also be cautioned about the possibility of development of valvular heart disease. The nurse should teach the patient to seek medical attention if symptoms such as excessive fatigue, dizziness, palpitations, or exertional dyspnea develop.

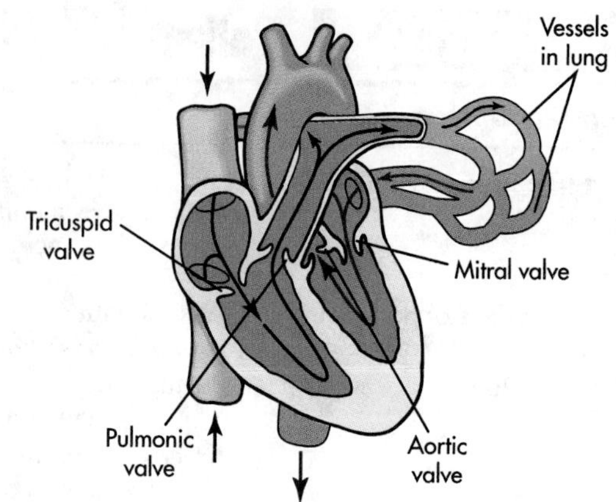

Fig. 34-7 Cross section of valves of the heart.

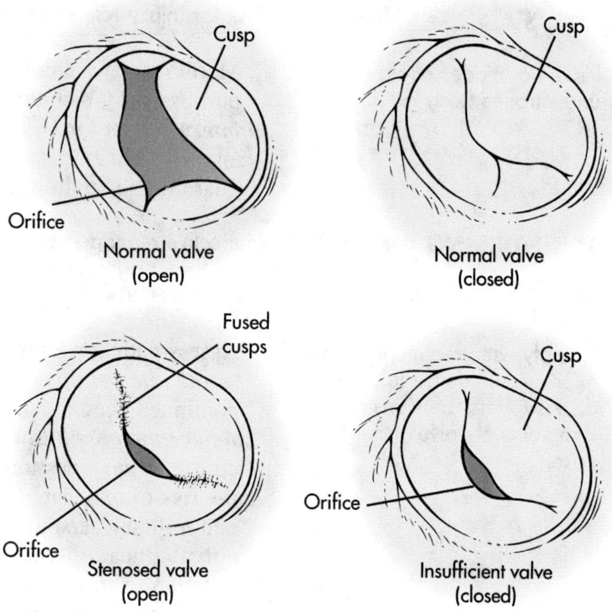

Fig. 34-8 A stenosed valve leads to decreased blood flow through the valve and gradual hypertrophy of the preceding chamber (e.g., a stenosed mitral valve leads to a hypertrophied left atrium). An insufficient valve leads to backward flow through the valve and dilatation of the preceding chamber (e.g., aortic insufficiency leads to a dilated left ventricle).

VALVULAR HEART DISEASE

The heart contains two atrioventricular valves, the mitral and the tricuspid, and two semilunar valves, the aortic and the pulmonic, which are located in four strategic locations to control unidirectional blood flow (Fig. 34-7). Types of valvular heart disease are defined according to the valve or valves affected and the two types of functional alterations, *stenosis* and *regurgitation* (Fig. 34-8).

The pressure on either side of an open valve is normally equal. However, in a stenotic valve the valve orifice is restricted, impeding the forward flow of blood and creating a pressure gradient difference across an open valve.[18] The degree of stenosis is reflected in the pressure gradient differences (i.e., the higher the gradient, the greater the stenosis). In regurgitation (also called *valvular incompetence* or *insufficiency*) incomplete closure of the valve leaflets results in the backward flow of blood.

Valvular disorders occur in children and adolescents primarily from congenital conditions such as tricuspid atresia, pulmonary stenosis, and aortic stenosis (Table 34-16). The incidence of congenital heart disease in the United States is 1 out of every 100 newborns, of which 15% to 20% have some type of congenital valvular heart defect.[19] Rheumatic heart disease is a common cause of adult valvular disease.

Table 34-16 Congenital Heart Lesions

Lesion	Description
Ventricular septal defect	Hole in septum between two ventricles
Atrial septal defect	Hole in septum between two atria
Patent ductus arteriosus	Persistence of opening between aorta and pulmonary artery, which normally closes shortly after birth
Pulmonic stenosis	Narrowing of pulmonic valve
Coarctation of aorta	Stricture and narrowing of aorta caused by infolding of wall of aorta
Aortic stenosis	Narrowing of aortic valve
Tetralogy of Fallot	Ventricular septal defect, pulmonic stenosis, aorta overriding two ventricles, and right ventricular hypertrophy
Transposition of great vessels	Reversal of position of aorta and pulmonary artery; origination of aorta from right ventricle, origination of pulmonary artery from left ventricle
Persistent truncus arteriosus	Single vessel exiting the heart to supply blood to pulmonary and systemic circulations
Tricuspid atresia	Absence of communication between right atrium and right ventricle

Mitral Stenosis

Etiology and Pathophysiology. The majority of adult cases of mitral stenosis result from rheumatic heart disease. Less common causes include congenital mitral stenosis, rheumatoid arthritis, and systemic lupus erythematosus. Rheumatic endocarditis causes scarring of the valve leaflets and the chordae tendineae. Contractures develop with adhesions between the commissures (the junctional areas) of the two leaflets.[20] The stenotic mitral valve assumes a funnel shape because of the thickening and shortening of the structures composing the mitral valve. Obstruction to flow through the mitral valve results from these structural deformities and creates a pressure gradient difference between the left atrium and the left ventricle during diastole. The flow obstruction increases left atrial pressure and volume resulting in increased pressure in the pulmonary vasculature. Hypertrophy of the pulmonary vessels occurs in cases of chronic left atrial pressure elevations. In chronic mitral stenosis, pressure overload occurs on the left atrium, the pulmonary vasculature, and the right ventricle.

Clinical Manifestations. Dyspnea, sometimes accompanied by hemoptysis, is the primary symptom of mitral stenosis because of reduced lung compliance (Table 34-17). Palpitations from atrial fibrillation and fatigue may also be present. Auscultatory findings generally include a loud or accentuated first heart sound, an opening snap (best heard at the apex with the stethoscope diaphragm), and a low-pitched, rumbling diastolic murmur (best heard at the apex with the stethoscope bell). Less frequently, patients with mitral stenosis may have hoarseness (from atrial enlargement), chest pain (from decreased CO), seizures (from emboli), or a cerebrovascular accident (from emboli) (see Table 34-17).

Mitral Regurgitation

Etiology and Pathophysiology. Mitral valve patency depends on the integrity of the mitral leaflets, the mitral annulus, the chordae tendineae, the papillary muscles, the left atrium, and the left ventricle. An anatomic or functional abnormality of any of these structures can result in regurgitation. Causes of chronic and acute mitral regurgitation are numerous and may be inflammatory, degenerative, infective, structural, or congenital in nature. The majority of cases may be attributed to chronic rheumatic heart disease, isolated rupture of chordae tendineae, mitral valve prolapse, ischemic papillary muscle dysfunction, and infectious endocarditis.

The regurgitant mitral orifice is parallel with the aortic valve, so the burden imposed on the left ventricle and the left atrium are determined by the etiology, severity, and duration of the mitral regurgitation. In chronic mitral regurgitation, volume overload on the left ventricle, the left atrium, and the pulmonary bed is created by the backward flow of blood from the left ventricle into the left atrium during ventricular systole, resulting in varying degrees of left atrial enlargement and left ventricular dilatation. Acute mitral regurgitation does not result in dilatation of the left atrium or left ventricle. Without dilatation to accommodate the regurgitant volume, pulmonary vascular pressures rise, ultimately causing pulmonary edema.

Clinical Manifestations. The clinical course of mitral regurgitation is determined by the nature of its onset (see Table 34-17). The left atrium is relatively noncompliant and when the atrium is abruptly distended, as occurs in papillary muscle rupture following a myocardial infarction, the sudden increases of volume and pressure are transmitted directly to the pulmonary vasculature. The resultant clinical picture in acute mitral regurgitation is that of pulmonary edema and shock. Patients will have thready, peripheral pulses and cool, clammy extremities. Auscultatory findings of a new systolic murmur may be obscured by a low cardiac output state.

Patients with chronic mitral regurgitation may remain asymptomatic for many years until the development of some degree of left ventricular failure. Initial symptoms include weakness, fatigue, and dyspnea that gradually progress to orthopnea, paroxysmal nocturnal dyspnea, and

Table 34-17 Clinical Manifestations and Diagnostic Findings of Valvular Heart Diseases

	Clinical Manifestations	Electrocardiogram	Echocardiogram	Cardiac Catheterization
Mitral Stenosis	Dyspnea, hemoptysis; fatigue; palpitations; loud, accentuated S_1; opening snap; low-pitched, rumbling diastolic murmur	Right axis deviation, left atrial enlargement, right ventricular hypertrophy, P "mitrale" (wide, M-shaped P wave), atrial flutter or fibrillation	Restricted movement of mitral valve leaflets decreased size of orifice	Left atrial pressure increased at end of diastole reduction in CO
Mitral Regurgitation	*Acute*—generally poorly tolerated with fulminating pulmonary edema and shock developing rapidly	Left atrial enlargement, left ventricular hypertrophy, atrial fibrillation	Hyperdynamic left ventricular contraction in association with shock; allows visualization of regurgitant jets and flail chordae	Dye injection in left ventricle showing regurgitation of blood into left atrium
	Chronic—Weakness, fatigue, exertional dyspnea, palpitations; an S_3 gallop, holosystolic or pansystolic murmur	P mitrale, left ventricular hypertrophy, atrial flutter or fibrillation	Left atrial enlargement	Dye injection in left ventricle showing regurgitation of blood into left atrium
Mitral Valve Prolapse	Palpitations, dyspnea, chest pain, activity intolerance, syncope, mobile, midsystolic nonejection click and a late or holosystolic murmur	Usually normal; occasionally T-wave inversion or biplasticity in leads II, III, and aVF are noted; complications of PVCs and tachydysrhythmias reported	On the M-mode echo, late systolic posterior motion or holosystolic billowing of the mitral leaflets; on 2-D echo, systolic billowing of the mitral leaflets	Left ventricular angiogram reveals mitral leaflets with prominent scalloping as the leaflets billow into the left atrium during systole
Aortic Stenosis	Angina pectoris, syncope, heart failure, normal or soft S_1, prominent S_4, crescendo-decrescendo murmur	Left ventricular hypertrophy, left bundle branch block, complete atrioventricular heart block	Restricted movement of aortic valve, diminished orifice	Left ventricular systolic pressure increased, reduction in CO
Aortic Regurgitation	*Acute*—abrupt onset of profound dyspnea, transient chest pain, progression to shock	Left ventricular hypertrophy	Normal-sized left ventricle with hyperdynamic systolic contraction; aortic dissection can be seen, if cause of acute process	Significant elevation of left ventricular diastolic pressure
	Chronic—fatigue, exertional dyspnea; Corrigan's pulse; heaving precordial impulse; diastolic high-pitched soft decrescendo diastolic murmur, characteristic Austin Flint murmur at diastolic rumble, systolic ejection click	Left ventricular hypertrophy	Enlarged left ventricle and dilated aortic root	Increase in left ventricular diastolic pressure, aortic root dye injection demonstrating regurgitation of blood into left ventricle

continued

Table 34-17 Clinical Manifestations and Diagnostic Findings of Valvular Heart Diseases—cont'd

	Clinical Manifestations	Electrocardiogram	Echocardiogram	Cardiac Catheterization
Tricuspid Stenosis and Regurgitation	Peripheral edema, ascites, hepatomegaly; diastolic low-pitched, decrescendo murmur with increased intensity during inspiration (stenosis), pansystolic murmur with increased intensity at inspiration (regurgitation)	Tall, peaked P waves; atrial fibrillation	Right ventricular dilatation and paradoxic septal motion, usually poor visualization of tricuspid valve itself	Pressure gradient across tricuspid valve and increased right atrial pressure (stenosis), reflux of contrast medium into right atrium (regurgitation)

CO, Cardiac output.

peripheral edema. Patients with chronic mitral regurgitation have brisk carotid pulses. Auscultatory findings reflect accentuated left ventricular filling leading to an audible third heart sound (S_3) even in the absence of left ventricular dysfunction. The murmur is a loud pansystolic or holosystolic murmur at the apex radiating to the left axilla.

Mitral Valve Prolapse

Etiology and Pathophysiology. Mitral valve prolapse (MVP) occurs when the mitral valve leaflets extend beyond the plane of the atrioventricular junction and into the left atrium during ventricular systole. The etiology of mitral valve prolapse is unknown but is related to diverse pathogenic mechanisms of the mitral valve apparatus. Mitral valve prolapse can occur in the presence of redundant mitral valve leaflets, elongated chordae tendineae, enlarged mitral annulus, and abnormally contracting left ventricular wall segments. Barlow, who first discussed MVP, contends that the use of the term "prolapse" is unfortunate because it is used even when the valve anomaly is functionally normal. He defines MVP as a failure of one or both leaflets to fit together resulting in displacement of an involved leaflet edge toward the atrium during systole.[21]

MVP is the most common form of valvular heart disease in the United States with prevalence ranging from 4% to 7% and reaching as high as 17% with detection by echocardiography alone. MVP has been noted in all ages but is most common in women of child-bearing age.[21] There is an increased familial incidence in some patients suggesting an autosomal dominant pattern of inheritance. In many patients the abnormality detected by echocardiography is not accompanied by any other clinical manifestations of cardiac disease, and the significance of the finding is uncertain.

Clinical Manifestations. MVP encompasses a broad spectrum of severity. Most patients are asymptomatic and remain so for their entire lives (see following Research box). Although severe mitral regurgitation is an uncommon complication of MVP, the latter has become the most common cause of isolated severe mitral regurgitation. A characteristic of MVP is a murmur from insufficiency that gets more intense through systole. This could be a late or holosystolic murmur. Another major sign is one or more clicks usually heard in midsystole to late systole [between first heart sound (S_1) and second heart sound (S_2)] and less frequently in early systole. The clicks may be constant or vary from beat to beat. MVP does not alter S_1 or S_2.

Dysrhythmias, most commonly ventricular premature contractions, paroxysmal supraventricular tachycardia, and ventricular tachycardia may cause palpitations, lightheadedness, and dizziness. Infective endocarditis may occur in patients with mitral regurgitation associated with MVP.

Patients may or may not have chest pain. If episodes of chest pain occur, the episodes tend to occur in clusters, especially during periods of emotional stress. The chest pain may occasionally be accompanied by dyspnea, palpitations, and syncope.

Patients with MVP generally have a benign, manageable course unless some severe problems associated with mitral regurgitation are present.[22] A teaching plan for patients with MVP is presented in Table 34-18.

Table 34-18 Teaching Plan for Patient with Mitral Valve Prolapse

1. Recommend antibiotic prophylaxis for endocarditis before undergoing certain dental or surgical procedures if the patient has MVP with regurgitation (refer to Tables 34-4 and 34-6).
2. Monitor the patient treated with β-blocker medications to control palpitations.
3. Advise the patient to adopt healthy eating patterns, such as avoiding caffeine because it is a stimulant and may exacerbate symptoms. Counsel the patient who uses diet pills containing stimulants that these preparations will exacerbate symptoms.
4. Instruct the patient to take over-the-counter drugs with caution and to check common ingredients, including caffeine, ephedrine, and pseudoephedrine.
5. Develop a planned aerobic exercise program and help the patient implement it.

RESEARCH

Implications for Nursing Practice

THE EFFECTS OF MITRAL VALVE PROLAPSE ON SELF-CARE

Citation Utz SW, Ramos MC: Mitral valve prolapse and its effects: a programme of inquiry within Orem's self-care deficit theory of nursing, *J Adv Nurs* 18: 742-751, 1993.

Purpose To determine the needs of patients with mitral valve prolapse.

Methods A multicomponent descriptive study involving patients with mitral valve prolapse and cardiovascular nurses. Medical record reviews of patients' charts, patient interviews, and a survey questionnaire of cardiovascular nurses were done.

Results and Conclusions Self-care needs of patients included acceptance by others of subjective discomfort, an understanding of the condition, and help with symptom management and lifestyle adjustment. The perceived impact of symptoms in the daily lives of those diagnosed with mitral valve prolapse was often dramatic. A review of the medical records indicated that physicians primarily focused their care on prescribing medications. The results of the nurses' survey indicated that methods of nursing assistance included teaching, supporting and guiding, and performing tasks for patients.

Implications for Nursing Practice This series of studies indicated that Orem's model of self-care can be used to identify health and self-care needs of patients with mitral valve prolapse. The proportion of health concerns reported by patients was much greater than the frequency of care sought. The nurse needs to be involved in identifying, teaching, and supporting the patient with mitral valve prolapse.

Aortic Stenosis

Etiology and Pathophysiology. Congenitally abnormal stenotic aortic valves are generally discovered in childhood, adolescence, or young adulthood. A patient seen later in life usually has aortic stenosis from traumatic heart disease, calcific degeneration of a bicuspid valve, or senile calcific degeneration of a normal valve. In contrast to mitral stenosis, isolated aortic valve stenosis is almost always nonrheumatic in origin. If it does occur secondary to rheumatic heart disease, mitral valve disease accompanies aortic stenosis.

Aortic stenosis results in obstruction of flow from the left ventricle to the aorta during systole. The effect is concentric left-ventricular hypertrophy and increased myocardial oxygen consumption because of the increased myocardial mass. As the disease course progresses and compensatory mechanisms fail, reduced cardiac output leads to pulmonary hypertension.

Clinical Manifestations. Symptoms of aortic stenosis (see Table 34-17) generally develop when the valve orifice becomes approximately one third its normal size and classically include angina pectoris, syncope, and heart failure. The prognosis is poor for a patient with symptoms and whose valve obstruction is not relieved. Survival from the time of onset of symptoms to the time of death is 2 years for the patient with heart failure, 3 years for one with syncope, and 5 years for the patient with angina. Auscultatory findings of aortic stenosis typically reveal a normal or soft first heart sound (S_1), a prominent fourth heart sound (S_4), and a systolic, crescendo-decrescendo murmur that ends before the second heart sound (S_2).

Aortic Regurgitation

Etiology and Pathophysiology. Aortic regurgitation may be the result of a primary disease of the aortic valve leaflets, the aortic root, or both. Acute aortic regurgitation is caused by bacterial endocarditis, trauma, or aortic dissection and constitutes a life threatening emergency. Chronic aortic regurgitation is generally the result of rheumatic heart disease, a congenital bicuspid aortic valve, syphilis, or chronic rheumatic conditions such as ankylosing spondylitis or Reiter's syndrome.

The basic physiologic consequence of aortic regurgitation is retrograde blood flow from the ascending aorta into the left ventricle resulting in volume overload. The left ventricle initially compensates for chronic aortic regurgitation by dilatation and hypertrophy. Myocardial contractility eventually declines and blood volumes increase in the left atrium and pulmonary vasculature. Ultimately, pulmonary hypertension and right ventricular failure develop.

Clinical Manifestations. Patients with acute aortic regurgitation have sudden clinical manifestations of cardiovascular collapse (see Table 34-17). The left ventricle is exposed to aortic pressure during diastole and the patient develops weakness, severe dyspnea, and hypotension that generally constitutes a medical emergency. Patients with chronic, severe aortic regurgitation have pulses that are of the water-hammer or collapsing type with abrupt distention during systole and quick collapse during diastole (*Corrigan's pulse*). Auscultatory findings may include a soft or absent S_1, presence of a S_3 or S_4, and a soft, decrescendo high-pitched diastolic murmur. A systolic ejection murmur may also be heard, and the *Austin-Flint murmur,* a low frequency diastolic rumble similar to that of mitral stenosis, may be auscultated.

The patient with chronic aortic regurgitation generally remains asymptomatic for years and is seen with exertional dyspnea, orthopnea, and paroxysmal nocturnal dyspnea only after considerable myocardial dysfunction has occurred (see Table 34-17). Angina pectoris occurs less frequently in aortic regurgitation than in aortic stenosis. However, a nocturnal angina accompanied by diaphoresis and abdominal discomfort may be present.

Tricuspid Valve Disease

Etiology and Pathophysiology. Tricuspid stenosis is extremely uncommon and occurs almost exclusively in patients with rheumatic mitral stenosis. It is also seen in IV drug users. Tricuspid regurgitation is usually the result of pulmonary hypertension or right ventricular dysfunction. In tricuspid stenosis, right atrial outflow is obstructed, resulting in right atrial enlargement and elevated systemic venous pressures. Volume overload of the right atrium and ventricle occurs in tricuspid regurgitation.

Clinical Manifestations. Both tricuspid stenosis and tricuspid regurgitation result in the backward flow of blood into the systemic circulation, and common manifestations, therefore, are peripheral edema, ascites, and hepatomegaly. The murmur of stenosis is presystolic (sinus rhythm) or midsystolic (atrial fibrillation), and a pansystolic murmur may be heard in regurgitation. Both types of murmurs dramatically increase in intensity with inspiration.

Pulmonic Valve Disease

Pulmonic valve disease is an uncommon entity and, in the case of pulmonary stenosis, is almost always congenital. Pulmonary regurgitation as an isolated abnormality has a benign course but is generally associated with disease of other valves.

Diagnostic Studies for Valvular Heart Disease

Diagnosis of valvular heart disease is generally based on the results of a history, a physical examination, an echocardiogram, and a cardiac catheterization (if surgery is considered) (Table 34-19). Chest x-ray results, electrocardiogram (ECG) findings, and the clinical manifestations exhibited by the patient also aid in establishing the correct diagnosis.

An echocardiogram provides information on the structure and function of the valves and on enlargement of the chambers. Transesophageal echocardiography and Doppler color flow imaging are particularly valuable in diagnosing and monitoring valvular heart disease. Cardiac catheterization detects pressure changes in the cardiac chambers, as well as pressure gradients across the valves. It also quantifies the size of the valve area. An ECG shows variation in the heart rate and rhythm and provides information about possible ischemia or chamber enlargement. Chest x-ray reveals the heart size, alterations in pulmonary circulation, and calcification of valves.

Therapeutic Management of Valvular Heart Disease

Conservative Management. An important aspect of conservative management of valvular heart disease (see Table 34-19) is prevention of recurrent rheumatic fever and infective endocarditis. Treatment of valvular heart disease depends on the valve involved and the severity of the disease. It focuses on preventing exacerbations of heart failure, acute pulmonary edema, thromboembolism, and recurrent endocarditis. If manifestations of CHF develop, digitalis, diuretics, and a low-sodium diet are recommended. Anticoagulant therapy is used to prevent and treat systemic or pulmonary embolization, and it is also used as a prophylactic measure in patients with atrial fibrillation. Dysrhythmias, especially atrial dysrhythmias, are common with valvular heart disease and are treated with digitalis, antidysrhythmic drugs, or electrical cardioversion. β-Adrenergic blocking drugs may be used to slow the ventricular rate in patients with atrial fibrillation.

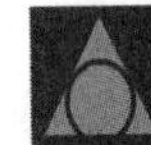

Table 34-19 Therapeutic Management: Valvular Heart Disease

Diagnostic
- History and physical examination
- Chest x-ray
- ECG
- Echocardiography
- Cardiac catheterization

Therapeutic

Nonsurgical
- Prophylactic antibiotic therapy
  - Rheumatic fever
  - Infective endocarditis*
- Digitalis[†]
- Diuretics[†]
- Sodium restriction
- Anticoagulant agents
  - Warfarin (Coumadin)
  - Dipyramidole (Persantine)
  - Aspirin
- Antidysrhythmic drugs
- Oral nitrates
- β-Adrenergic blockers
- Percutaneous transluminal balloon valvuloplasty

Surgical
- Valvuloplasty
- Closed commissurotomy
- Open commissurotomy
- Annuloplasty
- Valve replacement

ECG, Electrocardiogram.
*See Tables 34-4 and 34-5.
†See Tables 32-9 and 30-7.

Oral nitrates may be prescribed for patients with aortic valvular disease because the resulting peripheral vasodilatation reduces the blood volume returning to the heart and subsequently decreases the pressure gradient between the aorta and the left ventricle, allowing the ventricle to pump more effectively. In addition, nitrates improve coronary artery perfusion and reduce myocardial oxygen consumption.

Percutaneous transluminal balloon valvuloplasty. An alternative treatment for some patients with valvular heart disease is the *percutaneous transluminal balloon valvuloplasty* (PTBV) procedure (Fig. 34-9). Balloon valvuloplasty has been used for pulmonic, aortic, and mitral stenosis.[22] The procedure, performed in the cardiac catheterization laboratory, involves threading a balloon-tipped catheter from the femoral artery to the stenotic valve so that the balloon may be inflated in an attempt to separate the valve leaflets. A single- or double-balloon technique may be used for the PTBV procedure. A typical single balloon (the largest balloons available have a maximum inflation diameter of 25 mm) is shown inserted through the aortic valve orifice in Fig. 34-10. The double-balloon technique uses combinations of 10, 12, or 15 mm balloons inserted through each femoral artery to allow two balloons to be placed side

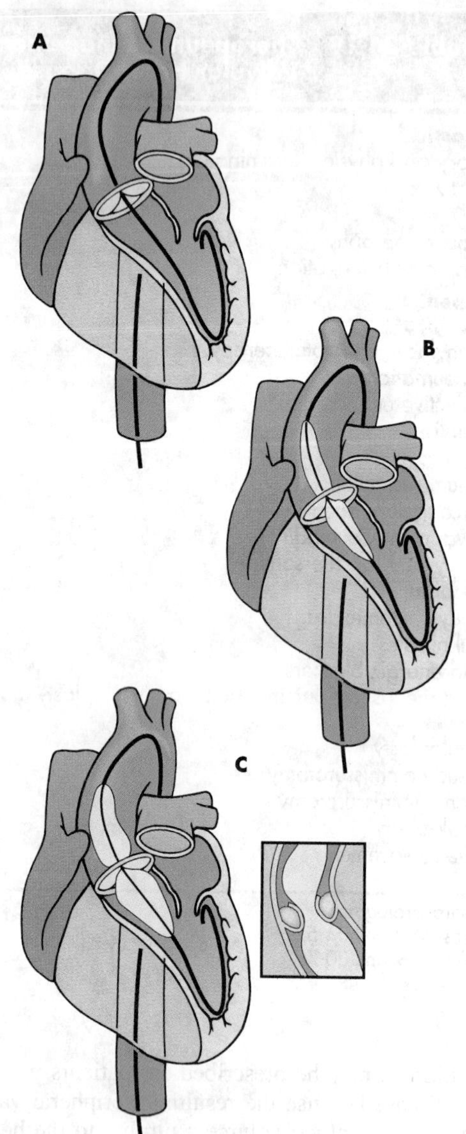

Fig. 34-9 Percutaneous transluminal balloon valvuloplasty procedure in a stenotic, calcific aortic valve. ***A,*** The loop of a wire guide, passed from the right femoral artery retrograde across the aortic valve, is seen nestling at the apex of the left ventricle. This positioning helps prevent perforation of the ventricular wall and minimizes ventricular ectopy. ***B,*** A 20 mm dilating balloon catheter, having been passed over the guide wire, is partially inflated; the indentation is caused by the stenosed valve. ***C,*** Full inflation of the balloon (*inset*) opens the aortic valve orifice.

by side into the valvular orifice, thus permitting a smaller arterial puncture and laceration.[23]

The PTBV procedure is generally indicated for older adult patients and for patients who are poor candidates for surgery. Complications and postprocedural care requirements are obviously lessened for those undergoing PTBV versus those undergoing valve replacement, but the long-term results of PTBV have not been determined.

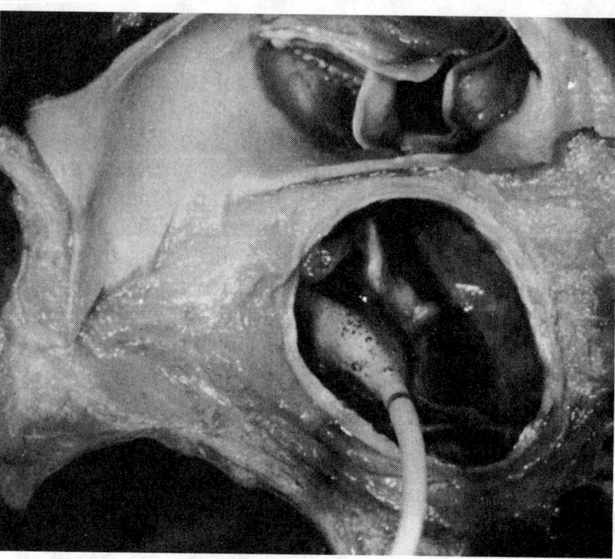

Fig. 34-10 Single balloon inflated through aortic valve orifice in the heart of a 73-year-old man with severe calcific aortic stenosis. Note that balloon does not occupy entire aortic valve opening, thereby allowing the patient to maintain perfusion throughout balloon inflation.

Surgical Interventions. The decision for surgical intervention is based on the clinical state of the patient as generally appraised through use of the New York Heart Association classification system for functional disability. The type of surgery used for a particular patient depends on the valves involved, the valvular pathology, the severity of the disease, and the patient's clinical condition. All types of valve surgery are palliative, and not curative, and patients will require lifelong health care.

Valve repair is becoming the surgical procedure of choice. Reparative or reconstructive procedures are often used in mitral or tricuspid valvular heart disease. Repair of these valves has a lower operative mortality than does replacement. *Mitral commissurotomy* (valvulotomy) is the procedure of choice for patients with pure mitral stenosis. The less precise *closed* (without cardiopulmonary bypass) method of commissurotomy has generally been replaced by the *open* method in the United States, Canada, and Western Europe.[20] The closed mitral commissurotomy is generally performed in developing nations where there is a higher number of younger patients with juvenile or third-decade mitral stenosis. Cost considerations are a significant factor.[20] The closed procedure is usually performed with the aid of a transventricular dilator inserted through the apex of the left ventricle into the ostium of the mitral valve (versus the previous use of a simple transatrial finger fracture). In contrast, the direct vision or open procedure entails the establishment of cardiopulmonary bypass, removal of thrombi from the atrium and its appendage, commissure incision, and as indicated, separation of fused chordae, splitting of underlying papillary muscle, and debriding the valve of calcium.

Further repair or reconstruction of the valve may be necessary and can be achieved by *annuloplasty,* a procedure

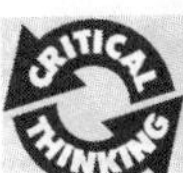

ETHICAL DILEMMAS

DO NOT RESUSCITATE

Situation A 68-year-old man has been admitted for a second mitral valve surgery and possible coronary artery bypass. He was noncompliant after his original surgery 5 years ago. The nurse was worried about his future compliance with medication to reduce blood clotting, appropriate diet, and exercise. His kidneys are failing and he is on dialysis, but not tolerating it well. Both the patient and family want complete therapeutic treatment and refuse to discuss Do Not Resuscitate (DNR) orders.

Discussion Lack of compliance in the past is not necessarily indicative of failure to comply in the future. As long as he can be maintained on medication, support, and dialysis, and no other organs fail, he has a good chance of survival. If during periods of competency, he tells the nurses that he wants to keep fighting, and he wants their help, then the nurses have the wishes of a competent adult regarding his treatment. His family agrees and seem to be supportive. A DNR order is a *physician's* order, not a patient's advance directive or expressed wish. It would reasonably follow that from certain advance directives and conversations with competent patients, a physician would place a DNR order in the chart, but that is the physician's decision. Legal problems could result if a DNR order were written against the expressed wishes of a patient and family, or if a non-terminally ill patient died as a result of not being resuscitated.

ETHICAL AND LEGAL PRINCIPLES

- DNR orders should be discussed with the patient or the patient's family.
- DNR orders should be reviewed periodically during a hospitalization or institutionalization, and should be reassessed if there are subsequent admissions.
- DNR orders should be detailed enough to cover a full range of emergency support treatments (e.g., intubation, drugs)

also used in cases of mitral or tricuspid regurgitation. Annuloplasty entails reconstruction of the valve leaflets and the annulus, with or without the aid of prosthetic rings (e.g., a Carpentier ring).

Open surgical *valvuloplasty* involves repair of the valve or suturing of torn leaflets. It is primarily performed to treat mitral regurgitation or tricuspid regurgitation. The main advantage of a reparative procedure is that it avoids the risks associated with valve replacement. The disadvantage is that it may not be possible to establish total valve competence.

Prosthetic valves. Valvular replacement may be required for mitral, aortic, tricuspid, and occasionally, pulmonic valvular disease. The surgical treatment of choice for combined aortic stenosis and aortic regurgitation is valvular replacement (Fig. 34-11, Table 34-20).

Prosthetic valves have improved since the first caged-ball valve was introduced in 1952. Early valves disintegrated, stuck, became incompetent, changed the structure of cardiac chambers, caused emboli, and traumatized blood cells. Newer valves and improved surgical techniques have made valve replacement safer and long-term valvular functioning more effective. A wide variety of valves has been introduced in an attempt to find the most sound, nonthrombogenic, and durable valve.

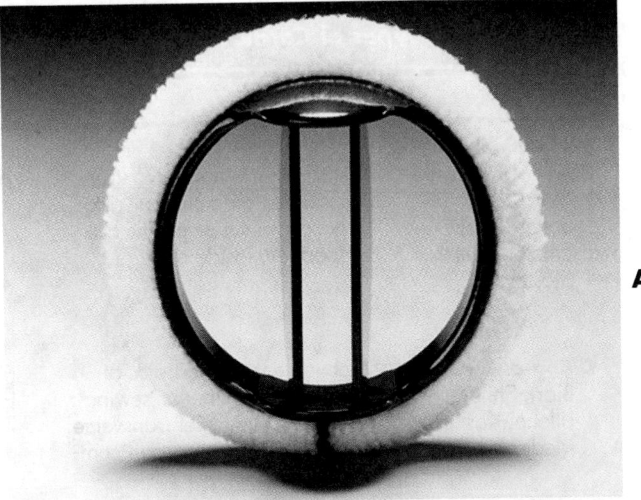

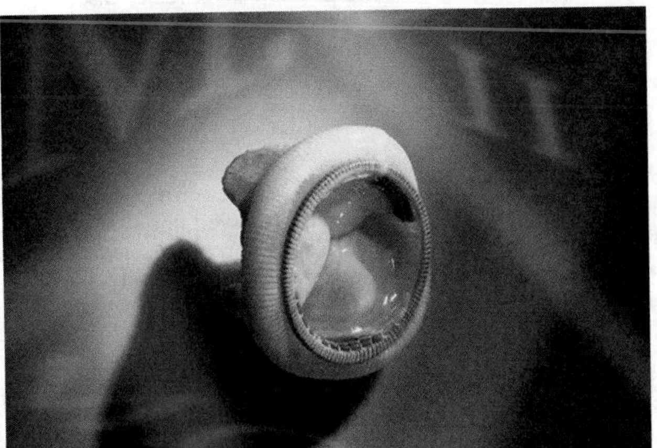

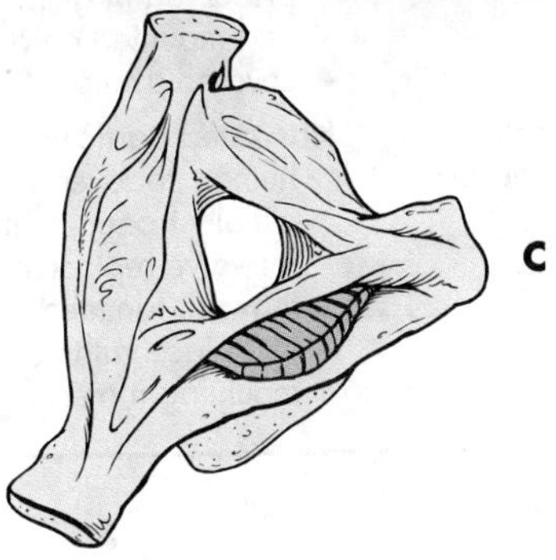

Fig. 34-11 Types of prosthetic and tissue valves. ***A,*** Bileaflet valve. ***B,*** Porcine xenograft. ***C,*** Pericardial xenograft.

Table 34-20 Types of Cardiac Prosthetic and Tissue Valves

Type	Description	Advantages	Disadvantages
Mechanical			
Caged-ball valve Starr-Edwards Sutter Silastic Smeloff-Cutter Magovern	Metal cage with several struts mounted on a circular ring; hollow metal or plastic ball *(poppett)* inside of cage	High durability (up to 20 yr)	Possibility of blood clots forming on or around valve (thrombogenic) with risk of embolism Need for long-term anticoagulation therapy Very large size
Tilting-disc valve Bjork-Shiley Lillehei-Kaster Medtronic Hall	Mobile, lens-shaped disc attached to a circular sewing ring by two offset transverse struts; pyrolytic carbon composition	Hemodynamic efficiency High durability	Tendency toward thrombogenicity and embolism Need for long-term anticoagulation therapy
Bileaflet valve St. Jude Medical Duromedics	Two pivoting semicircular discs that open centrally, mounted directly onto a sewing ring	Compact size; successful use in children and patients with small aortic roots	Possibility of thrombogenicity and embolism Need for long-term anticoagulation therapy
Biologic			
Porcine heterograft Hancock Carpentier-Edwards	Harvested aortic valve of pig that is preserved in glutaraldehyde and mounted on a specially designed sewing ring	Low thrombogenicity Need for anticoagulation therapy for only 3 mo after placement	Limited durability (failure rate increases sharply after 5-7 yr) Cumbersome structural design
Pericardial heterograph Ionescu-Shiley	Three leaflets composed of pericardium from 16- to 18-month-old calves that are preserved in glutaraldehyde and mounted on a Dacron-covered frame	Low thrombogenicity Need for only short-term anticoagulation therapy Less resistance to blood flow; useful in patients with small aortic roots	Limited durability
Homograft cadaver valve	Harvested aortic valve from human cadaver that is initially frozen until needed for valve replacement; then thawed, trimmed, and sewn into place with special mounting material	Excellent hemodynamics No hemolysis/low risk for embolism Only rare need for anticoagulation therapy	Limited durability Not useful for mitral or tricuspid valve replacement

The two categories of prosthetic valves are *mechanical* and *biologic* (tissue) valves. Mechanical valves are made of combinations of metal alloys, pyrolite carbon, and Dacron. Biologic valves are constructed from bovine, porcine, and human cardiac tissue. Within the past few years, major innovations in freezing and thawing techniques have enabled human grafts to be preserved for extensive periods without losing viability. Mechanical prosthetic valves are more durable and last longer than biologic tissue valves but have an increased risk of thromboembolism, which necessitates the use of long-term anticoagulant therapy. Biologic valves offer the patient freedom from anticoagulant therapy as a result of their low thrombogenicity. However, their durability is limited by the tendency for early calcification, tissue degeneration, and stiffening of the leaflets. Other problems associated with prosthetic valves include paravalvular leaks and endocarditis.

Long-term anticoagulation is recommended for all patients with mechanical prostheses and for patients with biologic tissue valves who are in atrial fibrillation. Some patients with biologic tissue valves or prosthetic rings may require anticoagulation during the first few months after surgery.

The choice of a valvular prosthesis depends on many factors. For example, if a patient cannot take anticoagulant therapy (e.g., women of childbearing age), a biological valve may be considered. A mechanical valve may be considered for a younger patient because it is more durable and lasts longer. For patients over the age of 65 the importance of

Table 34-21 Nursing Assessment: Valvular Heart Disease

Subjective Data

Important health information

Past health history: Rheumatic fever, endocarditis, congenital defects, myocardial infarction, chest trauma, cardiomyopathy, syphilis, Marfan's syndrome, staphylococcal or streptococcal infections

Medications: IV drug use

Functional health patterns

Health perception–health management: Fatigue

Activity-exercise: Palpitations; generalized weakness, activity intolerance; dizziness; dyspnea on exertion, cough, hemoptysis, orthopnea

Sleep-rest: Paroxysmal nocturnal dyspnea

Cognitive-perceptual: Angina or atypical chest pain

Objective Data

General

Fever

Integumentary

Diaphoresis, flushing, cyanosis, clubbing

Respiratory

Crackles, wheezes

Cardiovascular

Abnormal heart sounds, including opening snaps, clicks, thrills, systolic and diastolic murmurs, S_3, and S_4; dysrhythmias, including premature atrial contraction, atrial fibrillation; increase or decrease in pulse pressure; water-hammer pulse; peripheral edema

Neurologic

Visual field deficits

Possible findings

Cardiomegaly, valve calcification, pulmonary congestion on chest x-ray; decrease in excursion, calcification or vegetation of leaflets or prolapse, and chamber enlargement on echocardiogram; atrial and ventricular hypertrophy, dysrhythmias, conduction defects on ECG

ECG, Electrocardiogram; *IV,* intravenous; S_3 and S_4, third and fourth heart sounds.

durability is less of an issue, but the risks of noncompliance or hemorrhage from anticoagulants may be greater. (The care of the patient requiring cardiac surgery is discussed in Chapter 32.)

NURSING MANAGEMENT

VALVULAR DISORDERS

Nursing Assessment

Subjective and objective data should be obtained from an individual with valvular disease and are presented in Table 34-21.

Nursing Diagnoses

Nursing diagnoses are determined when the problem and etiologic factors are supported by clinical data. Nursing diagnoses related to valvular disease may include, but are not limited to, those presented in the following nursing care plan for the patient with valvular heart disease.

Planning

The overall goals are that the patient with valvular heart disease will have (1) normal cardiac function, (2) improved activity tolerance, and (3) an understanding of the disease process and preventive measures.

Nursing Implementation

Health Maintenance and Promotion. Prevention of acquired rheumatic valvular disease is achieved by diagnosing and treating streptococcal infection and providing prophylactic antibiotics for patients with a history of rheumatic fever. The patient at risk for endocarditis must also be treated with prophylactic antibiotics.

The patient must adhere to recommended therapies. The individual with a history of rheumatic fever, endocarditis, and congenital heart disease should know the symptoms suggestive of valvular heart disease so that early medical treatment may be obtained.

Acute Intervention and Chronic and Home Management. A patient with progressive valvular heart disease may require hospitalization or outpatient care for management of CHF, endocarditis, embolic disease, or dysrhythmias. CHF is the most common reason for ongoing medical care.

The role of the nurse is to implement and evaluate the effectiveness of therapeutic management. Activity should be designed after considering the patient's limitations. An appropriate exercise plan can increase cardiac tolerance. However, activities that regularly produce fatigue and dyspnea should be restricted, and an explanation should be provided to the patient. Smoking should be discouraged. Strenuous physical exercise should be avoided because damaged valves may not be able to handle the required increase in CO. The patient should be assisted in planning the activities of daily living, with an emphasis on conserving energy, setting priorities, and taking planned rest periods. Referral to a vocational counselor may be necessary if the patient has a physically or emotionally demanding job.

Auscultatory assessment of the heart should be performed to monitor the effectiveness of digitalis, β-adrenergic blocking agents, and antidysrhythmic drugs. Patients should be instructed to wear a Medic-Alert bracelet. The patient must understand the importance of prophylactic antibiotic therapy to prevent endocarditis (see Tables 34-4 and 34-5). If the valve disease was caused by rheumatic fever, prophylaxis to prevent recurrence is necessary.

Urinary output and daily weight should be monitored when diuretics are prescribed. The patient's diet should be well-balanced nutritionally, with sodium restriction to prevent fluid retention.

The nurse should help the patient with a valvular disorder achieve and maintain an optimal level of health. Extensive teaching regarding the actions and side effects of drugs is important to achieve compliance. When valvular heart disease can no longer be managed medically, surgical intervention is necessary (see Chapter 32). The patient who is on anticoagulation therapy after surgery for valve replacement needs to have the prothrombin time checked regularly (usually monthly) to assess the adequacy of therapy and to pre-

NURSING CARE PLAN Patient with Valvular Heart Disease

Planning: Outcome Criteria	Nursing Interventions and Rationales
➤ **NURSING DIAGNOSIS**	Activity intolerance *related to* insufficient oxygenation secondary to decreased cardiac output *as manifested by* weakness, fatigue, altered response to activity such as shortness of breath, dyspnea, weak pulse with increase or decrease in rate, BP changes
Demonstrate cardiac tolerance to increased activity (e.g., stable pulse, respirations, BP).	Assess and monitor patient responses to activity (e.g., pulse rate, respirations, BP) *to plan appropriate interventions.* Plan rest periods between activities *to conserve energy and decrease cardiac demands.* Organize care *to minimize unnecessary disturbance.* Assist patient with personal care as necessary *to minimize fatigue and dyspnea and ensure patient needs are met.* Progressively increase activity *to increase cardiac tolerance.*
➤ **NURSING DIAGNOSIS**	Ineffective management of therapeutic regimen *related to* lack of knowledge about disease process, signs and symptoms of congestive heart failure and infective endocarditis, and prevention and treatment strategies *as manifested by* lack of compliance with therapeutic regimen and clinical manifestations of valvular heart disease
Verbalize knowledge of disease process, complications, and preventive precautions; comply with therapeutic regimen	Explain nature and cause of disease process *to ensure patient has adequate knowledge base on which to make decisions.* Teach signs and symptoms of heart failure and infective endocarditis *to ensure early reporting and treatment of complications.* Teach the need to avoid all invasive surgical or diagnostic procedures that may predispose to bacteremia until prophylactic antibiotics given. Explain the importance of notifying the dentist, urologist, and gynecologist of valvular disease *so prophylactic antibiotics treatment can be initiated.** Explain need for good oral hygiene and avoidance of fatigue *to avoid increasing the opportunity for infection.* Discourage smoking *to prevent an increased cardiac work load and the oxygen-depleting effect of carbon monoxide from decreasing the oxygen available to the myocardium.* Discuss the name of prescribed medication, dosage, purpose, and side effects *to promote safe and accurate self-medication.* Instruct patient to wear a Medic-Alert bracelet.
➤ **NURSING DIAGNOSIS**	Sleep pattern disturbance *related to* pulmonary congestion *as manifested by* fatigue and paroxysmal nocturnal dyspnea
Verbalize satisfaction with sleep; feel rested on awakening.	Elevate head of bed 30 to 40 degrees *to decrease venous return, reduce oxygen demand, maximize respiratory excursion.* Administer oxygen as ordered *to increase oxygen saturation.* Reassure and remain with patient until respirations stabilize *to reduce anxiety which increases the cardiac work load.* Eliminate environmental noise *to promote a restful environment conducive to sleep.*
➤ **NURSING DIAGNOSIS**	Pain *related to* decreased coronary blood flow and increased myocardial oxygen demand secondary to decreased cardiac output *as manifested by* complaints of chest pain, nonverbal indicators of pain such as guarding and massaging painful areas
Verbalize satisfaction with level of pain; plan for pain control.	Monitor vital signs *to assess cardiac function.* Observe for verbal and nonverbal expressions of pain and discomfort *to evaluate effectiveness of pain control measures.* Decrease activity as ordered *to reduce tissue oxygen demands.* Administer analgesics as ordered *to provide pain relief.* Administer nitrates as ordered *to cause peripheral vasodilatation, improve coronary artery perfusion, and reduce myocardial oxygen consumption.*

continued

NURSING CARE PLAN Patient with Valvular Heart Disease—cont'd

COLLABORATIVE PROBLEMS

Nursing Goals	Nursing Interventions and Rationales
➤ POTENTIAL COMPLICATION Hypervolemia *related to* cardiac failure	
Assess for signs of hypervolemia, report deviations from acceptable parameters, and carry out medical and nursing interventions.	Monitor for manifestations of hypervolemia such as peripheral edema; taut, shiny skin; adventitious breath sounds *to detect hypervolemia.* Assess vital signs, auscultate breath sounds, assess for increased or decreased jugular distention, measure intake and output, palpate for edema, and assess for weight gain *to monitor indicators of hypervolemia.* Restrict sodium as ordered *to prevent fluid retention.* Monitor laboratory findings including electrolytes, hematocrit, BUN, and urinalysis *as changes can indicate hypervolemia.*
➤ POTENTIAL COMPLICATION Decreased cardiac output related to cardiac failure	
Assess for signs of decreased cardiac output, report deviations from acceptable parameters, and carry out medical and nursing interventions.	Monitor BP, apical pulse, respirations, breath and heart sounds *to assess for signs of decreased cardiac output* such as fatigue, malaise, shortness of breath, dyspnea on exertion, paroxysmal nocturnal dyspnea, palpitations, angina, vertigo, cardiac murmur, widened pulse pressure. Assess hemodynamic parameters (e.g., pulmonary artery pressure, pulmonary capillary wedge pressure, CO, central venous pressure) as ordered *as indicators of patient status.* Maintain bed rest as ordered *to decrease cardiac work load and oxygen demands.* Elevate head of bed 30 to 40 degrees *to reduce venous return, reduce oxygen demand, and maximize chest excursion.* Administer oxygen as ordered *to improve oxygen saturation.* Monitor cardiac rhythm *to detect changes from baseline.* Document and determine dysrhythmia. Administer parenteral therapy as ordered and measure intake and output *to assure appropriate fluid balance.* Administer inotropic medication as ordered *to increase myocardial contractility.*
➤ POTENTIAL COMPLICATION Systemic and pulmonary emboli related to thrombi development secondary to valve replacement	
Assess for signs of systemic or pulmonary emboli, report deviations from acceptable parameters, and carry out medical and nursing interventions.	Monitor for dyspnea, hemoptysis, pain, diminished or absent peripheral pulses, changes in skin color and temperature *to detect systemic and pulmonary emboli.* Monitor vital signs *as increases can indicate embolization* and neurologic status *as decreases in function can indicate embolization.* Auscultate breath sounds *to determine signs of pulmonary emboli such as crackles and accentuated pulmonic heart sounds.* Administer anticoagulants and oxygen as ordered. Assess peripheral pulses and lower extremities for color, warmth, and edema *as changes in status can indicate peripheral embolization.* Perform ROM exercises (active or passive) for extremities. Apply elastic compression gradient stockings *to promote venous return and prevent venous stasis.*

BP, Blood pressure; *BUN,* blood urea nitrogen; *CO,* cardiac output; *ROM,* range of motion.
*See Tables 34-4 and 34-5.

vent side effects. Teaching instructions related to anticoagulant therapy are listed in Table 35-14.

The patient needs to realize that valve surgery is not a cure, and that regular follow-up examinations by the healthcare provider will be required. The nurse also needs to teach the patient about when to seek medical care. Any manifestations of infection, congestive heart failure, signs of bleeding, and any planned invasive or dental procedures require the patient to notify the health care provider.

CRITICAL THINKING EXERCISES

CASE STUDY

VALVULAR HEART DISEASE

Patient Profile

Mrs. S., a 54-year-old woman, is admitted to the hospital for valvular heart disease.

Subjective Data

- Was told she had streptococcal sore throat as a child
- Was diagnosed 10 years ago with rheumatic heart disease
- Has shortness of breath at rest. Cannot get out of bed without becoming dyspneic
- Takes Digoxin (0.25 mg once a day)

Objective Data

Physical Examination

- Ankle edema
- Irregular pulse
- Crackles at lung bases
- Murmurs of mitral stenosis, mitral insufficiency, and aortic insufficiency

Diagnostic Studies

Chest x-ray and ECG indicate enlarged left atrium

Critical Thinking Questions

1. Explain the cause of Mrs. S.'s valvular heart disease. What valves are most likely to become involved with rheumatic heart disease?
2. Differentiate between the characteristics of mitral stenosis and mitral regurgitation.
3. What other conservative treatment measures might be initiated for this patient in addition to digoxin?
4. What are important nursing measures for Mrs. S.?
5. On the basis of the assessment data provided, write one or more nursing diagnoses. Are there any collaborative problems?

NURSING RESEARCH ISSUES

1. What are effective nursing measures to facilitate patient compliance with prophylactic antibiotic therapy for endocarditis?
2. How does the quality of life of a patient having valvular heart surgery differ preoperatively as compared to postoperatively?
3. Does a planned aerobic exercise program decrease symptoms associated with mitral valve prolapse?
4. What health problems are observed most frequently by the nurse caring for a patient with rheumatic heart disease?

REVIEW QUESTIONS

The number of the question corresponds to the same-numbered objective at the beginning of the chapter.

1. The microorganism most often responsible for acute infective endocarditis is

a. *Streptococcus viridans.*
b. *Staphylococcus aureus.*
c. *Escherichia coli.*
d. *Pseudomonas* species.

2. A patient with infective endocarditis would need instructions at discharge about which of the following signs and symptoms that indicate a relapse?

a. Fever
b. Restlessness
c. Right upper quadrant pain
d. Weight gain

3. Prophylactic antibiotics are indicated to prevent infective endocarditis for high-risk individuals who

a. are undergoing any dental procedure.
b. have acquired a viral respiratory tract infection.
c. are entering the third trimester of pregnancy.
d. are exposed to human immunodeficiency virus.

4. The most common cause of myocarditis is

a. myocardial infarction.
b. endocarditis.
c. viruses.
d. radiation.

5. Which of the following statements best characterizes the pathophysiology of rheumatic fever?

a. Viral infection of endocardium and valves
b. Sequela of β-hemolytic streptococcal infection
c. Sequela of *Streptococcus viridans* infection
d. Frequently triggered by immunosuppressive therapy

6. Management of rheumatic fever may include all of the following *except*

a. salicylates.
b. corticosteroids.
c. limited activity.
d. IV antibiotic therapy.

7. The most common cause of mitral valve disease is

a. rheumatic heart disease.
b. congenital heart disease.
c. infective endocarditis.
d. myocarditis.

8. A patient with chronic mitral regurgitation reflects accentuated left ventricular filling leading to

a. an audible third heart sound and a pansystolic or holosystolic murmur.
b. midsytolic click followed by an early systolic murmur.
c. audible third heart sound and a late diastolic murmur.
d. audible third heart sound and a middiastolic click with a late diastolic murmur.

9. All of the following are appropriate therapies for valvular heart disease *except*

a. percutaneous transluminal balloon valvuloplasty.
b. annuloplasty.
c. coronary artery bypass surgery.
d. valvulotomy.

10. The surgical splitting of valve leaflets is identified as a

a. curettage.
b. leaflet dilatation.
c. valvuloplasty.
d. commissurotomy.

REFERENCES

1. Scheld NM, Sande MA: Endocarditis and intravascular infections. In Mandell GL, Douglas RG, Bennett JE, editors: *Principles and practice of infectious disease,* ed 3, New York, 1990, Churchill-Livingstone.
2. Durack DT: Amenable infections-endocarditis, *Hosp Prac* (Suppl) 28:6, 1993.
3. Stekelberg JM, Wilson WR: Risk factors for infective endocarditis, *Infect Dis Clin North Am* 7:9, 1993.
4. Wahl MJ: Myths of dental-induced endocarditis, *Arch Intern Med* 154:137, 1994.
5. Dajani AS and others: Prevention of bacterial endocarditis: recommendation by the American Heart Association, *JAMA* 264:2929, 1990.
6. Simmons NS and others: Antibiotic prophylaxis of infective endocarditis: recommendations from the Endocarditis Working Party of the British Society for Antimicrobial Chemotherapy, *Lancet* 335:88, 1990.
7. Durack DT: Prophylaxis of infective endocarditis. In Mandell GL, Douglas RG, Bennett JE, editors: *Principles and practice of infectious disease,* ed 3, New York, 1990, Churchill-Livingstone.
8. Bisno AL: Antimicrobial prophylaxis for infective endocarditis, *Hosp Pract* 24:209, 1989.
9. Savoia MC, Oxman MN: Myocarditis, pericarditis and mediastinitis. In Mandell GL, Douglas RG, Bennett JE, editors: *Principles and practice of infectious diseases,* ed 3, 1990, New York, Churchill-Livingstone.
10. Pierce CD: Acute post-MI pericarditis, *J Cardiovasc Nurse* 6:46, 1992.
11. Bresler MJ: Acute pericarditis and myocarditis, *Emerg Med* 24:34, 1992.
12. Bisno AL: Medical practice: Group A streptococcal infections and acute rheumatic fever, *N Engl J Med* 325:11, 1991.
13. Burge DJ, DeHoratius RJ: Acute rheumatic fever, *Cardiovascular Clinics* 23:3, 1993.
14. Rheumatic fever: making a comeback, *Harvard Medical School Health Letter* 23:105, 1988.
15. Kavey RE, Kaplan EL: Resurgence of acute rheumatic fever, *Pediatrics* 84:585, 1989.
16. Conn HF and others: *Conn's current therapy,* Philadelphia, 1993, Saunders.
17. Kaplan EL: Acute rheumatic fever. In Schlant RE, Alexander RW, editors: *Hurst's the heart,* ed 8, New York, 1994, McGraw-Hill.
18. Khan SS, Gray RJ: Valvular emergencies, *Cardiol Clin* 9:689, 1991.
19. Anonymous: Recognizing valvular heart disease, *Emerg Med* 22:56, 1990. Cover story.
20. Feldman T: Rheumatic mitral stenosis, *Postgrad Med* 93:93, 1993.
21. Barlow JB: Mitral valve billowing and prolapse: an overview, *Aust N Z J Med* 22:541, 1992.
22. Scordo KA: Helping your patient cope with mitral valve prolapse syndrome, *Nursing* 22:34, 1992.
23. Nichols L and others: Percutaneous aortic valvuloplasty procedure and implications for nursing, *Heart Lung* 18:356, 1989.

Chapter 35

NURSING ROLE IN MANAGEMENT

Vascular Disorders

Diane Rudolphi **Jeanne Doyle**

Learning Objectives

1. Describe the pathophysiology, clinical manifestations, and surgical management of aortic aneurysms.
2. Discuss the perioperative nursing care of a patient having an aortic aneurysm repair.
3. Describe the pathophysiology, clinical manifestations, and management of aortic dissection.
4. Identify the risk factors associated with atherosclerosis.
5. Describe the pathophysiology, clinical manifestations, and therapeutic and surgical management of peripheral arterial occlusive disease.
6. Discuss the nursing management of the patient with acute arterial insufficiency affecting the lower extremities.
7. Identify three risk factors predisposing to the development of thrombophlebitis.
8. Differentiate between the clinical characteristics of superficial and deep vein thrombophlebitis.
9. Describe the nursing management of the patient with deep vein thrombophlebitis.
10. Explain the purpose and actions of commonly used anticoagulants and the nursing role for patients receiving them.
11. Describe the pathophysiology, clinical manifestations, and therapeutic and nursing management of pulmonary emboli.
12. Describe the pathophysiology and nursing management of venous stasis ulcers.

Problems of the vascular system include disorders of the aorta, arteries, veins, and lymphatic vessels. *Peripheral vascular disease* is a term used to describe a wide variety of conditions affecting these vessels in the neck, abdomen, and extremities.

DISORDERS OF THE AORTA

Aneurysms

Aneurysms are outpouchings or dilatations of the arterial wall and are a common problem involving the aorta. Aneurysms of peripheral arteries can also occur but are far less common. Aneurysms occur in men more often than in women, and their incidence increases with age.[1] They account for 1.7% of deaths in men 65 to 74 years of age.[2] Half of all aneurysms greater than 6 cm in diameter rupture within 1 year.[1,3]

Pathophysiology. Most aneurysms are found in the abdominal aorta below the level of the renal arteries. The aortic wall weakens and dilates with the turbulent blood flow. The growth rate of aneurysms is unpredictable, but the larger the aneurysm, the greater the risk of rupture. Thrombi are deposited on the aortic wall and can embolize.

Although the cause of aneurysms is unknown, there are several risk factors associated with the development of aneurysms, including hypertension, smoking, and atherosclerosis. A common cause of aortic aneurysm is atherosclerosis with plaques composed of lipids, cholesterol, fibrin, and other debris deposited beneath the intima or lining of the artery. This plaque formation causes degenerative changes in the media (middle layer of the arterial wall), leading to loss of elasticity, weakening, and eventual dilatation of the aorta.

Recently there have been several studies that have shown a strong genetic component in the development of abdominal aortic aneurysms.[4,5] Although the familial tendency to develop abdominal aortic aneurysms is primarily a genetic defect, no formal genetic analysis of family data has been performed.[4] Other less common causes of aneurysm formation include trauma, acute or chronic infections (e.g., tuberculosis, syphilis), and anastamotic disruptions.

Classification. Aneurysms are generally divided into two basic classifications: *true* and *false* (Fig. 35-1). A true aneurysm is one in which the wall of the artery forms the aneurysm, with at least one vessel layer still intact. Three

Reviewed by Jacqueline Helt, RN, BSN, Peripheral Vascular Nurse Specialist, New York University Medical Center, New York, NY.

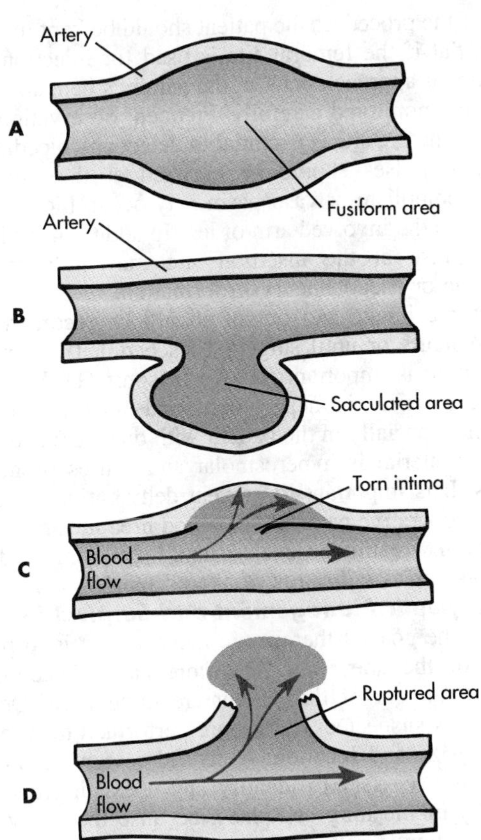

Fig. 35-1 ***A,*** True fusiform abdominal aortic aneurysm. ***B,*** True saccular aortic aneurysm. ***C,*** Dissecting aneurysm. ***D,*** False or pseudoaneurysm (pulsatile hematoma).

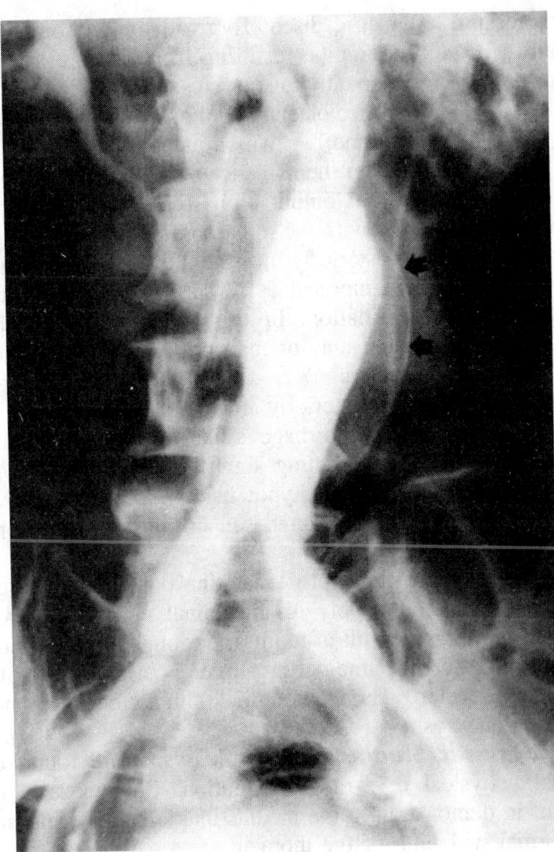

Fig. 35-2 Arteriogram demonstrating fusiform abdominal aortic aneurysm. Note calcification of the aortic wall (*arrows*) and extension of the aneurysm into the common iliac arteries.

fourths of true aneurysms occur in the abdomen (Fig. 35-2) and one fourth in the thoracic aorta. Popliteal artery aneurysms rank third in frequency.

True aneurysms can be further subdivided into fusiform and saccular dilatations. A *fusiform aneurysm* is circumferential and relatively uniform in shape. A *saccular aneurysm* is pouchlike and has a narrow neck connecting the bulge to one side of the arterial wall.

Aortic dissection is often misnamed "dissecting aneurysm" and occurs when there is a tear of the internal lining of the arterial wall that allows blood to enter between the intima and media, creating a false lumen. With arterial pulsations, the blood may continue to dissect down the artery, involving branch arteries along the way. This process may be acute and life threatening or self-limiting, resulting in a chronic and stable process for a period of time.[6] (Aortic dissection is discussed later in this chapter.)

A false aneurysm, or *pseudoaneurysm,* is not an aneurysm but a disruption of all layers of the arterial wall resulting in a leak of blood that is contained or tamponaded by surrounding structures. False aneurysms may result from trauma, infection, or disruption of an arterial suture line after surgery. They may also result from arterial leakage after removal of cannulae such as upper or lower extremity arterial catheters and intraaortic balloon pump devices.

Clinical Manifestations. Thoracic aneurysms are usually asymptomatic. When manifestations are present, they are varied. The most common manifestation is deep, diffuse chest pain. Aneurysms located in the ascending aorta and the aortic arch can produce hoarseness in the patient as a result of pressure on the recurrent laryngeal nerve. Pressure on the esophagus can cause dysphagia. If the aneurysm presses on the superior vena cava, it can cause distended neck veins and edema of the head and arms. Pressure of the aneurysm on pulmonary structures can lead to coughing, dyspnea, and airway obstruction.

Abdominal aneurysms are most often asymptomatic and are often detected on routine physical examination or coincidentally when the patient is being examined for an unrelated problem (e.g., abdominal x-ray, ultrasound, computed tomography scan, intravenous pyelogram, or abdominal surgery). On physical examination a pulsatile mass in the periumbilical area slightly to the left of the midline may be detected. Bruits (murmurlike sounds resulting from turbulent blood flow) may be audible with a stethoscope placed over the aneurysm.

Symptoms of an abdominal aortic aneurysm may mimic pain associated with any abdominal or back disorder. Symptoms may result from compression of nearby anatomic structures (e.g., back pain caused by lumbar nerve compression, epigastric discomfort with or without alteration in bowel elimination resulting from compression on the bowel). Occasionally aneurysms, even small ones, spontaneously embolize plaque and thrombi. This can cause the "blue toe syndrome," in which patchy mottling of the feet and toes occurs in the presence of pedal pulses.

Complications. Complications related to aneurysms can be catastrophic, with the most common being rupture. If rupture occurs posteriorly into the retroperitoneal space, bleeding may be tamponaded by surrounding structures, preventing exsanguination. In this case the patient has severe back pain and may or may not have back or flank ecchymosis (Turner's sign).

If rupture occurs anteriorly into the abdominal cavity, death from massive hemorrhage is likely. If the patient does reach the hospital, presenting signs are manifestations of shock such as tachycardia, hypotension, pale clammy skin, decreased urine output, altered sensorium, and abdominal tenderness on palpation.

Paraplegia is a rare but devastating possible complication. If the blood supply to the spinal cord is severely compromised as a result of rupture, prolonged hypotension, or prolonged clamp time during surgery, permanent paralysis may develop. This would most likely occur with a thoracic aneurysm.

Diagnostic Studies. Most aneurysms are found on routine physical or x-ray examination. Chest x-rays are useful in demonstrating the mediastinal silhouette and any abnormal widening of the thoracic aorta. A plain x-ray of the abdomen may show calcification within the wall of an abdominal aortic aneurysm.

When an electrocardiogram (ECG) is performed, it is used to rule out evidence of myocardial infarction (MI) because some persons may have symptoms suggestive of angina. Echocardiography assists in the diagnosis of aortic insufficiency related to ascending aortic dilatation. Ultrasonography is useful for screening. A computed tomography (CT) scan is the most accurate test to determine the anterior-to-posterior and cross-sectional diameter of the aneurysm and to identify the presence of thrombus in the aneurysm. Magnetic resonance imaging (MRI) may also be used to diagnose and assess the severity of aneurysms.

Aortography, anatomic mapping of the aortic system by contrast imaging, is performed only if arterial occlusive disease is suspected (e.g., absent peripheral pulses, uncontrolled hypertension) or the aneurysm extends above the renal arteries. Any structures receiving their arterial blood supply from the affected part of the aorta, which includes the distal circulation to the legs, can be carefully studied with aortography. Aortography is done with the use of a local anesthetic. A large needle with a stylet is inserted into the femoral artery, although a subclavian, axillary, brachial, or translumbar approach (through the back directly into the aorta) may also be used. A catheter is inserted and threaded through the needle into the artery. Contrast medium is then injected, and x-rays are taken with fluoroscopy. When all x-rays have been taken, the catheter is removed. Pressure is applied on the puncture site for 20 minutes or until the bleeding has stopped.

After the procedure the patient should be kept in bed and remain flat if the femoral site is used for injection. If the translumbar approach is used, the patient's hematocrit level should be monitored carefully. Frequent observation of the arterial puncture site is essential to detect any bleeding. The peripheral pulses should be checked at the same time because embolism or vasospasm may occur, blocking arterial flow to the involved arm or leg. In addition, a widening of the pulse at the insertion site may indicate either hematoma or pseudoaneurysm formation.

Accurate intake and output should be recorded for at least 24 hours or until surgery (if scheduled). Monitoring urine output is important for two reasons: (1) the injected contrast material is nephrotoxic and may impair renal function (especially in the patient with diabetes) and (2) the contrast material is hyperosmolar and causes pronounced diuresis. It is important to prevent dehydration, especially in the preoperative patient. The blood urea nitrogen (BUN) and serum creatinine levels should be compared with pretest values as indicators of altered renal function.

Therapeutic Management and Surgical Interventions. The goal of therapeutic management is to prevent rupture of the aneurysm. Therefore early detection and prompt treatment of the patient are imperative. Once an aneurysm is suspected, studies are performed to determine its exact size and location. A careful review of all body systems is necessary to identify any coexisting disorders, especially of the lung or kidney, because they may influence the patient's risk of surgery. The carotid and coronary arteries should be assessed for indications of atherosclerotic disease. If obstructions in these vessels are present, they may need to be corrected before the aneurysm is repaired. Generally, if coexisting problems are not severe, surgery is the treatment of choice. The type of surgery depends on the location of the aneurysm (Table 35-1).

The only effective treatment of an aortic aneurysm is surgery. Surgery to repair a fusiform aneurysm is known as *endoaneurysmorrhaphy.* The technique involves (1) incising the diseased segment of the aorta; (2) removing intraluminal thrombus or plaque; (3) inserting a synthetic arterial tube graft (Dacron or polytetrafluoroethylene), which is sutured to the normal aorta proximal and distal to the aneurysm; and (4) suturing the native aortic wall around the graft so that it will act as a protective cover (Fig. 35-3). If the iliac arteries are also aneurysmal, the entire diseased segment is replaced with a bifurcation graft (Fig. 35-4).

Before surgery, every effort is made to bring the patient to the best possible state of hydration and electrolyte balance. Any abnormalities in coagulation and blood cell count are corrected. The patient may receive antibiotics and baths with antiseptics before surgery. However, if the aneurysm has ruptured, the treatment of choice is immediate surgical intervention. Even with prompt care, the mortality rate is high (about 50%) after rupture and increases with the age of the patient. Aneurysms repaired electively have a surgical risk of 1% to 5%.

All aneurysm resections require cross-clamping of the aorta proximal and distal to the aneurysm. When aneurysms are repaired electively, the patient is systemically antico-

Table 35-1 Types of Aortic Aneurysm Resection

Location of Aneurysm	Incision Site	Use of Bypass or Hypothermia	Nursing Considerations
■ Ascending aorta with aortic valve insufficiency	Median sternotomy	Cardiopulmonary bypass and hypothermia are used.	Be aware that if aortic valvular insufficiency is severe, prosthetic valve replacement is performed.
■ Aortic arch	Median sternotomy	Cardiopulmonary bypass and hypothermia are used. If transverse aorta containing brachiocephalic vessels is involved, extracorporeal perfusion of brain is necessary.	Be aware that cold predisposes patient to dysrhythmias. Watch neurologic signs.
■ Descending thoracic aorta	Posterolateral at fourth intercostal space	Hypothermia is used. Cardiopulmonary bypass may be used.	Be aware that Carlen's tube (double-cuffed endotracheal tube) deflates either lung and causes pulmonary stress and atelectasis, that good pulmonary care is important, and that ischemia to spinal cord is common.
■ Abdominal aortic aneurysm	Xiphoid process to pubis	Bypass and hypothermia are not used. Arterial blood flow to lower extremities can be interrupted for time needed for surgical procedure.	Be aware that graft is placed within artery walls and that this technique prevents graft from eroding into surrounding structures such as bowel.
	Retroperitoneal (left flank, similar to nephrectomy incision)	Bypass and hypothermia are not used.	Be aware that because abdominal cavity is not entered, the patient often has fewer problems with gastrointestinal and pulmonary dysfunction and less pain.

agulated with intravenous (IV) heparin before cross-clamping the aorta. This prevents clotting of pooled blood distal to the aneurysm. If surgery is performed emergently (as in the case of rupture), no anticoagulation is indicated. Most resections can be completed in 30 to 45 minutes, after which time the clamps are removed and blood flow to the lower extremities is restored. Use of autotransfusion, which recycles the patient's own blood, has markedly reduced the need for blood transfusions. (Autotransfusions are discussed in Chapter 28.)

Fortunately most abdominal aortic aneurysms originate below the origin of the renal arteries. However, if the aneurysm extends above the renal arteries or if the cross clamp must be applied above the renal arteries, adequate renal perfusion after removal of the clamp should be ascertained before closure of the abdominal incision. The risk of renal complications postoperatively is significantly increased in patients who have surgical repair of aneurysms above the renal arteries.

With saccular aneurysms, it may be possible to excise only the bulbous lesion, repairing the artery by primary closure (suturing the artery together) or by application of an autogenous or synthetic patch graft over the arterial defect.

All patients undergoing aneurysmectomy should be placed in an intensive care unit (ICU) with appropriate support services and equipment postoperatively. When the patient arrives in the ICU, an endotracheal tube, an arterial line, a central venous pressure or pulmonary artery catheter, peripheral IV lines, an indwelling urinary catheter, and a nasogastric tube will likely be in place. If the thorax is entered during surgery, chest tubes will also be in place. Anesthesia may be done using a combination of general and epidural, with the epidural catheter left in place for epidural analgesia administration.

NURSING MANAGEMENT

ANEURYSMS

Nursing Assessment

The patient with an aneurysm may have a variety of manifestations or may be totally free of symptoms. There-

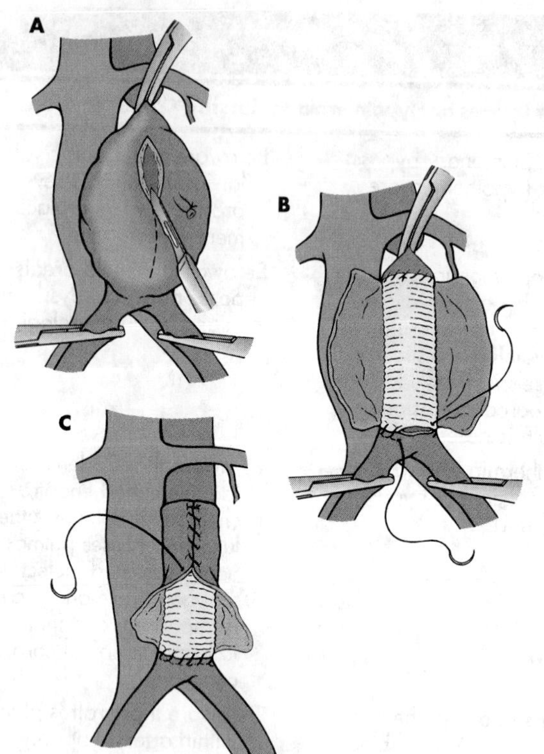

Fig. 35-3 Surgical repair of an abdominal aortic aneurysm. ***A,*** Incising the aneurysmal sac. ***B,*** Insertion of synthetic graft. ***C,*** Suturing native aortic wall over synthetic graft.

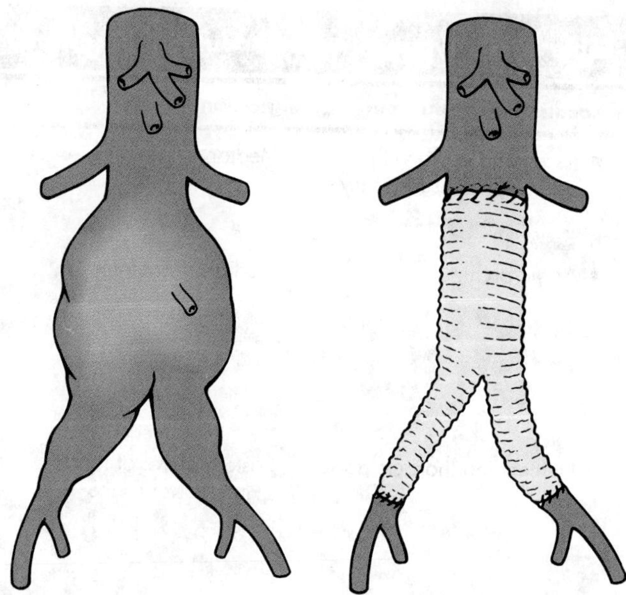

Fig. 35-4 Replacement of aortoiliac aneurysm with a bifurcated synthetic graft.

fore the nurse must use assessment skills to focus on early detection and treatment.

A thorough nursing history and assessment should be performed. Because most aneurysms are atherosclerotic and atherosclerosis is a systemic disease process, it is likely that the disease process is present throughout the body. Therefore it is important for the nurse to watch for signs of cardiac, pulmonary, cerebral, and peripheral vascular problems. The patient should be monitored for signs of rupture of the aneurysm, such as paleness, weakness, tachycardia, hypotension, abdominal pain, back pain, or groin pain.

Establishing baseline data is important for later postoperative assessment and intervention. In addition to gathering data, the nurse should observe the patient closely for subtle abnormalities. Special attention should be paid to the character and quality of the peripheral pulses and the neurologic status. Arterial pulse sites and skin lesions in the lower extremities should be marked and documented before surgery.

Planning

The overall goals are that a patient with an aneurysm will have (1) normal tissue perfusion, (2) intact motor and neurologic function, and (3) no complications related to surgical repair.

Nursing Implementation

Health Maintenance and Promotion. The nurse must be aware of cardiovascular disease risk factors and be alert for opportunities to teach health measures to patients in the hospital and the community (see Chapter 31). Special attention should be given to the patient with a strong family history of aneurysm or any evidence of other cardiovascular disease. A trauma victim should be urged to seek medical attention even in the absence of symptoms.

The patient should be encouraged to reduce risk factors known to be associated with the disease process. These should include controlling hypertension, stopping smoking, and following a diet low in fats and cholesterol. These measures are also done to ensure continued graft patency following surgical repair.

Acute Intervention and Postoperative Care. The nursing role during the preoperative period should include teaching, providing support for the patient and family, and carefully assessing all body systems. It is imperative that problems be identified early and proper intervention instituted.

In addition to maintaining adequate respiratory function, fluid and electrolyte balance, and pain control in the postoperative period, the nurse needs to monitor graft patency, pulmonary status, renal perfusion, and circulation. The nurse can also assist in preventing ventricular dysrhythmias, infections, and neurologic complications. Care of the patient with an aneurysm repair is described in the following nursing care plan.

Graft patency. Adequacy of systemic blood pressure (BP) is important to promote graft patency, but it does not ensure against thrombosis for other reasons (e.g., technical surgical defect). Prolonged hypotension may result in thrombosis of the graft as a result of decreased blood flow. Hypovolemia can be avoided by administration of IV fluids and blood components as indicated. Central venous pressure readings or pulmonary artery pressures should be monitored hourly to help assess the patient's state of hydration.

NURSING CARE PLAN Patient After Aortic Aneurysm Repair

Planning: Outcome Criteria	Nursing Interventions and Rationales
➤ **NURSING DIAGNOSIS** Risk for infection *related to* presence of a prosthetic vascular graft and invasive lines	
Have normal body temperature, no signs of infection.	Monitor for signs of infection, such as elevated body temperature; elevated WBC count, pulse, and RR; purulent drainage from incisions. Monitor sites of invasive lines. Administer broad-spectrum antibiotic as ordered *to maintain adequate blood levels of the drug.* Monitor temperature at least q4hr. Monitor WBC count *because a rising count may be the first sign of infection.* Use aseptic technique in caring for incision and any indwelling IV line, tubing, or catheter *because these sites are potential portals of entry for infection.* Ensure adequate nutrition *to promote healing.*
➤ **NURSING DIAGNOSIS** Risk for altered peripheral tissue perfusion *related to* bypass graft occlusion	
Have patent arterial graft with adequate distal perfusion.	Assess for absence of peripheral pulses in lower extremities; cool, pale extremities; sensory changes in extremities; return of ischemic pain *because these are indicators of altered peripheral perfusion.* Assess BP and all peripheral pulses hourly initially and then with decreasing frequency (e.g., q2hr, then q4hr) *to ensure adequacy of systemic blood pressure and peripheral perfusion.* Compare extremities for warmth and color *because differences may indicate occlusion of the graft.* Administer IV fluids at prescribed rates *to ensure adequate hydration and renal perfusion.*
➤ **NURSING DIAGNOSIS** Risk for sensory and perceptual alteration *related to* electrolyte imbalance, cerebral hypoxia, altered sensory input, and unfamiliar environment	
Return to baseline neurologic status.	Check chart for preoperative neurologic status *to provide baseline data for postoperative comparison.* Assess neurologic status, including level of consciousness, pupil size and response to light, movement of extremities, and hand grasp *to determine adequacy of cerebral perfusion.* Orient patient frequently to person, time, and place. Provide uninterrupted rest periods, especially while in ICU *to prevent sensory overload and exhaustion with subsequent decrease in mental acuity.* Monitor levels of serum electrolytes and ABGs *because deviations may result in sensory/perceptual alterations.*

continued

Severe hypertension may cause undue stress on the proximal and distal arterial anastomoses, resulting in leakage of blood or rupture at the suture line. Pharmacologic intervention with diuretics or antihypertensive agents may be indicated if severe hypertension persists.

Ventricular dysrhythmias. Ventricular dysrhythmias are usually caused by hypoxia, hypothermia, or unrecognized electrolyte imbalances. A patient with coexisting coronary artery disease is prone to dysrhythmias. Nursing interventions include cardiac monitoring and monitoring the results of electrolyte studies and arterial blood gas (ABG) determinations. The patient who returns from surgery with hypothermia should be placed on hyperthermia blankets.

Infection. The development of a prosthetic vascular graft infection can be a life-threatening complication. Nursing intervention to prevent infection should include ensuring that the patient receives a broad-spectrum antibiotic as prescribed to maintain adequate blood levels of the drug. It is important to assess body temperature regularly and to report any elevations. Laboratory data should be monitored because a rising white blood cell (WBC) count may be the first indication of an infection. In addition, the nurse should ensure adequate nutrition, monitor serum albumin levels, and observe the wound for evidence of poor healing, signs of infection, or any unusual drainage.

All IV, arterial, and central venous catheter insertion sites should be cared for carefully with the use of sterile technique because they are frequently a portal of entry for bacteria. Meticulous perineal care for the patient with an indwelling urinary catheter is also essential to minimize the risk of urinary tract infection. Incisions should be kept clean and dry.

Gastrointestinal status. After abdominal aneurysm resection, paralytic ileus may develop as a result of anesthesia and the manual manipulation and displacement of the bowel for long periods during surgery. The intestines may become swollen and bruised, and peristalsis ceases for variable intervals.

A nasogastric tube is inserted before surgery and connected to low, intermittent suction. This decompresses the stomach and duodenum, prevents aspiration of stomach contents, and decreases pressure on suture lines. The nasogastric tube should be irrigated with normal saline solution as needed, and the amount and character of the drainage

NURSING CARE PLAN Patient After Aortic Aneurysm Repair—cont'd

COLLABORATIVE PROBLEMS

Nursing Goals	Nursing Interventions and Rationales
➤ **POTENTIAL COMPLICATION**	Altered renal perfusion *related to* renal artery embolism, prolonged hypotension, or prolonged aortic cross-clamping intraoperatively
Assess signs of altered renal perfusion, report deviations from acceptable parameters, and carry out medical and nursing interventions.	Monitor hourly urinary output, daily weights, BUN, and serum creatinine *to detect signs of altered renal perfusion and renal failure.* Administer IV fluids and medications as ordered *to maintain adequate hydration, perfusion, and BP.*
➤ **POTENTIAL COMPLICATION**	Paralytic ileus secondary to bowel manipulation, pain medication, and immobility
Monitor for signs of paralytic ileus, report deviations from acceptable parameters, and carry out medical and nursing interventions.	Assess for absence of bowel sounds and flatus, abdominal distention, nausea, and vomiting *to detect signs of paralytic ileus.* Attach nasogastric tube to low suction *to decompress stomach and duodenum, prevent aspiration of stomach contents, and decrease pressure on suture line.* Irrigate with normal saline solution as needed *to ensure patency of the tube* and record drainage. Give frequent oral care while patient is receiving nothing orally *to stimulate salivary glands and provide for patient comfort.* Check all stools for guaiac *to detect occult bleeding.* Auscultate for bowel sounds q4-8hr *to determine return of peristalsis.* Palpate abdomen for distention. Encourage early ambulation (when possible) and turning q2hr while patient is awake *to foster return of peristalsis.*
➤ **POTENTIAL COMPLICATION**	Hypovolemia secondary to hemorrhage, extravascular fluid redistribution, or prolonged diuresis
Monitor for signs of hypovolemia, report deviation from acceptable parameters, and carry out medical and nursing interventions.	Administer packed RBCs (as ordered) *to use as replacement if hemorrhage should occur.* Observe drainage of chest tube (if inserted) *to detect excess bleeding.* Monitor BP and heart rate hourly and then with decreasing frequency *to detect changes indicating hypovolemia, such as decreased BP and increased heart rate.* Check Hb and Hct q4-6hr and as needed. Observe abdomen and record girth if abdominal distention appears to be developing *to assess for hemorrhage or extravascular fluid displacement.* Monitor intake and output and daily weights *to detect signs of hypovolemia.* Assess mental status frequently *to detect decreased cerebral perfusion.*
➤ **POTENTIAL COMPLICATION**	Cardiac dysrhythmia related to hypothermia, electrolyte imbalance, or coexisting coronary artery disease
Monitor for signs of cardiac dysrhythmias, report deviation from acceptable parameters, and carry out medical and nursing interventions.	Maintain temperature at about 37° C *to prevent hypothermia from causing a dysrhythmia.* Administer oxygen as ordered by ventilator or mask *to reduce hypoxia.* Monitor the results of ABGs and serum electrolytes *to prevent imbalance from initiating a dysrhythmia.* Keep lidocaine 100 mg IV bolus at bedside and administer as needed *to treat PVCs.*

ABGs, Arterial blood gases; *BP,* blood pressure; *BUN,* blood urea nitrogen; *Hb,* hemoglobin; *Hct,* hematocrit; *ICU,* intensive care unit; *IV,* intravenous; *PVC,* premature ventricular contraction; *RBC,* red blood cell; *RR,* respiratory rate; *WBC,* white blood cell.

should be recorded. The nurse should auscultate for the return of bowel sounds. The passing of flatus can also be a sign of returning bowel function and should be reported.

If the arterial blood supply to the bowel is disrupted during surgery, ischemia or death of intestinal tissue may result. This is evidenced by lack of bowel sounds, fever, abdominal distention, diarrhea, and bloody stools. Fortunately, this serious complication is uncommon.

It is unusual for paralytic ileus to persist beyond the fourth postoperative day. While the patient is receiving nothing orally (NPO), thorough mouth care should be given every few hours. In some situations ice chips may be given to the patient to soothe an irritated throat.

Neurologic status. Neurologic complications can occur after surgical procedures on the aorta, especially when the ascending aorta and aortic arch are involved. Nursing intervention should include assessment of neurologic signs (hourly initially after surgery and less frequently thereafter), including level of consciousness, pupil size and response to light, ability to move all extremities, and quality of hand grasps (see Chapter 53). These should be recorded in detail with a careful description of the patient's response. Any alteration from the baseline assessment should be reported to the physician immediately.

Circulatory status. The anatomic location of the aneurysm indicates the areas of major concern related to circulatory status. All peripheral pulses should be checked regularly and recorded. This should be done every hour for the first 24 hours and routinely thereafter at frequent intervals. Pulses to be assessed include the dorsalis pedis, posterior tibial, popliteal, and femoral, as well as the brachial, radial, carotid, and temporal pulses (see Fig. 29-8).

When checking the pulses, the nurse should mark the location lightly with a ballpoint or felt-tip pen so that others can locate them easily. It is also important to note the temperature, color, and movement of the extremities.

Occasionally pulses in the lower extremities may be absent for a short time following surgery. This is usually due to vasospasm and hypothermia. A decreased or absent pulse in conjunction with a cool, pale, mottled, or painful extremity may indicate embolization of thrombus or plaque from the aneurysm or occlusion of the graft. These findings should be reported to the surgeon immediately. In some patients the pulses may have been absent preoperatively because of coexistent arterial occlusive disease. Comparison with the preoperative status is essential to determine the etiology of a decreased or absent pulse and the proper treatment.

Renal perfusion. One of the causes of decreased renal perfusion is embolization of a fragment of thrombus or plaque from the aorta that subsequently lodges in both renal arteries. This can cause obstruction and ischemia of one or both kidneys. Hypotension, dehydration, prolonged aortic clamping, or blood loss can also lead to decreased renal perfusion.

The patient returns from surgery with an indwelling urinary catheter in place. An accurate record of fluid intake and urinary output should be kept until the patient resumes the preoperative diet. If hourly urine output drops below 30 ml per hour for 2 consecutive hours, the physician should be notified. Central venous pressure readings and pulmonary artery pressures also provide important information regarding hydration status. Daily BUN and serum creatinine studies are performed to evaluate renal function.

Chronic and Home Management. Most patients with aneurysms that are greater than two times the diameter of the normal artery are considered for operative repair. However, there are situations where operative repair is not performed. Examples of this are the presence of a very small aneurysm, a patient who is not a surgical candidate (e.g., severe lung or cardiac disease), or patient or family refusal to undergo repair. The patient who does not undergo surgical repair should be urged to receive regular routine physical examinations and should be reminded that any symptom, no matter how minor, must be investigated if it persists.

The patient may be apprehensive about returning home after major surgery involving the aorta. The nurse should encourage the patient to express any concerns and reassure the patient that normal activities of living can be resumed. The patient should be instructed to gradually increase activities. Fatigue, poor appetite, and irregular bowel habits are to be expected. Heavy lifting is avoided for at least 4 to 6 weeks following surgery. Observation of incisions for signs and symptoms of infection should be encouraged. Any redness, increased pain, or drainage from incisions should be reported to the physician. In addition, a fever greater than 100° F (37.8° C) should also be reported. Sexual dysfunction in male patients is not uncommon after aneurysm repair surgery. This may occur because the internal hypogastric artery is disrupted, leading to altered blood flow to the penis. The patient should also be taught to observe for changes in color or warmth of the extremities. The patient should be taught to palpate peripheral pulses and to assess changes in their quality. The patient who has received a synthetic graft should be aware that prophylactic antibiotics may be required before future invasive procedures.

Aortic Dissection

Aortic dissection, occurring most commonly in the thoracic aorta, is a longitudinal splitting of the medial layer of the artery by a column of blood. Aortic dissection affects men more often than women and occurs most frequently between the fourth and seventh decades of life. If not treated, acute aortic dissection has a 90% mortality rate.[6]

Pathophysiology. Aortic dissection results from a small tear in the intimal lining of the artery, allowing blood to "track" between the intima and media and creating a false lumen of blood flow. As the heart contracts, each systolic pulsation causes increased pressure on the damaged area, which further increases the dissection. As it extends proximally or distally, it may occlude major branches of the aorta, cutting off blood supply to areas such as the brain, abdominal organs, spinal cord, and extremities. Occasionally a small tear develops distally and the blood flow reenters the true vessel lumen.

Arterial dissection differs from an aneurysm in that a false lumen is formed by separation of the intima from the media in dissection. In contrast, a true aneurysm involves dilatation of the entire aortic wall.

The exact cause of dissection is uncertain. Many authorities believe cystic medial necrosis (destruction of the medial layer elastic fibers) to be the leading cause of the problem. Most people with dissection problems have hypertension. Persons with Marfan syndrome (a disease of the connective tissue) have a high incidence of dissection. Pregnancy also promotes vascular stress as a result of increased blood volume. Areas that seem to undergo the greatest amount of stress and are thus most prone to dissection are the ascending aorta, the aortic arch, and the descending aorta beyond the origin of the left subclavian artery.

Classification. Aortic dissections are usually identified by the Stanford classification scheme. *Type A* refers to dissections involving the ascending aorta, and *type B* involves the distal, descending aorta.[7]

Clinical Manifestations. The patient with aortic dissection usually has sudden, severe pain in the back, chest, or abdomen. The pain is described as "tearing" or "ripping." The severe pain may mimic that of an MI. As the dissection progresses, pain may be located both above and below the diaphragm. Dyspnea may also be present.

If the arch of the aorta is involved, the patient may exhibit neurologic deficiencies, including an altered level of consciousness, dizziness, and weakened or absent carotid and temporal pulses. An ascending aortic dissection usually produces some degree of aortic valvular insufficiency, and a murmur is audible on auscultation. Severe insufficiency may produce left ventricular failure with the development of dyspnea and orthopnea caused by pulmonary edema. When either subclavian artery is involved, pulse quality and BP readings may vary between the left and right arms. As the dissection progresses down the aorta, the abdominal organs and lower extremities may begin to demonstrate evidence of altered tissue perfusion and ischemia.

Complications. A severe complication of dissection of the ascending aortic arch is *cardiac tamponade,* which occurs when blood escapes from the dissection into the pericardial sac. Clinical manifestations include narrowed pulse pressure, distended neck veins, muffled heart sounds, and pulsus paradoxus (see Chapter 34).

Because the aorta is weakened by the medial dissection, it may rupture. Hemorrhage may occur into the mediastinal, pleural, or abdominal cavities.

Dissection can lead to occlusion of the arterial supply to many vital organs. The spinal cord, kidneys, and abdominal structures are the organs most commonly affected. Ischemia of the spinal cord produces symptoms varying from weakness to paralysis in the lower extremities and decreased pain sensation. Renal ischemia is usually manifested by low urinary output. Signs of abdominal ischemia include abdominal pain, decreased bowel sounds, and altered bowel elimination.

Diagnostic Studies. The diagnostic studies used to assess dissection of the aorta are similar to those performed for aneurysms (Table 35-2). An ECG is done to rule out the possibility of an MI. Left ventricular hypertrophy is a common finding on an echocardiogram and is possibly related to changes caused by systemic hypertension. A chest x-ray may show a widening of the mediastinal silhouette, and left pleural effusion is not uncommon. A CT scan provides valuable information on the presence and severity of the dissection. After the patient's condition has stabilized, aortography is necessary to assess the extent of the dissection.

Therapeutic Management. The goal of therapy for aortic dissection without complications is to lower the BP and myocardial contractility to diminish the pulsatile forces within the aorta (see Table 35-2). The use of trimethaphan (Arfonad) and nitroprusside (Nipride) IV rapidly reduces the BP. Intravenous β-blockers may also be used, such as propranolol (Inderal), or *A*-blockers and β-blockers such as labetalol (Normodyne). Propranolol is used to decrease the force of myocardial contractility.

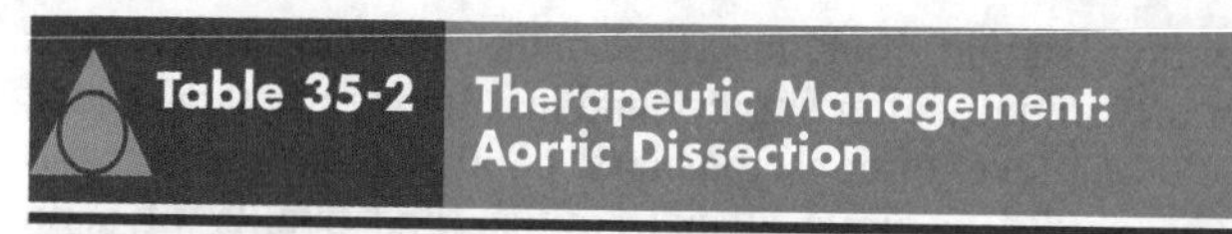

Table 35-2 Therapeutic Management: Aortic Dissection

Diagnostic
- Health history and physical examination
- ECG
- Chest x-ray
- CT scan
- Echocardiogram
- Aortography

Therapeutic
- Bed rest
- Pain relief with narcotics
- Control of blood pressure
  - Trimethaphan (Arfonad)
  - Sodium nitroprusside (Nipride)
- Propranolol (Inderal)
- Labetalol (Normodyne)
- Aortic resection and repair

CT, Computed tomography; *ECG,* electrocardiogram.

The patient with dissection without complications can safely be treated conservatively for an extended period. Supportive treatment is directed toward pain relief, blood transfusion (if required), and management of heart failure (if indicated). If the dissection is limited to the descending aorta, conservative therapeutic management is usually adequate to treat the problem. Success of the treatment is judged by relief of pain, which is an indication of stabilization of the dissection. If the dissection involves the ascending aorta (type A), surgery is usually indicated.

Surgery is also indicated when drug therapy is ineffective or when complications of aortic dissection (e.g., heart failure, leaking dissection, occlusion of an artery) are present. The aorta is fragile during the acute phase. Therefore surgery is delayed for as long as possible to allow time for edema in the area of dissection to clear, to permit clotting of the blood in the false lumen, and to allow the healing process to begin.

Surgery for aortic dissection involves resection of the aortic segment containing the intimal tear and replacement with a synthetic graft material. The extent of aortic replacement varies depending on the extent of the dissection.

NURSING MANAGEMENT

AORTIC DISSECTION

Nursing management related to an aortic dissection includes keeping the patient in bed in a semi-Fowler's position and maintaining a quiet environment. These measures assist in keeping the systolic BP at the lowest possible level. Narcotics and tranquilizers should be administered as ordered. Pain and anxiety must be managed for patient comfort and because they increase the BP.

Continuous IV administration of antihypertensive agents requires close nursing supervision. A cardiac monitoring device is used, and an intraarterial pressure line is usually inserted (see Chapter 61). The nurse should observe for changes in the quality of peripheral pulses and for signs of increasing pain, restlessness, and anxiety. Vital signs are taken frequently, sometimes as often as every 2 to 3 minutes. A widening pulse pressure may indicate increasing aortic valvular insufficiency. If the blood vessels branching off the aortic arch are involved, decreased cerebral blood flow may alter the sensorium and level of consciousness. Postoperative care after surgery to correct the dissection is similar to that after aneurysmectomy (see the section on Nursing Management of Aneurysms).

In preparation for discharge, the nurse needs to focus on patient and family teaching. The therapeutic regimen includes antihypertensive drugs, which are usually taken orally. The patient needs to understand that these drugs must be taken to control BP. Propranolol can be taken orally to continue to decrease myocardial contractility. It is important that the patient understand the drug regimen. The nurse should instruct the patient that if the pain returns or other symptoms progress, the patient must immediately return to the health care facility.

Aortitis

Aortitis (aortic arch syndrome, Takayasu's disease, pulseless disease) is a rare inflammatory disorder with occlusion of the aorta and one or more of the large arteries that branch off from the thoracic aorta. The terms aortic arch syndrome and pulseless disease are used to describe this clinical problem.

Occlusion of the carotid and subclavian arteries secondary to aortitis most commonly affects Asians, particularly young women less than 40 years of age. This disease syndrome is frequently called Takayasu's disease. Aortitis of the lower thoracic and abdominal aorta occurring in young women and children in the tropics is similar to Takayasu's disease.

Aortitis is not common in the United States. The most common infectious form is due to syphilis. Noninfectious aortitis has been associated with Hodgkin's disease, scleroderma, rheumatoid arthritis, and ankylosing spondylitis.

Clinical Manifestations. Clinical manifestations vary with the extent and location of the occlusion, the degree of collateral circulation, and the number of vessels involved. Initial manifestations of an acute disorder are fever, joint pain, weight loss, malaise, and headache.

After several years, symptoms of peripheral vascular insufficiency appear in the form of a nonspecific inflammatory process. The vessel intima is greatly proliferated, scarred, and fibrotic, and the media is thickened. Pulse deficits can be detected. Vascular bruits and hypertension are also present. Retinal changes and left ventricular failure may result from the hypertension. The mortality rate is about 18%, with the leading causes of death being congestive heart failure (CHF) and cerebrovascular accidents.[8]

Therapeutic Management. Management is symptomatic for hypertension and CHF. In general, treatment has not been satisfactory. The therapeutic role of corticosteroids has not been proven. Antibiotics and immunosuppression have not been effective. Surgery may be necessary if vascular insufficiency is severe, but the outcomes are poor.

ACUTE ARTERIAL OCCLUSIVE DISORDERS

Pathophysiology

Acute arterial occlusion occurs suddenly, without warning signs. It can be caused by embolism, thrombosis of an already narrowed artery, or trauma. Embolization of a thrombus from the heart or an atherosclerotic aneurysm is the most frequent cause of acute arterial occlusion. Heart conditions in which thrombi are prone to develop include infective endocarditis, MI, mitral valve disease, chronic atrial fibrillation, cardiomyopathies (see Chapter 32), and prosthetic heart valves. The thrombi become dislodged and may travel to the lungs if they originate in the right side of the heart or to anywhere in the systemic circulation if they originate in the left side of the heart.

Arterial emboli tend to lodge at sites of arterial branching or in areas of atherosclerotic narrowing. After an acute arterial occlusion the blood supply distal to the embolus decreases. The degree and extent of manifestations produced depend on the size and location of the obstruction, the occurrence of clot fragmentation with embolism to smaller vessels, and the degree of peripheral vascular disease already present.

Sudden local thrombosis may occur at the location of an atherosclerotic plaque. Traumatic injury to the extremity itself may produce partial or total occlusion of a vessel from compression, shearing, or laceration. Acute arterial occlusion may also develop as a result of arterial dissection in the carotid artery or aorta or as a result of iatrogenic arterial injury (e.g., after arteriography).

Clinical Manifestations

Symptoms usually have an abrupt onset. The exception is when a sudden occlusion is superimposed on preexisting chronic arterial insufficiency. In this case the symptoms may be insidious because collateral circulation is well developed.

Clinical manifestations of acute arterial occlusion include the "six *P*'s": *p*ain, *p*allor, *p*ulselessness, *p*aresthesia, *p*aralysis, and *p*oikilothermia (adaptation of the ischemic limb to its environmental temperature, most often cool). Without immediate intervention, ischemia may progress to tissue necrosis and gangrene within hours. It should be noted that paralysis is a very late sign of acute arterial ischemia and signals the actual death of nerves supplying the extremity. Because nerve tissue is extremely sensitive to lack of oxygen, limb paralysis or ischemic neuropathy may persist after revascularization and may be permanent.

Therapeutic Management

With true acute arterial occlusion in the absence of adequate collateral circulation to keep the limb viable, early treatment is essential to save the affected limb. Anticoagulant therapy is initiated immediately to prevent further enlargement of the thrombus and inhibit embolization. Continuous IV heparin is the agent of choice. The thrombus should be removed as soon as possible by embolectomy or thrombectomy. Balloon catheters can be used and are passed distal and proximal to the site to remove the clot material. This procedure can be done with the use of local anesthetics. Direct arteriotomy to perform an embolectomy or thromboendarterectomy may be necessary.

If the limb is stable on heparin, recently formed emboli may be effectively treated with an intraarterial infusion of a thrombolytic agent such as urokinase or streptokinase. In this procedure a percutaneous catheter is inserted into the femoral artery and threaded to the site of the clot. These drugs work by directly dissolving the clot over a period of 24 to 48 hours. Bed rest is maintained and periodic angiograms are performed. Although sometimes effective, this procedure is also associated with bleeding complications. Therefore patients are carefully selected and drug administration prescribed and monitored by experienced critical care providers.

If the patient remains at risk for further embolization from a persistent source such as chronic atrial fibrillation, long-term treatment includes oral anticoagulation to prevent further acute episodes.

CHRONIC ARTERIAL OCCLUSIVE DISEASE

Lower Extremity Disease

Chronic peripheral arterial occlusive disease involves progressive narrowing and degeneration and eventual obstruction of the arteries to the extremities, occurring predominantly in the legs. It may affect the aortoiliac, femoral, popliteal, tibial, peroneal vessels, or any combination of these areas (Fig. 35-5). Chronic arterial occlusion is a slowly progressive, insidious disease primarily attributed to the atherosclerotic process; hence the term *arteriosclerosis obliterans* is often used. It usually occurs in the sixth through eighth decades of life, primarily affects men, and has a familial tendency. It occurs at an earlier age in diabetic patients. Although the process may be slowed or arrested through risk factor modification, there is no cure. All treatments are palliative.

Etiology and Pathophysiology. The leading cause of chronic arterial occlusion is atherosclerosis, a gradual thickening of the intima and media, which leads to narrowing of the vessel lumen. Atherosclerosis primarily affects larger arteries. The involvement is generally segmental, with normal segments interspersed between involved ones. By the time symptoms occur, the vessel is about 75% narrowed.[9] The femoral-popliteal area is the site most commonly affected in the nondiabetic population. The patient with diabetes tends to develop disease in the arteries below the knee (specifically, the anterior tibial, posterior tibial, and peroneal arteries). In advanced stages, multiple levels of occlusions are seen.

The three most significant risk factors for peripheral arterial disease are cigarette smoking, hyperlipidemia, and hypertension. Others are diabetes mellitus, a positive family history, obesity, and a sedentary lifestyle.[10]

Chronic arterial obstruction leads to progressively inadequate oxygenation of the tissues supplied by the obstructed

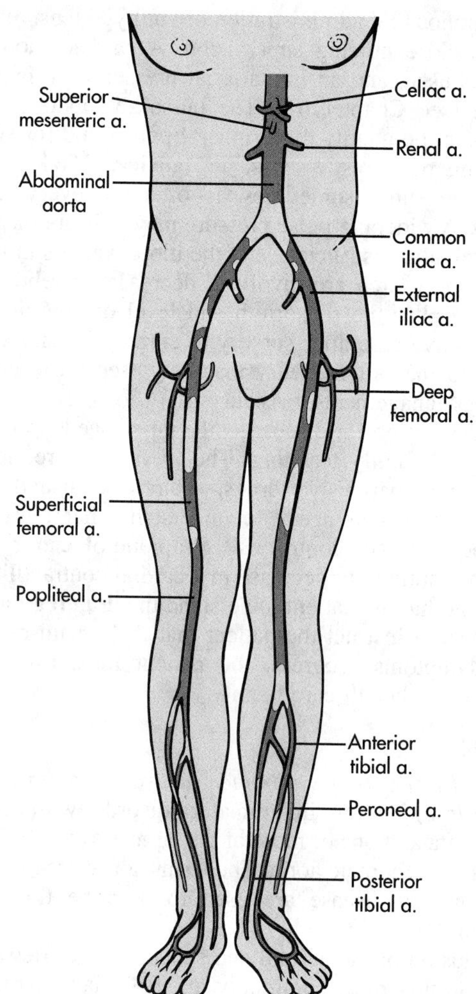

Fig. 35-5 Common anatomic locations of atherosclerotic lesions of the abdominal aorta and lower extremities.

arteries. The pain attributable to ischemia is produced by end products of anaerobic cellular metabolism, such as lactic acid. This usually occurs in the larger muscle groups of the legs (buttocks, thighs, or calves) during exercise. Once the patient stops exercising, the metabolites are cleared and the pain subsides. As the disease process becomes advanced, pain develops at rest. "Rest pain" most often occurs in the feet or toes and indicates insufficient blood flow to the nerves supplying the distal extremity. The patient may notice resting foot pain more often at night and achieve partial relief by lowering the limb below heart level (e.g., dangling the leg over the side of the bed).

Clinical Manifestations. The severity of the clinical manifestations depends on the site and extent of the occlusion and the adequacy of collateral circulation (Table 35-3). The classic symptom of peripheral arterial disease is *intermittent claudication,* ischemic muscle pain that is precipitated by a predictable amount of exercise and relieved by resting. Disease involving the femoral or popliteal arteries may cause claudication in the calf. Occlusive disease of the aortoiliac arteries may produce claudication in the buttocks

Table 35-3 Comparison of Chronic Arterial and Venous Insufficiency of the Lower Extremities

Characteristic	Arterial	Venous
Pulses	Decreased or absent peripheral pulses	Presence of peripheral pulses
Edema	No edema	Edema around ankles, sometimes feet
Hair	Loss of hair on legs, feet, toes	No hair loss
Ulcers	Ulceration or gangrene over bony prominences and pressure points on toes and feet	Ulceration around ankle, above or below medial malleoli; gangrene rare
Pain	Intermittent claudication (muscular leg or buttock pain with exercise)	Dull ache or heaviness in calf or thigh
Nails	Thickened; brittle	Normal
Skin color	Dependent rubor; pallor on elevation	Cyanotic if dependent; brown pigmentation
Skin texture	Thin, shiny, dry	Scaling eczema; stasis dermatitis; veins may be visible
Skin temperature	Cool	Warm

and upper part of the thighs. If disease extends into the internal iliac (hypogastric) arteries, impotence may result. Sexual dysfunction occurs in as many as 30% to 50% of patients with aortoiliac occlusion.[11]

Ischemic pain at rest occurs as the disease becomes more severe. This is an ominous symptom. Without revascularization the limb will progress to ulceration and gangrenous necrosis. Every attempt is made to save the limb, and surgery is always indicated unless the patient is at exceedingly high risk.

Paresthesia, manifested as numbness or tingling occurring in the toes or feet, may result from nerve tissue ischemia. True peripheral neuropathy occurs more commonly in patients with diabetes and in those with progressive long-standing ischemia. It produces excruciating shooting or burning pain in the extremity. It does not follow any particular nerve roots but may be present near ulcerated areas. Gradually diminishing perfusion to nerve tissue cells produces loss of both sensation and deep pain. Therefore injuries to the extremity often go unnoticed.

The physical appearance of the limb as a result of postural changes provides important information about the adequacy of blood flow. Pallor or blanching on elevation indicates significant arterial ischemia. Hyperemia (redness) and a bluish or dusky appearance are observed when the limb is allowed to hang in a dependent position (dependent rubor). The skin becomes shiny and taut and there is a loss of hair on the lower legs. Diminished or absent pedal, popliteal, or femoral pulses may be noted.

Complications. Chronic peripheral arterial disease progresses slowly. Prolonged ischemia leads to atrophy of the skin and underlying structures. Because of the decreased ability to heal, infection and necrosis may result from even minor trauma to the feet. Ischemic ulcers caused by arterial insufficiency most commonly occur over bony prominences on the toes and feet. (This contrasts to ulcers of venous insufficiency, which occur around the malleoli and lower parts of the leg [see Table 35-3]). If severe ischemia persists, gangrene can develop. Ischemic ulcers and gangrene are the most serious complications of chronic arterial disease and may result in lower extremity amputation if blood flow is not restored. Because most of these patients have diabetes, there is a risk for infection. If atherosclerosis has been present for an extended period, collateral circulation may prevent gangrene of the extremity.

Diagnostic Studies. Various tests have been developed to assess blood flow and to outline the vascular system (Table 35-4). Doppler ultrasound consists of a probe transducer containing a crystal that emits sound waves toward moving blood cells. It measures the velocity of blood flow through a vessel and emits an audible signal. Directional flow can be measured antegrade or retrograde. The Doppler is extremely sensitive to movement of blood. When arterial palpation is difficult or impossible because of severe occlusive disease, the Doppler can be useful in determining blood flow. A palpable pulse and a Doppler pulse are not equivalent and should not be used interchangeably. In addition, segmental blood pressures are also obtained (using a Doppler and sphygmomanometer) at the thigh, below the knee, and at ankle level. Pressures in the leg should equal pressures in the arm. As disease develops in the arteries of the legs the blood pressures drop. Dividing the ankle pressure by the highest brachial pressure yields the ankle-brachial index. A normal ankle-brachial index is 1.0. An ankle-brachial index between 0.8 and 0.95 indicates minimal disease, an index of 0.4 to 0.8 indicates moderate disease, and 0 to 0.4 indicates severe arterial disease. This technique is also used to follow patients postoperatively following revascularization to monitor patency of bypass grafts. This procedure has limited usefulness when arteries are calcified and noncompressive, as occurs in a diabetic patient. Plethysmography detects volume changes in limbs and is useful in detecting disease when vessels are calcified.

Duplex imaging, a newer noninvasive test, uses a Doppler system that can systematically map the entire region of an artery in which blood is flowing. It provides a picture similar to that of a conventional arteriogram and gives anatomic and physiologic information about the blood vessels.

Angiography (aortography and femoral arteriography) is used to further delineate the location and extent of the

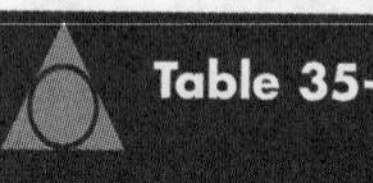

Table 35-4 Therapeutic Management: Chronic Arterial Occlusive Disease

Diagnostic
- Health history and physical examination, including palpation of peripheral pulses
- Doppler ultrasound studies
- Duplex imaging
- Angiography
- Magnetic resonance angiography

Therapeutic

Conservative
- Mild analgesic (e.g., codeine)
- Reverse Trendelenburg position 10 degrees while in bed
- Walking exercises 30 min twice daily as tolerated
- Foot care*
- Avoidance of thermal, chemical, and mechanical trauma
- No tobacco

Surgical
- Percutaneous transluminal angioplasty with or without stent
- Bypass graft
- Patch graft angioplasty, often in conjunction with bypass
- Thrombolytic therapy
- Atherectomy
- Endarterectomy (done rarely, with localized stenosis)
- Amputation

*See Table 46-17.

disease process. In addition, it provides information on inflow and outflow vessels to plan for surgery. Angiography is used only when an intervention (i.e., surgery or angioplasty) is indicated. Magnetic resonance angiography has also been used successfully in vascular imaging.[11]

Therapeutic Management. Conservative management objectives include protecting the extremity from trauma, slowing the progression of atherosclerosis, decreasing vasospasm, preventing and controlling infection, and improving collateral circulation[12] (see Table 35-4). The patient's risk factors should be assessed, and proper intervention should be begun regarding cessation of smoking, weight reduction (if indicated), and control of lipid disorders. Hypertension also needs to be properly managed (see Chapter 30).

Slow, progressive physical activity should be encouraged to help develop collateral circulation. For example, the patient should be out of bed at least four times per day, walk for 30 minutes twice a day, or as tolerated. Exercise should be stopped if pain occurs and resumed after a rest break when the pain subsides.

Careful inspection, cleansing, and lubrication of both feet is advised to prevent cracking of the skin and infection. Although cleansing is important, soaking of the affected foot should be avoided to prevent skin maceration (or breakdown). If ulceration is present, the affected foot should be kept clean and dry. Covering the ulcer with a dry, sterile dressing helps maintain cleanliness and protects the limb. Ulcers with any significant depth may be treated with a variety of wound care products, but without restoration of blood flow healing is unlikely. Footwear should be soft, roomy, and protective. Chemicals, heat, and cold should be avoided.

Interventional radiologic procedures or surgery is indicated when (1) the symptoms of intermittent claudication become incapacitating, (2) the limb is so ischemic that the patient experiences pain at rest, or (3) ulceration or gangrene is severe enough to threaten the viability of the limb. The latter problem will likely progress unless arterial circulation can be restored.

Interventional radiologic procedures. A technique known as *percutaneous transluminal angioplasty* involves the use of a special catheter with a cylindrical balloon. When inflated, the balloon dilates the vessel by cracking the confining atherosclerotic intimal shell while also stretching the underlying media[13] (Fig. 35-6). This procedure is used in certain patients who have localized, accessible lesions (less than 10 cm in length). Iliac artery lesions have responded most successfully to percutaneous transluminal angioplasty. Smaller vessels below the knee (tibial arteries) have the least favorable patency rates.

Laser technology in the lower extremity continues to be investigated. This technology uses laser energy to heat the tip of an intravascular catheter. The procedure basically bores a hole through an occluded artery. Although initially thought to have great potential in the area of vascular surgery, this technology has not proven to be of great benefit.

Newer devices, called *atherectomy catheters,* are also used inside the artery to "shave" or pulverize the plaque lining the arterial wall. Atherectomy is often performed in conjunction with angioplasty. Once the plaque is "debulked," dilatation is performed using a balloon catheter.[13]

Intravascular stents circumvent the problems of restenosis and arterial dissection following percutaneous balloon angioplasty. Stents are rigid or flexible and are positioned percutaneously within arteries. Stents are most frequently used in the iliac arteries when arterial dissection occurs following angioplasty.

Surgical interventions. Various surgical approaches can be used to improve arterial blood flow beyond a stenotic or occluded artery. The most common is an *arterial bypass* operation with autogenous vein or synthetic graft material to bypass or carry blood around the lesion (Fig. 35-7).

Other surgical options include *endarterectomy* (opening the artery and removing the obstructing plaque) and *patch graft angioplasty* (opening the artery, removing plaque, and sewing a patch to the opening to widen the lumen).

Amputation is the least desired surgical option, but it may be required if gangrene is extensive, infection is present in bone (osteomyelitis), or all major arteries in the limb are occluded, precluding the possibility of bypass surgery. Every effort is made to preserve as much of the limb as possible so that the potential for rehabilitation with an orthotic shoe or prosthesis is optimized (see Chapter 60).

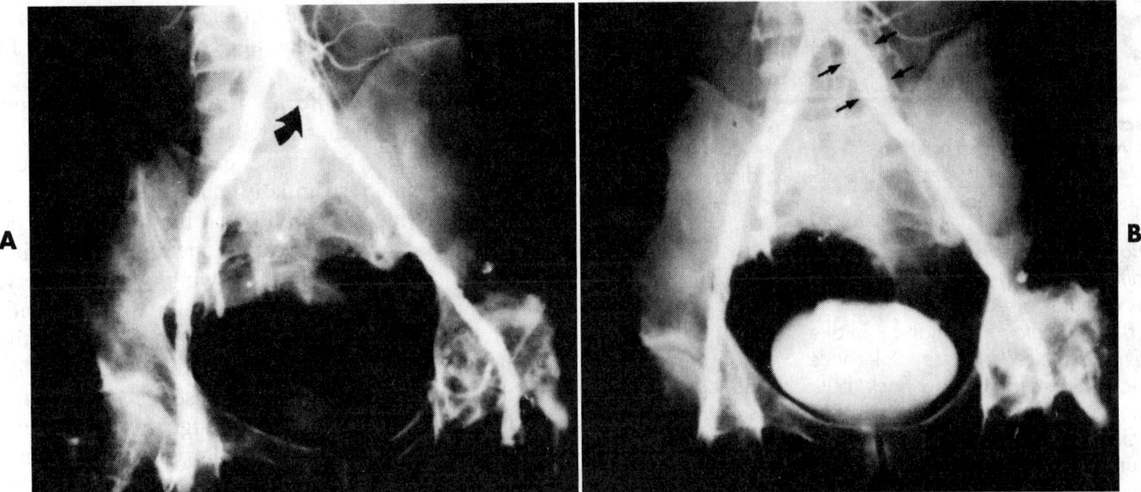

Fig. 35-6 ***A,*** Tight stenosis of the left common iliac artery (*arrow*). ***B,*** Dilatation of the left common iliac artery lumen following percutaneous transluminal angioplasty (*arrows*).

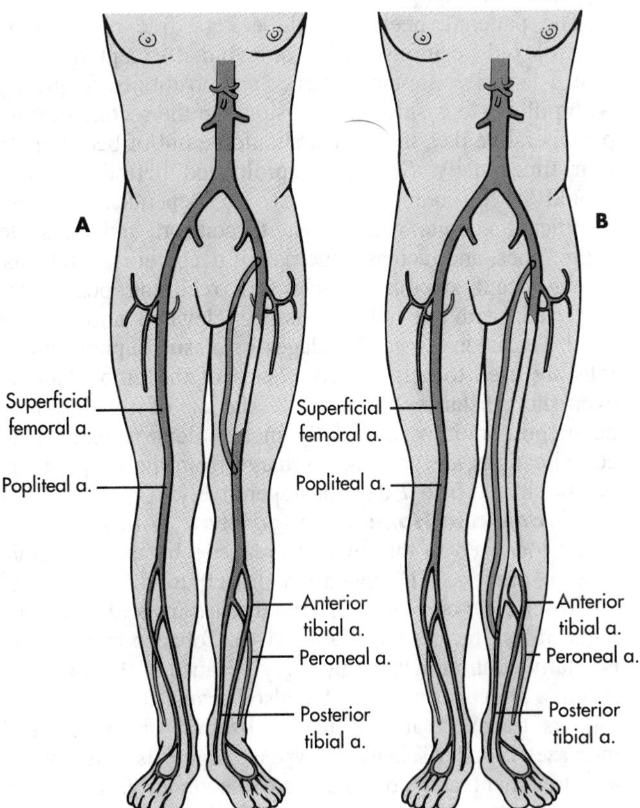

Fig. 35-7 ***A,*** Femoral-popliteal bypass graft around an occluded superficial femoral artery. ***B,*** Femoral-posterior tibial bypass graft around occluded superficial femoral, popliteal, and proximal tibial arteries.

Pharmacologic Management. Although various drugs are commonly prescribed to treat peripheral arterial occlusive disease, no specific agent is known to be effective except pentoxifylline (Trental), which increases erythrocyte flexibility and reduces blood viscosity, thus improving the supply of oxygenated blood to ischemic muscle.[14] Although it is not conclusive that antiplatelet aggregating agents such as aspirin improve circulation through diseased arteries or prevent intimal hyperplasia leading to stenosis, they are sometimes used after arterial bypass surgery to promote graft patency. Anticoagulation with warfarin (Coumadin) is sometimes instituted in the patient who has a propensity to occlude grafts secondary to a clotting abnormality. The effectiveness of anticoagulants and antiplatelet agents continues to be studied.

Nutritional Management. The patient with atherosclerosis should be taught and encouraged to do the following:

1. Adjust caloric intake so that optimum weight can be achieved and maintained
2. Decrease dietary cholesterol to less than 200 mg/day
3. Substantially reduce saturated dietary fat (see Table 31-5)
4. Restrict sodium to 2 g per day if edema is present (see Table 32-10)

NURSING MANAGEMENT

CHRONIC ARTERIAL OCCLUSIVE DISEASE

Nursing Assessment

Subjective and objective data that should be obtained from a patient with chronic arterial occlusive disease are presented in Table 35-5.

Nursing Diagnoses

Nursing diagnoses are determined when the problems and etiologic factors are supported by clinical data. Nursing diagnoses related to chronic arterial occlusive disease may

Table 35-5 Nursing Assessment: Chronic Arterial Occlusive Disease

Subjective Data
Important health information
Past health history: Hypertension, obesity, diabetes, smoking (pack years)
Medications: Use of any medications
Functional health patterns
Health perception–health management: Family history of vascular disease
Nutritional-metabolic: High fat intake
Activity-exercise: Exercise intolerance
Cognitive-perceptual: Low back, buttock, and leg pain that is precipitated by exercise and that subsides with rest (intermittent claudication); excruciating, burning pain in forefeet and toes that increases with activity and decreases with rest
Sexuality-reproductive: Impotence
Objective Data
Integumentary
Loss of hair on legs and feet; thick toenails; pallor with elevation; dependent rubor; thin, cool, glossy skin with muscle atrophy; ulcerations over bony areas; gangrene
Cardiovascular
Decreased or absent peripheral pulses; bruits present at pulse sites
Neurologic
Numbness, tingling, cold in legs or feet; mobility impairment, gait disorder
Possible findings
Positive plethysmography, Doppler pressures or angiography indicative of occlusive disease

include, but are not limited to, those presented in the following nursing care plan on chronic arterial occlusive disease.

Planning

The overall goals are that the patient with chronic arterial occlusive disease will have (1) adequate tissue perfusion; (2) relief of pain; (3) increased exercise tolerance; and (4) intact, healthy skin on extremities.

Nursing Implementation

Health Maintenance and Promotion. The patient should be assessed for risk factors and should be taught how to control them (see Table 31-4). The nursing role in patient education in the inpatient care facility is important in identifying high-risk patients. The nurse should also be involved at the community level, such as in screening clinics for peripheral arterial disease, hypertension, and diabetes. Young people and adults need to be educated about the hazards of cigarette smoking. The nurse should also assist in teaching diet modification to reduce the intake of animal fat and refined sugars, proper care of the feet, and the avoidance of injury to the extremities. Patients with positive family histories of cardiac, diabetic, or vascular disease need to be encouraged to obtain regular follow-up care.

Acute Intervention. After surgical intervention the patient is placed in an ICU or recovery area for close observation. The operative extremity should be checked every 15 minutes initially and then hourly for color, temperature, capillary refill, and the presence of peripheral pulses distal to the operative site. Ankle-brachial indices should also be monitored following bypass surgery. Ankle-brachial indices should increase above the patient's preoperative baseline. They should remain constant if the bypass remains patent. All of these findings should be compared with the patient's preoperative baseline and with findings in the opposite limb.[15] A Doppler signal is not equivalent to a palpable pulse. Loss of palpable pulses necessitates immediate intervention.

When the patient is transferred from the recovery room or ICU, nursing care should focus on continued circulatory assessment and monitoring for the development of potential complications. These include bleeding, hematoma, thrombosis, embolization, compartment syndrome, and deep vein thrombosis. Signs and symptoms of severe ischemic pain, loss of palpable pulse or pulses, decreasing ankle-brachial indices, numbness or tingling, or cold temperature may indicate occlusion of the bypass graft and should be reported to the surgeon immediately.

The patient's heels should be kept free of pressure. Knee-flexed positions should be avoided except for exercise. The patient should be turned and positioned frequently with pillows to cushion the incision. On the second or third postoperative day, the patient should be out of bed three to four times daily. Sitting for prolonged periods of time should be discouraged because leg dependency causes significant edema, resulting in discomfort and stress to suture lines, and increases the risk of deep vein thrombosis. If significant swelling develops, a reclining position is preferred, with the edematous leg elevated above heart level. Occasionally ace bandages or elastic support stockings are used to help control edema of the limb. Walking even short distances is desirable. The use of a walker may be helpful initially, especially in the older patient. If no complications are present, discharge from the hospital can be anticipated 5 to 7 days postoperatively.

Chronic and Home Management. Atherosclerosis is not localized to the lower extremities but is a systemic disease process. The overall approach to the control of atherosclerotic chronic occlusive disease involves management of risk factors (see Table 31-4). Tobacco in any form is totally contraindicated, not only because of the vasoconstrictive effects of nicotine, but also because tobacco smoke impairs transport and cellular utilization of oxygen and increases blood viscosity.[16] Bypass surgery is a symptomatic treatment and does not cure the underlying disease. Continuance of cigarette smoking adversely affects the long-term function of the bypass graft and also results in the development of symptomatic disease in other major arterial beds (e.g., carotid artery disease, coronary artery

NURSING CARE PLAN Patient with Chronic Arterial Occlusive Disease

Planning: Outcome Criteria	*Nursing Interventions and Rationales*
➤ **NURSING DIAGNOSIS**	Altered peripheral tissue perfusion *related to* decreased arterial blood flow *as manifested by* pain in hip, buttocks, thigh, or calf; diminished or absent peripheral pulses; paresthesia in toes or feet; pallor or blanching on elevation of limb; hyperemia when limb is dependent; shiny, taut skin and loss of hair on lower extremities
Verbalize medical care, diet, activities that promote vasodilatation; identify factors that impair peripheral circulation; report decreased pain.	Assess lower extremities for evidence of altered peripheral tissue perfusion *to provide appropriate interventions.* Explain the importance of smoking cessation *to increase patient cooperation and reduce vasoconstrictive and hypercoagulable effects of nicotine.* Encourage patient to change position every hour and to avoid crossing legs or knee-flexed position, and to perform range-of-motion exercises of feet *to promote circulation to extremities.* Encourage patient to walk to the point of pain *because this exercise decreases claudication.* Teach patient to avoid dependent position of lower extremities *because this position promotes venous stasis.* Teach patient to stop and rest if pain occurs while walking *to decrease oxygen needs of affected area.* Teach patient to avoid tight girdles, garters, or socks *because they impair collateral circulation.*
➤ **NURSING DIAGNOSIS**	Impaired skin integrity *related to* decreased peripheral circulation, altered sensation, and increased susceptibility to infection *as manifested by* scabs or wounds, edema, taut shiny skin on lower extremities
Have no wounds on lower extremities, no evidence of infection of wounds on lower extremities.	Prevent pressure on heels when hospitalized *to prevent decubiti.* Teach patient to avoid trauma to lower extremities *because tissue is very fragile and wounds heal poorly due to circulatory insufficiency.* Teach patient to check temperature of bath water with fingers rather than toes *because sensation may be diminished.* Teach proper foot care and inspection, including roomy, soft footwear and callus and toenail care by a professional only. Teach patient to inspect feet and lower extremities for evidence of trauma *so immediate care may be given.* Assess ulcers for signs of infection *because wound healing is delayed with impaired peripheral perfusion.* Teach patient or significant other wound care *to prevent infection and promote healing.* Treat the ulcer with topical antibiotics or dressings as ordered *to promote wound healing.* Teach patient to avoid use of chemicals on feet and to keep feet warm.
➤ **NURSING DIAGNOSIS**	Pain *related to* ischemia and exercise *as manifested by* complaints of pain during exercise, which is relieved by rest
Express fewer complaints of pain; have plan to relieve pain if it occurs.	Assess location, onset, degree, and duration of pain *so appropriate interventions are planned.* Encourage rest when pain occurs *so that tissue ischemia and pain are relieved or reduced.* Explain that pain is due to tissue ischemia *to increase patient cooperation with treatment plan.* Teach relaxation techniques *because stress increases vasoconstriction and pain.* Teach patient to report pain that continues at rest *because this is an indication of worsening of the occlusion.* Keep feet warm and dependent. Do *not* elevate feet if pain is present.
➤ **NURSING DIAGNOSIS**	Activity intolerance *related to* imbalance between oxygen supply and demand *as manifested by* pain on walking
Have improved ability to ambulate without pain.	Monitor the amount of exercise patient can perform before pain begins *to provide a baseline for evaluation.* Assist patient in developing a progressive exercise program *to promote development of collateral circulation and enhance venous return.* Explain that patient should walk to point of pain, rest until pain subsides, and resume walking *so endurance can be increased as collateral circulation develops.*

continued

NURSING CARE PLAN Patient with Chronic Arterial Occlusive Disease—cont'd

Planning: Outcome Criteria	Nursing Interventions and Rationales
➤ **NURSING DIAGNOSIS** Risk for injury *related to* decreased sensation and tissue hypoxia	
Have no evidence of injury; verbalize use of safety measures.	Assess neurovascular status of extremities *to determine risk factors for injury.* Inspect feet daily *to identify areas of irritation.* Teach patient methods of preventing injury to lower extremities, such as wearing soft, roomy shoes, arranging home environment *so that the patient will not injure lower legs on furniture*, protecting extremities from excessive cold, heat, or chemicals *because patient has diminished sensation.* Teach patient to seek professional footcare for corns, calluses, toenail care *because there is decreased sensation and impaired healing if tissues are nicked.* Teach patient to have heel protection when bedridden *to keep heels free of pressure.*
➤ **NURSING DIAGNOSIS** Anticipatory grieving *related to* potential loss of body part *as manifested by* withdrawal and verbalization of sadness about possible amputation	
Express grief; discuss possible loss with significant others.	Assess degree of patient's grief and how it is manifested *so that appropriate interventions may be initiated.* Provide opportunity for patient to discuss feelings *to offer support and demonstrate caring attitude.* Assist family members in supporting patient *to foster family cohesiveness.* Acknowledge reality of the situation, but also identify positive aspects of patient's condition *to maintain hope and a positive attitude.*
➤ **NURSING DIAGNOSIS** Ineffective management of therapeutic regimen *related to* lack of knowledge of self-care measures and prevention of complications *as manifested by* questioning about care of leg ulcers, fear of performing usual walking/exercise because of pain	
Describe disease and relate symptoms; demonstrate how to care for leg ulcers; make appropriate modifications in activity.	Assess patient's knowledge of disease and its treatment *to determine extent of the problem and plan appropriate interventions.* Identify factors that influence learning, such as perception of severity, available support systems, cognitive ability, and physical ability *so that teaching plan can be individualized.* Teach patient about the disease, treatment, activity restrictions, injury prevention, and ulcer treatment *so patient will be less anxious, be more cooperative with treatment plan, and make accurate adjustments in lifestyle.* Explain the importance of smoking cessation *so patient is informed of the effects of nicotine, such as vasoconstriction, impaired transport and cellular utilization of oxygen, and increased blood viscosity.* Emphasize the importance of meticulous foot care *to reduce the risk of trauma to feet.*

disease).[17] The health care team must consistently agree to inform the patient to abstain from smoking. The nurse needs to tell the patient about various community agencies and support groups, such as behavior modification and antismoking clinics, if the patient is unable to stop smoking.

If the patient is not a surgical candidate or decides not to have surgery, a plan of care can be implemented to optimize the patient's arterial circulation. A progressive exercise program often increases the patient's tolerance for exercise and enhances venous return. Collateral vessels—usually small, insignificant branches of major arteries—often enlarge and carry more blood "around" an occlusive lesion as a compensatory mechanism. The demand for blood and oxygen beyond an arterial blockage is believed to enhance collateral vessel development.

Walking is effective exercise. The patient should be instructed to walk only to the point of distress, to rest and allow the discomfort to subside, and then to resume walking until distress recurs. This exercise should be done for a prescribed time, usually 30 to 40 minutes a day, in addition to normal activity.

Both nonoperative and postoperative patients should be taught the importance of meticulous foot care to prevent injury. The patient should learn to inspect the extremities daily for skin color, mottling, scabs, alterations in the texture of the skin and subcutaneous fat, and reduction or absence of hair growth. Any ulceration or inflammation must be reported to the health care provider. Skin temperature should be noted, and capillary refill of the fingers and toes should be tested. In addition, the patient should be taught to palpate pulses and report any changes to their health care provider. Thick or overgrown toenails and calluses are potentially serious lesions that require regular attention by a skilled health care provider.

Emphasis on foot care is especially important in the patient with both arterial occlusive disease and diabetes, because diabetic neuropathy (i.e., diminished peripheral sensation) increases the susceptibility to traumatic injury and results in delay in seeking treatment (see Table 46-17). These measures also apply to the person with vascular disease who does not have diabetes.

The patient should be instructed to wear clean, all-cotton or all-wool socks. In addition, comfortable shoes with rounded (not pointed) toes and soft insoles should be worn. Shoes should not be laced tightly, and new shoes should be broken in gradually. Frequent inspection of the feet should be of paramount importance to this patient population so that prompt attention to problems can be facilitated. A patient with poor eyesight will need assistance with foot care.

Thromboangiitis Obliterans

Thromboangiitis obliterans (Buerger's disease) is an inflammatory, thrombotic disorder of the medium-sized arteries and veins of the upper or lower extremities. Occlusion of the vessel occurs with development of collateral circulation around areas of obstruction. The basic cause is not known. There is a direct relationship to cigarette smoking: the disease occurs only in smokers, and when smoking is stopped, the disease improves. Unlike atherosclerosis lipid accumulation does not occur in the vessel media. The disorder, generally asymmetrical, occurs predominantly in men between 25 and 40 years of age who smoke. A familial tendency has also been observed.

The symptom complex of Buerger's disease is often confused with that of atherosclerotic occlusive disease. The patient may have intermittent claudication. The development of rest pain is a premonitory sign of gangrene and may develop in advanced stages of the disease process. Other signs and symptoms may include color and temperature changes in the affected limb or limbs, paresthesia, thrombophlebitis, and cold sensitivity. Painful ulceration and gangrene may necessitate amputation of individual digits.

Treatment includes avoidance of trauma to the extremity and complete cessation of smoking. Patients are often told that they have a choice between their cigarettes and their legs; they cannot have both. Supportive psychotherapy and pharmacologic treatment of underlying anxiety disorders are sometimes helpful in assisting the patient to stop smoking. The disorder is difficult to treat. Anticoagulants and vasodilator therapy have met with little success. Amputation, generally below the knee, may be necessary in advanced cases.

Arteriospastic Disease

Arteriospastic disease (Raynaud's phenomenon) is an episodic vasospastic disorder of small cutaneous arteries, most frequently involving the fingers and toes. The exact etiology is not known. The condition occurs primarily in young women. It is seen frequently in association with collagen diseases such as rheumatoid arthritis, scleroderma, and lupus erythematosus. Other contributing factors include occupationally related trauma and pressure to the fingertips as noted in typists, pianists, and those who use handheld vibrating equipment. Exposure to heavy metals may also be a contributing etiologic factor. The symptoms are usually precipitated by exposure to cold, emotional upsets, caffeine, and tobacco use.

The disorder is characterized by three color changes (white, red, and blue) (Fig. 35-8). Initially the vasoconstrictive effect produces pallor (white), followed by cyanosis (bluish-purple). These changes are subsequently followed by rubor or hyperemia. Because Raynaud's phenomenon is a vasospastic disorder of small blood vessels, the wrist pulses are never lost. The patient usually describes cold and numbness in the vasoconstrictive phase and throbbing, aching pain; tingling; and swelling in the hyperemic phase. This type of episode usually lasts only minutes but in severe cases may persist for several hours. Complications include punctate (small hole) lesions of the fingertips and superficial gangrenous ulcers in advanced stages.

If the symptoms persist for several years in the absence of an associated underlying disorder, the diagnosis of primary Raynaud's disease may be made. It is of diagnostic importance to search for an underlying disease so that appropriate treatment can be instituted. Otherwise, treatment is generally not required because the symptoms are self-limiting. However, treatment of symptoms with certain calcium channel blockers has been encouraging. Oral vasodilators have been used with variable success. Sympathectomy is considered only in advanced cases.

Patient education should be directed toward reassurance that no serious underlying disorder is present and that prevention of recurrent episodes is possible. Loose, warm clothing should be worn as protection from the cold, including gloves when the refrigerator-freezer is used or when cold objects are being handled. Temperature extremes should be avoided. Moving to a warmer climate is not necessarily beneficial because symptoms may still occur during cooler weather and in an air-conditioned environ-

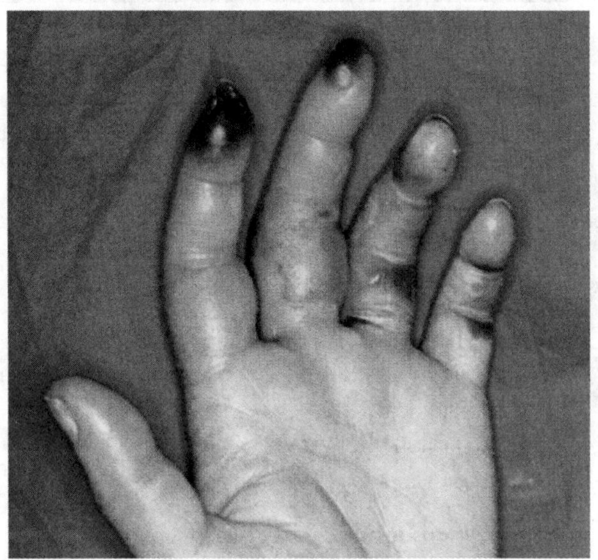

Fig. 35-8 Raynaud's phenomenon.

ment. The patient should stop smoking, avoid caffeine, and develop techniques to cope with anxiety-producing situations. Immersion of the hands in warm water often decreases the spasm.

DISORDERS OF THE VEINS

Thrombophlebitis

The most common disorder of the veins is thrombophlebitis, the formation of a thrombus (clot) in association with inflammation of the vein. The terms *phlebothrombosis* and *phlebitis* have been used to indicate whether the predominant process is thrombus formation or inflammation. In general, the preferred term is *thrombophlebitis* because both clots and inflammation are usually present. The initiating event is usually thrombus formation. Thrombophlebitis is classified as either *superficial* or *deep* (Table 35-6).

In about 65% of all patients receiving IV therapy, superficial thrombophlebitis develops, and in at least 5% of all surgical patients, deep vein thrombophlebitis develops. Superficial thrombophlebitis is often of minor significance and is treated with elevation, antiinflammatory agents, and warm compresses. Deep vein thrombophlebitis is of greater significance and can result in embolization of thrombi from deep veins to the lungs. This can be fatal and, at the least, results in prolonged hospitalization.

Etiology. Three important factors (Virchow's triad) in the etiology of thrombophlebitis are (1) stasis of venous flow, (2) damage of the endothelium (inner lining of the vein), and (3) hypercoagulability of the blood. The patient who is at high risk for the development of thrombophlebitis has predisposing conditions to any of these three disorders (Table 35-7).

Venous stasis. Normal blood flow in the venous system depends on the action of muscles in the extremities and on the functional adequacy of venous valves, allowing flow in one direction only. Venous stasis occurs if these valves are dysfunctional or if the muscles of the extremities are inactive. Venous stasis occurs in people who are obese, have CHF, have been on long trips without regular exercise, or are immobile for long periods (e.g., with spinal cord injuries or fractured hips). Also at risk are pregnant women and women in the postpartum period.[18]

The patient with atrial fibrillation is also at high risk because of stagnation of blood and the eddying in blood flow caused by irregular ventricular contractions in response to the fibrillation. Steroid and quinine therapy also predispose a patient to stasis and clot formation.

Endothelial damage. Damage to the lining of the vein is caused by trauma or external pressure and occurs any time a venipuncture is performed. Damaged endothelium has decreased fibrinolytic properties, predisposing to the development of thrombus. Increased endothelial damage is sustained when patients on IV therapy are receiving high-dose antibiotics, potassium, chemotherapeutic agents, or hypertonic solutions such as contrast media.

Other factors predisposing to endothelial inflammation and damage include the presence of an IV catheter in the same site for longer than 48 hours, the use of contaminated

Table 35-6 Clinical Manifestations of Thrombophlebitis

		Deep	
	Superficial	**Small Veins**	**Major Venous Trunks**
Usual causes	Varicose veins; direct trauma; IV catheters; thromboangiitis obliterans; caustic IV medications such as chemotherapy, radiopaque contrast material; IV drug use	Postoperatively, before and after childbirth, direct or distant trauma, congestive heart failure, prolonged bed rest, acute febrile disease, sepsis, debilitating disease, malignant disease, blood dyscrasias	Systemic lupus erythematosus, pressure of tumors on veins, estrogen therapy, malignant disease, blood dyscrasias, idiopathic cause
Usual location	Saphenous veins and their tributaries, forearm	Soleal; posterior tibial, other deep calf veins; popliteal; pelvis	Femoral, iliac, inferior or superior vena cava, axillary, subclavian
Clinical findings	Tender, red, inflamed induration along course of subcutaneous vein (visible and palpable)	Possible tenderness to deep pressure, induration of overlying muscle, minimal or no venous distention	Swelling, cyanosis, venous distention, mild to moderate pain, tenderness over involved vein (groin or axilla)
Edema of extremities	Almost never	Occasionally	Frequently
Embolization	Almost never	Always a threat	Always a threat
Chronic venous insufficiency	Almost never	Usually not	Frequently

IV, Intravenous.

IV equipment, a fracture that causes damage to the blood vessels, diabetes, blood pooling, burns, and any unusual physical exertion that results in muscular strain.

Hypercoagulability of blood. Hypercoagulability of blood occurs in many hematologic disorders, particularly polycythemia, severe anemias, various malignancies, and antithrombin III deficiency. A patient with systemic infections in which endotoxins are released also has hypercoagulability. Hypercoagulability also seems to be the contributing factor in idiopathic thrombophlebitis.

The patient who takes oral contraceptives (especially those containing estrogen) is at increased risk for thromboembolic disease. Recent studies show that women who take contraceptives and smoke double their risk because of the constricting effect of nicotine on the blood vessel wall. Smoking may also cause hypercoagulability.

Pathophysiology. Red blood cells (RBCs), WBCs, platelets, and fibrin adhere to form a thrombus. A frequent site of thrombus formation is the valve cusps of veins, where venous stasis allows accumulation of blood products. As the thrombus enlarges, increased amounts of blood cells and fibrin collect behind it, producing a larger clot with a "tail" that eventually occludes the lumen of the vein.

Table 35-7 Risk Factors for Deep Vein Thrombophlebitis and Thromboembolism

- History of thrombophlebitis
- Abdominal and pelvic surgery
- Suprapubic prostatectomy
- Obesity
- Neoplasms, especially hepatic and pancreatic
- Congestive heart failure
- Advanced age
- Atrial fibrillation
- Prolonged immobility
  - Bed rest
  - Long trip without adequate exercise
  - Spinal cord injury
  - Fractured hip
- Cerebrovascular disease
- Myocardial infarction
- Pregnancy
- Postpartum period
- Estrogen therapy, including oral contraceptives
- IV therapy
- Trauma
- Sepsis
- Venous cannulation or catheterization
- Drug abuse
- Cigarette smoking
- Excessive vitamin E intake
- Hypercoagulable states
  - Polycythemia vera
  - Severe anemias
  - Dehydration or malnutrition
- Antithrombin III deficiency

IV, Intravenous.

If a thrombus only partially occludes the vein and blood flow continues, the thrombus becomes covered by endothelial cells and the thrombotic process stops. If the thrombus does not become detached, it undergoes lysis or becomes firmly organized and adherent within 24 to 48 hours. The organized thrombi may detach and give rise to emboli. The turbulence of blood flow past the thrombus is a major factor contributing to its detachment from the vein wall. These emboli generally flow through the venous circulation, back to the heart, and into the pulmonary circulation.

Clinical Manifestations. Clinical manifestations of thrombophlebitis vary according to the size and location of the thrombus and the adequacy of collateral circulation around the obstructive process (see Table 35-6). The patient with superficial thrombophlebitis may have a palpable, firm, subcutaneous cordlike vein. The area surrounding the vein may be tender to the touch, reddened, and warm. A mild systemic temperature elevation and leukocytosis may be present. Edema of the extremity may or may not occur. The most common cause of superficial thrombophlebitis in the arms is IV therapy. The most common cause of superficial thrombophlebitis in the legs is related to varicose veins.

The patient with deep thrombophlebitis may have no symptoms or have unilateral leg edema, pain, warm skin, and a temperature greater than 100.4° F (38° C). If the calf is involved, tenderness may be present on palpation. *Homans' sign,* pain on dorsiflexion of the foot when the leg is raised, is a classic but unreliable sign because it is not specific for deep vein thrombosis. If the inferior vena cava is involved, both lower extremities may be edematous and cyanotic. If the superior vena cava is involved, both upper extremities and the neck, back, and face become edematous and cyanotic.

Complications. The most serious complications of thrombophlebitis are *pulmonary embolism, chronic venous insufficiency,* and *phlegmasia cerulea dolens.* Pulmonary embolism is the most feared complication of thrombophlebitis because of its lethal potential (see the section on Pulmonary Embolism).

Chronic venous insufficiency, a common complication resulting from recurrent thrombophlebitis, results in valvular destruction, allowing retrograde flow of blood. Persistent edema, increased pigmentation, secondary varicosities, ulceration, and cyanosis of the limb when it is placed in a dependent position may develop in a person with this complication.[19] Signs and symptoms of chronic venous insufficiency often do not develop for many years following deep thrombophlebitis.

Phlegmasia cerulea dolens (swollen, blue, painful leg) may develop in a patient with severe thrombophlebitis of the lower extremities. It presents as sudden, massive swelling and intense bluish discoloration of the extremity (Fig. 35-9). Gangrene may occur as a result of arterial occlusion resulting from obstruction of venous outflow.

Diagnostic Studies. Various diagnostic studies are used to determine the site and extent of the thrombus or emboli (Table 35-8).

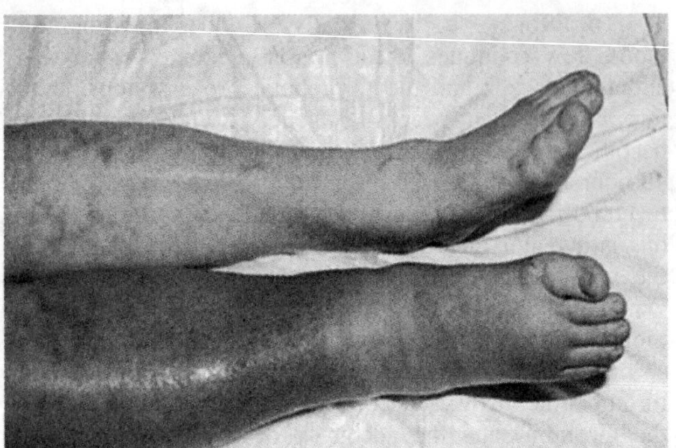

Fig. 35-9 Deep vein thrombosis.

Therapeutic Management

Conservative therapy. The patient with superficial thrombophlebitis is usually kept in bed with elevation of the affected extremity until the tenderness has subsided, usually for 5 to 7 days. Warm, moist heat may be used to relieve the pain and treat the inflammation. Mild oral analgesics such as aspirin and codeine are used to relieve pain. Nonsteroidal anti-inflammatory agents such as ibuprofen have been used to treat the inflammatory process and accompanying pain.

Anticoagulant therapy is usually not indicated for superficial thrombophlebitis but is routinely used for deep vein thrombophlebitis (Table 35-9). Heparin, administered by continuous IV infusion after an initial bolus dose, is given for up to 10 days and is followed by oral anticoagulants for 3 to 6 months. Bed rest with feet elevated above the level of the heart is indicated until therapeutic levels of anticoagulation are achieved and edema subsides.

If edema is present when the patient becomes ambulatory, graduated compression elastic stockings are recommended. Ideally they should be measured to fit the patient after some of the edema has resolved. The use of compression gradient stockings is recommended for several months to support the vein walls and valves and decrease pain on ambulation from swelling.

Surgical interventions. Most patients are treated conservatively, but a small percentage require surgical intervention (see Table 35-9). The primary indication for surgery is to prevent pulmonary emboli. Surgical procedures include venous thrombectomy (rarely performed) and inferior vena cava interruption. Venous thrombectomy involves the removal of an occluding clot through an incision in the vein. This procedure is done to prevent pulmonary embolism or to decrease the risk of the development of chronic venous insufficiency.

In the past extravascular interruption of the inferior vena cava to prevent pulmonary emboli involved abdominal surgery and application of a partitioning Teflon clip (Fig.

Table 35-8 Diagnostic Studies: Deep Vein Thrombophlebitis and Pulmonary Embolism

Study	Description and Abnormal Findings
■ Coagulation studies	
Platelet count, bleeding time, PT, PTT, APTT	Elevation if patient has underlying blood dyscrasia; decrease possible if patient has polycythemia; alteration possible because of previous medications
■ Noninvasive venous studies	
Venous Doppler evaluation	Determination of venous flow in deep femoral, popliteal, and posterior tibial veins; normal finding of spontaneous flow with variation transmitted by respiration cycle; abnormal finding of absence of flow augmentation with distal compression and proximal release
Duplex scanning	Combination of ultrasound imaging techniques and Doppler capabilities to determine location and extent of thrombus within veins (most widely used test to diagnose deep vein thrombosis)
Plethysmography	Measurement of increase in leg volume induced by obstruction of venous outflow by inflation of thigh cuff (maximum venous capitance), measurement of speed at which volume decreases on thigh cuff release (venous outflow), abnormal finding of slow outflow
Magnetic resonance imaging	Detection of deep vein thrombosis in leg veins; strong magnetic field is combined with radiofrequency waves to make a cross-sectional image of patient
■ Venogram (phlebogram)	X-ray determination (using contrast media) of location and site of clot, filling defect in vein lumen, and development of collateral circulation
■ Lung scan (ventilation and perfusion)	Means of determining presence of pulmonary embolism and extent of resulting lung damage, abnormal finding of mismatch between ventilation and perfusion components
■ Pulmonary arteriogram	X-ray determination (using contrast media) of location and size of pulmonary embolism

APTT, Activated partial thromboplastin time; *PT,* prothrombin time; *PTT,* partial thromboplastin time.

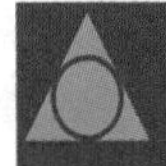

Table 35-9 Therapeutic Management: Deep Vein Thrombophlebitis

Diagnostic
- Health history and physical examination
- Chest x-ray
- CBC count with WBC differential
- PT, PTT, APTT, platelet count, bleeding time
- Electrocardiogram
- Venous studies (see Table 35-8)
- Venogram of affected limb (rarely performed)

Therapeutic

Conservative
- Continuous IV heparin
- Bed rest with bathroom privileges for bowel movement only
- Elevation of legs above heart level
- Oral anticoagulants
- Elastic compression gradient stockings
- Measurement and charting of size of both thighs and calves every morning
- Guaiac test on all stools while patient is on anticoagulant therapy

Surgical
- Venous thrombectomy (rarely done)
- Inferior vena cava interruption (rarely performed)
- Intracaval filter insertion

APTT, Activated partial thromboplastin time; *CBC,* complete blood count; *IV,* intravenous; *PT,* prothrombin time; *PTT,* partial thromboplastin time; *WBC,* white blood cell.

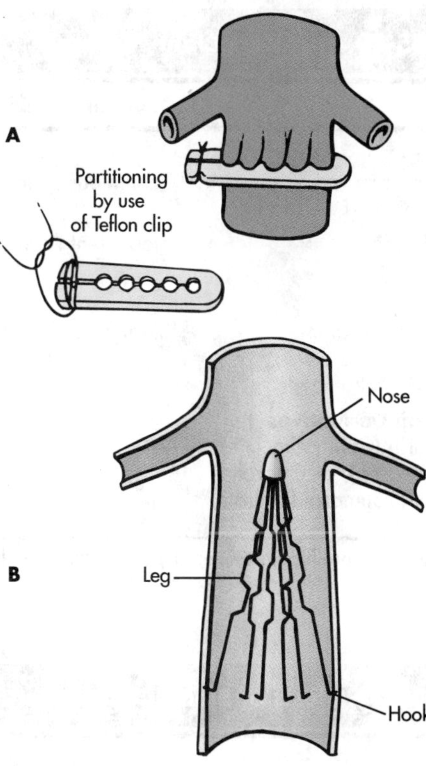

Fig. 35-10 Inferior vena caval interruption techniques to prevent pulmonary embolism. ***A,*** Partitioning extravascular Teflon clip. ***B,*** Intravascular Kimray-Greenfield stainless steel filter.

35-10, *A*). Although suture partitioning was once popular, it is rarely done currently.

Another procedure involves threading a caval filter device into the right internal jugular vein and into the inferior vena cava below the level of the renal veins (Fig. 35-10, *B*) using local anesthesia. The filter device is opened and the spokes penetrate the vessel walls. These devices result in "sieve-type" obstruction, permitting filtration of clots without interruption of blood flow. Newly developed catheters can be inserted percutaneously through superficial femoral veins.

Complications after the insertion of the intravascular filter device are rare. They include air embolism, improper placement, and migration of the filter more distally into the venous system. Venous congestion is common and is caused by accumulation of trapped clots at the filter site. At some point, these clots may clog the filter and completely occlude the vena cava. This process is usually so gradual that collateral vessels have a chance to develop and venous flow is maintained. However, development of large collateral venous pathways may provide an alternate route for pulmonary emboli.

Pharmacologic Management. The goals of anticoagulation therapy in the treatment of deep vein thrombophlebitis are to prevent propagation of the clot, development of a new thrombus, and embolization. Anticoagulant therapy does not dissolve the clot. Lysis of the clot begins spontaneously through the body's intrinsic fibrinolytic system (see Chapter 27).

The most commonly used anticoagulants are heparin and coumarin compounds (Table 35-10). Heparin acts directly on the intrinsic and common pathways of blood coagulation. Heparin inhibits thrombin-mediated conversion of fibrinogen to fibrin. It also potentiates the actions of antithrombin III, inhibits the activation of factor IX, and neutralizes activated factor X by activating factor X inhibitor.

Coumarin compounds, of which warfarin (Coumadin) is the most commonly used, exert their action indirectly on the coagulation pathway. Warfarin inhibits the hepatic synthesis of the vitamin K–dependent coagulation factors II, VII, IX, and X by competitively interfering with vitamin K. Vitamin K is normally required for the synthesis of these factors.

Oral anticoagulants are begun while heparin is still being administered. An overlap of 3 to 5 days is usually required to maintain therapeutic control of clotting. The clotting status is usually monitored by activated partial thromboplastin time (APTT) or partial thromboplastin time (PTT) for heparin therapy and prothrombin time (PT) for coumarin derivatives. However, other tests can be used (Table 35-11).

A careful history regarding childbearing status and drug history should be taken before initiating anticoagulation. Because coumarin compounds are contraindicated in pregnancy, patients requiring anticoagulation often receive subcutaneous heparin. Antiplatelet agents (e.g., aspirin) are also contraindicated while on anticoagulation. Other medi-

Table 35-10 Anticoagulant Therapy

Drug	Route of Administration	Comments
Heparin		
Panheprin	Continuous IV infusion by infusion pump	Initial bolus dose of heparin is required. Protamine sulfate should be available as an antidote.
Lipo-Hepin	Intermittent IV infusion q4hr	Clotting status is monitored by whole blood clotting time (Lee-White clotting time,), PTT, activated clotting time, and activated PTT.
Liquaemin sodium	Intermittent subcutaneous infusion q6hr	Aspirin should not be administered to a patient taking heparin. Low-dose prophylactic drugs do not alter clotting studies.
Coumarin Derivatives		
Warfarin (Coumadin, Panwarfin), dicumarol, acenocoumarol (Sintrom)	Oral	Vitamin K should be available as an antidote. Plasma levels may be maintained for up to 5 days. Clotting status is monitored by PT.

IV, Intravenous; *PT,* prothrombin time; *PTT,* partial thromboplastin time.

Table 35-11 Tests of Blood Coagulation

Test	Drug Monitored	Normal Value	Therapeutic Value
Lee-White whole blood clotting time	Heparin	9-14 min	20-30 min
PT	Warfarin	11-12 sec	17-24 sec
PTT	Heparin	60-90 sec	90-180 sec
APTT	Heparin	24-36 sec	48-60 sec
ACT	Heparin	80-135 sec	3 min

ACT, Activated clotting time; *APTT,* activated partial thromboplastin time; *PT,* prothrombin time; *PTT,* partial thromboplastin time.

cations that interact with coumarin compounds include ibuprofen (Advil, Motrin), phenytoin (Dilantin), and barbiturates (Table 35-12). Changes in diet can also interact with coumarin compounds. A diet high in vitamin K (e.g., green leafy vegetables) can make it difficult to maintain a patient within a therapeutic range. The patient should be instructed to follow a diet that includes foods containing vitamin K in moderate amounts. In addition, the patient should be instructed to avoid excessive amounts of vitamin E.

NURSING MANAGEMENT

THROMBOPHLEBITIS

Nursing Assessment

Subjective and objective data that should be obtained from a patient with thrombophlebitis are presented in Table 35-13.

Nursing Diagnosis

Nursing diagnoses are determined when the problems and etiologic factors are supported by clinical data. Nursing diagnoses related to thrombophlebitis may include, but are not limited to, those presented in the nursing care plan for thrombophlebitis on p. 1060.

Planning

The overall goals are that the patient with thrombophlebitis will have (1) relief of pain, (2) decreased edema, (3) no skin ulceration, and (4) no evidence of pulmonary emboli.

Nursing Implementation

Health Maintenance and Promotion. Thrombus formation can be prevented in many situations. Prophylactic measures include early ambulation and leg exercises postoperatively, use of elastic stockings (hose), avoidance of dehydration, and low-dose anticoagulant therapy. Heparin (5000 units subcutaneously every 8 to 12 hours) or oral anticoagulants are often recommended for the high-risk patient who is predisposed to thrombus formation.

Mechanical methods of prophylaxis, such as the use of intermittent pneumatic compression stockings or boots, help promote venous return and may also stimulate fibrinolytic activity within the vein. These devices are commonly used on a high-risk patient while hospitalized.

Another important preventive measure is to avoid prolonged standing or sitting in a motionless, leg-dependent position. Frequent knee flexion, ankle rotation, and active walking should be done during long periods of sitting or standing, especially on long trips.

Table 35-12 Drugs Interacting with Oral Anticoagulants

Drugs Potentiating Response	Drugs Diminishing Response
Anabolic steroids (e.g., Dianabol)	Barbiturates (e.g., secobarbital, phenobarbital)
Clofibrate (Atromid-S)	Cholestyramine (Cuemid, Questran)
Dextrothyroxine (Choloxin)	Ethchlorvynol (Placidyl)
Disulfiram (Antabuse)	Glutethimide (Doriden)
Metronidazole (Flagyl)	Griseofulvin (Grifulvin)
Neomycin	Rifampin (Rifadin, Rimactane)
Nonsteroidal anti-inflammatory drugs	
Oxyphenbutazone (Tandearil)	
Phenylbutazone (Butazolidin)	
Phenytoin (Dilantin)	
Phenyramidol (Analexin)	
Salicylates	
Sulfonamides (Gantrisin)	

The patient should be taught the importance of not smoking and to perform deep breathing and range-of-motion exercises. In addition, the nurse should identify the patient at high risk for deep vein thrombophlebitis and institute appropriate preventive measures.

Acute Intervention. Nursing care for the patient with thrombophlebitis is directed toward the reduction of inflammation and the prevention of emboli formation (see the nursing care plan for the patient with thrombophlebitis). Acute intervention for superficial thrombophlebitis involves the use of warm moist packs or soaks, elevation of the affected extremity, removal of an IV catheter if present, and provision of analgesia to minimize pain and inflammation. Some experts advocate surgical intervention if the greater saphenous system of the lower extremity is involved. The greater saphenous vein may be ligated to prevent extension of thrombus into the deep venous system.

Acute intervention for deep vein thrombophlebitis involves IV and oral anticoagulation, 5 to 7 days of bed rest with elevation of the affected extremity, and the use of elastic support (elastic bandages or compression gradient stockings) to promote venous return.

While the patient is receiving anticoagulation therapy, the nurse should closely observe for any indication of bleeding, including epistaxis and bleeding gingiva. Urine should be assessed for gross or microscopic hematuria. A smoky appearance to the urine is sometimes noted if blood is present. A specimen should be checked daily for hematuria. Particular attention should be paid to the protection of skin areas that may be traumatized. Surgical incisions should be closely observed for evidence of bleeding. Stools should be tested to determine the presence of occult blood from the gastrointestinal (GI) tract. Mental status changes, especially in the older patient, should be assessed as a possible indication of cerebral bleeding.

Table 35-13 Nursing Assessment: Thrombophlebitis

Subjective Data

Important health information

Past health history: Extremity trauma, varicosities, childbirth, bacteremia, smoking, obesity, prolonged bed rest, irregular heartbeat (e.g., atrial fibrillation), COPD, CHF, malignancies, systemic lupus erythematosus, MI, spinal cord injury, extensive travel

Medications: Use of estrogens (including oral contraceptives), steroids, quinine, excessive amounts of vitamin E, IV drug use, IV drug therapy (antibiotics, chemotherapy, potassium), IV contrast dyes

Surgery and other treatments: Any recent surgery, previous surgery involving veins, IV therapy

Functional health patterns

Cognitive-perceptual: Pain in area surrounding vein or on palpation or ambulation, positive Homan's sign

Objective Data

General

Fever, anxiety

Integumentary

Red, warm skin around involved vein; increased size of extremity when compared with other side; taut, shiny skin; tenderness to palpation; distention of superficial veins

Cardiovascular

Firm, palpable vein; edema and cyanosis of area

Possible findings

Leukocytosis, abnormal coagulation, anemia or elevated hematocrit and RBC count, positive venous plethysmographic or Doppler studies, positive venogram

CHF, Congestive heart failure; *COPD,* chronic obstructive pulmonary disease; *IV,* intravenous; *MI,* myocardial infarction.

The nurse should review with the patient any medications currently being taken that may interfere with anticoagulant therapy. The nurse should monitor the hemoglobin and hematocrit levels when a patient is receiving anticoagulant drugs. Medication doses are titrated according to the results of clotting studies. The nurse should be cautious about administering either heparin or coumarin without first checking the results of the clotting studies. The antidote for heparin is protamine sulfate, and vitamin K is used as the antidote for coumarin. These drugs must be immediately available if hemorrhage occurs.

Chronic and Home Management. Compression gradient stockings, properly measured, fitted, and evenly applied, should be worn when the patient becomes ambulatory. These stockings compress superficial veins and prevent venous stasis. The nurse should take care to prevent any pressure under the knee, such as by using pillows or bed gatches. The patient also should be taught to avoid crossing the legs at the knees. These measures will place pressure on the popliteal space and decrease venous return to the heart.

During all phases of care the nurse should evaluate the patient's psychologic response. Many patients are appre-

NURSING CARE PLAN Patient with Thrombophlebitis

Planning: Outcome Criteria	Nursing Interventions and Rationales
➤ **NURSING DIAGNOSIS**	Pain *related to* edema secondary to impaired circulation in extremities *as manifested by* complaints of pain in extremity; presence of edema in extremity; redness, tenderness, and warmth around affected vein
Have relief of pain and reduction of edema.	Administer analgesics as ordered *to relieve pain.* Apply continuous warm, moist heat (e.g., K-pad at low heat) if ordered *to relieve pain, reduce inflammation, and improve circulation by vasodilatation.* Keep affected leg elevated above heart level *to promote venous return and decrease swelling.* Instruct patient not to cross legs at knees *to prevent further restriction of circulation to legs.* Measure thighs and calves daily at a marked site *to provide quantitative measures to assess increase or decrease in edema.* Maintain bed rest or activity level in accordance with acuteness of condition *to reduce pain associated with activity and prevent increase in swelling.*
➤ **NURSING DIAGNOSIS**	Altered health maintenance *related to* lack of knowledge about disorder and its treatment *as manifested by* patient asking many questions or no questions about condition
Understand disease process and treatment, including anticoagulation management, diet and activity, and clothing to be avoided.	Instruct patient on need for routine monitoring of clotting studies *to provide data on response to treatment and to monitor the risk of bleeding.* Teach patient signs and symptoms of thrombophlebitis and of abnormal bleeding to report to physician *to enable early diagnosis and treatment.* Encourage patient to take anticoagulants according to prescribed schedule *to prevent overdosing or underdosing resulting in extension of the clot or hemorrhage.* Assist patient with obtaining Medic-Alert identification *to alert others to anticoagulant therapy.* Teach patient not to wear garters, girdles, or any constrictive clothing *to avoid restriction of blood flow and venous pooling.* Encourage dieting to lose weight if indicated *because obesity increases compression of vessels.* Teach patient to avoid rubbing or massaging extremity *to prevent dislodging a thrombus* and to avoid sitting with legs crossed, *which increases venous stasis.* Teach patient to minimize sitting with legs in dependent position *because this position increases stasis.*
➤ **NURSING DIAGNOSIS**	Risk for impaired skin integrity *related to* alteration in peripheral tissue perfusion and possible valvular destruction
Have no evidence of ulcer formation in legs.	Assess patient for altered skin pigmentation in lower extremity, pain, open ulcer, and edema of lower extremity *to identify signs of impaired skin integrity.* Teach patient to wear compression gradient stockings at all times except when sleeping *to provide compression of superficial veins and improve venous flow in deep veins* and to change positions when sitting or standing for prolonged periods *to reduce venous stasis.* Have patient elevate legs when sitting *to reduce venous pooling and promote venous return.* Lubricate skin regularly *to minimize itching which can lead to excoriation and infection.*

continued

hensive that clots will move to the heart or lungs and cause sudden death. Every patient should be allowed to verbalize concerns, and an attempt should be made to clarify misconceptions. The patient hospitalized for long periods of time should be provided with diversion.

Discharge teaching should stress the avoidance of contraceptives for the patient with recurrent thrombophlebitis, the hazards of smoking, the importance of compression gradient stockings, and the need to avoid constrictive girdles or garters. Exercise programs should be developed with an emphasis on swimming and wading, which are particularly beneficial because of the gentle, even pressure of the water. A balanced program of rest and exercise, along with proper posture and avoiding long periods of sitting, improves arterial filling and venous return. The older patient should be taught safety precautions to prevent falls.

Dietary considerations for the overweight patient are aimed at limiting caloric intake so that the desired weight can be attained. Fat intake should be reduced if lipid or triglyceride levels are above normal for the patient's age. Occasionally, sodium limitation is necessary if edema is present. Proper fluid balance is required to prevent additional hypercoagulability of the blood, which may occur in the presence of deficient fluid intake. A well-balanced diet

NURSING CARE PLAN Patient with Thrombophlebitis—cont'd

COLLABORATIVE PROBLEMS

Nursing Goals	Nursing Interventions and Rationales
➤ **POTENTIAL COMPLICATION** Pulmonary embolism *related to* dehydration, immobility, and embolization of thrombus	
Monitor patient for signs of pulmonary embolism, report deviations from acceptable parameters, and carry out appropriate medical and nursing interventions.	Monitor for signs of pulmonary embolism, such as sudden onset of dyspnea, tachypnea, tachycardia, hemoptysis; chest pain; change in mental status; shortness of breath *to identify the problem and ensure immediate treatment*. Take vital signs q4h *to provide data on patient's response*. Use laxative to reduce straining *because the Valsalva maneuver may cause a venous thrombosis to dislodge*. Maintain adequate hydration *to prevent increasing coagulability of the blood*. Maintain bed rest *to minimize risk of embolization of thrombus by promoting venous drainage with the recumbent position*. Administer anticoagulants as ordered *to prevent extension of thrombi*. Use compression gradient stockings when ambulation is started *to provide venous support and prevent pooling*.
➤ **POTENTIAL COMPLICATION** Hemorrhage *related to* anticoagulant medications	
Monitor for signs of hemorrhage and carry out medical and nursing interventions.	Assess for signs of hemorrhage, such as bright-red bleeding from any body orifice; decreased BP, increased pulse and respiration; restlessness or changes in mental status *to ensure early diagnosis and treatment*. Do not give any IM medication *to avoid the possibility of localized hemorrhage*. Check PT before giving warfarin and PTT or APTT before giving heparin *because values greater than two times normal can produce bleeding and hemorrhage*. Give anticoagulant therapy only if clotting studies are within prescribed limits *to prevent overdosing and increased risk of hemorrhage*. Observe patient closely for signs of bleeding, such as epistaxis, bleeding gingivae, petechiae, ecchymoses, painful joints, incisional bleeding, or melena *as indicators of hemorrhage at select sites*. Monitor Hb or Hct levels *to assess possible blood loss*. Avoid activities such as hard nose blowing and straining at stool *to prevent bleeding*. Avoid use of aspirin or other over-the-counter drugs *that increase the tendency to bleed*.

APTT, Activated partial thromboplastin time; *BP*, blood pressure; *Hb*, hemoglobin; *Hct*, hematocrit; *IM*, intramuscular; *PT*, prothrombin time; *PTT*, partial thromboplastin time.

is important because calcium, vitamin E, and vitamin K all play active roles in the clotting mechanism.

If the patient is to be discharged while receiving anticoagulant medication, both the patient and the involved family need careful explanations of its dosage, actions, and side effects, as well as the importance of routine blood tests and the need to report symptoms to the health care provider (Table 35-14).

Varicose Veins

Varicose veins, or varicosities, are dilated, tortuous subcutaneous veins most frequently found in the saphenous system. They may be small and innocuous or large and bulging. *Primary* varicosities are those in which the superficial veins are dilated and the valves may or may not be rendered incompetent. The condition tends to be familial, is characteristically found bilaterally, and is probably caused by congenital weakness of the veins. *Secondary* varicosities result from previous thrombophlebitis of the deep femoral veins, with subsequent valvular incompetence. Secondary varicose veins may also occur in the esophagus as varices, in the anorectal area as hemorrhoids, and as abnormal arteriovenous connections (also known as *fistulas* and *malformations*).

Pathophysiology. The basic cause of varicosities is unknown. Superficial veins in the lower extremities become dilated and tortuous, with increased venous pressure. The increased venous pressure may be due to congenital weakness of the vein structure, obesity, pregnancy, venous obstruction resulting from thrombosis or extrinsic pressure by tumors, or occupations that require prolonged standing. As the veins enlarge, the valves are stretched and become incompetent, allowing blood flow to be reversed. As back pressure increases and the venous pump (muscle movement that squeezes venous blood back toward the heart) fails, further venous distention results. The increased venous pressure is transmitted to the capillary bed, and edema develops.

Clinical Manifestations. Discomfort from varicose veins varies dramatically among people and tends to be wors-

Table 35-14 Patient Education Related to Anticoagulant Therapy

1. Reasons for and basic mechanism of action of anticoagulant therapy and how long anticipated therapy will last
2. Need to take medication at same time each day (preferably in afternoon or evening)
3. Close follow-up with blood tests to assess blood clotting and whether change in drug dosages required
4. Side effects and adverse effects of drug therapy requiring medical attention:
   Any bleeding that does not stop after a reasonable amount of time
   Blood in urine or stool, or black, tarry stools
   Unusual bleeding from gingivae, throat, skin, or nose
   Severe headaches or stomach pains
   Weakness, dizziness
5. Avoidance of any trauma or injury that might cause bleeding (e.g., vigorous brushing of teeth, contact sports, improperly fitted shoes)
6. Avoidance of aspirin-containing drugs, nonsteroidal anti-inflammatory drugs, and more than moderate intake of alcohol
7. Wearing of Medic-Alert bracelet or necklace indicating what anticoagulant is being taken
8. Use of electric razor when shaving
9. Avoidance of marked changes in eating habits, such as food fads and crash diets
10. Need to consult with physician before beginning or discontinuing any medication
11. Need to inform all health care providers that patient is on anticoagulant therapy

ened by superficial thrombophlebitis. In addition, many patients voice concern about cosmetic disfigurement (Fig. 35-11). The most common symptom of varicose veins is an ache or pain after prolonged standing, which is relieved by walking or by elevating the limb. Some patients feel pressure or a cramplike sensation. Swelling may accompany the discomfort. Nocturnal leg cramps, especially in the calf area, may occur.

Complications. Superficial thrombophlebitis is a serious consequence of varicose veins and may occur either spontaneously or after trauma, surgical procedures, or pregnancy. Rupture of varicose veins (although not common) occurs because of weakening of the vessel wall. Ulceration as a result of skin infections or trauma may also develop.

Areas of *chronic venous stasis ulceration* (damaged dermis as a result of decreased tissue perfusion) are usually located near the inner aspect of the ankle, above and behind the medial malleolus.

Diagnostic Studies. A duplex ultrasound examination can detect obstruction and reflux in the venous system with considerable accuracy and is the most widely used study in diagnosing deep vein thrombophlebitis.

Therapeutic Management. Treatment is usually not indicated if varicose veins are only a cosmetic problem. If incompetency of the venous system develops, therapeutic management involves rest with the feet elevated, compression gradient hose, and walking exercise.

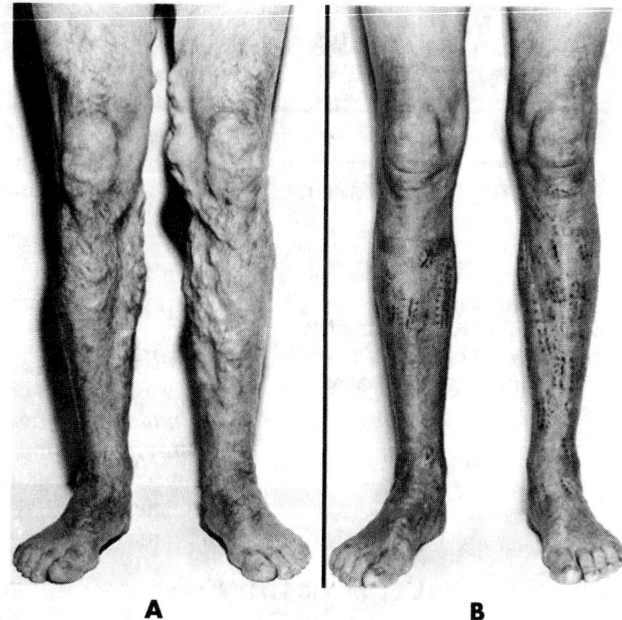

Fig. 35-11 Extensive varicosities (incompetency of the greater saphenous systems). ***A,*** Appearance preoperatively. ***B,*** Appearance 2 weeks postoperatively.

Injection sclerotherapy is used more commonly in the treatment of unsightly superficial varicosities.[19] Direct IV injection of a sclerosing agent such as Sotradecol induces inflammation and results in eventual thrombosis of the vein. This procedure can be performed safely in an office setting and causes minimal discomfort. After injection the leg is wrapped with an elastic bandage for 24 to 72 hours to maintain pressure over the vein. Local tenderness subsides within 2 to 3 weeks, and eventually the thrombosed vein disappears. After injection sclerotherapy the patient should be advised to wear compression stockings to help prevent the development of further varicosities.

Surgical intervention for varicose veins involves ligation of the entire vein (usually saphenous) and dissection and removal of its incompetent tributaries. Surgical interventions are indicated when chronic venous insufficiency cannot be prevented or controlled with therapy. Recurrent thrombophlebitis in varicose veins is another indication for surgery.

NURSING MANAGEMENT

VARICOSE VEINS

Prevention is a key factor related to varicose veins. The nurse should instruct the patient to avoid sitting or standing for long periods of time, to maintain ideal body weight, to take precautions against injury to the extremities, and to avoid wearing constrictive clothing.

After vein ligation surgery, the nurse should encourage deep breathing, which helps promote venous return to the right side of the heart. The extremities should initially be checked hourly for color, movement, sensation, temperature, the presence of edema, and pedal pulses. Bruising and discoloration are considered normal.

Postoperatively, elevation of the extremities at a 15-degree angle is encouraged (except for periods of ambulation) to prevent the development of venous stasis and edema. Compression gradient stockings are also used and should be removed once every 8 hours for short periods and reapplied.

Long-term management of varicose veins is directed toward improving circulation, relieving discomfort, improving cosmetic appearance, and avoiding complications, such as superficial thrombophlebitis and ulceration. Varicose veins can recur in other veins after the surgical procedure. The patient should be taught proper care of the lower extremities, including cleanliness and the use of individually fitted elastic hose. The patient should be taught to put on the hose while still lying down just before rising in the morning. The importance of periodic positioning of the legs above the heart should be stressed. The overweight patient will need assistance with weight reduction. The patient whose employment requires prolonged periods of standing or sitting should be encouraged to change position as frequently as possible. A pregnant patient with varicosities needs appropriate teaching as prescribed by the health care provider.

Venous Stasis Ulcers

Chronic venous insufficiency can lead to venous stasis ulceration, which may occur as a result of previous deep venous thrombosis. The basic dysfunction is incompetent valves of the deep veins. The ulcers usually develop around the ankles, especially in the area of the medial malleoli (Fig. 35-12). Loss of epidermis occurs, and portions of the dermal layer may also be involved, depending on the degree of venous stasis. A characteristic brownish coloration of the skin develops because of deposition of melanin and hemosiderin. When capillaries rupture, RBCs are released and disintegrate, with subsequent release of hemosiderin.

Clinical Manifestations and Complications. The skin texture of the lower leg is leathery, with a characteristic red-brown "brawny" appearance. Edema has usually been present for a prolonged period. The ulcer is a concave lesion below the margin of the skin surface and may become extensive. Pain may occur when the limb is in a dependent position or during ambulation. Pain is usually relieved by elevation of the foot.[20]

If the ulcer is untreated, the lesion becomes more extensive, eroding wider and deeper. The likelihood of infection is increased. Scar tissue formation around the rim of the ulcer is found. Poor hygiene, debilitation, and inadequate nutritional status contribute to the severity of the ulcerative lesion.

Therapeutic Management. The patient is instructed to elevate the extremity as much as possible. The key to facilitating healing is extrinsic compression to minimize venous stasis, venous hypertension, and edema. Extrinsic compression methods used include compression gradient

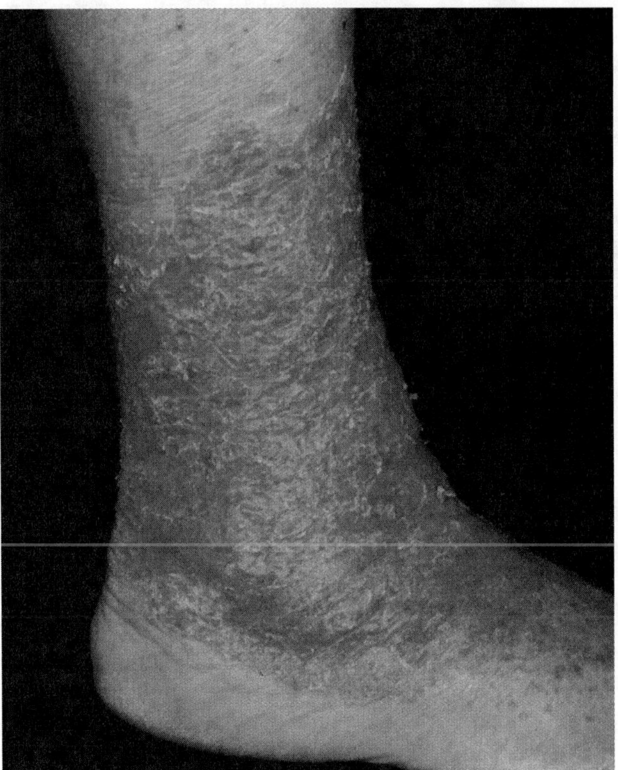

Fig. 35-12 Stasis dermatitis.

stockings, elastic bandages, and Unna's boot. The affected limb should be wrapped with an elastic bandage to provide compression. A dome paste (Unna's) boot, which hardens into a semirigid cast, is effective at promoting healing and works especially well as an outpatient therapy. It effectively controls edema and requires changes only once or twice weekly.[21]

Newer therapies, focused on promoting healing in a moist environment, are showing increasing promise.[22] Several adhesive hydrocolloid dressings are currently available and, when used in conjunction with extrinsic compression, have proved to be effective in hastening the healing of venous leg ulcers. (Hydrocolloid dressings are discussed in Chapter 9.)

Routine prophylactic antibiotic therapy is not indicated. If infection is evident as manifested by increased pain, temperature elevation, leukocytosis, or drainage from the site, cultures of the lesion are indicated and appropriate antibiotic therapy is then instituted.

If the ulcer fails to respond to several months of conservative therapy, skin grafting may be indicated. The ulcer is debrided and tissue from a donor site is used (see Chapter 21). Any varicosities in the area of the lesion are removed, and veins are ligated as necessary.

NURSING MANAGEMENT

VENOUS STASIS ULCERS

The patient with venous stasis ulcers should elevate the ulcerated leg as much as possible. The nurse should change the dressings as ordered and perform prescribed wound care measures, including observation for signs of infection. A balanced diet is encouraged, with protein and vitamin supplementation to promote wound healing.

Long-term management of venous stasis ulcers should focus on educating the patient in self-care measures because the incidence of recurrence is high. Discharge teaching should include avoidance of trauma to the limbs, proper skin care measures, and application of prescribed compression gradient stockings (after complete healing has occurred and swelling is minimized by elevation). Rest periods with elevation of the extremities should also be encouraged. A balanced nutritional program incorporating protein-vitamin supplementation should be instituted. Caloric limitation for weight reduction and diabetic diet management are taught when indicated. Once scar formation has occurred, the patient should return to a regimen of regular exercise (walking) and periods of leg elevation above the level of the heart.

PULMONARY EMBOLISM

Pathophysiology

Pulmonary embolism is the most common pulmonary complication in hospitalized patients. Although the actual incidence of mortality and morbidity from pulmonary embolism is unknown, it is estimated that nearly 50,000 people die of pulmonary embolism each year in the United States and another 650,000 have nonfatal pulmonary embolisms.[23]

Most pulmonary emboli arise from thrombi in the deep veins of the legs. Other sites of origin include the right side of the heart (especially with atrial fibrillation), upper extremities (rare), and the pelvic veins (especially after surgery or childbirth). Lethal pulmonary emboli originate most commonly in the femoral or iliac veins. Emboli are mobile clots that generally do not stop moving until they lodge at a narrowed part of the circulatory system. The lungs are an ideal location for emboli to lodge because of their extensive arterial and capillary network. The lower lobes are most frequently affected because they have a higher blood flow than the other lobes. Occasionally, the presence of deep vein thrombosis is unsuspected until a pulmonary embolism occurs.

Thrombi in the deep veins can dislodge spontaneously. However, a more common mechanism is jarring of the thrombus by mechanical forces, such as sudden standing, and changes in the rate of blood flow, such as those that occur with the Valsalva maneuver.

In addition to dislodged thrombi, rarer causes of pulmonary occlusion include fat emboli (from fractured long bones), air emboli (from improperly administered IV therapy), amniotic fluid, and tumors. Tumor emboli may originate from primary or metastatic malignancies.

Clinical Manifestations

The severity of clinical manifestations depends on the size of the emboli and the size and number of blood vessels occluded. The most common manifestation of pulmonary embolism is sudden onset of unexplained dyspnea, tachypnea, or tachycardia. Other manifestations are cough, chest pain, hemoptysis, crackles, fever, accentuation of the pulmonic heart sound, and sudden change in mental status as a result of hypoxemia.

Massive emboli may produce sudden collapse of the patient with shock, pallor, severe dyspnea, and crushing chest pain. However, some patients with massive emboli do not have pain. The pulse is rapid and weak, the BP is low, and an ECG indicates right ventricular strain. When rapid obstruction of 50% or more of the pulmonary vascular bed occurs, acute cor pulmonale may result because the right ventricle can no longer pump blood into the lungs. Death occurs in more than 60% of patients with massive emboli.

Medium-sized emboli often cause pleuritic chest pain accompanied by dyspnea, slight fever, and a productive cough with blood-streaked sputum. A physical examination may indicate tachycardia and a pleural friction rub.

Small emboli frequently are undetected or produce vague, transient symptoms. The exception to this is the patient with underlying cardiopulmonary disease, in whom even small or medium-sized emboli may result in severe cardiopulmonary compromise. However, repeated small emboli gradually cause a reduction in the capillary bed and eventual pulmonary hypertension. An ECG and chest x-ray may indicate right ventricular hypertrophy secondary to pulmonary hypertension.

Complications

Pulmonary Infarction. Pulmonary infarction (death of lung tissue) occurs in less than 10% of patients with emboli. Infarction is more likely when (1) occlusion of a large or medium-sized pulmonary vessel (greater than 2 mm in diameter), (2) insufficient collateral blood flow from the bronchial circulation, or (3) preexisting lung disease is present. Infarction results in alveolar necrosis and hemorrhage. Occasionally the infarcted tissue becomes infected and an abscess may develop. Concomitant pleural effusion is frequently found.

Pulmonary Hypertension. Pulmonary hypertension occurs when more than 50% of the cross-sectional area of the normal pulmonary bed is compromised. Pulmonary hypertension also results from hypoxemia. As a single event an embolus does not cause pulmonary hypertension unless it is massive. However, recurrent small to medium-sized emboli may result in chronic pulmonary hypertension. Pulmonary hypertension eventually results in dilatation and hypertrophy of the right ventricle. Depending on the degree of pulmonary hypertension and its rate of development, death may result rapidly or only mild or transient alterations may be produced (see Chapter 24).

Diagnostic Studies

An ECG is not a very sensitive or specific diagnostic measure to detect pulmonary embolism. With small to medium-sized pulmonary emboli it may remain normal or show a combination of changes transiently. As an isolated event, pulmonary embolism usually causes no ECG changes. Dysrhythmias are the most common finding related to pulmonary emboli. Recurrent small pulmonary emboli may eventually produce chronic pulmonary hypertension and ECG changes of right axis deviation with enlargement of the right atrium and right ventricle.

A chest x-ray is usually not diagnostic unless an infarction has occurred. Even with pulmonary infarction, the chest x-ray is nondiagnostic in about 50% of patients. Positive findings are best visualized 12 to 24 hours after embolism because variably shaped (round, linear, or, occasionally, wedge) areas of consolidation are sometimes found in the periphery or lower lobes. Pleural effusions are often noted. The chest x-ray can be valuable in assessing other pulmonary pathology, such as chronic obstructive pulmonary disease and tuberculosis.

A lung scan may be of value in screening for initial (or recurrent) pulmonary embolism, assessing the natural history of the lesion, and evaluating the effectiveness of therapeutic or surgical management. The lung scan has two components and is most accurate when both are performed:

1. *Perfusion scanning* involves IV injection of a radioisotope. A scanning device detects the adequacy of the pulmonary circulation.
2. *Ventilation scanning* involves inhalation of a radioactive gas such as xenon. Scanning reflects the distribution of gas through the lung. The ventilation component requires the cooperation of the patient and may be difficult or impossible to perform in the critically ill patient, particularly if the patient is intubated.

Venous studies (see Table 35-8) are helpful in diagnosing deep vein thrombosis as the likely source of a pulmonary embolism.

Pulmonary angiography is an invasive procedure that involves the insertion of a catheter through the antecubital or femoral vein and advancement to the pulmonary artery. Contrast medium is injected to visualize the pulmonary vascular system. This procedure remains the definitive diagnostic test for pulmonary embolism.[24]

ABG analysis is important. The arterial oxygen pressure (PaO_2) is always below normal because of inadequate oxygenation secondary to an occluded pulmonary vasculature. The arterial carbon dioxide pressure ($PaCO_2$) is usually below normal because of tachypnea and hyperventilation, which occur with pulmonary emboli. The pH remains normal unless respiratory alkalosis develops as a result of prolonged hyperventilation or to compensate for lactic acidosis caused by shock. ABGs may be greatly influenced by the presence of underlying cardiac and pulmonary disease.

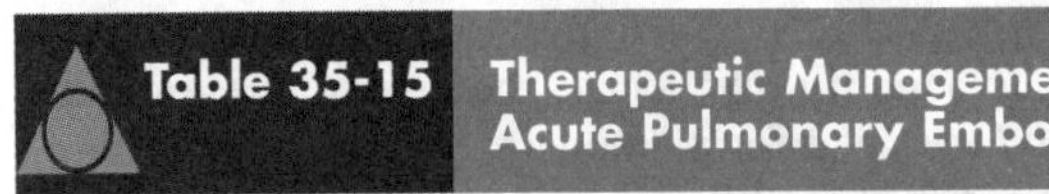

Table 35-15 Therapeutic Management: Acute Pulmonary Embolism

Diagnostic
- Health history and physical examination
- Lung scan (perfusion and ventilation)
- Chest x-ray
- Continuous ECG monitoring
- ABGs
- CBC count with WBC differential
- Pulmonary angiography
- Venous studies (Table 35-8)

Therapeutic
- Oxygen by mask or cannula
- Establishment of IV route for drugs and fluids
- Continuous IV heparin
- Bed rest
- Narcotics for pain relief
- Thrombolytic agents in certain patients
- Pulmonary embolectomy in life-threatening situations

ABGs, Arterial blood gases; *CBC,* complete blood count; *ECG,* electrocardiogram; *IV,* intravenous; *WBC,* white blood cell.

Therapeutic and Pharmacologic Management

When the diagnosis of thromboembolic disease has been made, treatment should be instituted immediately (Table 35-15). The objectives of therapeutic treatment are to prevent further growth or multiplication of thrombi in the lower extremities, prevent embolization from the upper or lower extremities to the pulmonary arteries, and provide cardiopulmonary support if indicated.

Conservative Therapy. Supportive therapy for the patient's cardiopulmonary status varies according to the severity of the pulmonary embolism. The administration of oxygen by mask or cannula may be adequate for some patients. Oxygen is given in a concentration determined by ABG analysis. In some situations, endotracheal intubation and mechanical ventilation may be needed to maintain adequate oxygenation. Respiratory measures such as turning, coughing, and deep breathing are necessary to prevent or treat atelectasis. If shock is present, vasopressor agents may be necessary to support systemic circulation (see Chapter 7). If heart failure is present, digitalis and diuretics are used (see Chapter 32). Pain resulting from pleural irritation or reduced coronary blood flow is treated with narcotics, usually morphine.

Properly managed anticoagulant therapy is effective in the treatment of many patients with pulmonary emboli. Heparin and warfarin (Coumadin) are the anticoagulant drugs of choice. Heparin should be started immediately and is continued as oral anticoagulants are initiated. The dosage of heparin is adjusted according to its effect on the PTT, and that of warfarin is regulated by the PT. Difficulties may be occasionally encountered in the patient in whom thrombosis or bleeding develops despite an apparently correct dosage.

Anticoagulant therapy for thromboembolic conditions may not be indicated in the presence of blood dyscrasias, hepatic dysfunction causing alteration in the clotting mechanism, injury to the viscera, overt bleeding, a history of hemorrhagic cerebrovascular accident, or neurologic conditions.

Surgical Interventions. If the degree of pulmonary arterial obstruction is severe (usually greater than 50%) and the patient does not respond to conservative therapy, an immediate embolectomy may be indicated. Pulmonary embolectomy is possible with the use of temporary cardiopulmonary bypass. Preoperative pulmonary angiography is necessary to identify and locate the site of the embolus. Fortunately, the need for pulmonary embolectomy is rare.

To prevent further pulmonary embolization, the surgical procedures appropriate for thrombophlebitis may be used (see the section on surgical interventions for thrombophlebitis, earlier in this chapter). These include insertion of intracaval filter devices and extravascular vena cava interruption (see Fig. 35-10).

Thrombolytic Agents. Thrombolytic agents such as urokinase and streptokinase have been shown to dissolve pulmonary emboli within 24 to 48 hours. Streptokinase, obtained from hemolytic streptococci, is thought to activate plasminogen, which is a fibrinolytic enzyme precursor. Urokinase also activates plasminogen. Both agents have been suggested for use in a patient with massive emboli or in whom surgery is contraindicated (see Chapter 31). Their use in the treatment of pulmonary emboli is undergoing investigation.

NURSING MANAGEMENT

PULMONARY EMBOLISM

Nursing Implementation

Health Maintenance and Promotion. Nursing measures aimed at prevention of pulmonary embolism parallel those for prophylaxis of deep vein thrombophlebitis (see earlier in this chapter).

Acute Intervention. The prognosis of a patient with pulmonary emboli is good if therapy is promptly instituted. The patient should be kept in bed in a semi-Fowler's position to facilitate breathing. A patent IV line should be maintained for medications and fluid therapy. The nurse should know the side effects of medications and observe for them. Oxygen therapy should be administered as ordered. Careful monitoring of vital signs, ECG, blood gases, and lung sounds is critical to assess the patient's status.

The patient is usually anxious because of pain, inability to breathe, and fear of death. The nurse should carefully explain the situation and provide emotional support and reassurance to help relieve the patient's anxiety. During the acute phase, someone should be with the patient as much as possible.

Many patients with pulmonary emboli have been hospitalized for a primary problem such as sepsis, acute respiratory failure, or surgical intervention. The nurse needs to focus on management of the problems caused by the primary disorder and those related to pulmonary emboli.

Chronic and Home Management. The patient affected by thromboembolic processes requires much psychologic and emotional support. In addition to the thromboembolic problems, the patient may have an underlying chronic illness requiring long-term treatment. To provide supportive therapy, the nurse must understand and differentiate between the various problems caused by the underlying disease and those related to thromboembolic disease.

Long-term management is similar to that for the patient with thrombophlebitis (see the nursing care plan for the patient with thrombophlebitis and Tables 35-9 to 35-14). Discharge planning is aimed at limiting progression of the condition and preventing complications. The nurse must reinforce the need for the patient to return to the health care facility for regular follow-up examination.

CRITICAL THINKING EXERCISES

CASE STUDY

ARTERIAL OCCLUSIVE DISEASE

Patient Profile

Mr. J., a 76-year-old male, was admitted to the hospital with rest pain of the right foot.

Subjective Data

- Has had a myocardial infarction, stroke, and arthritis
- Underwent a left femoral-popliteal bypass 5 years ago
- Has a smoking history of 45 pack years
- Complains of intense right foot pain for past 6 weeks
- Sleeps with leg dangling over side of bed

Objective Data

Physical Examination

- Has normal pulses in the left leg
- Has no palpable pulses in the popliteal, posterior tibial, or dorsalis pedis artery of the right leg
- Has small ulcer on right great toe

Critical Thinking Questions

1. What are Mr. J.'s risk factors for peripheral vascular disease?
2. What are the differences between acute as compared with chronic arterial ischemia?
3. What is the pathophysiology of rest pain?
4. What are the chances of Mr. J.'s foot ulcer healing?
5. What are the primary nursing responsibilities in caring for Mr. J.?
6. Based on the assessment data presented, write one or more appropriate nursing diagnoses. Are there any collaborative problems?

NURSING RESEARCH ISSUES

1. What changes in quality of life occur following vascular surgery (e.g., bypass surgery, aneurysm repair, or amputation)?
2. What is the effect of structured exercise programs in the rehabilitation of vascular surgery patients?
3. Can complications of peripheral vascular disease be prevented in high-risk patients?

REVIEW QUESTIONS

The number of the question corresponds to the same-numbered objective at the beginning of the chapter.

1. Which of the following statements accurately characterizes aortic aneurysms?
   a. There may be a genetic link in the development of abdominal aneurysms.
   b. They occur exclusively in the descending and abdominal aortas.
   c. They are most frequently caused by syphilis.
   d. They most commonly occur in young women after pregnancy.

2. An important nursing measure after an aneurysm repair is to
   a. administer anticoagulant therapy.
   b. position the legs in the Trendelenburg position.
   c. apply elastic stockings to both feet.
   d. palpate the peripheral pulses frequently.

3. Specific manifestations of aortic dissection vary depending on
   a. hypertension.
   b. extent of dissection and aortic branches affected.
   c. medications administered.
   d. respiratory status.

4. Which of the following is not considered a significant atherosclerotic risk factor?
   a. Sedentary lifestyle
   b. Cigarette smoking
   c. Hypertension
   d. Hyperlipidemia

5. Rest pain is a manifestation that occurs as a result of
   a. inadequate blood flow to the muscles during exercise.
   b. inadequate blood flow to the skin after application of heat.
   c. the beginning of gangrene in the toes.
   d. inadequate blood flow to the nerves of the feet.

6. All of the following statements characterize acute arterial ischemia *except* it
   a. is often an emergency requiring surgical intervention.
   b. presents suddenly with acute pain and pulselessness.
   c. can occur secondary to embolus from the heart.
   d. occurs as a consequence of deep vein thrombosis.

7. All the following predispose the patient to developing deep vein thrombophlebitis *except*
   a. elevated WBC count.
   b. endothelial damage.
   c. stasis.
   d. hypercoagulability.

8. Deep vein thrombophlebitis is often characterized by
   a. redness, heat, and tenderness of the affected area.
   b. generalized edema of the involved extremity.
   c. pallor and cyanosis of the involved extremity.
   d. paresthesia and coolness of the leg.

9. Which of the following nursing actions should be included in the plan of care for the patient with acute lower extremity deep vein thrombophlebitis?
   a. Encourage walking and leg exercises to promote venous return
   b. Apply compression gradient stocking
   c. Administer anticoagulants as ordered
   d. Administer vasodilator drug therapy

10. The patient discharged on anticoagulants should
   a. have blood drawn routinely to check fibrinolytic activity.
   b. be aware of and report signs or symptoms of bleeding.
   c. wear properly fitting, roomy shoes.
   d. report signs of nausea to the physician.

11. Pulmonary emboli often occur secondary to
   a. deep vein thrombophlebitis of the lower extremities.
   b. superficial thrombophlebitis.
   c. ventricular fibrillation.
   d. severe peripheral arterial disease.

12. Venous stasis ulcers
   a. are often chronic.
   b. are frequently infected.
   c. are associated with arterial disease.
   d. predispose to pulmonary emboli.

REFERENCES

1. Dalsing MC, Sawchuk AP: Surgery of the aorta. In Fahey VA, editor: *Vascular nursing,* ed 2, Philadelphia, 1994, Saunders.
2. Collin J, Murie J, Morris RJ: Two year prospective analysis of the Oxford experience with surgical treatment of abdominal aortic aneurysm, *Surg Gynecol Obstet* 169:527, 1989.
3. Doyle JE, Johantgen M, Vitello-Cicciu J: Vascular disease. In Kinney MR and others, editors: *AACN's clinical reference for critical-care nursing,* ed 3, St Louis, 1993, Mosby.
4. Webster NW and others: Abdominal aortic aneurysm: results of a family study, *J Vasc Surg* 13:366, 1991.
5. Powell J, Greenhalgh RM: Cellular enzymatic and genetic factors in the pathogenesis of abdominal aortic aneurysms, *J Vasc Surg* 9:297, 1989.
6. Cohn LH: Aortic dissection: new aspects of diagnosis and treatment, *Hosp Pract* 29:47, 1994.
7. Sarris GE, Miller DC: Peripheral vascular manifestations of acute aortic dissection. In Rutherford RD, editor: *Vascular surgery,* Philadelphia, 1989, Saunders.
8. Graham LM, Ford MB: Arterial disease. In Fahey VA, editor: *Vascular nursing,* ed 2, Philadelphia, 1994, Saunders.
9. Fellows E, Jocz AM: Getting the upper hand on lower extremity arterial disease, *Nursing* 21:34, 1991.
10. Bright LD, Georgi S: Peripheral vascular disease: is it arterial or venous? *Am J Nurs* 92:34, 1992.
11. Carpenter JP: Magnetic resonance angiography in peripheral artery disease, *Hosp Pract* 27:79, 1992.
12. Hiatt WR, Regensteiner JG: Nonsurgical management of peripheral arterial disease, *Hosp Pract* 27:59, 1992.
13. Ahn SS and others: Endovascular surgery, *Ann Surg* 216:1, 1992.
14. Nunnelee JD: Medications used in vascular patients. In Fahey VA, editor: *Vascular nursing,* ed 2, Philadelphia, 1994, Saunders.
15. Capasso VC, Cote K: The management of patients undergoing arterial reconstructive surgery, *Medsurg Nurs* 2:11, 1993.
16. Kannel WB: Cigarette smoking and peripheral arterial disease, *Prim Cardiol* 4:13, 1986.
17. Provan JL: The effect of cigarette smoking on the long-term success rates of aortofemoral and femoropopliteal reconstructions, *Surg Gynecol Obstet* 165:49, 1987.
18. Bachman JA: Pregnancy and thromboembolic disease, *J Soc Peripheral Vasc Nurs* 8:11, 1990.
19. Menzoian JO, Doyle JE: Venous insufficiency of the leg, *Hosp Pract* 24:109, 1989.
20. Margolis DJ. Management of venous ulcerations, *Hosp Pract* 27:32, 1992.
21. Mayberry JC and others: Nonoperative treatment of venous stasis ulcer. In Bergan JJ, Yao JST, editors: *Venous disorders,* Philadelphia, 1991, Saunders.
22. Cordts PR and others: A prospective, randomized trial of Unna's boot versus duoderm CGF hydroactive dressing plus compression in the management of venous leg ulcers, *J Vasc Surg* 15:480, 1992.
23. Goldhaber SZ: Managing pulmonary embolism, *Hosp Pract* 26:37, 1991.
24. Coffman JD: Venous thrombosis and the diagnosis of pulmonary emboli, *Hosp Pract* 27:99, 1992.

SECTION VII BIBLIOGRAPHY

Books

Birkenhager WH, editor: *Practical management of hypertension,* Boston, 1990, Kluwer Academic.

Douglas PS, editor: *Cardiovascular health and disease in women,* Philadelphia, 1993, WB Saunders.

Evans M J: *Cardiovascular nursing,* ed 2, Springhouse, Pa, 1994, Springhouse.

Ewy GA, Bressler, editors: *Cardiovascular drugs and the management of heart disease,* ed 2, New York, 1992, Raven.

Fardy PS: *Cardiac rehabilitation, adult fitness, and exercise testing,* ed 3, Baltimore, 1995, Williams & Wilkins.

Hurst JW and others, editors: *The heart, arteries, and veins,* ed 7, New York, 1990, McGraw-Hill.

Opie LH, editor: *Drugs for the heart,* ed 3, Philadelphia, 1991, WB Saunders.

Purdy RE: *Handbook of cardiac drugs,* ed 2, Boston, 1994, Little, Brown.

Singh BN, editor: *Cardiovascular pharmacology and therapeutics,* New York, 1994, Churchill Livingstone.

Zorb SL: *Cardiovascular diagnostic testing. A nursing guide,* Gaithersburg, Md, 1991, Aspen.

Journals

Akhtan M and others: Atrioventricular nodal reentry: clinical, electrophysiological, and therapeutic considerations, *Circulation* 88:282, 1993.

*Artinian NT and others: Age differences in patient recovery patterns following coronary artery bypass surgery, *Am J Crit Care* 2:453, 1993.

*Artinian NT: Spouse adaptation to mate's CABG surgery: 1-year follow up. *Am J Crit Care* 1:28, 1992.

*Ascherio A and others: A prospective study of nutritional factors and hypertension among US men, *Circulation* 86:1475, 1992.

Banasik JL: Endothelins: new players in cardiovascular physiology and disease, *J Cardiovasc Nurs* 8:87, 1994.

*Nursing research-based articles.

*Barkman A, Lunse CP: The effect of early ambulation on patient comfort and delayed bleeding after cardiac angiogram: a pilot study, *Heart Lung* 23:112, 1994.

Bennett B, Singh S: Management of ventricular arrhythmias: then and now, *Am J Crit Care* 1:107, 1992.

Bevans M, McLimore E: Intracoronary stents: a new approach to coronary artery dilatation, *J Cardiovasc Nurs* 7:34, 1992.

*Blohon RM, Tyrala M: Development of an instrument to assess patient knowledge of cardiac catheterization, *Can J Cardiovasc Nurs* 4:16, 1993.

Boehm J and others: Cardiopulmonary resuscitation standards: the 1992 Dartmouth experience in review, *AANA J* 61:463, 1993.

Boltz MA: Nurse's guide to identifying cardiac rhythms, *Nursing* 24:54, 1994.

Braun AE: Emergency cardiac care. A quick response to life-threatening arrhythmias, *RN* 57:54, 1994.

Braun AE: Emergency cardiac care: when arrest is imminent, *RN* 57:22, 1994.

*Brenner ZR: Patient's learning priorities for reoperative coronary artery bypass surgery, *J Cardiovasc Nurs* 7:1, 1993.

Brown KK: Boosting the failing heart with inotropic drugs, *Nursing* 23:34, 1993.

Charlton MR: A cardiac rehabilitation compliance assessment tool, *Rehabil Nurs* 18:179, 1993.

Christensen MA, Sutton KR: Myocardial contusion: new concepts in diagnosis and management, *Am J Crit Care* 2:28, 1993.

Clark BK: Beta-adrenergic blocking agents: their current status, *AACN Clin Issues Crit Care Nurs* 3:447, 1992.

Clements JV: Sympathomimetics, inotropes, and vasodilators, *AACN Clin Issues Crit Care Nurs* 3:395, 1992.

*Collins, MA: When your patient has an implantable cardioverter defibrillator, *Am J Nurs* 94:34, 1994.

Coombs M: Haemodynamic profiles and the critical care nurse, *Intensive Crit Care Nurs* 9:11, 1993.

Crammer MB, Carter V: Critical pathways—the pivotal tool, *J Cardiovasc Nurs* 7:30, 1993.

Cross JA: Pharmacologic management of heart failure: positive inotropic agents, *Crit Care Nurs Clin North Am* 5:589, 1993.

Crouch MA: Urokinase therapy in mesenteric venous thrombosis: a case study, *J Vasc Nurs* 11:99, 1993.

*Crumlish C: Coping and emotion in women undergoing cardiac surgery: a preliminary study, *MEDSURG Nurs* 2:283, 1993.

*Crumlish CM: Coping and emotional response in cardiac surgery patients, *West J Nurs Res* 16:57, 1994.

Cuny T, Enger EL: Medical management of chronic heart failure: direct acting vasodilation and diuretic agents, *Crit Care Nurs Clin North Am* 5:575, 1993.

Darling EJ: Overview of cardiac electrophysiologic testing, *Crit Care Nurs Clin North Am* 6:1, 1994.

*Davis TM and others: Preparing adult patients for cardiac catheterization: informational treatment and coping style interactions, *Heart Lung* 23:130, 1994.

Doering LV: The effect of positioning on hemodynamics and gas exchange in the critically ill: a review, *Am J Crit Care* 2:208, 1993.

*Dracup K and others: Is cardiopulmonary resuscitation training deleterious for family members of cardiac patients? *Am J Public Health* 84:116, 1994.

Dull S and others: Expected death and unwanted resuscitation in the prehospital setting, *Ann Emerg Med* 23:997, 1994.

*Engler MB: Vascular effects of omega-3 fatty acids: possible therapeutic mechanisms in cardiovascular disease, *J Cardiovasc Nurs* 8:53, 1994.

Epstein CD: Changing interpretations of angina pectoris associated with transient myocardial ischemia, *J Cardiovasc Nurs* 7:1, 1992.

Fabius DB: Diagnosing and treating ventricular tachycardia, *J Cardiovasc Nurs* 7:8, 1993.

*Ferguson JA: Pain following coronary artery bypass grafting: a exploration of contributing factors, *Intensive Crit Care Nurs* 8:153, 1992.

Fitzgerald CA: Current perspectives on prosthetic heart valves and valve repair, *AACN Clin Issues Crit Care Nurs* 4:228, 1993.

*Fitzsimmons L, Verderber A, Shively M: Enhancing sleep following coronary artery bypass graft surgery, *J Cardiovasc Nurs* 7:86, 1993.

Foley JJ: Significant changes in advanced cardiac life support medication guidelines, *J Emerg Nurs* 19:516, 1993.

Gavras I, Gavras H: ACE inhibitors: a decade of clinical experience, *Hosp Pract* 28:117, 1993.

*Gawlinski A: Effect of positioning on mixed venous oxygen saturation, *J Cardiovasc Nurs* 7:71, 1993.

Gilski DJ: Controversies in patient management after cardiac surgery, *J Cardiovasc Nurs* 7:1, 1993.

Goodliffe C, Sutcliffe R: Cardiac pacing: a clinical update, *Nurs Stand* 7:37, 1993.

*Goodnough-Hanneman SK: Multidimensional predictors of success or failure with early weaning from mechanical ventilation after cardiac surgery, *Nurs Res* 43:4, 1994.

*Gortner SR and others: Elders' expected and realized benefits from cardiac surgery, *Cardiovasc Nurs* 30:9, 1994.

*Grady KL: Quality of life in patients with chronic heart failure, *Crit Care Nurs Clin North Am* 5:661, 1993.

Grillo JA, Gonzalez ER: Changes in the pharmacotherapy of CPR, *Heart Lung* 22:548, 1993.

*Hanneman SK: Multidimensional predictors of success or failure with early weaning from mechanical ventilation after cardiac surgery, *Nurs Res* 43:4, 1994.

*Hawthorne MH: Gender differences in recovery after coronary artery surgery, *Image J Nurs Sch* 26:75, 1994.

*Hawthorne MH: Women recovering from coronary artery bypass surgery, *Scholar Inq Nurs Pract* 7:223, 1993.

*Hawthorne MH, Hixon ME: Functional status, mood disturbance and quality of life in patients with heart failure, *Prog Cardiovasc Nurs* 9:22, 1994.

Higgins SS, Reid A: Common congenital heart defects. Long-term follow-up, *Nurs Clin North Am* 29:233, 1994.

Hix CD: Magnesium in congestive heart failure, acute myocardial infarction, and dysrhythmias, *J Cardiovasc Nurs* 8:19, 1993.

*Holl RM: Role-modeled visiting compared with restricted visiting on surgical cardiac patients and family members, *Crit Care Nurs* 16:70, 1993.

*Jaeger AA and others: Functional capacity after cardiac surgery in elderly patients, *J Am Coll Cardiol* 24:104, 1994.

Joffres MR and others: Prevalence, control and awareness of high blood pressure among Canadian adults, *Can Med Assoc J* 146:1997, 1992.

Johannsen JM: Update: guidelines for treating hypertension, *Am J Nurs* 93:42, 1993.

*Keeling AW and others: Postcardiac catheterization time-in-bed study: enhancing patient comfort through nursing research, *Appl Nurs Res* 7:14, 1994.

*King KM, Jensen L: Preserving the self: women having cardiac surgery, *Heart Lung* 23:99, 1994.

Kuhn M: Angiotensin-converting enzyme inhibitors, *AACN Clin Issues Crit Care Nurs* 3:461, 1992.

Kuhn M: Nitrates, *AACN Clin Issues Crit Care Nurs* 3:409, 1992.

Lanuza DM, Dunbar SB: Circadian rhythms: implications for cardiovascular nursing and drug therapy, *J Cardiovasc Nurs* 8:63, 1993.

Ley SJ: Myocardial depression after cardiac surgery: pharmacologic and mechanical support, *AACN Clin Issues Crit Care Nurs* 4:293, 1993.

Low K: Recovery from myocardial infarction and coronary artery bypass surgery in women: psychosocial factors, *J Womens Health* 2:133, 1993.

Mackintosh C: Non-reporting of cardiac pain, *Nurs Times* 90:36, 1994.

*McKee DR, Wynne G, Evans TR: An evaluation of a training programme for third year student nurses in the use of an automatic external defibrillator, *Resuscitation* 27:35, 1994.

Moroney DA, Reedy JE: Understanding ventricular assist devices: a self-study guide, *J Cardiovasc Nurs* 8:1, 1994.

*Noll ML: Pulse oximetry in the postoperative care of cardiac surgical patients: a randomized clinical trial, *Heart Lung* 22:278, 1993.

Owen H: Cardiology update. Mobile cardiac catheterisation, *Nurs Stand* 8:55, 1994.

Packer M: Pathophysiology of chronic heart failure, *Lancet* 340:88, 1992.

Pier A: Using mixed venous oxygen saturation data to trend overall oxygenation in cardiothoracic surgical patients, *Crit Care Nurs Q* 16:72, 1993.

*Prevost S, Deshotels A: Quality of life after cardiac surgery, *AACN Clin Issues Crit Care Nurs* 4:320, 1993.

*Puntillo K, Weiss SJ: Pain: its mediators and associated morbidity in critically ill cardiovascular surgical patients, *Nurs Res* 43:31, 1994.

Radford KA: Wound complications after cardiac surgery: a new approach to healing by secondary intention, *J Cardiovasc Nurs* 7:82, 1993.

*Recker D: Patient perception of preoperative cardiac surgical teaching done pre- and postadmission, *Crit Care Nurse* 14:52, 1994.

Redberg R and others: Physiology of blood flow during cardiopulmonary resuscitation: a transesophageal echocardiographic study, *Circulation* 88:534, 1993.

*Rukholm E, McGirr M: A quality-of-life index for clients with ischemic heart disease: establishing reliability and validity, *Rehabil Nurs* 19:12, 1994.

Ruzevich S: Heart assist devices: state of the art, *Crit Care Nurs Clin North Am* 3:723, 1991.

Snyder SL: Nurses and clinical trials, *J Cardiovasc Nurs* 8:86, 1994.

Starr LM: Emergency oxygen: What? Who? When? *AAOHN J* 42:15, 1994.

Stewart S: Acute MI: a review of the pathophysiology, treatment, and complications, *Cardiovasc Nurs* 6:1, 1992.

Sullivan MJ: New trends in cardiac rehabilitation in patients with chronic heart failure, *Prog Cardiovasc Nurs* 9:13, 1994.

Tapp DM: Family protectiveness: a response to ischemic heart disease, *Can J Cardiovasc Nurs* 4:4, 1993.

Teplitz L, Siwik DA: Cellular signals in artherosclerosis, *J Cardiovasc Nurs* 8:28, 1994.

Trottier DJ, Kochar MS: Hypertension and high cholesterol: a dangerous synergy, *Am J Nurs* 92:40, 1992.

Vaska PL: The clinical nurse specialist in cardiovascular surgery: a new twist, *AACN Clin Issues Crit Care Nurs* 4:637, 1993.

Verderber A, Shively M, Fitzsimmons L: Preparation for cardiac catheterization, *J Cardiovasc Nurs* 7:75, 1992.

*Verderber A, Shively M, Fitzsimmons L: Post-cardiac surgery patterns of social and sexual activity, *J Cardiovasc Nurs* 7:88, 1993.

Warren JJ: Ethical concerns about noncompliance in the chronically ill patients, *Prog Cardiovasc Nurs* 7:10, 1992.

White P: Calcium channel blockers, *AACN Clin Issues Crit Care Nurs* 3:437, 1992.

Witherell CL: Cardiac rhythm control devices, *Crit Care Nurs Clin North Am* 6:85, 1994.

Wolfensperger-Bashford C: When a patient survives sudden cardiac death, *RN* 57:34, 1994.

Woo MA: Sudden cardiac death in patients with heart failure, *Crit Care Nurs Clin North Am* 5:609, 1993.

Woods SL, Osguthorpe S: Cardiac output determination, *AACN Clin Issues Crit Care Nurs* 4:81, 1993.

Yontz LL: Congestive heart failure: early recognition of congestive heart failure in the primary care setting, *J Am Acad Nurse Pract* 6:273, 1994.

Zeigler VL: Postoperative rhythm disturbances, *Crit Care Nurs Clin North Am* 6:227, 1994.

*Zeler KM, McPharlane TJ, Salamonsen RF: Effectiveness of nursing involvement in bedside monitoring and control of coagulation status after cardiac surgery, *Am J Crit Care* 1:70, 1992.

Organizations

American Association of Critical Care Nurses (AACN)
One Civic Plaza, Suite 330
Newport Beach, CA 92660
714-644-9310

American Heart Association
National Center
7320 Greenville Avenue
Dallas, TX 75231
214-373-6300

The Coronary Club
Cleveland Clinic Education Foundation
9500 Euclid Avenue, Ste. E4-15
Cleveland, OH 44195
216-444-3690

Council of Cardiovascular Nurses
American Heart Association
7320 Greenville Avenue
Dallas, TX 75231
214-373-6300

High Blood Pressure Information Center
4733 Bethesda Avenue, Ste. 530
Bethesda, MD 20814
301-951-3260

Medic Alert Foundation
P.O. Box 1009
Turlock, CA 95381-1009
209-668-3333

The Mended Hearts, Inc.
7320 Greenville Avenue
Dallas, TX 75231
214-373-6300

National Heart, Lung, and Blood Institute
National Institutes of Health
9000 Rockville Pike
Building 31, Room 4A21
Bethesda, MD 20892
301-496-4236

Society for Vascular Nursing
309 Winter Street
Norwood, MA 02062
617-762-3630
FAX: 617-762-5582

AHCPR Guidelines

Guides developed and published by The Agency for Health Care Policy and Research (AHCPR). The Patient Guides are available in English and Spanish. The guidelines can be obtained by writing to: Center for Research Dissemination and Liaison, AHCPR Clearinghouse, P.O. Box 8547, Silver Spring, Md 20907, or by calling 1-800-358-9295. The Guidelines are as follows:

Unstable angina: diagnosis and management, Clinical Practice Guideline. AHCPR Publ. No. 92-0602.

Diagnosing and managing unstable angina. Quick Reference Guide for Clinicians. AHCPR Pub. No. 92-0603.

Managing unstable angina. A Patient and Family Guide. AHCPR Pub. No. 92-0604.

Heart Failure: Management of Patients with Left-Ventricular Systolic Dysfunction. Guideline Overview. AHCPR Pub. No. 94-0610.

Heart Failure: Management of Patients with Left-Ventricular Systolic Dysfunction. Quick Reference Guide for Clinicians, No. 11. AHCPR Pub. No. 94-0613.

Living with Heart Disease: Is It Heart Failure? Patient Guide. AHCPR Pub. No. 94-0614.

PROBLEMS *of* INGESTION, DIGESTION, ABSORPTION, & ELIMINATION

Section Eight

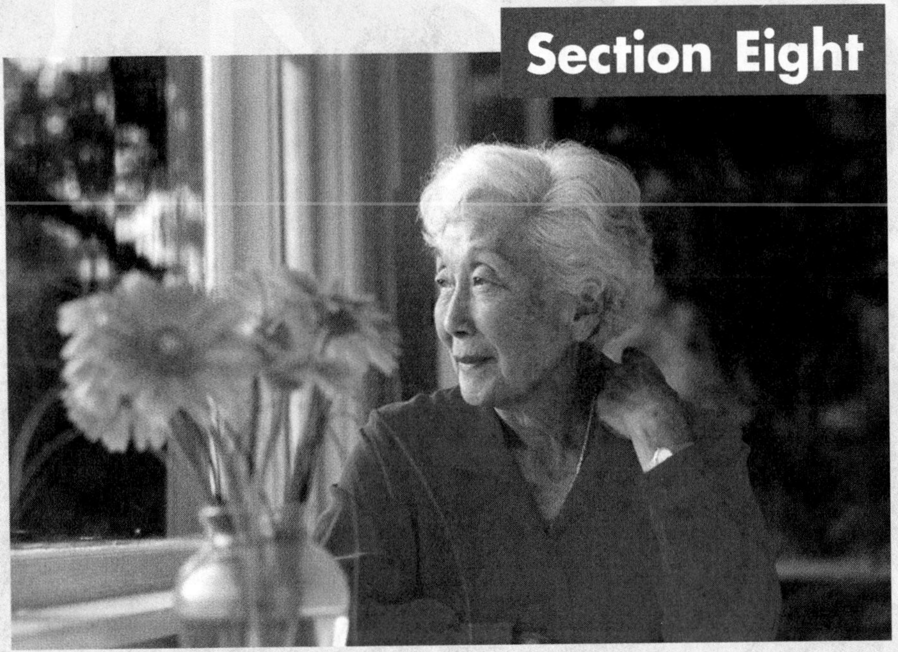

MEDICAL
SURGICAL
NURSING
MEDICAL
SURGICAL
NURSING
MEDICAL
SURGICAL
NURSING
MEDICAL
SURGICAL

Chapter 36

NURSING ASSESSMENT
Gastrointestinal System

Rachel Elrod

Learning Objectives

1. Describe the structures and functions of the organs of the gastrointestinal tract.
2. Describe the structures and functions of the liver, gallbladder, biliary tract, and pancreas.
3. Explain the processes of ingestion, digestion, absorption, and elimination.
4. Explain the processes of biliary metabolism, bile production, and bile excretion.
5. Describe age-related changes in the gastrointestinal system and differences in assessment findings.
6. Identify the significant subjective and objective data related to the gastrointestinal system that should be obtained from a patient.
7. Describe the appropriate techniques used in the physical assessment of the gastrointestinal system.
8. Differentiate normal from common abnormal findings of a physical assessment of the gastrointestinal system.
9. Describe the purpose, significance of results, and nursing responsibilities related to diagnostic studies of the gastrointestinal system.

The main function of the gastrointestinal (GI) system is to supply nutrients to body cells. This is accomplished through the processes of *ingestion* (taking in food), *digestion* (breakdown of food), and *absorption* (transfer of food products into circulation). *Elimination* is the process of excreting the waste products of digestion.

The GI system (also called the *digestive system*) consists of the GI tract and its associated organs. Included in the GI tract are the mouth, esophagus, stomach, small intestine, and large intestine. The associated organs are the liver, pancreas, and gallbladder (Fig. 36-1).

Psychologic or emotional factors, such as stress and anxiety, influence GI functioning in many people. Stress may be manifested as anorexia, epigastric and abdominal pain, or diarrhea. However, GI problems should never be solely attributed to psychologic factors. Organic and psychologically based problems can exist independently or concurrently. Physical factors, such as dietary intake, ingestion of alcohol and caffeine-containing products, cigarette smoking, and fatigue, may also affect GI function. Some organic diseases of the GI system, such as peptic ulcer disease and ulcerative colitis, may be aggravated by stress. Thus both physical and emotional factors affect GI function.

Reviewed by Peggi Guenter, PhD, RN, CNSN, Coordinator, Nutrition Support Service, The Graduate Hospital, Department of Surgery, Philadelphia, PA.

STRUCTURES AND FUNCTIONS OF THE GASTROINTESTINAL SYSTEM

The GI tract is a tube approximately 30 feet (9 m) long extending from the mouth to the anus. The entire tract is composed of four common layers. From the inside to the outside, these layers are (1) *mucosa,* (2) *submucosa,* (3) *muscle,* and (4) *serosa* (Fig. 36-2). In the esophagus the outer coat is fibrous tissue rather than serosa. The muscular coat consists of two layers: the *circular* (inner) and the *longitudinal* (outer).

The GI tract is innervated by the parasympathetic and the sympathetic branches of the autonomic nervous system. The parasympathetic system is mainly excitatory, and the sympathetic system is mainly inhibitory. For example, peristalsis is increased by parasympathetic stimulation and decreased by sympathetic stimulation. Pain is relayed through sensory fibers of the sympathetic nervous system.

The GI tract also has its own nervous system, the *enteric nervous system.* The enteric nervous system is composed of two nerve layers that lie between the mucosa and the circular muscle layer and the circular and longitudinal muscle layers. These neurons contribute to the coordination of GI motor and secretory activities.

The GI tract and accessory organs receive approximately 25% to 30% of the cardiac output. Circulation in the GI system is unique in that venous blood draining the GI tract organs empties into the portal vein, which then perfuses the liver. The upper portion of the GI tract receives its blood supply from the splanchnic artery. The small intestine receives

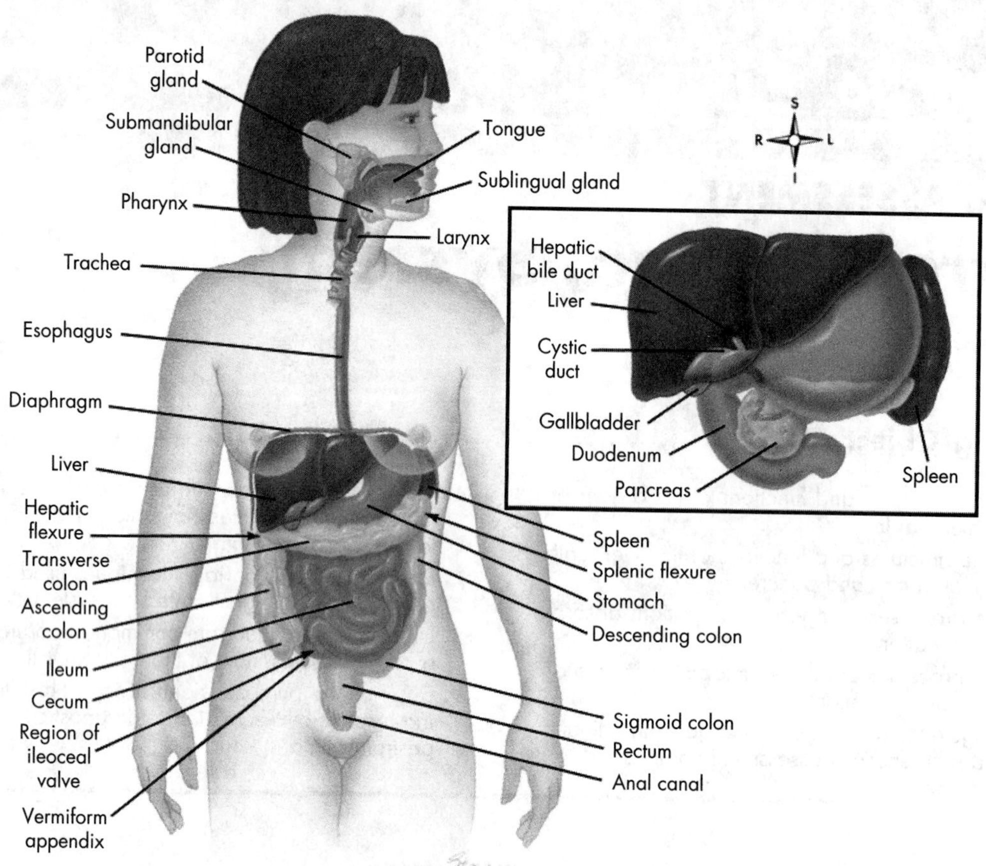

Fig. 36-1 Location of organs of gastrointestinal system.

its blood supply from branches of the hepatic and superior mesenteric artery. The large intestine receives its blood supply mainly from the superior and inferior mesenteric arteries. Because such a large percentage of the cardiac output perfuses these organs, the GI tract is a major source from which blood flow can be diverted during exercise or stress.

The two types of movement of the GI tract are *mixing* and *propulsion.* These movements are accomplished by segmentation and peristalsis. The secretions of the GI system consist of enzymes and hormones for digestion, mucus to provide protection and lubrication, and water and electrolytes.

The abdominal organs are almost completely covered by the *peritoneum.* The two layers of the peritoneum are the *parietal,* which lines the abdominal cavity wall, and the *visceral,* which covers the abdominal organs. The peritoneal cavity is the potential space between the parietal and visceral layers. The two folds of the peritoneum are the *mesentery* and *omentum.* The mesentery attaches the small intestine and part of the large intestine to the posterior abdominal wall and contains blood and lymph vessels. The lesser omentum goes from the lesser curvature of the stomach and upper duodenum to the liver, and the greater omentum hangs from the stomach over the intestines like an apron. The omentum contains fat and lymph nodes.

The primary functions of the GI system are (1) ingestion and propulsion (movement) of food, (2) digestion, (3) absorption, and (4) elimination. Each part of the GI system performs different activities to accomplish these functions.

Ingestion and Propulsion of Food

Ingestion is the intake of food. A person's appetite or desire to ingest food is a significant factor in how much food is eaten. Multiple factors are involved in the control of appetite. An appetite center is located in the hypothalamus. It is directly or indirectly stimulated by hypoglycemia, an empty stomach, decrease in body temperature, and input from higher brain centers. The sight, smell, and taste of food frequently stimulate appetite. Appetite may be inhibited by stomach distention, illness (especially accompanied by fever), hyperglycemia, nausea and vomiting, and certain drugs (e.g., amphetamines).

Deglutition (swallowing) is the mechanical component of ingestion. The organs involved in the deglutition of food are the mouth, pharynx, and esophagus.

Mouth. The mouth consists of the lips and oral (*buccal*) cavity. The lips surround the orifice of the mouth and function in speech. The roof of the oral cavity is formed by the hard and soft palate. The oral cavity contains the teeth, used in *mastication* (chewing), and the tongue. The tongue is a solid muscle mass and assists in mastication by keeping food between the teeth during chewing and moving the food to the back of the throat for swallowing (deglutition).

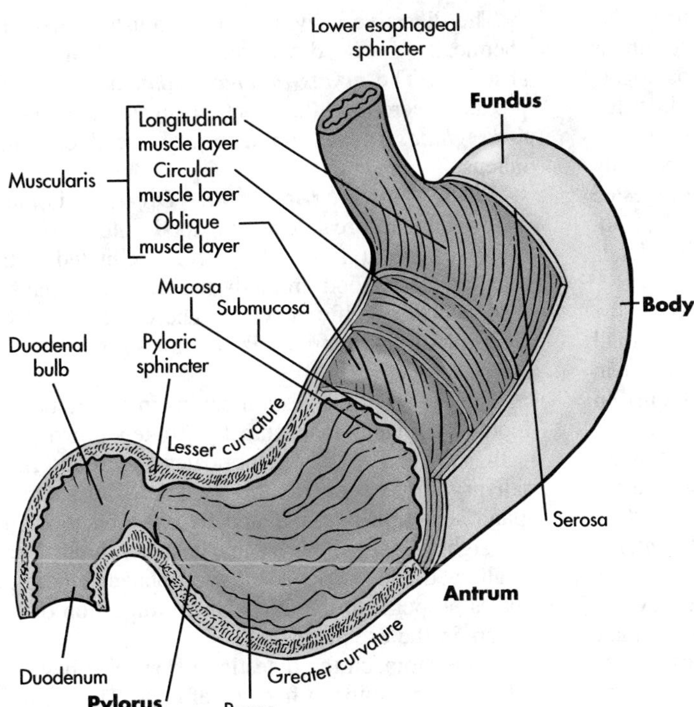

Fig. 36-2 Parts of the stomach.

Taste receptors are found on the sides and tip of the tongue. The tongue is also important in speech.

Within the oral cavity are three pairs of salivary glands: the *parotid, submaxillary,* and *sublingual.* These glands produce saliva, which consists of water, protein, mucin, inorganic salts, and salivary amylase. Approximately 1 liter of saliva is produced each day.

Pharynx. The pharynx is a musculomembranous tube that may be divided into the *nasopharynx, oropharynx,* and *laryngeal pharynx.* The mucous membrane of the pharynx is continuous with the nasal cavity, mouth, auditory tubes, and larynx. The oropharynx secretes mucus, which aids in swallowing. The *epiglottis* is a lid of fibrocartilage that closes over the larynx during swallowing. During ingestion the oropharynx provides a route for the food from the mouth to the esophagus. When receptors in the oropharynx are stimulated by food or liquid, the swallowing reflex is initiated.

Esophagus. The esophagus is a hollow, muscular tube that receives food from the pharynx and moves it to the stomach by peristaltic contractions. It is 9.2 to 10.0 inches (23 to 25 cm) long and 0.8 inches (2 cm) in diameter. The esophagus is located in the thoracic cavity and starts behind the trachea at the lower end of the pharynx and extends to the stomach. The upper one third of the esophagus is composed of striated skeletal muscle and the distal two thirds is composed of smooth muscle.

With swallowing, the *upper esophageal sphincter* (cricopharyngeal muscle) relaxes and a peristaltic wave moves the bolus into the esophagus. The muscular layers contract (peristalsis) and propel the food to the stomach. The *lower esophageal sphincter* (LES) at the distal end of the esophagus remains contracted except during swallowing, belching, or vomiting. The LES is an important barrier that prevents reflux of acidic gastric contents into the esophagus.

Digestion and Absorption

Mouth. Digestion begins in the mouth. It involves both mechanical (mastication) and chemical digestion. Saliva is the first secretion involved in digestion, and its main function is to lubricate and soften the food mass, thus facilitating swallowing. Saliva contains *amylase* (ptyalin), which hydrolyzes starches to maltose. However, salivary amylase is not necessary for the digestion of carbohydrates.

Stomach. The functions of the stomach are to store food, mix the food with gastric secretions, and empty contents into the small intestine at a rate in which digestion can occur. The stomach only absorbs small amounts of water, alcohol, electrolytes, and certain drugs.

The stomach lies obliquely in the epigastric, umbilical, and left hypochondriac regions of the abdomen (see Fig. 36-7). The shape and position of the stomach changes based on the degree of gastric distention. It always contains gastric fluid and mucus. The three main parts of the stomach are the *fundus, body,* and *antrum* (see Fig. 36-2). The pylorus is a small portion of the antrum that lies proximal to the pyloric sphincter. Sphincter muscles guard the entrance to and exit from the stomach. The LES is the opening between the esophagus and stomach; the pyloric sphincter is between the stomach and the duodenum.

The serous (outer) layer of the stomach is formed by the peritoneum. The muscular layer consists of the longitudinal (outer) layer, circular (middle) layer, and the oblique (inner) layer. The mucosal layer forms folds called *rugae* that contain many small glands. In response to nutrient intake, these glands secrete most of the gastric juice. In the fundus the glands contain chief cells, which secrete pepsinogen, and parietal cells, which secrete hydrochloric acid, water, and the intrinsic factor. The secretion of hydrochloric acid makes gastric juice acidic in comparison to other body fluids. This acidic pH aids in the protection against ingested organisms. The intrinsic factor promotes vitamin B_{12} absorption in the small intestine. Mucus is secreted by glands in the cardiac and pyloric areas.

Small Intestine. The two primary functions of the small intestine are digestion and absorption. The small intestine is a coiled tube approximately 23 feet (7 m) in length and from 1 to 1.1 inch (2.5 cm to 2.8 cm) in diameter, diminishing in diameter at the lower end. It extends from the pylorus to the ileocecal valve. The small intestine is composed of the *duodenum, jejunum,* and *ileum.* The ileocecal valve, which separates the small intestine from the large intestine, prevents reflux of colonic contents into the small intestine.

The serous coat of the small intestine is formed by the peritoneum. The mucosa is thick, vascular, and glandular. The circular folds in the mucous and submucous layers provide a greater surface area for digestion and absorption.

The functional units of the small intestine are *villi.* They are present in the entire small intestine. Villi are minute, fingerlike projections in the mucous membrane. They contain goblet cells that secrete mucus and epithelial cells that produce the intestinal digestive enzymes. The epithelial cells on the villi also have microvilli, which compose the *brush border.* Thus the presence of villi and microvilli greatly increases the surface area for absorption.

The digestive enzymes on the brush border of the villi chemically break down nutrients so that they can be absorbed. The *crypts of Lieberkühn,* or intestinal glands, produce secretions that contain digestive enzymes. *Brunner's glands* in the submucosa of the duodenum secrete mucus.

Physiology of Digestion. *Digestion* is the physical and chemical breakdown of food into absorbable substances. Digestion in the GI tract is facilitated by the timely movement of food through the various organs and the secretion of specific enzymes. These enzymes break down foodstuffs to appropriate size particles for absorption (Table 36-1).

The process of digestion begins in the mouth where the food is chewed, mechanically broken down, and mixed with saliva. The saliva lubricates the food. In addition, salivary amylase begins the breakdown of starch. Salivary gland secretion is stimulated by chewing movements and the sight, smell, thought, and taste of food. The food is swallowed and passes into the esophagus where peristaltic waves propel it to the stomach. No digestion or absorption occurs in the esophagus.

In the stomach the digestion of proteins begins with the release of pepsinogen from chief cells. The acidic environment of the stomach results in the conversion of pepsinogen to its active form, pepsin. Pepsin begins the initial breakdown of proteins. In the stomach there is minimal digestion of starches and fats. The food is mixed with gastric secretions, which are under neural and hormonal control (Tables 36-2 and 36-3). The stomach also serves as a reservoir for food, which is slowly expelled into the small intestine. The length of time food remains in the stomach

Table 36-1 Gastrointestinal Secretions Related to Digestion

Location	Daily Amount (ml)	Secretion/Enzymes	Action
Salivary glands	1000-1500	Salivary amylase (ptyalin)	Initiation of starch digestion
Stomach	2500	Pepsinogen	Protein digestion
		HCl	Protein digestion
		Lipase	Fat digestion
		Intrinsic factor	Essential for vitamin B_{12} absorption in ileum
Small intestine	3000	Enterokinase	Activation of trypsinogen to trypsin
		Amylase	Carbohydrate digestion
		Peptidases	Protein digestion
		Aminopeptidase	Protein digestion
		Maltase	Maltose to 2 glucose molecules
		Sucrase	Sucrose to glucose and fructose
		Lactase	Lactose to glucose and galactose
		Lipase	Fat digestion
Pancreas	700	Trypsinogen	Protein digestion
		Chymotrypsin	Protein digestion
		Amylase	Starch to disaccharides
		Lipase	Fat digestion
Liver and gallbladder	1000	Bile	Emulsification of fats and aid in absorption of fatty acids and fat-soluble vitamins (A, D, E, K)

Table 36-2 Phases of Gastric Secretion

Phase	Stimulus to Secretion	Secretion
Cephalic (nervous)	Sight, smell, taste of food (before food enters stomach); initiated in the CNS and mediated by the vagus nerve	Hydrochloric acid, pepsinogen, mucus
Gastric (hormonal and nervous)	Food in antrum of stomach, vagal stimulation	Release of gastrin hormone from antrum into circulation to stimulate gastric secretions and motility
Intestinal (hormonal)	Presence of chyme in small intestine	Acidic chyme (pH <2) release of secretin, gastric inhibitory polypeptide, cholecystokinin into circulation to decrease acid secretion Chyme (pH >3) release of duodenal gastrin to increase secretion

CNS, Central nervous system.

depends on the composition of the food, but average meals remain from 3 to 4 hours.

Digestion is completed in the small intestine, where carbohydrates are hydrolyzed to monosaccharides, fats to glycerol and fatty acids, and proteins to amino acids. The physical presence of *chyme* (food mixed with gastric secretions), along with its chemical nature in the small intestine, stimulates motility and secretion. Secretions involved in digestion include enzymes from the pancreas, bile from the liver (see Table 36-1), and intestinal secretions from glands in the small intestine. Both secretion and motility are under neural and hormonal control.

When food enters the stomach and small intestine, hormones are released into the bloodstream (Table 36-3). The hormone *secretin* stimulates the pancreas to secrete fluid with a high concentration of bicarbonate. This alkaline secretion enters the duodenum and neutralizes acid in the chyme. The duodenal mucosa also secretes mucus to protect against the hydrochloric acid. In response to the presence of chyme, the hormone *cholecystokinin* (CCK), produced by the duodenal mucosa, enters the bloodstream and stimulates contraction of the gallbladder and relaxation of the sphincter of Oddi. These actions permit bile to flow from the common bile duct into the duodenum. Bile is necessary for the digestion of fats. CCK also stimulates the pancreas to synthesize and secrete enzymes for enzymatic digestion of carbohydrates, fats, and proteins.

Enzymes present on the brush border of the microvilli complete the digestion process. These enzymes hydrolyze disaccharides to monosaccharides and peptides to amino acids for absorption.

Absorption is the transfer of the end products of digestion across the intestinal wall to the circulation. Most absorption occurs in the small intestine. The surface area of the small intestine is greatly increased by its circular folds, villi, and microvilli. The movement of the villi provides for exposure of the end products of digestion to be in contact with the absorbing membrane. Monosaccharides (from carbohydrates), fatty acids (from fats), amino acids (from proteins), water, electrolytes, and vitamins are absorbed.

Elimination

Large Intestine. The large intestine is a hollow muscular tube approximately 5 to 6 feet (1.5 to 2 m) long and 2 inches (5 cm) in diameter. The four parts of the large intestine are (1) the *cecum* and *appendix,* a narrow tube at

Table 36-3 Major Hormones Controlling Gastrointestinal Secretion and Motility

Hormone	Source	Activating Stimuli	Function
Gastrin	Gastric and duodenal mucosa	Stomach distention, partially digested proteins in pylorus	Gastric acid secretion, increased motility, maintenance of lower esophageal sphincter tone
Secretin	Duodenal mucosa	Acid entering small intestine	Inhibition of gastric motility and acid secretion, pancreatic bicarbonate secretion
Cholecystokinin	Duodenal mucosa	Fatty acids and amino acids in small intestine	Contraction of gallbladder and relaxation of sphincter of Oddi, allowing increased flow of bile into duodenum; release of pancreatic digestive enzymes
Gastric inhibitory peptide	Duodenal mucosa	Fatty acids and lipids in the small intestine	Inhibition of gastric acid secretion and gastric motility

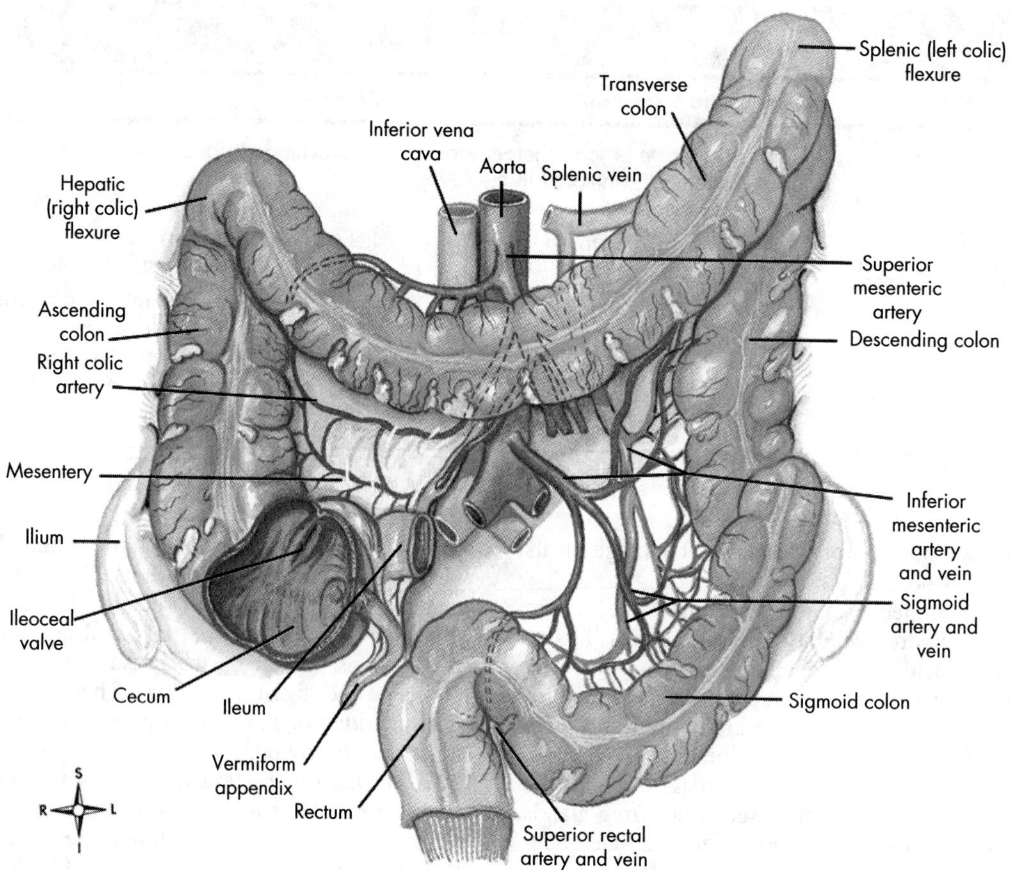

Fig. 36-3 Anatomic locations of the large intestine.

the end of the cecum; (2) the *colon* (ascending colon on the right side, transverse colon across the abdomen, descending colon on the left side, and the sigmoid colon); (3) the *rectum;* and (4) the *anus,* the terminal portion of the large intestine (Fig. 36-3).

The most important function of the large intestine is the absorption of water and electrolytes. It also forms feces and serves as a reservoir for the fecal mass until defecation occurs. Feces is composed of water (75%), bacteria, unabsorbed minerals, undigested foodstuffs, bile pigments, and desquamated epithelial cells. The large intestine secretes mucus, which acts as a lubricant and protects the mucosa.

Microorganisms in the colon are responsible for the breakdown of proteins not digested or absorbed in the small intestine. These amino acids are deaminated by the bacteria, leaving ammonia, which is carried to the liver and converted to urea. Bacteria in the colon also synthesize vitamin K and some of the B vitamins. Bacteria also play a part in the production of flatus.

The movements of the large intestine are usually slow. When the circular muscles contract, they produce an empty, kneading action called *haustral churning.* Propulsive (*mass movements*) peristalsis also occurs. When food enters the stomach and duodenum, the gastrocolic and duodenocolic reflexes are initiated, resulting in peristalsis in the colon. These reflexes are more active after the first daily meal and frequently result in bowel evacuation.

Defecation is a reflex action involving voluntary and involuntary control. Feces in the rectum stimulate sensory nerve endings that produce the desire to defecate. The reflex center for defecation is in the sacral portion of the spinal cord (parasympathetic nerve fibers). These fibers produce contraction of the rectum and relaxation of the internal anal sphincter. When the desire to defecate is felt, the external anal sphincter relaxes voluntarily. Defecation is controlled voluntarily by relaxing the external anal sphincter.

Defecation can be facilitated by the Valsalva maneuver. This maneuver involves contraction of the chest muscles on a closed glottis with simultaneous contraction of the abdominal muscles. These actions result in an increased intraabdominal pressure. The Valsalva maneuver is contraindicated in the patient with a head injury, eye surgery, cardiac problems, or liver cirrhosis with portal hypertension. Constipation is common in the older adult and is due to many factors including slower peristalsis, inactivity, decreased dietary fiber, decreased fluids, depression, constipating medications, and laxative abuse (see Chapter 40).[1]

Liver, Biliary Tract, and Pancreas

Liver. The liver is the largest internal organ in the body, weighing approximately 3 lb (1.36 kg) in the adult. It lies in the right hypochondriac and epigastric regions (see Fig. 36-7). Most of the liver is enclosed in peritoneum. It

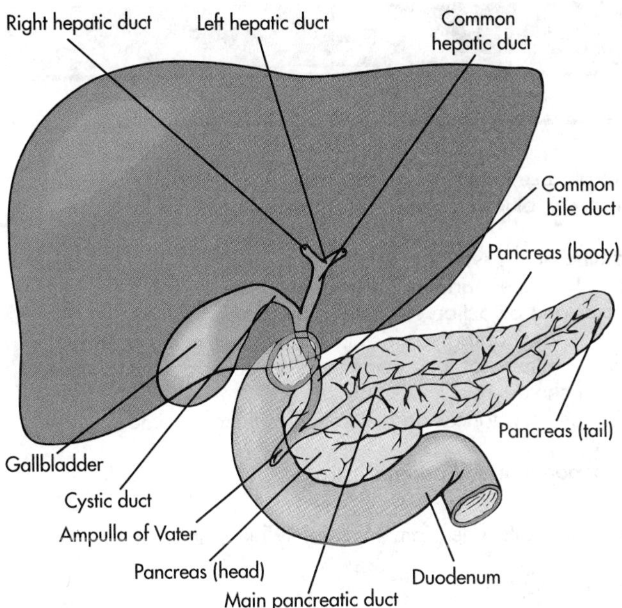

Fig. 36-4 Gross structure of the liver, gallbladder, pancreas, and the duct system.

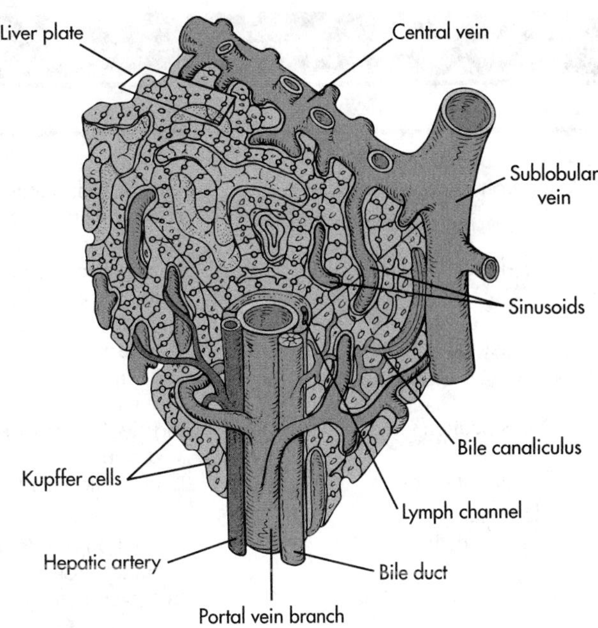

Fig. 36-5 Microscopic structure of liver lobule.

has a fibrous capsule that divides it into the right and left lobes (Fig. 36-4).

The functional units of the liver are lobules (Fig. 36-5). The lobule consists of rows of hepatic cells (*hepatocytes*) arranged around a central vein. The capillaries (*sinusoids*) are located between the rows of hepatocytes and are lined with *Kupffer cells,* which carry out phagocytic activity (removal of bacteria and toxins from the blood). Interlobular bile ducts form from bile capillaries (*canaliculi*). The hepatic cells secrete bile into the canaliculi.

The nerve supply to the liver is from the left vagus and sympathetic celiac plexus. About one third of the blood supply comes from the hepatic artery (branch of the celiac artery), and two thirds comes from the portal vein.

The portal circulatory system brings blood to the liver from the stomach, intestines, spleen, and pancreas. This blood enters the liver through the portal vein. In the liver the portal vein branches and comes in contact with each lobule. The blood in the sinusoids is a mixture of arterial and venous blood.

The liver is essential for life. It functions in the manufacture, storage, transformation, and excretion of a number of substances involved in metabolism. The functions of the liver are numerous but can be classified into four main areas, as identified in Table 36-4.

Biliary Tract. The biliary tract consists of the gallbladder and the duct system. The gallbladder is a pear-shaped sac located below the liver. The function of the gallbladder is to concentrate and store bile. It can hold approximately 45 ml of bile.

Bile is produced by the hepatic cells and secreted into the biliary canaliculi of the lobules. Bile then drains into the interlobular bile ducts, which unite into the two main left and right hepatic ducts. The hepatic ducts merge with the cystic duct from the gallbladder to form the common bile duct (see Fig. 36-4). This duct enters the duodenum at the ampulla of Vater. The sphincter of Oddi keeps the ampulla closed except when stimulated by the presence of food in the GI tract.

Bilirubin Metabolism

Bilirubin, a pigment derived from the breakdown of hemoglobin, is constantly produced (Fig. 36-6). Because it is insoluble in water, it is bound to albumin for its transport to the liver. This form of bilirubin is referred to as *unconjugated.* In the liver bilirubin is conjugated with glucuronic acid. Conjugated bilirubin is soluble and is excreted in bile. Bile also consists of water, cholesterol, bile salts, electrolytes, and phospholipids. Bile salts are needed for fat emulsification and digestion.

Bile initially enters the duct system in the canaliculi and flows through the interlobular ducts to the hepatic ducts. From the hepatic duct it can move to the cystic duct or down the common bile duct. Most bile is stored and concentrated in the gallbladder. It is then released into the cystic duct and moves down the common bile duct to enter the duodenum at the ampulla of Vater. In the intestines, most of the bilirubin is reduced to stercobilinogen and urobilinogen by bacterial action. Stercobilinogen accounts for the brown color of stool. A small amount of conjugated bilirubin is reabsorbed by the blood. Some urobilinogen is reabsorbed by the blood and returned to the liver through the portal circulation (enterohepatic) and excreted in the bile. An insignificant amount of urobilinogen is excreted in the urine.[2]

Pancreas. The pancreas is a long, slender gland lying behind the stomach and in front of the first and second lumbar vertebrae. It consists of the head, body, and tail. The anterior surface is covered by peritoneum. The pancreas contains lobes and lobules. The pancreatic duct extends

Table 36-4 Major Functions of the Liver

Function	Description
▪ **Metabolic functions**	
Carbohydrate metabolism	Glycogenesis (conversion of glucose to glycogen), glycogenolysis (process of breaking down glycogen to glucose), gluconeogenesis (formation of glucose from amino acids and fatty acids)
Protein metabolism	Synthesis of nonessential amino acids, synthesis of plasma proteins (except γ-globulin), synthesis of clotting factors, urea formation from NH_3 (NH_3 formed from deamination of amino acids and by action of bacteria on proteins in colon)
Fat metabolism	Synthesis of lipoproteins, breakdown of triglycerides into fatty acids and glycerol, formation of ketone bodies, synthesis of fatty acids from amino acids and glucose, synthesis and breakdown of cholesterol
Detoxification	Inactivation of drugs and harmful substances and excretion of their breakdown products
Steroid metabolism	Conjugation and excretion of gonadal and adrenal steroids
▪ **Bile synthesis**	
Bile production	Formation of bile, containing bile salts, bile pigments (mainly bilirubin), and cholesterol
Bile excretion	Bile excretion by liver about 1 L/day
▪ **Storage**	Glucose in form of glycogen; vitamins, including fat-soluble (A, D, E, K) and water-soluble (B_1, B_2, B_{12}, and folic acid); fatty acids; minerals (iron and copper); amino acids in form of albumin and β globulins
▪ **Mononuclear phagocyte system** Kupffer cells	Breakdown of old RBCs, WBCs, bacteria, and other particles, breakdown of hemoglobin from old RBCs to bilirubin and biliverdin

RBC, Red blood cell; *WBC*, white blood cell.

along the gland and enters the duodenum through the common bile duct (see Fig. 36-4). The pancreas has both *exocrine* and *endocrine* functions. It is the exocrine function of the pancreas that contributes to the process of digestion. Exocrine cells in the pancreas secrete pancreatic enzymes (see Table 36-1). The endocrine function is related to the islets of Langerhans, whose β cells secrete insulin and α cells secrete glucagon (see Chapter 45).

Effects of Aging on the Gastrointestinal System

The process of aging causes changes in the functional ability of the GI system (Table 36-5). Tooth enamel and dentin wear down and make the teeth susceptible to cavities. Periodontal disease can lead to the loss of teeth. Taste buds decrease, the sense of smell diminishes, and salivary secretions diminish, all of which can lead to a decrease in appetite and make eating less pleasurable.

As compared to other body systems the GI tract shows few age-related changes. Age-related changes in the esophagus include delayed emptying resulting from smooth muscle weakness and an incompetent LES.[1] Motility of the GI system decreases with age, but secretion and absorption are affected to a lesser extent. The elderly patient often experiences a decrease in hydrochloric acid secretion (*hypochlorhydria*), delayed gastric emptying, and constipation. With chronic atrophic gastritis there is a decrease in number of parietal cells and subsequent reduction in amount of acid and intrinsic factor secreted.

The liver size decreases after 50 years of age, but results of liver function tests remain within normal ranges. Enzyme changes in the liver that are age-related decrease the ability of the liver to metabolize medications and hormones. The size of the pancreas is unaffected by aging but does undergo structural changes such as fibrosis, fatty acid deposits, and atrophy. Aging does not cause changes in the structure and function of the gallbladder and bile ducts. However, with aging there is an increase in the incidence of gallstones.[3]

The economic inability to purchase food supplies may affect nutritional intake, especially in the older adult. Economic constraints may also reduce the number of fresh fruits and vegetables consumed and thus the amount of fiber. A reduction in dietary fiber may contribute to constipation.

ASSESSMENT OF THE GASTROINTESTINAL SYSTEM

Subjective Data

Important Health Information

Past health history. Information should be gathered from the patient about the history or existence of the following diseases or problems related to GI functioning: abdominal pain, gastritis, nausea and vomiting, diarrhea and constipation, hepatitis, colitis, peptic ulcer, abdominal distention, jaundice, anemia, hiatal hernia, gallbladder disease, dysphagia, heartburn, and dyspepsia.

The patient should be questioned about weight history. Any unexplained or unplanned weight loss or weight gain within the past 12 months should be explored in detail. A

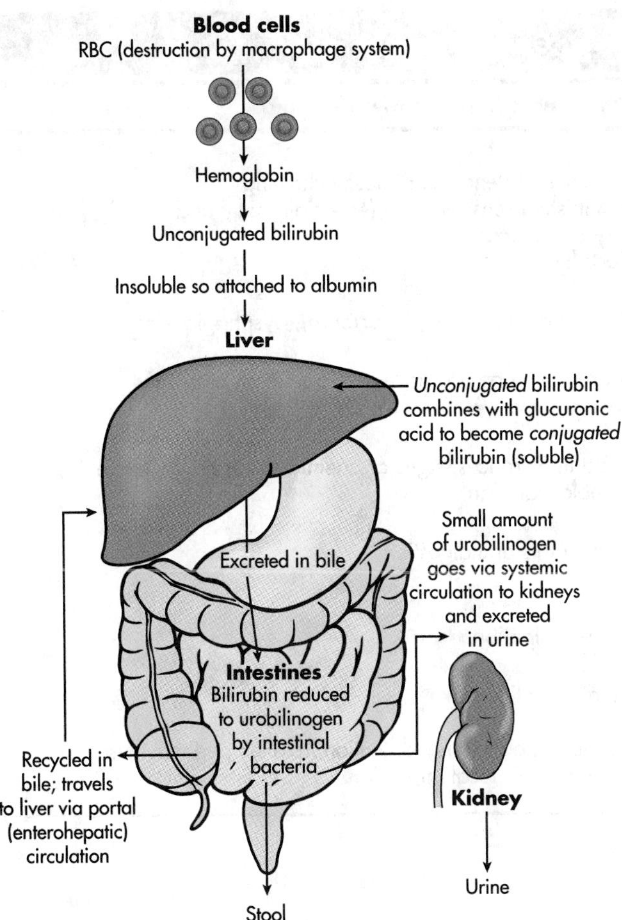

Fig. 36-6 Bilirubin metabolism and conjugation.

history of chronic dieting and repeated weight loss and gain should be documented.

Medications. The health history should include an assessment of the patient's past and current use of medications. This is an important part of the assessment, particularly in relation to liver problems. It should include over-the-counter and prescription drugs. Many chemicals and drugs are potentially hepatotoxic (Table 36-6). The nurse should ask the patient if antacids are taken, including the kind and frequency. Some people take baking soda (sodium bicarbonate) for an upset stomach. This can be dangerous because it is a systemic antacid that is readily absorbed and can cause metabolic alkalosis. Sodium bicarbonate is also in many over-the-counter effervescent drugs, such as Alka-Seltzer.

The use of prescription or over-the-counter appetite suppressant medication should be noted. The names of drugs and frequency and duration of use is also important.

Surgery or other treatments. Information should be obtained about hospitalizations for any problems related to the GI system. Data should also be obtained related to any abdominal or rectal surgery, including year, cause, postoperative course, and possible blood transfusions. Terminology related to surgery of the GI system is presented in Table 36-7.

Functional Health Patterns. Key questions to ask a patient with a GI problem are presented in Table 36-8.

Health perception–health management pattern. The nurse needs to ask about the patient's health practices related to the GI system, such as maintenance of normal body weight, attention to proper dental care, maintenance of adequate nutrition, and effective elimination habits.

The patient should be asked about exposure to hepatotoxic chemicals such as arsenic, phosphorus, and mercury. The nurse should also ask about foreign travel with possible exposure to hepatitis or parasitic infestation.

The patient should be assessed in relation to certain habits that have a direct effect on GI functioning. The consumption of alcohol in large quantities has detrimental effects on the mucosa of the stomach and also increases the secretion of hydrochloric acid and pepsinogen. Chronic alcohol exposure causes fatty infiltration of the liver. The nurse should obtain a history of cigarette smoking. Nicotine is irritating to the entire GI tract mucosa. Cigarette smoking is related to various GI cancers (especially mouth and esophageal cancers), esophagitis, and ulcers. Smoking will also delay the healing of ulcers.

Nutritional-metabolic pattern. A thorough nutritional assessment is essential. A dietary history should be taken and compared with the food pyramid. The nurse should ask open-ended questions that will allow the patient to express beliefs and feelings about the diet. The nurse may need to ask the patient to do a 24-hour dietary recall to analyze the adequacy of the diet. The nurse should assist the patient in recalling the preceding day's food intake, including early-morning and nighttime intake. The nurse should find out about the intake of snacks, liquids, and vitamin supplements. The nurse must then evaluate the diet in terms of the recommended groups and servings on the food pyramid and try to determine whether the 24-hour recall is typical of the patient's usual eating habits. If weekend eating habits vary greatly, the nurse should obtain a separate weekend diet history and assess the patient's intake for both quality and quantity of food.

The nurse should ask the patient about the use of sugar and salt substitutes, caffeine, and amount of fluid and fiber intake. The patient should be questioned about any changes in appetite, food tolerance, and weight. Anorexia and weight loss may indicate carcinoma. The nurse should ask the patient about allergies to any food and determine what GI symptoms such allergic responses cause.

Elimination pattern. A detailed account of the patient's bowel elimination pattern should be elicited. The frequency, time of day, and usual consistency of stool should be noted. The use of laxatives and enemas including type, frequency, and results should be documented. Any recent change in bowel patterns should be investigated.

The amount and type of fluid and fiber intake should be determined because they have an important effect on the frequency and consistency of stools. Inadequate intake of fiber can be associated with constipation. Analysis of fluid intake and output could indicate the presence of a urinary problem and the possibility of fluid retention.

Skin problems can be associated with GI problems. Food allergies can cause lesions, pruritus, and edema. Diarrhea

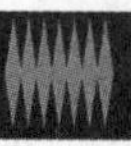

Table 36-5 Gerontologic Differences in Assessment: Gastrointestinal System

Changes	Differences in Assessment Findings
Mouth	
Loss of teeth	Presence of dentures, difficulty chewing
Decreased taste buds, decreased sense of smell	Diminished sense of taste (especially salty and sweet)
Decreased volume of saliva	Dry oral mucosa
Atrophy of gingival tissue	Poor-fitting dentures
Esophagus	
Decreased tone and motility	Complaints of pyrosis (heartburn), dysphagia, eructation
Abdominal Wall	
Thinner and less taut	More visible peristalsis, easier palpation of organs
Decrease in number and sensitivity of sensory receptors	Less sensitivity to surface pain
Stomach	
Decreased acid secretion, atrophy of gastric mucosa, hypochlorhydria	Food intolerances, signs of anemia as result of vitamin B_{12} malabsorption
Small Intestines	
Decreased secretion of most digestive enzymes, decreased motility	Complaints of indigestion
Liver	
Increased size and lowered in position	Easier palpation
Large Intestine, Anus, Rectum	
Decreased anal sphincter tone and nerve supply to rectal area	Fecal incontinence
Decreased muscular tone, decreased motility	Flatulence, abdominal distention, relaxed perineal musculature
Increase in transit time	Constipation, fecal impaction

Table 36-6 Hepatotoxic Chemicals and Drugs

Alcohol	Halothane
Arsenic	Isoniazid
Carbon tetrachloride	Propylthiouracil
Chloroform	Sulfonamides
Gold compounds	Thiazide diuretics
Mercury	6-Mercaptopurine
Phosphorus	Methotrexate
Anabolic steroids	Acetaminophen

can result in excoriation and pain in the perianal area. External drainage systems such as an ileostomy or ileal conduit can cause local skin irritation. The possible association between a skin problem and a GI problem should be investigated.

Activity-exercise pattern. The patient's ambulatory status should be assessed to determine if the patient is capable of securing and preparing food. If the patient is unable to do these tasks, it should be determined if family or an outside agency is meeting this need. Any limitation in the patient's ability to feed self independently should be noted.

Sleep-rest pattern. Many food-related events can interrupt and interfere with the quality of sleep. Nausea, vomit-

Table 36-7 Surgeries of the Gastrointestinal System

Antrectomy: Removal of antrum portion of stomach
Cecostomy: Opening into cecum
Cholecystectomy: Removal of gallbladder
Cholecystostomy: Opening into gallbladder
Choledochojejunostomy: Opening between common bile duct and jejunum
Choledocholithotomy: Opening into common bile duct for removal of stones
Colostomy: Opening into colon
Esophagoenterostomy: Removal of portion of esophgus with segment of colon attached to remaining portion
Esophagogastrostomy: Removal of esophagus and anastomosis of remaining portion to stomach
Gastrectomy: Removal of stomach
Gastrostomy: Opening into stomach
Glossectomy: Removal of tongue
Hemiglossectomy: Removal of half of tongue
Ileostomy: Opening into ileum
Mandibulectomy: Removal of mandible
Pyloroplasty: Enlargement and repair of pyloric sphincter area
Vagotomy: Resection of branch of vagus nerve

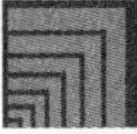

Table 36-8 Key Questions: Patient with a Gastrointestinal Problem

Health Perception–Health Management Pattern
- Describe any measures used to treat gastrointestinal symptoms such as diarrhea or vomiting.
- Do you smoke?* Do you drink alcohol?*
- Are you exposed to any chemicals on a regular basis?* Have you been exposed in the past?*
- Have you recently traveled outside the United States?*

Nutritional-Metabolic Pattern
- Describe your usual daily food and fluid intake.
- Do you take any supplemental vitamins or minerals?*
- Have you experienced any changes in appetite or food tolerance?*
- Has there been a weight change in the past?*
- Are you allergic to any foods?*

Elimination Pattern
- Describe the frequency and time of day you have bowel movements. What is the consistency of the bowel movement?
- Do you use laxatives or enemas?* If so, how often?
- Have there been any recent changes in your bowel pattern?*
- Describe any skin problems caused by gastrointestinal problems.
- Do you need any assistive equipment, such as ostomy equipment?

Activity-Exercise Pattern
- Do you have limitations in mobility that make it difficult for you to procure and prepare food?*
- Are you able to feed yourself?
- Do you have any gastrointestinal symptoms, such as vomiting or diarrhea, that affect your activity?*

Sleep-Rest Pattern
- Do you experience any difficulty sleeping because of a gastrointestinal problem?*
- Are you awakened by symptoms such as gas or esophageal burning?*

Cognitive-Perceptual Pattern
- Have you experienced any change in taste or smell that has affected your appetite?*
- Do you have any heat or cold sensitivity that affects eating?*
- Does pain interfere with food preparation, appetite, or chewing?*
- Do pain medications cause constipation or appetite suppression?*

Self-Perception–Self-Concept Pattern
- Describe any changes in your weight that have affected how you feel about ourself.
- Have you had any changes in normal elimination that have affected how you feel about yourself?*
- Have any symptoms of gastrointestinal disease caused physical changes that are a problem for you?*

Role-Relationship Pattern
- Describe the impact of any gastrointestinal problem on your usual roles and relationships.
- Have any changes in elimination affected your relationships?*
- Do you live alone? Describe how your family or others assist you with your gastrointestinal problems.

Sexuality-Reproductive Pattern
- Describe the effect of your gastrointestinal problem on your sexual activity.

Coping–Stress Tolerance Pattern
- Do you experience gastrointestinal symptoms in response to stressful or emotional situations?*
- Describe how you deal with any gastrointestinal symptoms that result.

Value-Belief Pattern
- Describe any culturally-specific health beliefs regarding food and food preparation that may influence the treatment of this gastrointestinal problem.

*If yes, describe.

ing, diarrhea, indigestion, bloating, and hunger can produce sleep problems and should be investigated. The patient should be questioned if GI symptoms affect sleep or rest. For example, a patient with a hiatal hernia may be awakened because of burning pain; sleep may be improved by elevating the head of the bed for this patient.

A patient often has a bedtime ritual that involves the use of a particular food or beverage. Warm milk is known to induce sleep through the effect of the serotonin precursor *L-tryptophan.* Herbal teas and melatonin are often sleep inducing. Individual routines should be noted and complied with whenever possible to avoid sleeplessness. Hunger can prevent sleep and should be relieved by a light, easily digested snack unless contraindicated.

Cognitive-perceptual pattern. Decreases in sensory adequacy can result in problems related to the acquisition, preparation, and ingestion of food. Changes in taste or smell can affect appetite and eating pleasure. Vertigo could make shopping and standing at a stove difficult and dangerous. Heat or cold sensitivity could make certain foods painful to eat. Problems in expressive communication could make it difficult and frustrating for the patient to make personal desires and preferences known. The nurse should assess the patient in this pattern to judge the effect of deficiencies on adequate nutritional intake. If the patient has been diagnosed as having a GI disorder, the nurse should ask questions to determine the patient's understanding of the illness as well as its treatment.

Pain is another area that needs careful assessment related to its effect on the GI system and nutrition. Relevant behaviors associated with chronic pain include avoidance of activity, fatigue, and disruption of eating patterns. The possible effects of pain medication related to constipation, sedation, and appetite suppression should be assessed.

Self-perception–self-concept pattern. Many GI and nutritional problems can have serious effects on the patient's self-perception. Overweight and underweight persons often have problems related to self-esteem and body image. Repeated attempts to achieve a personally acceptable weight can be discouraging and depressing for the patient. The affect associated with the recounting of an adult weight history can alert the nurse to potential problems in this area.

Another potentially problematic area is the need for external devices to manage elimination, such as a colostomy or ileostomy. The patient's willingness to engage in self-care and to discuss this situation should provide the nurse with valuable information related to body image and self-esteem.

The altered physical changes often associated with liver disease can be problematic for the patient. Jaundice and ascites cause significant changes in external appearance. The patient's attitude toward these changes should be assessed.

Role-relationship pattern. Problems related to the GI system such as cirrhosis, alcoholism, hepatitis, ostomies, obesity, and carcinoma can have a major impact on the patient's ability to maintain usual roles and relationships. A chronic illness may necessitate leaving a job or reducing the number of hours worked. Changes in body image and self-esteem can affect relationships. The availability and satisfaction with support should be determined. It is important that the nurse be aware of these possible consequences and assess for their presence.

Sexuality-reproductive pattern. Changes related to sexuality and reproductive status can result from problems of the GI system. For example, obesity, jaundice, anorexia, and ascites could decrease the acceptance of a potential sexual partner. The presence of an ostomy could affect the patient's confidence related to sexual activity. Chronic alcoholism could discourage a meaningful relationship that could develop into a sexual relationship. Sensitive questioning by the nurse could determine the presence of potential problems.

Anorexia can affect the reproductive status of a female patient. Alcoholism can affect the reproductive status of both men and women. A poor nutritional intake before and during pregnancy can result in a low-birth-weight infant. The nurse should determine the patient's desires in the area of reproduction and direct the assessment based on the patient's responses.

Coping–stress tolerance pattern. The nurse should try to determine what is a stressor for the patient and what coping mechanisms the patient uses to function with these stressors. GI symptoms such as epigastric pain, nausea, and diarrhea develop in many people in response to stressful or emotional situations. Some organic GI problems such as peptic ulcers are aggravated by stress.

Value-belief pattern. The patient's spiritual and cultural beliefs regarding food and food preparation should be assessed. Whenever possible, these preferences should be respected by the health care provider. In addition, it should be determined if any value-belief could interfere with planned interventions. For example, if the patient with anemia is a vegetarian, the prescription of a high meat diet would be met with patient resistance. Likewise, the recovering alcoholic could not take an alcohol-based cough medicine. Thoughtful assessment and consideration of the patient's beliefs and values will usually increase patient compliance and satisfaction.

Objective Data

In addition to collecting subjective data related to a diet history and functional health patterns, objective data related to a nutritional assessment should be collected. Anthropometric measurements (height, weight, skinfold thickness) and blood studies such as serum protein, albumin, and hemoglobin are examples of important objective data related to the GI system. A physical examination also adds valuable information.

Physical Examination

Mouth

INSPECTION. The lips should be inspected for symmetry, color, and size. They should be observed for abnormalities such as pallor or cyanosis, cracking, ulcers, or fissures. The dorsum (top) of the tongue should have a thin white coating; the undersurface should be smooth. The nurse should observe for any lesions. Using a tongue blade, the nurse should inspect the buccal mucosa and note the color, any areas of pigmentation, and any lesions. Dark-skinned people normally have patchy areas of pigmentation. In assessing the teeth and gums, the nurse should look for caries, loose teeth, abnormal shape and position of teeth, and swelling, bleeding, discoloration, or inflammation of the gingivae. Any distinctive breath odor should be noted.

The pharynx is inspected by tilting the patient's head back and depressing the tongue with a tongue blade. The tonsils, uvula, soft palate, and anterior and posterior pillars should be observed. The nurse should have the patient say "ah." The uvula and soft palate should rise and remain in the midline.

PALPATION. The nurse should palpate any suspicious areas in the mouth. Ulcers, nodules, indurations, and areas of tenderness should be palpated. The mouth of the older adult needs careful assessment. Particular attention should be given to dentures (e.g., fit, condition), ability to swallow, and lesions. The patient who has dentures must remove the dentures during an oral exam to allow for good visualization and palpation of the area.

Abdomen. Two systems are used to anatomically describe the surface of the abdomen. One system divides the abdomen into four quadrants by a perpendicular line from the sternum to the pubic bone and a horizontal line across the abdomen at the umbilicus (Fig. 36-7, *A* and Table 36-9). The other system divides the abdomen into nine regions (Fig. 36-7, *B*), but only the epigastrium, umbilical, and suprapubic or hypogastric regions are commonly addressed.

For the abdominal examination, good lighting should shine across the abdomen. The patient should be in the supine position and as relaxed as possible. To help relax the abdominal muscles, the patient should slightly flex the knees and the head of the bed should be raised slightly. The patient should have an empty bladder. The examiner should use warm hands when doing the abdominal examination to avoid eliciting muscle guarding. The patient should be asked to breathe slowly through the mouth.

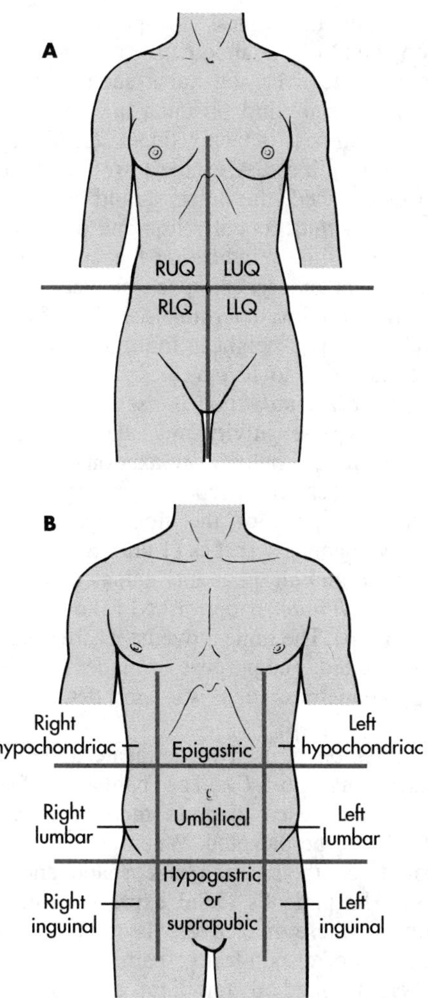

Fig. 36-7 ***A,*** Abdominal quadrants. ***B,*** Abdominal regions.

INSPECTION. The nurse should assess the abdomen for skin changes (color, texture, scars, striae, dilated veins, rashes, and lesions), umbilicus (location and contour), symmetry, contour (flat, rounded [convex], concave, protuberant, distention), observable masses (hernias or other masses), and movement (pulsations and peristalsis). A normal aortic pulsation may be seen in the epigastric area. The nurse should look across the abdomen tangentially (across the abdomen in a line) for peristalsis. Peristalsis is not normally visible in an adult but may be visible in a thin person.

AUSCULATION. During examination of the abdomen, auscultation is done before percussion and palpation because these latter procedures may alter the bowel sounds. Auscultation of the abdomen includes listening for increased or decreased bowel sounds and vascular sounds. The diaphragm of the stethoscope is used to auscultate bowel sounds because they are relatively high pitched. The bell of the stethoscope is used to detect lower-pitched sounds. Normal bowel sounds occur 5 to 35 times per minute and sound like high-pitched clicks or gurgles.[4] Before auscultation, warming the stethoscope in the hands helps prevent abdominal muscle contraction. The nurse should listen in the epigastrium and in all four quadrants. The nurse should listen for bowel sounds for 2 to 5 minutes. Bowel sounds cannot be described as absent until no sound is heard for 5 minutes (in each quadrant).[5] The frequency and intensity of bowel sounds will vary, depending on the phase of digestion. Normally they will sound relatively high pitched and gurgling. Loud gurgles indicate hyperperistalsis and are called *borborygmi* (stomach growling). The bowel sounds will be more high pitched (rushes and tinkling) when the intestines are under tension, such as in intestinal obstruction. The nurse should listen for decreased or absent bowel sounds. Terms used to describe bowel sounds include *present, absent, increased, decreased, high pitched, tinkling, gurgling,* and *rushing.* Normally no aortic bruits should be heard. A *bruit,* best heard with the bell of the stethoscope, is a swishing or buzzing sound and represents turbulent blood flow.

PERCUSSION. The purpose of percussion of the abdomen is to determine the presence of fluid, distention, and masses. Sound waves vary according to the density of underlying tissues; the presence of air produces a higher-pitched, hollow sound called *tympany*; the presence of fluid or masses produces a short, high-pitched sound with little resonance called *dullness.* The nurse should lightly percuss all four quadrants of the abdomen and assess the distribu-

Table 36-9 Abdominal Structures in Regions of the Abdomen

Right Upper Quadrant	Left Upper Quadrant	Right Lower Quadrant	Left Lower Quadrant
Liver and gallbladder	Left lobe of liver	Lower pole of right kidney	Lower pole of left kidney
Pylorus	Spleen	Cecum and appendix	Sigmoid flexure
Duodenum	Stomach	Portion of ascending colon	Portion of descending colon
Head of pancreas	Body of pancreas	Bladder (if distended)	Bladder (if distended)
Right adrenal gland	Left adrenal gland	Right ovary and salpinx	Left ovary and salpinx
Portion of right kidney	Portion of left kidney	Uterus (if enlarged)	Uterus (if enlarged)
Hepatic flexure of colon	Splenic flexure of colon	Right spermatic cord	Left spermatic cord
Portion of ascending and transverse colon	Portion of transverse and descending colon	Right ureter	Left ureter

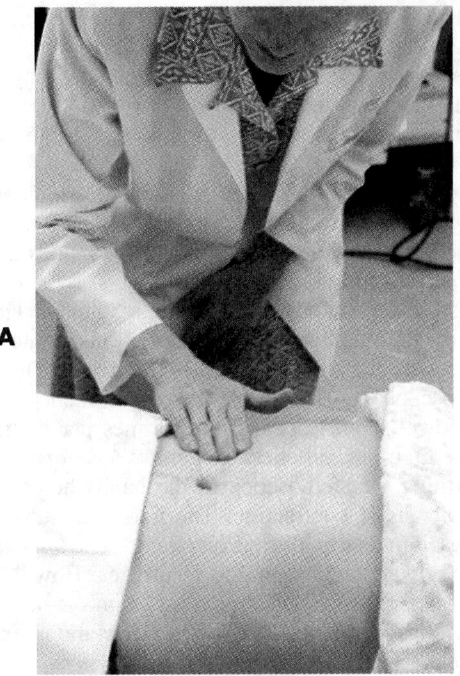

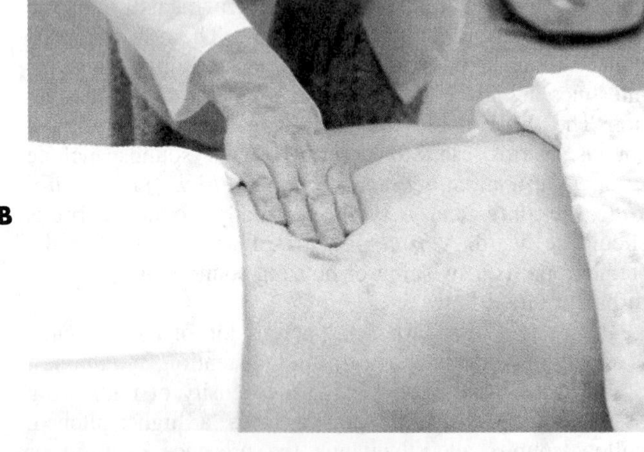

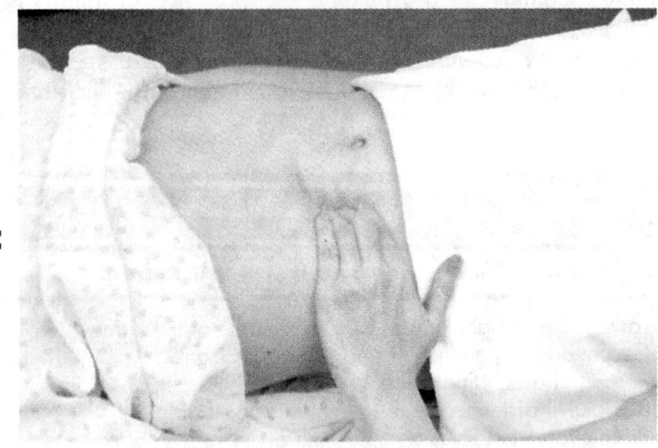

Fig. 36-8 ***A,*** Technique for light palpation of the abdomen. ***B,*** Technique for moderate palpation using the side of the hand. ***C,*** Technique for deep palpation.

tion of tympany and dullness. Tympany is the predominant percussion sound of the abdomen.

To percuss the liver, the nurse should start below the umbilicus in the right midclavicular line and percuss lightly upward until dullness is heard, thus determining the lower border of liver dullness. After the lower border of the liver has been determined, the nurse should start at the nipple line in the right midclavicular line and percuss downward to the area of dullness indicating the upper border of the liver. The height or vertical space between the two areas should be measured to determine the size of the liver. The normal range of liver height in the right midclavicular line is 2.4 to 5 inches (6 to 12 cm).

PALPATION. *Light palpation* is used to detect tenderness or cutaneous hypersensitivity, muscular resistance, masses, and swelling. It also helps in relaxation for deeper palpation. The nurse should keep fingers together and press gently with the pads of the fingertips, depressing the abdominal wall about .4 inches (1 cm). Smooth movements should be used and all quadrants palpated (Fig. 36-8 *A*).

Moderate palpation is performed following light palpation (Fig. 36-8 *B*). The same movements are used but greater pressure is exerted. The purpose of moderate palpation is to detect any tenderness that was not detectable by light palpation.

Deep palpation is used to delineate abdominal organs and masses (Fig. 36-8 *C*). The palmar surfaces of the fingers should be used to press more deeply. Again, all quadrants should be palpated. When palpating masses, the nurse should note the location, size, shape, and presence of tenderness. The patient's facial expression should be observed during these maneuvers because it will provide nonverbal cues of discomfort or pain.

An alternate method for light and deep abdominal palpation is the two-hand method. One hand is placed on top of the other. The fingers of the top hand apply pressure to the bottom hand. The fingers of the bottom hand feel for organs and masses. The nurse should practice both methods of palpation to determine which one is most effective.

A problem area on the abdomen can be checked for rebound tenderness by pressing in slowly and firmly over the painful site. The palpating fingers are withdrawn quickly. Pain on withdrawal of the fingers indicates peritoneal inflammation. Because assessing for rebound tenderness may produce pain and severe muscle spasm, it should be done at the end of the examination and only by an experienced practitioner.

To palpate the liver, the nurse's left hand is placed behind the patient to support the right eleventh and twelfth ribs (Fig. 36-9). The patient may relax on the nurse's hand. The nurse should press the left hand forward and place the right hand on the patient's right abdomen lateral to the rectus muscle. The fingertips should be below the lower border of liver dullness and pointed toward the right costal margin. The nurse should gently press in and up. The patient should take a deep breath with the abdomen so that the liver drops and is in a better position to be palpated. The

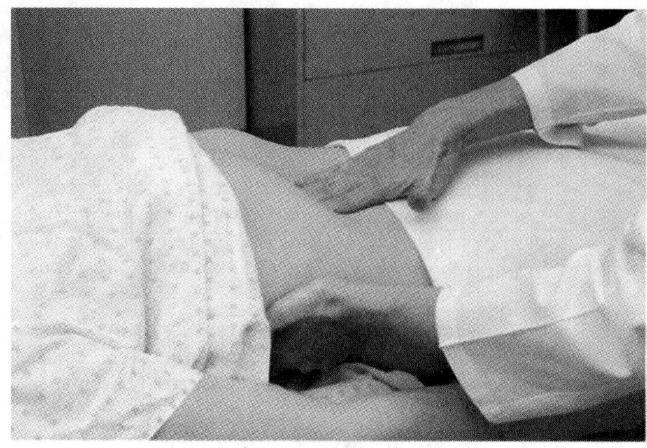

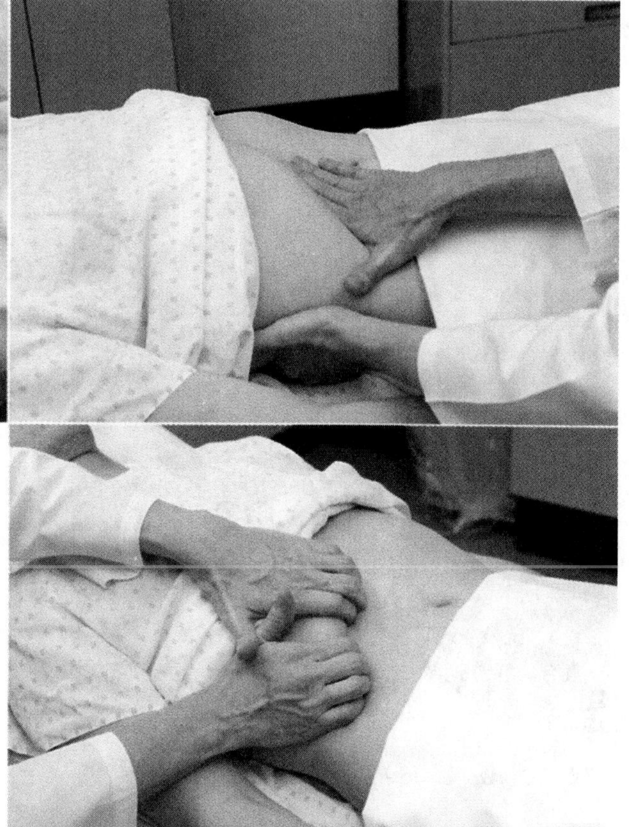

Fig. 36-9 ***A,*** Technique for liver palpation. ***B,*** Alternate technique. ***C,*** Palpating liver with fingers hooked over the costal margin.

nurse should try to feel the liver edge as it comes down to the fingertips. The liver edge should feel firm, sharp, and smooth. The surface and contour and any tenderness should be described.

To palpate the spleen, the nurse's left hand reaches over and under the patient and supports and presses the patient's left lower rib cage forward. The right hand is placed below the left costal margin and presses it in toward the spleen. The nurse should ask the patient to breathe deeply. The tip or edge of an enlarged spleen will be felt by the fingertips. The spleen is normally not palpable. If it is palpable, the nurse should not continue because manual compression of an enlarged spleen may cause it to rupture.

The standard approach for examining the abdomen can be used on the older adult. Palpation is important because it may reveal a tumor. The abdomen may be thinner and more lax unless the patient is obese. If the patient has chronic obstructive pulmonary disease, large lungs, or a low diaphragm, the liver may be palpated 0.4 to 0.8 inches (1 to 2 cm) below the right costal margin.

Rectum. The perianal and anal area should be inspected for color, texture, lumps, rashes, scars, excoriations, fissures, and external hemorrhoids. Any lumps or unusual areas should be palpated with a gloved hand.

For the digital examination of the rectum the gloved, lubricated index finger is placed against the anus while the patient strains (Valsalva maneuver). Then, as the sphincter relaxes, the finger is inserted. The finger is pointed toward the umbilicus. The nurse should try to get the patient to relax. The finger is inserted into the rectum as far as possible, and all surfaces are palpated. Nodules, tenderness, or any irregularities should be assessed. A check for occult blood should be included.

Recording of the normal physical assessment of the GI system is found in Table 36-10. Gerontologic differences in the GI system and differences in assessment findings are described in Table 36-5. Common abnormal assessment abnormalities are presented in Table 36-11.

DIAGNOSTIC STUDIES

Diagnostic studies provide important information to the nurse in monitoring the patient's condition and planning appropriate interventions. These studies are considered to be objective data. Table 36-12 presents diagnostic studies common to the GI system (see p. 1091).

Many of the diagnostic procedures of the GI system require measures to cleanse the GI tract as well as ingestion or injection of a contrast medium or a radiopaque dye. Often the patient has a series of GI diagnostic tests done. The nurse must monitor the patient closely to ensure adequate hydration and nutrition during the tests. Some diagnostic studies of the GI system are difficult and uncomfortable for the older adult. It may be necessary to individualize and make adjustments. It is particularly important to

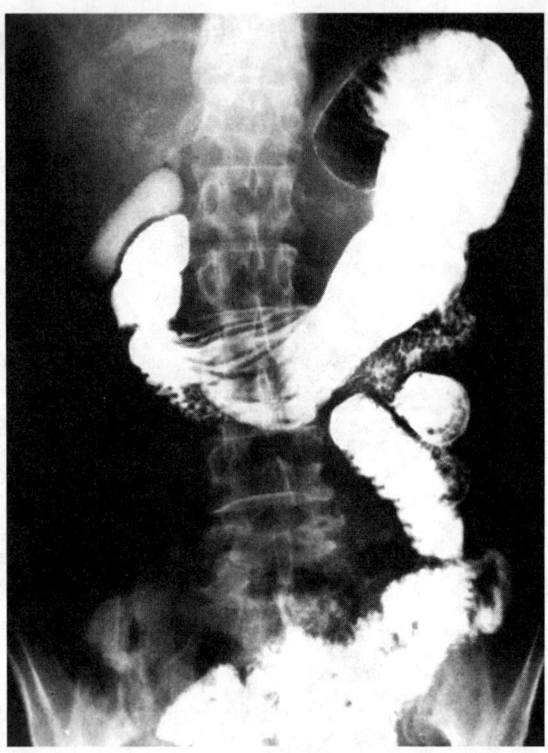

Fig. 36-10 Upper gastrointestinal tract x-ray.

prevent diarrhea from bowel cleansing procedures and dehydration from prolonged fluid restriction.

Many radiologic studies use either barium sulfate or meglumine diatrizoate (Gastrografin) as a contrast medium. Barium sulfate is more effective for visualizing mucosal detail. Gastrografin is water soluble and rapidly absorbed, so it is preferred when a perforation is suspected. Under other circumstances such as suspected aspiration, water-soluble media are contraindicated and barium is preferred because it is inert in the lung.

Radiologic Studies

Upper Gastrointestinal Series. The purpose of an upper GI series (barium swallow) is to observe the movement of a contrast medium through the esophagus and into the stomach by means of fluoroscopy and x-ray examination. It is used to identify esophageal and stomach disorders such as esophageal strictures, varices, polyps, tumors, hiatal hernia, and peptic ulcers in the stomach or duodenum (Fig. 36-10).

The procedure consists of the patient swallowing contrast medium and then assuming different positions on the x-ray table. The movement of the contrast medium is observed with fluoroscopy, and several x-rays are taken (see Table 36-12).

Lower Gastrointestinal Series. The purpose of a lower GI series (barium enema) x-ray examination is to observe by means of fluoroscopy the filling of the colon with contrast medium and to observe by x-ray the filled colon. This procedure identifies polyps, tumors, and other lesions in the colon. It consists of administering an enema of contrast medium to the patient. The air-contrast barium enema provides better visualization of an inflammatory bowel disease, polyps, and tumors (see Fig. 36-11 on p. 1096). It is not tolerated as well in an older or immobile patient.

Oral Cholecystogram. The purpose of an oral cholecystogram (gallbladder series) is to visualize the gallbladder. It is used to determine the gallbladder's ability to concentrate and store dye and to observe the patency of the biliary duct system. It is a common gallbladder test and may be used to detect gallstones, obstructions of the biliary tract, and other gallbladder disorders.

The procedure consists of an x-ray examination after the oral ingestion of a radiopaque dye. The radiopaque dye used is an organic insoluble iodide such as iopanoic acid (Telepaque, Priodax, or Oragrafin) (see Table 36-12).

Table 36-10 Normal Physical Assessment of the Gastrointestinal System

Mouth
Moist and pink lips; pink and moist buccal mucosa and gingivae without plaques or lesions; teeth in good repair; protusion of tongue in midline without deviation or fasciculations; pink uvula, soft palate, tonsils, and posterior pharynx

Abdomen
Flat without masses or scars, bowel sounds in all quadrants, nonpalpable liver and spleen, liver 10 cm in right midclavicular line, generalized tympany

Anus
Absence of lesions, fissures, hemorrhoids

Endoscopy

Endoscopy refers to the direct visualization of a body structure through a lighted instrument (scope). Most of the GI tract can be visualized by endoscopy, especially with the flexible fiberoptic scopes. The GI structures that can be examined by fiberoptic endoscopy include the esophagus, stomach, duodenum, colon, and, with the aid of fluoroscopy and x-rays, the pancreas and biliary tree. It is now possible to visualize the pancreatic, hepatic, and common bile ducts with side-viewing flexible endoscopes.[5]

The fiberscope is an instrument channel through which biopsy forceps and cytology brushes may be passed. Cameras may be attached and pictures taken. Endoscopy of the GI tract is frequently done in combination with biopsy and cytologic studies. The major complication of GI endoscopy is perforation through the structure being scoped. This complication is decreased with the use of the flexible fiberoptic scopes. All endoscopic procedures require informed, written consent. Specific endoscopy procedures are discussed in Table 36-12.

In addition to diagnostic procedures, many invasive and therapeutic procedures may be done with endoscopes. These include procedures such as polypectomy, sclerosis of

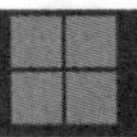

Table 36-11 Common Assessment Abnormalities: Gastrointestinal System

Finding	Description	Possible Etiology and Significance
Mouth		
Ulcer, plaque on lips or in mouth	Sore or lesion	Carcinoma, viral infections
Cheilosis	Softening, fissuring, and cracking of lips at angles of mouth	Riboflavin deficiency
Cheilitis	Inflammation of lips (usually lower) with fissuring, scaling, crusting	Often unknown
Geographic tongue	Scattered red, smooth (loss of papillae) areas on dorsum of tongue	Unknown
Smooth tongue	Red, slick appearance	Vitamin B_{12} deficiency
Leukoplakia	Thickened white patches	Premalignant lesion
Pyorrhea	Recessed gums, purulent pockets	Periodontitis
Herpes simplex	Benign vesicular lesion	Herpesvirus
Candidiasis	White, curdlike lesions surrounded by erythematous mucosa	Exposure to *Candida albicans*
Glossitis	Reddened, ulcerated, swollen tongue	Exposure to streptococci, irritation, injury, vitamin B deficiency, anemia
Acute marginal gingivitis	Friable, edematous, painful, bleeding gingivae	Irritation from ill-fitting dentures, calcium deposits on teeth, food impaction
Esophagus and Stomach		
Dysphagia	Difficulty in swallowing, sensation of food sticking in esophagus	Esophageal problems, cancer of esophagus
Hematemesis	Vomiting of blood	Esophageal varices, bleeding peptic ulcer
Pyrosis	Heartburn, burning in epigastric or substernal area	Hiatal hernia, esophagitis, incompetent lower esophageal sphincter
Dyspepsia	Burning or indigestion	Peptic ulcer, gallbladder disease
Odynophagia	Painful swallowing	Cancer of esophagus, esophagitis
Eructation	Belching	Gallbladder disease
Nausea and vomiting	Feeling of impending vomiting, expulsion of gastric contents through mouth	GI infections, common manifestation of many GI diseases; stress, fear, and pathologic conditions
Abdomen		
Distention	Excessive gas accumulation, enlarged abdomen; generalized tympany	Obstruction, paralytic ileus
Ascites	Accumulated fluid within abdominal cavity; eversion of umbilicus (usually)	Peritoneal inflammation, congestive heart failure, metastatic carcinoma, cirrhosis
Bruit	Humming or swishing sound heard through stethoscope over vessel	Partial arterial obstruction (narrowing of vessel), turbulent flow (aneurysm)
Hyperresonance	Loud, tinkling rushes	Intestinal obstruction
Borborygmi	Waves of loud, gurgling sounds	Hyperactive bowel as result of eating
Absent bowel sounds	No auscultation of bowel sounds	Peritonitis, paralytic ileus, obstruction
Absence of liver dullness	Tympany on percussion	Air from viscus (e.g., perforated ulcer)
Masses	Lump on palpation	Tumors, cysts
Rebound tenderness	Sudden pain when fingers withdrawn quickly	Peritoneal inflammation, appendicitis
Nodular liver	Enlarged, hard liver with irregular edge or surface	Cirrhosis, carcinoma
Hepatomegaly	Enlargement of liver, liver edge >1-2 cm below costal margin	Metastatic carcinoma, hepatitis, venous congestion
Splenomegaly	Enlargement of spleen	Chronic leukemia, hemolytic states, portal hypertension, some infections
Hernia	Bulge or nodule in abdomen, usually appearing on straining	Inguinal (in inguinal canal), femoral (in femoral canal), umbilical (herniation of umbilicus), or incisional (defect in muscles after surgery)

continued

Table 36-11 Common Assessment Abnormalities: Gastrointestinal System—cont'd

Finding	Description	Possible Etiology and Significance
Rectum		
Hemorrhoids	Thrombosed veins in rectum and anus (internal or external)	Portal hypertension, chronic constipation, prolonged sitting or standing, pregnancy
Mass	Firm, nodular edge	Tumor, carcinoma
Pilonidal cyst	Opening of sinus tract, cyst in midline just above coccyx	Probably congenital
Fissure	Ulceration in anal canal	Straining, irritation
Melena	Abnormal, black, tarry stool containing digested blood	Cancer, bleeding in upper GI tract from ulcers, varices
Tenesmus	Painful and ineffective straining at stool	Ulcerative colitis, diarrhea secondary to GI infection such as food poisoning
Steatorrhea	Fatty, frothy, foul-smelling stool	Chronic pancreatitis, biliary obstruction, malabsorption problems

GI, Gastrointestinal.

varices, laser treatment, cauterization of bleeding sites, papillotomy, common bile duct stone removal, and balloon dilatations. A new and valuable diagnostic procedure is video endoscopy. In this procedure an electronic video endoscope converts electronic signals that can be seen on a television screen.

Liver Biopsy

The purpose of a liver biopsy is to obtain hepatic tissue to be used in establishing a diagnosis such as cirrhosis, hepatitis, and neoplasms. It may also be useful for following the progress of liver disease.

The two types of liver biopsy are *open* and *closed.* The open method involves making an incision and removing a wedge of tissue. It is done in the operating room with the patient under general anesthesia, often concurrently with another surgical procedure. The closed or needle biopsy is an invasive procedure in which the site is infiltrated with a local anesthetic and a needle is inserted between the sixth and seventh or eighth and ninth intercostal spaces on the right side. The patient lies supine with the right arm over the head. The patient should be instructed to expire fully and not breathe while the needle is inserted. Nursing assessment before and after a liver biopsy is important (see Table 36-12).

Liver Function Studies

Liver function tests are usually described separately from other GI diagnostic studies. Liver function tests are basically biochemical determinations that reflect hepatic disease. Table 36-13 describes some common liver function tests (see p. 1097).

Table 36-12 Diagnostic Studies: Gastrointestinal System

Study	Description and Purpose	Nursing Responsibility
Radiologic		
■ Upper GI or barium swallow	Stomach is examined by x-ray study with fluoroscopy with contrast medium. Study is used to diagnose structural abnormalities of the esophagus, stomach, and duodenal bulb.	Explain procedure to patient and that patient will need to drink contrast medium and assume various positions on x-ray table. Keep patient NPO for 8-12 hr before procedure. Tell patient to avoid smoking after midnight the night before the study. After x-ray test, take measures to prevent contrast medium impaction (fluids, laxatives). Be aware that stool may be white up to 72 hr after test.
■ Small bowel series	Contrast medium is ingested and flat film taken q20 min until medium reaches terminal ileum.	Same as for upper GI.
■ Lower GI or barium enema	Fluoroscopic x-ray examination of colon uses contrast medium, which is administered rectally (enema). Double contrast or air contrast barium enema is test of choice. Air is infused after barium is evacuated.	Before the procedure, administer laxatives and enemas until colon is clear of stool evening before procedure. Administer clear liquid diet evening before procedure. Keep patient NPO for 8 hr before test. Instruct patient about being given barium by enema. Explain that cramping and urge to defecate may occur during procedure and that patient may be placed in various positions on tilt table. After the procedure, give fluids, laxatives, or suppositories to assist in expelling barium. Observe stool for passage of contrast medium.
■ Oral cholecystogram (GB series)	X-ray examination visualizes GB after radiopaque dye such as iopanoic acid (Telepaque) has been ingested orally. Study determines GB's ability to concentrate and store dye and patency of biliary duct system.	Assess patient for sensitivity to iodine. Administer radiopaque dye evening before test. Give 6 tablets (3g), 1 q5 min. Explain that patient may need 2 consecutive days of dye ingestion. Keep patient NPO after ingestion of dye. Observe for side effects of dye such as nausea, vomiting, diarrhea. May give fatty test meal after x-ray test to check for GB emptying.
■ Cholangiography IV cholangiogram	X-rays are used to visualize biliary duct system after IV injection of radiopaque dye.	Keep patient NPO for 8 hr. Assess sensitivity to iodine dye. During injection of dye, assess for urticaria, extreme flushing, respiratory distress.
Percutaneous transhepatic cholangiogram	After local anesthesia, liver is entered with long needle (under fluoroscopy), bile duct is entered, bile withdrawn, and radiopaque dye injected. Fluoroscopy is used to determine filling of hepatic and biliary ducts.	Observe patient for signs of hemorrhage or bile leakage.
Surgical cholangiogram	Study is performed during surgery on biliary structures, such as GB. Contrast medium is injected into common bile duct.	Explain to patient that anesthetic will be used.

continued

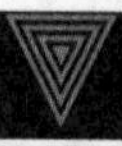

Table 36-12 Diagnostic Studies: Gastrointestinal System–cont'd

Study	Description and Purpose	Nursing Responsibility
Radiologic—cont'd		
▪ Ultrasound	This noninvasive procedure uses high-frequency sound waves (ultrasound waves), which are passed into body structures and recorded as they are reflected (bounded). A conductive gel (lubricant jelly) is applied to the skin and a transducer is placed on the area.	Be aware that bowel must be cleansed because presence of solid material in GI tract causes changes in reflected sounds and that ultrasound is not transmitted well through gas or air. Schedule test before upper GI or barium enema.
Abdominal ultrasound	Study detects abdominal masses (tumors and cysts) and is also used to assess ascites.	Same as above.
Hepatobiliary ultrasound	Study detects subphrenic abscesses, cysts, tumors, cirrhosis and is used to visualize biliary ducts.	Be aware that bowel must be cleansed. Explain procedure to patient.
GB ultrasound	Study detects gallstones (high degree of accuracy) and can be used for a patient with jaundice or allergic reaction to GB contrast media.	Administer clear liquids for 24 hr before examination. Give laxative evening before and cleansing enema morning of examination. Keep patient NPO 8 hr before procedure.
▪ Nuclear imaging scans	Purpose is to show size, shape, and position of organ. Functional disorders and structural defects may be identified. Radionuclide (radioactive isotope) is injected IV and a counter (scanning) device picks up radioactive emission, which is recorded on paper. Only tracer doses of radioactive isotopes are used.	Tell patient that substances contain only traces of radioactivity and pose little to no danger. Schedule no more than one radionuclide test on the same day. Explain to patient need to lie flat during scanning.
Gastric emptying studies	Radionuclide study is used to assess ability of stomach to empty solids or liquids. In solid-emptying study, cooked egg white containing Tc-99m is eaten. In liquid-emptying study, orange juice with Tc-99m is drunk. Sequential images from gamma camera are recorded q2 min for up to 60 min. Study is used in patients with emptying disorders from peptic ulcer, ulcer surgery, diabetes, or gastric malignancies.	Same as above.
Liver and spleen scans	Patient is given IV injection of Tc-99m and positioned under camera to record distribution of radioactivity in liver and spleen. In normal person, intensity of liver and spleen images is equal. Test is useful in detecting hepatomegaly, hepatocellular diseases, hepatic malignancies, and splenomegaly.	Same as above.
Endoscopic		
▪ Upper GI endoscopy Esophagoscopy	Technique directly visualizes mucosal lining of esophagus, stomach, and duodenum with flexible, fiberoptic endoscope. Test may use video imaging to visualize stomach motility. Inflammations, ulcerations, tumors, varices, or Mallory-Weiss tear may be detected.	Before the procedure, keep patient NPO for 8 hr. Make sure signed consent is on chart. Give preoperative medication if ordered (diazepam or meperidine). Explain to patient that local anesthetic may be sprayed on throat before insertion of scope, and that patient will be sedated during the procedure.

continued

Table 36-12 Diagnostic Studies: Gastrointestinal System–cont'd

Study	Description and Purpose	Nursing Responsibility
Endoscopic—cont'd		
Gastroscopy Gastroduodenoscopy		After the procedure, keep patient NPO until gag reflex returns. Gently tickle back of throat to determine reflex. Use warm saline gargles for relief of sore throat. Check temperature q15-30 min for 1-2 hr (sudden temperature spike is sign of perforation).
■ Proctosigmoidoscopy	Study directly visualizes rectum and sigmoid colon with lighted endoscope. It is usually done with rigid metal scope but may be done with flexible fiberscope. Sometimes special table is used to tilt patient into knee-chest position. Test may detec tu-mors, polyps, inflammatory and infectious diseases, fissures, hemorrhoids.	Administer enemas evening before and morning of procedure. Be aware that patient may have clear liquids day before or that no dietary restrictions may be necessary. Explain to patient knee-chest position (unless patient is older or very ill), need to take deep breaths during insertion of scope, and possible urge to defecate as scope is passed. Encour-age patient to relax—let abdomen go limp. Observe for rectal bleeding after polypectomy or biopsy.
■ Fiberoptic colonoscopy	Study directly visualize entire colon up to ileocecal valve with flexible fiberoptic scope. Patient's position is changed frequently during procedure to assist with advancement of scope to cecum. Test is used to diagnose inflammatory bowel disease, identify bleeding sites, and di-late strictures. Procedure allows for removal of colonic polyps without laparotomy.	Before the procedure, keep patient on clear liquids 1-3 days and NPO for 8 hr. Administer laxatives 1-3 days before and enemas night before. Explain to patient same information regarding insertion of scope as for sigmodoscopy. Explain to patient that sedation will be given. Administer alternate preparation of 1 gal of GoLytely or Colyte evening before (8 oz glass q10 min). On morning of procedure, allow clear liquids. After the procedure, be aware that patient may experience abdominal cramps caused by stimulation of peristalsis because the patient's bowel is constantly insufflated with air during procedure. Observe for rectal bleeding and signs of perforation (e.g. malaise, abdominal distention, tenesmus). Check vital signs.
■ Endoscopic retrograde cholangiopancreatography (ERCP)	Fiberoptic endoscope is inserted through the oral cavity into descending duodenum, then common bile and pancreatic ducts are cannulated. Contrast medium is injected into ducts and allows for direct visualization of structures. Technique can also be used to retrieve a gallstone from distal CBD, dilate strictures, biopsy tumors, diagnose pseudocysts.	Before the procedure, explain procedure to patient, including patient role. Keep patient NPO 8 hr before procedure. Ensure consent form signed. Administer sedation immediately before and during procedure. Administer antibiotics if ordered. After the procedure, check vital signs. Check for signs of perforation or infection. Be aware that pancreatitis is most common complication. Check for return of gag reflex

continued

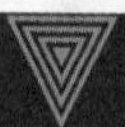

Table 36-12 Diagnostic Studies: Gastrointestinal System—cont'd

Study	Description and Purpose	Nursing Responsibility
Endoscopic—cont'd		
■ Computed tomography	Noninvasive radiologic examination combines special x-ray machine used for tomography (exposures at different depths) with computer. Study detects mainly biliary tract, liver, and pancreatic disorders. Use of contrast medium accentuates density differences and helps detect biliary problems.	Explain procedure to patient. Determine sensitivity to iodine if contrast material used.
■ Magnetic resonance imaging	Noninvasive procedure using radiofrequency waves and a magnetic field. Procedure is used to detect hepatic metastases, sources of GI bleeding, and to stage colorectal cancer.	Patient is NPO for 6 hr before procedure. Explain procedure to patient. Contraindicated in patient with metal implants, (e.g., pacemaker, or who is pregnant).
■ Peritoneoscopy (laparoscopy)	Peritoneal cavity and contents are visualized with laparoscope. Biopsy specimen may also be taken. Double-puncture peritoneoscopy permits better visualization of abdominal cavity, especially liver. Technique can eliminate need for exploratory laparotomy in many patients.	Make sure signed permit is on chart. Keep patient NPO 8 hr before study. Administer preoperative sedative medication. Ensure that bladder and bowel are emptied. Instruct patient that local anesthetic is used before scope insertion. Observe for possible complications of bleeding and bowel perforation after the procedure.
Blood Chemistries		
■ Serum amylase	Study measures secretion of amylase by pancreas and is important in diagnosing acute pancreatitis. Level of amylase peaks in 24 hr and then drops to normal in 48-72 hr. Depending on method, *normal finding* is 0-130 U/L (0-2.17 μkat/L).	Obtain blood sample in acute attack of pancreatitis. Explain procedure to patient.
■ Serum lipase	Study measures secretion of lipase by pancreas. Level stays elevated longer than serum amylase. *Normal finding* is 0-160 U/L (0-2.66 μkat/L).	Explain procedure to patient.
Invasive Procedures		
■ Liver biopsy	Invasive procedure uses needle inserted between sixth and seventh or eighth and ninth intercostal spaces on the right side to obtain specimen of hepatic tissue.	Before the procedure, check patient's coagulation status (PT, clotting or bleeding time). Ensure that patient is typed and cross-matched. Take vital signs as baseline data. Explain holding of breath after expiration when needle is inserted. Ensure that informed consent has been signed. After the procedure, check vital signs to detect internal bleeding q15 min × 2, q30 min × 4, q1hr × 4. Keep patient lying on right side for minimum of 2 hr to splint puncture site. Keep patient in bed in flat position for 12-14 hr. Assess patient for complications such as bile peritonitis, shock, pneumothorax.

continued

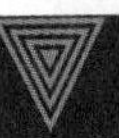

Table 36-12 Diagnostic Studies: Gastrointestinal System–cont'd

Study	Description and Purpose	Nursing Responsibility
Miscellaneous Tests		
▪ Gastric analysis	Purpose is to analyze gastric contents for acidity and volume. NG tube is inserted and gastric contents are aspirated. Contents are analyzed mainly for hydrochloric acid, but pH, pepsin, and electrolytes may be determined. Histalog and pentagastrin may be used to stimulate hydrochloric acid secretion. Exfoliative cytology may be done to determine whether malignant cells are present. With fasting, *normal acidity* is 2.5 mEq/L (2.5 mmol/L) and *normal volume* is 62 ml/hr; 30 min after Histalog or pentagastrin administration, normal acidity is 1.5 mEq/L (1.5 mmol/L) and normal volume is 110ml/hr.	Keep patient NPO for 8-12 hr. Explain insertion of NG tube. Withhold drugs affecting gastric secretions 24-48 hr before test. Ensure no smoking morning of test (nicotine increases gastric secretion).
▪ Fecal analysis	Form, consistency, color are noted. Specimen examined for mucus, blood, pus, parasites, and fat content. Tests for occult blood (guaiac test, Hemoccult, Hematest) are done.	Observe patient's stools. Collect stool specimens. Check stools for blood with Hemoccult or Hematest. Keep diet free of red meat for 24-48 hr before guaiac test.
▪ D-Xylose tolerance	Absorption test involves xylose, a monosaccharide, given orally in water. All urine is collected for 5 hr and amount of D-Xylose excreted is measured. *Normal finding* is 20% of xylose excreted in 5 hr.	Keep patient NPO for 10-12 hr before test. Ensure that patient empties bladder before xylose given orally.
▪ Duodenal drainage	Duodenal contents are aspirated by double-lumen NG tube—one lumen in stomach, the other in duodenum. Stimulant IV drug is given (usually CCK). Duodenal contents are analyzed for enzymes, blood, bile, malignant cells, cholesterol crystals, and volume.	Explain procedure to patient. Insert NG tube. Keep patient on NPO status.

CBD, Common bile duct; *CCK,* cholecystokinin *GB,* gallbladder; *GI,* gastrointestinal; *IV,* intravenous; *NG,* nasogastric; *Tc-99m,* technetium-99m.

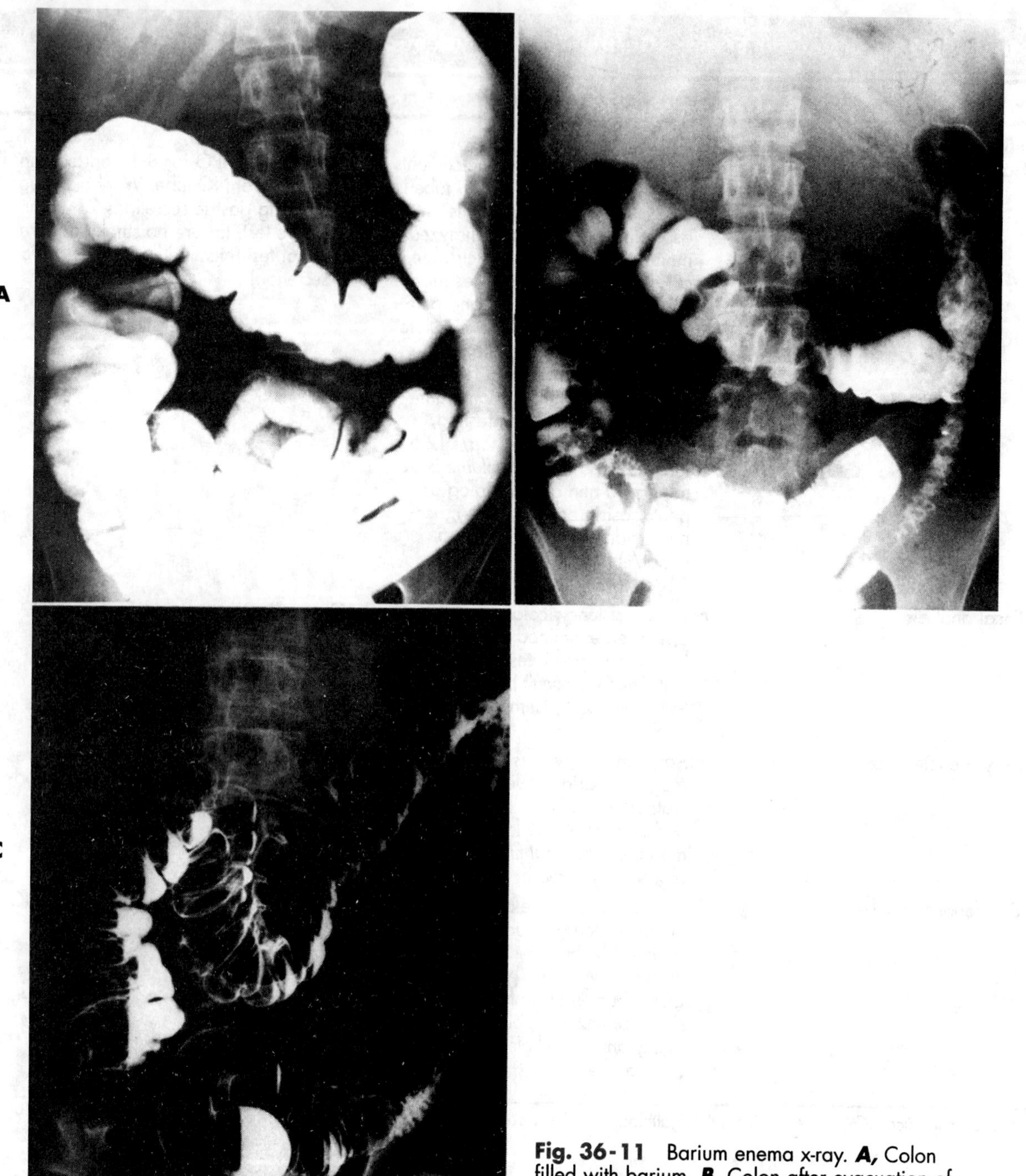

Fig. 36-11 Barium enema x-ray. ***A,*** Colon filled with barium. ***B,*** Colon after evacuation of barium. ***C,*** Air-contrast study of colon.

Table 36-13 Liver Function Tests

Test	Description and Purpose
Bile Formation and Excretion	
■ Serum bilirubin	Measurement of ability of liver to conjugate and excrete bilirubin, allowing differentiation between unconjugated (indirect) and conjugated (direct) bilirubin in plasma
Total	Measurement of direct and indirect total bilirubin *Normal finding* of 0.2-1.3 mg/dl (3.4-22.0 μmol/L)
Direct	Measurement of conjugated bilirubin, elevation in obstructive jaundice *Normal finding* of 0.1-0.3 mg/dl (1.7-5.1 μmol/L)
Indirect	Measurement of unconjugated bilirubin, elevation in hepatocellular and hemolytic conditions *Normal finding* of 0.1-1.0 mg/dl (1.7-17 μmol/L)
■ Urinary Bilirubin	Measurement of urinary excretion of conjugated bilirubin *Normal finding* of 0
■ Urinary urobilinogen	Measurement of urinary excretion of urobilinogen; maximum excretion midafternoon to early evening, collection of total urinary output for 2 hr in afternoon, sent to laboratory in dark container immediately because of oxidation of urobilinogen to urobilin on exposure to air. *Normal finding* of 0.5-4 mg/day (0.8-6.8 μmol/day)
■ Fecal urobilinogen	Measurement of fecal urobilinogen in stool specimen *Normal finding* of 30-220 mg/100 g stool (55-372 μmol/100 g of stool)
Dye Excretion Tests (Detoxification)	
■ Indocyanine green	Determination of liver's ability to take up and excrete dye given IV, drawing of blood samples every 5 min for 20-30 min *Normal finding* of 500-800 ml/m^2 of body surface/min
Protein Metabolism	
■ Serum protein levels	Measurement of serum proteins that are manufactured by the liver; measurement of albumin, *normal finding* of 3.5-5.0 g/dl (35-50 g/L); measurement of globulin, *normal finding* of 2.0-3.5 g/dl (20-35 g/L) *Normal total protein* of 6–8 g/dl (60-80 g/L) *Normal A/G ratio* of 1.5:1-2.5:1
■ α-Fetoprotein	Indication of hepatic cancer *Normal finding* of <25 ng/ml (<25 μg/L)
■ Blood ammonia levels	Conversion of ammonia to urea normally occurs in the liver, elevation can result in hepatic encephalopathy secondary to liver cirrhosis *Normal finding* of 30-70 μg/dl (17.6-41.1 μmol/L)
Hemostatic Functions	
■ Prothrombin	Determination of prothrombin activity *Normal finding* of 12-15 sec
■ Vitamin K production	Determination of response of liver to vitamin K, checking of PT necessary 24 hr after injection of vitamin K
Serum Enzyme Tests	
■ Alkaline phosphatase (ALP)	Normal presence of high concentrations, excretion in bile, elevation in obstructive jaundice *Normal finding* of 30-120 U/L (0.5-2.0 μkat/L), depending on method and age
■ Aspartate aminotrans ferase (AST) or serum glutamic-oxaloacetic transaminase (SGOT)	Elevation in liver damage and inflammation *Normal finding* of 7-40 U/L (0.12-0.67 μkat/L)
■ Alanine aminotransferase (ALT) or serum glutamic-pyruvic transaminase (SGPT)	Elevation in liver damage and inflammation *Normal finding* of 5-36 U/L (0.08-0.6 μkat/L)
■ δ-Glutamyl transpeptidase (GGT)	Present in biliary tract (not in skeletal muscle or cardiac), increase in hepatitis and alcoholic liver disease. More sensitive for liver dysfunction than ALP. *Normal finding* of 0-30 U/L (0-.5 μkat/L)

continued

Table 36-13 Liver Function Tests—cont'd

Test	Description and Purpose
Lipid Metabolism	
■ Serum cholesterol	Synthesis and excretion by liver, increase in biliary obstruction, decrease in extensive liver disease and malnutrition *Normal finding* of 140-200 mg/dl (3.6-5.2 mmol/L), varying with age
Serum Antigen and Antibody	
■ Hepatitis A antigen (HA Ag)	Present in serum and stool early in course of hepatitis A
■ Hepatitis A antibody (HA Ab)	Indicates past or present infection with hepatitis A
■ Hepatitis B surface antigen (Hb_s Ag)	Indicates current infection with hepatitis B or past infection with carrier state
■ Hepatitis B e antigen (Hb_e Ag)	Present in active and infective state of hepatitis B
■ Hepatitis B core antigen (Hb_c Ag)	Indicates ongoing infection with hepatitis B; higher titers in chronic carrier state
■ Hepatitis B surface antibody (Hb_s Ag)	Indicates previous hepatitis B infection or immunization
■ Hepatitis B e antibody (Hb_e Ab)	Present in cases of low-grade infectivity
■ Hepatitis B c antibody (Hb_c Ab)	Present in previous or ongoing infection with hepatitis B; high levels in chronic carrier state
■ Hepatitis C antibody (anti-HCV)	Indicates past or current infection with hepatitis C
■ Delta antigen	Present in serum in hepatitis D
■ Antibody to delta antigen	Present in cases of past or current infection with hepatitis D

IV, Intravenous; *PT,* prothrombin.

REVIEW QUESTIONS

The number of the question corresponds to the same-numbered objective at the beginning of the chapter.

1. Mrs. J., age 88 years, is admitted with a diagnosis of diarrhea with dehydration. Increased peristalsis resulting in diarrhea can be related to
   a. parasympathetic stimulation.
   b. sympathetic stimulation.
   c. sympathetic inhibition.
   d. mixing and propulsion.

2. The majority of the blood supply to the liver is from the
   a. hepatic artery.
   b. cephalic artery.
   c. renal artery.
   d. portal vein.

3. All of the following enzymes participate in the breakdown of proteins *except*
   a. amylase.
   b. trypsin.
   c. pepsin.
   d. peptidases.

4. Mrs. H. is jaundiced and her stools are clay-colored (gray). This is most likely related to
   a. increased production of cholecystokinin.
   b. decreased bile flow into the intestine.
   c. increased bile and bilirubin in the blood.
   d. increased production of urobilinogen.

5. Mr. S., age 80 years, states that although he adds a lot of salt to his food it still does not have much taste. The response by the nurse is based on which of the following facts regarding ingestion changes in the older adult?
   a. The older adult should not experience changes in taste.
   b. There is a loss of taste buds, especially for sweet and salty.
   c. There is a loss of taste buds for sweet only.
   d. There is some loss of taste but no difficulty chewing food.

6. Which of the following questions should the nurse ask the patient when assessing the health perception–health management pattern?
   a. What percentage of your income is spent on food?
   b. What is your usual bowel elimination pattern?

c. Have you traveled to a foreign country in the last year?
d. Do you have diarrhea when you are under a lot of stress?

7. Which of the following statements is correct related to an abdominal examination?

a. The patient should be in the supine position with the bed flat and knees straight.
b. The following order should be used: inspection, palpation, percussion, auscultation.
c. The nurse should listen in the epigastrium and all four quadrants for 2 to 5 minutes for bowel sounds.
d. Bowel sounds are described as absent if no sound is heard in the lower right quadrant after 2 minutes.

8. Which of the following is a normal physical assessment finding of the GI system?

a. Tympany on percussion of the abdomen.
b. Liver edge less than 1 to 2 cm below costal margin.
c. Finding of a firm, nodular edge on the rectal exam.
d. Easy palpation of the spleen edges with moderate pressure.

9. Which of the following is the correct explanation or instruction to a patient scheduled for colonoscopy?

a. Inform patient to eat lightly the day before the procedure.
b. Explain that sedation may be used during the procedure.
c. Explain that a signed permit is not necessary.
d. Inform patient that only one cleansing enema preparation is necessary.

REFERENCES

1. Eliopoulos C: *Caring for the elderly in diverse care settings,* Philadelphia, 1990, Lippincott.
2. Porth CM: *Pathophysiology concepts of altered health states,* ed 4, Philadelphia, 1994, Lippincott.
3. Burke MM, Walsh MB: *Gerontologic nursing care of the frail elderly,* St Louis, 1992, Mosby.
4. Doughty DB, Jackson DB: *Mosby's clinical nursing series: gastrointestinal disorders,* St Louis, 1993, Mosby.
5. Seidel HM and others: *Mosby's guide to physical examination,* ed 2, St Louis, 1991, Mosby.

Chapter 37

NURSING ROLE IN MANAGEMENT

Problems of Nutrition

Una Elizabeth Westfall   Gladys Elizabeth Deters

Learning Objectives

1. Describe the essential components of a nutritionally sound diet and their importance to good health.
2. Describe the common etiologic factors, clinical manifestations, and management of malnutrition.
3. Compare the etiologic factors, clinical manifestations, and therapeutic and nursing management of bulimia and anorexia nervosa.
4. Differentiate between central and peripheral total parenteral nutrition administration and tube feedings, including the indications for use, complications, and therapeutic and nursing management.
5. Discuss the multiple etiologies, complications, and therapeutic and surgical management of obesity.
6. Describe the nursing care related to conservative and surgical management of obesity.

The focus of this chapter is on problems related to nutrition. The primary nutritional problems discussed are malnutrition and obesity.

NUTRITIONAL PROBLEMS

Nutritional problems are present in all age groups, cultures, ethnic groups, and socioeconomic classes in all parts of the world. Intelligence and wealth do not necessarily preclude the development of poor nutritional habits. The nurse in the roles of caregiver, teacher, and resource person can have a profound influence on the nutritional practices of patients and their families. A strong foundation in the principles of sound nutrition is essential. Together with the physician and the dietitian, the nurse is in a strategic position to assess the dietary practices of the patient and provide important information, as well as link an individual with nutritional resources within and outside the institutional setting.

The nutritional state of a person or a family may be influenced by many factors. Attitudes toward the importance of food and eating habits are established early. Cultural or religious preferences and requirements are frequently reflected in dietary intake. The financial condition of a family or an individual often determines the type and amount of nutritionally sound food that can be purchased. Findings support that, generally, the lower the socioeconomic status, the poorer the nutritional state.[1] The availability of food sources also contributes to the nutritional state of people. This is usually not a problem in developed countries in which agriculture is well established and productive, but it may be a problem in underdeveloped countries.

Normal Nutrition

Nutrition is the process by which the body uses food for energy, growth, and maintenance and repair of body tissues. Good nutrition in the absence of any underlying disease process results from the ingestion of a balanced diet. The United States Department of Agriculture (USDA) has adopted the food guide pyramid that consists of food groups that are presented in proportions appropriate for a healthy diet. Figure 37-1 and Table 37-1 show these food groups with the daily requirements and examples of common sources.

The essential components of the basic food groups are *carbohydrates*, *fats*, *proteins*, *vitamins*, and *minerals*. Carbohydrates, the body's primary source of energy, yield approximately 4 kilocalories* per gram. Carbohydrates are either simple or complex. Simple carbohydrates come in two forms: monosaccharides (e.g., glucose and fructose), found in fruits and honey; and disaccharides (e.g., sucrose, maltose, and lactose), found in such substances as table sugar, malted cereal, and milk respectively. Complex carbohydrates or polysaccharides commonly appear in the diet as starches, such as cereal grains, potatoes, and legumes. Carbohydrates are the chief protein-sparing ingredient in a

Reviewed by Peggi Guenter, RN, PhD, CNSN, Coordinator, Nutrition Support Service, Department of Surgery, The Graduate Hospital, Philadelphia, PA.

*Kilocalories is the correct way to designate caloric intake and expenditure. However, calorie is more used commonly used.

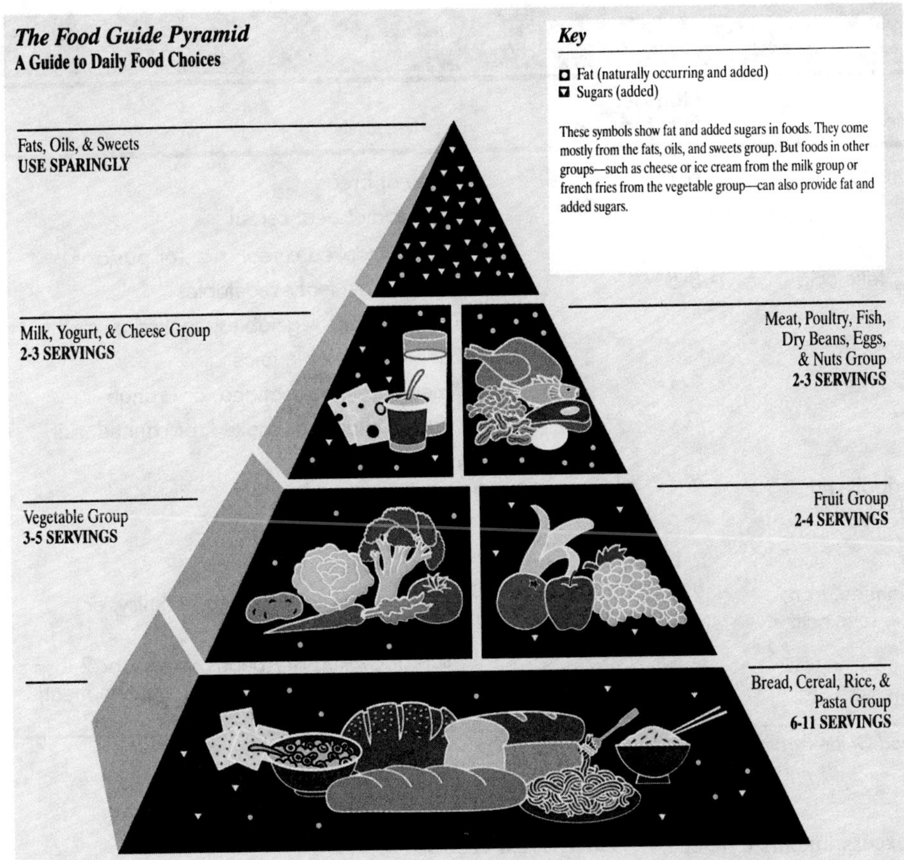

Fig. 37-1 Food guide pyramid: a guide to daily food choices and number of servings.

nutritionally sound diet and compose approximately 47% of the daily caloric needs of the body. The National Research Council recommends that, after infancy, at least half the energy level needed should come from carbohydrates, especially complex carbohydrates.[2]

Approximately 36% of the daily caloric intake in current American diets is derived from *fat*.[2] This level is considerably higher than that found in many other societies and is a cause for national concern. The Food and Nutrition Board's Committee on Diet and Health recommends that people reduce their fat intake to 30% of their total daily caloric intake.[3] One gram of fat yields 9 calories. Fats are stored in adipose tissue and in the abdominal cavity. Besides being a major source of energy, fats act as insulation, which reduces loss of body heat in cold environments, and provides padding and protection for vital organs. Fats also act as carriers of essential fatty acids and fat-soluble vitamins. Fats provide a feeling of satiety after eating, partly from the flavor added and partly from their slow rate of digestion, which delays hunger.

Proteins, another essential component of a well-balanced diet, are obtained from both animal and plant sources. They provide 15% to 20% of daily caloric needs of the body. The recommended daily protein intake is 0.8 g/kg of body weight. One gram of protein yields 4 calories. Proteins are complex nitrogenous organic compounds, of which *amino acids* are the fundamental units of structure. The 22 amino acids can be classified as *essential* and *nonessential*. The body is capable of synthesizing nonessential amino acids if an adequate supply of nitrogen is available. However, the essential amino acids, of which there are nine, cannot be synthesized, and their availability depends totally on dietary sources. Proteins containing all the essential amino acids are called *complete proteins*. Proteins that lack one or more of the essential amino acids are called *incomplete proteins*. Table 37-2 lists good sources of protein. Proteins are essential for tissue growth, repair, and maintenance; body regulatory functions; and energy production.

Vitamins are organic compounds required in small amounts by the body for normal metabolism. Vitamins function primarily in enzyme reactions that facilitate the metabolism of amino acids, fats, and carbohydrates. The body must rely on a dietary source to meet requirements for some vitamins, such as vitamin B_{12}. Vitamins are divided into two categories: *water-soluble* vitamins (vitamin C and the B complex vitamins) and *fat-soluble* vitamins (vitamins A, D, E, and K).

Mineral salts (e.g., magnesium, iron) make up approximately 4% of the total body weight. When minerals are present in minute amounts, they are referred to as *trace elements* or *micronutrients*. Minerals required in amounts greater than 100 mg a day are called *major minerals*. Table 37-3 lists the major minerals and trace elements. Minerals are necessary for the body to build tissues, regulate body fluids, and assist in various body functions. Some minerals are stored in a manner similar to that of the fat-soluble

Table 37-1 Pyramid Food Groups and Recommended Number of Servings

Group	Nutrients Provided	Number of Servings Daily	Serving Size
▪ Bread, cereal, rice, pasta	Thiamine, niacin, iron, protein	6-11	1 slice of bread 1 oz ready-to-eat cereal ½ cup of cooked cereal, rice, or pasta
▪ Vegetable	Vitamins A and C, folic acid	3-5	1 cup of raw leafy vegetables ½ cup of other vegetables, cooked or raw ¾ cup of vegetable juice
▪ Fruit	Vitamins A and C	2-4	1 medium apple, banana, or orange ½ cup of chopped, cooked, or canned fruit ¾ cup of fruit juice
▪ Milk, yogurt, cheese	Calcium, protein, riboflavin, vitamins B_6 and B_{12}	2-3	1 cup of milk or yogurt 1½ oz of natural cheese 2 oz of processed cheese
▪ Meat, poultry, fish, dry beans, eggs, nuts	Protein, niacin, thiamine, iron, zinc, vitamin B_{12}, folic acid	2-3	2-3 oz of cooked lean meat, poultry, or fish ½ cup of cooked dry beans, 1 egg, or 2 tbsp of peanut butter (count as 1 oz lean meat)

From Human Nutrition Information Service: *Food Guide Pyramid,* Hyattsville, MD, 1992, USDA.

vitamins and can be toxic if taken in excess amounts. The amount of minerals needed in the daily diet varies greatly from a few micrograms of trace minerals to a gram or more of the major minerals, such as calcium, phosphorus, and sodium. A well-balanced diet can usually meet the daily requirements of needed minerals. However, deficiency states can occur.

The daily caloric requirements of a person are influenced by body build, age, gender, physical activity, and level of physical and emotional health. Adjustments in caloric intake are necessary, depending on changes in health status and daily activity level. Table 37-4 summarizes the recommended daily caloric and protein intake. Table 37-5 gives an example of caloric and protein needs under normal and stress conditions.

Table 37-2 Good Sources of Protein

Complete Proteins	Incomplete Proteins
Milk and milk products (e.g., cheese) Eggs Fish Meats Poultry	Grains (e.g., corn) Legumes (e.g., navy beans, soybeans, peas) Nuts (e.g., peanuts) Seeds (e.g., sesame seeds, sunflower seeds)

Nutritional Needs

Children and Adolescents. Parents are responsible for setting an example of good nutritional habits for their children. Parental eating habits and attitudes toward food are readily passed on to their children. Parents who have little understanding of what constitutes a well-balanced diet or who cannot or will not learn good nutritional habits influence their children to follow the same poor dietary practices. The nurse is in a good position to help parents understand the changing food requirements of their children from infancy through adolescence.

Infants and children differ from adults in several ways. In the first months of life, the infant's gastrointestinal (GI)

Table 37-3 Major Minerals and Trace Elements

Major Minerals	Trace Elements
Calcium	Chromium
Chloride	Copper
Magnesium	Fluoride
Phosphorus	Iodine
Potassium	Iron
Sodium	Manganese
Sulfur	Molybdenum
	Selenium
	Zinc

Table 37-4 Recommended Daily Protein and Caloric Intake by Median Heights and Weights

Category	Age (yr)	Weight (lb)	Weight (kg)	Height (in)	Height (cm)	Protein (gm)	Average Daily Energy Allowance* (calories)
▪ Men	19-24	160	72	70	177	58	2900
	25-50	174	79	70	176	63	2900
	51 and over	170	77	68	173	68	2300
▪ Women	19-24	128	58	65	164	46	2200
	25-50	138	63	64	163	50	2200
	51 and over	143	65	63	160	50	1900

From Food and Nutrition Board, National Research Council, National Academy of Sciences: *Recommended dietary allowances*, ed 10, Washington, DC, 1989, National Academy Press.
*For light to moderate activity.

tract and kidneys are not functionally mature and, therefore are limited in the kinds and quantities of nutrients that should be given. In addition, an infant and a child operate at a high basal metabolic rate that leaves little in the way of nutritional reserves.

Adolescence is a particularly vulnerable time for the development of nutritional deficiencies because this is a time of rapid growth and bodily changes. It is a period during which there is extreme concern with body appearance and social acceptability. Teenage girls are often attracted to fad diets as a means of weight control. Unfortunately, fad diets are often nutritionally unsound. Unless good nutritional habits are encouraged and supervised by peers and parents during this developmental period, poor nutritional patterns may become established as a way of life. A state of chronic inadequate nutrition may result.

Socioeconomic Status. Because individuals and families from the lower socioeconomic class must spend a greater percentage of their limited income on food, there is a tendency to seek out cheaper foods as the cost of food increases. These foods may not provide adequate or balanced nutrition. In contrast, some lower income persons may prefer to select foods that are more expensive, but only marginally nutritious, because of their prestige value. The nurse and the dietitian can assist the poor in making food choices that meet nutritional requirements while staying within their limited resources. Table 37-6 presents low-cost protein supplements.

Older Adults. The unique nutritional requirements of an older adult are often overlooked. It is more common to find an undernourished older person than an obese one. As a person grows older there is a concomitant decrease in lean body mass, basal metabolic rate, and physical activity that lowers the caloric needs for energy. The older person frequently reduces the consumption of needed protein, vitamins, and minerals and may take in "empty calories," such as candy and pastries. The reasons given for such alterations are varied. Table 37-7 outlines factors affecting nutritional intake in older adults.

As a group, older adults may be less well informed about what constitutes a well-balanced diet. The older adult may be induced to purchase more costly "health foods" at specialty stores under the mistaken assumption that these foods offer more nutrients than foods bought at the local market.

When these factors are added to already existing medical problems, it is easy to see why poor dietary practices develop. In addition, poor dentition, ill-fitting dentures, anorexia, multiple losses affecting the social setting of meals, low income, and medical conditions involving the GI tract contribute to the type and amount of foods that can be eaten. The nurse, working with the nutritionist, must be aware of common medical and psychosocial factors in the

Table 37-5 Caloric and Protein Needs of a 150 lb (68 kg) Man

Activity	Calories	Protein (g)
Basal	1400	49
Moderate activity (activities of daily living)	2500	70
Postoperative (no complications)	3150	105
Stress response (e.g., to chemotherapy, radiation therapy)	3500	140
Infection	>4500	>175

Table 37-6 Low-Cost Protein Supplements*

Brewer's yeast	2⅓ tbs
Cheese	1-in cube
Cottage cheese	¼ cup
Egg	1
Milk (whole, low fat, or skim)	⅞ cup
Peanut butter	2 tbs
Pinto beans	¼ cup
Poultry	1 oz
Soybeans (cooked)	1 cup and 2 tsp
Split peas, lentils (cooked)	½ cup

Table 37-7 Factors Affecting Nutritional Intake in Older Adults

Age	Feelings of being valued
Degree of physical activity	Food fads
Anorexia	Food intolerance
Availability of desired foods	Gender
Availability of transportation to food stores	Health status
Available time for preparation and eating	Importance of food in the past
Chronic conditions	Income level
Decrease in number of taste buds	Lack of food preparation equipment
Dental problems	Loneliness or loss
Education level and nutritional knowledge	Mental awareness
	Physical disability
	Prescribed diets
	Prescribed or over-the-counter medicines
	Social isolation

older adult and should incorporate interventions for overcoming these problems in the teaching or plan of care.

Patients with Physical Illnesses. Regardless of the cause of the illness, the sick person has increased nutritional needs. Pathologic conditions are frequently aggravated by undernutrition, and an existing deficiency state is likely to become more severe during illness. Malnutrition is not an uncommon consequence of illness, surgery, injury, or hospitalization. Anorexia, nausea, vomiting, diarrhea, abdominal distention, and abdominal cramping may accompany diseases of the GI system. Any combination of these symptoms interferes with normal food consumption and metabolism. Additionally, a patient may restrict the dietary intake to a few foods or fluids that may not be nutritionally sound out of fear of aggravating the already disturbed GI function.

Malabsorption syndrome, which may result from decreased amounts of necessary enzymes or a reduced bowel surface area, can quickly lead to a deficiency state. Many pharmacologic agents may result in undesirable GI side effects and thus alter the normal digestive processes. For example, antibiotics change the normal flora of the intestines, decreasing the body's ability to synthesize some of the B complex vitamins.

Fever accompanies many illnesses, injuries, and infections, with a concomitant increase in the body's basal metabolic rate (BMR). Each degree of temperature increase on a Fahrenheit scale raises the BMR by 7%.[2] Without an increase in the amount of carbohydrates and fats ingested in the diet, body protein stores will be used to supply calories, and protein depletion can become a problem.

The hospitalized patient, especially the older adult, is at risk of becoming malnourished. Prolonged illness, major surgery, sepsis, draining wounds, burns, hemorrhage, fractures, and immobilization can all contribute to malnutrition. The nurse must assume responsibility, along with the physician and the dietitian, for meeting the patient's nutritional needs. The nurse must also be mindful of the requirements of a patient who is not overtly ill but who is undergoing diagnostic studies. This patient may be nutritionally fit on entering the hospital but can develop nutritional problems because of the dietary restrictions imposed by multiple diagnostic studies.

The role of nutrition in the development of diseases has long been studied. Studies of the association of personal dietary habits with the development of selected cancers and cardiovascular diseases have been widely published in recent years. There now appear to be strong links between some types of cancers and dietary intake [(e.g., high ingestion of fatty foods is linked with breast and endometrial cancer, and a low fiber intake is linked with some intestinal cancers ([see Chapter 12]))]. Further research in this area is needed for a better understanding of diet and the development of disease, especially cancer.

Vitamin Imbalances

Vitamin deficiencies are rare in most of the developed countries of the world. When vitamin deficiencies are present, several vitamins are usually involved rather than a single vitamin deficiency. In the United States the recommended dietary allowances (RDA) for essential vitamins and minerals can be obtained by eating a diet consisting of foods from the basic five food groups. RDAs from the Food and Nutrition Board have a safety margin because the levels exceed minimum daily requirements for most people. When vitamin imbalances do occur, they are usually found among persons such as alcoholics, drug addicts, and the poor, who follow poor dietary practices. Followers of fad diets or poorly planned vegetarian diets are also subject to a potential deficiency state. Clinical manifestations of vitamin imbalances are most commonly exhibited as neurologic manifestations (Table 37-8). In the growing child, the central nervous system (CNS) is primarily involved, while the peripheral nervous system is most affected in the adult.

Vegetarian Diets. The common element among all vegetarians is the exclusion of red meat from the diet. Vegetarianism cannot be considered a nutritional fad because it is found in all age groups, occupations, and lifestyles. A variety of reasons have been given for following this type of dietary practice, including religious or cultural beliefs, belief that it is a better way of attaining total health, respect for all living beings, ethical-ecologic ideals, and economics.

Vegetarian diets can result in a potential vitamin deficiency state. The two large classes of vegetarians are *vegans*, who are pure or total vegetarians and use only plant food, and *lacto-ovo-vegetarians*, who use plant foods and sometimes dairy products and eggs. There are several other types, including the *fruitarians*, but they constitute only a small percentage of the total group.

In well-planned vegetarian diets the essential vitamins and minerals are easily obtained. Plant protein, although of

Table 37-8 Recommended Dietary Vitamin Allowances and Signs of Imbalance

Vitamin	Recommended Dietary Allowances	Symptoms of Overdose	Manifestations of Deficiencies
Fat Soluble			
▪ A	Men: 1000 μg/Retinol equivalents* Women: 800 μg/Retinol equivalents	Hair loss, dry skin; headaches; dry mucous membranes; liver damage; bone and joint pain; blurred vision; nausea and vomiting	Dry, scaly skin; increased susceptibility to infection; night blindness; anorexia; eye irritation; xerosis; keratinization of respiratory and GI mucosa; bladder stones; anemia; retarded growth
▪ D	Adults 5-10 μg of cholecalciferol†	Deposits of calcium and phosphorus in soft tissue; kidney and heart damage; bone fragility; constipation; anorexia, nausea, vomiting; headache	Muscular weakness; excessive sweating; diarrhea and other GI disturbances; bone pain; active rickets; healed rickets; osteomalacia
▪ E	Men: 10 mg Women: 8 mg	Relatively nontoxic	Neurologic defects; hemolytic anemia (only in newborns)
▪ K	Men: 70-80 μg Women: 60 μg	Anemia	Defective blood coagulation
Water Soluble			
▪ B_1	Men: 1.2-1.5 mg Women: 1.0-1.1 mg	Not stored in body, therefore overdose does not occur	Loss of appetite; fatigue; nervous irritability; constipation; paresthesias; insomnia
▪ B_6	Men: 1.7-2.0 mg Women: 1.4-1.6 mg	Not stored in body, therefore overdose does not occur	Convulsions; dermatitis; anemia; neuropathy with motor weakness; anorexia
▪ B_{12}	Adults: 2-10 μg	Not stored in body, therefore overdose does not occur	Megaloblastic anemia; inadequate myelin synthesis; anorexia; glossitis; sore mouth and tongue; pallor; neurologic problems such as depression and dizziness; weight loss; nausea; constipation
▪ C	Adults: 50-60 mg	Not stored in body, therefore overdose does not occur	Bleeding gums; loose teeth; easy bruising; poor wound healing; scurvy; dry, itchy skin
▪ Folic acid	Men: 200 μg Women: 180 μg	Not stored in body, therefore overdose does not occur	Impaired cell division and protein synthesis; megloblastic anemia; anorexia; fatigue; sore tongue; diarrhea; forgetfulness

Modified from Food and Nutrition Board, National Academy of Sciences: National Research Council *Recommended dietary allowances,* ed 10, Washington DC, 1989, National Academy Press.
GI, Gastrointestinal.
*1 Retinol Equivalent = 10 IU Vitamin A activity from β-carotene or 3.33 IU Vitamin A activity from retinol.
†1 μg of cholecalciferol = 40 IU vitamin D.

a lesser quality than that of animal origin, fulfills most of the protein requirements. Combinations of vegetable protein foods (e.g., cornmeal, kidney beans) can increase the nutritional value. Lacto-ovo-vegetarians obtain additional protein sources from dairy products and eggs. Milk made from soybeans is an excellent protein source, especially for the true vegan. The primary deficiency of a strict vegan is lack of vitamin B_{12}. This vitamin can be obtained only from animal protein, special supplements, or foods that have been fortified with the vitamin. Vegans not using vitamin B_{12} supplements are susceptible to the development of megaloblastic anemia and the neurologic signs of vitamin B_{12} deficiency. Strict vegetarians and lacto-ovo-vegetarians are also at risk for iron deficiency. Iron-enriched foods or iron supplements are often prescribed during pregnancy, early childhood, adolescence, and after major blood loss. Table 37-9 lists examples of foods high in iron. Other deficiencies that may be present in a vegan include calcium, zinc, vitamins A and D, or protein.

Megavitamin Therapy. Megavitamin therapy refers to the administration of high doses of one or more vitamins, usually 10 to 20 times the RDA. Unless there are serious vitamin deficiencies, megavitamin therapy has a limited place in maintaining nutrition. The beneficial effects derived from the ingestion of commercially prepared daily vitamins are negligible if a balanced diet is eaten.

Table 37-9 Nutritional Management: Foods High in Iron

Food	Selected Serving Size	% of U.S. RDA
Breads, Cereals, and Grain Products		
Farina, regular or quick cooked (enriched)	⅔ cup	25-39
Oatmeal, instant, fortified, prepared (enriched)	⅔ cup	25-39
Ready-to-eat cereals, fortified (enriched)	1 oz	25-39
Meat, Poultry, Fish, and Alternatives		
Beef liver, braised	3 oz	25-39
Pork liver, braised	3 oz	>39
Chicken or turkey liver, braised	½ cup diced	25-39
Clams; steamed, boiled, or canned, drained	3 oz	>39
Oysters; baked, broiled, steamed or canned, undrained	3 oz	25-39
Soybeans, cooked	½ cup	25-39

From Human Nutrition Information Service *Good Sources of Nutrients,* Washington, DC, 1990, USDA.
RDA, Recommended dietary allowance.
Note: Vitamin C improves iron absorption.

The water-soluble vitamins (vitamins C and B complex) are absorbed only as needed by the body, and the excess is excreted rapidly in the urine. Toxicity from overdoses is rare. However, because the excess is excreted through the kidney and urinary tract, detrimental effects may occur. Vitamin C is uricosuric (increases the renal excretion of uric acid) and may cause the formation of urinary tract stones (uric acid stones) in susceptible persons when taken in megadoses. When taken in large doses, vitamins function as drugs rather than as nutrients and can cause toxic manifestations.

The fat-soluble vitamins (vitamins A, D, E, and K) are readily stored and can accumulate to toxic levels. Because most vitamins can be purchased without a prescription, high doses of vitamins A, D, and E can result in serious health hazards because the excess is not eliminated (see Table 37-8). Toxic levels of the fat-soluble vitamins can be reached within a matter of weeks, especially in infants and children.

Eating Disorders

Anorexia Nervosa. Anorexia nervosa, also called anorexia, is a specific psychiatric diagnosis. As a specific psychiatric disorder, anorexia nervosa is characterized by refusal to maintain body weight to greater than 85% of that expected for age and height.[4] This condition results in a severely malnourished state characterized by the vigorous pursuit of thinness and a morbid fear of becoming fat. Restricted intake occurs even in the presence of hunger.

The two subgroups of anorexia nervosa are the *bulimic* type and the *restrictive* type, depending on whether or not there are cycles of binging and purging.[5] This condition is found predominantly in adolescent girls. The disorder was first recorded in England in 1684 and was misnamed anorexia nervosa because it was thought to be secondary to severe sadness and anxiety. The name has persisted to the present day even though current research indicates a different cause. Anorexia nervosa usually begins during adolescence or early adulthood. It is a chronic illness that can place the patient at high risk for serious complications, affecting multiple systems such as the cardiovascular, the skeletal, the GI, and the endocrine systems. Life-threatening cardiac complications include hypotension, bradycardia, and malignant dysrhythmias. It is rare for the illness to occur for the first time in a woman who is more than 25 years old.

Anorexia nervosa is now recognized as occurring more often among persons whose sisters and mothers have the disorder than among the general population. Patients often come from a middle- or upper-class background. They often are perfectionists and tend to be high achievers. At the same time, they may be dependent and experience insecurity in social situations.[4] In some patients the disorder is associated with stressful life situations with which they are unable to cope. In addition, many patients are somewhat overweight at the onset of their illness.

Common physical signs and symptoms of anorexia nervosa include amenorrhea, bradycardia, orthostatic hypotension, cold intolerance, breast atrophy, lanugo (soft, downlike hair normally associated with a fetus), dry skin, hair loss, severe constipation, and edema with altered fluid balance. Diagnostic studies often show iron deficiency anemia, elevated total cholesterol levels, and an elevated blood urea nitrogen reflective of marked intravascular volume depletion and prerenal azotemia. Lack of potassium in the diet and loss of potassium in the urine lead to potassium deficiency in blood and tissues. This potassium deficiency can lead to weakness, cardiac dysrhythmias, and renal failure.

Once anorexia nervosa has developed, the person will go to almost any extreme to hide the eating behavior from parents or peers. Eating habits are severely disturbed. If purging is present, it is often accomplished by self-induced vomiting, or the use of cathartics or enemas.

If the eating pattern is permitted to continue for a prolonged time, body wasting and signs of severe malnutrition are evident. Multidisciplinary treatment must involve a combination of improved nutrition, and supportive and psychiatric care. Hospitalization may be necessary if there are severe physical complications that cannot be managed in an outpatient therapy program. Nutritional replenishment must be closely supervised, not merely for the few pounds the person can rapidly gain but for consistent and ongoing gains. The use of tube or parenteral feedings may be necessary. Improved nutrition, however, is not a cure for anorexia nervosa. The underlying psychiatric problem must be addressed by identification of the disturbed patterns of individual and family interactions, followed by individual and family counseling.

Bulimia. Bulimia is a chronic disorder that is often confused with anorexia nervosa. Concern about body image is a key feature in both bulimia and anorexia nervosa; however, the syndrome of bulimia is different from anorexia nervosa. Bulimia is characterized by compulsive binge eating and purging (through self-induced vomiting, laxative and exercise abuse, and diuretics). Food becomes an obsession and an addiction—an escape from the pressures of life. Unlike the person with anorexia, the patient caught up in the syndrome of bulimia usually maintains a normal or near-normal body weight, and the primary symptom is gorging rather than starvation.

Bulimia is increasing in incidence and may be even more prevalent than anorexia nervosa. Female students of college age are a population group that seems to be susceptible to this syndrome. The cause remains unclear but is thought to be similar to that of anorexia nervosa. Substance abuse, anxiety, affective disorders, and personality disturbances have been reported among persons with bulimia.

In addition to the psychologic considerations, bulimia may lead to some physical effects in those persons who binge and purge on a daily basis. Characteristic skin lesions on the back of the hand, which are often over the metacarpophalangeal joint and called *Russell's sign*, can result from repeated trauma to the skin from self-induced vomiting. In addition, dental problems may develop from constant vomiting. Swollen glands or salivary gland hypertrophy, sore throat, facial puffiness, chronic indigestion, irregular menstrual periods, electrolyte imbalances, and dehydration can also occur. Sudden death from cardiac arrest or fatal dysrhythmia is not uncommon. Although rare, esophageal tears and gastric rupture secondary to overdistention can occur. However, most bulimics have few, if any, noticeable signs of the illness.[6]

The patient with bulimia, similar to the one with anorexia nervosa, goes to great lengths to conceal abnormal eating habits. As the behavior persists, many problems associated with the condition become increasingly hard to deal with effectively.

Treatment of bulimia is similar to that described for anorexia nervosa. The multidisciplinary approach consists of strategies that include individual psychotherapy, nutritional counseling (including discussion of the dangers involved in binge eating and purging), cognitive behavior therapy, and drug therapy. Antidepressants (e.g., fluoxetine [Prozac], amitriptyline [Elavil]) are useful for the depression associated with both anorexia nervosa and bulimia. Vitamin, mineral, and iron supplements may be prescribed. However, iron supplementation is not generally required if amenorrhea is present. The return to normal eating habits may take several months to years to accomplish because relapses are frequent. Recovery is difficult; the abnormal eating behavior is hard to change because binge eating and purging provide the person with a feeling of satisfaction and of control over the body. Table 37-10 lists associations that offer help and support for persons with eating disorders.

Malnutrition

Malnutrition may be defined as an excess, deficit, or imbalance in the essential components of a balanced diet. Terms such as *undernutrition* and *overnutrition* are also used to describe malnutrition. Undernutrition describes a state of poor nourishment as a result of inadequate diet or diseases that interfere with normal appetite and assimilation of ingested food. Overnutrition refers to the ingestion of more food than is required for body needs, as in obesity.

Malnutrition is most prevalent in developing countries in which adequate food sources do not exist, the inhabitants are not well educated about their nutritional needs, and economic conditions often preclude the purchase of a balanced diet. As a result of federal nutritional studies, it is now known that undernutrition does exist in scattered parts of the United States. It is usually found in individuals or groups from the lower socioeconomic class.

Table 37-10 Support Organizations for Patients with Eating Disorders

American Anorexia/Bulimia Association
293 Central Park West
Suite 1R
New York, NY 10024
(312) 501-8351

Anorexia Nervosa and Related Eating Disorders, Inc.
Department P
PO Box 5102
Eugene, OR 97405
(503) 344-1144

National Eating Disorders Organization
Department P
5796 Karl Road
Columbus, OH 43229
(614) 436-1112

National Association of Anorexia Nervosa and Associated Disorders, Inc. (ANAD)
PO Box 7
Highland Park, IL 60035
(708) 831-3438

Overeaters Anonymous*
PO Box 44620
Rio Rancho, NM 87174-4020

*Consult the Yellow Pages for local chapters.

Types of Malnutrition

Protein-calorie malnutrition. Protein-calorie malnutrition (PCM) is the most common form of undernutrition and can result from either primary or secondary factors. Primary protein-calorie malnutrition is present when nutritional needs are not met as a result of poor eating habits. Secondary protein-calorie malnutrition is the result of an alteration or defect in ingestion, digestion, absorption, or metabolism. In this type of malnutrition, tissue needs are not met even though the dietary intake would be satisfactory under normal conditions. Secondary malnutrition may occur as a result of GI obstruction, surgical treatment (e.g., after peptic ulcer surgery), cancer, malabsorption syndromes, medications, and infectious diseases.

PCM may also be due to the ingestion of foods deficient in protein. In addition to decreased quantities of protein, the diet is generally low in necessary vitamins and minerals. PCM is a serious nutritional problem common throughout the world, affecting every socioeconomic and age group. In the United States, where protein intake is high and of good quality, severe malnutrition is less of a problem, but it can occur in high-risk groups.

Marasmus and kwashiorkor. Malnutrition has long been recognized in infants and children throughout the world by the terms marasmus and kwashiorkor. Adults may also be classified by this terminology. Marasmus is the result of a concomitant deficiency of both caloric and protein intake leading to generalized loss of body fat and muscle. Kwashiorkor is caused by a deficiency of protein intake that is superimposed on a catabolic stress event, such as a GI obstruction, a surgical procedure, cancer, a malabsorption syndrome, or an infectious disease.

Etiology. The following factors increase the potential for the development of malnutrition:

1. Major surgery, radiation therapy, or chemotherapy
2. Severe burns with exudate high in protein
3. Draining wounds
4. Chronic renal or liver diseases
5. Hemorrhage
6. Bone fractures with prolonged immobilization
7. Malabsorption syndrome
8. Draining pressure sores
9. Presence of infectious diseases such as tuberculosis or acquired immunodeficiency syndrome (AIDS)

The nitrogen loss after severe injury or major surgery may be as much as 20 g a day, excreted as urea, creatinine, and creatine.

Pathophysiology. Knowledge of the phases of the starvation process is essential to better understand the physiologic changes that occur in PCM. Initially, the body selectively uses carbohydrates (glycogen) rather than fat and protein to maintain metabolic function. These carbohydrate stores, found in the liver and muscles, are minimal and may be totally depleted within 18 hours. During this early phase of starvation, the only use of protein is in its obligatory participation in cellular metabolism. Once carbohydrate stores are depleted, protein begins to be converted to glucose for energy. Alanine and glutamine are the first amino acids to be used by the liver for the formation of glucose (*gluconeogenesis*). The resulting available plasma glucose allows the metabolic processes to continue. With these amino acids being used as energy sources, the person is in negative nitrogen balance (greater nitrogen excretion). However, within 5 to 9 days, body fat is fully mobilized to supply much of the needed energy. In prolonged starvation, up to 97% of calories are provided by fat, and protein is conserved. Fat stores are generally used up in 4 to 6 weeks. Depletion of these stores depends on the amount available. Once fat stores are used, body proteins can no longer be spared and rapidly decrease because they are the only remaining body source of energy available.

If the malnourished patient has surgery, experiences bodily trauma, or has an infection, the stress response is superimposed on the starvation response. These body insults cause an increase in the metabolic rate, with a subsequent increase in energy requirements. Protein stores are no longer spared and are used with increasing frequency for body energy because of the increased metabolic energy needs.

As the protein depletion continues, liver function is impaired, and synthesis of new plasma proteins is diminished. The plasma oncotic pressure is decreased because of decreased protein synthesis. A major function of plasma proteins, primarily of albumin, is the maintenance of the osmotic pressure of the blood. Because of this decreased pressure, a shift in body fluids occurs from the vascular space into the interstitial compartment. As protein ingestion decreases and body stores are depleted, albumin eventually leaks into the interstitial space along with the fluid. Edema becomes clinically observable. Often the edema present in the face and legs of the patient masks the muscle wasting that occurs. *Ascites* (abnormal intraperitoneal accumulation of fluid containing large amounts of protein and electrolytes) is a classic manifestation of kwashiorkor.

As the total blood volume is reduced, the skin appears dry and wrinkled. Along with the shift of fluids to the interstitial space, ions also move. Sodium (a predominant extracellular ion) is found in increased amounts within the cell, and potassium (a predominant intracellular ion) and magnesium are shifted to the extracellular space. The sodium-potassium exchange pump, which is dependent on adenosine triphosphatase (ATPase), has high energy needs, using 20% to 50% of all calories ingested. When the diet is extremely deficient in calories and essential proteins, the pump will fail, leaving sodium inside the cell (along with water), and the cell will expand.

The liver is the body organ that loses the most mass during protein deprivation. It gradually becomes infiltrated with fat secondary to decreased synthesis of lipoproteins. Immediate restoration to the diet of protein and other necessary constituents must be instituted or death will rapidly ensue. The most serious problem associated with PCM in the young is the probability of mental retardation. In severe malnutrition the development of brain cells is greatly slowed down. Brain cells increase most rapidly during fetal life and in the first 5 to 6 months after birth.

Once this critical time for brain development has passed, improvement in the nutritional state of the infant will not correct any mental deficiency already incurred.

Clinical Manifestations. The adult who is deprived of adequate protein and calories will have many of the clinical manifestations presented in Table 37-11. The most obvious clinical signs on physical examination are apparent in the skin, eyes, mouth, muscles, and CNS. The speed at which the protein deficiency develops depends on the quantity and quality of the protein intake, caloric value, and the age of the person.

The clinical manifestations of malnutrition are the result of numerous interactions occurring at the cellular level. As protein intake is severely reduced, the muscles, which make up the largest reservoir of protein in the body, become wasted and flabby, leading to weakness, fatigability, and decreased endurance. There is decreased protein available for repair, and as a result, wound healing may be delayed. Malnutrition in the hospitalized patient may result in delayed recovery and prolonged hospitalization. The person is more susceptible to all types of infections. Both humoral and cell-mediated immunity are deficient in PCM. There is a decrease in leukocytes in the peripheral blood. Phagocytosis is altered as a result of the lack of energy (ATP) necessary to drive the process. Most malnourished persons are anemic. Anemia resulting from PCM is usually caused by nutritional deficiencies such as iron and folic acid, the necessary building blocks for red blood cells (RBCs).

Diagnostic Studies. The diagnosis of PCM can be determined by a variety of laboratory studies used in conjunction with physical examination. Serum albumin is useful in the diagnosis of malnutrition. The degree of protein depletion can be identified with the use of the scale in Table 37-12. Serum albumin has a half-life of approximately 20 days. In the absence of marked fluid loss, such as from hemorrhage or burns, the serum albumin value lags behind actual protein changes by more than 2 weeks and therefore is not a good indicator of acute changes in nutrition status. Prealbumin, which has a half-life of 2 days, is a better indicator of recent or current nutritional status. Serum transferrin levels are another indicator of protein status. Transferrin, a protein synthesized by the liver and used as an iron-transport protein, decreases with the severity of protein deficiency. Serum electrolyte levels reflect changes taking place between the intracellular and the extracellular spaces. The serum potassium level is often elevated. The RBC count and the hemoglobin level will indicate the presence and degree of anemia. The total lymphocyte count will show a decreased number of lymphocytes. The total lymphocyte count is obtained from the differential white blood cell (WBC) count.

Liver enzyme studies reflect hepatic dysfunction and damage. The serum bilirubin level is usually elevated and this change is related to the fatty infiltration. Serum levels of both fat-soluble and water-soluble vitamins are usually diminished in malnutrition. The lowered levels of the fat-soluble vitamins correlate with the elevated serum bilirubin and the clinical signs of steatorrhea (fatty stools).

Therapeutic Management. PCM, even in its earliest phase, is an easily recognized condition. The affected person is obviously well below the ideal on weight-for-height scales according to age and gender. Inspection of the unclothed body reveals loss of muscle mass, muscle wasting, and little evidence of body fat. Diagnosis may be masked, however, in the patient where edema is disguising the deterioration of body muscle. The management of early uncomplicated PCM can be achieved without hospitalization by means of a diet high in calories and protein and by close supervision. Table 37-13 gives an example of a high-calorie, high-protein diet.

In severe PCM the patient may be hospitalized for correction of fluid and electrolyte imbalances and for treatment of infections secondary to a compromised immune system. Enteral feeding, both oral and tube feedings, can be used to supplement the diet. In cases of severe PCM, total parenteral nutrition (TPN) may be initiated.

NURSING MANAGEMENT

MALNUTRITION

Nursing Assessment

Regardless of the setting, the nurse needs to be aware of the nutritional status of the patient. Nursing assessment of the patient's nutritional status is presented in Table 37-14. The recording of the patient's height and weight is an important component of this assessment. When PCM is suspected, the patient's position on the height-for-weight chart should also be determined. If the assessment reveals that the patient is well below the average for age and gender, the nurse should get a record of the complete diet history from the patient or the family. The patient's nutritional state may not be the reason medical assistance was sought. However, it may well be a major factor in the outcome and perhaps may be the underlying reason for the patient's being ill. A dietitian should ultimately become involved in the plan of care. However, the nurse, as the first health professional dealing with the patient, should take the initiative in determining the seriousness of the nutritional problems.

The nurse should be aware that psychosocial problems have a direct effect on appetite. This is often overlooked as a cause of undernourishment. A diet history of foods eaten over the past week will reveal a great deal about the patient's dietary habits and knowledge of good nutrition. In addition to the height and weight and vital signs, the patient's physical state should be thoroughly assessed and documented. Each body system should be assessed. Table 37-15 summarizes conditions that can predispose persons to malnutrition.

Anthropometric measurements may be ordered. Skinfold thickness at various sites, an indicator of subcutaneous fat stores, and midarm muscle circumference, an indicator of protein stores, are compared to standards for healthy persons of the same age and gender. The nurse often performs these measurements. However, it requires practice to perform these measurements reliably. Sites most reflective of body fat are those over the biceps and the triceps, below the scapula, above the iliac crest, and the upper thigh. Both

Table 37-11 Signs of Protein-Calorie Malnutrition

Body System	Subclinical Signs	Clinical Signs
Integumentary	Slowed tissue turnover rate, surface temperature 1° F-2° F cooler, diminished febrile response to infection, delayed immune response	Brittle nails, decreased tone and elasticity of skin, xeroderma (dry skin), pigment changes (brown-gray), erythematous seborrheic dermatitis, scrotal dermatitis
Hair		Easy loss of hair, color changes, lack of luster
Visual	Night blindness	Blood vessel growth in cornea, Bitot's spots (gray keratinized epithelium on conjunctiva), dryness of conjunctiva and cornea, pale to red conjunctiva
Gastrointestinal		
Mouth and lips	Reduction in saliva production	Cheilosis (crusting and ulceration at angle of mouth)
Tongue	Mucosa more permeable to bacteria	Raw and beefy red, edematous and smooth, atrophy or hypertrophy of papillae
Teeth	Improper development, delayed eruption	Caries, loose teeth, discolored enamel
Gingivae		Periodontal disease, tendency to bleed easily, receding, pale, and soft
Stomach	Decreased gastric acidity, delayed gastric emptying	Constant hunger, increased incidence of ulcers
Intestines	Decreased motility and absorption, normal flora causing infection from increased permeability of mucosa	Diarrhea and flatulence, protruding abdomen, increased incidence of parasitic diseases
Liver-biliary	Fatty liver, decreased absorption of fat-soluble vitamins	Hepatomegaly
Cardiovascular	Decreased cardiac output, decreased circulation time, decreased hemoglobin, shift in heart position, increased risk of thrombophlebitis	Decreased blood pressure and pulse, slight cyanosis, anemia, body edema
Endocrine	Decreased insulin production	Thyroid enlargement, polydipsia, polyuria, increased sensitivity to cold
Immunologic	Decreased lymphocyte proliferation, decreased albumin levels, decreased antibody production, decreased total protein	Increased number of infections, decreased response to skin tests
Musculoskeletal	Decreased growth rate, decreased body stature with chronic PCM, decreased muscle mass	Prominence of bony structures such as face, clavicle, scapula, ribs, iliac crests, and spinal vertebrae, weak and spindly arms and legs, flat buttocks, weak and flabby muscles, decreased physical activity and ability to work, severe weight loss
Neurologic	Loss of ambition, feeling of being tired	Depression, confusion, decreased reflexes in legs and ankles, decreased position sense, decreased vibratory sense, paresthesias of hands and feet, syncope, motor weakness
Renal	Negative nitrogen balance, decreased BUN and creatinine levels	Nocturia, decreased urinary output
Reproductive	Decreased gonadotropin levels	Amenorrhea, impotence, atrophied breasts
Respiratory	Pulmonary edema, decreased strength of respiratory muscles	Proneness to respiratory infection, decreased respiratory rate, decreased vital capacity

BUN, Blood urea nitrogen; *PCM*, protein-calorie malnutrition.

Table 37-12 Serum Albumin Depletion Levels

Normal value	3.8-4.5 g/dl (38-45 g/L)
Mild depletion	3.0-3.7 g/dl (30-37 g/L)
Moderate depletion	2.5-2.9 g/dl (25-29 g/L)
Severe depletion	<2.5 g/dl (<25 g/L)

skinfold thickness and midarm muscle circumference measurements are decreased in chronic PCM and acute protein malnutrition. These measurements may also be influenced by shifts in hydration status. The exact relationship of the midarm circumference measure to body composition of functional protein, both muscle and nonmuscle, remains to be established.

Nursing Diagnoses

Nursing diagnoses specific to the patient with malnutrition include, but are not limited to, the following:

- Altered nutrition: less than body requirements related to decreased ingestion, digestion, or absorption of food or to anorexia

Table 37-13 Nutritional Management: High-Caloric, High-Protein Diet

General Principles

1. A normal diet is supplemented with larger portions to increase the protein and caloric content. It is used for patients with hypermetabolism, burns, excessive stress, and cancer.
2. It is important to eat regularly and not to skip meals or snacks.

Meal	Protein Content (g)	Sample Menu Plan 1	Sample Menu Plan 2	Sample Menu Plan 3
Breakfast				
Fruit		Large orange juice	Large apple juice	½ grapefruit
Starch, fat	2	1 toast with butter or jelly	Flour tortilla with butter	Biscuits and gravy
Starch, protein supplement	4	Cream of wheat with 2 tbs skim milk powder	Atole with 2 tbs skim milk powder	Grits with 2 tbs margarine
2 meat	14	2 poached eggs	2 fried eggs	Omelet with 2 eggs
Milk, protein supplement	10	High-protein milk shake (2 tbs skim milk powder added)	High-protein milk shake	High-protein milk shake
Lunch				
4 meat	28	Cheeseburger on bun with double meat patty, lettuce, tomato	2 burritos with extra cheese, meat	Split pea soup with ham hocks
4 starches	8			Grilled cheese sandwich
Vegetable	2		Lettuce and tomato salad with dressing	Watermelon wedge
4 fats		French fried potatoes	Biscochitos	Sugar cookies
Milk, protein supplement	10	High-protein milk shake	High-protein milk shake	High-protein milk shake
Dinner				
4 meat	28	Spaghetti with 4 oz meat sauce, Parmesan cheese	2 tamales with red chili sauce	4 oz fried chicken
3 starches	6			Sweet potato
Vegetable	2	Green beans with 2 tbs margarine	Spanish rice	Mustard greens with 2 tbs butter
7 fats		Bread with butter	Peas with 2 tbs butter	Biscuit
		Tapioca pudding	Custard	Vanilla ice cream
Milk, protein supplement	10	High-protein milk shake	High-protein milk shake	High-protein milk shake
Snack				
Milk	8	Fruit yogurt	Cottage cheese with fruit	½ sandwich with peanut butter
Fruit				Banana
	Total 132			

Table 37-14 Nursing Assessment: Malnutrition

Subjective Data
Important health information
Past health history: Diseases that affect nutritional status
Medications: Steroids, chemotherapeutic agents, diet pills, alcohol
Surgery: History of surgical procedures that affect nutritional status
Functional health patterns
Nutritional-metabolic: Recent weight changes, weight problems, appetite changes, number of meals and snacks a day, food preferences and aversions, any dietary problems, food allergies or foods that cause indigestion, gas, use of dentures, difficulty in chewing or swallowing, anorexia
Elimination: Constipation; diarrhea
Activity-exercise: Level of physical activity, fatigue
Cognitive-perceptual: Pain in mouth, paresthesias, loss of position and vibratory sense
Role-relationship: Change in financial status or family (e.g., loss of a spouse)
Sexual-reproductive: Menstrual irregularities in women, decreased libido

Objective Data
General
Height, weight, appearance (e.g., whether alert or listless, presence of cachexia, posture)
Mouth
Teeth: Dentures, caries, teeth missing or loose, teeth malpositioned
Buccal mucosa: Ulcerations, white patches or plaques, redness, swelling
Gingivae: Spongy, tend to bleed easily, inflamed, recessed, red, pale
Lips: Dry, scaly, swollen, red and swollen (cheilosis), presence of fever blisters, angular lesions at corners of mouth, fissures, or scars (stomatitis)
Tongue: Swollen, scarlet and raw, beefy appearance (glossitis), hyperemic, hypertrophic or atrophic papillae
Eyes
Pale or red conjunctivae, dry, red, and fissures at eyelid corners, dry eye membranes, soft cornea, dull cornea
Gastrointestinal
Liver or spleen enlargement
Cardiovascular
Tachycardia, decreased blood pressure, dysrhythmias
Musculoskeletal
Flaccidity, poor tone, underdeveloped or "wasted" appearance, bowlegs, knock-knees, beaded ribs, chest deformity, prominent scapulas
Neurologic
Decrease in or loss of reflexes, inattention, irritability, tremor
Integumentary
Hair: Dry, brittle, dull, stringy, thin, sparse, easily plucked, presence of alopecia or color changes
Skin: Rough, dry, scaly, pale, irritated, discolored, presence of petechiae or bruises, edema, darkness under eyes or over cheeks, greasy, scaly areas (nasolabial seborrhea)
Nails: Brittle, ridged, spoon shaped
Possible laboratory findings
Decreased hemoglobin and hematocrit values, decreased mean corpuscular volume or mean corpuscular hemoglobin (reflective of iron deficiency), increased mean corpuscular volume or mean corpuscular hemoglobin (reflective of folic acid or vitamin B_{12} deficiency), altered serum electrolyte levels, decreased BUN; decreased serum albumin, transferrin, and prealbumin, decreased peripheral lymphocytes.

BUN, Blood urea nitrogen.

- Deficit in self-feeding related to decreased strength and endurance, fatigue, and apathy
- Altered bowel elimination: constipation, diarrhea, or impaction related to poor eating patterns, immobility, or medication effects
- Risk for fluid volume deficit related to deviations affecting access to or absorption of fluids
- Risk for impaired skin integrity related to poor nutritional state
- Risk for noncompliance with treatment regimen related to alteration in perception, lack of motivation, or incompatibility of regimen with lifestyle or resources
- Activity intolerance related to weakness, fatigue, and inadequate caloric intake

Table 37-15 Conditions That Increase the Risk for Malnutrition

- Chronic alcoholism
- Drugs with antinutrient or catabolic properties, such as corticosteroids and oral antibiotics
- Gross underweight or overweight with recent weight loss exceeding 10% of usual body weight or 10 lbs (4.5 kg) a month for several months
- No oral intake or receiving standard intravenous solutions (5% Dextrose) for 10 days or in older adults, for 5 days
- Extreme need for nutrients because of hypermetabolism or stresses such as infection, burns, trauma or fever
- Nutrient losses from malabsorption, dialysis, fistulas, or wounds

Planning

The overall goals are that the patient with malnutrition will (1) achieve weight gain to within normal range for height and age, (2) consume a specified number of calories a day (with a diet individualized for the patient), and (3) have no adverse consequences related to malnutrition.

Nursing Implementation

Health Promotion and Maintenance. The nurse is in a good position to teach and reinforce healthy eating habits with individuals and groups of persons throughout their life span. The Surgeon General's Report on Nutrition and Health offers key recommendations for improving nutrition that are useful points for a teaching program.[7] The following recommendations are applicable to most people:

1. Reduce consumption of fat and cholesterol
2. Achieve and maintain a desirable weight
3. Increase energy expenditure through regular and sustained physical activity
4. Increase consumption of whole grain foods and cereal products, vegetables, and fruits
5. Reduce intake of sodium
6. Take alcohol only in moderation, if at all.

Acute Intervention. The nurse must avoid ignoring a patient's nutritional state and focusing attention on the other physical problems of the patient. The incidence of nutritional deficiency, especially PCM, is high in hospitalized patients. A number of nutritional studies have indicated that PCM may develop in as many as 50% of medical and surgical patients.[8] As a direct consequence of these findings, the nurse must become more aware of who is at risk, why, and how to intervene appropriately. In states of increased stress, such as surgery, severe trauma, sepsis, anxiety, or uncontrolled pain, more calories and protein are required. Wound healing requires increased protein synthesis. In cases of a malignant tumor, there are additional demands to meet tumor growth. Nitrogen loss is accelerated when fever is present. Despite the return of body temperature to normal, the rate of protein breakdown and resynthesis may be accelerated for several weeks. After major surgery a person is known to need several weeks of increased protein and calorie intake to promote healing and replenish body stores when intake is not sufficient to meet energy demands.

The nurse must have a thorough understanding of nutritional support and the rationale behind orders for such common tasks as recording the daily weight, intake, and output. Daily weights can give an accurate record of body weight gain or loss. However, rapid gains and losses are usually the result of shifts in fluid balance. The body weight, in conjunction with accurate recording of food and fluid intake, provides a clearer picture of the patient's fluid and nutritional state. To obtain an accurate weight, the nurse should weigh the patient at the same time each day, on the same scale, with the same type or amount of clothing, and preferably with the bladder recently emptied.

The protein and calorie intake required in the malnourished patient depends on the cause of the malnutrition, the treatment being employed, and other stressors affecting the patient. If the patient is able to take food by mouth, a daily calorie count and diet diary can be maintained to give an accurate record of food intake.

The nurse and the dietitian working with the patient and family can assist in the selection of high-caloric and high-protein foods. Preparation of foods preferred by the patient enhances the daily intake. Discussion with the patient and family about foods that should be eaten to provide high-protein, high-calorie content is important. The family can be encouraged to bring the patient's favorite foods from home while the patient is still hospitalized.

It is essential that the patient be encouraged to eat the meats and vegetables served at mealtimes. Drinking several cups of water, tea, or coffee with the meal may suppress the appetite for the more nutritious foods necessary for complete recovery. Visitors should be discouraged from bringing carbonated beverages or other types of drinks, unless they have high caloric value.

The undernourished patient usually receives between-meal supplements. These may consist of items prepared in the dietary department or commercially prepared products. Eating these items between meals increases the total daily intake and provides extra calories, proteins, fluids, and nutrients. In addition, multiple small feedings improve the tolerance for food intake by distributing the amount more evenly throughout the day.

Elemental diets are chemically defined, nutritionally sound diets that contain glucose, glucose derivatives, dextrins, amino acids, essential fatty acids, vitamins, and minerals. They are lactose free and leave little residue in the lower bowel. The nurse should be familiar with the commercial products being used in the particular setting, their ingredients, and whether the products can be used as complete meal replacements or only as dietary supplements (Table 37-16).

Chronic and Home Management. With shortened hospital stays, many patients are discharged home on a therapeutic diet. Discharge preparation for both the patient and the family is important. They must be carefully instructed on the cause of the undernourished state and ways to avoid the problem in the future. The patient must be made aware that undernourishment, whatever the cause, can recur and that adhering to a diet high in protein and calories for a few short weeks cannot restore a normal nutritional state. Many months are needed to reach this goal. Diet instruction is usually carried out by the dietitian, but it is important for the nurse to assess the patient's understanding and reinforce the information whenever possible. The patient's ability to comply with the dietary instructions must be examined in light of past eating habits, religious and ethnic preferences, age, income, other resources, and state of health.

Unless the patient and the family can be convinced of the necessity for dietary change and have the resources to effect change, it is likely that no long-term benefits will be

Table 37-16 Commonly Used Elemental Diets

Product	Protein (g)	Carbohydrates (% total Kcal)	Lipids (% total Kcal)	Protein (% total Kcal)	Kcal/ml
Criticare HN	38.0	83.0	3.0	14.0	1.1
Reabilan	31.5	52.0	35.0	13.0	1.0
Reabilan HN	58.0	47.0	35.0	18.0	1.3
Tolerex	20.6	91.0	1.0	8.0	1.0
Traum-Aid HBC	56.0	67.0	11.0	22.0	1.0
Vital HN	41.7	73.6	9.7	16.7	1.0
Vivonex T.E.N.	38.2	82.0	3.0	15.0	1.0

Modified from Feucht S: Enteral nutrition products. In Mahan L, Arlin M: *Krause's food, nutrition and diet therapy*, ed 3, Philadelphia, 1992, WB Saunders.

achieved. Ways should be found in which the patient can become involved in the recovery. Keeping a diet diary or a calorie count for a week at a time is one way to analyze eating patterns. These records are also helpful to the health care team in the follow-up care. Self-assessment of progress can be encouraged by having the patient weighed once or twice a week and keeping a weight record. The need for continuous follow-up care must be strongly emphasized if rehabilitation is to be accomplished and maintained.

The nurse is in an ideal position to determine the need for nutritious meals and snacks after discharge from the hospital. In addition, it is important to consider the availability and acceptability of nutritionally based community resources. Such aspects can be integrated into discharge planning and follow-up home visits by the nurse.

Gerontologic Considerations

The eating patterns established in youth and earlier years usually extend into old age. However, adjustments in the type of food ingested may be made as adaptations to age-related physiologic changes. These changes can result either in obesity or loss of weight depending on individual circumstances.

Some of the physiologic changes associated with aging affect the nutritional status of older adults. Of particular interest are the changes listed below:

1. Changes in the oral cavity (change in bite surfaces of the teeth, periodontal disease, drying of the mucous membrane of the mouth and tongue, poorly fitting dentures, decreased muscle strength for chewing, decreased number of taste buds, decreased saliva production)
2. Changes in digestion (decreased gastric secretion of hydrochloric acid, decreased absorption of vitamin B, vitamin B_{12}, vitamin A, carotene, and folic acid)
3. Changes in the endocrine system (decreased tolerance to glucose)
4. Changes in the musculoskeletal system (decreased bone density, degenerative joint changes)
5. Decrease in vision and hearing (procurement and preparation of food are more difficult)

Certain illnesses that are more prevalent in the older population are considered to be diet related. These include atherosclerosis, osteoporosis, diabetes mellitus, and diverticulitis. The need to treat these and other common chronic illnesses of the older patient often requires the use of multiple medications. These medications often have an adverse effect on the appetite of older adults increasing the possibility of inadequate intake.

To date, with the exception of calories, it has not been determined that older adults have requirements for specific nutrients that are different from those of middle-aged adults. Caloric intake needs to be decreased with age because there is a progressive loss of lean body mass and a decrease in basal metabolic rate. Fewer calories are, therefore, needed to meet nutritional needs. Unless caloric intake is decreased by careful attention to food intake, or energy expenditure is increased through greater physical activity and exercise, obesity will result.

Socioeconomic factors are important variables when assessing the nutritional status of an older adult. Because more than one third of older adults have incomes below the poverty level, it would follow that obtaining adequate and nutritious food can be an ongoing problem. In many cases the older person cannot afford to purchase meat, fresh vegetables, and fruit that provide many necessary nutrients.

Lifestyle changes such as relocation to a nursing home or retirement can have a significant impact on the eating habits of the older adult. Other important considerations that need to be assessed when evaluating the nutritional status of an older adult include the ethnic background, previous dietary practices, food preferences, knowledge of proper diet, availability and accessibility of food stores, transportation, and health status. Problems related to any or all of these areas can alert the nurse to the possibility of a nutritional problem.

Malnutrition can occur in an older person even though the caloric requirements decrease with age. If malnutrition is present, only approximately 10% of the malnourished older persons are able to ingest enough food to correct the malnourished state.[9] Special strategies, such as the use of soft diets for persons with chewing difficulties and adaptive devices such as a large handled spoon, often are helpful in increasing dietary intake. Some older persons may require enteral feeding until their strength and general health are improved.

Many community nutritional programs are available to the older person to make mealtime a pleasant, social event. Improving the social setting of a meal often improves the dietary intake. Home-delivered meals and meal sites in a central location are popular meal alternatives for many older adults. The use of food stamps is another alternative that allows low-income households, regardless of age, to buy more food of a greater variety.

TYPES OF SUPPLEMENTAL NUTRITION

Oral Feeding

High calorie supplemental oral feedings may be used in the patient whose nutritional intake is deficient. This may include dietary items such as milk shakes, puddings, eggnogs, or commercially available products (e.g., Ensure, Sustacal).

Tube Feeding

Tube feedings may be ordered for the patient who has a functioning GI tract but is unable to take oral nourishment. Indications for tube feeding, besides PCM, may include those persons with anorexia, orofacial fractures, head and neck cancer, neurologic or psychiatric conditions that prevent oral intake, extensive burns, and those who are receiving chemotherapy or radiation therapy. Tube feedings are easily administered, safer, more physiologically efficient, and less expensive than parenteral nutrition. They are used to provide nutrients by way of the GI tract (alone or as a supplement to oral or parenteral nutrition) or as a treatment for malnutrition.

A nasogastric (NG) tube is most commonly used for short-term feeding problems. If the feedings are necessary for an extended time, other means of feeding may be used, such as an esophagostomy tube, a gastrostomy tube (placed surgically, endoscopically, or percutaneously), or a jejunostomy tube that empties directly into the jejunum. Transpyloric (nasointestinal) tube placement or placement into the jejunum is used when physiologic conditions warrant feeding the patient below the pyloric sphincter. (Figure 37-2 shows the locations of commonly used enteral feeding tubes).

Recent advances in the manufacture of feeding tubes made of polyurethane or silicone materials (e.g., Dobbhoff, Duo-Tube, Entriflext, Keofeed, Vivonex tungsten tip) have added to the comfort level of the patient in tolerating extended periods of feeding. The older tubes made of rubber or polyvinyl chloride tend to stiffen with time. The new tubes are longer, smaller in diameter, softer, and more flexible, thereby decreasing the possibility of mucosal damage from prolonged placement. In addition, these newer tubes are generally radiopaque, making their position readily identified by x-ray. Many of these tubes also have weighted tips, allowing for easier passage of the tube through the pylorus into the duodenum. Placement into the intestine decreases the likelihood of regurgitation of contents into the esophagus and their subsequent aspiration. These tubes are also more easily placed in an uncooperative or comatose patient because the ability to swallow is not essential during insertion.

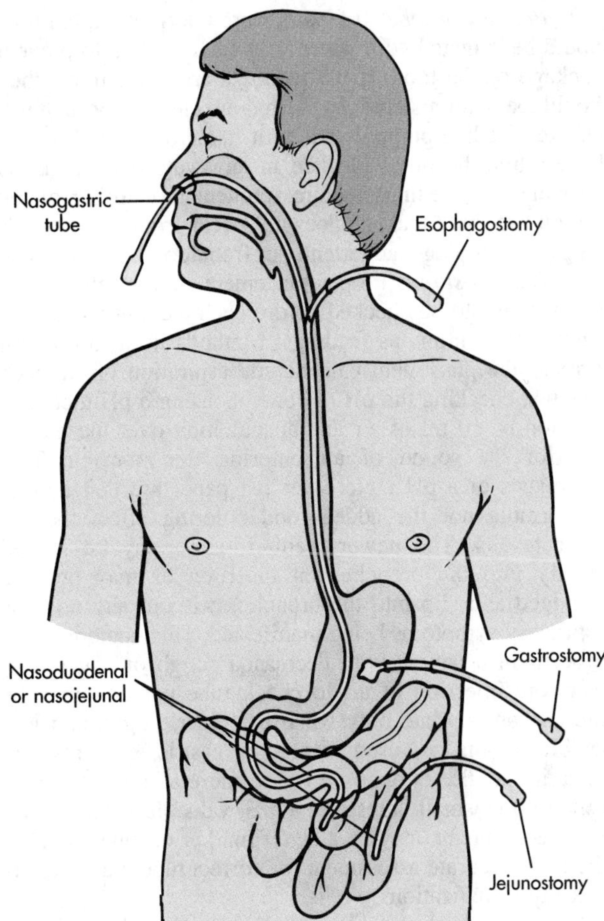

Fig. 37-2 Common placement locations for enteral feeding tubes.

Although the newer, smaller feeding tubes have many advantages over older tubes, such as the Levine tube, there are some disadvantages that the nurse must keep in mind. Because of the small diameter, these tubes are more easily blocked when feedings are thick and irrigation is more difficult. They are particularly prone to obstruction when oral medications have not been thoroughly crushed and dissolved in water before administration. They can become dislodged by vomiting or coughing and can also become knotted or kinked in the GI tract. Failure to flush the tubing after both medication administration and residual volume determinations can result in tube clogging. When the tube becomes clogged, it may necessitate removal and insertion of a new tube adding to cost and patient discomfort.

Procedure for Tube Feeding. The procedure for the administration of tube feeding through an NG tube is standard. The following principles apply:

1. *Patient position*: The patient should be sitting or lying with the head of the bed elevated 30 to 45 degrees to prevent aspiration.

2. *Patency of tube*: If feedings are intermittent, the tube should be irrigated with water after each feeding to prevent blockage of the tube. If the feedings are continuous, they should be administered by using an electric or battery-operated feeding pump with a built-in alarm that will sound if the tubing becomes blocked in any way. If no pump is available, the feedings require frequent monitoring of the drip rate so that blockage does not occur from the patient's lying on the tubing inadvertently or from too slow a drip rate.

3. *Tube position*: Proper placement of the tube in the stomach should be checked before each feeding or every 4 hours with continuous feedings. Methods used to confirm correct tube placement can include aspiration of stomach contents, checking the pH of contents using a pH meter, or injection of 10 ml of air and auscultation over the gastric area for the sound of air entering the stomach. Two advantages of a pH meter over pH paper are that neither the formula nor the added food coloring affect the pH meter results. The newer feeding tubes may be passed directly into the bronchus on insertion or may become dislodged and slip into the bronchus without any obvious respiratory symptoms being manifested. This is more likely to occur in a patient with decreased cough or gag reflex. Therefore injection of air to check tube position may be safe and appropriate only when the older, larger, and less flexible tubing is used. Because gastric contents are primarily acidic, as opposed to the more alkaline environment of the small intestine, a pH value less than 5 on aspirated contents may be a better marker of tube location. The most accurate assessment for correct tube placement is by x-ray visualization.

Frequent checking is necessary because the stomach may become atonic, and gastric residual volume may increase with any deterioration of the patient's condition. This is especially important when feedings are administered at high infusion rates. For example, when the infusion rate is 100 ml per hour, the total infused volume that may accumulate in 4 hours in an atonic stomach is 400 ml. Additionally, gastric secretions can swell the volume well beyond the 400 ml.[10] With increased residual volume there is increased risk for aspiration.

4. *Administration of feeding*: The principle of gravity is used with the drip method or with a bulb or plunger type of syringe. Applying pressure to force the feeding can damage the gastric mucosa. Pumps may be used. If the feedings have been refrigerated, they should be warmed to room temperature. The amount of the feeding is increased gradually for 1 to 3 days to minimize undue side effects, such as nausea or diarrhea. It is important to remember that the patient still needs water replacement, and at least 100 ml should be given every 4 to 6 hours (unless contraindicated).

5. *General nursing considerations*: The patient should be weighed daily or several times a week, and accurate intake and output records should be maintained. This permits monitoring of weight gain or loss and is an indicator of the tolerance of the feedings. If the patient is prone to development of nonketotic-hyperosmolar hyperglycemia, a serious condition that can arise as a result of high glucose intake from feeding formulas, frequent blood glucose checks should be performed at the bedside. An older patient who has glucose intolerance is particularly vulnerable to this problem. Feedings that have been opened and not refrigerated or feedings that have been infusing longer than 8 hours should be discarded to minimize bacterial growth and to prevent the administration of contaminated feeding. Feedings should, therefore, be labeled with the date and time they are initially used. If a pump is used, pump tubing should be changed every 24 hours.

RESEARCH

Implications for Nursing Practice

USE OF PH MEASUREMENT IN PREDICTING FEEDING TUBE PLACEMENT

Citation Metheney N and others: Effectiveness of pH measurements in predicting feeding tube placement: an update, *Nursing Research 42:324-331, 1993.*

Purpose To provide more definitive information on the ability of pH to differentiate between gastric and intestinal placement of feeding tubes, and between gastric and respiratory placement of feeding tubes.

Methods The sample consisted of 405 aspirates from small-bore nasogastric tubes and 389 aspirates from nasointestinal tubes. The aspirates were tested for pH by a pH meter and x-rays were taken to determine tube position.

Results and Conclusions The results showed that gastric placement of the tube was successfully distinguished from intestinal placement on the basis of pH-meter readings in the majority of cases. However, pH readings outside the normal expected ranges for the stomach and intestine occurred in 18% of the cases. Four tubes that were inadvertently placed in the respiratory system had pH values greater than 6.5.

When an x-ray is available, it is still the preferred method to check tube position initially in the high risk patient. In settings where x-ray is not available, an unequivocally acidic value obtained from a newly inserted feeding tube is a reasonable indicator of gastric versus respiratory placement.

Implications for Nursing Practice The nurse can be more certain of correct tube placement by determining the pH value from aspirates of newly inserted nasogastric tubes. Correct placement of the tube increases patient comfort and decreases the likelihood of aspiration.

Problems Related to Tube Feedings. The types of problems encountered in patients receiving tube feedings and corrective measures are presented in Table 37-17. The use of blenderized foods from a normal diet may be used as tube feedings. The patient may psychologically accept these feedings better than commercial products. Normal bowel function is promoted by fiber and residue content, which, in blenderized feedings, is similar to that of a normal diet.

Table 37-17 Common Problems of Patients Receiving Tube Feedings

Problems and Possible Causes	Corrective Measures
Vomiting	
Improper placement of tube	Replace tube in proper position. Check tube position before beginning feeding and every 4 hr if continuous feedings.
Initiation of feeding too soon after placement	Give patient time to get adjusted to tube before feeding.
Feeding too fast	Hold feeding 2-8 hr, then resume at slower rate. Give feeding by slow drip or via pump slowly. Avoid use of force.
Patient in wrong position	Keep head of bed elevated to 30- to 45-degree angle. Have patient lie on right side for ½ hr after feeding. Have patient sit up on side of bed or in chair. Encourage ambulation unless contraindicated.
Contamination of formula	Refrigerate unused formula and record date opened. Discard outdated formula every 24 hr. Discard formula left standing for a long time.
Air in stomach	Clear tubing of air before feeding. Keep tube feeding container filled so air does not enter through feeding set.
Diarrhea	
Feeding too fast, high concentration of formula	Decrease rate of feeding. Change to continuous drip feedings. Check for drugs that may cause diarrhea (e.g., antibiotics)
Lactose intolerance	Consult physician for change in formula to lactose-free solution.
Contamination of formula or tubing	Discard old tubing or other equipment. Change tubing every 24 hr.
Constipation	
No fiber in diet	Consult physician for change in formula to one with more fiber content. Obtain laxative order.
Inadequate fluid intake	Increase fluid intake if not contraindicated. Give free water as well as formula.
Drugs	Check for drugs that may be constipating.
Dehydration	
Excessive diarrhea, vomiting	Decrease rate or change formula. Check drugs patient is receiving, especially antibiotics. Take care to prevent bacterial contamination of formula and equipment.
Poor fluid intake	Increase intake and check amount and number of feedings. Increase amount of intake if appropriate.
High protein formula	Change formula.

When commercial products are used, the concentration, taste, lactose content, osmolarity, and amounts of protein, sodium, and fat vary according to the manufacturer. The standard concentration is generally 1 calorie per milliliter. A limited number of flavors is available, and the overuse of one or two flavors, even in tube feedings, can lead to dislike and less tolerance with time.

Osmolarity higher than normal (i.e., greater than 280 mOsm/L) may be poorly tolerated and results in symptoms of dumping syndrome (cold sweat, dizziness, distention, weakness, tachycardia, nausea, and diarrhea) (see Chapter 39). Protein content greater than 16% can lead to dehydration unless the patient is given supplemental fluids or is sufficiently alert to request additional fluids. The nurse must be aware of this potential problem and must provide extra fluids through the feeding tube or, if permitted, by mouth. Tube feedings with high sodium content are contraindicated in the patient with cardiovascular problems, such as congestive heart failure. High fat content is not advocated for a patient suffering from short bowel syndrome or ileocecal resections because of impaired fat absorption. Some elemental diets use predigested (hydrolyzed) protein that requires little digestion time and is rapidly absorbed. The disadvantages of the predigested protein are the chemical taste and the added expense.

The dietitian can be of considerable assistance to the nursing staff. When close consultation with the nursing staff occurs, existing problems with tube feedings can be quickly and efficiently addressed and resolved.

Gerontologic Considerations Related to Enteral Nutrition

Enteral nutrition strategies, including nasogastric, nasointestinal, and gastrostomy feedings, are frequently used in the older patient to improve nutritional status. Because of physiologic changes associated with aging, the older adult is more vulnerable to complications associated with these interventions, especially fluid and electrolyte imbalances. Complications such as diarrhea can leave the patient dehydrated. Decreased thirst perception or impaired cognitive function decrease the ability of the patient to seek additional fluids. With aging there is decreased ability to handle glucose loads. As a result, the older patient may be more susceptible to problems of hyperglycemia in response to the high carbohydrate load of most enteral feeding formulas. If the older adult has compromised cardiovascular function (e.g., congestive heart failure) there will be a decreased ability to handle large volumes of formula, in which case, the use of more concentrated formulas may be warranted. The older adult also is at increased risk for aspiration caused by an incompetent lower esophageal sphincter, hiatal hernia, or diminished gag reflex. Physical mobility, fine motor movement, and visual system changes associated with aging may contribute to difficulties in managing enteral nutrition equipment at home. In addition, age-related changes such as a decrease in lean muscle mass influence the reliability of measures used for nutritional assessment.

Total Parenteral Nutrition

When the GI tract cannot be used for the ingestion, digestion, and absorption of essential nutrients, TPN may be substituted. Parenteral nutrition (also called *hyperalimentation*) has become a relatively safe and practical method of delivering total nutritional needs by an IV route.

The goal of using TPN is to keep the patient in positive nitrogen balance and to allow for growth of new body tissue, which can be drastically depleted by prolonged inability to eat normally. Regular IV solutions of 5% dextrose (5 g dextrose/100 ml) in water (D_5W) or 5% dextrose in lactated Ringer's solution (D_5LR) contain no protein and have approximately 170 calories per liter. The normal adult requires a minimum of 1200 to 1500 calories a day to carry out normal physiologic functions. Patients who sustain severe injury, surgery, or burns, and those who are malnourished as a result of medical treatment or disease processes have greatly increased nutritional needs. Some patients (those with extensive trauma or burns) may require as many as 45 to 55 calories per kilogram per day. The volume of regular dextrose solutions needed to meet these high caloric requirements could exceed the capacity of the cardiovascular system. Table 37-18 lists common indications for the use of TPN.

Composition. Commercially prepared TPN base solutions are available for both central and peripheral use. These base solutions contain dextrose and nitrogen in the form of amino acids or protein hydrolysates. The hospital pharmacy adds the prescribed electrolytes (e.g., sodium, potassium, chloride, calcium, magnesium, and phosphate), vitamins, and trace elements (e.g., zinc, copper, chromium, and manganese) to customize the solution for the patient. Recently a three-in-one, or total nutrient, mixture containing an IV fat emulsion, dextrose, and amino acids, has become widely available. The development of suitable plastic containers for the mixture contributed to its availability.

Calories. Calories in TPN are supplied primarily by carbohydrates in the form of dextrose (20% to 50% of total calories). The administration of between 100 and 150 g of dextrose (1 g provides approximately 3.4 calories) daily has a protein-sparing effect. Protein should be provided at the rate of 1 g/kg per day. Because most patients receiving TPN are nutritionally depleted, their daily caloric needs are well above the average. Such needs include both calories for current energy needs and for replacing depleted reserves. Adequate nonprotein calories in the form of glucose and lipids must be provided to allow metabolism of amino acids to protein and not glucose. However, overfeeding can lead to multiple system impairments. To minimize these problems, an energy intake of 25 to 30 calories per kilogram per day in a nonobese patient is often recommended.[11] Providing both lipid and amino acid components meets the energy requirement while minimizing problems of overfeeding.

Nitrogen. The normal healthy man needs approximately 56 g of protein daily. In a nutritionally depleted patient under the stress of illness or surgery, requirements can exceed 150 g per day to ensure a positive nitrogen balance. However, protein intake levels of 1.5 to 1.75 g per kilogram per day are suggested for most patients with moderate to severe stress.[12]

Electrolytes. The assessment of individual requirements should take place daily at the beginning of therapy and then several times a week as the treatment progresses. The following are ranges for average daily electrolyte requirements for adult patients:

Sodium: 60 to 200 mEq
Potassium: 50 to 160 mEq
Chloride: 100 to 200 mEq
Magnesium: 20 to 30 mEq
Phosphate: 30 to 100 mEq

The exact amount needed is dependent upon the patient's health problem as well as on electrolyte levels as determined by blood testing.

Table 37-18 Common Indications for Total Parenteral Nutrition

Acute or chronic renal failure*
Alimentary tract anomalies and fistula
Burns
Chronic diarrhea and vomiting
Complicated surgery or trauma
Diverticulitis
Failure to thrive
Gastrointestinal obstruction
Granulomatous enterocolitis
Hepatic failure (reversible)*
Hypermetabolic states (sepsis, fractures)
Inflammatory bowel disease (Crohn's disease and ulcerative colitis)
Malabsorption
Malnutrition
Pancreatitis
Severe anorexia nervosa
Severe peptic ulcer disease
Short bowel syndrome

*TPN should be used with extreme caution in this situation.

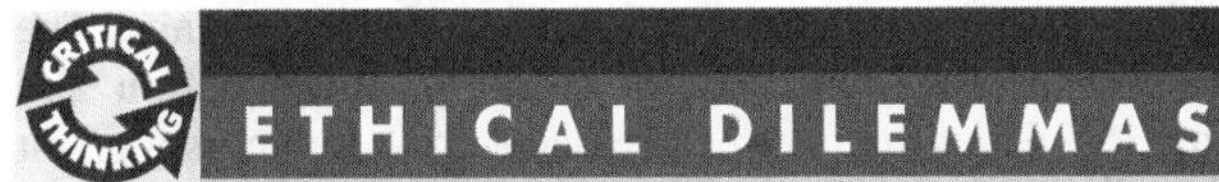

ETHICAL DILEMMAS

WITHHOLDING TREATMENT

Situation A 26-year-old patient in a permanent vegetative state is diagnosed with her fifteenth bladder infection. Her home care nurse must determine whether or not to seek antibiotics for this infection. The family has expressed a concern that no *heroic* measures be used to extend the biologic life of their daughter and sister, but they have been unwilling to withdraw the existing treatment, which is enteral nutrition. Should antibiotics be withheld?

Discussion The questions that arise when discussing *heroic measures* are of degree and intent. Is the intent not to prolong the patient's life or not to extend any suffering the patient might experience? Does antibiotic treatment constitute treatment above and beyond the normal care of the patient or is it simply appropriate treatment of a manageable condition? The familiy's resistance to the withdrawal of enteral nutrition may stem from discomfort and revulsion about starving the patient to death or from strong beliefs about the importance of maintaining her biologic existence. The nurse needs to clarify what the patient's wishes were, if they are known. The family's values and their concerns about the patient, about her ability to feel pain or discomfort, and about her quality of life also need to be discussed.

ETHICAL AND LEGAL PRINCIPLES

- Medical treatment may be withheld if a competent patient refuses to consent to it, if it is medically futile treatment, or if the burden of providing it outweighs its benefit.
- If withholding treatment or support leads to death, it is the underlying disease or condition that is the cause. Technologic intervention simply prolongs life.
- A patient in a permanent vegetative state cannot be cured of that brain damage. Any treatable comorbidities related to this condition will not lead to recovery from the permanent vegetative state.

Trace elements. Zinc, copper, manganese, cobalt, selenium, and iodine supplements must be ordered according to the patient's condition and needs. Levels of these elements are monitored in the patient receiving TPN. The physician may order additional amounts of these elements to be added to the solutions according to the patient's requirements.

Vitamins. The daily addition of a multivitamin preparation to 1 L of TPN generally meets the vitamin requirements. If multivitamin infusion is used, the vitamin B_{12} requirement may be met without the need for supplemental injections. It is necessary for the physician to order vitamin K and folic acid separately. Folic acid 500 μg is given daily. Intramuscular (IM) vitamin K may be ordered depending on the results of the prothrombin time.

Methods of Administration. TPN may be administered by two routes, *central* or *peripheral*. Central parenteral nutrition is given through a catheter most commonly threaded into the superior vena cava. The central catheter often originates at the subclavian vein. Recently *peripherally inserted central* (PIC) catheters are being placed, usually into the basilic or cephalic vein. Ease of placement, cost, and limited complications make this an attractive alternative to a centrally placed line. Central hyperalimentation is indicated when long-term nutritional support is necessary, when the patient has high protein and caloric requirements, and when suitable peripheral veins are not available. Peripheral parenteral nutrition (PPN) is administered through a large peripheral vein when (1) nutritional support is needed for only a short time (up to 2 weeks) because of limited patient tolerance, (2) protein and caloric requirements are not excessively high, (3) the risk of a central catheter is too great, or (4) nutritional support is used to supplement inadequate oral intake. Both central and peripheral TPN are used in a patient who is not a candidate for enteral support.

Central and peripheral parenteral nutrition differ in tonicity, which is measured in milliosmoles (mOsm), the concentration of particles in a fluid. Blood, which is isotonic, measures approximately 280 mOsm per liter. The standard IV solutions of D_5W and normal saline are essentially isotonic. Central hyperalimentation solutions are hypertonic measuring approximately 1600 mOsm per liter. The high glucose content ranges from 20% to 50%. Thus nutrients can be infused using smaller fluid volumes than PPN. Central hyperalimentation must be infused in a large central vein so that rapid dilution can occur. The use of a peripheral vein causes irritation and thrombophlebitis. PPN is less hypertonic (using as much as 20% glucose) and can be safely administered through a large peripheral vein, although phlebitis can occur. Another potential complication is fluid overload.

All TPN solutions should be prepared by a pharmacist or a trained technician using strict aseptic techniques under a laminar flow hood. Nothing should be added to hyperalimentation solutions after they are prepared in the pharmacy. The danger of drug incompatibilities and contamination is high. The fewer the personnel involved in the preparation and administration of TPN, the lower the danger of infection for the patient. In most hospitals the physician must order the TPN solution daily. In this way the solution and additives can be adjusted to the patient's current needs. Each bottle of solution indicates the glucose and protein content, all additives, the time mixed, and the date and time of expiration. In general, solutions are good for 24 to 36 hours and must be refrigerated until 1/2 hour before use.

Complications. Complications of TPN can be divided into three categories: (1) infectious, (2) metabolic, and (3) mechanical. The major complications of each category are presented in Table 37-19.

NURSING MANAGEMENT

TOTAL PARENTERAL NUTRITION

PPN is a form of IV nutrition that may be given concurrently with oral nourishment. A large peripheral vein can be used because the solution is less hypertonic and therefore

Table 37-19 Complications of Total Parenteral Nutrition

Infection
- Fungal
- Bacterial—both gram-positive and gram-negative bacteria

Metabolic Problems
- Glucose metabolism
  - Hyperglycemia, hypoglycemia, and hyperosmolar nonketotic coma
  - Glycosuria
  - Osmotic diuresis
  - Ketoacidosis
- Amino acid metabolism
  - Serum amino acid imbalances
  - Elevated serum ammonia
  - Prerenal azotemia
- Essential fatty acid deficiency
- Electrolyte and vitamin excesses and deficiencies
- Trace mineral deficiencies

Mechanical Problems
- Insertion
  - Air embolus
  - Pneumothorax, hemothorax, and hydrothorax
  - Hemorrhage
- Dislodgement
- Thrombosis of great vein

less irritating. The peripheral injection site should be observed for signs of phlebitis (redness and swelling). The site is changed at least every 48 hours, depending on established hospital policy. The preparation and administration of peripheral nutrition follow the same criteria as outlined for central hyperalimentation (see the nursing care plan on p. 1121).

Vital signs should be monitored every 4 hours in the patient receiving TPN. Daily weights give an indication of the patient's nutritional status as therapy progresses. Body weight is considered the sum of the changes in protein, fat, and water. On a daily basis, body water fluctuates more than protein or fat. Analysis must be made of whether gains or losses in weight are caused by fluid gained from edema, fluid lost through diuresis, or actual increase or decrease in tissue weight. Blood levels of glucose, electrolytes, protein, a complete blood count, and enzyme studies are followed daily or every other day. Assessment of these important values assists the nurse in assessing the patient's progress toward a more nutritionally balanced state.

Dressings covering the catheter site are changed according to institutional protocol, ranging from every other day to once a week. Frequently, specially trained nurses from the IV team or the nutritional support team are responsible for these dressing changes. Some institutions allow a staff nurse to do the dressing changes after special instruction. The procedure for changing the dressing is similar to that followed after catheter insertion. The institutional routine should be followed with respect to the appropriate use of acetone, betadine, and alcohol for the dressing change. The site is carefully observed for signs of inflammation and infection. Phlebitis can readily occur in the vein as a result of the hypertonic infusion and the area can become infected. Many patients receiving central TPN are immunosuppressed and are more susceptible to opportunistic infections. In this patient signs of inflammation or infection can be subtle, if present at all. Many are receiving chemotherapy, corticosteroids or antibiotics, which can mask signs of infection.

If sutures are used to anchor the catheter, they may become infected. If an infection is suspected during dressing change, a culture specimen of the site and drainage should be sent for analysis, and the physician should be notified immediately. The use of an occlusive dressing protects the wound from contamination.

Catheter Placement. The central placement of the catheter into a large main vein for TPN is performed by the physician. The vein most commonly used is the subclavian, although the innominate or the jugular vein may be used. The procedure is the same as for the insertion of a central venous pressure line and should be done under strict aseptic conditions.

A standard isotonic IV solution is infused through the central line until x-ray confirms proper placement of the catheter tip in the superior vena cava and not in the jugular vein or the heart. The catheter insertion site is covered with an iodine ointment, and an occlusive dressing is placed over it. The date is marked on the dressing.

Complications frequently associated with catheter placement are hemorrhage, hydrothorax and pneumothorax, hemothorax, air embolus, and venous thrombosis. It is important that the tip of the catheter not lie within the right atrium. TPN solution is hyperosmolar, and the catheter tip can cause erosions of the atrial tissue with subsequent infection.

Placement of a PIC line is done under sterile conditions, often by a specially trained nurse. A baseline measurement of the upper arm circumference is recommended. A tourniquet is then placed around the upper arm near the axilla to allow examination of the antecubital fossa and selection of a vein. If possible, the patient should be supine with the arm straight and at a 90-degree angle. Preparation of the insertion site should be done according to institutional policy. The sterile catheter will need to be cut to the predetermined length, depending on the vein selected.

A local anesthetic is usually used at the insertion site. This site should be cleaned, protected, and maintained according to institutional policy. As with the centrally placed line, chest x-ray is needed to verify proper tip placement before administering any TPN solution.

Proper placement of a catheter for central hyperalimentation is illustrated in Fig. 37-3 on p. 1123. Once established for TPN, a single lumen central catheter should not be used for the administration of blood or antibiotics, the drawing of blood samples, or the monitoring of central venous pressure.

Administration of Solution. Because TPN solutions are an excellent media for microbial growth, it is essential that proper aseptic techniques be followed. The FDA has

NURSING CARE PLAN Patient Receiving Total Parenteral Nutrition

Planning: Outcome Criteria	Nursing Interventions and Rationales
➤ NURSING DIAGNOSIS	Risk for infection *related to* placement of a central venous access catheter, inadequate aseptic practices, and decreased host defense mechanisms
Have no manifestations of infection, normal body temperature, negative blood cultures	Assess for altered defense mechanisms because of inadequate nutrition, compromised health status, wound for TPN line, and use of bacteriogenic solution *to plan for prevention of infection.* Refrigerate solution until ½ hour before using *to prevent bacterial growth in the solution.* Use aseptic technique when connecting IV tubing and filter to catheter; label tubing and filter with time and date; change filter q24hr and tubing with each bottle or according to institutional policy; check expiration date; change occlusive dressing over catheter site according to institutional policy, using aseptic technique (e.g., sterile gloves, mask) *to minimize the possibility of infection.* Observe for signs of inflammation and infection. Monitor vital signs q4hr *to ensure early detection of infection.*
➤ NURSING DIAGNOSIS	Impaired physical mobility of arm, shoulder, and chest *related to* muscle or nerve trauma secondary to catheter insertion and position restrictions and pain *as manifested by inability to move upper body at will, decreased muscle strength and control, neuromuscular impairment (e.g., brachial plexus injury), pain on movement.*
Have satisfactory movement of upper body; achieve ADLs; maintain satisfactory pain control.	Observe patient for pain in shoulder and sensory changes *to determine possible nerve damage or faulty catheter placement.* Assist with range-of-motion within position restrictions *to maintain normal range-of-motion of shoulder.* Assist with ADLs *to ensure patient's needs are met.* Administer pain medication as ordered *to maintain patient's comfort.*
➤ NURSING DIAGNOSIS	Anxiety *related to* inability to ingest food and fluids, uncertain outcome, lack of knowledge regarding catheter position and rationale, benefits, and management of TPN *as manifested by* restlessness and apprehension, expression of concern regarding changes in life events, frequent questioning regarding care of catheter and TPN line
State rationale for and demonstrate care of TPN line.	Instruct patient on rationale and benefits of TPN and care of line *because knowledge and facts may reduce anxiety.* Give approximate length of time TPN will be used *so patient can bolster resources to match the duration of the treatment.* Illustrate catheter position by drawings and pictures *to increase patient understanding. To relieve anxiety,* reassure patient the catheter will not move into the heart. Describe the advantages of physical activity *so patient will remain active and as independent as possible.* Provide range-of-motion exercises that patient can perform while in bed. Encourage ambulation *to maintain circulation and positive mental attitude.*

continued

recommended that Millipore filters be placed on all parenteral lines. When the filter is used, it should be placed proximal to the catheter hub. Filters are changed every 24 hours, and new IV tubing is changed with each new bottle of TPN. The tubing and the filter should be clearly labeled with the date and the time they are put into use.

Hyperglycemia is a metabolic complication of parenteral nutrition. At the beginning of TPN therapy, the solution is infused at a gradually increasing rate for 24 to 48 hours. This allows the pancreas to adapt to the increased amount of glucose in the circulation by producing more insulin. Blood glucose levels should be checked at the bedside every 4 to 6 hours with a glucose-testing meter (see Chapter 46). Some increase in blood glucose level is expected during the first few days after TPN is started. A sliding scale dose of insulin may be ordered to keep the level below 180 to 200 mg/dl (9.8 to 10.9 mmol/L). In the critical care patient it is recommended that insulin be administered to maintain blood glucose level below 220 mg/dl (12 mmol/L) whenever possible.[13] If blood glucose-testing meters are not available, the urine should be tested for glucose and acetone every 4 to 6 hours while the patient is receiving hyperalimentation. As with the blood glucose level, glycosuria of 1+ or 2+ is expected during the first few days of therapy. However, readings of 3+ or 4+ require either the addition of regular insulin to the solution or the administration of insulin on a sliding-scale schedule. (Sliding scale is explained in Chapter 46).

NURSING CARE PLAN Patient Receiving Total Parenteral Nutrition—cont'd

COLLABORATIVE PROBLEMS

Planning: Outcome Criteria	Nursing Interventions and Rationales
➤ POTENTIAL COMPLICATIONS Hyperglycemia, hypoglycemia, and electrolyte imbalances	
Monitor blood glucose and serum electrolytes; report deviations from acceptable parameters; carry out medical and nursing interventions.	Monitor for signs of hyperglycemia such as thirst, polyuria, confusion, elevated fasting blood glucose, blurred vision, dizziness, nausea and vomiting, dehydration, and deep labored breathing *to plan appropriate treatment.* Monitor for signs of hypoglycemia such as sweating, hunger, weakness, and tremors *to ensure early intervention.* Monitor serum electrolyte levels daily *to identify and treat complications early.* Check for symptoms of hyperkalemia (e.g., muscle weakness, flaccid paralysis, cardiac dysrhythmias, abdominal cramps, diarrhea) and hypokalemia (e.g., general weakness, decreased muscle tone, weak or irregular pulse, low BP, shallow respirations, abdominal distension, and ileus).* Check urine glucose and acetone q4hr. Notify physician of 3+ or 4+ readings *so that regular insulin may be added to the solution or administered on a sliding scale.* Administer regular insulin if ordered *to control the serum glucose level.* Initial TPN therapy must be gradually increased over 24 to 48 hr *so that the pancreas can adapt to the increased amount of glucose in the circulation by producing more insulin.* Maintain accurate infusion rate *to control the amount of glucose administered and prevent fluctuations.* Check every ½ hour or use an infusion pump (e.g., IVAC) *to ensure accurate administration.* Watch for kinks and obstruction or disconnected tubing *to prevent errors in administration.* Never increase or decrease flow rate by more than 10% *to prevent fluctuations in blood glucose levels.* Never stop TPN abruptly unless it is replaced by another glucose source *to prevent hypoglycemia.*
➤ POTENTIAL COMPLICATION Air embolus secondary to incorrect insertion position	
Monitor for and report signs of air embolus; carry out medical and nursing interventions.	On catheter insertion, place patient in Trendelenburg position with rolled towel between scapulae *to distend subclavian vein by increasing venous pressure.* Instruct patient to take a deep breath (Valsalva maneuver) and hold while needle is inserted into subclavian vein. Use the same position and Valsalva maneuver when changing tubing *to prevent air from being sucked into vein.* Reconnect catheter to IV tubing immediately *to prevent air entry.* If air embolism is suspected, place patient in Trendelenburg position with left side down *to trap "air" in right atria.* Continue to observe for shock, cough, and shortness of breath. Notify physician immediately *so definitive diagnosis and treatment can be initiated.* Monitor for signs of air embolus such as abnormal blood gases, cough, cyanosis, pain, anxiety, fatigue, respiratory rate and depth changes, altered chest excursion, shortness of breath *to assure early identification and treatment.*

ADLs, Activities of daily living; *BP,* blood pressure; *IV,* intravenous; *TPN,* total parenteral nutrition.
*Other manifestations of electrolyte imbalances are discussed in Chapter 13.

The nurse must be made aware that speeding or slowing the infusion rate is contraindicated. Speeding up the rate results in a large amount of glucose entering the circulation. Endogenous insulin levels often are not adequate to handle this increase in glucose, and a hyperosmolar state results. The renal tubules are unable to reabsorb the glucose and it spills into the urine. Conversely, slowing the rate may result in a hypoglycemic state because it takes time for the pancreatic islet cells to adjust to a reduced glucose level. Checking the amount infused and the rate every 1/2 to 1 hour is recommended. An infusion pump should be used during administration of TPN so that the infusion rate can be maintained, and an alarm will sound if the tubing becomes obstructed. Even when using an infusion pump, the nurse should periodically check the volume infused because pump malfunctions can alter the rate.

Before setting up and administering TPN, the nurse must check the label and ingredients in the solution to see that they are what the physician ordered. Solutions must also be examined for signs of contamination, such as a cloudy appearance. If contamination is suspected, the solution should be promptly returned to the pharmacy for replacement. It is the nurse's responsibility to ensure that the TPN solution is discontinued and replaced with a new solution if

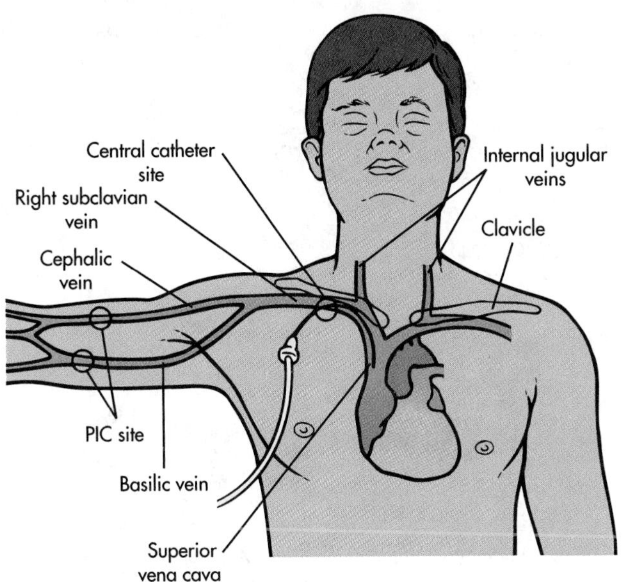

Fig. 37-3 Placement of catheter for total parenteral nutrition using subclavian vein. Peripherally inserted central (PIC) catheters can be inserted using the basilic or cephalic veins.

it is still infusing at the end of 24 hours. At room temperature, the solution is an excellent medium in which microorganisms grow.

If the patient exhibits signs and symptoms of a systemic infection, the catheter tip is usually suspect unless another cause can be found. Cultures of blood, sputum, urine, draining wound, and the catheter tip, if it has been removed, must be performed at once. A chest x-ray is taken to detect changes in pulmonary status. The current bottle of TPN solution with tubing and filter should also be cultured and replaced with an entirely new setup. When the catheter tip is the source of infection, antibiotic therapy is generally not necessary because removal of the catheter will eliminate the problem. A new central line may be immediately established or replaced by a peripheral route. It is important that a glucose source be maintained to prevent rebound hypoglycemia.

Weaning. The same precautions should be followed in weaning from TPN as when therapy is being initiated, except in the reverse order. The flow rate must be gradually decreased for 4 to 6 hours, while oral intake is increased. If an emergency situation precludes a slow weaning process, other dextrose-containing fluids should be administered without interruption. For the patient who will be undergoing surgery, the TPN should be discontinued ahead of the scheduled operation time. At the time the catheter is removed by the physician, the site is immediately covered with iodine ointment and an occlusive dressing is applied. The dressing should be changed daily until the wound heals. Oral nourishment should be encouraged, and a careful record of intake should be maintained. Daily weight recording and laboratory analysis of serum electrolyte and glucose levels may continue.

Table 37-20 Standard Contents of a 10% Intralipid Fat Emulsion in Water*

Soybean triglycerides	10.0%*
Egg yolk phospholipids	1.2%
Glycerin	2.25%
Electrolytes	0.0
Total kilocalories	100.0

*Another stock lipid solution is 20%.

Home Parenteral Nutrition. Home parenteral nutrition is now an accepted mode of nutritional therapy for the person who does not require hospitalization but who benefits from continued nutritional support. Some patients have been successfully treated at home for many months and even years. It is important to educate the patient or the family about catheter care, aseptic technique in mixing and handling of the IV solutions and tubing, and side effects.[11]

Intravenous Fat Emulsion

The first infusion of fat emulsions occurred during the 1920s in Japan. Further research was delayed until after World War II. The FDA has approved the use of 10% and 20% intralipid fat emulsion solutions. These lipid emulsions provide approximately 1 calorie per milliliter (10% solution) or 2 calories per milliliter (20% solution). The contents of intralipid fat emulsion are listed in Table 37-20. The use of IV fat is indicated for the following patients:

1. Those receiving peripheral hyperalimentation who require an additional source of calories
2. Those receiving long-term (more than 5 days) hyperalimentation who require a source of essential fatty acids
3. Those receiving central hyperalimentation who have excessive caloric needs

Using daily IV fat emulsions provides another nonprotein energy source. It is recommended that IV administered fat emulsions not provide more than 60% of the total energy or exceed a dose of 2.5 g/kg per day.[12] Nausea, vomiting, and elevated temperature have been reported, especially when lipids are infused quickly.

The administration of fat emulsion is contraindicated in the patient with a disturbance in fat metabolism. It should also be used with caution in the patient who is in danger of fat embolism and the patient with pancreatitis, liver damage, pulmonary disease, anemia, blood coagulation disorders, and allergic reaction to eggs.

Intralipid solution is isotonic and is used as the primary caloric substrate in complete peripheral TPN solutions. It can be infused separately. When it is used with TPN, the fat emulsion provides essential fatty acids that are not included in the standard dextrose-amino acid preparations of TPN. Prolonged use of TPN can lead to a fatty acid deficiency, which is manifested by dermatitis and loss of hair. Recent pharmacologic advances now permit the direct mixing of

CULTURAL & ETHNIC Considerations

NUTRITIONAL PROBLEMS

- Obesity has a higher incidence among African-American women as compared to Caucasian women.
- Anorexia nervosa is most common among women from middle and upper middle classes.
- Anorexia nervosa and bulimia have a higher incidence among Caucasians than among African-Americans and Asian-Americans.
- Lactase deficiency has a higher incidence among African-Americans than among Caucasians.

lipid emulsion with dextrose and amino acids in a single bag suitable for infusion.

Unopened intralipid solutions do not require refrigeration. However, those that have been opened or mixed with other nutrients do require refrigeration and should be refrigerated until 1 hour before administration. Special tubing is provided by the manufacturer, and new tubing is used with each bottle. Nothing is to be added to the solution before administration. Lipid solutions can be filtered but require a 1.2 μm filter. When peripheral hyperalimentation is being run concurrently, the fat emulsion should be connected below the filter through a Y-injection site as close as possible to the injection site. The preferred delivery method is a continuous low volume, such as 20% lipids delivered at 10 to 30 ml per hour depending on the patient needs.[14] Adverse reactions that can occur are allergic manifestations, dyspnea, cyanosis, fever, flushing, phlebitis, chest and back pain, and pain at the IV site. IV fat values may be determined daily or at least two to three times a week, depending on the caloric needs or fatty acid requirements of the patient. A major benefit derived from IV fat administration is that a large number of calories can be provided in a relatively small amount of fluid. This is especially beneficial when the patient is at risk for fluid overload.

OBESITY

Significance

Obesity is one of the major health problems in our society. In the United States obesity is the most common nutritional problem. Among adults 20 to 74 years of age, 24% of men and 27% of women are overweight, yielding an estimated total of 34 million overweight people in the United States.[15] The prevalence of overweight increases with age, for both men and women, but to a greater degree in women. African-Americans and Hispanics have a higher prevalence of being overweight than do Caucasians, especially among women.[16]

The calculated body mass index (BMI) is a common clinical index of obesity or altered body fat distribution. A scale has been developed to calculate BMI by gender using

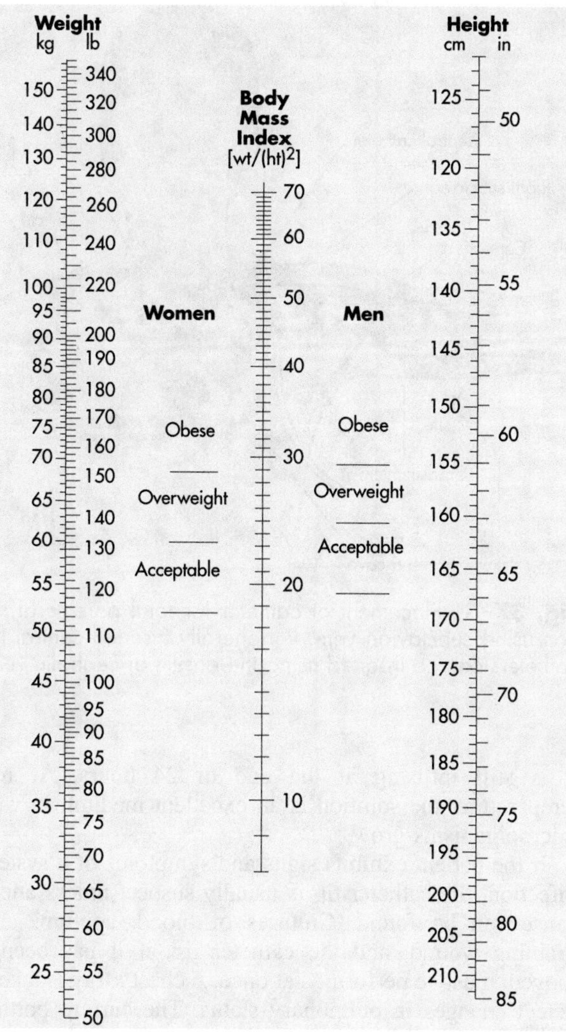

Fig. 37-4 A nomogram for determining body mass index (BMI). To use this nomogram, place a ruler or other straight edge between the column for height and the column for weight connecting an individual's numbers for these two variables. Read the BMI in kg/m^2 where the straight line crosses the middle lines when the height and weight are connected. Overweight: BMI of 25-30 kg/m^2; obesity: BMI over 30 kg/m^2. Heights and weights are without shoes or clothes.

weight-to-height ratios[17] (Fig. 37-4). Women with a BMI value of 23 to 29 are classified as being overweight and those with a value exceeding 29 as obese. Men with a BMI value of 25 to 30 are classified as overweight and those with a value exceeding 30 as obese.

The waist to hip ratio is another way to define obesity. This ratio is a method of describing the distribution of both subcutaneous and intrabdominal adipose tissue. The waist measurement is divided by the hip measurement to calculate the ratio. A number greater than 1.0 in men and 0.8 in women indicates overweight. This ratio increases with age and excessive weight.[17]

Anthropometric measurements can also be used to define the different levels of overweight. A patient with body weight 10% above the ideal for height and frame is termed overweight. A patient with body weight 20% above the ideal for height and frame is termed obese. Triceps skinfold greater than 15 mm in men and 25 mm in women would classify the person as overweight.[18] When body weight exceeds 100% of the ideal body weight it is classified as *morbid obesity*.

In obese persons a variety of problems occur at a rate higher than the expected rate. These include hypertension, hyperlipidemia, non–insulin-dependent diabetes mellitus (NIDDM), degenerative joint disease, gout, insulin resistance with hyperinsulinemia, cardiovascular disease, gallbladder disease, stroke, some kinds of cancer (breast, colon), and menstrual irregularities.[19] These conditions generally improve if weight loss occurs.

Formation of Adipose Tissue

The formation of adipose tissue, unless determined to be secondary to an organic cause, can occur only when a person consumes more food than is required to carry out normal physiologic functions and growth. The excess energy is converted to fat and is stored in adipose tissue in layers beneath the skin surface, the omentum, the mesentery, and in fat pads that normally surround the kidneys and the heart. The process of reaching an obese state is usually insidious. The person may be completely unaware of changes in eating habits, activity expenditure, or body size until looking in a mirror or discovering the need for a larger clothing size.

Adipose tissue present in obesity is of the same composition as fat tissue normally found in smaller amounts in the same areas. It consists of clumps of fat cells (adipocytes) together with supporting tissue, such as blood vessels, lymphatic vessels, and fibrous tissue. Although adipose tissue is high in neutral fat, it also contains water, protein, and a small amount of glycogen. The size of the adipose tissue mass reflects the number of adipocytes and the size of adipocytes, which is determined by the amount of triglyceride found within the cell.

Obesity research has demonstrated that expansion of the tissue mass occurs as a result of an increase in cell size (*hypertrophic obesity*) or an increase in cell number (*hyperplastic obesity*) or both (hypertrophic hyperplastic obesity). Until recently it was believed that fat cells increased in number only until puberty. After puberty, if a person absorbed more energy from food than was expended by metabolic processes or by physical activity, the excess energy was converted into fat and was stored in the existing adipocytes, which increased in size (hypertrophy). The adipocyte can increase 1000-fold in volume. It is now known that when faced with fat storage at any age, the fat cell first increases in size and, when a critical size is achieved, divides to form new fat cells.[20]

The adipose tissue mass in early-onset obesity is distributed universally over the entire body; the adipose tissue mass in adult-onset obesity is centrally distributed. How fat is distributed on the body frame can affect the severity of the health risk. Two commonly used classifications are the android pattern and the gynoid pattern (apple-and pear-shaped respectively). Table 37-21 presents characteristics of these two patterns of body fat distribution. A high waist-to-hip ratio, greater that 0.85, classifies one as *android*. A person with the *gynoid* pattern has a low waist-to-hip ratio. The android pattern is associated with a higher risk of coronary artery disease, hypertension, and disorders in glucose tolerance and hyperlipidemia.

Table 37-21 Body Fat Distribution Pattern Characteristics

Android (Apple-shaped)	Gynoid (Pear-shaped)
Upper-body involvement	Lower-body involvement
Waist-to-hip ratio >0.85	Waist-to-hip ratio <0.85
Abdominal prominence	Gluteal, femoral, visceral prominence
Central distribution	Peripheral distribution
Subscapular skin-fold thickness >25 mm	Subscapular skin-fold thickness <25 mm

Modified from Leaf D: Overweight assessment and management issues, *Am Fam Physician* 42:654, 1990.

An understanding of how adipose tissue is formed has considerable impact on methods of weight loss and of reduction of the adipose tissue mass in the adult. Severe dietary restrictions do not decrease the number of fat adipocytes present but do result in a decrease in the size of the cells.[19]

Pathophysiology

Many factors have been investigated in an effort to identify the critical elements in the development and maintenance of obesity. When assessing the obese patient, the nurse needs to consider several different types of questions, such as the following:

1. What is the psychologic importance of food to the patient?
2. Is the patient's food intake influenced by hunger?
3. Do the taste and appearance of food or other physical factors in the environment stimulate the patient to eat?
4. Is there an emotional problem that stimulates the patient to eat?
5. Are there any stressors influencing the patient's eating patterns?

The nurse must recognize that environmental and genetic factors are important. The children of obese parents tend to be obese. Obesity tends to affect several persons within a family. Evidence of a genetic component is suggested in twin and adoptive children studies.[21]

There are a growing number of theories related to the genetics of obesity.[22] It is likely that the human obesity genotypes will be complex multigenic systems with networks of gene-gene and gene-environment interactions. The complexity of the etiology of obesity is primarily caused by two reasons. First, the body fat content and, more specifically, an excess of body fat, results from an intricate network of additive and interactive causes that may be related to DNA sequence variation but may also be associated with behavior and lifestyle. Second, obesity is a heterogeneous phenotype, and evidence is growing that each phenotypic entity is modulated by a different set of causal factors. These factors include energy intake, resting metabolic rate, level of habitual physical activity, and nutrient partitioning (tendency to store ingested energy in the form of fat or lean tissue).

Research on the pathophysiology of obesity has focused on the role of the hypothalamus and energy balance.[23] The lateral and ventral-medial parts of the hypothalamus control appetite and, as a result, influence eating behavior. It is hypothesized that the hypothalamus has a set point for energy balance, above which energy conservation becomes increasingly less efficient and below which energy conservation becomes increasingly more efficient. This homeostatic mechanism accounts for the fact that most adults keep their weight remarkably constant, despite large swings in energy input and expenditure.

This ability of the body to conserve energy as dieting continues may account for the failure of sustained weight loss to occur even though caloric intake is drastically curtailed. It could also account for why the obese person, no matter what dietary regimen is followed, tends to remain overweight.

A sedentary lifestyle including a nonstrenuous indoor occupation and engagement in few, if any, spirited recreational activities is associated with the development of excess body weight and obesity. Thus an obese person with sedentary habits only adds to an already positive energy balance by not engaging in activities that burn off some excess fatty tissue through energy-consuming exercises.

The emotional component of the tendency to overeat is powerful. People use food for many reasons, including comfort and reward. Some people are triggered by specific foods to continue eating beyond satiety. The social component of eating develops early in life when food is associated with pleasure and fun at such events as birthday parties, Thanksgiving, and Christmas. All of these factors must be included when considering the etiology of obesity.

Complications

The medical and social problems associated with obesity are numerous. These problems are more common in a patient who exceeds ideal body weight by greater than 20%. The medical problems associated with obesity may be a direct result of too much fat. In addition, medical problems such as hypothyroidism can have an adverse effect on energy balance and result in excess body weight gain. Cardiovascular and respiratory problems are common in the obese person. Many patients experience dyspnea on exertion, orthopnea, paroxysmal nocturnal dyspnea, drowsiness, and somnolence. Obstructive sleep apnea is more prevalent in overweight or obese older men.

In addition, the obese patient is prone to the development of polycythemia secondary to low oxygenation of arterial blood. Polycythemia results in an increased viscosity of the circulating blood and sluggish flow through all vessels and capillaries. As a result, an obese patient may have occluded vessels and clotting abnormalities. Varicose veins, as well as venous leg ulcers, are common partly because of increased back pressure on the venous return from the lower limbs by excess intraabdominal adipose tissue. Heart size increases as body weight increases because the heart must work harder to maintain adequate circulation. Hypertension is the most common cardiovascular problem associated with obesity. The presence of polycythemia creates considerable strain on the heart because of the increased RBC count and plasma volume. Therefore obesity can precipitate hypertrophy of the heart, especially of the left ventricle.

The *Pickwickian syndrome*, which is known as obesity hypoventilation, has long been recognized as a result of morbid obesity. The bellows action of the chest wall is compromised, and there is dysfunction of the central respiratory control center. The movement of the muscles of the chest wall and the diaphragm is reduced because of the weight of the fatty tissue mass. Hypoventilation results in a state of chronic hypercapnia manifested by cyanosis, dyspnea, edema, and somnolence. In addition, most patients have a reduced vital capacity and polycythemia. Blood gas exchange is also directly affected. Although the Pickwickian syndrome is rare, caution should always be used when sedatives are used for the morbidly obese person because these drugs can precipitate severe respiratory complications.

Impaired glucose tolerance is common with obesity. The incidence of NIDDM is high in obese persons. Excessive food intake stimulates hyperinsulinemia. Through a negative-feedback mechanism, excessive insulin levels decrease the number of insulin-receptor sites on the cell membrane. The loss of insulin-receptor sites decreases the amount of glucose that can enter the cells. This promotes high levels of blood glucose. Thus the obese patient is often hyperglycemic and hyperinsulinemic. Weight reduction appears to reverse these effects by increasing insulin receptors and enhancing the movement of glucose into cells.

Gallstone formation in the obese patient is also common. The incidence of gallstones rises as the body weight increases. There is a concomitant rise in the serum cholesterol and triglyceride levels, as well as an increase in body weight. These substances precipitate in the gallbladder resulting in cholelithiasis and cholecystitis. With weight loss, cholesterol and triglyceride levels often decrease, resulting in decreased risk of gallstone formation. The high levels of cholesterol and triglycerides can also contribute to the development of coronary artery disease (Chapter 31).

Excessive weight on the weight-bearing joints (hips and knees) and the lower spine can cause pain and discomfort. Although obesity has not been implicated as a cause of degenerative joint disease, it is a predisposing factor. Obesity may contribute to the pathogenesis of osteoarthritis in multiple joints in which the disease process has already started.

Other complications associated with obesity are menstrual irregularities, infertility, endometrial cancer, and fatty liver infiltration. Understandably, the life expectancy of an obese person can be shortened as a result of the medical problems.

In addition to the many physical complications associated with obesity, the person may suffer from long-standing emotional and social problems. Society today puts great emphasis on attaining and maintaining a slim and vigorous look. Those who deviate from this prescribed standard often meet with discrimination and disdain. The morbidly obese person may find it difficult to obtain a desired job, social acceptance, or membership in organizations. Choice of clothing is often limited in style, color, size, and quantity. These socioemotional problems may be manifested in poor self-esteem and body image.

Diagnostic Studies

The overwhelming majority of obese persons have primary obesity, that is, excess calorie intake for the body's metabolic demands. Others have secondary obesity which is obesity resulting from various congenital or chromosomal anomalies or from metabolic or CNS lesions or disorders. A first step in the treatment process is to evaluate if any such physical conditions are present. A thorough history and physical examination are necessary and will reveal the extent and duration of the obese state.

There is no definite agreement on a technique for determining who is obese. Several methods are currently in use. One widely used method is to compare the patient's weight to a standardized weight-for-height chart and then designate the patient to be overweight by a certain percentage. Table 37-22 provides a standardized weight-for-height chart. Normal weight depends largely on body build. A limitation of this method of assessing obesity can be seen from the following example: A person who inherits a medium frame and bulky muscle mass may be considered 20% overweight according to the standardized chart and yet not be obese.

A more sensitive approach to determine the presence of obesity is the BMI discussed earlier in this chapter. The BMI (see Fig. 37-4) is not dependent on frame size. Because the BMI value rises with age, it has been suggested that age-specific guidelines for older adults be established. A more individualized method of determining the amount of body fat is by measuring skin fold thickness with special calipers at one or more of four body sites: the biceps, the triceps, the subscapular site, or the suprailiac site. Estimates of body fat are then derived as a result of correlations established with body density from anthropometric charts. Although considered a more exact technique, this method also has limitations. The disadvantage of this method of calculating the degree of obesity is that the standards for the skin fold thickness are generally obtained from healthy young men and women, 20 to 30 years of age, and do not consider age-related changes. As a person ages, the percent of total body fat increases, as does the skin fold thickness for the fatty tissue at each site. This measure is not as reliable in an obese individual as in midrange body weights. These measurements need to be performed by trained clinicians. The hip to waist ratio described earlier is another useful assessment technique.

Table 37-22 Desirable Weights for Men and Women*

	Frame Size		
Height	**Small**	**Medium**	**Large**
Men			
5′ 2″	128-134	131-141	138-150
5′ 3″	130-136	133-143	140-153
5′ 4″	132-138	135-145	142-156
5′ 5″	134-140	137-148	144-160
5′ 6″	136-142	139-151	146-164
5′ 7″	138-145	142-154	149-168
5′ 8″	140-148	145-157	152-172
5′ 9″	142-151	148-160	155-176
5′ 10″	144-154	151-163	158-180
5′ 11″	146-157	154-166	161-184
6′	149-160	157-170	164-188
6′ 1″	152-164	160-174	168-192
6′ 2″	155-168	164-178	172-197
6′ 3″	158-172	167-182	176-202
6′ 4″	162-176	171-187	181-207
Women			
4′ 10″	102-111	109-121	118-131
4′ 11″	103-113	111-123	120-134
5′	104-115	113-126	122-137
5′ 1″	106-118	115-129	125-140
5′ 2″	108-121	118-132	128-143
5′ 3″	111-124	121-135	131-147
5′ 4″	114-127	124-138	134-151
5′ 5″	117-130	127-141	137-155
5′ 6″	120-133	130-144	140-159
5′ 7″	123-136	133-147	143-163
5′ 8″	126-139	136-150	146-167
5′ 9″	129-142	139-153	149-170
5′ 10″	132-145	142-156	152-173
5′ 11″	135-148	145-159	155-176
6′	138-151	148-162	158-179

*From 1983 Metropolitan Life Insurance Company weight tables by height and size of frame for people aged 25 to 59, in 1-inch shoes and wearing 5 pounds of indoor clothing for men or 3 pounds for women.

The least reliable technique and yet perhaps the most frequently used is direct observation of the patient. A subjective assessment of total body fat is made. The ideal body is one that has only a thin layer of adipose tissue covering the skeletal frame. When a roll of excess subcutaneous adipose tissue is seen, the patient is considered obese.

More sophisticated measures of obesity utilize densitometry, dual photon absorption, magnetic resonance imaging, and ultrasonography. However, such measures are generally used only for research purposes.

The physician explores genetic and endocrine factors in the workup. Etiologic factors such as hypothyroidism, hypothalamic tumors, Cushing's syndrome, hypogonadism in men, or polycystic ovarian disease in women are studied. Laboratory tests of liver function, fasting glucose level, triglyceride level, and low- and high-density lipoprotein cholesterol levels assist in evaluating the cause and effects of obesity.

Conservative Therapeutic Management

When no organic cause can be found for obesity, it should be considered a chronic, complex illness. Any supervised plan of care should be directed at (1) successful weight loss, requiring a short-term energy deficit and (2) successful weight control, requiring long-term behavior changes. These are two different processes. A multipronged approach ought to be used with attention to dietary intake, physical activity, behavioral-cognitive modification, and perhaps drug therapy.

Nutritional Management. Restricted food intake is a cornerstone for any weight loss or maintenance program. A good weight loss plan should contain foods from the basic five food groups. Diets may be classified as low calorie (800-1200 calories/day) or very low calorie (<800 calories/day). Persons on low and very low calorie diets need frequent professional monitoring because the severe energy restriction places them at high risk for multiple nutrient deficiencies. A diet that includes adequate amounts of fruits and vegetables provides enough bulk to prevent constipation and meets daily vitamin A and vitamin C requirements. Lean meat, fish, and eggs provide sufficient protein, as well as the B complex vitamins. The caloric intake may need to be restricted to 800 to 1200 calories per day, depending on the patient's age, weight, nutritional status, activity level, and length of time estimated for the ideal weight to be achieved. Table 37-23 contains a sample 1200-calorie reducing diet.

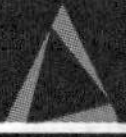

Table 37-23 Nutritional Management: 1200-Calorie-Restricted Weight-Reduction Diet*

General Principles

1. Eat regularly. Do not skip meals.
2. Measure foods to determine the correct portion size.
3. Avoid concentrated sweets, such as sugar, candy, honey, pies, cakes, cookies, and regular sodas.
4. Reduce fat intake by baking, broiling, or steaming foods.
5. Maintain a regular exercise program for successful weight loss.

Meal	Exchanges	Meal Plan 1	Meal Plan 2	Meal Plan 3
Breakfast	1 meat	1 scrambled egg	1 hard-boiled egg	1 oz ham
	2 bread	1 slice toast ¾ cup dry cereal (unsweetened)	1 flour tortilla ½ cup Cream of Wheat	2 griddle cakes with diet syrup
	1 fruit	½ small banana	⅓ cup orange juice	⅓ cup pineapple juice
	1 fat	1 tsp margarine 1 sausage link†	1 slice bacon	1 tsp margarine
	1 dairy	1 cup low-fat milk	1 cup low-fat milk	1 cup low-fat milk
	Beverage	Coffee	Coffee	Coffee
Lunch	2 meat	1 slice bologna 1 slice cheese	Cheese enchiladas (made with 2 oz cheese, 2 corn tortillas, chili sauce)	2 oz baked breaded pork chop
	2 bread	2 slices bread		1 corn muffin
	Vegetable	Lettuce, pickles	Tomato wedges	Spinach
	1 fruit	Fresh grapes (12)	2 canned peach halves (packed in water)	Fresh orange
	Beverage	Diet soda	Artifically sweetened lemonade	Unsweetened iced tea
Dinner	2 meat	2 oz roast beef	Chili con carne (made with ½ cup ground beef, ½ cup pinto beans, and chili powder)	2 oz baked chicken
	1 bread	Baked potato (with 1 tsp margarine†)		Corn on the cob with 1 tsp margarine
	Vegetable	Cooked carrots	Tossed salad and 1 tbs salad dressing†	Okra
	1 fruit	¾ cup strawberries	Fresh apple	Fruit cocktail (packed in water)
	1 milk	1 cup low-fat milk	1 cup low-fat milk	1 cup low-fat milk

*For 1000 calories, omit 1 fruit exchange and change low-fat milk to skim milk. For 1500 calories, add 1 meat, 1 fruit, and 2 fat exchanges; change low-fat milk to whole milk. For 1800 calories, add 2 bread, 3 meat, 3 fat, and 1 fruit exchanges; change low-fat milk to whole milk.
†One extra fat exchange allowed for each cup of 2% low-fat milk; 2 extra fat exchanges allowed for each cup of skim milk.

The only effective method of treating primary obesity is to restrict dietary intake so that it is below energy requirements. It is rare to find an overweight person who has not at some time attempted to lose weight. Some have met with limited and temporary success, and others have met only with failure. It is likely that the great majority of these persons attempted weight loss by trying out at least one of the many fad diets that offer the enticement to eat and get slim. Fad diets in general claim weight loss quickly and inexpensively. Although it is true that initially weight is lost, it is not fat but body water that is lost. The normal fat cell is composed of approximately 80% fat, 18% water, and 2% protein. It is also a storage area for small amounts of glycogen. Glycogen is known to bind with water. When reducing diets severely restrict carbohydrates, the body's glycogen stores become depleted within a few days. It is only when the glycogen-water pool is almost depleted of energy that protein and adipose tissue are burned to release energy for bodily functions.

An obese patient needs to understand that following a well-balanced, low-caloric diet is the most sensible approach to weight loss. Continuing to follow a well-balanced food plan will have a more satisfying and long-lasting result than fad diets.

The degree of success of any reducing diet depends in part on the amount of weight to be lost. A moderately obese person will obviously attain the goal more easily than will a massively obese person. Men are able to lose weight more quickly than women. Women have a higher percentage of metabolically less active body fat, whereas men have a higher percentage of metabolically more active lean body mass. Adult-onset obesity is often more amenable to successful treatment than the obesity of juvenile onset. In juvenile-onset obesity, the eating patterns have been present longer, and the number of fat cells is often higher. As a result, more drastic dieting efforts and perseverance are necessary to achieve weight reduction.

Motivation is an essential ingredient for achievement of success. The obese patient must see the need for weight loss and weight control and the advantages that will accrue. The nurse can assist by helping the patient track eating patterns by keeping a diet diary. A frank discussion of eating habits helps the patient realize that often eating is the result of bad habits picked up with time and not of hunger. The bad habits must be changed, or weight loss will be only temporary.

Setting a realistic goal, such as losing 1 to 2 pounds a week, must be agreed on at the outset. Trying to lose too much too fast usually results in a sense of frustration and failure for the patient. The nurse can help the patient understand that losing large amounts of weight in a short period of time causes skin and underlying tissue to lose elasticity and tone and become unsightly folds of flabby tissue. Slower weight loss offers better cosmetic results. Inevitably, the patient reaches plateau periods during which no weight is lost. These plateaus may last from several days to several weeks. It is especially important that the patient realize that these are normal occurrences during weight reduction, so that discouragement, frustration, and giving up of the prescribed dietary plan is prevented. A weekly check of body weight is a good method of monitoring progress. Daily weighing is not recommended because of the frequent fluctuations resulting from retained water (including urine) and elimination of feces. The patient should be instructed to record the weight at the same time each day, wearing the same type of clothing.

There is no firm agreement on the number of meals to be eaten when a person is on a diet. Some nutritionists advocate several small meals a day because the body's metabolic rate is temporarily increased immediately after eating. When several small meals a day are ingested, more calories are used. There seems to be general agreement that consumption of most of the daily caloric intake at a large evening meal results in less weight loss than when the calories are evenly distributed throughout the day.

When a person is first starting on a weight reduction program, food portions should be weighed in order to stay within the dietary guidelines. After a time, weighing may not be necessary because the patient can make more accurate judgments of size and weight. A list of permitted foods serves as a good reference and permits an occasional meal to be eaten at a restaurant. The patient who carefully follows the prescribed diet will not need to take vitamin supplements. Appropriate fluid intake should be encouraged. Alcoholic beverages are usually not permitted on a reducing diet because they increase the caloric intake and are low in nutritional value.

Exercise. Exercise is an important part of a weight control program. There is no evidence that increased activity promotes an increase in appetite or leads to dietary excess. In fact, exercise frequently has the opposite effect.

The addition of exercise to diet intervention produces more weight loss than does dieting alone. Exercise has a favorable effect on body fat distribution, with a reduction in waist-to-hip ratio with increased exercise.

Exercise is especially important in maintaining weight loss in overweight persons. Several prospective studies have shown that overweight men and women who are active and fit have lower rates of morbidity and mortality than overweight persons who are sedentary and unfit.[24] Therefore exercise is of benefit to overweight persons even if it does not make them lean.

Behavior-Cognitive Modification. For successful long-term weight loss management, behavior modification or cognitive therapy should be integrated into the management plan. Useful basic techniques include (1) self monitoring, (2) stimulus control, and (3) rewards. Self monitoring can focus on a record that shows what and when foods are eaten, as well as how the person was feeling when the foods were consumed. Stimulus control is aimed at separating events that trigger eating from the act of eating. Rewards may be used as incentive for weight loss. Short- and long-term goals are useful benchmarks for earning rewards. It is important that the reward for a specified weight loss not be associated with food, such as dinner out or a favorite treat. Reward items do not have to have a monetary component. For instance, time for a hot bath or an hour of pleasure reading would be an enjoyable reward for

Table 37-24 Pharmacologic Agents Used in Treatment of Obesity

Agent Category and Mechanism	Examples
Reduce nutrient digestibility	Tetrahydrolipstatin, olestra disaccharidase inhibitors
Disrupt micelle formation	Cholestyramine
Increase energy expenditure	
Calorigenic	Thyroid hormone, growth hormone, β-3-adrenergic agonists, ephedrine, caffeine
Alter palatability of food intake	
Sweeteners	Saccharin, aspartame
Topical anesthetic	Benzocaine
Taste altering	Capsaicin
Decrease food intake	
GI peptides	Cholecystokinin agonists, bombesin
Nutrients	Lactate, 3-hydroxybutyrate
Exert CNS effects—appetite suppression	
GABAergic antagonists	Picrotoxin
Adrenergic agonists	Phenethylamine derivatives
Serotonergic agonists	Fenfluramine, fluoxetine, sertraline
Peptides	Cholecystokinin agonists, opioid antagonists, β-3-adrenergic agonists

Modified from Bray G: Drug treatment of obesity, *Am J Clin Nutr* 55:539S, 1992.
CNS, Central nervous system; *GI*, gastrointestinal.

many people. People may participate in group or individual sessions, or both, as they work toward their goals.

Pharmacologic Management. Medications have been used in the treatment of obesity but only as adjuncts to a good diet and exercise program. Although effective and safe drugs are available for obesity treatment, multiple barriers exist to their proper and effective use. Historically, adverse experiences with "diet drugs" such as amphetamines have contributed to reluctance by health care providers and many in the public to explore newer pharmacologic agents that could be part of obesity treatment. (Table 37-24 shows the classification of drugs and the proposed mechanisms for obesity treatment.)

Appetite suppressant drugs reduce food intake through noradrenergic (drugs that mimic norepinephrine) or serotonergic mechanisms. Abuse of noradrenergic agents such as amphetamine, methamphetamine, and phenmetrazine has given the entire group of drugs a bad name. No clinical need exists for any of these drugs in the treatment of obesity.[25] The chemical manipulation of amphetamine has resulted in drugs that have less risk for CNS stimulation and abuse but that have retained the appetite-suppressing effects. Drugs such as benzphetamine (Didrex) and phendimetrazine (Anorex, Obalan) are examples of this type of drug. Adverse effects of these drugs include palpitations, tachycardia, overstimulation, restlessness, dizziness, insomnia, weakness, and fatigue.

Fenfluramine (Pondimin) is a serotonergic drug that acts as an appetite suppressant. The exact mechanism by which it suppresses the appetite has not been established. It may act by stimulating the satiety center in the hypothalamus, by altering brain levels or turnover of serotonin, or by increasing glucose utilization.[26] Increased brain serotonin levels depress the CNS and suppress appetite. The most common adverse effects of fenfluramine are drowsiness, diarrhea, and dry mouth. It is the drug of choice for the patient who is anxious and cannot tolerate CNS-stimulating drugs.

Because drugs will not cure obesity without substantial changes in food intake and increased physical activity, weight gain will occur when short-term drug therapy is stopped. Supervised long-term drug therapy with safe compounds can contribute to weight management as well as loss. As with any pharmacologic treatment, there are side effects. Careful evaluation for the presence of other medical conditions can help determine which drugs, if any, would be advisable for a given patient.

The role of the nurse in relation to drug therapy should center around teaching the patient about proper administration and side effects. The modification of dosage without consultation with the physician or the nurse can have detrimental effects. The nurse should reemphasize that the diet and exercise regimens are the cornerstones of permanent weight loss. Medications may be helpful but they do not help the patient change eating behavior. The purchase of over-the-counter diet aids should be discouraged. Emphasis here should be on the dangers of drug dependence and tolerance.

Even with a comprehensive action plan, there is a high rate of recidivism (weight regain) among all age groups. For successful management of obesity, it helps if obesity is viewed as a chronic condition that needs day-to-day attention to maintain weight loss.

Surgical Therapeutic Management

Many different types of surgical techniques have been described for treating obesity. These techniques can be classified as physical or mechanical (e.g., lipectomy, jaw wiring), malabsorptive (e.g., gastric bypass), and regulator (e.g., banding gastroplasty).

Lipectomy. Lipectomy (adipectomy) is performed to remove unsightly flabby folds of adipose tissue. The patient who chooses adipectomies does so for cosmetic reasons. In some patients, up to 15% of the total fat cells are removed from the breasts, abdomen, and lumbar and femoral areas. There is no evidence that a regeneration of adipose tissue occurs at the surgical sites. However, it must be emphasized to the patient that surgical removal does not prevent obesity from recurring, especially if lifetime eating habits remain the same. Although body image and self-esteem may be enhanced by such procedures, these operations are not without complications. The dangerous effects of general anesthesia and the potential for poor wound healing in the obese patient cannot be overemphasized. It is more useful for the majority of patients contemplating adipectomy to be instructed in preventive health measures, such as slow weight reduction to maintain and preserve tissue integrity, the value of exercise, and behavior-modification techniques.

Liposuction. Another surgical procedure is *liposuction* or *suction-assisted lipectomy*. The current use is for cosmetic purposes and not for weight reduction. This surgical intervention helps to improve facial appearance or body contours. A candidate for this type of surgery is one who has achieved weight reduction but who has excess fat under the chin, along the jawline, in the nasolabial folds, over the abdomen, or around the waist and upper thighs. The procedure is relatively easy to perform and generally free of major complications. A long, hollow, stainless steel cannula is inserted through a small incision over the fatty tissue to be suctioned (see Fig. 20-11). The purpose of this type of surgery is to improve body appearance, thereby enhancing body image and self-concept. It is not usually recommended for the older person because the skin is less elastic and will not accommodate to the new underlying shape.

Jaw Wiring. During the 1980s some obese patients had their mandible and maxilla wired together in an attempt to achieve weight reduction. The patient is able to speak after the procedure but is able to ingest only liquids. This type of obesity treatment does achieve weight loss but does not change the basic eating patterns of the person when the wires are removed. Weight is usually regained. While the jaw is wired, the patient must carry wire cutters at all times. Both the patient and the family need to be instructed in the use of wire cutters in times of emergency such as vomiting, choking, and cardiac arrest. Compliance with a meticulous oral hygiene regimen is essential while the wires are in place. Frequent dental checkups are advisable during this period because irritation to the cheeks and gingivae may occur from the wires. Routine brushing and gingival stimulation are encouraged. (The nursing care of patients with wired jaws is discussed in Chapter 38.) Jaw wiring may be more acceptable when performed before gastric bypass surgery or gastroplasty, when immediate weight loss is advantageous to the outcome of this more hazardous surgical intervention.

Intragastric Balloon. A recent innovation being used to control oral intake is a cylindrical plastic balloon in the stomach. Following introduction into the stomach by endoscopy, the balloon is inflated, thus reducing the stomach to a size similar to that achieved by gastroplasty. Significant side effects include stomach ulcers and the potential for perforation.[27] The bubble has been known to collapse spontaneously in the stomach, requiring surgical removal, and it has caused intestinal obstruction. The chief advantage of this weight-control measure is its ease of insertion. Long-term use of the gastric bubble will determine its proper place as a weight-control strategy.

For a patient to be selected for any of the operations for morbid obesity, the following criteria are considered:

1. Gross obesity for 5 years
2. Failure to reduce weight with other forms of therapy
3. Body weight 100% above the ideal for age, gender, and height
4. No serious endocrine problem causing the obesity
5. Absence of other medical conditions (liver disease, alcoholism, cardiovascular or pulmonary disease, inflammatory bowel disease, cancer)
6. Psychiatric and social stability and willingness to cooperate with long-term follow-up
7. Availability of a team of health care providers (nurses, physicians, dieticians) to provide immediate and long-term care
8. Presence of a high-risk condition (degenerative joint disease) that weight loss would ameliorate

Patients older than the age of 50 are frequently discouraged from seeking surgical treatment because the complications that accompany these procedures are more devastating with age. In 1991 the NIH Consensus Development Conference on GI surgery for severe obesity noted that many different types of surgery have been tried and rejected primarily because of complications or because they were not effective. However, two procedures endorsed for clinical use at the conference are vertical banded gastroplasty and Roux-en-Y gastric bypass (discussed later in the chapter).[28]

Gastrointestinal Surgeries. Vertical banded gastroplasty and Roux-en-Y gastric bypass are the main surgical procedures for treatment of obesity (see Table 37-25 and Fig. 37-5). Optimal weight loss or weight goals have not been defined, and outcome predictors are inadequate. Results depend more on motivation and behavior than on metabolic, GI, or technical factors.[29]

Through the years, surgical approaches within the GI tract have been directed toward either limiting food intake or producing malabsorption. An early surgery that led to malabsorption was the *jejunoileal bypass*. Approximately 100,000 of these procedures were performed in the United States.[27] This procedure resulted in excellent weight loss. However, because of frequent serious health-related complications including electrolyte imbalance, osteoporosis, bypass enteritis, and liver failure, this surgery is no longer performed. Many patients had surgical procedures done to reverse the bypass. Nonetheless, a group of patients may still have a jejunoileal bypass in place.

The *gastric bypass* operation now being performed leads to weight loss by reducing food intake and producing some

Table 37-25 Comparison of Surgical Interventions for Morbid Obesity

Procedure	Method of Weight Loss	Anatomic Changes	Advantages	Risks
▪ Roux-en-Y gastric bypass	Reduced gastric capacity Some malabsorption	Gastric pouch and gastrojejunostomy	Large and sustained weight loss Better state of health than with jejunoileal bypass	Staple line dehiscence Marginal ulceration Altered gastric histology Stomal stenosis Iron, calcium, and vitamin B_{12} deficiency Dumping syndrome with refined carbohydrates
▪ Vertical banding gastroplasty	Reduced gastric capacity	Small gastric pouch along lesser stomach curvature	Easy to perform procedure Anastomosis not necessary More normal anatomy and physiology maintained	Disrupted staple line Stomach stenosis Dilated pouch Erosion at band into stomach (rare) Maladaptive eating (calorically dense food intake)

malabsorption. With the Roux-en-Y surgical procedure, the stomach size is decreased. The procedure consists of stapling the stomach without transection to create a small pouch of approximately 30 to 45 ml capacity and a gastrojejunostomy. The chief contraindications to this surgical procedure are a history of peptic ulcer disease, coronary artery disease, malignant lesions, drug dependence, alcohol abuse, or psychiatric problems. A complication of this procedure is dumping syndrome in which gastric contents empty too rapidly into the small intestine, overwhelming its ability to digest nutrients. This operation is more likely to cause iron or calcium deficiency and B_{12} hypovitaminosis, which can require lifelong supplementation.

Vertical banded gastroplasty is the second type of GI surgical procedure that is currently being used to induce weight loss in the morbidly obese person. This approach leads to physical restriction of food intake. Previously, horizontal banding procedures were also done. However, lack of long-term weight loss coupled with complications such as disrupted staple lines, as well as dilated pouch and stoma led to discontinuing the use of horizontal banding in the treatment of morbid obesity. In the vertical banding gastroplasty, the stomach is partitioned into a small (usually about 10 to 15 ml) upper portion along the lesser curvature of the stomach. This small pouch drastically limits capacity. Additionally the stoma opening to the rest of the stomach is banded in order to delay emptying of solid food from the proximal pouch. This procedure has achieved considerable success in management of weight loss. Problems associated with gastric restriction operations are distention of the wall of the proximal pouch, rupture of the staple line, or erosion of the band into the stomach.

Gastroplasty has several advantages over the gastric bypass operation. It is technically easier to perform, especially when stapling is used. If reversal of the procedure is required, removal of the staples is easier than the difficult procedure of converting the gastric bypass. In addition, symptoms of the dumping syndrome and malabsorption are eliminated.

NURSING MANAGEMENT

OBESE PATIENT

Nursing Assessment

The nurse, working closely with the physician and dietitian, plays a major role in the planning and management of the obese patient. To be effective, the nurse must be aware of perceptions of and beliefs about obesity. If a care provider associates this condition with lack of willpower and gluttony, the patient can experience shame in a setting that claims to be a caring one. By being sensitive when asking specific and leading questions, the nurse can often obtain information that the patient may withhold out of embarrassment or shyness or because of being a poor historian. Information that can assist the nurse in understanding an obese patient and provide a basis for intervention is presented in Table 37-26. The nurse must provide acceptable reasons for such personally intrusive questions, respond to the patient's concerns about diagnostic tests, and interpret test outcomes. The patient's answers to questions must be treated with respect, understanding, and a nonjudgmental attitude, regardless of negative personal feelings the nurse may have about obesity and working with "fat" people.

Anthropometric measurements are an integral part of the assessment of an obese person. The nurse may perform these measurements and explain their significance to the patient. Measurements used with the obese person include skin fold thickness as well as height, weight, and BMI.

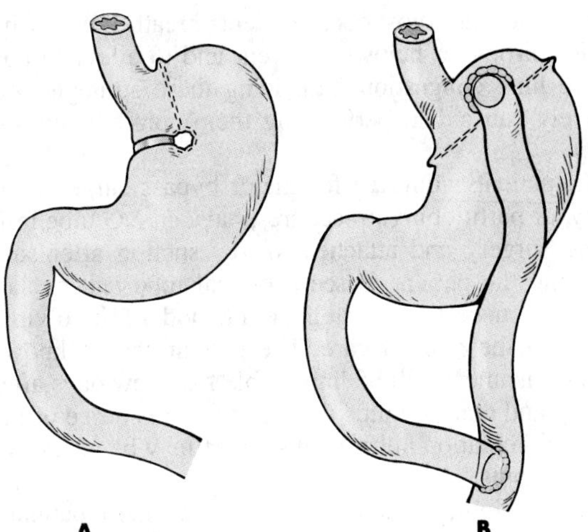

Fig. 37-5 Two gastrointestinal surgical procedures currently being used in the treatment of morbid obesity. ***A,*** Vertical banded gastroplasty consists of constructing a small pouch with a restricted outlet along the lesser curvature of the stomach. This outlet may be externally reinforced to prevent disruption or dilatation. ***B,*** Roux-en-Y gastric bypass procedure involves constructing a proximal gastric pouch whose outlet is a Y-shaped limb of small bowel.

Accumulation of fat cells in the gluteal-femoral area may be metabolically inert, except during the latter part of pregnancy and during lactation. Android obesity, in which fat is distributed over the abdomen and upper body (neck, arms, and shoulders), is associated with a greater cardiovascular risk of hypertension, NIDDM, dyslipidemia, ischemic heart disease, stroke, and death. The nurse should emphasize the importance of vigorous treatment of this type of obesity. The patient should be informed that gynecoid obesity carries a better prognosis but may be more difficult to reduce.

As part of the initial nursing physical assessment, each body system needs to be examined with particular attention to the organ system in which the patient has expressed a problem or concern. Providing specific documentation on these areas assists the physician with a more in-depth history and physical examination.

Table 37-26 Nursing Assessment: Obese Patient

Subjective Data

Important health information

Past health history: Time of obesity onset; diseases related to metabolism and obesity such as cardiac problems, chronic joint pain, respiratory problems, diabetes mellitus, cholelithiasis

Medications: Thyroid, diet pills

Surgery: Weight reduction procedures

Functional health patterns

Nutritional-metabolic: Frequency of eating; factors that contribute to overeating, such as boredom, time of day, stress

Elimination: Constipation

Activity-exercise: Level of physical activity

Sleep-rest: Sleep apnea

Cognitive-perceptual: Psychosocial problems related to obesity, such as feelings of rejection, isolation, guilt, or shame; compliance with prescribed reducing diets; attitude toward a long-term commitment to a weight-loss program

Role-relationship: Changes in financial status or family; resources to support a reducing diet, both personal and financial

Sexuality-reproductive: Menstrual irregularity, heavy menstrual flow in women; effect of obesity on sexual activity

Objective Data

General

Anthropometric measures including height, weight, body mass index, waist-hip ratio, appearance

Cardiovascular

Hypertension, serum cholesterol and triglyceride levels increased

Musculoskeletal

Decreased joint mobility

Nursing Diagnoses

Nursing diagnoses specific to the patient with obesity include, but are not limited to, the following:

- Altered nutrition: more than body requirements related to excessive intake in relation to metabolic need and decreased activity
- Impaired physical mobility related to excessive body weight
- Social isolation related to alterations in physical appearance and perceived unattractiveness
- Risk for impaired skin integrity related to alterations in nutritional state (obesity), immobility, excess moisture, and multiple skin folds
- Ineffective breathing pattern related to decreased lung expansion from obesity
- Risk for noncompliance with treatment regimen related to alteration in perception or lack of motivation
- Body-image disturbance related to deviation from usual or expected body size and inability to lose or retain weight loss

Planning

The overall goals are that the obese patient will (1) achieve weight loss to a specified level, (2) maintain weight loss at a specified level, (3) modify eating habits, and (4) participate in a regular physical activity program.

Nursing Implementation

Health Maintenance and Promotion. In collaboration with nutritionists, the nurse is in a prime position to participate in formal and informal health and nutritional teaching activities. This teaching can span the entire life span, including prenatal instruction. Targeting groups in the work setting is one way health promotion activities can be conducted and reinforced. Group competition within the work environment has been reported to offer moderate success for participants. Interrelated key factors are group support coupled with competition.

Acute Intervention

Preoperative care. Special considerations are necessary in the care of the patient who is admitted to the hospital for surgical treatment of obesity, especially the morbidly obese. Most nursing units are not prepared to meet the needs of a patient who is often too large for a typical hospital or recovery room bed or who has arms or legs that even a large-size blood pressure cuff will not fit. To eliminate embarrassment for the patient and frustration for the staff, plans for these special needs should be made before the patient's admission. Oversized blood pressure cuffs should be ready for use when the patient arrives. A private room may be necessary for privacy of the patient and to accommodate the bed and sitting arrangements. A strongly reinforced trapeze bar should be placed over the bed to facilitate movement and positioning. In some cases a specially constructed chair may have to be built and beds joined together to allow the patient to sit and sleep in comfort.

A care-planning conference should be a priority so that even simple nursing care measures do not become impossible tasks. Consideration should be given to questions such as how the patient will be weighed, how the patient will be transported throughout the hospital, and how simple physical assessment strategies may have to be adjusted to accommodate the morbidly obese patient. Anticipation of the need to use the hospital's meat or freight scales saves time and energy later for both the staff and the patient. Another need is a wheelchair with removable arms that is large enough to safely accommodate the patient and that will pass easily through doorways. Strategies for bathing, turning, and ambulating the patient, including the number of extra hands needed to carry out these measures, are invaluable when the actual need arises. Special gowns are also needed for the patient. Routine physical assessment strategies do not work well with a morbidly obese female patient who has numerous layers of skin folds covering the chest and abdomen in addition to huge, pendulous breasts obscuring the area to be assessed. Without identifying alternatives or unique methods of dealing with this problem, assessment of respiratory status and bowel sounds or even wound inspection could be awkward for the nurse and embarrassing for the patient.

Wound infection is one of the most common complications after surgery. Because of the many layers of flabby skin folds, especially in the abdominal area, preoperative skin preparation is important. Frequently the patient is instructed to take several showers a day for several days before admission to the hospital. Careful cleansing with soap and warm water of the abdominal area from the breasts to below the waist is emphasized.

The patient must be instructed in the proper coughing technique, deep breathing, and methods of turning and positioning to prevent pulmonary complications after surgery. The use of a spirometer may be introduced before surgery. Because most obese patients breathe shallowly, use of the spirometer helps to prevent and to alleviate postoperative lung congestion. Practicing these strategies preoperatively can aid in performing them correctly postoperatively.

All patients admitted for major bypass surgery, gastroplasty, or partitioning procedures, have an NG tube inserted during surgery and attached to low suction after surgery. Allowing the patient to see a typical tube and explaining why it is necessary is a good method of involving the patient in the plan of care. The patient should know that oral nourishment will be impossible for a few days after the surgery and that IV fluids will be the main source of intake. Hyperalimentation nutritional support may be necessary for some patients.

Early ambulation is mandatory for the obese patient. It is essential that the patient know that it is usually necessary to get out of bed soon after surgery and with increasing frequency thereafter, generally three to four times each day. The dangers of thrombophlebitis and measures to counteract its development are a routine part of preoperative teaching. The patient should know that elastic stockings, graduated compression stockings, or elastic wraps will be applied to the legs and that active and passive range-of-motion exercises will be a frequent part of daily care. Low-dose heparin often will be ordered. (General preoperative nursing care is discussed in Chapter 14.)

Postoperative care. The patient experiences considerable abdominal pain after surgery. Administration of pain medications should be given as frequently as necessary during the immediate postoperative period. If pain medication is not given by patient-controlled analgesia (PCA), the nurse must remember that IM medications must be given with an extra long needle, such as a spinal needle, so that the medication is administered into the muscle and not into the adipose or subcutaneous tissue, which will delay absorption. Because prevention of pulmonary complications is a major nursing goal, it must be anticipated that the patient will not fully cooperate with respiratory strategies. In addition, the large amount of truncal adipose tissue, especially on the abdomen and chest, compromises respiratory ability. Keeping the head of the bed elevated at a 30-degree angle at all times facilitates ventilatory efforts. Encouraging and assisting the patient to turn, cough, and deep breathe at least every 1 to 2 hours minimizes the risk for atelectasis and pneumonia. Frequent mouth and nose care also helps breathing efforts because the NG tube is inserted through one nostril.

Position changes and range-of-motion exercises are instituted immediately after surgery and carried out every 1 to 2 hours. Ambulatory efforts generally are begun on the evening of surgery. For patient safety, the nurse should enlist the assistance of other staff members during these initial efforts, while encouraging the patient to help.

The abdominal wound requires frequent observation for the amount and type of drainage, condition of the sutures, and signs of infection. The incision must be protected against undue straining that accompanies turning and coughing. Wound dehiscence and wound healing are potential problems with all obese patients. Monitoring the vital signs assists in identifying problems such as infection.

It is important that the NG tube be kept patent and in the correct position. Vomiting is common following gastroplasty bypass and gastric partitioning procedures. If patency is blocked or the tube requires repositioning, the physician should be notified at once. The upper gastric pouch is small (usually 15 to 40 ml), and irrigating the tube with too much solution or manipulating tube position can lead to disruption of the anastomosis or staple line. In most cases the NG tube can be removed in approximately 48 hours, or when bowel sounds have resumed.

Skin care should be carried out several times each shift. Perspiration may be excessive at times. The many layers of flabby skin should be kept clean and dry so that this source of irritation is eliminated. The patient who has gastric bypass may experience severe diarrhea early in the postoperative period. This is caused by malabsorption created by surgical shortening of the small intestine. Meticulous care should be taken of the skin around the anal area, and antidiarrheal medications should be administered immediately. For the patient who has an indwelling catheter, perineal care is important so that a urinary tract infection can be avoided.

Clear liquids are given orally when tolerance is established. The amount offered at first is necessarily limited to approximately 1 ounce, which is to be sipped slowly. More solid types of food are given to the patient who has had bypass surgery as progress is made through the postoperative recovery period. The patient who has had gastroplasty surgery is kept on a fluid diet for a longer time. The need for a liquid diet only is based on the rationale that the ingestion of too much fluid or foods can cause disruption of the staple or suture line, leading to leakage and possible peritonitis.

Discharge teaching. The patient who has undergone major surgical treatment for obesity has not, in the past, been successful in following or maintaining a prescribed diet. Now the patient is forced to reduce the oral intake as a result of the anatomic changes brought about by the operation. This patient finds adherence to a reduced intake is necessary because of the concern for abdominal distention, cramping abdominal pain, increased and foul-smelling flatus, and frequent diarrhea.

Weight loss is considerable during the first 6 to 12 months. More weight is lost by those who have bypass surgery than by those who undergo gastric reduction procedures. It is during this time that the patient must learn to adjust intake sufficiently to maintain a stable weight. Although behavior modification was not an intended outcome when these surgical procedures were devised, it becomes an unexpected secondary gain. The diet generally prescribed should be high in protein and low in carbohydrates, fat, and roughage and consist of six small feedings daily. Fluids should not be ingested with the meal, and in some cases, fluids should be restricted to less than 1000 ml per day. Fluids and foods high in carbohydrate tend to promote diarrhea and symptoms of the dumping syndrome. Generally calorically dense foods (foods high in fat) should be avoided to permit more nutritionally sound food to be consumed.

Vitamin deficiencies are a long-term concern after bypass surgery because of the induced malabsorption and the body's inability to absorb important vitamins such as vitamins A, C, and D. Parenteral vitamin B_{12} supplements are usually prescribed on a permanent basis because absorption of this vitamin takes place in the ileum. Ileal absorption capacity is drastically reduced by the surgical intestinal bypass. The patient should be aware of the signs and symptoms of vitamin deficiencies, as well as of electrolyte imbalances (see Table 37-8). It is often necessary to replace iron, calcium, and potassium to maintain required physiologic levels.

Proper diet and use of antidiarrheal medications must be clearly understood by the patient. Late complications can be anticipated after gastric bypass or gastroplasty, including anemia, vitamin deficiencies, diarrhea, and psychiatric problems. Failure to lose weight or loss of too much weight may be caused by the surgical formation of too large a stomach pouch or of an outlet that is much too small, respectively. Peptic ulcer formation, dumping syndrome, and small bowel obstruction may be seen late in the recovery and rehabilitative stage.

Long-term follow-up care must be stressed, in part because of complications late in the recovery period. The patient must be encouraged to adhere strictly to the prescribed diet and to keep the physician informed of any changes in physical or emotional condition. Some patients have been known to overeat when they return home and to gain rather than lose weight.

Reversal of the surgical procedures may be required for some patients. Reversal of the gastric bypass is extremely difficult because of the technical nature of the procedure. Reasons for revisional surgery include hepatic failure, weight loss below ideal weight, debilitating weakness, severe psychiatric problems, intractable electrolyte deficiencies, pulmonary tuberculosis, and renal failure.

The nurse must anticipate and recognize several potential psychologic problems after surgery. Some patients express guilt feelings concerning the fact that the only way they could lose weight was by surgical means rather than by the "sheer willpower" of reduced dietary intake. The nurse should be ready to provide support so that this patient does not dwell on negative feelings.

Many morbidly obese patients who blamed their feelings of social inferiority or inadequacies on their appearance before bypass surgery may suffer from episodes of depression. By 6 to 8 months after surgery, considerable weight loss has occurred, and they are able to see clearly how much their appearance has changed. Massive weight loss often leaves the patient with large quantities of flabby skin that result in problems of both body image and hygiene. Reconstructive surgery at least 1 full year after the initial surgery may alleviate this unsightly situation. Reduction of the breasts, upper arms, thighs, and excess abdominal skin folds are possible solutions. Discussion of this possible outcome with the patient before surgery and again during the rehabilitation phase of recovery helps facilitate the patient's adjustment to a new body image and social reintegration.

Chronic and Home Management

Physical activity teaching. Once a physical activity program has been outlined for the patient, the nurse can reinforce instruction and help individualize it to the patient's time schedule and physical limitations. The nurse should point out that engaging in weekend exercise only or in spurts of strenuous activity is not advantageous and can actually be dangerous. Joining a health spa can be one mechanism of getting exercise. However, sitting in a sauna and trying to spot-reduce a specific part of the body do not constitute an appropriate daily physical activity program. Walking, swimming, and cycling are more sensible forms of exercise and have more long-term benefits. The combination of a good reducing diet and an increased physical activity program can have profound effects on the patient's achievement of weight loss. When large muscles are involved in the exercise program, a primary benefit is cardiovascular conditioning.

Many psychologic benefits can be derived from an increased physical activity program. Reduction in tension and stress, better-quality sleep and rest, decreased desire to eat excessively, increased stamina and energy, improved self-concept and self-confidence, better attitudes toward work and play, and increased optimism about the future can be achieved.

Behavior-modification cognitive training. The person who is on any type of restrictive dietary program is often encouraged to join a group of other obese persons who are receiving professional counseling to help them modify their eating habits. The assumption behind behavior modification is that obesity is a learned disorder caused by overeating, and that the critical difference between an obese person and a nonobese person are the cues that stimulate eating behavior. Therefore most behavior-modification programs deemphasize the diet and focus on how and when the person eats. Participants often are taught to restrict their eating to designated meals and to increase the amount of physical activity in their lives. Persons who have undergone behavior therapy are more successful in maintaining their losses over an extended time than those who do not participate in such training.

Many self-help groups are available to the person who wants to learn more about successful dieting and who likes the support of others having the same problems and experiences. TOPS (Take Off Pounds Sensibly) is the oldest nonprofit organization of this type. Behavioral modification is an integral part of the program, along with nutrition education. Weight Watchers International, Inc. is probably the most successful commercial weight-reduction enterprise. Weight Watchers offers a food plan that is nutritionally balanced and practical to follow, and it has used behavior-modification techniques since 1974. Other self-help groups and organizations are Overeaters Anonymous, Weight Losers, Trim Clubs, Inc., and the Diet Workshop, Inc. These groups offer diet education, exercise plans, and behavior modification.

There has been a proliferation of commercial weight-reduction centers across the nation. Many of these programs are staffed by nurses or nutritionists, or both, and require an initial physical examination by a physician before a candidate is accepted for weight reduction. These weight-reduction centers are costly and are therefore out of reach of those with limited financial resources. Many of these programs also offer special prepackaged foods and supplements that must be purchased as part of the weight-reduction plan. Only these prescribed foods and drinks are to be consumed until an agreed-on amount of weight is lost. The patient is encouraged to buy the same type of foods for the maintenance phase of the program, lasting from 6 months to a year. Behavior-modification training is incorporated within these programs as well. Research has shown that, regardless of the commercial products used, successful weight loss and control were limited and required individualized programs consisting of restricted caloric intake, behavior modification, and exercise.[30] Although persons who follow this type of program are likely to lose weight, once they leave the program the weight is usually regained because they tend to resume previous eating behaviors and return to the foods previously eaten.

A new concept of influencing health behavior and better employee health has occurred recently. Programs on health teaching and maintenance have been started at places of employment. The rationale for such programs is that better health repays the cost of the programs through improved work performance, decreased absenteeism, and eventually less hospitalization. Weight-reduction and hypertension-reduction programs have been instituted and are popular with employees.

CRITICAL THINKING EXERCISES

CASE STUDY

OBESITY

Patient Profile

Mrs. R. is a 60-year-old woman who is 5′ 4″ tall and weighs 190 pounds.

Subjective Data

- Reports gradual weight gain during past 40 years
- Spends most of her free time watching television
- Reports health problems related to NIDDM, shortness of breath, hypertension, and chest pressure
- Had knee replacement surgery at age 56

Objective Data

Physical Examination

- Has obese, nontender, soft abdomen
- BP is 150/90

Laboratory Results

- Fasting blood glucose 250 mg/dl (13.9 mmol/L)
- Total cholesterol 205 mg/dl (5.3 mmol/L)
- Triglyceride 298 mg/dl (3.36 mmol/L)
- HDL cholesterol 31 mg/dl (0.8 mmol/L)

Critical Thinking Questions

1. What are Mrs. R.'s obesity risk factors?
2. What is her estimated BMI (use Fig. 37-4)?
3. What are the primary types of body fat distribution? Which type do you think Mrs. R. has, and why?
4. Of the possible complications of obesity, which ones does Mrs. R. have? What is the pathophysiology of Mrs. R.'s NIDDM? Of her cardiovascular symptoms? Of her knee replacement surgery?
5. What would you, as the nurse, include in a successful weight loss and weight management program for Mrs. R.?
6. Is Mrs. R. a candidate for surgical intervention for obesity? If so, why? If not, why not?
7. Based on the assessment data presented, write one or more appropriate nursing diagnoses. Are there any collaborative problems?

NURSING RESEARCH ISSUES

1. What impact does rapid gastric emptying of protein have on protein absorption, utilization, and subsequent nutritional status?
2. What mechanisms beyond physical activity maintain body weight in obese people when they generally consume fewer carbohydrates than do slender people?
3. How can fat-soluble vitamins be maintained within the RDA when population groups increase their use of fat substitutes in dietary patterns?
4. What happens to serum calcium and bone density in vegetarian patients over time?
5. What is the effect of surgical procedures for obesity on the quality of life or on functional abilities?
6. What is the most effective strategy to wean patients off of TPN?
7. Are there valid and reliable bedside methods for determining NG and NI tube placement?
8. What are the ways to reduce the risk of catheter sepsis in a patient receiving TPN?
9. What characteristics (medical condition, antibiotic therapy) are associated with diarrhea in the patient receiving tube feeding?

REVIEW QUESTIONS

The number of the question corresponds to the same-numbered objective at the beginning of the chapter.

1. Regardless of age, the most servings from any food group should come from
   a. the milk, yogurt, and cheese food group.
   b. the vegetable food group.
   c. the fruit food group.
   d. the bread, cereal, rice, and pasta food group.

2. During the first 24 hours of starvation, in which of the following orders does the body obtain substrate for energy?
   a. Glycogen, skeletal protein
   b. Liver protein, muscle protein, visceral protein
   c. Fat stores, skeletal protein, visceral protein
   d. Visceral protein, fat stores, glycogen

3. The diagnosis of bulimia is suspected in the presence of
   a. appetite loss.
   b. abdominal distension.
   c. enlarged parotid glands.
   d. fasting several days a week.

4. When infused into a peripheral vein, the glucose concentration of TPN should not exceed
   a. 5%.
   b. 10%.
   c. 25%.
   d. 50%.

5. Cardiovascular health problems are associated most often with which of the following obesity aspects?
   a. Primary obesity
   b. Gynoid fat distribution
   c. Android fat distribution
   d. Secondary obesity

6. A patient's daily caloric requirement is based on
   a. height, weight, age, and health status.
   b. duration of nutrient therapy, height and weight.
   c. activity level and body mass index.
   d. prior nutritional patterns, age, and stress level.

REFERENCES

1. Sobal J, Stunkard A: Socioeconomic status and obesity: a review of the literature. *Psych Bull* 105:260, 1989.
2. Townsend CD: *Nutrition and diet therapy,* Albany, NY, 1994, Delmar Publishers.
3. Food and Nutrition Board, National Research Council, National Academy of Sciences: *Recommended Dietary Allowances,* ed 10, Washington, DC, 1989, National Academy Press.
4. Behnke M, Grant M: Anorexia. In V Kohlman and others, editors: *Pathophysiological phenomena in nursing: human responses to illness,* ed 2, Philadelphia, 1993, WB Saunders.
5. Edwards K: Obesity, anorexia, and bulimia, *Med Clin North Am* 77:905, 1993.
6. Herzog DB: Eating disorders: new threat to health, *Psychosomatics* 33:10, 1992.
7. *Surgeon General's report on nutrition and health,* Rocklin, CA, 1989, Prima Publishing and Communications.
8. McWhirter JP, Pennington CR: Incidence and recognition of malnutrition in hospital patients. *Br Med J* 308:945, 1994.
9. Hoffman N: Diet in the elderly, *Med Clin North Am* 77:750, 1993.
10. McClave S and others: Use of residual volume as a marker for enteral feeding intolerance: prospective blinded comparison with physical examination and radiographic findings, *J Pediatr Nurs* 16: 102, 1992.
11. Sax HC, Souba WW: Enteral and parenteral feedings, *Med Clin North Am* 77:873, 1993.
12. McCrae JD, O'Shea R, Udine L: Parenteral nutrition: hospital to home, *J Am Diet Assoc* 93:665, 1993.
13. Guidelines for the use of parenteral and enteral nutrition in adult and pediatric patients, *J Parenteral Enteral Nutr* 17:21SA, 1993.
14. Grant JP: *Handbook of parenteral nutrition,* ed 2, Philadelphia, 1992, WB Saunders.
15. Williamson DF: Descriptive epidemiology of body weight and weight change in US adults, *Ann Intern Med* 119:646, 1993.
16. Kumanyika SK: Special issues regarding obesity in minority populations, *Ann Intern Med* 119:650, 1993.
17. Bray G: Obesity: part 1—pathogenesis, *West J Med* 149:431, 1988.
18. Fuller J, Schaller-Ayers J: *Health assessment: a nursing approach,* ed 2, Philadelphia, 1994, JB Lippincott.
19. Pi-Sunyer P: Short-term medical benefits and adverse effects of weight loss, *Ann Intern Med* 119:722, 1993.
20. Bray GA: An approach to the classification and evaluation of obesity. In P Bjorntorp, BN Brodoff, editors: *Obesity,* Philadelphia, 1992, JB Lippincott.
21. Allison DB and others: A genetic analysis of relative weight among 4,020 twin pairs with an emphasis on sex effects. *Health Psychol* 13:362, 1994.
22. Bochard C, Pérusse L: Genetics of obesity, *Ann Rev Nutr* 13:337, 1993.
23. Harris RB: Factors influencing body weight regulation, Digestive Diseases 11:133, 1993.
24. Blair SN: Evidence of success of exercise in weight loss and control, *Ann Intern Med* 119:702, 1993.
25. Bray G: Use and abuse of appetite-suppressant drugs in the treatment of obesity, *Ann Intern Med* 119:707, 1993.
26. Karch A, Boyd E: *Handbook of drugs and the nursing process,* Philadelphia, 1989, JB Lippincott.
27. Knol JA: Management of the problem patient after bariatrics surgery. *Gastroenterol Clin North Am* 23:345, 1994.
28. NIH Consensus Panel: Gastrointestinal surgery for severe obesity: National Institutes of Health Consensus Development Conference statement. *Am J Clin Nutr* 55:616S, 1992.
29. Kral JG: Overview of surgical techniques for treating obesity, *Am J Clin Nutr* 55:552S, 1992.
30. Hyman FN and others: Evidence for success of caloric restriction in weight loss and control, *Ann Intern Med* 119:681, 1993.

Chapter 38

NURSING ROLE IN MANAGEMENT

Problems of Ingestion

Margaret Heitkemper **Rachel Elrod**

Learning Objectives

1. Describe the etiology, prevention, and treatment of common dental problems.
2. Describe the etiology, clinical manifestations, and treatment of common oral inflammations and infections.
3. Describe the etiology, clinical manifestations, complications, and therapeutic and surgical management of carcinoma of the oral cavity.
4. Describe the nursing management after surgical stabilization of a mandibular fracture.
5. Explain the types, pathophysiology, clinical manifestations, complications, and therapeutic and surgical management of gastroesophageal reflux disease and hiatal hernia.
6. Describe the nursing management of the patient with gastroesophageal reflux disease and hiatal hernia.
7. Explain the pathophysiology, clinical manifestations, complications, and therapeutic and nursing management of cancer of the esophagus.
8. Describe the clinical manifestations and complications of esophageal diverticula, achalasia, esophageal strictures, and esophagitis.
9. Describe the types of gastrostomy tubes and related nursing care.
10. Identify the common types of food poisoning and the nursing responsibilities related to food poisoning.

Ingestion is the process of taking food and fluids into the body via the gastrointestinal (GI) tract. It begins in the mouth with mastication of food by the teeth. Food then passes down the esophagus and into the stomach. It is important that sufficient nutrients be ingested to meet bodily needs. Oral problems, such as poor dental health, infections and inflammations, and cancer, interfere with ingestion. Esophageal problems may also interfere with swallowing food and fluids and with passage of food to the stomach.

Many problems of ingestion make it necessary for the patient to use alternative methods of taking in nutrients, either temporarily or permanently. This involves physical and emotional adaptations. The mouth is associated with food, love, and pleasurable sensations. There are numerous social implications associated with not being able to eat. The older adult is particularly susceptible to many psychologic and physiologic problems related to alterations in ingestion.

Reviewed by Diane Britt, RN, MN, Medical-Surgical Clinical Nurse Specialist, University of Washington Medical Center and Barbara Albertson, RN, MN, University of Washington Medical Center, Seattle, WA.

DENTAL PROBLEMS

Dental Caries

Dental caries (decay of teeth) is a general term applied to the decalcification of the mineral components and dissolution of the organic matrix of the teeth. Cavity formation is the clinical evidence of the progression of this process. In the United States approximately 50% of all children, 96% of adults, and 99.5% of individuals more than 65 years of age have had dental caries.[1]

Caries development starts when *plaque* builds up and adheres to the teeth. Plaque is a gelatinous substance consisting of bacteria, saliva, and epithelial cells. The tight adherence of plaque to the teeth provides protection for the bacteria (usually *lactobacilli* and *Streptococcus mutans*). Within 30 minutes after eating, these bacteria produce acids from the breakdown of sugars contained in food deposits on the teeth. The acids destroy the outer enamel and later, the underlying dentin of the tooth (Fig. 38-1). The decay proceeds and can progress to the pulp of the tooth.

If the decay is not treated, a *pulpitis* develops and extends to the alveolar bone, forming an abscess. This results in pain, edema of facial structures, and sometimes malaise and fever. During the early stages of pulpitis, pain may be induced by temperature changes, especially cold

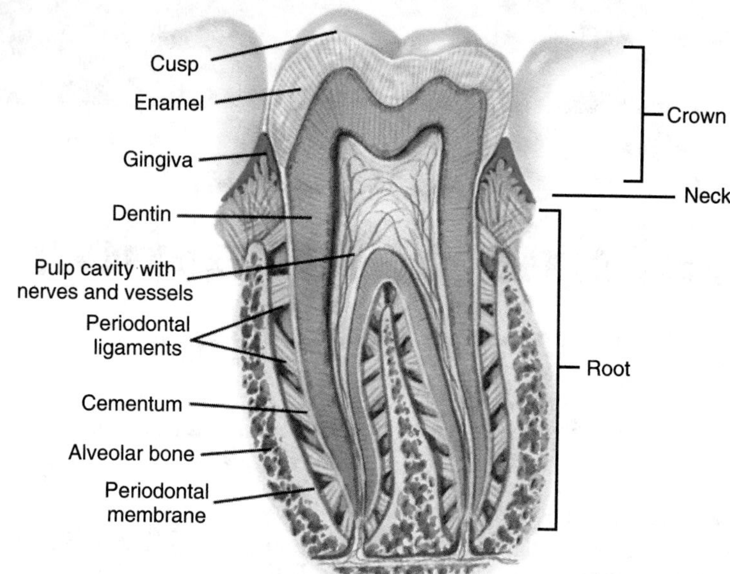

Fig. 38-1 Normal tooth structure.

drinks. In the later stages of pulpitis, heat or reclining may stimulate the onset of more severe pain. At this stage, damage to the pulp is irreversible. Treatment consists of tooth removal or root canal therapy (removal of the pulp and filling of the pulp canal with inert material).

Periodontal Disease

The *periodontium* is the tissue surrounding and supporting the teeth. It is composed of the gingivae (gums), cementum, alveolar bone, and periodontal ligament, which helps to fix the tooth firmly in its bony socket. Periodontal disease is the major cause of tooth loss in adults.[1] Approximately one out of three persons has some stage of periodontal disease.[2,3] Periodontal disease begins with gingivitis and eventually involves the periodontal ligament and the alveolar bone. Periodontal disease is the clinical result of a complex interaction between the host and plaque bacteria.

Dental plaque is the most important etiologic factor in periodontal disease. When plaque calcifies, it forms *calculus*, which is a hard, tenacious mass on the crowns of teeth. *Malocclusion* (faulty relationships between the teeth when the jaws are closed), margins of overextended fillings, and impacted food are other etiologic factors that can cause local irritation to the gingivae. Systemic conditions such as diabetes mellitus, thyroid diseases, pregnancy, and vitamin and nutritional deficiencies may modify the person's response to the local etiologic factors and make them more susceptible to periodontal disease. The exact role of systemic conditions is unknown.

Certain drugs cause changes, such as inflammation and hyperplasia of the gingiva, which may be related to periodontal disease. A common drug known to produce these effects is phenytoin (Dilantin).

When the gingivae are irritated from any of the local etiologic factors, they become inflamed (Fig. 38-2). The inflammation causes the gingiva to separate from the surface of the tooth. Pockets created between the teeth and

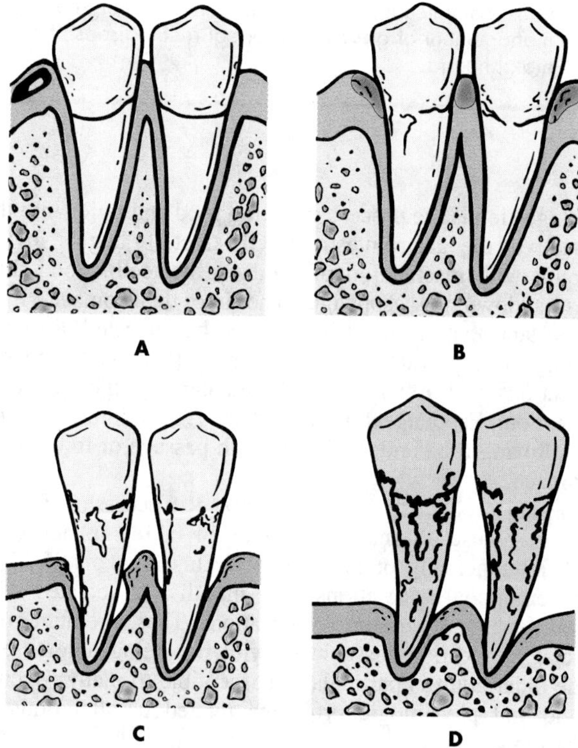

Fig. 38-2 Progression of periodontal disease. ***A,*** Calculus deposits on teeth at gingival line, causing gingivitis. ***B,*** Gingivae become swollen and tender with spread of inflammation. ***C,*** Inflammation spreads and pockets develop between teeth and gingivae, which are receding. ***D,*** The alveolar bone is destroyed and teeth become loose.

CULTURAL & ETHNIC
Considerations

ORAL, PHARYNGEAL, AND ESOPHAGEAL PROBLEMS

- Periodontal disease is more prevalent among African-Americans than among Caucasians.
- Cancers of the oral cavity and pharynx are the fourth leading cause of death in African-American men 35 to 54 years of age.
- Death rates as a result of oral cancer are decreasing in Caucasians but increasing in non-Caucasians.
- Esophageal cancer has a higer incidence among African-Americans and Asian-Americans than among Caucasians.

the gingivae can collect pus and bacteria (periodontitis). At this stage, bleeding occurs readily, and pus may ooze from the gingiva. Gradually the bone supporting the teeth is destroyed, and the teeth become loose. As the periodontal pockets deepen and seal themselves off, periodontal abscesses may occur (Fig. 38-3). At this stage the usual treatment is extraction of the involved tooth or teeth.

Early treatment of periodontal disease consists of *scaling* and *root planing*. Scaling is the removal of calculus, and root planing is the smoothing of root surfaces. Curettage may be combined with these procedures. This removes the soft tissue lining the pocket and helps the gums to heal. A *gingivectomy* and *gingivoplasty* may be necessary. In a gingivectomy, tissue and deep pockets are removed. A gingivoplasty involves reshaping of gingival tissue.

In the later stages of periodontal disease, the bone supporting the teeth is often destroyed. At this stage, treatment entails extraction of the teeth and wearing dentures or dental implants.

NURSING MANAGEMENT

DENTAL PROBLEMS

Nursing Assessment

The patient's teeth should be assessed for caries, missing teeth, displaced teeth, and dental appliances such as dentures, bridges, and crowns. The face is examined for symmetry, and the jaw is palpated for lumps. The gingivae (gums) should be assessed for redness, pallor, bleeding, recession, and ulcers. The patient should be asked questions regarding dental care and frequency of dental examinations.

Nursing Diagnoses

Nursing diagnoses specific to the patient with dental problems include, but are not limited to, the following:

- Altered oral mucous membrane related to caries, ineffective oral hygiene, periodontal disease, or ill-fitting dentures

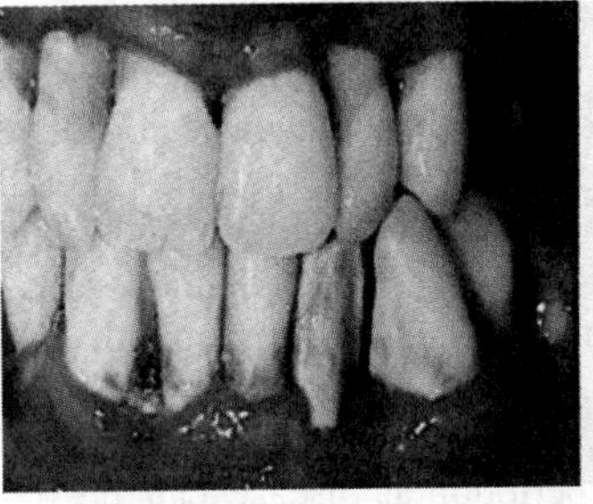
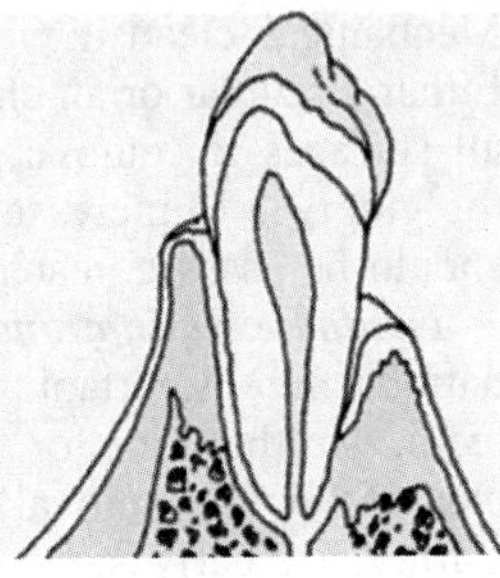

Fig. 38-3 Periodontitis. Signs include edema, periodontal abscess, hemorrhage on slight pressure, tissue recession with retraction of gingival margin, color change from light pink to deep red, loss of tissue in interdental area, horizontal bone loss, and widening of periodontal space.

- Altered nutrition: less than body requirements related to inability to ingest adequate nutrients because of ill-fitting dentures, displaced teeth, gingival disease, dental caries, sensitive teeth, edentulous condition, or oral pain
- Body image disturbance related to change in appearance of or unattractive teeth, difficulty with eating, or halitosis
- Risk for noncompliance with regular, periodic dental examinations related to altered perception, lack of motivation, inadequate finances, or lack of knowledge of consequences of noncompliance.

Planning

The overall goals are that the patient with dental caries and periodontal disease will (1) have a decrease in caries through improved dental hygiene, (2) be able to identify and reduce risk factors for caries and periodontal diseases, and (3) have a balanced nutritional intake.

Nursing Implementation

Health Promotion and Maintenance

Oral hygiene. Proper oral hygiene is essential to prevent caries and periodontal disease. This involves frequent complete cleaning of the teeth and gingivae with toothbrushing and flossing. The teeth should be brushed after each meal with a soft, rounded-bristle toothbrush. Brushing the teeth should remove food debris and plaque and stimulate the gingivae. The teeth should be brushed by first placing the bristles of the toothbrush next to the gum line and then brushing with a motion away from the gum line.

Flossing should be done at least once a day. It is a useful and important measure to remove plaque between teeth, an area that is not easily accessible when brushing. Flossing is done by gently forcing the floss between the teeth and moving the floss up and down the tooth surface a few times until it reaches the gum line.

During illness the patient may not salivate as usual, which reduces the natural cleaning process of the teeth and mouth. The nurse may need to assume responsibility for dental care and oral hygiene. Swabbing the patient's mouth and rinsing it with mouthwash are inadequate measures.

Mechanical cleansing is essential to remove the plaque. Either a regular or an electric toothbrush should be used on all surfaces to remove plaque and mechanically stimulate the gingivae to increase blood supply. The patient's mouth should be assessed each time oral care is given.

Dental examinations. Regular, periodic dental examinations are important to maintain a healthy mouth and teeth. At the time of a dental examination a thorough cleaning with removal of plaque and calculus is done. Caries and early signs of periodontal disease can be detected and treated. The mouth is examined for any signs of oral cancer. For most adults, an examination every 6 to 12 months is adequate. Some persons may require more frequent visits. Persons at risk for infective endocarditis (e.g., prolapsed mitral valve) require prophylactic antibiotics for dental procedures that may provoke bleeding such as teeth cleaning (see Chapter 34).

Nutrition. Caries develop with increasing frequency in persons who ingest diets high in refined carbohydrates. A prevention program should, therefore, include reduction in sugar intake. If sugars are eaten, the teeth should be brushed within 30 minutes of eating. There has been increasing interest in the development of sugar substitutes that are noncarinogenic.[4] Another aspect of diet therapy that seems to reduce plaque formation is increased vitamin C intake.

Fluoride. Fluoridation makes tooth enamel more resistant to the acids produced from the action of bacteria on sugars in the mouth. In drinking water, one part of fluoride per million results in a significant decrease in the decay rate.[5] Many communities consider the fluoridation of drinking water a municipal responsibility and have enacted the necessary legislation. A fluoride solution can be applied topically on the teeth during a dental office visit. In addition, many toothpastes have fluoride added to them, and they are recommended by the American Dental Association. Fluoride rinses and tablets are also available for at-home use.

Sealants. In addition to fluoride, sealants can be applied to the pits and fissures of teeth in children following the eruption of the teeth or in young adults to reduce caries. Sealant is a coating material that is applied directly to teeth surfaces in the dentist's office. Sealants reduce the attachment of plaque and have been found to be effective in reducing caries.[4]

New techniques. Some chemical methods to inhibit plaque formation and accumulation offer promise. Antimicrobial agents such as chlorhexidine have been used in mouthwashes and gels to reduce the *S. mutans* bacterial count in high risk individuals.[4,6]

Acute Intervention. The nurse may need to refer the patient for intervention and care of an acute dental problem. Local manifestations of dental problems include pain that is intermittent and caused by sensitivity to heat or cold stimulation, pain that is dull and continuous, facial swelling, halitosis, and bleeding or drainage of pus from the mouth. Systemic manifestations include fever, nausea, vomiting, and malaise.

If pulpitis and abscess develop, immediate dental care is needed to prevent further spread of infection to the bone. An opening may be drilled into the pulp chamber, or the gingivae may be incised to provide drainage for the abscess. Sometimes a root canal procedure or extraction of a tooth is necessary. After treatment of an abscess, the patient can use warm saline rinses. Analgesics may also be required to alleviate the pain.

A damaged or defective tooth or a tooth that has a severe abscess may need to be extracted. After the extraction, the patient should apply cold compresses (e.g., ice bag, cold washcloth) to the side of the face to reduce swelling and relieve discomfort. Some oozing of blood is expected the first 1 to 2 days. If there is loss of large amounts of bright-red blood, direct pressure should be applied to the bleeding site by the patient biting on a gauze pad, and the dentist should be notified. During the first 24 hours the patient should not suck (e.g., smoke or use a straw) because this increases the risk of clot disruption.

Sometimes day surgery is used for the extraction of several teeth, such as when impacted molars are excised or when dentures are required. Postoperatively the patient will experience pain and soreness. Ice packs and analgesics are used to relieve the discomfort. Nutrients should be liquid or semisoft for a few days. The dentist or oral surgeon may order mouthwashes for cleansing and relief of soreness.

Chronic and Home Management

Dentures. There are approximately 17 million Americans who are edentulous and, of these, 10 million are more than 65 years of age.[1] The decision to obtain dentures is not easy for most people. They are concerned about changes in cosmetic appearance and the ability to chew food. They need to be assured that dentures will usually decrease the spread of infection, improve nutritional intake, and improve appearance, especially if they have had multiple dental problems preceding the decision to obtain dentures.

Patience must be stressed in the adjustment phase to dentures. It does take time to get used to a different feel and way of chewing. The gingivae should be checked for proper fit and for any signs of gingival irritation. Dentures should be cleaned at least twice a day with salt and sodium bicarbonate or a dentifrice. When the dentures are removed, the patient should massage the gums for a few minutes. Some patients prefer to wear their dentures at all times, and there are generally no contraindications to this. In fact, facial contour is better maintained by this practice. If dentures are removed at night, they should be covered with water (especially if they are made of vulcanite) and stored in a safe place.

The patient who wears dentures should be encouraged to obtain regular dental care. Dentures may need to be modified because tissue changes occur from aging, weight changes, or disease processes.

Dental implants are being used in some patients who require tooth extractions. An implant involves insertion of a titanium post into the bone. The bone fuses with the post and then techniques of restorative dentistry are used to create a crown that is attached to the post. An advantage of dental implants is that the patient experiences less mandibular bone loss compared with dentures.[7]

ORAL INFLAMMATIONS AND INFECTIONS

Oral infections and inflammations may be specific mouth diseases, or they may occur in the presence of some systemic diseases such as leukemia or vitamin deficiency. When oral inflammations and infections are present, they can severely impair the ingestion of food and fluids. Common inflammations and infections of the oral cavity are presented in Table 38-1. The patient who is immunosuppressed (patient with acquired immunodeficiency syndrome or receiving chemotherapy) is most susceptible to oral infections.

CARCINOMA OF THE ORAL CAVITY

Carcinoma of the oral cavity may occur on the lips or anywhere within the mouth (e.g., tongue, floor of the mouth, buccal mucosa, hard palate, soft palate, pharyngeal walls, and tonsils). Oropharyngeal cancer is diagnosed in 30,000 Americans annually, and it is estimated that 8000 persons a year will die from the disease.[1] It is more common after 45

Table 38-1 Infections and Inflammations of the Mouth

Condition	Etiology	Clinical Manifestations	Treatment
■ Gingivitis	Neglected oral hygiene, malocclusion, missing or irregular teeth, faulty dentistry, eating of soft rather than fibrous foods	Inflamed gingivae and interdental papillae; bleeding during toothbrushing; development of pus, formation of abscess with loosening of teeth (periodontitis)	Prevention through health teaching, dental care, gingival massage, professional cleaning of teeth, fibrous foods, conscientious brushing habits with flossing
■ Vincent's infection (acute necrotizing ulcerative gingivitis, trench mouth)	Fusiform bacteria; Vincent spirochetes; predisposing factors of worry, excessive fatigue, poor oral hygiene, nutritional deficiencies (vitamins B and C)	Painful, bleeding gingivae; eroding necrotic lesions of interdental papillae; ulcerations that bleed; increased saliva with metallic taste; fetid mouth odor; anorexia, fever, and general malaise	Rest (physical and mental); avoidance of smoking and alcoholic beverages; soft, nutritious diet; correct oral hygiene habits; topical applications of antibiotics; mouth irrigations with hydrogen peroxide and saline solutions
■ Oral candidiasis (moniliasis or thrush)	*Candida albicans* (a yeast-like fungus), debilitation, prolonged high-dose antibiotic or corticosteroid therapy	Pearly, bluish white "milk-curd" membranous lesions on mucosa of mouth and larynx; sore mouth; yeasty halitosis	Nystatin or amphotericin B as oral suspension or buccal tablets, good oral hygiene
■ Herpes simplex (cold sore, fever blister)	Herpes simplex virus, type I or II; predisposing factors of upper respiratory infections, excessive exposure to sunlight, food allergies, emotional tension, onset of menstruation	Lip lesions, mouth lesions, vesicle formation (single or clustered), shallow, painful ulcers	Spirits of camphor, corticosteroid cream, mild antiseptic mouthwash, viscous lidocaine; removal or control of predisposing factors, antiviral agents (e.g., acyclovir)
■ Aphthous stomatitis (canker sore)	Recurrent and chronic form of infection secondary to systemic disease, trauma, stress, or unknown causes	Ulcers of mouth and lips, causing extreme pain; ulcers surrounded by erythematous base	Corticosteroids (topical or systemic), tetracycline oral suspension
■ Parotitis (inflammation of parotid gland, surgical mumps)	Usually *Staphylococcus* species, *Streptococcus* species occasionally, debilitation and dehydration with poor oral hygiene, NPO status for an extended time	Pain in area of gland and ear, absence of salivation, purulent exudate from duct of gland	Antibiotics, mouthwashes, warm compresses; preventive measures such as chewing gum, sucking on hard candy (lemon drops), adequate fluid intake
■ Stomatitis (inflammation of mouth)	Trauma; pathogens; irritants (tobacco, alcohol); renal, liver, and hematologic diseases; side effect of many cancer chemotherapy drugs	Excessive salivation, halitosis, sore mouth	Removal or treatment of cause, oral hygiene with soothing solutions, topical medications; soft, bland diet

Table 38-2 Oral Tumors

Location	Predisposing Factors	Clinical Manifestations	Treatment
▪ Lip	Constant overexposure to sun, ruddy and fair complexion, recurrent herpetic lesions, irritation from pipe stem, syphilis, immunosuppression	Indurated, painless ulcer	Surgical excision, radiation
▪ Tongue	Tobacco, alcohol, chronic irritation, syphilis	Ulcer or area of thickening; soreness or pain; increased salivation, slurred speech, dysphagia, toothache, earache (later signs)	Surgery (hemiglossectomy or glossectomy), radiation
▪ Oral cavity	Poor oral hygiene, tobacco usage (pipe and cigar smoking, snuff, chewing tobacco), chronic alcohol intake, chronic irritation (jagged tooth, ill-fitting prosthesis, chemical or mechanical irritants)	Leukoplakia; erythroplakia; ulcerations; sore spot; rough area; pain, dysphagia, difficulty in chewing and speaking (later signs)	Surgery (mandibulectomy, radical neck dissection, resections of buccal mucosa), internal and external radiation

years of age, with 60 being the average age at onset. Carcinoma of the oral cavity occurs in all ethnic groups. It is more common in men (male-to-female ratio of 2:1). Squamous cell carcinoma is the most common oral malignant tumor (more than 90%).[8] The 5-year survival rate for a patient with localized tumors is 70% to 90% and 0% to 60% for those with extensive primary oral cancer.[9]

Most of the malignant lesions occur on the lower lip in men. Other common sites are the lateral border and undersurface of the tongue, the labial commissure, and the buccal mucosa. Carcinoma of the lip has the most favorable prognosis of any of the oral tumors. This is probably because lip lesions are more apparent to the patient than other oral lesions and are usually diagnosed earlier.

Etiology

Although the cause of carcinoma of the oral cavity is not definitive, there are a number of predisposing factors (Table 38-2). Constant overexposure to ultraviolet radiation from the sun is definitely a factor in the development of cancer of the lip. Irritation from the pipe stem resting on the lip is a factor in pipe smokers. Factors that influence intraoral cancer include tobacco use (cigar, cigarette, pipe, snuff), excessive alcohol intake, and chronic irritation such as from a jagged tooth or poor dental care. A positive history of use of tobacco and alcohol, in the past or currently, is the most significant etiologic factor.[8]

Clinical Manifestations

Leukoplakia, called "white patch" or "smoker's patch," is frequently considered a precancerous lesion, although less than 5% of these lesions actually transform to malignant cells.[8] It is a whitish patch on the mucosa of the mouth or tongue. The patch becomes keratinized (hard and leathery) and is sometimes described as hyperkeratosis. Leukoplakia is the result of chronic irritation, especially from smoking. *Erythroplasia* (erythroplakia), which is seen as a red velvety patch on the mouth or tongue, is also considered a precancerous lesion. Areas of erythroplakia have a 90% chance of becoming malignant.[8]

Cancer of the lip usually appears as an indurated, painless ulcer on the lip. The first sign of carcinoma of the tongue is an ulcer or area of thickening. Soreness or pain of the tongue may occur, especially on eating hot or highly seasoned foods. Cancerous lesions are most likely to develop in the proximal half of the tongue. Some patients experience limitation of movement of the tongue. Later symptoms of cancer of the tongue include increased salivation, slurred speech, dysphagia, toothache, and earache. Approximately 30% of patients with oral cancer present with an asymptomatic neck mass.[10]

The common manifestations of carcinoma of the oral cavity are leukoplakia, erythroplakia, ulcerations, a sore spot, and a rough area (felt with the tongue). Later symptoms are pain, dysphagia, and difficulty in chewing and speaking.

Diagnostic Studies

Biopsy of the suspected lesion with cytologic examination is the best definitive diagnostic measure for oral cancer. Oral exfoliative cytology involves scraping of a suspicious lesion and spreading this scraping on a slide. Unlike biopsy, a negative cytologic smear does not reliably rule out the possibility of a malignant condition but may be used as a screening test. The toluidine blue test may also be used as a screening test for oral cancer. Toluidine blue is applied topically to stain an area of carcinoma.[8]

Therapeutic Management

Management of oral carcinoma usually consists of surgery, radiation, chemotherapy, or a combination of these (Table 38-3).

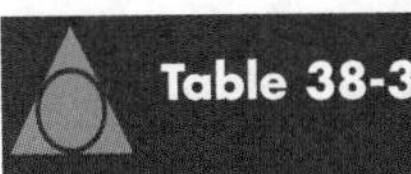

Table 38-3 Therapeutic Management: Oral Carcinoma

Diagnostic
- Biopsy
- Oral exfoliative cytology
- CT and MRI scans (for metastases)

Therapeutic*
- Surgical excision of the tumor
- Radical neck dissection
- Radiation (internal or external)
- Combined surgical resection with radiation
- Chemotherapy

CT, Computed tomography; *MRI,* magnetic resonance imaging.
*Any of the following approaches may be used, depending on the primary lesion and the extent of metastasis.

Surgical Interventions. Surgery remains the most effective treatment, especially for removing the central core of the tumor. Many of the operations are radical procedures involving extensive resections. Various surgical procedures may be performed, depending on the location and extent of the tumor. Some examples are partial *mandibulectomy* (removal of the mandible), *hemiglossectomy* (removal of half of the tongue), *glossectomy* (removal of the tongue), resections of the buccal mucosa and floor of the mouth, and radical neck dissection. Composite resections, which are combinations of the various surgical procedures, may be performed.

Because cancers of the oral cavity metastasize early to the cervical lymph nodes, a *radical neck dissection* is commonly performed. It includes wide excision of the involved primary lesion with removal of the regional lymph nodes, the deep cervical lymph nodes, and their lymphatic channels. In addition, the following structures may also be removed or transected (depending on the primary lesion and its extensiveness): the sternocleidomastoid muscle and other closely associated muscles, the internal jugular vein, the mandible, the submaxillary gland, part of the thyroid and parathyroid glands, and the spinal accessory nerve. A tracheostomy is commonly performed along with the radical neck dissection. Drainage tubes are inserted into the surgical area and connected to suction to remove fluid and blood (Fig. 38-4). Portable wound suction, as with a Hemovac, is usually used. The radical neck dissection usually involves one side of the neck. If the lesion is in the midline of the oral cavity, simultaneous bilateral neck dissection is done.

Modified neck dissection may be performed as an alternative to radical neck dissection. This procedure involves dissection of the major cervical lymphatic vessels and lateral cervical space, with preservation of several nerves and vessels, including the sympathetic and vagus nerves, the spinal accessory nerves, and the internal jugular vein.

Life-threatening complications, such as airway obstruction, hemorrhage, and tracheal aspiration, may occur. Airway obstruction must be prevented. Depending on the extent of surgery, a prophylactic tracheostomy is often performed. Hemorrhage can occur because of the vascularity of the head and neck area. Another complication is tracheal aspiration, the duration of which is dependent upon the extent of the surgery. It occurs because the patient is unable to swallow saliva or fluids and aspirates fluid. Other complications include infection, pneumothorax, subcutaneous emphysema or air leak under the skin flaps, and necrosis of the skin flaps. Neurologic complications can occur as a result of nerve severance during the surgical procedure. The nerves most commonly severed are the spinal accessory nerves and the cervical plexus. The facial nerve (cranial nerve III), which passes through the parotid gland, may be affected if this gland is removed. The patient undergoing radical neck dissection is also at risk for fluid and electrolyte imbalances secondary to syndrome of inappropriate antidiuretic hormone (SIADH). It is reported to occur is as many as 35% of patients undergoing this procedure.[11]

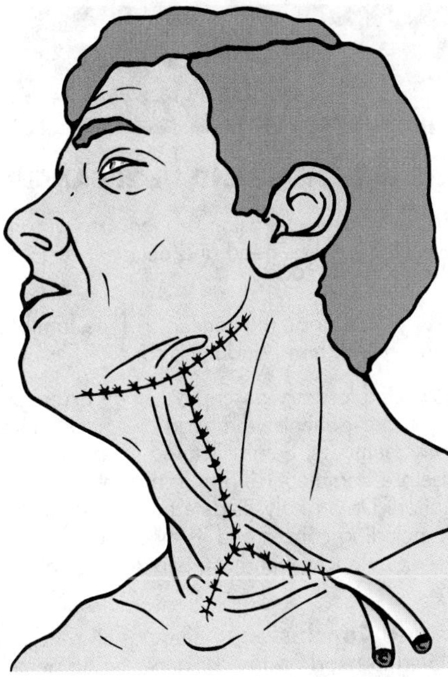

Fig. 38-4 Radical neck incision with suction tubing in place.

Radiation and Chemotherapy. Radiation is sometimes used before surgery to decrease the size of the tumor. Radiation may also be used postoperatively or palliatively. The type of radiation used may be internal or external. A common form of internal radiation (brachytherapy) is the implantation of seeds, such as radon seeds, in gold tubes or molds. This type of therapy is more effective in the early stages of the disease as compared with the later stages.[12] External radiation may also be used (see Chapter 12).

Chemotherapy and radiation are used together when the lesions are more advanced or involve several structures of the oral cavity. Chemotherapy may also be used when surgery and radiation fail or as the initial therapy for smaller tumors. Chemotherapeutic agents used include 5-fluorouracil (5-FU), cyclophosphamide, bleomycin, vinblastine, hydroxyurea, and cisplatin (see Chapter 12).

RESEARCH

IMPLICATIONS FOR NURSING PRACTICE

PATIENTS WITH HEAD AND NECK CANCER

Citation Mah MA, Johnston C: Concerns of families in which one member has head and neck cancer, *Cancer Nurs* 16:382-387, 1993.

Purpose To describe the concerns of the families and patients living with head and neck cancer

Methods Exploratory descriptive study examining the concerns of four patients with head and neck cancer and their family members. Semistructured interviews were performed before treatment, during treatment, and during rehabilitation. Data analyses determined five areas for concern, including cancer and its meaning, social relationships, experiences with hospitalization, treatment, and the future.

Results and Conclusions Findings showed the concerns related to head and neck cancer being perceived as threatening and harmful. Concerns about dying and the meaning of cancer were reported by all patients. Concerns among patients were different from those of their family members across the different periods.

Implications for Nursing Practice Head and neck cancer may be the most emotionally traumatic of any type of cancer because of disfigurement and functional impairment. The results of this study are useful in helping nurses understand the experience of head and neck cancer from the perspective of patients and family members. Understanding the concerns of patients and their families in their experiences with cancer can help nurses promote better quality of life and facilitate effective coping with cancer for patients and their families.

Palliative treatment may be the best management when the prognosis is poor, the cancer is inoperable, or the patient decides against surgery. Palliation aims to treat the symptoms and make the patient more comfortable. If it becomes difficult to swallow, a gastrostomy may be performed to allow for adequate nutritional intake (see Gastrostomy, later in this chapter). Analgesic medication should be given freely to this patient. Frequent suctioning of the oral cavity becomes necessary when swallowing becomes difficult. (Other nursing measures for the terminally ill patient are discussed in Chapter 12.)

Nutritional Management

Because of depression or presurgery radiation treatment, patients may be malnourished even before surgery. After radical neck surgery, the patient may be unable to take in nutrients through the normal route of ingestion because of swelling, the location of sutures, or difficulty with swallowing. Parenteral fluids will be given for the first 24 to 48 hours. After this time, tube feedings are usually given via a nasogastric or nasointestinal tube that was placed during surgery. (Nasogastric feedings are described in Chapter 37.) Sometimes a temporary feeding gastrostomy may be used (see Gastrostomy, later in this chapter). Cervical esophagostomy and pharyngostomy have also been used. The nurse must observe for tolerance of the feedings and adjust the amount, time, and formula if nausea, vomiting, diarrhea, or distention occurs. The patient is usually instructed about the tube feedings. When the patient can swallow, small amounts of water are given. Close observation for choking is essential. Suctioning may be necessary to prevent aspiration.

NURSING MANAGEMENT

CARCINOMA OF THE ORAL CAVITY

Nursing Assessment

Subjective and objective data that should be obtained from a patient with carcinoma of the oral cavity are presented in Table 38-4.

Nursing Diagnoses

Nursing diagnoses are determined when the problem and etiologic factors are supported by clinical data. Nursing diagnoses related to carcinoma of the oral cavity may include, but are not limited to, the following:

- Altered nutrition: less than body requirements related to oral pain, difficulty chewing and swallowing, surgical resection, and radiation treatment.
- Pain related to the tumor and surgical radiation

Table 38-4 Nursing Assessment: Cancer of the Mouth

Subjective Data

Important health information

Past health history: Use of alcohol and tobacco, pipe smoking, exposure to sunlight

Surgery and other treatments: Removal of previous tumors or lesions

Functional health patterns

Nutritional-metabolic: Reductions in oral intake, weight loss; difficulty in chewing food; increased salivation; intolerance to certain foods or temperatures of food

Cognitive-perceptual: Mouth pain, neck stiffness, dysphagia

Objective Data

Lips

Symmetry, color, size, cracking, ulcers, fissures

Tongue

Lesions, soreness, limitation of movement, leukoplakia, erythroplakia

Buccal mucosa

Color, pigmentation, lesions, areas of tenderness, leukoplakia, erythroplakia

Other

Breath odor, increased salivation, slurred speech, neck masses

- Anxiety related to diagnosis of cancer, uncertain future, potential for disfiguring surgery, potential for recurrence, and prognosis
- Altered health maintenance related to lack of knowledge of disease process and therapeutic regimen, and unavailability of a support system.

Planning

The overall goals are that the patient with carcinoma of the oral cavity will (1) have a patent airway, (2) be able to communicate, (3) have adequate nutritional intake to promote wound healing, and (4) have relief of pain and discomfort.

Nursing Implementation

Health Promotion and Maintenance. The nurse has a significant role in early detection and treatment of carcinoma of the oral cavity. The nurse needs to provide the patient with information regarding predisposing factors, such as constant overexposure to the sun, tobacco, and other irritants. Smoking and the long-term use of smokeless tobacco are the major risk factors for oral cancer. A patient identified as a smoker should be informed about smoking cessation programs available in the community. It is important that adolescents and teenagers be informed about the danger of using "snuff" and chewing tobacco. In addition, oral cancers have an increased chance of recurrence if risk factors are not reduced. The nurse should also teach correct oral hygiene and dental care and encourage the patient to seek preventive dental care. Risk factors need to be identified. Because early detection of oral carcinoma is important, the patient should be taught to examine the mouth and to recognize danger signals of oral cancer. If any of these signals are present, the patient should be instructed to visit a doctor. Danger signals are as follows:

- Unexplained pain or soreness in the mouth
- Unusual bleeding from the oral cavity
- Dysphagia
- Swelling or lump in the neck
- Any ulcerative lesion that does not heal within 2 to 3 weeks

The last sign is significant; a biopsy of the lesion should probably be performed. The nurse should inspect the patient's oral cavity to detect suspicious lesions.

Acute Intervention. Preoperative care for the patient who is to have a radical neck dissection involves consideration of the patient's physical and psychosocial needs (see the nursing care plan for the patient with a radical neck dissection on p. 1148). Physical preparation is the same as for any major surgery, with special emphasis on oral hygiene. Explanations and emotional support are of special significance and should include postoperative measures relating to communication and feeding. The surgical procedure should be explained to the patient, and the nurse should make sure that the information is understood by the patient.

Airway. Postoperatively, maintenance of a patent airway is a priority. The inflammation in the surgical area may compress the trachea. A tracheostomy is commonly done in conjunction with radical neck surgery to ensure an adequate airway. In addition, the patient has difficulty swallowing saliva and is at risk for aspiration. A gauze wick, placed to direct saliva into an emesis basin or a dental suction tip, may be used to remove secretions. If the patient has a tracheostomy, frequent suctioning may be necessary if the patient cannot clear secretions voluntarily (see Chapter 23). For the patient without a tracheostomy, oral or nasopharyngeal suctioning should be done when audible signs of fluid accumulation occur or when the patient indicates a need for suctioning. The patient should be observed for signs of respiratory distress.

Positioning. To facilitate drainage from the mouth and to prevent aspiration, proper positioning is essential. In the immediate and early postoperative period, the patient should be lying on the side or supine with the head turned to one side to prevent aspiration. As soon as the patient is awake, the head of the bed is usually elevated to promote venous and lymphatic drainage and to facilitate breathing and swallowing. The nurse should provide a basin and mouth wipes to help the patient manage the secretions. The basin should be emptied frequently because of the odor of the secretions.

Oral hygiene. Measures must be taken to prevent infection of the oral cavity. Accumulated mucus and old blood provides an excellent medium for microorganisms. Oral hygiene decreases the possibility of infection and also decreases the mouth odor and unpleasant taste for the patient. The oral care must be done carefully to prevent trauma. The mouth may be gently irrigated with sterile water, normal saline solution, or diluted hydrogen peroxide. A Water-Pik may be effective for oral irrigations. An applicator soaked with peroxide and saline solution may be used to cleanse the difficult-to-reach areas. However, such procedures may be contraindicated in a patient with large resections of the oral cavity because of the potential to injure the flap. The lips should be kept moist with lanolin or lubricant.

Wound care. It is important to observe the dressing for any signs of hemorrhage or constriction. When portable wound suction is used, the nurse should ensure that it is functioning properly. The drainage is serosanguineous and gradually diminishes from the initial 80 to 120 ml in 24 hours. Wound infection and flap necrosis are serious complications of radical neck dissection. The patient who is malnourished is particularly at risk for delayed wound healing.

Communication. One of the patient's postoperative fears is of not being able to talk and tell the nurse about pain and the need for help. Speech difficulties arise if the patient has a tracheostomy or if part of the tongue or palate has been resected. Speech difficulties may occur only temporarily or for a longer time, depending on the amount of tissue removed. Alternate means of communication, such as a pad and pencil, small chalkboard, or a picture board, should have been decided on preoperatively. Placing the call button within reach is essential. The nurse can provide added assurance and relieve anxiety by frequently visiting the patient.

NURSING CARE PLAN Patient After a Radical Neck Dissection

Planning: Outcome Criteria	Nursing Interventions and Rationales
➤ **NURSING DIAGNOSIS**	Ineffective airway clearance *related to* inability to maintain proper position and viscous secretions secondary to tracheostomy *as manifested by* abnormal breath sounds, respiratory distress, tachypnea, ineffective cough
Have patent airway, no aspiration of saliva	Assess for amount and viscosity of secretions *to plan appropriate interventions.* Position patient on side or supine with head turned to one side immediately after surgery *to prevent aspiration of secretions.* Position in a sitting position as soon as patient can tolerate it *to promote venous and lymphatic drainage and to facilitate breathing and swallowing.* Suction frequently and carefully *to remove secretions and to prevent trauma to surgical area.* Assess for early signs of respiratory distress *to provide immediate intervention.* Provide a basin and wipes for saliva and secretions *to help the patient manage the secretions.* Assist patient *to deep breath and cough effectively to prevent atelectasis.*
➤ **NURSING DIAGNOSIS**	Ineffective breathing pattern *related to* immobility and pain secondary to surgical incision *as manifested by* dyspnea, tachypnea, shortness of breath, cyanosis, cough, use of accessory muscles, abnormal breath sounds
Have clear lungs on auscultation, no respiratory distress.	Assess chest expansion and symmetry *to determine presence of lung complications.* Support patient's neck and head when deep breathing and coughing *to reduce pain and improve cooperation.* Auscultate lungs *to evaluate effectiveness of ventilation.* Reassure patient that measures are being taken to make breathing easier *so anxiety will not cause increased respiratory difficulty.*
➤ **NURSING DIAGNOSIS**	Acute pain *related to* surgical procedure and ineffective pain and comfort measures *as manifested by* communication of pain descriptors; guarding behavior; narrowed self-focus; behaviors indicative of pain, such as restlessness, crying, moaning; facial mask of pain; diaphoresis and changes in blood pressure, pulse, and respiratory rate
Express satisfaction with pain relief.	Administer mild analgesics *to reduce pain to a satisfactory level for patient.* Do not use narcotic analgesics *to prevent respiratory depression.* Support neck and head when moving patient *to reduce pain.* Use gentle suctioning *to prevent causing undue discomfort* and provide oral hygiene *to increase patient's comfort.*
➤ **NURSING DIAGNOSIS**	Altered nutrition: less than body requirements *related to* chewing and swallowing difficulties, nasogastric tube, and decreased taste and smell perceptions *as manifested by* inadequate food intake (less than recommended daily allowances), body weight 20% or more under ideal for height and frame, inability to ingest food
Have adequate intake of nutrients; maintain or attain desired body weight.	Administer tube feedings or total parenteral nutrition as ordered *to maintain required caloric and fluid intake while surgical wound heals.* Observe for tolerance of feedings *because feedings may produce diarrhea, nausea, vomiting.* Provide privacy when eating *because patient may be embarrassed with alterations in method of eating and chewing.* When patient starts taking fluids, observe for choking and have suction available *to prevent aspiration.* Offer small, frequent, attractively served meals with adequate fluid intake *to assist patient to meet nutritional requirements.* Monitor caloric intake and weight *to evaluate patient's response to the plan.*

continued

Self-image. The nurse should be aware of how the patient feels about body alterations. Many patients are sensitive about their appearance. Privacy is important to most patients, especially during eating. The patient may have a transparent dressing protecting the wound and therefore may be reluctant to go outside the room. The nurse should instruct the patient to tilt the head to the side to prevent drooling. Assistance with personal hygiene may lessen the patient's feelings of a poor body image. The nurse should convey acceptance through both verbal and nonverbal communication and not show negative feelings when caring for the patient.

NURSING CARE PLAN Patient After a Radical Neck Dissection—cont'd

Planning: Outcome Criteria	*Nursing Interventions and Rationales*
➤ **NURSING DIAGNOSIS**	Altered oral mucous membranes *related to* excessive secretions and inability to perform oral hygiene *as manifested by* oral pain or discomfort, edema, increased secretions, halitosis, weakness, inability or unwillingness to perform oral hygiene
Have clean oral cavity with no infection.	Provide frequent, gentle oral hygiene *to maintain clean, healthy oral mucosa and promote appetite.* Use mouth irrigations with sterile water, normal saline solution, or dilute peroxide *to remove accumulated mucus and old blood and prevent odors.* Suction *to remove pooled secretions* and provide tissues *to wipe away drooled saliva.* Use Water-Pik or power spray to clean hard-to-reach areas *to avoid accumulation of food particles in difficult-to-reach areas of the mouth.* Apply lubricant to dry lips. Reassure patient of your willingness to perform these tasks *to convey acceptance of patient.*
➤ **NURSING DIAGNOSIS**	Impaired verbal communication *related to* inability to speak secondary to tracheostomy *as manifested by* inability to communicate needs and anxiety
Use alternate means of communication.	Plan for and provide alternate means of communication (pad and pencil, small chalkboard, "Magic Slate") *to enable patient to communicate needs.* Place call button within reach *to provide patient with an easily accessible way to summon help when needed.* Visit frequently and assure patient that help is available to meet requests *to relieve anxiety associated with inability to verbalize needs.*
➤ **NURSING DIAGNOSIS**	Body-image disturbance *related to* disfiguring surgery, loss of oral communication, and drooling *as manifested by* withdrawal, depression, isolation, unwillingness to look at self or assist with care, refusal to see visitors
Acknowledge change in body structure and function; communicate feelings about surgery; participate in self-care.	Assess patient's body image concept *to identify patient at risk for unsuccessful adjustment.* Provide privacy *to respect patient's request while adjusting to change in body function and appearance.* If patient drools, instruct to tilt head to side *to allow collected secretions to flow easily from the mouth.* Encourage attention to personal hygiene *because improved appearance can boost self-esteem.* Encourage socialization with family and friends *because acceptance by significant others is a critical factor in patient's own acceptance.* Provide information about measures to help improve appearance such as wearing clothes with high collars, and wearing accessories that draw attention away from neck *to aid successful adjustment.* Answer questions honestly about changes in body image *to convey acceptance and to provide accurate information.* Involve patient in self-care *because participation in self-care is a sign of successful adjustment.* Assure patient of self-worth *to increase acceptance of altered physical appearance.*
➤ **NURSING DIAGNOSIS**	Anxiety *related to* lack of knowledge regarding possibilities of reconstructive surgery and prognosis *as manifested by* request for information, verbalization of problem, inappropriate or exaggerated behaviors
Discuss possibilities of reconstructive surgery; make realistic plans to resume lifestyle.	Provide information about prosthetic devices, speech therapy, and reconstructive surgery *to enable patient to select assistance in specific areas.* Cooperate with other members of the health care team *to facilitate interdisciplinary planning and total patient care.* Provide opportunities for patient to discuss fears about diagnosis and prognosis *to relieve patient's anxiety by correcting misinformation and providing accurate information.*

The patient may go through the grieving process. Support of family, significant others, and friends is important. The nurse should allow the patient to verbalize personal feelings about the surgery.

Depression. Depression is common in the patient who has had a radical neck dissection. The patient may not be able to speak because of the tracheostomy and cannot control saliva. The neck and shoulders are numb because of the transected nerves. The facial appearance may be significantly altered with swelling, edema, and deformities. The patient needs to understand that many of the physical changes are reversible as the edema subsides and the tracheostomy tube is removed (Fig. 38-5). Depression may also be related to the concern about the prognosis. The nurse can help the patient through the depression by allowing verbalization of feelings, conveying acceptance, and helping the patient regain an acceptable self-concept. Sometimes it is appropriate to obtain a psychiatric referral for the patient who is experiencing prolonged or severe depression.

Sexuality. The patient may feel less desirable sexually and may also feel inadequate. The nurse can assist the patient by allowing discussions regarding sexuality and encouraging the patient to discuss this problem with the sexual partner. It may be difficult for the patient to orally discuss sexual problems because of the alteration in communications. The nurse can allow the patient to plan how to communicate with the sexual partner and offer support and guidance to the sexual partner. Helping the patient see that sexuality involves much more than appearance may relieve some anxiety.

Chronic and Home Management. Facial disfigurement and other mutilating aspects of radical head and neck surgery may have a major long-term impact on the patient's body image and lifestyle. Many of these surgical procedures leave a deformity, both functionally and cosmetically. It may be difficult for the patient to eat and speak, and the altered physical appearance may be embarrassing and depressing. After surgery, there may be taste and sensation changes that may affect nutritional intake. The patient is taught to perform various exercises aimed at regaining maximum shoulder function and neck motion. Some patients may have to learn to swallow again. The patient may need information about prosthetic devices, speech therapy, and further reconstructive surgery.

The patient is often discharged with a tracheostomy and gastrostomy tube. The patient and the family need to be taught how to manage these tubes and who to call if there are problems. In addition, home health care may need to be provided initially to evaluate the family or the patient's ability to perform self-care activities.

Reconstructive surgery may be performed at the time of the initial surgery or soon after the tumor is removed. Various types of flaps and grafts are used. It may be necessary to rebuild the nose or the mandible or to close oral cutaneous openings. Prosthetic materials, such as Silastic and Plastigel (which is soft), are often used to reconstruct various deformities.

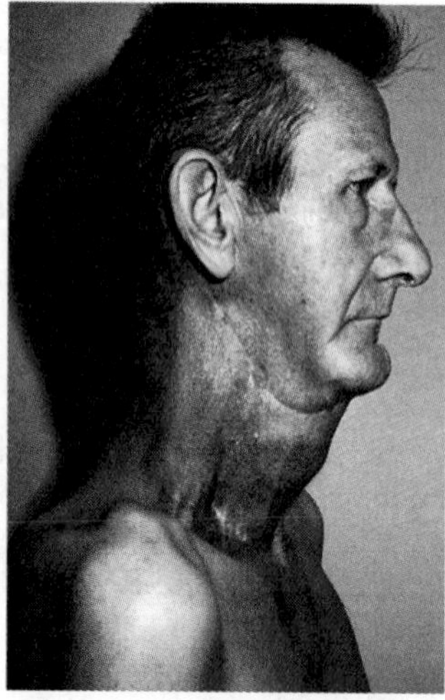

Fig. 38-5 Appearance of the neck following healing after a radical neck dissection. This patient also had postoperative external radiation therapy.

MANDIBULAR FRACTURE

Fracture of the mandible may result from trauma to the face or jaws. Maxillary fractures may also occur but are less common than mandibular fractures. The fracture may be simple, with no bone displacement, or it may involve loss of tissue and bone. The fracture may require immediate and sometimes long-term treatment to ensure survival and restore satisfactory appearance and function. Mandibular fracture may also be therapeutically performed to correct an underlying malocclusion problem that cannot be corrected by orthodontic procedures alone. In these conditions the mandible is split during surgery and moved forward or backward depending on the occlusion problem. For this patient, the procedure is performed on an elective basis.

Surgery consists of immobilization, usually by wiring the jaws (intermaxillary fixation). Internal fixation may be accomplished with screws and plates. In a simple fracture with no loss of teeth, the lower jaw is wired to the upper jaw. First, wires are placed around the teeth; then cross-wires or rubber bands are used to hold the lower jaw tight against the upper jaw (Fig. 38-6). Arch bars may be used and placed on the maxillary and mandibular arches of the

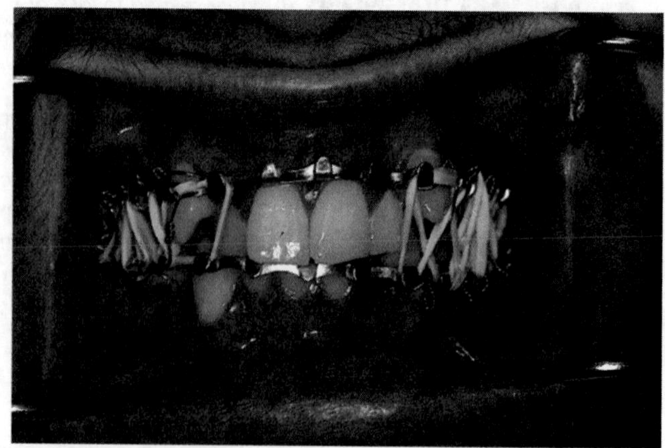

Fig. 38-6 Intermaxillary fixation.

teeth. Vertical wires are placed between the arch bars holding the jaws together. When teeth are missing or if there is bone displacement, other forms of fixation such as metal arch bars in the mouth or insertion of a pin in the bone may be used. The immobilization is usually necessary for only 4 to 5 weeks because the fractures heal rapidly.

NURSING MANAGEMENT

MANDIBULAR FRACTURE

Preoperative Care

The patient should be told preoperatively about the surgical procedure, including what it involves, how the face will look, and alterations the surgery will cause. The patient needs to be reassured about the ability to breathe normally, speak, and swallow liquids. Usually hospitalization is brief unless there are other injuries or problems.

Postoperative Care

Postoperative care should focus on a patent airway, oral hygiene, communication, and adequate nutrition. Two major potential problems in the immediate postoperative period are airway obstruction and aspiration of vomitus. Because the patient cannot open the jaws, measures to ensure an airway are essential. The nurse must observe for signs of respiratory distress. The patient should be placed on the side with the head slightly elevated immediately after surgery. A wire cutter or scissors (for rubber bands) must be taped to the head of the bed. These may be used to cut the wires or elastic bands in case of an emergency. The wires should be cut only as a last resort. Once the patient is awake the wires should be cut only in case of cardiac or respiratory arrest.

The physician should explain, by using a picture, the appropriate wire or wires to cut, and this should be included in the care plan. In some cases, cutting the wires may cause the entire facial and upper jaw structure to collapse and worsen the problem. A tracheostomy or an endotracheal tray should always be available.

If the patient begins to vomit or choke, the nurse should try to clear the mouth and airway. Suctioning may be necessary and may be done by the nasopharyngeal or oral route, depending on the extent of injury and the type of repair. A nasogastric tube may be used for decompression to remove fluids and gas from the stomach to help prevent aspiration. It will also help prevent vomiting. Antiemetics may also be used. The nasogastric tube can later be used as a feeding tube. The nurse should teach the patient to clear secretions and vomitus.

Oral hygiene is an important part of the nursing care. The mouth should be rinsed frequently, particularly after meals and snacks, to remove food debris. Warm normal saline solution, water, or alkaline mouthwashes may be used. A soft rubber catheter or a Water-Pik are effective for a thorough oral cleansing. The nurse should inspect the mouth several times a day to see that it is clean. A flashlight is necessary, and a tongue depressor is used to retract the cheeks. The lips and corners of the mouth should be kept moist.

Communication may be a problem, particularly in the early postoperative period. An effective way of communication must be established preoperatively (e.g., use of picture board, pad and pencil, small chalkboard) Usually the patient can speak well enough to be understood, especially after the first few postoperative days.

Ingestion of sufficient nutrients poses a real problem because the diet must be liquid. The patient easily tires of sucking through a straw or laboriously using a spoon. The diet must be planned to include adequate calories and protein. Liquid protein supplements may be helpful for improving the nutritional status. Adequate fluid intake must be included. The nurse needs to work with the dietitian and the patient to ensure adequate nutrition. The low-bulk, high-carbohydrate diet and the intake of air through the straw create a problem with flatus and constipation. Ambulation, prune juice, and bulk-forming laxatives may help relieve these problems.

The patient is usually discharged with the wires in place. The nurse needs to allow the patient to verbalize feelings about the altered appearance. Discharge teaching should include oral care, techniques of handling secretions, diet, and how and when to use wire cutters.

GASTROESOPHAGEAL REFLUX DISEASE

Pathophysiology

Gastroesophageal reflux disease (GERD) is not a disease, but a syndrome produced by conditions that result in reflux of gastric secretions into the esophagus. Predisposing conditions include hiatal hernia, incompetent lower esophageal sphincter (LES), decreased esophageal clearance, and decreased gastric emptying. In GERD there is confirmed evidence of reflux of gastric contents into the lower portion of the esophagus.[13] The acidity of the gastric secretion results in esophageal irritation and inflammation (esophagitis). In addition, the presence of intestinal secretions such as trypsin and bile salts are also corrosive to the esophageal mucosa.[14] The degree of inflammation is dependent on the amount of acid refluxed as well as on the ability of the esophagus to clear the acid (esophageal clearance).[15]

One of the primary factors in GERD is an incompetent LES. This is defined as a lack of high pressure in the distal portion of the esophagus. As a result gastric contents are able to move from an area of higher pressure (stomach) to an area of lower pressure (esophagus) when the patient is in a supine position or there is an increase in intraabdominal pressure. (Hiatal hernia is discussed in the next section).

Clinical Manifestations

Heartburn (*pyrosis*) from gastroesophageal reflux is the most common clinical manifestation. It is caused by irritation of the esophagus by the gastric acids. Heartburn is described as a burning, tight sensation that appears intermittently beneath the lower sternum and spreads upward to the throat or jaw. Heartburn occurs following ingestion of substances that decrease the LES pressure (Table 38-5). Heartburn is relieved with milk, alkaline substances, or water.

Regurgitation (effortless return of material from stomach into esophagus or mouth) is a fairly common manifestation of an incompetent LES. It is often described as hot, bitter, or sour liquid coming into the throat or mouth. Other

Table 38-5 Factors Affecting Lower Esophageal Sphincter Pressure and Reflux in Gastroesophageal Reflux Disease and Hiatal Hernia

Substances Affecting LES Pressure and Tone

Increase Pressure

Bethanechol (Urecholine)
Cisapride (Propulsid)
Metoclopramide (Reglan)

Decrease Pressure

Fatty foods	Theophylline
Chocolate (theobromine, caffeine)	Diazepam (Valium)
Peppermint, spearmint	Morphine sulfate
Alcohol	β-adrenergic blocking drugs
Nicotine	Calcium channel blockers
Anticholinergics	Nitrates
Progesterone	Prostaglandins
Tea, coffee (caffeine)	

Measures to Prevent Gastroesophageal Reflux

- *Do* eat high-protein, low-fat diet; eat small, frequent meals to prevent gastric distention; sleep with head of bed elevated on 4- to 6-in blocks (gravity fosters esophageal clearance); lose weight if overweight
- *Do not* lie down for 2 to 3 hr after eating, wear tight clothing around the waist, or bend over (especially after eating).
- *Avoid* alcohol, smoking (causes an almost immediate, marked decrease in LES pressure), and beverages that contain caffeine

LES, Lower esophageal sphincter.

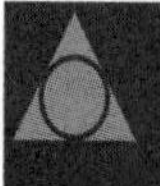

Table 38-6 Therapeutic Management: Gastroesophageal Reflux Disease and Hiatal Hernia

Diagnostic

Barium swallow
Esophagoscopy
pH monitoring (laboratory or 24 hr ambulatory)
Motility (manometry) studies

Therapeutic

Conservative

Elevation of head of bed on 4- to 6-in blocks
High-protein, low-fat diet with avoidance of foods that decrease LES pressure or irritate acid-senstive esophagus
Antacids/Gaviscon
Cholinergic drugs
Antisecretory agents
Prokinetic drug therapy*

Surgical

Nissen fundoplication
Hill gastroplexy
Belsey fundoplication
Antireflux prosthesis

LES, Lower esophageal sphincter.
*See Table 39-1.

symptoms include feelings of a lump in the throat or of food stopping, *dysphagia* (difficulty in swallowing), painful swallowing, and bleeding. An individual with GERD may also experience respiratory complications including bronchospasm, laryngospasm, and cricopharyngeal spasm because of movement of gastric contents into the upper airway.[14]

Complications

Complications of GERD are related to the direct local effects of gastric acid on the esophageal mucosa. As a result of repeated exposure, there may be scar tissue formation and decreased distensibility of the esophagus. This may result in dysphagia. In addition, esophageal metaplasia (Barrett's esophagus) may occur. There is also the potential for pulmonary complications (pneumonia) secondary to aspiration of gastric contents into the pulmonary system.

Diagnostic Studies

Diagnostic studies are performed to determine the cause of the GERD (e.g., hiatal hernia) (Table 38-6). Barium swallow is done to determine if there is protrusion of the gastric cardia. Radionucleotide tests may also be performed to detect reflux of gastric contents and the rate of esophageal clearance.[15] Esophagoscopy is useful in determining the incompetence of the LES and the extent of inflammation, potential scarring, and strictures. Biopsy and cytologic specimens can be taken to differentiate hiatal hernia from carcinoma of the stomach or esophagus and Barrett's esophagus. Esophageal motility studies are performed to measure pressure in the LES. The determination of pH using specially designed probes in the laboratory or using ambulatory monitoring systems may demonstrate the presence of acid in the normally alkaline esophagus.[16]

Therapeutic Management

Conservative management is focused on eliminating precipitating factors (see Tables 38-5 and 38-6) and using medications that reduce acid secretion and relieve symptoms.

Pharmacologic Management. Antacids are used to relieve heartburn by their neutralizing effect on hydrochloric acid. They should be taken 1 to 3 hours after meals and at bedtime. Alginic acid and an antacid (Gaviscon) are sometimes given together. The alginic acid reacts with sodium bicarbonate and forms a viscous solution that floats to the surface of the gastric contents and coats the esophagus, acting as a mechanical barrier to reflux. A summary of the pharmacologic management is shown in Table 38-7 on p. 1156.

Cholinergic drugs, such as bethanechol (Urecholine), may be used to increase LES pressure, improve esophageal clearance in the supine position, as well as increase gastric emptying. Metoclopramide (Reglan), a dopamine antagonist, increases LES pressure and gastric emptying. Another prokinetic agent that has been approved by the Food and Drug Administration (FDA) for the management of GERD is cisapride (Propulsid). Prokinetic agents are often admin-

Clinical Pathway for Laparoscopic Surgery

Procedure: ____________________
MD: ____________________
Patient Profile: ____________________

Laparoscopic Surgery CareMap®
Lakes Region General Hospital
Women and Children's Health Services Ad Hoc Committee/ General Surgery Committee
Reviewed with Patient: ____________ Initials/Date
Date Initiated: ____________

NOTE: Acceptable medical practice generally does include a variety of responses to a particular clinical problem.

Addressograph

Interventions	Preadmission (if applicable) Date:	AM admission via ODS Date:	Operative day—post PACU Date:	Postop day 1 to discharge Date:	Discharge day Date:
Assessment	Preop interview as indicated by MD	Nursing assessment completed Operative consent signed and on chart Patient able to verbalize postop expectations and plan of care for hospital course Reassurance/emotional support given	On admission and q4°: Patient easily aroused, oriented Skin color pale pink to pink, temperature warm and dry Vital signs Lungs clear without signs or symptoms of respiratory distress Pain controlled with prescribed analgesics If nausea/vomiting—controlled with prescribed antiemetics Bowel sounds present Dressing/bandaids dry and intact Voiding spontaneously within 8° postop. I & O q8°. Notify MD if <30 cc/hr (adult); < 15 cc/hr (pediatric) Coping mechanisms effective If applicable—parents attentive, assist in care	Assessment q shift: Patient alert, oriented Skin color pink, warm, and dry Vital signs q4° Lungs clear Pain controlled with prescribed analgesics If nausea/vomiting—controlled with prescribed antiemetics Bowel sounds positive. Passing flatus Dressing off, may cover if patient desires Incisions without signs or symptoms of infection Voiding spontaneously. I & O WNL Coping mechanisms effective If applicable—parents attentive, assist in care	Condition stable Patient alert, oriented Skin pink, warm, and dry Vital signs stable Lungs clear Pain controlled with PO analgesic No nausea, vomiting Bowel sounds present. Passing flatus Incision healing without signs or symptoms of infection. Voiding q shift Coping well If applicable—parents able to care for child
Treatments and interventions		Preop meds given as ordered IVs as ordered	Provide comfort measures: turning, relaxing, breathing technique, splinting abdomen when C + DB Skin care q shift Mouth care q2° while NPO IV as ordered	Assist with general comfort measures Skin care q shift IV DCd as ordered.	
Diet	Dietary teaching appropriate to procedure	NPO after MN except clear liquids until 3° before admission	Ice chips, and clear liquids as tolerated	Clear to full liquids tolerated well. Regular diet after flatus passed.	Tolerating regular diet

continued

Clinical Pathway for Laparoscopic Surgery—cont'd

Interventions	Preadmission (if applicable) Date:	AM admission via ODS Date:	Operative day—post PACU Date:	Postop day 1 to discharge Date:	Discharge day Date:
Activity		Side rails up on stretcher after preop meds Call bell in reach To OR via stretcher	T, C, DB q2° × 8, then q4°. Assist as necessary. Call bell in reach. Side rails as per standard. OOB with assistance. Personal hygiene with assistance.	C + DB q4° Call bell in reach. Side rails as per standard. Ambulate with minimal assist or ad lib. Self-care/shower independently.	Up ad lib. Patient up to ADLs/self-care
Lab tests/ other	Preop labs as ordered ECG if age ≥ 45 (male) ≥ 55 (female)	Preop testing done as ordered and results on chart			
Teaching and discharge planning	Preop teaching initiated Questions answered	Preop teaching reviewed/ completed Questions answered	Orient to room/unit and plan of care Reinforce preop and postop teaching Review needs identified on admission/ongoing assessment Begin discharge teaching: Activity, restrictions Diet Symptoms to notify MD Medications Follow-up appointment Care of incision	Review plan of care Review needs identified on admission/ongoing assessment Continue/complete discharge teaching: Activity, restrictions Diet Symptoms to notify MD Medications Follow-up appointment Care of incision	Discharge teaching completed and patient/SO verbalizes good understanding of all discharge instructions.

Check, initial, and sign. Note detours (deviations from normal) on next page	Signatures	Time	Date	Signatures	Time	Date	Signatures	Time	Date	Signatures	Time	Date	Signatures	Time	Date

continued

Clinical Pathway for Laparoscopic Surgery—cont'd

Detour Source Code

A. PATIENT/FAMILY
1. Patient condition
2. Patient/family decision
3. Patient/family availability
4. Patient/family other

B. CAREGIVER/CLINICIAN

5. Physician order
6. Caregiver(s) decision
7. Caregiver(s) response timely
8. Caregiver other

C. HOSPITAL/SYSTEM

9. Bed/appointment time availability
10. Inforrmation/data availability
11. Supplies/equipment availability
12. Department overbooked/closed
13. Hospital other

D. COMMUNITY

14. Placement/Home Care availabilty
15. Ambulance delay
16. Community other

Admission Criteria

Addressograph

Admission Date: ____
Actual Discharge Date: ____
Case Type: ____
Secondary Diagnosis: ____
Surgical Procedures: ____
DRG: ____
Expected LOS: ____

Detours

Detour record: code each entry with appropriate source code

Date	Time	Source code number	Description	Action taken	Intervention

A Detour Record is included with this Care Map®. Developed by Lakes Region General Hospital, Laconia, NH. Licensed by Center for Case Management, South Natick, MA.
ADLs, Activities of daily living; *C + DB*, coughing and deep breathing; *DC*, discontinue; *DRG*, diagnostic related group; *I & O*, intake and output; *IV*, intravenous; *LOS*, length of stay; *MN*, midnight; *NPO*, nothing by mouth; *ODS*, outpatient day surgery; *OOB*, out of bed; *OR*, operating room; *PACU*, postanesthesia care unit; *PO*, oral; *SO*, significant other; *T*, turn; *WNL*, within normal limits.

Table 38-7 Drug Therapy for Management of Gastroesophageal Reflux

Mechanism of Action	Examples
Increase LES Pressure	
Cholinergic	Bethanecol (Urecholine)
Dopamine antagonist	Metoclopramide (Reglan)
Serotonin antagonist	Cisapride (Propulsid)
Acid Neutralizing	
Antacids	Gelusil, Maalox, Mylanta
Antisecretory	
Histamine H_2 receptor antagonists	Ranitidine (Zantac) Cimetidine (Tagamet) Famotidine (Pepcid) Nizatidine (Axid) Omeprazole (Prilosec)
Acid-suppressing	
Cytoprotective	
Alginic acid-antacid	Gaviscon
Antacids	Gelusil, Maalox, Mylanta
Acid-protective	Sucralfate (Carafate)

LES, Lower esophageal sphincter.

istered with antisecretory agents to promote esophageal healing.[17]

Agents that decrease gastric hydrochloric acid secretion are also used in the management of reflux esophagitis. Histamine H_2-receptor blockers (e.g., ranitidine, cimetidine) have no effect on LES pressure but do decrease gastric acid production. They are particularly helpful for the patient with high acid outputs. Antisecretory drugs such as omeprazole (Prilosec) may also be used to decrease acid secretion that would then facilitate the healing of erosive reflux esophagitis. Sucralfate (Carafate), an antiulcer drug, may be used for its cytoprotective properties.

The nurse should observe for and instruct the patient about side effects of the medications being taken. Antacids have minimal side effects. Antacids that contain aluminum tend to cause constipation, whereas those that contain magnesium tend to cause diarrhea. Several of the antacids are combinations of aluminum and magnesium designed to minimize these side effects. If the patient is taking bethanechol, side effects to observe for include urinary urgency, increased salivation, abdominal cramping with diarrhea, nausea, vomiting, and hypotension. Side effects of metoclopramide include restlessness, anxiety, and insomnia. Side effects of sucralfate include drowsiness, dizziness, nausea, vomiting, constipation, urticaria, and rash. Cisapride has fewer side effects than metoclopramide.

Nutritional Management

A diet high in protein and low in fats is recommended for GERD. Fatty foods stimulate the release of cholecystokinin, which decreases LES pressure. Foods that decrease LES pressure, such as chocolate, peppermint, coffee, and tea (see Table 38-5), should be avoided because they cause reflux. Milk products should be avoided, especially at bedtime, because milk increases gastric acid secretion. Small, frequent meals are advised to prevent overdistention of the stomach. Fluids should be taken between rather than with meals to reduce distention. Certain foods (e.g., spicy tomato juice and orange juice) may irritate the acid-sensitive esophagus and thus may have to be avoided. No specific diet is necessary, but foods that cause reflux should be avoided. Weight reduction is recommended if the patient is obese.

NURSING MANAGEMENT

GASTROESOPHAGEAL REFLUX DISEASE

Patients with GERD need to avoid factors that cause reflux. (Measures to prevent reflux are outlined in Table 38-5.) The patient who is a smoker should definitely stop smoking. Smoking causes an almost immediate drop in LES pressure. The patient may need to be referred to other members of the health care team or to community resources for assistance in stopping smoking. Substances that decrease LES pressure and tone should be avoided (see Table 38-5). If stress seems to bring on symptoms, measures to cope with stress should be discussed.

Nursing care for the patient who is having acute symptoms consists mainly of teaching and encouraging the patient to follow the necessary regimen. The nurse should ensure that the head of the bed is elevated correctly (usually on 4- to 6-inch blocks) and that the patient does not lie down during the first 2 to 3 hours after eating. Teaching the patient to avoid food and activities that cause reflux is important (e.g., late-night eating should be avoided). The patient may be taking medications to relieve heartburn, so the nurse will need to observe for side effects and determine whether the medications are relieving symptoms. The patient should also be taught possible side effects of medications.

Surgical intervention may be necessary if conservative therapy fails, if a hiatal hernia is present, or if complications, such as stenosis, chronic esophagitis, and bleeding exist. The objective of surgery is to restore gastroesophageal integrity. Procedures used for the management of hiatal hernia are discussed below.

HIATAL HERNIA

Hiatal hernia is herniation of a portion of the stomach into the esophagus through an opening, or hiatus, in the diaphragm. It is also referred to as *diaphragmatic hernia* and *esophageal hernia.*

Types

Hiatal hernias are classified into two types (Fig. 38-7):

1. *Sliding*: The junction of the stomach and esophagus is above the hiatus of the diaphragm, and a part of the stomach slides through the hiatal opening in the diaphragm. It "slides" into the thoracic cavity when the patient is supine and usually goes back into the abdominal cavity when the patient is standing upright. This is the most common type.

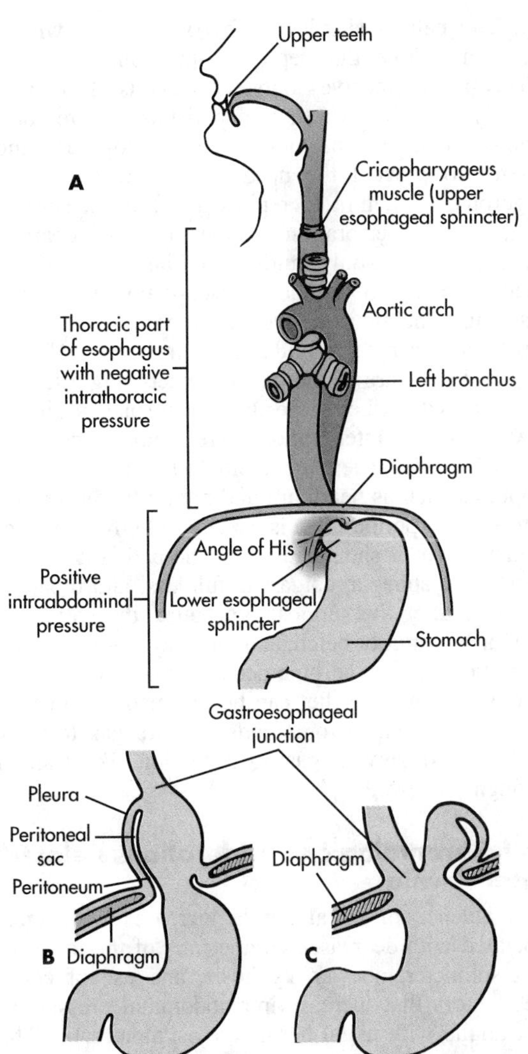

Fig. 38-7 ***A,*** Normal esophagus. ***B,*** Sliding hiatal hernia. ***C,*** Rolling or paraesophageal hernia.

2. *Paraesophageal or rolling*: The esophagogastric junction remains in the normal position, but the fundus and the greater curvature of the stomach roll up through the diaphragm, forming a pocket alongside the esophagus.

Significance

The incidence of hiatal hernia is difficult to determine. Although it is said to be the most common abnormality found on x-ray examination of the upper GI tract, the hernia is often asymptomatic. Hiatal hernias are common in older adults and occur more frequently in women than in men.

Etiology and Pathophysiology

The actual cause of hiatal hernia is unknown. Many factors contribute to the development of hiatal hernia. Structural changes, such as weakening of the muscles in the diaphragm around the esophagogastric opening, are usually contributing factors. Factors that increase intraabdominal pressure, including obesity, pregnancy, ascites, tumors, tight corsets, intense physical exertion, and heavy lifting on a continual basis, may also predispose to development of a hiatal hernia. Other predisposing factors are increased age, trauma, poor nutrition, and a forced recumbent position, as when a prolonged illness confines the person to bed. In some cases, congenital weakness is a contributing factor.

Clinical Manifestations

The signs and symptoms of hiatal hernia are similar to that described under GERD. Frequently the symptoms of hiatal hernia mimic gallbladder disease, peptic ulcer, and angina. However, some patients with hiatal hernia have no symptoms. Reflux and discomfort are also associated with position, occurring soon or several hours after lying down. Bending over may cause a severe burning pain, which is usually relieved by sitting or standing. Other common precipitating factors of pain include large meals, alcohol, and smoking. Nocturnal attacks are common, especially if the person has eaten before going to sleep.

Complications

Complications that may occur with hiatal hernia include problems such as hemorrhage from erosion, stenosis, ulcerations of the herniated portion of the stomach, strangulation of the hernia, and regurgitation with tracheal aspiration. Severe chronic esophagitis may follow reflux problems.

Diagnostic Studies

A barium swallow is an important diagnostic measure that may show the protrusion of gastric mucosa through the esophageal hiatus in the patient with hiatal hernia. Other tests are similar to those described in Table 38-6.

Therapeutic Management

Conservative Management. Conservative management of hiatal hernia includes administration of antacids and antisecretory agents, elimination of constricting garments, avoidance of lifting and straining, elimination of alcohol and smoking, and elevation of the head of the bed. Elevation of the bed on 4- to 6-inch blocks assists gravity in maintaining the stomach in the abdominal cavity and also helps prevent reflux and tracheal aspiration. If obese, the patient is encouraged to lose weight.

Surgical Interventions. The objective of surgical interventions for hiatal hernia is to reduce reflux. To accomplish this the LES must be reinforced. Surgical procedures are termed *valvuloplasties* or *antireflux* procedures. There are three slightly varied procedures: the Nissen fundoplication, the Hill gastroplexy, and the Belsey's fundoplication. These three surgical procedures are all variations of fundoplication, which involves "wrapping" the fundus of the stomach around the lower portion of the esophagus in varying degrees. These procedures reduce the hernia, provide an acceptable LES pressure, and prevent movement of the gastroesophageal junction. The Nissen fundoplication is shown in Fig. 38-8. A thoracic approach may also be used, but the abdominal approach is more common. The Nissen fundoplication procedure is being

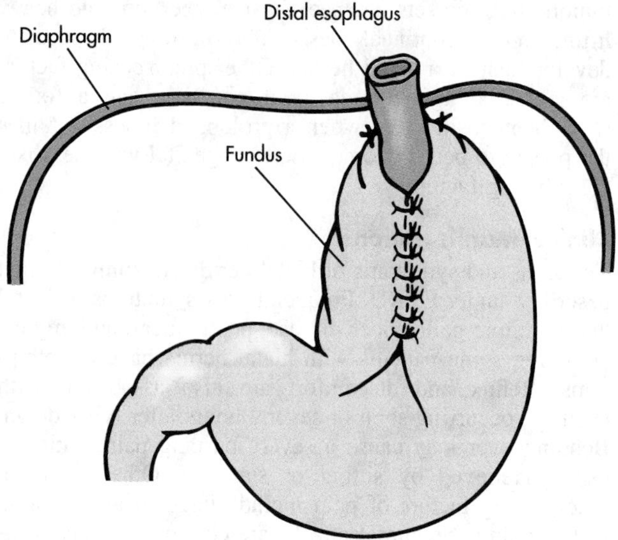

Fig. 38-8 Nissen fundoplication for repair of hiatal hernia. Fundus of stomach is wrapped around distal esophagus and sutured to itself.

performed laparoscopically with increasing frequency. The use of laparoscopic techniques has reduced the overall morbidity associated with abdominal surgery.[18,19]

Fundoplication prevents reflux in 90% of the patients. The success of fundoplication depends on achieving correct tightness of the fundal wrap. If it is too loose, reflux is not prevented. If it is too tight, dysphagia and the gas-bloat syndrome are problems.

An antireflux prosthesis, called the Angelchik antireflux prosthesis, is also available. This prothesis is a ring-shaped silicone gel with a tie strap attached. It is tied around the esophagus to prevent the stomach from sliding above the diaphragm. Complications of the Angelchik prosthesis include dysphagia, gas-bloat syndrome, and slipping or migration of the prosthesis.

NURSING MANAGEMENT

SURGICAL INTERVENTIONS FOR HIATAL HERNIA

Postoperative care focuses on concerns related to prevention of respiratory complications, maintenance of fluid and electrolyte balance, and prevention of infection. If a thoracic approach is used, a chest tube is inserted. Assessment and management related to closed chest drainage are important (see Chapter 24).

Respiratory complications can occur in a patient treated by an abdominal approach because of the high abdominal incision. Respiratory assessment should include respiratory rate and rhythm, chest reexpansion, pulse rate and rhythm, and signs of pneumothorax (e.g., dyspnea, chest pain, cyanosis). Coughing and deep breathing are essential to fully expand the lungs. Pulmonary physiotherapy is necessary. The patient should not be oversedated with drugs, such as morphine, that depress respiration.

The patient receives only intravenous (IV) fluids and electrolytes until the return of peristalsis. Care should be taken to maintain patency of the nasogastric tube (if present) to prevent the need to reinsert the tube. It is dangerous to attempt to replace the tube because of the possibility of perforation of the surgical repair. When peristalsis returns, only fluids are initially given. Solids are added gradually so that the stomach is not overloaded. The nurse must maintain an accurate recording of intake and output and observe for fluid and electrolyte imbalances (see Chapter 13). (Care of the patient undergoing a laparotomy procedure is described in the nursing care plan in Chapter 40.)

After surgical intervention, there should be no symptoms of gastric reflux. The patient should be instructed to report symptoms such as heartburn and regurgitation. In the early postoperative period there is usually mild dysphagia caused by edema, but it should resolve. The patient should report persistent dysphagia, epigastric fullness, and bloating. Immediately after the surgical procedure, the patient cannot voluntarily vomit or belch, and this may cause the gas-bloat syndrome. If this syndrome persists, medical advice should be sought. A normal diet can be resumed within 6 weeks. The patient should avoid foods that are gas forming and should try to prevent gastric distention. Food should be thoroughly chewed.

Gerontologic Considerations Related to Hiatal Hernia

The incidence of hiatal hernia increases with age. It is associated with decreased competency of the lower esophageal sphincter, obesity, kyphosis, and use of corsets or other factors that increase intraabdominal pressure. Some older adults with hiatal hernia are asymptomatic. The first indications may include esophageal bleeding secondary to esophagitis or pulmonary complications (e.g., aspiration, pneumonia) related to aspiration of gastric contents.

The clinical course and management of the problem are similar to that for the younger adult. With the increased use of laparoscopic procedures, surgical risks have been reduced. However, an older adult with cardiovascular and pulmonary problems may not be a good candidate for surgical intervention. In addition, changes in lifestyle, including elimination of dietary factors, such as caffeine-containing beverages and chocolate, and sleeping with additional pillows and elevating the head of the bed on blocks, may be more difficult.

MALIGNANT NEOPLASMS OF THE ESOPHAGUS

Significance

Carcinoma of the esophagus is unique in its geographic distribution. There are portions of Asia in which the rate of esophageal cancer is extremely high while in Western societies the incidence is low. The incidence of squamous cell esophageal cancer is currently decreasing in the United States, whereas the incidence of adenocarcinoma of the distal esophagus is increasing.[20] Squamous cell carcinoma, however, remains the most common form of esophageal cancer. The incidence of squamous cell carcinoma of the esophagus increases with age. There is a higher incidence of squamous cell carcinoma in African-Americans and in men. Because esophageal cancer is rarely diagnosed in early stages, the 5-year prognosis is poor.[21]

A condition called *Barrett's esophagus* is considered a metaplastic change and may progress to adenocarcinoma of the esophagus. This syndrome is characterized by replacement of areas of the normal squamous epithelium of the esophagus with columnar epithelium. It may result from severe reflux esophagitis and is considered a potential complication of GERD.[22]

Pathophysiology

The cause of cancer of the esophagus is unknown. Possible predisposing factors are cigarette smoking, excessive alcohol intake, chronic trauma, poor oral hygiene, and spicy foods. The two most important risk factors are smoking and excessive alcohol intake. Other risk factors include exposure to asbestos and metal and low intake of fresh fruits and vegetables.[20] Certain conditions of the esophagus, such as achalasia, diverticula, and lye burns, are considered premalignant lesions.

The malignant tumor usually appears as an ulcerated lesion. It may have advanced to this stage before the appearance of symptoms. The majority of tumors are located in the middle and lower portions of the esophagus. The tumor may penetrate the muscular layer and even extend outside the wall of the esophagus. Obstruction of the esophagus occurs in the later stages.

Clinical Manifestations

The onset of symptoms is usually late in relation to the extent of the tumor. Progressive dysphagia is the most common symptom and may be expressed as a substernal feeling as if food is not passing. Initially the dysphagia occurs only with meat, then with soft foods, and eventually with liquids.

Pain develops later and is described as occurring in the substernal, epigastric, or back areas and usually increases with swallowing. The pain may radiate to the neck, jaw, ears, and shoulders. If the tumor is in the upper third of the esophagus, symptoms such as sore throat, choking, and hoarseness may occur. Weight loss is fairly common. When esophageal stenosis is severe, regurgitation of blood-flecked esophageal contents is common.

Complications

Hemorrhage may occur if the cancer erodes into the aorta. Esophageal perforation with fistula formation into the lung or trachea sometimes develops. The tumor may enlarge enough to cause esophageal obstruction. Esophageal carcinoma has a poor prognosis because of early lymphatic spread and late development of symptoms. The liver and lung are common metastatic sites.

Diagnostic Studies

Barium swallow with fluoroscopy may demonstrate a narrowing of the esophagus at the site of the tumor (Table 38-8). Sometimes a crater is visible. Esophagoscopy with biopsy is necessary to make a definitive diagnosis of carcinoma by identification of malignant cells. Endoscopic ultrasonography is also used to detect tumor invasion into the muscle layer. A bronchoscopic examination may be performed to detect malignant involvement of the trachea. Computerized tomography scanning may be used to more accurately assess the extent of the disease.

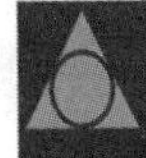

Table 38-8 Therapeutic Management: Carcinoma of the Esophagus

Diagnostic
- Barium swallow
- Esophagoscopy with biopsy
- Ultrasonography
- Bronchoscopy

Therapeutic
- Surgical resection
  - Esophagectomy
  - Esophagogastrostomy
  - Esophagoenterostomy
- Radiation
- Palliative
  - Dilatation
  - Stent or prosthesis
  - Gastrostomy
  - Laser therapy

Therapeutic Management

The treatment of carcinoma of the esophagus depends on the location of the tumor and whether invasion or metastasis has occurred (see Table 38-8). Surgical removal and radiation are the two methods used. Cancer of the esophagus has a poor prognosis, mainly because in most cases it is not diagnosed until the disease is advanced. Relatively few people are cured. The best results have been obtained with a combination of surgery and radiation. Chemotherapeutic agents are currently under investigation.[23]

If the tumor is in the cervical section (upper third) of the esophagus, radiation is usually indicated. A tumor in the lower third of the esophagus is usually resected surgically. In addition, radiation may be used either before or after surgery.

The types of surgical procedures that can be performed are (1) removal of part or all of the esophagus (*esophagectomy*) with use of a Dacron graft to replace the resected part; (2) resection of a portion of the esophagus and anastomosis of the remaining portion to the stomach (*esophagogastrostomy*); and (3) resection of a portion of the esophagus and anastomosis of a segment of colon to the remaining portion (*esophagoenterostomy*). The surgical approaches may be thoracic or both abdominal and thoracic.

Surgery may not be performed when the patient is an older adult or in poor physical health. Palliative therapy consists of restoration of the swallowing function and maintenance of nutrition and hydration. Palliation can be achieved by dilatation, stent placement, or both. Laser therapy or vaporization of the tumor by means of endoscopy may be used in combination with dilatation. Obstruction recurs as the tumor grows, but laser therapy can be repeated. Sometimes these procedures are combined with radiation therapy. Other measures for palliation include gastrostomy and esophagostomy.

Dilatation is done with various types of dilators (e.g., Celestin tube). Dilatation often relieves dysphagia and allows for improved nutrition. Placement of a stent or prosthesis may help when dilatation is no longer effective. The prostheses are composed of silicone rubber or nylon-reinforced latex tubes with distal and proximal collars. The prosthesis is placed in the esophagus so that food and fluids can pass through the stenotic segment of the esophagus. The prosthesis can be placed endoscopically.

Nutritional Management. After esophageal surgery, parenteral fluids are given for several days. When fluids are allowed after bowel sounds have returned, 30 to 60 ml of water are given hourly, with gradual progression to small, frequent bland meals. The patient should be in an upright position to prevent regurgitation of the fluid. The patient is observed for signs of intolerance to the feeding or leakage of the feeding into the mediastinum. Symptoms to report that indicate leakage are pain, increased temperature, and dyspnea. Symptoms of food intolerance include vomiting and abdominal distention.

A gastrostomy may be performed for the purpose of feeding the patient. It involves the insertion of a retention or mushroom catheter into the stomach.

NURSING MANAGEMENT

ESOPHAGEAL CANCER

Nursing Assessment

The patient should be assessed for progressive dysphagia and odynophagia (burning, squeezing pain while swallowing). The nurse should question the patient regarding the type of substances ingested that cause dysphagia, such as meat, soft foods, and liquids. The patient should also be assessed for pain (substernal, epigastric, or back areas), choking, hoarseness, cough, anorexia, weight loss, and regurgitation (sometimes bloody). The patient should also be questioned regarding tobacco and alcohol use.

Nursing Diagnoses

Nursing diagnoses specific to the patient with esophageal cancer include, but are not limited to, the following:

- Altered nutrition: less than body requirements related to dysphagia, odynophagia, weakness, and radiation therapy
- Pain related to tumor
- Anxiety related to diagnosis of cancer, uncertain future, and poor prognosis
- Anticipatory grieving related to diagnosis of life-threatening malignancy
- Altered health maintenance related to lack of knowledge of disease process and therapeutic regimen, unavailability of a support system, and chronic debilitating disease.

Planning

The overall goals are that the patient with esophageal cancer will (1) have relief of symptoms including pain and dysphagia, (2) achieve optimal nutritional intake, (3) understand the prognosis of the disease, and (4) experience a quality of life appropriate to disease progression.

Nursing Implementation

Health Promotion and Maintenance. Because the cause of esophageal cancer is not definitive, it is difficult to identify preventive measures. Health counseling needs to focus on elimination of smoking and of excessive alcohol intake. Maintenance of good oral hygiene and dietary habits (intake of fresh fuits and vegetables) may also be helpful.

Having the patient obtain treatment of esophageal problems, such as achalasia and diverticula, may be helpful, because these are considered premalignant problems. Early diagnosis of esophageal tumors is important but difficult because the onset of symptoms is usually late. The patient should be encouraged to have regular physical examinations and to seek medical attention for any esophageal problems, especially dysphagia. The patient who is at risk of esophageal adenocarcinoma, such as those with Barrett's esophagus, may need regular (yearly) endoscopic screening with biopsy and cytologic study.

Acute Intervention

Preoperative care. In addition to general preoperative teaching and preparation, particular attention to the patient's nutritional needs and oral care is important. Many patients are poorly nourished because of the inability to ingest adequate amounts of food and fluids before surgery. A high-caloric, high-protein diet should be provided. It may have to be in liquid form. Some patients may need IV fluid replacement or total parenteral nutrition. The nurse must keep an accurate intake and output record and assess the patient for signs of fluid and electrolyte imbalance.

Meticulous oral care is essential. A thorough cleaning of the mouth, including tongue, gingivae, and teeth or dentures, is necessary. It may be necessary to use swabs or a gauze pad and to really scrub the mouth, including the tongue. Milk of magnesia with mineral oil may be used to remove crust formation. A mixture of mouthwash, ice, and water makes a refreshing rinse for the patient.

Teaching should include information about chest tubes (if a thoracic approach is used), IV lines, nasogastric tube, gastrostomy feeding, turning, coughing, and deep breathing. (General preoperative care is presented in Chapter 14.)

Postoperative care. The patient usually has a nasogastric tube in place, and there may be bloody drainage for 8 to 12 hours. The drainage gradually changes to greenish yellow. Assessment of the drainage, maintenance of the tube, and oral and nasal care are nursing responsibilities.

Because of the location of the incision and the general condition of the patient, special emphasis must be placed on prevention of respiratory complications. Turning, coughing, and deep breathing should be done every 2 hours. Use of an incentive spirometer helps in preventing respiratory complications.

The patient should be positioned in a semi-Fowler's or Fowler's position to prevent reflux of gastric secretions. When the patient can drink fluids or eat, the upright position should be maintained for at least 2 hours after eating to assist the movement of food through the GI tract. Radiation therapy may be given as an adjunct to surgery or as primary therapy (see Chapter 12).

Chronic and Home Management. Many patients require long-term follow-up care after surgery or radiation for esophageal cancer. The patient needs encouragement and assistance in maintaining adequate nutrition. The patient may need a permanent feeding gastrostomy. The patient usually has fears and anxieties about a diagnosis of cancer. The nurse should know what the doctor has told the patient regarding the prognosis and then provide appropriate counseling. Some communities have resource groups consisting of persons with cancer who can serve as support systems. Groups can usually be contacted through the local chapter of the American Cancer Society.

Referral to a community health nurse may be necessary for continued care of the patient (e.g., gastrostomy teaching and follow-up wound care). (Management of the terminally ill patient is discussed in Chapter 12.)

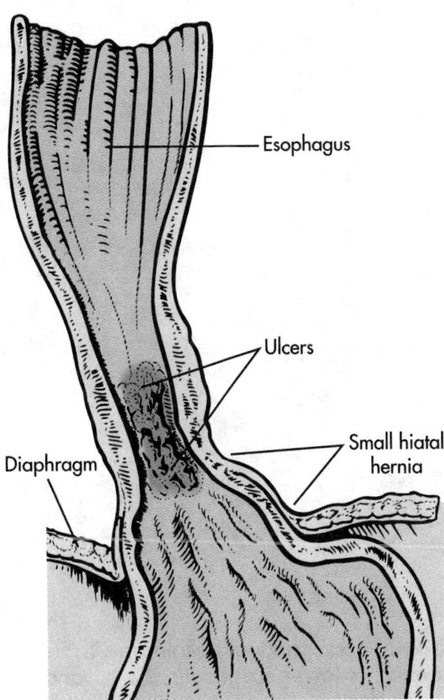

Fig. 38-9 Esophagitis with esophageal ulcerations.

OTHER ESOPHAGEAL DISORDERS

Esophagitis

Esophagitis (inflammation of the esophagus) is a frequent condition and may occur as a result of chemical irritation from lye or dust or physical irritants such as smoking, cold or hot liquids, and excessive alcoholic intake. Trauma to the esophagus may also produce inflammation. *Achalasia* (cardiospasm) and carcinoma may lead to esophagitis. (Esophagitis with esophageal ulcerations is shown in Fig. 38-9.)

Reflux esophagitis is common. It results from the reflux of gastric contents into the esophagus (see section on Gastrointestinal Reflux Disease, earlier in chapter). A sliding hiatal hernia is a common cause of reflux esophagitis (see section on Hiatal Hernia), although it occurs in many patients without hiatal hernia. Esophagitis results from an incompetent LES.

Treatment of esophagitis depends on the cause. If strong alkalis or acids cause acute esophagitis, prompt, vigorous treatment is necessary. The treatment of chronic esophagitis includes oral antacids, histamine H_2-antagonists, a bland diet, and sleeping with the head of the bed elevated. The goal of treatment is to prevent gastric juices from damaging the esophageal mucosa.

Diverticula

Diverticula are saclike outpouchings of one or more layers of the esophagus. They occur in three main areas: (1) above the upper esophageal sphincter (Zenker's diverticulum), which is the most common location; (2) near the esophageal midpoint (traction); and (3) above the LES (epiphrenic) (Fig. 38-10). The main symptoms are dysphagia and regurgitation, especially with Zenker's diverticulum. Traction diverticula may not cause signs and symptoms. The patient frequently complains of tasting sour food and smelling a foul odor caused by the stagnant food.

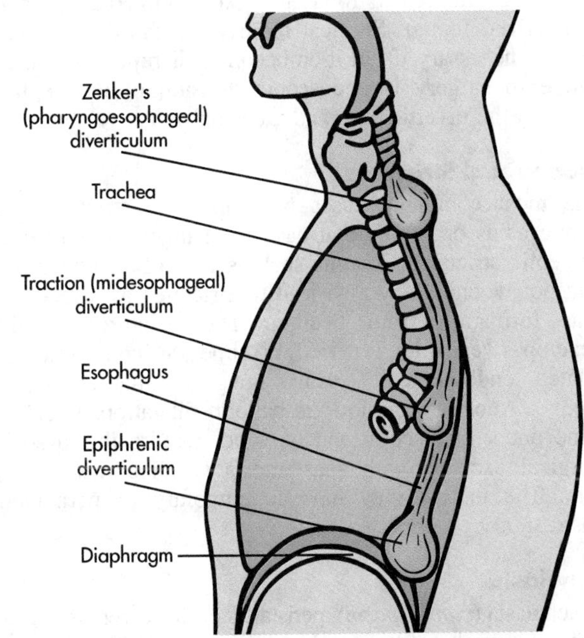

Fig. 38-10 Possible sites for the occurrence of esophageal diverticula. These hollow outpouchings may occur just above the upper esophageal sphincter (Zenker's, the most common type of pulsion diverticulum), near the midpoint of the esophagus (traction), and just above the lower esophageal sphincter (epiphrenic).

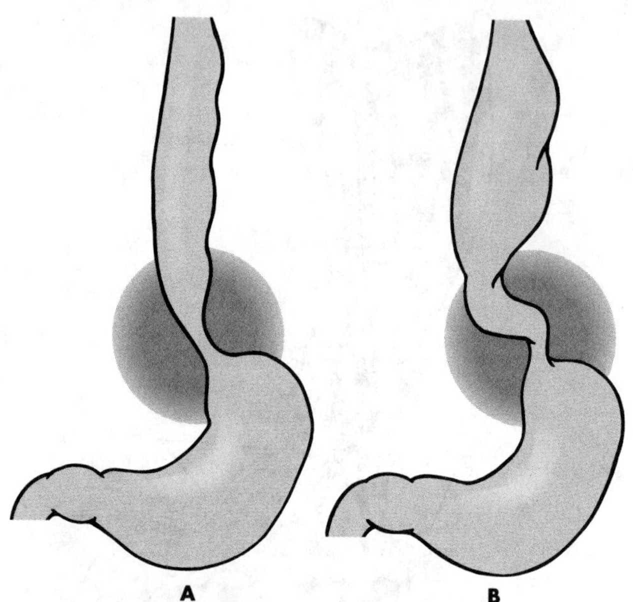

Fig. 38-11 Esophageal achalasia. ***A,*** Early stage, showing tapering of lower esophagus. ***B,*** Advanced stage, showing dilated, tortuous esophagus.

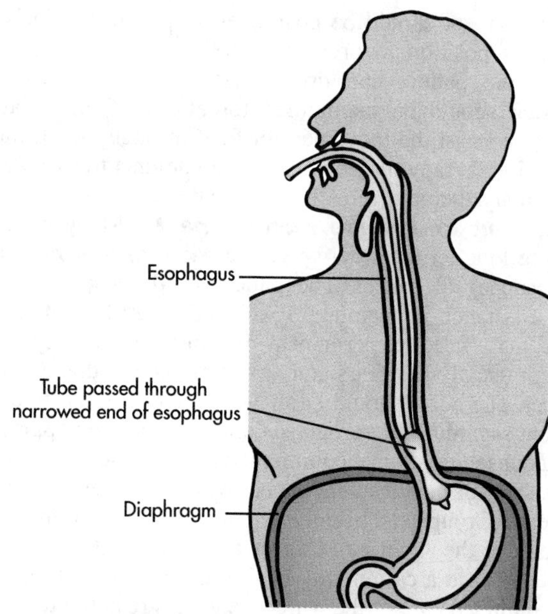

Fig. 38-12 Pneumatic dilatation attempts to treat achalasia by maintaining an adequate lumen and decreasing lower esophageal sphincter (LES) tone.

Complications include malnutrition, aspiration, and perforation.

There is no specific treatment for diverticula. Some patients find they can empty the pocket of food that collects by applying pressure at a point on the neck. The diet may have to be limited to foods that pass more readily (e.g., blenderized foods). Surgical removal of the diverticulum may be necessary if nutrition becomes disrupted. An alternative to surgery is endoscopic division of the septum between the diverticulum and the esophagus.

Esophageal Strictures

The most common causes of esophageal strictures are strong acids or alkalis that have been ingested and reflux or peptic strictures. Trauma such as throat lacerations and gunshot wounds may also lead to strictures as a result of scar formation from healing. The strictures usually develop over a long period of time. Strictures can be dilated endoscopically using bougies (dilating instruments). Another technique is balloon dilatation, which is done under endoscopy and does not require fluoroscopy. Surgical excision with anastomosis is sometimes necessary. The patient may have a temporary or permanent gastrostomy.

Achalasia

In achalasia (*cardiospasm*), peristalsis of the lower two thirds (smooth muscle) of the esophagus is absent. LES pressure is increased, along with incomplete relaxation of the lower esophageal sphincter. The result of this condition is dilatation of the lower esophagus (Fig. 38-11). Obstruction of the esophagus at or near the diaphragm also occurs. Food and fluid accumulate in the lower esophagus. The altered peristalsis is a result of impairment of the autonomic nervous system innervating the esophagus. Achalasia affects all ages and both genders. The course of the disease is chronic.

Dysphagia is the most common symptom and occurs more frequently with liquids. Substernal chest pain (similar to the pain of angina) occurs during or immediately after a meal. Halitosis and the inability to eructate are other symptoms. Another common symptom is regurgitation of sour-tasting food and liquids, especially when the patient is in a horizontal position. Weight loss is typical.

Treatment consists of dilatation, surgery, and use of drugs. All are directed at relieving the stasis caused by the increased LES pressure, nonrelaxing LES, and aperistaltic esophagus. The aim of therapeutic management is to relieve symptoms. Symptomatic treatment consists of a semisoft bland diet, eating slowly and drinking fluid with meals, and sleeping with the head elevated.

Esophageal dilatation (*bougienage*) is an effective treatment measure for many patients. Pneumatic dilatation of the LES with a balloon-tipped dilator passed orally is usually used. Commonly used dilators for pneumatic dilatation are the Mosher bag, the Tucker mercury dilator, and the Browne-McHardy dilator. They all depend on forcible expansion of a balloon in the LES (Fig. 38-12). The forceful dilatation does not restore normal esophageal motility but does provide for emptying of the esophagus into the stomach.

Surgical intervention may become necessary. An *esophagomyotomy* may be performed. In this procedure the muscle fibers that enclose the narrowed area of the esophagus are divided. This allows the mucosa to pouch out through the division in the muscle layer to allow food to be swallowed without obstruction.

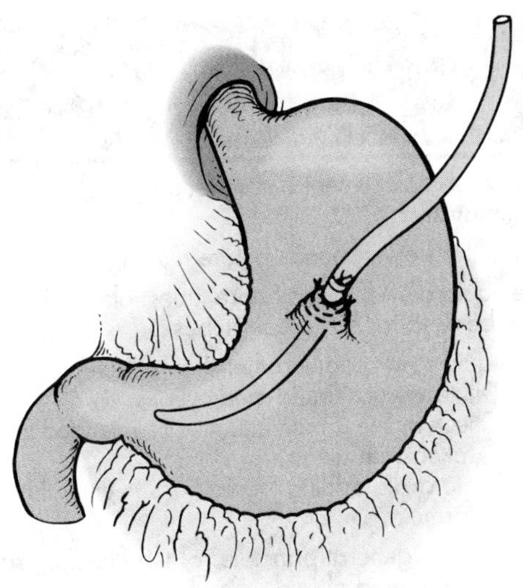

Fig. 38-13 Placement of a gastrostomy tube.

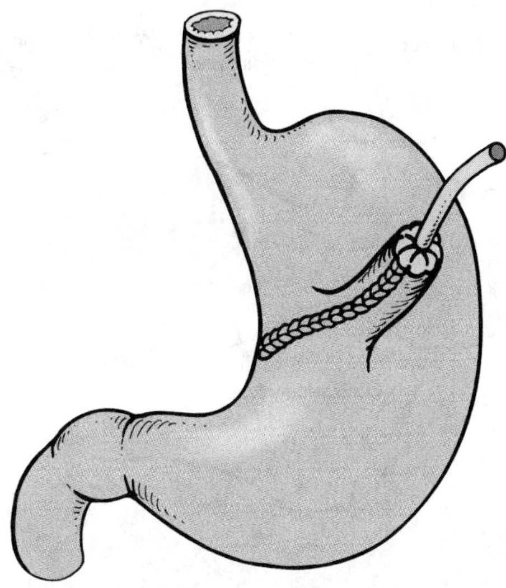

Fig. 38-14 Janeway gastrostomy.

A similar procedure is Heller's myotomy (cardiomyotomy), which disrupts the LES in a similar manner and reduces LES pressure. An antireflux procedure is frequently done with the myotomy.

Classes of drugs used in the treatment of achalasia include anticholinergics, calcium channel antagonists (nifedipine is one of the best), and long-acting nitrates.

Esophageal Varices

Esophageal varices are dilated, tortuous veins occurring in the lower portion of the esophagus as a result of portal hypertension (see Chapter 41).

GASTROSTOMY

Types of Gastrostomy Tubes

A gastrostomy bypasses the esophagus and allows feedings to maintain or restore the patient's nutrition. A catheter is placed in the stomach and sutured in place. The connecting end is brought to the surface and sutured to the skin (Fig. 38-13).

A permanent gastrostomy, such as a Janeway gastrostomy, may be used for a patient who requires tube feedings over an extended time. A permanent gastrostomy allows for removal of the feeding tube between feedings. A tube of gastric tissue is formed and brought out to form a stoma at the skin surface (Fig. 38-14). A small catheter (5 to 10F) is inserted at the skin surface. The stoma forms a seal when the catheter is removed. Problems of leakage and skin irritation are decreased or eliminated.[24]

Percutaneous Endoscopic Gastrostomy. A gastrostomy tube may be placed by means of *percutaneous endoscopic gastrostomy* (PEG) (Fig. 38-15). The patient must have an intact, unobstructed GI tract, and the esophageal lumen must be wide enough to pass the endoscope. A PEG has several advantages. The procedure itself has fewer risks (no general anesthesia or laparotomy), it can be done at a lower cost, and it requires minimum or no sedation in the patient who is severely compromised by the condition. The most frequent complications of gastrostomy feedings include aspiration pneumonia, accidental tube removal, wound cellulitis, and clogged tubes.[24]

Feedings can usually be started when bowel sounds are present, usually within 24 hours after catheter placement. Immediately after tube insertion, the tube length from the insertion site to the distal end should be measured and recorded. The tube is then marked at the skin insertion site.[24] Then at regular intervals the tube insertion length should be rechecked. The catheter is frequently connected to a pump for continuous feeding. Tap water may be infused within 2 hours after placement. For the patient with chronic reflux, a jejunostomy tube with jejunostomy feedings may be necessary to reduce reflux. Some important nursing implications for care and feeding of patients with PEGs are listed in Table 38-9.

Feedings

The first gastrostomy feeding consists of either water or glucose in water, 30 to 60 ml at a time with a gradual progression to food. The feeding may consist of blended foods or a special formula. Commercial formulas are preferable for small lumen tubes because of the risk of tube clogging. Blenderized feedings promote better bowel function and may be more acceptable psychologically. However, the milk content of these diets should be considered, because many adults have relative lactose intolerance. The feeding should be given at room or body temperature to decrease the likelihood of diarrhea and other GI complaints. Privacy should be provided. The head should be elevated in a normal eating position (or at least 30 degrees) and should remain elevated for 30 to 60 minutes after the feeding. This may be more difficult for a patient receiving continuous gastrostomy feedings.

Before introducing the feeding, the nurse should aspirate gastric contents and measure the amount. If greater than 100 ml is present, the next feeding should be delayed for 30 minutes. The aspirate should be reinstilled. A syringe or

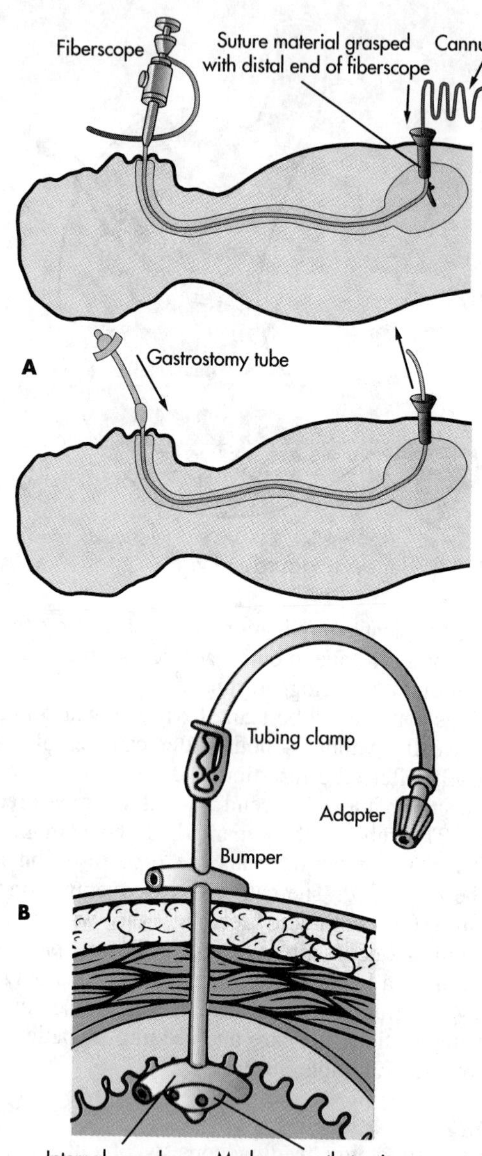

Fig. 38-15 Percutaneous endoscopic gastrostomy. ***A,*** Gastrostomy tube placement via percutaneous endoscopy. Using endoscopy a gastrostomy tube is inserted through the esophagus into the stomach and then pulled through a stab wound made in the abdominal wall. ***B,*** A retention disk and bumper secure the tube.

funnel is used to introduce the liquid into the tube. A small amount of water is first inserted to make sure the tube is patent. The catheter should be clamped at all times that feedings are not being given to prevent air from entering the tube. It should not be unclamped until the feeding is placed in a feeding bag or funnel. The feeding is usually 200 to 500 ml (depending on total caloric need) and if administered by gravity, should be administered over 15 to 30 minutes. After the feeding is finished, the tube should be cleared with water. The catheter is sometimes removed after approximately 2 weeks and reinserted for each feeding. It should be inserted approximately 4 to 6 inches.

Table 38-9 Nursing Management: Percutaneous Endoscopic Gastrostomy

- Check tube placement before feeding and drug administration.
- Assess for bowel sounds before feeding.
- Use liquid diets for small bore tubes; blenderized diets may be used for large bore tubes.
- Use liquid medications rather than pills.
  - Dilute viscous liquid medications.
  - Check to see if medications are intended to be taken with meals.
  - Try to avoid adding medications to enteral feeding formula.
- Follow other general principles of tube feeding such as elevating head of bed, checking for residual volumes, and flushing tube with water.
- Assess regularly for complications, such as aspiration, diarrhea, abdominal distention, hyperglycemia, constipation, and fecal impaction.

Rather than intermittent feedings, continuous feedings by means of an infusion pump are used frequently. A patient can remain at home with the infusion pumps.

The pleasurable aspects of eating, such as smelling, seeing, tasting, and chewing the food, are denied the patient with a gastrostomy. The patient should be allowed to smell, taste, and even chew small amounts of food before the feeding, then the chewed food must be spit out. The patient may hesitate to do this because it is not esthetic, but it stimulates salivary and gastric secretions and provides the pleasurable sensations associated with oral intake. The patient may become depressed and need frequent encouragement. The nurse should allow expression of feelings about being fed through a tube. Greater satisfaction may be experienced with self-feedings, and the patient should be taught self-feeding if possible. The patient should be encouraged to sit with the family during meals.

Complications Related to Gastrostomy Feedings. Complications related to gastrostomy feeding are similar to those outlined for tube feedings (see Table 37-17). A patient with a gastrostomy tube is at risk for pulmonary aspiration, particularly if there is diminished gag reflex, history of reflux, or delayed gastric emptying. Because of the powerful antral contractions there is a tendency for the tube to move distally if not properly secured. Therefore the position of the tube should be checked before each feeding or at least once each every 24 hours in the patient receiving continuous feeding. If the tube moves into the duodenum or jejunum and bolus feedings are administered, the patient will experience "dumping syndrome" and diarrhea.

Skin Care

Skin care around the gastrostomy is important because the action of the gastric juice is irritating to the skin. The nurse should try to prevent two possible problems: (1) skin irritation and (2) pulling out of the tube. The skin around the gastrostomy should be assessed daily for signs of redness and maceration. The skin should be kept clean and dry. It should be cleaned with sterile swabs moistened with hydrogen peroxide solution diluted to half strength with sterile water. Then the skin should be rinsed with sterile water and dried. Once the site has healed, it can be washed with mild soap and water. A protective ointment (zinc oxide, petrolatum gauze) or a skin barrier (karaya, Stomahesive) may be used on the skin around the gastrostomy. A small dressing may be placed around the tube. It needs to be changed promptly if it gets wet. Other types of drain or tube pouches may be used if there is a problem with skin irritation.

The patient and family members should be taught how to care for the gastrostomy. Teaching should include skin care, care of the tube, and complete information about feedings. (Additional information on tube feedings is presented in Chapter 37.)

FOOD POISONING

Food poisoning is a nonspecific term that describes acute GI symptoms, such as nausea, vomiting, diarrhea, and colicky abdominal pain caused by the intake of contaminated food. Food most commonly causes illness if it is contaminated with microorganisms or their products. The GI tract is frequently the portal of entry for the microorganisms. The two main types of food poisoning are (1) acute gastroenteritis from bacteria and (2) neurologic symptoms from botulism. The most common bacterial food poisonings are presented in Table 38-10.

Foods may be contaminated by poisonous chemicals, such as mercury, arsenic, zinc, and potassium chlorate. Poisoning can also occur from ingestion of poisonous plants (e.g., certain mushroom species).

The nursing role in relation to food poisoning is mainly health teaching to prevent its occurrence. Teaching should include correct food preparation and cleanliness, adequate cooking, and refrigeration. If the patient is hospitalized, nursing care focuses on correction of fluid and electrolyte imbalance from diarrhea and vomiting. With botulism, additional assessment and care relative to neurologic symptoms are indicated (see Chapter 57).

Table 38-10 Bacterial Food Poisoning

Type	Causative Agent	Sources	Onset of Symptoms (hr)	Symptoms	Treatment	Prevention
Staphylococcal	Toxin from *Staphylococcus aureus*	Meat, bakery products, milk; skin and respiratory tract of food handlers	1-6	Vomiting, abdominal cramping, diarrhea	Symptomatic, fluid and electrolyte replacement, antiemetics	Immediate refrigeration of foods, monitoring of food handlers
Clostridial	*Clostridium perfringens*	Meat or poultry dishes cooked at lower temperature (stew or pot pie), rewarmed meat dishes, improperly canned vegetables	8-24	Diarrhea, abdominal cramps, vomiting (rare); midepigastrium pain	Symptomatic, fluid replacement	Correct preparation of meat dishes, serving of food immediately after cooking or rapid cooling of food
Salmonella	*Salmonella typhimurium* (grows in gut)	Improperly cooked poultry, pork, beef, lamb, and eggs	8-24	Nausea and vomiting, diarrhea, abdominal cramps, fever and chills	Symptomatic, fluid and electrolyte replacement	Correct preparation of food
Botulism	Toxin from *Clostridium botulinum*, ingested toxin absorbed from gut and blocks acetylcholine at neuromuscular junction	Improperly canned or preserved food, home-preserved vegetables (most common), preserved fruits and fish, canned commercial products	12-36	GI symptoms of nausea, vomiting, abdominal pain, constipation, distention Central nervous system symptoms of headache, dizziness, muscular incoordination, weakness, inability to talk or swallow, diplopia, breathing difficulties, paralysis, delirium, coma	Maintenance of ventilation, polyvalent antitoxin, guanidine hydrochloric acid (enhances acetylcholine release)	Correct processing of canned foods, boiling of suspected canned foods for 15 min before serving
Escherichia coli	*E. coli* serotype 0157:H7	Contaminated beef	>16	Bloody stools, hemolytic uremic syndrome	Symptomatic, fluid and electrolyte replacement	Correct preparation of food.

CRITICAL THINKING EXERCISES

CASE STUDY

HIATAL HERNIA

Patient Profile

Mary, 63 years old, has had a sliding hiatal hernia for 10 years. Mary is admitted to the hospital for a hiatal hernia repair.

Subjective Data

- Reports increasing heartburn, especially at night
- Is currently on a bland diet and taking antacids
- Complains of substernal pain and heartburn
- Reports some problems with regurgitation

Objective Data

Physical Examination

- 5 feet 2 inches tall and weighs 195 pounds

Diagnostic Study

Barium swallow and an esophagoscopy revealed a large sliding hiatal hernia.

Therapeutic Management

Mary had a Nissen fundoplication through a laparoscopic approach.

Critical Thinking Questions

1. Explain the pathophysiology of a hiatal hernia. What is the difference between a sliding and a paraesophageal hiatal hernia?
2. What are the characteristic symptoms of a hiatal hernia? Which of these did Mary have?
3. Describe a Nissen fundoplication procedure. What is the objective of this surgical procedure?
4. What are potential postoperative complications, and what nursing measures prevent them?
5. What should be included in a teaching plan for Mary?
6. Based on the assessment data presented, write one or more nursing diagnoses. Are there any collaborative problems?

NURSING RESEARCH ISSUES

1. What are the most effective methods to get an individual to comply with dental and oral hygiene care?
2. What are the most effective topical methods to relieve pain related to stomatitis secondary to infection?
3. Are dietary interventions successful in improving symptoms in the patient with gastroesophageal reflux disease?
4. What are the best ways to make gastrostomy feedings seem like they are a "normal" diet?
5. What are the primary psychosocial problems for a patient with a gastrostomy?

REVIEW QUESTIONS

The number of the question corresponds to the same-numbered objective at the beginning of the chapter.

1. The most effective current method for removing plaque is
   a. physical removal by brushing and flossing.
   b. application of a fluoride solution.
   c. addition of antimicrobial agents to toothpaste.
   d. large doses of vitamin C.

2. Treatment of Vincent's infection includes
   a. topical application of antibiotics.
   b. smallpox vaccinations.
   c. viscous lidocaine rinses.
   d. amphotericin B suspension.

3. Which of the following is *not* considered a predisposing factor for carcinoma of the oral cavity?
   a. Pipe smoking
   b. Overexposure to the sun
   c. Poor dental care
   d. Use of lip balm

4. After surgical stabilization of a mandibular fracture the immediate postoperative goal is
   a. communication.
   b. patent airway.
   c. prevention of infection.
   d. nutritional intake.

5. The most characteristic symptom of a hiatal hernia is
   a. dysphagia.
   b. regurgitation.
   c. pyrosis.
   d. coughing.

6. All the following statements about the management of a patient with a hiatal hernia are true *except*
   a. the patient should be taught to avoid tight clothing and bending.
   b. the overweight patient should reduce body weight.
   c. the head of the bed may be elevated on blocks.
   d. the drug of choice is an anticholinergic.

7. The most common symptom of esophageal carcinoma is

a. sore throat.
b. dysphagia.
c. weight loss.
d. hemorrhage.

8. Which of the following is most likely to cause reflux esophagitis?

a. Outpouching of the muscular layer
b. Impairment of the autonomic nerve plexus
c. Incompetent LES
d. Stricture of the esophagus

9. All of the following statements about gastrostomy feedings are true *except*

a. the feeding may be blended foods or a special formula.
b. the feeding should be warmed to 104° F (38° C).
c. residual volumes should be checked before feeding.
d. water should be given before and after feedings.

10. The food poisoning in which vomiting is the prominent symptom and food sources are meat, bakery products, and milk is

a. staphylococcal.
b. salmonella.
c. botulism.
d. clostridial.

REFERENCES

1. Oral Health Coordinating Committee: Public Health Service, *Public Health Report* 108:657, 1993.
2. Stoltenberg JL and others: Prevalence of periodontal disease in a health maintenance organization and comparisons to the national survey of oral health. *J Periodontol* 64:853, 1993.
3. Douglas CW, Fox CH: Cross-sectional studies in periodontal disease: current status and implications for dental practice, *Adv Dent Res* 7:25, 1993.
4. Newbrun E: Preventing dental caries: breaking the chain of transmission, *Am J Dent Ass* 123:55, 1992.
5. Woodall I, Wefel J, Young NS: Fluoride therapy. In *Comprehensive dental hygiene care,* ed 4, St Louis, 1993, Mosby.
6. Sandham HJ and others: Clinical trials in adults of an antimicrobial varnish for reducing mutans streptococci, *J Dent Res* 70:1401, 1991.
7. von Wowern N and others: ITI implants with overdentures: a prevention of bone loss in edentulous mandibles, *Int J Oral Maxillofac Implants* 5:135, 1990.
8. Gullane P: Lip. In Gluckman JL, Gullane P, and Johnson J, editors: *Practical approaches to head and neck tumors,* New York, 1995, Raven Press.
9. Wolf GT, Hong WK: Induction chemotherapy as part of a new treatment strategy to preserve the larynx in advance laryngeal cancer. In Johnson JT, Didolkar MS, editors: *Head and neck cancer,* Vol III, Amsterdam, 1992, Elsevier Sciences Excerpta Medica.
10. Gluckman JL, Gullane P, Johnson J: *Practical approaches to head and neck tumors,* New York, 1995, Raven Press.
11. aWengen DF, Donald PJ: Complications of radical neck dissection. In Shockley WW, Pillsbury HC, editors: *The neck: diagnosis, and surgery,* St Louis, 1992, Mosby.
12. Podd TJ and others: Treatment of oral cancers using iridium-192 interstitial irradiation, *Br J Oral Maxillofac Surg* 32:207, 1994.
13. Hamilton SR: Esophagus. In Goldman H, Ming SC, editors: *Pathology of the gastrointestinal tract,* Philadelphia, 1992, WB Saunders.
14. Schulze-Delrieu KS, Summers RW: Esophageal diseases. In Stein JH, editor: *Internal Medicine,* ed 4, St Louis, 1994, Mosby.
15. DeVault KR, Castell DO: Current diagnosis and treatment of gastroesophageal reflux disease, *Mayo Clin Proc* 69:867, 1994.
16. Fass R, Mackel C, Sampliner RE: 24-hour pH monitoring in symptomatic patients without erosive esophagitis who did not respond to antireflux treatment, *J Clin Gastroenterol* 19:97, 1994.
17. Robinson M, Maton PN, Decktor DL: The pharmacologic treatment of gastroesophageal reflux disease. In Lewis JH, editor: *A pharmacological approach to gastrointestinal disorders,* Boston, 1994, Williams & Wilkins.
18. McKernan JB: Laparoscopic repair of gastroesophageal reflux disease: Toupet partical fundoplication versus Nissaen fundoplication, *Surg Endos* 8:581, 1994.
19. Hinder RA and others: Laparoscopic Nissen fundoplication is an effective treatment for gastroesophageal reflux disease, *Ann Surg* 220:472, 1994.
20. Blot WJ: Esophageal cancer trends and risk factors, *Semin Oncol* 21:403, 1994.
21. Tio LT and others: Staging and prognosis using endosonography in patients with inoperable esophageal cancer treated with combined intraluminal and external irradiation, *Gastrointest Endosc* 40:304, 1994.
22. Mayer RJ: Overview: the changing nature of esophageal cancer, *Chest* 103: 404S, 1993.
23. Kelsen DP: The role of chemotherapy in the treatment of esophageal cancer, *Chest Surg Clin N Amer* 4:173, 1994.
24. Caring for a gastrostomy: guidelines and troubleshooting tips, *Nursing* 24:48, 1994.

Chapter 39

NURSING ROLE IN MANAGEMENT

Problems of Digestion

Jane M. Georges   Gladys Elizabeth Deters

Learning Objectives

1. Describe the pathogenesis, complications, and therapeutic and nursing management of nausea and vomiting.
2. Differentiate between acute and chronic gastritis, including the causes, pathophysiology, and therapeutic and nursing management.
3. Explain the common causes, clinical manifestations, and therapeutic and nursing management of upper gastrointestinal bleeding.
4. Compare and contrast gastric and duodenal ulcers, including pathogenesis, clinical manifestations, complications, and therapeutic and nursing management.
5. Explain the anatomic and physiologic changes and the common complications that result from surgical procedures for gastric and duodenal ulcers.
6. Describe the clinical manifestations and therapeutic, surgical, and nursing management of cancer of the stomach.

NAUSEA AND VOMITING

Nausea and vomiting are the most common manifestations of gastrointestinal (GI) diseases. Although each symptom can occur independently, they are usually closely related and usually treated as one problem. They are also found in a wide variety of conditions that are unrelated to GI disease. These include pregnancy, infectious diseases, central nervous system (CNS) disorders (e.g., meningitis, CNS lesion), cardiovascular problems (e.g., myocardial infarction, congestive heart failure), side effects of drugs (e.g., digitalis, antibiotics), metabolic disorders (e.g., uremia), and psychological factors (e.g., stress, fear).

Nausea is a feeling of discomfort in the epigastrium with a conscious desire to vomit. Anorexia usually accompanies nausea and is brought on by unpleasant stimulation involving any of the five senses. Generally, nausea occurs before vomiting and is characterized by contraction of the duodenum and by slowing of gastric motility and emptying. A single episode of nausea accompanied by vomiting in an adult may not be significant. However, if vomiting occurs several times it is important that the cause be identified.

Vomiting is the forceful ejection of partially digested food and secretions from the upper GI tract. It occurs when the gut becomes overly irritated, excited, or distended. It can be a protective mechanism to rid the body of spoiled or irritating foods and liquids. Immediately before the act of vomiting, the person becomes aware of the need to vomit. The autonomic nervous system is activated resulting in both parasympathetic and sympathetic nervous system stimulation. Sympathetic activation produces tachycardia, tachypnea, and diaphoresis. Parasympathetic stimulation causes relaxation of the lower esophageal (cardiac) sphincter, an increase in gastric motility, and a pronounced increase in salivation. These manifestations are experienced immediately before vomiting.

Vomiting is a complex act that requires the coordinated activities of several structures, including closure of the glottis, deep inspiration with contraction of the diaphragm in the inspiratory position, closure of the pylorus, relaxation of the stomach and lower esophageal sphincter, and contraction of the abdominal muscles with increasing intraabdominal pressure. These simultaneous activities force the stomach contents up through the esophagus, into the pharynx, and out the mouth.

Pathophysiology

There is a vomiting center in the brainstem that coordinates the multiple components involved in vomiting. This center receives input from various stimuli. Neural impulses reach the vomiting center via afferent pathways through branches of the autonomic nervous system. Visceral receptors for these afferent fibers are located in the GI tract, kidneys, heart, and uterus. When stimulated, these receptors relay information to the vomiting center, which then initiates the vomiting reflex (Fig. 39-1).

In addition, the chemoreceptor trigger zone (CTZ) located on the floor of the fourth ventricle in the brain responds to

*Reviewed by Kathryn Hennessey, RN, MS, CNSN, Clinical Network Manager, Caremark Inc., Northbrook, IL.

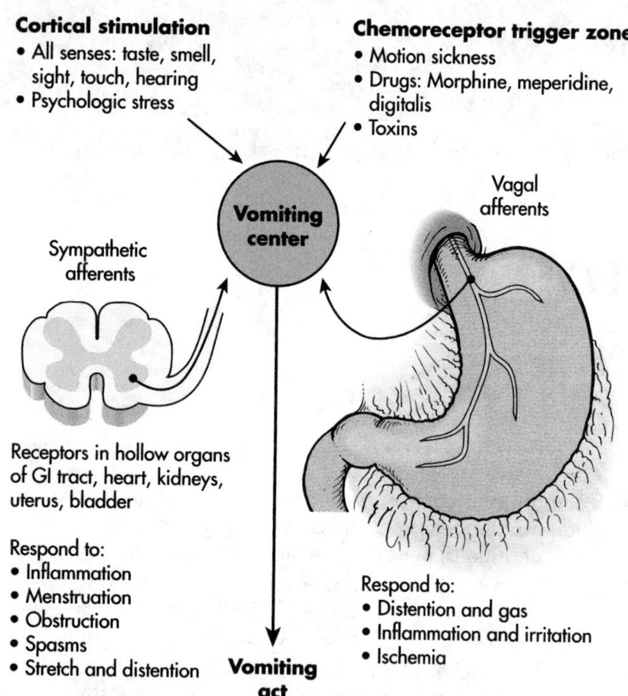

Fig. 39-1 Stimuli involved in the act of vomiting. *GI*, gastrointestinal.

chemical stimuli of drugs and toxins. The CTZ also plays a role in vomiting when it is due to labyrinthine stimulation (e.g., motion sickness). Once stimulated, the CTZ transmits impulses directly to the vomiting center. Emotions, stress, unpleasant sights and odors, and pain are all capable of triggering vomiting. Severe nausea and vomiting may also be caused by a metabolic crisis. For example, nausea and vomiting are frequently associated with uremia, hyperthyroidism, hyperparathyroidism and hypoparathyroidism, diabetic acidosis, Addison's disease, and hypertensive crisis.

When nausea and vomiting are prolonged, dehydration can rapidly occur. In addition to water, essential electrolytes (e.g., potassium) are also lost. As vomiting persists, there may be severe electrolyte imbalances, loss of extracellular fluid (ECF) volume, decreased plasma volume, and eventually circulatory failure. Metabolic alkalosis can result from loss of gastric hydrochloric acid. Metabolic acidosis can occur because of the loss of bicarbonate when contents from the small intestine are vomited. However, metabolic acidosis as a result of severe vomiting is less common than metabolic alkalosis. Weight loss is evident in a short time when vomiting is severe.

The threat of aspiration is a constant concern when vomiting is severe. Aspiration is especially a risk in the older adult and in the patient who is weak and debilitated. The patient who cannot adequately manage self-care should be put in a semi-Fowler's or side-lying position to prevent aspiration.

Therapeutic Management

The goals of therapeutic management are to determine and treat the underlying cause of the nausea and vomiting and to provide symptomatic relief of nausea and vomiting.[1] Determining the cause is often difficult because nausea and vomiting are manifestations of many conditions of the GI tract and of disorders of other body systems.

A careful history elicits important information regarding times when the vomiting occurs, precipitating factors, and a description of the contents of the vomitus. Differentiation must be made between vomiting, regurgitation, and projectile vomiting. *Regurgitation* is a process in which partially digested food is slowly brought up from the stomach. It is seldom preceded by retching or vomiting. *Projectile vomiting* is a very forceful projection of stomach contents without nausea and is characteristic of CNS lesions.

The presence of fecal odor and bile after prolonged vomiting is indicative of intestinal obstruction beyond the pylorus. A functioning ileocecal valve ordinarily prevents the backflow of fecal contents from the colon into the small intestine. The presence of bile may suggest obstruction below the ampulla of Vater or bile reflux gastritis. The presence of partially digested food several hours after a meal is indicative of gastric outlet obstruction or delay in gastric emptying.

The color of the emesis aids in determining the presence and source of bleeding. Vomitus with a "coffee ground" appearance is associated with bleeding in the stomach, which changes to dark brown as a result of its interaction with gastric acid. Bright red blood indicates active bleeding suggestive of a tear in the mucosal lining of the lower esophagus or fundus of stomach, bleeding gastric or duodenal ulcer or neoplasm, or bleeding esophageal varices.

The time of day at which the vomiting occurs is often helpful in determining the cause. Early-morning vomiting is a frequent occurrence in pregnancy and in uremia associated with renal disease. Emotional stressors with no evident functional disorder may elicit vomiting during or immediately after the ingestion of a meal.

The use of drugs in the treatment of nausea and vomiting depends on the cause of the problem. Many different drugs can be used (Table 39-1). Because the cause cannot always be readily determined, medications must be used with caution. The use of antiemetics before the cause of the vomiting is established can lead to masking of the underlying disease process and delay of diagnosis and treatment. Most of the antiemetic drugs act on the CNS at the level of the CTZ. In general, they block the neurochemicals that appear to trigger nausea and vomiting. Drugs which control nausea and vomiting include antimuscarinics (e.g., scopolamine), antihistamines (e.g., diphenhydramine), and phenothiazines (e.g., chlorpromazine, prochlorperazine). Because many of these drugs have anticholinergic actions, they are contraindicated for the patient with glaucoma, prostatic hyperplasia, pyloric or bladder neck obstruction, or biliary obstruction. They share many common side effects, which include dry mouth, hypotension, sedative effects, rashes, and GI disturbances such as constipation.

Table 39-1 Medications for Relief of Nausea and Vomiting

Classification	Generic Name	Trade Name
■ Antiemetic and antipsychotic	Chlorpromazine	Thorazine
	Haloperidol	Haldol
	Perphenazine	Trilafon
	Prochlorperazine	Compazine
	Promazine	Sparine
	Trifluoperazine	Stelazine
	Triflupromazine	Vesprin
■ Antihistamine	Buclizine	Bucladin-S
	Cyclizine	Marezine, meclizine
	Dimenhydrinate	Dramamine
	Diphenhydramine	Benadryl
	Promethazine	Phenergan
■ Prokinetics	Metoclopramide	Reglan
	Ondansetron	Zofran
	Granisetron	Kytril
	Cisapride*	Propulsid
■ Others	Benzquinamide	Emete-Con
	Diphenidol	Vontrol
	Scopolamine transdermal	Transderm-Scop
	Thiethylperazine	Torecan
	Trimethobenzamide	Tigan

*Approved for gastroesophageal reflux disease (see Chapter 38) and in clinical trials for other conditions.

Other drugs with antiemetic properties include metoclopramide (Reglan) and ondansetron (Zofran), which act peripherally to block serotonin receptors. These drugs are considered prokinetic agents because they stimulate gastric emptying and are used prophylactically to reduce nausea and vomiting associated with cancer chemotherapy. Consultation with a clinical pharmacist may be indicated before administering these medications to the patient with multiple medical problems.

Nutritional Management

The patient with severe vomiting requires intravenous (IV) fluid therapy with electrolyte replacement until able to tolerate oral intake. In some cases a nasogastric (NG) tube and suction are used to decompress the stomach. Once the symptoms have subsided, oral nourishment beginning with clear liquids is started. Extremely hot or cold liquids are not usually well tolerated. Carbonated beverages at room temperature and with the carbonation gone and warm tea are more easily tolerated. The addition of dry toast or crackers may alleviate the feeling of nausea and help prevent vomiting. Although broth and Gatorade have been used widely for the patient with severe vomiting, these substances are high in sodium and should be administered with caution. Water is the fluid of choice for rehydration by mouth.

As the patient's condition improves, a diet high in carbohydrates and low in fatty foods should be provided. Items such as a baked potato, plain gelatin, cereal with milk and sugar, and hard candy may be added. Foods that are known to be poorly tolerated include coffee, spicy foods, and highly acidic foods. Food should be eaten slowly and in small amounts so that overdistention of the stomach is avoided. When solid foods have been reintroduced, fluids should be taken between meals rather than with meals. It is advised that the patient remain quietly relaxed for approximately 1 hour after meals. A registered dietitian may be consulted regarding appropriate foods that have nutritional value and are well tolerated by the patient during the recovery process.

NURSING MANAGEMENT

NAUSEA AND VOMITING

Nursing Assessment

Each patient with a history of prolonged and persistent nausea or vomiting requires a thorough nursing assessment before a specific plan of care is developed. Although the conditions associated with nausea and vomiting are numerous, the nurse should have a basic understanding of some of the more common conditions and should be able to identify the patient who is at high risk. Knowledge of the physiologic mechanisms involved in nausea and vomiting and the demonstration of a genuine regard for the patient are essential. Table 39-2 presents subjective and objective data that should be obtained from a patient with nausea and vomiting, regardless of the underlying cause.

Nursing Diagnoses

Nursing diagnoses are determined when the problem and the etiologic factors are supported by clinical data. Nursing diagnoses for the patient with nausea and vomiting may include, but are not limited to, those presented in the nursing care plan for the patient with nausea and vomiting on p. 1173. In addition, there may be self-care deficits related to fatigue and discomfort of prolonged nausea and vomiting and altered oral mucous membranes related to prolonged and persistent vomiting and inadequate oral hygiene.

Planning

The overall goals are that the patient with nausea and vomiting will (1) experience minimal or no nausea and vomiting, (2) have normal electrolyte levels, and (3) return to a normal pattern of fluid balance and nutrient intake.

Nursing Implementation

Acute Intervention. The majority of individuals with nausea and vomiting can be managed at home. However, when nausea and vomiting persist regardless of home treatment strategies, hospitalization may be necessary for diagnosis of the underlying problem. Until a diagnosis is confirmed, the patient is kept on NPO status and given IV fluids. Antiemetic medications may be withheld or administered

Table 39-2 Nursing Assessment: Nausea and Vomiting

Subjective Data

Important Health Information

Past health history: GI disorders, chronic indigestion, food allergies, pregnancy, infection, CNS disorders, recent travel, bulimia, metabolic disorders, cancer, cardiovascular disease, renal disease

Medications: Use of antiemetics, digitalis, opiates, ferrous sulfate, aspirin, aminophylline, alcohol, antibiotics; general anesthesia; chemotherapy

Surgery and other treatments: Recent surgery

Functional Health Patterns

Nutritional-metabolic: Amount, frequency, character, and color of vomitus; anorexia; weight loss; abdominal tenderness; dry heaves

Activity-exercise: Weakness, fatigue

Coping-stress tolerance: Stress, fear

Objective Data

General

Lethargy, sunken eyeballs

Integumentary

Pallor, dry mucous membranes, poor skin turgor

Gastrointestinal

Amount, frequency, character (e.g., projectile), content (undigested food, blood, bile, feces), and color of vomitus (red, "coffee ground," green-yellow)

Urinary

Decreased output, concentrated urine

Possible findings

Altered serum electrolytes (especially hypokalemia), metabolic alkalosis, abnormal upper GI findings or abdominal x-rays

CNS, Central nervous system; *GI,* gastrointestinal.

with caution because they may mask the underlying condition. An NG tube connected to suction may be necessary for the patient with persistent vomiting. Keeping the stomach empty reduces the stimulus to vomit. The NG tube should be anchored to eliminate its movement in the nose and back of the throat because this can stimulate nausea and vomiting.

With prolonged vomiting, there is a possibility of dehydration and electrolyte imbalances. The nurse must plan care that includes an accurate record of intake and output, monitoring vital signs, assessment for signs of dehydration, proper positioning to prevent possible aspiration in the susceptible patient, and observation for changes in the patient's general physical comfort and mentation. The nurse must take responsibility for providing physical and emotional support, maintaining a quiet, odor-free environment, and giving explanations regarding any diagnostic tests or procedures performed.

Those who are already hospitalized for other health problems are also prone to episodes of nausea and vomiting. These individuals include the postoperative patient who is recovering from the effects of a surgical procedure, anesthesia, and pain, and who is experiencing adverse reactions to medications and treatment. Nausea and vomiting are common side effects in the cancer patient receiving chemotherapeutic drugs or radiation therapy. (A comprehensive review of nursing care for the patient who is receiving chemotherapy and radiation therapy is found in Chapter 12.)

Chronic and Home Management. The patient and family may need instructions on how to deal successfully with the unpleasant sensations of nausea, discussion of methods of preventing nausea and vomiting, and strategies to maintain fluid and nutritional intake during periods of nausea. The occurrence of nausea or vomiting may be minimized if measures are taken to keep the immediate environment quiet, free of noxious odors, and well ventilated. The avoidance of sudden changes of position and unnecessary activity is also helpful. Use of relaxation techniques, frequent rest periods, and diversional tactics help prevent nausea and vomiting or facilitate a more rapid recovery from their effects. Cleansing the face and hands with a cool washcloth and mouth care between episodes increase the person's comfort level. When the symptoms occur, all foods and medications should be stopped until the acute phase is past. If a medication is suspected as the cause, the physician should be notified immediately so that either the dosage can be altered or a new medication can be prescribed. The patient should be reminded that stopping the drug without consulting the physician may eliminate the immediate cause of the nausea and vomiting but that omission of the prescribed medication may have detrimental effects on health or the disease state.

When food is identified as the precipitating cause of nausea and vomiting, the nurse should help the patient solve the problem. What food was it? When was it eaten? Has this food caused problems in the past? Is anyone else in the family sick?

When the patient believes some foods and fluids can be tolerated, the nurse might suggest that it would be helpful to begin with clear liquids such as warm cola beverages, Gatorade, tea or broth, dry crackers or toast, and then plain gelatin. Bland foods, such as pasta, rice, and cooked chicken, are generally well tolerated in small amounts. An antiemetic drug should be taken only if prescribed by the physician. Taking over-the-counter drugs for relief of symptoms may make the condition worse.

Gerontologic Considerations

The older patient experiencing nausea and vomiting requires careful assessment and monitoring, particularly during periods of fluid loss and subsequent rehydration therapy. The older patient is at increased risk for preexisting conditions, such as cardiac or renal failure, and may experience a sudden compromise in renal or cardiac system functioning during episodes of fluid volume deficit.[2] In addition, the electrolyte imbalances that often accompany dehydration may result in life-threatening consequences for the elderly person who is already experiencing conditions such as congestive heart failure. Finally, the older adult with a decreased level of consciousness may be at high risk for aspiration of vomitus. Close monitoring of the patient's physical status and level of consciousness during episodes

NURSING CARE PLAN Patient with Nausea and Vomiting

Planning: Outcome Criteria	Nursing Interventions and Rationales
➤ **NURSING DIAGNOSIS**	Nausea and vomiting related to multiple etiologies *as manifested by* episodes of nausea and vomiting
Have minimal or no nausea or vomiting; verbalize satisfaction with care.	Treat specific etiology (when known) *to carry out problem-specific interventions.* Assess duration, frequency, and nature of vomitus, and aggravating and alleviating factors *to plan appropriate interventions.* Offer reassurance and explanations *to increase patient cooperation.* Remove visual stimuli and source of odors *to avoid precipitating factors of nausea and vomiting.* Provide mouth care; change soiled gown and linens *to ensure patient comfort.* Keep clean emesis basin and tissues within easy reach. Use diversional activities (if appropriate) *to decrease awareness of nausea.* Maintain quiet environment, restrict visitors, and avoid unnecessary procedures or activities *to minimize triggers of vomiting.* Administer antiemetics and pain medications as ordered. Instruct patient to take several deep breaths; prevent sudden changes in position; keep head of bed elevated *to decrease stimulation of the vomiting center.* Instruct patient to avoid foods and beverages *that stimulate nausea and vomiting*
➤ **NURSING DIAGNOSIS**	Fluid volume deficit *related to* prolonged vomiting and inability to ingest, digest, or absorb food and fluids *as manifested by* decreased urine output and increased urine concentration, increased pulse rate, hypotension (postural), decreased intake, nausea, decreased skin turgor, dry skin and mucous membranes, increased serum sodium, decreased serum potassium
Have no signs of dehydration.	Assess for signs of dehydration *to plan appropriate care.* Keep patient on NPO status until able to tolerate foods and fluids by mouth *to prevent stimulation of vomiting center.* Administer and monitor amount and type of IV fluid *to maintain fluid and electrolyte balance.* Administer antiemetic or pain medications as prescribed. Record amount and frequency of vomitus; maintain accurate intake and output records; weigh daily in acute phase *to accurately monitor fluid balance.* If ordered, maintain NG tube to low suction *to keep stomach empty and remove any stimulus for hydrochloric acid and pepsin secretion.* Check patency, type, and amount of drainage. Provide frequent mouth care. Assess skin tone and turgor *to assess degree of dehydration.* Monitor laboratory results of serum sodium, potassium, and chloride *as indicators of electrolyte and fluid balance.* Routinely test vomitus for pH, bile, blood; document amount, frequency, odor, and consistency of emesis *to assist in determining possible source of the problem.* Notify physician of results and changes in vomiting pattern *so treatment can be adjusted as appropriate.*
➤ **NURSING DIAGNOSIS**	Anxiety *related to* lack of knowledge of cause of problem, treatment plan, and follow-up care *as manifested by* verbalization of lack of knowledge, apprehension, tension; fear of nonspecific outcomes and recurrence of symptoms
Have early diagnosis of underlying disease process; develop trusting and helpful relationship; verbalize understanding of causative factors and purpose of therapeutic interventions.	Explain rationale for plan of care and diagnostic tests *to increase patient's understanding and reduce anxiety.* Teach about relationship between nausea and vomiting and foods, medications, treatment regimens, and psychosocial factors *to elicit patient's cooperation in avoiding potential causative factors.* Outline instructions or steps to take if nausea and vomiting recur *so patient will have a definite plan to follow.*
➤ **NURSING DIAGNOSIS**	Risk for altered nutrition: less than body requirements *related to* nausea and vomiting *as manifested by* lack of interest in or aversion to food, perceived or actual inability to ingest food, weight loss
Have gradual return to usual weight and eating habits.	Assess patient's interest in food, ability to ingest food, and weight *to determine if a problem is present.* Assure patient that appetite will return when nausea and vomiting are controlled. Maintain IV feedings or total parenteral nutrition until oral intake is possible *to provide necessary fluids, electrolytes, calories, and protein intake.* Instruct patient to resume eating cautiously with bland, nonirritating foods *to avoid irritating the stomach and initiating recurrence of nausea and vomiting.*

of nausea and vomiting must be a primary concern for the nurse.

GASTRITIS

Types

Gastritis, an inflammation of the gastric mucosa, is one of the most common problems affecting the stomach. Gastritis may be *acute* or *chronic* and may be diffuse or localized. Chronic gastritis can be further classified as type A (fundal) and type B (antral). Presently, the causes of gastritis and its relationship to other gastric disorders, such as gastric cancer, are the focus of intensive research.

Etiology and Pathophysiology

There is considerable evidence that gastritis is the result of a breakdown in the normal gastric barrier. A mucosal barrier normally protects the stomach tissue from autodigestion by acid. When the barrier is broken, acid can diffuse back into the mucosa. This allows hydrochloric (HCl) acid to enter and thereby increase the secretion of pepsinogen and the release of histamine from mast cells. The combined result of these occurrences is tissue edema, loss of plasma into the gastric lumen with disruption of capillary walls, and possible hemorrhage.

Causes of gastritis are listed in Table 39-3. Steroidal and nonsteroidal antiinflammatory drugs (NSAIDs) are known to inhibit the synthesis of prostaglandins, which then results in increased acid secretion in the stomach. Drugs such as aspirin, digitalis, and NSAIDs are directly irritating to the gastric mucosa. The ingestion of even small amounts of aspirin by the susceptible person is known to result in asymptomatic GI bleeding manifested by positive stool tests for occult blood. After an alcoholic drinking binge, acute damage to the gastric mucosa can range from local destruction of superficial epithelial cells to desquamation and destruction of the mucosa, with mucosal congestion, edema, and hemorrhage. Eating large quantities of spicy, irritating foods and metabolic conditions such as uremia can also cause acute gastritis.

Gastritis can occur from reflux of bile salts from the duodenum into the stomach as a result of anatomic changes following surgical procedures such as gastroduodenostomy and gastrojejunostomy. Reflux of bile salts may also be caused by prolonged vomiting. Intense emotional responses and CNS lesions may also produce inflammation of the mucosal lining as a result of hypersecretion of HCl.

Chronic gastritis may result from repeated episodes of acute gastritis. Chronic gastritis has an increasing incidence with age, with most cases occurring after the age of 50. Chronic exposure to the factors previously described (e.g., chronic alcohol abuse, excess ingestion of aspirin, reflux of duodenal contents after gastric surgery, uremia) will result in eventual loss of viable mucosal tissue. Chronic gastritis, in particular type A, may also be an autoimmune disorder. The high frequency of circulating antibodies in the patient with pernicious anemia suggests that atrophic gastritis may be an autoimmune disease. Approximately 95% of patients with pernicious anemia and 60% of patients with chronic atrophic gastritis have antibodies to parietal cells in their serum. Autoimmune atrophic gastritis affects both the fundus and body of the stomach and is associated with an increased risk of gastric malignancy.

Type B gastritis primarily involves the antrum of the stomach. The most common cause of type B gastritis is *Helicobacter pylori* (*H. pylori*). The presence of *H. pylori* also has been correlated with the presence of other gastric disorders, including gastric and duodenal ulcers and gastric cancer.[3] A description of the epidemiology of *H. pylori* and its proposed role in the promotion of gastric disorders is discussed in the sections on peptic ulcers and gastric cancer. This section will describe the current understanding of the mechanism by which *H. pylori* functions as a causative agent in chronic gastritis.

It is currently thought that *H. pylori* is acquired in childhood and is able to survive in the hostile environment of the gastric lumen. For reasons not clearly understood, *H. pylori* is capable of promoting the breakdown process of the gastric mucosal barrier, given certain "triggers" or conditions. Thus given time, *H. pylori* will eventually have a destructive effect on its host environment. This is congruent with the finding that the incidence of chronic gastritis increases with age. However, studies also have shown that not all persons infected with *H. pylori* go on to develop chronic gastritis. Thus it may be that a combination of factors is at work to "turn on" the virulent process by which *H. pylori* damages the gastric mucosal barrier.[3]

Progressive gastric atrophy from chronic alterations in the protective mucosal barrier causes the chief and parietal cells to eventually die. As the number of the acid-secreting parietal cells decreases with atrophy of the gastric mucosa, *hypochlorhydria* (decreased acid secretion) or *achlorhydria* (lack of acid secretion) occurs.

Table 39-3 Causes of Gastritis

Aspirin	Smoking
Nonsteroidal anti-inflammatory drugs	Physiologic stress
Corticosteroid drugs	Shock
Alcohol	Sepsis
Radiation	Burns
Helicobacter pylori	Psychologic stress
Staphylococcus organisms	Renal failure (uremia)
Salmonella	Spicy, irritating food
Bile and pancreatic secretions	Trauma
	Nasogastric suction
	Large hiatal hernia
	Endoscopic techniques

Clinical Manifestations

The symptoms of acute gastritis include anorexia, nausea and vomiting, epigastric tenderness, and a feeling of fullness. Hemorrhage is commonly associated with alcohol abuse and at times may be the only symptom. Acute gastritis is self-limiting, lasting from a few hours to a few days, with complete healing of the mucosa expected.

The manifestations of chronic gastritis are similar to those described for acute gastritis. Some patients have no symptoms directly associated with the gastric lesion. However, when the acid-secreting cells are lost or do not function as a result of atrophy, the source of intrinsic factor is also lost. Intrinsic factor, which normally combines with vitamin B_{12}, is unavailable, and thus vitamin B_{12} cannot be absorbed in the ileum. The intrinsic factor protects vitamin B_{12} from digestion by the GI enzymes. Eventually the body's storage of vitamin B_{12} in the liver is depleted and a deficiency state exists. Lack of this important vitamin, which is essential for the growth and maturation of red blood cells (RBCs), results in the development of anemia. (Vitamin B_{12} deficiency anemia is discussed in Chapter 28.)

Diagnostic Studies

Proper diagnosis of gastritis is frequently delayed or completely missed because the symptoms are nonspecific. Endoscopic examination with biopsy is necessary to obtain a definitive diagnosis. A specific analysis of gastric tissue for the presence of *H. pylori* may be performed. Radiographic studies are not helpful, since the superficial mucosa is generally involved, and changes will not show clearly on x-ray. A complete blood count (CBC) may demonstrate the presence of anemia from blood loss. Stools are tested for the presence of occult blood. A gastric analysis, although currently not used as much, demonstrates the amount of HCl acid present, with achlorhydria being a common sign of severe atrophic gastritis. Serum tests for antibodies to parietal cells and intrinsic factor may be performed. Cytologic examination is done to rule out gastric carcinoma.

Therapeutic Management

Elimination of the cause and preventing or avoiding it in the future are generally all that is needed to treat acute gastritis. The plan of care is supportive and similar to that described for nausea and vomiting. During the acute phase, bed rest, nothing by mouth, and IV fluids may be prescribed. Fluids and electrolytes lost through vomiting and occasionally diarrhea are replaced. In severe cases an NG tube may be used, either for lavage of the precipitating agent from the stomach or in conjunction with suction to keep the stomach empty and free of noxious stimuli. Antiemetics are given for nausea and vomiting. Antacids have proved beneficial in the relief of abdominal discomfort by raising intragastric pH to above 6. H_2 antagonists, such as ranitidine or cimetidine, may be prescribed to reduce gastric HCl acid secretion. Clear liquids are resumed when acute symptoms have subsided, with gradual reintroduction of solid, bland foods. Acute gastritis with hemorrhage is treated with blood transfusion and fluid replacement. Surgical intervention with partial gastrectomy, vagotomy, or pyloroplasty may be necessary if treatment fails.

The treatment of chronic gastritis focuses on evaluating and eliminating the specific cause (e.g., cessation of alcoholic intake, abstinence from drugs). Currently, various combinations of antibiotics and bismuth salt preparations (Pepto-Bismol) are being studied to eradicate infection with *H. pylori.* For the patient with pernicious anemia, regular injections of vitamin B_{12} are needed (see Chapter 28). An individualized bland diet and use of antacids are recommended. Smoking is contraindicated in all forms of gastritis. The patient undergoing treatment for gastritis may have to adapt to many lifestyle changes and adopt a strict adherence to a medication regimen.[4] An interdisciplinary team approach in which the physician, nurse, dietitian, and pharmacist provide consistent information and support may increase the patient's success in making these alterations.

NURSING MANAGEMENT

ACUTE GASTRITIS

Nursing Assessment

Dehydration can occur rapidly in severe gastritis accompanied by vomiting. Keeping the patient on NPO status and quiet and monitoring IV fluids is essential. If hemorrhage is considered likely, frequent checking of vital signs and testing the vomitus for blood are indicated. Elimination of the cause of the gastritis results in rapid improvement in the patient's condition. Identification of the causative agent is important to prevent future gastric irritation.

Nursing Diagnoses

The nursing diagnoses listed in the nursing care plan for the patient with nausea and vomiting (see p. 1173) are also applicable in gastritis.

Planning

The overall goals are that the patient with gastritis will (1) experience minimal or no symptoms of gastritis, (2) have no recurrent episodes of acute gastritis, and (3) achieve an optimal pattern of gastric function relative to the stage of the disease.

Nursing Implementation

The patient with gastritis should be encouraged to avoid causative factors and to follow the prescribed diet and medication regimen. Because the incidence of gastric cancer is higher in the patient who has a history of chronic gastritis, especially atrophic gastritis, close medical follow-up should be stressed.

The majority of patients with gastritis receive care in the home, and chronic management may be necessary for extended periods of time. A bland diet consisting of six small feedings a day and the use of an antacid after meals help the patient maintain normal gastric function. It is essential that the nurse have knowledge of the action and therapeutic effects of H_2 antagonists to teach the patient and to monitor drug effects. The care of the patient with chronic atrophic gastritis and gastric atrophy is also supportive. With advanced gastric atrophy, vitamin B_{12} injections may be necessary for the lifetime of the patient. Discussion of the continued need for this essential vitamin must be included in the plan of care.

The patient with severe dehydration and gastric bleeding may require acute intervention. All of the management strategies mentioned will apply in the inpatient setting. In addition, the nurse may wish to review the information on

RESEARCH

Implications for Nursing Practice

PERCEPTIONS OF CONTROL OVER HEALTH CARE

Citation Smith R and Draper P: Who is in control? An investigation of nurse and patient beliefs relating to control of their health care, *J Adv Nurs* 19:884-892, 1994.

Purpose To compare patient and nurse perceptions of how much control the patient has over own health care.

Methods Descriptive study that collected data from 21 nurses and 32 patients on a surgical unit using self-report questionnaires.

Results and Conclusions There were no differences between nurse and patient perceptions of patient control of health care. However, nurses were found to have a significantly greater desire for control over their own health care and a significantly weaker belief in the influence of doctors and nurses than did patients. Such differences in nurse and patient beliefs will have significant effects on how the nurse and patient feels about the care a patient receives.

Implications for Nursing Practice There are stress-reducing benefits of giving control to the patient who wants and expects it. Loss of control may have negative psychologic consequences, such as depression and feelings of helplessness, and may produce detrimental physiologic changes. Giving control that meets a patient's desire for control can produce better adjustment during treatment. The finding that nurse and patient beliefs differ in this area has significant implications for nursing care.

care of the patient with nausea and vomiting, as well as upper GI bleeding, which the patient with gastritis may also experience.

UPPER GASTROINTESTINAL BLEEDING

Etiology and Pathophysiology

Although the most serious loss of blood from the upper GI tract is characterized by a sudden onset, insidious occult bleeding can also be a major problem. The severity of bleeding depends on whether the origin is venous, capillary, or arterial. (Types of upper GI bleeding are presented in Table 39-4.) Bleeding from an arterial source is profuse, and the blood is bright red. The bright red color indicates that the blood has not been in contact with the stomach's acid secretions. In contrast, "coffee ground" vomitus reveals that the blood and other contents have been in the stomach for some time and have been changed by contact with gastric secretions. A massive upper GI hemorrhage is generally defined as a loss of more than 1500 ml of blood or a loss of 25% of intravascular blood volume. This type of bleeding may have come from the slower flow of a venous or capillary origin. *Melena* (black, tarry stools) indicates slow bleeding from an upper GI source. The longer the passage of blood through the intestines, the darker the color of the stool as a result of the degradation of hemoglobin and the release of iron.

Table 39-4 Types of Upper Gastrointestinal Bleeding

Type	Clinical Manifestations
Obvious bleeding	
▪ Hematemesis	Bloody vomitus appearing as fresh, bright red blood or "coffee ground" appearance (dark, grainy digested blood)
▪ Melena	Black, tarry stools (often foul smelling) caused by digestion of blood in the GI tract. The black appearance is from the presence of iron
Occult bleeding	Small amounts of blood in gastric secretions, vomitus, or stools not apparent by appearance; detectable by guaiac test

Discovering the cause of the bleeding is not always an easy task. A variety of areas in the GI tract may be involved, and there may be many different reasons for the blood loss. Table 39-5 lists the common causes of bleeding.

Esophageal Origin. Bleeding from an esophageal source is most likely the result of chronic esophagitis, bleeding from a tear in the mucosa near the esophago-gastric junction, or esophageal varices. Chronic esophagitis can be caused by the ingestion of chemicals irritating to the mucosa (e.g., lye) or hot, spicy, irritating foods. Alcohol and cigarettes are known irritants of the esophageal mucosa. An incompetent lower esophageal sphincter, which permits reflux of the acidic stomach contents back into the esophagus, can lead to chronic irritation and erosion. Severe retching and vomiting can cause a tear in the esophageal mucosa resulting in severe bleeding (Mallory-Weiss syndrome).

Esophageal varices usually occur secondary to cirrhosis of the liver. Branches of the vena cava and the azygos vein from the systemic circulation converge with the smaller vessels of the lower esophagus. These vessels are inelastic and become engorged and tortuous because of increased pressure exerted upon them secondary to portal hypertension. Anything that may increase the pressure (e.g., coughing, sneezing, trauma) or result in mechanical irritation (e.g., vomiting, irritation, erosion) may result in sudden, massive bleeding. (Esophageal varices are discussed in Chapter 41.)

Stomach and Duodenal Origin. Erosion of a blood vessel by a peptic ulcer located in the stomach or duodenum must always be considered as a possible cause of upper GI bleeding. Ulcers frequently penetrate blood ves-

Table 39-5 Common Causes of Upper Gastrointestinal Bleeding

Drug Induced	**Stomach and Duodenum**
Salicylates	Peptic ulcer disease
Corticosteroids	Stress ulcer
Phenylbutazone	Hemorrhagic gastritis
Indomethacin	Carcinoma
Esophagus	Polyps
Esophageal varices	**Systemic Diseases**
Esophagitis	Blood dyscrasias
Mallory-Weiss syndrome	Leukemia
	Uremia

sels. The left gastric artery may be penetrated by a gastric ulcer and the superior pancreaticoduodenal artery by a duodenal ulcer.

Some medications, either prescribed by the physician or self-administered, have been implicated as a cause of upper GI bleeding. The patient who regularly takes aspirin or aspirin-containing compounds may be at risk for bleeding episodes. Aspirin, NSAIDs (e.g., phenylbutazone, indomethacin), and corticosteroids, can cause irritation and erosion of the gastric mucosa. Aspirin-containing products are sold without prescriptions as over-the-counter drugs (see Table 28-15). It is not unusual for a patient to deny the use of aspirin yet be self-medicating with aspirin-containing drugs, such as Alka-Seltzer, Bufferin, and Excedrin. Erosion into the blood vessels is always a potential danger and a frequent cause of bleeding. A careful history of all commonly used medications is therefore necessary whenever upper GI bleeding is suspected.

Stress ulcers, which may occur after severe burn, trauma, or major surgery, erode more superficial blood vessels than does a peptic ulcer. They may also cause bleeding from erosion of a larger blood vessel. Gastritis produced by ingestion of drugs or alcohol or the reflux of bile contents commonly results in bleeding. Gastric carcinoma can be the cause of a steady blood loss as it grows and ulcerates through the mucosa and blood vessels located in its path. Hematemesis and melena are commonly associated with cancer of the stomach.

Systemic Diseases. Systemic diseases (e.g., leukemia, blood dyscrasias) that interfere with normal blood clotting must be considered whenever upper GI bleeding occurs.

Emergency Assessment and Management

Although approximately 75% of patients who have massive hemorrhage will spontaneously stop bleeding, the cause must be identified and treatment initiated immediately. In spite of advances in intensive care, hemodynamic monitoring, and fiberoptic endoscopy, there has been little change in the mortality rate for upper GI bleeding, which has remained approximately 10% for the past 40 years. This is due in part to the greater incidence of upper GI bleeding in older adults, especially women, related to the use of NSAIDs agents.

Although a complete history of events leading to the bleeding episode is important in discovering the cause of the blood loss, it should be deferred until emergency care has been initiated. The immediate physical examination must include a systemic evaluation of the patient's condition with emphasis on blood pressure, rate and character of pulse, peripheral perfusion with capillary refill, and observation for the presence or absence of neck vein distention. Vital signs should be monitored every 15 to 30 minutes. Signs and symptoms of shock must be evaluated, and treatment should be started as soon as possible (see Chapter 7). The patient's respiratory status is carefully assessed, along with a thorough abdominal examination. The presence or absence of bowel sounds should be assessed and noted. A tense, rigid, boardlike abdomen may indicate a perforation and peritonitis.

Once the immediate interventions have begun, the patient or family should answer the following questions. Is there a history of previous bleeding episodes? Has weight loss been a recent problem? Has the patient received blood transfusions in the past, and were there any transfusion reactions? Is there a religious preference that prohibits the use of blood or blood products? Are there any other illnesses that may contribute to bleeding or interfere with treatment (e.g., congestive heart failure, diabetes mellitus)?

Laboratory studies are ordered and include a CBC, blood urea nitrogen (BUN), serum electrolytes, blood glucose, prothrombin time, liver enzymes, arterial blood gases (ABGs), and a type and cross-match for possible blood transfusions. All vomitus and stools should be tested for the presence of gross and occult blood. A urinalysis provides information on the presence of blood in the urine, and the specific gravity gives an immediate indication of the patient's hydration status.

An open IV line with a 16- or 18-gauge needle should be established for fluid and blood replacement. The type and amount of fluids infused are dictated by physical and laboratory findings. It is generally best to begin with an isotonic crystalloid solution (e.g., lactated Ringer's solution). Whole blood, packed red blood cells, and fresh frozen plasma may be used for replacement of lost volume in massive hemorrhage. Packed red blood cells do not contain clotting factors that are depleted during major hemorrhagic events. (The use of blood transfusions and volume expanders is discussed in Chapter 28.) The hemoglobin and hematocrit values are not of immediate assistance in estimating the degree of blood loss but provide a baseline for guiding further treatment. The initial hematocrit may be normal and may not reflect the loss until 4 to 6 hours after fluid replacement has taken place, since initially the loss of plasma and RBCs is equal. When upper GI bleeding is less profuse, infusion of isotonic saline solution followed by packed red blood cells permits restoration of the hematocrit more quickly and does not create complications related to fluid volume overload.

For most patients who are bleeding profusely, an indwelling urinary catheter will be inserted so that urine volume can be accurately assessed hourly. A central venous pressure line may be inserted so that the patient's fluid volume status can be monitored easily. When a history of valvular heart disease, coronary artery disease, or congestive heart failure is elicited or when pulmonary edema is a factor, a pulmonary artery catheter may be necessary. A central venous pressure line is capable of monitoring right-sided heart pressure and function but does not reflect accurate left ventricular function. When the patient is vomiting blood, an NG tube is indicated. A large tube passed through the mouth may be more beneficial than a small one passed through the nose. Passage through the mouth is easier, but no tube should ever be advanced against resistance because of the likelihood of damaging the gastric mucosa or causing perforation. Aspiration of stomach contents through the tube facilitates the removal of clots from the stomach and alleviates the patient's need to vomit.

In most cases, bleeding ceases spontaneously without any intervention. However, for many years it has been common practice to lavage the stomach with cool or ice water or saline solution through an NG tube to induce local vasoconstriction of the bleeding vessel. The value of lavage is now in question. Recent studies indicate that ice water lavage has no effect on the rate of bleeding from gastric ulcers and may actually impede the body's normal coagulation mechanism by inhibiting platelet function.[5] Advocates of gastric lavage claim that when emergency endoscopy is necessary, lavage ensures that blood will not interfere with endoscopic visualization of the gastric mucosa.

If used, the usual procedure for gastric lavage is to instill 50 to 100 ml of water or saline solution each time, leave it in place for several minutes, and then aspirate it or allow drainage by gravity. The majority of patients who are bleeding from the stomach show diminished blood flow in about 30 to 45 minutes with this method. The addition of a vasoconstrictor to lavage solutions may also be used in some institutions. Drugs such as levarterenol (Levophed) diluted in saline solution have demonstrated the ability to help control hemorrhage from erosive gastritis.

The use of the endoscopic examination has recently expanded because of the ability to perform transendoscopic electrocoagulation.[6] Bleeding sites can be cauterized locally, which obviates the necessity of a surgical procedure. This procedure has proved useful in stopping the bleeding of gastritis, Mallory-Weiss syndrome, bleeding peptic ulcers, and polyps. Endoscopic thermal techniques now available to treat upper GI hemorrhage include (1) electrocoagulation, (2) heat probe, (3) argon laser, and (4) neodymium: yttrium-aluminum-garnet (Nd:YAG) laser. The heat probe is considered faster, safer, and more effective than the laser. It coagulates tissue by directly applying a heating element to the bleeding site.[5]

Diagnostic Studies

Fiberoptic Panendoscopy. In addition to using endoscopic procedures to stop bleeding, these procedures also allow for direct visualization of the bleeding site. Fiberoptic panendoscopy should be used before either angiography or barium studies. This diagnostic study is very accurate in identifying the specific source of the bleeding. When the procedure is performed by a skilled practitioner, bleeding from severe gastritis can be easily distinguished from that of a gastric or duodenal ulcer.

Angiography. Angiography has been used effectively in diagnosing upper GI bleeding. It is used when the bleeding site is not seen by endoscopic procedures. The procedure requires preparation and setup time and may not be appropriate for a high risk, unstable patient. In this procedure a catheter is placed into the left gastric or superior mesenteric artery and advanced until the site of bleeding is discovered. Angiography is an invasive procedure and should be undertaken only if the patient has no allergies to the contrast medium, has adequate hydration and urinary output, and has no cardiovascular contraindications.

Barium Contrast Studies. Barium contrast studies have less immediate value in the identification of major bleeding sites during the acute phase of treatment. These studies are of little value if the bleeding is the result of gastritis or a shallow superficial ulcer. Barium studies can document an actual lesion but cannot verify that it is the bleeding source. If barium is used initially as a diagnostic tool and the bleeding intensifies, the barium will obscure and delay endoscopy and angiography until it has been cleared from the stomach.

Therapeutic Management

Surgical Intervention. Surgical intervention is indicated when bleeding continues regardless of the therapy provided and when the site of the bleeding has been identified. A high percentage of patients are known to have another massive hemorrhage within 5 years after the first bleeding episode. Some physicians regard surgical therapy as necessary when the patient continues to bleed after rapid transfusion of up to 2000 ml of whole blood or remains in shock after 24 hours. The choice of operation is determined by the site of the hemorrhage. In addition, the surgeon must consider the age of the patient, since mortality rates increase considerably over the age of 60. It is essential that the operation be performed as soon as the need has been established.

Pharmacologic Management. During the acute phase, drugs are used to decrease bleeding, decrease HCl acid secretion, and neutralize the HCl acid that is present. Table 39-6 reviews their mechanism of action in relation to upper GI bleeding. Vasopressin (Pitressin), which is posterior pituitary extract, can produce vasoconstriction and is used to treat upper GI bleeding. It may be administered systemically through a vein or intraarterially at the local site of actual bleeding. It should be given with caution to the patient with a known history of vascular disease or hypersensitivity to vasopressin.

The injection of a sclerosing agent into the bleeding site holds promise in controlling upper GI bleeding. It is a simple procedure that requires little patient preparation. An agent such as epinephrine (a vasoconstrictor) is diluted and injected through the biopsy portal of the endoscope, causing the formation of submucosal deposits around the bleed-

Table 39-6 Drug Therapy for Gastrointestinal Bleeding

Drug	Source of GI Bleeding	Mechanism of Action
Antacids*	Duodenal ulcer, gastric ulcer, acute gastritis (corrosive, erosive, and hemorrhagic)	Neutralizes acid and maintains gastric pH above 5.5, elevated pH inhibits activation of pepsinogen
Histamine H_2-receptor antagonists Cimetidine (Tagamet), ranitidine (Zantac), famotidine (Pepcid), nizatidine (Axid)	Duodenal ulcer, gastric ulcer, esophagitis, acute gastritis (especially hemorrhagic)	Inhibits action of histamine at H_2 receptors of parietal cells and decreases acid secretion
Vasopressin	Acute gastritis (corrosive, erosive, and hemorrhagic)	Causes vasoconstriction and increases smooth muscle activity of the GI tract, reduces pressure in the portal circulation and arrests bleeding

*See Table 39-11.

ing site. The resultant vasoconstriction and local inflammation compress the site, and bleeding is controlled. Although further investigation is necessary, the use of thermal endoscopic techniques holds hope for the patient who is considered a poor surgical risk. The need for transfusions and the length of hospital stay are reduced, thus making these techniques attractive alternatives.

Histamine H_2-receptor antagonists cimetidine (Tagamet), ranitidine (Zantac), famotidine (Pepcid), and nizatidine (Axid) are well established in the treatment of peptic ulcer disease and in the prophylactic treatment of the patient at risk of stress-related upper GI hemorrhage. Although these drugs have no proven ability to control active bleeding, they have become part of standard treatment protocols. These drugs inhibit the action of histamine at the H_2 receptors of parietal cells and thereby decrease acid secretion. The neutralizing effects of each of these medications are much longer than those of regular antacid therapy (lasting up to about 5 hours for cimetidine and 13 hours for ranitidine).

Antacids have long been known to neutralize HCl acid and are used prophylactically in the management of peptic ulcer disease. Antacids are also beneficial to the healing process as well. Because antacids neutralize HCl acid and increase the pH of gastric contents to above 5, there is inhibition of the conversion of pepsinogen to its active form pepsin. The most frequently used antacid preparations are magnesium hydroxide, magnesium trisilicate, aluminum hydroxide, calcium carbonate, and sodium bicarbonate (see Table 39-10 later in this chapter). Aluminum hydroxide and magnesium trisilicates are the most useful because they are nonabsorbable. Calcium carbonate and sodium bicarbonate are absorbable, and prolonged use can lead to systemic alkalosis.

The neutralizing effects of antacids taken on an empty stomach last only 20 to 30 minutes. When antacids are taken after meals, the effects may last as long as 3 to 4 hours. After the acute phase of bleeding has diminished, antacids are generally administered hourly, either orally or through the NG tube. If the tube is in place, the stomach contents should be aspirated and tested periodically for pH. If pH is less than 5, intermittent suction may be used, or the frequency or dosage of the antacid may be increased.

For some patients, instillation of 60 to 180 ml of an antacid via the NG tube, clamping the tube for 15 minutes, and then testing gastric contents for pH may be prescribed. If the pH is below 7, antacid is again instilled, and the process is repeated until a neutral pH is attained. Antacids are then added regularly or intermittently to maintain a neutral pH. This regimen has demonstrated control of bleeding from a variety of causes.

Sedatives to control agitation and restlessness should be administered cautiously. They make accurate assessment of the patient's condition more difficult. Anticholinergic drugs are contraindicated in acute upper GI bleeding episodes.

NURSING MANAGEMENT

UPPER GASTROINTESTINAL BLEEDING

Nursing Assessment

As the nurse begins care of the patient admitted with upper GI bleeding, a thorough and accurate nursing assessment is an essential first step. Subjective and objective data that should be obtained from the patient or significant others are presented in Table 39-7.

The care of the patient who is bleeding from an unknown upper GI source requires continuous and diligent nursing care and assessment. The patient may not be able to provide specific information about the cause of the bleeding until the immediate physical needs are met. An immediate nursing assessment should be performed while getting the patient ready for initial treatment. The assessment should include the patient's level of consciousness, vital signs, appearance of neck veins, skin color, and capillary refill. The abdomen should be checked for distention, guarding, and peristalsis. Immediate determination of vital signs indicates whether the patient is in shock from blood loss and also provides a baseline blood pressure and pulse by

Table 39-7 Nursing Assessment: Upper Gastrointestinal Bleeding

Subjective Data
Important Health Information
Past health history: Precipitating events before bleeding episode, peptic ulcer disease, previous bleeding episodes and treatment, smoking or alcohol use
Medications: Use of aspirin, nonsteroidal antiinflammatory drugs, corticosteroids, anticoagulants
Functional Health Patterns
Health perception-health management: Family history of bleeding
Nutritional-metabolic: Vomiting, diarrhea; fever
Cognitive-perceptual: Epigastric pain, abdominal cramping pain
Coping-stress tolerance: Acute or chronic stressors
Objective Data
General
Vital signs, intake and output, bleeding from any site
Integumentary
Clammy, cool, pale skin; pale mucous membranes, nailbeds, and conjunctivae; spider angiomas; jaundice; ascites; edema
Possible findings
Decreased hematocrit and hemoglobin; hematuria; guaiac-positive stools, emesis, or gastric aspirate; decreased levels of clotting factors; elevated liver enzymes; abnormal upper GI studies or endoscopy results

which to monitor the progress of treatment. Signs and symptoms of shock include low blood pressure; rapid, weak pulse; increased thirst; cold, clammy skin; and restlessness. Vital signs should be monitored every 15 to 30 minutes, and the physician should be informed of any significant changes.

When obtaining vital signs, the nurse should consider the patient's age and physical condition. Taking the blood pressure and pulse with the patient laying down and then sitting will indicate postural changes that occur after acute blood loss. If the pulse rate increases more than 20 beats per minute (bpm) and the systolic blood pressure decreases 10 mm Hg, the blood loss is generally estimated to exceed 1 L. The older the patient, the more changes in vital signs should be expected.

Nursing Diagnoses

Nursing diagnoses specific to a patient with upper GI bleeding include, but are not limited to, the following:

- Fluid volume deficit related to acute loss of blood
- Altered peripheral tissue perfusion related to loss of circulatory volume
- Altered renal and cerebral tissue perfusion related to decreased blood volume
- Anxiety related to upper GI bleeding, hospitalization, uncertain outcome, source of bleeding
- Ineffective individual coping related to situational crisis and personal vulnerability
- Risk for aspiration related to active bleeding and altered level of consciousness
- Potential complication: hypovolemic shock related to loss of blood

Planning

The overall goals are that the patient with upper GI bleeding will (1) have no further GI bleeding, (2) have the cause of the bleeding identified and treated, (3) experience a return to a normal hemodynamic state, and (4) experience minimal or no symptoms of pain or anxiety.

Nursing Implementation

Health Promotion and Maintenance. Although not all cases of upper GI bleeding can be anticipated and prevented, the nurse shares responsibility with the physician in trying to identify the patient who is at high risk. The patient with a history of chronic gastritis or peptic ulcer disease should always be considered in the high-risk category because of the increased incidence of bleeding associated with chronic irritation or chronic ulcers. The patient who has had one major bleeding episode is likely to have another within a few years. This patient must be instructed to avoid irritating foods, prevent or decrease stress-inducing situations at home or at work, and take only prescribed medications. Over-the-counter medications can be harmful, since their contents may include drugs that are contraindicated because of their potentially irritating effects on the mucosa. This patient should be instructed in the methods of testing vomitus or stools for the presence of occult blood. Positive results should be promptly reported to the physician or the nurse. Close and frequent follow-up care is very important for all patients with ulcers because recurrence rates are high.

The patient who requires regular administration of ulcerogenic drugs, such as aspirin, corticosteroids, or NSAIDs (e.g., indomethacin), should receive instructions regarding the potential adverse effects these agents may have on the GI mucosa. These drugs should be avoided if at all possible. However, if aspirin must be prescribed, enteric-coated tablets can be substituted for regular tablets. Taking the medications with meals or snacks will lessen the potential irritating effects. The use of an antacid along with the prescribed medication is usually beneficial.

For the patient at risk for gastric ulcers because of NSAID use, misoprostol (Cytotec) may be prescribed. In addition to inhibiting acid secretion, this prostaglandin analog appears to have a protective effect on the gastric mucosal barrier. This drug can reduce upper GI bleeding episodes associated with NSAID use.

When the nurse is working with the patient who has a history of cirrhosis of the liver with esophageal varices, the instructions must be specific regarding the importance of avoiding known irritants, such as alcohol and hot, spicy, irritating foods. The prompt treatment of an upper respiratory tract infection should be stressed. Severe coughing or sneezing can create increased pressure on the already fragile varices and may result in massive hemorrhage.

The patient who is known to have blood dyscrasias or liver dysfunction or who is taking cancer chemotherapeutic drugs has a potential bleeding problem because of altered hemostasis caused by a decrease in clotting factors and platelets. When these patients also have a history of ulcer disease, gastritis, varices, or drug and alcohol abuse, they should be carefully instructed regarding their disease process and medications, and they should be closely observed for bleeding.

Acute Intervention. The patient should be approached in a calm and assured manner to help decrease the level of anxiety. Caution should be used before administering sedatives for restlessness because it is one of the warning signs of shock and may be masked by the medication.

Once an infusion has been started, the IV line must be maintained for fluid or blood replacement. An accurate intake and output record is essential so that the patient's hydration status can be assessed. Urine output should be measured hourly. A rate of at least 0.5 ml/kg per hour indicates adequate renal perfusion. Lesser amounts may indicate renal ischemia secondary to loss of blood volume. Urine specific gravity should be measured because it will give additional information regarding the patient's hydration status. Consistent readings greater than 1.025 (normal is 1.005 to 1.025) indicate that the urine is very concentrated and that there is probably a low blood volume. The physician needs to be kept informed of these important parameters so that the IV solutions can be increased or decreased accordingly. If the patient has a central venous pressure line or pulmonary artery catheter in place, readings should be recorded every 1 to 2 hours. Hemodynamic monitoring provides an accurate and quick assessment of blood flow and pressure within the cardiovascular system (see Chapter 61).

The older adult and patient with a history of cardiovascular problems should be observed closely for signs of fluid overload. However, the threat of volume overload and pulmonary edema must be a constant concern in all patients who are receiving large amounts of IV fluids within a short time. Therefore, auscultation of breath sounds and close observation of respiratory effort are important. Electrocardiographic (ECG) monitoring can also be used to evaluate cardiac function.

Foods such as beets or even swallowed mouthwash can give vomitus a bloody appearance. Unless the contents of the vomitus are checked for occult blood, false information may be recorded. Swallowed blood from a nosebleed must also be accurately noted to avoid misdiagnosis of an upper GI bleeding episode. When an NG tube is inserted, the nurse must pay special attention to keeping it in proper position and observing the aspirate for blood.

The majority of upper GI bleeding episodes cease spontaneously, even without intervention. Although the use of cool or iced gastric lavage has become standard treatment in many institutions, its effectiveness is of questionable value. Therefore the nurse must understand the rationale for this therapy and the results that are anticipated. Either cool or iced tap water or saline solution may be used. Water has the advantage of being able to break up large clots more easily than saline solution, is less expensive, and is always available. A disadvantage of tap water is that it may create more electrolyte imbalance than would an isotonic saline solution.

Instillation of approximately 50 to 100 ml of lavage fluid at a time into the stomach generally results in decreased bleeding if the blood is gastric in origin. Instilling too much can increase the patient's discomfort, especially if distention is already present. Instillation of too small an amount and aspirating too soon does not allow enough time for the cold fluid to cause vasoconstriction in the bleeding area.

The lavage fluid may be aspirated from the stomach or drained by gravity. When aspiration is the method used, it is important not to aspirate if resistance is felt. The tip of the NG tube may be up against the gastric mucosal lining. The constant pressure from attempts to aspirate the lavage fluid may cause erosion of the mucosa. When resistance is a factor, the nurse should use gravity as the alternative method of gastric drainage.

Close monitoring of vital signs, especially in the patient with a heart problem, is important because dysrhythmias may occur as a result of the close proximity of the cold, fluid-filled stomach to the heart. Keeping the patient warm and the head of the bed elevated provide comfort and prevent possible aspiration problems. The head of the bed should always be elevated when antacids are being instilled through an NG tube. Serious pulmonary complications can result if aspiration occurs. The nurse must chart the results of the lavages promptly and accurately.

The nurse caring for a patient with upper GI bleeding should be well informed as to what constitutes blood in the stools. Black, tarry stools are not usually associated with a brisk hemorrhage but indicate the presence of bleeding of prolonged duration. Bright red blood in the stool is usually from a source in the lower bowel. When vomitus contains blood but the stool contains no gross or occult blood, the hemorrhage is considered to have been of short duration.[7] Menses and bleeding hemorrhoids should be ruled out as possible sources of blood in the stools.

Monitoring the patient's laboratory studies enables the nurse to estimate the effectiveness of therapy. The hemoglobin and hematocrit are usually evaluated about every 4 to 6 hours and provide an accurate estimation of volume lost after rehydration has taken place. At first the hematocrit may not accurately reflect the amount of blood lost or the amount of blood replaced and will appear falsely high or low. Assessing the patient's BUN level also provides data on the degree of blood lost but not for about 24 to 48 hours. The BUN level is generally elevated with a significant hemorrhage, since blood proteins are subjected to bacterial breakdown in the GI tract. Renal disease as a cause of an elevated BUN level should be ruled out. Many patients receive oxygen by mask or nasally so that the circulating blood is ensured of an adequate oxygen content. The patient with chronic obstructive pulmonary disease should receive low flow rates of oxygen and be observed closely for signs of carbon dioxide narcosis when receiving oxygen (see Chapter 24).

When oral nourishment is begun, the patient is observed for symptoms of nausea and vomiting and a recurrence of bleeding. Feedings initially consist of clear fluids or milk and are given hourly until tolerance is determined. These feedings help neutralize the gastric secretions and assist in the mucosal repair. Gradual introduction of bland foods follows if the patient exhibits no signs of discomfort.

Antacids are one of the primary medications administered after upper GI bleeding. Anticipating the effects of the prescribed preparations can be helpful in providing better care. The nurse should know that preparations containing calcium or aluminum can result in constipation, whereas those with magnesium cause diarrhea. Although these preparations are nonabsorbable and result in fewer systemic problems, magnesium products must be used with care in the patient with renal insufficiency. Administering the antacid preparation accurately and on schedule is important if the stomach pH is to be maintained at a level no lower than 5.

The patient in whom hemorrhage was the result of chronic alcohol abuse requires close observation for the beginning of delirium tremens as withdrawal from alcohol takes place. Symptoms indicating the beginning of delirium tremens are agitation, uncontrolled shaking, sweating, and vivid hallucinations. (Alcohol withdrawal is discussed in Chapter 8.)

Chronic and Home Management. The patient and family need to be taught how to avoid future bleeding episodes. Ulcer disease, drug or alcohol abuse, and liver and respiratory diseases can all result in upper GI bleeding. The patient and family must be made aware of the consequences of noncompliance with diet and drug therapy. It must be emphasized that no medications (especially aspirin) other than those prescribed by the physician should be taken. Smoking and alcohol should be eliminated because they are sources of irritation and interfere with tissue repair. The need for long-term follow-up care may be necessary because of the possibility of another bleeding episode. The patient and family should be instructed on what to do if an acute hemorrhage occurs in the future.

PEPTIC ULCERS

Peptic ulcer is an erosion of the GI mucosa resulting from the digestive action of HCl acid and pepsin. Any portion of the GI tract that comes into contact with gastric secretions is susceptible to ulcer development, including the lower esophagus, stomach, duodenum, and margin of gastrojejunal anastomosis after surgical procedures. It is estimated that approximately 10% of men and 4% of women in the United States will have duodenal ulcers during their lifetime.[8]

Types

Peptic ulcers can be classified as *acute* or *chronic,* depending on the degree of mucosal involvement (Fig. 39-2), and *gastric* or *duodenal,* according to the location. The acute ulcer is associated with superficial erosion and minimal inflammation. It is of short duration and resolves quickly when the cause is identified and removed. A chronic ulcer is one of long duration, eroding through the muscular wall with the formation of fibrous tissue. It is present continuously for many months or intermittently throughout the person's lifetime. A chronic ulcer is at least four times as common as an acute erosion.[9] Gastric and duodenal ulcers, although defined as peptic ulcers, are distinctly different in their etiology and incidence (Table 39-8). Generally the treatment of all types of ulcers is quite similar.

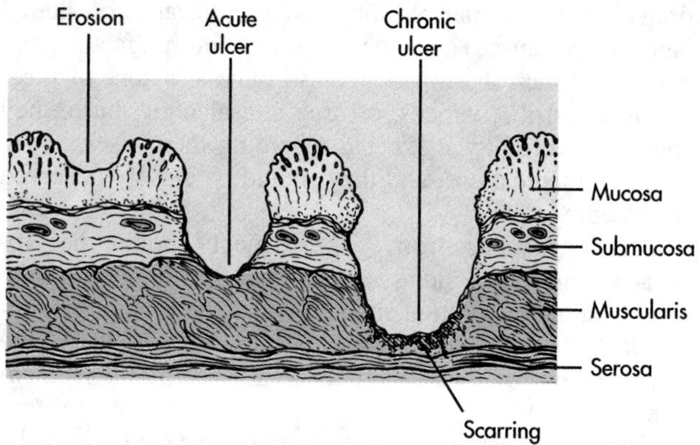

Fig. 39-2 Peptic ulcers, including an erosion, acute ulcer, and chronic ulcer. Both the acute and chronic ulcer may penetrate the entire wall of the stomach.

Pathophysiology

Pepsinogen, the precursor of pepsin, is activated to pepsin in the presence of HCl acid and a pH of 2 to 3. HCl acid is secreted by the parietal cells at a pH of 0.8. After mixing with the stomach contents, the pH reaches 2 to 3, a highly favorable range of acidity for pepsin activity. When the stomach acid level is neutralized by the presence of food or antacids, the pH is increased to 3.5 or more. At a pH of 3.5 or more, pepsin has little or no proteolytic activity.

Peptic ulcers develop only in the presence of an acid environment. It has been well established that the patient with pernicious anemia and achlorhydria rarely has gastric ulcers. An excess of gastric acid may not be necessary for ulcer development. The typical person with a gastric ulcer has normal to less than normal gastric acidity compared with the person with a duodenal ulcer. However, some intraluminal acid does seem to be essential for a gastric ulcer to occur.

The stomach is normally protected from autodigestion by the gastric mucosal barrier. The GI tract has a very high cell turnover rate, and the surface mucosa of the stomach is renewed about every 3 days. As a result of this high turnover rate, the mucosa can continually repair itself except in extreme instances when the cell breakdown surpasses the cell renewal rate. Normally, water, electrolytes, and water-soluble substances (e.g., glucose) can easily pass through the barrier. However, the mucosal barrier prevents the back diffusion of acid from the gastric lumen through the mucosal layers to the underlying tissue.

Under specific circumstances the mucosal barrier can be impaired and back-diffusion of acid can occur (Fig. 39-3). When the barrier is broken, HCl acid freely enters the mucosa and injury to the tissues occurs. This results in cellular destruction and inflammation. Histamine is released from the damaged mucosa, resulting in vasodilatation and

Table 39-8 Comparison of Gastric and Duodenal Ulcers

	Gastric Ulcers	Duodenal Ulcers
Lesion	Superficial; smooth margins; round, oval, or cone-shaped	Penetrating (associated with deformity of duodenal bulb from healing of recurrent ulcers)
Location of lesion	Predominantly antrum, also in body and fundus of stomach	First 1-2 cm of duodenum
Gastric secretion	Normal to decreased	Increased
Incidence	▪ Greater in women ▪ Peak age fifth to sixth decade ▪ More common in persons of lower socioeconomic status and in unskilled laborers ▪ Increased with smoking, drug, and alcohol use ▪ Increased with incompetent pyloric sphincter ▪ Increased with stress ulcers after severe burns, head trauma, and major surgery	▪ Greater in men, but increasing in women especially postmenopausal ▪ Peak age 35-45 yr ▪ Associated with psychologic stress ▪ Increased with smoking, drug, and alcohol use ▪ Associated with other diseases (e.g., chronic obstructive pulmonary disease, pancreatic disease, hyperparathyroidism, Zollinger-Ellison syndrome, chronic renal failure)
Clinical manifestations	▪ Burning or gaseous pressure in high left epigastrium and back and upper abdomen ▪ Pain 1-2 hr after meals; if penetrating ulcer, aggravation of discomfort with food ▪ Occasional nausea and vomiting, weight loss	▪ Burning, cramping, pressurelike pain across midepigastrium and upper abdomen; back pain with posterior ulcers ▪ Pain 2-4 hr after meals and midmorning, midafternoon, middle of night, periodic and episodic ▪ Pain relief with antacids and food; occasional nausea and vomiting
Recurrence rate	High	High
Complications	Hemorrhage, perforation, outlet obstruction, intractability	Hemorrhage, perforation, obstruction

increased capillary permeability. The released histamine is then capable of stimulating further secretion of acid and pepsin.

As described under gastritis, a variety of agents are known to destroy the mucosal barrier. By generating ammonia in the mucous layer, *H. pylori* may create a condition of chronic inflammation, which renders the mucosa especially vulnerable to other noxious substances.[10] Ulcerogenic drugs, such as aspirin and aspirin-like agents, inhibit synthesis of mucus and prostaglandins and cause abnormal permeability. Corticosteroids have the ability to decrease the rate of mucous cell renewal and thereby decrease its protective effects. Lipid-soluble cytotoxic drugs can pass through the barrier and destroy it.

When the mucosal barrier is disrupted, there is a compensatory increase in blood flow. This phenomenon can occur in several ways. Prostaglandin-like substances and histamine act as vasodilators, thus increasing capillary blood flow. As blood flow increases within the affected mucosa, hydrogen ions are rapidly removed from the area, buffers are delivered to help neutralize the hydrogen ions present, nutrients necessary for cell function arrive, and the rate of mucosal cell replication increases.[10] When blood flow is not sufficient to carry out these events, tissue injury results. When the increase is sufficient to dilute, buffer, and remove the excess, tissue damage may be minimal or may result in no injury at all. Figure 39-4 shows a representation of the interrelationship between the mucosal blood flow and disruption of the gastric mucosal barrier.

Although gastric ulcers are characterized by a normal to low secretion of gastric acid, the back-diffusion of acid is greater with chronic gastric ulcers than with duodenal ulcers or in the normal person. Therefore the critical pathologic process in gastric ulcer formation may not be the amount of acid that is secreted but the amount that is able to penetrate the mucosal barrier.

The gastric mucosa is also protected from the damage of ulceration by two other mechanisms. First, mucus is secreted by superficial mucous cells and forms a layer that can entrap or slow the diffusion of hydrogen ions across the mucosal barrier. Second, bicarbonate is secreted by the gastric and duodenal mucosa, and this helps neutralize HCl acid in the lumen of the GI tract.

Increased vagal nerve stimulation from a variety of causes (e.g., emotions) causes hypersecretion of HCl acid and pepsin. Increased concentrations of acid can alter the mucosal barrier. Duodenal ulcers are associated with high acid content. The fact that the person with duodenal ulcers is more vulnerable to the effects of emotional stressors may be one reason acid levels are above normal. It has been

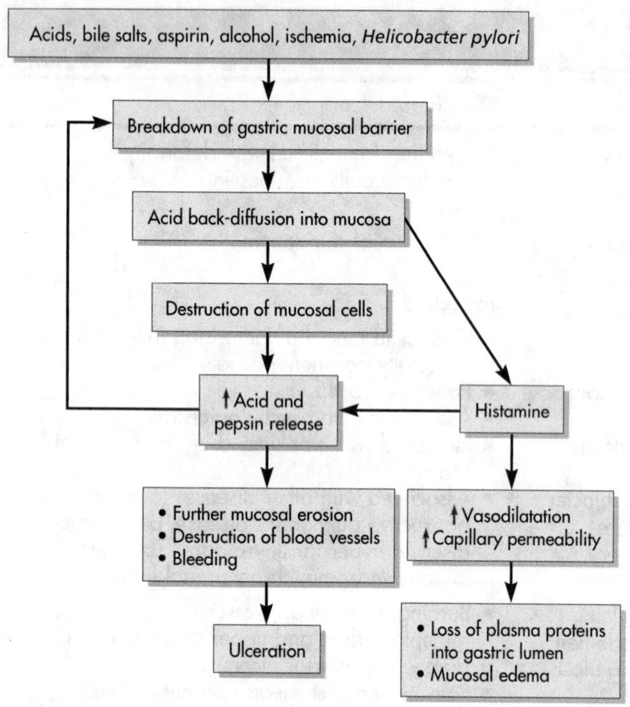

Fig. 39-3 Disruption of gastric mucosa and pathophysiologic consequences of back-diffusion of acids.

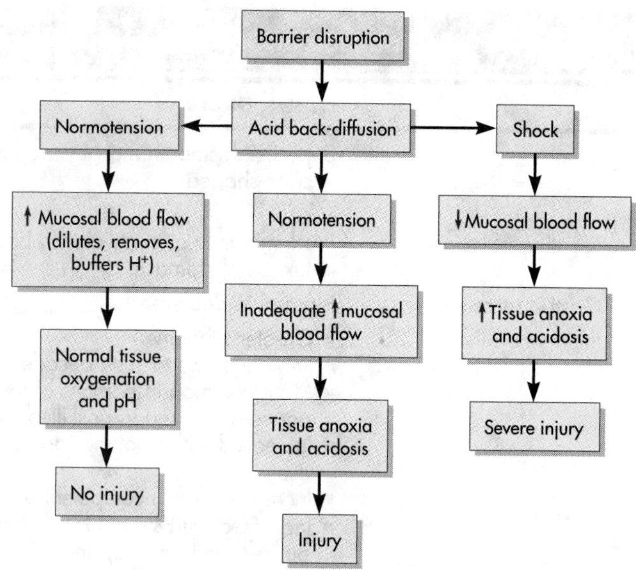

Fig. 39-4 The relationship between mucosal blood flow and disruption of the gastric mucosal barrier.

suggested that the continual response of the parietal cells to maximal stimulation results in hyperplasia of the cell mass. There is also an increase in gastrin levels in most persons with duodenal ulcers.

Gastric Ulcers. Although gastric ulcers can occur in any portion of the stomach, they are most commonly found on the lesser curvature in close proximity to the antral junction. Before 1900 gastric ulcers were more common than duodenal ulcers, and they were found predominantly in young women. Since the turn of the century, the incidence of gastric ulcers has decreased, and they are now surpassed in incidence by duodenal ulcers by a ratio of 4:1. Gastric ulcers remain more prevalent in women and in older adults.

The mortality rate from gastric ulcers is greater than that from duodenal ulcers because the peak incidence of gastric ulcers occurs in persons over 50 years of age. Contrary to common belief, gastric ulcers are not more prevalent among those in executive or managerial positions. Persons from the lower socioeconomic class and manual or unskilled workers are more prone to gastric ulcers.

Gastric ulcers have been attributed to various factors that can lead to acute episodes or to chronic involvement. Acute gastric lesions can be precipitated by stressful situations and drugs. A *stress ulcer* is a form of erosive gastritis.[11] It is believed that the gastric mucosa of the body of the stomach undergoes a period of transient ischemia in association with hypotension, severe injury, extensive burns, and complicated surgery. The ischemia is due to decreased capillary blood flow or shunting of blood away from the GI tract so that blood flow bypasses the gastric mucosa. This occurs as a compensatory mechanism in hypotension or shock. The decrease in blood flow produces an imbalance between the destructive properties of HCl acid and protective factors of the stomach's mucosal barrier, especially in the fundic portion, which results in ulceration. Multiple superficial erosions result, and these may bleed.

Medications can cause acute gastric ulcers and in some cases can lead to the development of chronic ulcers. Drugs most often implicated include aspirin, corticosteroids, NSAIDs (e.g., indomethacin, phenylbutazone), and reserpine. Other known causative factors of gastric ulcer formation are chronic alcohol abuse, gastritis, bile reflux gastritis from an incompetent pyloric sphincter, and coffee. Caffeine is known to stimulate gastric acid secretion. Cigarette smoking is positively linked with gastric ulcer. One proposed theory is that smoking causes a reduction of pancreatic bicarbonate secretion, thus creating a decreased pH in the duodenum. In addition, nicotine seems to enhance reflux of duodenal contents into the antrum of the stomach. The ingestion of hot, rough, or spicy foods has been suggested as a causative factor, but there is no evidence to substantiate this claim.

The understanding of the factors that contribute to ulcer formation is developing rapidly at the present time. As described previously under gastritis, the discovery of the bacterium, *H. pylori,* provides a new understanding of ulcer formation. *H. pylori* is thought to be a dominant factor in the promotion of peptic ulcer formation. Although many questions remain to be answered regarding *H. pylori,* it survives in the human upper GI tract for long periods of time as a result of its ability to move in mucus and attach to mucosal cells. In addition, it secretes a substance called urease, which buffers the area around the bacterium and protects it from destruction in an acidic environment.

Infection with *H. pylori* is highest in underdeveloped countries and in persons of low socioeconomic status. Although the routes of transmission are largely unknown, it is thought that infection occurs during childhood via transmission from family members to the child, possibly through an oral-oral route. In the United States and Canada, persons born before 1940 have a significantly higher risk of carrying *H. pylori* than persons in younger age groups. This enhanced prevalence in older persons has been attributed to the presence of crowded living conditions and poor sanitation practices, which were more common in the earlier part of the 1900s.

Research into a genetic cause for ulcers has shown that some members of the same family are more prone to develop gastric or duodenal ulcers. Evidence is not complete, however, and the ulcer development could just as well be due to the sharing of the same environment. For example, the transmission of *H. pylori* may be increased by crowded living conditions. Gastric ulcer personality has not been demonstrated, yet ulcer-prone persons do appear to react to stress with more frustration, fear, anxiety, and guilt than those who are less predisposed to ulcer formation. It is thought that destruction of the gastric mucosa by noxious agents such as drugs or smoking may be enhanced by the presence of *H. pylori,* which further promotes gastric mucosal destruction as described in the previous section on gastritis.

It is rare for gastric ulcers to become malignant, but transformation may occur in about 1% of all cases.[12] When there is any doubt, a biopsy of the gastric mucosa should be performed during endoscopy to differentiate between a benign ulcer and a malignant neoplasm.

Duodenal Ulcers. Duodenal ulcers account for about 80% of all peptic ulcers. Although duodenal ulcers still affect more men than women, the incidence of duodenal ulcers has followed a downward trend in men and a steady increase in women. The explanation for this change has not been clearly identified. However, it is possible that the overuse of aspirin and NSAIDs and increased consumption of alcohol by women may partially account for this increased incidence. Duodenal ulcers may occur at any age, but the incidence is especially high between the ages of 35 and 45 years.

Whereas many factors are thought to contribute to the formation of duodenal ulcers, *H. pylori* has been identified as playing a key role. The prevalence of *H. pylori* infection in duodenal ulcer patients has consistently been found to be between 95% and 100%. However, a clear-cut direct causal relationship between *H. pylori* and duodenal ulcer formation has not yet been proven.[8] Although duodenal ulcers often occur in persons susceptible to psychologic pressures and anxieties, this theory of causation requires more study. It is known that a duodenal ulcer can develop in anyone, regardless of occupation or socioeconomic group. The development of duodenal ulcers is associated with a high acid secretion by gastric parietal cells. Several diseases have been identified with a high risk of duodenal ulcer development; these include chronic obstructive pulmonary disease, cirrhosis of the liver, chronic pancreatitis, hyperparathyroidism, chronic renal failure, and the Zollinger-Ellison syndrome. A high gastric acid concentration is believed to be the factor common to all these conditions. It is possible that the treatment of these conditions may also have detrimental effects on the gastric mucosa. Alcohol ingestion and heavy smoking habits are also associated with duodenal ulcer formation since both are known irritants to the GI mucosa.

Pregnancy appears to protect women from developing ulcers. Estrogen and progesterone have demonstrated positive effects on ulcer healing. Progesterone has also been noted to lower acid secretion to a small degree. There is evidence that women past menopause, who no longer have this endocrine protection, develop ulcers at the same rate as men.

As with gastric ulcers, some persons in certain families are more prone to duodenal ulcer formation. Supporting a genetic etiology is the fact that persons with blood group O have an increased incidence of duodenal ulcers. This may be related to increased susceptibility to *H. pylori.*

Clinical Manifestations

It is common for the person with gastric or duodenal ulcers to have no pain or other symptoms. The gastric and duodenal mucosa do not have pain sensory fibers, which may account for this phenomenon. When pain does occur with duodenal ulcer, it is described as "burning" or "cramplike." It is most often located in the midepigastrium region beneath the xyphoid process. The pain associated with gastric ulcers is located high in the epigastrium and occurs spontaneously about 1 to 2 hours after meals. The pain is described as "burning" or "gaseous." The pain can occur when the stomach is empty or when food has been ingested. If the ulcer has eroded through the gastric mucosa, food tends to aggravate rather than alleviate the pain. Some persons do not experience any pain until the presence of the ulcer is demonstrated through a serious complication such as hemorrhage or perforation.

Ulcers located on the posterior aspect of the duodenum can be manifested by back pain. The pain usually occurs 2 to 4 hours after meals and is relieved by antacids and sometimes foods that neutralize and dilute the gastric acid. A characteristic of duodenal ulcer is its tendency to occur continuously for a few weeks or months and then disappear for a time, only to recur some months later. Some patients claim their symptoms worsen in the spring and fall of the year, thus strengthening the concept of a seasonal trend in occurrence. This course of events usually lasts throughout the entire life span of the ulcer.

Complications

The three major complications of chronic peptic ulcer disease are hemorrhage, perforation, and gastric outlet obstruction. All are considered emergency situations and are initially treated conservatively. However, surgery may become necessary at any time during the course of the therapy.

Hemorrhage. Hemorrhage is the most common complication of peptic ulcer disease. It develops from erosion of

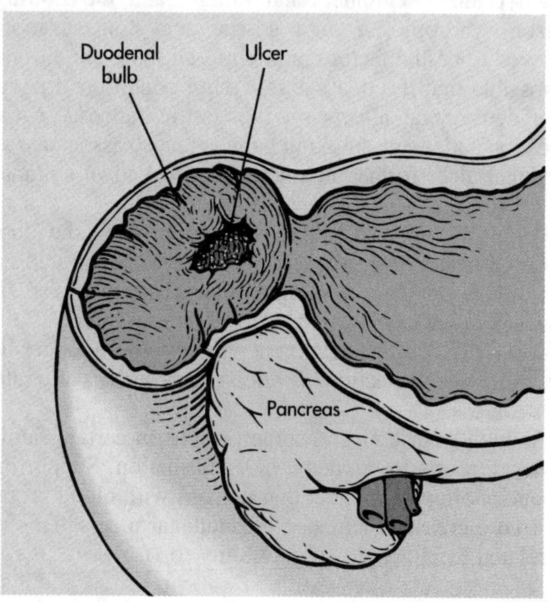

Fig. 39-5 Duodenal ulcer of the posterior wall penetrating into the head of the pancreas, resulting in a walled-off perforation.

the granulation tissue found at the base of the ulcer during healing or from erosion of the ulcer through a major blood vessel. Duodenal ulcers account for a greater percentage of upper GI bleeding episodes than gastric ulcers.

Perforation. Perforation is considered the most lethal complication of peptic ulcer. Perforation is commonly seen in large penetrating duodenal ulcers that have not healed and are located on the posterior mucosal wall (Fig. 39-5). Perforated gastric ulcers are most frequently located on the lesser curvature of the stomach. Even though duodenal ulcers are more prevalent and perforate more frequently, mortality rates associated with perforation of gastric ulcers are higher. The older age of the patient with gastric ulcers, who often has other concurrent medical problems, is thought to be the crucial factor.

Perforation of a peptic ulcer occurs when the ulcer penetrates the serosal surface, with spillage of either gastric or duodenal contents into the peritoneal cavity. The size of the perforation is directly proportional to the length of time the patient has had the ulcer. The larger the perforation, the longer the history of the ulcer. Small perforations seal themselves and result in a cessation of symptoms; larger perforations require immediate surgical closure. Spontaneous sealing occurs as a result of large amounts of fibrin being produced in response to the perforation. This leads to fibrinous fusion of the duodenum or gastric curvature to adjacent tissue, mainly the liver.

The clinical manifestations of perforation are characterized by their sudden and dramatic onset. The patient experiences sudden, severe upper abdominal pain that quickly spreads throughout the abdomen. The visceral and parietal layers of the peritoneum have an abundance of pain receptors, and this contributes to the abrupt, intense pain experienced. There may be shoulder pain if the spillage causes irritation to the phrenic nerve. The abdominal muscles contract, appearing rigid and boardlike as they attempt to protect the abdomen from further injury. The patient's respirations become shallow and rapid. Bowel sounds are usually absent. Nausea and vomiting may occur but are generally absent. Most patients have a history of ulcer disease or recent symptoms of indigestion.

The contents entering the peritoneal cavity from the stomach or duodenum contain a variety of ingredients that include air, saliva, food particles, HCl acid, pepsin, bacteria, bile, and pancreatic juices. A bacterial peritonitis may occur within 6 to 12 hours, followed by paralytic ileus. The intensity of the peritonitis is proportional to the amount and duration of the spillage through the perforation. It is difficult to determine from the sudden onset of symptoms whether gastric or duodenal ulcer is the cause, since the clinical characteristics of perforation are the same (see Chapter 40).

Gastric Outlet Obstruction. Ulcers located in the antrum and the prepyloric and pyloric areas of the stomach and the duodenum predispose to obstruction. In the early phase of obstruction (often referred to as the *compensated phase*), gastric emptying is normal to near normal. This phase may be associated with large peristaltic waves. Over time, excessive peristalsis creates hypertrophy of the stomach wall. After long-standing obstruction the stomach enters the *decompensated phase,* which results in dilatation and atony. The obstruction is not totally due to fibrous scar tissue because active ulcer formation is associated with edema, inflammation, and pylorospasm, all of which contribute to the narrowing of the pylorus.

The patient with gastric outlet obstruction generally has a long history of ulcer pain. Ulcerlike pain of short duration or complete absence of pain is more indicative of a malignant obstruction. The pain progresses to a more generalized upper abdominal discomfort that becomes worse toward the end of the day as the stomach fills and dilates. Relief may be obtained by belching or by self-induced vomiting. Vomiting is very common and often projectile. The vomitus contains food particles that were ingested many hours or even a day or two before the vomiting episode. There is often an offensive odor if the contents have been dormant in the stomach for a time. The patient who vomits frequently will be anorectic, with evident weight loss, and will complain of thirst and an unpleasant taste in the mouth. Constipation is a common complaint that usually results from dehydration and lack of roughage in the diet.

The patient with gastric outlet obstruction may show a swelling in the upper abdomen indicating dilatation of the stomach. Loud peristalsis can be heard, and visible peristaltic waves are often observed passing across the abdomen from left to right. If the stomach is grossly dilated, it is possible to palpate it as well.

An upper GI examination with barium as contrast medium is helpful in making a diagnosis and demonstrates the presence of an active ulcer crater or scarring from previously healed ulcers. Barium normally should pass from the stomach within 2 hours, but with gastric outlet obstruction, 50% of the barium remains on follow-up films up to 6 hours later.

Diagnostic Studies

The diagnostic measures used to determine the presence and location of a peptic ulcer are similar to those with acute upper GI bleeding. *Fiberoptic endoscopy* is the procedure most often used. It is more reliable than barium contrast studies because of the maneuverability of fiberoptic scopes for viewing the entire gastric and duodenal mucosa. This procedure can also be used to determine the degree of ulcer healing after treatment. During endoscopy, specimens can be obtained for identification of *H. pylori.* When gastric malignancy is a possibility, the endoscope also can be used in obtaining tissue specimens for biopsy.

Barium contrast studies, although widely used, are not accurate in identifying shallow, superficial ulcers because of failure of the barium to properly fill the ulcer crater. X-ray studies are also ineffective in differentiating a peptic ulcer from a malignant tumor. In addition, x-rays do not readily demonstrate the degree of healing that can be visually determined with the endoscope. Barium studies are of benefit in the diagnosis of pyloric obstruction caused by recurrent ulcers.

Exfoliative cytology is valuable when there is a need to distinguish between a benign and a malignant ulcer. The test consists of examining exfoliated cells that are found in various secretions or scraped from mucous membranes. A sample of these cells can be obtained during gastroscopic examination. Although the accuracy of this examination has proven value for determining the presence of a gastric tumor, it should not stand alone as a diagnostic tool because of the danger of false results.

Gastric analysis has questionable value in the diagnosis of peptic ulcer disease because in many patients gastric secretions are normal in amount and composition. However, it can provide important data in (1) identifying a possible gastrinoma (Zollinger-Ellison syndrome), (2) determining the degree of gastric hyperacidity, and (3) evaluating the results of therapy such as vagotomy and histamine H_2 -antagonist drug therapy. Several methods may be used to determine the amount of gastric secretions. An NG tube can be placed into the antrum with the use of fluoroscopy, and the secretions can be collected overnight for a 12-hour period. The HCl acid concentration is calculated and compared with equivalents already established for persons who do not have ulcers, those with gastric and duodenal ulcers, and those with Zollinger-Ellison syndrome. The accuracy of this method is not good because the NG tube may become plugged or aspiration methods may be inconsistent. Augmented histamine or pentagastrin stimulation may be more accurate in estimating the degree of acid secretion. In these tests the stomach's ability to secrete gastric juice is studied after stimulation with either betazole HCl (Histalog) or pentagastrin (a synthetic form of the hormone gastrin).

Laboratory analyses, including a CBC, urinalysis, liver enzyme studies, serum amylase determination, and stool examination, should be performed. A CBC may indicate the presence of anemia secondary to bleeding from the ulcer. Liver enzyme studies help determine any liver problems, such as cirrhosis, that may complicate the treatment of the ulcer. Urine and stool are routinely tested for the presence of blood. A serum amylase determination is frequently ordered if posterior penetration of the pancreas is suspected. It provides data on pancreatic function.

Therapeutic Management

Conservative Management. When the patient's clinical manifestations and health history suggest the diagnosis of a peptic ulcer and diagnostic studies confirm its presence, a medical regimen is instituted (Table 39-9). The regimen consists of adequate rest, dietary interventions, medications, elimination of smoking, and long-term follow-up care. The aim of the treatment program is to decrease the amount of gastric acidity, enhance mucosal defense mechanisms, and minimize the harmful effects on the mucosa. Hospitalization of the patient is not always necessary during the initial treatment phase.

Adequate rest, both physical and emotional, is important in the treatment process. A quiet, calm environment at home or on the job is not easy to achieve and may require some modifications in the patient's daily routine. The benefits derived from the elimination of stressors help decrease the stimulus for overproduction of gastric secretions. Moderation in daily activity is essential. Excessive physical activity can result in increased gastric secretions through increased motor activity.

Dietary changes are necessary so that foods and beverages irritating to the patient can be avoided or eliminated. An individualized bland diet consisting of six small meals a day is usually prescribed in the regimen. However, there is considerable controversy over the actual therapeutic benefits derived from this type of diet, since the rationale for a bland diet is not supported by scientific evidence. Therefore no specific diet seems totally appropriate in the treatment of ulcer disease. Each patient should be instructed to eat and drink foods and fluids that do not cause any distressing or harmful side effects. Alcohol and caffeine-containing products should be eliminated because of their irritating effects.

Smoking has an irritating effect on the mucosa, increases gastric motility, and delays mucosal healing. It should be eliminated completely or severely reduced. The combination of adequate rest and abstinence from smoking accelerates ulcer healing.

Medications are a vital part of therapy. The patient must be well informed about each drug prescribed, why it is ordered, and the expected benefits. Strict adherence to the prescribed regimen of drugs is mandatory. Drug therapy that includes the use of antacids, histamine H_2 -receptor antagonists, antisecretory agents, and anticholinergics is presented in Tables 39-10, 39-11, 39-12, 39-13. Aspirin and NSAIDs should be discontinued. When these medications must be continued, enteric coated or highly buffered preparations are more suitable. Antibiotics to eradicate *H. pylori* infection are prescribed. A major drawback to this therapy is the rapid emergence of resistance to antibiotics by the bacterium.[8]

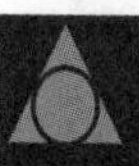

Table 39-9 Therapeutic Management: Peptic Ulcer Disease

Diagnostic
- Complete blood count
- Urinalysis
- Liver enzymes
- Serum electrolytes
- Fiberoptic endoscopy
- Upper GI barium-contrast study
- Gastric analysis
- Exfoliative cytology

Therapeutic

Conservative management
- Adequate rest
- Bland diet (six small meals a day)
- Cessation of smoking
- Medications
  - Antacids (Table 39-11)
  - H_2-receptor blocking agents (Table 39-10)
  - Anticholinergics (Table 39-13)
  - Cytoprotective drugs (sucralfate)
  - H^+, K^+-ATPase inhibitor (omeprazole)
  - Misoprostol (Cytotec)
- Stress reduction

Acute exacerbation without complications
- NPO
- NG suction
- Bed rest to moderate light activity
- Cessation of smoking
- IV fluid replacement
- Medications
  - Antacids
  - H_2-receptor blocking agents
  - H^+, K^+-ATPase inhibitor (omeprazole)
  - Anticholinergics
  - Sedatives

Acute exacerbation with complications (hemorrhage, perforation, obstruction)
- NPO
- NG suction
- Bed rest
- IV fluid replacement (lactated Ringer's solution)
- Blood transfusions
- Stomach lavage

Surgical intervention
- Perforation—simple closure with omentum graft
- Gastric outlet obstruction—pyloroplasty and vagotomy
- Ulcer cure
  - Billroth I and II
  - Vagotomy and pyloroplasty

GI, Gastrointestional; *IV*, intravenous; *NG*, nasogastric; *NPO*, nothing by mouth.

The healing of a peptic ulcer requires many weeks of therapy. Pain disappears after 3 to 6 days, but ulcer healing is much slower. Complete healing may take 3 to 9 weeks, depending on ulcer size and treatment regimen employed. Healing of the ulcer should be assessed by means of x-rays or endoscopic examination. Barium-contrast films can be used to adequately measure the healing of a gastric ulcer.

Table 39-10 Drug Therapy for Peptic Ulcer Disease

Antisecretory
- H_2-receptor antagonists
  - Cimetidine (Tagamet)
  - Ranitidine (Zantac)
  - Famotidine (Pepcid)
  - Nizatidine (Axid)
- H^+, K^+-ATPase inhibitor
  - Omeprazole (Prilosec)

Antisecretory and Cytoprotective
- Misoprostol (Cytotec)

Cytoprotective
- Sucralfate (Carafate)
- Bismuth subsalicylate (Pepto-Bismol)

Neutralizing
- Antacids*

Others
- Tricyclic antidepressants
  - Imipramine
  - Doxepin
- Antibiotics for *H. pylori*
  - Amoxicillin
  - Metronidazole
  - Tetracycline

*See Table 39-11.

However, it should be noted that endoscopic examination is the only accurate method to monitor for duodenal ulcer healing.

Because recurrence of peptic ulcer is frequent, interruption or discontinuation of therapy can have detrimental results. The patient must be encouraged to comply with therapy and continue with follow-up care for at least 1 year. If changes in lifestyle were part of the prescribed therapy, they should be maintained. Antacids and H_2-receptor antagonists may be stopped after the ulcer has healed or may be prescribed in the form of low-dose maintenance therapy. No other medications, unless prescribed by the physician, should be taken because they may have an ulcerogenic effect. Finally, the patient and family should be told what to do in the event pain and discomfort recur or blood is noted in the vomitus or stools.

Acute Exacerbation. The recurrence rate for both gastric and duodenal ulcers is high after treatment. The patient with an acute exacerbation of peptic ulcer can usually be treated with the same regimen used for conservative management. However, the situation is considered more serious because of the chronicity of the ulcer and the possible complications of perforation, hemorrhage, and obstruction.

An acute exacerbation is frequently accompanied by bleeding, increased pain and discomfort, and nausea and vomiting. One method of symptom relief involves the placement of an NG tube into the stomach, with intermittent suction for about 24 to 48 hours. The rationale is to keep the stomach empty and to remove any stimulus for HCl acid and pepsin secretion. Major disadvantages of this

Table 39-11 Composition of Antacid Preparations

Ingredient	Trade Name
Single Substance	
Aluminum carbonate	Basaljel
Aluminum hydroxide gel tablets	Amphojel, Alu-Cap
Aluminum phosphate	Phosphaljel
Calcium carbonate	Alka-2, Tums
Dihydroxyaluminum aminoacetate	Robalate
Dihydroxyaluminum sodium carbonate	Rolaids
Magaldrate	Riopan
Magnesium hydroxide	Mag-Ox, Maox
Sodium bicarbonate	Alka-Seltzer
Mixtures of aluminum hydroxide and magnesium salts	
	Aludrox
	A-M-T
	Cremalin
	Delcid
	Gaviscon
	Gelusil and Gelusil M
	Maalox
	Mylanta
	WinGel
Mixtures of calcium carbonate and aluminum and magnesium hydroxides	
	Camalox
	Ducon
Mixtures of calcium carbonate, magnesium carbonate, and magnesium oxide	
	Alkets

Table 39-12 Side Effects of Antacid Therapy

Antacid	Reactions
Aluminum hydroxide gels	Constipation, phosphorus depletion with chronic use
Calcium carbonate	Constipation or diarrhea, hypercalcemia, milk-alkali syndrome, renal calculi
Magnesium preparations	Diarrhea, hypermagnesemia
Sodium preparations	Milk-alkali syndrome if used with large amounts of calcium, used with caution in patients on sodium restrictions

Table 39-13 Anticholinergic Drugs Used in the Treatment of Peptic Ulcers

Trade Name	Generic Name
Antrenyl bromide	Oxyphenonium bromide, atropine sulfate
Banthine	Methantheline bromide
Bentyl	Dicyclomine
Cantil	Mepenzolate bromide
Darbid	Isopropamide iodide
Daricon	Oxyphencyclimine
Donnatol	Belladonna and phenobarbital
Pamine	Methscopolamine bromide
Pro-Banthine	Propantheline bromide
Robinul	Glycopyrrolate

intervention are esophageal and gastric mucosal irritation and erosion from the NG tube itself.

If there is a history of an incompetent pyloric sphincter allowing reflux of duodenal contents into the stomach, an NG tube will remove intestinal contents from the stomach. The maintenance of an empty stomach decreases the stimulus for pancreatic enzyme secretion as well. This period of stomach rest eliminates any causative factors that may have precipitated the acute exacerbation and permits the resolution of edema and inflammation of the mucosa. Fluids and electrolytes are replaced by IV infusion until the patient is able to tolerate oral feedings without distress.

Blood or blood products may be administered if bleeding has occurred. Careful monitoring of the vital signs, intake and output, laboratory studies, and signs of impending shock are important during this acute episode.

Endoscopic evaluation is performed to reveal the degree of inflammation or bleeding, as well as the ulcer location.[12,13] It is important to ascertain the presence of a prepyloric or pyloric ulcer that can cause gastric outlet obstruction. When endoscopic examination reveals no major problems and the patient's physical condition stabilizes, the plan of care for the patient should follow the same regimen of diet, activity, and medications used in conservative management. A 5-year follow-up program is recommended after acute exacerbation. An increase in the healing rate is achieved after conservative treatment, but the treatment plan cannot prevent the scar formation that can result in gastric outlet obstruction. Approximately 42% to 88% of ulcers recur.

Perforation. The immediate focus of therapeutic management of a patient with a perforation is to stop the spillage of gastric or duodenal contents into the peritoneal cavity and restore blood volume. An NG tube is inserted into the stomach to provide continuous aspiration and gastric decompression to halt spillage through the perforation. Although duodenal aspiration is not achieved as promptly, placement of the tube as near to the perforation site as possible facilitates decompression.

Circulating blood volume must be replaced with lactated Ringer's and albumin solutions. These solutions substitute for the fluids lost from the vascular and interstitial space as the peritonitis develops. Blood replacement in the form of packed RBCs may be necessary. Unless contraindicated, a central venous pressure line and an indwelling urinary catheter should be inserted and monitored hourly. The patient with a history of cardiac disease requires ECG monitoring or placement of a pulmonary artery catheter for more accurate assessment of left ventricular function. Broad-spectrum antibiotic therapy should be started immediately to treat bacterial peritonitis. Administration of pain medications provides comfort.

The operative procedure involving the least risk to the patient is simple oversewing of the perforation and reinforcement of the area with a graft of omentum. The excess gastric contents are suctioned from the peritoneal cavity during the surgical procedure. Before surgical closure some surgeons irrigate with warm lactated Ringer's solution or instill an antibiotic solution into the abdominal cavity to help counteract the peritonitis.

There is controversy regarding the need for more definitive surgical treatment of a perforated ulcer than can be achieved with simple closure. Other types of surgical procedures depend on the location of the peptic ulcer and the surgeon's preference. If cure of the ulcer is the ultimate goal, the surgical procedures may include gastric resection or vagotomy and pyloroplasty.

Gastric Outlet Obstruction. The aim of therapy for gastric outlet obstruction is to decompress the stomach, correct any existing fluid and electrolyte imbalances, and improve the patient's general state of health. An NG tube is inserted into the stomach and attached to continuous suction to remove excess fluids and undigested food particles. With continuous decompression for several days the stomach has the opportunity to regain its normal muscle tone, the ulcer can begin healing, and the inflammation and edema will subside.

The tube is clamped after several days of suction, and gastric residue is measured periodically. The frequency and amount of time the tube remains clamped are proportional to the amount of aspirate obtained and the comfort level of the patient. A method commonly followed is to clamp the tube overnight for approximately 8 to 12 hours and to measure the gastric residue in the morning. When the aspirate falls below 200 ml, it is considered to be within a normal range and the patient can begin oral intake of clear liquids. Initially, oral fluids are begun at 30 ml per hour and then gradually increased in amount. The patient must be watched carefully for signs of distress or vomiting. As the amount of gastric residue decreases, solid foods are added and the tube is removed.

IV fluids and electrolytes are administered according to the degree of dehydration, vomiting, and electrolyte imbalance indicated by laboratory studies. Pain relief results from the decompression measures, and analgesics are usually not necessary. Antacid and histamine H_2-receptor antagonist therapy is an integral part of treatment if the obstruction has been determined on endoscopic examination to be the result of an active ulcer. Pyloric obstruction may be removed nonsurgically by balloon dilatations performed through the endoscope. Surgical intervention may be necessary to remove scar tissue.

Pharmacologic Management

Antacids. Antacids are the initial drugs of choice in the treatment of peptic ulcers.[14] They decrease gastric acidity and the acid content of chyme reaching the duodenum. By raising the pH level to above 3.5, antacids effectively block the conversion of pepsinogen to its active form pepsin. In addition to their neutralizing effects, some antacids, such as aluminum hydroxide, can bind to bile salts, thus decreasing their detrimental effects on the gastric mucosa.

Antacids consist of systemic and nonsystemic types. Systemic antacids, such as sodium bicarbonate, are very soluble and are absorbed into the circulation. Their long-term use can lead to systemic alkalosis; therefore they are rarely used in ulcer treatment. The nonsystemic antacids are insoluble and poorly absorbed. The common commercial nonsystemic antacids consist of calcium carbonate, magnesium hydroxide, or aluminum hydroxide as single preparations or in various combinations (see Table 39-11).

The antacid preparation may be in liquid or tablet form. A large number of tablets may be required to equal the same dose of a liquid preparation. Since the tablets are chewable, much of the medication is left coating the teeth and gingivae instead of the stomach.

It has long been recognized that antacids ingested on an empty stomach are quickly evacuated and only partially used. Because the duration of action is only about 30 minutes, best results are obtained when they are prescribed 1 and 3 hours after meals and at bedtime. More frequent administration has resulted in poor tolerance and reduced long-term compliance. Acid secretion is also known to occur with higher doses and frequency by maintaining a high antral pH, which in turn stimulates release of gastrin.

The type and dosage of antacid prescribed depends on the adverse effects some of these preparations have on the health status or on other medications the patient may be taking (see Table 39-12). Preparations high in sodium, such as Titralac, Di-Gel, and Amphojel, should be used with caution in older adults and in the patient with cirrhosis of the liver, hypertension, congestive heart failure, and renal disease. Magnesium preparations should not be prescribed for the patient in renal failure because of the risk of magnesium toxicity. The most frequent side effect experienced with magnesium antacids is diarrhea. Aluminum hydroxide causes constipation. The combination of aluminum and magnesium salts seems to lessen the side effects of both.

Antacids have the capacity to interact unfavorably with some medications. They can enhance the absorption of drugs such as dicumarol and amphetamines. The action of digitalis preparations can be potentiated when taken in combination with calcium or magnesium antacids. In some instances, antacids may decrease the absorption rates of prescribed drugs, such as tetracycline. Therefore it is important to inform the physician of any drugs that are being taken before antacid therapy is begun.

The dosage of antacid must often be adjusted by the physician so that the amount prescribed has the capacity of neutralizing the acid present. It is generally recommended that each dose of an antacid be capable of neutralizing 100

Clinical Manifestations

The clinical manifestations exhibited by persons with gastric cancer can be categorized by signs and symptoms of anemia, peptic ulcer disease, or indigestion. Anemia is a common occurrence with stomach cancer. It is caused by chronic blood loss as the lesion erodes through the mucosa or as a direct result of pernicious anemia, which develops when intrinsic factor is lost. The person appears pale and weak and complains of fatigue, weakness, dizziness, and, in extreme cases, shortness of breath. The stool may be positive for occult blood.

The symptoms of gastric malignancy are sometimes identical to those of peptic ulcer disease. The pain and discomfort can actually be alleviated by belching and by the use of antacids and diet restrictions.

Manifestations related to indigestion include vague epigastric fullness with feelings of early satiety after meals. Weight loss, dysphagia, and constipation frequently accompany epigastric distress. When nausea, vomiting, and hematemesis occur, they may indicate obstruction at the gastric outlet or may be a warning of impending hemorrhage.

The early detection of gastric cancer is difficult because of the diversity of symptoms. On physical examination the patient may be pale and lethargic if anemia is present. When the appetite has been poor and weight loss has been considerable, the patient may appear cachectic. A mass can often be detected beneath the abdominal wall and is seen to move with each inspiration. On palpation the mass may be felt in the epigastrium. Masses that are predominantly in the antrum of the stomach are generally found to the left of the midline. Masses located to the right of midline usually tend to be metastases to the liver or indicate involvement of the perigastric lymph nodes. Supraclavicular lymph nodes that are hard and enlarged and located on the left side are suggestive of metastasis via the thoracic duct from the stomach lesion. The presence of ascites is an unfavorable sign.

Diagnostic Studies

The diagnostic studies for gastric malignancy include laboratory analysis of blood, stool, and gastric secretions. Blood chemistry studies assist in the determination of anemia and its severity. Liver enzymes and serum amylase may indicate liver and pancreatic involvement or other abnormalities related to their dysfunction. Stool examination provides evidence of occult or gross bleeding. A gastric analysis indicates the level of HCl acid present in the stomach after fasting. Washings obtained during the gastric analysis can be used for the exfoliative cytologic examination. The test demonstrates the histologic changes indicative of malignancy. However, this test should never be used as the sole diagnostic criterion because false readings are sometimes obtained.

The carcinoembryonic antigen (CEA) radioimmunoassay test is used as an adjunctive diagnostic tool for cancer of the GI tract. CEA is a glycoprotein that is found in significant amounts in embryonic life, especially in the large intestine. It is also found in some adult patients with GI carcinomas. Elevated levels of CEA may indicate malignancy, yet CEA may be elevated in persons who smoke and also in those with benign lesions. Therefore, whereas the CEA test may be of some use in the preoperative work-up of a patient with suspected cancer of the stomach, it should never be used as the only diagnostic tool. (CEA is also discussed in Chapters 12 and 40.)

Upper GI barium studies may demonstrate defects in peristalsis, tone, secretion, motility, and spasm of the stomach. On x-ray examination the malignant ulcer crater is more irregular around the edges and more elevated than the craters found with benign peptic ulcers. Barium studies do not always detect small lesions of the cardia and fundus.

Endoscopic examination of the stomach should be performed along with barium x-ray studies. Lesions that go undetected on x-ray can be more easily viewed and biopsied when the fiberoptic scope is used. The stomach can be distended with air during the procedure so that the mucosal folds can be stretched. Fixation of the mucosa is indicative of malignancy.

Therapeutic Management

When the diagnosis of gastric malignancy has been confirmed, the treatment of choice is surgical removal of the tumor. The preoperative management of the patient with gastric cancer focuses on the correction of nutritional deficits, transfusions for the treatment of anemia, and replacement of blood volume (Table 39-16).

Transfusions of packed RBCs correct the anemia. If a gastric lesion has been located at or near the pylorus and is causing gastric outlet obstruction, gastric decompression may be necessary before surgery. When the tumor has extended into the transverse colon and partial colon resec-

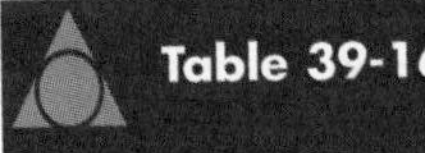

Table 39-16 Therapeutic Management: Gastric Cancer

Diagnostic
- History and physical examination
- Complete blood count
- Urinalysis
- Stool examination
- Liver enzymes
- Serum amylase
- Upper gastrointestinal barium study
- Carcinoembryonic antigen
- Exfoliative cytology
- Fiberoptic endoscopy and biopsy
- Gastric analysis

Therapeutic
- Surgery
  - Subtotal gastrectomy—Billroth I or II procedure
  - Total gastrectomy with esophagojejunostomy
- Adjuvant therapy
  - Radiation therapy
  - Chemotherapy
  - Combination radiation therapy and chemotherapy

tion is also required, special preparation of the bowel is necessary. This preparation may include a low-residue diet, enemas to cleanse the bowel, and the use of antibiotics to reduce the intestinal bacteria. The patient with achlorhydria who does not have gastric acid available to destroy the bacteria may also need antibiotic bowel preparation.

Correction of malnutrition is vital if surgery is planned. Malnutrition is associated with increased postoperative complications and mortality rates.

Surgical Interventions

The surgical intervention used in the treatment of stomach cancer may be the same surgical procedures used for peptic ulcer disease. The specific surgery employed is determined by the location and extent of the lesion, the patient's physical condition, and preference of the surgeon. When metastasis is widespread at the time of diagnosis, surgical intervention may be only palliative.

The surgical aim is to remove as much of the stomach as necessary to remove the tumor and a margin of normal tissue. When the lesion is located in the cardia or high in the fundus, a total gastrectomy with esophagojejunostomy is performed. This procedure involves anastomosis of the lower end of the esophagus to the jejunum (Fig. 39-7). Lesions located in the antrum or the pyloric region are generally treated by either a Billroth I or Billroth II procedure. When metastasis has occurred to adjacent organs, such as the spleen, ovaries, or bowel, the surgical procedures must be modified and extended as necessary.

The chance of a complete cure by surgical means is decreased considerably when the lymph nodes are involved. Survival rates are considerably shortened when organs adjacent to the stomach show evidence of invasion at the time of surgery.

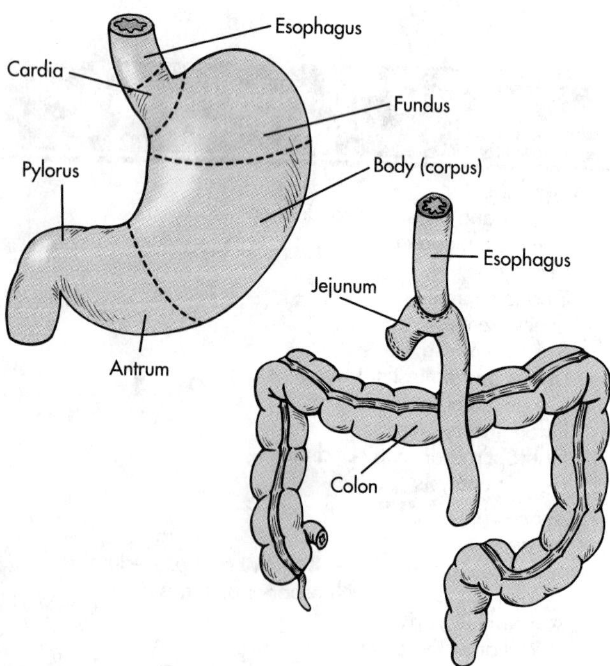

Fig. 39-7 A total gastrectomy for gastric cancer (total gastrectomy with esophagojejunostomy).

Adjuvant Therapy. Surgery is the only definitive means of achieving a cure. However, when the patient cannot physically withstand a surgical procedure or when surgical cure is not feasible, radiation or chemotherapy alone or in combination may be used. Neither radiation therapy nor chemotherapeutic agents have been very successful when used as the primary mode of treatment. Radiation therapy has proved to be of little value except in certain instances of obstruction of the cardia. The radiosensitivity of gastric cancers is low.

Preoperative radiation is usually not done because of the risk of poor wound healing of the anastomosis of the gastric stump to the bowel. When radiation is used as a palliative measure, the tumor mass can be decreased, with temporary relief of the cardia or pyloric obstruction. Postoperative radiation has not been widely used nor has it increased survival rates. The combination of chemotherapy and radiation is now being used for patients who are not candidates for surgical excision. Combination chemotherapy only causes a temporary relief of symptoms, and long-term survival rates have not shown significant improvement.

Until recently, single-agent chemotherapy for gastric cancer has proved of little value. Agents that have been identified as having some effect on gastric cancer are 5-FU, BCNU, methyl CCNU, doxorubicin (Adriamycin), and triazinate. A better response rate in patients with advanced gastric cancer is now found when chemotherapeutic agents are used in combination, such as FAT (5-FU, doxorubicin, and triazinate). The hope for better outcomes with the use of chemotherapy depends on finding new ways of administering old drugs, finding new drugs, and determining new drug combinations. The hope for the ultimate cure of patients with gastric cancer now seems to lie in the combined efforts of surgery, radiation, and chemotherapy. The role of biological response modifiers is still under investigation for use in gastric cancer. (These therapies are discussed in Chapter 12.)

NURSING MANAGEMENT

GASTRIC CANCER

Nursing Assessment

The assessment of a person with possible gastric cancer is similar to that for one with peptic ulcer disease (see Table 39-14). Important data to be obtained from the patient and the family should include a nutritional assessment, a psychosocial history, the patient's perceptions of the health problem and need for hospitalization, and the physical examination of the patient.

The nutritional assessment must elicit information regarding appetite, changes in eating patterns over the previous 6 months, and the role of highly seasoned or salty foods as a regular part of the diet. It is necessary to determine the patient's normal weight and any changes that may have occurred in the past few months. Unexplained weight loss is common in many types of cancer before diagnosis. A history of vague symptoms of dyspepsia, early satiety, feeling full after consuming even a small amount of food, or reporting symptoms of gas pain should help the nurse differentiate these typical gastric cancer symptoms from those of peptic ulcer. As with peptic ulcer patients, the nurse should determine whether pain is present, where and when it occurs, and how it is relieved. When the pain has been controlled with ingestion of foods, fluids, or antacids for a period of time but now continues or worsens regardless of interventions, gastric cancer may be the underlying cause.

Psychosocial and demographic data include age, present or previous occupation, and financial status. Gastric cancer can occur at any age, but the risk is more prevalent in men in the fifth to the sixth decade of life. A family history of cancer, especially gastric cancer, puts a person at greater than normal risk.

It is important to determine the patient's personal perception of the health problem and method of coping with hospitalization, diagnostic tests, and procedures and the way personal crisis was managed in the past. The possibility of a diagnosis of cancer and a treatment regimen that may include surgery, chemotherapy, or radiation treatment forecasts a prolonged stressful period and a possibly fatal outcome. Therefore it is essential that the nurse learn as much as possible about what the patient and the family understand and how well they will be able to handle and support the patient if tests result in an unfavorable diagnosis and complex treatment interventions are planned. If surgery is probable, the nurse should assess what the patient expects from surgery (cure or palliation) and how that patient has responded to any previous surgical procedures.

A complete physical examination reveals the patient's current functional abilities, the presence of other health problems, and an estimate on how well the patient may respond to therapy. Cachexia may be evident if the nutritional state has been compromised for an extended time. A malnourished patient does not respond well to chemotherapy or radiation therapy and is a poor surgical risk.

Nursing Diagnoses

Nursing diagnoses specific to the patient with gastric cancer include, but are not limited to, the following:

- Altered nutrition: less than body requirements related to inability to ingest, digest, or absorb nutrients
- Activity intolerance related to generalized weakness, abdominal discomfort, and nutritional deficits
- Anxiety related to lack of knowledge of diagnostic tests, unknown diagnostic outcome, disease process, and therapeutic regimen
- Pain related to underlying disease process and side effects of surgery, chemotherapy, or radiation therapy
- Anticipatory grieving related to perceived unfavorable diagnosis and impending death

Planning

The overall goals are that the patient with gastric cancer will (1) experience minimal discomfort, (2) achieve optimal nutritional status, and (3) maintain a degree of spiritual and psychologic well-being appropriate to the disease stage.

Nursing Implementation

Health Maintenance and Promotion. The nursing role in the early detection of cancer of the stomach is focused primarily on identification of the patient at risk because of specific disorders such as pernicious anemia and achlorhydria. The nurse should be aware of symptoms associated with gastric cancer, method of spread, and the significant findings on physical examination. The nurse should understand that the cure rate is often quite dismal because symptoms arise late in the course of the disease process, are vague, and often mimic other conditions, such as peptic ulcers.

The nurse must be alert to problems suggesting gastric cancer, such as poor appetite, weight loss, fatigue, and persistent gastric distress. If any of these manifestations are present, medical attention should be obtained and the necessary diagnostic tests performed. The role of diet in the causation of gastric cancer should be well understood by the nurse so that the patient at risk can be taught acceptable dietary alternatives. Changing dietary patterns may prevent stomach cancers.[18]

In addition, any patient with a positive family history of gastric cancer should be encouraged to undergo diagnostic evaluation if manifestations of anemia, peptic ulcer, or vague epigastric distress are present. It is imperative that the nurse recognize the possible existence of stomach cancer in a patient who is treated for peptic ulcer and who fails to gain relief after 3 weeks of diet and prescribed medications. The ulcer, if it is benign, should show signs of healing on x-ray examination.

Acute Intervention

Preoperative care. When the diagnostic tests confirm the presence of a malignancy, the patient and the family generally react with shock, disbelief, and depression, regardless of how thoroughly they may have been prepared for this possible outcome. The psychologic impact of the diagnosis, added to the physical distress already being experienced, can be quite devastating. Throughout this period the nurse must give emotional and physical support, provide information, clarify test results, and maintain a positive attitude with respect to the patient's immediate recovery and long-term survival.

On admission to the hospital, the patient may be in poor physical condition. Surgery may have to be delayed while the patient becomes more physically able to withstand the strain of major surgery. A positive nutritional state enhances wound healing as well as the ability to withstand infection and other possible postoperative complications. The nursing staff should recognize the necessity for surgical delay and the advantages to be gained for the patient. Many times the patient has been anorectic for a long time and has lost considerable body weight. The nutritional state is improved by a well-balanced diet, along with the administration of supplemental vitamins. Often the patient is better able to tolerate several small meals a day rather than three regular meals. The diet may be supplemented by a variety of commercial liquid supplements (see Chapter 37) and vitamins. The nurse is challenged to find innovative ways of persuading the patient to eat when lack of appetite and state of mind make eating difficult and unrewarding. Getting the patient's family to assist with meals and encourage intake may be beneficial. If the patient is unable to ingest oral feedings, it may be necessary to provide for nutritional needs with tube feedings or parenteral nutrition.

If needed, blood replacement and fluid volume restoration may be carried out in the preoperative period. Because anemia is usually present, packed RBCs may be administered. Close observation for reactions to the transfusions is important. Monitoring the hemoglobin and hematocrit levels provides information on the progress of therapy.

The preoperative teaching plan before gastric surgery for cancer is much the same as that for peptic ulcer surgery (see the previous section on Surgical Interventions Related to Peptic Ulcer).

Postoperative care. Postoperative care of the patient with gastric carcinoma is similar to that following a Billroth I or II procedure (see the previous section on Surgical Interventions Related to Peptic Ulcer). When the surgical intervention has involved a total gastrectomy, the plan of care is somewhat different. The operation performed usually requires some resecting of the lower esophagus along with the removal of the entire stomach and anastomosis of the esophagus to the jejunum. The chest cavity must be entered, and drainage is accomplished by the insertion of chest tubes. (Chest surgery and drainage tubes are discussed in Chapter 24.) After total gastrectomy, the NG tube does not drain a large quantity of secretions because removal of the stomach has eliminated the reservoir capacity. The NG tube is removed after several days, when peristalsis has resumed. Small amounts of clear fluid may then be started. The patient requires close observation for signs of leakage of the fluids at the anastomosis as evidenced by an elevation in the temperature and increasing dyspnea. When fluids are well tolerated without distress, the amount may be increased along with the addition of some solid foods. Meals consist of six to eight small feedings a day, and this pattern will be necessary for the lifetime of the patient.

As a consequence of a total gastrectomy, a patient experiences the symptoms of the dumping syndrome. Unfortunately, weight loss is very common, and these patients never do well nutritionally the rest of their lives. Postoperative wound healing may be impaired because of avitaminosis. This necessitates the IV or oral replacement of vitamins C, D, K, and the B complex vitamins and IM administration of vitamin B_{12}. Because these vitamins are absorbed primarily in the upper part of the small intestine, they must be replaced, since the duodenum has been bypassed in the surgical procedure.

A patient who has a Billroth I or II operative procedure should receive the same postoperative care as one who has had peptic ulcer surgery. This patient is also subject to the same type of postoperative complications as the dumping syndrome and postprandial hypoglycemia.

The patient with advanced malignant disease can be offered only palliative treatment. The chemotherapy agent found most useful for controlling symptoms of gastric cancer is 5-FU. When this medication or any of the combination drugs is prescribed, the nurse must have current information regarding the action and side effects of the drugs. The patient should be made aware of the potential benefits and hazards that can result from the chemotherapy. (The care of the patient receiving chemotherapy is discussed in detail in Chapter 12.)

Radiation therapy can be used as an adjuvant to surgery or for palliation. A patient is generally quite fearful of radiation and may develop many misconceptions regarding its value and dangers. To reassure the patient and ensure completion of the designated number of treatments, the nurse must provide detailed instruction. Because most therapy is completed on an outpatient basis, the nurse should assess the patient's knowledge of radiation, care of the skin, the need for good nutrition and fluid intake during therapy, and the appropriate use of antiemetic drugs. (Specific care of the patient receiving radiation therapy is discussed in Chapter 12.)

Chronic and Home Management. Before the patient is discharged, the need for teaching should be reviewed. Most dietary measures useful after peptic ulcer surgery are applicable after surgery for gastric carcinoma. Plans should be made for the relief of pain, including comfort measures and the judicious use of analgesics. Wound care, if needed, must be taught to the primary caregiver in the home situation. Dressings, special equipment, or special services may be required for the patient's continued care at home. A list of community agencies that are available for assistance can be provided before the patient goes home. The services of the American Cancer Society are especially helpful.

When treatment in the form of chemotherapy or radiation therapy is to be continued after discharge, a referral to the public health nurse may be beneficial. The public health nurse can assist with recovery, determine the degree of patient compliance, and be a sympathetic health care provider with whom the patient can consult.

Long-term follow-up must be stressed. The patient must be encouraged to comply with the prescribed dietary and medication regimens, keep appointments for chemotherapy administration or radiation treatments, and keep the physician informed of changes in physical condition. (Dealing with the long-term management of the cancer patient is discussed in Chapter 12.)

CRITICAL THINKING EXERCISES

CASE STUDY

NAUSEA AND VOMITING

Patient Profile

Roberta, a 40-year-old graduate student in nursing, is admitted to the emergency department with a history of continuous nausea and vomiting during the past 12 hours.

Subjective Data

- Has been experiencing occasional pain in right upper quadrant of abdomen
- Had three normal deliveries previously
- Has been vomiting all day
- Ate potato salad the previous day
- States she is very thirsty

Objective Data

Physical Examination

- Slightly decreased skin turgor
- Rigid RUQ during occasional pain spasms
- Vomitus is clear liquid

Laboratory Results

- Hb 17 g/dl (170 g/L); Hct 51%

Critical Thinking Questions

1. Discuss the concept of hemoconcentration as an indicator of depleted fluid status.
2. Outside the examining room, Roberta's husband asks you if there's a chance that Roberta might be seriously ill. What is your reply?
3. Discuss the importance of good oral care during periods of vomiting. What are the specific reasons that vomitus or regurgitated gastric contents are damaging to the teeth and oral mucosa?
4. Discuss proper positioning of the patient experiencing nausea and vomiting. What are your rationales for choosing a specific position?
5. Based on the assessment data presented, write one or more appropriate nursing diagnosis. Are there any collaborative problems?

NURSING RESEARCH ISSUES

1. What are optimal strategies to promote multiple life-style changes in a patient with peptic ulcer disease?
2. What are effective teaching methods to use in motivating a patient to make changes in smoking, alcohol, and food intake patterns?
3. What are environmental manipulations that could be used to promote decreased nausea in patients receiving chemotherapy?
4. What sensory stimuli in the environment, including sight, smell, and sound, could promote optimal nutrient intake in the chemotherapy patient who is experiencing nausea?
5. What is the most effective way to obtain a nutritional assessment from a patient with gastric carcinoma?
6. What indicators of poor nutritional status are the best markers of such problems as avitaminosis in a patient with gastric cancer?

REVIEW QUESTIONS

The number of the question corresponds to the same-numbered objective at the beginning of the chapter.

1. Mrs. J. calls to tell you that her elderly mother, age 85, has been nauseated all day and has vomited twice. Before you hang up and telephone the physician to communicate your assessment data, you instruct Mrs. Jones to

a. offer her mother a high-protein liquid supplement to drink to maintain her nutritional needs.
b. offer her mother large quantities of Gatorade to drink, since elderly people are at risk for sodium depletion.
c. give her mother sips of water and elevate the head of her bed to prevent aspiration.
d. administer antispasmodic medications and observe skin turgor.

2. The pernicious anemia which may accompany gastritis is due to which of the following?

a. Progressive gastric atrophy from chronic breakage in the mucosal barrier and blood loss
b. A lack of intrinsic factor normally produced by acid-secreting cells of the gastric mucosa
c. Hyperchlorhydria due to an increase in acid-secreting parietal cells and degradation of RBCs
d. Chronic autoimmune destruction of vitamin B_{12} stores in the body

3. Your teaching plan for the patient being discharged following an acute episode of GI bleeding will include information concerning the importance of

a. reading all over-the-counter medication labels to avoid medications containing stearic acid and calcium.
b. taking only medications prescribed by the physician.

c. taking all medications one hour before mealtime to prevent further bleeding.
d. avoiding taking aspirin with acidic beverages such as orange juice.

4. You are teaching your patient and her family about possible causative factors for peptic ulcers. You explain that ulcer formation is

a. promoted by a combination of possible factors which may result in erosion of the gastric mucosa, including certain medications, and alcohol.
b. caused by a stressful lifestyle and other acid-producing factors such as *C. pylori.*
c. inherited within families and reinforced by bacterial spread of *Staphylococcus aureus* in childhood.
d. promoted by factors which tend to cause oversecretion of acid, such as excess dietary fats, smoking, and *B. pylori.*

5. The dumping syndrome is associated with large

a. hyperosmolar volumes emptying rapidly into the intestine.
b. hypoosmolar volumes drawing fluid out of the plasma space and into the bowel.
c. isotonic volumes stimulating increased gastrointestinal motility.
d. hypertonic volumes promoting third-spacing in the intestinal cavity.

6. An optimal teaching plan for an outpatient with gastric carcinoma receiving radiation therapy should include information about

a. prosthetic devices, skin conductance, and grief counseling.
b. avitaminosis, ostomy care, and community resources.
c. cancer support groups, alopecia, and stomatitis.
d. wound and skin care, nutrition, medications, and community resources.

REFERENCES

1. Williams C: Causes and management of nausea and vomiting, *Nurs Times* 90:38, 1994.
2. Kauvar D: Treatment of common GI disorders in the elderly, *Physician Assist* 16:105, 1992.
3. Robert M, Weinstein W: *Helicobacter pylori*-associated gastric pathology, *Gastroenterol Clin North Am* 22:59, 1993.
4. Maier RV, Mitchell D, Gentilello L: Optimal therapy for stress gastritis, *Ann Surg* 220:353, 1994.
5. Kandel G: Management of nonvariceal upper GI hemorrhage, *Hosp Pract* 25:167, 1990.
6. Wiboltt KS, Petersson BG: Treatment of acute upper gastrointestinal bleeding: a retrospective study of the results in a surgical clinic, *Eur J Surg* 160:375, 1994.
7. Sleisenger MH and others: *Gastrointestinal disease: pathophysiology, diagnosis, management,* ed 5, Philadelphia, 1993, WB Saunders.
8. Tytgat G, Noach L, Rauws E: *Helicobacter pylori* infection and duodenal ulcer disease, *Gastroenterol Clin North Am* 22:127, 1993.
9. Pounder RE: Treatment of peptic ulcers from now to the millennium, *Baillieres Clin Gastroenterol* 8:339, 1994.
10. Dunn B: Pathogenic mechanisms of *Helicobacter pylori, Gastroenterology Clin North Am* 22:43, 1993.
11. Holland EG, Taylor AT: Practical management of stress-related gastric ulcers, *J Fam Pract* 33:625, 1991.
12. Parsonnet J: *Helicobacter pylori* and gastric cancer, *Gastroenterol Clin North Am* 22:89, 1993.
13. Ralph-Edwards A, Himal HS: Bleeding gastric and duodenal ulcers: endoscopic therapy versus surgery, *Can J Surg* 35:177, 1992.
14. Anonymous: Drugs for treatment of peptic ulcers, *Med Lett Drugs Ther* 36:65, 1994.
15. Andrews C: Ulcer-healing drugs and their actions and side-effects, *Nurs Times* 90:38, 1994.
16. Thompson GB: Gastric adenocarcinoma: where are we headed?, *Hosp Pract* 30:33, 1995.
17. Hoebler L, Irwin MM: Gastrointestinal tract cancer: current knowledge, medical treatment, and nursing management, *Oncol Nurs Forum* 19:1403, 1992.
18. Frank-Stromborg M: The epidemiology and primary prevention of gastric and esophageal cancer, *Cancer Nurs* 12:57, 1989.

Chapter 40

NURSING ROLE IN MANAGEMENT

Problems of Absorption and Elimination

Margaret Heitkemper **Lynda Sawchuck**

Learning Objectives

1. Explain the common etiologies and therapeutic and nursing management of diarrhea, fecal incontinence, and constipation.
2. Describe common causes of an acute abdomen and nursing care of the patient following an exploratory laparotomy.
3. Describe the nursing management of a patient with acute appendicitis.
4. Identify the therapeutic and nursing management of peritonitis.
5. Describe the common etiologies, clinical manifestations, and management of gastroenteritis.
6. Compare and contrast ulcerative colitis and Crohn's disease, including pathophysiology, clinical manifestations, complications, and therapeutic and nursing management.
7. Differentiate among mechanical, neurogenic, and vascular bowel obstructions, including causes and therapeutic and nursing management.
8. Describe the clinical manifestations and surgical and nursing management of cancer of the colon and rectum.
9. Explain the anatomic and physiologic changes that result from a sigmoid colostomy, a transverse colostomy, and an ileostomy.
10. Describe the preoperative and postoperative therapeutic and nursing management of a patient having bowel surgery.
11. Compare and contrast a colostomy and an ileostomy in relation to nursing care and patient teaching.
12. Differentiate between diverticulosis and diverticulitis, including clinical manifestations and therapeutic and nursing management.
13. Compare and contrast the types of hernias, including etiology and surgical and nursing management.
14. Describe the types of malabsorption syndrome and appropriate management of sprue syndrome and lactase deficiency.
15. Describe the types, clinical manifestations, and therapeutic and nursing management of anorectal conditions.

DIARRHEA, FECAL INCONTINENCE, AND CONSTIPATION

Diarrhea

Etiology. Diarrhea is not a disease but a symptom. The term *diarrhea* may mean different things to different patients. It is commonly used to denote an increase in stool frequency or volume and an increase in the looseness of stool. Causes of diarrhea can be divided into the general classifications of decreased fluid absorption, increased fluid secretion, motility disturbances, or a combination of these (Table 40-1). Causes of acute infectious diarrhea are listed in Table 40-2.

Reviewed by Diane Britt, RN, MN, Medical-Surgical Nurse Clinical Specialist, University of Washington Medical Center, Seattle, WA.

Clinical Manifestations and Complications. Diarrhea may be acute or chronic. *Acute* diarrhea most commonly results from infection. Bacterial or viral infection of the intestine may result in explosive watery diarrhea, *tenesmus* (spasmodic contraction of anal sphincter with pain and persistent desire to defecate), and abdominal cramping pain. Perianal skin irritation may also develop. Systemic manifestations include fever, nausea, vomiting, and malaise. Leukocytes, blood, and mucus may be present in the stool, depending on the causative agent (Table 40-2). Acute diarrhea is often self-limiting in the adult. Symptoms continue until the irritant or causative agent is excreted. The mucous membrane lining of the gastrointestinal (GI) tract is composed of epithelial cells, which regenerate following the inflammatory response.

Table 40-1 Causes of Diarrhea

Decreased Fluid Absorption
- Oral intake of poorly absorbable solutes (e.g., laxatives)
- Maldigestion and malabsorption
  - Mucosal damage: tropical sprue, Crohn's disease, radiation injury, ulcerative colitis, ischemic bowel disease
  - Pancreatic insufficiency
  - Intestinal enzyme deficiencies (e.g., lactase)
  - Bile salt deficiency
  - Decreased surface area (e.g., intestinal resection)

Increased Fluid Secretion
- Infectious: bacterial endotoxins (e.g., Cholera, *Escherichia coli, Shigella, Salmonella, Staphylococcus, Clostridium difficile,* viral agents [rotavirus], and parasitic agents [*Giardia lamblia*])
- Drugs: laxatives, antibiotics
- Hormonal: vasoactive intestinal polypeptide secretion from adenoma of the pancreas; gastrin secretion caused by Zollinger-Ellison syndrome; calcitonin secretion from carcinoma of the thyroid
- Tumor: villous adenoma

Motility Disturbances
- Irritable bowel syndrome
- Diabetic enteropathy
- Visceral scleroderma
- Carcinoid syndrome
- Vagotomy

Diarrhea is considered *chronic* when it persists for at least 2 weeks or when it subsides and returns more than 2 to 4 weeks after the initial episode. Severe diarrhea may be debilitating and life threatening. A patient may have severe dehydration (water and sodium loss) and electrolyte disturbances. Malabsorption and malnutrition are also sequelae of chronic diarrhea. Throughout the world diarrhea is one of the major causes of death, especially in infants.

Diagnostic Studies. Accurate diagnosis and management require a thorough history, physical examination, and, when indicated, laboratory tests. A history of travel, medication use, diet, previous surgery, and interpersonal contacts, as well as family history, should be obtained. Blood tests may identify anemia, elevated white blood cell (WBC) count, iron and folate deficiencies, liver enzyme increases, and electrolyte disturbances. Stools may be examined for the presence of blood, mucus, WBCs, and parasites. Stool cultures help in identifying infectious organisms.

In a patient with chronic diarrhea, measurement of stool electrolytes, pH, and osmolality may help determine whether the diarrhea is related to decreased fluid absorption or increased fluid secretion (secretory diarrhea). Measurement of stool fat and undigested muscle fibers may indicate fat and protein malabsorption conditions, including pancreatic insufficiency. Elevated serum levels of GI peptides such as vasoactive intestinal polypeptide (VIP) and gastrin may be present in some patients with secretory diarrhea. Endoscopy may be used to examine the mucosa and to obtain specimens for examination. Upper and lower barium studies may be helpful in detecting mucosal disease.

Therapeutic Management. The treatment of diarrhea is based on the cause and is aimed at replacement of fluid and electrolytes and decreasing the number, volume, and frequency of stools. Oral solutions containing glucose and electrolytes (e.g., Gatorade, Pedialyte) are often sufficient to replace losses from mild diarrhea. In situations of severe diarrhea, parenteral administration of fluids, electrolytes, vitamins, and potentially, nutrition is warranted.

Once the cause of the diarrhea has been ascertained antidiarrheal agents may be given to coat and protect mucous membranes, inhibit GI motility, decrease intestinal secretions, and decrease central nervous system (CNS) input to the GI tract (Table 40-3). Antiperistaltic agents are not given to a patient who has infectious diarrheal syndromes because of the potential of prolonging exposure to the infectious agent. Antidiarrheal medications should not be given for a prolonged time.

Antibiotics are usually not indicated in the treatment of diarrhea. Many antibiotics can cause diarrhea by altering the normal bowel flora. After administration of some antibiotics (e.g., clindamycin), *Clostridium difficile* may colonize the colon and produce pseudomembranous enterocolitis.[1] *C. difficile* releases a toxin that causes mucosal damage resulting in cramps, pain, and diarrhea that may be bloody. A patient with severe diarrhea may also have fever, leukocytosis, and dehydration. Health care workers who do not adhere to hand-washing procedures can transmit *C. difficile* from patient to patient.

NURSING MANAGEMENT

ACUTE INFECTIOUS DIARRHEA

Nursing Assessment

Nursing assessment should begin with a thorough history and physical examination (Table 40-4). The patient should be asked to describe the stool pattern and associated symptoms. Questions should focus on the duration, frequency, character, and consistency of stool. A medication history should include use of antibiotics, laxatives, and other drugs known to cause diarrhea. Recent travel, stress, and health and family history should be discussed. Dietary history should include questions about eating habits, appetite, and food intolerances, especially milk and dairy products.

Physical examination begins with obtaining vital signs and height and weight. The patient's skin should be inspected for decreased turgor, dryness, and areas of breakdown. The abdomen should be inspected for distention, auscultated for bowel sounds, and palpated for tenderness.

Nursing Diagnoses

Nursing diagnoses are determined when the problem and etiologic factors are supported by clinical data. Nursing diagnoses related to acute infectious diarrhea may include, but are not limited to, those presented in the nursing care plan for the patient with infectious diarrhea on p. 1211.

Table 40-2 Causes of Acute Infectious Diarrhea

	Onset	Duration	Symptoms and Signs
Viral			
Rotavirus, Norwalk	18-24 hr	24-48 hr	Explosive, watery diarrhea; nausea; vomiting; abdominal cramps
Bacterial			
Escherichia coli	4-24 hr	3-4 days	Four or five loose stools per day, nausea, malaise, low-grade fever
Shigella	24 hr	7 days	Watery stools containing blood and mucus, fever, tenesmus, urgency
Salmonellae	6-48 hr	2-5 days	Watery diarrhea, fever, nausea
Campylobacter species	24 hr	< 7 days	Profuse, watery diarrhea; malaise; nausea; abdominal cramps; low-grade fever
Clostridium perfringens	8-12 hr	24 hr	Watery diarrhea, abdominal cramps, vomiting
Clostridium difficile toxin	4-9 days after start of antibiotics	1-3 wk	Associated with antibiotic treatment; symptoms range from mild, watery diarrhea to severe abdominal pain, fever, leukocytosis, hypoalbuminemia, leukocytes in stool
Parasitic			
Giardia lamblia	1-3 wk	Few days to 3 months	Sudden onset; foul, explosive, watery diarrhea; flatulence; epigastric pain and cramping; nausea
Entamoeba histolytica	4 days	Weeks to months	Frequent soft stools with blood and mucus (in severe cases, watery stools), flatulence, distention, cramping, fever, leukocytes in stool

Table 40-3 Antidiarrheal Drugs

Type	Mechanism of Action	Examples
Demulcent	Soothes, coats, and protects mucous membranes	Bismuth subsalicylate (Pepto-Bismol; calcium polycarbophil (Mitrolan-OTC); activated charcoal; kaolin, pectin, hyoscyamine sulfate, atropine sulfate, and hyoscine hydrobromide (Donnagel)*; donnagel and opium (Donnagel-PG)*
Anticholinergic	Inhibits GI motility	Donnagel,* Donnagel-PG,* diphenoxylate with atropine sulfate (Lomotil, Colonaid), loperamide (Imodium)†
Antisecretory	Decreases intestinal secretion	Octreotide (Sandostatin), a synthetic analog of somatostatin
Narcotic	Decreases CNS stimulation of GI tract	Camphorated tincture of opium (paregoric); Donnagel-PG; paregoric, pectin, and kaolin (Parepectolin); tincture of opium, homatropine methylbromide, and pectin (Dia-Quel liquid OTC)‡

CNS, Central nervous system; *GI*, gastrointestinal.
* Also absorbent, which contributes to the adhesiveness of the stool.
† Has cholinergic and noncholinergic actions.
‡ Also an anticholinergic.

Planning

The overall goals are that the patient with diarrhea will (1) not transmit the microorganism causing the infectious diarrhea, (2) cease having diarrhea and resume normal bowel patterns, (3) have normal fluid and electrolyte and acid-base balance, (4) have normal nutritional intake, and (5) have no perianal skin breakdown.

Nursing Implementation

Adherence to precaution guidelines for infectious diseases (see Chapter 9) is important because some cases of acute diarrhea are infectious. All cases of acute diarrhea should be considered infectious until the cause is determined. The use of precautions is effective in reducing the spread of infectious diarrhea.

Table 40-4 Nursing Assessment: Diarrhea

Subjective Data

Important health information

Past health history: Usual bowel habits, ingestion of coarse and spicy foods, recent travel, infections, stress, diverticulitis or malabsorption, metabolic disorders, inflammatory bowel disease, irritable bowel syndrome

Medications: Use of laxatives, magnesium-containing antacids, antibiotics, methyldopa, digitalis, colchicine; over-the-counter antidiarrheal or cathartic medications

Functional health patterns

Health perception–health management: Weakness

Nutritional-metabolic: Anorexia, thirst; weight loss; bloating

Elimination: Amount, frequency, color, and character of stools

Cognitive-perceptual: Abdominal tenderness, abdominal pain and cramping; tenesmus

Objective Data

General

Lethargy, sunken eyeballs, fever, malnutrition

Integumentary

Pallor, dry mucous membranes, poor skin turgor, perianal irritation

Gastrointestinal

Amount, frequency, character (sudden onset, alternating diarrhea and constipation); color and consistency of stool; hyperactive bowel sounds; abdominal distention; presence of pus, blood, mucus, or fat in stools; fecal impaction

Urinary tract

Decreased output, concentrated urine

Possible findings

Abnormal serum electrolyte levels; anemia; leukocytosis; eosinophilia; positive stool cultures; presence of ova, parasites, leukocytes, blood, or fat in stools; abnormal sigmoidoscopic or colonoscopic findings; abnormal lower gastrointestinal series

Hand washing is the most important measure in prevention of the transfer of microorganisms. Hands should be washed before and after contact with each patient and when excretions of any kind are handled. The patient should be taught the principles of hygiene, infectious control precautions, and the potential dangers of an illness that is infectious to themselves and others. Proper handling, cooking, and storage of food should be discussed with the patient suspected of having infectious diarrhea.

Fecal Incontinence

Etiology and Pathophysiology. Knowledge of the mechanisms involved in fecal continence is helpful in understanding fecal incontinence. Normally fecal contents pass from the sigmoid colon into the rectum, causing rectal distention. Sensory (stretch) receptors in the muscles surrounding the rectum provide the sensation of rectal filling. This causes a reflex relaxation of the internal anal sphincter

Table 40-5 Causes of Fecal Incontinence

Traumatic	Inflammation
Obstetric	Infection
Postsurgical	Trauma
Hemorrhoidectomy	Radiation
Anterior resection	**Other**
Fistulectomy	Pelvic floor relaxation
Anorectal surgery	Perineal descent
Spinal cord injuries	Loss of elasticity of rectum (age-related)
Neurologic	Fecal impaction
Stroke	Diarrhea
Tumor	Medications
Degenerative disease	
Iatrogenic drug intoxication	
Multiple sclerosis	
Diabetes mellitus	
Dementia	

and contraction of the external anal sphincter. Sensory receptors in the epithelium of the anal canal can usually distinguish among solid, liquid, and gas. The combination of contraction of the abdominal muscles, relaxation of the pelvic muscles, squatting (which straightens the anorectal angle), and voluntary relaxation of the external anal sphincter allows for elimination of feces. *Fecal incontinence,* or the involuntary passage of stool, may be due to multiple causes (see Table 40-5). Treatment depends on the cause of the incontinence.

Diagnostic Studies and Therapeutic Management. The diagnosis and effective management of fecal incontinence require a thorough health history and physical examination with appropriate diagnostic studies. In all cases a rectal examination should be performed, followed by examination with a flexible sigmoidoscope. Fecal impaction, internal prolapse, increased perineal descent, and rectocele may be identified by rectal examination. If the impaction is higher in the colon, an abdominal x-ray may be helpful. Flexible sigmoidoscopy may identify inflammation, tumors, fissures, and other sigmoid-rectum pathology. Other studies may include barium enema, colonoscopy, and anorectal manometry.

Treatment of incontinence depends on the underlying cause. If fecal incontinence is related to noninfectious diarrhea, antidiarrheal agents may be prescribed. For example, loperamide (Imodium) may be useful in reducing diarrhea and increasing sphincter tone.

Fecal incontinence caused by fecal impaction can be a common problem in the older adult. Fecal impaction usually resolves after manual disimpaction and cleansing enemas. To prevent recurrence, a high-fiber diet (see Table 40-9 later in this chapter), along with increased fluid intake, should be given unless contraindicated.

Biofeedback therapy is effective in treating incontinence in the patient who has decreased sensory awareness or sphincter control. Biofeedback training requires intact

NURSING CARE PLAN Patient with Acute Infectious Diarrhea

Planning: Outcome Criteria	*Nursing Interventions and Rationales*
➤ NURSING DIAGNOSIS	Diarrhea *related to* acute infectious process *as manifested by* frequent loose, watery stools.
Have normal bowel elimination; be afebrile.	Monitor frequency, amount, color, consistency of stools *to determine severity of diarrhea and need for intervention.* Record intake and output *to monitor fluid balance.* Follow hospital procedure for enteric precautions; use strict medical asepsis when handling bedpan, linens, or patient *to prevent spread of infection.* Monitor vital signs q4hr *because changes can indicate development of hypovolemia.* Administer antiinfective and antidiarrheal medications as ordered *to treat bacterial infection and relieve diarrhea.*
➤ NURSING DIAGNOSIS	Fluid volume deficit *related to* excessive fluid loss and decreased fluid intake secondary to vomiting or diarrhea *as manifested by* dry skin and mucous membranes; poor skin turgor; hypotension; tachycardia; decreased urine output; electrolyte imbalance (e.g., decreased sodium, decreased potassium); decreased level of consciousness.
Have normal vital signs; normal skin turgor; pink, moist mucous membranes; urine output >0.5 ml/kg/hr; normal serum electrolytes; return to baseline mental status.	Assess for skin turgor changes, sunken eyes, rapid pulse, and anorexia *as indicators of fluid volume deficit.* Monitor intake and output *to determine fluid balance.* Monitor serum sodium and potassium levels *so abnormalities can be reported to physician.* Monitor vital signs q4hr. Weigh patient daily *to monitor fluid loss.* Administer IV fluids as ordered and increase intake of fluids as tolerated to at least 3000 ml/day *to replace fluids and electrolytes lost in stools.* Assess mouth for dryness and note patient's complaints of thirst *because dry mucous membranes and thirst are indicators of dehydration.* If patient is not vomiting, administer fluids, such as Gatorade or Pedialyte, *to replace glucose and electrolytes lost in stools.* Medicate with antidiarrheals as ordered *to decrease diarrhea.*
➤ NURSING DIAGNOSIS	Impaired skin integrity of perianal area *related to* contact with diarrheal stools and inadequate perianal hygiene *as manifested by* redness, swelling, possible ulceration of skin, pain during elimination.
Have no evidence of skin breakdown in perianal area.	Assess skin of perianal area *to plan appropriate interventions.* Cleanse area with warm water after each bowel movement, rinsing well and patting dry with a soft towel *to prevent skin excoriation and promote patient comfort.* Apply ointment *to promote healing.* Use an anesthetic ointment or spray foam *to decrease local discomfort.*
➤ NURSING DIAGNOSIS	Acute pain and abdominal cramping *related to* increased GI motility *as manifested by* guarding, doubling over, change in affect, verbal complaints, tachycardia, diaphoresis.
Verbalize satisfactory comfort level.	Provide quiet, stress-free environment *to reduce anxiety and promote rest.* Provide comfort measures such as hot packs *to promote comfort and decrease GI motility.* Administer antidiarrheals and anticholinergics as ordered *to decrease GI motility.*
➤ NURSING DIAGNOSIS	Risk for infection transmission *related to* lack of knowledge in prevention of reinfection or transmission of infectious disease.
Have no recurrence of symptoms; be knowledgeable about disease process and preventive measures.	Teach patient to be alert for recurrence of diarrhea, fever, and other symptoms; evidence of same symptoms in family members *as signs of possible infection transmission.* Assist patient in identifying factors that precipitated diarrhea *to avoid causing reinfection of self or transmission to others.* Stress importance of good hand-washing techniques *to prevent spread of diarrhea to others.* Explain importance of seeking medical care when diarrhea and other symptoms begin *so early treatment can be initiated.*

GI, Gastrointestinal; *IV*, intravenous.

sphincter function, adequate mental status, and motivation to learn.[2] Components of biofeedback include education, reinforcement, and concentration. It is a safe, painless, and inexpensive treatment for fecal incontinence. Bowel training programs are usually effective, even with the patient who lacks total sphincter function.[3]

Surgery should be considered only when conservative treatment fails, in cases of full-thickness prolapse, and when the sphincter needs repair.

NURSING MANAGEMENT

FECAL INCONTINENCE

Nursing Assessment

Fecal incontinence is not only an embarrassment to the patient but also a potential hazard to normal skin integrity. It is necessary to make an assessment of the patient's general condition to identify the best alternative for managing the patient with fecal incontinence. The nurse should identify normal bowel habits and current symptoms, including frequency and nature of the stools.

A neurologic assessment that includes evaluation of mental status can be helpful in identifying the most effective treatment for the patient. Assessment should also include history of multiple or traumatic childbirths, previous anorectal surgery, and injury.

Nursing Diagnoses

Nursing diagnoses specific to the patient with fecal incontinence include, but are not limited to, the following:

- Impaired skin integrity of the perianal area related to incontinence of stool
- Social isolation related to embarrassment and odor
- Self-esteem disturbance related to inability to control bowel functions
- Self-care deficit related to inability to manage bowel evacuation independently

Planning

The overall goals are that the patient with fecal incontinence will (1) have normal bowel control, (2) maintain perianal skin integrity, and (3) not suffer any self-esteem problems related to problems with bowel control.

Nursing Implementation

Prevention and treatment of fecal incontinence may be managed by implementing a bowel training program. The patient should be put on a bedpan, assisted to a bedside commode, or walked to the bathroom at a regular time daily to assist with reestablishment of bowel regularity. A good time to establish this pattern is within 30 minutes after breakfast. Most individuals experience an urge to defecate following the first meal of the day because of the gastrocolic reflex. If the usual bowel habits differ from this pattern, efforts should be made to adhere to the patient's individual timing.

If these techniques are ineffective in reestablishing bowel regularity, a bisacodyl (Dulcolax) or glycerin suppository may be inserted 15 to 30 minutes before the usual evacuation time. This stimulates the anorectal reflex and often can be discontinued when a regular pattern is reestablished.

Maintenance of skin integrity is of upmost importance, especially in the bedridden and older adult patient. Nursing management may necessitate drainage tubes or catheters, use of incontinence briefs, and meticulous skin care. Tubes and catheters are usually not recommended because their use for an extended period may decrease responsiveness of the rectal sphincter and cause ulceration of the rectal mucosa. Use of incontinence briefs may be helpful in maintaining skin integrity if changed frequently, but this can be demeaning and humiliating to the patient. Meticulous cleaning after each stool is required. Washing, rinsing, thorough drying, and application of a protective barrier are essential to the maintenance of skin integrity. Because the patient may have several stools each day, maintaining skin integrity is a time-consuming task for the nurse and the family.

Perianal pouching is an alternative in the management of fecal incontinence. Pouching provides skin protection and fecal containment as well as comfort and dignity. Because odor is often a problem, deodorant sprays and room deodorizers may be used. For the patient who is ambulatory, a chair (regular or special commode wheelchair) may be used. Regardless of the patient's mobility, the nurse must make sure the skin is clean, odorless, and intact.

Constipation

Etiology. Millions of persons suffer from constipation. Despite its prevalence, little is known about its pathophysiology.[4] *Constipation* may be defined as a decrease in frequency of bowel movements from what is "normal" for the individual; hard, difficult-to-pass stool; a decrease in stool volume; and retention of feces in the rectum. Normal bowel elimination may vary from three times a day to once every 3 days.[4] Because of this variability, it is important to determine the severity of constipation on the basis of the patient's normal pattern of elimination. It is important to remember that changes in bowel habits may also indicate bowel obstruction produced by a tumor.

Frequently constipation may be due to insufficient dietary fiber, inadequate fluid intake, medication use, and lack of exercise. If proper preventive measures are subsequently taken, constipation should not recur. Constipation may also be due to sociocultural beliefs, environmental constraints, ignoring the urge to defecate, chronic laxative abuse, and multiple organic causes (Table 40-6). Changes in diet, in mealtime, or in daily routines are a few environmental factors that may cause constipation. Depression and stress can also result in constipation.

Some patients believe that they are constipated if they do not have a daily bowel movement. This can result in chronic laxative use and subsequent *cathartic colon syndrome*. In this condition the colon becomes dilated and atonic.

Ignoring the urge to defecate for a period of time causes the muscles and mucosa in the rectal area to become

Table 40-6 Organic Causes of Constipation

Colonic Disorders	Systemic Disorders
Luminal or extra-luminal obstructing lesions	*Metabolic/endocrine*
Inflammatory strictures	Diabetes mellitus
Volvulus	Hypothyroidism
Intusussception	Pregnancy
Irritable bowel syndrome	Hypercalcemia/hyperparathyroidism
Diverticular disease	Pheochromocytoma
Rectocele	*Collagen vascular disease*
Drug Induced	Scleroderma
Antacids (calcium and aluminum)	Amyloidosis
Antidepressants	*Neurogenic disorders*
Anticholinergics	Hirschsprung's megacolon
Antipsychotics	Neurofibromatosis
Antihypertensives	Autonomic neuropathy (pseudoobstruction)
Barium sulfate	Multiple sclerosis
Iron supplements	Parkinson's disease
Bismuth	Spinal cord lesions or injury
Calcium supplements	Cerebrovascular accident
Laxative abuse	

insensitive to the presence of feces. In addition, the prolonged retention of feces in the rectum results in drying of stool because of the absorption of water. The harder and drier the feces, the more difficult it is to expel.

Clinical Manifestations and Complications. The clinical presentation of constipation may vary from a chronic discomfort to an acute event mimicking an "acute abdomen." Other clinical manifestations are presented in Table 40-7.

Hemorrhoids are the most common complication of chronic constipation. They result from venous engorgement caused by repeated *Valsalva maneuvers* (straining) and venous compression from hard impacted stool.

A Valsalva maneuver, which occurs during straining to pass a hardened stool, may cause serious problems in patients with congestive heart failure, cerebral edema, hypertension, and coronary artery disease. During straining, the patient takes a deep inspiration, the breath is held, and the glottis closes and traps the air. The abdominal muscles contract and try to push against the colon. Increases in intraabdominal pressure and intrathoracic pressure occur, reducing venous return to the heart. The heart slows temporarily (bradycardia), the cardiac output is decreased, and there is a transient drop in arterial pressure. When the patient relaxes, there is decreased thoracic pressure and a sudden flow of blood into the heart, causing distention and an increase in heart rate. Immediately the arterial pressure rises momentarily. These changes may be fatal for the patient who cannot compensate for sudden overload of blood flow returning to the heart.

Diverticulosis is another potential complication of chronic constipation. This is a relatively common complication in an older adult. Diverticuli or outpouchings of the colon wall are thought to be due to the increased intraluminal pressure needed to expel hard stool. Diverticulosis and diverticulitis are described later in this chapter.

Table 40-7 Clinical Manifestations of Constipation

Hard, dry stool	Increased flatulence
Abdominal distention	Nausea
Abdominal pain	Anorexia
Decreased frequency of bowel movements	Headache
Straining	Palpable mass
Rectal pressure	Stool with blood
Tenesmus	Dizziness
	Urinary retention

In the presence of *obstipation,* or fecal impaction secondary to constipation, colonic perforation may occur. Perforation, which is life threatening, causes abdominal pain, nausea, vomiting, fever, and an elevated WBC count. An abdominal x-ray shows the presence of free air, which is diagnostic of perforation. Rectal mucosal ulcers may also occur as a result of stool stasis or straining. These complications are most common in older patients.

Diagnostic Studies and Therapeutic Management. A thorough history and physical examination should be performed so that the underlying cause of constipation can be identified and treatment started. Abdominal x-rays barium enema, colonoscopy, sigmoidoscopy, and anorectal manometry may be helpful in the diagnosis. Most cases of constipation can be managed with diet therapy including fluids and an exercise program. Laxatives (Table 40-8) should always be used cautiously because with chronic overuse they may become a cause of constipation. Enemas are fast acting and are beneficial in the immediate treatment of constipation but should be limited in their use for long-term treatment of constipation. Soapsuds enemas should be avoided because they may lead to inflammation of colon mucosa. Oil-retention enemas may be used to soften fecal impactions.

For the patient in whom perceived constipation is related to rigid beliefs regarding bowel function, the nurse should initiate a discussion about these beliefs with the patient. Appropriate information on normal bowel function is given and discussed, along with the adverse consequences of excessive use of laxatives and enemas.

A patient with severe constipation related to a motility or mechanical disorder may require more intensive treatment. Studies such as anorectal manometry, radioactive transit studies, and sigmoidoscopic rectal biopsies should be performed before treatment. In a patient with unrelenting constipation, a subtotal colectomy with ileorectal anastomosis is the procedure of choice.[7]

Nutritional Management. Diet is an important factor in the prevention of constipation. Many patients experience an improvement in their symptoms when they simply increase their intake of dietary fiber and fluids. Dietary fiber

Table 40-8 Cathartic Agents

Category	Mechanisms of Action	Example	Onset of Action	Comments
▪ Bulk forming	Absorbs water; increases bulk, thereby stimulating peristalsis	Metamucil, Perdiem, Konsyl, Hydrocil	Usually within 24 hr	Contraindicated in patients with abdominal pain, nausea, and vomiting and in patients suspected of having appendicitis, biliary tract obstruction, or acute hepatitis; needs to be taken with fluids
▪ Stimulants	Increase peristalsis by irritating colon wall and stimulating enteric nerves	Antraquinone drugs Cascara sagrada, senna Phenolphthalein drugs Ex-Lax, Correctol, Feen-a-Mint, Bisacodyl, Dulcolax	Usually within 12 hr	Cause melanosis coli (brown or black pigmentation of colon), are most widely abused laxatives; should not be used in patients with impaction or obstipation
▪ Stool softeners and lubricants	Lubricate intestinal tract and soften feces, making hard stools easier to pass; do not affect peristalsis	Mineral oil, dioctyl sodium, sulfosuccinate, Colace, Peri-Colace, Doxidan	Softeners up to 72 hr, lubricants up to 8 hr	Can block absorption of fat-soluble vitamins such as vitamin K, which may increase risk of bleeding in patients on anticoagulants
▪ Saline and osmotic solutions	Cause retention of fluid in intestinal lumen caused by osmotic effect	Magnesium salts Magnesium citrate, Milk of Magnesia Sodium phosphates Fleets enema, Phospho-soda Lactulose Polyethylene glycol-saline solutions Go-Lytely, Colyte	15 min to 3 hr	Magnesium-containing products may cause hypermagnesemia in patients with renal insufficiency

is found in two forms: insoluble and soluble in water. Both are contained in most foods, but some foods are higher in soluble fiber (Table 40-9).

Insoluble fiber remains essentially unchanged by the time it reaches the colon, and it is found in higher concentrations in whole wheat and bran. *Soluble fibers* form gel-like substances that add viscosity to the digested contents, causing decreased gastric emptying and decreased transit time in the small intestine. This affects glucose absorption and cholesterol metabolism, which may be beneficial in the management of diabetes mellitus, atherosclerosis, and cholesterol gallstones. *Soluble fiber* is found in oat bran, fruits, vegetables, and psyllium. Patients should be told that initially fiber will increase gas production but that this effect decreases with time.

The diet should also include a fluid intake of at least 3000 ml per day, unless contraindicated by cardiac or renal disease. Increasing fiber intake without increasing fluids may predispose the patient to impaction or obstruction. The nurse should encourage the selection of foods the patient likes and is able to prepare and foods that are affordable. The patient's understanding of the diet and the importance of dietary fiber is important to ensure compliance.

NURSING MANAGEMENT
CONSTIPATION

Nursing Assessment

Subjective and objective data that should be obtained from a patient with constipation are presented in Table 40-10.

Nursing Diagnoses

Nursing diagnoses are determined when the problem and the etiologic factors are supported by clinical data. Nursing diagnoses related to constipation may include, but are not limited to, those presented in the nursing care plan for the patient with constipation on p. 1216.

Planning

The overall goals are that the patient with constipation will (1) increase dietary intake of fiber and fluids; (2) have the passage of soft, formed stools; and (3) not have complications, such as bleeding hemorrhoids.

Nursing Implementation

Nursing management should be based on the patient's symptoms (see Table 40-7) and the assessment of the patient (see

Table 40-9 Nutritional Management: High-Fiber Foods*

	Fiber Per Serving (g)	Size of Serving	Calories Per Serving
Vegetables			
Asparagus	3.5	½ cup	18
Beans			
Navy	8.4	½ cup	80
Kidney	9.7	½ cup	94
Lima	8.3	½ cup	63
Pinto	8.9	½ cup	78
String	2.1	½ cup	18
Broccoli	3.5	½ cup	18
Carrots, raw	1.8	½ cup	15
Corn	2.6	½ medium ear	72
Peas, canned	6.7	½ cup	63
Potatoes			
Baked	1.9	½ medium	72
Sweet	2.1	½ medium	79
Squash			
Acorn	7.0	1 cup	82
Tomato, raw	1.5	1 small	18
Fruits			
Apple	2.0	½ large	42
Banana	1.5	½ medium	48
Blackberries	6.7	¾ cup	40
Orange	1.6	1 small	35
Peach	2.3	1 medium	38
Pear	2.0	½ medium	44
Raspberries	9.2	1 cup	42
Strawberries	3.1	1 cup	45
Grain Products			
Bread			
Rye	0.8	1 slice	62
White	0.7	1 slice	64
Whole wheat	1.3	1 slice	59
Cereal			
All Bran (100%)	8.4	⅓ cup	70
Corn Flakes	2.6	¾ cup	70
Shredded Wheat	2.8	1 biscuit	70
Crackers			
Graham	1.4	2 squares	53
Popcorn	3.0	3 cups	62
Rice			
Brown	1.6	⅓ cup	72
White	0.5	⅓ cup	76

*Recommended for patients with diverticulosis, irritable bowel syndrome, constipation, hemorrhoids, colon cancer, atherosclerosis, hyperlipidemia, and diabetes mellitus.

Table 40-10). An important role of the nurse is teaching the patient the importance of dietary measures to prevent constipation. Emphasis should be placed on maintenance of a high-fiber diet, increasing fluid intake, and a regular exercise program. The patient should be taught to establish a regular time to defecate and not to suppress the urge to defecate. In many persons the urge to defecate occurs after breakfast because of the stimulation of the gastrocolic reflex. The patient should be discouraged from using laxatives and enemas to achieve fecal elimination.

Proper position is important when defecating. For a patient in bed, the bedpan should be placed and the head of the bed should be elevated as high as the patient can tolerate. For the person who can sit on a toilet, a footstool may be placed in front of the toilet. Placing the feet on the footstool promotes flexion of the thighs, which assists in defecation.

The patient with poor muscle tone should be encouraged to exercise the abdominal muscles and can be taught to contract the abdominal muscles several times a day. Sit-ups and straight leg raises can also be used to improve abdominal muscle tone.

Some patients may have to be encouraged to increase their social activities, as well as their physical activity; this is especially true of older adults, who may become depressed and socially isolated because of multiple factors. Inactivity can lead to constipation. This patient should be encouraged and assisted in establishing social contacts and activities outside the home.

Table 40-10 Nursing Assessment: Constipation

Subjective Data

Important health information

Past health history: Colorectal disease, neurologic dysfunction, bowel obstruction, environmental changes, cancer

Medications: Use of aluminum antacids, anticholinergics, antidepressants, antihistamines, antipsychotics, diuretics, narcotics, iron, laxatives, enemas

Functional health patterns

Health perception–health management: Malaise, weakness

Nutritional-metabolic: Fluid and food intake; anorexia; nausea; abdominal bloating

Elimination: Usual elimination patterns; frequency, amount, and consistency of stools; defecation difficulty; flatus; diarrhea (if impacted); tenesmus; rectal pressure

Activity-exercise: Immobility; sedentary lifestyle

Cognitive-perceptual: Dizziness, headache; anorectal pain; abdominal pain on defecation

Coping–stress tolerance: Acute or chronic stress

Objective Data

General

Lethargy

Integumentary

Anorectal fissures, hemorrhoids, abscesses

Gastrointestinal

Abdominal distention, fecal impaction, hypoactive or absent bowel sounds, stool consistency and amount

Possible findings

Guaiac-positive stools, abdominal x-ray study demonstrating stool in colon

NURSING CARE PLAN Patient with Constipation

Planning: Outcome Criteria	Nursing Interventions and Rationales
➤ **NURSING DIAGNOSIS**	Constipation *related to* inadequate dietary intake of fiber, inadequate fluid intake, and decreased physical activity *as manifested by* hard, dry stools; straining; painful defecation; abdominal distention; decreased frequency of defecation; headache; increased flatulence.
Consume diet of 20 to 30 g of fiber per day; increase fluid intake to 3000 ml/day; increase physical activity; establish regular pattern of elimination.	Assess pattern of bowel activity and character of stools *to plan appropriate interventions.* Provide patient with a list of high-fiber foods *to use as reference when selecting foods.* Encourage a minimum of 20 g of fiber intake daily *because fiber absorbs water, which adds softness and bulk to fecal mass, speeds up intestinal transit, and slows down rapid transit.* Teach role of fiber, fluid, and activity in prevention of constipation *so patient has knowledge base for participation in plan.* Encourage fluid intake of at least 3000 ml/day *to maintain bowel pattern and promote proper stool consistency and peristalsis.* Assist in establishing a regular exercise program *because exercise increases bowel motility and peristalsis.* Discuss importance of responding to urge to defecate *because ignoring the urge causes the muscles and membranes in rectal area to become insensitive to presence of feces.* Teach and assist in establishing regular elimination pattern *to develop a routine so the bowel reflex (urge) can be reestablished.* Provide privacy *so distractions will not override the urge to defecate.* Monitor and document bowel activity *to have a record for analyzing patient's pattern of elimination.* Administer and document results of prescribed agents *to evaluate patient's response and adjust plan if necessary.* Teach correct use of cathartics *because they may become a cause of constipation with chronic overuse.*

ABDOMINAL PAIN

Acute Abdominal Pain

Etiology. The patient with an *acute abdomen* has an acute onset of abdominal pain requiring prompt decision making. Causes of an acute abdomen are varied (Table 40-11). Although sometimes called "surgical" abdomen, acute abdominal pain does not always necessitate surgery.[5] Many disorders must be ruled out before a diagnosis is confirmed.

Clinical Manifestations. Pain is the most important presenting symptom. The patient may also complain of abdominal tenderness, vomiting, diarrhea, constipation, flatulence, fatigue, and an increase in abdominal girth.

Diagnostic Studies and Therapeutic Management. Diagnosis begins with a complete history and physical examination. Physical examination should include a rectal and pelvic examination. A complete blood count, (CBC) urinalysis, abdominal x-ray, and an electrocardiogram (ECG) are done initially. Pregnancy tests should be performed in women of childbearing age who have acute abdominal pain. The findings of these studies may provide some information as to the cause of the acute abdomen.

Emergency management of the patient with an acute abdomen is presented in Table 40-12. The goal of management is to identify and treat the cause. The physician attempts to make a differential diagnosis when the patient is seen with an acute abdomen because many causes of abdominal pain do not require surgery (see Table 40-11).

In addition to being a therapeutic measure, surgery can also be diagnostic. Operative exploration is usually done after a careful examination of the patient and is justified when "look and see" is better than "wait and see." The surgical procedure is an *exploratory laparotomy,* in which an opening is made through the abdominal wall into the peritoneal cavity to determine the cause of an acute abdomen. If the cause of the acute abdomen can be surgically removed (e.g., inflamed appendix) or surgically repaired (e.g., ruptured abdominal aneurysm), surgery is considered definitive therapy.

Table 40-11 Causes of Acute Abdomen

Abdominal penetrating trauma	Peptic ulcer
Acute ischemic bowel	Perforated gastrointestinal malignancy
Appendicitis	Peritonitis
Bowel obstruction with perforation or necrosis	Ruptured abdominal aneurysm
Cholecystitis	Ruptured ectopic pregnancy
Crohn's disease	Ruptured ovarian cyst
Diverticulitis with peritonitis	Ulcerative colitis
Foreign body perforation	Uterine rupture
Gastritis	Volvulus
Gastroenteritis	
Mesenteric adenitis	
Pancreatitis	
Pelvic inflammatory disease	

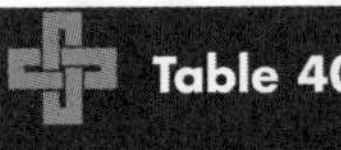

Table 40-12 Emergency Management: Acute Abdomen

Possible Etiologies

Inflammation (e.g., appendicitis, cholecystitis, pancreatitis, ulcerative colitis, gastritis, pyelonephritis, pelvic inflammatory disease), obstruction or perforation of an abdominal organ, gastrointestinal bleeding or vascular problems (e.g., ruptured aortic aneurysm, mesenteric vascular occlusion, ruptured ectopic pregnancy), infectious disease (*Giardia, Salmonella*)

Possible Assessment Findings

Abdominal pain or tenderness; diffuse, localized, dull, burning, sharp
Abdominal distention
Abdominal rigidity, rebound tenderness
Nausea, vomiting, diarrhea
Bleeding from gastrointestinal tract (e.g., hematemesis, melena)
Symptoms of hypovolemic shock (e.g., decreased blood pressure; tachycardia; cool, clammy skin; decreased pulse pressure; decreased level of consciousness)

Management

- Monitor airway; have airway equipment available, including suction and intubation supplies.
- Administer oxygen via nasal cannula or 100% nonrebreather mask if shock symptoms occur.
- Establish intravenous access with a large-bore catheter (14 or 16 gauge, two large bore lines if shock symptoms are present) with warm normal saline or lactated Ringer's solution.
- Monitor vital signs, including level of consciousness and oxygen saturation.
- Position in comfortable position, modified Trendelenburg if shock symptoms.
- Monitor pain.
- Obtain history and physical to determine underlying cause.
- Insert indwelling urinary catheter.
- Monitor intake and urinary output.
- Observe for vomiting; insert nasogastric tube if needed.

NURSING MANAGEMENT

ACUTE ABDOMEN

Nursing Assessment

Vital signs should be taken immediately. Blood pressure and pulse rate should be obtained to determine hypovolemic changes. An elevated temperature may indicate an inflammatory or infectious process. The abdomen should be inspected for distention, masses, abnormal pulsation, rashes, scars, and pigmentation changes. Bowel sounds should be auscultated. Bowel sounds that are diminished or absent in a quadrant may indicate a complete bowel obstruction, acute peritonitis, or paralytic ileus. Palpation should be gentle.

A thorough assessment of the patient's symptoms should be made to determine the onset, location, intensity, duration, frequency, and character of pain. The nurse should determine whether the pain has spread or moved to new locations (quadrants), as well as what makes the pain worse or better. It should also be determined whether the pain is associated with other symptoms, such as nausea, vomiting, changes in bowel and bladder habits, or vaginal discharge in women. Assessment of vomiting should include the amount, color, consistency, and odor of the vomitus. Bowel patterns and habits should also be carefully assessed.

Nursing Implementation

Nursing interventions are based on the diagnosis and medical or surgical management of the patient. General care for the patient involves management of fluid and electrolyte imbalances, pain, and anxiety.

Preoperative Care. Emergency preparation of the patient with an acute abdomen is usually limited to a CBC, typing and crossmatching of blood, and clotting studies. Catheterization, preparation of the abdominal skin, and the passage of a nasogastric (NG) tube may be done in the emergency department or operating room. (General care of the preoperative patient is discussed in Chapter 14.)

Postoperative Care. Postoperative care and management depends on the type of surgical procedure performed. The increased use of laparoscopic procedures has reduced the risk of postoperative complications related to wound care and altered gastrointestinal motility. These procedures generally result in shorter hospital stays.

A general nursing care plan for the postoperative patient is presented in Chapter 16. Nursing care for the patient following a laparotomy is presented in the nursing care plan on p. 1218.

An NG tube may or may not be present in the patient returning from surgery. If present, the NG tube is connected to suction as ordered. The purpose of the NG tube is to empty the stomach of secretions and gas to prevent gastric dilatation. GI peristaltic activity is often impaired because of the manipulative procedures of the surgery and anesthesia. Low intermittent suctioning is ordered to prevent trauma to the gastric mucosa.

Drainage from the NG tube may be dark brown to dark red for the first 12 hours. Later it should be light yellowish brown, or it may have a greenish tinge because of the presence of bile. If a dark red color continues or if bright red blood is observed, the physician should be notified at once of the possibility of hemorrhage. "Coffee ground" granules in the drainage are due to the presence of small amounts of blood that have been chemically acted on by gastric secretions.

The NG tube is checked frequently for patency. The tube may become obstructed with mucus, sediment, or old blood. An order is usually written to irrigate the tube with 20 to 30 ml of normal saline solution if needed. Repositioning the tube may facilitate drainage.

An accurate record of intake and output, including emesis and gastric drainage, is essential. The nurse should assess serum electrolyte values because prolonged gastric suctioning results in loss of sodium, chloride, potassium, and water.

NURSING CARE PLAN Patient After Laparotomy

Planning: Outcome Criteria	Nursing Interventions and Rationales
➤ NURSING DIAGNOSIS	Pain *related to* surgical incision and inadequate pain control measures *as manifested by* complaints of pain, body posturing and sounds indicative of pain, unwillingness to move in bed or to ambulate.
Verbalize satisfactory level of pain control.	Assess for pain and give pain medication q3-4hr as ordered for first 72 hr *to maintain satisfactory comfort level.* Splint incision with pillows during coughing, deep breathing, and moving *to relieve pain while performing these activities.* Position patient comfortably *to relieve pain.*
➤ NURSING DIAGNOSIS	Nausea and vomiting *related to* decreased GI motility, GI distention, and narcotics *as manifested by* complaints of nausea, vomiting of gastric contents, lack of or diminished bowel sounds, abdominal distention.
Have relief of nausea and vomiting.	Administer antiemetic medications (as ordered) *to relieve nausea and vomiting.* Assess response to pain medications *to determine if this is a possible cause of nausea and vomiting.* Maintain patency of NG tube (if present) *to prevent accumulation of gastric juices and subsequent vomiting.* Assess for bowel sounds and abdominal distention *to determine return of peristalsis.* Keep patient on NPO status until bowel sounds return *to prevent vomiting.* Limit unpleasant sights, smells, and stimuli *to prevent initiating episodes of nausea and vomiting.*
➤ NURSING DIAGNOSIS	Ineffective airway clearance *related to* effects of anesthesia, sedation, pain, immobility, and location of incision *as manifested by* shallow, labored respiratory pattern; decreased breath sounds; rhonchi; productive cough; fever.
Have lungs clear to auscultation; nonlabored, deep respirations; absence of fever.	Monitor vital signs q4hr *to assess cardiopulmonary function.* Report temperature elevation, labored respirations. Have patient cough and deep breathe 10 times q2hr for 72 hr *to prevent atelectasis.* Splint operative site with pillows during coughing and deep breathing *to assist patient with ventilation.* Turn patient q2hr *to mobilize secretions.* Auscultate lungs q4hr; assess breathing pattern and rate *to determine air exchange.* Ambulate patient at least three times a day, beginning the first postoperative day. Have patient assume semi-Fowler's position while in bed *to facilitate lung excursion.*
➤ NURSING DIAGNOSIS	Constipation *related to* immobility, pain, medication, and decreased motility *as manifested by* decreased or absent bowel sounds, abdominal pain, abdominal distention, inability to pass flatus or stool.
Have normal bowel sounds within 72 hours; soft, formed bowel movement within 4 days; abdomen soft to palpation.	Assess abdomen for distention and bowel sounds every shift *to determine need for intervention.* Check for passage of flatus and bowel movement and record. Administer cathartic as ordered if patient has not had bowel movement in 4 days *to soften fecal mass or promote elimination.* Encourage frequent position changes and ambulation as tolerated *to increase peristalsis.* Encourage increased fluid intake as tolerated *to soften fecal material.*

GI, Gastrointestinal; *NG*, nasogastric; *NPO*, nothing by mouth.

The NG tube is removed when intestinal peristalsis returns, usually 24 to 72 hours after surgery. Motility of the stomach normally returns within 24 to 48 hours. Motility of the small intestine usually resumes within 24 hours, whereas return of large intestine motility may take as long as 3 to 5 days. Peristaltic activity is assessed by auscultation for bowel sounds.

Mouth care and nasal care are essential. The patient tends to breathe through the mouth while the NG tube is in place. In addition, increased nasal secretions and crusting result from mechanical stimulation of the NG tube.

Parenteral fluids are administered to provide the patient with fluids and electrolytes until bowel sounds return. Occasionally, ice chips may be ordered because they aid in the flow of saliva and prevent dry mouth. When bowel sounds return, fluids and food are increased gradually. The diet may be supplemented with multivitamins and iron.

Nausea and vomiting are not uncommon after abdominal surgery. These problems are often self-limiting. Observation is important in determining the cause. Antiemetics such as promethazine (Phenergan), hydroxyzine (Vistaril), prochlorperazine (Compazine), or trimethobenzamide (Tigan) may be ordered.

Abdominal distention and gas pains are also common after surgery; these are due to swallowed air and impaired peristalsis resulting from immobility, manipulation of abdominal contents during surgery, and side effects of anesthesia. The pain can be so uncomfortable that medications to stimulate peristalsis, such as bethanechol (Urecholine) or neostigmine methylsulfate (Prostigmin), may be given. A rectal tube or moist heat on the abdomen may be effective in relieving distention. The physician should be informed of abdominal distention and rigidity. Gradually, as intestinal activity increases, distention and gas pains decrease.

Emotional support from the nursing staff is important. Honest, clear, concise explanations of all procedures in language the patient and the family can understand will assist in allaying anxiety.

Chronic and Home Management. Preparation for discharge begins when the patient returns from the operating room. Instructions to the patient and the family should include any modifications in activity, care of the incision, diet, and drug therapy. Small, frequent meals high in calories should be taken initially, with a gradual increase in intake of food as tolerated.

Normal activities should be resumed gradually, with planned rest periods. The patient should be aware of possible complications after surgery and should notify the physician immediately if vomiting, pain, weight loss, incisional drainage, or changes in bowel functions occur.

Chronic Abdominal Pain

Chronic abdominal pain may originate from abdominal structures or may be referred from a site with the same or a similar nerve supply. Some common causes are irritable bowel syndrome, peptic ulcer disease, diverticulitis, chronic pancreatitis, hepatitis, cholecystitis, pelvic inflammatory disease, and vascular insufficiency. Psychogenic pain should also be considered.

Diagnosis of chronic abdominal pain presents a challenge. Assessment should begin with a thorough history and identification of the specific pain pattern. Character and severity of pain, location, duration, and onset should be determined. The assessment should also include the relationship of pain to meals, defecation, activity, and factors that increase or decrease the pain. Deep pain, usually of visceral or somatic origin, is more characteristic of chronic abdominal pain. It is usually described as dull, aching, or diffuse.

Endoscopy, computed tomography (CT) scans, magnetic resonance imaging (MRI), laparoscopy, and radiographic barium studies have lessened the need for exploratory laparotomy but have not lessened the frustrations experienced by the clinician attempting to make a diagnosis.

ABDOMINAL TRAUMA

Etiology

Injuries to the abdominal area most often occur as a result of *blunt trauma* (e.g., motor vehicle accident) or *penetration injuries,* primarily gunshot wounds or stab wounds to the abdomen. (Blunt trauma is most common.) Regardless of whether it is a blunt or penetration injury, the result is often the same—damage to or alteration of the internal organs.

Common injuries of the abdomen include lacerated liver, ruptured spleen, pancreatic trauma, mesenteric artery tears, diaphragmatic rupture, urinary bladder rupture, great vessel tears, renal injury, and stomach or intestinal rupture. These injuries may result in massive blood loss and hypovolemic shock. Surgery must be performed as early as possible to repair the damaged organs and to stop the bleeding. Common sequelae of intraabdominal trauma are peritonitis and massive infection, particularly when the bowel is perforated.

Clinical Manifestations

Clinical manifestations of abdominal trauma are (1) guarding and splinting of the abdominal wall; (2) a hard, distended abdomen (indicating intraabdominal bleeding); (3) decreased or absent bowel sounds; (4) contusions, abrasions, or bruising over the abdomen; (5) abdominal pain; (6) pain over the scapula caused by irritation of the phrenic nerve by free blood in the abdomen; (7) hematemesis or hematuria; and (8) signs of hypovolemic shock. An ecchymotic discoloration around the umbilicus (Cullen's sign) can indicate intraabdominal or retroperitoneal hemorrhage.

Intraabdominal injuries are often associated with low rib fractures, fractured femur, fractured pelvis, and thoracic injury. If any of these injuries are present, the patient should be observed for abdominal trauma.

Diagnostic Studies

Specific diagnostic procedures include a complete blood count, urinalysis, x-ray examination of the abdomen, CT scan, and peritoneal lavage. In the peritoneal lavage procedure the abdomen below the umbilicus is locally anesthetized, and a large angiocatheter or peritoneal dialysis catheter is inserted into the abdomen. A syringe is attached to the catheter, and an attempt is made to gently aspirate any blood. A liter of saline solution is then infused into the abdomen and drained. The fluid is observed for gross abnormalities, especially blood, and is sent to the laboratory for microscopic evaluation. Positive findings include any of the following: (1) RBC count greater than 100,000/μl, (2) WBC count greater than 500/μl, (3) high amylase level, and (4) presence of bacteria, bile, or fecal material. If the results are positive, immediate surgery is indicated. If the results are negative, continued observation of the patient is warranted. An impaled object should never be removed until skilled care is available. Removal may cause further injury and bleeding.

THERAPEUTIC AND NURSING MANAGEMENT

ABDOMINAL TRAUMA

Emergency management of abdominal trauma focuses on fluid replacement and prevention of hypovolemic shock (Table 40-13). IV lines are inserted, and volume expanders or blood is given if the patient is hypotensive. A NG tube is inserted to decompress the stomach and prevent the aspiration of vomitus. No pain medication is given because analgesics can mask the progression of clinical manifestations.

Regardless of the mechanism of injury, physical evidence of abdominal trauma in a patient who is hemodynamically unstable mandates immediate laparotomy. In other cases the indications for laparotomy must be correlated with the mechanism of injury. For example, if an individual has a gunshot wound or impaled object, surgery is usually indicated.

If surgery is performed, the postoperative nursing care is for the patient after laparotomy (see the preceding nursing care plan for the patient after laparotomy).

INFLAMMATION

Appendicitis

Appendicitis is an inflammation of the appendix, a narrow blind tube that extends from the inferior part of the cecum.

Table 40-13 Emergency Management: Abdominal Trauma

Possible Etiologies

Blunt or penetrating abdominal trauma from acceleration or deceleration (e.g., falls, motor vehicle collisions, pedestrian vs. vehicle), crush injuries, knife, missiles

Possible Assessment Findings

Signs and symptoms of hypovolemic shock (e.g., tachypnea, tachycardia, decreased blood pressure, decreased pulse pressure, decreased level of consciousness)
Abrasions or ecchymoses on abdominal wall, flank, or peritoneum
Open wound on skin
Object impaled in abdomen
Rigid, distended abdomen with tender, rebound pain
Radiation of pain to shoulder and back
Nausea, vomiting
Bloody urine
Abdominal scars from previous surgeries or trauma

Management

- Monitor airway; have airway equipment available, including suction and intubation supplies.
- Administer oxygen via non-rebreather mask (100%) and monitor for respiratory distress.
- Control external bleeding with sterile pressure dressing.
- Establish intravenous access with a two large bore line (14 or 16 gauge catheters) with warm normal saline or lactated Ringer's solution.
- Remove patient's clothing and maintain patient warmth using warm blankets, warm intravenous fluids, overhead warming lights, warm humidified oxygen.
- Monitor vital signs, including level of consciousness and oxygen saturation.
- Do not remove penetrating objects; stabilize with bulky dressing.
- Cover protruding organs or tissue with sterile saline dressing.
- Anticipate need for indwelling urinary catheter (if no pelvic fracture, urethral tear, or high-riding prostate) and nasogastric tube.

It occurs in 6% of the general population. Peak incidence is between the ages of 11 and 30 years, and the condition occurs equally in both sexes.[6]

Etiology. The most common causes of appendicitis are obstruction of the lumen by a *fecalith* (accumulated feces) (Fig. 40-1), foreign bodies, intramural thickening caused by lymphoid hyperplasia, or tumor of the cecum or appendix. Obstruction results in distention, venous engorgement, and the accumulation of mucus and bacteria, which can lead to gangrene and perforation.

Clinical Manifestations. Appendicitis typically begins with periumbilical pain, followed by anorexia, nausea, and vomiting. The pain is persistent and continuous, eventually shifting to the right lower quadrant and localizing at McBurney's point (located halfway between the umbilicus and the right iliac crest). Further assessment of the patient reveals localized tenderness, rebound tenderness, and muscle guarding. The patient usually prefers to lie still, often with the right leg flexed. Low-grade fever may or may not be present, and coughing aggravates pain. Rovsing's sign may be elicited by palpation of the left lower quadrant, causing pain to be felt in the right lower quadrant. Complications of acute appendicitis are perforation, peritonitis, and abscesses.

Diagnostic Studies and Therapeutic Management. Examination of the patient includes a complete history and physical examination (particularly palpation of the abdomen) and a differential WBC count. A urinalysis may be done to rule out genitourinary (GU) conditions that mimic the manifestations of appendicitis.

The treatment of appendicitis is immediate surgical removal (*appendectomy*) if the inflammation is localized. If the appendix has ruptured and there is evidence of peritonitis or an abscess, conservative treatment, consisting of antibiotic therapy and parenteral fluids, may be used to prevent sepsis and dehydration for 6 to 8 hours before an appendectomy is performed.

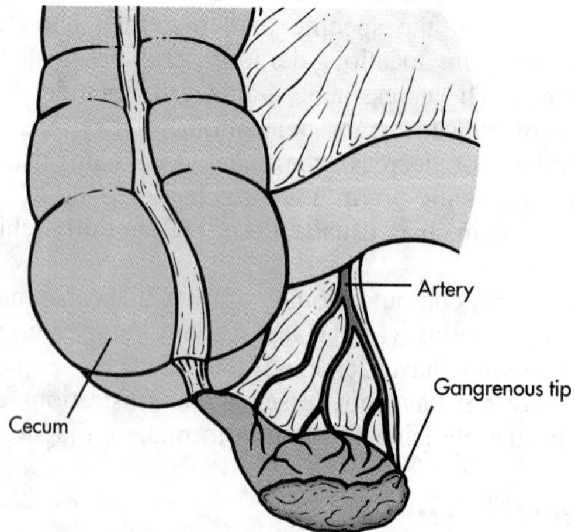

Fig. 40-1 In appendicitis the blood supply of the appendix is impaired by bacterial infection in the wall of the appendix, which may result in gangrene.

NURSING MANAGEMENT

APPENDICITIS

The patient with abdominal pain is encouraged to see a physician and to avoid self-treatment, particularly the use of laxatives and enemas. The increased peristalsis from these procedures may cause perforation of the appendix. Until the patient is seen by a physician, nothing should be taken by mouth (NPO) to ensure that the stomach will be empty in the event surgery is needed. An ice bag may be applied to the right lower quadrant to decrease the flow of blood to the area and impede the inflammatory process. Heat is never used because it may cause the appendix to rupture. Surgery is usually performed as soon as a diagnosis is made.

Postoperative nursing management is similar to postoperative care of the patient after laparotomy (see the preceding nursing care plan for the patient after laparotomy). In addition, the patient should be observed for evidence of peritonitis. Ambulation begins the day of surgery or the first postoperative day. The diet is advanced as tolerated. The patient is usually discharged on the first or second postoperative day, and normal activities are resumed 2 to 3 weeks after surgery.

Peritonitis

Peritonitis results from a localized or generalized inflammatory process of the peritoneum. (Table 40-14 lists causes of peritonitis.) It may appear in acute and chronic forms, and it may be caused by trauma or rupture of an organ containing chemical irritants or bacteria, which are released into the peritoneal cavity. Examples of a chemical peritonitis include gastric ulcer perforation and ruptured ectopic pregnancy. A chemical peritonitis is commonly followed by bacterial invasion. Bacterial peritonitis can be caused by a traumatic injury (e.g., gunshot wound, ruptured appendix), or it can be secondary to other diseases or conditions (e.g., pancreatitis, peritoneal dialysis).

Pathophysiology. The response of the peritoneum to the leakage of GI contents is localization of the offending agent by attempting to "wall it off." If that attempt fails, peritonitis worsens. The tissue begins to swell, and fibrinous exudate develops. Adhesions may form. These adhesions may shrink and disappear when the infection is eliminated. Normally, peritoneal injuries heal without formation of adhesions unless other factors, such as infection, ischemia, or foreign substances, are present.

Clinical Manifestations. Abdominal pain is the most common symptom of peritonitis, followed by ascites.[6] A universal sign is tenderness over the involved area. Rebound tenderness, muscular rigidity, and spasm are other major signs of irritation of the peritoneum. Abdominal distention, fever, tachycardia, tachypnea, nausea, vomiting, and altered bowel habits may also be present. These manifestations vary, depending on severity and acuteness of the underlying cause. Complications of peritonitis include hypovolemic shock, septicemia, intraabdominal abscess formation, paralytic ileus, and organ failure.

Diagnostic Studies. A CBC is done to determine leukocytosis and hemoconcentration (Table 40-15). Peritoneal aspiration may be performed and the fluid analyzed for blood, bile, pus, bacteria, fungus, and amylase content. An x-ray of the abdomen may show dilated loops of bowel consistent with paralytic ileus, free air if perforation has occurred, or air and fluid levels if an obstruction is present. Ultrasound and CT scans may be useful in identifying the presence of ascites and abscesses. *Peritoneoscopy* may be

Table 40-14 Causes of Peritonitis

Primary	Secondary
Blood-borne organisms	Appendicitis with rupture
Genital tract organisms	Blunt or penetrating trauma to abdominal organs
Cirrhosis with ascites	Diverticulitis with rupture
	Ischemic bowel disorders
	Obstruction in the gastrointestinal tract
	Pancreatitis
	Perforated peptic ulcer
	Peritoneal dialysis
	Postoperative (breakage of anastomosis)

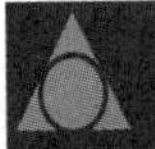

Table 40-15 Therapeutic Management: Peritonitis

Diagnostic
- CBC
- Serum electrolytes
- Abdominal x-ray
- Abdominal paracentesis and culture of fluid
- CT scan or ultrasound
- Peritoneoscopy

Therapeutic

Preoperative or nonoperative
- NPO status
- Fluid replacement
- Antibiotic therapy
- NG suction
- Analgesics
- Preparation for surgery to include the above and total parenteral nutrition

Postoperative
- NPO status
- NG tube to low-intermittent suction
- Semi-Fowler's position
- IV fluids with electrolyte replacement
- Total parenteral nutrition as needed
- Antibiotic therapy
- Blood transfusions as needed
- Sedatives and narcotics

CBC, Complete blood count; *CT*, computed tomography; *IV*, intravenous; *NG*, nasogastric; *NPO*, nothing by mouth.

helpful in the patient without ascites. Direct examination of the peritoneum can be obtained, along with biopsy specimens for diagnosis.

Therapeutic Management. The goals of management of peritonitis are to identify and eliminate the cause, combat infection, and prevent complications. Patients with milder cases of peritonitis or those who are poor surgical risks may be managed nonsurgically. Treatment consists of antibiotics, NG suction, analgesics, and IV fluid administration. Patients who require surgery need preoperative preparation as previously described. Those patients may be placed on total parenteral nutrition (TPN) because of increased nutritional requirements.

NURSING MANAGEMENT
PERITONITIS

Nursing Assessment

Assessment of the patient's pain, including the location, is important and may help in determining the cause of peritonitis. The patient should be assessed for the presence and quality of bowel sounds, increasing abdominal distention, abdominal guarding, nausea, fever, and manifestations of hypovolemic shock.

Nursing Diagnoses

Nursing diagnoses specific to the patient with peritonitis include, but are not limited to, the following:

- Abdominal pain related to inflammation of the peritoneum and abdominal distention
- Risk for fluid volume deficit related to collection of fluid in peritoneal cavity secondary to trauma, infection, or ischemia
- Altered nutrition: less than body requirements because of nausea and vomiting
- Anxiety related to uncertainty of cause or outcome of condition and pain
- Potential complication: hypovolemic shock related to loss of circulatory volume

Planning

The overall goals are that the patient with peritonitis will have (1) resolution of inflammation, (2) relief of abdominal pain, (3) freedom from complications (especially hypovolemic shock), and (4) normal nutritional status.

Nursing Implementation

The patient with peritonitis is very ill and needs skilled supportive care. The patient is monitored for pain and response to analgesic therapy. The patient may be positioned with knees flexed to increase comfort. The nurse should provide rest and a quiet environment. Sedatives may be given to allay anxiety.

Accurate monitoring of fluid intake and output and electrolyte status is necessary to determine replacement therapy. Vital signs are monitored frequently.

Antiemetics may be administered to decrease nausea and vomiting and further fluid losses. The patient is on NPO status and may have an NG tube in place to decrease gastric distention.

If the patient has an open surgical procedure, drains are inserted to remove purulent drainage and excessive fluid. Postoperative care of the patient is similar to the care of the patient with an exploratory laparotomy (see the nursing care plan on p. 1218).

Gastroenteritis

Gastroenteritis is an inflammation of the mucosa of the stomach and small intestine. Clinical manifestations include nausea, vomiting, diarrhea, abdominal cramping, and distention. Fever, leukocytosis, and blood or mucus in the stool may be present. Causative agents are varied (see Table 40-1). Most cases are self-limiting and do not require hospitalization. However, older adults and chronically ill patients may be unable to consume sufficient fluids orally to compensate for fluid loss. Until vomiting has ceased, the patient should be on NPO status. If dehydration has occurred, IV replacement of fluids may be necessary. As soon as tolerated, fluids containing glucose and electrolytes (e.g., Gatorade) should be given. If the causative agent is identified, appropriate antibiotic, antimicrobial, or antiinfective medication is given.

NURSING MANAGEMENT
GASTROENTERITIS

Accurate monitoring of intake and output is important for successful replacement of lost fluid. Strict medical asepsis and enteric precaution should be instituted when indicated. The patient should be instructed in the importance of proper food handling and preparation of food to prevent infections such as salmonellosis and trichinosis. The importance of rest and increased fluid intake as symptomatic treatment measures for gastroenteritis should be stressed.

Symptomatic nursing care is given for nausea, vomiting, and diarrhea. The nurse should assess complaints of pain, vomiting, and diarrhea because gastroenteritis is often confused with appendicitis. To allay the patient's apprehension, the nurse should explain that gastroenteritis usually runs an acute course with no sequelae.

IRRITABLE BOWEL SYNDROME

Irritable bowel syndrome (IBS) is a symptom complex characterized by intermittent and recurrent abdominal pain associated with an alteration in bowel function (diarrhea or constipation). Other symptoms commonly found include abdominal distention, excessive flatulence, urge to defecate, and sensation of incomplete evacuation. IBS is a common problem affecting approximately 10% to 17% of the population in the United States.[7] In western societies, approximately two times as many women than men seek health care services for IBS. Stress, psychologic factors, and specific food intolerances have been identified as major factors that precipitate IBS symptoms.

The key to accurate diagnosis is a thorough health history and physical examination. Emphasis should be on symptoms, past health history (including psychosocial aspects), family history, and drug and dietary history. Diagnostic tests should be selectively used to rule out more serious life-threatening disorders with symptoms similar to those of IBS, such as colon cancer, peptic ulcer disease, and malabsorption disorders.

The health care provider should establish a trusting relationship with the patient at the onset of treatment. The patient needs reassurance that the symptoms are functional. The patient should be encouraged to verbalize concerns and anxiety. A diet containing at least 20 g per day of dietary fiber should be initiated (see Table 40-9). This may also include the addition of psyllium-containing products (e.g., Metamucil).

The patient whose primary symptoms are abdominal distention and increased flatulence should be advised to eliminate common gas-producing foods such as broccoli and cabbage from the diet and to substitute yogurt for milk products if there is lactose intolerance. Anticholinergic agents, such as dicyclomine (Bentyl), may be helpful if taken before meals to alleviate the pain associated with ingestion of food. For the patient with a high level of anxiety, a mild sedative or tranquilizer may be ordered but should be prescribed for only a short time. Additional therapies include relaxation and stress management techniques, although no single therapy has been found to be effective for all patients with IBS.

INFLAMMATORY BOWEL DISEASE

Crohn's disease and *ulcerative colitis* are immunologically related disorders that are referred to as *inflammatory bowel disease* (IBD). These disorders are characterized by chronic, recurrent inflammation of the intestinal tract. For both conditions, the clinical manifestations are varied, with long periods of remission interspersed with episodes of acute inflammation. Both diseases can be debilitating.

Although there has been extensive research on the etiology of IBD, the cause of both ulcerative colitis and Crohn's disease remains unknown. Possible causes include (1) an infectious agent (e.g., virus, bacteria) because IBD produces mucosal changes in the colon similar to those of infectious diarrhea, although no consistent pathogen has been identified; (2) an autoimmune reaction from the presence of other immune-related disorders, such as systemic lupus erythematosus, ankylosing spondylitis, and erythema nodosum in patients with IBD; (3) food allergies (although this has not been substantiated); and (4) heredity (familial recurrences have been documented). In one study, 84% of identical twins of patients who had Crohn's disease also had the disorder.[8] Both Crohn's disease and ulcerative colitis run in related families.[9] For years IBD (especially ulcerative colitis) was thought to be due to psychosomatic factors, such as severe emotional stress. It is now believed that these emotional changes result from and are not the cause of the disease.

Ulcerative Colitis

Ulcerative colitis is characterized by inflammation and ulceration of the colon and rectum. It may occur at any age but peaks between the ages of 15 and 40 years. Ulcerative colitis affects both sexes but has a higher incidence in women. It is more common in Jewish and upper-middle-class urban populations.

Pathophysiology. The inflammation of ulcerative colitis is diffuse and involves the mucosa and submucosa, with alternate periods of exacerbations and remissions (Table 40-16). The disease usually begins in the rectum and sigmoid colon and spreads up the colon in a continuous pattern.

The mucosa of the colon is hyperemic and edematous in the affected area. Multiple abscesses develop in the crypts of Lieberkühn (intestinal glands). As the disease advances, the abscesses break through the crypts into the submucosa, leaving ulcerations. These ulcerations also destroy the mucosal epithelium, causing bleeding and diarrhea. Losses of fluid and electrolytes occur because of the decreased mucosal surface area for absorption. Breakdown of cells results in protein loss through the stool. Areas of inflamed, undermined mucosa form pseudopolyps. Granulation tissue develops, and the mucosa musculature becomes thickened, shortening the colon.

Clinical Manifestations. Ulcerative colitis may appear as an acute fulminating crisis or, more commonly, as a chronic disorder with mild to severe acute exacerbations that occur at unpredictable intervals over many years. The major symptoms of ulcerative colitis are bloody diarrhea and abdominal pain. Pain may vary from the mild, lower-abdominal cramping associated with diarrhea to the severe, constant abdominal pain associated with acute perforations. With mild disease, diarrhea may consist of one or two semiformed stools containing small amounts of blood per day. The patient may have no other systemic manifestations. In moderate ulcerative colitis there is increased stool output (4 to 5 stools per day), increased bleeding, and systemic symptoms (fever, malaise, anorexia). In severe fulminating cases, diarrhea is bloody, contains mucus, and occurs 10 to 20 times a day. In addition, fever, weight loss greater than 10% of total body weight, anemia, tachycardia, and dehydration are present. *Toxic megacolon* and perforation may ensue. Acute fulminant colitis is present in only 6% to 10% of patients with severe ulcerative colitis.[10]

Complications. Complications of ulcerative colitis may be classified into those that are *intestinal* and those that are *extraintestinal*. Intestinal complications of ulcerative colitis include hemorrhage, strictures, perforation, toxic megacolon, and colonic dilatation. Hemorrhage is a result of inflamed, ulcerated mucosa and is usually controlled with conservative therapy. Massive hemorrhage is unusual and requires emergency surgery. Strictures are less common in ulcerative colitis than in Crohn's disease and are seen most often in patients with severe, long-standing disease. Perforation is most often associated with toxic megacolon but may occur alone. Most cases of perforation occur in the left side of the colon. Toxic megacolon occurs in approximately 5% of patients with ulcerative colitis.[11] Colonic dilatation, most often in the transverse colon, occurs as a result of severe acute inflammation of the entire colon wall.

A patient who has had ulcerative colitis for more than 10 years is at greater risk of colon cancer. The risk of cancer depends on age at onset, duration, and extent of disease. The patient should be periodically screened with surveillance colonoscopy. During this procedure, biopsy speci-

Table 40-16 Comparison of Ulcerative Colitis and Crohn's Disease

Characteristic	Ulcerative Colitis	Crohn's Disease
Age	Young to middle age	Young
Location	Starts distally and spreads in a continuous pattern up the colon	Occurs anywhere along gastrointestinal tract in characteristic skip lesions; most frequent site is terminal ileum
Distribution	Continuous	Segmental
Depth of involvement	Mucosa and submucosa	Entire thickness of bowel wall (transmural)
Small-bowel involvement	Minimal	Common
Fistulas	Rare	Common
Strictures	Rare	Common
Anal abscesses	Rare	Common
Granulomas	Absent	Common
Perforation	Common	Common
Toxic megacolon	Common	Rare
Malabsorption	Minimal incidence	Common
Diarrhea	Common	Common
Abdominal crampy pain	Possible	Common
Fever (intermittent)	During acute attacks	Common
Weight loss	Common	Severe
Rectal bleeding	Common	Infrequent
Tenesmus	Severe	Rare
Pseudopolyps	Common	Rare
Cobblestoning of mucosa	Rare	Common
Carcinoma	Increased incidence after 10 yr of disease	Slightly greater then general population
Recurrence after surgery	Cure with colectomy	70% or more recurrence after segmental resections of small or large intestine

mens should be taken every 10 cm throughout the entire colon.

Extraintestinal complications may be directly related to the colitis and small intestine pathology (malabsorption), or they may be nonspecific complications[12] (Table 40-17). Colitis-related complications are associated with active inflammation and often respond to treatment of the underlying bowel disease. These manifestations can involve the joints, skin, mouth, and eyes. Skin lesions such as erythema nodosum and pyoderma gangrenosum are among the most frequently seen extraintestinal manifestations. Uveitis is the most common eye problem. Nonspecific complications occur in a small percentage of patients and have no correlation with the activity of the underlying disease.

Diagnostic Studies. Several studies are appropriate for diagnosis of ulcerative colitis (Table 40-18). Blood studies should include a CBC, serum electrolyte levels, and serum protein levels. A CBC typically shows iron deficiency anemia from blood loss. An elevated WBC count may indicate toxic megacolon or perforation. Decreases in serum electrolytes, such as sodium, potassium, chloride, bicarbonate, and magnesium, are due to fluid and electrolyte losses from diarrhea and vomiting. Hypoalbuminemia is present with severe disease and is due to protein loss from the bowel. The stool should be examined for blood, pus, and mucus. Stool cultures should be obtained to rule out infectious causes of inflammation.

Table 40-17 Extraintestinal Manifestations of Ulcerative Colitis

Colitis Related
- Joints
  - Peripheral arthritis (colitic)
  - Ankylosing spondylitis
  - Sacroiliitis
  - Finger clubbing
- Skin
  - Erythema nodosum
  - Pyoderma gangrenosum
- Mouth
  - Aphthous ulcers
- Eye
  - Conjunctivitis
  - Uveitis
  - Episcleritis

Related to Small-Bowel Pathology
- Malabsorption
- Gallstones
- Kidney stones

Nonspecific
- Liver disease—primary sclerosing cholangitis
- Osteoporosis
- Amyloidosis
- Peptic ulcer disease

Examinations with a flexible sigmoidoscope and a colonoscope allow direct examination of the mucosa of the large intestine. Using a sigmoidoscope the physician can view the rectum, the sigmoid colon, and the descending colon. The colonoscope allows for examination of the entire large intestine. The extent of inflammation, ulcerations, pseudopolyps, strictures, and lesions may be identified. Biopsy specimens should be taken for definitive diagnosis.

A double-contrast barium enema may show areas of granular inflammation with ulcerations. The colon may appear narrow and shortened, and pseudopolyps may be present. A double-contrast study (in which air is introduced into the bowel after the expulsion of barium) is effective in detecting mucosal abnormalities in ulcerative colitis.

Therapeutic and Pharmacologic Management. The goals of treatment are to (1) rest the bowel, (2) control the inflammation, (3) combat infection, (4) correct malnutrition, (5) alleviate stress, and (6) provide symptomatic relief using drug therapy (see Table 40-19). The mainstays of therapy are sulfasalazine (Azulfidine) and corticosteroids. Most patients can eventually be maintained on sulfasalazine alone. Corticosteroids are usually indicated for acute exacerbations of the disease. Hospitalization is indicated if the patient fails to respond to steroid therapy, if fever or abdominal pain develops, or if complications are suspected.

Drug therapy is an extemely important aspect of treatment (Table 40-19).[13] Sulfasalazine, a combination of sulfapyridine and 5-aminosalicylic acid (5-ASA), is the principal drug used. It is effective in the maintenance of clinical remission and in the treatment of mild to moderately severe attacks. After remission is obtained, therapy is continued with a gradual reduction over several months. The maintenance dose is usually continued for at least 1 year.

During active disease 5-ASA (the active form of sulfasalazine) and 4-ASA, given as retention enemas, are effective in the treatment of left-sided ulcerative colitis and proctitis. Topical salicylate therapy is the treatment of choice in patients with localized disease. 5-ASA (mesalamine [Rowasa]) can also be administered orally. The

Table 40-18 Therapeutic Management: Ulcerative Colitis

Diagnostic
- Fiberoptic colonoscopy
- Sigmoidoscopy
- Barium enema
- CBC
- Stool for blood, culture and sensitivity

Therapeutic

Mild and moderate disease
- Low-roughage diet and no milk or milk products
- Antimicrobial therapy
- Corticosteroids
- Anticholinergic therapy
- Antidiarrheal agents

Severe (fulminant) disease
- IV fluids with electrolytes
- Blood transfusions
- NPO status
- NG tube to low suction
- Antimicrobial therapy
- Corticosteroids
- Surgery if no improvement (colon resection with ileostomy)

CBC, Complete blood count; *IV,* intravenous; *NG,* nasogastric; *NPO,* nothing by mouth.

Table 40-19 Drugs Used to Treat Ulcerative Colitis

Category	Action	Examples
■ Antimicrobial	Prevention or treatment of secondary infection	Cephalothin sodium (Keflin) Sulfasalazine (Azulfidine)* Mesalamine (Rowasa)* Olsalazine (Dipentum)
■ Steroids	Antiinflammatory	Corticosteroids (cortisone, prednisone)
■ Anticholinergic	Decrease in GI motility and secretions and relief of smooth muscle spasms†	Methantheline bromide (Banthine) Propantheline (Pro-Banthine) Oxyphencyclimine (Daricon)
■ Sedatives	Quieting of CNS without inducing sleep or analgesia	Diazepam (Valium) Flurazepam (Dalmane)
■ Antidiarrheal	Decrease in GI motility	Diphenoxylate (Lomotil)
■ Immunosuppressives	Suppression of immune response	Azathioprine (Imuran)
■ Hematinics and vitamins	Correction of iron deficiency anemia and promotion of healing	Iron dextran injection (Imferon) Vitamin B_{12}

CNS, Central nervous system; *GI,* gastrointestinal.
*Mechanism of action unknown, likely to be antiinflammatory as well as antimicrobial.
†Used with caution during severe disease because of potential to produce toxic megacolon.

acrylic-coated tablets provide delivery of the drug more distally in the intestine.

Corticosteroids are of proven benefit in the management of active ulcerative colitis. Oral prednisone or prednisolone is effective in treatment of mild to moderate disease without systemic manifestations. If remission is not achieved, the patient requires hospitalization and IV therapy. A patient with severe attacks and systemic manifestations requires hospitalization and IV corticosteroid therapy. The patient is placed on a regimen of bowel rest. Fluids and electrolytes are administered IV. Hydrocortisone enemas and foams are effective in treatment of colitis limited to the rectosigmoid area. Rectal foams are usually administered in 5 ml volumes and are generally preferred over enemas because of the ease of administration. However, enemas are the preferred choice if the disease spreads beyond the sigmoid colon. Retention enemas have been shown to deliver medication into the descending colon and beyond in patients with active disease. Although steroids are reported to bring remission in 60% to 89% of cases, studies have also shown that they do not necessarily prolong remission.[14] The patient on corticosteroids is to be monitored for signs of Cushing's syndrome, hypertension, hirsutism, and mood swings. In some cases, psychosis may develop.

Immunosuppressive drugs (e.g., 6-mercaptopurine [6-MP]) have been used in severe cases of ulcerative colitis when a patient has failed to respond to any of the usual medications and before surgery is considered. Side effects of 6-MP, including bone marrow suppression and increased risk of infection, necessitate that it be used cautiously in these patients. Patients receiving this medication need to maintain an adequate fluid intake of 1800 to 2400 ml to reduce the risk of nephrotoxicity.[15] The drug should be taken with food and milk to reduce gastric irritation. More recently cyclosporine has been evaluated for its effectiveness in the treatment of severe ulcerative colitis that is unresponsive to corticosteroid treatment. (Cyclosporine is discussed in Chapter 44.)

Surgical Management. Approximately 85% of patients with ulcerative colitis go into remission with conservative therapy and nursing care, but 15% to 20% require surgery. Surgery is indicated if the patient fails to respond to treatment; exacerbations are frequent and debilitating; massive bleeding, perforation, strictures, obstruction, or changes that suggest dysplasia occur; or carcinoma develops.

Surgical procedures used to treat chronic ulcerative colitis include (1) total proctocolectomy with permanent ileostomy, (2) total proctocolectomy with continent ileostomy (Kock pouch), and (3) total colectomy with rectal mucosal stripping and ileoanal reservoir.

Total proctocolectomy with permanent ileostomy. Total proctocolectomy with an ileostomy, is a one-stage operation involving the removal of the colon, rectum, and anus with closure of the anus. The end of the terminal ileum is brought out through the abdominal wall and forms a stoma, or ostomy. The stoma is usually placed in the right lower quadrant below the belt line.

Total proctocolectomy with continent ileostomy. Kock pouch is a continent ileostomy, which is a variation from the traditional ileostomy (Fig. 40-2). This method eliminates the need for the patient to wear an external pouch over the stoma. The stoma is usually covered with a cap or dressing in case of mucus leakage. This procedure is considered curative for ulcerative colitis but has a higher complication rate than the traditional ileostomy.

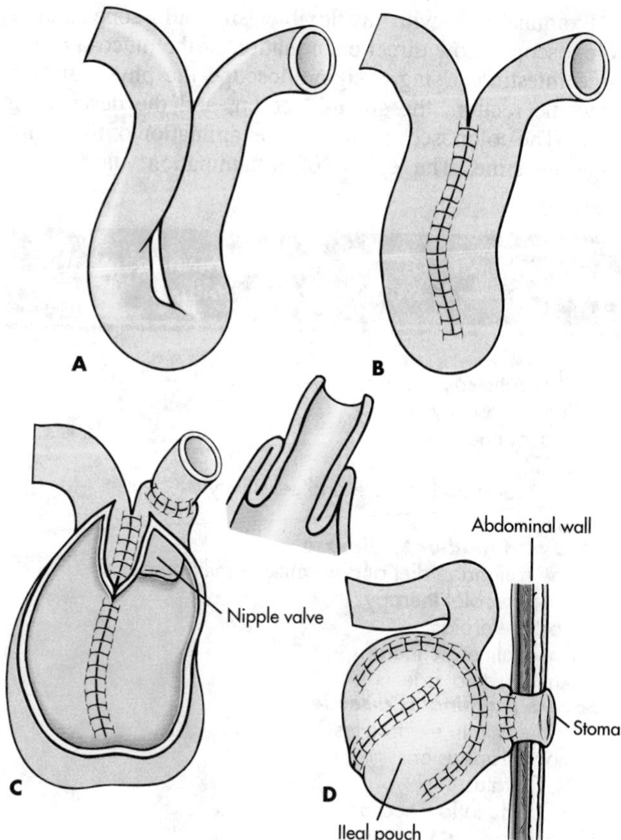

Fig. 40-2 Surgical formation of continent ileostomy (Kock pouch). ***A,*** Loop of terminal ileum. ***B,*** Both limbs sutured together and incised in a U shape. ***C,*** Pouch created with nipple valve. ***D,*** Pouch sutured to abdominal wall.

In this procedure an internal pouch in the distal segment of the ileum is made surgically, the intestine is split, a fold is made, and a one-way nipple valve is created and sutured into place on the abdomen. The pouch acts as a reservoir and is drained at regular intervals on insertion of a catheter. During surgery, a catheter is inserted into the pouch to allow suture lines to heal and to allow fixation of scar tissue around the valve to prevent slippage. Postoperative irrigations are performed every 2 to 4 hours to rinse mucus from the pouch. The catheter may stay in place for up to 3 to 4 weeks. Once the catheter is removed, insertion of a catheter to remove contents begins every 2 hours and is gradually decreased until it is needed only 3 to 6 times a day. The patient eventually determines the frequency by the changes in sensation of pressure in the pouch. A continuous leakage of fluid is prevented by the one-way valve created at the internal end of the ileum from the stoma to the ileal pouch. Pressure created when the pouch fills with feces forces the valve to close. The majority of complications that arise are a result of valve failure, which has been reported to be as high as 40%.

The primary late complications of the procedure include pouchitis, fistula development, and nipple valve extrusion. These complications affect function by increasing intubation frequency and compromising pouch continence. Manifestations of pouchitis are fever, malaise, and watery diarrhea. The lining appears red and inflamed, and biopsy shows nonspecific inflammation. Patients usually respond to treatment with metronidazole (Flagyl).

Total colectomy and ileal reservoir. A more widely performed procedure involves total colectomy and ileoanal anastomosis with the formation of an ileal reservoir (Fig. 40-3). The ileoanal surgical procedure is usually a combination of two procedures performed approximately 8 to 12 weeks apart. The initial procedure includes colectomy, rectal mucosectomy, ileal reservoir construction, ileoanal anastomosis, and temporary ileostomy. The second surgery involves closure of the ileostomy, which functionalizes the reservoir. Adaptation of the reservoir occurs over the next 3 to 6 months, which usually results in the ability to control and have decreased numbers of bowel movements over a 24-hour period.

Patient selection criteria include absence of colon cancer, small intestine free of disease (e.g., Crohn's), competent anal-rectal sphincter, and physical status adequate to permit lengthy surgery. In addition the patient needs to be motivated and capable of understanding self-care instructions.

Postoperative care. Postoperative care following surgical procedures to treat ulcerative colitis includes routine observations for patients who have had abdominal surgery. Stoma viability, mucocutaneous juncture, and peristomal skin integrity must be monitored. Because a more proximal portion of the bowel is used to create the ileostomy, output initially may be as high as 1500 to 2000 ml per 24 hours. The patient needs to be observed for signs of hemorrhage, abdominal abscess, small bowel obstruction, dehydration, and other related complications. If an NG tube is used, it will be removed when bowel function returns and oral intake is instituted. Drainage of serosanguineous fluid from the abdominal drain site may vary from 100 to 150 ml per 24 hours. The drain is usually removed within 4 days of surgery. The urinary catheter is removed 2 to 5 days after surgery. Systemic antibiotics are discontinued within 24 hours of the operation and corticosteroids, if used, are tapered.

Transient incontinence of mucus is a result of intraoperative manipulation of the anal canal. The patient should be reassured before the operation regarding this potential transient problem. Kegel exercises are recommended later on (several weeks postoperatively) to strengthen the pelvic floor and sphincter muscles. They are not recommended in the immediate postoperative period. Perianal skin care needs to be implemented to protect the epidermis from mucous drainage and maceration. The patient need to be instructed to gently rinse the skin with water and dry thoroughly. A moisture barrier ointment may be used, and a perineal pad may be required.

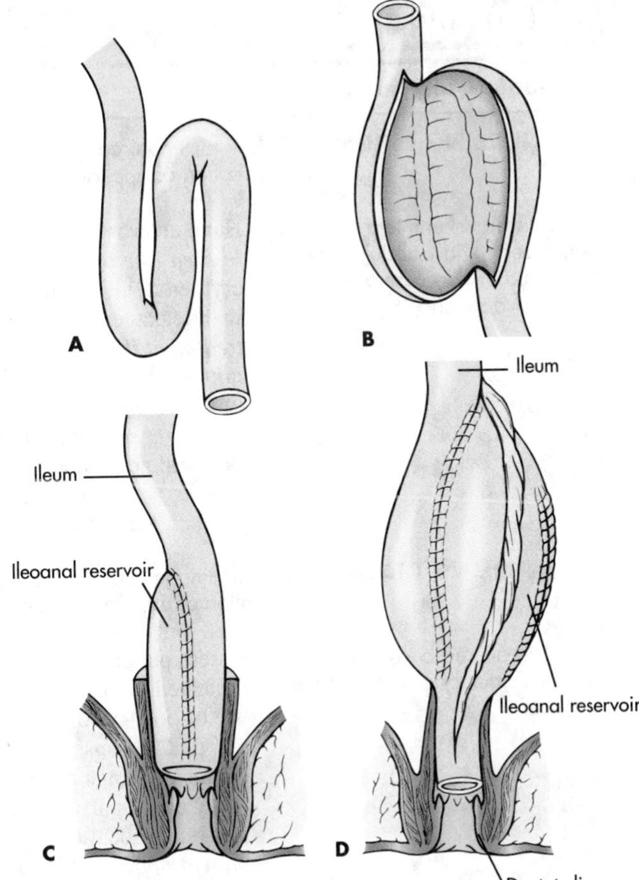

Fig. 40-3 Ileoanal reservoir. ***A,*** Formation of a reservoir. ***B,*** Posterior suture lines completed. ***C,*** S-shaped configuration for ileoanal reservoir. ***D,*** J-shaped configuration for ileoanal reservoir.

The most frequent type of ileostomy that is constructed is a loop. This frequently presents a pouching challenge because it retracts or drains inferiorly, resulting in effluent contact with the skin and predisposing to a denuded epidermis. An enterostomal therapy nurse is an appropriate referral for these challenging problems. Self-care instructions need to be reviewed and written information provided before discharge. Specific information is presented in the nursing care plan for the patient with a colostomy or ileostomy on p. 1228.

Nutritional Management. An important component in the treatment of ulcerative colitis is diet. The dietitian is an important member of the team and should be consulted regarding dietary recommendations. The goals of diet management are to provide adequate nutrition without exacerbating symptoms, to correct and prevent malnutrition, to replace fluid and electrolyte losses, and to prevent weight loss. The diet for each patient must be individualized.

Traditionally during the acute phase the patient may be on NPO status. When food is permitted, a high-calorie, high-protein, low-residue diet with vitamin and iron supplements is frequently prescribed. (A low-residue diet is presented in

NURSING CARE PLAN Patient with a Colostomy or Ileostomy

Planning: Outcome Criteria	Nursing Interventions and Rationales
➤ NURSING DIAGNOSIS	Risk for impaired skin integrity of peristomal area *related to* irritation from fecal drainage, irritation of appliance, and lack of knowledge of skin care.
Have normal skin integrity, intact pouch seal; know about proper technique of skin care and application of appliance.	Have enterostomal therapy nurse see patient before the operation *to mark stoma site in area free of creases and folds for better seal of the pouch.* After surgery assess for erythema, inflamed skin around stoma with burning and itching, poorly fitting pouch with leakage, lack of adequate skin care, and failure to use skin barrier *to initiate treatment if indicated.* During pouch change, assess skin for signs of breakdown *to initiate treatment if indicated.* Clean area with mild soap and water and dry thoroughly *to prevent irritation from intestinal contents or pouch adhesive.* Apply skin barrier *to protect skin and prevent direct contact with intestinal contents.* Teach patient proper skin and appliance care *to ensure proper technique for long-term care.* Plan for outpatient or home visit *for continued teaching.* Empty pouch when it is one-third full *to prevent seal from leaking.*
➤ NURSING DIAGNOSIS	Body-image disturbance *related to* presence of stoma and malodor *as manifested by* verbalization of embarrassment or shame because of malodor or presence of stoma.
Adjust to altered body image; have satisfactory plan for control of odor.	Assess patient's attitude toward colostomy *to determine if problem is present* and, if indicated, *plan appropriate intervention.* Instruct patient on measures for odor control, use of odor-proof pouch, pouch deodorants, use of room deodorants when pouch is emptied. Discuss normal emotional response to stoma and encourage patient to express feelings *to assist patient in adjusting to change in body.* Encourage family members to participate *to foster patient's support system.* Provide patient with information on local United Ostomy Association *to decrease sense of isolation and offer patient opportunity for education and support.* Prepare patient to do own stoma and pouch care *to increase independence and enhance self-esteem/image.*
➤ NURSING DIAGNOSIS	Altered nutrition: less than body requirements *related to* lack of knowledge of appropriate foods and decreased appetite *as manifested by* weight loss, vitamin and mineral deficiencies, inability to tolerate certain foods
Select and plan dietary intake to maintain weight at optimum level.	Assess nutritional intake *to determine need for intervention.* Reassure patient that a normal diet can be tolerated but that certain foods may need to be avoided *to prevent patient from needless avoidance of preferred food.* Gradually introduce foods one at a time *to identify individual foods that may be problematic* and begin with low-residue diet, *which is usually well tolerated.* Teach patient to chew food slowly and thoroughly *to facilitate digestion.* Give list of foods to avoid *so patient has a ready source of referral.* Arrange visit with dietitian if indicated.
➤ NURSING DIAGNOSIS	Altered sexuality patterns *related to* perceived loss of sexual appeal and possibility of accidental seepage of fecal material during sexual activity *as manifested by* verbalization of concern about intimate relations with spouse or significant other.
Have confidence in ability to resume previous sexual activity.	Assess patient's attitude about impact of stoma on sexual functioning *to determine if a problem exists and if there is a need to plan interventions.* Encourage discussion of meaning of sexuality to patient and significant other *to allow patient opportunity to discuss sensitive topic in a nonthreatening situation.* Discuss ways to avoid seepage and conceal stoma or pouch during intimate relations *to decrease fear of embarrassment or withdrawal from intimate situations because of anxiety over "accidents."* If appropriate, arrange visit with person of same sex and condition *to discuss sexual concerns and share potential solutions to provide patient with opportunity to ask questions and get practical, realistic answers from a supportive, understanding other.*

continued

NURSING CARE PLAN Patient with a Colostomy or Ileostomy—cont'd

Planning: Outcome Criteria	Nursing Interventions and Rationales
➤ NURSING DIAGNOSIS	Risk for fluid volume deficit *related to* excess fluid loss and inadequate oral intake secondary to ileostomy or diarrhea with a colostomy.
Have normal serum electrolytes; normal vital signs; good skin turgor; urine output >0.5 ml/kg/hr.	Assess for signs of weakness, poor skin turgor, sunken eyes, hypotension, tachycardia, hypokalemia, hyponatremia, oliguria *to determine presence of fluid volume deficit and, if present, plan appropriate interventions.* Record intake and output and include ileostomy drainage *to have an accurate record of fluid balance.* Monitor ileostomy drainage and notify physician of watery drainage *so treatment can be initiated.* Monitor vital signs q4hr *because hypotension can be an indicator of fluid volume deficit.* Report urine output <0.5 ml/kg/hr *so increased fluid intake can be initiated promptly.* Ensure fluid intake of at least 3000 ml/day in the initial postoperative period *to prevent dehydration.* Instruct patient to maintain high fluid intake and to increase during very hot weather, when patient is perspiring excessively, and during episodes of diarrhea *to ensure adequate fluid intake in various situations.* Monitor serum electrolytes *because inadequate fluid volume will be reflected in changed electrolyte values.* Instruct patient on signs and symptoms of sodium, potassium, and fluid deficits *to ensure early reporting and correction of underlying electrolyte problem.* Instruct patient on the definition of diarrhea in relation to anatomic location of stoma (i.e., normal output for an ileostomy is approximately 800 ml/ 24 hr.)
➤ NURSING DIAGNOSIS	Ineffective management of therapeutic regimen *related to* lack of knowledge of long-term management of stoma *as manifested by* frequent questioning about stoma care and concern about ability to manage self-care independently.
Be able to manage care or identify home-support system.	Assess patient's ability to manage self-care and instruct colostomy patient in irrigation procedure *if they meet criteria for learning irrigation to ensure appropriate long-term care.* Assess patient's ability to manage self-care *to plan appropriate interventions.* Teach patient and family stoma care related to pouch care, nutrition, personal hygiene, and emotional factors *to ensure appropriate long-term care.* Advise patient of problems such as fever or diarrhea that should be referred *so early intervention can be initiated.* Plan follow-up care and provide contact person if questions arise *to ensure patient is adequately managing long-term care.*

Table 40-20.) Special dietary restrictions are not usually necessary. Some physicians allow the patient to eat anything that does not cause symptoms. Cold foods, high-residue foods (whole-wheat bread, cereal with bran, nuts, raw fruit), and smoking increase GI motility and should be avoided.

Often enteral supplements and parenteral nutrition are necessary. Patients with systemic manifestations, significant fluid and electrolyte losses, or malabsorption may need parenteral hyperalimentation or enteral feedings, such as elemental diets. Elemental diets are high in calories and nutrients, lactose-free, and absorbed in the proximal small intestine, which allows the more distal bowel to rest. (Elemental diets are discussed in Chapter 37.)

Parenteral hyperalimentation allows for a positive nitrogen balance while resting the bowel. Vitamins, minerals, electrolytes, and other important nutrients can be administered to promote healing and correct nutritional deficiencies.

Iron dextran (Imferon) intramuscularly (IM) by Z-track or IV may be necessary if anemia is severe. In patients receiving long-term sulfasalazine therapy, folic acid deficiency may develop and supplementation may be necessary. Patients with small-bowel disease, ileal resection, or malabsorption, which affect the absorption of vitamin B_{12}, may need monthly injections of vitamin B_{12}. Potassium supplements may be necessary if corticosteroid therapy is used because hypokalemia can lead to toxic megacolon.

NURSING MANAGEMENT

ULCERATIVE COLITIS

Nursing Assessment

Subjective and objective data that should be obtained from a person with ulcerative colitis are presented in Table 40-21.

Nursing Diagnoses

Nursing diagnoses are determined when the problem and etiologic factors are supported by clinical data. Nursing diagnoses related to ulcerative colitis may include, but are

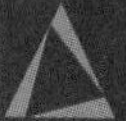

Table 40-20 Nutritional Management: Low-Residue Diet

Purpose

Low-residue diet provides foods low in fiber, which will result in a reduced amount of fecal material in the lower intestinal tract.

General Principles

1. This diet eliminates foods that are indigestible or stimulating to the intestinal tract to reduce the amount of residue in the colon. Foods should be included or excluded according to the following list.
2. Hot and cold foods should be eaten slowly.
3. Milk products are limited to 2 cups daily. For a more restricted-residue diet, milk should be eliminated.

Food	Foods Included	Foods Excluded
Beverages	Carbonated drinks, coffee, tea, cocoa, strained fruit juices	Alcohol, fruit juices with pulp
Bread	White bread, rolls, rusk, melba toast, crackers	Bread and crackers containing whole grain flour or bran; any hot breads such as biscuits, muffins, waffles, or pancakes
Cereals	Cooked, refined, or strained cereals: Cream of Wheat, Cream of Rice, farina, grits, dry cereals without bran, noodles, spaghetti, and macaroni	Whole grain cereals; cereals containing bran, nuts, and raisins; Shredded Wheat
Meat	Lean, tender ground beef, lamb, pork, veal or fish, broiled, stewed, or baked; canned tuna or salmon; shellfish; crisp bacon, chicken or turkey without skin, liver; creamy peanut butter	Fried, smoked, pickled, or cured meats, highly seasoned ham, fried fish, luncheon meats
Egg	All but fried	Fried or uncooked eggs
Cheese	Milk, cheese (American, cheddar), cottage cheese	All other cheeses
Milk	Limit to 1-2 cups (if tolerated), including that used in cooking; plain yogurt	Fruit yogurt
Fats	Butter, margarine, cream, oil, crisp bacon, mayonnaise, plain gravy	Any other; rich or spiced gravies
Soup	Cream and vegetable soups made from foods allowed and with milk allowed, bouillon, broth; strained vegetable juices	Cream and vegetable soups from foods not allowed (peas and dried beans)
Vegetables	Tender carrots, beets, or asparagus; strained vegetables; potatoes without skins; vegetable juices	Raw vegetables, all vegetables not strained, dried beans, peas, and legumes
Fruits	Strained fruit juices, ripe bananas, applesauce, pears, peaches, peeled apricots, Napoleon cherries, baked apple (no skin)	Raw fruits, fruits with skins, seeds
Desserts	Plain desserts (custards and puddings, plain ice cream from milk allowance), sherbet, plain gelatin desserts, angel food cake, sponge cake, plain butter cake, plain cookies	Nuts, coconut, raisins, rich desserts (pies, rich cakes, cobblers)
Condiments	Allspice, cinnamon, mace, paprika, salt, ground thyme, sugar, vinegar, lemon juice	All others

Breakfast	Lunch	Dinner
Sample Menu Plan		
½ cup applesauce ½ cup Cream of Wheat Scrambled egg White toast Butter or jelly 1 cup milk Coffee	Roast beef sandwich on 2 slices white bread (no lettuce or tomato) 1 tbs mayonnaise 2 sugar cookies Canned peach halves Coffee	Baked chicken Mashed potato Cooked carrots White bread Butter Angel food cake 1 cup milk Coffee

Table 40-21 Nursing Assessment: Ulcerative Colitis

Subjective Data

Important health information

Past health history: Ethnicity, infection

Medications: Use of antidiarrheal medications

Functional health patterns

Health perception–health management: Fatigue, malaise

Nutritional-metabolic: Nausea, vomiting; anorexia; weight loss

Elimination: Frequent bloody stools containing mucus and pus

Cognitive-perceptual: Lower abdominal pain (worse before defecation), cramping, tenesmus

Objective Data

General

Pallor, dry mucous membranes and poor skin turgor, emaciated appearance, intermittent fever

Integumentary

Anorectal excoriation

Gastrointestinal

Abdominal distention, hyperactive bowel sounds

Possible findings

Anemia; leukocytosis; electrolyte imbalance; guaiac-positive stool; abnormal proctosigmoidoscopic, colonoscopic, and barium enema findings.

not limited to, those presented in the nursing care plan for the patient with ulcerative colitis on p. 1232.

Planning

The overall goals are that the patient with ulcerative colitis will (1) experience a decrease in number and severity of acute exacerbations, (2) maintain normal fluid and electrolyte balance, (3) be free from pain or discomfort, (4) comply with medical regimens, and (5) maintain nutritional balance.

Nursing Implementation

During the acute phase, attention is focused on hemodynamic stability, pain control, fluid and electrolyte balance, and nutritional support. Accurate intake and output records need to be maintained. The number and appearance of stools are monitored. Nursing care of the patient with ulcerative colitis is directed toward an intensive therapeutic and supportive program. (See the nursing care plan on ulcerative colitis.) Emotional support is important because the patient with ulcerative colitis may feel insecure, dependent, and sensitive. It is important that the nurse establish a good working relationship and encourage the patient to talk about self and daily activities. Honesty, patience, and understanding are crucial in the relationship with the patient. An explanation of all procedures and treatment is necessary and may allay some apprehension. Appropriate diversional activity should be used to move the patient's attention away from the intestinal tract. Psychotherapy may be indicated if the patient is experiencing emotional problems, but the nurse needs to recognize that the patient's behavior may result from factors other than emotional ones. Any person who has 10 to 20 bowel movements a day and has rectal discomfort may be anxious, frustrated, discouraged, and depressed. Along with other team members, the nurse can assist the patient to accept the chronic condition and have an optimistic view with the possibility of cure after surgery. The nurse may find that inadequate coping mechanisms in the patient with ulcerative colitis are due to early onset of the disease (often at 10 to 15 years of age), which may have interfered with usual growth, development, and maturation.

Bed rest may be ordered if the patient has a severe exacerbation. Nursing interventions to prevent complications of immobility should be instituted. A sedative or tranquilizer may be prescribed to ensure rest. The nurse should allow the patient extra time to eat. In addition to teaching related to treatment, medications, diet, tests, and the disease and its management, discussion of everyday topics should also be a part of diversional therapy.

Rest is important in the management of ulcerative colitis. Patients may lose much sleep because of frequent episodes of diarrhea and abdominal pain. Nutritional deficiencies and anemia leave the patient feeling weak and listless. Activities should be scheduled around rest periods. The nurse should also set limits and follow through because the patient can be demanding. The patient needs to know and understand that the nurse wants to help and does not consider the care repugnant.

Until diarrhea is controlled, the patient must be kept clean, dry, and free of odor. A bedpan and wipes should be kept within reach of the patient. The bedpan should be emptied as soon as possible. A deodorizer should be placed in the room. Antidiarrheal agents should be administered as ordered. If the patient has continuous diarrhea, the enterostomal therapy nurse or therapist may give helpful suggestions. Meticulous perianal skin care using plain water (no harsh soap) is necessary to treat and prevent skin breakdown. Dibucaine (Nupercaine), witch hazel, or other soothing compresses or prescribed ointment and sitz baths may reduce irritation and relieve discomfort of the anus.

Crohn's Disease

Crohn's disease is a chronic, nonspecific inflammatory bowel disorder of unknown origin that can affect any part of the GI tract. It was once thought to be a disease specific to the small intestine and was called *regional enteritis.*

Crohn's disease may occur at any age but occurs most often between the ages of 15 and 30 years. When it occurs in older adults, the morbidity and mortality rates are higher because of other chronic problems that may be present. Both sexes are affected, with a slightly higher incidence in women. Similar to ulcerative colitis, it occurs more often in Jewish and upper-middle-class urban populations. The incidence of Crohn's disease is slightly lower than that of ulcerative colitis.

Pathophysiology. Crohn's disease is characterized by inflammation of segments of the GI tract. It can affect any part of the GI tract but is most often seen in the

NURSING CARE PLAN Patient with Ulcerative Colitis

Planning: Outcome Criteria	Nursing Interventions and Rationales
➤ **NURSING DIAGNOSIS**	Diarrhea *related to* irritated bowel and intestinal hyperactivity *as manifested by* frequent diarrheal stools (>10/day).
Have fewer, firmer stools.	Monitor frequency and character of stools *to evaluate effectiveness of antidiarrheal agents and dietary restrictions.* Maintain food and fluid restrictions *to rest bowl during exacerbations.* Teach patient to avoid nicotine, caffeine, and foods or fluids that *are irritating to bowel or cause increased motility.* Administer antidiarrheal medications as prescribed *to reduce incidence of diarrhea.*
➤ **NURSING DIAGNOSIS**	Sleep pattern disturbance *related to* frequent stools *as manifested by* numerous interruptions of sleep, fatigue during waking hours with resultant frequent naps
Verbalize feeling of being rested with improved sleep pattern.	Provide measures to reduce bowel irritability, such as prescribed medications *to reduce bowel movements during hours of sleep.* Instruct patient to refrain from nicotine *because it increases bowel motility* and caffeine *because it is a stimulant.* Encourage patient in use of usual sleeping routines *because deviations from usual pattern can cause anxiety and frustration with subsequent interference with sleep.*
➤ **NURSING DIAGNOSIS**	Anxiety *related to* possible social embarrassment, unfamiliar environment, diagnostic tests, and treatment *as manifested by* expression of concerns about effect of disease on social relationships, questions about hospitalization, treatment; withdrawal.
Verbalize less anxious feeling; have relaxed facial expression.	Monitor signs of anxiety *to plan appropriate interventions.* Encourage open discussion of feelings about diagnosis *to demonstrate acceptance and concern for patient.* Explain all treatments, diagnostic tests, and medications *because understanding may reduce anxiety.* Provide privacy *to reduce embarrassment and anxiety associated with frequent bowel movements.*
➤ **NURSING DIAGNOSIS**	Altered nutrition: less than body requirements *related to* decreased nutrient intake, increased nutrient loss through diarrhea, and decreased absorption in intestine *as manifested by* anorexia, nausea, and vomiting; weight loss; weakness, lethargy; anemia; change in hair, skin, and mucous membranes caused by nutrient and vitamin deficiencies
Maintain body weight within normal range; have adequate nutritional intake; have increased strength and activity tolerance.	Assess and document signs of malnutrition (e.g., hair loss, dry skin, bleeding, cracked gingivae, muscle weakness) *to direct plan for treating the problem.* Record daily weights *to evaluate nutritional status and response to treatment.* Monitor intake and output *to identify fluid intake needs.* Perform ongoing calorie counts *to determine adequacy of caloric intake.* Administer IV fluids and TPN as ordered to *allow for a positive nitrogen balance while resting the bowel.* Give and instruct patient on well-balanced, low-residue diet with small, frequent feedings *to reduce the amount of fecal material in the lower intestinal tract.* Administer nutritional supplements (as ordered) *to provide additional calories, protein, and fluid.* Assess patient's food likes and dislikes *so foods offered will have a higher likelihood of being eaten.* Assist in determining what foods are tolerated by patient *because irritating foods differ among patients and diet needs to be individualized.* Teach patient to take small bites, eat slowly, chew well *to facilitate digestion by slowing GI activity and breaking food down first in the mouth.*

continued

terminal ileum, jejunum, and colon. Involvement of the esophagus, stomach, and duodenum is rare. The inflammation involves all layers of the bowel wall (i.e., transmural). Areas of involvement are usually discontinuous, with segments of normal bowel occurring between diseased portions. Typically ulcerations are deep and longitudinal and penetrate between islands of inflamed edematous mucosa, causing the classic cobblestone appearance. Thickening of the bowel wall occurs, as well as narrowing of the lumen with stricture development. Abscesses or fistula tracts that communicate with other loops of bowel, skin, bladder, rectum, or vagina may develop. Histologically, granulomas

NURSING CARE PLAN Patient with Ulcerative Colitis—cont'd

Planning: Outcome Criteria	Nursing Interventions and Rationales
➤ NURSING DIAGNOSIS	Impaired skin integrity of perianal area *related to* diarrhea, immobility, and altered nutritional status *as manifested by* frequent loose, watery stools; erythema, redness of perianal area; discomfort around perianal area during and after evacuation; poor nutritional intake; prolonged bed rest.
Have no evidence of skin breakdown.	Assess skin for signs of breakdown *to ensure early intervention.* Cleanse perianal area after each bowel movement with mild soap and warm water and dry thoroughly *to remove bacteria, provide comfort, and stimulate circulation to treat and prevent skin breakdown.* Provide sitz baths *for comfort and hygiene.* Apply protective ointment. If patient is on bed rest, change position frequently (at least q2hr) *to minimize pressure over bony prominences.* Monitor fluid and nutrient intake *to identify fluid balance and negative nitrogen balance for early intervention.* Encourage increased intake of proteins *to promote healing.* Instruct patient and family on proper skin care techniques *to enable them to participate fully in treatment plan.*
➤ NURSING DIAGNOSIS	Ineffective individual coping *related to* chronic disease, lifestyle changes, stress, and chronic pain *as manifested by* inability to express feelings and concerns; display of dependent, attention-getting behavior.
Develop healthy coping behaviors.	Identify ineffective behaviors and institute plan *to assist patient in learning more effective behaviors.* Include other staff members and family in setting limits *to provide a consistent approach.* Encourage patient's expression of feelings *to provide support as patient explores areas of concern and add to patient's feelings of self-worth.* Discuss reasons for limitations *to enable patient to cooperate with plan.* Offer reassurance and psychological support *to demonstrate caring and concern.* Know personal limitations and refer to counseling when appropriate *because more intensive treatment may be required to deal with specific stress and problem areas.*
➤ NURSING DIAGNOSIS	Ineffective management of therapeutic regimen *related to* lack of knowledge of course of disease, appropriate lifestyle adjustments, and nutritional and pharmacologic interventions *as manifested by* questioning about disease and treatment, poor decisions about activities of daily living.
Repeat correct information about disease and treatment.	Provide information about the disease *to ensure patient has adequate knowledge about the disease and treatment.* Refer to dietitian if complex dietary changes are necessary *to provide patient with benefit of expert counseling.* Teach about the relationships of stress to the disease *because stress may stimulate hyperreactivity of the colon in susceptible persons.* Teach stress-reduction techniques *to assist patient in developing positive ways to reduce stress.*

COLLABORATIVE PROBLEMS

Nursing Goals	Nursing Interventions and Rationales
➤ POTENTIAL COMPLICATIONS	Hypovolemia and electrolyte imbalances
Monitor for signs of hypovolemia and electrolyte imbalances; report deviations from acceptable parameters; carry out medical and nursing interventions.	Monitor for tachycardia, hypotension, weakness, dizziness, poor skin turgor, pallor, sunken eyes, rectal bleeding, abnormal serum electrolytes, urine output <0.5 ml/kg/hr *to identify hypovolemia and electrolyte imbalances.* Assess and document skin turgor, color, and temperature q4hr *to provide ongoing evidence of patient's response to dehydration or hypovolemia.* Maintain accurate intake and output records; include stool volumes *to enable appropriate fluid replacement.* Monitor hourly urine outputs in severely ill patients and notify physician of output <0.5 ml/kg/hr *to ensure immediate treatment.* Monitor vital signs q4hr or more frequently if patient is unstable *to evaluate patient's response and guide treatment.* Monitor serum electrolyte values *to identify abnormal values and guide replacement therapy.* Notify physician of hypokalemia, hyponatremia *to ensure early medical intervention.* Administer IV fluids, blood products as ordered. Encourage oral intake (at least 3000 ml/day) when tolerated *to maintain fluid balance.*

GI, Gastrointestinal; *IV*, intravenous; *TPN*, total parenteral nutrition.

are present in 50% of patients and may be located in any layer of the bowel wall.[16]

Clinical Manifestations. The manifestations depend largely on the anatomical site of involvement, extent of the disease process, and presence or absence of complications. The onset of Crohn's disease is usually insidious, with nonspecific complaints such as diarrhea, fatigue, abdominal pain, weight loss, and fever. Early diagnosis may be more difficult than for ulcerative colitis. The principal symptoms of Crohn's disease are diarrhea and abdominal pain. Diarrhea is usually nonbloody and is a result of the inflammatory process or malabsorption. Pain may be severe and intermittent or constant, depending on the cause. Other manifestations include abdominal cramping and tenderness, abdominal distention, fever, and fatigue. Extraintestinal manifestations, such as arthritis and finger clubbing, may precede the onset of bowel disease. As the disease progresses, there is weight loss, malnutrition, dehydration, electrolyte imbalances, anemia, increased peristalsis, and pain around the umbilicus and right lower quadrant.

Crohn's disease is a chronic disorder with unpredictable periods of recurrence and remission. Attacks are intermittent, usually recurring over a period of several weeks to months, with diarrhea and abdominal pain subsiding spontaneously.

Complications. Complications, both gastrointestinal and extragastrointestinal, are common in Crohn's disease. Scar tissue from the inflammation narrows the lumen of the intestine and may cause strictures and obstruction, a frequent complication. Fistulas are a cardinal feature and may develop between segments of bowel. Cutaneous fistulas, common in the perianal area, and rectovaginal fistulas also occur. Fistulas communicating with the urinary tract may cause urinary tract infections. Inflammation of the intestines may involve all layers, predisposing the patient to perforation and the formation of intraabdominal abscesses and peritonitis.

Impaired absorption causing various nutritional abnormalities may occur as a result of damage to areas of the intestinal mucosa. Fat malabsorption causes a deficiency in the fat-soluble vitamins (A, D, E, and K). The patient may have an intolerance to gluten (a protein found in barley, rye, and wheat).

Systemic complications are similar to those of ulcerative colitis and include arthritis, liver disease, cholelithiasis (especially with ileal involvement), ankylosing spondylitis, pyoderma gangrenosum, erythema nodosum, and uveitis. Renal disorders are common, especially nephrolithiasis secondary to increased oxalate absorption.

Diagnostic Studies. Diagnosis of Crohn's disease can be made by means of a thorough history and physical examination to establish clinical signs and symptoms, barium studies, and endoscopy with biopsy (Table 40-22). Laboratory studies may determine electrolyte disturbances and the presence of anemia. Barium studies are useful in determining location and extent of the disease and may reveal classic findings, such as stricturing of the ileum (string sign), cobblestoning of the mucosa, fistulas, and areas of abnormal and normal mucosa. Endoscopic studies, such as colonoscopy and sigmoidoscopy, are useful in detecting such early mucosal changes as patchy inflammation, small ulcerations, and skip areas that may not be seen radiographically. Biopsies may be performed to determine the presence of granulomas. A small-bowel barium enema is preferred over an upper GI x-ray series, with small-bowel follow-through for defining mucosal abnormalities.

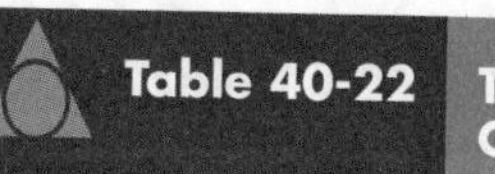

Table 40-22 Therapeutic Management: Crohn's Disease

Diagnostic
- Complete blood cell count
- Serum chemistries
- Stool for occult blood
- Barium enema of small and large intestine
- Proctosigmoidoscopic examination
- Flexible sigmoidoscopy and colonoscopy with biopsy

Therapeutic
- High-calorie, high-vitamin, high-protein, low-residue, milk-free diet
- Antimicrobial agents
- Corticosteroid drugs
- Supplementary parenteral nutrition
- Elemental diet
- Physical and emotional rest
- Surgery to treat complications (see Table 40-23)

Therapeutic Management. The goal of therapeutic management is to control the inflammatory process, relieve symptoms, correct metabolic and nutritional problems, and promote healing. Drug therapy and nutritional support are the mainstays of treatment.

Pharmacologic management. Sulfasalazine is effective when the disease involves the large intestine but is much less effective when only the small intestine is involved. Corticosteroid therapy is effective in reducing inflammation and suppressing disease. The dosage and the route of administration depend on the severity of the illness and the area involved. Once clinical symptoms subside, the dosage should be tapered. Immunosuppressive agents (6-MP, azathioprine) may be tried if repeated trials with corticosteroids fail. Patients require close monitoring because of the serious side effects of these drugs. Metronidazole (Flagyl) is useful in treating Crohn's disease of the perianal area. Marked exacerbations have been reported when the drug is stopped.

Balloon dilatation of strictures may be effective in relieving symptoms in some patients. This is usually performed through a colonoscope or under fluoroscopic guidance. Strictures most often dilated are those in the colon or small bowel.

Nutritional management. A major advance in nutrient therapy has been the elemental diet and TPN (see Chapter 37). Parenteral hyperalimentation may be given to patients with severe disease, small-bowel fistulas, or short-bowel syndrome. It is given before and after surgery to promote wound healing, reduce complications, and hasten recovery. The elemental diet provides a high-calorie, high-nitrogen, fat-free, no-residue substrate that is absorbed in the proxi-

Table 40-23 Indications for Surgical Management of Crohn's Disease

Drainage of abdominal abscess	Intestinal obstruction
Failure to respond to conservative therapy	Massive hemorrhage
Fistulas	Perforation
Growth retardation	Secondary hydronephrosis
Inability to decrease steroids	Severe anorectal disease
	Suspicion of carcinoma

mal small bowel. This diet can be given to most patients with Crohn's disease, even during acute exacerbations.

The diet should otherwise be low in residue, roughage, and fat but high in calories and protein. It may be difficult to maintain adequate absorption during periods of disease exacerbation and even during periods of remission. The patient usually responds favorably when milk and milk products are excluded from the diet. Lactose, the primary disaccharide found in milk, may not be adequately absorbed because of the inability of the damaged mucosa of the intestine to produce adequate amounts of lactase. High-fat diets are poorly tolerated because of the loss of absorbing mucosa and altered bile salt metabolism and absorption.

Vitamin deficiencies may develop as a result of malabsorption. Vitamin B_{12} injections every month may be needed because of the inability of the terminal ileum (if affected) to absorb this vitamin.

Surgical Interventions. Surgery is used in patients with severe symptoms that are unresponsive to therapy and in those with life-threatening complications. The majority of patients with Crohn's disease eventually require surgery at least once in the course of their disease. Indications for surgery are outlined in Table 40-23. Unlike ulcerative colitis, which can be cured by total proctocolectomy, Crohn's disease is not cured by surgery. The recurrence rate after surgery is high. The surgical procedure depends on the affected area and the condition of the patient. Conservative intestinal resection with anastomosis of healthy bowel is the procedure of choice.

NURSING MANAGEMENT
CROHN'S DISEASE

Acute care of the patient is similar to that of the patient with ulcerative colitis. As the patient's condition improves, the nurse should allow for more self-care, provide frequent rest periods, and advise the patient of the importance of rest and avoidance or control of emotional stress. Initially this may be difficult for the patient when told the nature of the disease and the limitations of the treatment. Special skin care may be needed by patients who have perianal fistulas or abscesses. Postoperative care should be the same as for exploratory laparotomy.

In the majority of patients with Crohn's disease the course is chronic and intermittent, regardless of the site of involvement. The patient and significant others may need help in setting realistic short-term and long-term goals. Teaching is important and should include (1) the importance of rest and diet management, (2) perianal care, (3) action and side effects of medications, (4) symptoms of recurrence of disease, (5) when to seek medical care, and (6) use of diversional activities to reduce stress.

Gerontologic Considerations

Although inflammatory bowel disease (i.e., ulcerative colitis and Crohn's disease) are considered diseases of young adults, a second peak in the distribution of these inflammatory conditions occurs around the age of 70. The pathogenesis, natural history, and clinical course of ulcerative colitis and Crohn's disease in older adults are similar to those observed in younger patients. However, the distribution of the inflammation appears to be somewhat different. In the older patient with ulcerative colitis the distal colon (proctitis) is usually involved. In the older patient with Crohn's disease the colon rather than the small intestine tends to be involved. There tends to be less recurrence of Crohn's disease in older patients treated with surgical resection. The degree of inflammation associated with both conditions tends to be less in the older adult than in the younger patient.

Medical management of the older patient with one of these conditions is similar to the younger patient. However, because of increased risk of cardiovascular and pulmonary complications, older adults tend to have increased morbidity associated with surgical procedures.

In addition to Crohn's disease and ulcerative colitis, older adults are also vulnerable to inflammation of the colon (colitis) from medication use and systemic vascular disease. Drugs such as nonsteroidal antiinflammatory drugs (NSAIDs), digitalis, vasopressin, estrogen, and allopurinol have been associated with colitis development in the elderly patient. Colitis may also be secondary to ischemic bowel disease related to atherosclerosis and congestive heart failure.

Inflammation of the colon as a result of inflammatory bowel disease or colitis results in diarrhea, which may be bloody. The loss of fluid and electrolytes and possibly blood may leave the older adult more vulnerable to problems related to volume depletion and dehydration. This may be particularly problematic in the patient with diminished renal and cardiovascular function. Thus nursing management is focused on careful assessment of fluid and electrolyte status and evaluation of the replacement therapies.

INTESTINAL OBSTRUCTION

Intestinal obstruction occurs when intestinal contents cannot pass through the GI tract, and it requires prompt treatment. The obstruction may be partial or complete. The causes of intestinal obstruction can be classified as *mechanical* or *nonmechanical.*

Types of Intestinal Obstruction

Mechanical. Mechanical obstruction may be caused by an occlusion of the lumen of the intestinal tract. Most

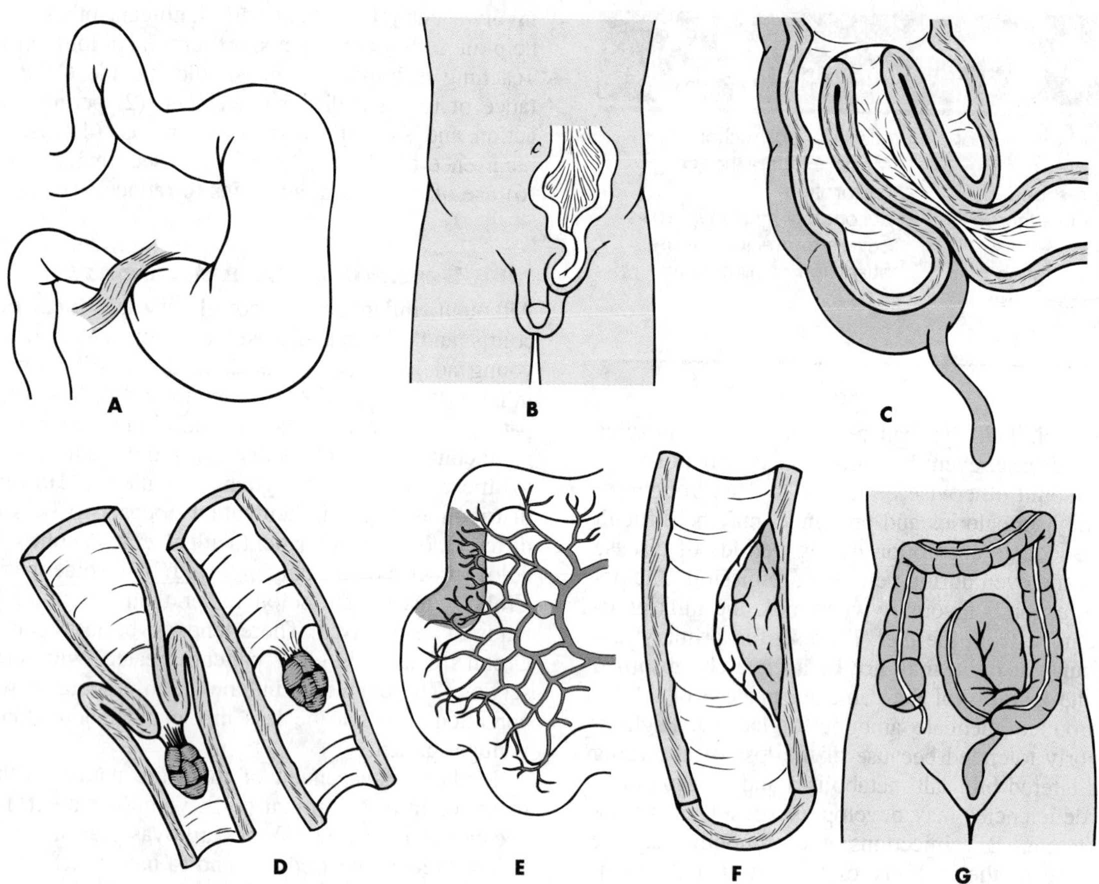

Fig. 40-4 Bowel obstructions. ***A,*** Adhesions. ***B,*** Strangulated inguinal hernia. ***C,*** Ileocecal intussusception. ***D,*** Intussusception from polyps. ***E,*** Mesenteric occlusion. ***F,*** Neoplasm. ***G,*** Volvulus of the sigmoid colon.

intestinal obstructions occur in the small intestine, most often in the ileum. Mechanical obstruction accounts for 90% of all intestinal obstructions (Fig. 40-4).[17] Adhesions account for 50%, hernias for 15%, and neoplasms for 15% of obstructions of the small intestine. Adhesions normally develop after abdominal surgery. Obstruction can occur within days of surgery or years later. Carcinoma is the most common cause of large bowel obstruction, followed by volvulus and diverticular disease.

Nonmechanical. A nonmechanical obstruction may result from a neuromuscular or vascular disorder. *Paralytic (adynamic) ileus* is the most common form of nonmechanical obstruction. It occurs to some degree after any abdominal surgery. Other causes of paralytic ileus include inflammatory reactions (e.g., acute pancreatitis, acute appendicitis), electrolyte abnormalities, and thoracic or lumbar spinal fractures.

Pseudoobstruction is an apparent mechanical obstruction of the intestine without demonstration of obstruction by radiographic methods. Pseudoobstruction may be caused by collagen vascular diseases and neurologic and endocrine disorders, but mostly it is found to be idiopathic.

Vascular obstructions are rare and are due to an interference with the blood supply to a portion of the intestines. The most common causes are emboli and atherosclerosis of the mesenteric arteries. The celiac, inferior, and superior mesenteric arteries supply blood to the bowel. Emboli may originate from thrombi in patients with chronic atrial fibrillation, diseased heart valves, and prosthetic valves. Venous thrombosis may be seen in low-blood-flow states, such as heart failure and shock.

Pathophysiology

Normally 6 to 8 L of fluid enters the small bowel daily. Most of the fluid is absorbed before it reaches the colon. Approximately 75% of intestinal gas is swallowed air. Bacterial metabolism produces methane and hydrogen gases. Fluid, gas, and intestinal contents accumulate proximal to the intestinal obstruction. This causes distention, and the distal bowel may collapse. The distention reduces the absorption of fluids and stimulates intestinal secretions. As the fluid increases, so does the pressure in the lumen of the bowel. The increased pressure leads to an increase in capillary permeability and extravasation of fluids and electrolytes into the peritoneal cavity. Edema, congestion, and necrosis from impaired blood supply and possible rupture of the bowel may occur. The retention of fluid in the intestine and peritoneal cavity can lead to a severe reduction in circulating blood volume and result in hypotension and hypovolemic shock.

The electrolyte-rich fluids, which are normally absorbed in the bowel, are retained in the bowel and subsequently lost into the peritoneal cavity. The location of the obstruction determines the extent of fluid, electrolyte, and acid-base imbalances. If the obstruction is high, as in the pylorus, metabolic alkalosis may result from the loss of hydrochloric acid from the stomach through vomiting or NG intubation.

When the obstruction is located in the small bowel, dehydration occurs rapidly. Dehydration and electrolyte imbalances do not occur early in large-bowel obstruction. If the obstruction is below the proximal colon, most GI fluids have been absorbed before reaching the point of the obstruction. Solid fecal material accumulates until symptoms of discomfort appear. Reverse peristalsis may cause vomiting of fecal material very late in the bowel obstruction.

Simple obstructions of the intestine involve blockage of the lumen in one spot. A closed-loop obstruction occurs when the lumen is blocked in two different spots (e.g., volvulus). This results in an isolated segment of bowel and obstruction proximal to that segment. Strangulation and gangrene are likely to develop if treatment is not immediate. A strangulated obstruction occurs when the circulation to the obstructed intestine is impaired. This is the most dangerous form of obstruction because it may lead to necrosis of the intestine (incarcerated). It is most commonly caused by volvulus, hernias, or adhesions.

Clinical Manifestations

The clinical manifestations of intestinal obstruction vary, depending on the location of the obstruction, and include nausea, vomiting, abdominal pain, distention, inability to pass flatus, and obstipation (Table 40-24). Obstruction located high in the small intestine produces rapid-onset, sometimes projectile vomiting with bile-containing vomitus. Vomiting from more distal obstructions of the small intestine is more gradual in onset. The vomitus may be orange-brown and foul smelling because of bacterial overgrowth. In some cases it may be feculent. Vomiting may be entirely absent in large-bowel obstruction if the ileocecal valve is competent; otherwise, the patient may eventually vomit feculent material.

Abdominal pain in high intestinal obstructions is usually relieved by vomiting. Persistent, colicky abdominal pain is seen with lower intestinal obstruction. A characteristic sign of mechanical obstruction is pain that comes and goes in waves. This is due to intestinal peristalsis trying to move bowel contents past the obstructed area. In contrast, paralytic ileus produces a more constant generalized discomfort. Strangulation causes severe, constant pain that is rapid in onset.

Abdominal distention is a common manifestation of intestinal obstructions. It is usually absent or minimally noticeable in high obstructions of the small intestine and greatly increased in lower intestinal obstructions. Abdominal tenderness and rigidity are usually absent unless strangulation or peritonitis has occurred.

Table 40-24 Clinical Manifestations of Small and Large Intestinal Obstructions

Clinical Manifestation	Small Intestine	Large Intestine
Onset	Rapid	Gradual
Vomiting	Frequent and copious	Rare
Pain	Colicky, cramplike, intermittent	Low-grade, crampy abdominal pain
Bowel movement	Feces for a short time	Absolute constipation
Abdominal distention	Minimally increased	Greatly increased

Auscultation of bowel sounds reveals high-pitched sounds above the area of obstruction. Audible borborygmi are often noted by the patient. The patient's temperature rarely rises above 100° F (37.8° C) unless strangulation or peritonitis has occurred.

Diagnostic Studies

A thorough history and physical examination should be performed. Abdominal x-rays are the most useful diagnostic aids. Upright and lateral abdominal x-rays show the presence of gas and fluid in the intestines. The presence of intraperitoneal air indicates perforation. Barium enemas are helpful in locating large intestinal obstructions. However, barium is not used if perforation is suspected. If the location is unknown, a lower GI tract study is done before an upper GI series. Sigmoidoscopy or colonoscopy may provide direct visualization of an obstruction in the colon.

Laboratory tests are important and provide essential information. A CBC and serum electrolyte, amylase, and blood urea nitrogen (BUN) determinations should be performed. An elevated WBC count may indicate strangulation or perforation; elevated hematocrit values may reflect hemoconcentration. Decreased hemoglobin and hematocrit values may indicate bleeding from a neoplasm or strangulation with necrosis. Serum electrolytes should be monitored frequently. They provide essential information on the patient's fluid and electrolyte balance. Serum sodium, potassium, and chloride concentrations are decreased in small-bowel obstruction. The BUN value may be increased because of dehydration. The stool should be checked for occult blood.

Therapeutic Management

Treatment is directed toward decompression of the intestine by removal of gas and fluid, correction and maintenance of fluid and electrolyte balance, and relief or removal of the obstruction.

NG or intestinal tubes (Fig. 40-5) may be used to decompress the bowel. NG tubes should be inserted before

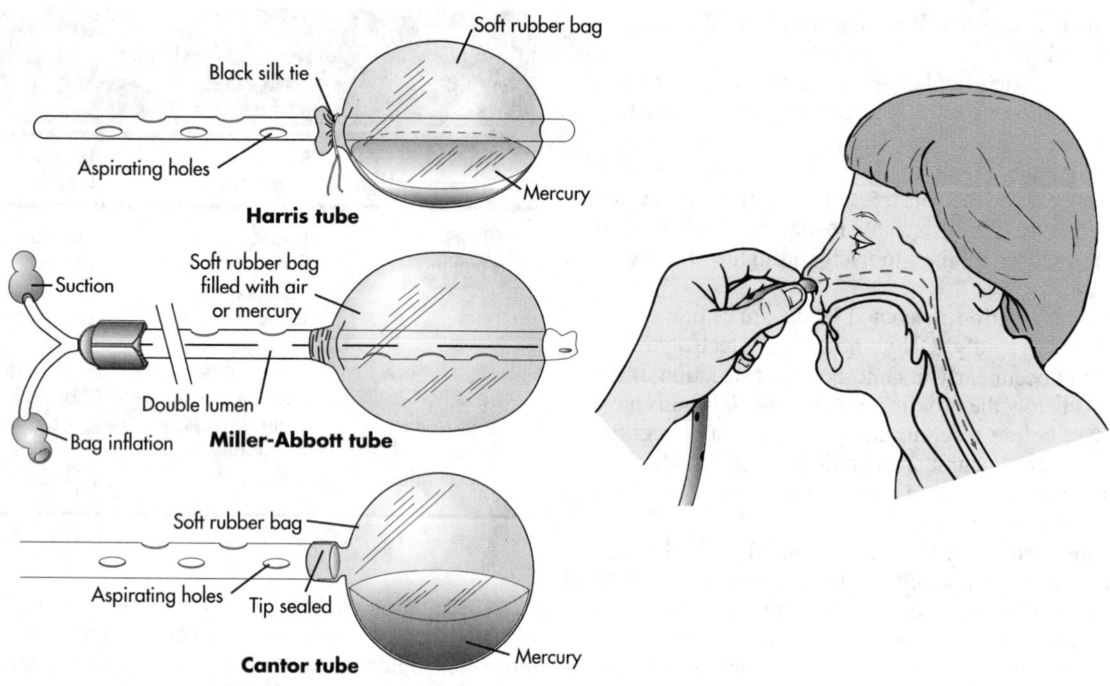

Fig. 40-5 Intestinal tubes used for decompression.

surgery to empty the stomach and relieve distention. They are also used instead of nasointestinal tubes to treat partial or complete small-bowel obstruction. Intestinal tubes, such as the Cantor or Miller-Abbott tubes, are passed into the small intestine. They are 10 feet (300 cm) long and mercury weighted. Insertion of an intestinal tube is controversial. Use of a long intestinal tube is difficult and time consuming. Some clinicians believe there is inadequate gastric decompression once the tube is in the small intestine. A higher incidence of postoperative complications and longer hospitalizations were noted in a group of patients treated with intestinal tubes as compared with those treated with NG tubes.[18] NG or intestinal tubes are effective in the treatment of patients with neurogenic obstruction who do not require surgery.

Decompression of the large intestine should not be attempted unless necrosis or perforation is present. Enemas, rectal tubes, sigmoidoscopy, and colonoscopy may be used. Sigmoidoscopy may successfully reduce a sigmoid volvulus. Colon-decompression catheters may be passed through partially obstructed areas via a colonoscope to decompress the bowel before surgery.

IV infusions that contain normal saline solution and potassium should be given to maintain fluid and electrolyte balance. Total parenteral hyperalimentation may be necessary in some cases to correct nutritional deficiencies, improve the patient's nutritional status before surgery, and promote postoperative healing.

Most mechanical obstructions are treated surgically. They may involve simply resecting the obstructed segment of bowel and anastomosing the remaining healthy bowel. Partial or total colectomy, colostomy, or ileostomy may be required when extensive obstruction or necrosis is present. Occasionally obstructions can be removed nonsurgically. A colonoscope can be used to remove polyps, dilate strictures, and remove and necrose tumors with a laser.

NURSING MANAGEMENT

INTESTINAL OBSTRUCTION

Nursing Assessment

Intestinal obstruction is a potentially life-threatening condition. Signs and symptoms are varied. Nursing assessment must begin with a detailed patient history and physical examination. The type and location of obstruction usually cause characteristic symptoms. The nurse should determine the location, duration, intensity, and frequency of abdominal pain and whether abdominal tenderness or rigidity is present. Onset, frequency, color, odor, and amount of vomitus should be recorded. Bowel function, including passage of flatus, needs to be determined. The nurse should auscultate for bowel sounds and document character and location; inspect the abdomen for scars, palpable masses, and distention; and observe for muscle guarding and tenderness.

Nursing Diagnoses

Nursing diagnoses specific to the patient with intestinal obstructions include, but are not limited to, the following:

- Pain related to abdominal distention and increased peristalsis
- Fluid volume deficit related to decrease in intestinal fluid reabsorption and loss of fluids secondary to vomiting
- Altered nutrition: less than body requirements related to intestinal obstruction and vomiting

Planning

The overall goals are that the patient with an intestinal obstruction will have (1) relief of the obstruction and return to normal bowel function, (2) minimal to no discomfort, and (3) normal fluid and electrolyte status.

Nursing Implementation

The patient should be monitored closely for signs of dehydration and electrolyte imbalance. A strict intake and output record should be maintained. All vomitus and tube drainage should be included. IV fluids should be administered as ordered. Serum electrolyte levels should be monitored closely. A patient with a high obstruction is more likely to have metabolic alkalosis; a patient with a low obstruction is at greater risk of metabolic acidosis. A patient is often restless and constantly changes position to relieve the pain. Analgesics may be withheld until the obstruction is diagnosed because they may mask other signs and symptoms and decrease intestinal motility. The nurse should provide comfort measures, promote a restful environment, and keep distractions and visitors to a minimum. Nursing care of the patient after surgery for an intestinal obstruction is similar to care of the patient after a laparotomy.

Care of Nasogastric and Intestinal Tubes. Although the physician usually inserts intestinal tubes, the nurse assists with the procedure. Insertion is easier if the patient relaxes, takes deep breaths, and swallows when instructed. If insertion of the tube to the small intestine is desired, the patient may be instructed or positioned to lie on the right side to facilitate tube passage through the pylorus. In some situations a prokinetic drug such as metoclopramide (Reglan) may be used to facilitate tube movement.

Once the tube is in place, mouth care is extremely important. Vomiting leaves a terrible taste in the patient's mouth, and fecal odor may be present. When an NG tube is in place, the patient breathes through the mouth, drying the mouth and lips. The nurse should encourage and assist the patient to brush the teeth frequently. Mouthwash and water for the patient to use in rinsing the mouth and petroleum jelly or water-soluble lubricant for the lips should be provided at the bedside.

The patient's nose should be checked for signs of irritation from the NG tube. This area should be cleaned and dried daily with application of a water-soluble lubricant and retaping of the tube. NG and intestinal tubes should be checked every 4 hours for patency. The patient may be placed on a schedule to clamp the tube every 2 hours for 1 hour, or for 3 out of every 4 hours before removal of the tube.

POLYPS OF THE LARGE INTESTINE

Colonic polyps arise from the mucosal surface of the colon and project into the lumen. They may be *sessile* (flat, broad-based, and attached directly to the intestinal wall) or *pedunculated* (attached to the intestinal wall by a thin stalk). Polyps tend to be sessile when small and become pedunculated as they enlarge, especially if they are in the left or descending colon.[19] They may be found anywhere in the large intestine but are most commonly found in the rectosigmoid area. Although most polyps are asymptomatic, rectal bleeding or occult blood in the stool are the most common symptoms.

Types

The most common types of polyp are *hyperplastic* and *adenomatous*. Hyperplastic polyps originate from the epithelium and are nonneoplastic growths. They rarely grow larger than 5 mm in size and never cause clinical symptoms. Other benign (nonneoplastic) polyps include inflammatory polyps, lipomas, and juvenile polyps (Table 40-25).

Adenomatous polyps are characterized by neoplastic changes in the epithelium. They are closely linked to colorectal adenocarcinoma. Structurally, there are three types, with tubular adenomas being the most prevalent. The risk of cancer in the polyp increases with polyp size and villous structure. Villous adenomas have a higher risk of turning cancerous than tubular adenomas.[19]

Although there are several polyposis syndromes, they are relatively rare. Of these, *familial adenomatous polyposis* (FAP) is the most common. This disorder is characterized by multiple polyps that at times number in the thousands and that are located in the large intestine and sometimes in other areas of the GI tract. Patients with a history of FAP have lifetime risk of developing colorectal cancer that approaches 100%. They also develop cancer at an earlier age (i.e., 40) than patients with non-FAP colon cancer. For children of patients with FAP, screening needs to be initiated at the age of 15 and then conducted annually. There is a 50% risk for these children to develop FAP. When there is indication of disease, total colectomy with ileostomy is the treatment of choice.[11]

Diagnostic Studies and Therapeutic Management

Diagnosis of polyps is made by barium enema, sigmoidoscopy, and colonoscopy. All polyps are considered abnormal and should be removed. In patients whose polyps are identified through barium enema, removal (polypectomy) should be done through a colonoscope or a sigmoidoscope. If the polyp is not removable, a biopsy specimen should be

Table 40-25 Types of Polyps of the Large Intestine

Neoplastic	Nonneoplastic
Epithelial polyps (adenomatous)	Epithelial polyps (hyperplastic)
Tubular adenoma	Hereditary polyposis syndromes (hamartomatous polyposis syndrome)
Tubular villous adenoma	Familial juvenile polyposis
Villous adenoma	Peutz-Jeghers syndrome
Hereditary polyposis syndromes (adenomatous polyposis syndrome)	Inflammatory polyps
Familial adenomatous polyposis	Pseudopolyps
Gardner syndrome	Benign lymphoid polyp
	Submucosal polyps
	Lipomas
	Leiomyomas
	Fibromas

taken for tissue examination. Surgery is not indicated unless carcinoma is present or in certain cases of polyposis syndromes. The patient should be observed for rectal bleeding, fever, severe abdominal pain, and abdominal distention, which may indicate hemorrhage or perforation.

CANCER OF THE COLON AND RECTUM

Significance

Colorectal cancer is the second most common cause of cancer death in the United States.[20] In 1994, there were approximately 149,000 new cases of colorectal cancer. In the United States, it accounts for approximately 56,000 deaths and about 20% of all deaths from cancer.[21] Cancer of the colon and rectum may occur at any age but is most prevalent over the age of 50. The 5-year survival rate for early, localized cancers is 92% for colon cancer and 85% for rectal cancer,[21] whereas it remains at 51% to 61% for cancer spread to adjacent organs and lymph nodes.

The incidence of cancer at specific sites in the colon varies (Fig. 40-6). In both sexes, the incidence of right colon cancers has increased and cancers in the rectum have decreased. The highest percentage of colorectal cancers in the United States are currently located in the cecum, ascending colon, and sigmoid colon. Approximately 20% of colorectal cancers are within reach of the examining finger, and 50% are within reach of the sigmoidoscope.

Pathophysiology

The causes of colorectal cancer remain unclear. Groups at high risk of colorectal cancer have been identified (Table 40-26). Age is a risk factor in both men and women. The risk for development in the general population increases slightly after the age of 40 and then rises rapidly in the following decades.

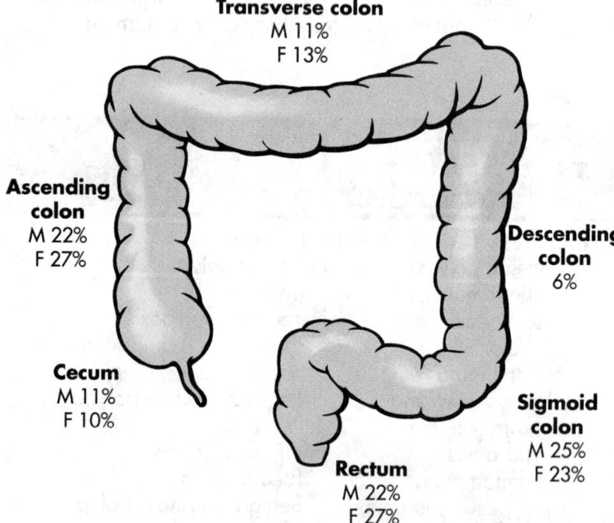

Fig. 40-6 Incidence of cancer. Approximately one half of all colon cancers occur in the rectosigmoid area and rectum. Percentages are listed for men and women.

Table 40-26 Risk Factors for Colorectal Cancer

Age	Family history of colorectal cancer
Familial polyposis	Previous history of colorectal cancer
Colorectal polyps	History of genital or breast cancer (women)
Chronic inflammatory bowel disease	

Diet is the most important environmental factor associated with colorectal cancer. The high-calorie, high-fat Western diet has been closely associated with development of colon cancer.

Adenocarcinoma is the most common type of colon cancer. Most colorectal cancers appear to arise from adenomatous polyps. All tumors tend to spread through the walls of the intestine and into the lymphatic system. Tumors commonly spread to the liver because the venous blood flow from the colorectal tumor is through the portal vein.

Clinical Manifestations

Clinical manifestations of colon cancer are usually nonspecific or do not appear until the disease is advanced. Cancer on the right side of the colon gives rise to clinical manifestations that are different from those on the left side of the colon.[22] Rectal bleeding, the most common symptom of colorectal cancer, is most often seen with left-sided lesions. Other commonly seen manifestations of left-sided lesions include alternating constipation and diarrhea, change in stool caliber (narrow, ribbonlike), and sensation of incomplete evacuation. Obstruction symptoms appear earlier with left-sided lesions because of the smaller lumen size.

Cancers of the right side of the colon are usually asymptomatic. Vague abdominal discomfort or crampy, colicky abdominal pain may be present. Iron deficiency anemia and occult bleeding dictate further investigation. Weakness and fatigue result from anemia.

CULTURAL & ETHNIC Considerations

COLON DISORDERS

- Inflammatory bowel disease is more common among Caucasians than African-Americans and Asian-Americans.
- Inflammatory bowel disease is more common among Jewish people and those of middle European origin.
- Colorectal cancer is higher in the United States and Canada than in Japan, Finland, or Africa.
- Incidence of colorectal cancer is declining in the United States except for African-American men.

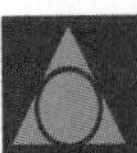

Table 40-27 Therapeutic Management: Cancer of the Colon

Diagnostic
- Sigmoidoscopy
- Barium enema
- Colonoscopy
- Rectal examination
- CBC
- Liver function studies
- Testing of stools for occult blood
- Carcinoembryonic antigen test
- CT scan of abdomen
- Ultrasound

Therapeutic
- Surgery
- Radiation therapy
- Chemotherapy

CBC, Complete blood count; *CT*, computed tomography.

Table 40-28 Dukes' Staging System for Colorectal Carcinoma

Classification	Description
A	Negative nodes, limitation of lesion to mucosa
B_1	Negative nodes, extension of lesion through mucosa but still within bowel wall
B_2	Negative nodes, extension through entire bowel wall
C_1	Positive nodes, limitation of lesion to bowel wall
C_2	Positive nodes, extension of lesion through entire bowel wall
D	Presence of distant, unresectable metastases

Diagnostic Studies

A thorough history with close attention to family history should be obtained, and a physical examination should be performed initially (Table 40-27). The digital rectal examination is the most important aspect of the physical examination because many rectal cancers are within reach of the finger.[23] If colorectal cancer is suspected, examination with the flexible sigmoidoscope and an air-contrast barium enema (in combination) are often performed. Colonoscopy is the procedure of choice if a questionable lesion is seen on barium enema or sigmoidoscopy. Other procedures include endorectal ultrasonography and a CT scan of the abdomen and pelvis to localize the lesion or determine its size. Synchronous lesions may be present at other sites in the colon, and tissue diagnosis may be made by brushing or biopsy during the procedure.

Laboratory studies should include a CBC to check for anemia, clotting studies, and liver function tests. A CT scan of the abdomen may be helpful in detecting liver metastases, retroperitoneal and pelvic disease, and depth of penetration of tumor into the bowel wall. A CT scan should be done before surgery. Liver function tests are performed to determine liver metastases.

A carcinoembryonic antigen (CEA) test is often performed, although it is not specific for colon cancer. A normal level of CEA does not exclude the possibility of a malignant condition. This test is used most effectively in following the progress of a patient after surgery. Return to normal of a previously elevated CEA indicates successful removal of the tumor. In contrast, persistent postoperative elevated or increasing CEA levels suggest residual tumor or tumor spread.

Therapeutic Management

Prognosis and treatment correlate with pathologic staging of the disease. Several methods of staging are currently being used. The most widely known is Dukes' classification (Table 40-28). Surgical removal of the primary lesion is the treatment for Dukes' stages A, B, and C. Prognosis for Dukes' stage A is 90% to 100% 5-year survival compared with less than 15% with Dukes' stage D.

The most recent classification of colorectal cancer is the TNM system, which is based on pathologic assessment and includes data from the history and physical examination and presurgical endoscopic and laboratory evaluations. *T* describes the extent of the primary tumor; *N* represents the location and number of lymph nodes involved; and *M* indicates the presence of distant metastasis. Cancer of the colon can also be divided into stages, with *stage 0* representing cancer in situ, *stage I* corresponding to Dukes' A and B_1, *stage II* corresponding to B_2, *stage III* corresponding to C_1 and C_2, and *stage IV* corresponding to Dukes' D.

Several noninvasive procedures may be performed through a colonoscope to treat certain types of colorectal cancer effectively. Endoscopic polypectomy is a highly effective and safe procedure. Adequate treatment is thought to be obtained if the resected margin of the polyp is free of cancer, the cancer is well differentiated, and there is no apparent lymphatic or blood vessel involvement. Laser therapy may be used to ablate nonresectable tumors. This is usually used only as palliative therapy in patients with obstructive symptoms.

Surgical Interventions. Surgery is the only curative treatment of colorectal cancer. The type of surgery performed is determined by the location and extent of the cancer. Success of surgery depends on resection of the tumor with an adequate margin of healthy bowel and resection of the regional lymph nodes.

Right hemicolectomy is performed when the cancer is located in the cecum, ascending colon, hepatic flexure, or transverse colon to the right of the middle colic artery. A portion of the terminal ileum, the ileocecal valve, and the appendix are removed, and an ileotransverse anastomosis is performed. A *left hemicolectomy* involves resection of the left transverse colon, the splenic flexure, the descending colon, the sigmoid colon, and the upper portion of the rectum.

Clear margins are most difficult to obtain with rectal carcinoma. Location of the rectal lesion determines the surgical procedure to be performed. There must be enough rectum left to ensure a secure anastomosis, or an abdominal-perineal resection is indicated. *Abdominal-perineal resection* is most often performed when the cancer is located within 5 cm of the anus.

In the abdominal-perineal resection, an abdominal incision is made and the proximal sigmoid is brought through the abdominal wall in a permanent colostomy. The distal sigmoid, rectum, and anus are removed through a perineal incision. The perineal wound may be closed around a drain or left open with packing to allow healing by granulation. Complications that can occur are delayed wound healing, hemorrhage, persistent perineal sinus tracts, infections, and urinary tract and sexual dysfunctions.

Low anterior resection may be indicated for tumors of the rectosigmoid and the mid to upper rectum. The use of EEA staplers has allowed lower and more secure anastomoses. The stapler is passed through the anus, where the colon is stapled to the rectum. This technique has made it possible to resect lesions as low as 5 cm from the anus.

Sphincter-sparing procedures are being performed on the patient who is a poor operative risk and for the patient with early disease. The number of these procedures may increase with continued early detection and surveillance. In these procedures a local resection is performed and the anal sphincters are left intact.

Radiation Therapy and Chemotherapy. Radiation may be used preoperatively or as a palliative measure for patients with advanced lesions. As a palliative measure, its primary objective is to reduce tumor size and provide symptomatic relief. (For discussion on radiation therapy, see Chapter 12.) Chemotherapy is recommended when a patient has positive lymph nodes at the time of surgery or has metastatic disease. No drug is available that can cure malignant colon or rectal tumors. The most commonly used drugs are 5-fluorouracil (5-FU) and methotrexate. Nitrosoureas, BCNU, levamisole, and MeCCNU are sometimes used in combination with 5-FU.

Table 40-29 Nursing Assessment: Colorectal Cancer

Subjective Data

Important health information

Past health history: Previous breast or gynecologic cancer; familial polyposis; villous adenoma; adenomatous polyps; Gardner's syndrome; chronic ulcerative colitis or Crohn's disease

Medications: Use of any medications affecting bowel function (e.g., cathartics, antidiarrheal medication)

Functional health patterns

Health perception–health management: Family history of cancer, especially colon or breast; weakness, fatigue

Nutritional-metabolic: Anorexia, weight loss; nausea and vomiting

Elimination: Change in bowel habits; alternating diarrhea and constipation; rectal bleeding; mucoid stools; black, tarry stools; increased flatus, decrease in stool caliber; feelings of incomplete evacuation; urgency

Cognitive-perceptual: Abdominal and low back pain, tenesmus

Objective Data

General

Pallor, cachexia, lymphadenopathy (later signs)

Gastrointestinal

Palpable abdominal mass, distention, ascites and hepatomegaly (liver metastasis)

Possible findings

Anemia; guaiac-positive stools; palpable mass on digital rectal exam; positive proctosigmoidoscopy, colonoscopy, or barium enema; positive biopsy

NURSING MANAGEMENT

COLON AND RECTAL CANCER

Nursing Assessment

Subjective and objective data that should be obtained from a patient with cancer of the colon or rectum are presented in Table 40-29.

Nursing Diagnoses

Nursing diagnoses specific to the patient with cancer of the colon or rectum include, but are not limited to, the following:

- Diarrhea or constipation related to altered bowel elimination patterns
- Abdominal pain related to difficulty in passing stools because of partial or complete obstruction from tumor
- Fear related to diagnosis of colon cancer, surgical or therapeutic interventions, and possible terminal illness
- Ineffective individual coping related to diagnosis of cancer and side effects of treatment

Planning

The overall goals are that the patient with cancer of the colon or rectum will have (1) no metastasis or recurrence of the cancer, (2) normal bowel elimination patterns, (3) quality of life appropriate to disease progression, (4) relief of pain, and (5) feelings of comfort and well-being.

Nursing Implementation

Health Promotion and Maintenance. The current recommendations from the American Cancer Society for colorectal cancer screening in patients who are not at high risk include annual digital rectal examination and fecal testing for occult blood beginning at the age of 40. Starting at the age of 50, flexible sigmoidoscopy should be done every 3 to 5 years, after two negative examinations 1 year apart. Positive findings should be followed with colonoscopy or air-contrast barium enema.

High-risk patients should be screened differently. Screening usually begins with colonoscopy and fecal occult blood testing, and continued follow-up varies according to risk factors.[24,25]

Acute Intervention

Preoperative care. Acute nursing care for the patient with a colon resection is similar to care of the patient having a laparotomy (see the preceding nursing care plan for the patient after laparotomy, p. 1218). In addition to general preoperative teaching and ostomy care instructions, the patient undergoing abdominal-perineal resection should be informed of the extent of the surgical procedure and the amount of care necessary to facilitate complete wound healing. The patient should be taught side-to-side positioning and made to understand that short walks are better than sitting. The nurse should teach and assist the patient in proper positioning for taking a sitz bath. The patient may not know that the sitz bath and positioning are sources of comfort. The patient may experience phantom rectal sensation because the sympathetic nerves responsible for rectal control are not severed during the surgery. The nurse must be astute in distinguishing phantom sensations from perineal abscess pain.

A well-developed, consistent nursing plan of care should be coordinated early. The implementation of this plan will facilitate the healing process and hasten the patient's rehabilitation.

Postoperative care. After an abdominal-perineal resection, there are two wounds and a stoma is surgically constructed in the left lower quadrant. There is an abdominal incision through which the colon is resected and an incision in the perineum. The management of a perineal incision differs depending on the type of wound. Three techniques are used: (1) packing of the entire open wound; (2) partial closure with Penrose drains for open drainage; and (3) primary closure of the perineal wound with closed-suction drainage of the pelvic cavity. The type of management of the perineal wound is individualized. The open and packed method is used in patients with extensive surgery or uncontrollable bleeding in the pelvic wound. When infection or contamination is minimal, a partial closure with drains is used. Wound sites connected to low intermittent suction or a Jackson Pratt or Hemovac suction placed in the perineal wound is commonly used to provide drainage of the operative site during the early postoperative period. This usually remains until drainage is less that 50 ml per 24 hours, which occurs after approximately 3 to 5 days.

A patient who has open and packed wounds requires meticulous postoperative care. During the immediate postoperative period the perineal dressing is reinforced and changed frequently because drainage can be profuse for several hours after surgery. All drainage is carefully assessed for amount, color, and consistency. The drainage is usually serosanguineous.

The packing is usually left in place for 2 to 3 days. Packing the pelvic cavity for prolonged periods may result in sepsis and rigidity of the cavity wall and thus impede the healing process. The nurse should examine the wound regularly and record bleeding, excessive drainage, and unusual odor. The perineal wound is usually irrigated with a normal saline solution when the dressings are changed. Dressings are changed several times a day, and aseptic technique is always used.

If the wound is partially closed and drains are in place, the nurse assesses the incision for suture integrity and signs and symptoms of wound inflammation and infection. The drainage is examined for amount, color, and characteristics. When the primary closure technique is used, the catheters are left in place for approximately 3 to 5 days, and during this time the drainage is examined and observations recorded. The area around the catheter is observed for signs of inflammation and kept clean and dry. The nurse should observe for signs of edema, erythema, drainage around the suture line, fever, and elevated WBC count. If the perineal wound was not closed, warm sitz baths at 100.4° to 106° F (38° to 41° C) for 10 to 20 minutes three to four times a day assist in tissue debridement, provide comfort, and increase circulation to the area. Moist heat causes vasodilatation, which allows more oxygen to flow to the affected area. Sitz baths of more than 20 minutes may result in too much vasodilatation, causing congestion and discomfort.

The patient may complain of pain and itching in and around the wound. There is no physiologic explanation of sensations that are felt, but a careful examination should be made to rule out delayed wound healing. Antipruritic agents and sitz baths are usually ordered. Use of a pressure-reducing chair cushion provides comfort when sitting. Sitting on a toilet for prolonged periods is discouraged until the perineal wound is well healed.

Sexual dysfunction is a possible complication of an abdominal-perineal resection and should be included in the plan of care. Although the effect of the procedure depends on the technique used, the subject should be discussed intelligently and tactfully by the surgeon, with follow-up as necessary by other members of the health care team. The nurse should understand that erection, ejaculation, and orgasm involve different nerve pathways and that a dysfunction of one does not mean total sexual dysfunction. The enterostomal therapy nurse is an important member of the team and can often provide correct and factual information concerning sexual dysfunction resulting from an abdominal-perineal resection.

Chronic and Home Management. Psychologic support for the patient and family is important. The recovery period is long, and the possibility of recurrence of cancer is always present. The overall 5-year survival rate for all patients undergoing resection for colon cancer is less than 50%. This presents a problem for the patient and health care providers because of the often painful, debilitating, and demoralizing manifestations produced by the recurrent disease and the lack of any effective palliative therapy. Chemotherapy may be used as an adjuvant measure for the patient with evidence of local or distant metastasis. (The special needs of the cancer patient are discussed in Chapter 12.)

The perineal wound may not be completely healed before discharge. After discharge the patient is usually seen by the physician, the home health nurse, and the enterostomal therapist in an outpatient clinic. The wound is usually irrigated and débrided. The skin around the wound should be assessed for loose hair. Shaving may be necessary to prevent the development of a chronic draining sinus. The

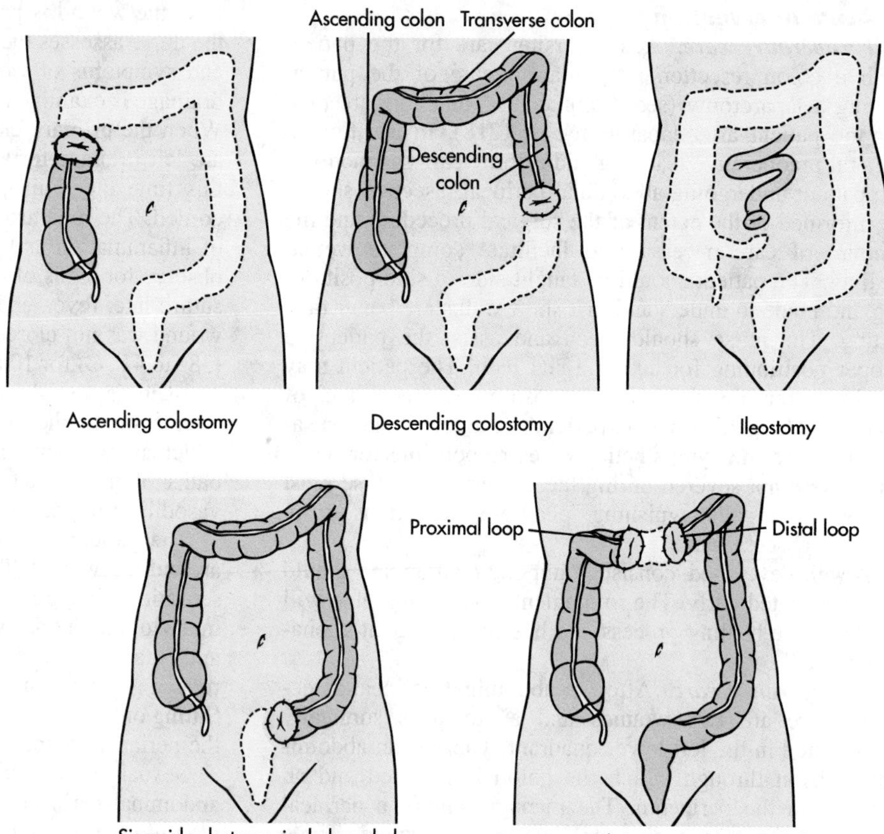

Fig. 40-7 Types of ostomies.

nurse should report the drainage because it may also indicate the presence of a foreign body, fistula, osteomyelitis, or rectal tissue not removed during surgery. The patient and significant others are taught management of the wound and the procedure to take a sitz bath at home. The patient and the family should be aware of all community services available for assistance.

STOMA SURGERY

Types

A *stoma* is created when the intestine is brought through the abdominal wall and sutured to the skin. It may be permanent or temporary. Fecal matter is diverted through the stoma to the outside of the abdominal wall.

An *ileostomy* is an opening from the ileum through the abdominal wall and is also referred to as a *conventional* or *Brooke* ileostomy (Fig. 40-7). It is most commonly used in surgical treatment of ulcerative colitis, Crohn's disease, and familial polyposis.

A *cecostomy* is an opening between the cecum and the abdominal wall. Both cecostomies and ascending colostomies are uncommon. They are usually temporary and most often are used for fecal diversion before surgery or for palliation.

A *colostomy* is an opening between the colon and the abdominal wall. The proximal end of the colon is sutured to the skin. Locations for colostomies are shown in Fig. 40-7. A *temporary colostomy* is usually performed to protect an end-to-end anastomosis after a bowel resection or is an emergency measure following bowel obstruction (e.g., malignant tumor), abdominal trauma (e.g., gunshot wound), or a perforated diverticulum. Temporary colostomies are usually located in the transverse colon. *Loop colostomy* (Fig. 40-8) and *double-barrel colostomy* (see Fig. 40-7) are most commonly performed as temporary colostomies, but they may be permanent (Fig. 40-8). A comparison of colostomies and ileostomy is shown in Table 40-30.

Surgical Interventions

End stoma. An end stoma is surgically constructed by dividing the bowel and bringing out the proximal end as a

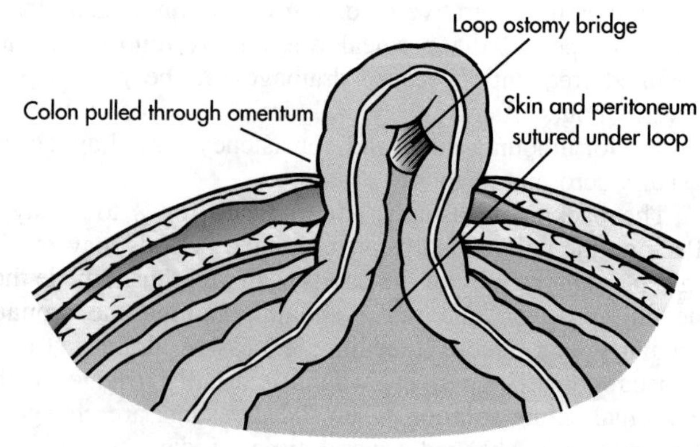

Fig. 40-8 Loop colostomy.

Table 40-30 Comparison of Colostomies and Ileostomy

	Colostomy			
	Ascending	**Transverse**	**Sigmoid**	**Ileostomy**
Stool consistency	Semiliquid	Semiformed	Formed	Liquid to semiliquid
Fluid requirement	Increased	Possibly increased	No change	Increased
Bowel regulation	No	Uncommon	Yes (if there is a history of a regular bowel pattern)	No
Appliance and skin barriers	Yes	Yes	Dependent on regulation	Yes
Irrigation	No	No	Possible every 24-48 hr (if patient meets criteria)	No
Indications for surgery	Perforating diverticulitis in lower colon; trauma; inoperable tumors of colon, rectum, or pelvis; rectovaginal fistula	Same as for ascending; birth defect	Cancer of the rectum or rectosigmoidal area; perforating diverticulum; trauma	Ulcerative colitis, Crohn's disease, diseased or injured colon, birth defect, familial polyposis, trauma, cancer

single stoma. The distal portion of the GI tract is surgically removed, or the distal segment is oversewn and left in the abdominal cavity with its mesentery intact. An end colostomy or ileostomy is then constructed. When the distal bowel is oversewn rather than removed, the procedure is known as a *Hartmann's pouch* (Fig. 40-9). If the distal bowel is removed, the stoma is permanent; if the distal bowel remains intact and oversewn, the potential exists for the bowel to be reanastomosed and the stoma to be closed (referred to as a *takedown*).

Loop stoma. A loop stoma is constructed by bringing a loop of bowel to the abdominal surface and then opening the anterior wall of the bowel to provide fecal diversion. This results in one stoma with a proximal and distal opening and an intact posterior wall that separates the two openings. The loop of bowel is frequently held in place with a plastic rod for 7 to 10 days after surgery to prevent it from slipping back into the abdominal cavity (see Fig. 40-8). A loop stoma is usually temporary.

Double-barrel stoma. When the bowel is divided, both the proximal and distal ends are brought through the abdominal wall as two separate stomas (see Fig. 40-7). The proximal one is the functioning stoma; the distal, nonfunctioning stoma is referred to as the *mucus fistula*. The double-barrel stoma is usually temporary.

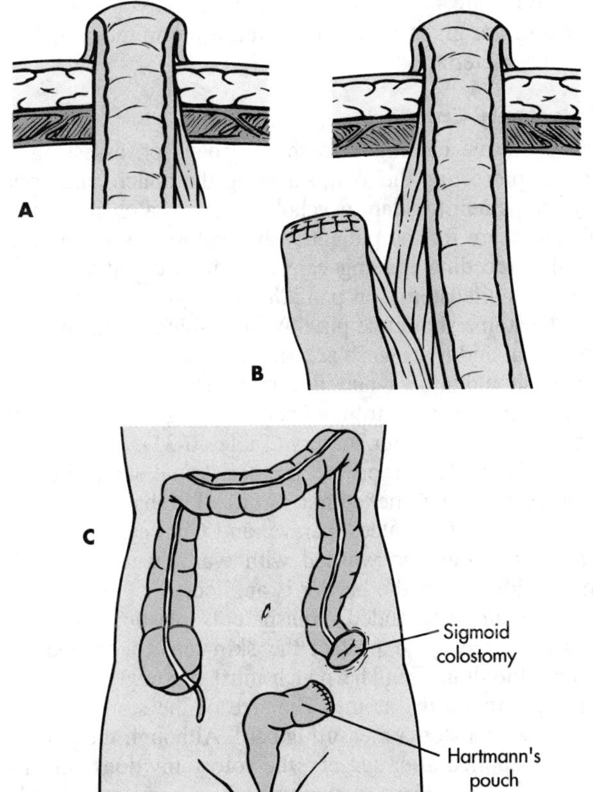

Fig. 40-9 ***A,*** Cross-sectional view of end stoma. ***B,*** Cross-sectional view of end stoma with distal bowel oversewn and secured to anterior peritoneum at stoma site. ***C,*** Sigmoid colostomy. Distal bowel is oversewn and left in place to create Hartmann's pouch.

NURSING MANAGEMENT

STOMA SURGERY

Preoperative Care

It is important to review the information the patient has received from the physician. Psychologic preparation is very important. The family and the patient usually have many questions concerning the procedures. If available, an enterostomal therapy nurse or therapist should visit with the patient and the family. The nurse or enterostomal therapy (ET) nurse must determine the patient's ability to perform self-care, identify support systems, and determine potential adverse factors that could be modified to facilitate learning during rehabilitation. Preoperative assessment must be comprehensive and include physical, psychologic, social, cultural, and educational components. Assessment is ongoing, including both the patient and family. In some institutions the ET nurse marks the stoma site before surgery. An improperly placed stoma complicates rehabilitation by increasing time and expense of pouch change routine. It can also contribute to skin irritation and poor adaptation. The patient and the family should understand the extent of surgery and the type of stoma and its care.

If the patient desires a referral and the physician agrees, a trained ostomy visitor from the United Ostomy Association can provide meaningful psychologic support. The patient has the opportunity to see a person who has adjusted well and who has experienced some of the same feelings and concerns. The family will also benefit from the visit.

Bowel preparation before surgery decreases the chance of a postoperative infection by cleansing the bowel of feces and bacteria. Orally administered osmotic lavages (e.g., Go-Lytely) have shortened the classic 72-hour preparation with clear liquids, cathartics, and enemas. IV and oral antibiotics are given. Nonabsorbable neomycin and erythromycin are given orally to decrease the number of intracolonic bacteria.

Colostomy Care

Postoperative nursing care should focus on assessing the stoma, protecting the skin, selecting the pouch, and assisting the patient to adapt psychologically to a changed body. Nursing care for the patient with a colostomy is presented in the preceding nursing care plan for the patient with a colostomy/ileostomy on p. 1228.

The stoma should be pink. A dusky-blue stoma indicates ischemia, and a brown-black stoma indicates necrosis. The nurse should assess and document stoma color every 8 hours. There is mild to moderate swelling of the stoma the first 2 to 3 weeks after surgery (Table 40-31). A skin barrier should be applied to protect the peristomal suture line and skin surrounding the stoma. Solid skin barriers include Stomahesive (Convatec), karaya, and Comfeel (Coloplast). The skin should be washed with warm water and dried thoroughly before the barrier is applied.

With an open-ended, transparent, plastic, odor-proof pouch it is easy to protect the skin and to observe and collect the drainage. The pouch must fit snugly to prevent leakage around the stoma. The size of the stoma is determined with a stoma measuring card. Although the pouch is usually applied after surgery, the colostomy does not function until 2 to 4 days postoperatively, when peristalsis has been adequately restored. An exception to this is when a temporary colostomy is performed and the stoma is opened in the operating room with no bowel preparation being done previously.

The volume, color, and consistency of the drainage are recorded. Each time the pouch is changed, the condition of the skin is observed for irritation. A pouch should *never* be placed directly on irritated skin without the use of a skin barrier.

Table 40-31 Characteristics of Stoma

Characteristic	Description or Cause
Color*	
Rose to brick red	Viable stoma mucosa
Pale	May indicate anemia
Blanching, dark red to purple	Indicates inadequate blood supply to the stoma or bowel from adhesions, low flow state, or excessive tension on the bowel at the time of construction
Edema†	
Mild to moderate edema	Normal in the initial postoperative period Trauma to the stoma Any medical condition that results in edema
Moderate to severe edema	Obstruction of the stoma Allergic reaction to food Gastroenteritis
Bleeding	
Small amount	Oozing from the stoma mucosa when touched is normal because of its high vascularity
Moderate to large amount‡	Moderate to large amount‡ of bleeding from the stoma mucosa could indicate coagulation factor deficiency; stomal varices secondary to portal hypertension Moderate to large amount from intestinal stoma opening could indicate lower gastrointestinal bleeding

*Sustained color changes must be reported to surgeon.
†Closely observe and report to the surgeon and adjust the stoma opening size in the pouch.
‡Report moderate to large amounts of bleeding to surgeon.

A colostomy in the ascending and transverse colon has semiliquid stools and is more difficult to regulate than a colostomy on the left side of the colon. The patient needs to be instructed to use a drainable pouch. A colostomy in the sigmoid or descending colon has semiformed or formed stools and can sometimes be regulated by the irrigation method. The patient may or may not wear a drainage pouch. A nondrainable pouch should have a gas filter.

For most patients with colostomies, there are few, if any, dietary restrictions. A well-balanced diet and adequate fluid intake is important. The patient's medical and surgical history need to be considered when individualizing dietary

Table 40-32 Effects of Food on Stoma Output

Odor Producing	Diarrhea Causing
Eggs	Alcohol
Garlic	Beer
Onions	Cabbage family
Fish	Spinach
Asparagus	Green beans
Cabbage	Coffee
Broccoli	Spicy foods
Alcohol	Fruits (raw)
Gas Forming	**Potential Obstruction in Ileostomy**
Beans	Nuts
Cabbage family	Raisins
Onions	Popcorn
Beer	Seeds
Carbonated beverages	Chocolate
Cheeses, strong	Vegetables (raw)
Sprouts	Celery
	Corn

instructions. Table 40-32 lists foods and their effects on stoma output.

Colostomy Irrigations

Colostomy irrigations are intended to regulate bowel function, treat constipation, or prepare the bowel for surgery. When irrigating to achieve a regular bowel pattern, the irrigations stimulate the bowel to function at a specific time every day or every other day. If control is achieved, there should be little or no spillage between irrigations. The patient who establishes regularity may need to wear only a pad or cover over the stoma. The patient who cannot or chooses not to establish regularity by irrigations must wear a pouch at all times. The procedure for colostomy irrigation is presented in Table 40-33.

All equipment should be assembled before the irrigation. A commercially obtained irrigation set usually has all the equipment needed. The nurse should encourage the patient to watch the procedure and should explain each step to the patient. The cone tip on the tubing controls the depth of insertion and prevents the water from coming out from the stoma and not going into the colon. If resistance is met, force should not be used because perforation of the intestine can result. However, this is unlikely when using a stoma cone. A hard plastic catheter is not recommended because of the risk of intestinal perforation. The procedure should not be rushed; the patient should feel relaxed. The patient or family member must be instructed in the procedure and must be able to demonstrate the ability to irrigate before being independent. This can be done in the outpatient setting.

The patient should be able to perform skin care, control odor, care for the stoma, and identify signs and symptoms of complications. The patient should know the importance of fluids and food in the diet, have names and addresses of the United Ostomy Association, and know when to seek medical care. Outpatient follow-up by an ET nurse is highly recommended. Patients need to be discharged with written pouch change instructions, teaching literature relevant to the type of stoma they have, a list of equipment they use (including names and phone numbers), a list of equipment retailers, outpatient follow-up appointments with the surgeon and ET nurse, and the phone numbers of the surgeon and nurse.

Table 40-33 Equipment and Procedure for Colostomy Irrigation

Equipment

- Lubricant
- Irrigation set (1000-2000 ml container, tubing with irrigating cone, clamp)
- Irrigating sleeve with adhesive or belt
- Toilet tissue to clean around the stoma
- Disposal sack for soiled dressing

Procedure

1. Place 500-1000 ml of lukewarm water (not to exceed 105° F) [40.5° C] in container. The volume is titrated for the individual; use enough irrigant to distend the bowel but not enough to cause cramping pain. Most adults use 500-1000 ml of water.
2. Ensure comfortable position. Patient may sit in chair in front of toilet.
3. Clear tubing of all air by flushing it with fluid.
4. Hang container on hook or intravenous pole (18-24 in) above stoma (about shoulder height).
5. Apply irrigating sheath and place bottom end in bed pan or toilet bowl.
6. Lubricate cone and insert cone tip gently into the stoma and hold tip securely in place to prevent back flow.
7. Allow irrigation solution to flow in steadily for 5-10 min.
8. If cramping occurs, stop the flow of solution for a few seconds, leaving the cone in place.
9. Clamp the tubing and remove irrigating cone when the desired amount of irrigant has been delivered or when the patient senses colonic distention.
10. Allow 30-45 min for the solution and feces to be expelled. Initial evacuation is usually complete in 10-15 min. Close off the irrigating sheath at the bottom to allow ambulation.
11. Clean, rinse, and dry peristomal skin well.
12. Replace the colostomy drainage pouch or desired stoma covering.
13. Wash and rinse all equipment and hang to dry.

Ileostomy Care

Care of the ileostomy is presented in the preceding nursing care plan for the patient with a colostomy or ileostomy on p. 1228. An ileostomy stoma protrusion of at least 1 to 1.5 cm makes care easier. When the stoma is flat, seepage occurs and the skin becomes denuded. Drainage is constant and extremely irritating to the skin. Regularity cannot be established. A pouch must be worn at all times. An open-ended, drainable pouch is worn by the patient so that drainage can be emptied as needed. The drainable pouch is usually worn for several days before being changed as long as leakage does not occur around the stoma. If pouch leakage occurs, the pouch should be promptly removed and the skin should be cleansed and a new pouch placed. A solid skin barrier should always be used. A transparent pouch should be used in the initial postoperative period to facilitate assessment of stoma viability.

Immediately after surgery, intake and output must be accurately monitored. The patient should be observed for signs and symptoms of fluid and electrolyte imbalance, particularly potassium, sodium, and fluid deficits. In the first 24 to 48 hours after surgery the amount of drainage from the stoma may be negligible. A person with an ileostomy has lost the absorptive functions provided by the colon, as well as the delay feature provided by the ileocecal valve. Once peristalsis returns, the patient may experience a period of high-volume output of 1000 to 1800 ml per day. Later on, the average amount can be 800 ml daily because the proximal small bowel adapts. If the small bowel has been shortened as a result of surgical resections in Crohn's or other disease, the drainage from the ileostomy may be greater. The importance of fluid and electrolyte balance must be understood by the patient.

The patient should be instructed to drink at least 1 to 2 L of fluid daily; more may be necessary when diarrhea occurs and in the summer, when perspiration is increased. Diarrhea from an ileostomy produces acidosis from the loss of bicarbonate. The physician may instruct the patient to take an electrolyte solution at home (e.g., 1 teaspoon of salt and 1 teaspoon of baking soda in 1 quart of water). Fluids rich in electrolytes should be encouraged.

Usually a low-roughage diet is ordered initially. Fiber-containing foods are reintroduced gradually. Later there are no dietary restrictions except for foods that are troublesome (e.g., high-roughage popcorn) for the patient. Return to a normal, presurgical diet is the goal.

The ileal stoma often bleeds easily when it is touched because it has a high vascular supply. The patient should be told that minimal oozing of blood is normal. If the terminal ileum has been removed, the patient may need to return to the clinic for vitamin B_{12} injections every 3 months.

Adaptation to a Stoma

Adaptation to the stoma is a gradual process. The patient experiences a grief reaction to the loss of a body part and an alteration in body image. Each person uses different coping mechanisms. The adjustment period for the person depends on the individual. Psychologic support during the grieving process is needed. There are concerns about body image, sexual activity, family responsibilities, and changes in lifestyle. The patient may become resentful and have fears of odor or soiling. Supportive measures by nurses include helping the patient acquire knowledge, providing or recommending support services, and identifying coping mechanisms that are effective. The nurse provides support by responding to the physiologic needs of stoma care and the psychosocial needs of self-esteem.

RESEARCH
Implications for Nursing Practice

BODY IMAGE IN STOMA PATIENTS

Citation Salter MJ: What are the differences in body image between patients with a conventional stoma compared with those who have had a conventional stoma followed by a continent pouch? *J Adv Nurs* 17:841-848, 1992.

Purpose To attempt to identify if perceived body image problems were decreased in a person with a continent pouch who does not have to wear an external device.

Methods Qualitative study of seven patients. The study explored the perceptions of body image in patients with a conventional stoma compared with those who have had a conventional stoma followed by a continent pouch. A phenomenologic approach, a qualitative research method, was used to obtain information from the patients.

Results and Conclusions The results of this study indicated that patients with a stoma expressed difficulty in coming to terms with a stoma, with perceived negative feelings of their body image. In contrast, patients with a continent pouch were of the opinion that such a procedure enhanced their lives over an ileostomy. However, the majority of the patients with continent pouches still found their experience traumatic.

Implications for Nursing Practice If people are happy with the physical aspects of themselves, they are more likely to experience positive feelings of self-esteem. Part of the rehabilitative process for ulcerative colitis surgery includes encouraging patients to view themselves as normal after surgery. Patients should be encouraged to view the stoma as an inconvenience rather than a handicap. Although the patient needs to come to terms with the loss of a body part, the emphasis needs to be placed on normality.

The patient should not be forced to learn to care for the stoma. The nurse should watch for clues that the patient is ready. Teaching at the appropriate time is an important part of the care and can contribute to a smooth adjustment process.

Activities of daily living are resumed within 6 to 8 weeks. Heavy lifting should be avoided. The patient's physical condition determines when sports may be resumed. Bathing and swimming are not prohibited. Water does not harm the stoma.

Sexual Dysfunction after Stoma Surgery

Discussion of sexuality and sexual function needs to be incorporated in the plan of care. The nurse can help the patient understand that sexual function or sexual activity may be affected, but sexuality does not have to be altered.

Pelvic surgery can disrupt nerve and vascular supply to the genitals. Radiation, chemotherapy, and medications can also alter sexual function. Desire is influenced by hormones and overall physical health of the patient. Certain pain medications and antiemetics can lower the sex drive. Generalized fatigue caused by illness can also influence desire. By communicating this information to patients, they can plan sexual activity around a medication schedule and energy levels. Any pelvic surgery that removes the rectum has the potential of damaging the parasympathetic nerve plexus. Arousal in men depends on the parasympathetic nerves that control blood flow and vascular supply to the pelvis and the pudendal nerves that transmit sensory responses from the genital area. Nerve-sparing surgical techniques are used when possible to preserve sexual function. Radiation therapy to the pelvis can reduce blood vascularity to the pelvis by causing scarring in the small blood vessels. A woman's arousal includes expansion and lubrication of the vagina. Pelvic surgery usually does not affect a woman's arousal unless part or all of the vagina is removed. Radiation therapy can affect the small blood vessels, which reduces available blood supply and can affect vaginal expansion and lubrication.[25]

Muscular contraction and genital pleasure that occur during orgasm are not disrupted by pelvic surgery. If the sympathetic nerves in the presacral area are damaged, the male mechanism of emission can be disrupted. This can occur in an abdominal-perineal resection. Orgasms can occur in both men and women with stoma surgery, although other aspects of the response cycle may be affected.[25]

The psychologic impact of the stoma and how it affects the patient's body image and self-esteem need to be discussed. Emotional factors can contribute to sexual problems. A life-threatening illness can override concerns about sexual function. The nurse can assist a patient to identify ways of coping with depression and anxiety resulting from illness, surgery, or postoperative problems.

The social impact of the stoma is interrelated with the psychological, physical, and sexual aspects. Concerns of people with stomas include the ability to resume sexual activity, altering clothing styles, the effect on daily activities, sleeping while wearing a pouch, passing gas, the presence of odor, cleanliness, and deciding when or if to tell others about the stoma. The fear of rejection from a partner or the fear that others will not find them desirable as a sexual partner can be a concern. The nurse should encourage open communication about feelings and should realize that the patient needs time to adjust to the pouch and to body changes before feeling secure in his or her sexual functioning.

Although pregnancy is possible, a limit to the number of pregnancies may be recommended by the physician on the basis of the patient's physical condition. The person with a stoma who becomes pregnant should have regular medical care.

DIVERTICULOSIS AND DIVERTICULITIS

A diverticulum is a saccular dilatation or outpouching of the mucosa through the circular smooth muscle of the intestinal wall. Clinically, diverticular disease occurs in two forms: diverticulosis and diverticulitis. Multiple noninflamed diverticula are present with diverticulosis. The patient is most often free of symptoms but may have some

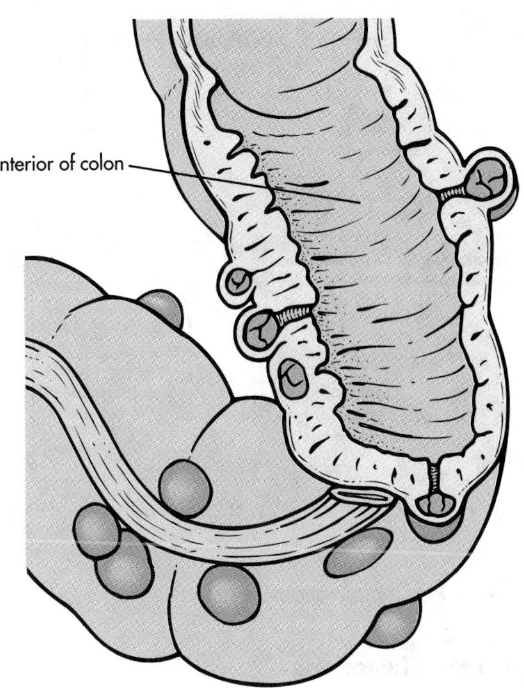

Fig. 40-10 Diverticula are outpouchings of the colon. When they become inflamed, the condition is diverticulitis. The inflammatory process can spread to the surrounding area in the intestine.

abdominal discomfort. In diverticulitis, inflammation of the diverticula occurs (Fig. 40-10). Diverticula may occur at any point within the GI tract but are most commonly found in the sigmoid colon.

Etiology and Pathophysiology

Diverticular disease is a common GI disorder that affects 5% of the population by the age of 40, and 50% are affected by the age of 80.[26] It affects men and women equally, but men seem to have a higher complication rate. Although it affects almost 30 million Americans, most are asymptomatic.

There is no known cause of diverticular disease, but deficiency in dietary fiber has been associated with it. The disease is more prevalent in Western populations that consume diets low in fiber and high in refined carbohydrates, and it is virtually unknown in areas of the world, such as rural Africa, where high-fiber diets are consumed.

When diverticula form, the smooth muscle of the colon wall becomes thickened. Lack of dietary fiber slows transit time and more water is absorbed from the stool, making it more difficult to pass through the lumen. Decreased bulk of the stool, combined with a more narrowed lumen in the sigmoid colon, causes high intraluminal pressures. These factors are believed to contribute to the formation of diverticula.

The cause of diverticulitis is related to the retention of stool and bacteria in the diverticulum, forming a hardened mass called a *fecalith*. This causes inflammation and usually small perforations. Inflammation of the diverticulum spreads to the surrounding area in the intestines (Fig. 40-11), causing the tissue to become edematous. Abscesses may form, or complete perforation with peritonitis may occur.

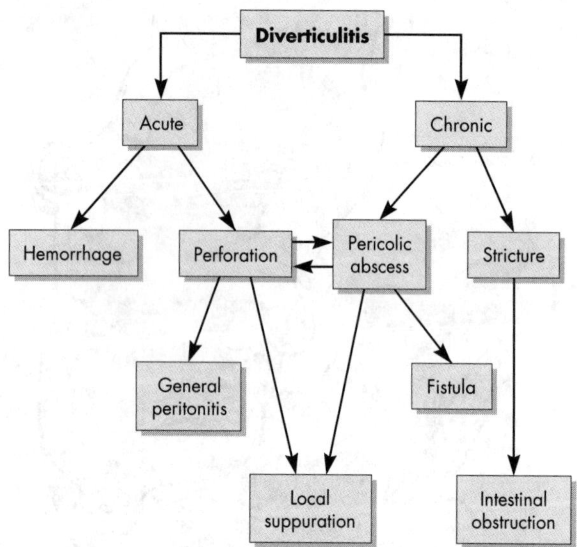

Fig. 40-11 Complications of diverticulitis.

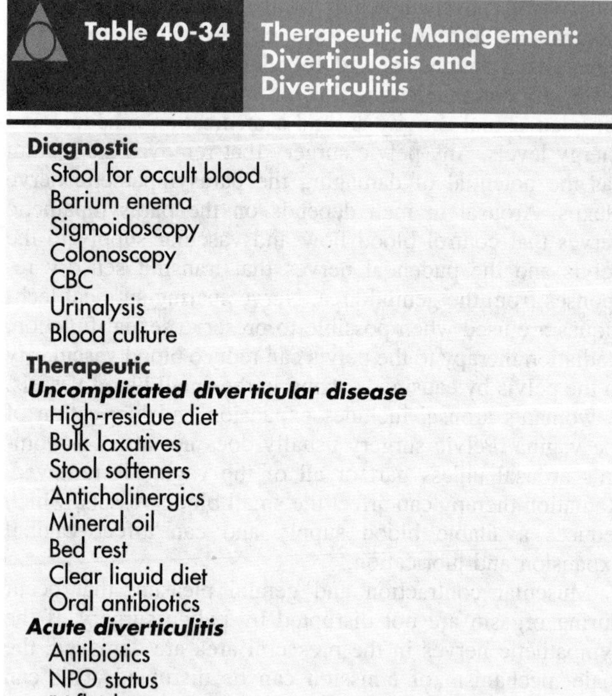

Table 40-34 Therapeutic Management: Diverticulosis and Diverticulitis

Diagnostic
Stool for occult blood
Barium enema
Sigmoidoscopy
Colonoscopy
CBC
Urinalysis
Blood culture
Therapeutic
Uncomplicated diverticular disease
High-residue diet
Bulk laxatives
Stool softeners
Anticholinergics
Mineral oil
Bed rest
Clear liquid diet
Oral antibiotics
Acute diverticulitis
Antibiotics
NPO status
IV fluids
Possible colon resection for obstruction or hemorrhage
Bed rest
NG suction

CBC, Complete blood count; *IV,* intravenous; *NG,* nasogastric; *NPO,* nothing by mouth.

Clinical Manifestations

The majority of patients with diverticulosis have no symptoms. Those with symptoms typically have crampy abdominal pain located in the left lower quadrant that is usually relieved by passage of flatus or bowel movement. Alternating constipation and diarrhea may be present.

Approximately 15% of patients with diverticulosis progress to acute diverticulitis. In patients with diverticulitis, abdominal pain is localized over the involved area of the colon. A tender, left lower quadrant mass may be felt on palpation of the abdomen. Fever, chills, nausea, anorexia, and leukocytosis may be present. Elderly patients with diverticulitis are frequently afebrile, with a normal WBC, and little, if any, abdominal tenderness.[26]

Complications of diverticulitis include perforation with peritonitis, abscess and fistula formation, bowel obstruction, ureteral obstruction, and bleeding. Bleeding is a common complication of diverticulitis and is manifested by *hematochezia* (maroon stools). Bleeding usually stops spontaneously.

Diagnostic Studies

A barium enema is typically used to diagnose diverticular disease. A CBC, urinalysis, and fecal occult blood test should be performed (Table 40-34). A colonoscopy should be performed on patients with symptoms to rule out possible hidden polyps or lesions. A patient with acute diverticulitis should not have a barium enema or colonoscopy because of the possibility of perforation and peritonitis.

Therapeutic Management

Uncomplicated diverticular disease is treated with a high-fiber diet and bulk laxatives, such as psyllium hydrophilic mucilloid (Metamucil). Anticholinergic drugs such as dicyclomine (Bentyl) and Donnatol may be used to relieve discomfort from spasm of the bowel.

In acute diverticulitis, broad-spectrum antibiotic therapy is required. The patient is maintained on bed rest to decrease intestinal motility and is kept on NPO status. The WBC count is monitored. An NG tube may be necessary.

Approximately 30% of patients with acute diverticulitis require surgical intervention.[26] Patients with complicated diverticular disease often require surgery. Surgical intervention is necessary to drain abscesses or to resect an obstructing inflammatory mass. The usual surgical procedures involve resection of the involved colon with a temporary diverting colostomy. The colostomy is reanastomosed after the colon is healed.

NURSING MANAGEMENT

DIVERTICULOSIS AND DIVERTICULITIS

The patient should be provided with a full explanation of the condition. The better the patient understands the disease process and adheres to the prescribed regimen, the less likely the exacerbation of the disease and the onset of complications.

Uncomplicated diverticular disease is primarily treated by a high-fiber diet (see Table 40-9). Fluids should be increased because fibers retain water, thus decreasing the amount absorbed by the body. If the patient is obese, a reduction in weight is needed.

Increased intraabdominal pressure should be avoided because it may precipitate an attack. Factors that increase intraabdominal pressure are straining at stool, vomiting, bending, lifting, and tight, restrictive clothing.

In acute diverticulitis, the goal of treatment is to allow the colon to rest and the inflammation to subside. The patient is kept on NPO status and bed rest and given parenteral fluids. The patient should be observed for signs of possible peritonitis.

When the acute attack subsides, oral fluids progressing to a semisolid diet are allowed. Ambulation is also permitted. At this stage the patient should be observed for a recurrent attack. If the patient has a bowel resection or colostomy, the nursing care is the same as for these procedures.

HERNIAS

A hernia is a protrusion of a viscus through an abnormal opening or a weakened area in the wall of the cavity in which it is normally contained. A hernia may occur in any part of the body, but it usually occurs within the abdominal cavity. If the hernia can be placed back into the abdominal cavity, it is known as *reducible*. The hernia can be reduced by manipulation, or it can occur without manipulation when the person lies down. If the hernia cannot be placed back into the abdominal cavity, it is known as *irreducible,* or *incarcerated.* In this situation the intestinal flow may be obstructed. When the hernia is irreducible and the intestinal flow and blood supply are obstructed, the hernia is *strangulated.* The result is an acute intestinal obstruction.

Types

The *inguinal* hernia is the most common type of hernia and occurs at the point of weakness in the abdominal wall where the spermatic cord in men and the round ligament in women emerge (Fig. 40-12). When the protrusion escapes through the inguinal ring and follows the spermatic cord or the round ligament, it is termed an *indirect* hernia. When it escapes through the posterior inguinal wall, it is a *direct* hernia. An inguinal hernia is more frequent in men.

A *femoral* hernia occurs when there is a protrusion through the femoral ring into the femoral canal. It occurs below the inguinal (Poupart's) ligament as a bulge. It becomes strangulated easily and occurs more frequently in women. The *umbilical* hernia occurs when the rectus muscle is weak or the umbilical opening fails to close after birth. This type is found most commonly in children.

Ventral, or *incisional,* hernia is due to weakness of the abdominal wall at the site of a previous incision. It is found most commonly in patients who are obese, who have had multiple surgical procedures in the same area, and who have had inadequate wound healing because of poor nutrition or infection.

Clinical Manifestations

A hernia commonly occurs over the involved area when the patient stands or strains. There may be some discomfort as a result of tension. Severe pain is caused if the hernia becomes strangulated. In this situation the clinical manifestations of a bowel obstruction, such as vomiting, crampy abdominal pain, and distention, are found.

Therapeutic Management

Diagnosis is based on history and physical examination findings. Surgery is the treatment of choice for hernias to prevent the possible complication of strangulation. An umbilical hernia is not usually repaired surgically because it may reduce itself if left alone until the child gets older. The surgical repair of a hernia is known as a *herniorrhaphy*. The reinforcement of the weakened area with wire, fascia, or mesh is known as a *hernioplasty*. When there is strangulation, necrosis and gangrene may develop if immediate care is not given. A bowel resection of the involved area or a temporary colostomy may be needed to treat a strangulated hernia.

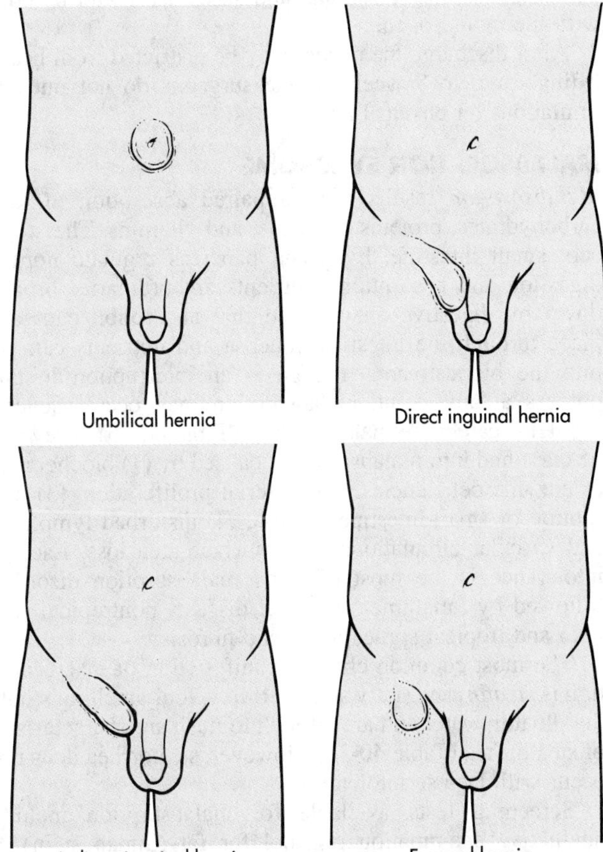

Fig. 40-12 Types of hernias.

NURSING MANAGEMENT

HERNIAS

Some patients with hernias wear a *truss,* a pad placed over the hernia and held in place with a belt. The truss is worn to keep the hernia from protruding. If a patient wears a truss, the nurse should check for skin irritation caused by the continual rubbing of the truss.

After a hernia repair, the patient may have difficulty voiding. Therefore the nurse should observe for a distended bladder. An accurate intake and output record is important. Scrotal edema is a painful complication after an inguinal hernia repair. A scrotal support with application of an ice bag may help relieve pain and edema. Coughing is not encouraged, but deep breathing and turning should be done. If the patient needs to cough or sneeze, the incision should be splinted during coughing, and sneezing should be done with the mouth open.

After discharge the patient may be restricted from heavy lifting for 6 to 8 weeks. Some surgeons do not put any limitations on physical activities.

MALABSORPTION SYNDROME

Malabsorption results from impaired absorption of fats, carbohydrates, proteins, minerals, and vitamins. The stomach, small intestine, liver, and pancreas regulate normal digestion and absorption. Nutrients are ordinarily broken down by digestive enzymes so that absorption can take place through the intestinal mucosa and nutrients can get into the bloodstream. If there is an interruption in this process at any point, malabsorption may occur. Several problems can cause malabsorption (Table 40-35). They can be classified into malabsorptions caused by (1) biochemical or enzyme deficiencies, (2) bacterial proliferation, (3) disruption of small-intestine mucosa, (4) disturbed lymphatic and vascular circulation, or (5) surface area loss. Lactose intolerance is the most common malabsorption disorder, followed by inflammatory bowel disease, nontropical (celiac) and tropical sprue, and cystic fibrosis.

The most common clinical manifestation of malabsorption is *steatorrhea* (fatty stools). Bulky, foul-smelling stools that float in water and are difficult to flush are characteristic of steatorrhea (Table 40-36). However, steatorrhea does not occur with lactose intolerance.

Screening tests available for malabsorption include qualitative examination of stool for fat (Sudan stain), a

Table 40-35 Common Causes of Malabsorption

Biochemical or Enzyme Deficiencies
Lactase deficiency
Biliary tract obstruction
Pancreatic insufficiency
Cystic fibrosis
Chronic pancreatitis
Zollinger-Ellison syndrome
Bacterial Proliferation
Tropical sprue
Parasitic infection
Small Intestinal Mucosal Disruption
Celiac disease
Whipple's disease
Crohn's disease
Disturbed Lymphatic and Vascular Circulation
Lymphoma
Ischemia
Lymphangiectasia
Congestive heart failure
Surface Area Loss
Billroth II gastrectomy
Short-bowel syndrome
Distal ileal resection, disease, or bypass

Table 40-36 Clinical Manifestations of Malabsorption

Manifestations	Pathophysiology
Gastrointestinal	
Weight loss	Malabsorption of fat, carbohydrates, and protein leading to loss of calories; marked reduction in caloric intake or increased use of calories
Diarrhea	Impaired absorption of water, sodium, fatty acids, bile, or carbohydrates
Flatulence	Bacterial fermentation of unabsorbed carbohydrates
Steatorrhea	Undigested and unabsorbed fat
Glossitis, cheilosis, stomatitis	Deficiency of iron, riboflavin, vitamin B_{12}, folic acid, and other vitamins
Hematologic	
Anemia	Impaired absorption of iron, vitamin B_{12}, and folic acid
Hemorrhagic tendency	Vitamin C deficiency Vitamin K deficiency inhibiting production of clotting factors II, VII, IX, and X
Musculoskeletal	
Bone pain	Osteoporosis from impaired calcium absorption Osteomalacia secondary to hypocalcemia, hypophosphatemia, inadequate vitamin D
Tetany	Hypocalcemia, hypomagnesemia
Weakness, muscle cramps	Anemia, electrolyte depletion (especially potassium)
Muscle wasting	Protein malabsorption
Neurologic	
Altered mental status	Dehydration
Paresthesias	Vitamin B_{12} deficiency
Peripheral neuropathy	Vitamin B_{12} deficiency
Night blindness	Thiamine deficiency Vitamin A deficiency
Integumentary	
Bruising	Vitamin K deficiency
Dermatitis	Fatty acid deficiency, zinc deficiency, niacin and other vitamin deficiencies
Brittle nails	Iron deficiency
Hair thinning and loss	Protein deficiency
Cardiovascular	
Hypotension	Dehydration
Tachycardia	Hypovolemia, anemia
Peripheral edema	Protein malabsorption, protein loss in diarrhea

72-hour stool collection for quantitative measurement of fecal fat, and the D-xylose absorption-excretion test, which is a good screening test for carbohydrate absorption (see Table 36-11). Other diagnostic studies include three different kinds of breath test: (1) the bile acid breath test, which is used to evaluate bile-salt malabsorption or malabsorption from bacterial overgrowth; (2) the triolein breath test, which measures carbon dioxide excretion after ingestion of a radioactive triglyceride; and (3) the excretion of breath hydrogen after ingestion of lactose, which is a sensitive, specific, and noninvasive test for detection of lactase deficiency. The rationale for the hydrogen breath test is that bacterial metabolism is the only source of hydrogen production in humans, and most of this occurs in the colon.

A pancreatic secretion test using secretion may be performed to rule out pancreatic insufficiency. Endoscopy may be used to obtain a small bowel biopsy specimen for diagnosis. Radiographic studies of the esophagus, stomach, and small intestine may be indicated. A small-bowel barium enema is frequently performed to identify abnormal mucosal patterns.

Laboratory studies that are frequently ordered include a CBC, determinations of prothrombin time, serum vitamin A and carotene levels, serum electrolytes, cholesterol, and calcium.

Sprue

Two closely related malabsorption conditions are *nontropical sprue* and *tropical sprue*. Tropical and nontropical sprue are found in adults. Nontropical sprue is most commonly referred to as *celiac sprue* (especially in children) but is also called *adult celiac disease* and *gluten-induced enteropathy*.

Etiology. In celiac disease there is marked atrophy and flattening of the villi. As a result, absorption within the small intestine is reduced. The proposed reason for the injury to the villi is a hypersensitivity response initiated by gluten and gliadin (a breakdown product of gluten). Gluten is a protein found in wheat, rye, barley, and oats. The hypersensitivity leads to an inflammatory response of the mucosa.

Tropical sprue is a chronic disorder acquired in endemic tropical areas. The exact cause is unknown, but the disorder has been linked to an infectious agent. Folate deficiency is also believed to play a role in the development of this disease. Clinically, it resembles nontropical sprue.

Clinical Manifestations. A patient may become symptomatic at any age with celiac sprue, but the incidence peaks in childhood when gluten is first introduced and then during the fourth and fifth decades.[27] Symptoms include steatorrhea (bulky, foul-smelling, yellow-gray, greasy stools with putty-like consistency), diarrhea, weight loss, abdominal distention, and excessive flatulence. There may also be signs of multiple vitamin deficiencies (e.g., glossitis, cheilosis).

Diagnostic Studies and Therapeutic Management. Diagnosis of sprue may be made by stool content analyses or intestinal biopsy. Barium enema may demonstrate abnormalities, including obliteration of intestinal folds. Treatment of sprue syndrome is based on the underlying cause. In nontropical sprue, a gluten-free diet usually leads to clinical recovery. Wheat, barley, oats, and rye products should be avoided. Soybean flours may be used. Foods must be scrutinized for the gluten content. Additives such as hydrolyzed vegetable proteins are often derived from cereal grains, including wheat. For those patients who are unresponsive to dietary exclusion therapy (gluten-free diet), corticosteroids may be used to treat nontropical sprue. The basis for this treatment is that the inflammatory response is mediated by an immunologic response.

Tropical sprue is treated with broad-spectrum antibiotics (e.g., tetracycline) in conjunction with folic acid therapy. The patient who responds to this therapy and achieves a remission is usually maintained on folic acid.

Lactase Deficiency

Lactase deficiency is a condition in which the lactase enzyme is deficient or absent. Lactase is the enzyme that breaks down lactose into two simple sugars—glucose and galactose. Although primary lactase deficiency seems to be hereditary, milk intolerance may not become clinically evident until late adolescence or early adulthood. About 5% of the adult population has primary lactase deficiency. The highest incidence is found in African-Americans, Native Americans, Mexican-Americans, and persons of Jewish descent. Acquired lactase deficiency is often seen in other GI diseases in which the mucosa has been damaged, including ulcerative colitis, Crohn's disease, gastroenteritis, and sprue syndrome.

Clinical Manifestations. The symptoms of lactose intolerance include bloating, flatulence, crampy abdominal pain, and diarrhea. They may occur within one half hour to several hours after drinking a glass of milk or ingesting a milk product. The diarrhea of lactose intolerance results from fluid secretion into the small intestines, responding to the osmotic action of undigested lactose.

THERAPEUTIC AND NURSING MANAGEMENT

LACTASE DEFICIENCY

Many lactose-intolerant persons are aware of their milk intolerance and avoid milk. A lactose intolerance test can be performed to rule out milk allergies. The patient is given 50 g of lactose orally. Blood samples are drawn before the consumption of lactose and at 15-, 30-, 60-, and 90-minute intervals. Failure of the blood glucose level to increase more than 20 mg/dl is suggestive of lactase deficiency. Results of the hydrogen breath test after ingestion of lactose are abnormal.

Treatment consists of eliminating lactose from the diet by avoiding milk and milk products. A lactose-free diet is given initially and is gradually advanced to a low-lactose diet as tolerated by the patient. The objective of care is to teach the importance of adherence to the diet. Many lactose-intolerant persons may not exhibit symptoms if lactose is taken in small amounts. In some persons, lactose may be tolerated better if taken with meals.

The patient needs to be aware that milk, ice cream, cottage cheese, and cheese have a high lactose content. If

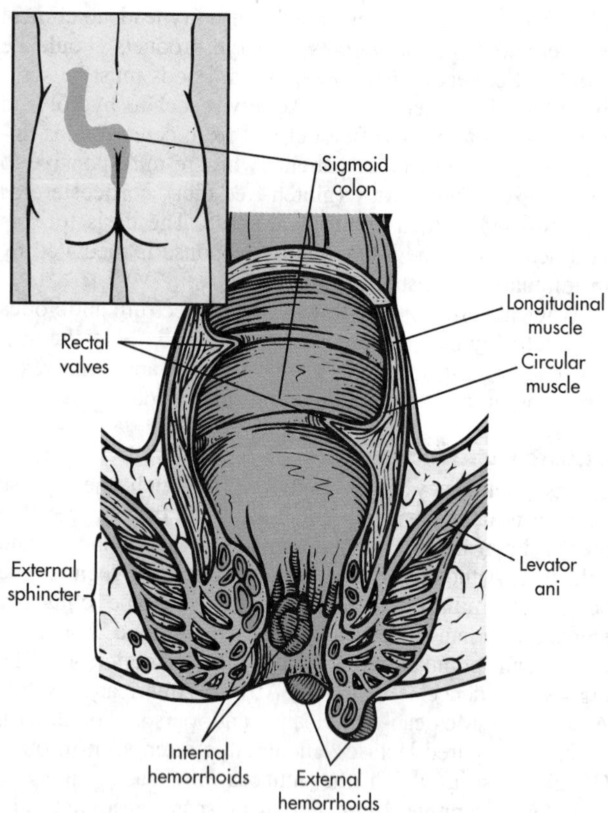

Fig. 40-13 Anatomic structures of the rectum and anus with external and internal hemorrhoids.

the milk has been fermented (e.g., cultured buttermilk, yogurt, sour cream), the patient with low lactase levels may tolerate it better.

Lactase enzyme (Lactaid) is available commercially as an over-the-counter product. It is mixed with milk and breaks down the lactose before the milk is ingested.

ANORECTAL PROBLEMS

Hemorrhoids

Hemorrhoids are dilated hemorrhoidal veins. They may be *internal* (occurring above the internal sphincter) or *external* (occurring outside the external sphincter) (Fig. 40-13). Symptoms of hemorrhoids, including bleeding, pruritis, prolapse, and pain, are common in all age groups. In affected persons, hemorrhoids appear periodically, depending on amount of anorectal pressure.

Pathophysiology. Hemorrhoids develop when the flow of blood through the veins of the hemorrhoidal plexus is impaired. Internal hemorrhoids may become constricted and painful. They are the most common cause of bleeding with defecation. The amount of blood lost at one time may be small but may lead to iron deficiency anemia over time. External hemorrhoids are reddish blue and seldom bleed or cause pain unless a vein ruptures. If the blood clots in external hemorrhoids, they become inflamed, painful, and are said to be *thrombosed.*

Hemorrhoids may be caused by many factors, including pregnancy, prolonged constipation, straining in an effort to defecate, heavy lifting, prolonged standing and sitting, and portal hypertension (as found in cirrhosis).

Therapeutic Management. Hemorrhoids are diagnosed by inspection, digital examination, proctoscopy, or examination with the flexible sigmoidoscope. Therapy should be directed toward the causes and the patient's symptoms. A high-fiber diet and increased fluid intake will prevent constipation and reduce straining, which allows engorgement of the veins to subside. Ointments such as Nupercaine, creams, suppositories, and impregnated pads that contain anti-inflammatory agents (e.g., hydrocortisone) or astringents and anesthetics (e.g., witch hazel, pramoxine, benzocaine) may be used to shrink the mucous membranes and relieve discomfort. Stool softeners may be ordered to keep the stools soft, and sitz baths may be ordered to relieve pain.

Application of ice packs for a few hours, followed by warm packs, may be used for thrombosed hemorrhoids. Another conservative treatment involves use of a sclerosing solution, such as 5% phenol in oil, or a combined solution of quinine and urea may be injected into the submucous tissue surrounding the hemorrhoids, causing a fibrosing and shrinking of the supporting tissues.

Internal hemorrhoids may be ligated with a rubber band. The constrictive effect impairs circulation, and the tissue becomes necrotic, separates, and sloughs off. There is some local discomfort with this procedure, but no anesthetic is required. Aspirin or propoxyphene (Darvon) is usually given for discomfort. Anal dilatation and lateral sphincterotomy may be performed to reduce vascular engorgement by reducing sphincter pressure. Other methods, such as infrared photocoagulation, bipolar diathermy, and cryotherapy, are used to treat the mucosa.

A *hemorrhoidectomy* is the surgical excision of hemorrhoids. Surgery is indicated when there is prolapse, excessive pain or bleeding, or large hemorrhoids. In general, hemorrhoidectomy is reserved for patients with severe symptoms related to multiple thrombosed hemorrhoids or marked protrusion. Surgical removal may be done by cautery, clamp, or excision. One surgical approach is to leave the area open so that healing takes place by secondary intention. In another approach the hemorrhoids are removed, the tissue is sutured, and healing takes place by primary-intention wound healing.

NURSING MANAGEMENT

HEMORRHOIDS

Conservative nursing management for the patient with hemorrhoids includes teaching measures to prevent constipation, avoidance of prolonged standing or sitting, proper use of over-the-counter medications available for hemorrhoidal symptoms, and the need to seek medical care for severe symptoms of hemorrhoids (e.g., excessive pain and bleeding, prolapsed hemorrhoids) when necessary.

Pain is a common problem after a hemorrhoidectomy. The nurse must be aware that although the procedure is minor the pain is severe, and narcotics are usually given initially.

Sitz baths are started 1 to 2 days after surgery. A warm sitz bath provides comfort and keeps the anal area clean. A sponge ring in the sitz bath helps relieve pressure on the area. Initially the patient should not be left alone because of the possibility of weakness or fainting.

Packing may be inserted into the rectum to absorb drainage. A T-binder may hold the dressing in place. If packing is inserted, it usually is removed the first or second postoperative day. The nurse should assess for rectal bleeding. The patient may be embarrassed when the dressing is changed, and privacy should be provided. The patient usually dreads the first bowel movement and often resists the urge to defecate. Pain medication may be given before the bowel movement to reduce discomfort.

A stool softener such as docusate (Colace) is usually ordered the first few postoperative days. If the patient does not have a bowel movement within 2 to 3 days, an oil retention enema is given.

Discharge teaching includes the importance of the diet, care of the anal area, symptoms of complications (especially bleeding), and avoidance of constipation and straining. Sitz baths are recommended for 1 to 2 weeks. The physician may order a stool softener to be taken for a time. Hemorrhoids may recur. Occasionally anal strictures develop and dilatation is necessary. Regular checkups are important in the prevention of any further problems.

Anal Fissure

An *anal fissure* (*fissura in ano*) is a skin ulcer or a crack in the lining of the anal wall that is caused by trauma or local infection. It is frequently associated with constipation and subsequent stretching of the anus from hard feces. The most common clinical manifestations are painful spasms of the anal sphincter and severe, burning pain during defecation. Some bleeding may occur, and constipation results because of fear of pain associated with bowel movements.

Conservative treatment consists of bowel regulation with mineral oil and stool softeners. Sitz baths and anal anesthetic suppositories (Anusol) are also ordered. Surgical treatment usually consists of excision of the fissure. Postoperative nursing care is the same as the care for the patient who has had a hemorrhoidectomy.

Anorectal Abscess

Anorectal abscesses are defined as undrained collections of perianal pus (Fig. 40-14). They are due to perirectal infections in patients who have compromised local circulation or active inflammatory disease. The most common causative organisms are *Escherichia coli*, staphylococci, and streptococci. Clinical manifestations include local pain and swelling, foul-smelling drainage, tenderness, and elevated temperature. Sepsis can occur as a complication.

Surgical treatment consists of drainage of abscesses. If packing is used, it should be impregnated with petroleum jelly and the area should be allowed to heal by granulation. The packing is changed every day, and moist, hot compresses are applied to the area. Care must be taken to avoid soiling the dressing during urination or defecation. A low-residue diet is given. The patient may leave the hospital with the area open. Discharge teaching should include wound care, the importance of sitz baths, thorough cleaning after bowel movements, and follow-up visits to the physician.

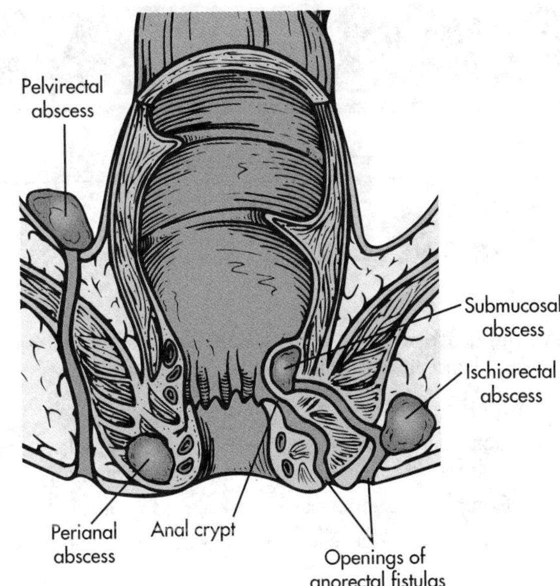

Fig. 40-14 Common sites of anorectal abscesses and fistula formation.

Anorectal Fistula

An anal fistula is an abnormal tunnel leading out from the anus or rectum. It may extend to the outside of the skin, vagina, or buttocks. Anorectal fistulas are a complication of Crohn's disease. This condition often precedes an anorectal abscess.

Feces may enter the fistula and cause an infection. There may be persistent, blood-stained, purulent discharge or stool leakage from the fistula. The patient may have to wear a pad to prevent staining of clothes.

Surgical treatment involves a fistulotomy or a fistulectomy. In a fistulotomy the fistula is opened and healthy tissue is allowed to granulate. A fistulectomy is an excision of the entire fistulous tract. Gauze packing is inserted and the wound is allowed to heal by granulation. Care is the same as after a hemorrhoidectomy.

Pilonidal Sinus

A *pilonidal sinus* is a small tract under the skin between the buttocks in the sacrococcygeal area. It is thought to be of congenital origin. It may have several openings and is lined with epithelium and hair, thus the name pilonidal ("a nest of hair").

The skin is moist, and movement of the buttocks causes the short, wiry hair to penetrate the skin. The irritated skin becomes infected and forms a pilonidal cyst or abscess. There are no symptoms unless there is an infection. If it becomes infected, the patient complains of pain and swelling at the base of the spine.

The formed abscess requires incision and drainage. The wound may be closed or left open to heal by secondary intention. The wound is packed and sitz baths are ordered.

Nursing care includes hot, moist heat applications when an abscess is present. The patient is usually more comfortable lying on the abdomen or side. The patient should be instructed to avoid contaminating the dressing when urinating or defecating and to avoid straining whenever possible.

CRITICAL THINKING EXERCISES

CASE STUDY

ULCERATIVE COLITIS

Patient Profile

Marie, a 37-year-old woman, is admitted for the fifth time in an 11-month period with acute ulcerative colitis.

Subjective Data

- Complains of severe diarrhea (10 to 15 stools a day with blood and mucus) and intestinal cramping
- Complains of anorexia, nausea, and vomiting
- States she takes sulfasalazine (Azulfidine) and prednisone
- Has not taken any medication in past 72 hours because of nausea and vomiting

Objective Data

Physical Examination

- Temperature of 100.4° F (38° C)
- Is crying
- Palpation over the colon reveals abdominal tenderness

Laboratory Tests

- Hct 26%; Hb 9 g/dl (90 g/L); serum albumin 2.3 g/dl (23 g/L).

Critical Thinking Questions

1. Explain the pathophysiologic changes that occur in ulcerative colitis.
2. How does ulcerative colitis differ from Crohn's disease?
3. Explain the reason for Marie's anemia and low serum albumin.
4. What would a proctosigmoidoscopic examination reveal during the acute phase?
5. What are effective nursing interventions for Marie at this stage of her illness?
6. What are the complications of ulcerative colitis and the role of the nurse in preventing their occurrence?
7. Based on the assessment data presented, write one or more nursing diagnosis. Are there any collaborative problems?

NURSING RESEARCH ISSUES

1. What are the primary problems related to sexuality and sexual function in patients with colostomies and ileostomies?
2. What can a nurse do to help improve the self-image of patients with ostomies?
3. What is the quality of life for a patient after a continent ileostomy?
4. Do psychosocial factors have a significant role in the exacerbation of inflammatory bowel disease?
5. Do relaxation therapy strategies decrease the symptoms for a patient with irritable bowel syndrome?
6. What are the barriers to health care for a patient experiencing chronic problems with fecal incontinence or constipation?

REVIEW QUESTIONS

The number of the question corresponds to the same-numbered objective at the beginning of the chapter.

1. Common treatment measures for the patient with constipation are
   a. low-residue diet and anticholinergic drugs.
   b. stool softeners and high-residue diet.
   c. antiemetics and low-fiber diet.
   d. enemas and high fluid intake.

2. During the first 12 hours after an exploratory laparotomy for manifestations of an acute abdomen, drainage from the nasogastric tube is likely to be
   a. bright red with blood clots.
   b. clear gastric secretion.
   c. dark brown to dark red.
   d. yellowish in color.

3. Which of the following is not a common clinical manifestation of acute appendicitis?
   a. Prolonged diarrhea
   b. WBC of 18,000/μl (18×10^9/L)
   c. Nausea and vomiting
   d. Constipation

4. For which of the following should the physician be notified with regard to potential ruptured appendix?
   a. Nausea and vomiting
   b. Tenderness in the right lower quadrant
   c. Sudden, sharp pain in the right lower quadrant
   d. Elevated temperature of 100° F (37.8° C)

5. Common clinical manifestations of gastroenteritis are
   a. abdominal cramps, nausea, and vomiting.
   b. fever, diarrhea, and leukopenia.
   c. anorexia, pain, and constipation.
   d. vomiting, fever, and constipation.

6. Which of the following statements regarding a comparison between ulcerative colitis and Crohn's disease is accurate?

a. Crohn's disease is more likely to be treated with a colectomy.
b. Ulcerative colitis is characterized by skip lesions.
c. Crohn's disease is more likely than ulcerative colitis to result in cancer.
d. Both diseases are characterized by remissions and exacerbations.

7. Intestinal obstruction can occur due to

a. adhesions and paralytic ileus.
b. intussusception and dehydration.
c. volvulus and varices.
d. atresias and telangiectasia.

8. In carcinoma of the large intestine there is a higher incidence of bowel obstruction in the

a. ascending colon because of its narrow lumen.
b. transverse colon because of its semisolid content.
c. ileocecal valve because of the semiliquid content.
d. sigmoid region because of the narrow lumen and fecal consistency.

9. Physiologic changes occurring after an ileostomy necessitate

a. stoma irrigations.
b. skin care around the stoma.
c. avoidance of low-residue diets.
d. the need to wear a belted appliance.

10. Bowel preparation for a colostomy with nonabsorbable antibiotics is done primarily to

a. reduce the bacterial flora in the colon.
b. prevent diarrhea.
c. prevent constipation.
d. prevent additional formation of ammonia.

11. During a colostomy irrigation the patient may experience cramping. If this occurs, the nurse should

a. slow the flow by lowering the container.
b. discontinue the irrigation at once.
c. reduce the temperature of the irrigation solution.
d. insert the catheter about 1 inch farther

12. In contrast to diverticulitis, the patient with diverticulosis

a. often has no symptoms.
b. has rectal bleeding.
c. has localized crampy pain.
d. has abscesses.

13. Hernias are commonly found in any of the following sites *except*

a. epigastrium.
b. inguinal ring.
c. umbilicus.
d. femoral ring.

14. In nontropical sprue the patient's diet must be a

a. gluten-free, high-protein, high-caloric diet.
b. gluten-free, low-fat, low-protein diet.
c. milk-free, high-protein, high-caloric diet.
d. low-caloric, low-protein, high-fat diet.

15. Hemorrhoids are characterized by all of the following *except*

a. tendency toward constipation.
b. internal or external.
c. bleeding after bowel movement.
d. dilatation of the rectal arteries.

REFERENCES

1. Handerhan B: Complications: pseudomembranous enterocolitis, *Nursing* 23:6, 1993.
2. Whitehead WE: Biofeedback treatment of gastrointestinal disorders, *Biofeedback Self Regul* 17:59, 1992.
3. Bassotti G, Whitehead WE: Biofeedback as a treatment approach to gastrointestinal tract disorders, *Am J Gastroenterol* 89:158, 1994.
4. Tremaine WJ: Chronic constipation: causes and management, *Hosp Pract* 25:89, 1990.
5. Jess LW: Acute abdominal pain, *Nursing* 23:34, 1993.
6. Tang CK: Disorders of the vermiform appendix. In Ming S, Goldman H, editors: *Pathology of the gastrointestinal tract,* Philadelphia, 1992, Saunders.
7. Drossman DA and others: US householder survey of functional gastrointestinal disorders: prevalence, sociodemography, and health impact, *Dig Dis Sci* 38:1569, 1993.
8. Toyoda H and others: Distinct associations of HLA class II genes with inflammatory bowel disease, *Gastroenterology* 104:741, 1993.
9. Lashner BA: Inflammatory bowel disease: family patterns and risks, *Compr Ther* 18:2, 1992.
10. Carpani de Kaski M, Hodgson HJ: Rolling review: inflammatory bowel disease, *Aliment Pharmacol Ther* 7:567, 1993.
11. Doughty DB, Broadwell-Jackson D: *Gastrointestinal disorders,* St Louis, 1993, Mosby.
12. Goldman H: Ulcerative colitis and Crohn's disease. In Ming S, Goldman H, editors: *Pathology of the gastrointestinal tract,* Philadelphia, 1992, Saunders.
13. Hanauer SB, D'Haens G: Pharmacotherapy of inflammatory bowel diseases. In Lewis J, editor: *A pharmacologic approach to gastrointestinal disorders,* Baltimore, 1994, Williams & Wilkins.
14. Greenfield SM and others: Review article: the mode of action of the aminosalicylates in inflammatory bowel disease, *Aliment Pharmacol Ther* 7:369, 1993.
15. Doughty DB: What you need to know about inflammatory bowel disease, *Am J Nurs* 94:24, 1994.
16. Goldman H: Systemic and miscellaneous disorders. In Ming S, Goldman H, editors: *Pathology of the gastrointestinal tract,* Philadelphia, 1992, Saunders.
17. McConnell E: Loosening the grip of intestinal obstructions, *Nursing* 24:39, 1994.
18. Brolin R, Crosna M: Mast B: Use of tubes and radiographs in the management of small bowel obstruction, *Ann Surg* 206:126, 1987.
19. Bond J: Managing colon polyps, *Hosp Pract* 28:149, 1993.
20. Bleiberg H: Natural history of the colorectal cancer, *Bull Cancer (Paris)* 80:1051, 1993.
21. American Cancer Society: *Cancer facts and figures—1994,* Altlanta, 1994, American Cancer Society.
22. Witt ME: Current management of adults with colorectal cancer, *Med Surg Nurs* 2:105, 1993.
23. Ransohoff DF: The case for colorectal cancer screening, *Hosp Pract* 29:25, 1994.
24. Ransohoff DF, Lang CA: Screening for colorectal cancer, *N Engl J Med* 325:37, 1992.
25. Smith D: Psychosocial adaptation. In Hampton BG, Bryant RA, editors: *Ostomies and continent diversions,* St Louis, 1992, Mosby.
26. Van Ness M, Peller C: Acute diverticulitis: diagnosis and management, *Hosp Pract* 26:83, 1991.
27. Trier JS: Diagnosis and treatment of celiac sprue, *Hosp Pract* 28:41, 1993.

Chapter 41

NURSING ROLE IN MANAGEMENT

Problems of the Liver, Biliary Tract, and Pancreas

Rachel Elrod

Learning Objectives

1. Define jaundice and describe signs and symptoms that may occur with the different types of jaundice.
2. Differentiate among the types of viral hepatitis, including etiology, pathophysiology, clinical manifestations, complications, and therapeutic management.
3. Describe the nursing management of the patient with viral hepatitis.
4. Explain the etiology, pathogenesis, clinical manifestations, complications, and therapeutic and surgical management of cirrhosis of the liver.
5. Describe the nursing management of the patient with cirrhosis.
6. Describe the clinical manifestations and management of carcinoma of the liver.
7. Describe the pathophysiology, clinical manifestations, complications, and therapeutic and surgical management of acute and chronic pancreatitis.
8. Describe the nursing management of the patient with pancreatitis.
9. Explain the clinical manifestations and management of carcinoma of the pancreas.
10. Explain the pathophysiology, clinical manifestations, complications, and therapeutic and surgical management of gallbladder disorders.
11. Describe the nursing management of the patient undergoing therapeutic or surgical treatment of cholecystitis and cholelithiasis.

JAUNDICE

Jaundice, a yellowish discoloration of body tissues, results from an alteration in normal bilirubin metabolism or flow of bile into the hepatic or biliary duct systems. It is a symptom rather than a disease. Jaundice results when the concentration of bilirubin in the blood becomes abnormally increased. The bilirubin level has to be approximately three times normal levels (total serum bilirubin is normally 2 to 3 mg/dl [34 to 51 μmol/L]) for jaundice to occur. Jaundice can usually first be detected in the sclera and skin (Fig. 41-1).

Most of the body's bilirubin is formed from the breakdown of hemoglobin (from erythrocytes) by macrophages (see Fig. 36-6). This unconjugated (indirect) bilirubin is released into the circulation and is not water soluble, so it is bound to albumin. Because unconjugated bilirubin is not water soluble and cannot be filtered in the kidneys, it is not excreted in the urine. In the liver the unconjugated bilirubin is conjugated with glucuronic acid to form conjugated (direct) bilirubin, which is water soluble. Conjugated bilirubin is secreted into bile, which flows through the hepatic and biliary duct system into the small intestine. In the large intestine, bilirubin is converted to stercobilinogen and urobilinogen by bacterial action. Stercobilinogen gives the characteristic brown color to feces. Some urobilinogen is reabsorbed into the portal circulation and returned to the liver. Normally a very small amount of urobilinogen is excreted in urine.

The three types of jaundice are classified as hemolytic, hepatocellular, and obstructive.

Hemolytic Jaundice

Hemolytic (prehepatic) *jaundice* is due to an increased breakdown of red blood cells (RBCs), which produces an increased amount of unconjugated bilirubin in the blood. The liver is unable to handle this increased load. Causes of hemolytic jaundice include blood transfusion reactions, sickle cell crisis, and hemolytic anemia.

Hepatocellular Jaundice

Hepatocellular (hepatic) *jaundice* results from the liver's altered ability to take up bilirubin from the blood or to conjugate or excrete it. Both unconjugated and conjugated

Reviewed by Deborah L. Martin, RN, MN, Chief Executive Officer, Infection Control and Prevention Analysis, Inc., Austin, TX.

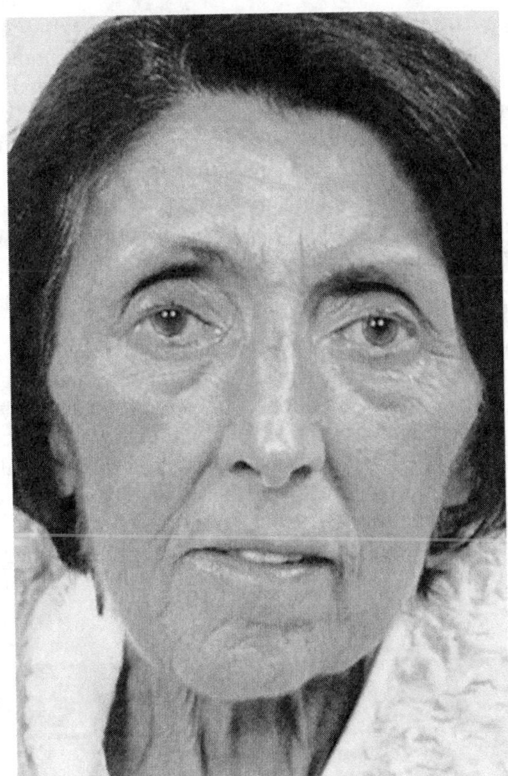

Fig. 41-1 Severe jaundice.

bilirubin serum levels increase. Because conjugated bilirubin is water soluble, it is excreted in the urine. The most common causes of hepatocellular jaundice are hepatitis, cirrhosis, and hepatic carcinoma.

Obstructive Jaundice

Obstructive (posthepatic) *jaundice* is due to impeded or obstructed flow of bile through the liver or biliary duct system. The obstruction may be intrahepatic or extrahepatic. Intrahepatic obstructions are due to swelling or fibrosis of the liver's canaliculi and bile ducts. This can be caused by damage from liver tumors, hepatitis, or cirrhosis. Causes of extrahepatic obstruction include common bile duct obstruction from a stone, sclerosing cholangitis, and carcinoma of the head of the pancreas. Laboratory findings show an elevation of both unconjugated and conjugated bilirubin and urine bilirubin. Because bilirubin does not enter the intestines, there is decreased to no fecal or urinary urobilinogen and stercobilinogen. With complete obstruction, the stools are clay colored.

VIRAL HEPATITIS

Hepatitis is an inflammation of the liver. *Acute viral hepatitis* is the most common cause of hepatitis. The types of infectious viral hepatitis are A, B, C (formerly called posttransfusion non-A, non-B), D, and E. Noninfectious hepatitis may also be caused by drugs and other chemicals (see Table 36-6). Rarely, hepatitis is caused by bacteria, such as streptococci, salmonellae, and *Escherichia coli*.

CULTURAL & ETHNIC Considerations

DISORDERS OF THE LIVER, PANCREAS, AND GALLBLADDER

- Mortality from cirrhosis occurs more frequently among African-Americans than in other ethnic groups.
- Primary hepatic cancer has a higher incidence among African-Americans, Asian-Americans, and Eskimos than Caucasians.
- Pancreatic cancer occurs more frequently among African-Americans and Asian-Americans than Caucasians.
- Caucasians and Native Americans have a higher incidence of gallbladder disease than African-Americans or Asian-Americans.

In the United States, approximately 45,000 to 60,000 cases of all types of viral hepatitis are reported annually.[1] Hepatitis A occurs worldwide. It is nearly universal during childhood in developing countries. Approximately 25,000 cases of hepatitis A occur annually in the United States.[1] By adulthood up to 50% of individuals in the United States have been infected with the hepatitis A virus. Although the reported incidence of acute hepatitis B increased by 37% from 1979 to 1989, the reported numbers of cases declined from 1990 to 1992. In 1992 16,126 new cases of hepatitis B were reported in the United States. About 5000 new cases of hepatitis C were reported in 1993.[1] Active cases of hepatitis A, B, and C are typically underreported. In addition, many cases are asymptomatic and therefore never diagnosed.

Etiology

Viral hepatitis can be caused by one of five viruses: A, B, C, D, and E.[2] Other viruses known to damage the liver include cytomegalovirus, Epstein-Barr virus, herpes virus, coxsackievirus, and rubella virus.

The only definitive way to distinguish the various forms of viral hepatitis is by the presence of the antigens and antigenic subtypes and the subsequent development of antibodies to them. Outbreaks of hepatitis are consistently caused by hepatitis A virus; 20% to 60% of episodic or sporadic hepatitis is caused by hepatitis B virus or C virus.[3] Infection with each virus provides immunity to that virus (homologous immunity). However, the patient can still develop another type of viral hepatitis. Characteristics of hepatitis viruses are summarized in Table 41-1.

Hepatitis A Virus. The hepatitis A virus (HAV) is an RNA virus that is transmitted through the fecal-oral route. It frequently occurs in small outbreaks caused by fecal contamination of food or drinking water. The incubation period is 15 to 50 days. It is found in feces 2 or more weeks before the onset of symptoms and up to 1 week after the onset of jaundice (Fig. 41-2). It is present in the blood only briefly. Anti-HAV (antibody to hepatitis A virus) IgM appears in the serum as the stool becomes negative for the virus. The finding of anti-HAV IgG in the serum indicates that the patient has had a prior sensitization to hepatitis A virus, and the presence of this antibody provides lifelong immunity.

Hepatitis B Virus. Hepatitis B virus (HBV) is a DNA virus that is transmitted by percutaneous (e.g., IV drug use, accidental needle stick punctures) or permucosal exposure to infectious blood, blood products, or other body fluids (semen, vaginal secretions, saliva). Perinatal transmission is also possible. HBV is a complex structure with three distinct antigens: the surface antigen (HBsAg), the core antigen (HBcAg), and the e-antigen (HBeAg).

Each antigen has a corresponding antibody that may be elicited during an attack of acute viral hepatitis. These antibodies can be detected in the serum of persons with prior exposure to the antigenic virus (Fig. 41-3). The presence of anti-HBs indicates immunity to hepatitis B. The persistence of HBsAg in the serum for 6-12 months or longer indicates a carrier state of hepatitis B.

Hepatitis C Virus. Hepatitis C virus (HCV) is an RNA virus that is primarily transmitted percutaneously. Other routes of transmission are sexual or perinatal. Forty percent of cases have no known source.[4] HCV was formerly one type of hepatitis non-A, non-B. In the United States and Canada hepatitis B and C occur most frequently in drug abusers, patients in chronic care institutions, health care workers, hemodialysis patients, and transplant recipients.[5]

Hepatitis D Virus. Hepatitis D virus (HDV), also called delta virus, is a defective RNA virus that cannot survive on its own. The importance of HDV relates to its clinical virulence. It can transform asymptomatic or mild chronic hepatitis B infection to severe, progressive chronic active hepatitis and cirrhosis and can accelerate the course of chronic active hepatitis B. Delta virus is also a contributing factor in a substantial number of cases of fulminant hepatitis B. Delta hepatitis can occur as a primary infection along with HBV (coinfection) or in a

Table 41-1 Characteristics of Hepatitis Viruses

	Incubation Period	Mode of Transmission	Sources of Infection and Spread of Disease	Infectivity
Hepatitis A (HAV)	15-50 days (average 28)	Fecal-oral (fecal contamination and oral ingestion)	Crowded conditions; poor personal hygiene; poor sanitation; contaminated food, milk, water, and shellfish; persons with subclinical infections; infected food handlers; sexual contact	Most infectious during 2 wk before onset of symptoms; infectious until 1-2 wk after symptoms start
Hepatitis B (HBV)	45-180 days (average 60-90)	Percutaneous (parenteral)/permucosal exposure to blood or blood products Sexual contact Perinatal contact	Contaminated needles, syringes, and blood products; sexual activity with infected partners; asymptomatic carriers	Before and after symptoms appear; infectious for 4-6 mo; in carriers continues for patient's lifetime
Hepatitis C (HCV)	14-180 days (average 56)	Percutaneous (parenteral)/permucosal exposure to blood or blood products	Blood and blood products, needles and syringes, sexual activity with infected partners	1-2 wk before symptoms; continues during clinical course; indefinitely with carriers
Hepatitis D (HDV)	Not firmly established HBV must precede HDV; chronic carriers of HBV are always at risk	Can cause infection only together with HBV; routes of transmission same as for HBV	Same as HBV	Blood is infectious at all stages of HDV infection
Hepatitis E (HEV)	15-64 days (average 26-42 days in different epidemics)	Fecal-oral	Contaminated water; poor sanitation; found in Asia, Africa, and Mexico; not common in the United States and Canada	Not known; may be similar to HAV

carrier of hepatitis B (superinfection). HDV is transmitted percutaneously.

Hepatitis E Virus. Hepatitis E virus (HEV) is an RNA virus that is transmitted by the fecal-oral route. Hepatitis E is also called enteric non-A, non-B hepatitis. Hepatitis E occurs primarily in developing countries. There have been reported epidemics in India, Asia, Mexico, and Africa. There are currently no serologic tests available for hepatitis E so its diagnosis is one of exclusion.

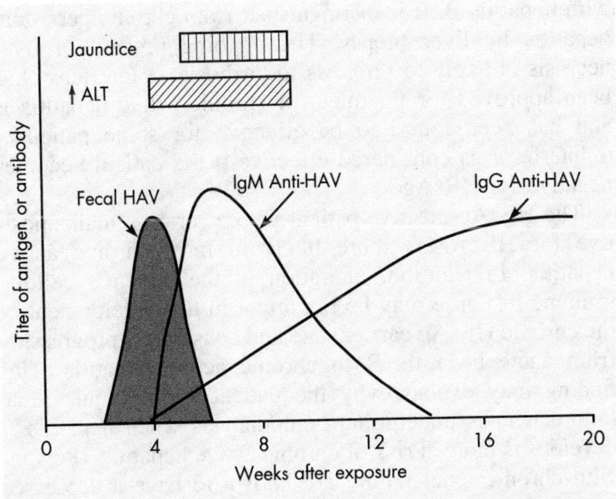

Fig. 41-2 Clinical and serologic events of a typical patient infected with hepatitis A virus (HAV). Elevated alanine aminotransferase (ALT) levels are present by 4 weeks and jaundice appears by about 5 weeks after exposure to the virus.

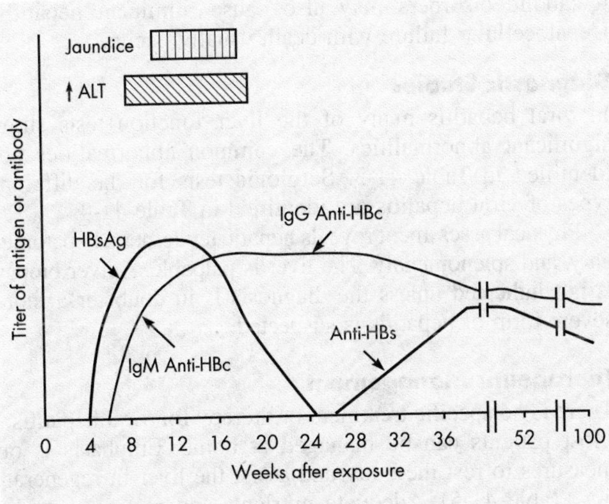

Fig. 41-3 Clinical and serologic events of a typical patient infected with acute hepatitis B (HB). Elevated alanine aminotransferase (ALT) levels are present by about 8 weeks and jaundice appears by about 10 weeks after exposure to the virus. HBc, hepatitis B core (antigen); HBs, hepatitis B surface (antigen).

Pathophysiology

Liver. The pathophysiologic changes in the various types of viral hepatitis are similar. Hepatitis involves widespread inflammation of liver tissue. Liver cell damage consists of hepatic cell degeneration and necrosis. There is proliferation and enlargement of the Kupffer cells. Inflammation of the periportal areas may interrupt bile flow. Cholestasis may occur. The liver cells regenerate in an orderly manner, and if no complications occur, they should resume their normal appearance and function during convalescence.

Systemic Effects. The antigen-antibody complexes between the virus and its corresponding antibody form a circulating immune complex in the early phases of hepatitis. The presence of circulating immune complexes activates the complement system (see Chapter 10). The clinical manifestations of this activation are rash, angioedema, arthritis, fever, and malaise. Glomerulonephritis and vasculitis have also been found secondary to immune complex disease.[6]

Clinical Manifestations

A large number of patients, especially the younger ones, have no symptoms. The clinical manifestations of viral hepatitis may be classified into three phases: (1) preicteric or prodromal phase, (2) icteric phase, and (3) posticteric or convalescent phase (Table 41-2).

Preicteric Phase. The preicteric phase precedes jaundice and lasts from 1 to 21 days. This is the period of maximal infectivity for hepatitis A. Hepatitis B patients who are HBcAg positive can be infective for years. Gastrointestinal (GI) symptoms include anorexia, nausea, ab-

Table 41-2 Clinical Manifestations of the Phases of Hepatitis

Preicteric	Icteric	Posticteric
Anorexia	Jaundice	Malaise
Nausea, vomiting	Pruritus	Easy fatigability
Right upper quadrant discomfort	Dark urine	Hepatomegaly
Constipation or diarrhea	Bilirubinuria	
Decreased sense of taste and smell	Light stools	
Malaise	Fatigue	
Headache	Continued hepatomegaly with tenderness	
Fever	Weight loss	
Arthralgias		
Urticaria		
Hepatomegaly		
Splenomegaly		
Weight loss		

dominal (right upper quadrant) discomfort, and sometimes vomiting, constipation, or diarrhea. The anorexia is frequently severe and is thought to be caused by a toxin produced by the diseased liver. The patient may find food repugnant and, if a smoker, have a distaste for cigarettes. There is also a decreased sense of smell. Weight loss occurs during the preicteric phase. Other symptoms during this phase are malaise, headache, fever (low-grade), arthralgias, and skin rashes. Physical examination reveals hepatomegaly, lymphadenopathy, and sometimes splenomegaly.

Icteric Phase. The icteric phase lasts 2 to 4 weeks and is characterized by jaundice. Jaundice results when bilirubin diffuses into the tissues. The urine may darken because of excess bilirubin being excreted by the kidneys. If conjugated bilirubin cannot flow out of the liver because of obstruction or inflammation of the bile ducts, the stools will be light or clay colored. Pruritus sometimes accompanies the jaundice, especially if cholestasis is present. The pruritus occurs as a result of the accumulation of bile salts beneath the skin.

When jaundice occurs, the fever usually subsides. The GI symptoms usually remain, and some fatigue may continue. The liver is usually enlarged and tender.

Posticteric Phase. The convalescent stage of the posticteric phase begins as jaundice is disappearing and lasts weeks to months, with an average of 2 to 4 months. During this period the patient's major complaint is malaise and easy fatigability. Hepatomegaly remains for several weeks, but splenomegaly subsides during this period. Relapses may occur, and the disappearance of jaundice does not mean the patient has totally recovered.

General Considerations. Not all patients with viral hepatitis have jaundice. This is referred to as *anicteric hepatitis* and occurs more frequently in children. A high percentage of persons with HAV are anicteric and do not have symptoms.

There is some slight variation in manifestations between the types of hepatitis. In hepatitis A the onset is more acute and the symptoms are usually mild, flulike manifestations. In hepatitis B the onset is more insidious and the symptoms are usually more severe. There may be fewer GI symptoms. Extrahepatic manifestations of HBV include glomerulonephritis and polyarteritis nodosa. These manifestations are thought to be caused by the deposition of circulating HBsAg and its antibody in tissue and subsequent complement activation.

Complications

Most patients with viral hepatitis recover completely with no complications. The mortality rate is 0.6% in hepatitis A, 0.5% to 2.0% in hepatitis B, and 1% to 2% in hepatitis C. The mortality rate is higher in older adults and those with underlying debilitating diseases.[3] Complications that can occur include chronic persistent hepatitis, chronic active hepatitis, fulminant viral hepatitis, and cirrhosis of the liver.

Chronic Persistent Hepatitis. The most common complication of viral hepatitis is *chronic persistent hepatitis* in which there is a delayed convalescent period. It is usually benign and is characterized by fatigue and hepatomegaly. However, no treatment is required. Liver function tests may remain abnormal for several years.

Chronic Active Hepatitis. Chronic active hepatitis is characterized by the persistence of signs and symptoms of hepatitis and abnormal liver function tests for more than 6 months. Chronic active hepatitis is seen in hepatitis B and C but not in hepatitis A or E. It is only seen in patients with hepatitis D if they also have hepatitis B. HBsAg persists longer than 6 months in approximately 10% of patients with hepatitis B. It is distinguished from chronic persistent hepatitis by liver biopsy. The ongoing process of liver necrosis is likely to progress to cirrhosis. α-Interferon has been approved for treatment of chronic active hepatitis B and has been found to be effective for some patients.[7] α-Interferon is considered effective if the patient becomes negative for HBsAg.

The HBsAg-positive patient whose serum remains positive for HBeAg is more likely to have chronic active hepatitis. In addition, alteration in the patient's cellular immune response may be important in the development of the chronic HBsAg carrier state and consequent progression from acute hepatitis B to chronic active hepatitis. This finding may explain why the patient with chronic renal failure who is undergoing hemodialysis when hepatitis B develops is more at risk of chronic active hepatitis. (Persons with chronic renal failure are known to have a depressed cellular immune response.)

Fulminant Hepatitis. Fulminant viral hepatitis is a clinical syndrome that results in severe impairment or necrosis of liver cells and potential liver failure. Fulminant viral hepatitis develops in a small percentage of patients. The disorder may occur as a complication of hepatitis B or C, particularly hepatitis B accompanied by infection with delta virus (HDV). Toxic reactions to drugs and congenital metabolic disorders may also cause fulminant hepatitis. Hepatocellular failure with death usually occurs.

Diagnostic Studies

In viral hepatitis many of the liver function tests show significant abnormalities. The common abnormalities are identified in Table 41-3. Serologic tests for the different types of viral hepatitis are identified in Table 41-4.

Physical assessment reveals hepatic tenderness, hepatomegaly, and splenomegaly. The liver is palpable. A liver biopsy is not indicated unless the diagnosis is in doubt or a more severe form of hepatitis is suspected.

Therapeutic Management

There is no specific treatment or therapy for viral hepatitis.[8] Most patients can be managed at home. Emphasis is on measures to rest the body and assist the liver in regenerating (Table 41-5). Adequate nutrients and rest seem to be most beneficial for healing and liver cell (hepatocyte) regeneration. Dietary emphasis is on a well-balanced diet that the patient can tolerate.

Rest reduces the metabolic demands on the liver and promotes cell regeneration. Bed rest may be indicated while the patient is symptomatic. The degree of rest ordered de-

Table 41-3 Diagnostic Findings in Hepatitis

Test	Abnormal Finding	Etiology
Transaminases (aminotransferases)		
Aspartate aminotransferase (AST) or serum glutamic-oxaloacetic transaminase (SGOT)	Elevation in preicteric phase; decrease as jaundice disappears	Liver cell injury
Alanine aminotransferase (ALT) or serum glutamic-pyruvic transaminase (SGPT)	Elevation in preicteric phase; decrease as jaundice disappears	Liver cell injury
γ-Glutamyl transpeptidase (GGT)	Elevation	Liver cell injury
Alkaline phosphatase	Some elevation	Impaired excretory function of the liver
Serum proteins		
γ-Globulin	Normal or increased	Impaired clearance of the liver
Albumin	Normal or decreased	Liver damage
Serum bilirubin (total)	Elevation to about 8-15 mg/dl (137-257 μmol/L)	Hepatocellular damage
Urinary bilirubin	Elevation	Conjugated hyperbilirubinemia
Urinary urobilinogen	Elevation 2-5 days before jaundice	Diminished reabsorption of urobilinogen
Prothrombin time	Prolonged	Decreased absorption of vitamin K in intestine with decreased production of prothrombin by liver

Table 41-4 Serologic Tests for Viral Hepatitis

Virus	Tests	Significance
A	Anti-HAV IgM	Acute infection
	Anti-HAV IgG	Previous infection and long-term immunity
B	HBsAg (hepatitis B surface antigen)	Current infection (but not necessarily acute)* Positive in chronic carriers
	Anti-HBs (antibody to surface antigen)	Indicates immunity to hepatitis B. Marker for response to vaccine
	HBeAg (hepatitis B e antigen)	Indicates high infectivity; present in acute, active infection
	Anti-HBe (antibody to e antigen)	Indicates previous infection
	Anti-HBc IgM	Acute infection*
	Anti-HBc IgG (antibody to HB core antigen)	Indicates previous infection Does not appear after vaccination
	HBV-DNA	Indicates viral replication Best indicator of viral replication
C	Anti-HCV (antibody to hepatitis C)	Marker for acute or chronic infection with HCV
D	Anti-HDV	Coexisting infection with HBV
E	Serologic tests are under development	

DNA, Deoxyribonucleic acid; *HAV*, hepatitis A virus; *HBV*, hepatitis B virus; *HCV*, hepatitis C virus; *HDV*, hepatitis D virus.
*If positive HBsAg and anti-HBc IgM, it indicates the presence of acute infection.

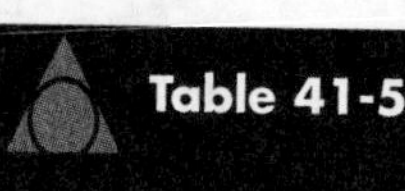

Table 41-5 Therapeutic Management: Viral Hepatitis

Diagnostic
- Liver function studies
- Hepatitis serology
  - HBsAg (HBeAg in some cases)
  - Anti-HBs
  - Anti-HBc—IgM and IgG
  - Anti-HAV—IgM and IgG
  - Anti-HCV

Therapeutic
- High-calorie, high-protein, high-carbohydrate, low-fat diet
- Vitamin supplements
- Rest—degree of strictness varying
- Avoid alcohol intake and drugs detoxified by the liver

HAV, Hepatitis A virus; *HB,* hepatitis B; *HCV,* hepatitis C virus.

pends on the severity of symptoms, but usually alternating periods of activity and rest are adequate.

Pharmacologic Management. There are no specific drug therapies for the treatment of acute viral hepatitis. Steroid therapy is controversial. Supportive drug therapy may include antiemetics, such as dimenhydrinate (Dramamine) or trimethobenzamide (Tigan). Phenothiazines should not be used because of their possible cholestatic and hepatotoxic effects. If the patient requires a sedative or hypnotic drug, diphenhydramine (Benadryl) or chloral hydrate may be used.

Immune globulin is used in the prevention and modification of viral hepatitis. Immune globulin (IG) is effective for hepatitis A if given up to 2 weeks after exposure. It provides temporary passive immunity. IG is recommended in cases of exposure to hepatitis A from close (household, day care center) contact in persons who are not positive for anti-HAV and for travelers to foreign countries with high endemic levels of Hepatitis A. Hepatitus A vaccine is discussed later in this chapter.

The first line of defense against Hepatitis B is the Hepatitis B vaccine.[9] Vaccines available for hepatitis B are discussed further later in this chapter. For acute one-time exposure to the virus, Hepatitis B immune globulin (HBIG) plus the vaccine can be administered. HBIG is prepared from plasma of donors with a high titer of anti-HBs. It is very expensive. HBIG provides temporary passive immunity and is recommended for postexposure prophylaxis in cases of needle stick, mucous membrane contact, or sexual exposure.

Nutritional Management. An important measure in assisting hepatocytes to regenerate is adequate nutrition. No special diet is required in the treatment of viral hepatitis. However, a diet high in carbohydrates and proteins with low fat content is usually recommended. Adequate calories are important because the patient usually loses weight. If fat content is poorly tolerated because of decreased bile production, it should be reduced. Basically the specific foods in the diet are dictated by the patient. Vitamin supplements, particularly B complex and vitamin K, are frequently used.

Ensuring that the patient receives adequate nutrients is not always easy. The anorexia and extreme distaste for food cause nutritional problems. Dietary assessment must be considered. The nurse should try to determine whether there is something that appeals to the patient in spite of the anorexia. Small, frequent meals may be preferable to three large ones and may also help prevent nausea. Frequently, a patient with hepatitis finds that anorexia is not as severe in the morning, so it is easier to eat a good breakfast than a large dinner. Measures to stimulate the appetite, such as mouth care, antiemetics, and attractively served meals in pleasant surroundings, should be included in the nursing care plan. Other measures that may be tried to counteract the anorexia are carbonated beverages and avoidance of very hot or very cold foods. Adequate fluid intake is important (2500 to 3000 ml per day).

If anorexia, nausea, and vomiting are severe, intravenous (IV) solutions of glucose or supplemental tube feedings may be used. Fluid and electrolyte balance must be maintained.

NURSING MANAGEMENT

HEPATITIS

Nursing Assessment

Subjective and objective data that should be obtained from a person with hepatitis are presented in Table 41-6.

Nursing Diagnoses

Nursing diagnoses are determined when the problem and etiologic factors are supported by clinical data. Nursing diagnoses related to hepatitis may include, but are not limited to, those presented in the following nursing care plan for the patient with hepatitis.

Planning

The overall goals are that the patient with viral hepatitis will (1) have relief of discomfort, (2) be able to resume normal activities, and (3) return to normal liver function without complications. Specific outcomes are identified in the nursing care plan for viral hepatitis on p. 1266.

Nursing Implementation

Health Promotion and Maintenance. Viral hepatitis is a community health problem. The nurse must assume a significant role in the control and prevention of this disease. It is helpful to first understand the epidemiology of the different types of viral hepatitis before considering appropriate control measures.

Hepatitis A. Outbreaks of viral hepatitis are usually due to HAV. The mode of transmission of HAV is predominantly fecal-oral (mainly by ingestion of food or liquid infected with the virus) and rarely parenteral. Poor hygiene, crowded situations, and poor sanitary conditions are all factors related to hepatitis A.

Transmission occurs between family members, institutionalized individuals, and from common-source outbreaks.

Table 41-6 Nursing Assessment: Hepatitis

Subjective Data

Important health information

Past health history: IV drug and alcohol abuse; hemophilia; exposure to infected persons; ingestion of contaminated food or water; sexual promiscuity; exposure to benzene or carbon tetrachloride; ingestion of poisonous mushrooms; crowded, unsanitary living conditions; exposure to contaminated needles; recent travel

Medications: Use and misuse of acetaminophen, phenytoin, halothane, methyldopa

Functional health patterns

Health perception–health management: Malaise, fatigue; distaste for cigarettes (in smokers)

Nutritional-metabolic: Weight loss, anorexia; feeling of fullness in right upper quadrant; pruritis, urticaria

Elimination: Dark urine; light-colored stools, diarrhea

Activity-exercise: Arthralgias, myalgias

Cognitive-perceptual: Right upper quadrant pain and tenderness, headache

Objective Data

General

Low-grade fever, lethargy, lymphadenopathy

Integumentary

Rash, angioedema, jaundice, icteric sclera, injection sites

Gastrointestinal

Hepatomegaly, splenomegaly

Possible findings

Abnormal liver function tests; anemia; serologic tests positive for hepatitis, including HBsAg, anti-HBs, anti-HBc, anti-HAV IgM, anti-HCV, elevated serum bilirubin; abnormal liver scan; positive liver biopsy

HAV, Hepatitis A virus; *HB,* hepatitis B; *HCV,* hepatitis C virus; *IV,* intravenous.

The disease occurs more frequently in underdeveloped countries. Certain foods, such as contaminated milk, water, and shellfish, are other sources of infection. The eating of raw shellfish from contaminated waters can also be a source of infection. Food-borne hepatitis A outbreaks are usually due to contamination of food during preparation by an infected food handler.

There is no chronic carrier state for HAV. The virus is present in feces during the incubation period, so it can be carried by persons who have undetectable, subclinical infections. The greatest risk of transmission occurs before clinical symptoms are apparent. It can also be transmitted by patients with anicteric hepatitis A.

Preventive measures include personal and environmental hygiene and health education to promote good sanitation. Hand washing is essential and is probably the most important precaution. Health teaching should include careful hand washing after bowel movements and before eating. When hepatitis A occurs in a food handler, IG should be administered to all other food handlers at the establishment. Patrons may also need to be given IG.

Isolation is not required for hepatitis A. For a patient with hepatitis A, infection control procedures should be used (see Tables 9-18 and 9-19). A private room is indicated if the patient is incontinent of stool or has poor personal hygiene. Hand washing is essential.

A major preventive measure for hepatitis A is administration of immune globulin (IG). Because patients with hepatitis A are most infectious just before the onset of symptoms, those exposed through household contact or food-borne outbreaks should be given IG within 1 to 2 weeks of exposure. If the exposed person has anti-HAV antibodies, the IG is not necessary. When given within 2 weeks of exposure, IG can prevent infection in most people. Although IG may not prevent infection in all persons, it may modify the illness to a subclinical infection. IG provides 6 to 8 weeks of passive protection. It may also be used as a prophylactic measure for travelers to foreign countries that have a high incidence of hepatitis A.

Hepatitis A vaccine (Havrix) became available in 1995. Primary immunization consists of a single dose administered intramuscularly in the deltoid. A booster is recommended any time between 6 and 12 months after the initiation of the primary dose in order to ensure adequate antibody titers. However, a primary immunization provides immunity within 15 days after a single dose. The vaccine may be administered concomitantly with IG, although the ultimate antibody titer obtained is likely to be lower than if the vaccine is given alone. The side effects of the vaccine are mild and are usually limited to soreness and redness at the injection site. There are still questions as to who should receive the hepatitis A vaccine, but people who are most likely to benefit from it include workers in day care centers, residents in institutions with close living conditions, those in the military, travelers to endemic areas, and persons engaging in high-risk sexual activities.[10]

Hepatitis B. HBV is transmitted percutaneously, sexually, through mucous membranes or nonintact skin, and perinatally. HBsAg has been detected in almost every body fluid, including vaginal secretions, menstrual fluids, semen, saliva, respiratory secretions, tears, gastric juice, synovial fluid, and cerebrospinal fluid. Infected semen and saliva contain much lower concentrations of HBV than blood, but the virus can be transmitted via these secretions. If GI bleeding occurs, feces can be contaminated with the virus from the blood. There is no evidence that urine, feces, breast milk, tears, or sweat are infective. Sometimes HBV is transmitted by unidentified means. In some patients with acute hepatitis B there are no readily identifiable risk factors.

Hepatitis B is a sexually transmitted disease. One third to two thirds of the new annual hepatitis B infections in the United States during the past 10 years were sexually transmitted.[11] Male homosexuals (especially with anal intercourse) and heterosexuals with multiple partners are at risk for HBV infection. Although there is a much lower risk of transmission, kissing and sharing of food items may spread the virus via saliva.

Six percent to 10% of adults who become infected with hepatitis B virus become chronic HBV carriers and may transmit the virus.[11] The HBsAg level remains elevated in

NURSING CARE PLAN Patient with Viral Hepatitis

Planning: Outcome Criteria	*Nursing Interventions and Rationales*
➤ **NURSING DIAGNOSIS**	Altered nutrition: less than body requirements *related to* anorexia, nausea, and reduced metabolism of nutrients by liver *as manifested by* inadequate food intake; perceived inability to ingest food; lack of interest in food; aversion to eating; actual or potential metabolic needs in excess of intake with or without weight loss
Have adequate nutritional intake; maintenance of normal body weight.	Assess patient's appetite and adequacy of intake *so appropriate interventions can be planned.* Offer frequent small feedings, provide oral care before meals *to enhance patient's dietary intake.* Allow patient to choose food items; serve high-carbohydrate and high-protein foods at time of day patient feels most like eating *to increase likelihood of adequate intake.* Provide attractively served meals in pleasant surroundings *to stimulate patient's appetite.* Take weight daily on same scale, at same time, with same clothing *to monitor weight loss secondary to poor appetite.*
➤ **NURSING DIAGNOSIS**	Activity intolerance *related to* fatigue, weakness, increased energy utilization associated with increased basal metabolic rate caused by viral infection, and inadequate nutritional status *as manifested by* verbal report of fatigue or weakness, altered response to activity (as measured by BP, pulse, respiratory rate)
Have increased tolerance for activity.	Plan rest periods. Increase patient's activity gradually as allowed and tolerated *so previous activity pattern can be resumed.* Conserve patient's strength by careful monitoring activity *to prevent increasing weakness and fatigue.* Teach patient to monitor and control activities that provoke fatigue *so patient can be an active participant in plan.*
➤ **NURSING DIAGNOSIS**	Anxiety *related to* lack of understanding of diagnosis, anticipated changes in lifestyle, and fear of prognosis and complications *as manifested by* increased tension, apprehension, restlessness, insomnia, expression of concern, and frequent questioning regarding changes in health status
Be aware of own anxiety and coping patterns; verbalize increase in psychologic and physiologic comfort.	Assess level of anxiety *to plan appropriate interventions.* Provide reassurance and comfort and convey sense of empathic understanding (e.g., touch, quiet presence) *to foster effective coping.* Ascertain and support current coping skills. Encourage verbalization of fear and anxiety *to provide patient with opportunity to express concerns and organize thoughts.* Explain tests, procedures, and health maintenance behaviors *because knowledge can decrease anxiety and foster effective coping.*
➤ **NURSING DIAGNOSIS**	Upper abdominal pain *related to* inflammation of the liver *as manifested by* communication of pain descriptors, guarding behavior, narrowed self-focus, behaviors indicative of pain (e.g., reluctance to move)
Verbalize decreased discomfort; have absence of objective signs of discomfort or pain, relaxed demeanor.	Assess pain *to plan appropriate interventions.* Administer mild analgesic not metabolized by the liver as ordered *to promote comfort and decrease possibility of further liver damage.* Use nursing care measures *to help relieve the discomfort or pain* (e.g., position changes, back rub, relaxation, diversion, guided imagery).

continued

carriers (HBsAg-positive on at least two occasions at least 6 months apart). With carrier status, liver enzyme values may be normal. The carriers of hepatitis B may have low-grade disease, a normal liver, or severe chronic active liver disease. α-Interferon is now being used to try to eliminate the chronic HBV carrier state. A positive test for anti-HBs in adults indicates that they have had hepatitis B or the vaccine.

Control and prevention of hepatitis B focuses on identification of possible exposure via percutaneous and sexual transmission. The nurse must be aware of the groups at high risk of contracting hepatitis B and teach methods to reduce risks. These include patients receiving frequent transfusions or hemodialysis, workers in hemodialysis units and blood chemistry laboratories, IV drug users, persons with multiple sexual partners, prison inmates, and household members and sexual partners of HBV carriers.

Good hygienic practices, including hand washing and the use of gloves when expecting contact with blood, are important. A condom is advised for sexual intercourse, and

NURSING CARE PLAN Patient with Viral Hepatitis—cont'd

Planning: Outcome Criteria	Nursing Interventions and Rationales
➤ **NURSING DIAGNOSIS**	Body-image disturbance *related to* stigma of having a communicable disease, change in appearance (jaundice), and possible alterations in lifestyle and roles (alcohol consumption, drug use, restriction of sexual activity) *as manifested by* negative verbal or nonverbal response to actual or perceived change in structure or function
Make a positive adaption to changes in appearance; verbalize understanding of body changes; seek information as needed.	Assess patient's feelings about disease process and appearance *to plan appropriate interventions.* Clarify misconceptions regarding limitations *to avoid unnecessary restrictions on patient's activities.* Encourage participation in self-care *to foster independence and self-esteem.* Instruct patient in ways to prevent spread of hepatitis *to reduce fear and guilt associated with potential for infecting others.* Assist patient in expressing feelings. Encourage patient to ask questions *because accurate information fosters good decision making.*
➤ **NURSING DIAGNOSIS**	Ineffective management of therapeutic regimen *related to* lack of knowledge of follow-up care *as manifested by* frequent questions about transmission of disease, activities allowed, and general follow-up care
Verbalize understanding of follow-up care; have plan for follow-up visit with health-care provider.	Teach patient basic facts about illness, modes of transmission, diet, activities allowed, avoidance of alcohol, and need for follow-up care *so appropriate follow-up care will be planned and carried out.*
➤ **NURSING DIAGNOSIS**	Fatigue *related to* viral infection *as manifested by* malaise, decreased interest in participating in activities of daily living, expression of tiredness, sleepiness
Verbalize increased ability to carry out usual activities.	Apply heat to aching muscles and joints as ordered *to cause vasodilatation and subsequent decrease in pain.* Medicate as needed *to reduce fever and promote comfort and rest.* Provide periods of uninterrupted rest *to promote recovery and sense of well-being.* Plan activities and care to patient's tolerance *to avoid exacerbating symptoms and increasing fatigue.* Monitor appetite, fluids, and food intake *so inadequate intake does not increase fatigue or hinder recovery.*

BP, Blood pressure.

the partner should be vaccinated. Razors, toothbrushes, and other personal items should not be shared. Close contacts of the patient with hepatitis B who are HBsAg negative and antibody negative should be vaccinated.

According to Centers for Disease Control and Prevention (CDC) guidelines, infection control precautions should be followed for the patient with hepatitis B. This includes the use of disposable needles and syringes, which should be disposed of in puncture-resistant disposal units without recapping, bending, or breaking. (See Tables 9-18 and 9-19 for various types of infection control precautions.)

Immunization with hepatitis B vaccine is the most effective method of preventing HBV infection. Recommendations of the CDC's Immunization Practices Advisory Committee include making hepatitis B vaccine a part of routine vaccination schedules for all infants. The objective of the Childhood Immunization Initiative is that by 1998 at least 90% of 2-year-old children will have received hepatitis B vaccine as part of routine vaccination.[12]

In addition to immunizing infants, it is important to vaccinate adolescents and adults in the major risk groups (Table 41-7). It may be helpful to screen for the antibody before vaccination because past infection is high in sexually active homosexual men and IV drug users. It is hoped that universal vaccination will lead to eventual prevention and control of hepatitis B.

Hepatitis B vaccine is produced through recombinant DNA technology (see Fig. 10-12). The vaccines are Recombivax HB and Engerix-B. The vaccine is given in a series of three intramuscular (in the deltoid) injections. The second dose is administered within 1 month of the first one, and the third one within 6 months after the first. The cost is about $150 for the series. The vaccine is 90% to 95% effective.[10] Successful vaccination should result in anti-HBs titers of 10 mIU/ml or greater. Only minor adverse reactions have been reported with vaccination, including transient fever and soreness at the injection site.

The vaccine is not contraindicated in pregnancy. Currently a booster (fourth dose) has not been recommended by the CDC's Immunization Practices Advisory Committee. This committee has also stated that the vaccine should last at least 7 years in an individual with a normal immune system.

For postexposure prophylaxis, the vaccine and HBIG are used. HBIG contains antibodies to HBV and confers tem-

Table 41-7 Preventive Measures for Viral Hepatitis

Hepatitis A	Hepatitis B and C
General Measures Hand washing Proper personal hygiene Environmental sanitation Control and screening (signs, symptoms) of food handlers Serologic screening while carrying virus Active immunization: HAV vaccine *Use of Immune Globulin* Early administration (1-2 wk after exposure) to those exposed Use of prophylaxis for travelers to areas where hepatitis A is common	*Percutaneous Transmission* Screening of donated blood B—HbsAg C—anti-HCV Use of disposable needles and syringes *Sexual Transmission* Acute exposure: HBIG administration to sexual partner of HbsAg-positive person Administer hepatitis B vaccine series to uninfected sexual partners Use condoms for sexual intercourse *General Measures* Hand washing Avoid sharing toothbrushes and razors HBIG administration for one-time exposure (needle stick, contact of mucous membranes with infectious material) Active immunization: HBV vaccine

HAV, Hepatitis A virus; *HBV*, hepatitis B virus; *HCV*, hepatitis C virus.

porary passive immunity. HBIG is given to persons who have been exposed to HBV (needle stick, sexual exposure, infants born to mothers who are positive for HBsAg), and who have not been vaccinated. It should be given after exposure, preferably within 24 hours. The vaccine series should also be started. Preventive and control measures for hepatitis A and B are summarized in Table 41-8.

Hepatitis C. Risk factors for HCV infection include intravenous drug use, needlestick accidents, hemophilia, and hemodialysis. Posttransfusion HCV infection is best prevented through routine screening for anti-HCV (antibody to hepatitis C).[13] At this time there is no test commercially available for the HCV virus (antigen). There is no vaccine for hepatitis C.

Control of Hepatitis in Health Care Personnel

Hepatitis A. Hepatitis A is rarely transmitted from patients to health care personnel. When this does occur, it is associated with patients with undiagnosed hepatitis who are treated for other problems. Usually these patients are incontinent of feces. The use of infection control precautions should prevent transmission of HAV to health care personnel.

Hepatitis B. Before the use of hepatitis B vaccine approximately 18,000 health care workers contracted hepa-

Table 41-8 Measures to Prevent Transmission of Hepatitis Viruses from Patients to Health Care Personnel*

Hepatitis A	Hepatitis B	Hepatitis C
Always maintain good personal hygiene. Wash hands after contact with a patient or removal of gloves. Use infection control precautions.†	Use infection control precautions.† Wash hands. Reduce contact with blood or blood-containing secretions. Handle the blood of patients as potentially infective. Dispose of needles properly. Administer HBV vaccine to all health care personnel. Use needleless IV access devices when available.	Use infection control precautions.† Wash hands. Reduce contact with blood or blood-contaminated secretions. Handle the blood of patients as potentially infective. Dispose of needles properly. Use needleless IV access devices when available.

HBV, Hepatitis B virus; *IV*, intravenous.

*A suggested guideline for general practice to prevent the nurse from contracting viral hepatitis from diagnosed and undiagnosed patients and carriers is for the nurse to wear disposable gloves, goggles, gowns (sometimes) when fecal or blood contamination is likely in handling (1) soiled bedpans, urinals, and catheters and (2) patient's bed linens soiled by body excreta or secretions.

†See Tables 9-18 and 9-19.

titis B annually from occupational exposure. Currently, fewer health care workers now contract the disease. Health care workers may be exposed to HBV from needle sticks or blood contamination to mucous membranes or nonintact skin. If a health care worker is exposed to HBV through a needle stick and does not receive the vaccine, there is a 6% to 30% chance of infection with hepatitis B.[2] Vaccination is the most effective method to prevent hepatitis B in health care workers. Employers are required by the Occupational Safety and Health Administration (OSHA) to provide free HBV immunization to employees at risk for infection.

The principal mode of transmission of HBV for health care personnel is parenteral. Examples of parenteral transmission include accidental needle sticks and, rarely, transfusion of contaminated blood or blood products. Because all blood and blood products are tested for HBV and anti-HCV, there is diminishing risk of this latter mode of transmission. Other forms of transmission include contamination of fresh cutaneous scratches or abrasions, burns, and contamination of mucosal surfaces with infective blood, blood products, saliva, or semen.

Hepatitis C. Transmission is usually due to percutaneous needle exposure or other blood exposure and undetected parenteral transmission. Measures to prevent transmission of the viruses from patients to health care personnel are presented in Table 41-8. Very rarely do health care workers infect patient contacts.

Acute Intervention

Jaundice. The nurse should assess for the degree of jaundice. In light-skinned persons the jaundice is usually observed first in the sclera of the eyes and later in the skin. In dark-skinned persons, jaundice is observed in the hard palate of the mouth and inner canthus of the eyes. Ictotest reagent tablets may be used to detect urinary bilirubin. The urine may be cola-colored or mahogany because of the presence of bilirubin. Comfort measures to relieve pruritus (if present), headache, and arthralgias are helpful (see the nursing care plan for the patient with hepatitis, p. 1266).

Rest. Rest is essential and is an important factor in promoting liver cell regeneration. The nurse must assess the patient's response to the rest and activity plan and modify it accordingly. The care plan should include appropriate time schedules for rest and activity, with scheduled rest periods uninterrupted by visitors or nursing staff. If the patient is on strict bed rest, measures to prevent respiratory and circulatory complications should be initiated. Assessment of the liver function tests and symptoms should continue as a guide to activity.

Psychologic and emotional rest are as essential as physical rest. Strict bed rest may produce anxiety and extreme restlessness in some patients and may be more damaging than reasonable ambulation. Diversional activities, such as reading and hobbies (e.g., knitting, stamp collecting), may help the patient. The patient should be assisted to understand the temporary nature of symptoms, especially sexual abstinence, during the period of communicability.

Chronic and Home Management. Most patients with viral hepatitis will be cared for at home, so the nurse must assess the patient's knowledge of nutrition and provide the necessary dietary teaching. Rest and adequate nutrition are especially important until studies show that liver function has returned to normal. The patient must be cautioned about overexertion and the need to follow the physician's advice about when it is safe to return to work. The nurse must also teach the patient and family about preventive measures and how to prevent transmission to other family members. The patient should know what symptoms need to be reported to the physician.

The patient should be assessed for any manifestations indicative of complications. Bleeding tendencies with increasing prothrombin time values, symptoms of encephalopathy, or greatly abnormal liver function tests indicate problems, and the patient should be assessed and treated promptly.

The patient should be instructed to have regular follow-up for at least 1 year after the diagnosis of hepatitis. Because relapses are fairly common with hepatitis B and C, the patient should be instructed about symptoms of recurrence. Alcohol should be avoided for 1 year because it is detoxified in the liver and may interfere with recovery.

A patient who remains positive for HBsAg is a carrier and should never be a blood donor. The patient with hepatitis B should also be instructed to use condoms when engaging in sexual intercourse until tests for HBsAg are negative.

The patient who is receiving α-interferon for the treatment of hepatitis B or C requires education regarding the medication. α-interferon needs to be administered IM or subcutaneously, and thus the patient or family member needs to be taught how to administer the drug. There are numerous side effects with the therapy, including flulike symptoms (fever, malaise, fatigue, chills).[14] The physician may recommend that acetaminophen be administered 30 to 60 minutes before injection to reduce these symptoms. Other significant side effects include thrombocytopenia, neutropenia, psychologic disturbances (mood swings, depression) and limited alopecia. (Additional information on α-interferon is presented in Chapters 10 and 12.)

TOXIC AND DRUG-INDUCED HEPATITIS

Liver injury and death may occur after the inhalation, parenteral injection, or ingestion of certain chemical substances (see Table 36-6). The two major types of chemical hepatotoxicity are toxic and drug-induced hepatitis. Agents producing *toxic hepatitis* are generally systemic poisons (e.g., carbon tetrachloride, gold compounds) or are converted in the liver to toxic metabolites (e.g., acetaminophen). Liver necrosis generally occurs within 2 to 3 days of acute exposure to a toxic substance.

Idiosyncratic drug reactions produce *drug-induced hepatitis*. Such agents as halothane, isoniazid, chlorothiazides, methotrexate, and methyldopa may produce idiosyncratic reactions because of patient susceptibility (metabolic reactivity) to these agents or immunologically mediated hypersensitivity responses. Liver injury may occur at any time during or shortly after exposure. Some responses occur 2 to 5 weeks after exposure.

Toxic and drug-induced hepatitis are similar to viral hepatitis in the pathophysiologic changes in the liver and the clinical manifestations. The usual presenting clinical findings are anorexia, nausea, vomiting, hepatomegaly, splenomegaly, and abnormal liver function studies. Treatment is largely supportive, as in acute viral hepatitis. Recovery may be rapid if the hepatotoxin is identified and removed. Liver transplantation may be necessary.

IDIOPATHIC HEPATITIS

Chronic active hepatitis may also occur in a number of patients who have no known risk factors for the development of viral hepatitis. The cause of this form of hepatitis is idiopathic. However, because many of these patients often have a number of systemic problems, including glomerulonephritis and arthritis, the disease is thought to be autoimmune.[6] The presenting signs and symptoms are variable, similar to viral hepatitis. Laboratory tests (elevation of liver enzymes) reveal liver inflammation without evidence of viral antigens. The majority (70% to 80%) of patients who are diagnosed with autoimmune hepatitis are women. The course of the disease is also variable, with the majority of the patients exhibiting chronic active hepatitis.

Unlike viral hepatitis, autoimmune hepatitis (in which there is evidence of necrosis and cirrhosis) is treated with corticosteroids or other immunosuppressive agents. Daily treatment with methylprednisone is the first line of therapy for nonviral chronic active hepatitis. Azathioprine (Imuran) may also be used to treat the disease.

CIRRHOSIS OF THE LIVER

Cirrhosis is a chronic progressive disease of the liver characterized by extensive degeneration and destruction of the liver parenchymal cells. The liver cells attempt to regenerate, but the regenerative process is disorganized, resulting in abnormal blood vessel and bile duct relationships from the fibrosis. The overgrowth of new and fibrous connective tissue distorts the liver's normal lobular structure, resulting in lobules of irregular size and shape with impeded vascular flow. Cirrhosis may have a very insidious, prolonged course.

Cirrhosis is ranked as the fifth leading cause of all deaths and the third leading cause of death in persons 25 to 65 years of age.[15] The highest incidence occurs between the ages of 40 and 60, and it is twice as common in men as in women. Excessive alcohol ingestion is the single most common cause of cirrhosis.

Etiology

The four types of cirrhosis, in order of incidence, are as follows:

1. *Alcoholic* (previously called *Laennec's*), also called portal or nutritional cirrhosis, is usually associated with alcohol abuse. The first change in the liver from excessive alcohol intake is an accumulation of fat in the liver cells. Uncomplicated fatty changes in the liver are potentially reversible if the person stops drinking alcohol.[16] If the alcohol abuse continues, widespread scar formation occurs throughout the liver.
2. *Postnecrotic cirrhosis* is a complication of viral, toxic, or idiopathic (autoimmune) hepatitis. Broad bands of scar tissue form within the liver.
3. *Biliary cirrhosis* is associated with chronic biliary obstruction and infection. There is diffuse fibrosis of the liver with jaundice as the main feature.
4. *Cardiac cirrhosis* results from long-standing severe right-sided heart failure in patients with cor pulmonale, constrictive pericarditis, and tricuspid insufficiency.

Pathophysiology

In cirrhosis, cell necrosis occurs, and the destroyed liver cells are replaced by scar tissue. The normal lobular architecture becomes nodular. Eventually irregular, disorganized regeneration, poor cellular nutrition, and hypoxia caused by inadequate blood flow and scar tissue result in decreased functioning of the liver.

The specific cause of cirrhosis may not be determined in all patients. It is known that cirrhosis occurs with greatest frequency among alcoholics. There continues to be some controversy as to whether the cause is the alcohol or the malnutrition that frequently coexists with chronic ingestion of alcohol. A common problem in alcoholics is protein malnutrition. There have been cases of nutritional cirrhosis resulting from extreme dieting or malnutrition. It is believed that the combined impact of malnutrition and alcohol is especially damaging to hepatocytes. Alcohol alone has a direct hepatotoxic effect. It is known to produce necrosis of cells and fatty infiltration with formation of fibrous septa. Some persons seem to have a predisposition to cirrhosis, regardless of their dietary or alcohol intake.

Clinical Manifestations

Early Manifestations. The onset of cirrhosis is usually insidious. Occasionally there is an abrupt onset of symptoms. GI disturbances are common early symptoms and include anorexia, dyspepsia, flatulence, nausea and vomiting, and change in bowel habits (diarrhea or constipation). These symptoms occur as a result of the liver's altered metabolism of carbohydrates, fats, and proteins. The patient may complain of abdominal pain described as a dull, heavy feeling in the right upper quadrant or epigastrium. The pain may be due to swelling and stretching of the liver capsule, spasm of the biliary ducts, and intermittent vascular spasm. Other early manifestations are fever, lassitude, slight weight loss, and enlargement of the liver and spleen. The liver is palpable in many patients with cirrhosis.

Later Manifestations. Later symptoms may be severe and result from liver failure and portal hypertension. Jaundice, peripheral edema, and ascites develop gradually. Other late symptoms include skin lesions, hematologic disorders, endocrine disturbances, and peripheral neuropathies (Fig. 41-4). In the advanced stages the liver becomes small and nodular.

Jaundice. Jaundice results from the functional derangement of liver cells and compression of bile ducts by connective tissue overgrowth. Jaundice occurs as a result of

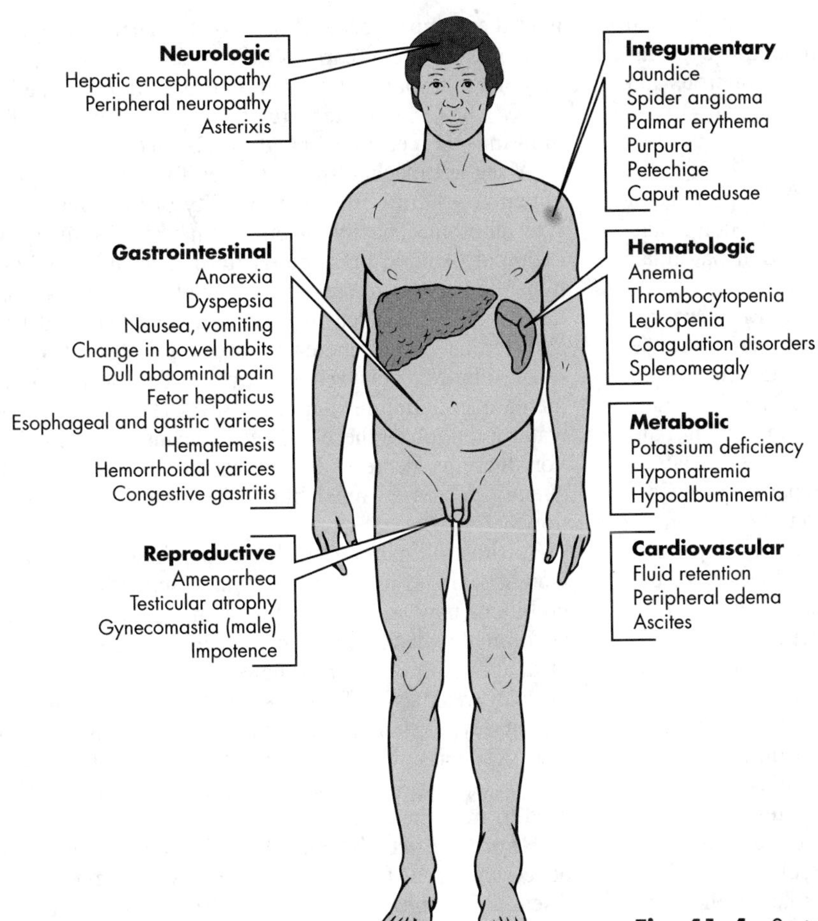

Fig. 41-4 Systemic clinical manifestations of liver cirrhosis.

the decreased ability to conjugate and excrete bilirubin (hepatocellular jaundice). The jaundice may be minimal or severe, depending on the degree of liver damage. If obstruction of the biliary tract occurs, obstructive jaundice may also occur and is usually accompanied by pruritus. The pruritus is due to an accumulation of bile salts underneath the skin.

Skin lesions. Various skin manifestations are commonly seen in cirrhosis. *Spider angiomas* (*telangiectasia* or *spider nevi*) are small, dilated blood vessels with a bright red center point and spiderlike branches. They occur on the nose, cheeks, upper trunk, neck, and shoulders. *Palmar erythema* (red areas that blanch with pressure) is located on the palms of the hands. Both of these lesions are attributed to an increase in circulating estrogen as a result of the damaged liver's inability to metabolize steroids.

Hematologic problems. Hematologic problems include thrombocytopenia, leukopenia, anemia, and coagulation disorders. Thrombocytopenia, leukopenia, and anemia are probably caused by the splenomegaly. Splenomegaly results from backup of blood from the portal vein into the spleen. Overactivity of the enlarged spleen results in increased removal of blood cells from circulation. The anemia is also due to inadequate red blood cell production and survival. Other factors involved in the anemia relate to poor diet, poor absorption of folic acid, and bleeding from varices.

The coagulation problems result from the liver's inability to produce prothrombin and other factors essential for blood clotting. Coagulation problems are manifested by hemorrhagic phenomena or bleeding tendencies, such as epistaxis, purpura, petechiae, easy bruising, gingival bleeding, and heavy menstrual bleeding.

Endocrine disturbances. Several signs and symptoms relating to the metabolism and inactivation of adrenocortical hormones, estrogen, and testosterone occur in cirrhosis. Normally the liver metabolizes these hormones. When the damaged liver is unable to do this, various manifestations occur. In men, gynecomastia, loss of axillary and pubic hair, testicular atrophy, and impotence with loss of libido may occur as a result of estrogen accumulation. In younger women amenorrhea may occur, and in older females there may be vaginal bleeding. The liver fails to metabolize aldosterone adequately, and this results in hyperaldosteronism with subsequent sodium and water retention and potassium loss.

Peripheral neuropathy. Peripheral neuropathy is a common finding in alcoholic cirrhosis. It is probably due to a dietary deficiency of thiamine, folic acid, and vitamin B_{12}.

The neuropathy usually results in mixed nervous system symptoms, but sensory symptoms may predominate. Clinical manifestations of cirrhosis of the liver are numerous and may eventually involve the total body (see Fig. 41-4).

Complications

Major complications of cirrhosis are portal hypertension with resultant esophageal varices, peripheral edema and ascites, hepatic encephalopathy (coma), and hepatorenal syndrome.

Portal Hypertension and Esophageal Varices. Because of the structural changes in the liver from the cirrhotic process, there is compression and destruction of the portal and hepatic veins and sinusoids. These changes result in obstruction to the normal flow of blood through the portal system, resulting in portal hypertension. Many pathophysiologic changes result from portal hypertension. Collateral circulation develops in an attempt to reduce this high portal pressure and also to reduce the increased plasma volume and lymphatic flow. The common areas where the collateral channels form are in the lower esophagus (the anastomosis of the left gastric vein and the azygos veins), the anterior abdominal wall, the parietal peritoneum, and the rectum. Varicosities may develop in areas where the collateral and systemic circulations communicate, resulting in esophageal and gastric varices, caput medusae (ring of varices around the umbilicus), and hemorrhoids.

Esophageal varices (graded I to IV) are a common complication, occurring in two thirds to three fourths of patients with cirrhosis. These collateral vessels contain little elastic tissue and are quite fragile. They tolerate the high pressure poorly, and the result is distended, tortuous veins that bleed easily. Large varices are more likely to bleed.

Patients with bleeding esophageal varices have a high mortality rate. These varices are the most life-threatening complication of cirrhosis. The mortality rate for the first bleeding episode averages 50%. Recurrence of bleeding is very high.[17]

The varices rupture and bleed in response to ulceration and irritation. Factors producing ulceration and irritation include alcohol ingestion; swallowing of poorly masticated food; ingestion of coarse food; acid regurgitation from the stomach; and increased intraabdominal pressure caused by nausea, vomiting, straining at stool, coughing, sneezing, or lifting heavy objects. The patient may have melena or hematemesis. There may be slow oozing or massive hemorrhage. Massive hemorrhage is a medical emergency.

Peripheral Edema and Ascites. Peripheral edema sometimes precedes ascites, but in some patients its development coincides with or occurs after ascites. Edema results from decreased colloidal osmotic pressure from impaired liver synthesis of albumin and increased portocaval pressure from portal hypertension. Peripheral edema occurs as ankle and presacral edema.

Ascites is the accumulation of serous fluid in the peritoneal or abdominal cavity. It is a common manifestation of cirrhosis. When the blood pressure is elevated in the liver, as occurs in portal cirrhosis, proteins move from the blood vessels via the larger pores of the sinusoids (capillaries) into the lymph space (Fig. 41-5). When the lymphatic system is unable to carry off the excess proteins and water, they leak through the liver capsule into the peritoneal cavity. The osmotic pressure of the proteins pulls additional fluid into the peritoneal cavity (Table 41-9).

A second mechanism of ascites formation is hypoalbuminemia resulting from the inability of the liver to synthesize albumin. The hypoalbuminemia results in decreased colloidal osmotic pressure. A third mechanism of ascites, hyperaldosteronism, results when aldosterone is not metabolized by damaged hepatocytes. The increased level of aldosterone causes increased sodium reabsorption by the renal tubules. This retention of sodium, as well as an increase in antidiuretic hormone (ADH), causes additional water retention in these patients. Because of edema formation there is decreased intravascular volume and subsequently decreased renal blood flow and glomerular filtration.

Ascites is manifested by abdominal distention with weight gain (Fig. 41-6). If the ascites is severe, the umbilicus may be everted. Abdominal striae with distended abdominal wall veins may be present. The patient has signs of dehydration (e.g., dry tongue and skin, sunken eyeballs, muscle weakness). There is also a decrease in urinary output. Hypokalemia is common and is due to an excessive loss of potassium because of the effects of aldosterone. Low potassium levels can also result from diuretic therapy used to treat the ascites.

Hepatic Encephalopathy. Hepatic encephalopathy, or coma, is a frequent terminal complication in liver disease. Encephalopathy is a more descriptive term than coma. Hepatic encephalopathy can occur in any condition in which liver damage causes ammonia to enter the systemic circulation without liver detoxification. There is a high mortality rate associated with hepatic encephalopathy.

The pathogenesis of hepatic encephalopathy is incompletely understood at this time. A number of etiologic factors may be involved. It is basically a disorder of protein metabolism and excretion. The main pathogenic agents appear to be nitrogenous ammonia and aromatic amino acids. A major source of ammonia is the bacterial and enzymatic deamination of amino acids in the intestines. The ammonia that results from this deamination process normally goes to the liver via the portal circulation and is converted to urea, which is then excreted by the kidneys. When the blood is shunted past the liver via the collateral anastomoses or the liver is unable to convert ammonia to urea, large quantities of ammonia remain in the systemic circulation. The ammonia crosses the blood-brain barrier and produces neurologic toxic manifestations. A number of factors may precipitate hepatic encephalopathy, mostly because they increase the amount of circulating ammonia (Table 41-10).

Other metabolic products that may contribute to hepatic encephalopathy are mercaptans (such as methionine) and short-chain fatty acids. Another theory is that the liver may produce substances necessary for normal brain functioning. When the diseased liver can no longer produce these substances, encephalopathy may result.

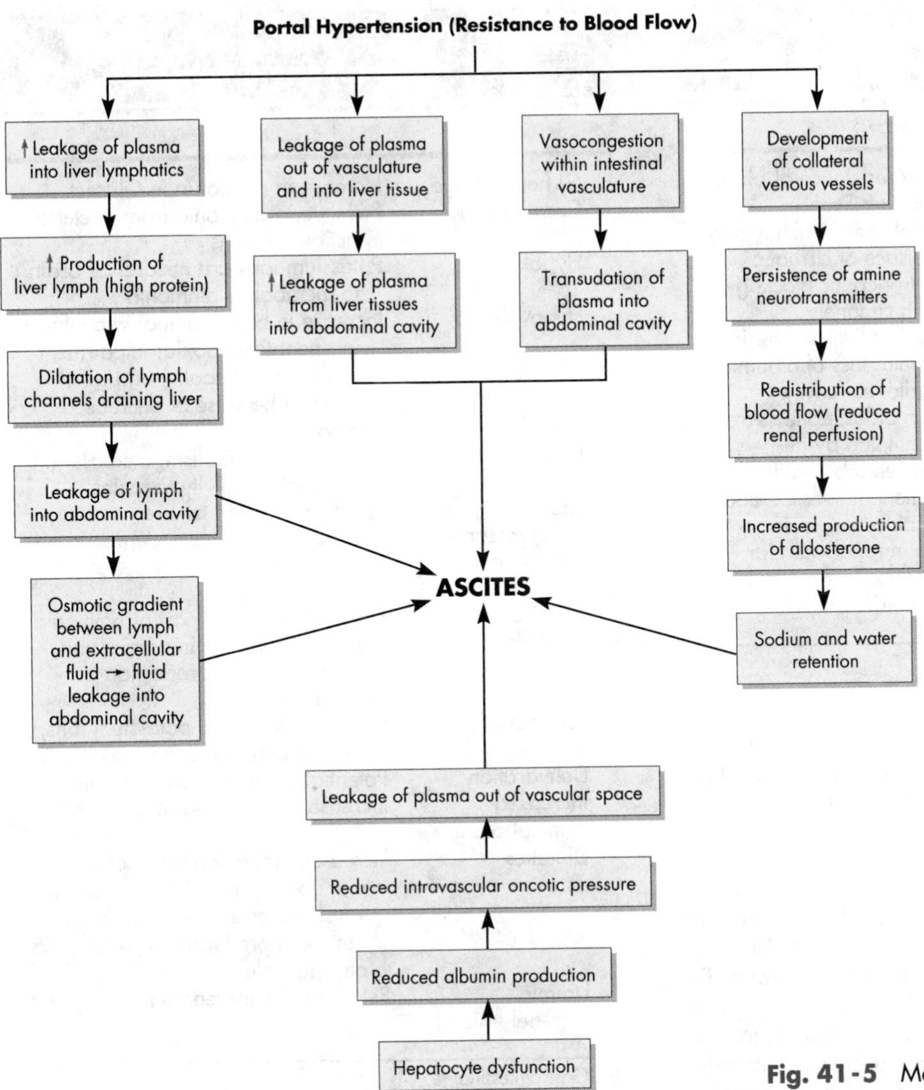

Fig. 41-5 Mechanisms for development of ascites.

Clinical manifestations of encephalopathy are changes in neurologic and mental responsiveness, ranging from lethargy to deep coma. Changes may occur suddenly because of an increase in ammonia in response to bleeding varices or gradually as blood ammonia levels slowly increase. In the early stages, manifestations include euphoria, depression, apathy, irritability, memory loss, confusion, yawning, drowsiness, insomnia, agitation, slow and slurred speech, emotional lability, impaired judgment, hiccups, slow and deep respirations, hyperactive reflexes, and a positive Babinski reflex.

Clinical manifestations of impending coma include disorientation as to time, place, or person. A characteristic symptom is *asterixis,* or flapping tremors (liver flap). This may take several forms, the most common involving the arms and hands. When asked to hold the arms and hands stretched out, the patient is unable to hold this position and there will be a series of rapid flexion and extension movements of the hands. Other signs of asterixis are rhythmic movements of the legs with dorsiflexion of the foot and rhythmic movements in the face with strong closure of the eyelids. Impairments in writing involve difficulty in moving the pen or pencil from left to right and apraxia (the inability to construct simple figures). Other signs include hyperventilation, hypothermia, and grimacing and grasping reflexes.

Fetor hepaticus occurs in some patients with encephalopathy. It is a musty, sweet odor of the patient's breath. This odor is from the accumulation of digestive byproducts that the liver is unable to degrade.

Hepatorenal Syndrome. Hepatorenal syndrome is a serious complication of cirrhosis.[18] It is characterized by functional renal failure with advancing azotemia, oliguria, and intractable ascites. There is no structural abnormality of the kidneys. The exact cause of the decreased renal function is unknown but is thought to be related to a redistribution of blood flow from the kidneys to peripheral and splanchnic circulations or hypovolemia secondary to ascites. In the patient with cirrhosis the syndrome frequently follows diuretic therapy, GI hemorrhage, or paracentesis. Hepatic

Table 41-9 Factors Involved in the Development of Ascites

Factor	Mechanism
Portal hypertension	Increase in resistance of blood flow through liver
Increased flow of hepatic lymph	Weeping of protein-rich lymph from surface of cirrhotic liver, intrahepatic blockage of lymph channels
Decreased serum colloidal oncotic pressure	Impairment of liver synthesis of albumin, loss of albumin into peritoneal cavity
Hyperaldosteronism	Increase in aldosterone secretion stimulated by decreased renal blood flow, impairment of liver metabolism of aldosterone
Impaired water excretion	Reduction in renal vascular flow and excessive serum levels of ADH

ADH, Antidiuretic hormone.

encephalopathy is also associated with the deterioration in renal function. Treatment measures include salt-poor albumin, salt and water restrictions, and diuretic therapy. However, treatment is usually unsuccessful.

Diagnostic Studies

A liver profile in cirrhosis demonstrates abnormalities in most of the liver function studies (see Table 36-13). Enzyme levels, including alkaline phosphatase, AST (SGOT), ALT (SGPT), and GGT, are elevated because of the release of these enzymes from damaged liver cells. Protein metabolism tests show decreased total protein, decreased albumin, and increased globulin levels. The liver does not synthesize γ-globulins but does synthesize albumin. γ-Globulins (antibodies) are produced by B lymphocytes in the lymphatic system and spleen. The globulin level often increases in cirrhosis and indicates increased synthesis or decreased removal. Fat metabolism abnormalities are reflected by decreased cholesterol levels. Dye excretory tests, such as the indiocyanine green (ICG) test, show retention of the dye. The prothrombin time is prolonged, and bilirubin metabolism is altered (Table 41-11). Liver biopsy may be performed to identify liver cell changes and alterations in the lobular structure. Differential analysis of ascitic fluid may be helpful in establishing a diagnosis.

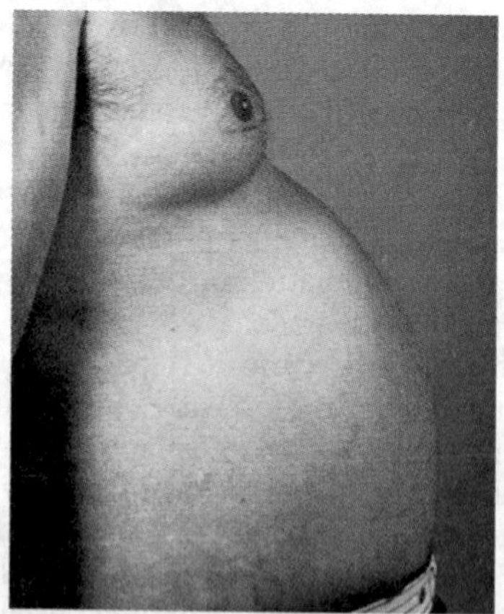

Fig. 41-6 Ascites and gynecomastia associated with cirrhosis of the liver. Photograph was taken after a paracentesis was performed.

Table 41-10 Factors Precipitating Hepatic Encephalopathy

Factor	Mechanism
GI hemorrhage	Increase in ammonia in GI tract
Constipation	Increase in ammonia from bacterial action on feces
Hypokalemia	Potassium ions are needed by brain to metabolize ammonia
Hypovolemia	Increase in blood ammonia by causing hepatic hypoxia; impairment of cerebral, hepatic, and renal function because of decreased blood flow
Infection	Increase in catabolism, increase in cerebral sensitivity to toxins
Cerebral depressants (e.g., narcotics)	No detoxification by liver, causing increase in cerebral depression
Metabolic alkalosis	Facilitation of transport of ammonia across blood-brain barrier, increase in renal production of ammonia
Paracentesis	Loss of sodium and potassium ions, decrease in blood volume
Dehydration	Potentiation of ammonia toxicity
Increased metabolism	Increase in workload of liver
Diuretics	Increase in renal formation of ammonia, possibly resulting in azotemia, which increases endogenous ammonia production; hypokalemia also possible
Uremia (renal failure)	Retention of nitrogenous metabolites

GI, Gastrointestinal.

Therapeutic Management

Rest. Although there is no specific therapy for cirrhosis, certain measures can be taken to promote liver cell regeneration and prevent or treat complications (Table 41-12). Rest is significant in reducing metabolic demands of the liver and allowing for recovery of liver cells. At various times during the progress of cirrhosis the rest may have to take the form of complete bed rest.

Table 41-11 Bilirubin Metabolism Abnormalities in Cirrhosis*

Type	Finding
Serum bilirubin	
Unconjugated	↑
Conjugated	↑
Urine bilirubin	↑
Urobilinogen	
Stool	Normal, ↓
Urine	Normal, ↑

*These are bilirubin metabolism abnormalities occurring with *hepatocellular jaundice,* the most frequent type of jaundice with cirrhosis.

Ascites. Management of ascites is focused on sodium restriction, diuretics, and fluid removal. A low-sodium diet is prescribed (250 to 500 mg per day). The patient is usually not on restricted fluids unless severe ascites develops. There should be accurate assessment and control of fluid and electrolyte balance. Bed rest initially produces diuresis, which increases fluid excretion. However, complete bed rest may not be necessary unless the patient has severe ascites. Salt-poor albumin may be used to help maintain intravascular volume and adequate urinary output by increasing plasma colloid osmotic pressure.

Diuretic therapy is an important part of management. Frequently a combination of drugs that work at multiple sites in the nephron is more effective. Spironolactone (Aldactone) is an effective diuretic, even in patients with severe sodium retention. Spironolactone is an antagonist of aldosterone and is potassium sparing. Other potassium-sparing diuretics are amiloride (Midamor) and triamterene (Dyrenium). A high-potency loop diuretic, such as furosemide (Lasix), is frequently used in combination with a potassium-sparing drug. Chlorothiazide (Diuril) or hydrochlorothiazide may also be used, but the thiazide diuretics are not as potent as the loop diuretics.

A *paracentesis* (needle puncture of the abdominal cavity) may be performed to remove ascitic fluid. However, it is reserved for the patient with impaired respiration or abdominal pain caused by severe ascites. It is only a temporary measure as the fluid tends to reaccumulate.

Peritoneovenous shunt. A surgical procedure, peritoneovenous shunt, provides for the continuous reinfusion of ascitic fluid into the venous system. One type is called the *LaVeen peritoneovenous shunt* and consists of a tube and a one-way valve. The tube runs from the abdominal cavity through the peritoneum, under the subcutaneous tissue, and into the jugular vein or superior vena cava (Fig. 41-7). The valve opens when the pressure in the peritoneal cavity is 3 to 5 cm H_2O higher than that in the superior vena cava. This allows the ascitic fluid to flow into the venous system. The patient's inspiration increases the intraperitoneal pressure, causing the valve to open. Another shunt, the *Denver shunt,* has a subcutaneous pump that irrigates the tubing when manually compressed. This shunting of the ascitic fluid causes an improvement in hemodynamic factors and

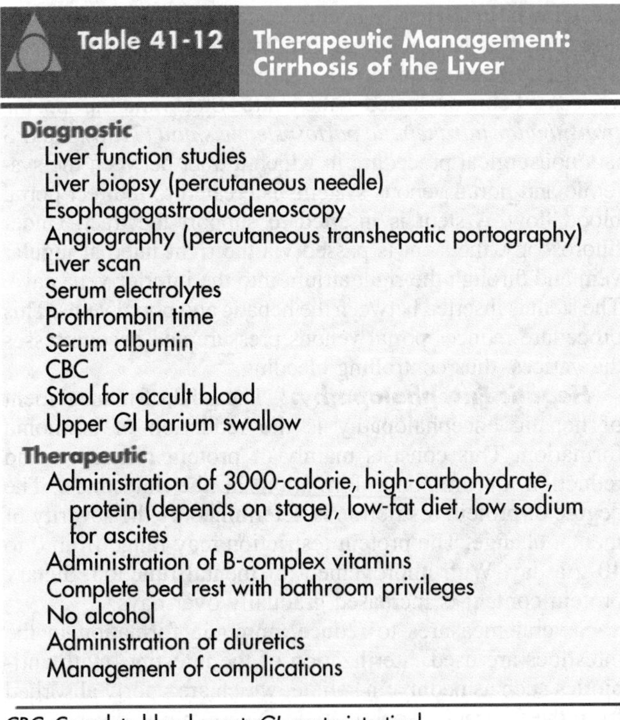
Table 41-12 Therapeutic Management: Cirrhosis of the Liver

Diagnostic
Liver function studies
Liver biopsy (percutaneous needle)
Esophagogastroduodenoscopy
Angiography (percutaneous transhepatic portography)
Liver scan
Serum electrolytes
Prothrombin time
Serum albumin
CBC
Stool for occult blood
Upper GI barium swallow
Therapeutic
Administration of 3000-calorie, high-carbohydrate, protein (depends on stage), low-fat diet, low sodium for ascites
Administration of B-complex vitamins
Complete bed rest with bathroom privileges
No alcohol
Administration of diuretics
Management of complications

CBC, Complete blood count; *GI,* gastrointestinal.

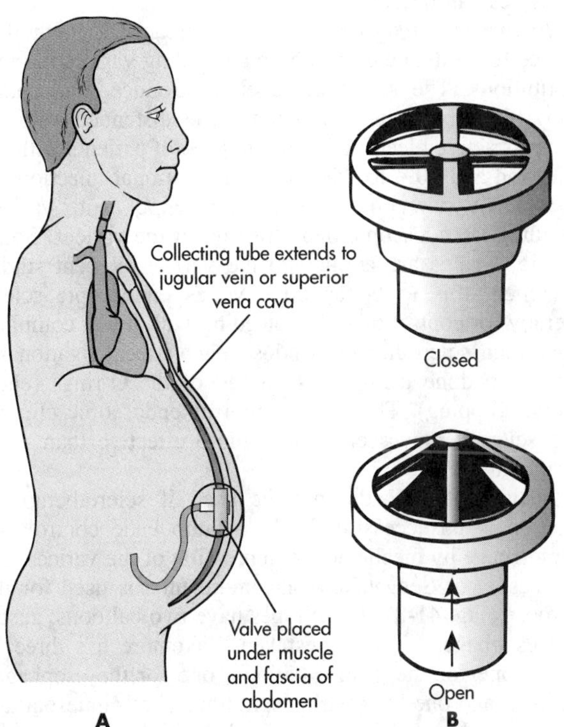

Fig. 41-7 LaVeen continuous peritoneovenous shunt. ***A,*** Collecting tube. ***B,*** Valve in closed and open positions.

increases sodium and fluid excretion. Urine output is also increased.

Esophageal Varices. The main therapeutic goal related to esophageal varices is avoidance of bleeding and hemorrhage. The patient who has esophageal varices should avoid ingesting alcohol, aspirin, and irritating foods. Upper respiratory infections should be treated promptly, and coughing should be controlled.

Management related to bleeding esophageal varices includes emergency, therapeutic, and prophylactic interventions.[19] Management measures used are vasopressin (VP) and nitroglycerin (NTG), β-blockers, balloon tamponade, sclerotherapy, ligation of varices, and shunt therapy.

When esophageal variceal bleeding occurs, the first step is to make a definitive diagnosis. This is important because patients with cirrhosis can also bleed from erosive gastritis, peptic ulcers, and Mallory-Weiss tears. The diagnosis is made by endoscopic examination as soon as possible. Lavage with a wide-bore nasogastric (NG) tube (e.g., Ewald) may be done to remove blood and clots to prepare the patient for endoscopy.

The initial measures to stop the bleeding include the intravenous administration of vasopressin (VP). VP produces vasoconstriction of the splanchnic arterial bed, decreased portal blood flow, and decreased portal hypertension. It has many side effects, including decreased coronary blood flow and heart rate and increased blood pressure. Current drug therapy in some institutions is a combination of VP and NTG. The NTG reduces the detrimental effects of the VP while enhancing its beneficial effect. The main goal of drug therapy is to stop bleeding so treatment measures can be done.

Endoscopic sclerotherapy is the treatment method of choice for both acute and chronic bleeding varices in many institutions. The sclerosing agent, introduced via endoscopy, thromboses and obliterates the distended veins. It controls active bleeding in 70% to 80% of patients with one injection and 90% to 95% with an additional injection.

A fairly new procedure for managing acute variceal bleeding is endoscopic band ligation of the varices. Small, elastic O-rings are applied to the varices. Recent studies document this to be as effective as endoscopic sclerotherapy for control of active bleeding with fewer complications than sclerotherapy. Endoscopic variceal ligation has also been done using clips instead of the O-rings (endoscopic clipping). The combination of endoscopic clipping and sclerotherapy seems to be more effective than either treatment alone.[20]

Balloon tamponade may be used if sclerotherapy or ligation is unsuccessful. Balloon tamponade controls the hemorrhage by mechanical compression of the varices. The Minnesota or Sengstaken-Blakemore tube is used for this purpose (Fig. 41-8). These tubes have two balloons: gastric and esophageal. The Sengstaken-Blakemore has three lumens: one for the gastric balloon, one for the esophageal balloon, and one for gastric aspiration. The Minnesota tube has an esophageal aspiration port. When inflated, the gastric and esophageal balloons put mechanical compression on the varices. The gastric balloon anchors the tube in position and also applies pressure to any bleeding gastric varices.

Supportive measures during an acute variceal bleed include administration of fresh frozen plasma and packed RBCs, vitamin K (Aquamephyton), and histamine (H_2) blockers such as cimetidine (Tagamet). Neomycin administration may be started to prevent hepatic encephalopathy from breakdown of blood and the release of ammonia in the intestine.

Long-term management. Long-term management of patients who have had an episode of bleeding includes repeated sclerotherapy, endoscopic ligation, β-blockers, and portosystemic shunts. There is a high incidence of recurrent bleeding with a high mortality risk with each bleeding episode, so continued therapy is necessary. Repeated endoscopic sclerotherapy is commonly used. Endoscopic ligation or a combination of it with sclerotherapy is continuing to be evaluated.

Propranolol (Inderal), a β-blocker, can be given orally to prevent recurrent GI bleeding. It reduces portal venous pressure. This effect is due to reduced cardiac output and possibly constriction of splanchnic vessels. However, because it reduces hepatic blood flow, it can enhance the possibility of hepatic encephalopathy.

Various surgical shunting procedures may be used to decrease portal hypertension by diverting some of the portal blood flow while at the same time allowing adequate liver perfusion. Currently, the shunts most commonly used are the *portacaval shunt* and the *distal splenorenal shunt* (Fig. 41-9). Shunts are indicated more after a second major bleeding episode than an initial bleeding episode. Although a prophylactic portacaval shunt lessens bleeding, it does not prolong life. Patients die of hepatic encephalopathy caused by the diversion of the ammonia past the liver and into the systemic circulation. The distal splenorenal shunt (Warren shunt) leaves portal venous flow intact (see Fig. 41-9), so it has a lower incidence of hepatic encephalopathy. With time, however, the flow of blood through the liver decreases.

An experimental procedure for the treatment of esophageal varices is being evaluated in the United States and Europe: the *transjugular intrahepatic portosystemic shunt (TIPS).*[21] TIPS is a nonsurgical procedure in which a tract between the systemic and portal venous systems is created to redirect portal blood flow. A stent is inserted to support the tract. Under fluoroscopy, the stent is passed via the right internal jugular vein and through the right atrium into the inferior vena cava. The stent is inserted between the hepatic and portal veins. This procedure reduces portal venous pressure and decompresses the varices, thus controlling bleeding.[22]

Hepatic Encephalopathy. The goal of management of hepatic encephalopathy is the reduction of ammonia formation. This consists mainly of protein restriction and reduction of ammonia formation in the intestines. The degree of protein restriction is determined by the severity of mental change. The protein restriction may range from 0 to 40 g a day. With improvement of mental function, dietary protein content is increased gradually over days.

Several measures to reduce ammonia formation in the intestines are used. Sterilization of the intestines with antibiotics such as neomycin sulfate, which are poorly absorbed from the GI tract, is one method. Neomycin is given orally or rectally. This reduces the bacterial flora of the colon.

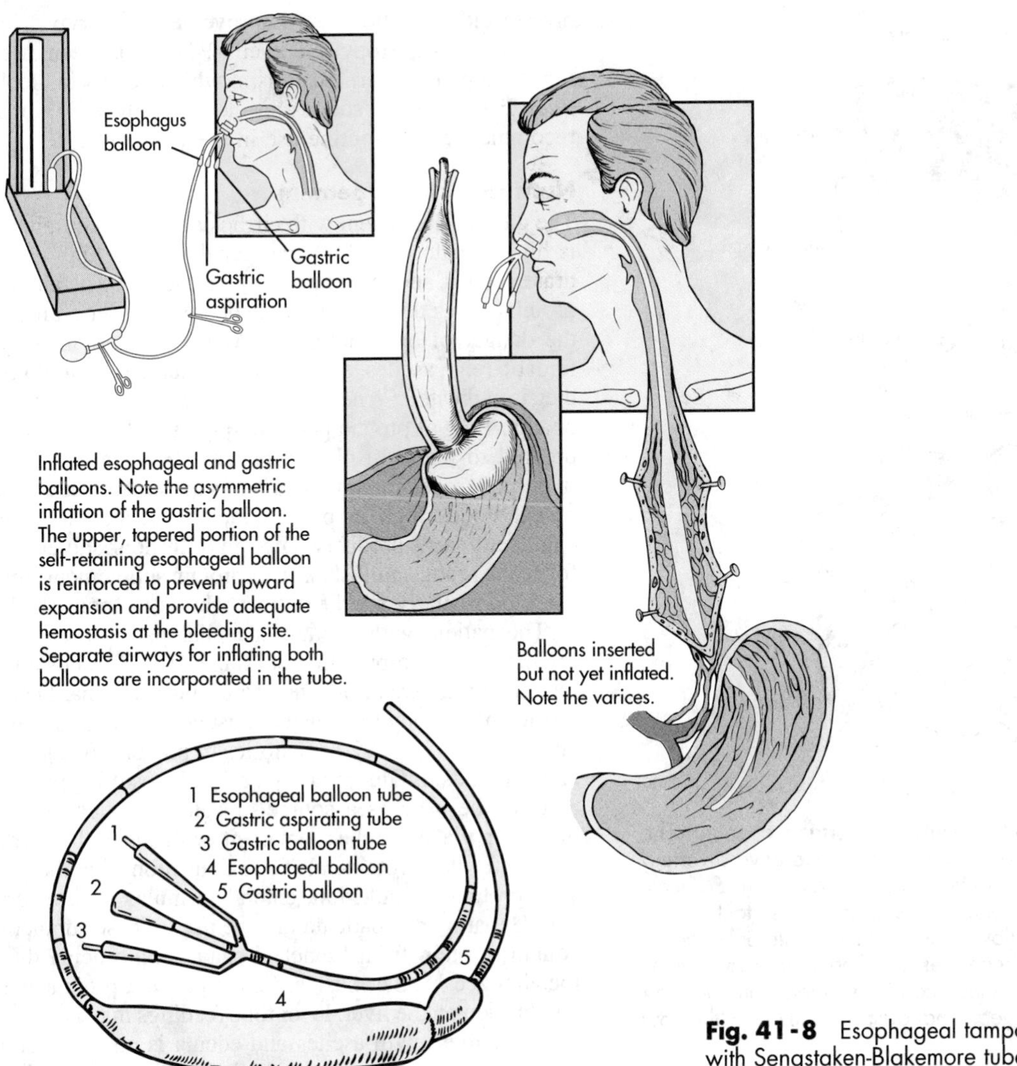

Fig. 41-8 Esophageal tamponade accomplished with Sengstaken-Blakemore tube.

Bacterial action on protein in the feces results in ammonia production. Cathartics and enemas are also used to decrease bacterial action. Constipation should be prevented.

Lactulose (Cephulac) may also be used to treat hepatic encephalopathy. This is a synthetic ketoanalog of lactose. In the colon, it is split into lactic acid and acetic acid, which decreases the pH from 7.0 to 5.0. The acidic environment discourages bacterial growth. The lactulose traps the ammonia in the gut, and the laxative effect of the drug expels the ammonia from the colon. It is usually given orally but may be given as a retention enema or via NG tube. Because neomycin may cause renal toxicity and hearing impairments, lactulose is frequently the preferred drug.

Levodopa has been used in the treatment of hepatic encephalopathy. It is a precursor of dopamine and norepinephrine. Use of levodopa is based on the theory that there is a deficiency of dopamine and norepinephrine in encephalopathy because they are replaced by false transmitters (amines from breakdown of dietary proteins). Normally these false transmitters are destroyed by liver enzymes, but when the liver is diseased, this no longer happens. There is limited evidence that the use of levodopa prolongs the lives of patients with coma resistant to other measures.

Control of hepatic encephalopathy also involves treatment of precipitating causes (see Table 41-10). This involves controlling GI hemorrhage and removing the blood from the GI tract to decrease the protein in the intestine. Electrolyte and acid-base imbalances and infections should also be treated.

Liver transplantation should be considered in patients with recurring hepatic encephalopathy and end-stage liver disease. The use of liver transplantation depends on a number of factors, including the cause of the cirrhosis and other systemic medical problems.[23]

Pharmacologic Management

There is no specific drug therapy for cirrhosis. However, a number of medications are used to treat symptoms and complications of advanced liver disease (Table 41-13). Some drug therapy is being used in the treatment of cirrhosis to try to prevent or reverse the fibrosis that occurs in the liver. The use of Colbenemid (combination of colchicine and

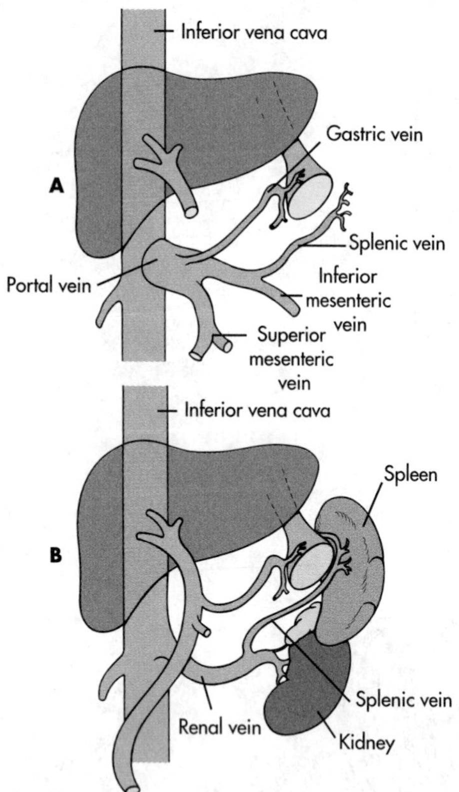

Fig. 41-9 Portosystemic shunts. ***A,*** Portacaval shunt. The portal vein is anastomosed to the inferior vena cava diverting blood from the portal vein to the systemic circulation. ***B,*** Distal splenorenal shunt. The splenic vein is anastomosed to the renal vein. The portal venous flow remains intact while esophageal varices are selectively decompressed. (The short gastric veins are decompressed.) The spleen conducts blood from the high pressure of the esophageal and gastric varices to the low pressure renal vein.

probenecid) has shown an improvement in survival in cirrhotic patients. Propylthiouracil (PTU) has been used to reduce hepatic hypermetabolism, which occurs in alcoholic liver disease. More studies are needed before PTU can be recommended for routine use in these patients.

Nutritional Management

The diet for the patient with cirrhosis without complications is high in calories (3000 kcal per day) with high carbohydrate content and moderate to low fat levels. The amount of protein varies depending on the degree of liver damage and the danger of encephalopathy. When the patient is symptomatic (e.g., ascites, edema, mental changes), a low-protein diet is indicated. When there is reduced risk of encephalopathy, 1.5 g of protein per kilogram of body weight may be ordered to maintain plasma osmotic balance and promote liver cell regeneration. Vitamin supplements are usually given. Foods high in protein include meat, fish, poultry, eggs, and dairy products. High-protein nourishment in the form of eggnogs, milkshakes, or protein supplements may be used, particularly for the patient who is malnourished.

The patient with hepatic encephalopathy is on a very-low-protein to no-protein diet (Table 41-14). Foods allowed include toast, cereal, rice, tea, fruit juices, and hard candies. Sufficient carbohydrate intake must be provided to maintain an intake of 1500 to 2000 calories to prevent hypoglycemia and catabolism. Glucose polymer (Polycose) is protein free and can be used as a source of calories. It can be given orally or via NG tube. A patient with alcoholic cirrhosis frequently has protein-calorie malnutrition. For the patient with protein malnutrition, enteral formulas such as Travasorb Hepatic or Hepaticaid may be used. These supplements contain protein from branched-chain amino acids that are metabolized by the muscles. They provide protein but put less burden on the liver. IV or tube feedings may be required.

The patient with ascites and edema is on a low-sodium diet. The degree of sodium restriction varies depending on

Table 41-13 Medications Used in Cirrhosis

Medication	Mechanism of Action
Vasopressin (Pitressin)	Hemostasis and control of bleeding in esophageal varices, constriction of splanchnic arterial bed
Propranolol (Inderal)	Reduction of portal venous pressure, prevention of gastrointestinal bleeding
Neomycin sulfate	Decrease in bacterial flora, decreasing formation of ammonia
Lactulose (Cephulac)	Acidification of feces in bowel and trapping of ammonia, causing its elimination in feces
Levodopa	Conversion to dopamine, which has been displaced with amines from protein breakdown, to increase vascular resistance
Cimetidine (Tagamet)	Decrease in gastric acidity
Diuretics	
Spironolactone (Aldactone)	Blocking of action of aldosterone, potassium sparing
Chlorothiazide (Diuril)	Thiazide that acts on proximal tubule to decrease reabsorption of sodium and potassium ions and water
Furosemide (Lasix)	Rapid action on distal tubule and loop of Henle to prevent reabsorption of sodium and potassium ions and water
Magnesium sulfate	Magnesium replacement; hypomagnesemia occurs with liver dysfunction
Vitamin K (Synkavite)	Correction of clotting abnormalities

Table 41-14 Nutritional Management: Low-Protein Diet for Hepatic Failure

General Principles
Limit protein to 20 g per day at onset of severe hepatic failure.
Protein must be from protein sources with high biologic value.
Diet must be high in calories.
Fat is limited only to prevent early satiety.
Protein is increased in diet by 10 g increments as tolerated without causing signs and symptoms of hepatic encephalopathy.
Sodium is also usually restricted as well as fluid when edema and ascites are present.

Meal	Menu Plan 1	Menu Plan 2	Menu Plan 3
Breakfast 1 fruit, calorie supplement 1 low-protein bread 1 egg (protein) Fat, calorie supplement ¼ cup milk (2 g protein)	½ cup grape juice with 2 tbs Polycose powder[†] French toast made with low-protein bread, 1 egg, 3 tsp salt-free butter and syrup ¼ cup milk	¼ cup cranberry juice with 2 tbs Polycose powder Low-protein toast with 3 tsp salt-free butter and 2 tsp jelly 1-egg omelet with 3 tsp salt-free butter ¼ cup milk	¼ cup prune juice with 2 tbs Polycose powder Low-protein toast with 3 tsp salt-free butter 1 egg fried in 3 tsp salt-free butter ¼ cup milk
Snack Calorie supplement	Jelly beans	Hard candy	Sugar mints
Lunch 2 starch (4 g protein) 1 vegetable (2 g protein) 1 fruit, calorie supplement Fat, calorie supplement	¼ cup half and half ½ cup Cream of Wheat with 3 tsp salt-free butter Applesauce with whipped topping or Lipomul[‡] Small tossed salad with 3 tbs oil and vinegar[§] Peas with 3 tsp salt-free butter	¼ cup half and half ½ cup cornmeal (atole) with 3 tsp salt-free butter Small guacamole salad Gelatin with whipped topping or Lipomul Corn with 3 tsp salt-free butter.	¼ cup half and half ½ cup grits with 3 tsp salt-free butter Cucumbers in sour cream Peaches with whipped topping or Lipomul Sweet potatoes with brown sugar and 3 tsp salt-free butter
Snack Calorie supplement	Low-protein cookies	Low-protein bread cubes with whipped cream and strawberries	Popsicles made with Polycose
Dinner 1 starch (2 g protein) 1 vegetable (2 g protein) 1 low-protein bread ¼ cup milk (2 g protein) Fat, calorie supplement	½ baked potato 3 tsp salt-free butter Low-protein bread ¼ cup sour cream ½ cup green beans with 3 tsp salt-free butter and 2 tsp jelly ¼ cup milk	½ cup fried potatoes with 1 tsp melted salt-free butter ½ cup zucchini with 3 tsp salt-free butter Low-protein toast with 3 tsp salt-free butter and 2 tsp marmalade ¼ cup milk	½ cup mashed potatoes ½ cup fried okra Low-protein toast with 3 tsp salt-free butter and 2 tsp jam ¼ cup milk

*The diet plan contains approximately 20 g protein.
[†]Polycose is a brand-name product made by Ross Laboratories.
[‡]Lipomul is a fat emulsion made by Upjohn.
[§]Crisp food should be avoided because of the possibility of esophageal varices.

the patient's condition. The patient needs instruction regarding the degree of restriction. Table salt is the most common source of sodium. Sodium is also present in baking soda and baking powder. Foods that are high in sodium content include canned soups and vegetables, salted snacks such as potato chips, nuts, smoked meats and fish, crackers, breads, olives, pickles, catsup, and beer.

Sodium is also present in many over-the-counter medications (e.g., antacids). However, most antacids are now lower in sodium than previously. Carbonated beverages tend to be high in sodium, and low-sodium and sodium-free carbonated drinks are available. The patient should be advised to read labels. Foods high in protein usually have large amounts of sodium. Alternative protein supplements that are low in sodium may have to be used. The patient and the family need assistance to make the diet more palatable by the use of seasonings such as garlic, parsley, onion, lemon juice, and spices.

NURSING MANAGEMENT

CIRRHOSIS

Nursing Assessment

Subjective and objective data that should be obtained from an individual with cirrhosis are presented in Table 41-15.

Nursing Diagnoses

Nursing diagnoses are determined when the problem and the etiologic factors are supported by clinical data. Nursing diagnoses related to cirrhosis may include, but are not limited to, those presented in the nursing care plan for the patient with cirrhosis on p. 1281.

Table 41-15 Nursing Assessment: Cirrhosis

Subjective Data

Important health information

Past health history: Alcohol abuse; previous hepatitis; chronic biliary obstruction and infection; severe right-sided heart failure; exposure to carbon tetrachloride, benzene derivatives, or other hepatotoxic agents

Medications: Adverse reaction to any medication; use of anticoagulants, aspirin, acetaminophen

Functional health patterns

Health perception–health management: Weakness, fatigue

Nutritional-metabolic: Anorexia, weight loss, dyspepsia, nausea and vomiting; pruritis, dry skin; bleeding and bruising tendencies

Elimination: Dark urine; light-colored stools, change in bowel habits

Cognitive-perceptual: Dull, right upper quadrant or epigastric pain; numbness, tingling of extremities

Sexuality-reproductive: Impotence, amenorrhea

Objective Data

General

Cachexia, wasting of extremities

Integumentary

Icteric sclera, jaundice, petechiae, ecchymoses, spider angiomas, alopecia, edema, palmar erythema, loss of axillary and pubic hair

Cardiovascular

Peripheral edema, ascites

Gastrointestinal

Abdominal distention, palpable liver and spleen, foul breath, GI bleeding, red tongue, hemorrhoids

Reproductive

Gynecomastia and testicular atrophy (men), impotence (men), loss of libido, amenorrhea or heavy menstrual bleeding (women)

Neurologic

Altered mentation, asterixis

Possible findings

Anemia, thrombocytopenia; leukopenia; abnormal liver function studies; elevated coagulation studies, ammonia, and bilirubin levels; abnormal abdominal ultrasound and liver scan; positive liver biopsy

GI, Gastrointestinal.

Planning

The overall goals are that the patient with cirrhosis will (1) have relief of discomfort; (2) have minimal to no complications (ascites, esophageal varices, hepatic encephalopathy); and (3) return to as normal a lifestyle as possible. Specific outcomes are identified in the nursing care plan for the patient with cirrhosis on p. 1281.

Nursing Implementation

Health Promotion and Maintenance. The common etiologies of cirrhosis are alcohol, malnutrition, hepatitis, biliary obstruction, and right-sided heart failure. Prevention and early treatment of cirrhosis must focus on the primary etiology. Alcoholism must be treated (see Chapter 8). Adequate nutrition, especially for the alcoholic and other individuals at risk for cirrhosis, is essential to promote liver regeneration. Hepatitis must be identified and treated early so that it does not progress to chronic hepatitis. Biliary disease must be treated so that the stones do not cause obstruction and infection. The underlying cause (e.g., chronic lung disease) of right-sided heart failure must be treated so that the heart failure does not lead to cirrhosis.

Acute Intervention. The focus of nursing care for the patient with cirrhosis is on conserving the patient's strength (see the nursing care plan for the patient with cirrhosis). Rest enables the liver to restore itself. Complete bed rest may not always be necessary. When the patient requires complete bed rest, measures to prevent pneumonia, thromboembolic problems, and pressure ulcers should be taken. The activity and rest schedule may be modified according to signs of clinical improvement (e.g., decreasing jaundice, improvement in liver function studies). Major concerns of the nurse in determining appropriate nursing care measures to meet the need for rest involve regulation of the physical, emotional, and social climate.[24]

Anorexia, nausea and vomiting, pressure from ascites, and poor eating habits all create problems in maintenance of an adequate intake of nutrients. The nursing measures relating to nutrition for patients with hepatitis also apply here. Oral hygiene before meals may improve the patient's taste sensation. Between-meal nourishments should be available so that they can be provided at times when the patient can best tolerate them. Food preferences should be provided whenever possible. Explanations to the patient and the family of the reason for any dietary restrictions should be provided.

Nursing assessment and care should include the patient's physiologic response to cirrhosis. Is jaundice present? Where is it observed—sclera, skin, hard palate? What is the progression of jaundice? If the jaundice is accompanied by pruritus, measures to relieve itching should be carried out. Cholestyramine (Questran) may be ordered to help relieve the pruritus. The color of the urine and stools should be noted. With jaundice the urine is often cola-colored or mahogany and the stool gray or tan.

Edema and ascites are frequent manifestations of cirrhosis and require nursing assessments and interventions. Accurate calculation and recordings of intake and output, daily weights, and measurements of extremities and ab-

NURSING CARE PLAN Patient with Cirrhosis

Planning: Outcome Criteria	Nursing Interventions and Rationales
➤ **NURSING DIAGNOSIS**	Altered nutrition: less than body requirements *related to* anorexia, impaired utilization and storage of nutrients, nausea, and loss of nutrients from vomiting *as manifested by* lack of interest in food, aversion to eating, reported inadequate food intake, perceived inability to ingest food
Have adequate intake of nutrients; maintain normal body weight.	Monitor weight *to determine if weight loss occurs.* Provide oral care before meals *to remove foul taste and improve taste of food.* Administer antiemetics as ordered *to relieve vomiting by depressing the chemoreceptor trigger zone.* Provide small, frequent meals with nourishments at times the patient can best tolerate them *to prevent feeling of fullness and maintain nutritional status.* Determine food preferences and allow these whenever possible *to increase nutritional appeal for patient because a low-protein or no-protein diet is unpalatable.*
➤ **NURSING DIAGNOSIS**	Impaired skin integrity *related to* edema, ascites, and pruritis *as manifested by* complaints of itching; areas of excoriation caused by scratching; taut, shiny skin over edematous areas; areas of skin breakdown
Maintain skin integrity; have relief of pruritus.	Restrict sodium intake as ordered *to prevent additional fluid retention.* Restrict fluids if ordered *to reduce fluid retention.* Administer prescribed diuretics *to prevent fluid retention and promote diuresis.* Observe for side effects *that may result from diuretic therapy.* Monitor intake and output *to maintain necessary fluid restrictions and assess renal function.* Assess location and extent of edema by weighing patient at the same time each day, taking daily measurements of extremities and abdominal girth (same location each time) *to measure patient's response to treatment.* Provide meticulous skin care *because edematous tissues are easily traumatized and subject to breakdown.* Reposition patient at least q2hr *to relieve pressure over bony prominences.* Do range-of-motion exercises *to maintain joint function and muscle strength.* Elevate edematous areas *to promote venous drainage, increase the patient's comfort and ability to breathe.* Have patient use special mattress, such as alternating-air pressure or egg crate mattress *to reduce the risk of skin breakdown from prolonged pressure.* Clip patient's nails short and keep clean *to prevent excoriation caused by pruritus secondary to deposit of bile salts in skin.* Administer antipruritic medication as ordered *to relieve itching.* Provide diversions and distractions *to assist patient in coping with the discomfort of itching and edema.*
➤ **NURSING DIAGNOSIS**	Ineffective breathing pattern *related to* pressure on diaphragm and reduced lung volume secondary to ascites *as manifested by* dyspnea, shortness of breath, tachypnea, cyanosis, cough, changes in pulse or respiratory rate, depth, or pattern
Be able to breathe with minimal difficulty; have effective breathing pattern, absence of cyanosis and other signs and symptoms of hypoxia.	Place patient in semi-Fowler's or Fowler's position; support patient's arms and chest with pillows *to facilitate breathing by relieving pressure on diaphragm.* Auscultate chest for crackles *to identify collection of fluid in lungs.* Assess respiratory rate and rhythm *to identify increasing dyspnea.*
➤ **NURSING DIAGNOSIS**	Risk for injury *related to* diminished sensory perception secondary to peripheral neuropathy
Have no injury caused by decreased sensory perception.	Assess for numbness and tingling of lower extremities, decreased sensation in lower extremities *to determine risk of injury.* Prevent excess stimulation or trauma to extremities *because patient may not be able to detect harmful stimuli.* Do not use restrictive bed linens, *which reduce circulation and place pressure on edematous tissue.* Instruct patient to avoid tight clothing, *which impedes circulation.* Use care with heat and cold applications *because patient's ability to perceive temperature is impaired.* Assist with ambulation *to assess patient's ability to safely ambulate and to prevent injury.*

continued

NURSING CARE PLAN Patient with Cirrhosis—cont'd

Planning: Outcome Criteria	Nursing Interventions and Rationales
➤ **NURSING DIAGNOSIS**	Activity intolerance *related to* fatigue, anemia, ascites, dyspnea, treatment schedule, and cardiac deconditioning *as manifested by* fatigue or weakness, abnormal heart rate or blood pressure, altered response to activity and weakness
Feel rested; have increased tolerance for activity.	Assess patient's ability to perform activities *to plan appropriate interventions.* Conserve patient's strength *to minimize cardiac and respiratory work.* Provide activity and rest as required by regulating physical, emotional, and social climate *to reduce metabolic demands on the liver, reduce hepatic blood flow, and allow for recovery of liver cells.* Monitor hemoglobin and hematocrit levels *to detect GI hemorrhage.* Plan scheduled rest periods for patient *to promote liver cell regeneration and decrease fatigue.* Assist with activities of daily living as needed *to ensure patient's needs are met.*
➤ **NURSING DIAGNOSIS**	Body-image disturbance *related to* changes in appearance and body function *as manifested by* verbalization of dissatisfaction with appearance, avoidance of contact with others, disparaging remarks about self and body, preoccupation with body
Accept altered body image.	Assess patient's response *to determine extent of patient's body image disturbance.* Present an accepting attitude *because patient is very sensitive to body changes.* Be a supportive listener *to help the person feel valued.* Care for the patient with concern and warmth *to convey nonjudgmental attitude.* Explain changes in body image *to promote patient's understanding and sense of control and cooperation.* Assure patient and family that jaundice is not permanent *to relieve anxiety.* Encourage actions to promote appearance, such as use of makeup, *to enhance the person's self-esteem.*
➤ **NURSING DIAGNOSIS**	Risk for infection *related to* leukopenia and increased susceptibility to environmental pathogens
No signs or symptoms of infections.	Use appropriate infection control measures. Assess patient for evidence of risk factors, including leukopenia, altered immune response, and altered circulation *to ensure early identification of infection.* Monitor patient's temperature q2-4 hr *because fever is an indicator of infection.* Observe for any local and systemic manifestations of infection *to enable early diagnosis and treatment.* Protect patient from others with infections *to reduce the risk of infection secondary to decreased resistance.* Monitor WBC count *to assess patient's response to treatment.*
➤ **NURSING DIAGNOSIS**	Ineffective management of therapeutic regimen *related to* lack of knowledge regarding importance of consistent follow-up care, signs, and symptoms of complications, proper diet, and alcohol restrictions *as manifested by* reports or demonstrations of an unhealthy practice or lifestyle (e.g., substance abuse, alcohol), expressions of inaccurate perception of health status, verbalization of deficiency in knowledge or skill
Maintain state of wellness at highest level possible for patient; verbalize understanding of disease process; initiate necessary changes in lifestyle.	Explain to patient and family importance of continuous health care *so problems can be detected early and treatment initiated.* Teach patient and family symptoms of complications and when to seek medical attention *to enable prompt treatment of complications.* Teach proper diet *because a low-protein, high-carbohydrate diet is usually indicated and can be difficult to follow.* Teach patient to avoid potentially hepatotoxic over-the-counter drugs *because diseased liver is unable to metabolize these medications.* Encourage abstinence from alcohol *because continued use of alcohol will increase the risk of liver complications.* Instruct patient to avoid aspirin and control cough *to prevent hemorrhage in the patient with esophageal varices.* Have patient avoid spicy and rough foods and activities that increase portal pressure, such as straining at stool, coughing, sneezing, and retching and vomiting *because hemorrhage is a danger because of inability of liver to produce factors necessary for coagulation.*

continued

NURSING CARE PLAN Patient with Cirrhosis—cont'd

Planning: Outcome Criteria	*Nursing Interventions and Rationales*
➤ **NURSING DIAGNOSIS**	Total self-care deficit *related to* weakness, fatigue, balance and gait disturbances, and dyspnea *as manifested by* inability to initiate or complete self-care activities
Have care needs met by self or others.	Assess patient's ability to care for self *to plan amount of assistance required.* Perform activities of care patient cannot do *to ensure that care is provided and fatigue minimized.* Maintain positive caring attitude while giving care *to enhance patient's sense of self-esteem.* Encourage patient to resume self-care activities when able *because self-care enhances feelings of self-worth.*
➤ **NURSING DIAGNOSIS**	Sleep pattern disturbance *related to* frequent assessments and treatments, discomfort, and inability to assume usual sleep position because of orthopnea *as manifested by* interruption in sleep cycles, complaints of tiredness, frequent napping
Verbalize feeling of being rested; have longer periods of uninterrupted sleep.	Plan care to allow uninterrupted period for sleep *so patient can experience full cycles of sleep.* Assist patient to assume comfortable position for sleep such as side-lying or semi-Fowler's position *to relieve discomfort caused by abdominal pressure.*
➤ **NURSING DIAGNOSIS**	Ineffective airway clearance *related to* inability to remove and swallow secretions and bleeding from esophageal varices *as manifested by* ineffective cough; inability to remove airway secretions; abnormal breath sounds; abnormal respiratory rate, rhythm, depth
Have patent airway, normal breath sounds.	Suction patient (oral and pharyngeal areas) frequently *to reduce risk of aspiration because patient is unable to swallow with Sengstaken-Blakemore (SB) tube in place.* Place in semi-Fowler's position *to facilitate drainage from mouth and ease breathing by reducing intraabdominal pressure.* Have scissors near bed to cut SB tube (if necessary) *to prevent a displaced esophageal balloon from obstructing the airway.* (Indications include increased respiratory rate, cyanosis, dyspnea.) Encourage patient to expectorate *because the patient is unable to swallow saliva while the inflated esophageal balloon occludes the esophagus.* Offer frequent oral and nasal care to provide relief from taste of blood and irritation from mouth bleeding.

COLLABORATIVE PROBLEMS

Nursing Goals	*Nursing Interventions and Rationales*
➤ **POTENTIAL COMPLICATION**	Hepatic encephalopathy *related to* increased formation of ammonia and aromatic amino acids
Monitor for signs of hepatic encephalopathy; report deviation from acceptable parameters and carry out appropriate medical and nursing interventions.	Monitor for encephalopathy by assessing patient's general behavior, orientation to time and place, speech, blood pH and ammonia levels *because liver is unable to convert accumulating ammonia to urea for renal excretion.* Encourage fluids (if not restricted) and give laxatives and enemas as ordered *to decrease production of ammonia.* Provide low-protein or no-protein diet as ordered *because ammonia (a breakdown product of protein) is responsible for mental changes.* Limit physical activity *because exercise produces ammonia as a byproduct of metabolism.* Control factors known to precipitate coma.

continued

dominal girth help in the ongoing assessment of the location and extent of the edema. If the patient can assume a kneeling position when abdominal girth measurement is taken, the abdominal fluid will go to the most dependent part of the abdomen. This gives the best measurement of abdominal girth. For many patients, girth must be measured in the standing or lying position. Where the measurements are taken should be recorded and should be a part of the nursing care plan.

When a paracentesis is done the nurse must have the patient void immediately before the procedure to prevent puncture of the bladder. The patient should sit on the side of the bed or be placed in high Fowler's position. Following the procedure the nurse should monitor for hypovolemia,

NURSING CARE PLAN Patient with Cirrhosis—cont'd

Nursing Goals	Nursing Interventions and Rationales
➤ **POTENTIAL COMPLICATION** Hemorrhage *related to* bleeding tendency secondary to altered clotting factors	
Monitor for signs of hemorrhage and initiate appropriate medical and nursing interventions.	Monitor for hemorrhage by assessing for epistaxis, purpura, petechiae, easy bruising, gingival bleeding, heavy menstrual bleeding, hematuria, melena *because liver disease results in impaired synthesis of clotting factors.* Provide gentle nursing care *to minimize the risk of tissue trauma.* Provide assistance with ambulation as needed *to prevent injury.* Observe for bleeding from body orifices, urine, and stool *to detect bleeding early and allow prompt intervention.* Use smallest-gauge needle possible when giving injection and apply gentle but prolonged pressure after injection *to minimize risk of bleeding into tissue.* Advise use of soft-bristle toothbrush *to reduce trauma to mouth because mucous membranes have increased risk of injury resulting from high vascularity.* Teach patient to avoid straining at stool, vigorous blowing of nose, coughing *to reduce risk of hemorrhage from these areas.* Observe for signs of thrombocytopenia such as purpura on the forearms, axillae, and skin *because subacute DIC may develop secondary to altered clotting factors.* Monitor laboratory results (hematocrit, hemoglobin, and prothrombin time) *as indicators of anemia, active bleeding, or impending complications (e.g., DIC).*

DIC, Disseminated intravascular coagulation; *GI*, gastrointestinal; *WBC*, white blood cell.

electrolyte imbalances, and check the dressing for bleeding and leakage.

Dyspnea is a frequent problem for the patient with ascites. A semi-Fowler's or Fowler's position allows for maximal respiratory efficiency. Pillows can be used to support the arms and chest and may increase the patient's comfort and ability to breathe.

Meticulous skin care is essential because the edematous tissues are subject to breakdown. An alternating–air pressure mattress or other special mattress should be used. A turning schedule (minimum of every 2 hours) must be adhered to rigidly. The abdomen may be supported with pillows. If the abdomen is taut, cleansing must be done very gently. This patient tends to move very little because of the abdominal discomfort and dyspnea. Therefore range-of-motion exercises are helpful, and measures such as coughing and deep breathing to prevent respiratory problems should be implemented. The lower extremities may be elevated. If scrotal edema is present, a scrotal support provides some comfort.

When the patient is taking diuretics, the serum levels of sodium, potassium, chloride, and bicarbonate should be monitored. The patient should be observed for signs of fluid and electrolyte imbalance, especially hypokalemia. Hypokalemia may be manifested by cardiac dysrhythmias, hypotension, tachycardia, and generalized muscle weakness. Water excess is manifested by muscle cramping, weakness, lethargy, and confusion.

Observations and nursing care in relation to hematologic disorders (bleeding tendencies, anemia, increased susceptibility to infection) are the same as for the patient with advanced liver disease (see the nursing care plan for the patient with cirrhosis, p. 1281).

The nurse must assess the patient's response to altered body image resulting from jaundice, spider angiomas, palmar erythema, ascites, and gynecomastia. The patient may experience a great deal of anxiety regarding these changes. The nurse should explain these phenomena and should be a supportive listener. Nursing care with concern and warmth regardless of physical changes helps the patient maintain self-esteem.

Bleeding esophageal varices. If the patient has esophageal varices in addition to cirrhosis, the nurse must be observant of any signs of bleeding from the varices, such as hematemesis and melena. If hematemesis occurs, the nurse should assess the patient for hemorrhage, call the physician, and be ready to assist with whatever treatment is used to control the bleeding. The patient will be admitted to the ICU. The patient's airway must be maintained.

When balloon tamponade is used, the initial nursing task related to insertion of the tube is to explain the use of the tube and how it will be inserted. The balloons should be checked for patency. Sometimes the stomach is lavaged with saline solution before insertion of the tube. It is usually the physician's responsibility to insert the tube. It may be inserted via the nose or the mouth (see Fig. 41-8). The placement of the tube is ascertained by x-ray. Then the gastric balloon is inflated with approximately 250 ml of air and the tube is retracted until resistance (gastroesophageal junction) is felt. The tube is secured by placement of a piece of sponge or foam rubber at the nostrils (nasal cuff). This protects the mucosal surfaces from irritation and injury. For continued bleeding the esophageal balloon is then inflated. A sphygmomanometer is used to maintain and measure the desired pressure at 20 to 40 mm Hg. The position of the balloons is verified by x-ray. Sometimes it is

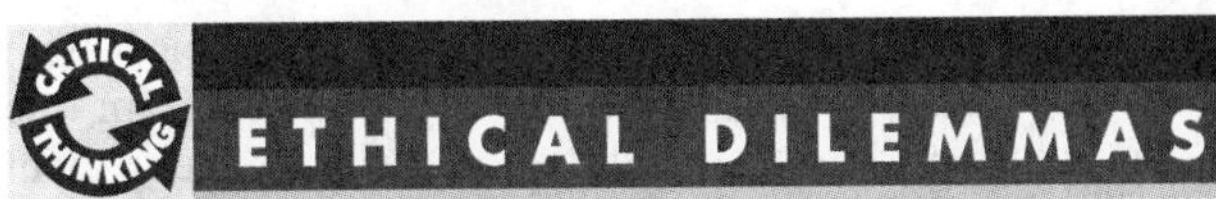

RATIONING

Situation A 43-year-old woman with cirrhosis of the liver is frequently admitted to the hospital. She has been told that her continued drinking will inevitably lead to her death. Now she has been admitted for GI bleeding and needs blood transfusions. She has a rare blood type and it is frequently difficult to get compatible blood. Should the nurse call for an ethics consultation?

Discussion A noncompliant patient whose behavior has led to a worsening of the disease process raises difficult ethical problems regarding rationing care. Rationing treatment of a manageable presenting problem probably would not be discussed for a cancer or a trauma patient. However, because alcoholism is understood as a disease with a behavioral component, this patient could be seen to be both noncompliant and unworthy of additional treatment. If the GI problem can be treated and transfusions are integral to that treatment, will that change the overall condition of the patient with regard to her cirrhosis? Will it extend her life or improve the quality of her life? If her underlying disease and quality of life cannot be treated or improved, this treatment could be seen as medically futile and therefore not required. Rationing decisions should be made based on triage, when necessary, rather than assessments of compliance or moral depravity. If the blood supply is very low and desperately needed by a patient whose disease or condition can be effectively treated by transfusions, rationing treatment to the patient with cirrhosis might be appropriate. However, if the blood supply is sufficient and no other patients are in competition for it, this is not a rationing decision. However, this continues to be a medical futility issue, and may eventually be the basis for decisions about which treatments can be withheld for the greater benefit of all patients.

ETHICAL AND LEGAL PRINCIPLES

- Rationing is the distribution of scarce resources to an individual patient or a class of patients and the denial of those resources to others. It is based on a limited amount of technology, specific resources (e.g., blood, organs, ICU beds), or financing allocated at the macro or societal level.
- Prior noncompliant behavior should not be grounds for denying care of the present, acute problem. If the noncompliance is expected to continue and will affect the goals of this medical treatment, it can be grounds for decisions about whether or how to treat the presenting problem.
- Triage is the priority of care given to patients in an emergency or disaster situation based on the utility of providing the greatest good for the greatest number of patients.

helpful to have the patient wear a football helmet with the tube secured to the mouth guard. This stabilizes the tube and applies traction. Traction may also be applied (0.75 to 1.25 pounds [0.3 to 0.6 kg]) to hold the tube securely in place and prevent downward movement. Traction causes ulceration of the nasal mucosa and can be used only for short intervals (2 to 3 hours) at a time.

Sometimes iced or room temperature saline lavage is used to remove blood from the stomach. (Nursing care of upper GI bleeding is discussed in Chapter 39.) This helps prevent the blood from degrading to ammonia, leading to encephalopathy. The nurse must ensure that the right amount of pressure is maintained for the correct time. Constant tension and an upward pull on the stomach initiate contraction of the stomach, which may lead to retching and increased portal pressures. The esophageal balloon should be deflated every 8 to 12 hours to avoid necrosis. Each lumen must be labeled to avoid confusion. The NG lumen may be connected to suction to remove blood and keep the stomach empty to reduce the risk of aspiration. The most common complication of balloon tamponade therapy is aspiration pneumonia.

Nursing care includes monitoring for complications of rupture or erosion of the esophagus, regurgitation and aspiration of gastric contents, and occlusion of the airway by the balloon. If the gastric balloon breaks or is deflated, the esophageal balloon will slip upward, obstructing the airway and causing asphyxiation. If this happens, the nurse must cut the tube or deflate the esophageal balloon. Scissors should be kept at the bedside. Regurgitation can be minimized by oral and pharyngeal suctioning and by keeping the patient in a semi-Fowler's position.

The patient is unable to swallow saliva because of the inflated esophageal balloon occluding the esophagus. With the Minnesota tube, which has an esophageal aspiration lumen, this problem can be alleviated. The nurse should encourage the patient to expectorate and should provide an emesis basin and tissues. Frequent oral and nasal care provides relief from the taste of blood and irritation from mouth breathing.

The patient is extremely ill at this stage. The crisis of the bleeding and the ordeal of the tube create a great deal of psychologic trauma. Emotional support and gentle caring must be provided.

Hepatic encephalopathy. The focus of nursing care of the patient with hepatic encephalopathy is on sustaining life and assisting with measures to reduce the formation of ammonia. The nurse should assess (1) the patient's level of responsiveness (e.g., reflexes, pupillary reactions, orientation); (2) sensory and motor abnormalities (e.g., hyperreflexia, asterixis, motor coordination); (3) fluid and electrolyte imbalances; (4) acid-base imbalances; and (5) the effect of treatment measures.

The neurologic status, including an exact description of the patient's behavior, should be assessed and recorded at least every 2 hours. Care of the patient with neurologic problems should be based on the severity of the encephalopathy.

Nursing measures to prevent constipation should be instituted to decrease ammonia production. Drugs, laxatives, and enemas should be given as ordered. Encouragement of fluids may also help if not contraindicated. The patient should not strain at stool because this may cause bleeding of hemorrhoidal varices. Any GI bleeding may worsen the coma. The patient who is taking lactulose should be assessed for diarrhea. Some physicians have diarrhea as a goal when treating with lactulose. The drug's laxative action expels the ammonia from the colon. Because lactulose can cause severe purging, the nurse should observe the patient for excessive fluid and electrolyte loss.

Factors that are known to precipitate coma should be controlled as much as possible (see Table 41-10). Because exercise produces ammonia as a by-product of metabolism, the physical activity of the patient must be limited. Hypokalemia should be controlled.

The patient is on either a very-low-protein or a no-protein diet, neither of which is very palatable. Vegetable protein is better tolerated than meat protein. Foods and fluids high in carbohydrate should be given because the liver is not synthesizing and storing glucose. The patient may require tube feedings if an adequate diet cannot be ingested.

Chronic and Home Management. The patient with cirrhosis may be faced with a very prolonged course and the possibility of serious, life-threatening problems and complications. The nurse should be a resource person in helping the patient achieve the highest level of wellness. The patient and the family need to understand the importance of continuous health care and medical supervision. They should be taught symptoms of complications and when to seek medical attention. Patients with cirrhosis should refrain from eating raw shellfish and avoid activities that place them at risk for contracting viral hepatitis.

Measures to achieve and maintain a remission should be encouraged. These include proper diet, rest, avoidance of potentially hepatotoxic over-the-counter drugs such as acetaminophen, and abstinence from alcohol. Abstinence from alcohol is important and results in improvement in most patients. The nurse must realize the difficulty this poses for some patients. The nurse's own attitude regarding the patient whose cirrhosis is attributed to alcohol abuse should be explored. Care should be given without rejection and moralizing. The alcoholic patient should be treated with a caring attitude.

Cirrhosis is a chronic disease. The patient is affected not only physically but also psychologically, socially, and economically. Major adjustments may be required to make lifestyle changes, especially if alcohol abuse is the primary etiologic factor. The nurse should provide information regarding community support programs, such as Alcoholics Anonymous, for help with alcohol abuse.

Adequate explanations, along with written instructions, related to fluid or dietary restrictions should be given to the patient and the family. Other health teaching should include instruction about adequate rest periods, how to detect early signs of complications, skin care, drug therapy precautions, observation for bleeding, and protection from infection. Counseling information regarding sexual problems may be needed. Referral to a community or home health nurse may be helpful to ensure adequate patient compliance with prescribed therapy. The emphasis of home care for the patient with cirrhosis should be on helping the patient maintain the highest level of wellness possible and initiate and maintain necessary lifestyle changes.

CARCINOMA OF THE LIVER

Primary carcinoma (originating in the liver) is quite rare. Metastatic carcinoma of the liver is more common. Hepatocellular carcinoma is the most common malignant tumor of the liver.[25] The remaining primary tumors are cholangiomas or bile duct carcinomas. A high percentage of patients with primary cell carcinoma have cirrhosis of the liver. Some cases of hepatocellular carcinoma are associated with chronic hepatitis B or C.[26] Men have a higher incidence of primary liver cancer than women.

The liver is a common site of metastatic growth because of its high rate of blood flow and extensive capillary network. Cancer cells in other parts of the body are commonly carried to the liver via the portal circulation.

The malignant cells cause the liver to be enlarged and misshapen. Hemorrhage and necrosis in the liver are common. Lesions may be singular or numerous and nodular or diffusely spread over the entire liver. Some tumors infiltrate into other organs such as the gallbladder or into the peritoneum or diaphragm. Primary liver tumors commonly metastasize to the lung.

Clinical Manifestations

It is difficult to diagnose carcinoma of the liver. It is particularly difficult to differentiate it from cirrhosis in its early stages because many of the clinical manifestations (e.g., hepatomegaly, weight loss, peripheral edema, ascites, portal hypertension) are similar. Other common manifestations include dull abdominal pain in the epigastric or right upper quadrant region, jaundice, anorexia, nausea and vomiting, and extreme weakness. Patients frequently have pulmonary emboli. Tests used to assist in the diagnosis are a liver scan, hepatic arteriography, endoscopic retrograde cholangiopancreatography (ERCP), and a liver biopsy. The test for α-fetoprotein (AFP) may be positive in hepatocellular carcinoma. AFP helps distinguish primary cancer from metastatic cancer.

THERAPEUTIC AND NURSING MANAGEMENT

CANCER OF THE LIVER

Treatment of cancer of the liver is largely palliative. Surgical excision (lobectomy) is sometimes performed if the tumor is localized to one portion of the liver. Only 30% to 40% of patients have surgically resectable disease. Usually surgery is not feasible because the cancer is too far advanced when it is detected. Surgical excision offers the only chance for cure of liver cancer. Management is very similar to that for cirrhosis. Chemotherapy may be used, but there is usually a poor response. Portal vein or hepatic artery perfusion with 5-fluorouracil may be attempted.

Nursing intervention for the patient with liver carcinoma focuses on keeping the patient as comfortable as possible. Because this patient manifests the same problems as any patient with advanced liver disease, the nursing interventions discussed for cirrhosis of the liver apply. (See Chapter 12 for care of the patient with cancer.)

The prognosis for cancer of the liver is poor. The cancer grows rapidly, and death may occur within 4 to 7 months as a result of hepatic encephalopathy or massive blood loss from GI bleeding.

LIVER TRANSPLANTATION

The first human liver transplant was performed in 1963 at the University of Colorado by Thomas Starzl. In the last decade, liver transplantation has become a practical therapeutic option for many adults and children with irreversible liver disease. It improves the quality of life for end-stage liver patients and is an accepted treatment modality for these patients. Indications for liver transplantation include congenital biliary abnormalities, inborn errors of metabolism, hepatic malignancy (confined to the liver), sclerosing cholangitis, and chronic end-stage liver disease.[27] Cirrhosis of the liver is a major indication in adults. Liver transplants are not recommended for the patient with widespread malignant disease.

The major postoperative complications are rejection and infection.[28] Rejection is not as major a problem as in kidney transplants. The liver seems to be less susceptible to severe rejection than the kidney. Cyclosporine is an effective immunosuppressant drug. The use of cyclosporine has been a major factor in the success rates of liver transplantation. Cyclosporine depresses T-helper cell function and preserves T-suppressor cell function (see Chapter 44). It does not cause bone marrow suppression and does not impede wound healing. Side effects of cyclosporine include hypertension, headaches, hirsutism, and nephrotoxicity. Other immunosuppressants used include azathioprine (Imuran), corticosteroids, and the monoclonal antibody OKT3 (see Table 44-10). Other factors in the improved success rate are advances in surgical techniques, better selection of potential recipients, and improved management of the underlying liver disease before surgery.

The patient who has had a liver transplant requires competent and highly skilled nursing care, either in an ICU or in some other specialized unit. Postoperative nursing care includes assessing neurologic status, monitoring for signs of hemorrhage, preventing pulmonary complications, and monitoring drainage, electrolytes, urinary output, and for signs and symptoms of infection and rejection. Common respiratory problems are pneumonia, atelectasis, and pleural effusions. The nurse should have the patient use measures such as coughing, deep breathing, incentive spirometry, and repositioning to prevent these complications. Drainage from the Jackson-Pratt drain, NG tube, and T-tube should be measured and the color and consistency of drainage noted. A critical aspect of nursing care following liver transplantation is monitoring for infection. The first 2 months after the surgery are critical. Infection can be viral, fungal, or bacterial. Fever may be the only sign of infection. Emotional support and teaching the patient and family are essential.

RESEARCH

IMPLICATIONS FOR NURSING PRACTICE

QUALITY OF LIFE OF LIVER TRANSPLANT RECIPIENTS

Citation Leyendecker B and others: Quality of life for liver transplant recipients: a pilot study, *Transplantation* 56:561-567, 1993.

Purpose To provide an understanding of the quality of life of patients receiving a liver transplant.

Methods Cross-sectional survey of the quality of life of 45 liver transplant recipients included the following parameters: physical and psychologic status, physical complaints, ability to participate in daily life, social support, and global quality of life. The average time of follow-up was 9 months after transplantation.

Results and Conclusions Although physical complaints were higher than in the general population, most patients were able to participate in activities of daily living. Most reported good social support and psychologic adjustment. Sixty percent reported their quality of life as very high and 9% felt very bad. This survey shows that during the first year after transplantation recipients reported a relatively high quality of life despite physical complaints.

Implications for Nursing Practice The positive results obtained by this study can be explained in part by the fact that most patients are chronically ill long before the liver transplant. Success of transplantation surgery should be evaluated not just by survival rates but also by quality of life data related to one's subjective perception of one's own physical and emotional state.

ACUTE PANCREATITIS

Significance

Acute pancreatitis is an acute inflammatory process of the pancreas. The degree of inflammation varies from mild edema to severe hemorrhagic necrosis.

Acute pancreatitis is most common in middle-aged men and women, but affects more men than women. The severity of the disease varies according to the extent of pancreatic destruction. Some patients recover completely, others have recurring attacks, and chronic pancreatitis develops in others. Acute pancreatitis can be life threatening.

Etiology and Pathophysiology

Many factors can cause injury to the pancreas. The primary etiologic factors are biliary tract disease and alcoholism.[29] In the United States the most common cause is alcoholism, followed by gallbladder disease. Other, less common, causes of acute pancreatitis include trauma (postsurgical, abdominal); viral infections (mumps, coxsackievirus B); penetrating duodenal ulcer; cysts; abscesses; cystic fibrosis; Kaposi's sarcoma; certain drugs (corticosteroids, thiazide diuretics, oral contraceptives, sulfonamides, nonsteroidal

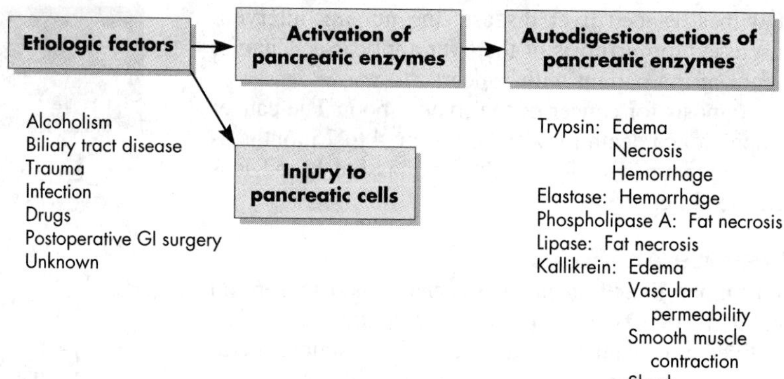

Fig. 41-10 Pathogenic process of acute pancreatitis. *GI*, Gastrointestinal.

antiinflammatory drugs); and metabolic disorders such as hyperparathyroidism, hyperlipidemia, and renal failure. Pancreatitis may occur after surgical procedures on the pancreas, stomach, duodenum, or biliary tract. Pancreatitis can also occur after endoscopic retrograde cholangiopancreatography (ERCP) (see Table 36-12). In some cases the cause is not known (idiopathic).

The most common pathogenic mechanism is believed to be autodigestion of the pancreas (Fig. 41-10). The etiologic factors cause injury to pancreatic cells or activation of the pancreatic enzymes in the pancreas rather than in the intestine. It is not clear how the activation of pancreatic enzymes occurs. One possible cause is believed to be the reflux of bile acids into the pancreatic ducts through an open or distended sphincter of Oddi. This reflux may occur because of gallstones impacted at the ampulla of Vater, atony and edema of the sphincter, or obstruction of pancreatic ducts and pancreatic ischemia.

Trypsinogen is an inactive proteolytic enzyme produced by the pancreas. Normally it is released into the small intestine via the pancreatic duct. In the intestine it is activated to trypsin by enterokinase. Normally, trypsin inhibitors in the pancreas and plasma bind and inactivate any trypsin that is inadvertently produced. In pancreatitis, activated trypsin is present in the pancreas. This enzyme can digest the pancreas and also activate other proteolytic enzymes such as elastase and phospholipase.

Elastase and phospholipase A play a major role in autodigestion of the pancreas. Elastase is activated by trypsin and causes hemorrhage by producing dissolution of the elastic fibers of blood vessels. Phospholipase A is probably activated by trypsin and bile acids and causes fat necrosis.

It is not entirely clear how alcohol causes acute pancreatitis. One theory is that it stimulates secretion and excess production of hydrochloric acid. A decrease in the gastric pH results in the release of the hormone secretin from the intestinal mucosa. This hormone then stimulates pancreatic secretions. Alcohol may also cause regurgitation of duodenal contents into the pancreatic duct, resulting in inflammation.

The pathophysiologic involvement of acute pancreatitis ranges from edematous pancreatitis (which is mild and self-limiting) to necrotizing pancreatitis (in which the degree of necrosis correlates with the severity of manifestations).

Clinical Manifestations

Abdominal pain is the predominant symptom of acute pancreatitis. The pain is usually located in the left upper quadrant but may be in the midepigastrium. It commonly radiates to the back because of the retroperitoneal location of the pancreas. The pain has a sudden onset and is described as severe, deep, piercing, and continuous or steady. It is aggravated by eating and frequently has its onset when the patient is recumbent; it is not relieved by vomiting. The pain may be accompanied by flushing, cyanosis, and dyspnea. The patient may assume various positions involving flexion of the spine in an attempt to relieve the severe pain. The pain is due to distention of the pancreas, peritoneal irritation, and obstruction of the biliary tract.

Other manifestations of acute pancreatitis include nausea and vomiting, low-grade fever, leukocytosis, hypotension, tachycardia, and jaundice. Abdominal tenderness with muscle guarding is common. Bowel sounds may be decreased or absent. Ileus may occur and causes marked abdominal distention. The lungs are frequently involved, with crackles present. Intravascular damage from circulating trypsin may cause areas of cyanosis or greenish to yellow-brown discoloration of the abdominal wall. Other areas of ecchymoses are the flanks (*Grey Turner's spots* or *sign*, a bluish flank discoloration) and the periumbilical area (*Cullen's sign*, a bluish periumbilical discoloration). These result from seepage of blood-stained exudate from the pancreas and may occur in severe cases.

Shock may occur because of hemorrhage into the pancreas or toxemia from the activated pancreatic enzymes. The increased formation of kinin peptides (activated by trypsin), such as kallikrein and bradykinin, causes vasodilatation, increased capillary permeability, and altered vasomotor tone. Hypovolemia also occurs as a result of exudation of blood and plasma proteins into the retroperitoneal space (massive fluid shifts).

Complications

Two significant local complications of acute pancreatitis are pseudocyst and abscess. A pancreatic *pseudocyst* is a cavity continuous with or surrounding the outside of the pancreas. The pseudocyst is filled with necrotic products and liquid secretions, such as plasma, pancreatic enzymes, and inflammatory exudates. As pancreatic enzymes escape from the pseudocyst, the serosal surfaces next to the pancreas become inflamed, with subsequent formation of granulation tissue leading to encapsulation of the exudate. Symptoms of pseudocyst are abdominal pain, palpable epigastric mass, nausea, vomiting, and anorexia. The serum amylase level frequently remains elevated. These cysts usually resolve spontaneously within a few weeks but may perforate, causing peritonitis, or rupture into the stomach or duodenum. Treatment consists of an internal drainage procedure with a Roux-en-Y anastomosis between the pancreatic duct and the jejunum.

A pancreatic *abscess* is a large fluid-containing cavity within the pancreas. It results from extensive necrosis in the pancreas. It may become infected or perforate into adjacent organs. Manifestations of an abscess include upper abdominal pain, abdominal mass, high fever, and leukocytosis. Pancreatic abscesses require prompt surgical drainage to prevent sepsis.

The main systemic complications of acute pancreatitis are pulmonary complications (pleural effusion, atelectasis, and pneumonia) and tetany caused by hypocalcemia. The pulmonary complications are probably caused by the passage of the exudate containing pancreatic enzymes from the peritoneal cavity through transdiaphragmatic lymph channels. When hypocalcemia occurs, it is a sign of severe disease. It is due in part to the combining of calcium and fatty acids during fat necrosis. The exact mechanisms of how or why hypocalcemia occurs are not well understood.

Diagnostic Studies

The primary diagnostic tests for acute pancreatitis are serum amylase (pancreatic isoamylase) and lipase and urinary amylase levels (Table 41-16). The serum amylase level is the criterion most commonly used. It may elevate to levels greater than 200 U/L (3.34 μkat/L). The serum amylase is usually elevated early and remains elevated for 24 to 72 hours.

The serum lipase is also elevated in acute pancreatitis and is a helpful complementary test because other disorders (e.g., mumps, cerebral trauma, renal transplantation) may also cause an increase in serum amylase.

There is an increase in urinary amylase, which may persist several days beyond the elevation of serum amylase. Urinary amylase may be increased to more than 3600 U per day. Normally a timed collection (e.g., a 2-hour collection) is a more dependable measure than a randomly collected urinary specimen.

The renal amylase-creatinine clearance test estimates the amount of blood cleared of amylase by the kidney per minute. The finding that the renal clearance of amylase is higher than the creatinine clearance in acute pancreatitis has led to the suggestion that the amylase-creatinine clearance ratio is a more specific test than urinary amylase levels alone.

Other laboratory abnormalities include hyperglycemia, hyperlipidemia, and hypocalcemia (Table 41-16). There is a high incidence of hyperlipidemia with recurrent pancreatitis.

ERCP is diagnostic for gallstones, pancreatic cysts, and abscesses. A combination of laboratory studies and ERCP is usually used to help make the diagnosis.[30] Abdominal x-ray and ultrasound scan of the pancreas may also be performed.

Table 41-16 Diagnostic Studies: Acute Pancreatitis

Laboratory Test	Abnormal Finding	Etiology
Primary Tests		
Serum amylase	Increased (>200 U/L [3.34 μkat/L])	Pancreatic cell injury
Serum lipase	Elevated	Pancreatic cell injury
Urinary amylase	Elevated	Pancreatic cell injury
Secondary Tests		
Blood glucose	Hyperglycemia	Impairment of carbohydrate metabolism due to β-cell damage and release of glucagon
Serum calcium	Hypocalcemia	Saponification of calcium by fatty acids in areas of fat necrosis
Serum triglycerides	Hyperlipidemia	Release of free fatty acids by lipase

Therapeutic Management

Objectives of therapeutic management of acute pancreatitis include (1) relief of pain; (2) prevention or alleviation of shock; (3) reduction of pancreatic secretions; (4) control of fluid and electrolyte imbalance; (5) prevention or treatment of infections; and (6) removal of the precipitating cause, if possible (Table 41-17).

A primary consideration is the relief and control of pain.[31] Meperidine (Demerol) is preferred because it causes less spasm of the smooth muscles of the ducts than morphine. It may be combined with an antispasmodic. However, atropine-like drugs should be avoided when paralytic ileus is present because they may contribute to the problem. Other medications that relax smooth muscles (spasmolytics), such as nitroglycerin or papaverine, may be used.

If shock is present, blood volume replacements are used. Plasma or plasma volume expanders such as dextran or albumin may be given. Fluid and electrolyte imbalances are corrected with lactated Ringer's solution or other electrolyte solutions. Central venous pressure readings may be used to assist in determination of fluid-replacement requirements.

It is important to reduce or suppress pancreatic enzymes to decrease stimulation of the pancreas and allow it to rest. This is accomplished in several ways. First, the patient is allowed to take nothing by mouth (NPO). Second, NG suction may be used to reduce vomiting and gastric distention and to prevent gastric acidic contents from entering the duodenum. These measures suppress pancreatic secretion. Certain drugs may also be used for this purpose (Table 41-18).

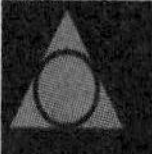

Table 41-17 Therapeutic Management: Acute Pancreatitis

Diagnostic
Serum amylase
Serum lipase
2-hour urinary amylase and renal amylase clearance
Blood glucose
Serum calcium
Triglycerides
Flat plate of the abdomen
Pancreatic ultrasound scan
CT scan of the pancreas
ERCP
Therapeutic
Meperidine IM
NPO with NG tube to suction
Cimetidine or ranitidine IV
Albumin (if shock present)
IV calcium gluconate (10%) (if tetany present)
Lactated Ringer's solution

CT, Computed tomography; *ERCP,* endoscopic retrograde cholangiopancreatography; *IM,* intramuscular; *IV,* intravenous; *NG,* nasogastric; *NPO,* nothing by mouth.

The inflamed and necrotic pancreatic tissue is a good media for bacterial growth. Therefore it is important to prevent infections. There is some controversy about the prophylactic use of antibiotics. It is important to monitor the patient closely so that antibiotic therapy can be instituted early if infection occurs.

Peritoneal lavage or dialysis has been used to remove the kinin and phospholipase A–containing exudate from the peritoneal cavity. This has proved beneficial in some cases of severe acute pancreatitis. It prevents early death but has little effect on overall mortality. Endoscopic papillotomy may be used to remove an impacted gallstone from the common bile duct when the pancreatitis is due to the stone.

Surgical intervention may be indicated when the diagnosis is uncertain and in patients who do not respond to conservative therapy.[32] Surgery is necessary for an abscess, acute pseudocyst, and severe peritonitis. Percutaneous drainage of a pseudocyst can be performed, and a drainage tube is left in place. Surgical treatment of associated biliary tract disease may be necessary.

Pharmacologic Management. Several different drugs may be used in the treatment of both acute and chronic pancreatitis (Table 41-18). A number of drugs are used in an effort to suppress pancreatic secretion, but these drugs have not proved very effective in the management of pancreatitis.

Nutritional Management. Initially the patient with acute pancreatitis is on NPO status to reduce pancreatic secretion. When food is allowed, small, frequent feedings are given. The diet is usually high in carbohydrate content because that is the least stimulating to the exocrine portion

Table 41-18 Drugs Used in Treatment of Acute and Chronic Pancreatitis

Drug	Mechanisms of Action
Acute Pancreatitis	
Meperidine (Demerol)	Relief of pain
Nitroglycerin or papaverine	Relaxation of smooth muscles and relief of pain
Antispasmodics (e.g., dicyclomine [Bentyl], propantheline bromide [Pro-Banthine])	Decrease of vagal stimulation, motility, pancreatic outflow (inhibition of volume and concentration of bicarbonate and enzymatic secretion); contraindicated in paralytic ileus
Carbonic anhydrase inhibitor (acetazolamide [Diamox])	Reduction in volume and bicarbonate concentration of pancreatic secretion
Antacids	Neutralization of gastric secretions; decrease in hydrochloric acid stimulation of secretin, which stimulates production and secretion of pancreatic secretions
Histamine H_2-receptor antagonists (cimetidine [Tagamet], ranitidine [Zantac])	Decrease in hydrochloric acid by inhibiting histamine (hydrochloric acid stimulates pancreatic activity)
Calcium gluconate	Treatment of hypocalcemia to prevent or treat tetany
Adrenocortical steroids	Use only for seriously ill patients with hypotension or shock
Aprotinin (Trasylol)	Antitryptic and antikallikreinic actions
Glucagon	Reduction in pancreatic inflammation and decrease in serum amylase, suppression of pancreatic secretions
Somatostatin	Inhibition of pancreatic secretions
Chronic Pancreatitis	
Pancreatin (Viokase)	Replacement therapy for pancreatic enzymes
Insulin	Treatment for diabetes mellitus if it occurs or for hyperglycemia

of the pancreas. The diet combines high carbohydrate intake with low fat and high protein intake. It is bland, with no stimulants (e.g., caffeine) or alcohol. Supplemental fat-soluble vitamins may be given. The patient may require supplemental commercial liquid preparations. If severe nutritional deficiencies exist, total parenteral nutrition (TPN) may be used (see Chapter 37).

NURSING MANAGEMENT

ACUTE PANCREATITIS

Nursing Assessment

Subjective and objective data that should be obtained from a person with acute pancreatitis are presented in Table 41-19.

Nursing Diagnoses

Nursing diagnoses are determined when the problem and the etiologic factors are supported by clinical data. Nursing diagnoses related to acute pancreatitis may include, but are not limited to, those presented in the nursing care plan for the patient with acute pancreatitis on p. 1292.

Table 41-19 Nursing Assessment: Acute Pancreatitis

Subjective Data
Important health information
Past health history: Alcohol abuse, biliary tract disease, abdominal trauma, duodenal ulcers, infection, metabolic disorders
Medications: Use of thiazides, estrogens, corticosteroids, azathioprine, sulfonamides, opiates, furosemide
Surgery and other treatments: Surgical procedures on the pancreas, stomach, duodenum, or biliary tract
Functional health patterns
Health perception–health management: Weakness
Nutritional-metabolic: Nausea and vomiting; anorexia
Activity-exercise: Dyspnea
Cognitive-perceptual: Severe midepigastric or left upper quadrant pain that may radiate to the back, aggravation with food and alcohol intake

Objective Data
General
Restlessness, anxiety, flushing, low-grade fever, diaphoresis
Integumentary
Discoloration of abdomen and flanks, jaundice; decreased skin turgor, dry mucous membranes
Respiratory
Tachypnea, basilar crackles, dyspnea
Cardiovascular
Tachycardia, hypotension
Gastrointestinal
Abdominal distention and tenderness, diminished bowel sounds
Possible findings
Elevated serum amylase and lipase, leukocytosis, hyperglycemia, elevated urine amylase, abnormal ultrasound and CT scans of pancreas

CT, Computed tomography.

Planning

The overall goals are that the patient with acute pancreatitis will have (1) relief of pain, (2) return of fluid and electrolyte balance, (3) minimal to no complications, and (4) no recurrent attacks. Specific outcomes are identified in the nursing care plan for the patient with acute pancreatitis.

Nursing Implementation

Health Promotion and Maintenance. The major factors involved in health promotion are assessment of the patient for predisposing and etiologic factors of pancreatitis and encouragement of early treatment of these factors to prevent occurrence of acute pancreatitis. The nurse should encourage the early diagnosis and treatment of biliary tract disease, such as cholelithiasis. The patient should be encouraged to eliminate alcohol intake, especially if there have been any previous episodes of pancreatitis. Attacks of pancreatitis become milder or disappear with the discontinuance of alcohol use.

Acute Intervention. Because abdominal pain is a prominent symptom of pancreatitis, a major focus of nursing care is the relief of pain (see the nursing care plan for the patient with acute pancreatitis). Giving the prescribed medications before the pain becomes too severe makes the medication more effective. The nurse should ascertain how long the pain medication provides relief. Measures such as comfortable positioning, frequent changes in position, and relief of nausea and vomiting assist in reducing the restlessness that usually accompanies the pain. Some patients experience lessened pain by assuming positions that flex the trunk and draw the knees up to the abdomen. A side-lying position with the head elevated 45 degrees decreases tension on the abdomen and may help ease the pain. It is important to control the pain and restlessness because they increase body metabolism and subsequent stimulation of pancreatic secretions.

Nursing measures for the patient who is on NPO status or has an NG tube should be employed. Frequent oral and nasal care to relieve the dryness of the mouth and nose is comforting to the patient. Oral care is essential to prevent parotitis. If the patient is taking anticholinergics to decrease GI secretions, there will be additional dryness of the mouth caused by the side effects of the drug. If the patient is taking antacids to suppress secretions, they should be sipped slowly or inserted in the NG tube. The nurse must regularly assess the functioning of the suction.

A vital part of the nursing care plan for this patient is observation for electrolyte imbalances. Frequent vomiting, along with gastric suction, may result in decreased chloride, sodium, and potassium levels. Because hypocalcemia can also occur, the nurse must observe for symptoms of tetany, such as jerking, irritability, and muscular twitching. Numbness or tingling around the lips and in the fingers is an early indicator of hypocalcemia. The patient should be assessed for a positive Chvostek's or Trousseau's sign. Calcium gluconate as ordered should be given to treat symptomatic hypocalcemia.

NURSING CARE PLAN Patient with Acute Pancreatitis

Planning: Outcome Criteria	Nursing Interventions and Rationales
➤ **NURSING DIAGNOSIS**	Pain *related to* distention of pancreas, peritoneal irritation, obstruction of biliary tract, and ineffective pain and comfort measures *as manifested by* communication of pain descriptors, guarding behavior, narrowed self-focus, behaviors indicative of pain (e.g., moaning), diaphoresis, changes in blood pressure, pulse, and respiratory rate
Report satisfaction with pain control.	Assess degree and nature of pain *to plan appropriate interventions.* Give ordered analgesic and antispasmodic medications before pain gets too severe *to ensure more effective relief of pain.* Ascertain how long the medication provides relief *to adjust pain medication administration in order to provide ongoing relief of pain.* Provide comfort measures, such as positioning patient comfortably with frequent changes in position and diversional activities *to assist in reducing the restlessness that usually accompanies the pain and to demonstrate caring behaviors by the nurse.*
➤ **NURSING DIAGNOSIS**	Fluid volume deficit *related to* nausea, vomiting, NG suction, and restricted oral intake *as manifested by* thirst, increased fluid output, altered intake, dry skin and mucous membranes, decreased skin turgor, decreased oral intake
Maintain adequate intake of fluids and electrolytes as evidenced by normal skin turgor; moist mucous membranes; stable weight; normal electrolyte studies.	Give antiemetics as ordered *to reduce fluid loss by preventing vomiting.* Measure and describe emesis *as indicator of replacement needs and effectiveness of treatment.* Provide oral hygiene after emesis *to enhance patient's comfort.* Observe for manifestations of metabolic alkalosis such as confusion, irritability, tachycardia, nausea, vomiting, muscle cramps *so appropriate replacements can be started promptly.*
➤ **NURSING DIAGNOSIS**	Altered oral mucous membranes *related to* NG tube and NPO status *as manifested by* dry mouth, oral pain or discomfort, coated tongue, stomatitis, halitosis, oral lesions or ulcers, lack of or decreased salivation
Have moist lips and nares, absence of parotitis and stomatitis.	Assess oral mucosa *to monitor condition of mouth and plan appropriate interventions.* Give oral and nasal care q1-2 hr *to prevent parotitis, relieve dryness caused by anticholinergics, and increase patient's comfort.* Moisten patient's nostrils and lips with water-soluble lubricant *to relieve dryness and enhance patient comfort.*
➤ **NURSING DIAGNOSIS**	Altered nutrition: less than body requirements *related to* anorexia, dietary restrictions, nausea, loss of nutrients from vomiting, and impaired digestion resulting in decreased use of nutrients *as manifested by* weight loss, weakness, fatigue, weight below normal for height and age
Have weight appropriate for height; no further weight loss; adequate energy to perform activities of daily living.	Monitor weight and laboratory values *as indicators of patient's response to treatment.* Observe stools for steatorrhea, *which may develop from incomplete digestion of fats.* Administer total parenteral nutrition if ordered *to provide carbohydrates, lipids, and amino acids to prevent negative nitrogen balance.* Implement measures to reduce pain and nausea *to increase patient's desire to eat.* Provide oral care before and after meals *to decrease foul taste and odor that inhibit appetite.* If oral intake is allowed, provide small portions of appealing foods *to reduce malabsorption and distention by decreasing the amount of protein metabolized at one time.* Obtain dietary consult if indicated *to provide new information and ideas to improve patient's nutritional status.*

continued

The patient with acute pancreatitis is susceptible to infections. The nurse should observe for fever and other manifestations of infection. Respiratory infections are common because the retroperitoneal fluid raises the diaphragm, which causes the patient to take shallow, guarded abdominal breaths. Measures to prevent respiratory infections include turning, coughing, deep breathing, and assuming a semi-Fowler's position.

Other important assessments are observation for signs of paralytic ileus, renal failure, and mental changes. Glucometer determination of the blood glucose level should be done to assess damage to the β-cells of the islets of Langerhans in the pancreas.

After pancreatic surgery the patient may require special wound care for an anastomotic leak or a fistula. Measures

NURSING CARE PLAN Patient with Acute Pancreatitis—cont'd

Planning: Outcome Criteria	Nursing Interventions and Rationales
➤ NURSING DIAGNOSIS	Ineffective management of therapeutic regimen *related to* lack of knowledge of preventive measures, diet restrictions, restriction of alcohol intake, and follow-up care *as manifested by* verbalization of the problem, request for information, inaccurate follow-through of instruction
Verbalize understanding of condition or disease process and treatment; initiate lifestyle changes and participate in treatment regimen; plan for follow-up care.	Teach patient (1) to abstain from alcohol *to prevent the patient from experiencing future attacks of acute pancreatitis and development of chronic pancreatitis;* (2) to restrict fats and avoid rich, rough, and stimulating foods *to decrease stimulation of the pancreas and allow it to rest;* (3) to use more carbohydrates in diet *because these are less stimulating to pancreas* and (4) to correctly measure blood glucose levels and to observe for steatorrhea *because high blood glucose and fatty stools indicate destruction of pancreatic tissue.* Assess patient's understanding of prescribed regimen; provide details on follow-up care *to increase likelihood of successful convalescence and to minimize the possibility of recurrence.* Suggest follow-up if alcohol use problematic *because continued use of alcohol will result in additional attacks of acute pancreatitis and eventual chronic pancreatitis.*

COLLABORATIVE PROBLEMS

Nursing Goals	Nursing Inverventions and Rationales
➤ POTENTIAL COMPLICATION	Fluid and electrolyte imbalance *related to* loss of fluids into peritoneal cavity
Monitor for signs of hypokalemia, hyponatremia, hypocalcemia, and hypochloremia; report deviations from acceptable parameters; carry out medical and nursing interventions.	Observe for signs of fluid and electrolyte imbalance such as confusion, anorexia, diarrhea, seizures, muscle weakness, paralytic ileus, dysrhythmias, metabolic alkalosis, muscle cramps, mental changes, tetany; monitor serum laboratory reports *to aid in early detection and prompt intervention.* Give calcium gluconate as ordered *to treat symptomatic hypocalcemia.*
➤ POTENTIAL COMPLICATION	Hemorrhagic shock *related to* destruction of blood vessel walls by proteolytic enzymes
Monitor for signs of hemorrhagic shock, report deviations from acceptable parameters; carry out appropriate medical and nursing interventions.	Assess for continuing or increasing signs of shock, such as pallor; cool, clammy skin; hypotension; tachycardia; increased respirations *to ensure prompt detection and intervention.* Monitor vital signs q1-2 hr *to evaluate patient's response to treatment.* Assess hourly for decreased urinary output *as an indicator of circulating blood volume as well as renal perfusion.*

NG, Nasogastric; *NPO,* nothing by mouth.

to prevent skin irritation should be used. These include skin barriers such as Stomahesive, karaya paste or Colley-Seel, pouching, and drains. In addition to protecting the skin, pouching also provides a more accurate determination of fluid and electrolyte losses and increases patient comfort. Sterile pouching systems are available. The nurse may want to consult with a clinical specialist or an enterostomal therapist, if available.

Chronic and Home Management. After acute pancreatitis most patients will need home care follow-up. The patient may have lost physical reserve and muscle strength. Physical therapy may be needed. Continued care to prevent infection and detect any complications is important. Because frequent doses of narcotics may be required for this patient during the acute stage, follow-up for assessment of possible narcotic addiction may be indicated. This is a more likely problem with chronic pancreatitis than in the patient with acute pancreatitis. Counseling regarding abstinence from alcohol is important to prevent the patient from experiencing future attacks of acute pancreatitis and development of chronic pancreatitis. Beverages with caffeine should not be consumed. Because smoking and stressful situations can overstimulate the pancreas, they should be avoided.

Dietary teaching should include restriction of fats because they stimulate the secretion of cholecystokinin, which then stimulates the pancreas. Carbohydrates are less stimulating to the pancreas, so they should be encouraged. The patient should be instructed to avoid crash dieting and binging because these can precipitate attacks.

Early detection makes it possible to correct mental changes by treating the cause before overt psychotic behavior is manifested. Possible causes of mental changes include sepsis, anorexia, toxicity from cellular breakdown products, and withdrawal from alcohol.

The patient and the family should be given instructions regarding the recognition and reporting of symptoms of infection, diabetes mellitus, or steatorrhea (foul-smelling, frothy stools). These changes indicate possible destruction of pancreatic tissue. The nurse should make sure the patient fully understands the prescribed regimen. Each aspect must be explained. The importance of taking the required medications and following the recommended diet should be stressed.

CHRONIC PANCREATITIS

Pathophysiology

Chronic pancreatitis is progressive destruction of the pancreas with fibrotic replacement of pancreatic tissue. Strictures and calcifications may also occur in the pancreas. There are several types of chronic pancreatitis, but they all have a common underlying pathophysiologic disorder. The two major types are chronic obstructive pancreatitis and chronic calcifying pancreatitis. Chronic pancreatitis may follow acute pancreatitis, but it may also occur in the absence of any history of an acute condition.

Chronic obstructive pancreatitis is associated with biliary disease. The most common cause is inflammation of the sphincter of Oddi associated with cholelithiasis. Cancer of the ampulla of Vater, duodenum, or pancreas can also cause this type of chronic pancreatitis.

In chronic calcifying pancreatitis there is inflammation and sclerosis, mainly in the head of the pancreas and around the pancreatic duct. This type of chronic pancreatitis is the most common form. It is also called alcohol-induced pancreatitis. Increases in heavy social drinking have produced a higher incidence in countries in which the disease was previously considered rare. In the United States chronic pancreatitis is found almost exclusively in alcoholics. As with cirrhosis there seems to be a metabolic abnormality that predisposes a person who drinks to the direct toxic effect of the alcohol on the pancreas.

In chronic calcifying pancreatitis the ducts are obstructed with protein precipitates. These precipitates block the pancreatic duct and eventually calcify. This is followed by fibrosis and glandular atrophy. Pseudocysts and abscesses commonly develop.

Clinical Manifestations

As with acute pancreatitis, a major manifestation of chronic pancreatitis is abdominal pain. The patient may have episodes of acute pain, but it usually is chronic (recurrent attacks at intervals of months or years). The attacks may become more and more frequent until they are almost constant, or they may diminish as the pancreatic fibrosis develops. The pain is located in the same areas as in acute pancreatitis but is usually described as a heavy, gnawing feeling or sometimes as burning and cramplike. The pain is not relieved with food or antacids.

Other clinical manifestations include symptoms of pancreatic insufficiency, including malabsorption with weight loss, constipation, mild jaundice with dark urine, steatorrhea, and diabetes mellitus. The steatorrhea may become severe, with voluminous, foul, fatty stools. Urine and stool may be frothy. Some abdominal tenderness may be present.

Diagnostic Studies

Laboratory findings in chronic pancreatitis include increased serum amylase (200 to 600 U/L [3.34 to 10.0 μkat/L]), increased serum bilirubin, and increased alkaline phosphatase levels. There is usually mild leukocytosis and an elevated sedimentation rate.

The secretin stimulation test is probably the most useful test in diagnosing chronic pancreatitis. Secretin is given IV, and gastric-duodenal secretions are collected with a double-lumen tube for separate gastric and duodenal aspiration. In chronic pancreatitis there is reduced volume of secretions and reduced bicarbonate concentration (less than 90 mEq/L). Normally, secretin stimulates the production of pancreatic fluid high in bicarbonate content.

Other abnormal diagnostic findings are hyperglycemia and fatty stools (steatorrhea) found in fecal fat determination. Neutral fat indicates maldigestion. Arteriography and x-rays may demonstrate fibrosis and calcification.

ERCP involves cannulation and visualization of the pancreatic and common bile ducts through a fiberoptic endoscope that is inserted into the esophagus and then into the duodenum. The common bile duct and the pancreatic duct are then cannulated. Contrast dye can be injected into the ducts for visualization. Changes in the pancreatic ductal system, such as gross dilatation and microcysts, can be visualized through the use of ERCP.

Therapeutic and Pharmacologic Management

When the patient with chronic pancreatitis is experiencing an acute attack, the therapeutic management is identical to that for acute pancreatitis. At other times the focus is on prevention of further attacks, relief of pain, and control of pancreatic exocrine and endocrine insufficiency. It sometimes takes large, frequent doses of analgesics to relieve the pain, and narcotic addiction may become a problem.[33]

Diet, pancreatic enzyme replacement, and control of the diabetes are measures used to control the pancreatic insufficiency. The diet is a bland, low-fat, high-carbohydrate, and high-protein diet. The patient does not tolerate fatty, rich, and stimulating foods, and these should be avoided to decrease pancreatic secretions and demands on the pancreas. Alcohol must be totally eliminated.

Antacids and anticholinergic drugs may be given to decrease hydrochloric acid, which stimulates pancreatic activity. Cimetidine (Tagamet) and ranitidine (Zantac), which block histamine receptors and thus decrease hydrochloric acid secretion, may be used for the same purpose. Pancreatic enzymes such as pancreatin (Viokase) and pancrelipase (Cotazym) contain amylase, lipase, and trypsin and are used to replace the deficient pancreatic enzymes. They are usually enteric coated to prevent their breakdown or inactivation by gastric acid. Bile salts are sometimes given to facilitate the absorption of the fat-soluble vitamins (A, D, E, and K) and prevent further fat loss. If diabetes develops, it is controlled with insulin or oral hypoglycemic drugs.

Treatment of chronic pancreatitis sometimes requires surgery. When biliary disease is present or if obstruction or pseudocyst develops, surgery may be indicated. Operations performed are procedures to divert bile flow or relieve ductal obstruction. A choledochojejunostomy diverts bile around the ampulla of Vater, where there may be spasm or hypertrophy of the sphincter. In this procedure the common bile duct is anastomosed into the jejunum. If the pancreatic sphincter is fibrotic, a sphincterotomy enlarges it. Pancreatic drainage procedures relieve ductal obstruction. One type is the Roux-en-Y pancreatojejunostomy, in which the pancreatic duct is opened and an anastomosis is made with the jejunum. Total pancreas transplantation and islet cell transplantation are experimental techniques currently being studied in clinical trials to provide long-term replacement of endocrine function.

NURSING MANAGEMENT

CHRONIC PANCREATITIS

Except during an acute episode, the focus of nursing management is on chronic care and health promotion. The patient should be instructed to take measures to prevent further attacks. Dietary control, along with consistency of other treatment measures such as taking pancreatic enzymes, is essential. The pancreatic extracts are usually given with meals or can be given with a snack. The nurse should observe the patient's stools for steatorrhea to help determine the effectiveness of the enzymes. The patient and the family need instructions regarding observation of stools.

If diabetes has developed, the patient will need instruction regarding testing of blood glucose levels and medications (see Chapter 46). The patient who is taking liquid antacids should be instructed to sip the medication slowly, and the nurse should make certain it is taken as ordered to help control gastric acidity. Antacids should be taken after meals. Both the antacid and the pancreatic enzymes may be left at the bedside to prepare the patient for self-management at home.

Alcohol must be avoided, and the patient may need assistance with this problem. If the patient has developed a dependence on alcohol or narcotics, referral to other agencies or resources may be necessary (see Chapter 8).

CARCINOMA OF THE PANCREAS

The incidence of carcinoma of the pancreas is increasing. There were an estimated 27,000 new cases and 25,900 deaths in the United States in 1994. It is the fourth leading cause of death from cancer. It is more common in men and more common in African-Americans than Caucasians. The risk increases with age, with the peak incidence occurring between 65 and 79 years of age.[34]

Most of the tumors are adenocarcinomas originating from the epithelium of the ductal system. More than half the tumors occur in the head of the pancreas. As the tumor grows, the common bile duct becomes obstructed and obstructive jaundice develops. Tumors starting in the body or tail often remain silent until their growth is advanced. The majority of cancers have metastasized at the time of diagnosis. The signs and symptoms of pancreatic cancer are often similar to chronic pancreatitis. The prognosis of a patient with cancer of the pancreas is poor. Most patients die within 5 to 12 months of the initial diagnosis, and the 5-year survival rate is low (3%).[34] The prognosis is related to the location of the tumor.

Etiology

The cause of cancer of the pancreas remains unknown. There may be some relationship between cancer, diabetes mellitus, and chronic pancreatitis. However, it is not clear whether the cancer follows these diseases or whether these diseases occur as a result of pancreatic cancer. It is known that pancreatic cancer can be induced with chemicals such as nitrosoureas. Major risk factors seem to be cigarette smoking, high-fat diet, diabetes, and exposure to chemicals such as benzidine and coke. Pancreatic cancer develops twice as frequently in persons with a history of heavy cigarette use (more than two packs a day) than in nonsmokers. The carcinogens from the tobacco probably reach the pancreatic ducts by bile reflux or via the bloodstream. Another risk factor is the Western diet, particularly the high fat content. High consumption of meat has also been implicated. Methods of processing foodstuffs may also be involved as a possible risk factor for cancer of the pancreas.

Clinical Manifestations

Common manifestations of pancreatic cancer include abdominal pain (dull, aching), anorexia, rapid and progressive weight loss, nausea, and jaundice. Pain is common and is related to the location of malignancy. Extreme, unrelenting pain is related to extension of the cancer into the retroperitoneal tissues and nerve plexuses. The pain is frequently located in the upper abdomen or left hypochondrium and frequently radiates to the back. It is commonly related to eating, and it also occurs at night. Weight loss is due to poor digestion and absorption caused by lack of digestive juices from the pancreas.

Diagnostic Studies

Better diagnostic measures are needed for detection of pancreatic cancer because most of the current methods detect only advanced stages. Cytologic examination of the pancreatic juice may reveal malignant cells. The secretin test frequently indicates a decreased volume of pancreatic juice with normal bicarbonate and enzyme production. Carcinoembryonic antigen (CEA) is elevated in a high percentage of patients with advanced disease, but it is also increased with other types of cancers and even some benign conditions. The CEA plasma level is therefore probably more useful in assessing the patient's response to treatment than in diagnosis. CA 19-9 is a more specific tumor marker because it is associated with pancreatic cancer in particular.

Ultrasonography detects abnormalities of the pancreas but cannot distinguish cancer from other pancreatic disorders such as pancreatitis. Since this is a noninvasive procedure, it may be used in some situations. CT scans are effective in identifying a solid tumor mass and changes such as lymph node spread. Pancreatic arteriography demonstrates occlusion of the celiac axis and the superior mesenteric artery.

With ERCP it is possible to get excellent x-ray visualization of the pancreatic ducts. In pancreatic cancer, findings include obstruction or narrowing of a major duct and, frequently, saccular dilatations of smaller peripheral ducts. Material for cytology and biopsy may show malignant cells. ERCP is usually considered to be the best diagnostic test.

Therapeutic Management

Surgery provides the most effective treatment of cancer of the pancreas. The classic surgery is a *radical pancreaticoduodenectomy,* or *Whipple's procedure* (Fig. 41-11). This entails resection of the proximal pancreas (proximal pancreatectomy), the adjoining duodenum (duodenectomy), the distal portion of the stomach (partial gastrectomy), and the distal segment of the common bile duct. An anastomosis of the pancreatic duct, common bile duct, and stomach to the jejunum is done. A total pancreatectomy is performed in some institutions for cancers of the head of the pancreas. Sometimes a simple bypass procedure, such as a cholecystojejunostomy to relieve biliary obstruction, may be used as a palliative measure. Some surgeons suggest a more radical resection, such as a total pancreaticoduodenectomy with splenectomy. Biliary stents (e.g., Cotton-Leung stent) can be used as a palliative measure when tumors compress the bile duct.

Radiation therapy alters survival rates little but is effective for pain relief. External radiation is usually used, but implantation of internal radiation seeds into the tumor has also been used. Chemotherapy has limited success. Combinations of drugs such as 5-FU and BCNU produce a better response than single chemotherapeutic agents. Biologic response modifiers are sometimes attempted (see Chapter 12). Adjuvant therapy, which uses surgical resection, radiation, and chemotherapy, is believed by some to be the most effective way to manage the almost always fatal cancer of the pancreas.

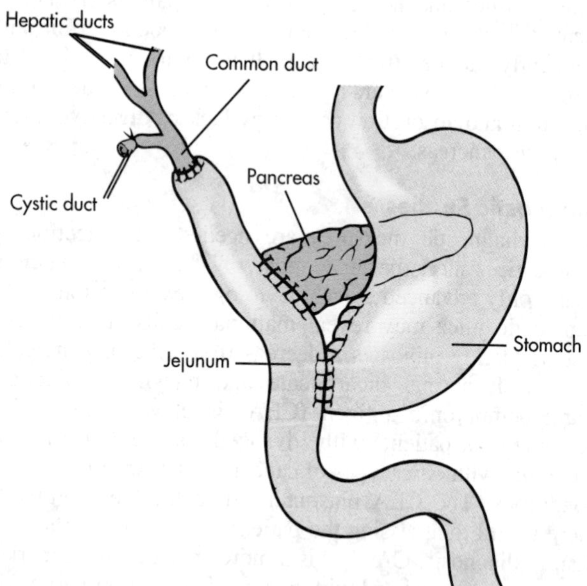

Fig. 41-11 Whipple procedure or radical pancreaticoduodenectomy. This surgical procedure involves resection of the proximal pancreas, adjoining duodenum, distal portion of the stomach, and distal portion of the common bile duct. An anastomosis of the pancreatic duct, common bile duct, and stomach to the jejunum is done.

NURSING MANAGEMENT

CARCINOMA OF THE PANCREAS

Because the patient with carcinoma of the pancreas has many of the same problems as the patient with pancreatitis, nursing care includes the same measures (see the nursing care plan for the patient with acute pancreatitis on p. 1292). The nurse should provide symptomatic and supportive nursing care. Medications and comfort measures to relieve pain should be provided before the patient reaches the peak of pain. Psychologic support is essential, especially during times of anxiety or depression, which seem to occur frequently in these patients.

Adequate nutrition is an important part of the nursing care plan. Frequent and supplemental feedings may be necessary. Measures to stimulate the appetite as much as possible and to overcome anorexia, nausea, and vomiting should be included in the nursing care. Because bleeding can result from impaired vitamin K production, the nurse should assess for bleeding from body orifices and mucous membranes. If the patient is undergoing radiation therapy, the nurse must observe for adverse reactions, such as anorexia, nausea, vomiting, and skin irritation.

The prognosis for a patient with pancreatic cancer is not good. A significant component of the nursing care is helping the patient and the family or significant others through the grieving process.

DISORDERS OF THE BILIARY TRACT

The most common disorder of the biliary system is *cholelithiasis* (stones in the gallbladder) (Fig. 41-12). *Cholecystitis* (inflammation of the gallbladder) is usually associated with cholelithiasis. The stones may be lodged in the neck of the gallbladder or in the cystic duct. Cholecystitis may be acute or chronic. These conditions usually occur together.

Significance

Gallbladder disease is a common health problem in the United States. It is estimated that 8% to 10% of the adults in the United States have cholelithiasis. The actual number is not known because many persons are aysmptomatic with stones. *Cholecystectomy* (removal of the gallbladder) ranks among the most common surgical procedures performed in the United States. The incidence of cholelithiasis is higher in women, multiparous women, and persons over 40 years of age. Postmenopausal women on estrogen therapy are at somewhat greater risk of having gallbladder disease than are women who are taking birth control pills. Oral contraceptives alter the character of bile, resulting in increased cholesterol saturation. Other factors that seem to increase the occurrence of gallbladder disease are a sedentary lifestyle, a familial tendency, and obesity. Obesity causes increased secretion of cholesterol in bile. Gallbladder disease is more common in Caucasians than in Asians and African-Americans. There is an especially high incidence in the Native American population, particularly in the Navajo and Pima tribes.

Pathophysiology

Cholecystitis. Cholecystitis is most commonly associated with stones. When it occurs in the absence of stones, it is thought to be caused by bacteria reaching the gallbladder via the vascular or lymphatic route or chemical irritants in the bile. *Escherichia coli* is the most common bacterium involved. Streptococci and salmonellae are also common causative bacteria. Other etiologic factors include adhesions, neoplasms, extensive fasting, frequent weight fluctuations, anesthesia, and narcotics.

Inflammation is the major pathophysiologic condition and may be confined to the mucous lining or involve the entire wall of the gallbladder. During an acute attack of cholecystitis the gallbladder is edematous and hyperemic. It may be distended with bile or pus. The cystic duct is also involved and may become occluded. The wall of the gallbladder becomes scarred after an acute attack. Decreased functioning occurs if large amounts of tissue are fibrosed.

Cholelithiasis. The actual cause of gallstones is unknown. Basically, cholelithiasis develops when the balance that keeps cholesterol, bile salts, and calcium in solution is altered so that precipitation of these substances occurs. Conditions that upset this balance include infection and disturbances in the metabolism of cholesterol.

It is known that in patients with cholelithiasis the bile secreted by the liver is supersaturated with cholesterol (lithogenic bile). The bile in the gallbladder also becomes supersaturated with cholesterol. Whenever bile is supersaturated with cholesterol, precipitation of cholesterol will occur.

A high percentage of gallstones are precipitates of cholesterol. Other components of bile that precipitate into stones are bile salts, bilirubin, calcium, and protein. The stones sometimes have a mixed consistency. Mixed cholesterol stones, which are predominantly cholesterol, are the most common gallstones.

The changes in the composition of bile are probably significant in the formation of gallstones. Stasis of bile leads to progression of the supersaturation and changes in the chemical composition of the bile. Immobility, pregnancy, and inflammatory or obstructive lesions of the biliary system decrease bile flow. Hormonal factors during pregnancy may cause delayed emptying of the gallbladder.

The stones may remain in the gallbladder or migrate to the cystic duct or to the common bile duct. They cause pain as they pass through the ducts and may lodge in the ducts and produce an obstruction. Small stones are more likely to move into a duct and cause obstruction. Table 41-20 depicts the changes and manifestations that occur when the stones obstruct the common bile duct. If the blockage occurs in the cystic duct, the bile can continue to flow into the duodenum directly from the liver. When the bile in the gallbladder

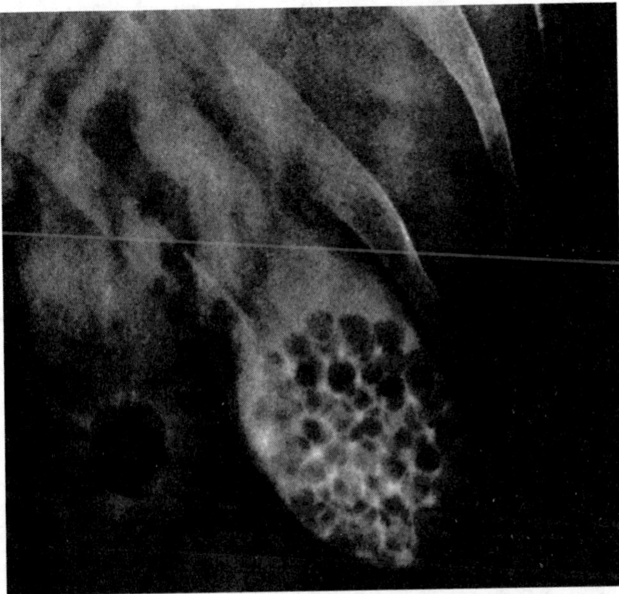

Fig. 41-12 X-ray of a gallbladder with gallstones.

Table 41-20 Clinical Manifestations Caused by Obstructed Bile Flow

Clinical Manifestation	Etiology
Obstructive jaundice	No bile flow into duodenum
Dark amber urine, which foams when shaken	Soluble bilirubin in urine
No urobilinogen in urine	No bilirubin reaching small intestine to be converted to urobilinogen
Clay-colored stools	Same as above
Pruritus	Deposition of bile salts in skin tissues
Intolerance for fatty foods (nausea, sensation of fullness, anorexia)	No bile in small intestine for fat digestion
Bleeding tendencies	Lack of or decreased absorption of vitamin K, resulting in decreased production of prothrombin
Steatorrhea	No bile salts in duodenum, preventing fat emulsion and digestion

cannot escape, however, this stasis of bile may lead to cholecystitis.[35]

Clinical Manifestations

Manifestations of cholecystitis vary from indigestion to moderate to severe pain, fever, and jaundice.[36] Initial symptoms of acute cholecystitis include indigestion and pain and tenderness in the right upper quadrant, which may be referred to the right shoulder and scapula. Manifestations of inflammation, such as leukocytosis and fever, occur. Acute cholecystitis may be present, with sudden onset of midepigastric or right upper quadrant pain radiating to the back and right shoulder. The pain is accompanied by restlessness, diaphoresis, and nausea and vomiting. Physical findings include right upper quadrant tenderness and abdominal rigidity. Symptoms of chronic cholecystitis include a history of fat intolerance, dyspepsia, heartburn, and flatulence.

Cholelithiasis may produce severe symptoms or none at all. Many patients have "silent cholelithiasis." The severity of symptoms depends on whether the stones are stationary or mobile and whether obstruction is present. When a stone is lodged in the ducts or when stones are moving through the ducts, spasms may result. The spasms are the tissues' responses to the stone in an attempt to move it forward. This sometimes produces severe pain, which is termed *biliary colic* even though the pain is rarely colicky; it is more often steady. The pain can be excruciating and accompanied by tachycardia, diaphoresis, and prostration. The severe pain may last up to an hour, and when it subsides there is residual tenderness in the right upper quadrant. The attacks of pain frequently occur 3 to 6 hours after a heavy meal or when the patient assumes a recumbent position. When total obstruction occurs, symptoms related to bile blockage are manifested (see Table 41-20).

Complications

Complications of cholecystitis include subphrenic abscess, pancreatitis, *cholangitis* (inflammation of biliary ducts), biliary cirrhosis, fistulas, and rupture of the gallbladder, which can produce bile peritonitis.

Many of the same complications can occur from cholelithiasis, including cholangitis, biliary cirrhosis, carcinoma, and peritonitis. *Choledocholithiasis* (stone in the common bile duct) may occur, producing symptoms of obstruction.

Diagnostic Studies

Ultrasonography is probably the best means of diagnosing gallstones (see Table 36-12). It is 90% to 95% accurate in detecting stones. It is especially useful for patients with jaundice (because it does not depend on liver function) and for patients who are allergic to contrast medium.

An oral cholecystogram allows for the detection of stones when they are radiopaque. An IV cholangiogram outlines both the gallbladder and the ducts, so gallstones that have moved into the ductal system can be detected. Percutaneous transhepatic cholangiography may be used to diagnose obstructive jaundice and to locate stones within the bile ducts. Bile taken during ERCP is sent for culture to identify any possible infecting organism.

Laboratory tests may demonstrate abnormalities in some of the liver function tests and an increased WBC count as a result of inflammation. Both the direct and indirect bilirubin levels are elevated, as is the urinary bilirubin level if there is an obstructive process present. If the common bile duct is obstructed, no bilirubin will reach the small intestine to be converted to urobilinogen. Serum enzymes, such as alkaline phosphatase and AST (SGOT) may be elevated. The serum amylase is increased if there is pancreatic involvement.

Therapeutic Management

Cholecystitis. During an acute episode of cholecystitis the focus of treatment is on control of pain, control of possible infection with antibiotics, and maintenance of fluid and electrolyte balance (Table 41-21). Treatment is mainly supportive and symptomatic. If nausea and vomiting are severe, gastric decompression may be used to prevent further gallbladder stimulation. Anticholinergics to decrease secretions (which prevents biliary contraction) and counteract smooth muscle spasms may be administered. Analgesics are given to decrease the pain.

Cholelithiasis. There are currently several options for therapeutic management of cholelithiasis. These include cholesterol solvents such as methyl tertiary terbutyl ether (MTBE), oral drugs that dissolve stones, endoscopic sphincterotomy, extracorporeal shock-wave lithotripsy (ESWL),

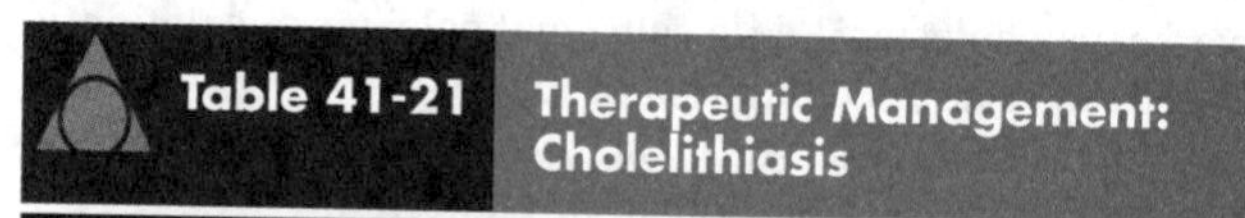

Table 41-21 Therapeutic Management: Cholelithiasis

Diagnostic
- Ultrasound
- Cholecystogram or IV cholangiogram
- Liver function studies
- WBC count

Therapeutic

Conservative treatment
- IV fluid
- NPO with NG tube, later progressing to low-fat diet
- Antiemetics
- Analgesics (e.g., meperidine)
- Fat-soluble vitamins (A, D, E, and K)
- Anticholinergics (antispasmodics)
- Bile salts
- Antibiotics
- ERCP with sphincterotomy (papillotomy)
- Cholesterol solvents
- Bile acid therapy
- Extracorporeal shock-wave lithotripsy

Surgical treatment
- Laparoscopic cholecystectomy
- Incisional cholecystectomy
- See Table 41-22

ERCP, Endoscopic retrograde cholangiopancreatography; *IV*, intravenous; *NG*, nasogastric; *NPO*, nothing by mouth; *WBC*, white blood cell.

and surgery. Supportive treatment, similar to that given for cholecystitis, may also be necessary. If the stones cause an obstruction, additional treatment consists of replacement of fat-soluble vitamins, administration of bile salts to facilitate digestion and vitamin absorption, and a low-fat diet.

A direct contact dissolving agent such as MTBE can be instilled into the gallbladder via a percutaneous catheter. MTBE dissolves cholesterol stones within hours. The gallstones may reoccur. The instillation of MTBE has not been approved by the Food and Drug Administration (FDA). Oral bile acids are also used to dissolve stones.

Endoscopic sphincterotomy (papillotomy) is especially effective in removing common bile duct stones (Fig. 41-13). The endoscope is passed to the duodenum. With an electrodiathermy knife attached to the endoscope, the sphincter of Oddi is widened by incision of the sphincter muscle (sphincterotomy). A basket is used to retrieve the stone. The stone may be removed in the basket, but more commonly it is left in the duodenum and will be passed naturally in the stool.[37]

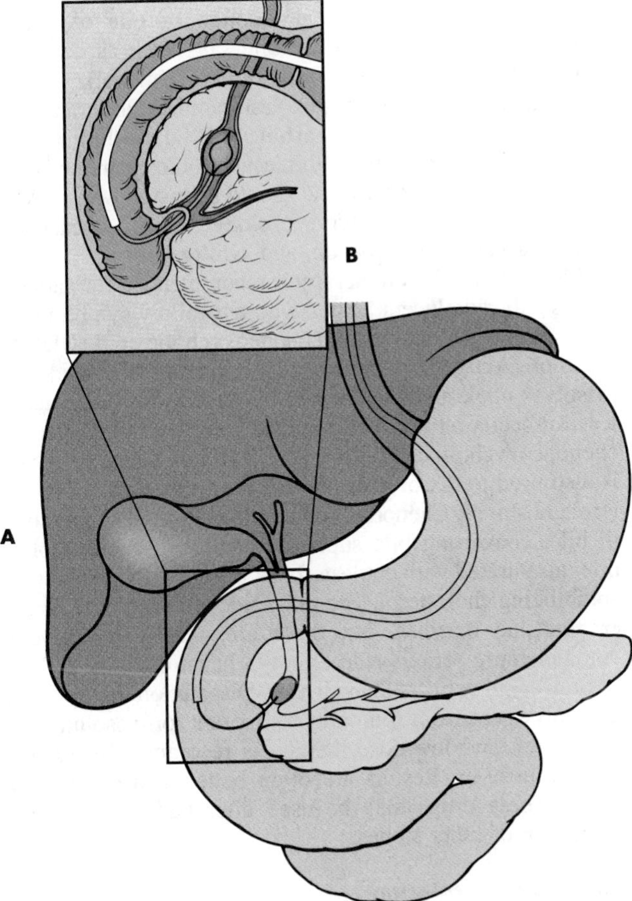

Fig. 41-13 ***A,*** During endoscopic sphincterotomy, a flexible endoscope is advanced through the mouth and stomach until its tip sits in the duodenum opposite the common bile duct. ***B,*** After widening the duct mouth by incising the sphincter muscle, the physician advances a basket attachment into the duct and snags the stone.

In ESWL a biliary lithotriptor uses high-energy shock waves to disintegrate gallstones. The patient must have a functioning gallbladder. An ultrasound scan is first done to locate the stones and to determine where to direct the shock waves. The shock waves are directed through the abdomen as a water-filled cushion is pressed against the area. It usually takes 1 to 2 hours to disintegrate the stones. After they are broken up, the fragments pass through the common bile duct and into the small intestine. There has been mixed success with ESWL. It is not currently approved by the FDA in the United States.

Surgical intervention. Surgical intervention for cholelithiasis is frequently indicated and may consist of any one of several procedures (Table 41-22). The procedure of choice for most patients is still a cholecystectomy. This is a safe procedure with minimal morbidity, and it requires only a brief hospitalization. One procedure is removal of the gallbladder through a right subcostal incision. A T-tube is inserted into the common bile duct during surgery when a common bile duct exploration is part of the surgical procedure (Fig. 41-14). This ensures patency of the duct until the edema produced by the trauma of exploring and probing the duct has subsided. It also allows the excess bile to drain while the small intestine is adjusting to receiving a continuous flow of bile.

The laparoscopic cholecystectomy is considered by many surgeons to be the preferred surgical procedure.[38] This procedure is done instead of the open surgical procedure about 80% to 85% of the time. In this procedure the gallbladder is removed through one of four small punctures in the abdomen. A 1-cm puncture is made slightly above the umbilicus, and the surgeon inflates the abdominal cavity with 3 to 4 L of carbon dioxide to improve visibility. A laparoscope, which has a camera attached, is then inserted into the abdomen. Two additional punctures are made just

Table 41-22 Gallbladder Surgery Procedures

Name	Description
Cholecystectomy	Removal of gallbladder
Cholecystostomy (usually an emergency)	Incision into gallbladder (usually for removal of stones)
Choledocholithotomy	Incision into common bile duct for removal of stones
Cholecystogastrostomy	Anastomosis between stomach and gallbladder
Cholecystoduodenostomy	Anastomosis between gallbladder and duodenum to relieve obstruction at distal end of common bile duct
Laparoscopic cholecystectomy	Removal of gallbladder via laparoscopy using a dissecting laser

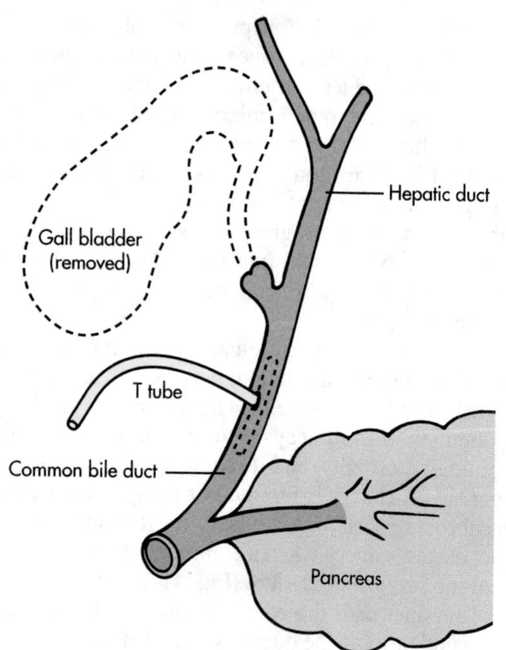

Fig. 41-14 Placement of T tube. *Dotted lines* indicate parts removed.

below the ribs, one on the right anterior axillary line and the other on the right midclavicular line. These punctures are used for insertion of grasping forceps. A dissection laser is inserted into the fourth puncture, which is made just right of the midsection. (The incision sites may vary.) Using closed-circuit monitors to view the abdominal cavity, the surgeon retracts and dissects the gallbladder and removes it with grasping forceps.

This procedure is relatively minor with few complications. Most patients experience minimal postoperative pain and are discharged the day of surgery or the day after. In most cases they are able to resume normal activities and return to work after 2 or 3 days.

Advantages to the laparoscopic cholecystectomy include decreased postoperative pain, shorter hospital stay, and earlier return to work and full activity. The main complication is injury to the common bile duct. There are few contraindications to laparoscopic cholecystectomy. The primary ones are peritonitis, cholangitis, gangrene or perforation of the gallbladder, portal hypertension, and serious bleeding disorders.

Transhepatic Biliary Catheter. The transhepatic biliary catheter can be used preoperatively in biliary obstruction and in hepatic dysfunction secondary to obstructive jaundice. It can also be inserted when inoperable liver, pancreatic, or bile duct carcinoma obstructs bile flow. The catheter is inserted under fluoroscopy and involves percutaneous insertion across the liver parenchyma into the common bile duct and duodenum. It decompresses obstructed extrahepatic bile ducts so that bile can flow freely. After insertion, the catheter is connected to a drainage bag. The skin around the catheter insertion site has to be cleansed daily with an antiseptic. It is important to observe for bile leakage at the insertion site. Depending on the reason the catheter was inserted, the patient may be discharged with it in place.

Pharmacologic Management

The most common drugs used in the treatment of gallbladder disease are analgesics, anticholinergics (antispasmodics), fat-soluble vitamins, and bile salts. Meperidine (Demerol) is used if a narcotic analgesic is required. This causes less spasm in the ducts than opiates such as morphine sulfate.

Anticholinergics such as atropine and other antispasmodics may be used to relax the smooth muscle and decrease ductal tone. Nursing observations for side effects of drugs and relief of the pain should be made.

If the patient has chronic gallbladder disease or any biliary tract obstruction, fat-soluble vitamins (A, D, E, and K) will probably be given. Bile salts may be administered to facilitate digestion and vitamin absorption.

Hydrocholeretic drugs, which stimulate the production of bile with a low specific gravity, may be administered following gallbladder surgery when a T-tube is in place or with conservative therapy as long as there is no obstruction. These drugs stimulate the production of bile of a low specific gravity. Examples are bile salts such as dehydrocholic acid (Decholin) and florantyrone (Zanchol).

For treatment of pruritus, cholestyramine (Questran) may provide relief. This is a resin that binds bile salts in the intestine, increasing their excretion in the feces. Cholestyramine is administered in powder form and should be mixed with milk or juice. The nurse should observe for side effects of nausea, vomiting, diarrhea or constipation, and skin reactions.

Medical dissolution therapy is recommended for patients with small radiolucent stones who are mildly symptomatic and are poor surgical risks. Ursodeoxycholic acid (UDCA) ursodiol (Actigall) is a naturally occurring bile acid that dissolves cholesterol gallstones by decreasing biliary cholesterol secretion and desaturating bile. A similar agent is chenodeoxycholic acid (CDCA, chenodiol, Chenix), which is also used to dissolve or prevent the formation of cholesterol gallstones. Chenodiol reduces the cholesterol secretion in bile, converting bile supersaturated with cholesterol to bile unsaturated with cholesterol. It also dissolves stones by solubilizing cholesterol. The main side effects of CDCA are cramps and diarrhea, but these are usually not severe. Another more serious side effect is hepatotoxicity. UDCA has fewer side effects than CDCA. Dissolution therapy may take anywhere from 6 months to 2 years for dissolution of the stones, and low-dose therapy is recommended to prevent recurrence. Results are often better in nonobese patients. These drugs may be used after ESWL to prevent formation of other stones.

Nutritional Management

The major dietary modification for a patient with cholelithiasis and cholecystitis is a low-fat diet (see Table 31-5). If obesity is a problem, a reduced-calorie diet is indicated. The low-fat diet decreases stimulation of the gallbladder. Foods that are avoided include dairy products such as whole milk, cream, butter, whole milk cheese, and ice cream; fried foods;

rich pastries; gravies; and nuts. Many patients have fewer problems if they eat smaller, more frequent meals.

After a laparoscopic cholecystectomy the patient is instructed to have liquids for the rest of the day and eat light meals for a few days. If an incisional cholecystectomy is done, the patient will progress from liquids to a bland diet once bowel sounds have returned. The amount of fat in the postoperative diet depends on the patient's tolerance of fat. A low-fat diet may be helpful if the flow of bile is reduced (usually only in the early postoperative period) or if the patient is overweight. Sometimes the patient is instructed to restrict fats for 4 to 6 weeks. Otherwise no special dietary instructions are needed other than to eat nutritious meals and avoid excessive fat intake.

NURSING MANAGEMENT

GALLBLADDER DISEASE

Nursing Assessment

Subjective and objective data that should be obtained from a person with gallbladder disease are presented in Table 41-23.

Table 41-23 Nursing Assessment: Cholecystitis or Cholelithiasis

Subjective Data

Important health information

Past health history: Obesity, multiparity, infection, cancer, extensive fasting, pregnancy, diabetes, cirrhosis

Medications: Use of estrogen or oral contraceptives

Surgery and other treatments: Previous abdominal surgery

Functional health patterns

Health perception–health management: Positive family history; chills

Nutritional-metabolic: Weight loss, anorexia; indigestion, fat intolerance, nausea and vomiting, dyspepsia, pyrosis

Elimination: Clay-colored stools, flatulence; dark urine

Cognitive-perceptual: Moderate to severe pain in right upper quadrant that may radiate to the back or scapula

Objective Data

General

Fever, restlessness

Integumentary

Jaundice, icteric sclera

Respiratory

Tachypnea, splinting during respirations

Cardiovascular

Tachycardia

Gastrointestinal

Palpable gallbladder, abdominal guarding and distention

Possible findings

Elevated liver enzymes and bilirubin, leukocytosis, abnormal gallbladder ultrasound, positive oral cholecystogram or IV cholangiogram

IV, Intravenous.

Nursing Diagnoses

Nursing diagnoses are determined when the problem and the etiologic factors are supported by clinical data. Nursing diagnoses related to the surgical management of gallbladder disease include, but are not limited to, those presented in the nursing care plan for the patient with a cholecystectomy.

Planning

The overall goals are that the patient with gallbladder disease will (1) have relief of pain and discomfort, (2) no complications postoperatively, and (3) no recurrent attacks of cholecystitis or cholelithiasis. Specific outcomes are identified in the nursing care plan for gallbladder disease.

Nursing Implementation

Health Promotion and Maintenance. The nurse should assume responsibility for recognition of predisposing factors of gallbladder disease in general health screening. Ethnic groups in which the disease is more common, such as Native Americans, should be taught initial manifestations and instructed to seek medical care if these manifestations occur. The patient with chronic cholecystitis does not have acute symptoms and may not seek help until jaundice and biliary obstruction occur. Earlier detection in these patients is beneficial so that they can be treated with a low-fat diet and monitored more closely.

Acute Intervention. Nursing objectives for the patient undergoing conservative therapy include relieving pain, relieving nausea and vomiting, providing comfort and emotional support, maintaining fluid and electrolyte balance and nutrition, making accurate assessments for effectiveness of treatment, and observing for complications.

The patient with cholecystitis or cholelithiasis is frequently experiencing severe pain. The medications ordered to relieve the pain should be given as required by the patient and before the pain becomes more severe. The nurse should assess what medications relieve the pain and how much medication is required. Observations for side effects of the medications must be part of the continued assessment. Nursing comfort measures, such as a clean bed, comfortable positioning, and oral care, are appropriate.

Some patients have more severe nausea and vomiting than others. For these patients it may be necessary to use gastric decompression. The elimination of intake of food and fluids also prevents further stimulation of the gallbladder. Oral hygiene, care of nares, accurate intake and output measurements, and maintenance of suction should be a part of the nursing care plan for this patient. For patients with less severe nausea and vomiting, antiemetics are usually adequate. When the patient is vomiting, comfort measures such as frequent mouth rinses should be provided. Any vomitus should be immediately removed from the patient's view.

If pruritus occurs with jaundice, measures to relieve itching are necessary. Such measures include baking soda or Alpha Keri baths; lotions, such as those containing calamine; antihistamines; soft, old linen; and control of the temperature (not too hot and not too cold). The patient's nails should be kept short and clean. Patients should be

NURSING CARE PLAN Patient with an Incisional Cholecystectomy

Planning: Outcome Criteria	Nursing Interventions and Rationales
➤ **NURSING DIAGNOSIS**	Pain *related to* surgical incision and presence of drains and bulky dressing *as manifested by* communication of pain descriptors, guarding behavior, narrowed self-focus, behaviors indicative of pain (e.g., moaning), diaphoresis, and changes in blood pressure, pulse, and respiratory rate
Report satisfaction with pain control; understand temporary nature of drains and dressing.	Administer ordered analgesic frequently enough *to ensure that the patient will move about.* Provide comfort measures such as good positioning and a quiet environment *to prevent unnecessary pain.* Help patient support incision when coughing and deep breathing and getting out of bed *to decrease pain from stress on incision line.*
➤ **NURSING DIAGNOSIS**	Ineffective breathing pattern *related to* splinted or guarded respirations secondary to pain *as manifested by* dyspnea, shortness of breath, tachypnea, cyanosis, cough, respiratory depth changes, changes in respiratory rate or pattern, changes in pulse
Have normal breath sounds, respiratory rate of 12-16/min.	Assist patient to cough and deep breathe every hour *to remove secretions and prevent pooling of secretions.* Auscultate lung sounds q2-4hr *to monitor patient's status and response to treatment.* Plan a schedule with patient and ensure that analgesia is given as needed *to make it easier to cough, deep breathe, and move about.* Support incision with pillow or hands *to reduce incisional pain caused by coughing and deep breathing.* Encourage early ambulation *to prevent respiratory complications associated with bed rest.* When patient is in bed, place in low Fowler's position *to facilitate breathing by decreasing pressure on diaphragm and preventing aspiration of vomitus or secretions.*
➤ **NURSING DIAGNOSIS**	Risk for impaired skin integrity *related to* irritating drainage from surgical area
Have surgical area free from signs of irritation and inflammation.	Assess patient for disruption of epidermal and dermal tissue, erythema, denuded skin, lesions, pruritus, drainage from surgical area *to determine status of skin.* Keep dressing dry and clean *to protect skin from irritation and reduce risk of infection.* Use Montgomery straps *to reduce skin irritation from frequent removal of tape.* Observe and record type of drainage *to detect complications associated with abnormal volume or type of drainage.* Cleanse skin carefully with warm water and pat dry *to remove irritating bile drainage and prevent additional trauma.*

continued

taught to rub with their knuckles rather than scratch with their nails when they cannot resist the scratching.

A significant portion of the nursing care plan for this patient centers on accurate assessment of progression of the symptoms and development of complications. The nurse must be knowledgeable of and observe for signs of obstruction of the ducts by stones. These include jaundice; clay-colored stools; dark, foamy urine; steatorrhea; fever; and increased WBC count.

When symptoms of obstruction are present (see Table 41-20), the nurse must be aware of the possibility of bleeding as a result of decreased prothrombin production. Common sites to observe for bleeding are the mucous membranes of the mouth, nose, gingivae, and injection sites. If injections are given, a small-gauge needle should be used and gentle pressure applied after the injection. The nurse should know what the patient's prothrombin time is and use this as a guide in the assessment process.

Assessment for infections includes monitoring of vital signs. A temperature elevation with chills and jaundice may indicate choledocholithiasis.

Nursing care of the patient after endoscopic papillotomy includes assessment to detect complications such as pancreatitis, perforation, infection, and bleeding. The patient's vital signs should be monitored. Abdominal pain and fever may indicate pancreatitis. The patient should be on bed rest for several hours and should have nothing by mouth until the gag reflex returns.

Care after surgical intervention. Postoperative nursing care following a laparoscopic cholecystectomy includes monitoring for complications such as bleeding, making the patient comfortable, and preparing the patient for discharge. A common postoperative problem is referred pain to the shoulder because of the CO_2 that was not released or absorbed by the body. The CO_2 can irritate the phrenic nerve and the diaphragm, causing some difficulty breathing. Placing the patient in Sim's position (left side with right knee flexed) helps move the gas pocket away from the diaphragm. Deep breathing should be encouraged. There is usually minimal pain that can be relieved by narcotic analgesics such as oxycodone and acetaminophen (Percocet). The patient is allowed clear liquids and can walk to the

NURSING CARE PLAN Patient with an Incisional Cholecystectomy—cont'd

Planning: Outcome Criteria	Nursing Interventions and Rationales
➤ **NURSING DIAGNOSIS**	Impaired management of therapeutic regimen *related to* lack of knowledge of postoperative management, diet, and activity restrictions *as manifested by* verbalization of problem, request for information, inaccurate follow-through of instruction
Know activity level and dietary restrictions; plan for follow-up care.	Instruct patient to avoid heavy lifting for 4-6 wk *as a precaution to prevent dehiscence of wound or herniation into the wound.* Provide dietary teaching plan if patient is required to remain on low-fat diet or if put on a weight-reduction program *to provide information that will enable patient to follow prescribed diet.* Assist patient to arrange necessary follow-up care *to ensure monitoring of convalescence.*

COLLABORATIVE PROBLEMS

Nursing Goals	Nursing Interventions and Rationales
➤ **POTENTIAL COMPLICATION**	Paralytic ileus *related to* decreased peristalsis secondary to surgery and immobility
Monitor for signs of paralytic ileus; report deviations from acceptable parameters; carry out appropriate medical and nursing interventions.	Assess for signs of paralytic ileus such as failure to pass gas or feces, abdominal distention and tenderness, absence of bowel sounds *to ensure early intervention.* Keep patient on NPO status until bowel sounds are present *because absence of bowel sounds means peristalsis has not returned.* Maintain IV fluid administration at prescribed rate *to maintain fluid and electrolyte balance.* Provide oral care q1-2hr *to stimulate salivation and prevent parotitis.* Auscultate for bowel sounds q4hr *to detect resumption of peristalsis.* Encourage ambulation 3 or 4 times a day if not contraindicated *because movement stimulates the return of peristalsis.*

IV, Intravenous; *NPO,* nothing by mouth.

bathroom to void. Many patients go home the same day, but some will stay overnight.

Postoperative nursing care for incisional surgery (cholecystectomy) is discussed in the nursing care plan for the patient with cholecystectomy. Adequate ventilation and prevention of respiratory complications are important objectives for this patient. The high incision in the right subcostal region is near the diaphragm, and the patient is reluctant to take deep breaths because of the pain this causes. When bowel sounds are heard, the patient is given clear liquids with progression to a surgical soft diet and then to a low-fat or regular diet. The nurse should observe tolerance to the diet and assist in any required dietary instruction.

The patient may have a Penrose drain or a Jackson-Pratt drain inserted into a stab wound near the incision. This allows for drainage and prevents accumulation of fluid and serous drainage in the area from which the gallbladder was removed. If there is serosanguineous bile-tinged drainage, the dressing should be changed frequently. The wound should be kept dry and clean because bile is irritating to the skin. When changing the dressing, the nurse should use sterile technique, clean around the drain (if indicated), and take special care not to dislodge the drain. Currently many patients have no drains and may have a dressing for only 24 to 48 hours.

If the patient has a T-tube, part of the nursing care plan is related to maintaining bile drainage and observation of the T-tube functioning and drainage. The T-tube is connected to a closed gravity drainage system. If the Penrose or Jackson-Pratt drain or the T-tube is draining large amounts, it is helpful to use a sterile pouching system to protect the skin.

Chronic and Home Management. When the patient is on a conservative therapy, long-term nursing management depends on symptoms and on whether surgical intervention is being planned. Dietary teaching is usually necessary. The diet is usually low in fat, and sometimes a weight-reduction diet is also recommended. The patient may need to take fat-soluble vitamin supplements. The nurse should provide instructions regarding observations the patient should make indicating obstruction (stool and urine changes, jaundice, and pruritus). Continued health care is important, and its significance should be explained and stressed.

The patient who undergoes a laparoscopic cholecystectomy is discharged soon after the surgery, so home care is important. Teaching is essential. The patient should be instructed to remove the bandages on the puncture sites the day after surgery and bathe or shower. The patient should be instructed to report signs and symptoms of complications such as redness, swelling, or bile-colored drainage or pus from any incision; severe abdominal pain, nausea, vomiting, fever, chills. The patient can gradually return to normal activity and return to work within a week after the surgery.

The patient may be discharged as soon as 3 to 5 days after an open incision cholecystectomy. The patient should be instructed to avoid heavy lifting for 4 to 6 weeks. Usual

CRITICAL THINKING EXERCISES

CASE STUDY

CIRRHOSIS OF THE LIVER

Patient Profile

Mr. R. is a 55-year-old man admitted with a diagnosis of cirrhosis of the liver.

Subjective Data

- Has had cirrhosis for 12 years
- Acknowledges that he had been drinking heavily for 20 years but has been sober for the past 2 years
- Complains of anorexia, nausea, and abdominal discomfort

Objective Data

Physical Examination

- Thin and malnourished
- Has moderate ascites
- Has jaundice of sclera and skin
- Has 4+ pitting edema of the lower extremities
- Liver and spleen are palpable

Laboratory Values

- Total bilirubin 15 mg/dl (257 μmol/L)
- Serum ammonia 220 μg/dl (122 μmol/L)
- AST 190 U/L (3.2 μkat/L)
- ALT 210 U/L (3.5 μkat/L)

Critical Thinking Questions

1. What are possible causes of cirrhosis? What type of cirrhosis does Mr. R. have?
2. Describe the pathophysiologic changes that occur in the liver as cirrhosis develops.
3. List Mr. R.'s clinical manifestations of liver failure. For each manifestation, explain the pathophysiologic bases.
4. Explain the significance of the results of his laboratory values.
5. If Mr. R. begins to manifest signs and symptoms of hepatic encephalopathy, what would you monitor? What measures should be instituted to control or decrease the ammonia level?
6. Mr. R. was being closely observed for the possibility of gastrointestinal bleeding. Why is this considered a possible complication?
7. In the early stages of cirrhosis, what can be done to control the disease?
8. Based on the assessment data presented, write one or more nursing diagnoses. Are there any collaborative problems?

NURSING RESEARCH ISSUES

1. What is the most effective way to assess jaundice in a dark-skinned person?
2. What are the most significant psychosocial problems experienced by a patient with viral hepatitis?
3. What are the best ways to treat pruritis associated with jaundice in patients with hepatitis?
4. What is the quality of life for a patient after a liver transplant?
5. Can nutritional support improve outcomes in patients with alcohol-related cirrhosis?
6. What support resources are needed by the family of a patient with pancreatic cancer?

sexual activities, including intercourse, can be resumed as soon as the patient feels ready unless given other instructions by the physician.

Sometimes the patient is required to remain on a low-fat diet for 4 to 6 weeks. If so, a dietary teaching plan is necessary. A weight-reduction program may be helpful if the patient is overweight. Most patients tolerate a regular diet with no difficulties but should avoid excessive fats.

CANCER OF THE GALLBLADDER

Primary cancer of the gallbladder is rare. The majority of gallbladder carcinomas are adenocarcinomas. There seems to be a definite relationship between cancer of the gallbladder and chronic cholecystitis and cholelithiasis. Approximately 80% of patients with gallbladder malignancy also have gallstones.[39]

The early symptoms of carcinoma of the gallbladder are insidious and are similar to those of chronic cholecystitis and cholelithiasis, which makes diagnosis difficult. Later symptoms are usually those of biliary obstruction. Cancer of the gallbladder has a poor prognosis.

Treatment is mainly symptomatic and supportive. Sometimes the tumor is resected. Chemotherapy and radiotherapy are seldom used because they are neither curative nor palliative.

Nursing management involves supportive care with special attention to nutrition, hydration, skin care, and pain relief. Many of the nursing care measures used for patients with cholecystitis and cholelithiasis are frequently applied, as well as nursing care measures for the patient with cancer (see Chapter 12).

REVIEW QUESTIONS

The number of the question corresponds to the same-numbered objective at the beginning of the chapter.

1. Which of the following signs or symptoms would be found in a patient with obstructive jaundice?

a. Serum bilirubin 1 mg/dl
b. Dark urine and clay-colored stools
c. Elevated urinary urobilinogen
d. Pyrexia and severe pruritis

2. Ms. H. is in the prodromal (preicteric) phase of viral hepatitis. Which of the following would be expected during this phase?

a. Sudden onset of jaundice
b. Weight loss
c. Flulike symptoms
d. Acute yellow atrophy

3. Mr. B. has hepatitis B. He is being discharged in 2 days. Which of the following should be included in his discharge teaching plan?

a. Use of a condom for sexual intercourse
b. Have family members get an injection of immunoglobulin
c. Follow a low-protein, moderate-carbohydrate, moderate-fat diet
d. Avoid alcohol for 3 weeks

4. Which of the following clinical manifestations would the nurse expect to assess in the patient with advanced cirrhosis of the liver?

a. Infection and metabolic alkalosis
b. Dyspepsia and flatulence
c. Ascites, spider angiomas, bleeding tendencies
d. Leukocytosis, abdominal discomfort, nausea

5. When caring for a patient with hepatic encephalopathy the nurse may give enemas, provide a low-protein diet, and limit physical activity. These measures are done to

a. eliminate potassium ions.
b. decrease the production of ammonia.
c. increase the production of ammonia.
d. decrease portal pressure.

6. Which of the following statements about carcinoma of the liver is true?

a. Nursing intervention focuses on symptomatic and comfort measures.
b. Surgical excision of the tumor is highly successful.
c. The prognosis is very good.
d. Primary carcinoma is more common than metastatic carcinoma.

7. The most common pathogenic mechanism in acute pancreatitis is

a. cellular disorganization.
b. lack of secretion of enzymes.
c. autodigestion of the pancreas.
d. overproduction of enzymes.

8. In a patient with acute pancreatitis nursing management should include which of the following?

a. Monitoring for infection, particularly respiratory infection
b. Observing stools for signs for steatorrhea
c. Checking for signs of hypercalcemia
d. Providing a diet low in carbohydrates with moderate fat

9. Identify the true statement about carcinoma of the pancreas.

a. Cigarette smoking is a major risk factor.
b. Pain is a common early symptom.
c. The most effective treatment is external radiation.
d. With surgical treatment there is a good prognosis.

10. Identify the true statement regarding gallbladder disease.

a. A significant factor in the formation of gallstones seems to be an increase in the bile acid pool concentration.
b. All individuals with cholelithiasis experience symptoms such as pain, nausea, and dyspepsia.
c. Oral bile acids are very effective for dissolving gallstones.
d. The patient who has a laparoscopic cholecystectomy will be discharged the same day of the surgery or the following day.

11. Teaching in relation to home management after a laparoscopic cholecystectomy should include

a. keeping the bandages on the puncture sites for 48 hours.
b. reporting any bile-colored drainage or pus from any incision.
c. staying on clear liquids for 48 hours.
d. expecting a lot of abdominal pain.

REFERENCES

1. Centers for Disease Control and Prevention: Summary of notifiable disease, United States, *MMWR* 42:53, 1993.
2. Jackson MM, Rymer TE: Viral hepatitis: anatomy of a diagnosis, *Am J Nurs* 94:43, 1994.
3. Alter MJ, Mast EE: The epidemiology of viral hepatitis in the United States, *Gastroenterol Clin North Am* 23:437, 1994.
4. Steen ID, Gill JS, Hall R: Hepatitis C, *Aust Fam Physician* 23:1747, 1994.
5. Alter HJ: Transfusion transmitted hepatitis C and non-A, non-B, non-C, *Vox Sanguinis* 67 (suppl 3):19, 1994.
6. Czaja AJ: Autoimmune hepatitis and viral infection, *Gastroenterol Clin North Am* 23:547, 1994.
7. Saracco G, Rizzetto M, Verme G: Interferon in chronic hepatitis B, *Antiviral Res* 24:137, 1994.
8. Hoofnagle JH: Therapy of acute and chronic viral hepatitis, *Adv Intern Med* 15:241, 1994.
9. Perrillo RP, Mason AL: Therapy for hepatitis B virus infection, *Gastroenterol Clin North Am* 23:581, 1994.
10. Ellis RW, Douglas G: New vaccine technologies, *JAMA* 271:929, 1994.
11. Centers for Disease Control: Sexually transmitted diseases treatment guidelines, *MMWR* 42:RR-14, 91, 1993.
12. Centers for Disease Control: Reported vaccine-preventable diseases, US, 1993, and the Childhood Immunization Initiative, *MMWR* 43:59, 1994.
13. van der Poel CL: Hepatitis C virus infection from blood and blood products, *FEMS Microbiol Rev* 14:241, 1994.
14. Van Thiel DH: Current and future uses of biological response modifiers in the treatment of viral hepatitis, *J Okla State Med Assoc* 87:319, 1994.

15. Blendis LM: Review article: the treatment of alcoholic liver disease, *Aliment Pharmacol Ther* 6:541, 1992.
16. el-Newihi HM, Mihas AA: Alcoholic hepatitis: recent advances in pathogenesis and therapy, *Postgrad Med* 96:61, 1994.
17. Pierce JD: Acute esophageal bleeding and endoscopic injection sclerotherapy, *Crit Care Nurse* 10:67, 1990.
18. Mudge C, Carlson L: Hepatorenal syndrome, *AACN Clin Issues Crit Care Nurs* 3:614, 1992.
19. Burroughs AK: Acute management of bleeding esophageal varices, *Drugs* 44(suppl 2):14, 1992.
20. Koutsomanis D: Endoscopic clipping for bleeding varices, *Gastrointest Endosc* 40:126, 1994.
21. Doherty MM, Carver DK: Transjugular intrahepatic portosystemic shunt: new relief for esophageal varices, *Am J Nurs* 93:58, 1993.
22. Thomas S: A new development in radiology: TIPS, *Nurs Stand* 7:25, 1992.
23. Killeen TL: Alchoholism and liver transplantation: ethical and nursing implications, *Perspect Psychiatr Care* 29:7, 1993.
24. Covington H: Nursing care of patients with alcoholic liver disease, *Crit Care Nurse* 13:47, 1993.
25. Tsukuma H and others: Risk factors for hepatocellular carcinoma among patients with chronic liver disease, *N Engl J Med* 328:1797, 1993.
26. Kew MC: Hepatitis C virus and hepatocellular carcinoma, *FEMS Microbiol Rev* 14:205, 1994.
27. Webberley M, Neuberger J: Changing indications in liver transplantation, *Baillieres Clin Gastroenterol* 8:495, 1994.
28. Thomas DJ: Risking infection: an issue of control for liver transplant recipients, *AACN Clin Iss Crit Care Nurs* 4:471, 1993.
29. Marshall JB: Acute pancreatitis: a review with an emphasis on new developments, *Arch Intern Med* 153:1185, 1993.
30. Sherman S, Lehman GA: Endoscopic therapy of pancreatic disease, *Gastroenterologist* 1:5, 1993.
31. Domingues-Munoz JE, Malfertheiner P: Management of severe acute pancreatitis, *Gastroenterologist* 4:248, 1993.
32. McFadden DW, Reber HA: Indications for surgery in severe acute pancreatitis, *Int J Pancreatol* 15:83, 1994.
33. Malfertheiner P, Dominguez-Munoz JE, Buchler MW: Chronic pancreatitis: management of pain, *Digestion* 55(suppl 1):29, 1994.
34. Murr MM and others: Pancreatic cancer, *CA Cancer J Clin* 44:304, 1994.
35. O'Donnell LJ, Fairclough PD: Gall stones and gall bladder motility, *Gut* 34:440, 1993.
36. Diehl AK: Symptoms of gallstone disease, *Bailleres Clin Gastroenterol* 6:635, 1992.
37. Sauerbruch T: Endoscopic management of bile duct stones, *J Gastroenterol Hepatol* 7:328, 1992.
38. Cappuccino H, Cargill S, Nguyen T: Laparoscopic cholecystectomy: 563 cases at a community teaching hospital and a review of 12,201 cases in the literature, Monmouth Medical Center Laparoscopic Cholecystectomy Group, *Surg Laparosc Endosc* 4:213, 1994.
39. Deehan DJ and others: Carcinoid tumor of the gall bladder: two case reports and a review of published works, *Gut* 34:1274, 1993.

SECTION VIII BIBLIOGRAPHY

Books

Burtis G, Davis J, Martin S: *Applied nutrition and diet therapy,* ed 2, Philadelphia, 1994, WB Saunders.

Corman ML: *Colon and rectal surgery,* ed 3, Philadelphia, 1993, JB Lippincott.

Schiff L, Schiff ER, editors: *Diseases of the liver,* ed 7, Philadelphia, 1993, JB Lippincott.

Sherlock S, Dooley J: *Diseases of the liver and biliary system,* ed 9, London, 1993, Blackwell Scientific.

Sleisenger MH, Fordtran JS: *Gastrointestinal disease, pathophysiology, diagnosis and management,* ed 5, Philadelphia, 1993, WB Saunders.

Zakim D, Bayer TD, editors: *Hepatology: a textbook of liver disease,* ed 2, Philadelphia, 1990, WB Saunders.

Journals

Ahmed F: Effect of nutrition on the health of the elderly, *J Am Diet Assoc* 92:1102, 1992.

Anand A and others: Epidemiology, clinical manifestations, and outcome of Clostridium difficile-associated diarrhea, *Am J Gastroenterol* 89:519, 1994.

Bennett RG, Greenough WB: Approach to acute diarrhea in the elderly, *Gastroenterol Clin North Am* 22:517, 1993.

Berry SM, Lacy J: Nutrition management of the hepatic transplant patient, *Nutr Clin Pract* 8:36, 1993.

*Bingham S: The use of 24-h urine samples and energy expenditure to validate dietary assessment, *Am J Clin Nutr* 59(suppl):227S, 1994.

Blanford NL: The involvement of the pulmonary system in liver failure, *Crit Care Nurse* 14:19, 1994.

*Bond EF, Heitkemper MM, Jarrett M: Intestinal transit and body weight responses to ovarian hormones and dietary fiber in rats, *Nurs Res* 43:18, 1994.

Bray G: Barriers to the treatment of obesity, *Ann Intern Med* 115:152, 1991.

Brown A: Acute pancreatitis: pathophysiology, nursing diagnoses, and collaborative problems, *Focus Crit Care* 18:121, 1991.

Buckner E: Do you have patients with anorexia or bulimia? *Postgrad Med* 89:209, 1991.

Butler L: Hepatitis: A nurse's story, *RN* 55:66, 1992.

Butler RW: Managing the complications of cirrhosis, *Am J Nursing* 94:46, 1994.

Buzzard IM and others: Diet intervention methods to reduce fat intake: nutrient and food group composition of self-selected low-fat diets, *J Am Diet Assoc* 90:42, 1990.

Buzzard IM, Sievert Y: Research priorities and recommendations for dietary assessment methodology, *Am J Clin Nutr* 59(suppl):275S, 1994.

Camp D and others: How to insert and remove nasogastric tubes quickly and easily, *Nursing* 20:59, 1990.

Cassidy C: Walk a mile in my shoes: culturally sensitive food-habit research, *Am J Clin Nutr* 59(suppl):190S, 1994.

Centers for Disease Control: Postexposure prophylaxis for hepatitis B, *MMWR* 40:RR-13, 21, 1991.

Chase SL: OTC. GI remedies, *RN* 56:30, 1993.

Coats K and others: Hospital-associated malnutrition: a reevaluation 12 years later, *J Am Diet Assoc* 93:27, 1993.

Cohen D: Dementia, depression, and nutritional status, *Prim Care* 21:107, 1994.

Cope KA: Nutritional status: a basic "vital sign," *Home Healthc Nurse* 12:29, 1994.

Covington H: Nursing care of patients with alcoholic liver disease, *Crit Care Nurse* 13:47, 1993.

DeChicco RS, Matarese LE: Selection of nutrition support regimens, *Nutr Clin Pract* 7:239, 1992.

Deitel M, Shahi B: Morbid obesity: selection of patients for surgery, *J Am Coll Nutr* 11:457, 1992.

Doherty MM, Carver DK: New relief for esophageal varices, *Am J Nurs* 93:58, 1993.

Dolan MB, Robinson JH, Roberts S: When the doctor delays pain relief, *Nursing* 23:46, 1993.

Driscoll DW: Perinatal transmission of hepatitis B, *RN* 55:65, 1992.

Eisenberg PG: Causes of diarrhea in tube-fed patients: a comprehensive approach to diagnosis and management, *Nutr Clin Pract* 8:119, 1993.

Estoup M: Approaches and limitations of medication delivery in patients with enteral feeding tubes, *Crit Care Nurse* 14:68, 1994.

*Flynn M and others: Aging in humans: a continuous 20-year study of physiologic and dietary parameters, *J Am Coll Nutr* 11:660, 1992.

Forseter G and others: Hepatitis C in the health care setting. II. Seroprevalence among hemodialysis staff and patients in suburban New York City, *Am J Infect Control* 21:5, 1993.

Front ME, Wise SR, Carey LC: Common bile duct strictures: diagnosis, management, follow-up, *AORN J* 57:57, 1990.

Gauwitz DF: Endoscopic cholecystectomy: the patient-friendly alternative, *Nursing* 20:58, 1990.

Gilchrist E: Hepatitis B—it will never happen to me, *Todays OR Nurse* 13:15, 1991.

Greifzu S, Dest V: When the diagnosis is pancreatic cancer, *RN* 54:38, 1991.

Gruber M, Byrd R: Post-traumatic stress disorder and GI endoscopy: a case study, *Gastroenterol Nurs* 16:17, 1993.

*Hankin J, Wilkens L: Development and validation of dietary assessment methods for culturally diverse populations, *Am J Clin Nutr* 59(suppl):198S, 1994.

Henderson C and others: Prolonged tube feeding in long-term care: nutritional status and clinical outcomes, *J Am Coll Nutr* 11:309, 1992.

Herzog D: Eating disorders: new threats to health, *Psychosomatics* 33:10, 1992.

Herzog D and others: Questions and answers: recent advances in bulimia nervosa, *J Clin Psychiatry* 52(10 suppl):39, 1991.

*Hirsch S and others: Nutritional status of surgical patients and the relationship of nutrition to postoperative outcome, *J Am Coll Nutr* 11:21, 1992.

Hoffman N: Diet in the elderly: needs and risks, *Med Clin North Am* 77:745, 1993.

Huber D, Hemstrom M: GI nursing: the community health aspect, *Gastroenterol Nurs* 16:219, 1994.

Jackson MM, McPherson DC: Hepatitis A through E: current and future trends, *Todays OR Nurse* 13:7, 1991.

Jackson MM, Pugliese G: The OSHA bloodborne pathogens standard, *Todays OR Nurse* 14:11, 1992.

Jackson MM, Rymer TE: Viral hepatitis: anatomy of a diagnosis, *Am J Nurs* 94:43, 1994.

Johnson MH: Observing radiation safety practices in GI nursing, *Gastroenterol Nurs* 16:166, 1994.

Jurf JB and others: Cholecystectomy made easier, *Am J Nurs* 90:38, 1990.

*Kaw M, Sekas G: Long-term follow-up of consequences of percutaneous endoscopic gastrostomy (PEG) tubes in nursing home patients, *Dig Dis Sci* 39:738, 1994.

Kayman S and others: Maintenance and relapse after weight loss in women: behavioral aspects, *Am J Clin Nutr* 52:800, 1990.

Kennedy S, Garfinkel P: Advances in diagnosis and treatment of anorexia nervosa and bulimia nervosa, *Can J Psychiatry* 37:309, 1992.

Kenny MJ, Malem F: Gastrointestinal emergencies, *Br J Nurs* 2:588, 1993.

Kerstetter J and others: Malnutrition in the institutionalized older adult, *J Am Diet Assoc* 92:1109, 1992.

Killeen TK: Alcoholism and liver transplantation: ethical and nursing implications, *Perspect Psychiatr Care* 29:7, 1993.

Kohn CL, Brozenec S, Foster PF: Nutritional support for the patient with pancreatobiliary disease, *Crit Care Nurs Clin North Am* 5:37, 1993.

Korula J: Investigative studies in portal hypertension, *Gastroenterol Nurs* 15:233, 1993.

Kral J: Overview of surgical techniques for treating obesity, *Am J Clin Nutr* 55(suppl):552S, 1992.

Kushner R: Bioelectrical impedance analysis: a review of principles and applications, *J Am Coll Nutr* 11:199, 1992.

Lancaster S, Stockbridge J: PV shunts relieve ascites, *RN* 55:58, 1992.

Lehmann S, Barber J: Giving medications by feeding tube: how to avoid problems, *Nursing* 21:58, 1991.

Leigh JP, Jiang WY: Liver cirrhosis deaths within occupations and industries in the California occupational mortality study, *Addiction* 88:767, 1993.

Lettau LA: The A, B, C, D, and E of hepatitis: spelling out the risks for health care workers, *Infect Control Hosp Epidemiol* 13:77, 1992.

Lockhart JS, Hoelsken R: Abdominal hemorrhage, *Nursing* 23:33, 1993.

Makaroff RJ: Liver failure: a case study of a complex problem, *Crit Care Nurse* 14:19, 1994.

MacFie H: Assessment of the sensory properties of food, *Nutr Rev* 48:87, 1990.

Martin FL: When the liver breaks down, *RN* 55:52, 1992.

McConnell EA: Auscultating bowel sounds, *Nursing* 24:20, 1994.

McConnell EA: Managing a nasoenteric-decompression tube, *Nursing* 24:18, 1994.

McCrae J and others: Parenteral nutrition: hospital to home, *J Am Diet Assoc* 93:664, 1993.

Medeiros L and others: Dietary practices and nutrition beliefs through the adult life cycle, *J Nutr Ed* 25:201, 1993.

Merta W: Food intake measurements: is there a "gold standard"? *J Am Diet Assoc* 92:1463, 1992.

*Metheny N and others: Effectiveness of pH measurements in predicting feeding tube placement: an update, *Nurs Res* 42:324, 1993.

Monaghan D: Community nutrition and dietetics, *Prof Nurse* 9:482, 1994.

Morgan S: Rational weight loss programs: a clinician's guide, *J Am Coll Nutr* 8:186, 1989.

Monroe D: Patient teaching for x-ray and other diagnostics: Patient instructions—ERCP and oral cholecystogram, *RN* 53:52, 1990.

Murphy D: Managing patient stress in endoscopy, *Gastroenterol Nurs* 16:72, 1993.

Murray M, Blaylock B: Maintaining effective pressure ulcer prevention programs, *MEDSURG Nurs* 3:85, 1994.

Nader P: The role of the family in obesity prevention and treatment, *Ann N Y Acad Sci* 699:147, 1993.

Negus E: Stroke-induced dysphagia in hospital: the nutritional perspective, *Br J Nurs* 3:263, 1994.

NIH Technology Assessment Conference Panel: methods for voluntary weight loss and control, *Ann Intern Med* 116:942, 1992.

Parker K and others: Community resources in obese care, *J Fla Med Assoc* 79:389, 1992.

Pearson S, Watson R: Chemoembolisation: treating liver cancer, *Nurs Stand* 8:25, 1994.

Ragan JA: Lasers in gastroenterology, *Nurs Clin North Am* 25:685, 1990.

Ratnasuriya RH and others: Anorexia nervosa: outcome and prognostic factors after 20 years, *Br J Psychiatry* 158:495, 1991.

Reishtein J: Liver failure: case study of a complex problem, *Crit Care Nurse* 13:46, 1993.

Renkes J: GI endoscopy—managing the full scope of care, *Nursing* 23:50, 1993.

Robison J et al: Obesity, weight loss, and health, *J Am Diet Assoc* 93:445, 1993.

*Rolandelli RH, Ullrich JR: Nutritional support in the frail elderly surgical patient, *Surg Clin North Am* 74:79, 1994.

Russell R, Suter P: Vitamin requirements of elderly people: an update, *Am J Clin Nutr* 58:4, 1993.

Saffel-Shrier S, Athas B: Effective provision of comprehensive nutrition case management for the elderly, *J Am Diet Assoc* 93:439, 1993.

Scanlan F, Dunne J, Toyne K: Introducing a nutritional assessment tool and action plan, *Prof Nurse* 9:382, 1994.

Shuster MH, Mancino JM: Ensuring successful home tube feeding in the geriatric population, *Geriatr Nurs* 15:67, 1994.

Smith G, Gibbs J: Are gut peptides a new class of anorectic agents? *Am J Clin Nutr* 55:283S, 1992.

Spielman A and others: The cost of losing: an analysis of commercial weight-loss programs in a metropolitan area, *J Am Coll Nutr* 11:36, 1992.

Spollett GR: Nutritional management of common gastrointestinal problems, *Nurse Pract Forum* 5:24, 1994.

*Springett J, Murray C: Parenteral nutrition, *Nurs Times* 90:48, 1994.

*Stanford JL: Comparison of two methods of measuring gastric pH, *Heart Lung* 23:180, 1994.

Stunkard AJ, Wadden R: Restrained eating and human obesity, *Nutr Rev* 48:78, 1990.

Taylor M: Total parenteral nutrition, *Nurs Stand* 8:25, 1994.

Thompson C: Managing acute pancreatitis, *RN* 55:52, 1992.

van Staveren WA and others: Assessing diets of elderly people: problems and approaches, *Am J Clin Nutr* 59(suppl):221S, 1994.

Walsh BT, Devlin M: The pharmacologic treatment of eating disorders, *Psychiatr Clin North Am* 15:149, 1992.

Walsh S and others: How to insert a small-bore feeding tube safely, *Nursing* 20:55, 1990.

Webber-Jones J and others: How to declog a feeding tube, *Nursing* 22:62, 1992.

Weigley ES: Nutrition in nursing education and beginning practice, *J Am Diet Assoc* 94:654, 1994.

Whiteman K and others: Liver transplantation, *Am J Nurs* 90:68, 1990.

Whitney R: Comparing long-term central venous catheters, *Nursing* 21:70, 1991.

Wing R: Behavioral treatment of severe obesity, *Am J Clin Nutr* 55(suppl):545S, 1992.

Wretlind A: Recollections of pioneers in nutrition: landmarks in the development of parenteral nutrition, *J Am Coll Nutr* 11:366, 1992.

Yen J: General overview and treatment considerations of anorexia and bulimia, *Compr Ther* 18:26, 1992.

Young C, White S: Preparing patients for tube feeding at home, *Am J Nurs* 92:46, 1992.

Young LM: Managing the patient with liver failure, *Medsurg Nurs* 2:275, 1993.

*Zbar RI: Liver laceration after cardiopulmonary resuscitation: a case report, *Heart Lung* 22:463, 1993.

Organization

Alcoholics Anonymous World Services
P.O. Box 459
Grand Central Station
New York, NY 10163
212-870-3400

American Cancer Society (ACS)
1599 Clifton Road NE
Atlanta, GA 30329
404-320-3333

Crohn's and Colitis Foundation of America (CCFA)
444 Park Avenue South
New York, NY 10016-7374
212-685-3440
800-343-3637

Help for Incontinent People (HIP)
P.O. Box 544
Union, SC 29379
803-579-7900

Society of Gastroenterology Nurses and Associates, Inc.
1070 Sibley Tower
Rochester, NY 14604
716-546-7241

United Ostomy Association (UOA)
36 Executive Park, Suite 120
Irvine, CA 92714-6744
714-660-8624
800-8262-0826

Wound Ostomy and Continence Nurses Society
2755 Bristol Street, Ste. #110
Costa Mesa, CA 92626
712-476-0268

*Nursing research–based articles.

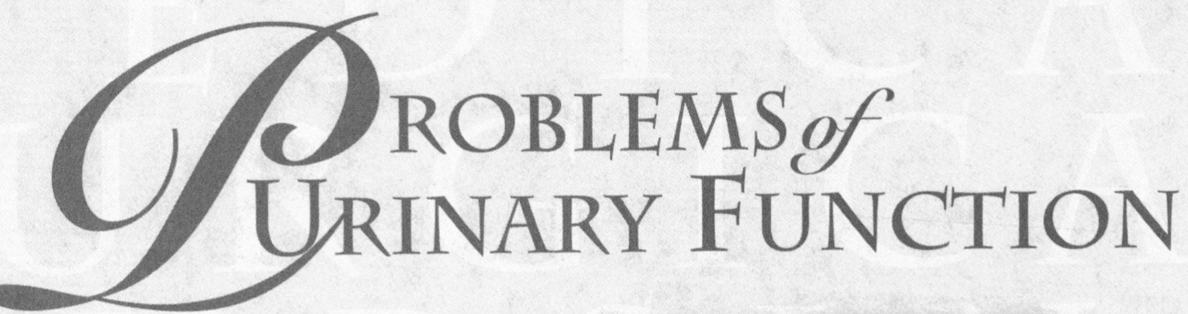

Problems of Urinary Function

Section Nine

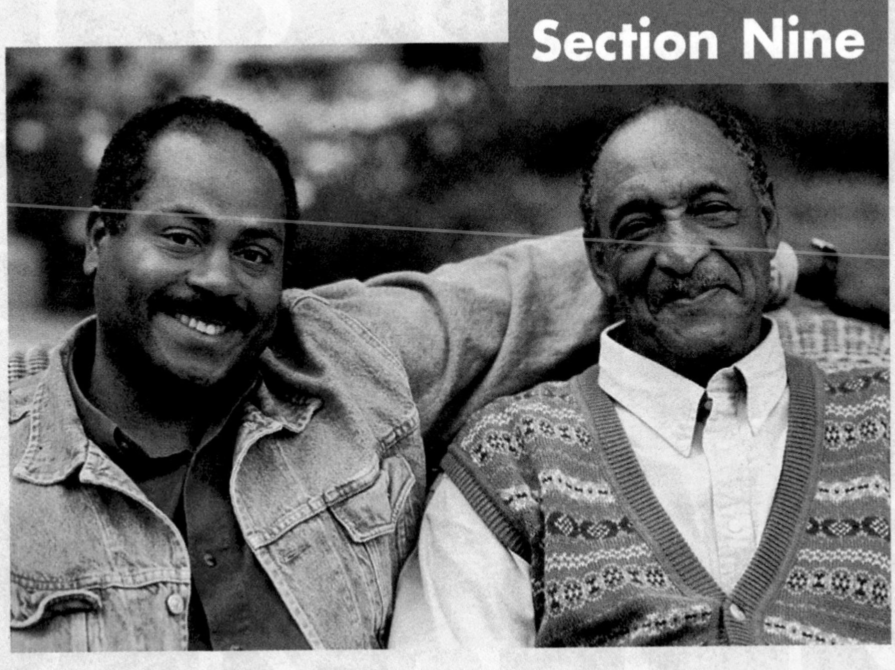

MEDICAL
SURGICAL
NURSING
MEDICAL
SURGICAL
NURSING
MEDICAL
SURGICAL
NURSING
MEDICAL
SURGICAL

Chapter 42

NURSING ASSESSMENT Urinary System

Patricia Bates **Sharon L. Lewis**

Learning Objectives

1. Describe the anatomic location and functions of the kidneys, ureters, bladder, and urethra.
2. Explain the physiologic events involved in the formation and passage of urine from glomerular filtration to voiding.
3. Identify the significant subjective and objective data related to the urinary system that should be obtained from a patient.
4. Describe age-related changes in the urinary system and differences in assessment findings.
5. Describe the appropriate techniques used in the physical assessment of the urinary system.
6. Differentiate normal from common abnormal findings of a physical assessment of the urinary system.
7. Describe the purpose, significance of results, and nursing responsibilities related to diagnostic studies of the urinary system.
8. Describe the normal physical and chemical characteristics of urine.

"Bones can break, muscles can atrophy, glands can loaf, even the brain can go to sleep without immediate danger to survival. But should the kidneys fail . . . neither bone, muscle, gland, nor brain could carry on."[1] This statement underlines the importance of kidneys to our lives. Adequate functioning of the kidneys is essential to the maintenance of a healthy body. If there is complete kidney failure and treatment is not given, death is inevitable.

The kidneys are the principal organs of the urinary system. Besides the two kidneys, there are two ureters, a urinary bladder, and a urethra in the urinary system (Fig. 42-1). The other organs can be thought of as storage and drainage channels for the urine after it is formed by the kidneys.

The primary function of the kidneys is to regulate the volume and composition of extracellular fluid (ECF). The excretory function of kidneys is secondary to this regulatory function. Other major functions of the kidneys include renin secretion and blood pressure control, erythropoietin production, vitamin D activation, and acid-base balance regulation.

STRUCTURES AND FUNCTIONS OF THE URINARY SYSTEM

Kidneys

Macrostructure. The kidneys are bean-shaped organs that are retroperitoneal (behind the peritoneum) on either side of the vertebral column at about the level of the twelfth thoracic (T12) vertebra to the third lumbar (L3) vertebra. Each kidney weighs 4 to 6 ounces (120 to 170 g) and is about 5 inches (12 cm) long. The right kidney, with the liver above it, is lower than the left. The right kidney is at the level of the twelfth rib. An adrenal gland lies on top of each kidney.

Each kidney is surrounded by a considerable amount of fat and connective tissue that serve to support and maintain its position. The surface of the kidney is covered by a thin, smooth layer of fibrous membrane called the *capsule*. The *hilus* on the medial side of the kidney serves as the entry site for the renal artery and nerves, as well as the exit site for the vein and ureter.

On a longitudinal section of the kidney (Fig. 42-2), the internal structures can be visualized. The outer layer is referred to as the *cortex*, and the inner layer is called the *medulla*. The medulla consists of a number of *pyramids*. The apices of these pyramids are called *papillae*, through which urine passes to enter the *calyces*. The minor calyces widen and merge to form major calyces, which form a funnel-shaped sac called the *renal pelvis*. The minor and major calyces and the renal pelvis are holding areas for urine before it exits the kidney via the ureter. The capacity of the renal pelvis is about 3 to 5 ml. The lumen of the pelvis decreases to form the ureter.

Microstructure. The functional unit of the kidney is the *nephron*. Each kidney has more than 1 million nephrons. A nephron is composed of a glomerulus, Bowman's

Reviewed by Mary Jo Holechek, RN, MS, CNN, Senior Transplant Coordinator for Kidney, Liver, and Pancreas, Johns Hopkins Hospital, Baltimore, MD.

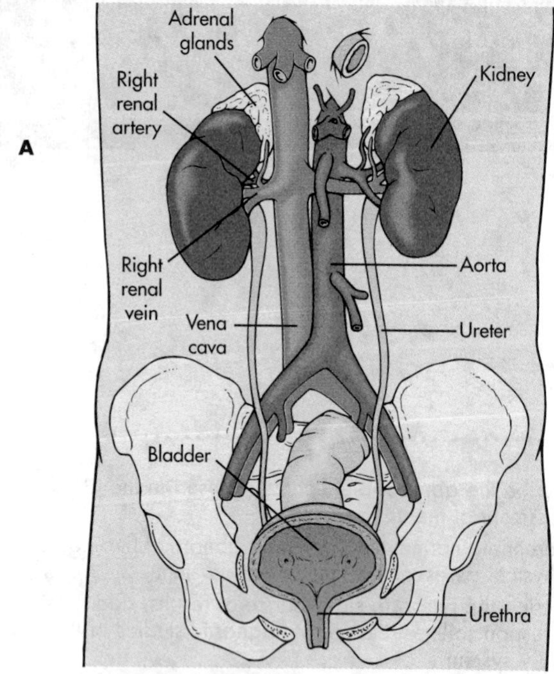

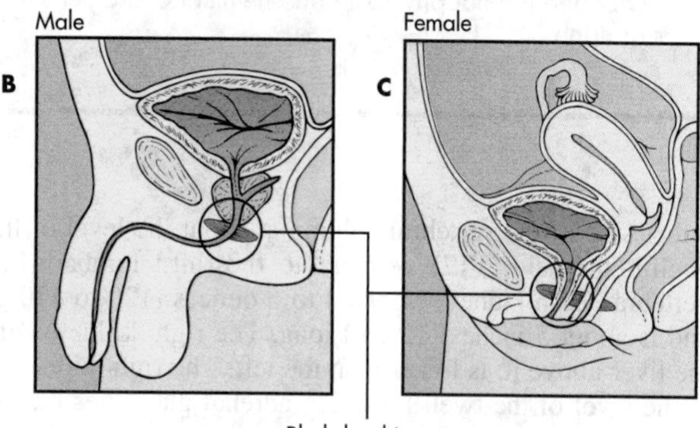

Fig. 42-1 Organs of the urinary system. ***A***, Upper urinary tract in relation to other anatomic structures. ***B***, Male urethra in relation to other pelvic structures. ***C***, Female urethra.

capsule, and tubular system. The tubular system consists of the proximal convoluted tubule, the loop of Henle, and the distal convoluted tubule (Fig. 42-3). Several nephrons converge into a collecting duct, which eventually merges into a pyramid and empties via the papilla into a minor calyx.

The glomeruli, Bowman's capsule, proximal tubule, and distal tubule are located in the cortex of the kidney. The loop of Henle and the collecting ducts are located in the medulla.

Blood Supply. A blood supply of about 1200 ml/min, which is 20% to 25% of the cardiac output, flows to the two kidneys. Blood reaches the kidneys via the renal artery, which arises from the aorta and enters the kidney through the hilus. The renal artery divides into secondary branches and then into still smaller branches, each of which eventually forms an *afferent arteriole* (Fig. 42-4). The afferent

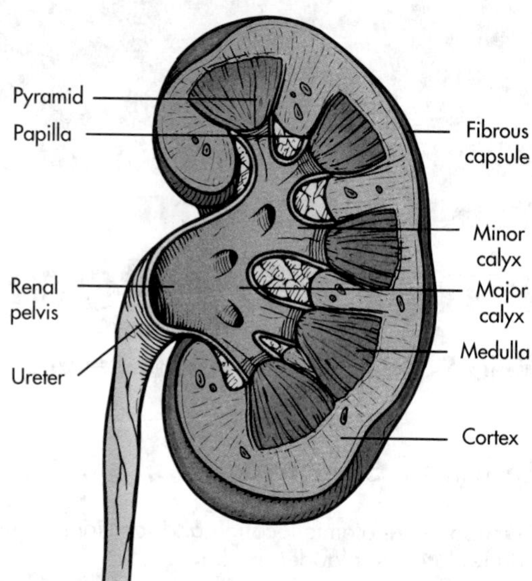

Fig. 42-2 Longitudinal section of the kidney.

arteriole divides into a capillary network called the *glomerulus*, which is a tuft of up to 50 capillaries. The capillaries of the glomerulus eventually unite in the efferent arteriole. This arteriole splits to form a capillary network called the *peritubular capillaries*, which, as the name suggests, surround the tubular system. All peritubular capillaries eventually drain into the venous system. The renal vein empties into the inferior vena cava.

Physiology of Urine Formation

Normal Glomerular Function. Urine formation starts at the glomerulus where blood is filtered. The glomerulus, which is a semipermeable membrane, allows for filtration (see Fig. 42-3). The hydrostatic pressure of the blood within the glomerular capillaries cause a portion of blood to be filtered across the semipermeable membrane into Bowman's capsule, where the filtered portion of the blood called the *glomerular filtrate* begins to pass down to the tubule. Filtration is more rapid in the glomerulus than in ordinary tissue capillaries because of the porosity of the glomerular membrane. The ultrafiltrate is similar in composition to blood except that it lacks blood cells, platelets, and large plasma proteins. Under normal conditions the capillary pores are too small to allow the loss of these large blood components. Capillary permeability is increased in many renal diseases, permitting plasma proteins to pass into the urine.

The amount of blood filtered by the glomeruli in a given time is referred to as the *glomerular filtration rate* (GFR). The normal GFR is about 125 ml per minute. However, on the average only 1 ml per minute is excreted as urine because most glomerular filtrate is reabsorbed by the peritubular capillary network before it reaches the end of the collecting duct.

Tubular Function. Because the glomerular membrane is a selective filtration membrane that filters primarily by size, provision is made for the reabsorption of essential

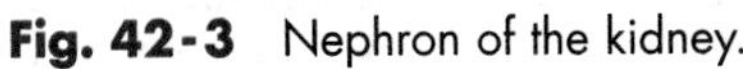

Fig. 42-3 Nephron of the kidney.

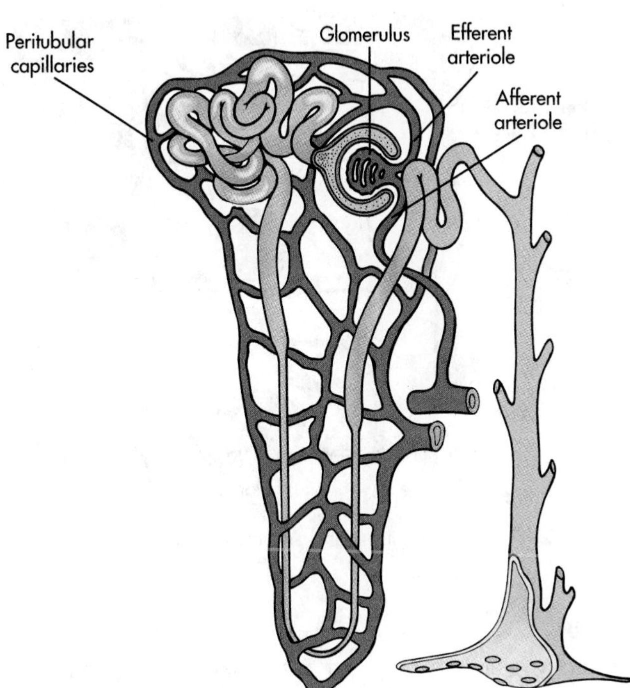

Fig. 42-4 Blood supply of the nephron.

materials and the excretion of nonessential ones (Table 42-1). The tubules and collecting ducts carry out these functions by means of reabsorption and secretion (Fig. 42-5). *Reabsorption* refers to the passage of a substance from the lumen of the tubules through the tubule cells and into the capillaries. This process involves both active and passive transport. *Tubular secretion* refers to the passage of a substance from the capillaries through the tubular cells into the lumen of the tubule. Reabsorption and secretion occur along the entire length of the tubule, causing numerous changes in the composition of the glomerular filtrate as it moves through the tubules.

In the proximal convoluted tubule, about 80% of the electrolytes are reabsorbed. Normally, all the glucose, amino acids, and protein are reabsorbed. For the most part reabsorption occurs by active transport. Hydrogen ions (H^+) and creatinine are secreted into the filtrate.[2]

The loop of Henle is important in conserving water and thus concentrating the filtrate. In the loop of Henle, reabsorption continues. The descending loop is permeable to water and moderately permeable to sodium, urea, and other solutes. In the ascending limb, chloride ions (Cl^-) are actively reabsorbed, followed passively by sodium ions (Na^+). About 25% of the filtered sodium is reabsorbed here.

Two important functions of the distal convoluted tubules are final regulation of water balance and acid-base balance. Antidiuretic hormone (ADH), released by the posterior

Table 42-1 Functions of the Segments of the Nephron

Component	Function
▪ Glomerulus	Selective filtration
▪ Proximal tubule	Reabsorption of 80% of electrolytes and water, reabsorption of all glucose and amino acids, reabsorption of HCO_3^-, secretion of H^+ and creatinine
▪ Loop of Henle	Reabsorption of Na^+ and Cl^- in ascending limb, reabsorption of water in descending loop, concentration of filtrate
▪ Distal tubule	Secretion of K^+, H^+, ammonia; reabsorption of water (regulated by ADH); reabsorption of HCO_3^-; regulation of Ca^{2+} and PO_4^{2-} by parathormone; regulation of Na^+ and K^+ by aldosterone
▪ Collecting duct	Reabsorption of water (ADH required)

ADH, Antidiuretic hormone; *Ca^{2+}*, calcium ions; *Cl^-*, chloride ions; *H^+*, hydrogen ions; *HCO_3^-*, bicarbonate ions; *K^+*, potassium ions; *Na^+*, sodium ions; *PO_4^{2-}*, phosphate ions.

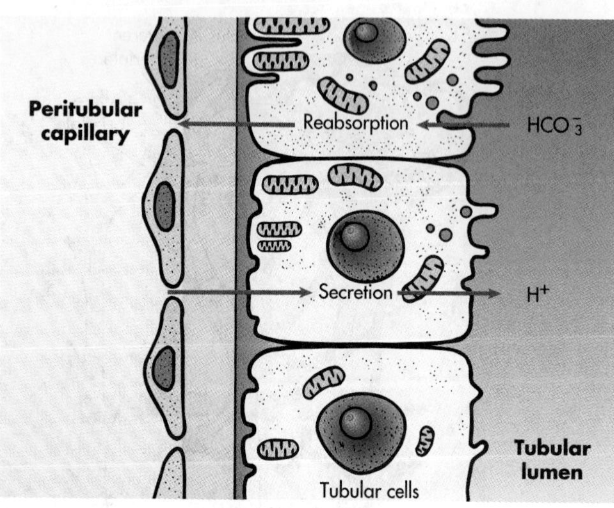

Fig. 42-5 Reabsorption and secretion in the tubules.

pituitary gland, is required for water reabsorption. The stimulus for ADH release is increased serum osmolality and decreased blood volume. ADH makes the distal convoluted tubules and the collecting ducts permeable to water, allowing it to be reabsorbed into the peritubular capillaries and to be eventually returned to circulation. In the absence of ADH the tubules are practically impermeable to water, and any water in the tubules leaves the body as urine.

In the presence of aldosterone (released from the adrenal cortex) acting on the distal tubule, reabsorption of Na^+ and water occurs. In exchange for Na^+, potassium ions (K^+) are excreted. The secretion of aldosterone is influenced by both circulating blood volume and plasma concentrations of Na^+ and K^+.

Acid-base regulation involves reabsorbing and conserving most of the bicarbonate (HCO_3^-) and secreting excess H^+. The distal tubule functions in different ways to maintain the pH of ECF within a range of 7.35 to 7.45 (see Chapter 13).

Atrial natriuretic factor (ANF) is a hormone secreted from cells in the right atrium when right atrial blood pressure increases. ANF inhibits the secretion and effect of ADH and results in a large volume of dilute urine that decreases blood volume and blood pressure.

Parathyroid hormone (parathormone) is released from the parathyroid gland in response to low serum calcium levels. It causes increased tubular reabsorption of calcium ions (Ca^{2+}) and decreased tubular reabsorption of phosphate ions (PO_4^{2-}). Therefore serum Ca^{2+} levels are increased.

The basic function of nephrons is to clean or clear blood plasma of unnecessary substances. After the glomerulus has filtered the blood, the tubules separate the unwanted from the wanted portions of tubular fluid. The necessary portions are returned to the blood, and the unnecessary portions pass into urine.

Other Renal Functions

In addition to their function in regulating the volume and composition of ECF, the kidneys also have other vital functions including the production of erythropoietin, production and secretion of renin, and activation of vitamin D.

Erythropoietin is produced and released in response to decreased oxygen tension in the renal blood supply, which is usually caused by a loss of red blood cells (RBCs). Erythropoietin stimulates the production of RBCs in the bone marrow. A deficiency of erythropoietin leads to anemia in renal failure.[3]

Vitamin D is a hormone that can be obtained in the diet or synthesized by the action of ultraviolet radiation on cholesterol in the skin. These forms of vitamin D are inactive and require two more steps to become metabolically active. The first step in activation occurs in the liver. The second step occurs in the kidneys. Active vitamin D is essential for the absorption of calcium from the gastrointestinal (GI) tract. The patient with renal failure has a deficiency of the active metabolite of vitamin D and manifests problems of altered calcium and phosphate balance (see Chapter 44).

Renin is important in the regulation of blood pressure (Fig. 42-6). It is released from the granular cells of the afferent arteriole. These cells, together with the macula densa cells of the distal convoluted tubule and the mesangial cells, form the *juxtaglomerular apparatus.* Renin is released in response to decreased arterial blood pressure, renal ischemia, ECF depletion, increased norepinephrine, and increased urinary Na^+ concentration. Renin catalyzes the splitting of the plasma protein angiotensinogen into angiotensin I, which is subsequently converted to angiotensin II by a converting enzyme made in the lungs. Angiotensin II stimulates the release of aldosterone from the adrenal cortex, which causes Na^+ and water retention, leading to an increased ECF volume. Angiotensin II also causes increased peripheral vasoconstriction. The increase in ECF and vasoconstriction causes an elevation in blood pressure, which should inhibit renin release. Excessive renin production caused by impaired renal perfusion may be a contributing factor in the etiology of renal hypertension (see Chapter 30).

Prostaglandins. Prostaglandins (PGs) are synthesized by most body tissues from the precursor, arachidonic acid, in response to appropriate stimuli. PGs, which are involved in the regulation of cell function and host defenses, exert their influence primarily on cells or tissues that are close to the site where they are synthesized. (See Chapter 9 for a more detailed discussion of prostaglandins.)

In the kidney, PG synthesis (primarily PGE_2 and PGI_2) occurs primarily in the medulla. These PGs have a vasodilating action in addition to increasing renal blood flow and promoting Na^+ excretion. They counteract the vasoconstrictor effect of substances such as angiotensin and norepinephrine. Renal PGs may have a systemic effect in lowering blood pressure by decreasing systemic vascular resistance.[4]

The significance of these PGs is related to the role of the kidneys in causing hypertension. In renal failure with a loss

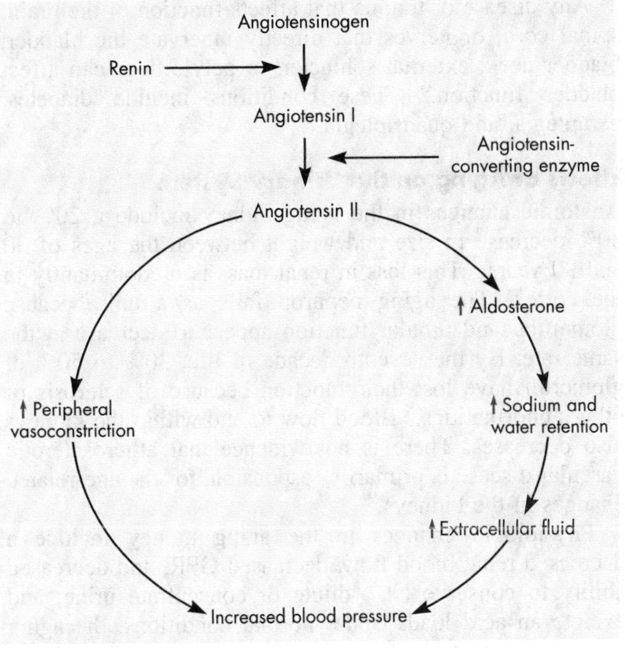

Fig. 42-6 Renin-angiotensin mechanism.

of functioning tissue, these renal vasodilator factors are also lost. This may be one factor that contributes to the common finding of hypertension in renal failure (see Chapter 44).

Ureters

The ureters are tubes approximately 10 to 12 inches (25 to 35 cm) long and 0.08 to 0.3 inch (0.2 to 0.8 cm) in diameter that carry urine from the renal pelvis to the bladder. The narrow area where the ureter joins the renal pelvis is known as the *ureteropelvic junction* (UPJ). After coursing down along the psoas muscle, the ureter crosses over the pelvic brim and iliac artery and inserts into the base of the bladder at the *ureterovesical junction* (UVJ). The ureteral lumen is narrowest at these junctions; consequently, they are often the sites of urinary stone (calculi) obstruction. Since the lumen of the ureter is narrow, it can be easily occluded internally (e.g., calculi) or externally (e.g., tumors, adhesions, inflammation).

Sympathetic and parasympathetic nerves, along with the vascular supply, surround the mucosal lining of the ureter. Circular and longitudinal smooth muscle fibers are arranged in a meshlike outer layer and contract to promote the peristaltic one-way flow of urine. These muscle contractions can be affected by distention and neurologic, endocrine, and pharmacologic factors. Stimulation of these nerves during passage of a stone or clot may cause acute, severe pain known as *renal colic*.

Because the renal pelvis holds only 3 to 5 ml of urine, kidney damage can result from a backflow of more than that amount of urine. The UVJ relies on the ureter's angle of bladder penetration and muscle fiber attachments with the bladder to prevent the backflow of urine (reflux) and ascending infection. The distal ureter entering the bladder has more longitudinal muscle fibers than the upper ureter. This segment enters the bladder laterally at its base, courses along obliquely through the bladder wall for about 1.5 cm, and intermingles with muscle fibers of the bladder base. Circular and longitudinal bladder muscle fibers adjacent to the imbedded ureter help secure it. When bladder pressure rises (e.g., during voiding or coughing), muscle fibers that the ureter shares with the bladder base contract first to help promote ureteral lumen closure. The bladder then contracts against its base to further close the UVJ and prevent urine from moving back through the junction.

Bladder

The urinary bladder is a distensible organ positioned behind the symphysis pubis and anterior to the vagina and rectum. Its primary functions are to serve as a reservoir for urine and to help the body eliminate waste products. Normal adult urine output is approximately 1500 ml per day, which varies with food and fluid intake. The volume of urine produced at night is less than half of that formed during the day because of hormonal influences (e.g., ADH). This diurnal pattern of urination is normal. Most persons urinate five to six times during the day and occasionally at night.

The triangular area formed by the two ureteral openings and the bladder neck at the base of the bladder is known as the *trigone*. It is affixed to the pelvis by many ligaments, and it does not change its shape during bladder filling or emptying. The bladder muscle, the *detrusor*, is composed of layers of intertwined smooth muscle fibers and is capable of considerable distention during bladder filling and contraction during emptying. It is affixed to the abdominal wall by an umbilical ligament. Consequently, as the bladder fills, it rises toward the umbilicus. The dome, anterior, and lateral aspects of the bladder expand and contract. When the bladder is empty, it appears as multiple folds within the pelvis.

On the average, 200 to 250 ml of urine in the bladder causes moderate distention and the urge to urinate. When the quantity of urine reaches about 400 to 600 ml, the person feels uncomfortable. Bladder capacity varies with the individual, ranging from 600 to 1000 ml. Evacuation of urine is called urination, micturition, or voiding.

The bladder has the same mucosal lining as that of the renal pelvis, ureter, and bladder neck. It is called *transitional cell epithelium* or *urothelium* and is unique to the urinary tract. Transitional cell epithelium resists urine secretion or absorption. Therefore urinary wastes produced by the kidneys do not leak out of the urinary system after they leave the kidneys. Microscopically, transitional cell epithelium is several cells deep. These cells stretch out in the bladder to only a few cells deep as it accommodates filling. As the bladder empties, the epithelium resumes its multicell layer formation.

Because the lining is the same, transitional cell tumors that occur in one section of the urinary tract can easily metastasize to other urinary tract areas. Malignant cells may move down from upper urinary tract tumors and imbed in the bladder, or large bladder tumors can invade the ureter. Tumor recurrence within the bladder is common. Intact urothelium also has phagocytic properties, although the exact mechanism is unknown.

Urethra

The urethra is a small muscular tube that leads from the bladder neck to the external meatus. Its primary functions are to prevent urinary leakage between voidings and serve as a conduit for urine to the outside of the body.

The urothelium and submucosal layers are the same as that of the bladder. Smooth muscle fibers extend from the bladder neck down into the urethra and are further supported by circular smooth muscle fibers around the urethra. Special C-shaped striated muscle fibers (the *rhabdosphincter* or external sphincter) surround a portion of the urethra and voluntarily contract and prevent leaking when bladder pressure increases.

The female urethra is 1 to 2 inches (3 to 5 cm) long and lies behind the symphysis pubis but anterior to the vagina. The rhabdosphincter encircles the middle third of the urethra. The short urethra is a contributing factor to the increased incidence of urinary tract infections in women.

The male urethra, which is about 8 to 10 inches (20 to 25 cm) long, originates at the bladder neck and extends the length of the penis. It is often separated into three parts. The *prostatic urethra* extends from the bladder neck through the prostate to the urogenital diaphragm. The *membranous urethra* passes through the urogenital diaphragm. The rhabdosphincter encircles this portion. Because of the concentrated muscular support, this short portion is not as expandable; consequently, stricture formation in this area after instrumentation is common. The *penile urethra* continues through the corpora spongiosum, a cavernous penile body, from the urogenital diaphragm to a distal dilated area, the fossa navicularis, before terminating at the meatus.

Urethrovesical Unit Function

Together, the bladder, bladder neck, urethra, and pelvic floor muscles form what is called the *urethrovesical unit.*[5] Normal voluntary control of this unit is defined as continence. Various areas of the brain send stimulating and inhibiting impulses to the thoracolumbar (T11-L2) and sacral (S2-S4) areas of the spinal cord to control voiding. Distention of the bladder stimulates stretch receptors within the bladder wall. Impulses are transmitted to the sacral spinal cord and then to the brain, causing a desire to urinate. If the time to void is not appropriate, inhibitor impulses in the brain are stimulated and transmitted back to the thoracolumbar and sacral nerves innervating the bladder. In a coordinated fashion, the detrusor accommodates to the pressure (does not contract) while the sphincter and pelvic floor muscles tighten to resist bladder pressure. If voiding is appropriate, cerebral inhibition is voluntarily suppressed, and impulses are transmitted via the spinal cord for the bladder neck, sphincter, and pelvic floor muscles to relax and for the bladder to contract. The sphincter closes and the detrusor muscle relaxes when the bladder is empty.

Any disease or trauma that affects function of the brain, spinal cord, or nerves that directly innervate the bladder, bladder neck, external sphincter, or pelvic floor can affect bladder function.[6] These conditions include diabetes, paraplegia, and quadriplegia.

Effects of Aging on the Urinary System

Anatomic changes in the aging kidney include a 20% to 30% decrease in size and weight between the ages of 30 and 90 years.[7] This loss in renal mass is predominantly in the cortex. The aging nephron fails as a unit because glomerular and tubular function appear to decrease at the same rate. By the seventh decade of life, 30% to 50% of glomeruli have lost their function because of sclerosis or other abnormalities.[8] Blood flow to and within the kidneys also decreases. There is no evidence that atherosclerotic vascular disease is primarily responsible for the age-related changes in the kidneys.[9]

Physiologic changes in the aging kidney include a decreased renal blood flow, decreased GFR, and decreased ability to conserve Na^+, dilute or concentrate urine, and excrete an acid load. Under normal conditions, the aging kidney is able to maintain homeostasis, but after abrupt changes in blood volume, acid load, or other insults, the kidneys may not be able to function effectively because much of its renal reserve has been lost.

ASSESSMENT OF THE URINARY SYSTEM

Subjective Data

Important Health Information

Past health history. The patient should be questioned about the presence or history of diseases that are known to be related to renal or other urologic problems. Some of these diseases are hypertension, diabetes mellitus, gout and other metabolic problems, connective tissue disorders (e.g., systemic lupus erythematosus, scleroderma), skin or upper respiratory infections of streptococcal origin, tuberculosis, viral hepatitis, congenital disorders, neurologic conditions (e.g., stroke, back injury), or trauma. Specific urinary problems such as cancer, infections, benign prostatic hyperplasia, and calculi should be noted.

Medications. An assessment of the patient's current and past use of medication is important. This should include over-the-counter drugs, as well as prescription medications. Drugs affect the urinary tract in several ways. Many drugs are known to be nephrotoxic (Table 42-2). Certain drugs may alter the quantity and character of urine output (e.g., diuretics). Numerous drugs such as phenazopyridine (Pyridium) and nitrofurantoin (Macrodantin) change its color.[10] Anticoagulants may cause hematuria. Many antidepressants, calcium channel blockers, antihistamines, and medications used for neurologic and musculoskeletal disorders affect the ability of the bladder or sphincter to contract or relax normally.

Surgery or other treatments. The patient should also be questioned about any previous hospitalization related to renal or urologic diseases and all urinary problems during past pregnancies. The duration, severity, and patient's perception of any problem and its treatment should be elicited.

Table 42-2 Nephrotoxic Agents

Antibiotics	Other Agents
Amikacin	Captopril
Amphotericin B	Cimetidine
Bacitracin	Cisplatin
Cephalosporins	Cocaine
Colistin	Contrast medium
Gentamicin	Cyclosporine
Kanamycin	Ethylene glycol
Neomycin	Gold
Polymyxin B	Heavy metals
Streptomycin	Heroin
Sulfonamides	Lithium
Tobramycin	Methotrexate
Vancomycin	Nitrosoureas (e.g., carmustine)
	Nonsteroidal antiinflammatory agents (e.g., ibuprofen, indomethacin)
	Phenacetin
	Quinine
	Rifampin
	Salicylate (large quantities)

Past surgeries, particularly pelvic surgeries, or urinary tract instrumentation should be documented. Information should be obtained from the patient about any radiation or chemotherapy treatment for cancer.

Functional Health Patterns. Key questions to ask a patient with problems related to the urinary system are listed in Table 42-3.

Health perception–health management pattern. The nurse may want to ask about the patient's general health. Sometimes responses such as "feeling tired all of the time," changes in weight or appetite, excess thirst, fluid retention, and complaints of headache, pruritis, or blurred vision may be related to abnormal kidney function.

An occupational history should be taken. Exposure to certain chemicals can affect the kidneys and urinary tract system. Phenol and ethylene glycol are examples of nephrotoxic chemicals. Aromatic amines and certain organic chemicals may increase the risk of bladder cancers. Textile workers, painters, hairdressers, and industrial workers have a high incidence of bladder tumors.[11]

A smoking history should be obtained. Cigarette smoking is a major factor in the risk for bladder cancer. Tumors occur four times more frequently in cigarette smokers than in nonsmokers.[12]

Places where a patient has lived may be important information to obtain. It has been shown that persons living in certain parts of the United States (Great Lakes, Southwest, Southeast) have a higher than normal incidence of urinary calculi. This may be caused by the higher mineral content of the soil and water. A person living in Middle Eastern countries or Africa can acquire certain parasites that can cause cystitis or bladder cancer.[12]

The presence of certain renal or urologic problems in a family history increases the likelihood of similar problems occurring in the patient. The nurse should ask about family members who have had any of the diseases referred to in the past health history, as well as polycystic renal disease, congenital urinary tract abnormalities, and Alport's syndrome (hereditary nephritis).

Nutritional-metabolic pattern. The usual quantity and types of fluid a patient drinks are important information related to urinary tract disease. Dehydration may contribute to urinary infections, calculi formation, and renal failure. Large intake of particular foods, such as dairy products or foods high in proteins, may also lead to calculi formation. Coffee or spicy foods often aggravate urinary inflammatory diseases. An unexplained weight gain may be the result of fluid retention secondary to a renal problem. Anorexia and nausea and vomiting can dramatically affect fluid status and require careful assessment. Information on vitamin and mineral supplements should be obtained. The patient may not think of these supplements when listing over-the-counter drugs; supplements are often considered part of nutritional intake.

Elimination pattern. The patient should be questioned about urinary patterns such as frequency or urgency and the amount of urine output. Table 42-4 lists some of the common clinical manifestations of urinary tract disorders. Changes in the color and appearance of urine are often significant and should be evaluated. If blood is visible in the urine, it should be determined if it occurs at the beginning, throughout, or at the end of urination.

Bowel function should also be investigated. Problems with fecal incontinence may signal neurologic causes for bladder problems because of shared nerve pathways. Constipation and fecal impaction can partially obstruct the urethra, causing inadequate bladder emptying and overflow incontinence.[13]

The nurse should find out the patient's method of handling a urinary problem. A patient may already be using a catheter or collection device. Sometimes a patient has to assume a particular position to urinate or perform such maneuvers as pressing on the abdomen (*Valsalva*), straining, or stretching the rectum to empty the bladder.

Activity-exercise pattern. The patient's level of activity should be assessed. A sedentary person is more likely than an active one to have stasis of urine, which can predispose to infection and calculi. Demineralization of bones in a person with limited physical activity causes increased urine calcium precipitation.

An active person may find that increasing activity aggravates the urinary problem. The patient who has had prostate surgery or who has weakened pelvic floor muscles may leak urine when attempting particular activities such as running. Some men may develop chronic inflammatory prostatitis or epididymitis after heavy lifting or long-distance driving.

Sleep-rest pattern. Lower urinary tract disorders, such as infections, neurologic conditions, or bladder outlet obstructions, often necessitate a person getting up as much as every hour at night. This situation can lead to sleep deprivation. Sleep problems associated with a urinary dis-

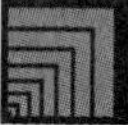

Table 42-3 Key Questions: Patient with a Urinary Problem

Health Perception–Health Management Pattern
- How is your energy level compared with a year ago?
- Do you notice any visual changes?*

Nutritional-Metabolic Pattern
- How is your appetite?
- Has your weight changed over the past year?*
- Do you take vitamin or mineral supplements?*
- How much and what kinds of fluids do you drink daily?
- How much dairy products or meat do you eat?
- Do you drink coffee? Colas?
- Do you eat chocolate?
- Do you spice your food heavily?*

Elimination Pattern
- How often do you urinate during the day and night?
- Is the color normal for you?
- Do you ever notice blood in your urine?* If so, at what point in the urination does it occur?
- Do you find it difficult to postpone urination when you feel the urge to urinate?*
- Do you ever leak urine? If so, when does it occur?
- Do you ever have pain when you urinate?*
- Have you ever experienced urinary incontinence? If so, please describe specifically.
- Do you use special devices or supplies for urine elimination or control?*
- Do your bowels move regularly?

Activity-Exercise Pattern
- Have you noticed any changes in your ability to do your usual daily activities?*
- Do certain activities aggravate your urinary problem?*
- Has your urinary problem caused you to alter or stop any activity or exercise?*
- Do you require assistance in moving or getting to the bathroom?*

Cognitive-Perceptual Pattern
- Describe any pain you have in relation to urination

Self-Perception–Self-Concept Pattern
- How does your urinary problem make you feel about yourself
- Do you perceive your body differently since you have developed a urinary problem

Role-Relationship Pattern
- Does your urinary problem interfere with your relationships with family or friends?*
- Has your urinary problem caused a change in your job status or affected your ability to carry out job-related responsibilities?*

Sexuality-Reproductive Pattern
- Has your urinary problem caused any change in your sexual pleasure or performance?*
- Do you have hygiene problems related to sexual activities that cause you concern?*

Coping-Stress Tolerance Pattern
- Do you feel able to manage the problems associated with your urinary problem? If not, explain.
- What strategies are you using to cope with your urinary problem?

Values-Beliefs Pattern
- Has your present illness affected your belief system?*
- Are your treatment decisions related to your urinary problem in conflict with your value system?*

*If yes, describe.

order should be documented. The older adult may awaken many times during the night to urinate and may need to be assured that this may be normal. However, a complete assessment should be made to rule out any problem.

Cognitive-perceptual pattern. Level of mobility, visual acuity, and dexterity are important factors to determine for a patient with urologic problems when managing his own care at home, particularly when bladder retention or incontinence is a problem. It should be determined if the patient is alert, is able to understand instructions, and can recall the instructions when necessary.

If urinary incontinence is present, a thorough history of the problem should be elicited to assist in determining the type of incontinence. It is important to document what the patient has tried to manage the problem. Incontinence is a distressing problem and calls for great sensitivity on the part of the nurse if accurate information is to be obtained.

Pain is a frequent symptom of urinary tract disease. Types of pain associated with renal and urologic problems include dysuria, groin pain, costovertebral pain, and suprapubic pain. If present, the location, character, and duration should be assessed. The absence of pain when other urinary symptoms exist is also significant. Many urinary tract tumors are painless in the early stages.

Self-perception–self-concept pattern. Problems associated with the urinary system, such as incontinence, urinary diversion tubes, and chronic fatigue, can result in loss of self-esteem and a negative body image. Sensitive questioning may elicit cues to problems in this area.

Role-relationship pattern. Urinary problems can affect many aspects of a person's life including the ability to work and relationships with others. These factors will have important implications on future treatment and management. The nurse needs to be aware of cues from the patient.

Urinary system problems may be serious enough to cause problems in job and social-related situations. Long-term dialysis often makes regular employment or full-time homemaking impossible. Also, the concurrent poor health and negative body image can seriously alter existing roles. The nurse needs to assess this area to plan appropriate interventions.

Sexuality-reproductive pattern. The patient should be questioned about the effect of a renal or urologic problem

Table 42-4 Clinical Manifestations of Disorders of the Urinary System

General Manifestations	
Fatigue	Itching
Headaches	Excess thirst
Blurred vision	Chills
Elevated blood pressure	Change in body weight
Anorexia	Change in mentation
Nausea and vomiting	
Related to Urinary System	
Pain	***Changes in urine output***
Dysuria	Polyuria
Flank or costovertebral angle	Oliguria
	Anuria
Groin	***Changes in urine consistency***
Suprapubic	
Changes in patterns of urination	Hematuria
	Pyuria
Frequency	Concentrated
Nocturia	Dilute
Dysuria	Color (red, brown, yellowish green)
Hesitancy of stream	
Change in stream	***Edema***
Urgency	Facial (periorbital)
Retention	Ankle
Incontinence	Ascites
Stress incontinence	Anasarca
Enuresis	Sacral

on their sexual patterns and satisfaction. Problems related to personal hygiene and fatigue can seriously affect a sexual relationship. Counseling of both the patient and partner may be indicated.

Objective Data

Physical Examination

Inspection. The nurse should assess for changes in the following:

Skin: Pallor, yellow-gray cast, excoriations, changes in turgor, bruises, texture (e.g., rough, dry skin)
Mouth: Stomatitis, ammonia breath odor
Face, abdomen, and extremities: Generalized edema, peripheral edema, bladder distention, masses, enlarged kidneys
Weight gain: Secondary to edema
General state of health: Fatigue, lethargy, and diminished alertness

Palpation. The kidneys are posterior organs protected by the abdominal organs, the ribs, and the heavy back muscles. A landmark useful in locating the kidneys is the *costovertebral angle* (CVA) formed by the rib cage and the vertebral column. The normal-sized left kidney is rarely palpable because it is overlain by the spleen. Occasionally the lower pole of the right kidney is palpable.

To palpate the right kidney, the examiner's left hand is placed behind and supports the patient's right side between the rib cage and the iliac crest (Fig. 42-7). The right flank is elevated with the left hand, and the right hand is used to palpate deeply for the right kidney. The lower pole of the right kidney may be felt as a smooth, rounded mass that descends on inspiration. If the kidney is palpable, its size, contour, and tenderness should be noted. Kidney enlargement is suggestive of severe hydronephrosis, neoplasm, polycystic disease, or a renal abscess.[14]

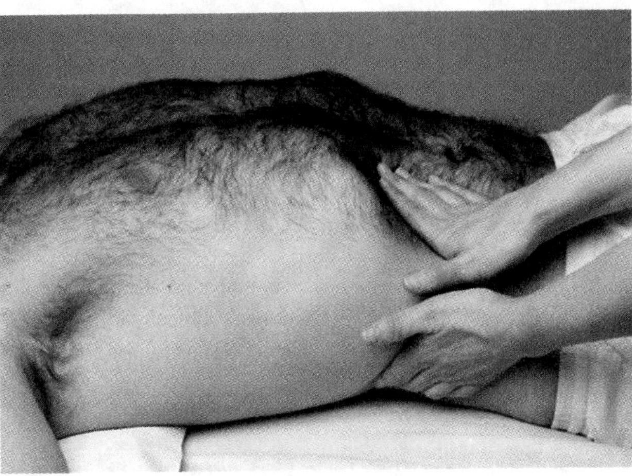

Fig. 42-7 Palpating the right kidney.

The urinary bladder is normally not palpable unless it is distended with urine. If the bladder is full, it may be felt as a smooth, round, firm organ and is sensitive to palpation.

Percussion. Tenderness in the flank area may be detected by fist percussion. This technique is performed by striking the fist (kidney punch) of one hand against the dorsal surface of the other hand, which is placed flat along the posterior CVA margin. Normally a firm blow in the flank area should not elicit pain. If CVA tenderness and pain are present, it may indicate a kidney infection or polycystic kidney disease.

Normally a bladder is not percussible until it contains 150 ml of urine. If the bladder is full, dullness is heard above the pubic symphysis. A distended bladder may be percussed as high as the umbilicus.

Auscultation. The diaphragm of the stethoscope may be used to auscultate over both CVAs and in the upper abdominal quadrants. With this technique, the abdominal aorta and renal arteries are auscultated for a bruit (an abnormal murmur), which indicates impaired blood flow to the kidneys.

Table 42-5 shows how to record the normal physical assessment findings of the urinary system. Table 42-6 pre-

Table 42-5 Normal Physical Assessment of the Urinary System

No costovertebral angle tenderness
Nonpalpable kidney and bladder
No palpable masses

Table 42-6 Common Assessment Abnormalities: Urinary System

Finding	Description	Possible Etiology and Significance
■ Dysuria	Painful or difficult urination	Sign of urinary tract infection and wide variety of pathologic conditions
■ Frequency	Increased incidence of urinating	Acutely inflamed bladder, retention with overflow, excess fluid intake
■ Enuresis	Involuntary nocturnal urinating	Symptomatic of lower urinary tract disorder
■ Hesitancy	Delay or difficulty in initiating urinating	Partial urethral obstruction
■ Urgency	Strong desire to urinate	Inflammatory lesions in bladder or urethra, acute bacterial infections
■ Hematuria	Blood in the urine	Cancer of genitourinary tract, blood dyscrasias, renal disease, urinary tract infection, stones in kidney or ureter, medications (anticoagulants)
■ Burning on urination	Stinging pain in urethral area	Urethral irritation, urinary tract infection
■ Pneumaturia	Passage of urine containing gas	Fistula connections between bowel and bladder, gas-forming urinary tract infections
■ Retention	Inability to urinate, even though bladder contains excessive amount of urine	Finding after pelvic surgery, childbirth, catheter removal; urethral stricture or obstruction; neurogenic bladder; postanesthesia
■ Pain	Presence over suprapubic area (related to bladder), urethral pain (irritation of bladder neck), flank (CVA) pain	Infection, urinary retention, foreign body in urinary tract, urethritis, pyelonephritis, renal colic or stones
■ Incontinence	Inability to voluntarily control discharge of urine	Neurogenic bladder, bladder infection, injury to external sphincter
■ Stress incontinence	Involuntary urination with increased pressure (sneezing or coughing)	Weakness of sphincter control
■ Nocturia	Frequency of urination at night	Renal disease with impaired concentrating ability, bladder obstruction, congestive heart failure, diabetes mellitus, finding after renal transplant
■ Polyuria	Large volume of urine in a given time	Diabetes mellitus, diabetes insipidus, chronic renal failure, diuretics, excess fluid intake
■ Anuria	Technically no urination (24-hr urine output <100 ml)	Acute renal failure, end-stage renal disease, bilateral ureteral obstruction
■ Oliguria	Diminished amount of urine in a given time (24-hr urine output of 100-400 ml)	Severe dehydration, shock, transfusion reaction, kidney disease, end-stage renal disease

CVA, Costovertebral angle.

sents common assessment abnormalities of the urinary system. Normally, assessment findings may vary in the older adult. Table 42-7 shows the assessment changes in the urinary system that are associated with aging.

Diagnostic Studies. Diagnostic studies provide important information to the nurse in monitoring the patient's condition and in planning appropriate interventions. These studies are considered to be objective data. Table 42-8 contains diagnostic studies common to the urinary system.

DIAGNOSTIC STUDIES

Diagnostic studies are important in locating and understanding problems of the urinary system. The accuracy of the study findings is influenced by (1) adherence to the proper procedures related to the study and (2) cooperation of the patient in restricting fluids, collecting urine specimens, and lying quietly on the examination table.

Many radiologic studies require the use of a bowel preparation the evening before the study to clear the lower GI tract of feces and gas. Because the kidneys lie in a retroperitoneal location, the contents of the colon may obstruct visualization of the urinary tract. If a bowel preparation is not properly done, the study may be unsuccessful and have to be rescheduled. Commonly used bowel preparations include enemas, castor oil, magnesium citrate, and bisacodyl (Dulcolax) tablets or suppositories. Sometimes a further bowel preparation is required the morning of the study. Some bowel preparations, such as magnesium citrate and Fleets are contraindicated in the patient with renal failure.

Table 42-7 Gerontologic Differences in Assessment: Urinary System

Changes	Differences in Assessment Findings
Kidney	
Decrease in amount of renal tissue	Less palpable
Decrease in number of nephrons and renal vascular bed; thickened basement membrane of Bowman's capsule and glomeruli	Decrease in creatinine clearance, increase in BUN level
Decrease in function of loop of Henle and tubules	Alterations in drug excretion; nocturia; loss of normal diurnal excretory pattern because of decreased ability to concentrate urine; less concentrated urine
Ureter, Bladder, and Urethra	
Decrease in elasticity and muscle tone	Palpable bladder after urination because of retention
Weakening of urinary sphincter	Stress incontinence (especially during Valsalva maneuver), dribbling of urine after urination
Decrease in bladder capacity and sensory receptors	Frequency, urgency, nocturia, overflow incontinence
Estrogen deficiency leading to thin, dry vaginal tissue; prostatic enlargement; uninhibited bladder contractions	Stress incontinence, dribbling

BUN, Blood urea nitrogen.

When a patient has repeated diagnostic studies on consecutive days, it is important to prevent dehydration. It is not uncommon to have a patient take nothing by mouth (NPO) after midnight, spend all morning in the x-ray department, return too late for lunch or too tired to eat, sleep all afternoon, and be on NPO status after midnight again because of studies the next day. Severe dehydration, especially in a diabetic, debilitated, or older patient, may lead to acute renal failure. The nurse is responsible for ensuring that a patient undergoing diagnostic studies is properly hydrated and given adequate nourishment between studies. The nurse should also check with the physician regarding the insulin dose for the diabetic patient who is NPO.

Another important nursing responsibility related to diagnostic studies is providing the patient with an adequate explanation of the procedure. The period during a diagnostic workup is typically an anxious one for most patients. The fear inherent in not knowing what is wrong is often worse than the diagnosis itself. Additional anxiety is caused by the unknown nature of the procedure. The patient needs to know what the procedure involves and its basic purpose, where it will be done, how long it will take, and whether it will hurt. These things should be explained at a level appropriate to the patient's understanding. The patient should also be instructed on personal responsibility during a particular study (e.g., to lie flat on the table or to keep the legs straight).

Diagnostic studies of the urinary system often cause embarrassment and emotional stress. Examination of the urinary system may be perceived as an intrusion on a personal body area. The nurse should alleviate anxiety by providing privacy and protecting the patient's modesty.

Urine Studies

Urinalysis. In evaluating disorders of the urinary tract, one of the first studies done is a urinalysis (Tables 42-8 and 42-9). This test may provide information about possible abnormalities, indicate what further studies need to be done, and supply information on the progression of a diagnosed disorder (e.g., diabetes mellitus).

For a routine urinalysis, a specimen may be collected at any time of the day. However, it is best to obtain the first specimen urinated in the morning. This concentrated specimen is more likely to contain abnormal constituents if they are present in the urine. The specimen should be examined within 1 hour of urinating. If it is not, bacteria multiply rapidly, RBCs hemolyze, casts disintegrate, and the urine becomes alkaline as a result of urea-splitting bacteria. If it is not possible to send the specimen to the laboratory, it should be refrigerated. However, to obtain the best results, the nurse should coordinate specimen collection with routine laboratory hours.

The results of a urinalysis usually include a description of the appearance, specific gravity (mass and density), pH, glucose, ketones, and protein in the urine and a microscopic examination of urine sediment for white blood cells (WBCs), RBCs, crystals, and casts (see Table 42-9).

Composite Urine Collections. Composite urine specimens are collected over a period that may range from 2 to 24 hours. The purpose of a composite specimen is to examine or measure specific components, such as electrolytes, sugar, protein, 17-ketosteroids, catecholamines, creatinine, and minerals. These specimens may have to be refrigerated, or preservatives may have to be added to the container used for collecting urine.

For collection of a composite urine specimen, the patient is instructed to urinate and discard this first urine specimen. This time is noted as the start of the test. All urine from subsequent urinations is saved in a container for the designated period. Finally, at the end of the period, the patient is asked to urinate and this urine is added to the container. Incomplete collections do not provide valid results.

Table 42-8 Diagnostic Studies: Urinary System

Study	Description and Purpose	Nursing Responsibility
Urine Studies		
■ Urinalysis	Study is a general examination of urine to establish baseline information or provide data to establish a tentative diagnosis and determine whether further studies are to be ordered.*	Try to obtain first urinated morning specimen. Ensure that specimen is examined within 1 hr of urinating. Wash perineal area if soiled with menses or fecal material.
■ Creatinine clearance	Creatinine is a waste product of protein breakdown (primarily body muscle mass). Clearance of creatinine by the kidney approximates the GFR. *Normal finding* is 85-135 ml/min.	Collect 24-hr urine specimen. Discard first urination when test is started. Save urine from all subsequent urinations for 24 hr. Instruct patient to urinate at end of 24 hr., and add specimen to collection. Ensure that serum creatinine is determined during 24-hr period.
■ Urine culture ("clean catch")	Study is done to confirm suspected urinary tract infection and identify causative organisms. *Normally,* bladder is sterile, but urethra contains bacteria and a few WBCs. If properly collected, stored, and handled: <10,000 organisms/ml usually indicates no infection; 10,000-100,000/ml is usually not diagnostic, and test may have to be repeated; >100,000/ml indicates infection.	Use sterile container for collection of urine. Touch only outside of container. For women, separate labia with one hand and clean meatus with other hand, using at least three sponges (saturated with cleansing solution) in a front-to-back motion. For men, retract foreskin (if present) and cleanse glans with at least three cleansing sponges. After cleaning, instruct patient to start urinating, stop, and then continue voiding in sterile container. (The initial voided urine flushes out most contaminants in the urethra and perineal area.) Inform physician of need for catheterization if patient is unable to cooperate with this procedure.
■ Concentration test	Study evaluates renal concentration ability. Concentration is measured by specific gravity readings. *Normal finding* is 1.020-1.035.	Instruct patient to fast after given time in evening (in usual procedure). Collect three urine specmens at hourly intervals in morning.
■ Residual urine	Study determines amount of urine left in bladder after urinating. Finding may be abnormal in problems with bladder innervation, sphincter impairment, BPH, or urethral strictures. *Normal finding* is ≤50 ml urine (increases with age).	If residual urine test is ordered, catheterize patient immediately after urinating. If a large amount of residual urine is obtained, physician may want catheter left in bladder.
■ Protein determination—Dipstick (Albustix, Combistix)	Test detects protein (primarily albumin) in urine. *Normal finding* is 0-trace.	Dip end of stick in urine, and read result by comparison with color chart on label as directed. Grading is from 0 to 4+. Interpret with caution. A positive result may not indicate significant proteinuria; some medications may give false-positive readings.
Quantitative test for protein	A 12- or 24-hr collection gives a more accurate indication of the amount of protein in urine. Persistent proteinuria usually indicates glomerular renal disease. *Normal finding* is <150 mg/24 hr (<0.15 g/24 hr), consisting mainly of albumin.	Perform 12- or 24-hr urine collection.
Blood Chemistries		
■ BUN	Study is most commonly used to identify presence of renal problems. Concentration of urea in blood is regulated by rate at which kidney excretes urea. *Normal finding* is 10-30 mg/dl (1.8-7.1 mmol/L).	Be aware that when interpreting BUN, nonrenal factors may cause increase (e.g., rapid cell destruction from infections, fever, GI bleeding, trauma, athletic activity with excessive muscle breakdown, steroid therapy).
■ Creatinine	Study is more reliable than BUN as a determinant of renal function. Creatinine is end-product of muscle and protein metabolism and is liberated at a constant rate. *Normal finding* is 0.5-1.5 mg/dl (44-133 μmol/L). Results are higher in men.	Explain test, and watch for postpuncture bleeding.
■ BUN/creatinine ratio	*Normal finding* is 10:1.	

continued

Table 42-8 Diagnostic Studies: Urinary System—cont'd

Study	Description and Purpose	Nursing Responsibility
Blood Chemistries—cont'd		
■ Uric acid	Study is used as a screening test primarily for disorders of purine metabolism but can indicate kidney disease as well. Values depend on renal function and rate of purine metabolism and dietary intake of food rich in purines. *Normal finding* is 2.5-5.5 mg/dl (149-327 μmol/L) for women and 4.5-6.5 mg/dl (268-387 μmol/L) for men.	Explain test, and watch for postpuncture bleeding.
■ Sodium	Sodium is main extracellular electrolyte determining blood volume. Usually, values stay within normal range until late stages of renal failure. *Normal finding* is 135-145 mEq/L (135-145 mmol/L).	Explain test, and watch for postpuncture bleeding.
■ Potassium	Kidneys are responsible for excreting majority of body's potassium. In renal disease, K^+ determinations are critical because K^+ is one of the first electrolytes to become abnormal. Elevated K^+ levels of >6 mEq/L can lead to muscle weakness and cardiac dysrhythmias. *Normal finding* is 3.5-5.5 mEq/L (3.5-5.5 mmol/L).	Explain test, and watch for postpuncture bleeding.
■ Calcium	Calcium is main mineral in bone and aids in muscular contraction, neurotransmission, and clotting. In renal disease, decreased absorption of Ca^{2+} leads to renal osteodystrophy. *Normal finding* is 9-11 mg/dl (4.5-5.5 mEq/L, 2.25-2.74 mmol/L).	Explain test, and watch for postpuncture bleeding.
■ Phosphorus	Phosphorus balance is inversely related to Ca^{2+} balance. In renal disease, phosphorus levels are elevated because the kidney is the primary excretory organ. Soft tissue calcification may occur if both Ca^{2+} and phosphorus are elevated. *Normal finding* is 2.8-4.5 mg/dl (0.9-1.45 mmol/L).	Explain test, and watch for postpuncture bleeding.
■ Bicarbonate	Most patients in renal failure have metabolic acidosis and low serum HCO_3 levels. *Normal finding* is 20-30 mEq/L (20-30 mmol/L).	Explain test, and watch for postpuncture bleeding.
Radiologic Procedures		
■ Kidneys, ureters, bladder (KUB)	Study involves flat-plate x-ray examination of abdomen and pelvis and delineates size, shape, and position of kidneys.	Perform bowel preparation (if ordered).
■ IVP or excretory urogram	X-ray examination visualizes urinary tract after IV injection of contrast material.	Evening before procedure, give cathartic or enema to empty colon of feces and gas. Keep patient on NPO status 8 hr before procedure. Before procedure, assess patient for iodine sensitivity to avoid anaphylactic reaction. Inform patient that procedure involves lying on table and having serial x-rays taken. After procedure, force fluids (if permitted) to flush out contrast material.
■ Nephrotomogram	X-ray is taken with rotating tubes. Test delineates segments of the kidney at different levels. Multiple exposures are taken to visualize specific sections of the kidney after IV injection of contract material.	Explain procedure, and prepare patient as for IVP.

continued

Table 42-8 Diagnostic Studies: Urinary System—cont'd

Study	Description and Purpose	Nursing Responsibility
Radiologic Procedures—cont'd		
▪ Retrograde pyelogram	X-ray of urinary tract is taken after injection of contrast material into kidneys. Cystoscope is inserted, and ureteral catheters are inserted through it into renal pelvis. Contrast material is injected through catheters.	Prepare patient as for IVP. Inform patient that pain may be experienced from distention of pelvis and discomfort from cystoscope. Inform patient that general anesthesia may be given for procedure.
▪ Cystogram	Contrast material is instilled into bladder via cystoscope or catheter. Purpose is to visualize bladder and evaluate vesicoureteral reflux.	Explain procedure to patient. If done via cystoscope, follow nursing care related to cystoscopy.
▪ Renal arteriogram (angiogram)	Study is performed by injecting contrast material into renal artery via catheter inserted into femoral artery. Purpose is to visualize renal blood vessels.	Prepare patient evening before procedure by giving cathartic or enema. The morning of the procedure, give preoperative medication to sedate and relax patient. Before injection of contrast material, test for iodine sensitivity. After procedure, check insertion site for bleeding, and take peripheral pulses in involved leg every 30-60 min to detect occluded blood flow.
▪ Ultrasound	Small external ultrasound probe is attached to patient. Conductive gel is applied to the skin. Noninvasive procedure involves passing sound waves into body structures and recording images as they are reflected back. Computer interprets tissue density based on sound waves and displays it in picture form. Study is most valuable in detection of renal or perirenal masses, differential diagnosis of renal cysts, solid masses, and identification of obstructions. It can be used safely in patients with renal failure.	Explain procedure to patient.
▪ CT scan	Study provides excellent visualization of kidneys. Kidney size can be evaluated; tumors, abscesses, suprarenal masses (e.g., adrenal tumors, pheochromocytomas), and obstructions can be detected. Advantage of CT over ultrasound is its ability to distinguish subtle differences in density. Use of IV-administered contrast material during CT accentuates density of renal tissue and helps differentiate masses.	Explain procedure to patient.
▪ MRI	Computer-generated films rely on radiowaves and alteration in magnetic field. Useful for visualization of kidneys. Not proven useful for detecting urinary calculi or calcified tumors.	Explain procedure to patient. Have patient remove all metal objects. Patients with a history of claustrophobia may need to be sedated.
Renal Radionuclide Imaging		
▪ Renal scan	Radioactive isotopes are injected IV. Radiation detector probes are placed over kidney, and scintillation counter monitors radioactive material in kidney. Purpose is to show blood flow, glomerular filtration, tubular function, and excretion. Radioisotope distribution in kidney is scanned and mapped. Test is useful in showing location, size, and shape of kidney and, in general, assessing blood perfusion and its ability to secrete urine. Abscesses, cysts, and tumors may appear as cold spots because of presence of nonfunctioning tissue.	Requires no dietary or activity restriction. Inform patient that no pain or discomfort should be felt during test.

continued

Table 42-8 Diagnostic Studies: Urinary System—cont'd

Study	Description and Purpose	Nursing Responsibility
Endoscopy		
■ Cystoscopy	Study involves use of tubular lighted scope to inspect bladder. Lithotomy position is used. It may be done using local or general anesthesia.	Before procedure, force fluids or give IV fluids if general anesthesia is to be used. Ensure consent form is signed. Explain procedure to patient. Give preoperative medication. After procedure, explain that burning on urination, pink-tinged urine, and urinary frequency are expected effects after cystoscopy. Do not let patient walk alone immediately after procedure because orthostatic hypotension may occur. Offer warm sitz baths, heat, mild analgesics to relieve discomfort.
Urodynamics		
■ Cystometrogram	Study involves insertion of catheter and instillation of water or saline solution into bladder. Measurements of pressure exerted against bladder wall are recorded. Purpose is to evaluate bladder tone, sensations of filling, and bladder (detrusor) stability.	Explain procedure to patient. Observe patient for manifestations of urinary infection after procedure.
Invasive Procedure		
■ Renal biopsy	Technique is usually done as a skin (percutaneous) biopsy through needle insertion into lower lobe of kidney. Purpose is to obtain renal tissue for examination to determine type of renal disease or to follow progress of renal disease.	Before procedure, ascertain coagulation status through patient history, medication history, CBC, hematocrit, prothrombin time, and bleeding and clotting time. Type and crossmatch patient for blood. Ensure consent form is signed. Be aware that IVP or ultrasound study is done before biopsy. After procedure, apply pressure dressing to biopsy site, and check frequently for bleeding. Keep patient on bed rest up to 24 hrs. Take vital signs frequently. Observe urine for gross bleeding. Determine microscopic bleeding by use of dipstick. Assess patient for flank pain. Monitor hematocrit levels.

BPH, Benign prostatic hyperplasia; *BUN,* Blood urea nitrogen; *CBC,* complete blood count; *CT,* computed tomography; *GFR,* glomerular filtration rate; *GI,* gastrointestinal; *IV,* intravenous; *IVP,* intravenous pyelogram; *KUB,* kidneys, ureters, bladder; *MRI,* magnetic resonance imaging; *NPO,* nothing by mouth; *WBC,* white blood cell.
*See Table 42-9
†See Chapter 44.

Reminding the patient to save all urine during the study period is critical.

Creatinine Clearance. One of the most common composite indicators used to analyze urinary system disorders is creatinine clearance. Creatinine is a waste product produced by muscle breakdown. Urinary excretion of creatinine is a measure of the amount of active muscle tissue in the body, not of body weight. Therefore, people with larger muscle mass have higher values. Because almost all creatinine in the blood is normally excreted by the kidneys, creatinine clearance is the most accurate indicator of renal function. The result of a creatinine clearance closely approximates that of the GFR. A blood specimen for serum creatinine determination should be obtained during the period of urine collection. Creatinine clearance is calculated as follows:

$$\text{Creatinine clearance (ml/min)} = \frac{\text{Urine creatinine (mg/ml)} \times \text{Urine volume (ml/min)}}{\text{Serum creatinine (mg/ml)}}$$

Creatinine levels remain remarkably constant for each person because they are not significantly affected by protein ingestion, muscular exercise, water intake, or rate of urine production. Normal creatinine clearance values range from 85 to 135 ml per minute. After the age of 40, the creatinine clearance rate decreases at a rate of about 1 ml per minute per year.

Radiologic Studies

Kidney, Ureter, and Bladder Film. The kidney, ureter, and bladder (KUB) film is an abdominal view taken without using a contrast medium to show the renal outline,

Table 42-9 Urinalysis Findings

Test	Normal	Abnormal Finding and Significance
Color	Amber yellow	■ Dark, smoky color suggests hematuria. Yellow brown to olive green indicates excessive bilirubin. Orange red or orange brown caused by phenazopyridine (Pyridium) or urobilin in excess. Cloudiness of freshly voided urine indicates infection. Colorless urine indicates excessive fluid intake, renal disease, or diabetes insipidus.
Smell	Aromatic	■ On standing, urine becomes more ammonia-like in smell. In urinary tract infections, urine smells unpleasant.
Protein	0-150 mg/24 hr 0-18 mg/dl	■ Persistent proteinuria is characteristic of acute and chronic renal disease, especially involving glomeruli. In absence of disease, positive reading may be caused by high-protein diet, strenuous exercise, dehydration, fever, or emotional stress. Vaginal secretions may contaminate urine specimen and give positive reading.
Glucose	None	■ Glycosuria indicates diabetes mellitus or low renal threshold for glucose reabsorption (if blood glucose level is normal). Small amounts may be found after glucose loading (e.g., glucose tolerance test).
Ketones	None	■ Altered carbohydrate and fat metabolism indicates diabetes mellitus and starvation. Findings can also be seen in dehydration, vomiting, and severe diarrhea.
Bilirubin	None	■ Presence of bilirubinuria is as significant as jaundice in detection of liver disorders. Bilirubin may appear in urine before jaundice becomes visible or may be present in persons with hepatic disorders who do not have recognizable jaundice.*
Specific gravity	1.003-1.030	■ Specific gravity of morning urine specimen reflects maximum concentrating ability of kidney and is 1.025-1.030. Low specific gravity indicates dilute urine and possibly excessive diuresis. High specific gravity indicates dehydration. If it becomes fixed at about 1.010, this indicates renal inability to concentrate urine, suggesting that kidney is progressing to end-stage renal disease.
Osmolality	300-1300 mOsm/kg (300-1300 mmol/kg)	■ Measurement is a more accurate method than specific gravity for determining diluting and concentrating ability of kidneys. Deviations from normal indicate tubular dysfunction. Findings indicate if kidney has lost ability to concentrate or dilute urine. (Not part of routine urinalysis.)
pH	4.0-8.0 (average, 6.0)	■ If >8.0, finding may be the result of standing of urine or urinary tract infections because bacteria decompose urea to form ammonia. If <4.0, may indicate respiratory or metabolic acidosis.
RBC	0-4/hpf	■ Bleeding in urinary tract is caused by calculi, cystitis,neoplasm, glomerulonephritis, tuberculosis, kidney biopsy, or trauma.
WBC	0-5/hpf	■ Increased number of WBCs in urine (pyuria) indicates urinary tract infection or inflammation.
Casts	None-occasional hyaline	■ Casts are molds of the renal tubules and may contain protein, WBCs, RBCs, or bacteria. Noncellular casts are hyaline in appearance, and a few may be found in normal urine. Casts indicate renal dysfunction or urinary tract infections.
Culture for organisms	No organisms in bladder, $<10^4$ organisms/ml result of normal urethral flora	■ Bacteria counts $>10^5$/ml indicate urinary tract infection. Organisms most commonly found in urinary tract infections are *Escherichia coli*, enterococci, *Klebsiella*, *Proteus*, and streptococci.

hpf, High powered field; *RBC*, red blood cell; *WBC*, white blood cell.
*See Chapter 41 for further discussion.

psoas shadow, and the bladder, if full. Radiopaque stones and foreign bodies can be seen on this x-ray. The form, size, and position of the kidneys can also be seen. Abscesses, tumors, and cysts may distort anatomic relationships on the KUB. Sometimes tomograms (sectional views that focus on a single plane of the kidney) are ordered at the same time as the KUB x-ray.

Intravenous Pyelogram. The purpose of an intravenous pyelogram (IVP), or excretory urogram, is to visualize the urinary tract. The presence, position, size, and shape of the kidneys, ureters, and bladder can be evaluated. Cysts, tumors, lesions, and obstructions cause a distortion in the normal appearance of these structures. The IVP also gives clues to renal function since sequential films are taken, but other tests (discussed later) are more accurate for this purpose.

The procedure consists of injecting an intravenous (IV) dose of contrast material, which circulates in the blood and is excreted by the kidneys into the urine. During injection, the patient may experience warmth, a flushed face, and a salty taste. After injection, films are taken sequentially. (A *rapid-sequence IVP* has x-ray films taken every minute for the first 5 minutes.) The sequencing of films is planned so that contrast excretion can be followed from the cortex of the kidney to the bladder. A film taken at 45 minutes allows visualization of the bladder. The presence of bladder atony or outlet obstruction also can be detected by a film taken after urination, which shows the residual volume of urine in the bladder. Sometimes abdominal compression (e.g., using abdominal binders) is used to enhance the clarity of kidney images.

Preparation of the patient the evening before the test includes giving a cathartic or an enema to eliminate feces and air from the colon. The patient with neurologic bowel dysfunction may require more vigorous routines. Fluids are withheld for 8 hours before testing to produce slight dehydration so that the contrast material will concentrate and therefore improve visualization. The patient with significantly decreased renal function should not have an IVP because the contrast material will not be properly excreted by the kidneys. Contrast medium can also be nephrotoxic and can worsen renal function. An IVP should be avoided on a pregnant patient, particularly in the first trimester, because of radiation exposure and harm to the fetus.

The patient should be assessed for any possible allergic reactions to the contrast material. The contrast medium is typically an iodine derivative or shellfish. A person with iodine sensitivity may have an anaphylactic reaction after contrast material is injected. If known to have an allergy to iodine or seafood, the patient should not have an IVP, or it can be done using prophylactic diphenhydramine (Benadryl) and corticosteroids.

During contrast material injection, the patient should be observed for signs of respiratory distress, urticaria, decrease in blood pressure, and other signs of anaphylaxis. Emergency drugs such as diphenhydramine (Benadryl), corticosteroids, epinephrine (Adrenalin), and cardiopulmonary resuscitation equipment should be available. A patient may experience transient hypersensitivity reactions (e.g., nausea, itching), but these are not considered serious reactions contraindicating future IVPs.

After the procedure, the nurse should encourage the patient to force fluids to dilute and flush out the contrast material. Dilution of the contrast medium makes it less nephrotoxic. The patient should be monitored for delayed reactions such as itching, nausea, respiratory problems, and decreased urine output.

Retrograde Pyelogram. A retrograde pyelogram evaluates the same structures as an IVP. This is an x-ray visualization of the kidneys, ureter, and bladder after direct injection of a contrast material into the kidney via a ureteral catheter introduced through a cystoscope. It may be done if an IVP does not visualize the urinary tract or if the patient is allergic to the contrast material or has decreased renal function. The dangers associated with a retrograde pyelogram are similar to those related to cystoscopy, including the risk of infection and the use of anesthesia.

Renal Ultrasound. A renal ultrasound uses high-frequency waves to image the kidneys, ureter, and bladder. Because radiation exposure is avoided, a number of images can be obtained, and repeat studies over a brief period of time can be done. Images can be obtained from both the prone and supine positions. A bowel preparation is not required for a renal ultrasound.

Computed Tomography Scan. Computed tomography (CT) of the abdomen and pelvis may be done to detect tumors and possible metastases. The CT scan can differentiate these from cysts or abscesses. Contrast material may be used to help visualize urinary structures more clearly in the computer-generated images produced by the machine. The patient is instructed to lie very still during the procedure while the machine takes precise transaxial images. Sedation may be required if the patient is unable to cooperate.

Magnetic Resonance Imaging. Specific structures such as the kidney or prostate can be visualized by disturbing the electromagnetic fields generated by different body tissues and converting this to computer-generated images. This is done using radiofrequency waves. Magnetic resonance imaging (MRI) helps to evaluate genitourinary tumors and abdominal or pelvic masses. The patient must lie still in an enclosed cylinder while these images are being produced. Sedation may be required. Some patients cannot tolerate being in the small MRI chamber. All metal objects must be removed because they interfere with the radiofrequency. The MRI is contraindicated in a patient with a pacemaker or with certain kinds of metallic vascular surgery clips.

Cystogram. The purpose of a cystogram is to outline and visualize the bladder and evaluate the UVJ for reflux. In addition to suspected vesicoureteral reflux, indications for a cystogram include a neurogenic bladder and recurrent urinary tract infections. A cystogram can also delineate abnormalities of the bladder, such as diverticuli, calculi, and tumors. The procedure involves instillation of a contrast material into the bladder, which may be done via a cystoscope or catheter.

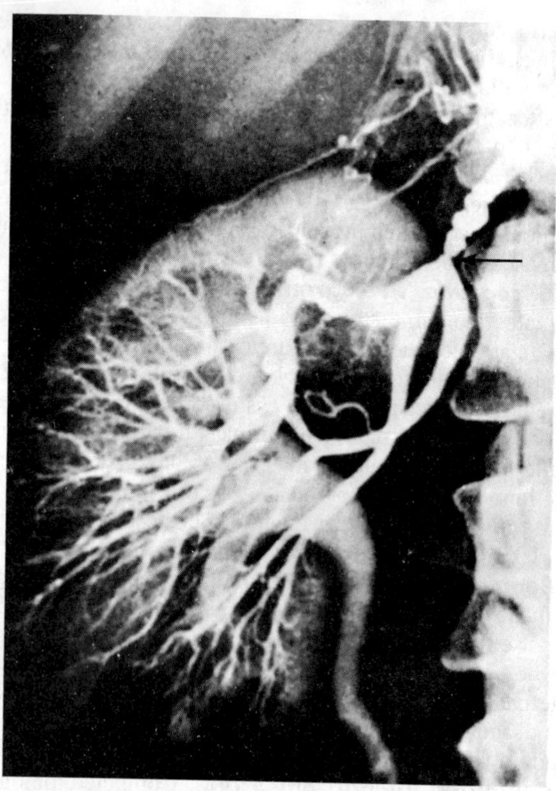

Fig. 42-8 Renal arteriogram showing stenosis of the right renal artery.

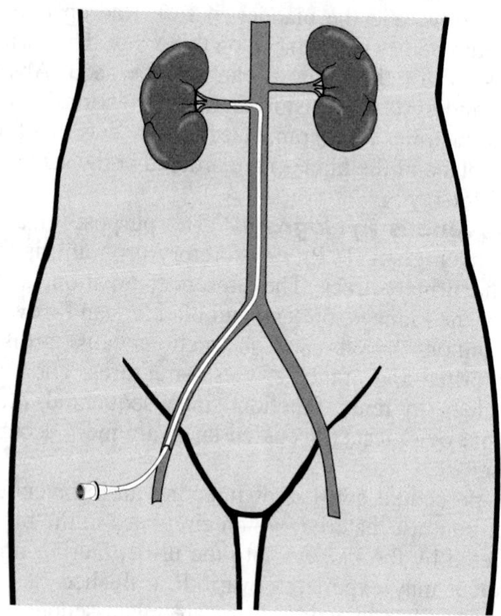

Fig. 42-9 Catheter insertion for a renal arteriogram.

A voiding cystourethrogram is a voiding study of the bladder opening and urethra. The bladder is filled with contrast material. During urination, films are taken to visualize the bladder and urethra. After urination, another film is taken to assess for residual urine. A voiding cystourethrogram can detect abnormalities of the lower urinary tract, urethral stenosis, bladder neck obstruction, and prostatic enlargement.

Renal Arteriogram. The purpose of a renal arteriogram (angiogram) is to visualize the renal blood vessels. The findings of an arteriogram can assist in diagnosing renal artery stenosis (Fig. 42-8), additional or missing renal blood vessels, and renovascular hypertension and can assist in differentiating between a renal cyst and a renal tumor. Renal arteriograms are also included in the workup of a potential renal transplant donor.

The evening before the procedure, the patient is given a cathartic to eliminate fecal material from the colon. The morning of the procedure, a preoperative medication is given to relax and sedate the patient.

Most arteriograms are done in the x-ray department by a specially trained physician. The patient is given a local anesthetic at the site of catheter insertion. A catheter is usually inserted into the femoral artery and passed up the aorta to the level of the renal arteries (Fig. 42-9). Contrast material is then injected to outline the renal blood supply, and x-rays are taken. The patient may experience a transient warm feeling along the course of the blood vessel when the contrast material is injected. As with all contrast studies, possible iodine and shellfish allergies should be determined before the study.

After the catheter is removed, a pressure dressing is placed over the femoral injection site. It is important to observe the site for bleeding. Bed rest is usually prescribed with the affected leg straight for 12 to 24 hours. Peripheral pulses in the involved leg should be taken at least every 30 to 60 minutes to detect occlusion of blood flow caused by a thrombus. Complications that may result from a renal arteriogram include thrombus, embolus, local inflammation, and hematoma. The patient with baseline renal insufficiency may experience a decrease in renal function secondary to the nephrotoxic contrast material.

Digital Subtraction Angiography. Because of potential complications, the renal arteriogram is sometimes replaced by digital subtraction angiography (DSA) in many hospitals that have the facilities to perform this procedure. Using computer technology, this procedure permits visualization of the arteries after an IV injection of contrast material. A primary advantage of DSA is that it requires small peripheral venous injections of contrast medium compared with the relatively large doses that must be injected via arterial cannulation for a renal arteriogram. (See Table 29-7 for a further description of DSA.)

Renal Radionuclide Imaging. Renal scans involving the use of radionuclides are useful in evaluating the anatomic structures, perfusion, and function of the kidneys. Different institutions use different imaging techniques. In general, the following radionuclides are used for these purposes:

Anatomic structures: Technetium 99m (^{99m}Tc)-labeled compounds such as dimercaptosuccinic acid (DMSA) or glucoheptonate

Perfusion and function: Iodine 131-labeled orthiodohippurate (Hippuran) and ^{99m}Tc-labeled diethylenetriamine pentaacetic acid (DTPA)
Infection or abscesses: Gallium-67 citrate

For this procedure a radioactive isotope is injected intavenously. Radiation detector probes are placed over the kidneys, and a scintillation counter monitors the appearance and disappearance of the radioactive material in the kidney.

The results reveal the difference between the two kidneys with respect to blood flow, tubular function, and excretion. A normal scan shows symmetrical functioning of both kidneys. Normally the distribution of activity is recorded throughout the kidneys. A lesion (e.g., a tumor) is indicated by the absence of radioactivity in the involved area and the appearance of the resultant defect on the scan. In renovascular disease, an area with decreased blood flow can be readily visualized. This study is particularly useful in detecting renal vascular disease, acute renal failure, and upper urinary tract obstruction, as well as useful in monitoring the function of a transplanted kidney.

Usually there are no dietary or activity restrictions related to preparation of the patient. During the test the patient should feel no pain or discomfort. No special precautions are needed in the use of radioactive material since only tracer doses are used.

Renal Biopsy. The purpose of a renal biopsy is to determine the nature and extent of renal disease. This information can be used in establishing a diagnosis and following the progress of a disease, as well as determining the treatment. Biopsy material can be obtained through an open biopsy or a closed percutaneous needle biopsy. An open biopsy is rarely performed because it requires a surgical procedure with anesthesia. A percutaneous needle biopsy is more common. It is usually done in the x-ray department or in the patient's room, although it may be done in the operating room.

Absolute contraindications to a percutaneous renal biopsy are bleeding disorders, the presence of a single kidney, and uncontrolled hypertension. Relative contraindications include suspected renal infection, hydronephrosis, and possible vascular lesions.

Because hemorrhage is one danger of biopsy, the patient's coagulation status should be assessed before the procedure. This includes a health history, complete blood count (CBC), hematocrit, prothrombin time, and bleeding or clotting time determinations. The patient may also be typed and crossmatched for blood. The patient who is to be biopsied should not be taking aspirin or warfarin (Coumadin) before the procedure.

An IVP or ultrasound examination is done to determine the position and location of the kidneys as a guide to needle insertion. Preparation also includes explaining the procedure to the patient and discussing all concerns. A signed consent form is required before a biopsy is performed.

The procedure consists of having the patient lie prone with a pillow or sandbag to elevate the abdomen and kidneys. Using the IVP or ultrasound findings as a guide, the position of the kidney is marked on the body. Local anesthesia is used, and a biopsy needle is inserted into the kidney just below the twelfth rib. The patient is instructed to hold his breath while the biopsy specimen is being taken.

After the procedure, a pressure dressing is applied, and the patient is kept prone for 30 to 60 minutes. Usually bed rest is prescribed for 24 hours. Vital signs should be taken every 5 to 10 minutes during the first hour and then with decreasing frequency, if no problems are noted. The biopsy site should be inspected frequently for bleeding. Serial urine specimens should be assessed for gross and microscopic hematuria. A dipstick can be used to test for bleeding, even when hematuria is not obvious. The physician may order all urine sent for laboratory analysis to detect possible hematuria. The patient should also be assessed for flank pain, hypotension, decreasing hematocrit, and temperature elevation. The patient should be observed for chills, urinary frequency, and dysuria.

Complications of a renal biopsy include renal hemorrhage, hematoma, and infection. Even if no complications occur, the patient should be instructed to avoid lifting heavy objects for 5 to 7 days. The patient should be instructed not to take any anticoagulant medication until permission is given by the physician who performed the biopsy.

Endoscopy

Cystoscopy. The main purpose of cystoscopy is to inspect the interior of the bladder with a tubular lighted scope called a cystoscope (Fig. 42-10). Cystoscopes can be used to insert ureteral catheters, remove calculi, obtain biopsy specimens of bladder lesions, and treat bleeding lesions. In most cases, bladder disorders can be determined by cystoscopic examination. Although rigid instruments still are used, newer flexible cystoscopes (and ureteroscopes) make visualization easier for the urologist and the procedure more comfortable for the patient.

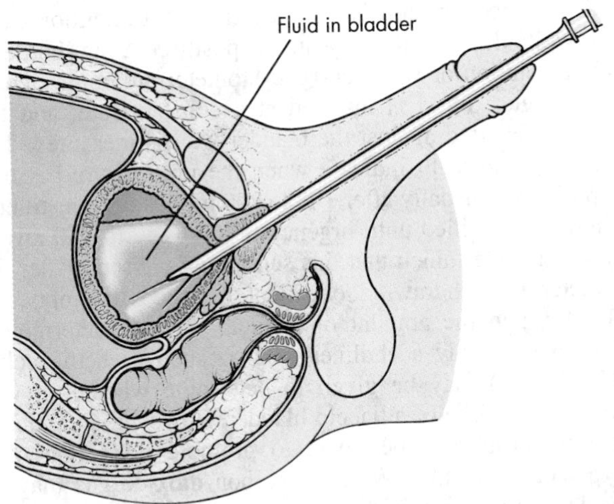

Fig. 42-10 Cystoscopic examination of the bladder in a man.

The patient may be given a preoperative medication for sedation about 1 hour before the procedure. Cystoscopy is usually done in a cystoscopy room in the x-ray department or in the operating room. A signed consent form is required. To ensure a continuous flow of urine, fluids may be forced before the procedure. If general anesthesia is given, IV fluids may be used to maintain adequate fluid intake.

The cystoscopic examination may be performed with local or general anesthesia, depending on the needs and condition of the patient. The patient is put in a lithotomy position. Most of the pain associated with cystoscopy results from spasms and contractions of bladder and sphincter. Relaxation and deep breathing by the patient alleviate some of the bladder and sphincter spasms. A local anesthetic is instilled into the urethra before scope insertion. During the examination, water or saline solution is inserted slowly to distend the bladder. This allows better visualization but causes an urge to urinate.

After the procedure the patient can expect to have some burning on urination, blood-tinged urine, and urinary frequency from the irritation of scope insertion and manipulation. The nurse should observe for bright red bleeding, which is not normal. The patient should not be allowed to walk without assistance immediately after the procedure because postural hypotension may result from blood flow back to the legs after the patient has been in a lithotomy position. After the procedure the nurse is responsible for keeping the patient well hydrated, administering mild analgesics, providing sitz baths, and applying heat to decrease the patient's discomfort. Complications that may result from cystoscopy include urinary retention, urinary tract hemorrhage, bladder infection, and perforation of the bladder.

Urodynamics

Cystometrogram. The purpose of a cystometrogram is to evaluate bladder tone and neurologic bladder dysfunction. It is usually ordered if a patient has incontinence or neurogenic dysfunction of the bladder.

The procedure consists of insertion of a retention catheter while the patient is in a supine position. A liter bottle of saline solution or water and a cystometer are connected to the catheter. Fluid is instilled at a constant rate, and the pressure exerted against the bladder wall is measured. The patient is asked to indicate when the urge to void is first experienced (usually after 100 to 200 ml has been instilled). Fluids are instilled until urgency occurs (350 to 450 ml) or until it is determined that this sensation is absent. After the catheter is withdrawn the patient is asked to empty the bladder, and the amount of residual urine is determined. During the study a cholinergic drug such as bethanechol (Urecholine) may be given to determine whether it will enhance the tone of a flaccid bladder. However, an anticholinergic drug may be given to promote relaxation of a hyperactive bladder. Water or carbon dioxide gas may be used for this examination. Complete urodynamic studies are often done simultaneously using specialized equipment and catheters.

REVIEW QUESTIONS

The number of the question corresponds to the same-numbered objective at the beginning of the chapter.

1. The main function of the pelvis of the kidney is to
   a. give structural support to the kidney.
   b. serve as a collecting chamber for urine.
   c. regulate the concentration of the filtrate.
   d. serve as the entry and exit site for blood vessels.

2. The action of ADH causes
   a. increased sodium reabsorption.
   b. decreased sodium reabsorption.
   c. increased water reabsorption.
   d. decreased water reabsorption.

3. A patient related a history of the following diseases. Which is known to be related to urinary calculi?
   a. Measles
   b. Diabetes mellitus
   c. Hyperparathyroidism
   d. Gastric ulcer

4. Normal changes associated with aging of the urinary system include
   a. decreased amount of renal tissue.
   b. increased bladder capacity.
   c. decreased normal levels of BUN.
   d. more easily palpable kidneys.

5. Which of the following statements regarding the physical assessment of the urinary system is accurate?
   a. An empty bladder is palpable as a small nodule.
   b. Auscultation is used to listen to urine in the bladder.
   c. The patient lies prone when the kidneys are palpated.
   d. The flank area is percussed with a firm blow.

6. Which of the following findings of a physical assessment of the urinary system is considered normal?
   a. Easily palpable left kidney
   b. CVA tenderness elicited by a kidney punch
   c. Nonpalpable left kidney
   d. Palpable bladder to the level of the pubic symphysis

7. An important nursing responsibility after an IVP is to
   a. encourage ambulation 2 to 3 hours after the study.
   b. observe urine for remaining contrast material.
   c. monitor breathing and voiding.
   d. keep the patient on NPO status for 4 hours after the study.

8. Which of the following is considered a normal constituent of urine?
   a. Ketones
   b. Creatinine
   c. Amino acids
   d. Bacteria

REFERENCES

1. Smith HW: *Fish to philosopher,* Boston, 1953, Little, Brown.
2. McCance KL, Huether SE: *Pathophysiology: the biologic basis for disease in adults and children,* ed 2, St Louis, 1994, Mosby.

3. Lundin AP: Recombinant erythropoietin and chronic renal failure, *Hosp Pract* 26:61, 1991.
4. Smith MC, Dunn MJ: Role of kidney in blood pressure regulation. In Jacobson HR and others, editors: *The principles and practice of nephrology,* Philadelphia, 1993, BC Decker.
5. Gray M: *Genitourinary disorders,* St Louis, 1992, Mosby.
6. Steele D: Neurophysiology of voiding, *Innovations in Urology Nursing* 4:2, 1993.
7. Christiansen JL, Grzybouski JM: *Biology of aging,* St Louis, 1993, Mosby.
8. Fliser D and others: Renal functional reserve in healthy elderly subjects, *J Am Soc Nephrol* 3:1371, 1993.
9. Roy AT and others: Renal failure in older people: UCLA grand rounds, *J Am Geriatr Soc* 38:239, 1990.
10. Cohen MS, Thill JR: What's the cause of abnormally colored urine? *Contemp Urol* 4:25, 1992.
11. Brettschneider NR, Orihuela E: Carcinoma of the bladder, *Urol Nursing* 10:14, 1990.
12. Catalona WJ: Urothelial tumors of the urinary tract. In Walsh PC and others, editors: *Campbell's urology,* ed 6, Philadelphia, 1992, Saunders.
13. Duffy LM: Continence management for the frail elderly and cognitively impaired, *Urol Nursing* 12:66, 1992.
14. Sökeland J: *Urology—a pocket reference,* ed 2, New York, 1989, Thieme Medical Publishers.

Chapter 43

NURSING ROLE IN MANAGEMENT

Renal and Urologic Problems

Patricia Bates **Sharon L. Lewis**

Learning Objectives

1. Describe the pathophysiology, clinical manifestations, and therapeutic and pharmacologic management of cystitis, urethritis, and pyelonephritis.
2. Explain the nursing management of urinary tract infections.
3. Describe the immunologic mechanisms involved in glomerulonephritis.
4. Explain the clinical manifestations and therapeutic and nursing management of acute poststreptococcal glomerulonephritis, Goodpasture's syndrome, and chronic glomerulonephritis.
5. Describe the common causes, clinical manifestations, and therapeutic and nursing management of nephrotic syndrome.
6. Compare and contrast the etiology, clinical manifestations, and therapeutic and nursing management of various types of urinary calculi.
7. Explain the common causes and management of renal trauma, renal vascular problems, congenital abnormalities, and hereditary renal problems.
8. Describe the mechanisms of renal involvement in metabolic and connective tissue disorders.
9. Describe the clinical manifestations and therapeutic management of renal and bladder cancer.
10. Describe the common causes and management of bladder dysfunctions.
11. Differentiate among ureteral, suprapubic, nephrostomy, and urethral catheters with regard to indications for use and nursing responsibilities.
12. Explain the nursing management of the patient undergoing nephrectomy or urinary diversion surgery.

Renal and urologic disorders encompass a wide spectrum of clinical problems. The diverse causes of these disorders may involve infectious, immunologic, obstructive, metabolic, collagen-vascular, traumatic, congenital, neoplastic, and neurologic mechanisms. This chapter discusses the therapeutic and nursing management of patients with specific disorders of the kidneys, ureters, bladder, and urethra. An effective management plan must deal with the significant psychosocial problems that may arise for these patients. These issues include anxiety about discussing problems related to the genitalia or urination, embarrassment related to exposure during examination and treatment, and fear of changes in body image or body function. (Acute and chronic renal failure are discussed in Chapter 44. Female reproductive problems are discussed in Chapter 51. Male genitourinary problems are discussed in Chapter 52.)

Reviewed by Mikel Gray, RN, PhD, CURN, CCCN, UroHealth, PSC; Director of Urodynamics, Suburban Medical Center, Louisville, KY; Adjunct Professor, Lansing School of Nursing, Bellarmine College, Louisville, KY.

INFECTIOUS DISORDERS OF THE URINARY SYSTEM

Significance

Urinary tract infections (UTIs) are the second most common bacterial disease. Sexually active younger women outnumber men 30 to 1 in prevalence of UTIs, but with increasing age the female-to-male ratio becomes 2 to 1.[1] At least 8000 persons die each year of infections of the kidney. In addition, more than 100,000 persons are hospitalized annually for an average of 6 to 7 days because of renal infections. Nosocomial urinary infections are responsible for 35% to 45% of all hospital-acquired infections.[2] More than 15% of patients who develop gram-negative bacteremia die, and one third of these are caused by bacteria originating in the urinary tract.[3]

Infections of the urinary tract may appear as a variety of disorders. The common factor is a microbial invasion of the tissues of the urinary tract, most often by *Escherichia coli (E. coli)* (Table 43-1). Bacterial counts of 10^5 organisms or more generally indicate a UTI. However, bacterial counts as low as 10^2 to 10^3 in a person with symptoms are indicative of UTI. Viral, fungal, and parasitic infections are not as common but are seen most frequently in the patient

Table 43-1 Common Microorganisms Causing Urinary Tract Infections

*Escherichia coli**	*Proteus*
Enterococci	*Pseudomonas*
Klebsiella	*Staphylococci*
Enterobacter	*Candida*
Serratia	

*Causes about 80% of cases in persons who do not have urinary tract structural abnormalities or calculi.

who is immunosuppressed, has diabetes mellitus, or has taken courses of antibiotics.

Classification

Infections may be broadly classified as upper and lower UTIs (Fig. 43-1) based on the patient's symptoms. Terminology may specifically delineate the site of inflammation or infection. Examples of terms are *pyelonephritis* (involvement of kidney and kidney pelvis) or *cystitis* (involvement of bladder). However, it may be difficult to determine the specific location of a UTI. A patient may have a simultaneous infection in both the upper and lower urinary tract, an infection of adjacent organs causing urinary infection-like symptoms, or no symptoms at all.

Determining whether a UTI is complicated or uncomplicated will be a significant factor in determining the treatment plan. Uncomplicated infections are those that occur in an otherwise normal urinary tract. Complicated infections include coexisting presence of obstruction, stones, or catheters, when diabetes or neurologic diseases exist, or when an infection is a recurrent one. The individual with a complicated infection is often the one at highest risk for renal damage.

Only about one fourth of individuals who develop an acute infection go on to develop a recurrent UTI.[4] Recurrent UTIs can be classified as *relapses* (recurrence with the same strain of bacteria from within the urinary tract that occurs within 1 to 2 weeks of stopping antibiotic therapy) or *reinfections* (recurrence with a new strain from outside the urinary tract).

Relapse can be further defined as states of *unresolved bacteriuria* or true *bacterial persistence.* Unresolved bacteriuria occurs when bacteria are resistant to the antibiotic used to treat an infection or when the infection is undertreated. Some bacteria, although initially sensitive to a drug, can mutate during therapy. Insufficient antibiotic concentrations in the urinary system may be attributed to renal insufficiency or an inability of the antibiotic to infiltrate the tissues (such as the prostate or urethra). Often the patient feels better and stops medication before an adequate course is completed. Bacterial persistence occurs when there is a high concentration of persistent bacteria. Stones are a common cause. Urine cultures may be negative immediately following antibiotic therapy but will show growth again when cultured about 1 week after treatment.

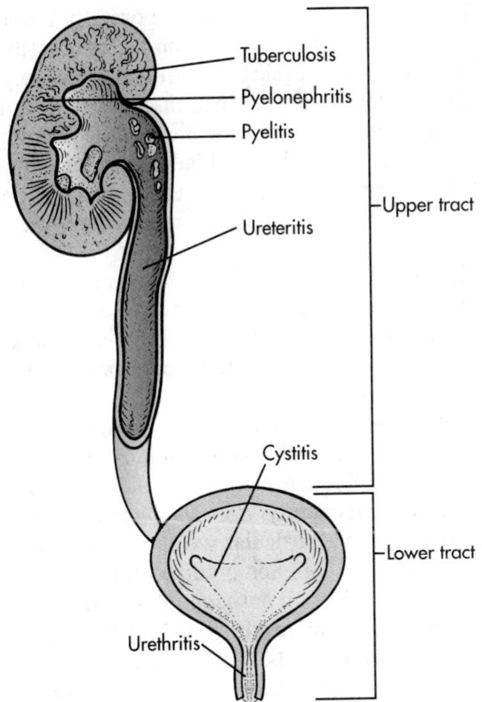

Fig. 43-1 Sites of infectious processes in the urinary tract.

Etiology

Defense Mechanisms. The urinary tract above the urethra is normally sterile. Several physiologic and mechanical defense mechanisms assist in maintaining sterility and preventing UTIs. These defenses include normal voiding with complete emptying of the bladder, normal antibacterial ability of the bladder mucosa and urine, ureterovesical junction competence, and peristaltic activity that propels urine toward the bladder. An alteration in any of these defense mechanisms increases the risk of contracting a UTI. The following factors may predispose a patient to a urinary tract infection:

1. Renal scarring from previous infections
2. Diminished ureteral peristalsis during pregnancy
3. Urinary retention for any reason
4. Presence of a foreign body such as a urinary catheter
5. Vesicoureteral reflux of urine in a retrograde direction from the bladder toward the kidney
6. Humoral or cellular immunodeficiency in an otherwise normal urinary tract
7. Female gender—shorter urethra that is in close proximity to the vagina and rectum
8. Presence of calculi
9. Clinical disorder such as neurogenic bladder

Source of Urinary Tract Infections. The organisms that usually cause UTIs are introduced via the ascending route from the urethra. Other less common routes are via the bloodstream or lymphatic system. Most infections are due to gram-negative aerobic bacilli normally found in the gastrointestinal (GI) tract. A common factor contributing to ascending infection is urologic instrumentation (e.g., catheterization, cystoscopic examinations). Instrumentation allows bacteria that are normally present at the opening of the urethra to enter the urethra or bladder. Sexual intercourse promotes milking of bacteria from the vagina and perineum and may cause minor urethral trauma that predisposes women to UTIs.

Rarely do UTIs result from a hematogenous route, where blood-borne bacteria secondarily invade the kidneys, ureters, or bladder from elsewhere in the body. For a kidney infection to occur from hematogenous transmission, there must be prior injury to the urinary tract, such as obstruction of the ureter, damage caused by stones, or renal scars.

An important source of UTIs is hospital-acquired, or *nosocomial,* infection. The cause of nosocomial infection is often *E. coli* and, less frequently, *Pseudomonas* organisms. Urologic instrumentation, particularly with an indwelling urinary catheter, is the most common predisposing factor. UTIs account for about 40% of all nosocomial infections, and about 80% of these infections result from catheterization.[2]

The occurrence of UTIs is often related to the presence of abnormalities of the urinary tract, such as strictures and obstructions. An untreated UTI can lead to chronic pyelonephritis and a progressive decrease in renal function. If no abnormality exists, uncomplicated pyelonephritis rarely leads to progressive renal damage and renal failure.

Cystitis

Pathophysiology. Although the majority of patients with cystitis are women, other groups with a high incidence are older men and young children (especially girls). These age and sex variations in the frequency of cystitis are related to anatomic differences or pathologic changes in the groups at risk. The adult female urethra is short, and its proximity to the rectum and vagina predisposes women to the risk of bladder contamination. Bacterial contamination of the bladder can be the result of poor personal hygiene practices and sexual intercourse.

In children and older men, UTIs are often associated with other preexisting problems. In children, vesicoureteral reflux is usually the preexisting abnormality. In men, the longer urethra (of which the proximal two thirds is normally sterile) and the antibacterial property of prostatic secretions provide protection from bacterial infections unless there are predisposing causes. In older men, the infection is usually related to obstruction caused by benign prostatic hyperplasia (see Chapter 52).

Not all bacterial invasions of the bladder result in lower UTI or cause spread to the upper urinary tract (pyelonephritis). Once cystitis has occurred, it may remain localized in the urinary bladder for years without ascension to the kidneys or may be completely resolved after initial treatment. Although the bacterial infection may be self-limiting, the urinary tract should be evaluated if there is recurrence, even in the patient who has no symptoms. The risk of recurrent symptomatic infection is increased when there are urinary tract abnormalities.

Asymptomatic bacteriuria can occur and is not synonymous with UTI. It indicates that bacteria are present in the urine. Tissue invasion must occur for an infection to exist. *Pyuria* (the presence of white blood cells [WBCs] in the urine) usually signals this occurrence. Asymptomatic bacteriuria occurs in about 10% of women over 65 years of age.[5] Asymptomatic bacteriuria may be important in a patient of any age if that person is at risk for complicated urinary infection and resultant renal damage.

Clinical Manifestations. The manifestations of cystitis are frequency and urgency of urination, suprapubic pain, dysuria, and foul-smelling urine. In some persons, hematuria and pyuria may be present. The presence of fever, nausea and vomiting, and flank tenderness usually indicates pyelonephritis. About one half of all persons with significant bacteriuria have no symptoms or may report nonspecific signs such as increased fatigue, anorexia, or changes in cognitive ability. The incidence of asymptomatic bacteriuria increases greatly with age.[1]

Diagnostic Studies. Examining the urine for the presence of WBCs by means of either a microscope or a urine dipstick is important in evaluating a person who complains of dysuria. The definitive diagnosis of cystitis is made on examination of a urine Gram stain or by urine culture. The best method for obtaining the urine culture is the midstream technique called *clean-catch urine.* (See Table 42-8 for an explanation of this technique.) If a satisfactory specimen cannot be obtained with this method, catheterization may be used. This procedure carries a 1% to 2% risk of introducing microorganisms into the bladder and causing a UTI.[5]

As an alternative to standard overnight culture methods, rapid methods to detect bacteriuria have been developed to provide results in 1 to 2 hours.[6] Antibody coating and other tests used to differentiate upper from lower UTIs were initially promising, but they are expensive and not 100% specific or sensitive.[5]

The nurse needs to be aware that noninfectious agents also cause irritative bladder symptoms similar to UTI. The patient with a bladder tumor or the individual receiving intravesical chemotherapy or pelvic radiation often experience urinary frequency, urgency, and dysuria. Nonbacterial inflammatory lesions such as interstitial cystitis, cystitis cystica, and cystitis glandularis also cause these symptoms.

Therapeutic and Pharmacologic Management. Once cystitis has been diagnosed, appropriate antimicrobial therapy is initiated. The therapeutic management of cystitis is summarized in Table 43-2.

Many drugs are effective against organisms that cause UTIs. These include sulfonamides, including sulfisoxazole (Gantrisin); sulfamethoxazole (Gantanol); nitrofurantoin (Furadantin, Macrodantin, Macrobid); ampicillin; and amoxicillin. Sulfamethoxazole combined with trimethoprim (Bactrim, Septra) has proved to be effective in treating UTIs, especially recurrent ones. When these drugs are combined, resistance seems to develop less rapidly. Systemic antibiotics such as cephalosporins, aminoglycosides (gentamicin, tobramycin), and fluoroquinolones (ciprofloxacin, norfloxacin) can also be used.

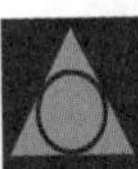

Table 43-2 Therapeutic Management: Cystitis

First Infection—Symptomatic
Diagnostic
Urinalysis
Urine for culture and sensitivity
Therapeutic*
Administration of antimicrobials for 5-10 days
Administration of single high dose of oral antibiotic (amoxicillin, ampicillin, sulfisoxazole, trimethoprim-sulfamethoxazole, or fluoroquinolone)
Administration of 3-day course of oral antibiotics (trimethoprim-sulfamethoxazole or fluoroquinolone)
Encouragement of high fluid intake
Repeat of urine culture
Recurrent Infection
Diagnostic
Urinalysis
Urine for culture and sensitivity
Evaluation of urinary tract (e.g., IVP, voiding cystourethrogram, cystoscopy, pelvic examination)
Therapeutic*
Administration of antimicrobials for 10-14 days based on sensitivity testing
Administration of prophylactic drug (e.g, trimethoprim-sulfamethoxazole or nitrofurantoin) for repeated recurrent infections
Encouragement of high fluid intake
Repeat of urine culture

IVP, Intravenous pyelogram.
*See text for description of different treatment protocols.

Phenazopyridine (Pyridium) may be used in cystitis to provide an analgesic effect on the urinary mucosa. This drug should relieve the burning sensation. The azo dye in the drug stains the urine reddish orange. It is important to tell the patient about the color change so that he does not think it is related to the infection. Phenazopyridine stain is also fairly permanent on underclothing.

Other drugs that may be used are nalidixic acid (Neg-Gram), methenamine mandelate (Mandelamine), hyoscyamine sulfate (Cystospaz), and flavoxate hydrochloride (Urispas). Methenamine achieves its desired effect by decomposing to formaldehyde and ammonia. The urinary pH should be less than 6 for methenamine to be effective, so urinary pH should be tested to ensure the activity of the drug. Hyoscyamine and flavoxate help decrease bladder muscle irritability and spasm.

High single-dose therapy has been effective when the infection is localized to the bladder and the organism is sensitive to antibiotics. Single-dose therapy results in lowered cost, increased compliance, and decreased potential for resistant organisms. If there is involvement of the kidney or if the patient is an older adult or has diabetes, single-dose therapy is not appropriate. All patients should have follow-up cultures, but it is especially important for the patient treated with a single course of antibiotics. The patient who has a positive culture after single-dose therapy may be assumed to have upper UTI or a persistent source of bacteria in the bladder or prostate and should be appropriately evaluated and treated.

Many clinicians are now treating uncomplicated lower UTI with a 3-day course of antibiotics. As with single-dose therapy, the candidate for 3-day therapy must be chosen to exclude the patient with febrile UTI.

Antibiotic therapy is not usually recommended for asymptomatic bacteriuria unless symptoms develop or there is evidence of obstructive uropathy in the symptom-free patient. The risk of developing bacterial resistance and the inability to treat the patient when symptoms do occur is great. In general, asymptomatic bacteriuria in the older adult should not be treated. Prophylactic antibiotics may be ordered when a patient with asymptomatic bacteriuria undergoes surgery or genitourinary instrumentation.

NURSING MANAGEMENT

CYSTITIS

Nursing Assessment

Subjective and objective data that should be obtained from a patient with cystitis are presented in Table 43-3.

Nursing Diagnoses

Nursing diagnoses are determined when the problem and etiologic factors are supported by clinical data. Nursing diagnoses for cystitis may include, but are not limited to, those presented in the nursing care plan on p. 1341.

Planning

The overall goals are that a patient with cystitis will have (1) relief from dysuria, (2) no upper urinary tract complications, and (3) no recurrent episodes of UTI.

Nursing Implementation

Health Promotion and Maintenance. Health promotion and maintenance measures include recognizing the groups with a higher than normal incidence of UTIs. Especially for these individuals, health promotion activities can help decrease the frequency of infections and promote early detection of infection. These activities include teaching preventive measures, such as emptying the bladder regularly and completely, wiping the perineal area from front to back after urination and defecation, and drinking an adequate amount of liquid each day. The standard adult requirement for daily liquid intake is approximately 15 ml per pound of body weight.[7] For example, a 135-pound person would require a minimum 2025 ml or over 8 8-ounce glasses of liquids each day. In addition, it is important to teach the patient to seek early treatment once symptoms are identified.

The nurse can play a major role in the prevention of nosocomial infections. Debilitated persons, older adults, patients with severe underlying disease (cancer, cirrhosis, diabetes), and patients treated with immunosuppressive drugs, long-term corticosteroid therapy, or radiation are at

Table 43-3 Nursing Assessment: Urinary Tract Infection

Subjective Data
Important health information
Past health history: Previous urinary tract infections; urinary calculi, stasis, reflux, strictures, or retention; neurogenic bladder; pregnancy; prostatic hyperplasia; sexually transmitted disease; renal failure; bladder cancer; polycystic kidney disease
Medications: Antibiotics, anticholinergics, antispasmodics
Surgery and other treatments: Recent urologic instrumentation (catheterization, cystoscopy, surgery)
Functional health patterns
Health perception–health management: Fever, chills, lassitude, malaise
Nutritional-metabolic: Nausea, vomiting, anorexia; fever, chills
Elimination: Frequency, urgency, hesitancy, dysuria, nocturia, burning on urination
Cognitive-perceptual: Suprapubic or low back pain; bladder spasms

Objective Data
Gastrointestinal
Abdominal rigidity with upper UTI
Urinary
Hematuria, foul-smelling urine
Upper UTI: Tender, enlarged kidney; decreased urinary output
Possible findings
Leukocytosis; urinalysis positive for bacteria, pyuria, RBCs, and WBCs; positive urine culture; antibody-coated bacteria test (positive in pyelonephritis, negative in cystitis); IVP, CT scan, ultrasound, voiding cystourethrogram and cystoscopy demonstrating abnormalities of urinary tract

CT, Computed tomography; *IVP,* intravenous pyelogram; *RBCs,* red blood cells; *UTI,* urinary tract infection; *WBCs,* white blood cells.

high risk of UTIs. The patient undergoing instrumentation of the urinary tract is also at risk of developing nosocomial infections, and the aseptic technique should always be followed for these procedures. Washing hands before and after contact with each patient and wearing gloves for care involving the urinary system are especially important. In general, catheterization of the bladder should be avoided if possible.

For the patient at risk of a nosocomial UTI, it is important to provide good perineal hygiene, especially after a bedpan is used. Incontinence should be avoided by answering the call light quickly or offering the bedpan or urinal at frequent intervals to the bedridden patient. If a catheter has been inserted, special catheter care measures must be employed as explained in the section on Urethral Catheterization.

Acute Intervention. Acute intervention for a patient with cystitis includes an adequate fluid intake if this is not contraindicated. This means drinking more than the standard daily requirement. It is sometimes difficult to get the patient to maintain an adequate fluid intake because the person may think it will increase a feeling of urgency. Explain to the patient that fluids will increase frequency at first but will also dilute the urine, making the bladder less irritable. Fluids will help flush out bacteria before they have a chance to colonize in the bladder. Caffeine, alcohol, citrus juices, chocolate, and highly spiced foods or beverages should be avoided because they are potential bladder irritants. A heating pad or sitz bath may also help reduce discomfort. Treatment of cystitis does not usually require hospitalization.

The patient needs to be instructed about the prescribed drug therapy. Common side effects of the drugs should be explained, and the patient should be told to notify the physician if they occur. It is important for the patient to take the full course of antibiotics. Sometimes a second medication or a reduced dose of medication is ordered after the initial course to suppress bacterial growth in certain patients susceptible to recurrent UTI.

The urine should be examined for gross or microscopic hematuria, presence of WBCs, malodor, and sediment. The patient should be instructed to watch for any changes in the color or consistency of the urine and a decrease in or cessation of symptoms as a sign of the effectiveness of therapy.

Chronic and Home Management. Chronic management of a patient with a UTI emphasizes the need for the patient's compliance with the medication regimen. It is the nurse's responsibility to educate the patient about the need for ongoing care. This includes taking antimicrobial medication as ordered, maintaining more than an adequate daily fluid intake, emptying the bladder when the urge to urinate occurs or at least every 2 to 3 hours, urinating after intercourse, and discontinuing use of a diaphragm (if used).

The patient must understand the need for follow-up care with urine culture to determine that the infection has been adequately treated. Relapse with bacteria of the same species usually occurs within 1 to 2 weeks after completion of therapy. If the patient has been compliant, relapse suggests possible renal involvement in the infectious process. For the individual who has more than two infections every 6 months, the use of long-term antibiotic therapy may be ordered.

Urethritis

Urethritis (inflammation of the urethra) is often difficult to diagnose, but the clinical manifestations are the same as those of cystitis. The female urethra may be extremely tender, or there may be a discharge, especially in men. Inflammatory changes may make recovery of bacteria difficult because they become entrapped in urethral tissue and do not appear in the urine. Urethritis may coexist with cystitis. Cultures on split urine collections or any urethral discharge may confirm a diagnosis of urethral infection. Causes of urethritis include a bacterial or viral infection, *Trichomonas* and monilial infection (especially in women), Chlamydia, and gonorrhea (especially in men). (Gonococcal urethritis is discussed in Chapter 50.)

Treatment is based on identifying and treating the cause and providing symptomatic relief. Sulfamethoxazole with trimethoprim or nitrofurantoin are examples of medications used for bacterial infections. Tinidazole, nimorazol, or metronidazole may be used for Trichomonas. Medications such as nystatin (Mycostatin) may be prescribed for monilial infections. In Chlamydial infections, doxycycline may be used. Women with negative urine cultures and no pyuria do not usually respond to antibiotics. Hot sitz baths without perfumed bath oil or bath salts may relieve the symptoms. The patient should be instructed to avoid the use of vaginal deodorant sprays, to properly cleanse the perineal area after bowel movements and urination, and to avoid intercourse until symptoms subside.

Urethral Syndrome

Symptoms of dysuria, urgency, and frequency unaccompanied by significant bacteriuria (i.e., less than 10^2 to 10^3 per ml of urine) have been called the acute *urethral syndrome.* Clinically these patients cannot be readily distinguished from those with cystitis. When present, bacteria are usually *E. coli,* enterococci, or staphylococci. If few or no bacteria are detected, *Chlamydia trachomatis* or *Neisseria gonorrhoeae* (both sexually transmitted pathogens) may be the cause. Detection of Chlamydial organisms requires tissue culture or immunologic testing for Chlamydial antigen in urethral or cervical specimens. Chlamydial infection is less likely to cause hematuria and suprapubic pain than bacterial infection.

Vaginitis needs to be ruled out. If vaginitis is the cause, the symptoms may have a more gradual onset, and pruritis or vaginal discharge may be present.

Treatment depends on the causative agent. If bacteria are involved, the treatment is similar to that for cystitis. This patient responds well to single-dose therapy. Simultaneous treatment of the individual's sexual partner may be recommended. Heat or sitz baths may help to alleviate symptoms. Acute symptoms of urethral syndrome tend to recur. The patient needs a great deal of reassurance.

Interstitial Cystitis

Interstitial cystitis is a chronic bladder condition that most commonly occurs in women. The etiology is unknown. Once thought to be psychologic in etiology, interstitial cystitis is now considered a physiologic syndrome with multifactorial etiologies.[8] The classic symptom complex includes continuous frequency and urgency and suprapubic pain relieved by voiding. Pyuria and hematuria are sometimes present. The diagnosis is made following cystoscopy with the characteristic findings of reduced bladder capacity and the presence of superficial, often stellate, ulcers. In the earlier stages of the disease, only multiple petechiae-like hemorrhages may be found and the bladder capacity may be normal.

Specific treatments do not help everyone, but they are based on theories of physiologic causes and directed to improvement of symptoms. Hydraulic distention of the bladder under anesthesia, intravesical instillation of dimethyl sulfoxide (DMSO) and other medications, and medications such as amitriptyline, sodium pentosanpolysulfate, nifedipine, and hydroxyzine bring symptom relief to many patients. Dietary and activity changes, biofeedback, application of heat, diversional activities, and involvement in interstitial cystitis support groups are also helpful approaches for decreasing symptoms.

Acute Pyelonephritis

Etiology. Pyelonephritis is an acute or chronic inflammatory process of the renal pelvis and parenchyma of the kidney. Generally the inflammatory process is caused by bacterial invasion. Most infections are caused by the normal inhabitants of the intestinal tract (e.g., *E. coli*).

Pyelonephritis can develop via the ascending route following cystitis. In this situation another preexisting factor is often present. In children it is usually associated with vesicoureteral reflux or other urinary tract abnormalities. In adults the common preexisting factors are bladder tumors, prostatic hyperplasia, strictures, urinary stones, and pregnancy. Repeated attacks of acute pyelonephritis, especially in the presence of these abnormalities, can result in chronic pyelonephritis. The infection commonly starts in the renal medulla and spreads to the adjacent cortex. The infected portion of the kidney heals, resulting in fibrosis and scarring.

Clinical Manifestations. The clinical manifestations of acute pyelonephritis vary from mild lassitude to the sudden onset of chills, fever, vomiting, malaise, flank pain, dysuria, and frequent urination. Symptoms of cystitis may or may not be present. Costovertebral tenderness will be present on the affected side. The clinical manifestations usually subside within a few days, even without specific therapy. However, bacteriuria or pyuria may persist.

Bacteremia (presence of bacteria in blood) can occur secondary to a urinary tract infection ascending to the kidney and can result in sepsis. The patient will have a high fever and elevated WBC count. Some patients develop septic shock syndrome as a result of endotoxins produced by gram-negative bacteria that are released in the blood. (Septic shock is discussed in Chapter 7.) If bacteremia is a possibility, close observation and vital sign monitoring are essential. Prompt recognition and treatment of septic shock may prevent irreversible damage.

Therapeutic Management. The diagnostic and therapeutic management of acute pyelonephritis is summarized in Table 43-4 (see p. 1340). Urine cultures should always be obtained when pyelonephritis is suspected. Intravenous pyelograms (IVPs) or excretory urograms are usually not obtained in the early stages of pyelonephritis to prevent the possible spread of infection.

An essential principle of therapeutic management is to consider factors that may be contributing to the infection, such as an obstruction or urinary tract anomaly. In addition to an IVP, other diagnostic procedures such as a cystourethrogram and cystoscopy may be used to evaluate any uropathies. It is essential to obtain follow-up urine cultures to determine the effectiveness of therapy.

Pharmacologic Management. The patient with mild symptoms may be treated for 14 days (see Table 43-4).

CLINICAL PATHWAY FOR URINARY TRACT INFECTION WITH SYSTEMIC INVOLVEMENT (PYELONEPHRITIS)

Admit Date: ______ Diagnostic Related Group 320 Length of Stay 5 Days Discharge Date: ______

Pathway	Day 1	Day 2	Days 3-4	Day 5
Critical path implemented (initial):				
Diagnostic Studies	■ CBC ■ UA, Urine C&S ■ Chem 7 ■ CXR ■ Blood culture × ____ Consider: ■ KUB/Abd x-ray if flank pain present	Consider: ■ CBC ■ Electrolytes	Consider: ■ CBC ■ Electrolytes ■ Repeat blood culture if pain and fever persist past 72 hr of therapy ■ Ultrasound or CT to R/O urologic pathology, otherwise D/C	■ Repeat urine culture 2 wk after therapy as outpatient
Treatments	■ Strain all urine if flank pain present			
IV/Meds	■ IV ___ at ___ cc/hr ■ Antibiotics ■ Analgesic/Antipyretic ■ Antiemetic		■ Transition to p.o. meds if afebrile ×48h ■ Heplock IV	
Consults	■ Social Services if indicated			
Nursing	■ Physical assessment q shift/prn, especially fluid volume parameters (turgor, electrolytes, I & O, mucous membranes) ■ VS q2hr×6hr, then q4hr×24hr, then q8hr, monitor temperature and notify physican of spike > ___ ° ■ I & O q4hr×24hr, then q shift, notify MD of UO < 600 cc/24hr, admission weight ■ Skin care, assist with ADLs, daily reevaluation of skin risk assessment with appropriate interventions, obtain skin care evaluation if indicated ■ Collaborate with patient on pain management, use 1-5 pain scale ■ Provide emotional support to patient/family to help reduce anxiety			
Diet	■ Clear liquids, advance as tolerated			
Activity and Safety	■ OOB as tolerated ■ Routine safety measures	■ OOB as tolerated	■ Consider discharge if stable	■ Discharge
Teaching Patient and Family	■ Teach 1-5 pain scale ■ Orient to environment ■ Explain tests/procedures to patient/family ■ Explain diet, meds, activity	■ Explain relationship between disease process, resulting symptoms, and therapy prescribed ■ Implement UTI teaching plan ■ Implement related procedural teaching plans		
Discharge Planning	■ Initial assessment ■ Advance Directives reviewed ■ Assess educational needs	■ Facilitate physican/RN/family conference for discharge planning and medical follow-up		

continued

Intravenous (IV) antibiotics are often given initially in the hospital to achieve quick, high serum and urinary drug levels. If this treatment appears to be successful, the patient may be discharged on an oral form of the antibiotic. Relapses may be treated with a 6-week course of antibiotics. Reinfections may be treated as individual episodes of disease or managed with long-term antibiotic therapy. Antibiotic prophylaxis may also be used for recurrent infections. The effectiveness of therapy is evaluated in accordance with the presence or absence of bacterial growth on urine culture.

NURSING MANAGEMENT
PYELONEPHRITIS
Nursing Assessment

Subjective and objective data that should be obtained from a patient with a UTI are presented in Table 43-3.

Nursing Diagnoses

Nursing diagnoses are determined when the problem and the etiologic factors are supported by clinical data. Nursing diagnoses specific to the patient with a UTI include, but are not limited to, those presented in the nursing care plan on p. 1341.

CLINICAL PATHWAY FOR URINARY TRACT INFECTION—cont'd

Diagnostic Related Group 320 Length of Stay 5 Days

Problem List	Day 1	Day 2	Days 3-4	Day 5
Meets expected outcome (initial):				
Fever from UTI: ■ T >101° and/or ■ WBC >15,000 and/or ■ Signs and symptoms of sepsis, toxic appearance	■ Antipyretics stabilizing temp ■ Patient expressing sense of comfort after medication	■ Temperature returning to normal ■ Patient comfortable ■ Skin warm and dry	■ Temperature WNL ■ WBC (if done) <15,000	■ Afebrile
Fluid volume deficit: ■ Altered intake ■ c/o thirst ■ Altered vital signs ■ Poor skin turgor, tenting ■ Hemo concentration of lab values (BUN >20, urine specific gravity >1.025)	■ UO >30 cc/hr ■ Vital signs stabilizing after 6 hr of IV fluids ■ c/o thirst	■ Vital signs stable ■ Skin, color, temperature WNL ■ No c/o thirst ■ Skin turgor improved from admission	■ Intake equals output – 200 cc ■ Electrolytes WNL ■ Skin turgor WNL	■ Fluid volume stable
Pain and discomfort: ■ Altered urinary pattern ■ Urinary frequency ■ Patient verbalizes pain site ■ Self-focused	■ Patient identifies/ describes characteristics of pain ■ Patient describes pain on 1-5 scale ■ Patient expresses feeling of comfort after medication	■ Pain managed ■ Urinary frequency subsiding ■ Patient able to focus, concentrate, and participate in therapeutic regime	■ Pain managed ■ No urinary frequency	■ Pain/discomfort managed with oral medications ■ Urinary pattern WNL
Potential alteration in skin integrity: ■ High risk for skin breakdown (fever, perspiration, urinary excretion)	■ Maintains adequate skin circulation ■ Maintains adequate fluid intake ■ Skin maintained clean and dry	■ Maintains adequate food and fluid intake ■ No evidence of skin breakdown	■ Skin clean, warm, and dry	■ No evidence of skin breakdown
Knowledge deficit: ■ Home care needs ■ Meds ■ Medical follow-up	■ Patient/family understand disease process and treatment plan	■ Patient/family understand medication regime ■ Patient/family understand signs and symptoms of impending UTI	■ Patient/family understand the importance of medical follow-up and know when and how to contact the doctor	■ Patient/family understand discharge instructions
Other				

Other parts of this Critical Path include Patient Pathways, Patient Education Documentation Record, and Physician's orders. Developed by Nanticoke Hospital, Seaford, DE. Licensed by the Center for Case Management, Inc., South Natick, MA.
Abd, Abdominal; *ADLs*, activities of daily living; *BUN*, blood urea nitrogen; *C & S*, culture and sensitivity; *CBC*, complete blood count; *CT*, computed tomography; *CXR*, chest x-ray; *D/C*, discontinue; *I & O*, intake and output; *KUB*, kidneys, ureter, bladder; *OOB*, out of bed; *R/O*, rule out; *UA*, urinalysis; *UO*, urinary output; *UTI*, urinary tract infection; *WBC*, white blood cell; *WNL*, within normal limits.

Table 43-4 Therapeutic Management: Acute Pyelonephritis

Diagnostic
Urinalysis
Urine for culture and sensitivity, Gram stain
IVP, ultrasound, or CT scan
WBC count
Blood culture (if bacteremia suspected)
Palpation for flank pain
Therapeutic
Mild symptoms
Bed rest
Outpatient management or short hospitalization for IV antibiotics
Administration of oral antibiotics (e.g., trimethoprim-sulfamethoxazole, fluoroquinolone) for 14 days
High fluid intake
Follow-up urine cultures
Severe symptoms
Hospitalization
Parenteral antibiotics (e.g., aminoglycoside [amikacin, gentamycin], cephalosporin [cefoxitin, cefoperazone])
High fluid intake
Follow-up urine cultures

CT, Computed tomography; *IV*, intravenous; *IVP*, intravenous pyelogram; *WBC*, white blood cell.

Planning

The overall goals are that the patient with pyelonephritis will have (1) relief of pain, (2) normal body temperature, (3) no complications, and (4) no recurrence of symptoms.

Nursing Implementation

Health Promotion and Maintenance. Health promotion and maintenance measures are similar to those for cystitis (see Health Promotion and Maintenance under Cystitis). In addition, it is important that the patient receive early treatment for cystitis to prevent ascending infections. Because the patient with structural abnormalities of the urinary tract is at high risk for infection, the need for regular medical care should be stressed.

Acute and Chronic Intervention. Nursing interventions vary depending on the severity of symptoms. These interventions include teaching the patient about the disease process with emphasis on (1) the need to continue medications as prescribed, (2) the need for a follow-up urine culture to ensure proper management, and (3) identification of recurrence of infection or relapse. In addition to antibiotic therapy, the patient should be encouraged to drink at least eight glasses of fluid every day. Increased fluid intake should be continued, even after the infection has been treated. Bed rest is often indicated to increase patient comfort. The patient with frequent relapses or reinfections may be treated with long-term, low-dose antibiotics. Understanding the rationale for therapy is important to enhance patient compliance. The nursing care plan for a patient with a UTI is on p. 1341.

Chronic Pyelonephritis

Chronic pyelonephritis (also called *chronic interstitial nephritis*) is not the result of an isolated episode of acute pyelonephritis unless there are predisposing factors such as obstruction, neurogenic bladder, or vesicoureteral reflux. Chronic pyelonephritis is usually the end result of longstanding UTIs with relapses and reinfections.

The pathologic changes indicate that there have been repeated episodes of chronic inflammation and scarring. Grossly, both kidneys are irregularly and asymmetrically scarred. The renal pelvis and calyces are deformed, blunted, and dilated.

Clinical features of chronic pyelonephritis include a history of recurrent acute infections leading to progressive destruction of functioning nephrons resulting in chronic renal insufficiency. During active infection, urine cultures are positive and leukocyte casts are found on urinalysis. End-stage chronic pyelonephritis is not easily distinguished from other causes of chronic renal failure. IVP, renal biopsy, renal ultrasound, or computed tomography (CT) scan may be useful in delineating the severity of renal involvement after the infection has been resolved.

The level of renal function can vary in chronic pyelonephritis. The patient may have improvement in function after an acute exacerbation. Chronic pyelonephritis may progress to chronic renal failure. (Therapeutic and nursing care of the patient with chronic renal failure is discussed in Chapter 44.)

Renal Tuberculosis

Renal tuberculosis (TB) is rarely a primary lesion. It is usually secondary to TB of the lung. In 4% to 8% of patients with pulmonary TB, the tubercle bacilli reach the kidneys via the bloodstream. Onset occurs 5 to 8 years after the primary infection. The patient is often asymptomatic when the kidney is initially infiltrated with bacilli. Sometimes the patient complains of fatigue and develops a low-grade fever. As the lesions ulcerate, infection descends to the bladder, and the patient experiences frequent urination, burning on voiding, and epididymitis (in men). Symptoms of cystitis are the first sign in 65% of all cases of renal TB.[9] Renal lesions may calcify as they heal. Infrequently, renal colic, lumbar and iliac pain, and hematuria may be present. A diagnosis is based on localization of tubercle bacilli in the urine and on IVP findings.

Long-term complications of renal TB depend on the duration of the disease before treatment. Scarring of the renal parenchyma and the development of ureteral strictures occur. The earlier treatment is initiated, the less likely renal failure will develop. Reduced bladder volume may be irreversible in advanced disease.[10] The patient may require long-term urologic follow-up. (Nursing and therapeutic management for the patient with TB is discussed in Chapter 24.)

NURSING CARE PLAN Patient with a Urinary Tract Infection

Planning: Outcome Criteria	Nursing Interventions and Rationales
NURSING DIAGNOSIS	Altered comfort: fever *related to* infection *as manifested by* elevation in temperature, tachycardia, tachypnea, chills, malaise
Have normal temperature, no chills.	Assess vital signs q2-4hr *to plan appropriate intervention.* Administer antipyretics and antibiotics as ordered *to control fever and infection and promote comfort.* Ensure adequate hydration via oral or IV route *as fever increases fluid loss.* Monitor intake and output *to ensure adequate hydration and monitor renal function.* Cover patient lightly and keep patient dry *to prevent chilling and promote comfort.* Provide cooling sponge baths or compresses *to assist in temperature reduction by evaporation of moisture on skin.*
NURSING DIAGNOSIS	Pain *related to* dysuria, urgency, frequency, and bladder spasms secondary to inflammation and tissue trauma *as manifested by* pain on urination, flank pain, suprapubic pain, lower back pain, bladder spasms; statement that pain is present
Be satisfied with pain control or have no pain.	Assess pain for location and severity *to plan appropriate interventions.* Palpate abdomen and percuss flank *to identify painful area.* Position patient *for comfort.* Administer analgesics, antispasmodics, and azo dyes as ordered *to promote comfort,* and note their effectiveness. Apply heating pad to painful area *as heat relieves pain associated with UTI.* Alert patient that azo dyes will color urine *to prevent concern over unusual appearance of urine.* Encourage fluid intake *to promote a high output and subsequent improvement in symptoms.* Encourage bed rest during acute phase *to promote physical and mental recovery.*
NURSING DIAGNOSIS	Altered patterns of urinary elimination: frequency, urgency, incontinence, or nocturia related to UTI *as manifested by* urgency, frequency, nocturia, incontinence, hematuria; verbalization of concern over altered elimination pattern
Have no evidence of infected urine; have normal urination pattern.	Assess for changes in usual voiding pattern *to determine presence of UTI.* Instruct patient regarding reason for symptoms *to promote understanding and cooperation.* Encourage high fluid intake or administer IV fluids as ordered *to maintain a dilute, nonirritating urine and to decrease bacterial concentration.* Obtain urine for culture and sensitivity *to determine cause of UTI, or to monitor effectiveness of treatment.* Administer antimicrobial medication as ordered *to eliminate symptoms by inhibiting bacterial synthesis.* Instruct patient about good perineal care and cleansing after each bowel movement *to prevent reintroducing infection.* Observe urine for color, odor, amount, and frequency *to evaluate effectiveness of treatment plan.* Reassure patient that symptoms are temporary and may take 24-48 hr to subside *to alleviate patient's anxiety.*
NURSING DIAGNOSIS	Risk for reinfection *related to* lack of knowledge regarding prevention of recurrence and signs and symptoms of recurrence
Have negative urine culture and no manifestations of UTI.	Assess for recurrent UTI and the patient's lack of knowledge of measures to prevent reinfection *to determine risk for reinfection;* assess patient's knowledge of prevention and recurrence *to plan appropriate teaching.* Instruct patient about the need to maintain high fluid intake unless contraindicated *to maintain a dilute, nonirritating urine.* Explain rationale for use of medications, times, and method of administration *to promote adherence to medication regimen.* Explain importance of taking all antibiotics as prescribed *to prevent the development of resistant organisms.* Explain need for follow-up care. Instruct patient on appropriate hygiene, including careful cleansing of perineal region, wiping from front to back after urinating, cleansing with soap and water after each bowel movement *to prevent reinfection.* Explain the importance of emptying the bladder before and after intercourse *to eliminate a possible source of reinfection.* Instruct patient to urinate when the urge occurs or at least q2-3hr *to prevent urinary stasis and overdistention of the bladder, which increases susceptibility to infection.* Instruct patient to avoid bath salts, oils, and vaginal sprays, *which can irritate the urethral meatus;* instruct patient to observe for symptoms of recurrence such as changes in urinating habits, character of urine, flank pain, or incontinence.

IV, Intravenous; *UTI,* urinary tract infection.

IMMUNOLOGIC DISORDERS OF THE KIDNEY

Glomerulonephritis

Significance. Immunologic processes involving the urinary tract predominantly affect the renal glomerulus. The disease process results in *glomerulonephritis* (inflammation of the glomeruli). It affects both kidneys equally. Although the glomerulus is the primary site of inflammation, tubular, interstitial, and vascular changes also occur. Glomerulonephritis is divided into a number of classifications, which may describe (1) the extent of damage (diffuse or focal), (2) the initial cause of the disorder (systemic lupus erythematosus, scleroderma, streptococcal infection), or (3) the extent of changes (minimal or widespread).

Etiology and Pathophysiology. Two types of antibody-induced injury can initiate glomerular damage. In the first type, the antibodies have specificity for antigens within the glomerular basement membrane (GBM). These are called *anti-GBM antibodies.* Immunoglobulins and complement are deposited along the basement membrane. The mechanism that causes a person to develop antibodies against its GBM is not known. Production of *autoantibodies* (antibodies to one's own tissue) may be stimulated by a structural alteration in the GBM or by a reaction of the basement membrane with an exogenous agent (e.g., hydrocarbon, viruses).

In the second type of immune process, the antibodies react with circulating nonglomerular antigens and are randomly deposited as immune complexes along the GBM. On electron microscopy of renal tissue sections, the deposits appear "lumpy-bumpy." In this immune complex process, the antigens do not come from the glomeruli but from either endogenous circulating native deoxyribonucleic acid (DNA) or exogenous sources (e.g., bacteria, viruses, chemicals, drugs). Bacterial products appear to be important in poststreptococcal glomerulonephritis and in endocarditis. Viral agents have been recognized in certain cases of glomerulonephritis that develop after hepatitis and measles.

All forms of immune complex disease are characterized by an accumulation of antigen, antibody, and complement in the glomeruli, which can result in tissue injury. The immune complexes activate complement (see Chapter 10). Complement activation results in the release of chemotactic factors that attract polymorphonuclear leukocytes and causes the release of histamine and other vasoactive amines. The intrinsic clotting pathway may also be activated. The end result of these processes is glomerular injury as a result of inflammation.

Clinical Manifestations. There are many clinical manifestations of glomerulonephritis. They may include varying degrees of hematuria (ranging from microscopic to gross) and urinary excretion of various formed elements, including red blood cells (RBCs), WBCs, and some granular casts. Proteinuria and elevated blood urea nitrogen (BUN) and serum creatinine levels are other manifestations. In most cases, recovery from the acute illness is complete. However, if progressive involvement occurs, the result is destruction of renal tissue and marked renal insufficiency.

The patient's history provides important information related to glomerulonephritis. It is necessary to assess exposure to drugs, immunizations, microbial infections, and viral infections such as hepatitis. It is also important to evaluate the patient for more generalized conditions involving immune disorders, such as systemic lupus erythematosus and systemic progressive sclerosis (scleroderma).

Acute Poststreptococcal Glomerulonephritis

Acute poststreptococcal glomerulonephritis (APSGN) is most common in children and young adults, but all age groups can be affected.[11] APSGN develops 5 to 21 days after an infection of the pharynx or skin (e.g., streptococcal sore throat, impetigo) by certain nephrotoxic strains of group A β-hemolytic streptococci. The person produces antibodies to the streptococcal antigen. Although the specific mechanism is not known with certainty, the antigen-antibody complexes are deposited in the glomeruli and activate complement. Complement activation causes an inflammatory reaction to the injury. The response to the injury is also a decrease in the filtration of metabolic waste products from the blood and an increase in the permeability of the glomerulus to larger protein molecules.

Clinical Manifestations and Complications. The clinical manifestations of APSGN appear as a variety of signs and symptoms, which may include generalized body edema, hypertension, oliguria, hematuria with a smoky or rusty appearance, and proteinuria. Fluid retention occurs as a result of decreased glomerular filtration. The edema appears initially in low-pressure tissues, such as around the eyes (periorbital edema), but later progresses to involve the total body as ascites or peripheral edema in the legs. Smoky urine is indicative of bleeding in the upper urinary tract. The degree of proteinuria varies with the severity of the glomerulonephropathy. Hypertension primarily results from increased extracellular fluid volume.

The patient with APSGN may have abdominal or flank pain. At times the patient has no symptoms, with the problem found with routine urinalysis.

More than 95% of patients with APSGN recover completely or improve rapidly with conservative management. The prognosis for adults is less favorable than for children. Chronic glomerulonephritis develops in 5% to 15% of the affected persons, and irreversible renal failure occurs in less than 1% of patients.[11]

Diagnostic Studies. The diagnosis of APSGN is based on a complete history and physical examination and laboratory studies (Table 43-5) to determine the presence or history of a group A β-hemolytic streptococcus in a throat or skin lesion. An immune response to the streptococcus is often demonstrated by assessment of antistreptolysin O (ASO) titers. The finding of decreased complement components (especially C1q, C3, and C4) is indicative of an immune-mediated response. A renal biopsy may be performed to confirm the presence of the disease.

Dipstick and urine sediment microscopy will reveal the presence of erythrocytes in significant numbers. Erythrocyte casts are highly suggestive of acute glomerulonephritis. Proteinuria may range from mild to severe. Screening blood tests include BUN and serum creatinine to assess the extent of renal impairment.

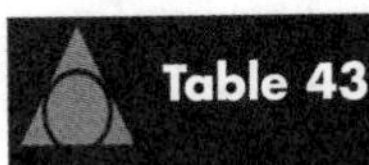

Table 43-5 Therapeutic Management: Acute Glomerulonephritis

Diagnostic
History and physical examination
Urinalysis
CBC
BUN, serum creatinine and albumin
Complement levels and ASO titer
Renal biopsy (if indicated)
Therapeutic
Bed rest
Sodium and fluid restriction
Administration of loop diuretics (furosemide, ethacrynic acid)
Antihypertensive therapy
Adjustment of dietary protein intake to level of proteinuria and uremia

ASO, Antistreptolysin; *BUN*, blood urea nitrogen; *CBC*, complete blood count.

Therapeutic Management. The therapeutic management of APSGN focuses on symptomatic relief (Table 43-5). Bed rest is recommended until the signs of glomerular inflammation (proteinuria, hematuria) and hypertension subside. Edema is treated by restricting sodium and fluid intake and by administrating loop diuretics such as furosemide (Lasix), ethacrynic acid (Edecrin), and bumetanide (Bumex). Severe hypertension is treated with antihypertensive drugs. Dietary protein intake may be restricted if there is evidence of an increase in nitrogenous wastes (e.g., elevated BUN value). The restriction varies with the degree of proteinuria.

Penicillin or erythromycin should be given only if the streptococcal infection is still present. Steroids and cytotoxic drugs have not been shown to be of value.

NURSING MANAGEMENT

ACUTE POSTSTREPTOCOCCAL GLOMERULONEPHRITIS

One of the most important ways to prevent the development of APSGN is to encourage early diagnosis and treatment of sore throats and skin lesions. If streptococci are found in the culture, treatment with appropriate antibiotic therapy (usually penicillin) is essential. The patient needs to be encouraged to take the full course of antibiotics to ensure that the bacteria have been eradicated. Good personal hygiene is an important factor in preventing the spread of cutaneous streptococcal infections.

The nursing management of acute glomerulonephritis is specific to the patient's symptoms. An important nursing measure is helping the patient plan adequate rest to allow the kidneys to heal. The patient may need assistance in the management of fluid and dietary restrictions. (Low-protein, low-sodium, fluid-restricted diets are discussed in Chapter 44.)

Goodpasture's Syndrome

Goodpasture's syndrome, an example of cytotoxic (type II) autoimmune disease, is characterized by the presence of circulating antibodies against GBM and alveolar basement membrane.[12] Although the primary target organ is the kidney, the lungs are also involved. The pathologic nature of the syndrome results when binding of the antibody causes an inflammatory reaction mediated by complement fixation and activation (see Chapter 10). Type A_2 influenza viruses, hydrocarbons, penicillamine, and unknown genetic factors stimulate autoantibody production.

Goodpasture's syndrome is a rare disease that is seen mostly in young men. The clinical manifestations include hemoptysis, pulmonary insufficiency, crackles, rhonchi, renal involvement with hematuria and renal failure, weakness, pallor, and anemia. Pulmonary hemorrhage usually occurs and may precede glomerular abnormalities by weeks or months. Abnormal diagnostic findings include low hematocrit and hemoglobin readings, elevated BUN and serum creatinine levels, hematuria, and proteinuria.

THERAPEUTIC AND NURSING MANAGEMENT

GOODPASTURE'S SYNDROME

Until recently, the prognosis for the patient with Goodpasture's syndrome was poor. Therapeutic management consists of corticosteroids, immunosuppressive drugs (e.g., cyclophosphamide, azathioprine), plasmapheresis (see Chapter 10), and dialysis. Renal transplantation can be attempted once the circulating anti-GBM antibody titer decreases. Although recurrences may develop, the disease is not a contraindication to transplantation. In selected patients with severe pulmonary hemorrhage, bilateral nephrectomy has been helpful. The exact mechanism for improvement has not been proved.

Nursing management appropriate for a critically ill patient who is experiencing symptoms of acute renal failure and respiratory distress is instituted. Death is often secondary to respiratory hemorrhage. (Nursing interventions for a patient in acute renal failure are discussed in Chapter 44, and nursing interventions for a patient with respiratory failure are discussed in Chapter 26.) Because this syndrome is rare and primarily affects previously healthy young men, support and understanding of the patient and family are of major importance. The patient and family need instructions concerning current therapy, medications, and complications of the disease process.

Rapidly Progressive Glomerulonephritis

Rapidly progressive glomerulonephritis (RPGN) is characterized by sudden onset of symtoms and rapid deterioration of renal function. Renal failure may occur within weeks to months in contrast to chronic glomerulonephritis, which develops insidiously and progresses over many years.

RPGN can occur in a variety of situations: (1) as a complication of inflammatory or infectious disease (e.g., APSGN), (2) as a complication of a multisystemic disease (e.g., systemic lupus erythematosus, Goodpasture's syndrome), (3) as an idiopathic disease, or (4) in association with the use of certain drugs (e.g., penicillamine).

NURSING CARE PLAN Patient with Acute Urinary Calculus

Planning: Outcome Criteria	Nursing Interventions and Rationales
➤ **NURSING DIAGNOSIS**	Pain *related to* irritation of stone, obstruction of urine flow, and inadequate pain control or comfort measures *as manifested by* complaints of pain, facial grimacing, restlessness
Have minimal or no pain; verbalize decrease in pain and satisfaction with pain control.	Assess for pain location and severity *to plan appropriate interventions.* Encourage high fluid intake unless contraindicated *to promote passage of stone, dilute the urine, and reduce risk of additional stone formation.* Administer pain medication as ordered *to promote comfort.* Apply moist heat to flank area as needed *as heat reduces inflammation and reflex muscle spasm and promotes comfort.* Schedule activity as tolerated between attacks of renal colic *to promote as much activity as possible to help with passage of stones.*
➤ **NURSING DIAGNOSIS**	Anxiety *related to* uncertain outcome and lack of knowledge regarding possible surgery *as manifested by* expressions of concern about future treatments, withdrawn demeanor, emotional lability
Express relief of anxiety and confidence in treatment plan.	Assess cause and level of anxiety *to plan appropriate interventions.* Explain surgical or nonsurgical procedure (include insertion of ureteral catheter or stent) *as accurate information often decreases anxiety and fosters control.* Encourage patient to express feelings of anxiety, fear of surgery *to validate feelings and provide support.*
➤ **NURSING DIAGNOSIS**	Ineffective management of therapeutic regimen *related to* lack of knowledge about prevention of recurrence, diet, fluid requirements, and symptoms of recurrence *as manifested by* questions that indicate inadequate knowledge of disorder
Verbalize correct self-care measures and knowledge of symptoms of recurrence.	Instruct patient during initial hospital stay regarding increasing fluids, unless contraindicated, and diet restrictions and rationale *to prepare for home self-care.* Inform patient about rationale, dose, frequency, and side effects of medication *to foster adherence to medication regimen.* Tell patient to strain all urine through a piece of gauze or commercial device (if necessary) *to determine if stones are passed,* and to bring stone to physician *for analysis.* Educate patient about symptoms of recurrence (e.g., hematuria, flank pain) *to ensure early reporting and initiation of treatment.*

COLLABORATIVE PROBLEMS

Nursing Goals	Nursing Interventions and Rationales
➤ **POTENTIAL COMPLICATION**	Urinary obstruction *related to* presence of stone in path of urine flow
Monitor for signs of urinary obstruction, report occurrence, and carry out medical and nursing interventions.	Assess patient for signs and symptoms of urinary obstruction such as complaints of persistent pain, urgency along with inability to void, and bladder distention *to ensure early identification of the problem.* Monitor urine output and fluid intake *as decreased output relative to intake can suggest urinary obstruction.* Notify physician of oliguria *so treatment can be started promptly.* Strain all urine *to determine if stones are passed.* Save stones *so they can be sent for analysis to determine chemical composition.*

Treatment of RPGN has included corticosteroids, cytotoxic agents, anticoagulants, and antithrombotic agents. Plasmapheresis has recently been used.[13] More than one half of patients with RPGN progress to end-stage renal disease within 6 months after the diagnosis of the illness. Dialysis therapy and transplantation are used to maintain the patient with RPGN. Following renal transplantation, RPGN may recur.

Chronic Glomerulonephritis

Chronic glomerulonephritis is a syndrome that reflects the end stage of glomerular inflammatory disease. Most types of glomerulonephritis and nephrotic syndrome can eventually lead to chronic glomerulonephritis.

The syndrome is characterized by proteinuria, hematuria, and the slow development of uremic syndrome (see Chapter 44) as a result of decreasing renal function. Chronic glomerulonephritis does not usually follow an acute course. It progresses insidiously toward renal failure over a few to as many as 30 years.

Chronic glomerulonephritis is often found coincidentally when an abnormality on a urinalysis or elevated blood pressure is detected. It is quite common to find that the patient has no recollection or history of acute nephritis or any renal problems. A renal biopsy may be performed to determine the exact cause and nature of the glomerulonephritis. However, many institutions now prefer to use ultrasound and CT scanning as diagnostic measures.

Treatment is supportive and symptomatic. Hypertension and urinary tract infections should be treated vigorously. Protein and phosphate restrictions may slow the rate of progression of renal failure. (Management of chronic renal failure is discussed in Chapter 44.)

NEPHROTIC SYNDROME

Etiology and Clinical Manifestations

The *nephrotic syndrome* describes a clinical course that can be associated with a number of disease conditions. Some of the more common causes of nephrotic syndrome are listed in Table 43-6. The characteristic manifestations include edema, massive proteinuria, hyperlipidemia, and hypoalbuminemia.[14] The increased glomerular membrane permeability found in nephrotic syndrome is responsible for the massive excretion of protein in the urine. This results in decreased serum protein and subsequent edema formation.

The diminished plasma oncotic pressure from the decreased serum proteins stimulates hepatic lipoprotein synthesis, which results in hyperlipidemia. Initially, cholesterol and low-density lipoproteins are elevated. Later the triglyceride level is also increased. Fat bodies (fatty casts) commonly appear in the urine.

Immune responses, both humoral and cellular, are altered in nephrotic syndrome. As a result, infection is an important cause of morbidity and mortality. Skeletal abnormalities may occur, including hypocalcemia, blunted calcemic response to parathyroid hormone, hyperparathyroidism, and osteomalacia.

Hypercoagulability with thromboembolism is potentially the most serious complication of nephrotic syndrome. The renal vein is the site most commonly involved for thrombus formation. Pulmonary emboli occur in about 40% of nephrotic patients with thrombosis.

Therapeutic Management

Treatment of nephrotic syndrome is symptomatic. The goals are to relieve edema and cure or control the primary disease. Therapeutic management of the edema includes the cautious use of loop diuretics and a low-sodium (2 to 3 gm per day), high-protein diet (1.5 to 2.0 g/kg per day). IV albumin may be of value in the patient with symptomatic hypovolemia and hypotension or in the patient with edema resistant to therapy with diuretic drugs. The combined use of IV albumin and a loop diuretic may be useful, although it produces only a transient increase in plasma albumin concentration because most of the albumin is lost in the urine. Therefore long-term therapy with albumin is not a practical approach. However, an increase in dietary protein or IV albumin may ameliorate the hypoalbuminemia if either angiotensin-converting enzyme (ACE) inhibitors or nonsteroidal antiinflammatory drugs (NSAIDs) are administered concomitantly.

Table 43-6 Causes of Nephrotic Syndrome

Primary Glomerular Disease
Membranous proliferative glomerulonephritis
Primary nephrotic syndrome
Focal glomerulonephritis
Inherited nephrotic disease
Extrarenal Causes
Multisystem disease
Systemic lupus erythematosus
Diabetes mellitus
Amyloidosis
Infections
Bacterial (streptococcal, syphilis)
Viral (hepatitis, human immunodeficiency virus infection)
Protozoal (malaria)
Neoplasms
Hodgkin's disease
Solid tumors of lungs, colon, stomach, breast
Leukemias
***Allergens* (e.g., bee sting, pollen)**
Drugs
Penicillamine
Nonsteroidal antiinflammatory drugs
Captopril
Heroin

The treatment of hyperlipidemia is frequently unsuccessful. However, treatment with lipid-lowering agents, such as colestipol (Colestid), probucol (Lorelco), and lovastatin (Mevacor), may result in moderate decreases in serum cholesterol levels.

Corticosteroids and cyclophosphamide (Cytoxan) may be used for the treatment of severe cases of nephrotic syndrome. Prednisone has been effective to varying degrees in persons with lipoid nephrosis, membranous glomerulonephritis, proliferative glomerulonephritis, and lupus nephritis. Management of diabetes and treatment of edema are the only measures used for diabetic nephrosis.

NURSING MANAGEMENT

NEPHROTIC SYNDROME

A major nursing intervention for a patient with nephrotic syndrome is related to edema. It is important to assess the edema by weighing the patient daily, accurately recording intake and output, and measuring abdominal girth or extremity size. Comparing this information daily provides the nurse with a tool for assessing the effectiveness of treatment. The edematous skin needs careful cleaning. Trauma should be avoided, and the effectiveness of diuretic therapy must be monitored.

The patient has the potential to become malnourished from the excessive loss of protein in the urine. Maintaining a high-protein diet that is also low in sodium is not always easy. The protein intake should be 1.0 to 1.5 g/kg of body weight. The patient is usually anorexic. Serving small, frequent meals in a pleasant setting may encourage better dietary intake.

Because the patient is susceptible to infection, measures should be taken to avoid exposure to persons with known infections. The person with nephrotic syndrome is often ashamed of an edematous appearance and needs support in dealing with an altered body image.

RENAL DISEASE AND ACQUIRED IMMUNODEFICIENCY SYNDROME

The patient with human immunodeficiency viral (HIV) infection can have a variety of renal manifestations, ranging from mild fluid and electrolyte abnormalities to progressive renal impairment resulting in end-stage renal disease.[15] The incidence of renal disease associated with HIV infection is about 10% and is highest among IV drug users.[16]

HIV-associated renal syndromes include the following:

1. *Proteinuria and nephrotic syndrome,* which occurs in about 10% of patients with HIV infection.[15] It may be the initial sign of HIV infection in some persons.
2. *HIV-associated nephropathy* (HIVAN), which is characterized by proteinuria, progressive azotemia, absence of hypertension, large kidney size on renal imaging studies, and unusually rapid progression to end-stage renal disease.
3. *Acute renal failure,* which is most commonly seen in the patient with acquired immunodeficiency syndrome (AIDS) who is critically ill with HIV-related infection or malignancy. Both oliguric and nonoliguric forms of renal failure can occur. The natural cause of acute renal failure secondary to AIDS is similar to acute renal failure associated with other acute illnesses (see Chapter 44). Survival and recovery usually depend on the treatment of the primary cause of renal failure and support of renal function by dialysis. (HIV infection is discussed in Chapter 11.)

OBSTRUCTIVE UROPATHIES

Obstruction of the urinary system may occur at any point from the kidney to the urethral meatus (Fig. 43-2). It may be congenital or acquired. Obstruction may be due to intrinsic causes such as anomalies, diverticuli, tumors, or benign growth within the urinary tract; extrinsic causes such as tumors, adhesions, retroperitoneal fibrosis, or prolapsed adjacent organs; or functional causes as a result of neurologic or psychogenic factors. Some common intrinsic obstructions are narrowing of the ureteropelvic junction, bladder neck contracture, benign prostatic hyperplasia, urethral stricture, and meatal stenosis. Common extrinsic causes include pelvic and abdominal tumors or a prolapsed uterus. Examples of functional causes are vesicosphincter dyssynergia after spinal cord injury or neurogenic bladder secondary to diabetes.

Damaging effects from urinary tract obstruction affect the system above the level of the obstruction. The severity of these effects depends on the location, duration of obstruction, amount of pressure or dilatation, presence of urinary stasis, and whether infection is present. Infection increases the risk of irreversible consequences.

Although obstruction distal to the prostate in men or the bladder neck in women causes mucosal scarring and a slower stream, it rarely results in major obstructive uropathy because the urethral wall pressure is less than that of the bladder neck and bladder. Urethral obstruction may contribute to outlet resistance and cause lower or upper urinary tract damage when other obstructive or dysfunctional factors are also present. For example, there is an increased risk of compromised renal function in the patient with a spinal cord injury with vesicosphincter dyssynergia.

When obstruction occurs at the level of the bladder neck or prostate, significant bladder changes can occur. Detrusor muscle fibers *hypertrophy* (increase in size) in order to contract harder to push urine out a narrower pathway. Over a long period of time, the detrusor loses its ability to compensate for this resistance. Muscle bundles separate and become less compliant. This separation is called *trabeculation.* The areas between these muscle bundles are called *cellules.* Because these areas have no muscle support, the bladder mucosa can herniate between detrusor muscle bundles, forming sacs that drain poorly, called *diverticuli.* Residual urine can be very high in a noncompensating bladder.

Pressure increases during bladder filling or storage and can be transmitted to the ureter when *bladder outlet obstruction* is present. This pressure overcomes the normal peristaltic pressure and leads to *reflux* (a backflow of urine); ureteral dilatation, kinking, and tortuosity; *hydroureter* (di-

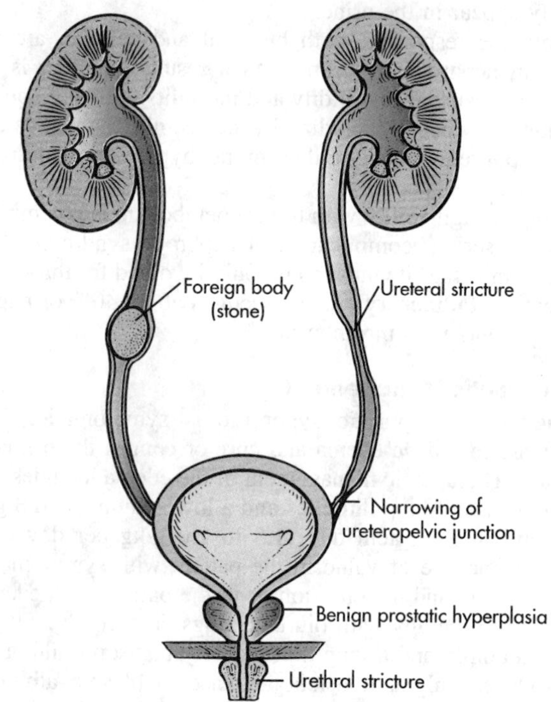

Fig. 43-2 Common causes of urinary tract obstruction.

latation of the renal pelvis); and *hydronephrosis* (dilatation of the calyces), and consequent chronic pyelonephritis, and renal atrophy (Fig. 43-3). If only one kidney is obstructed, the other kidney may try to compensate by hypertrophy, but the ureter will not be dilated on this contralateral side.

Partial obstruction may occur in the ureter or at the ureteropelvic junction (UPJ). If the pressure remains low or moderate, the kidney may continue to dilate with no noticeable loss of function. There is an increased risk of pyelonephritis because of urinary stasis and reflux. If only one kidney is involved and the other kidney is functioning, the patient may be free of symptoms. If both kidneys or only one functioning kidney is involved (e.g., if the patient has only one kidney), disturbances in renal function (e.g., increased BUN or serum creatinine levels) are found. If the obstruction progresses, oliguria or anuria develops. Often episodes of oliguria are followed by polyuria if the obstruction is a stone that becomes dislodged. Treatment requires location and relief of the blockage. This can include insertion of a tube (e.g., urethral or ureteral), surgical correction of the disease process, or diversion of the urinary stream above the level of blockage.

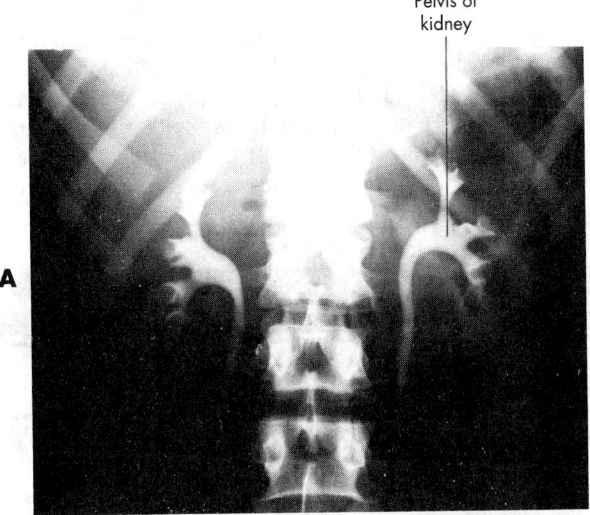

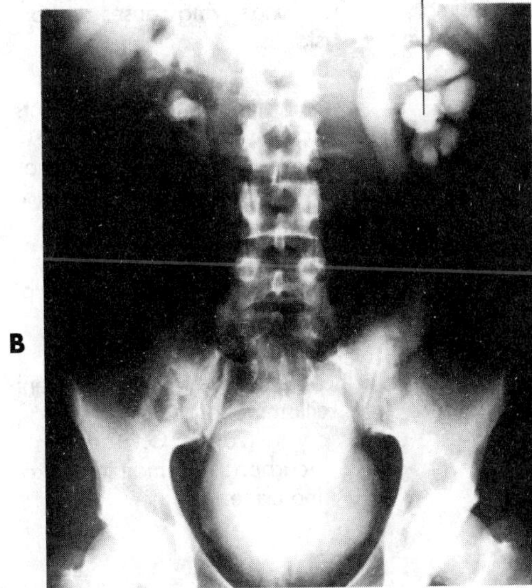

Fig. 43-3 ***A,*** Normal intravenous pyelogram (IVP). ***B,*** IVP showing hydronephrosis and hydroureter.

Urinary Tract Calculi

Significance. Each year an estimated 500,000 people in the United States have *nephrolithiasis* (kidney stone disease), and 1% to 5% experience a kidney stone at some time during their lives.[17] Many of these people require hospitalization. In the United States the incidence of urinary stone disease is highest in the Southeast and Southwest, followed by the Midwest. Except for *struvite,* stones (magnesium-ammonium-phosphate stones associated with UTI), are more common in women; stone disorders are more common in men. The majority of patients are between 20 and 55 years of age. Stone formation is more frequent in Caucasians than in African-Americans. The incidence is also higher in persons with a family history of stone formation. Recurrence of stones can occur in up to 80% of patients. There is seasonal variation, with stone formation occurring more often in the summer months, thus raising the question of the role of dehydration in this process. Stone formation in the kidney also seems to increase in incidence as countries become more industrialized, whereas the incidence of bladder stones decreases.[18]

Etiology. Many factors are involved in the incidence and type of stone formation, including metabolic, dietary, genetic, climatic, lifestyle, and occupational influences (Table 43-7). Many theories have been proposed to explain

Table 43-7 Risk Factors in the Development of Urinary Tract Calculi

Metabolic
Abnormalities that result in increased urine levels of calcium, oxaluric acid, uric acid, or citic acid
Climate
Warm climates that cause increased fluid loss, low urine volume, and increased solute concentration in urine
Diet
Large intake of dietary proteins that increases uric acid excretion
Excessive amounts of tea or fruit juices that elevate urinary oxalate level
Large intake of calcium and oxalate
Low fluid intake that increases urinary concentration
Genetic Factors
Family history of stone formation, cystinuria, gout, or renal acidosis
Lifestyle
Sedentary occupation, immobility

the formation of stones in the urinary tract. No single theory can account for stone formation in all cases. Crystals, when in a supersaturated concentration, can precipitate and unite to form a stone. Keeping urine dilute and free-flowing reduces the risk of recurrent stone formation in many individuals. It is known that a mucoprotein is formed (the matrix for the stone) in the kidneys that form stones. Urinary pH, solute load, and inhibitors in the urine affect the formation of stones. The higher the pH, the less soluble are calcium and phosphate. The lower the pH, the less soluble are uric acid and cystine.

Other important factors in the development of stones include obstruction with urinary stasis and urinary infection with urea-splitting bacteria (e.g., *Proteus, Klebsiella, Pseudomonas,* and some species of staphylococci). These bacteria cause the urine to become alkaline and contribute to the formation of calcium-magnesium-ammonium phosphate stones (struvite or triple phosphate stones). Infected stones, when they are entrapped in the kidney, may assume a staghorn configuration as they enlarge. Infected stones are frequent in the patient with an external urinary diversion, long-term indwelling catheter, neurogenic bladder, or urinary retention.

CULTURAL & ETHNIC Considerations

UROLOGIC DISORDERS

- Urinary tract calculi are more common among Caucasians than African-Americans.
- Jewish men have a high incidence of uric acid stones.
- Bladder cancer has a higher incidence among Caucasian men than African-American men. In all ethnic groups it affects men about three times more often than women.

Types. The term *calculus* refers to the stone and *lithiasis* refers to stone formation. There are five major categories of stones: (1) calcium phosphate, (2) calcium oxalate, (3) uric acid, (4) cystine, and (5) struvite (magnesium-ammonium phosphate) (Table 43-8). Stone composition may be mixed, although calcium stones are the most common.

Table 43-8 Types of Urinary Tract Calculi

Urinary Stone	Incidence (%)	Characteristics	Predisposing Factors	Therapeutic Measures
Calcium oxalate*	35-40	Small, often possible to get trapped in ureter; more frequent in men than in women	Idiopathic hypercalcuria, hyperoxaluria, independent of urinary pH, family history	Increase hydration. Reduce dietary oxalate.‡ Give thiazide diuretics, phosphate therapy. Give cholestyramine to bind oxalate. Give calcium lactate to precipitate oxalate in gastrointestinal tract.
Calcium phosphate	8-10	Mixed stones (typically), with struvite or oxalate stones	Alkaline urine, primary hyperparathyroidism	Treat underlying causes and other stones.
Struvite ($MgNH_4PO_4$)	10-15	Three to four times as common in women than men, always in association with urinary tract infections, large staghorn type (usually)†	Urinary tract infections (usually *Proteus* organisms)	Administer antimicrobial agents, acetohydroxamic acid. Use surgical intervention to remove stone. Take measures to acidify urine.
Uric acid	5-8	Predominant in men, high incidence in Jewish men	Gout, acid urine, inherited condition	Reduce urinary concentration of uric acid. Alkalinize urine. Administer allopurinol.
Cystine	1-2	Genetic autosomal recessive defect, defective absorption of cystine in gastrointestinal tract and kidney, excess concentrations causing stone formation	Acid urine	Increase hydration. Give α-penicillamine to prevent cystine crystallization. Give sodium bicarbonate to maintain alkaline urine.

*Calcium stones can exist as calcium oxalate, calcium phosphate, or a mixture of both. Calcium stones account for the majority of all stones.
†See Fig. 43-4.
‡See Table 43-9.

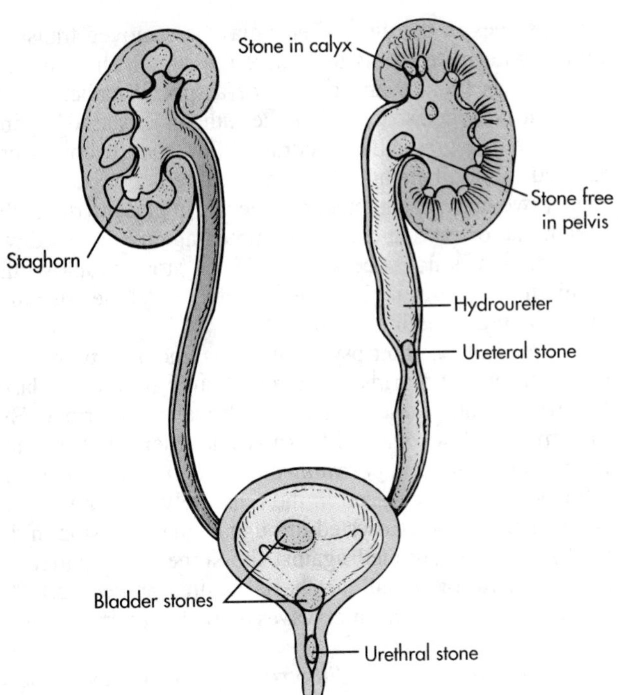

Fig. 43-4 Location of calculi in the urinary tract.

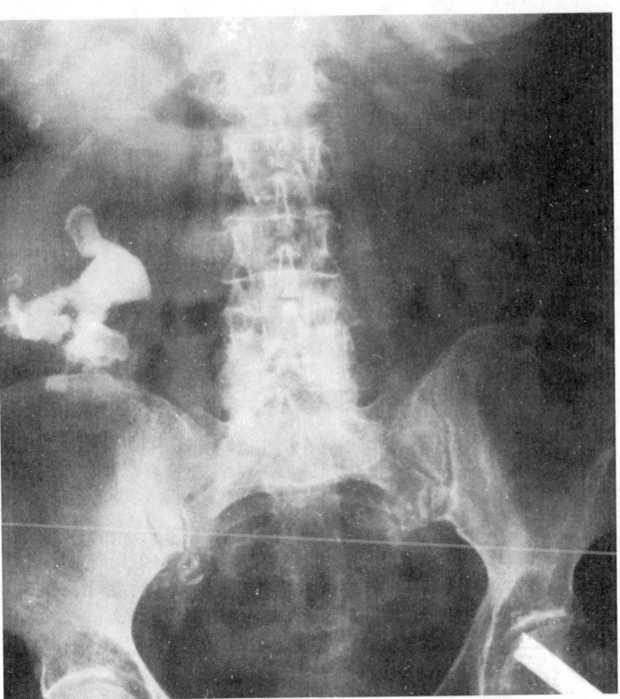

Fig. 43-5 X-ray of a staghorn calculus.

Clinical Manifestations. Urinary stones cause clinical manifestations when they cause obstruction to urinary flow. Common sites of complete obstruction are at the UPJ, in the ureter at the point it crosses the iliac vessels, and at the ureterovesical junction (UVJ). Symptoms include hematuria, abdominal or flank pain, and renal colic. The type of pain is determined by the location of the stone (Fig. 43-4). If the stone is nonobstructing, pain may be absent. If it produces obstruction in a calyx or at the UPJ, the patient may experience dull costovertebral flank pain or even colic. Pain resulting from the passage of a calculus down the ureter is intense and colicky. The patient may be in mild shock with cool, moist skin. As a stone nears the UVJ, pain will be felt in the lateral flank and sometimes down into the testicles, labia, or groin. Other clinical manifestations include the presence of urinary infection accompanied by fever, vomiting, nausea, and chills.

Diagnostic Studies. Diagnostic studies useful in the evaluation and management of renal lithiasis include urinalysis, urine culture, IVP, retrograde pyelogram, ultrasound, and cystoscopy. CT scans may be used to differentiate a nonopaque stone from a tumor. Measurement of the urine and serum levels of various substances involved in stone formation (e.g., calcium, phosphate, oxalate, uric acid) is often done after a stone is discovered to determine possible metabolic causes and preventive management strategies. BUN and serum creatinine are determined to assess renal function. A careful history, including previous stone formation, prescribed and over-the-counter medications and dietary supplements, and familial stone formation, is useful. Measurement of urine pH is useful in the diagnosis of struvite stones and renal tubular acidosis (tendency to alkaline pH) and uric acid stones (tendency to acidic pH). X-ray examination of kidneys, ureters, and bladder (KUB) with tomograms may be done to pinpoint the location, number, and size of radiopaque stones (Fig. 43-5). An IVP or retrograde pyelogram can further localize the degree and site of obstruction and confirm the presence of nonradiopaque stones (uric acid, cystine). Retrieval and analysis of the stones are important in the diagnosis of the underlying problem contributing to stone formation. Chemical and crystallographic analyses are done.

Therapeutic Management. Evaluation and management of a patient with renal lithiasis consist of two concurrent approaches. The first approach is directed toward management of the acute attack. This involves treating the symptoms of pain, infection, or obstruction as indicated for the individual patient. At frequent intervals, narcotics are typically required for relief of renal colic pain. A high fluid intake (e.g., 3-4 L per day) is recommended to produce enough urine output to assist stone movement down through the urinary tract. About 90% of stones pass spontaneously. However, stones larger than 4 mm are unlikely to pass through the ureter.

The second approach is directed toward evaluation of the etiology of the stone formation and the prevention of further development of stones. Information to be obtained from the patient includes family history of stone formation, geographic residence, nutritional assessment including the intake of vitamins A and D, activity pattern (active or sedentary), history of periods of prolonged illness with immobilization or dehydration, and any history of disease or surgery involving the GI or genitourinary (GU) tract.

Proper therapy for active stone formers requires a concerted therapeutic and nursing management approach, with primary emphasis on teaching and on developing a thera-

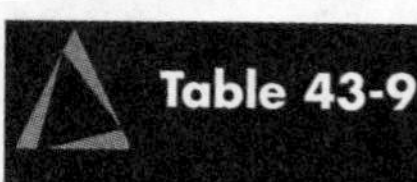

Table 43-9 Nutritional Management: Urinary Tract Calculi

The following is a list of foods high in purine, calcium, or oxalate content

Purine

High: Sardines, herring, mussels, liver, kidney, goose, venison, meat soups, sweetbreads

Moderate: Chicken, salmon, crab, veal, mutton, bacon, pork, beef, ham

Calcium

Milk, cheese, ice cream, yogurt, sauces containing milk; foods containing flour; all beans (except green beans), lentils; fish with fine bones (e.g., sardines, kippers, herring, salmon); dried fruits, nuts; chocolate, cocoa, Ovaltine

Oxalate

Spinach, rhubarb, asparagus, cabbage, tomatoes, beets, nuts, celery, parsley, runner beans; chocolate, cocoa, instant coffee, Ovaltine, tea; Worcestershire sauce

peutic regimen with which the patient can reasonably comply (see Table 43-8). Adequate hydration, dietary changes (Table 43-9), and the use of medications minimize urinary stone formation. Various medications are prescribed, depending on the specific problem underlying stone formation. Some examples are thiazides, sodium cellulose phosphate, orthophosphate, allopurinol, and potassium citrate. These medications prevent stone formation in various ways including altering urine pH, preventing excessive urinary excretion of a substance, or correcting a primary disease (e.g. hyperparathyroidism).

Treatment of struvite stones requires control of infection. This may be difficult if the stone remains in place. In addition to antibiotics, acetohydroxamic acid may be used in the treatment of kidney infections that result in the continual formation of struvite stones. Acetohydroxamic acid, an inhibitor of the chemical action caused by the persistent bacteria, can be used effectively to retard struvite stone formation. If the infection cannot be controlled, the stone may have to be removed surgically.

Indications for surgical, endoscopic, or lithotripsy stone removal include the following:

1. Stones too large for spontaneous passage
2. Stones associated with bacteriuria or symptomatic infection
3. Stones causing impaired renal function
4. Stones causing persistent pain, nausea, or ileus
5. Inability of patient to be treated medically
6. Patient with solitary kidney

If the stone is located in the bladder, *a transurethral litholapaxy* may be performed. In this operation an instrument is inserted into the bladder via the urethra, and the stone is crushed and then washed out with irrigating solution. Small stones in the distal ureter may be removed transurethrally with instruments that snare the stone. These are referred to as *baskets* and consist of a special catheter with filaments attached so that when the catheter is passed beyond the stone and gradually withdrawn, the stone becomes entangled in the filaments. If this procedure is not successful, one or two ureteral catheters may be left in place to dilate the ureter, and extraction can be attempted again in a few days. If extraction is not successful or if the stone is above the manipulation range in the ureter, *lithotripsy* (stone crushing) or open surgery is indicated.

Lithotripsy. Lithotripsy techniques include percutaneous ultrasonic lithotripsy, electrohydraulic lithotripsy, laser lithotripsy, and extracorporeal shock-wave lithotripsy. Extracorporeal shock wave lithotripsy and laser lithotripsy are the most common. In *percutaneous ultrasonic lithotripsy* an ultrasonic probe is placed in the renal pelvis via a percutaneous nephroscope (inserted through a small incision in the flank) and is positioned against the stone. (The patient is given general or spinal anesthesia for this procedure.) The probe produces ultrasonic waves, which break the stone into sandlike particles.

The *electrohydraulic lithotripsy* probe is also placed directly on a stone, but it breaks the stone into small fragments that are removed by forceps or by suction. A continuous saline irrigation flushes out the stone particles, and all outflow drainage is strained so that the particles can be analyzed. The calculi can also be removed by forceps or basket extraction. Complications are rare but include hemorrhage, sepsis, and abscess. Postoperatively, the patient usually complains of moderate to severe colicky pain. The first few voidings are bright red; as the bleeding subsides, the urine becomes dark red or turns a smoky color. Antibiotics are usually given for 2 weeks to reduce the risk of infection.

Laser lithotripsy probes are used to fragment lower ureteral and large bladder stones. The medium used, a coumarin-based pulsed dye, works on a wavelength that fragments stones but does not injure the surrounding tissue.[19,20]

In *extracorporeal shock-wave lithotripsy,* a noninvasive procedure, the patient is anesthetized (spinal or general) and placed in a water bath. Anesthesia is necessary to keep the patient very still during the procedure. Some of the newer generation lithotripters do not require submersion and use other means of initiating shock waves. The lithotripters are categorized as electrohydraulic, electromagnetic, and pizoelectric.[21] The second generation lithotripters use less power to fragment stones. Lower power reduces a patient's pain, but usually some sedation or analgesia is necessary.[22,23]

Fluoroscopy or ultrasound is used to focus the lithotripter on the affected kidney, and a high-voltage spark generator produces high-energy acoustic shock waves that shatter the stone without damaging the surrounding tissues. The stone is broken into fine sand, which is excreted into the patient's urine within a few days after the procedure.

Hematuria is common after lithotripsy procedures. A self-retaining ureteral stent is often placed after the procedure to promote passage of this sand and to prevent obstruction caused by *steinstrasse* (a buildup of sand in the ureter). The stent is removed 1 to 2 weeks after lithotripsy. A primary advantage of these techniques compared with open surgery is the decrease in the length of hospitalization and the patient's earlier return to normal activities.

Surgical intervention. There are a small group of select patients who need open surgical procedures, such as the very obese patient or the individual with complex abnormalities in the calyces or at the UPJ. The type of open surgery needed depends on the location of the stone. A *nephrolithotomy* is an incision into the kidney to remove a stone. A *pyelolithotomy* is an incision into the renal pelvis to remove a stone. If the stone is located in the ureter, a *ureterolithotomy* is performed. A *cystotomy* may be indicated for bladder calculi. For open surgery on the kidney or ureter, a flank incision directly below the diaphragm and across the side is usually the preferred surgical approach.

Nutritional Management. A high fluid intake (at least 3000 ml per day) is recommended after an episode of urolithiasis to produce a urine output of at least 2 L per day. High urine output prevents supersaturation of minerals (i.e., dilutes the concentration) and flushes them out before the minerals have a chance to precipitate. Increasing the fluid intake is especially important for the patient who is active in sports, lives in a dry climate, performs physical exercise, has a family history of stone formation, or works in an occupation that requires outdoor work or a great deal of physical activity that can lead to dehydration.

Dietary intervention may be important in the management of urolithiasis. In the past, calcium restriction was routinely implemented for the patient with kidney stones. Recent research suggests that a high dietary calcium intake, which was previously thought to contribute to kidney stones, may actually lower the risk by reducing the urinary excretion of oxalate, a common factor in many stones.[24] Initial nutritional management should include limiting oxalate-rich foods and thereby reducing oxalate excretion. Foods high in calcium, oxalate, and purines are presented in Table 43-9.

Table 43-10 Nursing Assessment: Urinary Tract Calculi

Subjective Data

Important health information

Past health history: Recent or chronic UTI, bed rest; immobilization; previous obstruction or kidney disease with urinary stasis; gout, prostatic hyperplasia

Medications: Use of antibiotics, phosphates, thiazides, antihypertensives, sodium bicarbonate, allopurinol, analgesics

Functional health patterns

Health perception–health management: Family history of renal calculi; fever, chills

Nutritional-metabolic: Nausea, vomiting, diarrhea; dietary intake of purines, calcium, oxalates, phosphates; low fluid intake

Elimination: Decreased urinary output, feeling of bladder fullness, burning with urination, urgency, frequency

Cognitive-perceptual: Acute, severe, colicky pain in flank, back, abdomen, groin, or genitalia; dysuria

Objective Data

General

Anxiety, guarding

Integumentary

Warm, flushed skin or pallor with cool, moist skin (mild shock)

Gastrointestinal

Abdominal distention, absence of bowel sounds

Urinary

Oliguria, hematuria, tenderness on palpation of renal areas, passage of stone or stones

Possible findings

Elevated BUN and serum creatinine levels; RBCs, WBCs, pyuria, crystals, casts, minerals, bacteria on urinalysis; elevated creatinine, uric acid, calcium, phosphorus, oxalate, or cystine values on 24-hr urine sample; calculi or anatomic changes on IVP or KUB x-ray; direct visualization of obstruction on cystour-eteroscopy

BUN, Blood urea nitrogen; *IVP,* intravenous pyelogram; *KUB,* kidneys, ureters, bladder; *RBCs,* red blood cells; *UTI,* urinary tract infection; *WBCs,* white blood cells.

NURSING MANAGEMENT

RENAL CALCULI

Nursing Assessment

Subjective and objective data that should be obtained from a patient with renal lithiasis are presented in Table 43-10.

Nursing Diagnoses

Nursing diagnoses are determined when the problem and etiologic factors are supported by clinical data. Nursing diagnoses related to a patient with urinary tract lithiasis include, but are not limited to, those presented in the nursing care plan for the patient with urinary calculus (on p. 1344) and the nursing care plan for the patient following lithotripsy (on p. 1352).

Planning

The overall goals are that the patient with urinary tract calculi will have (1) relief of pain, (2) no urinary tract obstruction, and (3) an understanding of measures to prevent further recurrence of stones.

Nursing Implementation

Preventive measures relate to the person who is on bed rest or is relatively immobile for a prolonged time. It is important to maintain a high fluid intake and to prevent urinary stasis by turning the patient every 2 hours and helping the patient to sit or stand if possible. In the acute phase it is important to retrieve the stone if passed. All urine voided by the patient should be strained through gauze or a special urine strainer in an effort to detect the stone. Increased intake of fluids and ambulation help the stone pass down the urinary tract. The patient should not walk if pain is present during an attack of renal colic.

NURSING CARE PLAN Patient Following Lithotripsy

Planning: Outcome Criteria	Nursing Interventions and Rationales
➤ NURSING DIAGNOSIS	Altered patterns of urinary elimination: decreased output and hematuria *related to* trauma or blockage of ureters or urethra *as manifested by* decrease in urinary output, bloody urine
Have free flow of urine and minimal to no hematuria.	Monitor urine amount and character *to ensure patency in urinary system and to ensure that hematuria is not excessive.* Encourage increased fluid intake *as increased hydration flushes bacteria and blood and may facilitate passage of stone fragments.*
➤ NURSING DIAGNOSIS	Risk for infection *related to* introduction of bacteria following manipulations of the urinary tract
Have no urinary tract infections.	Assess for elevation in temperature, chills, and cloudy, foul-smelling urine *as indicators of potential infection.* Monitor vital signs and observe for fever *as abnormalities may indicate infection.* Report any fever or chills to physician *so prompt treatment can be initiated.* Administer antipyretics if indicated *to reduce fever and increase comfort.* Encourage high fluid intake unless contraindicated *as stones form more readily in concentrated urine, and increased fluids help the stone fragments pass down urinary tract.* Note character and color of urine *to identify abnormalities and to plan for prompt intervention.* Observe for cloudy, foul-smelling urine *as an indicator of infection.* Administer antibiotics as ordered *to maintain constant blood level and treat infection.*
➤ NURSING DIAGNOSIS	Pain *related to* trauma and inflammation and inadequate pain control or comfort measures *as manifested by* complaints of pain
Have absence of or relief from pain; express satisfaction with pain control.	Maintain patency of urinary system *as obstruction of urinary flow will put pressure on kidneys and increase pain.* Monitor urinary output *to detect obstruction, pyuria, or hematuria.* Assess pain *to determine appropriate nursing intervention.* Administer medication for pain as ordered. Explain cause of pain or spasms to patient *to reduce anxiety.* Be aware that pain is more severe after percutaneous approach than extracorporeal lithotripsy.
➤ NURSING DIAGNOSIS	Risk for recurrence of lithiasis *related to* lack of knowledge regarding prevention of recurrence.
Have no recurrence of urinary calculi.	Teach patient to drink plenty of fluids (at least 2-3 L daily), especially during warm weather or during strenuous exercise *to dilute concentrates in urine.* Instruct patient to void frequently and always when they have the urge *to prevent stasis of urine.* If ordered, patient needs to take the whole course of prescribed antibiotics *to prevent growth of resistant bacteria.*

Narcotics will be required for renal colic because the pain is excruciating. Pain management and patient comfort are primary nursing responsibilities (see the nursing care plan for the patient with urinary calculus, p. 1344).

Stones that do not pass spontaneously must be removed. See the nursing care plan for the patient following lithotripsy, above.

Stone formation can be prevented, and the recurrence rate can be greatly reduced. After the acute phase, it is important for the nurse to teach the patient ways to prevent recurrence. Dietary restriction of oxalate is important for the patient who has calcium oxalate stones. Diets that restrict purines may be helpful to the patient at risk for developing uric acid stones. Follow-up care includes monitoring the patient's compliance with fluid and dietary recommendations. Periodic urine cultures may be indicated. Testing the pH of the urine is important, especially to assess the effectiveness of acidifying or alkalinizing agents. It is important to emphasize the need to avoid inadvertent dehydration from excessive exercise and to increase fluid needs during illness.

Strictures

A *stricture* is a narrowing of the lumen and is sometimes congenital but is usually acquired. Strictures may occur in the bladder neck, urethra, or ureters. Strictures of the bladder neck may be congenital or may result from chronic prostatitis in men or cystitis in women. Causes of urethral strictures include trauma from accidents (e.g., those resulting in fractured pelvis), gonorrheal infections, and urethral instrumentation. The membranous urethra is a common site of stricture caused by instrumentation because of its location (the urethral curve just below the prostatic urethra) and because the surrounding rhabdosphincter muscles prevent easy distention. Meatal stenosis, a narrowing of the urethral opening, is also common. Ureteral strictures may be caused by severe or chronic infection, radiation therapy, and retroperitoneal abscess formation from inflammatory bowel disease and perforation.

Strictures can sometimes be avoided by the proper management of inflammatory processes or traumatic injuries. Treatment of existing strictures includes dilatation, use of a catheter for temporary or permanent drainage for ureteral or urethral strictures, and surgery. Some patients are taught to dilate the urethra themselves between office visits to keep strictured areas open. Nursing interventions include preparing and informing the patient about the procedure and assessing the patient's need for management, education, and follow-up care.

RENAL TRAUMA

A continual increase in the incidence of traumatic renal injuries is related to an increase in the mechanization and speed of transportation and to the increase in violent crimes and injuries.[25] The majority of incidents occur in men younger than 30 years of age. Blunt trauma is the most frequent cause. Injury to the kidney should be considered in multiple or sports injuries, traffic accidents, and falls. It is especially likely when the patient injures the abdomen, flank, or back. Penetrating injuries may result from violent encounters (e.g. gunshot or stabbing incidents), or from surgical errors.

Clinical findings include a history of trauma to the area of the kidneys. Gross or microscopic hematuria may be present. Diagnostic studies include urinalysis, IVP with cystography, ultrasound, or CT evaluation. Renal arteriography may also be used. Both the injured kidney and the noninvolved kidney should be evaluated to provide information for further management.

The severity of renal trauma depends on the extent of the injury. There are five classifications: renal contusion, cortical laceration, calyceal laceration, complete renal tear, and vascular pedicle injury.[26] Each require different treatments that range from bed rest, fluids, and analgesia to surgical exploration and repair or nephrectomy.

Nursing interventions vary with the type and extent of associated injuries. Specific interventions related to renal trauma include assuring increased fluid intake, providing comfort measures, monitoring intake and output, observing for hematuria, determining the presence of myoglobinuria, assessing the cardiovascular status, and monitoring potentially nephrotoxic antibiotics.

RENAL VASCULAR PROBLEMS

Vascular problems involving the kidney include (1) nephrosclerosis, (2) renal artery stenosis, and (3) renal vein thrombosis.

Nephrosclerosis

Nephrosclerosis consists of sclerosis of the small arteries and arterioles of the kidney. There is decreased blood flow, which results in patchy necrosis of the renal parenchyma. Ischemic necrosis and destruction of glomeruli with subsequent fibrosis also occur.

Benign nephrosclerosis usually occurs in adults 30 to 50 years of age. It is caused by vascular changes resulting from hypertension and from the arteriosclerotic process. Arteriosclerotic vascular changes account for most of the loss of renal function associated with aging. There is a direct relation between the degree of nephrosclerosis and the severity of hypertension. The patient with benign nephrosclerosis may have normal renal function in the early stages. The only detectable abnormality may be hypertension.

Accelerated nephrosclerosis, or *malignant nephrosclerosis,* is associated with malignant hypertension, a complication of hypertension characterized by a sharp increase in blood pressure with a diastolic pressure greater than 130 mm Hg. The patient is usually a young adult, with a male predominance of 2:1. Renal insufficiency progresses rapidly.

Treatment of benign nephrosclerosis is the same as that of essential hypertension (see Chapter 30). Malignant nephrosclerosis is treated with aggressive antihypertensive therapy (see Chapter 30). The availability and use of antihypertensives have improved the prognosis for the patient with benign nephrosclerosis. Renal dysfunction and renal failure (in some persons) constitute two of the major complications of hypertension. The prognosis for the patient with malignant hypertension is poor, with the major cause of death related to renal failure.

Renal Artery Stenosis

Renal artery stenosis is a partial occlusion of one or both renal arteries and their major branches. It can be due to atherosclerotic narrowing or fibromuscular dysplasia. Renal artery stenosis accounts for 2% to 5% of all cases of hypertension.

Renal artery stenosis is considered a major cause of hypertension when it develops abruptly, especially in the patient under 20 or over 50 years of age and in the patient with no familial history of hypertension. This contrasts with the age distribution for essential hypertension, which is 30 to 50 years of age. A renal arteriogram is the best diagnostic tool for identifying renal artery stenosis.

Surgical revascularization of the kidney is indicated when blood flow is decreased enough to cause renal ischemia or when evidence indicates that renovascular hypertension is present and surgical intervention may result in the patient becoming normotensive. The surgical procedure usually involves anastomoses between the kidney and another major artery, usually the splenic artery or aorta. Percutaneous transluminal angioplasty may be an alternative for the patient who is not a good candidate for surgery. In selected cases of unilateral renal involvement with high renin production, unilateral nephrectomy may be indicated.

Renal Vein Thrombosis

Renal vein thrombosis may occur unilaterally or bilaterally. Glomerulonephritis, amyloidosis, diabetic glomerulosclerosis, and thrombophlebitis resulting from excessive use of diuretics predispose the patient to bilateral vein thrombosis. Unilateral thrombosis may result from external trauma, perinephric abscess, retroperitoneal tumors, renal biopsy, renal tumors, surgery near or on the renal hilus, and nephrotic syndrome as a result of membranous glomerulonephritis.

The patient has symptoms of flank pain, hematuria, or fever or has nephrotic syndrome. Anticoagulation is important in treatment because there is a high incidence of pulmonary emboli. Steroids may be used in the patient with nephrosis. Surgical thrombectomy may be performed instead of or along with anticoagulation.

HEREDITARY RENAL DISEASES

Hereditary renal diseases involve developmental abnormalities of the renal parenchyma. These abnormalities are either isolated or part of more complex malformation syndromes. The majority of inherited structural abnormalities are cystic. However, cysts may also develop as a result of obstructive uropathies, metabolic derangements, or neurologic diseases. Cysts may be evaluated to rule out any tumor content.

Polycystic Renal Disease

There are two forms of hereditary polycystic renal disease. It may be manifested in childhood or adulthood. The childhood form of polycystic disease is a rare autosomal recessive disorder that is often rapidly progressive.

The adult form of polycystic disease is an autosomal dominant disorder. It is latent for many years and is usually manifested at about 40 years of age. It involves both kidneys and occurs in both men and women. The cortex and the medulla are filled with thin-walled cysts that are several millimeters to several centimeters in diameter (Fig. 43-6). The cysts enlarge and destroy surrounding tissue by compression. They are filled with fluid and may contain blood or pus.

Clinical Manifestations. In the patient with polycystic disease, symptoms appear when the cysts begin to enlarge. A common early symptom of adult cystic disease is flank pain, which is either steady and dull or abrupt in onset, as well as episodic and colicky. On physical examination, palpable bilateral enlarged kidneys are often found. Other clinical manifestations include hematuria, UTI, and hypertension. Diagnosis is based on clinical manifestations, family history, IVP, ultrasound, or CT scan. Usually the disease progresses to chronic renal failure.

Therapeutic Management. There is no specific treatment for polycystic kidney disease. A major aim of treatment is to prevent infections of the urinary tract or to treat them with appropriate antibiotics if they occur. Nephrectomy may be necessary if pain, bleeding, or infection becomes a chronic, serious problem.

When the patient begins to experience progressive renal failure, the therapeutic and nursing interventions are determined by the remaining renal function. Nursing measures are those used for management of end-stage renal disease (see Chapter 44). They include diet modification, fluid restriction, medications, assisting the patient to accept the chronic disease process, and assisting the patient and family to deal with altered body image, financial concerns, and other issues related to the hereditary nature of the disease.

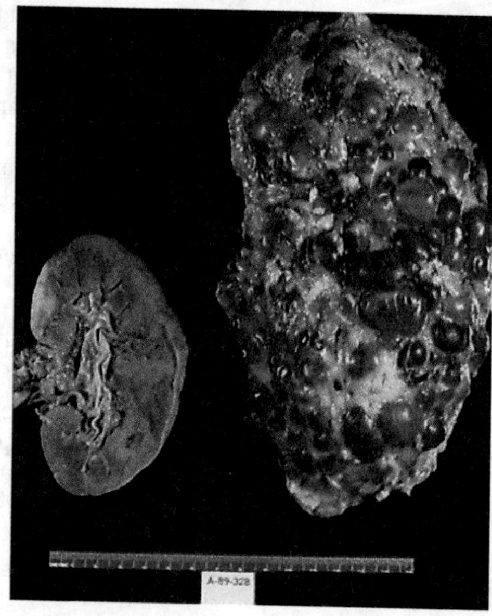

Fig. 43-6 Polycystic kidneys.

The patient who has adult polycystic disease often has children by the time the disease is diagnosed. Each child of a parent with polycystic kidney disease has a 50% chance of having the disease. The patient will need appropriate counseling regarding plans for having more children. In addition, genetic counseling resources should be provided for the children.

Medullary Cystic Disease

Medullary cystic disease is a hereditary disorder that occurs in two forms. The *recessive* form is associated with renal failure before the age of 20; the *dominant* form is associated with renal failure after the age of 20. Most cysts are located in the medulla. The kidneys are asymmetric in shape and are significantly scarred. There are defects in the concentration ability of the kidneys. Polyuria, progressive renal failure, severe anemia, metabolic acidosis, and poor sodium conservation are common. Hypertension can be a terminal event. Genetic counseling may be helpful in family planning. Treatment measures are those related to end-stage renal disease (see Chapter 44).

Alport's Syndrome

Alport's syndrome is also known as *chronic hereditary nephritis.* Two forms of the disease exist: (1) classic Alport's syndrome, which is inherited as a sex-linked disorder with hematuria, sensorineural deafness, and deformities of the anterior surface of the lens; and (2) nonclassical Alport's syndrome, which is inherited as an autosomal trait that causes hematuria but not deafness or lens deformities. Men are affected earlier and more severely than women. The disease is frequently diagnosed in the first decade of life. The basic defect is altered synthesis of the GBM. The patient most commonly has hematuria and progressive uremia. Treatment is supportive. Steroids and cytotoxic drugs are not effective. The disease does not recur after kidney transplantation.

CONGENITAL ABNORMALITIES OF THE URINARY SYSTEM

Congenital malformations of the urinary system are of concern for several reasons. These malformations may be the preexisting causes of infection, hypertension, or the development of calculi. Congenital disorders of the kidneys involve abnormalities in the amount, position, form, and differentiation of renal tissue. Congenital disorders include: (1) horseshoe kidney, (2) solitary kidney, (3) anomalies of origin and termination of the renal blood vessels, (4) an abnormal number or structure of the ureters, (5) an abnormal position of the urethral meatus, and (6) exstrophy of the bladder. These and many other serious congenital abnormalities of the urinary tract are discovered and treated when the patient is a child. These disorders are discussed in more detail in pediatric urology textbooks.

Horseshoe kidney involves fusion of both kidneys. The condition can result in a number of problems. The patient may have episodes of abdominal pain or the abnormality may be entirely asymptomatic. The horseshoe kidney is more susceptible in abdominal trauma. The areas of the kidneys that are fused have poor drainage of urine, and this can predispose to stasis of urine, infection, and formation of calculi. Nursing interventions include teaching follow-up health care, symptoms to be reported, and the proper treatment and prevention of UTIs and the development of calculi.

Exstrophy of the bladder is a rare condition that can include anomalies of the bladder (everted on the abdominal wall), pubic bones, and GU system. Initially the upper urinary tract is not involved. However, if the condition is not corrected, obstruction with resulting hydronephrosis and hydroureter develops. Surgical closure should be performed within the first 48 hours of life. Depending on the anomalies involved, some type of urinary diversion surgery may be required.

RENAL INVOLVEMENT IN METABOLIC AND CONNECTIVE TISSUE DISEASES

Various metabolic and connective tissue disease processes may have an effect on renal function. The pathophysiologic effects on the renal parenchyma are not always specific to each process. The clinical course of renal involvement is that of chronic progressive nephropathy, which can result in uremia and death. Therapeutic management includes treatment of the primary disorder along with symptomatic relief of renal involvement. If renal involvement progresses to chronic renal failure, management includes dialysis or transplantation (see Chapter 44). Nursing interventions include teaching the patient about the primary disease process, the renal involvement, and the resulting need to comply with dietary and fluid restrictions and medication.

Diabetes mellitus may affect the kidneys in several ways. Microangiopathic changes in diabetes consist of diffuse glomerulosclerosis, involving thickening of the GBM and nodular glomerulosclerosis (Kimmelstiel-Wilson syndrome), which is characterized by nodular lesions. Nodular glomerulosclerosis is reasonably specific for type I diabetes mellitus. The diabetic patient prone to glomerulonephropathy (e.g., the presence of trace proteinuria or retinopathy) requires careful monitoring of glucose levels and insulin requirements. Diabetic glomerulopathy can result in chronic renal failure. The patient with diabetes is especially susceptible to UTIs. Primary nursing interventions include teaching the patient about the increased risk of UTIs, the appropriate preventive measures, and when to seek additional medical care (see Chapter 46).

Gout is a syndrome of acute attacks of arthritis caused by hyperuricemia (see Chapter 60). Monosodium urate crystals deposited in joints are responsible for the syndrome. Renal disease may develop as a result of damage caused by deposition of uric acid crystals in the renal interstitium and tubules.

Amyloidosis is a disease manifested by altered structure and function caused by deposition of a hyaline substance (amyloid) in a variety of organs. The hyaline consists largely of protein. Kidney involvement is very common in amyloidosis. Proteinuria is often the first clinical manifestation.

Systemic lupus erythematosus is a connective tissue disorder characterized by the involvement of several tissues and organs, particularly the joints, skin, and kidneys (see Chapter 60). Clinical manifestations of lupus nephritis are similar to those of other forms of glomerulonephritis. Most frequently found are microscopic hematuria and significant proteinuria. Renal failure frequently occurs in systemic lupus erythematosus and has a poor prognosis. The long-term course of the disorder is extremely variable. Steroids are effective for the patient with severe renal disease. Recently, plasmapheresis therapy has been used.

Scleroderma (progressive systemic sclerosis) is a disease of unknown etiology characterized by widespread alterations of connective tissue and by vascular lesions in many organs (see Chapter 60). In the kidney, vascular lesions are associated with fibrosis. An immune complex mechanism has been postulated as a possible etiologic factor. The severity of renal involvement varies. The patient who develops severe renal lesions has a poor prognosis. Once uremia develops, about 70% die within 3 years.

NEOPLASTIC DISORDERS OF THE URINARY TRACT

Renal Tumors

Tumors of the kidney are responsible for approximately 8000 deaths per year. They arise from the cortex or pelvis (and calyces). Tumors arising from both areas may be benign or malignant. However, malignant tumors are more frequent. *Renal cell carcinoma* (adenocarcinoma) is the most common type. Adenocarcinoma is twice as frequent in men as in women and is typically discovered when the

Table 43-11 Robson's System of Staging Renal Carcinoma

Stage	Description
I	Limitation to renal capsule
II	Spreading to perirenal fat, but confined within fascia; includes metastasis to adrenal gland
III	Regional lymph node involvement, tumor thrombus in renal vein or vena cava, involvement of lymph nodes and renal vein or vena cava
IV	Presence of distant metastases

person is 50 to 70 years old. Risk factors include cigarette smoking, gender, family history, and exposure to cadmium.

There are no characteristic early symptoms. Generalized symptoms of weight loss, weakness, and anemia are the earliest manifestations. The classic manifestations of gross hematuria, flank pain, and a palpable mass are those of advanced disease. The most common sites of metastases include the lungs, liver, and long bones. Local extension of renal cancer into the renal vein and vena cava is common. Renal cystic disease and renal-associated carcinomas may develop in the patient with end-stage renal disease on maintenance renal dialysis (see Chapter 44).

Several studies are used to diagnose adenocarcinoma of the kidney. IVP with nephrotomography is the primary examination by which most masses are detected and evaluated. Ultrasounds have improved the ability to differentiate between a tumor and a cyst. Arteriography, percutaneous needle aspiration, CT, and magnetic resonance imaging (MRI) are also used in the diagnosis of renal tumors. Small renal tumors are found earlier because of the increased use of CT scans and MRI.

Robson's system of staging renal carcinoma is presented in Table 43-11. Tumor, node, metastases (TNM) classification is also used for renal cancer staging. The treatment of choice is a radical nephrectomy. Radical nephrectomy is the removal of the kidney, adrenal gland, surrounding fascia, part of the ureter, and draining lymph nodes. Radiation therapy is used palliatively in inoperable cases and when there are metastases to bone or lungs. At present, chemotherapy or hormonal therapy is not effective. Biologic response modifiers, including α interferon, tumor necrosis factor (TNF), and interleukin-2, are under investigation in the treatment of metastatic disease.[27]

The course is variable, and the extent of metastases may be prognostic as to survival. The patient with metastasis only into the perinephric fat may have a 5-year survival rate of 45%, whereas the patient with metastasis to lymph nodes or adjacent organs have a 0% to 30% 5-year survival rate.[28]

Wilms' Tumor

Wilms' tumor is a common renal tumor of infants and children. Of these tumors, 40% are hereditary, with an autosomal dominant mode of transmission. The most common clinical manifestation is abdominal swelling or distention. This distention is often noticed by the parents or is found on a routine examination. Other symptoms include pain, fever, hematuria, and hypertension. Diagnostic studies for Wilms' tumor include ultrasound and renal arteriography.

These tumors respond well to multimodality therapy. Therapeutic treatment includes surgical removal of the involved kidney and radiation therapy. Radiation therapy is used postoperatively and for inoperable tumors, bilateral tumors, and metastases. Chemotherapy with actinomycin D and vincristine is also frequently used.

Cancer of the Bladder

Bladder cancer accounts for nearly 1 in every 20 cancers diagnosed in the United States. The most frequent malignant tumor of the urinary tract is transitional cell carcinoma of the bladder. Most bladder tumors are papillomatous growths within the bladder. Cancer of the bladder is most common between the ages of 60 and 70 years and is at least three times as common in men as in women. Risk factors for bladder cancer include cigarette smoking, exposure to dyes used in the rubber and cable industries, and chronic abuse of phenacetin-containing analgesics. Individuals with chronic, recurrent nephrolithiasis and recurrent upper urinary tract infections also have an increased incidence of bladder cancer.[29]

Gross, painless hematuria is the most common clinical finding and the first in 75% of patients. Bladder irritability with dysuria, frequent urination, and intermittent bleeding may also be noted. When cancer is suspected, urine specimens for cytology can be obtained to determine the presence of neoplastic or atypical cells.

Bladder cancer can be classified as superficial, invasive, or metastatic. Superficial carcinomas are seen in patients with carcinoma in situ, mucosal involvement, and submucosal involvement. The patient with invasive disease has cancer that has progressed into the muscle, surrounding fat, or both. Bladder tumors are staged using the Jewett-Strong-Marshall system or the TNM system. The Jewett-Strong-Marshall classification system broadly classifies bladder cancer as superficial (CIS, O, A), invasive (B1, B2, C), or metastatic (D1–D4) disease. Pathologic grading systems are also used to classify the malignant potential of tumor cells, indicating a scale from well-differentiated to anaplastic categories. Low-stage, low-grade bladder cancers are the most responsive to treatment and are more easily cured.

THERAPEUTIC AND NURSING MANAGEMENT

BLADDER CANCER

Therapeutic management is outlined in Table 43-12. Surgical interventions include five possible procedures. *Endoscopic resection and fulguration* (electrocautery) is used for the diagnosis and treatment of superficial lesions with a low recurrence rate. This procedure is also used to control bleeding in the patient who is a poor operative risk or who has advanced tumors. With this technique the tumor mass is

Table 43-12 Therapeutic Management: Carcinoma of the Bladder

Diagnostic
- Urinalysis
- Intravenous pyelogram
- Cystoscopy with biopsy
- Cytology studies
- CT scan

Therapeutic
- Surgical treatment
  - Endoscopic resection and fulguration
  - Laser photocoagulation
  - Open loop resection and fulguration
  - Segmental resection
  - Total cystectomy
- Radiation
- Chemotherapy (intravesical or systemic when metastastic)

CT, Computed tomography.

excised by means of a blade inserted through the cystoscope. The remaining portions of the tumor are cauterized.

A second technique, *laser photocoagulation,* is also used to treat superficial bladder cancers. This procedure can be repeated a number of times for recurrence. The advantages of laser include bloodless destruction of the lesion, minimal risk of perforation, and lack of need for a urinary catheter. Because laser destroys tumor tissue, pathologic evaluation cannot be done after this procedure.

A third technique used is *open loop resection* (snaring of polyp types of lesion) *and fulguration.* It is used for the control of bleeding, for large superficial tumors, and for multiple lesions. Treatment of large lesions entails a *segmental resection* of the bladder.

Postoperative management of the patient who has had one of these three surgical procedures includes instructions to drink large amounts of fluid each day, measurement of intake and output, avoidance of alcoholic beverages, use of analgesics and stool softeners (if necessary), and sitz baths to promote muscle relaxation and reduce urinary retention. The nurse should also help the patient and family cope with fears about cancer, surgery, and sexuality and should emphasize the importance of regular follow-up care. Frequent routine cystoscopies are required.

When the tumor is invasive or involves the trigone (the area where the ureters insert into the bladder) and the patient otherwise has a good life expectancy and has demonstrated no metastases beyond the pelvic area, a *total cystectomy* with urinary diversion is the treatment of choice (see the following section on Urinary Diversion).

Radiation therapy is used with cystectomy or as the primary therapy when the cancer is inoperable or when surgery is refused. Sometimes, combination systemic chemotherapy is used for bladder cancer, usually preoperatively or preradiation therapy, or is used to treat distant metastases.

Chemotherapy with local instillation of thiotepa is of some use in the treatment of superficial recurring lesions. Thiotepa is an alkylating agent that is pharmacologically related to nitrogen mustard. It is instilled directly into the patient's bladder and retained for about 2 hours. The position of the patient may be changed every 15 minutes for maximum contact in all areas of the bladder, especially if the tumor occurred on the bladder dome.

Other intravesical chemotherapeutic agents include doxorubicin (Adriamycin), mitomycin (Mutamycin), and bacillus Calmette-Guérin (BCG). BCG is the drug of choice for carcinoma in situ of the bladder. Protocols vary, but intravesical therapy is usually initiated at weekly intervals for a number of weeks before the intervals are increased. Most patients have irritative bladder symptoms following intravesical therapy. Thiotepa can significantly reduce WBC and platelet counts in some individuals. Mitomycin may cause contact dermatitis, and BCG may cause flulike symptoms, hematuria, or systemic infection.[30] Systemic side effects usually associated with chemotherapy, such as nausea, vomiting, and hair loss, are not experienced with intravesical chemotherapy. Cyclophosphamide (Cytoxan), vinblastine (Velban), doxorubicin (Adriamycin), methotrexate, and cisplatin (Platinol) are systemic chemotherapeutic agents used in treating invasive bladder cancer.

Nursing responsibilities include encouraging the patient to increase the daily fluid intake and to quit smoking, assessing the patient for secondary urinary tract infection, and stressing the need for routine urologic follow-up. The patient may have fears or concerns about sexual activity or bladder function that will need to be addressed.

URINARY INCONTINENCE AND RETENTION

An estimated 10 million people in the United States suffer from urinary incontinence or the involuntary loss of urine that is sufficient to be a problem.[31] Incontinence exacts physical (infection, pressure sores, perineal rashes), psychosocial (embarrassment, isolation, depression), and economic costs. However minor the problem, incontinence can cause severe psychologic distress. Incontinence is not an inevitable consequence of aging; in most cases among older adults, it can be significantly improved or corrected.[32] Retention is the inability to urinate in spite of the presence of urine in the bladder. Both incontinence and retention may occur in the same person.

Normal Bladder Function

Storage of urine in the bladder is mediated by relaxation of the detrusor muscle (which provides the propulsive force for emptying the bladder) and closure of the sphincters. The detrusor muscle is controlled by the parasympathetic nervous system through the pelvic nerves from sacral spinal cord segments S2, S3, or S4. These spinal segments are modulated by the pons (brainstem) and cortical centers in the brain. The smooth muscle of the trigonal portion of the bladder between the ureteral orifices and the posterior area of the bladder outlet is innervated by the sympathetic nervous system, in which α receptors predominate. This layer of muscle acts as an involuntary internal sphincter.

The external urethral sphincter and perineal muscles are under voluntary control.

The sensation of bladder fullness is transmitted via sensory nerves to the sacral cord. If not suppressed by cortical control, the sacral cord discharges motor impulses by reflex that cause powerful sustained detrusor contraction. Urination can be prevented by means of cortical suppression of the reflex arc or voluntary contraction of the external sphincter and perineal muscles. Urination occurs when detrusor contraction is coordinated with sphincter relaxation.

Causes of Urinary Incontinence and Retention

Anything that interferes with bladder or urethral sphincter control can result in *urinary incontinence.* Causes may be transient (e.g. caused by confusion or depression, infection, medications, restricted mobility, or stool impaction). Congenital disorders that produce incontinence include exstrophy of the bladder, epispadias, spina bifida with myelomeningocele, and ectopic ureteral orifice. Acquired disorders are described in Table 43-13. *Neurogenic bladder* is a general term referring to any bladder dysfunction resulting from a central nervous system (CNS) neurologic disorder. There are numerous causes of this condition, including such problems as CNS tumors, cerebrovascular accidents, multiple sclerosis, diabetic neuropathy, and spinal cord injury. A person with a neurogenic bladder may have problems with urgency, frequency, incontinence, inability to urinate, and obstruction-like symptoms. Long-term problems include formation of calculi, urinary tract infection, and progressive deterioration in renal function.

A simple way to classify neurogenic dysfunction is to identify whether there is a failure to store, failure to empty, or both problems and whether the dysfunction is of the bladder or urethra. Either or both problems lead to urinary tract damage if not treated. The type of dysfunction usually depends on where the problem affects the brain or spinal cord (e.g., cerebral centers, suprasacral spinal cord, sacral cord area). Lesions in the brain or upper spinal cord usually cause hyperreflexic symptoms, whereas lesions in the sacral cord cause arreflexia. Detrusor sphincter dyssynergia (the bladder and sphincter contract at the same time) is often associated with lesions in the suprasacral spinal cord.[33] (A more detailed description of neurogenic bladder is found in Chapter 57.)

Retention can be found in association with incontinence but can also be independent of incontinence. Drugs that may cause retention include (1) antihypertensives (methyldopa [Aldomet], hydralazine [Apresoline]), (2) antiparkinsonian drugs (levodopa), (3) antihistamines, (4) anticholinergics (atropine, belladonna), (5) antispasmodics, (6) sedatives, and (7) anesthesia (especially spinal anesthesia).

Postoperative urinary retention is not uncommon and is related to preoperative medication (atropine and sedatives are frequently used), anesthesia, supine position after surgery, and low fluid intake. Postoperative retention may also be related to the effects of surgical manipulation of the bladder nerves.

Another cause of retention is urethral obstruction, which may be caused by congenital urethral stenosis, benign prostatic hyperplasia, fecal impaction, or tumors (involving bladder outlet or large, displaced uterine myomas). Psychologic problems may also contribute to urinary retention. Psychogenic urinary retention is found more commonly in women than in men.

Diagnostic Studies

A complete history and physical examination (with particular attention to the GU system) are essential to obtain information on the patient's past and current urination patterns, current physical health, and underlying reasons for incontinence or retention. A drug history, including both prescription and over-the-counter drugs, should be obtained.

Diagnostic tests of urologic dysfunction are essential in the evaluation of the function and structure of the urinary tract, especially the bladder. These tests may include IVP, cystoscopy (including urethroscopy), urodynamic studies (to assess sphincter, perineal, and muscle activity), and catheterization for residual urine.

Therapeutic Management

Treatment should correct the factors responsible for incontinence or retention, if possible (see Table 43-13). Treatment includes behavioral techniques, medications, electrostimulation, and surgery. (Bladder training programs are described in Chapter 57.)

Surgical approaches vary, depending on the underlying problem. For example, a transurethral resection of the prostate is used to treat benign prostatic hyperplasia. Urethral strictures are dilated. Several surgical procedures help correct anatomic malposition of the bladder neck and urethra that causes female stress incontinence. The Marshall-Marchetti procedure involves suspending the urethra and bladder neck by suturing the anterior vaginal wall on each side to the periosteum of the pubic bones and lower rectum through an abdominal incision. The Pereyra procedure and subsequent modifications involve suspending the tissues adjacent to the bladder neck to the abdominal fascia, mainly through a transvaginal approach.

Injection of urethral bulking agents, such as teflon or collagen, and implantation of a prosthetic urethral sphincter, are also done for stress incontinence in selected cases. There is risk of teflon particles migrating to lungs; consequently, alternatives are more favorable. Augmentation enterocystoplasty (enlarging the bladder with a segment of bowel or stomach) may be attempted for severe urge incontinence when the disorder does not respond to other treatment measures and when kidney function may be compromised as a result of reflux.

Pharmacologic Management

Vaginal or oral estrogen replacement is often prescribed for postmenopausal women to restore urethral suppleness. Anticholinergic agents such as propantheline (Pro-Banthine), oxybutynin (Ditropan), and dicyclomine hydrochloride (Bentyl), are used to treat hyperreflexic bladders by suppressing the unwanted contractions that occur when the bladder has only a small volume of urine. Anticholinergic drugs are contraindicated in the patient with narrow-angle

Table 43-13 Acquired Disorders Causing Urinary Incontinence

Type	Description	Causes	Treatment
■ Stress incontinence	Sudden increase in intraabdominal pressure causes involuntary passage of urine. It can occur during coughing, heavy lifting, straining, or laughing.	Condition is found most commonly in women with relaxed pelvic musculature (frequently from obstetric complications or multiple pregnancies). Structures of the female urethra atrophy when estrogen decreases. Condition is found in men after prostate surgery for benign prostatic hyperplasia or prostatic carcinoma.	Perineal muscle exercises (e.g., Kegel exercises), weight loss if patient is obese, insertion of vaginal pessary, estrogen vaginal creams, condom catheters or penile clamp
■ Urge incontinence	Condition occurs randomly when involuntary urination is preceded by warning of few seconds to few minutes. Leakage is periodic but frequent. Nocturnal frequency and incontinence are common. Condition may appear with varying severity during psychologic stress.	Condition is caused by uncontrolled contraction or overactivity of detrusor muscle. Bladder escapes central inhibition and contracts reflexively. Conditions include central nervous system disorders (e.g., cerebrovascular disease, Alzheimer's disease, brain tumor, Parkinson's disease), bladder disorders (e.g., carcinoma in situ, radiation effects, interstitial cystitis), interference with spinal inhibitory pathways (e.g., malignant growth in spinal cord, spondylosis), and bladder outlet obstruction, as well as conditions of unknown etiology.	Treatment of underlying cause, instruction to have patient urinate more frequently, anticholinergic drugs (e.g., propantheline), imipramine at bedtime, calcium channel blockers, condom catheters, vaginal estrogen creams
■ Overflow (paradoxical) incontinence	Condition occurs when the pressure of urine in overfull bladder overcomes sphincter control. Leakage of small amounts of urine is frequent throughout the day and night. Urination may also occur frequently in small amounts. Bladder remains distended and is usually palpable.	Disorder is caused by outlet obstruction (prostatic hyperplasia, bladder neck obstruction, urethral stricture) or by underactive detrusor muscle caused by myogenic or neurogenic factors (e.g., herniated disk, diabetic neuropathy). It may also occur after anesthesia and surgery (especially procedures such as hemorrhoidectomy, herniorrhaphy, cystoscopy). Neurogenic bladder (flaccid type) is another cause.	Urinary catheterization to decompress bladder, implementation of Credé or Valsalva maneuver, prazosin (α-adrenergic blocker) to decrease outlet resistance, bethanechol to enhance bladder contractions, intermittent catheterization, surgery to correct underlying problem
■ Reflex incontinence	Condition occurs when no warning or stress precedes periodic involuntary urination. Urination is frequent, is moderate in volume, and occurs equally during the day and night.	Spinal cord lesion above S2 interferes with central nervous system inhibition. Disorder results in detrusor hyperreflexia and interferes with pathways coordinating detrusor contraction and sphincter relaxation.	Treatment of underlying cause, bladder decompression to prevent ureteral reflux and hydronephrosis, intermittent self-catheterization, α-adrenergic blocker (e.g., prazosin) to relax internal sphincter, diazepam or baclofen to relax external sphincter, prophylactic antibiotics, surgical sphincterotomy
■ Incontinence after trauma or surgery	Vesicovaginal or urethrovaginal fistula may occur in women. Alteration in continence control in men involves proximal urethral sphincter (bladder neck and prostatic urethra) and distal urethral sphincter (external striated muscle).	Fistulas may occur during pregnancy, after delivery of baby, as a result of hysterectomy or invasive cancer of cervix, or after radiation therapy. Incontinence is found as postoperative complication after transurethral, perineal, or retropubic prostatectomy.	Surgery to correct fistula, urinary diversion surgery to bypass urethra and bladder, external condom catheter, penile clamp, placement of artificial implantable sphincter

glaucoma (acceptable if wide-angle glaucoma is present). Parasympathomimetics (cholinergics) such as bethanechol (Urecholine) and neostigmine (Prostigmin) are used to treat flaccid bladders by stimulating bladder contractions. Alpha-adrenergic blockers such as prazosin (Minipress) and phenoxybenzamine (Dibenzyline) can be used to relax spastic bladder necks. Sympathomimetics such as ephedrine and phenylephrine may be used to increase bladder neck and urethral tone (which may decrease in stress incontinence). Alpha-adrenergic agonists such as phenylpropanolamine and imipramine (Tofranil) also increase urethral resistance. Imipramine and calcium channel blockers (nifedipine) reduce detrusor contractions and improve continence. Side effects from these drugs are common, especially in the older patient.

NURSING MANAGEMENT

URINARY INCONTINENCE

The nurse must recognize both the physical and the emotional problems that accompany incontinence. The patient's dignity, privacy, and feelings of self-worth must be maintained or enhanced. Most persons suffering from incontinence can be helped with proper diagnosis and modern therapeutic approaches.

A patient with stress incontinence can be taught to do pelvic floor (perineal) muscle exercises (Kegel exercises). The patient should contract the pelvic muscles, as though trying to stop the flow of urine, while relaxing the abdomen, thighs, and buttocks. These exercises should be repeated in sets of 10 or more contractions and done four to five times each day over several weeks. Consistency and persistence are necessary for success, and exercise regimens have to be individualized. Vaginal cones[34] or biofeedback may help the patient to identify correct pelvic muscles, avoid using incorrect muscles, and realize progress in regaining continence.

The nurse has a major responsibility to help the patient with incontinence problems in a variety of settings. In the hospital, nursing measures aimed at maintaining urinary continence include identifying transient causes and assessing the patient for signs of bladder infection, fecal impaction, or bladder distention. The nurse should offer the urinal or bedpan or help the patient to the bathroom every 2 hours or at scheduled times.

Assuming the usual position for urination (standing for the man and sitting and leaning forward for the woman) or using relaxation techniques often help a patient to urinate successfully, particularly in unfamiliar settings. Applying pressure over the bladder area (Credé maneuver) may be helpful when bladder outlet obstruction is not a problem. The nurse should be sure the patient has privacy and is not rushed when trying to urinate. Techniques to stimulate urination include running water in the sink, placing hands in water, and pouring warm water over the perineum. Fluid intake patterns can be monitored and fluids encouraged at a goal of 15 ml per pound of body weight in 24 hours, the minimum daily requirement.

The patient should be taught that incontinence is not a normal part of aging and that it can be eliminated or controlled in most cases. Local medical supply resources and suggestions for improving urinary control, including having the problem further evaluated, are helpful in discharge planning. The patient may feel more comfortable talking about incontinence when given this kind of permission to talk about a problem that is embarrassing to most people.

Fluid restriction, incontinence pads, and keeping a urinal in place at all times are only temporary measures to reduce the occurrence or effects of incontinence. Long-term use of these measures discourages continence and can lead to dehydration and skin problems.

If bladder retraining cannot be achieved, external appliances or intermittent self-catheterization may be indicated. Several external appliances that prevent soiling, decrease odor, and improve body image are available for men. External appliances for women are not useful in most situations. Intermittent self-catheterization using a clean technique can be taught to selected patients. Keeping the skin clean and dry is essential to prevent skin irritation and breakdown.

RESEARCH

IMPLICATIONS FOR NURSING PRACTICE

URINARY INCONTINENCE

Citation Burgio LD and others: The effects of changing prompted voiding schedules in the treatment of incontinence in nursing home residents, *J Am Geriatr Soc* 42:315-320, 1994.

Purpose To determine the effects of different prompted voiding schedules on urinary incontinence in a continence unit and the effects of maintenance of benefits on normal nursing units.

Methods Multiphase study with both intrasubject and intersubject comparisons. Incontinent nursing home residents (n = 41) were assigned to one of four treatment groups that varied as to the schedule of prompted voiding. The study used chart reviews, Katz Activities of Daily Living, and Mini-Mental Status Examination. Urologic status, self-initiated toileting, urine volumes voided, and incontinence assessed by pads and pants check data were collected. The effects of different prompted voiding schedules were evaluated.

Results and Conclusions Prompted voiding is an effective treatment for urinary incontinence. A less intense 3-hour schedule was superior to the standard 2-hour schedule for some residents. The improvements in dryness can be maintained by nursing home staff if formal staff management procedures are used by nurse supervisors.

Implications for Nursing Practice Dryness can be improved in nursing home residents with the use of prompted voiding schedules. The results of this study and other guidelines addressing quality of care suggest that nursing homes need to deemphasize custodial care and adopt a rehabilitation model.

INSTRUMENTATION

A catheter is a tubular instrument made of rubber, plastic, metal, or other material used to drain or inject gases or fluids through a body passage. The process of inserting the catheter into a body cavity or passage is termed *catheterization.* Indwelling catheters often have self-retaining balloons to keep the catheter in place. Nursing responsibility includes understanding the reason for catheterization, the scientific principles involved, aseptic technique, and the appropriate care of the patient after catheterization.

The reasons for urinary catheterization are listed in Table 43-14. Two reasons that are *not* indications for catheterization are (1) routine acquisition of a sterile specimen for laboratory analysis and (2) convenience of the nursing staff or the patient's family. The risks of nosocomial infection are too high to allow catheterization of a patient for the convenience of hospital personnel or family members. A catheter should be the final means of providing the patient with a dry environment for prevention of skin breakdown and protection of dressings or skin lesions.

Urinary catheterization is commonly used in the management of the hospitalized patient. However, it is not without serious risks. The urinary tract is the most common site of nosocomial infections. Urinary catheterization is a major cause of UTIs. Scrupulous aseptic technique is mandatory when a urinary catheter is inserted. After insertion, maintenance and protection of the closed drainage system are major nursing responsibilities. Irrigation of the catheter should *not* be routinely performed.

While the patient has a catheter in place, nursing actions should include maintaining patency of the catheter, managing fluid intake, providing for the comfort and safety of the patient, and preventing infection. Attention should be given to the psychologic implications of urinary drainage. Concerns of the patient can include embarrassment related to exposure of the body, an altered body image, and fear concerning the care of the catheter that results in increased dependency.

Catheters vary in construction materials, tip shape (Fig. 43-7), and size of the lumen. Catheters are sized according to the French scale. Each French unit equals 0.33 mm of diameter. The diameter measured is the internal diameter of the catheter. The size used varies with the size of the individual and the purpose for catheterization. In women, urethral catheter sizes 14 to 16 F are the most common; in men, sizes 16 to 18 F are used. Problems resulting from too small a catheter include possible obstruction of the urinary flow by blood clots, mineral sediment, or mucous plugs and difficulty in passing the catheter if resistance is met in the urethra. The primary problem resulting from too large a catheter is tissue erosion secondary to excessive pressure on the meatus or urethra. Four routes are used for urinary tract catheterization: urethral, ureteral, suprapubic, and via a nephrostomy tube.

Table 43-14 Indications for Urinary Catheterization

1. Relief of urinary retention caused by lower urinary tract obstruction, paralysis, or inability to void
2. Bladder decompression preoperatively and operatively for lower abdominal or pelvic surgery
3. Facilitation of surgical repair of urethra and surrounding structures
4. Splinting of ureters or urethra to facilitate healing after surgery or other trauma in area
5. Instillation of medications into bladder
6. Accurate measurement of urinary output in critically ill patient
7. Measurement of residual urine after urination
8. Study of anatomic structures of urinary system
9. Urodynamic testing

Urethral Catheterization

The most common route of catheterization is insertion of the catheter through the external meatus into the urethra, past the internal sphincter, and into the bladder. Several principles that should be considered in the management of the patient with a urethral catheter include the following:

1. The indwelling urinary catheter should be used *only* when absolutely necessary and never solely for the convenience of the caregivers. Its use should be discontinued as early as possible.
2. The catheterized patient, particularly the person who is ambulatory, should receive appropriate instruction regarding catheter care.
3. A sterile, closed drainage system should always be used in short-term catheterization. The distal urinary catheter and the proximal drainage tube should not be discon-

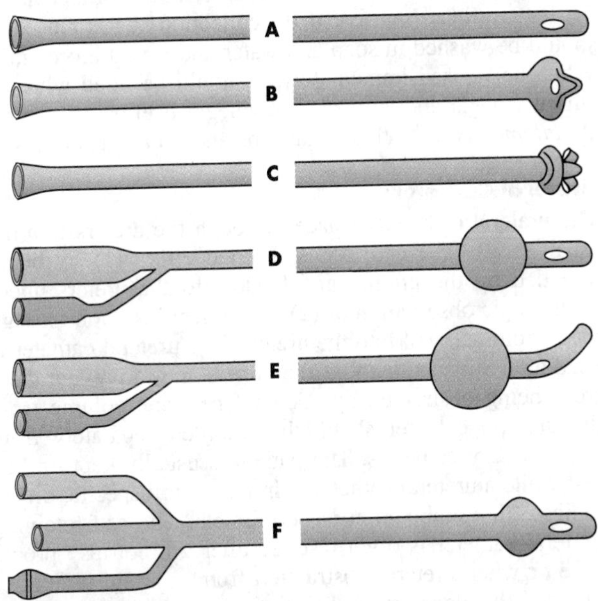

Fig. 43-7 Different types of commonly used catheters. ***A,*** Simple urethral catheter. ***B,*** Mushroom or dePezzar (can be used for suprapubic catheterization). ***C,*** Winged-tip or Malecot. ***D,*** Indwelling with inflated balloon. ***E,*** Indwelling with Coudé tip. ***F,*** Three-way indwelling (the third lumen is used for irrigation of the bladder).

nected except for necessary catheter irrigation. Unobstructed downhill flow must be maintained. The collecting bag should be emptied regularly and kept below the level of the bladder. A poorly functioning catheter should be replaced. The leg bag should not be used for the short-term patient because the risk of bacterial infection is great.

4. Perineal care (one to two times per day and when necessary) should include cleaning of the meatus-catheter junction with soap and water. Following this, an antimicrobial ointment may be applied. Lotion or powder should not be used near the catheter. The catheter should be properly secured to the leg to prevent movement and urethral traction.

5. Sterile technique must be used whenever the collecting system is opened. Catheter irrigation is performed only when obstruction or blood clots are suspected or, in the case of long-term catheterization, to reduce sediment buildup. If frequent irrigations are necessary in short-term catheterization for catheter patency, a triple-lumen catheter is preferable, permitting continuous irrigations within a closed system. Small volumes of urine for culture can be aspirated from the distal catheter by means of a sterile syringe and a 21-gauge needle. The puncture site must first be prepared with a tincture of iodine or alcohol solution. Many drainage systems are now equipped with a sampling port. Silicone or plastic catheters do not self-seal. Urine for chemical analysis (e.g., electrolytes) can be obtained from the drainage bag.

6. When the patient is catheterized for less than 2 weeks, routine catheter change is not necessary. For long-term use of an indwelling catheter, replacement is necessary when concretions can be palpated in the catheter or when the catheter malfunctions. With long-term use of a catheter, the leg bag may be used. If the collection bag is reused, it should be washed in soap and water and rinsed thoroughly. When not reused immediately, it should be filled with 1/2 cup of vinegar and drained. The vinegar is effective against *Pseudomonas* and other organisms and eliminates odors.

Ureteral Catheters

The ureteral catheter is placed through the ureters into the renal pelvis. The catheter is inserted either (1) by being threaded up the urethra and bladder to the ureters under cystoscopic observation or (2) by surgical insertion through the abdominal wall into the ureters. The ureteral catheter is used after surgery to splint the ureters and to prevent them from being obstructed by edema. The urine volume from the ureteral catheter should be recorded separately from other urinary catheters. The patient is usually kept on bed rest while a ureteral catheter is in place until specific orders indicate that ambulation is permissible. The self-retaining ureteral catheter is often inserted after a lithotripsy procedure or when ureteral obstruction from adjacent tumors or fibrosis threatens renal function. The double-J ureteral catheter is often used and allows the patient to ambulate. One end coils up in the kidney pelvis, while the other coils in the bladder.

The placement of the ureteral catheter should be checked frequently, and tension on the catheter should be avoided. The catheter drains urine from the renal pelvis, which has a capacity of 3 to 5 ml. If the volume of urine in the renal pelvis increases, tissue damage to the pelvis will result from pressure. Therefore the ureteral catheter should not be clamped. If the physician orders irrigation of the ureteral catheter, strict aseptic technique is required. If output is decreased, the physician should be notified immediately. Drainage should be checked often (at least every 1 to 2 hours). It is normal for some urine to drain around the ureteral catheter into the bladder. Accurate recording of urine output from both the ureters and the urethral catheter is essential. Sometimes a ureteral catheter may be used as a stent and is not expected to drain. It is important to check with the physician as to the type of catheter and what to expect.

Suprapubic Catheters

Suprapubic catheterization is the simplest and oldest method of urinary diversion. The two methods of insertion of a suprapubic catheter into the bladder are (1) through a small incision in the abdominal wall and (2) by the use of a trocar. A suprapubic catheter is placed while the patient is under general anesthesia for another surgical procedure or at the bedside with a local anesthetic. The catheter is usually sutured into place, but a Foley catheter may also be used. The nursing responsibility includes taping the catheter to prevent dislodgment. The care of the tube and catheter is similar to that of the urethral catheter. A pectin-base skin barrier (e.g., Stomahesive) is effective around the insertion site in protecting the skin from breakdown.

The suprapubic catheter is used in temporary situations such as bladder, vesical neck, prostate, and urethral surgery. Suprapubic catheterization may be used instead of urethral catheterization, especially in the young or infant boy and when a urethral catheter cannot be inserted. The suprapubic catheter is also used long-term in selected patients (e.g., male quadraplegic patient who tends to form penoscrotal fistulas).

A suprapubic catheter is prone to poor drainage because of mechanical obstruction of the catheter tip by the bladder wall, sediment, and clots. Nursing interventions to ensure patency of the tube include (1) preventing tube kinking by coiling the excess tubing and maintaining gravity drainage, (2) having the patient turn from side to side, and (3) milking the tube. If these measures are not effective, the catheter is irrigated with sterile technique after a physician's order has been obtained.

If the patient experiences bladder spasms that are difficult to control, urinary leakage may result. Oxybutinin (Ditropan) or other oral antispasmodics, or belladonna and opium (B + O) suppositories may be prescribed to decrease bladder spasms.

Nephrostomy Tubes

The nephrostomy tube (catheter) is inserted on a temporary basis to preserve renal function when a complete obstruction of the ureter is present. It is inserted directly into the pelvis of the kidney and attached to connecting tubing for closed drainage. The principle is the same as with the ureteral catheter; that is, the catheter should never be kinked, laid upon, or clamped. If the patient complains of excessive pain in the area or if there is excessive drainage around the tube, the catheter should be checked for patency. If irrigation is ordered, strict aseptic technique is required. No more than 5 ml sterile saline solution is gently instilled at one time to prevent overdistention of the kidney pelvis and renal damage. Infection and secondary stone formation are complications associated with the insertion of a nephrostomy tube.

Intermittent Catheterization

An alternative approach to a long-term indwelling catheter is intermittent catheterization. It is being used with increasing frequency in conditions characterized by neurogenic bladder (e.g., spinal cord injuries, chronic neurologic diseases). This type of catheterization may also be used in the oliguric and anuric phases of acute renal failure to reduce the possibility of infection from an indwelling catheter. Intermittent catheterization is also used postoperatively, often after a surgical procedure for female incontinence. The main goal of intermittent catheterization is to prevent urinary retention, stasis, and compromised blood supply to the bladder, that is due to prolonged pressure.

The technique consists of inserting a urethral catheter into the bladder every 3 to 5 hours. The bladder is emptied and the catheter is removed. Lubricant is necessary for men and may make catheterization more comfortable for women. The catheter may be inserted by the patient or the care provider.

In the hospital, sterile technique is used. For home care, a clean technique that includes good hand washing with soap and water is used. There has been no significant increase in infection with the use of an appropriate clean technique as compared with sterile technique. The patient is taught to observe for signs of UTI so that treatment can be instituted early. If indicated, some patients are placed on a regimen of prophylactic antibiotics.

SURGERY OF THE URINARY TRACT

Renal and Ureteral Surgery

The most common indications for nephrectomy are a renal tumor, polycystic kidneys that are bleeding or severely infected, massive traumatic injury to the kidney, and the elective removal of a kidney from a donor. Surgery involving the ureters and kidneys is most commonly performed to remove calculi that become obstructive, correct congenital anomalies, and divert urine when necessary.

Preoperative Management. The basic needs of the patient undergoing renal and ureteral surgery are similar to those of any patient who experiences surgery (see Chapters 14 to 16). In addition, it is especially important preoperatively to ensure adequate fluid intake and a normal electrolyte balance. The patient should be told that there will probably be a flank incision on the affected side and that surgery will require a hyperextended, side-lying position. This position frequently causes the patient to experience muscle aches after surgery. If a nephrectomy is planned, the patient needs to be assured that one working kidney is sufficient to maintain normal renal function.

Postoperative Management. Specific postoperative needs of a patient are related to urine output, respiratory status, and abdominal distention.

Urine output. In the immediate postoperative period, urine output should be determined at least every 1 to 2 hours. Drainage from various catheters should be recorded separately. The catheter or tube should not be clamped or irrigated without a specific order. The total urine output should be at least 30 to 50 ml per hour. It is also important to assess for urine drainage on the dressing and to estimate the amount. Daily weighing of the patient is important. The same scale should be used, properly balanced, and the patient should wear similar clothing and dressings each time.

It is important to observe and monitor the color and consistency of urine. Urine with increased amounts of mucus, blood, or sediment may occlude the drainage tubing or catheter.

Respiratory status. Renal surgery is usually performed through a flank incision just below the diaphragm and frequently involves removal of the twelfth rib. Postoperatively, it is important to ensure adequate ventilation. The patient is often reluctant to turn, cough, and deep breathe because of the incisional pain. Adequate pain medication should be given to ensure the patient's comfort and ability to perform coughing and deep-breathing exercises. Frequently, additional respiratory devices such as an incentive spirometer are used every 2 hours while the patient is awake. In addition, early and frequent ambulation assists in maintaining adequate respiratory function.

Abdominal distention. Abdominal distention is present to some degree in most patients who have had surgery on their kidneys or ureters. It is most commonly due to paralytic ileus caused by manipulation and compression of the bowel during surgery. Oral intake is restricted until bowel sounds are present (usually 24 to 48 hours after surgery). IV fluids are given until the patient can take oral fluids. Progression to a regular diet follows.

Laparoscopic Nephrectomy. Laparoscopic nephrectomy has recently been performed in selected situations to remove a kidney. In contrast to the open incision of about 7 in (18 cm) required in a standard nephrectomy, a laparoscopic nephrectomy is performed using 5 puncture sites of less than .5 in (12 mm). One incision is to view the kidney and the others to dissect it. Once dissected, the kidney is maneuvered into a nylon impermeable sack; while still in the patient, it is chopped up with a tiny rotating blade. The sack and its contents can then be safely removed from the patient.

Urinary Diversion

Removal of the urinary bladder (cystectomy) with diversion of the urine to an external device may be performed in several conditions, including cancer of the bladder, neurogenic bladder, congenital anomalies, strictures, trauma to the bladder, and chronic infections with deterioration of renal function. Several types of surgical procedures are performed (Table 43-15 and Fig. 43-8). The most common type of surgery is the *ileal conduit (ileal loop)*. In this procedure a

Table 43-15 Types of Urinary Diversion Surgery

Type	Description	Advantages	Disadvantages	Special Considerations
▪ Ileal conduit	Ureters are implanted into part of ileum or colon that has been resected from intestinal tract. Abdominal stoma is created.	Relatively good urine flow with few physiologic alterations	External appliance necessary to continually collect urine	Surgical procedure is more complex. Postoperative complications may be increased. Reabsorption of urea by ileum occurs. Meticulous attention is necessary to care for stoma and collecting device.
▪ Cutaneous ureterostomy	Ureters are excised from bladder and brought through abdominal wall, and stoma is created. Ureteral stomas may be created from both ureters, or ureters may be brought together and one stoma created.	No need for major surgery as required with ileal conduit	External appliance necessary because of continuous urine drainage; possibility of stricture or stenosis of small stoma	Periodic catheterizations may be required to dilate stomas to maintain patency.
▪ Nephrostomy	Catheter is inserted into pelvis of kidney. Procedure may be done to one or both kidneys and may be temporary or permanent. It is most frequently done in advanced disease as palliative procedure.	No need for major surgery	High risk of renal infection; predisposition to calculus formation from catheter	Nephrostomy tube may have to be changed every month. Catheter must never be clamped.

6 to 8 in (15 to 20 cm) segment of the ileum is converted into a conduit for urinary drainage. The colon is used (colon conduit) instead of the ileum with increasing frequency. The ureters are anastomosed into one end of the conduit, and the other end of the bowel is brought out through the abdominal wall to form a stoma (Fig. 43-9). Although the segment of bowel remains supported by the mesentery, it is completely isolated from the intestinal tract. The bowel is anastomosed and continues to function normally. Because there is no valve and no voluntary control over the stoma, drops of urine flow from the stoma every few seconds, requiring the use of a permanent external collecting device.

Continent diversions are internal pouches created similarly to the ileal conduit. Large segments of bowel are altered to prevent peristaltic action. A continence mechanism is formed between this large, low-pressure reservoir and the stoma by intussuscepting a portion of bowel. In this way, a patient does not leak involuntarily. The patient with a continent reservoir needs to self-catheterize every 4 to 6 hours but does not need to wear external attachments. Examples of continent diversions are the Kock (Fig. 43-10), Mainz, Indiana, and Florida pouches. A main difference between the various diversions are the segments of bowel used.

All urinary diversions have disadvantages. Strictures often develop with ureterostomies. Pyelonephritis and obstruction occur when tubes drain the kidney. Infection, calculi formation, reabsorption of electrolytes, stomal and skin problems, and increased postoperative complications occur after surgeries for conduit and continent diversions. Incontinence, vesicoureteral reflux, fistula, and bowel dysfunction are additional risks after continent diversion surgery.

Preoperative Management. The patient awaiting cystectomy and ileal conduit or continent diversion needs to be given a great deal of information. The nurse must assess ability and readiness to learn before initiating a teaching program. If the patient is not ready to learn, the teaching plan should be adjusted. The patient's anxiety and fear may be decreased by the information. However, the anxiety and fear may also interfere with learning. The patient's family should be involved in the teaching process. A discussion of the social aspects of living with a stoma (including clothing, changes in body image and sexuality, exercise, and odor) provides the patient with facts that may allay some fears. The patient who will have a continent diversion must be taught to catheterize and irrigate the pouch and be able to adhere to a strict catheterization schedule. Concerns about the effect on sexual activities should be discussed.

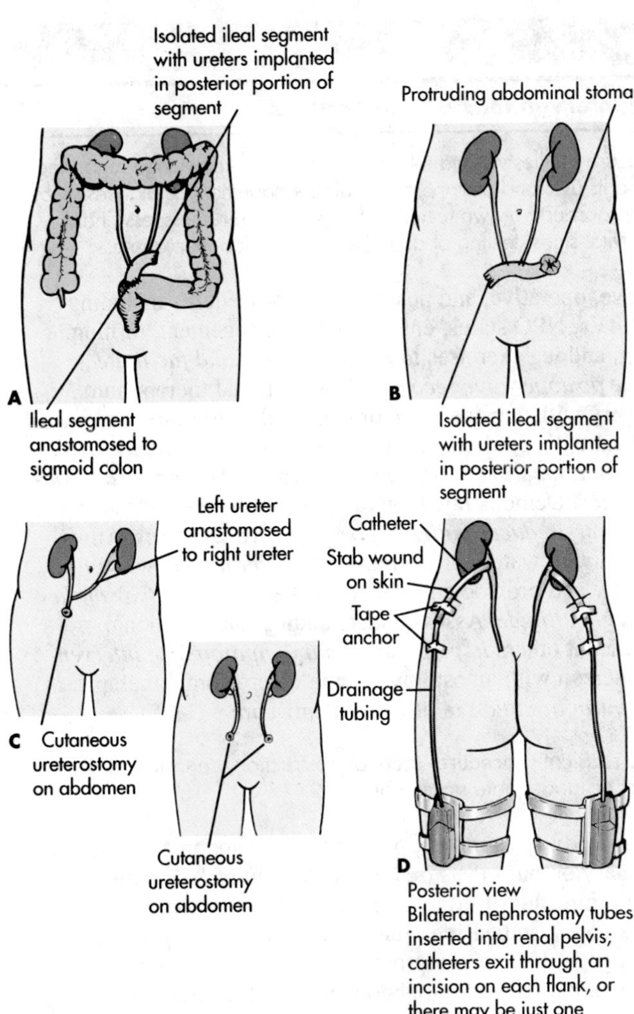

Fig. 43-8 Methods of urinary diversion. ***A,*** Ureteroileosigmoidostomy. ***B,*** Ileal loop (or ileal conduit). ***C,*** Ureterostomy (transcutaneous ureterostomy and bilateral cutaneous ureterostomies). ***D,*** Nephrostomy.

The enterostomal therapy nurse should be involved in the preoperative phase of the patient's care. A visit from an ostomate or enterostomal therapy nurse may be helpful. Additional interventions are presented in the nursing care plan on p. 1366.

Postoperative Management. Nursing interventions during the postoperative period (see the following nursing care plan) should be planned to prevent surgical complications such as postoperative atelectasis and shock (see Chapter 16). After pelvic surgery, there is an increased incidence of thrombophlebitis. With removal of part of the bowel, there is an increased incidence of paralytic ileus and small-bowel obstruction, the patient is NPO, and a nasogastric tube is necessary for 3 to 5 days.

Specific attention should be given to preventing injury to the stoma and maintaining urine output. Mucus is present in the urine because it is secreted by the intestines as a result of the irritating effect of the urine. The patient should be told

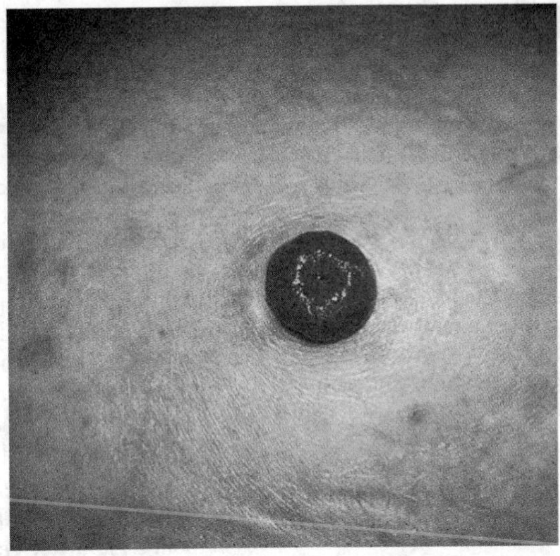

Fig. 43-9 Ideal urinary stoma. It is symmetric, has no skin breakdown, and protrudes about 1.5 cm; the mucosa is a healthy red and the configuration is flat when the patient is upright and supine.

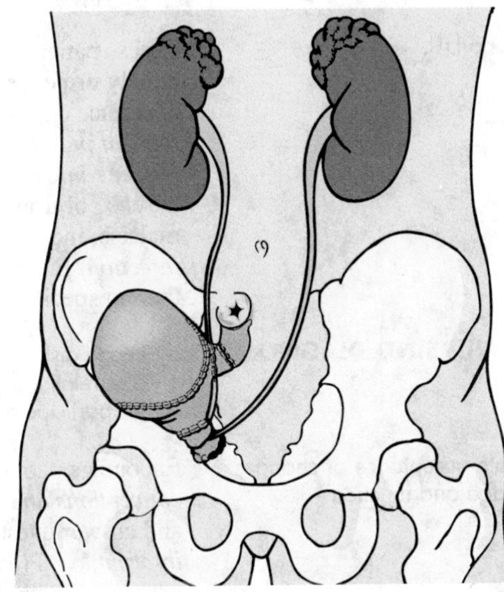

Fig. 43-10 Creation of a Kock pouch with implantation of ureters into one intussuscepted portion of the pouch and creation of a stoma with the other intussuscepted portion.

that this is a normal occurrence. A high fluid intake is encouraged to "flush" the ileal conduit or continent diversion.

When an ileal conduit is created, the skin around the stoma requires meticulous care. Alkaline encrustations with dermatitis may occur when alkaline urine comes in contact with exposed skin (Fig. 43-11). Other common peristomal skin problems include yeast infections, product allergies,

NURSING CARE PLAN Patient with an Ileal Conduit

Planning: Outcome Criteria	Nursing Interventions and Rationales
➤ **NURSING DIAGNOSIS**	Anxiety *related to* effects of procedure on lifestyle and relationships; lack of knowledge regarding surgical procedure, appliance, and its use; and postoperative pain management *as manifested by* frequent questions about surgical procedure; drawn facies; pallor, sweating, restlessness, inability to sleep, talkativeness; increase in vital signs; feeling of apprehension, tension, nervousness
Demonstrate knowledge about preoperative, operative, and postoperative procedures, including both stoma and appliance.	Instruct patient in preoperative, operative, and postoperative procedures including diet, medications, NG tubes, IVs, NPO status, enemas, pain management, turning, coughing and deep breathing, and leg exercises *to reduce anxiety and facilitate patient's progress through the postoperative recovery.* Enterostomal therapy nurse marks stoma site before surgery with consideration of skin folds, old scars, abdominal muscles, clothing lines, and patient's predominant use of right or left hand *to assist surgeon in placing the stoma in a location most convenient for patient and most conducive to a well-fitting appliance.* Demonstrate how to apply appliance and use equipment *as knowledge before surgery reduces patient's postoperative concerns.* Allow patient to wear appliance filled with water under clothing *to determine how it will feel.* Answer questions honestly and provide emotional support *to reduce fear of the unknown and to convey a caring attitude.* Assess understanding and emotional response of patient and significant others *to guide in planning appropriate interventions.* Arrange for visit with person with an ostomy or with enterostomal therapist *to provide patient with significant information related to ostomy care.*
➤ **NURSING DIAGNOSIS**	Risk for ascending UTI *related to* surgical procedure, ureteral obstruction, chronic use of external appliance, and incorrect or inadequate stoma care
Have no UTI.	Assess patient for elevation in body temperature, pain in back or abdomen, bloody or cloudy urine, decrease in urinary output *to ensure early detection of UTI.* Empty appliance q2-3hr or when one-third full of urine *to reduce risk of urinary reflux and to prevent pull on the appliance seal.* Use bedside drainage bag at night *to prevent reflux of urine into conduit.* Instruct patient about symptoms to be reported, including absence of urine, blood in urine, pain in back or abdomen, elevated temperature, malaise, increase in abdominal girth, nausea and vomiting *as indicators of possible infection.* Encourage high fluid intake *to maintain adequate urine flow.* Inform patient that no specific diet is required.
➤ **NURSING DIAGNOSIS**	Body-image disturbance *related to* effects of loss of body parts and change in body function on lifestyle or relationships *as manifested by* negative feelings about self, refusal to look at or touch stoma or participate in self-care, expression of concern about effect on family and lifestyle
Indicate acceptance of changes in image and function.	Encourage patient to share feelings *to provide opportunity to assist with issues and misconceptions and to plan appropriate interventions.* Demonstrate willingness to listen and answer questions *to convey interest in the patient's concerns and to provide needed information.* Provide information about surgery and expected effects *to reduce anxiety associated with the unknown and altered body function.* Determine the need for additional support (e.g., psychiatric support, visit by an ostomate) *as these persons may provide new information and suggestion of ways to modify lifestyle.* Encourage gradual involvement in self-care *as independence in self-care helps to improve self-esteem.*
➤ **NURSING DIAGNOSIS**	Ineffective management of therapeutic regimen *related to* lack of knowledge regarding stoma and appliance care *as manifested by* expression of concern about how to manage ileal conduit and frequent questions or inaccurate responses regarding stoma care
Demonstrate ability to change stoma bag and cleanse stoma; demonstrate ability to maintain permanent appliance.	Demonstrate proper method of changing stoma bag, and have patient give return demonstration *to teach correct care and to evaluate learning.* Have patient change temporary bag under supervision *to gain confidence and ability to manage self-care.* Teach measures such as high fluid intake, regular activity, and urine acidification *to prevent urinary calculi and infection.* Teach practices such as proper care of stoma and pouch; empty or change pouch when ⅓ to ½ full; avoid odor-producing foods such as onions, fish, eggs, cheese; drink cranberry juice or use a liquid appliance deodorant *to reduce odor.*

continued

NURSING CARE PLAN Patient with an Ileal Conduit—cont'd

Planning: Outcome Criteria	*Nursing Interventions and Rationales*
➤ **NURSING DIAGNOSIS**	Risk for impaired skin integrity *related to* ill-fitting appliance, inadequate hygiene, and lack of knowledge regarding stoma care
Have intact, viable stoma; clean and intact skin surrounding stoma.	Assess skin for improperly fitted appliance and reddened and irritated skin around stoma *to ensure prompt identification of the problem.* Check appliance position *to prevent leakage of caustic drainage onto skin.* Observe stoma for any bleeding or eroded areas *for early identification and treatment of complications.* Cleanse stoma as ordered *to reduce encrustations and bacterial contact with the stoma and surrounding skin.* Allow no tight clothing or binders over stoma *to enable unobstructed circulation of blood and flow of urine.*
➤ **NURSING DIAGNOSIS**	Risk for altered sexuality patterns *related to* perceived or actual effects of surgery on sexual activity
Verbalize feelings about changes in sexuality and sexual function; verbalize satisfaction with sexual practices.	Assess patient's concerns related to sexuality such as future sexual functioning and lack of understanding by significant other *to determine presence and extent of problem.* Provide accurate information related to sexual activity *so patient will know the effect of this surgery on sexual activities and practices.* Provide information about penile implant to the male patient when appropriate *so patient can consider this alternative.* Inform female patient about water-based vaginal lubricant for intercourse *to reduce dyspareunia related to inadequate vaginal lubrication*; teach Kegel exercises *to promote control of the pubococcygeal muscles around the vagina to ease dyspareunia.* Provide information and support for spouse or significant other *to reduce concerns and facilitate resumption of sexual relationship as appropriate.*

COLLABORATIVE PROBLEMS

Nursing Goals	*Nursing Interventions and Rationales*
➤ **POTENTIAL COMPLICATION**	Thrombophlebitis *related to* surgery involving pelvic manipulation
Monitor for signs of thrombophlebitis; report deviations from acceptable parameters; and initiate appropriate medical and nursing interventions.	Assess for signs of thrombophlebitis such as diminished or absent lower extremity pulses; assess for swelling, warmth, and pain in legs *to assure early identification and treatment.* Teach patient method to do range-of-motion exercises for legs while in bed, and instruct patient to keep legs uncrossed *to improve circulation in legs and reduce venous stasis.* Turn or help patient turn q2hr while in bed *to improve circulation to all body systems.* Gradually increase activity level and have patient ambulate as soon as possible *to improve circulation, especially in lower extremities.* Provide elastic wraps or elastic gradient compression stockings for legs as ordered *to provide support around veins and improve venous return of blood.* Administer anticoagulants if ordered *to reduce risk of thrombophlebitis by increasing clotting time.*
➤ **POTENTIAL COMPLICATION**	Paralytic ileus *related to* surgical manipulation of bowel
Monitor for signs of paralytic ileus; report deviations from acceptable parameters; initiate appropriate medical and nursing interventions.	Assess patient for signs of paralytic ileus such as absence of bowel sounds, abdominal distention, cramping pain, nausea and vomiting *to enable early identification and treatment.* Maintain patency of NG tube *to prevent accumulation and assure removal of GI secretions.* Encourage early ambulation *to promote peristalsis.* Administer IV fluids as ordered *to maintain fluid and electrolyte balance.* Monitor fluid and electrolyte levels *to identify imbalance and enable prompt treatment.* Assess for presence of bowel sounds, flatus, and bowel movements *as indicators of peristalsis.*

GI, Gastrointestinal; *IV,* intravenous; *NG,* nasogastric; *NPO,* nothing by mouth; *UTI,* urinary tract infection.

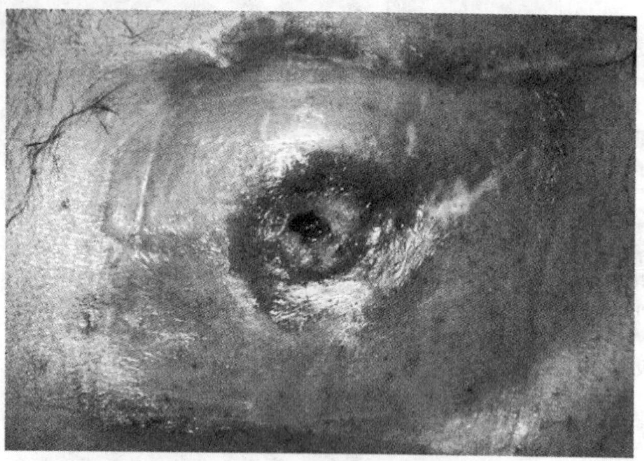

Fig. 43-11 Ammonia salt encrustation secondary to alkaline urine.

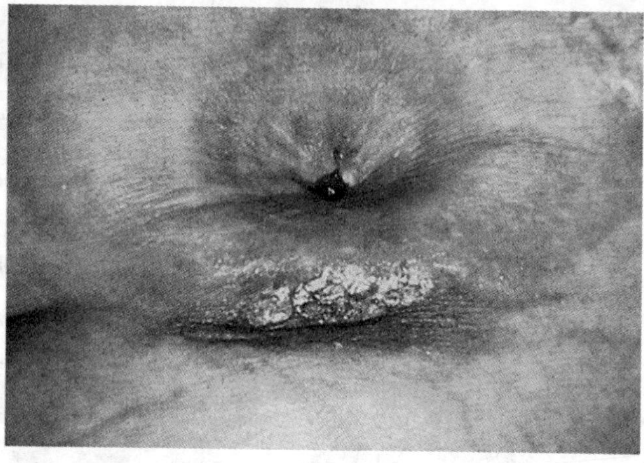

Fig. 43-12 Retracted urinary stoma with pressure sore from faceplate above stoma.

Table 43-16 Guidelines for Changing Ileal Conduit Appliances

Temporary Appliance

1. Cut hole in pouch to fit over stoma (pouch 3.2 mm [⅛ in] larger than stoma).
2. Remove old pouch.
3. Clean area gently and remove old adhesive.
4. Wash area with warm water.
5. Place wick (rolled-up 4 × 4 in pad) over stoma to keep area dry during rest of procedure.
6. Dry skin around stoma.
7. Apply tincture of benzoin or other skin protectant around stoma to area where pouch will be placed.
8. Apply pouch by first smoothing its edges toward side and lower portion of body.
9. Remove wick and complete application of bag.
10. If patient is usually in bed, apply bag so that it lies toward side of body.
11. If patient is ambulatory, apply bag so that it lies vertically.
12. Connect drainage tubing to pouch.
13. Keep drainage pouch on same side of bed as stoma.

Permanent Appliance*

1. Keep appliance in place for 2-14 days.
2. Change appliance when fluid intake has been restricted for several hours.
3. Have patient sit or stand in front of mirror.
4. Moisten edge of faceplate with adhesive solvent and gently remove.
5. Clean skin with adhesive solvent.
6. Wash skin with warm water. (Patient may shower.)
7. Dry skin and inspect.
8. Place wick (rolled up 4 × 4 in pad) over stoma to keep skin free of urine.
9. Apply skin cement to faceplate and skin.
10. Place appliance over stoma.
11. Wash removed appliance with soap and lukewarm water; soak in distilled vinegar; rinse with lukewarm water and air dry.

*Many disposable appliances with self-adhesive backing are used as permanent appliances.

and shearing effect excoriations.[35] Changing appliances is discussed in Table 43-16. A properly fitting appliance is essential to prevent skin problems. The appliance should be about 0.1 inch (0.2 cm) larger than the stoma. It is normal for the stoma to shrink within the first few weeks after surgery. The urine is kept acidic to prevent alkaline encrustations.

Acceptance of the surgery and of alterations in body image is needed to ensure the patient's best adjustment. Concerns of the patient include fear that the stoma will be offensive to others and will interfere with sexual, personal, professional, and recreational activities. The patient should know that few activities, if any, will be restricted as a result of the urinary diversion.

Discharge planning includes teaching the patient symptoms of obstruction or infection and care of the ostomy. The patient with an ileal conduit is fitted for a permanent appliance 7 to 10 days after surgery and may need to be refitted at a later time, depending on the degree of stoma shrinkage. Appliances are made of a variety of products, including natural and synthetic rubbers, plastics, and metals. Most appliances have a faceplate that adheres to the skin, a collecting pouch, and an opening to drain the pouch. The faceplate may be secured to the skin with glues, adhesives, or adhering synthetic wafers. Some appliances do not require adhesives, but their design relies on pressure to keep the pouch in place. If improperly fitted or applied, the faceplate may cause skin problems (Fig. 43-12). The patient needs information on where to purchase supplies, emergency telephone numbers, location of ostomy clubs, and follow-up visits with an enterostomal therapist. Physician follow-up is imperative to monitor and correct homeostatic abnormalities and to prevent complications or renal function deterioration.

CRITICAL THINKING EXERCISES

CASE STUDY

URINARY TRACT INFECTION

Patient Profile

Sue, a 28-year-old woman, was seen in the nurse practitioner's office for a history of painful, frequent urination.

Subjective Data

- Has had a history of painful, frequent urination with passage of small volumes of urine for 3 days
- Has had intermittent fever, chills, and back pain during these 3 days
- Was frightened when she saw blood in her urine
- Is anxious because her father died of kidney cancer

Objective Data

Physical Examination

- Complains of bilateral flank pain and abdominal tenderness to palpation
- Temperature is 100.4° F (38° C)

Diagnostic Study

- Urine culture was positive for *E. coli*

Critical Thinking Questions

1. What are the most common organisms that cause UTIs?
2. What factors predispose a patient to a UTI?
3. What is the difference between upper and lower UTIs?
4. What nursing interventions will help Sue cope with her symptoms?
5. What can the nurse do to help Sue prevent another UTI?
6. Based on the data presented, write one or more appropriate nursing diagnoses. Are there any collaborative problems?

NURSING RESEARCH ISSUES

1. In the patient with UTI, what are the most effective methods to ensure compliance with therapy and follow-up care?
2. What therapeutic measures are most effective in treating stress incontinence?
3. What are the differences in quality of life of the patient with an ileal conduit as compared with the patient with a continent urinary diversion?
4. What are the most effective ways to manage pain following lithotripsy?

REVIEW QUESTIONS

The number of the question corresponds to the same-numbered objective at the beginning of the chapter.

1. The organisms that cause pyelonephritis most commonly reach the kidneys by which of the following means?

a. Descending infection
b. Ascending infection
c. Bloodstream
d. Lymphatic system

2. Women who are especially susceptible to UTIs should

a. take prophylactic sulfonamides for the rest of their lives.
b. drink at least 2 to 3 L of fluid per day.
c. take tub baths with bubble bath.
d. cleanse themselves from the rectum to the urethra after toileting.

3. The immunologic mechanisms involved in glomerulonephritis include all of the following *except*

a. activation of complement resulting in release of chemotactic factors.
b. deposition of immune complexes along the GBM.
c. destruction of glomeruli by proteolytic enzymes contained in the GBM.
d. release of kinins and vasoactive amines.

4. Clinical manifestations of acute pyelonephritis include

a. elevated blood pressure.
b. albuminuria and edema.
c. bacteria and WBCs in the urine.
d. immune complexes in the blood.

5. The edema that occurs in nephrotic syndrome is due to

a. increased hydrostatic pressure caused by sodium retention.
b. decreased colloidal osmotic pressure caused by loss of serum albumin.
c. decreased aldosterone secretion from adrenal insufficiency.
d. increased colloidal osmotic pressure caused by increased serum albumin.

6. Clinical manifestations of renal calculi include

a. dribbling at the end of urination and pyuria.
b. severe flank pain and hematuria.
c. frequency of urination and polyuria.
d. urgent, uncontrollable urination.

7. Which of the following is inherited as an autosomal dominant disorder?

a. Adult-onset polycystic renal disease
b. Horseshoe kidney
c. Malignant nephrosclerosis
d. Exstrophy of the bladder

8. Renal tissue changes that may occur in diabetes mellitus include
   a. glomerulosclerosis and pyelonephritis.
   b. renal sugar-crystal calculi and cysts.
   c. lipid deposits in the glomerulus and nephrons.
   d. uric acid calculi and nephrolithiasis.

9. The classic manifestations of advanced renal adenocarcinoma include all the following *except*
   a. palpable mass.
   b. gross hematuria.
   c. flank pain.
   d. renal colic.

10. Which of the following measures is not appropriate for a bladder-training program for incontinence?
   a. Limiting fluid intake at bedtime
   b. Muscle-strengthening exercises
   c. Scheduled voiding times
   d. Clamping and releasing catheter to increase bladder tone

11. A patient with a ureterolithotomy returns from surgery with a nephrostomy tube in place. Which of the following should be included in nursing care?
   a. Notify the physician if nephrostomy tube drainage is more than 30 ml per hr.
   b. Irrigate the nephrostomy tube with 10 ml of normal saline solution as needed.
   c. After nausea has subsided, encourage fluids of at least 2 to 3 L per day.
   d. Encourage patient to drink fruit juices and milk.

12. A patient has had a cystectomy and ileal conduit diversion performed. Four days postoperatively, mucous shreds are seen in the drainage bag. The nurse should
   a. notify the physician.
   b. notify the charge nurse.
   c. chart it as a normal observation.
   d. irrigate the drainage tube.

REFERENCES

1. Yoshikawa TT: Chronic urinary tract infections in elderly patients, *Hosp Pract* 28:103, 1993.
2. Stamm WE: Nosocomial urinary tract infection. In Bennett JV, Brachman PS, editors: *Hospital infections,* ed 3, Boston, 1992, Little, Brown, & Co.
3. Levine FS, Staskin DR: Genitourinary infection. In Siroky MB, Crane RJ: *Manual of urology diagnosis and therapy,* ed 1, Boston, 1990, Little, Brown, & Co.
4. Schaeffer AJ: Infections of the urinary tract. In Walsh PC and others, editors: *Campbell's urology,* ed 6, Philadelphia, 1992, WB Saunders.
5. Kunin CM: *Detection, prevention, and management of urinary tract infections,* ed 4, Philadelphia, 1987, Lea and Febiger.
6. Johnson JR, Stamm WE: Urinary tract infections in women: diagnosis and treatment, *Ann Intern Med* 111:906, 1989.
7. Pearson BD: Liquidate a myth: reducing liquid intake is not advisable for elderly with urine control problems, *Urol Nurs* 13:86, 1993.
8. Batra AK, Wein AJ, Hanno PM: *Interstitial cystitis* (AUA Update Series), Houston, 1993, American Urological Association, Inc.
9. Gow JG: Genitourinary tuberculosis. In Walsh PC and others, editors: *Campbell's urology,* ed 6, Philadelphia, 1992, WB Saunders.
10. Gray M: *Genitourinary disorders,* St Louis, 1992, Mosby.
11. Tejani A, Inguilli E: Poststreptococcal glomerulonephritis: current clinical and pathologic changes, *Nephron* 55:1, 1990.
12. Wiseman KC: New insights on Goodpasture's syndrome, *ANNA J* 20:17, 1993.
13. Cole E: Plasma exchange in rapidly progressive glomerulonephritis, *Apheresis* 1:257, 1990.
14. Bernard DB: Nephrotic syndrome: a clinical approach, *Hosp Pract* 25:114, 1990.
15. Seney FD and others: Acquired immunodeficiency syndrome and the kidney, *Am J Kidney Dis* 16:1, 1990.
16. Schoenfeld P, Feduska NJ: Acquired immunodeficiency syndrome and renal disease: report of the National Kidney Foundation—National Institutes of Health Task Force on AIDS and Kidney Disease, *Am J Kidney Dis* 16:14, 1990.
17. Pak CYC: The many facets of kidney stone disease, *Contemp Urol* 2:56, 1990.
18. Preminger GM: Is there a need for medical evaluation and treatment of nephrolithiasis in the "Age of lithotripsy?" *Semin Urol* 12:51, 1994.
19. Freeman NL: Ureteroscopic laser lithotripsy and extracorporeal shock wave lithotripsy: the advantage of both in a lithotripsy center, *Urol Nurs* 11:28, 1991.
20. Marshall B: Laser lithotripsy: a nursing perspective, *Urol Nurs* 11:25, 1991.
21. Zhong P, Preminger GM: Differing modes of shock-wave generation, *Semin Urol* 12:2, 1994.
22. Wilson WT, Preminger GM: Extracorporeal shock wave lithotripsy—an update, *Urol Clin North Am* 17:231, 1990.
23. Segura JW: Extracorporeal shock wave lithotripsy. In JF Glenn, editor: *Urologic surgery,* ed 4, Philadelphia, 1991, Lippincott.
24. Curhan GC and others: A prospective study of dietary calcium and other nutrients and the risks of symptomatic kidney stones, *N Engl J Med* 328:833, 1993.
25. Sox MA, Fabian TC: The pelvis. In Moore EE and others, editors: *Early care of the injured patient,* ed 4, Philadelphia, 1990, BC Decker.
26. Blank CA, Irwin GH, Mascitti-Mazur JE: Genitourinary trauma: Part 1, diagnostic testing, renal and ureteral trauma, *Urol Nurs* 11:11, 1991.
27. Debruyne FMJ and others: *New prospects in the management of metastatic renal cell carcinoma: experimental and clinical data, Urooncology: current status and future trends,* 1990, Willey-Liss.
28. de Kernion JB: Renal tumors. In Walsh PC and others, editors: *Campbell's urology,* ed 6, Philadelphia, 1992, WB Saunders.
29. Moore S and others: Treating bladder cancer: new methods, new management, *AJN* 93:32, 1993.
30. Switters DM, Soares SE, deVere White RW: Nursing care of the patient receiving intravesical chemotherapy, *Urol Nurs* 12:136, 1992.
31. McCormick KA and others: A practical guideline for urinary incontinence: the challenge to nurses, *Urol Nurs* 12:40, 1992.
32. Urinary Incontinence Guideline Panel: *Urinary incontinence in adults: clinical practice guideline.* AHCPR Pub. No. 92-0038. Rockville, MD, Agency for Health Care Policy and Research, Public Health Service, US Department of Health and Human Services, 1992.
33. Steele D: Neurophysiology of voiding, *Innovations Urol Nurs* 4:2, 1993.
34. Moore K, Metcalfe JB: Effectiveness of vaginal cones in treatment of urinary incontinence, *Urol Nurs* 12:69, 1992.
35. Maidl L: Stomal and peristomal skin complications with urostomies, *Urol Nurs* 10:17, 1990.

Chapter 44

NURSING ROLE IN MANAGEMENT

Acute and Chronic Renal Failure

Tricia McCarley Sharon L. Lewis

Learning Objectives

1. Differentiate between acute and chronic renal failure.
2. Differentiate among the causes of prerenal, intrarenal, and postrenal acute renal failure.
3. Describe the clinical course of reversible acute renal failure.
4. Explain the therapeutic and nursing management for a patient in the oliguric and diuretic phases of acute renal failure.
5. Describe the systemic effects of chronic renal failure.
6. Explain the conservative management and the related nursing management of the patient with chronic renal failure.
7. Differentiate between peritoneal dialysis and hemodialysis in terms of purpose, indications for use, advantages and disadvantages, and nursing responsibilities.
8. Compare common vascular access sites used for hemodialysis.
9. Compare dialysis and renal transplantation as methods of treatment for end-stage renal disease.
10. Describe the nursing management of patients in the preoperative, intraoperative, and postoperative stages of kidney transplantation.
11. Explain the long-term problems of the patient with a kidney transplant.

Renal failure is severe impairment or total lack of kidney function. In renal failure there is an inability to excrete metabolic waste products and water, as well as functional disturbances of all body systems. Renal failure is classified as *acute* or *chronic*. Acute renal failure most commonly has a rapid onset. In contrast, chronic renal failure usually develops insidiously over time and necessitates the initiation of dialysis or transplantation for long-term survival.

Although acute renal failure is potentially reversible, the mortality rate remains distressingly high in spite of advances in treatment. The focus in chronic renal failure has changed from treating a terminally ill patient to dealing with a person who has a manageable chronic disease that requires long-term care. The change in focus is a result of the technical advances in dialysis and improved surgical techniques, as well as immunosuppressive therapy in renal transplantation.

ACUTE RENAL FAILURE

Acute renal failure is a clinical syndrome characterized by a rapid decline in renal function with progressive *azotemia* (an accumulation of nitrogenous waste products such as blood urea nitrogen [BUN]) and increasing levels of serum creatinine. *Uremia* is the condition in which azotemia progresses to a symptomatic state. Acute renal failure is usually associated with a decrease in urinary output to less than 400 ml per day (oliguria), although it is possible to have normal or increased urinary output. There is no correlation between the amount of urine produced and the severity of the renal failure.

Acute renal failure usually develops over hours or days with progressive elevations of BUN, creatinine, and potassium with or without oliguria. Most commonly, acute renal failure follows prolonged hypotension or hypovolemia or contact with a nephrotoxic agent.

Etiology and Pathophysiology

The etiologies of acute renal failure are multiple and complex. They are categorized according to similar pathogenesis into prerenal, intrarenal (or renal parenchymal), and postrenal causes (Table 44-1).

Prerenal causes consist of factors outside the kidneys that impair renal blood flow and lead to decreased glomerular perfusion and filtration. Prerenal disease can lead to intrarenal disease (tubular necrosis) if renal ischemia is prolonged. Prerenal causes are the most common, accounting for 50% to 70% of all cases of acute renal failure.[1]

Intrarenal causes include conditions that lead to actual damage to the renal tissue (parenchyma) resulting in mal-

Reviewed by Mary Jo Holechek, RN, CNN, MS, Senior Transplant Coordinator for Kidney, Liver, and Pancreas, Johns Hopkins Hospital, Baltimore, MD.

Table 44-1 Common Causes of Acute Renal Failure

Prerenal	Intrarenal	Postrenal
▪ Hypovolemia caused by: Hemorrhage Burns Dehydration Prolonged diarrhea or vomiting ▪ Decreased cardiac output caused by: Myocardial infarction Cardiac dysrhythmias Congestive heart failure Cardiogenic shock Pericardial tamponade Surgery (e.g., open heart) ▪ Decreased peripheral vascular resistance caused by: Septic shock Anaphylaxis ▪ Renal vascular obstruction caused by: Thrombosis of renal arteries Bilateral renal vein thrombosis Embolism	▪ Nephrotoxic injury from the following: Drugs (aminoglycosides [gentamicin, tobramycin, amikacin], amphotericin B, cisplatin) Radiographic contrast agents Hemolytic blood transfusion reaction (hemoglobin blocks tubules) Severe crushing injury (myoglobin released from muscles blocks tubules) Chemicals (ethylene glycol, mercuric chloride, carbon tetrachloride, lead, arsenic) ▪ Acute glomerulonephritis ▪ Acute pyelonephritis ▪ Toxemia of pregnancy ▪ Malignant hypertension ▪ Systemic lupus erythematosus ▪ Interstitial nephritis Allergic (antibiotics [sulfonamides, rifampin], nonsteroidal anti-inflammatory drugs, ACE inhibitors) Infection (bacterial [e.g., acute pyelonephritis], viral [e.g., CMV], fungal [e.g., candidiasis])	▪ Calculi formation ▪ Benign prostatic hyperplasia ▪ Prostate cancer ▪ Bladder cancer ▪ Trauma (to back, pelvis, or perineum) ▪ Strictures ▪ Spinal cord disease

ACE, Angiotensin-converting enzyme; *CMV*, cytomegalovirus.

functioning of nephrons. Primary renal diseases such as acute glomerulonephritis and acute pyelonephritis may lead to acute renal failure. More commonly, acute tubular necrosis (ATN) is the predisposing insult. ATN may be caused by ischemia, nephrotoxins (e.g., antibiotics), hemoglobin released from hemolyzed red blood cells (RBCs), or myoglobin released from necrotic muscle cells. Nephrotoxic chemicals and drugs can cause obstruction of intrarenal structures by crystallization or actual damage to the epithelial cells of the tubules. The most common pharmacologic agents that cause nephrotoxic injury are aminoglycoside antibiotics, radiocontrast agents, angiotensin-converting enzyme (ACE) inhibitors, and nonsteroidal antiinflammatory drugs. Hemoglobin and myoglobin block the tubules and cause renal vasoconstriction. Intrarenal causes account for 20% to 30% of all cases of acute renal failure.[1]

Postrenal causes involve mechanical obstruction of urinary outflow. As the flow of urine is blocked, urine backs up into the renal pelvis, ultimately resulting in renal failure. The most common causes are prostate cancer, benign prostatic hyperplasia, calculi, trauma, and tumors. Postrenal causes of acute renal failure account for 1% to 10% of cases with a higher incidence among the elderly.[1] These causes are almost always treatable.

The two major mechanisms that lead to acute renal failure are renal ischemia and nephrotoxic injury (Fig. 44-1). Acute renal failure that results from these two causes is usually referred to as ATN. Severe renal ischemia causes a disruption in the basement membrane and patchy destruction of the tubular epithelium. Nephrotoxic agents cause necrosis of tubular epithelial cells, which slough off and plug the tubules. Nephrotoxic injury usually leaves the basement membrane intact. ATN is potentially reversible if the basement membrane is not destroyed and if the necrotic tubular epithelium regenerates.

Possible pathologic processes involved in acute renal failure include the following:[2,3]

1. *Renal vasoconstriction:* Hypovolemia and decreased renal blood flow stimulate renin release, which activates the angiotensin-aldosterone system (see Fig. 42-6) and results in constriction of the peripheral arteries and the renal afferent arterioles. With decreased blood flow, there is decreased glomerular capillary pressure and glomerular filtration rate

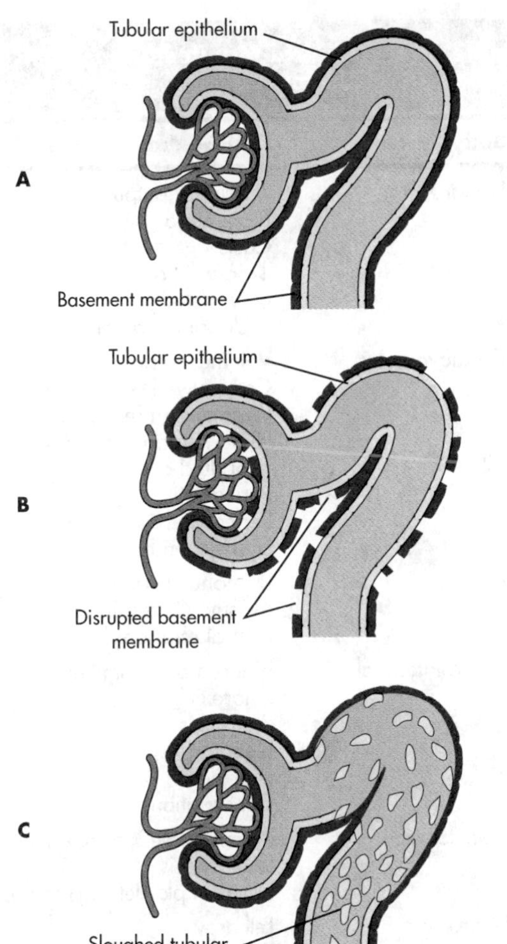

Fig. 44-1 Nephron destruction in acute renal failure. ***A,*** Normal nephron. ***B,*** Damage from renal ischemia results in patchy necrosis of the tubule. The lumen may also be blocked by casts. ***C,*** Damage from nephrotoxic agents.

(GFR), as well as tubular dysfunction and, ultimately, oliguria.

2. *Cellular edema:* Ischemia causes anoxia, which leads to endothelial cell edema. Cellular edema raises tissue pressures above capillary flow pressure; consequently, blood flow through the arterioles may still be altered after treatment of the underlying condition. Inadequate renal blood flow further depresses the GFR.

3. *Decreased glomerular capillary permeability:* Ischemia alters glomerular epithelial cells and thus decreases glomerular capillary permeability. This in turn reduces the GFR, which significantly reduces tubular blood flow and leads to tubular dysfunction.

4. *Intratubular obstruction:* When tubules are damaged, interstitial edema occurs, and necrotic epithelial cells accumulate in the tubules. This accumulated debris also lowers the GFR by obstructing the tubules and increasing intratubular pressure.

5. *Leakage of glomerular filtrate:* Glomerular filtrate leaks back into plasma through holes in the damaged tubular membranes, which decreases intratubular fluid flow.

Clinical Course

Clinically acute renal failure may progress through the phases of oliguria, diuresis, and recovery. In some situations the patient does not recover from acute renal failure, and chronic renal failure results.

Oliguric Phase. The most common initial manifestation of acute renal failure is oliguria caused by a reduction in the GFR. The oliguria usually occurs within 1 to 7 days of the causative event. If the cause is ischemia, oliguria may occur within 24 hours, but when nephrotoxic drugs are involved, the onset may be delayed for as long as a week. Initially, the presence of anuria is rare unless the precipitating cause is a urinary obstructive disorder. (*Acute nonoliguric renal failure* may also occur. In this situation, the onset may be less obvious with hypervolemia or an elevated BUN as the first presenting abnormality.) The duration of the oliguric phase may range from a few days to several weeks. Some cases have lasted for several months. The average duration is about 10 to 14 days, but it rarely exceeds 4 weeks. The longer the oliguric phase lasts, the poorer the prognosis for recovery of renal function.

It is important to distinguish prerenal oliguria from oliguria of acute intrarenal failure. In prerenal oliguria there is no damage to the renal tissue. The oliguria is caused by a decrease in circulating blood volume (e.g., as a result of shock, burns, severe dehydration, decreased cardiac output) and is potentially reversible. (Many causes of intrarenal failure are also potentially reversible.) Prerenal oliguria is characterized by urine with a high specific gravity and a low sodium concentration. In contrast, oliguria of intrarenal failure is characterized by urine with a low specific gravity and a high sodium concentration. Prerenal oliguria can be potentially reversed by correcting the precipitating factor. For example, fluid replacement can be used to treat hypovolemia.

The manifestations of the oliguric phase are changes in urinary output, fluid and electrolyte abnormalities, and uremia. The nurse must be alert for the signs and symptoms of these changes.

Urinary changes. Urinary output decreases to less than 400 ml per 24 hours. The urine may be bloody. A urinalysis may show casts, RBCs, white blood cells (WBCs), a specific gravity fixed at around 1.010, and urine osmolality at about 300 mOsm/kg. This is the same specific gravity and osmolality as for plasma, reflecting tubular damage with a loss of concentrating ability by the kidney. Proteinuria may be present if the renal failure is related to glomerular membrane dysfunction.

Fluid volume excess. When urinary output decreases, fluid retention occurs. The neck veins become distended, the pulse becomes more bounding, and edema and hypertension may develop. Fluid overload can eventually lead to congestive heart failure, pulmonary edema, and pericardial and pleural effusions.

Metabolic acidosis. In renal failure the kidneys cannot synthesize ammonia, which is needed for H^+ excretion, or excrete acid metabolites. The bicarbonate level decreases because bicarbonate is used up in buffering hydrogen ions. In addition, defective reabsorption and regeneration of bicarbonate occur. The patient may develop Kussmaul's (rapid, deep) respirations to increase the excretion of carbon dioxide.

Sodium balance. Damaged tubules cannot conserve sodium. Consequently, the urinary excretion of sodium may increase, resulting in normal or below normal levels of serum sodium. However, excessive intake of sodium should be avoided as it can lead to volume expansion, hypertension, and congestive heart failure.

Potassium excess. The serum potassium levels increase since the normal ability of the kidneys to excrete 80% to 90% of the body's potassium is impaired. If the acute renal failure was caused by massive tissue trauma, the damaged cells release additional potassium to the extracellular fluid. Thus the patient with tissue injury may have a higher serum potassium level. In addition, acidosis enhances the movement of potassium from intracellular to extracellular fluid.

When potassium levels exceed 6 mEq/L (6 mmol/L), treatment must be initiated immediately to prevent cardiac dysrhythmias. Before clinical signs of hyperkalemia are apparent, the electrocardiogram (ECG) will show tall, peaked T waves, widening of the QRS complex, and ST depression. Progressive changes in the ECG, which are related to increasing potassium levels, are depicted in Fig. 13-13.

Calcium deficit and phosphate excess. A low serum calcium level results from decreased gastrointestinal (GI) absorption of calcium. To absorb calcium from the GI tract, activated vitamin D must be present. Only functioning kidneys can activate vitamin D, allowing absorption to occur. Elevated serum phosphate levels are a result of its decreased excretion by the kidneys. Normally most plasma calcium is found ionized (physiologically active form) or bound to protein. In renal failure it is unusual for hypocalcemia to be symptomatic because acidosis keeps more calcium in an ionized form. Sometimes a low serum level of ionized calcium can lead to tetany.

Nitrogenous product accumulation. The kidneys are the primary excretory organs for urea, an end-product of protein metabolism and creatinine, an end-product of endogenous muscle metabolism. The BUN and serum creatinine levels are elevated in renal failure. Catabolism, caused by factors such as infections, fever, severe injury, or GI bleeding, will cause further elevations of BUN.

Eventually all body systems become involved in the acute uremic syndrome (Table 44-2). The extrarenal manifestations are generally similar to those found in the patient with chronic uremia (Fig. 44-2).

Table 44-2 Clinical Manifestations of Acute Uremia

Body System	Clinical Manifestations
Urinary	↓ Urinary output Proteinuria Casts ↓ Specific gravity ↓ Osmolality ↑ Urinary sodium
Cardiovascular	Volume overload Congestive heart failure Hypotension (early) Hypertension (after development of fluid overload) Pericarditis Pericardial effusion Dysrhythmias
Respiratory	Pulmonary edema Kussmaul's respiration Pleural effusions
Gastrointestinal	Nausea and vomiting Anorexia Stomatitis Bleeding Diarrhea Constipation
Hematologic	Anemia (development within 48 hr) Leukocytosis Defect in platelet functioning
Neurologic	Lethargy Convulsions Asterixis Memory impairment
Others	↑ Susceptibility to infection ↑ BUN ↑ Creatinine ↑ Potassium ↓ pH ↓ Bicarbonate ↓ Calcium ↑ Phosphate

BUN, Blood urea nitrogen.

Diuretic Phase. The diuretic phase begins with a gradual increase in daily urine output of 1 to 3 L per day but may reach 3 to 5 L per day or more. Although urine output is increasing, the kidneys are still not completely healed.[4] The high urine volume is caused by osmotic diuresis from the high urea concentration in the glomerular filtrate and the inadequate concentrating ability of the tubules. In this phase the kidneys have recovered their ability to excrete wastes but not to concentrate the urine.

At this stage the uremia may still be severe, as reflected by low creatinine clearances and elevated serum creatinine and BUN levels. Because of the large losses of fluid and electrolytes, the patient must be monitored for hyponatremia, hypokalemia, and dehydration. The diuretic phase may last 1 to 3 weeks. Near the end of this phase the patient's acid-base, electrolyte, and waste product parameters begin to normalize.

Recovery Phase. The recovery phase begins when the GFR increases so that BUN and serum creatinine levels start to stabilize and then decrease. Although the major improvements occur in the first 1 to 2 weeks of this phase, renal function can continue to improve for up to 12 months after acute renal failure.

The outcome of acute renal failure is influenced by the patient's overall health, the severity of renal failure, and the number and type of complications. The mortality rate from acute renal failure varies from 30% to 60%, depending on the cause. Patients with ATN and oliguria have a 50% risk

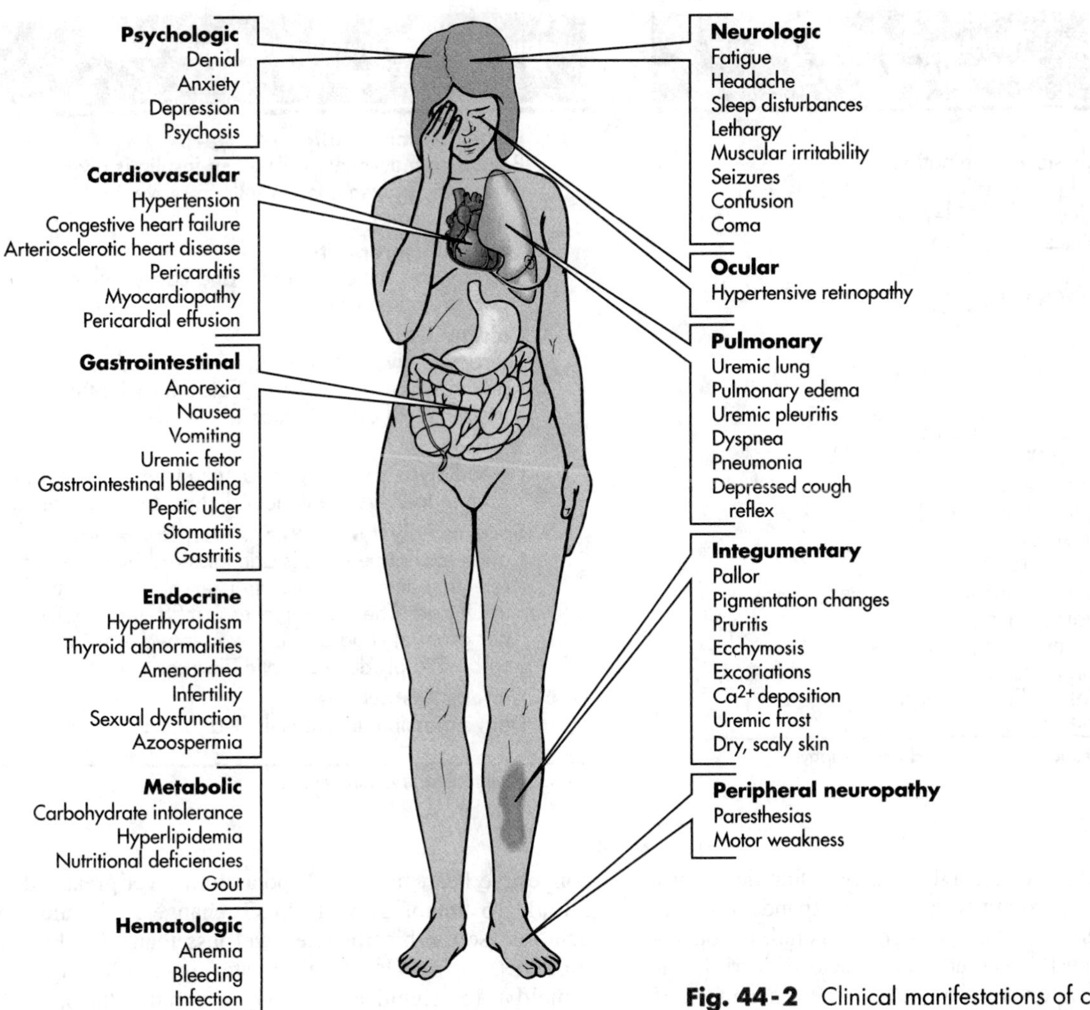

Fig. 44-2 Clinical manifestations of chronic uremia.

of mortality, especially when there is an underlying disease.[1] Many deaths are related to the underlying disease. However, the most common cause of death is infection. Infection occurs in 30% to 70% of individuals who develop acute renal failure.[5] The incidence of infection is highest in the individual in whom surgery or traumatic injury contributed to renal failure.

Some individuals do not recover and progress to chronic renal failure. The older adult patient recovers normal renal function less frequently than the younger patient. Among the individuals who recover, the vast majority achieve clinically normal renal function with no complications (e.g., hypertension).

Diagnostic Studies

The most important tool for distinguishing prerenal, intrarenal, and postrenal causes is the history, including a thorough review of recent clinical events and drug therapy. Prerenal causes should be suspected when there is a history of heart disease or extracellular fluid volume loss or depletion. Intrarenal causes may be suspected if the patient has been taking potentially nephrotoxic medication or has a history of systemic disorders such as systemic lupus erythematosus. Postrenal causes are suggested by a history of changes in urinary stream, hematuria or pyuria, or cancer of the bladder or prostate.

Urinalysis is an important diagnostic test. Urine sediment containing abundant cells, casts, or proteins suggests intrarenal disorders. ATN is associated with abundant urinary casts. Normal urine sediment is possible in both prerenal and postrenal causes. Hematuria, pyuria, and crystals may be associated with postrenal causes.

If the cause of acute renal failure is difficult to determine from the history and physical examination, further testing may be necessary such as a renal scan, renal ultrasound, retrograde pyelogram, computed tomography (CT) scan, or magnetic resonance imaging (MRI).

Therapeutic Management

Because acute renal failure is potentially reversible, the primary goal of treatment is to maintain the patient in as normal a state as possible while the kidneys are repairing themselves (Table 44-3). The precipitating cause is determined and corrected if possible. Management is focused on controlling the patient's symptoms and preventing complications. The first step is to correct hypovolemia and maintain cardiac output

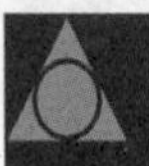

Table 44-3 Therapeutic Management: Acute Renal Failure

Diagnostic
- History and physical examination
- Identification of precipitating cause
- Serum creatinine and BUN levels
- Serum electrolytes
- Urinalysis
- Retrograde pyelogram
- Renal scan
- Renal ultrasound
- CT scan

Therapeutic
- Treatment of precipitating cause
- Fluid restriction (500-600 ml plus fluid loss)
- Nutritional management
  - Adequate protein provision (1.0-1.5 g/kg)
  - Phosphate restriction
  - Sodium restriction
- Measures to lower potassium (if elevated)*
- Phosphate-binding agents
- Total parenteral nutrition (if indicated)
- Enteral nutrition (if indicated)
- Initiation of dialysis (if necessary)

BUN, Blood urea nitrogen; *CT,* computed tomography.
*See Table 44-4.

Table 44-4 Therapies to Lower Serum Potassium Levels

1. **Insulin Administration IV**
   Potassium moves into cells when insulin is given. Glucose is given concurrently to prevent hypoglycemia.
2. **Sodium Bicarbonate**
   Therapy can correct acidosis and cause shift of potassium into cells.
3. **Calcium Gluconate IV**
   Therapy is given IV and is generally used in advanced cardiac toxicity. Calcium raises the threshold for dysrhythmias.
4. **Dialysis**
   Hemodialysis can bring potassium levels to normal in 30 min to 2 hrs. Peritoneal dialysis takes longer.
5. **Sodium Polystyrene Sulfonate (Kayexalate)**
   Cation-exchange resin is administered by mouth or retention enema. Potassium is exchanged for Na^+ in GI tract. Therapy removes 1 mEq of potassium per gram of drug and is mixed in water with sorbitol to produce osmotic diarrhea.
6. **Dietary Restrictions**
   Daily potassium intake is limited to 2 g (50 mEq).

GI, Gastrointestinal; *IV,* intravenous.

to ensure adequate perfusion of the kidneys. Diuretic therapy is often administered along with volume expanders to prevent volume overload. Diuretic therapy includes loop diuretics (furosemide [Lasix], ethacrynic acid [Edecrin], bumetanide [Bumex]) or an osmotic diuretic (mannitol). If acute renal failure is already established, forcing fluids and diuresis is not effective and may in fact be harmful. Conservative therapy may be all that is necessary until renal function resumes. However, the general trend is to initiate early and frequent dialysis to keep the patient as free of symptoms as possible and to prevent complications.

Fluid intake must be closely monitored during the oliguric phase. The common rule for calculating fluid replacement is to consider all losses (e.g., urine, diarrhea, vomitus, blood) plus 500 to 600 ml for insensible losses in a 24-hour period. For the next 24-hour period, the patient's fluid intake is restricted to the previous day's losses. For example, if a patient excreted 300 ml of urine on Tuesday with no other losses, fluid replacement on Wednesday would be 800 to 900 ml.

Hyperkalemia is one of the most dangerous complications in acute renal failure because it can cause life-threatening cardiac dysrhythmias. The various therapies used to decrease potassium levels are listed in Table 44-4. The first three measures described in the table constitute only temporary treatment and do not result in a decrease in total body potassium. The fourth and fifth measures result in actual loss of potassium from the body.

The most common indications for the use of dialysis in acute renal failure include (1) volume overload resulting in congestive heart failure, (2) potassium level greater than 6 mEq/L (6 mmol/L) with ECG changes, (3) metabolic acidosis (serum bicarbonate level less than 15 mEq/L [15 mmol/L]), (4) BUN level greater than 120 mg/dl (43 mmol/L), (5) significant change in mental status, and (6) pericarditis, pericardial effusion, or cardiac tamponade.

Hemodialysis (HD) has the advantage of efficiency and shorter duration compared with peritoneal dialysis (PD). However, it is technically more complicated and may require anticoagulation therapy. Rapid biochemical changes on HD may induce side effects such as hypotension and dialysis disequilibrium syndrome. PD is simpler than HD but carries the risk of peritonitis, is less efficient in the catabolic patient, and takes longer. PD may be preferred for the individual with intracranial bleeding or cardiovascular instability. HD is preferred for the hypercatabolic patient and for the individual who has had abdominal or thoracic trauma or surgery. (HD and PD are discussed later in this chapter.)

Continuous renal replacement therapy (CRRT) may also be used in the treatment of acute renal failure. (CRRT is discussed later in this chapter.) In the hemodynamically unstable patient, CRRT provides gradual removal of excess fluid and solutes. It is technically similar to HD and requires extracorporeal blood circulation via cannulation of an artery and vein. Blood removed from the artery or vein passes through a hemofilter where solutes and water are removed, and then the blood is returned to the patient. CRRT is used continuously and requires at least 12 to 24 hours. Larger amounts of fluid may be removed than with intermittent HD. It is the preferred treatment in the hemodynamically unstable patient with mild to moderate acute renal failure or fluid overload.[6]

Nutritional Management

In the past the regimen of fluid restriction and nutritional therapy was designed so that body weight would decrease by 0.25 to 0.5 kg per day from the loss of body tissue catabolized on the low-protein diet. Today, these severe restrictions are usually not necessary except during the interval between the diagnosis of oliguria and the establishment of dialysis and a nutritional regimen. However, a stable weight or a weight gain during this interval usually indicates hypervolemia.

If the patient does not receive adequate nutrition, catabolism of body protein will occur. This process causes increased urea, phosphate, and potassium levels. The major goal of nutritional management is to decrease catabolism of the body's protein. Adequate energy must be provided from carbohydrate and fat sources to prevent ketosis from fat breakdown and gluconeogenesis from protein breakdown. Nonprotein calories (35 to 55 kcal/kg body weight) should be provided daily.[7] Protein intake is generally 1.0 to 1.5 g/kg. Essential amino acid supplements (e.g., Amin-Aid) may be given for amino acid and caloric supplementation, either orally or through tube feedings. Potassium and sodium are regulated in accordance with plasma levels. Sodium is restricted as needed to prevent edema, hypertension, and congestive heart failure. Dietary fat intake is increased so that the patient receives at least 30% to 40% of total calories from fat.[7] Intralipid (fat emulsions) infusions can also be given as a nutritional supplement, and it provides a good source of nonprotein calories (see Chapter 37). If a patient cannot obtain an adequate oral intake, enteral nutrition is the preferred route for nutritional support (see Chapter 37). When the GI tract is not functional, total parenteral nutrition (TPN) is necessary for the provision of adequate nutrition. TPN is most commonly used in the patient who has had extensive surgical procedures or multiple trauma. The patient treated with TPN may need daily HD or CRRT to remove the accumulation of excess fluid. However, concentrated TPN formulas are available to minimize fluid volume.

NURSING MANAGEMENT

ACUTE RENAL FAILURE

Nursing Assessment

An assessment of the patient in acute renal failure includes the specific areas presented in Table 44-2. It is important to monitor the blood pressure, pulse, respiratory rate and pattern, and temperature. The patient's general appearance should be assessed including skin color, peripheral edema, neck vein distention, and bruises.

The vascular access site should be observed for signs of inflammation. The patient's mental status and level of consciousness should also be determined. The oral mucosa should be examined for dryness and presence of inflammation. The lungs should be auscultated for the presence of crackles and rhonchi. Heart sounds should be monitored for the presence of S_3 sounds and murmurs. If a pulmonary artery catheter is inserted, the pulmonary artery pressures should be obtained.

Any urine output should be assessed including volume, color, sediment, specific gravity, and the presence of blood, glucose, or protein. ECG readings should be obtained to assess for the presence of dysrhythmias.

Nursing Diagnoses

Nursing diagnoses specific to the patient with acute renal failure include, but are not limited to, the following:

- Fluid volume excess related to renal failure and fluid retention
- Risk for infection related to invasive lines, uremic toxins, and altered immune responses secondary to renal failure
- Altered nutrition: less than body requirements related to altered metabolic state and dietary restrictions
- Sensory-perceptual alteration related to uremic toxins and fluid and electrolyte and acid-base imbalances
- Altered thought processes related to effects of uremic toxins on central nervous system (CNS)
- Impaired skin integrity related to vascular access sites or peritoneal dialysis catheter
- Fatigue related to anemia and uremic toxins
- Anxiety related to disease process, therapeutic interventions, and uncertainty of prognosis
- Potential complication: renal insufficiency related to loss of renal function
- Potential complication: hyperkalemia related to decreased renal excretion of potassium
- Potential complication: dysrhythmias related to electrolyte imbalances
- Potential complication: metabolic acidosis related to the inability of the kidneys to excrete hydrogen ions

Planning

The overall goals are that the patient with acute renal failure will completely recover with no residual loss of kidney function, be maintained in normal fluid and electrolyte balance, have decreased anxiety, and comply with and understand the need for careful follow-up care.

Nursing Implementation

Health Maintenance and Promotion. Prevention of acute renal failure is essential because of the high mortality rate and is primarily directed toward identifying and monitoring high-risk populations, controlling industrial chemicals and nephrotoxic drugs, and preventing prolonged episodes of hypotension and hypovolemia. In the hospital the patient at greatest risk for developing acute renal failure is the person who has experienced massive trauma, major surgical procedures, extensive burns, cardiac failure, sepsis, obstetrical complications, or the individual who has a baseline renal insufficiency as a result of chronic diseases such as hypertension, diabetes mellitus, or systemic lupus erythematosus. This patient must be monitored carefully for intake and output, fluid and electrolyte balance, and possible blood transfusion reactions. Extrarenal losses of fluid from vomitus, diarrhea, hemorrhage, and increased insensible losses must be assessed and recorded. Prompt replacement of lost extracellular fluids will help prevent ischemic tubular damage associated with trauma, burns, and extensive surgery. Intake and output records and the patient's weight provide valuable indicators of fluid volume status. Aggressive diuretic therapy for the patient with fluid overload as a result of any cause can lead to inadequate renal vascular perfusion.

Streptococcal infections must be identified and treated with antibiotics. Compliance with the antibiotic regimen is critical to eliminate the source of infection. Complications of streptococcal infections include acute poststreptococcal glomerulonephritis and rheumatic heart disease.

The older adult patient or the individual with diabetes who is undergoing multiple diagnostic studies, especially those requiring IV dye injection, need special attention to prevent the patient from sustaining a nephrotoxic injury secondary to the dye. Adequate hydration is critical. The individual with urinary tract infections needs prompt treatment and careful follow-up care. Other persons who are considered at risk are those taking chemotherapeutic drugs that cause hyperuricemia.

Industrial and agricultural chemicals and products (organic solvents, insecticides, cleaning agents) need to be monitored regularly regarding their safety for both the employee and the general population. The individual who is taking drugs that are potentially nephrotoxic (see Table 42-2) needs to have renal function monitored with serum creatinine and BUN determinations. Nephrotoxic medications should be used sparingly in the high-risk patient. When they need to be used, nephrotoxic medications should be given in the smallest effective doses for the shortest possible periods. The patient should be cautioned about the abuse of over-the-counter analgesics (especially nonsteroidal antiinflammatory drugs), since some of these are also potentially nephrotoxic drugs in the patient with borderline renal insufficiency.

Acute Intervention. The patient with acute renal failure is critically ill and suffers not only from the effects of a renal disease but often from those effects of the nonrenal disease or condition (e.g., trauma, cardiac disease) that contributed to the renal failure. The nursing staff may become overly concerned with the patient's urinary output and forget to focus on the patient as a total person with many physical and emotional needs. Usually the changes caused by renal failure come on suddenly. Both the patient and the family need assistance in understanding that the functioning of the whole body can be disrupted by renal failure. These changes are potentially reversible, since the kidneys can repair themselves.

The nursing role in managing fluid and electrolyte balance is important during the oliguric and diuretic phases. Observing and recording the accurate intake and output of fluids cannot be overemphasized. Daily weights measured with the same scale at the same time each day are essential in evaluating and detecting excessive gains or losses of body fluid (one pound is equivalent to about 500 ml of fluid). The nurse must be knowledgeable about the common signs and symptoms that result from hypervolemia (in the oliguric phase) or hypovolemia (in the diuretic phase), hypernatremia or hyponatremia, hyperkalemia or hypokalemia, and other electrolyte imbalances that may occur in acute renal failure (see Chapter 13). Hyperkalemia is a leading biochemical cause of death in the oliguric phase of acute renal failure. Most typically, hyperkalemia is manifested by impairment of neuromuscular function and dysrhythmias. Muscle weakness, abdominal cramps, flaccid paralysis, and absence of deep tendon reflexes are signs of neuromuscular impairment. Cardiac conduction abnormalities to watch for include a prolonged PR interval, prolonged QRS interval, peaked T wave, and depressed ST segment.

Because infection is the leading cause of death in acute renal failure, meticulous aseptic technique is critical. The use of an indwelling catheter should be avoided. If acute renal failure is diagnosed in a patient, the catheter may need to be removed. The patient should be protected from other individuals with infectious diseases. The nurse should be alert for local manifestations of infection (e.g., swelling, redness, pain) and systemic manifestations (e.g., anorexia, malaise, leukocytosis) because an elevated temperature may not be present in the patient with renal failure. If antibiotics are used to treat an infection, the type and dosage must be carefully considered because the kidneys are the route of excretion for many antibiotics.

Respiratory complications, especially pneumonitis, can be prevented. Humidified oxygen, intermittent positive-pressure breathing, turning, coughing, deep breathing, and ambulation are measures the nurse can use to help the patient maintain adequate respiratory ventilation.

Skin care and measures to prevent pressure ulcers should be performed, since the patient usually develops edema, as well as loss of muscle tone. Mouth care is important to prevent stomatitis, which develops when urea in saliva irritates the mucous membranes.

Chronic and Home Management. Recovery from acute renal failure is highly variable and depends on the underlying illness, the general condition and age of the patient, the length of the oliguric phase, and the management of the patient. The rest of the body, as well as the kidneys, have experienced a major insult. Good nutrition, rest, and limited activity are necessary to restore the patient to a functioning state. The diet should be high in calories, and protein intake should be regulated in accordance with renal function. Follow-up care and regular evaluation of renal function are necessary. The patient should be taught the signs and symptoms of recurrent renal disease, especially manifestations of fluid and electrolyte imbalances. Measures to prevent the recurrence of acute renal failure must be emphasized.

The long-term convalescence of 3 to 12 months may cause social and financial hardships for the family, and appropriate counseling and referrals should be done. Occasionally, renal function deteriorates, and manifestations of chronic renal failure develop. If the kidneys do not recover, the patient progresses to chronic renal failure.

Gerontologic Considerations

The older adult is more susceptible than the younger adult to acute renal failure. Although decreased renal reserve function in advancing age is the primary risk factor, age itself and impaired function of other organ systems are independent risk factors. The aging kidney is less able to withstand changes in hydration, solute load, and cardiac output. Common causes of acute renal failure in the older adult include dehydration, hypotension, diuretic therapy, aminoglycoside therapy, obstructive disorders (e.g., prostatic hyperplasia), surgery, infection, and radiocontrast agents. The prognosis after acute renal failure is generally worse in the older adult than in the younger person. The mortality rate after acute renal failure is 5% to 25% higher in the older adult than in the younger person, and death is usually caused by infection, GI hemorrhage, or myocardial infarction.[8]

CHRONIC RENAL FAILURE

Chronic renal failure involves progressive, irreversible destruction of both kidneys. The disease process progresses until many nephrons are destroyed and replaced by nonfunctional scar tissue. Although there are many different causes of chronic renal failure (Fig. 44-3), the end result is a systemic disease involving every body organ. (The specific disease processes are discussed in Chapter 43.)

The kidneys have remarkable functional reserve. Up to 80% of the GFR (reflected in creatinine clearance measurements) may be lost with few overt changes in the functioning of the body. A person is born with 2 million nephrons and can survive (albeit with difficulty) with as few as 20,000.[9] In the vast majority of cases the individual passes through the early stages of chronic renal failure without recognizing the disease state because the remaining nephrons hypertrophy to compensate. The prognosis and course of chronic renal failure are highly variable. Some individuals live normal, active lives with compensated renal failure, whereas others may rapidly progress to end-stage renal failure. When the creatinine clearance falls below 10 ml per minute (from the norm of 85 to 135 ml per minute for the average adult), some form of dialysis or transplantation is required for survival.

Although there are no distinct stages in chronic renal failure, the disease progression may be divided into three stages:

1. *Diminished renal reserve:* This stage is characterized by normal BUN and serum creatinine levels and an absence of symptoms.
2. *Renal insufficiency:* This stage occurs when the GFR is about 25% of normal. BUN and serum creatinine levels are increased. Easy fatigue and weakness are common symptoms. As the renal failure progresses, headaches, nausea, and pruritis may occur. Nocturia and polyuria occur as a result of the kidneys' loss of ability to concentrate urine.
3. *End-stage renal disease* (ESRD) *or uremia:* The last stage occurs when the GFR is less than 5% to 10% of normal or when creatinine clearances are less than 5 to 10 ml/min. It is at this stage that most patients are no longer able to carry out basic activities of daily living (ADLs) because of the progressive nature of symptoms.

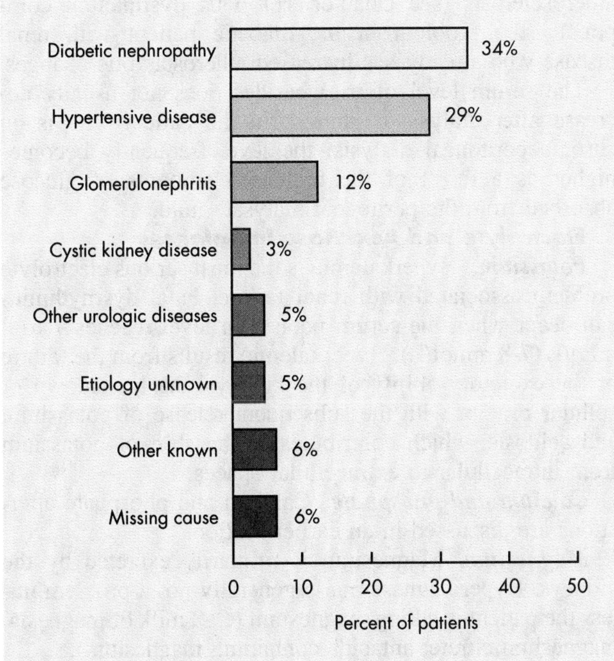

Fig. 44-3 Primary renal disease leading to end-stage renal failure.

CULTURAL & ETHNIC Considerations

END-STAGE RENAL DISEASE

- End-stage renal disease (ESRD) is more common among African-Americans and Native Americans than Caucasians. A history of hypertension and diabetes is also more common in these high risk groups.
- Risk of ESRD from hypertension is significantly increased in African-Americans.
- Risk of ESRD from diabetes is significantly increased in Native Americans.
- African-Americans live longer and have better outcomes on chronic dialysis than Caucasians.

Significance

In the United States over 220,000 individuals have ESRD. This number could double in the next 7 years if current trends continue. Each year over 30,000 people die from various diseases of the kidneys.[10] During the 1970s, dramatic changes in the focus of treatment of chronic renal disease occurred. In July 1973 the federal government enacted a law that provided financial assistance through Medicare for all eligible persons who had ESRD and required treatment.*

*Medicare pays 80% of the cost of dialysis when the patient has been on chronic dialysis for 3 months or has begun home training.

Since 1973 many deaths have been prevented through the use of maintenance dialysis and renal transplantation. The majority of patients (more than 160,000) are treated with dialysis because (1) there is a lack of donated organs, (2) many patients do not want transplants, or (3) patients are medically unsuitable for the transplantation procedure.[10] With the expansion of dialysis programs each year, an increasing percentage of older individuals and patients with systemic disease (diabetics and patients with stable cancer) are being maintained on dialysis.

Because of the End-Stage Renal Disease Medicare Program in the United States, almost every patient, regardless of age, is offered dialysis. The incidence of patients being treated for ESRD is rising by an average of 7.8% per year. Older patients remain the fastest growing group entering the Medicare Renal Disease Program with 55% of patients now over age 60.[10]

The increasing number of older adults with ESRD has changed the data related to the most common causes of chronic renal failure. Before the mid 1970s, glomerulonephritis and interstitial nephritis were the most common causes. Currently, diabetes and hypertension are the leading causes of chronic renal failure in the United States. In Canada the leading causes of ESRD are diabetes and glomerulonephritis.[11]

Clinical Manifestations

As renal function progressively deteriorates, every body system becomes involved. The clinical manifestations are a result of retained substances including urea, creatinine, phenols, hormones, abnormal electrolyte concentrations, and many other substances. Uremia is a syndrome that causes disturbances in the various systems throughout the body (see Fig. 44-2). It is important to recognize that the manifestations of uremia vary among patients, according to the etiology of the renal failure, comorbid conditions, age, and degree of compliance with the prescribed medical regimen.

Urinary System. In the stage of renal insufficiency, the most noticeable sign is polyuria that is caused by the inability of the kidneys to concentrate urine. The patient will notice this most frequently at night when he must arise several times to urinate (nocturia). Because of the decrease in renal concentrating ability, the specific gravity of urine gradually becomes fixed at around 1.010 (the osmolar concentration of plasma). As renal failure progresses, oliguria develops, and later, anuria may develop. If the patient is still producing urine, common findings are proteinuria with casts, pyuria, and hematuria.

Metabolic Disturbances

Nitrogenous product accumulation. As GFR decreases, the BUN and serum creatinine levels increase. The BUN levels are influenced by protein intake, fever, and catabolic rate. For this reason serum creatinine and creatinine clearance determinations are more accurate indicators of renal function than BUN. As BUN increases, nausea, lethargy, fatigue, vomiting, diarrhea, and headaches become common complaints.

The serum creatinine level in an older adult patient with ESRD is lower than the level expected in a younger person with the same degree of renal dysfunction. Decreased muscle mass and decreased muscle activity account for this finding.

The initial treatment for nitrogenous product accumulation is protein restriction. As BUN decreases, nausea, vomiting, and fatigue usually become less noticeable.

Altered carbohydrate metabolism. Defective carbohydrate metabolism is caused by impaired glucose use resulting from cellular insensitivity to the normal action of insulin. The exact nature of this insulin resistance is unclear but may be related to circulating insulin antagonists, alterations in hormone receptors, or abnormalities of transport mechanisms. Moderate hyperglycemia, hyperinsulinemia, and abnormal glucose tolerance tests are common findings. Insulin and glucose metabolism may improve (but not to normal values) after the initiation of dialysis. The individual who has diabetes mellitus and then becomes uremic may require less insulin than before the onset of chronic renal failure. The insulin doses of insulin-dependent diabetics must be individualized and monitored carefully.

Elevated triglycerides. The hyperinsulinemia stimulates hepatic production of triglycerides, and the assimilation of triglycerides by peripheral tissues is diminished. Almost all patients with uremia develop hyperlipidemia, which is usually a type IV profile with elevated very low-density lipoproteins (VLDLs), normal or decreased low-density lipoproteins (LDLs), and lowered high-density lipoproteins (HDLs). The reason for the altered lipid metabolism is related to decreased levels of the enzyme lipoprotein lipase, which is important in the breakdown of lipoproteins. Type IV hyperlipidemia is a definite risk factor for accelerated atherosclerosis (see Chapter 31). This dysfunction compounds the problem in the diabetic patient with renal disease who already has increased atherosclerotic changes.

The serum level of triglycerides does not usually decrease after dialysis is started. In the patient who is on chronic peritoneal dialysis, the level frequently becomes higher as a result of the increased amounts of glucose absorbed from the peritoneal dialysate fluid.

Electrolyte and Acid Base Imbalances

Potassium. Hyperkalemia is the most serious electrolyte problem associated with renal failure. Fatal dysrhythmias can occur when the serum potassium level reaches 7 to 8 mEq/L (7-8 mmol/L). Hyperkalemia results from the failure of the excretory ability of the kidneys, the breakdown of cellular protein with the subsequent release of potassium, and acidosis, which contributes to the shift of potassium from intracellular to extracellular spaces.

Calcium and phosphate. Calcium and phosphate alterations are discussed in an earlier section.

Magnesium. Magnesium is primarily excreted by the kidneys. Hypermagnesemia is generally not a problem unless the patient is taking magnesium (e.g., milk of magnesia, magnesium citrate, antacids containing magnesium).

Sodium. Sodium levels can range from low to normal. Hypernatremia is unusual because whenever sodium is retained, so is water resulting in a dilutional hyponatremia. Sodium retention can contribute to edema, hypertension, and congestive heart failure. Sodium intake needs to be individually determined but is generally restricted in all patients.

Metabolic acidosis. Metabolic acidosis results from the impaired ability of the kidneys to excrete the acid load (primarily ammonia) and from defective reabsorption and regeneration of bicarbonate. The average adult produces 80 to 90 mEq of acid per day, and the kidneys are responsible for excreting this acid load. Plasma bicarbonate usually stabilizes at a new steady state at around 16 to 20 mEq/L (16 to 20 mmol/L). It generally does not progress below this level because hydrogen ion production is usually balanced by buffering from demineralization of the bone (the phosphate buffering system). Although Kussmaul's respiration is less prominent in chronic than in acute renal failure, it reduces the severity of acidosis by increasing carbon dioxide excretion.

Hematologic System

Anemia. The anemia associated with chronic renal failure is classified as normocytic and normochromic and is a result of the hypoproliferative bone marrow. The main cause of anemia is decreased production of erythropoietin by the kidneys, resulting in decreased erythropoiesis by the bone marrow. Other factors contributing to anemia are nutritional deficiencies, decreased RBC life span, increased hemolysis of RBCs, frequent blood samplings, and bleeding from the GI tract.[12] Sufficient iron stores are needed for erythropoiesis. Many patients with renal failure are iron deficient. For the patient on maintenance HD, blood loss in the dialyzer may also contribute to the anemic state. Folic acid, which is essential for RBC maturation, is dialyzable. If it is not adequately replaced in the diet or by drugs, megaloblastic anemia may develop in a patient on chronic HD. Elevated levels of parathyroid hormone (produced to compensate for low serum calcium levels) can inhibit erythropoiesis, shorten survival of RBCs, and stimulate bone marrow fibrosis, which can result in decreased numbers of hematopoietic cells.

Bleeding tendencies. The most common cause of bleeding in uremia is a qualitative defect in platelet function. This dysfunction is caused by impaired platelet aggregation and impaired release of platelet factor 3. The altered platelet function, hemorrhagic tendencies, and GI bleeding are usually reversible by HD or PD. In addition, there are alterations in the coagulation system with increased concentrations of both factor VIII and fibrinogen found in the serum of these patients.

Infection. Infectious complications are caused by changes in leukocyte function and altered immune response and function. A diminished inflammatory response occurs as a result of an altered chemotactic response by both neutrophils and monocytes. This impairment significantly decreases the accumulation of WBCs at the site of injury or infection. Both cellular and humoral immune responses are also suppressed. Characteristic clinical findings include lymphopenia, lymphoid atrophy (especially of the thymus), decreased antibody production, and suppression of the delayed hypersensitivity response. Other factors contributing to the increased risk of infection include protein malnutrition, the uremic effect on mucous membranes, hyperglycemia, and external trauma (e.g., catheters, needle insertions into vascular access sites).

Cardiovascular System. The most common cardiovascular abnormality is hypertension, which is usually caused by sodium retention and increased extracellular fluid volume. In some individuals, increased renin production contributes to the problem (see Fig. 42-6). Hypertension accelerates atherosclerotic vascular disease, produces intrarenal arterial spasm, and eventually leads to left ventricular hypertrophy and congestive heart failure. Hypertension also causes retinopathy and encephalopathy.

Congestive heart failure from left ventricular hypertrophy can lead to pulmonary edema. Peripheral edema is also commonly present. Cardiac dysrhythmias may result from hyperkalemia, hypocalcemia, and decreased coronary artery perfusion.

Uremic pericarditis develops and occasionally progresses to pericardial effusion and cardiac tamponade. Pericarditis is manifested by a friction rub, chest pain, and low-grade fever.

The vascular changes from long-standing hypertension and the accelerated atherosclerosis from elevated triglyceride levels are responsible for many of the cardiovascular complications (e.g., myocardial infarction, cerebrovascular accident), which are the leading causes of death for patients on chronic dialysis. Diabetes mellitus is also a major risk factor in the development of vascular problems.

Respiratory System. Respiratory changes include Kussmaul's respiration, dyspnea from congestive heart failure, pulmonary edema, uremic pleuritis (pleurisy), pleural effusion, and a predisposition to respiratory infections, which may be related to decreased pulmonary macrophage activity. The sputum is thick and tenacious. The cough reflex is depressed. "Uremic lung," or uremic pneumonitis, is typically found in chronic renal failure and shows up as an interstitial edema on chest x-ray. This condition usually responds to vigorous fluid removal during dialysis treatments.

Gastrointestinal System. Every part of the GI system is affected as a result of inflammation of the mucosa caused by excessive urea. Mucosal ulcerations, found throughout the GI tract, are caused by the increased ammonia produced by bacterial breakdown of urea. Stomatitis with exudations and ulcerations, a metallic taste in the mouth, and a urinous odor of the breath are commonly found. Anorexia, nausea, and vomiting caused by GI irritation contribute to weight loss. Diarrhea may occur because of hyperkalemia and altered calcium metabolism. Constipation is a frequent complication of aluminum hydroxide and calcium-containing phosphate binders, which are taken to facilitate phosphate excretion.

Neurologic System. Neurologic changes are expected as renal failure progresses. The exact cause of these changes is unknown, but they may be partially attributed to increased nitrogenous waste products, electrolyte imbalances, and axonal atrophy and demyelination of nerve fibers.

High levels of uremic toxins have been implicated in axonal damage.

In renal failure a general depression of the CNS results in lethargy, apathy, decreased ability to concentrate, fatigue, and altered mental ability. Convulsions and coma may result from hypertensive encephalopathy and a rapidly increasing BUN. Dialysis encephalopathy (dialysis dementia) is a condition associated with aluminum toxicity.

Peripheral neuropathy is initially manifested by a slowing of nerve conduction to the extremities. The patient complains of a restless leg syndrome and may describe it as "bugs crawling inside the leg." Paresthesias, especially of both feet and legs, may be described by the patient as a burning sensation. Eventually, motor involvement may lead to bilateral footdrop, muscular weakness and atrophy, and loss of deep tendon reflexes. Muscle twitching, jerking, asterixis (hand-flapping tremor), and nocturnal leg cramps also occur.

The treatment for neurologic problems is dialysis and, ultimately, transplantation. Altered mental status is often the signal that dialysis needs to be initiated. Dialysis should improve the general CNS symptoms and may halt the progression of neuropathies but not necessarily. Motor neuropathy may not be reversible. The problem of uremic neuropathy is compounded in the diabetic patient who has diabetic neuropathy as well.

Musculoskeletal System. Renal osteodystrophy is a syndrome of skeletal changes found in chronic renal failure.[13] This syndrome is a result of alterations in calcium and phosphate metabolism (Fig. 44-4). Normally the calcium/phosphate ratio maintains the electrolytes in an

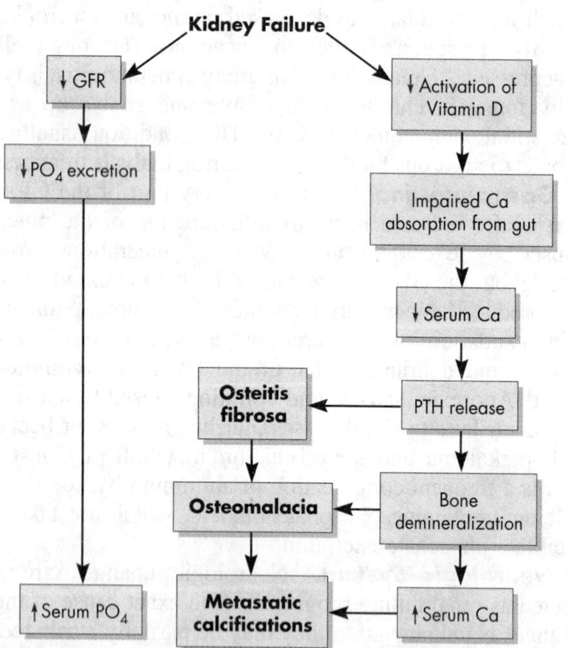

Fig. 44-4 Mechanisms of renal osteodystrophy. *GFR,* Glomerular filtration rate; *PTH,* parathyroid hormone.

insoluble state. As the GFR decreases, phosphate cannot be excreted by the kidneys, thus increasing the serum phosphate. Normally the kidneys metabolize vitamin D (formed in the skin or ingested) to its active form. The active form of vitamin D is needed for calcium absorption from the GI tract. In renal failure the kidneys fail to activate vitamin D, and calcium absorption is impaired, thus lowering serum calcium. Low serum calcium stimulates the release of parathyroid hormone (PTH), which causes resorption of calcium and phosphate from the bone. This release increases serum calcium, as well as serum phosphate. When the phosphate level is high, it complexes with calcium, leading to the formation of metastatic calcifications that are deposited throughout the body.

The changes resulting from increased phosphate retention, bone resorption of calcium, inadequate calcium absorption, and elevated PTH levels lead to the following conditions:

1. *Osteomalacia:* This condition results from lack of mineralization of newly formed bone. It can be a result of hypocalcemia. It can also be caused by aluminum accumulation, since the primary route for excretion is through the kidneys. The primary source of aluminum is aluminum-based phosphate binders.
2. *Osteitis fibrosa:* This condition results from calcium resorption from the bone and replacement with fibrous tissue. Osteitis fibrosa is primarily a result of elevated levels of PTH that causes bone resorption.
3. *Metastatic calcification* (soft-tissue calcification): This condition results from calcium phosphate deposits in soft tissues of the body. Common sites are the blood vessels, joints, lungs, muscles, myocardium, and eyes. "Uremic red eye" is caused by the irritation of the deposits in the eye. Metastatic calcifications in the arteries of the fingers and toes may cause gangrene.

Integumentary System. The most noticeable change in the integumentary system is a yellowish discoloration of the skin. This change is a result of the absorption and retention of urinary chromogens that normally give the characteristic color to urine. The skin also appears pale as a result of anemia and is dry and scaly because of a decrease in oil and sweat gland activity. Decreased perspiration results from a decrease in the size of the sweat glands.

Pruritus most commonly results from a combination of the dry skin, calcium-phosphate deposition in the skin, and sensory neuropathy. The itching may be so intense that it can lead to bleeding or infection secondary to scratching. Uremic frost is a condition in which urea crystallizes on the skin and is usually seen only when BUN levels are extremely high.

The hair is dry and brittle and may fall out. The nails are thin, brittle, and ridged. Petechiae and ecchymoses may be present and are caused by clotting abnormalities.

Reproductive System. Both sexes characteristically experience infertility and a decreased libido. Women usually have decreased levels of estrogen, progesterone, and luteinizing hormone, causing anovulation and menstrual changes (usually amenorrhea). Menses and ovulation may return after dialysis is started. Men experience loss of testicular consistency, decreased testosterone levels, and low sperm counts. Sexual dysfunction in both sexes may also be caused by anemia, which causes fatigue and decreased libido. In addition, peripheral neuropathy can cause impotence in men and anorgasmy in women. Additional factors that may cause changes in sexual function are psychologic problems (e.g., anxiety, depression), physical stress, and side effects of medication.

Sexual function may improve with maintenance dialysis and may return to normal with successful transplantation. In rare cases pregnant dialysis patients have been able to carry a fetus to term, but there is significant risk to the mother and infant. Pregnancy in transplant patients is more common, but in this situation there is also a risk to both the mother and fetus.

Endocrine System. All patients with chronic renal failure exhibit some clinical manifestations of hypothyroidism. Tests of thyroid function yield low to low-normal levels for serum triiodothyronine (T_3) and thyroxine (T_4) levels. Neither the clinical significance nor the exact reason for these findings is known.

Psychologic Changes. Personality and behavior changes, emotional lability, withdrawal, and depression are commonly observed. Fatigue and lethargy contribute to the patient's feeling of sickness. The changes in body image caused by edema, integumentary disturbances, and access devices (e.g., fistulas, catheters) lead to further anxiety and depression. Decreased ability to concentrate and lessened mental activity make the patient appear dull and disinterested in the environment. The patient is faced with significant changes in lifestyle, occupation, family responsibilities, and financial status. The patient's future depends on drugs, dietary restrictions, dialysis, and possibly another person's kidney. The patient will grieve the loss of renal function. This can be a prolonged process for some individuals.

Conservative Management

When a patient is diagnosed as having chronic renal insufficiency, conservative management is attempted before maintenance dialysis begins (Table 44-5). Every effort is made to detect and treat potentially reversible causes of renal failure (e.g., cardiac failure, dehydration, pyelonephritis, nephrotoxins, lower urinary tract obstruction, renal artery stenosis). Conservative management is directed toward preserving existing renal function, treating the symptoms, preventing complications, and providing for the patient's comfort. Conservative management primarily consists of pharmacologic and nutritional management and supportive care.

Pharmacologic Management

Hyperkalemia. Acute hyperkalemia is usually treated with intravenous (IV) glucose and insulin or IV 10% calcium gluconate (see Table 44-4). Dietary restrictions of foods high in potassium are needed. (Foods high in protein content are usually high in potassium.) Sodium polystyrene sulfonate (Kayexalate), a cation-exchange resin, is commonly used to lower potassium levels. The exchange resin,

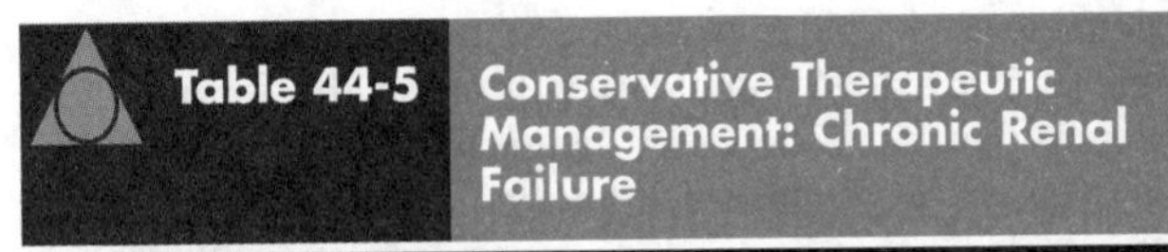
Table 44-5 Conservative Therapeutic Management: Chronic Renal Failure

Diagnostic
- Identification of reversible renal disease
  - Renal scan
  - CT scan
  - Renal ultrasound
- Hematocrit and hemoglobin levels
- BUN, serum creatinine, and creatinine clearance levels
- Serum electrolytes
- Urinalysis and urine culture

Therapeutic
- Correction of extracellular fluid volume overload or deficit
- Nutritional management*
- Erythropoietin therapy
- Administration of phosphate binders
- Antihypertensive therapy
- Measures to lower potassium†
- Adjustment of drug dosages to degree of renal function

BUN, Blood urea nitrogen; *CT,* computed tomography.
*See Tables 44-6, 44-7, 44-8.
†See Table 44-4.

administered orally or rectally, exchanges 1 mEq of sodium for 1 mEq of potassium. The potassium is bound to the resin, which is excreted in the stool. To ensure excretion of potassium, a bulk laxative (usually sorbitol) is mixed with Kayexalate. The patient should be told to expect some diarrhea. Kayexalate should never be given to a patient with hypoactive bowels because fluid shifts could lead to bowel necrosis.

Hypertension. The progression of chronic renal failure can be delayed by controlling hypertension. Treatment of hypertension initially consists of sodium and fluid restriction and the administration of antihypertensives. The antihypertensive drugs most commonly used are calcium channel blockers (e.g., nifedipine [Procardia], nicardipine [Cardene]), and ACE inhibitors (e.g., captopril [Capoten], enalapril [Vasotec]) (see Chapter 30). ACE inhibitors should be used cautiously when ESRD occurs as they can further decrease GFR. The blood pressure should be measured in supine, sitting, and standing positions to effectively monitor the antihypertensive drugs. Treatment that is too vigorous can cause a hypotensive reaction in a patient who has compensated for long-standing hypertension. Blood pressure control is essential to slow atherosclerotic changes that could further impair renal function.

Renal osteodystrophy. Phosphate intake is generally restricted to less than 1000 mg/day. Aluminum hydroxide gels or antacids (e.g., Alu-Cap, Amphojel, Basaljel, and Alternagel) are used to bind the phosphate, which is then excreted in the stool. Because of dementia associated with excessive absorption of aluminum, calcium-based phosphate binders such as calcium carbonate (e.g., Tums) and calcium acetate (e.g., PhosLo) are being used more frequently.[14,15] Giving a calcium-based binder when the phosphate levels are still high (>6 mg/dl [6 mmol/L]) will cause the formation of calcium-phosphate deposits. Magnesium-containing antacids (Maalox, Mylanta) should not be given because magnesium is dependent on the kidneys for excretion. Phosphate binders should be administered with each meal to be effective. Aluminum or calcium binders are available in liquid, tablet, or capsule form. If the patient finds one form unpalatable, another form may be substituted. Because phosphate binders contribute to constipation, stool softeners are usually prescribed. Excessive absorption of aluminum can also lead to aluminum bone disease (osteomalacia). Hypercalcemia may occur with calcium binders.

If hypocalcemia persists in spite of controlled serum phosphate levels and supplemental calcium, the active form of vitamin D may be given. It is commercially available in oral preparations such as calcitriol (Rocaltrol) and in IV form as calcitriol (Calcijex). It is important to lower the phosphate level before administering calcium or vitamin D because these drugs may contribute to soft-tissue calcification if both calcium and phosphate levels are elevated. If renal osteodystrophy remains severe, a subtotal parathyroidectomy may be performed to decrease the synthesis and secretion of PTH. In some situations a total parathyroidectomy is performed and some parathyroid tissue is implanted into the forearm so there is easy access if additional tissue needs to be removed.

The most common methods for evaluating the status of the bone disease are skeletal x-ray, bone scans, bone biopsy, and bone densitometry. PTH and alkaline phosphatase levels should also be done. This enzyme is elevated when there is demineralization of the bone.

Anemia. The most important cause of renal anemia is a decreased production of erythropoietin. With the use of recombinant deoxyribonucleic acid (DNA) technology (see Chapter 10), human erythropoietin can now be made in large amounts and is available for the treatment of anemia.[16,17] It can be administered IV at the end of HD or subcutaneously for the PD patient. Erythropoietin has been effective in treating anemia. Clinically, a significant increase in hematocrit is usually not seen for 2 to 3 weeks. The patient who is receiving erythropoietin has an improved cardiac performance and exercises tolerance and an enhanced quality of life.[18]

A common adverse effect of exogenous erythropoietin is the development or aggravation of hypertension. The underlying mechanism is related to the hemodynamic changes (e.g., increased whole blood viscosity) that occur as the patient's anemia is corrected. Another side effect of erythropoietin therapy is the development of functional iron deficiency as a result of the increased demand for iron to support erythropoiesis. Most patients receive oral iron supplements. Parenteral iron is used if iron deficiencies persist in spite of oral iron intake. Orally administered iron should not be taken at the same time as phosphate binders because the aluminum and calcium binds the iron. Supplemental folic acid (1 mg or more daily) is usually given as it is needed for RBC formation, and it is usually deficient in these patients.

Blood transfusions should be avoided in treating anemia unless the patient experiences an acute blood loss or has symptomatic anemia (i.e., dyspnea, excess fatigue, tachycardia, palpitations, chest pain). Undesirable effects of transfusions are the suppression of erythropoiesis as a result of a decrease in the hypoxic stimulus, the possible transmission of hepatitis, and the possibility of an iron overload.

Complications of Drug Therapy. Most drugs are excreted partially or totally by the kidneys. Drug dosages must be adapted to the degree of renal failure. Drug toxicity is a serious problem in the patient with uremia. Delayed and decreased elimination leads to an accumulation of drugs in the body. Increased sensitivity to the drug may result as drug levels increase in the blood and tissues.

Digitalis preparations are excreted largely by the kidneys. Loading doses may not have to be changed, but maintenance dosages may have to be adjusted. Dialysis does not affect body levels of digoxin, but it does affect potassium levels, which can potentiate the action of digitalis.

Aminoglycosides (gentamicin, kanamycin, tobramycin), penicillin in high doses, and tetracyclines are potentially nephrotoxic. The frequency of doses or the dose of many antibiotics, such as vancomycin and gentamicin, must be decreased because they are dependent on the kidney for excretion. These drugs can accumulate to toxic levels if appropriate precautions are not taken. Meperidine should never be administered because the liver metabolizes it to normeperidine, which is dependent on the kidneys for excretion. If normeperidine accumulates, seizures can result. Other pain medications are appropriate, but they may need to be given less frequently and in smaller doses.

Nutritional Management

Protein restriction. Before the use of maintenance dialysis, Giovannetti and Giordano designed a 20 g, high-quality protein diet to prevent the accumulation of nitrogenous waste products. This diet provided the essential amino acids from eggs and milk. No meat was allowed. In addition to eggs and milk, low-protein vegetables, noodles, butter balls, and high carbohydrate foods were included. Patient acceptance of this dietary regimen was poor, and patients were malnourished and vitamin deficient.

The current diet is designed to be as normal as possible to maintain good nutrition (Table 44-6). For the patient who is not undergoing dialysis, one guide is to restrict protein intake to 0.6 to 0.8 g/kg of ideal body weight (IBW) when the creatinine clearance is less than 20 ml per minute. Some treatment centers use a routine 40 g protein diet (Table 44-7). Because this diet is deficient in vitamins, multivitamins are prescribed. Once the patient is started on dialysis, protein intake can be increased to 1.0 to 1.5 g/kg of IBW. Dietary protein guidelines for the patient on PD differ from those for the patient on HD. Because excessive amounts of protein are lost in the dialysate during peritoneal dialysis, the protein intake must be high enough to compensate for the losses so that the nitrogen balance is maintained. The recommended protein intake is 1.2 to 2.0 g/kg of IBW, depending on the individual needs of the patient. For all patients with renal failure, at least 70% of protein intake

Table 44-6 Nutritional Management: Daily Requirements for the Patient with Chronic Renal Failure

	Conservative Management	Hemodialysis	Peritoneal Dialysis
Fluid allowance	Urine output plus 500-600 ml	Urine output plus 1000 ml	No restriction
Protein*	.6-.8g/kg body weight	1.0-1.5 g/kg IBW	1.2-2.0 g/kg IBW
Calories	35-40 kcal/kg EDW	35-40 kcal/kg EDW*	35-40 kcal/kg IBW*
Fat	Determined by caloric requirement	Determined by caloric requirement	Determined by caloric requirement
Carbohydrate	Unlimited intake of sugars and starches; bread and cereal products limited because of protein limit	Same as for conservative management	Dependent on individual patient needs
Iron	No supplementation	900 mg supplement	500-900 mg supplement
Potassium	2-3 g	2-3 g	3-4 g, no restrictions
Sodium	1-3 g	2 g	2-4 g
Phosphorus	700-1200 mg	700-1200 mg	700-1200 mg
Calcium	1000-2000 mg	1000-1500 mg	1000-1500 mg
Folic acid	1.0 mg supplement	1.0 mg supplement	1.0 mg supplement

EDW, Estimated dry weight; *IBW*, ideal body weight.
*At least 70% of protein intake should be of high biologic value (e.g., coming from eggs, milk, and meat).
†Includes dialysate calories.

should come from eggs, milk, poultry, and meat; these foods are considered to have high biologic value because they contain all of the essential amino acids.

Sufficient calories from carbohydrates and fat are needed to minimize catabolism of body protein and to maintain body weight. Therefore 100 g of carbohydrates and an appropriate amount of fat are prescribed to maintain an intake of 2000 to 2500 calories per day (35 kcal/kg body weight/day). See Table 44-6 for specific guidelines.

Lowering the protein intake decreases the metabolic end-products of urea, potassium, phosphate, and hydrogen. As the BUN level decreases, the symptoms of nausea, vomiting, fatigue, and headache become less troublesome.

Commercially prepared products that are high in calories and low in protein, sodium, and potassium are available. Liquid and powder preparations include Microlipid, SumaCal, Suplena, and Polycose. Products containing only the essential amino acids (Amin-Aid) can also be used as dietary supplements.

Water restriction. Water intake depends on the daily urine output. Generally, 500 to 600 ml (from insensible loss) plus an amount equal to the urine output is allowed for a patient with chronic renal failure who is not on dialysis. This amount of fluid is in addition to the fluid found in food. Foods that are liquid at room temperature (e.g., Jell-O and ice cream) should be counted as fluid intake. The fluid allotment should be spaced throughout the day so that the patient does not become uncomfortable from thirst. During chronic HD, fluid intake is adjusted so that ideally the patient gains no more than 1.0 to 1.5 kg between dialyses.

Sodium and potassium restriction. The amount of sodium and potassium restriction depends on the ability of the kidneys to excrete these electrolytes. Sodium-restricted diets may vary from 1000 to 4000 mg (1 mEq = 23 mg of sodium), depending on the degree of edema and hypertension. (The average daily intake of sodium is 3 g to 7 g.) Sodium and salt should not be equated because the sodium content in 1 g of sodium chloride is equivalent to 400 mg of sodium. The patient should be instructed to avoid foods known to be high in sodium such as cured meats, pickled foods, canned soups and stews, frankfurters, cold cuts, soy sauce, and salad dressings (see Table 32-11). Most salt substitutes should not be used because most contain potassium chloride.

Controlled dietary restrictions of potassium range from 1500 to 4000 mg (1 mEq = 39 mg of potassium). Some PD patients do not need restrictions. For every 20 g increase in dietary protein, the potassium intake is increased by 500 mg. This makes it virtually impossible to restrict potassium to 40 mEq (1.6 g) in an 80 g protein diet because most foods that are high in protein are also high in potassium. Foods with high potassium levels that should be avoided are dried fruits, legumes, oranges, bananas, melons, deep green and deep yellow vegetables, beans, and peas (see Table 44-8).

Low-protein diets. Protein restriction may reduce the decline of renal function in the patient with chronic renal insufficiency. A low-protein (0.6 g/kg body weight), low-phosphorus diet supplemented with amino acids and their ketoanalogues can slow the progression of renal failure.[19] Keto acids of essential amino acids are a dietary supplement. The rationale for using this treatment is that in the body, nonessential amino acids transfer amine groups to the essential keto acids synthesizing essential amino acids. Thus the nitrogen present in nonessential amino acids is used, and the total nitrogen intake is kept to an absolute minimum. Keto acid supplements are available in liquid preparations. A large multicenter study on protein-restricted diets demonstrated that some patients benefitted from a low protein diet.[20] Modest protein restric-

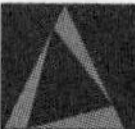

Table 44-7 Nutritional Management: Chronic Renal Failure*

General Principles
1. Protein, sodium, potassium, phosphorus, and fluids are controlled to meet each patient's needs.
2. Protein sources should be of high biologic value.
3. High-sodium and high-potassium foods should be avoided.
4. Sufficient calories and nutrients are provided to meet daily requirements.

Meal	Exchanges	Sample Menu 1	Sample Menu 2	Sample Menu 3
Breakfast	1 fruit 1 bread 1 meat 3 fats	60 ml grape juice Toast or corn flakes Scrambled egg 2 tsp margarine or butter 30 ml cream Jelly	60 ml apple juice Tortilla Fried egg 2 tsp butter 30 ml cream Jam	Applesauce Grits Poached egg 2 tsp butter 30 ml cream Jam
	Beverage Dairy	250 ml decaf coffee 120 ml milk	250 ml decaf coffee 120 ml milk	250 ml decaf coffee 120 ml milk
Lunch	1 meat 2 breads	Salt-free tuna (¼ cup) 2 slices bread	2 enchiladas (using ¼ cup ground beef, 2 corn tortillas, and shredded lettuce)	Fried chicken leg Cornbread ½ cup rice
	Vegetable Fruit 2 fats	Lettuce and cucumber Canned plums 2 tbs salt-free mayonnaise Hard candy	Chili sauce Canned pears 2 tbs oil for cooking Jelly beans	Zucchini Canned peaches 1 tsp butter 1 tbs oil for cooking Hard candy
	Beverage	250 ml carbonated beverage	250 ml carbonated beverage	250 ml carbonated beverage
Dinner	1 meat 1 bread	1 oz fried fresh fish ½ cup mashed potatoes (using presoaked potatoes)	1 oz chicken 1 salt-free corn or flour tortilla to make chicken taco	1 oz pork Salt-free corn on the cob
	Vegetable Fruit 3 fats	Salt-free green peas Fruit cocktail 30 ml cream 1 tbs fat for cooking 1 tsp butter	Tossed salad Canned pineapple 30 ml cream 2 tbs salt-free dressing	Salt-free green beans Grapes 2 tsp butter
	Beverage	250 ml fruit punch 250 ml decaf coffee	250 ml fruit punch 250 ml decaf coffee	250 ml fruit punch 250 ml decaf coffee
Snack		120 ml gelatin dessert with whipped topping 140 ml carbonated beverage†	180 ml Popsicle 80 ml carbonated beverage	Butter balls 320 ml carbonated beverage

*Each diet plan contains 40 g protein, 40 mEq potassium, 2 g sodium, and 1500 ml fluid. To increase the protein to 60 g, the dietitian can add 3 oz meat; 1 egg and 2 oz meat; 120 ml milk, 1 egg, and 1½ oz meat; or 120 ml milk and 2½ oz meat. With the increase in protein, the potassium level also increases to 60 mEq.
†Coke is an acceptable beverage.

tion (.6 to .8 g/kg per day) appears to be a relatively safe therapeutic option for patients with moderate renal insufficiency.[21]

NURSING MANAGEMENT

CONSERVATIVE THERAPY OF CHRONIC RENAL FAILURE

Nursing Assessment

The nurse should obtain a complete history of any existing renal disease or family history of renal disease because many renal disorders have a hereditary basis. Information on long-term health problems such as hypertension, diabetes, recurrent urinary tract infections, and systemic lupus erythematosus need to be obtained. Because many medications are potentially nephrotoxic, both current and past use of prescription and over-the-counter medications need to be determined.

The nurse should assess the patient's dietary habits and discuss any problems. Accurate height and weight assessment and information about recent weight gain or loss need to be obtained.

Table 44-8 High-Potassium Foods

100-250 mg K^+	250-350 mg K^+	>350 mg K^+
Fruits		
1 medium tangerine	½ cup prune juice	⅒ honey dew melon
½ cup fresh pineapple	3 apricots	1 medium banana
1 medium orange	1 fresh peach	10 dried prunes
1 dried fig	½ fresh papaya	10 dates
½ grapefruit	¼ cantaloupe	½ cup raisins
1 fresh pear		½ avocado
½ cup grapefruit juice		1 nectarine
½ cup orange juice		
½ cup pineapple juice		
½ cup apricot nectar		
Cooked Vegetables		
½ cup broccoli	½ cup tomato juice	½ cup parsnips
½ cup rutabagas	½ cup vegetable juice	Artichokes
½ cup pared and boiled potatoes	½ cup rhubarb	1 baked potato
½ cup yams	½ cup pumpkin	
2½-in diameter tomato	½ cup winter squash	
½ cup brussels sprouts		
½ cup pinto beans		
Miscellaneous		
2 tbs wheat germ	1 oz chocolate	1 cup milk
2 slices whole grain bread		1 tbsp dark molasses
2 ounces meat		
2 tbs cocoa		
1 cup bran cereal		
20 pecans		
10 peanuts		
10 walnuts		
1 tbsp light molasses		

Clinical manifestations of chronic renal failure are related to alterations in multiple body systems (see Fig. 44-3). The nurse needs to be aware of the wide diversity of problems in the patient. Fatigue and lethargy are often the early symptoms of chronic renal failure; hypertension and changes in urine characteristics are often the first signs.

Family and other support systems need to be assessed. The chronicity of renal disease and the long-term nature of treatment modalities impact every area of a person's life including family relationships, social and work activities, and self-image. The choice of treatment modality may be related to support systems available to the patient.

Nursing Diagnoses

Nursing diagnoses are determined when the problem and etiologic factor are supported by clinical data. Nursing diagnoses for chronic renal failure may include, but are not limited to, those presented in the following nursing care plan.

Planning

The overall goals are that a patient with chronic renal failure will (1) demonstrate knowledge and ability to comply with therapeutic regimen, (2) participate in decision making for plan of care and future treatment modality, (3) demonstrate effective coping strategies, and (4) continue with activities of daily living within physiologic limitations.

Nursing Implementation

Health Promotion and Maintenance. Individuals need to be instructed on the importance of maintaining an adequate fluid intake each day (at least 2 L). Any changes in urine appearance (color, odor), frequency, or volume need to be reported to the health care provider. Routine urinalysis should be an essential part of a physical examination.

If a patient has a history of renal disease, hypertension, diabetes mellitus, or a family history of renal disease, regular check-ups including serum creatinine, BUN, and urinalysis are essential. When a patient is prescribed potentially nephrotoxic drugs, it is important to monitor renal function with serum creatinine and BUN determinations.

Acute Intervention. The specific nursing management related to various problems is included in the following nursing care plan for the patient with chronic renal failure. In addition, it is important to educate the patient and family because diet, medications, and follow-up medical care are the responsiblities of the patient. The patient should weigh daily, learn to take daily blood pressures, and be able to identify signs and symptoms of edema, hyperkalemia, and

(Text continued on p. 1392.)

NURSING CARE PLAN Patient with Chronic Renal Failure

Planning: Outcome Criteria	***Nursing Interventions and Rationales***
➤ **NURSING DIAGNOSIS**	Fluid volume excess *related to* inability of kidney to excrete fluid, inadequate dialysis, excessive fluid intake, and elevated plasma sodium levels *as manifested by* edema, hypertension, bounding pulse, peripheral venous distention, weight gain, shortness of breath, pulmonary edema
Have absence or control of edema; no evidence of dyspnea; dry weight remaining within 2 lb (1 kg) of patient's established dry weight; blood pressure within limits defined for patient.	Restrict fluid and sodium intake as ordered *to decrease excess fluid retention.* Maintain a low-sodium diet *to control edema and hypertension.* Weigh patient daily *to monitor fluid loss or gain and to use as a guide for treatment plan.* Teach patient fluid control measures and low sodium diet *to promote compliance.* Monitor fluid intake and output *to provide data to regulate fluid replacement.* Observe and record blood pressure and amount of periorbital, sacral, and peripheral edema *as indicators of the extent of fluid retention.* Provide skin care with special emphasis on edematous areas *as these areas are prone to breakdown.* Auscultate chest for crackles *to identify possible fluid in the lungs.* Monitor for dyspnea, jugular venous distention, and pericardial friction rub, *which are indicators of fluid excess.*
➤ **NURSING DIAGNOSIS**	Impaired skin integrity *related to* decrease in oil and sweat gland activity, deposition of calcium-phosphate precipitates, capillary fragility, excess fluid, and neuropathy *as manifested by* itching, bruising, dry skin, yellow-gray skin, edema, skin inflammation or infection, excoriation.
Have no itching or skin dryness; intact, clean skin that is free from infection.	Assess skin for changes in color, texture, turgor, and vascularity *to identify areas of poor circulation and to provide direction for appropriate interventions.* Inspect patient for bruises, purpura, and signs of infection *that may indicate trauma from scratching.* Provide skin care with tepid water, xipamide (Aquaphor), or bath oils *to relieve itching and to moisturize dry, cracked skin.* Apply ointments or creams (lanolin, Aquaphor) following bath or shower *to relieve itching and promote comfort.* Administer antihistamines and antipruritics as prescribed *to relieve itching.* Trim patient's nails short and keep them clean *to reduce tissue damage from scratching and to prevent infection.* Monitor serum calcium and phosphate levels *since elevated blood levels may lead to calcium-phosphate precipitation in the skin.*
➤ **NURSING DIAGNOSIS**	Risk for injury: fracture *related to* alterations in the absorption of calcium and excretion of phosphate; altered vitamin D metabolism and metastatic calcifications
Have slowing of bone disease; serum calcium levels > 8mg/dl (2.0 mmol/L) and phosphate levels <5.5 mg/dl (1.8 mmol/L), no bone fractures.	Assess for hypocalcemia, elevated serum phosphate levels, muscle pain, limited mobility of joints, deposition of calcium-phosphate in joints and other places, and demineralization of bone *to detect potential risks for injury.* Observe for manifestations of bone pain *as a possible indicator of bone injury.* Provide range-of-motion exercises and encourage ambulation *to foster osteoblast activity and decrease bone resorption.* Administer aluminum hydroxide binders, calcium binders or supplements, and vitamin D as ordered *to prevent or treat the bone demineralization.* Give calcium supplements or phosphate binders with meals *to increase effectiveness by binding dietary phosphorus to form insoluble calcium phosphate or aluminum phosphate, which is excreted in feces.* Instruct patient in the importance of taking these drugs with meals *to facilitate compliance with therapeutic regimen.* Ensure that patient understands and follows dietary restrictions of phosphate. Observe for and prevent constipation when calcium phosphate or aluminum hydroxide is used *as this is a common complication.* Observe for hypercalcemia when using calcium supplements. Explain to patient the potential for fracture *to reduce the risk of unsafe practices that might result in a traumatic or pathologic fracture.* Assist with ambulation *as exercise helps maintain strength and mobility and decreases bone resorption.* Provide safe environment *to reduce the risk of injury.*

continued

NURSING CARE PLAN Patient with Chronic Renal Failure—cont'd

Planning: Outcome Criteria	Nursing Interventions and Rationales
➤ **NURSING DIAGNOSIS**	Activity intolerance *related to* anemia secondary to uremia, bleeding, and blood loss during dialysis *as manifested by* fatigability, poor tolerance for activity, shortness of breath, pallor, dyspnea, tachycardia
Maintain hematocrit in acceptable range; perform activities of daily living without undue fatigue.	Administer iron between meals and erythropoietin as ordered *to maintain normal erythropoiesis and stimulate production of RBCs.* Do not administer folic acid before or during hemodialysis *as folic acid is dialyzable and would be lost in the dialysate.* Assess patient's response to activity *to make appropriate adjustments in plan of care.* Provide adequate periods of rest *to enable patient to recuperate from past activities and participate in future activity.* Teach patient to plan activities *to avoid fatigue.* Minimize blood loss during dialysis and watch for any bleeding sites *as bleeding reduces RBCs and can result in decreased O_2 at cellular level and subsequent decrease in activity.* Monitor hematocrit and hemoglobin levels *as an indicator of the patient's O_2-carrying capacity.*
➤ **NURSING DIAGNOSIS**	Altered nutrition: less than body requirements *related to* restricted intake of nutrients (especially protein), nausea and vomiting, anorexia, stomatitis, and altered metabolism of nutrients *as manifested by* loss of appetite, loss of weight, alterations in electrolyte balance, unpleasant taste in mouth
Maintain ideal body weight; maintain albumin and total protein within acceptable limits.	Administer antiemetics as ordered *to control nausea and vomiting.* Provide frequent mouth care *to prevent stomatitis, remove foul tastes, and increase patient's comfort.* Provide small, frequent meals *as smaller, more frequent feedings reduce nausea and vomiting.* Allow patient freedom in choosing food and fluid intake within limitations *to increase the patient's sense of control.* Provide at least 2000 to 2500 kcal/day with a high carbohydrate intake *to minimize catabolism of body protein and maintain body weight.* Restrict protein and phosphate to prescribed amount *to decrease the metabolic end-products of urea, potassium, phosphate, and hydrogen.* Provide hard candy, gum, and lollipops *to improve taste and increase carbohydrate intake if individual is not a diabetic patient.* Monitor weight, BUN, serum creatinine, albumin, total protein, and serum electrolytes *as indicators of effectiveness of dialysis and response to treatment.*
➤ **NURSING DIAGNOSIS**	Constipation *related to* decreased mobility, antacid intake, fluid restrictions, dietary modification, or electrolyte imbalances *as manifested by* lack of usual bowel elimination
Resume usual bowel elimination pattern.	Administer stool softeners as prescribed *to prevent constipation by maintaining soft stools.* Teach patient to avoid over-the-counter laxatives that contain magnesium *since hypermagnesemia could develop.* Encourage ambulation to patient's ability *to increase bowel peristalsis.*
➤ **NURSING DIAGNOSIS**	Diarrhea *related to* GI inflammation secondary to urea or hyperkalemia or as side effect of sorbitol-Kayexalate treatment *as manifested by* frequent, loose-to-watery stools
Resume usual bowel elimination pattern.	Record and measure stool *to monitor fluid and electrolyte losses.* Monitor electrolytes (especially potassium, calcium, and bicarbonate levels) when patient has persistent diarrhea *as altered levels can result in significant problems.* Encourage oral intake of fluids containing electrolytes *to replace losses.* Clean perianal area gently, and apply lotions *to maintain perianal skin integrity.* Increase oral fluid intake to prescribed maximum, and return to normal diet as tolerated *to promote return to normal bowel functioning.*
➤ **NURSING DIAGNOSIS**	Anticipatory grieving *related to* loss of kidney function *as manifested by* expression of feelings of sadness, anger, inadequacy, hopelessness
Progress toward acceptance of chronic disease.	Listen to concerns of patient *to convey a caring attitude and foster the nurse-patient relationship and to determine how patient is handling the situation.* Allow patient time to mourn loss of body function *so patient can deal with feelings and identify ways of coping with losses more effectively.* Include family members in discussions of patient's concerns *to enable them to assist the patient and foster their support and understanding.*

continued

NURSING CARE PLAN Patient with Chronic Renal Failure—cont'd

Planning: Outcome Criteria	*Nursing Interventions and Rationales*
➤ **NURSING DIAGNOSIS**	Self-esteem disturbance *related to* enforced lifestyle changes, dependency on dialysis, chronic fatigue, body image changes, occupational problems, and role maintenance *as manifested by* expression of feelings of inadequacy and unworthiness and concerns about family finances and functioning
Express positive feelings about self; participate in treatment regimen; adapt lifestyle to changing health status.	Provide opportunity for patient to discuss concerns *to determine how patient is dealing with life changes.* Refer patient to social worker and for counseling if indicated *to provide additional assistance for management of chronic illness.* Assure patient of self-worth *to raise self-esteem by reinforcing positive attributes.* Encourage patient and significant others to share feelings *as verbalization helps to clarify feelings and may provide insight into solutions.*
➤ **NURSING DIAGNOSIS**	Sensory and perceptual alterations *related to* CNS changes induced by uremic toxins *as manifested by* confusion, slowing of thought processes, decreased attention and memory span, disorientation, changes in sensorium (e.g., somnolence, stupor), changes in mood (e.g., irritability, depression), changes in behavior (e.g., withdrawal)
Have mental alertness and appropriate interaction with environment.	Provide explanation to patient and family of effects of uremia on CNS *to reduce anxiety over changes in mentation.* Assess patient's level of consciousness and mental status at regular intervals *as minor confusion and irritability can progress and indicate a worsening condition.* Discuss significant material for brief rather than long time periods *to reduce confusion and increase possibility that information will be understood and retained.* Allow patient time to respond. Validate patient's understanding of what is discussed *to provide feedback regarding patient's understanding and need for further discussion.* Provide aids such as calendars and clocks *to aid in patient orientation.* Teach family how to evaluate mental changes and when to refer to physician *to enable early identification and treatment for deteriorating status.* Provide calm, nonstimulating environment *to prevent increasing patient's confusion and agitation.*
➤ **NURSING DIAGNOSIS**	Risk for sexual dysfunction *related to* effects of uremia on reproductive and endocrine systems and the psychosocial impact of renal failure and its treatment
Express satisfaction with sexual relationship by patient and significant other.	Assess female patient for amenorrhea, failure to ovulate, and decreased libido; assess male patient for impotence, atrophy of testicles, gynecomastia, and azoospermia *to determine presence and extent of risk factors for sexual dysfunction and to plan appropriate interventions.* Discuss birth control measures if woman is menstruating *to prevent unplanned pregnancy.* Discuss meaning of sexuality with patient and significant other *to determine significance of problem.* Encourage patient and partner to discuss feelings openly and to use other means of sexual expression besides intercourse; explore new patterns of sexual activity if previous patterns lead to anxiety *to assure continued expression of sexual feelings.* Emphasize importance of giving and receiving love and affection as opposed to performing *to reduce patient's anxiety.*
➤ **NURSING DIAGNOSIS**	Risk for infection *related to* suppressed immune system, access sites, and malnutrition secondary to dialysis and uremia
Have no infections, WBC count within normal range.	Assess for chills, fever, and tachycardia; redness, swelling, or drainage in area of break in skin *to detect signs of possible infection.* Provide frequent oral and personal hygiene *to reduce risk of self-contamination.* Instruct patient to avoid exposure to people with infections *as the patient has an altered immune response and therefore has an increased risk of infection.* Watch for local and systemic manifestations of infection *to promote early identification and treatment.* Maintain aseptic technique when performing dialysis *to prevent the introduction of organisms.* Avoid invasive procedures such as catheterization *to avoid introduction of organisms.*

continued

NURSING CARE PLAN Patient with Chronic Renal Failure—cont'd

Planning: Outcome Criteria	*Nursing Interventions and Rationales*
➤ **NURSING DIAGNOSIS**	Ineffective management of therapeutic regimen *related to* lack of knowledge of treatment plan and prevention of complications *as manifested* by expressed difficulty in following diet and inability to recognize signs and symptoms of complications
Describe dietary restrictions, medications, and reportable signs and symptoms.	Teach patient dietary and fluid restrictions, medication therapy including side effects, methods to record intake and output and weight, signs and symptoms of complications *to ensure patient understanding and to enhance cooperation.* Teach alternative ways of reducing thirst (e.g., sucking on lemon or ice cube) *so thirst is reduced without significant increase in fluid intake.* Encourage discussion of difficulties in modifying diet and fluid intake *to assist in identifying helpful suggestions and to explore patient's feelings and ability to cope.* Explain signs and symptoms of electrolyte imbalance to patient and significant other *to enable early identification and prompt intervention.* Teach patient and significant other to report weight gain >2 lb (1 kg), shortness of breath, increasing fatigue or weakness, and confusion or lethargy *as these are complications of the disease or a failure to comply with therapeutic regimen.* Teach methods *to prevent localized bleeding,* (e.g, using soft toothbrush and electric razor), to avoid constipation, and to avoid strenuous exercise. Provide information on community resources such as the National Kidney Foundation *to assist in coping with home care and adjustments in lifestyle.*

COLLABORATIVE PROBLEMS

Nursing Goals	*Nursing Interventions and Rationales*
➤ **POTENTIAL COMPLICATION**	Hypertension *related to* sodium and water retention and alterations of renin-angiotensin system
Monitor for hypertension, report deviations from acceptable parameters, and carry out appropriate medical and nursing interventions.	Assess patient for elevated blood pressure, headache, dizziness, shortness of breath, chest pain, edema *to identify the presence of hypertension.* Take vital signs q4hr *to provide a data base for ongoing analysis of patient's response to treatment.* Administer antihypertensive medications as ordered. Observe for orthostatic hypotension and other side effects of medication *as overtreatment may cause problems in the compensated patient.* Instruct patient to change positions slowly *to minimize dizziness caused by orthostatic hypotension.* Explain the actions and side effects of drugs and the risks of uncontrolled hypertension (e.g., stroke) *to foster adherence to medication regimen.*
➤ **POTENTIAL COMPLICATION**	Hyperkalemia *related to* decreased renal function, increased tissue catabolism, and shift of potassium into extracellular fluid *secondary to* metabolic acidosis
Monitor for signs of hyperkalemia, report deviations from acceptable parameters, and carry out appropriate medical and nursing interventions.	Assess for signs of hyperkalemia such as serum potassium >5.5 mEq/L (5.5 mmol/L), muscle weakness, dysrhythmias, paresthesias, intestinal colic and diarrhea, peaked T waves on ECG *to assure early identification and treatment.* Discuss importance of following prescribed diet and avoiding foods high in potassium *to prevent complications of hyperkalemia.* Monitor serum potassium, and notify physician of elevated levels and ECG results *as elevated potassium can cause life-threatening cardiac dysrhythmias.* Be prepared to administer treatment for hyperkalemia *as this is a medical emergency requiring prompt treatment.*
➤ **POTENTIAL COMPLICATION**	Peripheral neuropathy *related to* effects of uremia on peripheral nerves
Monitor for peripheral neuropathies, report deviations from acceptable parameters, and carry out appropriate medical and nursing interventions.	Assess patient for decreased sensation in feet, numbness and burning of feet, muscle cramps, restlessness of legs, loss of muscle strength, and footdrop *to identify the presence of peripheral neuropathy so early treatment can be initiated.* Explain to patient reason for neuropathy *to increase understanding and decrease anxiety.* Prevent trauma and excess stimulation to extremities *as areas with diminished sensation are extremely prone to injury.* Instruct patient to avoid tight clothing and restricting bed linens *to prevent inadvertent injury since the affected areas have decreased sensation.* Teach patient to examine areas of decreased sensation *to observe for injury.* In collaboration with physical therapy department, develop exercise regimen *to maintain prescribed level of activity.* Assess adequacy of dialysis therapy *as dialysis may reduce the symptoms and halt the progress of neuropathies.*

BUN, Blood urea nitrogen; *CNS,* central nervous system; *ECG,* electrocardiogram; *GI,* gastrointestinal; *RBC,* red blood cells; *WBC,* white blood cells.

other electrolyte imbalances. The patient and family need to understand the importance of strict dietary adherence. The dietitian and the nurse need to meet with the patient and family on a continuing basis to assist in diet planning. A diet history and consideration of cultural variations make diet planning and adherence more easily achieved goals.

The patient needs a complete understanding of the drugs, the dosages, and the common side effects. It may be helpful to make a list of the medications and the times of administration that can be posted in the home in a convenient location. The patient needs to be instructed to avoid certain over-the-counter drugs such as laxatives and antacids that contain magnesium.

It is important that the patient be motivated to assume the primary role in the management of the disease. The period of conservative management provides a good opportunity to evaluate each patient's ability to manage the disease. This is a critical factor in considering each patient as a candidate for home dialysis or transplantation.

Chronic and Home Management. The length of time a patient can be maintained on conservative management is highly variable and depends on the progression of renal failure. When conservative therapy is no longer effective, dialysis and transplantation are the only measures that can be used to prolong life.

While the patient is being maintained on conservative management, the decision regarding future therapies, if any, should be made. This should be done before complications such as mental status changes, bleeding, progressive neuropathies, and persistent congestive heart failure occur.

The patient and family need a clear explanation of what is involved in dialysis and transplantation. If alternative treatments are presented early in the course of therapy, the patient will have an opportunity to carefully consider choices. The patient will feel more control over his life and health care when educated about treatment and treatment options and when active in the decision-making process. The patient needs to be informed that if dialysis is chosen, the option of transplantation still remains. If transplantation does not work, the patient can return to dialysis. Many individuals with chronic renal failure have received more than one kidney transplant.

DIALYSIS

Dialysis refers to the movement of fluid and molecules across a semipermeable membrane from one compartment to another. Clinically, dialysis is a technique in which substances move from the blood through a semipermeable membrane and into a dialysis solution (dialysate). Dialysis is used to correct fluid and electrolyte imbalances and to remove waste products in renal failure. Dialysis can also be used to treat drug overdoses (see Chapter 62). The two methods of dialysis are *peritoneal dialysis* (PD) and *hemodialysis* (HD) (Table 44-9). In PD the peritoneal membrane is used as the semipermeable membrane. In HD an artificial membrane (usually made of cellulose-based or synthetic materials) is used as the semipermeable membrane that is in contact with the patient's blood.

Dialysis is begun when the patient's uremic state can no longer be adequately managed conservatively. A general guideline is to start dialysis when the GFR (or creatinine clearance) is less than 5 to 10 ml per minute. However, this criterion varies widely in different clinical situations, and the physician determines when to start dialysis on an individual basis. Certain uremic complications, including encephalopathy, neuropathies, uncontrollable hyperkalemia, pericarditis, and accelerated hypertension, indicate a need for immediate dialysis.

General Principles

Solutes and water move across the membrane from the blood to the dialysate or from the dialysate to the blood in

Table 44-9 Comparison of Peritoneal Dialysis and Hemodialysis

Peritoneal Dialysis		Hemodialysis	
Advantages	**Disadvantages**	**Advantages**	**Disadvantages**
Immediate initiation in almost any hospital Less complicated than hemodialysis Portable system with CAPD Fewer dietary restrictions Relatively short training time Usable in the patient with vascular access problems Less cardiovascular stress Home dialysis possible Preferable for the diabetic patient	Bacterial or chemical peritonitis Protein loss into dialysate Exit-site and tunnel infections Self-image problems with catheter placement Hyperglycemia Aggravated hyperlipidemia Surgery for catheter placement Contraindication in the patient with multiple abdominal surgery or trauma	Rapid fluid removal Rapid removal of urea and creatinine Effective potassium removal Less protein loss Lowering of serum triglycerides Home dialysis possible	Vascular access problems Dietary and fluid restrictions Heparinization necessary Extensive equipment necessary Disequilibrium and hypotension during dialysis Added blood loss that contributes to anemia Specially trained personnel necessary

CAPD, Continuous ambulatory peritoneal dialysis.

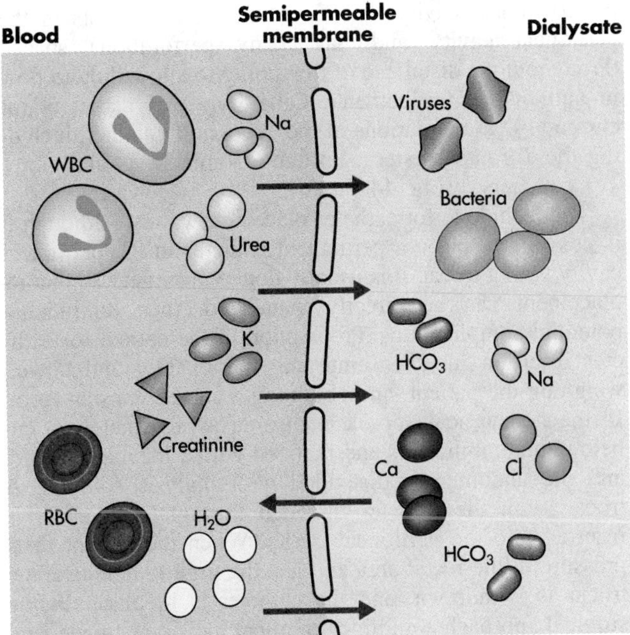

Fig. 44-5 Osmosis and diffusion across a semipermeable membrane. *RBC*, Red blood cell; *WBC*, white blood cell.

accordance with concentration gradients. The principles of diffusion, osmosis, and ultrafiltration are involved in dialysis (Fig. 44-5). *Diffusion* is the movement of solutes from an area of greater concentration to an area of lesser concentration. In renal failure, urea, creatinine, uric acid, and electrolytes (potassium, phosphate) move from the blood to the dialysate with the net effect of lowering their concentration in the blood. RBCs, WBCs, and large plasma proteins are too large to diffuse through the membrane.

Osmosis is the movement of fluid from an area of lesser to an area of greater concentration of solutes. Glucose is added to the dialysate bath and creates an osmotic gradient across the membrane to remove excess fluid from the blood.

Ultrafiltration (water and fluid removal) results when a pressure gradient across the dialyzer membrane is created by an increased pressure in the blood compartment (positive pressure) or a decreased pressure in the dialysate compartment (negative pressure). Extracellular fluid moves into the dialysate because of the pressure gradient. In peritoneal dialysis, excess fluid is removed by increasing the osmolality of the dialysate with the addition of glucose. In HD, excess fluid is removed by creating a pressure differential between the blood and the dialysate solution with a combination of positive pressure in the blood compartment or a negative pressure in the dialysate compartment.

The dialysate solution usually contains an electrolyte composition similar to that of normal plasma except that potassium is not in the solution. The concentration of the dialysis solution may be individually determined on the basis of the patient's needs.

RESEARCH

Implications for Nursing Practice

QUALITY OF LIFE FOR THE SPOUSE OF A DIALYSIS PATIENT

Citation Dunn SA and others: Quality of life for spouses of CAPD patients, *ANNA J* 21:237-247, 1995.

Purpose To describe the quality of life for the spouse of a continuous ambulatory peritoneal dialysis (CAPD) patient.

Methods A descriptive, correlational method was used to study 38 spouses of CAPD patients. The spouses completed a demographic data form, the Jalowiec Coping Scale, the Dyadic Adjustment Scale, and a Quality of Life Index. The primary nurse completed the End Stage Renal Disease Severity Index on the patients.

Results and Conclusions Twenty-one percent of the spouses perceived their quality of life as high, 55% as moderate, and 24% as fair to poor. The results indicated that the quality of life for the spouse was similar to that of the patient. Marital adjustment and income status were the best predictors of quality of life for the spouse.

Implications for Nursing Practice End-stage renal disease (ESRD) presents a life crisis not only for the patient but for the significant other as well. Understanding the effect that a chronic illness has on the spouse will assist the nurse in providing quality care for both the patient and the spouse. Spouse support groups may be beneficial and provide a social network that may have been missing from their lives.

Peritoneal Dialysis

Although PD was first used in 1923, it did not come into widespread use for chronic treatment until the 1970s with the development of soft, pliable peritoneal solution bags and the introduction of the concept of continuous PD. In the United States, approximately 13% of patients receiving ESRD treatment are on peritoneal dialysis. In Canada, approximately 36% of patients are on home PD because of the decreased availability of HD.[11] In recent years the use of PD to treat both acute and chronic renal failure has increased considerably. The large surface area of the peritoneum makes it a good semipermeable membrane for performing clinical dialysis.

Catheter Placement. Peritoneal access is obtained by inserting a catheter through the anterior abdominal wall (Fig. 44-6). The prototype of the catheter that is used was developed by Tenckhoff in 1968 and is made of silicone rubber tubing (see Fig. 44-6). The current version of this catheter is about 25 cm long and has one or two Dacron cuffs at the subcutaneous and peritoneal ends of the catheter that anchor it securely and prevent the migration of microorganisms down the shaft from the skin. Within a few weeks, fibrous tissue grows into the Dacron cuff, anchors the catheter in place, and prevents bacterial penetration into

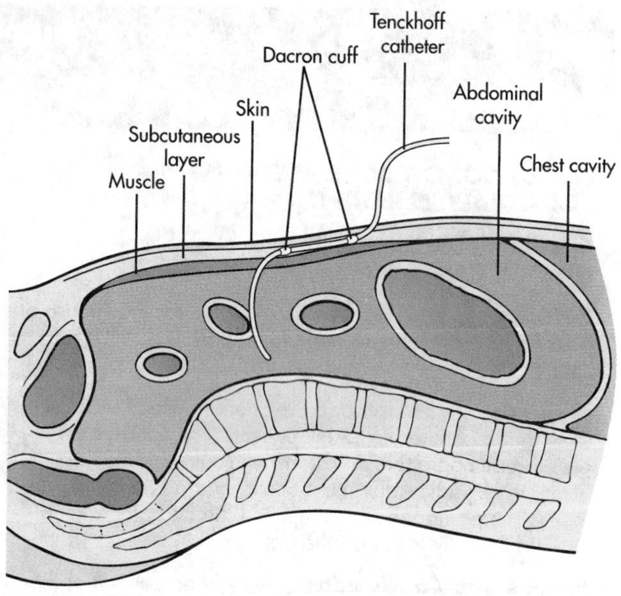

Fig. 44-6 Tenckhoff catheter used in peritoneal dialysis.

the peritoneal cavity. The tip of the catheter rests in the peritoneal cavity and has many perforations spaced throughout the distal end of the tubing to allow fluid to flow in and out of the catheter. Other types of catheters for chronic PD are variations of the Tenckhoff catheter, including the Toronto-Western, Purdue-Column Disc, and Gore-Tex catheters[22] (Fig. 44-7).

The technique for catheter placement varies. Although it is possible to place a permanent catheter in the peritoneal cavity with a trocar, it is usually done via surgery so that its placement can be directly visualized, thus minimizing potential complications. Preparation of the patient for catheter insertion includes emptying the bladder and bowel, weighing the patient, and obtaining a signed consent form. In the nonsurgical approach an area approximately 2 cm below the umbilicus is anesthetized with a local anesthetic, and the abdomen is distended with dialysis solution. A trocar, with the catheter threaded through or over it, is inserted into the peritoneal cavity. When the patient feels pressure in the rectal area and has the urge to defecate, the trocar is withdrawn, and the catheter is in place. In the surgical approach a midline umbilical incision is made, and a small puncture is made to one side and below this incision. The catheter is tunnelled under the skin to the puncture site, and the distal end is placed in the peritoneum. After the catheter is inserted, the skin is cleaned with an

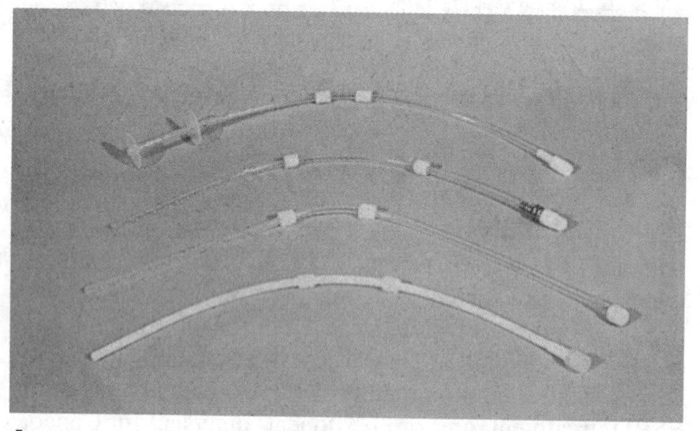

A

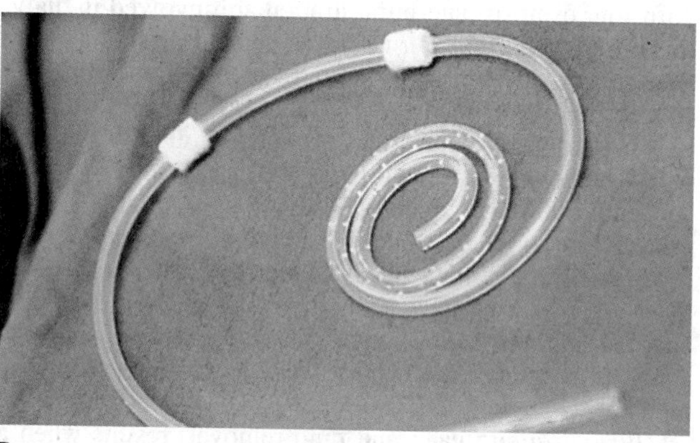

B

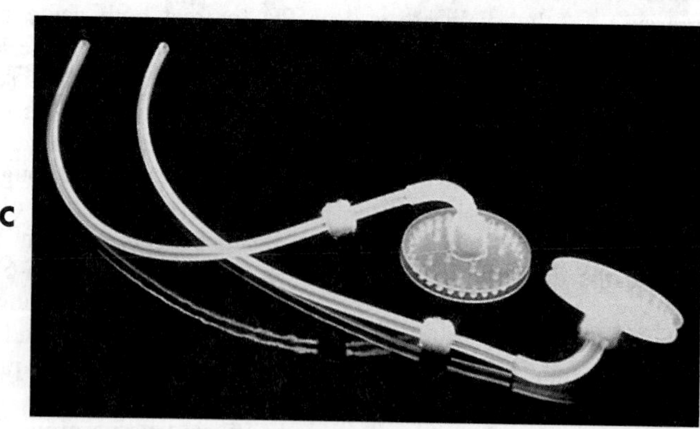

C

Fig. 44-7 ***A,*** Peritoneal catheters used for peritoneal dialysis. ***B,*** Bent neck curl catheter. ***C,*** Disc catheters.

antiseptic solution, and a sterile dressing is applied. Complications of catheter insertion include perforation of the bladder, bowel, or a blood vessel and the introduction of bacteria.

The catheter is connected to a sterile tubing system and anchored to the abdomen with tape. The catheter is irrigated immediately with heparinized dialysate (usually 500 ml) to clear blood and fibrin from it. The irrigations may continue for 12 to 24 hours using small volumes of dialysate. This procedure helps prevent the catheter from clogging, resulting in poor drainage and inflow.

Before the start of PD, it is preferable to allow a waiting period of 7 to 14 days for proper sealing of the catheter and for tissue ingrowth into the cuffs. However, some centers start dialysis 5 to 7 days after catheter insertion. About 2 to 4 weeks after catheter implantation, the exit site should be clean, dry, and free of redness and tenderness (Fig. 44-8). Once the catheter incision site is healed, the patient may shower and then pat the catheter and exit site dry. Daily catheter care includes the application of an antiseptic solution and a sterile dressing, as well as examination of the catheter site for signs of infection.

Dialysis Solutions and Cycle. Dialysis solutions are available commercially in 1- or 2-liter (and sometimes smaller or larger volumes) plastic bags (Dianeal, Inpersol) with glucose concentrations of 1.5%, 2.5%, and 4.25%. The electrolyte composition is similar to that of plasma except there is no potassium in the dialysate. The dialysis solution is warmed to body temperature to increase peritoneal clearance, prevent hypothermia, and make the patient more comfortable.

Ultrafiltration (fluid removal) during PD depends on osmotic forces with glucose being the most effective osmotic agent currently used. However, the problems arising from high rates of peritoneal glucose absorption such as obesity, hypertriglyceridemia, and control of blood glucose levels in the diabetic patient have led to a search for alternative osmotic agents, including amino acid solutions. Many of these agents are currently under investigation.

The three phases of the peritoneal dialysis cycle are *inflow* (fill), *dwell* (equilibration), and *drain*. (The three phases are called an *exchange*). The patient dialyzing at home will recieve about four exchanges per day. An acutely ill hospitalized patient may receive 12 to 24 exchanges per day. During inflow, a prescribed amount of solution, usually 2 L, is infused over about 10 minutes. The flow rate may be decreased if the patient becomes uncomfortable. After the solution has been infused, the inflow clamp is closed before air enters the tubing.

The next part of the cycle is the dwell phase, or equilibration, during which diffusion and osmosis occur between the patient's blood and the peritoneal cavity. The duration of the dwell time can last 20 to 30 minutes to 8 or more hours, depending on the method of PD. Drain time takes 15 to 30 minutes and may be facilitated by gently massaging the abdomen or changing the patient's position. The cycle starts again with the infusion of another 2 L of solution. For manual PD, a period of about 30 to 50 minutes is required to complete an exchange.

Peritoneal Dialysis Systems. Two types of PD currently being used are automated peritoneal dialysis (APD) and continuous ambulatory peritoneal dialysis (CAPD).[23]

Automated peritoneal dialysis. Cycler equipment is used to deliver the dialysate for ADP (Fig. 44-9). The automated cycler times and controls the fill, dwell, and drain phases. The machine cycles four to eight exchanges per night with 1 to 2 hours per exchange. Alarms and monitors are built into the system to make it safe for the patient to dialyze while sleeping. It may be easier to teach the patient and family to use the PD machine at home compared with the HD equipment. APD includes the following variations: continuous cyclic peritoneal dialysis (CCPD), intermittent peritoneal dialysis (IPD), and nightly peritoneal dialysis (NPD). In CCPD the dialysis solution can be left in the peritoneal cavity during the day between nightly cycling, or the peritoneal cavity can be left "dry" during the day. With IPD and NPD, cycling is performed five to seven nights per week, and the abdomen is left empty between dialysis.

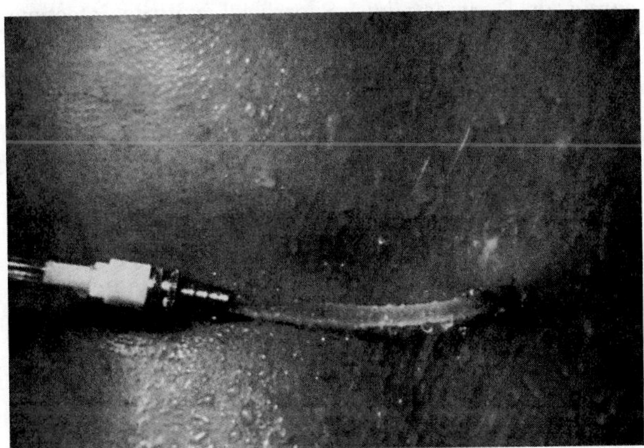

Fig. 44-8 Placement of peritoneal catheter.

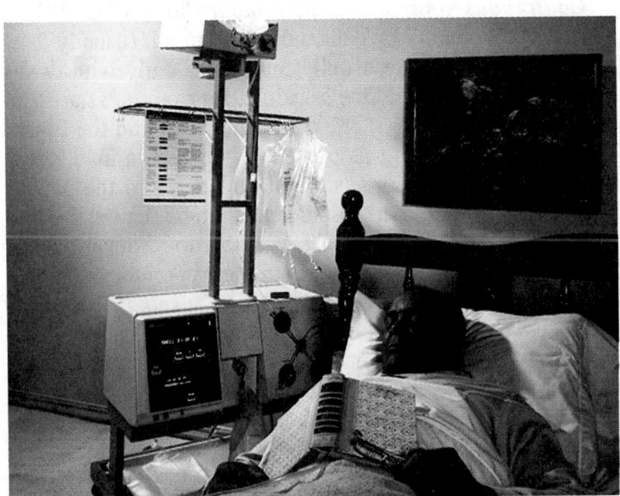

Fig. 44-9 Automated peritoneal dialysis cycler, which is used while the patient is sleeping at night.

ETHICAL DILEMMAS

WITHDRAWING TREATMENT

Situation A patient with chronic renal failure tells the nurse he wants to discontinue his dialysis. His quality of life has diminished during the 2 years he has been on dialysis. He is not a prospective transplant patient. How should the nurse respond to the patient's request?

Discussion The first concern about a patient's wish to discontinue life support treatment should be his or her mental state. Is the patient clinically depressed, mentally affected by the progress of the disease or condition, or affected by the medication or treatment? If a psychiatric consultation finds the patient is not impaired, then a competent adult patient has expressed a legally valid treatment directive. As the case manager, the nurse should explain the consequences to the patient and to the family of withdrawing treatment and offer a referral to hospice care. The physician should be contacted to confer with the patient and family and should offer palliative support.

ETHICAL AND LEGAL ISSUES

- There is no ethical responsibility to continue or finish a treatment once it has begun, especially if the patient no longer consents to it or if it is no longer having the intended outcome.
- Dialysis therapy may control, but it cannot cure renal failure. The goal of technologic intervention is to relieve undue burdens on the patient, as the patient defines burden. However, once the patient perceives that the burden of the treatment outweighs the benefits, a competent adult patient may decide to request the withdrawal of treatment.
- The competent adult has the legal right to forego any form of treatment, including life-sustaining treatment.

Continuous ambulatory peritoneal dialysis. CAPD is carried out manually by exchanging 1.5 to 3 L (usually 2 L) of peritoneal dialysate usually four times daily with dwell times of 4 to 10 hours. One schedule, for example, starts the three exchanges at 7 AM, 12 noon, and 5 PM, and the fourth exchange at 10 PM. In this procedure the person instills 2 L of dialysate from a collapsible plastic bag into the peritoneal cavity through a disposable plastic tube (called the *line* or *transfer set*). The tube is secured to the permanent catheter on one end and attaches to the bag on the other end by means of a device (commonly called a *spike*). Technical advances in CAPD systems, including Y sets and twin bag systems, allow the bag and line to be disconnected after the instillation of the fluid. After the equilibration period the line is reconnected to the catheter, and the dialysate (effluent) is drained from the peritoneal cavity, and a new 2 L bag of dialysate solution is infused (Fig. 44-10). It is critical in PD to maintain aseptic technique. Several tubing connections and devices are commercially available to help maintain an aseptic system.

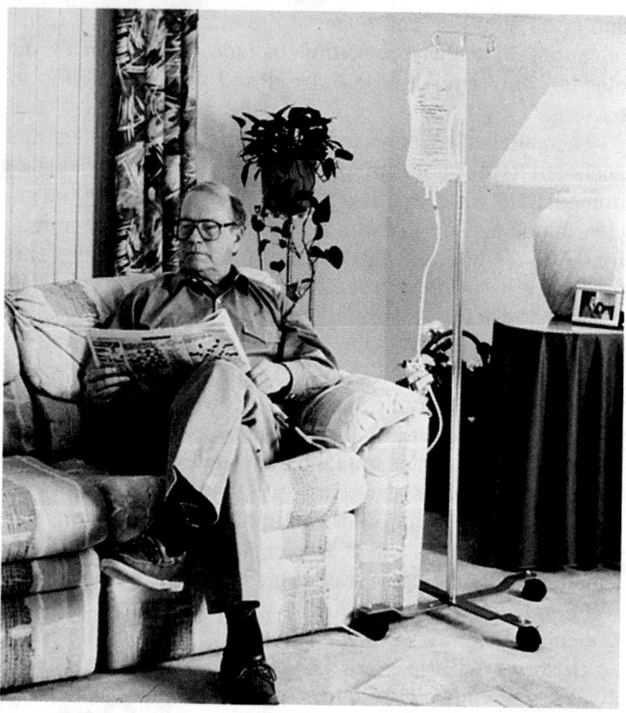

Fig. 44-10 Infusion period for a continuous ambulatory peritoneal dialysis patient.

Contraindications for PD include the following:

1. History of multiple abdominal surgical procedures or severe pathology (e.g., severe pancreatitis, diverticulitis)
2. Recurrent abdominal wall or inguinal hernias
3. Excessive obesity with large abdominal wall and fat deposits
4. Preexisting vertebral disease (e.g., chronic back problems)
5. Severe obstructive pulmonary disease

Complications

Exit site infection. Infection of the peritoneal catheter exit site is most commonly caused by *Staphylococcus aureus* or *S. epidermidis*. Superficial exit-site infections caused by these organisms are generally resolved with antibiotic therapy. Clinical manifestations of an exit-site infection include redness at site, tenderness, and drainage. If not treated immediately, subcutaneous tunnel infections usually result in abscess formation and may cause peritonitis and thus necessitate catheter removal.[24]

Peritonitis. Peritonitis results from contamination of the dialysate or tubing or from progression of exit-site or tunnel infections. Peritonitis is usually caused by *S. aureus* or *S. epidermidis* (from skin flora). The primary clinical manifestation of peritonitis is a cloudy peritoneal effluent that has a WBC count of over 100 cells per microliter (particularly neutrophils). GI manifestations may also be present, including diffuse abdominal pain, diarrhea, vomiting, abdominal distention, and hyperactive bowel sounds. Fever may or may not be present. Cultures, Gram's stain, and a cell count and a differential of peritoneal effluent are used to confirm the diagnosis of peritonitis. Antibiotics are given by mouth, IV, or intraperitoneally. The patient is usually treated on an outpatient basis. Repeated infections may necessitate the removal of the peritoneal catheter and termination of dialysis. The formation of adhesions in the peritoneum can result from repeated infections and can interfere with the peritoneal membrane's ability as a dialyzing surface.

Abdominal pain. Although not severe, pain is a common complication caused by the low pH of the dialysate solution, peritonitis, intraperitoneal irritation (which usually subsides in 1 to 2 weeks), and placement of the catheter. Pain can also occur when the tip of the catheter touches the bladder, bowel, or peritoneum. A change in the position of the catheter should correct this problem. Accidental infusion of air or infusing the dialysate too rapidly may cause referred pain in the shoulder. If the infusion rate is decreased, the pain usually subsides.

Outflow problems. When outflow is less than 80% of inflow immediately after catheter placement, it may be caused by a kink in the tunnel segment of the catheter, omentum wrapped around the catheter, or migration of the catheter out of the pelvic region. Outflow problems after the catheter has settled into place are often a result of a full colon; bowel evacuation frequently relieves the problem.

Hernias. Because of increased intraabdominal pressures secondary to the dialysate infusion, hernias develop in predisposed individuals such as multiparous women and older men. However, in most situations after hernia repair, peritoneal dialysis can be restarted after several days using small dialysate volumes and keeping the patient supine.

Lower back problems. Increased intraabdominal pressure can cause or aggravate lower back pain. The lumbosacral curvature is increased by intraperitoneal infusion of dialysate. Orthopedic binders and a regular exercise program for the back muscles have been beneficial for some patients.

Bleeding. Effluent drained after the first few exchanges may be pink or slightly bloody because of the trauma of catheter insertion. Bloody effluent over several days or the new appearance of blood in the effluent can indicate active intraperitoneal bleeding. If this occurs, the blood pressure and hematocrit need to be determined. Blood may also be present in the effluent of women who are menstruating.

Pulmonary complications. Atelectasis, pneumonia, and bronchitis may occur from repeated upward displacement of the diaphragm, resulting in decreased lung expansion. The longer the dwell time, the greater the likelihood of pulmonary complications. Frequent repositioning and deep-breathing exercises can help alleviate pulmonary complications. When lying in bed, elevation of the head of the bed may prevent these problems.

Protein loss. The peritoneal membrane is permeable to plasma proteins, amino acids, and polypeptides. Therefore these substances are lost in the dialysate fluid. The amount of loss may be as much as 9 to 12 g per day. This protein loss may be increased up to 40 g per day during episodes of peritonitis. The patient can maintain a positive nitrogen balance with satisfactory protein intake.

Carbohydrate and lipid abnormalities. Dialysate glucose is absorbed via the peritoneum and may amount to as much as 100 to 150 g per day. Continuous absorption of glucose results in increased insulin secretion and increased plasma insulin levels. The hyperinsulinemia stimulates hepatic production of triglycerides (see p. 1380).

Encapsulating sclerosing peritonitis. *Encapsulating sclerosing peritonitis* is a term applied to the development of a thick fibrous membrane that surrounds and compresses the bowel. Intestinal obstruction and strangulation are common complications. This condition generally necessitates changing the patient to HD because of the loss of ultrafiltration.

Loss of ultrafiltration. Loss of ultrafiltration is associated with encapsulating sclerosing peritonitis. It can also occur as a result of unknown reasons or accidental infusion of disinfecting agents. Loss of ultrafiltration is associated with rapid glucose absorption.

Effectiveness of and Adaptation to Chronic Peritoneal Dialysis. The use and popularity of chronic PD is increasing. The technique is associated with a short training program, independence, and ease of traveling. Clinically, the patient on PD does at least as well as the patient on HD and sometimes better. There are fewer dietary restrictions, and greater mobility is possible than with conventional HD. The major disadvantage is the possibility of developing peritonitis. As further improvements in techniques are made (e.g., improved connecting and sterilizing devices, inline filters, improved catheters), the incidence of peritonitis should decrease.

PD is especially indicated for the individual who has vascular access problems and responds poorly to the hemodynamic stresses of HD (e.g., the older adult patient with diabetes and cardiovascular disease). The diabetic patient with ESRD does better on PD than on HD. The advantages of PD for the diabetic patient includes better blood pressure control, stable cardiovascular status without rapid fluid shifts, better control of blood sugars by intraperitoneal insulin (which can often eliminate the need for subcutaneous insulin), and avoidance of the risk of retinal hemorrhage from heparin use during HD.

Hemodialysis

In 1943, Willem Kolff in the Netherlands performed the first successful dialysis on a human being with the use of a rotating-drum dialyzer. He established dialysis treatment in the United States in the 1950s.

Vascular Access Sites. Vascular access is one of the major problems with HD. To carry out HD, a high blood flow is required. Before 1960, HD required the insertion of needles into arteries and veins for each dialysis. Chronic dialysis was not possible with this technique. In 1960 Scribner developed a Teflon silicone rubber cannula that could be inserted into the radial artery and into an adjacent forearm vein (Fig. 44-11, *A*). The cannula is implanted subcutaneously in both the artery and vein and is connected to a silicone rubber tubing that exits from the skin. The two ends are connected by a U-shaped shunt that has a connector at its midpoint. This connection can be opened after

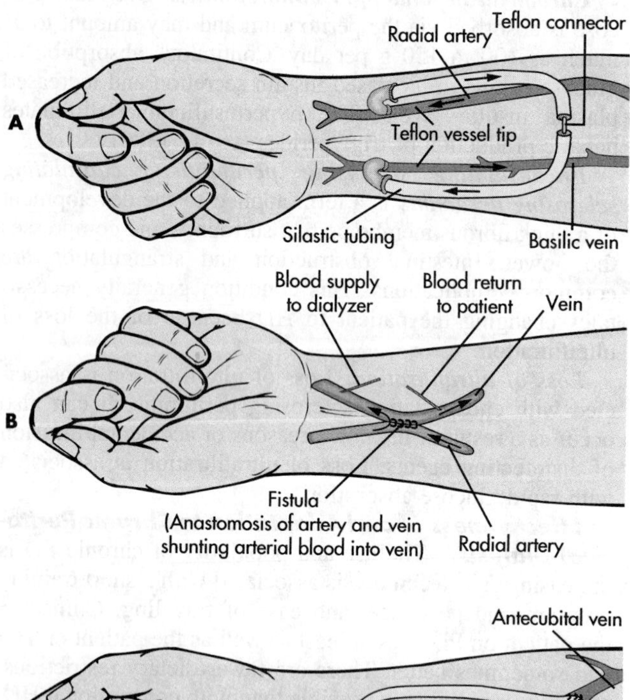

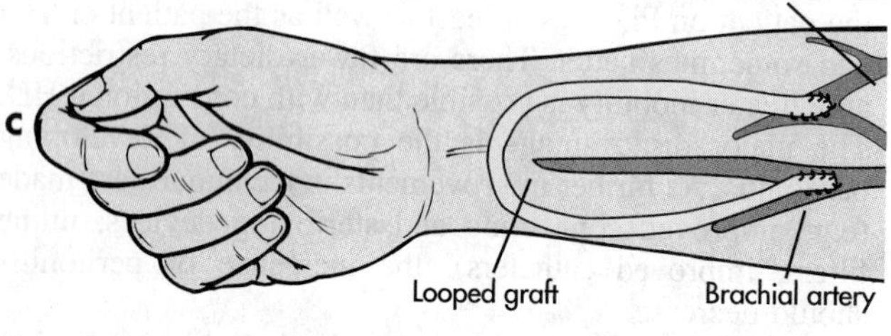

Fig. 44-11 Methods of vascular access for hemodialysis. ***A,*** External cannula or shunt. ***B,*** Internal arteriovenous fistula. ***C,*** Looped graft in forearm.

clamping on both sides to attach the patient to the dialysis machine. The external access cannula is commonly referred to as an *external shunt* and can be used immediately. The external shunt is associated with many complications including infection and bleeding. Therefore it is rarely used for chronic dialysis. Its primary use is as a temporary access for continuous renal replacement therapy (see later discussion).

Internal arteriovenous fistulas and grafts. In 1966 the use of the subcutaneous internal arteriovenous native fistula (Fig. 44-11, *B*) was introduced by Cimino and Brescia. An arteriovenous (AV) fistula is created in the forearm or thigh by a side-to-side, end-to-side, or end-to-end anastomosis between an artery (usually radial or ulnar) and a vein (usually cephalic). The fistula provides for arterial blood flow through the vein. The increased pressure of the arterial blood flow through the vein makes the vein dilate and become tough making it accessible for repeated venipuncture and allowing it to handle the high blood flows required for HD. The vein is accessed using two large gauge needles.

Native (using the person's own blood vessels) fistulas are suitable only for the patient with relatively healthy blood vessels. Therefore native fistulas are often not created in the patient with severe hypertension, diabetes, or history of IV drug abuse. For these individuals a synthetic graft is usually required. The grafts are made of synthetic materials (PTFE, polytetrafluoroethylene/Teflon) and form a "bridge" between the arterial and venous blood supplies.[25] Grafts are surgically anastomosed between an artery (usually brachial) and a vein (usually antecubital) (Fig. 44-11, *C*). The graft, like the fistula, is under the skin and accessed using two large gauge needles. Because grafts are made of manmade materials, they can become infected easily and are thrombogenic.

The native fistula requires 4 to 6 weeks to mature (dilate and toughen) sufficiently for use. Similarly, when a graft is created, an interval of 2 to 4 weeks is usually necessary to allow for healing. Some institutions use the graft earlier. Two 14- to 16-gauge needles are inserted into the engorged vein or graft (with the use of local anesthesia) to obtain vascular access. The needles are attached via tubing to dialysis lines. Normally, a thrill can be felt by palpating the area of anastomosis, and a bruit can be heard with a stethoscope. The bruit and thrill are created by arterial blood rushing into the vein. Blood pressures, IV insertion, and venipuncture should not be performed on the affected extremity.

The subcutaneous AV fistula is much less likely to clot and become infected than a graft. Native fistulas seem to get better as the years go by. Thrombosis in grafts is common. Grafts can lead to the development of distal ischemia (steal syndrome) because arterial blood is being shunted. This is usually seen soon after surgery. Another complication is the development of an aneurysm at the fistula site. When a graft becomes infected, it is a serious problem that is frequently associated with bacteremia and often requires the removal of the graft.

Temporary vascular access. In some situations when temporary vascular access is required, percutaneous cannulation of the subclavian, internal jugular, or femoral vein is used. A flexible Teflon, silicone rubber, or polyurethane catheter is inserted into one of these large veins and provides easy immediate access to circulation without the need for the patient to have surgery or to sacrifice a peripheral artery or vein. The catheters usually have a double lumen (Fig. 44-12). The procedure for percutaneous cannulation is similar to the method of insertion of a pulmonary artery catheter (see Chapter 61).

Percutaneous cannulas in the subclavian or jugular veins can be left in place for 1 to 3 weeks. Femoral-vein cannulas can remain in place for up to 1 week. A disadvantage of femoral-vessel cannulization is the short time the catheter can remain in place. If these vessels are used for vascular access, repeated venipunctures are needed for the course of acute dialysis. Complications of femoral catheterization consist of femoral-vein thrombosis with pulmonary emboli (especially if the treatment is prolonged), infections, immobility, and inadvertent blood-vessel punctures with hematoma formation. Technical complications of subclavian vein catheterization include brachial plexus problems, hemothorax, and pneumothorax. A moderate risk of infection also exists. While the catheter is in place, the patient is

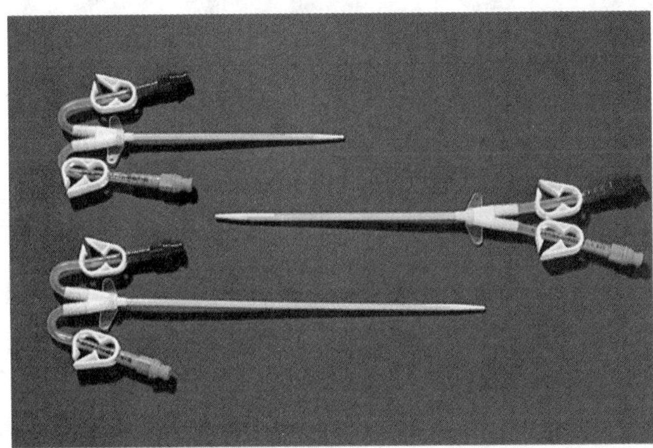

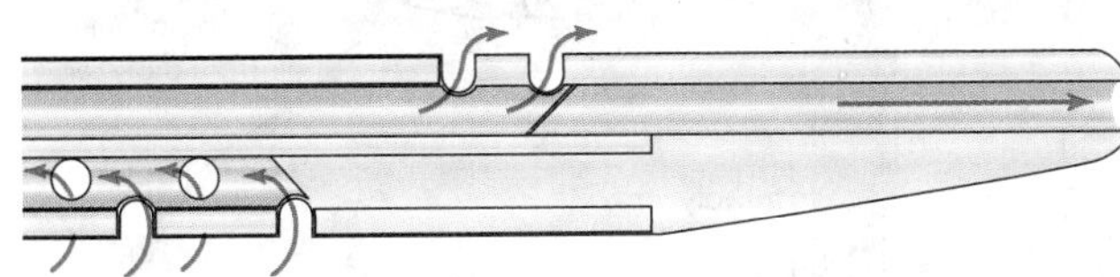

Fig. 44-12 Temporary double-lumen-single-needle vascular access catheter for acute hemodialysis. ***A,*** The soft, flexible dual-lumen polyurethane tube is attached to a Y hub. ***B,*** Blood is withdrawn continuously through the outer lumen upstream and returned through the inner lumen downstream, thus reducing recirculation.

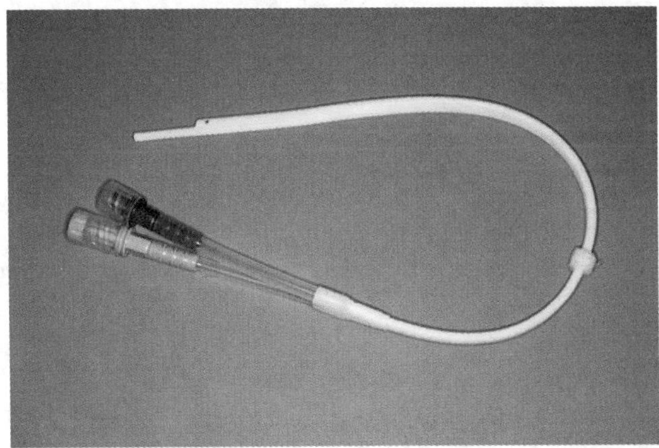

Fig. 44-13 Silastic permanent catheter used for permanent or temporary access.

usually comfortable and can be ambulatory. No medications should be administered or blood withdrawn from this catheter by nondialysis staff. Trained dialysis staff may inject heparin into the lumen of the catheter at the end of dialysis and remove the heparin before starting dialysis. Subclavian vein thrombosis and stenosis is a complication of subclavian cannulation. Although jugular cannulation is associated with a low incidence of jugular vein thrombosis, short-term jugular vein access with stiff catheters is often unacceptable to the patient since the catheter is in the patient's neck and can cause pain and restrict movement.

A permanent, soft, flexible Silastic double-lumen catheter is being used more commonly (Fig. 44-13). It exits on the upper chest wall and is tunneled subcutaneously to the internal or external jugular vein. It has two Dacron cuffs, which reside subcutaneously to prevent infection and anchor the catheter, thus eliminating the need for sutures. A disadvantage is that the catheter must be placed radiologically. It is used as a temporary access while awaiting fistula placement and development or long-term access when other forms of vascular access have failed.[26]

When dialysis is indicated, a permanent access is created, and a temporary access is used until the permanent access becomes available to use. A subcutaneous AV fistula is created or a graft inserted, and the patient is hemodialyzed via a subclavian or jugular catheter until the AV fistula or graft is ready. Preferably the AV fistula or graft is surgically created while the patient is being maintained on conservative therapy, well in advance of ESRD.

Dialyzers. The coil dialyzer was the first type of dialyzer used in which blood flowed through a series of cellophane tubes. Historically, this was later replaced by a flat plate dialyzer (Kiil) in which blood flowed between sheets of membrane outside of which the dialysate passed. Today the dialyzer is a hollow fiber tube that contains thousands of parallel fibers packed in a cylinder (Fig. 44-14). The fibers are the semipermeable membrane made of cellulose-based or other synthetic materials. The blood is pumped through the fibers, and dialysis fluid bathes the outside of them with dialysis, and ultrafiltration occurs through the pores of the semipermeable membrane. Various dialyzers differ in regard to surface area, membrane composition and thickness, clearance of waste products, and removal of fluid.

Most chronic dialysis units now reprocess and reuse the dialyzers for the same patient after cleaning and subsequent disinfection. Reprocessing and reusing dialyzers allows for significant cost savings. With reuse the dialyzers become more biocompatible so that there are fewer side effects from blood-membrane interactions during the dialysis procedure. A major concern with reprocessing and reuse is potential residual contamination from the disinfectant used to clean the dialyzer.

Procedure. To initiate chronic dialysis, two needles are placed in the fistula or graft. The needle closest to the fistula is used to obtain "arterial" blood from the patient and send it to the dialyzer with the assistance of a blood pump. The dialyzer is usually primed with saline solution. The saline solution is infused into the patient as blood fills the dialyzer circuit. Heparin is added to the blood as it flows into the dialyzer to prevent clotting. Once the blood enters the extracorporeal circuit, it is propelled through the dialyzer by a blood pump at a flow rate of 200 to 500 ml/min, while the dialysate (warmed to body temperature) circulates in the opposite direction at a rate of 300 to 900 ml/min. Blood is returned from the dialyzer to the patient via the "venous" line through the second needle.

In addition to the dialyzer, there is a dialysate delivery and monitoring system (Fig. 44-15). This system pumps the dialysate through the dialyzer, countercurrent to the blood flow. Adjustments can be made for ultrafiltration by creating a positive pressure in the blood side or a negative

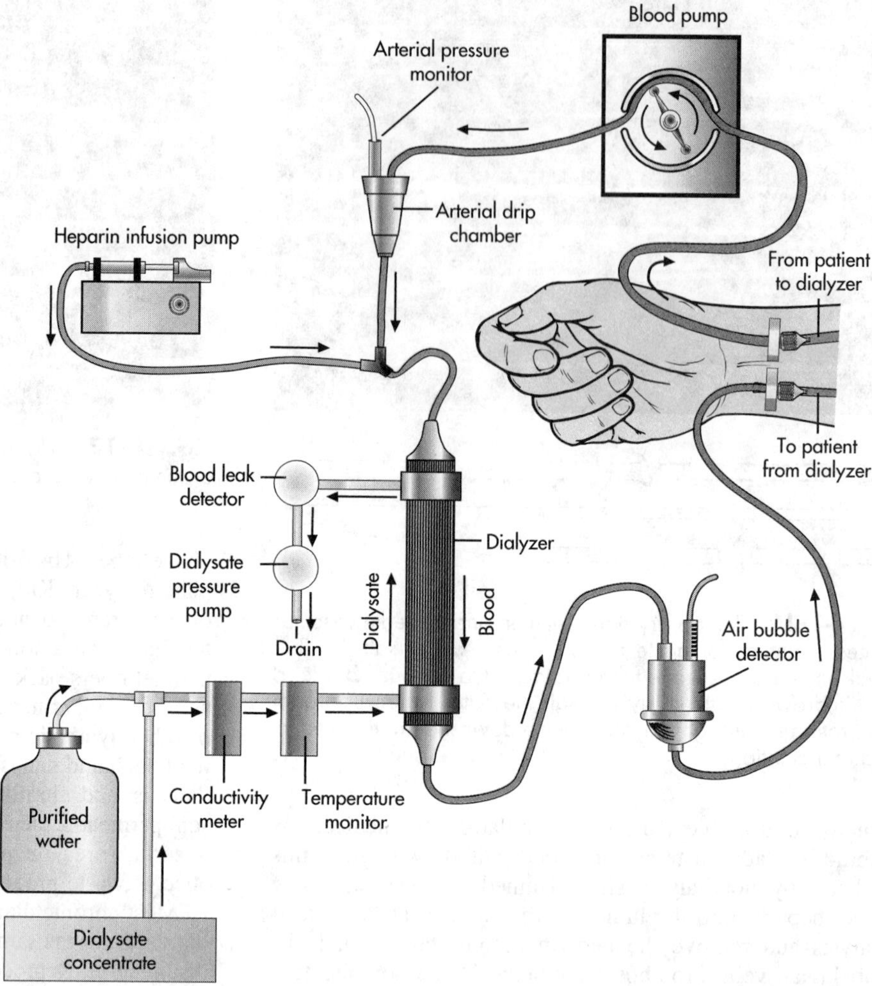

Fig. 44-14 Components of a hemodialysis system.

pressure on the dialysate side or by a combination of both. The newest dialysis delivery systems have ultrafiltration controllers that equalize negative and positive pressures for the removal of the precise amount of fluid per hour. The dialysis system has an alarm system to warn of blood leaking into the dialysate or air leaking into the blood; alterations in dialysate temperature, concentration, or pressure; and extremes in blood pressure readings.

Dialysis is terminated by flushing the dialyzer with saline solution to return all blood to the patient. The needles are then removed from the patient, and firm pressure is applied to the venipuncture sites until the bleeding stops.

Before beginning treatment, the nurse must complete an assessment that includes fluid status (weight, blood pressure, peripheral edema, lung and heart sounds), condition of vascular access, temperature, and general condition of the skin. The difference between the last postdialysis weight and the present predialysis weight determines the ultrafiltration or the amount of weight to be removed. Ideally, no more than 1.0 to 1.5 kg should be gained between treatments to avoid causing hypotension associated with the removal of larger volumes of fluid. While the patient is on dialysis, vital signs should be taken at least every 30 to 60 minutes, since rapid changes may occur in the blood pressure.

Most maintenance dialysis units use reclining chairs in an attempt to create a nonhospital environment. Most people sleep, read, talk, or watch television during dialysis. HD usually lasts 3 to 4 hours and occurs three times per week. While patients are attached to dialysis machines, they can engage in meaningful interaction with the staff.

Settings for Hemodialysis. HD can be done in an inpatient (hospital) or outpatient (clinic or hospital) setting. Inpatient dialysis is used for treating seriously ill patients. In outpatient dialysis the patient comes to the hospital or a satellite unit for treatment. The patient may choose self-care in either setting with backup support from trained personnel if needed. The patient who self-cares often puts in the needles and sets up the machines.

Another choice of setting for HD is the home. In 1963 home HD training was started. Today only about 2% of patients on HD use it. One of the main advantages of home HD is that it allows greater freedom in choosing dialysis times. Today home PD is the treatment choice for more patients because it is less technically demanding.

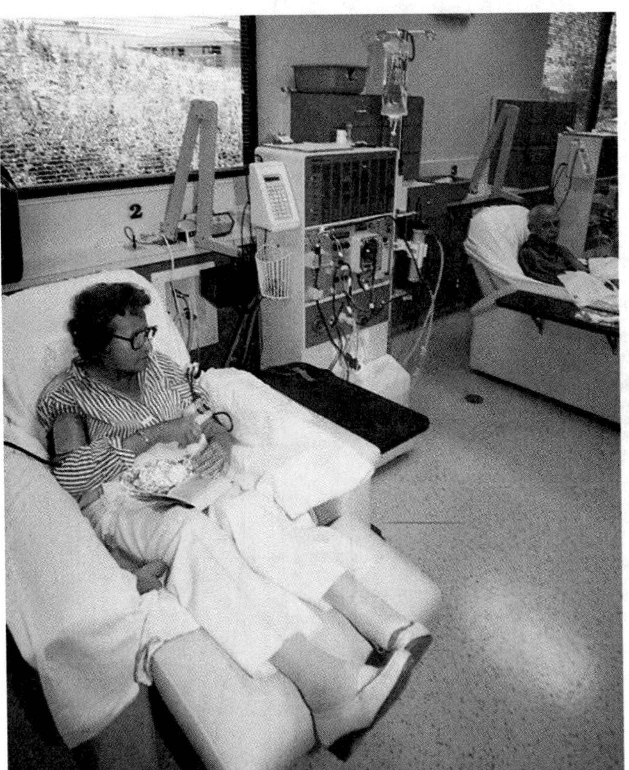

Fig. 44-15 Hemodialysis delivery system.

Complications of Hemodialysis

Disequilibrium syndrome. *Disequilibrium syndrome* develops as a result of rapid changes in the composition of the extracellular fluid. Urea, sodium, and other solutes are removed more rapidly from the blood than from the cerebrospinal fluid and the brain. This creates a high osmotic gradient in the brain resulting in the shift of fluid into the brain, causing cerebral edema. Manifestations include nausea, vomiting, confusion, restlessness, headaches, twitching and jerking, and seizures. In addition, the rapid changes in osmolality may cause muscle cramps and contribute to hypotension. Treatment consists of slowing or stopping dialysis and infusing hypertonic saline solution, albumin, or mannitol to draw fluid from the brain cells back into circulation. It is more commonly observed in the initial treatment of the patient when the BUN level is high. First dialyses are purposely short and inefficient to limit total solute removal.

Hypotension. Hypotension that occurs during HD primarily results from rapid removal of vascular volume (hypovolemia), decreased cardiac output, and decreased systemic vascular resistance. The drop in blood pressure during dialysis may precipitate lightheadedness, nausea, vomiting, seizures, and coronary ischemia. The usual treatment for hypotension includes decreasing the volume of fluid being removed, infusion of 0.9% saline solution (100 to 300 ml), and placement of the patient in Trendelenburg position to improve cerebral blood flow and increase blood pressure. If a patient experiences recurrent hypotensive episodes, a reassessment may have to be done of dry weight, dialyzer size, and blood pressure medications. Blood pressure medications may be held before dialysis if there is hypotension during dialysis.

Muscle cramps. Muscle cramps are a common problem in the patient on dialysis and are associated with significant discomfort and pain. They result from too rapid removal of sodium and water or from neuromuscular hypersensitivity. Treatment includes reducing the ultrafiltration rate and administering a hypertonic solution or normal saline bolus.

Loss of blood. Blood loss may result from residual blood not being rinsed from the dialyzer, from accidental separation of blood tubing or dialysis membrane rupture, or from bleeding after the removal of needles at the end of dialysis. In a patient who has received too much heparin or has clotting problems, there can be significant postdialysis bleeding.

Hepatitis. The cause of hepatitis in the patient on dialysis is related to blood transfusions, IV drug abuse, or the lack of adherence to precautions used to prevent the spread of infection. Although the patient is frequently free of symptoms if he develops hepatitis B as a result of his immunocompromised state, the patient does become a carrier of hepatitis B. The incidence of hepatitis B has decreased with frequent testing for hepatitis B surface antigen (HB_sAg), isolation of the infected dialysis patient, the use of disposable equipment, and the use of universal precautions. In addition, hepatitis B vaccine is now available to patients and personnel in dialysis units.

Currently hepatitis C is responsible for the majority of cases of hepatitis in dialysis patients. (Hepatitis is discussed in more detail in Chapter 41.) Currently the Centers for Disease Control and Prevention (CDC) does not recommend isolation of the HD patient positive for hepatitis C antibody. Universal precautions are mandated in the care of the patient with hepatitis C to protect the patient and staff.[27] Further evaluation of the clinical importance of hepatitis C is needed.

Sepsis. Sepsis is most often related to infections of vascular access sites. Bacteria can also be introduced during the dialysis treatment as a result of poor technique or interruption of blood tubings or dialyzer membranes. Bacterial endocarditis can occur because of the frequent and prolonged access to the vascular system.

Dialysis encephalopathy. Dialysis encephalopathy, a progressive neurologic impairment, is characterized by speech disturbances, dementia, lack of muscle coordination, and myoclonic seizures. A frequent cause of this problem is aluminum toxicity, which may result from ingestion of aluminum-containing antacids and a decreased ability of the kidneys to excrete aluminum. Phosphate-binding antacids (e.g., calcium acetate, calcium carbonate) that are not aluminum-based are being administered.

Increased incidence of cancer. There is a significant increase in the incidence of neoplasms in the patient with renal failure who has not had transplants as compared with the general population. Lung, breast, uterus, colon, prostate, and skin malignancies are most commonly found.[28]

Effectiveness of and Adaptation to Hemodialysis. HD is still an imperfect technique in treating ESRD. It

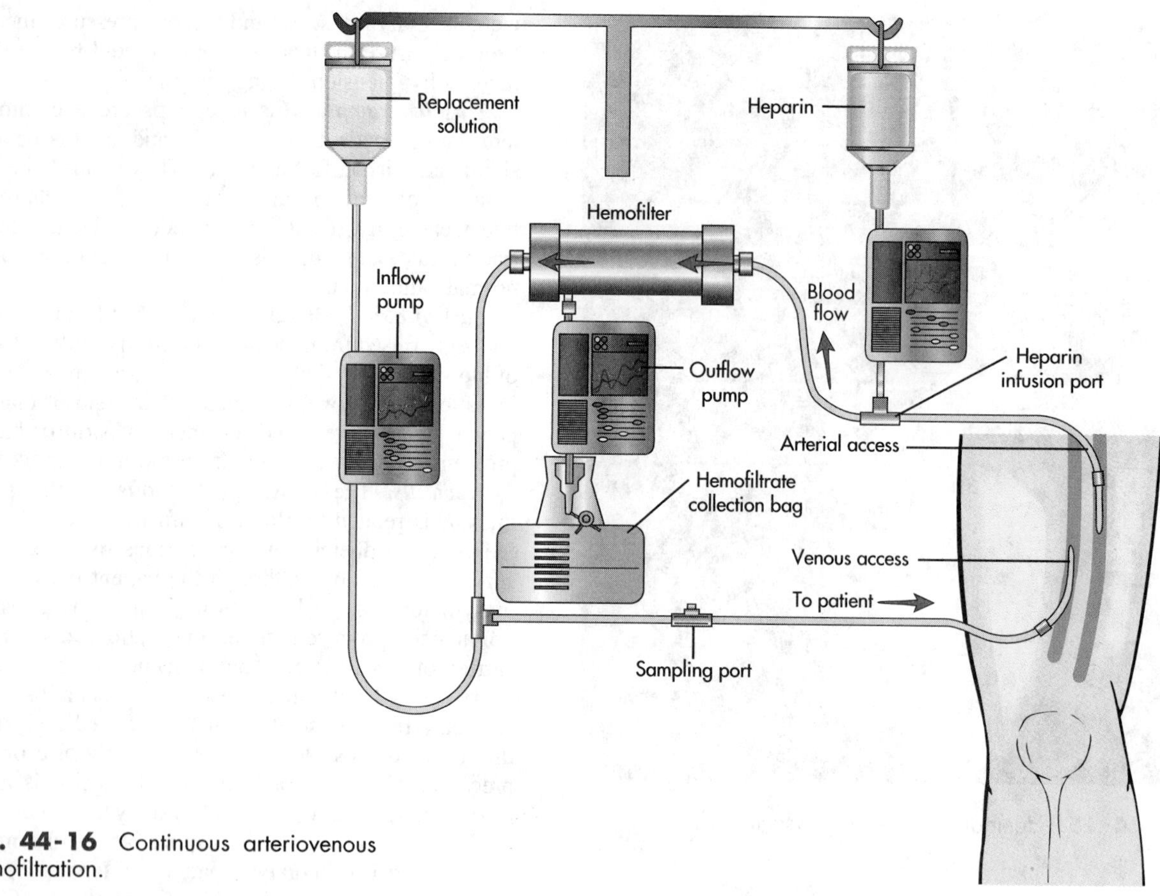

Fig. 44-16 Continuous arteriovenous hemofiltration.

cannot replace the metabolic and hormonal functions of the kidneys. HD can relieve most of the symptoms of chronic renal failure and, if started early, can prevent certain complications. However, it does not alter the accelerated atherosclerosis and may only partially correct anemia.

The yearly death rate of patients on maintenance dialysis has increased from about 10% to close to 20%.[10] The major reason for this is the increased proportion of older adult patients who are now receiving dialysis as maintenance therapy. The majority of deaths are caused by cardiovascular-related disease (cerebrovascular accident or myocardial infarction); infectious complications are the second leading cause of death. Many of the complications associated with chronic renal failure continue after the transplantation period and can affect the success of a kidney transplant.

Individual adaptation to maintenance HD varies considerably. Initially many patients feel positive about the machine because it makes them feel better. Some people come to hospitals or satellite units for dialysis because they know that if they are not treated, they will get sick and die. Dependence on a machine is a reality. Many patients have dreams about being tied to the machine. Depression and suicidal tendencies may be manifested in noncompliance with diet or drug therapy or in a large weight gain. A primary nursing goal is to help the patient regain or maintain positive self-esteem and continue to be productive in society.

Continuous Renal Replacement Therapy

CRRT is an alternative or adjunctive method of treating acute renal failure (Fig. 44-16). CRRT provides a means by which solutes and fluids can be removed slowly and continuously in the hemodynamically unstable patient.[29] CRRT is especially useful in the individual with fluid overload regardless of the cause of the overload (e.g., acute renal failure with or without hemodynamic instability, pulmonary edema). If a patient with acute renal failure has severe manifestations of uremia (e.g., hyperkalemia, pericarditis), HD is indicated for therapy rather than any of the continuous therapies. However, CRRT can be used in conjunction with HD for continuous fluid removal.

There are several technical variations of CRRT. In ultrafiltration techniques, fluid is removed but not replaced. In hemofiltration, fluid and solutes are removed, and fluid is replaced. One type of CRRT is continuous arteriovenous therapies (CAVT), which include slow continous ultrafiltration (SCUF), continuous arteriovenous hemofiltration (CAVH), and continuous arteriovenous hemodialysis (CAVHD). Continuous venovenous therapies (CVVT) achieve the same goals of CAVT but do not require arterial access.

In CAVH a highly permeable hollow fiber hemofilter removes plasma water and nonprotein solutes, which are collectively called *ultrafiltrate*. Vascular access is achieved by means of an AV Scribner external shunt or cannulation of the femoral artery and vein or a subclavian vein. The systemic blood pressure provides the force to achieve sufficient blood flow through the hemofilter. When the hydrostatic pressure exceeds the oncotic pressure, water and nonprotein solutes pass out of the filter into the extracapillary space and drain through the ultrafiltrate port into a collection device. The remaining fluid continues through the filter and returns to the patient through the venous access site. While the ultrafiltrate pours out of the hemofilter, fluid and electrolyte replacements can be infused into the venous port. This fluid is designed to replace volume and solutes such as sodium, chloride, bicarbonate, and glucose and is free of unwanted solutes such as creatinine, urea, potassium, and phosphates. Total parenteral nutrition can also be infused to provide essential nutrients. The infusion rate of replacement fluids is determined in accordance with the ultrafiltration rate to control weight reduction and fluid and electrolyte elimination. Replacement fluid may also be infused into the arterial port and is called *predilutional fluid replacement*. This method of fluid replacement allows for greater clearance of urea and can decrease filter clotting. Like HD, CAVH provides for the removal of fluid, electrolytes, and solutes. However, several of its features differ from HD, including the following:

1. It is continuous rather than intermittent.
2. Solute removal occurs by means of convection rather than by osmosis and diffusion (no dialysate required).
3. It relies on a patient's blood pressure rather than a pump to propel blood through the circuit.
4. It has fewer or no effects on cardiovascular stability (e.g., hypotension).
5. It does not require the specialized skills of a HD nurse.
6. It does not require complicated HD equipment.

CAVH can be continued as long as 30 to 40 days, but the hemofilter is changed about every 24 to 48 hours because of loss of filtration efficiency or clotting. The ultrafiltrate should be clear yellow, and specimens may be obtained for evaluation of serum chemistries. If the ultrafiltrate becomes bloody or blood-tinged, a possible rupture in the filter membrane should be suspected, and changing the hemofilter is necessary.

During CAVH the nurse must monitor fluid and electrolyte balance. Hourly intake and output measurements and daily weights must be recorded. Vital signs and hemodynamic status should be monitored hourly. Although reductions in central venous pressure and pulmonary artery pressure are expected, there should be little change in mean arterial pressure or cardiac output. Assessment and care of the vascular access sites are important.

An alternative to CAVH is CAVHD. During CAVHD a bag of PD solution is connected to the end of the hemofilter opposite the ultrafiltration port and infused, creating a diffusion gradient. The advantage of CAVHD is that urea and creatinine clearances are greater than during CAVH. The increased rate of solute removal can reduce the incidence of uremia, acidosis, and electrolyte imbalances. High ultrafiltration rates can be achieved by changing the glucose concentration of the dialysis solution to create a greater osmotic gradient.

In CVVT both output and input vascular access sites are venous. For the hemodynamically unstable patient with no arterial access, low platelet count, or coagulation problems, CVVT may be the only treatment option. One double-lumen catheter is inserted into a large vein, usually the subclavian or femoral. A blood pump is used to regulate blood flow. Because the blood flow rate remains constant, there is less clotting in the filter.[30]

TRANSPLANTATION

The first kidney transplant in the United States was performed in 1954 in Boston between identical twins. Today in the United States, over 100,000 individuals have received kidney transplants. The limited availability of living related donors (LRDs) has turned the focus to cadaveric donors. Although there are over 160,000 people on maintenance dialysis, only about 9000 kidney transplants are performed each year. Currently, more than 20,000 people are waiting for kidney transplants.[31]

Preoperative Period

Living Related Donor Selection and Preparation. LRDs provide 15% to 20% and cadaveric donors provide 80% to 85% of all donated kidneys. LRDs are usually parents, siblings, or children. Only one donor kidney is needed to provide adequate renal function. Physiologic and psychologic assessments of a potential donor are done. Histocompatibility (tissue typing) studies and blood typing are done first. A donor must have a compatible blood type with the recipient and have a similar tissue type to prevent rejection. If the donor and recipient's blood type and tissue type are compatible, the prospective donor's complete history is taken, and a complete physical examination is performed, including chest x-ray, urinalysis, urine culture, intravenous pyelogram (IVP), ECG, complete blood count (CBC), electrolyte studies, glucose tolerance tests, BUN, serum creatinine, creatinine clearance, aortogram, and renal arteriogram. An individual can donate a single kidney since the remaining kidney will provide adequate renal function for the donor.

Cadaveric Donors. Cadaveric donors are most commonly trauma victims. The kidneys are suitable only if they have not been subjected to prolonged ischemia or trauma. The generally accepted age for cadaveric donors is 5 to 55 years, although suitable kidneys have been obtained from younger and older donors. Donors must be free of systemic disease (e.g., diabetes mellitus, malignancies) and infection (including hepatitis, HIV) and must have normal kidney function. Permission from the donor's immediate family is required after determination of brain death. Even if the donor carries a signed donor card, consent from the closest relative is required.

A nationwide computerized service is used to distribute cadaveric organs. The computer can identify patients whose tissue and blood types match that of the donor. The kidneys will then be distributed to patients based on a number of factors including current health status, amount of time on the waiting list, and geographic proximity to the donor's hospital.

After the kidneys are removed from the cadaveric donor, they are flushed with an electrolyte solution and can then be transported in a sterile environment in a compact watertight container filled with ice. This method is called *cold preservation* or *hypothermic storage*. With this method, kidneys can be preserved for up to 48 hours allowing for transport to other facilites.

Recipient Selection and Preparation. A successful transplant can now be achieved in circumstances previously thought to carry too high a risk of failure or death (e.g., in a patient with diabetes mellitus). The age range within which transplants are performed continues to widen. At the lower end, it now extends into the first year of life, and, at the higher end, there is no well-defined or widely agreed on cutoff point. Contraindications to transplantation include disseminated malignancies, refractory cardiac failure, chronic respiratory failure, extensive vascular disease, chronic infection, and unresolved psychosocial disorders (e.g., alcoholism, drug addiction). A hepatitis B carrier state is an adverse factor but not a contraindication to transplantation.

In addition to a determination of ABO blood type and human leukocyte antigens (HLAs) as baseline screening data, the potential recipient's serum should be screened regularly for cytotoxic (anti-HLA) antibodies (see later discussion). These antibodies often appear transiently or permanently after blood transfusion or rejection of a transplanted kidney. An individual with a high antibody level may have more difficulty finding a matching donor kidney.

Histocompatibility studies. Histocompatibility testing is performed to determine the degree of similarity between donor and recipient antigens. ABO blood group antigens are important in determining histocompatibility and must be matched. In addition, the HLAs, which determine the acceptance or rejection of transplanted tissue, are determined (see Chapter 10). All recipients and donors express HLA antigens on all nucleated cells. The HLA antigens initiate the process of rejection and serve as targets of the immunologic attack against the grafted organ (Fig. 44-17).

The HLA complex is located on chromosome 6 in humans. Major HLA loci that have been identified in this region include A, B, C, D, and D-related (DR) (see Fig. 10-10). Each locus may have multiple alleles (antigens). Each person has two antigens for each locus, one inherited from each parent. Because the genes that code for HLA are closely linked, they are inherited as a group or haplotype. One haplotype is inherited from each parent (see Fig. 10-10). After HLA testing, the potential kidney to be transplanted is considered an *HLA-one haplotype match, HLA-identical (two-haplotype match*), or *non-HLA-identical* (*HLA mismatch*).

The purpose of histocompatibility testing is to identify the antigens at each locus. A serologic test is used to type for the antigens at HLA-A, HLA-B, and HLA-C loci with lymphocytes taken from peripheral blood. The total time required for HLA typing is about 4 hours for HLA-A and HLA-B.

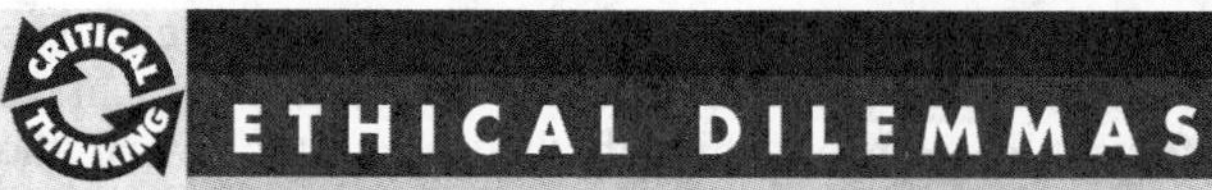

ALLOCATION OF RESOURCES

Situation The nurse on the transplant team has just been called about an available kidney that would be a possible match for two of her patients on the waiting list. One is a 58-year-old alcoholic who has spent most of his adult life in and out of prison. The other patient is a 40-year-old school teacher who is married and has two children. Which patient should she call?

Discussion It is tempting to believe that we can be neutral, basing our allocation of scarce resources on need rather than worth. Medical necessity rather than societal contribution should be the basis. However, it is difficult to practice patient-neutral care in life and death situations such as this. Before renal dialysis was covered by federal funding and before machines were as available as they are now, there were committees that decided which patients would receive dialysis. Out of this difficult process has grown a national organ procurement system, which is, in itself, set up to be neutral about the patient in all respects except those biologic and psychologic areas relevant to transplantation. If a patient is placed on the list for transplantation, no single patient is deemed of greater or lesser worth than any other patient. In cases of kidney transplantation, there is no option but to transplant the organ into the best matched patient, regardless of her or his position on the list or the health professional's opinion of the patient's *worth*.

ETHICAL AND LEGAL ISSUES

- Blaming the patient for his disease and his lifestyle choices does not contribute to the appropriate professional detachment owed to all patients. Unless medical history or current compliance will affect treatment decisions, they are best left out of consideration for allocation of scarce resources.
- Organ transplantation systems are based on medical necessity, prognosis, and need. If two patients of equal medical standing are on the list of those awaiting transplantation, the first one on the list has priority unless the patient's tissue type does not appropriately match that of the donor kidney.
- Any attempt to bring moral judgments about the worth of patients into the selection process for allocation of scarce resources raises the questions of criteria and authority. Finally, since organ donation is voluntary and altruistic in the United States, any concerns that the system of procurement and transplantation is not fair may negatively affect the pool of available organs.

A mixed lymphocyte culture assesses the antigen match at the D locus. In this test, lymphocytes from the recipient are incubated for 5 to 7 days with lymphocytes from the donor. The degree of proliferation of lymphocytes correlates with the degree to which the donor cells are recognized as foreign. This is the in vitro equivalent of the

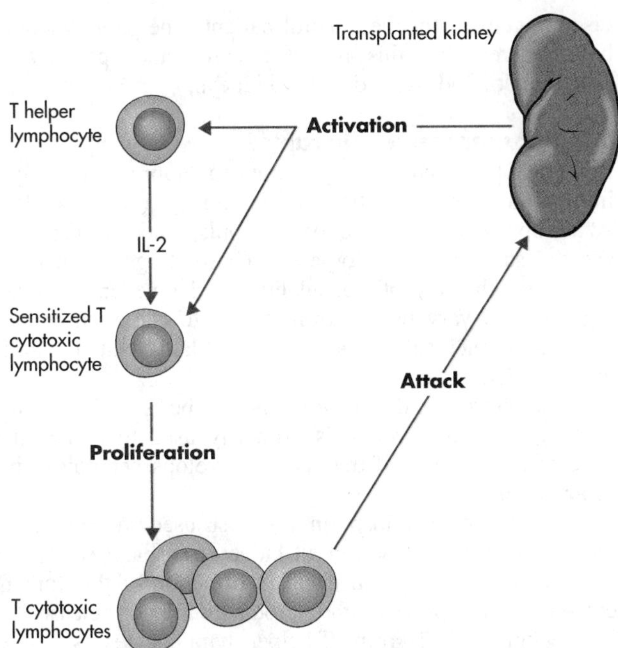

Fig. 44-17 The mechanism of action of T-cytotoxic lymphocyte activation and attack of renal transplanted tissue. The transplanted kidney is recognized as foreign and activates the immune system. T helper cells are activated to produce interleukin-2 and T cytotoxic lymphocytes are sensitized. After these T cytotoxic cells proliferate, they attack the transplanted kidney.

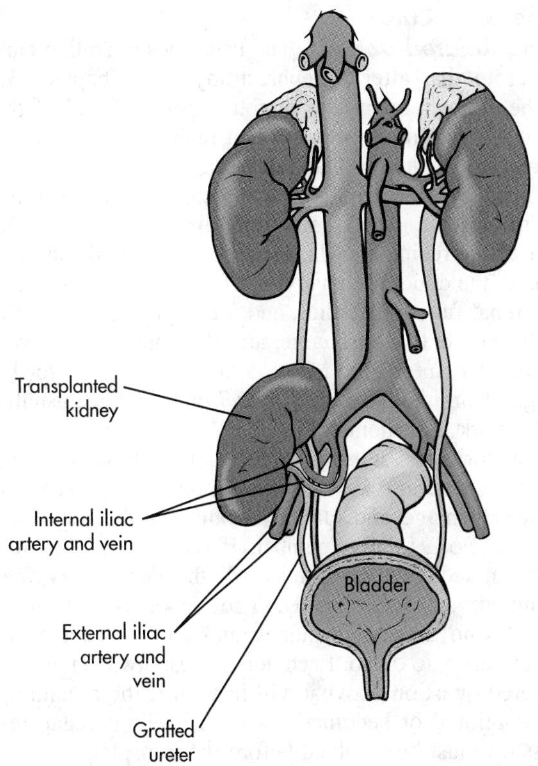

Fig. 44-18 Surgical placement of transplanted kidney.

response expected in vivo. Because this test takes so long, it is not used for cadaveric donors. HLA-DR typing is done by means of a serologic test similar to HLA-A and HLA-B typing to assess for D-antigen compatibility in cadaveric transplant situations. Since D and DR loci are so closely linked on the chromosome, the products of these two loci are probably inherited together. Typing for DR takes about 4 to 6 hours.

A tissue typing crossmatch uses serum from the recipient mixed with donor lymphocytes to test for any preformed cytotoxic (anti-HLA) antibodies to the donated kidney. The recipient may have been exposed to antigens similar to those of the donor by means of previous blood transfusions, pregnancy, or a previous kidney transplant. This procedure takes about 3 to 5 hours and is used in both LRDs and cadaveric donors. A positive crossmatch indicates that the recipient has cytotoxic antibodies to the donor and is an absolute contraindication to transplantation. If transplanted, this type of kidney will immediately undergo hyperacute rejection.

In cadaveric transplantation an attempt is made to match as many antigens as possible between the HLA-A, HLA-B, and HLA-DR loci. The effect of a good match is less important in the era of new immunosuppressive medication. However, this is a matter of controversy.

Preoperative dialysis. In the patient on HD, preoperative dialysis is usually required unless the last routine dialysis was completed within the previous 24 hours. The main purpose of dialysis in this situation is to correct hyperkalemia and hypervolemia. Possible sites of infection, including the lungs, urinary tract, and vascular access sites, should be carefully assessed and treated with appropriate antibiotics.

Surgical Procedure

For a LRD kidney transplant, two surgical teams are used. One team carefully removes the donor kidney including the artery, vein, and ureter. After the kidney is removed, it is core-cooled by flushing with an electrolyte solution at approximately 50° F (10° C). Frequently, mannitol is added to this solution to increase osmolality. The kidney is then carried to the operating room where the recipient is located.

The donated kidney, whether LRD or cadaveric, is surgically implanted in the iliac fossa because the iliac blood vessels are easy to expose (Fig. 44-18). When either kidney from the donor is equally satisfactory, the left is usually chosen because it has a longer renal vein. The renal artery is anastomosed to the internal iliac (hypogastric) artery or the external iliac artery. The renal vein is attached to the external iliac vein. The donor's ureter is implanted into the recipient's bladder.

Bilateral nephrectomies of the recipient's kidneys are not performed unless the patient has uncontrollable hypertension, chronic kidney infections, bleeding in the kidneys, or ureteral reflux, which leads to chronic kidney infections.

Postoperative Care

Living Related Donor. The usual postoperative care is similar to that after a nephrectomy (see Chapter 43). Often the donor remains the forgotten person as all of the attention is focused on the transplant recipient. The pain of a nephrectomy is greater than that of the iliac fossa incision experienced by the recipient. Nephrectomy often requires partial rib resection and entry into the pleural space. In contrast to the recipient, who feels better as renal function is restored, the donor feels very sick for 2 to 3 days. A urine culture, renal function studies, and a complete blood count are performed before discharge, and the donor is followed up at regular intervals. Most donors are ready to be discharged from the hospital in 6 or 7 days and can usually return to work in a month.

The majority of related kidney donors have positive psychologic reactions because the donation provides a boost in self-image and elation because of the improved health of a close family member. If the kidney does not function immediately or is rejected, the donor may feel disappointed, angry, or guilty. The donor is a healthy individual who donated a kidney and took a leave from work and family to do so. Each donor must always face the unanswered question of what will happen if the remaining kidney is injured or becomes diseased. Feelings regarding these issues must be resolved before the transplant.

Recipient. The nursing care for a recipient is similar to that for any patient who has had major surgery. The immediate postoperative care includes careful monitoring of fluid and electrolyte balance and intake and output. Diuresis generally occurs if the transplanted kidney begins to function. IV fluids are adjusted hourly according to the urine output and the state of hydration. An indwelling catheter is used to monitor urine output hourly. The catheter is removed as soon as possible to decrease the risk for infection but may be left in place up to 3 days to allow the suture line in the bladder to become more stable. While the catheter is in place, observing for patency of the tubing, assessing for urinary tract infection, and providing catheter care are important. Urine in the immediate postoperative period is blood-tinged but this usually clears in a few days.

The abdominal dressing should be checked for both blood and urine drainage. Urinary leakage may be present if the ureteral anastomosis is not securely implanted in the bladder. It may also result from ureteral obstruction of the newly implanted ureter. Careful, frequent monitoring of vital signs is also critical. A low-grade fever may be a sign of rejection or infection. Hypotension can lead to impaired perfusion of the transplanted kidney.

Preventing pulmonary infections is important. Coughing and deep breathing can be combined with the use of incentive spirometry to enhance ventilation and facilitate the movement of secretions. The patient should be turned every few hours in the immediate postoperative period. Frequent and early ambulation is encouraged.

Most patients feel good as their renal function returns. Occasionally the new kidney does not produce urine immediately. If this occurs, the patient must be dialyzed until adequate renal function begins. This is often a time of great discouragement for the hopeful patient. The patient should be reassured that this is not uncommon, especially in recipients of cadaveric donated kidneys.

Immunosuppressive Therapy

Immunosuppressive therapy is used to suppress the body's immune response to the foreign kidney (Table 44-10). Azathioprine (Imuran), corticosteroids, and cyclosporine are the standard drugs ordered. These drugs are usually started on the day of transplantation. However, the drug regimen can vary widely from center to center. Immunosuppressive medications must be taken daily while the graft is still functioning.

Cyclophosphamide (Cytoxan) can be substituted for azathioprine. However, it is primarily used to reduce the dose of azathioprine if the patient develops hepatotoxicity to azathioprine.

Cyclosporine (cyclosporin A), first used in Europe in 1978, is now being used in all kidney transplant centers in the United States. The mechanism of action of this fungus extract is to prevent the production and release of interleukin-2 (IL-2) from T-helper lymphocytes (see Fig. 44-17). Since the proliferation and maturation of T-cytotoxic lymphocytes is mediated by IL-2, cyclosporine alters the cell-mediated immune attack against the transplanted kidney. This drug does not cause bone marrow depression or alter the normal inflammatory response. Cyclosporine is used in conjunction with steroids or with a combination of steroids and azathioprine. Many of the side effects of cyclosporine are dose-related. Cyclosporine is nephrotoxic. For this reason, drug levels are followed closely to prevent toxicity.

Antilymphocyte globulin (ALG) and antithymocyte globulin (ATG) are also used as immunosuppressive therapy in many transplant centers. These agents are prepared by immunizing horses, rabbits, or goats with lymphoblasts (for ALG) or thymocytes (for ATG). Human thymocytes are obtained from the thymic tissue of cadavers or from patients who are undergoing cardiac surgery. The ALG or ATG is then purified and given to humans. The actual mechanism of action of ALG and ATG is not known. These polyclonal antibody preparations, which are directed against lymphocytes, induce lymphopenia and decrease the proliferative response of T lymphocytes, possibly as a result of the generation of T-suppressor lymphocytes. Current experience suggests that ALG and ATG should be used at the onset of an acute rejection rather than as maintenance immunosuppressive therapy.

In contrast to the polyclonal antibody preparations of ALG and ATG, monoclonal antibodies are used for treating acute rejection episodes (monoclonal antibodies are discussed in Chapter 10). OKT3 was the first of these monoclonal antibodies to be used in clinical transplantation.[32] OKT3 is a mouse monoclonal antibody that reacts with the T3 antigen found on the surface of human thymocytes and mature T cells. Thus OKT3 is an antiantigen-receptor antibody that interferes with the function of the T lymphocyte, the pivotal cell in the response to graft rejection. This agent reverses 95% of acute rejection episodes. OKT3 is administered IV push daily for 10 to 14 days.

Table 44-10 Immunosuppressive Therapy for Renal Transplant Recipients

Agent	Route of Administration	Mechanism of Action	Adverse Side Effects
Azathioprine (Imuran)	IV, PO	Is derivative of 6-mercaptopurine, interferes with purine synthesis and inhibits DNA and RNA synthesis, inhibits proliferation of T lymphocytes	Bone marrow suppression (leukopenia, anemia, thrombocytopenia), drug-induced hepatitis, oral lesions, increased susceptibility to infection
Corticosteroids Prednisone Methylprednisolone (Solu-Medrol)	 PO IV	Suppresses inflammatory response, prevents proliferation of T-cytotoxic lymphocytes	Cushingoid syndrome (peptic ulcer, GI bleeding, aseptic necrosis, sodium and water retention, acne, muscle weakness, fat dystrophy, capillary fragility, delayed healing, hyperglycemia, mood alterations); bacterial, fungal, and viral infections
Cyclophosphamide (Cytoxan)	PO	Is alkylating agent; interferes with DNA, RNA, and protein synthesis	Alopecia, leukopenia, hemorrhagic cystitis
ALG, ATG (ATGAM)	IV, IM	Has unknown mechanism, is directed against lymphocytes, reduces circulating lymphocytes, decreases lymphocyte proliferation	Serum sickness, fever and chills, anaphylactic shock, rash, local phlebitis, thrombocytopenia
Cyclosporine (cyclosporin A, Sandimmune)	PO, IV	Prevents production and release of interleukin 2, inhibits maturation of T-cytotoxic lymphocyte precursors	Hepatotoxicity, nephrotoxicity, lymphomas, infections, skin rashes, hirsutism, hypertension, tremors, gingival hyperplasia, breast fibroadenoma, nausea, and anorexia
OKT3 (Orthoclone, OKT3)	IV	Masks T-cell receptor for foreign antigens that recognize HLA mismatch between donor and recipient	Fever, tachycardia, headache, vomiting, chills, diarrhea, hypertension, hypotension, bronchospasm, infection, aseptic meningitis

ALG, Antilymphocytic globulin; *ATG*, antithymocytic globulin; *DNA*, deoxyribonucleic acid; *GI*, gastrointestinal; *HLA*, human leukocyte antigen; *IM*, intramuscular; *IV*, intravenous; *PO*, oral; *RNA*, ribonucleic acid.

Unfortunately all T cells are affected rather than just the subset active in graft rejection. Within minutes after the initial infusion of OKT3, circulating T cells become essentially undetectable. Adverse reactions are usually experienced with the first, second, and third injections and include a febrile response beginning 30 to 60 minutes after infusion. The most exciting aspect of monoclonal antibody therapy is the possibility of developing immunosuppressive protocols with highly uniform activity directed toward only selected T-cell subsets rather than toward the entire lymphocyte population.

FK506, one of several new investigational drugs, is being evaluated in clinical trials. It is similar to cyclosporine in action but much more potent.[33] Currently a number of other drugs are being developed and tested. These include brequinar (an inhibitor of T and B cell DNA synthesis), rapamycin (a blocker of cytokine action on T and B cells), and mycophenolate mofetil (an agent that prevents DNA synthesis in T and B cells).

Immunosuppressive agents affect the entire body, not just the transplanted kidney. This puts the patient at great risk for infection and the development of malignancies. More specific immunosuppressive therapy aimed only at the foreign kidney, not the total body, is needed.

Complications of Transplantation

Rejection

Hyperacute rejection. Hyperacute (humoral-mediated) rejection occurs minutes to hours after transplantation. Renal vessels thrombose and the kidney dies. Preformed cytotoxic antibodies from pregnancy, blood transfusions, or previous transplants react with recipient antigens in the donor kidney. There is no treatment and the transplanted kidney is removed. Hyperacute rejection can usually be prevented by avoiding the transplantation of a kidney with HLA-antigens to which the recipient has been sensitized.

Acute rejection. Acute rejection most commonly occurs 4 days to 4 months after transplantation. This type of rejection is mediated by the recipient's T-cytotoxic cells, which attack the foreign kidney. It is not uncommon to have at least one rejection episode, especially with cadaveric-donated kidneys. These episodes are usually reversible with additional immunosuppressive therapy, which usually consists of increased doses of steroids and ALG, ATG, or OKT3.

Signs of rejection include decreasing creatinine clearance, increasing serum creatinine, elevated BUN levels, fever, weight gain, decreased urine output, increasing blood pressure, and a swollen and painful transplant site. It is sometimes difficult to distinguish between acute rejection and nephrotoxicity as a side effect of cyclosporine.

Chronic rejection. Chronic rejection is a process that occurs over months or years. The kidney is infiltrated with large numbers of T and B cells characteristic of an ongoing, low-grade immunologically mediated injury. Chronic rejection is associated with a gradual occlusion of the renal blood vessels. Signs include proteinuria, hypertension, steady weight gain, and increasing serum creatinine levels. There is no definitive therapy for this type of rejection. Treatment is mainly supportive. This type of rejection is difficult to manage and is not associated with the optimistic prognosis of acute rejection.

Infections. Infections are common and serious complications of immunosuppressive therapy.[34] Respiratory infections are the most frequent cause of death from infection. The patient is at greatest risk during the early months when maximum dosages of immunosuppressives are administered. The patient with a compromised immune system is susceptible to infection from opportunistic organisms. Bacterial infections (lung, urinary tract, and wound) are usually caused by endogenous organisms. *Pneumocystis carinii* (a parasitic protozoan), *Legionella* organisms (gram-negative bacteria), and *Mycobacterium tuberculosis* are also common causes of respiratory infections. Fungal infections (e.g., *Candida*, *Cryptococcus* organisms) can occur anywhere in the body and are difficult to treat. Viral infections (e.g., cytomegalovirus [CMV]) occur frequently after prolonged immunosuppressive therapy. Administration of IV hyperimmune anti-CMV globulin is somewhat protective in preventing CMV disease. Ganciclovir can also be used to prevent or treat CMV infection.

Malignancies. The incidence of malignancies (5% to 6% of patients) in kidney transplant recipients is 100 times greater than that in the general population. In general, the primary reason for this increased incidence is related to an altered immune system caused by the effect of immunosuppressive therapy. The malignancies include cancer of the skin and lips, lymphomas, and cervical cancer.

Chronic Liver Disease. Chronic liver disease has become an increasingly important complication of kidney transplantation.[34] Chronic infection with hepatitis B and C viruses are major causes of progressive liver disease in the transplant recipient. Morbidity and mortality result from the development of chronic active hepatitis, cirrhosis, hepatocellular carcinoma, and superimposed bacterial infection.

Recurrence of Renal Disease. Recurrence of the same type of renal disease that destroyed the original kidney takes place in 15% of kidney transplant recipients. It is most common with certain types of glomerulonephritis and can result in the eventual loss of a functioning kidney transplant.

Vascular Disease. Patients who receive transplants and those who remain on HD have an increased incidence of atherosclerotic vascular disease. Coronary artery disease is a leading cause of death after renal transplantation. The exact reasons for this are not known. It may be because of an inability to alter the process that started with renal failure or because hypertension and hyperlipidemia are present and enhanced by steroid therapy.

Aseptic Bone Necrosis. Aseptic necrosis of the hips, knees, or both can occur in kidney transplant recipients. This problem is primarily the result of the side effects of chronic steroid therapy and may be potentiated by altered calcium metabolism. Currently, there is no intervention to prevent this complication.

Effectiveness of and Adaptation to Transplantation

If a transplant is successful, the patient has the potential to return to nearly normal functioning. Most patients feel so improved that euphoria predominates for a while. Some of the euphoria is a result of the effect of the steroids. The possibility of rejection (if and when) is a continual fear. The longer a person goes without rejection, the better the prognosis. Even if a kidney is rejected, the alternatives of dialysis and another transplant are available.

Most people who have successful transplants believe that it was worth all the risks to feel so good. These individuals suffer the greatest depression when the kidney is rejected after many months or years. They need to be reassured that they have done nothing (other than possibly failing to comply with drug therapy) to cause the rejection.

The prolongation of life in chronic renal failure puts the patient in an unusual situation. First the patient wonders whether it is possible to learn to accept death. Then there is hope for life with dialysis. The patient next asks a healthy relative to donate a kidney, or the patient receives cadaveric kidney transplant. Then the patient lives through months wondering how long this new kidney will last.

The leading causes of death after transplantation are infection and cardiovascular disease. If the transplant is successful, the quality of life is much better than that offered by maintenance dialysis.

The use of cyclosporine and OKT3 has dramatically improved graft survival in the past 5 years. The 3-year patient and graft survival rates for LRD transplant recipients are about 95% and 85%, respectively; for cadaveric transplant recipients, 3-year patient and graft survival rates are 80% and 70%, respectively.

When the transplant fails, the patient usually returns to dialysis and can continue on dialysis or wait for another transplant. Because immunosuppressive therapy is still inadequate, a major research goal is to develop more specific and less toxic drugs.

Gerontologic Considerations

The incidence of ESRD in the United States and Canada is increasing most rapidly in older patients. According to the U.S. Renal Data Systems (USRDS), 31% of new cases of ESRD in 1993 were in individuals 65 years or older.

Currently the average age of the patient on dialysis is 62 years.[10] The most common diseases leading to renal failure in the older adult are hypertension and diabetes.

The health problems of the older ESRD patient differ significantly from the younger patient. For example, the incidence of other chronic illnesses increases with advancing age.[35] Physiologic changes of clinical importance in the older ESRD patient include diminished cardiopulmonary function, bone loss, immunodeficiency, altered protein synthesis, and altered drug metabolism. Malnutrition is common in the older ESRD patient for a variety of reasons, including lack of mobility, lack of understanding of basic nutritional requirements, social isolation, physical disability, impaired cognitive function, and malabsorption problems.

The older patient and the family need to consider what is the best form of dialysis. Home peritoneal dialysis allows the patient to be more mobile and to enjoy an increased sense of control over the illness. Peritoneal dialysis is not as hemodynamically stressful as HD. On the other hand, PD requires self-care or assistance from a family member. The older adult may not want to burden the family to get involved in their medical care.

Withdrawal from dialysis accounts for 9% of deaths in United States and Canadian dialysis patients.[36] For patients over 70 years old, voluntary withdrawal is the most common cause of death in U.S. patients. If a patient decides to withdraw from dialysis, it is crucial to support the patient, family, and dialysis staff (see Ethical Dilemmas). In the early years of the ESRD program, the older adult was not placed on dialysis. The availability of chronic PD changed this situation. The increasing number of elderly, debilitated ESRD patients on dialysis has raised a number of ethical concerns about the appropriateness of using scarce technical resources in a population with limited life expectancy.

On the other hand, substantial evidence exists showing success of dialysis (especially PD) in the elderly. Quality of life has also been reported to be good to excellent in many older ESRD patients. There appears to be no justification for excluding the older adult from dialysis programs. Rationing dialysis on the basis of age alone is not supported based on currently available outcome and quality of life data.[37]

CRITICAL THINKING EXERCISES

CASE STUDY

CHRONIC RENAL FAILURE

Patient Profile

Sue, a 46-year-old female, has been treated for Type I diabetes since the age of 15. She met with her doctor, complaining of anorexia, nausea, vomiting, and headache for 3 days.

Subjective Data

- Complains of swelling in her feet and hands
- Has gained 10 pounds (4.5 kg) in the past 2 weeks
- Complains of dyspnea and weakness when walking

Objective Data

Laboratory Data

▪ Creatinine clearance	8.2 ml/min
▪ Serum creatinine	12.8 mg/dl (1132 μmol/L)
▪ BUN	125 mg/dl (45 mmol/L)
▪ K	6 mEq/L (6 mmol/L)
▪ Hematocrit	20%

Chest X-ray

- Pulmonary edema and cardiomegaly

Critical Thinking Questions

1. Explain the basic pathologic changes that resulted in the development of diabetic nephropathy.
2. What are the indications for dialysis in this patient?
3. Identify the abnormal diagnostic study results and why each would occur.
4. Explain why Sue developed each of her clinical manifestations.
5. What are important nursing interventions for Sue and her family?
6. Based on the assessment data provided, write one or more nursing diagnoses. Are there any collaborative problems?

NURSING RESEARCH ISSUES

1. What is the psychosocial impact of home peritoneal dialysis on the spouse and family?
2. What nursing strategies promote compliance in the dialysis patient?
3. Are the stressors for older (>65 years) dialysis patients different from those of younger patients?
4. What is the impact of kidney transplantation on rehabilitation and functional capacity?
5. What is the quality of life for a living-related donor following surgery?
6. What are the needs of the family when a patient chooses to withdraw from dialysis treatment?

REVIEW QUESTIONS

The number of the question corresponds to the same-numbered objective at the beginning of the chapter.

1. Which of the following best describes chronic renal failure?
 a. Rapid decrease in urinary output with azotemia
 b. Progressive irreversible destruction of both kidneys
 c. Sudden decrease in urinary output to less than 400 ml/day
 d. Creatinine clearance increases as urinary output decreases

2. Prerenal causes of acute renal failure include
 a. myocardial infarction and calculi formation.
 b. hypovolemia and cardiogenic shock.
 c. acute glomerulonephritis and neoplasms.
 d. septic shock and nephrotoxic injury from drugs.

3. The nurse must be alert for what signs and symptoms during the oliguric phase of acute renal failure?
 a. Urine with high specific gravity and low sodium concentration
 b. Hypotension and fluid volume deficit
 c. Fluid volume excess and hypertension
 d. Kussmaul's respiration and increased appetite

4. If a patient is in the diuretic phase of acute renal failure, the nurse must monitor for which serum electrolyte imbalances?
 a. Hyperkalemia and hyponatremia
 b. Hyperkalemia and hypernatremia
 c. Hypokalemia and hyponatremia
 d. Hypokalemia and hypernatremia

5. Anemia occurs in renal failure because there is
 a. decreased production of erythropoietin
 b. decreased level of parathyroid hormone
 c. increased erythropoiesis in bone marrow
 d. decreased hemolysis of red blood cells

6. Which of the following measures is appropriate in the conservative management of chronic renal failure?
 a. Increase fluid intake, decrease carbohydrate intake and protein intake
 b. Decrease fluid intake and carbohydrate intake, increase protein intake
 c. Decrease fluid intake and protein intake, increase carbohydrate intake
 d. Decrease fluid intake, carbohydrate intake, and protein intake

7. Complications for a patient on PD include all the following except
 a. infection.
 b. protein loss.
 c. pulmonary complications.
 d. risk of hemorrhage.

8. A common complication associated with internal graft vascular access devices is
 a. infection.
 b. bleeding.
 c. palpable thrill.
 d. rupture.

9. Management of hypotension during dialysis includes all of the following except
 a. placement of patient in Trendelenburg position.
 b. infusion of bolus saline.
 c. increasing rate of fluid removal.
 d. reassess dry weight.

10. Nursing care for the transplant recipient includes teaching the patient which of the following signs of rejection?
 a. Fever, weight loss, increased urinary output, decreased blood pressure
 b. Fever, weight loss, increased urinary output, increased blood pressure
 c. Fever, weight gain, increased urinary output, increased blood pressure
 d. Fever, weight gain, decreased urinary output, increased blood pressure

11. The following immunosuppressive drugs are used in the management of the transplant patient. For which one is the correct adverse side effect given?
 a. OKT3—fever
 b. Azathioprine—increased RBC production
 c. Prednisone—hypoglycemia
 d. Cyclosporine—bone marrow depression

REFERENCES

1. Anderson RJ: Prevention and management of acute renal failure, *Hosp Pract* 28:61, 1993.
2. Baer CL: Acute renal failure: recognizing and reversing its deadly course, *Nursing* 20:34, 1990.
3. Baer CL, Lancaster L: Acute renal failure, *Crit Care Nurs Q* 14:1, 1992.
4. Humes H: The recovery phase of acute renal failure: the cellular and molecular biology of regenerative repair, *The Kidney* 24:1, 1991.
5. Toto KH: Acute renal failure: a question of location, *Am J Nurs* 92:44, 1992.
6. Price C: Chronic renal replacement therapy: the treatment of choice for acute renal failure, *ANNA J* 18:239, 1991.
7. Butler B: Nutritional management of catabolic acute renal failure requiring renal replacement therapy, *ANNA J* 18:247, 1991.
8. Porcush JG, Faubert PF: *Renal disease in the aged,* Boston, 1991, Little Brown.
9. Maher JF: *Replacement of renal function by dialysis,* ed 3, Boston, 1989, Kluwer Academic Publishers.
10. United States Renal Data System, 1994.
11. Mendelssohn DC and others: A comparison of dialysis in the US and Canada, *Cont Dial Neph* 10:27, 1993.
12. Paganini EP: Erythropoietin therapy in renal failure, *Intern Med* 38:223, 1993.
13. Brunier GM: Calcium/phosphate imbalances, aluminum toxicity, and renal osteodystrophy, *ANNA J* 21:171, 1994.
14. Fournier A and others: Use of alkaline calcium salts as phosphate binders in uremic patients, *Kidney Int* (Suppl)38:550, 1992.
15. Delmez JA and others: Calcium acetate as a phosphorous binder in hemodialysis patients, *J Am Soc Neph* 3:96, 1992.
16. Levine N, Ameling R: Erythropoietin update, *The Kidney* 26:1, 1993.
17. Eschbach JW: Erythropoietin 1991—an overview, *Am J Kid Dis* 18:3, 1991.

18. Laupacis A, Wong C, Churchill D: The use of generic and specific quality-of-life measures in hemodialysis patients treated with erythropoietin, *Controlled Clinical Trials* 12:168S, 1991.
19. Wasserman AG: Changing patterns of medical practice; protein restriction for chronic renal failure, *Ann Intern Med* 199:79, 1993.
20. Klahr S and others: The effects of dietary protein restriction and blood pressure control on the progression of chronic renal disease, *N Engl J Med* 330:877, 1994.
21. Michael B, Burkie JF: Chronic renal disease: new therapies to delay kidney replacement, *Geriatrics* 49:33, 1994.
22. Gokal R and others: Peritoneal catheters and exit-site practices: toward optimum peritoneal access, *Peritoneal Dial Int* 13:29, 1993.
23. Daugirdas JT, Ing TS: *Handbook of dialysis,* ed 2, Boston, 1994, Little Brown.
24. Keane W and others: Peritoneal dialysis—related peritonitis treatment recommendations, 1993 update, *Peritoneal Dial Int* 13:14, 1993.
25. Boger MP: A brief historical development of vascular access for hemodialysis, *J Vasc Nurs* 8:13, 1990.
26. Nissenson AR, Fine RN: *Dialysis therapy,* Philadelphia, 1993, Hanley and Belfus.
27. Salai PB: Hepatitis C: implications for nurses and patients, *Nephrol Nursing Today* 3:1, 1993.
28. Marple JT, McDougall M: Development of malignancy in the end-stage renal disease patient, *Semin Neph* 13:306, 1993.
29. Bosworth C: SCUF/CAVH/CAVHD critical differences, *Crit Care Nurs Q* 14:45, 1992.
30. Dirkes S: How to use the new CVVH renal replacement systems, *Am J Nurs* 94:67, 1994.
31. Hull A: 1990 Transplant statistics show more hard times ahead, *Neph News Issues* 6:22, 1992.
32. Shaefer MS, Collier DS: Immunosuppression for solid organ transplantation, *Dial Transplant* 22:541, 1993.
33. Duffy MM, Uber L: Immunosuppressive medications, *Dialysis and Transplantation* 23:571, 1994.
34. First MR: Long-term complications after transplantation, *Am J Kid Dis* 22:477, 1993.
35. Kutner NG and others: Dialysis in elderly patients: outcome differences related to race, *Dialysis Transplantation* 23:496, 1994.
36. Mailloux LU and others: Death by withdrawal from dialysis: a 20-year experience, *J Am Soc Nephrol* 3:1631, 1993.
37. Nissenson AR: Peritoneal dialysis in the elderly patient. In Gokal R, Nolph KD, editors: *The textbook of peritoneal dialysis,* Dordrecht, The Netherlands, 1994, Kluwer Academic Publishers.

SECTION IX BIBLIOGRAPHY

Books

Burrows-Hudson S, editor: *Standards of clinical practice for nephrology nursing;* Pitman, NJ, 1993, American Nephrology Nurses Association.

Daugirdas JT, Ing TS: *Handbook of dialysis,* Boston, 1992, Little, Brown.

Glassock RJ: *Current therapy in nephrology and hypertension,* ed 3, St Louis, 1992, Mosby.

Gray M: *Genitourinary disorders,* St Louis, 1992, Mosby.

Gutch CF, Stoner MH, Corea AL: *Review of hemodialysis for nurses and dialysis personnel,* St Louis, 1993, Mosby.

Jacobson HR, Striker GE, Klahn S: *The principles and practice of nephrology,* St Louis, 1991, Mosby.

Jeter K, Faller N, Norton C: *Nursing for continence,* Philadelphia, 1990, WB Saunders.

Karlowicz KA, editor: *Urologic nursing: principles and practices,* Philadelphia, 1995, WB Saunders.

Smith SL, editor: *Tissue and organ transplantation,* St Louis, 1990, Mosby.

Solez K, Racusen L: *Acute renal failure, diagnosis, treatment and prevention,* New York, 1991, Marcel Kekken.

Tanagho EA, McAninch JW, editors: *Smith's general urology,* ed 13, Norwalk, Conn, 1992, Appleton & Lange.

Twardowsky ZJ, Nolph KD, Khanna R: *Peritoneal dialysis: new concepts and applications,* New York, 1990, Churchill Livingstone.

Walsh PC and others, editors: *Campbell's urology,* ed 6, Philadelphia, 1992, WB Saunders.

Journals

Bailey S: Using bladder wash-outs, *Nurs Times* 87:75, 1991.

Bennett WM, Elzinga LW, Barry JM: Polycystic kidney disease: II. Diagnosis and management, *Hosp Pract* 27:61, 1992.

Blanford NL: Renal transplantation: a case study of the ideal, *Crit Car Nurs* 13:46, 1993.

Brennan DE: Diabetes and end stage renal disease: issues in diabetic nephropathy, *Nephrol Nurs Today* 7:1, 1991.

Carr M, Carr M: Dangerous brew, *Can Nurse* 90:34, 1994.

Chambers JK, Boggs DL: Development of an instrument to measure knowledge about kidney function, kidney failure and treatment options, *ANNA J* 20:637, 1993.

Chambers JK: Renal insufficiency: implications for the care of the medical surgical patient, *Medsurg Nurs* 2:33, 1993.

Collins JW: The treatment of mild to moderate hypertension in patients with diabetes mellitus, *Nurs Pract* 16:28, 1991.

Chmielewski C: Renal anatomy and overview of nephron function, *ANNA J* 19:34, 1992.

Counts C: Potential complications of the internal vascular access: implications for nursing care, *Dialysis Trans* 22:75, 1993.

Cummings JM, Houston K: The treatment of urinary incontinence, *Hosp Pract* 29:97, 1994.

Cunningham N, Boteler S, Windham S: Renal transplantation, *Crit Care Nurs Clin North Am* 4:79, 1992.

Dunn S: How to care for the dialysis patient, *Am J Nurs* 93:26, 1993.

Eberle CM, Winsemius D, Garibaldi RA: Risk factors and consequences of bacteriuria in non-catheterized nursing home residents, *J Gerontol* 48:M266, 1993.

Fedric TN: Immunosuppressive therapy in renal transplantation, *Crit Care Nurs North Am* 2:23, 1990.

*Ferrans CE, Powers MJ: Quality of life of hemodialysis patients, *ANNA J* 20:575, 1993.

*Gallagher N, Lepak S: Functional capacity and activity level before and after renal transplantation, *ANNA J* 18:378, 1991.

Graham-Macaluso MM: Complications of peritoneal dialysis: nursing care plans to document teaching, *ANNA J* 18:479, 1991.

Grantham JJ: Polycystic kidney disease: I. Etiology and pathogenesis, *Hosp Pract* 27:51, 1992.

Gross PA and others: Quality standard for the treatment of bacteremia, *Infect Control Hosp Epidemiol* 15:189, 1994.

Hagland MR: The management of acute renal failure in the intensive therapy unit, *Intensive Crit Care Nurs* 9:237, 1993.

*Hauser M and others: Predicted and actual quality of life changes following renal transplantation, *ANNA J* 18:295, 1991.

Hockenberry B: Multiple drug therapy in the treatment of essential hypertension, *Nurs Clin North Am* 26:417, 1991.

Hoffart N, editor: Directory of nephrology nurse researchers, *ANNA J* 19:291, 1992.

Holechek MJ, Burrell-Diggs D, Navarro MO: Renal transplantation: an option for end stage renal disease patients, *Crit Care Nurs Q* 13:62, 1991.

Hutteri H, Locking-Cusolito H: Retirement to renal failure: the management of the elderly dialysis patient, *J CAANT* 2:14, 1992.

Innerarity SA: Electrolyte emergencies in the critically ill renal patient, *Crit Care Nurs Clin North Am* 2:89, 1992.

Kee CC: Age-related changes in the renal system: causes, consequences, and nursing implications, *Geriatr Nurs* 13:80, 1992.

Kelleher BM: Dialysis in the surgical intensive care patient: a case study, *Crit Care Nurs Q* 14:72, 1992.

Lafrades AR: Percussion after extracorporeal shock wave lithotripsy, *Urol Nurs* 12:112, 1992.

Leese D: An overview of urologic complications in diabetes mellitus, *Urol Nurs* 11:17, 1991.

Lieske JC, Toback FG: Autosomal dominant polycystic kidney disease, *J Am Soc Nephrol* 3:1442, 1993.

Molzahn A: An evaluation of the nephrology nursing research literature, *ANNA J* 20:395, 1993.

McConnell E: Managing the patient with acute renal failure, *Nursing* 22:84, 1992.

McCormick KA and others: Urinary incontinence in adults, *Am J Nurs* 92:75, 1992.

McCormick RA, Palmer MH: Urinary incontinence in older adults, *Annu Rev Nurs Res* 10:25, 1992.

Moore S and others: Treating bladder cancer, *Am J Nurs* 93:32, 1993.

Neskey KL, Loehner D: Urinary diversion with an Indiana pouch, *Nursing* 24:32C, 1994.

Palmer J, Shook P: Successful use of orthoclone OKT3 for steroid resistant acute rejection in pediatric renal allograft recipients, *ANNA J* 19:375, 1992.

Paola AS: Hematuria: Essentials of diagnosis, *Hosp Pract* 25:144, 1990.

Paschall FE: Thrombotic thrombocytopenic purpura: the challenges of a complex disease process, *AACN Clin Issues Crit Care Nurs* 4:655, 1993.

Pearson BD, Larson J: Improving elders continence state, *Clin Nurs Res* 1:430, 1992.

Pinkerman ML: Indwelling urinary catheters, *Nursing* 24:66, 1994.

Price CA: Issues related to the care of critically ill patients with end stage renal failure, *Crit Car Nurs* 3:585, 1992.

Prowant B and others: Nephrology nursing care plan and patient education plan for the patient receiving Epogen, *ANNA J* 18:188, 1991.

Prowant BF, Warardy BA, Nolph KD: Peritoneal dialysis catheter exit site care: results of an international survey, *Perit Dial Int* 13:149, 1993.

Resnick B: Retraining the bladder after catheterization, *Am J Nurs* 93:46, 1993.

Resnick NM: Urinary incontinence in older adults, *Hosp Pract* 27:139, 1992.

Riehmann M and others: Risk factors for bacteriuria in men, *Urology* 43:617, 1994.

Rimmer JM: The consequences of renal artery stenosis, *Hosp Pract* 29:29, 1994.

Shellenbarger T, Krouse A: Treating and preventing kidney stones, *Medsurg Nurs* 3:389, 1994.

Stark J: Acute renal failure in trauma-current perspectives, *Crit Care Nurs Q* 16:49, 1994.

Stark JL: Acute tubular nerosis: differences between oliguria and non oliguria, *Crit Care Nurs Q* 14:22, 1992.

Steele D: Neurophysiology of voiding, *Innovations Urol Nurs* 23:2, 1993.

Thayer D: How to assess and control urinary incontinence, *Am J Nurs* 94:42, 1994.

White M, McNatt G: Early transplantation for patients with diabetic nephropathy, *ANNA J* 19:457, 1992.

Wiseman KC: New insights on Goodpasture's syndrome, *ANNA J* 20:17, 1993.

Organizations

Agency for Health Care Policy and Research (AHCPR)
Office of the Forum
Executive Office Center, Suite 401
2101 East Jefferson Street
Rockville, MD 20852

The American Association for Nephrology Nurses and Technicians
Middle City Station
P.O. Box 2368
Philadelphia, PA 19103

American Council on Transplantation
700 N. Fairfax Street, Suite 505
Alexandria, VA 22314

American Kidney Fund
7315 Wisconsin Avenue
Bethesda, MD 20814-3266
800-638-8299

American Nephrology Nurses Association
North Woodbury Road, Box 56
Pitman, NJ 08071
609-589-2187
FAX: 609-589-7463

American Urological Association Allied
11512 Allecingie Parkway
Richmond, VA 23235
804-379-1306

American Urological Association Allied
6845 Lake Shore Drive
P.O. Box 9397
Raytown, MO 64133

Interstitial Cystitis Association
P.O. Box 1553
Madison Square Station
New York, NY 10159
212-979-6057

National Association for Patients on Hemodialysis and Transplantation (NAPHT)
211 East 43rd Street, Suite 301
New York, NY 10017
212-867-4486

National Kidney Foundation
2 Park Avenue
New York, NY 10016
212-889-2210

National Kidney and Urologic Diseases
Information Clearinghouse (NKUDIC)
9000 Rockville Pike
Bethesda, MD 20892
301-468-6345

United Ostomy Association
2001 West Beverly
Los Angeles, CA 90057

AHCPR Guidelines

Guides developed and published by The Agency for Health Care Policy and Research (AHCPR). The Patient Guides are available in English and Spanish. The guidelines can be obtained by writing to: Center for Research Dissemination and Liaison, AHCPR Clearinghouse, P.O. Box 8547, Silver Spring, MD 20907, or by calling 1-800-358-9295. The Guidelines are as follows:

Urinary incontinence in adults. Clinical Practice Guideline. AHCPR Pub. No. 92-0038.

Urinary incontinence in adults. Quick Reference Guide for Clinicians. AHCPR Pub. No. 92-0041.

Urinary incontinence in adults. A Patient's Guide. AHCPR Pub. No. 92-0040.

---

*Nursing research-based articles.

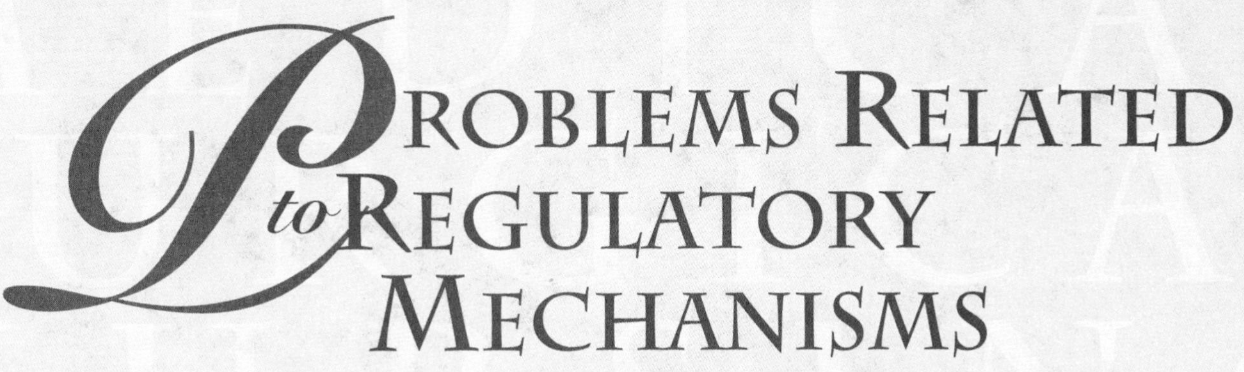

Problems Related to Regulatory Mechanisms

Section Ten

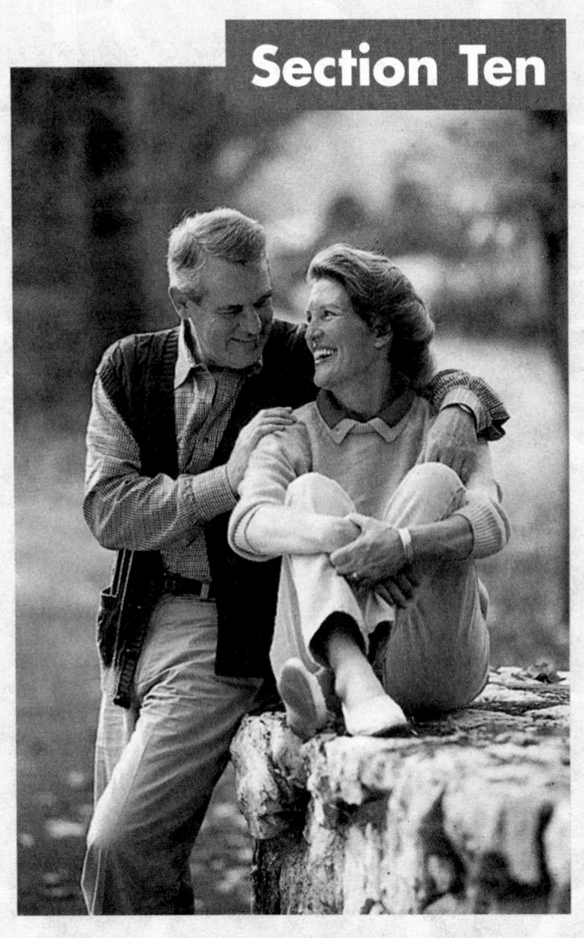

MEDICAL
SURGICAL
NURSING
MEDICAL
SURGICAL
NURSING
MEDICAL
SURGICAL
NURSING
MEDICAL
SURGICAL

Chapter 45

NURSING ASSESSMENT
Endocrine System

Linda B. Haas

Learning Objectives

1. Identify the common characteristics and functions of hormones.
2. Identify the locations of the endocrine glands.
3. Describe the functions of hormones secreted by the pituitary, thyroid, parathyroid, and adrenal glands and the pancreas.
4. Describe the locations and roles of hormone receptors.
5. Identify the significant subjective and objective assessment data related to the endocrine system that should be obtained from a patient.
6. Describe the appropriate technique used in the physical assessment of the thyroid gland.
7. Describe age-related changes in the endocrine system and differences in assessment findings.
8. Differentiate normal from common abnormal findings in the assessment of the endocrine system.
9. Describe the purpose, significance of results, and nursing responsibilities related to diagnostic studies of the endocrine system.

The endocrine system is an integrated chemical communication and coordination system that enables reproduction, growth and development, and regulation of energy. With the nervous and immune systems, the endocrine system maintains the internal homeostasis of the body and coordinates responses to external and internal environmental changes. The endocrine system is composed of glands or glandular tissues that synthesize, store, and secrete chemical messengers (hormones) that travel through the blood to specific target cells throughout the body. The specificity of this system is determined by the affinity of receptors on the target organs and tissues for a particular hormone, the "lock and key" mechanism (Fig. 45-1). The endocrine glands include the hypothalamus, pituitary, thyroid, parathyroids, adrenals, pancreas, ovaries, testes, pineal, and thymus[1] (Fig. 45-2). The pineal gland is not discussed, as the significance of the hormones secreted by this gland in humans is unclear.[2] The thymus gland, important in the development of the immune system, is discussed in Chapter 10. In addition to the glands mentioned above, other organs of the body secrete hormones. For example, the kidneys secrete erythropoietin, the heart secretes atrial natriuretic factor, and the gastrointestinal tract secretes numerous peptide homones (e.g., gastrin). These hormones are discussed in the respective assessment chapters.

Reviewed by Florencetta Hayes Gibson, BSN, MEd, MSN, Associate Professor, Northeast Louisiana University, Monroe, LA.

STRUCTURES AND FUNCTIONS OF THE ENDOCRINE SYSTEM

Glands

Exocrine Glands. Exocrine glands pass along their secretions through ducts that empty outside the body or into the lumen of the organ lined with the same embryonic epithelium as the gland. For example, the exocrine secretions of the sweat glands are discharged directly onto the surface of the skin. Exocrine secretions of the pancreas, called enzymes, are secreted into the pancreatic duct and transported to the intestine.

Endocrine Glands. Endocrine organs (glands and cells) are ductless but highly vascularized. They synthesize hormones and secrete them into blood, where they eventually affect specific target tissues. For instance, the thyroid (gland) synthesizes thyroxine (the hormone), which influences all body tissues (target tissue).

Hormones

Characteristics. A *hormone* is a chemical substance synthesized and secreted by a specific organ or tissue. Hormones are carried by the blood to other sites in the body where their actions are exerted. Most hormones have common characteristics, including circulation through the blood; secretion in minute but effective amounts at variable, but predictable rates; binding to specific cellular receptors to change intracellular metabolism; and variable effects on the rates of physiologic responses of target tissues. A newly discovered chemical messenger believed to

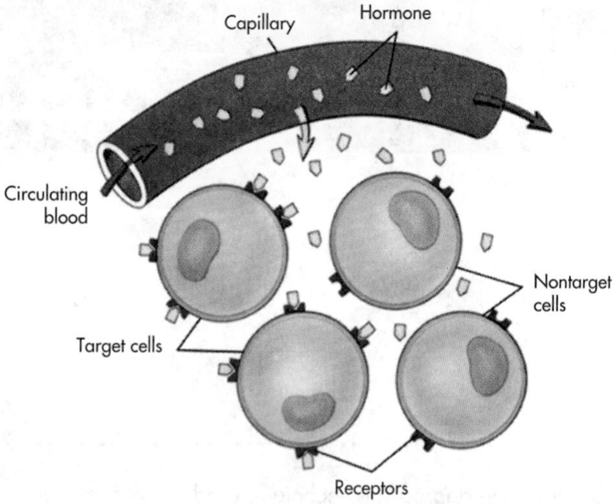

Fig. 45-1 The target cell concept. A hormone acts only on cells that have receptors specific to that hormone, because the shape of the receptor determines which hormone can react with it. This is an example of the lock-and-key model of biochemical reactions.

be a hormone is called a *factor* until its chemical structure has been determined.

Many hormones (e.g., somatostatin, vasoactive intestinal peptide) are synthesized and secreted by several tissues and stimulate different physiologic responses depending on the source and target tissue. For example, somatostatin is found in several areas of the brain, including the part of the hypothalamus that controls the anterior pituitary. In this instance, somatostatin inhibits growth hormone and thyroid-stimulating hormone (TSH) release. Somatostatin is also synthesized and secreted by the delta cells of the pancreas where it inhibits insulin and glucagon release.

Structure. Structurally the major hormones are amines, peptides (proteins), and steroids. Amine hormones, derived from the amino acid tyrosine, include the catecholamines, which bind to cell membrane receptors, and thyroid hormones, which bind to receptors in the cell nucleus. Peptide hormones bind to cell membrane receptors because they are unable to penetrate cell membranes because of their large size and lipid insolubility. Steroid hormones, secreted by the adrenal cortices and gonads, are synthesized from cholesterol, are lipid soluble, and are able to diffuse into cells and bind with cytoplasmic receptors. This hormone-receptor complex then translocates to the cell nucleus to produce changes.

Transport. Steroid and thyroid hormones are not water soluble. Therefore the majority of these hormones are bound to plasma proteins for transport in the blood. This bound state decreases or prevents liver breakdown. However, only the unbound hormone is active. Peptides and catecholamines are water soluble. Thus they do not need to be bound to proteins, and circulate freely in blood.

Functions. Hormones alter the rate of many physiologic activities. Important hormonal functions are related

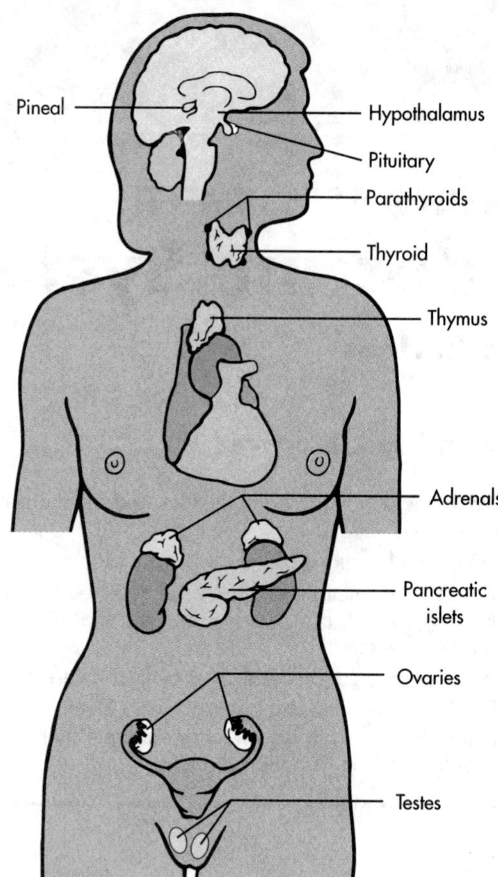

Fig. 45-2 Location of the major endocrine glands. The parathyroid glands actually lie on the posterior surface of the thyroid.

to reproduction, responses to stress and injury, electrolyte balance, energy metabolism, growth, maturation, and aging. Table 45-1 summarizes the major hormones, glands or tissues from which they are synthesized, target organs or tissues, and functions.

Hormone-Receptor Interaction

Hormone Receptors. The specificity of hormone-target cell interaction is determined by receptors. *Receptors* or *hormone-binding sites* are glycoprotein macromolecules of the target cell that interact with a hormone in the first step of the hormone's action. The receptor allows the hormone to recognize the cell. Steroid and thyroid hormone receptors are in the cytoplasm of the target cell, whereas receptors for other hormones are in the cell membrane.[1]

Intracellular hormone-receptor complexes, such as those seen in steroid hormone action, translocate to the cell nucleus where they stimulate or inhibit the synthesis of messenger ribonucleic acid (mRNA). This mRNA migrates to the cytoplasm, where it stimulates the synthesis of new protein at the ribosomes. The new proteins produce specific effects in the target cell[2] (Fig. 45-3). This process requires minutes to days. Peptide hormone and catecholamine recep-

Table 45-1 Major Endocrine Glands and Hormones

Hormones	Target Tissue	Functions
Posterior Pituitary (Neurohypophysis)		
▪ Oxytocin (pitocin)*	Uterus, mammary glands	Stimulates milk secretion; uterine motility
▪ Antidiuretic hormone (ADH) or vasopressin*	Renal tubules, vascular smooth muscle	Promotes reabsorption of water
Anterior Pituitary (Adenohypophysis)		
▪ Growth hormone (GH) or somatotropin	All body cells	Promotes protein anabolism (growth, tissue repair), lipid mobilization, and catabolism
▪ Thyroid-stimulating hormone (TSH) or thyrotropin	Thyroid gland	Stimulates synthesis and release of thyroid hormones, growth and function of thyroid (stimulation of thyroidal iodine uptake)
▪ Adrenocorticotropic hormone (ACTH) or corticotropin	Adrenal cortex	Fosters growth of adrenal cortex; stimulates secretion of glucocorticoids
▪ Prolactin or lactogen	Ovary and mammary glands in females	Stimulates milk production, protein synthesis, mammary gland development; unclear function in males
▪ Gonadotropic hormones (e.g., follicle-stimulating [FSH] and luteinizing hormones [LH])	Reproductive organs	Stimulates sex hormone secretion, reproductive organ growth, reproductive processes
▪ Melanocyte-stimulating hormone (MSH)	Melanocytes in skin	Increases melanin production in melanocytes to make skin darker in color
▪ Prolactin	Ovary and mammary glands in females	Stimulates milk production in lactating women; increases response of follicles to LH and FSH; increase causes gynecomastia in men
Thyroid		
▪ Thyroxine (T_4)	All body tissues	Precursor to T_3
▪ Triiodothyronine (T_3)	All body tissues	Regulates metabolic rate of all cells and processes of cell growth and tissue differentiation
▪ Calcitonin (CT)	Bone tissue	Regulates calcium and phosphorus blood levels, lowering of blood Ca^{++} levels
Parathyroids		
▪ Parathyroid hormone (PTH) or parathormone	Bone, intestine, kidneys	Regulates calcium and phosphorus blood levels (bone demineralization, increased intestinal absorption)
Pancreas (Islets of Langerhans)		
▪ Insulin (from beta cells)	Liver, fat, and liver cells	Promotes utilization and storage of fuels (carbohydrates, protein, fats)
▪ Glucagon (from alpha cells)	Liver	Promotes hepatic glucogenolysis and gluconeogenesis
▪ Somatostatin (from delta cells)	Pancreas	Inhibits insulin and glucagon secretion

continued

tors are located in the cell membrane. The hormone-receptor complex is then linked to effector molecules via coupling by G-proteins. The effector molecules can stimulate or inhibit secondary messengers within the cell, which in turn alter the cell's metabolism or gene expression. These intracellular effector molecules activate secondary messengers such as cyclic adenosine monophosophate (cAMP). cAMP exerts its action by activating kinases to regulate intracellular activity (Fig. 45-4).

Thyroid hormones act at several cellular sites. Specific receptors exist on the cell membranes and within the mitochondria and nucleus. At the cell membrane, the hormone-receptor complex stimulates nutrient transport; in the mitochondria, the complex increases metabolic energy;

Table 45-1 Major Endocrine Glands and Hormones—cont'd

Hormones	Target Tissue	Functions
Adrenal Medulla		
▪ Epinephrine (adrenalin)	Sympathetic effectors	Enhances and prolongs effects of sympathetic division of ANS
▪ Norepinephrine	Sympathetic effectors	Responds to stress; enhances and prolongs effects of sympathetic division of ANS
Adrenal Cortex		
▪ Corticosteroids (e.g., cortisol, hydrocortisone)	All body tissues	Promotes organic metabolism, response to stress
▪ Androgens (e.g., testosterone, androsterone) or estrogen	Sex organs	Promotes masculinization in men, growth and sexual activity in women
▪ Mineralocorticoids (e.g., aldosterone)	Kidney	Regulates sodium and potassium balance and thus water balance
Gonads		
Women: ovaries		
▪ Estrogen	Reproductive system, breasts	Stimulates development of secondary sex characteristics, preparation of uterus for fertilization and fetal development; stimulates bone growth
▪ Progesterone	Reproductive system	Maintains lining of uterus necessary for successful pregnancy
Men: testes		
▪ Testosterone	Reproductive system	Stimulates development of secondary sex characteristics; stimulates epiphyseal closure

ANS, Autonomic nervous system.
*These hormones are synthesized in the hypothalamus; the posterior pituitary stores and secretes them.

and at the nuclear level, it promotes synthesis of structural and functional cellular components.

Regulation of Hormonal Secretion

The regulation of endocrine activity is controlled by specific mechanisms of varying levels of complexity. These mechanisms stimulate or inhibit hormone synthesis and secretion. One such mechanism, *simple feedback,* which may be negative or positive, is based on the blood level of a particular substance. This substance may be a hormone or other chemical compound regulated by, or responsive to, a hormone.

In *negative feedback,* high levels of the substance inhibit hormone synthesis and secretion, and low levels stimulate hormone synthesis and secretion. Negative feedback is similar to the functioning of a thermostat in which cold air in a room activates the thermostat to release heat, and hot air turns off the thermostat to prevent more warm air from entering the room. A physiologic example of this is the relationship between calcium and parathyroid hormone (PTH). Low blood calcium levels stimulate the parathyroid glands to release PTH, which acts on bone, the intestine, and the kidneys to increase blood calcium levels. The increased blood calcium levels then inhibit further PTH release (Fig. 45-5).

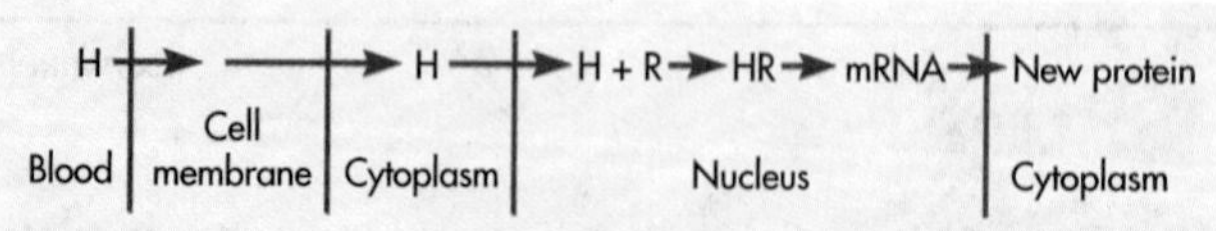

Fig. 45-3 Hormone-receptor action: steroid hormones. Hormone (*H*) diffuses through the cell membrane and cytoplasm and combines with its receptor (*R*) in the nucleus to form a hormone-receptor complex (*HR*), which affects formation of new messenger ribonucleic acid (*mRNA*). This mRNA then diffuses to the cytoplasm where it codes for the synthesis of new protein.

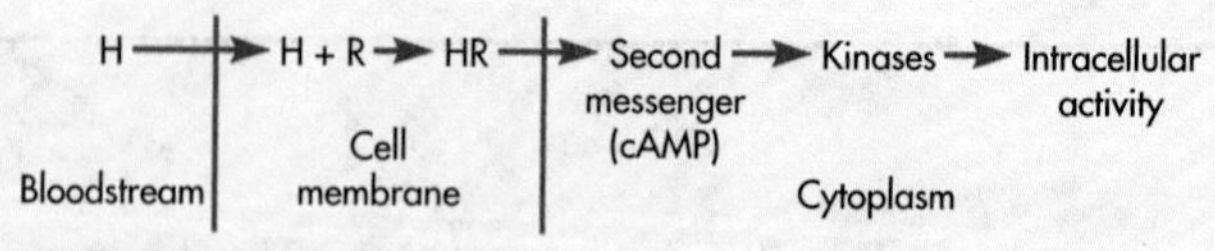

Fig. 45-4 Hormone-receptor action: peptide hormones and catecholamines. Hormone (*H*) binds to receptor (*R*) in the cell membrane to form hormone-receptor complex (*HR*). The HR activates secondary messengers (e.g., cyclic adenosine monophosphate [cAMP]) at the membrane's inner surface. The secondary messenger activates kinases in the cytoplasm. The kinases regulate intracellular activity.

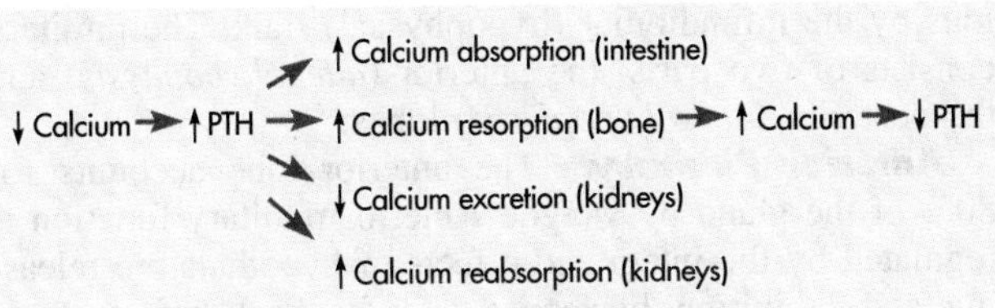

Fig. 45-5 Simple negative feedback: calcium and parathyroid hormone (PTH).

In *positive feedback,* high levels of a substance stimulate hormone synthesis and secretion, and low levels inhibit hormone synthesis and secretion. An example of positive feedback is the stimulatory effect of increased luteinizing hormone (LH) levels on ovarian estradiol secretion during the menstrual cycle.

Another level of complexity exists in feedback systems. An example of this is regulation of thyroid hormones (Fig. 45-6). The synthesis and release of TSH or thyrotropin from the anterior pituitary is stimulated by thyrotropin-releasing hormone (TRH), which is secreted by the hypothalamus. T_3 and T_4 have an inhibitory effect on the secretion of both TRH from the hypothalmus and TSH from the anterior pituitary.

An example of a complex feedback system is insulin regulation (Table 45-2). High levels of circulating glucose, amino acids, and fats (as seen after a meal) stimulate insulin secretion. In addition, gastrointestinal or enteric hormones such as gastrin and gastric inhibitory polypeptide enhance insulin release after a meal, as does vagal stimulation. After a high protein meal, the secretion of both glucagon and insulin increases. Glucagon increases gluconeogenesis and insulin causes target tissue to accept the amino acids for protein synthesis. Insulin secretion is inhibited by low circulating levels of glucose and amino acids, high circulating levels of steroids and catecholamines (as seen in stress), hypokalemia, and other pancreatic hormones such as glucagon and somatostatin.

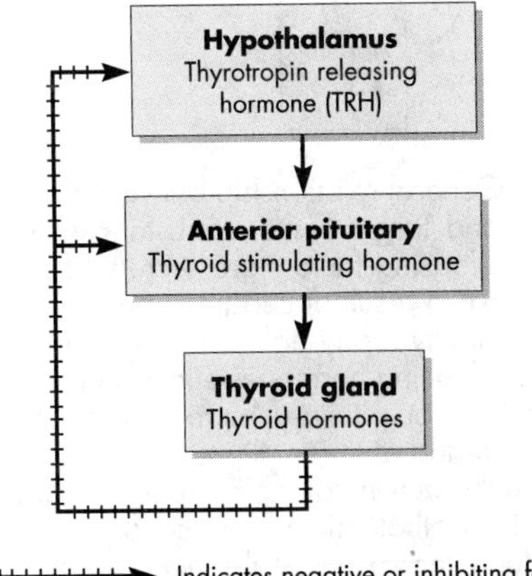

Fig. 45-6 Hypothalamic-pituitary-target gland feedback loop.

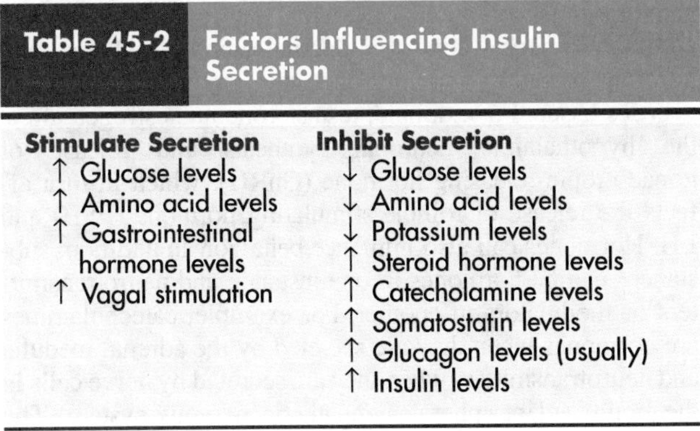

Table 45-2 Factors Influencing Insulin Secretion

Stimulate Secretion	Inhibit Secretion
↑ Glucose levels	↓ Glucose levels
↑ Amino acid levels	↓ Amino acid levels
↑ Gastrointestinal hormone levels	↓ Potassium levels
↑ Vagal stimulation	↑ Steroid hormone levels
	↑ Catecholamine levels
	↑ Somatostatin levels
	↑ Glucagon levels (usually)
	↑ Insulin levels

In addition to chemical regulation, some endocrine glands are directly affected by the activity of the nervous system. Pain, emotion, sexual excitement, and stress can stimulate the nervous system to modulate hormone secretion. Neural involvement is initiated by the central nervous system (CNS) and implemented by the autonomic nervous system (ANS).

Another regulatory mechanism affecting many hormonal secretions involves the *rhythms* of secretions. These rhythms originate in brain structures. A common physiologic rhythm is the *diurnal (circadian) rhythm,* in which a hormone level fluctuates predictably during a 24-hour period. These rhythms may be related to sleep-wake or dark-light cycles. For example, cortisol rises early in the day, declines toward evening, and rises again toward the end of sleep to peak by morning (Fig. 45-7). Growth hormone (GH) and prolactin secretion peak during sleep. TSH secretion is also maximum during sleep and ebbs 3 hours after a person awakens in the morning. The menstrual cycle is an example of a body rhythm that is longer than 24 hours (*ultradian*). These rhythms must be considered when interpreting hormone levels on laboratory results.

Neuroendocrine System

The ANS and endocrine system are interrelated and interdependent, and together integrate stimuli to allow a coordi-

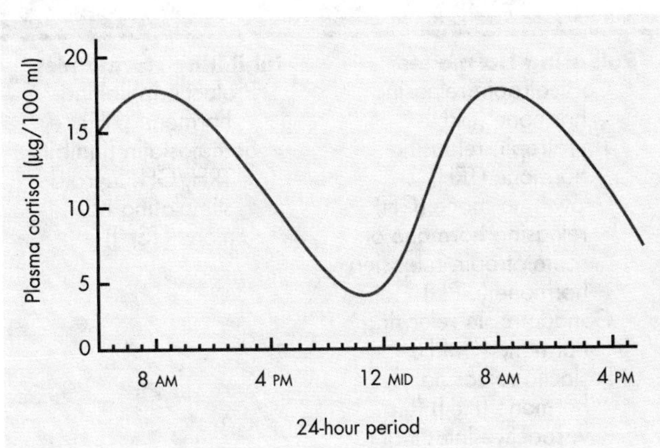

Fig. 45-7 Circadian rhythm of cortisol secretion.

nated response to internal or external environmental changes. Autonomic nerves control endocrine gland blood flow and hormone secretion, and hormones have a regulatory effect on nervous tissue. For example, testosterone and estrogen affect the hypothalamic neuronal synthesis and release of gonadotropin-releasing hormone (GnRH), which in turn affects the release of follicle-stimulating hormone (FSH) and LH. Hormones can also influence behavior. In addition, substances can be hormones in one instance and neurotransmitters or modulators in another. For example, catecholamines are hormones when they are secreted by the adrenal medulla and neurotransmitters when they are secreted by nerve cells in the brain and peripheral sympathetic nervous system. The differentiating factor is the mode of transport. When epinephrine travels through the blood, it is a hormone. When it travels across synaptic junctions, it is a neurotransmitter.

Hypothalamus

The hypothalamus and the pituitary gland integrate communication between the nervous and endocrine systems. CNS input is mediated by hypothalamic hormones and neurotransmitters (norepinephrine, dopamine, serotonin, and acetylcholine), which helps to regulate pituitary hormone secretion and has effects outside of the pituitary (e.g., influences secretion, metabolism, and transport of protein in the target organ). Hypothalamic hormones can stimulate or inhibit the synthesis and release of anterior pituitary hormones (Table 45-3).

The hypothalamus and pituitary gland communicate via veins called the median eminence portal system (Fig. 45-8). The hypothalamus secretes releasing and inhibiting hormones that travel through this portal system to the anterior pituitary, where they interact with specific receptors and rapidly stimulate or inhibit the synthesis and release of anterior pituitary hormones (see Table 45-3).

Pituitary Gland

The pituitary gland (*hypophysis*) weighs approximately 0.6 g and is located in the sella turcica at the base of the brain above the sphenoid bone. It is connected to the hypothalamus by the infundibular (hypophyseal) stalk. The pituitary consists of two parts, the anterior (*adenohypophysis*) and the posterior (*neurohypophysis*) lobes.

Anterior Pituitary. The anterior lobe accounts for 80% of the gland by weight. Anterior pituitary function is regulated by the integrated effects of hypothalamic releasing and inhibiting hormones and feedback effects from circulating hormones. Hormones secreted by the anterior pituitary include GH, TSH, adrenocorticotropic hormone (ACTH), prolactin, gonadotropic hormones (e.g., FSH and LH), and β-lipotropin (see Table 45-1).

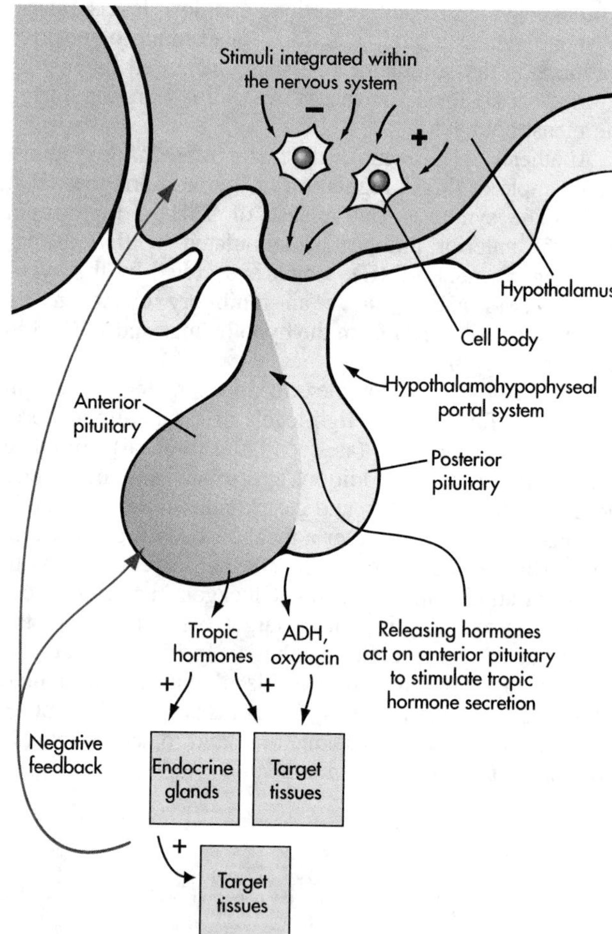

Fig. 45-8 General relationship between the hypothalamus, the pituitary, and target tissues. Substances called releasing hormones or releasing factors are secreted from the hypothalamic neurons as a result of certain stimuli. They pass through the hypothalamo-hypophyseal portal system to the anterior pituitary. The releasing hormones either stimulate or inhibit the secretion of anterior pituitary hormones. Secreted hormones from cells within the anterior pituitary pass through the blood and influence the activity of their target tissues. In response to stimulation of hypothalamic neurosecretory cells, action potentials pass along the axons of the neurosecretory cells to the posterior pituitary. The action potentials cause the release of neurohormones from the posterior pituitary and pass through the blood to target tissues. *ADH,* Antidiuretic hormone.

Table 45-3 Hormones of the Hypothalamus

Releasing Hormones	Inhibiting Hormones
Corticotropin-releasing hormone (CRH)	Prolactin-inhibiting hormone (PIH)
Thyrotropin-releasing hormone (TRH)	Somatostatin (inhibits TRH, GH, thyroid-stimulating hormone [TSH])
Growth hormone (GH)—releasing hormone or somatotropin-releasing hormone (GRH)	
Gonadotropin-releasing hormone (GnRH)	
Prolactin-releasing hormone (PRH) (e.g., vasoactive intestinal peptide)	

Posterior Pituitary. The posterior pituitary is an extension of the hypothalamus. The cell bodies of neurons that carry posterior pituitary hormones are in the hypothalamus, and the axons terminate in the posterior pituitary. The posterior pituitary lies behind the anterior pituitary and consists of pituicytes, unmyelinated nerve fibers, and the terminals of axons. The hormones of the posterior pituitary, antidiuretic hormone (ADH) or vasopressin and oxytocin, are produced in the hypothalamus as prohormones, travel down the nerve fibers, and are stored in the posterior pituitary near capillaries. The hormones are released into the general circulation after appropriate stimulation.

The major physiologic role of ADH is regulation of fluid volume by stimulating reabsorption of water in the renal tubules. ADH can also be a potent vasoconstrictor, and potentiates the effects of corticotropin-releasing hormone (CRH). The most important stimulus to ADH secretion is increased osmotic pressure of body fluid as reflected by increased plasma osmolality (a measure of solute concentration of circulating blood). Plasma osmolality is increased by decreased extracellular fluid or increased sodium concentration. The increased plasma osmolality activates osmoreceptors, which are extremely sensitive, specialized neurons near the supraorbital nucleus of the hypothalamus. These activated osmoreceptors then stimulate ADH release. Therefore when body fluids become highly concentrated, osmoreceptors cause ADH release. In the absence of ADH, dilute urine is excreted.

Nonosmotic stimuli to ADH secretion include decreased blood volume, orthostatic changes in blood pressure, hypotension, pain, nausea, vomiting, hypoglycemia, and many pharmacologic agents. ADH release is inhibited by an increase in fluid volume, hypothermia, β-adrenergic agonists, and alcohol.[3]

Oxytocin stimulates ejection of milk into mammary ducts, contraction of uterine smooth muscle, and possibly prolactin release. Secretion of oxytocin is increased by stimulation of touch receptors in the nipples and manipulation or distention of the female genital tract, as well as by hemorrhage and psychologic stress. Oxytocin secretion is inhibited by endorphins and alcohol.[1]

Thyroid Gland

The thyroid gland is located in the anterior portion of the neck in front of the trachea. It consists of two encapsulated lateral lobes connected by a narrow isthmus. It is a highly vascular organ.

The major function of the thyroid gland is the production, storage, and release of the thyroid hormones, T_4 (thyroxine) and T_3 (triiodothyronine). T_4 is the precursor for T_3, which is the more active hormone. About 10% of circulating T_3 is secreted directly by the thyroid gland, and the remainder is obtained by peripheral conversion of T_4.

Iodine is necessary for the synthesis of thyroid hormones. T_4 and T_3 affect metabolic rate, caloric requirements, oxygen consumption, carbohydrate and lipid metabolism, growth and development, brain functions, and nervous system activity. More than 99% of thyroid hormones circulate bound to plasma proteins, the majority to thyroxine-binding globulin synthesized by the liver and the remainder to prealbumin and albumin. Only the unbound, "free" hormones are biologically active.

Thyroid hormone production and release is stimulated by TSH. Low circulating levels of thyroid hormone stimulate the release of TRH by the hypothalamus and TSH by the anterior pituitary. High circulating thyroid hormone levels have an inhibitory effect on the secretion of both TRH from the hypothalamus and TSH from the adenohypophysis.

Calcitonin is a hormone produced by thyroid C cells (*parafollicular* cells) in response to high circulating calcium levels. Secretion is inhibited by somatostatin. In pharmacologic doses, calcitonin inhibits calcium resorption from bone, increases calcium storage in bone, and increases renal excretion of calcium and phosphorus, thereby lowering serum calcium levels.[3]

Parathyroid Glands

The *parathyroid glands* are small, oval structures arranged in pairs behind each thyroid lobe. Occasionally they are found in the chest. There are usually four glands. The major cell type of the glands is epithelial, and the gland is richly supplied with blood by fenestrated capillaries from the inferior and superior thyroid arteries. The parathyroids secrete *parathyroid hormone* (PTH), or *parathormone.* Its major role is to regulate the blood level of calcium. PTH acts on bone, the kidneys, and indirectly, the gastrointestinal (GI) tract. In bone, PTH stimulates bone resorption and inhibits bone formation, resulting in the release of calcium and phosphate into the blood. In the kidney, PTH increases calcium reabsorption and phosphate excretion. In addition, PTH stimulates the renal conversion of vitamin D to its most active form (1,25-dihydroxyvitamin D_3). This active vitamin D then enhances the intestinal absorption of calcium.

PTH is free of pituitary and hypothalamic control. The secretion of this hormone is directly regulated by a feedback system. When the serum calcium level is low, PTH secretion increases; when the serum calcium level rises, PTH secretion falls (see Fig. 45-5). In addition, high levels of active vitamin D inhibit PTH and low levels of magnesium stimulate PTH secretion.

Adrenal Glands

The *adrenal glands* are small, paired, highly vascularized glands located near the upper poles of each kidney and lateral to the lower thoracic and upper lumbar vertebrae. Each gland weighs about 4 g and consists of two parts, the inner medulla and the outer cortex. Each has distinct functions.

Adrenal Medulla. The adrenal medulla constitutes 10% to 20% of the gland, and consists of sympathetic postganglionic neurons. The medulla secretes the catecholamines—epinephrine (the major hormone [75%]), norepinephrine (25%), and dopamine. Catecholamines, usually considered neurotransmitters, are hormones when secreted by the adrenal medulla. They are considered hormones as they are released into the circulation and transported to their target organs. Catecholamines exert their effects after binding to adrenergic receptors on cells, and have widespread effects on all body systems (see Chapters 5 and 50).

Adrenal Cortex. The adrenal cortex, the outer part of the adrenal gland, constitutes 80% to 90% of the gland. It secretes more than 50 steroid hormones, which are classified as glucocorticoids, mineralocorticoids, and androgens. Glucocorticoids (e.g., cortisol) are named for their effects on glucose metabolism. Mineralocorticoids are essential for the maintenance of fluid and electrolyte balance. Adrenal androgens and estrogens (sex steroids) are produced and secreted in small but significant amounts.

Glucocorticoids. *Cortisol,* the most abundant and potent glucocorticoid, is necessary to maintain life. Approximately 75% to 80% of circulating cortisol is bound to transcortin (corticosteroid-binding globulin) and about 15% to albumin. The free cortisol (*5% to 10% of total*) binds with receptors in the cytoplasm and nucleus of a target cell. The hormone-receptor complex exerts cortisol's effects within the nucleus of the target tissue. Cortisol is episodically secreted in a diurnal pattern (see Fig. 45-7). Major functions of cortisol are to facilitate hepatic gluconeogenesis by facilitating conversion of protein to glucose and inhibiting protein synthesis, and to decrease peripheral glucose use in the fasting state. In addition, cortisol contributes to lipid and nucleic acid metabolism and physiologic responses to many hormones. Cortisol is also critical in the body's response to stress.[1] Glucocorticoids stimulate lipolysis in adipose tissue, thereby mobilizing glycerol and free fatty acids.

Other effects of glucocorticoids include their antiinflammatory action and supportive actions in stressful situations. Cortisol decreases the inflammatory response by stabilizing the membranes of cellular lysosomes and preventing increased capillary permeability. The lysosomal stabilization reduces the release of proteolytic enzymes and thereby their destructive effects on surrounding tissue. Cortisol can also inhibit production of prostaglandins, thromboxanes, and leukotrienes, and decrease the cell-mediated immune response. Cortisol helps maintain vascular integrity and responsiveness and fluid volume, and has mineralocorticoid effects because it can bind to mineralocorticoid receptors. A marked increase in the rate of cortisol secretion by the adrenal cortex can aid the body in coping more effectively with stressful situations (see Chapter 5). The major control of cortisol is by means of a negative feedback mechanism that involves the secretion of CRH from the hypothalamus. CRH stimulates the secretion of ACTH by the anterior pituitary. Cortisol levels are also increased by surgical stress, burns, infection, fever, psychoses, acute anxiety, and hypoglycemia.

Mineralocorticoids. *Aldosterone,* a potent mineralocorticoid, maintains extracellular fluid volume. It acts at the renal tubule to promote renal reabsorption of sodium and excretion of potassium and hydrogen ions. Aldosterone synthesis and secretion are stimulated by angiotensin II (see Fig. 42-6), hyponatremia, and hyperkalemia, and inhibited by atrial natriuretic factor and hypokalemia.

Androgens and other sex hormones. Adrenal androgens are the third class of steroids synthesized and secreted by the adrenal cortex. The normal adrenal cortex secretes small amounts of both male hormones (androgens) and female hormones (estrogen). Adrenal androgens stimulate pubic and axillary hair growth and sex drive in females. In women, adrenal androgens may function in sexuality and libido. In postmenopausal women, the adrenal cortex is the major source of endogenous estrogen (see Chapters 48 and 49). Their effects in men are negligible in comparison to testosterone secreted by the testes.

Pancreas

The pancreas, a long, tapered, lobular, soft gland that weighs between 60 and 90 g, lies behind the stomach, anterior to the first and second lumbar vertebrae. The pancreas performs exocrine and endocrine functions. The islets of Langerhans are the areas of endocrine activity; they release their secretions into the portal circulation. The secretions are also paracrine. (Paracrine secretions diffuse to neighboring cells to exert their action, rather than traveling to their target tissues through the blood like endocrine secretions.) The islets account for less than 2% of the gland and consist of alpha, beta, and delta cells. Glucagon is synthesized by the alpha cells, insulin by the beta cells, and gastrin and somatostatin by the delta cells.

Glucagon. Glucagon is synthesized and released from pancreatic alpha cells in response to low levels of blood glucose, protein ingestion, and exercise. Glucagon stimulates hepatic glycogenolysis and gluconeogenesis and enhances adipose tissue lipolysis. Usually, glucagon and insulin function in a reciprocal manner to maintain normal blood glucose levels (*euglycemia*). The exception is after ingestion of a high-protein carbohydrate-free meal, in which case both hormones are secreted. In this instance, glucagon counteracts the inhibitory effect of insulin on gluconeogenesis, and euglycemia is maintained.[4]

Insulin. Insulin is the principal regulator of the metabolism and storage of ingested carbohydrates, fats, and proteins. Insulin facilitates glucose transport across cell membranes in most tissues. However, the brain, nerves, the lens of the eye, hepatocytes, erythrocytes, and cells in the intestinal mucosa and kidney tubules are not dependent on insulin for glucose uptake. An increased blood glucose level is the major stimulus for insulin synthesis and secretion. Other stimuli to insulin secretion are increased amino acid levels; specific GI hormones, which enhance the response to glucose; and vagal stimulation. Insulin secretion is usually inhibited by low blood glucose levels, glucagon, somatostatin, hypokalemia, and catecholamines.

A major effect of insulin on glucose metabolism occurs in the liver, where the hormone enhances glucose incorporation into glycogen and triglyceride by altering enzymatic activity and inhibiting gluconeogenesis. In peripheral tissues, insulin facilitates glucose transport into cells, transport of amino acids across muscle membranes and their synthesis into protein, and transport of triglyceride into adipose tissue. Thus insulin is a storage, or anabolic, hormone.

The endocrine system is concerned with the regulation of body processes and the maintenance of internal homeostasis despite vastly changing substrates, as is seen in glucose homeostasis after food ingestion. After a meal, insulin is responsible for the storage of nutrients (*anabolism*). In the fasting state (during which ingested glucose is not readily available), hormones such as cortisol and glucagon break down stored complex fuels (*catabolism*) to provide simple glucose as fuel for energy.

Heart

Atrial natriuretic factor (ANF) is a hormone produced by atrial myocytes; it helps maintain fluid homeostasis. Its release is stimulated by an increase in the stretch of the atrial wall caused by abnormally high blood volume or blood pressure. These receptors in the atrial myocytes are also stimulated by cold water immersion, increased plasma osmolality, and sodium intake. ANF acts on the kidneys to inhibit the reabsorption of sodium ions. When sodium is lost, water follows, resulting in a decrease in blood volume and a decrease in blood pressure. ANF also inhibits renin, ADH, and the action of angiotensin II on the adrenal glands.[3]

Gerontologic Considerations

Normal aging has many effects on the endocrine system (Table 45-4). General changes include increased connective tissue in the glands, decreased blood supply, and decreased metabolism resulting in increased half-life. This can be manifested by events such as changes in a hormone's basal

Table 45-4 Effects of Aging on the Endocrine System

Hormone	Basal Level	Secretion	MCR	Target Organ Response	Clinical Significance
Posterior Pituitary					
ADH	—	↑	—	↓ (renal)	Sodium imbalance, syndrome of inappropriate ADH
Anterior Pituitary					
GH	↓	↓	—	—	
TSH	—	—	—	—	
ACTH	—	—	—	—	Decreased response to surgical stress
Prolactin	↑	↑	?	?	
LH and FSH	↑	↑	?	↓	
Thyroid					
T_4	—	↓	↓	↓	Atypical presentation of hyperthyroidism
T_3	—	—	↓	↓	Increased hypothyroidism
Parathyroids					
PTH	↑	↑	?	?	Hypercalcemia, hypercalciuria
Adrenal Cortex					
Cortisol	—	↓	↓	↓	
Androgens	↓	↓	?	?	
Aldosterone	↓	—	↓	?	Decreased response to sodium restriction and upright posture
Adrenal Medulla					
Epinephrine	—		—	↓	Decreased response to β-blockers (e.g., less of a decrease in heart rate and cardiac output)
Norepinephrine	↑	↑	↑	↓	Increased peripheral and α-adrenergic sympathetic nerve activity
Pancreas					
Insulin	↑	↓	—	↓	Impaired glucose tolerance
Gonads					
Estrogen	↓	↓	—	?	Increased hot flashes, osteoporosis, decreased vaginal secretions
Testosterone	↓	↓	?	?	Decreased ejaculatory force
Kidneys					
Renin	↓	↓	?	?	Decreased response to sodium restriction, upright posture
Vitamin D	↓	N/A	?	?	Decreased intestinal absorption of calcium

ACTH, Adrenocorticotropic hormone; *ADH*, antidiuretic hormone; *FSH*, follicle-stimulating hormone; *GH*, growth hormone; *LH*, luteinizing hormone; *MCR*, metabolic clearance rate; *T_3*, triiodothyronine; *T_4*, thyroxine, *TSH*, thyroid-stimulating hormone.

level, response to stimuli, transport of the hormone, target organ responsiveness, and catabolism. Often one change such as decreased response to stimuli is offset by another such as decreased metabolic clearance rate so that the net effect is normal hormone levels. Because radioimmunoassays of hormone levels have become widely available, problems previously attributed to age-related endocrine changes have been found to be the effects of specific illnesses, health problems, or nutritional deficits affecting the endocrine system.

Assessment of the effects of aging on the endocrine system is difficult because the subtle changes of aging often mimic symptoms of endocrine disorders. However, there are endocrine changes with clinical significance. Aging is associated with altered hypothalamic neurotransmitters, and the hypothalamus is less sensitive to feedback inhibition. In addition, increased PTH secretion is often seen and may be related to the bone changes seen in older adults. In addition to endocrine changes related to aging, the nurse must be aware that endocrine problems may occur differently in an older adult than in a younger person. Altered PTH secretion usually manifests as hyperparathyroidism. However, the older adult often has altered mental status, fatigue, and generalized weakness rather than the kidney stones and peptic ulcers seen in a younger person.

Some symptoms of hypothyroidism in the older adult are similar to those in a younger person but are more likely to be overlooked because the symptoms—fatigue, mental impairment, sluggishness, and constipation—are often attributed solely to aging.[6] The older person with hypothyroidism has symptoms unique to the age set including more disturbances of the CNS, such as syncope, convulsions, dementia, and coma. There is often pitting edema and deafness. The older patient with hyperthyroidism frequently has manifestations related only to the cardiovascular system, such as palpitations, angina, atrial fibrillation, and breathlessness. The older adult may also have depression, anorexia, and constipation (apathetic hyperthyroidism). Thus signs and symptoms often attributed to "old age" may actually indicate an endocrine problem.

ASSESSMENT OF THE ENDOCRINE SYSTEM

Hormones affect every body tissue and system, causing great diversity in the signs and symptoms of endocrine dysfunction. Therefore assessment of the endocrine system is often difficult and requires keen clinical skills to detect manifestations of disorders (Table 45-5). Endocrine dysfunction may result from deficient or excessive hormone secretion, transport abnormalities, an inability of the target tissue to respond to a hormone, or inappropriate stimulation of the target-tissue receptor. If the patient has a specific problem, an appropriate history should be taken and the system involved should be assessed. For instance, a chief complaint of tachycardia indicates the need for a cardiovascular assessment and for information related to stress, diet, exercise, and sleep. The nurse must also remember the possibility of endocrine dysfunction and assess for hyperthyroidism.

Endocrine disorders may have nonspecific or specific manifestations. For example, weight loss may be a sign of panhypopituitarism, hyperthyroidism, occasionally hypothyroidism, Addison's disease, pheochromocytoma, relative or absolute insulin deficiency, or hyperparathyroidism. Alternatively, it may be due to malignancy, GI or emotional problems, or a well-planned weight reduction program. A careful health history will yield data to help sort out possible causes. Some signs of endocrine dysfunction are specific, such as the classic "polys" (polyuria, polydipsia, and polyphagia) in diabetes mellitus and exophthalmos in hyperthyroidism. Specific signs make the assessment easier while nonspecific signs and symptoms such as tachycardia and fatigue are more problematic. The lack of clear-cut manifestations of endocrine problems requires a conscientious and detailed health history.

Certain guidelines (see Chapter 4) should be used in the assessment of endocrine dysfunction. Nonspecific changes should alert the clinician to the possibility of an endocrine disorder. The most common nonspecific symptoms are fatigue and depression, often accompanied by other manifestations. The latter includes changes in energy level, alertness, sleep patterns, mood, affect, weight, skin, hair, personal appearance, and sexual function (Table 45-6).

Subjective Data

Important Health Information

Past health history. During an assessment, the patient should be questioned about the general state of health and if there have been any changes. In addition, the patient or significant other should be specifically questioned about previous or concurrent endocrine abnormalities. The presence of delay or acceleration in growth and development and abnormal secondary sex characteristics (e.g., facial hair in a woman or decreased need for shaving in a man) should also be documented.

Medications. The patient should be questioned as to whether any hormone replacements are being taken, and the reasons for these hormones. This is particularly important if the patient is taking large doses of glucocorticoids, as abrupt discontinuance of these medications may cause an Addisonian crisis. In addition, regular long-term glucocorticoid therapy can result in potentially serious side effects and complications (see Table 47-19).

Insulin replacement should be identified in terms of type, amount, and timing of replacement. In addition, some medications may adversely affect endocrine function. Corticosteroids may cause glucose intolerance in the susceptible patient by increasing glycogenolysis and insulin resistance. There is a greater glucose lowering effect of sulfonylureas and insulin when taken with large doses (>2 g per day) of aspirin. Dicumarol can cause adrenal hemorrhage and resultant adrenal insufficiency. Lithium carbonate has many adverse effects on the endocrine system including diffuse nontoxic goiter, hypercalcemia, hyperparathyroidism, transient hyperglycemia, and impotence or sexual dysfunction. Many medications affect blood glucose levels (see Table 46-10).

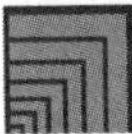

Table 45-5 Key Questions: Patient with an Endocrine Problem

Health Perception–Health Management Pattern
- What is your usual day like?
- Have you noticed any changes in your ability to perform your usual activities compared to last year and five years ago?*

Nutritional-Metabolic Pattern
- What is your weight and height?
- How much do you want to weigh?
- Have there been any changes in your appetite or weight?*
- Have you noticed any changes in the distribution of hair anywhere on your body?*
- Have you noticed any changes in the color of your skin, particularly on your face, neck, hands, or body creases?*
- Has the texture of your skin changed? For example, does it seem thicker and drier than it used to?*
- Have you noticed any difficulty swallowing, or are your shirts more difficult to button?*
- Do you feel more nervous than you used to? Do you notice your heart pounding, or that you sweat when you do not think you should be sweating?*
- Do you have difficulty holding things because of shakiness of your hands?*
- Do you feel that most rooms are too hot or too cold? Do you frequently have to put on a sweater, or feel as though you need to open windows when others in the room seem comfortable?*

Elimination Pattern
- Do you have to get up at night to urinate? If so, how many times? Do you keep water by your bed at night?
- Have you ever had a kidney stone?*
- Describe your usual bowel pattern. Have you noted any bowel changes?*
- Do you use anything, such as laxatives, to help you move your bowels?*

Activity-Exercise Pattern
- What is your usual activity pattern during a typical day?
- Do you have a planned exercise program? If yes, what is it and have you had to make any changes in this routine lately? If so, why and what kinds of changes?
- Do you experience fatigue with or without activity?*

Sleep-Rest Pattern
- How many hours do you sleep at night? Do you feel rested on awakening?
- Are you ever awakened by sweating during the night?*
- Do you have nightmares?*
- Does anyone in your family complain about your snoring?*

Cognitive-Perceptual Pattern
- How is your memory? Have you noticed any changes?*
- How long can you concentrate on any one thing? Has this changed lately?*
- Have you experienced any blurring or double vision?*
- When was your last eye examination?

Self-Perception–Self-Concept Pattern
- Have you noticed any changes in your physical appearance or size?*
- Are you concerned about your weight?*
- Do you feel you are able to do what you think you should be capable of doing? If not, why not?
- Does your health problem affect how you feel about yourself?*

Role-Relationship Pattern
- Are you married? Do you have any children? Do you think you are able to take care of your family and home? If no, why not?
- Have there been any changes in your ability to function at work or at school?*

Sexuality-Reproductive Pattern

Females:
- When did you start to menstruate? Was this earlier or later than other women in your family? Do you have scant, heavy, or irregular menstrual flows?
- How many children have you had? How much did they weigh at birth? Were you told you had diabetes during any pregnancy?*
- Were you able to nurse your children if you wanted to?
- Are you attempting to get pregnant but cannot?

Males:
- Have you noticed any changes in your ability to have an erection?*
- Are you trying to have children but cannot?*

Coping-Stress Tolerance Pattern
- Where do you work? What kind of work do you do? Are you able to do what is expected of you and what you expect of yourself?
- What kind of stressors do you have at work or school?
- If retired, what do you do with your time? What did you do before you retired?
- If unemployed, are you looking for work?
- Is your income adequate for your needs?
- How do you deal with stress or problems?
- What is your support system? Whom do you turn to when you have a problem?

Value-Belief Pattern
- Do you think medicine should still be taken even though you feel okay?
- Does your health plan cause any conflict in your value-belief system?*

*If yes, describe.

Table 45-6 Nonspecific Manifestations of Hormone Dysfunction

Manifestations	Panhypopituitary Hormone	ADH	Thyroid Hormone	Cortisol	Mineralocorticoids	Insulin	PTH
■ Nutrition and							
elimination	↓	↑↓	↑↓	↑↓	↑↓	↑↓	↑↓
Weight	↓		↓↑	↑↓	↑	↓↓	↓
Appetite	↓		↑↓	↑↓		↑↓	↓
Growth abnormality							
(children)	+		+	++		+	+
Abdominal pain			++	+		+	+
Stool output	↓		↑↓				↓
Urine output		↓↑			↑	↑	↑
■ Cardiovascular system							
Blood pressure		↑↓		↑	↑	↑	
Heart rate			↑↓	↑		↑	
Anemia	+		++	+			+
■ Neurologic system							
Temperature			↑↓	↑		↓↑	
Sleep disturbances	+	+	+	++		+	+
Convulsions	+	+	+	+		+	+
■ Mood							
Depression or apathy	+	++	+	++		+	++
■ Skin							
Body hair	↓		↓↓	↑			↓
Pigmentation	↓		↓	↑↓			↓
■ Reproductive or sexual							
system				++			
Male dysfunction	+		++		+	+	+
Female dysfunction	+		++	++		+	

ADH, Adrenocorticotropic hormone; *PTH*, parathyroid hormone; ↑, increased; ↓, decreased; +, present.

Surgery or other treatments. The nurse should inquire about previous hospitalizations, surgeries, chemotherapies, and radiation treatments (especially of the neck). A history of a severe blow to the head could indicate pituitary or hypothalamic trauma.

Functional Health Patterns

Health perception–health management pattern. The nurse needs to ask about energy levels, particularly as compared to the patient's past energy level. Fatigue and hyperactivity are two common problems associated with endocrine problems. Inquiry should also be made about the patient's general health care and health care behaviors. Such an inquiry might result in the identification of vague, nonspecific symptoms that could suggest an endocrine problem.

Heredity and general health can play a major role in the occurrence of endocrine problems. The patient should be questioned about the following conditions in family members: diabetes mellitus or insipidus; hyperthyroidism or hypothyroidism, goiter; hypertension or hypotension; obesity; infertility; growth problems; pheochromocytoma (neoplastic tumor of the adrenal medulla or sympathetic ganglia); autoimmune diseases (e.g., Addison's disease); and adrenal hyperplasia. Further information may be elicited by asking additional questions such as the following: Are there any other members of your family who have, or have had, a similar problem? This frequently uncovers evidence of a familial tendency that cannot be found in any other way.

Nutritional-metabolic pattern. Because a major function of the endocrine system is regulating metabolism and maintenance of homeostasis, the patient with endocrine dysfunction will often experience alterations in nutritional-metabolic patterns. Changes in appetite and weight can indicate endocrine dysfunction. Weight loss with increased appetite may indicate hyperthyroidism or diabetes mellitus, particularly type I. Weight loss with decreased appetite may indicate hypopituitarism, hypocortisolism, or gastroparesis from diabetes mellitus. Weight gain may indicate hypothyroidism and, if the weight gain is concentrated in the truncal area, hypercortisolism. In addition, weight gain in a genetically susceptible patient may increase the risk for type II diabetes.

Assessment of the endocrine system includes growth and development patterns, weight distribution and changes, and comparisons of these factors with normal findings. Height should be measured in all patients. The charts used should be race-specific because significant racial differences exist in normal children. For example, Caucasian children usually are smaller than African-American children, but are larger than those from Asian races. Familial patterns should always be assessed. A helpful guide in growth assessment is that approximate normal growth rates are 3 inches per year (7.5 cm) from ages 1 to 7 and 2 inches per year (5 cm) from ages 8 to 15. Heights more than three standard deviations below the mean should be investigated.[7] Approximate average heights for children and young teenagers can be estimated on the basis of age using the following formula:

$$\text{Height (inches)} = 2.5 \times \text{Age (years)} + 30$$

In adults, weight changes may indicate endocrine dysfunction. A patient's percentage of ideal body weight (IBW) may be obtained by dividing the actual weight by the ideal or optimal weight for height and multiplying by 100.

Body mass index (BMI) is a common way to assess obesity.[7] This estimation takes height into account. It is derived by dividing the weight (in kg) by the height (in meters squared) [BMI = Wt(kg)/ht(m^2)]. A BMI of 25 is the upper limits of normal, one of 25 to 29.9 indicates a patient is overweight, and a BMI of 30 and above indicates obesity. A weight increase of more than 1 kg per day usually indicates fluid retention.

Changes in hair distribution and skin and hair color and texture can all indicate endocrine dysfunction. Hair loss can indicate hypopituitarism, hypothyroidism, hypoparathyroidism, or increased testosterone and androgens. Increased body hair may indicate hypercortisolism. Decreased skin pigmentation can occur in hypopituitarism, hypothyroidism, and hypoparathyroidism, whereas increased skin pigmentation, particularly in sun exposed areas, can indicate hypocortisolism. A patient with hypothyroidism or excess growth hormone may complain of coarse, leathery skin. A patient with hyperthyroidism may comment about fine, silky hair. A history of hypertension may indicate excess ADH, aldosterone, or cortisol.

Difficulty swallowing or a change in neck size may indicate thyroid hyperplasia or inflammation. Questions related to increased sympathetic nervous system activity (e.g., nervousness, palpitations, sweating, tremors) may assist the nurse in identifying a thyroid disorder or pheochromocytoma. Heat or cold intolerance may indicate hyper- or hypothyroidism, respectively. The patient should be questioned about dietary intake. This record should be examined for the presence of foods that contain thyroid-inhibiting substances (goitrogens) (see Table 47-8).

Elimination pattern. Because maintenance of fluid balance is a major role of the endocrine system, questions related to elimination patterns may uncover endocrine dysfunction. For instance, increased thirst and urination can indicate diabetes mellitus or insipidus. A history of nephrolithiasis (kidney stones) may indicate excess PTH. The patient should be asked about the frequency and consistency of bowel movements. Hyperdefecation may indicate hyperthyroidism. Large volume, watery stools, or fecal incontinence may indicate autonomic gastroenteropathy of diabetes mellitus. Constipation is also seen in the gastroenteropathy of diabetes mellitus as well as in hypothyroidism, hypoparathyroidism, and hypopituitarism.

Activity-exercise pattern. The major effect of endocrine dysfunction on activity-exercise pattern will be an inability to maintain previous activity levels. Although a patient with hyperthyroidism may seem to have excess energy, fatigue is common. A patient with an endocrine dysfunction will almost always manifest apathy and, frequently depression. This indicates the need for the nurse to specifically question the patient or significant other to describe current activity in relation to previous activity patterns. In addition, in diabetes mellitus, the patient's activity-exercise patterns will help determine diabetes management, including insulin therapy.

Sleep-rest pattern. It is important that the nurse obtain a detailed sleep history. Sleep disturbances are frequently seen in endocrine dysfunction. The patient with diabetes mellitus or insipidus will complain of nocturia, which can severely disrupt normal sleep patterns. The patient with tightly controlled type I diabetes mellitus who complains of sweating or nightmares may be experiencing hypoglycemia. The hyperthyroid patient may complain of inability to sleep, as may one with hypercortisolism. The patient with hypothyroidism, hypocortisolism, or hypopituitarism may tell the nurse of sleeping all the time, yet still being fatigued. The significant other of a patient with excess growth hormone may tell the nurse of an inability to sleep because of the patient's snoring.

Cognitive-perceptual pattern. The nurse can question both the patient and significant others to determine if any cognitive changes are present. Memory deficits, inability to concentrate, and decreased energy levels are common in endocrine disorders. As mentioned earlier, depression and apathy are frequent in endocrine disorders. Visual changes can also occur. A patient with hyperglycemia may complain of blurred vision. Diplopia may indicate pressure from a pituitary tumor. Exophthalmos secondary to hyperthyroidism can cause corneal drying as well as other visual disturbances.

Self-perception–self-concept pattern. Endocrine disorders may affect the patient's self-perception because of associated physical changes. Changes in weight, size, and level of fatigue should be determined. Weight changes often occur, and both increases and decreases can affect self-perception. Increases in the size of the head, hands, or feet in the adult (e.g., change in ring, glove, or shoe size) may indicate excess growth hormone. In addition, the fatigue so often experienced by a patient with an endocrine disorder often affects feelings about self.

The chronicity of many endocrine disorders and need for continued therapy can affect the patient's self-perception. The patient can be asked to describe the effects of the present illness on self-perception.

Role-relationship pattern. The nurse should ask whether there have been any changes in the patient's ability to maintain roles at home, at work, or in the community. Often the patient with an endocrine disorder will be unable to sustain life's roles. However, in most cases the patient can be advised that, with adequate management, previous roles can be resumed. This can be very reassuring for the patient and family.

Sexuality-reproductive pattern. Problems with menstruation and pregnancy in a woman may indicate an endocrine disorder. Consequently, a detailed history of menstruation and pregnancy should be obtained. Menstrual irregularities are seen in disorders of the ovaries, pituitary, thyroid, and adrenal glands. A female patient with a history of large babies may have had undiagnosed gestational diabetes, which may put her at a higher risk to develop type II diabetes. A history of inability to lactate may indicate a pituitary disorder.

Male sexual dysfunction is also frequently seen in endocrine disorders. It usually takes the form of impotence, although retrograde ejaculation can occur in diabetes mellitus. Infertility in either sex warrants a full reproductive and endocrine work-up.

Coping–stress tolerance pattern. Stressors of all kinds affect the endocrine system. Areas that can cause a great deal of stress should be investigated. The patient should be asked about place of employment, kind of work, ability to meet job requirements, and the amount of stress involved. The nurse asks whether the job provides an adequate income to identify financial stressors. Usual coping patterns are also discussed. The nurse then determines whether previous coping patterns are still successful. It is often useful to ask family members or a significant other about the patient's coping strategies and reaction to stress.

Value-belief pattern. When dealing with a patient with a chronic condition, identification of the patient's value-belief patterns can assist the health care team to identify appropriate regimens. This is particularly important in a condition such as diabetes mellitus, which may require major lifestyle changes for successful management. Other endocrine disorders, such as hypothyroidism or hypercortisolism, can be easily managed with oral medication taken faithfully. Identification of a patient's ability to make lifestyle changes or take daily medication, and increase this medication as indicated, is an important nursing function.

Objective Data

Physical Examination

Mental-emotional status. Throughout the examination the patient's orientation, alertness, memory, affect, personality, anxiety, and speech pattern should be objectively assessed. Endocrine disorders commonly cause changes in mental status and level of consciousness.

Inspection. The nurse should observe the patient's general appearance, including physical growth and development, level of consciousness and orientation, and appearance and appropriateness of dress for ambient temperature. Endocrine dysfunction can subtly or markedly affect the size, shape, color, and maturation of the body. Assessment should include the following:

1. *Body size:* Height and weight compared with a table of standards or estimation of normality; size of head and extremities, proportionality and posture; facial features
2. *Integumentary system:* Skin color, pigmentation, texture, coarseness, leathery texture, excessive thinness, size of sweat glands, diaphoresis, acne, striae, ecchymosis, vitiligo (patchy loss of pigmentation)
3. *Hair:* Texture, distribution, brittleness, alopecia (patchy baldness)
4. *Face:* Color; erythema, especially on cheeks (plethora); pained, anxious expression
5. *Eyes:* Eyebrows, hair distribution; visual acuity, lens opacity; shape, position, movement of eyelids; lid lag; visual fields; extraocular movements; edema
6. *Nose:* Mucosa, noisy breathing
7. *Mouth:* Buccal mucosa, condition of teeth, malocclusion and mottling, tongue size and fasciculations (localized, uncoordinated, uncontrollable twitching of a single muscle group), size and shape of jaw
8. *Voice:* Huskiness or hoarseness, volume, pitch, slurring
9. *Neck:* Symmetry, alignment; forceful carotid pulsations; unusual bulging of the thyroid lobes behind the sternocleidomastoid muscles; trachea in midline; dullness, thickening, flabbiness of vocal chords; polyps; gray-brown hyperpigmentation on posterior neck and axillae (acanthosis nigricans). When inspecting the thyroid gland, observation should be made first in the normal position, preferably with side lighting, then in slight extension, and then as the patient swallows some water.
10. *Extremities:* Size, shape, symmetry, proportionality (distance from symphysis pubis to foot: approximately half of total height), edema
    a. *Hands:* Tremors (a piece of paper is placed on outstretched fingers, palm down, to assess fine tremors); muscle strength, grip, thenar (ball of the thumb) wasting, Dupuytren's contracture, clubbing, muscle wasting
    b. *Legs:* Muscle weakness (assessed by having the seated patient extend one leg to a horizontal position; ability to hold this position for 2 minutes usually indicates normal muscle strength), bowing, color and amount of hair, size of feet, corns, calluses, pedal pulses
    c. *Toes:* Maceration, fissures, deformities, toenails with fungal infection
11. *Reflexes:* Particularly deep tendon reflexes, relaxation time
12. *Pulses:* Rate and force
13. *Thorax:* Gynecomastia in men
14. *Abdomen:* Increased pigmentation of scars, purplish striae, pain on light palpation
15. *Genitalia:* Decreased hair distribution (diamond pattern in women may indicate virilizing adrenal tumor), size of testes, clitoral enlargement

Palpation. The thyroid is the only palpable endocrine gland. Thyroid palpation requires considerable practice, as well as validation by an experienced examiner. Palpation can cause the release of thyroid hormone into the circulation, increasing the patient's symptoms and potentially causing a thyroid storm (see Chapter 47). In the patient with a visibly enlarged thyroid, palpation of the thyroid should be deferred if a more experienced clinician will be examining the patient.

To palpate the thyroid, the nurse identifies other midline neck structures (Fig. 45-9). The thyroid can be palpated

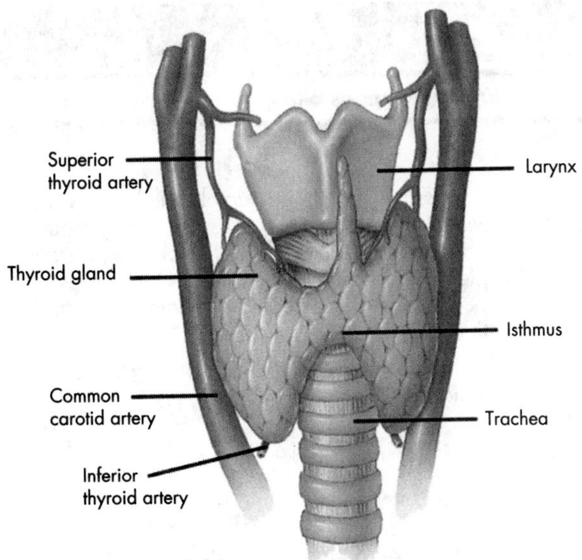

Fig. 45-9 Frontal view of thyroid gland.

anteriorly and posteriorly. Water should always be available for the patient to swallow as part of this examination.

Anterior Palpation. Standing in front of the patient, with the patient's neck flexed, the nurse places the thumb horizontally with the upper edge along the lower border of the cricoid cartilage. The thumb is then moved over the isthmus as the patient swallows water. The fingers are then placed laterally to the anterior border of the sternocleidomastoid muscle, and each lateral lobe is palpated before and while the patient swallows water.

Posterior Palpation. The examiner stands behind the patient. With the thumbs of both hands resting on the nape of the patient's neck, the nurse uses the index and middle fingers of both hands to feel for the thyroid isthmus and for the anterior surfaces of the lateral lobes. To facilitate the examination of each lobe and to relax the neck muscles, the nurse asks the patient to flex the neck slightly forward and to the right. The thyroid cartilage is displaced to the right by the left hand and fingers. The nurse palpates with the right hand after placing the thumb deep and behind the sternocleidomastoid muscle with the index and middle fingers in front of it; the area is palpated with the right hand (Fig. 45-10). While this is done, the patient is asked to swallow water. This procedure is then repeated on the left side. The thyroid is palpated for its size, shape, symmetry, tenderness, and for any nodules. In the average person the thyroid is often not palpable. If palpable, it usually feels smooth with a firm consistency and is not tender with gentle pressure. Nodules, enlargement, asymmetry, or hardness is abnormal, and the patient should be referred for further evaluation.

Other assessment skills. Percussion and auscultation are not normally part of an endocrine assessment. When an enlarged thyroid has been noted, however, the lateral lobes should be auscultated with the stethoscope bell to determine the presence of a bruit.

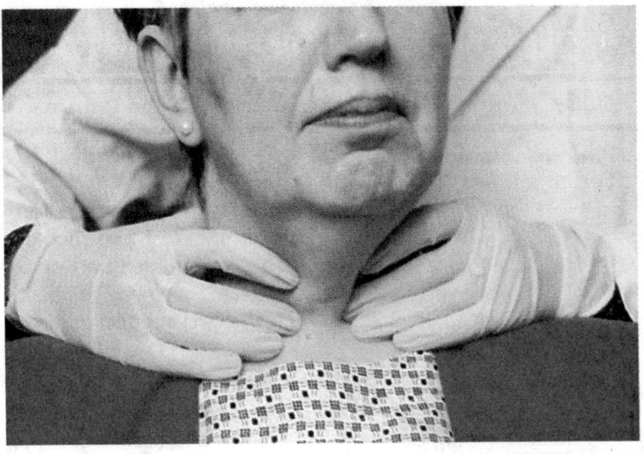

Fig. 45-10 Posterior palpation of the thyroid gland.

Assessment of vital signs should include the following:

1. Temperature: Elevation or hypothermia
2. Pulse: Rate and rhythm
3. Respirations: Change in rate or rhythm
4. Blood pressure: Widening of the pulse pressure, hypotension, hypertension, or orthostatic hypotension (see Chapter 30)
5. Heart sounds: Systolic murmur at apex or pulmonic area (possible indication of increased blood flow as a result of hyperthyroidism)

Diagnostic Studies. Diagnostic studies provide important information to the nurse in monitoring the patient's condition and planning appropriate interventions. These studies are considered to be objective data. Diagnostic studies common to the endocrine system are presented in Table 45-7.

DIAGNOSTIC STUDIES

Accurately performed laboratory tests aid and confirm diagnoses of problems of the endocrine system. These tests can measure absolute hormone levels and estimate the production, transport, and catabolism of hormones. Hormones with fairly constant basal levels (e.g., T_4) require only a single measurement. Hormones with pulsatile secretion (e.g., LH) may require multiple samples with a measurement taken from pooled aliquots. Notation of sample time on the laboratory slip and sample is important for hormones with circadian or sleep-related secretion (e.g., cortisol, GH).

On occasion, multiple blood sampling is indicated, such as in suppression tests (e.g., dexamethasone suppression) and stimulation tests (e.g., glucose tolerance). To decrease patient discomfort and minimize the effects of stress hormones, the nurse initiates an intravenous (IV) infusion of normal saline solution with a stopcock between the extension and the infusion tubing. After insertion of the infusion,

(Text continued on p. 1436.)

Table 45-7 Diagnostic Studies: Endocrine System

Study	Description and Purpose	Nursing Responsibility
Pituitary Studies		
Serum studies		
■ GH (Somatotropin)	Evaluates GH hypersecretion. After an overnight fast, GH should be <5 ng/ml (5 μg/L) in men and <10 ng/ml (10 μg/L) in women. Values >50 ng/ml (50 μg/L) suggest acromegaly.	Inform patient that blood sample will be drawn. Make sure that patient takes nothing by mouth after midnight and does not smoke. Send samples to laboratory immediately. Observe venipuncture site for bleeding or hematoma formation.
■ Somatomedin C (Insulin-like growth factor I [IGFI], Growth Factor I)	Evaluates GH; it is less variable than GH because it is not subject to circadian rhythm and fluctuations. *Normal values* are 135-250 ng/ml; low levels indicate GH deficiency, and high levels indicate GH excess. Values increase during puberty and pregnancy.	Observe venipuncture site for bleeding or hematoma formation.
■ GH release after exercise	Evaluates GH reserve in suspected hypopituitarism. Exercise stimulates GH secretion. Patient exercises vigorously for ½ hr before blood sample drawn. GH values should rise above 20 ng/ml (20 μg/L) after exercise.	Have patient fast for 12 hr. Explain procedure. Monitor pulse rate before and after exercise. May be contraindicated in patient with coronary artery insufficiency or exercise-induced asthma. Send sample to laboratory immediately.
■ Insulin-induced hypoglycemia	Used in examination of patient with suspected hypopituitarism. IV injection of regular insulin is given, based on body weight (usually 0.1 U/kg). Basal samples of GH, cortisol, and glucose are drawn. Blood samples are drawn at 30, 45, 60, and 90 min after injection. If test is terminated because of hypoglycemia (glucose level <40 mg/dl [2.22 mmol/L]), samples are drawn for GH and cortisol levels 30 min after IV dextrose. GH level should rise 2-3 times over baseline levels. Response is subnormal or absent in GH deficiency.	Ensure that patient fasted overnight (water is allowed) and that bed rest was maintained. Have 5% cortisone, 20 ml of 50% dextrose, and IV solution of 5% glucose at bedside for use if severe hypoglycemia occurs and test will continue. Weigh patient. Continually assess patient's mental status because seizures, cardiac dysrhythmias, and coma can result from hypoglycemia (test is contraindicated in patient with seizure disorders, cardiac disease, hypocortisolism, and hypothyroidism.) Assess capillary glucose levels immediately with BGM. Note on laboratory slips times that blood is drawn. Provide 25 g glucose and breakfast after last sample.
■ Prolactin level	Evaluates prolactin levels. Decreased levels in postpartum woman attempting to nurse may be associated with Sheehan's syndrome. *Normal values* are <20 ng/ml (<20 μg/L) (nonlactating); levels >200 ng/ml (200 μg/L) indicate pituitary tumors.	Have patient fast. Inform patient that blood sample will be drawn. Draw blood within 3-4 hr after patient awakens. Observe venipuncture site for bleeding or hematoma formation.

continued

Table 45-7 Diagnostic Studies: Endocrine System—cont'd

Study	Description and Purpose	Nursing Responsibility
Pituitary Studies		
Serum studies—cont'd		
▪ Gonadotropin levels: FSH, LH	Useful in distinguishing primary gonadal problems from pituitary insufficiency. Normal levels vary according to age and sex. In women, there are marked differences during menstrual cycle and in postmenopausal period. Levels are low in pituitary insufficiency and high in primary gonadal failure. In women, values for FSH are: basal rate—2-15 mIU/ml (2-15 IU/L); ovulatory surge—8-40 mIU/ml (8-40 IU/L); and postmenopausal level—>50 mIU/ml (50 IU/L). In women, values for LH are: basal rate—2-20 mIU/ml (2-20 IU/L); ovulatory surge—30-140 mIU/ml (30-140 IU/L); and postmenopausal level—>50 mIU/ml (50 IU/L). In men, values for FSH are 2-15 mIU/ml (2-15 IU/L) and LH 3-25 mIU/ml (3-25 IU/L).	Ensure that patient has fasted. Inform patient that 3 blood samples may be drawn 30 min apart for FSH. For women, note on laboratory slip time of menstrual cycle or whether she is postmenopausal.
▪ Water deprivation test	Used to differentiate causes of polyuria, including pituitary DI, nephrogenic DI, syndrome of inappropriate ADH, and psychogenic polydipsia. Two units of ADH or vasopressin diluted in saline solution are administered IV over a 2-hr period. With a normal patient and with a patient with psychogenic DI, urine osmolality is >600 mOsm/kg and plasma osmolality is <300 mOsm/kg after ADH administration. With a patient with pituitary DI, plasma osmolality is >300 mOsm/kg; with dilute urine, it is <270 mOsm/kg. With a patient with nephrogenic DI, there is little or no response to ADH.	Have patient discontinue tea, coffee, alcohol, and smoking after midnight. Obtain baseline weight and urine and plasma osmolality. Ensure that fluid is withheld. Weigh patient and take 3 postural BP measurements (lying and standing BP measurements separated by 2 min) hourly. Assess urine hourly for volume and specific gravity. Send hourly samples for urine osmolality. Draw sample for plasma osmolality when (1) urine samples are collected and (2) orthostatic hypotension and postural tachycardia appear. Assess weight at 4, 6, 7, and 8 hr. The patient must be very closely supervised during this test.
Radiologic studies		
▪ Skull x-ray, CT scan, MRI scan	Useful in evaluating sella turcica for volume, enlargement, or erosion when disease of hypothalamic-pituitary axis is suspected. Compare with normal measurement of sella turcica in relation to patient's height.	Inform patient of the need to lie as still as possible during test; explain that tests are painless and noninvasive. Explain procedure.
Thyroid Studies		
Serum studies		
▪ T_4 (Thyroxine)	Measures total serum level of T_4. Useful in evaluating thyroid function and monitoring thyroid therapy. *Normal values* are 5-12 μg/dl (51-142 nmol/L)	Inform patient that fasting is not necessary. Inform patient that blood samples will be drawn. Observe venipuncture site for bleeding or hematoma formation.
▪ T_3 (Triiodothyronine)	Measures serum levels of T_3. It is helpful in diagnosing hyperthyroidism if T_4 levels are normal. *Normal values* are 65-195 ng/dl (1.0-3.0 nmol/L).	Same as above.

continued

Table 45-7 Diagnostic Studies: Endocrine System—cont'd

Study	Description and Purpose	Nursing Responsibility
Thyroid Studies		
Serum studies—cont'd		
▪ T_3 resin uptake (T_3RU)	This study indirectly measures binding capacity of thyroid-binding globulin. *Normal values* are 25-35% (0.25-0.35).	Same as above.
▪ Free T_4	Measures active component of total T_4. *Normal values* are 1.0-3.5 ng/dl (12.9-45.0 pmol/L)	Same as above.
▪ Free T_3	Measures active component of total T_3. *Normal values* are 0.26-0.65 ng/dl.	Same as above.
▪ Thyroid ^{131}I uptake (radioactive iodine uptake)	Provides direct measure of thyroid activity. Useful for evaluation of functional activity of solitary thyroid nodules. Small tracer dose of ^{131}I is given orally or IV. Serum uptake measurements are drawn at 2-4 and 24 hr. *Normal serum values* for 2-4 hr are 3-10% and for 24 hr, they are 5-30%. Values are affected by drugs, seafood, certain radiographic contrast media, and antiseptics containing iodine.	Instruct patient to discontinue thyroid medication and to start T_3 (Cytomel) 2-3 times/day for 4 wk. Tell patient to report for further testing in 10-14 days. Collect 24-hr urine specimen.
▪ TSH (immunoradiometric)	This test measures level of TSH, which is markedly elevated in primary hypothyroidism. *Normal values* are 0.3-5.4 μU/ml (0.3-5.4 mU/L).	Inform patient that fasting is not necessary. Inform patient that blood sample will be drawn. Observe venipuncture site for bleeding or hematoma formation.
▪ Calcitonin	High calcitonin level with normal serum calcium level is associated with medullary thyroid carcinoma. *Normal values* are ≤0.155 pg/ml (0.155 ng/L) for men and 0.105 pg/ml (0.105 ng/L) for women.	Ensure that patient has fasted. Inform patient that blood sample will be drawn. Observe venipuncture site for bleeding or hematoma formation.
Radiologic studies		
▪ Thyroid scan	Used to evaluate nodules of the thyroid. Tracer dose of technetium is given IV. Scanner passes over thyroid and makes graphic record of radiation emitted. Normal thyroid scan reveals homogeneous pattern with symmetric lobes.	Determine whether other tests requiring iodine preparation (IV pyelogram, saturated solution of potassium iodine, or barium enema) have been done within 30 days (can invalidate test). Explain procedure to patient.
Parathyroid Studies		
Serum studies		
▪ PTH	Measures PTH level in serum. Normal range depends on assay used, (Check with laboratory.) This study must be interpreted in terms of concomitantly drawn serum calcium level.	Fasting specimen preferred. Inform patient that blood sample will be drawn. Sample must be kept on ice. Observe venipuncture site for bleeding or hematoma formation.
▪ Total calcium	Measures total serum calcium to help detect bone and parathyroid disorders. Hypercalcemia can indicate primary hyperparathyroidism, and hypocalcemia can indicate hypoparathyroidism. *Normal values* are 9.0-11.0 mg/L or 4.5-5.5 mEq/L (2.25-2.74 mmol/L).	Fasting specimen preferred. Inform patient that blood sample will be drawn. Observe venipuncture site for bleeding or hematoma formation. Ensure that prolonged tourniquet application does not cause falsely elevated values. Adjust total calcium for albumin levels, using following formula: Total serum calcium (mg/dl) − albumin (g/dl) + 4.0 = adjusted total serum calcium.

continued

Table 45-7 Diagnostic Studies: Endocrine System—cont'd

Study	Description and Purpose	Nursing Responsibility
Parathyroid Studies		
Serum studies—cont'd		
▪ Phosphorus	Measures inorganic phosphorus. Hyperphosphatemia indicates primary hypoparathyroidism or secondary causes (e.g., renal failure); hypophosphatemia indicates hyperparathyroidism. Phosphorus and calcium levels are inversely related. *Normal values* are 2.8-4.5 mg/dl (0.9-1.45 mmol/L).	Need for fasting varies with laboratory. Determine fasting requirement. Inform patient that blood sample will be drawn. Observe venipuncture site for bleeding or hematoma formation.
▪ 1,25-Dihydroxyvitamin D_3	This test is used to evaluate calcium and phosphorus levels and bone disease. *Normal values* are 15-60 pg/ml (39-176 nmol/L).	Inform patient that blood sample will be drawn. Observe venipuncture site for bleeding or hematoma formation.
Radiologic studies		
▪ Skeletal x-ray, CT scans	Used to determine bone disease and osteoporosis. Fractures or deformities can be caused by the demineralization produced by excessive PTH.	Monitor patient's exposure to radiation. Inform patient that tests are painless and noninvasive and that no special preparation is required for x-ray studies. For CT scan, give patient radiolabeled agent 4 hr before scan.
Adrenal Studies		
Serum studies		
▪ Cortisol	Measures amount of cortisol in serum and evaluates status of adrenocortical function. *Normal values* are 5-25 μg/dl (138-690 nmol/L) at 8 AM, <10 μg/dl (<276 nmol/L) at 8 PM.	Inform patient that blood sample will be taken. Observe venipuncture site for bleeding and hematoma formation. Ensure collection of properly timed blood sample. Draw specimen early in morning when cortisol levels are highest. Mark time on laboratory slip. Minimize stress to avoid raising level.
▪ Aldosterone	Normal values are 5-20 ng/dl (139.7-555.8 pmol/L) upright position and 8.5 ng/dl (236.8 pmol/L) supine position.	Increases with low salt diet (<2g/day), stress, an upright position, and diuretics; decreases with a high salt diet, ACE inhibitors such as captopril, and supine position. Determine which maneuvers will be done and advise patient.
▪ ACTH stimulation	Used to evaluate adrenal function. After baseline samples are drawn, 250 μg synthetic ACTH is given as IV or IM bolus; samples are drawn 30 and 60 min after bolus. Baseline ACTH sample is often drawn in case results are abnormal. Plasma cortisol at 60 min should be (1) > baseline and (2) >20 μg/dl.	Inject ACTH with a plastic syringe and collect samples for ACTH in plastic, heparinized tubes. Administer test with continuous-infusion method. Monitor site and rate of IV infusion. Ensure sample collection at appropriate times.
▪ Dexamethasone suppression (overnight)	Assesses adrenal function and is especially helpful if hyperactivity is suspected. Useful in evaluation of Cushing's syndrome. Dexamethasone (Decadron) 2 mg is given @ 2300 hr to suppress secretion of corticotropin-releasing hormone. Plasma cortisol sample is drawn @ 0800 hr. Cortisol level <5 μg/dl (138 nmol/dl) indicates normal adrenal response (50% decrease in cortisol production).	Ensure that patient has fasted. Inform patient that blood sample will be taken. Observe venipuncture site for bleeding and hematoma formation. Do not test acutely ill patient or patient under stress. ACTH may override suppression. Screen patient for drugs such as estrogen and glucocorticoids, which may give false-positive results. Ensure accurate timing of medication and sample collection.

continued

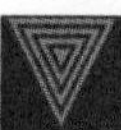

Table 45-7 Diagnostic Studies: Endocrine System—cont'd

Study	Description and Purpose	Nursing Responsibility
Adrenal Studies		
Serum studies—cont'd		
▪ Metyrapone suppression	Used to evaluate feedback response of hypothalamus and pituitary and adrenal glands and to differentiate causes of endogenous glucocorticoid overproduction. Metyrapone (30 mg/kg) is given at 1200 hr. Sample is drawn at 0800 hr for plasma 11-deoxycortisol (Compound S), cortisol, and ACTH. Normal response is 11-deoxycortisol: 7-232 μg/dl (202-6696 nmol/L) and ACTH >250 pg/mL (55.1 pmol/L). To validate blockage by metyrapone, cortisol must be (1) <8 μg/dl (220 nmol/dl) and (2) <45% of Compound S level.	Weigh patient. Administer metyrapone with milk and snack at midnight. (Note that metyrapone can cause gastrointestinal distress and confusion.) Draw ACTH into heparinized plastic tube with plastic syringe. Ensure that patient has not ingested estrogens, phenytoin, and phenobarbital because these substances invalidate test.
Urine studies		
▪ 17-Ketosteroids	Measures androgen metabolites in urine and evaluates adrenal cortical and gonadal function. *Normal values* are 10-22 mg/day (35-76 μmol/day) for men and 6-16 mg/day (21-55 μmol/day) for women.	Instruct patient regarding 24-hr urine collection. Tell patient that specimen must be kept refrigerated or iced during collection. Determine whether preservative is required for assay method used.
▪ Aldosterone	Measures urinary aldosterone level to evaluate adrenal function. Useful in determining therapy for hypertension. *Normal values* are 2-26 μg/24 hr (5.5-72 nmol/day).	Ensure that patient is on unrestricted diet with normal salt intake and no medication for 3 wk before collection. Instruct patient regarding 24-hr urine collection.
▪ Free cortisol	Preferred test to evaluate hypercortisolism. Can also be used to screen for endogenous glucocorticoids. *Normal values* are <100 mg/24 hr.	Instruct patient regarding 24-hr urine collection and avoidance of stressful situations and excessive physical exercise. Tell patient that some drugs (e.g., reserpine, diuretics, phenothiazines, amphetamines) may elevate levels. Ensure that patient is on low-sodium diet.
▪ Vanillylmandelic acid	Measures urinary excretion of catecholamine metabolite and is helpful in diagnosing pheochromocytoma. *Normal values* are <8 mg/24 hr (40 μmol/day); pheochromocytoma is indicated with values of 10-250 mg/24 hr (51-126 μmol/day).	Keep 24-hr urine collection at pH of <3.0 with hydrochloric acid as preservative. Know that newer methods are not affected by dietary intake. Consult with laboratory or physician about patient discontinuing any drugs 3 days before urine collection.

continued

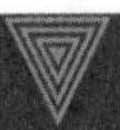

Table 45-7 Diagnostic Studies: Endocrine System—cont'd

Study	Description and Purpose	Nursing Responsibility
Pancreatic Studies		
Serum studies		
▪ FBS levels	Measures circulating glucose level. *Normal serum values* for adult are 70-110 mg/dl (3.9-6.1 mmol/L) and for pregnant woman 60-90 mg/dl (3.3-5 mmol/L).	Ensure that patient has fasted at least 4 hr. Inform patient that blood sample will be drawn. Observe venipuncture site for bleeding or hematoma formation.
▪ Oral glucose tolerance	Two-hr test used to diagnose diabetes mellitus if FBS is equivocal. Patient drinks 75 g of glucose; samples for glucose are drawn immediately and at 30, 60, and 120 min. *Normal values* are <200 mg/dl (11.1 mmol/L) at 30, 60, and 90 min and <140 mg/dl (7.8 mmol/L) at 120 min. Five-hr test used to evaluate hypoglycemia. Patient drinks 100 g of glucose; samples of glucose are drawn immediately and at 30, 60, 90, 120, 180, 240, and 300 min. Baseline cortisol level test is done if patient becomes symptomatic. The patient with reactive hypoglycemia has adrenergic symptoms and glucose <60 mg/dl (3.3 mmol/L) between 30 min and 5 hr after glucose ingestion.	Ensure that tests are not done on patient who is malnourished, confined to bed for over 3 days, or severaly stressed. Instruct patient to refrain from smoking and caffeine and to fast for 12 hours before test. Ensure that patient's diet 3 days before test included 150-300 g of carbohydrate with intake of at least 1500 calories/day. Screen for estrogens, phenytoin, and corticosteroids, and check for hypokalemia, which may impair glucose tolerance. Simultaneously monitor glucoses with capillary BGM.
▪ Capillary glucose monitoring	Used to give immediate glucose values with glucose oxidase or electrochemical methods. Capillary values (whole blood) are usually 10-15% < serum values.	Obtain large drop of blood from clean finger, touch strip to drop of blood (not finger), time accurately, and compare colors in good lighting, if using visual method. Use digital readout if available. Use automatic fingerpuncture device if available. Be sure to change section of device that touches patient's fingers between patients.
▪ Glycosylated hemoglobin	Measures degree of glucose control during previous 3 mo (life span of hemoglobin molecule). *Normal values* are <7% (values vary widely, check with laboratory.)	Inform patient that fasting is not necessary and that blood sample will be drawn. Observe venipuncture site for bleeding or hematoma formation.
Urine studies		
▪ Glucose (Clinistix, Labstix, Multistix, Clinitest)	Estimates amount of glucose in urine by using reducing substance. Results have wide range from negative (no glucose) to 2% (large amount of glucose).	Use freshly voided urine specimen collected at appropriate time. Know that many different drugs alter glucose readings and that errors are great if directions for timing are not followed exactly. Follow package directions.
▪ Ketone (Acetest, Ketostix, Labstix, Multistix)	Measures amount of acetone excreted in urine as result of incomplete fat metabolism. Positive result can indicate lack of insulin and diabetic acidosis.	Use freshly voided urine specimen. Test is often done with glucose test. Directions must be followed exactly. Certain drugs can produce false-positive and false-negative results.
▪ Glucose and acetone (Ketodiastix)	Measures glucose and acetone levels.	Know that large amounts of urinary acetone may depress glucose measurement.

ACE, Angiotensin-converting enzyme; *ADH*, antidiuretic hormone; *BP*, blood pressure; *BGM*, blood glucose monitoring; *CT*, computed tomography; *DI*, diabetes insipidus; *FBS*, fasting blood sugar; *FSH*, follicle-stimulating hormone; *GH*, growth hormone; *IM*, intramuscular; *IV*, intravenous; *LH*, luteinizing hormone; *MRI*, magnetic resonance imaging; *PTH*, parathyroid hormone; T_3, triiodothyronine; T_4, thyroxine; *TSH*, thyroid-stimulating hormone.

15 to 30 minutes should be allowed for stress hormones to normalize. Baseline samples are then drawn, the appropriate medication is given through the stopcock, and samples are withdrawn through the stopcock at the appropriate times. A heparin lock may be used in place of the saline infusion. It is necessary to draw and discard 1.5 to 3 ml of blood from the patient before drawing the sample for measurement. This prevents saline or heparin dilution.

In general, tests of endocrine function require patient fasting and the elimination of as many environmental stimuli as possible. This necessitates inactivity throughout the test; such inactivity can be achieved with bed rest with the head of the bed elevated or through the use of a recliner chair. The patient should refrain from smoking or taking food or fluids by mouth. A thorough explanation of the test and the reasons for reducing environmental stimuli reassures patients and helps them cooperate. The patient should be monitored frequently during the test, not just when samples are being taken.

During endocrine testing there are instances in which simultaneous blood and urine samples or special preservatives are needed for samples. The nurse ensures thorough patient instruction, as well as correct and complete sample collection. When a patient is having multiple endocrine testing, such as with suspected pituitary disease, a fluid volume deficit may occur. Nursing interventions in this instance include recording the amount of blood and urine taken per test, assessing for dehydration, and promptly notifying the physician if blood loss through sample collection is excessive or the patient becomes dehydrated. Using the saline infusion method helps offset fluid volume deficit.

Several types of laboratory tests are used to determine endocrine status, including *radioimmunoassay, immunometric assay, radioreceptor assay,* and *in vitro bioassays.*[8] The radioimmunoassay, a displacement assay, uses antibodies specific for a hormone or parts of a hormone and can measure very small amounts of circulating hormones. It is used for peptide, steroid, and thyroid hormones. Immunometric assays can measure minute hormone levels and are used for TSH measurements. Radioreceptor assays measure the ability of a hormone to bind to its receptor. Receptor measurements are useful in states of hormone resistance such as those seen with insulin, PTH, and vitamin D.

Specific diagnostic studies related to the endocrine system are summarized in Table 45-7. Because of the interrelatedness of the endocrine system, nursing interventions are focused on reducing the stress and anxiety often associated with diagnostic testing. Unless nursing measures related to patient instruction and expectations are initiated, the effect of stress hormones can produce inaccurate and misleading results.

Normal values and collection procedures vary among laboratories. It is therefore important to check with the laboratory doing the testing to determine the correct collection and transport procedures and normal values.

REVIEW QUESTIONS

The number of the question corresponds to the same-numbered objective at the beginning of the chapter.

1. The need to bind to receptors to initiate cellular activity is a characteristic of

a. glands.
b. proteins.
c. enzymes.
d. hormones.

2. The pituitary gland is located in the

a. sella turcica at the base of the brain.
b. anterior portion of the neck.
c. upper poles of the kidneys.
d. area behind the stomach.

3. Mineralocorticoids are involved in

a. maintenance of extracellular fluid volume.
b. modulation of the stress response.
c. metabolism and storage of carbohydrates.
d. maintenance of blood level of calcium.

4. The function of a hormone receptor is to

a. receive and store hormones until needed.
b. prevent the hormone from entering the cell.
c. allow the hormone to recognize the cell.
d. alter a gene's expression.

5. Which is the most important information to obtain from a patient if an endocrine problem is suspected?

a. Intake of vitamin C
b. Employment history
c. Frequency of sexual intercourse
d. Energy level

6. When a normal thyroid gland is palpable, it should feel

a. hard.
b. nodular.
c. smooth.
d. asymmetric.

7. There is a relationship between bone changes seen in aging and

a. T_4.
b. PTH.
c. insulin.
d. ADH.

8. Which of the following is an abnormal finding in an endocrine assessment?

a. BP 100/70
b. Soft, formed stool every other day
c. Knee reflex 2+
d. Nocturia

9. Before having a blood test of T_4, the patient should be informed that

a. thyroid medication must be stopped.
b. fasting is not necessary.
c. multiple venipunctures are required.
d. a concurrent 24-hour urine is collected.

REFERENCES

1. Genuth SM: The endocrine system. In Berne RM, Levy MN, editors: *Physiology,* ed 3, St Louis, 1993, Mosby.
2. Seeley R, Stephens T, Tate P: *Anatomy and physiology,* ed 2, St Louis, 1992, Mosby.
3. Ganong WF: *Review of medical physiology,* ed 15, Norwalk, CT, 1991, Appleton & Lange.
4. Unger RH, Orci L: Glucagon. In Rifkin H, Porte D, editors: *Diabetes mellitus: theory and practice,* ed 4, New York, 1990, Elsevier.
5. Thibodeau G, Patton K: *Anatomy and physiology,* ed 2, St Louis, 1993, Mosby.
6. Miller M: Disorders of the thyroid. In Brockhurst JC, Tallis RC, Fillit HM, editors: *Textbook of geriatric medicine,* ed 4, Edinburgh, 1992, Churchill Livingstone.
7. Horton, ES, Jeanrenaud B: Obesity and diabetes mellitus. In Rifkin H, Porte D, editors: *Diabetes mellitus: theory and practice,* ed 4, New York, 1990, Elsevier.
8. Corbett J: *Laboratory tests and diagnostic procedures with nursing diagnoses,* ed 3, Norwalk, CT, 1992, Appleton & Lange.

Chapter 46

NURSING ROLE IN MANAGEMENT

Patient with Diabetes

Virginia Valentine

Learning Objectives

1. Describe the pathophysiology and clinical manifestations of diabetes mellitus.
2. Describe the differences between insulin-dependent (type I) diabetes and non–insulin-dependent (type II) diabetes.
3. Identify the pathophysiology and manifestations of the acute and chronic complications of diabetes mellitus.
4. Describe the components of the management plan for diabetes mellitus.
5. Describe the role of nutrition in the management of diabetes.
6. Describe the nursing management of a patient with newly diagnosed diabetes mellitus.
7. Describe the nursing responsibilities in the chronic and home management of the patient with diabetes.

SIGNIFICANCE

Diabetes mellitus is a serious health problem throughout the world. An estimated 14 million people have diabetes in the United States alone. It is estimated that, counting both diagnosed and undiagnosed diabetes, as many as 5.2% of the U.S. population have diabetes mellitus. It is the fourth leading cause of death by disease in this country and the leading cause of new cases of blindness. One in four African-Americans between the ages of 65 to 74 has diabetes.[1] It increases the risk of coronary artery disease twofold or more. More than 50 percent of people with non–insulin-dependent diabetes mellitus have hypertension.[1] The staggering cost of diabetes-related expenses was estimated in 1992 at $45.2 billion for direct medical costs and $46.6 billion for productivity losses. Hospitalization costs accounted for the greatest proportion of direct medical costs.[2] These dollar amounts do not reflect the impact that the diagnosis of diabetes has on the lives of patients and their families.

PATHOPHYSIOLOGY

Diabetes mellitus is not a single disease. Rather, it is a group of genetically and clinically heterogeneous disorders characterized by abnormalities in glucose homeostasis resulting in hyperglycemia. The hyperglycemia of diabetes is caused by a decrease in the secretion or activity of insulin. These insulin alterations result in disordered metabolism of carbohydrate, fat, and protein. In time, structural abnormalities in a variety of organs and organ systems, especially the heart, kidneys, and eyes, develop. The complications arise primarily from microangiopathy, macroangiopathy, and neuropathy. Chronic hyperglycemia is generally recognized as contributing to the development of these complications. In addition, diabetes mellitus is associated with complications in pregnancy.

Normal Insulin Metabolism

Insulin is a hormone produced by the β cells in the islets of Langerhans of the pancreas. In normal conditions, insulin is continuously released into the bloodstream in small pulsatile increments (a basal rate), with increased release (bolus) when food is ingested (Fig. 46-1). The activity of released insulin lowers blood glucose and facilitates a stable, normal glucose range of approximately 70 to 120 mg/dl (3.9 to 6.7 mmol/L). The average amount of insulin secreted daily by an adult is approximately 40 to 50 units or 0.6 U/kg of body weight. Other hormones (glucagon, epinephrine, growth hormone, cortisol, and somatostatin) work to counter the effects of insulin and are often referred to as *counterregulatory hormones* because they stimulate glycogen release and breakdown and thereby increase blood glucose levels. Insulin and these counterregulatory substances provide a sustained but regulated release of glucose for energy during food intake and periods of fasting and usually maintain blood glucose levels within the normal range. Some researchers believe that an abnormal production of any or all these hormones may be present in diabetes.[3]

Reviewed by Gail D'Eramo Melkus, PN, ANP, EdD, CDE, Associate Professor, Yale University School of Nursing, New Haven, CT.

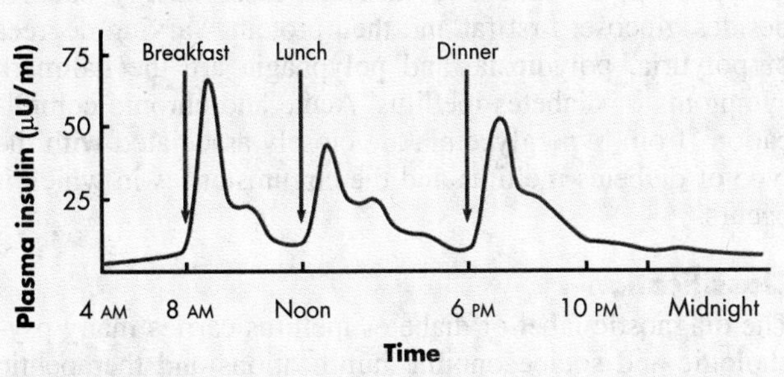

Fig. 46-1 Normal endogenous insulin secretion. In the first hour or two after meals, insulin concentrations rise rapidly in blood and peak at about 1 hour. After meals, insulin concentrations promptly decline toward preprandial values as carbohydrate absorption from the gastrointestinal tract declines. After carbohydrate absorption from the gastrointestinal tract is complete and during the night, insulin concentrations are low and fairly constant with a slight increase at dawn.

Once insulin is released into the bloodstream from the β cells as proinsulin, it is routed through the liver. Within the liver, approximately 50% to 70% of received insulin is extracted from the blood. Insulin is formed from proinsulin after cleavage of the C-peptide chain.[4] The presence of C peptide in serum and urine is a useful indicator of β-cell function. The remaining insulin (now active A- and B-peptide chains) functions to promote glucose transport from the bloodstream across the cell membrane to the cytoplasm of the cell. The rise in plasma insulin after a meal stimulates storage of glucose as glycogen in liver and muscle, enhances fat deposition in adipose tissue, inhibits protein degradation, and accelerates the processes of amino acid transport into cells and protein synthesis. The fall in insulin level during normal overnight fasting facilitates the release of stored glucose from the liver, protein from muscle, and fat from adipose tissue.[5] For this reason insulin is known as the *storage hormone*.

Skeletal muscle and adipose tissue have specific receptors for insulin and are considered to be insulin-dependent tissues. Other tissues (e.g., brain, liver, and blood cells) do not directly depend on insulin for glucose transport but require an adequate glucose supply.

As shown in Fig. 46-2 there are altered mechanisms in type I and type II diabetes in different tissue sites. The development of hyperglycemia arises from different causes.

CULTURAL & ETHNIC Considerations

DIABETES MELLITUS

- The highest incidence of diabetes is among Native Americans.
- There is a higher incidence of diabetes among African-Americans and Hispanics than Caucasians.
- Complications of diabetes are more common in Native Americans and African-Americans than Caucasians.
- Type II diabetes tends to affect a younger age population in non-Caucasians than Caucasians.

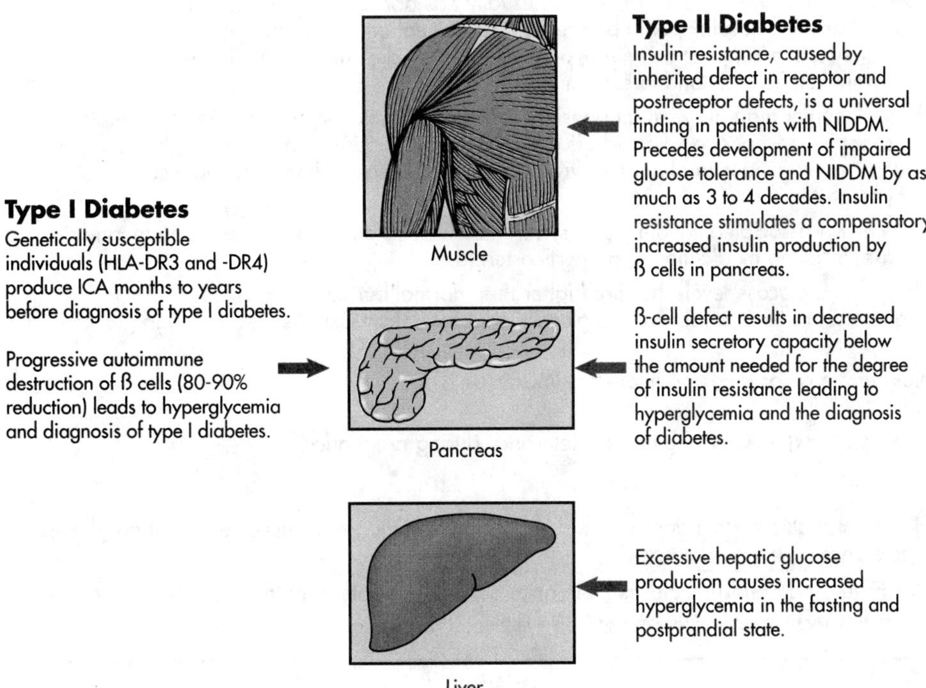

Fig. 46-2 Altered mechanisms in the type I and type II diabetes. *ICA,* Islet cell antibodies; *NIDDM,* non–insulin-dependent diabetes mellitus.

Type I diabetes results from progressive destruction of β-cell function as a result of an autoimmune process in a susceptible individual. Islet cell antibodies and insulin autoantibodies cause a reduction in β cells of 80% to 90% of normal before hyperglycemia and symptoms occur. Type II diabetes is a combination of genetically determined defects in skeletal muscle, fat, and liver receptors for insulin and β cell secretory exhaustion. Excessive hepatic glucose production eventually adds to the fasting and post-prandial hyperglycemia.[5] Because of these possibilities for malfunctioning, diabetes mellitus must be considered a heterogeneous disease that cannot be managed by only one treatment regimen.

Clinical Manifestations

Normally, insulin and its counterregulatory hormones maintain blood glucose within a range of 70 to 120 mg/dl (3.9 to 6.7 mmol/L). Elevated blood glucose levels produce symptoms related to the degree of actual or relative insulin deficiency. When an absolute insulin deficiency or decreased insulin activity occurs, glucose is not used properly. Glucose remains in the bloodstream and produces an osmotic effect on intracellular and interstitial fluid. This shift in fluid balance results in clinical symptoms of frequent urination (*polyuria*) and thirst (*polydipsia*). Without sufficient insulin the patient may experience hunger (*polyphagia*) as the body turns to other energy sources besides glucose: first fat and then protein. Varying degrees of polyuria, polydipsia, and polyphagia are the hallmark symptoms of diabetes mellitus. Acute and chronic complications from hyperglycemia are closely associated with the type of diabetes mellitus and the circumstances in which it occurs.

Classification

The diagnostic label of diabetes mellitus carries many psychologic and socioeconomic ramifications and therapeutic requirements. Therefore accurate classification of the degree of glucose intolerance and the type of diabetes is important. Based on knowledge about diabetes, a system for the diagnosis and classification of degree and type was developed by the National Diabetes Data Group of the National Institutes of Health in 1979.[6] The classification system is based not only on the presence and degree of hyperglycemia but also the presenting history and symptoms (see Table 46-1). The classification scheme also includes the person who has had or who is having glucose intolerance without overt signs of diabetes mellitus. Recognition of this difference allows a person at risk for diabetes to be followed up without being misclassified or mismanaged.

The diagnosis of diabetes mellitus is made when the fasting plasma glucose level exceeds 140 mg/dl (7.8 mmol/L) on at

Table 46-1 Types of Diabetes Mellitus and Other Categories of Glucose Intolerance

Classes	Distinguishing Characteristics
Clinical	
▪ Insulin-dependent diabetes mellitus, type I	May be of any age, is usually thin, and usually has abrupt onset of signs and symptoms with insulinopenia before age 30. Patient often has strongly positive urine ketone tests in conjunction with hyperglycemia and depends on insulin therapy to prevent ketoacidosis and to sustain life.
▪ Non–insulin-dependent diabetes mellitus, type II (obese or nonobese)	Is usually older than 30 yr at diagnosis, is obese, and has relatively few classic symptoms. Patient is not prone to ketoacidosis except during periods of stress. Although not dependent on exogenous insulin for survival, patient may require it for adequate control of hyperglycemia.
▪ Secondary forms of diabetes mellitus	Has certain associated conditions or syndromes such as pancreatic disease, endocrine disease, is taking medication (e.g., corticosteroids).
▪ Impaired glucose tolerance (obese or nonobese)	Has plasma glucose levels that are higher than normal but not diagnostic for diabetes mellitus. In response to glucose challenge, has sustained level of high glucose.
▪ Other types of impaired glucose tolerance	Has certain associated conditions or syndromes.
▪ Gestational diabetes mellitus	Has onset or discovery of glucose intolerance during pregnancy.
At Risk	
▪ Previous abnormality of glucose tolerance	Has normal glucose tolerance and history of transient diabetes mellitus or impaired glucose tolerance.
▪ Potential abnormality of glucose tolerance	Has never had abnormal glucose tolerance but has a greater than normal risk of diabetes mellitus or impaired glucose tolerance developing.

least two occasions or when a random blood glucose measurement exceeds 200 mg/dl (11.1 mmol/L). *Impaired glucose tolerance* is classified as a fasting plasma glucose level higher than normal but lower than that considered diagnostic for diabetes mellitus.

ETIOLOGY

Diabetes mellitus is not a single disease. It is a heterogeneous syndrome for which several theories of etiology have been proposed. Current theories link the causes of diabetes, singly or in combination, to genetic, autoimmune, viral, and environmental factors such as obesity and stress. There are primarily two types of diabetes mellitus: *type I,* in which insulin production by the β cells is reduced or completely absent and for which the management requires insulin replacement; and *type II,* which is the more prevalent type of diabetes mellitus (approximately 90% of patients). Table 46-2 depicts the distinguishing characteristics of type I and type II diabetes mellitus.

Type I: Insulin-Dependent Diabetes Mellitus

In type I diabetes, also called insulin-dependent diabetes mellitus (IDDM) autoimmune β-cell destruction is attributed to a genetic predisposition coupled with one or more viral agents and possibly chemical agents. It is not known conclusively that these are the only factors involved.

The complexity may be better appreciated in relationship to information about human leukocyte antigens (HLAs), which are proteins on the cell surface controlled by genes on chromosome 6. (See Chapter 10 for a discussion of HLA antigens and disease associations.) Five groups of these antigens—A, B, C, D, and DR—have been recognized, and these groups can appear in many variations. Results of family studies confirm that susceptibility to type I diabetes is strongly linked to the HLA-DR3 and DR4 loci.[7] The individual at highest risk for type I diabetes has one or more of the following HLA types: B8, DR3, B15, DR4.[7] Theoretically, when an individual with these genetic characteristics is exposed to viral infections, the β cells are destroyed directly, or an autoimmune process is triggered, which in turn destroys the β cells. A combination of both processes may occur. Current research continues to seek genetic markers to identify a person at risk for type I diabetes who is free of symptoms and to study immunologic parameters that may be manipulated to prevent or cure type I diabetes.

Genetic counseling for parents is based on statistical risk. If one child has type I diabetes, other siblings have a 5% to 10% chance of type I diabetes developing (up to 45% if the sibling is an identical twin). The offspring of a father with type I diabetes has a risk of 4% to 6%, double that of offspring of IDDM mothers (2% to 3%).[8]

The onset and progression of hyperglycemic symptoms are usually more rapid and acute in type I diabetes, and successful treatment depends on insulin replacement. If the disease process is allowed to progress without treatment, diabetic ketoacidosis with nausea and vomiting, electrolyte

Table 46-2 Characteristics of Type I and Type II Diabetes Mellitus

Factor	Type I	Type II
▪ Age at onset	Usually in young person but possible at any age	Usually >age 35 yr but possible at any age
▪ Type of onset	Signs and symptoms abrupt, but disease process may be present for several years	Insidious
▪ Genetic susceptibility	HLA-DR3, -DR4, and others	Frequent genetic background, no relation to HLA
▪ Environmental factors	Virus, toxins	Obesity, nutrition
▪ Islet cell antibody	Present at onset	Absent
▪ Endogenous insulin	Minimal or absent	Possibly excessive, adequate but delayed secretion or reduced but not absent secretion
▪ Nutritional status	Thin, catabolic state	Obese or possibly normal
▪ Symptoms	Thirst, polyuria, polyphagia, fatigue	Frequently none or mild
▪ Ketosis	Prone at onset or during insulin deficiency	Resistant except during infection or stress
▪ Control of diabetes	Often difficult with wide glucose fluctuation	Variable, control with diet and exercise
▪ Dietary management	Essential	Essential, possibly sufficient for glycemic control
▪ Insulin	Required for all	Required for 30-40%
▪ Sulfonylurea	Not efficacious	Efficacious
▪ Vascular and neurologic complications	In majority of patients after ≥5 yr diabetes	Frequent

HLA, Human leukocyte antigens.

imbalance, weight loss, and muscle wasting may develop. Without treatment (i.e., insulin) ketoacidosis can progress to coma and death.

Once treatment is initiated, the patient with type I diabetes may go into a remission (often called the *honeymoon phase*). During this time, the patient needs very little insulin to control blood glucose. The honeymoon period occurs because, even as insulin islet cell antibodies destroy the β cells, β cells continue to produce insulin. Eventually, blood glucose levels climb, more insulin is needed, and the honeymoon period ends. The honeymoon period may last up to a year, depending on the patient.[9]

Type II: Non-Insulin-Dependent Diabetes Mellitus

Approximately 90% of diabetes mellitus is type II non–insulin-dependent diabetes mellitus (NIDDM). There are two recognized subtypes of type II: obese and nonobese (see Table 46-1). Type II diabetes has a strong genetic influence (almost 100% concordance in monozygotic twins), but no correlation with HLA type has been found.

Genetic counseling for the type II group is based on a known higher familial risk. The siblings of a person with type II diabetes are at a 7% to 14% risk for type II diabetes developing. The offspring of parents who both have type II diabetes have a 15% to 45% chance of the disease developing. Children and young adults with type II diabetes have a 50% chance of transmitting the disease to their children.[8]

Prevalence of diabetes increases with age, with about half of cases in people older than 55. It was formerly called maturity or adult onset diabetes. Prevalence also varies by race and is highest among Native Americans such as the Pima tribe (1 out of 2 adults has NIDDM). Hispanic populations are two times as likely to develop diabetes as non-Hispanic whites. Overall, the prevalence of diagnosed and undiagnosed diabetes in adults is about 30% higher in African-Americans than in Caucasians.[1]

In addition to older age at onset, this type of diabetes mellitus is distinguished by an endogenous insulin supply sufficient to inhibit the development of diabetic ketoacidosis (DKA), which occurs when endogenous insulin is markedly reduced or absent. The pathophysiologic factors that have been identified in type II diabetes include decreased tissue (e.g., fat, muscle) responsiveness to insulin as a result of receptor or postreceptor defects; and overproduction of insulin in the early phase, but eventual decreased secretion of insulin from β-cell exhaustion; and abnormal hepatic glucose regulation. Obesity appears to play a major role in type II diabetes by downregulating insulin receptors in skeletal muscle and fat cells; that is, the number of available insulin receptors is decreased. The development of these events is often referred to as *peripheral insulin resistance*. This resistance stimulates increased insulin production as a compensatory response, which may also predispose the patient to weight gain. A reduced-calorie diet for the obese type II patient tends to reverse this phenomenon.[5] The type II patient may benefit from oral hypoglycemic agents, which have been found to be physiologically effective in several ways, including increasing insulin production, improving cell receptor binding, and regulating hepatic glucose production.

In type II diabetes mellitus the onset of hyperglycemic symptoms may occur over a long period. The person may "adjust" to the persistent feelings of fatigue, thirst, polyuria, and blurred vision without realizing that the diabetic disease process is producing the symptoms.[10] If the patient with type II diabetes has marked hyperglycemia (e.g., 500 to ≥1000 mg/dl [27.6 to ≥55.1 mmol/L]), a sufficient endogenous insulin supply may prevent DKA from occurring, but fluid and electrolyte loss may become severe and lead to hyperosmolar coma. (See Fig. 46-13 for the sequence of events associated with hyperosmolar hyperglycemia.) During precipitating and acute situations (such as acute illness), the patient with type II diabetes may briefly require insulin administration. It is also possible for the type II patient to have DKA if a precipitating stress event is severe and strains the available endogenous insulin supply. The fact that some persons with type II diabetes may require insulin during times of stress or for treatment of hyperosmolar hyperglycemia does not mean that these persons are insulin-dependent or will require long-term insulin treatment.[11]

DIAGNOSTIC STUDIES

The classification of diabetes depends on appropriate and accurate diagnostic studies (Table 46-3). Urine tests are not sufficient for diagnosing diabetes mellitus because variables such as age, medications, and a normally low renal threshold for glucose may show glycosuria without the presence of diabetes or glucose intolerance.

When overt symptoms of hyperglycemia—polyuria, polydipsia, and polyphagia—together with fasting blood glucose levels of 140 mg/dl (7.8 mmol/L) or greater are present, further glucose tolerance tests are usually not warranted. However, when oral glucose tolerance tests are used, the accuracy of test results depends on adequate

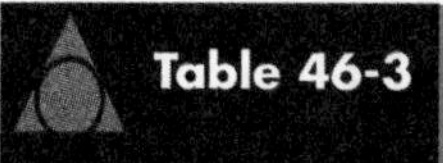

Table 46-3 Therapeutic Management: Diabetes Mellitus

Diagnostic
- Complete history and physical examination
- Blood tests, including fasting blood glucose, postprandial blood glucose, glycosylated hemoglobin, cholesterol and triglyceride levels, blood urea nitrogen and serum creatinine, electrolytes
- Urine for complete urinalysis, microalbuminuria, culture and sensitivity, glucose and acetone
- Funduscopic examination
- Neurologic examination
- Blood pressure
- Monitoring of weight
- Doppler scan

Therapeutic
- Calculated food plan
- Exercise plan
- Insulin or oral hypoglycemia agent (if indicated)
- Dental examination
- Podiatric examination
- Specific teaching and follow-up programs

patient preparation and attention to the many factors that may influence the outcome of such tests. For example, factors that can cause falsely elevated values include recent severe restrictions of dietary carbohydrate, acute illness, medications such as contraceptives and glucocorticosteroids, and restricted activity such as bed rest. A patient with impaired gastrointestinal (GI) absorption may also have false-negative test results.

Because diabetes is a multisystem, multiproblem disease, all laboratory studies must be correlated with clinical findings. The most common finding in overt diabetes mellitus is an elevated blood glucose level (>140 mg/dl [7.8 mmol/L]). Glucose values differ depending on the source of the sample and the site from which it is taken, the timing in relation to meals, and the time of day. Arterial and capillary plasma values tend to be higher than whole blood and venous blood samplings. Postprandial (after meals) and late afternoon values also tend to be higher.

In the presence of abnormal insulin use, fat metabolism is altered. This results in elevations of lipid, cholesterol, and triglyceride levels that are associated with the vascular disorders of diabetes.

The results of urine tests for glucose and acetone depend on age, severity of diabetes, and renal function. Blood glucose is a better measurement of glycemic status because glycosuria may not be evident when hyperglycemia is present. The presence of ketonuria and elevated serum ketones accompanied by marked hyperglycemia is the heralding sign of DKA. When a person without diabetes fasts, ketonuria also develops as a result of fat breakdown but without accompanying hyperglycemia.

Glycosylated hemoglobin is a measurement that is useful in determining glycemic levels over time. The hemoglobin of red blood cells (RBCs) attracts a certain amount of glucose (approximately 5% to 7% in the nondiabetic person). When blood glucose is elevated over time, or when the person has frequent wide fluctuations in glycemic levels, the amount of glucose attached to the hemoglobin molecule increases. The glucose remains attached to the RBC for the life of the cell (120 days). Therefore a glycosylated hemoglobin test indicates the overall glucose control for the past 120 days. Laboratory methods may differ in this assay because some methods measure the entire glycosylated hemoglobin molecule, whereas other methods measure only a specific glycosylated hemoglobin, hemoglobin A_1, or hemoglobin A_{1c}. The ideal goal range for glycosolated hemoglobin is a value that is less than 1% to 2% above the lab normal. Diseases affecting RBCs (e.g., sickle cell anemia) also affect the glycosylated hemoglobin results and should be taken into consideration in the interpretation of this test result. The glycosylated albumin (fructosamine), a glycosylated serum protein test, reflects blood glucose control over the preceding 7 to 10 days. The reliability and clinical applicability of these tests is under evaluation.[11]

Proteinuria is a sign of early nephropathy. Analysis for microalbuminuria may show early nephropathy long before routine urinalysis displays proteinuria.[12] Microalbuminuria tests are now the recommended method for early detection of nephropathy. The presence of protein in the urine as detected by microalbuminuria urinalysis should be followed with a 24-hour urine collection for determination of creatinine clearance and serum creatinine. It is important to monitor renal function because the patient with diabetes in the later stages of renal disease may require a reduction in insulin dose as a result of both a decrease in caloric intake and an alteration in insulin function and metabolism in chronic renal failure.[12] Diagnostic tests requiring the use of fluorescein dyes should be approached with extreme caution in the patient with proteinuria. The patient with serum creatinine levels of 4 to 6 mg/dl (353.6 to 530.4 μmol/L) or greater may have irreversible deterioration of renal function and oliguria after an intravenous (IV) pyelogram or angiogram.

The Doppler instrument is used to diagnose the presence or degree of peripheral vascular disease. It is a device similar to an electronic stethoscope that amplifies sound. The procedure is noninvasive and can measure blood pressure in the lower extremities and blood flow velocity. It can indicate areas of stenosis or occlusion and is useful as an indicator of the need for additional vascular tests.

THERAPEUTIC MANAGEMENT

Management of diabetes mellitus is primarily aimed at achieving a balance of diet, activity, and medications together with appropriate monitoring and patient and family education (Fig. 46-3 and Table 46-3). These components are equally necessary for good control of diabetes.

Nutritional Management

Nutritional therapy is the cornerstone of care for the person with diabetes. Achieving nutritional goals requires a coordinated team effort that includes the person with diabetes. Today there is no one "diabetic" or "ADA" diet. In an institutional setting, the prescribed diet is often labeled "ADA," indicating that the meal plan follows the American Diabetes Association's current nutritional recommendations.

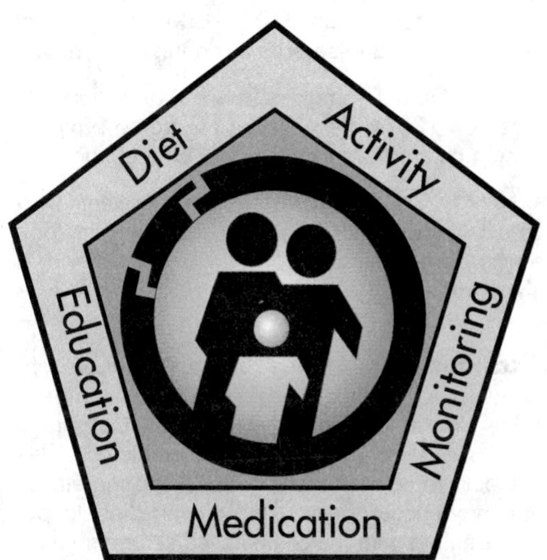

Fig. 46-3 The five aspects of diabetes management make up the complete program for good control.

The recommended diet can only be defined as a dietary prescription based on nutritional assessment and goals. Because of the complexity of nutritional issues, it is recommended that a registered dietitian, with expertise in diabetes management, be a member of the treatment team. Effective self-management training requires an individualized approach, appropriate for the personal lifestyle and diabetes management goals of the patient. Monitoring of glucose and glycosolated hemoglobin, lipids, and renal status is essential to evaluate nutrition-related outcomes. Nutritional assessment is used to determine what the individual with diabetes is able and willing to do. Sensitivity to cultural, ethnic, and financial considerations is important when developing individual meal planning approaches.

Goals of Therapy. The overall goal is to assist people with diabetes in making changes in nutrition and exercise habits leading to improved metabolic control. Additional specific goals include:

1. Maintenance of as near-normal blood glucose levels as possible by balancing food intake with insulin (either endogenous or exogenous) or oral glucose-lowering medications and activity levels.
2. Achievement of optimal serum lipid levels.
3. Provision of adequate calories for maintaining or attaining reasonable weights for adults, normal growth and development rates in children and adolescents, increased metabolic needs during pregnancy and lactation, or recovery from catabolic illnesses. Reasonable weight is defined as the weight an individual and health care provider acknowledge as achievable and maintainable, both short-term and long-term. This may not be the same as the usually defined desirable or ideal body weight.
4. Prevention and treatment of the acute complications such as hypoglycemia, and long-term complications such as renal disease, neuropathy, hypertension, and cardiovascular disease.
5. Improvement of overall health through optimal nutrition. Dietary Guidelines for Americans and the Food Guide Pyramid summarize and illustrate nutritional guidelines and nutrient needs for all healthy Americans, and can be used by the patient with diabetes (see Chapter 37).

RESEARCH

IMPLICATIONS FOR NURSING PRACTICE

DEPRESSION AND SMOKING AMONG PERSONS WITH DIABETES

Citation Haire-Joshu D and others: Depressive symptomatology and smoking among persons with diabetes, *Res Nurs Health* 17:273-282, 1994.

Purpose To determine whether (1) symptoms of depression are more prevalent and severe among diabetic smokers than nondiabetic smokers, (2) smoking is related to depressive symptomatology among diabetic patients, and (3) there is a positive relationship between number of cigarettes smoked and severity of depressive symptoms.

Methods Diabetic smokers (n = 83) and diabetic nonsmokers (n = 103) were surveyed regarding symptoms of depression as measured by the Beck Depression Inventory.

Results and Conclusions Diabetic patients who smoke exhibit significantly more depressive symptoms than those who do not smoke. In addition, as severity of depressive symptoms increases, so does patients' use of cigarettes.

Implications for Nursing Practice Diabetic patients should be routinely assessed as to the number of cigarettes smoked, which may provide a clue to the presence and severity of depressive symptomatology. The nurse should remember that the mood-altering effects of nicotine may encourage smoking among diabetic patients who are dealing with the complicated self-management tasks associated with diabetes.

Type I Diabetes. Meal planning should be based on the individual's usual food intake with insulin therapy integrated into the usual eating and exercise patterns. It is recommended that the individual using insulin therapy eat meals at consistent times synchronized with the time-action of the insulin preparation used. Additionally, the individual needs to monitor blood glucose levels and adjust insulin doses for the amount of food eaten. Intensified insulin therapy, such as multiple daily injections or use of an insulin pump, allows considerable flexibility in food selection and can be adjusted for deviations from usual eating and exercise habits (Fig. 46-4).

Type II Diabetes. The emphasis for nutritional therapy in type II diabetes should be placed on achieving glucose, lipid, and blood pressure goals. Weight loss and hypocaloric diets usually improve short-term glycemic levels and have the potential to increase long-term metabolic control. However, traditional dietary strategies and even very-low-calorie diets have usually not been effective in achieving long-term weight loss, and focus should now be placed on glucose and lipid goals. Although weight loss is desirable, and some individuals are able to lose and maintain weight loss, several strategies can be implemented to improve metabolic control. There is no one proven strategy or method that can be uniformly recommended. A nutritionally adequate meal plan with a reduction of total fat, especially

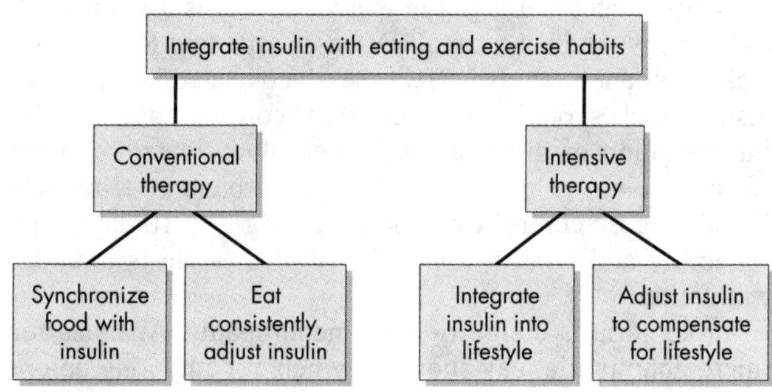

Fig. 46-4 Nutrition therapy for type I diabetes.

saturated fats, can be employed. Spacing meals is another strategy that can be adopted to spread nutrient intake throughout the day. A weight loss of 11 to 22 lbs (5 to 10 kg) has been shown to improve diabetes control, even if desirable body weight is not achieved. Weight loss is best attempted by a moderate decrease in calories and an increase in caloric expenditure. Regular exercise and learning new behaviors and attitudes can help facilitate long-term lifestyle changes. Monitoring of blood glucose levels, glycosolated hemoglobin, lipids, and blood pressure is essential (Fig. 46-5). Table 46-4 describes dietary strategies for type I and type II diabetes.

Food Composition. Distribution of nutrients is based on guidelines for all Americans. There is limited data on which to establish firm nutritional recommendations for protein. Dietary protein derived from both animal and vegetable sources should make up about 10% to 20% of calories. The remaining 80% to 90% of calories should be distributed between dietary fat and carbohydrates. Less than 10% of these calories should be from saturated fats. The distribution of calories from fat and carbohydrates can vary and can be individualized based on the nutritional assessment and treatment goals. Consideration of the individual's usual eating habits, lifestyle, body weight, and quality of life is essential for successful meal planning.

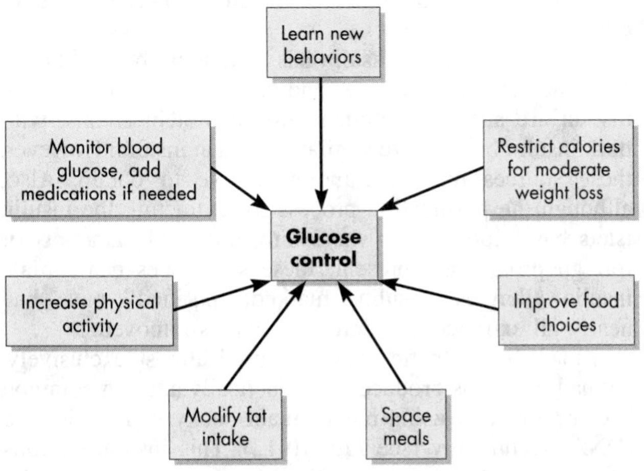

Fig. 46-5 Nutrition therapy for type II diabetes.

An area receiving increased attention and research is "glycemic indices," which refer to the ranking of foods by comparing the glycemic effect on blood glucose in reference to white bread. This type of information is useful in considering ways to select and prepare foods for more predictable glycemic control. It has been concluded that starches and sucrose do not act differently in the context of a mixed meal when it comes to glycemic effect. It is important for patients to understand the principles underlying glycemic index, or how foods of different composition affect blood glucose. Mixed meal, method of food preparation, and fiber content also play an important role.[13]

Scientific research has not supported the belief that simple sugars should be avoided and replaced with complex carbohydrates. Fruits and milks have been shown to have a lower glycemic response than most starches, and sucrose produces a glycemic response similar to that of bread, rice, and potatoes. Even though various starches do have different glycemic responses, from a clinical perspective, priority should be given to the total amount of carbohydrate consumed rather than the source of carbohydrate. The 1994 Nutrition Recommendations and Principles for People with Diabetes from the American Diabetes Association advise that the use of sucrose as a part of the meal plan does not impair blood glucose control in individuals with type I or type II diabetes. Sucrose and sucrose-containing foods must

Table 46-4 Nutritional Management: Dietary Strategies for Type I and Type II Diabetes Mellitus

Factor	Type I	Type II
▪ Total calories	Increase in caloric intake possibly necessary to achieve desirable body weight and restore body tissues	Reduction in caloric intake desirable for the obese patient
▪ Effect of diet	Diet and insulin necessary for glucose control	Diet alone possibly sufficient for glucose control
▪ Distribution of calories	Equal distribution of carbohydrates through meals or adjustment of carbohydrates for insulin activity	Equal distribution not essential. Low-fat desirable
▪ Consistency in daily intake	Necessary for glucose control	Desirable for weight reduction
▪ Uniform timing of meals	Crucial for NPH/Lente insulin programs, flexibility with multidose regular insulin	Desirable but not essential
▪ Intermeal and bedtime snacks	Frequently necessary	Not recommended
▪ Supplement for exercise programs	Carbohydrates 20 g/hr for moderate physical activities	Necessary if patient controlled on sulfonylurea or insulin

be substituted for other carbohydrates and not simply added to the meal plan. In making such substitutions, the nutrient content of concentrated sweets and sucrose-containing foods, as well as the presence of other nutrients frequently ingested with sucrose such as fat, must be considered.[14]

Diet Education. Most often the dietitian initially teaches the principles of the dietary prescription. However, the nurse should be knowledgeable about diabetes dietary principles to answer questions and to help the patient make appropriate selections and decisions. The nurse should include the family of the patient when teaching the diet plan. Particular attention and teaching efforts should be directed to the person who will be cooking. It is important, however, that the responsibility for maintaining a diabetic diet not fall to someone other than the patient with diabetes. Reliance on another person to make health decisions fosters dependence and should be avoided except in special situations.

Principles that both the nurse and dietitian should teach and reinforce include the following:

1. Eat according to the prescribed meal plan. A dietary prescription is individualized to reflect the dietary needs related to a specific patient's body weight, occupation, age, activities, and type of diabetes. Individual responses to a dietary prescription should be monitored, and appropriate adjustments should be made when necessary.
2. Never skip meals. This is particularly important for the patient taking insulin or oral hypoglycemic agents (OHAs). The body requires food at regularly spaced intervals throughout the day. Insulin and OHAs are prescribed to fit this schedule. Omission or delay of meals can result in hypoglycemia.
3. Learn to recognize appropriate food portions. Practice can result in accurate portion allotments.

Areas of Concern

Alcohol. Alcohol is high in calories, has no nutritive value, and promotes hypertriglyceridemia. In addition, it has detrimental effects on the liver (see Chapter 41). The inhibitory effect of alcohol on gluconeogenesis can cause severe hypoglycemia in patients on glucose-lowering agents. A patient can reduce this risk by eating carbohydrates when drinking alcohol. Alcohol may produce a disulfiram (Antabuse) effect (nausea and vomiting, flushing, respiratory distress, chest pain) proportional to the amount ingested with certain OHAs.

However, if the patient chooses, a drink can be included in the meal plan. One drink has approximately 135 calories. When possible, the patient with diabetes should drink on a full stomach, use sugar-free mixes, and drink dry, light wines.

Dietetic foods. The word *dietetic* is confusing because it does not always refer to a lack of calories. The caloric value of dietetic foods should be considered if weight loss is a dietary goal.

Dietetic foods are expensive and, although convenient, are not necessary. The patient can be taught to make intelligent decisions regarding the use of nondietetic foods by reading labels. The increasing availability of foods prepared with artificial sweeteners allows greater freedom in the diet. Recipes that use artificial sweeteners are also available.

Pharmacologic Management

The two types of glucose-lowering agents used in the treatment of diabetes are insulin and OHAs.

Insulin

Indications for use. Exogenous insulin is needed when a patient has inadequate insulin to meet specific metabolic needs, and the combination of dietary management, exercise, and OHAs cannot maintain a satisfactory blood glucose level. Exogenous insulin is required for the management of type I diabetes. Exogenous insulin may be prescribed for the patient with type II diabetes during periods of severe stress, such as illness or surgery, or when attempts at glycemic control by means of diet, exercise, or OHAs fail.

Types. Exogenous insulin has commonly been obtained from the pancreases of pigs and cows. These two forms of insulin are similar to human insulin protein chains, with pork insulin being more similar to human insulin. However, these sources have become expensive to obtain. Also, although the purification process for extracting the insulin islets has improved to where only minuscule amounts of foreign protein are present, these substances can initiate insulin allergies. Insulins marked "purified" have had nearly all extraneous pancreatic proteins removed.

Today, biosynthetic insulin is used almost exclusively. Human insulin is produced by genetically altering common bacteria or yeast using recombinant deoxyribonucleic acid (DNA) technology (see Fig. 10-12). This insulin exhibits chemical and biologic properties identical to human insulin produced by human β cells. The advantage of these new insulins is a reduced allergic response and a more predictable insulin activity. The purified and human insulins are the preferred type of drug.

In addition to origin and purity, insulins differ in regard to onset, peak action, and duration (Fig. 46-6). The specific properties of each type of insulin are matched with the patient's diet and activity. Not all patients respond to insulin exactly as shown in Table 46-5. The action times are listed as approximate guidelines. Human insulin may have slightly less activity time.

By adding zinc, acetate buffers, and protamine to insulin in various ways, the onset of activity, peak, and duration times can be manipulated.[15] Different combinations of these insulins can be used to tailor treatment to the patient's specific pattern of blood glucose levels. Formulas are classified as short-acting (e.g., regular insulin), intermediate-acting (e.g., NPH insulin), and long-acting (ultralente insulin).

All insulin preparations start with regular insulin as a base; zinc is added to make Lente insulin, and zinc and protamine are added to make NPH to prolong the action of insulin. These binding agents can cause an allergic reaction at the injection site. Regular insulin is prescribed when a rapid onset of glucose-lowering action is needed, such as before meals and during periods of acute illness, surgery, or

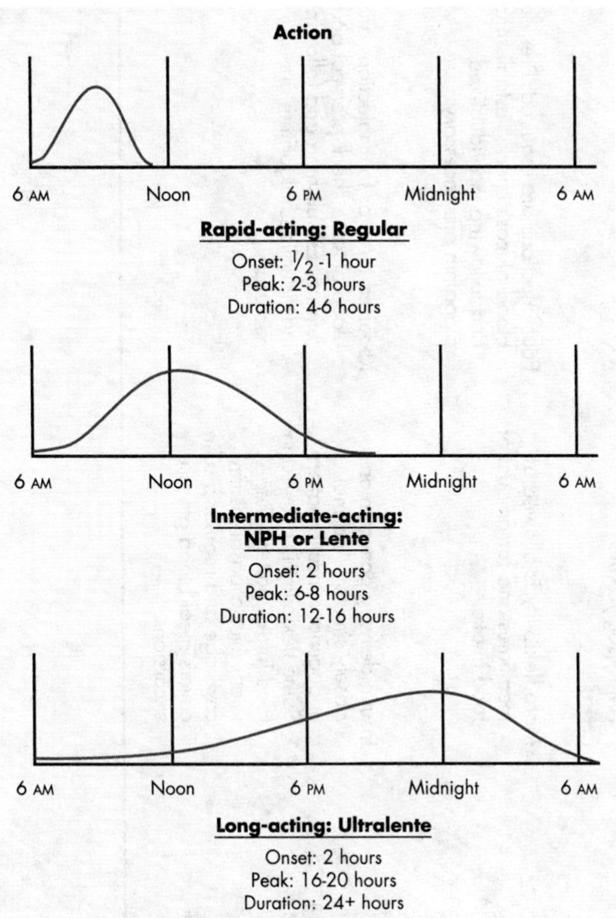

Fig. 46-6 Commercially available insulin preparations showing onset, peak, and duration.

stress. Only regular insulin can be administered IV; thus it is used in emergencies.

Insulins are commonly used in combination to mimic the normal endogenous insulin secretion (see Fig. 46-1). The timing of insulin administration in relation to meals is important. Regular insulin should be taken 30 to 45 minutes before meals to ensure the onset of action in conjunction with meal absorption. A variety of approaches to alter the time action of regular insulin is under investigation. Fast-acting insulin analogs suitable for subcutaneous injection are in clinical trials. These insulins may make the premeal timing issue moot with an onset in 10 to 15 minutes and peak action in 1 to 2 hours. Examples of insulin combination regimens, onset, peak, and descriptions of the advantages and disadvantages of each regimen are presented in Table 46-5. Ideally, regimens should be mutually selected by the patient and the health care provider. The criteria for selection are based on the type of diabetes and the required, desired, and feasible levels of glycemic control.

Because a single injection of a modified insulin rarely provides adequate glycemic control for most insulin-dependent patients, regular insulin is mixed with the modified insulin in the same syringe to avoid unnecessary injections. On the basis of current insulin formulations and use, the effect of NPH and regular insulin mixed in any proportion is the same as if the two were injected separately. The commercially available 70/30 or 50/50 mixtures of NPH and regular insulin appear to have the same activity as their component insulins given at separate injection sites.

Mixing human regular and Lente insulins results in blunting of the usual peak action of the regular insulin, presumably because the excess zinc in the Lente insulin binds regular insulin. A patient is sometimes given the option to mix regular and Lente or Ultralente and should be instructed to give the injection immediately after mixing if combining a Lente insulin and regular in the same syringe.

As a protein, insulin requires special storage considerations. Heat and freezing alter the insulin molecule. Insulin in use may be left at room temperature for up to 4 weeks unless the room temperature is higher than 85° F (30° C) or below freezing. Extra insulin may be stored in the refrigerator. The same principles apply for a patient with diabetes who is traveling. Insulin can be stored in a thermos or cooler to keep it cool (not frozen) if the patient is traveling in hot climates.

Administration of insulin

INJECTION. Because insulin is inactivated by gastric juices, it must be administered by injection. Daily administration of insulin is most commonly done by means of subcutaneous (SC) injection, although intramuscular (IM) or IV administration of regular insulin can be done when immediate onset of action is desired. The half-life of regular insulin in the circulation is 4 minutes, necessitating a continuous IV infusion for administration rather than a bolus IV injection. The steps in administering a SC insulin injection are outlined in Table 46-6. The technique should be taught to new insulin users and reviewed periodically with long-term users. It should never be assumed that because insulin is being used, the patient knows and practices the correct insulin injection technique. Inaccurate preparation is often caused by poor eyesight. Air bubbles in the syringe may not be seen, or the scale on the syringe may be read improperly. Administration systems, such as the insulin "pen," or "prefilled syringe," are available for patient convenience and are sometimes useful for visually or manually impaired persons.

The patient receiving mixed insulins (e.g., regular and an intermediate-acting insulin) needs to learn the proper technique for combining both in the same syringe if commercially prepared premixed insulins cannot be used (Fig. 46-7). Insulins should not be mixed if they differ in purity or species origin.

Recommended sites for insulin injection are noted in Fig. 46-8. The speed with which peak serum concentrations are reached varies with the anatomic site for injection. The fastest absorption is from the abdomen, then the arm, thigh, and buttock. Because of the variability in absorption and the decreased frequency of lipoatrophy in a patient treated with human or purified pork insulins, rotation of injection sites is no longer the recommended injection technique when these types of insulin are used. The patient should rotate the injection sites within a particular area, such as the

Table 46-5 Insulin Regimens

Regimen	Type of Insulin Used	Time Administered and Expected Time-Action Curve*	Advantages	Disadvantages
Single dose	Intermediate insulin (I)	7 AM (I); Noon; 6 PM; Midnight; 7 AM	One injection should cover noon and PM meal. Hypoglycemia during sleep is not a problem.	No fasting, breakfast, or nighttime coverage of hyperglycemia is available.
Split-mixed dose (20/30 premix)	Intermediate and regular insulin (I + R)	7 AM (I + R); Noon; 6 PM; Midnight; 7 AM	Two injections provide coverage for 24 hr.	Two injections are required. Patient must adhere to a set meal pattern.
Split-mixed dose	Intermediate and regular insulin (I + R)	7 AM (I + R); Noon; 7 PM (R); 9 PM (I); Midnight; 7 AM	Three injections provide coverage for 24 hr, particularly during early AM hours. Potential is reduced for 2-3 AM hypoglycemia.	Three injections are required.
Multiple dose	Intermediate and regular insulin (I + R)	7 AM (R); Noon (R); 7 PM (R); 9 PM (I); 7 AM	More flexibility is allowed at mealtimes and for amount of food intake.	Four injections are required. Premeal blood glucose checks, establishing and following individualized algorithm are necessary.
Multiple dose† (split dose long-acting insulin [Ultra Lente])	Regular insulin and longest-acting insulin (R + LA)	7 AM (R + LA); Noon (R); 7 PM (R); Midnight; 7 AM	Insulin delivery pattern more closely simulates normal endogenous insulin pattern. Some flexibility is allowed in food intake pattern. Regimen gives a basal insulin coverage and regular insulin covers meal blood glucose excursions.	Required three or four injections and blood glucose check premeal and on retiring. Establishing and following individualized algorithm are necessary.

*Regular insulin ——; intermediate insulin ---------.
†Insulin delivery through a pump is similar to this regimen.

Table 46-6 Administering an Insulin Injection

1. Wash hands thoroughly.
2. Roll intermediate insulin bottle between palms of hands to mix insulin. *Note:* Always inspect insulin bottle before using it for first time. Make sure that it is of proper type and concentration, expiration date has not passed, and top of bottle is in perfect condition.
3. Prepare insulin injection in same manner as for any injection.
4. Select proper injection site and inject following procedure for any SC injection.* In sites where SC tissue is adequate, inject commercial insulin needles at 90-degree angle. For sites with minimal SC tissue, pinch up skin and insert needle at 45-degree angle.
5. If blood appears in syringe after needle is inserted, select new site for injection. Aspiration of syringe is not necessary.
6. After injecting insulin, apply some pressure with alcohol swab or cotton ball at site when withdrawing needle.
7. Hold swab in place for few seconds but do not massage.
8. Destroy and dispose of single-use syringe safely. *Note:* When instructing patient to self-inject insulin, use the following guidelines (if appropriate): (1) syringe does not need to be aspirated before injection and (2) disposable syringes can be reused for several injections.

SC, Subcutaneous.
*See Fig. 46-8.

1. Wash hands.
2. Gently rotate NPH insulin bottle.
3. Wipe off tops of insulin vials with alcohol sponge.
4. Draw back amount of air into the syringe that equals total dose.

5. Inject air equal to NPH dose into NPH vial. Remove syringe from vial.

6. Inject air equal to regular dose into regular vial.

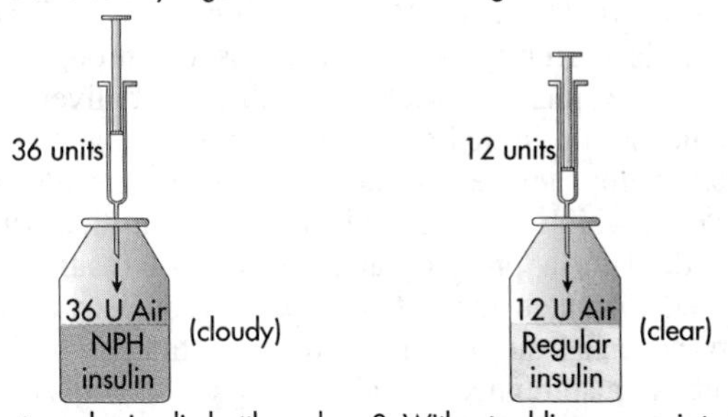

7. Invert regular insulin bottle and withdraw regular insulin dose.

8. Without adding more air to NPH vial, carefully withdraw NPH dose.

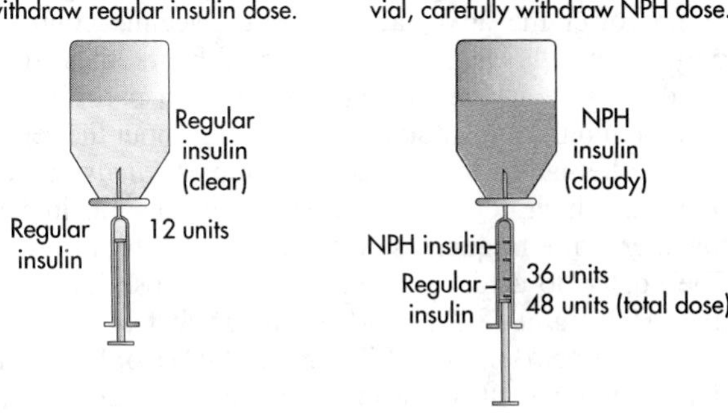

Fig. 46-7 Mixing insulins. This step-order process avoids the problem of contaminating regular insulin with intermediate-acting insulin.

abdomen, for a period, and then, if rotation to the thigh is desired, the patient can adjust the regimen to the new peak and action times for the new site.

The patient should also be cautioned about injecting into a site that is to be exercised. For example, the patient should not inject insulin into the thigh and then go jogging. Exercise of the area containing the injection site together with the increased body heat generated by the exercise may increase the rate of absorption and speed the onset of insulin action.

Insulin administration also requires the appropriate syringe. Most commercial insulin is available as U100, indicating that each milliliter contains 100 U of insulin. U100 insulin must be used with a U100-marked syringe. For a user taking smaller doses of insulin, insulin syringes with larger black lines are marked for 25, 30, or 50 U and are available for use with U100 insulin. One important distinction regarding the different size syringes is that the 100 unit syringe is marked in 2 unit increments, whereas the 50 unit and 30 unit are marked in one unit increments. It is important that the patient gets the right sized syringe and not switch back and forth with different size syringes to avoid serious dosing errors. Before the development of U100 insulin, insulin was available in concentrations of U40 and U80.

Some patients may prefer to use their syringe more than once. Insulin preparations have bacteriostatic additives that inhibit growth of bacteria commonly found on the skin. Many studies have shown that it is both safe and practical for the syringe to be reused if the patient desires. The syringe should be discarded when the needle becomes dull, has been bent, or has come in contact with any surface other than the skin. If reuse is planned, the needle must be recapped after each use.[16]

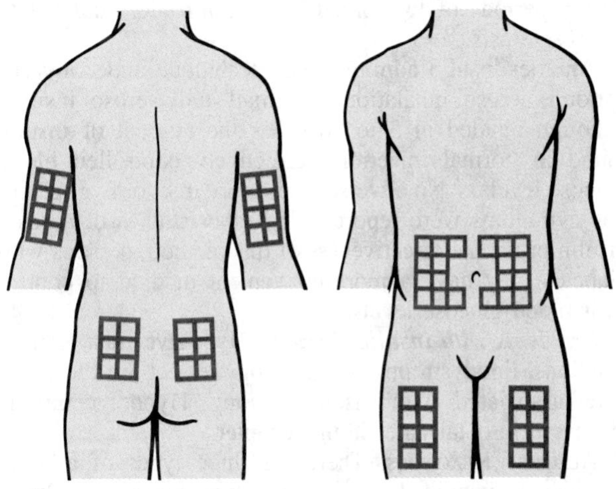

Fig. 46-8 Injection sites for insulin.

Another change in the insulin injection routine relates to the use of the alcohol swab on the skin before injection. When instructing a patient on the technique of insulin injection, the use of the alcohol wipe is optional. Routine hygiene such as washing with soap and rinsing with water is adequate.[17]

ALTERNATE DELIVERY METHODS. Continuous SC insulin infusion is currently being accomplished through *insulin pumps*. The pump devices are able to deliver insulin continuously in titrated amounts through tubing attached to a small pump device on one end and to a needle on the other end, which is placed subcutaneously in the skin. The pump delivers a pre-programmed dose of insulin that is designed to match the patient's basal profile to achieve a nearly normal insulin delivery on a continuous basis. The patient can also regulate meal coverage with bolus doses of insulin given at the patient's discretion. Although insulin pumps offer the advantage of tight glycemic control and only one needle change every 48 to 72 hours, these devices are expensive and require vigorous patient participation in glucose monitoring and decision making about the regimen.

An alternative to the insulin pump is *intensive insulin therapy,* which consists of several daily insulin injections together with frequent self-monitoring of blood glucose. The goal is to achieve a near normal glucose level of less than 150 mg/dl (8.3 mmol/L). The Diabetes Control and Complications Trial (DCCT) proved that people who have tight glucose control through intensive management, develop fewer and less severe complications.[18] Studies have shown comparable control outcomes in patients receiving intensive therapy and patients with an insulin pump. Because the required patient participation is similar, intensive therapy may be instituted before the initiation of pump use.[19] Because of the specialized nature of these insulin delivery systems and devices, expert guidance from a physician and a nurse educator is essential.

Intensive insulin therapy is not for everyone. Children are already at increased risk for low blood sugar (hypoglycemia), which can impair normal brain development. This risk is increased with intensive insulin therapy. In the elderly, intensive insulin therapy increases the risk of hypoglycemia, which could result in heart attacks or strokes during periods of low blood glucose in older adults with atherosclerosis.[20]

Another insulin administration technique under investigation is aerosol inhalation. In a small study aerosol insulin, although inhaled in 5 to 10 times the amount of insulin found in normal injections, effectively controlled blood glucose levels.[21] No adverse respiratory tract or hypoglycemic symptoms were reported. If further studies of aerosol insulin prove the effectiveness of this method, persons with diabetes may have a more convenient method to control their blood glucose levels.

Problems with insulin therapy. Hypoglycemia, allergic reactions, lipodystrophy, and Somogyi effect are the problems associated with insulin therapy. Hypoglycemia is discussed in detail later in this chapter.

ALLERGIC REACTIONS. There are three types of allergic reactions to insulin. Local reactions may occur as itching, erythema, and burning around the injection site. Local reactions may be self-limiting within 1 to 3 months or may improve with a low dose of antihistamine.

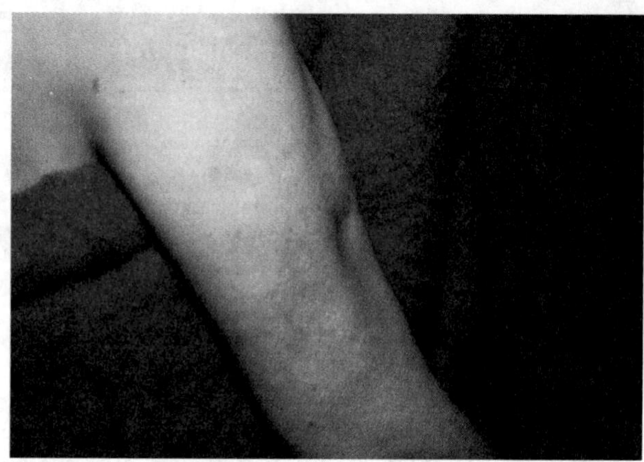

Fig. 46-9 Lipodystrophy of the arm.

A "true" insulin allergy is a systemic response with urticaria and possibly anaphylactic shock generally resulting from the use of animal insulins. Fortunately, this type of allergy is rare, particularly since human insulin has become available. A more common type of allergy is *insulin resistance*, in which antibodies are formed against the insulin and actually bind to the insulin molecules and render them inactive. The insulin molecule may be released at a later, unpredictable time to trigger unanticipated peaks in insulin action. An insulin allergy may be the suspected problem when insulin requirements approach 100 U per day. This type of allergy is seen more often in a patient who starts insulin therapy, enters a brief remission in diabetes, and then resumes insulin when the remission is over. For this reason the patient may receive a low dose of insulin (<10 U) during the honeymoon period. Most of these reactions can be avoided through the use of insulin with greater purity.

LIPODYSTROPHY. *Lipodystrophies* (hypertrophy or atrophy of SC tissue [lipoatrophy]) may occur if the same injection sites are used frequently without a daily or weekly rotation (Fig. 46-9). Hypertrophy, a thickening of the SC tissue, eventually regresses if the patient does not use the site for at least 6 months. The use of hypertrophied sites may result in erratic insulin absorption. Lipoatrophies have been most commonly associated with beef or beef and pork insulin and rarely with human insulin. Purified pork or human insulin may be used to treat the lipoatrophy by injecting at the edge of the lipoatrophic area. This stimulates fat cells to regenerate tissue. Site rotation on a daily or weekly basis is not necessary with human insulin.

SOMOGYI EFFECT AND DAWN PHENOMENON. The *Somogyi effect* is characterized by wide differences in early morning (low) and postprandial (high) glucose levels (Fig. 46-10). The blood glucose level drops below normal in response to too much insulin (see Table 46-16 for the causes of hypoglycemia). Counterregulatory hormones are released, stimulating lipolysis, gluconeogenesis, and glycogenolysis,

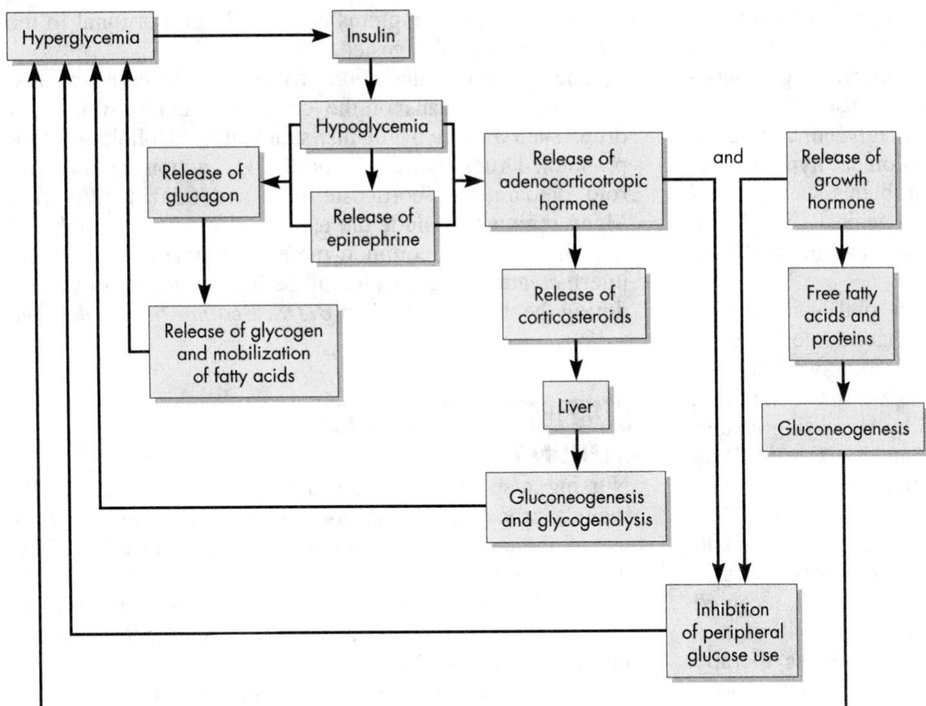

Fig. 46-10 The Somogyi effect.

which in turn produce rebound hyperglycemia and ketosis. The danger of this effect is that, when blood glucose is measured, the patient (or the health care professional) may assess the situation as hyperglycemia and increase the insulin dose. The Somogyi effect is associated with the occurrence of undetected hypoglycemia during sleep, although it can happen at any time. The patient may report headaches on awakening and may recall night sweats or nightmares. When the Somogyi effect occurs at night, the patient's blood glucose is elevated on awakening in the morning.

With *dawn phenomenon*, hyperglycemia is also present on awakening in the morning and ketonuria may be present. The cause is theorized to be a dawn release of endogenous growth hormone or cortisol, diurnal variation of insulin clearance, and insulin sensitivity. Both growth hormone and cortisol are counterregulatory hormones to insulin and raise the blood glucose level. The dawn phenomenon affects the majority of diabetics and tends to be most severe when growth hormone is at its peak in adolescence and young adulthood.

Careful assessment is required to document each phenomenon because the treatment for each differs. The treatment for Somogyi effect is less insulin. The treatment for dawn phenomenon is an adjustment in the timing of insulin administration or an increase in insulin. The assessment must include insulin dose, injection sites, and variability in the time of meals or insulin administration. In addition, the patient is asked to measure and document bedtime, between 2 to 4 AM, and morning fasting blood glucose levels on several occasions. If the predawn levels are below 60 mg/dl (3.3 mmol/L) and signs and symptoms of hypoglycemia are present, the insulin dosage should be reduced. If the 2 to 4 AM blood glucose is high, the insulin dosage should be increased.[22] In addition, the patient should be counseled on appropriate bedtime snacks.

Oral Hypoglycemic Agents. Sulfonylureas were found to have blood glucose-lowering effects during research on their antibiotic properties in the 1940s. They are called first generation or second generation depending on when they were introduced into clinical use in the United States. The first generation of these drugs used in the treatment of diabetes mellitus included tolbutamide (Orinase), acetohexamide (Dymelor), tolazamide (Tolinase), and chlorpropamide (Diabinese). A second generation of sulfonylureas, approved for use in the United States more recently, includes glipizide (Glucotrol), and glyburide (Micronase, DiaBeta, Glynase).

Second generation drugs have fewer adverse effects, are about 100 times more potent by weight, and have more predictable time actions and half-lives.[23] Also, their drug interaction potential is lower because they bind to circulating proteins differently. The main disadvantage of second-generation drugs is their increased expense. Metformin (Glucophage) is a biguanide glucose-lowering agent. Worldwide, metformin is widely used as a monotherapy and in combination with a sulfonylurea. Unlike sulfonylureas, metformin is not bound to plasma proteins, is not metabolized, and is eliminated rapidly by the kidney. The glucose-lowering effect occurs without stimulation of insulin secretion and results mainly from increased glucose utilization. The presence of insulin is required, and enhancement of insulin action at the postreceptor level occurs in peripheral tissues such as muscle. Metformin also increases glucose utilization by the intestine, primarily via nonoxidative metabolism. Metformin may also act by decreasing the rate of hepatic glucose production (gluconeogenesis). Because metformin does not cause clinical hypoglycemia, it is actually an antihyperglycemic drug. It does not cause weight gain and helps combat hypertriglyceridemia.[24] Side effects include GI problems such as nausea, diarrhea, and flatulence. Lactic acidosis is also a potential side effect for which the patient and nurse should monitor.

Indication for use. OHAs are not oral insulin or a substitute for insulin. The patient must have some functioning endogenous insulin for OHAs to be effective. They are thought to act by stimulating the β cells' insulin secretion in response to rising blood glucose and by increasing insulin sensitivity to receptors on insulin-sensitive tissue. They may also reduce hepatic glucose production.[25]

The patient who is most likely to respond well to OHAs is over 40 years of age at the onset of diabetes, has had diabetes for less than 5 years, is obese or of normal weight, has a consistent dietary intake, and has never received insulin or has been well controlled on less than 40 units a day.[23] In the patient with newly diagnosed diabetes, therapy with OHAs may not be started until the patient has been given an opportunity to try dietary control. Even if OHA therapy is initially successful, the patient may eventually fail to maintain control and insulin therapy may have to be initiated. The results of the DCCT related to decreasing complications with the use of intensive blood glucose control for type I diabetics may not be applicable to type II diabetics.[26] Further study is needed.

A study in 1970 indicated that cardiovascular deaths were more frequent in patients treated with OHAs (e.g., tolbutamide) than in those treated with insulin or diet therapy alone.[27] Although the results of this study have been disputed, many physicians are still reluctant to prescribe oral agents and prefer to use methods of treatment such as diet, exercise, and insulin.

Types of OHAs. As with insulin, the sulfonylureas differ in terms of dosage, absorption time, peak action, and duration. Second-generation sulfonylureas offer the advantages of lower doses, fewer side effects, and partial biliary excretion. The action, dosage, and side effects of first- and second-generation OHAs are listed in Table 46-8. Additional OHAs that are currently in use in Europe and may be introduced in the United States in the next few years include glimiprimide and acarbose.[28]

Disadvantages of OHAs. OHAs, which are broken down by the kidney, should be used cautiously in the patient with renal disease. Sulfonylureas, which are metabolized by the liver, should also be avoided in cases of impaired liver function. The patient with allergies to sulfonamides should use OHAs cautiously if at all. The sulfonylureas can cause side effects such as nausea and vomiting, diarrhea, skin allergies, and hematologic disorders, although these effects are less common in second-generation OHAs. A small percentage of patients taking alcohol while receiving an OHA may have an Antabuse-like effect (i.e., nausea, vomiting, flushing, respiratory distress, and chest pain). Symptoms are usually proportional to the amount of alcohol ingested.

The hypoglycemic action of OHA can be enhanced and prolonged by means of the concurrent administration of drugs such as anticoagulants, salicylates, alcohol, and propranolol. Drugs that can oppose OHA action include thyroid preparations, corticosteroids, and thiazide diuretics. Many regimens include the use of sulfonylureas combined with insulin. One common method of treatment is to use intermediate-acting insulin at bedtime and sulfonylureas during the day, this is called ***BIDS, B****edtime* ***i****nsulin* ***d****aytime* ***s****ulfonylureas*.[29]

NURSING MANAGEMENT

INSULIN THERAPY

Nursing responsibilities for the patient receiving insulin include proper administration, assessment of the patient's use of and response to insulin therapy, and education of the patient regarding administration, adjustment to, and side effects of insulin. Table 46-7 lists guidelines for the nurse assessing a patient using glucose-lowering agents, including insulin and OHAs.

The patient with newly diagnosed diabetes should be assessed for the ability to understand the purpose of insulin therapy; the interaction of insulin, diet, and activity; and the ways side effects may be manifested. The patient or significant other also has to be able to prepare and inject the insulin. If the patient or family lacks the psychomotor skills to prepare insulin, the nurse may have to find additional resources to assist the patient.

Some patients find it difficult to inject themselves. This may be due to fear of the needle or anger and lack of acceptance of the disease. The nurse needs to determine the emotions and attitude of the patient and family regarding insulin therapy.

Follow-up assessment of the patient who has been using insulin therapy also includes an inspection of injection sites for allergic reactions, a review of insulin preparation and injection technique, a history pertaining to the occurrence of hypoglycemic episodes, and the patient's method for handling hypoglycemic episodes. A review of the patient's record of urine and blood glucose tests is also important in assessing overall glycemic control.

ORAL HYPOGLYCEMIC AGENTS

Nursing responsibilities for the patient taking OHAs are similar to those for the patient taking insulin. Proper administration, assessment of the patient's use of and response to the OHA, and education of the patient and the family about OHAs are all part of the nurse's function. Table 46-7 lists guidelines for the nurse assessing a patient starting therapy with OHAs and the follow-up assessment.

The assessment done by the nurse can be invaluable in determining the most appropriate oral agent for a patient. The assessment includes the patient's mental status, eating habits, home environment, attitude toward diabetes, and use of oral agents. For example, if the patient is older, lives alone, or has difficulty remembering to follow a medication

Table 46-7 Assessing the Patient Treated with Glucose-Lowering Agents

For patient with newly diagnosed diabetes or for reevaluation of GLA regimen	
Cognitive	Is patient or responsible other able to understand why insulin or OHAs are being used as part of diabetes management? Is patient or responsible other able to understand concepts of asepsis, combining insulins, insulin-OHA actions, and side effects? Is patient able to remember to take >1 dose/day? Does patient take medications at right times in relation to meals?
Psychomotor	Is patient or responsible other physically able to prepare and administer accurate doses of GLA?
Affective	What emotions and attitudes are patient and responsible others displaying in regard to diagnosis of diabetes and insulin or OHA treatment?
For follow-up of GLA-treated patient	
Effectiveness of therapy	Is patient having symptoms of hyperglycemia? Does blood glucose and urine record show good or poor control? Is glycosylated hemoglobin consistent with glucose records?
Side effects of GLA therapy	Is atrophy or hypertrophy present at injection sites? Has patient had hypoglycemic episodes? If so, how often? What time of day? Are there complaints of nightmares, night sweats, or early morning headaches? Has patient had skin rash or GI upset since taking OHA?
Self-management behaviors	If patient is having hypoglycemic episodes, how are those episodes managed? How much insulin or OHA is patient taking and at what times of day? Is patient adjusting insulin or OHA dose? Under what circumstances and by how much? Has exercise pattern changed? Is patient adhering to number of prescribed calories? Are meals taken at times corresponding to peak insulin action?

GI, Gastrointestinal; *GLA*, glucose-lowering agent; *OHA*, oral hypoglycemic agent.

and diet schedule, a shorter-acting OHA may be preferable. Some patients may assume that their diabetes is not a serious condition if they are taking only a pill for glycemic control. The patient needs to understand the importance of diet and not skipping meals. The patient should not take extra pills if overeating has occurred and should not take a dose any later than the evening meal. The patient also needs to know that hypoglycemic reactions may be severe and prolonged and that health care provider supervision may be necessary, particularly for the older patient.

The patient should also be instructed to contact a physician if periods of illness or extreme stress occur. During such a period, insulin therapy may be required to prevent or treat hyperglycemic symptoms and hyperglycemic hyperosmolar nonketosis (HHNK).

Other Drugs Affecting Blood Glucose Levels

The patient with diabetes may be concurrently taking other medications. Both the patient and the health care provider must be aware of drug interactions that can potentiate hypoglycemic and hyperglycemic effects. For example, β-adrenergic drugs block the hepatic glycogenolytic response that occurs in response to hypoglycemia. Thiazide diuretics can also potentiate hyperglycemia by inducing potassium loss. A list of medications that may influence glycemic control is presented in Table 46-9. Medications may have to be changed or dosages adjusted if the patient is also taking glucose-lowering agents (GLAs).

Exercise

Regular, consistent exercise is considered an essential part of diabetic management. Exercise contributes to weight loss, reduces triglycerides and cholesterol, increases muscle tone, and improves circulation. In type I diabetes, exercise may increase insulin sensitivity, thereby allowing a lowering of the insulin dose. In type II diabetes, exercise contributes to weight loss and improves insulin binding on cell receptors. However, the patient should be aware that exercise is perceived by the body as a stress, and that counterregulatory hormones are increased to ensure that adequate glucose is readily available. As a result, hyperglycemia may occur in situations of poorly controlled diabetes or in insulin-dependent patients who exercise at a time of day when insufficient insulin is available. Additional information about exercise and diabetes that is important for both the patient and the health care provider to know includes the following:

1. Exercise does not have to be vigorous to be effective. The blood glucose-reducing effects of exercise can be attained with mild exercise such as brisk walking. The exercises selected should be enjoyable to foster regularity.
2. Exercise is best done after meals, when the blood glucose level is rising.
3. Exercise plans should be individualized for each patient and monitored by the health care provider.
4. The patient should be encouraged to self-monitor blood glucose levels before, during, and after exercise to determine the effect exercise has on blood glucose level at particular times of the day.
5. The patient should be alerted to the possibility of delayed exercise-induced hypoglycemia, which may occur several hours after the completion of exercise.

Table 46-8 Oral Hypoglycemic Agents

Name	Dosage	Duration of Action	Metabolism and Excretion
First-Generation Sulfonylureas			
Tolbutamide (Orinase)	500-3000 mg 2-3 times/day	6-12 hr (half-life of 4-5 hr)	Rapidly metabolized in liver, 100% excreted in urine
Acetohexamide (Dymelor)	250-1500 mg 2 times/day	12-24 hr (half-life of 1-2 hr)	Rapidly metabolized in liver, 60% excreted in urine
Tolazamide (Tolinase)	100-1000 mg 1-2 times/day	12-24 hr (half-life of 7 hr)	Metabolized in liver, 85% excreted in urine
Chlorpropamide (Diabinese)	100-500 mg/day	36-60 hr (half-life of 36 hr)	99% excreted in urine, virtually nonmetabolized by liver
Second-Generation Sulfonylureas			
Glipizide (Glucotrol)	2.5-40 mg/day	10-24 hr (half-life of 2-4 hr)	Metabolized in liver, excreted in urine (60-90%) and bile (5-20%)
Glyburide (Micronase, DiaBeta Glynase)	1.25-20 mg/day	24 hr (half-life of 10 hr)	Metabolized in liver, excreted in urine (50%) and bile (50%)
Biquanide Metformin (Gluophage)	500-2550 mg/day	12-24 hr	Excreted in urine as active drug

*Side effects can be minimized if OHA choice is matched appropriately to patient's needs. OHAs are not appropriate for ketosis-prone patients and pregnant patients and should be used cautiously if at all in patients with renal or hepatic dysfunction. There is <5% incidence of side effects.

Table 46-9 Medications That Affect Blood Glucose Levels

Glucose-Lowering Effect		
Acetaminophen	Clofibrate	Potassium salts
Alcohol	Dicumarol	Probenecid
Allopurinol	Fenfluramine	Salicylates in large doses
Anabolic steroids	Histamine antagonists	Sulfonylureas
β-Blockers	Insulin	Tricyclic antidepressants
Biguanides	Monoamine oxidase inhibitors	Urinary acidifiers
Chloramphenicol	Phenylbutazone	
Occasional Glucose-Raising Effect		
Acetazolamide	Ethacrynic acid	Marijuana
Asparaginase	Morphine	Nicotine
Caffeine in large doses	Epinephrine	Nifedipine
Arginine hydrochloride	Furosemide	Phenobarbital
Barbiturates	Glucagon	Phenothiazines
β-Blockers	Glucose	Phenytoin
Birth control pills	Glycerin	Rifampin
Cholestyramine	Glycerol	Thiazide diuretics
Corticosteroids	Levodopa	Urinary alkalizing agents
Calcitonin	Lithium	

6. The patient taking a GLA should not have to forego the enjoyment of planned or spontaneous exercise. The patient can be taught to compensate for extensive planned and spontaneous activity by monitoring blood glucose level to make adjustments in the insulin dose (if taken) and food intake.

Hypoglycemia is likely to occur if the insulin-dependent patient exercises at a time when the GLA action is peaking or if exercise is strenuous and prolonged and carbohydrate is not replaced. This can also occur if a normally sedentary patient with diabetes has an unusually active day. Exercise can be scheduled about 1½ hours after a meal or a 10 to 15 g carbohydrate snack can be eaten before exercising to avoid hypoglycemia. For every 45 minutes to 1 hour of strenuous exercise such as tennis, the patient should repeat the 10 to 15 g carbohydrate snack. (See Table 46-10 for guidelines on calories burned per hour for different activities.)

Table 46-10 Activities That Affect Caloric Expenditure

Light Activity (100-200 cal/hr)	Moderate Activity (200-350 cal/hr)	Vigorous Activity (400-900 cal/hr)
Driving a car	Active housework	Aerobic exercise
Fishing	Bicycling	Bicycling
Light housework	Bowling	Hard labor
Secretarial work	Brisk walking	Ice skating
Teaching	Dancing	Outdoor sports
Walking casually	Gardening	Running
	Golf	Soccer
	Roller skating	Tennis
		Wood chopping

Hyperglycemia may occur if exercise is scheduled at a time when insulin action is waning. When the insulin dose is insufficient to cover the amount of exercise, the increase in blood glucose created by the counterregulatory hormones may not be curtailed. Again, the patient can guard against this situation by scheduling exercise when sufficient insulin is available. Some patients may have to inject a small bolus of regular insulin if the blood glucose level is elevated before exercising to prevent progressive hyperglycemia.[30]

MONITORING BLOOD GLUCOSE

Glucose levels must be determined daily to monitor the interactions and effect of diet, exercise, and medication on an individual diabetic regimen. Detection of extreme or episodic hyperglycemia is necessary to avoid DKA and HHNK. Traditionally, monitoring has been accomplished by checking for the presence and degree of glycosuria. This technique provides only gross, semiquantitative information. Many factors affect urine test results, such as age, medications, disease, and the individual renal threshold. Urine testing also cannot measure the presence or degree of hypoglycemia. Urine testing for ketonuria, however, is a valuable aid in determining the advent of DKA and is recommended for every patient with type I diabetes when the patient is experiencing hyperglycemia or acute illness. Second voided specimens, which were previously recommended for the patient using urine testing, have been shown to constitute an unnecessary step.

Self-Monitoring

Self-monitoring of blood glucose using *capillary blood glucose monitoring* (CBGM) technology is a more reliable technique for measuring blood glucose. Commercially available glucose-testing products, including disposable lancets and lancet holders, are widely available. A small drop of capillary blood (usually from a finger stick) is dropped onto a reagent strip. After a specified time, the strip is read either visually or by a machine. The machines are either reflectance meters or sensors. Reflectance meters work by measuring the amount of light reflected onto a strip that has reacted with a color change in response to the reaction of glucose with the reagent strip. Sensors use the measurement of conductivity of electricity as it is affected by the glucose in the blood. The technology of CBGM is a rapidly changing field with newer and more convenient systems being introduced every year. Blood glucose monitoring technology using a noninvasive spectroscopy, or the use of laser light on a skin surface such as the forearm or web space between finger and thumb is being researched for possible use in the future. Implantable sensors for continuous glucose monitoring are also being considered in research trials.[31] A diabetes educator should be consulted to learn the latest in monitoring technology.

Many meters are computerized and are becoming increasingly sophisticated. Some models are capable of storing "memory" of previous blood glucose tests. These tests can be retrieved to provide a more complete picture of blood glucose fluctuations over time and to guide adjustment to the regimen.

The blood glucose level reported by a laboratory is often lower than the patient's home glucose monitor or the hospital's portable meter. This is because a finger stick is based on a capillary rather than a venous sample so it may be 20 to 70 mg/dl (3.9 mmol/L) higher. Also, portable meters test whole blood, while most laboratories test plasma or serum glucose. Plasma or serum gives a lower glucose reading.[32] Finally, home-monitoring equipment needs to be cleaned and calibrated regularly to maintain its accuracy.

The technique for using a blood glucose-monitoring product accompanies each product. Because errors in monitoring technique can cause errors in clinical management strategies that may be based on erroneous CBGM information, patient training should be emphasized at not only the initial session, but at follow-up visits with any member of the health care team. Patient technique should be reassessed at 30 to 180 days after initial training and yearly thereafter.[33] The major source of variability in results obtained with CBGM devices is attributable to the user.[34] The following steps should be taught to every patient performing CBGM:

1. Hands are washed in warm water. Cleaning the site with alcohol is not necessary and may even interfere with test results.
2. If it is difficult to obtain an adequate drop of blood for testing, the patient should warm the hands in warm water or let the arms hang dependently for a few minutes before the finger puncture is made.
3. The puncture is made on the side of the finger pad rather than near the center. Fewer nerve endings are along the side of the finger pad.
4. The puncture should be only deep enough to obtain a sufficiently large drop of blood. Unnecessarily deep punctures may cause pain and bruising.

The advantages of CBGM are that it ensures immediate information about blood glucose levels and produces accurate records with daily glucose fluctuations and trends. CBGM is the preferred glucose-monitoring method for the patient with type I diabetes. The type II diabetic patient may also benefit from CBGM by seeing the correlation between dietary choices and blood glucose levels. As weight is lost and blood glucose levels are lowered, the obese type II patient may also gain reinforcement from CBGM.[35]

The frequency of monitoring depends on the glycemic goals the patient and health care provider set and the intensity of the treatment regimen. The patient receiving two or more injections per day may want to test before meals every day. If the glycemic control is relatively stable, the patient may elect to test two or more times a day on certain days of the week. Testing is most often done before meals but can be done any time the patient needs to know the way a factor, such as exercise or stress, is affecting the blood glucose level. The frequency of recording CBGM results to guide therapy decisions should be mutually determined by the health care provider and the patient.

Ideally, a patient should be motivated to learn not only CBGM technique but also how to interpret the results. Most patients find that CBGM brings about physiologic and emotional benefits as well as a willingness to be an active partner in the treatment. Achieving the desired level of patient participation also requires time and effort from the health care professional. The nurse involved in this aspect of management should anticipate a close working relationship with the patient for a period of 3 to 6 months as the patient learns refinements of the technique and appropriate decision making regarding changes in diet, medication, and exercise. A patient who is visually impaired, color blind, or limited in manual dexterity needs careful evaluation of the glucose-monitoring method most appropriate for that patient's needs. Reflectance meters are now commercially available for the visually impaired.

NURSING MANAGEMENT

DIABETES MELLITUS

Nursing Assessment

Initial subjective and objective data that should be obtained from a person with diabetes mellitus are presented in Table 46-11. After the initial assessment, periodic patient assessments should be done on a schedule as outlined in Table 46-12.

Table 46-11 Nursing Assessment: Diabetes Mellitus

Subjective Data

Important health information

Past health history: Mumps, rubella, coxsackievirus or other viral infections; recent trauma, infection, or stress; pregnancy, gave birth to infant >9 lbs; chronic pancreatitis; Cushing's syndrome, acromegaly

Medications: Use of and compliance with insulin or oral hypoglycemic agents; use of glucocorticoids, diuretics, phenytoin (Dilantin)

Surgery and other treatments: Any recent surgery

Functional health patterns

Health perception–health management: Positive family history; fatigue, malaise

Nutritional-metabolic: Obesity; compliance with diet; thirst, hunger; nausea and vomiting; weight loss (in type I), weight gain (in type II); itching, skin infections, poor healing especially involving the feet

Elimination: Constipation or diarrhea; frequent urination, nocturia, incontinence

Activity-exercise: Muscle weakness

Cognitive-perceptual: Abdominal pain, headache; blurred vision; numbness or tingling of extremities; irritability

Sexuality-reproductive: Impotence; frequent vaginal infections; decreased libido

Objective Data

General

Fruity breath, dehydration

Integumentary

Dry, inelastic skin; pigmented lesions (on legs); ulcers (especially on feet); skin infection

Cardiovascular

Cool extremities, loss of hair on toes

Neurologic

Cataracts, vitreal hemorrhages, altered reflexes

Musculoskeletal

Muscle wasting

Possible findings

Serum electrolyte abnormalities; fasting blood glucose level >140 mg/dl (7.8 mmol/L); glucose tolerance test >200 mg/dl (11.1 mmol/L); leukocytosis; elevated blood urea nitrogen, serum creatinine, triglycerides; dyslipidemia, glycosylated hemoglobin; glycosuria; ketonuria; albuminuria

Nursing Diagnoses

Nursing diagnoses are determined when the problem and etiologic factors are supported by clinical data. Nursing diagnoses related to diabetes mellitus may include, but are not limited to, those found in the nursing care plan for the patient with diabetes on p. 1458.

Planning

The overall goals are that the patient with diabetes mellitus will (1) be an active participant in the management of the diabetes regimen; (2) experience minimal or no episodes of DKA, HHNK, or hypoglycemia; (3) prevent or delay the occurrence of chronic complications of diabetes; and (4) adjust lifestyle to accommodate diabetes regimen with a minimum of stress.

Nursing Implementation

Health Promotion and Maintenance. The role of the nurse in health promotion and maintenance relates to the identification, monitoring, and education of the patient at risk for the development of diabetes mellitus. This group includes persons with a genetic predisposition to diabetes, obese persons, persons with high stress, and older adults. Native Americans are at greatly increased risk and need regular evaluation. A person with impaired glucose tolerance with plasma levels of glucose that are higher than normal are also at increased risk for diabetes. In addition, the presence of pancreatic or endocrine disease or the use of

Table 46-12 Periodic Assessment for a Patient with Diabetes

Item	Initial Visit	Every 3 Mo	Every 12 Mo
Assessment of Glycemic Control			
Symptoms of hypoglycemia	X	X	
Symptoms of hyperglycemia	X	X	
Record of blood tests	X	X	
Glycosylated hemoglobin	X	X	
Assessment for Complications			
Postural blood pressure and pulse	X	X	
Weight	X	X	
Funduscopic	X	X	
Primary provider	X		
Ophthalmologist			X
Cardiac examination	X		X
Neurologic examination			
Sensory: pinprick vibration sense	X		X
Motor: ankle reflexes, muscle bulk and tone	X		X
Pelvic examination as indicated for vaginal discharge		As needed	
Extremities			
Feet: calluses, toenails, ulcers	X	X	
Peripheral pulses			
Dorsalis pedis	X		X
Posterior tibial	X		X
Popliteal	X		X
Femoral	X		X
Assessment of Educational Needs			
Diet	X	X	
Medication management	X	X	
Monitoring skills	X	X	
Diagnostic Studies			
Blood glucose level	X	X	
Blood urea nitrogen and creatinine level	X		X
Urinalysis for microalbuminuria	X		X
Electrocardiogram	X*		X
Lipid profile	X		X
Fasting triglyceride level	X		X

*If appropriate to age and history.

certain medications such as corticosteroids also alerts the nurse to evaluate this person for diabetes.

Acute Intervention. The nurse is involved with the care of a patient with diabetes in many acute situations, such as DKA, hypoglycemia, and HHNK. Other areas of acute intervention relate to management during stress, such as during acute illness and surgery.

Stress of acute illness and surgery. Both emotional and physical stress can increase the blood glucose level and result in hyperglycemia. However, it is impossible to avoid stress totally in life situations such as deaths in the family, job interviews, and final examinations. These situations may require extra insulin to avoid hyperglycemia.*

*Gestational diabetes mellitus and management of the pregnant patient with diabetes is a specialized area not covered in this chapter. The reader is advised to consult an obstetric text for information about this area.

Common stress-evoking situations include acute illness and the controlled stress of surgery. The patient with diabetes who has a minor illness such as a cold or the flu should continue drug therapy and food intake. A carbohydrate liquid substitution such as regular soft drinks, gelatin dessert, or beverages such as Gatorade may be necessary. The patient should understand that food intake is important during this time because the body requires extra energy to deal with the stress of the illness. Extra insulin may be necessary to meet this demand without DKA concurrently developing.

Blood glucose monitoring should be done every 1 to 2 hours by either the patient or a person who can assume responsibility for care during the illness. Urine output and the presence and degree of ketonuria should be monitored, particularly when fever is present. Fluid intake should be increased to prevent dehydration, with a minimum of 4 oz per hour for an adult.

NURSING CARE PLAN Patient with Diabetes*

Planning: Outcome Criteria	Nursing Interventions and Rationales
Chronic Management	
➤ **NURSING DIAGNOSIS**	Ineffective management of therapeutic regimen *related to* lack of knowledge of adequate exercise program, diet and weight control, administration and potential side effects and complications of GLA, glucose monitoring, and care during acute minor illness *as manifested by* frequent questioning regarding all aspects of diabetic management, inaccurate responses to direct questions about diabetic management
Participate in exercise program to meet therapeutic goals (e.g., weight loss, improved insulin sensitivity, improved muscle tone, endurance).	Complete diabetes assessment with special attention to exercise behaviors *to provide information to plan interventions related to activity.* Plan individualized exercise program with patient *as exercise is an integral part of diabetic management.* Review steps to prevent hyperglycemia and hypoglycemia *as activity changes can cause changes in insulin needs.*
Practice dietary preparation and intake appropriate for GLA and patient.	Complete diabetes assessment with specific attention to diet *to provide information to plan intervention related to diet.* Review diet and problem areas with patient *to provide teaching in problem areas.* Counsel on weight loss if appropriate *as excess weight complicates diabetic management.* Refer to dietitian *as dietary management of diabetes can be complex and requires ongoing monitoring.*
Practice safe, effective administration of GLA with minimal or no side effects.	Complete diabetes assessment with special attention to GLA administration *to provide information to plan interventions related to GLA.* Review administration; have patient give return demonstration of insulin injection *to ensure proper technique.* Assess injection sites *to determine need for changing sites or initiating treatment to problematic areas.* Review symptoms and treatment of hypoglycemia *so early treatment can be initiated.*
Demonstrate proper blood glucose testing, recording of measurements, appropriate use of records to alter regimen.	Complete diabetes assessment and review patient glucose record *to provide information to plan interventions.* Demonstrate glucose testing; have patient give return demonstration *to ensure proper technique.* Review glucose records with patient and explain how to identify trends *to improve glucose levels and prevent wide fluctuations.* Remind patient to call physician if blood glucose is >250 mg/dl (13.9 mmol/L) and ketonuria is present *so appropriate adjustments can be made to prevent development of DKA.*
Verbalize steps for sick-day care; have plan of action for self in event of illness, and symptoms lasting >24 hr that require immediate physician attention including fever, nausea, and vomiting.	Review effect of stress on glycemic control *so patient is aware that stress increases glucose level.* Review sick-day care *so patient can make appropriate adjustments in diabetic management.* Assist patient in devising a sick-day plan, including foods to have on hand, and family member or friend who can be with patient during illness episode *to be ready to properly manage diabetes when illness occurs.* Review symptoms needing attention of physician, including blood glucose level >250 mg/dl (13.9 mmol/L), ketonuria, fever, nausea and vomiting *so patient can contact physician when necessary to prevent occurrence of DKA and HHNK.*
➤ **NURSING DIAGNOSIS**	Risk for infection *related to* depressed immune system, inadequate circulation, and environmental pathogens
Verbalize steps of prevention (skin care; foot care, regular dental care); verbalize and demonstrate care for minor cuts and burns; verbalize signs of infection and need for intervention.	Assess for signs of infection such as redness, swelling, or pus at trauma or pressure site; fever *to ensure early recognition and treatment.* Assess oral cavity, skin, pulses, particularly lower extremities and pedal pulses *to detect areas of infection or poor circulation.* Review skin and foot care; have patient give return demonstration of foot care *to ensure patient knows proper technique.* Review signs of infection, including redness, swelling, pus and when to contact physician *to ensure patient can recognize infection and notify physician if indicated so treatment can be initiated.*

continued

NURSING CARE PLAN Patient with Diabetes*—cont'd

Planning: Outcome Criteria	*Nursing Interventions and Rationales*
➤ **NURSING DIAGNOSIS**	Self-esteem disturbance *related to* lifestyle changes imposed by diabetes and its treatment, stigma of having a chronic illness, and frustration at progression of disease despite careful management *as manifested by* negative feelings about self, resistance to incorporating treatment regimen into lifestyle, refusal to acknowledge diagnosis
Verbalize positive attitude about self and ability to manage disease, plan for continued contact with health care provider for health monitoring.	Encourage patient to discuss diagnosis and its implications *so appropriate counseling and interventions can be planned.* Suggest individualized diabetes education and support group *to increase patient's knowledge base and meet other people with diabetes.* Suggest creative approaches to problems with patient *as patient may be overwhelmed initially by complexity of disease management.* Assure patient of continued value and self-worth *to minimize impact of diabetes on patient's self-esteem.*

COLLABORATIVE PROBLEMS

Acute Management

➤ **POTENTIAL COMPLICATION**	Diabetic ketoacidosis and hyperglycemic hyperosmolar nonketosis *related to* inadequate insulin and excess blood glucose secondary to increased caloric intake, physical or emotional stress, or undiagnosed diabetes
Monitor for signs of DKA and HHNK, report deviations from acceptable parameters, and carry out appropriate medical and nursing interventions.	Assess for signs of DKA such as increase in urination; vomiting; somnolence; dehydration; dry, loose skin; hypotension with weak, rapid pulse; coma; hyperglycemia >250 mg/dl (13.9 mmol/L); presence of urine ketones; pH <7.3 *to ensure early recognition and intervention.* Assess for signs of HHNK such as hyperglycemia >500 mg/dl (27.8 mmol/L), serum osmolality >300 mOsm/kg (300 mmol/kg), absence of ketonuria *to detect signs of HHNK.* Administer insulin per physician's order *to stabilize blood glucose level.* Administer fluid and electrolyte replacement as ordered *to correct dehydration.* Monitor input and output and vital signs *to detect signs of inadequate tissue perfusion.* Assess for precipitating factors *to prevent recurrence and identify teaching needs.* Monitor cardiac activity *to detect cardiac problems associated with dehydration.*
➤ **POTENTIAL COMPLICATION**	Hypoglycemia *related to* low blood glucose secondary to too much insulin
Monitor for signs of hypoglycemia, report deviations from acceptable parameters, and carry out appropriate medical and nursing interventions.	Assess for signs of hypoglycemia such as cold sweats; weakness; trembling; nervousness; irritability; pallor; increase in heart rate; confusion; fatigue; abnormal behavior *to ensure prompt identification and treatment.* Check blood glucose if time permits (e.g., when symptoms are mild) *to provide indicator for treatment.* Provide quick-acting carbohydrate source such as 6-8 oz orange juice, 1 cup milk, or 6-8 oz soft drink *to quickly reverse hypoglycemia*; give orally only if patient is alert enough to swallow *to prevent aspiration.* Repeat oral dose in 10-15 min if no improvement. If no improvement or patient is comatose, per physician's order give 1 mg glucagon subcutaneously *to stimulate hepatic response to convert glycogen to glucose* or 30-50 ml 50% IV dextrose *to increase blood glucose level.* When patient improves and is alert, provide long-acting carbohydrate or next scheduled meal *to keep blood glucose level within acceptable range.* Assess for precipitating factors such as history of too much insulin, too little food, unusual amounts of exercise, or delayed eating *to prevent recurrence and identify teaching needs.*

DKA, Diabetic ketoacidosis; *GLA,* glucose-lowering agent; *HHNK,* hyperglycemic hyperosmolar nonketosis; *IV,* intravenous.
*This care plan is intended to be used for the person with newly diagnosed diabetes.

The patient should be instructed to contact the health care provider when a blood glucose level more than 250 mg/dl (13.9 mmol/L), fever, ketonuria, and nausea and vomiting occur. The health care provider should supervise the necessary adjustments in the treatment regimen during times of stress. Eventually, the well-informed patient will be able to make most adjustments independently on the basis of past successful experiences.

Surgery is controlled stress, and adjustments in the diabetes regimen can be planned to ensure glycemic control. The patient is given IV fluids and insulin immediately before, during, and after surgery when there is no oral intake. The type II diabetic patient receiving OHAs usually has the OHAs discontinued 48 hours before surgery and is treated with insulin during the surgical period. The patient should understand that this is a temporary measure and is not to be interpreted as a worsening of diabetes.

The nurse caring for an unconscious surgical patient receiving insulin must be alert for hypoglycemic signs such as sweating, tachycardia, and tremors. The nurse should be aware that blood glucose monitoring must also be done frequently.

Chronic and Home Management. The nurse may be involved in any or all aspects of management, but the focus of nursing care has two aims: to care for the patient during acute episodes and to assist the patient in learning to live with diabetes every day. Both aims require the nurse to be thoroughly familiar with diabetes and its management and to educate the patient with diabetes about all aspects of the disease.

The nurse may request consultation with a diabetes educator who is certified by the American Association of Diabetes Educators. Certified diabetes educators have met stringent preparation and experience criteria and have demonstrated expertise in the field of diabetes education. Nurses, dietitians, pharmacists, physicians, and other health care professionals who make up the diabetes management team are eligible to apply for the CDE credential. The certified diabetes educator is designated with the initials CDE after the name.*

The effect of the diagnosis of diabetes cannot be overestimated. An assessment of the patient's perception of what it means to have diabetes must be carefully assessed before patient education is designed and implemented. The nurse should foster a positive attitude about the prescribed regimen and assist the patient in developing an individualized management plan. Learning goals should be mutually determined by the patient and the nurse on the basis of individual needs as well as therapeutic requirements. The nurse needs to assess the patient's feelings and facilitate acceptance of diabetes mellitus and its treatment over time.

Personal hygiene. The potential chronic complications of infections, neuropathy, and microangiopathy require the patient with diabetes to participate in good hygiene practices related to skin and dental care. Because of susceptibility to periodontal disease and pyorrhea, daily brushing and flossing should be encouraged. When dental work must be done, the dentist should be informed that the patient has diabetes.

Daily baths should be part of routine care, with particular emphasis given to foot care. If cuts, scrapes, or burns occur, they should be treated promptly. The area should be washed, and a nonabrasive or nonirritating antiseptic ointment must be applied. The area should be covered with a dry, sterile pad. If the injury does not begin to heal within 24 hours or if signs of infection develop, the health care provider should be notified immediately.

Medical identification and travel. The patient should be instructed to carry medical identification at all times indicating diabetes. An identification card (Fig. 46-11) can supply valuable information, such as the name of the health care provider and the type and dose of insulin or OHA. A medical alert bracelet or necklace should be worn by every person with diabetes. Police, paramedics, and many private citizens are aware of the need to look for this identification when working with sick or unconscious persons.

Travel for a patient with diabetes requires planning in advance. The patient should have all supplies in carry-on luggage and keep them at hand at all times. This includes insulin, syringes, quick-acting carbohydrate, and glucagon. Extra insulin should be available in case a bottle breaks or gets lost. If the patient is planning a trip out of the country,

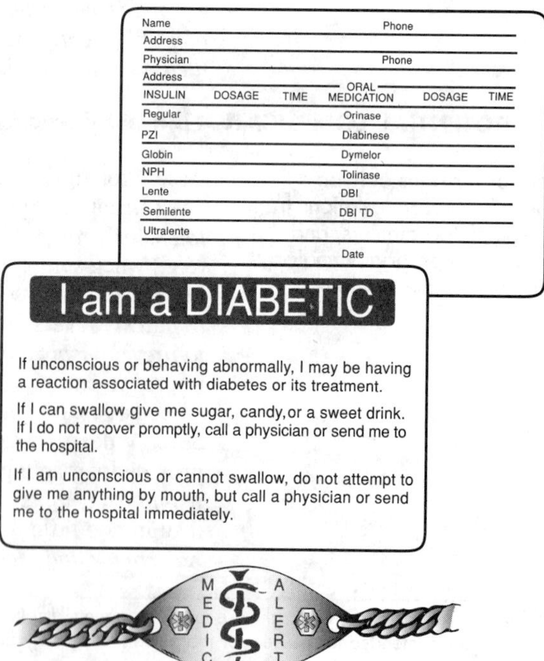

Fig. 46-11 Medical alerts: A patient with diabetes should carry a card and wear a bracelet or necklace that indicates diabetes. If the patient with diabetes is unconscious, these measures will ensure prompt and appropriate attention.

*For information regarding certified diabetes educators in your area or regarding the certification process, contact The American Association of Diabetes Educators, 444 N Michigan Ave, Suite 1240, Chicago, IL 60611. Phone: 800-338-DMED.

it is wise to have a letter from the physician explaining that the patient has diabetes and requires all the materials, particularly syringes, for ongoing health care.

Some travel involves time changes such as traveling coast to coast or across the international date line. The patient should contact the health care provider to plan an appropriate insulin schedule. Many patients find it easier and more predictable to take only regular insulin every 4 to 6 hours to cover insulin needs while on long airplane trips instead of trying to anticipate the peak of intermediate insulin and the availability of meals. During travel, most patients find it helpful to keep watches set to the time of the city of origin until they reach their destination. The key to travel when taking insulin is to know the type of insulin being taken, its onset of action, and the anticipated peak time. Meals or carry-along food can then be planned around this schedule.

Diabetes Education

The major educational objective is a level of self-management appropriate to the individual patient. Ideally, the patient should be taught about the disease and encouraged to achieve self-management with guidance only from the health care provider. The more in control the patient with diabetes can feel, the more likely the patient is to accept and adhere to the management program. The basis of self-management is a sound educational program related to diabetes. A knowledgeable patient should be able to make minor adjustments in insulin dosage and diet prescription to compensate for special circumstances, such as illness or increased exercise.

Not all patients with diabetes are capable of self-management. If the patient is not able to manage the disease, a family member may be able to assume this role. If the patient or the family cannot make decisions related to diabetes management, the nurse may identify appropriate resources outside the family. These resources can assist the patient and the family in outlining a feasible treatment program that meets their capabilities. Patient and health care provider resources are listed at the end of this chapter.

The American Diabetes Association offers pamphlets, booklets, and a bimonthly magazine called *Diabetes Forecast* for patients of all ages. Affiliates of the American Diabetes Association are located in all states. The American Diabetes Association also publishes materials and sponsors conferences for health care professionals concerned with diabetes research and management. It gives recognition to education programs that meet the national standards of diabetes education and can provide a list of these programs. Drug companies manufacturing diabetes-related products also have free educational material for patients and health care providers.

Treatment programs take time to learn. The theory and textbook information are only the beginning. The information must then be incorporated into the patient's lifestyle. The health care provider who educates the patient and family understands that the education process initially takes weeks to months and provides periodic reassessment after the basics have been learned and integrated.

Another useful strategy is to divide the teaching content into the level that must be learned right away and the level that can be scheduled for another time. Levels of diabetes education include survival, home management, and improvement of lifestyle. These levels are outlined in Table 46-13. The levels provide the diabetes educator with some structure for patient education and relieve the expectation that the patient will have to be taught everything in a short time.

In 1984 the National Diabetes Advisory Board established a set of standards to be used for ensuring the quality of diabetes patient education programs. The American Diabetes Association then developed a set of review criteria that specify the conditions under which each standard is to be met for a diabetes education program to be "recognized." It is believed that meeting the national standards and obtaining recognition will result in improvement in the overall quality of diabetes patient education programs. In addition, recognition is seen as a prerequisite to obtaining third-party reimbursement for patient education services nationally.[48]

Assessment of Learning Needs. After the initial diagnosis of diabetes has been made, the lifelong process of patient education begins. The nurse's understanding of diabetes mellitus is central to a successful teaching program. An assessment of the patient's knowledge of diabetes and lifestyle preferences is useful in planning the teaching program. Table 46-14 is an example of a diabetes patient education record that can provide the nurse with a framework related to the patient's learning needs. Based on the information obtained from the record, an educational plan can be developed to meet the patient's individual needs. Table 46-15 is a summary of educational needs that can be used to track the progress of the patient's educational program. The nurse should assess the patient's knowledge base frequently so that gaps in knowledge or incorrect or inaccurate ideas can be quickly corrected. The record can be reviewed with the patient to outline and contract for additional educational information. The record can also provide an efficient way for other health care providers to be aware of what the patient knows or needs to learn.

Patients are often treated in outpatient diabetes clinics. Frequently these clinics are staffed by diabetes nurse specialists. These specialists have preparation beyond the baccalaureate degree in diabetes and work collaboratively with physicians to manage patients with diabetes. The diabetes nurse specialist is also often available to the nursing staff for consultation in the acute-care setting. The diabetes outpatient clinic can provide specialized instruction, group interaction, and contact with other persons with diabetes. Often such clinics are run in accordance with the team concept. Consequently, an endocrinologist, a diabetes nurse specialist, diabetes nurse educator, dietitian, podiatrist, counselor, and social worker may be available to the patient at one visit.

Follow-Up Nursing Management

Although the educational emphasis is on self-care, the patient should be encouraged to also be a partner in care with the health care provider. In addition to carrying out the daily management routines, maintaining a schedule of

Table 46-13 Levels of Diabetes Education

Level 1
Educational guidelines for initial management of diabetes
Provide content required at time of diagnosis and represents basic or survival needs. Level is based on limitations of patient and family to accept and assimilate all there is to know about diabetes at time of diagnosis and limitations of some settings to provide additional education. *Example:* Capillary blood glucose monitoring and insulin administration and hypoglycemia prevention and management.
Aims
Educational activities provide patient and family with initial knowledge and skills to enable person to get along (survive) at time of initial diagnosis of diabetes.

Level 2
Educational guidelines for home management of diabetes
Place emphasis on increasing knowledge and flexibility as some experience is gained in living with diabetes. This is perceived as essential for every patient but must be tailored to individual needs and capacity. This type of educational experience is preferably offered in a nonhospital environment as close to home as possible. *Example:* Goals for control, diabetes diet management, and sick day guidelines.
Aims
Educational activities provide patient and family with diabetes skills and knowledge to participate in home management of tasks. Goal is to enable patient and family to become self-sufficient in daily management of diabetes. Patient and family members play an integral role in diabetes care and should be regarded as equal members of the health care team.

Level 3
Education guidelines for improvement of lifestyle
Present form of advanced learning viewed as enriching patient's life with flexibility, insight, and self-determination. Most patients are forced to discover this information by trial and error through experience. Although no educational program can or should entirely replace personal experience, the process need not be experienced by each person. *Example:* Exercise, adjusting insulin and lifestyle, stress management.
Aims
Educational offerings are aimed at increasing patient's and family's understanding of diabetes and focus on individual needs. Improved lifestyle suggests intelligent participation by patient in management of needs. Flexibility in management enables patient to participate in activities and ultimately leads to greater self-determination.

regular follow-up to assess the progress of the disease and additional education are necessary. Table 46-12 outlines a suggested follow-up schedule to aid in the long-term care of a patient with diabetes (see p. 1457).

COMPLICATIONS OF DIABETES

With the discovery and initial administration of insulin, it was believed that a cure for diabetes had been found. However, 70 years of insulin therapy has proved that insulin is not the total answer in the treatment of diabetes. Hyperglycemia-related problems do not cause death as often as they did before insulin was discovered. Other chronic complications of long-term therapy are responsible for more than 75% of all diabetic deaths.

The acute problems of diabetes are associated with severe, untreated hyperglycemia (e.g., DKA, HHNK) or the hypoglycemic side effects of treatment with GLAs. Chronic problems are primarily those of end organ disease from microangiopathy, macroangiopathy, and neuropathy. Hyperglycemia also plays a role in these complications, but the extent of this role has not yet been determined. Hyperglycemia may damage cells and tissue in at least two ways:

1. Metabolic dysfunction in the breakdown of glucose may lead to accumulation of damaging byproducts (e.g., sorbitol).

2. Glucose becomes abnormally bound to protein structures of the body and produces deleterious effects in nerves and blood vessels over time.

In June of 1993 the National Institute of Diabetes and Digestive and Kidney Diseases announced the results of a landmark medical study that began in 1983. Called the Diabetes Control and Complications Trial (DCCT), it compared different forms of diabetes treatment in preventing or slowing the complications of diabetes. The trial included more than 1400 people with insulin-dependent diabetes at 29 medical centers in the United States and Canada, half with no retinopathy at base line (the primary-prevention cohort) and the other half with mild retinopathy (the secondary intervention cohort). Patients were randomly assigned to one of two groups: *intensive* or *standard* treatment. The intensive treatment group took three or more insulin injections a day or used an insulin pump. The patients in the standard treatment group took one to two injections a day and tested their blood glucose once or twice a day. The intensive group was distinguished from the standard treatment group in terms of glycosylated hemoglobin levels and capillary blood glucose values throughout the study (average glycosylated hemoglobin in the intensive treatment group was about 7.2% and the standard treatment group was about 9% on a normal range 4.0% to 6.05%).

Table 46-14 Diabetes Patient Education Record

1. Demographic information Date: ____________
Name: ______________________________ Age: ______________________________
Race: ________ Sex (circle): M F Participant status (circle): Inpatient Outpatient
Level of education: __________ Occupation: ______________________________
Physician's name: ______________________________ Marital status (circle): Single Married Widowed Divorced

2. General medical condition
Height: ____________ Weight: ____________ % Ideal weight: ____________ Blood pressure: ____________
Hb_{A1c}: ________ Total cholesterol level: ____________ HDL: ____________ Triglycerides level: ____________
Allergies: ______________________________
Other medications: ______________________________
Other medical problems: ______________________________
Present health status: ______________________________

3. Diabetes history
Type of diabetes: ____________ Duration of diabetes: ____________
Treatment plan (check): _____ Insulin _____ OHAs _____ Diet alone
Monitoring system: Type: _______ Test times: _______ Product: _______ Usual AM glucose level: ____________
Attach monitoring log, if appropriate.
Name and type of insulin or OHA: Dose Times taken
______________ ______________ ______________
______________ ______________ ______________
Describe any side effects to OHAs/insulin: ____________
Complications (check):
___Retinopathy ___ Neuropathy ___ Renal ___ Foot ___ Macrovascular ___ Other (specify)
Describe: ______________________________
Incidences of DKA, hypoglycemia, hyperglycemia (date, etc.): ______________________________

4. Dietary habits
If prescribed, daily caloric intake: ____________ Food or foods to avoid: ____________
Indicate times of Breakfast ____________ Lunch ____________ Dinner ____________
Attach dietary recall data or nutrition workup, if appropriate.

5. Physical activity habits
Does patient have regular exercise program (20 min, 3 days/wk)? Yes ________ No ________
If yes, indicate:

Type	Duration	Intensity (Circle)
____________	____________	Light Medium Heavy
____________	____________	Light Medium Heavy
		Light Medium Heavy

6. Diabetes education history
Prior diabetes education? Patient/NP___ Yes ___ No Significant Other ___ Yes ___ No
Prior education: ______________________________
Special educational needs: ______________________________
Will significant other participate in program? Yes ____ No ____ Relationship: ____________

7. Source of referral (check one)
___ Physician /NP ___ Self-referred ___ Facility staff ___ Community agency ___ Other (specify): ____________

8. Social history
Cigarettes/day: ________ Alcoholic drinks/wk: ________
No. in household: ________ Relationship: ______________________________
Types of health/medical insurance: ______________________________

Modified from *Meeting the standards: a manual for completing the ADA application for recognition,* ed 3, Alexandria, VA, 1991, American Diabetes Association.

Table 46-15 Summary of Educational Needs Assessment and Progress Form

Content Area	Preprogram*		Taught†	Postprogram‡	
Patient			**Date/initial/method**		
1. Understands general facts of diabetes	Y	N		Y	N
2. Is well adjusted psychologically in relation to diabetes	Y	N		Y	N
3. Adequately or appropriately involves family in diabetes care	Y	N		Y	N
4. Understands and practices effective nutritional management	Y	N		Y	N
5. Understands benefits of and engages in appropriate exercise	Y	N		Y	N
6. Monitors blood or urine glucose levels appropriately	Y	N		Y	N
7. Properly uses insulin or OHAs	Y	N		Y	N
8. Knows relationship among nutrition, exercise, and medication	Y	N		Y	N
9. Recognizes and responds appropriately to symptoms of hypoglycemia and hyperglycemia	Y	N		Y	N
10. Understands effects of illness on diabetes management and responds appropriately	Y	N		Y	N
	Y	N		Y	N
11. Practices proper hygiene (skin care, foot care, dental care) to prevent complications of diabetes	Y	N		Y	N
12. Cooperates in therapeutic management and rehabilitation of diabetes complications	Y	N		Y	N
13. Understands benefits and responsibilities of self-management in diabetes	Y	N		Y	N
14. Effectively uses available health care systems	Y	N		Y	N
15. Makes appropriate use of community resources	Y	N		Y	N

Modified from *Meeting the standards: a manual for completing the American Diabetes Association application for recognition,* ed 3, Alexandria, VA, 1991, American Diabetes Association.
OHAs, Oral hypoglycemic agents; *N,* no; *Y,* yes.
*Preprogram: Did patient know content before education?
†Taught: Was content taught? Put date, initials (instructor's name must accompany initials at least once); method of instruction (L, lecture; D, demonstration; R, return demonstration; V, video; X, other); and format (1/1, one to one; CL, classroom; G, group; SI, self-instruction module).
‡Postprogram: Did patient know content after education?

The results found that in the primary prevention cohort, intensive therapy reduced the adjusted mean risk for the development of retinopathy by 76%, as compared with conventional therapy. In the secondary-intervention cohort, intensive therapy slowed the progression of retinopathy by 54%. In the two cohorts combined, intensive therapy reduced the occurrence of microalbuminuria by 39% and of albuminuria (urinary albumin excretion of ≥300 mg per 24 hours) by 54%, and that of clinical neuropathy by 60%. The chief adverse event associated with intensive therapy was a two- to-threefold increase in severe hypoglycemia.[40]

The American Diabetes Association issued a position statement regarding the DCCT:

> A primary treatment goal in insulin-dependent diabetes mellitus (IDDM) should be blood glucose control at least equal to that achieved in the intensively treated cohort. This goal may not apply to all patients with IDDM and must be based on clinical judgment. Of importance, intensively treated patients had a three-fold greater risk of hypoglycemia than did patients in the control group. Because serious hypoglycemia is dangerous, "tight" control goals may have to be sacrificed in people in whom frequent or severe hypoglycemia cannot be avoided by treatment modification.[41]

Acute Metabolic Complications

The acute problems of DKA and HHNK coma arise from events associated with hyperglycemia and insufficient insulin. A problem that may arise from too much insulin or an excessive dose of an OHA is *hypoglycemia* (also referred to as *insulin reaction* or *low blood glucose*), which occurs when the level of available blood glucose falls. It is important for the health care provider to be able to distinguish between hyperglycemia and hypoglycemia because hypoglycemia can constitute a serious threat and requires immediate attention. Table 46-16 compares the manifestations, causes, management, and prevention of hyperglycemia and hypoglycemia.

Diabetic Ketoacidosis. DKA, also referred to as *diabetic acidosis* and *diabetic coma,* may develop quickly or over several days or weeks. It can be caused by too little insulin accompanied by increased caloric intake, physical or emotional stress, or undiagnosed diabetes. DKA is most likely to occur in type I diabetes but may be seen in type II in conditions of severe illness or stress when extra demand for insulin cannot be met by the pancreas.

When the insulin supply is insufficient, glucose cannot be properly used for cellular energy. In response to cellular starvation, the body releases and breaks down stored fats and protein to provide the needed energy. Free fatty acids from stored triglycerides are released and metabolized in the liver in such large quantities that ketones are formed (ketonemia). Excess ketones alter the pH balance, and acidosis develops. More water is lost as ketones are excreted (ketonuria) in an attempt to balance the pH (Fig. 46-12).

Table 46-16 Comparison of Hyperglycemia and Hypoglycemia

Hyperglycemia	Hypoglycemia	Hyperglycemia	Hypoglycemia
Manifestations* Blood glucose >500mg/dl (27.8 mmol/L) Increase in urination Increase in appetite followed by lack of appetite Weakness, fatigue Blurred vision Headache Glycosuria Nausea and vomiting Abdominal cramps Progression to DKA or HHNK	Blood glucose <50 mg/dl (2.8 mmol/L) Cold, clammy skin Numbness of fingers, toes, mouth Rapid heartbeat Emotional changes Headache Nervousness, tremors Faintness, dizziness Unsteady gait, slurred speech Hunger Changes in vision Seizures, coma	**Treatment** Physician's attention Continuance of diabetes medication as ordered Frequent checking of blood and urine specimens and recording of results Hourly drinking of fluids	Immediate ingestion of 5-20 g of simple carbohydrates Ingestion of another 5-20 g of simple carbohydrates in 15 min if no relief obtained Contacting of physician if no relief obtained Discussion with physician about medication dosage
Causes Too much food Too little or no diabetes medication Inactivity Emotional, physical stress Poor absorption of insulin	Alcohol intake with food Too little food—delayed, omitted, inadequate intake Too much diabetic medication Too much exercise without compensation Diabetes medication or food taken at wrong time Loss of weight with change in medication Use of β-blockers interfering with recognition of symptoms	**Preventive Measures** Taking of prescribed dose of medication at proper time Accurate administration of insulin Maintenance of diet Maintenance of good personal hygiene Adherence to sick-day rules when ill Checking of blood for glucose as ordered Contacting of physician regarding ketonuria Wearing of diabetic identification	Taking of prescribed dose of medication at proper time Accurate administration of insulin Ingestion of all ordered diet foods at proper time Provision of compensation for exercise Ability to recognize and know symptoms and treat them immediately Carrying of simple carbohydrates Education of friends, family, fellow employees about symptoms and treatment Checking blood glucose as ordered

*There is usually a gradual onset of symptoms in hyperglycemia and a rapid onset in hypoglycemia.

Gluconeogenesis from protein is the last resource used by the body as a compensatory response to provide a cellular energy source. The result is an increase in blood glucose and nitrogen. However, because of the prevailing insulin deficiency, this glucose resource cannot be used and the blood glucose level rises further, adding to the osmotic diuresis. Dehydration and loss of electrolytes, particularly potassium, ensue. The patient's skin becomes dry and loose, and the eyeballs become soft and sunken. Hypotension with a weak, rapid pulse may develop.

Vomiting caused by the acidosis results in more fluid and electrolyte losses. The continual bicarbonate loss adds to the acidosis. Finally, Kussmaul respirations (rapid, deep breathing associated with dyspnea) begin to remove carbonic acid through the exhalation of carbon dioxide. Acetone is noted on the breath as a sweet, fruity odor.

Renal failure may eventually occur from hypovolemic shock. This failure causes the retention of ketones and glucose, and the acidosis progresses. The patient becomes comatose as a result of the neurologic stressors of dehydration, electrolyte imbalance, and acidosis. If the condition is not treated, death is inevitable.

Therapeutic management. Before the advent of self-monitoring of blood glucose, patients with DKA required hospitalization for treatment. Today, hospitalization may not be required. In instances where fluid and electrolyte imbalance is not severe and self-monitoring of blood glucose can be done by the patient or someone in the household, less severe forms of DKA may be managed on an outpatient basis. However, other factors, such as presence of fever, nausea and vomiting, or diarrhea; altered mental status; nature of the cause of the ketoacidosis; and availability of frequent communication with the physician (every few hours), must also be considered in this decision.

Regardless of the setting in which it occurs, DKA is a serious condition that proceeds rapidly and must be treated promptly. See Table 46-17 for the emergency management of a patient with DKA. Treatment is aimed at immediate administration of insulin, replacement of fluid to correct hypovolemia, and replacement of electrolytes to correct imbalances.

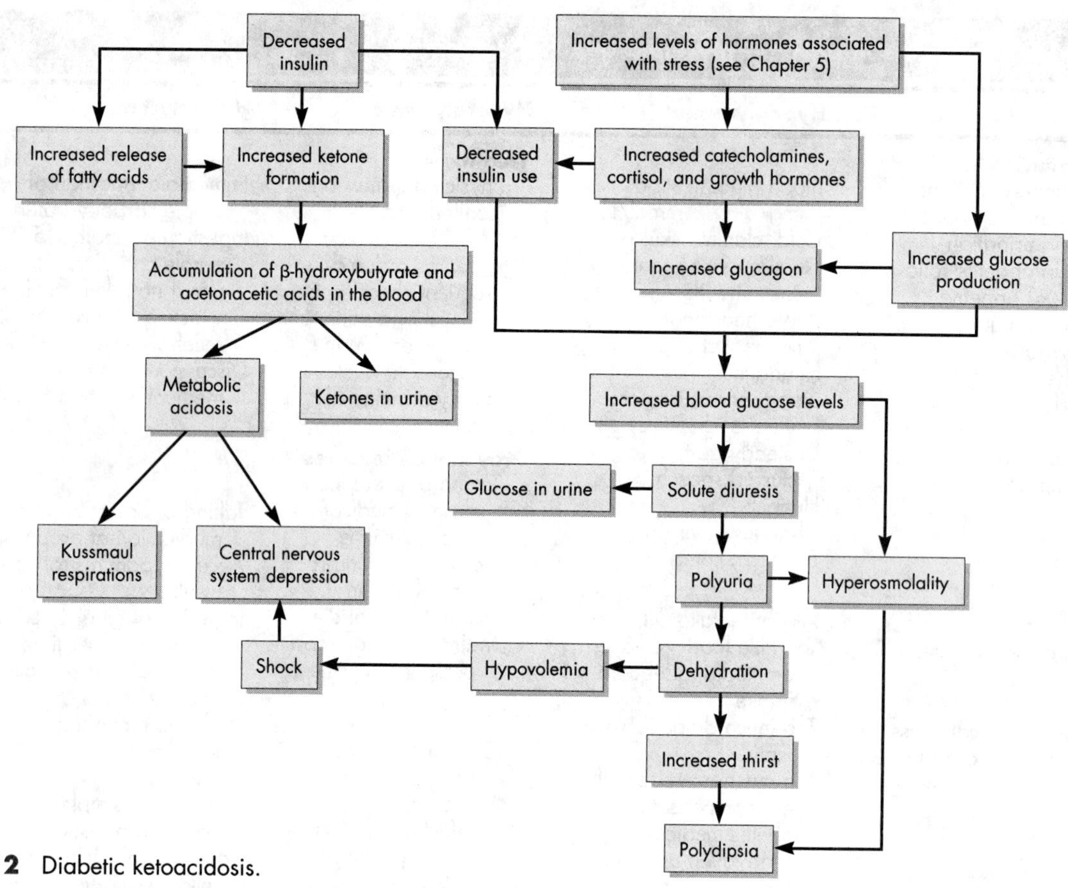

Fig. 46-12 Diabetic ketoacidosis.

The preferred treatment for DKA is the low-dose insulin IV infusion method. In this method a loading dose of 25 to 50 units of insulin is administered as a bolus, then 5 to 10 units per hour in normal saline solution are administered until ketoacidosis is reversed.[38] This insulin therapy is continued until a blood glucose level of 250 mg/dl (13.9 mmol/L) is reached. When the blood glucose level reaches 250 mg/dl (13.9 mmol/L), a solution containing 5% to 10% glucose (e.g., 5% dextrose in saline solution) is given to prevent hypoglycemia along with IV or SC insulin as needed to maintain blood glucose control.

Fluid and electrolyte therapy is aimed at replacing extracellular and intracellular water and deficits of sodium, chloride, bicarbonate, potassium, phosphate, magnesium, and nitrogen. The principal goal of potassium therapy is to prevent hypokalemia. Regardless of the initial plasma potassium value, the total body potassium deficit is large. Early potassium replacement is essential because hypokalemia remains a significant cause of unnecessary and avoidable mortality during treatment of DKA.

Assessment of blood pressure, pulse, and tissue turgor; cardiac monitoring; and determination of central venous pressure give some indications of the degree of hypovolemia. Bicarbonate is usually not given to correct acidosis unless the condition is severe (pH <7.0). Indiscriminate use of bicarbonate may reverse acidosis too quickly and result in severe hypokalemia, which can produce potentially fatal cardiac dysrhythmias.

Hyperglycemic Hyperosmolar Nonketosis. HHNK occurs in the patient with diabetes who is able to produce enough insulin to prevent DKA but not enough to prevent severe hyperglycemia, osmotic diuresis, and extracellular fluid depletion (Fig. 46-13). The increasing hyperglycemia causes intracellular dehydration because of a shift of fluid from the intracellular to the extracellular space. This causes neurologic abnormalities such as somnolence, coma, seizures, hemiparesis, and aphasia. HHNK often occurs in the older adult patient with type II diabetes. There is usually a history of inadequate fluid intake, increasing mental depression, and polyuria.

Therapeutic management. HHNK constitutes a medical emergency. This acute complication has a mortality rate greater than 50%.[42] The immediate therapy to reverse this hyperosmolar state consists of the rapid administration of IV solutions. From 6 to 20 L of fluid may have to be given during the first 24 to 48 hours. Depending on the degree of dehydration, either 0.9% or 0.45% sodium chloride is used. Regular insulin is given IV to aid in reducing the hyperglycemia. When blood glucose levels fall to 250 mg/dl (13.9 mmol/L), IV fluids containing glucose should be administered. Electrolytes are monitored and replaced as needed. Vital signs, intake and output, tissue turgor, and

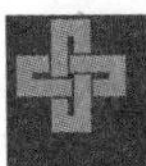

Table 46-17 Emergency Management: Diabetic Ketoacidosis

Possible Etiologies

Undiagnosed or untreated diabetic condition, insulin not taken as prescribed, presence of infection

Possible Assessment Findings

Dry mouth, thirst
Abdominal pain
Nausea and vomiting
Gradually increasing restlessness, confusion, stupor
Red, dry, warm skin; eyes that appear sunken
Breath odor of acetone
Rapid, weak pulse
Labored breathing

Management

- Administer O_2 via nasal cannula or non-rebreather mask and monitor for respiratory distress.
- Establish IV access with one large gauge catheter and administer normal saline.
- Determine whether patient has diabetes, time of last food intake, and time and amount of last insulin injection.
- Do not administer anything by mouth unless patient is fully alert.
- Monitor vital signs including level of consciousness and O_2 saturation.
- If patient has blood glucose monitoring equipment available, check blood glucose level. If glucose level is <70 mg/dl (3.9 mmol/L) and patient is alert, administer high-carbohydrate treatment such as juice, or sugar drink. If blood glucose is elevated >400 mg/dl (22.2 mmol/L) or meter reads "high," seek emergency medical assistance.
- If no monitoring equipment is available and patient is unconscious, give glucagon l mg IM or SC or 50 ml of 50% Dextrose IV. If blood glucose is high, patient will not be harmed but if blood glucose is low, further deterioration of mental status can be prevented.

IM, Intramuscular; *IV*, intravenous; *SC*, subcutaneous.

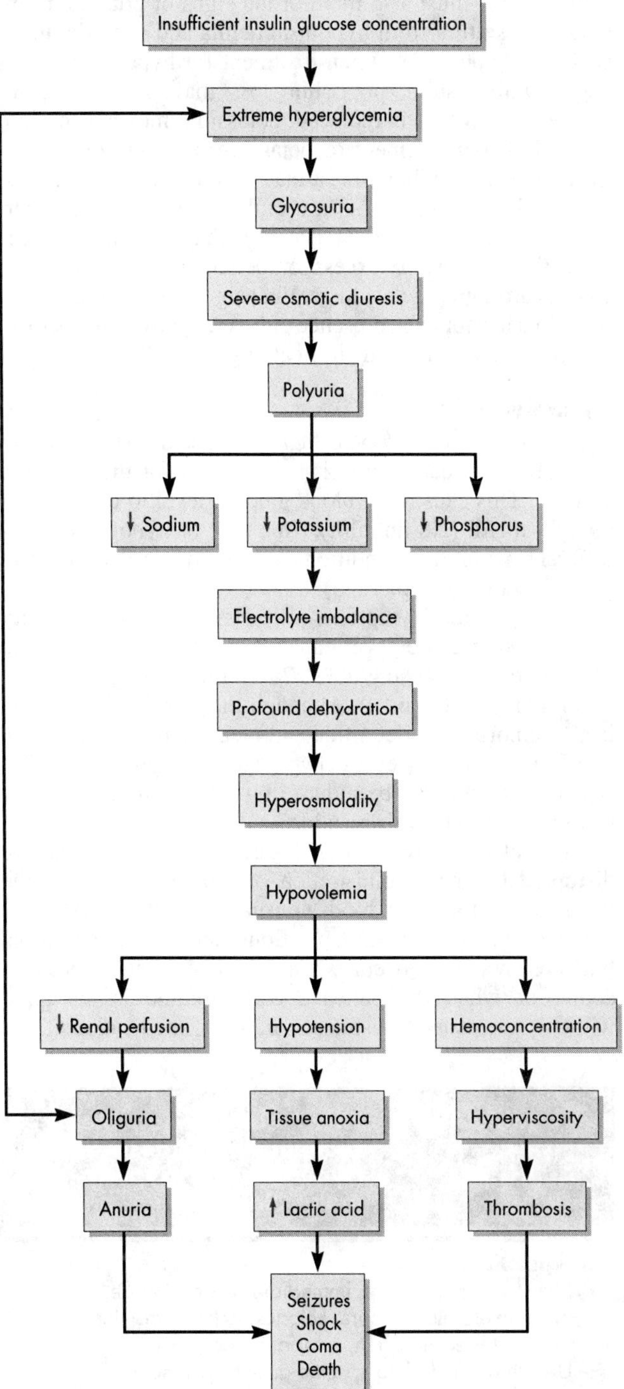

Fig. 46-13 Pathophysiology of hyperglycemic hyperosmolar nonketosis.

cardiac monitoring are assessed to monitor fluid and electrolyte loss.

The management for both DKA and HHNK is similar except that HHNK requires greater fluid replacement (Table 46-18). Once the patient is stabilized, attempts to detect and correct the underlying precipitating cause should be initiated.

NURSING MANAGEMENT

DIABETIC KETOACIDOSIS AND HYPERGLYCEMIC HYPEROSMOLAR NONKETOSIS

When hospitalized, the patient is closely monitored with appropriate blood and urine tests. The nurse is responsible for monitoring blood glucose and urine for output and ketones as well as using laboratory data to direct care.

Areas that need monitoring are administration of IV fluids to correct dehydration, administration of insulin therapy to reduce blood glucose and serum acetone, administration of electrolytes to correct electrolyte imbalance, assessment of renal status, assessment of the cardiopulmonary status related to hydration and electrolyte levels, and monitoring of the level of consciousness.

The nurse must also monitor the signs of potassium imbalance resulting from hypoinsulinemia and osmotic diuresis (see Chapter 13). When treatment for hyperglycemia is begun with insulin, potassium loss may initially be increased. As insulin is replaced, potassium moves back into the cell. This movement of potassium into and out of extracellular fluid influences cardiac functioning. For this reason, cardiac monitoring is a useful aid in detecting hyperkalemia and hypokalemia because characteristic changes indicating potassium excess or deficit are observable on electrocardiographic readings. Vital signs should be assessed often to determine the presence of fever, hypovolemic shock, tachycardia, and Kussmaul breathing.

Hypoglycemia

Hypoglycemia, or *low blood glucose*, occurs when proportionately too much insulin is in the blood for the available glucose. This causes the blood glucose level to drop to less than 50 mg/dl (2.8 mmol/L). This type of hypoglycemia is different from the condition commonly termed reactive hypoglycemia (see p. 1473).

Hypoglycemic symptoms may also occur when a very high blood glucose level falls too rapidly (e.g., a blood glucose level of 300 mg/dl [16.7 mmol/L] falling quickly to 180 mg/dl [10 mmol/L]). Although the blood glucose level is above normal by definition and measurement, the sudden metabolic shift can evoke hypoglycemic symptoms. This type of situation can be induced by too vigorous treatment of hyperglycemia with insulin.

The balance between blood glucose and insulin can be disrupted by the administration of too much insulin, the ingestion of too little food, unusual amounts of exercise, and delayed eating. Insulin reactions can occur at any time, but most reactions occur when the GLA is at its peak of action or when the patient's daily routine is disrupted without adequate adjustments in diet, medications, and activity. Although hypoglycemia is more common with insulin therapy, it can occur with OHAs and may be severe and persist for an extended time as a result of the longer half-lives of active metabolites of some OHAs.

A decrease in available blood glucose can result in sympathetic nervous system activation with the release of epinephrine. This results in manifestations of cold sweats, weakness, trembling, nervousness, irritability, pallor, and increased heart rate. The clinical manifestations of hypoglycemia vary with each patient. The brain depends on a constant supply of glucose because it is unable to store glucose or glycogen. If that supply is inadequate, the patient will experience confusion, fatigue, and abnormal behavior that can resemble alcohol intoxication.

In recent years the physiology of glucose recovery has been shown to depend on glucagon and epinephrine. In type I diabetes, secretion and use of one or both of these substances may be impaired. As a result, some type I patients do not have the early warning symptoms produced by epinephrine. Rather, they have neuroglycopenia, that is, the more advanced symptoms of cerebral glucose deficit. The symptoms of this condition are irritability, irrational behavior, dizziness, tremors, and loss of consciousness. This may result from the development of autonomic neuropathy or from treatment with β-adrenergic blocking agents.[43] These patients must be managed with intensive education and instruction in the prevention of hypoglycemia.

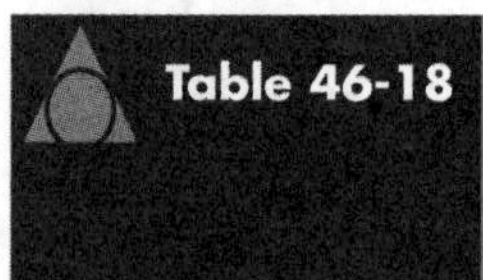

Table 46-18 Therapeutic Management: Diabetic Ketoacidosis and Hyperglycemic Hyperosmolar Nonketosis

Diagnostic
- Blood work, including immediate blood glucose, complete blood count, ketones, pH, electrolytes, blood urea nitrogen, arterial blood gases
- Urinalysis, including specific gravity, pH, sugar, acetone

Therapeutic
- Administration of regular insulin
- Administration of intravenous fluids
- Electrolyte replacement
- Assessment of mental status
- Recording of intake and output
- Central venous pressure monitoring (if indicated)
- Assessment of blood glucose level
- Assessment of blood and urine for ketones
- Cardiac monitoring

THERAPEUTIC AND NURSING MANAGEMENT

HYPOGLYCEMIA

The preferred treatment of hypoglycemia is prevention. However, if hypoglycemia occurs, the patient should be able to reverse the situation before medical assistance is required. The patient's ability to do this depends on the state of alertness and ability to swallow and the availability of a quick-acting carbohydrate source.

At the first sign of hypoglycemia the patient should ingest 5 to 20 g of a simple (fast-acting) carbohydrate, such as 120 to 180 ml of orange juice, 180 to 240 ml of regular soft drink, two packets of sugar, or five or six hard candies. Overtreatment with large quantities of quick-acting carbohydrates such as a whole candy bar should be avoided.

If the symptoms are still present after 10 to 15 minutes, ingestion of 5 to 20 g of carbohydrate should be repeated.[44] Once the symptoms have improved, the patient should eat a longer-lasting carbohydrate such as bread or milk to prevent symptoms from recurring. Commercial products such as gels or tablets containing specific amounts of quick-acting carbohydrate are convenient for carrying in a purse or pocket to be used in such situations. High-fat foods and high-protein foods should not be used initially to correct hypoglycemia. These food sources are metabolized too slowly to be effective as immediate treatment.

If there is little discernible improvement in the patient's condition after two to three doses of 5 to 20 g of simple carbohydrate within 30 minutes or if the patient is not alert enough to swallow, 1 mg of glucagon may be administered with the same technique used for an insulin injection, although an IM injection in a site such as the deltoid will result in a quicker response. Glucagon stimulates a strong hepatic response to convert glycogen to glucose making glucose rapidly available. Once the patient is receiving medical care, a concentrated glucose solution may also be administered slowly IV until the patient regains consciousness. Blood glucose level must be carefully monitored during the treatment. (See Table 46-19 for a summary of therapeutic and nursing management.)

With effective treatment, hypoglycemia can be quickly reversed. Once the acute hypoglycemia has been reversed, the nurse should explore with the patient the reasons why the situation developed. This assessment may indicate the need for additional education of the patient and the family to avoid future episodes of hypoglycemia. The danger of hypoglycemic reactions must be stressed because memory and learning impairment can result from repeated episodes of severe hypoglycemia.

DKA, HHNK, and hypoglycemia constitute potentially life-threatening situations and may be frightening to the patient and the family. The nurse should attempt to keep the family members informed about the patient's progress to relieve their anxiety. The nurse's calm, competent manner in caring for the patient can provide assurance to the acutely ill patient and the family.

Chronic Complications

Angiopathy. Angiopathy, or blood vessel disease, is estimated to account for the majority of deaths among patients with diabetes. Many factors are being investigated in the development of angiopathy. These chronic blood vessel dysfunctions are divided into two categories: macroangiopathy and microangiopathy.

Macroangiopathy. Macroangiopathy, or disease of large and medium-sized blood vessels, is essentially atherosclerosis and arteriosclerotic vascular disease characterized by a higher frequency and earlier onset than in the nondiabetic population. The degree of vascular damage appears to be related to the duration of the diabetes, not to its severity. Although atherosclerotic plaque formation is believed to have a genetic origin, its development seems to be promoted by the altered lipid metabolism common to diabetes (Table 46-20). Tight glucose control may help delay the atherosclerotic process.[40]

The complications resulting from macroangiopathy are cerebrovascular, cardiovascular, and peripheral vascular disease. Although genetic makeup cannot be altered, a patient with diabetes can diminish other risk factors associated with macroangiopathy, such as obesity, smoking, hypertension, high fat intake, and low activity level.

In addition to the association of type I and type II diabetes with ischemic heart disease, recent data suggest that hyperinsulinemia is itself an independent risk factor for

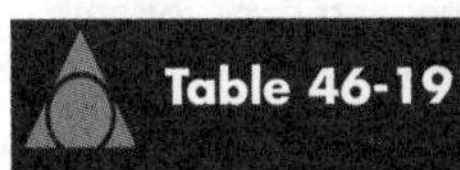

Table 46-19 Therapeutic Management: Hypoglycemia

Diagnostic
- Stat blood glucose
- History (if possible)

Therapeutic
- Determination of cause of hypoglycemia (after correction of condition)

Conscious patient
- Administration of 5-20 g of quick-acting CHO (e.g., 6-8 oz regular soda, 1 tbs syrup or honey, 4 tsp jelly, 4-6 oz orange juice, 8 oz milk, 2½ tsp sugar, commercial dextrose products [per label instructions])
- Repetition of treatment in 15 min (if no improvement)
- Administration of additional food of longer-acting CHO (e.g., slice of bread, crackers) after subsiding of symptoms
- Immediate notification of physician or emergency service (if patient outside hospital) if symptoms not subsiding after 2 to 3 administrations of quick-acting CHO

Worsening symptoms or unconscious patient
- SC or IM injection of 1 mg of glucagon
- Administration of 50 ml 50% IV glucose

CHO, Carbohydrate; *IM,* intramuscular; *IV,* intravenous; *SC,* subcutaneous.

Table 46-20 Mechanisms of Macrovascular Disease in Diabetes

Cellular Mechanisms
- Arterial endothelial cell injury (sorbitol accumulation, hypoxia, hypertension, immune complexes)
- Foam cell activation (smooth muscle cell migration, monocyte/macrophage activation)

Hemostatic Mechanisms
- Platelet dysfunction (aggregation, thromboxane production, growth factor release)
- Clotting factor abnormalities (raised fibrinogen, factor VII, factor VIII, reduced fibrinolysis)
- Cell-cell forces (RBC rigidity)

Lipoprotein Abnormalities
- Hypertriglyceridemia (increased VLDL, remnant particles, reduced lipoprotein lipase activity, reduced HDL in type II diabetes mellitus)
- Hypercholesterolemia (increased LDL in type II diabetes mellitus)
- Apolipoprotein abnormalities (e.g., glycosylation)

Other Mechanisms
- Chronic renal disease secondary to diabetes (raised VLDL, LDL; lowered HDL; hypertension)
- Increased arterial wall proteoglycans (trapping of lipoproteins, local cell activation)
- Abnormalities of collagen, fibronectin (synthesis, glycosylation)
- Insulin-induced lipogenesis, esterification
- Intramural coronary vascular (macro and micro) disease

HDL, High-density lipoproteins; *LDL,* low-density lipoproteins; *VLDL,* very-low-density lipoproteins; *RBC,* red blood cell.

cardiovascular disease. Insulin resistance has also been implicated in the pathogenesis of essential hypertension and dyslipidemia. The term *Syndrome X* is applied to the clinical association of insulin resistance, hypertension, and increased very-low-density lipoprotein (VLDL) and decreased high-density lipoprotein (HDL) cholesterol concentrations. The role of hyperinsulinemia in the pathogenesis of hypertension is not well understood but it may directly promote hepatic VLDL production even when there is resistance to the effect of insulin.[45]

Microangiopathy. Microangiopathy, or disease of the small blood vessels, is different from macroangiopathy in that it is specific to diabetes. Microangiopathy is the result of thickening of the basement membranes in the capillaries and arterioles, a highly characteristic concomitant of long-term diabetes mellitus. Although microangiopathy can be found throughout the body, the areas most noticeably affected are the eyes (*retinopathy*), the kidneys (*nephropathy*), and the skin (*dermopathy*). Thickening of the basement membrane has been found in some persons with diabetes before or at the time of diagnosis or before the onset of symptoms of diabetes mellitus. However, clinical manifestations usually do not appear until 15 to 20 years after the onset of diabetes.[46]

Peripheral vascular disease. Peripheral vascular disease (PVD) is a combination of microangiopathy and macroangiopathy as well as clotting abnormalities. The legs and feet are most often affected in diabetes mellitus, and associated problems account for 20% of hospitalizations of patients with diabetes. The sequelae of PVD can lead to infection, gangrene, and amputation. Signs of PVD include intermittent claudication, pain at rest, cold feet, loss of hair, delayed capillary filling, and dependent rubor. The disease is diagnosed by history, Doppler findings, and angiography. Management centers on control or reduction of risk factors, particularly smoking, high cholesterol intake, and hypertension. Antibiotics are necessary when infection is present. If the infection cannot be reversed with antibiotic therapy, amputation may be necessary. Proper care of the feet is crucial for the patient with PVD; guidelines for foot care are listed in Table 46-21. Approximately 6% of the U.S. diabetic population (14 million) experience lower extremity amputation because of diabetic foot ulcers.[47]

Table 46-21 Guidelines for Foot Care

1. Wash feet daily with a mild soap and *warm* water. Test water temperature with hands first.
2. Pat feet dry gently, especially between toes.
3. Examine feet daily for cuts, blisters, swelling, and red, tender areas. Do not depend on feeling sores. If eyesight is poor, have others inspect feet.
4. Use lanolin on feet to prevent skin from drying and cracking. Do not apply between toes.
5. Use mild foot powder on sweaty feet. Powder feet only, not shoes.
6. Do not use commercial remedies to remove calluses or corns.
7. Cleanse cuts with *warm* water and mild soap, covering with clean dressing. Do not use iodine, rubbing alcohol, or strong adhesives.
8. Report skin infections or nonhealing sores to health care provider immediately.
9. Cut toenails even with rounded contour of toes. Do not cut down corners. Soak nails before cutting.
10. Separate overlapping toes with cotton or lambswool.
11. Break in new shoes slowly. Avoid open-toe, open-heel, and high-heel shoes. Leather shoes are preferred to plastic ones. Wear slippers with soles. Do not go barefoot. Shake out shoes before use.
12. Wear clean, absorbent (cotton or wool) socks or stockings that have not been mended. Colored socks must be colorfast.
13. Do not wear clothing that leaves impressions, hindering circulation.
14. Do not use hot water bottles or heating pads to warm feet. Wear socks for warmth.
15. Guard against frostbite.
16. Exercise feet daily either by walking or by flexing and extending feet in suspended position. Avoid prolonged sitting, standing, and crossing of legs.

Diabetic retinopathy. The term retinopathy literally means disease of the retina; however, *diabetic retinopathy* refers to the microangiopathic process seen in a patient with diabetes. After 10 years with diabetes mellitus, 50% of patients demonstrate diabetic retinopathy; after 15 years, approximately 80% of patients have some retinal disease.

The primary problems in diabetic retinopathy are microvascular damage and occlusion of retinal capillaries. Retinopathy is classified as background retinopathy, preproliferative retinopathy, and proliferative retinopathy. The types are outlined in Table 46-22. In *background retinopathy*, the most common form, partial occlusion of the small blood vessels in the retina causes the development of microaneurysms in the capillary walls. These microaneurysms are so weak that capillary fluid leaks out, causing retinal edema and eventually hard exudates or intraretinal hemorrhages. Vision may be affected if the macula is involved. *Preproliferative retinopathy* is distinct from background retinopathy and indicates further destruction of retinal capillaries.

Proliferative retinopathy, the most severe form, involves the retina and the vitreous. When retinal capillaries become occluded, new blood vessels are formed (*neovascularization*) to supply the retina with blood. These new vessels hemorrhage easily and may produce vitreous contraction. The vessels are torn and bleed into the vitreous cavity, preventing light from reaching the retina. The patient sees black or red spots or lines. If these new blood vessels pull the retina while the vitreous contracts, causing a tear, partial or complete retinal detachment will occur. If the macula is involved, vision is lost. Without treatment, more than half of patients with proliferative diabetic retinopathy will be blind within five years.[48]

The two most common forms of treatment of diabetic retinopathy are photocoagulation and vitrectomy. *Photocoagulation* by laser converts light energy into heat and

Table 46-22 Types of Diabetic Retinopathy

Type	Pathologic Alteration
Background	Microvasculature of retina of eye is damaged. Capillaries become damaged, resulting in development of microaneurysms (seen as tiny red dots on retina).
Preproliferative	Possible progression from background retinopathy represents further destruction of retinal capillaries and development of capillary dropout.
Proliferative	Abnormal blood vessels (neovascularization) grow on surface of retina. Vessels can grow into chamber of vitreous surface and can hemorrhage, filling vitreous chamber with blood.

Modified from Peragallo V: *A core curriculum for diabetes education,* Chicago, 1993, American Association of Diabetes Educators.

coagulates the tissue in the area where the light is directed. It is particularly useful with neovascularization because the laser obliterates new vessels, stopping the hemorrhage. It can be done on an outpatient basis in a short time.

Vitrectomy is the aspiration of blood, membrane, and fibers from the inside of the eye through a small incision just behind the cornea. This form of surgery is particularly useful for the treatment of organized vitreous hemorrhage and traction retinal detachments.

Persons with diabetes are also prone to other visual problems. Glaucoma occurs as a result of the occlusion of the outflow channels secondary to neovascularization. This type of glaucoma is difficult to treat and often results in blindness. Cataracts occur with increasing frequency in the patient with diabetes. Although the process is similar to that of senile cataracts, it occurs at an earlier age in the patient with diabetes. Diabetic retinopathy may occur concurrently with nephropathy and parallel its progression. Although the vast majority of diabetic patients have some degree of retinopathy, nephropathy develops in only 35% to 45% of patients with IDDM.[46]

Nephropathy. Diabetic nephropathy is now the leading cause of end-stage renal disease (ESRD) in the United States.[49] Mild proteinuria develops in 70% of persons with diabetes mellitus and may progress to more serious involvement and ESRD. This occurs as a result of microvascular abnormalities associated with diabetes mellitus, but these processes are not clearly understood.

Microangiopathy in the kidneys causes diffuse and nodular glomerulosclerosis. Diffuse glomerulosclerosis affects the basement membranes of all glomerular capillaries, usually in both kidneys. The basement membranes become thickened and leaky. Sclerosis of glomerular vascular tufts leads to progressive renal failure. In nodular glomerulosclerosis (Kimmelstiel-Wilson lesions), nodules develop in the glomeruli. In advanced cases most glomeruli are involved. In more than 70% of patients, the course of diabetes nephropathy is complicated by the presence of hypertension. The monitoring and treatment of hypertension is an important part of diabetes management and is believed to be a significant factor in controlling the progression of nephropathy. (See Chapter 30 for a discussion of hypertension and Chapter 44 for a discussion of acute and chronic renal failure.) The majority of insulin-dependent diabetics with diabetic nephropathy die of cardiovascular disease. The risk of cardiovascular disease is 30 to 40 times higher in patients with nephropathy than in those diabetics who did not develop renal diseases.[49]

ESRD requires treatment by either dialysis or kidney transplantation. A patient in the later stages of nephropathy may require an adjustment in insulin and OHAs because of a loss of the insulin-degradative function of the kidneys and an abnormal peripheral insulin response.

Another treatment option for ESRD resulting from type I diabetes is a kidney-pancreas transplantation. The goals of transplantation are to eliminate the need for exogenous insulin and dietary restrictions and to prevent or stabilize microvascular and neuropathic complications of diabetes.[50] Current 1 year graft survival rates are nearing 80%. Evidence is accumulating that improvement occurs in microvascular and neuropathic complications of diabetes after transplantation. The most common complications are associated with fluid and electrolyte imbalances that can be managed with careful attention to replacement.

Neuropathy. Neuropathy is probably one of the most common complications of diabetes in adults. However, its cause is unclear. Mononeuropathic conditions (i.e., single nerve branch involvement) are theorized to develop from microangiopathy, whereas the more diffuse neuropathic conditions are attributed to metabolic defects and the accumulation of by-products in the nerve tissue. The result is reduced nerve conduction and demyelinization. Neuropathy can precede, accompany, or follow the diagnosis of diabetes.

The two major categories of diabetic neuropathy are neuropathic conditions of the peripheral nervous system, including symmetric peripheral polyneuropathy, mononeuropathic disorders, and diabetic amyotrophy; and autonomic neuropathic conditions, including cardiovascular abnormalities, GI abnormalities, urinary bladder abnormalities, and sexual dysfunction. Symmetric peripheral polyneuropathy affects all the extremities but most often affects the legs. Symmetric peripheral polyneuropathy is usually bilateral and symmetric and is thought to be due to both metabolic and vascular mechanisms. The patient has pain and paresthesias. The pain, described as burning, cramping, crushing, or tearing, is usually worse at night and may occur only at that time. It may be relieved by walking.

The paresthesias are associated with tingling, burning, and itching sensations. Complete or partial loss of sensitivity to touch and temperature is common. Foot injury and ulcerations can occur without the patient ever having pain (Fig. 46-14). The patient may report a feeling of walking on pillows or numb feet. At times the skin becomes so

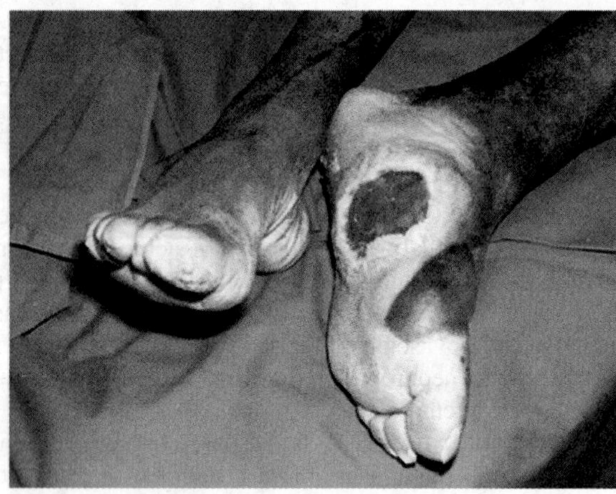

Fig. 46-14 Neuropathy: neurotrophic ulceration.

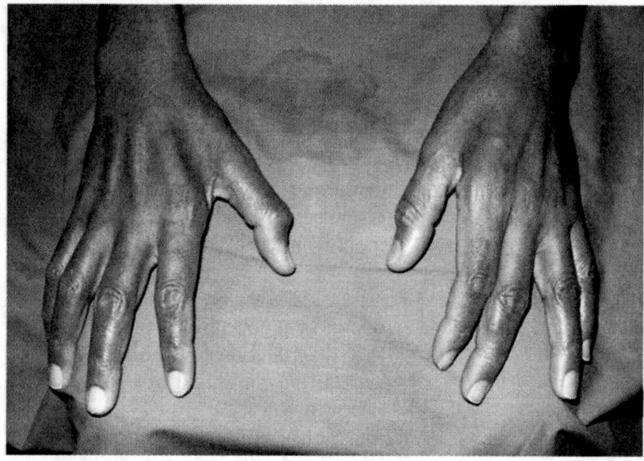

Fig. 46-15 Diabetic neuropathy: muscle atrophy.

sensitive (hyperesthesia) that even light pressure from bed sheets cannot be tolerated. Neuropathy in the hands causes atrophy of the small muscles, limiting fine movement (Fig. 46-15).

Mononeuropathic conditions tend to occur unilaterally and are characterized by a sudden onset of pain with weakness or paralysis. Although the extremities are most often affected, cranial nerves III, IV, and VI may be involved.

No direct treatment for neuropathy is known. Treatment is aimed at relief of symptoms, particularly pain. Medications commonly used include tricyclic antidepressants and topical creams (e.g., capsaicin [Zostrix]). Better glucose control may also aid in the reduction of symptoms. As nerve conduction improves, the pain may initially increase before relief is noted. A class of drugs referred to as aldose-reductase inhibitors is currently under investigation for treatment of complications of diabetes such as neuropathic disorders, retinopathy, and nephropathy. These drugs reverse some of the biochemical and physiologic changes believed to underlie these complications.[43] It is hoped that they will block the development of complications as well as relieve symptoms.[51]

Neuropathy affecting the autonomic nervous system may produce nocturnal diarrhea, postural hypotension, impotence, and neurogenic bladder. Nocturnal diarrhea is not associated with abdominal cramping. It affects few persons with diabetes and does not disturb diabetic control. *Gastroparesis diabeticorum* is delayed gastric emptying that can produce anorexia, nausea, vomiting, and persistent feelings of fullness. Gastroparesis can trigger hypoglycemia by delaying food absorption. Metoclopramide (Reglan), a dopamine receptor antagonist and serotonin antagonist, stimulates esophageal and gastric emptying and has been used in the treatment of gastroparesis. Other drugs that are sometimes useful to increase intestinal mobility are domperidone (Motillium) and cisapride (Propulsid).

The cardiovascular abnormalities associated with autonomic neuropathy are postural hypotension, resting tachycardia, and painless myocardial infarction. A patient with postural hypotension should be instructed to change from a lying or sitting position slowly. If postural hypotension is severe, medication may have to be prescribed.

Reports of the prevalence of impotence among men with diabetes vary from 30% to 60%. Impotence associated with diabetes mellitus is believed to result from damage to the sacral parasympathetic nerves. Determining whether impotence is of organic or psychologic origin is an important part of the assessment. Organic impotence usually develops insidiously, whereas psychologic impotence is often acute in onset. Measuring nocturnal penile tumescence (extent and duration of penile erection) during rapid eye movement phases of sleep is one assessment method to establish the presence of organic disease. Nonsurgical devices and surgical prosthetic implantations have been developed that make vaginal penetration possible. Decreased libido is a problem with some women with diabetes. Monilial and nonspecific vaginitis are also common. Organic impotence or sexual dysfunctioning in either the male or the female patient requires sensitive therapeutic counseling for both the patient and the patient's partner. (See Chapter 48 for a further discussion of impotence.)

A neurogenic bladder develops as sensation in the inner bladder wall decreases, causing urinary retention. A patient with retention has infrequent voiding, difficulty in voiding, and a weak stream of urine. Emptying the bladder every 3 hours in a sitting position helps prevent stasis and subsequent infection. Tightening the abdominal muscles during voiding and using the Credé maneuver (mild massage downward over the lower abdomen and bladder) may also help with complete bladder emptying. Cholinergic drugs such as bethanechol (Urecholine) may be used. The patient may also have to learn self-catheterization (see Chapter 43).

Neuropathic arthropathy, or Charcot's joints, results in ankle and foot changes that ultimately lead to joint dysfunction and foot-drop. These changes occur gradually and promote an abnormal distribution of weight over the foot. New pressure points emerge, and neuropathic ulcers often develop. The ulcers resemble a "BB shot" or "punched out" wound and are initially painless when peripheral polyneuropathy is present. Infection is a danger and may penetrate to underlying bone tissue, necessitating the long-term use of antibiotics and weeks of avoidance of weight bearing on the affected limb. The ideal treatment is prevention. Table 46-21 outlines rules for foot care that can reduce the patient's risk for infection and possible amputation.

The treatment of neuropathic disorders involves good diabetic control and supportive care. There is no known cure. The patient under relatively good glycemic control appears to have a lower incidence of neuropathy than one with poorly controlled disease. However, neuropathy can occur despite good control.

Skin changes. Skin disorders such as diabetic dermopathy and necrobiosis lipoidica diabeticorum are attributed to microangiopathy. *Shin spots* are brown spots located on the anterior surfaces of the lower extremities. They are harmless and painless and initially measure less than 1 cm in diameter. *Necrobiosis lipoidica diabeticorum*, which is believed to be the result of trauma, consists of lesions similar to those of diabetic dermopathy but is more likely to be associated with ulcerations and necrosis. The lesions are reddish yellow and atrophic. Skin grafts are sometimes required because of the slow healing of the lesions. Necrobiosis lipoidica diabeticorum is present most often in insulin-dependent women and may precede the onset of overt diabetes.

Infection. A patient with diabetes is more susceptible to infections than other patients. The mechanisms for this phenomenon include a defect in the mobilization of inflammatory cells and an impairment of white blood cells (WBCs) in the process of phagocytosis. Recurring or persistent infections such as *Candida albicans* as well as boils and furuncles in the undiagnosed patient often lead the health care provider to suspect diabetes. Loss of sensation (neuropathy) may delay the detection of an infection.

Persistent glycosuria may encourage bladder infections, especially in a neurogenic bladder. Decreased circulation as a result of angiopathy can prevent or delay the healing process. Protein waste during hyperglycemia and DKA is also responsible for poor healing. Antibiotic therapy has prevented infection from being a major cause of death in diabetic patients. The treatment of infections must be prompt and vigorous.

Gerontologic Considerations

The prevalence of diabetes is about 18% in persons between age 65 and 74. The increased blood glucose levels and decreased glucose tolerance make diabetes more difficult to diagnose in the older adult. Aging is also associated with an increase in the prevalence of other factors that tend to impair carbohydrate metabolism and are more likely to be treated with medications that impair insulin action (e.g., steroids, antihypertensives, phenothiazines). The clinical manifestations of renal, retinal, and neurologic complications of diabetes generally take 10 to 20 years to develop. Attempts to normalize glucose are associated with an increased frequency of hypoglycemia. Therefore, in the older patient, there is less reason for treatment of hyperglycemia based on the prevention of these specific diabetic complications. Whereas it is generally agreed that treatment is usually indicated for this patient, the goals for control probably do not need to be as near normoglycemia as in the younger population.[37] Because of the physiologic changes that occur with aging, the therapeutic outcome for the older adult with diabetes who receives OHAs may be altered. The second-generation OHAs such as glyburide and glipizide have increased potency but appear to have fewer side effects and fewer drug interaction problems when compared to the first-generation agents. Insulin therapy may be instituted if OHAs fail, recognizing the limitations among some individuals for manual dexterity and visual acuity required for accurate insulin administration.[38]

The patient education issues for the older patient that should be addressed are self-care in terms of vision, mobility, mental status, functional ability, and finances; the effect of multiple medications; eating habits; undetected hypoglycemia; and quality of life issues.

Patient instructions should be based on the individual's needs, using a slower pace with simple printed or audio materials. It is important to include family or a support person in the teaching.

REACTIVE HYPOGLYCEMIA

Many people claim to have reactive hypoglycemia. However, reactive hypoglycemia occurs infrequently in persons other than those with diabetes treated with insulin or sulfonylureas. Reactive hypoglycemia results from an uncompensated reduction in blood glucose level. The symptoms are similar to those of the hypoglycemia of diabetes: sudden onset of hunger, diaphoresis, tremulousness, weakness, nervousness (adrenergic) and headache, confusion, slurred speech, behavioral aberrations, focal neurologic signs, and coma (neuroglycopenic). These symptoms mimic the effects of anxiety and stress and are often misinterpreted.

Idiopathic hypoglycemia (i.e., hypoglycemia of no known cause) is particularly difficult to document. Various physiologic disturbances have been suggested, but subtle abnormalities of insulin response to food (particularly excessive or delayed secretion) seem the most likely possibilities.[39] A definite diagnosis can be made only if the plasma glucose concentration is less than 50 mg/dl (2.8 mmol/L) accompanied by symptoms of hypoglycemia and relieved by eating. The usual treatment is a diet balanced in protein and carbohydrate with frequent small meals.

If a patient claims to have reactive hypoglycemia, it should be determined whether this has been medically diagnosed or self-diagnosed. Because of the similarity to symptoms of anxiety reaction, careful assessment of the symptoms and the treatment is important.

CRITICAL THINKING EXERCISES

CASE STUDY

DIABETES KETOACIDOSIS

Patient Profile

John, a 34-year-old man, was admitted to the emergency department after he was found comatose in his apartment by his wife.

Subjective Data (provided by wife)

- Was diagnosed with diabetes mellitus 12 months ago
- Was taking 48 U of insulin daily: 12 U of regular insulin plus 20 U of NPH before breakfast, 8 U of regular insulin before dinner, and 8 U of NPH at bedtime
- Has history of flu for one week with vomiting and anorexia
- Stopped taking insulin 2 days ago when he was unable to eat

Objective Data

Physical Examination

- Breathing is deep and rapid
- Acetone smell on breath
- Skin flushed and dry

Diagnostic Studies

- Blood glucose level of 730 mg/dl (40.5 mmol/L)
- Serum acetone of 3^{+} with Acetest tablets
- Blood pH of 7.26

Discussion Questions

1. Briefly explain the pathophysiology of the development of DKA in this patient.
2. What clinical manifestations of DKA does this patient exhibit?
3. What factors precipitated this patient's DKA?
4. What distinguishes this case history from one of HHNK or hypoglycemia?
5. What educational needs must be met before the patient's discharge?
6. What role does John's wife play in the management of his diabetes?
7. Based on the assessment data presented, write one or more appropriate nursing diagnoses. Are there any collaborative problems?

NURSING RESEARCH ISSUES

1. What degree of pain does the patient associate with capillary blood glucose monitoring?
2. How often does the patient make phone contact with a diabetes patient educator when this service is available free as compared to when there is a charge?
3. Is the patient willing to maintain tight glycemic control in the present to forestall chronic complications from diabetes in the future?
4. Does the frequency of review of major diabetes education issues affect the frequency of occurrence of acute complications of diabetes?

REVIEW QUESTIONS

The number of the question corresponds to the same-numbered objective at the beginning of the chapter.

1. The normal release of insulin could best be described as
   a. pulsatile in response to food ingestion.
   b. circadian with maximum release between 2 AM and 4 AM.
   c. pulsatile with a bolus when food is ingested.
   d. variable based on carbohydrate ingestion and exercise.

2. Insulin-dependent diabetes is characterized by all of the following *except*
   a. islet cell antibody.
   b. catabolic state.
   c. minimal or absent endogenous insulin.
   d. patient is usually older than 35 years at onset.

3. Hyperglycemic hyperosmolar nonketosis is characterized by all of the following manifestations *except*
   a. cessation of all insulin production.
   b. severe hyperglycemia.
   c. extracellular fluid depletion.
   d. osmotic diuresis.

4. The type of insulin with the longest duration suitable for basal coverage is
   a. NPH.
   b. regular.
   c. Lente.
   d. Ultralente.

5. A diabetic diet is designed
   a. to normalize blood glucose by elimination of sugar.
   b. only for type I diabetes.
   c. for use during periods of high stress.
   d. to teach the patient how foods affect blood glucose.

6. "Survival skills" education should include
   a. an exercise program.
   b. diet control.
   c. capillary blood glucose monitoring.
   d. weight loss measures.

7. Appropriate instruction for the patient with diabetes related to skin care of the feet is
   a. use of heat to increase blood supply.
   b. avoidance of softening lotions and creams.
   c. daily inspection of all surfaces of the feet.
   d. use of iodine on cuts and abrasions.

REFERENCES

1. *Diabetes 1993 vital statistics,* Alexandria, VA, 1993, American Diabetes Association.
2. *Direct and indirect costs of diabetes in the United States in 1992,* Alexandria, VA, 1993, American Diabetes Association.
3. Peragallo-Dittko V: *A core curriculum for diabetes education,* ed 2, Chicago, 1993, American Association of Diabetes Educators.
4. Kitabchi AE, Duckworth WC, Stentz FB: Insulin synthesis, proinsulin and C-peptides. In Rifkin H, Porte D, editors: *Ellenberg and Rifkins diabetes mellitus theory and practice,* ed 4, New York, 1990, Elsevier.
5. DeFronzo R, Bonadonna RC, Ferrannini E: Pathogenesis of NIDDM: a balanced overview, *Diabetes Care* 15:318, 1992.
6. National Diabetes Data Group classification and diagnosis of diabetes mellitus and other categories of glucose intolerance, *Diabetes* 28:1039, 1979.
7. Fajans S: Classification and diagnosis of diabetes. In Rifkin H, Porte D, editors: *Ellenberg and Rifkins diabetes mellitus theory and practice,* ed 4, New York, 1990, Elsevier.
8. Rotter JI, Vadheim CM, Rimoin DL: Genetics of diabetes mellitus. In Rifkin H, Porte D, editors: *Ellenberg and Rifkins diabetes mellitus theory and practice,* ed 4, New York, 1990, Elsevier.
9. Gusek A: 10 commonly asked questions about diabetes, *Am J Nurs* 94:19, 1994.
10. Leahy JL, Bonner-Weir S, Weir GC: β-cell dysfunction induced by chronic hyperglycemia, *Diabetes Care* 15:442, 1992.
11. Gebhart SS and others: A comparison of home glucose monitoring with determinations of hemoglobin A_{1c} total glycate hemoglobin, fructosamine and random serum glucose in diabetic patients, *Arch Intern Med* 151:1133, 1991.
12. Mahnensmith RL: Diabetic nephropathy: a comprehensive approach, *Hosp Pract* 28:129, 1993.
13. American Diabetes Association Position Statement: Nutritional recommendations and principles for people with diabetes mellitus, *Diabetes Care* 18:16, 1995.
14. Bantle JP and others: Metabolic effects of dietary sucrose on type II diabetic subjects, *Diabetes Care* 16:1301, 1993.
15. Kestel F: Are you up to date on diabetes medications? *Am J Nurs* 94:48, 1994.
16. Position statement on insulin administration by the American Diabetes Association, *Diabetes Care* 16 (Suppl):31, 1993.
17. McCarthy JA, Covarrubias B, Sink P: Is the traditional alcohol wipe necessary before an insulin injection? Dogma disputed, *Diabetes Care* 16:402, 1993.
18. McCarren M: And: it works, *Diabetes Forecast* 16:49, 1993.
19. Hirsch IB, Farkas-Hirsch R, Skyler JS: Intensive insulin therapy for treatment of type I diabetes, *Diabetes Care* 13:1265, 1990.
20. Steinburg C: Is intensive therapy for everyone? *Diabetes Forecast* 16:52, 1993.
21. Diabetes update 93, *Nursing* 23:59, 1993.
22. Macheca MK: Diabetic hypoglycemia: how to keep the threat at bay, *Am J Nurs* 9:26, 1993.
23. Steil CF, Deakin DA: Oral hypoglycemics, *Nursing* 22:34, 1992.
24. Bailey DJ: Biguanides and NIDDM, *Diabetes Care* 16:755, 1992.
25. Wilson BA: What nurses don't know about managing NIDDM, *Medsurg Nurs* 3:152, 1994.
26. Schrier RW, Savage S: On recent advances in diabetes management, *Hosp Pract* 29:11, 1994.
27. University Group Diabetes Program: A study of the effects of hypoglycemic agents on vascular complications in patients with adult onset diabetes: mortality results, *Diabetes* 19 (Suppl 2):747, 1970.
28. Bihm B, Wilson BA: Metformin (Glucophage): new treatment for NIDDM, *Medsurg Nurs* 4:236, 1995.
29. White J, Campbell RK: Pharmacologic therapies in the management of diabetes mellitus. In Haire-Joshu D, editor: *Management of diabetes mellitus,* St Louis, 1992, Mosby.
30. Maynard T: Exercise: Part I; Physiological response to exercise in diabetes mellitus, *Diabetes Educator* 17:196, 1991.
31. Pickup JC: Invivo glucose monitoring: sense and sensorbility, *Diabetes Care* 16:535, 1993.
32. Gusek A: 10 commonly asked questions about diabetes, *Am J Nurs* 94:19, 1994.
33. The National Steering Committee for Quality Assurance in Capillary Blood Glucose Monitoring: Proposed strategies for reducing user error in capillary blood glucose monitoring, *Diabetes Care* 16:493, 1993.
34. Self-monitoring of blood glucose, *Diabetes Care* 16:60, 1993.
35. Consensus statement of the American Diabetes Association: Self-monitoring of blood glucose, *Diabetes Care* 13 (suppl):41, 1990.
36. Meeting the standards: *A manual for completing the American Diabetes Association application for recognition of diabetes patient education programs,* ed 3, Alexandria, VA, 1991, American Diabetes Association.
37. LeMone P: Response of the older adult to the effects and management of diabetes mellitus, *Medsurg Nurs* 3:122, 1994.
38. Lun WS: Oral agents in the elderly, *Practical Diabetology* 12:10, 1993.
39. Amiel SA, Gale E: Physiological response to hypoglycemia: counterregulation and cognitive function, *Diabetes Care* 16:48, 1993.
40. The Diabetes Control and Complications Trial Research Group: The effect of intensive treatment of diabetes on the development and progression of long-term complications in insulin-dependent diabetes mellitus, *N Engl J Med* 329:977, 1993.
41. American Diabetes Association Position Statement: Implications of the Diabetes Control and Complications Trial, *Clin Diabetes* July/August:1993.
42. Foster DW: Diabetes mellitus. In Isselbacker KJ and others, editors: *Harrison's principles of internal medicine,* ed 13, New York, 1994, McGraw-Hill.
43. Cryer PE: Hypoglycemia unawareness in IDDM, *Diabetes Care* 16 (Suppl 3):40, 1993.
44. Reising DL: Acute hypoglycemia, *Nursing* 25:41, 1995.
45. Moller DE, Flier JS: Insulin resistance: mechanisms, syndromes and implications, *N Engl J Med* 325:931, 1991.
46. Nathan DM: Long-term complications of diabetes mellitus, *New Engl J Med* 328:1676, 1993.
47. Kaufman MW, Bowsher JE: Preventing diabetic foot ulcers, *Medsurg Nurs* 3:204, 1994.
48. Ferris FL: Issues in management of diabetic retinopathy, *Hosp Pract* 28:79, 1993.

49. Jacobson EJ: Diabetic nephropathy, *Dialysis and Transplantation* 22:616, 1994.
50. Bartucci MR, Loughman KA, Moir EJ: Kidney-pancreas transplantation: a treatment option for ESRD and type I diabetes, *ANNA J* 19:467, 1992.
51. Passariello N and others: Effect of aldose reductase inhibitor (Tolrestat) on urinary albumin excretion rate and glomerular filtration rate in IDDM subjects with nephropathy, *Diabetes Care* 16:789, 1993.

DIABETES INFORMATION RESOURCES

American Diabetes Association National Service Center
1660 Duke Street
Alexandria, VA 22314
Phone: (800) ADA-DISC.

American Association of Diabetes Educators
444 N Michigan Ave, Suite 1240
Chicago, IL 60611
Phone: (800) 338-DMED.

Juvenile Diabetes Foundation
23 E 26th Street
New York, NY 10010

Chapter 47

NURSING ROLE IN MANAGEMENT

Endocrine Problems

Linda B. Haas

Learning Objectives

1. Describe the pathophysiology, clinical manifestations, and therapeutic and nursing management of the patient with an imbalance of hormones produced by the anterior pituitary gland.
2. Describe the pathophysiology, clinical manifestations, and therapeutic and nursing management of the patient with an imbalance of hormones produced by the posterior pituitary gland.
3. Describe the pathophysiology, clinical manifestations, and therapeutic and nursing management of the patient with thyroid enlargement or dysfunction.
4. Describe the pathophysiology, clinical manifestations, and therapeutic and nursing management of the patient with an imbalance of the hormone produced by the parathyroid glands.
5. Describe the pathophysiology, clinical manifestations, and therapeutic and nursing management of the patient with an imbalance of hormones produced by the adrenal cortices.
6. Describe the pathophysiology, clinical manifestations, and therapeutic and nursing management of the patient with an excess of hormones produced by the adrenal medullae.
7. Name the endocrine disorders characterized by excesses and deficits in fluid volume, and describe the appropriate nursing interventions.
8. Describe the systemic effects of replacement and pharmacologic use of corticosteroid therapy.
9. List the nursing assessments, interventions, rationales, and expected outcomes related to patient education for chronic management of endocrine problems.

This chapter deals with problems related to hormones produced by the anterior and posterior pituitary, thyroid, parathyroid, and adrenal glands. (Diabetes mellitus is discussed in Chapter 46, problems related to the reproductive system are discussed in Chapters 51 and 52, and the concept of stress is discussed in Chapter 5.)

HEALTH MAINTENANCE AND PROMOTION

The goal of health maintenance activities is to maintain or restore the highest level of health and to promote a healthy lifestyle for the individual. For the patient with an endocrine problem, the nursing process should be directed toward (1) careful assessment to detect the early and subtle changes that indicate dysfunction, particularly when caring for the patient with a condition that may predispose him to endocrine dysfunction; (2) prevention of hormone imbalance; (3) education and support when irreversible dysfunction or its manifestations occur or when lifestyle changes are indicated; and (4) reduction of future risks or complications. The nurse performs the meticulous assessment of the usual and potential stressors that interact with the endocrine system, notes subtle changes in biopsychosocial parameters, and plans interventions that focus on the maintenance of homeostasis and patient education. The patient and significant others should be included in the plan of care whenever possible.

The nurse's role in the management of the patient with endocrine dysfunction includes the following actions:

1. Assessment
   a. Physical, psychologic, and social parameters related to endocrine function
   b. Usual coping patterns and support systems
   c. Emotional, physical, and environmental stressors (past, current, and potential)
   d. Familial patterns
2. Development of nursing diagnoses on the basis of nursing assessment
3. Establishment of expected outcomes related to each diagnosis within the realm of the patient's psychobiologic and social limitations
4. Interventions

Reviewed by Florencetta Hayes Gibson, RN, MEd, MSN, Associate Professor, Northeast Louisiana University, Monroe, LA.

Table 47-1 Patient Information Related to Drug Therapy

- Correct dosage and time schedule
- Correct route and technique for administration
- Side effects
- Extraneous influences that may interfere with response to medication (e.g., stress)
- Signs and symptoms that indicate need to increase, decrease, or discontinue prescribed medication
- Signs and symptoms that indicate need to contact primary care provider
- Knowledge that lifetime replacement is usually necessary
- Plan for regular follow-up care
- Necessity of wearing an identification or medical alert device at all times

a. Preparation, support, and encouragement in the management of diagnostic and acute phases to ensure accurate testing and promote effective coping
b. Education for long-term medication therapy for health maintenance, including verbal and appropriate written instructions, with demonstrations and return demonstrations, if applicable (Table 47-1)
c. Information about when and how to seek help and the availability of community resources for optimal health maintenance
d. Education, referral, and support for nutritional modification (if applicable)
e. Education in the most appropriate methods of dealing with present and potential stressors (building on the patient's past and current coping strengths)
f. Problem solving to identify strategies that may help resolve problems that inevitably arise when an individual has a chronic condition

Education and assistance in developing new strategies for coping with a chronic disease and the alterations involved in a patient's self-image, behavior, and lifestyle are major areas of focus for the nursing care for a patient with an endocrine dysfunction.

Often the signs and symptoms of endocrine dysfunction are vague (Table 45-5) and could be caused by many unrelated physical and psychologic disorders, including hypochondriasis. The signs and symptoms are often overlooked by the patient, family, and clinician until obvious symptoms occur, sometimes with irreversible pathologic results. A nurse with a sound knowledge base related to endocrine problems and good assessment skills may detect endocrine problems early. (See Chapter 45 for a discussion of the assessment of the endocrine system.)

Promotion and maintenance of endocrine health require adequate nutrients for hormone production. The importance of adequate nutrition is illustrated by the thyroid enlargement and marginal hypothyroidism that can develop in the individual with iodine deficiencies (endemic goiter). However, iodine is only one of many substances required for normal hormone production. Protein and thyroid hormones incorporate amino acids into their structure. To maintain adequate endocrine function, the dietary intake must contain adequate protein, minerals, and vitamins.

Although steroid hormones are synthesized from cholesterol, the nutritional (exogenous) cholesterol requirements are uncertain. Cholesterol is produced endogenously in the liver. Research has shown a strong positive correlation between high serum cholesterol levels and atherosclerosis, which contributes to cardiovascular disease, the leading cause of death in Western societies.[1] The patient on a typical American diet is likely to consume excess cholesterol (>300 mg/day). All persons except cachectic individuals and those suffering from malabsorption and debilitating diseases, such as cancer and anorexia nervosa, should monitor dietary cholesterol intake to avoid excess.

Disruptions in rhythmic patterns produce disharmony between body requirements and hormone production. The distress experienced by jet travelers and shift workers is characteristic of this disharmony. Changes in the routine of living should be minimized. If sudden significant alterations are unavoidable, the individual should attempt to minimize other life stressors as much as possible to lessen the total stress load.

Stress greatly alters the rate and patterns of hormone production and disrupts natural rhythms. Strategies should be developed to keep stress within manageable limits. Stress is also a potent stimulus to the endocrine system. Many acute endocrine conditions first appear after a major stressor, such as the death of a close family member. Unusual stress is also a factor in exacerbations of chronic endocrine conditions. (See Chapter 5 for a discussion of techniques for stress management.)

Most endocrine problems are chronic, with signs and symptoms that may subside with proper treatment, care, education, and self-management by the patient or family. Consistent adherence to daily self-management regimens and follow-up care can frequently prevent acute episodes. Whereas some individuals require only continuing treatment with medications and periodic evaluation, others have exacerbations or concurrent illness and require hospitalization. Careful assessment, management, and education of the patient and family can have a positive effect on the course and outcome of problems associated with the endocrine system.

In general, endocrine problems are caused by overproduction or underproduction of hormones, hormone transport abnormalities, inability of target tissues to respond to hormones, or problems with feedback mechanisms. Endocrine disorders are often described as primary or secondary. In *primary disorders* the defect is in the gland producing the hormone. Examples are tumors that cause abnormal hormone secretion (pituitary adenoma), autoimmune disease in which antibodies attack the gland (Hashimoto's thyroiditis), and inborn errors of metabolism. *Secondary disorders* are related to increased or decreased stimulation of the glands, usually by a tropic hormone. This is illustrated by hypothyroidism, which can be caused by a lack of thyroid-stimulating hormone (TSH), or Cushing's disease, which can be a result of excess cortisol secretion by the adrenal glands caused by excess adrenocorticotropic hormone (ACTH) from a pituitary adenoma.

PITUITARY GLAND

Disorders of the Anterior Pituitary Gland

Growth Hormone Excess. Growth hormone (GH), an anabolic hormone, promotes protein synthesis and mobilizes glucose and free fatty acids. Overproduction of GH, which is usually caused by a benign pituitary adenoma (tumor), causes gigantism or acromegaly characterized by soft tissue and bony overgrowth. *Gigantism* results when the onset occurs before closure of the epiphyses, while the long bones are still capable of longitudinal growth. The onset usually occurs in early childhood but may occur at puberty. The excessive growth is usually proportional. These children may grow as tall as 8 feet (240 cm) and weigh more than 300 lb (136 kg). These tumors are rare, and affected children are not healthy and usually die in early adulthood.[2]

Acromegaly, although also rare, is the more common abnormality caused by GH excess. Symptoms begin insidiously in the third and fourth decades of life, and both genders are affected equally. When the problem develops after epiphyseal closure, bones increase in thickness and width. Physical features include enlargement of the hands, feet, and paranasal and frontal sinuses; and deformities of the spine and mandible (Fig. 47-1). In addition, enlargement of soft tissue (e.g., tongue, skin, abdominal organs) causes manifestations such as speech difficulties and hoarseness, coarsening of facial features, sleep apnea, and abdominal distention. Persons with acromegaly may exhibit hypertension, cardiomegaly, left ventricular hypertrophy, diaphoresis, oily skin, peripheral neuropathy, proximal muscle weakness, and joint pain.

The enlarged pituitary gland can exert pressure on surrounding structures, leading to visual disturbances and headaches. Because GH mobilizes stored fat for energy, it increases free fatty acids levels in the blood and predisposes the patient to atherosclerosis. The hormone also antagonizes the action of insulin and can cause hyperglycemia. Prolonged stimulation by GH is diabetogenic (see Chapter 46).

Diagnostic Studies. In addition to the history and physical examination, diagnosis of GH excess requires evaluation of plasma GH and somatomedin C (insulin-like growth factor) levels and GH response to an oral glucose challenge. Skull x-rays may show a large sella turcica and increased bone density. Computerized tomography (CT) scanning with contrast media and magnetic resonance imaging (MRI) are used for further evaluation and tumor localization, with MRI being the more sensitive method for identification, localization, and determination of invasion. The patient with a macroadenoma (>10 mm) will require a complete ophthalmologic examination, including visual fields.[3]

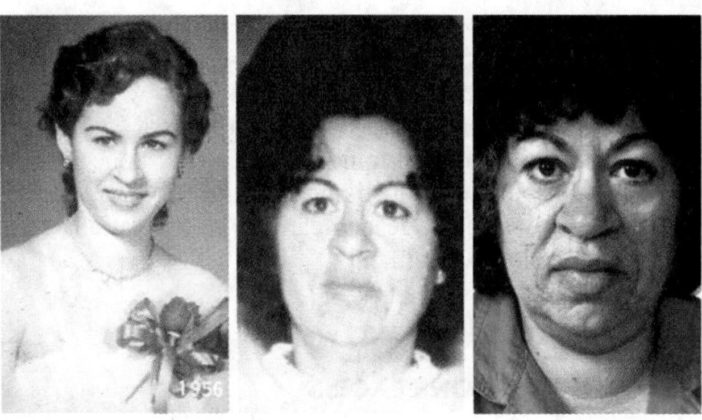

Fig. 47-1 Progressive development of facial features of acromegaly.

Therapeutic Management. The therapeutic goal in gigantism and acromegaly is to return GH levels to normal. This may be accomplished by surgery, radiation, pharmacologic intervention, or a combination of these three. Surgery is the usual treatment and offers the best hope for a cure, especially for microadenomas (<10 mm). Surgery is most commonly accomplished with the transsphenoidal approach, in which an incision is made in the inner aspect of the upper lip and gingiva. The sella turcica is entered through the floor of the nose and sphenoid sinuses. The goal of transsphenoidal microsurgery is to remove only the GH-secreting adenoma. However, the pituitary gland may be destroyed or removed in some instances. Removal of the entire gland results in permanent deficiencies of hormones of the anterior pituitary. Rather than replacing the tropic hormones, which requires parenteral administration, the essential hormones produced by target organs (glucocorticoids, thyroid hormone, and certain sex hormones) can be given orally. Testosterone can be administered to men via a transdermal patch or self-administered intramuscularly (IM) every 2 weeks. Hormone replacement must be continued throughout life.

External radiation normalizes GH levels in 30% to 70% of patients treated in this manner, although it may be months to years before GH levels normalize.[4] If a tumor is large or has a great deal of supersellar extension, surgery may be followed by radiation. Depending on the amount of radiation and the patient's susceptibility, the patient may experience local skin changes, alopecia, or oral complications.[5] Hypopituitarism is a common sequela that often requires replacement therapy.

Stereotactic radiosurgery (gamma surgery) may be applied to small, surgically inaccessible pituitary tumors. This procedure consists of radiation delivered to a single site from multiple angles and can be used to occlude blood vessels feeding the tumor, thereby starving it. The radiation source is arranged on a helmet device on the patient's head and focused on the tumor.

Pharmacologic treatment is accomplished with bromocriptine, a dopamine agonist, or with octreotide, a somatostatin analog, that reduces GH levels to within the normal range in many patients. The GH-lowering effects of these drugs are seldom complete or permanent, and they are often used as adjuncts to other therapies or to reduce tumor size before surgery.

The prognosis depends on age at onset, age when treatment is initiated, and tumor size. Usually bone growth can be arrested, and soft-tissue hypertrophy can be reversed. However, diabetic and cardiac complications may continue in spite of treatment.

NURSING MANAGEMENT

GROWTH HORMONE EXCESS

The nurse should assess for signs and symptoms of abnormal tissue growth and evaluate the physical size of each patient. Assessment of children includes evaluation of growth and development with the use of growth charts (see Chapter 45).

Notably accelerated growth, especially if greater than 5 to 6 inches (12 to 15 cm) per year and if inconsistent with familial patterns, constitutes cause for medical referral. The adult should be questioned about increases in hat, ring, glove, and shoe sizes. The patient can be questioned about changes in appearance noted in serial photographs.

When first seen, the patient usually has experienced undesirable changes in appearance and may have substantial alterations in self-image. The individual also commonly exhibits symptoms of diabetes mellitus such as polydipsia, polyuria, and blurred vision. Cardiovascular disease may be present. The patient needs unconditional acceptance by health care workers and considerable emotional support during the periods of diagnosis and treatment. Referral to the Acromegaly Network Association ([619] 431-2625) may be helpful. The patient should be carefully monitored for hyperglycemia and cardiovascular signs and symptoms such as angina pectoris, hypertension, and congestive heart failure.

The individual treated surgically needs skilled neurosurgical nursing care and must be prepared before surgery for postoperative care. Nursing interventions include discussion of mouth breathing, mouth care, ambulation, pain control, activity, and hormone replacement. The patient should be instructed to avoid vigorous coughing, sneezing, and straining at stool (Valsalva maneuver) to prevent cerebrospinal fluid leakage from the point at which the sella turcica was entered.[6]

After surgery in which a transsphenoidal approach has been used, the head of the patient's bed should be elevated at a 30-degree angle at all times. This elevation avoids pressure on the sella turcica and decreases headaches, a frequent postoperative problem. Mild analgesia is given for headaches. The nurse should perform mouth care every 4 hours to keep the surgical area clean and free of debris and to promote patient comfort. Tooth brushing should be avoided to prevent disrupting the suture line and to avoid discomfort.

Any clear nasal drainage should be sent to the laboratory to be tested for glucose. A level greater than 30 mg/dl (1.67 mmol/L) indicates cerebrospinal fluid leakage from an open connection to the brain, which places the patient at an increased risk for meningitis. Complaints of persistent and severe generalized or supraorbital headache may indicate cerebrospinal fluid leakage into the sinuses. A cerebrospinal fluid leak usually resolves within 72 hours when treated with head elevation and bed rest. If the leak persists, daily spinal taps may be done to reduce pressure to below normal levels and allow the fossa to heal. Intravenous (IV) antibiotics are usually administered when there is a cerebrospinal fluid leak to prevent meningitis. If the leak does not respond to treatment in 48 to 72 hours, surgical intervention may be required.

If stereotactic radiosurgery is used, the patient is usually moved from the specialized radiation center to the neurosurgical nursing unit for overnight observation. Vital signs, neurologic status, and fluid volume status must be carefully monitored. Possible complications include increased headaches, seizures, nausea and vomiting, and discomfort at the pin sites. All staff should know how to remove a stereotactic frame in case of an emergency. The patient with a history of seizures is at increased risk for seizures for 24 hours after the procedure. The anterior pin sites should be cleaned with hydrogen peroxide and covered with clean dressings. The posterior pin sites should be cleaned with 3% peroxide every 6 hours for 48 hours. Family members can be instructed in pin-site care if the patient is discharged the day after the procedure.[7]

If a *hypophysectomy* (removal of pituitary gland) is performed, hormone replacement is necessary. Immediately after surgery the patient may exhibit signs of diabetes insipidus (discussed later in chapter) because of the loss of antidiuretic hormone (ADH), which is stored in the posterior lobe of the pituitary gland. Vasopressin (Pitressin) is given IM as needed if the urine output exceeds 800 to 900 ml over 2 hours or if the urine specific gravity is less than 1.004. This is temporary, unless the entire pituitary gland is removed. In this case, permanent ADH replacement will be needed.

Because the source of ACTH may have been removed, cortisol replacement may be needed. Careful patient education is necessary when cortisone must be taken regularly.

Hypopituitarism causes infertility because of deficient sex hormones secondary to loss of gonadotropins. In addition, gamete (ova and sperm) production ceases because of a lack of stimulation from the gonadotropins, follicle-stimulating hormone (FSH) and luteinizing hormone (LH). However, if an individual with deficient FSH and LH wishes to have children, these hormones can be replaced with intermittent subcutaneous injections with possible restoration of fertility.

Because surgery may result in pituitary destruction with permanent hormone deficiencies and possible altered fertility, the patient needs assistance in working through the grieving process associated with these losses. It is important that the patient be aware of the consequences if surgery is not done so that an informed decision can be made. The need for continued drug therapy reduces the patient's perception of independence and requires considerable emotional adjustment. The nurse must consider the emotional impact of a hypophysectomy when counseling the patient and planning the educational program related to hormone replacement.[5]

Excesses of Other Tropic Hormones. Excesses of other tropic hormones and overproduction of a single anterior pituitary hormone usually produce syndromes related to hormone excess from the target organ. If ACTH is involved, Cushing's disease (ACTH excess) results; if TSH levels are excessive, hyperthyroidism develops.

In some instances, excess secretion of a pituitary hormone may be appropriate, such as when there are alterations in the negative feedback system. (See Chapter 45 for a discussion of negative feedback.) In the adult, hypersecretion of FSH and LH occurs in primary gonadal failure. The resultant low levels of sex hormones cause oversecretion of gonadotropins by the pituitary gland and are not indicative of intracranial disease. Thus excess FSH and LH may indicate a pathologic gonadal process such as orchitis, or the excess may be a normal consequence of aging such as menopause. Sex hormone replacement therapy normalizes gonadotropin activity but does have side effects (see Chapters 51 and 52).

Sometimes symptoms of excess gonadotropins signify pituitary disease and require prompt referral for a definitive diagnosis. This is true of inappropriate lactation in either gender and precocious puberty in children.

Prolactin-secreting adenomas (prolactinomas) are the most frequently occurring pituitary tumor. The affected patient may experience headaches and visual problems. The visual problems are secondary to pressure on the optic chiasm. Women may have galactorrhea, menstrual abnormalities, or infertility. In men, impotence and decreased libido and sperm density may result. Treatment is achieved with surgery, radiation, or pharmacologic intervention.

Hypofunction of the Pituitary Gland. *Hypopituitarism* is a rare disorder and involves a decrease in one or more of the anterior pituitary hormones. Primary hypofunction may be a result of infections, autoimmune disorders, tumors, vascular diseases, or destruction of the gland. Failure to secrete GH is the most common abnormality, followed by deficiencies of the gonadotropins, TSH, ACTH, and prolactin.[8] The manifestations of hypopituitarism depend on the specific pituitary hormones that are lacking. Thus infertility may be caused by primary gonadal failure or may be the first indication of pituitary hypofunction. In the latter case the gonads lack tropic hormone stimulation. The most common cause of pituitary hypofunction is a tumor, but destruction of the pituitary can also result from trauma, radiation, and surgical procedures. Cranial radiation used in the treatment of other conditions may cause hypothalamic dysfunction, which often results in pituitary dysfunction.

In women, hypofunction can follow a postpartum hemorrhage. This is called *postpartum pituitary necrosis,* or *Sheehan's syndrome.* Sheehan's syndrome should be suspected when failure to lactate and amenorrhea occur in a patient with a history of postpartum hemorrhage. The vascularity of the pituitary gland increases during pregnancy making it vulnerable to hemorrhage. If hemorrhagic shock occurs during childbirth, the pituitary gland can become hypoxic causing a slow degeneration and necrosis of the gland.[2] Panhypopituitarism may develop over a span of 10 to 15 years. The patient does not lactate secondary to postpartum hemorrhage after childbirth and is subsequently infertile because of prolactin, FSH, and LH deficiencies. Later, hypothyroidism develops and is followed by glucocorticoid deficiency. Because lethargy and apathy are characteristic of these two hormone deficiencies, affected women rarely seek treatment. Many women with Sheehan's syndrome are diagnosed only after an acute Addisonian crisis (discussed later in chapter). Some are never diagnosed or treated and succumb to this life-threatening condition.

Decreased pituitary hormone secretion is associated with anorexia nervosa and bulimia (see Chapter 38). This condition usually affects young women with distorted body images. The patient decreases caloric intake and may increase exercise levels to the point where body weight and body fat percentage fall below a critical level for normal hypothalamic-pituitary gonadotropin function, leading to amenorrhea. Decreased circulating thyroid hormone with inadequate TSH response and glucocorticoid and androgen abnormalities can also occur.

Clinical manifestations. Clinical findings associated with pituitary hypofunction vary with the degree and speed of onset of pituitary dysfunction and are related to hyposecretion of the target glands. The symptoms are often nonspecific and commonly include weakness, fatigue, headache, sexual dysfunction, fasting hypoglycemia, dry and sallow skin, diminished tolerance for stress, and poor resistance to infection. In the adult, premature, fine wrinkling around the eyes and mouth is common. Psychiatric symptoms include apathy, mental slowness, and delusions. Orthostatic hypotension may also occur. If a pituitary tumor exerts pressure on the optic chiasm, there may be asymmetric visual field changes. If the tumor is large, blindness in one or both eyes may occur.

Hyposecretion of GH during childhood results in growth retardation. Growth may be normal for the first 1 or 2 years but then slows progressively. Intelligence is usually normal. Replacement therapy with recombinant GH is available. Prepubertal children respond better than postpubertal children. This therapy is costly, up to $20,000 per year. Controversy exists as to whether the constitutionally "short" child should be treated with recombinant GH to increase height and improve self-image.[9] There are no obvious manifestations of GH deficiency in the adult, although short-term replacement therapy results in improved exercise tolerance, decreased body fat, and increased body mass.

When pituitary hypofunction affects FSH and LH, sexual development is impaired and features remain childlike. FSH and LH deficiencies in the adult woman are first manifested as menstrual irregularities, diminished libido, and changes in secondary sex characteristics (e.g., decreased breast size). If the cause is Sheehan's syndrome, lactation fails and infertility occurs. Men with FSH and LH deficiencies experience testicular atrophy, diminished spermatogenesis, loss of libido along with impotence, and decreased facial hair and muscle mass.

If hypopituitarism is not detected and treated, the patient eventually develops deficiencies of thyroid hormone and the adrenal corticosteroids. The latter deficiency causes a tendency toward shock and may result in an episode of acute adrenal insufficiency (refractory and life-threatening shock from sodium and water depletion).

Therapeutic management. Treatment of hypopituitarism consists of surgery or radiation for tumor removal, permanent target gland hormone replacement, and a nutritious dietary plan. Replacement therapy is carried out with corticosteroids, thyroid hormone, and sex hormones. Gonadotropins can sometimes restore fertility.

NURSING MANAGEMENT

ANTERIOR PITUITARY INSUFFICIENCY

A primary nursing role in anterior pituitary insufficiency is assessment and recognition of subtle signs and symptoms. The patient with hypopituitarism may first exhibit symptoms in stressful situations such as trauma or surgery. In addition, hypopituitarism may be detected in the patient with symptoms of failure to grow, infertility, or amenorrhea. Failure to grow may indicate pituitary dwarfism, and infertility and amenorrhea can be signs of Sheehan's syndrome or a pituitary adenoma.

Children affected by pituitary dwarfism exhibit slow but proportional growth. Except for their small size, they may appear completely normal. When the age of puberty is reached, however, sexual maturation may not occur. If it does occur, the epiphyses will close, ending the possibility of further longitudinal bone growth despite hormone replacement. For this reason and because normal stature and psychosocial development are more likely to be achieved with early initiation of treatment, these children must be identified and treated early. (See a pediatric text for a complete discussion of pituitary dwarfism.)

The nurse should be alert for the possibility of Sheehan's syndrome and refer any woman with the following characteristics for diagnosis and treatment:

1. History of hemorrhage or other hypoxic episode during the birth of youngest child
2. Failure to lactate after birth—this is usually the prominent clue
3. Scanty, irregular, or absent menses
4. Decrease in secondary sex characteristics (or complaints of being "less womanly" than before)
5. Signs and symptoms of hypothyroidism
6. Signs and symptoms of glucocorticoid insufficiency without the "bronzing" of the skin associated with the condition

Although Sheehan's syndrome has been considered a relatively rare condition, there is evidence that it has been seriously underdiagnosed. The disease is devastating to affected women but is largely reversible with hormone replacement.

If the disease is not detected and treated early, the woman is likely to need considerable help in rebuilding her life. Marital, vocational, or psychologic counseling may be needed, and appropriate referrals should be made. The nature of the physiologic problem should be explained to significant others, and their help should be enlisted in the rehabilitative process.

Disorders of the Posterior Pituitary

The hormones secreted by the posterior pituitary are *ADH,* also called *arginine vasopressin* (AVP), and *oxytocin.* These hormones are formed in the hypothalamus and stored in the posterior pituitary. ADH contributes to fluid balance by controlling renal reabsorption of free water (Fig. 47-2). It also has potent vasoconstrictive properties. Oxytocin controls lactation and uterine contractions. Oxytocin excess is not recognized as a clinical problem. This hormone is administered pharmacologically in the management of labor.

Syndrome of Inappropriate Antidiuretic Hormone. The syndrome of inappropriate antidiuretic hormone (SIADH) occurs when ADH is released in amounts far in excess of those indicated by the plasma osmotic pressure (Fig. 47-3). This syndrome is associated with diseases that affect osmoreceptors in the hypothalamus. SIADH is characterized by fluid retention, serum hypoosmolality, dilutional hyponatremia, hypochloremia, concentrated urine greater than 120 to 150 mOsm/kg in the presence of normal or increased intravascular volume, and normal renal function.

Causes and clinical manifestations. SIADH has various causes (Table 47-2). Ectopic ADH production by carcinomas is not a primary pituitary disorder but has similar manifestations and nursing care. Bronchogenic carcinoma is the most common ADH-secreting tumor. Other pulmonary conditions, such as pneumonia, tuberculosis, lung abscess, and positive pressure breathing have been associated with SIADH. The syndrome is also associated with such diverse conditions as trauma (all types but most frequently head trauma), meningitis, subarachnoid hemorrhage, peripheral neuropathy, delirium tremens, Addison's disease, psychoses, vomiting, stress, and many medications.[10]

The excess ADH increases renal tubular permeability and reabsorption of water into the circulation. Consequently, extracellular fluid (ECF) volume expands, plasma osmolality declines, the glomerular filtration rate rises, and sodium levels decline (dilutional hyponatremia).

Problems related to SIADH include low urinary output and weight gain without edema. As plasma osmolality and serum sodium levels continue to decline, cerebral edema may occur, leading to lethargy, anorexia, confusion, headache, convulsions, and coma. Other effects of hyponatremia include muscle cramps and weakness.

Therapeutic management. The diagnosis of SIADH is made by simultaneous measurements of urine and serum osmolality. The serum osmolality is much lower than the urine osmolality, indicating the inappropriate excretion of concentrated urine in the presence of very dilute serum. Associated manifestations correlate with the serum sodium level. Initially, thirst, dyspnea on exertion, fatigue, and dulled sensorium may be evident. As the serum sodium level falls, symptoms become more severe and include vomiting, abdominal cramps, muscle twitching, and convulsions.

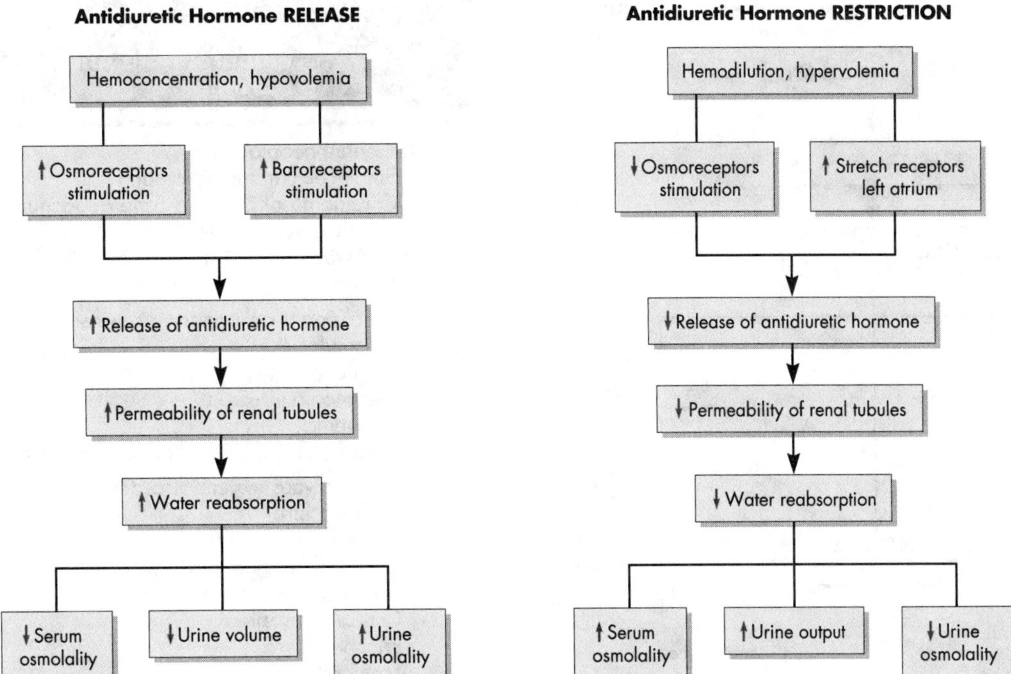

Fig. 47-2 Physiology of the release and restriction of antidiuretic hormone.

The treatment goal is to restore normal fluid volume and osmolality. Fluids may be restricted to 800 to 1000 ml per day. This should result in gradual, daily reductions in weight, a progressive rise in serum sodium concentration and osmolality, and symptomatic improvement. If fluid restriction alone does not improve the symptoms, an IV of 3% to 5% (hypertonic) saline solution may be administered. A diuretic such as furosemide may be used to promote diuresis if cardiac symptoms develop. Because furosemide increases potassium excretion, potassium supplements may be needed. SIADH tends to be self-limiting when caused by head trauma or drugs but chronic in nature when associated with tumors or metabolic diseases. Treatment of the underlying cause or discontinuing the causal medication is indicated to improve the clinical course.

In chronic, symptomatic SIADH, demeclocycline (Declomycin), a tetracycline that causes nephrogenic diabetes insipidus, is useful. This drug blocks the action of ADH at the level of the distal and collecting tubules, regardless of the ADH source. Other therapeutic measures in chronic management include furosemide and the use of urea, an osmotic diuretic.

NURSING MANAGEMENT

SYNDROME OF INAPPROPRIATE ANTIDIURETIC HORMONE

Careful nursing assessment of the patient who has had surgery or is susceptible to the syndrome (Table 47-2) can help in the early detection of SIADH. The nurse should be alert for low urinary output with a high specific gravity, a sudden weight gain, or a serum sodium decline. If a patient has SIADH, nursing measures include the assessments and interventions presented in Table 47-3.

When SIADH is chronic, the patient must learn to self-manage treatment regimens. Fluids are restricted to 800 to 1000 ml per day. Sucking on hard candy or ice chips can help decrease thirst. If drinking liquids is an aspect of socialization, the patient should be assisted in planning fluid intake so liquid allowances are saved for social occasions. The patient may be treated with a diuretic to remove excess fluid volume. The diet should be supplemented with sodium and potassium, especially if diuretics are prescribed. Salts of these electrolytes must be well diluted to prevent gastrointestinal (GI) irritation or damage. They are best taken at mealtime to allow mixing with and dilution by food. If urea is prescribed, the patient should be instructed to mix it with juice for palatability. The patient should be taught the symptoms of fluid and electrolyte imbalances, especially those involving sodium and potassium, so that responses to treatment can be monitored (see Chapter 13). If a patient is to be treated with demeclocycline, the need for close follow-up care should be stressed because of the nephrotoxic side effects and the potential for fungal infections associated with this drug.

Diabetes Insipidus. Central diabetes insipidus (DI) is characterized by increased thirst (polydipsia) and increased urination (polyuria) (see Fig. 47- 4 on p. 1486). It occurs when any organic lesion of the hypothalamus, infundibular stem, or posterior pituitary interferes with ADH synthesis, transport, or release. An estimated 30% of cases have no apparent cause (i.e., idiopathic).[11] The remainder are due to brain tumors, pituitary or other cranial surgery, closed head trauma, granulomatous disease, central nervous system

Syndrome of Inappropriate Antidiuretic Hormone (SIADH)

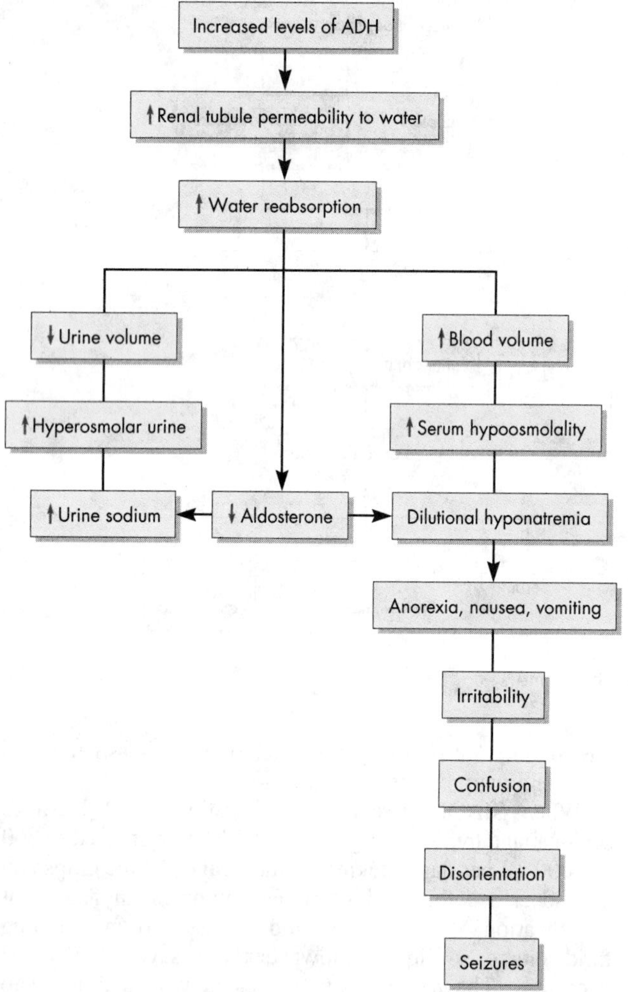

Fig. 47-3 Pathophysiology of syndrome of inappropriate antidiuretic hormone (SIADH).

Table 47-2 Causes of Syndrome of Inappropriate Antidiuretic Hormone

- Malignant neoplasms
  - Small-cell carcinoma of lung
  - Carcinoma of pancreas and duodenum
  - Lymphosarcoma, reticulum cell sarcoma, Hodgkin's disease
  - Thymoma
- Nonmalignant pulmonary diseases
  - Tuberculosis
  - Lung abscess
  - Pneumonia
  - Empyema
  - Chronic obstructive pulmonary disease
- Central nervous system disorders
  - Skull fracture
  - Subdural hematoma
  - Subarachnoid hemorrhage
  - Cerebral vascular thrombosis
  - Cerebral atrophy
  - Encephalitis
  - Meningitis
  - Guillain-Barré syndrome
  - Systemic lupus erythematosus
- Drugs
  - Chlorpropramide
  - Vincristine
  - Vinblastine
  - Cyclophosphamide
  - Carbamazepine
  - Oxytocin
  - General anesthesia
  - Narcotics
  - Tricyclic antidepressants
- Miscellaneous causes
  - Hypothyroidism
  - Positive pressure mechanical ventilation

From Moses A, Streeten D: Disorders of the neurohypophysis. In Isselbacher K and others, editors: *Harrison's principles of internal medicine,* ed 13, New York, 1994, McGraw-Hill.

(CNS) infections, and vascular disorders. Central DI may also be caused by osmoreceptor destruction.

Clinical manifestations. The primary characteristic of DI is the excretion of large quantities of urine (5 to 20 L per day) with a very low specific gravity. In the milder form, urinary output may be lower (2 to 4 L per day). Most patients compensate for fluid loss by drinking great amounts of water so that serum osmolality is normal or only moderately elevated. The patient with central DI particularly favors cold or iced drinks. The patient is usually fatigued from nocturia. If oral fluid intake cannot keep up with urinary losses, severe fluid volume deficit results. This deficit is manifested by weight loss, poor tissue turgor, hypotension, tachycardia, constipation, and shock. In addition, the patient shows CNS manifestations, ranging from irritability and mental dullness to coma. These symptoms are related to rising serum osmolality and hypernatremia. Central DI usually occurs suddenly. After intracranial surgery, central DI usually has a triphasic pattern: the acute phase, with abrupt onset of polyuria; an interphase, where urine volume apparently normalizes; and a third phase, where central DI is permanent. The third phase is usually apparent within 10 to 14 days postoperatively.

Therapeutic management. Because polydipsia and polyuria (usually defined as output greater than 250 ml of urine per hour with a specific gravity of less than or equal to 1.005 and urine osmolarity of 2100 mOsm/kg) may be pituitary (central), renal (nephrogenic), or psychologic (psychogenic) in origin, identification of the cause of the DI is the initial step in therapeutic management. A complete history is taken, and a complete physical is done. An attempt is made to rule out psychogenic DI related to emotional disturbances. Psychogenic DI is associated with overhydration and hypervolemia rather than with the dehydration and hypovolemia seen in other forms of DI. A water

Table 47-3 Nursing Management: Syndrome of Inappropriate Antidiuretic Hormone

Assessment*
- Accurate hourly intake (oral and parenteral) and output
- Hourly measurement of urine specific gravity
- Daily weights
- Level of consciousness
- Observation for signs of hyponatremia every 2 hr (decreased neurologic function, convulsions, nausea and vomiting, muscle cramping)
- Monitoring of heart and lung sounds and blood pressure

Interventions
- Restriction of total fluid intake to no more than 1000 ml/day (including that taken with medications); restriction of oral intake to 700 ml < urine output until normalization of serum sodium (if appropriate)
- Positioning head of bed flat or with no more than 10° of elevation to enhance venous return to heart and increase left atrial filling pressure, reducing antidiuretic hormone release
- Positioning side rails up because of potential alterations in mental status
- Turning of patient every 2 hr, proper positioning, range-of-motion exercise, massage (if patient bedridden)
- Use of seizure precautions such as padded side rails and dim lighting
- Assistance with ambulation
- Provision of frequent oral hygiene

*Use a flow sheet for assessment documentation.

deprivation test is usually done to confirm the diagnosis of central DI (see Table 45-8).

Neurogenic DI that results from head trauma is usually self-limiting and improves with treatment of the underlying problem. DI following cranial surgery is more likely to be permanent. The goal of treatment is maintenance of fluid and electrolyte balance. This goal may be accomplished by IV administration of fluid (saline and glucose) and by hormone replacement, with ADH administered by injection or inhalation. In acute DI, fluids should be administered at a rate that decreases the serum sodium by about 1 mEq/L every 2 hours. Chlorpropamide, clofibrate, carbamazepine, and thiazide diuretics may be prescribed for symptomatic DI. For long-term therapy, desmopressin acetate, an analog of ADH that is administered as a nasal preparation and does not have the vasoconstrictive effect, is the preferred therapy.

NURSING MANAGEMENT

DIABETES INSIPIDUS

Nursing care of the patient with DI is based on the clinical symptoms. Because of the polyuria, severe dehydration and hypovolemic shock may occur. Fluids must be replaced orally or intravenously, depending on the patient's condition and ability to drink copious amounts of fluids. Adequate fluids should be kept at the bedside. If IV glucose is used, urine should be assessed for glucose. If positive, the physician should be notified, because glucosuria causes an osmotic diuresis, which increases the fluid volume deficit. Accurate records of intake and output, urine specific gravity, and daily weights are mandatory in the assessment of fluid volume status. Fluid volume deficit manifested by hypotension, tachycardia, and rapid, shallow respirations can be detected early by frequent assessment. Polyuria and nocturia can cause disturbances in rest and sleep patterns. The patient is often listless, tired, and discouraged. Support and reassurance that the sleep disturbances are temporary are helpful. Perineal care should be done at least twice daily for the bedridden female patient to cleanse urine from the perineum.

If a water deprivation test is done, the patient's baseline weight, pulse, urine and plasma osmolarities, specific gravity of urine, and blood pressure are obtained. All fluids are withheld for 8 to 16 hours. The patient may be anxious and should be reassured that the test will be stopped if fluid volume deficit becomes severe. The patient should be observed throughout the test because of the craving to drink. During the test, the patient's blood pressure, weight, and urine osmolality are assessed hourly. The test continues until urine osmolalities stabilize (hourly increase less than 30 mOsm/kg [30 mmol/kg] in 2 consecutive hours) or body weight declines by 3%. Aqueous vasopressin (5 U) is then given subcutaneously (SC), and urine osmolality is measured 1 hour later. In central DI, the rise in urinary osmolality after vasopressin exceeds 9%.[12]

When the patient affected by DI is hospitalized, often for emergency treatment of hypertonic encephalopathy, the therapeutic goal is to restore fluid balance. Desmopressin acetate is administered as a nasal or subcutaneous preparation. Overmedication can precipitate volume excess. The patient should be assessed for weight gain, headache, restlessness, and chest pain. The adequacy of treatment is assessed by monitoring fluid intake and output and by urine specific gravity. Increased urine volume with lower specific gravity is related to an inadequate pharmacologic effect, and the physician should be notified immediately.

The patient who requires long-term ADH replacement needs instruction in self-management. Desmopressin acetate is usually taken intranasally twice daily. Nasal irritation, headache, and nausea may indicate overdosage, whereas failure to improve may indicate underdosage.

THYROID GLAND

Thyroid hormones—thyroxine (T_4) and triiodothyronine (T_3), which is the more active form—regulate energy metabolism and growth and development. Thyroid disorders are manifested as hyperfunction, hypofunction, inflammation, or enlargement (goiter). A goiter may interfere with surrounding structures and can be associated with increased, normal, or decreased hormone production.

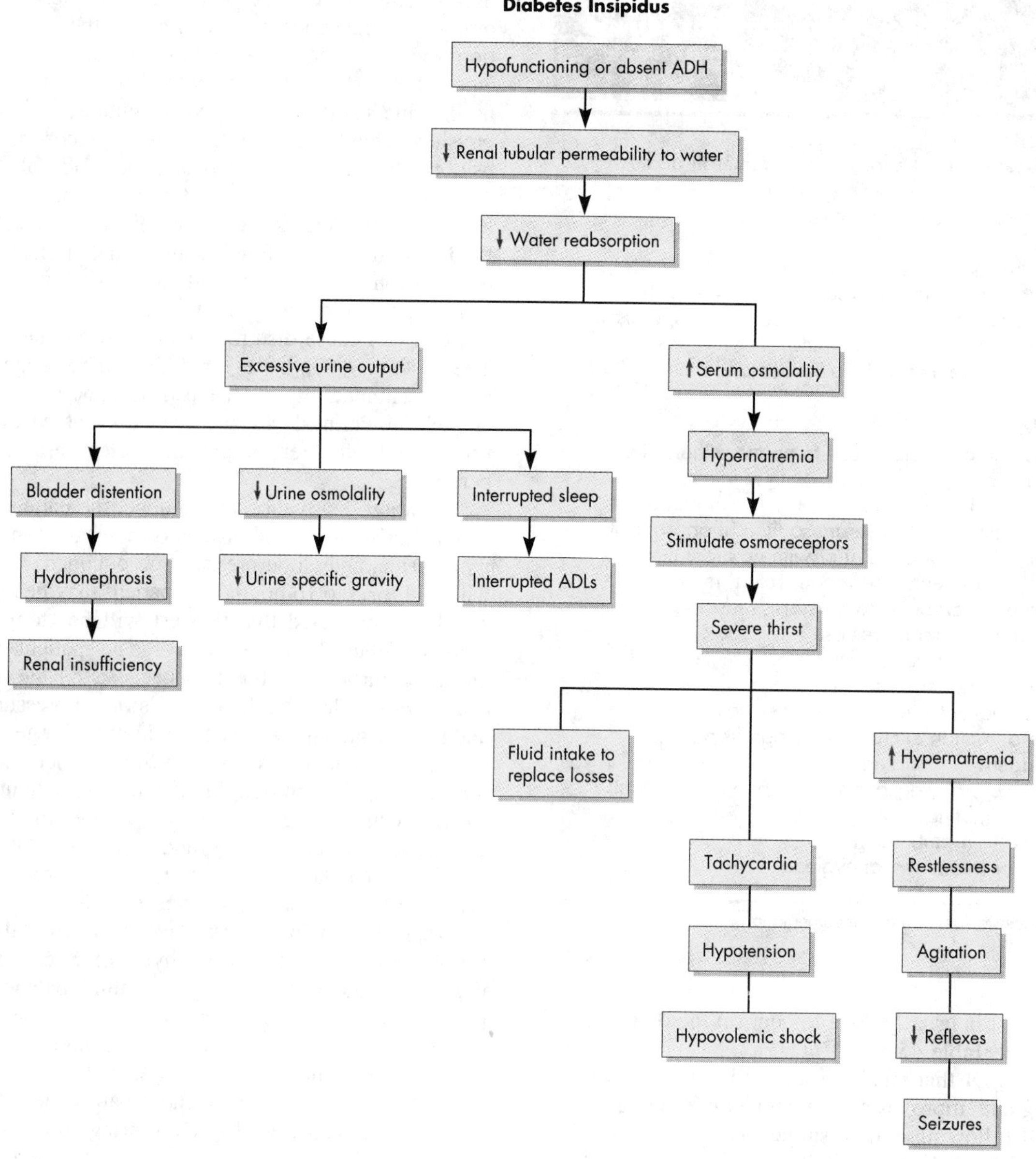

Fig. 47-4 Pathophysiology of diabetes insipidus (DI). *ADH,* Antidiuretic hormone; *ADLs,* activities of daily living.

Hyperthyroidism

Hyperthyroidism (hyperfunction of the thyroid) results from excess circulating levels of T_4, T_3, or both. It is second only to diabetes mellitus among noniatrogenic-occurring endocrine diseases. The incidence of hyperthyroidism is six times greater in women, and the highest frequency is in the 30- to 50-year-old age group. Iodine deficiency is believed to predispose the patient to hyperthyroidism and other thyroid diseases with a greater incidence in iodine-poor geographic locations (goiter belt). The most common form of hyperthyroidism is Graves' disease, followed by multinodular goiter.

Types

Graves' disease. Graves' disease is an autoimmune disease of unknown etiology marked by increased production of thyroid hormone. The patient who is genetically susceptible becomes sensitized to and develops antibodies against various antigens within the thyroid gland and often to other tissues as well. Most patients with Graves' disease have hyperthyroidism and diffuse thyroid hyperplasia caused by antibodies that attack thyroid tissue and thus stimulate hyperplasia. These antibodies are found in the serum of the individual with Graves' disease. These antibodies, known collectively as *thyroid-stimulating antibodies* (TSAbs), stimulate the TSH receptor on the thyroid and inappropriately activate the production of thyroid hormones.

Graves' disease occurs more frequently in women in their third and fourth decades. A concordance rate of 40% to 60% in identical twins indicates genetic and environmental components in the expression of the disease. The disease

CRITICAL THINKING ETHICAL DILEMMAS

ALTERNATIVE HEALERS

Situation Although thyroid replacement therapy is the planned treatment, the patient's cultural healer tells her not to take the medication; she should begin an herbal regimen instead. Should the nurse intervene?

Discussion Knowledge of a patient's cultural background and setting is important to a successful treatment plan. If the nurse can learn about the healing practices and come to know the healers in the community, a partnership can develop between traditional and allopathic medicine. Education can be conducted in both directions, and the cultural healer's methods can be used in conjunction with the prescribed treatment. However, if the nurse reacts negatively and downplays or condemns traditional healing, the patient may be forced to choose between what is culturally appropriate, acceptable, and known, and that which is required by the Western medical establishment. Hostility between Western medical professionals and traditional, cultural healers does not benefit the patient and may, in fact, dissuade the community from seeking medical attention. It is always in the patient's best interest for health care providers to be knowledgeable of the cultures of the people they serve and to develop relationships with cultural healers.

ETHICAL AND LEGAL PRINCIPLES

- Patient autonomy (the right of a patient to decide for himself or herself) must be upheld.
- Plan appropriate and effective health care that takes into consideration a patient's cultural values and beliefs.
- In some situations, Western (allopathic) medicine can no longer provide definitive care (e.g., terminally ill cancer patient), and alternative medicine may provide hope and support to the patient.

is characterized by remissions and exacerbations, with or without treatment. It may progress to destruction of thyroid tissue, causing hypothyroidism. Precipitating factors such as insufficient iodine supply, infections, and emotions may interact with genetic factors that control immunologic and metabolic abnormalities to cause Graves' disease.[13]

Multinodular goiter. Multinodular goiter is characterized by small, discrete, autonomously functioning nodules that secrete thyroid hormone. If associated with signs of hyperthyroidism, a nodule is termed *toxic adenoma.* The frequency of toxic multinodular goiter is highest in women in the sixth and seventh decades of life. There is usually a history of preexisting simple goiter for years before the onset of demonstrable hyperthyroidism. The manifestations are slower to develop and usually less severe than in Graves' disease. Multinodular goiter is usually not associated with exophthalmos (eyeball protrusion from the orbit). These nodules may be benign or malignant.

Clinical Manifestations. The clinical manifestations of hyperthyroidism are related to the effects of excess thyroid hormones in two ways. The first is their direct effect of increasing metabolism. The second is an increased tissue sensitivity to stimulation by the sympathetic division of the autonomic nervous system. Thyroid hormones increase the number of β-adrenergic receptors, thereby increasing sensitivity to the activity of catecholamines, even though the absolute levels of these hormones (epinephrine and norepinephrine) are not elevated.[14] (The manifestations of hyperthyroidism are summarized in Table 47-4.) A patient with advanced disease may exhibit many of the symptoms, whereas a patient in the early stages of hyperthyroidism, may only exhibit weight loss and increased nervousness. In the elderly patient, this disorder is an exaggeration of an underlying disease rather than a hyperthyroid state.[15] Table 47-5 compares features of hyperthyroidism in young and geriatric patients.

Exophthalmos. Exophthalmos (proptosis), in which the eyeballs protrude from the orbits, is due to impaired venous drainage from the orbit leading to increased deposits of fat and fluid (edema) in the retroorbital tissues (Fig. 47-5). This sign, which is seen in 20% to 40% of patients with Graves' disease, is autoimmune in nature. In exophthalmos the upper lids are usually retracted and elevated, and the eyeballs are forced outward with the sclera above the iris visible. This produces the characteristic stare and protrusion of the eyeball. Exophthalmos is usually bilateral but can be unilateral or asymmetric. When the eyelids do not close completely, the exposed corneal surfaces become dry and irritated. Serious consequences, such as corneal ulcers and eventual loss of vision, can occur.

Complications. *Hyperthyroid crisis* (thyrotoxic crisis) is an acute but rare condition where all hyperthyroid manifestations are heightened. It is potentially fatal, but death is rare when treatment is vigorous and initiated early. The cause is presumed to be stressors such as infection, trauma, or surgery in a patient with preexisting hyperthyroidism, either diagnosed or undiagnosed. The physiologic factor or factors that initiates thyrotoxic crisis are unknown. It may represent a shift from protein-bound to free hormone secondary to circulating inhibitors to binding in systemic illness. Manifestations include severe tachycardia, heart failure, shock, hyperthermia (up to 105.3° F) [40.7° C], restlessness, agitation, abdominal pain, nausea, vomiting, diarrhea, delirium, and coma. Measures must be taken to prevent death. Treatment is aimed at reducing circulating thyroid hormone levels and the clinical manifestations of this disorder by appropriate drug therapy and extracorporeal removal of thyroid hormone. Therapy is directed at fever reduction, fluid replacement, and elimination or management of the initiating stressor(s).[16]

Diagnostic Studies. Serum T_4 and T_3 can be measured with radioimmunoassay techniques (see Table 45-8) and will be elevated. T_3 resin uptake (T_3RU) is also elevated. T_3RU varies inversely with the amount of thyroid hormone that is protein bound and therefore inactive; that is, a high T_3RU indicates that more hormone than normal is biologically active. Free T_4 and T_3 are usually elevated in hyperthyroidism, and TSH is subnormal or undetectable. In the nonpregnant, nonlactating patient, a 6- or 24-hour radioactive iodine uptake (RAIU) may be done. This test is

Table 47-4 Clinical Manifestations: Thyroid Hormone Dysfunction

Hypofunction	Hyperfunction
Cardiovascular System	
Increased capillary fragility Decreased pulse rate Varied changes in blood pressure Cardiac hypertrophy, weak contractility Distant heart sounds Anemia Tendency to develop congestive heart failure, angina, myocardial infarction	Systolic hypertension Increased rate and force of cardiac contractions Bounding, rapid pulse Increased cardiac output Cardiac hypertrophy Systolic murmurs Dysrhythmias Palpitations Atrial fibrillation (more common in the older adult) Angina
Respiratory System	
Dyspnea Decreased breathing capacity	Increased respiratory rate Dyspnea on mild exertion
Gastrointestinal System	
Decreased appetite Nausea and vomiting Weight gain Constipation Distended abdomen Enlarged, scaly tongue	Increased appetite, thirst Weight loss Increased peristalsis Diarrhea, frequent defecation Increased bowel sounds Splenomegaly Hepatomegaly
Integumentary System	
Dry, thick, inelastic, cold skin Thick, brittle nails Dry, sparse, coarse hair Poor turgor of mucosa Generalized interstitial edema Puffy face Decreased sweating Pallor	Warm, smooth, moist skin Thin, brittle nails detached from nail bed (onchyolysis) Hair loss (may be patchy) Acropachy (clubbing) Palmar erythema Fine silky hair Premature graying (in men) Diaphoresis Vitiligo
Musculoskeletal System	
Fatigue Weakness Muscular aches and pains Slow movements Arthralgia	Fatigue Muscle weakness (especially proximal) Proximal muscle wasting Pretibial myxedema Dependent edema Osteoporosis
Nervous System	
Apathy Lethargy Forgetfulness Slowed mental processes Hoarseness Slow, slurred speech Prolonged relaxation of deep tendon muscles Stupor, coma Paresthesias Anxiety, depression Polyneuropathy	Difficulty in focusing eyes Nervousness Fine tremor (of fingers and tongue) Insomnia Lability of mood, delirium Restlessness Personality changes of irritability, agitation Exhaustion Hyperreflexia of tendon reflexes Depression, fatigue, apathy (in the older adult) Lack of ability to concentrate Stupor, coma
Reproductive System	
Prolonged menstrual periods or amenorrhea Decreased libido Infertility	Menstrual irregularities Amenorrhea Decreased libido Impotence in men Gynecomastia Decreased fertility
Other	
Increased susceptibility to infection Increased sensitivity to narcotics, barbiturates, anesthesia Intolerance to cold Decreased hearing Sleepiness Goiter	Intolerance to heat Increased sensitivity to stimulant drugs Elevated basal temperature Lid lag, stare Eyelid retraction Exophthalmos Goiter Rapid speech

not appropriate for pregnant or lactating women because radioactive iodine can cross the placenta and destroy the fetal thyroid or enter breast milk and destroy the newborn thyroid. This test can differentiate Graves' disease from other forms of thyroiditis. The patient with Graves' disease will show a diffuse, homogeneous uptake of 25% to 95%, whereas the patient with another form of thyroiditis will show an uptake of less than 5%.[17] In addition, the electrocardiogram (ECG) may show tachycardia, atrial fibrillation, and alterations in P and T waves.

Therapeutic and Pharmacologic Management. The therapeutic goals are to block the adverse effects of thyroid hormones and stop their oversecretion. Therapy involves pharmacotherapy with antithyroid drugs and β-adrenergic receptor blockers, thyroid ablation with radioactive iodine, and subtotal thyroidectomy after adequate preparation (Table 47-6). The choice of treatment is influenced by the patient's age, severity of the disorder, complicating features (including pregnancy), and patient's preferences. If surgery is to be performed, the patient is usually given antithyroid drugs to produce a euthyroid state and possibly iodine and β-adrenergic blockers to relieve symptoms preoperatively. Any other associated disorders, such as cardiac disease or diabetes mellitus, must also be controlled before surgery.

Table 47-5 Comparison of Hyperthyroidism in Younger and Older Patients

	Young Adult	Older
▪ Common causes	Graves' disease in >90% of cases	Graves' disease or toxic nodular goiter
▪ Syndrome	Nervousness, irritability, weight loss, palpitations, heat intolerance, and warm, fine skin	Cardiac (angina, dysrhythmia, congestive heart failure) Gastrointestinal (weight loss) Myopathy
▪ Goiter	In >90% of cases	In about 50% of cases
▪ Eye signs	Endocrine exophthalmos reflects autoimmune pathogenesis of Graves' disease	Eye signs less frequent
▪ Cardiac features	Tachycardia without heart disease	Underlying cardiac disease common
▪ Thyroxine (T_4)	Elevated in >90% of cases	Elevated somewhat less often
▪ Triiodothyronine (T_3)	Elevated	Elevated
▪ Thyroid stimulating hormone	Low	Low

From Federman D: Hyperthyroidism in the geriatric population, *Hosp Pract* 26:61, 1991.

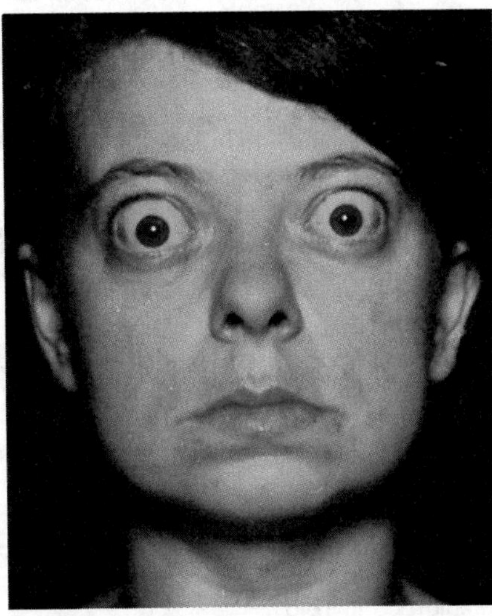

Fig. 47-5 Exophthalmos secondary to Graves' disease.

For thyroidectomy to be effective, approximately 90% of thyroid tissue must be removed. If too much tissue is taken, the gland will not regenerate after surgery and hypothyroidism will develop. Occasionally the recurrent laryngeal nerve or parathyroid glands may be damaged during surgery.

Antithyroid drugs. The most commonly used antithyroid drugs are classified as thioamides. Propylthiouracil (PTU) and methimazole (Tapazole) are clinically the most commonly used drugs. These drugs inhibit the synthesis of thyroid hormones. PTU also blocks peripheral conversion of T_4 to T_3. Although there is considerable individual variation, improvement usually begins 1 to 2 weeks after the initiation of therapy, and good results are seen within 4 to 8 weeks. Therapy is usually continued for 6 months to 2 years to allow for spontaneous remission. Two major disadvantages of antithyroid drugs are patient noncompliance and a high rate of recurrence of hyperthyroidism when the drugs are discontinued. In addition, agranulocytosis may occur in rare situations. Indications for use of antithyroid drugs include Graves' disease in the young patient, thyrotoxicosis during pregnancy, and the need to make a patient euthyroid before surgery or irradiation.

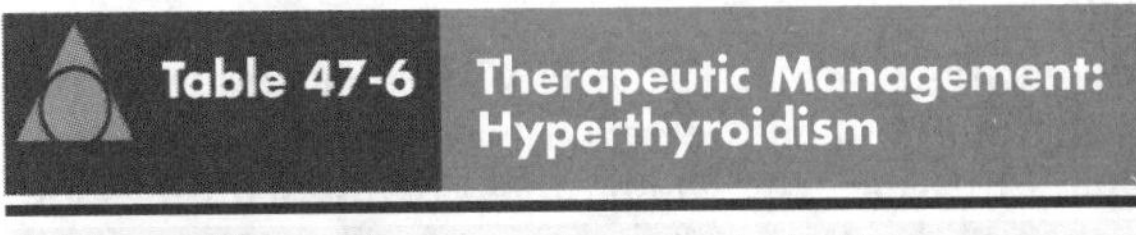

Table 47-6 Therapeutic Management: Hyperthyroidism

Diagnostic
- History and physical examination
- Ophthalmologic examination
- ECG
- Laboratory tests
  - Serum T_3RU, T_4, free T_3, TSH levels
  - TRH stimulation test
- Nuclear medicine-thyroid scan

Therapeutic

Graves' disease
- Antithyroid drugs
  - Propylthiouracil
  - Methimazole
- β-Adrenergic blockers such as propranolol (Inderal)
- Ablation of thyroid tissue
  - Radioactive iodine (^{131}iodine)
  - Subtotal thyroidectomy
- High-caloric diet

Multinodular goiter
- Antithyroid drugs
  - Propylthiouracil
  - Methimazole
- Ablation of thyroid tissue by radioactive iodine

ECG, Electrocardiogram; *TRH*, thyrotropin-releasing hormone; *T_3RU*, T_3 resin uptake; *TSH*, thyroid-stimulating hormone.

Iodine. Iodine (e.g., Lugol's solution, potassium iodide) in large doses inhibits synthesis of active thyroid hormones T_3 and T_4 and blocks the release of these hormones into circulation. Its maximal effect is usually seen within 1 to 2 weeks. After that time a reduction in the therapeutic effect may be seen, and long-term iodine therapy is not effective in controlling hyperthyroidism. Usually one drop of a saturated solution of potassium iodide is administered three times daily before surgery. Iodine decreases the size and vascularity of the thyroid, making resection safer and easier. Administration of PTU, with iodine therapy added 10 days before surgery, is a common method for surgical preparation of a patient with hyperthyroidism.

β-Adrenergic blockers. Propranolol (Inderal) is the most frequently used β-adrenergic blocker. It relieves the symptoms of hyperthyroidism that result from increased β-adrenergic receptors caused by excess thyroid hormones. These symptoms include heat intolerance, palpitations, nervousness, tremor, and muscle weakness. Propranolol is used with other antithyroid treatment and rapidly relieves the symptoms that cause such discomfort to the patient with hyperthyroidism. Propranolol is not used in the patient with asthma or heart disease. Atenolol (Tenormin) may be used instead.

Radioactive iodine. Radioactive iodine (radioiodine) limits thyroid hormone secretion by damaging or destroying thyroid tissue. It is administered orally, with the dose determined by estimated thyroid weight. This treatment is effective but often results in hypothyroidism with a frequency that increases with time.[18] Radioactive iodine has a delayed response, and maximum effects may not be seen for 2 to 3 months. However, it is effective and inexpensive and can be administered on an outpatient basis. The patient is treated with PTU or propranolol before and during the first 3 months after the initiation of radioactive iodine therapy and for relief of hyperthyroid symptoms until the effects of irradiation become apparent. Thyroid ablation with ^{131}I is not indicated in children because carcinogenesis may be increased nor in pregnant women because radioactive iodine crosses the placenta and destroys the fetal thyroid. It is not used in men or women in their childbearing years because of the potential for chromosome damage.

Nutritional Management. The potential for nutritional deficits is high when an increased metabolic rate is present. A high-caloric diet (4000 to 5000 kcal/day) may be ordered to satisfy hunger and prevent tissue breakdown. This is accomplished with six full meals a day and snacks high in protein, carbohydrates, minerals, and vitamins (particularly vitamin A), thiamin, B_6, and ascorbic acid. The protein allowance should be 1 to 2 g/kg of ideal body weight. Increased carbohydrates should compensate for disturbed metabolism, provide energy, and spare protein. Recommended foods should be kept readily available. The nurse should weigh the patient daily to monitor adequacy of diet, since weight increases are usually desirable. Offering fluids frequently prevents volume deficit related to diaphoresis and insensible loss. Highly seasoned and high-fiber foods should be avoided because they stimulate the already hypermotile GI tract. Substitutes should be provided for caffeine-containing liquids such as coffee, tea, and cola because the stimulating effects of these fluids increase the restlessness and sleep disturbances. Milk is an excellent food source that provides both calcium and protein. A dietitian should be consulted for guidance in meeting the nutritional needs of a patient with hyperthyroidism.

NURSING MANAGEMENT

HYPERTHYROIDISM

Nursing Assessment

Subjective and objective data that should be obtained from an individual with hyperthyroidism are presented in Table 47-7.

Table 47-7 Nursing Assessment: Hyperthyroidism

Subjective Data

Important health information

Past health history: Preexisting goiter; recent infection
Medications: Use of thyroid hormones
Surgery, trauma, treatments: Exposure to head and neck radiation; recent trauma or surgery

Functional health patterns

Health perception–health management: Positive family history of thyroid disorders or pernicious anemia; emotional lability, irritability, fatigue
Nutritional-metabolic: Weight loss; increased appetite; increased iodine intake; nausea; itching; sweating; heat sensitivity
Elimination: Diarrhea; polyuria
Activity-exercise: Dyspnea on exertion; palpitations; muscle weakness
Sexuality-reproductive: Decreased libido; impotence; gynecomastia (in men); amenorrhea (in women)

Objective Data

General
Exophthalmos, infrequent blinking, restlessness, agitation, rapid speech and body movements, hyperthermia, enlarged thyroid

Integumentary
Warm, diaphoretic, velvety skin; thin, loose nails; hair loss; palmar erythema; diffuse increased pigmentation

Respiratory
Tachypnea

Cardiovascular
Tachycardia, bounding pulse, systolic murmurs, hypertension, diffuse edema of legs and feet, dysrhythmias

Neurologic
Hyperreflexia, diplopia, tremors (of hands, tongue, eyelids)

Musculoskeletal
Muscle wasting

Possible findings
Elevated serum T_3, T_4, and T_3 resin uptake and iodine levels; negative serum thyrotropin-releasing hormone (TRH) stimulation test; chest x-ray showing cardiac hypertrophy

Nursing Diagnoses

Nursing diagnoses are determined when the problem and etiologic factors are supported by clinical data. Nursing diagnoses related to hyperthyroidism may include, but are not limited to, those presented in the nursing care plan on p. 1492.

Planning

The overall goals are that the patient with hyperthyroidism will (1) experience relief of symptoms, (2) have no serious complications related to the disease or treatment, and (3) cooperate with the therapeutic plan.

Nursing Implementation

Acute Intervention. A restful, calm, quiet room should be provided because increased metabolism causes sleep disturbances. Provision of adequate rest may be a challenge because of the patient's irritability and restlessness. Interventions may include placing the patient in a cool room, away from very ill patients and noisy, high-traffic areas; using light bed coverings and changing the linen frequently if the patient is diaphoretic; encouraging and assisting with exercise involving large muscle groups (tremors can interfere with small-muscle coordination) to allow the release of nervous tension and restlessness; restricting visitors who upset the patient; and establishing a supportive, trusting relationship to help the patient cope with aggravating events and lessen anxiety.

Nursing interventions with the patient's significant others include assisting them to perform the nursing interventions, instructing them in the nature of the patient's illness to enable them to understand the physical and emotional manifestations the patient experiences, exploring or suggesting ways they can help reduce stressful situations, and providing a nonjudgmental atmosphere for them to express difficulties in accepting and dealing with the patient's demands and behavior.

If exophthalmos is present, there is a potential for corneal injury related to irritation and dryness. The patient may also have orbital pain. Nursing interventions to relieve eye discomfort and prevent corneal ulceration include applying artificial tears to soothe and moisten conjunctival membranes. Salt restriction may help reduce periorbital edema. Elevation of the patient's head promotes fluid drainage from the periorbital area; the patient should sit upright as much as possible. Dark glasses reduce glare and prevent irritation from smoke, air currents, dust, and dirt. If the eyelids cannot be closed, they should be lightly taped shut for sleep. To maintain flexibility, the patient should be taught to exercise the intraocular muscles several times a day, by turning the eyes in the complete range of motion. Good grooming can be helpful in reducing the loss of self-esteem that can result from an altered body image. If the exophthalmos is severe, treatment may involve suturing the eyelids together, administering corticosteroids, radiation of retroorbital tissues, orbital decompression, or corrective lid or muscle surgery.

NURSING MANAGEMENT

RADIOACTIVE IODINE THERAPY

Radioactive iodine therapy (ablation) is usually administered on an outpatient basis and is the therapy of choice for the adult beyond childbearing years. Because the usual therapeutic dose of radioactive iodine is only 7 to 10 mCi, no radiation safety precautions are necessary. The patient should be instructed that radiation thyroiditis and parotiditis are possible and may cause dryness and irritation of the mouth and throat. Relief may be obtained with frequent sips of water, ice chips, or the use of a salt and soda gargles three to four times per day. This gargle is made by dissolving 1 teaspoon of salt and 1 teaspoon of baking soda in 2 cups of warm water. The discomfort should subside in 3 to 4 days. If dryness and irritation persist, the patient should contact a clinician. Because of the high frequency of hypothyroidism after radioactive iodine therapy, the patient and significant others should be taught the symptoms of hypothyroidism and instructed to seek medical help if these symptoms occur.

NURSING MANAGEMENT

THYROID SURGERY

Preoperative Care

When subtotal thyroidectomy is the treatment of choice, the patient must be adequately prepared to avoid postoperative complications. The signs and symptoms of hyperthyroidism must be alleviated as much as possible, and cardiac problems must be controlled before surgery. If iodine is used to relieve hyperthyroid symptoms, it should be mixed with water or juice, sipped through a straw, and administered after meals. The patient must be assessed for signs of iodine toxicity such as swelling of buccal mucosa and other mucous membranes, excessive salivation, nausea and vomiting, and skin reactions. If toxicity occurs, iodine administration should be discontinued and the physician notified.

Preoperative teaching should include comfort and safety measures in which the patient can participate. Coughing, deep breathing, and leg exercises should be practiced, and their importance explained. The patient should be taught how to support the head manually while turning in bed, since this maneuver minimizes stress on the suture line after surgery. Range-of-motion exercises of the neck should be practiced. The nurse should explain routine postoperative care such as IV infusions. The patient should be told that talking is likely to be difficult for a short time after surgery.

Postoperative Care

The hospital room must be prepared before the patient's return from surgery. Oxygen, suction equipment, and a tracheostomy tray should be readily available. A tracheostomy tray is required in case airway obstruction occurs. Although this happens rarely, it is an emergency situation. Recurrent laryngeal nerve damage leads to vocal cord paralysis. If there is paralysis of both cords, spastic airway obstruction will occur, requiring an immediate tracheostomy.

Respiration may also become difficult because of excess swelling of the neck tissues, hemorrhage, and hematoma formation. Laryngeal stridor (harsh, vibratory sound) may occur during respiration as a result of tetany, which occurs

NURSING CARE PLAN Patient with Hyperthyroidism

Planning: Outcome Criteria	Nursing Interventions and Rationales
➤ **NURSING DIAGNOSIS**	Sleep pattern disturbance *related to* anxiety, environmental stimulation, disruption of normal sleep pattern, and caffeine intake *as manifested by* complaints of restlessness, irritability, insomnia, fatigue; awakening during the night
Decrease purposeless movements; verbalize feeling of being rested on awakening.	Promote continuation of usual practices related to rest and sleep unless contraindicated *to promote maximal rest and sleep.* Decrease environmental stimuli *to decrease contributing to patient's restlessness and irritability and to promote rest and sleep.* Administer frequent back rubs with effleurage *because this activity is calming and soothing to the patient.* Approach patient with calm, unhurried demeanor; work efficiently when with patient; encourage quiet diversions *to avoid increasing irritability.* Encourage frequent short walks during the day *to defuse restlessness and promote sleep.* Administer antithyroid drugs as ordered *to decrease thyroid hormone production and relieve symptoms.* Administer sedatives as needed *to relieve CNS stimulation.* Eliminate caffeine (e.g., coffee, tea, cola, chocolate) from diet *to avoid stimulating the patient and increasing restlessness and sleep problems.*
➤ **NURSING DIAGNOSIS**	Activity intolerance *related to* fatigue, exhaustion, and heat intolerance secondary to hypermetabolism *as manifested by* complaints of weakness, inability to perform usual activities, short attention span, memory lapses, dyspnea, tachycardia, irritability
Have decrease in perception of weakness and fatigue.	Assess for signs of activity intolerance *because hyperthyroidism results in protein catabolism, overactivity, and increased metabolism leading to exhaustion.* Monitor vital signs q4hr and before and after activities *because tachycardia and blood pressure elevations can indicate excessive activity.* Assist patient with self-care as needed *to make certain patient's daily needs are met.* Limit ambulation to short walks *to avoid fatiguing patient.* Schedule activities of daily living and treatments *to promote adequate rest periods.*
➤ **NURSING DIAGNOSIS**	Risk for injury: corneal ulceration *related to* decreased blinking or inability to close eyelids secondary to exophthalmos
Have no evidence of corneal damage.	Assess patient for complaints of eye pain, feeling of grittiness or "sand" in eyes; proptosis; inability to close eyelids completely; lid lag; lid retraction; visible sclera above iris; "stare" *to determine if risk factors are present and to initiate appropriate interventions.* Instruct patient to wear dark glasses *to reduce glare and reduce irritation from dust and dirt.* Restrict patient's salt intake *to reduce periorbital edema.* Raise head of bed at night *to promote fluid drainage.* Teach patient to exercise extraocular muscles daily *to maintain flexibility.* Cover patient's eyes with mask or tape shut if eyes will not close if exophthalmos is severe *to prevent corneal drying and, at night, to promote sleep.* Apply methylcellulose eyedrops (artifical tears) *to soothe and moisten conjunctival membranes.*
➤ **NURSING DIAGNOSIS**	Risk for trauma *related to* fine muscle tremors, fatigue, inattentiveness, incoordination
Have no accidental injury.	Assess ability to perform tasks requiring small muscles; restlessness, fatigue; fine-muscle tremors; uncoordinated movements; pretibial myxedema *to determine risk for trauma and to plan appropriate interventions.* Assist patient as necessary with tasks requiring fine motor skills; reduce environmental hazards *to reduce exposure to high risk activities.* Assist patient with ambulation *to prevent trauma from falling or bumping into items.* Teach patient safety practices *to reduce possibility of trauma and to increase patient's sense of control.*

continued

NURSING CARE PLAN Patient with Hyperthyroidism—cont'd

Planning: Outcome Criteria	Nursing Interventions and Rationales
➤ **NURSING DIAGNOSIS**	Altered nutrition: less than body requirements *related to* hypermetabolism and inadequate diet *as manifested by* complaints of weight loss, hunger, clothing too large; less than optimal body weight
Maintain weight (or gain weight); alleviate (or prevent) nutritional deficiency; verbalize satisfaction with diet.	Assess patient's eating habits and weight pattern *to determine extent of the problem and to plan appropriate interventions.* Teach and provide high-caloric, high-vitamin, high-mineral diet that includes between-meal and bedtime snacks *because hyperthyroidism increases metabolic rate with resulting need to prevent muscle breakdown and weight loss.* Weigh patient daily *to evaluate effectiveness of nutritional plan.* Monitor blood urea nitrogen and albumin levels *to evaluate protein levels to determine extent of protein malnutrition.* Arrange dietary consultation if indicated.
➤ **NURSING DIAGNOSIS**	Anxiety *related to* lack of knowledge about management and course of disease, hypermetabolism, and presence of hypertension *as manifested by* inability to verbalize information regarding medication and low-sodium foods and inability to cope with stresses and increased metabolic activities
Verbalize knowledge of management and course of disease; verbalize decrease in anxiety.	Teach patient about disease management, including medication regimen, potential for hypertension, chronic nature of disease, and dietary implications *because knowledge decreases anxiety and increases a sense of control.* Assist patient to develop strategies for behavior change *to incorporate medication regimen into lifestyle.* Promote rest and relaxation *because anxiety often causes difficulty with rest and sleep.* Teach patient strategies for coping with stress *to prevent increasing anxiety.* Administer medications as ordered *because decrease in disease activity will relieve anxiety.*
➤ **NURSING DIAGNOSIS**	Altered comfort: hyperthermia *related to* impaired temperature adaptation and altered perception of ambient temperature *as manifested by* verbalization of feelings of excess warmth; wearing of inappropriately scant amount of clothing; elevated temperature; warm, moist skin; diaphoresis
Have decrease in perspiration and increase in comfort.	Assess for elevated temperature, diaphoresis, and heat intolerance *to determine extent of problem and to plan interventions.* Maintain cool environmental temperature; provide light, loose clothing *to reduce patient's perception of being overheated.* Bathe patient frequently; change linen frequently *to promote patient comfort.* Encourage fluids to 3 L/day *to replace fluid lost if diaphoretic.*

COLLABORATIVE PROBLEMS

Nursing Goals	Nursing Interventions and Rationales
➤ **POTENTIAL COMPLICATION**	Congestive heart failure related to increased cardiac workload secondary to hypermetabolism
Monitor for signs of congestive heart failure, report deviations from acceptable parameters, and carry out appropriate medical and nursing interventions.	Assess complaints of dyspnea, fatigue, chest pain, edema; cardiac enlargement; atrial fibrillation; diaphoresis *to determine presence of congestive heart failure.* Reduce environmental stressors; promote rest and relaxation *to reduce cardiac workload.* Assess tolerance to activity *so appropriate assistance can be provided.* Discourage physical activity that is not well tolerated *to prevent stressing heart beyond its limit to respond.* Administer cardiotonics as ordered *to stabilize cardiac status.* Monitor vital signs and cardiac status frequently *to evaluate effectiveness of plan.*

if the parathyroid glands are removed or damaged during surgery. To treat tetany, calcium salts such as calcium gluconate and calcium chloride should be readily available for IV administration.

After a thyroidectomy the nurse should do the following:

1. Assess the patient every 2 hours for 24 hours for signs of hemorrhage or tracheal compression such as irregular breathing, neck swelling, frequent swallowing, sensations of fullness at the incision site, choking, and blood on the anterior or posterior dressings.
2. Place the patient in a semi-Fowler's position and support the head with pillows, avoiding flexion of the neck and any tension on the suture lines.
3. Monitor vital signs. Complete the initial assessment by checking for signs of tetany secondary to hypoparathyroidism (e.g., tingling in toes, fingers, or around the mouth; muscular twitching; apprehension) and by evaluating difficulty in speaking and hoarseness. Some hoarseness is to be expected for 3 to 4 days after surgery because of edema.
4. Control postoperative pain by giving medication. Meperidine (Demerol) and morphine are commonly prescribed.

The neck incision should be lubricated and range-of-motion exercises should be carried out three or four times daily to promote comfort and the return of full range of motion. The patient should be taught movements that cause flexion, extension, rotation, and lateral bending of the neck. The appearance of the incision may be quite distressing. The patient can be reassured that the scar will fade in color and eventually look like a normal neck wrinkle. A scarf, jewelry, high collar, or other covering can effectively camouflage a fresh scar.

If postoperative recovery is uneventful, the patient is ambulated the first day, takes fluid as soon as tolerated, and eats a soft diet by the second day after surgery.

Chronic and Home Management

Follow-up care is important for the patient who has undergone thyroid surgery. Hyperthyroidism may recur after a period of time, requiring further treatment. Hormone balance should be monitored periodically to ensure that normal function has returned. Most patients experience a period of relative hypothyroidism soon after surgery because of the substantial reduction in the size of the thyroid. The remaining tissue usually hypertrophies, recovering the capacity to produce the hormone needed by the body; but this takes time. The administration of thyroid hormone is avoided because exogenous hormone inhibits pituitary production of TSH and delays or prevents the restoration of normal gland function and thyroid tissue regeneration.

The patient can do a great deal to prevent complications and promote a return to normal function during the hypothyroid period after surgery. Caloric intake must be reduced substantially below the amount that was required before surgery to prevent weight gain. The surgeon may suggest avoiding foods that contain thyroid-inhibiting substances (goitrogens) (Table 47-8). Adequate iodine is necessary to promote thyroid function, but excesses inhibit the thyroid. Seafood once or twice a week or normal use of iodized salt should provide sufficient intake. Regular exercise helps stimulate the thyroid and should be encouraged. Exposure to alternating extremes of temperature, such as hot and cold showers, also promotes thyroid hyperplasia but is not acceptable to many individuals because of cold intolerance. High environmental temperature should be avoided because it inhibits thyroid regeneration.

Regular follow-up care is necessary. The patient should be seen biweekly for a month and then at least semiannually to assess for the development of hypothyroidism. If a complete thyroidectomy has been performed, the patient needs instruction in lifelong pharmacologic thyroid replacement. Failure of thyroid function is considered by some authorities to be the normal endstage of Graves' disease. The patient should be taught the signs and symptoms of progressive thyroid failure and instructed to seek medical care if these develop. Hypothyroidism is relatively easy to control with oral administration of thyroid preparations.

Table 47-8 Common Exogenous Goitrogens

Foods
- Potent goitrogens
  - Turnips
  - Rutabagas
  - Soybeans (especially when fed to infants in formula)
  - Skins of peanuts
  - Milk from kale-fed cattle
- Less potent goitrogens
  - Seafood
  - Green leafy vegetables
  - Peanuts
  - Peaches
  - Peas
  - Strawberries
  - Carrots
  - Cabbage
  - Mustard seed
  - Radishes

Drugs
- Thyroid inhibitors
  - Propylthiouracil
  - Methimazole
  - Carbimazole
  - Iodine in large doses
- Others
  - Sulfonamides
  - Salicylates
  - p-Aminosalicylic acid
  - Phenylbutazone
  - Lithium
  - Amiodarone

Thyroid Enlargement

Enlargement of the thyroid gland is called *goiter* (Fig. 47-6). Goiter may result from hypertrophy caused by excess TSH stimulation, which in turn can be caused by

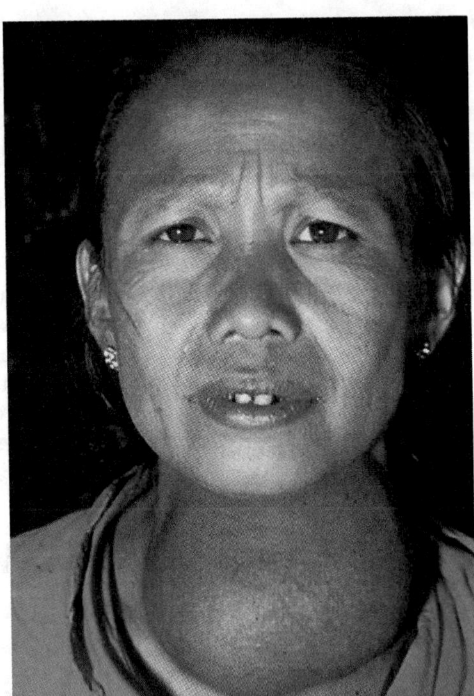

Fig. 47-6 Simple goiter.

inadequate circulating thyroid hormones. Goiter may also be caused by growth-stimulating immunoglobulins and other growth factors. Goitrogens (see Table 47-8), which inhibit synthesis of thyroid hormone, can cause goiter but usually only in the individual who lives in an iodine-deficient area (endemic goiter).

TSH and T_4 are measured to determine whether a goiter is associated with hyperthyroidism, hypothyroidism, or normal thyroid function. Thyroid antibodies are measured to assess for thyroiditis. Treatment with thyroid hormone may prevent further thyroid enlargement. Surgery to remove large goiters may be necessary.

Thyroid Nodules. A thyroid nodule, a palpable deformity of the thyroid gland, may be benign or malignant. Malignant tumors of the thyroid gland are rare. The major sign of thyroid cancer is the appearance of a hard, painless nodule in an enlarged thyroid. A thyroid scan shows whether nodules on the thyroid are "hot" or "cold." When a person is given tracer doses of ^{131} I, thyroid tumors on the thyroid may or may not take up the radioactive iodine. Tumors that take up the radioactive iodine are called hot nodules and are nearly always benign. If the nodule does not take up the radioactive iodine, it appears as "cold" and has a higher risk of being malignant. Ultrasonography and MRI may also be used to aid in diagnosis. Needle biopsy of the nodule is usually done to identify malignant tissue. Measurement of serum calcitonin is also helpful in diagnosis, since increased levels are associated with medullary thyroid carcinoma. Benign nodules are usually not dangerous, but they can cause tracheal compression if they become too large.

Neoplasms are treated by surgical removal. Surgical procedures may range from unilateral total lobectomy with removal of the isthmus to total thyroidectomy with bilateral neck dissection. Many thyroid cancers are TSH-dependent, and thyroid hormone in hyperphysiologic doses is often prescribed to inhibit pituitary secretion of TSH. External radiation may be used to prolong survival. Nursing care for the patient with thyroid tumors is similar to care for the patient who has undergone thyroidectomy and also includes general nursing measures for the patient with cancer (see Chapter 12).

Thyroiditis. Thyroiditis is an inflammatory process in the thyroid and can have several causes. *Subacute granulomatous thyroiditis* (de Quervain's thyroiditis), which presents with hyperthyroidism, is thought to be caused by a viral infection. *Acute thyroiditis* is due to bacterial or fungal infection. Subacute and acute forms of thyroiditis have abrupt onsets. Silent thyroiditis, a form of lymphocytic thyroiditis, has a variable onset. This condition may occur in the postpartal period. In addition, two epidemics have been noted to be related to contamination of ground beef with thyroid tissue. *Autoimmune thyroiditis* (Hashimoto's thyroiditis), leading to hypothyroidism, is insidious in onset. Hashimoto's thyroiditis is a chronic autoimmune disease in which thyroid tissue is replaced by lymphocytes and fibrous tissue. It is the most common cause of goiterous hypothyroidism in the United States.

T_4 and T_3 are initially elevated in subacute, acute, and silent thyroiditis but may become depressed with time. TSH levels are low and then elevated. Thyroid hormone levels are usually low in chronic Hashimoto's thyroiditis and TSH is high. Suppression of RAIU is seen in subacute and silent thyroiditis. Antithyroid antibodies are present in Hashimoto's thyroiditis.

Recovery from thyroiditis may be complete in weeks or months without treatment. If the condition is bacterial in origin, treatment may include specific antibiotics or surgical drainage. In subacute and acute forms, salicylates and nonsteroidal antiinflammatory drugs (NSAIDs) are used. If there is no response to these drugs in 48 hours, corticosteroids are given. Propranolol or atenolol may be used for the cardiovascular symptoms of a hyperthyroid condition. Thyroid hormone is used if the patient is hypothyroid.

Nursing care of the patient with thyroiditis includes education regarding normal thyroid function and what is happening in the patient's specific instance. Other nursing interventions depend, in part, on the therapeutic management. Nursing interventions include reassurance, support, and assistance during the recovery period. The patient should be instructed to remain under close health supervision so that progress can be monitored and to report any change in symptoms to the health care provider.

The patient with thyroiditis of autoimmune origin may be susceptible to other autoimmune diseases such as Addison's disease, pernicious anemia, or premature gonadal failure or Graves' disease. The patient should be taught the signs and symptoms of these disorders, particularly Addison's disease. Because stress may aggravate these autoimmune diseases, stress management is an important part of patient education (see Chapter 5). The patient should also be given a list of common goitrogens (see Table 47-8) and encouraged to avoid them as much as possible.

A patient receiving thyroid hormone replacement or corticosteroids must be taught the expected side effects of these drugs and measures to manage them. The patient should also be instructed in unexpected side effects and told when and to whom these should be reported. Toxic symptoms should be clearly defined, and the patient should be instructed to report them. Table 47-4 lists signs of hyperthyroidism that are the same as toxic symptoms of thyroid hormone replacement. Table 47-14 lists signs of hypercortisolism that are similar to corticosteroid toxicity. Patient handouts written in understandable language should accompany verbal instruction. The handouts should be reviewed with the patient to assess understanding, and information should be clarified when necessary. The patient treated surgically needs care similar to that given to the person undergoing thyroidectomy.

Hypothyroidism

Hypothyroidism usually results from insufficient circulating thyroid hormone as a result of a variety of abnormalities. All hypothyroid states have certain features in common, regardless of the cause. Some differences depend on the patient's age at onset of the deficiency.

Causes. Hypothyroidism may occur in infancy (*cretinism*), childhood, or adulthood. Cretinism is caused by thyroid hormone deficiencies during fetal or early neonatal life. It can be caused by maternal iodine deprivation or congenital thyroid abnormalities. Juvenile hypothyroidism has causes similar to those seen in the adult and requires prompt diagnosis and treatment to prevent developmental retardation.

In the adult the most common cause of primary hypothyroidism is atrophy of the thyroid gland, considered to be the end result of both Hashimoto's thyroiditis and Graves' disease. These autoimmune diseases destroy the thyroid gland. Thyroid deficiency also occurs when pituitary TSH production is inadequate. Iatrogenic causes of hypothyroidism include surgical removal of the thyroid, destruction of the thyroid gland by radiation, and surgical removal of the pituitary gland. Occasionally, hypothyroidism develops as a result of the ingestion of excessive amounts of goitrogens (Table 47-8). The person with underlying autoimmune disease is particularly susceptible to goitrogens.

Although the typical patient with hypothyroidism is a woman over 50, the disease can occur at any age and in either sex. An increased incidence has been correlated with the previous therapeutic use of radioactive iodine. Hypothyroidism is more common in iodine-deficient areas of the world, such as Zaire and Nepal.

Clinical Manifestations. The major manifestations of cretinism are defective physical development and mental retardation. Although affected infants usually appear normal at birth, cretinism should be suspected when there is a long gestational period and a large infant who fails to thrive. Affected infants may exhibit a large posterior fontanel, squinting, excessive sleeping, thickened skin and lips, enlarged tongue, abdominal distention with vomiting, a hoarse cry, dull facial expression, feeding and respiratory difficulty, peripheral cyanosis, supraclavicular and periorbital edema, umbilical hernia, and hypothermia.

Cretinism occurs in 1 of 4500 births in the United States. Early recognition is essential for normal physical and mental development. All states require neonatal screening for cretinism with a simple heel capillary blood test of T_4 or TSH. Cretinism causes irreversible mental retardation and dwarfism. When treatment with hormone replacement is begun soon after birth, normal physical and intellectual development will ensue.[19]

Hypothyroidism in childhood is usually due to autoimmune thyroiditis. A prevalence of 1.3% to 6% has been reported in school-aged children. Intellectual development is normal, but the child may seem mentally sluggish. Physical and sexual development are altered. Although there is generalized muscle hypertrophy, the face remains childlike, and eruption of permanent teeth, linear growth, and sexual maturation are delayed. In addition, there is a high frequency of other autoimmune diseases.[20]

Hypothyroidism in the adult is characterized by an insidious and nonspecific slowing of body processes, personality changes, fatigue, and lethargy. Mental changes seen in hypothyroidism include impaired memory, slowed speech, decreased initiative, and somnolence. In addition, cold intolerance, hair loss, dry and coarse skin, brittle nails, hoarseness, muscle weakness and swelling, overall weakness, constipation, weight gain, and menorrhagia are common.

Unless hypothyroidism occurs after thyroidectomy or thyroid ablation, or during treatment with antithyroid drugs, the onset of symptoms may occur over months to years. The symptoms are so insidious that medical attention is seldom sought. The patient's family and friends are often unaware of the changes. The severity of the symptoms depends on the degree of thyroid hormone deficiency.

The clinical manifestations of hypothyroidism result from the long-term physiologic effects of thyroid hormone deficiency. They may involve any body system but are more pronounced in cardiovascular, GI, reproductive, and hematopoietic systems.

Hypothyroid heart disease includes cardiomyopathy, pericardial effusion, and coronary atherosclerosis. Bradycardia and weakened cardiac contractility lead to decreased cardiac output. Pericardial effusion, however, seldom results in hemodynamic compromise. Increased serum cholesterol and triglyceride levels and the accumulation of mucopolysaccharides in the intima of small blood vessels can result in coronary atherosclerosis. This accumulation is seldom symptomatic (i.e., characterized by angina) because of the decreased myocardial oxygen consumption that has been observed in hypothyroidism.

GI motility is decreased in hypothyroidism and achlorhydria (absence of hydrochloric acid) is common. Constipation, which is a common complaint, may progress to obstipation and, rarely, to intestinal obstruction. The underlying metabolic disease makes the individual a high-risk candidate for intestinal surgery.

Women with hypothyroidism frequently complain of menorrhagia. Some affected individuals have been treated for menorrhagia for years and may have undergone hysterectomy before the hypothyroidism was diagnosed. In addition, anovulatory cycles with subsequent infertility may occur.

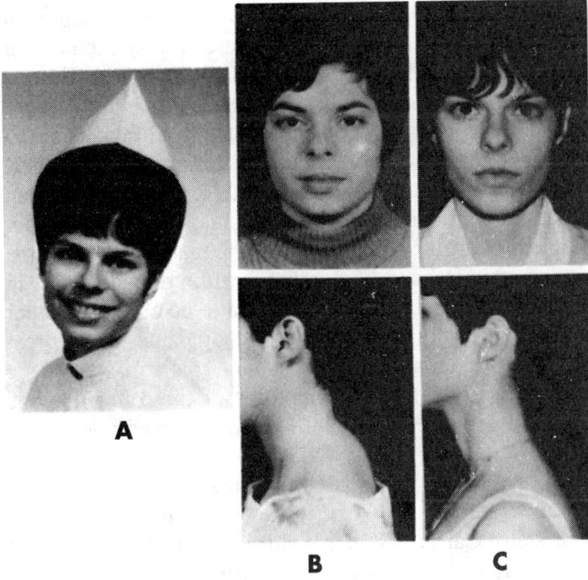

Fig. 47-7 A woman with Cushing's syndrome resulting from right adrenal cortical adenoma. ***A,*** Patient at age 18, 2 years before surgery. ***B,*** Patient at age 20, 1 month before surgery. ***C,*** Patient at age 21, 1 year after surgery.

Anemia is a common feature of hypothyroidism. Erythropoietin levels may be low or normal. Oxygen demand is decreased in the periphery, and there is hypocellular bone marrow. The result is a low hematocrit. Other hematopoietic problems are vitamin B_{12}, iron, and folate deficiencies, and a predisposition to bruising.

The brain is affected by diminished cerebral blood flow related to decreased cardiac output. This is manifested by mental sluggishness, inattentiveness, memory loss, lethargy, and changes in affect. Although some individuals with hypothyroidism exhibit a jocular air regarding their condition, others appear depressed. They express distress and describe an impaired self-image in regard to their disabilities and altered appearance. Although the patient with hypothyroidism sleeps long hours, stage 3 and stage 4 sleep are reduced.

The term *myxedema* is often used synonymously with hypothyroidism but actually connotes severe, long-standing hypothyroidism. With myxedema there is accumulation of hydrophilic mucopolysaccharides in the ground substance of the dermis and other tissues. This mucinous edema causes the characteristic facies of hypothyroidism and puffiness, periorbital edema, and masklike affect (Fig. 47-7).

Clinical diagnosis of hypothyroidism in the elderly adult can be difficult. The typical manifestations of hypothyroidism are often considered normal changes of aging—fatigue, cold dry skin, hoarseness, hair loss, constipation, cold intolerance, depression, or dementia.

Complications. The mental sluggishness, drowsiness, and lethargy of hypothyroidism may progress gradually or suddenly to a notable impairment of consciousness or coma. This situation, termed *myxedema coma,* constitutes a medical emergency. Myxedema coma can be precipitated by infection, drugs (especially narcotics, tranquilizers, and barbiturates), exposure to cold, and trauma. It is characterized by subnormal temperature, hypotension, and hypoventilation. For the patient to live, vital functions must be supported, and IV thyroid hormone must be administered.

Table 47-9 Diagnostic Studies: Hypothyroidism

Study	Finding
Serum T_3RU	Low
Serum T_3	Low
Serum T_4	Low
Serum cholesterol	Increased
ECG	Bradycardia, low voltage
Serum TSH	High (if thyroid diseased), low (if pituitary diseased)
TRH stimulation test	Increase in TSH if hypothalamus diseased, no change in TSH if pituitary diseased

ECG, Electrocardiogram; *TRH,* thyrotropin-releasing hormone; *T_3RU,* T_3-resin uptake; *TSH,* thyroid-stimulating hormone.

Diagnostic Studies. T_4, T_3, and T_3RU levels are usually low in hypothyroidism. These values, correlated with symptoms gathered from the history and physical examination, confirm the diagnosis. Serum TSH levels help determine the cause of hypothyroidism. Serum TSH is high when the defect is in the thyroid and low when it is in the pituitary or hypothalamus. An increase in TSH after TRH injection suggests hypothalamic dysfunction, whereas no change suggests anterior pituitary dysfunction (Table 47-9). In the well elderly, T_3, T_4, and TSH levels are unchanged.

Therapeutic Management. The therapeutic objective in hypothyroidism is restoration of a euthyroid state as safely and rapidly as possible with hormone replacement therapy. In the adult a low-calorie diet is indicated to promote weight loss. Lifelong thyroid replacement therapy is usually required for both adults and children.

Pharmacologic Management. Synthetic oral thyroxine (Synthroid, Levothroid, Noroxine) is the drug of choice to treat hypothyroidism. In the young, otherwise healthy patient, the maintenance replacement dose can be started at once. In the older adult patient and the person with compromised cardiac status, a small initial dose is recommended because the usual dose may increase myocardial oxygen consumption. The resultant oxygen demand may cause angina and cardiac dysrhythmias. Any chest pain experienced by a patient starting thyroid replacement should be reported immediately, and ECG and serum cardiac enzyme tests must be performed. The dose is increased at 1- to 4-week intervals. It is important that the patient take replacement medication regularly.

NURSING MANAGEMENT

HYPOTHYROIDISM

Nursing Assessment

Assessment of the patient who is suspected of having hypothyroidism should include questions about weight gain, mental changes, fatigue, slowed and slurred speech, cold intolerance, skin changes such as increased dryness or thickening, constipation, and dyspnea. The patient should be assessed for bradycardia; distended abdomen; dry, thick, cold skin; thick, brittle nails; paresthesias; and muscular aches and pains.

Nursing Diagnoses

Nursing diagnoses are determined when the problem and etiologic factors are supported by clinical data. Nursing diagnoses related to hypothyroidism may include, but are not limited to, those presented in the nursing care plan on p. 1499.

Planning

The overall goals are that the patient with hypothyroidism will (1) experience relief of symptoms, (2) maintain an euthyroid state, (3) maintain a positive self-image, (4) and comply with lifelong thyroid replacement therapy.

Nursing Implementation

Acute Intervention. The following nursing interventions contribute to the recovery of a patient with hypothyroidism:

1. Provide a comfortable, warm environment because of the patient's intolerance to cold.
2. Take measures to prevent skin breakdown. Use soap sparingly, and apply an emollient or lotion. An alternating-pressure mattress may be helpful.
3. Avoid using sedatives. If they must be given, give the lowest possible dose, and closely monitor mental status, level of consciousness, and respirations.
4. Prevent constipation by gradually increasing exercise, increasing fiber in the meal plan, administering stool softeners, and promoting regular bowel habits. Avoid enemas because they produce vagal stimulation, which can be hazardous to the patient with cardiac disease.
5. Teach the patient the nature of the thyroid hormone deficiency, self-care practices necessary to recovery, and signs and symptoms to monitor.

For assessment of the patient's progress, vital signs, body weight, fluid intake and output, and visible edema should be monitored. Cardiac assessment is especially important because the cardiovascular response to the hormone determines the medication regimen. Energy level and mental alertness should be noted. These should increase within 2 to 14 days and continue to rise steadily to normal levels.

Chronic and Home Management. Repeated patient education is imperative. Initially the hypothyroid patient needs more time than usual to comprehend all of the necessary information. It is important to provide written instructions, repeat the information often, and assess the patient's comprehension level regularly. The need for lifelong drug therapy must be stressed. The signs and symptoms of hypothyroidism or hyperthyroidism that indicate hormone imbalance should be included in the teaching plan. It is sometimes difficult for the patient to recognize signs of overdosage or underdosage; therefore a family member or friend should be included in the instruction process. Forgetfulness is an early indication of thyroid deficiency.

The patient must be taught to contact a clinician immediately if signs of overdose such as orthopnea, dyspnea, rapid pulse, palpitations, nervousness, or insomnia appear. The patient with diabetes mellitus should test his or her capillary blood glucose at least daily because return to the euthyroid state frequently increases insulin requirements. In addition, thyroid preparations potentiate the effects of other common drug groups, such as anticoagulants, antidepressants, and digitalis compounds. The patient should be taught the toxic signs and symptoms of these medications and should remain under close medical observation until stable.

With treatment, striking transformations occur in both appearance and mental function. Most adults return to a normal state. Cardiovascular conditions and (occasionally) psychosis may persist despite corrections of the hormonal imbalance. Relapses occur if treatment is interrupted.

PARATHYROID GLANDS

Hyperparathyroidism

Hyperparathyroidism is a condition involving increased secretion of parathyroid hormone (PTH). PTH helps regulate calcium and phosphate levels by stimulating bone resorption, renal tubular reabsorption of calcium, and activation of vitamin D. Until recently, this dysfunction was considered rare. With the increased use of routine evaluation of serum calcium levels, however, the prevalence in the general population is estimated to be 0.04%, and the annual incidence in persons over 40 years of age ranges between 0.1% and 0.5%.[21]

Hyperparathyroidism is classified as primary, secondary, or tertiary. *Primary hyperparathyroidism* is due to an increased secretion of PTH leading to disorders of calcium, phosphate, and bone metabolism. The excessive concentration of circulating hormone usually leads to hypercalcemia and hypophosphatemia. The most common cause is a benign neoplasm or a single adenoma (80% of cases). *Secondary hyperparathyroidism* appears to be a compensatory response to states that induce or cause hypocalcemia, the main stimulus of PTH secretion. Disease conditions associated with secondary hyperparathyroidism include vitamin D deficiencies, malabsorption, chronic renal failure, and hyperphosphatemia. *Tertiary hyperparathyroidism* occurs when there is hyperplasia of the parathyroid glands and a loss of circulating calcium levels that cause autonomous secretion of PTH, even with normal calcium levels. It is observed in the patient who has had a kidney transplant after a long period of dialysis treatment for chronic renal failure (see Chapter 44).

Primary hyperparathyroidism is more common in women and usually occurs between 30 and 70 years of age. The peak incidence is in the fifth and sixth decades of life. Previous head and neck radiation may predispose a patient to the development of parathyroid adenoma.[22] Increased PTH has a multisystem effect (Table 47-10). In the bones,

NURSING CARE PLAN Patient with Hypothyroidism

Planning: Outcome Criteria	Nursing Interventions and Rationales
NURSING DIAGNOSIS	Altered comfort *related to* cold intolerance *as manifested by* complaints of feeling cold, shivering
Express satisfaction with temperature of environment and personal comfort.	Provide extra clothing, blankets, warm environment *to increase patient's comfort.* Explain to patient and significant others that decreased heat production causes discomfort *to increase understanding and empathy of patient's condition.*
NURSING DIAGNOSIS	Altered nutrition: more than body requirements *related to* hypometabolism *as manifested by* weight gain
Maintain weight in normal range.	Provide low-calorie, high-protein diet; include foods high in vitamin B_{12}, folic acid, iron, and vitamin C *to reduce tendency for weight gain while preventing muscle wasting and anemia.* Explain the need for fewer calories *so patient will be more agreeable to dietary restrictions.* Assist patient to develop method of monitoring weight and caloric intake *so excess weight gain can be avoided.* Encourage small, frequent meals *because early satiety and decreased gastrointestinal motility can cause gas and discomfort.*
NURSING DIAGNOSIS	Constipation *related to* gastrointestinal hypomotility *as manifested by* irregular, hard stools
Have daily soft, formed stool.	Assess bowel pattern and characteristics *to plan appropriate interventions.* Provide 2 to 3 L of fluids per day *to maintain soft stool.* Encourage activity *to stimulate peristalsis.* Administer laxatives if necessary *to increase stool output.* Offer foods high in bulk and roughage *to increase fecal mass.*
NURSING DIAGNOSIS	Activity intolerance *related to* decreased metabolic rate and mucin deposits in joints and interstitial spaces *as manifested by* generalized weakness and muscle and joint stiffness
Be able to participate in self-care activities with minimal discomfort and fatigue.	Assess ability to participate in self-care activities *to determine extent of problem and plan appropriate interventions.* Monitor vital signs and comfort level *to determine effect of activities and plan activity increases.* Administer thyroid hormone as ordered *to correct hypometabolic state.* Plan frequent rest periods *to improve patient's tolerance and comfort level.* Apply splints and hot packs if appropriate *to relieve joint stiffness and pain by immobilization.* Pace activities to match patient's abilities *to allow maximum participation.*
NURSING DIAGNOSIS	Altered thought processes *related to* diminished cerebral blood flow secondary to decreased cardiac output *as manifested by* forgetfulness, impaired ability to conceptualize, and personality changes
Maintain orientation to reality at highest level possible.	Assess thinking processes such as memory, attention span, orientation to time, person and place *to enable appropriate planning.* Repeat information to patient *because this patient requires more time to comprehend.* Explain cause of symptoms to patient and family *to reduce anxiety and frustration.* Provide clock and calendar *to maintain orientation to time and day.* Provide written handouts with all instructions *to help patient remember and thereby enhance adherence to regimen.*

subperiosteal bone resorption, decreased bone density, cyst formation, and general weakness can occur as a result of the effect of PTH on osteoclastic (bone resorbers) and osteoblastic (bone formers) activity.

In the kidneys the excess calcium cannot be reabsorbed, leading to hypercalciuria. This urinary calcium, along with a large amount of urinary phosphate, can lead to calculi formation. In addition, the glomerular filtration rate decreases, and proximal renal tubular acidosis may occur. Also in the kidneys, PTH stimulates the synthesis of a biologically active form of vitamin D, a potent stimulator of calcium transport in the intestine. In this way, PTH apparently increases GI absorption of calcium.

Clinical Manifestations and Complications. Hyperparathyroidism has varying symptoms, including weakness, loss of appetite, constipation, increased need for sleep,

Table 47-10 Clinical Manifestations of Parathyroid Dysfunction

System	Hypofunction	Hyperfunction
Cardiovascular	Decreased contractility of heart muscle Decreased cardiac output Prolongation of QT and ST intervals on ECG Dysrhythmias	Dysrhythmias Shortened QT interval on ECG Hypertension
Gastrointestinal	Abdominal cramps Urinary and fecal incontinence (in older adult)	Vague abdominal pain Anorexia Nausea and vomiting Constipation Pancreatitis Peptic ulcer disease Cholelithiasis Weight loss
Integumentary	Dry, scaly skin Hair loss on scalp and body Brittle nails, transverse ridging Changes in developing teeth, lack of tooth enamel	Skin necrosis Moist skin
Musculoskeletal	Fatigue Weakness Painful muscle cramps Skeletal x-ray changes, osteosclerosis Soft-tissue calcification Difficulty in walking	Skeletal pain Backache Weakness, fatigue Pain on weight bearing Osteoporosis Pathologic fractures of long bones Compression fractures of spine Decreased muscle tone
Neurologic	Personality changes Psychiatric manifestations of depression, anxiety Irritability Memory impairment Headache Convulsions Positive Chvostek's sign or Trousseau's phenomenon Tremor Paresthesias of perioral area, hands, feet Hyperactive deep-tendon reflexes Disorientation, confusion (in older adult)	Personality disturbances Emotional irritability Memory impairment Psychosis Delirium, confusion, coma Incoordination Hyperactive deep-tendon reflexes Abnormalities of gait Psychomotor retardation Headache
Renal	Urinary frequency	Hypercalciuria Kidney stones (nephrolithiasis) Urinary tract infections Polyuria
Other	Eye changes, including lenticular opacities, cataracts, papilledema	Corneal calcification on slit-lamp examination

ECG, Electrocardiogram.

and shortened attention span. Major signs include loss of calcium from bones (osteoporosis), broken bones, and kidney stones (nephrolithiasis). Neuromuscular abnormalities are characterized by muscle weakness, particularly in the proximal muscles of the lower extremities. Asymptomatic cases are being identified with increasing frequency with routine calcium screening. Serious complications of hyperparathyroidism are renal failure, pancreatitis, collapse of vertebral bodies, cardiac changes, and long bone and rib fractures.

Diagnostic Studies. PTH, as measured by radioimmunoassay, will be elevated. Serum calcium levels usually exceed 10 mg/dl (2.50 mmol/L). Because of its inverse relation with calcium, the serum phosphorus level is usually below 3 mg/dl (0.1 mmol/L). Elevations in other laboratory tests include urine calcium, serum chloride, uric acid, creatinine, amylase (if pancreatitis is present), and alkaline phosphatase (if bone disease has begun). If bone changes are present, radiologic studies may reveal subperiosteal resorption, bone cysts, bone demineralization, tumors of the long bones, and loss of the lamina dura of the teeth. ECG studies may reveal shortened QT intervals, prolonged QR intervals, and abnormal QRS complexes.

Therapeutic Management. The treatment objectives are to relieve symptoms and prevent complications caused by excess PTH. The choice of therapy depends on the urgency of the clinical situation, the degree of hypercalcemia, the underlying disorder, the status of renal and hepatic function, the clinical presentation of the patient, and the particular advantages and disadvantages of the different therapeutic modalities.

Parathyroid tumors should be removed surgically. The parathyroid glands occasionally lie in ectopic sites such as the mediastinum. This situation requires a highly skilled surgeon to open the chest and explore the area behind the sternum. Generally, a single gland is removed if an adenoma is the cause of the hyperparathyroidism. When cancer is the cause, all the parathyroid glands are removed.

If the symptoms are mild or if the patient is elderly or at increased surgical risk from other health problems, a conservative management approach is used. This includes an annual examination with tests for serum PTH, calcium, phosphorus, and alkaline phosphatase levels and renal function, x-rays to assess for metabolic bone disease, and measurement of urinary calcium excretion.

Specific management measures include maintenance of a high fluid intake, a moderate calcium intake, a sodium intake of 8 to 10 g per day to replace losses from increased urine output, and phosphorus supplementation, unless contraindicated by an increased risk for urinary calculi formation. Diuretics may be given to increase the urinary excretion of calcium. Continued ambulation and the avoidance of immobility are critical aspects of management.

Pharmacologic Management. Mithramycin, an antihypercalcemic agent, lowers serum calcium within 48 hours. However, because of toxic side effects, its use is limited to the patient with metastatic parathyroid carcinoma and severe bone disease. Estrogen therapy can reduce serum and urinary calcium levels in the postmenopausal woman and may retard demineralization of the skeleton.[23]

In severe hyperparathyroidism, normal saline is given IV to correct fluid volume deficit and promote calcium excretion. Furosemide (Lasix) is given orally or IV to promote sodium loss and decrease renal tubular reabsorption of calcium. Propranolol (Inderal) may be used to inhibit the action of catecholamines at β_2 receptors, which stimulate PTH secretion.

NURSING MANAGEMENT

HYPERPARATHYROIDISM

Nursing Assessment

Subjective and objective data that should be obtained from an individual with hyperparathyroidism are presented in Table 47-11.

Nursing Diagnoses

Nursing diagnoses are determined when the problem and etiologic factors are supported by clinical data. Nursing diagnoses related to hyperparathyroidism may include, but are not limited to, those presented in the nursing care plan on p. 1502.

Table 47-11 Nursing Assessment: Hyperparathyroidism

Subjective Data

Important health information

Past health history: Vitamin D deficiency; malabsorption, malnutrition; chronic renal failure

Medications: Compliance with renal failure medications (e.g., phosphate binders, calcium supplements)

Surgery, trauma, or treatments: Previous head or neck x-ray examinations

Functional health patterns

Health perception–health management: Family history of multiple endocrine neoplasias, familial hyperparathyroidism; malaise, fatigue

Nutrional-metabolic: Anorexia, weight loss

Elimination: Polyuria, dysuria; constipation

Activity-exercise: Weakness

Sleep: Increase in sleeping

Cognitive-perceptual: Irritability, depression; generalized skeletal pain, abdominal pain, arthralgias; renal colic

Objective Data

General

Apathy

Cardiovascular

Hypertension, dysrhythmias (especially bradycardias)

Neurologic

Drowsiness, slow mentation, confusion, delirium, poor coordination

Musculoskeletal

Osteoporosis, fractures, decreased muscle tone

Possible findings

Elevated serum calcium (>10 mg/dl), parathyroid hormone, chloride, alkaline phosphatase, uric acid, creatinine; decreased serum phosphate (<3 mg/dl); bicarbonate; guaiac positive stool and emesis (peptic ulcer); subperiosteal bone resorption on x-ray examinations; enlarged parathyroids on ultrasonography

Planning

The overall goals are that the patient with hyperparathyroidism will (1) maintain satisfactory activity level, (2) keep a consistently high fluid intake, (3) not experience any serious complications related to the disease or its treatment, (4) maintain a positive self-image, and (5) accept and comply with the long-term nature of the problem.

Nursing Implementation

If surgery is performed, close monitoring of the patient's vital signs is required. Other aspects of care are similar to that after thyroidectomy. The major postoperative complications are tetany and fluid and electrolyte disturbances. Tetany is usually apparent early in the postoperative period but may develop over several days. Mild tetany, characterized by unpleasant tingling of the hands and around the

NURSING CARE PLAN Patient with Hyperparathyroidism

Planning: Outcome Criteria	Nursing Interventions and Rationales
➤ **NURSING DIAGNOSIS**	Activity intolerance *related to* muscle weakness and fatigue secondary to low calcium levels *as manifested by* complaints of weakness and fatigue; inability to use stairs, arise from chairs; pain on weight bearing
Have decrease in perception of fatigue and weakness; have ADL needs met by self or others.	Assist with ambulation and limit ambulation to short walks *to demonstrate a caring attitude and to prevent fatigue.* Assist patient with self-care as needed *to ensure ADL needs are met and to conserve energy.* Plan ADLs and treatment *to allow for adequate rest periods.* Provide patient with walker or cane as necessary *as aids to safe ambulation and to keep patient ambulatory.*
➤ **NURSING DIAGNOSIS**	Ineffective management of therapeutic regimen *related to* lack of knowledge of need for high fluid intake *as manifested by* hypercalciuria, urinary tract infection; verbalized desire to manage required fluid intake
Have no renal stones; have prompt detection and early treatment of renal stones; verbalize a plan by patient and family to adhere to dietary instructions.	Consult dietitian *to provide expert instruction.* Instruct patient about symptoms of renal stones *to ensure early reporting of symptoms.* Strain urine *to detect stones.* Keep fluids within easy reach and offer frequently; encourage fluid intake to point of moderate overhydration (4000 ml plus fluid output per day) *to keep fluid level high so kidneys are flushed and stone formation is less likely.* Assess patient for flank pain and hematuria and report immediately *because these symptoms can indicate renal calculi.*
➤ **NURSING DIAGNOSIS**	Altered nutrition: less than body requirements *related to* loss of appetite, nausea, vomiting, and personality disturbances *as manifested by* complaints of loss of appetite, nausea; refusal to socialize; inability to recall instructions; vomiting, guarding of abdominal area; irritability; self-isolation
Maintain adequate food and fluid intake; maintain stable weight.	Administer mouth care frequently with use of flavored mouthwash or toothpaste *to keep mouth fresh.* Eliminate noxious odors from environment *to prevent this potential cause of a decreased appetite.* Encourage eating with others in a sitting or dining room *because socialization during meals often increases intake.* Serve small amounts of food frequently *to prevent bloating and early satiety.*
➤ **NURSING DIAGNOSIS**	Constipation *related to* dehydration and inactivity *as manifested by* complaints of less than usual number of stools, rectal fullness and pressure, pain on defecation; hard stools, less than 3 stools per week; diminished bowel sounds
Have regular evacuation (preferably daily) of soft, formed stools, prompt detection of constipation or impaction.	Encourage fluid intake to point of moderate overhydration *to increase fluid content of fecal mass.* Administer prune juice daily *because it contains dihydroxyphenyl isatin, which acts as a laxative.* Maintain diet high in bulk *to increase fecal mass.* Request stool softener from physician. Encourage frequent, short walks *to promote increased peristalsis and movement of fecal mass.* Promote maintenance of regular habit of defecation consistent with preadmission pattern *to foster bowel regularity.*

continued

mouth, may be present but should abate without problems. If tetany becomes more severe (e.g., muscular spasms or laryngospasms develop), IV calcium may be given. Strict monitoring of intake and output is necessary to evaluate fluid status. Calcium, potassium, phosphate, and magnesium levels are assessed frequently. Mobility is encouraged to promote bone calcification. If surgery is not performed, treatment to relieve symptoms and prevent complications is carried out.

Hypoparathyroidism

Hypoparathyroidism, or inadequate circulating PTH, is uncommon. It is characterized by hypocalcemia resulting from a lack of PTH to maintain serum calcium levels. PTH resistance at the cellular level may also occur (pseudohypoparathyroidism). This is caused by a genetic defect resulting in hypocalcemia in spite of normal or high PTH levels and is often associated with hypothyroidism and hypogonadism.

NURSING CARE PLAN Patient with Hyperparathyroidism—cont'd

Planning: Outcome Criteria	*Nursing Interventions and Rationales*
➤ **NURSING DIAGNOSIS**	Risk for injury: fractures and joint contractures *related to* decreased bone density, weakness, improper body alignment, immobility
Have no occurrence of deformity or accidental injury.	Monitor for complaints of bone and joint pain, weakness, backache; impaired mobility, unsteady gait, uncoordinated movements; decrease in mental status *to detect potential for injury.* Maintain patient in good body alignment *to foster musculoskeletal health.* Assist patient with ambulation, reduce safety hazards in environment, maintain bed in low position *to reduce potential for injury.* Alert other hospital departments about handling and positioning patient during tests *to avoid accidental injury as a result of unawareness of patient's musculoskeletal fragility.*
➤ **NURSING DIAGNOSIS**	Body image disturbance *related to* weight loss, weakness, fatigue, and mental status changes *as manifested by* verbalization of negative feelings about self; weakness, fatigue; inability to cope with usual activities; expression of feelings of hopelessness; hostile, angry behavior; self-isolation; weight loss
Make statements and actions indicative of improved self-image; have more positive mental outlook.	Encourage patient to express feelings about physical and emotional changes *because venting of feelings helps to clarify issues.* Compliment patient when appropriate *to promote a positive body image.* Reassure patient that fatigability and depression will improve when hormone imbalance is corrected *to foster hope and a positive attitude.* Encourage short walks to social areas *to prevent isolation.* Ascertain which activities the patient has enjoyed in the past; encourage continued involvement in those activities that are appropriate to setting and patient's condition.
➤ **NURSING DIAGNOSIS**	Sensory and perceptual alterations *related to* slowed mentation, depression, and drowsiness *as manifested by* disorientation, inappropriate behavior or response, difficulty in concentrating
Maintain reality-based orientation; make appropriate actions and reactions.	Assess sensory and perceptual status *to plan appropriate interventions.* Orient patient as indicated *to assist with reality orientation.* Provide calm, restful environment *to minimize confusion and foster rest.* Explain actions in simple language *to avoid increasing patient's confusion.* Monitor and record level of consciousness and orientation every shift *to evaluate effectiveness of plan and alter as appropriate.*

ADLs, Activities of daily living.

Causes. The most common cause of hypoparathyroidism is accidental removal of the parathyroids or damage to the vascular supply of the glands during neck surgery (e.g., thyroidectomy, radical neck surgery).[24] Idiopathic hypoparathyroidism resulting from absence, fatty replacement, or atrophy of the glands is a rare disease that usually occurs early in life and may be associated with other endocrine disorders. Affected patients may have antiparathyroid antibodies. Hypomagnesemia is increasingly being recognized as a cause of hypoparathyroidism. Hypomagnesemia, as seen in alcoholism or malabsorption, impairs PTH secretion and its action on bone and kidneys.

Clinical Manifestations. The clinical features of acute hypoparathyroidism are due to a low serum calcium level (see Table 47-10). Sudden decreases in calcium concentration give rise to a syndrome called *tetany.* This state is characterized by tingling of the lips, fingertips, and occasionally feet and increased muscle tension leading to paresthesias and stiffness. Dysphagia, painful tonic spasms of smooth and skeletal muscles (particularly of the extremities and face), a constricted feeling in the throat, and laryngospasms are also present. Chvostek's sign (facial muscle spasm when the face is tapped below the temple) and Trousseau's phenomenon (carpopedal spasm when arterial circulation is interrupted by applying a blood pressure cuff for 3 minutes [see Fig. 13-14]) are usually positive. Respiratory function may be severely compromised by accessory muscle spasm and laryngeal spasm–induced airway obstruction. Patients are usually anxious and apprehensive. Abnormal laboratory findings include decreased serum calcium and PTH levels and increased serum phosphate levels. Other causes of chronic hypocalcemia include chronic renal failure, vitamin D deficiency, and hypomagnesemia.

Therapeutic and Pharmacologic Management. The main objectives of treatment are to treat tetany when present and prevent long-term complications by maintaining eucalcemia. Tetany is treated with IV infusion or slow push of calcium salts. Long-term therapy consists of the administration of vitamin D and possibly supplemental calcium and oral phosphate binders.

Emergency treatment of tetany requires the administration of IV calcium. Generally, in adults, 10 to 20 ml of a 10% solution of calcium gluconate is infused over 10 minutes. Calcium salts can cause hypotension and cardiac arrest; thus a slow IV push is required.[21] In addition, these salts can cause venous irritation and inflammation if leakage occurs into extravascular tissues. For long-term management, oral calcium supplements may be prescribed. Calcium carbonate, an antacid, is readily available but may alter acid-base balance. It also stimulates secretion of hydrochloric acid, which could be a problem for the patient with an ulcer. Calcium gluconate, which is available in tablet form, should be chewed into fine particles. Acid aids in the gastrointestinal absorption of calcium gluconate, so it should be taken at the end of a meal. Oral calcium supplements are given four times a day.

Specific hormone replacement of PTH is not used to treat hypoparathyroidism because of antibody formation to the PTH, expense, and the need for parenteral administration. Vitamin D is used in chronic and resistant hypocalcemia to enhance intestinal calcium absorption and bone resorption. The preferred preparations are Hytakerol and 1, α25 dihydroxycholecalciferol (calcitriol, Rocaltrol). These drugs are more potent, raise calcium levels rapidly, and are quickly metabolized. Rapid metabolism is desired because vitamin D is a fat-soluble vitamin and toxicity can cause irreversible renal impairment.

NURSING MANAGEMENT

HYPOPARATHYROIDISM

Nursing Assessment

Nursing care of a patient with hypoparathyroidism requires close assessment for signs of tetany. The patient should be observed closely for carpopedal spasm (Trousseau's phenomenon) while blood pressures are being taken because this is an early sign of tetany. Periodic assessment for Chvostek's sign is advisable. Tingling in the fingertips and around the mouth, irritability, anxiety, apprehension, muscular hypertonicity, and cramps may precede acute tetany. It is important to note any allergy to iodine because it may be used in associated diagnostic testing such as an IVP.

Nursing Diagnoses

Nursing diagnoses specific to the patient with hypoparathyroidism include, but are not limited to, the following:

- Impaired skin integrity related to dry, scaly skin
- Activity intolerance related to fatigue, weakness, and painful muscle cramps
- Altered thought processes related to personality and psychiatric changes and memory impairment
- Ineffective management of therapeutic regimen related to lack of knowledge regarding signs and symptoms of calcium deficiency, calcium-rich foods and supplements, and chronic nature of the problem
- Potential complication: dysrhythmia
- Potential complication: tetany

Planning

The overall goals are that the patient with hypoparathyroidism will (1) develop no complications such as tetany or dysrhythmias, (2) recognize signs and symptoms of hypoparathyroidism and hyperparathyroidism, and (3) comply with periodic assessment of calcium level.

Nursing Implementation

Acute Intervention. If tetany or generalized muscle cramps develop, rebreathing may partially alleviate the symptoms. The patient who can cooperate should be instructed to breathe in and out of a paper bag or breathing mask. This reduces carbon dioxide excretion from the lungs, increases carbonic acid levels in the blood, and lowers body pH. Because an acidic environment enhances both solubility and the degree of ionization of calcium, the proportion of total body calcium available in physiologically active form (i.e., ionized calcium) is increased, temporarily relieving the functional hypocalcemia.

IV calcium salts should be available at the bedside for treatment of acute tetany. Calcium salts must be infused slowly because high blood levels can cause serious cardiac dysrhythmias or cardiac arrest. The patient who has been digitalized is particularly vulnerable. Because calcium-induced ventricular standstill occurs in systole, this type of arrest is less likely than other types to respond to resuscitation. ECG monitoring is indicated. Side rails should be padded as a seizure precaution. The patient should be kept in a nonstimulating environment, assisted with hygienic needs, and given support and encouragement until free of symptoms.

Chronic and Home Management. The patient with hypoparathyroidism needs instruction in the management of long-term nutrition and drug therapy. A high-calcium meal plan includes foods such as dark green vegetables, soy beans, and tofu. The patient should be told that foods containing oxalic acid (e.g., spinach and rhubarb), phytic acid (e.g., bran and whole grains), and phosphorus reduce calcium absorption. Calcium supplements of at least 1 g/day for the patient under 40 years of age and 2 g per day for the patient more than 40 years of age are usually prescribed. These supplements are best administered 2 to 3 hours after meals. Although calcium carbonate often leads to constipation and flatulence, bran and whole grain foods should not be used for treatment. Alternative nursing interventions include providing stool softeners, adequate fluids, and fresh fruits.

The patient should be instructed with written handouts about the signs and symptoms of hypocalcemia and hypercalcemia and to report these to a clinician as soon as possible if they occur. If manifestations of hypocalcemia occur, calcium supplementation should be increased. The need for lifelong treatment and health supervision should be stressed. The patient's calcium levels should be monitored three to four times a year. Treatment modification is often necessary because hypercalcemia can develop without apparent cause. Thorough patient instruction and frequent serum calcium assessment should allow a normal life expectancy. The patient needs support and encouragement to continue with the regimen. The patient may dislike taking so many pills.

ADRENAL CORTEX

Cushing's Syndrome

Cushing's syndrome is a spectrum of clinical abnormalities caused by excess corticosteroids, particularly glucocorticoids. There are three main classifications of adrenal steroid hormones. *Glucocorticoids* regulate metabolism and are critical in the physiologic stress response. *Mineralocorticoids* regulate sodium and potassium balance. *Androgens* contribute to growth and development in both genders and to sexual activity in adult women. Several conditions can cause Cushing's syndrome (Table 47-12). The most common cause is iatrogenic administration of exogenous cortisone. The most common cause of endogenous Cushing's syndrome is an ACTH-secreting pituitary tumor (*Cushing's disease*). Other causes include adrenal tumors and ectopic ACTH production by tumors outside the hypothalamic-pituitary-adrenal axis (usually of the lung or pancreas). Cushing's disease and primary adrenal tumors are more common in females, whereas ectopic ACTH production is more common in males.[25]

Clinical Manifestations. The clinical manifestations of Cushing's syndrome can be seen in most body systems and are related to excess levels of corticosteroids (Table 47-13). Although manifestations of glucocorticoid excess usually predominate, symptoms of mineralocorticoid and androgen excess may also be seen.

Glucocorticoid excess causes pronounced changes in personal appearance (Fig. 47-8). These signs and symptoms logically flow from the known actions of glucocorticoids. Weight gain, the most common feature, results from the accumulation of adipose tissue in the trunk, face, and cervical area. Transient weight gain from sodium and water retention may be present because of the mineralocorticoid effects of cortisol. Glucose intolerance occurs because of cortisol-induced insulin resistance and increased gluconeogenesis by the liver.

Protein wasting is caused by the catabolic effects of cortisol on peripheral tissue. Muscle wasting leads to muscle weakness, especially in the extremities. Loss of protein matrix in bone leads to osteoporosis with subsequent pathologic fractures, vertebral compression fractures, and bone and back pain. Loss of collagen makes the skin weaker and thinner; therefore it bruises easier. The skin and mucous membranes may take on a bronze or brownish color because of the melanotropic activity of ACTH.

Mineralocorticoid excess may cause hypertension, whereas adrenal androgen excess may cause pronounced acne, virilization in women, and feminization in men. Menstrual disorders and hirsutism in women and gynecomastia and impotence in men are seen more commonly in adrenal carcinomas. Catabolic processes predominate, and wound healing is delayed. Mood disturbances (irritability, anxiety, euphoria), insomnia, irrationality, and occasionally psychosis may occur.

The clinical presentation, as revealed by the history and physical examination, is the first indication of Cushing's syndrome. Of particular importance are (1) a combination of centripedal obesity and protein wasting as indicated by slender extremities and thin, friable skin; (2) "moon facies" (fullness of the face); (3) purplish red striae, which are usually depressed below the skin surface, on the abdomen, breast, or buttocks; (4) premenopausal osteoporosis; and (5) unexplained hypokalemia.

Diagnostic Studies. Abnormal findings include granulocytosis, lymphocytopenia, eosinopenia, polycythemia, hypokalemia, hyperglycemia, glycosuria, hypercalciuria, and osteoporosis (as observed on x-rays). Plasma cortisol levels may be elevated, with loss of diurnal variation. Plasma ACTH may be low, normal, or elevated depending on the underlying problem. High or normal levels indicate ACTH-dependent Cushing's, whereas low or undetectable levels indicate an adrenal or exogenous etiology. When Cushing's syndrome is suspected, a 24-hour urine collection for free cortisol and a low-dose dexamethasone suppression test (see Chapter 45) are done. If these results are abnormal, a high-dose dexamethasone suppression test is done. False-positive results can occur in depressed patients, those under acute stress, and those who are active alcoholics. CT scanning and MRI may be used for tumor localization.

Therapeutic Management. The treatment of choice for Cushing's disease is transsphenoidal surgical removal of the pituitary adenoma (hypophysectomy). Adrenalectomy is indicated for adrenal tumors or hyperplasia. Patients with ectopic ACTH-secreting tumors are managed with treatment of the neoplasm. In inoperable cases or in cases in which residual disease remains, treatment with *o, p'-DDD* (mitotane) may be used. This drug suppresses cortisol production, alters peripheral metabolism of steroids, and decreases plasma and urine steroid levels by actually killing adrenocortical cells. The action of this drug results in a "medical adrenalectomy." Metyrapone, ketoconazole, and aminoglutethimide may be used to inhibit cortisol synthesis. Occasionally, bilateral adrenalectomy is necessary (Table 47-14). The relatively common side effects of these agents include anorexia, nausea and vomiting, GI bleeding, depression, vertigo, skin rashes, and diplopia. Ketoconazole, which inhibits synthesis of gonadal and adrenal steroids, may also be used. The side effects from this medication are fewer than those of other adrenal suppressants.

Table 47-12 Causes of Cushing's Syndrome

Prolonged administration of high doses of corticosteroids
ACTH-secreting pituitary tumor (Cushing's disease)
Cortisol-secreting neoplasm within the adrenal cortex that can be either carcinoma or adenoma
Excess secretion of ACTH from carcinoma of lung or other malignant growth outside pituitary or adrenals

ACTH, Adrenocorticotropic hormone.

Table 47-13 Clinical Manifestations of Adrenal Cortical Hormone Dysfunction

System	Hypofunction	Hyperfunction
Glucocorticoids		
General appearance	Weight loss	Truncal (centripedal) obesity, thin extremities, rounding of face (moon face), fat deposits on back of neck and on shoulders ("buffalo hump")
Integumentary	Bronzed or smoky hyperpigmentation of face, neck, hands (especially creases), buccal membranes, nipples, genitalia, and scars (if pituitary function normal); vitiligo, alopecia	Thin, fragile skin; purplish-red striae; petechial hemorrhages; bruises; florid cheeks (plethora); acne; poor wound healing
Cardiovascular	Hypotension, tendency to develop refractory shock, vasodilatation	Hypervolemia, hypertension, edema of lower extremities
Gastrointestinal	Anorexia, nausea and vomiting, cramping abdominal pain, diarrhea	Increase in secretion of pepsin and hydrochloric acid, anorexia
Urinary		Glycosuria, hypercalciuria, kidney stones
Musculoskeletal	Fatigability	Muscle wasting in extremities, proximal muscle weakness, fatigue, osteoporosis, awkward gait, back and joint pain, weakness, growth retardation (in children)
Immune	Propensity toward autoimmune diseases	Inhibition of immune response, suppression of allergic response, inhibition of inflammation
Hematologic	Anemia, lymphocytosis	Leukocytosis, lymphopenia, polycythemia, increased coagulability
Fluids and electrolytes	Hyponatremia, hypovolemia, dehydration, hyperkalemia	Sodium and water retention, edema, hypokalemia
Metabolic	Hypoglycemia, insulin sensitivity, fever	Glucose intolerance, negative nitrogen balance, dyslipidemia
Emotional	Neurasthenia, depression, exhaustion or irritability, confusion, delusions	Psychic stimulation, euphoria, irritability, hypomania to depression, emotional lability
Mineralocorticoids		
Fluid and electrolytes	Sodium loss, decreased volume of extracellular fluid, hyperkalemia, salt craving	Marked sodium and water retention, tendency toward edema, marked hypokalemia
Cardiovascular	Hypovolemia, tendency toward shock, decreased cardiac output, decreased heart size	Hypertension, hypervolemia
Androgens		
Integumentary	Decreased axillary and pubic hair (in women)	Hirsutism, acne
Reproductive	No effect in men, decreased libido in women	Menstrual irregularities and enlargement of clitoris (in females); gynecomastia and testicular atrophy (in males)
Musculoskeletal	Decrease in muscle size and tone	Increase in muscle development

If Cushing's syndrome has developed during the course of prolonged administration of steroids, one or more of the following alternatives may be tried: (1) gradual discontinuance of steroid therapy, (2) reduction of the steroid dose, and (3) conversion to an alternate-day regimen. Gradual discontinuance of the causative drug is necessary to avoid potentially life-threatening adrenal insufficiency. An alternate-day regimen is one in which twice the daily dosage of a shorter-acting corticosteroid is given every other morning to minimize hypothalamic-pituitary-adrenal suppression, growth suppression, and altered appearance. This regimen is not used when the corticosteroids are given as physiologic replacements.

NURSING MANAGEMENT

CUSHING'S SYNDROME

Nursing Assessment

Subjective and objective data that should be obtained from a patient with Cushing's syndrome are presented in Table 47-15.

Nursing Diagnoses

Nursing diagnoses are determined when the problem and etiologic factors are supported by clinical data. Nursing diagnoses related to Cushing's syndrome may include, but are not limited to, those presented in the nursing care plan on p. 1509.

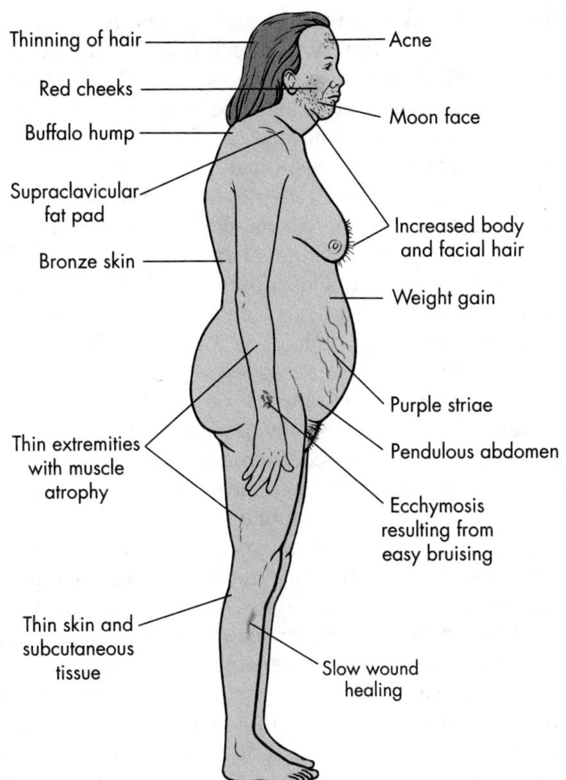

Fig. 47-8 Common characteristics of Cushing's syndrome.

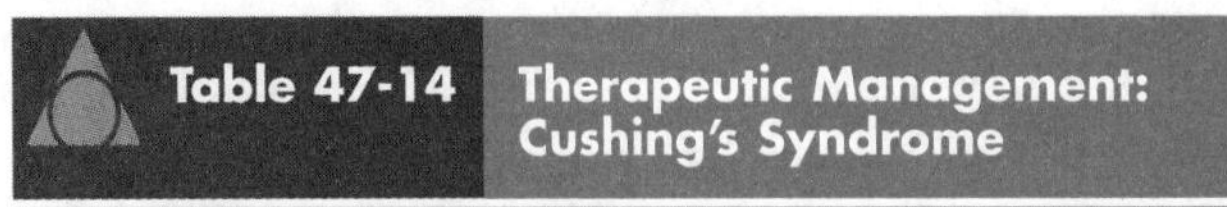

Table 47-14 Therapeutic Management: Cushing's Syndrome

Diagnostic
- History and physical examination
- Mental status examination
- Plasma cortisol levels for diurnal variations
- Plasma ACTH level
- Complete blood count
- Blood chemistries for sodium, potassium, glucose
- Dexamethasone suppression test
- 24-hour urine for free cortisol
- Examination of visual fields
- CT scan, MRI

Therapeutic
- Adrenal cortical adenoma, carcinoma, or hyperplasia
  - Surgical adrenalectomy
  - Medical adrenalectomy
- Pituitary corticotropin (ACTH) hypersecretion
  - Transsphenoidal resection of microadenoma
  - Radiation
  - Treatment with hypothalamic serotonin antagonist (cyproheptadine)
- Surgical removal of nonendocrine corticotropin-producing tumors, adrenalectomy (if pituitary tumor inoperable)
- Discontinuance of or alteration in administration of exogenous corticosteroids

ACTH, Adrenocorticotropic hormone; *CT*, computed tomography; *MRI*, magnetic resonance imaging.

Planning

The overall goals are that the patient with Cushing's syndrome will (1) experience relief of symptoms, (2) experience no serious complications, (3) maintain a positive self-image, and (4) actively participate in the therapeutic plan.

Nursing Implementation

Acute Intervention. The patient with Cushing's syndrome is seriously ill. Because the therapeutic interventions have many side effects, the focus of daily assessment is on signs and symptoms of hormone and drug toxicity and complicating conditions such as cardiovascular disease, diabetes mellitus, infection, nephrolithiasis, and pathologic fractures. Daily nursing assessment includes the following:

1. Vital signs every 4 hours, particularly blood pressure
2. Daily weights (gain possibly indicates volume excess)
3. Signs and symptoms of infection, especially pain, loss of function, and purulent drainage, because other signs and symptoms of inflammation such as fever and redness may be minimal or absent
4. Location, time, and duration of abdominal pain
5. Signs and symptoms of abnormal thromboembolic phenomena, such as sudden chest pain, dyspnea, or tachypnea
6. Glucose monitoring
7. Bone pain or limitations of range of motion, especially in the lower back
8. Changes in mental status, particularly depression

The patient needs a great deal of emotional support. Changes in appearance such as centripedal obesity, multiple bruises, hirsutism in females, and gynecomastia in males can be distressing. The patient may feel unattractive, repulsive, or unwanted. The nurse can help by remaining sensitive to those feelings and offering respect and unconditional acceptance. The patient can be reassured that the physical changes and much of the emotional lability are related to side effects of drug therapy and will resolve when hormone levels return to normal.

Interventions Related to Surgery. If treatment involves surgical removal of a pituitary adenoma, an adrenal tumor, or one or both adrenal glands, nursing care will have an additional focus on preoperative and postoperative care. Surgery on glandular structures poses risks beyond those of other types of operations. Because glands are highly vascular, the risk of hemorrhage is increased. Manipulation of glandular tissue during surgery may release large amounts of hormone into the circulation, producing marked fluctuations in the metabolic processes affected by these hormones.

Preoperative management. Before surgery the patient should be brought to optimal physical condition. Hypertension and hyperglycemia need to be controlled and hypokalemia is corrected with diet and potassium supplements. A high-protein meal plan helps correct the protein depletion.

Although adrenalectomy is uncommon, patients experiencing this procedure should be aware that IV infusions and

Table 47-15 Nursing Assessment: Cushing's Syndrome

Subjective Data

Important health information

Past health history: Pituitary tumor (Cushing's disease); adrenal, pancreatic, or pulmonary neoplasms; GI bleeding; alcoholism; frequent infections

Medications: Use of corticosteroids

Functional health patterns

Health perception–health management: Fatigue

Nutritional-metabolic: Increased appetite, weight gain; prolonged wound healing, easy bruising

Elimination: Polyuria

Activity-exercise: Weakness

Sleep: Insomnia, poor sleep quality

Cognitive-perceptual: Headache; back, joint, and rib pain; emotional lability; poor concentration and memory

Sexuality-reproductive: Amenorrhea, impotence, decreased libido

Coping–stress tolerance: Anxiety

Objective Data

General

Truncal obesity, supraclavicular fat pads, buffalo hump, moon facies

Integumentary

Plethora; hirsutism; thin, friable skin; acne; petechiae; purpura; hyperpigmentation; purplish red striae on breasts, buttocks, and abdomen

Cardiovascular

Hypertension, edema

Reproductive

Gynecomastia (in men), enlarged clitoris (in women)

Neurologic

Poor coordination

Musculoskeletal

Muscle wasting, thin extremities

Possible findings

Hypokalemia, hyperglycemia, leukocytosis, polycythemia, elevated plasma cortisol and ACTH levels; abnormal dexamethasone suppression test; elevated free cortisol, 17 ketosteroids on urine testing; osteoporosis on chest x-ray

ACTH, Adrenocorticotropic hormone; *GI,* gastrointestinal.

nasogastric suctioning are likely after surgery. Information and instruction about exercises, coughing, and deep breathing are particularly important because patients are prone to thrombosis and infection. If the surgical approach is abdominal, the incision will be high in the abdomen, increasing the difficulty of coughing and deep breathing.

Postoperative management. Because of hormone fluctuations, blood pressure, fluid balance, and electrolyte levels tend to be unstable after surgery. High doses of cortisone are administered IV during surgery and for several days afterward to ensure adequate responses to the stress of the procedure. If large amounts of endogenous hormone have been released into the systemic circulation during surgery, the patient is likely to develop hypertension, increasing the risk of hemorrhage. High levels of cortisone also increase susceptibility to infection and delay healing.

Any rapid or significant changes in blood pressure, respirations, or heart rate should be reported. Fluid intake and output should be monitored carefully and assessed for potential imbalance. The critical period for circulatory instability ranges from 24 to 48 hours after surgery. IV corticosteroids are given, and the dose and rate of flow are adjusted to the patient's clinical manifestations and fluid and electrolyte balance. Oral doses are given as tolerated. The IV line may be kept in place after IV corticosteroids are withdrawn to keep a line open for quick administration of corticosteroids or vasopressors.

If cortisone dosage is tapered too rapidly after surgery, acute adrenal insufficiency may develop. Vomiting after the nasogastric tube is removed, increased weakness, dehydration, and hypotension may indicate hypocortisolism. In addition, the patient may complain of painful joints, pruritus, or peeling skin and may experience severe emotional disturbances. These signs and symptoms should be reported so that drug doses can be adjusted. The nurse must constantly be alert for signs of glucocorticoid imbalance. After surgery the patient is usually maintained on bed rest until the blood pressure stabilizes. The nurse must be alert for subtle signs of postoperative infections because the usual immune and inflammatory responses are suppressed. Meticulous care must be used when changing the dressing and during any other procedures that necessitate access to body cavities, circulation, or areas under the skin so that infection is prevented.

Chronic and Home Management. The discharge instructions are based on the patient's lack of endogenous cortisol and resulting inability to react to stressors physiologically. Patients should wear Medic-Alert bracelets at all times and carry medical identification and instructions in a wallet or purse. Exposure to extremes of temperature, infections, and emotional disturbances should be avoided as much as possible. Stress may produce or precipitate acute adrenal insufficiency because the remaining adrenal tissue cannot meet an increased hormonal demand. Many patients can be taught to adjust their corticosteroid replacement therapy in accordance with their stress levels. The nurse should consult with each patient's physician to determine the parameters for dosage changes if this plan is feasible. If the patient cannot adjust his or her own medication or if weakness, fainting, fever, or nausea and vomiting occur, the patient should contact the clinician for a possible adjustment in corticosteroid dosage. Lifetime replacement therapy is required by many patients, but it may take several months to adjust the hormone dose satisfactorily, and patients should be prepared for this.

Adrenocortical Insufficiency

Adrenocortical insufficiency (hypofunction of the adrenal cortex) may be primary (*Addison's disease*) or secondary, from a lack of pituitary ACTH. In Addison's disease, all three classes of adrenal steroids (glucocorticoids, mineralocorticoids, and androgens) are reduced. In secondary adrenocortical insufficiency, corticosteroids and androgens

NURSING CARE PLAN Patient with Cushing's Syndrome

Planning: Outcome Criteria	*Nursing Interventions and Rationales*
➤ **NURSING DIAGNOSIS**	Risk for infection *related to* exposure to environmental pathogens and suppression of immune system secondary to hypercortisolism
Have no infection; detect and treat any infectious process, verbalize signs and symptoms of infection, plan to eat high-protein diet.	Assess for inadequate protein stores, proteinuria, muscle wasting, poor wound healing *as indicators of risk for infection.* Assess potential infection sites such as urinary and respiratory tracts, skin, and IV lines *so infection can be detected early and treatment initiated promptly.* Note pain, loss of function, and purulent drainage *because other signs and symptoms of infection may be minimal or absent.* Provide private room, if possible; maintain meticulous asepsis and prevent contact with contagious individuals *to reduce the risk of cross-contamination because patient has an increased susceptibility to infection.* Instruct patient in self-care practices *to avoid infection* (e.g., hand washing). Refer patient to dietitian for high-protein diet instruction *to help correct the protein depletion caused by excess glucocorticoids.* Instruct patient and family in signs and symptoms of infection *because the usual immune and inflammatory responses are suppressed* and to report these to clinician immediately *so treatment can be initiated promptly.*
➤ **NURSING DIAGNOSIS**	Risk for injury: fracture *related to* decreased muscle strength, fatigue, osteoporosis, and increased protein catabolism
Have no accidental injury; be able to list high-calcium foods.	Assess for complaints of weakness, fatigue, back and rib pain; difficulty in ambulating, impairment in mobility; impairment in judgment; drowsiness; hypocalcemia *to detect injury risk factors.* Assist patient as necessary with ambulation and self-care *to ensure patient safety.* Provide cane or walker as necessary *to provide patient with stabilizing device.* Keep side rails up if patient's judgment is impaired *to reduce possibility of falls.* Provide quiet environment and rest periods as indicated *because stress may produce or precipitate acute adrenal insufficiency.* Reinforce dietary instructions. Instruct patient in high-calcium diet *to replace lost calcium and prevent increasing the severity of osteoporosis.* Reinforce dietary instructions. Instruct patient and family in provisions of a safe environment (e.g., nonskid surfaces in wet areas, use of railings, good lighting). Orient patient to new surroundings *to prevent falling over items in unfamiliar environments.*
➤ **NURSING DIAGNOSIS**	Altered nutrition: more than body requirements *related to* increased appetite, and intake of high-calorie foods and inactivity *as manifested by* statement of increased appetite; preference for fatty, sweet foods; weight 10% or more than optimum for height; inappropriate menu choices
Maintain body weight if appropriate or no more than 1- to 2-lb loss per week; be satisfied with food intake; make good food selections.	Obtain dietary consult for instruction in low-calorie, high-nutrition diet (including protein and calcium) *because excess glucocorticoids produce weight gain and calcium and protein loss.* Assist with appropriate menu choices *to reinforce dietary instructions.* Provide low-calorie, high-vitamin snacks. Instruct in or refer to psychologist for instruction in behavior modification techniques related to eating *because these techniques aid in changing eating behaviors.*

continued

are deficient but mineralocorticoids rarely are. ACTH deficiency may be caused by pituitary disease or suppression of the hypothalamic-pituitary axis as a result of the administration of exogenous glucocorticoids.[26]

Addison's Disease. In the United States, the most common cause of primary Addison's disease (which is a rare condition) is autoimmune—adrenal tissue is destroyed by antibodies against the patient's own adrenal cortex. Often, other endocrine conditions are present and Addison's disease is considered a component of *polyendocrine deficiency syndrome.* Tuberculosis can cause Addison's disease, but this is now rare in areas in which tuberculosis is controlled. Less common causes include hemorrhage, infarction, fungal infections (e.g., histoplasmosis), acquired immunodeficiency syndrome (AIDS), and metastatic cancer. Iatrogenic Addison's disease may be due to anticoagu-

NURSING CARE PLAN Patient with Cushing's Syndrome—cont'd

Planning: Outcome Criteria	Nursing Interventions and Rationales
➤ **NURSING DIAGNOSIS**	Self-esteem disturbance *related to* altered body image, emotional lability, and diminished physical capabilities secondary to hormone imbalance *as manifested by* verbalization of negative feelings regarding personal appearance, inability to perform usual activities, poor grooming and hygiene, truncal obesity, moon facies, acne, plethora, buffalo hump, excess body hair, bruises, edema
Verbalize acceptance of appearance by patient and family; use self-care methods to improve appearance.	Explain to patient and family that physical and emotional changes are related to hormone imbalance and that most will disappear when hormone imbalance is corrected *to increase their understanding and assist with coping.* Accept and respect patient as a person *to maintain patient's self-worth.* Encourage good grooming and use of attractive attire *to improve patient's appearance and self-esteem.* Compliment patient when appropriate *to boost morale by providing positive feedback.*
➤ **NURSING DIAGNOSIS**	Impaired skin integrity *related to* excess steroids, immobility, and altered skin fragility *as manifested by* edema; thin, fragile skin; impaired healing
Have intact skin without signs of trauma.	Assess skin every shift *for early detection of trauma.* Protect patient from bumping and bruising *to prevent injury to easily traumatized tissue.* Change patient's position frequently *to minimize pressure over bony prominences and improve circulation in edematous tissue.* Provide good skin care, particularly to edematous areas and areas over bony prominences *because these areas have decreased circulation.* Assist patient with ambulation as tolerated *to foster mobility and improve circulation.*

lant therapy (causing adrenal hemorrhage), antineoplastic chemotherapy, ketoconazole therapy for AIDS, or bilateral adrenalectomy.

Progressive weakness, fatigue, weight loss, and anorexia are primary features. Skin hyperpigmentation, a striking feature, is seen primarily in sun-exposed areas of the body, at pressure points, over joints, and in creases, especially palmar creases. It is most likely due to increased secretion of β-lipotropin, which contains MSH, or ACTH, caused by hypocortisolism and the resultant lack of negative feedback on these tropic hormones. Other frequent manifestations are hypotension, hyponatremia, hyperkalemia, nausea and vomiting, and diarrhea. The most dangerous feature of Addison's disease is hypotension, which may cause shock, especially during stress. Circulatory collapse from this cause is unresponsive to the usual treatment (vasopressors and fluid replacement) and requires glucocorticoid administration to reverse the hypotension. Patients with secondary adrenocortical hypofunction may have many signs and symptoms in common with patients with Addison's disease but are characteristically not hyperpigmented because ACTH and related peptide levels are low. When severe dehydration, hyponatremia, and hyperkalemia are present, a diagnosis of primary adrenocortical insufficiency is favored because of the severe mineralocorticoid insufficiency associated with this disorder.

Acute Adrenal Insufficiency. Patients with adrenocortical insufficiency are at risk for *acute adrenal insufficiency* (Addisonian crisis), which is a life-threatening emergency caused by insufficient adrenocortical hormones or a sudden sharp decrease in these hormones. It may occur during stress (e.g., from infection, surgery, trauma, hemorrhage, or psychologic distress); sudden withdrawal of adrenocortical hormone replacement therapy (which is often done by a patient who lacks knowledge of the importance of replacement therapy); adrenal surgery; or sudden pituitary gland destruction (pituitary apoplexy).

Severe manifestations of cortisol and aldosterone deficiencies are exhibited, including hypotension (particularly postural), tachycardia, dehydration, hyponatremia, hyperkalemia, hypoglycemia, fever, weakness, and confusion. GI manifestations include nausea, vomiting, diarrhea, and vague abdominal pain.

Diagnostic studies. In addition to clinical features, a diagnosis of Addison's disease can be made when cortisol levels are subnormal or fail to rise over basal levels with an ACTH stimulation test. Other abnormal laboratory findings include hyperkalemia, hypochloremia, hyponatremia, hypoglycemia, anemia, and increased blood urea nitrogen levels. Urine levels of free cortisol are low. A failure of cortisol levels to rise in response to ACTH stimulation indicates primary adrenal disease. A positive response to ACTH stimulation indicates a functioning adrenal gland and points to probable pituitary disease (see Table 45-8). CT scan and MRI are used to localize tumors or identify adrenal calcifications or enlargement.

Therapeutic and Pharmacologic Management. Treatment of adrenocortical insufficiency is focused on management of the underlying cause when possible. Regardless of etiology, the mainstay of treatment is replace-

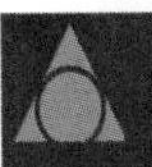

Table 47-16 Therapeutic Management: Addison's Disease

Diagnostic
- Health history and physical examination
- Plasma cortisol levels
- Serum electrolytes
- ACTH-stimulation test
- Tuberculin test
- CT scan, MRI

Therapeutic
- Daily cortisone replacement (two thirds on awakening in morning, one third in late afternoon)*
- Daily fluorocortisone in morning*
- Salt additives for excess heat or humidity

ACTH, Adrenocorticotropic hormone; *CT,* computed tomography; *MRI,* magnetic resonance imaging.
*For conditions of normal daily stress in individuals with usual daytime activity.

ment therapy with glucocorticoids. Hydrocortisone, the most commonly used form of replacement therapy, also has mineralocorticoid properties (Table 47-16). Glucocorticoids are usually given in divided doses, two thirds in the morning and one third in the afternoon. Mineralocorticoids are given once daily, preferably in the evening. This dosage schedule reflects normal circadian rhythm in endogenous hormone secretion and decreases the side effects associated with steroid replacement therapy. When any illness or stress occurs, whether mild or acute, glucocorticoid dosage must be increased to prevent adrenal crisis. Examples of situations requiring steroid adjustment are fever, influenza, extraction of teeth, and rigorous physical activity, such as playing tennis on a hot day or running a marathon. The patient should take two to three times the usual dose and notify the clinician. When in doubt, it is better to err on the side of overreplacement. If vomiting or diarrhea occurs, as may happen with influenza, the clinician must be notified immediately because electrolyte replacement may be necessary. In addition, these symptoms may be early indicators of crisis. Overall, however, patients who take their medications consistently can anticipate a normal life expectancy.

Management of Addisonian crisis requires immediate glucocorticoid replacement therapy. Treatment must be vigorous and directed toward shock management. IV hydrocortisone 100 mg every 6 hours, sodium, fluids, and dextrose (for hypoglycemia) are necessary for 24 hours or until blood pressure returns to normal.[27]

NURSING MANAGEMENT

ADDISON'S DISEASE

Nursing Assessment

Nursing assessment related to the patient with Addison's disease includes assessment of subjective data such as weight loss, hyperpigmentation, loss of body hair, anorexia, salt craving, nausea and vomiting, cramping abdominal pain, and diarrhea. Patients may also complain of exhaustion, profound weakness, inability to perform usual activities, muscle aches, light-headedness, lack of interest in usual activities and relationships, confusion, inability to tolerate any stress, decreased libido, and amenorrhea.

Objective data noted during the physical examination include emaciation, pale skin (but bronzed in sun-exposed areas, scars, buccal mucosa, and genitalia), and sparse body hair (particularly axillary and genital). Irritability, confusion, disorientation, or depression may also be noted. Skin tenting (delayed return of skin to flat position after pinching) may be observed with poor skin turgor. Hypotension (particularly postural), decreased cardiac output and heart size, muscle wasting, and weakness may also be present. Laboratory values may indicate hyponatremia, hyperkalemia, hypoglycemia, low serum cortisol, increased serum ACTH, decreased 24-hour urine free cortisol, and lack of response to an ACTH stimulation test (see Table 45-8).

Nursing Diagnoses

Nursing diagnoses related to the patient with Addison's disease include, but are not limited to, the following:

- Activity intolerance related to weakness and hypotension
- Self-care deficit related to weakness, lack of interest, and depression
- Altered nutrition: less than body requirements related to weakness, anorexia, and nausea and vomiting
- Self-esteem disturbance related to inability to perform usual activities, loss of hair, skin hyperpigmentation, and diagnosis of chronic illness
- Altered health maintenance related to lack of knowledge of management of lifelong hormone replacement therapy
- Decreased cardiac output related to hypotension and volume depletion
- Altered sexuality patterns related to weakness, malaise, depression, and changing self-concept
- Potential complication: hypotension related to volume depletion

Planning

The overall goals are that the patient with Addison's disease will (1) manage self-care activities, (2) experience relief of symptoms, (3) learn to adjust medication dosage to life situations, (4) avoid acute adrenocortical insufficiency, and (5) actively participate in long-term therapeutic plan.

Nursing Implementation

Acute Intervention. When the patient with Addison's disease is hospitalized, whether for diagnosis, an acute crisis, or some other health problem, frequent nursing assessment is necessary. Vital signs and signs of fluid volume deficit and electrolyte imbalance should be assessed every 30 minutes to 4 hours for the first 24 hours depending on the patient's instability. In addition, the following nursing assessments and orders should be included: daily weights, diligent steroid administration, protection against exposure to infection (reverse isolation), and complete assistance with daily hygiene. The patient should be protected from noise, light, and environmental temperature

Table 47-17 Patient Education Related to Addison's Disease

1. Names and dosages of drugs
2. Actions of drugs
3. Symptoms of overdosage and underdosage
4. Conditions requiring increased medication (e.g., trauma, infection, surgery, emotional crisis)
5. Course of action to take relative to changes in medication
   Increase in dose of glucocorticoid
   Administration of large dose of glucocorticoid IM—including demonstration and return demonstration
   Consultation with clinician
6. Prevention of infection and need for prompt and vigorous treatment of existing infections
7. Need for lifelong replacement therapy
8. Need for lifelong medical supervision
9. Need for medical identification device

IM, Intramuscularly.

extremes. The patient cannot cope with these stresses because he or she cannot produce corticosteroids.

If the hospitalization was due to adrenal crises, the patient usually responds by the second day and can start oral corticosteroid replacement. Because discharge frequently occurs before the usual maintenance dose of corticosteroids is reached, the patient should be instructed on the importance of keeping scheduled follow-up appointments.

Chronic and Home Management. The nurse has an important role in the long-term management of Addison's disease. Because of the serious nature of the disease and the need for lifelong replacement therapy, a well-organized and carefully presented teaching plan is vital to the health of the patient. Table 47-17 outlines the major areas that must be included in the teaching plan.

Because the patient with Addison's disease is unable to tolerate physical or emotional stress, long-term care revolves around recognizing the need for additional replacement medication and techniques for stress management. Patients who can control or manage the degree of stress they experience maintain better hormone balance than those who cannot. The nurse should help the patient develop effective coping skills and techniques for handling stress or make appropriate referrals.

A hormone-deficient patient receiving glucocorticoid replacement is less apt to exhibit harmful symptoms from the medication than a patient receiving pharmacologic doses of these drugs. Because the aim of replacement therapy is to return to normal hormone levels, nursing care is designed to help the patient maintain hormone balance and manage the medication regimen.

Because glucocorticoids are stimulating to the CNS, they may cause insomnia if taken late in the evening. The need for glucocorticoid hormone is proportional to stress levels. A patient who cannot produce endogenous hormone must adjust the dose of exogenous hormone to the stress level. Doses are usually doubled when minor stress occurs (e.g., a respiratory infection or dental work) and tripled when major stress occurs.

Patients must be taught the signs and symptoms of glucocorticoid deficiency and excess. These should be reported to their clinicians so that dosages can be adjusted to each patient's need. It is also important that the patient wear an identification band stating that the patient has Addison's disease so that appropriate therapy can be initiated in case of an unexpected trauma, accident, or crisis. The patient should be instructed and given handouts related to other medications that cause a need to increase steroid dosage (e.g., phenytoin, barbiturates, rifampin, and antacids).[28] Patients using mineralocorticoid therapy should be instructed how to take their blood pressure and given parameters to report to their clinicians, because untoward changes may indicate a need for dosage adjustment.

The patient should carry an emergency kit at all times. The kit should consist of 100 mg of IM hydrocortisone, syringes, and instructions for use. The patient and significant others should be instructed in how to give an IM injection in case the replacement therapy cannot be taken orally. The patient should verbalize instructions, practice IM injections with saline, and have written instructions as to when to alter the dose.[29]

Glucocorticoid Therapy

Cortisone and related glucocorticoids are used to relieve the signs and symptoms associated with many diseases (Table 47-18). The long-term administration of glucocorticoids in therapeutic doses often leads to serious complications and side effects (see Table 47-19); therefore glucocorticoid therapy is not recommended for minor chronic conditions. Rather, therapy should be reserved for diseases in which there is a risk of death or permanent loss of function and conditions in which short-term therapy is likely to produce remission or recovery. The potential benefits of treatment must always be weighed against the risks.

Effects. The therapeutic actions of glucocorticoids include the following:

1. Antiinflammatory action: glucocorticoids decrease the number of circulating lymphocytes, monocytes and macrophages, and eosinophils; enhances the release of polymorphonuclear leukocytes from bone marrow; inhibits the accumulation of leukocytes at the site of inflammation; and inhibits the release of substances involved in the inflammatory response (e.g., kinins, prostaglandins, and histamine) from the leukocytes. Therefore manifestations of inflammation, including redness, tenderness, heat, swelling, and local edema, are suppressed.
2. Immunosuppression: glucocorticoids cause atrophy of lymphoid tissue, suppress cell-mediated immune responses, and decrease production of antibodies.
3. Maintenance of normal blood pressure: glucocorticoids potentiate the vasoconstrictor effect of norepinephrine and act on the renal tubules to increase sodium reabsorption and enhance potassium and hydrogen excretion. Retention of sodium (and subsequently water) increases blood volume and helps maintain blood pressure.

Table 47-18 Pharmacologic Uses of Glucocorticoids

Hormone Replacement
- Adrenal insufficiency
- Congenital adrenal hyperplasia

Therapeutic Effect
- Allergic reactions
  - Anaphylaxis
  - Bee stings
  - Contact dermatitis
  - Drug reactions
  - Serum sickness
  - Urticaria
- Collagen diseases
  - Giant cell arteritis
  - Mixed connective tissue disorders
  - Polymyositis
  - Polyarteritis nodosa
  - Systemic lupus erythematosus
- Eye disease
  - Inflammation
- Gastrointestinal diseases
  - Inflammatory bowel disease
  - Nontropical sprue
- Hypercalcemia
  - Thyroid storm
- Endocrine diseases
  - Hypercalcemia
  - Hashimoto's thyroiditis
  - Thyroid storm
- Immunosuppression (after organ transplantation)
- Liver diseases
  - Alcoholic hepatitis
  - Autoimmune hepatitis
  - Subacute necrotic necrosis
- Nephrotic syndrome
- Neurologic disease
  - Prevention of cerebral edema and increased intracranial pressure
  - Malignancies, leukemia, lymphoma
  - Head trauma
- Pulmonary diseases
  - Aspiration pneumonia
  - Asthma
  - Chronic obstructive pulmonary disease
- Rheumatoid arthritis
- Skin diseases

4. Carbohydrate and protein metabolic effects: glucocorticoids antagonize the effects of insulin and can induce glucose intolerance by increasing hepatic glycogenolysis and insulin resistance. They also stimulate the breakdown of protein for gluconeogenesis, which can lead to skeletal muscle wasting. Although corticosteroids mobilize free fatty acids and redistribute fat in cushingoid patterns, the mechanism for this process is unknown. Corticosteroids also decrease the conversion of T_4 to T_3.

Table 47-19 Side Effects of Glucocorticoid Therapy

- Susceptibility to infection is increased. Infection develops more rapidly and spreads more widely in the cushingoid individual.
- Blood pressure is increased because of excess blood volume and potentiation of vasoconstrictor effects. Hypertension in turn predisposes patient to cardiac failure.
- Glucose intolerance affects more than 90% of individuals with cushingoid patterns.
- Protein depletion decreases bone formation, density, and strength and predisposes patient to pathologic fractures, especially compression fractures of the vertebrae (osteoporosis).
- Hypocalcemia related to anti–vitamin D effect may occur.
- Decreased mucus production predisposes patient to stomach and duodenal ulceration (peptic ulcer).
- Patients undergoing surgery are at increased risk for dehiscence and evisceration. Healing is delayed.
- Hypokalemia may develop, and potassium supplements may be indicated.
- Skeletal muscle atrophy occurs, and muscle weakness predisposes patient to accidental injury.
- Suppression of pituitary ACTH synthesis occurs. Glucocorticoid deficiency is likely if hormones are withdrawn abruptly.
- Mood and behavior changes (feelings of invulnerability and depression) may be observed.
- Fat from extremities is redistributed to trunk and face.

ACTH, Adrencorticotropic hormone.

Complications. Beneficial and harmful effects of the glucocorticoids relate to their physiologic actions. A beneficial effect in one situation may be a harmful one in another. Thus the vasopressive effect of the hormone is critical in enabling the organism to function in stressful situations but can produce hypertension when the substance is used for drug therapy. Inhibition of cell division is therapeutic and sometimes curative in the treatment of malignancies, but it slows healing after trauma or surgery. Suppression of inflammation and the immune response may help save the lives of the victim of anaphylaxis and the transplant recipient, but it causes reactivation of latent tuberculosis and greatly reduces resistance to other infections. Specific side effects related to glucocorticoid therapy are listed in Table 47-19.

NURSING MANAGEMENT

GLUCOCORTICOID THERAPY

Many patients receive glucocorticoid therapy for nonendocrine reasons (see Table 47-18), and thorough instruction is necessary to ensure patient cooperation. Steroids are taken once daily or once every other day. They should be taken early in the morning with food to decrease gastric irritation. Because exogenous corticosteroid administration may suppress endogenous ACTH and therefore endogenous cortisol (suppression is time and dose dependent), the danger of abrupt cessation of glucocorticoid therapy must be emphasized to patients and significant others. Further instruction and interventions to minimize the side effects and complications of glucocorticoid therapy include the following:

1. A diet plan high in protein, calcium (at least 1500 mg per day), and potassium but low in fat and concentrated simple carbohydrates such as sugar, honey, syrups, and candy
2. Assistance in identifying measures to ensure adequate rest and sleep, such as daily naps and avoidance of caffeine late in the day
3. Assistance in developing and maintaining an exercise program to help maintain bone integrity
4. Instruction in how to recognize edema and ways to restrict sodium intake to less that 2000 mg per day if edema occurs
5. Instruction in glucose monitoring, symptoms and signs of hyperglycemia (e.g., polydipsia, polyuria, blurred vision), and glycosuria (glucose in the urine) and the need to report hyperglycemic symptoms or capillary glucose levels greater than 180 mg/dl (10 mmol/L) or urine positive for glucose.
6. Instruction to notify a clinician if the patient experiences postprandial heartburn or epigastric pain that is not relieved by antacids
7. Instruction to see an eye specialist yearly to assess development of posterior subcapsular cataract
8. Instruction in safety measures, such as getting up slowly and using good lighting to avoid accidental injury
9. Instruction about maintaining good hygiene practices and avoiding contact with persons with colds or other contagious illnesses to avoid infection

Disorders of Aldosterone Secretion

Primary Hyperaldosteronism. Primary hyperaldosteronism (aldosteronism) is characterized by excessive aldosterone secretion caused by an adenoma of the adrenal zona glomerulosa or bilateral adrenal hyperplasia. This disorder is seen in approximately 0.05% of patients with hypertension. It is more common in women, and the usual age of diagnosis is between 20 and 50 years. The main effects of aldosterone are sodium retention and potassium and hydrogen ion excretion. Thus the hallmark of this disease is hypertension with hypokalemic alkalosis.

The sodium retention leads to hypernatremia, hypertension, and headache. Edema does not usually occur because the rate of sodium excretion is reset, which prevents more severe sodium retention. However, there is an increased loss of potassium. The potassium wasting leads to hypokalemia, which causes generalized muscle weakness, tiredness, cardiac dysrhythmias, glucose intolerance, and metabolic alkalosis that may lead to tetany.[30]

The diagnosis of hyperaldosteronism should be suspected in all patients with hypokalemia and hypertension who are not being treated with diuretics. Diagnostic tests show increased plasma aldosterone and serum sodium levels and decreased serum potassium levels and plasma renin activity. An IV saline infusion test is often performed. In this test, 2 L of normal saline are infused over 4 hours, with plasma aldosterone levels measured at the beginning and end of the infusion. If aldosterone fails to suppress (i.e., is >10 ng/dl [277 pmol/L]), the patient probably has hyperaldosteronism. Adenomas are localized by means of a CT scan. If a tumor is not found, plasma 18-hydroxycorticosterone is measured after overnight bed rest. A level greater than 50 ng/dl (1387 pmol/L) indicates an adenoma.

The treatment for adenoma is unilateral adrenalectomy. Before surgery, patients should be treated with a low-sodium diet, potassium-sparing diuretics, and antihypertensive agents to control serum potassium levels and blood pressure. Spironolactone (Aldactone) binds to the mineralocorticoid receptor in the terminal distal tubules and collecting ducts of the kidney and increases excretion of sodium and water and retention of potassium. Potassium supplements and sodium restrictions are also necessary. Potassium supplementation and a potassium-sparing diuretic should not be started simultaneously because of the danger of hyperkalemia. Patients with bilateral hyperplasia are treated with spironolactone; amiloride (Midamor), another potassium-sparing diuretic; or aminoglutethimide, which blocks aldosterone synthesis. Calcium channel blockers may also be used.[31]

Nursing care includes careful assessment for signs of hypokalemia, tetany, fluid and electrolyte balance, and cardiovascular status. Blood pressure should be monitored frequently before and after surgery because unilateral adrenalectomy is successful in controlling hypertension in only 50% of patients with adenoma.

Patients receiving maintenance therapy with spironolactone or amiloride need instruction about the possible side effects of gynecomastia, impotence, and menstrual disorders, as well as knowledge about the signs and symptoms of hypokalemia and hyperkalemia. Patients should be taught how to monitor their own blood pressure and the need for frequent monitoring. The need for continued health supervision should be stressed.

Secondary Hyperaldosteronism. Secondary hyperaldosteronism occurs in response to an extraadrenal stimulus (often angiotensin), renal artery stenosis, or juxtaglomerular cell tumors. If treatment of the primary disorder is not possible, angiotensin-converting enzyme (ACE) inhibitors are useful in inhibiting the powerful mineralocorticoid.

Congenital Adrenal Hyperplasia Syndromes. The adrenal glands normally produce small amounts of androgens. Overproduction of these hormones can be caused by *adrenogenital syndromes.*[32] Causes of these syndromes are congenital enzymatic deficiencies leading to hypocortisolism. The hypocortisolism causes increased ACTH secretion, which overstimulates the adrenals and causes hypertrophy and excess androgen production.[33] The onset of symptoms may occur from birth to early adult life and depends on the enzymes affected. In some deficiencies, males show precocious sexual development, whereas in others, sexual development may fail to occur. Females can show signs of masculinization and menstrual irregularities.

Adrenal Medulla

Pheochromocytoma. Disorders of the adrenal medulla are uncommon. There are no specific diseases caused by insufficiency of catecholamines (epinephrine and norepinephrine). The most common disorder of the adrenal medulla is pheochromocytoma, a neoplasm that produces excessive catecholamines. Most of these tumors (95%) are benign and encapsulated.[34] Pheochromocytoma can occur at any age and in either gender, but it is found most commonly in patients between 40 and 60 years of age.

The most striking clinical features of pheochromocytoma are severe, episodic hypertension; severe, pounding headache; and profuse sweating. Attacks of episodic hypertension are due to sympathetic nervous system stimulation usually from norepinephrine and are often accompanied by anxiety, palpitations, and profuse sweating. Attacks may be provoked by exercise, hypoglycemia, sexual activity, postural change, emotional distress, hyperventilation, compression or palpation of the tumor, surgery, and major trauma.[35] Additional symptoms may include vasomotor changes (e.g., pallor, facial flushing, pupil dilatation), orthostatic hypotension, and visual blurring. The duration of the attacks may vary from a few minutes to several hours. Untreated, pheochromocytoma may lead to diabetes mellitus, cardiomyopathy, and manifestations of uncontrolled hypertension and death.

THERAPEUTIC AND NURSING MANAGEMENT

PHEOCHROMOCYTOMA

Measurement of urinary metanephrines (catecholamine metabolites) is the simplest and most reliable test. Values are elevated in at least 90% of persons with pheochromocytoma. Plasma catecholamines are also elevated. It is preferable to measure catecholamines during an "attack." CT scans and MRI are used for tumor localization. Case finding is an important nursing function. Any patient with hypertension accompanied by symptoms of sympathoadrenal discharge should be referred to a physician for definitive diagnosis.

Treatment consists of surgical removal of the tumor. This is one of the few conditions in which dangerously high blood pressure can be corrected surgically.

Before surgery the patient is hospitalized for treatment to correct hypovolemia and cardiovascular complications to decrease the risk of surgery. Sympathetic blocking agents (e.g., phenoxybenzamine [Dibenzyline], propranolol [Inderal]) are administered to reduce the blood pressure and alleviate other symptoms of catecholamine excess. Because this management may result in orthostatic hypotension, the patient must be advised to make postural changes cautiously. Patients need rest, nourishing food, and emotional support during this period. Preoperative and postoperative care is similar to that for any patient undergoing adrenalectomy except that blood pressure fluctuations from catecholamine imbalances tend to be severe and must be carefully monitored. If surgery is not an option, metyrosine is used to diminish catecholamine production by the tumor and simplify chronic management.

Complete removal of the tumor cures the hypertension in three fourths of the cases. In the others, hypertension persists or returns but is usually well controlled by standard therapy.

CRITICAL THINKING EXERCISES

CASE STUDY

GRAVES' DISEASE

Patient Profile

Sally C., a 43-year-old woman, was admitted to the hospital with a high fever. Following an endocrine workup, she was diagnosed as having Graves' disease.

Subjective Data

- Reports recent job loss because of inability to cope with job stress
- Reports symptoms which include fatigue, unintentional weight loss, insomnia, palpitations, and heat intolerance

Objective Data

Physical examination

- Has a fever of 105° F (40.6° C)
- Has blood pressure of 150/78, pulse of 118, and respiratory rate of 24
- Has hot, moist skin
- Has fine tremors of the hands
- Has 4+ deep tendon reflexes and muscle strength of 1 to 2

Therapeutic Management

- Subtotal thyroidectomy planned for 2 months later
- Started on propylthiouracil and propranolol

Critical Thinking Questions

1. What is the etiology of the patient's symptoms?
2. What diagnostic studies were probably ordered? What would the results have been to establish the diagnosis of Graves' disease?
3. Why was surgery delayed?
4. What was the purpose of the pharmacologic intervention?
5. What are the patient's immediate learning needs and her learning needs preoperatively and postoperatively?
6. What are the nursing interventions for successful long-term management of this patient after the subtotal thyroidectomy?
7. Based on the assessment data presented, write one or more appropriate nursing diagnoses pertinent to this patient while hospitalized. Are there any collaborative problems?

NURSING RESEARCH ISSUES

1. Is sucking on hard candy or ice chips more effective in decreasing the subjective sensation of thirst in patients with SIADH?
2. Do patients with hyperthyroidism sleep better in a private hospital room than in a hospital room shared with another patient?
3. What is the difference in the mental status of hypothyroid patients before and after thyroid replacement therapy?
4. What are the presenting symptoms of infection in patients with Cushing's syndrome?
5. Is a nurse-directed dosage adjustment more effective in preventing symptoms in the patient lacking endogenous cortisol who is exposed to stress than a patient-directed dosage adjustment?
6. Does regular exercise prevent bone loss in patients receiving glucocorticoid therapy?

REVIEW QUESTIONS

The number of the question corresponds to the same-numbered objective at the beginning of the chapter.

1. The adult patient with growth hormone excess exhibits all of the following *except*

a. hypoglycemia.
b. abnormal bone growth.
c. headaches.
d. visual changes.

2. SIADH is characterized by all of the following *except*

a. low urine output.
b. weight gain.
c. edema.
d. decline in plasma osmolality.

3. A commonly used drug in the treatment of hyperthyroidism that inhibits the synthesis of thyroid hormones is

a. propranolol.
b. propylthiouracil.
c. corticosteroids.
d. potassium iodide.

4. If the parathyroid glands are removed accidentally during neck surgery, the patient may develop

a. kidney stones.
b. difficulty in swallowing.
c. thyroid crisis.
d. tetany.

5. An important nursing intervention when caring for a patient with Cushing's syndrome is to

a. administer steroids in equal doses.
b. protect the patient from exposure to infection.
c. restrict protein intake.
d. observe for signs of hypotension.

6. After an adrenalectomy for pheochromocytoma the patient is most apt to experience

a. hyperglycemia.
b. pronounced sodium and water retention.
c. hypokalemia.
d. pronounced fluctuations in blood pressure.

7. Nursing assessment for fluid volume imbalance includes all of the following *except*

a. urine acetone.
b. intake and output.
c. urine specific gravity.
d. daily weights.

8. A common pharmacologic use of steroid therapy is in the treatment of

a. peptic ulcers.
b. migraine headaches.
c. asthma.
d. osteoporosis.

9. The patient needs to know that the best time to take cortisone for replacement purposes is

a. every other day on awakening.
b. regularly by the clock, at 6- or 8-hour intervals.
c. on arising and in the late afternoon.
d. once a day at bedtime.

REFERENCES

1. Lipid Research Clinics Program: The Lipid Research Clinics coronary primary prevention trial results. I. Reduction in incidents of coronary heart disease, *JAMA* 25:1351, 1984.
2. Thorner MO and others: The anterior pituitary. In Wilson JD, Foster DW, editors: *Williams textbook of endocrinology,* ed 8, Philadelphia, 1992, Saunders.
3. Thapar K and others: Pituitary adenomas: current concepts in classification, histopathology, and molecular biology, *Endocrinologist* 3:39, 1993.
4. Melmed S: Management choices in acromegaly, *Endocrinologist* 1:331, 1991.
5. Smith-Rooker J, Garrett A, Hodges LC: Case management of the patient with pituitary tumor, *Medsurg Nurs* 2:265, 1993.
6. Chipps E: Transsphenoidal surgery for pituitary tumors, *Crit Care Nurse* 12:30, 1992.
7. Krause EA and others: Radiosurgery: a nursing perspective, *J Neurosci Nurs* 23:24, 1991.
8. Findling JW, Tyrrell JB: Anterior pituitary gland. In Greenspan FS, editor: *Basic and clinical endocrinology,* ed 3, Norwalk, CT, 1991, Appleton & Lange.
9. Underwood LE, Van Wyk JJ: Normal and aberrant growth. In Wilson JD, Foster DW, editors: *Williams textbook of endocrinology,* ed 8, Philadelphia, 1992, Saunders.
10. Lindeman C: S.I.A.D.H. Is your patient at risk? *Nursing* 22:60, 1992.
11. Reeves WB, Andreoli TE: The posterior pituitary and water metabolism. In Wilson JD, Foster DW, editors: *Williams textbook of endocrinology,* ed 8, Philadelphia, 1992, Saunders.
12. Moses A, Streeten D: Disorders of the neurohypophysis. In Isselbacher K and others, editors: *Harrison's principles of internal medicine,* ed 13, New York, 1994, McGraw-Hill.
13. Volpe R: Graves' disease: pathogenesis. In Braverman LE, Utiger RD, editors: *Werner and Ingbar's the thyroid: a fundamental and clinical text,* ed 6, Philadelphia, JB Lippincott, 1991.
14. Coffland FI: Thyroid-induced cardiac disorders, *Crit Care Nurse* 25, 1993.
15. Federman D: Hyperthyroidism in the geriatric population, *Hosp Prac* 26:61, 1991.
16. Spittle L: Diagnoses in opposition: thyroid storm and myxedema coma, *AACN Clin Issues Crit Care Nurs* 3:300, 1992.
17. Ladenson PW: Diagnosis of thyrotoxicosis. In Braverman LE, Utiger RD, editors: *Werner and Ingbar's the thyroid: a fundamental and clinical text,* ed 6, Philadelphia, 1991, JB Lippincott.
18. Cooper DS: Treatment of thyrotoxicosis. In Braverman LE, Utiger RD, editors: *Werner and Ingbar's the thyroid: a fundamental and clinical text,* ed 6, Philadelphia, 1991, JB Lippincott.
19. Tiwary CM: Neonatal screening for metabolic and endocrine diseases, *Nurse Pract* 12:28, 1987.
20. Hung W: Thyroid disorders of infancy and childhood. In Becker KL and others, editors: *Principles and practice of endocrinology and metabolism,* Philadelphia, 1990, JB Lippincott.
21. Arnaud CD, Kolb FO: The calciotropic hormones and metabolic bone disease. In Greenspan FS, editor: *Basic and clinical endocrinology,* Norwalk, CT, 1991, Appleton & Lange.
22. Fitzpatrick LA, Bilezikian JP: Primary hyperparathyroidism. In Becker KL and others, editors: *Principles and practice of endocrinology and metabolism,* Philadelphia, 1990, JB Lippincott.
23. Avioli LV: Hyperparathyroidism, estrogens, and osteoporosis, *Hosp Pract* 26: 115, 1991.
24. Downs RW, Levine MA: Hypoparathyroidism and other causes of hypocalcemia. In Becker KL and others, editors: *Principles and practice of endocrinology and metabolism,* Philadelphia, 1990, JB Lippincott.
25. Loriaux DL: Cushing's syndrome. In Becker KL and others, editors: *Principles and practice of endocrinology and metabolism,* Philadelphia, 1990, JB Lippincott.
26. Loriaux DL: Adrenocortical insufficiency. In Becker KL and others, editors: *Principles and practice of endocrinology and metabolism,* Philadelphia, 1990, JB Lippincott.
27. Epstein CD: Adrenocortical insufficiency in the critically ill patient, *AACN Clin Issues Crit Care Nurs* 3:705, 1992.
28. Axelrod L: Corticosteroid therapy. In Becker KL and others, editors: *Principles and practice of endocrinology and metabolism,* Philadelphia, 1990, JB Lippincott.
29. Braatvedt GD, Newrick PG, Corrall RJM: Patient's self administration of hydrocortisone, *Br Med J* 301:1312, 1990.
30. Biglieri EG, Kater CE: Mineralocorticoids. In Greenspan FS, editor: *Basic and clinical endocrinology,* Norwalk, CT, 1991, Appleton & Lange.
31. Gill JR: Primary hyperaldosteronism, *Endocrinologist* 1:365, 1991.
32. Laue L, Cutler GB: 21-Hydroxylase deficiency: overview of treatment, *Endocrinologist* 2:291, 1992.
33. Hughes IA: Congenital adrenal hyperplasia, *Trends Endocrinol Metab* 1:123, 1990.
34. Golub MS, Tuck ML: Diagnostic and therapeutic strategies in pheochromocytoma, *Endocrinologist* 2:101, 1992.
35. Agana-Defensor R, Proch M: Pheochromocytoma: a clinical review, *AACN Clin Issues Crit Care Nurs* 3:309, 1992.

Chapter 48

NURSING ASSESSMENT
Reproductive Systems

Nancy MacMullen Laura Dulski

Learning Objectives

1. Describe the structures and functions of the male and female reproductive systems.
2. Explain the functions of the major hormones essential for the structure and function of the reproductive systems.
3. Describe the physiologic and psychologic changes of a man and of a woman during the stages of sexual response.
4. Describe age-related changes in the reproductive systems and differences in assessment findings.
5. Identify significant subjective and objective data related to the reproductive systems and information about sexual function that should be obtained from a patient.
6. Describe noninvasive techniques used in the physical assessment of the reproductive systems.
7. Differentiate normal from abnormal findings obtained from a physical assessment of the reproductive systems.
8. Describe the purpose, significance of results, and nursing responsibilities related to diagnostic studies of the reproductive systems.

STRUCTURES AND FUNCTIONS OF THE MALE AND FEMALE REPRODUCTIVE SYSTEMS

The reproductive system is interrelated with other systems, including the neurologic, endocrine, and urinary systems, and also with general physiologic function. For example, estrogen (produced primarily in a woman's ovaries) influences bone density and testosterone (produced in a man's testes) influences muscle mass. The reproductive system is responsible for the perpetuation of the species through fertilization, implantation, maintenance of pregnancy, and birth of a baby. The reproductive system is also directly related to sexual function and is therefore intricately interwoven into the complex, sensitive, and frequently stress-laden area of psychosocial mores and cultural values regarding sex.

Male Reproductive System

The male reproductive system consists of the external structures—the penis and the scrotum—and the internal structures, including the prostate gland, the seminal vesicles, and several ducts (Fig. 48-1). The *scrotum* lies within the scrotal sac, which is a thin, loose outer layer of skin over a more muscular internal layer. The scrotum consists of two halves divided by a septum; each half contains a testis, an epididymis, and a spermatic cord. The testis is an ovoid, smooth, firm organ measuring 2 to 2.5 cm in depth and 2 to 3 cm in width. Within the testes are the *seminiferous tubules,* where spermatozoa (sperm) are formed at a rate of 10 to 30 billion per month. The tubules lead into a system of small ducts that conduct sperm to the *epididymis.*

The epididymis is a soft, cordlike structure that measures almost 212 inches (530 cm) in length if stretched out. It lies in the anterior plane and along the posterolateral surface of each testis. This organ may be considered to be a large duct. It stores the sperm as they mature and until they are released by ejaculation or until they disintegrate and are reabsorbed by the body (Fig. 48-2). The *ductus deferens* extends from the epididymis to a point close to the prostate gland, where it becomes the *ejaculatory duct* and enters the urethra. The duct system emerging from each testis conveys sperm into the urethra.

The spermatic cord contains not only the ductus deferens but also the arteries, veins, and lymph vessels that supply the testis and epididymis. All of these structures are enclosed by the cremaster muscle and by layers of fascia. The cord enters the inguinal canal through the external inguinal ring. The cord ends there, and its components, primarily the ductus deferens, continue along a backward course toward the scrotum.

The prostate gland, the seminal vesicles, and Cowper's (bulbourethral) glands are the accessory glands of the male reproductive system. These glands produce and secrete seminal fluid, which contains the sperm. The *prostate gland*

Reviewed by Mary C. Brucker, CNM, DNSc, Director, Parkland School of Nurse-Midwifery, Dallas, TX.

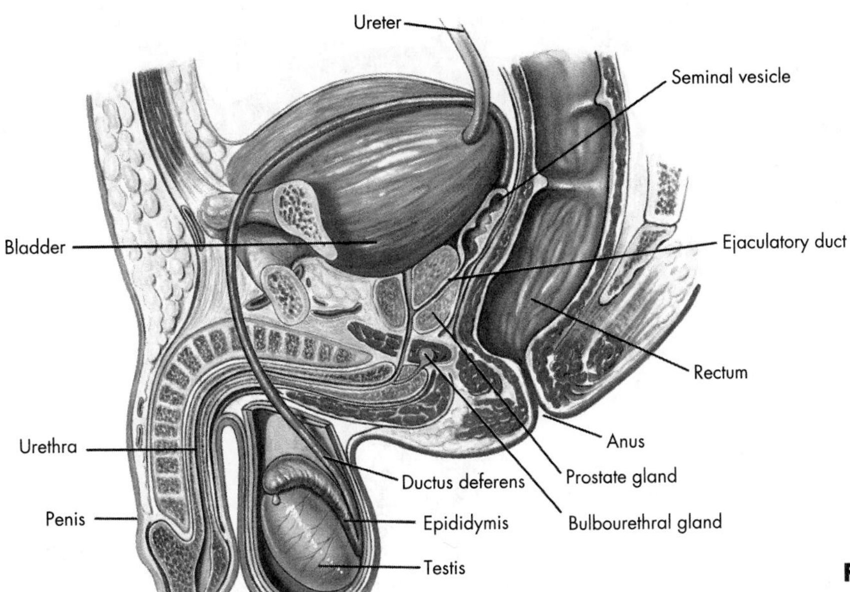

Fig. 48-1 External and internal male sex organs.

lies underneath the bladder. Its posterior surface approximates the rectal wall. The normal prostate measures 2 cm in width and 3 cm in length and is divided into the right and left lateral lobes and an anteroposterior median lobe. As the ejaculate passes through the urethra, it receives an alkaline secretion from the prostate gland. The *seminal vesicles* lie just behind the bladder and between the rectum and the bladder. The ducts of the seminal vesicles fuse with the ductus deferens to form the ejaculatory ducts that enter

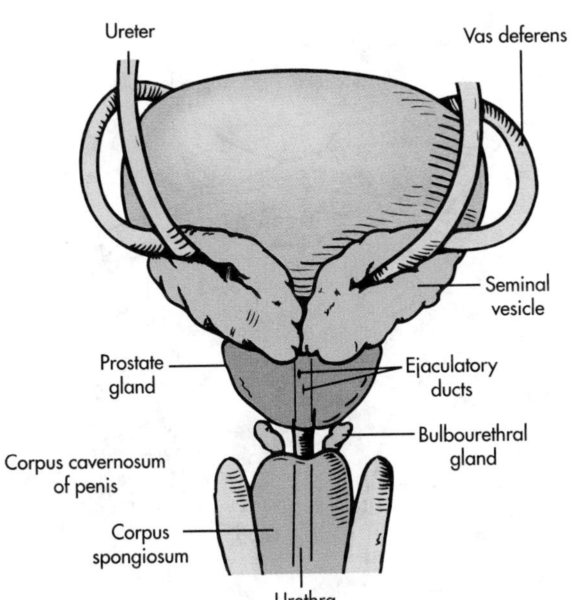

Fig. 48-2 Formation of the ejaculatory ducts by union of the seminal vesicles with the ductus deferens just before entrance into the prostate gland. The ejaculatory ducts open into the prostatic portion of the urethra.

the prostate gland. *Cowper's glands* lie on each side of the urethra and slightly posterior to it, just below the prostate. The ducts of these glands enter directly into the urethra. The secretion from the prostate makes up most of the fluid in the ejaculate. By comparison, the seminal vesicles and Cowper's glands contribute a minimum amount of fluid to the ejaculate. These various secretions serve as a medium for the transport of sperm and create an alkaline, nutritious environment that promotes sperm motility and survival. Figure 48-2 follows the route of sperm from production to ejaculation.

The urethra extends from the bladder, through the prostate, and ends in a slitlike opening (the meatus) on the ventral side of the *glans,* the end of the penis. The glans is covered by a fold of skin, the prepuce (or foreskin), which forms at the junction of the glans and the shaft of the penis. There is no prepuce in the circumcised male. The broadened segment of the glans at the junction is the *corona.* The shaft of the penis consists of erectile tissue composed of the corpus cavernosum and corpus spongiosum; the fibrous sheath that encases the erectile tissue; and the urethra. The skin covering the penis is thin, loose, and essentially hairless.

Female Reproductive System

The female reproductive system consists of the breasts, the uterus, the ovaries, the fallopian tubes, the vagina, and the external genitalia (the vulva), as well as ligaments and pelvic bones.

Breasts. The breasts are a secondary sex characteristic that develops during puberty in response to estrogen and progesterone. Cyclic hormonal changes lead to regular changes in breast tissue to prepare it for lactation when fertilization and pregnancy occur. The breasts are also considered a major organ of sexual stimulation and response among some cultures.

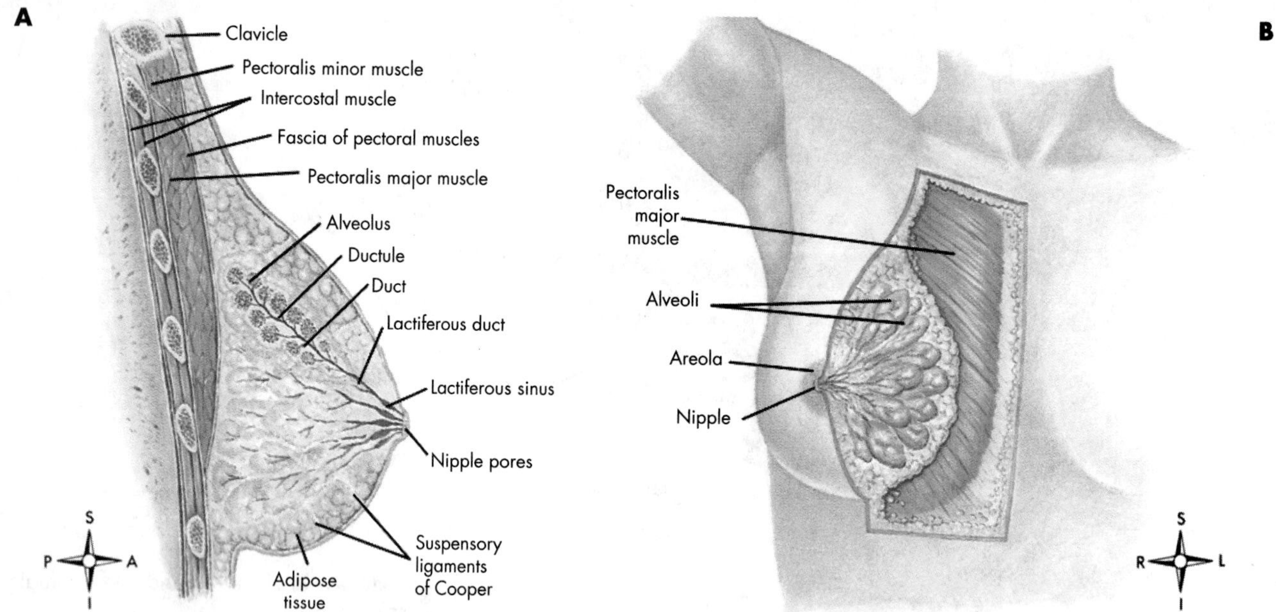

Fig. 48-3 The female breast. ***A,*** Sagittal section of a lactating breast. Notice how the glandular structures are anchored to the overlying skin and to the pectoral muscles by suspensory ligaments of Cooper. Each lobule of glandular tissue is drained by a lactiferous duct that eventually opens through the nipple. ***B,*** Anterior view of a lactating breast. In nonlactating breasts the glandular tissue is much less prominent, with adipose tissue comprising most of each breast.

The breasts extend from the second to the sixth ribs, with the tail reaching the axilla (Fig. 48-3). The fully mature breast is dome shaped and contains a pigmented center called the *areola.* The areolar region contains *Montgomery's tubercles,* which are similar to sebaceous glands and assist in moistening the nipple. The nipple itself contains 15 to 20 tiny openings that lead into ducts forming the *lactiferous sinuses,* where milk is stored during lactation. Ducts (secondary tubules) extend and branch from the lactiferous sinuses outward, eventually ending in lobules called *alveoli* or *acini* of the breasts. The alveoli secrete milk during lactation. The breast's rich lymphatic network drains primarily into the axillary, the infraclavicular, and the supraclavicular channels. This system is often responsible for the metastasis of a malignant tumor from the breast to other parts of the body (Fig. 48-4). The fibrous and fatty tissue that supports and separates the channels of the mammary duct system is primarily responsible for the varying sizes and shapes of the breasts in different individuals.

Pelvic Organs

Ovaries. The ovaries are usually located on either side of the uterus, just behind and below the fallopian (uterine) tubes (Fig. 48-5). The ovaries are firm and solid, averaging 1.5 cm in width, 3 cm in length, and 2 cm in depth. Their functions include ovulation, as well as secretion of the two major reproductive hormones, estrogen and progesterone. The outer zone of the ovary contains follicles with germ cells, or oocytes. Each follicle contains a primordial (immature) oocyte surrounded by granulosa and theca cells. These two layers protect and nourish the oocyte until the follicle reaches maturity and ovulation occurs. However, not all follicles reach maturity. In a process called *atresia* the primordial follicles become smaller and are reabsorbed by the body; thus the number of follicles declines from 2 to 4 million at birth to approximately 300,000 to 400,000 at menarche. This number continues to decrease throughout a woman's reproductive years.[1] The vast majority of oocytes are destroyed by atresia. Fewer than 500 are actually re-

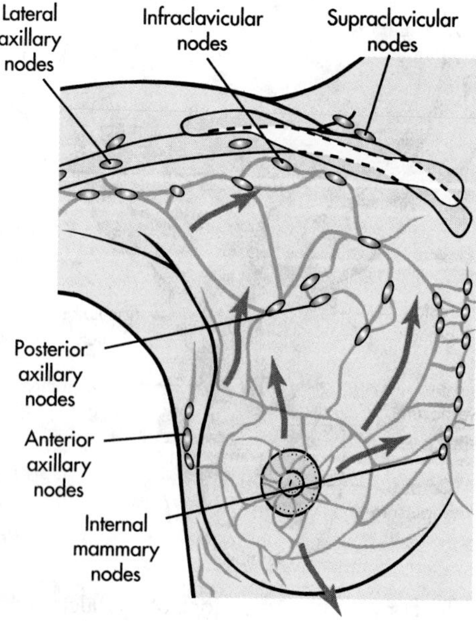

Fig. 48-4 Lymphatic drainage of the breast. *Arrows* indicate direction of drainage.

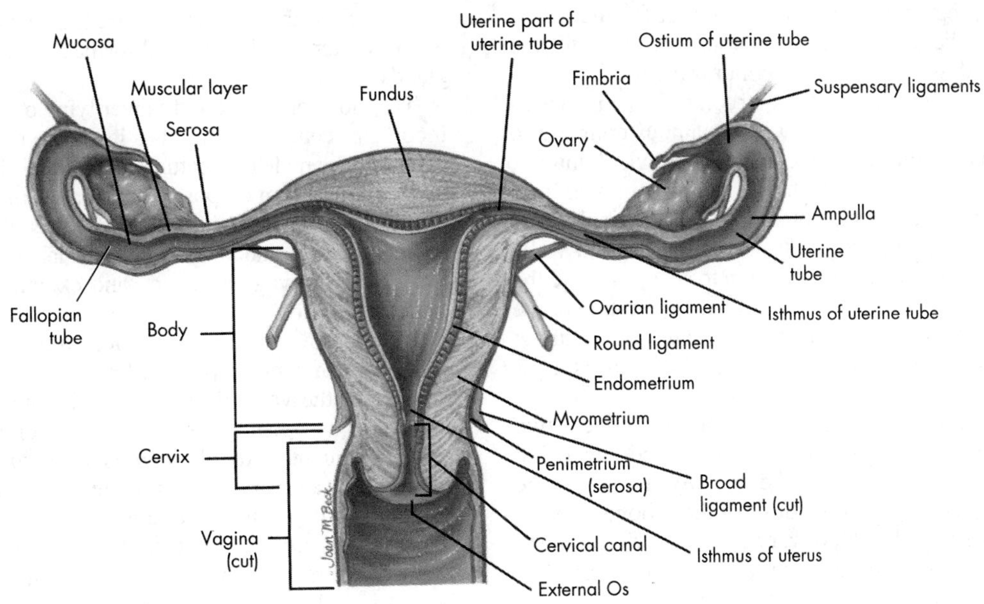

Fig. 48-5 Anatomy of the female reproductive tract.

leased by ovulation during the reproductive years of the normal healthy woman.

Fallopian tubes. Normally, each month during a woman's reproductive years, one ovarian follicle reaches maturity, and the ovum is ovulated, or expelled, from the ovary through the stimulus of the gonadotropic hormones, follicle-stimulating hormone (FSH) and luteinizing hormone (LH). The ovum then travels up a fallopian tube where fertilization by a sperm occurs, assuming that sperm are present. An ovum can be fertilized up to 72 hours after its release. Sperm are viable for 24 to 48 hours.[2]

The distal ends of the fallopian tubes consist of fingerlike projections called *fimbriae* that "massage" the ovaries at ovulation to help extract the mature ovum. The tubes, which average 4.8 inches (12 cm) in length, extend from the fimbriae to the superior lateral borders of the uterus. Fertilization usually takes place within the outer one third of the tubes.

Uterus. The uterus is a pear-shaped, hollow, muscular organ (Fig. 48-5). It is located between the bladder and the rectum. In the mature nulliparous (never pregnant) female the uterus is approximately 6 cm in length and 4 cm in width. The uterine walls consist of an outer or serosal layer, a middle muscular layer, the *myometrium,* and an inner mucosal layer, the *endometrium.*

The uterus consists of the fundus, the body (or the corpus), and the cervix. The body makes up about 80% of the uterus and connects with the cervix at the isthmus, or the neck.

The *cervix* is the lower portion that invaginates (projects) into the anterior wall of the vaginal canal. It makes up about 15% to 20% of the uterus in the nulliparous female. The cervix consists of the *ectocervix,* or the outer portion that protrudes into the vagina, and the *endocervix,* or the canal in the opening of the cervix. The ectocervix is covered with squamous epithelial cells, which give it a smooth, pinkish appearance. The endocervix contains a lining of columnar epithelial cells, which give it a rough, reddened appearance. The junction at which the two types of epithelial cells meet is called the *squamocolumnar junction* and contains the optimal types of cells needed for an accurate Papanicolaou (Pap) smear to screen for malignancies. The presence of endocervical cells in the sample taken for a Pap smear ensures that the squamocolumnar junction, or the transformation zone, has been sampled. Cells taken from the vagina provide a less accurate diagnosis and, therefore, are not included in the routine Pap smear.[2] The cervical canal is 2 to 4 cm long and is relatively tightly closed. The cervix, however, allows sperm to enter the uterus and also allows menses to be expelled. The columnar epithelium, under hormonal influence, provides enough elasticity at labor for the cervix to stretch so that a fetus can pass. The entrance of sperm into the uterus is facilitated by mucus produced by the cervix under the influence of estrogen. Under normal conditions, the cervical mucus becomes watery and more abundant at ovulation. This mucus can stretch several inches (*spinnbarkheit*) and allows for the easy entrance of sperm into the uterus. The postovulatory cervical mucus, under the influence of progesterone, is thick and inhibits sperm passage. Knowledge of these physiologic changes is used in natural approaches to family planning.

The anterior and posterior peritoneal covering of the uterus is called the *broad ligament.* It separates the uterus from the bladder and the rectum but does not provide support for the uterus or the adnexa (ovaries and tubes). The cardinal ligaments, which extend from the isthmus of the uterus to the pelvic wall, also offer only minimal support. The round ligament, which extends anteriorly to the labia majora, provides some support but is easily weakened by pregnancy. The firmest support for the uterus is provided by the uterine sacral ligaments, which pull the uterus back and away from the vaginal orifice.

Vagina. The vagina is a tubular structure 3 to 4 inches (8 to 10 cm) in length that is lined with squamous epithelium. The secretions of the vagina consist of cervical mucus, desquamated epithelium, and, during sexual stimulation, a direct transudate. These fluids protect against vaginal infection. The muscular and erectile tissue of the vaginal walls allow enough dilatation and contraction to accommodate the passage of the fetus during labor as well as penetration of the penis during intercourse. The anterior vaginal wall lies along the urethra and bladder. The posterior vaginal wall is adjacent to the rectum.

Pelvis. The female pelvis consists of four bones: two hipbones (also called the *innominate bones* and consisting of the *ilium,* the *ischium,* and the *symphysis pubis*), the sacrum, and the coccyx. The sections of these bones that lie below the iliopectineal line are very important during birth and are often a factor determining the ability of a woman to deliver a child vaginally. Knowledge of these bones and the landmarks that they form in the pelvis allows the practitioner to estimate pelvic measurements and the potential for a woman's pelvis to accommodate the birth of a full-term fetus. Specialty references discuss the specific techniques of clinical pelvimetry.

The pelvis is also divided into the true pelvis and the false pelvis. The true pelvis encompasses the brim, the cavity, and the outlet and is the bony passageway through which the fetus passes during birth. The false pelvis consists of the superior portion of the iliac bones, above the brim or the iliopectineal line.[1]

External Genitalia. The external portion of the female reproductive system (Fig. 48-6), commonly called the *vulva,* consists of the mons pubis, the labia majora, the labia minora, the clitoris, the urethral meatus, the ducts of Skene's glands, the vaginal orifice, and the Bartholin's glands.

The mons pubis is a fatty layer lying over the pubic bone. It contains coarse hair that lies in an upside-down triangular pattern. (The male hair pattern is diamond shaped.) The labia majora are folds of adipose tissue that form the outer borders of the vulva. These hair-covered folds contain sweat glands and sebaceous glands. The hairless labia minora form the borders of the vaginal orifice and extend anteriorly to enclose the clitoris.

In a virgin the vaginal orifice usually but not always contains a thin membrane called the *hymen,* which varies the size of the vaginal orifice in individuals from that of a pinhole to an opening large enough to allow two fingers to enter. Frequently, the hymen is torn during first sexual intercourse, and only tags remain. In many societies, the bleeding that occurs with this tearing has been used to validate virginity. However, not all hymens are torn by the first intercourse. Some are already well stretched or are torn because of childhood activity, tampon usage, or accidents.

The *clitoris* is homologous (similar) to the male penis; it is the erectile tissue that becomes engorged during sexual excitation. It lies anterior to the urethral meatus and the vaginal orifice and is usually covered by the prepuce or hood. Clitoral stimulation is an important part of sexual activity for many women.

Skene's glands and ducts lie alongside the urethral meatus and have no known function. They are homologous to the male prostate. Bartholin's glands, which are at the posterior and lateral aspects of the vaginal orifice, secrete a thin, mucoid material believed to contribute slightly to lubrication during sexual intercourse. These glands are not usually palpable unless sebaceous-like cysts form or an infection, especially a sexually transmitted disease, arises.

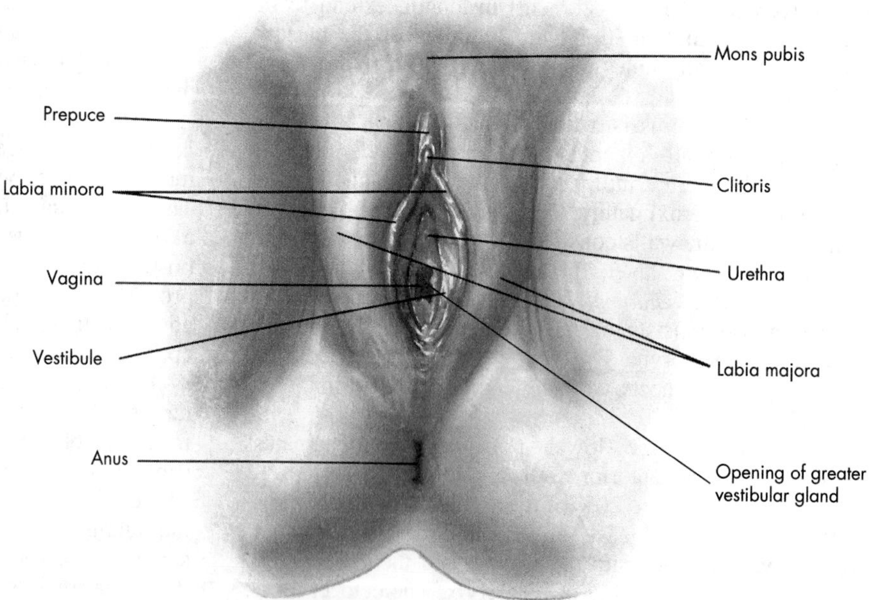

Fig. 48-6 External female genitalia.

Neuroendocrine Regulation

The hypothalamus and pituitary gland (see Chapter 45) and the gonads (organs of reproduction) secrete numerous hormones (Fig. 48-7). These hormones regulate the processes of ovulation, spermatogenesis (formation of sperm), and fertilization, as well as the formation and function of the secondary sex characteristics. The cyclic changes in the amounts of these hormones secreted by the anterior pituitary gland cause cyclic changes in the ovaries. The hypothalamus secretes gonadotropin-releasing hormones (GnRHs), which stimulate the pituitary gland to secrete its hormones, including FSH, LH, and luteotropic hormone (LTH) or prolactin. LH in males is sometimes called interstitial cell stimulating hormone (ICSH). The gonadal hormones are estrogen, progesterone, and testosterone.

In women, FSH production by the pituitary stimulates the growth and maturity of the ovarian follicles to cause ovulation. The mature follicle produces estrogen, which in turn suppresses the release of FSH. Another hormone, inhibin, is also secreted by the ovarian follicle and inhibits both GnRH and FSH secretion. In men FSH stimulates the seminiferous tubules to produce sperm.

LH contributes to the ovulatory process because it causes follicles to complete maturation and undergo ovulation. It also causes the development of the ruptured follicle into a corpus luteum, from which progesterone is secreted. Progesterone maintains the rich vascular state of the uterus (secretory phase) in preparation for fertilization and implantation. In men, ICSH is responsible for the production of testosterone by the interstitial cells of the testes and thus is essential for the full maturation of sperm. Prolactin has no known function in men but, with other hormones, stimulates the development and growth of the mammary glands in women. During lactation, it initiates and maintains milk production.

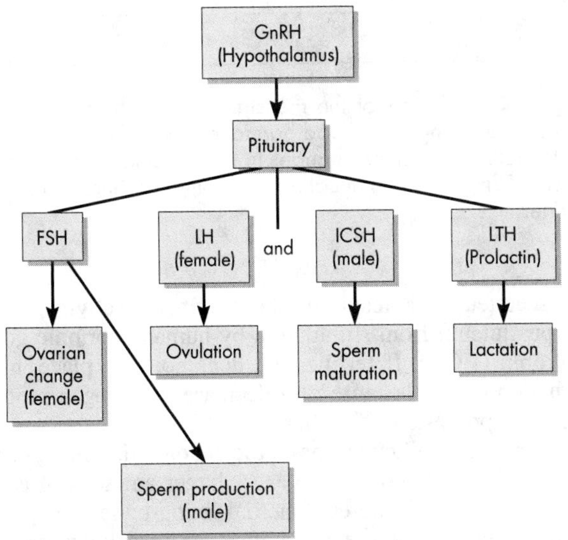

Fig. 48-7 The hypothalamic-pituitary-gonadal axis. Only the major pituitary hormone actions are depicted. *FSH,* Follicle-stimulating hormone; *GnRH,* gonadotropin-releasing hormone; *ICSH,* interstitial cell–stimulating hormone; *LH,* luteinizing hormone; *LTH,* luteotropic hormone.

The gonadal hormones, estrogen and progesterone, in women are produced by the ovaries. Small amounts of an estrogen precursor are also produced in the adrenal cortices of women. Estrogen is essential to the development and maintenance of the secondary sex characteristics, the phase of the menstrual cycle immediately after menstruation (proliferative phase), and the uterine changes essential to pregnancy. Estrogen has also been found in the urine of men, although its role and importance are not well understood. In men, this hormone is produced predominantly in the adrenal cortex.

Progesterone plays a major role in the menstrual cycle but most specifically in the secretory phase. Like estrogen, progesterone is involved in the bodily changes associated with pregnancy. Adequate progesterone is necessary to maintain an implanted egg.

The major gonadal hormone of men, testosterone, is produced by the testes. Testosterone is responsible for the development and maintenance of secondary sex characteristics, as well as for adequate spermatogenesis.

The circulating levels of gonadal hormones are controlled primarily by a negative feedback process. Receptors within the hypothalamus and pituitary are sensitive to the circulating blood levels of the hormones (Table 48-1). Increased levels of hormones stimulate a hypothalamic response to decrease the high circulating levels. Likewise, low circulating levels provoke a hypothalamic response that increases the low circulating levels. For example, if the circulating level of testosterone is low, the hypothalamus is stimulated to secrete GnRH. This stimulates the pituitary to secrete greater amounts of FSH and ICSH, which in turn causes an increase in the production of testosterone. The high levels of testosterone then stimulate a decrease in the production of GnRH and, thus, of FSH and ICSH.

In women, however, there is a slight variation. The circulating levels are controlled through a combination of both a negative and a positive feedback system. A negative feedback control mechanism exists, as in men. When circulating estrogen levels are low, the hypothalamus is stimulated to increase its production of GnRH. GnRH

Table 48-1 Gonadal Feedback Mechanisms

Negative Feedback			
↓ Estrogen	→ ↑ GnRH (hypothalamus)	→ ↑ FSH (pituitary)	→ ↑ Estrogen (ovaries)
Positive Feedback			
↑ Estrogen	→ ↑ GnRH (hypothalamus)	→ ↑ LH (pituitary)	
Testes (Negative Feedback)			
↓Testosterone	→↑ GnRH (hypothalamus)	→↑ FSH and ICSH (pituitary)	→↑ Testosterone (testes)

FSH, Follicle stimulating hormone; *GnRH,* gonadotropin-releasing hormone; *ICSH,* interstitial cell–stimulating hormone; *LH,* luteinizing hormone.

stimulates the pituitary to secrete greater amounts of FSH and LH, resulting in higher levels of estrogen production by the ovaries. Reciprocally higher levels of circulating estrogen result in a decreasing secretion of GnRH and thus a decrease in the secretion of FSH by the pituitary.

There is also a positive feedback control mechanism in women. Thus, with increasing levels of circulating estrogen, a greater level of GnRH is produced, resulting in an increased level of LH from the pituitary. Likewise, lowered levels of estrogen result in a lowered level of LH.

Menarche

Menarche is the first episode of menstrual bleeding, indicating a female has reached puberty. This usually occurs around 13 years of age, although there is individual variation according to race, nutrition, health, and heredity.

As puberty approaches, there are changes associated with the elevated rate of estrogen and progesterone secretion by the ovaries. These changes include the development of breast buds, the development of pubic hair, and later, the development of axillary hair. During this time, there is a decrease in the sensitivity of the hypothalamic-pituitary axis that allows for increased secretion of FSH and LH and a resultant increase in estrogen. It is during this time that the adult pattern of gonadotropin secretion occurs, resulting in the menstrual cycle. Menstrual cycles are often irregular during the first few years of menarche because of anovulation.

Menstrual Cycle

The major functions of the ovaries are ovulation and the secretion of hormones. These functions are accomplished during the normal menstrual cycle, a monthly process mediated by the hormonal activity of the hypothalamus, the pituitary gland, and the ovaries. Menstruation occurs during each month in which an egg is not fertilized (Fig. 48-8). The endometrial cycle is divided into three phases labeled in relation to uterine and ovarian changes: (1) the proliferative or follicular phase, (2) the secretory or luteal phase, and (3) the menstrual phase or ischemic phase. The length of the menstrual cycle ranges from 20 to 40 days, the average being 28 days.

The menstrual cycle begins on the first day of menstruation, which usually lasts 3 to 5 days. During this time, estrogen and progesterone levels are low, but FSH levels begin to increase. During the follicular phase, a single follicle matures fully under the stimulation of FSH. (The mechanism that ensures that usually only one follicle reaches maturity is not known.) The mature follicle stimulates estrogen production, causing a negative feedback with resulting decreased FSH secretion.

Although the initial stage of follicular maturation is stimulated by FSH, complete maturation and ovulation occur only with the presence of LH. When estrogen levels peak on about the twelfth day of the cycle, there is a surge of LH, which triggers ovulation a day or two later. After ovulation (maturation and release of an ovum), LH promotes the development of the corpus luteum.

The fully developed corpus luteum continues to secrete estrogen and initiates progesterone secretion. If fertilization occurs, high levels of estrogen and progesterone continue to

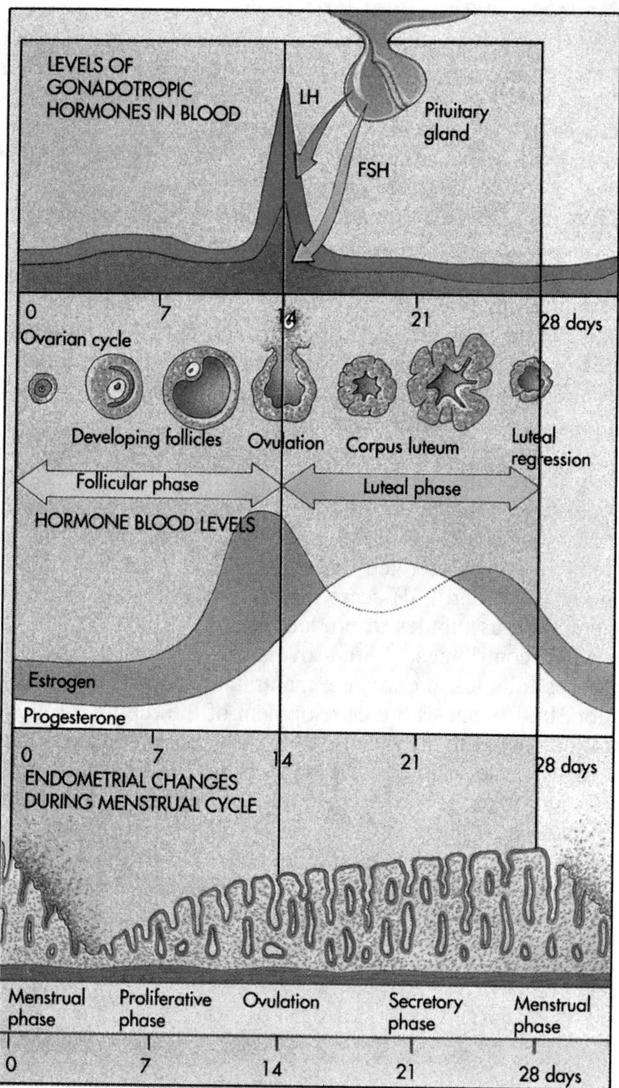

Fig. 48-8 Events of the menstrual cycle. The various lines depict the changes in blood hormone levels, the development of the follicles, and the changes in the endometrium during the cycle. *FSH,* Follicle-stimulating hormone; *LH,* luteinizing hormone.

be secreted as a result of the continued activity of the corpus luteum from stimulation by human chorionic gonadotropin (HCG). If fertilization does not take place, menstruation occurs because of a decrease in estrogen production and progesterone withdrawal.

During the follicular phase, the endometrial lining of the uterus also undergoes change. As larger amounts of estrogen are produced, the endometrial lining undergoes proliferative changes—there is an increase in cellular growth, including an increase in the length of blood vessels and glandular tissue.

With ovulation and the resulting increased levels of progesterone, the luteal, or secretory, phase begins. In this phase, the blood vessels begin to coil, increasing the surface area of the vascular supply. The glandular tissues mature and secrete a glycogen-rich substance, and the glandular ducts dilate. If the corpus luteum regresses (when fertilization does not occur) and estrogen and progesterone levels fall, the endometrial lining can no longer be supported. As a result, the blood vessels contract, and tissue begins to slough (fall away). This sloughing results in the menses and the start of the menstrual phase.

Menopause

Menopause is the cessation of the menses for the remainder of a woman's lifetime. It is usually considered complete after one year of *amenorrhea* (absence of menstruation). The average age at which menopause occurs is 52 years, but this can vary.[3] The climacteric, also commonly known as the *perimenopause,* is the period during which symptoms of approaching menopause begin, menopause actually occurs, and equilibrium after menopause is established (Table 48-2). Ovulation decreases over a period of years. In a way, the factors that result in menopause are established during fetal life. Approximately 2 to 4 million oocytes are present by the 20th week of gestation, after which time the number begins to decline. The average female ovulates 400 to 500 times during a lifetime. Most follicles undergo *atresia* and are then called atretic follicles.[1] In 40 to 50 years after birth the full store of oocytes is greatly depleted. Because the number of oocytes decreases during the climacteric, the amount of estrogen produced also begins to decrease.

The decreasing level of estrogen causes a gradual increase in FSH and LH as a result of the negative feedback process. By the time menopause occurs, there is a ten- to twentyfold increase in FSH. These elevated FSH levels may take several years to return to premenopausal levels. The reduced estrogen level also causes a decrease in the frequency of ovulation and results in atrophy of the secondary sex characteristics.

The reason for "hot flashes" or vasomotor instability is not clearly understood. It has been theorized that temperature regulators in the brain are in proximity to the area where GnRH is released. However, lowered estrogen levels are correlated with dilatation of cutaneous blood vessels, resulting in "hot flashes" and increased sweating. The more sudden the withdrawal of estrogen (as associated with surgical removal of the ovaries, for example), the more likely that the symptoms will be severe (if no replacement is provided). These symptoms subside over time, with or without hormone replacement therapy. Autonomic nervous system instability may also be related to emotional irritability during the climacteric, but this "symptom" has been greatly exaggerated in literature and myth. Atrophy of the vaginal epithelium often causes vaginal dryness that is responsible for mild to moderate *dyspareunia* (painful intercourse). This can lead to unnecessary and premature cessation of sexual activity. Dryness is a problem that can be easily corrected with water soluble lubricants or, if needed, with hormonal creams or systemic hormone replacement therapy. In general, the extent and severity of the symptoms of the climacteric vary and are not easily predicted, even with a detailed history of family patterns.

Osteoporosis, a condition in which the bone mass is decreased because of increased bone resorption, is quite prevalent in menopausal women. This condition puts women at a much greater risk for sustaining fractures of the spine, vertebrae, wrists, and hips. Such fractures can be life-threatening in older women. Although the exact mechanism is not known, cessation of estrogen production is associated with accelerated bone loss. Estrogen replacement in the postmenopausal period retards this bone loss. Estrogen replacement therapy has also been associated with a decreased incidence of coronary artery disease and a slightly increased risk of breast cancer with long-term use.[4]

The changes of menopause and particularly the risk of osteoporosis create a dilemma in the care of menopausal women. The use of estrogen replacement therapy often reduces the risk of such symptoms but can create other potentially serious side effects. Adequate calcium intake and exercise both before and after menopause are also important factors in the prevention of osteoporosis (see Chapter 59).

Table 48-2 Common Manifestations During the Climacteric

Premenopausal / Menopausal	Postmenopausal
Premenopausal	**Postmenopausal**
Irregular menses	Atrophic vaginitis
Vasomotor instability (hot flashes)	Occasional vasomotor symptoms
Nervousness	Atrophy of genitourinary tissue with decreased support
Menopausal	Osteoporosis
Cessation of menses	
Frequent vasomotor symptoms	
Atrophy of genitourinary tissue (e.g., vaginal epithelium)	
Stress and urge incontinence	

Phases of the Sexual Response

It is helpful to look at the structural homologues in the male and female reproductive systems to understand the sexual response (Table 48-3). Masters and Johnson described the sexual response in terms of the excitement, plateau, orgasmic, and resolution phases.[5]

Orgasm does not occur in every sexual encounter. In addition, orgasm does not depend on anatomic features such as the size of the penis or of the vaginal canal. The sexual response is a complex interplay of psychologic and physiologic phenomena and is therefore influenced by daily stress, as well as by illness and crisis.

Male Sexual Response. The penis and the urethra are essential to the transport of sperm into the vagina and the cervix during intercourse. This transport is facilitated by penile erection in response to sexual stimulation during the excitement phase. Erection results from the filling of the large venous sinuses within the erectile tissue of the penis. In the flaccid state the sinuses hold only a small amount of

Table 48-3 Structural Homologues of the Male and Female Reproductive Systems

Male	Female
Penis	Clitoris
Scrotal ridge	Labia minora
Scrotum	Labia majora
Testes	Ovaries
Cowper's glands	Bartholin's glands
Prostate gland	Skene's ducts
Prostatic utricle (blind pouch of urethra)	Vagina

blood, but during the erection stage they are congested with blood. Because the penis is richly endowed with sympathetic, parasympathetic, and pudendal nerve endings, it is readily stimulated to erection. The loose skin of the penis becomes taut as a result of the intense venous congestion. This erectile tautness allows for easy insertion into the vagina.

As the man reaches the plateau phase, the erection is maintained, and a small increase in diameter occurs as a result of a slight increase in vasocongestion. There is also an increase in testicular size. Sometimes a change in color occurs in the glans penis, which becomes more reddish-purple.

The subsequent contraction of the penile and urethral musculature during the orgasmic phase propels the sperm outward through the meatus. In this process, termed *ejaculation,* sperm are released into the ductus deferens during contractions. They advance through the urethra, where fluids from the prostate and seminal vesicles are added to the ejaculate. The sperm continue their path through the urethra, receiving a small amount of fluid from the Cowper's glands, and are finally ejaculated through the urinary meatus. Orgasm is characterized by the rapid release of the vasocongestion and myotonia that have developed. The rapid release of muscular tension (through rhythmic contractions) occurs primarily in the penis, the prostate gland, and the seminal vesicles.

After ejaculation, a man enters the resolution phase. During this phase the penis undergoes involution, gradually returning to its unstimulated, flaccid state.

Female Sexual Response. The changes that occur in a woman during sexual excitation are similar to those in a man. In response to stimulation the clitoris swells (becomes congested, as does the penis in a man) and vaginal lubrication increases from secretions from the cervix and Bartholin's glands and sweating of the vaginal walls. This initial response is the excitation phase.

As excitation is maintained in the plateau phase, the vagina expands and the uterus is elevated (in the male, correspondingly, there is an increase in testicular size). In the orgasmic phase, contractions occur in the uterus from the fundus to the lower uterine segment. There is a slight relaxation of the cervical os, which helps the entrance of the sperm, and rhythmic contractions of the vagina. Muscular tension is rapidly released through rhythmic contractions in the clitoris, the vagina, and the uterus. This phase is followed by a resolution phase in which these organs return to their preexcitation state. However, women do not have to go through the resolution (refractory) recovery state before they can be orgasmic again. They can be multiorgasmic without resolution between orgasms.

Effects of Aging on Sexual Responses

With advancing age, changes occur in the male and female reproductive systems. In women, many of these changes are related to the altered estrogen production that is associated with menopause. Table 48-4 lists age-related changes that should be considered when caring for an older adult.

Gradual changes resulting from advancing age occur in the sexual responses of men and women (Table 48-5). These changes occur at different rates and to varying degrees. The cumulative effects of these changes, as well as the negative social attitude toward sexuality in older adults, can affect the sexual practices of people in this age group. Nurses have an important role in providing accurate and unbiased information about sexuality and age. Nurses should emphasize the normalcy of sexual activity in older adults. Counseling may be necessary to help older patients accommodate to these normal physiologic changes.[6]

ASSESSMENT OF THE MALE AND FEMALE REPRODUCTIVE SYSTEMS

Subjective Data

Important Health Information. Problems in other systems are often interrelated with problems and stresses within the reproductive system. The nurse must elicit general information as well as information specifically relating to the reproductive system.

Past health history. Every woman who enters the health care system should have a complete obstetric and gynecologic history taken (Table 48-6). The gynecologic history provides information related to such problems as pelvic pain, exposure to sexually transmitted diseases, vaginal infections, and the presence of symptoms such as vaginal discharge and dyspareunia that need treatment. An obstetric history provides important information related to family planning and fertility counseling most relevant to the individual.

In addition, the nurse should obtain data related to inutero exposure to diethylstilbestrol (DES). DES was frequently administered to women to prevent spontaneous abortions during the 1940s and 1950s, with a national decline in use during the 1960s. It is associated with cervical adenosis and cervical and vaginal adenocarcinoma in women who were exposed to it in utero. Male offspring of mothers given DES experience congenital anomalies such as structural defects of the genitourinary tract and decreased sperm levels, as well as an increase in the incidence of penile cancer.

Common pediatric illnesses that affect reproductive function are mumps and rubella. The occurrence of mumps in young men has been associated with an increase in

Table 48-4 Gerontologic Differences in Assessment: Reproductive System

Changes	Differences in Assessment Findings
Male	
Penis	
Decreased subcutaneous fat, decreased skin turgor	Easily retractable foreskin (if uncircumcised), decrease in size, fewer sustained erections
Testes	
Decreased testosterone production	Decrease in size, change in position (lower), increase in firmness
Prostate	
Benign hyperplasia	Enlargement
Breasts	
Enlargement	Gynecomastia (abnormal enlargement)
Female	
Breasts	
Decreased subcutaneous fat, increased fibrous tissue, decreased skin turgor	Less resilient, looser, more pendulous tissue
Vulva	
Decreased skin turgor	Atrophy, decreased amount of pubic hair, decreased size of clitoris
Vagina	
Atrophy of tissue, decreased muscle tone	Pale mucosa, dryness of mucosa, less intense sexual response, relaxation of outlets
Urethra	
Decreased muscle tone	Cystocele (protrusion of bladder through vaginal wall)
Uterus	
Decreased thickness of myometrium	Decrease in size
Ovaries	
Decreased ovarian function	Nonpalpable ovaries

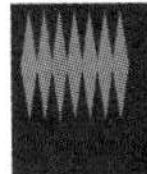

Table 48-5 Gerontologic Differences in Assessment: Sexual Function

Male
- Increased stimulation necessary for erection
- Decreased need to ejaculate
- Decreased ability to attain erection
- Negative attitude by society toward sexual relations by older adults
- Possible decreased response to sexual stimuli

Female
- Decreased vaginal lubrication
- Possible decreased response to sexual stimuli
- Negative attitude by society toward sexual relations by older adults

sterility because of bilateral testicular atrophy secondary to orchitis. In the health history, the nurse should elicit whether male patients have had mumps, been immunized, or had any indications of sterility.

Rubella is of primary concern to women of childbearing age. If rubella occurs during the first 3 months of pregnancy, the possibility of congenital anomalies is increased. For this reason, nurses should encourage immunization for all women of childbearing age who have not been immunized for rubella or have not already had the disease. However, women should not be immunized if they are already pregnant. Women are also advised not to conceive for at least 3 months after immunization.

The presence of a chronic disease such as diabetes mellitus that can affect the functioning of the reproductive system must be determined. Men who have diabetes mellitus frequently experience impotency problems because of associated neuropathies. Impotence and retrograde ejaculation are additional manifestations of diabetes in men. In women with uncontrolled diabetes, pregnancy and the use of oral contraceptives may constitute significant risks to health. Likewise, in women, a history of cardiovascular disease, including hypertension, thrombophlebitis, and angina, causes a higher incidence of morbidity and mortality with pregnancy or oral contraceptive use. Anemia is also relevant to women's reproductive health. Anemia can result from or be aggravated by menstrual flow. Fear of painful intercourse can occur in women because of the physiologic changes of vaginal atrophy and decreased vaginal lubrication.

A history of a stroke (cerebrovascular accident [CVA]) should be determined. In men, strokes may cause physiologic or psychologic impotence. Men who have suffered heart attacks frequently experience impotence. This impotence is often caused by the fear of precipitating another

Table 48-6 Gynecologic and Obstetric History Format

General Gynecologic Information

External genitalia

_____ Pain
_____ Rashes
_____ Lesions
_____ Other
_____ Vaginal discharge

Amount __________
Color __________
Consistency __________
Odor __________
Past history of vaginal infection _____ Yes _____ No
If yes, type __________

_____ Pain during intercourse
_____ Bleeding after intercourse

Sexually transmitted diseases (STDs)

_____ Chlamydia
_____ Genital herpes
_____ Gonorrhea
_____ HIV
_____ Other (specify) __________
_____ Syphilis
_____ Yeast infection *(Candida albicans)*

Gynecologic history

Last Pap Smear _____ Abnormal _____ (Yes or No)
_____ Uterine fibroids Treatment if any __________
_____ Endometriosis Treatment if any __________
_____ Ovarian cyst __________
Did your mother take hormones when she was pregnant with you? (Yes, No, or Not Sure)
Any difficulties in getting pregnant? (Yes, No, or Has not attempted)
Gynecologic surgery (e.g., D&C, cryosurgery)
Type __________
Reason __________
Year __________

Obstetric Information

_____ Number of pregnancies
_____ Number of full-term births
_____ Number of preterm births
_____ Number of live births
_____ Number of spontaneous abortions (miscarriages)
_____ Number of therapeutic abortions
_____ Number of ectopic (tubal) pregnancies
_____ Number of cesarean sections

Problems during pregnancy, if any __________

Menstrual Information

Age at onset __________
Last menstrual period __________
Cycle (frequency) _____ Irregular periods _____ Length _____
Duration of each menses __________
Number of pads or tampons used on heaviest days _____
Clots _____ Spotting (other than during menses) _____
Dysmenorrhea (describe) __________
Treatment __________
Change in flow or amount (yes or no)
Explain __________
Menopause _____ Menopausal symptoms _____
Hormonal replacement __________ (yes or no)
What __________ Dose __________
If menopausal, have you noticed any vaginal bleeding? __________
Birth control method (if applicable)
Length _____ Previous methods __________

Breast Information

_____ Monthly breast self-exam (yes or no)
Breast lumps (location) __________
Treatment, if any __________
_____ Mammogram (date) __________
_____ Breast pain
Onset __________
Severity __________
Previous occurrence __________
_____ Breast discharge
Onset __________
Amount __________
Color __________
Odor and consistency __________
Breastfeeding __________ (yes or no)
Where are you in your menstrual cycle (in case any breast abnormality is found)? __________

heart attack as a result of the increased heart rate associated with sexual activity. This same concern is shared by the woman both as a partner and as the person recovering from a heart attack. The interviewer must be sensitive to this concern. Questions asked about the original cardiac event may elicit fear and thus indicate a need for counseling and support regarding safe sexual practices related to cardiac health.

Questions relating to endocrine disorders, particularly hypothyroidism and hyperthyroidism, must also be asked because these disorders directly interfere with women's menstrual cycles and with sexual performance in men. Finally, men and women should be assessed for kidney and urinary tract disorders because sexual functioning and reproductive capacity can be affected by genitourinary problems.

Medications. A pharmacologic profile of prescribed and over-the-counter drugs is necessary for all patients. Particularly relevant in assessment of the reproductive system is the use of diuretics (sometimes prescribed for premenstrual

Table 48-7 Surgeries of the Reproductive Systems

Surgery	Definition
Men	
Herniorrhaphy	Repair of hernia
Orchiectomy	Removal of a testis
Prostatectomy	Removal of prostate gland
Repair of testicular torsion	Correction of axial rotation of spermatic cord, which cuts off blood supply to the testicle, epididymis, and other structures
Varicocelectomy	Repair of varicose vein of scrotum
Vasectomy	Removal of part of ductus deferens
Women	
Cryosurgery	Use of subfreezing temperature to destroy tissue, especially in treatment of malignancy
Dilatation and curettage (D and C)	Dilatation of uterus and scraping of endometrium, performed to diagnose disease of uterus, correct heavy or prolonged vaginal bleeding, or empty uterus of products of conception; also used in the treatment of infertility to correlate state of endometrium and time of cycle
Hysterectomy	Removal of uterus
Oophorectomy	Removal of one or both ovaries
Repair of cystocele	Correction of protrusion of urinary bladder through vaginal wall
Repair of rectocele	Correction of protrusion of rectum and posterior vaginal wall into vagina
Salpingectomy	Removal of one or both fallopian tubes
Tubal sterilization	Ligation of fallopian tubes

edema), psychotropic agents (which may interfere with sexual performance), and antihypertensives (some of which have been implicated in impotence). Thus patients who use drugs such as methyldopa (Aldomet), clonidine (Catapres), guanethidine (Ismelin), and hydralazine (Apresoline) must be closely assessed for these problems. All drugs taken by female patients should be evaluated for possible teratogenic effects in women of childbearing age.

In women, the use of oral contraceptives or other hormones should be noted. The use of estrogen replacement therapy is relevant for women because of its effect on the prevention of osteoporosis and coronary artery disease. In women with a uterus, the concurrent use of a progestational agent should be documented. The use of estrogen alone has been shown to increase the incidence of uterine cancer. The nurse must also note the use of drugs such as marijuana, barbiturates, amphetamines, and phencyclidine hydrochloride (PCP) or "angel dust," which can have serious behavioral or physiologic impacts on the functioning of the reproductive system.

Oral contraceptive use can aggravate the symptoms of neurologic dysfunction, such as seizures or migraine headaches. However, the use of lower doses in current contraceptives makes these side effects less problematic. A history of cholecystitis and hepatitis is important information because these conditions may be contraindications for oral contraceptives; cholecystitis is often aggravated by oral contraceptives, and chronic active inflammation of the liver generally precludes the use of estrogen products because they are metabolized by the liver. Other contraindications to oral contraceptive use may be chronic obstructive respiratory problems because progesterone thickens respiratory secretions.

Surgery and other treatments. Any hospitalizations or surgeries should be noted in the health history. In particular, certain types of surgeries should be noted (Table 48-7). Therapeutic or spontaneous pregnancy interruptions are also documented at this time.

Functional Health Patterns. The key questions to ask a patient with a reproductive problem are presented in Table 48-8.

Health perception–health management pattern. The patient's sexual and contraceptive practices are important aspects of health management (Table 48-9). The patient's knowledge of safe sexual practices should be determined. Exposure to environmental toxins and sexually transmitted diseases can adversely affect fertility and reproductive health. Monthly breast self-examination (BSE), mammography according to age-specific guidelines, and routine Pap smears are integral to a woman's health. Testicular self-examination (TSE) should be practiced by all men. Prostate examination should be done annually by a health care professional for all men over 40.

Initial questions asked of the patient usually refer to the breast. The nurse asks the patient whether she performs a monthly BSE (see Chapter 49). If a lump is present, its onset, size, and consistency should be noted. The nurse also asks whether there has been an increase or a decrease in the size and shape of the lump since its onset or discovery. The patient is also questioned about breast pain or tenderness. She should describe the degree and severity of pain; breast pain or tenderness is not usually present with a malignant mass, particularly in the early stages.

The nurse should also inquire about a history of breast cancer in a woman's mother, maternal aunt, or sister because such a history increases the patient's risk of developing breast cancer. A family history of cancer, particularly cancer of the reproductive organs, is important information related to health counseling. Determination of a familial tendency for diabetes mellitus, hypothyroidism, hyperthyroidism, hy-

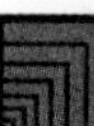

Table 48-8 Key Questions: Patient with a Reproductive Problem†

Health Perception–Health Management Pattern
- Have you had or been immunized for rubella?
- Are you currently attempting to become pregnant?
- Do you practice BSE? TSE?
- When was your last mammogram? Pap test? Rectal exam? Results?
- Do you have any chronic diseases?*
- Do you have any vaginal or urethral discharge?*

Nutritional-Metabolic Pattern
- Do you have a problem with anemia?*
- What is your daily calcium intake? Do you take calcium supplements?*
- If pregnant or lactating, what is your average daily caloric intake?

Elimination Pattern
- Do you have any problems related to urination? Bowel elimination?*
- Do you have frequent urinary tract infections?*

Activity-Exercise Pattern
- Describe your usual activity and exercise.
- Are you able to carry out your activities of daily living? If no, explain.

Cognitive-Perceptual Pattern
- If pregnant, do you have any balance problems?*
- Do you have any pain associated with your reproductive organs or with intercourse?*

Self-Perception–Self-Concept Pattern
- Has the problem in your reproductive system affected how you feel about yourself as a woman or as a man?*

Role-Relationship Pattern
- What effect has your reproductive problem or pregnancy had on your work, family, or social life?
- Are you experiencing any role-associated problems in your family?*

Sexuality-Reproductive Pattern
- Are you satisfied with your present means of sexual expression? If no, explain.
- Have you had any recent changes in your sexual practices?*
- Does the problem of your reproductive system affect your ability to have a satisfactory sex life?*

Coping–Stress Tolerance Pattern
- Is your health problem causing you stress?*
- Do you feel able to cope with your current health problem? If no, explain.
- Do your have people from whom you can get support? If yes, identify.

Value-Belief Pattern
- Do you have a conflict between your planned treatment and your system of values and beliefs?*

BSE, Breast self-examination; *TSE,* testicular self-examination.
†Some questions apply only to a woman or only to a man.
*If yes, describe.

pertension, stroke, angina, myocardial infarction, endocrine disorders, or anemia is also important.

The nurse must determine if the patient is allergic to sulfonamides, penicillin, rubber, or latex. Sulfonamides and penicillin are used frequently in the treatment of reproductive and genitourinary problems such as vaginitis and gonorrhea. Rubber or latex are commonly used in diaphragms and condoms. An allergy to these substances precludes their use as contraceptive methods.

Assessment of the reproductive system is incomplete without a knowledge of the patient's lifestyle choices. The nurse should know whether a woman uses cigarettes, alcohol, caffeine, or other drugs because these substances can be detrimental to both mother and fetus. Cigarette smoking may delay conception. Maternal smoking during pregnancy may result in an infant of low birthweight and increases the risk of spontaneous abortion, fetal death, neonatal death, and sudden infant death syndrome (SIDS). Cigarette smoking can increase the risk of morbidity in women using contraceptives and is associated with early menopause. These substances may also adversely affect sperm count in men and cause impotence or decreased libido.

Table 48-9 Sexual History Format

- How long have you been sexually active?
- How frequently do you have penile-vaginal intercourse?
- How frequently do you masturbate?
- How many sexual partners do you have?
- What is your sexual preference?
- How frequently do you have oral sex?
- How frequently do you have rectal intercourse?
- Have you ever had an STD? If yes, what?
- Are you using a contraceptive method? If yes, what kind? How often? Is it satisfactory?
- Do you consider your sex life satisfactory?
- How often have you experienced impotence or difficulty with vaginal lubrication or pain with intercourse?
- Has your sex life changed? If yes, how?
- Would you like to see your sex life change? If yes, how?
- How would your partner rate your sex life?

STD, Sexually transmitted disease.

Nutritional-metabolic pattern. Anemia is a common problem in women in their reproductive years, particularly during pregnancy and the postpartum period. The adequacy of the diet should be evaluated with this problem in mind. Women should be encouraged to gain adequate but not excessive weight during pregnancy. The nurse should determine whether specific dietary recommendations from the health care provider are being followed throughout pregnancy.

A thorough nutritional and psychologic history should be taken to assess for the presence of an eating disorder. Anorexia can cause amenorrhea and the subsequent problems, such as osteoporosis, that are related to estrogen cessation. From early adolescence, women must be counselled regarding calcium intake for the prevention of osteoporosis. The patient's daily calcium intake should be estimated to determine whether there is a need for supplementation. Folic acid intake for women in their reproductive years should be evaluated because a deficiency can result in spina bifida and other neural tube defects in the fetus.[7]

Elimination pattern. Many gynecologic problems can result in genitourinary problems. Stress and urge incontinence are common in older women because of relaxation of the pelvic musculature caused by multiple births or advancing age. Vaginal infections predispose patients to chronic or recurrent urinary tract infections. The proximity of the reproductive organs and the genitourinary tract make metastasis of malignant tumors to this site a possibility to be considered. Benign prostatic hyperplasia is a common problem of aging in men. It can impede normal urination, causing retention and difficulty in initiating the stream.

Activity-exercise pattern. Weight-bearing exercise decreases the risk of osteoporosis in women. The amount, type, and intensity of exercise should be documented. Lack of stress on bones, secondary to lack of exercise, is an important factor in the development of osteoporosis. Anemia, secondary to menorrhagia, can result in fatigue and activity intolerance and can interfere with satisfactory performance of the activities of daily living. Exercise should be encouraged during pregnancy, following guidelines regarding the type of exercise, the intensity, and the frequency of workouts.

Sleep-rest pattern. Sleep disturbances occur during pregnancy because of nocturia and the woman's inability to find a comfortable sleeping position. Sleep patterns may be affected during the postpartum period and also while raising young children. The hot flashes and sweating often present during the perimenopause can cause serious sleep interruption when the woman is awakened in a drenching sweat. The need to change her nightgown and bedding further disrupts her sleep. Insomnia is also a common complaint of perimenopausal women. Daytime fatigue often results from such nighttime awakenings.

Cognitive-perceptual pattern. Changes in balance and sensory perception accompany normal pregnancy. Aches and pains during gestation are caused by stretching of muscles and ligaments to accommodate the growing fetus. Pelvic pain is associated with various gynecologic disorders such as pelvic inflammatory disease, ovarian cysts, and endometriosis.

Reproduction and sexual issues are often considered very personal and private and are not easily discussed by many patients. The nurse must strive to develop trust and must maintain a professional demeanor when eliciting a reproductive history.

Dyspareunia (painful intercourse) can be particularly problematic for a woman. The pain associated with intercourse can make her reluctant to participate in sexual activity and strain her relationship with her sexual partner. The woman should be referred to her health care provider if dyspareunia is present.

Self-perception–self-concept pattern. For both men and women, there may be body image changes associated with developmental changes. Menarche and puberty herald the appearance of secondary sexual characteristics which may result in either pride or embarrassment. Adolescent problems related to body image include acne, myopia, obesity, anorexia nervosa, bulimia, and scoliosis.

Pregnancy may affect a woman's body image in a negative way as her size increases and her functional abilities decrease. Changes in body shape become more threatening to the woman as the pregnancy progresses.

The reproductive changes of aging such as pendulous breasts and vaginal dryness in women and decreased size of the penis in men may lead to emotional distress. The subtle changes associated with sexuality and advancing age may challenge the self-concept of many persons.

Role-relationship pattern. The addition of a new baby into the family may change family dynamics. Indeed, one maternal task is to integrate the new member of the household into the family.

The changes occurring during adolescence and the need to challenge parental authority may lead to stress among family members. Conflicts that arise during the adolescent's quest for identity can add further tension. Risk-taking behaviors, such as smoking and substance abuse on the part of the adolescent, are often symptomatic of the problem.

As the years go by, role relationship patterns again change as children begin their careers and move away from home. This again rearranges the family configuration.

The nurse seeks information about the type of family to which the patient belongs. Questions regarding recent changes or family conflicts should be asked. It is important to ascertain the patient's role in the family as a starting point in determining family dynamics.

A thorough health history also includes information about the patient's occupation and potential hazards associated with it. For example, exposure to toxic chemicals can affect sexual functioning and reproductive capacity.

Sexuality-reproductive pattern. The extent and depth of the interview about a patient's sexuality depend primarily on the expertise of the interviewer and on the needs and the willingness of the patient. Before taking a sexual history, interviewers should assess their comfort with their own sexuality, because any discomfort in questioning becomes obvious to the patient. Interviews must be carried out in an environment that provides reassurance, confidentiality, and a nonjudgmental attitude. It is best to begin with the least sensitive areas and then move to more sensitive areas. For this reason, sexual histories are frequently initiated during the review of the genitourinary and gynecologic systems. Early questioning can thus relate to menstruation, the onset of puberty, and the presence or absence of symptoms of genitourinary problems. These questions thus serve as an introduction for both the care provider and the patient before they move into more sensitive areas. Questions about sexuality should always be asked in a straightforward and nonjudgmental manner. Table 48-9 outlines questions appropriate for an initial assessment or annual examination. Both men and women should be asked about their general satisfaction with sexuality. Indications of sexual dysfunction may require referral or consultation with a sex counselor. A thorough genitourinary history must also be collected for the assessment of the reproductive system to be complete.

Problems of the reproductive system can cause physiologic or psychologic problems that can lead to painful intercourse, impotence, sexual dysfunction, or infertility. Both the cause and the effect of such problems should be determined.

The patient should be questioned about sexual beliefs and practices and whether orgasm is achieved. The patient's satisfaction with the opportunities for sexual gratification is important information that should be elicited. Any unexplained change in sexual practices or performance should be explored. This is an appropriate time to discuss methods of birth control and safe sex.

Menstrual history data are used in the detection of pregnancy, infertility, and numerous other gynecologic concerns. Changes in the usual menstrual pattern must be explicitly described to determine whether the change is transient and unimportant or connected with a more serious gynecologic problem. Metrorrhagia (spotting or bleeding between menstruations), menorrhagia (excessive menstrual bleeding), amenorrhea (lack of menstruation), and postcoital bleeding are examples of such problems. Changes in menstrual patterns associated with the use of contraceptive pills, intrauterine devices (IUDs), subdermal estrogen-only implant (Norplant), or medroxyprogesterone acetate (Depo Provera) must be identified. Contraceptive pills usually decrease the amount and duration of flow, whereas IUDs may cause an increase in the amount and duration. IUDs also frequently increase the severity of dysmenorrhea.

Patterns of sexual relationships also provide important information. A history of multiple sex partners increases the risk of contracting a sexually transmitted disease (STD). For a woman, this can increase the risk of pelvic inflammatory disease (PID), which can compromise her ability to become pregnant.

Coping–stress tolerance pattern. The stress related to situational or maturational crises such as pregnancy, menopause, or the climacteric may cause an increased dependence upon support systems. It is essential for the nurse to ascertain who the support people are in the patient's life. The diagnosis of an STD can cause stress to the patient and the partner. Means to manage such stress should be explored.

Value-belief pattern. Sexual and reproductive functioning is closely related to cultural, religious, moral, and ethical values. The nurse should be aware of her own beliefs in these areas. She should recognize and sensitively react to the patient's personal beliefs associated with reproductive issues.

Objective Data

Physical Examination. The examination of the external genitalia uses inspection and palpation.

Male genitalia. An examination may be performed with the patient lying or standing. The standing position is generally preferred. The examiner should be seated in front of the standing patient. Gloves should be used during examination of the male genitalia.

PUBES. The nurse observes the diamond-shaped pattern of hair distribution. The absence of hair is not normal. The skin is also evaluated.

PENIS. The nurse notes the size and skin texture of the penis and any lesions, scars, or swelling. The location of the urethral meatus, as well as the presence or absence of a foreskin, should be noted. If present, the foreskin should be retracted to note cleanliness and replaced over the glans after observation. The glans are compressed to note any discharge and its amount, color, and odor if present. The nurse also palpates the penile shaft for tenderness or masses and observes the ventral and dorsal aspects.

SCROTUM AND TESTES. The nurse performs a complete skin examination by lifting each testis to inspect all sides of the scrotal sac. Palpation of the scrotum is done to note changes in consistency or the presence of masses. The patient should also be taught TSE (see Chapter 52).

INGUINAL REGION AND SPERMATIC CORD. The examiner inspects the inguinal regions for rashes, lesions, or lymphadenopathy, which may suggest pelvic organ infection. The nurse has the patient cough or bear down and notes any conspicuous bulging in the inguinal canals. The nurse also palpates the area for any bulging as the patient again coughs or bears down.

The spermatic cord is located posteriorly in the scrotal sac. The nurse follows the cord on each side. The inguinal region is gently palpated using the forefinger or small finger and by pushing up through the loose scrotal skin to the abdominal wall along the inguinal region. The internal inguinal ring meets and impedes the finger. At this point, the patient again bears down and coughs. The nurse determines whether the strain produces a bulging of the intestines through the ring, indicating the presence of a hernia, a condition that requires follow-up.

ANUS AND PROSTATE. The anal sphincter and perineal regions are inspected for lesions, masses, and hemorrhoids. A digital examination is required for all patients who have symptoms of prostate trouble, such as difficulty in initiating the flow and the urge to void frequently; this examination should be performed annually for all men over 40 years of age.

Female breasts and external genitalia. Physical examination of women often begins with inspection and palpation of the breasts and then proceeds to the abdomen. Examination of the abdomen provides an opportunity to detect pain or any masses that may involve the genitourinary system.

BREASTS. Breasts are examined first by visual inspection. The nurse, with the patient seated, observes the breasts for symmetry, size, shape, skin color and texture, vascular patterns, and the presence of unusual lesions. The patient is asked to put her arms at her sides, arms overhead, lean forward, and press hands on hips. The nurse observes for any abnormalities during these maneuvers. The axillae and the clavicular areas are then palpated for enlarged lymph nodes.

After the patient assumes a supine position, a pillow is placed under the back on the side to be examined. The patient is asked to put the arm above and behind the head. These maneuvers flatten breast tissue and make palpation easier. The breast is then palpated in a systematic fashion using a vertical line, a clockwise, or a spoke approach. The nurse should use the distal finger pads for palpation. The tail of Spence should be included in the examination as this area and the upper outer quadrant are the areas where most breast malignancies develop.

Finally, the nurse should palpate the area around the areolae for masses. The nipple should be compressed to determine the presence of discharge or any masses. The color, consistency, and odor of any discharge should be documented.

EXTERNAL GENITALIA. The mons pubis, the labia majora, the labia minora, the perineum, and the anal region are inspected for characteristics of skin, hair distribution, and contour. Lesions, swelling, and discharge are noted.

The nurse separates the labia to fully inspect the clitoris, the urethral meatus, the vaginal orifice, the hymen, the perineum, and the anal region. Any inflammation or cysts on Bartholin's glands or Skene's glands are noted.

INTERNAL PELVIC EXAMINATION. During the speculum examination, the nurse observes the walls of the vagina and the cervix for inflammation, discharge, polyps, and suspicious growths. During this examination, it is possible to take a Pap smear and collect secretions for culture and study under the microscope (i.e., wet smears).

After the speculum examination, a bimanual examination is performed to allow assessment of the size, shape, and consistency of the uterus, ovaries, and tubes. The tubes are not normally palpable. Details of the pelvic and bimanual examinations are described in physical assessment textbooks. Because these skills are not usually within the scope of the nurse generalist, they are not described here.

Table 48-10 illustrates a recording format for the physical assessment findings of the male and female reproductive systems. Tables 48-11 through 48-13 summarize common assessment abnormalities of the breasts, the female reproductive system, and the male reproductive system.

Diagnostic Studies. Diagnostic studies provide important information to the nurse in monitoring the patient's condition and planning appropriate interventions. These studies are considered to be objective data. Table 48-14 contains diagnostic studies common to both the male and the female reproductive systems.

Table 48-10 Recording the Normal Physical Assessment of the Reproductive Systems

Male	Female
Penis and scrotum	***Breasts***
Diamond-shaped hair distribution	Symmetric
Skin	Nipples everted, no dimpling
No lesions, redness, swelling, masses, or inflammation	No nipple discharge
Circumcised penis	No masses, lesions, or tenderness
Meatus patent, no discharge	No axillary nodes palpable
Testes smooth, firm, 2 cm in width and 3 cm in length	Appropriate for age and parity
No masses, slight tenderness	***Vulva***
Epididymis	Triangular hair distribution
Nontender	No lesions, redness, swelling, masses, or inflammation
No masses	Patent vaginal orifice, no discharge
No inguinal hernias	Nonpalpable Skene's ducts and Bertholin's glands, no tenderness
Rectum	Intact clitoris and urethral meatus
No hemorrhoids	

DIAGNOSTIC STUDIES

Many diagnostic tests that are performed to assess problems occurring in other body systems also provide valuable data on the condition of the reproductive systems. Table 48-14 summarizes the most commonly used diagnostic studies in the assessment of the reproductive systems and the nurse's responsibility regarding these diagnostic tests.

In order to understand many of the diagnostic studies of the reproductive system, it is important to understand the concepts of sensitivity and specificity. *Sensitivity* addresses the issue of how well a test identifies people with a particular disease. The goal of sensitivity testing is to avoid the occurrence of false negative results, that is, to avoid saying that someone does not have a particular health problem when, in fact, the disease is present. It is considered a screening test. *Specificity* testing answers the question of how well a test eliminates those individuals without the disease. The goal of sensitivity testing is to avoid false positive results. It is specifically the nurse's responsibility to ensure that the patient understands the purpose of any test being performed.

Urine Studies

Pregnancy Testing. Occurrence of pregnancy is generally validated by measuring the output of human chorionic gonadotropin (HCG) in the urine by means of an immunologic test. A solution containing monoclonal antibodies specific for HCG is mixed with a small amount

Table 48-11 Common Assessment Abnormalities: Breast

Finding	Description	Possible Etiology and Significance
■ Nipple inversion or retraction	Recent onset, erythematous, pain, unilateral	Abscess, inflammation, cancer
	Recent onset (usually within past year), unilateral presentation, lack of tenderness	Neoplasm
■ Nipple secretions		
Galactorrhea (female)	Milky, no relationship to lactation, unilateral or bilateral or intermittent or consistent presentation	Drug therapy, particularly phenothiazines, tricyclic antidepressants, methyldopa; hypofunction or hyperfunction of thyroid or adrenal glands; tumors of hypothalamus or pituitary gland; excessive estrogen; prolonged suckling or breast foreplay
Galactorrhea (male)	Milky, bilateral presentation	Chorioepithelioma of testes
Purulent	Gray-green or yellow color; frequent unilateral presentation; association with pain, erythema, induration, nipple inversion	Puerperal (after birth) mastitis (inflammatory condition of breast) or abscess
	Same as above but usually without nipple inversion	Infected sebaceous cyst
Serous discharge	Clear appearance, unilateral or bilateral or intermittent or consistent presentation	Intraductal papilloma
Dark green or multicolored discharge	Thick, sticky, and frequently bilateral	Mammary duct ectasia (dilatation of mammary ducts)
Serosanguineous or bloody drainage	Unilateral presentation	Papillomatosis (widespread development of nipplelike growths), intraductal papilloma, carcinoma (male and female)
■ Scaling or excoriation of nipple	Unilateral or bilateral presentation, crusting, possible ulceration	Paget's disease, eczema, infection
■ Nodules, lumps, or masses	Multiple, bilateral, well-delineated, soft or firm, mobile cysts; pain; premenstrual occurrence	Fibrocystic changes
	Rubbery consistency, fluid-filled interior, pain	Mammary duct ectasia
	Soft, mobile, well-delineated cyst, absence of pain	Lipoma, fibroadenoma
	Erythema, tenderness, induration	Infected sebaceous cysts, abscesses
	Usually singular, hard irregularly shaped, poorly delineated, nonmobile	Neoplasm

of urine. The presence of HCG causes a change in color of the urine. To reduce cross-reactivity with LH and other pituitary hormones, the beta subunit of HCG is measured.

Home pregnancy test kits use the same assay principle as described above. Positive results are based on the presence of HCG in urine. Some tests can detect pregnancy as early as the first day after the expected period. These tests are 97% accurate, but a negative test should be repeated in 2 weeks to achieve the greatest accuracy.[8] Serum pregnancy tests have also been developed. They are almost 100% accurate.

Hormone Studies. Although estrogen studies are performed on urine, the results are frequently inaccurate because of variable estrogen levels during the normal cycle and the difficulty in estimating the day of the cycle in women with irregular menses. Adrenal androgens are precursors of estrogens and can be measured in the urine of both men and women. FSH can be measured in a 24-hour urine specimen. Increased and decreased FSH levels can indicate gonad failure resulting from pituitary dysfunction.

Blood Studies

Recently, serum pregnancy tests using radioimmunoassays have been developed. One test, a radioimmunoassay for the beta subunit of HCG, is so sensitive that a pregnancy can be detected before a woman misses her menstrual period.

Table 48-12 Common Assessment Abnormalities: Female Reproductive System

Finding	Description	Possible Etiology and Significance
■ Vulvar discharge	Plaque-like consistency, frequent itching and inflammation, lack of odor	Candidiasis (*Candida* or yeast infection), vaginitis
	Grayish color, copious flow, frothy appearance, vulvar irritation	Bacterial vaginosis infection
	Purulent odor, grayish-green or yellow color	*Trichomonas vaginalis*
	Bloody color	*Chlamydia trachomatis* or *Neisseria gonorrhoeae* infection, menstruation, trauma, cancer
■ Vulvar erythema	Bright or beefy red color, itching	*Candida albicans,* allergy, chemical vaginitis
	Reddened base, painful vesicles or ulcerations	Genital herpes
	Macules or papules, itching	Chancroid (STD), contact dermatitis, scabies, pediculosis
■ Vulvar growths	Soft, fleshy growth; nontender	Condyloma acuminatum
	Flat and warty appearance, nontender	Condyloma latum
	Same as either of above, possible pain	Neoplasm
	Reddened base, vesicles, and small erosions; pain	Lymphogranuloma venereum, genital herpes, chancroid
	Indurated, firm ulcers; lack of pain	Chancre (syphilis), granuloma inguinale
■ Abdominal pain or tenderness	Intermittent or consistent tenderness in right or left lower quadrant	Salpingitis (infection of fallopian tube), ectopic pregnancy, ruptured ovarian cyst, PID, tubal or ovarian abscess
	Periumbilical location, consistent occurrence	Cystitis, endometritis (inflammation of endometrium), ectopic pregnancy

PID, Pelvic inflammatory disease; *STD,* sexually transmitted disease.

The prolactin assay is used primarily in the workup of a patient with amenorrhea. High levels of prolactin are normally associated with low levels of estrogen, such as those that occur during lactation. However, the same finding can occur with pituitary adenomas, especially with otherwise unexplained galactorrhea.

Serum progesterone and estradiol are sometimes tested in ovarian function assessment, particularly for amenorrhea. In addition, hormonal blood studies are essential components of a thorough fertility workup.

Biologic tumor markers are often secreted by germinal cell cancers of the testis. The two most common markers are alpha-fetoprotein (AFP) and HCG. Measurement of these markers is useful in monitoring therapy (marker levels rise as disease progresses and fall with disease regression) because marker levels may rise months before new disease or metastasis is evident.

Syphilis Studies

The types of tests performed to diagnose syphilis can be classified as *nontreponemal* or *treponemal.* Nontreponemal tests such as the Venereal Disease Research Laboratory (VDRL) test and the rapid plasma reagin (RPR) test are inexpensive and reliable, but have high levels of false-positive results (i.e., good sensitivity but poor specificity). These tests detect the presence of antibodies in the serum of infected patients. Nonspecific antibodies can be produced during many pathologic processes, especially some types of autoimmune diseases, and can yield false-positive test results.

Treponemal tests such as the fluorescent treponemal antibody absorption (FTA-ABS) test are highly reliable and should be used after a positive nontreponemal test, even if it is weakly positive or questionable. This test measures specific antibodies to *Treponema pallidum.* The FTA-ABS test does not assess the adequacy of treatment of syphilis; the test remains reactive even after treatment. Antibody titers obtained with a VDRL test are used to measure the adequacy of therapy.

The most specific and direct examination for syphilis is dark-field microscopy of a specimen obtained from a potential syphilitic lesion (chancre). Unfortunately, the chancre is frequently gone by the time other symptoms occur, so the test cannot be performed. Other miscellaneous tests of secretions involve wet mounts, cultures, and stains to detect specific reproductive problems (see Table 48-14).

Cytologic Studies

The Pap smear is a screening test to detect abnormal cells obtained from the cervix, vagina, or nipple. It is performed by obtaining cells from the cervical canal, preferably the endocervix, as well as from the vagina, and placing these cells in a fixative for examination by a cytologist for cellular abnormalities. Pap smears are more accurate if performed at midcycle or during the secretory phase of the menstrual cycle because there is a greater likelihood that

Table 48-13 Common Assessment Abnormalities: Male Reproductive System

Finding	Description	Possible Etiology and Significance
■ Penile growths or masses	Indurated, smooth, disklike appearance; absence of pain; singular presentation	Chancre
	Papular to irregularly shaped ulceration with pus, lack of induration	Chancroid
	Ulceration with induration and nodularity	Cancer
	Flat, wartlike nodule	Condyloma latum
	Elevated, fleshy, moist, elongated projections with single or multiple projections	Condyloma acuminatum
	Localized swelling with retracted, tight foreskin	Paraphimosis (inability to replace foreskin to its normal position after retraction), trauma
■ Vesicles, erosions, or ulcers	Painful, erythematous base; vesicular or small erosions	Genital herpes, balanitis (inflammation of glans penis), chancroid
	Painless, singular, small erosion with eventual lymphadenopathy	Lymphogranuloma venereum, cancer
■ Scrotal masses	Localized swelling with tenderness, unilateral or bilateral presentation	Epididymitis (inflammation of epididymis), testicular torsion, orchitis (mumps)
	Swelling, tenderness	Incarcerated hernia
	Unilateral or bilateral presentation; swelling without pain; translucent, cordlike or wormlike appearance	Hydrocele (accumulation of fluid in outer covering of testes), spermatocele (firm, sperm-containing cyst of epididymis), varicocele (dilatation of veins that drain testes), hematocele (accumulation of blood within scrotum)
	Firm, nodular testes or epididymis; frequent unilateral presentation	Tuberculosis, cancer
■ Penile discharge	Clear to purulent color, minimal to copious flow	Urethritis or gonorrhea, *Chlamydia trachomatis* infection, trauma
■ Penile or scrotal erythema	Macules and papules	Scabies, pediculosis
■ Inguinal masses	Bulging, unilateral presentation during straining	Inguinal hernia
	Shotty, 1-3 cm nodules	Lymphadenopathy

abnormal cells will be detected during these times. A Pap smear should be performed annually or more frequently in women with a history of dysplasia or exposure to DES. Pap smears are necessary in women who have had a hysterectomy because abnormal vaginal cells can sometimes be detected.

Although a Pap smear is very accurate in detecting cervical cancer, a negative Pap test does not rule out endometrial cancer. Specific tests are available to obtain a smear directly from the endometrium. Uterine aspiration and cannulation into the uterine cavity make it possible to obtain endometrial tissue. Cytologic studies are also performed on any nipple discharge.

Radiologic Examinations

Mammography has become one of the most frequently used diagnostic tools in reproductive system assessment (see Chapter 49). Unfortunately, its frequent use has been highly criticized because of the potential risks of radiation. However, increased awareness of the risks from radiographic studies has resulted in valuable improvements in the technique of mammography, particularly in lowering the exposure per examination. The American Cancer Society recommends that a screening mammogram be performed every 1 to 2 years for women between the ages of 40 and 49, and yearly after 50 years of age.[9]

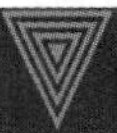

Table 48-14 Diagnostic Studies: Male and Female Reproductive Systems

Study	Description and Purpose	Nursing Responsibility
Urine Studies		
Pregnancy testing	HCG is detected in urine to ascertain whether a woman is pregnant. Hydatidiform mole and chorioepithelioma (in men and women) may also be detected.	Obtain thorough menstrual history from patient, including birth control methods. Determine presence or absence of presumptive signs of pregnancy (e.g., breast changes or increased whitish vaginal discharge).
Hormone Testing		
Testosterone levels	Tumors and developmental anomalies of the testes can be detected.	Instruct patient to collect 24-hr urine specimen. Keep it refrigerated. Obtain genitourinary and reproductive system history.
FSH assay	Test indicates gonadal failure because of pituitary dysfunction. Female: Follicular phase: 2-5 IU/24 hr (2-5 IU/d); midcycle: 8-40 IU/24 hr (8-4 IU/d); luteal phase: 2-10 IU/24 hr (2-10 IU/d); menopause: 35-100 IU/24 hr (35-100 IU/d) Male: 2-15 IU/24 hr (2-15 IU/d)	Instruct patient to collect 24-hr urine specimen. Indicate phase of menstrual cycle, if menopausal, and if taking oral contraceptives or any hormone.
Blood Studies		
Prolactin assay	This test detects pituitary dysfunction that can cause amenorrhea.	Ensure that patient has fasted. Inform patient that blood sample will be drawn in morning. Observe venipuncture site for bleeding or hematoma formation.
Serum HCG radioimmunoassay	Same as pregnancy testing.	Instruct patient to have blood drawn in laboratory. Elicit where she is in her menstrual cycle, whether she has missed menses, and if so, how late she is.
Serum androstenedione and testosterone levels	These tests ascertain whether elevated androgens are due to adrenal or ovarian dysfunction. Serum testosterone is also measured to assess cause of amenorrhea.	Collect health history to eliminate potential sources of interference with accuracy of results (i.e., use of steroids or barbiturates, presence of hypothyroidism or hyperthyroidism).
Serum progesterone	This test is frequently used to detect functioning corpus luteum cyst. It may also be used for determining adrenal pathology.	Ensure that woman has fasted. Inform patient that blood sample will be drawn in morning. Observe venipuncture site for bleeding or hematoma formation. Instruct woman that blood must be drawn around day 24 or 25 of cycle for greatest accuracy.
Serum estradiol	This test measures ovarian function. It is particularly useful in assessing estrogen-secreting tumors and states of precocious female puberty. Normal values depend on laboratory that performs test and should be obtained from that laboratory. May be used to confirm perimenopausal period.	Ensure that patient has fasted. Inform patient that blood sample will be drawn in morning. Observe venipuncture site for bleeding or hematoma formation.
Serum FSH	The test indicates gonadal failure because of pituitary dysfunction; used to validate menopause Female: Folicular phase: 4-30 mIU/ml (4-30 IU/L); midcycle: 10-90 mIU/ml (10-90 IU/L); luteal phase: 4-30 mIU/ml (4-30 IU/L); menopause: 40-250 mIU/ml (40-250 IU/L) Male: 4-25 mIU/ml (4-25 IU/L)	No food or fluid restrictions required. State phase of menstrual cycle, if menopausal, or if on oral contraceptive or hormones.

continued

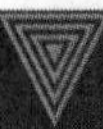

Table 48-14 Diagnostic Studies: Male and Female Reproductive Systems—cont'd

Study	Description and Purpose	Nursing Responsibility
Syphilis Studies		
Nontreponemal serologic tests: Wassermann; Venereal Disease Research Laboratory (VDRL); Rapid plasma reagin (RPR)	These tests are nonspecific antibody tests used to screen for syphilis. Positive readings can be made within 1-2 wk after appearance of primary lesion (chancre) or 4-15 wk after initial infection.	Tell the patient that fasting is unnecessary. Inform patient that blood sample will be drawn. Observe venipuncture site for bleeding or hematoma formation. Obtain data to determine presence or absence of problems such as hepatitis, pregnancy, and autoimmune diseases that may interfere with the accuracy of results.
Treponemal test: Fluorescent treponemal antibody absorption (FTA-ABS)	This test detects antitreponema antibodies. It also detects early syphilis with great accuracy. It is usually performed if results of nontreponemal testing are questionable.	Tell the patient that fasting is unnecessary. Inform patient that blood sample will be drawn. Observe venipuncture site for bleeding or hematoma formation.
Miscellaneous Studies		
Dark-field microscopy	Direct examination of specimen obtained from potential syphilitic lesion (chancre) is performed to detect treponema.	Avoid direct skin contact with open lesion.
Wet mounts	Direct microscopic examination of specimen of vaginal discharge is performed immediately after collection. This determines presence or absence and number of *Trichomonas*, bacteria, white and red blood cells, and candidal buds or hyphae. Other clues or causes of inflammation or infection may be determined.	Explain procedure and purpose to patient. Instruct patient not to douche before examination. Prepare for collection of specimens (glass slide, 10-20% potassium hydroxide [KOH] solution, sodium chloride [NaCl] solution, and cotton-tipped applicators).
Cultures	Specimens of vaginal, urethral, or cervical discharge are taken for culture to assess presence of gonorrhea or chlamydia. Rectal and throat cultures may also be performed, depending on data obtained from sexual history.	Obtain specific contact and sexual history inclusive of oral and rectal intercourse. Instruct against douching before examination. Obtain urethral specimen from men before they void. Instruct women who are sexually active with multiple partners to have at least a yearly culture for gonorrhea and chlamydia. Instruct sexually active men to have any discharge evaluated immediately to rule out gonorrhea strains that do not cause classic symptoms of dysuria.
Gram stain	This presumptive test is used for rapid detection of gonorrhea. Presence of gram-negative intracellular diplococci generally warrants initiation of treatment. Not very accurate for women.	Same as above.
Cytologic Studies		
Pap smear	Microscopic study of exfoliated cells by special staining and fixation technique detects malignancy. Cells most commonly studied are those obtained directly from endocervix, cervix, vaginal pool, and endometrial lining of uterine cavity.	Instruct women who are sexually active and who are over 18 to have Pap smears according to American Cancer Society guidelines. Arrange for smear at midcycle time. Instruct patients not to douche for at least 24 hr before examination. Obtain careful menstrual and gynecologic history.
Nipple discharge test	Cytologic study of nipple discharge is performed.	Indicate whether hormonal preparations or other drugs are being taken, breastfeeding, or history of amenorrhea. Instruct patient during demonstration of breast self-examination or examination of breasts that nipple discharge should always be evaluated.

continued

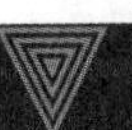

Table 48-14 Diagnostic Studies: Male and Female Reproductive Systems—cont'd

Study	Description and Purpose	Nursing Responsibility
Radiologic Studies		
Soft tissue mammography	Low dose x-ray image of breast tissue on photographic film is used to assess breast masses, recent breast enlargement, and nipple discharge to detect malignancy. It is usually an outpatient procedure.	Instruct patient about risks (radiation) and advantages of the examination. Instruct regarding American Cancer Society recommendations.
Contrast mammography	This test is used to evaluate abnormal nipple discharge. It is particularly effective in detecting nonpalpable intraductal papillomas. Test consists of injection of radiopaque dye in breast duct.	Determine actual or possible allergy to contrast medium.
Ultrasound	This test measures and records high-frequency sound waves as they pass through tissues of variable density. It is very useful in detecting masses greater than 3 cm such as ectopic pregnancies, IUDs, ovarian cysts, and hydatidiform moles.	Instruct patient that a full bladder may be required depending on the reason for the study.
Surgical Procedures		
Breast biopsy	Histologic examination of excised breast tissue is performed.	Before surgery instruct patient about operative procedures and sedation. After surgery perform wound care and instruct patient about breast self-examination.
Colposcopy	Direct visualization of cervix with binocular microscope that allows magnification and study of cellular dysplasia and vascular and tissue abnormalities of cervix. This test is used as a follow-up study for abnormal Pap smears and for examination of women exposed to DES in utero. Biopsy of cervix may be taken during colposcopic examination. This test is valuable in decreasing number of false-negative cervical biopsies.	Instruct patient about this outpatient procedure. Inform patient that this examination is similar to speculum examination. Explain purpose of procedure and prepare patient for it.
Conization	Cone-shaped sample of squamocolumnar tissue of cervix is removed for direct study.	Explain purpose and method of procedure and that it requires use of surgical facilities and anesthesia. Instruct patient to rest for at least 3 days after procedure. Also discuss necessity for 3 wk follow-up check.
Culdotomy, culdoscopy, and culdocentesis	Culdotomy is an incision made through posterior fornix of cul-de-sac and allows visualization of peritoneal cavity (specifically, uterus, tubes, and ovaries). Culdoscope can then be used to study these structures closely. This technique is valuable in fertility evaluations. Withdrawal of fluid (culdocentesis) allows examination of fluid characteristics.	Explain purpose and method of procedure. Prepare patient for vaginal operation with preoperative instruction and sedation. Perform assessment of bleeding and discomfort after surgery.

continued

Table 48-14 Diagnostic Studies: Male and Female Reproductive Systems—cont'd

Study	Description and Purpose	Nursing Responsibility
Surgical Procedures—cont'd		
Laparoscopy (peritoneoscopy)	This method of entry into the abdomen allows visualization of pelvic structures via fiberoptic scopes inserted through small abdominal incisions. Instillation of carbon dioxide into cavity improves visualization. This technique is used in diagnostic assessment of uterus, tubes, and ovaries. Can be used in conjunction with tubal sterilization.	Explain purpose and method of procedure. Before surgery, instruct patient about procedure, prepare abdomen, and reassure patient about sedation. Tell patient to rest for 1-3 days after surgery. Inform patient of probability of shoulder pain because of air in the abdomen.
Dilatation and Curettage (D&C)	The operative procedure dilates cervix and allows curetting of endometrial lining. This test is used in assessment of abnormal bleeding patterns and cytologic evaluation of lining.	Before surgery, instruct patient about procedure and sedation. Tell patient that overnight hospitalization is occasionally required. Perform postoperative assessment of degree of bleeding (frequent pad check during first 24 hr).
Fertility Studies		
Semen analysis	Semen is assessed for volume (2-5 ml), viscosity, sperm count (>20 million/ml), sperm motility (60% motile), and percent of abnormal sperm (60% with normal structure).	Instruct patient to bring in fresh specimen within 2 hr after ejaculation.
Basal body temperature assessment	This measurement indicates indirectly whether ovulation has occurred. (Temperature rises at ovulation and remains elevated during secretory phase of normal menstrual cycle.)	Instruct woman to take her temperature using special basal temperature thermometer (calibrated in tenths of degrees) every morning before getting out of bed. Tell woman to record temperature on graph.
Huhner test or Sims-Huhner	Mucus sample of cervix is examined within 2-8 hr after intercourse. Total number of sperm is assessed in relation to number of live sperm. This test is performed to determine whether cervical mucus is "hostile" to passage of sperm from vagina into uterus.	Instruct couples to have intercourse at estimated time of ovulation and be present for test within 2-8 hr after intercourse.
Endometrial biopsy	In this outpatient procedure, small curette is used to obtain piece of endometrial lining to assess endometrial changes resulting from progesterone secretion after ovulation.	Tell patient that test must be performed postovulation. Explain that procedure should cause only short period of uterine cramping.
Hysterosalpingogram	This test involves instillation of radioscopic dye through cervix into uterine cavity and subsequently through and out of fallopian tubes. Spot x-ray images are taken to detect abnormalities of uterus and its adnexa (ovaries and tubes) as dye progresses through them. Test may be most useful in diagnostic assessment of fertility (e.g., to detect adhesions near ovary, an abnormal uterine shape, or blockage of tubal pathways).	Inform patient about procedure and that it may be fairly uncomfortable, especially shoulder pain. Determine possibility of dye allergy.
Serum progesterone	Same as blood studies.	Same as blood studies.

DES, Diethylstilbesterol; *FSH,* follicle-stimulating hormone; *HCG,* human chorionic gonadotropin; *IUD,* intrauterine device.

REVIEW QUESTIONS

The number of the question corresponds to the same-numbered objective at the beginning of the chapter.

1. Which of the following structures make up the accessory organs of the male reproductive system?
   a. Scrotum, ductus deferens, seminal vesicles, urethra
   b. Penis, testes, epididymis, spermatic cord
   c. Prostate, Cowper's glands, seminal vesicles
   d. Testes, spermatic cord, prostate, seminal vesicles

2. Which of the following hormones are produced by the gonadal organs?
   a. LTH, progesterone, testosterone, and FSH
   b. GnRH, estrogen, and testosterone
   c. FSH, LH, and ICSH
   d. Estrogen, progesterone, and testosterone

3. Female orgasm is the result of which of the following events?
   a. Clitoral swelling and increased vaginal lubrication
   b. Rapid release of vasocongestion and myotonia in the reproductive structures
   c. Clitoral swelling, vaginal lubrication, and uterine elevation
   d. Vaginal enlargement and secretion with penile insertion

4. Decreased muscle tone in the aging female reproductive system can result in
   a. nonpalpable ovaries.
   b. gynecomastia.
   c. cystocele.
   d. pendulous breasts.

5. Which of the following are not significant to data collection regarding past health history for the assessment of male and female reproductive systems?
   a. Stature, physical strength, and appearance
   b. Presence or absence of measles, mumps, and rubella immunizations
   c. Hypertension, prostate surgery, and dilatation and curettage
   d. Allergies to rubber, breast surgery, and vasectomy

6. Which of the following is not a part of the physical examination of a man?
   a. Palpation of testes and epididymis
   b. Palpating for Bartholin's glands and Skene's ducts
   c. Palpation for inguinal hernia
   d. Palpation of spermatic cord

7. Vaginal discharge and penile discharge may indicate which of the following diseases?
   a. Syphilis
   b. Gonorrhea
   c. Balanitis
   d. Epididymitis

8. Which of the following criteria should be followed for mammography according to the American Cancer Society?
   a. Women should have a baseline mammogram at age 50.
   b. Women over the age of 40 should have a mammogram every 1 to 2 years only if they are at high risk for breast cancer.
   c. Women between 40 and 49 years of age should have a mammogram every 1 to 2 years and women over the age of 50 should have a yearly mammogram.
   d. Mammography should be performed only when a discernible mass is found.

REFERENCES

1. Seeley R, Stephens T, Tate P: *Anatomy and physiology,* ed 3, St Louis, 1995, Mosby.
2. Thibodeau G, Patton K: *Anatomy and physiology,* ed 2, St Louis, 1993, Mosby.
3. Benson R, Pernall M: *Handbook of obstetrics and gynecology,* ed 9, New York, 1994, McGraw-Hill.
4. Piepho R and others: Clinical therapeutic conference, *J Clin Pharmacol* 32:776, 1992.
5. Masters WH, Johnson E: *Human sexual response,* Boston, 1966, Little, Brown & Co.
6. Bolten A and others: Love and sex after 60: how physical changes affect intimate expression, *Geriatrics* 49:21, 1994.
7. Editorial, Folic acid and neural tube defects, *Lancet* 338:153, 1991.
8. Munroe W: Home diagnostic kits, *Am Pharm* 34:50, 1994.
9. Brown HG: The messages primary care physicians should convey to their patients about mammography, *Women's Health Issues* 1:74, 1991.

Chapter 49

NURSING ROLE IN MANAGEMENT
Breast Disorders

Cynthia L. Vorpahl

Learning Objectives

1. Assess breast tissue by inspection and palpation using appropriate examination techniques.
2. Teach breast health awareness and breast self-examination, including rationale, technique, and reasons for referral.
3. Describe the types, causes, clinical manifestations, and appropriate therapeutic and nursing management of common benign breast disorders.
4. Identify the known risk factors for breast cancer.
5. Describe the pathophysiology, clinical manifestations, and therapeutic management of breast cancer.
6. Identify the types, indications for, and complications of surgical interventions for breast cancer.
7. Explain the physical and psychologic preoperative and postoperative aspects of nursing management for the patient undergoing a mastectomy.
8. Describe the indications for, types, potential risks, complications, and nursing management after reconstructive surgery of the breast.

Breast disorders represent a significant health concern to women. In a woman's lifetime, there is a one in nine chance that she will be diagnosed with a malignant breast disorder before menopause and then a one in eight chance after menopause. Whether benign or malignant, intense feelings of shock, fear, and denial often accompany the initial discovery of a lump or change in the breast. These feelings are associated both with the fear of survival and with the possible loss of a breast. Throughout history, the female breast has been regarded as a symbol of beauty, sexuality, and motherhood. The potential loss of a breast, or part of a breast, may be devastating for many women because of the significant psychologic, social, sexual, and body-image implications associated with it.

HEALTH PROMOTION AND MAINTENANCE
Early Detection

Health promotion and maintenance practices apply to all women, regardless of their age or menstrual status. It is critical that breast disorders be detected early, diagnosed accurately, and treated promptly. A variety of factors influence the potential for cure, the length of a disease-free period, and the overall length of survival after a diagnosis of breast cancer. Research indicates that 85% of patients diagnosed with early-stage breast cancer with little or no axillary node involvement will be alive in 5 years. Conversely, only 10% of patients diagnosed with advanced-stage breast cancer will survive 5 years.[1] The essential factors in the early detection of breast cancer and other breast-related problems are the regular performance of breast self-examination (BSE), regular clinical breast examination (CBE), and routine mammography. The frequency of these examinations is determined by the woman's age, the presence of significant risk factors, and her past medical history (Table 49-1). Current guidelines accepted by the American Cancer Society, the National Cancer Institute, and the American College of Radiology regarding breast surveillance practices include the following:

1. Monthly BSE starting by age 20
2. Physical examination of the breasts by a trained health professional (CBE) every 3 years between ages 20 and 40 and every year thereafter
3. Screening mammography for asymptomatic women between the ages of 40 and 49 every 1 to 2 years and an annual mammogram for women 50 years of age or older[2]

The benefits of early detection of breast cancer are well established. BSE is an important tool in early detection because approximately 90% of palpable lesions in the breast are found by the woman herself coincidentally or while doing BSE.[3] In recent years there has been some controversy regarding the value of BSE and its role in reducing mortality from breast cancer in women under 50.[3]

Reviewed by Mary C. Brucker, RN, CNM, DNSc, Director, Parkland School of Nurse-Midwifery, Dallas, TX.

Table 49-1 Risk Factors for Breast Cancer

Increased Risk	Comments
Being female	99% of breast cancer cases are in women
Age 55 yr or over	Nearly two thirds of breast cancers are found in post-menopausal women
Onset of menarche at age 12 yr or younger; onset of menopause at age 55 yr or older	Active menstruation for 40 yr or more results in twice the breast cancer risk
First full-term pregnancy after age 30; nulliparity	Prolonged exposure to unopposed estrogen increases risk for breast cancer
Benign breast disease with atypical epithelial hyperplasia	Atypical changes in breast biopsy increase the risk of breast cancer five times
Family history	Breast cancer in a maternal first-degree relative, particularly when premenopausal or bilateral, increases risk; 85-90% of women with breast cancer have no family history
Personal history of breast cancer, colon cancer, endometrial cancer	Personal history significantly increases risk of breast cancer, risk of cancer in other breast; or recurrence
Obesity	Fat cells store and release estrogen
Exposure to ionizing radiation	Radiation damages DNA

Studies are currently underway to evaluate the impact of BSE on breast cancer mortality.

Although the reasons that women report for failing to practice regular BSE have changed somewhat over the years, 65% of women still do not regularly examine their breasts.[4] Some reasons cited by women for not practicing BSE are embarrassment, lack of confidence in ability to do BSE, complexity of the procedure, and not remembering to do BSE. Factors that increase BSE compliance include a reminder system, confidence in BSE skill, encouragement from health care providers and significant others, and BSE instruction that involves the woman's active participation.[5]

The nurse who is teaching BSE must emphasize that early detection and treatment enhance survival rates. Efforts must be directed toward teaching women the importance of BSE, how to perform it, what to do if a problem is detected, and the importance of clinical examination and mammography. BSE teaching techniques should include allowing time for the woman to ask questions about the procedure and to perform a return demonstration. The technique for BSE has been established by the American Cancer Society and the National Cancer Institute (Fig. 49-1). BSE should be done monthly at a regular time when the breasts are not tender. In premenopausal women, the best time is 7 days

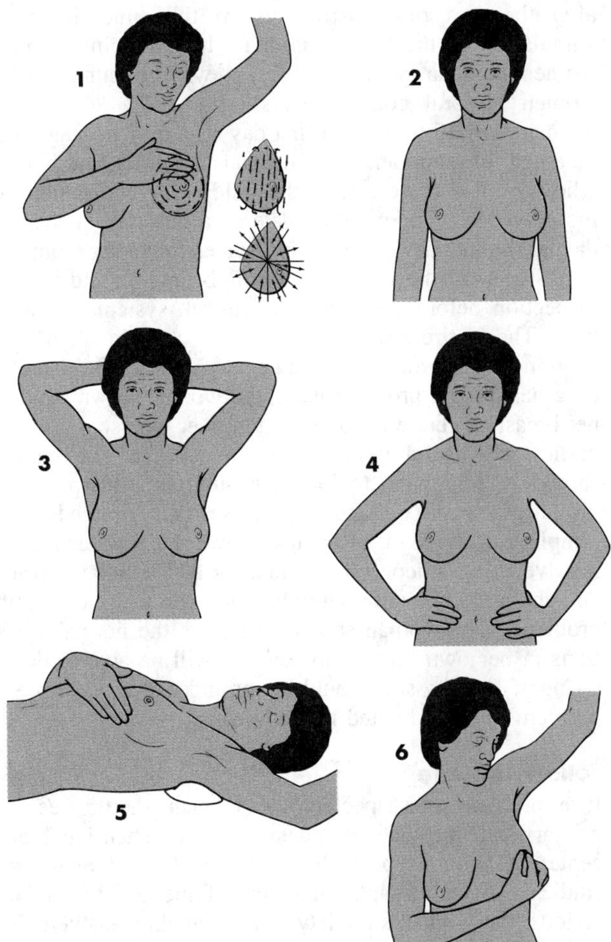

Fig. 49-1 Breast self-examination and patient instruction. (1) While in the shower or bath, when the skin is slippery with soap and water, examine your breasts. Use the pads of your second, third, and fourth fingers to firmly press every part of the breast. (While examining your left breast, use your right hand, and use your left hand to examine your right breast.) Check for any lump, hard knot, or thickening of the tissue. (2) Look at your breasts in a mirror. Stand with our arms at your side. (3) Raise your arms overhead and check for any changes in the shape of your breasts, dimpling of the skin, or any changes in the nipple. (4) Next, place your hands on your hips and press down firmly, tightening the pectoral muscles. Observe for asymmetry or changes, keeping in mind that your breasts probably do not exactly match. (5) Feel your breasts while lying down. When examining your right breast, place a folded towel under your right shoulder and put your right hand behind your head. Using the pads of the fingers on your left hand, examine the entire breast using small circular motions in a spiral, or in an up-and-down motion so that the entire breast area is examined. Repeat the procedure using your right hand to examine your left breast. (6) Finally, gently squeeze the nipple of each breast between your thumb and index finger to check for any discharge.

after the start of menstruation. At this time, hormonal stimulation of the breasts is at its lowest point. In most women, nodularity and tenderness will be minimal. For women on oral contraceptives (about 20% to 25% of women ages 15 to 45) the first day of a new package may be a helpful reminder. Postmenopausal women and women who have had hysterectomies should set a regular date for monthly BSE. The monthly date of a birthday or the first day of the month are common choices for many women.

BSE should be done in good light and should include inspection before a mirror and careful, systematic palpation. The entire breast, axilla, and clavicle should be examined. The woman should be taught the BSE procedure by a health care provider using the woman's own hand on her breast. A gentle circular motion over wet, soapy skin is particularly useful if she is in the shower. The woman should be told what to look for, such as a lump, nipple discharge, nipple retraction, redness, pain or tenderness, dimpling of the skin, or edema. Some teaching techniques involve using silicone breast models that simulate normal and abnormal breast tissue to help women learn to identify problems. The woman should be shown the normal variations in her own breasts so that she will be able to detect changes. Finally, she should be reminded that most breast problems are not related to malignancy.

Follow-Up Care

If a problem is suspected, the woman should see her primary care provider or contact a comprehensive breast center as soon as possible so that additional diagnostic studies can be promptly initiated. If the problem is not serious, the woman's anxiety can be quickly relieved. If a serious problem is suspected or diagnosed, definitive treatment is not delayed. Even when the woman faithfully practices BSE, she should have an annual breast examination by a qualified health care provider and a mammogram if age appropriate. The care and attention to detail shown by the clinician in performing BSE reinforces the practice of BSE by the patient.

ASSESSMENT OF BREAST DISORDERS

The most frequently encountered breast disorders in women are fibrocystic changes, carcinoma, fibroadenoma, intraductal papilloma, and ductal ectasia including dilated ducts (Table 49-2). In men, gynecomastia is overwhelmingly the most frequently observed breast disorder.

Many factors must be considered when the nurse is assessing a breast problem. Gender and age are important variables. Only 1% of breast carcinomas occur in males. Benign lesions occur more frequently in premenopausal women. Breast cancer is predominantly found in postmenopausal women, and the incidence increases with age. Family history is also a significant risk factor. Although not as frequent, premenopausal breast cancer tends to be more aggressive.

Risk factors in the woman's history must be evaluated. The history of the breast disorder assists in establishing the diagnosis. The presence of nipple discharge, pain, rate of growth, and correlation with the menstrual cycle should all be investigated (Table 49-2).

The size and location of the lump or lumps should be carefully documented, and the physical characteristics of the lesion, such as consistency, mobility, and shape, should be assessed. If nipple discharge is present the color and consistency should be noted, as well as whether it occurs from single or multiple ducts or from one or both breasts.

Diagnostic Studies

Several techniques can be used to screen for breast disease or provide a diagnosis of a suspicious physical finding. *Mammography* is an x-ray technique used to visualize the internal structure of the breast (Fig. 49-2). Approximately 2 million women have mammograms annually. Mammography can detect tumors that cannot be felt by palpation. The minimum size detectable by physical examination is 1 cm. It takes 10 or more years to grow a tumor this size. Mammography can detect masses of 0.5 cm. Because tumors usually metastasize late in the preclinical course, earlier detection by mammography may prevent metastasis of these smaller lesions.

Comparative mammography may show early cancer tissue changes. The diagnostic accuracy of mammography in combination with physical examination has significantly improved early and accurate detection of breast malignancies.[6] In younger women mammography is less sensitive because of the greater density of breast tissue, resulting in more false-negatives. Ten percent to 25% of breast cancers cannot be seen on mammography. Suspicious masses should be biopsied even if mammogram findings are unremarkable.

Definitive diagnosis of a mass can be made only by means of histologic examination of biopsied tissue. Biopsy technique may be either fine-needle aspiration (FNA) biopsy and cytologic examination or open surgical biopsy. Even if the lesion is nonpalpable, an FNA biopsy can be used. FNA and cytologic evaluation should be done only if an experienced cytologist is available and all suspicious lesions read as negative are followed with a more definitive biopsy procedure. If the aspirated specimen is positive for malignancy, the patient can be given this information at the same visit and begin learning about the treatment issues.

Improved imaging techniques have reduced the radiation exposure that accompanies mammography to insignificant levels. Therefore, the benefits of mammography outweigh the risks from radiation exposure. Ultrasound (echogram, sonogram) is another diagnostic procedure that can be used to differentiate a benign cyst (fluid filled) from a malignant mass (solid). An ultrasound will not detect microcalcifications, which are often the only indicators of very small tumors. Thermography is not currently recommended as a screening method for a breast mass because the results are inconclusive. (See Table 48-14 for a more detailed discussion of diagnostic studies of the breast.)

BENIGN BREAST PROBLEMS

Breast Infections

Mastitis. Mastitis is an inflammatory condition that occurs most frequently in lactating women. *Lactational mastitis* presents as a localized area that is erythematous, painful, and tender to palpation. Fever is usually present.

Table 49-2 Differential Diagnosis of Selected Breast Masses

Condition	Risk Factors	Clinical Picture
■ Breast cancer	Genetic predisposition Radiation Age in general Menarche/menopausal ages Proliferative breast disease (atypia) Alcohol intake	Breast mass (movable or fixed) Abnormal breast findings may also accompany mass, such as increase in breast size, dimpling, nipple inversion, or bloody discharge
■ Puerperal mastitis	Lactating woman Occurs spontaneously in approximately 2% of all postpartum lactating mothers (both primipara and multipara), usually 2-4 wk after birth	Warm to touch Indurated Usually unilateral Most common etiology is *Staphylococcus aureus*
■ Nonpuerperal mastitis	Rare condition Usually women in late adolescence or midyears	Palpable mass Usually an obscure organism Should rule out syphilis or tuberculosis
■ Galactocele	Resolved lactation (caused by obstruction of lactiferous ducts culminating in distention with milk and desquamation of epithelial cells)	Single or multiple lesions Usually subareolar Often accompanied by nipple discharge (initially white, later green or yellow)
■ Ductal ectasia (plasma cell mastitis or comedomastitis)	Perimenopausal woman—most common in 50s age group Previous lactation Inverted nipples	Fixation of nipple Usually accompanied by nipple discharge of thick gray material Often associated with breast pain
■ Physiologic nodularity (fibrocystic breast changes)	Most common between the ages of 35 and 50	Not usually discrete masses, nodularity instead; usually accompanied by cyclic pain and tenderness; mass(es) usually cyclic in occurrence
■ Fibroadenoma	Peak age range between 21 and 25 Most occur before age 30 Most common among African-American women	Often bilateral Most common size at diagnosis is 2-3 cm Rapid growth Accounts for 2-3% of all breast masses
■ Fat necrosis	Any age 50% report previous history of trauma to breast	Usually a hard, tender, mobile, indurated mass with irregular borders
■ Mondor's disease (thrombosis of superficial veins)	Most common during the ages of 30 and 50 (also reported among men)	Breast pain common with reddened, tender, hard cord usually unilateral on or near the breast; not associated with nipple discharge
■ Cystosarcoma phillodes	Most common between the ages of 40 and 50	Most commonly unilateral with irregular edges (leaflike appearance—hence the name); rapid growing
■ Intraductal papilloma (benign lesion of lactiferous duct)	Peak age at 40	Usually associated with serous, serosangineous, or bloody nipple discharge on affected side

From Brucker MC, Scharbo-DeHaan: Breast disease: the role of the nurse-midwife, *Nurse Midwifery* 36:1, 1991.

The infection develops when organisms, usually staphylococci, gain access to the breast through a cracked nipple. In its early stages, mastitis can be cured with antibiotics. Breastfeeding should continue unless an abscess is forming or a purulent drainage is noted. The mother may wish to use a nipple shield or to hand-express milk from the involved breast until the pain subsides. The woman should see her health care provider promptly to begin a course of antibiotic therapy.

Lactational Breast Abscess. If lactational mastitis persists after several days of antibiotic therapy, a *lactational breast abscess* may have developed. In this condition the skin may become red and edematous over the involved breast, often with a corresponding palpable mass, and the

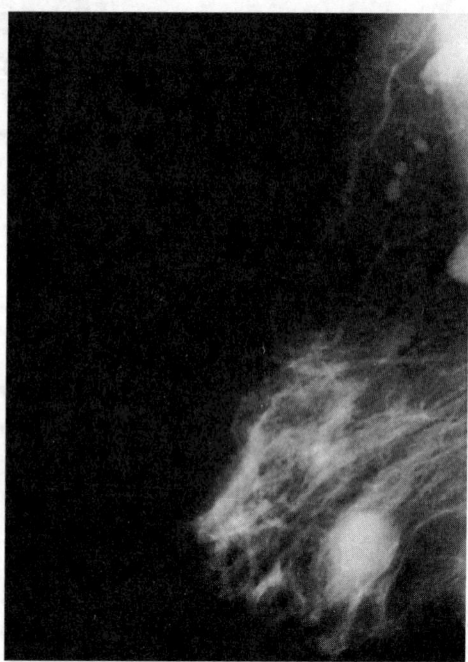

Fig. 49-2 Mammogram indicating the presence of carcinoma. Note enlarged axillary lymph nodes from tumor involvement.

patient may have an elevated temperature. Antibiotics alone constitute insufficient treatment for a breast abscess. Surgical incision and drainage is necessary. The drainage is cultured, sensitivities are obtained, and therapy with an appropriate antibiotic is begun. Often the woman will find it necessary to express and discard milk from the affected breast until the abscess is resolved.

Fibrocystic Changes

Fibrocystic changes in the breast constitute a benign condition characterized by changes in breast tissue. The changes include the development of excess fibrous tissue, hyperplasia of the epithelial lining of the mammary ducts, proliferation of mammary ducts, and cyst formation. These changes produce pain by nerve irritation from connective tissue edema and by fibrosis from nerve pinching. The use of the term *fibrocystic disease* is incorrect because the cluster of problems is actually an exaggerated response to hormonal influence. It has been suggested that the term *fibrocystic condition* or *fibrocystic complex* be used given the high prevalence of fibrocystic changes and the lack of increased risk of cancer for the majority of patients.[7] Masses or nodularities can appear in both breasts and are often found in the upper, outer quadrants and usually occur bilaterally. It is the most frequently occurring breast disorder.

Fibrocystic changes occur most frequently in women between 35 and 50 years of age but often begin in women as young as 20 years of age. Pain and nodularity often increase over time but tend to subside after menopause unless high doses of estrogen replacement are used. The cause of these fibrocystic changes is thought to be heightened responsiveness of breast parenchyma and stroma to circulating estrogens and progesterones. Predominantly affected are women with premenstrual abnormalities, nulliparous women, women with a history of spontaneous abortion, nonusers of oral contraceptives, and women with early menarche and late menopause.[8] Fibrocystic changes often exacerbate in the premenstrual phase and subside after menstruation.

Symptoms of fibrocystic breast changes include one or more palpable lumps that are usually round, well delineated, and freely movable within the breast. Some lumps are fibrous and do not contain cysts. There may be accompanying discomfort ranging from tenderness to pain. The lump is usually observed to increase in size and perhaps in tenderness before menstruation. Cysts may enlarge or shrink rapidly. Nipple discharge associated with fibrocystic breasts is often milky, watery-milky, yellow, or green.

THERAPEUTIC AND NURSING MANAGEMENT

FIBROCYSTIC CHANGES

With the initial discovery of a discrete mass in the breast by a woman or her provider, aspiration or surgical biopsy may be indicated. A wait of 7 to 10 days may be planned if the nodularity is recurrent to note changes as the menstrual cycle changes. With large or frequent cysts, surgical removal may be favored over repeated aspiration. An excisional biopsy should be done if no fluid is found on aspiration, if the fluid that is found is hemorrhagic, or if a residual mass remains. This surgery is performed in an office or day surgery unit under local anesthesia.

Biopsies in women with fibrocystic disease may indicate an increased risk for breast cancer. About 4% of biopsy specimens contain hyperplastic changes approximating the histologic appearance of carcinoma in situ and are called atypical hyperplasia.

The woman with cystic changes should be encouraged to return regularly for follow-up examinations throughout life. She should also be taught BSE to self-monitor the problem. Severe fibrocystic changes may make palpation of the breast more difficult. Any new lumps should be evaluated, and changes in symptoms should be reported and investigated.

Many types of treatment have been suggested for a fibrocystic condition. These include dietary (low-salt diet, restriction of methylxanthines such as coffee and chocolate, vitamin therapy), therapeutic (analgesics, danocrene [Danazol], diuretics, hormone therapy, antiestrogen therapy), and surgical (subcutaneous mastectomy). Most of these treatments have not been proven efficacious.

In the United States, danocrene has been approved as a treatment for fibrocystic changes. Danocrene decreases follicle-stimulating hormone (FSH) and luteinizing hormone (LH), which will ultimately culminate in anovulation and amenorrhea. The ensuing reduction of estrogen stimulation by this drug results in decreased pain and nodularity. It may take 3 to 6 months for the effects of danocrene to be noted. Side effects can be severe, including masculinization, hypoestrogenic effects, and hepatic dysfunction. However, these side effects do not usually occur with the dosage used to treat fibrocystic changes.

Abstention from all forms of methylxanthines (e.g., caffeine, theophylline, and theobromide) is commonly prescribed. However, the bulk of research evidence does not support an etiologic role for caffeine as a cause of breast pain or a therapeutic benefit from caffeine restriction.[7] In spite of these research findings, many women report that reduction of caffeine provides relief in reducing premenstrual breast tenderness. A woman can actively participate in reducing caffeine in the diet to see if it brings symptomatic relief.

Because stress can be a contributing factor in breast discomfort, efforts should be directed toward the reduction of stress. Many of these approaches are considered experimental. The large number of possible interventions indicates the uncertainty surrounding the causes and treatment of fibrocystic condition.

The role of the nurse in the care of the patient with fibrocystic breast changes is primarily one of teaching. A woman with fibrocystic breasts should be told that she may expect recurrence of the cysts in one or both breasts until menopause and that cysts may enlarge or become painful just before menstruation. Additionally, she should be reassured that cysts do not "turn into" cancer. Any new lump that does not respond in a cyclic manner over 1 to 2 weeks should be examined promptly. The woman should be carefully instructed in BSE, using her own breasts. Teaching breast models can also be helpful.

Fibroadenoma

Fibroadenoma is a common tumor of the breast in American women. It generally occurs in women between 15 and 25 years of age and is the most frequent cause of breast tumors in women under 25 years of age. Fibroadenomas tend to develop more frequently in African-American women. The possible cause of fibroadenoma may be increased estrogen sensitivity in a localized area of the breast.[9] Fibroadenomas are usually small, painless, round, well delineated, and very mobile. They may be soft but are usually solid, firm, and rubbery in consistency. There is no accompanying retraction or nipple discharge. The lump is usually painless. The tumor may appear as a single unilateral mass, although multiple bilateral fibroadenomas have been reported. The tumor grows slowly and often stops growing when it reaches a size of 2 to 3 cm. Tumor size is not affected by menstruation. However, pregnancy can stimulate dramatic growth. Fibroadenomas are rarely associated with cancer.

THERAPEUTIC AND NURSING MANAGEMENT

FIBROADENOMA

Fibroadenomas are easily detected by physical examination and are often visible on mammography. Definitive diagnosis, however, requires biopsy and tissue examination by a pathologist. Treatment is by excision, which is not urgent in women under 25 years of age. In women over 35 years of age, all new lesions should be examined using an excisional biopsy. Fibroadenomas are not reduced by radiation and are not affected by hormone therapy. The nurse frequently has the opportunity to counsel a young woman with fibroadenomas. During this contact the benign nature of the lesion should be stressed, follow-up examinations should be encouraged, and BSE should be carefully taught.

Nipple Discharge

Nipple discharge may occur spontaneously or as a result of nipple manipulation. A milky secretion is due to inappropriate lactation (*galactorrhea*) as a result of such problems as drug therapy, endocrine problems, and neural disorders. It may also be idiopathic.

Secretions can also be serous, grossly bloody, or brown to green. These may be caused by either benign or malignant disease. A slide can be made of the secretion to detect specific disease. Diseases associated with nipple discharge include malignancies, cystic disease, intraductal papilloma, and ductal ectasia. Treatment depends on identification of the cause. In most cases, nipple discharge is not related to malignancy. If galactorrhea is accompanied by amenorrhea, various gynecologic endocrinopathies should be explored.

Intraductal Papilloma. Intraductal papillomas are benign, wartlike growths found in the mammary ducts, usually near the nipple. Typically, there is an associated bloody nipple discharge, a mass, or both. Intraductal papillomas usually affect women 40 to 60 years of age. A single duct or several ducts may be involved. Treatment includes excision of the papilloma and the involved duct or duct system.

Ductal Ectasia. Ductal ectasia is a benign breast disease of perimenopausal and postmenopausal women involving the ducts in the subareolar area. It usually involves several bilateral ducts. Nipple discharge is the primary symptom. This discharge is multicolored and sticky. Ductal ectasia is initially painless but may progress to burning, itching, and pain around the nipple, as well as swelling in the areolar area. Inflammatory signs are often present, the nipple may retract, and the discharge may become bloody in more advanced disease. Ductal ectasia is not associated with malignancy. If an abscess develops, warm compresses and antibiotics are usually effective treatments. Therapy consists of close follow-up examinations or surgical excision of the involved ducts.

Gynecomastia in Men

Gynecomastia, a transient enlargement of one or both breasts, is the most common breast problem in men. The condition is usually temporary and benign. Gynecomastia in itself is not an established risk factor for breast cancer. The most common cause of gynecosmastia is a disturbance of the normal ratio of active androgen to estrogen in plasma or within the breast itself. Other causes include tumor of the testes or pituitary, medication with estrogen or steroidal compounds, or failure of the liver to inactivate circulating estrogen, as in liver failure (e.g., cirrhosis).

Pubertal Gynecomastia. Pubertal gynecomastia caused by increased estrogen production is seen most often in boys between the ages of 13 and 17. It is usually limited, although occasionally the localized hyperplasia may measure 2 to 3 cm in size. Pubertal gynecomastia is almost always self-limiting, and disappears within 4 to 6 months of onset. Parents and the affected boy should be reassured that in almost all cases this is a normal physiologic phenomenon that will disappear spontaneously and will require no treatment. Rarely, unilateral gynecomastia in the young male may be marked and fail to regress. This is the only indication for surgical intervention.

Senescent Gynecomastia. Senescent gynecomastia occurs in 40% of older men.[10] A probable cause is the elevation in plasma estrogen in older adult men as the result of an increase in the peripheral conversion of androgens to estrogens with age. Although initially unilateral, the tender, firm, centrally located enlargement may become bilateral. When gynecomastia is characterized by a discrete, circumscribed mass, it must be diagnosed to differentiate it from the rarer breast cancer in males. Senescent hyperplasia requires no treatment and generally regresses within 6 to 12 months.

Other Types of Gynecomastia. Gynecomastia may also be a symptom of other problems. It is seen accompanying developmental abnormalities of the male reproductive organs. It may also accompany organic diseases, including testicular tumors, cancer of the adrenal cortex, pituitary adenomas, hyperthyroidism, and liver disease. Gynecomastia may occur as a side effect of drug therapy, particularly with administration of estrogens and androgens, digitalis, isoniazid, ranitidine, and spironolactone. Use of heroin and marijuana can also cause gynecomastia.

Age-Related Breast Changes

Loss of subcutaneous fat and structural support and atrophy of mammary glands often result in pendulous breasts in the postmenopausal woman. The nurse should encourage older women to wear a well-fitting bra. Adequate support can improve physical appearance and reduce pain in the back, shoulders, and neck. It can also prevent *intertrigo* (dermatitis caused by friction between opposing surfaces of skin). Surgical lifting of sagging breasts is possible and may be desirable when reconstruction after a mastectomy is performed.

The decrease in glandular tissue in older women makes a breast mass easier to palpate. This decreased density is probably age related and occurs even with women on hormone replacement therapy. Rib margins may be palpable in the older adult woman and can be confused with a mass. As a woman becomes more familiar with her own breasts and is reassured about her findings, the anxiety about this finding should decrease. The nurse should encourage the older woman to continue BSE and to have annual mammograms and clinical examinations because the incidence of breast cancer increases with age.

BREAST CANCER

Significance

Breast cancer is the most common malignancy in American women. This disease develops in one in eight postmenopausal women. It is second only to lung cancer as the leading cause of death from cancer in women. Although the actual number of women diagnosed with breast cancer is increasing, the probability of surviving the disease is also increasing.[4] Each year in the United States, approximately 180,000 cases of breast cancer occur and about 46,000 women die of the disease.[9]

Although the vast majority of breast problems occur in women, men can have breast problems. Therefore, it is critical that men know the importance of examining their breasts. One out of every 100 cases of breast cancer occurs in men. Predisposing risk factors include states of hyperestrogenism, schistosomiasis, a family history of breast cancer, and radiation exposure. A thorough examination of the male breast should be a routine part of a physical examination.

Etiology and Risk Factors

Although the etiology is not completely understood, a number of factors are thought to relate to the cause of breast cancer. Heredity or genetically related susceptibility is considered to play a role. Hormonal regulation of the breast is related to the development of breast cancer, but the mechanisms are poorly understood. Sex hormones may act as tumor promoters if initiating agents have induced malignant changes. A number of external factors have been

RESEARCH

IMPLICATIONS FOR NURSING PRACTICE

BREAST SELF-EXAMINATION COMPLIANCE IN OLDER WOMEN

Citation Lierman LM and others: Effects of education and support on breast self-examination in older women, *Nurs Res* 43:158-163, 1994.

Purpose To determine the effects of a breast self-examination (BSE) teaching program and support on the frequency, proficiency, and perceived skill of BSE in middle-aged and older women.

Methods Quasi-experimental using 57 women assigned to a no-support control group, 54 to the peer support group, and 53 to the selected partner support group; mean age of sample was 61.41 years. Frequency, proficiency, and perceived skill of BSE were measured at 6 and 12 months after instruction. All women were taught BSE.

Results and Conclusions There were significant differences between the initial interview and 6-month scores on all three BSE measures. Self and expert ratings of proficiency and perceived skill continued to increase at 12 months postinstruction. No significant differences in frequency, proficiency, and perceived skill were found among the three groups.

Implications for Nursing Practice Nurses should focus on expert instruction of women related to BSE technique. Presence or absence of a support partner to increase motivation does not make a difference in compliance or proficiency rate of BSE in well-trained women.

CULTURAL & ETHNIC
Considerations

BREAST CANCER

- African-American women are more than twice as likely to die from breast cancer as Caucasian women.
- African-American women are diagnosed at a later stage of breast cancer than Caucasian women, but this fact alone does not account for the higher mortality rate.
- There is a high incidence of breast cancer among Jewish women.

considered as contributory, including diet, obesity, viruses, and use of alcohol. Environmental factors such as chemicals and radiation may play a role.

Some factors that place a woman at higher risk for breast cancer have been identified (see Table 49-1). Women are at far greater risk than men because 99% of breast cancers occur in women. Increasing age also increases the risk of developing breast cancer. The incidence of breast cancer in women under 25 years of age is very low and increases gradually until age 60. After the age of 60 the incidence increases dramatically.[9] Positive family history is an important risk factor, especially if the involved member with breast cancer was premenopausal, had bilateral disease, and was a first-degree relative (i.e., mother, sister, daughter). Having any first-degree relative with breast cancer increases a woman's risk of breast cancer 1.5 to 3 times, depending on age.[11] Risk factors appear to be cumulative; therefore, the presence of other risk factors may greatly increase the overall risk, especially for those with a positive family history.[12] Identification of risk factors indicates an increased need for careful surveillance of the patient and careful instruction in BSE. However, about 75% of women who develop breast cancer have none of the identifiable risk factors.[13]

As many as 5% of all breast cancer patients may have inherited a specific genetic abnormality contributing to the development of their breast cancer. The BRCA1 gene, located on chromosome 17, has been identified as one genetic alteration.[10] As many as 1 in 200 to 400 women in the United States may be carriers. A blood test for BRCA1 is some years off. When available, routine screening for genetic abnormalities in women without evidence of a strong family history of breast cancer diagnosed at an early age is not warranted.

Pathophysiology

The majority of breast cancers (70% to 80%) arise from lobular or ductal epithelium. Tumors originating from ductal epithelium but confined to ductal lumen without invasion into surrounding tissue are called intraductal tumors. They rarely metastasize and have a high cure rate. Carcinomas invading adjacent tissues are called infiltrating ductal carcinomas. They have a propensity for early metastasis and have a poor prognosis.

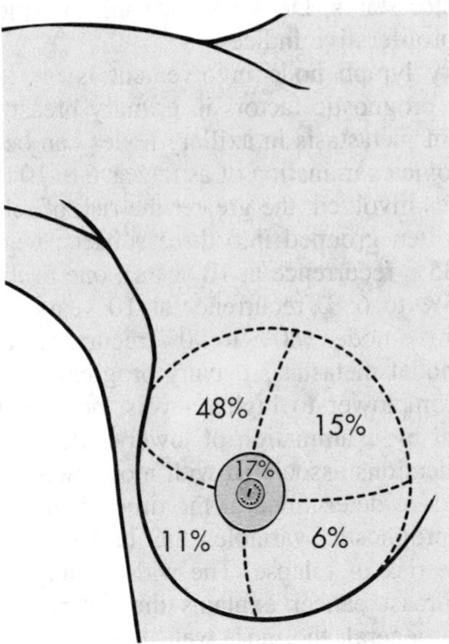

Fig. 49-3 Distribution of carcinomas in different areas of the breast.

The natural history of breast cancer varies considerably from patient to patient. The cancer can range from slowly progressive to rapidly growing. Factors that affect growth are axillary node involvement (the more nodes involved, the worse the prognosis); tumor differentiation (morphology of malignant cells); estrogen and progesterone receptor status; tumor site; and abnormal DNA content.

Clinical Manifestations

Breast cancer is usually first detected as a single lump in the breast. It occurs most often in the upper, outer quadrant of the breast because most of the glandular tissue is there (Fig. 49-3). The rate at which the lesion grows varies considerably. Slow-growing lesions are often associated with a lower mortality rate. On palpation, breast cancer is characteristically hard, irregularly shaped, poorly delineated, and nonmobile. Malignant lesions are characteristically painless and nontender.

A small percentage of breast cancers present as nipple discharge. The discharge is usually unilateral and may be clear or bloody. Nipple retraction may occur. Plugging of the dermal lymphatics can cause skin thickening and exaggeration of the usual skin markings, giving the skin the appearance of an orange peel (*peau d'orange*). In late stages, infiltration, induration, and dimpling (pulling in) of the overlying skin may occur.

Diagnostic Studies

In addition to biopsy and FNA used to diagnose breast cancer, there are other tests available that are useful in predicting the risk of recurrence or metastatic breast disease. These tests include axillary lymph node status, tumor size and histologic characteristics, estrogen and progesterone receptor status, DNA content analysis (ploidy status), and cell proliferative indices.

Axillary lymph node involvement is one of the most important prognostic factors in primary breast cancer. The presence of metastasis in axillary nodes can be determined by pathologic examination of as few as 6 to 10 nodes.[14] The more nodes involved, the greater the risk of relapse. Nodal status is often grouped into three subsets: negative nodes (30% to 35% recurrence at 10 years), one to three positive nodes (55% to 65% recurrence at 10 years), and four or more positive nodes (80% to 90% recurrence at 10 years). Because nodal metastasis usually progresses in an orderly fashion from lower to higher levels, nodal status can be determined by examination of lower nodes, thus avoiding the complications associated with more radical dissection.

Tumor size determined at the time of lumpectomy is a valuable prognostic variable: the larger the tumor, the greater the risk of relapse. The wide variety of histologic types of breast cancer explains the heterogeneity of the disease. In general, the more well differentiated the tumor, the less aggressive it is. Poorly differentiated tumors appear morphologically disorganized and aggressive.

Another diagnostic test useful both for treatment decisions and prediction of prognosis is estrogen and progesterone receptor status. Receptor-positive tumors commonly show histologic evidence of being well-differentiated, frequently have a diploid DNA content and low proliferative indices, have a low propensity for visceral recurrence, and are frequently hormone dependent and responsive to hormonal therapy. Receptor-negative tumors (1) are frequently poorly differentiated histologically, (2) have a high incidence of aneuploidy (abnormally high or low DNA content) and higher proliferative indices, (3) frequently recur on visceral sites, and (4) are usually unresponsive to hormonal therapy.[14]

Flow cytometry can be used to measure DNA content (ploidy status) and cell proliferation. The technique uses a laser-powered flow cytometer to measure certain characteristics of malignant cells that are difficult to measure by microscopy. This test quantifies cellular DNA content and determines if a tumor is diploid (DNA content equal to that in normal cells) or aneuploid (abnormally high or low DNA content). Ploidy correlates with tumor aggressiveness. Diploid tumors have been shown to have a significantly lower risk of relapse than aneuploid tumors.[15]

Cell proliferative indices indirectly measure the rate of tumor cell proliferation. The percent of tumor cells in the S phase of the cell cycle (see Fig. 12-1) is another important prognostic indicator. Cells with high S-phase fractions have a higher risk for recurrence and can produce earlier cancer death.

Another prognostic indicator is a genetic marker termed HER-2 (also called c-erbB-2 or neu).[14] Amplification and overexpression of this gene have been noted in breast cancer tissue and are associated with a worse prognosis. People with this gene have tumors that are routinely resistant to some forms of chemotherapy and more responsive to others.

Complications

The main complication of breast cancer is recurrence (Table 49-3). Recurrence may be local or regional (skin or soft tissue near the mastectomy site, axillary or internal mammary lymph nodes) or distant (most commonly bone, lung, brain, and liver). However, metastatic disease can be found in any distant site.

About 50% to 75% of patients with node-positive disease have recurrences, compared with about 25% to 33% of those with negative nodes.[16] Seventy percent of all recurrences occur during the 3 to 4 years following diagnosis.

Widely disseminated or metastatic disease involves the growth of colonies of cancerous breast cells in parts of the body distant from the breast. Metastases primarily occur through the lymphatic chains, principally those of the axilla (see Fig. 48-4). However, the cancer can spread to other parts of the body without invading the axillary nodes even when the primary breast tumor is small. Even in node-negative breast cancer, there is a possibility of distant metastasis. Prognosis is directly related to the number of nodes involved and other factors discussed in the section on Diagnostic Studies.

Chemotherapy is the usual treatment for recurrent disease. Hormonal therapy or irradiation may be used alone or in combination with chemotherapy when recurrent disease occurs.

Therapeutic Management

Historically, radical ablative surgery was the standard of care. Presently there is a wide range of treatment options available to both the patient and the care providers attempting to make critical decisions about what treatment to select (Table 49-4). Many prognostic factors are considered when treatment decisions are made about a specific breast cancer. These factors include lymph node status, tumor size, histologic classification, and the identification of special histologic subtypes. All of these factors enter into the *staging* of breast cancer. The most widely accepted staging method is the American Joint Committee on Cancer's (AJCC) TNM system. This system uses tumor size (T), nodal involvement (N), and presence of metastasis (M) to determine the stage of disease. The stages range from I to IV, with stage I being very small tumors (less than 2 cm) with no lymph node involvement and no metastasis. Stages II and III are broken down into IIA, IIB, IIIA, and IIIB. Classification within these stages depends on the size of the tumor and the number of lymph nodes involved. Stage IV indicates the presence of metastatic spread, regardless of tumor size or lymph node involvement.[17] The therapeutic regimen is often dictated by the clinical stage classification of the cancer. (Side effects and appropriate nursing management of general treatment modalities for cancer are discussed in Chapter 12.)

In spite of the advent of new prognostic indicators such as flow-cytometric determination of DNA content and analysis of cell-cycle fractions, the single most powerful prognostic factor related to local recurrence or metastasis after primary therapy is still the presence or absence of metastatic carcinoma in axillary lymph nodes.

Table 49-3 Common Sites of Breast Cancer Recurrence and Metastasis

Site	Clinical Presentation
Local recurrence	
Skin	Firm, discrete nodules; occasionally pruritic, usually painless
Regional recurrence	
Lymph nodes	Enlarged nodes in axilla or supraclavicular area, usually nontender, superior vena caval obstruction from enlarged supraclavicular nodes (oncologic emergency), pain in shoulder and arm of affected side
Distant metastases	
Skeletal metastasis	Localized pain of gradually increasing intensity, percussion tenderness at involved sites, pathologic fracture caused by involvement of bone cortex, hypercalcemia from skeletal metastasis or endocrine therapy
Spinal cord metastasis	Progressive back pain, localized and radicular; muscular weakness, usually in lower extremities; paresthesias in one or more extremities; bowel or bladder sphincter dysfunction; paralysis from epidural spinal cord compression
Brain metastasis	Headache, unilateral sensory loss, focal muscular weakness, hemiparesis, incoordination (ataxia), visual defects, speech disorder (dysphasia), impaired cognition, behavioral or mental changes, loss of sphincter control, papilledema, persistent nausea and vomiting, seizure activity, progressive decrease in level of consciousness
Pulmonary metastasis (including lung nodules and pleural effusions)	Dependent on sites and extent of pulmonary metastases; chest pain, dyspnea on exertion, shortness of breath, tachypnea, nonproductive cough (not present in all patients); adventitious breath sounds, dullness to percussion, restricted chest-wall expansion on affected side with pleural effusion
Liver metastasis	Abdominal distention; right lower quadrant abdominal pain sometimes with radiation to scapular area; nausea and vomiting, anorexia, weight loss; weakness and fatigue; hepatomegaly, ascites, jaundice; peripheral edema; elevated liver enzymes
Bone marrow metastasis	Anemia; infection; increased bleeding, bruising, petechiae; weakness and fatigue; mild confusion, lightheadedness; dyspnea

Surgical Interventions. Breast conservation surgery with radiotherapy and modified radical mastectomy with or without reconstruction are currently the most common options for resectable breast cancer. Most women diagnosed with early-stage breast cancer (tumors <4 to 5 cm) are candidates for either treatment choice (75% to 80% of new cases).[7] Ten-year overall survival with lumpectomy and radiation is about the same as that with modified radical mastectomy.[6]

Axillary node dissection. Axillary lymph node dissection is usually performed regardless of the treatment option selected. Examination of nodes provides the most powerful prognostic data currently available. Also, removal of axillary nodes is highly effective in preventing axillary recurrence, aids in decision making regarding adjuvant chemotherapy or hormonal therapy, and eliminates the need for axillary nodal radiation. If other promising techniques such as microvascular counts could establish breast cancer prognosis adequately, the role of axillary node dissection in any stage of breast cancer would be questioned. Radiation of the axilla is equally effective in decreasing the incidence of axillary recurrence.[20]

Lymphedema (accumulation of lymph in soft tissue) can occur as a result of the excision or radiation of lymph nodes. When the axillary nodes cannot return lymph fluid to the central circulation, the fluid accumulates in the arm, causing obstructive pressure on the veins and venous return. The patient may experience heaviness, pain, impaired motor function in the arm, and numbness and paresthesia of the fingers as a result of lymphedema. Cellulitis and progressive fibrosis can result from lymphedema.

Although lymphedema is not always preventable, it can be controlled somewhat after surgery or irradiation. Frequent and sustained elevation of the arm, regular use of a custom-fitted pressure sleeve, and treatment with an inflatable sleeve (pneumomassage) are all helpful in preventing or reducing lymphedema.

Breast conservation surgery. Breast conservation surgery (lumpectomy) involves the removal of the entire tumor along with a margin of normal tissue. A nodal dissection may be done. Following surgery, radiation therapy is delivered to the entire breast, ending with a boost to the tumor bed. This treatment method is an option when the tumor is less than 4 cm and can be totally removed. If there is evidence of systemic disease, chemotherapy may be given before radiation therapy. Contraindications to breast conservation surgery include breast size too small to yield an acceptable cosmetic result, tumor exceeding 4 cm, masses and calcifications that are multifocal (within the same breast quadrant), masses that are multicen-

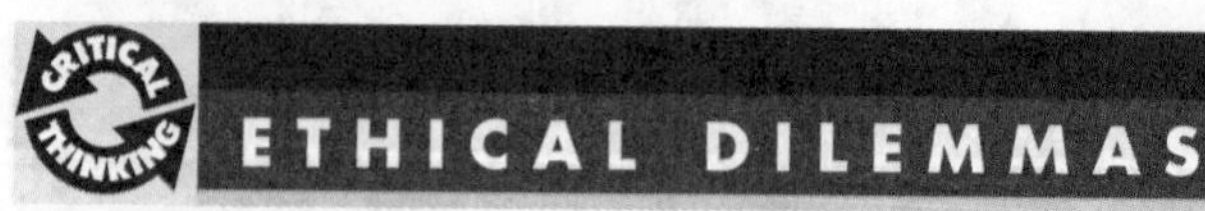

PASSIVE EUTHANASIA AND SUFFERING

Situation A 50-year-old woman with metastatic breast cancer resistant to chemotherapy and radiation has developed severe bone pain that is not being managed adequately by her present dose of morphine. The patient has told her care team she no longer wants to live because of this pain. Her physician increases her dose of morphine. Even though the increased dose of morphine seems excessive, it is appropriate.

Discussion A medical intervention for the purpose of causing death in order to reduce a patient's suffering is *active euthanasia* and is not legal in the United States. The *intent* in active euthanasia is that the patient die. In *passive euthanasia,* the intent is to reduce pain and suffering and to allow the disease to take its course; the *consequence* may be a hastened death. Although most cancer pain can be managed by health care professionals trained in pain management, a specific patient's pain may be very challenging to manage. Relieving this patient's pain and suffering is the goal of her drug therapy.

ETHICAL AND LEGAL PRINCIPLES

- *Euthanasia* (good death) can be defined as active or passive. *Active euthanasia* involves the intentional act to cause the death of another; *passive euthanasia* results from the omission of treatment that would sustain life or the provision of pain medication at a dose that could hasten death. The difference is ambiguous and is often felt to be irrelevant.
- In the theory of double effect, it is permissible to provide acceptable levels of medication to provide pain relief even if the effect of that medication is a hastened death.
- The principles of beneficence and nonmaleficence may be considered to conflict in this case. Providing pain relief is beneficent, but hastening a death by an increased dosage could be viewed as harmful. Refusing to give adequate pain relief is harmful to the patient, but not hastening the patient's death is beneficent.

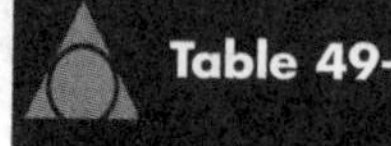

Table 49-4 Therapeutic Management: Breast Cancer

Diagnostic
- History of risk factors
- Physical examination of breast and lymphatics
- Mammography
- Ultrasound
- Biopsy
- Estrogen-progesterone receptor assays or analysis

Staging work-up
- Complete blood count
- Calcium and phosphate levels, liver function tests
- Chest x-ray
- Liver scan
- Bone scan

Therapeutic
- Surgery
  - Breast-conserving*
  - Modified radical mastectomy
- Radiation therapy
  - Primary radiotherapy
  - Adjuvant radiotherapy
  - Palliative radiotherapy
- Chemotherapy
  - Adjuvant chemotherapy
  - Chemotherapy for recurrent disease
- Hormonal therapy†
  - Hormones (e.g., tamoxifen, megestrol acetate, aminoglutethimide)
- Surgical ablation therapy

*With or without axillary node sampling or dissection.
†If estrogen receptor positive.

tric (in more than one quadrant), or diffuse calcifications in more than one quadrant.

One of the main advantages of breast conservation surgery and radiation is that it preserves the breast, including the nipple. The goal of the combined surgery and radiation is to maximize the benefits of both cancer treatment and cosmetic outcome while minimizing risks. Disadvantages of this surgery include the increased cost of the surgery plus radiation over surgery alone and the possible side effects of radiation. Table 49-5 describes treatment options, side effects, complications, and patient issues related to the most common surgical procedures currently used to treat breast cancer.

Modified radical mastectomy. The modified radical mastectomy includes removal of the breast and axillary lymph nodes, but it preserves the pectoralis major muscle. This surgery would be selected over breast conservation therapy if the tumor is too large to excise with good margins and attain a reasonable cosmetic result. Some patients may select this surgical procedure over lumpectomy when presented with the choice of either procedure.

When a modified radical mastectomy is performed, the patient has the option of breast reconstruction. If the patient chooses to have reconstructive surgery, it can be performed immediately following the mastectomy or it can be delayed until postoperative recovery is complete (about 6 months).

Follow-up care. After surgery, the woman must be followed up for the rest of her life at regular intervals. Most women have professional examinations every 3 months for 2 years, every 6 months for the next 3 years, and then annually thereafter. In addition, the woman must continue to practice a monthly BSE on both breasts or the remaining breast and the mastectomy site. The most common sites of recurrence of breast cancer are at the surgical site and in the opposite breast. The woman should also have yearly mammography of the remaining breast or breast tissue.

Adjuvant Therapy. The decision to recommend adjuvant (additional) therapy after surgery depends on the number of involved nodes, menstrual status, age, cell type, size and extent of the cancer, presence or absence of

Table 49-5 Breast Cancer: Treatment Options, Side Effects, Complications, and Patient Issues

Procedure	Description	Hospitalization	Side Effects	Potential Complications: Short Term	Potential Complications: Long Term	Patient Issues
Modified radical mastectomy	Removal of breast, preservation of pectoralis muscle, axillary dissection	Hospital stay is 1-4 days	Chest wall tightness Phantom breast sensations Arm swelling Sensory changes	Skin flap necrosis Seroma Hematoma Infection	Muscle atrophy Muscle weakness Lymphedema	Loss of breast Incision Body image Need for prosthesis Impaired arm mobility
Breast conservation surgery with radiation therapy	Wide excision of tumor, axillary dissection, radiation therapy	Hospital stay is 1-3 days Radiation 6-7 weeks	Breast soreness Breast edema Skin reactions Arm swelling Sensory changes (surgery–arm) Sensory changes (breast–x-ray treatment) Fatigue	Moist desquamation Hematoma Seroma Infection	Fibrosis Rib fractures Lymphedema Myositis Pneumonitis	Prolonged treatment Impaired arm mobility Change in texture and sensitivity of breast
Immediate reconstruction—implant	Implantation of prosthesis under musculofascial layer of chest wall	Hospital stay is 1-4 days	Discomfort (greater than mastectomy alone because of elevation and stretching of muscles)	Skin flap necrosis Wound separation Seroma, hematoma Infection	Capsular contractions Loss of implant Risks of silicone implants	Body image Prolonged physician visits (expander implants)
Immediate reconstruction—flap procedures	A musculocutaneous flap (muscle, skin, blood supply) is transposed to chest wall area	Hospital stay is 5-7 days	Pain related to two surgical sites and extensive of the surgery	Delayed wound healing Cellulitis		Prolonged postoperative recovery

From Knobf MT: Treatment options for early stage breast cancer, *Medsurg Nurs* 3:249, 1994.

estrogen receptors, and other preexisting health problems that can complicate treatment. Adjuvant therapies include radiation therapy and systemic therapies such as chemotherapy, hormonal manipulation, and biological response modifiers.

Radiation therapy. The three situations in which radiation therapy may be used for breast cancer are (1) as the primary treatment to destroy the tumor or as a companion to surgery to prevent local recurrence, (2) to shrink a large tumor to operable size, and (3) as the palliative treatment for pain caused by local recurrence and metastases. Lumpectomy is almost always followed by radiation.

PRIMARY RADIATION THERAPY. When radiation therapy is the primary treatment, it is usually performed after local excision of the breast mass. The breast (and the regional lymph nodes in some cases) are radiated daily over the course of approximately 4 to 5 weeks. An external beam of radiation is used to deliver an approximate total dose of 4500 to 5000 cGy (4500 to 5000 rads; 1 rad = 1 cGy). A "boost" treatment to the full breast may also be given, either before or after therapy has been completed. The boost is a dose of radiation delivered to the area in which the original tumor was located. It can be given by external beam and usually adds 10 treatments to the total number given. Esophagitis, tracheitis, fatigue, skin changes, and breast edema may be temporary side effects of external beam radiation therapy. Chemotherapy may be used systemically to enhance the local effects of irradiation. (Nursing management of the patient receiving radiation therapy is discussed in Chapter 12).

RADIATION THERAPY AS ADJUNCT TO SURGERY. Although an uncommon treatment mode, preoperative radiation therapy can be used to reduce the size of a large tumor mass to operable proportions by destroying the cancer cells. Additionally, because the malignant cells are partially or completely destroyed, the rate of local recurrence decreases. The disadvantages of potential delayed wound healing and increased lymphedema do not seem to outweigh the advantages of preoperative radiation in cases in which the cancer is locally advanced.

The decision to use radiation therapy after mastectomy is based on the probability of the presence of local residual cancer cells. Radiating the area will not prevent the appearance of distant metastasis at a later date. The site of radiation therapy (lymph nodes, chest wall, or both) depends on the degree of possible spread of the cancer.

PALLIATIVE RADIATION THERAPY. In addition to reducing the primary tumor mass with a resultant decrease in pain, radiation therapy is also used to stabilize symptomatic metastatic lesions in such sites as bone, soft-tissue organs, the brain, and the chest. Radiation therapy relieves pain and is often successful in controlling recurrent or metastatic disease for long periods.

Systemic therapy. The goal of systemic therapy is to destroy or control tumor cells that have spread to distant sites. The vast majority of women with breast cancer have no evidence of metastatic disease at the time of diagnosis. However, micrometastases have probably occurred even in stage I disease and especially in stage II disease, making breast cancer a systemic disease at the time of diagnosis. Because of the high risk for recurrent disease, nearly all women with evidence of node involvement, particularly those who are hormone-receptor negative, will have some type of systemic therapy. Certain women, particularly those who are premenopausal, are known to be at higher risk for recurrent or metastatic disease. These women are often recommended for systemic therapy even when no evidence of node involvement is found. Weighing the different risk factors to determine the need for adjuvant therapy in a node-negative patient is a complex process.

After analyzing the results of 133 worldwide clinical studies, the Early Breast Cancer Trialists' Collaborative Group concluded that systemic therapy as an adjuvant to primary local treatment, in the absence of demonstrable metastases, significantly decreases tumor recurrence rates and increases survival, the extent of the benefit depending on a number of variables in the patient population and type of therapy.[19]

Current types of systemic therapy available for breast cancer treatment include chemotherapy, hormonal manipulation, and biologic response modifiers.

CHEMOTHERAPY. *Chemotherapy* refers to the use of cytotoxic drugs to destroy cancer cells. The greatest benefits from chemotherapy have been achieved among premenopausal women with node findings that are positive for malignancy. Some studies indicate improved outcomes for postmenopausal women as well.[20]

In some instances chemotherapy is being used preoperatively. Preoperative chemotherapy may be more convenient than postoperative administration and can decrease the size of the primary tumor, possibly permitting less extensive surgery. Also, it has been shown that preoperative chemotherapy suppresses tumor growth and prolongs survival.[21,22]

Breast cancer is one of the solid tumors that is most responsive to chemotherapy. The use of combinations of drugs is clearly superior to the use of a single drug. The benefit of combination treatment results from the use of drugs that have different actions on cell growth and division. Two common combination-therapy protocols are cyclophosphamide, methotrexate, 5-fluorouracil, vincristine, and prednisone (CMFVP); and cyclophosphamide, doxorubicin (Adriamycin), and 5-fluorouracil (CAF).

Because healthy cells are also affected by chemotherapy, a variety of side effects accompany this treatment modality. The incidence and severity of predictable and commonly observed side effects will be influenced by the specific drug combination, drug schedule, and dose intensity of the drug or drugs. Usually body organs with rapidly growing cells are the most strongly affected. The most common side effects involve the gastrointestinal (GI) tract, bone marrow, and hair follicles, resulting in nausea, anorexia, weight loss, bone marrow suppression and subsequent fatigue, and alopecia. When prednisone is added to the chemotherapy regimen, the side effects related to myelosuppression and GI toxicity are reduced.

HORMONAL THERAPY. Estrogen can promote growth of breast cancer cells if the cells are estrogen-receptor positive.

If the source of estrogen is removed, tumor regression may occur. The source of estrogen (especially estradiol) can be greatly reduced by surgical ablation (e.g., oophorectomy, adrenalectomy, and hypophysectomy) or with additive hormonal therapy. Hormonal therapy is widely used to treat recurrent or metastatic cancer but may occasionally be used as an adjuvant to primary treatment.[23]

Two advances have increased the use of hormone therapy. First, reliable tests (hormone receptor assays) have been developed to identify women who are likely to respond to hormone therapy. Both estrogen and progesterone receptor status of the tumor can be determined. The importance of these assays is their ability to predict whether hormone manipulation is a treatment option for women with breast cancer, either at the time of initial therapy or if the cancer recurs. Second, drugs have been developed that can inactivate the hormone-secreting glands as effectively as surgery or radiation, without the side effects of these therapies or the need to supplement other hormones no longer secreted by the ablated gland.

Not all breast malignancies are estrogen dependent. Although normal breast tissue contains receptor sites for hormones, malignant cell transformation alters these receptor sites in some cells. If a malignant cell retains hormone receptor sites, it continues to depend on estrogen for cell division. The receptor sites that are altered as a result of malignant transformation are no longer controlled by hormones. Premenopausal and perimenopausal women are more likely to have tumors that are not hormone dependent, whereas women who are past menopause are likely to have hormone-dependent tumors.[5] Chances of tumor regression observed with hormone manipulation are minimal in women whose tumors are lacking estrogen and progesterone receptors. Receptor status probably has no relation to response to chemotherapy. Receptor status may change following hormonal therapy, radiotherapy, or chemotherapy.

Tamoxifen citrate is the usual first choice of treatment in postmenopausal, estrogen receptor–positive women with or without nodal involvement. Tamoxifen, an antiestrogen, blocks the estrogen-receptor sites of malignant cells and is commonly used to prevent or treat recurrent breast cancer. Side effects of tamoxifen are minimal but include hot flashes, nausea, vomiting, dry skin, vaginal bleeding, menstrual irregularities, and other effects commonly associated with decreased estrogen.

Women with breast cancer have an increased risk of a second primary breast tumor. Tamoxifen reduces not only the risk of recurrent breast cancer but also that of new primary tumors. Although originally prescribed for 1 to 2 years, it is often used now for longer periods of time, even indefinitely.[26] It has been shown that the risk for endometrial cancer increases following tamoxifen therapy for invasive breast cancer.[24] However, it is generally agreed that the net benefit greatly outweighs the risk. Endometrial cancers occurring after tamoxifen therapy do not appear to be of a different type than endometrial cancers in nontamoxifen-treated patients.

National clinical trials have begun on the use of tamoxifen as a modality to prevent breast cancer in high-risk individuals. Results of these trials can be anticipated in the next 3 to 5 years.[25]

Additional drugs that may be used to suppress hormone-dependent breast tumors include megestrol acetate (Megace), diethylstilbestrol (DES), fluoxymesterone (Halotestin), and aminoglutethimide (Cytadren). Less common hormone-deprivation strategies include bilateral oophorectomy, adrenalectomy, and hypophysectomy.

Biologic Response Modifiers. The use of biologic response modifiers represents an attempt to stimulate the body's natural defenses to recognize and attack cancer cells. The use of high-dose chemotherapy and bone marrow transplant are other potential treatments. The use of these therapies is discussed in Chapter 12.

NURSING MANAGEMENT

BREAST CANCER

Nursing Assessment

Subjective and objective data that should be obtained from an individual suspected of having or diagnosed as having breast cancer are presented in Table 49-6.

Nursing Diagnoses

Nursing diagnoses related to the care of a patient diagnosed with breast cancer vary. Following diagnosis and before a treatment plan has been selected, the following diagnoses would apply:

- Decisional conflict related to lack of knowledge about treatment options and their effects
- Fear related to diagnosis of breast cancer
- Risk of body image disturbance related to anticipated physical and emotional effects of treatment modalities.

If breast conservation surgery is selected as the initial therapy, the nursing diagnoses appropriate for the care of the preoperative patient (see Chapter 14) and for the patient receiving radiation therapy (see Chapter 12) would apply as well as those indicated in the nursing care plan for the patient after a modified radical mastectomy on p. 1557. If a modified radical mastectomy is planned, the nursing diagnoses may include, but are not limited to, those presented in the nursing care plan on p. 1557.

Planning

The overall goals are that the patient with breast cancer will (1) actively participate in the decision-making process related to treatment options, (2) fully comply with the therapeutic plan, (3) manage the side effects of adjuvant therapy, and (4) be satisfied with the support provided by significant others and health care providers.

Nursing Implementation

Acute Intervention. The time between diagnosis of breast cancer and the selection of a treatment plan is a difficult period for the woman and her family. Although the primary care provider has discussed treatment options, the woman often relies on the nurse to clarify and expand on

Table 49-6 Nursing Assessment: Breast Cancer

Subjective Data
Important health information
Past health history: Previous unilateral breast cancer; menstrual history (early menarche with late menopause); parity, age when first child born; previous endometrial, ovarian, or colon cancer; Klinefelter's syndrome; testicular atrophy (in men); infertility treatment
Medications: Use of estrogens, especially as postmenopausal hormone replacement therapy and in oral contraceptives
Surgery and other treatments: Exposure to excessive radiation
Functional health patterns
Health perception–health management: Positive family history (especially mother or sister); palpable lump found on BSE
Nutritional-metabolic: Alcohol intake; obesity; anorexia (possible indicator of metastasis)
Cognitive-perceptual: Headache, bone, head, or arm pain (possible indicators of metastasis)
Sexuality-reproductive: Unilateral nipple discharge (clear, milky, or bloody); change in breast contour, size, or symmetry
Coping–stress tolerance: Chronic psychologic stress

Objective Data
General
Anxiety, axillary and supraclavicular lymphadenopathy
Respiratory
Pleural effusions (possible indicator of metastasis)
Gastrointestinal
Hepatomegaly, jaundice; ascites, edema (possible indicators of liver metastasis)
Reproductive
Hard, irregular, nonmobile breast lump most often in upper, outer sector, possibly fixated to fascia or chest wall; nipple retraction, erosion; edema ("orange peel"), erythema, induration, infiltration, or dimpling (in later stages)
Possible findings
Finding of lump on breast examination; positive results of mammography, thermography, or ultrasonography; positive results of FNA or surgical biopsy

BSE, Breast self-examination; *FNA,* fine-needle aspiration.

these options. During this time, the woman may be very self-focused, verbalizing her conflict and indecision frequently. Appropriate nursing interventions during this period include exploring the woman's usual decision-making patterns, helping the woman accurately evaluate the advantages and disadvantages of the options, providing information relevant to the decision, and supporting the patient once the decision is made.

During this period the woman may exhibit signs of distress or tension, such as tachycardia, increased muscle tension, and restlessness, whenever she focuses on the decision to be made. The nurse should assess the woman's body language, motor activity, and affect during periods of high stress and indecision so appropriate interventions can be carried out.

Regardless of the surgery planned, the patient must be provided with sufficient information to ensure informed consent. Some patients need extensive, detailed information. For others, this only increases anxiety. Sensitivity to individual needs is essential. Preoperative diagnostic studies must be completed. Teaching in the preoperative phase includes instruction in turning, coughing and deep breathing, a review of postoperative exercises, and explanation of the recovery period from the time of surgery until discharge.

The woman who has breast conservation surgery usually has an uneventful postoperative course with only a moderate amount of pain. The woman who has had a modified radical mastectomy needs nursing interventions specific to this surgery.

Restoring arm function on the affected side after mastectomy is one of the most important goals of nursing activities. The woman should be placed in a semi-Fowler's position with the arm on the affected side elevated on a pillow. Flexing and extending the fingers should begin in the recovery room with daily increases in activity. (Information pertaining to arm exercises and care also apply to women who have had an axillary node dissection after lumpectomy or simple mastectomy.) Postoperative mastectomy exercises are instituted gradually at the surgeon's direction (see Fig. 49-4 on p. 1559). These exercises are designed to prevent contractures and muscle shortening, maintain muscle tone, and improve lymph and blood circulation. The difficulty and pain encountered by the woman in performing the previously simple tasks included in the exercise program may cause frustration and depression.

Postoperative discomfort can be minimized by administering analgesics about 30 minutes before initiating exercises. If showering is appropriate, the flow of warm water over the involved shoulder often has a soothing effect and reduces joint stiffness. Whenever possible, the same nurse should work with the woman so that progress can be commended and problems can be identified.

Measures to prevent or reduce lymphedema must be used by the nurse and taught to the woman. The affected arm should never be dependent, even while the person is sleeping. Blood pressure readings, venipunctures, and injections should not be done on the affected arm. Elastic bandages should not be used in the early postoperative period because they inhibit collateral lymph drainage. The woman must be instructed to protect the arm on the operative side from even minor trauma such as a pinprick or sunburn. If trauma to the arm occurs, the area should be washed thoroughly with soap and water. A topical antibiotic ointment and a bandage or other sterile dressing should be applied. The surgeon must be advised of the trauma, and the site of injury must be observed closely for evidence of inflammation. The patient must know and understand that she is at risk of developing lymphedema for the rest of her life.

When lymphedema is acute, an intermittent pneumatic compression sleeve can be used. This device applies me-

NURSING CARE PLAN Patient After A Modified Radical Mastectomy

Planning: Outcome Criteria	Nursing Interventions and Rationales
➤ NURSING DIAGNOSIS	Pain *related to* surgical incision and manipulation of tissue *as manifested by* verbalization regarding presence and degree of pain at operative area*
Have absence of or tolerable level of pain; express satisfaction with pain control.	Administer analgesics as prescribed *to relieve pain.* Position arm *to prevent tension on suture line and provide support.* Encourage use of noninvasive pain management strategies such as distraction, guided imagery, and relaxation *to complement analgesics and decrease need for analgesia.*
➤ NURSING DIAGNOSIS	Ineffective management of therapeutic regimen *related to* lack of knowledge regarding BSE and signs and symptoms to report to health care provider *as manifested by* acknowledgement of lack of information about or confidence in performing BSE; lack of information about plans for follow-up care, signs and symptoms of recurrent or metastatic disease*
Have early recognition of recurrent or metastatic disease; practice monthly BSE.	Teach or evaluate BSE performance *to ensure that patient is performing correctly.* Reinforce importance of annual mammogram *because it is a recommended screening technique for early identification of recurrence both locally and in other breast.* Provide information about signs and symptoms to report to health care provider (e.g., new and persistent bone pain, weakness, constipation, visual disturbances, confusion, localized rash at surgical site, new lump in breast or chest wall) *so necessary treatment can be initiated promptly.*
➤ NURSING DIAGNOSIS	Altered sexuality patterns *related to* loss of body part, fatigue, surgical procedure, medication, and anxiety regarding diagnosis *as manifested by* decrease in sexual desire and responsiveness, perception of sexual activities as undesirable
Adapt to altered body image; have satisfying sexual relationships.	Assess degree of problem, adaptation to loss, and personal ability to cope *to identify individual's response and plan appropriate interventions.* If appropriate, refer woman and partner for therapy, counseling, or support *to provide additional specialized assistance for resolution of problems.*
➤ NURSING DIAGNOSIS	Fear *related to* diagnosis of cancer *as manifested by* questioning, insomnia, reduced attention span, crying*
Verbalize fear, have support of significant others; express confidence in ability to cope.	Encourage woman to talk about feelings and diagnosis of cancer *to promote successful resolution of fear and establish effective coping mechanisms.* Provide accurate information *to promote understanding, clarify information, and reduce anxieties.* Provide opportunity for significant others to discuss situation and learn about support groups *because their fear about diagnosis and outcome can decrease their effectiveness as a support system.*

continued

chanical massage to the arm. Manual massage is also effective in mobilizing subcutaneous accumulations of fluid. Elevation of the arm so that it is level with the heart, diuretics, and isometric exercises may be recommended to reduce the fluid volume in the arm. The patient may need to wear an elastic pressure-gradient sleeve during waking hours to maintain maximum volume reduction.

Psychologic care. Throughout interactions with a woman with breast cancer, the nurse must keep in mind the extensive psychologic impact of the disease. It is important that the nurse is aware that the major psychologic distress experienced by a woman is primarily related to the cancer diagnosis, and not the loss of the breast.[27] All aspects of care must include sensitivity to the woman's efforts to cope with a life-threatening disease. An open relationship in which the woman can express her fears and feelings is essential. The nurse can help meet the woman's psychologic needs by doing the following:

1. Assisting her to develop a positive but realistic attitude
2. Helping her identify sources of support and strength to her, such as her partner, family, and spiritual practices
3. Encouraging her to verbalize her anger and fears about her diagnosis and the impact it will have on her life
4. Promoting open communication of thoughts and feelings between the patient and her family

NURSING CARE PLAN Patient After A Modified Radical Mastectomy—cont'd

Planning: Outcome Criteria	Nursing Interventions and Rationales
➤ **NURSING DIAGNOSIS**	Self-esteem disturbance *related to* altered body image and loss of body part *as manifested by* verbalization of concern about appearance and feelings of loss of femininity, depression, refusal to view incision, fear of intimacy
Verbalize feelings about surgery and change in body image; indicate beginning resolution of negative feelings toward self; accept altered body image.	Assess degree of self-esteem disturbance *so appropriate interventions can be initiated.* Arrange for Reach to Recovery visitor or similar community resource, if available, *to serve as a role model and provide hope for recovery and a normal future.* Provide information regarding prosthesis fitting and breast reconstruction (if patient is interested) *so patient can make informed decisions regarding options.* Assist patient to verbalize feelings and encourage open communication with significant others *to promote grief work and maintain support from family and friends.* Share information regarding community resources (e.g., support groups, information services) *to enable patient to find a place to exchange concerns and feelings about the experience.*
➤ **NURSING DIAGNOSIS**	Impaired physical mobility *related to* decreased arm and shoulder mobility *as manifested by* limitation in movement of upper extremity on surgical side
Return to usual arm and shoulder function.	Assess degree of mobility impairment *to provide baseline data* for evaluation of plan and *to plan appropriate interventions.* Flex and extend fingers in postoperative care area and continue throughout postoperative period *to maintain range of motion and promote arm circulation.* Carry out postmastectomy exercises to *prevent contractures and muscle shortening, maintain muscle tone, and improve lymph and blood circulation.* Assist woman to resume activities of daily living as tolerated or as directed by physician *to reduce dependent behaviors, raise self-esteem, and maintain mobility of affected arm.* Emphasize bilateral activity of upper extremities *to prevent guarding of operative side and loss of function.*

COLLABORATIVE PROBLEMS

Nursing Goals	Nursing Interventions and Rationales
➤ **POTENTIAL COMPLICATION**	Lymphedema *related to* edema on operative side and lack of knowledge of preventive measures
Monitor for signs of lymphedema; report deviations from acceptable parameters; carry out appropriate medical and nursing interventions.	Assess woman for signs of lymphedema such as edema in hand or arm on operative side, heaviness, or localized pain *to enable early diagnosis and intervention to prevent/treat the complication.* Instruct patient about self-care strategies and precautions to reduce risk of lymphedema *so patient will be an active, informed participant in self-care.* Do not perform venipunctures or take blood pressure measurements in affected arm *to reduce risk of constriction, infection, and lymphedema in affected arm.* Avoid dependent arm position *to allow proper wound healing and decrease stress to incision site.* Elevate arm and hand on pillow *to use gravity to assist with drainage of fluid.* Restrict abducting arm for first week *to allow proper wound healing and prevent incisional stress.* Perform hand and wrist movements, elbow flexion, and extension hourly or as indicated *to maintain circulation and range of motion of affected arm.* Encourage participation in activities of daily living and self-care as much as possible *to promote patient's independence and maintain use of affected arm.* Use elastic sleeve if ordered *to apply mechanical pressure to reduce fluid collection in affected arm and promote venous return.*

BSE, Breast self-examination.
*Also applies to the patient following breast conservation therapy.

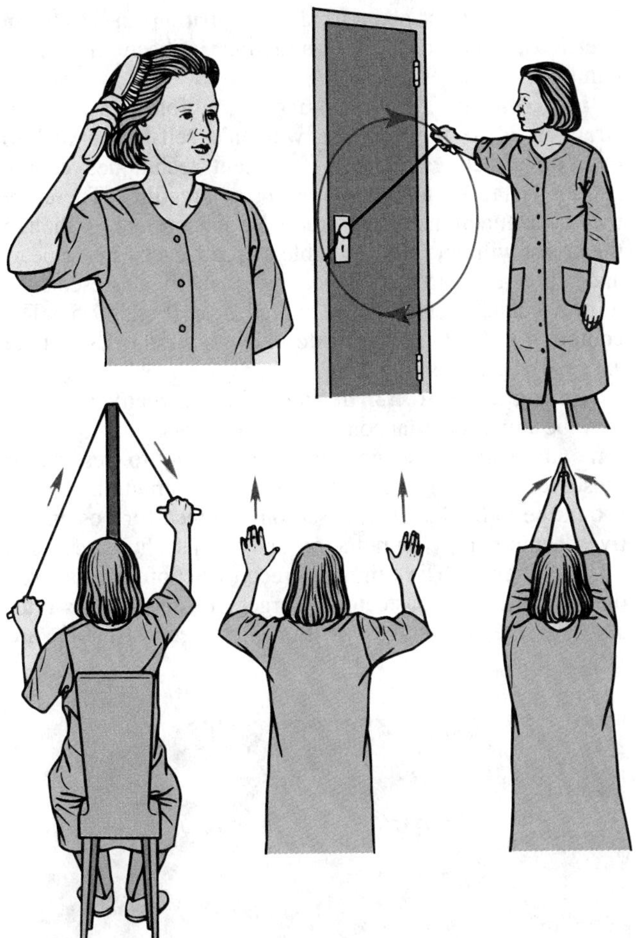

Fig. 49-4 Postoperative mastectomy exercises.

5. Providing accurate and complete answers to questions about her disease, treatment options, and reproductive/lactation issues (if appropriate)
6. Offering information about community resources, such as Reach to Recovery, Encore, and local support organizations and groups

The nurse can promote the woman's recovery by arranging a visit from a woman who had similar treatment, such as a Reach to Recovery volunteer, if the service is available. The Reach to Recovery Program of the American Cancer Society is a rehabilitation program for women who have had breast surgery. It is designed to help them meet their psychologic, physical, and cosmetic needs. The volunteers, who are all women who have had breast cancer, can answer questions about what to expect at home, how to tell people about the surgery, and what prosthetic devices are available. If a Reach to Recovery volunteer is not available, it is the nurse's responsibility to be knowledgeable about the needs of the woman after breast surgery. The American Cancer Society and the National Cancer Institute can provide excellent materials to assist the nurse in meeting the special needs of women with breast cancer.

The professional staff must never underestimate the tremendous psychologic impact that a diagnosis of cancer and subsequent breast surgery can have on a woman. Emotional complications are common. The nurse's accepting, concerned attitude can do a great deal to relieve the feelings of anger and depression experienced by many patients.

Chronic and Home Management. The nurse should explain the follow-up routine to the patient and emphasize the importance of beginning and continuing BSE and annual mammography. Symptoms that should be reported to the clinician include new back pain, weakness, constipation, shortness of breath, and confusion. If adjuvant therapy is to be used, the woman should have specific instructions about appointment times and treatment locations.

The nurse should stress the importance of wearing a well-fitting prosthesis. A variety of products are available to meet the specific needs of the individual woman. A well-trained salesperson can help the woman select a suitable prosthesis. There are both physical and psychologic advantages to the use of a prosthesis; the return of a normal external appearance is especially important to most women.

The implications of loss of a breast on the sexual identity and relationships of the woman vary.[28] A preoperative sexual assessment provides helpful baseline data that the nurse can use to plan postoperative interventions. Often the husband, sexual partner, or family members may need assistance in dealing with their emotional reactions to the diagnosis and surgery for them to act as effective means of support for the patient.[29] There are no physical reasons for a mastectomy to prevent sexual satisfaction. The woman taking tamoxifen may have a decreased sexual drive or vaginal dryness. She may need to use lubrication to prevent discomfort during intercourse. If difficulty in adjustment or other problems develop, counseling may be necessary to deal with the emotional component of a mastectomy and the diagnosis of cancer.

Initial coping mechanisms often begin to lose effectiveness at about 3 months, and a period of depression ensues. It is important that the nurse provide anticipatory guidance for this eventuality. Special nursing interventions are necessary, in terms of both psychologic support and self-care education, if a recurrence of cancer is found. Participation in a cancer support group is important and has been found to have a clinically significant impact on survival.

Paget's Disease

Paget's disease is a breast malignancy characterized by a persistent eczematoid lesion of the nipple and areola with or without a palpable mass. Itching, bloody nipple discharge, erosion, and ulceration may be present. Diagnosis of Paget's disease is confirmed by pathologic examination of the surgical specimen. (Paget disease of the bone is discussed in Chapter 59.) The treatment of Paget's disease is a simple or modified radical mastectomy. The nursing care for the patient with Paget's disease is the same as the care for a patient with any breast carcinoma.

MAMMOPLASTY

Mammoplasty is the surgical change in the size or shape of the breast. It may be done electively for cosmetic purposes to either enlarge or reduce the size of the breasts. It may also be done to reconstruct the breast after a mastectomy.

Health care providers should remain nonjudgmental toward women who desire mammoplasty. The desire to alter the appearance of the breasts has special significance for each woman as she attempts to alter or re-create her body image. It is important for the nurse to be aware of the cultural value placed on the breast by the woman. The U.S. "Playboy" mentality invests a great deal of sexuality with the female breast. This is not necessarily a shared cross-cultural attitude.

The woman's motives should not be questioned. It is important, however, that the woman have a realistic idea about what mammoplasty can accomplish and about possible complications, such as hematoma formation, hemorrhage, and infection. If an implant is involved, capsular contracture and loss of the implant are possible.

Breast Augmentation

In *augmentation mammoplasty* (the procedure to enlarge the breasts) an implant is placed in a surgically created pocket between the capsule of the breast and the pectoral fascia. Most implants are silicone envelopes filled with a fluid such as dextran, saline, or silicone. Because of their resemblance to the human breast, implants filled with silicone were the most widely used. In April of 1992, the Food and Drug Administration (FDA) suspended the use of silicone implants in response to potential hazards related to silicone leakage. However, the FDA has approved silicone implants for use in postmastectomy reconstructive surgery for breast cancer patients. Their use in breast augmentation not related to breast cancer is still limited to clinical trials.

Breast Reduction

For some women, large breasts can be a source of pain and embarrassment. They can interfere with normal daily activities such as walking, typing, and driving a car. Overly large breasts can interfere with self-esteem and self-image and can lead to back, shoulder, and neck problems. They may make stylish dressing more difficult. Reduction in the size of the breasts can have positive effects on both the psychologic and the physical health of the patient. Reduction mammoplasty is performed by resecting wedges of tissue from the upper and lower quadrants of the breast. The excess skin is removed, and the areola and nipple are relocated on the breast. Lactation can usually be accomplished if massive amounts of tissue are not removed and the nipples are left connected during surgery.

Breast Reconstruction

Breast reconstruction can be done at the time of mastectomy or any time after mastectomy. Recent advances in techniques have made breast reconstruction a satisfactory alternative for many women. The possibility of breast reconstruction may encourage women to seek professional help if a breast lump is detected. Women are demanding more information about and participation in treatment decisions, and breast reconstruction is becoming more common and accepted.

Indications. The main indication for breast reconstruction is to improve the woman's self-image and to overcome feelings of loss.[30] Present techniques cannot restore lactation, nipple sensation, or erectility. Therefore the erotic functions of the breast are not present. Although the breast will not fully resemble its premastectomy appearance, the reconstructed appearance usually represents an improvement over the mastectomy scar (Fig. 49-5). The contour of the breast is restored without the use of an external prosthesis.

Timing of Reconstruction. Reconstructive surgery may be done simultaneously with a mastectomy or some time afterward to achieve symmetry and to restore or preserve body image. The timing of reconstruction surgery should be individualized, based on the need for postoperative chemotherapy or radiation and the psychologic needs of the patient.[12] The timing of reconstruction ranges from during the initial mastectomy surgery to many years after surgery. The advantages to immediate reconstruction are

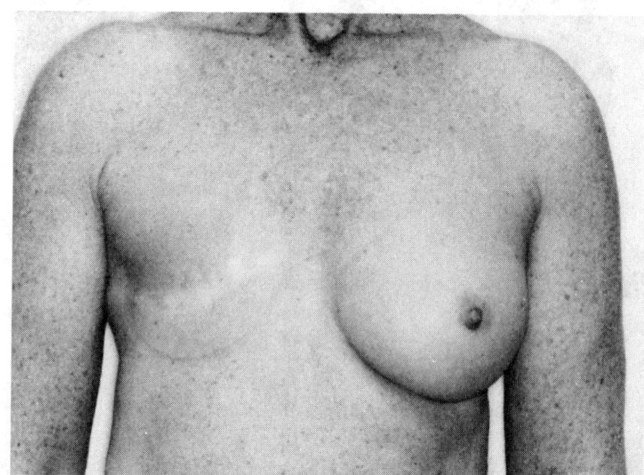

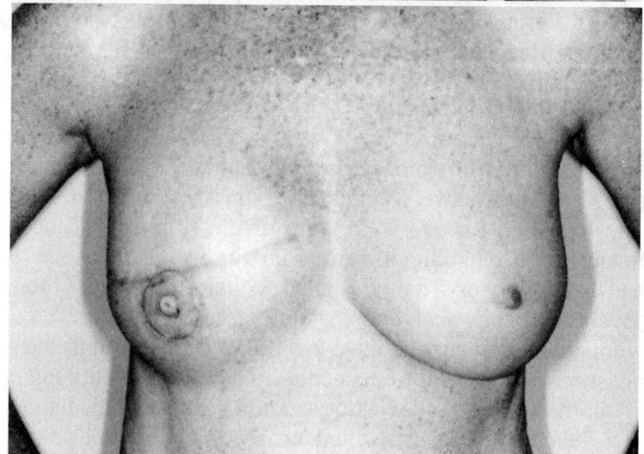

Fig. 49-5 ***A,*** Appearance of chest following right modified radical mastectomy. ***B,*** Appearance of chest following breast reconstruction using a tissue expander.

one hospital admission, one trip to surgery, one anesthesia induction, and one recovery period. Also, surgery takes place before the development of scar tissue or adhesions. The disadvantages are more incisions, more blood loss, more surgical drains, more time under anesthesia, a longer recovery period, and a slightly longer hospitalization.[31] Early reconstruction does not retard or influence further treatment or adversely affect predicted survival. Timing of reconstruction may depend on insurance coverage. Some plans reimburse only within a specified period of time.

Techniques of Reconstruction. The extent of the reconstruction depends on the type of mastectomy done. If extensive chest-wall defects are not present, a tissue expander can be used to stretch the skin and muscle at the mastectomy site. Placement of the expander can be performed at the time of mastectomy or at a later date. The tissue expander, which is fully deflated at the time of surgery, is gradually filled by weekly injections of sterile water or saline solution, which stretch the skin and muscle. Once the tissue is adequately stretched, the expander is surgically removed and the permanent implant is inserted. Some expanders are designed to remain in place and become the implant, eliminating the need for a second surgical procedure.

The silicone gel implant came under the scrutiny of the media and the government in 1992. Allegations of associated immune-related diseases caused or exacerbated by the presence of silicone gel implants have caused considerable controversy and litigation. Since 1992, the FDA has placed restrictions on the use of silicone gel implants. Patients must sign an informed consent stating that the patient is aware of all the risks involving silicone and that the patient agrees to be included in all FDA-mandated research.[32]

If insufficient muscle is left after mastectomy or if the chest wall has been radiated, myocutaneous flaps may be used to repair the soft-tissue defects. Flaps are most often taken from the back (latissimus dorsi muscle) or the abdomen (transverse rectus abdominis muscle). An implant may be used in addition to the flap if the flap does not provide the desired cosmetic result alone. If sufficient abdominal tissue is present, it may be used to reconstruct the breast in place of an implant. The nipple-areolar complex may be reconstructed. Tissue to construct a nipple may be taken from the ear or great toe. The areola may be grafted from the labia or may be tattooed with a permanent pigmented dye. If the nipple-areolar complex is completely free of malignancy and is to be saved, it can be sutured to the groin or abdomen to continue adequate blood supply until the reconstructive process is performed.

The body's natural response to the presence of a foreign substance is the formation of a fibrous capsule around the implant. If excessive capsular formation occurs as a result of infection, hematoma, trauma, or reaction to a foreign body, a contracture can develop, resulting in a deformed breast. Surgeons differ in their approaches to the prevention of contracture formation, although gentle manual massage around the implant is routine. Prevention of the problems that cause excessive capsule formation is critical. Other postoperative complications include skin ulceration, hypertrophic scar formation, intercostal neuralgia, and wound infection.

NURSING MANAGEMENT

MAMMOPLASTY

Mammoplasty may be done in the outpatient surgical area, or it may involve overnight hospitalization. General anesthesia is used. Drains are generally placed in the surgical site to prevent hematoma formation and then removed 2 to 3 days after surgery or when drainage is under 20 ml per day. The drainage must be examined for color and odor to detect postoperative infection or hemorrhage. The woman's temperature should also be monitored. Dressings should be changed as necessary using sterile technique. In cases in which a nipple graft has been performed, the dressings should not be disturbed for 7 to 10 days. After surgery the woman needs to be assured that the appearance of the breast will improve when sutures are removed and healing is completed. Blackening of the reimplanted nipple immediately after the operation is expected. The patient should be instructed to wear a bra that provides good support continuously for 2 to 3 days after mammoplasty. Depending on the extent of the operation, most women can resume normal activities within 2 to 3 weeks. Strenuous exercise may not be appropriate until several weeks later.

CRITICAL THINKING EXERCISES

CASE STUDY

BREAST CANCER

Patient Profile

Sara J., a 42-year-old woman, discovered a large lump in the upper outer quadrant of her right breast while showering.

Subjective Data

- Has family history of breast cancer
- Had onset of menarche at age 11
- Has two daughters, first birth at age 33
- Has no previous history of breast cancer
- States she is afraid she has cancer

Objective Data

- Large fixed palpable mass in upper outer quadrant of right breast and 2 palpable lymph nodes
- 4-5 cm mass in her right breast confirmed by mammogram
- Otherwise normal physical examination
- Incisional biopsy and one axillary node positive for cancer

Therapeutic Management

- Scheduled for modified radical mastectomy and axillary lymph node dissection

Critical Thinking Questions

1. What characteristics of malignancy could be determined by palpation of Sara's breast mass?
2. What information would the nurse provide to Sara about her planned therapy?
3. What information about breast cancer risks is important for the nurse to provide to Sara and her daughters? What early detection measures are important for them to know?
4. What are the possible complications the patient may face after a modified radical mastectomy?
5. What are common postoperative exercises that Sara will need to practice?
6. What community resources are available to help Sara and her family adjust to the change in her body and to cope with the diagnosis of cancer? How can the nurse access these resources?
7. Based on the assessment data presented, write one or more appropriate nursing diagnoses. Are there any collaborative problems?

NURSING RESEARCH ISSUES

1. What are the major concerns of women who are diagnosed with breast cancer?
2. Does use of a skin film increase sensitivity when performing a breast self-examination?
3. Does attendance at a cancer support group decrease anxiety in women who elect to have breast conservation surgery and radiation?
4. What influence does immediate versus delayed reconstruction have on the psychosocial adjustment of a woman after a mastectomy?
5. What effect does dietary intake of caffeine have on a woman's perception of the severity of fibrocystic changes in the breast?
6. Does perceived susceptibility to breast cancer increase a woman's motivation to practice breast self-examination?
7. What is the influence of individualized teaching by a health professional on the frequency of breast self-examination practice in women?

REVIEW QUESTIONS

The number of the question corresponds to the same-numbered objective at the beginning of the chapter.

1. BSE involves both the palpation of the breast tissue and

a. a physical examination.
b. inspection of the breasts for changes in the skin.
c. mammographic evaluation of the breast tissue.
d. squeezing the breast tissue.

2. In addition to an annual CBE, all women over 50 years of age should

a. have mammographic evaluation every 1 to 2 years.
b. perform monthly BSE and have mammography done yearly.
c. avoid harmful radiation exposure from frequent mammograms.
d. have no additional examination.

3. A woman experiencing lactational mastitis will have the clinical symptoms of

a. a painless, round, well-delineated lesion in the breast.
b. firm, rubbery breast lesions bilaterally.
c. a localized area of erythema, painful to palpation.
d. bloody discharge from the nipple with no palpable lesions in the breast.

4. The incidence of breast cancer

a. remains unchanged throughout the life span.
b. decreases after the age of 60.
c. increases after the age of 60.
d. is equal in men and women.

5. Classification of cancer into stages allows

a. for increased recovery from surgery.
b. for a more accurate determination of prognosis and treatment options.
c. the patient to select treatments.
d. for constant surveillance of disease progression.

6. The definitive test for a breast malignancy is

a. mammogram.
b. ultrasound.
c. incisional biopsy.
d. staging.

7. Measures to prevent or reduce lymphedema include all of the following *except*

a. never position the affected arm in a dependent position.
b. protection of the affected arm from trauma.
c. treatment with an inflatable sleeve.
d. early postoperative use of elastic bandages.

8. Postoperative complications associated with breast reconstruction include all of the following *except*

a. skin ulceration.
b. intercostal neuralgia.
c. metastatic spread of the breast cancer.
d. wound infection.

REFERENCES

1. Grier S: Breast cancer: prevention and detection, *Oncol Patient Care* 3:5, 1993.
2. Mettlin C and others: Defining and updating the American Cancer Society guidelines for the cancer related checkup: prostate and endometrial cancers, *CA Cancer J Clin* 43:42, 1993.
3. Scanlon EF: Breast cancer. In Holleb AI, Fink DJ, Murphy GP, editors: *American Cancer Society textbook of clinical oncology,* Atlanta, 1991, American Cancer Society.
4. Steinberger C: Breast self-examination: how nurses can influence performance, *Medsurg Nurs* 3:367, 1994.
5. Goodman M, Harte N: Breast cancer. In Groenwald SL and others, editors: *Cancer nursing principles and practice,* ed 2, Boston, 1990, Jones & Bartlett.
6. Freundlich IM: Mammographic screening for breast cancer, *Cancer Bulletin* 44:17, 1992.
7. Marrow M: Breast pain. In Harris JR and others, editors: *Breast diseases,* ed 2, Philadelphia, 1991, Lippincott.
8. Miller AB and others: Canadian national breast screening study, 1. Breast cancer detection and death rates among women aged 40 to 49 years. 2. Breast cancer detection and death rates among women aged 50 to 59 years, *Can Med Assoc J* 147:459, 1992.
9. Deckers PJ, Ricci A: Pain and lumps in the female breast, *Hosp Pract* 27:67, 1992.
10. Lynch H: Hereditary breast cancer and family cancer syndromes, *World J Surg* 18:21, 1994.
11. Thompson WD: Genetic epidemiology of breast cancer, *Cancer Supplement* 74:279, 1994.
12. Harris JR and others: Breast cancer, *N Engl J Med* 327:319, 1992.
13. Shapiro CL, Hayes DF: Cancer screening and prevention, *Contemp Intern Med* 5:60, 1993.
14. Osborne CK: Prognostic factors in breast cancer, *Principles Pract Oncol* 4:1, 1990.
15. Kallioniemi O and others: Tumour DNA ploidy as an independent prognostic factor in breast cancer, *Br J Cancer* 56:367, 1987.
16. Stewart J: Breast cancer: recurrent disease, *Hosp Pract* 29:59, 1994.
17. Beahrs OH and others: *Manual for staging of cancer,* ed 4, Philadelphia, 1992, Lippincott.
18. Madeya ML, Pfab-Tokarsky JM: Flow cytometry: an overview, *Oncol Nurs Forum* 19:459, 1992.
19. Early breast cancer trialists; collaborative group: systemic treatment of early breast cancer by hormonal, cytotopic, or immune therapy: 133 randomized trials involving 31,000 recurrences and 24,000 deaths among 75,000 women (parts 1 and 2), *Lancet* 339:71, 1992.
20. Steward JA: Breast cancer I: screening and early management, *Hosp Pract* 29:83, 1994.
21. Boring CC, Squires TS, Tong T: Cancer statistics, *CA Cancer J Clin* 43:7, 1993.
22. Dorr FA: Adjuvant therapy of breast cancer: current clinical trials and future decisions. In Fowble and others, editors: *Breast cancer treatment,* St Louis, 1991, Mosby.
23. Honig SF, Swain SM: Hormonal manipulation in the adjuvant treatment of breast cancer. In DeVita VT, Hellman S, Rosenberg SA, editors: *Important advances in oncology 1993,* Philadelphia, 1993, Lippincott.
24. Fisher AB and others: Endometrial cancer in tamoxifen-treated breast cancer patients: findings from the National Surgical Adjuvant Breast and Bowel Project, *J Natl Cancer Inst* 86:478, 1994.
25. Gould K, Gates ML, Miaskowski C: Breast cancer prevention: a summary of the chemoprevention trial with tamoxifen, *Oncol Nurs Forum* 21:835, 1994.
26. Jordan VC: Targeted hormone therapy for breast cancer, *Hosp Pract* 28:58, 1993.
27. Dudas S: Altered body image and sexuality. In Groenwald SL and others, editors: *Cancer nursing principles and practice,* ed 3, Boston, 1993, Jones & Bartlett.
28. Knoff MT: Treatment options for early stage breast cancer, *Medsurg Nurs* 3:252, 1994.
29. Snodgrass SE, editor: *Communicating about breast cancer: help me to tell you,* monograph, Research Triangle Park, NC, 1992, Burroughs Welcome.
30. Johnson JR: Caring for the woman who's had a mastectomy, *Am J Nurs* 94:26, 1994.
31. Hidalgo DA: Are breast prostheses safe for use in breast reconstruction? Yes. In DeVita VT, Hellman S, and Rosenberg SA, editors: *Important advances in oncology,* Philadelphia, 1993, Lippincott.
32. Geomieso CB, Suster V: Free flap breast reconstruction, *Medsurg Nurs* 3:11, 1994.

Chapter 50

NURSING ROLE IN MANAGEMENT

Sexually Transmitted Diseases

Janis Luft **Linda C. Carnago**

Learning Objectives

1. Identify the factors contributing to the high incidence of sexually transmitted diseases.
2. Explain the etiology, clinical manifestations, complications, and diagnostic abnormalities of gonorrhea, syphilis, genital herpes, chlamydial infections, and condylomata acuminata.
3. Compare primary genital herpes with recurrent genital herpes.
4. Explain the therapeutic and pharmacologic management of gonorrhea, syphilis, genital herpes, chlamydial infections, and condylomata acuminata.
5. Identify nursing assessment and nursing diagnoses for patients who have a sexually transmitted disease.
6. Describe the nursing role in the prevention and control of sexually transmitted diseases.
7. Describe the nursing management of patients with sexually transmitted diseases.

SEXUALLY TRANSMITTED DISEASES

Sexually transmitted diseases (STDs) are infectious diseases usually associated with intimate sexual contact. Historically they have been referred to as *venereal diseases.* The existence of syphilis and gonorrhea is generally known, but there are many other diseases that can be sexually transmitted (Table 50-1). Some STDs, such as chancroid and granuloma inguinale, are more common in tropical and semitropical areas. However, with the mobility of modern society, their occurrence in other areas of the world is increasing. Diseases that are associated with sexual transmission can also be contracted by other routes such as through blood, blood products, and accidental inoculation. Common STDs are discussed in this chapter. Human immunodeficiency virus (HIV) infection and related problems are discussed in Chapter 11.

Significance

In the United States all cases of gonorrhea and syphilis must be reported to the state or local health officer. In spite of this requirement, there are many unreported and undiagnosed cases. Often, various STDs coexist; for instance, if a person has gonorrhea, chlamydial infection may also be present. Gonorrhea ranks first and syphilis ranks third among the communicable diseases reported in the United States. The incidence of gonorrhea steadily increased after 1966 but began to decline in 1975. This trend continued throughout the 1980s, possibly influenced by more focused control activities, changes in surveillance and reporting procedures, and changes in host factors. While the overall number of cases of gonorrhea has been declining since 1975, the prevalence of resistant strains of gonorrhea, primarily penicillinase-producing *Neisseria gonorrhoeae* (PPNG), has been increasing steadily during the same time period.[1] Teenagers and young adults account for 25% to 40% of all gonorrhea cases reported. Most states have enacted laws that permit examination and treatment of minors without parental consent.

The incidence of primary and secondary syphilis has changed since 1941 (Fig. 50-1), mainly because of the availability of penicillin. Between 1986 and 1990 syphilis infections in the United States rose dramatically. The Centers for Disease Control (CDC) received reports of more than 50,000 cases of primary and secondary syphilis, the highest number of cases since 1948. But in 1991, a 15% decline in infections over the previous year was seen, the first decline since 1985.[2] The reasons for this decline are unclear but the recognition of the epidemic rise of syphilis and a renewed priority in screening, treating, and educating at-risk populations by health care providers may have been a factor.

Because genital herpes, *Chlamydia trachomatis* infections, and condylomata acuminata (genital warts) are not reportable diseases in most states, their true incidence is difficult to determine. It is estimated that more than 30 million people in the United States are infected with genital herpes and that an

---

Reviewed by Mary Ann Faucher, BSN, MS, MPH, CNM, Faculty Associate, University of Texas Southwestern Medical Center, Dallas, TX.

Table 50-1 Microorganisms Responsible for Diseases Transmitted by Sexual Activity

Organism	Disease
Chlamydia trachomatis	Nongonococcal urethritis (NGU); cervicitis; lymphogranuloma venereum
Cytomegalovirus (CMV)	Multiple diseases
Hepatitis B virus	Hepatitis B
Herpes simplex virus (HSV)	Genital herpes
Human immuno-deficiency virus (HIV)	HIV infection, acquired immuno-deficiency syndrome (AIDS)
Human papillomavirus	Genital and anal warts
Molluscum contagiosum virus	Molluscum contagiosum
Neisseria gonorrhoeae	Gonorrhea
Treponema pallidum	Syphilis

additional 50,000 new cases occur each year.[3] Infections caused by *C. trachomatis* are the most prevalent bacterial STDs in the United States today.[4] Chlamydia is found to be the causative organism in one third to one half of all cases of nongonococcal urethritis in men, and is also found concurrently in 15% to 35% of men with gonococcal urethritis.[5] Chlamydial infections are a common cause (25% to 40%) of pelvic inflammatory disease (PID).[6] Genital warts, the primary clinical manifestation of human papilloma virus (HPV), have become increasingly common with an estimated annual incidence of 500,000 to 1 million cases. There is a relationship between certain strains of HPV and genital cancer.

Factors Affecting Incidence of Sexually Transmitted Diseases

There are contributing factors to the increased incidence of STDs. Earlier reproductive maturity and increased longevity have resulted in a longer sexual life span. The increase in the total population has resulted in an increase in the number of susceptible hosts. Other factors include greater sexual freedom, changing roles of women, changes in the institutions of marriage and the family, decreased social control by religious institutions, and an increased emphasis on sexuality on the part of the media. In many studies, the incidence of drug abuse is closely correlated with increasing numbers of cases of STDs.[8,9] In addition, increased leisure time, inexpensive travel, and urbanization have brought together people of varying cultural backgrounds and value systems.

Changes in the methods of contraception are also reflected in the incidence of STDs. The condom is considered to be the only contraceptive device that is prophylactic in regard to STDs. Although condom use is increasing in selected populations, it is not used frequently in the general population.[10,11] Commonly used oral contraceptives cause the secretions of the cervix and the vagina to become more alkaline. This change produces a more favorable environment for the growth of organisms that cause STDs at these sites. Women who take oral contraceptives have a lower risk of PID as a result of the ability of the cervical mucus to act as a barrier against bacteria. However, the proliferation of chlamydia, the leading cause of nongonococcal PID, may be enhanced by oral contraceptive use.[11] Whether or not intrauterine device users are at increased risk of PID is controversial,[12,13] but it is clear that IUDs confer no protection against STDs. The impact of long-acting contraception such as Norplant and Depo Provera on the incidence of STDs is unknown. However, they confer no protection against STDs. Lack of awareness of this fact may be a factor leading to STDs in persons using these products.

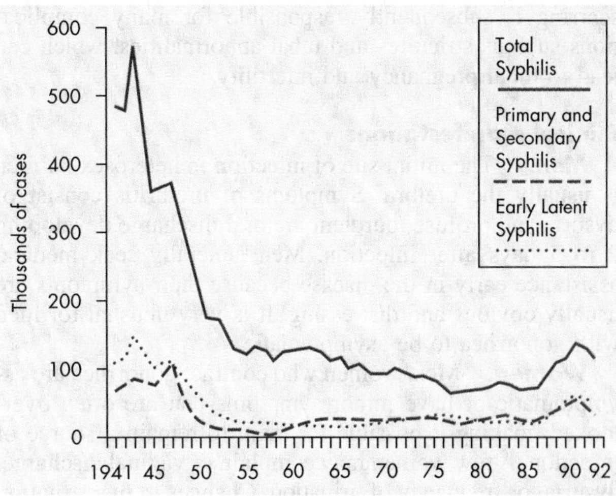

Fig. 50-1 Syphilis. Reported cases by stage of illness: United States, 1941 to 1992.

GONORRHEA

Pathophysiology

Gonorrhea is caused by *Neisseria gonorrhoeae,* a gram-negative diplococcus. Mucosa with columnar epithelium is susceptible to gonococcal infection. This tissue is present in the genitalia (the urethra in men, the cervix in women), the rectum, and the oropharynx. The disease is spread by direct physical contact with an infected host, usually during sexual activity. Neonates can develop a gonococcal infection after passage through an infected birth canal. The delicate gonococcus is easily killed by drying, heating, or washing with an antiseptic solution. Consequently, indirect transmission by instruments or linens is rare. The incubation period is 3 to 4 days. The disease confers no immunity to subsequent reinfection. Gonococcal infection elicits an inflammatory response, which, if left untreated, leads to the formation of fibrous tissue and adhesions. This fibrous scarring is subsequently responsible for many complications such as strictures and tubal abnormalities, which can lead to tubal pregnancy and infertility.

Clinical Manifestations

Men. The initial site of infection in heterosexual men is usually the urethra. Symptoms of urethritis consist of dysuria and profuse, purulent urethral discharge developing 2 to 5 days after infection. Men generally seek medical assistance early in the disease because their symptoms are usually obvious and distressing. It is very unusual for men with gonorrhea to be asymptomatic.

Women. Most women who contract gonorrhea are asymptomatic or have minor symptoms that are often overlooked, making it possible for them to remain a source of infection. A few women may complain of vaginal discharge, dysuria, or frequency of urination. Changes in menstruation may be a symptom, but these changes are often disregarded by the woman. After the incubation period, redness and swelling occur at the site of contact, which is usually the cervix or urethra. A purulent exudate often develops with a potential for abscess formation. The disease may remain local or can spread by direct tissue extension to the uterus, fallopian tubes, and ovaries. Although the vulva and vagina are uncommon sites for a gonorrheal infection, they may become involved when little or no estrogen is present, as is the case in prepubertal girls and postmenopausal women. Because the vagina acts as a natural reservoir for infectious secretions, transmission is often more efficient from men to women than it is from women to men.

General. Anorectal gonorrhea may be present, particularly in homosexual men, and is usually caused by anal intercourse. Gonococcal proctitis in women probably results from rectal coitus as well as contamination from infected vaginal secretions. Most patients with rectal infections have no significant symptoms. A small percentage of individuals develop gonococcal pharyngitis resulting from orogenital sexual contact. When the gonococcus can be demonstrated by culture, individuals of either gender are infectious to their sexual partners.

Complications

Because men often seek treatment early in the course of the disease, they are less likely to develop complications. The complications that do occur in men are prostatitis, urethral strictures, and sterility from orchitis or epididymitis. Because women who are free of symptoms seldom seek treatment, complications are more common and usually constitute the reason for seeking medical attention. PID, Bartholin abscess, ectopic pregnancy, and infertility are the main complications of gonorrhea in women. A small percentage of infected persons, mainly women, may develop a disseminated gonococcal infection (DGI). In disseminated infection the appearance of skin lesions, fever, arthralgia, or arthritis usually causes the patient to seek medical help.

Eye Infections in Newborns. Almost all states have a health department regulation or law requiring the instillation of a prophylactic drug such as erythromycin (0.5%) or silver nitrate into the eyes of all newborns.[14] The incidence of gonorrheal eye infections in newborns (*ophthalmia neonatorum*) is, therefore, relatively rare today. Untreated infected infants develop permanent blindness.

Diagnostic Studies

The most reliable way to confirm gonococcal infection is to isolate the organism in culture. The immediate identification of *N. gonorrhoeae* is usually made with a Gram stain of smears made from the exudate. The slides should be interpreted by an experienced technician so that a correct diagnosis is made initially, since some patients fail to return for follow-up care. Cultures of the discharge or secretion can provide a definitive diagnosis after incubation for 24 to 48 hours. No effective blood test is available for the diagnosis of gonorrhea.

For men, a presumptive diagnosis of gonorrhea is made if there is a history of sexual contact with an infected individual followed within a few days by a urethral discharge. Typical clinical manifestations, combined with a positive finding in a Gram-stained smear of the purulent discharge from the penis, gives an almost certain diagnosis. Culture of the discharge is indicated for men whose smears are negative in the presence of strong clinical evidence.

Making a diagnosis of gonorrhea in women on the basis of symptoms is difficult because most women are symptom free or have complaints that may be confused with other conditions. Smears and purulent discharge do not establish a diagnosis of gonorrhea because the female genitourinary (GU) tract normally harbors a large number of organisms that resemble *N. gonorrhoeae.* A culture must be performed to confirm the diagnosis. Although the cervix is the most common site of sampling, specimens may also be taken from the urethra, anus, or oropharynx to confirm the diagnosis. The CDC recommends that all women treated for gonorrhea have a rectal culture done.

For culture, a specific medium (Thayer-Martin), which encourages the growth of the gonococcus, is used. If laboratory facilities are not readily accessible, special holding media are available. Alternative techniques for identification of gonococci have recently become available. These newer methods, including gene probe techniques and polymerase chain reaction, do not involve bacterial culture and are useful in situations where culture facilities are unavailable. The new tests, however, are currently only recommended as alternatives to culture as their specificity and sensitivity are inferior to that of culture methods.

Therapeutic and Pharmacologic Management

A history of sexual contact with a partner known to have gonorrhea is considered good evidence for the presence of gonorrhea. Because of a short incubation period and high infectivity, treatment is instituted without awaiting culture results, even in the absence of any signs or symptoms. The treatment of gonorrhea in the early stage is curative. Traditionally, the drug of choice for gonorrheal therapy had been penicillin, but changes have been made because of resistant strains of *N. gonorrhoeae* and the presence of coexisting chlamydial infection (Table 50-2).

Recently, a rapid increase in the number of cases of gonorrhea caused by resistant strains of *N. gonorrhoeae* has been identified (Fig. 50-2). The three most important

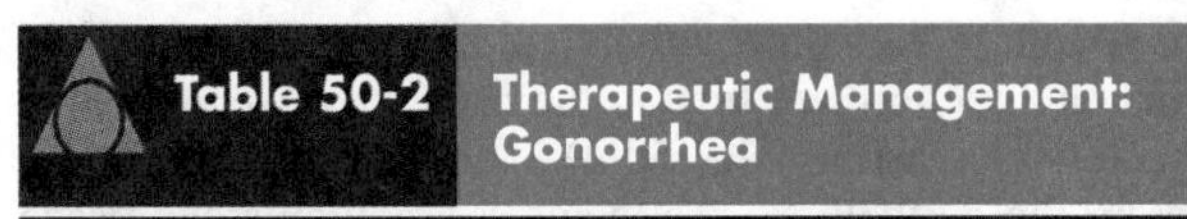

Table 50-2 Therapeutic Management: Gonorrhea

Diagnostic
- History and physical examination
- Gram-stained smears of urethral or endocervical exudate
- Cultures for *N. Gonorrhea*
- Testing for other STDs (syphilis, HIV, chlamydia)

Therapeutic*
- Uncomplicated gonorrhea: ceftriaxone (single dose IM) plus doxycycline
- Alternate therapy: doxycycline plus cefixime or ofloxacin or spectinomycin
- Follow-up cultures after completion of treatment (usually 7 days)
- Case finding
- Treatment of contacts
- Instruction on abstinence from sexual intercourse and alcohol
- Reexamination if symptoms persist or recur after completion of treatment
- Repeat of serologic test for syphilis at one month

Modified from Centers for Disease Control: STD treatment guidelines, *MMWR* 42:14, 1993.
HIV, Human immunodeficiency virus; *IM*, intramuscular; *STDs*, sexually transmitted diseases.

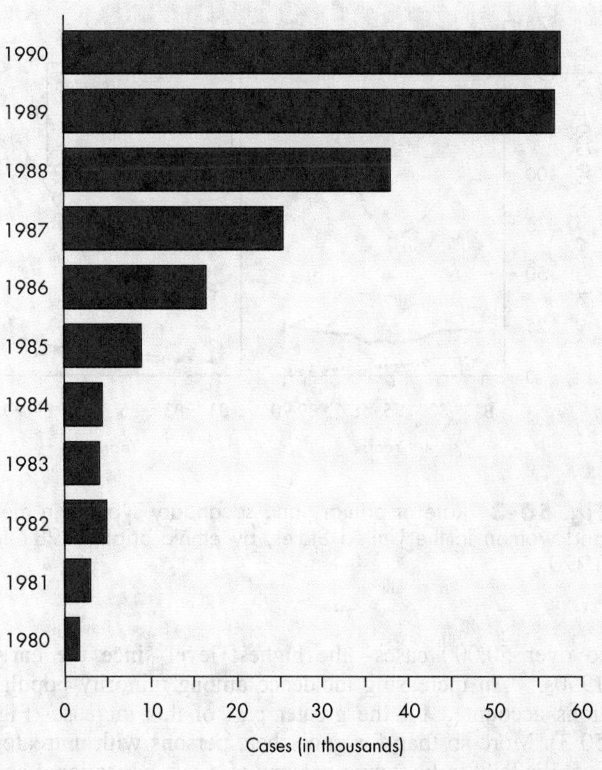

Fig. 50-2 Antibiotic-resistant gonorrhea. Reported cases: United States, 1980 to 1990.

mechanisms of antibiotic resistance from a public health standpoint are penicillinase producing (these strains first appeared in 1976), chromosomally mediated resistance to penicillin (strains displaying this mechanism first appeared in 1983), and plasmid-mediated high-level tetracycline resistance (these strains first appeared in 1985). In 1987 an outbreak of *N. gonorrhea* with chromosomally mediated resistance to spectinomycin was reported in American military personnel in Korea, but this strain remains rare in the United States and North America.[15]

There is no clinical distinction between infections caused by resistant or sensitive strains of *N. gonorrhoeae*. It was therefore anticipated that there would be increased numbers of disease-related complications (e.g., PID, DGI), extended periods of infectiveness resulting in increased numbers of sex partners becoming infected, and increased cost of treatment. As a result, ceftriaxone, a penicillinase-resistant cephalosporin, became part of the treatment plan. The high frequency (45%) of coexisting chlamydial and gonococcal infections has led to the addition of doxycycline or tetracycline to the treatment regimen. The expense of diagnosing chlamydial infection and the sequelae of chlamydial infection make this strategy cost effective. Patients with coincubating syphilis are likely to be cured by the same drugs.

All sexual contacts of patients with gonorrhea must be treated to prevent reinfection after resumption of sexual relations. The "ping-pong" effect of reexposure, treatment, and reinfection can cease only when infected partners are treated simultaneously. Additionally, the patient should be counseled to abstain from sexual intercourse and alcohol for 2 to 4 weeks. Sexual intercourse allows the infection to spread and can retard complete healing as a result of vascular congestion. Alcohol has an irritant effect on the healing urethral walls. Men should be cautioned against squeezing the penis to look for further discharge. Follow-up examination and reculture should be done at least once after treatment, usually in 4 to 7 days. Relapse, reinfection, and complications should be treated appropriately.

SYPHILIS

Etiology and Pathophysiology

The causative organism of syphilis is *Treponema pallidum*, a spirochete. It is extremely fragile and easily destroyed by drying, heating, or washing. The organism is thought to enter the body through very small breaks in the skin or mucous membranes. Its entry is facilitated by the minor abrasions that often occur during intercourse. Not all people who are exposed to syphilis acquire the disease; about one third become infected after intercourse with an infected person. In addition to sexual contact, syphilis may be spread through contact with infectious lesions and sharing of needles among drug addicts. Congenital syphilis is transmitted from an infected mother to the fetus in utero.

The incubation period for syphilis ranges from 10 to 90 days but is usually considered to be 3 weeks. Immunity to reinfection may develop if the disease is not eradicated during the primary stage.

Between 1984 and 1990, the number of reported cases of primary and secondary syphilis in the United States doubled

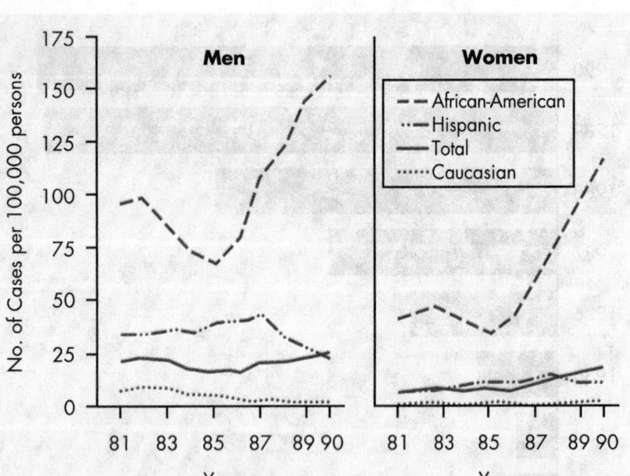

Fig. 50-3 Rate of primary and secondary syphilis in men and women in the United States, by ethnic origin, 1981 to 1990.

to over 50,000 cases—the highest level since the early 1950s.[16] An increasing incidence among minority populations accounted for the greater part of this increase (Fig. 50-3). More so than for gonorrhea, persons with untreated syphilis tend to be young persons of a low educational and socioeconomic level, a group that also has high rates of prostitution and drug abuse. This section of the population has proved to be extremely hard to reach for education and case finding.

Syphilis is a disease of the blood vessels. The tissue reaction to the presence of *T. pallidum* multiplying in the lymphatics and the perivascular spaces is characterized by dilatation and swelling of the capillaries and proliferation of the endothelium and a perivascular infiltration of lymphocytes, giant cells, and fibroblasts, with the formation of new blood vessels. Scar tissue formation is the method of healing in syphilis. The severity and extent of the damage varies.

There is an association between syphilis and HIV infection. Persons at highest risk for acquiring syphilis are also at high risk for acquiring HIV. Often, both infections are present in the same person. The presence of syphilitic lesions on the genitals enhances HIV transmission. HIV-infected patients with syphilis appear to be at greatest risk for clinically significant central nervous system (CNS) involvement and may require more intensive treatment with penicillin than do other patients with syphilis. Therefore, the evaluation of all patients with syphilis should also include serologic testing for HIV with the patient's consent.

Clinical Manifestations

Syphilis presents with a variety of signs and symptoms that can mimic a number of less serious diseases. Consequently, compared to other venereal diseases, it is more difficult to recognize syphilis. If it is not treated, specific clinical stages are characteristic of the progression of the disease (Table 50-3). *Chancres,* which are painless indurated lesions found on the penis, vulva, and lips, and in the mouth, vagina, and rectum, are seen in the *primary stage* at the site of bacterial invasion (Fig. 50-4). There, *T. pallidum* multiples in the epithelium, producing a granulomatous tissue reaction (chancre). Some of these microorganisms drain with the lymph into adjacent lymph nodes.

Secondary syphilis is systemic. During this stage bloodborne bacteria spread to all major organ systems. Manifestations characteristic of the secondary stage include cutaneous eruptions, alopecia (hair loss), and generalized adenopathy. The cutaneous eruptions include a bilateral, symmetrical rash usually involving the palms and soles; mucous patches in the mouth, tongue, or cervix; and *condyloma lata* (moist papules) in the anal and genital area (Fig. 50-5). *Latent syphilis* follows the secondary stage and is a period during which the immune system is able to suppress the infection. There are no signs or symptoms of syphilis during this time. The diagnosis is established by the finding of a positive specific treponemal antibody test for syphilis together with a normal cerebrospinal fluid (CSF) examination and the absence of clinical manifestations of syphilis on physical examination and chest radiograms. About 70% of untreated patients with latent syphilis never develop clinically evident late syphilis, but the occurrence of a spontaneous cure is in doubt.[17]

Late syphilis (also called tertiary syphilis) is the most severe stage of the disease. Because antibiotics can cure syphilis, manifestations of late syphilis are rare. However, when it does occur, it is responsible for significant morbidity and mortality. The pathogenesis of the manifestations of this stage is unclear. *Gummas* (destructive skin, bone, and soft tissue lesions associated with late syphilis) are probably caused by a severe hypersensitivity reaction to the microorganism. Within the cardiovascular system late syphilis may cause aneurysms, heart valve insufficiency, and heart failure. Within the CNS the presence of *T. pallidum* in CSF may cause manifestations of neurosyphilis (see Table 50-3).

Complications

Complications of the disease occur chiefly in late syphilis. The gummas of benign late syphilis may produce irreparable damage to bone, liver, or skin but seldom result in death. In cardiovascular syphilis, the resulting aneurysm may press on structures such as intercostal nerves, resulting in pain. The possibility of rupture exists as the aneurysm increases in size. Scarring of the aortic valve results in aortic valve insufficiency and, eventually, heart failure.

Neurosyphilis (general paresis) is responsible for degeneration of the brain with mental deterioration. Evidence of other neurologic deficits may be present. Problems related to sensory nerve involvement are a result of *tabes dorsalis* (progressive locomotor ataxia). There may be sudden attacks of pain anywhere in the body, which can confuse the diagnosis of conditions such as peptic ulcer. Loss of vision and sense of position in the feet and legs can also occur. Walking may become even more difficult as joint stability is lost. (Late syphilis is also discussed in Chapter 56.)

Table 50-3 Stages of Syphilis

Clinical Stage	Characteristic Findings	Communicability	Duration of Stage
Primary	Chancre	Exudate from chancre highly infectious; blood is infectious	3-8 wk
Secondary	Cutaneous eruptions, alopecia, systemic symptoms (malaise, arthralgia, headache, occasionally liver and kidney dysfunction), regional adenopathy 6-12 wk after chancre	Exudate from skin and mucous membrane lesions highly infectious	1-2 yr
Latent	Absence of signs or symptoms	Noninfectious after 4 yr, possible placental transmission	Throughout life or progression to late stage
Late*	Appearance 3-20 yr after initial infection	Noninfectious	Chronic (without treatment), possibly fatal
Benign	Gummas (chronic, destructive lesions affecting any organ of body, especially skin, bone, liver, mucous membranes)	Spinal fluid possibly containing organism	
	Aortic valve insufficiency or saccular aneurysm of thoracic aorta, aortitis		
Cardiovascular	General paresis (personality changes from minor to psychotic, tremors, physical and mental deterioration)		
Neurosyphilis	Tabes dorsalis (ataxia, areflexia, paresthesias, lightning pains, damaged joints [Charcot's joints])		

*Several forms such as cardiovascular and neurosyphilis occur together in approximately 25% of untreated cases.

Diagnostic Studies

The first step in diagnosis is to obtain a detailed history of sexual behavior. A physical examination should be done to identify any suspicious lesions as well as to note other significant signs and symptoms.

The presence of spirochetes on dark-field microscopy of tissue scrapings from primary or secondary lesions can confirm a clinical diagnosis of syphilis. However, syphilis is more commonly diagnosed by a serologic test. Tests for syphilis may be classified as those performed for screening and those performed for confirmation of a positive screening test. Nonspecific antitreponemal antibodies can be detected by tests such as the Venereal Disease Research Laboratory (VDRL) test and the rapid plasma reagin (RPR) test. These nontreponemal tests are suitable for screening purposes and usually become positive 10 to 14 days after the appearance of a chancre. The fluorescent treponemal antibody absorption (FTA-ABS) test and the microhemagglutination (MHA) test detect specific antitreponemal antibodies and are suitable for confirming the diagnosis.

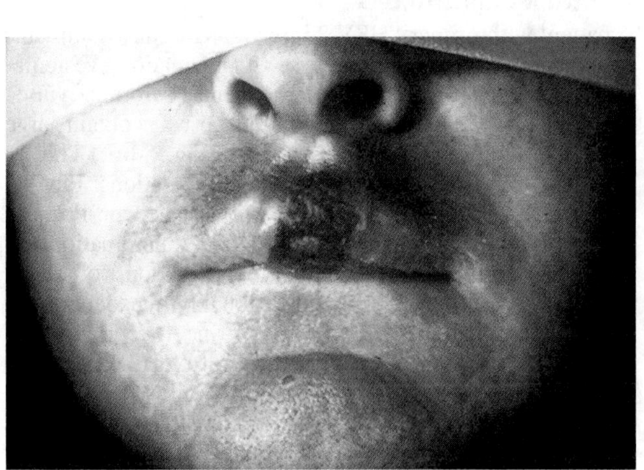

Fig. 50-4 Primary syphilis chancre on upper lip.

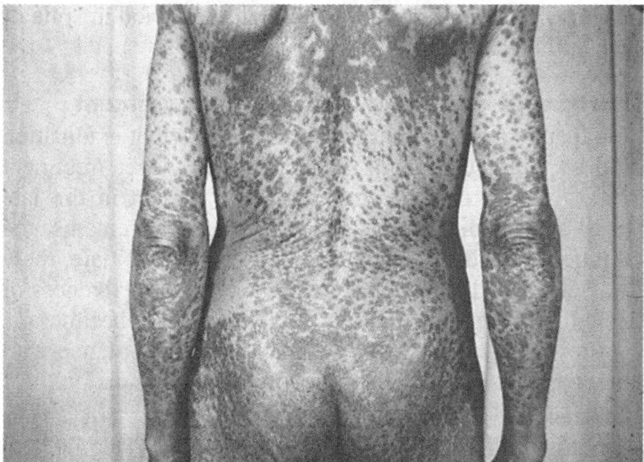

Fig. 50-5 Generalized posterior cutaneous eruptions in secondary syphilis. Distribution of lesions is bilateral and symmetric.

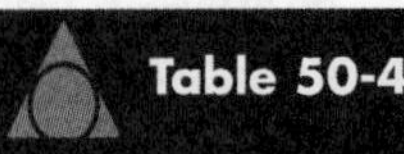

Table 50-4 Therapeutic Management: Primary Syphilis

Diagnostic
- History and physical examination
- Dark-field microscopy
- Nontreponemal or treponemal serologic testing
- Testing for other STDs (HIV, gonorrhea, chlamydia)

Therapeutic
- Appropriate drug therapy*
- Confidential counseling and testing for HIV infection
- Case finding
- Surveillance
  - Repeat of quantitative nontreponemal tests at 3, 6, and 12 mo
  - Examination of cerebrospinal fluid at 1 yr if treatment involves alternative antibiotics

HIV, Human immunodeficiency virus; *STDs,* sexually transmitted diseases.
*See Table 50-5.

False negative and false positive test results do occur with the nontreponemal tests (VDRL, RPR). A false negative result may be obtained during primary syphilis if the test is done before the individual has had time to produce antibody. A false positive finding may occur with other diseases or conditions such as hepatitis, infectious mononucleosis, after smallpox vaccination, collagen diseases, narcotic addiction, pregnancy, or aging. Positive nontreponemal test results should be confirmed by more specific treponemal tests to rule out other causes. In the CSF, changes such as increased white blood cell (WBC) count, increased total protein, and a positive treponemal antibody test are diagnostic of asymptomatic neurosyphilis.

If a patient is treated with antibiotics early in the course of the disease on the basis of the history and the symptoms, the serologic testing may not indicate the presence of syphilis. Once a person has positive serologic findings for syphilis, indicating the presence of antibodies, these findings may remain positive for an indefinite period in spite of successful treatment.

Therapeutic and Pharmacologic Management

Therapeutic management of syphilis is aimed at eradication of all syphilitic organisms (Table 50-4). However, treatment cannot reverse damage that is already present in the late stage of the disease. Parenteral penicillin remains the treatment of choice for all stages of syphilis. To date, there is no evidence to suggest a decrease in the effectiveness of penicillin against *T. pallidum.* Table 50-5 describes therapy for the various stages of syphilis and is in accordance with United States Public Health Service recommendations. All stages of syphilis should be treated.

Appropriate antibiotic treatment of maternal syphilis before the 18th week of pregnancy prevents infection of the fetus. Appropriate treatment after 18 weeks of pregnancy cures both mother and fetus because the antibiotics can cross the placental barrier. Treatment administered in the second half of pregnancy may pose a risk of premature labor. Some authorities recommend hospitalization and fetal monitoring of women at 20 weeks of gestation or greater.[18] All patients with neurosyphilis must be carefully monitored, with periodic serologic testing, clinical evaluation at 6-month intervals, and repeat CSF examinations for at least 3 years. Specific therapeutic management is based on the presenting symptoms.

GENITAL HERPES

Etiology and Pathophysiology

There are two different strains of herpes simplex virus (HSV) that cause infection—type 1 and type 2. In general, HSV type 1 (HSV-1) causes infection above the waist, involving the gingivae, the dermis, the upper respiratory tract, and the CNS. HSV type 2 (HSV-2) most frequently infects the genital tract and the perineum (i.e., locations below the waist). However, either strain can cause disease on the mouth or the genitals. HSV-1 can be transmitted from mouth to genitals, and HSV-2 can be transmitted from genitals to mouth through oral-genital contact.

In the course of the primary infection, HSV is established in the sensory nerve ganglion innervating the primary site. The virus remains dormant within sensory and autonomic nerve ganglia and can cause recurrence of the disease. Upon activation, the virus travels down the nerve axon to the skin or to the mucous membrane. Additional sexual contact is, therefore, not necessary for a recurrence of HSV infection. The recurrent infection produces a syndrome similar to but less intense than the primary infection.

Because HSV is readily inactivated at room temperature and by drying, airborne and fomitic spread have not been documented as significant means of transmission. The virus enters through the mucous membrane or through breaks in the skin during contact with an infected person. When a person is infected with HSV, the virus usually persists within the individual for life. Approximately 500,000 people a year contract genital herpes. The incubation period ranges from 1 to 45 days with an average of 6 days.[19]

Clinical Manifestations

A patient with primary HSV-2 infections initially complains of burning or tingling at the site of inoculation. Vesicular lesions, which may occur on the penis, scrotum, vulva, perineum, perianal region, vagina, or cervix, contain large quantities of infectious viral particles (Fig. 50-6). The lesions rupture and form shallow, moist ulcerations. Finally, crusting and epithelialization of the erosions occur. Primary infections tend to be associated with local inflammation and pain, accompanied by systemic manifestations of fever, headache, malaise, myalgia, and regional lymphadenopathy.

Urination may be painful from urine touching active lesions. Retention may occur as a result of HSV urethritis or cystitis. A purulent vaginal discharge may develop with HSV cervicitis. The duration of symptoms is longer and the frequency of complications is greater in women. Many HSV-2 infections, both primary and secondary, are asymptomatic; the exact percentage is unknown. Transmission of

Table 50-5 Drug Therapy for Syphilis

Stage	Benzathine Penicillin G (IM)	Aqueous Crystalline Penicillin G (IV)	Other Antibiotics*
▪ Early syphilis (primary, secondary, and early latent)	At single visit		Doxycycline, tetracycline, erythromycin
▪ Syphilis lasting >1 yr	Three weekly infections		
▪ Symptomatic neurosyphilis		Daily for 14 days followed by penicillin G benzathine weekly for 3 doses	Doxycycline, tetracycline, erythromycin

Modified from Centers for Disease Control: *STD treatment guidelines of USPHS*, Atlanta, 1993, Centers for Disease Control.
IM, Intramuscular; *IV*, intravenous.
*Given when penicillin is contraindicated.

genital herpes, therefore, can occur by sexual contact with an excretor of virus who is free of symptoms. Primary lesions are generally present for 17 to 20 days, but new lesions sometimes continue to develop for 6 weeks.

After the first infection, HSV-2 establishes latency in the sacral ganglia and may be reactivated periodically. Recurrent attacks occur in about 50% to 80% of all cases during the year following the primary episode. Stress, sexual activity, sunburn, and fever tend to trigger recurrence. Many patients can predict a recurrence by noticing early symptoms of tingling, burning, and itching at the site where lesions eventually arise. The symptoms of recurrent episodes are less severe, and the unilateral lesions heal within 8 to 12 days. With time the recurrent lesions generally occur less frequently.

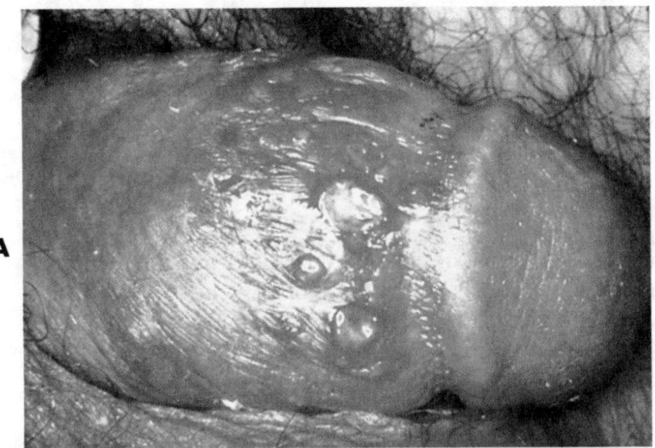
A

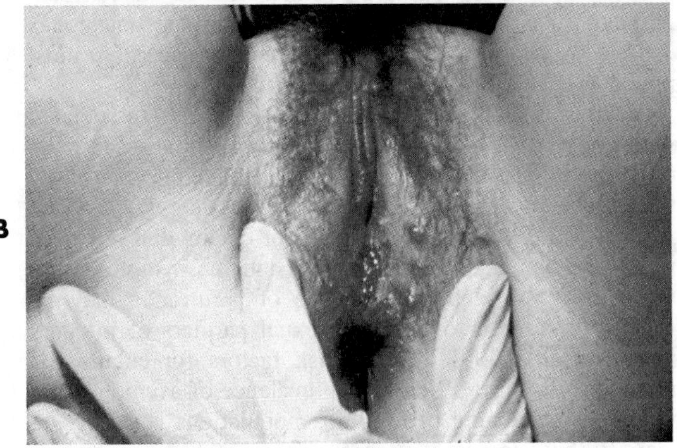
B

Fig. 50-6 Herpes simplex virus type 2 in a male and a female patient. Vesicular lesions on ***A,*** penis, and ***B,*** perineum.

Although viral transmission is easier when overt genital lesions are present, there does not appear to be any period of time when viral transmission is not possible once the primary HSV-2 infection has occurred. It has been shown that women with recurrent symptomatic genital herpes shed the virus up to 1% of the time even when no visible lesions are present.[20] The person with HSV is capable of transmitting the virus at any time. Barrier forms of contraception, especially condoms, used during asymptomatic periods, decrease transmission of the disease. When lesions are present, the patient should avoid sexual activity altogether as even barrier protection is not satisfactory in eliminating disease transmission.

Complications

Although most infections are of a relatively benign nature, complications of genital herpes may involve the CNS, causing aseptic meningitis and lower motor neuron damage.[21] Neuron damage may result in atonic bladder, impotence, and constipation. The most common complication is autoinoculation of the virus to extragenital sites such as fingers (whitlow), lips, and breasts.

HSV Infection in Pregnancy. Recent studies indicate no difference in the length or severity of symptoms in pregnant or nonpregnant women.[22] The incidence of abortion is higher if a primary HSV-2 infection is contracted during the first 20 weeks of pregnancy. Neonatal HSV and prematurity are most common in infants of women who contracted a primary infection in the third trimester. The development of disseminated neonatal herpes virus infections carries a high incidence of infant mortality. Although women with recurrent HSV infections are not at higher risk for transmitting the virus to their infants, an active genital lesion at the time of delivery usually indicates the need for cesarean section delivery, since most infections to neonates occur during passage through an infected birth canal.

Diagnostic Studies

Diagnosis of genital herpes is usually based on the patient's symptoms and history. The diagnosis can be confirmed through isolation of the virus from active lesions by means of tissue culture. Tzanck- or Pap-stained smears from lesions may show the cellular characteristics of viral infection, including multinucleated giant cells and intranuclear inclusions. Rapid testing using anti-HSV antibodies in direct immunofluorescence tests or in an enzyme linked immunosorbant assay (ELISA), and DNA hybridization is now available with sensitivity ranging from 75% to 90%. Herpes antibody tests are unreliable for distinguishing between HSV-1 and HSV-2 antibodies. Highly accurate serologic methods have been developed, based on identification of specific antibody to the glycoprotein G component of the outer membrane of the virus. These tests, however, have limited availability.

Therapeutic and Pharmacologic Management

The skin lesions of genital herpes heal spontaneously unless secondary infection occurs. Symptomatic treatment such as good genital hygiene and the wearing of loose-fitting cotton undergarments should be encouraged (Table 50-6). The lesions should be kept clean and dry. To ensure complete drying of the perineal area, women may use a hair dryer set on a cool setting. Frequent sitz baths may soothe the area and reduce inflammation. Pain may require a local anesthetic such as lidocaine (Xylocaine) or systemic analgesics such as codeine and aspirin. Patients are advised to abstain from sexual contact while lesions are present. However, sexual transmission of HSV has been documented even in the absence of clinical lesions, and the use of condoms should be encouraged.

Currently, acyclovir (Zovirax), a purine analogue that inhibits herpetic viral replication, is being prescribed for primary infections or for suppression of frequent recurrences (more than 6 episodes per year.) Although not a cure, acyclovir shortens the duration of viral shedding and the healing time of genital lesions and suppresses 75% of recurrences with daily use. Continued use of oral acyclovir for up to 5 years is safe and effective, but should be interrupted after one year to assess the patient's rate of recurrent episodes. Adverse reactions to acyclovir are mild and include headache, occasional nausea and vomiting, and diarrhea. The safety of systemic acyclovir for treatment of pregnant women has not been established. Acyclovir ointment appears to be of no clinical benefit in the treatment of recurrent lesions, either in speed of healing or in resolution of pain, and is not commonly recommended.[20] IV acyclovir is reserved for severe or life-threatening infections. Hospitalization is required, and nephrotoxicity has been observed with its use.

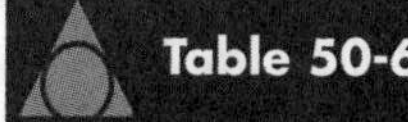

Table 50-6 Therapeutic Management: Genital Herpes

Diagnostic
- History and physical examination
- Viral isolation by tissue culture
- Cytologic examination of vesicular exudate for multinucleated giant cells

Therapeutic

Primary infection
- Acyclovir 200 mg orally 5 times a day for 7-10 days or until clinical resolution

Recurrent infection
- Acyclovir 200 mg orally 5 times a day for 5 days or acyclovir 800 mg orally 2 times a day for 5 days*
- Daily suppressive therapy for frequent recurrence (>6 episodes/yr). Acyclovir 200 mg 2-5 times a day or acyclovir 400 mg 2 times a day for up to 5 yr
- Attempt to identify trigger mechanisms
- Yearly Pap smear
- Abstinence from sexual contact while lesions are present
- Provision of symptomatic interventions
- Confidential counseling and testing for HIV

Modified from Centers for Disease Control: STD treatment guidelines, *MMWR* 42:14, 1993.
HIV, Human immunodeficiency virus.
*Most episodes of recurrent herpes do not benefit from treatment with acyclovir. In severe recurrent disease, patients who begin therapy at the beginning of prodrome or within 2 days of onset of lesions may benefit.

CHLAMYDIAL INFECTIONS

Urogenital Infections

Chlamydia trachomatis, a gram-negative bacterium, is recognized as a genital pathogen that is responsible for an increasing variety of clinical illnesses. There are numerous different serotypes, or strains, of *C. trachomatis,* which cause urogenital infection (e.g. nongonococcal urethritis [NGU] in men and cervicitis in women); ocular trachoma; and lymphogranuloma venereum. Consequently, more than 4 million chlamydial infections occur annually, particularly among adolescents.[23] Symptoms however, may be absent or minor in most infected women and in many men. Although it is not a reportable disease in most states, it is estimated that *C. trachomatis* infections are the most prevalent STDs in the United States.[24]

Because chlamydial infections are closely associated with gonococcal infections, clinical differentiation may be difficult (Table 50-7). Both infections are, therefore, usually treated concurrently even without diagnostic evidence. The incubation period of 1 to 3 weeks for chlamydial infection is longer than that for gonorrhea, and the symptoms are often milder. The high incidence of recurrence may be because of failure to treat the sexual partners of infected persons. Table 50-8 lists the risk factors for chlamydial infection. Because of the high prevalence of asymptomatic infections, screening of high-risk populations is needed to identify those infected.

Clinical Manifestations and Complications. As with gonorrhea, chlamydial infections result in a superficial mucosal infection that can become more invasive. Infec-

Table 50-7 Comparison of Gonorrhea and Chlamydia

Site of Infection	N. Gonorrhoeae	C. Trachomatis
Men		
Urethra	Urethritis	Nongonococcal urethritis; postgonococcal urethritis
Epididymis	Epididymitis	Epididymitis
Rectum	Proctitis	Proctitis
Conjunctiva	Conjunctivitis	Conjunctivitis
Systemic	Disseminated gonococcal infection	Reiter syndrome
Women		
Urethra	Acute urethral syndrome	Acute urethral syndrome
Bartholin's gland	Bartholinitis	Bartholinitis
Cervix	Cervicitis	Cervicitis; atypical cervical cells
Fallopian tube	Salpingitis	Salpingitis
Conjunctiva	Conjunctivitis	Conjunctivitis
Liver capsule	Perihepatitis	Perihepatitis
Systemic	Disseminated gonococcal infection	Arthritis-dermatitis syndrome

From McCance K L, Huether S E: *Pathophysiology: the biologic basis for disease in adults and children*, ed 2, St. Louis, 1995, Mosby.

Table 50-8 Risk Factors for Chlamydial Infection

Age <25 yr
Multiple sex partners
Sex partners who have had multiple partners
History of STDs
Use of nonbarrier contraception
Bleeding inducible by swabbing of cervical mucosa

STDs, Sexually transmitted diseases.

tions and associated signs and symptoms in men include urethritis (dysuria, urethral discharge), epididymitis (unilateral scrotal pain, swelling, tenderness, fever), and proctitis (rectal discharge and pain during defecation). Infections and associated signs and symptoms in women include cervicitis (mucopurulent discharge and hypertrophic ectopy [area that is edematous and bleeds easily]), urethritis (dysuria, frequent urination, and pyuria), bartholinitis (purulent exudate), pelvic inflammatory disease (abdominal pain, nausea, vomiting, fever, malaise, abnormal vaginal bleeding, and menstrual abnormalities), and perihepatitis (fever, nausea, vomiting, and right upper quadrant pain).[26] A large number of women with chlamydial cervicitis have been found to have a male partner with NGU.

Complications often develop from poorly managed, inaccurately diagnosed, or undiagnosed chlamydial infections. Infection in men may result in epididymitis, with possible infertility and Reiter's disease (a systemic condition characterized by urethritis, conjunctivitis, arthritis, and mucocutaneous lesions). Women may develop hypertrophic erosion of the cervix, salpingitis leading to PID, and infertility. Proctitis is associated with rectal intercourse. *Chlamydial* infection may be transmitted from a mother to the newborn, causing inclusion conjunctivitis or pneumonia.

Diagnostic Studies and Therapeutic Management. Chlamydial infections in men can be diagnosed by excluding gonorrhea. If no gram-negative intracellular diplococci are found on the Gram-stained smear of male urethral discharge or the sediment of first-catch urine specimen, a culture is done. If both are negative and signs of inflammation are present (e.g., polymorphonuclear leukocytes [PMNs] on the Gram-stained smear), a diagnosis of NGU-*Chlamydia* infection can be made. The availability of nonculture tests has made the screening of women more effective. Direct fluorescent antibody (DFA) tests, enzyme immunoassay (EIA), and DNA hybridization tests (using specific DNA probes) do not require special handling of specimens, are less expensive, and are easier to perform than are cell cultures. However, these tests are less specific than are cultures, and may produce false-positive results. Culturing for chlamydial organisms should be done if the laboratory facilities are available.

Chlamydial infections respond to treatment with tetracycline, doxycycline, or azithromycin. For tetracycline, the dosage is 500 mg orally four times a day for at least 7 days. For doxycycline, the dosage is 100 mg two times a day. Doxycycline is more expensive than tetracycline. Azithromycin (1 gm in a single dose) offers the advantage of ease of administration, but the safety and efficacy in patients under 15 years of age has not been established. All of the above medications are contraindicated in pregnancy. Erythromycin is the drug of choice for use in pregnant patients. Follow-up care should include advising the patient to return if symptoms persist or recur, treatment of sex partners, and encouraging the use of condoms during all sexual contacts.

Lymphogranuloma Venereum

Lymphogranuloma venereum (LGV) is a chronic sexually transmitted disease caused by *C. trachomatis.* LGV is rare in the United States; during 1990 only 277 cases were reported.[25] LGV is endemic in other areas of the world, including Africa, India, Southeast Asia, South America, and the Caribbean.

The strain of *C. trachomatis* that causes LGV probably enters the skin and mucous membranes through tiny abrasions. LGV begins as a skin lesion and spreads via the regional lymphatics. It may also spread systemically through the bloodstream and enter the CNS. Penile, vulvar, and anal infection can lead to inguinal and femoral lymphadenopathy. Marked inflammation occurs, resulting in necrosis, buboes (greatly enlarged, inflamed lymph nodes), abscesses of inguinal lymph nodes, and infection of surrounding tissue.

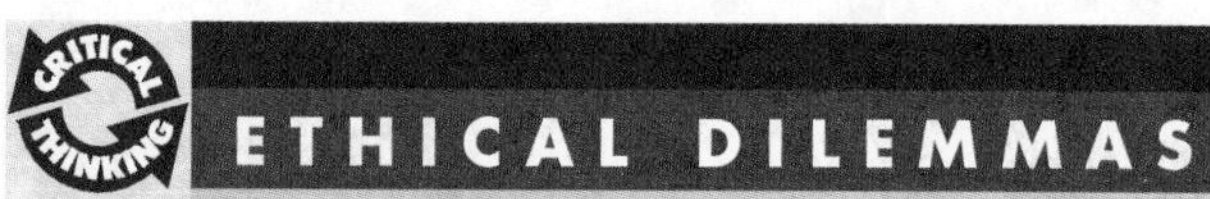

CONFIDENTIALITY

Situation A nurse in a clinic gives the positive results of a test for *Chlamydia* to a patient and advises her to tell her sexual partners that she has this disease. The patient refuses to tell her boyfriend because he will know that she has had sex with another partner. Should the nurse contact the boyfriend?

Discussion A patient has the right to confidential diagnosis and treatment. However, if the boyfriend is not treated and continues to have sex with this (treated) patient, she will be reinfected. And if he has additional partners, he could transmit the disease to them which, if left untreated, could cause sterility. While this disease could potentially endanger others, it is not life threatening nor is it a public health issue. At this time, chlamydial infection is not a sexually transmitted disease in all states, which must, by law, be reported to and tracked by public health officials. Education, not violation of confidentiality or coercion, is the key issue. The patient needs to be educated about reinfection as well as the long-term effects on others that this disease may have. The nurse should discuss the potential for reinfection if the boyfriend is not treated and encourage the patient to inform her partners of her diagnosis.

ETHICAL AND LEGAL PRINCIPLES

- Providers of health care have a legal obligation to maintain their patient's confidentiality unless required by law to report those who pose a risk to the health or life of innocent parties.
- Health care professionals have an ethical obligation to do no harm.
- Health care professionals have a primary responsibility to their patients. If trust cannot be maintained between health care professionals and their patients, patients may choose *not* to seek medical attention.

Healing occurs by fibrosis after several weeks or months and results in scarring, which damages the lymph nodes and disrupts nodal function.

Constitutional symptoms that occur during the stage of regional lymphadenopathy include fever, chills, headache, meningismus (meningitus-like symptoms), anorexia, myalgia, and arthralgia. Complications of untreated anorectal infection include perirectal abscess, fistula in ano, and rectovaginal, rectovesical, and ischiorectal fistulas. LGV is treated with a 2 week course of tetracycline. Sex partners should also be treated.

CONDYLOMATA ACUMINATA

Condylomata acuminata (genital warts), which are caused by human papillomavirus (HPV), is a highly contagious STD seen frequently in young, sexually active adults. It is often found in conjunction with other STDs. Accurate incidence data are not available because it is not a reportable condition. The genitalia and anorectal region as well as the urethral, bladder, and oral mucosa may be affected. The incubation period of the virus is 1 to 6 months. Prevention is hampered by a high proportion of asymptomatic infections and lack of curative treatment.

Minor trauma during intercourse can cause abrasions that allow HPV to enter the body. The epithelial cells infected with HPV undergo transformation, proliferate, and form a warty growth. Immunosuppressed persons, pregnant women, and diabetics are the individuals most susceptible to HPV.

Clinical Manifestations and Complications

Condylomata acuminata lesions are discrete single or multiple papillary growths that are white to gray. The warts may grow and coalesce to form large, cauliflower-like masses. In men, the warts may occur on the penis and scrotum, around the anus, or in the urethra. In women, the warts may be located on the vulva, the vagina, and the cervix, and in the perianal area.

During pregnancy, genital warts tend to grow rapidly. An infected mother may transmit the condition to her newborn. Cesarean delivery is not routinely indicated unless the birth canal becomes blocked by massive warts. Bleeding on defecation may occur with anal warts.

Subclinical HPV Infections. Recent research has linked HPV infection with cervical and vulvar cancer in women and with anorectal and squamous cell carcinoma of the penis in men. A direct causal relationship is suspected but has not yet been established.[20] To date more than 60 molecular types of HPV have been identified, at least 15 of which invade the genital tract. Some of these types appear to be harmless and self-limiting (e.g., types 6 and 11 commonly found in genital warts), while others seem to have oncogenic (cancer causing) potential (e.g., types 16, 18, and 31).[27] Up to two thirds of the early lesions caused by these viruses are undetectable by visual examination. Flat subclinical lesions are commonly found on the cervix, introitus, and perianal and intraanal mucosa of women and on the penis, perianal, and anal mucosa of men[28] and are strongly associated with the development of dysplasia and neoplasia at these sites.

Diagnostic Studies and Therapeutic Management

Diagnosis of condylomata can be made on the basis of the gross appearance of the lesions. However, the warts may be confused with condylomata lata of secondary syphilis, carcinoma, or benign neoplasms. Serologic and cytologic testing should be done to rule out these conditions. If dysplasia is confirmed by the Pap smear, a biopsy should be performed. Virapap, a test that uses DNA hybridization techniques, determines the presence of some types of HPV. Currently, HPV virus cannot be confirmed by culture.

Genital warts are difficult to treat and often require multiple office visits with a variety of treatment modalities. One common treatment is the use of 80% to 90% trichloroacetic acid applied directly to the wart surface. Petroleum jelly is applied to the surrounding normal skin to minimize irritation before a small amount of trichloroacetic acid is applied to the wart with a cotton swab. A sharp stinging pain is often felt with initial acid contact but this quickly subsides. Trichloroacetic acid is not washed off after treatment. It can be used in pregnant women.

Podophyllin (10% to 25%), a cytotoxic agent, is recommended therapy for small external genital warts. When podophyllin is used, it is applied carefully to each wart, with normal tissue being avoided, and is then thoroughly washed off in 1 to 4 hours. This substance encourages the sloughing off of skin containing viral particles. Podophyllin has local (e.g., pain, burning) and systemic (e.g., nausea, dizziness, leukopenia, respiratory distress) toxic symptoms. It is contraindicated in pregnant women. If the warts do not regress, treatments such as cryotherapy with liquid nitrogen, electrocautery, laser therapy, 5-fluorouracil (5% cream), and surgical excision may be indicated. Because treatment does not destroy the virus, merely the infected tissue, recurrences or reinfection are possible and careful long-term follow-up is advised.

Table 50-9 Nursing Assessment: Sexually Transmitted Disease

Subjective Data
Important health information
Past health history: Contact with individuals with STDs, multiple partners, pregnancy
Medications: Use of oral contraceptives; allergy to any antibiotics, especially penicillin
Functional health patterns
Health perception–health management: Malaise
Nutritional-metabolic: Pharyngitis, oral lesions, itching at infected site, alopecia, fever, chills
Elimination: Dysuria, frequency, urinary retention, urethral discharge; tenesmus
Cognitive-perceptual: Arthralgia; headache; painful, burning lesions
Sexuality-reproductive: Dyspareunia, vaginal discharge, presence of genital or perianal lesions

Objective Data
General
Lymphadenopathy (generalized or inguinal)
Integumentary
Syphilis: Primary—painless, indurated genital or perianal lesions; secondary—bilateral, symmetric rash on palms, soles, or entire body
Genital herpes: Painful genital or anal vesicular lesions or shallow ulcers
Condylomata: Single or multiple gray or white genital or anal warts (possibly becoming massive)
Gastrointestinal
Purulent rectal discharge (indicator of gonorrhea), rectal lesions, proctitis
Urinary
Urethral discharge, erythema
Reproductive
Cervical discharge, lesions, inflamed Bartholin's glands
Possible findings
Gonorrhea: Positive Gram stain, smears, (gram-negative diplococci within PMNs), and cultures
Syphilis: Positive findings on VDRL and RPR tests, spirochetes on dark-field microscopy
Genital Herpes: Positive tissue culture for HSV-2
Chlamydia: Positive culture for *Chlamydia* organisms

HSV, Herpes simplex virus; *PMNs,* polymorphonuclear neutrophils; *RPR,* rapid plasma reagin; *STDs,* sexually transmitted diseases; *VDRL, Venereal Disease Research Laboratory.*

NURSING MANAGEMENT

SEXUALLY TRANSMITTED DISEASES

Nursing Assessment

Subjective and objective data that should be obtained from a person with a sexually transmitted disease are presented in Table 50-9.

Nursing Diagnoses

Nursing diagnoses specific to the patient with a sexually transmitted disease include, but are not limited to, those listed in the nursing care plan on p. 1576.

Planning

The overall goals are that the patient with a sexually transmitted disease will (1) demonstrate understanding of the mode of transmission of STDs and the the risk posed by STDs, (2) complete treatment and return for appropriate follow-up, (3) notify or assist in notification of contacts about their need for testing and treatment, (4) abstain from intercourse until infection is resolved, and (5) demonstrate knowledge of safe sex practices.

Nursing Implementation

Health Promotion and Maintenance. Many approaches to curtailing the spread of STDs have been advocated and have met with varying degrees of success. Nurses should be prepared to discuss safe sex practices such as abstinence, monogamy with an uninfected partner, avoidance of certain high risk sexual practices, and use of condoms and other barriers to limit contact with potentially infectious body fluids or lesions. Sexual abstinence is a certain method of avoiding all sexually transmitted diseases, but few adults consider this a feasible alternative to sexual expression. Limiting sexual intimacies outside of a well-established monogamous relationship can reduce the risk of contracting a sexually transmitted disease.

Nurses should also be knowledgeable about the connection between some strains of HPV and cervical intraepithelial neoplasia (CIN). CIN is a precancerous lesion that appears to be an STD itself. It is now commonly believed that carcinomas of the cervix originate from CIN. Therefore, an annual Pap smear is an important health practice for sexually active women.

Measures to prevent infection. An inspection of the sexual partner's genitals before coitus is recommended. The presence of discharge, sores, blisters, or rash should be viewed with concern. A patient who is aware of specific signs and symptoms of infection can intelligently make the decision to continue the sexual interaction with modifica-

NURSING CARE PLAN Patient with a Sexually Transmitted Disease*

Planning: Outcome Criteria	Nursing Interventions and Rationales
➤ NURSING DIAGNOSIS	Risk for infection transmission *related to* lack of knowledge about mode of transmission, inadequate personal and genital hygiene, and failure to practice precautionary measures
Describe mode of transmission; practice appropriate hygienic measures; have no spread of infection to others.	Assess knowledge of hygienic precautions and mode of transmission and presence of infectious lesions *to determine extent of problem and plan appropriate interventions.* Instruct patient in hygienic measures, especially good hand washing *to destroy causative organisms on the hands and to avoid this source of disease transmission.* Treat with appropriate antibiotics *to eradicate infection.* Investigate need for treatment of sexual partners with antibiotics *to prevent ping pong effect;* instruct patient regarding abstinence or use of condoms *to prevent transmission of disease.* Explain mode of transmission *so patient can take necessary precautions to prevent spread of disease.* Teach patient to abstain from sexual intercourse during treatment and to use condoms when sexual activity is resumed *to prevent spread of infection and prevent reinfection.* Advise follow-up examination and reculture at least once after treatment if appropriate *to confirm complete cure and prevent relapse.*
➤ NURSING DIAGNOSIS	Anxiety *related to* impact of condition on relationships, disease outcome, and lack of knowledge of disease *as manifested by* emotional response of anger and restlessness, requesting of information about signs and symptoms of complications
Have decreased or absence of anxiety related to diagnosis; know signs and symptoms of recurrence.	Allow patient and sexual partner to verbalize concerns *to clarify areas that need explanation.* Investigate need for counseling *so the appropriate level of help is offered.* Instruct patient about symptoms of complications and need to report problems *to ensure proper follow-up and early treatment of reinfection.*
➤ NURSING DIAGNOSIS	Altered health maintenance *related to* lack of knowledge and questions about disease process, appropriate follow-up measures, and possibility of reinfection *as manifested by* questions about disease process, hygienic precautions, and follow-up procedure
Have no reinfection; comply with follow-up protocol.	Explain precautions to take, such as being monogamous, asking potential partners about sexual history, using condoms, voiding and washing genitalia after coitus *to reduce the occurrence of reinfection.* Inform patient regarding state of infectivity *to prevent a false sense of security from resulting in careless sexual practices and poor personal hygiene.* Assist with case finding *since many STDs are easily transmitted and sexual partners need to be treated.* Instruct patient on time frame if follow-up testing is indicated *to ensure eradication of the disease.*
➤ NURSING DIAGNOSIS	Pain *related to* clinical manifestations of an STD *as manifested by* verbal report of pain
Be satisfied with level of pain relief.	Assess location, intensity, and etiology of the pain *to determine an appropriate treatment plan.* Provide or teach problem-specific pain relief measures such as high fluid intake for dysuria and warm compresses for lesions *to promote patient comfort and sense of being cared for.* Administer analgesia as ordered *to reduce pain.*
➤ NURSING DIAGNOSIS	Body image disturbance *related to* symptoms associated with an STD *as manifested by* self-deprecating comments and reluctance to view self or participate in self-care
Have an accepting attitude toward body changes; participate in self-care activities.	Assess patient's perception of bodily changes *to determine if a problem is present and plan appropriate interventions.* Be truthful with patient about disease outcome on personal appearance *to establish a trusting relationship and help patient have realistic expectations.*
➤ NURSING DIAGNOSIS	Risk for noncompliance *related to* lack of knowledge of possible complications and confusion about therapy
Complete course of treatment as prescribed; understand and comply with treatment plan.	Teach patient about the etiology, treatment plan, mode of transmission, and consequences of noncompliance *to foster cooperation* and compliance with planned therapy. Allow time to answer questions *to prevent confusion and treatment error.* Write out instructions for patient *to avoid confusion and misunderstanding.*

STDs, Sexually transmitted diseases.
*This general care plan can be adapted when caring for a patient with a specific STD.

tions or elect not to have sexual relations. The patient should remember that, when engaging in sex, there is exposure to the infections of everyone with whom the partner has ever had sex. Men should be told that some protection is provided if they void immediately following intercourse and wash their genitalia and the adjacent areas with soap and water. Women may also benefit from post-coital voiding and washing. Spermicidal jellies and creams have a mild detergent effect that may reduce the risk of contracting STDs. These same barriers can serve as supplementary lubrication, thereby decreasing irritation and friction and chances for development of a minor laceration which could serve as an entry point for the organism.

Proper use of a latex condom provides a highly effective mechanical barrier to infection. The condom should be undamaged and correctly in place throughout all phases of sexual activity. The use of a spermicide, such as nonoxynol-9 (which inactivates most STD organisms) in the vagina and concurrent use of a condom can further reduce risk of disease.[29] Some studies have shown that misinformation or lack of knowledge about proper usage strongly contributes to negative experiences and dissatisfaction with condoms.[30,31] The patient should be given specific verbal and written instructions on the proper use of condoms (see Chapter 11). The objections to condom usage, such as interference with spontaneity and the presence of a barrier, should be discussed by the partners. Information about the mechanics of sexual arousal and incorporating a condom into lovemaking can help in overcoming patient or partner resistance to its use. The Reality female condom is a lubricated polyurethane sheath with a ring at each end designed for vaginal wear (see Chapter 11). Laboratory studies indicate that it is an effective barrier to microorganisms including viruses, but clinical trials are currently lacking for STDs.[32]

Sexual contact with persons known or suspected to have HIV infection should be avoided (see Chapter 11). A sexually active homosexual man can reduce risk by minimizing the number of sexual contacts. Anal intercourse should be eliminated, and condoms should be used if sexual contact continues.

The nurse can initiate an interview to establish the patient's risk for contracting a STD. Questions to ask include number of partners, type of birth control used, use of condoms, use of IV drugs, and sexual preference. Patient education can be planned based on the response to these questions.

Screening programs. Screening programs that are used to detect infected patients can also help prevent certain STDs. For many years, there have been various screening programs to find cases of syphilis. According to the 1993 *World Almanac,* 30 states and the District of Columbia require premarital blood testing for syphilis. A total of 49 states require prenatal testing for syphilis, but often those women at highest risk have the least access to prenatal care. At present, only two states, California and New Hampshire, mandate offering HIV screening and AIDS information to couples applying for marriage licenses. Many institutions offer prenatal HIV testing and counseling for pregnant women.

Screening programs have been developed and implemented for detection of gonorrhea. These programs are targeted to women because women are more likely to have asymptomatic gonorrhea and thereby serve as sources of infection. Routine gonorrheal cultures during pelvic examinations and prenatal visits are being performed as a major part of these programs. Their effectiveness is well documented. Mass application of screening programs for genital chlamydial infections, genital herpes, and HPV infections (warts) may also be possible when rapid, cost-effective tests are developed.

Case finding. Interviewing and case finding are other processes used to control venereal disease. These activities are directed toward locating and examining all contacts of each known patient with an STD as soon after sexual exposure as possible, so that effective treatment can be initiated. Trained interviewers may often find cases even if they are supplied with only limited information. The caseworkers, who are often nurses, are aware of the social implications of these diseases and the need for discretion. Sexual contacts are often not informed about the origin of the information naming them as a contact so that greater cooperation and privacy is ensured.

Educational and research programs. Nurses can actively encourage their communities to provide better education about STDs for their citizens. Teenagers, who are known to have a high incidence of infection, should be a prime target for such educational programs. Hot-line services, school nurses, nurse practitioners, nurse midwives, and outreach programs sponsored by the CDC are effective. The National Gay Task Force and the Herpes Resource Center were established to provide education and support where needed. Knowledge and understanding of the disease can decrease the STD epidemic. Currently, efforts are being made to develop a serologic test for gonorrhea and effective immunizing agents for syphilis, gonorrhea, genital herpes, HPV, and HIV. The development of effective vaccines is viewed by many clinicians as a prerequisite for eradication of sexually transmitted diseases.

Acute Intervention

Psychologic support. The diagnosis of an STD may be met with a variety of emotions such as shame, guilt, anger, and a desire for vengeance. The nurse should provide counseling and try to help the patient verbalize feelings. Couples in marital or committed relationships are confronted with an added problem when an STD is diagnosed. The implication of sexual activity by one of the partners with a person outside the relationship must be faced. Other concerns relative to their relationship are present, and the acute problem may serve as an incentive for further problem solving. Support and counseling for the couple are needed. A referral for professional counseling to explore the ramifications of an STD in their relationship may be indicated.

A patient who has contracted genital herpes is faced with the fact that repeated infections can occur and that no cure is available. This can be frustrating and disruptive to the patient's physical, emotional, social, and sexual lives. Helping the patient identify and avoid any factors that may precipitate the condition is indicated. Informing the patient that the incidence and severity of recurrences will decrease over time may provide a degree of support.

HPV infections involve a prolonged course of treatment. The patient can become frustrated and distressed because of frequent office visits, associated costs, potential for unpleasant side effects as a result of treatment, and effects of the infection on future health and sexual relationships. Tremendous support and a willingness to listen to the patient's concerns are needed.

Compliance and follow-up. A nurse working in public health facilities, clinics, or other outpatient settings may care for a patient with an STD more often than a nurse in a hospital. This nurse is in a position to explain and interpret treatment measures such as the purpose and possible side effects of prescribed drugs and the need for follow-up care.

Fortunately, single-dose treatment for gonorrhea, chlamydial infection, and syphilis helps prevent the problems associated with noncompliance with drug therapy. The patient requiring multiple-dose therapy should be given special instructions in completing the prescribed regimen and should be informed about problems resulting from noncompliance. All patients should return to the treatment center for a repeat culture from the infected sites or for serologic testing at designated times to determine the effectiveness of the treatment. Informing the patient that cures are not always obtained on the first treatment can reinforce the need for a follow-up visit. The patient should also be advised to inform sexual partners of the need for treatment, regardless of whether they are free of symptoms or experiencing symptoms.

Hygiene measures. The patient with an STD should have certain hygiene measures emphasized. An important measure is frequent hand washing and bathing; this results in the destruction of many of the causative organisms of STDs. Bathing and cleaning of the involved areas can provide local comfort and prevent secondary infection. Douching may spread the infection and is therefore contraindicated. The synthetic materials used in most undergarments frequently increase or exacerbate local irritations by trapping moisture. Cotton undergarments provide better absorption and are cooler and more comfortable for the patient with an STD.

Sexual activity. Sexual abstinence is indicated during the communicable phase of the disease. If sexual activity occurs before treatment of the patient has been completed, the use of condoms may prevent the spread of infection and reinfection. The patient can also choose to relate to a partner in an intimate way that avoids both coitus and oral-genital contact.

Chronic and Home Management. Because many STDs are cured with a single dose or short course of antibiotic therapy, many persons are casual about the outcome of these diseases. The consequences of this attitude can include delays in treatment, noncompliance with instructions, and subsequent development of complications. The complications are serious and costly; they can result in disfigurement and destruction of important tissues and organs.

Surgery and prolonged therapy are indicated for many patients with disease-related deformity. Major surgical procedures such as resection of an aneurysm or aortic valve replacement may be necessary to treat cardiovascular problems. Pelvic surgery and procedures to correct fertility problems secondary to an STD may include lysis of adhesions, dilatation of strictures, reconstructive tuboplasty, and in vitro fertilization.

CRITICAL THINKING EXERCISES

CASE STUDY

CHLAMYDIA

Patient Profile

Sara M. is a 17-year-old female who visits the outpatient Teen Clinic seeking birth control pills.

Subjective Data

- Had first time intercourse with boyfriend 2 weeks ago
- Did not use condom or spermicide
- Has not asked boyfriend about his sexual practices
- Denies any symptoms

Objective Data

- Has hypertrophic ectopy noted during Pap test
- Tested positive for chlamydia
- Crying and very upset when informed of positive test result

Treatment

- Doxycycline 100 mg bid for 10 days

Critical Thinking Questions

1. What were Sara's risk factors for acquiring chlamydial infection?
2. What complications could have occurred if Sara's infection had not been detected?
3. What impact is her diagnosis likely to have on Sara's self-image? On her relationship with her boyfriend?
4. What instructions should Sara receive to ensure successful treatment? To prevent reinfection? To prevent further transmission of the infection?
5. What does she need to know about other STDs? What other testing would you recommend?
6. Based on the assessment data presented, write one or more nursing diagnoses. Are there any collaborative problems?

NURSING RESEARCH ISSUES

1. What are the best strategies for encouraging safe sex practices and condom use among high risk populations?
2. What is the level of teens' knowledge of risk, transmission, and impact of STDs? How can teaching about STDs best be adapted to their developmental level?
3. Does education about safe sex practices increase preventive behaviors?

REVIEW QUESTIONS

The number of the question corresponds to the same-numbered objective at the beginning of the chapter.

1. Factors that have contributed to an increase in STDs include all of the following *except*

a. longer sexual life span.
b. decreased influence of religious groups.
c. use of barrier methods of contraception.
d. greater sexual freedom.

2. Symptoms of chlamydial infections in women

a. mimic those of genital herpes.
b. include a macular palmar rash in later stages.
c. may be absent.
d. are more virulent in primary infections.

3. The patient with gonorrhea is treated with ceftriaxone and tetracycline or doxycycline because

a. no single agent successfully eradicates all strains of gonorrhea.
b. the high rate of coexisting chlamydial infection or syphilis necessitates dual coverage.
c. most patients do not respond to ceftriaxone alone.
d. longer coverage with oral medications prevents reinfection.

4. A primary HSV infection differs from recurrent episodes in that

a. symptoms may include more systemic manifestations such as fever and myalgia.
b. only primary infections are sexually transmissible.
c. it is of shorter duration than recurrent episodes.
d. the patient may complain of burning and tingling prior to lesion formation.

5. The nursing diagnosis least applicable to the patient with an STD is

a. self-esteem disturbance.
b. pain related to lesions.
c. risk for noncompliance.
d. difficulty with ambulation.

6. Counseling regarding measures to prevent infections with and transmission of STDs should include

a. an explanation of the appropriate use of birth control pills.
b. a discussion of sexual positions used to avoid infection.
c. an explanation of safe sex practices.
d. only adolescents because mature adults are not at risk.

7. Emotional support is best given to the patient with a sexually transmitted disease through
   a. offering of many alternatives.
   b. concerned listening.
   c. isolation from others.
   d. emphasis on duration of disease.

REFERENCES

1. Centers for Disease Control: Sentinel surveillance for antimicrobial resistance in *Neisseria gonorrhea*: United States, 1988–1991, *MMWR* 42:3, 1993.
2. Centers for Disease Control: Surveillance for primary and secondary syphilis: United States, 1991, *MMWR* 42:3, 1993.
3. United States Department of Health and Human Services: 1991 Annual report, Division of STD/HIV prevention, Atlanta, 1992, Centers for Disease Control.
4. Centers for Disease Control: An evaluation of surveillance for *Chlamydia trachomatis* infections in the United States, 1987–1991, *MMWR* 42:3, 1993.
5. Zenilman JM: Update on bacterial sexually transmitted disease, *Urol Clin North Am* 19:1, 1992.

*6. Jossens MOR, Sweet RL: Pelvic inflammatory disease: risk factors and microbial etiologies, *JOGNN*, 22:2, 1993.

7. Stone K: Epidemiologic aspects of genital HPV infections, *Clin Obstet Gynecol* 32:114, 1989.
8. Ernst AA, Martin DH: High syphilis rates among cocaine abusers identified in an emergency department, *Sex Trans Dis* 20:2, 1993.
9. Finelli L and others: Early syphilis: relationship to sex, drugs, and changes in high-risk behavior from 1987-1990, *Sex Trans Dis* 20:2, 1993.
10. Mosher WD: Contraceptive practice in the United States 1982-1988, *Fam Plann Perspect* 22:83, 1990.
11. Louv WC and others: Oral contraceptive use and the risk of chlamydial and gonococcal infections, *Am J Obstet Gynecol* 160:2, 1989.
12. Kronmal RA and others: The intrauterine device and pelvic inflammatory disease: the Women's Health Study reanalyzed, *J Clin Epidemiol* 44:2, 1991.
13. Burkman RT and others: Response to "The intrauterine device and pelvic inflammatory disease: the Women's Health Study reanalyzed." *J Clin Epidemiol* 44:2, 1991.
14. U.S. Department of Health Education and Welfare, Public Health Services: *Venereal disease control laws: summary,* Atlanta, 1972, Centers for Disease Control.
15. Zenilman JM: Gonorrhea: clinical and public health issues, *Hosp Pract* 28:40, 1993.
16. Handsfield HH: Recent developments in STDs. I Bacterial diseases, *Hosp Pract* 26:50, 1991.
17. Lukehart SA, Holmes KK: Syphilis. In *Harrison's principles of internal medicine,* ed 13, New York, 1994, McGraw-Hill.
18. Brunham RC and others: Sexually transmitted diseases in pregnancy. In Holmes KK, editor: *Sexually transmitted diseases,* ed 2, New York, 1990, McGraw-Hill.
19. Smith MA, Singer C: Sexually transmitted viruses other than HIV and papillomavirus, *Uro Clin North Am* 19:1, 1992.
20. Handsfield HH: Recent developments in STDs. II Viral and other syndromes, *Hosp Pract* 27:175, 1992.
21. Catotti DN and others: Herpes revisited, *Sex Trans Dis* 20:2. 1993.
22. Corey L: Genital herpes. In Holmes KK, editor: *Sexually transmitted diseases,* ed 2, New York, 1990, McGraw-Hill.
23. U.S. Department of Health and Human Services, Public Health Service: Recommendations for the prevention and management of *Chlamydia trachomatis* infections, 1993, Atlanta, 1993, Centers for Disease Control.
24. Greener DL: Sexually transmitted diseases. In McCance K, Huether S, editors: *Pathophysiology: the biologic basis for disease in adults and children,* ed 2, St Louis, 1995, Mosby.
25. Stamm W, Holmes K: Chlamydial infections. In Isselbacher K and others, editors: *Harrison's principles of internal medicine,* New York, 1994, McGraw-Hill.
26. Erickson MF: Chlamydial infections: combating the silent threat, *AJN* 94:16B, 1994.

*27. Kelley KF and others: Genital human papillomavirus infection in women, *JOGNN* 21:6, 1992.

28. Spitzer M, Krumholz BA: Human papillomavirus-related diseases in the female patient, *Urol Clin North Am* 19:1, 1992.
29. Centers for Disease Control: Update: barrier protection against HIV infection and other sexually transmitted diseases, *MMWR* 42:30, 1993.

*30. Norris AE, Ford K: Urban, low-income, African-American and Hispanic youths' negative experiences with condoms: implications for nursing intervention, *Nurse Prac* 18:5, 1993.

31. Trussell J and others: Condom slippage and breakage rates, *Fam Plann Perspect* 24:1, 1992.
32. U.S. Department of Health and Human Services, Public Health Service: 1993 sexually transmitted diseases treatment guidelines, Atlanta, 1993, Centers for Disease Control.
33. Centers for Disease Control: *Prenatal examination laws,* Atlanta, 1979, Centers for Disease Control.

---

* Nursing research-based articles.

Chapter 51

NURSING ROLE IN MANAGEMENT

Female Reproductive Problems

Kathryn A. Patterson Linda Carnago

Learning Objectives

1. Describe the etiology, clinical manifestations, and therapeutic and nursing management of common problems of menstruation.
2. Identify the purposes of and preoperative and postoperative care for the patient having a dilatation and curettage.
3. Explain the physical and psychologic alterations and appropriate management during the climacteric and menopause.
4. Compare the advantages and disadvantages of common contraceptive and birth control methods.
5. Differentiate between spontaneous and induced abortion, including therapeutic and nursing management.
6. Describe the effects of rape and appropriate therapeutic, legal, and nursing interventions.
7. Differentiate among the common vaginal, vulvar, and cervical inflammations and infections including therapeutic and nursing management.
8. Describe the etiology, complications, and therapeutic and nursing management of pelvic inflammatory disease.
9. Describe the clinical manifestations, complications, and therapeutic and nursing management of endometriosis.
10. Explain the manifestations and management of benign tumors of the uterus and ovaries.
11. Identify the clinical manifestations, diagnostic studies, therapeutic management, and surgical interventions of malignant tumors of the uterus, ovaries, and vulva.
12. Describe the preoperative and postoperative nursing interventions for the patient requiring major surgery of the female reproductive system.
13. Identify the nursing responsibilities related to internal radiation therapy for uterine cancer.
14. Explain the etiology, clinical manifestations, and therapeutic management of uterine displacements.
15. Identify the clinical manifestations and therapeutic and nursing management of cystoceles, rectoceles, and fistulas.

PROBLEMS RELATED TO MENSTRUATION

Menstruation is a periodic discharge of blood and disintegrating endometrium at the conclusion of a normal ovulatory cycle. This process is a normal event, occurring approximately every 28 days. However, there may be considerable variation in the days between cycles and in the duration, amount, and character of bleeding. Some of these variations are associated with reproductive problems.

Health Maintenance and Promotion

Before the nurse plans any health teaching, the patient's knowledge related to the menstrual cycle should be assessed. Table 51-1 includes characteristics of the menstrual cycle and related patient education. When this information is discussed and explained, the patient becomes aware that variations do exist for the normal menses. This knowledge can help dispel apprehension and misconceptions. If the patient's menstrual cycle pattern does not fall within the range of normal, the nurse should urge her to seek medical attention.

Many myths are told concerning activities allowed during menstruation. The nurse should be prepared to clarify the facts. The patient should be assured that bathing and hair washing are safe. A daily warm tub bath may actually relieve some of the associated pelvic discomfort. Women can swim, exercise, have intercourse, and basically continue their usual daily activities.

Frequent changing of tampons or pads meets comfort and hygiene needs during menstruation. The selection of internal or external sanitary protection is a matter of personal preference. Tampons are convenient and make menstrual hygiene easier, whereas pads may provide better protection.

Reviewed by Kay D. Sedler, MSN, CNM, Chief, Nurse-Midwifery Division, University of New Mexico, School of Medicine, Albuquerque, NM.

Table 51-1 Characteristics of Menstrual Cycle and Related Patient Education

Characteristic	Patient Education
Menarche	
Occurs between ages of 9 and 18 yr, average age at onset is 12 or 13 yr	See physician regarding possible endocrine or developmental abnormality when delayed.
Interval	
Usually is 27-31 days, but regular cycles as short as 17 or as long as 45 days are considered normal if pattern is consistent for individual	Keep written record to identify own pattern of menstrual cycle. Expect some irregularity in premenopausal period. Be aware that drugs (phenothiazines, narcotics, contraceptives) and stressful life events can result in missed periods.
Duration	
Menstrual flow generally lasts 2-8 days	Realize that pattern is fairly constant but that wide variations do exist.
Amount	
Average menstrual flow is 30-100 ml per period; amount varies among women and in the same woman at different times; it is usually heaviest first 2 days	Count pads or tampons used per day. The average tampon or pad completely saturated absorbs 20-30 ml. Very heavy flow is indicated by complete soaking of 2 pads in 1-2 hr. Know that flow increases and then gradually decreases in premenopausal period. IUD or drugs such as anticoagulants and thiazides can produce heavy menses.
Composition	
Menstrual discharge is mixture of endometrium, blood, mucus, and vaginal cells; it is dark red and less viscous than blood and usually does not clot	Realize that clots indicate heavy flow or vaginal pooling.

IUD, Intrauterine device.

Premenstrual Syndrome

Premenstrual syndrome (PMS) constitutes a group of physical, psychologic, and behavioral changes distressing enough to impair interpersonal relationships or interfere with usual activities. PMS symptoms occur cyclically, usually 7 to 14 days before the onset of menstruation, and are not present at other times of the month. PMS is difficult to define because of the range of symptoms described by women and the variable severity of symptoms from cycle to cycle in the same woman.[1] The syndrome can occur at any time between menarche and menopause, but women who seek treatment for PMS are usually 30 to 40 years of age.[2]

Etiology. Although the specific etiology of PMS is unknown, the proposed etiologic factors are as diverse as the symptoms. It is thought to involve cyclic fluctuations of ovarian hormone levels or fluctuations of endogenous opiate peptides and serum glucose levels. Deficiencies of vitamin B and magnesium, prostaglandin excess, and changes in the hypothalamic-pituitary axis have also been suggested as the etiology of PMS. There is support for each of the potential causes, but none seems to explain PMS completely. The sociocultural context of the woman's life may contribute significantly to the manifestation of symptoms. Women are having fewer children and therefore experience more periods during their reproductive years. Life stressors may make it difficult to balance biological processes with the demands of contemporary society.[3]

Clinical Manifestations. PMS is diagnosed by exclusion. A complete health, gynecologic, obstetric, and psychologic history and a thorough physical examination are necessary to rule out any underlying conditions, such as thyroid dysfunction, uterine fibroids, or psychopathology, that may account for the premenstrual symptoms. In addition, no helpful biomedical or laboratory markers are available in establishing the diagnosis.

Commonly occurring physical symptoms include breast discomfort, peripheral edema, abdominal bloating, episodes of binge eating, and headache. Abdominal bloating and breast swelling are apparently caused by local fluid shifts because total body weight does not generally change. Anxiety, depression, irritability, and mood swings are some of the emotional changes women may experience.

The number and severity of symptoms that should be present to confirm the diagnosis have not been established. The patient's symptoms and her menstrual cycle can be correlated through the use of a prospective daily diary in which menstrual experiences and basal body temperature are recorded. The menstrual diary must show identical symptoms in at least two consecutive cycles to support the diagnosis of PMS.[4] A slight rise in the basal body temperature identifies the timing of ovulation. Comparison of the two records generally shows an absence of symptoms in the follicular phase (first part of menstrual cycle) and the presence of complaints in the luteal phase (phase of menstrual cycle after release of an ovum from a mature ovarian follicle), which resolve with the onset of menstruation.

Therapeutic Management. Nonpharmacologic and pharmacologic strategies aid in relieving some PMS symp-

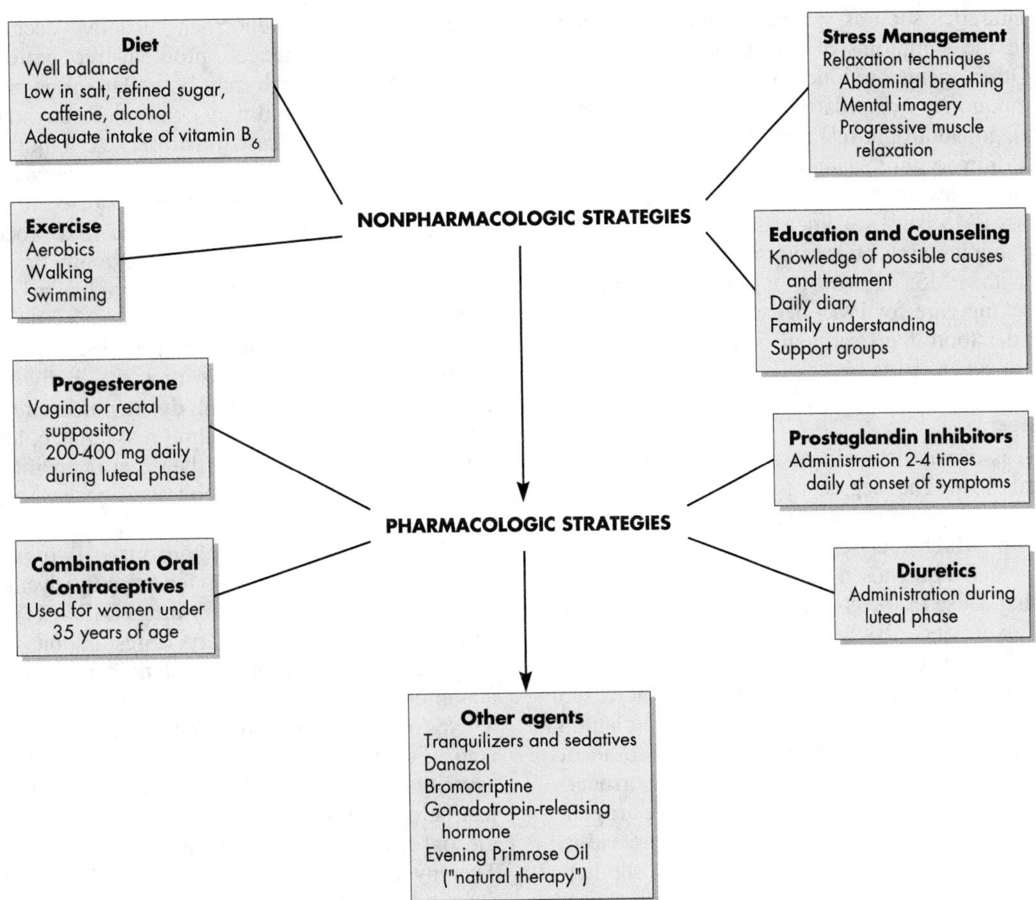

Fig. 51-1 Treatment strategies for premenstrual syndrome.

toms (Fig. 51-1). The nonpharmacologic approaches emphasize diet manipulation, exercise, stress management, education, and counseling. The patient who eats a nutritious, well-balanced diet and limits salt, refined sugar, and caffeine intake notes that symptoms of edema, increased appetite, and irritability lessen. Vitamin supplementation, especially vitamin B_6 (pyridoxine), is recommended. A dosage of 100 mg of vitamin B_6 daily partially relieves symptoms of dizziness, nausea, and withdrawal behavior. Because excess vitamin B_6 increases the risk of peripheral neuropathy (characterized by ataxia and profound changes in vibratory and position sensation), regular evaluation to assess symptoms of neuropathy is needed.[5] Most of the symptoms of peripheral neuropathy are reversible when vitamin B_6 is discontinued. Naturally occurring vitamin B_6 may be found in such foods as pork, milk, egg yolk, and legumes. Oral contraceptives can cause deficiencies in both vitamin B_6 and magnesium.

Exercise results in a release of endorphins, leading to mood elevation. Aerobic exercises have a tranquilizing effect on muscular tension. The patient's lifestyle and interests should be considered when an exercise program is being planned. Because fatigue tends to exaggerate the symptoms of PMS, adequate rest in the premenstrual period is a priority. Explanation, reassurance, and exploration of any psychologic aspects should also be done. The use of recognized techniques for stress reduction, including yoga, meditation, imaging, and biofeedback training, should be encouraged.

The patient should be educated and counseled regarding PMS and the current theories on its etiology and treatment. Counseling should involve listening and reassurance, as well as provision of factual information. The spouse or significant other needs to be informed about the nature of PMS because understanding and support will be important in the patient's daily life. Joining a PMS support group can also be beneficial for some women.

Pharmacologic Management. Pharmacologic treatment strategies should be considered when symptoms persist. Presently, no single drug is being prescribed for the treatment of PMS symptoms. One therapy is used for a time, and if no improvement is observed, another approach is tried. Progesterone has been widely advocated, but its use remains controversial because results have not been as beneficial as originally thought. The precise role of ovarian hormones in PMS is still unclear.

Excessive synthesis of prostaglandins is thought to trigger PMS symptoms, and prostaglandin inhibitors such as ibuprofen (Motrin, Advil) have been used. These medications are effective in reducing depression, pain, headache, and tension. Diuretics such as spironolactone (Aldactone) have improved the symptoms of abdominal bloating and weight gain. Other agents used include combined oral contraceptives, tranquilizers or sedatives, bromocriptine (Parlodel), danazol, gonadotropin-releasing hormone analogues, and Evening Primrose Oil ("natural therapy").

An increasingly aware public is demanding assistance with the distress PMS causes women and their families. As a result, many clinics now offer counseling and treatment for patients with PMS. However, a woman should be cautious in seeking care for PMS because the cause is not completely understood, the treatment is not definitive, and the potential for quackery is high.

Dysmenorrhea

Dysmenorrhea is defined as pain or discomfort associated with menstrual flow. The degree of pain and discomfort varies with the individual. The two types of dysmenorrhea are *primary,* in which pelvic organs are normal, and *secondary,* in which a diagnosed pelvic disease or condition is the underlying cause of the problem. Approximately 50% of all women experience dysmenorrhea, making it one of the most common gynecologic problems.[6]

Etiology. Current evidence suggests that increased production of prostaglandin $F_{2\alpha}$ ($PGF_{2\alpha}$) and prostaglandin E_2 (PGE_2) released from the endometrium at the time of menstruation are associated with primary dysmenorrhea.[7] The sequential stimulation of the endometrium by estrogen, followed by progesterone, results in a dramatic increase in prostaglandin production by the endometrium. Prostaglandins increase myometrial contractions and cause constriction of small endometrial blood vessels, with consequent tissue ischemia, endometrial disintegration, bleeding, and pain. Prostaglandins are also known to cause headaches, diarrhea, and vomiting, which are secondary manifestations of dysmenorrhea. Dysmenorrhea may be caused by excessive tissue ischemia resulting from increased intrauterine pressure, vessel constriction, and decreased uterine blood flow. Dysmenorrhea usually occurs in ovulatory cycles, although it has been noted in anovulatory cycles. Primary dysmenorrhea occurs in some women on oral contraceptives, but most women experience few or no symptoms while "on the pill."

Secondary dysmenorrhea often occurs well before the onset of menses and may persist for a longer time during the flow than primary dysmenorrhea. Secondary dysmenorrhea is due to pelvic diseases such as endometriosis, chronic pelvic inflammatory disease, uterine leiomyomas, and adenomyosis. Various diagnostic and therapeutic measures are used when secondary dysmenorrhea is suspected.

Clinical Manifestations. Primary dysmenorrhea usually occurs within 3 years of menarche. Characteristic manifestations include lower, midabdominal pain that is colicky in nature, with radiation to the lower back and upper thighs. The abdominal pain is often accompanied by nausea, diarrhea or loose stools, fatigue, headache, and a general sense of malaise. The pain usually begins at the onset of menstruation and lasts for 12 to 72 hours, with the most severe pain occurring on the first day.

Secondary dysmenorrhea usually occurs after the woman has experienced problem-free periods for some time. The pain, which may be unilateral, is generally more constant in nature and may continue throughout the period.

Therapeutic Management. A major management goal is to distinguish primary from secondary dysmenorrhea.[6] Taking a complete health history and performing a physical examination should be the first procedure. If the history is suggestive and pelvic examination findings are normal, the problem is usually treated as primary dysmenorrhea.

Treatment of dysmenorrhea varies depending on the severity of the symptoms and the individual patient's response. Many patients with dysmenorrhea respond well to symptomatic therapy, including reassurance, local heat, and mild analgesics. Dysmenorrhea is a recurring problem, so the use of narcotics is discouraged because addiction is a possibility.

Pharmacologic Management. Two groups of drugs considered highly effective for primary dysmenorrhea are nonsteroidal antiinflammatory drugs (NSAIDs) and oral contraceptives. Antiinflammatory drugs inhibit production of prostaglandins in the menstrual fluid and their subsequent action on the uterus.

NSAIDs such as ibuprofen, naproxen, and mefenamic acid (Ponstel) significantly decrease the frequency and severity of symptoms. NSAIDs are prescribed to be taken just before menses (for women who can accurately predict the onset of menses) or at the time of onset of menses. Therapy usually continues four times daily for the first 3 to 4 days of the period. If there is a possibility of pregnancy, the use of NSAIDs is precluded.

The most common side effects of NSAIDs include dizziness and gastrointestinal (GI) distress. Taking food with the drug may relieve the latter problem. A history of asthma or peptic ulcers should be reported to the physician because NSAIDs are contraindicated in these situations.

Oral contraceptives may be the first line of treatment if they are also the woman's contraception choice. With the suppression of ovulation by oral contraceptives, the production of prostaglandins is also suppressed. Because dysmenorrhea occurs most frequently in young women, there are few contraindications to the use of oral contraceptives.

Acupuncture, exercise, and transcutaneous nerve stimulation provide varying degrees of relief. These methods may be used for women who obtain inadequate relief from medications or who prefer not to take medications. Patients who are unresponsive to these treatments should be evaluated for chronic pelvic pain.

NURSING MANAGEMENT

DYSMENORRHEA

Patients often ask nurses what can be done when minor discomforts associated with cycles sometimes occur. Women should be aware that during acute pain, relief may be obtained by lying down for short periods, drinking hot beverages, applying heat to the abdomen, and taking an antiinflammatory drug for mild analgesia. The nurse should instruct the woman about the use of these modalities. The nurse can also suggest noninvasive pain-relieving practices such as distraction and guided imagery (see Chapter 6). These practices may increase the patient's feeling of control and self-reliance.

Other health care measures that can decrease the discomfort of dysmenorrhea are known and should be used. These include regular exercise, maintenance of proper nutritional habits, avoidance of constipation, maintenance of good body mechanics, and avoidance of stress and overfatigue, particularly during the time preceding menstrual periods. Staying active and interested in activities may also help. The nurse's approach to the problem of dysmenorrhea must be thoughtful and sensitive. The counsel and supportive therapy given can provide a foundation for coping with this common problem.

Menstrual Irregularities

The ovarian cycle is more unstable and vulnerable to disruptive influences in its early (adolescence) and late phases (premenopausal). Therefore abnormal bleeding is more common at the beginning and end of the active menstrual life. When irregular bleeding becomes problematic for the patient, whether amenorrhea, menorrhea, or metrorrhagia, a systematic investigation will lead to the cause of dysfunctional uterine bleeding. When menorrhagia (increased amount or duration of menstrual bleeding) or metrorrhagia (bleeding or spotting between periods) occurs, the possibility of pelvic neoplasm must always be considered.

Types of Dysfunctional Uterine Bleeding

Amenorrhea. The absence of menses refers to the failure to menstruate before 18 years of age (*primary amenorrhea*) and cessation of menses for 6 months or more after they have become established (*secondary amenorrhea*). Amenorrhea probably occurs in less than 5% of patients. The common causes of amenorrhea are listed in Table 51-2.

Reasons for changes in the usual pattern of menstruation vary, as does the associated degree of concern. Changes in lifestyle such as marriage, recent moves, a death in the family, financial stress, and other emotional crises can cause amenorrhea or unusual bleeding. These effects demonstrate the strong influences that psychologic factors have on endocrine function and should be considered when the patient is evaluated.

Menorrhagia. Menorrhagia is an increased duration or amount of menstrual bleeding at the time of a normal period. In the early reproductive years, it may be associated with anovulatory cycles or uterine growths. A single episode of excessive bleeding may indicate a spontaneous abortion or ectopic pregnancy. Uterine tumors, including carcinoma, are common causes of menorrhagia. Pelvic inflammatory disease, endometriosis, the use of an intrauterine device (IUD), and drugs such as anticoagulants and thiazides (secondary to thrombocytopenia) can also produce heavy menses.

Metrorrhagia. Metrorrhagia is bleeding or spotting between menstrual periods. The most common cause of intramenstrual bleeding is the use of hormonal contraceptives. This is referred to as *breakthrough bleeding.* Intramenstrual blood loss may also be caused by uterine lesions such as fibroids, polyps, hyperplasia, and carcinoma; cervical inflammation or lesions; and pelvic inflammatory disease.

Table 51-2 Causes of Amenorrhea
Hypothalamic-Pituitary Axis
Reversible CNS-mediated insults (e.g., emotional stress, anorexia nervosa or severe dieting, strenuous exercise, postpill syndrome, chronic or acute illness)
Prolactinoma and other causes of hyperprolactinemia (e.g., drugs)
Craniopharyngioma and other brain stem or parasellar tumors
Congenital conditions (e.g., isolated gonadotropin deficiency)*
Trauma (e.g., head injury with hypothalamic contusion)
Infiltrative processes (e.g., sarcoidosis)
Vascular disease (e.g., hypothalamic vasculitis)
Pituitary tumors
Sheehan's syndrome
Ovaries
Autoimmune disease (often involving thyroid, adrenal, and islet cells)
Premature menopause (idiopathic) or resistant-ovary syndrome
Polycystic ovary disease
Tumors
Congenital or genetic conditions (e.g., Turner's syndrome)*
Infection (e.g., mumps oophoritis)
Toxins (especially alkylating chemotherapeutic agents)
Irradiation
Trauma, torsion (rare)
Uterovaginal Outflow Tract
Asherman's syndrome (postcurettage loss of endometrium)
Müllerian dysgenesis*
Hormonal Synthesis and Action
Male pseudohermaphroditism (e.g., testicular feminization)*
17-Hydroxylase deficiency*

CNS, Central nervous system.
*Usually presents as primary amenorrhea.

Therapeutic Management. Because the causes of menstrual irregularities are multiple and varied, diagnostic and therapeutic measures vary as well. A detailed health history and a careful physical examination, including a pelvic examination, will limit the possible diagnoses and lead to a logical selection of laboratory tests and diagnostic procedures. For menstrual irregularity caused by inflammation and infection, see the discussion in this chapter on pelvic inflammatory disease.

Treatment of menstrual irregularities depends on the woman's need for contraception, her desire to conceive, or her wish to regulate irregular bleeding.[7] The treatment goal is to stop the current episode of bleeding, to prevent recurrence, and to preserve ovulation if pregnancy is desired. Conservative treatment consists of hormonal therapy. For a woman wishing to conceive, progesterone given in a single course for a problem of short duration or for three to four menstrual cycles may result in the return of normal ovarian function and control of excessive bleeding. For recurrent irregular bleeding, low-dose oral contraceptives are the treatment of choice.

For chronic recurrent bleeding, microsurgical techniques using a laser or electrocautery have demonstrated excellent results. It is a safe and effective alternative to hysterectomy when conservative therapy has failed. However, this therapy may result in no return of menses (60%), return of normal menses (30%), or no change in bleeding (10%).[8]

When treating amenorrhea, pregnancy should first be ruled out before any further endocrine workup is undertaken. Depending on the cause of the amenorrhea, treatment may involve hormone replacement therapy (e.g., estrogens, thyroid hormone, glucocorticoids, clomiphene citrate, gonadotropins, bromocriptine) or a corrective procedure, such as surgical removal of a pituitary tumor.

Surgical Interventions. Surgical interventions for the treatment of menstrual irregularities include a variety of procedures such as dilatation and curettage (D & C), polypectomy, cauterization (destruction of tissue by a chemical or by heat), myomectomy (removal of uterine tumor without removal of the uterus), and hysterectomy. These procedures may be performed using standard surgical techniques, but more often microsurgical techniques, using a hysteroscope or a laparoscope and laser or electrocautery, are done. Microsurgery reduces bleeding and postoperative infection. Patients have fewer recovery days from these less invasive techniques.

D & C is the most frequently performed gynecologic procedure. *Dilatation* is the widening of the cervical canal with a dilator. *Curettage* is the scraping of the lining of the uterus with a curette. A D & C is considered both a diagnostic and a therapeutic measure. A diagnostic D & C is performed to identify a lesion in the endocervix or endometrium. A therapeutic D & C is done for an incomplete abortion or to correct excessive or prolonged bleeding. Dilatation of the cervix may be done to treat dysmenorrhea or sterility caused by cervical stenosis. A D & C is most often done as an outpatient procedure, but overnight hospitalization may be indicated.

NURSING MANAGEMENT
MENSTRUAL IRREGULARITIES
Nursing Implementation

Acute Intervention. The amount of vaginal bleeding the patient experiences should be accurately assessed. The number and size of pads or tampons used and the degree of saturation should be reported and recorded. The patient's fatigue level, along with variations in blood pressure and blood count, should be noted because anemia and hypovolemia may be present.

When a patient is scheduled for a D & C, food intake is restricted after midnight the evening before the procedure. The procedure may be done in the operating room, in a free-standing surgery center, or in the physician's office, using either local or general anesthesia. Even if the choice is local anesthesia, the patient should be prepared to receive general anesthesia if it becomes necessary.

Postoperatively, the patient's vital signs should be checked every 15 minutes until stable. The amount of vaginal bleeding should be noted, and a pad count should be kept. Some abdominal cramping, pelvic discomfort, or back pain is usual. These problems should be relieved with mild antiinflammatory analgesics (e.g., aspirin, ibuprofen). Persistent pain should be reported to the physician because the uterus is occasionally perforated during the procedure.

Because the patient is discharged within 1 to 6 hours after the operation, teaching is an especially important aspect of nursing care. Specific instructions for self-care must be provided, including the following:

1. Avoid the use of tampons or douching and refrain from intercourse until examination the second week after the operation.
2. Expect a vaginal discharge during the healing process. It should be lighter in amount than the usual menses and from dark red to dark brown, and it should last no longer than 1 week.
3. Avoid strenuous activity for 1 week, but a return to usual activities 2 days after recovery from anesthesia is usually appropriate.
4. Report any signs of infection, such as fever, chills, foul-smelling discharge, heavy bleeding, and pelvic pain.

The patient should also be told that the subsequent menstrual period is not usually affected.

Chronic and Home Management. Treatment of menstrual problems is not always adequate. For example, a D & C for metrorrhagia may be helpful for a time, but the problem may recur. Continued use of contraceptives may become undesirable because of the patient's age or state of health. If abnormal bleeding persists, the patient generally becomes frustrated and worried and wants something done to correct the condition. It is common for adolescent women to experience anovulatory cycles as dysfunctional uterine bleeding during the first years of menstruation. It is critical that the nurse take time to provide an extensive explanation of common variations of menstruation. Irregular menstruation during adolescence should not be construed as something abnormal. Young women in particular need reassurance that this does not indicate future reproductive problems.

If fibroids are noted and abdominal bleeding persists, hysterectomy may be the treatment of choice. The nurse may play an important role in addressing the concerns some women express about physical, sexual, and emotional changes after a hysterectomy. The woman who does not wish to become pregnant may be relieved to have an end to persistent bleeding. Assessment of the individual woman provides the direction for the counseling.

Menopause

In 1900 fewer than 5 million American women were over 50 years of age. In 1991 1.3 million women turned 50 years old. They joined the 35 million other women who have reached menopause. With the current life expectancy approaching 80 years, women can expect to live more than one third of their lives during their postmenopausal years.[9]

Historically, before the physiology of menopause was understood, many cultures attached negative meaning to the loss of reproduction. Although some women continue to feel that way today, many women find that it is during these years that they can care for themselves and achieve lifetime desires that were delayed during child-rearing years.

Menopause occurs during the years known as the *climacteric* or *perimenopause*. The climacteric refers to the phase of aging for a woman during which reproductive function gradually diminishes and then ceases. It lasts approximately 15 to 20 years, from about the ages of 40 to 60. During this period, monthly menses occur less frequently and are irregular. The *menopause* is the physiologic cessation of menses associated with decreased ovarian function. Menopause is defined by 1 year without menstruation. Natural menopause usually occurs between 47 and 52 years of age. Menopause results from radiation of the ovaries or is surgically induced following removal of both ovaries, with or without a hysterectomy. Menopause results from a decrease in estrogen. The signs and symptoms of diminishing estrogen are listed in Table 51-3.

Clinical Manifestations

Physical. When discussing clinically noticeable menopausal changes, it is important to remember that menopause is a normal physiologic occurrence. The hallmark of the menopausal transition is the appearance of irregular menses. In addition, the most common physical changes directly related to menopause are hot flashes and atrophic vaginal changes. These changes are physiologic responses to a rapid decrease in estrogen levels with an increase in plasma levels of gonadotropins, especially FSH.[10] *Hot flashes* are described as a sensation of warmth in the upper part of the chest, neck, and face followed by profuse perspiration and sometimes chilling. These sensations last from several seconds to 5 minutes and occur most often at night, thereby disturbing sleep. Hot flashes can be triggered by situations that affect body temperature, such as eating a hot meal, hot weather, drinking an alcoholic beverage, stress, or warm clothing.

Atrophic vaginal changes secondary to decreased estrogen include thinning of the vaginal mucosa and disappearance of rugae. Vaginal secretions also decrease and become more alkaline. Because of these changes, the vaginal canal is easily traumatized and susceptible to infection. Dyspareunia may be a problem.

Atrophic changes also occur postmenopausally in the lower urinary tract because of a decrease in estrogen. These changes include thinning of the urethra, atrophy of the periurethral tissues and blood vessels, lowered bladder sensory threshold to void, and loss of pelvic tone. These anatomic and physiologic changes in the lower urinary tract lead to symptoms such as dysuria, urgency, frequency, suprapubic discomfort, and urge and stress incontinence.[11]

The loss of estrogen plays a significant role in the cause of age-related pathology. Changes that are most critical to a woman's well-being are the increased risk of heart attack from cardiovascular changes and the risk of developing osteoporosis secondary to bone density loss.[12,13] Other changes include a redistribution of fat, a tendency to gain weight more easily, muscle and joint pain, loss of skin elasticity, and atrophy of external genitalia and breast tissue.

Obese women experience few menopausal symptoms. The large number of adipocytes provides a source of estrogen through the conversion of adrenal androgens to estrogen in the adipocytes.

Psychologic. Estrogen and progesterone have much to do with a women's sense of well-being.[13] Decreasing estrogen also alters the time spent in rapid eye movement (REM) sleep. Because of these changes and the interruption of sleep caused by hot flashes, sleep deprivation develops in many menopausal women. This can result in complaints of irritability, anxiety, nervousness, fatigue, and forgetfulness. Although family, social, and personal changes may also be factors influencing a woman's life during this time, double-blind studies reveal that estrogen replacement significantly reduces these symptoms when compared with placebo treatment.[14]

Therapeutic and Pharmacologic Management. Significant beneficial effects as well as potential risks are associated with the use of hormonal replacement therapy (HRT) in menopausal women. HRT has been advocated in the management of the physical and emotional symptoms of menopause, osteoporosis prevention and treatment, and cardiovascular disease prevention. The decision as to whether, when, and how to use HRT and the duration of its use are controversial. The lowest effective dose of estrogen for the shortest possible time is prescribed by some providers, whereas others advocate long-term therapy to 70 years

Table 51-3 Signs and Symptoms of Estrogen Deficiency

- Vasomotor
  - Hot flashes
- Genitourinary
  - Atrophic vaginitis
  - Dyspareunia secondary to poor lubrication
  - Dysuria
- Psychologic
  - Emotional lability
  - Change in sleep pattern
  - Decreased REM sleep
- Skeletal
  - Increased fracture rate, particularly of vertebral bodies but also of humerus, distal radius, and upper femur
- Cardiovascular
  - Decreased high-density lipoproteins
  - Increased low-density lipoproteins
- Dermatologic
  - Diminished collagen content of skin
  - Breast tissue changes

REM, Rapid eye movement.

of age or beyond.[14] Low-dose estrogen effectively controls disabling vasomotor symptoms. Most women can accept and tolerate hot flashes without treatment if they are assured that the hot flashes will stop within 1 to 5 years.

When atrophic vaginal changes occur, estrogen vaginal creams or suppositories (e.g., Premarin) provide effective and rapid relief. These are administered daily for about a week and thereafter once or twice a week, depending on the patient's response. Because substantial systemic absorption of estrogen occurs with vaginal use, the risks are the same as those associated with systemic estrogen therapy.

HRT is effective in preventing cardiovascular disease. Estrogen is capable of reducing low-density lipoproteins and increasing high-density lipoproteins. Estrogen replacement is associated with a greater than 50% reduction in the risk of cardiovascular disease.[15] However, progestins may adversely affect lipoproteins, thereby reducing some of the cardiovascular benefits provided by estrogen.

Prevention of osteoporosis results in arresting or slowing the process of demineralization from bone. The loss of minerals, especially calcium, from bone begins with the onset of the climacteric at around 40 years of age. Effective therapy should begin before demineralization occurs and should continue throughout the menopausal and postmenopausal periods. Adequate calcium supplementation and regular weight-bearing exercise are needed to maintain bone and prevent further bone loss,[16] regardless of whether HRT is used. (See Chapter 59 for a discussion of osteoporosis.)

The risks of estrogen replacement use are the suspected increase in endometrial cancer and some types of breast cancer. Endometrial cancer is a high-risk potential for women taking only estrogen replacement because unopposed estrogen may induce endometrial hyperplasia and ultimately adenocarcinoma. The addition of a progestin in a cyclic or daily regimen reduces this risk. However, the cycling of estrogen and progesterone mimics the normal menstrual cycle, resulting in the reestablishment of menses. Women who prefer not to continue menstruation under the influence of HRT may be prescribed a daily dose of both estrogen (Premarin, Estinyl, and Ogen) 0.625 mg and progesterone (Norlutin and Provera) 2.5 mg. Under this regimen, menstruation should cease within 6 to 9 months. The use of progestins in a woman who has no uterus is unnecessary and possibly detrimental.

Because women are still producing some level of estrogen in a cyclic fashion, menstrual irregularities may occur while taking HRT. A distinction between the menstrual irregularities that are basically physiologic features of menopause and the development of pathologic conditions such as polyps or cancer must be made. This entails careful physical and pelvic examinations, cervical cytologic study, and endometrial biopsy. Once pathologic conditions are ruled out, women should be advised of the expected menstrual irregularities and provided with options for natural or hormonal management.

A woman's cumulative lifetime exposure to estrogen is strongly related to her risk of developing breast cancer.[17] Therefore, it is suspected that continued use of estrogen in the postmenopausal years will increase the risk of breast cancer. However, it has been extremely difficult to demonstrate in clinical trials that taking estrogen during the menopausal years actually increases that risk. Furthermore, a recent analysis of many studies suggests that estrogen in doses of 0.625 mg or less probably does not pose a substantial increased risk of breast cancer.[18] The role of estrogen-progesterone therapy in the prevention of breast cancer is inconclusive and deserves further long-term study.[14]

Hormone Replacement Therapy. If a woman chooses HRT, a careful health history should be obtained to document whether a family tendency for cancer, hypertension, cardiovascular disease, or osteoporosis exists. A complete physical examination, including breast and pelvic examinations, a Papanicolaou's (Pap) smear, endometrial biopsy, and a baseline blood pressure, is also done. Estrogen is given cyclically in a dosage ranging from 0.3 to 1.25 mg per day, with the medication omitted 5 to 7 days per month. Progestins are added in a dosage of 2.5 to 10 mg per day

RESEARCH

IMPLICATIONS FOR NURSING PRACTICE

OSTEOPOROSIS PREVENTION IN PERIMENOPAUSAL AND ELDERLY WOMEN

Citation Ali NS, Twibell KR: Barriers to osteoporosis prevention in perimenopausal and elderly women, *Geriatr Nurs* 15:201-205, 1994.

Purpose To describe osteoporosis-preventive behaviors in a sample of perimenopausal and elderly women and to examine perceived benefits and barriers related to the performance of these behaviors.

Methods Descriptive study using 100 perimenopausal and elderly women. Participants provided information about their daily calcium intake, exercise participation, and whether or not they took estrogen replacement therapy (ERT). They also completed three barriers/benefits scales related to calcium intake, exercise participation, and ERT.

Results and Conclusions Results indicated that the sample lacked proper information about the age-related need for daily calcium intake. Although half of the sample performed exercise, none of the participants expressed the benefit of exercise in influencing bones and the prevention of osteoporosis. Only 11% of the sample took ERT. Nontakers of ERT indicated a lack of knowledge about ERT, confusion about therapy, lack of understanding of reasons to take the therapy for the rest of their lives, and economic barriers to continuing the therapy.

Implications for Nursing Practice Nurses' recognition of women's perceptions toward calcium, exercise, and ERT may facilitate the design of effective interventions to change the behaviors. Positive lifestyle changes could delay or prevent osteoporosis.

during the last 7 to 10 days of estrogen. With this schedule, shedding of the endometrium (menses) continues. For women choosing not to continue monthly menstruation, both estrogen and a progestin are given daily through the entire month within the aforementioned dose range sufficient to suppress any breakthrough bleeding. An increase in the incidence of gallstones and hypertension has been noted in women taking HRT. Because HRT involves lower doses of estrogen, the risk of thrombophlebitis and stroke is not observed, as it may be in women who use oral contraceptives.

Estrogen may also be administered through a skin patch. Transdermal estradiol (Estraderm 0.05 to 0.1 mg) is applied to a clear, dry area on the trunk of the body and is worn either continuously or for the first 21 days of the cycle. Each patch delivers a lower dose of estrogen than oral estrogens. Because the dose is absorbed in 3 to 3.5 days, the patch must be changed *only* twice a week. Studies show that the patch relieves menopausal symptoms, has a low incidence of skin irritation, and is acceptable to the patient.[17] Transdermal estradiol treatment is also effective in postmenopausal women with osteoporosis. The cardioprotective effect of transdermal estrogen has not been definitively determined.[19] Progestin should be given as discussed previously if the uterus is still present.

A woman's decision to initiate HRT must be an informed one. The therapeutic use of replacement therapy for menopausal changes, osteoporosis prevention, and cardiovascular protection must be discussed. The woman should be reexamined every 6 months to 1 year, at which time the HRT dosage can be adjusted as needed. An endometrial biopsy should be performed after 2 years of treatment or if any unexpected vaginal bleeding occurs. Estrogen should not be used by patients with unexplained vaginal bleeding, known or suspected estrogen-dependent neoplasia, acute liver disease or chronic impaired liver function, renal insufficiency, acute vascular thrombosis, or neuroophthalmologic vascular diseases.[20] The side effects of HRT include weight gain, breast and pelvic discomfort from engorgement, headache, GI disturbances, vaginal discharge, and skin pigmentation. These symptoms usually result from an excessive estrogen dosage or are an initial response to therapy. They can be reduced by decreasing the dosage, or they may resolve spontaneously with continued use of the drugs.

Nutritional Management. Nutrition is an important area of health education for the perimenopausal woman. A daily intake of about 30 cal/kg body weight with maintenance of sound nutrition is recommended. A decrease in metabolic rate and careless eating habits and not menopause itself can be the causes for weight gain and related fatigue.

An adequate intake of calcium and vitamin D can help maintain healthy bones and thereby counteract the effect of decreased estrogen that tends to make bones grow lighter and more fragile. The recommended daily allowance (RDA) of calcium for the average menstruating woman and the postmenopausal woman on HRT is 800 to 1000 mg per day. It is recommended that postmenopausal women not on HRT have a daily calcium intake of 1500 mg.[6] However, a study of upper-middle-class women between 50 and 79 years of age showed a daily calcium intake of less than 800 mg.[6] For women with low calcium intake or lactose intolerance, supplemental calcium to the recommended level should be taken daily. Dairy products are an excellent source of dietary calcium. Use of low-fat dairy products eliminates the concern over the high caloric and fat content of many dairy products. Intake of junk foods, soft drinks, and protein should be decreased because these foods raise phosphate levels and therefore lower free calcium levels. Vitamin E and the B complex vitamins have been associated with a decrease in physical and emotional menopausal symptoms; therefore moderate supplementations are recommended.

NURSING MANAGEMENT

MENOPAUSE

When the perimenopause period begins, women have almost as many years of their adult lives ahead of them as behind them. During this period a woman can choose to foster good health, vitality, and attractiveness, or she can perceive that menopause is the beginning of a prolonged degenerative process. The nurse can help the woman work through changes that occur by providing health teaching and reassurance.

The patient's understanding of the physiology of menopause should be assessed because this may affect reactions to the changes and compliance with the therapeutic approach. The patient should be made aware that the symptoms she is experiencing are normal and will pass after a time. Many misconceptions about menopause have been perpetuated and should be clarified by the nurse to reduce unnecessary anxiety.

A regular program of exercise and physical activity can improve circulation, maintain good muscle tone, and delay some aspects of aging for women in menopause. Exercising for 20 to 60 minutes at least 3 times a week stimulates osteoblastic activity, thereby stimulating calcium deposition into bone and delaying osteoporosis. Activities such as brisk walks, bicycling, and gardening are healthy and enjoyable. Development of new interests can help ease tension and anxiety.

Sexual function can continue with little change in the vast majority of postmenopausal women. Cessation of menstruation and ability to bear children should not be equated with cessation of sexual capability. Femininity and libido do not disappear with menopause. An older woman often displays greater warmth and sensitivity in her sexual relationships than she did as a younger woman.[13] Atrophic changes in vaginal epithelium associated with inadequate lubrication may lead to *dyspareunia* (painful coitus). A water-soluble lubricant (e.g., Replens) is often effective in managing this problem. An active sex life helps increase lubrication and maintain the pliability of vaginal tissues. The patient should be given an opportunity to discuss concerns related to sexual functioning candidly.

The nurse should be alert to the risks, benefits, and possible side effects of the drugs that the patient is taking and should be able to interpret them for the patient. Hormonal replacement may be continued indefinitely as part of a plan to prevent the development or worsening of osteoporosis.

CONTRACEPTION AND BIRTH CONTROL

Many social changes have been brought about and encouraged by the women's liberation movement. Women have more options in pursuing careers in addition to family and childbearing roles. With the advent of effective methods of contraception and abortion, pregnancy is seen as a choice. Women can now make choices about family size and spacing in keeping with their lifestyle. Poor health or genetic problems of either partner and the mutual desire for fewer children may be motivators for the use of current methods of family planning. These practices can result in planned pregnancies at desired intervals.

Significance

The rapid growth in the world population has been identified as a threat to natural resources and to the quality of life for all. Consequently, the issue of population control is influenced by political and economic factors balanced against sociocultural constraints for each social group. Because of this situation, women may expect a high priority to be placed on the development of contraceptives with a high degree of safety, effectiveness, and availability. However, sociocultural constraints often inhibit actions that appear to be logical and practical approaches to the problem of population growth. For example, despite increasing pregnancies among adolescents, adequate and accurate contraceptive information is rarely provided to teenagers. Despite growing concern over the number of children born into an adverse socioeconomic environment, there are efforts to restrict the option of abortion for poor women. Women are often left to consider the health consequences and economic risk-benefit ratio between pregnancy and contraception. These factors often leave women in a moral dilemma in their decision making about contraceptives.

Contraceptive Methods

An ideal contraceptive is one that is safe, simple to use, inexpensive, reversible, and does not interfere with the act of intercourse. No single method that meets all these criteria is yet available. *Temporary* contraceptives provide protection for individuals who wish to avoid or delay pregnancy. To be effective, they must be used correctly and consistently. *Permanent* methods of birth control such as sterilization are becoming increasingly acceptable to men and women. Sterilization is often chosen by persons who have completed their families or who wish to remain childless. Table 51-4 summarizes the common contraceptive methods, their use, their side effects, and related patient education. Selected methods are discussed in the following.

Female Contraception

Hormonal contraception. Hormonal contraceptives continue to be the form of contraception that is most widely used in the United States and Canada. Advances in the combined estrogen and progesterone pill have resulted in lower hormone levels and levels of doses to more closely mimic the natural fluctuations occurring in the body. During the last 5 years the greatest development has occurred in progestin-only contraception. Research has shown that progestins are more effective when absorbed in the skin rather than orally. Table 51-4 list methods of birth control and all forms of progestins that are currently approved by the FDA. POPS (progestin-only pills) or Minipills have the highest rate of failure, but the injectable and subdermal methods have effectiveness rates greater than the combined oral contraceptives. Improvements in Norplant (subdermal progestin-only implant) are directed at reducing the number of capsules from six to two and making them biodegradable so that they do not have to be surgically removed.[21]

Other contraceptive methods are used widely in Europe and Asia but are not approved for use in the United States. Monthly combined contraceptive injectables, progestin vaginal rings, and RU 486 are some examples. RU 486 is a progesterone antagonist that causes the onset of menses whether or not fertilization has occurred. It is used as a postcoital contraceptive and therefore regarded by some as inducing abortion. For this reason it has been controversial in the United States, although the FDA did approve the use of RU 486 in clinical trials in 1994.[22]

Female condom. The female condom is another option for contraception and preventing transmission of HIV and some other sexually transmitted diseases.[23] The female condom consists of two flexible polyurethane rings and a soft loose-fitting polyurethane sheath that lines the vagina (see Fig. 51-2 on p. 1594). Results of clinical trials on the female condom have concluded that it is 88% effective in preventing pregnancy. Also, HIV, cytomegalovirus, and hepatitis B do not penetrate the sheath. Less than 1% incidence of breaks and tears and no significant adverse reactions were reported.[23] Specific instructions for use are included with the product, which is available over the counter.

Male Contraception. Male contraception is possible by several different methods.[24] The only device is the condom (a barrier) (Fig. 51-2). This form of contraception has attracted renewed interest for the protection it provides against sexually transmitted diseases and HIV. Research on steroidal contraceptives continues. The combined use of GnRH and testosterone to suppress gonadotropins and inhibin (hormone that inhibits activity of FSH) is being studied. It is not known whether this suppression will persist during a longer treatment period or whether it will reliably induce azoospermia. There have been no reported side effects.[25] Male sterilization is discussed in Chapter 52.

Gossypol, a cottonseed derivative, alters sperm structure and motility and decreases sperm production. However, problems associated with gossypol include potassium depletion with cardiac dysrhythmias, slow onset of action, and slow return of fertility. Most researchers agree that the product will not be ready for marketing for at least 5 years.[21]

NURSING MANAGEMENT

CONTRACEPTION AND BIRTH CONTROL

Persons desire to prevent conception for a number of reasons related to personal convenience, economics, social

Table 51-4 Methods of Birth Control

Description	Side Effects and Complications	Patient Education
TEMPORARY		
Combined		
Combination pill contains both estrogen and progesterone (standard and low-dose) taken usually on fifth through twenty-fifth day of each cycle. Prevents ovulation, causes changes in endometrium, alterations in cervical mucus, and tubal transport. Simple and unobtrusive in use, 99% effective. Failure from irregular or incorrect use.	Side effects of weight gain, nausea and vomiting, spotting and breakthrough bleeding, postpill amenorrhea, breast tenderness, headache, chloasma, irritability, nervousness, depression, and decreased libido; complications of benign liver tumors, gallstones, myocardial infarction, thromboembolism, stroke (smokers over age 35 at higher risk); contraindications of history of cardiovascular or liver disease, hypertension, breast or pelvic cancer and caution with diabetes mellitus, sickle cell anemia. Provides no protection against HIV transmission.	Instruct patient in correct use of pills. Tell patient to take pill same time each day; if forgotten one day, take two next day. Review side effects, contraindications. Explain that patient should report cramps or swelling of legs, chest pain. Discuss need for periodic (every 6-12 mo) checkup that involves weight, BP, Pap smear, hematocrit. Review danger signs of drug. Take drug history, asking about use of phenytoin, phenobarbital, antibiotic (e.g., ampicillin), which decrease contraceptive action. Inform patient that method is usually not recommended for persons over age 35. Discourage smoking.
Morning-after pill (Ovral) ethinyl estradiol 50 μg and norgestrel 0.5 mg. Another use of combined hormonal contraception. 98.4% effective. Fewer side effects than DES. Creates hostile uterine lining and alters tubal transport.	Nausea for 1 or 2 days. Would not prevent an ectopic pregnancy. At risk for usual hormonal complications of ACHES.	Take two Ovral within 72 hr of coitus. Repeat if vomiting occurs. Take second dose 12 hr later. Menses should begin within 2-3 wk. Start an ongoing method of contraception immediately after menses.
Progestin Only		
Progestin-only pills (POPS or Minipills) are taken daily, with no pill-free days. Preferred for women who are breast feeding. Does not suppress lactation. Inhibits ovulation.Thickens cervical mucus. Alters uterine lining. Lower cardiovascular risk than combined pills.	Menstrual changes; breakthrough bleeding, prolonged cycles or amenorrhea. Increase in functional cysts of the ovary. Increase in ectopic pregnancy.	Use alternate contraception when starting POPS or if pill is missed. Take pill at same time every day. Keep record of menses and get pregnancy test if 2 wk late.
Depoprovera (DMPA) is a progestin-only drug given by injection every 3 mo. A private, convenient, and highly effective method.	May cause amenorrhea, headaches, bloating, and weight gain. Return of fertility may be delayed for several months.	Return every 3 mo for injection. Discontinue method for several months before planning to conceive.
Norplant is a progestin-only subdermal implant. Six silicone capsules provide protection for 5 yr. Continuous, long-term contraception. Failure rate is extremely low. Does not suppress lactation.	Surgical removal of capsules after 5 yr. Menstrual irregularities, especially during the first year. Later may cause amenorrhea. May cause abdominal pain, headaches, weight gain.	Is effective after 24 hr. Keep arm dry for 48 hr after insertion. Report arm pain. Implants are soft and flexible and cannot break. Expect some irregular bleeding. Report any other changes. Remove implants in 5 yr. Continue to protect against STDs.

continued

Table 51-4 Methods of Birth Control—cont'd

Description	Side Effects and Complications	Patient Education
Barrier Method		
Vaginal sponge		
Cup-shaped disposable polyurethane sponge that is impregnated with spermicide. Removal loop located on bottom; provision of 24-hr mechanical and chemical barrier that traps and absorbs sperm; one size; available without prescription. 89-90% effective; failure caused by improper placement.	Allergy or irritation to sponge or spermicide; risk of toxic shock syndrome uncertain but with no greater incidence than for tampon use	Ascertain patient's ability to palpate cervix, properly place moistened sponge over cervix, and remove (gently to avoid tearing). Inform patient that removal is aided by bearing down and that sponge remains in place 5 hr after coitus. Advise patient that it is not suitable if severe pelvic relaxation is present or during menses.
Cervical cap		
Rubber thimble-shaped shield covering cervix held in place only by suction. Spermicide in inner surface provides mechanical barrier to sperm. Fitting by professional. Effectiveness similar to diaphragm; failure from dislodgement and improper fit.	Allergy to rubber or spermicide, possible cervical irritation or erosion from suction.	Provide sufficient time for practice with insertion and removal (more time than for diaphragm). Give instruction for cleaning, storing, and inspecting for damage. Inform patient that it can be used with abnormalities of vaginal canal but not with cervical inconsistencies or pelvic inflammatory disease.
Condom		
Male: thin rubber sheath fitting over erect penis and providing mechanical barrier to sperm. Simple method to use, no prescription necessary. 85% effective; failure from tearing or slipping during coitus. Used with spermicide. Affords some protection against STDs and HIV transmission.	Possible allergy to rubber, possible decrease in sensation and interference with foreplay.	Advise patient to roll sheath along entire penis, leaving slack at end to receive semen. Inform patient that sharp object (e.g., fingernails) may tear condom. Tell patient to hold sheath in place when penis is withdrawn to prevent emptying of sperm in or near vagina.
Female: double ring system fitted into vagina up to 8 hr before intercourse. No prescription necessary; 88% effective. Affords protection against HIV, cytomegalovirus, and hepatitis B.	No significant side effects; generally acceptable to couple.	Discuss insertion, lubrication, method of removal. More expensive than male condom.
Diaphragm		
Dome-shaped latex cup with flexible metal ring (varies in size) covering cervix. Inner surface coated with spermicide before insertion. Provides mechanical barrier to sperm. Prescription method; fitting by professional; recurrent motivation to use necessary. 87% effective; failure from improper fitting or placement of device.	Allergy to latex, spermicide.	Demonstrate how to hold, insert, and remove device, using model. Allow for insertion and removal practice sessions. Advise patient that insertion may be any time before coitus, but removal should be 6-8 hr after coitus. Tell patient that bowel and bladder should be emptied before insertion. Give instructions for cleansing and storing, checking for holes or deterioration. Advise patient that diaphragm must be refitted following pregnancy, weight loss, or weight gain. Advise patient that it is not suitable if severe pelvic relaxation is present.

continued

Table 51-4 Methods of Birth Control—cont'd

Description	Side Effects and Complications	Patient Education
Other Methods		
IUD		
Insertion into uterus of flexible objects made of plastic or copper wire (nonmedicated or medicated with substance altering uterine environment), usually with attached string that protrudes into vagina. Contraception probably prevented by inflammatory response in endometrium, preventing implantation. After insertion, no additional equipment necessary; 97-99% effective; failure mainly from undetected expulsion. Most common type used today is Progestsert (contains progestins).	Increased menstrual flow, intramenstrual bleeding and cramping, especially during early months of use; possible complications of ectopic pregnancy, pelvic infection, perforation of uterus, infertility. Undetected expulsion of IUD resulting in pregnancy.	Discuss techniques and experience of insertion and removal. Inform patient that insertion may be more difficult and expulsion and complications greater in nulliparous patients. Instruct patient to check for string in vagina after each period; report to physician if unable to locate. Discuss need for annual pelvic examination and Pap smear.
Rhythm method		
Periodic abstinence during fertile portion of menstrual cycle. Requires strong motivation, self-control; complies with all religious doctrines; 60-65% effective; failure from difficulty in determining precise day of ovulation, irregularity of menses.	Inaccurate or incomplete knowledge of menstrual cycle.	Discuss methods to establish baseline menstrual patterns and identify ovulation. Give instructions in use of calendar or basal body temperature method to determine ovulation and fertile period.
PERMANENT		
Tubal		
Variety of abdominal and vaginal surgical procedures (laparotomy, laparoscopy, culdoscopy) that permanently prevent sperm and ovum from meeting. Crushing, ligating, clipping, or plugging of fallopian tubes (potentially reversible procedure); 99.96% effective; failure due to recanalization of fallopian tubes, erroneous ligation.	Bowel injury, hemorrhage, or infection.	Determine whether temporary contraceptives were used and reason for patient's dissatisfaction. Counsel regarding effects of procedure on physiology and sexual performance. Assist in obtaining written informed consent for procedure. Inform patient that procedure requires short-term hospitalization or can be done on outpatient basis.
Hysterectomy		
Surgical removal of uterus. 100% effective.	Bladder infection, vascular disorders, infection, hemorrhage, pain, psychologic adjustment.	Assess or counsel regarding understanding of extent of surgery, altered physiology, complications, and sexual performance. Hysterectomy done for other reason; sterility is secondary benefit when desired.
Vasectomy		
Bilateral surgical ligation and resection of ductus deferens, 100% effective.	Hematoma, swelling, psychologic adjustment.	Inform patient that procedure is usually done as outpatient procedure and takes 15-30 min. Tell patient that alternative form of contraception is needed until no sperm is seen on examination. Explain that procedure does not affect masculinity.

ACHES, see p. 1594; *BP*, blood pressure; *DES*, diethylstilbestrol; *HIV*, human immunodeficiency virus; *IUD*, intrauterine device; *STDs*, sexually transmitted diseases.

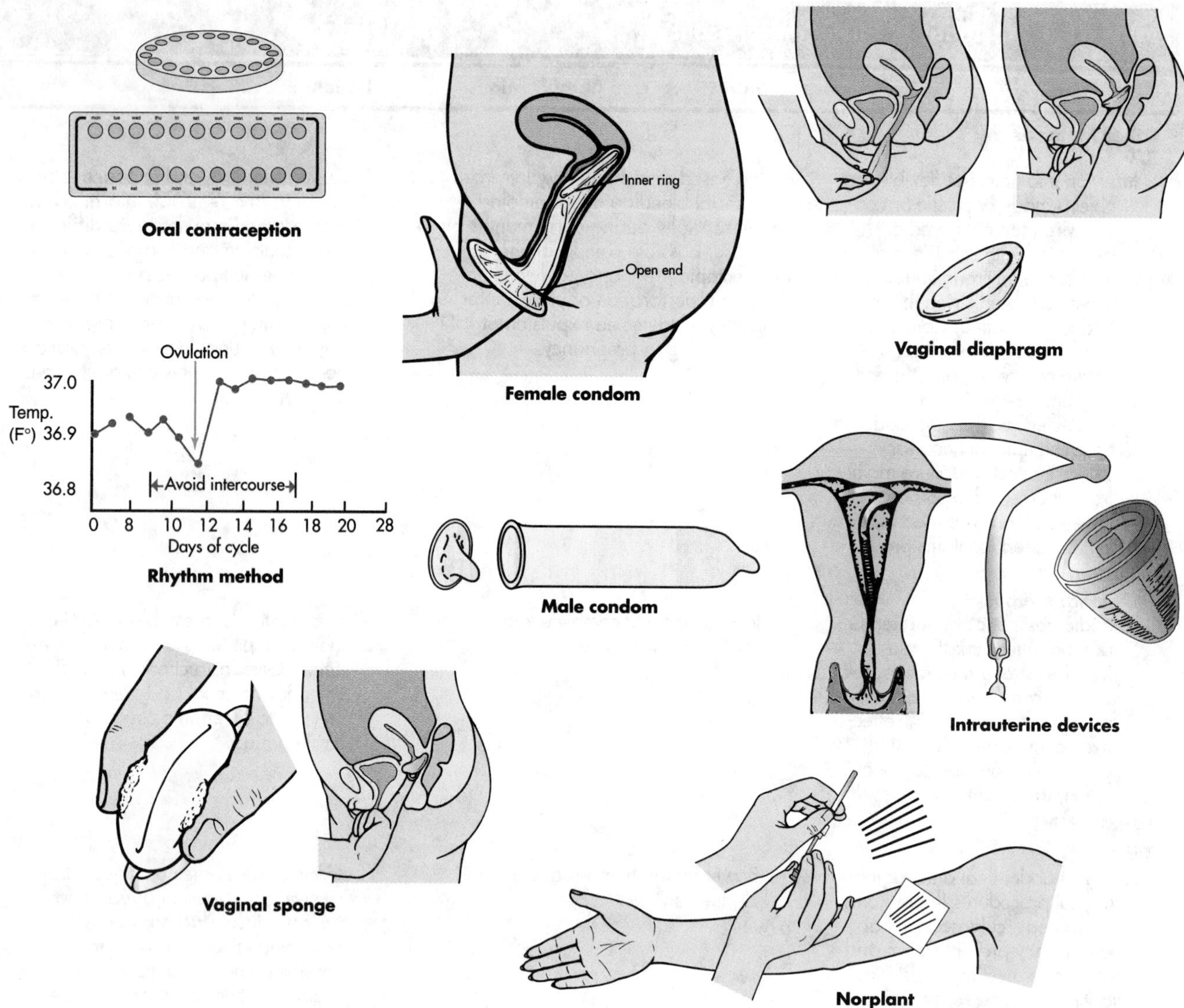

Fig. 51-2 Temporary contraceptive methods and devices.

values, and lifestyle. The nurse is in a position to counsel individuals and couples about birth control methods. The nurse can assist them by presenting concise, factual, unbiased information about methods available, including their benefits and risks. The couple should choose a method that is most compatible with their personal circumstances.

Women who are considering sterilization as a contraceptive method have common concerns about pain associated with the procedure, the effects of sterilization, and possible complications. Counseling should provide accurate information about these concerns and allow the individuals to explore their feelings about ending reproductive functioning. When motives are healthy and the woman is well adjusted, sterilization will not adversely affect sexual functioning, physiology, or self-concept.

With the increased interest in family planning, nurses should know the available resources for contraceptive referral within their communities. *Planned Parenthood* is a resource that is available in most areas. Literature dealing with contraception should also be provided for persons who demonstrate an interest in it.

When the person has made a decision on the method of contraception, counseling in the proper use of the method must be given. If the woman selects "the pill" (the most common form of contraception) she should be aware of early danger signs. The acronym ACHES is used for these signs: *A,* abdominal pain; *C,* chest pain, cough, shortness of breath; *H,* headache, dizziness, weakness, or numbness; *E,* eye problems, speech problems; *S,* severe leg pain.[26] If any of these danger signs are present, the woman should contact her health care provider promptly. The nurse should evaluate the patient's understanding of the method chosen and provide explanations and interpretation if necessary. The patient should also be aware of an alternative method of contraception if emergencies such as misplacing a diaphragm occur at an inopportune time. Specific counseling strategies are beyond the scope of this text.

Persons who use contraceptives but wish to eventually have a family should understand the risks of deferring pregnancy. Fertility for women peaks at 24 years of age and then declines, with a rapid fall after age 35. Men who are 25 years old are three times more likely to initiate a pregnancy than men who are age 40.[27] Fetal and maternal risks also increase with age. Women with progressive medical conditions such as heart disease should be advised to have their families as early as possible.

INFERTILITY

Infertility is the failure to conceive after a year or more of unprotected, appropriately timed intercourse. Approximately 15% of couples in the United States are involuntarily infertile. Professional intervention can help about 40% of these couples achieve a pregnant state.

In determining the cause of infertility and in treating it, both the man and woman must be evaluated. A causative factor for the infertility relating to the woman is found in no more than one half of couples who are evaluated. Proper study and the subsequent therapeutic measures require time (often a year or more) and patience for results to be obtained. A trusting relationship between the health professionals and the infertile couple should be established early in the investigative process.

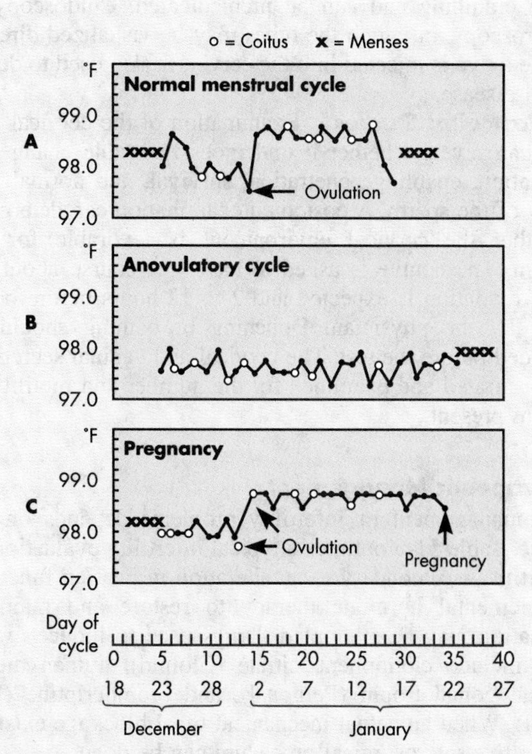

Fig. 51-3 Basal body temperature chart. ***A,*** Typical biphasic temperature curve indicative of ovulation and normal progesterone effect. ***B,*** Irregular monophasic curve characteristic of anovulatory cycles. ***C,*** Ovulatory curve with sustained temperature elevation following conception and the first missed period.

Etiology

A complete list of the causes of female infertility is extensive. The following problems are found most frequently in women: anovulation, tubal or uterine disease, and abnormalities of the cervical mucus. Other possible causes include systemic illnesses, marital and sexual difficulties, and lack of knowledge about reproductive functioning. (Male infertility is discussed in Chapter 52.) In 15% of instances the fertility problem can be attributed to the couple rather than to one of the partners. Immune factors (antisperm agglutinating and immobilizing antibodies found in either partner), infrequent intercourse, and suboptimal sexual techniques may be implicated.

Diagnostic Studies

After a detailed history is obtained and a general physical examination of the woman is performed to rule out any related medical or gynecological disease, several basic tests are performed to evaluate whether the cause is female infertility. These tests include ovulatory studies, tubal patency studies, and postcoital studies.[20]

Ovulatory Studies. A basal body temperature record is kept to determine whether there is regular ovulation. The woman is instructed to take and record her temperature on awakening, before any activity. The same site (e.g., oral) should be used each time. Any cause for variation, such as sleeplessness or illness, should be noted. As ovulation approaches, the production of estrogen increases and may cause a drop in temperature. When ovulation occurs, progesterone is produced, causing a rise in temperature. The temperature graph and the readings (Fig. 51-3) therefore detect ovulation and suggest the timing of intercourse if pregnancy is desired. Rigid adherence to a schedule can produce psychologic stress sufficient to inhibit sexual relations.

Simple rapid ovulation prediction kits are now available for use by patients at home. These kits are generally used daily to measure luteinizing hormone (LH) levels in urine samples. Ovulation occurs about 28 to 36 hours after the first rise of LH, so intercourse can be properly timed.[22] Other tests for ovulation include cervical and vaginal smears, endometrial biopsy, and plasma progesterone levels.

Tubal Patency Studies. Tubal disease (occlusion, anomaly, or deformity) is assessed most commonly by means of hysterosalpingogram. This procedure consists of the radiologic visualization of the uterus and tubes by injection of a radiopaque dye through the cervix. Tubal patency, shape, position, and any distortions of the endometrial cavity can be determined. Chlamydial infections and gonorrhea can cause tissue scarring even after successful treatment.[29] During the procedure the patient may experience cramping and can be premedicated. Culdoscopy or laparoscopy, in which the tubes may be visualized directly while a dye is injected into the cervix, is also used to detect tubal disease.

Postcoital Studies. Examination of the cervical mucus can reveal whether it undergoes favorable changes at ovulation, enabling penetration, survival, and normal motility of the sperm. A postcoital examination can determine whether the cervical environment is favorable for the sperm. The couple is asked to have intercourse about the time ovulation is expected and 2 to 12 hours before being seen by the physician. Douching or bathing should be avoided before the test. The cervical and vaginal secretions are aspirated and examined for the number and motility of sperm present.

Therapeutic Management

The management of infertility problems depends on the cause. Table 51-5 outlines a typical infertility evaluation. If infertility is secondary to an alteration in ovarian function, supplemental hormone therapy to restore and maintain ovulation may be attempted. Drugs used to induce ovulation include clomiphene citrate (Clomid), human menopausal gonadotropin (Pergonal), and bromocriptine (Parlodel). When an actual mechanical tubal blockage exists, a reparative microsurgical procedure can be done.

Poor cervical mucus may be a result of chronic cervicitis or inadequate estrogenic stimulation. Careful cauterization of the cervix may eradicate the chronic cervicitis, and the administration of estrogens can improve the quantity and quality of the cervical mucus.

Improving the patient's general health may help, especially when a debilitating or chronic illness is present. Removing or reducing psychologic stress can improve the emotional climate, making it more conducive to achieving a pregnancy. Education of the couple regarding the probable time of ovulation and appropriate coital technique may also be indicated.

When a couple has not succeeded in conceiving while under infertility management, another option is intrauterine insemination with the husband's or donor's sperm. If this technique does not succeed, *in vitro fertilization* (IVF) may be used. IVF is the removal of mature oocytes from the woman's ovarian follicle via laparoscopy, followed by fertilization of the ova with the partner's sperm in a petri dish. When fertilization and cleavage have occurred, the resulting embryos are transferred into the woman's uterus. The procedure requires 2 to 3 days to complete and is used in cases of fallopian tube obstruction, oligospermia, and unexplained infertility. IVF is costly and emotionally stressful, but it has become a recognized and accepted method of therapy for infertile couples.

Assisted reproductive technologies (ART) have developed rapidly since the first IVF baby was born in 1978. ARTs consist of IVF, *gamete intrafallopian transfer* (GIFT), *zygote intrafallopian transfer* (ZIFT), *cryopreserved embryo transfer* (CPE), and *donor oocyte programs* (DOP). Current research successes predict a rapid expansion of these techniques in the next decade. With the increased knowledge of freezing techniques for embryos (CPE), couples will have an increased pregnancy potential. Research is also investigating the replication of normal tubal secretions. This important tubal factor is recognized because there is a higher pregnancy rate with GIFT and ZIFT than with IVF. Finally, the development of embryo biopsy and genetic engineering may allow for preconception techniques for those couples with identified genetic abnormalities. It also poses the possibility of gender selection. Noncoital reproduction poses many ethical, legal, and social concerns.[30] All decisions related to infertility are influenced by the age of the couple, their wishes, and the length of time they have been attempting to conceive.[31]

Table 51-5 Evaluation of the Infertile Couple

Initial Visit
- ***Clinical***
  - History/physical for both partners
  - Extensive review of menstrual pattern
- ***Laboratory***
  - Testing to assess specific medical findings
  - Assess for sexually transmitted diseases
  - Papanicolaou smear
  - Semen analysis
- ***Education***
  - Health maintenance (breast and scrotal self-examinations)
  - Discussion of possible future testing options and cost
- ***Ovulation monitoring***
  - Instruction for at-home ovulation testing using basal body temperature, cervical mucus evaluation, and urinary LH test kit

Second Visit (at preovulatory part of cycle)
- ***Clinical***
  - Postcoital test
- ***Laboratory***
  - Sperm penetration assay
- ***Education***
  - Review ovulation monitoring data and techniques
  - Review laboratory findings from last visit

Third Visit (at postovulatory part of cycle)
- ***Clinical***
  - Endometrial biopsy
- ***Laboratory***
  - Draw midluteal progesterone/prolactin
- ***Education***
  - Discuss need to assess tubal/uterine integrity (hysterosalpingogram vs. laparoscopy)

Fourth Visit (conclusion of initial work-up)
- ***Education***
  - Outline biochemical/physiologic bases of couple's infertility
  - Outline management plans with time and cost for each
  - Discuss referral for possible assisted reproductive technologies (ART)

Modified from Stenchever MA: *Office gynecology,* St Louis, 1992, Mosby.

NURSING MANAGEMENT

INFERTILITY

The nurse has a major responsibility for teaching and providing emotional support throughout the infertility testing and treatment period. Feelings of anger, frustration, sadness, and helplessness between partners and between the couple and health care providers may heighten as more and more tests are performed. The problem of infertility can generate great tension in a marriage as the couple exhaust their financial and emotional resources. Few insurance carriers cover the cost of infertility testing or the therapeutic measures associated with infertility. Shame and guilt may be precipitated when other persons become involved in this intimate area of a relationship. Recognizing and taking steps to deal with the psychologic and emotional factors that surface can assist the couple to better cope with the situation. Couples should be encouraged to participate in a support group for infertile couples as well as individual therapy.

Provisions for giving information and emotional support by the nurse continue as therapeutic measures are attempted. Couples should be given ample opportunities to plan what is financially realistic—each GIFT and ZIFT can exceed $10,000 per attempt. Pergonal treatment costs about $3000 per month, and each IVF treatment costs $4500 to $6000.[32]

ABORTION

An abortion is the termination of a pregnancy before 20 weeks or a fetal weight of less than 500 g. Abortions are classified as *spontaneous,* occurring naturally, or *induced,* occurring as a result of mechanical or medicinal interruption. *Miscarriage* is the lay term indicating the unintended termination of a pregnancy. *Habitual abortion* is defined by a history of three or more previous abortions.

Spontaneous Abortion

Spontaneous abortion occurs in about 30% to 40% of all conceptions. Fetal or maternal abnormalities are the chief causes of these abortions. The cause of spontaneous abortions is multifactorial and includes genetic factors (43%), endocrine factors (25%), uterine factors (12%), and other causes, including endometriosis, infection, immunologic factors, and environmental factors (20%).[7]

Therapeutic Management. The presence of uterine cramping serves as an aid to diagnose vaginal bleeding as a spontaneous abortion. This symptom is usually absent in vaginal bleeding caused by other conditions, such as polyps. Serial serum β-hCGs and vaginal ultrasound examination of the pelvis are the most reliable indicators of an early abortion. The gestational sac can be visualized using ultrasound as early as 6 weeks of gestation.

Treatment for a spontaneous abortion is limited. Although bed rest and abstention from sexual activity are often recommended, there is no evidence that these measures or any active medical management improves the outcome. The woman is advised to report any bleeding to the physician. An estimated 80% of patients proceed to abortion regardless of management. A D & C is generally performed after spontaneous abortion to minimize blood loss, reduce the chance of secondary infection, and shorten convalescence. For women who habitually abort in the second trimester because of an incompetent cervical os, the cervix may be tightened surgically. The patient must be monitored closely for preterm labor. Bed rest may be indicated to reduce gravity's pressure on the cervix. At delivery the suture is removed by the physician to allow a vaginal delivery, or the suture is retained and delivery is by cesarean birth.

NURSING MANAGEMENT

SPONTANEOUS ABORTION

It may be necessary for the patient who is threatening to abort to be admitted to the hospital. Vital signs are monitored, and an estimation of blood loss is made. Measures are taken to restrict activity and reduce stress to provide the needed physical and mental rest. Any tissue or suspicious clots that are passed are saved to be examined for traces of fetus and placenta. The possibility of losing the pregnancy may be distressing to the patient. If the pregnancy is aborted, the nurse should arrange for the family to be present for emotional support. The nurse should offer other resources for support of the grieving process that may result from this loss.

Induced Abortion

Abortion for medical and social reasons is now available to more than half the world's population, making it one of the most commonly performed surgical procedures. Therapeutic abortions are most commonly performed during the first trimester by menstrual extraction or suction curettage in an outpatient office or hospital.

In 1973 the U.S. Supreme Court reached a decision (*Roe v. Wade*) establishing that abortion is a matter between the woman and her physician, within certain limits. In 1989 the Supreme Court gave control of abortion to the states (*Webster decision*). For women who rely on state-supported abortion funding, restrictions and accessibility of abortion may be prohibitive (*Casey Decision, 1992*). The Supreme Court ruled that it was the woman's right to exercise her choice, but also that the state may try to persuade her to continue the pregnancy by making it more costly and less accessible.[33]

Techniques. The decision about which technique to use to terminate a pregnancy depends on the length of the pregnancy and the woman's condition. Early abortion methods include menstrual extraction, suction curettage, and D & C. Late or second-trimester abortions include intrauterine instillation of drugs and hysterotomy. Table 51-6 summarizes the methods of abortion in current use, including the advantages and disadvantages of each.

NURSING MANAGEMENT

INDUCED ABORTIONS

Because physical and psychologic complications can arise after abortion procedures, the decision to have an abortion

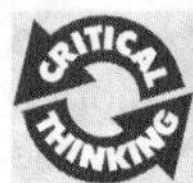

ETHICAL DILEMMAS

ABORTION

Situation A recently married 39-year-old woman, after amniocentesis, is informed that her fetus has major chromosomal abnormalities and is expected to have severe physical and mental disabilities. The patient has no children, but her husband has three children from a previous marriage. She asks the nurse what she should do. How would the nurse respond?

Discussion The patient has three choices: (1) continue the pregnancy and raise the child, (2) terminate the pregnancy, or (3) continue the pregnancy and relinquish the child for adoption. Although these are all legal and morally acceptable decisions, each is extremely difficult. The patient and her family need support, information, and as much time as is practical to make their decision. Appropriate pregnancy counseling would involve clarification about the nature of this pregnancy (e.g., was it a desired pregnancy), the patient's concerns and desires about having a child with her husband, how she feels about both abortion and the prospects of raising a child with severe disabilities, and education about future pregnancy risks, both to the fetus and to the patient. The nurse might suggest counseling for the patient and her husband and a meeting with the physician to answer questions they have about the diagnosis, the prognosis, and their alternatives. It also might be helpful to refer them to agencies that deal with children with disabilities for additional information.

ETHICAL AND LEGAL PRINCIPLES

- Abortion was legalized in the United States in 1973 in the *Roe v. Wade* case heard before the Supreme Court. Abortion in the first trimester is a private matter between a woman and her physician. In the second trimester the state may regulate abortion services for safety concerns. Third-trimester abortions may be performed in cases where the life or health of the woman is endangered by the pregnancy.
- Patient autonomy requires that a woman decide for herself whether or not to continue a pregnancy. She may consult with her family or physician before this decision is made.
- Coercion occurs when a health care provider attempts to influence a patient to act in a way that the health care provider would act in the situation.

warrants careful consideration. The woman and her significant others need support and acceptance. Most patients benefit from counseling before the procedure, especially when the decision to have an abortion involves conflict. The specific procedure planned must be explained to each patient. At times the overriding need to have the pregnancy terminated does not allow detailed explanations or teaching to be absorbed. Anxiety, loneliness, and fear are emotions often experienced before and during the procedure. Friends or family may not be present to support the patient. The nurse can be an important factor in the patient's experience of the event.

Follow-up care includes instructions on signs and symptoms of possible complications, including increase in vaginal flow, severe abdominal cramping, and signs associated with infection, such as fever and drainage. The importance of avoiding intercourse, use of tampons, and douching until reexamination should be stressed. The patient is instructed to return for reexamination in 2 weeks. Grief and depression are common, and the patient should be prepared for this before discharge. Contraception can be initiated during the patient's return visit in accordance with her needs and desires.

ECTOPIC PREGNANCY

An *ectopic pregnancy* is the implantation of the fertilized ovum anywhere outside the uterine cavity. The number of ectopic pregnancies recorded by hospital admissions has steadily decreased for the past 3 years.[34] The most frequent site is the fallopian tube, but the location may be ovarian, abdominal, or cervical (Fig. 51-4). Any blockage of the tube or reduction of tubal peristalsis impedes or delays the passage of the zygote to the uterine cavity and can result in tubal fertilization. The four strongest risk factors for ectopic pregnancy are current IUD use, history of infertility, history of pelvic inflammatory disease, and prior tubal surgery.[7] However, approximately 50% of all ectopic pregnancies are not explained by these factors. Although implantation occurs, the thin tubal wall can expand only minimally with growth of the gestational sac before it ruptures. Symptoms usually occur 6 to 8 weeks after the last normal menstrual period. Tubal pregnancy has been known to interfere with future reproductive ability because of strictures and scarring.

Clinical Manifestations

A woman may be asymptomatic and seek care because she missed her menses. However, the majority of women with tubal pregnancy exhibit subacute symptoms. Symptoms may range from menstrual irregularity, vaginal spotting (which occurs after fetal death and estrogen withdrawal), and crampy pain in the lower abdomen (caused by tubal distention). Significant pelvic or abdominal tenderness may not be present on physical examination. Generally there is a gradual drop in the hemoglobin level.

The more dramatic occurrence is a woman who has had intermittent abdominal cramping with an acute exacerbation. She may faint or feel faint with pain radiating into her shoulder. The referred pain to the shoulder results from intraabdominal bleeding. The profuse bleeding that occurs with ruptured ectopic pregnancy is the reason that ectopic pregnancy is one of the leading causes of maternal death. Hypovolemic shock may result, as manifested by its classic signs and symptoms (see Chapter 7). An obvious emergency situation exists.

Therapeutic Management

Ectopic pregnancy generally represents a diagnostic challenge not only because of its vague manifestations, but also because of its similarity to a wide variety of other pelvic

Table 51-6 Induced Abortion

Method	Length of Pregnancy	Procedure	Advantages	Disadvantages
Early Abortion				
▪ Menstrual extraction or regulation	Usually up to 2 wk after first missed period	Catheter is inserted through cervix into uterus, and suction is applied. Endometrium and contents of uterus are aspirated.	Low cost, simple, done at outpatient facility without anesthesia or cervical dilatation, minimally traumatic	Continuation of pregnancy possible, potential for uterine injury and bleeding
▪ Suction curettage	10-12 wk	Cervix is usually dilated, uterine aspirator is introduced, and suction is applied, removing endometrial tissue and implanted pregnancy.	Outpatient procedure, most often involving local anesthesia, 1- to 2-day recovery period	Infection, uterine perforation possible
▪ D & C	10-16 wk (approximate)	Cervix is dilated, and products of conception are removed by scraping uterine walls with a curet.	Safe and effective procedure for more advanced pregnancy, outpatient procedure with general anesthesia, 2-day recovery period	More psychologic trauma, more expensive, greater risk with general anesthesia and more invasive procedure
Late Abortion				
▪ Instillation of drugs Hypertonic saline solution	After 16 wk	About 200 ml of amniotic fluid is withdrawn, and a similar amount of 20% normal saline solution is injected. Uterus is apparently irritated and begins to contract within 12-36 hr. Contractions may be assisted with IV oxytocin.	Inexpensive, readily available, feticidal	Hypernatremia, infection, hemorrhage, disseminated intravascular coagulation, more emotional trauma because of time required
Prostaglandins	After 16 wk	Amniocentesis is done, and 8 ml of prostaglandin is inserted into amniotic sac, resulting in stimulation of smooth muscle of uterus. Expulsion of uterine contents occurs within 24 hr.	Fast induction, no need for surgery	Nausea and vomiting, abdominal cramps, cervical laceration, possible delivery of live fetus, high cost
▪ Hysterotomy	16-20 wk	Miniature cesarean section is performed. Incision is made into uterus and contents are removed.	Concurrent sterilization procedure possible	More difficult and expensive in time and money, surgical incision with possible complications

D & C, Dilatation and curettage; *IV,* intravenous.

and abdominal disorders, such as salpingitis, spontaneous abortion, rupture of a cyst, appendicitis, and peritonitis. Vaginal ultrasonography, which determines the presence or absence of an intrauterine gestational sac in early pregnancy, and serum radioimmunoassay for human chorionic gonadotropin (hCG) level, which is used as an indication of pregnancy, are the first diagnostic tests performed. When the signs and symptoms are more pronounced, culdocentesis (aspiration of the cul-de-sac) for unclotted blood or a laparoscopy is used to confirm the diagnosis.

Once a definitive diagnosis of ectopic pregnancy is made, surgery should proceed immediately. If the tube has ruptured, the patient may be given a blood transfusion and supplemental IV therapy fluid to relieve shock and restore a satisfactory blood volume for safe anesthesia and surgery. A salpingectomy or salpingostomy may be done to remove

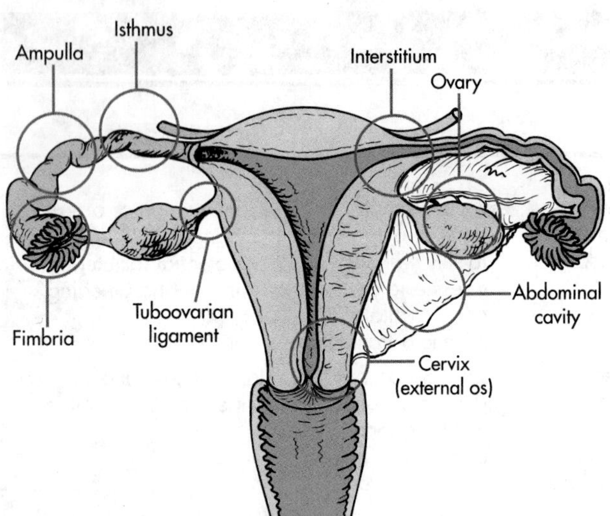

Fig. 51-4 Sites of implantation of ectopic pregnancies. Order of frequency of occurrence is ampulla, isthmus, interstitium, fimbria, tuboovarian ligament, ovary, abdominal cavity, and cervix (external os).

the products of conception from an unruptured tubal pregnancy. Salpingectomy is more commonly performed, especially if the contralateral tube appears normal. All gross abdominal blood and clots are removed to prevent intraperitoneal adhesions. The use of microsurgery techniques has resulted in fewer repeated ectopic pregnancies and a higher rate of future successful pregnancies.

An alternative method to surgery is drug-induced pregnancy termination. Even fewer complications are predicted with the use of a single intramuscular injection of methotrexate (MTX). MTX has been reported successful in terminating ectopic pregnancies that are hemodynamically stable with an enlargement of 3.5 cm or less.[34]

NURSING MANAGEMENT

ECTOPIC PREGNANCY

Nursing care depends on the condition of the patient. Before diagnosis has been confirmed the nurse should be alert to signs of increasing pain and vaginal bleeding, which may indicate that rupture of the tube has occurred. Vital signs are monitored closely, along with observation for signs of shock. Explanations and preparation for diagnostic procedures are given when appropriate. Preparation of the patient for abdominal surgery may follow rapidly. The patient's emotional status should be assessed. Reassurance and support for the surgery should be given to both the patient and her family. Postoperatively, the patient may express a fear of future ectopic pregnancies and have many questions about the impact of this experience on her future fertility.

RAPE

Significance

Rape may be defined as any nonconsensual sexual act. The number of rapes, particularly against women, is increasing at an alarming rate. The Federal Bureau of Investigation reported 94,504 cases of rape in 1989, representing 6% of all crimes of violence. In 1990 there was a 2.2% increase over 1989, and in 1991 the number increased another 3.9%.[35] At the same time, the projection is that two unreported rapes occur for every rape reported because of the fear and embarrassment of the victims. There is no legal requirement that the rape of an adult be reported. Some women feel that they would not be able to withstand the stresses of prosecution or that they would be met with disbelief and humiliation from the police, the medical staff, or their peers.

Clinical Manifestations

Physical Injuries. Rape may result in genital and extragenital injuries, pregnancy, and sexually transmitted diseases. Genital injuries appear less frequently and include bruises and lacerations to the perineum, hymen, vulva, vagina, cervix, and anus. Some women have sustained lacerations of the ligaments supporting the uterus, resulting in uterine displacement, and severe lacerations of the vagina, requiring extensive surgical reconstruction and repair. Dyspareunia and vaginismus (painful spasms of the vagina) have developed as a consequence. In 1991 there were 176 homicides related to rape and sex offenses.[36]

In general, the more serious injuries involve extragenital areas, such as the face, neck, and extremities, and often occur after the rape. Fractures, subdural hematomas, cerebral concussions, and intraabdominal injuries have resulted in the need for hospitalization. Rape is an act of violence with sex as the weapon; it is not a sexual act. Table 51-7 outlines the emergency management of the patient who has been sexually assaulted. Most emergency departments (ED) have identified personnel who work with women who have been raped. Special procedures are followed in taking the history and conducting the examination in order to preserve all evidence in case of future prosecution.

Emotional Trauma. The emotional trauma of a rape survivor often affects the survivor's future sexual functioning and intimate relationships. The initial reaction of most women to rape is shock, disbelief, and emotional breakdown, including crying, agitation, and incoherence. Feelings of fear, humiliation, degradation, embarrassment, anger, and the need for revenge and self-blame are commonly expressed. Within several days to weeks after the rape the woman displays controlled behavior and a return to normal life patterns. It is believed that the survivor's real feelings at this time may be hidden under her calm, composed affect. The long-term results of the rape include the integration and resolution of the experience. This progressive pattern of behavior has been described as the *rape trauma syndrome*. Rape trauma syndrome is an accepted NANDA nursing diagnosis. Some time is needed for the woman to complete this process; not all women are able to achieve full resolution of the rape experience. Many victims develop phobias, such as fear of crowds. Others are unable to resume their usual sexual patterns or have frightening dreams that persist for long periods. Counseling and rape support groups are recommended for assistance with resolution.

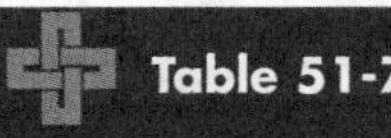

Table 51-7 Emergency Management: Sexual Assault

Possible Etiologies
Sexual molestation, sodomy, or assault involving genitalia (male or female) without consent

Possible Assessment Findings
Emotional or physical manifestations of shock
Hysteria, crying, anger
Decreased level of consciousness
Hyperventilation
Pain in genital area or from extragenital injuries
Signs of trauma

Management
- Treat for shock and treat urgent medical problems (e.g., head injury, bleeding wounds, fractures).
- Assess emotional state.
- Contact support person for survivor (e.g., social worker, rape advocate, sexual assault nurse examiner).
- *Do not* cleanse the patient; keep the patient from cleansing, douching, or urinating.
- Collect sexual assault evidence per protocol (e.g., clothing, body hair, tissue, blood samples).
- Maintain chain of evidence for all legal specimens; clearly label evidence and keep in locked cabinet until turned over to law enforcement agency.
- Monitor vital signs.
- Consider prophylactic antibiotics and pregnancy prophylaxis.
- Counsel patient about confidential HIV and STD testing.

HIV, Human immunodeficiency virus; *STD*, sexually transmitted disease.

Social Effects. The support and acceptance offered rape survivors by their significant others are important in reducing the emotional crisis of rape. The men in the woman's life take on a greater significance. How they respond to the situation will affect her future relations with them and with all men. The men may have serious problems resolving the incident and need as much help as the survivor.

Changes in residency and place of employment may occur as a consequence of the experience because of fear or inability to maintain previous relationships. Rape trauma dramatically disrupts the homemaking and parenting roles normally performed by the adult woman. The survivor's husband and family have a tremendous potential for both negative and positive influence. They can revictimize her and increase her burden in resolving the rape, or they can provide her with support and find support themselves in resolving a shared crisis.[37]

Therapeutic Management

When the survivor of a rape is admitted to the ED or clinic, a specific chain of events occurs (Table 51-8). A signed informed consent is obtained from the victim before rape data are collected. All materials gathered are well documented, labeled, and given to the appropriate person, such as the pathologist or a police officer. The materials are handled by as few people as possible, and signatures of all responsible for keeping and handling the data are obtained. Many items can be used as evidence if the victim chooses to file a complaint. Consequently, the integrity of the material must be maintained. The nurse's involvement in the medicolegal process depends on the policies of the individual institution and state law.

A gynecologic and sexual history and an account of the assault (who, what, when, where, why), as well as a general physical and pelvic examination, add further information about the rape incident. Laboratory tests are done primarily to determine the presence of sperm in the vagina and to rule out the possibility of venereal disease and pregnancy.

During the treatment period the patient's physical injuries are attended to and prophylaxis for venereal disease and pregnancy are administered. The patient's immediate and long-term need for emotional support is given special consideration.

The health care provider cannot legally state that rape occurred. However, the provider can swear that the findings show that sexual intercourse took place and that injury was inflicted. These findings, along with others such as the police report and examination of the rape scene, can form the foundation for the rapist's conviction.

NURSING MANAGEMENT

RAPE

All women should be aware of rape prevention tactics (Table 51-9). They should also be encouraged to learn some basic techniques of self-defense. Local high schools and the YWCA usually have self-defense classes in which formal instruction is given. Practicing the various techniques with a friend builds up a woman's confidence in her ability to fight back. Learning self-defense can make the woman less vulnerable and more self-reliant.

When a rape survivor is brought to the clinic or emergency room, she should be given the highest priority for care and treatment. A quiet, private area should be used for the initial assessment and the examinations that follow. The patient should not be left alone. Whenever possible, the same nurse should remain with her throughout her stay and provide needed emotional support. The patient's actions and words as she describes the rape incident may be inconsistent, confused, and inappropriate. The nurse should maintain a nonjudgmental attitude.

The patient usually has many feelings and thoughts about the rape and generally wants to talk about them to an interested listener. Talking may help the patient feel better and gain understanding of her reactions to the incident. When the nurse listens carefully, the patient feels that she is not alone and is better able to gain control over the situation.

The nurse should assess the patient's stress level before preparing her for the various procedures that will follow. The patient's coping mechanisms are supported when she knows what to expect and what is expected of her, as well

Table 51-8 Checklist for Evaluation of Alleged Rape

1. **Medicolegal**
   Valid written consent for examination, photographs, laboratory tests, release of information, and laboratory samples
   Appropriate "chain of evidence" documentation
2. **History**
   Current health status and past history
   Age, parity, and gravidity
   Menstrual and contraceptive history
   Time of last coitus before assault
   Activities performed after assault (e.g., changed clothes, bathed, douched, urinated, brushed teeth)
   History of assault (who, what, when, where, why)
   Penetration, ejaculation, condom, extragenital acts
3. **General physical examination**
   Vital signs and general appearance
   Extragenital trauma—mouth, breasts, neck
   Cuts, bruises, scratches (photograph taken)
4. **Pelvic examination**
   Vulvar trauma, erythema, hymen, anal, and rectal status
   Matted hairs or free hairs
   Vaginal examination with unlubricated speculum for foreign body, discharge, blood, lacerations
   Uterine size
   Adnexa, especially hematomas
5. **Laboratory samples**
   Saline irrigation of vagina with 2 ml solution and swab; acid phosphatase, blood groups
   Vaginal smears—Pap and Gram stain
   Oral or rectal swabs and smears, if indicated
   Blood samples—VDRL serology, blood group and type, pregnancy test, alcohol; serologic testing for HIV and hepatitis B infection, if appropriate, with repetition 8-12 wk later
   Cultures—cervix and other areas if indicated (gonococcal and chlamydial)
   Combing and clipping of scalp hairs
   Fingernail scrapings
   Combing of pubic hairs
   Clipping of matted pubic hairs
   Clipping of pubic hair
6. **Treatment**
   Care of injuries and emotional trauma
   Antibiotic prophylaxis for venereal disease, if appropriate; ceftriaxone 250 mg IM followed by doxycycline 100 mg orally bid for 7 days
   Protection against pregnancy if any risk with diethystilbestrol (DES), 25 mg bid for 5 days or ethinyl estradiol, 0.5 mg daily for 5 days
   Protection of legal rights
   Recommendation of continued follow-up and services of rape crisis center
   Repetition of gonorrhea and chlamydial culture 14 to 21 days later
   Repetition of serologic testing for HIV and hepatitis B 8 to 12 wk later
   Pregnancy test if appropriate

HIV, Human immunodeficiency virus; *IM*, intramuscular; *VDRL*, Venereal Disease Research Laboratory.

Table 51-9 Rape Prevention Tactics

- See that there are lights at all entrances to your home.
- Keep your doors locked and do not open them to a stranger; ask for identification if a service person comes to the door.
- Do not advertise that you live alone; list only your initials with your last name in the telephone directory or on the mailbox; never reveal to a caller that you are home alone.
- Avoid walking alone in deserted areas; walk to the parking lot with a friend; be sure you see each other leave.
- Have your keys ready as you approach your car or home.
- Keep all doors locked and windows up when driving.
- Never get on an elevator with a suspicious person; pretend you have forgotten something and get off.
- Say what you mean in social situations; be sure your voice and body language reflect your response.
- Carry a loud whistle and use it when you think you are in danger.
- Yell "fire" if you are attacked and run toward a lighted area.

as why the particular procedure must be done. Because the pelvic examination may trigger a flashback of the rape, the nurse should answer all related questions before the examination and urge the patient to relax as much as possible.

Following the examinations, the patient's physical comfort needs should be considered. She may need safety pins or needle and thread for her torn clothing or a cool drink to relieve her thirst. Most women who have been raped feel dirty and would appreciate a place to wash as well as use a mouthwash, especially if oral sex was involved.

The nurse can also further emphasize and elaborate on any prescribed treatment. The patient's understanding of the possible side effects of the medications given should be assessed. The patient is urged to see her own physician or to return for a follow-up examination and venereal disease testing. Many rape victims are unaware of the availability of financial compensation (a law in most states) and appreciate information about the application process. This compensation is to assist them in paying for emergency services and for emotional injuries that may temporarily interfere with their ability to work.

When the patient is discharged, the nurse should make certain the patient has transportation home. If friends or family members are not available, the hospital or clinic should make arrangements with an appropriate community resource. The patient should not be sent home alone.

Many communities today have rape crisis centers. These public service organizations have trained professional and nonprofessional volunteers who provide an emotional support system for rape survivors on request. Their programs provide advocacy to ensure dignified treatment throughout

Table 51-10 Infections of the Lower Genital Tract

Infection/Etiology	Clinical Manifestations and Diagnostic Methods	Management
▪ Bacterial vaginitis *Escherichia coli* and *Staphylococcus aureus*	Vulvar irritation, heavy yellowish discharge; microscopic examination—many WBCs, Gram stain—short rods or cocci	Triple sulfa vaginal cream, vinegar douche; sitz bath for vulvitis
▪ Monilial vaginitis *Candida albicans* (fungus)	Commonly found in mouth, gastrointestinal tract, and vagina; pruritus, thick white curdy discharge; KOH microscopic examination—pseudohyphae; pH 4.0-4.7	Monistat, Gyne-Lotrimin, Myclex (available over the counter); available in cream or suppository
▪ Trichomoniasis *Trichomonas vaginalis* (protozoa)	Sexually transmitted; pruritus, frothy greenish or gray discharge; hemorrhagic spots on cervix or vaginal walls; saline microscopic examination—swimming trichimonads; pH 5.0-7.0.	Flagyl 2 g orally in single dose for patient and partner
▪ Bacterial vaginosis *Gardnerella vaginalis* *Corynebacterium vaginale*	Watery discharge with fishy odor; may or may not have other symptoms; saline microscopic examination—epithelial cells; pH 5.0-5.5	Sexually transmitted; metronidazole (Flagyl) 500 mg orally or clindamycin (Cleocin) 300 mg orally bid for 7 days; examine and treat partner
▪ Cervicitis *Chlamydia trachomatis* *Neisseria gonorrhoeae* *Staphylococcus aureus*	Sexually transmitted; mucopurulent discharge with postcoital spotting from cervical inflammation; culture for chlamydia and gonorrhea.	Doxycycline 100 mg for 7 days or tetracycline 500 mg for 7 days; examine and treat partner
▪ Severe recurrent vaginitis: *Candida albicans* (most often)	May be first indication of HIV infection; all women who are unresponsive to first-line treatment should be counseled and offered HIV testing	Drug appropriate to opportunistic organism

HIV, Human immunodeficiency virus; *WBCs*, white blood cells.

the medical and police procedures, short-term counseling for the woman and her family, and court assistance and public education on rape-related issues. The nurse should be able to give the patient the names and local telephone numbers of such organizations.

INFLAMMATION AND INFECTIONS OF THE VAGINA, CERVIX, AND VULVA

Etiology

Infection and inflammation of the vagina, cervix, and vulva tend to occur when the natural defenses of the acid vaginal secretions (maintained by sufficient estrogen levels) and the presence of *Lactobacillus* are disrupted. The woman's resistance may also be decreased as a result of aging, poor nutrition, and the use of drugs that alter the mucosa. Organisms gain entrance to the areas through contaminated hands, clothing, and douche nozzles and during intercourse, surgery, and childbirth. Table 51-10 relates the specific etiologic factors, clinical manifestations and diagnostic methods, and therapeutic management of common inflammations and infections.

Drugs such as oral contraceptives, antibiotics, and steroids may produce changes in the vaginal discharge, which can trigger an overgrowth of the organisms present. For example, *Candida albicans* may be present in small numbers in the vagina. An overgrowth of this organism causes Monilial or yeast vaginitis.

Transmission

Most lower genital tract infections are transmitted through sexual contact. Vulvar infections, such as herpes and genital warts, and vaginal infections, such as trichomoniasis, bacterial vaginosis, and chlamydial cervicitis, are common gynecologic conditions. Other lower genital tract infections, such as human papillomavirus, gonorrhea, and syphilis, are occurring with increasing frequency[38] (Table 51-10). The increased sexual freedom since the 1960s, younger age of first intercourse, and the use of hormonal contraceptives are largely responsible for the increased occurrence of sexually transmitted diseases (STDs). Barrier contraceptives (such as condoms and diaphragms) with spermicides provide the best protection against sexual transmission. The realization and acceptance of the relevance of STD protection has never been more important because AIDS has become a major cause of death in women in the United States.[39] (STDs are discussed in Chapter 50. AIDS is discussed in Chapter 11.)

It is estimated that 80,000 to 125,000 women have been infected with HIV but are not yet symptomatic.[40] For women, the first symptoms of HIV infection are often gynecologic problems. Common symptoms are yeast vaginitis, pelvic inflammatory disease, cervical abnormalities, and herpes infection.

MEDICAL AND NURSING MANAGEMENT

INFLAMMATION AND INFECTIONS OF VAGINA, CERVIX, AND VULVA

Normally the endocervical glands secrete a clear exudate, which may become cloudy and take on a slight odor as it passes through the vagina. The amount of discharge may increase (*physiologic leukorrhea*) at ovulation, just before menstruation, during pregnancy and sexual excitement, and during use of oral contraceptives. When changes in the amount, color, character, or odor of the discharge occur, they usually indicate an infection (*pathophysiologic leukorrhea*).

Risk Factors. Women need to know what situations increase the risk of vaginal, cervical, and vulvar infections. Douching more than once every week or two, for example, can be harmful because it destroys the vagina's balance of naturally occurring organisms. Many other organisms have been cultured from vaginal discharge even when the woman is asymptomatic. One study of vaginal cultures of asymptomatic women reported *Lactobacilli* to be the most common with 95% occurrence. *Mycoplasma hominis* was present in 20% to 50% of the cultures, and *Escherichia coli, Streptococcus, Staphylococcus, Gardnerella,* and *Candida* were recovered 20% of the time.[6] Anaerobes and viruses have also been identified from vaginal cultures. HIV is cultured most frequently from blood, semen, and vaginal discharge.

It is important that the nurse be well informed about inflammation and infection of the genitals and STDs and to pass that information on to the patient without making assumptions about the patient's lifestyle. Without adequate information treatment may fail, resulting in an infection that may be recurrent (such as herpes), impaired fertility if the patient develops pelvic inflammatory disease, or death if the patient is infected with HIV. The nurse plays a vital role in providing information about the type of infection diagnosed, its treatment, and how to prevent its recurrence.

Treatment. A variety of treatment measures are prescribed for vaginal, cervical, and vulvar infections. Vaginal suppositories, ointments, and creams are often used when infection occurs. Instructions in their use are best given with the aid of a model of the pelvis. The importance of hand washing before and after their insertion should be stressed. The patient should be advised to use the medication at bedtime; the patient should remain recumbent for more than 30 minutes after insertion to allow for absorption and to prevent loss of the medication from the vagina. Once the patient rises, there will be expulsion of much of the cream from the vagina. The woman should be advised to wear a minipad during the day for any residual drainage. During treatment the patient should refrain from intercourse or request that her partner use a condom. If it is a sexually transmitted disease, the woman should be counseled and offered HIV testing. The partner should be examined and treated as well. Because treatment measures are usually carried out by the patient, her understanding of them and her ability to perform the treatment correctly must be assessed.

Heat in the form of a sitz bath, perineal irrigation, and douching are often prescribed to reduce inflammation, promote healing, and provide comfort. Instructions in their use should be given as indicated. Disposable sitz baths that fit over the toilet bowl are available, although the bathtub serves the same purpose. (A nursing fundamentals textbook should be consulted for correct douching technique.)

Local measures, such as scratching, excessive moisture (including too frequent bathing), and tight clothing, should be avoided, and wearing of underpants or pantyhose with a cotton crotch is advocated. Chafing, increased heat and moisture, and interference with normal ventilation promote favorable conditions for the growth of fungal, protozoan, and bacterial agents. Cleanliness after urinating and defecating should be stressed. It may be necessary to review the importance of using daily health and hygienic practices with some patients. Instructions to seek care when symptoms occur should also be given.

Reinfection. When reinfection occurs readily, the possibility of a symptom-free male carrier or the presence of undiagnosed diabetes mellitus or HIV infection should be investigated. A review of the prescribed treatment measures for possible misunderstandings and a check on compliance with drug therapy may also be indicated.

If the patient has cauterization or cryosurgery for chronic cervicitis, specific instructions are necessary. These instructions are similar to those following a D & C. The patient should also know that an unpleasant vaginal discharge caused by the sloughing of destroyed cells may persist for up to 3 weeks. Cryosurgery involves the freezing and removal of abnormal cervical tissue through the use of a probe and liquid nitrogen. The treatment is quick and almost painless. The patient will have a watery discharge for up to 2 weeks. Topical antiseptic creams may be prescribed during the 7- to 8-week healing period.

TOXIC SHOCK SYNDROME

Toxic shock syndrome (TSS) is an example of an opportunistic infection by an organism that is common in the vagina. It is an acute condition caused by the toxin of a local infection of *Staphylococcus aureus,* which can develop into a systemic infection. TSS usually occurs in women who are menstruating and using tampons or who have chronic vaginal infections.

TSS typically begins suddenly with high fever, vomiting, and profuse watery diarrhea. Within 48 hours, hypotensive shock and a characteristic rash develop. In the recovery phase, there is a desquamation of varying skin surfaces.[41] A variety of organ systems can be involved.

There is no definitive test for TSS. However, cervical-vaginal isolates of *Staphylococcus aureus* have been present 90% of the time with TSS.[41] Once diagnosed by presumptive signs, prompt treatment with antistaphylococcal B lactamase–resistant antibiotics and fluid replacement therapy is initiated.

Because TSS has been linked to the use of tampons during menstruation, it is recommended that superabsorbent tampons not be used. They provide a favorable milieu for bacterial growth because they can absorb a large amount of menstrual blood and may be left in place longer than other tampons. The nurse should advise patients to alternate tampons with sanitary napkins, using the latter at night. When tampons are used, they should be changed several times a day and inserted carefully to avoid abrasions. Good handwashing techniques should always be used. Organisms gain entrance into the circulatory system through abrasions in the vagina. Women who have had TSS are at risk of recurrence and should be instructed not to use tampons until *Staphylococcus aureus* is no longer present in the vaginal flora.[7] Treatment is symptomatic and supportive.

PELVIC INFLAMMATORY DISEASE

Pelvic inflammatory disease (PID) is an infectious condition of the pelvic cavity that may involve the fallopian tubes (salpingitis), ovaries (oophoritis), pelvic peritoneum, and pelvic vascular system.

Etiology

The frequent causative organisms of PID are *Neisseria gonorrhoeae* and *Chlamydia trachomatis*. These organisms, as well as mycoplasma, streptococci, and anaerobes, may gain entrance during sexual intercourse or after abortion, pelvic surgery, or childbirth. Users of IUDs or women with multiple sexual partners have an increased risk of getting the condition. PID is a common complication of gonorrhea and chlamydial infections. The infection can be acute, subacute, or chronic.

Clinical Manifestations

The patient with *acute PID* seeks medical attention because of crampy or continuous, bilateral lower abdominal pain. In acute cases, movement or ambulation increases the pain. Irregular menstrual bleeding and a vaginal discharge, occasionally greenish or brownish yellow and foul smelling, frequently accompany the pain. Dysuria, dyspareunia, fever, and chills may also be present. Nausea and vomiting are seen in advanced cases. Women with *subacute or chronic PID* may have increased cramps with menses, irregular bleeding, and moderate pain with intercourse. Women who do not develop the classic signs of an acute infection with chills and fever may not seek medical care or may be misdiagnosed and go untreated. Chronic PID can result if the acute phase of the condition does not respond to treatment or if treatment is not initiated or is inadequate.

Once introduced, the infection spreads by two typical routes. One route is along the uterine endometrium to the tubes and into the peritoneum (Fig. 51-5). Salpingitis, pelvic peritonitis, or tuboovarian abscess may result. The second route is primarily through the uterine or cervical lymphatics, across the parametrium, to the tubes or ovaries. In long-term untreated cases, pelvic cellulitis and sometimes thrombophlebitis of the pelvic veins can occur.

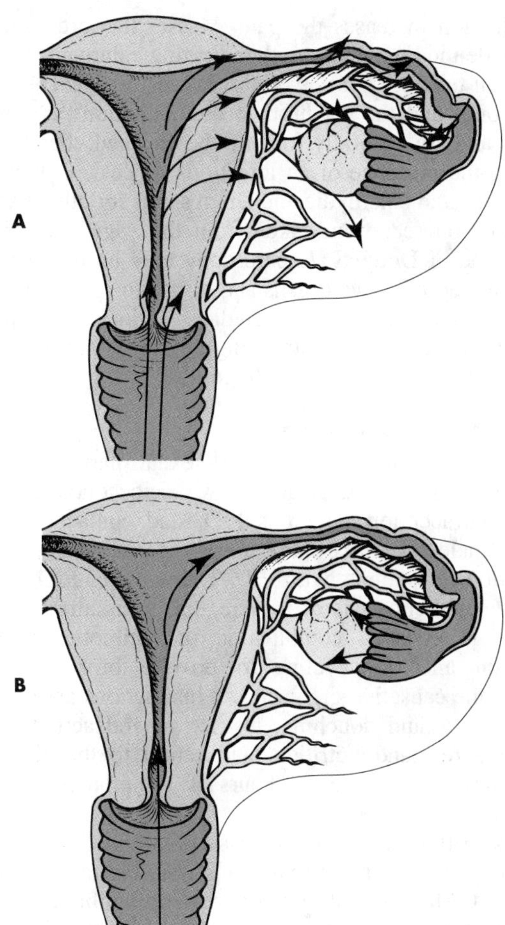

Fig. 51-5 Common routes of the spread of pelvic inflammatory disease. ***A,*** Direct spread of bacterial infection other than *Neisseria gonorrhoeae*. ***B,*** Direct spread of *Neisseria gonorrhoeae*.

Complications

Frequently the patient is rendered sterile as a result of adhesions and strictures that may develop in the fallopian tubes. This can result in closure of the fallopian tubes because of scarring and adhesions. Ectopic pregnancy may result when a tube is partially obstructed because the sperm can pass through the stricture but the fertilized ovum cannot reach the uterus. Pelvic and tubal ovarian abscesses may "leak" or rupture, resulting in pelvic or generalized peritonitis. Embolic episodes may occur after thrombophlebitis of the pelvic veins. As the general circulation is flooded with bacterial endotoxins from the infected areas, septic shock may result.

Diagnostic Studies

The first step in the diagnosis of PID is obtaining a careful health history and performing a physical examination. Often there is a history of a recent acute infection of the lower genital tract. An abdominal examination usually reveals the presence of pain and tenderness in both lower quadrants. Movement of the pelvic organs during vaginal examination increases the pain. Masses that are fixed and poorly defined may be found, indicating enlargement of the fallopian tubes or ovaries or abscess formation. The leukocyte count and the erythrocyte sedimentation rate are assessed and are generally found to be elevated, thereby confirming the presence of an infectious process. Cultures for gonorrhea and chlamydia and Gram stains for other bacteria are done on secretions taken from the vagina, cervix, or cul-de-sac of Douglas. Laparoscopy may be performed to view the reproductive organs and to obtain specimens from the tubal mucosa for culture studies. Vaginal ultrasonic examinations can aid in diagnosing abscesses and following the progress of healing with treatment.

Therapeutic Management

Risk factors, such as multiple sexual partners, sexual activity in female teenagers, low socioeconomic status, IUD contraception, previous PID, and contact with untreated male sexual partners, are considered when planning education for patients with PID. Treatment of PID may be on an outpatient basis or may require hospitalization. The patient is given a combination of antibiotics such as cefoxitin and doxycycline to provide broad coverage against the causative organisms.[38] Instructions are given to avoid coitus and douching, restrict general activities, get adequate rest and nutrition, and return to the clinic for reevaluation in 48 to 72 hours if symptoms persist or increase.

If outpatient treatment is not successful or if the patient is acutely ill or in severe pain, admission to the hospital is indicated. Maximum doses of parenteral antibiotics can be given in the hospital. Some providers believe the addition of cortisone to the antibiotics serves to reduce the inflammation, allowing for faster recovery and improvement in subsequent fertility. Application of heat to the lower abdomen or sitz baths may be used to improve circulation and decrease pain. Bed rest in the semi-Fowler's position promotes drainage of the pelvic cavity by gravity and may prevent the development of abscesses high in the abdomen. Analgesics to relieve pain and IV fluids to prevent dehydration are also prescribed. Sexual partners of women with PID should also be treated as possible sources of infection.

Indications for surgery include the presence of residual masses (abscesses) with the potential for rupture and peritonitis, failure of the patient to respond to conservative management, and a history of frequent exacerbations. The abscess may be drained without laparotomy, or it may be necessary to remove the infected areas along with the uterus, tubes, and ovaries. The extent of the disease and the age and condition of the patient determine the extent of the surgery. The childbearing function in young women is preserved whenever possible.

NURSING MANAGEMENT

PELVIC INFLAMMATORY DISEASE

Nursing Assessment

Subjective and objective data that should be obtained from a patient with PID are presented in Table 51-11.

Table 51-11 Nursing Assessment: Pelvic Inflammatory Disease

Subjective Data

Important health information

Past health history: Use of IUD; previous PID or STD; multiple sexual partners; exposure to partner with urethritis; infertility; recent childbirth, abortion, or pelvic surgery

Medications: Use of and allergy to any antibiotics

Functional health patterns

Health perception–health management: Malaise, fever, chills

Nutritional-metabolic: Nausea, vomiting

Elimination: Frequency, urgency

Cognitive-perceptual: Lower abdominal and pelvic pain; low back pain; pain on fundal palpation and cervical motion; onset of pain just after a menstrual cycle; dysmenorrhea, dyspareunia, dysuria

Sexuality-reproductive: Abnormal vaginal bleeding and menstrual irregularity; vulvar pruritus; vaginal discharge

Objective Data

Reproductive

Mucopurulent cervicitis, vulval maceration, vaginal discharge (heavy and purulent to thin and mucoid), tenderness on motion of cervix and uterus

Gastrointestinal

Tenderness, presence of inflammatory masses

Possible findings

Leukocytosis, elevated erythrocyte sedimentation rate, positive culture of secretions or endocervical fluid, pelvic inflammation and positive endometrial biopsy on laparoscopic examination, abscess or inflammation on ultrasonography

IUD, Intrauterine device; *PID,* pelvic inflammatory disease; *STD,* sexually transmitted disease.

Nursing Diagnoses

Nursing diagnoses are determined when the problem and the etiologic factors are supported by clinical data. Nursing diagnoses related to PID may include, but are not limited, to those presented in the nursing care plan on p. 1607.

Planning

The overall goals are that the patient with pelvic inflammatory disease will (1) experience relief of symptoms, (2) practice good perineal hygiene and safe sex, (3) not become infertile as a result of the disease, and (4) comply with the treatment regimen to prevent the disease from becoming chronic.

Nursing Implementation

Health Maintenance and Promotion. Prevention, early recognition, and prompt treatment of vulvar, vaginal, and cervical infections can help prevent PID and its serious complications. If the nurse knows the factors that predispose a person to the development of PID, patients who are at risk can be identified and appropriate interventions planned.

NURSING CARE PLAN Patient with Pelvic Inflammatory Disease

Planning: Outcome Criteria	*Nursing Interventions and Rationales*
➤ **NURSING DIAGNOSIS**	Acute pain *related to* infectious process *as manifested by* crampy, continuous, bilateral lower abdominal pain, guarding behavior, altered muscle tone
Verbalize satisfactory level of pain control.	Assess degree of pain *to plan appropriate interventions.* Provide comfort measures (e.g., backrub, nonstimulating environment, heat to lower abdomen) *to increase patient comfort.* Administer analgesics as ordered *to relieve the pain.* Instruct patient to restrict movement *to avoid increasing pain.*
➤ **NURSING DIAGNOSIS**	Risk for infection transmission *related to* vaginal discharge and lack of knowledge of proper hygiene and appropriate sexual practices regarding precautionary measures
Know and use principles of medical asepsis; avoid practices that could lead to transmission of disease.	Assess for purulent vaginal discharge, inadequate hand washing, improper disposal of perineal pads, unsafe sexual practices *as possible sources of transmission of infection.* Use and teach strict medical asepsis when in contact with discharge (e.g., proper hand washing, careful handling and disposal of perineal pads); explain need for precautions related to vaginal discharge and encourage patient's participation in them; advise patient against sexual contact while infected *to prevent transmission of infection.* Provide frequent perineal care *to remove infectious drainage and increase patient comfort.*
➤ **NURSING DIAGNOSIS**	Anxiety *related to* imposed activity restrictions, perceived loss of control, and lack of knowledge of outcome on reproductive status and course of disease *as manifested by* restlessness, frequent questioning about restricted activity and outcome, few visitors, irritability, impatience, crying spells
Accurately discuss possible outcomes of disease process on reproductive status and course of disease; accept possible outcome and restrictions.	Assess degree of anxiety and areas of questioning and concern *to plan appropriate interventions.* Maintain bed rest in semi-Fowler's position *to promote drainage of pelvic cavity by gravity and possibly prevent development of an abscess.* Explain need for limited activity *to improve patient's understanding and increase cooperation.* Provide diversional activities; provide stimulation and orientation (e.g., radio, clock); place in room with patients who are oriented to and interested in surroundings *to reduce anxiety and aid in tolerance of enforced rest.* Allow patient to help in planning care *to improve cooperation and foster a sense of personal control.* Discuss possible outcomes of disease process *to assist patient in considering a realistic outcome.* Provide time for patient to express feelings; listen and interact therapeutically *to allow patient opportunity to clarify concerns and begin problem solving.* Provide counsel for patient and significant others *to demonstrate caring and understanding.* Clarify course of disease *so patient can prepare herself and be an informed partner in the plan of care.*
➤ **NURSING DIAGNOSIS**	Impaired skin integrity *related to* vaginal drainage *as manifested by* irritated, painful, reddened perineal area
Perform correct perineal care and have no excoriation in perineal area.	Assess and record the color, amount, and character of the drainage *to determine degree of problem and direct interventions.* Provide and teach gentle perineal cleansing technique q3-4hr *to decrease irritation and promote healing.* Avoid excessive warmth from covers or clothing *to prevent perspiration and increased moisture from causing further irritation to the perineal area.* Teach front-to-back wiping technique *to avoid contaminating the perineum with infectious drainage or fecal matter.*

Gynecologic surgery, childbearing, and abortion may predispose to infection. In these instances, careful medical and surgical asepsis is imperative to prevent the introduction of organisms into the pelvis and reproductive tract. The nurse should counsel the patient to seek medical attention for any unusual vaginal discharge or possible infection of the reproductive organs. The patient should be encouraged by the awareness that some discharges are not indicative of infection and that early diagnosis and treatment of an infection can prevent complications. Routine cultures for *Neisseria gonorrhoeae* and chlamydia should be taken at the time a pelvic examination is being done on every sexually active woman. Women should be informed of the methods of preventing infection and the signs of infection in their partners.

Acute Intervention. During the acute phase of PID, frequent perineal cleansing is indicated to prevent the spread of the infection. The character, amount, color, and odor of the vaginal discharge are recorded. Irritation of the vulva may occur from the vaginal discharge. An explanation of the need for limited activity (bed rest in a semi-Fowler's position) increases patient cooperation. Frequent checks of the vital signs and the degree of abdominal pain can give clues about the effectiveness of therapy.

The nurse should assess the patient's pain level and plan appropriate interventions such as heat to the lower abdomen, sitz baths, and administration of analgesics. Usually the pain is dull and achy in character. The location and intensity of the pain varies according to the underlying pathology. Midline abdominal pain is caused from endometritis. Bilateral lower abdominal pain and pelvic pain is secondary to salpingitis. Peritonitis causes increased abdominal pain, nausea, and vomiting. Pain gradually subsides as the treatment become effective.

Efforts must be made to prevent spread of the infection to others. Proper hand washing with a germicidal soap and use of precautions when handling and disposing of soiled perineal pads are required. Disinfection of utensils, bedpans, and all items in direct contact with the patient is an additional measure that can be used to contain the infection. The need for these precautions should be explained to the patient, and her participation in them should be encouraged.

Chronic and Home Management. The patient with chronic PID experiences chronic pelvic discomfort and requires repeated treatment. Her emotional response to the disease and the therapy should be assessed. The patient may feel well one day and develop distressing discomforts the next. She may become discouraged and depressed. The nurse should be aware of these feelings and provide the patient with emotional support, as well as clarification about the course of the disease.

The patient may have guilt feelings about the problem, especially if it was associated with an STD. She may also be concerned about the complications associated with PID, such as adhesions and strictures of the fallopian tubes, sterility, and the increased incidence of ectopic pregnancy. Discussion with the patient and significant others regarding these feelings and concerns can assist her to cope more effectively with them.

ENDOMETRIOSIS

Endometriosis is a condition characterized by the presence and proliferation of endometrial tissue in sites outside the endometrial cavity. The most frequent sites are in or near the ovaries, the uterosacral ligaments, and the uterovesical peritoneum (Fig. 51-6). Endometrial tissues can be in many other locations, however, such as the stomach, lungs, intestines, and spleen. The tissue responds to the hormones of the ovarian cycle and undergoes a minimenstruation similar to the uterine endometrium. Endometriosis appears to cause infertility in 30% to 60% of cases.[6]

Etiology

Although many theories about the cause of endometriosis have been advanced, the etiology remains unknown. Various theories have been proposed, including a polygenic or multifactorial inheritance and environmental stimuli. Immunologic and hormonal explanations for the ectopic implantation of endometrium have been proposed more recently. Another theory investigated an "increased sensitivity to estrogen," and others looked at unruptured luteinizing follicles as producing an inhibitor for extrauterine implantation.[42] Each theory identifies a component of the etiology, but none offers a complete understanding of what causes endometriosis.

Clinical Manifestations

The symptoms may be vague and diffuse because of the multiple sites affected. Some patients have no symptoms, and the disease is discovered incidental to abdominal surgery. More commonly, the patient complains of pelvic pain that takes the form of secondary dysmenorrhea. The pain is described as dull, aching, or cramping in the lower abdominal region, occurring 1 to 2 days before menses and dimin-

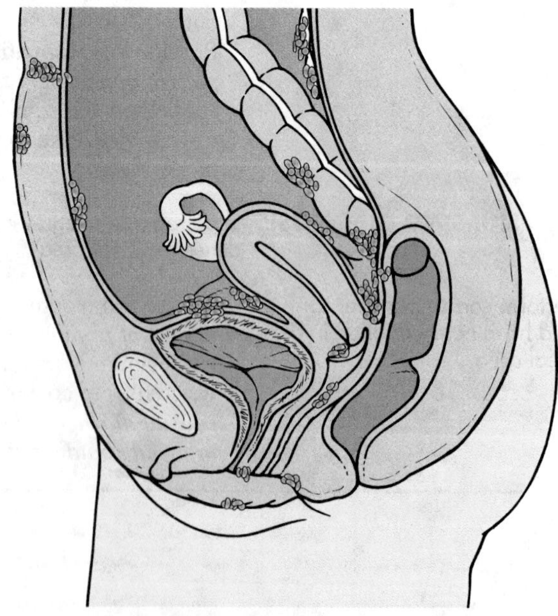

Fig. 51-6 Common sites of endometriosis.

NURSING CARE PLAN Patient with a Total Abdominal Hysterectomy

Planning: Outcome Criteria	Nursing Interventions and Rationales
➤ **NURSING DIAGNOSIS**	Altered patterns of urinary elimination: retention *related to* loss of bladder tone, uncomfortable urinating position, and pain *as manifested by* distention of bladder, voiding of small amounts, difficulty using bedpan and commode
Urinate in sufficient quantities without difficulty.	Measure intake and output *to determine if satisfactory balance is present.* Encourage fluids orally within limitations of diet *to ensure adequate quantity of urine to stimulate urge to urinate.* Palpate bladder *to detect distention.* Catheterize as ordered. Provide privacy during patient's attempts to urinate *to avoid inhibition secondary to embarrassment.* Give perineal care every shift *to assess external genitalia and promote patient comfort.* Report any complaints of backache and decreased output *because these are signs of a possible ligation of a ureter.* Provide routine catheter care if indwelling catheter is in place *to ensure catheter patency and free flow of urine.*
➤ **NURSING DIAGNOSIS**	Body-image disturbance *related to* perceived loss of femininity and future inability to conceive *as manifested by* crying, weeping, depression; verbalization of perceived loss of femininity or ability to conceive
Make accurate statement of effects of hysterectomy; verbalize confidence in ability to adjust to postsurgical state.	Assess depth of impact of surgery on body image *to determine need and plan for intervention.* Provide factual information regarding anticipated bodily changes *so patient will have accurate information.* Provide information on hormone replacement *so patient is informed about possible treatment of surgical menopause.* Encourage discussion with patient, significant others, and health professionals *to minimize emotional impact of hysterectomy through open discussion.*
➤ **NURSING DIAGNOSIS**	Altered sexuality patterns *related to* perceived lack of desirability and fatigue secondary to surgery and lack of knowledge regarding resumption of sexual activity *as manifested by* frequent questioning about future sexual response, lack of desire to resume presurgical sexual practices
Be optimistic that satisfactory sexual practices can be resumed when indicated by surgeon.	Facilitate discussion of sexuality with significant other *to clarify areas of misunderstanding and foster mutual approach to any problems.* Reassure patient that energy and desire will return after a period of convalescence *to prevent discouragement and depression.* Explain psychologic and physiologic implications of hysterectomy related to a woman's sexuality *to provide accurate facts and decrease fear of consequences of hysterectomy.*
➤ **NURSING DIAGNOSIS**	Altered health maintenance *related to* lack of knowledge regarding activity restrictions and hormone replacement therapy (HRT) *as manifested by* questioning about postdischarge plans *pertaining to* presurgery occupational and leisure activity and advisability of HRT
Have confidence in ability to make appropriate decisions related to occupational and leisure activity and HRT.	Encourage expression of concerns *to clarify areas of concern.* Assess knowledge level. Provide information regarding HRT *so patient has accurate information on which to make decisions.* Provide timetable for gradual resumption of presurgery activity *so patient does not resume activities too soon or delay resumption of activities unnecessarily.*

continued

ishing after the onset of flow. It may be related to hemorrhagic distention of the cystlike nodules or to escape of bloody discharge into the peritoneal cavity. Other symptoms include backache, abnormal uterine bleeding, dyspareunia, and painful defecation.

As the ectopic endometrium menstruates, the blood collects in cystlike nodules that have a characteristic bluish black look. Nodules in the ovaries are sometimes called *chocolate cysts* because of the thick, chocolate-colored material they contain. When a cyst ruptures, the pain may be acute and the resulting irritation promotes the formation of adhesions, which fix the affected area to another pelvic structure. The adhesions may become severe enough to cause a bowel obstruction or painful micturition. Adhesions involving the uterus, tubes, or ovaries may result in infertility.

NURSING CARE PLAN Patient with a Total Abdominal Hysterectomy—cont'd

Planning: Outcome Criteria	Nursing Interventions and Rationales
➤ **NURSING DIAGNOSIS** Acute pain *related to* incision and manipulation of internal organs *as manifested by* statements about pain, guarding of incision, reluctance to ambulate, facial grimacing	
Verbalize satisfactory level of pain control.	Assess degree of pain *to plan appropriate interventions.* Provide comfort measures (e.g., backrub, nonstimulating environment, heat to lower abdomen) *to increase patient comfort.* Administer analgesics as ordered *to relieve the pain.* Instruct patient on methods for moving and coughing while supporting abdominal incision.

COLLABORATIVE PROBLEMS

Nursing Goals	Nursing Interventions and Rationales
➤ **POTENTIAL COMPLICATION** Paralytic ileus *related to* surgical manipulation of bowel and immobility	
Monitor for signs of paralytic ileus, report if present, and carry out appropriate medical and nursing interventions.	Assess for distended abdomen, complaints of gas pains, decreased bowel sounds *to detect presence of paralytic ileus.* Encourage ambulation q4hr *to promote bowel peristalsis.* Insert rectal tube as ordered *to expel flatus and promote patient comfort.* Withhold food and fluids if paralytic ileus is present *to prevent nausea and vomiting.* Insert and monitor nasogastric tube as ordered *to prevent accumulation of gas and fluids.*
➤ **POTENTIAL COMPLICATION** Thromboembolic phenomenon *related to* immobility and irritation of vessels of pelvis and upper thigh	
Monitor for signs of thromboembolism, report if present, and carry out appropriate medical and nursing interventions.	Assess lower extremities for warmth, color, blanching, pain, and sensation q8hr *to detect impaired circulation.* Report and record positive signs *so early treatment can be initiated.* Carry out active-passive exercises q2hr; ambulate q4hr *to promote good circulation and prevent stasis.* Reapply elastic compression gradient stockings every shift *to apply even pressure to veins to prevent venous stasis.*

Therapeutic Management

Diagnosis is frequently confirmed by a history of the characteristic symptoms of the condition and the palpation of firm nodular lumps in the adnexa on bimanual examination. Visualization of the typical bluish nodes with culdoscopy, laparoscopy, or during a laparotomy establishes a definite diagnosis. The treatment of endometriosis is influenced by the patient's age, her desire to bear children, and the severity of the symptoms. With menopause, ovarian atrophy begins and hormonal stimulation declines, usually leading to the disappearance of the symptoms.

Observation and mild analgesia are used initially when symptoms are not severe or incapacitating. Regular follow-up examinations at least once yearly to check on further progression of the disease are needed so that necessary changes in the plan of management can be made. Pregnancy and lactation often result in the relief of symptoms because menstruation ceases during this time.

Management with drugs is directed at imitating a state of pregnancy or menopause because both natural conditions relieve symptoms. Continuous use (for 9 months) of combined progestin and estrogen softens and causes regression of endometrial tissue. Ovulation is suppressed and *pseudopregnancy* (hyperhormonal amenorrhea) is produced. However, because of troublesome side effects, this treatment modality is used less frequently today. Another approach to hormonal treatment is danazol (Danocrine), a synthetic androgen that inhibits the anterior pituitary. When given in dosages of up to 800 mg/day for 6 to 9 months, the drug produces a pseudomenopause (ovarian suppression), with consequent atrophy of ectopic endometrial tissue. Subjective relief of symptoms is noted within 6 weeks of danazol use. Side effects include weight gain, acne, hot flashes, and hirsutism. The associated cost is a major drawback.

The newest and most expensive drug therapy is injectable gonadotropin-releasing hormone analog (Lupron Depot). It causes a hypoestrogenic state resulting in amenorrhea. The side effects reported by patients are usually the same as menopause (hot flashes, vaginal dryness, and emotional lability). Loss of bone density has also been reported in women who remain on the therapy longer than 6 months.

Endometriosis is controlled but not cured by hormonal therapy. Persistent lesions give rise to subsequent recurrences once the menstrual cycle is reestablished.

Surgical Interventions. Surgical treatment may be conservative or radical. Conservative surgery is usually used in the management of young women who are concerned about infertility. It involves removal or destruction of endometrial implants and lysing or excision of adhesions by means of laparoscopic laser surgery and laparotomy. GnRH agonist therapy (e.g., leuprolide acetate [Lupron]) can be administered for 4 to 6 months to reduce the size of the lesions before surgery. By reducing the extent of the surgery, this preoperative drug treatment helps reduce the development of adhesions that may further threaten fertility.[29] Efforts are made to conserve all tissues necessary to maintain fertility. Radical surgery is generally performed in women approaching menopause. It involves removal of the uterus, tubes, ovaries, and as many endometrial implants as possible. Hysterectomy with removal of as many implants as possible but with preservation of all or part of the ovarian tissue is recommended for the young woman who does not want children but wishes to have cyclical ovarian function.

NURSING MANAGEMENT

ENDOMETRIOSIS

Nurses should encourage women to have regular physical examinations in an effort to identify early symptoms of endometriosis. Patient education about the disease process can clarify and dispel false ideas and fears. Dysmenorrhea after years of relatively pain-free menses and the inability to achieve pregnancy may serve as clues to the presence of this disease and should be reported and investigated.

When the symptoms are less severe, treatment for dysmenorrhea and a "wait-and-see" approach may be used. Education of the patient and reassurance that a health-threatening situation does not exist may permit her to accept a conservative and progressive treatment. The nurse is often the person who counsels the patient in the use of drugs. The action of the prescribed hormones should be explained, as well as the possible side effects. Psychologic support may be needed for the patient who is experiencing severe disabling pain, sexual difficulties secondary to dyspareunia, and infertility.

If conservative surgery is the treatment selected, the nursing care is similar to the general preoperative and postoperative care of a patient undergoing laparotomy. If radical surgery is planned, the nursing care is similar to the patient undergoing an abdominal hysterectomy (see the nursing care plan on p. 1609). The nurse must know the extent of the procedure so that appropriate postoperative teaching can be done.

BENIGN TUMORS OF THE FEMALE REPRODUCTIVE SYSTEM

Leiomyomas

Etiology. *Leiomyomas* (fibroids, myomas, fibromyomas, fibromas) are the most common benign tumors of the female genital tract. By 30 years of age, 10% of Caucasian women and 30% of African-American women will have uterine leiomyomas. The cause of leiomyomas is unknown, but they are thought to depend on ovarian hormones, growing slowly during the reproductive years and undergoing atrophy with the advent of menopause. These tumors are composed mainly of smooth muscle and fibrous connective tissue.

Clinical Manifestations. Twenty percent to 50% of women with leiomyomas develop symptoms, the most common being menorrhagia. Although rarely experienced with leiomyomas, pain is associated with infection or twisting of the pedicle from which the tumor is growing. Dysmenorrhea and dyspareunia may occasionally occur. Pressure on surrounding organs may result in rectal, bladder, and lower abdominal discomfort. Large tumors may cause a general enlargement of the lower abdomen. These tumors are sometimes associated with abortion and infertility.

Therapeutic Management. Diagnosis is usually based on the characteristic pelvic findings of an enlarged uterus distorted by nodular masses. The presence of a malignant tumor is ruled out before treatment is begun. Treatment depends on the symptoms, the age of the patient, her desire to bear children, and the location and size of the tumor or tumors. An intravenous pyelogram should be obtained to detect urethral compression with resulting hydronephrosis. If the symptoms are minor, the provider may elect to follow the patient closely for a time. If the woman is experiencing menorrhagia, the use of aspirin is discouraged because of its effect on platelets. In the young woman who wishes to have children, a myomectomy is performed. In cases of large leiomyomas, the treatment is hysterectomy. Gonadotropin-releasing hormone agonist (Lupron) may be used preoperatively to shrink the size of the leiomyomas. However, this medication is expensive and, when used over 6 months, leads to the onset of menopausal signs and symptoms, including osteoporotic changes and hot flashes.

Cervical Polyps

Cervical polyps are benign pedunculated lesions that generally arise from the endocervical mucosa and are seen protruding through the external os on speculum examination of the cervix and vagina. Polyps are a characteristic bright cherry red and are soft and fragile in consistency. They are generally small, measuring less than 3 cm in length, and may be single or multiple. Their origin is unknown. Symptoms are usually not present, but metrorrhagia and bleeding after straining and coitus can occur. Polyps are prone to infection. When the polyp is small, it can be excised in an outpatient procedure. If the point of attachment of the polyp cannot be identified and is not accessible to cautery, a polypectomy is performed in an operating room. All tissue removed is sent for pathologic review because polyps occasionally undergo malignant changes.

Benign Ovarian Tumors

Benign tumors of the ovary are many and varied. The cause of most of them is unknown. For purposes of clarity, they are divided into nonneoplasms and neoplasms. *Nonneoplasms* are usually simple cysts surrounded by a thin capsule and are seen mainly during the reproductive years. *Neoplasms* of the ovaries are fluid-filled cysts that are primarily bilateral.

CULTURAL & ETHNIC Considerations

CANCER OF FEMALE REPRODUCTIVE SYSTEM

- Ovarian cancer is seen more frequently among Caucasian women than among African-American women.
- Endometrial cancer occurs more frequently among Caucasian women than among African-American women.
- Cervical cancer has a higher incidence among Hispanic, African-American, and Native American women than Caucasians. Mortality rate from cervical cancer is more than twice as high among African-American women than among Caucasian women.
- There is a low incidence of cervical cancer among Jewish women.

Ovarian tumors are often asymptomatic until they are large enough to cause pressure in the pelvis. Constipation, menstrual irregularities, urinary frequency, a full feeling in the abdomen, anorexia, and peripheral edema may occur, depending on the size and location of the tumor. There may be an increase in abdominal girth. Pelvic pain may be present if the tumor is growing rapidly. Severe pain results when the cyst twists on its pedicle (twisted ovarian cyst).

Pelvic examination reveals a mass or an enlarged ovary that demands further investigation. Laparoscopy or exploratory laparotomy is often performed to confirm the diagnosis. During surgical treatment, attempts are made to save as much ovarian function as possible. If follicular cysts are found, surgery may involve aspiration of the fluid; if not, removal of one or both ovaries may be necessary.

MALIGNANT TUMORS OF THE FEMALE REPRODUCTIVE SYSTEM

Cervical Cancer

Carcinoma of the cervix is the sixth most frequent malignancy in women, behind cancer of the breast, colon, rectum, endometrium, lung, and ovary.[43] It occurs predominantly in women between 30 and 50 years of age. The incidence is higher among African-American and Hispanic women than among Caucasian women. An increased risk of cervical cancer is associated with low economic status, early marriage, early sexual activity, several partners (particularly those with poor penile hygiene), multiple pregnancies, a history of untreated chronic cervicitis, venereal disease (e.g., venereal warts), viral infections, papilloma, HSV II infection, and smoking. Nearly 29% of deaths from cervical cancer are associated with cigarette smoking.[43]

The number of deaths from cervical cancer has fallen steadily over the past 40 years. This is attributable to better and earlier diagnosis with the widespread use of the Pap test. Its high detection efficiency permits treatment at a time (stage 0) when cure is almost certain. The American Cancer Society recommends that annual Pap tests begin with the onset of sexual activity. Following three negative Pap tests, less frequent tests may be recommended by the provider.

In the late 1960s, several cases of cervical (and vaginal) carcinoma were reported in adolescent girls. Subsequent studies revealed that diethylstilbestrol (DES) had been administered to their mothers during pregnancy. Enough evidence has accumulated to recommend that DES not be used during pregnancy. Daughters of women who were treated with DES are encouraged to have regular gynecologic examinations.

Currently, there is a resurgence of cervical carcinoma in young women. Risk varies directly with an increase in number of sexual partners and with early incidence of first intercourse. These circumstances, along with certain serotypes of papilloma virus, have resulted in detection of cervical cancer in women in their early twenties. Preventive education should be directed toward counseling on delaying sexual activity and the use of barrier and spermicidal contraceptives.

The fears and anxieties that arise in relation to cancer are many and varied. Women have seen and heard accounts of the disfigurement and disabilities that may follow the diagnosis of cancer. Nurses should emphasize the positive fact that early discovery improves the prognosis and hinders the occurrence of more serious outcomes. The important goal of disease prevention is again the major concern.

Women at high risk with family histories of cervical cancer should be sought out and encouraged to have frequent examinations for the appearance of cancer. An annual pelvic examination and Pap testing are a woman's best insurance for early detection and treatment of cervical cancer.

Pathophysiology. The World Health Organization has developed an international classification of cancer of the cervix with stages from 0 to IV (Table 51-12). Stage 0, the preinvasive stage of carcinoma in situ of the cervix, is limited to the epithelial layer. A period of 5 to 10 years may elapse between the preinvasive stage and a stage I lesion, making the prognosis good for early diagnosis. Stage IV involves cancer that has extended outside the reproductive tract.

Clinical Manifestations. Early cervical cancer is generally asymptomatic, but leukorrhea and intermenstrual bleeding eventually occur. The discharge is usually thin and watery but becomes dark and foul smelling as the disease advances, suggesting the presence of an infection. The vaginal bleeding is initially only spotting, but as the tumor enlarges, it becomes heavier and more frequent. Pain is a late symptom and is followed by weight loss, anemia, and cachexia.

Diagnostic Studies. A Pap test, the Schiller iodine test (see Chapter 48), colposcopy, and a biopsy may be used to diagnose cancer of the cervix. (Details of the Pap test are given in Chapter 48.) The classification for cytologic findings used by many laboratories is given in Table 51-13. The current trend is to use the Bethesda system because it improves accuracy and quality of diagnosis by standardizing diagnostic reports.[44]

Table 51-12 International Classification of Clinical Stages of Carcinoma of the Cervix

Stage	Extent	Treatment	5-Year Survival Rate (%)*
Stage 0	In situ, intraepithelial	Cervical conization, total hysterectomy, cryosurgery, laser surgery	95-100
Stage I	Strict confinement to cervix (no consideration of extension to corpus)		75-85
Stage IA	Microinvasive (early stromal invasion)	Radiation or surgery	
Stage IB	All other cases of stage I	Radiation, Wertheim's hysterectomy	
Stage II	Extension beyond cervix but not to pelvic wall, involvement of vagina, but not as far as lower third		
Stage IIA	No obvious parametrial involvement	Radiation, Wertheim's hysterectomy	65-75
Stage IIB	Obvious parametrial involvement	Radiation; if this fails, pelvic exenteration may be required	50-65
Stage III	Extension to pelvic wall, no cancer-free space between tumor and pelvic wall on rectal examination, involvement of lower third of vagina, hydronephrosis or nonfunctioning kidney	Radiation	20-30
Stage IIIA	No extension to pelvic wall		
Stage IIIB	Extension to pelvic wall or hydronephrosis or nonfunctioning kidney		
Stage IV	Extension beyond true pelvis or clinical involvement of the mucosa of bladder or rectum, no stage IV classification with bullous edema alone	Radiation, surgery (e.g., exenteration)	1-10
Stage IVA	Spread to adjacent organs		
Stage IVB	Spread to distant organs		

*Statistics are compiled from a variety of references. Those most generally agreed on are used here.

The finding of an abnormal Pap smear (with the exception of class V) indicates the need for additional procedures, such as colposcopy and biopsy, before a definitive diagnosis of cancer can be made. Colposcopy involves examination of the cervix with a binocular microscope with low levels of magnification (10× to 40×). The procedure discloses epithelial abnormalities and suggests areas for biopsy. As a result, it improves the rate of detection for cervical cancer and can lead to more focused treatment.

The type and extent of the biopsy vary with the abnormality seen. A punch biopsy may be done on an outpatient basis with special punch biopsy forceps. The excision of a cone-shaped section of the cervix may be used for both diagnosis and treatment. Conization is accomplished using one of several techniques. The choice of procedure is determined by the provider's experience and the availability of the equipment. *Cryotherapy* (freezing) and laser cone vaporization destroy the tissue. Laser cone excision and *loop electrosurgery excision procedure* (LEEP) remove the identified tissue and allow for histologic examination to ensure that all microinvasive tissue has been removed. These procedures can be performed in the office with some mild analgesics or relaxants. Complications of these procedures include excessive bleeding and possible cervical stenosis with healing.

Therapeutic Management. Treatment of cancer of the cervix is guided by the stage of the tumor and the patient's age and general state of health (see Table 51-13). Conization may be the only type of therapy needed for cervical intraepithelial neoplasia (CIN) if analysis of the removed tissue demonstrates that a wide area of normal tissue surrounds the excised malignancy. Laser treatments, in which a directed infrared beam causes the boiling and vaporization of intracellular water, is effective in the destruction of dysplastic tissue. Cautery and cryosurgery may also be used. Fertility is preserved with these four procedures. Invasive cancer of the cervix is treated with surgery, radiation, or a combination of the two to remove or destroy

Table 51-13 Classification of Cytologic Findings of Pap Tests

Papanicolaou Class	Dysplasia	CIN	Bethesda System
Class I			
Normal smear	Negative	Negative	Within normal limits
Class II			
Atypical cells, no dysplasia	Reactive atypia Koilocytosis or HPV Mild dysplasia	Koilocytosis or HPV CIN 1	Regeneration, repair Inflammation Low-grade squamous intraepithelial lesion
Class III			
Abnormal cells consistent with dysplasia	Moderate dysplasia	CIN 2	
Class IV			
Abnormal cells consistent with CIS	Severe dysplasia, CIS	CIN 2 CIN 3	High-grade squamous intraepithelial lesion
Class V			
Abnormal cells consistent with invasive or squamous cell origin	Squamous cell carcinoma	Squamous cell carcinoma	Squamous cell carcinoma

From Stenchever MA: *Office gynecology,* St Louis, 1992, Mosby.
CIN, Cervical intraepithelial neoplasia; *CIS,* carcinoma in situ; *HPV,* human papilloma virus.

the involved areas and lymphatic drainage. Surgical procedures commonly carried out include hysterectomy, radical hysterectomy (Wertheim procedure), and rarely pelvic exenteration. Radiation may be external (e.g., cobalt) or internal (e.g., cesium or radium). Standard radiation treatment is 5 to 6 weeks of external radiation followed with 1 or 2 treatments with internal implants.

Systemic or regional chemotherapy has been disappointing in most cases of recurrent cervical cancer. Previously radiated areas are especially difficult to treat because the capillary blood supply is diminished, resulting in poor drug delivery to the tumor bed.

Endometrial Cancer

Significance. Cancer of the endometrium has become the most common gynecologic malignancy, accounting for about 50% of female genital tract neoplasms. However, it has a relatively low mortality, with approximately 75% survival.[45] It is associated with women who are between 50 and 70 years of age, nulliparous, obese, hypertensive, or diabetic or who had a late menopause or prolonged unopposed estrogen-only replacement therapy. Possible external factors contributing to the increased incidence include aging of the population, better reporting of cases, and more widespread prescribing of estrogens for postmenopausal women.[7] Obesity is the most important risk factor because it increases endogenous estrogen production and availability.

Pathophysiology. Cancer arises from the lining of the endometrium. The precursor may be a hyperplastic state that progresses to invasive carcinoma. Direct extension develops into the cervix and through the uterine serosa. As invasion of the myometrium occurs, regional lymph nodes, including the paravaginal and paraaortic, become involved. Hematogenous metastases develop concurrently. The usual sites of metastases are lung, bone, liver, and eventually brain. Malignant cells can be found in the peritoneal cavity, presumably by tubal transport, and their presence is included in staging. Prognostic factors include histologic differentiation, uterine size at time of diagnosis, myometrial invasion, peritoneal cytology, lymph node and adnexal metastases, and tumor size.

Most tumors are pure adenocarcinomas. Endometrial cancer grows slowly, metastasizes late, and is amenable to therapy if diagnosed early. The first sign of endometrial cancer is abnormal uterine bleeding, usually in postmenopausal women. Because perimenopausal women have sporadic periods for a time, it is important that this sign not be ignored or automatically blamed on menopause. Pain occurs late in the disease process, and other symptoms that may arise are related to metastasis to other organs.

Diagnostic Studies and Therapeutic Management. D & C, endometrial biopsy, and smears are used to diagnose endometrial cancer. D & C and endometrial biopsy can be done as an office procedure in which endometrial tissue is "aspirated" from the uterus. Occurrence of breakthrough bleeding in a postmenopausal woman mandates obtaining a tissue sample to exclude endometrial cancer. The Pap test is not a reliable diagnostic tool for endometrial cancer, but it can rule out cervical cancer. Treatment is by total hysterectomy, which includes bilateral salpingooophorectomy with selective node biopsies. Surgery may be followed by radiation, either externally with cobalt or internally with intracavitary radium.

Chemotherapy is reserved for recurrences or distant metastases. Progesterone therapy (e.g., Provera, Megace) is the treatment of choice when the progesterone receptor status is positive and the tumor is well differentiated. Chemotherapy is considered when progesterone therapy is unsuccessful.

Ovarian Cancer

Because most patients with ovarian cancer have advanced disease at diagnosis, it is the most deadly gynecologic malignancy in the United States, ranking third among the gynecologic cancers.[7] Cancer of the ovary seems to be linked to multiparity, infertility, advanced age, long history of menstrual irregularities, and higher socioeconomic group. Breast feeding, multiple pregnancies, oral contraceptives, and early age at first birth seem to reduce the risk of ovarian cancer. It occurs more frequently in women between 40 and 65 years of age and has a high familial incidence.

Pathophysiology. Eighty percent to 85% of ovarian cancers are epithelial carcinomas. Germ cell tumors account for another 10%. Histologic grading is an important prognostic determinant. Generally, tumors are divided into well differentiated (grade I), moderately well differentiated (grade II), and poorly differentiated (grade III). Grade III lesions carry a worse prognosis than the other grades.

Ovarian cancer has two patterns of metastasis: lymphatic and direct. Primary lymphatic drainage of the ovary is through the retroperitoneal nodes surrounding the renal hilum. Secondary drainage is through the iliac lymphatics. Tertiary drainage is through the inguinal lymphatics. Ovarian cancer also metastasizes directly to the abdominal cavity, the diaphragm, and the omentum.

Careful staging is critical in making rational treatment decisions. Because of the numerous metastatic pathways for ovarian cancer, accurate staging usually involves multiple biopsies. Stage I describes disease limited to the ovaries; stage II, disease limited to the true pelvis; stage III, disease limited to the abdominal cavity; and stage IV, distant metastatic disease.

Clinical Manifestations. In its early stages, ovarian cancer is asymptomatic. As the malignancy grows, a variety of symptoms, such as an increase in abdominal girth, bowel and bladder dysfunction, pain, menstrual irregularities, and ascites, can occur. An ovarian malignancy should be considered when abnormal uterine bleeding occurs.

Diagnostic Studies. Serum CA-125 is a specific marker for ovarian cancer. It is useful both in detecting disease in its early stages and in following the response to treatment. CA-125 is positive in 80% of women with epithelial ovarian cancer.[46] CA-125 antigen levels in the blood will decrease as the cancer cells decrease.[47]

The bimanual pelvic examination, ultrasonography, and laparoscopy remain the only reliable diagnostic tools. When a suspicious mass in the ovarian area is palpated, ultrasound, CT scan, or laparoscopy is performed to establish the diagnosis. If the mass is malignant, treatment depends on the surgical staging of the disease.

Therapeutic Management. The usual treatment for stage I malignancies is a total abdominal hysterectomy and bilateral salpingooophorectomy with removal of as much of the tumor as possible (i.e., tumor debulking). The remaining tissues in the abdomen and pelvis are carefully scrutinized. Ascitic fluid is submitted for cytologic study, and appropriate biopsies are performed to determine the stage of the disease.

The addition of chemotherapy or the instillation of intraperitoneal radioisotopes is usually suggested for stage I disease. The patient with stage II disease may receive external abdominal and pelvic radiation, intraperitoneal radiation, or systemic combined chemotherapy after tumor-reducing surgery. After completion of systemic chemotherapy, in the patient who is clinically free of symptoms, a "second-look" surgical procedure is often performed to determine whether there is any evidence of disease. This option does not necessarily improve the outcome. If no disease is found, the chemotherapy is stopped and the patient is monitored for recurrent disease. Chemotherapy (e.g., cisplatin, carboplatin) is one of the mainstays of treatment for stage III and stage IV diseases. Altretamine (Hexalen) is used for palliative treatment of persistent, recurrent ovarian cancer. Pacletaxel (Taxol) is used to treat metastatic ovarian cancer. Surgical debulking is often done in conjunction with chemotherapy for advanced disease. Intraperitoneal chemotherapy, although associated with substantial side effects, is coming into wider use for the patient who has minimum residual disease after surgery. Unfortunately, the malignancy may have metastasized to the peritoneum, omentum, or bowel surface before discovery of the tumors. In these situations the prognosis is poor. Recurrent pleural effusion causing shortness of breath and discomfort may require frequent paracenteses, but the fluid accumulates again. Irradiation and chemotherapy may be used to shrink the size of the tumor, relieving pressure and pain.

Vaginal Cancer

Primary vaginal cancers are rare. The most common symptoms include abnormal bleeding, discharge, pain, urinary frequency, constipation, and tenesmus. The most common type of vaginal cancer is squamous cell carcinoma.

Treatment of vaginal cancer depends on the type of cells involved and the stage of the disease, the size of the tumor, and the location of the tumor. Squamous cell carcinomas can be treated with both surgery and radiation. Surgery is the preferred treatment in younger women. A radical hysterectomy, partial vaginectomy, and pelvic lymphadenectomy are usually effective. Both internal and external radiation is used, but proximity to the bladder and rectum makes this problematic.

An association between intrauterine exposure to diethylstilbestrol and clear cell adenocarcinoma of the vagina has been established. This type of vaginal cancer can spread locally, as well as by the lymphatic or hematogenous routes. Metastasis to regional pelvic nodes has been found, particularly in higher stage tumors. Both surgery and radiation (intracavitary implant and full pelvic radiation) are used to treat this type of vaginal cancer. In both types of vaginal cancer, chemotherapy using multiagents has been used to treat metastatic disease.

Nursing care of the patient with vaginal cancer requires expert and sensitive care. Often, the surgery is extensive, painful, and mutilating. Vaginal sexual activity may not be possible without vaginal reconstruction. Important points for the nurse to discuss with the patient with vaginal cancer include (1) possible impact of surgery and radiation on vaginal sex; (2) potential problems, such as dyspareunia and decreased libido (caused by radiation therapy); (3) effect of surgery or radiation on her feelings about her sexuality and personhood; and (4) need to continue regular health follow-up to detect metastasis should it occur.

Vulvar Cancer

Cancer of the vulva is relatively rare, occurring mainly among women over 50 years of age with a peak incidence over age 70. The malignancy is visible and accessible, making early diagnosis more likely.

Although the exact cause is not known, cancer of the vulva may follow *leukoplakia* (irregular white patches on vulva mucosa that produce intense pruritus) or other conditions causing chronic irritation of the area. The patient may initially experience pruritus, soreness of the vulva, unusual odor, discharge, or bleeding but tends to ignore these symptoms. Edema of the vulva and pelvic lymphadenopathy develop as the disease progresses.

Diagnosis of vulvar cancer is done by means of pelvic examination and biopsy. The treatment for vulvar cancer is vulvectomy. The extent of the surgery depends on the size and site of the malignancy. If it is in situ, a simple vulvectomy (surgical excision of the vulva) is done. If the cancer is invasive, a radical vulvectomy with superficial and deep lymph node dissection is indicated. Irradiation is not generally used in this area because the tissues do not tolerate it well.

NURSING MANAGEMENT
MALIGNANT TUMORS

Nursing Assessment

Malignant tumors of the female reproductive system can be found in the cervix, endometrium, ovaries, vagina, and vulva. The patient with any of these malignant tumors may experience a variety of clinical manifestations, including leukorrhea (white discharge from the vagina), irregular vaginal bleeding, vaginal discharge, increase in abdominal pain and pressure, bowel and bladder dysfunction, and vulvar itching and burning. Assessment for these signs and symptoms is an important nursing responsibility.

Nursing Diagnoses

Nursing diagnoses specific to the female patient with malignant tumors of the reproductive system include, but are not limited to, the following:

- Anxiety related to threat of a malignancy and lack of knowledge related to disease process and prognosis
- Pain related to pressure secondary to enlarging tumor
- Body-image disturbance related to loss of body part and loss of good health
- Altered sexuality patterns related to physiologic limitations and fatigue
- Ineffective breathing pattern related to presence of ascites and effusions
- Anticipatory grieving related to poor prognosis of advanced disease

Planning

The overall goals are that the patient with a malignant tumor will (1) actively participate in treatment decisions, (2) achieve satisfactory pain and symptom management, (3) recognize and report problems promptly, (4) maintain preferred lifestyle as long as possible, and (5) continue to practice cancer detection strategies.

Nursing Implementation

Health Maintenance and Promotion. Although early diagnosis and treatment of cancer of the female reproductive tract have improved, a relatively high associated death rate remains. The chief reason may be that women do not sufficiently participate in good preventive care. In their many contacts with women, nurses can play a major role in advocating preventive care. To carry out this mission successfully, nurses have to be well informed about reproductive tract screening schedules and malignancies, especially the early signs and symptoms and the various diagnostic studies and treatment measures available.

SURGICAL PROCEDURES INVOLVING THE FEMALE REPRODUCTIVE SYSTEM

Types

A variety of surgical procedures (Table 51-14) are carried out when benign or malignant tumors of the genital tract are found. A hysterectomy may be done either vaginally or abdominally. A vaginal route is often used when vaginal repair is to be done in addition to removal of the uterus. The abdominal route is used when large tumors are present and the pelvic cavity is to be explored or when the tubes and ovaries are to be removed at the same time (Fig. 51-7). The abdominal route can present more postoperative problems because it involves an incision and the opening of the abdominal cavity. In both vaginal and abdominal hysterectomies the ligaments that support the uterus are attached to the vaginal cuff so that normal depth of the vagina is maintained.

NURSING MANAGEMENT
TUMORS

Surgical Intervention

All patients experience a degree of anxiety when surgery is contemplated, but the prospect of major gynecologic surgery may heighten these concerns. Some women may fear a loss of femininity and worry about possible changes in their secondary sex characteristics. Others may experience feelings of guilt, anger, or embarrassment. Still others may focus on the effect surgery will have on their reproductive and sexual functions. There are also women who view the whole process as annoying or who are relieved by the thought of no longer having to worry about becoming pregnant. Each patient must be understood in light of her fears and concerns and must be approached and evaluated

Table 51-14 Surgical Procedures on the Female Reproductive Tract

Type of Surgery	Description
Subtotal hysterectomy	Removal of uterus without cervix (rarely done today)
Total hysterectomy	Removal of uterus and cervix
Panhysterectomy (TAH-BSO)	Removal of uterus, cervix, fallopian tubes, and ovaries
Simple vulvectomy	Excision of vulva and wide margin of skin
Radical vulvectomy	Excision of tissue from anus to few cm above symphysis pubis (skin, labia majora and minora, and clitoris) with superficial and deep lymph node dissection
Vaginectomy	Removal of vagina
Radical hysterectomy (Wertheim)	Panhysterectomy, partial vaginectomy, and dissection of lymph nodes in pelvis
Pelvic exenteration	Radical hysterectomy, total vaginectomy, removal of bladder with diversion of urinary system and resection of bowel with colos-tomy
Anterior pelvic exenteration	Above operation without bowel resection
Posterior pelvic exenteration	Above operation without bladder removal

individually. The nurse who exhibits interest and a willingness to listen can provide considerable psychologic support.

Hysterectomy. Preoperatively, the patient is prepared physically for surgery with the standard perineal or abdominal preparation and shave. A vaginal douche and enemas may be given, according to the preference of the surgeon. The bladder should be emptied before the patient is sent to the operating room. An indwelling catheter is often inserted preoperatively.

Surgical dressing. After surgery the patient who has had a hysterectomy will have an abdominal dressing (abdominal hysterectomy) or a sterile perineal pad (vaginal hysterectomy). (See the preceding nursing care plan for the patient after a total abdominal hysterectomy.) The dressing should be observed frequently for any sign of bleeding during the first 8 hours after surgery. A moderate amount of serosanguineous drainage on the perineal pad is expected following a vaginal hysterectomy.

Urinary considerations. The patient may experience urinary retention postoperatively because of temporary bladder atony resulting from edema or nerve trauma. This problem is more acute when a radical hysterectomy has been performed. At times an indwelling catheter is used for 1 to 2 days postoperatively to maintain constant drainage of the bladder and prevent strain on the suture line. If an indwelling catheter is not used, catheterization may be necessary if the patient has not urinated for 8 hours postoperatively. If residual urine is suspected after the removal of an indwelling catheter, catheterization is done to prevent bladder infection caused by pooling of urine. Accidental ligation of a ureter is

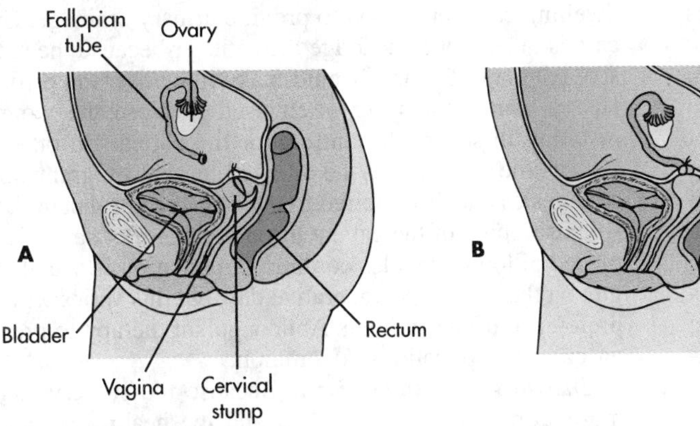

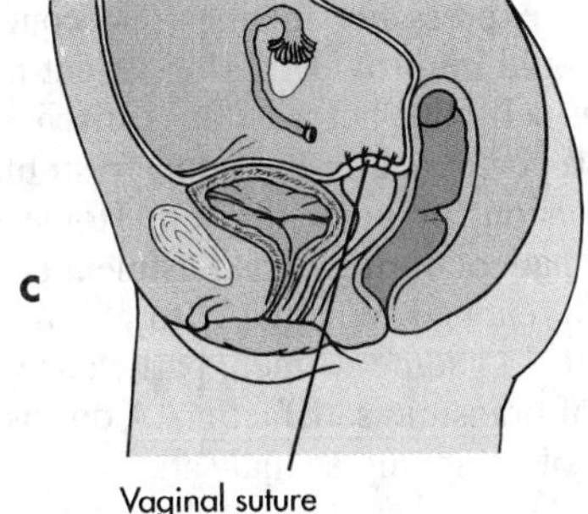

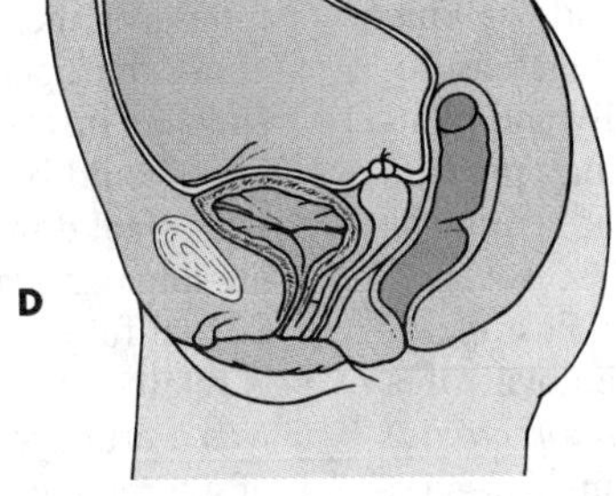

Fig. 51-7 ***A,*** Cross section of subtotal hysterectomy. Note that cervical stump, fallopian tubes, and ovaries remain. ***B,*** Cross section of total hysterectomy. Note that fallopian tubes and ovaries remain. ***C,*** Cross section of vaginal hysterectomy. Note that fallopian tubes and ovaries remain. ***D,*** Total hysterectomy, salpingectomy, and oophorectomy. Note that uterus, fallopian tubes, and ovaries are completely removed.

a serious surgical complication. Any complaint of backache or decreased urine output should be reported to the surgeon.

Abdominal distention. Abdominal distention may develop from the sudden release of pressure on the intestines when a large tumor is removed or from paralytic ileus secondary to anesthesia and pressure on the bowel. Food and fluids may be restricted if the patient is nauseated. A rectal tube may be prescribed to relieve abdominal flatus, and ambulation is encouraged. A Fleets enema or suppository is frequently given on the third postoperative day.

Thrombophlebitis. Special care must be taken to prevent the development of thrombophlebitis of the veins in the pelvis or legs. Frequent changes of position and the avoidance of high Fowler's position and pressure under the knees minimize stasis and pooling of blood. Special attention must be given to patients with varicosities. Leg exercises to promote circulation and the use of elastic gradient compression stockings or elastic bandages can be helpful.

Emotional response. If the ovaries are removed, the patient may feel depressed for several weeks, possibly because of hormonal changes. She may experience periodic crying spells, sometimes called "hysterectomy blues," resulting from wide vacillation in estrogen and progesterone levels. Hormone replacement therapy is usually initiated in the early postoperative period. The loss of a body part may bring about grieflike responses that occur when any great personal loss is sustained. Sympathetic understanding and care are needed during this period. Families, especially partners, must understand and accept these responses.

Discharge considerations. Before discharge the nurse should be certain that the patient knows what changes will occur in her body because of the surgery (e.g., she will not menstruate if a total hysterectomy was performed). If the ovaries have been removed, she may experience hot flashes within days and other menopausal changes gradually. Her discharge planning should include immediate and long-term restrictions. Intercourse should be avoided until the wound is healed (about 4 to 6 weeks). However, intercourse is not contraindicated once healing is complete. Sutures at the top of the vagina can tear and produce considerable bleeding if genital sex is engaged in too early or is too unrestrained. Secondary sex characteristics are not affected unless the ovaries have been removed. If a vaginal hysterectomy is performed, the woman needs to know that there may be a temporary loss of vaginal sensation. She should be reassured that sensation will return in several months.

Physical restrictions are limited for a short time. Heavy lifting should be avoided for 2 months. Activities that may increase pelvic congestion, such as dancing and walking swiftly, should be avoided for several months, whereas activities such as swimming may be both physically and mentally helpful. Wearing a girdle is allowed and may provide comfort. Once the patient has been assured that healing is complete, all previous activity can be resumed.

Salpingectomy and Oophorectomy. Postoperative care of the woman who has undergone removal of a fallopian tube (*salpingectomy*) or an ovary (*oophorectomy*) is similar to that for any patient having abdominal surgery. One exception is that if a large ovarian cyst is removed, there may be abdominal distention caused by the sudden release of pressure in the intestines. An abdominal binder may provide relief until the distention subsides.

When both ovaries are removed (*bilateral oophorectomy*), surgical menopause results. The symptoms are similar to those of regular menopause but may be more severe because of the sudden withdrawal of hormones. Attempts are made to leave at least a portion of an ovary. Replacement therapy with estrogen is given to most patients to preserve secondary sex characteristics, avoid symptoms of menopause, and to prevent bone loss and the development of osteoporosis.

Vulvectomy. Although cancer of the vulva is relatively uncommon, the extent of the required surgery and the psychologic implications for the patient demand the best in nursing management. It is important that the nurse recognize the extent of the vulvectomy and the impact it will have on the patient's life. An honest, open attitude with the patient and her partner preoperatively can be most helpful in the postoperative period.

Wound care. After a vulvectomy the patient returns to the unit with a wound in the perineal area extending to the groin. The wounds may be covered or left exposed and frequently have drains attached to portable suction (e.g., Hemovac). A heavy pressure dressing is often in place for the first 24 to 48 hours. The wounds are cleaned with normal saline solution or an antiseptic twice daily. Solutions can be applied with an aseptic bulb syringe or a Water Pic machine. A heat lamp or a hair dryer is then used to dry the area. Wound care must be meticulous to prevent infection, which results in delayed healing.

Bowel and bladder care. Special attention to bowel and bladder care is needed. A low-residue diet and fecal softeners prevent straining at stool and wound contamination. An indwelling catheter is used to provide urinary drainage. Great care is taken not to dislodge the catheter because the extensive edema in the area would make its reinsertion difficult. Heavy, taut sutures are often used to close the wounds, resulting in severe discomfort for the patient. In other instances the wound may be allowed to heal by granulation. Analgesics may be required frequently to control pain. Careful positioning of the patient through the use of strategically placed pillows provides comfort. Ambulation is usually begun on the second postoperative day, but this varies with the preference of the surgeon. Anticoagulant therapy to prevent vascular complications is common.

Discharge considerations. Because the surgery causes mutilation of the perineal area and the healing process is slow, the patient is likely to become discouraged. Opportunities for the patient to express her feelings and concerns about the operation should be provided. The patient needs specific instructions in self-care before she is discharged. She should be told to report any unusual odor, fresh bleeding, breakdown of incision, or perineal pain. Home care nursing can benefit the patient during her adjustment period. Sexual function is often retained. Whether clitoral sensation is retained may be critical to some women, particularly if it was a primary source of orgasmic satisfaction. A discussion of alternative methods of achieving sexual satisfaction may also be indicated.

Pelvic Exenteration. When other forms of therapy are ineffective in checking the spread of cancer and no metastases have been found outside of the pelvis, pelvic exenteration may be performed. Although different types are done, this radical surgery usually involves removal of the uterus, ovaries, fallopian tubes, vagina, bladder, urethra, and pelvic lymph nodes. In some situations, the descending colon, rectum, and anal canal may also be removed. Candidates for this procedure are selected on the basis of their likelihood of surviving the surgery and their ability to adjust to and accept the resulting limitations.

The postoperative care involves that of a patient who has had a radical hysterectomy, an abdominal perineal resection, and an ileostomy or colostomy (Fig. 51-8). The physical, emotional, and social adjustments to life on the part of the woman and her family are great. There are urinary or fecal diversions in the abdominal wall, a reconstructed vagina, and the onset of menopausal symptoms.

The patient's rehabilitative process should keep pace with her acceptance of the situation. Much understanding and support is needed from the nursing staff during a long hospital stay. The patient should be gently encouraged to regain her independence. She needs to verbalize her feelings about her altered body structure to an interested and concerned listener. The family must be included in the plan of care.

The patient is told to return to her physician or clinic at specified intervals. Early recurrence of the cancer may then be identified and treated. At this time the patient's physical and emotional adjustment to the changes in body image produced by the surgery and her ability to carry out any treatment measures can also be assessed. Additional teaching and counseling can then be provided.

RADIATION THERAPY FOR UTERINE CANCER

Internal Radiation

Internal radiation is used in the management of cervical and endometrial cancer because of the accessibility of these body parts and the favorable results obtained. Radium and cesium are two commonly used isotopes. In preparation of the patient for the treatment, a cleansing enema is given to prevent straining at stool, which could cause displacement of the isotope. An indwelling catheter is inserted to prevent a distended bladder from coming into contact with the radioactive source.

A variety of applicators have been developed for intracavitary treatment. Some are inserted as multiple small irradiators (e.g., Heyman's capsules, Fig. 51-9, *A*), whereas others consist of a central tube (tandem) with irradiators placed on each side of the cervix (vaginal ovoids).

The applicator may contain the radioactive material when it is inserted into the endometrial cavity and vagina of an anesthetized patient in the operating room. This is known as *preloading*. In the *afterloading* technique (Fig. 51-9, *B*) the applicator is implanted in the operating room but is not loaded with the radioactive material until its correct placement is checked by x-ray and the patient has been returned to her room. Radiation exposure to the patient is precisely controlled. The radiation exposure to the physician and other personnel involved in the implantation is reduced when the afterload technique is used. The applicator is secured with vaginal packing and is left in place for 24 to 72 hours (Fig. 51-9, *C*). The radiologist determines the exact amount of radioactive substance to be used and the length of time it will be left in place so that destruction of cancer cells can occur with minimal damage to normal cells.

During the treatment the patient is placed in a lead-lined private room and is on absolute bed rest. She may be turned from side to side. The presence of an intrauterine applicator produces uterine contractions that may require analgesics. The destruction of cells results in a foul-smelling vaginal discharge, and a deodorizer is helpful. Nausea, vomiting, diarrhea, and malaise may develop as a systemic reaction to the radiation.

The nurse should not stay in the immediate area any longer than is necessary to give proper care and attention. No individual nurse should attend the patient for more than 30 minutes per day. The nurse may stay at the foot of the bed or at the entrance to the room to minimize radiation exposure. Visitors should stay 6 feet away from the bed and limit visits to less than 3 hours a day. The reasons for these precautions should be explained to the patient and her visitors. (A more detailed discussion of nursing care of the patient with an internal implant is given in Chapter 12.)

At the end of the prescribed period of radiation, the radioactive material and the catheter are removed. The patient is allowed to ambulate and is usually discharged from the hospital the next morning. Late complications that may arise after radiation of the uterus include fistulas (vesicovaginal, ureterovaginal), cystitis, phlebitis, hemorrhage, and fibrosis. If fibrosis occurs, the vaginal wall becomes smaller in diameter and shorter. Dilatation of the vagina through intercourse or the use of an obturator is indicated. The patient is urged to report any unusual symptoms or complaints to her physician.

After internal radiation the patient may be concerned about resumption of sexual activity. Application of a water-

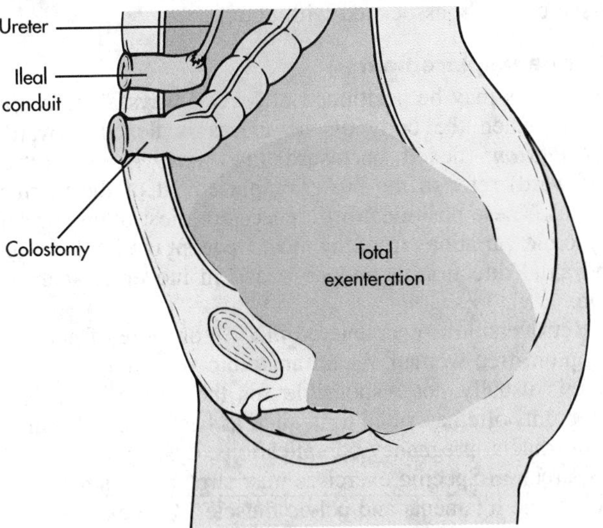

Fig. 51-8 Total exenteration is removal of all pelvic organs with creation of an ileal conduit and colostomy.

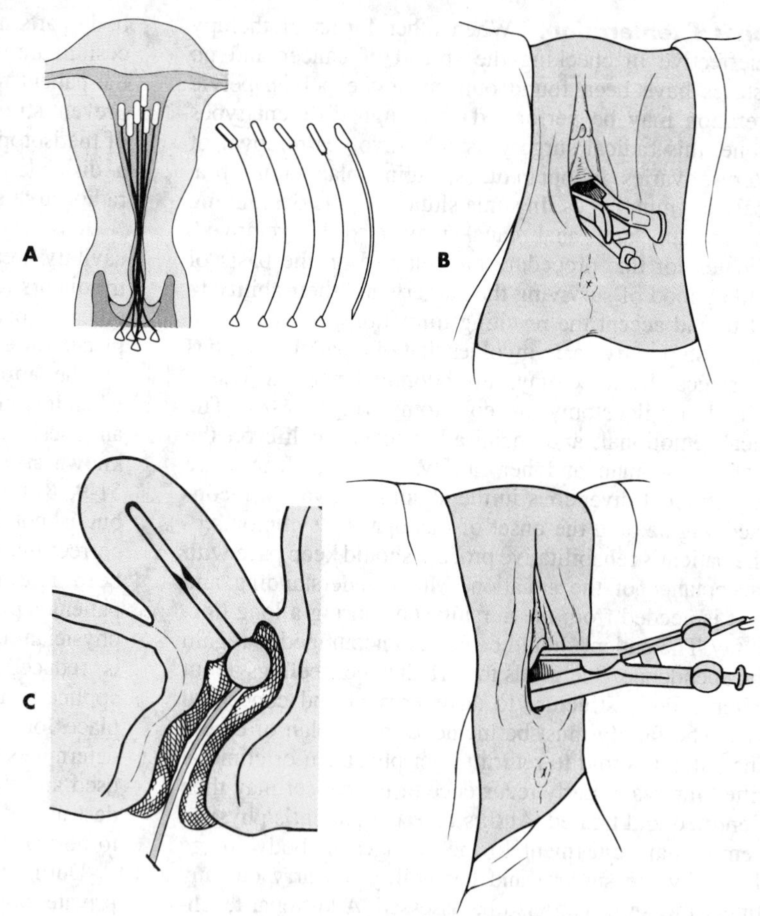

Fig. 51-9 Intracavitary radiation for uterine cancer. ***A,*** Heyman's capsules: various sizes and capsules in place. ***B,*** Applicator in position ready to be loaded (afterloading). ***C,*** Applicator secured with vaginal packing.

soluble lubricant and increased foreplay can aid in vaginal lubrication. Reassurance that intercourse is not contraindicated for either party is important.

External Radiation

Pelvic radiation is delivered by supervoltage equipment, such as a linear accelerator and cobalt 60. The treatment period usually extends for 4 to 6 weeks. The care of the patient receiving external pelvic radiation is the same as it is for treatment elsewhere in the body (see Chapter 12). The patient should be told to urinate immediately before the treatment to minimize radiation exposure to the bladder. Radiation side effects, including enteritis and cystitis, may occur. These are natural reactions to radiotherapy and do not indicate an overdose. Informing the patient in advance of the possible side effects and what measures to use lessens the impact when side effects do occur.

UTERINE STRUCTURAL ABNORMALITIES

The uterus commonly flexes anteriorly about 45 degrees and is movable. The cervix points downward and posteriorly. The filling of the bladder or bowel may cause a change in uterine position. Displacement of the uterus, bladder, and rectum can be either congenital or acquired as a result of stretching and weakness of muscles of the pelvic floor and the ligaments that support the uterus. The acquired displacement of these structures is frequently due to injuries sustained during childbirth or surgery, closely occurring pregnancies, tumors, inflammatory disease, and the loss of tissue elasticity associated with aging.

Uterine Displacement

The uterus may be positioned in several ways. *Anteflexion* occurs when the body of the uterus is flexed forward. *Retroflexion* (flexed backward) and *retroversion* (tilted backward) refer to the posterior placement of the uterine fundus. These positional differences are most often normal anatomic variations from the most frequent uterine location and axial direction in midpelvis and in moderate anteversion.

Retroversion is encountered in 20% or more of normal, symptom-free women. As an anatomic variation, retroversion is usually not responsible for the variety of pelvic symptoms often ascribed to it, such as backache, infertility, menorrhagia, pregnancy complications, dysmenorrhea, and dyspareunia. Specific exercises may stretch and strengthen the uterine ligaments and pelvic muscles. One exercise has the woman assume the knee-chest position, causing the uterus to fall forward for a few minutes several times a day. There is no evidence that this will permanently alter the

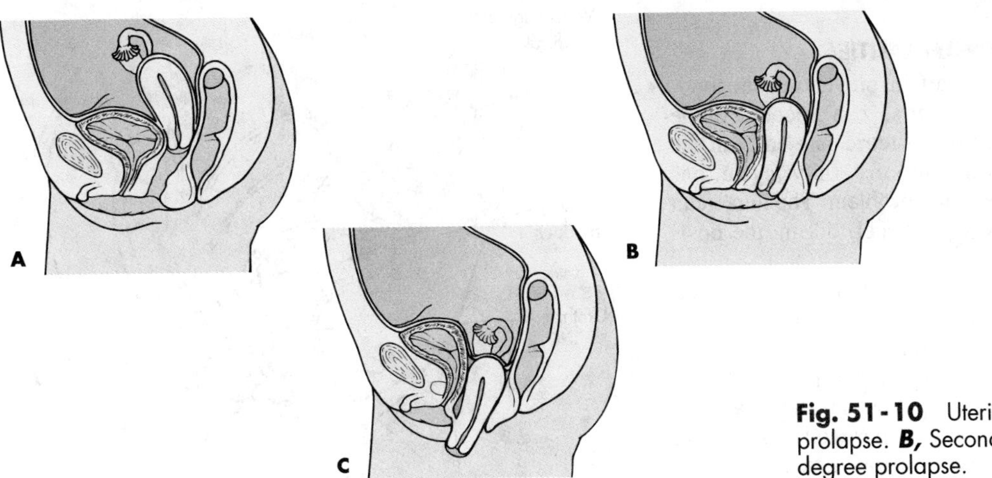

Fig. 51-10 Uterine prolapse. ***A,*** First-degree prolapse. ***B,*** Second-degree prolapse. ***C,*** Third-degree prolapse.

uterine position. A more beneficial exercise is called Kegel exercises, in which the woman tightens the muscles of the perineum as if to stop the flow of urine. The tension should be maintained for 5 seconds at a time, with the exercise repeated in sets of 10 and repeated 10 times during the day. Strengthening of these muscles helps support the pelvic floor and bladder. Kegel exercises are most appropriate after childbirth.

However, if the uterus is retroverted and adherent posteriorly, it is noted as secondary or acquired retroversion and is often associated with PID, endometriosis, or other conditions that may cause scarring. Treatment is directed toward resolving the underlying cause, if it can be found. A uterine suspension (shortening of the round ligaments) may be the treatment of choice for acquired retroversion. This surgery brings the uterus into an anteverted position.

Uterine Prolapse

Downward displacement, or *prolapse,* of the uterus through the pelvic floor and vaginal outlet is traditionally rated as first-degree (the cervix comes down to the introitus), second-degree (the cervix protrudes through the introitus), or third-degree (procidentia—the entire uterus protrudes through the introitus) prolapse (Fig. 51-10). The patient complains of a feeling of "something coming down." She may have dyspareunia, a dragging or heavy feeling in the pelvis, backache, and bowel or bladder problems if cystocele or rectocele are also present. Stress incontinence is a common and troubling problem. When second-degree or third-degree uterine prolapse occurs, the protruding cervix and vaginal walls are subjected to constant irritation, and tissue changes may occur.

Surgery generally involves a vaginal hysterectomy with anterior and posterior repair of the vagina and underlying fascia. In situations in which surgery is contraindicated, pessaries are used to correct the prolapse. A *pessary* (a rubber or plastic donut-shaped ring placed in the vagina) will provide uterine support. Before insertion of the vaginal pessary, the uterus is manually replaced in its normal position. Once inserted, the pessary holds the cervix in a posterior position, thus allowing the uterus to be in an anteflexed position. When the pessary is properly positioned, the woman is unaware of its presence and experiences no difficulty in voiding or during intercourse. A variety of pessaries are available for the different degrees of prolapse. Every 3 to 4 months the pessary is cleaned and replaced by the woman, if possible, or by her health care provider. She is also checked for signs of excessive irritation. Pessaries that are unattended for long periods are associated with erosion, fistulas, and an increased incidence of vaginal carcinoma.

Cystocele and Rectocele

Cystocele occurs when support between the vagina and bladder is weakened. Similarly, a *rectocele* results from weakening between the vagina and rectum. This weakening occurs most frequently during the process of childbirth. Further relaxation of these muscles results from decreasing hormones during menopause.

A cystocele or a rectocele may cause a dragging pain in the back and in the pelvis. A cystocele often causes urinary symptoms such as frequency, urgency, and incontinence, especially with activities that increase intraabdominal pressure (e.g., coughing, exercising, lifting). A rectocele may cause bowel symptoms such as constipation and incontinence of gas or liquid feces. Infection, hemorrhoids, and cystitis may occur as complications of these conditions.

In the early stages of cystocele or rectocele, Kegel exercises may be used to strengthen the weakened perineal muscles. Surgery is usually deferred until the woman has completed childbearing. A pessary may be placed when surgery is contraindicated or refused. Surgery designed to tighten the vaginal wall is generally the method of treatment. A cystocele is corrected with a procedure called an *anterior colporrhaphy,* whereas a *posterior colporrhaphy* is done for a rectocele. If further surgery is needed to relieve stress incontinence, procedures to support the urethra and restore the proper angle between the urethra and the posterior bladder wall are used.

NURSING MANAGEMENT

UTERINE STRUCTURAL ABNORMALITIES

The nurse can play an active part in preventing the incidence of uterine prolapse. The nurse can encourage the pregnant patient to seek qualified obstetric care early in the pregnancy. Better care during the maternity cycle has helped reduce the occurrence of the problem. The nurse can also teach perineal exercises (e.g., Kegel) during the postpartum period.

As part of the preoperative preparation for vaginal surgery, a cleansing douche may be ordered the morning of surgery. A cathartic and a cleansing enema are usually given when a rectocele repair is scheduled. A perineal shave is done. The nurse can assist the patient in understanding any limitations that surgery may impose on sexual and reproductive capacity because misunderstandings frequently occur.

In the postoperative period, the goals of care are to prevent wound infection and pressure on the vaginal suture line. This necessitates perineal care at least twice a day and after each urination or defecation.

A heat lamp may be used to help dry the area and enhance the healing process. An ice pack applied locally may relieve the initial perineal discomfort and swelling. A disposable glove filled with ice and covered with a cloth works well in these instances. Later, sitz baths are generally used.

After an anterior colporrhaphy, an indwelling catheter is usually left in the bladder for 4 days to allow the local edema to subside. The catheter keeps the bladder empty, thereby preventing strain on the sutures. Catheter care with an antiseptic is generally done twice daily. After posterior colporrhaphy, straining at stool is avoided by means of a low-residue diet and the prevention of constipation. Mineral oil is usually given each night.

Discharge instructions should be reviewed before the patient leaves the hospital. They include the use of douches or mild laxatives as needed; restriction of heavy lifting and prolonged standing, walking, or sitting; and avoidance of intercourse until the physician gives permission. There may be a loss of vaginal sensation, which can last for several months. The patient needs to be reassured that this situation is temporary.

FISTULAS

A fistula is an abnormal opening between internal organs or between an organ and the exterior of the body. Gynecologic procedures have been reported to cause 75% of urinary tract fistulas. Other causes include injury during delivery, surgery, radiation therapy, and disease processes, such as carcinoma. They may develop between the vagina and the bladder, urethra, ureter, or rectum. When *vesicovaginal fistulas* (between the bladder and the vagina) develop, some urine leaks into the vagina, whereas with *rectovaginal fistulas* (between the rectum and the vagina), flatus and feces escape into the vagina (Fig. 51-11). In both instances, excoriation and irritation of the vaginal and vulvar tissues occur and may lead to severe infections. In addition to wetness, offensive odors may develop, causing embarrassment and severely limiting socialization.

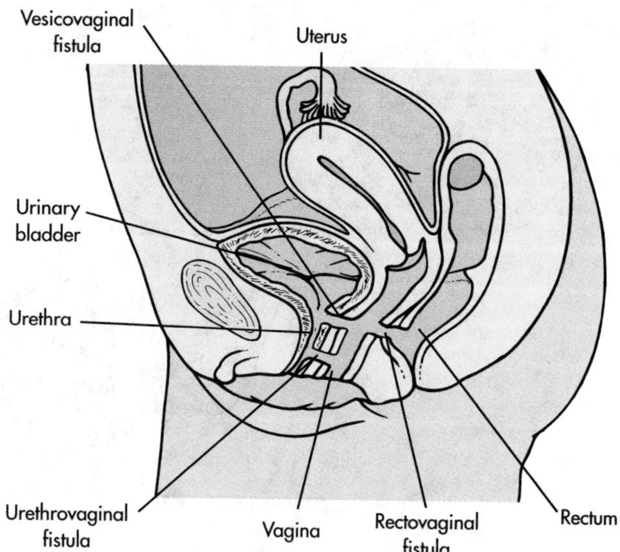

Fig. 51-11 Common fistulas involving the vagina.

THERAPEUTIC AND NURSING MANAGEMENT

FISTULAS

Because small fistulas may heal spontaneously within a matter of months, treatment can be postponed. If the fistula does not heal, surgical excision is required. Inflammation and tissue edema must be eliminated before surgery is attempted. This may involve a wait of up to 6 months for the surgery. The fistulectomy may result in the patient's having an ileal conduit or temporary colostomy.

Perineal hygiene is of great importance, both preoperatively and postoperatively. The perineum should be cleansed every 4 hours. Warm sitz baths should be taken 3 times daily if possible. Perineal pads should be changed frequently. Deodorizing and comfort measures such as douches and local heat are used. Douches should be given with low pressure to avoid further damage to the tissues. A low-residue diet and high enemas may be given to reduce the constant flow of feces. The patient should be encouraged to maintain an adequate fluid intake. Encouragement and reassurance by the staff are needed in helping the patient cope with her problems.

Postoperatively, nursing care emphasis is on avoidance of stress on the repaired areas and prevention of infection. Care should be taken so that the indwelling catheter, usually in place for 7 to 10 days, is draining at all times. Oral fluids should be urged to provide for internal catheter irrigation. Minimal pressure and strict asepsis are used if catheter irrigation becomes necessary. The first stool after bowel surgery may be purposely delayed to prevent contamination of the wound. Later, stool softeners or mild laxatives may be given. (See Chapter 43 for care of a patient with an ileal conduit and Chapter 40 for care of a

CRITICAL THINKING EXERCISES

CASE STUDY

TOTAL ABDOMINAL HYSTERECTOMY

Patient Profile

Marion P., a 40-year-old woman with two children, consulted her care provider about experiencing menorrhagia and occasionally metrorrhagia for the past 5 months. She was diagnosed with leiomyomas, and a total abdominal hysterectomy was recommended.

Subjective Data

- Was initially reluctant about surgery
- States family is complete
- Concerned that she may actually have uterine cancer

Objective Data

Physical Examination

- Has several large, firm masses in body of uterus thought to be leiomyomas
- Had otherwise normal physical examination

Postoperative Status

- Returned to room with indwelling urinary catheter in place
- Legs wrapped in full-length elastic compression gradient stockings

Critical Thinking Questions

1. What are the common causes of menorrhagia and metrorrhagia?
2. What clinical manifestations may result from leiomyomas?
3. What physical and psychologic preoperative preparation should be given to this patient?
4. What observation should be made in the patient's immediate postoperative period?
5. What possible complications, including their basis for development, can arise after abdominal hysterectomy?
6. Based on the assessment data, write one or more appropriate nursing diagnoses. Are there any collaborative problems?

NURSING RESEARCH ISSUES

1. Do women who exercise regularly experience less dysmenorrhea than women who do not exercise regularly?
2. Do working or nonworking women experience more episodes of vasomotor instability during the perimenopausal period?
3. Are women who use a female condom satisfied with this form of birth control?
4. Does the emotional response of the nurse caring for a rape victim help or hinder effective intervention?
5. What parameters can a nurse use in deciding how much information to provide to a woman who is to have a pelvic exenteration?

patient with a colostomy.) Surgical repair of fistulas is not always effective, even in the best conditions. Supportive nursing care for the patient and her significant others therefore is especially important.

REVIEW QUESTIONS

The number of the question corresponds to the same-numbered objective at the beginning of the chapter.

1. Secondary dysmenorrhea is usually
   a. due to overexertion.
   b. rare in the teenager.
   c. idiopathic.
   d. due to a pelvic disease or condition.

2. Postoperative care following a D & C includes
   a. observing the suture line.
   b. checking on bowel activity.
   c. doing a pad count.
   d. planning interventions for severe cramps.

3. Menopausal changes that may occur include all of the following *except*
   a. vasomotor reactions.
   b. irregular menstrual periods.
   c. thickening of the urethra.
   d. decreased vaginal secretions.

4. The use of oral contraceptives may result in
   a. weight loss.
   b. thromboembolic disorders.
   c. infection of the uterus.
   d. sterility.

5. An induced abortion
   a. occurs without apparent cause.
   b. occurs with mechanical intervention.
   c. is always illegal.
   d. produces few psychologic effects.

6. The first nursing intervention for the patient who has been raped is to
a. document bruises and lacerations of the perineum and cervix.
b. contact support person for the patient.
c. treat urgent medical problems.
d. provide supplies for the patient to cleanse self.

7. A prominent symptom of cervicitis is
a. leukorrhea.
b. urinary frequency.
c. severe perineal pain.
d. vaginal hemorrhage.

8. A serious complication of PID is
a. polyps.
b. sterility.
c. renal failure.
d. hepatitis B.

9. A common management strategy for endometriosis is
a. chemical suppression of ovulation.
b. long-term administration of an NSAID.
c. vitamin therapy, especially A and E.
d. fluid restriction during menses.

10. The most common symptom of a leiomyoma is
a. constant cramping pain.
b. increased abdominal girth.
c. menorrhagia.
d. sterility.

11. The diagnosis of endometrial cancer is best made by
a. D & C.
b. Schiller iodine test.
c. Pap smear.
d. culdoscopy.

12. Abdominal distention commonly associated with a hysterectomy can be treated by all of the following *except*
a. restriction of food and fluids.
b. use of rectal tube.
c. early ambulation.
d. bed rest.

13. Nursing responsibilities related to intracavitary radiation for uterine cancer include
a. allowing the patient bathroom privileges only.
b. maintaining absolute bed rest for the patient.
c. remaining at the bedside 1 hour a day for care.
d. limiting visitors to 5 hours a day.

14. The nursing care of the postoperative gynecologic cancer patient includes all of the following *except*
a. monitoring flow from indwelling catheter.
b. providing support and counseling for episodes of depression.
c. teaching pelvic exercises.
d. avoiding discussion of the diagnosis and prognosis.

15. A vesicovaginal fistula results in
a. fecal incontinence.
b. leakage of urine from the bladder.
c. leakage of fecal material into the vagina.
d. leakage of urine from the vagina.

REFERENCES

1. Hsia LS, Long MH: Premenstrual syndrome, *J Nurs Midwifery* 35:351, 1990.
2. Brancroft J and others: Perimenstrual complaints in women complaining of PMS, menorrhagia, and dysmenorrhea: toward a dismantling of the premenstrual syndrome, *Psychosom Med* 55:133, 1993.
*3. Taylor D, Woods NF, editors: *Menstruation, health, and illness*, New York, 1991, Hemisphere.
4. Pirie M, Halliday-Smith L: Coping with PMS, *Can Nurse* 88:24, 1992.
5. Mortola JF: Assessment and management of premenstrual syndrome, *Curr Opin Obstet Gynecol* 4:877, 1992.
6. Stenchever MA: *Office gynecology*, St Louis, 1992, Mosby.
7. Copeland LJ: *Textbook of gynecology*, Philadelphia, 1993, Saunders.
8. Goldfarb HA: A review of 35 endometrial ablations using the Nd:YAG laser for recurrent menometrorrhagia, *Obstet Gynecol* 76:833, 1990.
9. US Congress, Office of Technology Assessment: *The menopause, hormone therapy, and women's health*, Washington, DC, 1992, OTA-BP-BA-88.
10. Freedman RR, Woodward S, Sabharwal SC: α-Adrenergic mechanism in menopausal hot flashes, *Obstet Gynecol* 76:573, 1990.
11. Greendale G, Judd H: The menopause: health implications and clinical management, *J Am Geriatr Soc* 41:427, 1993.
12. Samsioe G: Hormone replacement therapy and cardiovascular disease, *Int J Fertil Menopausal Stud* 38S:23, 1993.
13. Meschia M and others: Effect of hormone replacement therapy and calcitonin on bone mass in postmenopausal women, *Eur J Obstet Gynecol Reprod Biol* 47:53, 1992.
14. Rosenberg L: Hormone replacement therapy: the need for reconsideration, *Am J Public Health* 38:1670, 1993.
15. Wood AJ: The prevention and treatment of osteoporosis, *N Engl J Med* 327:620, 1992.
16. Sardana R: Nutritional management of osteoporosis. To slow the advancement of osteoporosis, nurses must encourage their patients to increase their intake of calcium. For geriatric nurses, this may be a challenge, *Geriatr Nurs* 13:315, 1992.
17. Transdermal HRT Investigator Group: A randomized study to compare the effectiveness, tolerability, and acceptability to two different transdermal estradiol replacement therapies, *Int J Fertil Menopausal Stud* 38:5, 1993.
18. Dupont WD, Page DL: Menopausal estrogen replacement therapy and breast cancer, *Arch Intern Med* 151:67, 1991.
19. Lufkin EG and others: Treatment of postmenopausal osteoporosis with transdermal estrogen, *Ann Intern Med* 117:7, 1992.
20. Miller VT, Ravinkar VA, Timmons MC: ERT: weighing the risks and benefits, *Patient Care* 25:30, 1990.
21. Mastroianni L, Robinson J: Contraception in the 1990s, *Patient Care* 29:107, 1994.
22. Hatcher RA and others: *Contraceptive technology, 1990-92*, New York, 1990, Irvington.
23. Anastasi JK: What to tell patients about the female condom, *Nursing* 93:71, 1993.
24. Waites GM: Male fertility regulation: the challenges for the year 2000, *Br Med Bull* 49:210, 1993.
25. Bagatell CJ and others: Comparison of gonadotropin releasing hormone plus testosterone versus testosterone alone as potential male contraceptive regimens, *J Clin Endocrinol Metab* 77:427, 1993.
26. Hatchen RA and others: *Contraceptive technology*, ed 15, New York, 1992, Irvington.
27. Jaffe SB, Jewelewicz R: The basic infertility investigation, *Fertil Steril* 56:599, 1991.

28. Jaffe SB, Jewelewicz R: The basic infertility investigation, *Fertil Steril* 56:602, 1991.
29. Shane JM: Evaluation and treatment of infertility, *Clin Symp* 45:2, 1993.
30. Society for Assisted Reproductive Technology: Assisted reproductive technology in the U.S. and Canada, *Fertil Steril* 59:956, 1993.
31. Lobo R: Unexplained infertility, *J Reprod Med* 38:241, 1993.
32. Halpren S: Infertility: playing the odds, *Ms.* 1:154, 1989.
33. Mariner WK: The Supreme Court, abortion and the jurisprudence of class, *Am J Public Health* 82:1556, 1992.
34. Crenin MD, Washington AE: Cost of ectopic pregnancy management: surgery vs. methotrexate, *Fertil Steril* 60:963, 1994.
35. Cherner LL: *The universal healthcare almanac,* Phoenix, 1993, Silver & Cherner.
36. U.S. Department of Justice: *Sourcebook of criminal justice statistics—1992,* ed 20, Washington, DC, 1993, US Government Printing Office.
37. Dunn SF, Gilchrist VJ: Sexual assault, *Prim Care* 20:359, 1993.
38. MacKay HT: Treatment of common gynecologic infections, *Female Pt* 17:55, 1992.
39. Clark R and others: HIV: what's different for women? *Patient Care* 28:119, 1993.
40. Update: acquired-immunodeficiency syndrome—US, 1992, *MMWR* 42:547, 1993.
41. Hanrahan SN: Historical review of menstrual toxic shock syndrome, *Women Health* 2:141, 1994.
42. Lichtman R, Papera S: *Gynecology: well-woman care,* Norwalk, CT, 1990, Appleton & Lange.
43. Centers for Disease Control: Chronic disease reports: deaths from cervical cancer—United States, 1984–86, *MMWR* 38:652, 1989.
44. Herbst AL and others: Interpreting the new Bethesda classification system, *Contrib Gynecol Obstet* :86, 1993.
45. Weiss GR: *Clinical oncology,* Norwalk, CT, 1993, Appleton & Lange.
46. Dillon P: Ovarian cancer: confronting the silent killer, *Nursing* 24:66, 1994.
47. Bischof P: What do we know about the origin of CA 125? *Eur J Obstet Gynecol Reprod Biol* 49:93, 1993.

---

*Nursing research-based articles.

Chapter 52

NURSING ROLE IN MANAGEMENT

Male Genitourinary Problems

Cindy Meredith

Learning Objectives

1. Describe the pathophysiology, clinical features, and therapeutic management of benign prostatic hyperplasia.
2. Describe the nursing management of benign prostatic hyperplasia.
3. Describe the pathophysiology, clinical features, and therapeutic management of cancer of the prostate.
4. Describe the nursing management of cancer of the prostate.
5. Describe the pathophysiology, clinical features, and therapeutic and nursing management of problems of the penis, scrotum, and prostatitis.
6. Explain the nursing management of problems related to male sexual functioning.
7. Identify the psychologic and emotional implications of problems related to the male genitourinary organs.

Problems of the male genitourinary system can involve a variety of structures (Fig. 52-1) and are a source of anxiety for many men. This anxiety may be related to manipulation and exposure of the genitalia, discussion of intimate topics, and fear of possible pathologic conditions related to the male genitourinary organs. Anxiety and fear may cause the patient to delay seeking help for a problem or practicing health-promoting behaviors. The nurse should be particularly sensitive to the possible embarrassment associated with seeking health care for a genitourinary problem.

PROBLEMS OF THE PROSTATE GLAND

Benign Prostatic Hyperplasia or Hypertrophy

Significance. The most common problem of the adult male reproductive system is *benign prostatic hyperplasia* or *hypertrophy* (BPH), a term referring to new growth of epithelial and especially stromal elements within the prostate gland. Although hypertrophy is a misnomer because it refers to enlargement of existing cells, it is commonly used to describe this problem. Hyperplasia is the correct term because it refers to an increase in the number of cells. This problem occurs in about 50% of men over 50 years of age and 75% of men over 70 years of age. BPH is most likely to develop in the innermost part of the prostate,[1] and cancer is most likely to develop in the outer part of the prostate[2] (Fig. 52-2). Prostatic hyperplasia does not predispose to the development of cancer of the prostate.

Etiology and Pathophysiology. BPH begins with enlargement of the glandular tissue. Although the cause is not completely understood, it is thought that the increased number of cells results from endocrine changes associated with aging. Excessive accumulation of dihydroxytestosterone (the principal intraprostatic androgen), stimulation of estrogen, and local growth hormone action are proposed causes. Other factors under investigation include diet, race, and lifestyle issues.

Clinical Manifestations. The patient seeks assistance for relief of the symptoms related to urinary obstruction. Symptoms are usually gradual in onset and may not be noticed by the patient until prostatic enlargement has been present for some time. There is no direct relationship between the degree of obstruction and the size of the prostate. Mild hyperplasia can cause severe obstruction, whereas severe hyperplasia can result in few bladder symptoms. Treatment is generally based on the degree to which the symptoms bother the patient rather than on the size of the prostate alone.

Early symptoms can be minimal because compensatory hypertrophy of the detrusor musculature of the bladder can compensate for the resistance to urine flow.[3] With increasing blockage, *obstructive symptoms* of BPH develop, including diminution in the caliber and force of the urinary stream, hesitancy in initiating voiding, dribbling at the end of urination, and a feeling of incomplete bladder emptying

Reviewed by Jane Blackwell, RN, DNSc, CNM, Director, Certified Nurse Midwives of Toledo, Toledo, OH.

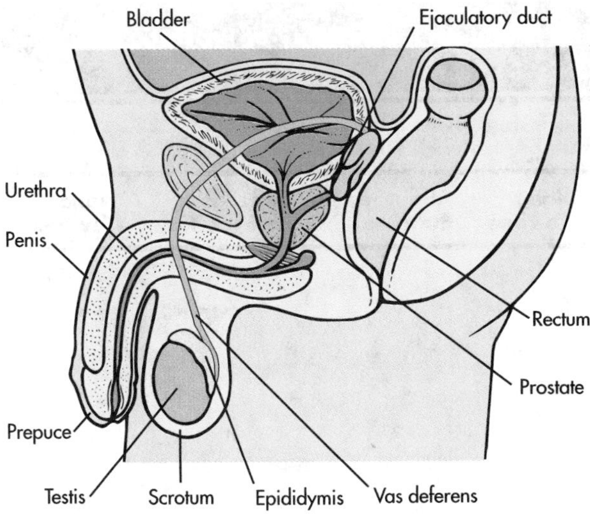

Fig. 52-1 Areas of the male reproductive system in which problems are likely to develop.

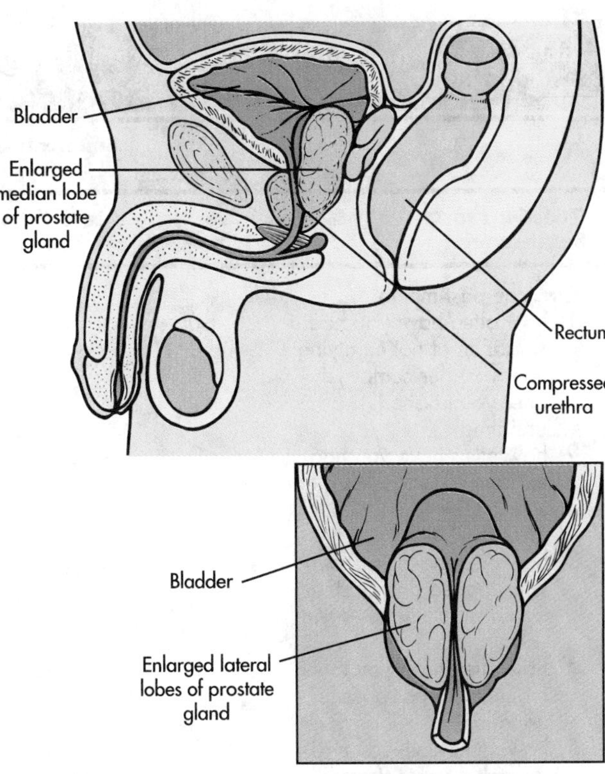

Fig. 52-2 Benign prostatic hyperplasia.

because of urinary retention. *Irritative symptoms,* including nocturia, dysuria, and urgency, can develop from inflammatory, infectious, or neoplastic causes.

A new system called the AUA Symptom Index has been developed by the American Urological Association (AUA). The AUA is recommending the scale be utilized at an initial interview for all patients presenting with symptoms and after treatment as a means of gathering standardized data (Table 52-1). The patients' score is based on a 0 to 5 scale with mild (total score, 0 to 7), moderate (total score, 8 to 19), and severe (total score, 20 to 35) categories.

Complications. The patient with BPH is at increased risk for urinary tract infection because of failure of the bladder to empty completely owing to partial or complete obstruction of the proximal urethra. The residual urine provides a favorable environment for bacterial growth. Calculi may develop because of the alkalinization of the residual urine. Breakage of tiny overstretched blood vessels in the bladder may produce hematuria.

More serious complications resulting from urinary retention are abnormally distended ureters (hydroureters), destruction of the kidney's parenchyma from the back pressure of the urine (hydronephrosis), and infection (pyelonephritis). These complications can lead to renal failure.

Diagnostic Studies. The most common sign of BPH is enlargement of the prostate on rectal palpation. In the early stages of BPH, the specific gravity of the urine may be unchanged or elevated because the patient may restrict fluid intake to decrease the need to void. If hydronephrosis with renal impairment has occurred, the specific gravity will be about 1.010, which is the specific gravity of plasma. If BPH has been a long-standing problem, the blood urea nitrogen (BUN) and serum creatinine levels may be elevated because of renal involvement. The presence of bacteria, white blood cells, or microscopic hematuria may indicate the presence of infection or inflammation.

Cystourethroscopy is indicated to evaluate vesicle neck obstruction. Postvoiding catheterization is helpful in determining the extent of obstruction. Residual urine over 100 ml is considered abnormally high. Measuring the urinary flow rate also helps to gauge blockage. A maximum flow rate greater than 15 ml per second is normal, whereas a flow rate of less than 10 ml per second points to obstruction.[4]

In 1994, the clinical practice guidelines for BPH were developed by a national panel of health care experts and published by the U.S. Department of Health and Human Services. A brief overview of the guidelines is presented in Table 52-2.

Therapeutic Management. The goals of therapeutic management are to restore bladder drainage, relieve the patient's symptoms, and prevent or treat the complications of BPH. Although these goals may be temporarily accomplished by catheterization, it does not resolve the underlying problem of prostatic enlargement. The treatment of asymptomatic BPH is now referred to as "watchful waiting." There are numerous treatment options for BPH which can be categorized as pharmacologic, nonsurgical invasive, and surgical invasive options.

Pharmacologic management. Hormone manipulation is used to cause regression of hyperplastic tissue[5] through suppression of androgens. There are numerous ways to

Table 52-1 American Urologic Association Symptom Index to Determine Severity of Prostatic Problems

	American Urologic Association (AUA) Symptom Score* (Circle 1 number on each line)					
Questions to Be Answered	**Not At All**	**Less Than 1 Time in 5**	**Less Than Half the Time**	**About Half the Time**	**More Than Half the Time**	**Almost Always**
Over the past month, 1. how often have you had a sensation of not emptying your bladder completely after you finished urinating?	0	1	2	3	4	5
2. how often have you had to urinate again, less than 2 hr after you finished urinating?	0	1	2	3	4	5
3. how often have you found you stopped and started again several times when you urinated?	0	1	2	3	4	5
4. how often have you found it difficult to postpone urination?	0	1	2	3	4	5
5. how often have you had a weak urinary stream?	0	1	2	3	4	5
6. how often have you had to push or strain to begin urination?	0	1	2	3	4	5
7. how many times did you most typically get up to urinate from the time you went to bed at night until the time you got up in the morning?	0 (None)	1 (1 Time)	2 (2 times)	3 (3 times)	4 (4 times)	5 (5 times or more)
Sum of circled numbers (AUA Symptom Score):* ________						

From Barry B and others: The American Urological Association symptom index for benign prostatic hyperplasia, *J Urol* 148:1547, 1992. Used with permission.
*Score is interpreted as: 0-7, mild; 8-19, moderate; and 20-35, severe.

suppress androgen formation. Drugs that block the testosterone metabolite dihydroxytestosterone, the principal intraprostatic androgen, are popular approaches at present. Finasteride (Proscar) is a new agent that blocks this conversion by inhibiting the converting enzyme 5α-reductase. This drug is probably of most benefit to men with a predominantly glandular hyperplasia. Studies have shown a 30% decrease in prostate size and a similar increase in urine flow. It has been found to be extremely safe with about a 4% incidence of erectile dysfunction and no reported gynecomastia.[6] These medications must be taken on a long-term basis to achieve therapeutic results. Finasteride was approved in 1992 by the Food and Drug Administration (FDA) for use in the treatment of BPH.

α-Adrenergic receptor blockade is another drug treatment option in the treatment of BPH. This type of drug causes smooth muscle relaxation that ultimately facilitates urinary flow through the prostatic urethra.[7] Three selective α-adrenergic blockers, prazosin (Minipress), doxazosin (Cardura), and terazosin (Hytrin) are currently being used. Only terazosin is approved by the Food and Drug Administration (FDA) for treatment of BPH. Side effects, including postural hypotension, dizziness, and fatigue can be problematic. These antagonists are not believed to have a significant effect on prostate size or volume.[6]

Nonsurgical invasive management. If BPH becomes symptomatic, nonsurgical invasive options may be tried before surgery. These options include heat, a prostatic balloon device, laser ablation, and stents or coils. Localized application of heat is used in an attempt to reduce the size of the prostatic tissue. Although experimental, this approach appears to be a promising alternative for patients with mild disease, who are poor candidates for surgery or drug therapy. When target temperatures are below 113° F (45° C), the treatment is called *hyperthermia*; when target temperatures exceed 113° F (45° C), the strategy is termed

Table 52-2 Therapeutic Management: Benign Prostatic Hyperplasia

Diagnostic
Primary Screening
Health history including AUA Symptom Index score
Physical examination including digital rectal exam
Urinalysis with culture
Serum creatinine and BUN
Prostate specific antigen (PSA) (if indicated)
Secondary Screening
Urodynamic flow studies
Transrectal ultrasound
Cystoscopy (for surgical candidates)
Therapeutic
"Watchful waiting" and patient education (asymptomatic BPH)
Catheterization (intermittent or indwelling)
High fluid intake
Antibiotics
Alpha adrenegic blockers
- Prazosin (Minipress)
- Doxazosin (Cardura)
- Terazosin (Hytrin)

Finasteride (Proscar) therapy
Balloon dilatation
Transurethral incision of prostate (TUIP)(<30 g)
Transurethral resection of prostate (TURP)
Open prostatectomy (>50 g)
- Suprapubic
- Retropubic
- Perineal

Experimental procedures
Thermoregulatory procedures
Laser ablation
Coil or stent placement

AUA, American Urological Association; *BPH,* benign prostratic hyperplasia; *BUN,* blood urea nitrogen.

thermotherapy. One technique to achieve a desired temperature of 109.4° F (43° C) or greater involves the intracavitary placement in the urethra of a radiating microwave antenna that emits heat. This procedure results in a significant increase in urine flow rate, decrease in postvoid residual urine capacity, and decrease in frequency of nocturia.[8] Mild side effects include occasional problems of bladder spasm, hematuria, dysuria, and retention.

An alternative treatment is a *prostatic balloon device* that dilates the urethra by stretching, fracturing, or compressing the gland to enlarge the passage and allow for free flow of urine.[9] The balloon is inflated for approximately 10 to 20 minutes, during which time the patient may experience mild pain and urinary urgency. After dilatation the balloon is removed, and the urethra is assessed for an increase in diameter. If the procedure is successful, an indwelling catheter is left in place for the first 24 hours to monitor urinary output and the extent of hematuria. The dilatation procedure may be repeated if the first attempt is unsuccessful. Complications resulting from this procedure have been rare, and the short-term results are encouraging. The procedure is not a permanent solution to the problem of an enlarged prostate but does offer a nonsurgical, cost-saving option to appropriate patients, particularly those at high risk for surgery. The efficacy of the treatment varies considerably and does not have the same level of satisfactory results as reported for a transurethral resection.[5] The balloon technique is contraindicated in patients with atonic bladder because dilatation alone will not allow proper emptying of the bladder.

Laser ablation is another experimental approach to the treatment of BPH. A *transurethral, ultrasound-guided, laser-induced prostatectomy* (TULIP) is the usual treatment approach. A specially designed laser is used to improve directional control of the beam.

Another therapeutic option is the placement of *stents* (stainless steel) or *coils* (titanium) in the prostatic urethra. These devices hold back the walls of the prostate to allow for the unobstructed flow of urine. In the majority of cases the stents become completely covered by epithelium, thus reducing the risk of encrustation and infection.[10] The procedure is used most often for men who have medical contraindications to anesthesia and surgery because only local anesthesia is required for this procedure. The advantages and disadvantages of the various nonsurgical invasive treatment options are compared in Table 52-3.

Surgical invasive management. Surgery is indicated when there is a decrease in urine flow of a magnitude sufficient to cause discomfort, persistent residual urine, acute urinary retention because of obstruction with no reversible precipitating cause, or hydronephrosis. Treatment of symptomatic BPH primarily involves resection of the prostate. The selection of a surgical approach to remove the adenomatous tissue depends on the size and position of the prostatic enlargement (Fig. 52-3). No correlation has been found between symptoms and the size of the prostate.

The type of surgery selected depends on the degree of debility and the reproductive outlook of the patient. The nurse can help the patient ask appropriate questions regarding the impact of a particular type of surgery on sexual functioning.

TRANSURETHRAL RESECTION. The transurethral resection (TUR or TURP) approach is the most common route for partial removal of the prostate. This approach is useful for removal of the medial lobe surrounding the urethra. No external surgical incision is made because a resectoscope is passed through the urethra to excise and cauterize prostatic tissue. A large (No. 18 to No. 22) three-way indwelling catheter with a 30 ml balloon containing 30 to 60 ml of sterile water is usually inserted into the bladder after the procedure to provide hemostasis and facilitate urinary drainage. The bladder is irrigated, either continuously or intermittently, for at least 24 hours to prevent obstruction from mucous threads and blood clots. A TUR is often the surgery of choice for the debilitated patient or for the patient with moderate prostatic enlargement. The advantages of a TUR are that it does not involve an external incision and is less likely to result in erectile dysfunction or long-term incontinence. A disadvantage is that it does not completely remove all prostatic tissue, leaving the potential

Table 52-3 Invasive Treatment Options for Benign Prostatic Hyperplasia

Treatment Option	Advantages	Disadvantages
Nonsurgical		
Laser (Transurethral, ultrasound-guided, laser-induced prostatectomy [TULIP])	Short operating time Little bleeding No fluid absorption Shorter hospitalization Decreased incidence of retrograde ejaculation or bladder-neck contracture	Postoperative urinary retention Tissue sample unavailable for histologic examination
Stents and coils	Local anesthesia Minimal bleeding Short operating time Usually an outpatient procedure	Short-term incontinence
Heat	Thermotherapy only a 1-hr treatment No retrograde ejaculation Decrease in postvoid residual urine capacity Decrease in nocturia	Cell death in normal tissue, as well as in benign and malignant neoplasms Potential for urinary retention
Balloon dilatation	Less expensive Simple, short procedure Topical or local anesthesia used Minimal hospitalization Outpatient procedure No impotence or retrograde ejaculation	Later treatment not ruled out Long-term effectiveness unknown Tissue sample unavailable for histologic examination
Surgical		
Transurethral resection (TUR or TURP)	No external incision Erectile dysfunction and long-term incontinence unlikely	Not all prostatic tissue removed Regular follow-up less likely
Transurethral incision of the prostate (TUIP)	Maintenance of antegrade ejaculation Short operating time Minimal complications	Temporary solution Effective only on small masses (<20 g) No histologic examination Possible rectal injury
Suprapubic resection	Allows better exploration Procedure of choice for larger masses (>60 g)	Increased risk of urinary tract infection, spasms, incontinence, and hemorrhage Recovery time longer than with TURP
Retropubic resection	Allows removal of large mass high in pelvic area Direct visualization of prostate possible Bladder not incised Voiding problems rare	Difficult in obese patients High risk of hemorrhage Slight risk of erectile dysfunction
Perineal resection	Allows removal of a large mass low in pelvic area and lymph nodes	High incidence of erectile dysfunction Possible urinary incontinence Greater risk of infection

for recurrence of hyperplasia, and sometimes the false impression that there is no need for yearly rectal exams.

Transurethral Incision of the Prostate. A transurethral incision of the prostate (TUIP) can be performed in high-risk patients, those with mild obstruction, or in younger patients. Transurethral slits or incisions are made into the prostatic tissue to relieve bladder neck obstruction.[11] This method is usually used to treat intravesical obstruction related to BPH. The incision can be made unilaterally or bilaterally with a variety of instruments (including laser) at different locations around the bladder neck. The patient is discharged with an indwelling catheter for the first 24 hours to monitor urinary output and hematuria. Table 52-3 lists the advantages and disadvantages of this procedure.

Suprapubic Resection. A suprapubic resection is done when an extremely large mass of tissue (>60 g) obstructs the urethra. The prostate is approached through a low midline abdominal incision that cuts through the bladder to the anterior aspect of the prostate. This technique removes the gland completely. After surgery, a suprapubic catheter is

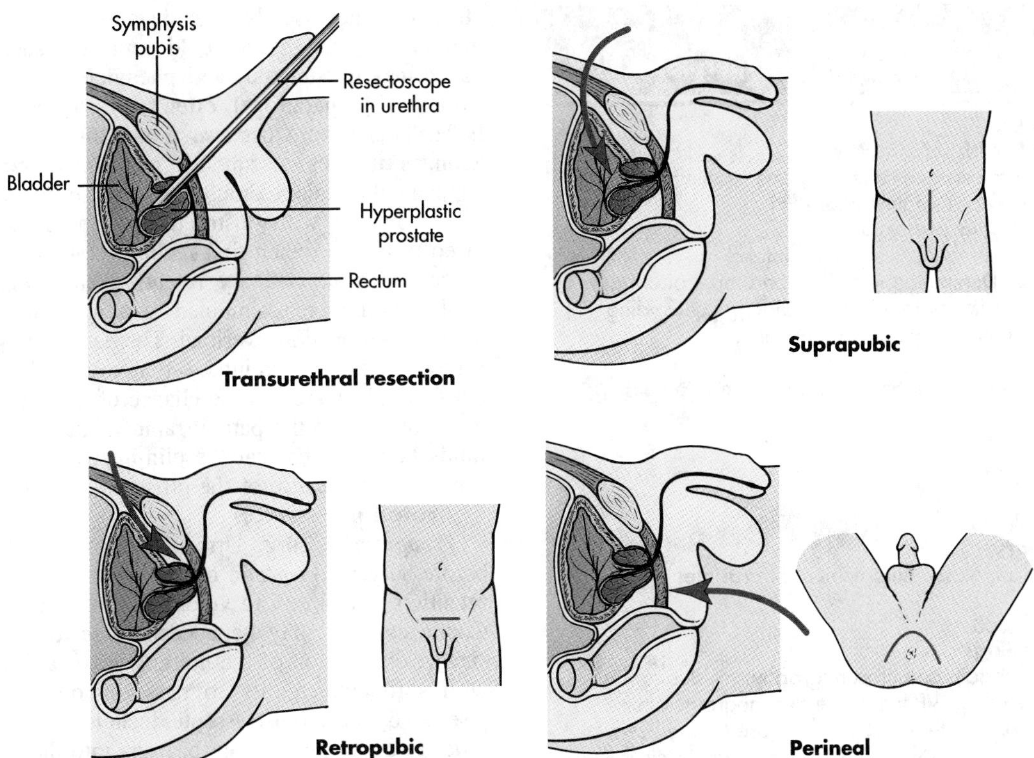

Fig. 52-3 Four types of prostatectomy.

often required and left in place through the abdominal incision to prevent pressure on the suture line and to aid in bladder healing. An indwelling catheter with a 30 ml balloon is placed in the bladder via the urethra. The bladder is irrigated continuously through the urethral catheter for 24 hours. This approach allows better exploration, but it has an increased risk of urinary tract infections, incontinence, bladdar spasms, and hemorrhage. The postoperative recovery phase is significantly longer than after a TURP.

Retropubic Resection. The retropubic approach is used to remove a massive gland located high in the pelvic area. This approach is more commonly used for a radical prostatectomy with lymph node dissection for cancer of the prostate.[12] A low midline abdominal incision is made into the prostate gland. After surgery, the patient has a large indwelling catheter with a 30 ml balloon placed in the bladder via the urethra. A Penrose drain may be left at the site of the abdominal incision to aid in the removal of drainage from the area. Although the bladder is not incised in this approach, direct visualization of the prostate is possible. The risk of hemorrhage remains high. Both suprapubic and retropubic resections are difficult in the obese patient.

Perineal Resection. The perineal approach is used to remove a mass located low in the pelvic area and is more commonly used with cancer of the prostate. It is used for BPH when the gland is extremely large. The incision is made between the scrotum and the anus. Because of the possibility of inadvertently entering the rectum, the bowel is prepared with enemas, antibiotics, and a low-residue diet. After surgery, an indwelling catheter with a 30 ml balloon is left in the urethra. A Penrose drain may be placed in the incision site to promote drainage of the area. Although all open procedures carry some risk of erectile dysfunction, the perineal approach is most likely to result in impotence. Urinary incontinence may also be a problem.

Complications of Prostatic Surgery. The major postoperative complications of these types of surgery are hemorrhage, infection, bladder spasm, and erectile problems.The Campbell-Walsh procedure is a nerve-sparing surgical technique that greatly reduces the incidence of erectile dysfunction, and it is used primarily with the retropubic approach. The patient should be encouraged to discuss this procedure with the surgeon before surgery.[13] A prophylactic vasectomy may be done with an open prostatectomy to decrease the risk of epididymitis.

NURSING MANAGEMENT

BENIGN PROSTATIC HYPERPLASIA

Because the primary treatment for BPH continues to be surgical resection of the hyperplastic tissue, nursing care will focus on preoperative and postoperative care of the patient having prostatic surgery.

Nursing Assessment

Subjective and objective data that should be obtained from a patient with BPH are presented in Table 52-4.

Table 52-4 Nursing Assessment: Benign Prostatic Hyperplasia

Subjective Data
Important health information
Medications: Estrogen or testosterone supplementation
Surgery: Previous treatment for BPH
Functional health patterns
Nutritional-metabolic: Usual fluid intake
Elimination: Diminution in caliber and force of urinary stream; hesitancy in initiating voiding; postvoiding dribbling; urinary retention; incontinence
Sleep: Nocturia
Cognitive-perceptual: Sensation of incomplete voiding; bladder discomfort
Self-perception: Anxiety
Objective Data
General
Older adult male
Genitourinary
Smooth, firm, elastic enlargement of prostate
Abdomen
Palpable bladder
Possible findings
Enlarged prostate on ultrasonography; residual urine on postvoiding IVP film or renal sonogram with sonographic determination; decreased urine flow rate; elevated BUN and serum creatinine levels if renal involvement

BHP, Benign prostatic hyperplasia; *BUN,* blood urea nitrogen; *IVP,* intravenous pyelogram.

Nursing Diagnoses

Nursing diagnosis specific to a patient with BPH include, but are not limited to, those presented in the nursing care plan on p. 1633.

Planning

The overall preoperative goals are that the patient having prostatic surgery will have (1) restoration of urinary drainage, (2) treatment of any urinary tract infection, and (3) understanding of the upcoming surgery and implications for sexual functioning and urinary control. The overall postoperative goals are that the patient, after prostate surgery, will have (1) no complications, (2) restoration of urinary control, (3) complete bladder emptying, and (4) satisfying sexual expression.

Nursing Implementation

Health Maintenance and Promotion. Because the cause of BPH is poorly understood, the focus of health promotion is on early detection and treatment. The American Cancer Society, along with the AUA, recommends a yearly medical history and digital rectal examination for men over 40 years of age in an effort to provide early detection of prostate problems. After 50 years of age, and when symptoms of prostatic hyperplasia become evident, further diagnostic screening may be necessary (see Tables 52-1 and 52-2).

Some men find that the ingestion of alcohol and caffeine tends to increase prostatic symptoms because of the diuretic effect that increases bladder distention. Compounds found in common cough and cold remedies such as pseudoephedrine (in Sudafed) and phenylephrine (in Allerest or Coricidin preparations) often worsen the symptoms of BPH. This occurs because these drugs are α-adrenergic agonists that cause smooth muscle contraction. If this happens, the patient should avoid these drugs.

The patient with obstructive symptoms should be advised to urinate when first feeling the urge so that urinary stasis and acute urinary retention are minimized. Fluid intake should be maintained at a normal level to avoid dehydration or fluid overload. The patient may believe that if he restricts his fluid intake, symptoms will be less severe, but this only increases the chance of an infection developing. However, if the patient rapidly increases his intake of fluids beyond what can be eliminated, bladder distention can develop because of the prostatic obstruction.

Acute Intervention

Preoperative care. Urinary drainage must be restored before surgery. Prostatic obstruction may have resulted in retention or inability to void. A urethral catheter such as a Coudé catheter may be needed to restore drainage. If a sizable obstruction of the urethra exists, a filiform catheter with sufficient rigidity to pass the obstruction may be inserted by a urologist. Aseptic technique is important at all times to avoid introducing bacteria into the bladder.

Any infection of the urinary tract must be treated before surgery. Restoring drainage, encouraging a high fluid intake, and providing a diet high in acid ash-producing foods are helpful in clearing the infection. Antibiotics are usually given.

The patient is usually concerned about the impact of the impending surgery on his sexual functioning. Data gathered from the health history relating to sexual activities will identify possible problem areas. The nurse should provide an opportunity for the patient to express his concerns. The patient needs to know how the surgery will affect sexual functioning and whether a vasectomy is planned.[14] The consequences of this in regard to his ability to father children should be explored. The surgical consent form should indicate whether a vasectomy is to be performed. A prostatectomy does not usually result in erectile dysfunction except with the perineal approach. All types of prostatic surgery generally result in some degree of retrograde ejaculation. The patient should be informed that the ejaculate may be decreased in amount or totally absent. Retrograde ejaculation is not harmful because the semen is simply eliminated during the next urination, but it can affect fertility.

Postoperative care. The main complications of prostatectomy are hemorrhage, bladder spasms, and infection. The plan of care should be adjusted to the type of surgery, the reasons for surgery, and the patient's response to surgery. Discharge planning and home care issues are important aspects of postprostatectomy care. Instructions include caring for an indwelling catheter, if one is in place; maintaining oral fluids between 2000 to 3000 ml per day; observing for signs and symptoms of urinary tract and wound infection; preventing constipation; avoiding heavy

NURSING CARE PLAN Patient Undergoing Transurethral Resection

Planning: Outcome Criteria	*Nursing Interventions and Rationales*
PREOPERATIVE	
➤ **NURSING DIAGNOSIS**	Acute pain *related to* bladder distention secondary to enlarged prostate *as manifested by* complaints of need to void, palpable bladder, no urine output, diaphoresis, facial appearance of pain, restlessness
Have no complaints of pain because of bladder distention.	Assist with insertion of indwelling catheter (usually done by urologist) *to reduce pain by providing urinary drainage.* Monitor intake and output *to evaluate renal function and adequacy of bladder drainage.* Percuss bladder every shift for distention *to validate adequate emptying of the bladder.* Assess comfort status *to continue or revise plan as necessary.* Maintain patency of catheter *to ensure continuous flow of urine from the bladder.*
➤ **NURSING DIAGNOSIS**	Risk for urinary infection *related to* indwelling catheter, environmental pathogens, and urinary stasis
Have no evidence of urinary tract infection.	Assess for elevated temperature and cloudy, foul-smelling urine with every shift *to identify symptoms of infection and initiate appropriate interventions.* Collect urine for culture *to determine presence and cause of infection.* Give patient 8 oz of water every waking hour *to prevent urinary stasis and dilute the urine.* Observe strict aseptic technique for catheter care *to minimize the risk of introducing an infectious organism.* Maintain closed system with catheter securely anchored to inner thigh or abdomen *to decrease risk of ascending infection.* Observe color and characteristics of urine because *cloudy, foul-smelling urine can indicate the presence of infection.*
➤ **NURSING DIAGNOSIS**	Fear *related to* actual or potential sexual dysfunction, possible diagnosis of cancer, and lack of knowledge regarding surgical procedure and postoperative care *as manifested by* verbalization of fear about impact of surgery on sexuality, questioning, or inaccurate comments about surgical course
Have decrease in fear about effect of surgery on sexuality and surgical course as shown by accurate knowledge base, correct responses to questions, calm demeanor.	Perform standard preoperative teaching *to provide information regarding the preoperative and postoperative routines.* Assess patient's concerns related to sexual functioning and correct misconceptions and inaccuracies *to plan appropriate interventions that address unique concerns.* Provide opportunity for private conversation for patient to ask personal questions *because a private setting facilitates open discussion.* Inform patient about retrograde ejaculation *as this occurs in prostatic surgery and is not harmful because the fluid is eliminated during the next urination.*
POSTOPERATIVE	
➤ **NURSING DIAGNOSIS**	Acute pain: bladder spasms *related to* irrigations and clots, presence of catheter, and surgical procedure *as manifested by* expression of pain from spasms, nonverbal signs of pain such as moaning, crying, and legs drawn to abdomen, inability to irrigate catheter, blood or urine expressed from catheter meatal junction
Report a decrease in pain; be satisfied with comfort level.	Maintain patency of catheter *because clots cause obstruction of urine flow resulting in bladder spasms.* Irrigate catheter if occluded with clots (according to aseptic technique and institution protocols) *so urine can flow freely.* Instruct patient to try not to urinate around catheter *as this increases the occurrence of spasm.* Give belladonna and opium suppository as needed; instruct patient in relaxation techniques such as deep breathing exercises and distraction therapy or visual imagery *to relieve pain and decrease spasm.*
➤ **NURSING DIAGNOSIS**	Ineffective management of therapeutic regimen *related to* lack of knowledge regarding need for follow-up care and activity restriction postoperatively *as manifested by* unawareness of potential for prostatic cancer, questioning, or inaccurate comments about postoperative activity
Have no postoperative bleeding because of performing activities that increase intraabdominal pressure; have annual prostate examination.	Teach patient that some prostatic tissue is present that could become malignant *so patient understands need for annual prostatic examination.* Instruct patient to avoid heavy lifting (> 10 pounds [4.5 kg]), straining during defecation, prolonged periods of travel, stair climbing, driving, and sexual activity until surgeon approves such activity (usually 6 wk) *to prevent increases in intraabdominal pressure and the possibility of bleeding.*

continued

NURSING CARE PLAN Patient Undergoing Transurethral Resection—cont'd

Planning: Outcome Criteria	*Nursing Interventions and Rationales*
➤ **NURSING DIAGNOSIS**	Urge incontinence *related to* poor sphincter control *as manifested by* inappropriate leakage of urine.
Have absence or satisfactory control of dribbling.	Teach patient exercises *to strengthen sphincter tone* (e.g., Kegel exercises). Advise patient about devices to control dribbling *so patient is aware of various devices and can make an informed decision among alternatives.*
➤ **NURSING DIAGNOSIS**	Risk for urinary infection *related to* indwelling catheter, bladder irrigations, environmental pathogens, inadequate oral intake, and poor catheter care
Have no evidence of infection.	Assess for fever, diaphoresis, presence of indwelling catheter, self-restriction of fluid intake, cloudy urine *to determine if risk factors or signs and symptoms of infection are present.* Monitor temperature q4hr for the first 48 hr postoperatively *because fever is a good indicator of infection.* Give patient 8 oz of water hourly while awake *to maintain good urine flow and dilute the urine.* Observe strict aseptic technique for catheter care and bladder irrigations *to prevent introducing infectious organisms.*

COLLABORATIVE PROBLEMS

Nursing Goals	*Nursing Interventions and Rationales*
➤ **POTENTIAL COMPLICATION**	Hemorrhage *related to* surgical procedure
Monitor for and report signs of hemorrhage and carry out appropriate medical and nursing interventions.	Observe urinary drainage and report bright red bleeding in larger than expected quantities immediately *as this could indicate hemorrhage and the need for immediate intervention.* Monitor blood pressure (BP), pulse, and respirations and report abnormalities *as increasing pulse and respirations and decreasing BP can indicate hemorrhage.* Maintain catheter drainage *to prevent obstruction and allow monitoring of bleeding and urine flow.* Do not perform rectal treatments such as enemas or rectal temperatures (except belladonna and opium suppositories for bladder spasms) *as bleeding could be initiated.* Teach patient not to strain during bowel movement; limit ambulation and chair sitting to 15 min TID *to decrease pressure on operative area.*

lifting (>10 pounds [4.5 kg]); and refraining from driving or intercourse for 6 weeks after surgery as directed by the surgeon.

After prostatectomy the bladder may be continuously irrigated with sterile normal saline solution or another prescribed solution to remove clotted blood from the bladder and ensure drainage of urine. Some form of irrigation (continuous or intermittent) may be used for 24 hours or until no clots are noted draining from the bladder.

Blood clots are normal after a prostatectomy for the first 24 to 36 hours. However, large amounts of bright red blood in the urine can indicate hemorrhage. Postoperative hemorrhage may occur from displacement of the catheter or from increases in abdominal pressure. Release or displacement of the catheter dislodges the balloon that provides counterpressure on the operative site. Traction on the catheter may be applied to provide counterpressure (tamponade) on the bleeding site in the prostate, decreasing bleeding. Such traction can result in local necrosis if pressure is applied for too long. Pressure should therefore be relieved on a scheduled basis by qualified personnel. Activities that increase abdominal pressure, such as sitting or walking for prolonged periods and straining to have a bowel movement (Valsalva maneuver), should be avoided in the postoperative recovery period.

Bladder spasms are a distressing complication for the patient after transurethral and suprapubic prostatectomy. They occur as a result of irritation of the bladder mucosa from the insertion of the resectoscope, the presence of a catheter, or clots leading to obstruction of the catheter. The patient should be instructed not to attempt to urinate around the catheter because this increases the likelihood of spasm. If bladder spasms develop, the catheter should be checked for clots. If present, the clots should be removed by irrigation so urine can flow freely. Belladonna and opium suppositories, along with relaxation techniques, are used to relieve the pain and decrease spasm. The catheter is removed 2 to 4 days after surgery. The patient should urinate within 6 hours after catheter removal. If he cannot, a catheter is reinserted for a day or two. If the problem continues, the nurse may need to instruct the patient in self-catheterization.

Sphincter tone may be poor immediately after surgery, resulting in incontinence or dribbling. This is a common but distressing situation for the patient. Sphincter tone can be strengthened by having the patient practice Kegel exercises (pelvic floor muscle technique) 10 to 20 times per hour. The patient should be encouraged to practice starting and stopping the stream several times during urination. This facilitates learning the pelvic floor exercises.[15] It usually takes several weeks to achieve urinary continence. In some instances, control of urine may never be fully regained. Continence can improve for up to 12 months. If continence has not been achieved by that time, the patient may be referred to a continence clinic; a variety of methods, including biofeedback, have been used to achieve positive results. The patient can also be instructed to use a penile clamp, condom catheter, or incontinence briefs to avoid embarrassment from dribbling.[16] In severe cases, an occlusive cuff that serves as an artificial sphincter can be surgically implanted to restore continence. The nurse should assist the patient with a continence problem in developing practices that will allow him to socialize and interact with relatives and friends.[17,18]

The patient should be observed for signs of postoperative infection. If an external wound is present, the area should be observed for redness, heat, swelling, and purulent drainage. Special care must be taken if a perineal incision is present because of the proximity of the anus. Rectal procedures, such as taking rectal temperatures and administering enemas should be avoided because they may initiate bleeding. The insertion of belladonna and opium suppositories is acceptable. Careful aseptic technique should be used when irrigating the bladder because bacteria can be introduced into the urinary tract. Proper care of the catheter is important. The catheter should be connected to a closed drainage system and should not be disconnected unless it is being removed, changed, or irrigated.[19] The secretions that accumulate around the meatus should be cleansed daily with soap and water.

Dietary intervention and stool softeners are important in the postoperative period to prevent the patient from straining while moving his bowels. Straining increases the intraabdominal pressure, which can lead to bleeding at the operative site. A diet high in fiber facilitates the passage of stool.

Chronic and Home Management. After prostatic surgery the patient may be concerned about erectile dysfunction. Physiologic impotence may occur when nerves are cut or damaged during surgery. The patient often experiences anxiety over the loss of his sex role, his self-esteem, and the quality of sexual interaction with his sexual partner. Sexual counseling and treatment options may be necessary if erectile dysfunction becomes a chronic or permanent problem.[20,21] Patients may also require counseling regarding treatment options.

Many men experience retrograde ejaculation after prostatectomy because of trauma to the internal sphincter. Semen is discharged into the bladder at orgasm and may produce cloudy urine when the patient urinates after orgasm. The nurse should discuss these changes with the patient and his partner and allow them to ask questions and express their concerns.

The bladder may take up to 2 months to return to its normal capacity. The patient should be instructed to drink at least 1 to 2 L of fluid per day and to urinate every 2 to 3 hours to flush the urinary tract. Because the patient may be experiencing incontinence or dribbling, he may incorrectly believe that decreasing fluid intake will relieve this problem. Urethral strictures may result from instrumentation or catheterization. Treatment ranges from teaching the patient intermittent clean catheterization to urethral dilatation.

The patient must be advised that he should continue to have yearly rectal examinations if he has had any procedure other than complete removal of the prostate. Hyperplasia and/or cancer can occur in the remaining prostatic tissue.

CULTURAL & ETHNIC *Considerations*

CANCER OF MALE GENITOURINARY SYSTEM

- Prostate cancer occurs twice as frequently among African-American men as among Caucasian men.
- African-American men tend to be diagnosed with prostate cancer at an earlier age, have more advanced disease at the time of diagnosis, and have a higher mortality rate than do Caucasian men.
- Hispanic and Asian-American men have a lower incidence of prostate cancer and lower mortality rate as compared with Caucasian men.
- Testicular cancer occurs most frequently among Caucasians and is rare in African-Americans.

Cancer of the Prostate

Significance. Although rarely found in men less than 60 years of age, cancer of the prostate is the most common cancer in men. It is the second leading cause of cancer death in men, after lung cancer.[22] Current studies indicate that 80% of prostate cancers are diagnosed in men over 65 years of age. Because of the lack of symptoms, 75% of first-time patients over 65 years of age are diagnosed at Stage C or D (discussed later).[23] It is estimated that by the year 2000, there will be a 90% increase in prostate cancer cases per year and a 37% increase of deaths from prostate cancer. Projected increases are primarily because of an aging population.[24]

Pathophysiology. Prostate cancer is an androgen-dependent adenocarcinoma. Factors such as sexual activity, socioeconomic class, or alcohol use have not been shown to be significant risk factors. Researchers are now investigating high fat diets, family histories, and environmental factors for possible links to prostate cancer. A higher incidence exists in men 60 years of age or older, in African-American men, and in married men. African-Americans have the highest incidence of prostate cancer.

The tumor is slow growing and usually begins in the posterior or lateral portions of the prostate. It spreads by three routes: by direct extension, via the lymphatics, and via the bloodstream. Direct extension is by continuity to the seminal vesicles, urethral mucosa, bladder wall, and external sphincter. The cancer later spreads through the perineural lymphatic system to the regional lymph nodes. The veins from the prostate seem to be the mode of spread to the pelvic bones, head of the femur, lower lumbar spine, liver, and lungs.

Clinical Manifestations and Complications. Prostate cancer is asymptomatic in the early stages. Eventually the patient may have symptoms similar to those of BPH, including dysuria, hesitancy, dribbling, frequency, urgency, hematuria, nocturia, and retention. The prostate feels hard, enlarged, and fixed on rectal examination. The enlargement is usually unilateral. Pain in the lumbosacral area, which radiates down to the hips or legs, when coupled with urinary symptoms, is strongly indicative of metastasis.

Early recognition and treatment of this tumor is required to control growth and prevent metastasis. The tumor can spread to pelvic lymph nodes, bones, bladder, lungs, and liver. Once the tumor has spread to distant sites, the major problem becomes the management of pain. As the cancer spreads to the bones, pain can become severe, especially in the back and the legs because of compression of the spinal cord (see Chapter 6).

Diagnostic Studies. Improved diagnostic techniques have greatly enhanced the physician's ability to detect cancer of the prostate at an earlier stage. Screening for prostate cancer consists of palpation of the gland during rectal examination, a blood test for prostate specific antigen (PSA ([a glycoprotein that is detected only in the epithelial cells of the prostate]), and transrectal ultrasound. The carcinoma is characteristically hard, nodular, and irregular, but induration may also be a result of fibrous areas in BPH, focal infarcts, or calculi, as well as of the tumor itself. The American Cancer Society and the AUA recommend yearly digital rectal exams for all men over the age of 40.[25] Current evidence strongly suggests that the combination of digital rectal examination and serum PSA level measurement increases the chances of early detection of prostate cancer.[3] Ultrasonography of the prostate allows the physician to visualize the outer lobes of the prostate and pinpoint potential cancer sites. When a suspicious area is located, a special biopsy needle can be inserted and the specimen examined. Ultrasonography with guided-needle biopsy provides a method of early detection and treatment of prostatic cancer.[26,27]

Elevated levels of PSA (normal level, 0-4 ng/ml [0-4 μg/L]) and the prostatic isoenzyme of acid phosphatase (prostatic acid phosphatase [PAP]) are both indicative of cancer of the prostate. Elevated PSA levels indicate prostatic pathology, although not necessarily cancer of the prostate. Mild elevations in PSA may occur in BPH, in acute or chronic prostatitis, or in infarction of the prostate. In addition, cystoscopy, indwelling urethral catheters, and prostate biopsies may produce an elevation for several weeks. A routine rectal examination does not falsely elevate the PSA level.[28] An elevated PSA alerts the physician to the possibility of cancer of the prostate. PSA is useful in following patients after definitive treatment for localized disease. When treatment has been successful in removing all prostatic tissue, the PSA should fall to undetectable levels.

Elevated PAP is indicative of cancer of the prostate. In stage D, serum alkaline phosphatase is increased as a result of metastasis.[29] Other tests used to determine the location and extent of the spread of the cancer may include a biopsy, computed tomography (CT), or magnetic resonance imaging (MRI).

Therapeutic Management. The therapeutic management of cancer of the prostate depends upon the stage of the cancer. Prostatic cancer is staged on the basis of growth of the tumor (Table 52-5). Surgery is the most accurate method of staging because the extent of the tumor growth and the lymph node involvement can be assessed most accurately by means of inspection during the operation and evaluation of the pathology reports. At all stages, there is more than one possible treatment option. The decision on which treatment course to pursue is made jointly by the patient and the physician based on a careful analysis of the facts and the patient's unique situation. Table 52-6 summarizes the various treatment options available.

Surgery. Surgery is often the first line of treatment, particularly in the earlier stages of the disease. A TURP or total prostatectomy may be the treatment, or the patient may be observed carefully, with annual rectal exams and PSA testing. For patients with Stage C tumor, surgery is usually a radical prostatectomy involving resection of the prostate gland, seminal vesicles, and part of the ampulla of the vas deferens. Surgery is usually not considered an option for Stage D cancer except to relieve obstruction because metastasis outside the prostate has already occurred.

A nerve-sparing technique is sometimes used to prevent erectile dysfunction. This surgery is useful only for patients

Table 52-5 Whitmore-Jewett Staging Classification of Prostate Cancer

Stage A: Clinically Unrecognized	
A1	<5% of prostatic tissue neoplastic
A2	>5% of prostatic tissue neoplastic, all high-grade tumors
Stage B: Clinically Intracapsular	
B1	Nodule <2 cm and surrounded by palpably normal tissue
B2	Nodule >2 cm or multiple nodules
Stage C: Clinically Extracapsular, Localized to Periprostatic Area	
C1	Minimal extracapsular extension
C2	Large tumors involving seminal vesicles and/or adjacent structures
Stage D: Metastatic Disease	
D1	Pelvic lymph node metastases or ureteral obstruction causing hydronephrosis
D2	Distant metastases to bone, viscera, or other soft tissue structures

who have negative lymph nodes, no elevation of serum alkaline phosphatase levels, and no clinical evidence of extracapsular extension. Thus, while patients with extensive disease may not benefit from the nerve-sparing operation, a patient with a localized nodule or with small-volume disease may. In these latter situations, up to 70% of the patients undergoing a nerve-sparing operation will retain potency postoperatively.[30]

Hormonal therapy. A unique feature of prostate cancer is that cell growth initially depends on the presence of androgens. Surgical removal of the prostate followed by orchiectomy (removal of the testes) removes the source of 90% of circulating androgens. Orchiectomy often provides rapid relief of bone pain and may induce sufficient shrinkage of the prostate to relieve urinary obstruction in later stages of disease when surgery is not an option.[31]

Estrogen (e.g., diethylstilbestrol) treatment can be substituted for orchiectomy. It causes regression of the size of the prostate and of metastatic bone lesions. The minimum dose that is capable of suppressing plasma testosterone to castration levels is used. Estrogen therapy often results in gynecomastia, mood swings, decreased libido, hot flashes, and total loss of erectile functioning.[32-34]

Estrogen treatment is declining in popularity because of the side effects and the reduced effectiveness in decreasing androgen levels. Agents such as leuprolide (Lupron) and goserelin (Zoladex) that are agonists of luteinizing hormone-releasing hormone (LHRH [plays a major role in controlling release of luteinizing hormone and follicle stimulating hormone]), block androgens at the pituitary level and are being used increasingly. The medication is given by monthly subcutaneous injections, requires monitoring, and must be taken indefinitely. Side effects include hot flashes, loss of libido, and erectile dysfunction.

Other therapies. Recent studies now indicate that external beam radiation therapy for early stages of prostate cancer matches the survival rates of radical surgery, offering yet another treatment option.[35] Radiation therapy is also used in disseminated prostate cancer. Spot radiation can be extremely helpful in alleviating pain associated with isolated osseous metastasis. Side effects of radiation include diarrhea, cystitis, and erectile dysfunction.

Chemotherapy is occasionally used in late-stage disease with some success. However, it has not been shown to improve survival.

Prostatic cryosurgery is an experimental but promising approach to treating cancer of the prostate.[36] The treatment takes about 2 hours under general or spinal anesthesia and does not involve a major abdominal incision. Liquid nitrogen is circulated in probes inserted into the prostate gland through tiny punctures in the perineum. Possible complications of prostatic cryosurgery include the development of a urethrorectal fistula (an opening between the urethra and the rectum) or a urethrocutaneous fistula (an opening between the urethra and the skin), tissue sloughing, erectile dysfunction, urinary incontinence, or hemorrhage.

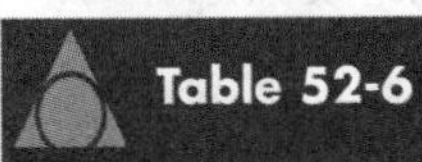

Table 52-6 Therapeutic Management: Prostate Cancer

Diagnostic
- Rectal examination
- PSA level determination
- PAP level determination in advanced stages
- Transrectal ultrasound
- Biopsy, needle aspiration, open biopsy
- Bone scan
- Grading and staging

Therapeutic

Stage A
- Medical follow-up, observation, TURP or total prostatectomy

Stage B
- TURP
- Total prostatectomy with or without lymphadenectomy
- Radiation therapy

Stage C
- Hormone manipulation, luteinizing hormone–releasing hormone analogues, or orchiectomy
- Radical resection of prostate
- External beam radiation therapy

Stage D
- Hormone therapy
- Radiation to metastatic bone areas
- Chemotherapy

PAP, Prostatic acid phosphatase; *PSA,* prostate specific antigen; *TURP,* transurethral resection of prostate.

NURSING MANAGEMENT

PROSTATIC CANCER

Nursing Assessment

Subjective and objective data that should be obtained from an individual with cancer of the prostate are presented in Table 52-7.

Nursing Diagnoses

Nursing diagnoses specific to the patient with cancer of the prostate depend upon the stage of the cancer. General nursing diagnoses, which may or may not apply to every patient with cancer of the prostate, include, but are not limited to, the following:

- Decisional conflict related to numerous alternative treatment options
- Pain related to surgery, prostatic enlargement, bone metastasis, and bladder spasms
- Urinary retention related to obstruction of urethra or bladdar neck by the prostate, blood clots, and loss of bladder tone
- Sexual dysfunction related to effects of treatment
- Anxiety related to uncertain outcome of disease process on life and lifestyle and effect of treatment on sexual functioning

Planning

The overall goals are that the patient with cancer of the prostate will (1) be an active participant in the treatment plan, (2) have satisfactory pain control, (3) follow the therapeutic plan, (4) accept the effect of the therapeutic

RESEARCH

IMPLICATIONS FOR NURSING PRACTICE

FATIGUE IN PATIENTS RECEIVING TREATMENT WITH CHEMOTHERAPY AND RADIOTHERAPY

Citation Irvine D and others: The prevalence and correlates of fatigue in patients receiving treatment with chemotherapy and radiotherapy, *Cancer Nursing* 17:367-378, 1994.

Purpose To compare the prevalence and correlates of fatigue between healthy individuals and patients receiving chemotherapy or radiotherapy.

Method A total of 104 patients and 53 healthy individuals participated in the study. Data on various illness and treatment variables and demographic data were collected. Instruments were used to measure fatigue, mood disturbance, symptom distress, and functional abilities. Chemotherapy patients were surveyed before treatment and 10-14 days after treatment. Radiotherapy patients were surveyed 1 week and 6 weeks after treatment. Control subjects were surveyed at a single point in time.

Results and Conclusions Cancer patients experienced a significant increase in fatigue after treatment when compared to healthy individuals. The best predictors of fatigue were their symptom distress and mood disturbance. Symptom distress and fatigue were significant predictors of impairment in functional activities related to illness.

Implications for Nursing Practice Men with testicular or prostate surgery may receive chemotherapy or radiotherapy as part of their treatment. It would be anticipated that their level of fatigue would increase and their functional abilities would decrease over the course of their treatment.

Knowing that the level of fatigue will increase and that functional abilities will decrease following cancer treatment would assist the nurse in planning appropriate interventions for this group of patients. The nurse could also provide anticipatory guidance pertaining to fatigue and functional abilities that could positively affect the quality of life and role function.

plan on sexual function, and (5) find a satisfactory way to achieve sexual expression.

Nursing Implementation

Health Promotion and Maintenance. One of the most important roles for nurses in relation to prostate cancer is to encourage patients to have an annual prostate examination to facilitate early detection of this malignant tumor. Men should have an annual rectal examination beginning at 40 years of age.

Acute Intervention. Preoperative and postoperative phases of therapy are the same as for BPH. Nursing interventions for the patient who undergoes radiation therapy and chemotherapy are discussed in Chapter 12. An additional consideration is the psychologic response of the patient to a diagnosis of cancer. The nurse needs to provide psychologic support for the patient and his family to help them cope with the diagnosis of cancer[37] (see Chapter 12).

Chronic and Home Management. If the patient is discharged with an indwelling catheter in place, the nurse must teach appropriate catheter care. The patient should be instructed to clean the urethral meatus with soap and water once a day; maintain a high fluid intake; keep the collecting bag lower than the bladder at all times; keep the catheter securely anchored to the inner thigh or abdomen; and report any signs of bladder infection, such as bladder spasms, fever, or hematuria.

Cancer of the prostate has a high cure rate if detected and treated early. However, prognosis for Stage D prostate cancer is very unfavorable. Pain control is the primary nursing intervention for this terminally ill patient. Hospice care is often appropriate and most beneficial to the patient and family. (Hospice care is discussed in Chapter 12.)

Table 52-7 Nursing Assessment: Cancer of the Prostate

Subjective Data

Important health information

Past health history: Positive family history, prostatic hypertrophy, sexually transmitted diseases

Medications: Use of any medications affecting urinary tract, such as morphine, anticholinergics, MAO inhibitors, and tricyclic antidepressants

Functional health patterns

Health perception–health management: Increasing fatigue and malaise

Nutritional-metabolic: Possible indicators of metastasis—weight loss, anorexia; high fat intake

Elimination: Hesitancy or straining to start stream, urgency, retention with dribbling, frequency, weak stream, hematuria

Sleep: Nocturia

Cognitive-perceptual: Possible indicators of metastasis such as dysuria, bone pain, low back pain radiating to legs or pelvis

Role-relationship: Exposure to environmental toxins

Objective Data

General

Age, race, pelvic lymphadenopathy (late sign)

Urinary

Distended bladder on palpation; hard, enlarged, and fixed prostate on rectal examination

Musculoskeletal

Pathologic fractures (metastasis)

Lab Findings

Elevated serum PSA or PAP (metastasis), positive biopsy results

MAO, Monoamine oxidase; *PAP,* prostatic acid phosphatase; *PSA,* prostate specific antigen.

Prostatitis

Pathophysiology. A number of inflammatory conditions can affect the prostate gland. The three most common forms of prostatitis are acute bacterial prostatitis, chronic bacterial prostatitis, and non-bacterial prostatitis. Bacterial infections generally result from organisms reaching the prostate gland by one of the following routes: ascending from the urethra, descending from the bladder, and invasion via the bloodstream or the lymphatic channels.[38]

Bacterial prostatitis is primarily a disease of older men and is the most common urinary tract infection in this age group.[39] It is frequently associated with urethritis or an infection of the lower urinary tract. It can also be associated with an indwelling urethral catheter. Common causative organisms are *Escherichia coli, Pseudomonas, Enterobacter, Proteus, Chlamydia trachomatis,* and group D streptococci. Chronic bacterial prostatitis should be considered in men with a history of recurrent bacteriuria.

Nonbacterial prostatitis may occur after a viral illness or may be secondary to a sudden decrease in sexual activity, particularly in a younger adult. The cause of this problem is not known, and a culture reveals no causative organisms.

Clinical Manifestations and Complications. Acute bacterial prostatitis results in manifestations of fever, chills, dysuria, urethral discharge, increased urinary frequency and urgency, low back and perineal pain, and acute cystitis with cloudy, smelly urine. The prostate is extremely swollen, tender, firm, and warm to touch. The complications of prostatitis are epididymitis and cystitis. Chronic prostatitis can predispose the patient to recurrent urinary tract infections. Sexual functioning may be affected as manifested by postejaculation pain, libido problems, and erectile dysfunction. Prostatic abscess is a rare complication.

The symptoms of chronic prostatitis may be absent or are generally milder than those of acute prostatitis. These include backache, perineal pain, mild dysuria, and increased frequency of urination. Factors that may contribute to chronic prostatitis include urethral obstruction, persistent infections above the urethra, and prostatic pathologic conditions such as hyperplasia and prostatic calculi. The prostate feels irregularly enlarged, firm, and slightly tender on palpation.

Diagnostic Studies. If a patient with prostatitis has a fever, the white blood cell (WBC) count may be elevated. The urine is often cloudy with a foul odor. The patient may be instructed to void into two or three separate containers for a split specimen urinalysis. The first container shows many more WBCs and bacteria than subsequent containers. On palpation, the prostate gland may be normal or may appear enlarged, tender, and in long-standing cases, reveal the presence of calculi. Cystoscopy and catheterizations are avoided during the acute phase to minimize the risk of introducing the organisms into the bladder and to avoid further pain.

Therapeutic Management. Therapeutic management of acute bacterial prostatitis usually consists of administering an antibiotic that concentrates in the prostate. Most antibiotics cannot penetrate the prostate because the low pH of the gland precludes solubility of the drugs. The exceptions are tetracycline and the combination of sulfamethoxazole and trimethoprim. Other interventions include increasing fluid intake, use of stool softeners, and rest. Therapeutic management of chronic prostatitis may consist of long-term administration of antibiotics, antiinflammatory agents, frequent prostatic massage and ejaculations, sitz baths, and stool softeners.

Nonbacterial prostatitis is difficult to treat because no bacteria are found in the urine or prostatic fluid. Treatment generally consists of antiinflammatory agents, hot sitz baths, and sexual activities that result in ejaculation.

NURSING MANAGEMENT

PROSTATITIS

The patient with acute bacterial prostatitis experiences prostate pain, especially when standing. Nursing interventions are aimed at relief of pain and fever, bed rest, and the maintenance of adequate hydration. The patient with chronic prostatitis should be instructed regarding the long-term nature of the problem. Because the prostate can serve as a source of urinary tract infection, fluid intake should be kept at a high level. Antibiotics may have to be taken for a number of months. Activities that drain the prostate, such as intercourse, masturbation, and prostatic massage, are often helpful in the long-term management of this problem. Chronic prostatitis may eventually lead to erectile dysfunction, for which the patient may need to seek treatment.

PROBLEMS OF THE PENIS

Health problems of the penis are rare if sexually transmitted infectious diseases are excluded (see Chapter 50). The problems may be classified as congenital problems, problems of the prepuce, problems with the erectile mechanism, and cancer.

Congenital Problems

Hypospadias is present when the urethral meatus is located on the ventral surface of the penis anywhere from the corona to the perineum. It is thought that hormonal influences, along with environmental and genetic factors, may play a part in this urologic anomaly.[40] Surgical repair of hypospadias is usually not necessary unless it is severe or there is an associated chordee or curvature of the penis during erection, which may prevent intercourse. Surgery may also be done for cosmetic reasons or emotional well-being.

Epispadias, opening of the urethra on the dorsal surface of the penis, is a complex birth defect that is usually associated with other genitourinary tract defects. Corrective surgery to place the urethra in a normal position in the penis is usually done in early childhood.

Problems of the Prepuce

Problems of the prepuce have been a rare occurrence because circumcision has been so widely practiced in the United States for the past 40 to 60 years. However, the trend is now shifting away from routine circumcision, which may result in an increased incidence of problems.[41]

Circumcision, the removal of the foreskin of the penis, may be done for religious, cultural, or hygienic reasons. The American Academy of Pediatrics currently does not recommend routine circumcision because of the potential risk of infection and penile trauma. However, parents are encouraged to make the final decision after consideration of the advantages and disadvantages.

Phimosis is caused by edema or inflammation of the foreskin. This results in the foreskin constricting around the opening and making retraction difficult. *Paraphimosis* is edema of the retracted foreskin, preventing normal return over the glans. In both cases, circumcision or dorsal slit of the prepuce may be required. Careful cleaning and replacement of the foreskin generally prevent these problems.

Problems of the Erectile Mechanism

Priapism is a painful erection, lasting longer than 6 hours. The patient may be unable to urinate. Causes of priapism include thrombosis of the veins of the corpora cavernosa, leukemia, sickle cell anemia, diabetes mellitus, degenerative lesions of the spine, neoplasms of the spinal cord, prolonged foreplay, injection of vasoactive medications into the corpus cavernosa, and cocaine use. Treatment may include sedatives, injection of vasoconstrictors directly into the penis, aspiration of the corpora cavernosa with a large-bore needle, or the surgical creation of a shunt to drain the corpora.[42] After an episode of priapism, the patient may be unable to achieve a normal erection.

Peyronie's disease is caused by plaque formation in one of the corpora cavernosa of the penis. The plaque formation may result from trauma to the penile shaft or may occur spontaneously. The plaque prevents adequate blood flow into the spongy tissue which results in a curvature on erection. If conservative measures do not correct the problem, surgery may be necessary.[43]

Cancer of Penis

Cancer of the penis is rare and is usually seen only in men who were not circumcised as infants. The tumor begins as a warty lesion that may be mistaken for a venereal wart. The majority of malignancies (95%) are well-differentiated squamous cell carcinomas.[44] Treatment in the early stages is laser removal of the growth or a partial penectomy. A radical resection may be done if the cancer has spread. The 5-year survival rate for tumors confined to the penis is 60% to 90%. The survival rate drops to 10% to 30% with distant metastasis.[45]

PROBLEMS OF THE SCROTUM AND ITS CONTENTS

External Problems

The skin of the scrotum is susceptible to a number of common dermatoses. The most common conditions of the scrotal skin are fungal infections, dermatitis (neurodermatitis, contact dermatitis, and seborrheic dermatitis), and parasitic infections (scabies and lice). These conditions involve discomfort for the patient but are associated with few, if any, severe complications (see Chapter 20).

Congenital Problems

Cryptorchidism (undescended testicles) is the most common congenital testicular condition.[46] It may occur bilaterally or unilaterally and may be the cause of infertility if corrective surgery is not done by 2 years of age. The incidence of testicular cancer is also high if the condition is not corrected before puberty.

Absence of the vas deferens is a rare condition associated most often with cystic fibrosis. With the advent of advanced techniques to treat infertility, this defect can be circumvented.

"*DES sons*" refers to the male children of women who took diethylstilbestrol (DES) during pregnancy. Until recently it was felt that only females were affected in utero if their mothers took DES during pregnancy. The impact on males is now seen in the form of undescended or underdeveloped testicles, a micro or small penis, varicocele, or epididymal cysts. These males also have an increased rate of infertility.

Acquired Problems

Problems that develop within the scrotum usually are first noticed as a mass or as scrotal edema. Some problems produce pain, whereas others do not. Acquired conditions affecting scrotal contents in the adult include epididymitis, hydrocele, spermatocele, varicocele, orchitis, torsion, and testicular cancer (Fig. 52-4).

Epididymitis. Epididymitis is an inflammatory process of the epididymis, usually secondary to an infectious process (sexually or nonsexually transmitted), trauma, or urinary reflux down the vas deferens. Swelling may progress to the point that the epididymis and testis are indistinguishable. The problem may be associated with prostatitis and is usually painful. The use of antibiotics is important for both partners if the transmission is through sexual contact. Conservative treatment consists of bed rest with elevation of the scrotum, use of ice packs, and analgesics. Ambulation places the scrotum in a dependent position and increases pain. Most tenderness subsides within 1 week, although swelling may last for weeks or months.

Hydrocele. A hydrocele results from interference with lymphatic drainage of the scrotum, with swelling of the tunica vaginalis that surrounds the testis. Diagnosis is fairly simple because the mass can be transilluminated with a bright light. No treatment is indicated unless the swelling becomes very large and uncomfortable in which case aspiration or surgical drainage of the mass is performed.

Spermatocele. A spermatocele is a firm, sperm-containing cyst of the epididymis that may be visible with transillumination. The cause is unknown, and surgical removal is the treatment. It is important for the patient to see his doctor as he would be unable to distinguish this cyst from cancer when performing self-examination.

Varicocele. A varicocele is a dilatation of the veins that drain the testes. The scrotum feels wormlike when palpated. The cause of the problem is unknown. The varicocele is usually located on the left side of the scrotum as a consequence of retrograde blood flow from the left renal vein. Surgery is indicated if the patient is infertile, since persistent varicoceles are associated with 40% to 50% of the causes of infertility. Repair of the varicocele may be through injection of a sclerosing agent or by surgical ligation of the spermatic vein.[47]

Orchitis. Orchitis is a rare testicular inflammation, generally occurring after an episode of mumps, pneumonia, tuberculosis, or syphilis. It can also be a side effect of epididymitis, prostatectomy, catheterization, or complicated urinary tract infection (UTI).[48] Mumps orchitis is a condition contributing to infertility and could easily be decreased by childhood vaccination against mumps.

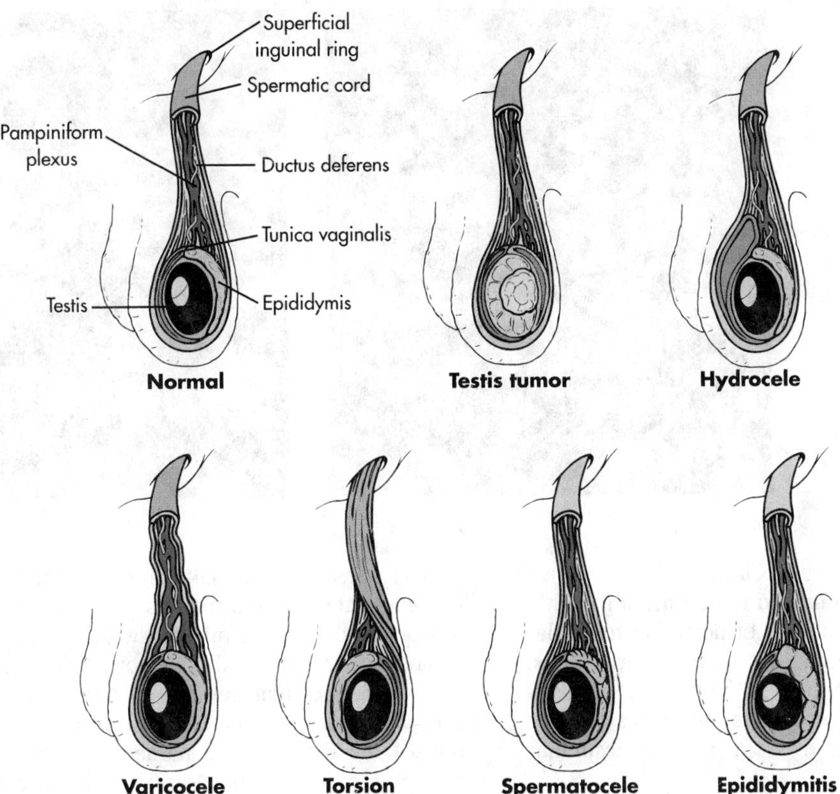

Fig. 52-4 Scrotal masses.

Torsion. Testicular torsion involves a twisting of the spermatic cord that supplies blood to the testes and epididymis. It is most commonly seen at puberty. Torsion constitutes a surgical emergency. The patient experiences severe pain, tenderness, swelling, nausea, and vomiting. Urinary complaints, fever, and WBCs or bacteria in the urine are absent. The pain does not subside with rest or elevation of the scrotum. Unless surgery to untwist the cord and restore the blood supply is performed quickly, the testicle atrophies and becomes useless.

Testicular Cancer

Significance and etiology. Testicular tumors make up about 0.7% of all forms of cancer in men. They occur in 2 of 100,000 men per year, with the peak age of incidence between 20 and 40 years of age.[49] Testicular tumors are much more common in males who have had undescended testicles (cryptorchidism). Other predisposing factors include a history of mumps, orchitis, inguinal hernia in childhood, and testicular cancer in the contralateral testis. The etiology of testicular neoplasms is unknown.

Testicular tumors may develop from the cellular components of the testis or from the embryonal precursors (germinal tumors). Nongerminal tumors are very rare, are usually benign, and can occur at any age. Germinal tumors are almost always malignant.

Diagnostic studies. Palpation of the scrotal contents is the first step in diagnosing testicular cancer. Additional tests that aid in diagnosis include a testicular sonogram and MRI. Once the diagnosis of a testicular neoplasm is suspected, a blood sample should be set aside before orchiectomy for subsequent determination of the tumor marker glycoproteins alpha fetoprotein (AFP) and human chorionic gonadotropin (HCG).

Following orchiectomy, tumor staging is done on the biopsy specimen. Testicular cancer is histologically classified as seminoma or nonseminoma. AFP is not produced by a pure seminoma. After diagnosis and staging, AFP and HCG will continue to be monitored, if appropriate, to detect metastases and assess the response to therapy. These measures are repeated only if initial levels are elevated.

Clinical manifestations. Germinal tumors may have a slow or rapid onset depending on the type of tumor. The patient may notice a lump in his scrotum, as well as scrotal swelling and a feeling of heaviness. The scrotal mass is usually nontender, very firm, and cannot be transilluminated. Manifestations associated with metastasis to other systems include back pain, cough, dyspnea, hemoptysis, dysphagia (difficulty swallowing), alterations in vision or mental status, papilledema, and seizures.

THERAPEUTIC AND NURSING MANAGEMENT

TESTICULAR CANCER

As with many forms of cancer, the survival of the patient is closely associated with early recognition of the tumor. The scrotum is easily examined, and beginning tumors are

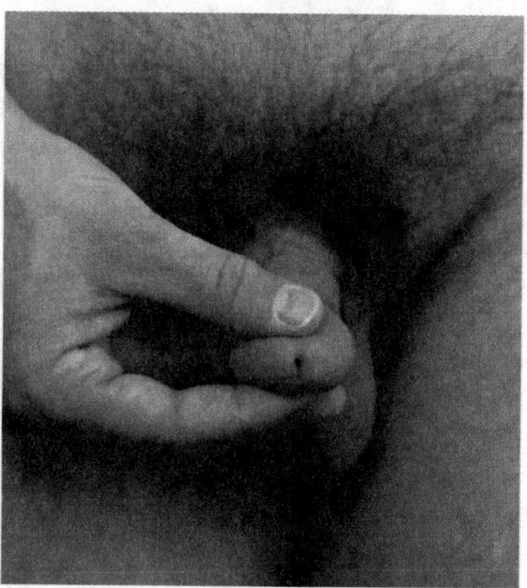
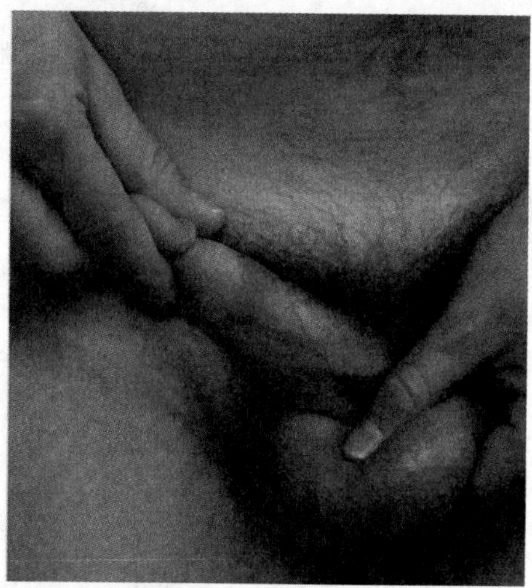

Fig. 52-5 Testicular self-examination.

usually palpable. Every male between 20 and 40 years of age should be taught and encouraged to perform a monthly testicular self-exam for the purpose of detecting testicular tumors or other scrotal abnormalities such as varicoceles. The nurse should teach the patient how to do a self-examination with particular emphasis on males with a history of an undescended testis or a previous testicular tumor.

The procedure for self-examination is not difficult. The patient may indicate some reluctance to examine his own genitals. With encouragement the patient can learn this simple procedure. He should be encouraged to perform self-examinations frequently until he is comfortable with the procedure. The scrotum should be examined once a month. Videotapes are now available as teaching aids and ideally, are shown during high school or college physical education classes.

The guidelines for self-examination of the scrotum are as follows:

1. Perform the examination while the scrotum is warm because the testes retract toward the perineum when cold. During a shower or bath is a good time for examination (Fig. 52-5).
2. Use both hands to palpate the scrotal contents. Roll each testicle between the thumb and first three fingers until the entire surface has been covered.
3. Identify the structures. The testicles should feel round and smooth, like hard-boiled eggs. Differentiate the testis from the epididymis. The epididymis is not as smooth as the egg-shaped testis. One testis may be larger than the other. Size is not as important as texture. Check for lumps, irregularities, pain in the testicles, and a dragging sensation. Locate the spermatic cord, which is usually firm and smooth.
4. Choose a consistent day of the month that is easy to remember to examine the testicles. The examination can be performed more frequently if desired.
5. Notify the doctor at once if any abnormalities are found.

The nurse should make this procedure as simple and uncomplicated for the man as possible. The man needs to practice to develop familiarity with his body, and whatever means he chooses for this, is correct for him.

Therapeutic management of testicular cancer involves surgical removal of the affected testis and cord and resection of the regional and paraaortic lymph nodes. A high radical inguinal orchiectomy is the usual treatment to prevent local recurrence and metastases to the inguinal lymphatics. Radiation of the remaining lymph nodes and single or multiple chemotherapeutic agent regimens, including bleomycin-vincristine-cisplatin-vinblastine are also used after surgery, depending on the histologic conditions and disease stage.

The prognosis for patients with testicular cancer has improved and 75% of the patients obtain complete remission of the disease if it is detected in the early stages. All patients with testicular cancer, regardless of pathology or stage, require meticulous follow-up and regular physical examinations, chest radiography, CT scan, and assessment of HCG and AFP (if appropriate). The goal is to detect relapse when the tumor burden is minimal. The man with testicular cancer should have the opportunity to discuss fertility and sperm banking during the preoperative period.

SEXUAL FUNCTIONING

Vasectomy

Vasectomy is the bilateral surgical ligation or resection of the vas deferens performed for the purpose of sterilization (Fig. 52-6). The procedure requires only 15 to 30 minutes and is usually performed with the patient under local anesthesia on an outpatient basis. Vasectomy is considered a permanent form of sterilization, although some successful reversals (*vasovasotomy*) have been reported.

After vasectomy, the patient should not notice any difference in the look or feel of the ejaculate, because its major component is seminal fluid. The patient will need to use an alternative form of contraception until semen examination reveals no sperm. This usually requires at least 10 ejaculations or 6 weeks to evacuate sperm distal to the

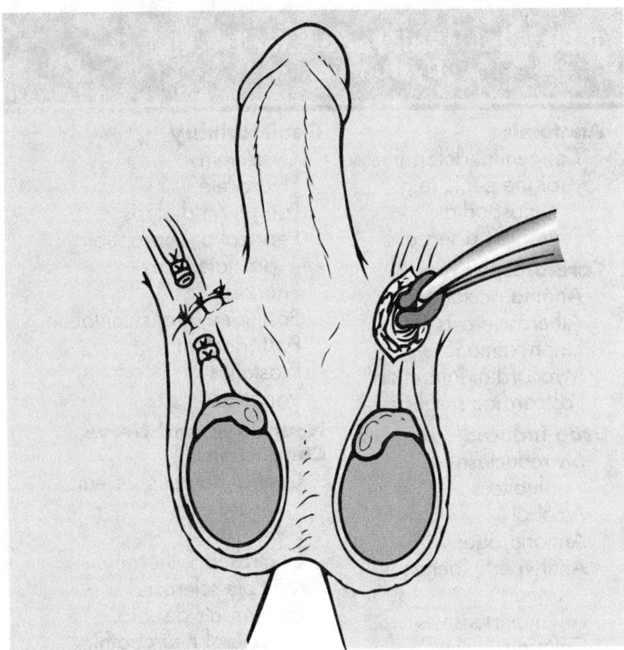

Fig. 52-6 Vasectomy procedure. The vas deferens is ligated or resected for the purpose of sterilization.

anastomotic site. Sperm cells continue to be produced by the testes but are absorbed by the body rather than being passed through the vas deferens.

Vasectomy does not affect the production of hormones, ejaculation, or the physiologic mechanisms related to sexual functioning. Occasionally postoperative hematoma and swelling of the scrotum occur. Psychologic adjustment may be a problem after surgery. It may be very difficult for the patient to separate vasectomy from castration at a subconscious level. Some men may develop erectile dysfunction or may feel the need to become much more sexually active than they were in the past to prove their masculinity. Careful discussion of the procedure and its outcome before the surgery can be helpful in detecting patients who may have problems with psychologic adjustment. Surgery should be delayed for these patients.

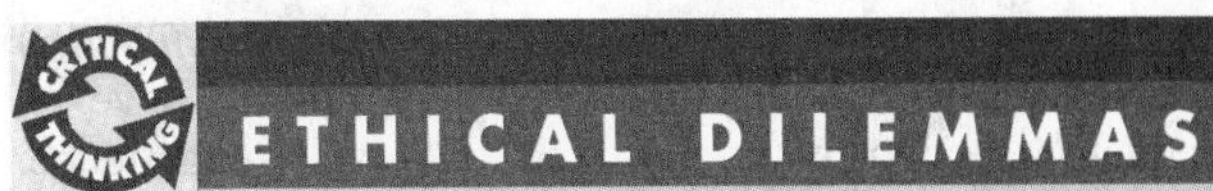

ETHICAL DILEMMAS

STERILIZATION

Situation A 43-year-old male patient is requesting a vasectomy and informs the nurse that he does not wish to discuss this with his wife. The physician's policy is to have the spouse or partner sign a form acknowledging the patient's desire to be sterilized. This patient explains that while his wife wants to have more children, the one they already have is all he wants.

Discussion Physician practice rather than state law dictates the need for disclosure to the patient's spouse or significant other of the intent to sterilize a patient. Had the patient not informed the physician that he was married, this would not be an issue. As it is, he is perfectly able to seek another physician to perform this procedure, one who has no such reservations, or he may choose not to disclose his marital status. Women in most states are not required to prove that their husbands or significant others are aware of their intention to terminate a pregnancy, but the (intended) finality of a vasectomy is considered different. Professional ethics require that the nurse explain to the patient that he cannot have a vasectomy with this physician without obtaining the needed consultation with his wife. The patient would then be free to determine how to handle this problem.

ETHICAL AND LEGAL PRINCIPLES

- Patient autonomy would require that matters relating to reproduction be left to the privacy and discretion of the individual.
- Nonmaleficence and truthtelling, however, would require informing the patient's wife of the patient's intention to permanently render himself unable to procreate. If the patient is unwilling to discuss the matter with her, and the physician is unable to convince him that this is crucial to the integrity of his marriage, the physician can refuse to be party to this deception.
- Competent adults may legally choose to be sterilized either for convenience or for medical reasons.

Erectile Dysfunction

Significance. Ten to 20 million men in the United States experience erectile dysfunction.[50] The problem is increasing in all segments of the sexually active male population. In younger men the increase is attributed to an increase in substance abuse, such as recreational drugs and alcohol. Middle-aged men are affected by modern medical technology, such as major organ transplants, bypass surgeries, and chemotherapeutic agents. The older population (men over 70 years of age) are living longer, fuller lives and expect to remain sexually active, regardless of any existing medical conditions. Stress factors associated with modern lifestyles are affecting men of all ages and contribute greatly to the psychologic causes of erectile failure.[51]

Pathophysiology. Erectile dysfunction is the inability to attain or maintain an erect penis that allows satisfactory sexual performance. This problem occurs at some time or other for almost all sexually active males. The problem can occur at any age, although it is most common among males between 55 and 65 years of age. When the problem occurs during more than 25% of sexual encounters, intervention is appropriate.

Erection is a parasympathetic reflex initiated mainly by certain tactile, visual, and mental stimuli. It consists of dilation of the arteries and arterioles of the penis, which in turn fills and distends spaces in its erectile tissue and compresses veins. Therefore, more blood enters the penis through the dilated arteries then leaves it through the constricted veins.[52] Hence, the penis becomes larger and rigid, or, in other words, erection occurs. Problems occur when these spaces (corporeal bodies) fail to fill when desired, or when they empty before orgasm. There are two classifications of erectile dysfunction. *Primary dysfunction* occurs when the patient has never been able to have an adequate erection with any type of sexual experience. *Secondary dysfunction* occurs when the patient has lost the ability to achieve an erection or is able to have an erection in only a particular way. Some men can only have an erection with a full bladder or masturbation; others have an erection with a particular partner but not with others. A functional erection requires not only the desire but also adequate blood supply, nerve innervation, and hormone balance.

Clinical Manifestations and Complications. The risk factors for the disorder may be physiologic, psychologic, or both (Table 52-8). The major complication of this problem is that the man's inability to perform sexually can cause stress in his interpersonal relationships and may preclude sex-role functioning. Table 52-9 lists normal age-related changes in sexual performance. Explanation of these age-related changes may be all that is necessary to reassure an anxious older man regarding his sexuality.

Table 52-8 Risk Factors for Erectile Dysfunction

Anatomic
- Congenital deformities of the penis (e.g., hypospadias)
- Peyronie's disease

Cardiorespiratory
- Angina pectoris
- Atherosclerosis
- Emphysema
- Myocardial infarction
- Postcardiac surgery

Drug-induced
- 5α-reductase inhibitors
- Alcohol
- Antiandrogens
- Antihyperlipidemic agents
- Antihypertensives
- Caffeine
- Diuretics
- Drugs for Parkinson's disease
- Estrogen
- Histamine-receptor antagonists
- Hypertension
- LHRH analogues
- Major tranquilizers
- Marijuana, cocaine, LSD
- Narcotics
- Nicotine
- Tricyclic antidepressants

Endocrine
- Addison's disease
- Diabetes mellitus
- High levels of prolactin
- Myxedema
- Obesity
- Pituitary tumor
- Testosterone deficiency
- Thyrotoxicosis

Genitourinary
- Cystectomy
- Hydrocele
- Long-term dialysis
- Perineal or suprapubic prostatectomy
- Phimosis
- Postkidney transplantation
- Postpriapism
- Prostatitis
- Varicocele

Neurologic and Nerve Conduction
- Central nervous system disorders
- CVA
- Electroshock therapy
- Multiple sclerosis
- Parkinson's disease
- Peripheral neuropathic conditions
- Spina bifida
- Sympathectomy
- Trauma to spinal cord
- Tumors or transection of spinal cord

Psychogenic
- Depression
- Excessive stress in family, work, or interpersonal relationships
- Fatigue
- Fear of failure to perform

Vascular
- Aortic aneurysm
- Aortofemoral bypass
- Arteriosclerosis of pelvic blood vessels
- High levels of cholesterol

CVA, Cerebrovascular accident; *LHRH,* luteinizing hormone–releasing hormone; *LSD,* lysergic acid diethylamide.

Diagnostic Studies. Rapid advances have been made in the diagnosis and treatment of erectile dysfunction in the past 10 years. Until 15 years ago, a man's problem was generally labeled as "psychological" unless he had severe diabetes or total paralysis. With the advent of modern technology, 80% to 90% of the causes are being attributed to physiologic reasons and can be determined by diagnostic studies.[53] Diagnostic testing is now divided into primary and secondary levels based on findings during the initial assessment (Table 52-10).

Therapeutic Management. The treatment for erectile dysfunction is based on the cause. Treatment of psychologic causes of erectile dysfunction should be carried out by a qualified therapist. The approach may be behavioral or psychologic, or in some patients it may also involve therapeutic intervention to temporarily restore self-confidence. The goal of therapy is to have the man and his partner develop a satisfactory sexual relationship after treatment.

When the problem is physical, interventions are directed at correcting or eliminating the cause or restoring function by medical means. The results of these interventions are usually quite satisfactory when both partners are involved in the decision-making process and have realistic expectations of the treatment. Many treatment options are available to the male experiencing erectile dysfunction because of physiologic causes. The National Institutes of Health (NIH) issued a consensus statement in 1992 indicating noninvasive treatment methods should be the primary approach to care.[50] Invasive and experimental techniques should be limited to research centers.

Nonsurgical management

PHARMACOLOGIC MANAGEMENT. Whenever possible, collaboration should occur between the primary physician providing the medical care and the urologist treating the erectile dysfunction. Elimination of or substitution for a medication that causes erectile dysfunction (e.g., methyldopa, propranolol) is sometimes all that is necessary to alleviate the problem.

Yohimbine (Yocan), an oral medication, is a mild vasodilator and a reported aphrodisiac. It is often used in conjunction with other forms of therapy and may serve to provide a placebo effect or boost the confidence of the man.

When there is an established diagnosis of testicular failure (hypogonadism) androgen replacement therapy may sometimes be effective in improving erectile function. It should be given as an intramuscular (IM) injection of testosterone enanthate or testosterone cypionate. Oral androgens that are currently available are not indicated. The effectiveness of testosterone supplementation for older men experiencing a normal, gradual decline is doubtful. For men with hyperprolactinemia, bromocriptine therapy is often

Table 52-9 Gerontologic Considerations: Sexual Performance*

1. Time lag between perceiving sexual opportunity and full erection
2. Diminished size and rigidity of the penis at full erection
3. Increased time interval to ejaculation
4. Changed nature of ejaculation with less spurting and lessened intensity of feeling
5. Shortened period between ejaculation and flaccidity
6. Increase in time to next reaction to sexual stimulation

*For almost all men by the age of 45 to 50 years.

Table 52-10 Diagnostic Studies: Erectile Dysfunction

Primary
- Medical history and physical examination
- Detailed sexual history, including practices and techniques
- Psychosocial evaluation
- Testosterone levels; blood chemistry
- PSA levels
- Intracavernosal vasoactive drug testing

Secondary
- Blood profile (e.g., prolactin, FSH, LH)
- Vascular flow studies (e.g., duplex Doppler, cavernosogram)
- Neurologic evaluation
- Sleep tumescence studies
- Tests to exclude unrecognized systemic disease: CBC, urinalysis, creatinine, lipid profile, FBS, thyroid function studies

CBC, Complete blood count; *FBS*, fasting blood sugar; *FSH*, follicle stimulating hormone; *LH*, luteinizing hormone; *PSA*, prostate specific antigen.

effective in normalizing the prolactin level and improving sexual functioning.[54] Careful evaluation of the man's serum testosterone level and prostate condition must precede introduction of this therapy. Administration of testosterone to a man with normal levels of hormone production may actually suppress the body's natural ability to produce testosterone. Testosterone is contraindicated in men with cancer of the prostate because of its ability to cause proliferation of the prostate cancer cells.

Intracavernosal injection therapy is an innovative diagnostic and treatment option that is gaining in popularity. Vasoactive medications (e.g., papaverine, prostaglandin E_1, phentolamine, or combinations of these) are injected directly into the corporeal body using a 25- to 27-gauge syringe.[54,55] Several new combinations of vasoactive medications and smooth muscle relaxants are presently in clinical trials. Within 15 to 30 minutes after injection an erection is obtained, which may last for up to 2 hours. The dose is regulated on an individual basis to prevent the side effect of priapism. Other side effects may include pain, penile corporal fibrosis, fibrotic nodules, and hypotension. Home injection therapy instruction is given to those men who are suitable candidates for the therapy.[56] This treatment is not suitable for men with severe vascular problems, intolerance for transient hypotension, severe psychiatric disease, poor manual dexterity, poor vision, or those receiving anticoagulant therapy. The injection is nearly painless and produces a more natural erection than a vacuum device or implant. Success rates have been very high when there is adequate patient teaching and follow-up, but dropouts rates, often early in treatment, are also high.

Aids or Devices. Suction devices applied to the flaccid penis produce a vacuum within a cylinder, thereby pulling blood up into the corporeal bodies producing an erection. A penile ring or other device placed around the base of the penis causes vasoconstriction and prevents detumescence (subsidence of swelling).[57] Special care must be taken in using these devices to prevent tissue damage. Suction devices are sometimes used in conjunction with intracorporeal injection therapy in those patients with moderate-to-severe venous leaks of the penile veins.

Alternative Methods. Some patients do not require penetration for satisfactory sexual expression and a vibrator or dildo (rubber penis) could be used. Patients experiencing temporary loss of erection or who are awaiting surgical interventions use a variety of methods to achieve sexual satisfaction. Sexual counselors or therapists acting as consultants can provide support and suggest alternative forms of sexual expression.

Electronic stimulators in the form of rectal probes provide direct stimulation to damaged nerve endings that innervate the sympathetic and parasympathetic pathways involved in producing an erection. Their primary use is in patients with spinal cord injuries and multiple sclerosis. Presently, the devices have limited availability.

Surgical interventions (Fig. 52-7)

Penile Implants. Penile implants have provided surgical management of erectile dysfunction for more than 20 years.[58] The paired devices can be semirigid, malleable, or inflatable. They are implanted into the corporeal bodies to provide an erection firm enough for penetration. All implants provide a usable erection and should be chosen carefully based on the man's mental and physical capabilities, surgical risk factors, personal lifestyle, and insurance and financial resources. The main problems associated with penile prostheses are mechanical failure, infection, and erosions. The ability to please both partners enhances satisfaction levels.

For essentially healthy men the surgical procedure may be performed on an outpatient basis, with patients being monitored by home care nurses. Complete recovery time varies from 4 to 6 weeks. Patients considered to be at high risk for complications include those with uncontrolled diabetes mellitus and those with severe circulatory problems. Patients should be advised that a prosthesis will not restore ejaculation or tactile sensations if they were absent before surgery. Sexual counseling is often recommended before and after surgery to deal with unrealistic expectations and to restore or promote techniques of communication.

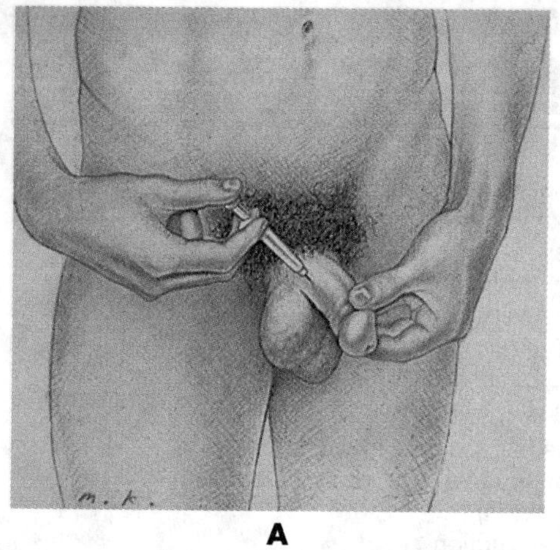

A

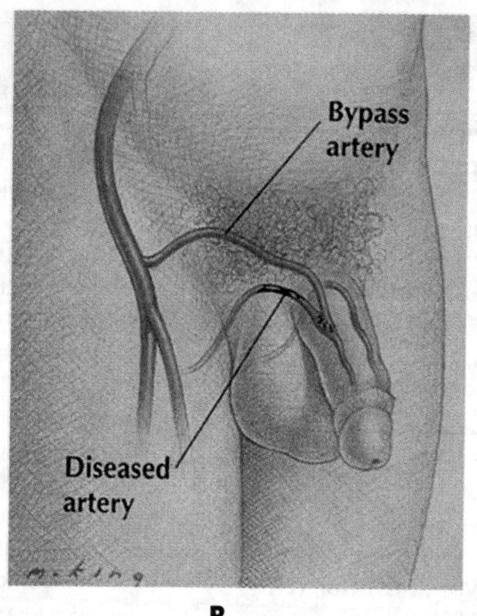

B

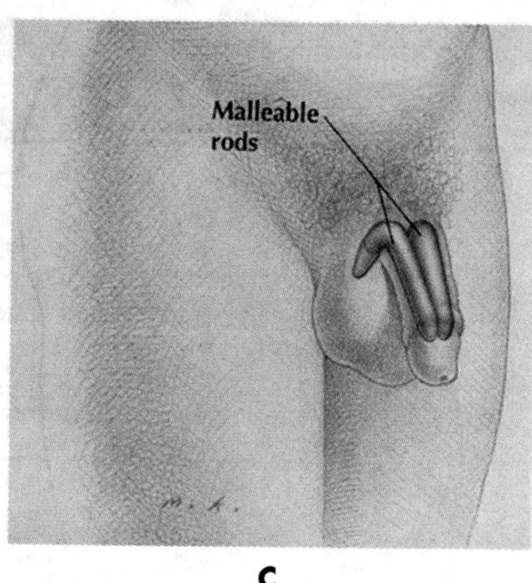

C

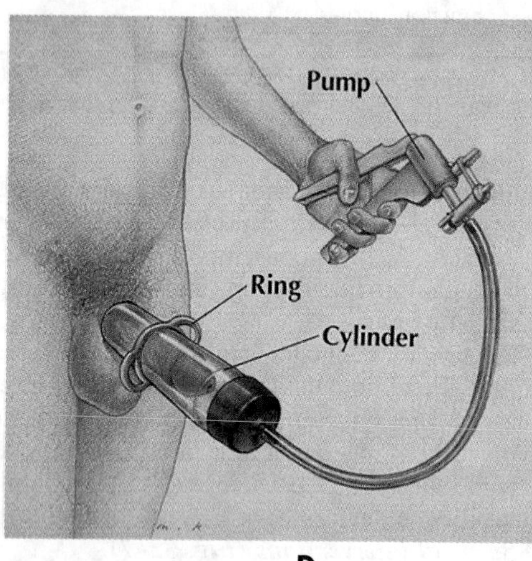

D

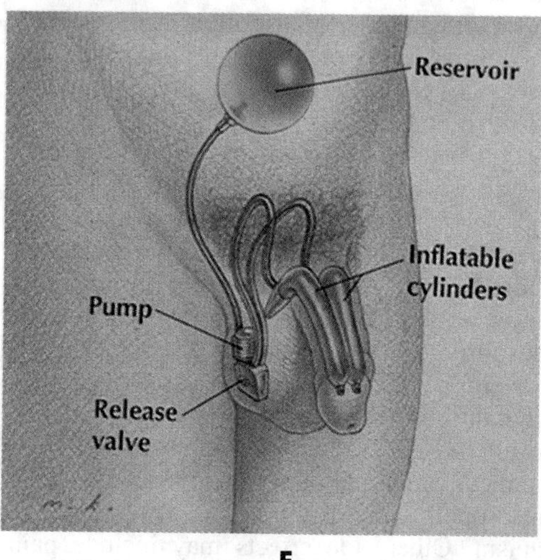

E

Fig. 52-7 ***A,*** Self-injection therapy involves injecting a medication directly into the penis. This increases blood flow and causes an erection. ***B,*** A bypass operation can restore blood flow and sometimes cure erectile dysfunction. Unfortunately, it is rarely appropriate and long-term success has been disappointing. ***C,*** A malleable implant is always erect but can be bent close to the body for concealment. ***D,*** With the vacuum device in place, blood can be drawn into the penis by means of a hand pump. This creates an erection. For intercourse, the ring is slipped to the base of the penis and the cylinder removed. ***E,*** Inflatable implants consist of cylinders in the penis, a small pump in the scrotum, and a reservoir in the lower abdomen. When activated, the pump fills the cylinders with fluid from the reservoir. A small release valve permits the fluid to drain back into the reservoir after intercourse.

Vascular Surgery. When impotence occurs because of inadequate blood flow into the penis, revascularization of the corporeal bodies may be beneficial. If a venous leak occurs, ligation of the affected veins may provide a solution. Careful vascular diagnostic studies are completed first to determine whether the problem is insufficient blood flowing into the corporeal bodies or a rapid loss of blood from the area that prevents the maintenance of an erection. Bypass grafts and venous ligation have limited success in older men because of the rapid obstruction of the graft and the natural tendency to form collateral circulation around the ligated vessel.[59] The NIH consensus statement on impotence recommends that surgery of the penile vascular system only be attempted in investigational settings because of poor outcomes on long-term follow-up.[50]

NURSING MANAGEMENT

ERECTILE DYSFUNCTION

The patient experiencing erectile dysfunction requires a great deal of emotional support for both himself and his partner. Men often do not feel comfortable discussing their problems with others because of society's expectations of a man's sexual abilities. The man may experience and demonstrate isolation from support systems, and he may also lose self-esteem, which can eventually lead to loss of role functions.

The patient needs reassurance that confidentiality will be maintained. In conjunction with therapeutic treatment, it often becomes necessary to provide counseling and therapy for the couple to establish realistic expectations and develop meaningful communication patterns. The majority of men wait an average of 2 years before seeking medical assistance. They are often highly motivated and expect immediate solutions to their problems. The health care team should provide a support system and accurate information as soon as possible.

Pain management of patients experiencing surgical interventions generally consists of administration of prescribed analgesics and elevation and application of ice to the scrotum for the first 48 hours postoperatively. The normal course for healing ranges from 4 to 6 weeks. Resumption of sexual activities before complete healing may result in infection, extrusion, erosion, or rupture. Patients should also be instructed to use a water-soluble lubricant and approach penetration slowly and at a comfortable angle.

Infertility

In about one third of childless marriages, the primary cause of infertility can be ascribed to the male.[60] Infertility can be caused by disorders of the hypothalamic-pituitary system, disorders of the testes, and abnormalities of the ejaculatory system. The physical causes are generally divided into three categories: the pretesticular or endocrine (this occurs only rarely, in about 3% of the cases); testicular (this comprises 50% of the cases, with varicocele being the major cause); and post-testicular (approximately 5% to 7% of the cases, with obstruction, infection or vasectomy being the chief causes). The remaining 40% are classified as idiopathic or of unknown causes. A careful health history, including sexual practices, and a physical examination are the initial diagnostic measures in an infertility study. Examination can disclose a varicocele, a treatable cause of male infertility. The use of drugs, such as chemotherapeutic drugs, ketoconazole, sulfasalazine, and cimetidine, which have a known effect on testicular function, should also be documented.

The first test in an infertility study is usually a semen analysis to determine the number and motility of sperm. Additional tests helpful in determining the etiology include plasma testosterone and serum LH and FSH measurements. A test for sperm penetration abilities may also be done. The specific cause of infertility is often not determined.

The nurse should be concerned and tactful in dealing with the male patient undergoing infertility studies. For many men, fertility and masculinity are equated. The nurse must be sensitive to the problem of gender identity in the infertile male. Treatment options for the male range from conservative lifestyle changes (e.g., avoidance of scrotal heat, substance abuse, high stress) to in vitro fertilization techniques and corrective surgery. Achievement of pregnancy varies from 8% to 60% and ranges in cost from several hundreds to several thousands of dollars. Infertility can seriously strain a marriage, and the couple may require counseling and discussion of alternatives if conception will never be possible. (Female infertility is discussed in Chapter 51.)

CRITICAL THINKING EXERCISES

CASE STUDY

BENIGN PROSTATIC HYPERPLASIA

Patient Profile

Mr. R.K., a 71-year-old married man, presents in the emergency department because of an inability to void for the past 12 hours.

Subjective Data

- Complains of severe bladder pain and pressure
- Is very restless and agitated
- Relates history of three cans of beer at party the previous evening; has not voided since then.

Objective Data

Physical Examination

- Has prostate enlargement on rectal examination
- Has hematuria and WBCs in urine
- Has palpable bladder above umbilicus

Laboratory Studies

- PSA: 8 ng/ml (normal, 0-4 ng/ml)

Therapeutic Management

- An indwelling catheter was inserted by a urology resident and Mr. R.K. was admitted to the hospital

Critical Thinking Questions

1. What risk factors for acute urinary retention and BPH are present in Mr. R.K.?
2. Explain the etiology of the objective symptoms Mr. R.K. exhibited.
3. Discuss the pharmacologic options available to Mr. R.K.
4. Discuss the invasive options available to Mr. R.K.
5. Mr. R.K. asks you about the effect of the various treatment options on his ability to have sex. How would you respond?
6. Write one or more appropriate nursing diagnoses based on the assessment data presented. Are there any collaborative problems?
7. Upon further assessment, you note that Mr. R.K. has a nursing diagnosis of decisional conflict. How would you help him to resolve this conflict related to treatment options?

NURSING RESEARCH ISSUES

1. Is a man more likely to report problems related to prostatic enlargement directly to the health care provider or via a printed questionnaire?
2. What percentage of patients presenting with prostatic enlargement have a concurrent urinary tract infection?
3. What is the best strategy to get men over 40 years of age to get an annual digital rectal examination?
4. What relaxation techniques are most effective in relieving bladder spasms after a transurethral or suprapubic prostatectomy?
5. How receptive are men with an erectile dysfunction to the idea of a prosthetic device to accomplish an erection?
6. What is the compliance rate for testicular self-examination at 3, 6, and 12 months following a training program for high school boys?
7. Does awareness of behaviors that can cause acute urinary retention in men with BPH alter the practice of these behaviors?

REVIEW QUESTIONS

The number of the question corresponds to the same-numbered objective at the beginning of the chapter.

1. The most common problem of the adult male genitourinary system is
   a. benign prostatic hyperplasia.
   b. erectile dysfunction.
   c. prostate cancer.
   d. testicular cancer.

2. In teaching health promoting activities related to benign prostatic hyperplasia, the nurse should recommend all the following *except*
   a. cautious use of alcohol.
   b. avoidance of a low fluid intake.
   c. high caffeine intake.
   d. urinating when the urge is first felt.

3. In order to detect cancer of the prostate early, it is important that a man have which of the following tests annually?

a. Prostatic acid phosphatase (PAP)
b. Prostatic ultrasound
c. Serum creatinine
d. Rectal examination

4. Assessment findings that could alert the nurse to the possibility of cancer of the prostate include all of the following *except*

a. positive family history.
b. patient below 35 years of age.
c. low back pain radiating to legs or pelvis.
d. elevated PSA.

5. Important nursing activities after transurethral resection include all of the following *except*

a. monitoring intake and output.
b. removing catheter if it becomes clogged.
c. teaching Kegel exercises.
d. encouraging a high fluid intake.

6. The nurse can inform the patient that after vasectomy the patient will be

a. immediately sterile.
b. unable to ejaculate in a normal manner.
c. unable to contract venereal disease.
d. able to resume his usual sexual functioning.

7. The nurse can decrease the patient's discomfort regarding care involving his reproductive organs by all of the following actions *except*

a. ensuring privacy for personal care.
b. maintaining a nonjudgmental attitude toward his sexual practices.
c. relating his sexual concerns to his sexual partner.
d. making sure he understands the terminology being used for body parts.

REFERENCES

1. McConnell JD and others: Benign prostatic hyperplasia: diagnosis and treatment. *Clinical practice guideline,* no. 8, AHCPR publication no. 94-0582, Rockville, MD, February 1994. Agency for Health Care Policy and Research, Public Health Service, US Department of Health and Human Services.
2. Prostate Health Council: *Prostate cancer. What every man over 40 should know,* Baltimore, 1991, American Foundation for Urologic Disease.
3. Gagalowski AI, Wilson JD: Hyperplasia and carcinoma of the prostate. In Isselbacher KJ and others, editors: *Harrison's principles of internal medicine,* ed 13, New York, 1994, McGraw-Hill.
4. Willis D: Taming the overgrown prostate, *Am J Nurs* 92:34, 1992.
5. Riehmann M, Bruskewitz R: New options in benign prostatic hyperplasia, *Hosp Pract* 28:17, 1993.
6. Stone NN: Treatment options in benign prostatic hypertrophy, *Hosp Pract* 27:85, 1992.
7. Lepor H: The role of alpha blockage in BPH, *J Androl* 12:389, 1991.
8. Baum N: Alternatives to TURP for the management of enlarged prostate, *Geriatr Med Today* 9:43, 1990.
9. McLaughlin J and others: Dilation of the prostatic urethra with 35 mm balloon, *Br J Urol* 67:177, 1991.
10. Bruskewitz RC: Benign prostatic hyperplasia: intervene or wait? *Hosp Pract* 27:99, 1992.
11. Grunert RT, Bruskewitz M: Choose TUIP for the younger patient, *Contemp Urol* 3:13, 1991.
12. Orandi A: Transurethral resection versus transurethral incision of the prostate, *Urol Clin North Am* 17:601, 1990.
13. Walsh PC: Radical retropubic prostatectomy. In Walsh PC and others, editors: *Campbell's urology,* ed 6, Philadelphia, 1992, Saunders.
14. Smith DB, Babaian RJ: The effect of treatment for cancer on male fertility and sexuality, *Cancer Nurs* 15:271, 1992.
15. Newman DK, Smith DA: Pelvic muscle reeducation as a nursing treatment for incontinence, *Urol Nurs* 12:9, 1992.
16. Wanich CK, Reilly NJ: Incontinence care products: non-surgical management of urinary incontinence, *Ostomy Wound Management* 34:45, 1991.
17. Jeter KF, Faller N, Norton C: *Nursing for continence,* Philadelphia, 1990, Saunders.
18. Wells T: Conquering incontinence, *Geriatr Nurs* 11:133, 1990.
19. Sant GR, Meares EM: Catheter. In Suki WN, Massy SG, editors: *Therapy of renal diseases and related disorders,* ed 2, Hingham, MA, 1991, Kluwer Academic Publishers.
20. Meredith CE: Treatment options for men with erectile dysfunction, *Innov Urol Nurs* 3:2, 1991.
21. Einhorn C: Helping the prostate surgery patient face sexual dysfunction, *Innov Urol Nurs* 3:1, 1991.
22. American Cancer Society, *Cancer facts and figures,* Pub No 5008-93, Atlanta, 1993.
23. Littrup PJ, Goodman AC, Mettlin CJ: The benefit and cost of prostate cancer early detection, *Cancer* 43:134, 1993.
24. Lind J: Genitourinary cancers. In Clark JC, McGee RF, editors: *Core curriculum for oncology nursing,* ed 2, Philadelphia, 1992, Saunders.
25. Klimaszewski AD, Karlowicz KA: Cancer of the male genitalia. In Karlowicz KA, editor: *Urologic nursing: principles and practice,* Philadelphia, 1995, Saunders.
26. Hernandez AD, Smith JA: Transrectal ultrasonography for early detection and staging of prostate cancer, *Urol Clin North Am* 17:745, 1990.
27. Naragon P: Neoplasms of the prostate gland. In Tanagho EA, McAninch JW, editors: *Smith's general urology,* ed 14, Norwalk, CT, 1991, Appleton and Lange.
28. Edelstein RA, Babayan RK: Managing prostate cancer. I. Localized disease, *Hosp Prac* 28:61, 1993.
29. Taylor TK: Endocrine therapy for advanced stage D prostate cancer, *Urol Nurs* 11:22, 1991.
30. Moore S and others: Nerve-sparing prostatectomy, *Am J Nurs* 92:59, 1992.
31. Edelstein RA, Babayan RK: Managing prostate cancer. II. Disseminated disease, *Hosp Pract* 28:25, 1993.
32. Polomano RC: Quality of life issues with metastatic prostate cancer, *Innov Urol Nurs* 2:2, 1991.
33. Smith DB, Babaian RJ: The effect of treatment for cancer on male fertility and sexuality, *Cancer Nurs* 15:271, 1992.
34. Fallon B, Williams RD: Current options in the management of clinical stage C prostatic carcinoma, *Urol Clin North Am* 17:853, 1990.
35. National Cancer Institute, *Cancer of the prostate: research report,* NIH Pub No 91-528, Bethesda, MD, 1990, National Institutes of Health.
36. Razanauzskas M, Hoebler L: Treating prostate cancer with cryosurgery, *Nursing* 94:66, 1994.
37. Kumasaka LM, Dungan JM: Nursing strategy for initial emotional response to cancer diagnosis, *Cancer Nurs* 16:296, 1993.
38. Thin RN: Diagnosis of prostatitis: a review, *Genitourin Med* 67:279, 1991.

39. Cunha BA, Marx J, Gingrich D: Managing prostatitis in the elderly, *Geriatrics* 46:60, 1991.
40. Sugar EC, Hoyler-Grant C: Disorders of the external genitalia in children. In Karlowicz DA, editor: *Urologic nursing: principles and practice,* Philadelphia, 1994, Saunders.
41. American Academy of Pediatrics: Report of task force on circumcision, *Pediatrics* 84:388, 1989.
42. Winter CC: Priapism. In Glenn JF, editor: *Urologic surgery,* ed 4, Philadelphia, 1991, JB Lippincott.
43. Devine PC: Peyronies' disease. In Glenn JF, editor: *Urologic surgery,* ed 4, Philadelphia, 1991, Lippincott.
44. Burgers JK, Badalament RA, Drago JR: Penile cancer: clinical presentation, diagnosis and staging, *Urol Clin North Am* 19:247, 1992.
45. Schellhammer PF, Jordan GH, Schlossberg SM: Tumors of the penis. In Walsh PC and others, editors: *Campbell's urology,* ed 6, Philadelphia, 1992, Saunders.
46. Kogan S: Cryptorchidism. In Kelalis PP, King LR, Belman AB, editors: *Clinical pediatric urology,* ed 3, Philadelphia, 1992, Saunders.
47. Parsch EM and others: Semen parameters and conception rates after surgical treatment and sclerotherapy of varicocele, *Andrologia* 22:275, 1990.
48. Giroux J: Urinary tract infections in adults. In Karlowicz KA, editor: *Urologic nursing: principles and practice,* Philadelphia, 1995, Saunders.
49. Richie JP: Detection and treatment of testicular cancer, *Cancer* 43:151, 1993.
50. National Institutes of Health: *Impotence, NIH consensus statement,* Bethesda, MD, 1992, National Institutes of Health. 10(4).
51. Meredith CE: Erectile dysfunction. In Karlowicz KA, editor: *Urologic nursing: principles and practice,* Philadelphia, 1995, Saunders.
52. Thibodeau GA, Patton KT: *Anatomy and physiology,* ed 2, St Louis, 1993, Mosby.
53. Lue TF: Erectile impotence: diagnostic methods, *Prob Urol* 5:520, 1991.
54. Bennett AH, Carpenter AJ, Barada JA: An improved vasoactive drug combination for a pharmacological erection program, *J Urol* 146:1564, 1991.
55. Virag R and others: Intracavernous self-injection of vasoactive drugs in the treatment of impotence: 8 year experience with 615 cases, *J Urol* 145:287, 1991.
56. Benard F, Lue TF: Self-administration in the pharmacological treatment of impotence, *Drugs* 39:394, 1990.
57. Cookson MS, Nadig PW: Long-term results with vacuum constriction device, *J Urol* 14:290, 1993.
58. Petrou SP, Barrett DM: Current penile prosthesis available for the treatment of erectile dysfunction, *Prob Urol* 5:594, 1991.
59. Furlow WL, Knoll LD: Arteriogenic impotence: diagnosis and management, *Prob Urol* 5:577, 1991.
60. Elmer-Dewitt P: Making babies, *Time* 138:57, 1991.

SECTION X BIBLIOGRAPHY

Books

Boston Women's Health Book Collective: *The new our bodies, ourselves. A book by and for women,* New York, 1992, Simon & Schuster.

Conte JE, Barriere SL: *Manual of antibiotics and infectious diseases,* ed 7, Philadelphia, 1992, Lea & Febiger.

Davidson JK: *Clinical diabetes mellitus: a problem oriented approach,* ed 2, New York, 1993, Thieme Medical.

Davita VT, Hellman S, Rosenberg SA, editors: *Cancer: principles and practice,* ed 4, Philadelphia, 1993, JB Lippincott.

Glass RH, editor: *Office gynecology,* ed 4, Baltimore, 1993, Williams & Wilkins.

Griffin JE, Ojeda RO: *Textbook of endocrine physiology,* ed 2, New York, 1992, Oxford University Press.

Jawetz E: Antiviral chemotherapy and prophylaxis. In Katzung BG, editor: *Basic and clinical pharmacology,* ed 5, Norwalk, CT, 1992, Appleton & Lange.

Ledger W and others, editors: *Obstetrics and gynecology,* ed 9, St Louis, 1991, Mosby.

Long JW: *The essential guide to prescription drugs,* New York, 1993, Harper Collins.

May KA, Mahlmeister LR, editors: *Comprehensive maternity nursing,* ed 3, Philadelphia, 1994, JB Lippincott.

Scott J and others: *Danforth's obstetrics and gynecology,* ed 7, Philadelphia, 1994, JB Lippincott.

Vander AJ, Sherman JH, Luciano DS: *Human physiology: the mechanisms of body function,* ed 5, New York, 1990, McGraw-Hill.

Wilson JD, Foster DM, editors: *Williams textbook of endocrinology,* ed 8, Philadelphia, 1992, WB Saunders.

Journals

Andrews EB and others: Acyclovir in pregnancy registry: six years' experience, *Obstet Gynecol* 79:7, 1992.

Boehm S and others: Behavioral analysis and behavioral strategies to improve self-management of type II diabetes, *Clin Nurs Res* 2:327, 1993.

Chantelau E and others: Outpatient treatment of unilateral diabetic foot ulcers with "half shoes," *Diabet Med* 10(3):267, 1993.

Coffland FI: Thyroid-induced cardiac disorders, *Crit Care Nurse* 13:25, 1993.

Davis ED and others: Implementing a nursing care quality program to improve diabetes patient education, *J Nurs Care Q* 6:67, 1992.

Degroote NE, Pieper B: Blood glucose monitoring at triage, *J Emerg Nurs* 19:131, 1993.

DiJanni NK, McCallum WL: A systems approach to capillary blood glucose monitoring: a joint nursing/patient education effort, *J Nurs Staff Dev* 8:175, 1992.

Edelstein EL, Cesta TG: Nursing case management: an innovative model of care for hospitalized patients with diabetes, *Diabetes Educ* 19:517, 1993.

Frenkel and others: Pharmacokinetics of acyclovir in the term human pregnancy and neonate, *Am J Obstet Gynecol* 164:569, 1991.

Govindji A: Diabetes and food—the positive approach: dietary advice for people with diabetes, *Prof Nurse* 9:561, 1994.

Gregory E: Nursing practice management: insulin-dependent diabetes mellitus, *J School Nurs* 8:44, 1992.

Haas LB: Chronic complications of diabetes mellitus, *Nurs Clin North Am* 28:71, 1993.

Haddad J and others: Oral acyclovir and recurrent genital herpes during late pregnancy, *Obstet Gynecol* 82:102, 1993.

Hentinen M, Kyngas H: Compliance of young diabetics with health regimens, *J Adv Nurs* 17:530, 1992.

Joseph DH, Patterson B: Risk taking and its influence on metabolic control: a study of adult clients with diabetes, *J Adv Nurs* 19:77, 1994.

LeMone P: Human sexuality in adults with insulin-dependent diabetes mellitus, *Image J Nurs Sch* 25:101, 1993.

Martinez NC: Diabetes and minority populations: focus on Mexican Americans, *Nurs Clin North Am* 28:87, 1993.

Meehan CD, Bove LA, Jennings AS: Comparison of first-generation and second-generation blood glucose meters for use in a hospital setting, *Diabetes Educ* 18:228, 1992.

*Shaw CR, Wilson SA, O'Brien ME: Information needs prior to breast biopsy, *Clin Nurs Res* 3:119, 1994.

*Nursing research-based article.

Thompson A, Gibbon C: Setting standards in diabetes education, *Nurs Stand* 7:25, 1993.

Walton J, Brand S: Diabetes mellitus: implications for nursing care, *Br J Nurs* 3:442, 1994.

Organizations

American Association of Diabetes Educators
500 N. Michigan Avenue
Suite 1400
Chicago, IL 60611

American College of Nurse-Midwives
1522 K Street, NW, Suite 1000
Washington, DC 20005

American Diabetes Association
505 8th Avenue
New York, NY 10018

American Diabetes Association
National Service Center
1660 Duke Street
Alexandria, VA 22314

Juvenile Diabetes Foundation
23 East 26th Street
New York, NY 10010

Nurse Association of the American College of Obstetricians and Gynecologists
409 12th Street, SW
Washington, DC 20024

AHCPR Guidelines

Guide developed and published by The Agency for Health Care Policy and Research (AHCPR). The Patient Guides are available in English and Spanish. The guidelines can be obtained by writing to: Center for Research Dissemination and Liaison, AHCPR Clearinghouse, P.O. Box 8547, Silver Spring, MD 20907, or by calling 1-800-358-9295. The Guidelines are as follows:

Benign prostatic hyperplasia: diagnosis and treatment. Clinical Practice Guideline. AHCPR Pub. No. 92-0582.

Benign prostatic hyperplasia: diagnosis and treatment. Quick Reference Guide for Clinicians. AHCPR Pub No 92-0583.

Treating your enlarged prostate. A Patient's Guide. AHCPR Pub No 92-0584.

Quality determinants of mammography. Guideline overview, AHCPR Pub No 95-0630.

High-quality mammography: information for referring providers. Quick reference guide for clinicians, AHCPR Pub No 95-0633.

Things to know about quality mammograms. A woman's guide, 950634.

Acute low back problems in adults. Guideline overview, 950640.

Acute low back problems in adults: Assessment and treatment. Quick reference guide for clinicians, 950643.

Understanding acute low back problems. Patient guide, 950644.

Problems Related to Movement and Coordination

Section Eleven

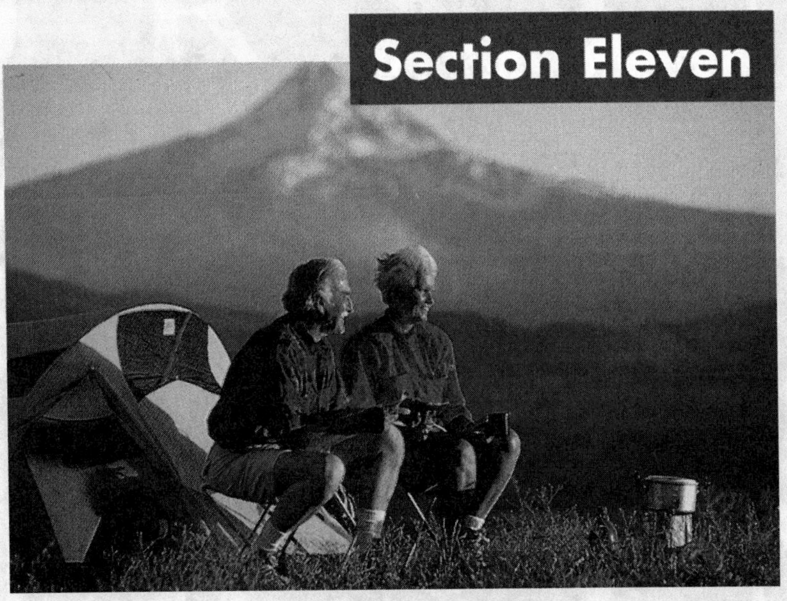

Chapter 53

NURSING ASSESSMENT
Nervous System

Judith M. Ozuna

Learning Objectives

1. Describe the functions of neurons and neuroglia.
2. Explain the electrochemical aspects of nerve impulse transmission.
3. Explain the anatomic location and functions of the cerebrum, brainstem, cerebellum, spinal cord, peripheral nerves, and cerebrospinal fluid.
4. Identify the major arteries supplying the brain.
5. Describe the functions of the 12 cranial nerves.
6. Compare the functions of the two divisions of the autonomic nervous system.
7. Describe age-related changes in the neurologic system and differences in assessment findings.
8. Identify the significant subjective and objective data related to the nervous system that should be obtained from a patient.
9. Describe the techniques used in the physical assessment of the nervous system.
10. Differentiate normal from common abnormal findings of a physical assessment of the nervous system.
11. Describe the purpose, significance of results, and nursing responsibilities related to diagnostic studies of the nervous system.

STRUCTURES AND FUNCTIONS OF THE NERVOUS SYSTEM

The human nervous system is a highly specialized system responsible for the control and integration of the body's many activities. The nervous system can be divided into the central nervous system (CNS) and the peripheral nervous system (PNS). The CNS consists of the brain and spinal cord. The PNS consists of the cranial and spinal nerves and the peripheral components of the autonomic nervous system (ANS). Before considering higher-order structures and their functions, cellular elements and nerve impulse transmission are discussed.

Cells of the Nervous System

The nervous system is made up of two types of cells, *neurons* and *neuroglia.* Although neuroglial cells are more numerous, they are mainly supportive to the neuron, the primary functional unit of the nervous system. Neurons are nonmitotic; that is, they do not replicate and cannot replace themselves if they are irreversibly damaged. Neuroglia, however, are mitotic and can replicate themselves.

Neurons. The neurons of the nervous system come in many different shapes and sizes, but they all share common characteristics: (1) excitability, or the ability to generate a nerve impulse; (2) conductivity, or the ability to transmit the impulse to other portions of the cell; and (3) the ability to influence other neurons, muscle cells, and glandular cells by transmitting nerve impulses to them.

A typical neuron consists of a cell body, an axon, and several dendrites (Fig. 53-1). The *cell body* containing the nucleus and cytoplasm is the metabolic center of the neuron. *Dendrites* are short processes extending from the cell body. They receive nerve impulses from the axons of other neurons and conduct impulses toward the cell body. The nerve *axon* projects varying distances from the cell body, ranging from several micrometers to more than a meter. Its function is to carry nerve impulses to other neurons or to end organs. The end organs are smooth and striated muscles and glands. Axons may be myelinated or unmyelinated. Many axons present in the CNS and the PNS are covered by a segmentally interrupted myelin sheath composed of a white, lipid substance that acts as an insulator for the conduction of impulses. Generally, the smaller fibers are unmyelinated.

Neuroglia. Neuroglia, or glial cells, provide support, nourishment, and protection to neurons. They comprise almost half the brain and spinal cord mass and are five to ten times more numerous than neurons. Different types of glial cells, including oligodendroglia, astrocytes, ependymal cells, and microglia, have specific functions. *Oligoden-*

Reviewed by Mary Lou Muwaswes, RN, MS, Clinical Nurse Specialist, University of California Hospital and Clinics, San Francisco, CA.

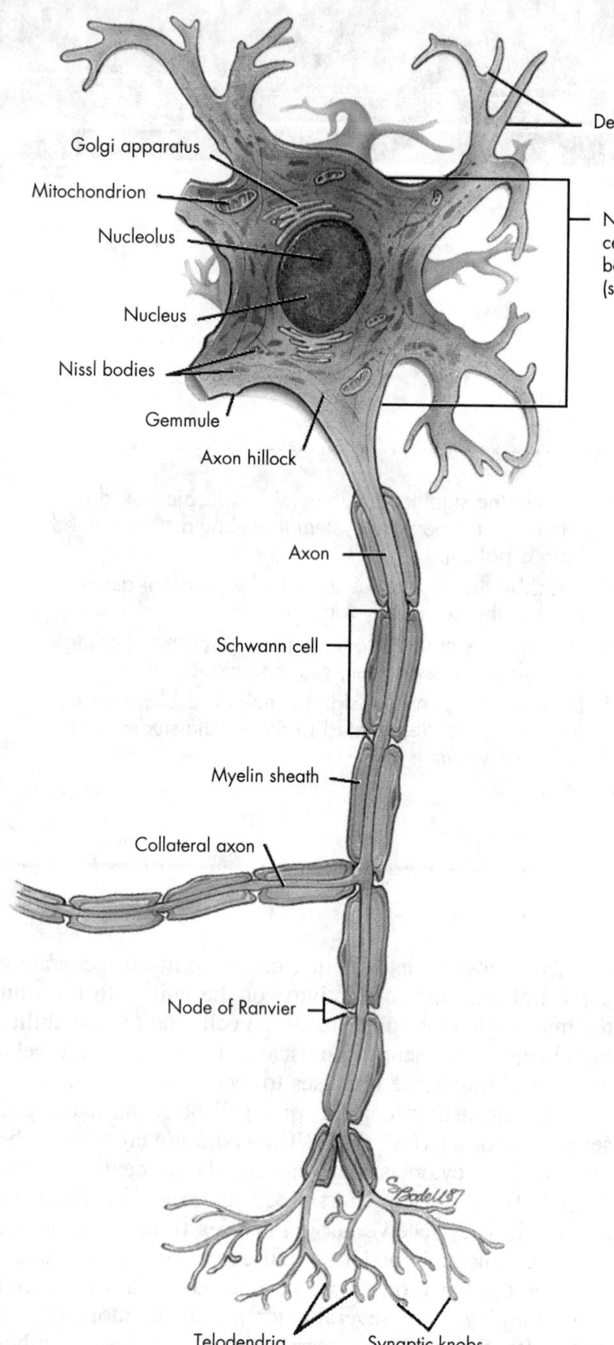

Fig. 53-1 Structural features of neurons: dendrites, cell body, and axons.

droglia produce the myelin sheath of nerve fibers in the CNS (Schwann cells myelinate the nerve fibers in the periphery) and are primarily found in the white matter of the CNS. *Astrocytes* are found primarily in gray matter; however, their physiologic importance is not well understood. They are thought to provide structural support to neurons and their delicate processes, form the blood-brain barrier with the endothelium of the blood vessels, and play an indirect role in synaptic transmission (conduction of impulses between neurons). When the brain is injured, astrocytes act as phagocytes for neuronal debris. They help to restore the neurochemical milieu as well as provide support for repair. Proliferation of astrocytes contributes to the formation of scar tissue (*gliosis*) in the CNS. *Ependymal cells* line the brain ventricles and aid in the secretion of cerebrospinal fluid. *Microglia,* a type of macrophage, are relatively rare in normal CNS tissue. They migrate to areas of CNS damage, act as phagocytes, and are important in host defense.

Most primary CNS tumors involve neuroglia. Primary malignancies involving neurons are rare because these cells are not mitotic.

Nerve Regeneration

Once a neuron dies, it is not replaced. At birth the human body contains all the nerve cells it will ever have. The body cannot make new nerve cells. If only the axon of the nerve cell is damaged, the cell attempts to repair itself. When damaged, all nerve cells attempt to grow back to their original destinations by sprouting many branches from the damaged ends of their axons. Unfortunately, axons in the CNS are less successful than peripheral axons in regenerating. This difference may be because of dense scar tissue that develops in the CNS and forms a barrier. Regenerating nerve fibers grow 4 mm per day.[1]

In the PNS (outside the brain and the spinal cord), injured nerve fibers can successfully regenerate by growing within the protective myelin sheath of the supporting Schwann cells if the cell body is intact. The final result of nerve regeneration depends on the number of axon sprouts that join with the appropriate Schwann cell columns and reinnervate appropriate end organs.[2]

Nerve Impulse

The purpose of a neuron is to initiate, receive, and process messages about events both within and outside the body. The initiation of a neuronal message (nerve impulse) involves the generation of an action potential. Once an action potential is initiated, a series of *action potentials* travel along the axon. When the impulse reaches the end of the nerve fiber, it is transmitted across the junction between nerve cells (*synapse*) by a chemical interaction involving neurotransmitters. This chemical interaction generates another set of action potentials in the next neuron. These events are repeated until the nerve impulse reaches its destination.

Action Potential. When nerve cells are in a resting (nonactive) state, the inside of the cell carries a negative electric charge relative to the outside of the cell. Sodium ions (Na^+) are in high concentration outside the cell, and potassium ions (K^+) are in high concentration inside the cell. The difference in electric charge across the cell membrane is called the *resting membrane potential* (Fig. 53-2). An action potential occurs when a stimulus is of sufficient magnitude to alter the membrane potential.

During the action potential, the cell membrane becomes more permeable to Na^+, allowing the Na^+ to move readily into the cell. The resulting change in the voltage across the

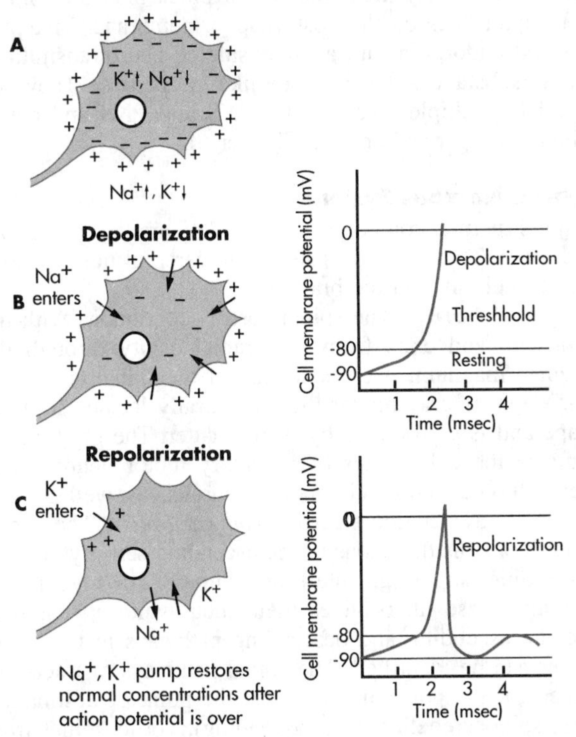

Fig. 53-2 ***A,*** Resting membrane potential. ***B,*** Depolarization. ***C,*** Repolarization.

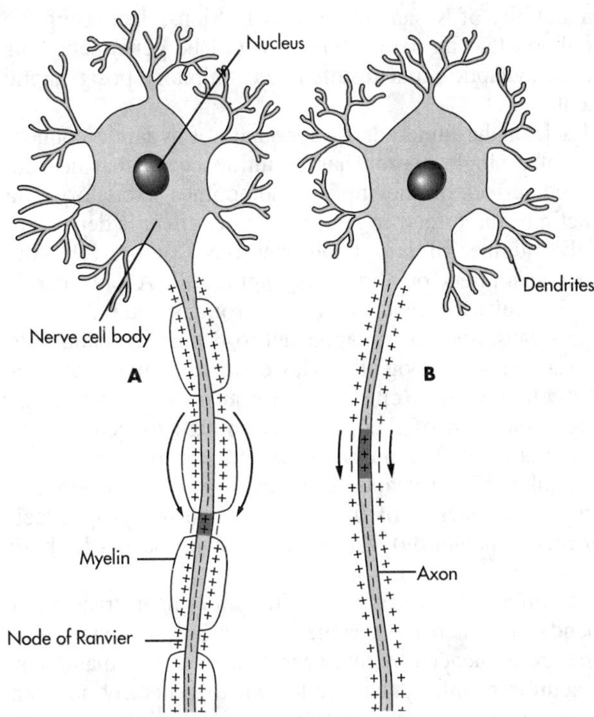

Fig. 53-3 ***A,*** Saltatory conduction in a myelinated nerve fiber. ***B,*** Depolarization in an unmyelinated fiber.

cell membrane is called *depolarization.* The inside of the cell temporarily becomes positive relative to the outside. After rapid depolarization, *repolarization* (the inside of the cell becoming negative relative to the outside) is facilitated by a slower increase in K^+ permeability, which in turn is caused by the depolarization associated with entry of Na^+ into the cell. The whole process of depolarization and repolarization of the nerve cell membrane takes only 1 to 2 milliseconds. With repeated action potentials the cells accumulate Na^+. An active metabolic process within the cell is required to move Na^+ out of and K^+ back into the cell. This metabolic process is accomplished by the Na^+- K^+ pump which requires energy from the breakdown of adenosine triphosphate (ATP).

The action potential has an all-or-none quality; that is, once the cell depolarizes enough to cause an action potential, the size of the action potential is independent of the strength of the stimulus. When an action potential is initiated at one point of a neuron, it is transmitted along the axon without losing its intensity.

Because of its insulating capacity, myelination of nerve axons facilitates the conduction of an action potential. Many peripheral nerve axons have gaps, called *nodes of Ranvier,* at regular intervals in the myelin sheath surrounding them. An action potential traveling down one of these axons hops from node to node without traversing the insulated membrane segment between nodes, making the action potential travel much faster than it would otherwise. This is called *saltatory* (hopping) *conduction.* In an unmyelinated fiber the wave of depolarization traverses the entire length of the axon, each portion of the membrane becoming depolarized in turn. Figure 53-3 compares nerve impulse transmission of myelinated and unmyelinated fibers.

Synapse. A synapse is the structural and functional junction between two neurons. It is the point at which the nerve impulse is transmitted from one neuron to another or from neuron to efferent organ. The essential structures of synaptic transmission are a *presynaptic terminal,* a *synaptic cleft,* and a *receptor site* on the postsynaptic cell (Fig. 53-4). When a nerve impulse reaches the end of the axon (presynaptic terminal), it causes release of a chemical substance (neurotransmitter) from tiny vesicles within the axon terminal. This release depends on influx of calcium (Ca^{++}), initiated by depolarization of the nerve terminal. The neurotransmitter then crosses the microscopic space (synaptic cleft) between the two neurons and attaches to receptor sites of the receiving (postsynaptic) neuron. This causes a change in the permeability of the postsynaptic cell membrane to specific ions such as Na^+ and K^+ and a change in the electric potential of the membrane.

Neurotransmitters. Neurotransmitters are chemical agents involved in the transmission of an impulse across the synaptic cleft. Some neurotransmitters are *excitatory:* they cause an increase in Na^+ permeability at the postsynaptic cell membrane, increasing the likelihood that an action potential will be generated. This type of synaptic input results in an excitatory postsynaptic potential. Other neurotransmitters are *inhibitory:* they cause an increase in permeability of K^+ and chloride (Cl^-) ions, decreasing the likelihood that an action potential will be generated. This type of synaptic input results in an inhibitory postsynaptic potential.

Each of the hundreds to thousands of synaptic connections of a single neuron has an influence on that neuron. The net effect of the input is sometimes excitatory and sometimes inhibitory. In general, the net effect is dependent on the number of presynaptic neurons that are releasing neurotransmitters on the postsynaptic cell. A presynaptic cell that releases an excitatory neurotransmitter does not always cause the postsynaptic cell to depolarize enough to generate an action potential. However, when many presynaptic cells release excitatory neurotransmitters on a single neuron, the sum of their input is enough to generate an action potential. The presynaptic input can be summed by the number of presynaptic cells firing (*spatial summation*) or by the frequency of firing of a single presynaptic cell (*temporal summation*). Summation usually occurs by both events.

The effect of an excitatory or inhibitory neurotransmitter depends on which ion channels in the postsynaptic membrane are influenced by that neurotransmitter. In mammals, the neurotransmitters that are known to generally have an excitatory influence are acetylcholine, norepinephrine, serotonin, dopamine, glutamate, and histamine. The neurotransmitters that generally have an inhibitory influence are gamma-aminobutyric acid and glycine.

Neurotransmitters continue to combine with the receptor sites at the postsynaptic membrane until they are inactivated by enzymes, are taken up by the presynaptic endings, or diffuse away from the synaptic region. In addition, neurotransmitters can be affected by drugs and toxins, which can modify their function or block their attachment to receptor sites on the postsynaptic membrane. Enkephalins and endorphins are also considered neurotransmitters. These substances have opiate-like properties. They are found in multiple areas of the CNS and PNS and act to inhibit pain perception (see Chapter 6).

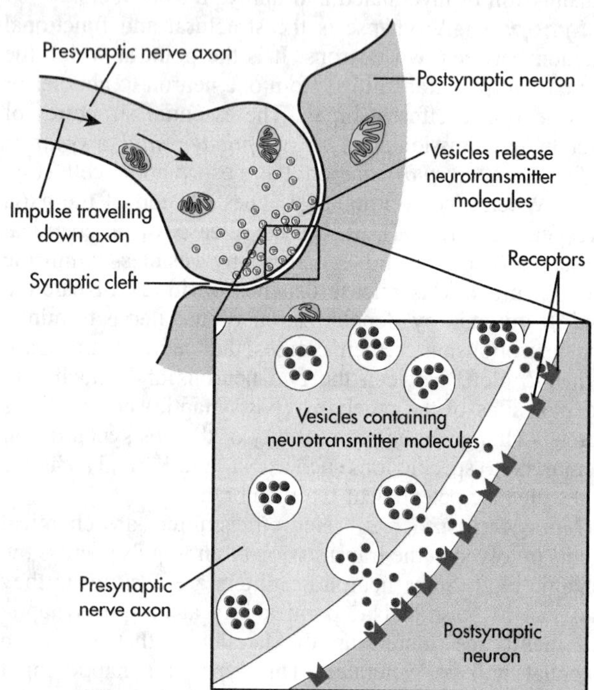

Fig. 53-4 A synapse.

Central Nervous System

Major structural components of the CNS are the spinal cord and brain. The brain consists of the cerebral hemispheres, the cerebellum, and the brainstem.

Spinal Cord. The spinal cord is continuous with the brainstem and exits from the cranial cavity through the foramen magnum. A cross section of the spinal cord (Fig. 53-5) reveals gray matter that is centrally located in an H shape and is surrounded by white matter. The gray matter contains the cell bodies of voluntary motor neurons and preganglionic autonomic motor neurons, as well as cell bodies of association neurons (*interneurons*). The white matter contains the axons of the ascending sensory and the descending (suprasegmental) motor fibers. The myelin surrounding these fibers gives them their white appearance. Specific ascending and descending pathways in the white matter can be identified. The spinal pathways or tracts are named for the point of origin and the point of destination [e.g., spinocerebellar tract (ascending), corticospinal tract (descending)]. The major spinal pathways are presented in Fig. 53-5.

Ascending tracts. In general, the ascending tracts carry specific sensory information to higher levels of the CNS. This information comes from special sensory endings (receptors) in the skin, muscles and joints, viscera, and blood vessels, and enters the spinal cord by way of the dorsal roots of the spinal nerves. The *fasciculus gracilis* and the *fasciculus cuneatus* (commonly called the *dorsal* or *posterior columns*) carry information and transmit impulses

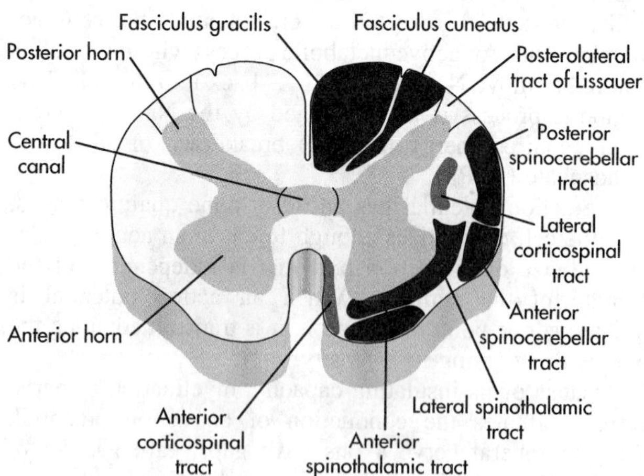

Fig. 53-5 Schematic cross section of spinal cord showing arrangement of gray matter and white matter. Major ascending (sensory) tracts of the white matter are indicated in *black;* major descending (motor) tracts are in *red.*

concerned with touch, deep pressure, vibration, position sense, and kinesthesia (appreciation of movement, weight, and body parts). The *spinocerebellar tracts* carry subconscious information about muscle tension and body position to the cerebellum for coordination of movement. This information is not consciously perceived. The *spinothalamic tracts* carry pain and temperature sensations. Therefore, the ascending tracts are organized by sensory modality as well as by anatomy.

Although the functions of these pathways are generally accepted, other ascending tracts may also carry sensory modalities. The symptoms of various neurologic diseases suggest that additional pathways for touch, position sense, and vibration exist.

Descending tracts. Descending tracts carry impulses that are responsible for muscle movement. Among the most important descending tracts are the *corticobulbar* and *corticospinal tracts,* collectively called the *pyramidal tract.* These tracts carry volitional (voluntary) impulses from the cortex to the cranial and peripheral nerves, respectively. Another group of descending motor tracts carries impulses from the *extrapyramidal system,* which includes all motor systems (except the pyramidal system) concerned with voluntary movement. It includes descending pathways originating in the brainstem, the basal ganglia, and the cerebellum. The motor output exits the spinal cord by way of the ventral roots of the spinal nerves.

Lower and upper motor neurons. *Lower motor neurons* (LMNs) are the final common pathway through which descending motor tracts influence skeletal muscle, the effector organ for movement. The cell bodies of LMNs, which send axons to innervate the skeletal muscles of the arms, trunk, and legs, are located in the anterior horn of the corresponding segments of the spinal cord (e.g., cervical segments contain LMNs for the arms). LMNs for skeletal muscles of the eyes, face, mouth, and throat are located in the corresponding segments of the brainstem. These cell bodies and their axons make up the somatic motor components of the cranial nerves. LMN lesions generally cause weakness or paralysis, denervation atrophy, hyporeflexia or areflexia, and decreased muscle tone (flaccidity).

Upper motor neurons (UMNs) include all supraspinal motor neurons that influence skeletal muscle movement. These neurons are located in the brainstem and cerebral cortex. UMN lesions generally cause weakness or paralysis, disuse atrophy, hyperreflexia, and increased muscle tone (spasticity).

Reflex arc. A reflex is defined as an involuntary response to a stimulus. The components of a monosynaptic reflex arc (the simplest kind of reflex arc) are a receptor organ, an afferent neuron, an effector neuron, and an effector organ (e.g., skeletal muscle). The afferent neuron synapses with the efferent neuron in the gray matter of the spinal cord. A reflex arc is shown in Fig. 53-6. More complex reflex arcs have other neurons (interneurons) in addition to the afferent neuron influencing the effector neuron. In the spinal cord, reflex arcs play an important role in maintaining muscle tone, which is essential for body posture.

Brain. The brain can be divided into three major components including the cerebrum, the brainstem, and the cerebellum.

Cerebrum. The cerebrum is composed of the right and left hemispheres. Both hemispheres can be further divided into four major lobes: frontal, temporal, parietal, and occipital (Fig. 53-7). These divisions are useful to delineate portions of the neocortex (gray matter), which makes up the outer layer of the cerebral hemispheres. Neurons in specific parts of the neocortex are essential for various highly complex and sophisticated aspects of mental functioning, such as language, memory, and appreciation of visual-spatial relationships.

The functions of the cerebrum are multiple and complex. Specific areas of the cerebral cortex are associated with specific functions. Table 53-1 summarizes the location and function of the parts of the cerebrum.

The *basal ganglia,* the *thalamus,* the *hypothalamus,* and the *limbic system* are also located in the cerebrum. The

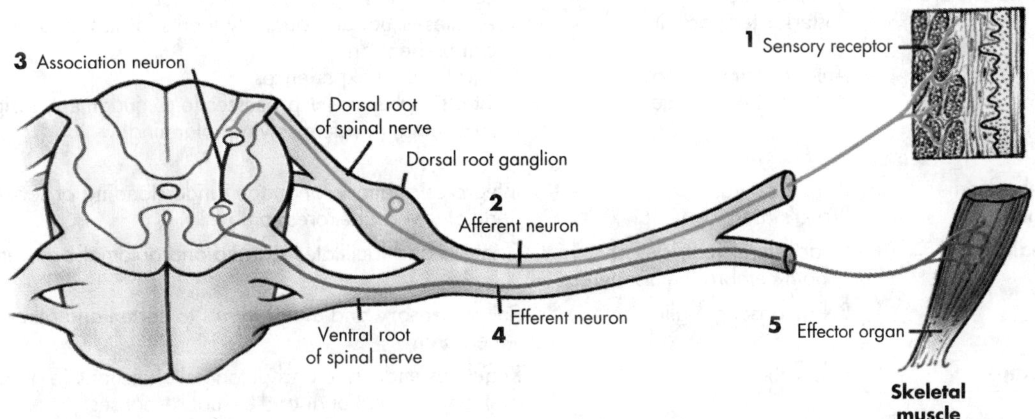

Fig. 53-6 Basic diagram of a reflex arc, including the (1) sensory receptor, (2) afferent neuron, (3) association neuron, (4) efferent neuron, and (5) effector organ.

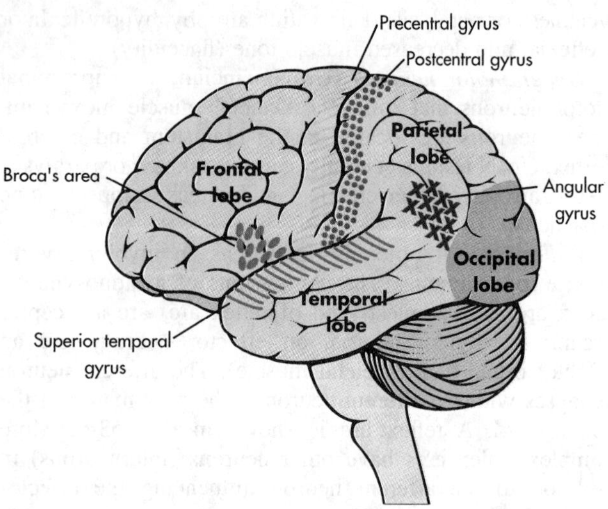

Fig. 53-7 Right hemisphere of cerebrum, lateral surface, showing major lobes and areas of the brain.

basal ganglia are a group of paired structures located centrally in the cerebrum and midbrain; most of them are on both sides of the thalamus. The function of the basal ganglia is to modulate the initiation, execution, and completion of voluntary movements and automatic movements associated with skeletal muscle activity, such as swinging of the arms while walking, swallowing saliva, and blinking.

The thalamus (part of the diencephalon) lies directly above the brainstem (Figs. 53-8 and 53-9) and is the major relay center for sensory and other afferent (i.e., cerebellar) inputs to the cerebral cortex. The hypothalamus is located just inferior to the thalamus and slightly in front of the midbrain. It regulates the autonomic nervous system and the endocrine system. The limbic system is, phylogenetically, an old part of the human cerebrum. It is located near the inner surfaces of the cerebral hemispheres (Fig. 53-10) and is concerned with emotion, aggression, feeding behavior, and sexual response.

Brainstem. The brainstem includes the *midbrain, pons,* and *medulla* (see Figs. 53-8 and 53-9). Ascending and descending fibers pass through the brainstem going to and from the cerebrum and cerebellum. The cell bodies, or nuclei, of cranial nerves III through XII are in the brainstem. Also located in the brainstem is the *reticular formation,* a diffusely arranged group of neurons and their axons that extends from the medulla to the thalamus and hypothalamus. The functions of the reticular formation include relaying sensory information, influencing excitatory and inhibitory control of spinal motor neurons, and

Table 53-1 Location and Function of the Parts of the Cerebrum

Part	Location	Function
Cortical areas		
Motor		
Primary	Precentral gyrus	Controls initiation of movement on opposite side of body
Supplemental	Anterior to precentral gyrus	Facilitates proximal muscle activity, including activity for stance and gait, and spontaneous movement and coordination
Sensory		
Somatic	Postcentral gyrus	Registers body sensations (e.g., temperature, touch, pressure, pain) from opposite side of body
Visual	Occipital lobe	Registers visual images
Auditory	Superior temporal gyrus	Registers auditory inputs
Association areas	Parietal lobe	Integrates somatic and special sensory inputs
	Posterior temporal lobe	Integrates visual and auditory inputs for language comprehension
	Anterior temporal lobe	Integrates past experiences
	Anterior frontal lobe	Controls higher-order processes (e.g., judgment, insight, reasoning, problem solving, planning)
Language		
Comprehension	Angular gyrus	Integrates auditory language (understanding of spoken words)
Expression	Broca's area	Regulates verbal expression
Basal ganglia	Near lateral ventricles of both cerebral hemispheres	Controls and facilitates learned and automatic movements
Thalamus	Below basal ganglia	Relays sensory and motor inputs to cortex and other parts of cerebrum
Hypothalamus	Below thalamus	Regulates endocrine and autonomic functions (e.g., feeding, sleeping, emotional and sexual responses)
Limbic system	Lateral to hypothalamus	Influences affective (emotional) behavior and basic drives such as feeding and sexual behavior

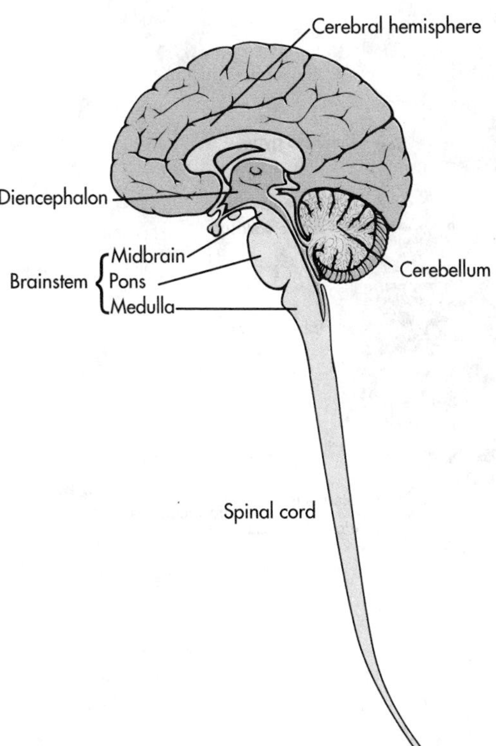

Fig. 53-8 Major divisions of the central nervous system.

controlling vasomotor and respiratory activity. The *reticular activating system* is part of a reticular formation and is the regulatory system for arousal, a component of consciousness.

The vital centers concerned with respiratory, vasomotor, and cardiac function are located in the medulla. The brainstem also contains the centers for sneezing, coughing, hiccupping, vomiting, sucking, and swallowing.

Cerebellum. The cerebellum is located in the posterior part of the cranial fossa, along with the brainstem, under the occipital lobe of the cerebrum. The function of the cerebellum is to coordinate voluntary movement and to maintain trunk stability and equilibrium. It influences motor activity through its axonal connections to the motor cortex, brainstem nuclei, and their descending pathways. To perform these functions, the cerebellum receives information from the cerebral cortex, muscles, joints, and inner ear.

Ventricles and cerebrospinal fluid. Several supporting structures located within the CNS are important in regulating neuronal function and physical support of the brain. The *ventricles* are four fluid-filled cavities within the brain that connect with one another and with the spinal canal. The lower portion of the fourth ventricle becomes the spinal canal in the lower part of the brainstem. The spinal canal is located in the center and extends the full length of the spinal cord. Figure 53-11 shows the ventricles and the flow of cerebrospinal fluid in the CNS.

The ventricles and spinal canal are filled with an average of 135 ml of *cerebrospinal fluid* (CSF). CSF circulates within the subarachnoid space that surrounds the brain, brainstem, and spinal cord. This fluid provides cushioning for the brain and spinal cord, allows fluid shifts from the cranial cavity to the spinal cavity, and carries nutrients. The formation of CSF in the choroid plexus in the ventricles seems to involve both passive diffusion and active transport of substances.[3] CSF resembles an ultrafiltrate of blood plasma. Although CSF is continually being formed, many physiologic factors influence its rate of absorption and formation.

The CSF circulates throughout the ventricles and seeps into the subarachnoid space surrounding the brain and spinal cord. It is absorbed primarily through the arachnoid villi (tiny projections into the subarachnoid space) and into

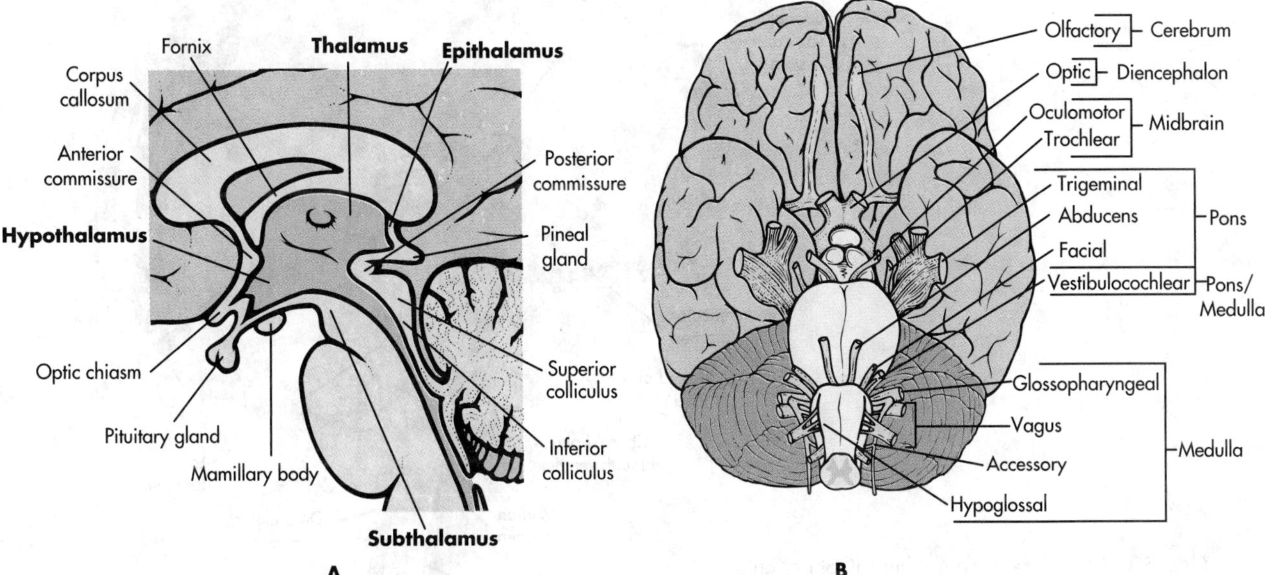

Fig. 53-9 ***A,*** Diencephalon (thalamus and hypothalamus). ***B,*** Cranial nerves.

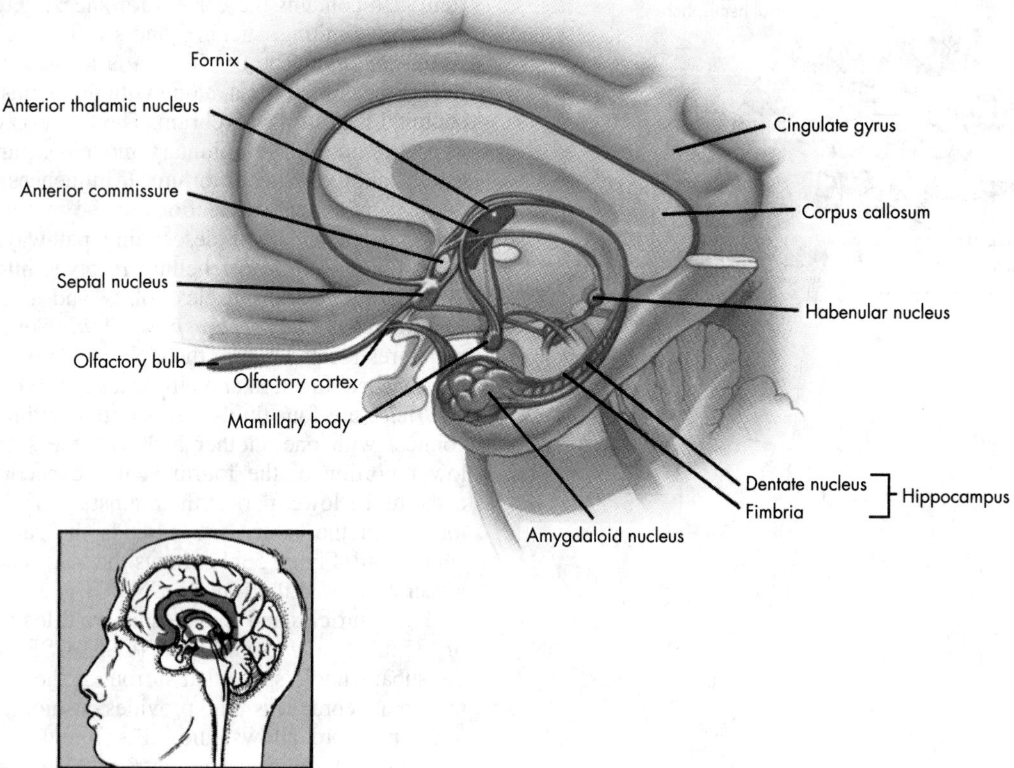

Fig. 53-10 Limbic system.

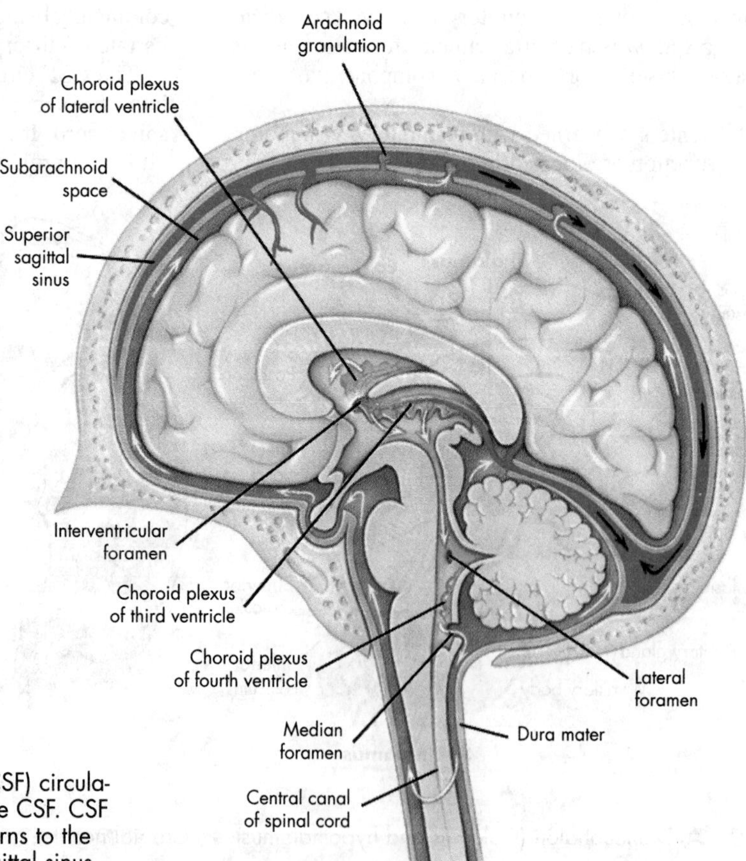

Fig. 53-11 Cerebrospinal fluid (CSF) circulation. *Arrows* represent the route of the CSF. CSF is produced in the ventricles and returns to the venous circulation in the superior sagittal sinus.

the intradural venous sinuses and eventually into the venous system. The analysis of CSF composition provides useful diagnostic information relating to certain nervous system diseases. CSF pressure is sometimes measured in patients with actual or suspected intracranial diseases. Increases in intracranial pressure, indicated by increased CSF pressure, can lead to herniation of the brain and compression of vital brainstem structures. The signs marking this event are part of the herniation syndrome (see Chapter 54).

Peripheral Nervous System

The PNS includes all the neuronal structures that lie outside the CNS. It consists of the spinal and cranial nerves, their associated ganglia (groupings of cell bodies), and portions of the ANS.

Spinal Nerves. The spinal cord can be seen as a series of spinal segments, one on top of another. In addition to the cell bodies, each segment contains a pair of dorsal (afferent) sensory nerve fibers or roots and ventral (efferent) motor fibers or roots, which innervate a specific region of the neck, trunk, or limbs. This combined motor-sensory nerve is called a *spinal nerve* (Fig. 53-12). The cell bodies of the voluntary motor system are located in the anterior horn of the spinal cord gray matter. The cell bodies of the autonomic (involuntary) motor system are located in the anterolateral portion of spinal cord gray matter. The cell bodies of sensory fibers are located in the dorsal root ganglia just outside the spinal cord. On exiting the spinal column, each spinal nerve divides into *ventral and dorsal rami,* a collection of motor and sensory fibers that eventually goes to peripheral structures (e.g., skin, muscles, viscera). The sympathetic ganglia are attached to the ventral rami of the spinal nerves by gray and white *rami communicans.*

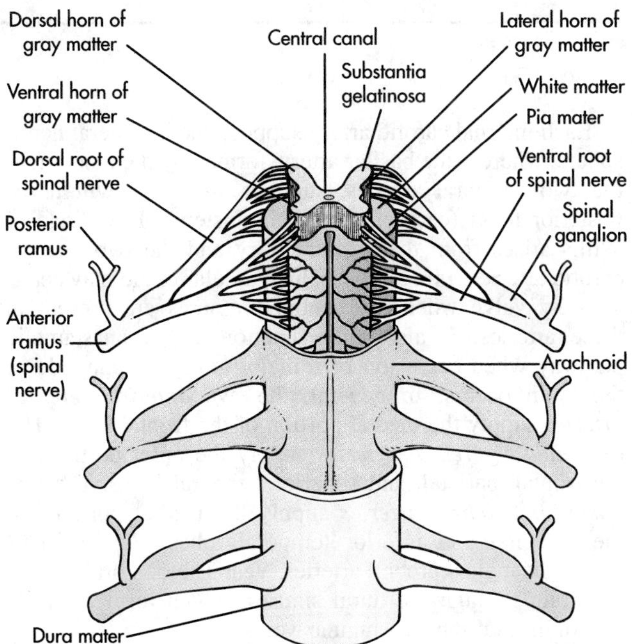

Fig. 53-12 Cross section of spinal cord showing attachments of spinal nerves.

A *dermatome* is the area of skin innervated by the sensory fibers of a single dorsal root of a spinal nerve. A *myotome* is a muscle group innervated by the primary motor neurons of a single ventral root. These are simple components in the embryonic stage of human development. However, the dermatomes and myotomes of a given spinal segment overlap with those of adjacent segments in the adult because of the development of ascending and descending collateral branches of nerve fibers. The dermatomes give a general picture of somatic sensory innervation by spinal segments.

Cranial Nerves. The cranial nerves (CNs) are the 12 paired nerves composed of cell bodies with fibers that exit from the cranial cavity. Unlike the spinal nerves, which always have both afferent sensory and efferent motor fibers, some CNs have only afferent and some only efferent fibers; others have both. Table 53-2 summarizes the motor and sensory components of the CNs. Figure 53-9 shows the position of the CNs in relation to the brain and spinal cord. Just as the cell bodies of the spinal nerves are located in specific segments of the spinal cord, so are the cell bodies (nuclei) of the cranial nerves located in specific segments of the brain. Exceptions are the nuclei of the olfactory and optic nerves. The primary cell bodies of the olfactory nerve are located in the nasal epithelium and those of the optic nerve are in the retina. CN XI is a spinal nerve, and its efferent fibers migrate upward before exiting the neuroaxis at the level of the medulla.

Autonomic Nervous System. The ANS governs involuntary functions of cardiac muscle, smooth (involuntary) muscle, and glands. Until recently it was thought that these functions could not be consciously controlled. However, research in biofeedback and studies of Asian cultures indicate that many of these "involuntary" functions can be voluntarily affected.

The ANS is divided into two components, *sympathetic* and *parasympathetic,* which are anatomically as well as functionally different. These two systems function together to maintain a relatively balanced internal environment. The ANS is primarily considered an efferent system and consists of preganglionic nerves and postganglionic nerves.

The preganglionic cell bodies of the sympathetic nervous system (SNS) are located in spinal segments T1 to L2. The sympathetic ganglia, which contain the cell bodies of the postganglionic neurons, lie close to the spinal column, along the vertebral bodies in the rami communicans. These ganglia and the connecting nerves are called the *paravertebral chain.* The major neurotransmitter released by the postganglionic fibers of the SNS is norepinephrine, whereas the neurotransmitter released by the preganglionic fibers is acetylcholine.

In contrast, the preganglionic cell bodies of the parasympathetic nervous system (PSNS) are located in the brainstem and in the sacral spinal segments (S2 to S4). The parasympathetic ganglia are located in or near the structures that they innervate. Acetylcholine is the neurotransmitter released at both preganglionic and postganglionic nerve endings.

The ANS provides dual and often reciprocal innervation to many structures. For example, the SNS increases the rate

Table 53-2 Cranial Nerves

Nerve	Connection with Brain	Function
I. Olfactory nerves and tract	Anterior ventral cerebrum	Sensory: from olfactory epithelium of superior nasal cavity
II. Optic nerve	Lateral geniculate body of the thalamus	Sensory: from retina of eyes
III. Oculomotor nerve	Midbrain	Motor: to four eye-movement muscles and levator palpebrae Parasympathetic: smooth muscle in eyeball
IV. Trochlear nerve	Midbrain	Motor: to one eye-movement muscle, the superior oblique
V. Trigeminal nerve		
Ophthalmic branch	Pons	Sensory: from forehead, eye, superior nasal cavity
Maxillary branch	Pons	Sensory: from inferior nasal cavity, face, upper teeth, mucosa of superior mouth
Mandibular branch	Pons	Sensory: from surfaces of jaw, lower teeth, mucosa of lower mouth, and anterior tongue Motor: to muscles of mastication
VI. Abducens nerve	Pons	Motor: to one eye-movement muscle, the lateral rectus
VII. Facial nerve	Junction of pons and medulla	Motor: to facial muscles of expression and cheek muscle, the buccinator
VIII. Vestibulocochlear nerve	Junction of pons and medulla	Sensory: taste from anterior two thirds of tongue
Vestibular branch		Sensory: from equilibrium sensory organ, the vestibular apparatus
Cochlear branch	Junction of pons and medulla	Sensory: from auditory sensory organ, the cochlea
IX. Glossopharyngeal nerve	Medulla	Sensory: from pharynx and posterior tongue, including taste Motor: superior pharyngeal muscles
X. Vagus nerve	Medulla	Sensory: much of viscera of thorax and abdomen Motor: larynx and middle and inferior pharyngeal muscles Parasympathetic: heart, lungs, most of digestive system
XI. Accessory nerve	Medulla and superior spinal segments	Motor: to several neck muscles, sternocleidomastoid and trapezius
XII. Hypoglossal nerve	Medulla	Motor: to intrinsic and extrinsic muscles of tongue

From Guyton AG: *Basic neuroscience: anatomy and physiology,* Philadelphia, 1991, Saunders.

and force of the heart contraction, and the PSNS decreases the rate and force. The SNS dilates bronchi and bronchioles of the lungs, and the PSNS constricts them. Some structures are innervated by only one system (e.g., the hair follicles and the sweat glands, which are innervated only by the SNS). Table 53-3 compares the SNS and PSNS.

The result of SNS stimulation is activation of mechanisms required for the "fight or flight" response that occurs throughout the body. In contrast, the PSNS is geared to act in localized and discrete regions. It serves to conserve and restore the energy stores of the body.

Cerebral Circulation

The blood supply of the brain arises from the *internal carotid arteries* (anterior circulation) and the *vertebral arteries* (posterior circulation), which are shown in Fig. 53-13. Knowledge of the distribution of the major arteries of the brain and the area supplied is essential for understanding and evaluating the signs and symptoms of cerebral vascular disease and trauma.

Each internal carotid artery supplies the ipsilateral hemisphere, whereas the basilar artery, formed by the junction of the two vertebral arteries, supplies structures within the posterior fossa (cerebellum and brainstem). The Circle of Willis arises from the basilar artery and the two internal carotid arteries (Fig. 53-14). This vascular circle may act as a safety valve when differential pressures are present in these arteries. It also may function as an anastamotic pathway when occlusion of a major artery on one side of the brain occurs. In general, the two *anterior cerebral arteries* supply the medial portion of the frontal lobes. The two *middle cerebral arteries* supply the outer portions of the frontal, parietal, and superior temporal lobes. The two *posterior cerebral arteries* supply the medial portions of the occipital and inferior temporal lobes. Figure 53-13 shows the major cerebral arteries. Venous blood drains from the brain through the dural sinuses, which form channels that drain into the two jugular veins.

Blood-Brain Barrier. The blood-brain barrier is a physiologic barrier between blood capillaries and brain tis-

Table 53-3 Effect of Sympathetic and Parasympathetic Nervous Systems

Visceral Effector	Effect of Sympathetic Nervous System*	Effect of Parasympathetic Nervous System†
Heart	Increase in rate and strength of heartbeat (β receptors)	Decrease in rate and strength of heartbeat
Smooth muscle of blood vessels		
Skin blood vessels	Constriction (α receptors)	No parasympathetic fibers
Skeletal muscle blood vessels	Dilatation (β receptors)	No parasympathetic fibers
Coronary blood vessels	Dilatation (β receptors)	No parasympathetic fibers
Abdominal blood vessels	Constriction (α receptors)	No parasympathetic fibers
Blood vessels of external genitals	Ejaculation (contraction of smooth muscle in male ducts [e.g., epididymis, ductus deferens])	Dilatation of blood vessels causing erection in male
Smooth muscle of hollow organs and sphincters		
Bronchi	Dilatation (β receptors)	Constriction
Digestive tract, except sphincters	Decrease in peristalsis (β receptors)	Increase in peristalsis
Sphincters of digestive tract	Contraction (α receptors)	Relaxation
Urinary bladder	Relaxation (β receptors)	Contraction
Urinary sphincters	Contraction (α receptors)	Relaxation
Eye		
Iris	Contraction of radial muscle, dilatation of pupil	Contraction of circular muscle, constriction of pupil
Ciliary	Relaxation, accommodation for far vision	Contraction, accommodation for near vision
Hairs (pilomotor muscles)	Contraction producing goose pimples or piloerection (α receptors)	No parasympathetic fibers
Glands		
Sweat	Increase in sweat (neurotransmitter, acetylcholine)	No parasympathetic fibers
Digestive (e.g., salivary, gastric)	Decrease in secretion of saliva; not known for others	Increase in secretion of saliva and gastric HCl acid
Pancreas, including islets	Decrease in secretion	Increase in secretion of pancreatic juice and insulin
Liver	Increase in glycogenolysis (β receptors), increase in blood glucose level	No parasympathetic fibers
Adrenal medulla‡	Increase in epinephrine secretion	No parasympathetic fibers

Modified from Thibodeau GA, Patton KT: *Anatomy and physiology,* ed 2, St Louis, 1993, Mosby.
*Neurotransmitter is norepinephrine unless otherwise stated.
†Neurotransmitter is acetylcholine unless otherwise stated.
‡Sympathetic preganglionic axons terminate in contact with secreting cells of the adrenal medulla. Thus the adrenal medulla functions as a "giant sympathetic postganglionic neuron."

sue. The structure of brain capillaries differs from that of other capillaries. Some substances that normally pass readily into most tissues are prevented from entering brain tissue. This barrier protects the brain from certain potentially harmful agents, while allowing nutrients and gases to enter. Because the blood-brain barrier affects the penetration of pharmaceutical agents, only certain drugs can enter the CNS from the bloodstream. Lipid-soluble compounds enter the brain easily, whereas water-soluble and ionized drugs enter the brain and spinal cord slowly. Damage to the blood-brain barrier results in the penetration of drugs and other substances into brain tissue.

Protective Structures

Meninges. The meninges are three layers of protective membranes that surround the brain and spinal cord. The thick *dura mater* forms the outermost layer, with the *arachnoid layer* and *pia mater* being the next two layers. The falx cerebri is a fold of the dura that separates the two cerebral hemispheres and prevents expansion of brain tissue in situations such as the presence of a rapidly growing tumor or acute hemorrhage. The expanding brain must squeeze under this structure, causing displacement toward the side opposite the lesion. The *tentorium cerebelli* is a fold of dura that separates the cerebral hemispheres from

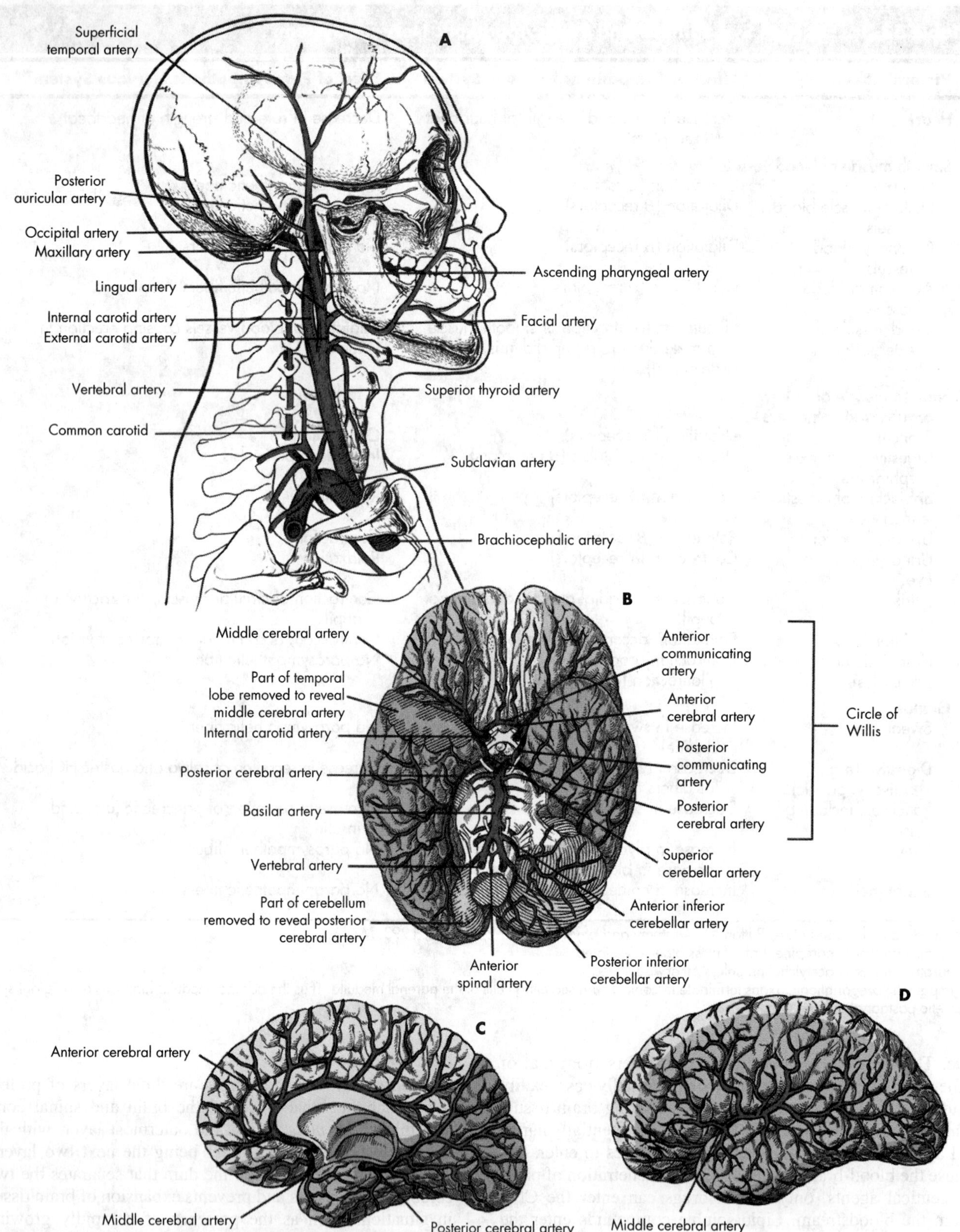

Fig. 53-13 Arteries of the head and neck. ***A,*** The brachiocephalic artery, the right common carotid artery, the right subclavian artery, and their branches. The major arteries to the head are the common carotid and vertebral arteries. ***B,*** Inferior view of the brain showing the vertebral, basilar, and internal carotid arteries and their branches. ***C,*** Medial view of the brain showing middle, anterior, and posterior cerebral arteries. ***D,*** Lateral view of the brain showing the distribution of the middle cerebral artery. (***B*** to ***D***: Colors indicate brain regions supplied by various arteries—*yellow,* anterior cerebral; *orange,* middle cerebral; *purple,* posterior cerebral.)

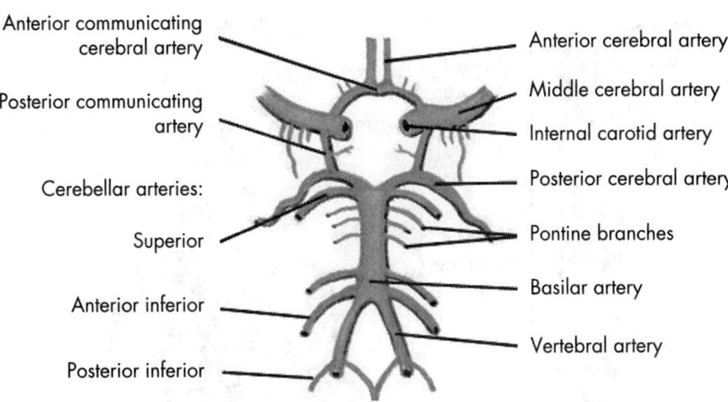

Fig. 53-14 Arteries at the base of the brain. The arteries that compose the Circle of Willis are the two anterior cerebral arteries joined to each other by the anterior communicating cerebral artery and to the posterior cerebral arteries by the posterior communicating arteries.

the posterior fossa (which contains the brainstem and cerebellum). Expansion of mass lesions in the cerebrum forces the brain to herniate through the opening created by the brainstem. This is referred to as *tentorial herniation.*

The arachnoid layer is a delicate, impermeable membrane that lies between the thick dura mater and the pia mater and directly covers the brain and spinal cord. The subarachnoid space lies between the arachnoid layer and the pia mater. This space is filled with CSF. Structures passing to and from the brain and the skull or its foramina (holes through which blood vessels and nerves enter and exit the intracranial compartment) must pass through the subarachnoid space. Therefore all cerebral arteries and veins lie in this space, as do the cranial nerves. A larger subarachnoid space is present in the region of the third and fourth lumbar vertebrae, which is the area penetrated to obtain CSF during a lumbar puncture. (The spinal cord itself ends between the first and second lumbar vertebrae.)

Skull. The bony skull protects the brain from external trauma. It is composed of 8 cranial bones and 14 facial bones. The structure of the skull cavity explains the physiology of head injuries (see Chapter 54). Although the top and sides of the inside of the skull are relatively smooth, the bottom surface is uneven. It has many ridges, prominences, and foramina. The largest hole is the *foramen magnum,* through which the brainstem extends to the spinal cord. This foramen offers the only major space for the expansion of brain contents when increased intracranial pressure occurs.

Vertebral Column. The vertebral column protects the spinal cord, supports the head, and provides for flexibility. The vertebral column is made up of 33 individual vertebrae: 7 cervical, 12 thoracic, 5 lumbar, 5 sacral (fused into one), and 4 coccygeal (fused into one). Each vertebra has a central opening through which the spinal cord passes. The vertebrae are held together by a series of ligaments. Intervertebral disks occupy the spaces between vertebrae. Figure 53-15 shows the vertebral column in relation to the trunk.

Effects of Aging on the Nervous System

The high rate of metabolic activity of neurons and their inability to replicate make them particularly vulnerable to change over time. One associated age-related change involves the decline in brain concentration of neurotransmitter substances. Age-related changes in the biosynthetic capabilities of neurons affect neurotransmitter levels and neuronal activity. Changes in the neuronal membranes influence the interaction of neurotransmitters with their receptors.[4]

Across the life span, brain weight decreases from loss of neurons. The number of synapses, axons, and dendrites also decreases. There is a decrease in cerebral blood flow. In addition, CSF production declines. Clinically relevant changes are decreases in memory, vision, hearing, taste, smell, vibration and position senses, muscle strength, and reaction time.[5]

Changes in assessment findings result from age-related alterations in the various components of the nervous system. Table 53-4 lists these alterations and associated assessment changes.

ASSESSMENT OF THE NERVOUS SYSTEM

Subjective Data

Important Health Information

Past health history. Three points should be considered in taking the history of a patient with neurologic problems.[6] The first is to avoid suggesting symptoms to the patient. Caution must be used not to suggest certain symptoms to the patient or ask leading questions such as "Is your headache throbbing?" or "Are you weak on the right side?" It is better to ask open-ended questions such as "What is your headache like?" or "Is there anything about your right side that bothers you?" A second point is that the mode of onset and the course of the illness are especially important aspects of the history. Often the nature of a neurologic disease process can be described by these facts alone, and the nurse should elicit all pertinent data in the history of the present illness, especially data related to the characteristics and progression of the symptoms. The third point is that because many neurologic diseases affect a patient's mental functioning, mental status must be accurately assessed before assuming that the history is factual. If the patient is not considered a reliable historian, the health history should be obtained from a person who has firsthand knowledge of the patient's problems and complaints. In many instances a health history cannot be obtained, and the clinician must proceed with objective data only.

The health history helps guide the approach for the neurologic examination; that is, it can direct the clinician toward the parts of the nervous system that need to be closely assessed. If the patient's primary complaint is dizziness, the examination may be focused on visual, vestibular, and cerebellar functions rather than on somatic motor and sensory functions.

Many complaints, including behavioral changes, alteration in level of consciousness, developmental problems, paroxysmal disorders, infectious processes, pain, motor or sensory aberrations, and trauma, should alert the clinician

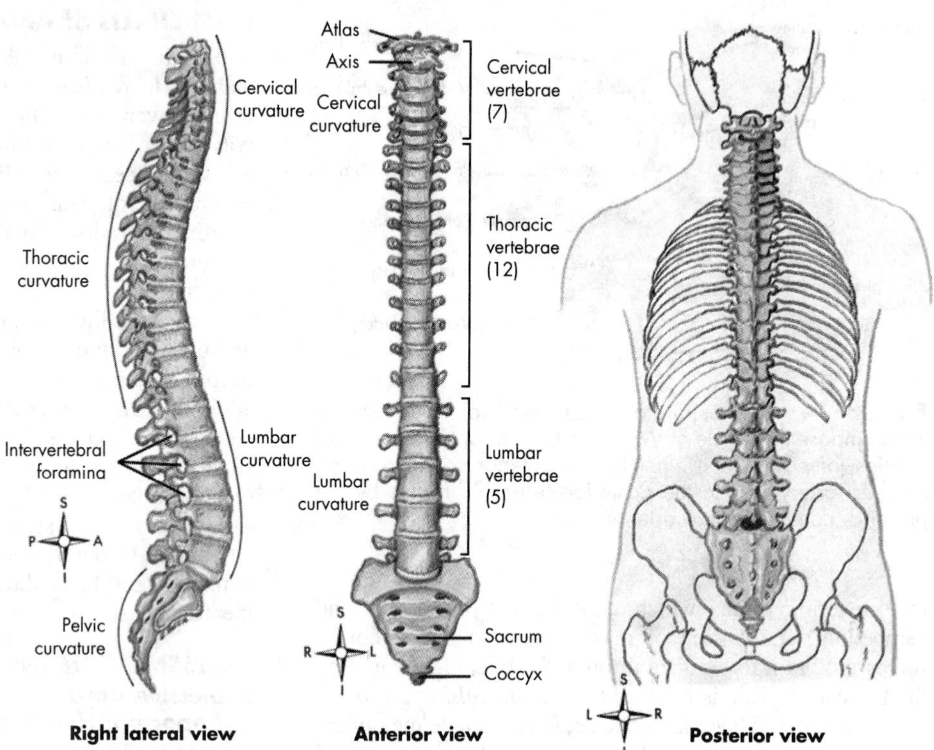

Fig. 53-15 The vertebral column (*three views*).

to the need for a detailed neurologic examination. In addition to being a primary complaint, neurologic problems often result from other problems, such as alcoholism or metastatic lesions.

When eliciting data about the health history, the nurse should ask the patient specific questions about diabetes mellitus, pernicious anemia, cancer, infections, thyroid disease, substance abuse, and hypertension because these conditions can affect the nervous system. Any hospitalizations, injuries, or surgeries related to the nervous system should be noted.

Medications. Particular attention should be given to eliciting a careful medication history, especially the use of sedatives, narcotics, tranquilizers, and mood-elevating drugs. If the patient experiences dizziness as a side effect of a medication, it should be noted. If the drug cannot be changed, the patient will need to be instructed in strategies to cope with dizziness and prevent falls.

Many patients with neurologic problems will be taking antiseizure medications such as phenytoin (Dilantin), carbamazepine (Tegretol), and phenobarbital. The nurse should inquire about the occurrence of common side effects such as diplopia, drowsiness, ataxia, and mental slowing.

If the patient experiences headaches, the medications taken most commonly for the problem should be investigated. Many headache medications have potentially dangerous side effects such as gastric bleeding and coagulation abnormalities. The occurrence of these side effects should be noted.

Surgery or other treatment. The nurse should inquire about any surgery involving any part of the nervous system such as the head, spine, or sensory organs. If a patient had surgery, the date, cause, procedure, convalescence, and current status should be investigated.

The perinatal history may reveal exposure to toxic agents such as viruses, alcohol, tobacco, drugs, and radiation, which are known to adversely influence the development of the nervous system. The history may reveal a difficult labor and delivery, which can cause brain damage as a result of hypoxia, forceps delivery, or Rh incompatibility. If the patient is elderly, this line of questioning may be unnecessary.

Growth and developmental history can be important in ascertaining whether nervous system dysfunction was present at an early age. The nurse should specifically inquire about major developmental tasks such as walking and talking. Success at school or identified problems in an educational setting are other important developmental data to gather. Often this information is not available when the older patient is interviewed. If the patient cannot provide a detailed developmental history, the nurse should proceed with the history gathering and avoid distressing the patient by further probing.

Functional Health Patterns. Key questions to ask a patient with a neurologic problem are presented in Table 53-5.

Health perception–health management pattern. The nurse should ask about the patient's health practices related to the nervous system, such as avoidance of substance abuse and smoking, maintenance of adequate nutrition, safe participation in physical and recreational activities, use of seat belts and helmets, and control of hypertension. The nurse should ask about previous hospitalizations for neurologic problems. A careful family history may determine whether

Table 53-4 Gerontologic Differences in Assessment: Nervous System

Component	Changes	Differences in Assessment Findings
Central Nervous System		
Brain*	Reduction in cerebral blood flow and metabolism	Alterations in selected mental functioning
	Decrease in efficiency of temperature-regulating mechanism	Decrease in body temperature, impairment of ability to adapt to environmental temperature
	Decrease in neurotransmitter content, disruption in integration as result of loss of neurons	Repetitive movements, tremors
	Decrease in oxygen supply, changes in basal ganglia caused by vascular changes	Changes in gait and ambulation (e.g., extrapyramidal, Parkinson-like gait); diminished kinesthetic sense
Peripheral Nervous System		
Cranial and spinal nerves	Loss of myelin and decrease in conduction time in some nerves	Decrease in reaction time in specific nerves
	Cellular degeneration, death of neurons	Decrease in speed and intensity of neuronal reflexes
Functional Divisions		
Motor	Decrease in muscle bulk	Diminished strength and agility
	Decrease in electrical activity	Decrease in reactions and movement time
Sensory†	Decrease in sensory receptors caused by degenerative changes and involution of fine corpuscles of nerve endings	Diminished sense of touch; inability to localize stimuli; decrease in appreciation of touch, temperature, and peripheral vibrations
	Decrease in electrical activity	Slowing of or alteration in sensory reception
	Atrophy of taste buds	Signs of malnutrition, weight loss
	Degeneration and loss of fibers in olfactory bulb	Diminished sense of smell
	Degenerative changes in nerve cells in vestibular system of inner ear, cerebellum, and proprioceptive pathways in nervous system	Poor ability to maintain balance, widened gait
Reflexes	Possible decrease in deep tendon reflexes	Below-average reflex score
	Decrease in sensory conduction velocity as result of myelin sheath degeneration	Sluggish reflexes, slowing of reaction time
Reticular Formation		
Reticular activating system	Modification of hypothalamic function, reduction in stage IV sleep	Increase in frequency of spontaneous awakening together with tiredness, interrupted sleep, insomnia
Autonomic Nervous System		
SNS and PSNS	Morphologic features of ganglia, slowing of ANS responses	Orthostatic hypotension, systolic hypertension

ANS, Autonomic nervous system; *PSNS*, parasympathetic nervous system; *SNS*, sympathetic nervous system.
*See Table 2-2 for the effects of aging on adult mental functioning.
†Specific changes related to the eye are in Table 17-1 and specific changes related to the ear are in Table 17-7.

the neurologic problem has a hereditary or congenital background. Specifically, the patient should be questioned about a family history of such disorders as epilepsy, amyotrophic lateral sclerosis, multiple sclerosis, Huntington's disease, muscular dystrophy, mental retardation, dementia, stroke, and cancer.

If the patient has an existing neurologic problem, the nurse should ask about how it affects daily living and the ability to carry out self-care. After a careful review of information, the nurse should ask someone who knows the patient well whether any mental or physical changes have been noticed in the patient. The patient with a neurologic problem is often not aware of it or is unable to provide enough specific data to aid in the diagnosis.

Nutritional-metabolic pattern. Neurologic problems can result in problems of inadequate nutrition. Problems related to chewing, swallowing, facial nerve paralysis, and muscle coordination could make it difficult for the patient to ingest adequate nutrients. Also, certain vitamins such as thiamine (B_1), niacin, and pyridoxine (B_6) are essential for the main-

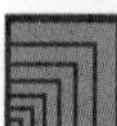

Table 53-5 Key Questions: Patient with a Neurologic Problem

Health Perception–Health Management Pattern
- What are your usual daily activities?
- Do you use any recreational drugs?*
- What safety practices do you perform in a car? On a motorcycle? On a bicycle?
- Do you have hypertension? If so, is it controlled?
- Have you ever been hospitalized for a neurologic problem?*
- How does it affect your daily living?

Nutrition-Metabolic Pattern
- Give a 24-hr dietary recall.
- Do you have any problems getting adequate nutrition because of chewing or swallowing difficulties, facial nerve paralysis, or poor muscle coordination?*
- Are you able to feed yourself?

Elimination Pattern
- Do you have incontinence of bowel or bladder? If yes, explain in detail the onset and pattern of the problem.
- What measures have you used to control the incontinence?
- Do you ever experience problems with hesitancy, urgency, retention?*
- Do you postpone defecation?*
- Does a neurologic problem make it difficult to reach a toilet when needed?
- Do you take any medication to manage neurologic problems? If so, what?

Activity-Exercise Pattern
- Describe any problems you experience with usual activities and exercise as a result of a neurologic problem.
- Do you have weakness or lack of coordination due to a neurologic problem?*
- Does a neurologic problem keep you from performing your personal hygiene needs independently?*

Sleep-Rest Pattern
- Describe any problems you have with sleep.
- If you have trouble falling asleep, what do you do about it? (Ask specifically about use of sleep-inducing medications.)

Cognitive-Perceptual Pattern
- Have you noticed any changes in your memory?*
- Do you experience vertigo, heat or cold sensitivity, numbness, or tingling?*
- Describe any pain you have experienced during the past 6 mo.
- Do you have any difficulty with verbal or written communication?*

Self-Perception–Self-Concept Pattern
- What effect has your neurologic problem had on how you feel about yourself? Your abilities? Your body?
- Describe your general emotional pattern.

Role-Relationship Pattern
- Have you experienced changes in roles such as spouse, parent, breadwinner because of neurologic disease?*
- How do you feel about these changes?

Sexuality-Reproductive Pattern
- Are you satisfied with sexual functioning? Describe any problems you experience related to your sexuality and sexual functioning.
- Are problems related to sexual functioning causing tension in an important relationship?*
- Do you feel the need for professional counseling related to your sexual functioning?*
- Do you use alternative methods of achieving sexual satisfaction?

Coping–Stress Tolerance Pattern
- Describe your usual coping pattern.
- Do you think your present coping pattern is adequate to meet the stressors of your neurologic problem?*
- Is your support system adequate to meet your needs? If not, what needs are unmet?

Value-Belief Pattern
- Describe any culturally-specific beliefs and attitudes which may influence the treatment of this neurologic problem.

*If yes, describe.

tenance and health of the CNS. Deficiencies in one or more of these vitamins could result in such nonspecific complaints as depression, apathy, neuritis, weakness, mental confusion, and nervous irritability.

Elimination pattern. Bowel and bladder problems are often associated with neurologic problems, such as stroke, head injury, spinal cord injury, multiple sclerosis, and dementia. It is important to determine if the bowel or bladder problem was present before or after the neurologic event in order to plan appropriate interventions. Incontinence of urine and feces and urinary retention are the most common elimination problems associated with a neurologic problem. Careful documentation of the detail of the problem such as number of episodes, accompanying sensations or lack of sensations, and measures to control the problem is important.

Activity-exercise pattern. Many neurologic disorders can cause problems in the patient's mobility, strength, and coordination. These problems can result in changes in the patient's usual activity and exercise patterns. Falls can also result from such problems. Many aspects of daily living such as getting out of a bed or chair, ambulating, preparing meals, and performing personal hygiene can be affected and should be assessed. The ability to perform fine motor tasks may be affected, which increases the possibility of personal injury.

Sleep-rest pattern. Sleep can be disrupted by many neurologically-related factors. Discomfort from pain and inability to move and change to a position of comfort because of muscle weakness and paralysis could interfere with sound sleep. Hallucinations resulting from dementia or medications can also interrupt sleep. The nurse should carefully document the sleep problem and the patient's methods of dealing with the problem.

Cognitive-perceptual pattern. Because the nervous system controls cognition and sensory integration, many neurologic disorders affect these functions. The nurse should assess memory, language, calculation ability, problem-solving, insight, and judgment. Often a structured mental status questionnaire will be used to evaluate these functions and provide baseline data.

Information about sensory changes related to hearing, sight, and touch should be sought. In addition, the patient should be questioned about problems with vertigo and sensitivity to heat and cold.

Ability to both use and understand language is a cognitive function that the nurse should also assess. Appropriateness of responses is a useful indicator of cognitive and perceptual ability.

Pain is a common event associated with many health problems. It is often the reason a patient seeks health care. A careful assessment of the patient's pain should be carried out (see Chapter 6).

Neurologic problems and their treatment can be complex and confusing. The patient's understanding and ability to carry out necessary treatments should be determined. Cognitive changes associated with the problem can also interfere with understanding and compliance.

Self-perception–self-concept pattern. Neurologic disease can drastically alter control over one's life and create dependency on others for daily needs. Also, the patient's physical appearance and emotional control can be affected. The nurse should ask about the patient's evaluation of self-worth, perception of abilities, body image, and general emotional pattern.

Role-relationship pattern. The patient should be asked if changes in roles, such as spouse, parent, or breadwinner, resulting from a neurologic problem have occurred. Physical impairments, such as weakness and paralysis can alter or limit participation in usual roles and activities. Cognitive changes, however, can permanently change a person's ability to maintain previous roles. These changes can dramatically affect both the patient and significant others. Spousal relationships often change to dependent relationships.

Sexuality-reproductive pattern. The ability to participate in sexual activity should be assessed because many nervous system disorders can affect sexual response. Cerebral lesions may inhibit the desire phase or the reflex responses of the excitement phase. Brainstem and spinal cord lesions may partially or completely interrupt the connections between the brain and effector systems necessary for intercourse.

Neuropathies and spinal cord lesions that affect sensation, especially in the erotic zones, may decrease desire. Finally, autonomic neuropathies and lesions of the sacral cord and cauda equina may prevent reflex activities of the sexual response. The nurse should determine if the patient and the spouse or significant other are satisfied with their sexual activity. The use or need for alternative methods of achieving sexual satisfaction should be explored. Despite neurologic-related changes in sexual functioning, many persons can achieve satisfying expression of intimacy and affection.

Coping–stress tolerance pattern. The physical sequelae of a neurologic problem can seriously strain a patient's coping patterns. Often the problem is chronic and may require that the patient learn new coping skills. The nurse needs to assess the patient's usual coping pattern to determine if coping skills are adequate to meet the stress of a problem.

When the problem is a decrease in cognitive functioning, both the patient and the caregiver can be seriously stressed. The nurse needs to assess for the potential for suicide, abuse, and burnout of the involved parties. The presence of an adequate support system in this type of situation needs to be assessed.

Value-belief pattern. Many neurologic problems have serious, long-term, life-changing effects. These effects can strain the patient's belief system and should be assessed. The nurse should also determine if any religious or cultural beliefs could interfere with the planned treatment regimen.

Objective Data

Physical Examination. The standard neurologic examination was developed by physicians and clinicians to help determine the presence, location, and nature of disease of the nervous system. The examination assesses six categories of functions: mental status, function of cranial nerves, motor function, cerebellar function, sensory function, and reflex function.[7] The choice of particular parts of the examination depends on the purpose for which it is done. If a comprehensive baseline assessment of neurologic functioning is desired, all components of the examination are done. However, if a specific problem is to be evaluated, only certain components may be assessed. For example, if a patient's primary complaint is lack of feeling in the feet, the examination may be focused only on movement and sensation of the lower limbs. Similarly, if a patient comes into the emergency department after a head injury and is unconscious, a limited examination is conducted because the patient is not able to respond to verbal instructions.

A different approach to the neurologic examination has been proposed for nursing purposes. The primary purposes of the nursing neurologic examination are to determine the effects of neurologic dysfunction on daily living in relation to the patient's and the family's ability to cope with the neurologic deficits. Although the method of gathering data may be the same, the interpretation of the data is different from the medical model. The standard medical model of the neurologic examination can also be used for nursing purposes. Nurses and physicians share the responsibility for assessing life-threatening neurologic dysfunction.

Mental status. Assessment of mental status (cerebral functioning) gives an indication of how the patient is functioning as a whole and how the patient is adapting to the environment. It involves determination of complex and high-level cerebral functions that are governed by many areas of the cerebral cortex. Much of the area covered in this part of the examination is assessed during the history and therefore does not need to be evaluated further. For example, language and memory can be assessed when the patient is asked for details of the illness and significant past events. The patient's cultural and educational background should be taken into account when evaluating mental status.

The components of the mental status examination are as follows:

1. *General appearance and behavior:* This component includes motor activity, body posture, dress and hygiene, facial expression, and speech.
2. *State of consciousness:* The patient must be conscious before other functions can be determined. The nurse should note orientation to time, place, person, and situation, as well as memory, general knowledge, insight, judgment, problem solving, and calculation. Common questions are "Who were the last three presidents?" "What does 'a stitch in time saves nine' mean?" "Subtract 7 from 100, and keep subtracting 7." The nurse should consider whether the patient's plans and goals match the physical and mental capabilities.
3. *Mood and affect:* The nurse should note agitation, anger, depression, or euphoria and the appropriateness of these states. Questions should be directed to bring out the feelings of the patient.
4. *Thought content:* The nurse should note illusions, hallucinations, delusions, or paranoia.
5. *Intellectual capacity:* The nurse should note retardation, dementia, and intelligence.

Cranial nerves. Testing of each CN is an essential component of the neurologic examination (see Table 53-2).

Olfactory Nerve. After determining that both nostrils are patent, the olfactory nerve (CN I) is tested by asking the patient to close one nostril, close the eyes, and sniff from a bottle containing coffee, spice, soap, or some other readily recognized odor. The same is done for the other nostril. Generally, olfaction is not tested unless the patient has some disturbance with smell. Chronic rhinitis, sinusitis, and heavy smoking can often decrease the sense of smell. Disturbance in ability to smell may be associated with a tumor involving the olfactory bulb, or it may be the result of a basilar skull fracture that has damaged the olfactory fibers as they pass through the delicate cribriform plate of the skull.

Optic Nerve. Visual fields and visual acuity are assessed to test the function of the optic nerve (CN II). Visual fields are assessed by confrontation. The examiner, positioned directly opposite the patient, asks the patient to close one eye, look directly at the bridge of the examiner's nose, and indicate when an object (finger, pencil tip, head of pin) presented from the periphery of each of the four visual field quadrants is seen (Fig. 53-16). The same test is repeated for the other eye. The examiner is used as a control because both examiner and patient are sharing the same visual field. It is important to remember that the nasal side of the visual field is narrower because of the nasal bridge. Visual field defects may arise from lesions of the optic nerve, optic chiasm, or tracts that extend through the temporal, parietal, or occipital lobes. Visual field changes resulting from brain lesions are usually either a *hemianopsia* (one half of the visual field is affected), a *quadrantanopsia* (one fourth of the visual field is affected), or *monocular.*

Visual acuity is tested by asking the patient to read a Snellen chart from 20 feet away. The number on the lowest line that the patient can read with 50% accuracy is recorded. The patient who wears glasses should wear them during testing, unless they are used only for reading. The eyes should be tested individually and together. If a Snellen chart is not available, the patient should be asked to read newsprint for a gross assessment of acuity. The distance from the patient to the newsprint, required for accurate reading should be recorded. Acuity may not be testable by these means if the patient does not read English, is retarded, or is aphasic.

Fundoscopy reveals the physical condition of the optic disk (head of the optic nerve), as well as the retina and

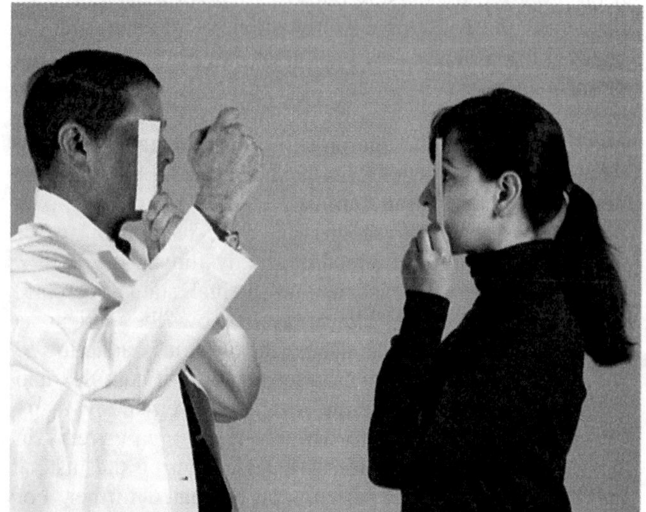

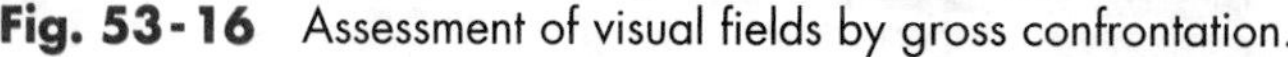

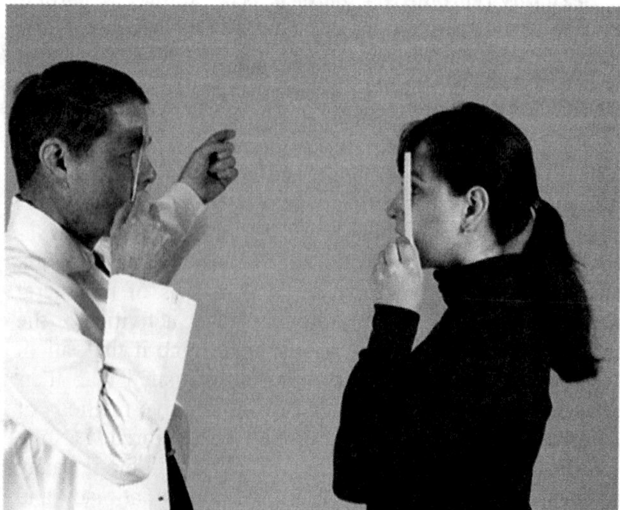

Fig. 53-16 Assessment of visual fields by gross confrontation.

blood vessels. This procedure is routinely performed when the optic nerve is tested. Optic nerve atrophy and papilledema can be detected by this method.

OCULOMOTOR, TROCHLEAR, AND ABDUCENS NERVES. Because the oculomotor (CN III), trochlear (CN IV), and abducens (CN VI) nerves all help to move the eye, they are tested together. The patient is asked to follow the examiner's finger as it moves horizontally and vertically (making a cross) and diagonally (making an X). If there is weakness or paralysis of one of the eye muscles, the eyes do not move together, and the patient has a disconjugate gaze. The presence and direction of *nystagmus* (fine, rapid jerking movements of the eyes) is observed at this time, even though it is most often indicative of vestibulocerebellar problems.

Other functions of the oculomotor nerve are tested by checking for pupillary constriction and for *convergence* (eyes turning inward) and *accommodation* (pupils constricting with near vision). To test pupillary constriction, the examiner shines a light into the pupil of one eye and looks for ipsilateral constriction of the same pupil and contralateral (consensual) constriction of the opposite eye. The size and shape of the pupils are also noted. The optic nerve must be intact for this reflex to occur. Testing for pupillary constriction is an important component of the neurologic assessment of patients at risk for herniation syndrome (see Chapters 54 and 55). Because the oculomotor nerve exits at the top of the brainstem at the tentorial notch, it can be easily compressed by expanding mass lesions in the cerebral hemispheres. The result is a pupil that does not constrict to light; it may become dilated because the sympathetic input to the pupil acts unopposed. Convergence and accommodation are tested by having the patient focus on the examiner's finger as it moves toward the patient's nose. Another function of the oculomotor nerve is to keep the eyelid open. Damage to the nerve can cause *ptosis* (drooping eyelid), pupillary abnormalities, and eye muscle weakness.

TRIGEMINAL NERVE. The sensory component of the trigeminal nerve (CN V) is tested by having the patient identify light touch (cotton) and pinprick in each of the three divisions (ophthalmic, maxillary, and mandibular) of the nerve on both sides of the face. The patient's eyes should be closed during this part of the examination. The motor component is tested by asking the patient to clench the teeth and palpating the masseter muscles just above the mandibular angle. The corneal reflex test evaluates CN V and CN VII simultaneously. It involves applying a cotton wisp strand to the cornea. The sensory component of this reflex (corneal sensation) is innervated by the ophthalmic division of CN V. The motor component (eye blink) is innervated by the facial nerve (CN VII). This reflex is not normally tested in patients who are awake and alert because other tests evaluate these two nerves. However, for patients with a decreased level of consciousness, the corneal reflex test provides an opportunity to evaluate the integrity of the brainstem at the level of the pons because the fibers of CN V and CN VII have connections in this area.

FACIAL NERVE. The facial nerve (CN VII) innervates the muscles of facial expression. Its function is tested by asking the patient to raise the eyebrows, close the eyes tightly, purse the lips, draw back the corners of the mouth in an exaggerated smile, and frown. The examiner should note any asymmetry in the facial movements because they can indicate damage to the facial nerve. Although taste discrimination of salt and sugar in the anterior two thirds of the tongue is a function of this nerve, it is not routinely tested unless a peripheral nerve lesion is suspected.

ACOUSTIC NERVE. The cochlear portion of the acoustic (vestibulocochlear) nerve (CN VIII) is tested by having the patient close the eyes and indicate when a ticking watch or the rustling of the examiner's fingertips is heard as the stimulus is brought closer to the ear. Each ear is tested individually, and the distance from the patient's ear to the sound source when first heard is recorded. This test identifies only gross deficits in hearing. For more precise assessment of hearing, an audiometer is used (see Chapter 17). The vestibular portion of this nerve is not routinely tested unless the patient complains of dizziness, vertigo, or unsteadiness or has auditory dysfunction. If this is the case, caloric testing, which is beyond the scope of routine testing, may be done.

GLOSSOPHARYNGEAL AND VAGUS NERVES. The glossopharyngeal and vagus nerves are tested together because both innervate the pharynx. The glossopharyngeal nerve (CN IX) is primarily sensory. In the gag reflex (bilateral contraction of the palatal muscles initiated by stroking or touching either side of the posterior pharynx or soft palate with a tongue blade), the sensory component is mediated by CN IX and the major motor component by the vagus nerve (CN X). It is important to assess the gag reflex in patients who have a decreased level of consciousness, a brainstem lesion, or a disease involving the throat musculature. If the reflex is weak or absent, the patient is in danger of aspirating food or secretions. The strength and efficiency of swallowing is important to test in these patients for the same reason. Another test for the awake, cooperative patient is to have the patient phonate by saying "ah" and to note the bilateral symmetry of elevation of the soft palate. Any asymmetry can indicate weakness or paralysis. Swallowing is also assessed by lightly holding the examiner's hands on either side of the patient's throat and asking the patient to swallow. Once again, any asymmetry is noted.

SPINAL ACCESSORY NERVE. The spinal accessory nerve (CN XI) is tested by asking the patient to shrug the shoulders against resistance and to turn the head to either side against resistance. There should be smooth contraction of the sternomastoid and trapezius muscles. Symmetry, atrophy, or fasciculation of the muscle should also be noted.

HYPOGLOSSAL NERVE. The hypoglossal nerve (CN XII) is tested by asking the patient to protrude the tongue. It should protrude in the midline. The patient should also be able to push the tongue to either side against the resistance of a tongue blade. Again, any asymmetry, atrophy, or fasciculation should be noted.

Motor system. The motor system examination includes assessment of bulk, tone, and power of the major muscle groups of the body, as well as assessment of balance and coordination. The examiner tests strength by asking the patient to push and pull against the resistance of the examiner's arm as it opposes flexion and extension of the patient's muscle. The patient should be asked to offer resistance at the shoulder, elbow, wrist, hips, knees, and ankles. The patient's grip strength can also be tested. Mild weakness of the upper extremities may be tested by having the patient extend both arms forward at shoulder height with palms up while the eyes are closed. Mild weakness of the arm is demonstrated by downward drifting of the arm or pronation of the palm (pronator drift). Any weakness or asymmetry of strength between the same muscle groups of the right and left side should be noted.

Tone is tested by passively moving the limbs through their range of motion; there should be a slight resistance to these movements. Abnormal tone is described as *hypotonia* (flaccidity) or *hypertonia* (spasticity). Involuntary movements (e.g., tics, tremor, myoclonus, athetosis, chorea, dystonia) should be noted.

Cerebellar function is tested by assessing balance and coordination. A good screening test for both balance and muscle strength is to observe the patient's stature (posture while standing) and gait. The examiner should note the pace and rhythm of the gait and observe the arm swing. (The arms should move symmetrically and in the opposite direction of the leg on the same side.) The patient's ability to ambulate is a key factor in determining the amount of nursing care that is needed and the risk of injury from falling. A patient with cerebellar disease may have an *ataxic* or staggering gait, in which the feet are placed wide apart and the steps are unsteady.

Coordination can be easily tested in several ways. The finger-to-nose test involves having the patient alternately touch the nose with the index finger, then touch the examiner's finger. The examiner repositions the finger while the patient is touching the nose so that the patient must adjust to a new distance each time the examiner's finger is touched. These movements should be performed smoothly and accurately. Other tests include asking the patient to pronate and supinate both hands rapidly and to do a shallow knee bend, first on one leg, and then on the other. Dysarthria or slurred speech should be noted because it is a sign of uncoordination of the speech muscles.

The heel-to-shin test involves having the patient place one heel on the opposite shin below the knee and moving the heel down the shin to the ankle. This is repeated for the other leg. These movements should flow smoothly without jerking or hesitation.

Sensory system. Several modalities are tested in the somatic sensory examination. Each modality is carried by a specific ascending pathway in the spinal cord before it reaches the sensory cortex.

There are some general guidelines for performing the sensory examination. The patient should always have the eyes closed to avoid visual clues. The examiner should avoid giving verbal cues such as, "Is this sharp?" The sensory stimulus should be applied in such a way that the patient does not expect it; that is, the examiner should avoid rhythmical application of the stimulus. In the routine neurologic examination, sensory testing of the four extremities is sufficient. However, if a disturbance in sensory function of the skin is identified, the boundaries of that dysfunction should be carefully delineated.

LIGHT TOUCH. Light touch is usually tested first. The examiner gently strokes a cotton wisp over each of the four extremities and asks the patient to indicate when the stimulus is felt by saying "touch." (The sensory examination of the trigeminal nerve may be delayed until this time because the same material for testing sensation is used.)

PAIN AND TEMPERATURE. Pain is tested by touching the skin with the sharp end of a pin. This stimulus is irregularly alternated with a simple touch stimulus with the dull end of the pin to determine whether the patient can distinguish the two stimuli. Extinction or inhibition is assessed by simultaneously stimulating opposite sides of the body symmetrically with either a pain or a touch stimulus. Normally, the simultaneous stimuli are perceived (sensed); perception of only one may indicate a parietal lobe lesion.

The sensation of temperature is tested by applying tubes of warm and cold water to the skin and asking the patient to identify the stimuli with the eyes closed. If pain sensation is intact, assessment of temperature sensation may be omitted because both sensations are carried by the same ascending pathways.

VIBRATION SENSE. Vibration sense is assessed by applying a vibrating C-128 tuning fork to the fingernails and the bony prominences of the hands, legs, and feet with the patient's eyes closed. The examiner asks the patient if the vibration or "buzz" is felt. The examiner then asks the patient to indicate when the vibration ceases. The examiner stops the vibration with the hand as desired.

POSITION SENSE. Position sense is assessed by placing the thumb and forefinger on either side of the patient's forefinger or great toe and gently moving the finger up or down. The patient is asked to indicate the direction in which the digit is moved.

Another test of position sense of the lower extremities is the *Romberg test.* The patient is asked to stand with the feet together and then close his eyes. If the patient is able to maintain balance with the eyes open, but sways or falls with the eyes closed (i.e., a positive Romberg test), this may indicate disease in the posterior columns of the spinal cord. It is important that the nurse be aware of patient safety during this test.

CORTICAL SENSORY FUNCTIONS. Several tests evaluate cortical integration of sensory perceptions (which occurs in the parietal lobes). *Two-point discrimination* is assessed by placing the two points of a calibrated compass on the tips of the fingers and toes. The minimum recognizable separation is 4 to 5 mm in the fingertips and a greater degree of separation elsewhere. This test is important in diseases of the sensory cortex and in peripheral nerve disease.

Graphesthesia is tested by having the patient identify numbers traced on the palm of the hands. *Stereognosis* is tested by having the patient identify the size and shape of easily recognized objects (e.g., coins, keys, a safety pin) placed in the hands. *Sensory extinction* or *inattention* is evaluated by touching both sides of the body simultaneously. An abnormal response occurs when the patient

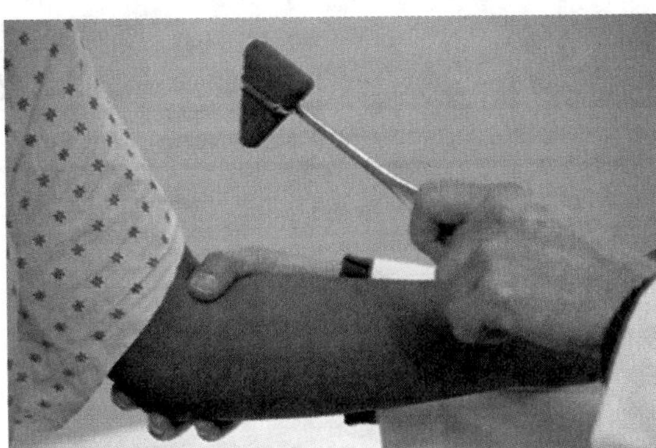

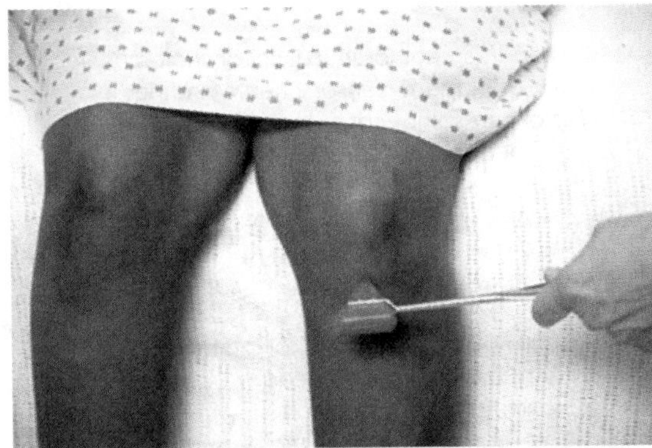

Fig. 53-17 The examiner strikes a swift blow over a stretched tendon to elicit a stretch reflex.

Table 53-6 Recording the Normal Neurologic Examination*
Mental Status
Alert and oriented, orderly thought processes, appropriate mood and affect
Cranial Nerves†
Smell intact to soap and coffee; visual fields full to confrontation; visual acuity 20/20 in both eyes; intact extraocular movements; no nystagmus; pupils equal, round, reactive to light and accommodation; intact facial sensation to touch and pinprick; facial movements full; intact gag and swallow reflexes; symmetric elevation of soft palate; full strength with head turning and shrugging of shoulders against resistance; midline protrusion of tongue
Motor System
Normal gait and station; normal tandem walk; negative Romberg test; normal and symmetric muscle bulk, tone, strength; smooth performance of finger-nose, heel-shin movements
Sensory System
Intact sensation to light touch, position sense, vibration, pinprick, heat and cold, two-point discrimination; intact stereognosis and graphesthesia
Reflexes‡
Biceps, triceps, brachioradialis, patellar, and Achilles tendon reflexes 2+ bilaterally; downgoing toes with plantar stimulation

*If some portion of the neurologic examination was not done, this should be indicated (e.g., "Smell not tested").
†May also be recorded as "CN I to XII intact."
‡May also be recorded as drawing of stick figure indicating reflex strength at appropriate sites.

perceives the stimulus only on one side. The other stimulus is "extinguished."

Reflexes. Tendons attached to skeletal muscles have receptors which are sensitive to stretch. A *reflex* contraction of the skeletal muscle occurs when the tendon is stretched. A simple muscle stretch reflex is initiated by briskly tapping the tendon of a stretched muscle, usually with a reflex hammer (Fig. 53-17). The response (muscle contraction of the corresponding muscle) is measured as follows: 0 = absent, 1 = weak response, 2 = normal response, 3 = exaggerated response, 4 = hyperreflexia with clonus. *Clonus,* an abnormal response, is a continued rhythmic contraction of the muscle after the stimulus has been applied.

In general, the biceps, triceps, brachioradialis, and patellar and Achilles tendon reflexes are tested. The examiner elicits the biceps reflex by placing the thumb over the biceps tendon in the antecubital space and striking the thumb with a hammer. The patient should have the arms partially flexed at the elbow with the palms up. The normal response is flexion of the arm at the elbow or contraction of the biceps muscle that can be felt by the examiner's thumb.

The triceps reflex is elicited by striking the triceps tendon above the elbow while the patient's arm is flexed. The normal response is extension of the arm or visible contraction of the triceps.

The brachioradialis reflex is elicited by striking the radius 3 to 5 cm above the wrist while the patient's arm is relaxed. The normal response is flexion and supination at the elbow or visible contraction of the brachioradialis muscle.

The patellar reflex is elicited by striking the patellar tendon just below the patella. The patient can be sitting or lying as long as the leg being tested hangs freely. The normal response is extension of the leg with contraction of the quadriceps.

The Achilles tendon reflex is elicited by striking the Achilles tendon while the patient's leg is flexed at the knee and the foot is dorsiflexed at the ankle. The normal response is plantar flexion at the ankle.

Table 53-6 is an example of how to record a normal neurologic assessment. Common abnormal assessment findings of the neurologic system are presented in Table 53-7.

Nursing Approach. The premise of the nursing approach is that the primary purpose of nursing is to help patients cope effectively with deficits in self-care and in activities of daily living.[8] Consequently, the neurologic examination should be viewed in terms of functional disabilities rather than dysfunction of component parts of the nervous system. The effects of the disabilities on the patient's

Table 53-7 Common Assessment Abnormalities: Nervous System

Finding	Description	Possible Etiology and Significance
Altered consciousness	Inability to speak, obey commands, open eyes appropriately with verbal or painful stimulus	Intracranial lesions, metabolic disorder, psychiatric disorders
Anisocoria	Inequality of pupil size	Lesion, injury, or intracranial pressure in area of midbrain
Agnosia	Inability to determine meaning or significance of sensory stimulus	Cerebral cortex lesion
Apraxia	Inability to perform learned movements, defect in motor planning	Cerebral cortex lesion
Aphasia	Loss of language faculty (language comprehension, language expression, or both)	Cerebral cortex lesion
Analgesia	Loss of pain sensation	Lesion in spinothalamic tract or thalamus, lack of or damage to sensory nerve endings
Anesthesia	Absence of sensation	Lesions in spinal cord, thalamus, sensory cortex, or peripheral sensory nerve
Hyperesthesia	Increase in sensation	
Hypoesthesia	Decrease in sensation	
Anosognosia	Inability to recognize bodily defect or disease	Lesions in right parietal cortex, common in right-brain stroke
Astereognosis	Inability to recognize form of object by touch	Lesions in parietal cortex
Ataxia	Lack of coordination of movement	Lesions of sensory or motor pathways, cerebellum; anticonvulsant, sedative, hypnotic drug toxicity (including alcohol)
Muscle atrophy (disuse or denervation atrophy)	Wasting away or diminution in size of muscle	Suprasegmental (upper motor neuron) lesions, segmental (lower motor neuron) lesions
Bladder dysfunction		
Atonic (autonomous)	Absence of muscle tone and contractility, enlargement of capacity, no sensation of discomfort, overflow with large residual, inability to voluntarily empty or empty by reflex	Early stage of spinal cord injury
Hypotonic	More ability than atonic bladder but less than normal	Interruption of afferent pathways from bladder
Hypertonic	Increase in muscle tone, diminished capacity, reflex emptying, dribbling, incontinence	Lesions in pyramidal tracts (efferent pathways)
Diplopia	Double vision	Lesions affecting nerves of extraocular muscles, cerebellar toxicity
Dysarthria	Lack of coordination in articulating speech	Lesions in cerebellum or pathway of cranial nerves (including brainstem); anticonvulsant, sedative, or hypnotic drug toxicity (including alcohol)
Dyskinesia	Impairment of power of voluntary movement, resulting in fragmentary or incomplete movements	Disorders of basal ganglia, idiosyncratic reaction to psychotropic drugs
Dysphagia	Difficulty in swallowing	Lesions involving motor pathways of CN IX, X (including lower brainstem)
Extensor plantar response (Babinski sign)	Upgoing toes with plantar stimulation	Suprasegmental or upper motor neuron lesion

continued

Table 53-7 Common Assessment Abnormalities: Nervous System—cont'd

Finding	Description	Possible Etiology and Significance
Homonymous hemianopsia	Loss of vision in one side of visual field	Injury or lesions in area of optic tract or its radiations to occipital cortex
Hemiplegia	Paralysis on one side	Stroke and other lesions involving motor cortex
Nystagmus	Jerking or bobbing of eyes as they track moving object	Lesions in cerebellum, brainstem, vestibular system; anticonvulsant, sedative, hypnotic toxicity (including alcohol)
Ophthalmoplegia	Paralysis of eye muscles	Lesions in brainstem or CN III, IV, VI
Opisthotonus	Extreme arching of back with retraction of head	Meningitis, tonic phase of grand mal seizure
Papilledema	"Choked disk," swelling of optic nerve head	Increase in intracranial pressure
Paraplegia	Paralysis of lower extremities	Spinal cord transection or mass lesion (thoracolumbar region)
Quadriplegia	Paralysis of all extremities	Spinal cord transection or mass lesion (cervical region) or brainstem

potential for self-care, movement, and desired activities of daily living should be the focus. This includes understanding, communicating, remembering, seeing, speaking, feeling, moving, walking, and using integrated regulatory functions, such as elimination and temperature regulation. In addition, based on knowledge of the location of the problematic area and the functions it controls, the nurse should ask specific questions and perform certain exams to determine what other effects the lesion may have on daily functioning.

All functions of the nervous system can be categorized in six areas: consciousness, mentation, movement, sensation, integrated regulation, and coping with disability. Table 53-8 lists the functions involved in each of these categories and thus forms the basis of a nursing neurologic assessment.

Diagnostic Studies. Diagnostic studies provide important information to the nurse in monitoring the patient's condition and planning appropriate interventions. These studies are considered to be objective data. Diagnostic studies common to the nervous system are presented in Table 53-9.

DIAGNOSTIC STUDIES

Cerebrospinal Fluid Analysis

CSF analysis provides information about a variety of CNS diseases. Normal CSF fluid is clear, colorless, and free of red blood cells (RBCs) and contains little protein. Normal CSF values are listed in Table 53-10.

Lumbar Puncture. Lumbar puncture is the most common method of obtaining CSF for analysis. It is contraindicated in the presence of increased intracranial pressure or infection at the site of puncture.

Nurses often assist in this procedure because it is usually performed in the patient's room. Before the procedure, the nurse should have the patient empty the bladder. The patient should lie in the lateral recumbent position, with the back as near as possible to the edge of the bed. The nurse should assist the patient to draw up the knees to the abdomen and flex the head to the chest. This helps separate the vertebrae so that the needle can be inserted more easily.

Using strict sterile technique, the physician inserts a long needle below the third lumbar vertebra. This may cause some local discomfort. There is no danger of injuring the spinal cord, since the cord terminates between the first and

Table 53-8 Functional Categories in Nursing Neurologic Assessment

Consciousness	
Arousal	Self-awareness
Mentation	
Thinking	Language
Remembering	Problem solving
Perceiving	
Movement	
Expressing (facial)	Transferring
Speaking	Eating (chewing, swallowing)
Walking	Blinking (combined movement and sensation)
Sensation	
Seeing	Feeling (e.g., touch, temperature, pain, pressure, position, form, shape)
Smelling	
Hearing	
Integrated Regulatory Function	
Eating (ingesting, digesting)	Circulation
	Temperature control
Eliminating	Sexual response
Breathing	Emotion
Coping with Disability	
Self-care competence	Coping (e.g., adapting, supporting, growing)
Role competence	

Table 53-9 Diagnostic Studies: Nervous System

Study	Description and Purpose	Nursing Responsibility
Cerebrospinal Fluid Analysis		
Lumbar puncture	CSF is aspirated by needle insertion in L4-5 interspace to assess many CNS diseases. (See Table 53-10.)	Assist patient to assume and maintain lateral recumbent position with knees flexed. Ensure maintenance of strict aseptic technique. Ensure labeling of CSF specimens in proper sequence. Keep patient flat for at least a few hours depending on physician preference. Encourage fluids. Monitor neurologic and VS. Administer analgesia as needed.
Radiologic		
Skull and spine x-rays	Simple x-ray of skull and spinal column is done to detect fractures, bone erosion, calcifications, abnormal vascularity.	Explain that procedure is noninvasive. Explain positions to be assumed.
Cerebral angiography	Serial x-ray visualization of intracranial and extracranial blood vessels is performed to detect vascular lesions and tumors of brain. Radiopaque contrast medium is used.	Withhold preceding meal. Explain that patient will have hot flush of head and neck when dye is injected. Administer premedication. Explain need to be absolutely still during procedure. Monitor neurologic and VS every 15-30 min first 2 hr, every hr next 6 hr, then every 2 hr for 24 hr. Maintain pressure dressing and ice to injection site. Maintain bed rest until patient is alert and VS are stable. Report any signs of change in neurologic status.
Computed tomography (CT) scan	Computer-assisted x-ray of several levels or thin cross sections of body parts are done to detect problems such as hemorrhage, tumor, cyst, edema, infarction, brain atrophy, hydrocephalus.	Explain that procedure is noninvasive (if no dye used). Observe for allergic reaction and note puncture site (if dye used). Explain appearance of scanner. Instruct patient on need to remain absolutely still during procedure.
Myelography	X-ray of spinal cord and vertebral column after injection of dye into subarachnoid space is used to detect spinal lesions (e.g., ruptured disk, tumor).	Administer preprocedure sedation as ordered. Instruct patient to empty bladder. Inform patient that test is performed with patient on tilting table that is moved during test. Note that specific postprocedural management depends on whether oil- or water-based contrast medium is used. Encourage fluids. Monitor neurologic and VS.
Magnetic resonance imaging (MRI)	Internal body parts are visualized by means of magnetic energy. No invasive procedures are required unless dye is used.	Screen patient for metal parts in body. Instruct patient on need to lie very still for up to 1 hr. Sedation may be necessary if patient is claustrophobic.
Electrographic		
Electroencephalography	Electrical activity of brain is recorded by scalp electrodes to evaluate cerebral disease, CNS effects of systemic diseases, brain death.	Inform patient that procedure is painless and without danger of electric shock. Withhold stimulants. Inform that patient may be asked to perform various activities such as hyperventilation during test. Determine whether any medications (e.g., tranquilizers, anticonvulsants) should be withheld. Resume medications after test. Assist patient to wash electrode paste out of hair.
Electromyography	Electrical activity associated with innervation of skeletal muscle is recorded by insertion of needle electrodes to detect myopathic conditions and peripheral nerve disease.	Inform patient of slight discomfort associated with insertion of needles.

continued

Table 53-9 Diagnostic Studies: Nervous System—cont'd

Study	Description and Purpose	Nursing Responsibility
Evoked potentials	Electrical activity associated with nerve conduction along sensory pathways is recorded by electrodes placed on skin and scalp. Stimulus generates the impulse. Procedure is used to diagnose disease, locate nerve damage, and monitor function intraoperatively.	Explain procedure to patient.
Visual evoked potentials	Electrical activity in visual pathway is recorded with rapidly reversing checkerboard pattern on television screen. One eye is tested at a time.	Explain procedure to patient.
Brainstem auditory evoked potentials	Electrical activity in auditory pathway is recorded with earphones that produce clicking sounds. One ear is tested at a time.	Explain procedure to patient.
Somatosensory evoked potentials	Electrical activity in certain peripheral nerves is recorded with mild electrical pulse (several per sec).	Inform patient that stimulus may cause mild discomfort or muscle twitch.
Ultrasound		
Carotid duplex studies	Sound waves determine blood flow velocity which indicates presence of occlusive vascular disease.	Explain procedure to patient.
Transcranial Doppler	Same technology as carotid duplex, but evaluates intracranial vessels.	Explain procedure to patient.

CNS, Central nervous system; *CSF*, cerebrospinal fluid; *VS*, vital signs.

Table 53-10 Normal Cerebrospinal Fluid Values

Parameter	Normal Value
Specific gravity	1.007
pH	7.35
Appearance	Clear, colorless
RBCs	None
WBCs	0-8/μL (0-0.008/L)
Protein	
Lumbar	15-45mg/dl (0.15-.45 g/L)
Cisternal	15-25 mg/dl (0.15-0.25 g/L)
Ventricular	5-15 mg/dl (0.05-0.15 g/L)
Glucose	45-75 mg/dl (2.5-4.2 mmol/L)
Microorganisms	None
Opening pressure with lumbar puncture	60-150 mm H_2O

RBCs, Red blood cells; *WBCs*, white blood cells.

second lumbar vertebrae. However, the patient may have some pain radiating down the leg or muscle twitching if the spinal root is irritated by the needle. The nurse can assure the patient that this is temporary, and that the patient is not in danger of being paralyzed.

A manometer is attached to the needle, and CSF pressure is determined *after* the patient is asked to relax and extend the legs. If this is not done, the pressure appears abnormally high. CSF is withdrawn in a series of tubes and sent for analysis. Some examiners believe that the patient should be kept lying flat for at least a few hours after the procedure to avoid a spinal headache, which is presumably caused by loss of the cushioning effect of CSF as a result of leakage of CSF at the puncture site. The prone position may be effective in preventing CSF leakage. Other clinicians do not believe that the lying position is necessary because headache seems to develop in some patients despite precautions. Meningeal irritation (nuchal rigidity) or signs and symptoms of local trauma (hematoma, pain) may develop in some patients.

Radiologic Studies

Cerebral Angiography. Cerebral angiography is indicated when vascular lesions or tumors are suspected. A catheter is inserted into the femoral (sometimes brachial) artery. It is then passed up the artery to the aortic arch and into the base of a carotid or a vertebral artery for injection of radiopaque dye. A series of x-rays is taken in a timed sequence so that pictures of the arteries, smaller vessels, and veins can be obtained (Fig. 53-18). This study can help localize and determine the presence of abscesses, aneurysms, hematomas, arteriovenous malformations, arterial spasm, and certain tumors.

Because this is an invasive procedure, adverse reactions may occur. The patient may have an allergic (anaphylactic) reaction to the contrast medium. This reaction usually occurs immediately after injection of the contrast medium and may require emergency resuscitation measures in the procedure room. The most common precaution for nurses to take in caring for the patient after the return to the room is observation for bleeding at the catheter puncture site (usually the groin). A pressure dressing and ice are usually placed on the site to promote hemostasis and prevent swelling.

Computed Tomography. Computed tomography (CT) scan is a noninvasive procedure, although intravenous (IV) injection of contrast medium may be used to enhance

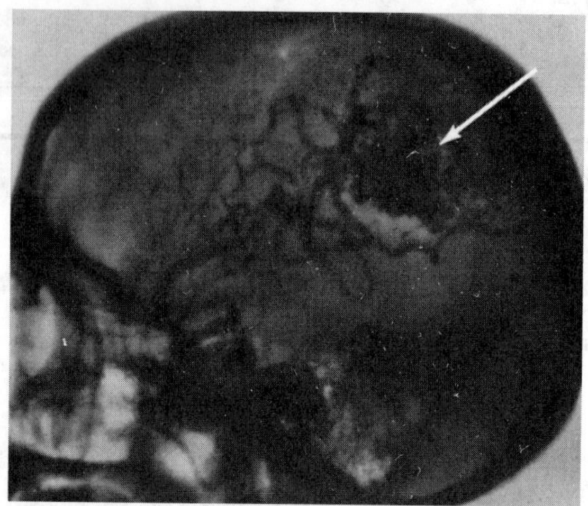

Fig. 53-18 Cerebral angiogram illustrating an arteriovenous malformation (*arrow*).

visualization of the blood vessels and identify disruptions in the blood-brain barrier. CT scans can be done on an outpatient basis. A series of x-rays scanning different levels of the brain are compiled with computer assistance and presented in a series of black-and-white pictures. These pictures, which illustrate "slices" of the brain, can show hemorrhages, tumors, cysts, edema, infarction, brain atrophy, and hydrocephalus. CT scans do not illustrate structures in the posterior fossa and the base of the brain as clearly as does magnetic resonance imaging (MRI).

Magnetic Resonance Imaging. Magnetic resonance imaging (MRI) became available in the mid-1980s. Rather than using x-rays, this method involves two kinds of magnetism. The patient is placed within a giant magnetic field that aligns the protons of the hydrogen ions in the cells of the body (Fig. 53-19). Bursts of radiofrequency magnetism are introduced to flip the protons out of alignment. When the radiofrequency magnetism is turned off, the protons realign. The resulting magnetic field change is picked up by the machine and is processed by a computer. A vivid black-and-white picture of slices of the brain is then produced.

MRI is useful in evaluating brain and spinal cord edema, hemorrhage, infarction, blood vessels, neoplasms, and bone lesions. Because MRI yields greater contrast in the images of soft-tissue structures than does the CT scan, it is the diagnostic test of choice for many neurologic diseases.

Myelography. Myelography is used to visualize the spinal column and the subarachnoid space when a spinal lesion is suspected. The most common lesion for which this test is used is a herniated or protruding intervertebral disk. Other lesions include spinal tumors, adhesions, syringomyelia, bony deformations, and arteriovenous malformations. The test involves x-rays of the spinal column after injection of the contrast medium into the subarachnoid space via a catheter. Water-soluble iodine dyes such as iopamidol (Isovue) are used most often because they are absorbed into the bloodstream and excreted by the kidneys.

Preparation for this procedure is the same as for lumbar puncture. Before the dye is injected, patients must be asked whether they have any allergies, specifically whether they have had any anaphylactic or hypotensive episodes from other dyes. After myelography, the head of the patient's bed should be kept elevated at a 30-degree angle for a few hours so that the dye does not accumulate in the brain.

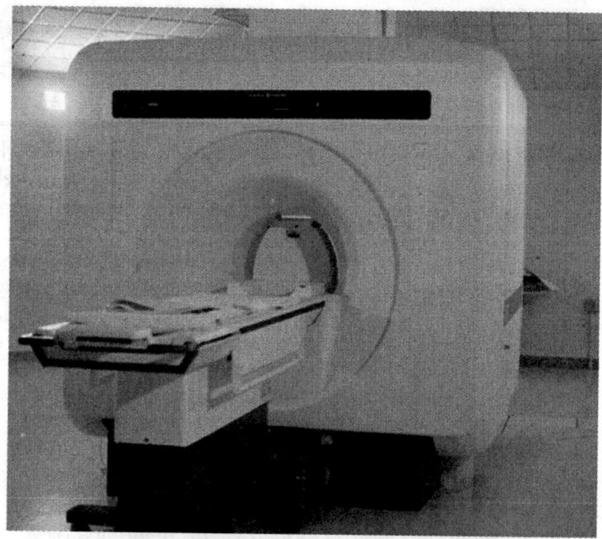

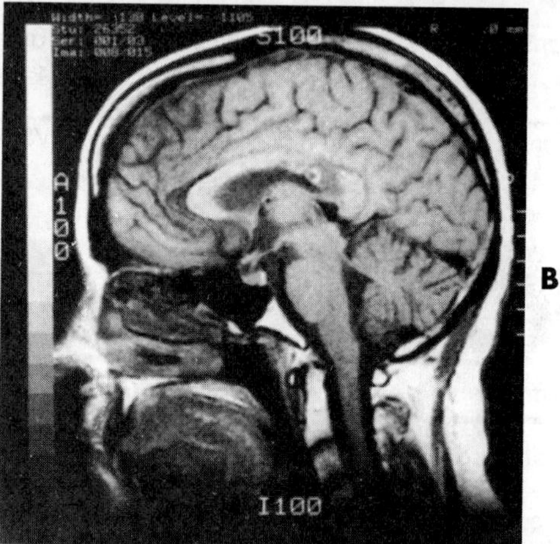

Fig. 53-19 ***A,*** Clinical setting for magnetic resonance imaging (MRI). ***B,*** Midline sagittal view of the brain using MRI.

Headache is the most common complaint after myelography. It may be accompanied by nausea and occasionally by vomiting. The nurse should observe the patient for any changes in neurologic status and provide a quiet, comfortable environment after the procedure.

Electrographic Studies

Electroencephalography. The technique of electroencephalography (EEG) involves the recording of the electrical activity of the surface cortical neurons of the brain by 8 to 16 electrodes placed on specific areas of the scalp. This test is done to evaluate not only cerebral disease but also the CNS effects of many metabolic and systemic diseases and to determine brain death. Among the cerebral diseases assessed by EEG are epilepsy, mass lesions (e.g., tumor, abscess, hematoma), cerebrovascular lesions, and brain injury (Fig. 53-20). The procedure is noninvasive. Patients

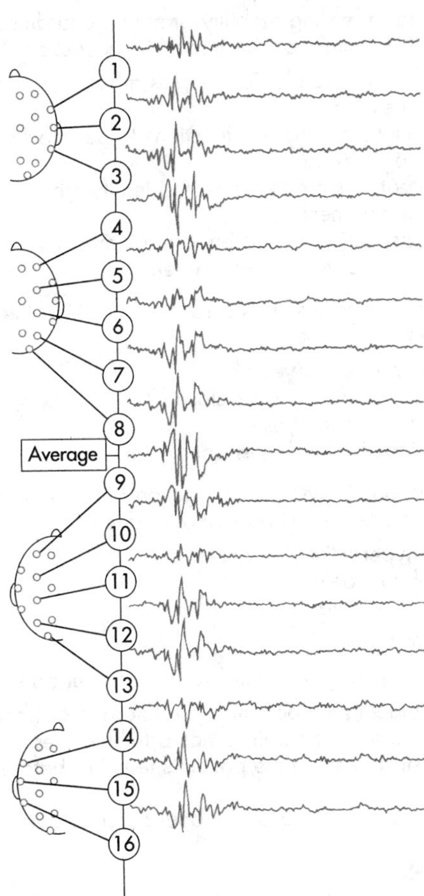

Fig. 53-20 Electroencephalogram showing a generalized epileptic discharge.

sometimes have the misconception that the recording electrodes will give them an electric shock. They should be assured that this is not true and that the procedure is similar to electrocardiography.

Electromyography and Nerve Conduction Studies. Electromyography (EMG) is the recording of electrical activity associated with innervation of skeletal muscle. The recording is displayed on a cathode-ray oscilloscope and may be played on a loudspeaker for simultaneous analysis. Needle electrodes are inserted into the muscle to record specific motor units because recording from the skin is not sufficient. Normal muscle at rest shows no electrical activity. Typical electrical activity occurs when the muscle contracts. This activity may be altered in diseases of muscle itself (e.g., myopathic conditions) or in disorders of muscle innervation (e.g., segmental or lower motor neuron lesions, peripheral neuropathic conditions). Fibrillations are spontaneous, independent contractions of individual muscle fibers that can be detected only by EMG. They appear on EMG 1 to 3 weeks after a muscle has lost its nerve supply.

Nerve conduction studies involve application of a brief electrical stimulus to a distal portion of a sensory or mixed nerve and recording the resulting wave of depolarization at some point proximal to the stimulation. For example, a stimulus can be applied to the forefinger and a recording electrode placed over the median nerve at the wrist. The time between the onset of the stimulus and the initial wave of depolarization at the recording electrode is measured. This is called the nerve conduction velocity. Damaged nerves have slower conduction velocities.

Evoked Potentials. Evoked potentials are recordings of electrical activity associated with nerve conduction along sensory pathways. The activity is generated by a specific sensory stimulus related to the type of study (e.g., checkerboard patterns for visual evoked potentials, clicking sounds for auditory evoked potentials, and mild electrical pulses for somatosensory evoked potentials). Electrodes placed on specific areas of the skin and scalp record the electrical activity, which is stored and averaged by a computerized instrument. A wave pattern appears on a screen and is printed on paper. Peaks in the wave pattern correspond to conduction of the stimulus through certain points along the sensory pathway (e.g., peripheral nerve, brainstem, and cortical areas). Increases in the normal time from stimulus onset to a given peak (latency) indicate slowed nerve conduction or nerve damage. Indications for these tests include evaluation of the optic nerve in conditions such as multiple sclerosis (optic neuritis) and the vestibulocochlear nerve in acoustic neuroma.

Combined Doppler and Ultrasound (Duplex) Studies

Carotid Duplex. A carotid duplex study uses combined ultrasound and pulsed Doppler technology. A technician places a probe on the skin over the carotid artery and slowly moves the probe along the course of the common carotid to the bifurcation of the external and internal carotid arteries. The ultrasound signal emitted from the probe reflects off the moving blood cells within the vessel. The frequency of the reflected signal corresponds to the blood velocity. This response is amplified and is registered on a graphic record and also as sound. The graphic record registers blood velocity. Increased blood flow velocity can indicate stenosis of a vessel. Carotid duplex scanning is a noninvasive study which evaluates carotid occlusive disease.

Transcranial Doppler Sonography. Transcranial doppler (TCD) sonography uses the same technology as carotid duplex studies, except that it records blood flow velocities of the intracranial blood vessels. The probe is placed on the skin at various "windows" in the skull (areas in the skull which have only a thin bony covering) in order to register velocities of the middle cerebral artery, anterior cerebral artery, posterior cerebral artery, terminal carotid artery, and occasionally, the anterior and posterior communicating arteries. The temporal, orbital, and suboccipital sites are used. The ultrasound signal received is recorded graphically as a wave form. Peak blood flow velocities and systolic-diastolic ratios can be calculated from this information. TCD sonography is a noninvasive technique which is useful in assessing vasospasm associated with subarachnoid hemorrhage, altered intracranial blood flow dynamics associated with occlusive vascular disease, cerebral autoregulation, presence of emboli, and brain death.

REVIEW QUESTIONS

The number of the question corresponds to the same-numbered objective at the beginning of the chapter.

1. Glial cells responsible for producing myelin in the central nervous system are
   a. astrocytes.
   b. microglia.
   c. oligodendroglia.
   d. ependymal cells.
2. An action potential involves
   a. changes in cell membrane permeability to sodium and potassium.
   b. restoration of neurotransmitters in the nerve terminal.
   c. inactivation of the sodium-potassium pump.
   d. maintenance of the resting membrane potential.
3. Two functions of cerebrospinal fluid are
   a. carrying nutrients and preventing infection.
   b. providing cushioning and carrying nutrients.
   c. forming myelin and preventing infection.
   d. providing cushioning and forming myelin.
4. The anterior arteries supply
   a. the medial portion of the frontal lobes.
   b. the outer portions of the frontal, parietal, and superior temporal lobes.
   c. the posterior fossa.
   d. the occipital lobes.
5. Paralysis of lateral gaze indicates a lesion of cranial nerve
   a. II.
   b. III.
   c. IV.
   d. VI.
6. Evacuation of contents from the bowel and bladder is controlled by the
   a. parasympathetic nervous system.
   b. sympathetic nervous system.
   c. hypothalamus.
   d. thalamus.
7. Assessment of the muscle strength of older adults cannot be compared to that of younger adults because
   a. most young people exercise more than older people.
   b. aging leads to a decrease in muscle bulk and strength.
   c. nutritional status is better in young adults.
   d. stroke is more common in older adults.
8. Data regarding mobility, strength, coordination, and activity tolerance are important because
   a. many neurologic diseases affect one or more of these areas.
   b. these are the first functions to be affected by neurologic disease.
   c. patients are less able to identify other neurologic impairments.
   d. aspects of movement are the most important functions of the nervous system.
9. The Romberg sign is assessed by asking the patient to stand with feet
   a. apart and eyes closed.
   b. together and eyes closed.
   c. apart and eyes open.
   d. together and eyes open.
10. Continued rhythmic contraction of a muscle after it has been stretched is abnormal and is called
    a. hyperactive response.
    b. hypertonia.
    c. hypotonia.
    d. clonus.
11. Nursing responsibilities for lumbar puncture include
    a. placing the patient in the lateral recumbent position.
    b. ensuring the patient has a full bladder.
    c. straightening the patient's legs just before the puncture.
    d. warning the patient about possible paralysis.

REFERENCES

1. Phillips JO, Fuchs AF: Somatic sensation: central processing. In Patton HD and others, editors: *Textbook of physiology,* Philadelphia, 1989, Saunders.
2. Mackinnon SE, Dellon AL: *Surgery of the peripheral nerve,* New York, 1988, Thieme Publishers.
3. Lyons MK, Meyer FB: Cerebrospinal fluid physiology and the management of increased intracranial pressure, *Mayo Clin Proc* 65:684, 1990.
4. Christiansen JL, Grzybowski JM: *Biology of aging,* St Louis, 1993, Mosby.
5. Barclay L, Wolfson L: Normal aging: pathophysiologic and clinical changes. In Barclay L, editor: *Clinical geriatric neurology,* Philadelphia, 1993, Lea & Febiger.
6. Adams R, Victor M: *Principles of neurology,* New York, 1993, McGraw-Hill.
7. Haerer AF: *DeJong's the neurologic examination,* ed 5, Philadelphia, 1992, JB Lippincott.
8. Hickey JV: *The clinical practice of neurological and neurosurgical nursing,* ed 3, Philadelphia, 1992, JB Lippincott.

Chapter 54

NURSING ROLE IN MANAGEMENT

Intracranial Problems

Mary E. Kerr   Connie A. Walleck

Learning Objectives

1. Define unconsciousness.
2. Explain the mechanisms of unconsciousness.
3. Describe the nursing management of the unconscious patient.
4. Define intracranial pressure, including normal values.
5. Identify the physiologic mechanisms of accommodation that maintain normal intracranial pressure.
6. Identify the common etiologies, clinical manifestations, and therapeutic management of increased intracranial pressure.
7. Describe the nursing management of the patient with increased intracranial pressure.
8. Differentiate types of head injury by mechanism of injury, clinical manifestations, and treatments.
9. Describe the therapeutic and nursing management of head injury.
10. Compare the types, clinical manifestations, and therapeutic management of intracranial tumors.
11. Identify the nursing diagnoses and nursing management of the patient with an intracranial tumor.
12. Describe the nursing management of the patient undergoing cranial surgery.
13. Compare the primary causes, therapeutic management, and prognosis of common cerebral inflammatory problems.
14. Explain the general nursing management of the patient with a cerebral inflammatory problem.

UNCONSCIOUSNESS

Unconsciousness is a state caused by many different health problems. Intracranial problems are the focus of this chapter because they often result in unconsciousness. The same general principles of care of an unconscious patient apply, regardless of the cause of the unconscious state.

Unconsciousness is an abnormal state in which the patient is unaware of self or environment. Unconsciousness can range from a brief episode, such as fainting, to the prolonged unconsciousness of coma from which the person cannot be roused, even with vigorous external stimuli. Between these two extremes are degrees of unconsciousness varying in length and severity. Unconsciousness itself is not a diagnosis or a disease but rather a manifestation of a large number of pathophysiologic processes, including trauma, metabolic disturbances, mass lesions, and infections. Therapeutic and nursing management is aimed at determining and correcting the cause of the unconsciousness, maintaining the bodily functions of the patient, supporting the vital functions, and protecting the patient from injury and the hazards of immobility.

Reviewed by Karen March, MN, RN, Clinical Nurse Specialist, Harborview Medical Center, Seattle, WA.

Etiology

Consciousness involves two aspects: arousal and content. The *arousal component* of consciousness refers to a state of wakefulness dependent on the activity of the reticular activating system (RAS), a network of nerve fibers and cell bodies that is located in the reticular formation in the central part of the brainstem and that has neural connections to many parts of the nervous system. An intact RAS can maintain a state of wakefulness, even in the absence of a functioning cortex. The *content component* of consciousness refers to the ability to reason, think, and feel and to react to stimuli with purpose and awareness. These activities are mediated by the cerebral hemispheres, commonly called the higher centers. Intellect and emotional functions are also controlled by these centers.

Interruption of impulses from the RAS or alteration of the functioning of the cerebral hemispheres can cause unconsciousness. Any condition that widely alters the function of the hemispheres or that depresses or destroys the upper brainstem results in an impaired consciousness. Many specific etiologic events can result in unconsciousness. Causes can be grouped according to pathophysiologic mechanisms, such as supratentorial mass lesions, subtentorial mass lesions, destructive lesions, or metabolic and diffuse cerebral disorders (Table 54-1). Psychiatric disor-

Table 54-1 Causes of Unconsciousness

Supratentorial Mass Lesions	Metabolic and Diffuse Cerebral Disorders
Epidural hematoma	Hypoxia or anoxia (decreased cardiac output)
Subdural hematoma	Postictal states and concussion
Intracerebral hematoma	Infection (meningitis, encephalitis)
Cerebral infarction	Subarachnoid hemorrhage
Brain tumor	Exogenous toxins
Brain abscess	Drug overdose
Subtentorial Lesions	Alcohol intoxication
Brainstem infarction	Lead poisoning
Brainstem tumor	Endogenous toxins and deficiencies
Brainstem hemorrhage	Hypoglycemia
Cerebellar hemorrhage	Uremia
Cerebellar abscess	Hepatic encephalopathy
	Thiamine deficiency

ders such as depression, catatonia, and schizophrenia can also result in failure to respond to the environment.

Supratentorial mass lesions generally interfere with consciousness by compressing and shifting the cerebral contents and causing pressure on the upper brainstem containing the RAS. These lesions, occurring above the tentorium, may include those resulting from trauma (e.g., lacerations or contusions, subdural or epidural hematomas), subarachnoid hemorrhage, intracerebral hemorrhage or infarction, tumors, and abscesses. The most serious consequence of a supratentorial mass lesion is the possibility of herniation of the cerebral hemisphere through the tentorial notch, causing compression of the brainstem. Another form of herniation can occur if the brain shifts laterally, forcing the cingulate gyrus under the falx and compressing the blood vessels of the opposite hemisphere.

Subtentorial masses or destructive lesions occur below the tentorium and interfere with consciousness by compressing or destroying the RAS above the midpons. Pontine or cerebellar hemorrhage, infarction, tumor, or abscess can affect the subtentorial area of the brain.

Metabolic and diffuse cerebral disorders of either intracranial or extracranial origin can cause alterations in the conscious state. These disorders can cause disturbances in the cerebral metabolism that regulates cellular nutrition, electrolyte balance, oxygen and carbon dioxide regulation, and enzymatic functions. Specific metabolic problems that can cause unconsciousness include uremia, diabetes, hypoglycemia, alcohol intoxication, drug (e.g., barbiturate) overdose, and lead poisoning.

Regardless of the cause of the unconscious state, two major reactions affecting cerebral metabolism generally occur: cerebral ischemia-anoxia and cerebral edema. The most common physiologic problem of metabolic brain disease is a decreased oxygen uptake. Cerebral ischemia-anoxia, both focal and global, is managed by instituting measures to ensure adequate systemic circulation. Cerebral edema and the resulting increased intracranial pressure may be treated by hyperventilation, hyperosmotic drugs, dehydration, and corticosteroids.[1]

Psychiatric or psychogenic disorders can cause unconsciousness. Although the neurologic system is intact, the patient does not react to the environment. A psychiatric referral is appropriate when the possibility of organic disease has been ruled out.

Unconscious State

The patient's state of consciousness is defined by both the behavior and the pattern of brain activity recorded by an electroencephalogram (EEG). In the deepest state of unconsciousness, the patient does not respond to painful stimuli. Corneal and pupillary reflexes are absent. The patient cannot swallow or cough and is incontinent of urine and feces. The EEG pattern demonstrates decreased or absent neuronal activity. This patient is in a coma.

Behavior. The nurse may find it helpful to conceptualize states of consciousness as a continuum. This continuum of electrical activity in the brain ranges from the hyperexcitable state of seizure to the hypoexcitable state of coma. The normal level of alertness is between these two states, with abnormalities ranging from slight disorientation to coma. A variety of terms have been used to describe points on the continuum, but they tend to be confusing (e.g., the term lethargy has a variety of meanings). Rather than relying on these terms, the nurse needs to learn appropriate assessment techniques and to describe the level of consciousness by noting the specific behaviors observed. When a deviation from the normal state of consciousness occurs, a more structured method of observation should be initiated. This type of systematic approach to nursing assessment is illustrated in Fig. 54-1 and consists of assessing the level of consciousness by the Glasgow Coma Scale (GCS) and by body functions.

Glasgow Coma Scale. Because of the confusion and ambiguity that surround terms describing altered states of consciousness, the GCS was developed in 1974. The three areas assessed in this method correspond to the definition of coma as the inability of a patient to speak, obey commands, or open the eyes when a verbal or painful stimulus is applied.[2] Specific assessments evaluate the patient's response to varying degrees of stimuli. Three indicators of response are evaluated, including opening of the eyes, the best verbal response, and the best motor response (Table 54-2). Specific behaviors that are seen as responses to the testing stimulus in each of these three areas are given a numerical value and can be plotted on a graph. The clinician's responsibility is to elicit the best response on each of the scales: the higher the scores, the higher the level of brain functioning. The graph visually plots a place on the consciousness continuum to determine whether the patient is stable, improving, or deteriorating. The subscale scores are particularly important if a patient is untestable in one area. For example, severe periorbital edema may make eye opening impossible. In addition, the score for each can

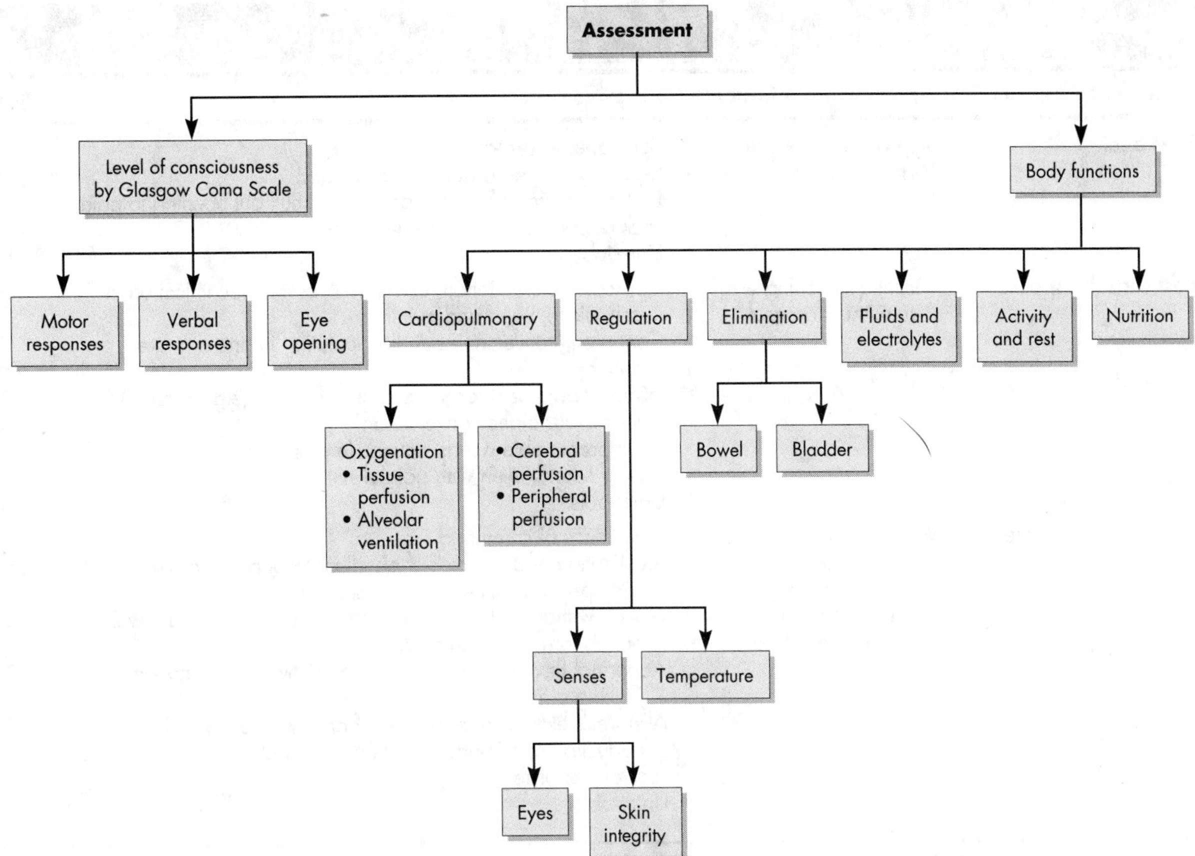

Fig. 54-1 A systematic approach to nursing assessment of the unconscious patient.

be added to give a sum. This sum can be interpreted by comparing it to the highest score of 15, for a fully alert person, and the lowest possible score of 3. A score of 8 or less is generally indicative of coma.

The GCS offers several advantages in the assessment of the unconscious patient. It is specific and structured, allowing different clinicians to arrive at the same conclusion regarding the patient's status. It saves time for the assessor because the ratings are done with numbers rather than with lengthy descriptions. The GCS is also specific enough to discriminate between different or changing states.

The GCS is used to assess the level of consciousness only. Other components of the neurologic assessment include pupillary checks, extremity strength testing, and, if appropriate, corneal reflex testing.

Monitoring of Body Functions. In addition to assessing the neurologic state of the unconscious patient, various body functions, such as respiration and elimination, also need to be monitored (Fig. 54-1). Adequate circulation and respiration are the most vital and should always be the first body functions evaluated.

INTRACRANIAL PRESSURE

Understanding the mechanisms associated with intracranial pressure (ICP) is important in caring for patients with many different neurologic problems. The skull is like a closed box with three essential volume components: brain tissue, blood, and cerebrospinal fluid (CSF) (Fig. 54-2). The total volume in the skull is 1900 ml. The intracellular and extracellular fluids of brain tissue comprise approximately 78% of this volume. Blood in the arterial, venous, and capillary network makes up 12% of the volume, and the remaining 10% is the volume of the cerebrospinal fluid (CSF). Under normal conditions, in which intracranial volume remains relatively constant, the balance between these components maintains the ICP. The modified Monro-Kellie doctrine explains the relatively constant volume of these three components within the rigid skull structure. If the volume added to the cranial vault equals the volume displaced from it, the total intracranial volume will not change. This hypothesis is not applicable in situations where the skull is not rigid (e.g., in neonates and in adults with unfused skull fractures).

Other factors that influence ICP under normal circumstances are changes in (1) arterial pressure, (2) venous pressure, (3) intraabdominal and intrathoracic pressure, (4) posture, and (5) temperature (especially hypothermia). The degree to which these other factors increase or decrease the ICP depends on the ability of the brain to accommodate to the changes.

Regulation and Maintenance of Intracranial Pressure

Normal Intracranial Pressure. Normal ICP is the pressure exerted by the total volume from the three compo-

Table 54-2 Glasgow Coma Scale

Category of Response	Appropriate Stimulus	Response	Score
■ Eyes open	Approach to bedside	Spontaneous response	4
	Verbal command	Opening of eyes to name or command	3
	Pain	Lack of opening of eyes to previous stimuli but opening to pain	2
		Lack of opening of eyes to any stimulus	1
		Untestable	U
■ Best verbal response	Verbal questioning with maximum arousal	Appropriate orientation, conversant, correct identification of self, place, year, and month	5
		Confusion, conversant, but disorientation in one or more spheres	4
		Inappropriate or disorganized use of words (e.g., cursing), lack of sustained conversation	3
		Incomprehensible words, sounds (e.g., moaning)	3
		Lack of sound, even with painful stimuli	1
		Untestable	U
■ Best motor response	Verbal command (e.g., "raise your arm, hold up two fingers")	Obedience of command	6
		Localization of pain, lack of obedience but presence of attempts to remove offending stimulus	5
	Pain (pressure on proximal nail bed)	Flexion withdrawal,* flexion of arm in response to pain without abnormal flexion posture	4
		Abnormal flexion, flexing of arm at elbow and pronation, making a fist	3
		Abnormal extension, extension of arm at elbow usually with adduction and internal rotation of arm at shoulder	2
		Lack of response	1
		Untestable	U

*Added to the original scale by many centers.

nents within the skull; brain tissue, blood, and CSF. ICP can be measured in the ventricles, subarachnoid space, subdural space, epidural space, or brain parenchymal tissue using a water manometer or a pressure transducer. With the patient in the lateral recumbent position, the pressure is generally recorded at 80 to 180 cm H_2O with the use of the water manometer. When the patient is lying with a 30-degree elevation of the head and the pressure is measured intracranially, it is 0 to 15 mm Hg with the use of the pressure transducer. A sustained pressure above the upper limit is considered abnormal.

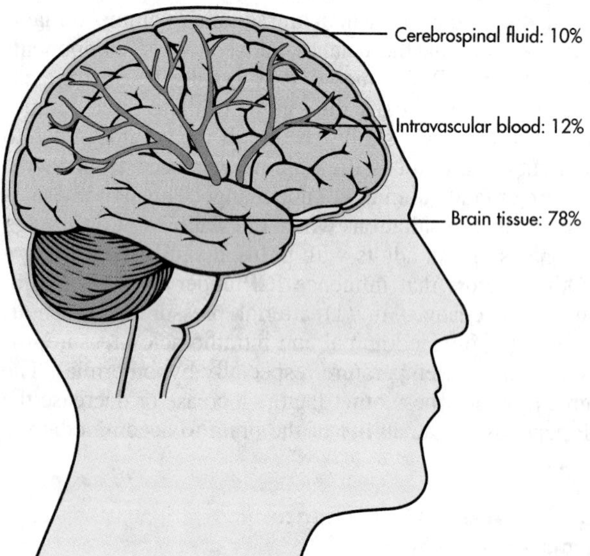

Fig. 54-2 Components of the brain.

Normal Compensatory Adaptations. In applying the modified Monro-Kellie doctrine, the body can compensate for changes in the volume of components of the skull to maintain a normal ICP. The body does this by making small changes in any of the three components. Initial compensatory mechanisms include increased CSF absorption, displacement of CSF into the spinal subarachnoid space, and collapse of the cerebral veins and dural sinuses. Other mechanisms that assist in compensation are (1) distensibility of the dura, (2) increased venous outflow, (3) decreased CSF production, (4) changes in intracranial blood volume, and (5) slight compression of brain tissue.[3]

Initially, an increase in volume produces no increase in ICP as a result of the compensatory mechanisms. However, these compensatory adaptations to changes in volume are limited, and as the volume increase continues, the ICP rises and decompensation occurs.[3]

Cerebral Blood Flow

Cerebral blood flow is the amount of blood in milliliters passing through 100 g of brain tissue in 1 minute. The global cerebral blood flow is approximately 50 ml per minute per 100 g of brain tissue. There is a difference in flow between the white and gray matter of the brain. The white matter has a slower blood flow, approximately 25 ml per minute per 100 g and the gray matter has a faster blood flow, approximately 75 ml per minute per 100 g. The maintenance of blood flow to the brain is critical because the brain requires a constant supply of oxygen and glucose. The brain uses 20% of the body's oxygen and 25% of its glucose.[4]

Autoregulation of Cerebral Blood Flow. The brain has the ability to regulate its own blood flow in response to its metabolic needs in spite of wide fluctuations in systemic arterial pressure. *Autoregulation* is defined as the automatic alteration in the diameter of the cerebral blood vessels to maintain a constant blood flow to the brain during changes in systemic arterial pressure. The purpose of autoregulation is to ensure a consistent cerebral blood flow and to maintain cerebral perfusion pressure within normal limits. The lower limit of systemic arterial pressure at which autoregulation is effective in a normotensive person is a mean arterial pressure (MAP) of 50 mm Hg. Below this, cerebral blood flow decreases and symptoms of cerebral ischemia, such as syncope and blurred vision, occur. The upper limit of systemic arterial pressure at which autoregulation is effective is 150 mm Hg. When this pressure is exceeded, the vessels are maximally constricted. Thus, further vasoconstrictor response is lost and the blood-brain barrier is disrupted; the result is an increase in cerebral edema.

The *cerebral perfusion pressure* (CPP) is the pressure needed to ensure blood flow to the brain. Its pressure is equal to the MAP minus the ICP (CPP = MAP – ICP). This formula is clinically useful, although it does not consider the effect of systemic vascular resistance.[1] As the CPP decreases, autoregulation fails and cerebral blood flow decreases. A CPP below 30 mm Hg results in cellular ischemia and is incompatible with life. Table 54-3 shows how to calculate the CPP. Under normal circumstances, autoregulation maintains an adequate cerebral blood flow and perfusion pressure by three physiologic mechanisms: changes in intracranial pressure, cerebral vasodilatation, and metabolic factors.

Pressure Changes. The relationship of pressure to volume is depicted in the pressure-volume curve. The curve is affected by the brain's elastance and compliance. *Elastance* is the brain's ability to accommodate changes in volume. It represents the stiffness of the brain. With high elastance, large increases in pressure occur with small increases in volume.

$$\text{Elastance} = \frac{\text{pressure}}{\text{volume}}$$

Compliance is the inverse of elastance and is the expansability of the brain. It is represented as the volume increase for each unit increase in pressure. Low compliance is the same as high elastance. With low compliance, high changes in pressure result from small changes in volume.

$$\text{Compliance} = \frac{\text{volume}}{\text{pressure}}$$

The concept of the pressure-volume curve can be used to represent the stages of increased ICP (intracranial hypertension) (Fig. 54-3). At stage 1 on the curve, there is high compliance and low elastance. The brain is in total compensation, with accommodation and autoregulation intact. An increase in volume does not increase the ICP. At stage 2, the compliance is lower and elastance is increasing. An increase in volume places the patient at risk of increased ICP. At stage 3, there is high elastance and low compliance. Any small addition of volume causes a great increase in pressure. There is a loss of autoregulation, and there may be symptoms indicating increased ICP, such as systolic hypertension with an increasing pulse pressure, bradycardia, and slowing of respiratory rate (*Cushing's triad*). With the loss of autoregulation and the rise in the systolic blood pressure as a result of the Cushing response, decompensation occurs. The ICP passively mimics the blood pressure. Finally, when the patient is in stage 4, the ICP rises to terminal levels with little increase in volume. Herniation occurs as the brain tissue shifts from the compartment of greater pressure to a compartment of lesser pressure.

Factors Affecting Cerebral Blood Flow. Oxygen tension, carbon dioxide tension, and hydrogen ion concen-

Table 54-3 Calculation of Cerebral Perfusion Pressure

CPP = MAP – ICP

MAP = DBP + ⅓(SBP-DBP) or $\frac{\text{SBP} + 2(\text{DBP})}{3}$

Example: Systemic blood pressure = 122/84

MAP = 97

ICP = 12 mm Hg

CPP = 85 mm Hg

CPP, Cerebral perfusion pressure; *DBP,* diastolic blood pressure; *ICP,* intracranial pressure; *MAP,* mean arterial pressure; *SBP,* systolic blood pressure.

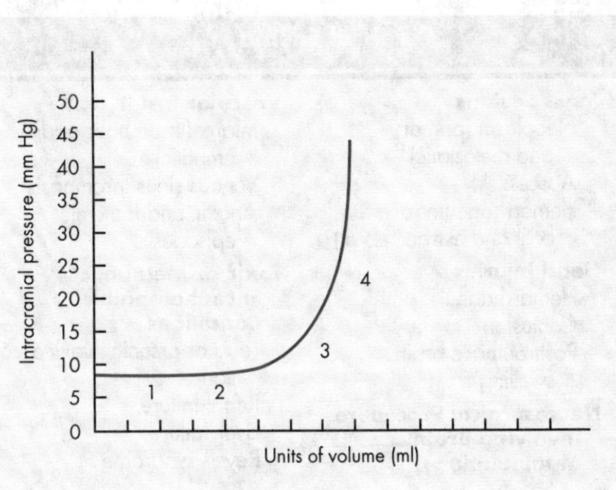

Fig. 54-3 Intracranial volume-pressure curve. (See text for descriptions of 1, 2, 3, and 4.)

tration affect cerebral vessel tone. Cerebral arteries dilate when the cerebral oxygen tension falls below 50 mm Hg. This dilatation decreases cerebral vascular resistance and increases cerebral blood flow in an effort to raise oxygen tension. If oxygen tension is not raised, anaerobic metabolism begins, resulting in an accumulation of lactic acid. In an acid environment, an increase in vasodilatation and a further increase in blood flow occur. An increase in the partial pressure of arterial carbon dioxide ($PaCO_2$) is the most potent vasodilator. An increase in $PaCO_2$ relaxes the smooth muscles. This decreases cerebrovascular resistance and increases cerebral blood flow. A severely low arterial oxygen pressure (PaO_2) and a high hydrogen ion concentration (acidosis) are also potent cerebral vasodilators.[4]

Extreme cardiovascular changes such as asystole and pathophysiologic states such as diabetic coma can alter or abolish autoregulation globally. Trauma and tumors can alter autoregulation focally. When autoregulation is lost, cerebral blood flow is no longer maintained at a constant level but is directly influenced by changes in systemic blood pressure, hypoxia, or the effects of catecholamines. Increasing ICP can progress to loss of consciousness, changes in neurologic function, brain herniation, and death.

Increased Intracranial Pressure

Increased ICP is a life-threatening situation that results from an increase in any or all of the three components of the skull-brain tissue, blood, and CSF. Cerebral edema is an important factor related to increased ICP.

Cerebral Edema. A variety of conditions are associated with cerebral edema (Table 54-4). Regardless of the cause, cerebral edema results in an increase in tissue volume that carries the potential for increased ICP. The extent and severity of the original insult are the factors that determine the degree of cerebral edema.

Three types of cerebral edema, vasogenic edema, cytotoxic edema, and interstitial edema, have been distinguished. More than one type may result from a single insult in the same patient.[5] *Vasogenic cerebral edema,* the most common type of edema, occurs mainly in the white matter, and is attributed to changes in the endothelial lining of cerebral capillaries. These changes allow leakage of macromolecules from the capillaries into the surrounding extracellular space, resulting in an osmotic gradient that favors the flow of water from the intravascular to the extravascular space. A variety of insults, such as brain tumors, abscesses, and ingested toxins, may cause an increase in the permeability of the blood-brain barrier and produce an increase in the extracellular fluid volume. The speed and extent of the spread of the edema fluid are influenced by the systemic blood pressure, the site of the brain injury, and the extent of the blood-brain barrier defect. This edema may manifest as focal neurologic deficits, disturbances in consciousness, and severe increased ICP.

Cytotoxic cerebral edema results from local disruption of the functional or morphologic integrity of cell membranes and occurs most often in the gray matter. Cytotoxic cerebral edema develops from destructive lesions or trauma to brain tissue resulting in cerebral hypoxia or anoxia, sodium depletion, and syndrome of inappropriate antidiuretic hormone (SIADH). Cerebral edema results as fluid and protein shift from the extracellular space directly into the cells, with subsequent swelling and loss of cellular function.

Interstitial cerebral edema is the result of periventricular diffusion of ventricular CSF in a patient with uncontrolled hydrocephalus. It can also be caused by enlargement of the extracellular space as a response to systemic water excess (hyponatremia). Osmotic particles and fluid move into the cells to equilibrate with the hypoosmotic interstitial fluid. Regardless of the cause of cerebral edema, manifestations of increased ICP result, unless compensation is adequate.

Mechanisms of Increased Intracranial Pressure. Increased ICP can be caused by several clinical problems, including a mass lesion, such as a hematoma, contusion, or rapidly growing tumor; cerebral edema associated with brain tumors, hydrocephalus, head injury, or brain inflammation; or metabolic coma. These cerebral insults may result in hypercapnia, cerebral acidosis, impaired autoregulation, and systemic hypertension, which promote the formation and spread of cerebral edema. This edema distorts brain tissue, further increasing the ICP, which leads to even more tissue hypoxia and acidosis. Figure 54-4 illustrates the progression of increased ICP.

Unless there is a reduction in the ICP, brainstem compression occurs. As the intracranial mass continues to increase, herniation of the brain from one compartment to another can occur.

Complications. The major complication of uncontrolled increased ICP is cerebral herniation (Fig. 54-5). The three major patterns of supratentorial brain shift are *cingulate* (lateral, beneath the falx) herniation, *central* or *transtentorial* (downward) herniation, and *uncal* (lateral and downward) herniation. These patterns are distinguished by the direction of the shift and by the cerebral structures involved. Regardless of the specific intracranial shift, displacement and herniation cause a potentially reversible pathophysiologic process to become irreversible. Ischemia

Table 54-4 Conditions Associated with Cerebral Edema

Mass Lesions Neoplasm (primary and metastatic) Abscess Hemorrhage (intracerebral and extracerebral) **Head Injuries** Hemorrhage Contusion Posttraumatic brain swelling **Neurosurgical Procedures Involving Brain Manipulation** **Infections**	**Vascular Insult** Infarct (thrombolic and embolic) Venous sinus thrombosis Anoxic and ischemic episodes **Toxic or Metabolic Encephalopathic Conditions** Lead or arsenic intoxication Renal failure Liver failure Reye's syndrome

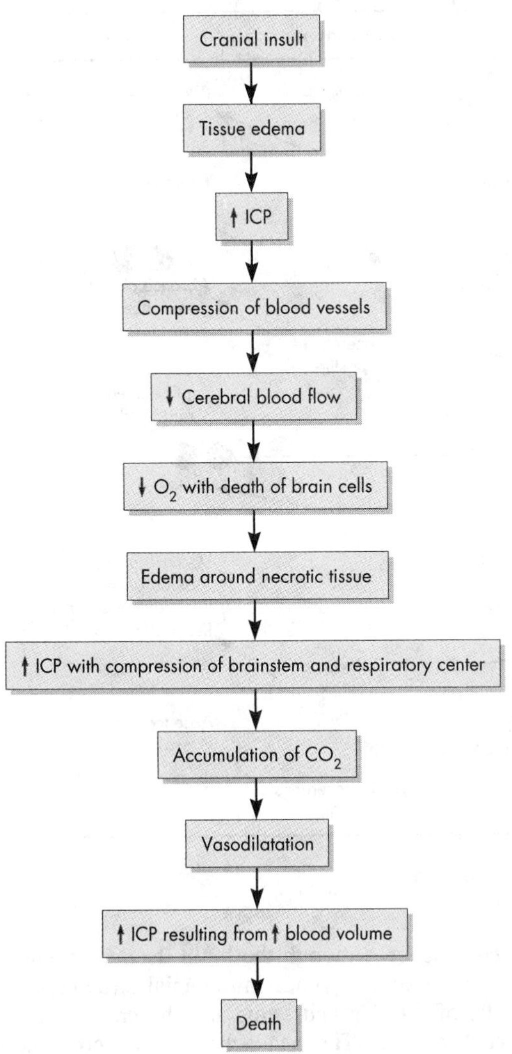

Fig. 54-4 Progression of increased intracranial pressure (ICP).

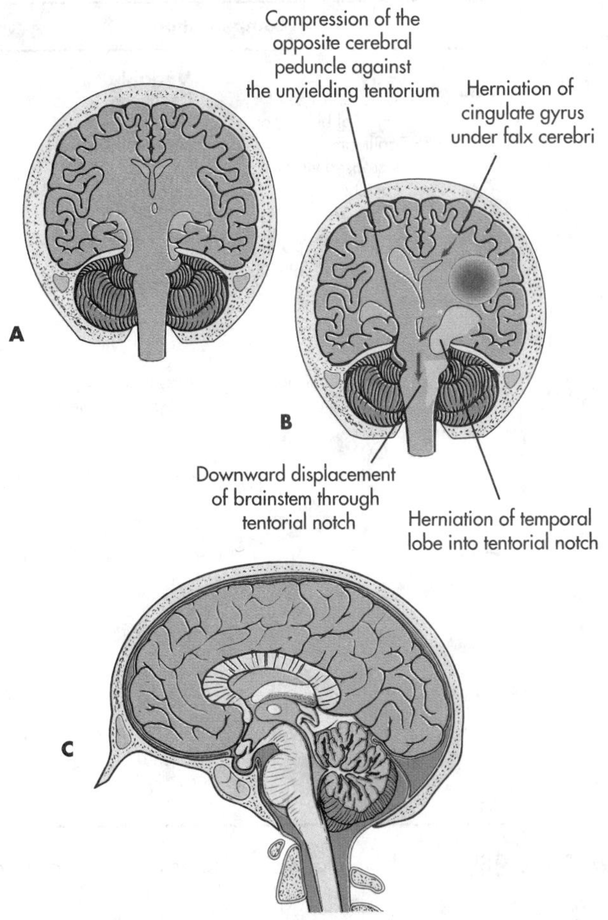

Fig. 54-5 Herniation. ***A,*** The normal relationship of intracranial structures. ***B,*** Shift of intracranial structures. ***C,*** Downward herniation of the cerebellar tonsils into the foramen magnum.

and edema are further increased, compounding the preexisting problem. Compression of the brainstem and cranial nerves may be fatal. Figure 54-6 illustrates symptoms of supratentorial increased ICP from the early phase through herniation of the brain.

Subtentorial and infratentorial herniations force the cerebellum and brainstem downward through the foramen magnum. If compression of the brainstem is unrelieved, respiratory arrest may occur.

Clinical Manifestations. The clinical manifestations of increased ICP can take many forms, depending on the cause, location, and rate at which the pressure increase occurs. The earlier the condition is recognized and treated, the better the prognosis. The clinical manifestations of increased ICP associated with supratentorial lesions include the following:

1. *Change in level of consciousness*: The level of consciousness (LOC) is a sensitive and important indicator of the patient's neurologic status. A decreasing LOC should always be investigated carefully. The change in consciousness may be dramatic, as in coma, or subtle, such as a flattening of affect, change in orientation, or decrease in level of attention. Changes in LOC are a result of impaired cerebral blood flow, which affects the cells of the cerebral cortex and the RAS.
2. *Changes in vital signs*: Although the complex of increasing systolic pressure (widening pulse pressure), bradycardia with a full and bounding pulse, and irregular respiratory pattern (Cushing's triad) may be present, these symptoms often do not appear until ICP has been increased for some time. Changes in vital signs are caused by increasing pressure on the thalamus, hypothalamus, pons, and medulla. A change in body temperature may also be noted.
3. *Ocular signs*: Compression of the oculomotor nerve (CN III) results in dilatation of the ipsilateral pupil, sluggish or no response to light, inability to move the eye upward, and ptosis of the eyelid. These signs can be the result of a shifting of the brain from the midline, a process

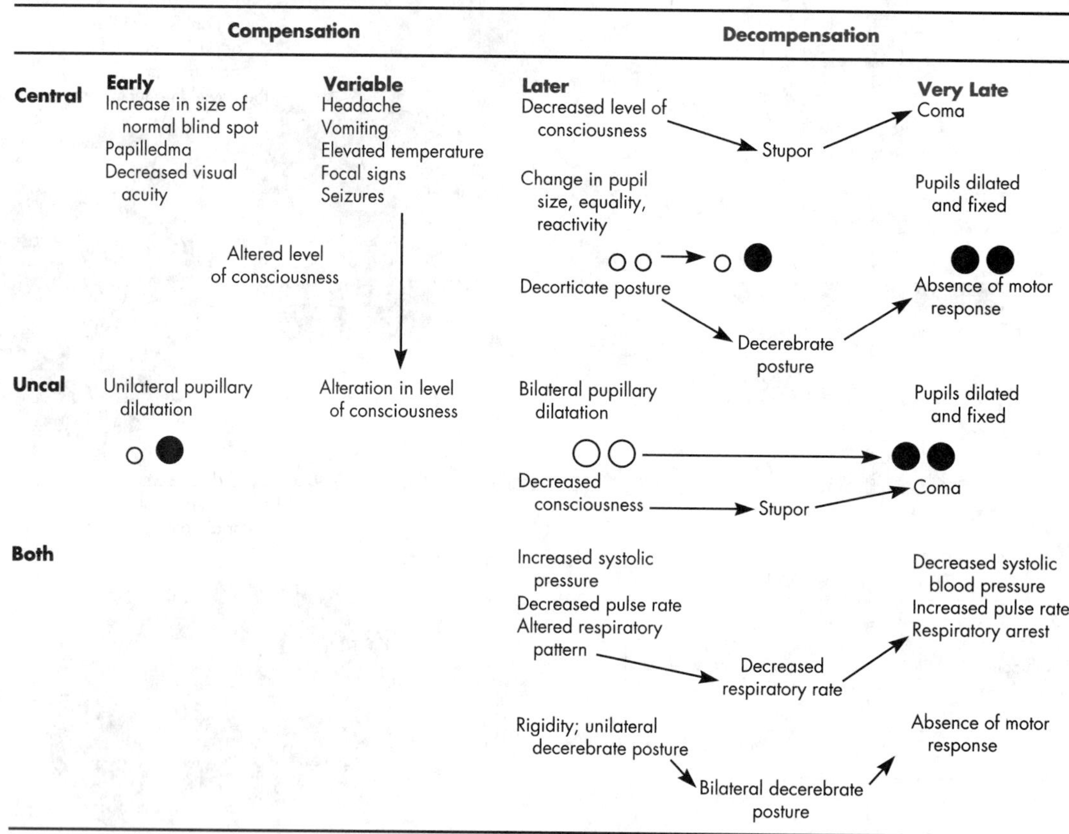

Fig. 54-6 Signs and symptoms of supratentorial increased intracranial pressure.

that compresses the trunk of CN III, paralyzing the pupil sphincter. A fixed, unilaterally dilated pupil is a neurologic emergency that indicates transtentorial herniation of the brain. Other cranial nerves may also be affected, such as the optic (CN II), trochlear (CN IV), and abducens (CN VI) nerves. Signs of dysfunction of these cranial nerves include blurred vision, diplopia, and changes in extraocular eye movements. Papilledema, a choked optic disk seen on retinal examination, is also seen and is a nonspecific sign that is associated with long-standing increased ICP.

4. *Decrease in motor function*: As the ICP continues to rise, the patient manifests changes in motor ability. A contralateral hemiparesis or hemiplegia may be seen, depending on the location of the source of the increased ICP. If painful stimuli to elicit a motor response are used, the patient may exhibit a localization to the stimuli or a withdrawal from it. *Decorticate* (flexor) and *decerebrate* (extensor) posturing may also be elicited by noxious stimuli (Fig. 54-7). A decorticate posture consists of internal rotation and adduction of the arms with flexion of the elbows, wrists, and fingers as a result of interruption of voluntary motor tracts. Extension of the legs may also be seen. A decerebrate posture may indicate more serious damage and results from disruption of motor fibers in the midbrain and brainstem. In this position, the arms are stiffly extended, adducted, and hyperpronated. There is also hyperextension of the legs with plantar flexion of the feet.

5. *Headache*: Although the brain itself is insensitive to pain, compression of other intracranial structures such as the walls of arteries and veins and the cranial nerves can produce headache. The headache is often continuous but worse in the morning. Straining or movement may accentuate the pain.

6. *Vomiting*: Vomiting, usually not preceded by nausea, is often a nonspecific sign of increased ICP. This is called *unexpected vomiting* and is related to pressure changes in the cranium. Projectile vomiting may also be seen in children and is related to increased ICP.

It is often difficult to identify increased ICP as the cause of coma. Loss of consciousness also confuses the interpretation of clinical signs, making it difficult to follow the progression of the increasing ICP.

Diagnostic Studies. Diagnostic studies are aimed at identifying the presence and the underlying cause of increased ICP (Table 54-5). Computed tomography (CT) has revolutionized the diagnosis of increased ICP. It is usually the initial test and can be used to differentiate the many conditions that can cause increased ICP and to evaluate therapeutic options. CT scans are particularly helpful in patients who have experienced trauma or who have tumors. Other tests that may be used include cerebral angiography, EEG, cerebral blood flow and transcranial Doppler studies, and evoked potential studies. New diagnostic tests, such as positron emission tomography (PET) and magnetic reso-

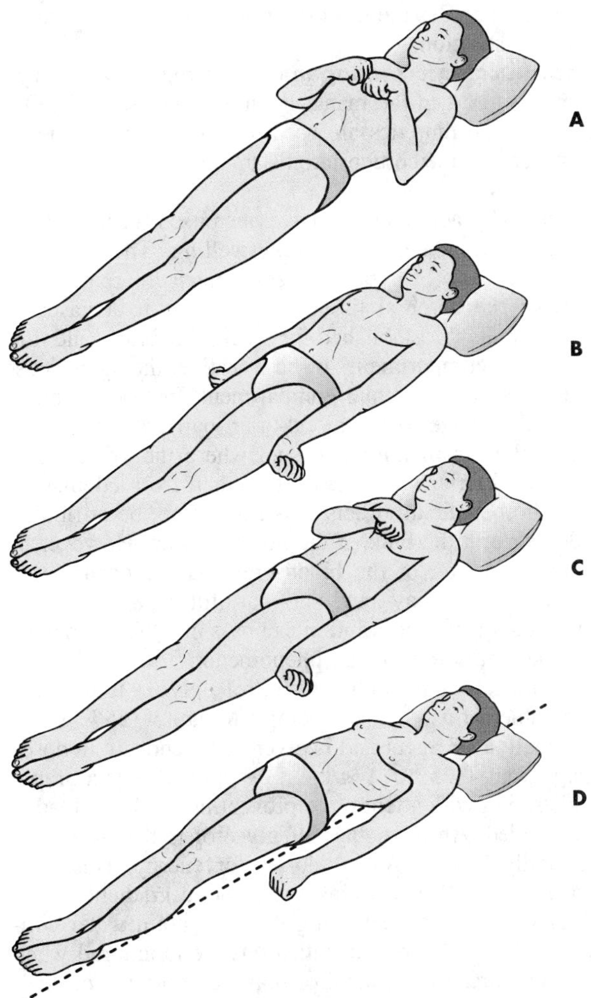

Fig. 54-7 Decorticate and decerebrate posturing. ***A,*** Decorticate response. Flexion of arms, wrists, and fingers with adduction in upper extremities. Extension, internal rotation, and plantar flexion in lower extremities. ***B,*** Decerebrate response. All four extremities in rigid extension, with hyperpronation of forearms and plantar extension of feet. ***C,*** Decorticate response on right side of body and decerebrate response on left side of body. ***D,*** Opisthotonic posturing.

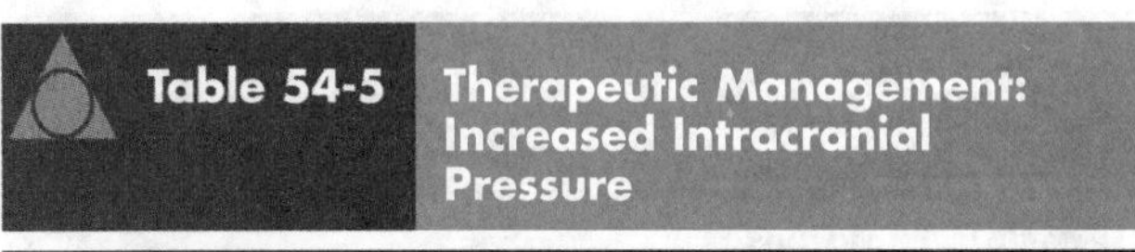

Table 54-5 Therapeutic Management: Increased Intracranial Pressure

Diagnostic
History and physical examination
Vital signs, neurologic checks, ICP measurements (via intraventricular catheter, subdural bolt, or epidural transducer) every hour
Skull, chest, and spinal x-ray studies
CT scan, EEG, angiography
Cerebral blood flow and velocity studies, MRI, PET
Laboratory studies, including CBC, coagulation profile, electrolytes, creatinine, ABGs, ammonia level, general drug and toxicology screen, CSF protein, cells, and glucose
ECG
Therapeutic
Elevation of head of bed to 30 degrees with head in neutral position
Intubation and controlled ventilation to $PaCO_2$ of 30 to 35 mm Hg
Good pulmonary toilet
Maintenance of fluid balance with 0.5 normal saline solution, assessment of osmolality
Maintenance of systolic arterial pressure between 100 and 160 mm Hg
Maintenance of CPP >70 mm Hg
Maintenance of PaO_2 at 100 mm Hg or greater
Maintenance of normothermia
Adequate sedation
Drug therapy
Osmotic diuretics (mannitol)
Loop diuretics (furosemide, ethacrynic acid)
Corticosteroids (methylprednisolone, dexamethasone)
ICP monitoring

ABGs, Arterial blood gases; *CBC,* complete blood count, *CPP,* cerebral perfusion pressure; *CT,* computed tomography; *CSF,* cerebrospinal fluid; *ECG,* electrocardiogram; *EEG,* electroencephalogram; *ICP,* intracranial pressure; *MRI,* magnetic resonance imaging; *$PaCO_2$,* partial pressure of arterial carbon dioxide; *PaO_2,* partial pressure of arterial oxygen; *PET,* position emission tomography.

nance imaging (MRI), may prove to be even more helpful in diagnosing the cause of increased ICP. Transcranial Doppler studies may be used to determine cerebral blood flow and velocity. In general, a lumbar puncture is not performed when increased ICP is suspected because of the possibility of cerebral herniation from the sudden release of the pressure in the skull from the area above the lumbar puncture.

Therapeutic Management. The goals of therapeutic management (Table 54-5) are to identify and treat the underlying cause of increased ICP and to support brain function. A careful history is an important diagnostic aid that can direct the search for the underlying cause.

The emergency management of the patient with actual or potential increased ICP is important to prevent secondary injury to the brain (Table 54-6). Once the patient has been transported to a hospital, aggressive therapeutic management is needed.

While the cause of increased ICP is being sought, the condition itself must be treated aggressively to interrupt the cycle. Ensuring adequate oxygenation to support brain function is the first step in the management of increased ICP. An endotracheal tube or tracheostomy may be necessary to maintain adequate ventilation. Arterial blood gas (ABG) analysis guides the oxygen therapy. The goal is to maintain the PaO_2 at 100 mm Hg or greater. It may be necessary to maintain the patient on a ventilator to ensure adequate oxygenation.

A mild hyperventilation to maintain a $PaCO_2$ of 30 to 35 mm Hg can have an effect on cerebral blood flow. The lowering of the $PaCO_2$ leads to constriction of the cerebral blood vessels, reducing cerebral blood flow and thereby

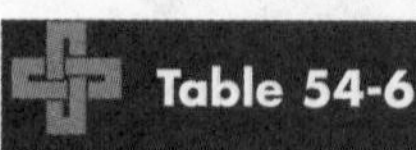

Table 54-6 Emergency Management of the Unconscious Patient

Possible Etiologies

Head and neck trauma, drug overdose, meningitis, encephalitis, metabolic conditions (e.g., diabetic coma, insulin shock, liver failure, uremia, carbon dioxide narcosis), cardiac arrest, exogenous toxins (e.g., ethylene glycol, salicylates), cerebrovascular accident

Possible Assessment Findings

Unable to arouse
Altered neurologic and vital signs
Pupillary changes (dilated or pinpoint)
Involuntary movements
Flaccidity or rigidity of muscles
Depressed or hyperactive reflexes
Decerebrate or decorticate posturing
Diaphoresis
Unresponsive to deep stimuli
Glasgow Coma Score <12
Odor of alcohol or acetone on breath
Use of combative, abusive language; forgetfulness

Management

- Monitor airway. Have airway equipment available, including suction and intubation supplies. Anticipate need for intubation if gag reflex is absent.
- Administer oxygen via nasal cannula or non-rebreather mask (100%) and monitor for respiratory distress. If not breathing, ventilate with bag-valve mask.
- Establish IV access with one large-bore catheter and normal saline.
- Obtain history, attempt to determine underlying cause (e.g., drug overdose, medical problem, trauma).
- Monitor vital signs including level of consciousness, oxygen saturation, cardiac rhythm, Glasgow Coma Score, pupil size
- Administer IV naloxone (if possibility of narcotic overdose) and thiamine (e.g., to treat Wernicke's syndrome)
- Check blood glucose and administer one vial of 50% dextrose if blood glucose <60 mg/dl (3.3 mmol/L); if glucose >400 mg/dl (22.2 mmol/L) notify physician and prepare to administer subcutaneous or IV insulin and start an insulin drip
- Anticipate need for gastric lavage if drug overdose

IV, Intravenous.

decreasing the ICP.[6] This positive effect assumes that the brain will respond to hypocapnia by vasoconstriction. Lowering the $PaCO_2$ below 20 mm Hg can cause ischemia and a worsening of the increased ICP.

If the condition is caused by a mass lesion, such as a tumor or hematoma, surgical removal of the mass is the best management (see Intracranial Tumors, later in this chapter). Nonsurgical intervention for the reduction of tissue volume related to cerebral tissue swelling and cerebral edema includes the use of diuretics and corticosteroids and fluid restriction.

Pharmacologic Management. Drug therapy plays an important part in the management of increased ICP. Osmotic and loop diuretics are used to reduce the volume of brain water, and the corticosteroids are thought to control the cerebral edema.

Osmotically active agents have been used for more than 50 years to treat cerebral tissue swelling. The principle governing the use of hypertonic solutions is the removal of fluid from the cerebral tissues in response to a vascular osmotic gradient established between the brain and the intravascular compartment. To be effective, the agent must remain in the intravascular compartment. In cases of brain injury and damage to the blood-brain barrier, the osmotic withdrawal is from normal tissue, where the vessels and blood-brain barrier are intact, rather than from edematous tissue. The beneficial effects must, therefore, be attributed to a decrease in the bulk of the normal tissue. However, if a major disruption of the blood-brain barrier occurs, this form of therapy may be more harmful than beneficial, because the hypertonic solution can pass into the edematous tissue and lead to a rebound phenomenon.[5]

Agents such as mannitol (Osmitrol), glycerol, and urea are available for use in osmotherapy. Mannitol (25%) is the most widely used agent and is given intravenously in doses ranging from 0.25 to 1 g/kg. For optimal effect, rapid administration with attention to preventing fluid overload is recommended. An advantage of glycerol is that it can be given orally and provides calories for energy. This drug decreases the ICP by altering the osmotic gradient across cerebral vessels and decreasing the total brain water content.[7] Fluid and electrolyte status must be monitored when these drugs are used. Mannitol may be contraindicated if renal disease is present and if serum osmolality is elevated. The effect of these hypertonic solutions is rapid and short lived.

Recent studies have demonstrated the positive effect on increased ICP of loop diuretics such as furosemide (Lasix) and ethacrynic acid (Edecrin). These diuretics inhibit sodium and chloride reabsorption in the ascending limb of the loop of Henle and cause a reduction in the rate of CSF production by 40% to 70%, thus reducing the ICP.[4] This lowering of pressure enhances the clearance of tissue fluid.

Despite the controversy over the value of corticosteroid therapy in certain forms of cerebral edema, corticosteroids have been used extensively in the treatment of cerebral edema. Dexamethasone (Decadron), a semisynthetic steroid, is the most commonly used steroid, and studies have demonstrated that it effectively reduces vasogenic cerebral edema.

The mode of action of corticosteroids is not completely known. It is theorized that they act by their stabilizing effect on the cell membrane. Corticosteroids are also thought to improve neuronal function by improving cerebral blood flow and restoring autoregulation. Corticosteroids are most beneficial in patients who have brain tumors with peritumoral edema. High-dose dexamethasone treatment is not effective in improving the outcome of severe head injuries.[8]

Complications associated with the use of corticosteroids include hyperglycemia, increased incidence of infections, and gastrointestinal (GI) bleeding. Patients receiving corticosteroids should concurrently be given antacids or histamine H_2 receptor blockers such as cimetidine (Tagamet) to prevent GI bleeding. Fluid intake should be monitored because of the potential for hyponatremia. Since hyperglycemia has also been associated with corticosteroid use, glucose levels of the blood and urine should be monitored regularly.

Pharmacologic management of the cerebral metabolic rate is effective in controlling the ICP. The reduction in the metabolic rate decreases the cerebral blood flow and, therefore, the ICP. High-dose barbiturates (e.g., pentobarbital and thiopental) are used in patients with increased ICP because they produce a decrease in cerebral metabolism and a subsequent decrease in increased ICP. A secondary effect is a reduction in cerebral edema and a more uniform blood supply to the brain.[6] Capabilities to monitor the patient should be available when this treatment is used.

Research into other agents that may be useful in controlling the metabolic rate and the ICP following injury is ongoing. These agents include phenytoin, lidocaine, calcium channel blockers, and antioxidants.[9] Their mechanisms are not well understood, but their effect on preventing the formation of cerebral edema and controlling ICP is promising.

Nutritional Management. All patients must have their nutritional needs met, regardless of their state of consciousness or health. The patient with increased ICP is in a hypermetabolic and hypercatabolic state and in need of glucose to provide the necessary fuel for the metabolism of the injured brain. If the patient cannot maintain an adequate oral intake, other means of meeting the nutritional requirements, such as an enteral feeding tube or total parenteral nutrition should be initiated (see Chapter 37). Because certain types of feedings are low in sodium, added salt may be necessary. In addition to added minerals, free water may also be needed to meet the fluid needs of the patient. Because malnutrition promotes continued cerebral edema, maintenance of optimal nutrition is imperative.

It is controversial as to whether patients should be maintained in a state of moderate dehydration. On one hand, moderate dehydration is thought to be effective in reducing cerebral edema; in this case fluids are restricted to 65% to 75% of normal requirements. However, the concern is that hypovolemia may result in a decrease in cardiac output and blood pressure which may have an impact on cerebral perfusion and the amount of oxygen delivered to the brain. There is additional concern that dehydrated patients do not respond well to vasoactive drugs. Because of this it is recommended by some clinicians that patients be kept normovolemic with a pulmonary wedge pressure of 4 to 6 mm Hg.[10] The use of fluid restriction to reduce tissue volume should be evaluated on the basis of clinical factors such as urine output, insensible fluid loss, serum and urine osmolality, and the condition of the patient.

A lowering of serum osmolarity and an increase in cerebral edema occur if 5% dextrose in water is used for the administration of piggyback medications. If an intravenous (IV) drug routine is used, 0.45% or 0.9% sodium chloride is the preferred solution.[6]

NURSING MANAGEMENT

INCREASED INTRACRANIAL PRESSURE

Regardless of the cause of unconsciousness, the unconscious patient is managed with the assumption that the ICP is increased or has the potential to increase. The primary goals of nursing management are to (1) prevent secondary cerebral damage, (2) maintain function, and (3) prevent complications secondary to immobility and the decreased LOC.

Nursing Assessment

Subjective data about the unconscious patient can be obtained from family members or other persons who are familiar with the patient. Events preceding the unconscious state should be investigated. Figure 54-1 presents a systematic approach to assessment of the unconscious patient. This information, together with data for the GCS (see Table 54-2), provides the base of knowledge on which a nursing care plan can be formulated.

Ongoing assessment and recording of the ICP is important for evaluating trends and responses to nursing care. Figure 54-8 illustrates a typical neurologic clinical flow sheet used to display a patient's neurologic status over time.

The general plan of the neurologic assessment is to evaluate the patient's mental status, cranial nerve functioning, motor functioning, sensory status, cerebellar functioning, and reflexes. This schema helps the nurse organize the assessment to gather the data needed (see Chapter 53 for a discussion of the neurologic assessment). If the patient is critically ill, an abbreviated neurologic assessment using the GCS, pupillary checks, and certain cranial nerve evaluations is made by the nurse on an ongoing basis.

The pupils are compared to one another for size, movement, and response (Fig. 54-9). If the oculomotor nerve is compressed by supratentorial pressure, the pupil on the affected side (ipsilateral) becomes larger until it fully dilates. If ICP continues to increase, both pupils dilate.

Pupillary reaction is tested with a flashlight. The normal reaction is brisk constriction when the light is shone directly into the eye. A consensual response (a slight constriction in the opposite pupil) should also be noted at the same time. A sluggish reaction can indicate early pressure on CN III. A fixed pupil shows no response to light stimulus, which usually indicates increased ICP.

Evaluation of other cranial nerves can be included in the neurologic check. Eye movements controlled by cranial nerves III, IV, and VI can be examined in the patient who is awake and can be used to assess the function of the brainstem. In the unconscious patient, extraocular eye movements are not specifically tested. Testing the corneal reflex gives information on the functioning of cranial nerves V and VII. If this reflex is absent, routine eye care should be initiated to prevent corneal abrasion (see Chapter 18).

Eye movements of the uncooperative or unconscious patient can be elicited by reflex with the use of head move-

Neurologic Assessment Record

Coma scale

	Date ⟶															
	Time ⟶															
Eyes open	Spontaneously															Eyes closed by swelling = C
	To speech															
	To pain															
	None															
Best verbal response	Oriented															Endotracheal tube or tracheostomy = T
	Confused															
	Inappropriate															
	Incomprehensible															
	None															
Best motor response	Obey commands															Usually record the best arm response Agitated = A
	Localize pain															
	Flexion to pain															
	Extension to pain															
	None															
Vital signs	Blood pressure															1 2 3 4 5 6 7 8
	Pulse															
	Respiration															
	Temperature															**Pupil scale (mm)**
Pupils react = + No reaction = − Eye closed = C	**R** Size															
	Reaction															0. No evidence of muscle contraction.
	L Size															
	Reaction															1. Palpable muscle movement — no joint motion.
Limb movement	Right upper															
	Right lower															2. Complete motion without gravity.
	Left upper															3. Barely complete motion against gravity.
	Left lower															
	Intake															4. Complete motion against gravity with some resistance.
	Output															5. Complete motion against gravity with full resistance.
																F — Abnormal flexion
																E — Abnormal extension

Fig. 54-8 Neurologic clinical flow sheet.

ments (oculocephalic) and caloric stimulation (oculovestibular) (see Chapters 17 and 18).[11] To test the oculocephalic reflex ("doll's-head" or "doll's-eyes" phenomenon), the nurse rotates the patient's head briskly while holding the eyelids open. A positive response is movement of the eyes across the midline in the direction opposite to that of the rotation. Next, the nurse quickly flexes and then extends the neck. Eye movement should be opposite to the direction of head movement—up when the neck is flexed and down when it is extended. Abnormal responses can aid in locating the intracranial lesion. This test should not be attempted if a cervical spine problem is suspected. (The oculovestibular reflex is discussed in Chapters 17 and 18.)

Motor strength is tested by asking the patient who is awake to squeeze the nurse's hands to compare strength in the hands. The palmar drift test is an excellent measure of strength in the upper extremities. The patient raises the arms in front of the body with the palmar surface facing upward. If there is any weakness in the upper extremity, the palmar surface turns downward and the arm drifts downward. Asking the patient to raise the foot from the bed or to bend the knees up in bed is a good assessment of lower extremity strength. All four extremities should be tested for

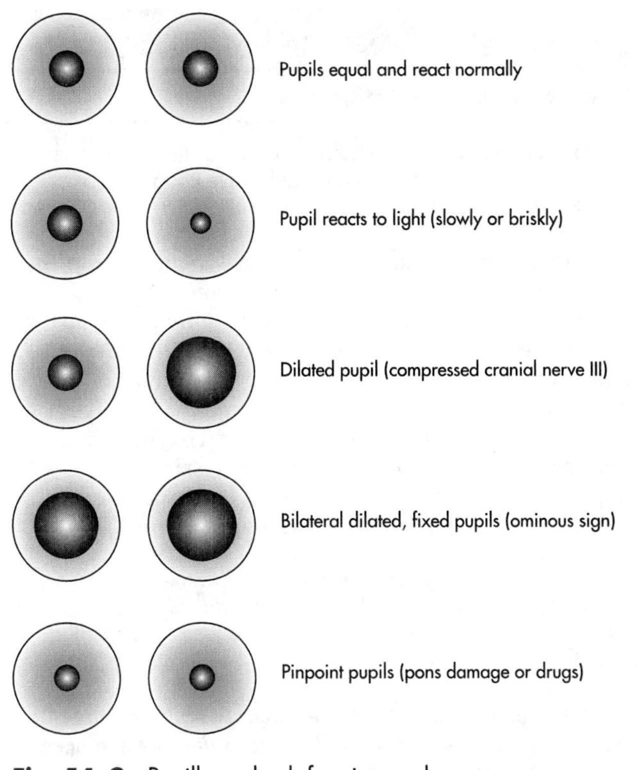

Fig. 54-9 Pupillary check for size and response.

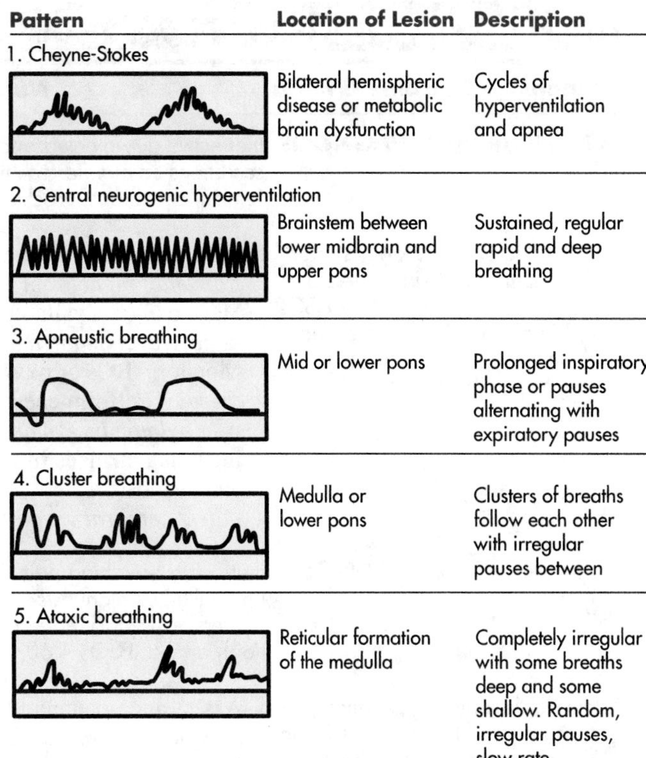

Fig. 54-10 Common abnormal respiratory patterns associated with coma.

strength and evaluated for any asymmetry in strength or movement.

The motor strength of the unconscious or uncooperative patient can be assessed by observation of spontaneous movement. If no spontaneous movement is possible, a pain stimulus should be applied to the patient, and the response should be noted. Resistance to movement during passive range-of-motion exercises is another measure of strength.

The vital signs, including blood pressure, pulse, respiratory rate, and temperature, should also be systematically recorded. The nurse needs to be aware of the Cushing triad, since this indicates severe increased ICP. Besides recording respiratory rate, the nurse should also note the respiratory pattern (Fig. 54-10).

Nursing Diagnoses

The nursing diagnoses are supported by the data obtained on assessment and include those associated with increased ICP and unconsciousness. Patients with one or both of these serious problems require the highest level of nursing care because they are usually totally dependent on the nurse. Nursing diagnoses related to the unconscious patient are presented in the nursing care plan for the unconscious patient on p. 1696.

Planning

The overall goals are that the patient with increased ICP and unconsciousness will (1) have decreased ICP to within normal limits, (2) maintain a patent airway, and (3) demonstrate normal fluid and electrolyte balance.

Nursing Implementation

Maintenance of Respiratory Function. Maintenance of a patent airway is critical in the patient with increased ICP and is a primary nursing responsibility. As the LOC decreases, the patient is at increased risk of airway obstruction from the tongue dropping back and occluding the airway or from accumulation of secretions. Altered breathing patterns may become evident. Airway patency can be aided by keeping the patient lying on one side, with frequent position changes. Snoring sounds, which may indicate obstruction, should be noted. Accumulated secretions should be removed by suctioning, as needed. An oral airway facilitates breathing and provides an easier suctioning route in the comatose patient.

The nurse must use measures to prevent hypoxia and hypercapnia. Proper positioning of the head is important. Elevation of the head of the bed by 30 degrees enhances respiratory exchange and aids in decreasing cerebral edema. Suctioning and coughing can cause transient increases in the ICP and decreases in the PaO_2. Suctioning should be kept to a minimum and should be less than 10 seconds in duration, with administration of 100% oxygen before and after to prevent decreases in the PaO_2.[12] To avoid cumulative increases in the ICP with suctioning, suctioning should be limited to two passes per suction procedure. Patients with elevated ICP are at risk for lower CPP during suctioning.[13]

Abdominal distention can interfere with respiratory function and should be prevented. Insertion of a nasogastric

NURSING CARE PLAN Unconscious Patient

Planning: Outcome Criteria	Nursing Interventions and Rationales
➤ **NURSING DIAGNOSIS**	Ineffective airway clearance *related to* unconsciousness, immobility, and inability to mobilize secretions *as manifested by* inability to maintain proper position, ineffective cough, inability to clear secretions, crackles on auscultation, thick secretions
Have decreased risk of aspiration; demonstrate increased air exchange as measured by ABGs within normal limits; have clear chest x-ray; have clear breath sounds in all lobes of the lungs.	Maintain patient's side-lying position, keeping head of bed elevated *to prevent aspiration and tongue from blocking airway and to assist in decreasing cerebral edema.* Have oxygen available *to treat cerebral hypoxia if necessary.* Suction frequently *to remove accumulated secretions, reduce risk of aspiration, and ensure patent airway.* Monitor ABGs or oxygen saturation by pulse oximetry *to evaluate effectiveness of therapy.* Perform chest physical therapy at least q4hr *to improve ventilation and prevent pulmonary complications.* Monitor patient for signs of decreased oxygenation, including changes in LOC, decreased PaO_2 or SaO_2, and increased respiratory rate and cyanosis *as low PaO_2 and a high hydrogen ion concentration (acidosis) are potent cerebral vasodilators which increase cerebral flow and may increase ICP.*
➤ **NURSING DIAGNOSIS**	Ineffective breathing patterns *related to* loss of central nervous system integrative function and immobility *as manifested by* hypoventilation or hyperventilation as measured by ABGs, altered respiratory pattern (e.g., Cheyne-Stokes respiration, central neurogenic hyperventilation), apnea, PaO_2 <60 mm Hg, $PaCO_2$ >45 mm Hg
Have adequate oxygenation as demonstrated by PaO_2 >80 mm Hg, clear chest x-ray finding, normal breathing pattern.	Assess and document breathing pattern and breath sounds *to identify abnormalities and plan appropriate interventions.* Monitor ABGs *to guide oxygen therapy* and need for ventilatory support. Implement ventilatory support as ordered *to ensure adequate oxygenation.* Suction patient as needed *to reduce risk of aspiration and maintain patent airway.* Provide frequent rest periods *to prevent respiratory fatigue.* Monitor use of drugs (e.g., barbiturates and narcotics) *as they may depress respirations and reduce the patient's LOC.*
➤ **NURSING DIAGNOSIS**	Altered cerebral tissue perfusion *related to* cerebral tissue swelling *as manifested by* Glasgow Coma Scale <8, agitation, altered thought processes, elevated systolic blood pressure, bradycardia, widened pulse pressure, intracranial pressure >20 mm Hg, CPP <60 mm Hg
Have no further deterioration in LOC, ICP <20 mm Hg, CPP >60 mm Hg, stable vital signs.	Monitor patient's neurologic status at least every hour initially; assess level of consciousness and document *to evaluate patient's response to treatment and modify if necessary.* Monitor ICP and calculate CPP *to evaluate adequacy of cerebral blood perfusion, detect patient's response to treatment, and provide information necessary for clinical decisions.* Limit care activities that increase intracranial pressure (e.g., suctioning, hip flexion) *to avoid raising intraabdominal pressure which can restrict movement of the diaphragm and cause respiratory distress leading to increased ICP.* Provide comfort measures *as pain or agitation increase ICP.* Elevate head of bed 30 to 45 degrees *to facilitate reduction of cerebral edema.* Hyperventilate patient to $PaCO_2$ of 30 to 35 mm Hg when ICP >20 mm Hg *as CO_2 is a potent cerebral vasodilator and hyperventilation reduces $PaCO_2$.* Monitor reactions to all medications (especially diuretics and sedatives) *to evaluate reduction of cerebral edema and level of consciousness.* Calibrate and maintain intracranial monitoring device *to provide an accurate indicator of intracranial pressure.*

continued

tube to aspirate the stomach contents can prevent distention, vomiting, and possible aspiration.

ABGs should be measured and evaluated regularly (see Chapter 22). The appropriate ventilatory support can be ordered on the basis of the PaO_2 and $PaCO_2$ values. The nurse should be aware if moderate hyperventilation ($PaCO_2$ of 30 to 35 mm Hg) is desired.

Unless the patient is on ventilatory support, the use of narcotic sedatives and opiates should be evaluated on an individual basis. Besides depressing respirations, these agents can also cloud the patient's LOC. A narcotic that does not increase the ICP, depress respiration, or cloud LOC should be selected to control pain. A nonnarcotic analgesic can be used in the patient with an increased ICP

NURSING CARE PLAN Unconscious Patient—cont'd

Planning: Outcome Criteria	*Nursing Interventions and Rationales*
➤ **NURSING DIAGNOSIS**	Altered nutrition: less than body requirements *related to* hypermetabolism and inability to ingest food and fluids *as manifested by* further decrease in LOC, self-care deficit for feeding, hyperthermia (body temperature >101° F [38.3° C]), metabolic needs in excess of intake, weight loss
Have adequate caloric intake to maintain weight and promote healing; maintain weight within 5 lb (2.3 kg) of admission weight; have normal electrolyte levels.	Assess fluid status and document intake and output hourly initially *to evaluate adequacy of renal perfusion and indicators of fluid balance.* Check skin turgor *as an indicator of fluid balance.* Monitor electrolytes *to identify electrolyte imbalance and initiate treatment.* Weigh patient daily *as an indicator of effectiveness of nutritional therapy.* Maintain fluid restrictions as ordered *to prevent exacerbating cerebral edema.* Evaluate swallowing abilities *to reduce risk of aspiration if oral intake is maintained.* Advance patient to high-protein, high-caloric feedings (enteral or oral as indicated) *to provide nutrients needed to prevent wasting and negative nitrogen balance.* Auscultate bowel sounds before feeding *to assure presence of peristalsis.* Elevate head of bed during and after feedings *to reduce risk of regurgitation and aspiration.* Provide adequate free water if not contraindicated *to maintain a high fluid intake.*
➤ **NURSING DIAGNOSIS**	Impaired skin integrity *related to* nutritional deficit, self-care deficit, and immobility *as manifested by,* pressure sores, irritated areas, dry skin, fever, weight loss >10 lb (4.5 kg), abrasions or lacerations
Have absence of skin breakdown.	Assess skin frequently, especially over bony prominences and around genitalia and buttocks *to identify potential or actual skin problems and initiate a plan of care.* Turn patient at least q2hr as indicated *as prolonged pressure decreases capillary circulation and leads to tissue hypoxia and necrosis.* Provide fluids *to prevent dehydration.* Use low-air-loss beds as indicated *to reduce pressure to bony prominences by distributing body weight evenly.* Cleanse all irritated skin areas; massage skin as indicated *to reduce risk of infection and stimulate circulation.*
➤ **NURSING DIAGNOSIS**	Risk for infection *related to* immobility, invasive monitoring devices and lines, and compromised immune system
Be free of wound infections; have normal temperature and white blood cell count, and no abnormal chest x-ray findings.	Assess for hyperthermia (temperature >101° F [38.4° C]), exudate around catheter insertion sites (IV, indwelling, intracranial), lethargy, abnormal chest x-ray findings and breath sounds, foul-smelling urine *to determine if factors indicating infection are present.* Observe strict sterile technique when assisting with insertion and maintenance of ICP-monitoring devices and all invasive lines; maintain integrity of all closed systems *to prevent introduction of bacteria and subsequent infection.* Monitor and record any leakage of fluid from nose (rhinorrhea), ears (otorrhea), or around ICP monitoring site and invasive lines *since fluid can introduce bacteria into a site.* Take temperature rectally at least q4hr *as one indicator of infection.* Monitor for signs of meningitis (e.g., change in LOC, fever, increased WBC count, nuchal rigidity, photophobia) *to enable prompt initiation of treatment.* Obtain cultures of exudate or as ordered *to identify causative organism so specific treatment can be initiated.*
➤ **NURSING DIAGNOSIS**	Self-care deficit (total) *related to* altered mental state *as manifested by* inability to follow commands or move purposefully, use of sedation to control metabolic rate, inability to perform ADLs
Have all ADLs met by caregivers until self-care is possible.	Assess level of motor and sensory abilities at least q4hr *to determine level of care needed.* Bathe patient daily *to maintain hygiene needs.* Turn patient q2hr as indicated *to promote skin integrity.* Perform ROM exercises at least q4hr as tolerated *to maintain joint ROM and muscle strength.* Begin bowel program as soon as possible *to resume bowel elimination pattern and prevent impaction.* Allow family to participate in care when appropriate *to make them feel like a part of the treatment team and to provide diversion for them.* Allow patient to participate in care when able *to promote self-esteem and physical activity.* Monitor intake and output *to evaluate patient's fluid balance and renal function.*

continued

NURSING CARE PLAN Unconscious Patient—cont'd

Planning: Outcome Criteria	Nursing Interventions and Rationales
➤ **NURSING DIAGNOSIS**	Risk for injury *related to* seizure activity, environmental hazards, and inability to monitor personal safety
Have no injury; have a safe environment provided by caregiver.	Assess for decreased LOC, motor or sensory deficits or loss, and seizure activity *to determine if risk for injury is present.* Assess hospital and home environment *to identify safety hazards.* Make sure side rails are up at all times; maintain bed in low position; monitor for seizure activity; pad side rails *to protect patient from inadvertent self-injury.* Place airway at bedside *for use during seizure to reduce oral trauma and help maintain airway.* Document all seizure activity *so a record of trends of seizure activity is available.* Assess patient's motor and sensory abilities frequently *so injury-prevention intervention will be appropriate to current status.* Orient patient to environment when appropriate *to minimize risk of injury due to unfamiliarity with environment.* Stay with patient during any seizure activity *so injury-prevention strategies can be initiated as appropriate.*
➤ **NURSING DIAGNOSIS**	Anxiety of family members *related to* lack of knowledge concerning nature and prognosis of coma *as manifested by* frequent questioning by family regarding patient's condition, unrealistic expectations for recovery, expressions of anxiety over lack of knowledge
Family will have increased knowledge and adequate information on which to make decisions about future care; express tolerable anxiety level.	Encourage family members to ask questions of health care team *to promote understanding, lessen fears of unknown, and reduce anxiety.* Spend time with family members (especially when they are at the bedside) *to provide support, answer questions, and demonstrate appropriate interventions.* Explain all procedures thoroughly to them *to reduce fears of unknown.* Encourage regular family conferences with physicians, nurses, and other health care team members *to provide information about patient's condition, enable family to be integral part of patient's care, and provide sense of control.*
➤ **NURSING DIAGNOSIS**	Altered family processes *related to* comatose family member *as manifested by* inability to adapt to health crisis of family member, lack of communication or miscommunication among family members
Family members will verbalize feelings, participate in care of ill member, use appropriate referrals, support each other in positive manner.	Assess effect of ill family member on family as a whole *to determine extent of problems and to plan appropriate interventions.* Teach and assist family members to provide care to ill family members when appropriate *to enable the family to be an integral part of patient's care.* Facilitate family communication and realistic planning for needs of ill family member *so patient's care needs are met with minimal disruption to lives of other family members.* Provide accurate information to family regarding patient's situation *to promote understanding and facilitate effective coping.* Initiate referrals as indicated *so specialized care and instruction are provided as needed.*

ABGs, Arterial blood gases; *ADLs,* activities of daily living; *CPP,* cerebral perfusion pressure; *ICP,* intracranial pressure; *LOC,* level of consciousness; *$PaCO_2$,* partial pressure of arterial carbon dioxide; *PaO_2,* partial pressure of arterial oxygen; *ROM,* range of motion.

for an extended period of time. Agitation and restlessness should be evaluated, and appropriate drugs should be used, if indicated. Narcotics and opiates may be used in a patient on a mechanical ventilator who is also undergoing ICP monitoring. At times it may even be necessary to use paralytic agents such as pancuronium (Pavulon) or curare to ensure optimal ventilatory support (see Chapter 26). The patient should then be fully monitored.

Fluid and Electrolyte Balance. Fluid and electrolyte disturbances can have an adverse effect on ICP. IV fluids should be closely monitored with the use of a limited-volume device or a volume-control apparatus for accuracy. Intake and output, with insensible losses and daily weights taken into account, are important parameters in the assessment of fluid balance.

Electrolyte determinations should be made daily, and any abnormal values should be discussed with the physician. It is especially important to monitor serum glucose, sodium, potassium, and osmolality. Urinary output is monitored to detect problems related to diabetes insipidus (e.g., increased urinary output related to a decrease in antidiuretic hormone secretion) and SIADH, which results in decreased urinary output. Besides urinary output, the serum sodium and osmolality are also used to diagnose diabetes insipidus and SIADH. Diabetes insipidus may result in severe dehydration unless treated. The usual treatment is fluid replacement, vasopressin (Pitressin), or desmopressin acetate (see Chapter 47). SIADH results in a dilutional hyponatremia that may produce cerebral edema, changes in LOC, seizures, and coma. (Treatment of SIADH is described in Chapter 47.)

Monitoring of Intracranial Pressure. In 1960 Lundberg refined a technique for the continuous monitoring of ICP by insertion of a catheter into the ventricles.[14] Over the last 35 years, the technology for monitoring ICP has improved greatly and is now regularly used in patients with suspected increased ICP who may benefit from treatment and in whom the underlying process is thought to be self-limiting. Patients with irreversible pathologic processes or advanced neurologic decline caused by primary or metastatic lesions may not be monitored. The measurement of ICP is valuable in detecting the early rise of ICP and the patient's response to treatment and in providing information necessary for clinical decisions.

There are three ways to monitor ICP: by an epidural sensor, by a subdural subarachnoid bolt, or by an intraventricular catheter. These methods are discussed in detail in Chapter 61.

The nursing care of the patient with increased ICP who is being monitored is complex. Prevention of infection by use of strict aseptic technique during dressing changes is imperative. Maintenance of the intactness of the system is also critical to ensure that the ICP readings are accurate, since treatment is generally based on the pressures.

Body Position. The patient with increased ICP should be maintained in the head-up position. The nurse must take care to prevent extreme neck flexion, which can cause venous obstruction and contribute to increased ICP. The body position should be adjusted to decrease the ICP maximally and to improve the CPP. Traditional practice has been to elevate the head of the bed to at least 30 degrees, unless a concurrent cervical neck injury has been identified. Research now suggests there is an inconsistent response of the ICP and the CPP to head elevation.[15] Elevation of the head of the bed reduces sagittal sinus pressure, promotes venous drainage from the head via the valveless jugular system, and decreases the vascular congestion that can produce cerebral edema. However, raising the head of the bed may decrease the CPP. Careful evaluation of the effects of elevation of the head of the bed on both the ICP and the CPP is required. The bed should be positioned so that it lowers the ICP while maintaining the CPP.

Care should be taken to turn the patient with slow, gentle movements because rapid changes in position may increase the ICP. Continuous rotation bed therapy allows for frequent position changes and does not increase ICP.[16] Caution should be used to prevent discomfort in turning and positioning the patient because pain or agitation also increases pressure. Increased intrathoracic pressure also contributes to increased ICP by impeding the venous return; thus coughing, straining, and the Valsalva maneuver should be avoided. Extreme hip flexion should be avoided in order to decrease the risk of raising the intraabdominal pressure, which can restrict movement of the diaphragm and cause respiratory distress. The patient should be turned at least every 2 hours.

Decorticate or decerebrate posturing is a reflex response in some patients with increased ICP. Turning, skin care, and even passive range of motion can elicit the posturing reflexes. Attempts should be made to provide needed physical care activities to minimize complications of immobility, such as atelectasis and contractures. In cases of severe posturing reflexes, these activities may have to be done less frequently because posturing can cause increases in ICP.

Protection from Injury and Environmental Management. The patient with increased ICP and a decreased LOC needs protection from self-injury. Confusion, agitation, and the possibility of seizures can put the patient at risk of injury. Restraints should be used judiciously in the agitated patient. If restraints are absolutely necessary to keep the patient from removing tubes or falling out of bed, they should be secure enough to be effective, and the skin area under the restraints should be observed regularly for irritation. Agitation may increase with the use of restraints, which indicates the need for other measures to protect the patient from injury. Light sedation with agents such as haloperidol (Haldol) or lorazepam (Ativan) may be needed. Having a family member stay with the patient may have a calming effect. For the patient with seizures or the patient at risk of seizure activity, seizure precautions should be instituted. They include padded side rails, an airway at the bedside, accurate and timely administration of anticonvulsants, and close observation.

The patient can benefit from a quiet, nonstimulating environment. The nurse should always use a calm, reassuring approach. Touching and talking to the patient, even one who is in a coma, is always an appropriate care approach. The nurse needs to create a balance between sensory deprivation and sensory overload for the patient with increased ICP.

Contributory Factors. There is a relationship between nursing care activities and increases in ICP. Table 54-7 lists some of the factors that have been identified as contributors to increased ICP.[17] Nurses should be alert to these factors and should attempt to minimize them. Nursing management of the patient with increased ICP is one of the most important aspects of the care provided these patients.

Psychologic Considerations. Besides the carefully planned physical care provided patients with increased ICP, the nurse must also be aware of the psychologic well-being of the patients and their families. Anxiety over the diagnosis and the prognosis for the patient with neurologic problems can be distressing to the patient, the family, and the nursing staff. The nurse's competent and assured manner in performing the care needed by the patient is reassuring to everyone involved. Short, simple explanations are appropriate and allow the patient and the family to acquire the amount of information they desire. There is a need for support, information, and education of both patients and families that begins with the traumatic event and continues for years after the event.[18] The nurse should assess the family members' desire and need to assist in providing care for the patient and allow for their participation as appropriate.

Table 54-7 Etiologic Factors for Increased Intracranial Pressure

- Hypercapnia ($PaCO_2$ >45 mm Hg)
- Hypoxemia (PaO_2 <60 mm Hg)
- Cerebral vasodilating agents (e.g., halothane, antihistamines)
- Valsalva maneuver
- Body positions (e.g., prone position, flexion of neck, extreme hip flexion)
- Isometric muscle contractions
- Coughing or sneezing
- Rapid-eye-movement sleep
- Emotional upset
- Noxious stimuli
- Arousal from sleep
- Clustering of activities

Modified from Hickey J: *The clinical practice of neurological and neurosurgical nursing,* Philadelphia, 1992, Lippincott.

Table 54-8 Types of Skull Fractures

Description	Cause
Linear	
Break in continuity of bone without alteration of relationship of parts	Low-velocity injuries
Depressed	
Inward indentation of skull	Powerful blow
Simple	
Linear or depressed skull fracture without fragmentation or communicating lacerations	Low to moderate impact
Comminuted	
Multiple linear fractures with fragmentation of bone into many pieces	Direct, high-momentum impact
Compound	
Depressed skull fracture and scalp laceration with communicating pathway to intracranial cavity	Severe head injury

HEAD TRAUMA

Head injury includes any trauma to the scalp, skull, or brain. The term *head trauma* is used primarily to signify craniocerebral trauma, which includes an alteration in consciousness, no matter how brief.

Head trauma has a high potential for poor outcome. Deaths from head injury trauma occur at three time points after injury: immediately after the injury, within 2 hours after injury, and at 3 weeks after injury.[20] The majority of deaths after a head injury occur immediately after the injury, either from the direct head trauma or from massive hemorrhage and shock. Deaths occurring within a few hours of the trauma are caused by progressive worsening of the head injury or from internal bleeding. An immediate note of changes in neurologic status, together with surgical intervention are critical in the prevention of deaths at this point. Deaths occuring 3 weeks or more after injury result from multisystem failure. Expert nursing care in the weeks following the injury are crucial in decreasing mortality. Factors that predict a poor outcome include the presence of an intracranial hematoma, increasing age of the patient, abnormal motor responses, impaired or absent eye movements or pupil light reflexes, early sustained hypotension, hypoxemia or hypercapnia, and ICP levels higher than 20 mm Hg despite artificial ventilation.[20]

Significance

Statistics regarding the occurrence of head injuries are incomplete because many victims die at the scene of the accident or because the condition is considered minor and health care is not sought. An estimated 3 million persons suffer head injuries each year in the United States.[21] Mortality related to head injury is approximately 24 per 100,000 persons in the United States. Seventy thousand work-related accidents from head injuries resulted in compensation for lost work time in 1990.[22] Motor vehicle accidents remain the most common cause of head injury. Other causes include falls, assaults, sports-related injuries, and recreational accidents.

Types of Head Injuries

Scalp Lacerations. Scalp lacerations are the most minor of the head traumas. Because the scalp contains many blood vessels with poor constrictive abilities, most scalp lacerations are associated with profuse bleeding. The major complication associated with scalp laceration is infection.

Skull Fractures. Skull fractures frequently occur with head trauma. There are several ways to describe skull fractures: (1) linear or depressed, (2) simple, comminuted, or compound, and (3) closed or open (Table 54-8). Fractures may be closed or open, depending on the presence of a scalp laceration or extension of the fracture into the air sinuses or dura. The type and severity of a skull fracture depend on the velocity, the momentum, the direction of injuring agent, and the site of impact. Specific manifestations of a skull fracture are generally associated with the location of the injury (Table 54-9).

The location of the fracture alters the presentation of the clinical symptoms. For example, a specialized type of linear fracture is seen when the fracture occurs at the base of the skull, a basilar skull fracture. This fracture generally crosses a sinus and tears the dura (e.g., the frontal or the temporal) and is associated with leakage of CSF. Rhinorrhea (CSF leakage from the nose) or otorrhea (CSF leakage from the ear) generally confirms that the fracture has traversed the dura (Fig. 54-11). Two methods of testing can be used to determine whether the fluid leaking from the nose or ear is CSF. The first method is to test the leaking fluid with a Dextrostik or a Testape strip to determine

Table 54-9 Clinical Manifestations of Skull Fractures by Location

Location	Syndrome or Sequelae
▪ Frontal fracture	Exposure of brain to contaminants through frontal air sinus; possible association with air in forehead tissue, CSF rhinorrhea, or pneumocranium
▪ Orbital fracture	Periorbital ecchymosis (raccoon eyes)
▪ Temporal fracture	Boggy temporal muscle because of extravasation of blood, benign oval-shaped bruise behind ear in mastoid region (Battle's sign), CSF otorrhea
▪ Parietal fracture	Deafness, CSF or brain otorrhea, bulging of tympanic membrane caused by blood or CSF, facial paralysis, loss of taste, Battle's sign
▪ Posterior fossa fracture	Occipital bruising resulting in cortical blindness, visual field defects; rare appearance of ataxia or other cerebellar signs
▪ Basilar skull fracture	CSF or brain otorrhea, bulging of tympanic membrane caused by blood or CSF, Battle's sign, tinnitus or hearing difficulty, facial paralysis, conjugate deviation of gaze, vertigo

CSF, Cerebrospinal fluid.

whether glucose is present. CSF gives a positive reading for glucose. If blood is present in the fluid, however, testing for the presence of sugar is unreliable because blood contains glucose. In this event, the nurse should look for the "halo" or "ring" sign (Fig. 54-11, *C*). To perform this test, the nurse allows the leaking fluid to drip onto a white pad (4 × 4) or towel and observes the drainage. Within a few minutes the blood coalesces into the center, and a yellowish ring encircles the blood if CSF is present. The color, appearance, and amount of leaking fluid must be noted because both tests can give false-positive results.

The major potential complications of skull fractures are intracranial infections and hematoma as well as meningeal and brain tissue damage. A frontal or orbital fracture may also have CSF leakage, but periorbital ecchymosis (raccoon eyes) may also be present. A basal skull fracture may result in ecchymosis of the mastoid process of the temporal bone (Battle's sign) (Fig. 54-11, *B* and Fig. 54-12), conjunctival hemorrhage, or periorbital edema.

Minor Head Trauma. Brain injuries are categorized as being minor or major. *Concussion* (a sudden transient mechanical head injury with disruption of neural activity and a change in the LOC) is considered a minor head injury. The patient may not lose total consciousness with this injury.

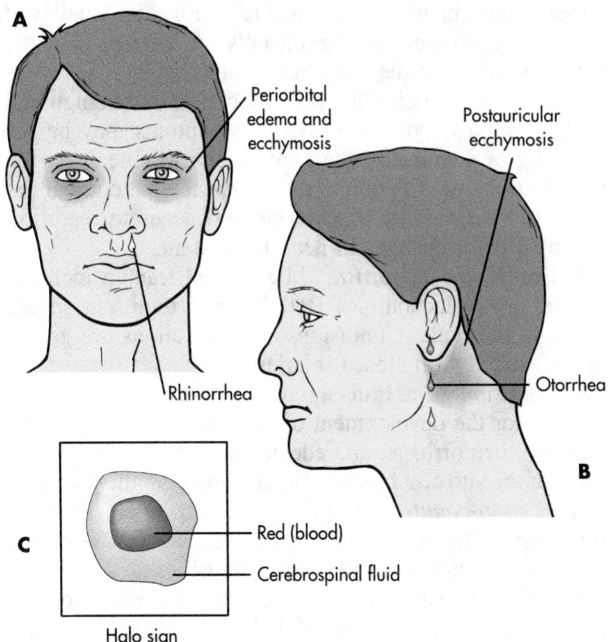

Fig. 54-11 ***A,*** Raccoon eyes and rhinorrhea. ***B,*** Battle's sign (postauricular ecchymosis) with otorrhea. ***C,*** Halo or ring sign (see text).

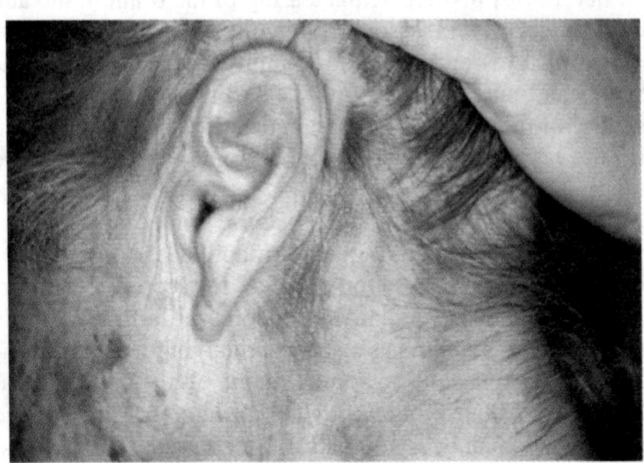

Fig. 54-12 Battle's sign.

Signs of concussion include a brief disruption in LOC, amnesia regarding the event (retrograde amnesia), and headache. The manifestations are generally of short duration. If the patient has not lost consciousness, or if the loss of consciousness lasts less than 5 minutes, the patient is usually discharged from the care facility with instructions to notify the physician if symptoms persist or if behavior changes are noted.

The *postconcussion syndrome* is seen anywhere from 2 weeks to 2 months after the concussion. Symptoms include persistent headache, lethargy, personality and behavior changes, shortened attention span, decreased short-term memory, and changes in intellectual ability. It is believed that this syndrome can significantly affect the patient's abilities to perform the activities of daily living.

Although concussion is generally considered benign and usually resolves spontaneously, the symptoms may be the beginning of a more serious, progressive problem. At the time of discharge it is important to give the patient and the family instructions for observation and accurate reporting of symptoms or changes in neurologic status.

Major Head Trauma. Major head trauma includes contusions and lacerations. Both injuries represent severe trauma to the brain. Contusions and lacerations are generally associated with closed injuries.

A *contusion* is a bruising of the brain tissue with a potential for the development of areas of necrosis, pulping infarction, hemorrhage, and edema. A contusion frequently occurs at the site of a fracture. With contusion, the phenomenon of *coup-countrecoup* injury is often noted. Damage from coup-contrecoup injury occurs because of mass movement of the brain inside the skull. Contusions or lacerations occur both at the site of the direct impact of the brain on the skull and at a secondary area of damage on the opposite side away from injury, leading to multiple contused areas. Bleeding around the contusion site is generally minimal, and the blood is reabsorbed slowly. Neurologic assessment demonstrates focal findings and a generalized disturbance in the LOC. Seizures are a common complication of brain contusion.

Lacerations involve actual tearing of the brain tissue and occur frequently in association with depressed and compound fractures and penetrating injuries. Tissue damage is severe, and surgical repair of the laceration is impossible because of the texture of the brain tissue. If bleeding is deep into the brain parenchyma, focal and generalized signs are noted.

When major head trauma occurs, many delayed responses are seen, including hemorrhage, hematoma formation, seizures, and cerebral edema. Intracerebral hemorrhage is generally associated with cerebral laceration. This hemorrhage is manifest as a space-occupying lesion accompanied by unconsciousness, hemiplegia on the contralateral side, and a dilated pupil on the ipsilateral side. As the hematoma expands, symptoms of increased ICP become more severe. Prognosis is generally poor for the patient with a large intracerebral hemorrhage. Subarachnoid hemorrhage and intraventricular hemorrhage can also occur secondary to head trauma.

Diffuse Axonal Injury. Diffuse axonal injury (DAI) is widespread axonal damage occuring after a mild, moderate, or severe traumatic brain injury. The damage occurs primarily around axons in subcortical white matter of the basal ganglia, thalamus, and brain stem.[23] Initially, DAI was believed to occur from the tensile forces of trauma that sheared axons resulting in axonal disconnection. There is increasing evidence that axonal damage is not preceded by an immediate tearing of the axon from the traumatic impact but rather the trauma changes the function of the axon, resulting in axon swelling and disconnection. This injury is difficult to diagnose from a CT scan because of the lack of obvious pathologic changes in brain tissue and is normally diagnosed from the severity of clinical symptoms. The clinical signs and symptoms include a decreased LOC, increased ICP, decerebration or decortication, and global cerebral edema.

Pathophysiology

Epidural Hematoma. An epidural hematoma results from bleeding between the dura and the inner surface of the skull. An epidural hematoma is a neurologic emergency and is usually associated with a linear fracture crossing a major artery in the dura, causing a tear. It can have a venous or an arterial origin. Venous epidural hematomas are associated with a tear of the dural venous sinus and develop slowly. With arterial hematomas, the middle meningeal artery lying under the temporal bone is frequently torn. Hemorrhage occurs into the epidural space, which lies between the dura and the inner surface of the skull (Fig. 54-13, *A*). Because this is an arterial hemorrhage, the hematoma develops rapidly and under high pressure. Symptoms typically include unconsciousness at the scene, with a brief lucid interval followed by a decrease in LOC. Other symptoms may be a headache, nausea and vomiting, or focal findings. Rapid surgical intervention to prevent cerebral herniation dramatically improves outcomes.[24] Patients over 65 years of age with increased ICP have an even higher mortality rate than younger patients.[25]

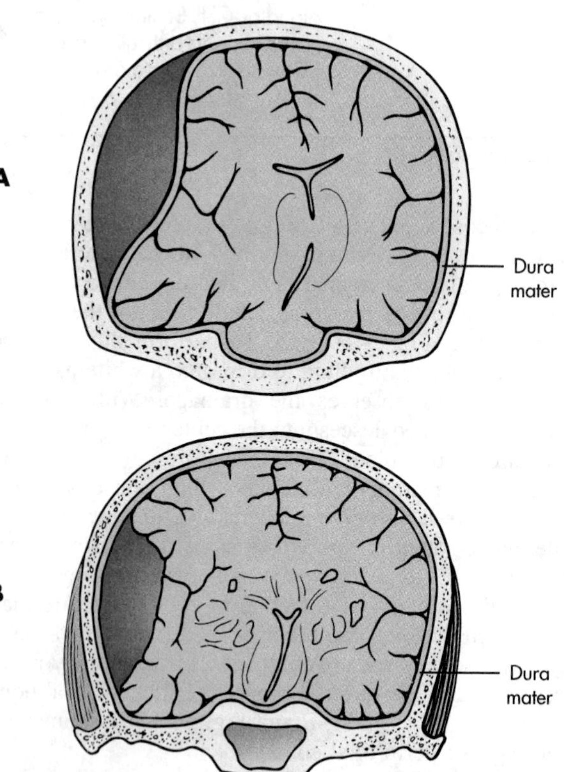

Fig. 54-13 ***A,*** Epidural hematoma in the temporal fossa, usually a result of laceration of the middle meningeal artery. ***B,*** Subdural hematoma, usually a result of laceration of the subdural veins.

Subdural Hematoma. A subdural hematoma occurs from bleeding between the dura mater and the arachnoid layer of the meningeal covering of the brain. A subdural hematoma usually results from injury to the brain substance and its parenchymal vessels (Fig. 54-13, *B*). The veins that drain from the surface of the brain into the sagittal sinus are the source of most subdural hematomas. Because a subdural hematoma is usually venous in origin, the hematoma is much slower to develop into a mass large enough to produce symptoms. However, a subdural hematoma may be caused by an arterial hemorrhage, in which case it develops more rapidly. Subdural hematomas may be acute, subacute, or chronic (Table 54-10).

After the initial bleeding of the veins, a subdural hematoma may appear to enlarge over time as the breakdown products of the blood draw fluid into the subdural space to reach isotonicity. An acute subdural hematoma manifests signs within 48 hours of the injury. The signs and symptoms are similar to those associated with brain tissue compression in increased ICP and include decreasing LOC and headache. The patient appears drowsy and confused. The ipsilateral pupil dilates and becomes fixed. A subacute subdural hematoma usually occurs within 2 to 14 days of the injury. Failure to regain consciousness may point to this possibility.

A chronic subdural hematoma develops over weeks or months after a seemingly minor head injury. The peak incidence of chronic subdural hematoma is in the sixth and seventh decades of life when a potentially larger subdural space is available as a result of brain atrophy. With atrophy, the brain remains attached to the supportive structures, but tension is increased, and it is subject to tearing. The larger size of the subdural space also accounts for the presenting complaint to be the focal symptoms, rather than the signs of increased ICP. Chronic alcoholics are also prone to cerebral atrophy and subsequent development of subdural hematoma.

Delay in diagnosis in the older adult can be attributed to the fact that the symptoms mimic other health problems in persons of this age group, such as vascular disease and senile dementia. Somnolence, confusion, lethargy, and memory loss are associated with health problems other than subdural hematoma. The patient has a history of head trauma in only 60% to 70% of cases.

Diagnostic Studies and Therapeutic Management

Skull x-rays are routinely ordered on any patient with a craniocerebral trauma. This is done to rule out a skull fracture. Skull x-rays are also useful in identifying orbital fractures and other facial fractures. CT scans are considered the best diagnostic test to determine craniocerebral trauma. CT scans allow for rapid diagnosis and intervention. MRI, PET, and evoked potential studies may also be used in the diagnosis and differentiation of head injuries. Transcranial Doppler studies allow for the measurement of cerebral blood flow and velocity. In general, the diagnostic studies are similar to those used for a patient with increased ICP (see Table 54-5).

Emergency management of the patient with a head injury is presented in Table 54-11. In addition to measures to prevent secondary injury by treating cerebral edema and managing increased ICP, the principal treatment of head injuries is timely diagnosis and surgery if necessary. For the patient with concussion and contusion, observation and management of increased ICP are the primary management strategies.

The treatment of skull fractures is usually conservative. For depressed fractures and fractures with loose fragments, a craniotomy is necessary to elevate the depressed bone and remove the free fragments. If large amounts of bone are destroyed, the bone may be removed (craniectomy) and a cranioplasty will be needed at a later time (see Cranial Surgery, later in this chapter).

In cases of acute subdural and epidural hematomas the blood must be removed. A craniotomy is generally per-

Table 54-10 Acute, Subacute, and Chronic Subdural Hematomas

Occurrence after Injury	Progression of Symptoms	Treatment	Type of Trauma
Acute 24-48 hr	Immediate deterioration	Craniotomy, evacuation and decompression	Severe
Subacute 48 hr-2 wk	Initial unconsciousness, gradual improvement, deterioration over hours, dilation of pupils, ptosis	Evacuation and decompression	Severe
Chronic Weeks, months (>20 days)	Nonspecific, nonlocalizing progression; progressive alteration in LOC	Evacuation and decompression, membranectomy	Trivial, nonexistent, or forgotten (recollection of incident by only 60-70% of patients)

LOC, Level of consciousness.

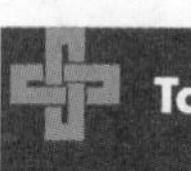

Table 54-11 Emergency Management: Head Injury

Possible Etiologies

Head trauma secondary to motor vehicle accident, assault, fall, or sports injury causing shearing, venous or arterial tears with subsequent increase in intracranial pressure and decreased cerebral blood flow

Possible Assessment Findings

Obvious scalp lacerations
Breaks or depressions in skull
Bruises or contusions on face, Battle's sign (bruising behind ears), or raccoon eyes (dependent bruising around eyes)
Unequal or dilated pupils
Asymmetric facial movements
Garbled speech, confusion, abusive speech
Decreased level of consciousness, inability to arouse, combativeness
Altered neurologic and vital signs
Involuntary movements, seizure activity
Loss of bowel and bladder control
Flaccidity or rigidity of muscles
Depressed or hyperactive reflexes
Decerebrate or decorticate posturing
Glasgow Coma Score <12
Cerebrospinal fluid leaking from ears or nose

Management

- Monitor airway. Have airway equipment available, including suction and intubation supplies. Anticipate need for intubation if gag reflex is absent.
- Maintain cervical spine precautions. Always assume neck injury with head injury.
- Administer oxygen via nasal cannula or nonrebreather mask (100%) and monitor for respiratory distress. If not breathing, ventilate with bag valve mask.
- Establish IV access with one large-bore catheter (14 or 16 gauge; if multiple trauma, two large-bore lines with blood tubing) with saline should be used.
- Control external bleeding with sterile pressure dressing.
- Obtain history, attempt to determine underlying cause (e.g., assault, fall, motor vehicle accident).
- Remove patient's clothing and keep patient warm using warm blankets, warm intravenous fluids, overhead warming lights, warm humidified oxygen.
- Monitor vital signs including level of consciousness, oxygen saturation, cardiac rhythm, Glasgow Coma Score, pupil size
- Assess for rhinorrhea, otorrhea, scalp wounds

IV, Intravenous.

formed to visualize the bleeding vessels so that the bleeding can be controlled. Burr-hole openings may be used in an extreme emergency for a more rapid decompression, followed by a craniotomy to stop all bleeding. A drain is generally placed postoperatively for several days to prevent any reaccumulation of blood. Treatment of chronic SIADH is described in Chapter 47.

NURSING MANAGEMENT

HEAD TRAUMA

Nursing Assessment

The patient with a head injury is always considered to have the potential for development of increased ICP. Increased ICP is associated with greater mortality and poorer functional outcomes.[26] The data collected generally include information gathered for the unconscious patient (see Fig. 54-1). The most important aspects of the objective data are noting the GCS score (see Table 54-2), monitoring the neurologic status (see Fig. 54-8), and determining whether a CSF leak has occurred.

Nursing Diagnoses

Nursing diagnoses specific to the patient who has sustained a head injury include, but are not limited to, the following:

- Altered cerebral tissue perfusion related to interruption of cerebral blood flow associated with cerebral hemorrhage, hematoma, and edema
- Risk for increased ICP and altered intracranial adaptive capacity secondary to cerebral edema.
- Hyperthermia related to increased metabolism, infection, and loss of cerebral integrative function secondary to possible hypothalamic injury
- Sensory or perceptual alterations related to cerebral injury and intensive care unit environment
- Pain related to headache, nausea, and vomiting
- Impaired physical mobility related to decreased LOC and treatment-imposed bed rest
- Risk for eye injury related to loss of protective reflexes
- Risk for infection related to environmental contamination secondary to open wound
- Anxiety related to abrupt change in health status, hospital environment, and lack of knowledge of seriousness of health problem
- Self-esteem disturbance related to altered appearance of head and face and dependence on others

Planning

The overall goals are that the patient with an acute head injury will (1) maintain adequate cerebral perfusion, (2) remain normothermic, (3) be free from pain, discomfort, and infection, and (4) attain maximal motor and sensory function.

Nursing Implementation

Health Promotion and Maintenance. One of the best ways to prevent head injuries is to prevent car and motorcycle accidents. The nurse can be active in campaigns that promote driving safety and can speak to driver education classes regarding the dangers of unsafe driving and of driving after drinking alcohol. The use of seat belts in cars and the use of helmets for riding on motorcycles are the most effective measures for increasing survival after accidents. Increasingly, individual states are passing legislation requiring the use of automobile safety devices for both children and adults. The wearing of protective helmets by lumberjacks, construction workers, miners, horseback riders, bicycle riders, and sky divers is also recommended. The nurse should be familiar with data on outcomes with and without safety devices in working with groups who oppose safety legislation as an infringement of personal freedom. Young parents should be educated in the proper use of car seats and restraints for their children. The nurse should also teach younger children about safety precautions for bicycle riding, skateboarding, and contact sports.

Acute Intervention. Action taken at the scene of the accident can have an important impact on the outcome of the head injury. Emergency management of head injury is discussed in Table 54-11.

The general nursing management of the head-injured patient may initially consist only of observation for changes in neurologic status. This action is critically important because the patient's condition may deteriorate rapidly, necessitating emergency surgery. Appropriate preoperative and postoperative nursing interventions are initiated if surgery is anticipated.

The nurse should explain the need for frequent neurologic assessments to both the patient and the family. Behavioral manifestations associated with head injury can result in a frightened, disoriented patient who is combative and resists help. The nurse's approach should be calm and gentle. Restraints should be avoided if possible because they often produce agitation, which further increases ICP. A family member may be available to stay with the patient and thus prevent increasing anxiety and fear.

The nurse should perform neurologic assessments at intervals, based on the patient's condition. The GCS is useful in assessing the level of arousal (see Table 54-2). Indications of a deteriorating neurologic state, such as a decreasing LOC or a lessening of motor strength, should be reported to the physician, and the patient's condition should be closely monitored.

Much of the nursing care for the brain-injured patient relates to the unconscious state and increased ICP (see Nursing Management of Increased Intracranial Pressure). However, there may be specific problems that require nursing intervention.

Eye problems may include loss of the corneal reflex, periorbital ecchymosis and edema, and diplopia. Loss of the corneal reflex may necessitate administering lubricating eye drops, taping the eyes shut, or suturing the eyelids to prevent abrasion. Periorbital ecchymosis and edema disappear spontaneously, but cold and, later, warm compresses provide comfort and hasten the process. Diplopia can be relieved by use of an eye patch.

Hyperthermia may occur from infection or injury to the hypothalamus. Increased metabolism secondary to hyperthermia increases metabolic waste, which in turn produces further cerebral vasodilatation.

Nursing measures specific to the care of the immobilized patient, such as those related to bladder and bowel function, skin care, and infection, are also indicated. If CSF rhinorrhea or otorrhea occurs, the nurse should inform the physician immediately. The patient should lie flat in bed unless this is contraindicated because of increased ICP. The head of the bed may be raised to decrease the CSF pressure so that a tear can seal. A loose collection pad may be placed under the nose or over the ear. No dressing should be placed into the nasal or ear cavities. The patient should be cautioned not to sneeze or blow the nose. Nasogastric tubes should not be used, and nasotracheal suctioning should not be performed on these patients.

Nausea and vomiting may be a problem and can be alleviated by antiemetic medication. Headache can usually be controlled with aspirin or small doses of codeine.

If the patient's condition deteriorates, intracranial surgery may be necessary (see Cranial Surgery, later in this chapter). A burr-hole or craniotomy may be indicated, depending on the underlying injury that is causing the symptoms.

The patient is often unconscious before surgery, making it necessary for a family member to sign the consent form for surgery. This is a difficult and frightening time for the patient's family and requires sensitive nursing management. The suddenness of the situation makes it especially difficult for the family to cope.

The emergency nature of the surgery may prevent the usual careful preoperative preparation. The nurse should consult with the neurosurgeon to determine specific preoperative nursing measures.

Chronic and Home Management. Once the condition has stabilized, the patient is usually transferred to a general neurologic unit for rehabilitation. As with any craniocerebral problem, there may be chronic problems related to motor and sensory deficits, communication, memory, and intellectual functioning. Many of the principles of nursing management of the patient with a stroke are appropriate (see Chapter 55). With time and patience, many of the chronic problems subside or disappear. Outward appearance is not a good indicator of how well the patient will function in the home or work environment.

Seizure disorders are seen in approximately 5% of patients with a nonpenetrating head injury. The most vulnerable period of time for seizures to develop is during the first week after the head injury. In 25% of patients who develop a seizure disorder, the onset is at 4 or more years after the initial injury. Anticonvulsants are not used prophylactically but are generally instituted after a witnessed seizure, or if an EEG demonstrates subclinical seizure activity. However, some clinicians recommend that anticonvulsants be used during the first week and then be discontinued if no seizure activity is observed. Phenytoin (Dilantin) is the anticonvulsant of choice in posttraumatic seizure activity.

The mental and emotional sequelae of brain trauma are often the most incapacitating problems. It is estimated that more than 60% of patients with head injuries who have been comatose for more than 6 hours undergo some personality change. They may suffer loss of concentration and memory and defective memory processing. Personal drive may decrease; apathy and apparent laziness may increase. Euphoria and lability, along with a seeming lack

RESEARCH

IMPLICATIONS FOR NURSING PRACTICE

LONG-TERM PROBLEMS OF TRAUMA PATIENTS

Citation Van Dongen S and others: Trauma patient outcomes: six-month follow-up, *Rehabil Nurs* 18:76-81, 1993.

Purpose To determine the length of time before trauma patients discharged home were able to return to their pre-injury activity levels.

Methods Descriptive study involving 146 trauma patients discharged home from an acute-care setting. These patients were followed during a 6-month period after discharge to determine functional problems they experienced and the time required to return to normal activity levels.

Results and Conclusions At 1 week, 58% were unable to drive a car, 59% experienced difficulty with lifting, and 76% were unable to return to work. At 1 month, 27% continued to have trouble driving, 32% had trouble lifting, and 37% had not yet returned to work. Head injury patients and those with orthopedic injuries of the extremities or pelvis experienced problems returning to work. The head injury group also experienced vocational problems.

Implications for Nursing Practice The findings of this study suggest that a return to normal functioning levels is a long-term process. Patients with head injuries are at high risk for experiencing difficulty returning to normal vocational roles and activities of daily living. Results of this study reinforce the need to follow patients after discharge.

of awareness of the seriousness of the injury, mark their affect. The patient's behavior may indicate a loss of social restraint, judgment, tact, and emotional control.

Progressive recovery may continue for 6 months or more before a plateau is reached and a prognosis for recovery can be made.[27] Specific nursing management in the posttraumatic phase depends on specific residual deficits.

In all cases the family must be given special consideration. They need to understand what is happening, and they must be taught appropriate interaction patterns. The nurse must give guidance and referrals for financial aid, child care, and other personal needs and must assist the family in involving the patient in family activities whenever possible. Assisting the patient and family in developing and maintaining hope and keeping communication open are strategies perceived as supportive by families.[29]

The family often has unrealistic expectations of the patient as the coma begins to recede. The family expects full return to pretrauma status. In reality, the patient experiences a reduced awareness and ability to interpret environmental stimuli. The nurse needs to prepare the family for the emergence of the patient from coma and must explain that the process of awakening often takes several weeks.

When the time for discharge planning arrives, the family and the patient may benefit from very specific posthospital instructions to avoid family-patient friction. Special "no" policies that may be appropriately suggested by the neurosurgeon, neuropsychologist, and nurse include *no* drinking of alcoholic beverages, *no* driving, *no* use of firearms, *no* work with hazardous implements and machinery, and *no* unsupervised smoking.[29] Family members, particularly spouses, go through role transition as the role changes from one of spouse to that of caregiver.[29]

INTRACRANIAL TUMORS

Significance

Tumors within the cranial cavity cause approximately 2% of all deaths. In 1990 in the United States, 41,200 cases of brain tumor were diagnosed, including 20,500 cases of primary tumors and 20,700 cases of metastatic brain tumors. This is an incidence rate of 8.2 per 100,000 for primary brain tumors and 8.3 per 100,000 for metastatic brain tumors.[30] Brain tumors rank tenth in men and twelfth in women as the cause of death from cancer.

Types

Tumors of the brain may be primary, arising from tissues within the brain, or secondary, resulting from a metastasis from a malignant neoplasm elsewhere in the body. Brain tumors arise from within the brain and may be found in any location. They are generally classified according to the tissue from which they arise. If malignant, the tumor is graded according to general cancer staging procedures. Brain tumors may be classified as those arising inside the brain substance (e.g., gliomas, vascular tumors) or those arising outside the brain substance (e.g., meningiomas, cranial nerve tumors). Probably more than half of the intracranial tumors are malignant; they infiltrate the brain parenchyma and are not amenable to complete surgical removal. Other tumors may be histologically benign but are so located that complete removal is not possible. Brain tumors are more commonly seen in middle-aged persons, but they may occur at any age.

Unless treated, all intracranial tumors eventually cause death from increasing tumor volume leading to increased ICP. Brain tumors rarely metastasize outside the central nervous system (CNS) because they are contained by structural (meninges) and physiologic (blood-brain) barriers. Table 54-12 compares the major intracranial tumors. An astrocytoma is shown in Fig. 54-14 on p. 1708.

Clinical Manifestations

The clinical manifestations of intracranial tumors are generally caused by the local destructive effects of the tumor, the resulting accumulation of metabolites, the displacement of structures, the obstruction of CSF flow, and the effects of edema and increased ICP on cerebral function. The rate of growth and the appearance of manifestations depend on the location, size, and rate of growth of the tumor. Figure 54-15 (p. 1708) illustrates the functional areas of the cerebral cortex and can be used as a guide to correlate local manifestations with the location of the tumor.

Table 54-12 Major Intracranial Tumors

Tumor	Tissue of Origin	% of Brain Tumors	Usual Locations	Malignant or Benign
■ Gliomas				
Astrocytoma	Supportive tissue, glial cells and astrocytes	20	White matter of frontal and temporal lobes in adults, lateral cerebellar lobes in children	Moderately malignant, grades I and II
Glioblastoma multiforme	Primitive stem cell (glioblast)	20	Cerebral hemispheres	Highly malignant and invasive, grades III and IV
Oligodendroglioma	Glial cells and dendrites	2	Cerebral hemispheres, most in frontal lobe, some in basal ganglia and cerebellum	Benign (encapsulation and calcification)
Ependymoma	Ependymal epithelium	1	Lateral and fourth ventricles in children and young adults (usual)	Benign to highly malignant, most benign and encapsulated
Medulloblastoma	Supportive tissue	1	Posterior fossa, fourth ventricle, brainstem in children	Highly malignant and invasive, metastatic to spinal cord and remote areas of brain
■ Meningioma	Endothelial cells, fibrous tissue elements, transitional cells, angioblasts	20	Arachnoid villi, dura, half over convexity of hemisphere and half at base of hemisphere	Benign, encapsulation outside brain substance
■ Acoustic neuroma (neurofibroma)	Sheath of vestibular portion of CN VIII	5	Site between pons and cerebellum	Benign or low-grade malignancy, encapsulation
■ Pituitary adenoma	Pituitary glandular tissue	10	Pituitary gland	Usually benign
■ Vascular tumors Hemangioblastoma Arteriovenous malformation	Overgrowth of arteries and veins enlarging from feeder vessels	3	Parietal cortex near middle cerebral vessels	Benign
■ Metastatic tumors	Lungs, breast, kidney, thyroid, prostate	8	Cerebral cortex, diencephalon	Malignant

A wide range of possible clinical manifestations are associated with brain tumors. In some circumstances, a slight decrease in mental acuity may be the only symptom. In other cases there may be a dramatic event such as a seizure. In others the manifestations of increased ICP may be apparent. Finally, manifestations may clearly indicate the location of the tumor by an alteration in the function controlled by the affected area (Table 54-13).

Complications

If the tumor mass obstructs the ventricles or occludes the outlet, ventricular enlargement (*hydrocephalus*) can occur. Surgical treatment is needed to relieve the pressure and involves placement of a ventriculoatrial, a ventriculopleural, or a ventriculoperitoneal shunt. A catheter is placed in the ventricle to provide the drainage, and a distal catheter is tunneled through the skin to drain into the right atrium, the pleural cavity, or the peritoneum. Rapid decompression can cause prostration and headache, so the patient is gradually introduced to the upright position. The patient should be instructed to avoid contact sports that may result in a blow to the valve or shearing of the catheter. The physician should be notified if signs of increased ICP, such as headache, blurred vision, vomiting without nausea, decreasing LOC, or restlessness, occur. Signs of an infected shunt, such as high fever, persistent headache, and stiff neck, warrant investigation.

Diagnostic Studies

An extensive history and a comprehensive neurologic examination need to be done in the work-up of a patient with a suspected brain tumor. A careful history and physical examination may provide data with respect to location. Diagnostic studies are similar to those used for a patient with increased ICP (see Table 54-5). The sensitivity of MRI allows detection of very small tumors. Other diagnostic studies include CT scan, skull x-rays, cerebral angiography, EEG, brain scan, PET, lumbar puncture, or myelogram. CT and brain scanning are used to diagnose the location of the lesion. Newer diagnostic tools such as PET and MRI provide more reliable diagnostic information. The EEG is useful but of less importance. A lumbar puncture is seldom

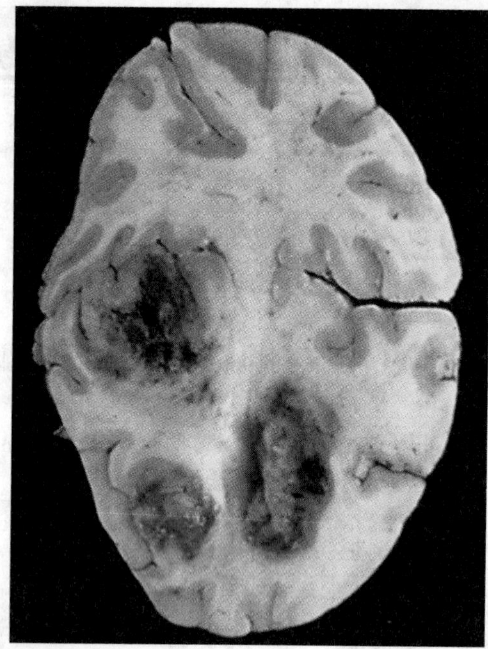

Fig. 54-14 Astrocytoma.

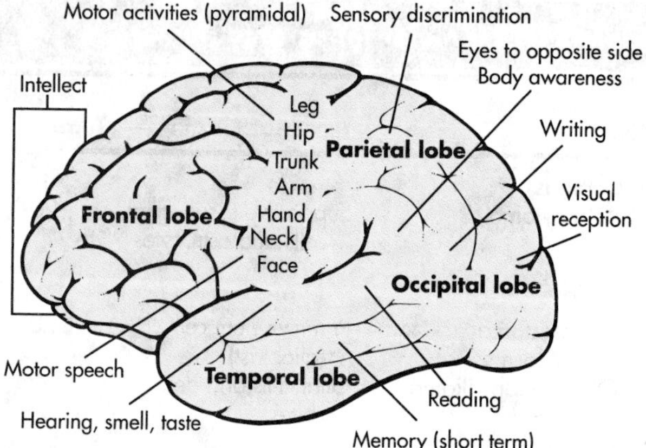

Fig. 54-15 Each area of the brain controls a particular activity.

diagnostic and carries with it the risk of cerebral herniation. Angiography can be used to determine blood flow to the tumor and further localize the tumor.

Therapeutic Management

Treatment goals are aimed at (1) identifying the tumor type and location, (2) removing or decreasing tumor mass, and (3) preventing or managing increased ICP.

Surgical Interventions. Surgical removal is the preferred treatment for brain tumors (see Cranial Surgery, later in this chapter). However, the outcome depends on the type and location of the tumor. Meningiomas and oligodendrogliomas can usually be completely removed, whereas the more invasive gliomas and medulloblastomas can be only partially removed. Surgery reduces tumor mass, which decreases ICP and provides relief of symptoms with an extension of survival time. Tumors located in the deep central areas of the dominant hemisphere, the posterior corpus callosum, or the upper brainstem cause extensive neurologic damage and are considered inoperable.

Radiation and Chemotherapy. Radiation therapy lengthens survival in patients with malignant gliomas, especially when it is combined with partial surgical removal. Patients with less malignant tumors respond to radiation with a longer survival time and decreased recurrence of tumor. Cerebral edema and rapidly increasing ICP may be a complication of radiation therapy, but they can be managed with high doses of corticosteroids.

Normally the blood-brain barrier prohibits the entry of most drugs into the brain parenchyma. The most malignant tumors cause a breakdown of the blood-brain barrier in the area of the tumor, allowing chemotherapeutic agents to be used to treat the malignancy.[6] A group of chemotherapeutic drugs called the nitrosoureas (e.g., carmustine [BCNU], lomustine [CCNU]) are particularly effective in treating brain tumors. Other drugs being used include methotrexate and procarbazine (Matulane). Brain tumors that cannot be totally removed may be treated with a combination of corticosteroids, surgery, radiation, and chemotherapy (see Chapter 12).

Many techniques to control and treat brain tumors are currently under investigation; these include radium implants into the tumor bed, local hyperthermia, and biological response modifiers. Although progress in treatment has increased length and quality of survival of patients with gliomas, death is almost always inevitable.

NURSING MANAGEMENT

INTRACRANIAL TUMOR

Nursing Assessment

The subjective and objective data of the patient with a brain tumor include the data the nurse collects for the unconscious patient. In addition to the assessment data listed in Fig. 54-8, the initial assessment should be structured to provide baseline data of the neurologic status and the information needed to design a realistic, individualized care plan. Areas to be assessed include the LOC and content of consciousness, motor abilities, sensory perception, integrated function (including bowel and bladder function), balance and proprioception, and the coping abilities of the patient and family. Watching a patient perform activities of daily living and listening to the patient's conversation are convenient ways to perform part of the neurologic assessment. Having the patient or the family explain the problem can be very helpful in determining the patient's limitations and can also provide the nurse with information about the patient's insight into the problems. All initial data should be accurately recorded to provide a baseline for comparison to determine whether the patient's condition is improving or deteriorating.

Interview data are as important as the actual physical assessment. Questions concerning medical history, intellec-

Table 54-13 Tumor Location and Associated Presenting Symptoms

Tumor Location	Presenting Symptoms
▪ Cerebral hemisphere	
Frontal lobe (unilateral)	Unilateral hemiplegia; seizures; memory deficit; personality and judgment changes; visual disturbances
Frontal lobe (bilateral)	Symptoms associated with unilateral frontal lobe tumors; ataxic gait
Parietal lobe	Speech disturbance (if tumor is in the dominant hemisphere, inability to write, spatial disorders, unilateral neglect)
Occipital lobe	Blindness and seizures
Temporal lobe	Few symptoms; seizures, dysphagia
▪ Subcortical	Hemiplegia; other symptoms may depend on area of infiltration
▪ Meningeal tumors	Symptoms are associated with compression of the brain and depend on tumor location
▪ Metastatic tumors	Headache, nausea or vomiting because of ICP; other symptoms depend on tumor location
▪ Thalamus and sellar tumors	Headache, nausea, vision disturbances, papilledema, nystagmus occurs from an increase in ICP; diabetes insipidus may occur
▪ Fourth ventricle and cerebellar tumors	Headache, nausea, and papilledema from increased ICP; ataxic gait and changes in coordination
▪ Cerebellopontine tumors	Tinnitus and vertigo, deafness
▪ Brainstem tumors	Headache upon awakening, drowsiness, vomiting, ataxic gait, facial muscle weakness, hearing loss, dysphagia, dysarthria, "crossed eyes" or other visual changes, hemiparesis
▪ Spinal cord tumors	Depend on the nerves involved Cervical: pain, weakness or muscle wasting in arms, back, neck, or legs Thoracic area: pain accentuated with deep breathing and coughing, lack of bowel or bladder control may occur depending on tumor location

ICP, Intracranial pressure.

tual abilities and educational level, and history of nervous system infections and trauma should be asked. Determination of the presence of seizures, syncope, nausea and vomiting, pain, and headaches or other pain is important in planning care for the patient.

Nursing Diagnoses

Nursing diagnoses specific to the patient with a brain tumor include, but are not limited to, the following:

- Altered cerebral tissue perfusion related to cerebral edema
- Pain (headache) related to cerebral edema and increased ICP
- Self-care deficit related to altered neuromuscular function secondary to tumor growth and cerebral edema
- Anxiety related to diagnosis and treatment
- Potential complication: seizures related to abnormal electrical activity of the brain
- Potential complication: increased ICP from presence of tumor and failure of normal compensatory mechanisms

Planning

The overall goals are that the patient with a brain tumor will (1) maintain normal ICP, (2) maximize neurologic functioning, (3) be free from pain and discomfort, and (4) be aware of the long-term implications with respect to prognosis and cognitive and physical functioning.

Nursing Implementation

Behavioral Changes. A primary or metastatic tumor of the frontal lobe can cause behavioral and personality changes. Loss of emotional control, confusion, disorientation, memory loss, and depression may be signs of a frontal lobe lesion. These behavioral changes are often not perceived by the patient but can be very disturbing and even frightening to the family. These changes can also cause a distancing to occur between the family and the patient. Assisting the family in understanding what is happening to the patient and supporting the family through this diagnostic phase are very important roles for the nurse.

The confused patient with behavioral instability can be a challenge. Protecting the patient from self-harm is an important part of nursing care. At times when the patient manifests rage and aggression, the nurse must also be concerned about self-protection. Close supervision of activity, use of side rails, judicious use of restraints, padding of the rails and the area around the bed, and a calm, reassuring approach to care are all essential techniques in the care of these patients.

Perceptual problems associated with frontal lobe and parietal lobe tumors contribute to a patient's disorientation and confusion. Minimization of environmental stimuli, creation of a routine, and use of reality orientation can be incorporated into the care plan for the confused patient.

Physical Changes. Seizures frequently occur with brain tumors. These are managed with anticonvulsant drugs.

Seizure precautions should be instituted for the protection of the patient. Some behavioral changes seen in the patient with a brain tumor are a result of seizure disorders and can improve with control of the seizures by means of drugs (see Chapter 56).

Motor and sensory dysfunctions are problems that interfere with the activities of daily living. Alterations in mobility must be managed, and the patient needs to be encouraged to provide as much self-care as physically possible. Self-image often depends on the patient's ability to participate in care within the limitations of the physical deficits.

Language deficits can also occur in patients with brain tumors. Motor (expressive) or sensory (receptive) dysphasias may occur. The disturbance in communication can be frustrating for the patient and may interfere with the nurse's ability to meet the patient's needs. Attempts should be made to establish a communication system that can be used by both the patient and the staff.

Nutritional intake may be decreased because of the patient's inability to eat, loss of appetite, or loss of desire to eat. Assessing the nutritional status of the patient and ensuring adequate nutritional intake are important aspects of care. The patient may need encouragement to eat or, in some cases, may have to be fed orally, parenterally, by gastrostomy or nasogastric tube, or by total parenteral nutrition. The patient with a brain tumor who undergoes cranial surgery requires complex nursing care. This is discussed in the next section.

CRANIAL SURGERY

The cause or indication for cranial surgery may be related to a brain tumor, CNS infection or abscess, vascular abnormalities, craniocerebral trauma, epilepsy, and intractable pain (Table 54-14).

Surgical Procedures

Various types of cranial surgical procedures are presented in Table 54-15.

Stereotactic Surgery. Stereotactic surgery is surgery targeted by three-dimensional coordinates identified through imagery (usually CT scan or MRI). These coordinates indicate

Table 54-14 Indications for Cranial Surgery

Indication	Cause	Manifestations	Procedure
Intracranial infection	Bacteria	Early findings: stiff neck, headache, fever, weakness, seizures; later findings: seizures, hemiplegia, speech disturbances, ocular disturbances, change in LOC	Excision or drainage of abscess
Hydrocephalus	Overproduction of CSF, obstruction to flow, defective reabsorption	Early findings: mental changes, disturbances in gait; later findings: memory impairment, urinary incontinence, increased tendon reflexes	Placement of ventriculovenous, ventriculopleural, or ventriculoperitoneal shunt
Intracranial tumors	Benign or malignant cell growth	Change in LOC, pupillary changes, sensory or motor deficit, papilledema, seizures, personality changes	Excision or partial resection of tumor
Intracranial bleeding	Rupture of cerebral vessels because of trauma or cardiovascular accident	Epidural: momentary unconsciousness; lucid period, then rapid deterioration; subdural: headache, seizures; pupillary changes	Surgical evacuation through burr holes or craniotomy
Skull fractures	Trauma to skull	Headache, CSF leakage, cranial nerve deficit	Debridement of fragments and necrotic tissue, elevation and realignment of bone fragments
Arteriovenous malformation	Congenital tangle of arteries and veins (frequently in middle cerebral artery)	Headache, intracranial hemorrhage, seizures, mental deterioration	Excision of malformation
Aneurysm repair	Dilatation of weak area in arterial wall (usually near anterior portion of Circle of Willis)	Before rupture: headache, lethargy, visual disturbance; after rupture: violent headache, decreased LOC, visual disturbances, motor deficit	Dissection and clipping of aneurysm

CSF, Cerebrospinal fluid; *LOC*, level of consciousness.

where biopsy, radiosurgery, or dissection should occur. It is a procedure used frequently as part of the initial diagnostic work-up. For example, *stereotactic biopsy* can be performed to obtain tissue samples for histologic examination. CT scans establish the sites for precise tumor sampling. With the patient under general or local anesthesia, the surgeon drills a burr hole or creates a bone flap for an entry site, and then introduces a probe and biopsy needle.

Stereotactic radiosurgery is a procedure that involves closed-skull destruction of an intracranial target using ionizing radiation focused with the assistance of an intracranial guiding device. The three radiosurgical techniques make use of a stereotactic Bragg peak proton beam, a linear accelerator, or a gamma knife. In the gamma knife procedure, a single, high dose of cobalt radiation is delivered to precisely targeted tumor tissue.

Craniotomy. Depending on the location of the pathologic condition, a craniotomy may be frontal, parietal, occipital, temporal, or a combination of any of these. A set of burr holes is drilled, and a saw is used to connect the holes to remove the bone flap. Sometimes operating microscopes are used to magnify the site. After surgery the bone flap is wired or sutured. Sometimes drains are placed to remove fluid and blood. Patients are usually cared for in a critical care unit until stable.

Table 54-15 Types of Cranial Surgery

Type	Description
▪ Burr hole	Opening into the cranium with a drill; used to remove localized fluid and blood beneath the dura
▪ Craniotomy	Opening into the cranium with removal of a bone flap and opening the dura to remove a lesion, repair a damaged area, drain blood, or relieve increased ICP
▪ Craniectomy	Excision into the cranium to cut away a bone flap
▪ Cranioplasty	Repair of a cranial defect resulting from trauma, malformation, or previous surgical procedure; artificial material used to replace damaged or lost bone
▪ Stereotaxis	Precision localization of a specific area of the brain using a frame or a frameless system based on 3-dimensional coordinates; procedure is used for biopsy, radiosurgery, or dissection
▪ Shunt procedures	These procedures provide an alternate pathway to redirect cerebrospinal fluid from one area to another using a tube or implanted device. Examples include ventriculoperitoneal shunt and Ommaya reservoir

ICP, Intracranial pressure.

NURSING MANAGEMENT

CRANIAL SURGERY

Nursing Assessment

The nursing assessment of the patient undergoing cranial surgery would be similar to that for the patient with increased ICP (see Intracranial Pressure, earlier in this chapter) or that for the patient with an intracranial tumor. (see Intracranial Tumors, earlier in this chapter).

Nursing Diagnoses

Nursing diagnoses are determined when the problem and the etiologic factors are supported by clinical data. Nursing diagnoses for patient with cranial surgery may include, but are not limited to, those presented in the nursing care plan for the patient with cranial surgery on p. 1712.

Planning

The overall goals are that the patient with cranial surgery will (1) return to normal consciousness, (2) be free from pain and discomfort, (3) maximize neuromuscular functioning, and (4) be rehabilitated to maximum ability.

Nursing Implementation

Acute Intervention. The general preoperative and postoperative nursing care for the patient undergoing cranial surgery is similar, regardless of the cause. Nursing management is presented in the nursing care plan for the patient with cranial surgery on p. 1712.

The patient (if conscious and coherent) and the family will be gravely concerned about the potential physical and emotional problems that can result from surgery. The uncertainty regarding prognosis and outcome requires compassionate nursing care in the preoperative period.

Preoperative teaching is important in allaying the fears of the patient and the family and also in preparing them for the postoperative period. The patient and the family should be given general information concerning the type of operation that will be performed and what can be expected immediately after the operation. Explaining that the patient's hair will be shaved to allow for better exposure and prevention of contamination may prevent unnecessary concern over this task. The head is usually shaved in the operating room after induction of anesthesia. The family should also be informed that the patient will be taken to an intensive care unit or to a special care unit after the operation.

The primary goal of care after cranial surgery is prevention of increased ICP. The turning and positioning of the patient sometimes depends on the site of the operation. If the surgical approach is in the posterior fossa, the patient is generally kept flat or at a slight elevation (10 to 15 degrees). Lying on the back will be prevented as much as possible, and flexion of the neck will be avoided to protect the suture line. The maximum swelling in the operative area occurs within 24 to 48 hours after the surgery.

With an incision over the skull in the anterior or middle fossae, the patient will return from the operating room with the head elevated at an angle of 30 to 45 degrees. If a bone flap has been removed (craniectomy), care should be taken not to have the patient positioned on the operative side.

NURSING CARE PLAN Patient with Cranial Surgery

Planning: Outcome Criteria	Nursing Interventions and Rationales
➤ **NURSING DIAGNOSIS**	Ineffective breathing pattern *related to* decreased LOC, immobility, positioning, and impaired coughing *as manifested by* change in pulse and respiratory rates from baseline, adventitious breath sounds
Have patent airway, absence of crackles or rhonchi, ABGs within normal limits; have no respiratory distress or infection.	Assess all respiratory parameters q2hr for 72 hr, then q4-8hr *to provide a baseline for comparison to determine if breathing problems occur.* Draw and evaluate ABGs regularly *to guide oxygen therapy and evaluate response to treatment.* Give oxygen by nasal catheter, prongs, or mechanical ventilator until ABGs are stable for at least 24-72 hr *to maintain stable cerebral oxygenation.* Encourage gentle coughing and turning and position patient on side with head slightly hyperextended if LOC is decreased *to improve ventilation, prevent atelectasis, and prevent aspiration of secretions or obstruction of airway.* Suction gently and for <10-15 seconds duration when necessary *to avoid increasing ICP and minimize hypoxemia.* Hyperoxygenate before and after each coughing or suctioning session *to prevent hypoxia which adversely affects cerebral perfusion.* Observe for gastric distention; insert nasogastric tube (if indicated) and maintain patency *to reduce pressure on the diaphragm and risk of aspiration.* Report any alterations in breathing patterns such as apnea or central neurogenic hyperventilation *to assure immediate medical intervention.* Be aware of possible need for intubation so artificial ventilation *can be started promptly if condition deteriorates.* Culture any abnormal secretions *to determine source of infection and direct therapy.*
➤ **NURSING DIAGNOSIS**	Pain *related to* craniotomy, position, and environmental stimuli *as manifested by* report of headache, behaviors indicative of head pain, such as shielding eyes, holding head, pained expression
Have decrease in complaints of pain; able to rest; express satisfaction with pain relief.	Assess location, type, duration, degree, and severity of pain *to evaluate patient's need for and response to treatment.* Administer ordered analgesics, and evaluate effects of analgesics *to maintain LOC and decrease pain.* Position as comfortably as possible *to relieve positional discomforts related to the location of incision.* Keep environment quiet, darken room, put cool cloth on patient's eyes *to promote comfort by reducing environmental stimuli.*
➤ **NURSING DIAGNOSIS**	Altered nutrition: less than body requirements *related to* inability to feed self, difficulty swallowing, and decreased LOC *as manifested by* weight loss, poor skin turgor, abnormal electrolyte levels
Have normal electrolyte levels, absence of negative nitrogen balance or excessive weight loss.	Evaluate ability to swallow *as feeding route is determined by swallowing ability.* Advance patient to high-protein, high-caloric, small frequent feedings as tolerated *to prevent negative nitrogen balance and excessive weight loss and to prevent pressure on the diaphragm and premature feeling of bloating.* Feed patient if necessary *to ensure adequate nutritional intake if self-feeding is not possible.* If patient is unable to eat, administer tube feedings q3-4hr or total parenteral nutrition as ordered *to provide necessary fluids, electrolytes, calories, and protein until patient can eat.*
➤ **NURSING DIAGNOSIS**	Risk for infection *related to* presence of incision, drains, invasive monitoring devices, and environmental pathogens
Have no signs of local or systemic infection.	Assess for fever, drainage, redness at tube sites and incision *as indicators of infection.* Use meticulous aseptic technique *to prevent wound infection.* Provide catheter and drain care *to validate correct placement, evaluate drainage, and prevent contamination.* Monitor vital signs and laboratory values *to identify indicators of infection and notify physician.* Maintain adequate nutritional and fluid intake *to improve patient's ability to fight off infection.* Observe dressing for color, odor, and amount of drainage *to detect infection and initiate early intervention.*

continued

NURSING CARE PLAN Patient with Cranial Surgery—cont'd

Planning: Outcome Criteria	Nursing Interventions and Rationales
➤ **NURSING DIAGNOSIS**	Self-esteem disturbance *related to* physical appearance resulting from surgery *as manifested by* refusal to look at self or participate in self-care, crying, anger about appearance, social withdrawal
Accept temporary nature of appearance; maintain normal activities.	Encourage patient to express feelings about appearance *to enable patient to recognize and begin to deal with feelings.* Explain the rate of hair regrowth of about ¾ in per month *so patient will have realistic expectation.* Provide information about wigs or hairpieces *so patient is aware of this alternative.* Encourage the use of scarves in women and hats in men *to boost their appearance and self-esteem and minimize embarrassment.* Reassure patient about self-worth *to bolster patient's self-esteem and coping ability.*
➤ **NURSING DIAGNOSIS**	Sensory or perceptual alteration *related to* altered sensory reception, transmission, or integration secondary to neurologic surgery *as manifested by* possible disorientation, decreased LOC, altered sight, hearing, taste, or smell
Maintain highest possible level of contact with environment.	Assess patient's ability to speak, see, hear, taste, and smell *to enable appropriate planning of care.* Orient patient to surroundings; describe surroundings when sight is impaired *to increase patient's awareness and reduce anxiety and risk of injury.* Eliminate extraneous noise *to reduce anxiety and confusion caused by sensory overload.* Provide stimulation for all senses *to aid in retraining sensory pathways to integrate reception and interpretation of stimuli.*
➤ **NURSING DIAGNOSIS**	Self-care deficit (total) *related to* decreased LOC, weakness, or postoperative status *as manifested by* inability or unwillingness to perform activities of daily living
Have all self-care needs met.	Assess patient's self-care abilities *to determine level of care needed and plan appropriate interventions.* Provide for total self-care requirements of the patient, including hygiene and skin care and tube feeding or total parenteral nutrition *to ensure that all ADLs needs are met.* Turn patient at least q2hr *to promote effective circulation, ventilation, and to prevent skin breakdown.* Maintain indwelling catheter patency, assess need for enema or suppository *to promote adequate bowel and bladder elimination.* Maintain range of motion of all joints *to prevent contractures.* Provide oral hygiene q2hr *to prevent stomatitis and promote comfort.* Keep patient's eyes closed if unconscious or unable to blink *to prevent corneal damage.*

continued

The dressing should be observed for color, odor, and amount of drainage. The physician should be notified immediately of any excessive bleeding or clear drainage. Checking drains for placement and assessing the area around the dressing are also important.

Frequent assessment of the neurologic status of the patient is essential during the first 48 hours. In addition to the neurologic functions, fluids, electrolyte levels, and osmolality are monitored closely to detect changes in sodium regulation, the onset of diabetes insipidus, or severe hypovolemia.

The dressing is usually in place for 3 to 5 days. Scalp care should include meticulous care of the incision to prevent wound infection. The area should be cleansed with povidone-iodine (Betadine) or a similar antiseptic-disinfectant. Cleansing should be followed by application of an antibiotic ointment according to procedure. Once the dressing is removed, use of an antiseptic soap for washing the scalp may also be beneficial. The psychologic impact of baldness can be alleviated by the use of a wig, turban, or cap after the incision has completely healed. For the patient who is receiving radiation, use of a sunblock and head covering should be advocated if any exposure to the sun is anticipated.

Chronic and Home Management. The rehabilitative potential for a patient after cranial surgery depends on the reason for the surgery, the postoperative course, and the patient's general state of health. Nursing interventions must be based on a realistic appraisal of these factors. An overall goal for the nurse is to foster independence for as long as possible and to the highest degree possible.

Specific rehabilitation potential cannot be determined until cerebral edema and increased ICP subside postoperatively. Care must be taken to maintain as much function as

NURSING CARE PLAN Patient with Cranial Surgery—cont'd

COLLABORATIVE PROBLEMS

Nursing Goals	Nursing Interventions and Rationales
➤ **POTENTIAL COMPLICATION** Increased ICP *related to* cerebral edema	
Monitor for signs of increased ICP, report deviations from acceptable parameters, and carry out appropriate medical and nursing interventions.	Assess for signs of increased ICP such as altered LOC, dysphagia, headache, pupil inequality, decreased respirations and pulse rate, elevated systolic blood pressure with widened pulse pressure, swelling around surgical site, elevation of bone flap *to enable immediate reporting and initiation of treatment.* Assess neurologic function immediately on patient's return from operating room *to establish baseline parameters.* Perform neurologic checks every hour until the patient stabilizes; then q4hr for at least 72 hr postoperatively *to evaluate status of ICP.* Report significant changes *to enable prompt intervention and to prevent serious complications.* Continuously monitor ICP *to promptly determine increasing ICP so interventions can be initiated.* Calibrate and maintain monitoring equipment in functioning condition *to ensure accurate readings.* Provide aseptic care of insertion site *to prevent infection and subsequent increase in ICP from exudate.* Protect equipment from being dislodged *to enable accurate readings and modifications of treatment.* Administer diuretics and corticosteroids as ordered *to reduce cerebral edema.* Position patient with head of bed elevated to 30 degrees *to promote venous drainage from head, reducing cerebral edema.* Avoid neck and hip flexion *to prevent venous obstruction and decrease risk of increasing intraabdominal pressure which restricts diaphragm movement, increasing* $PaCO_2$*, which increases cerebral blood flow and ultimately results in cerebral edema.* Prevent constipation and straining with defecation *to prevent increased ICP caused by Valsalva maneuver.* Manage elevated temperature *as elevated temperature increases cerebral metabolism and causes increased ICP.* Use measures to decrease agitation and hyperactivity *to reduce risk of self-injury and to prevent increased ICP.* Assess surgical site for signs of elevation of flap during dressing change *as a symptom of increased ICP or infection of flap.*
➤ **POTENTIAL COMPLICATION** CSF leak from nose or ears *related to* surgical incision	
Monitor and report signs of CSF leak and carry out appropriate medical and nursing interventions.	Assess for clear or slightly yellow drainage from ears or nose *as indicators of CSF leaks with risk of infection.* Test drainage for glucose or CSF ring, report to physician if positive *to confirm drainage is CSF.* Culture drainage of ears and nose *to rule out possibility of infectious drainage.* Do not plug nose or ears with cotton; use loose "snuffer" type of gauze dressing for comfort (change frequently) *to allow free drainage until injured area is repaired.* Watch for temperature elevation, irritability, headache, or nuchal rigidity and report immediately *as these are key indicators of meningitis.* Administer antibiotics if ordered *as treatment for infection.*

ABGs, Arterial blood gas; *ADLs,* activities of daily living; *CSF,* cerebrospinal fluid; *ICP,* intracranial pressure; *LOC,* level of consciousness.

possible through measures such as careful positioning, meticulous skin and mouth care, regular range-of-motion exercises, bowel and bladder care, and adequate nutrition.

Referrals may be made to other specialists on the health care team. For example, the speech therapist may be helpful to the patient who has a speech problem. The needs and problems of each patient should be addressed individually because many variables affect the plan.

Mental and emotional residual deficits are often more difficult for the patient and the family to accept than are motor and sensory losses. The nurse can provide much help and support during the adjustment phase and in long-range planning.

The mental and physical deterioration of the patient, including seizures, personality disorganization, apathy, and wasting, is difficult for both family and health professionals to endure. Although progress is continuously being made to help the patient with a brain tumor by means of chemotherapy, conventional and interstitial radiation, and biological response modifiers, the prognosis remains grim.

INFLAMMATORY CONDITIONS OF THE BRAIN

Meningitis, encephalitis, and brain abscesses are the most common inflammatory conditions of the brain and spinal cord. Inflammation can be caused by bacteria, viruses, fungi, and chemicals (e.g., contrast media used in diagnos-

Table 54-16 Cerebral Inflammatory Conditions

	Meningitis	Encephalitis	Brain Abscess
Causative Organisms	Bacteria, (pneumococci, meningoccoci, streptococci) yeasts, fungi, viruses,	Bacteria, fungi, parasites, herpes simplex virus, other viruses	Streptococci, staphylococci through bloodstream
CSF			
Pressure (normal, 60-150 mm H_2O)	Increased	Normal to slight increase, increase with increased ICP	Increased
WBC count (normal, 0-8/μl)	500/μl (mainly PMN)	<500/μl, PMN (early), lymphocytes (later)	25-300/μl (PMN)
Protein (normal, 15-45 mg/dl [0.15-0.45g/L])	High	Slight increase	Normal
Glucose (normal, 45-75 mg/dl [2.5-4.2 mmol/L])	Low or absent	Normal	Low or absent
Appearance	Turbid	Clear	Clear
Diagnostic Studies	Stained smears and cultures	Viral studies	CT scan, EEG, skull x-ray
Treatment	Antibiotics with sensitivity tests	Supportive, prevention of symptoms of increased ICP, vidarabine (Vira-A)	Antiobiotics, incision and drainage

CSF, Cerebrospinal fluid; *CT,* computed tomography; *EEG,* electroencephalogram; *ICP,* intracranial pressure; *PMN,* polymorphonuclear cells; *WBC,* white blood cell.

tic tests or blood in the subarachnoid space) (Table 54-16). CNS infections may occur via the bloodstream, by extension from a primary site, by extension along cranial and spinal nerves, or in utero. Bacterial infections are the most common, and the organisms usually involved are *Streptococcus pneumoniae, Haemophilus influenzae, Neisseria meningitides, Staphylococcus aureus,* and *Meningococci.* The mortality rate is high and 50% of the survivors experience long-term neurologic deficits.[31] Bacterial meningitis carries the highest mortality and is considered a medical emergency.[32]

Meningitis

Pathophysiology. Meningitis is an acute inflammation of the pia mater and the arachnoid membrane surrounding the brain and the spinal cord. Therefore, meningitis is always a cerebrospinal infection. The organisms usually gain entry to the CNS through the upper respiratory tract or the bloodstream, but they may enter by direct extension from penetrating wounds of the skull or through fractured sinuses in basal skull fractures.

Meningitis usually occurs in the fall, winter, or early spring and is often secondary to viral respiratory disease. Children under 6 years of age, older adults, and persons who are debilitated are more often affected than is the general population. *S. pneumoniae* causes about 30% of the infections.

The inflammatory response to the infection tends to increase CSF production, with a moderate increase in pressure. The purulent secretion produced quickly spreads to other areas of the brain through the CSF. If this process extends into the brain parenchyma, or if a concurrent encephalitis is present, cerebral edema and increased ICP become more of a problem. All patients with meningitis must be observed closely for manifestations of increased ICP, which is thought to be a result of swelling around the dura, increased CSF volume, and endotoxins produced by the bacteria.

Clinical Manifestations. Fever, severe headache, nausea, vomiting, and nuchal rigidity (resistance to flexion of the neck) are key signs of meningitis. A positive Kernig's sign, a positive Brudzinski's sign (see Chapter 53), photophobia, a decreased LOC, and signs of increased ICP may also be present. Coma is associated with a poor prognosis and occurs in 5% to 10% of patients with bacterial meningitis. Seizures occur in 20% of all cases.[33] With meningitis, the headache becomes progressively worse and may be accompanied by vomiting and irritability. If the infecting organism is a meningococcus, a skin rash is common and petechiae may be seen.

Complications. The most common complication of meningitis is residual neurologic dysfunction. Cranial nerve dysfunction often occurs with cranial nerves III, IV, VI, VII, or VIII in bacterial meningitis. The dysfunction usually disappears within a few weeks. Hearing loss may be permanent after bacterial meningitis, but it is not a complication of viral meningitis.

Cranial nerve irritation can have serious sequelae. The optic nerve (CN II) is compressed by increased ICP. Papilledema is often present, and blindness may occur. When the oculomotor (CN III), trochlear (CN IV), and abducens (CN VI) nerves are irritated, ocular movements

NURSING CARE PLAN Patient with an Inflammatory Condition of the Brain

Planning: Outcome Criteria	Nursing Interventions and Rationales
➤ **NURSING DIAGNOSIS**	Sensory or perceptual alteration *related to* decreased level of consciousness *as manifested by* inaccurate interpretation of environment, signs of fear or anxiety, disorientation, restlessness, reports of auditory or visual hallucinations
Have minimal disorientation, no evidence of agitation.	Assess LOC *to determine extent of the problem.* Administer sedative medication as ordered *to reduce fear and anxiety.* Keep room quiet and lights dim; use calm, reassuring approach *to avoid stimulating or frightening the patient.* Avoid use of restraints *to avoid increasing patient's disorientation and initiating combative behavior.* Assist and support patient during uncomfortable or frightening diagnostic procedures; have family member at bedside when possible *to assist with orientation and reduce anxiety.*
➤ **NURSING DIAGNOSIS**	Pain *related to* headache, muscle and joint aches, and malaise secondary to pressure on nerves and presence of infectious exudate *as manifested by* general discomfort of head, joints, and muscles, apathy, grimacing on movement, reluctance to talk or move, noncompliance with treatment measures
Express satisfaction with pain relief; increase participation in treatment plan.	Administer mild analgesia as needed; assist patient to position of comfort in bed *to relieve pain.* Encourage gentle range of motion and leg exercises *to reduce joint stiffness and promote circulation.* Control environment to encourage rest *as pain can be exhausting to the patient.*
➤ **NURSING DIAGNOSIS**	Ineffective management of therapeutic regimen *related to* possible sequelae of condition *as manifested by* problems involving senses, activity, and cognitive status and anxiety over outcome by patient and others
Have satisfactory management of condition following acute phase by self or others.	Monitor for residual effects such as vision, hearing, activity, and cognitive problems *to determine appropriate referrals.* Inform patient and others that residual problems often improve over time *to reduce anxiety.* Arrange for postdischarge care if required *so patient's needs are met.*
➤ **NURSING DIAGNOSIS**	Hyperthermia *related to* infection and abnormal temperature regulation by hypothalamus from increased ICP *as manifested by* extremely high body temperature
Have normal body temperature.	Carry out general measures of care for patient with a fever.* Use hypothermia blanket if other measures unsuccessful to reduce temperature, *because an elevated temperature increases brain metabolism and increases the risk of seizures or increased ICP.* Reduce temperature gradually *to prevent shivering which can cause a rebound effect and raise rather than lower the temperature.* When using a hypothermia blanket, protect extremities with sheepskin or by wrapping in towels *to prevent tissue damage from prolonged cold.*

COLLABORATIVE PROBLEMS

Nursing Goals	Nursing Interventions and Rationales
➤ **POTENTIAL COMPLICATION**	Seizure activity *related to* cerebral irritation
Monitor for seizure activity, carry out appropriate medical and nursing interventions, and report and record event.	Monitor for seizure activity *so interventions can be initiated immediately.* Keep side rails up and padded *to protect patient if a seizure occurs.* Administer sedative and anticonvulsant medications as ordered *to control or prevent seizure activity.* Initiate vigorous nursing interventions *to reduce fever.* Carry out interventions to treat underlying causes of inflammatory brain condition *to prevent seizure activity.*
➤ **POTENTIAL COMPLICATION**	Increased ICP *related to* presence of infectious exudate, increased production of CSF†

CSF, Cerebrospinal fluid; *ICP,* intracranial pressure; *LOC,* level of consciousness.
*See the nursing care plan for the patient with a fever (Chapter 9).
†See the nursing care plan for the patient with cranial surgery (p. 1712).

are affected. Ptosis, unequal pupils, and diplopia are common. Irritation of the trigeminal nerve (CN V) is evidenced by sensory losses and loss of the corneal reflex, and irritation of the facial nerve (CN VII) results in facial paresis. Irritation of the vestibulocochlear nerve (CN VIII) causes tinnitus, vertigo, and deafness.

Hemiparesis, dysphasia, and hemianopsia may also occur. These signs usually resolve over time. If resolution does not occur, then a cerebral abscess, subdural empyema, subdural effusion, or a persistent meningitis is suggested. Acute cerebral edema may occur with bacterial meningitis, causing seizures, CN III palsy, bradycardia, hypertensive coma, and death.

A noncommunicating hydrocephalus may occur if the exudate causes adhesions that prevent the normal flow of the CSF from the ventricles. CSF reabsorption by the arachnoid villi may also be obstructed by the exudate. Surgical implantation of a shunt is the only treatment.

A complication of meningococcal meningitis is the *Waterhouse-Friderichsen syndrome.* The syndrome is manifest by petechiae, disseminated intravascular coagulation, and adrenal hemorrhage. Disseminated intravascular coagulation is a serious complication of meningitis (see Chapter 28). It is the cause of death in about 1% of patients with meningitis.

Diagnostic Studies. A major diagnostic tool is examination of the CSF. Diagnosis is verified in 90% of the cases by a positive CSF culture. Variations in the CSF depend on the causative organism. Protein levels in the CSF are usually elevated and are higher in bacterial than in viral cases. Decreased CSF glucose concentration is common in bacterial meningitis and may be normal in viral meningitis. The CSF is purulent and turbid in bacterial meningitis; it may be the same or clear in viral meningitis. The predominant white blood cell (WBC) type in the CSF during inflammatory disorders of the brain is polymorphonuclear (PMN) cells (see Table 54-16). Specimens of blood, sputum, and nasopharyngeal secretions are taken for culture before the start of antibiotic therapy to identify the causative organism.

X-rays of the skull may demonstrate infected sinuses. CT scans are usually normal in uncomplicated meningitis. In other cases, CT scans may reveal evidence of increased ICP or hydrocephalus.

Therapeutic Management. Rapid diagnosis based on history and physical examination is crucial because the patient is usually in a critical state when health care is sought (Table 54-17). When meningitis is suspected, antibiotic therapy is instituted after the collection of specimens for cultures, even before the diagnosis is confirmed. Diagnostic measures include lumbar puncture and analysis of CSF. The fundus of the eye should be examined via ophthalmoscope for papilledema before lumbar puncture for identification of possible increased ICP.

Ampicillin, penicillin, and a third-generation cephalosporin, usually cefotaxime, are the drugs of choice for treating meningitis. These drugs are effective because of their ability to penetrate the blood-brain barrier.

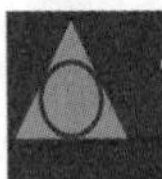

Table 54-17 Therapeutic Management: Cerebral Inflammatory Problems

Diagnostic
- History and physical examination
- Analysis of CSF
- CBC, electrolyte levels, glucose, prothrombin time, platelet count
- Routine urinalysis
- Blood cultures (twice)
- Urine specific gravity (q4hr)
- CT scan
- EEG
- Skull x-ray studies
- Brain scan

Therapeutic
- Strict bed rest
- IV fluids
- Ampicillin, penicillin IV
- Cefotaxime, ceftriaxone IV
- Codeine for headache
- Aspirin for temperature above 100.4° F (38° C)
- Hypothermia
- Clear liquids as desired/tolerated
- Phenytoin IV

CBC, Complete blood count; *CSF,* cerebrospinal fluid; *CT,* computed tomography; *EEG,* electroencephalogram; *IV,* intravenous.

NURSING MANAGEMENT

MENINGITIS

Nursing Implementation

Health Promotion and Maintenance. Prevention of respiratory infections through vaccination programs for pneumococcal pneumonia and influenza should be supported by nurses. In addition, early and vigorous treatment of respiratory and ear infections is important. Persons who have close contact with anyone who has meningitis should be given prophylactic antibiotics.

Acute Intervention. The patient with meningitis is usually acutely ill. The fever is high and head pain is severe. Irritation of the cerebral cortex may result in seizures. The changes in mental status and LOC depend on the degree of increased ICP.

Initial assessment should include vital signs, neurologic evaluation, fluid intake and output, and evaluation of lung fields and skin. These should be reassessed at intervals based on the patient's condition and recorded carefully.

Head pain and neck pain secondary to movement require attention. Codeine provides some pain relief without undue sedation for most patients. The patient should be assisted to a position of comfort, often curled up with the head slightly extended. The head of the bed should be slightly elevated, when permitted after lumbar puncture. A darkened room and a cool cloth over the eyes relieve the discomfort of photophobia.

For the delirious patient, additional low lighting may be necessary to decrease hallucinations. All patients suffer some degree of mental distortion and hypersensitivity and may be frightened and misinterpret the environment. Every attempt should be made to minimize environmental stimuli and the resulting exaggerated perception. Restraints should be avoided. Padded side rails with sheets tied to the four corners to keep the patient from getting out of bed may be used to prevent injury. Arm boards, secured with multiple layers of stretch gauze (e.g., Kerlix), protect the IV infusion site. The presence of a familiar person at the bedside has a calming effect. The nurse needs to be efficient with care but also needs to project an attitude of caring and of unhurried gentleness. The use of touch and a soothing voice to give simple explanations of activities is helpful. If seizures occur, appropriate observations should be made and protective measures should be taken. Anticonvulsant medications are administered as ordered. Problems associated with increased ICP are also managed (see Intracranial Pressure, earlier in this chapter).

Fever must be vigorously managed because it increases cerebral edema and the frequency of seizures. In addition, neurologic damage may result from an extremely high temperature over a prolonged time. Aspirin may be used to reduce fever, and its antiinflammatory effects are therapeutic. However, if the fever is resistant to aspirin, more vigorous means are necessary. The automatic cooling blanket is an efficient way to reduce high fever. Care should be taken not to reduce the temperature too rapidly because shivering may result, causing a rebound effect and increasing the temperature. The extremities should be wrapped in sheepskin, soft towels, or a blanket covered with a sheet to protect them from "frostbite." Care of the skin should be frequent to prevent breaks in the skin. If a cooling blanket is not available or desirable, tepid sponge baths with water may be effective in lowering the temperature. The skin needs to be protected from excessive drying or injury.

Because high fever greatly increases the metabolic rate and thus insensible fluid loss, the patient should be assessed for dehydration and adequacy of fluid intake. Diaphoresis further increases fluid losses, which should be estimated and included in an intake and output record. Replacement fluids should be calculated as 800 ml for respiratory losses and 100 ml for each degree of temperature above 100.4° F (38° C). Supplemental feeding to maintain adequate nutritional intake via tube or oral feedings may be necessary. The designated antibiotic schedule must be followed to maintain therapeutic blood levels. Observations should be made for side effects of the drugs used.

In most cases, meningitis no longer requires isolation, with the exception of meningococcal meningitis. However, good aseptic technique is essential to protect the patient and the nurse.

Chronic and Home Management. After the acute period has passed, the patient requires several weeks of convalescence before normal activities can be resumed. In this period, good nutrition should be stressed, with an emphasis on a high-protein, high-caloric diet in small, frequent feedings. Muscle rigidity may persist in the neck and the backs of the legs. Progressive range-of-motion exercises and warm baths are useful. Activity should be gradually increased as tolerated, but adequate bed rest and sleep should be encouraged. Quiet activities that are based on an assessment of individual interests should be encouraged to prevent boredom.

Residual effects are uncommon in meningococcal meningitis but pneumococcal meningitis can result in sequelae such as dementia, seizures, deafness, hemiplegia, and hydrocephalus. Vision, hearing, cognitive skills, and motor and sensory abilities should be assessed after recovery, with appropriate referrals as indicated. Meningitis in infancy may have "silent" neurologic sequelae, which are manifest as learning and behavior problems when the child reaches school age.

Throughout the acute and convalescent periods the nurse should be aware of the anxiety and stress experienced by individuals close to the patient. Meningitis is generally considered a serious and usually fatal illness by the general public. The family needs to be supported and involved in care as much as possible.

Encephalitis

Encephalitis is an acute inflammation of the brain and is usually caused by a virus. Many different viruses have been implicated in encephalitis, some of them associated with certain seasons of the year and endemic to certain geographical areas. Epidemic encephalitis is transmitted by ticks and mosquitoes. Nonepidemic encephalitis may occur as a complication of measles, chickenpox, or mumps.

Encephalitis is a serious, and sometimes fatal, disease. Mortality ranges from 5% to 20%, with the highest fatality in encephalitis caused by herpes simplex virus and the eastern and Venezuelan equine viruses. Manifestations resemble those of meningitis, but they have a more gradual onset. They include headache, high fever, seizures, and a change in LOC. Therapeutic and nursing management is symptomatic and supportive. Cerebral edema is a major problem, and hypertonic solutions and corticosteroids are used to control it. The disease is characterized by diffuse damage to the nerve cells of the brain, perivascular cellular infiltration, proliferation of glia, and increasing cerebral edema. The sequelae of encephalitis include mental deterioration, amnesia, personality changes, and hemiparesis.

Vidarabine suspension (Vira-A) is used in the treatment of herpes simplex encephalitis. It has been shown to reduce mortality from 70% to 28%, although neurologic complications may not be reduced. For maximal benefit, the medication must be started before the onset of coma. The potential toxicity of vidarabine requires that nurses be knowledgeable about the method of administration and the side effects. Acyclovir is also used for the treatment of herpes simplex encephalitis. It has fewer side effects than vidarabine and is often the preferred treatment.

Brain Abscess

Brain abscess is an accumulation of pus within the brain tissue that can result from a local or a systemic infection

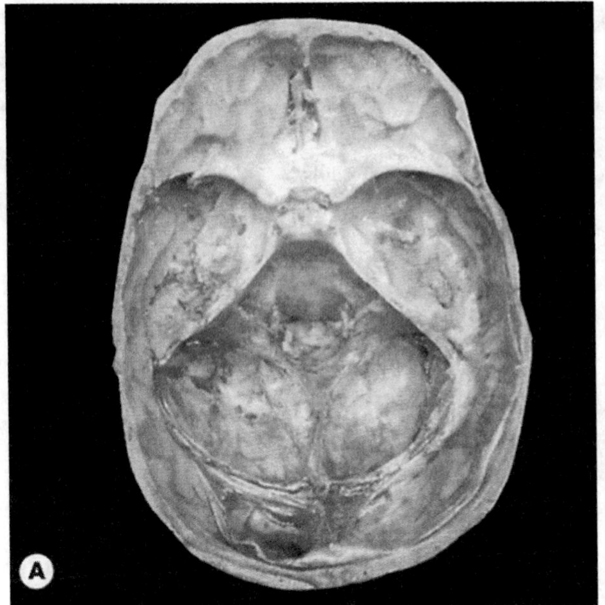

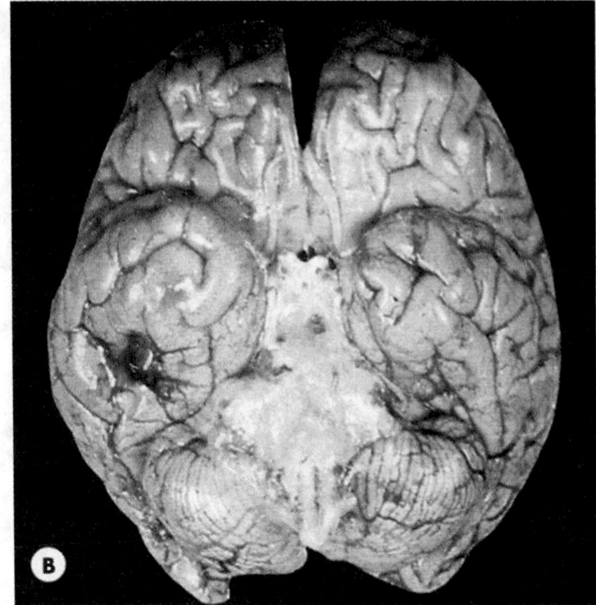

Fig. 54-16 ***A,*** Normal brain. ***B,*** Brain with abscess.

(Fig. 54-16). Direct extension from ear, tooth, mastoid, or sinus infection is the primary cause. Other causes for brain abscess formation include septic venous thrombosis from a pulmonary infection, bacterial endocarditis, skull fracture, and a nonsterile neurologic procedure. Streptococci and staphylococci are the primary infective organisms.

Manifestations are similar to those of meningitis and encephalitis and include headache and fever. Signs of increased ICP may include drowsiness, confusion, and seizures. Focal symptoms may be present and reflect the local area of the abscess. For example, visual field defects or psychomotor seizures are common with a temporal lobe abscess, whereas an occipital abscess may be accompanied by visual impairment and hallucinations.

Antimicrobial therapy is the primary treatment for brain abscess. Other manifestations are treated symptomatically. If pharmacologic management is not effective, the abscess may need to be drained, or removed if it is encapsulated. In untreated cases, mortality approaches 100%. Seizures occur in approximately 30% of the cases. Nursing measures are similar to those for management of meningitis or increased ICP.

Other infections of the brain include subdural empyema, osteomyelitis of the cranial bones, epidural abscess, and venous sinus thrombosis after periorbital cellulitis.

CRITICAL THINKING EXERCISES

CASE STUDY

HEAD INJURY

Patient Profile

George S, a 27-year-old man, is admitted to the emergency department with a diagnosis of traumatic brain injury from a pedestrian–motor vehicle accident. Mr. S was crossing a two-lane highway when he was struck by an oncoming car.

Subjective Data

The paramedic reported that he was unconscious at the scene

Objective Data

At the Scene

- Pulls away from painful stimuli, moving upper extremities and lower right extremity

In the ED

- Pupils are equal, 3-4 mm and react sluggishly
- Vital signs remain within normal limits
- Glasgow Coma Scale = 5, ICP and CPP average 20 mm Hg and 60 mm Hg, respectively
- Fractured left femur and humerus
- Multiple lacerations and contusions

Diagnostic Studies

- Brain CT scan was unremarkable, revealing some generalized brain swelling, small, scattered intraparenchymal hemorrhages but no significant impending subdural or epidural hematomas

Critical Thinking Questions

1. What could be the cause of Mr. S's nonresponsive neurologic condition based on his initial clinical condition and CT scan?
2. Discuss conditions of the injury and the pathophysiologic changes that can occur from the injury in relation to Mr. S.'s neurologic status.
3. What do the signs and symptoms suggest for Mr. S.'s area of brain involvement?
4. What are the priority interventions based on the nursing assessment?
5. Write one or more appropriate nursing diagnoses based on the assessment data. Are there any collaborative problems?

NURSING RESEARCH ISSUES

1. What type of information and education do families need at each stage of recovery for the head-injured patient?
2. What are the temporal changes in brain compliance associated with mortality and poor functional outcomes?
3. Are there any age-related differences in brain compliance associated with poor outcomes?
4. What is the effect of nursing activities or interventions on intracranial pressure, cerebral perfusion pressure, cerebral blood flow, and cerebral tissue oxygenation?
5. What is the most valid noninvasive or continuous method for real-time monitoring of cerebral tissue perfusion and oxygenation?
6. What is the best method to sample cerebrospinal fluid from the ventricles without increased risk of infection?
7. Do neuromuscular blockers or other anesthetic agents (e.g., opioids, benzodiazepines) alter the patient's response to nursing care activities?
8. Do cognitive stimulation programs decrease the frequency of cognitive and behavior changes that occur after minor head injury?

REVIEW QUESTIONS

The number of the question corresponds to the same-numbered objective at the beginning of the chapter.

1. An unconscious patient

a. is unaware of self or environment.
b. shares an underlying mechanism common to all unconscious patients.
c. arouses easily to external stimuli.
d. may be aroused with painful stimuli.

2. Consciousness involves

a. activation of a network of fibers located in the cerebral cortex.
b. an arousal component that functions if the cerebral cortex remains intact.
c. the ability to reason, think, feel, and react to stimuli in a purposeful manner.
d. adequate functioning of the autonomic nervous system.

3. In caring for an unconscious patient, the nurse needs to do all of the following *except*

a. place the patient on the side with the head of the bed elevated.
b. pad siderails for safety.
c. suction as needed.
d. limit care activities that increase the intracranial pressure.

4. Normal intracranial pressure is

a. 0 to 15 mm Hg.
b. 16 to 20 mm Hg.
c. 21 to 30 mm Hg.
d. >30 mm Hg.

5. Vasogenic cerebral edema increases intracranial pressure by

a. shifting fluid in the gray matter.
b. changing the endothelial lining of cerebral capillaries.
c. leaking molecules from the intracellular fluid to the capillaries.
d. altering the osmotic gradient flow into the intravascular compartment.

6. Clinical manifestations of a rising intracranial pressure include all of the following *except*

a. nausea and vomiting.
b. headache.
c. tinnitus.
d. change in level of consciousness.

7. The best way to position the patient with increased intracranial pressure is to

a. raise the head of the bed 30° with patient on left side.
b. keep the head of the bed flat.
c. maintain head alignment at a 30°-angle.
d. use a continuous rotation bed to continuously change patient position.

8. An epidural hematoma occurs

a. from bleeding between the dura mater and arachnoid.
b. frequently from a linear fracture crossing a major artery.
c. usually within 2 to 14 days after injury.
d. most often in men 60 to 80 years of age.

9. The nursing diagnoses of patients experiencing a head injury includes all of the following *except*

a. altered cerebral tissue perfusion.
b. self-care deficit.
c. hyperthermia.
d. hypothermia.

10. A patient is suspected of having a cranial tumor. The signs and symptoms include memory deficits, visual disturbances, weakness of right upper and lower extremities, and personality changes. In which lobe is the tumor most likely located?

a. Frontal
b. Parietal
c. Occipital
d. Temporal

11. The nursing management of a patient with a brain tumor includes

a. assisting and supporting the family in understanding any changes in behavior.
b. using diversion techniques to keep the patient stimulated and motivated.
c. discussing with the patient methods to control inappropriate behavior.
d. limiting self-care activities until the patient has regained maximum physical functioning.

12. The primary goal of nursing care after a craniotomy is

a. prevention of infection.
b. avoiding need for secondary surgery.
c. ensuring patient comfort.
d. preventing increased intracranial pressure.

13. Meningitis is an acute infection of the

a. lateral third and fourth ventricles.
b. cranial sinuses.
c. pia mater and arachnoid membrane.
d. subarachnoid cisterns.

14. In monitoring a patient for possible meningitis, the most critical signs and symptoms to note are

a. headache, fever, heart palpitations.
b. nausea, vomiting, restlessness.
c. irritability, headache, anorexia.
d. headache, fever, nuchal rigidity.

REFERENCES

1. Drummond BL: Preventing increased intracranial pressure: nursing can make a difference, *Focus Crit Care* 17:116, 1990.
2. Jennett B, Teasdale G: Aspects of coma after severe head injury, *Lancet* 23:878, 1977.
3. Hickey JV: Increased intracranial pressure. In Hickey JV, editor: *The clinical practice of neurologic and neurosurgical nursing,* ed 2, Philadelphia, 1992, Lippincott.
4. Ginsberg MD: Cerebral circulation: Its regulation, pharmacology and pathophysiology. In Asbury AK and others, editors: *Diseases of the nervous system: clinical neurobiology,* Philadelphia, 1992, Saunders.
5. Betz AL, Crockard A: Brain edema and the blood-brain barrier. In Crockard A and others, editors: *Neurosurgery: the scientific basis of clinical practice,* Boston, 1992, Blackwell Scientific Publications.
6. Marshall SB and others: *Neuroscience critical care: pathophysiology and patient management,* ed 2, Philadelphia, 1990, Saunders.
7. Ropper AH: Coma and acutely raised intracranial pressure. In Asbury AK and others, editors: *Diseases of the nervous system: clinical neurobiology,* Philadelphia, 1992, Saunders.
8. Sefrin P: Current level of prehospital care in severe head injury: potential for improvement, *Acta Neuroch Suppl* 57:141, 1993.
9. Meyer F: The intensive care management of cerebral ischemia. In Andrews B, editor: *Neurosurgical intensive care,* New York, 1993, McGraw-Hill.
10. Vos HR: Making headway with intracranial hypertension, *Am J Nurs* 93:28, 1993.
11. Mitchell PH: Neurologic data acquisition. In Kinney MR, Packa DR, Dunbar SB, editors: *AACN's clinical reference for critical-care nursing,* St Louis, 1993, Mosby.

*12. Rudy EB and others: Endotracheal suctioning in adults with head injury. *Heart Lung* 20:667, 1991.

*13. Kerr ME and others: Head injured adults: recommendations for endotracheal suctioning, *J Neurosci Nurs* 25:86, 1993.

14. Lundberg N: Continuous recording and control of ventricular fluid pressure in neurosurgical practice, *Acta Psychiatr Neurol Scand* 36:1, 1960.

*15. March K and others: Effect of backrest position on intracranial and cerebral perfusion pressures, *J Neurosci Nurs,* 22:375, 1990.

16. Tillett JM and others: Effect of continuous rotational therapy on intracranial pressure in the severely brain-injured patient, *Crit Care Med,* 21:1005, 1993.

17. Andrus C: Intracranial pressure: dynamics and nursing management, *J Neurosci Nurs,* 23:85, 1991.

*18. Resnick C: The effect of head injury on family and marital stability, *Soc Work Health Care,* 18:49, 1993.

19. Wisner D: The intensive care management of multisystem injury. In Andrews BT, editor: *Neurosurgical intensive care,* New York, 1993, McGraw-Hill.

20. Marmarou A and others: Impact of ICP instability and hypotension on outcome in patients with severe head trauma, *J Neurosurgery* 75:S59, 1991.

21. US Consumer Product Safety Commission: *National electronic injury surveillance system: data highlights,* CPSC, Washington DC, 14, 1990.

22. National Safety Council: *Accident Facts,* Chicago, 1991, National Safety Council.

23. Povlishock JT: Traumatic brain injury: the pathobiology of injury and repair. In Gorio A, editor: *Neuroregeneration,* New York, 1993, Raven Press.

24. Walleck C: Patients with head injury and brain dysfunction. In Clochesy JM and others, editors: *Critical care nursing,* Philadelphia, 1993, Saunders.

*25. Ross AM and others: Prognosticators of outcome after major head injury in the elderly, *J Neurosci Nurs* 24:88, 1992.

26. Marmarou A and others: NINDS Traumatic Coma Bank: intracranial pressure monitoring methodology, *J Neurosurgery* 75:S21, 1991.

*27. VanDongen S and others: Trauma patient outcomes: six-month follow-up, *Rehabil Nurs* 18:76, 1993.

*28. Acorn S, Roberts E: Head injury: impact on the wives, *J Neurosci Nurs* 24:324, 1992.

29. Hickey J: *The clinical practice of neurologic and neurosurgical nursing,* ed 3, Philadelphia, 1992, Lippincott.

30. Mahaley S: National survey of patterns of care for brain tumor patients, *J Neurosurg* 71:8, 1989.

31. Tunkel AR, Scheld WM: Bacterial infections in adults. In Asbury AK and others, editors: *Diseases of the nervous system: clinical neurobiology,* Philadelphia, 1992, Saunders.

32. Sapien GM and others: *Pediatric nursing care,* St Louis, 1990, Mosby.

33. McGillicuddy JE, Hoff JT: Infections of the central nervous system. In Crockard A, Hayward R, and Hoff JT, editors: *Neurosurgery: the scientific basis of clinical practice,* ed 2, vol 2, Boston, 1992, Blackwell Scientific Publications.

*Nursing research-based articles.

Chapter 55

NURSING ROLE IN MANAGEMENT

Stroke Patient

Christina M. Mumma

Learning Objectives

1. Describe the incidence of and risk factors for stroke.
2. Explain the mechanisms that affect cerebral blood flow.
3. Compare and contrast the pathophysiology of strokes caused by thrombosis, embolism, and intracranial hemorrhage.
4. Correlate the clinical manifestations of stroke with the underlying pathophysiology.
5. Describe diagnostic study abnormalities commonly found in stroke.
6. Describe the therapeutic, pharmacologic, and dietary management of the stroke patient.
7. Describe the acute nursing management of the stroke patient.
8. Describe the rehabilitative nursing management of the stroke patient.
9. Explain the psychosocial impact of a stroke on the patient and the patient's family.

A *cerebrovascular accident* (CVA), or stroke, is the abrupt or rapid onset of a neurologic deficit resulting from disease of the blood vessels that supply the brain.[1] The term *stroke* is used to describe an event that can be caused by a number of different pathologic processes.[1,2] For most persons who experience a stroke, it seems to "just happen" without warning. However, a warning sign or symptom may have occurred and gone unrecognized.

Regardless of the cause, the parts of the brain damaged by the loss of blood supply can no longer perform their specific cognitive, sensory, motor, or emotional functions. The resulting impairments can be slight or severe and temporary or permanent.

SIGNIFICANCE

Stroke is ranked third among all causes of death in the United States, exceeded only by heart disease and cancer. A 30% decrease in the incidence of stroke has occurred during the past 20 years. However, stroke continues to be a major public health problem in terms of both mortality and permanent disability. An estimated 500,000 first strokes occur each year, of which one fourth to one third are fatal.[2] In Canada there were approximately 15,000 deaths from cerebrovascular disease in 1991, representing 7% of all deaths.[3] Stroke is often considered a disease of the older adult because approximately 60% to 75% of all strokes occur in persons over 65 years of age. From a global perspective, stroke is likely to become an increasingly important health problem as the population continues to age. Approximately 30% to 50% of those who survive a stroke are left with moderate to severe disability and require assistance with activities of daily living (ADLs).[4]

Stroke has significant economic effects on the patient and family and on the total economy. The combined direct and indirect costs of stroke are estimated to be greater than $18 billion per year in the United States.[5] The heavy toll in terms of human suffering and disruption of lives must also be considered, although this figure is not calculable in economic terms. The need for continued improvement in the control of risk factors and the prevention of stroke is critical.

RISK FACTORS

The risk factors most closely associated with stroke can be divided into two categories: nonmodifiable and potentially modifiable. Risk of stroke increases for persons with more than one risk factor.

The nonmodifiable risk factors include gender, age, race, and heredity. The overall incidence of stroke is higher for men than for women. The risk of stroke greatly increases with advancing age. African-Americans are more likely than Caucasians to have a stroke, probably because they have a higher incidence of hypertension. There is sometimes a hereditary pattern to the occurrence of strokes, although the inherited factor or factors are not clear.

Reviewed by Karen March, RN, MN, Clinical Nurse Specialist, Harborview Medical Center, Seattle, WA.

CULTURAL & ETHNIC
Considerations

CEREBROVASCULAR DISEASE

- A high mortality rate from CVAs exists among African-American men, possibly as a result of the high frequency of hypertension in this group.
- Ischemic strokes are twice as common among African-Americans as Caucasians.
- Hemorrhagic strokes are three times more common among African-Americans than Caucasians.

The risk factors that are potentially modifiable include hypertension, cardiac disease, diabetes mellitus, blood lipid abnormalities, and certain lifestyle habits. The most important risk factor associated with stroke is hypertension.[6,7] Available evidence suggests that treatment of hypertension is the most significant contributor to the prevention of stroke.[8,9] The evidence of a link between stroke and the other potentially modifiable risk factors has been growing in recent years but remains inconclusive. There is general agreement about the increased risk of stroke associated with cardiac disease and diabetes mellitus.[9,10] There is, however, little agreement about the effects of the other potentially alterable risk factors on stroke proneness. Most of the lifestyle risk factors associated with coronary artery disease (see Chapter 31) are not as clearly linked to stroke. These risk factors include obesity, cigarette smoking, alcohol use, and a diet high in saturated fats and cholesterol.

Excessive intake of alcohol may indirectly increase the risk of stroke because of the association between alcohol use and hypertension. Cigarette smoking may also indirectly affect stroke risk because of the association between cigarette smoking and coronary artery disease. Female cigarette smokers have a threefold increase in the risk of stroke compared with nonsmokers.[11] Obesity may contribute to the risk of stroke because of the higher blood pressure associated with excess body weight. There is no conclusive evidence of higher risk of stroke from dietary intake of fats, inactivity, salt intake, or stress. There may be an increased risk of stroke among women who use oral contraceptives.[11] Additional risk factors for stroke among young adults include migraine headache and mitral valve prolapse.

PATHOPHYSIOLOGY

Regulation of Cerebral Blood Flow

Because the neurons of the brain do not divide, the prevention of cerebral damage is important. For adequate cerebral functioning, blood flow must be maintained at 750 to 1000 ml/min, which is one fifth of the cardiac output. If this blood flow is interrupted, as in a stroke, neuronal metabolism is altered in 30 seconds, metabolism ceases in 2 minutes, and cellular death occurs in 5 minutes. Once the neuron is dead, its function is lost unless another part of the brain can adapt to take over the lost function.

The cerebrovascular system is very adaptive. It maintains a constant blood flow to the brain in spite of pronounced changes in the systemic circulation. The factors that affect cerebral blood flow can be divided into extracranial and intracranial factors.

Extracranial Factors. The extracranial factors are primarily related to the circulatory system. They include systemic blood pressure, cardiac output, and viscosity of the blood. During ADLs there are great variations in local oxygen requirements. Alterations in cardiac output, vasomotor tone, and distribution of blood flow are effective in maintaining constant cerebral perfusion. The mean arterial blood pressure has to fall below 70 mm Hg or rise above 160 mm Hg before the cerebral blood flow is altered, and cardiac output has to be reduced by one third before cerebral blood flow is reduced. Changes in blood viscosity increase or decrease cerebral blood flow. Anemia increases flow and polycythemia reduces it.

Intracranial Factors

Metabolic factors. Metabolic alterations are important intracranial factors involved in the regulation of cerebral blood flow. Metabolic factors that result in vasodilatation with restoration of blood flow toward normal include high carbon dioxide concentration and low oxygen tension. Carbon dioxide, however, is the most potent regulator of cerebral blood flow. An increase in hydrogen ion concentration also increases cerebral blood flow. Alone or in combination, these metabolic factors can maintain adequate cerebral blood flow in normal situations.

Blood vessels. The condition of the blood vessels supplying the brain also influences the cerebral blood flow (see Chapter 53). Many persons have congenital anomalies in the cerebrovascular system. These anomalies include tortuosity, coiling, kinking, and arteriovenous malformations. These congenital anomalies may interfere with cerebral blood flow and are common sites for the development of atherosclerotic diseases. Atherosclerosis from any cause increases resistance in the blood vessels and further reduces blood flow.

Collateral circulation is another factor related to cerebral blood flow. Collateral circulation develops in response to a decrease in normal blood flow. The Circle of Willis contains many collateral circulatory connections and is responsible for the greater part of collateral circulation (Fig. 55-1).

Collateral vessels should maintain cerebral blood flow in the event of damage to the main blood supply. However, they cannot always do so. Individual differences in the state of the collateral circulation when a stroke occurs are the factors that determine whether major loss of function results.

Intracranial pressure. Intracranial pressure (ICP) is another factor that influences cerebral blood flow (see Chapter 54). Among the causes of increased ICP are stroke, neoplasms, inflammation, trauma, and hydrocephalus. Increased ICP compresses the brain and reduces cerebral blood flow. Greatly reduced cerebral blood flow may result in cerebral infarction.

Both extracranial and intracranial factors may be involved in a stroke. The initial insult may be related to one

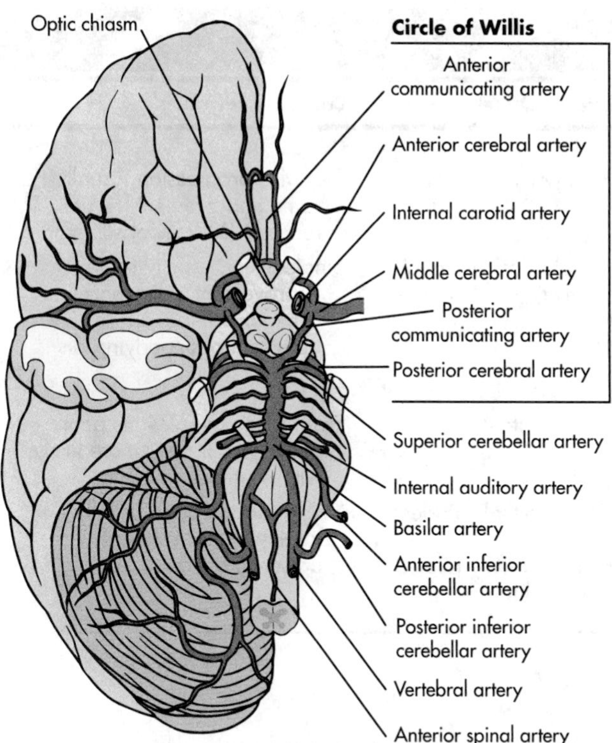

Fig. 55-1 Circle of Willis and vertebrobasilar circulation. Temporal lobes have been removed to show the course of the middle cerebral artery.

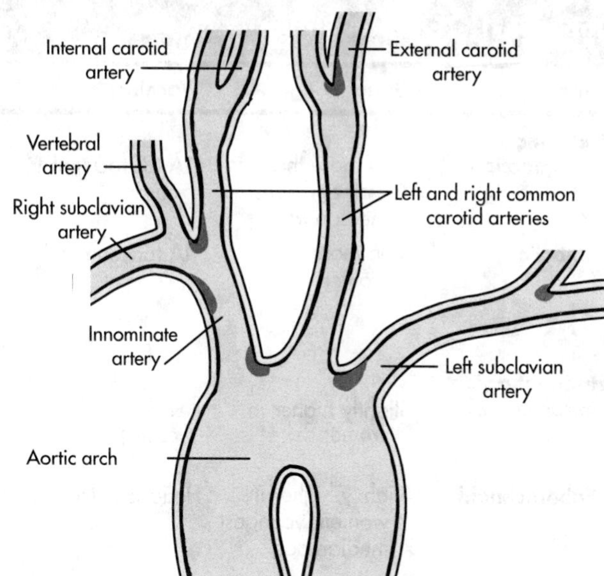

Fig. 55-2 Common sites for the development of atherosclerosis in extracranial and intracranial arteries. The main locations are just above the common carotid bifurcation (most common site) and the start of the branches from the aorta, innominate, and subclavian arteries.

or more of these factors. For example, when an intracranial hemorrhage occurs, the continuity of the vascular system is interrupted. The lost blood and the edema secondary to the inflammatory process cause an increase in ICP. This interferes with cerebral perfusion, and carbon dioxide and hydrogen ion concentration increase, leading to a further increase in blood flow and ICP.

Atherosclerosis

Atherosclerosis, a common pathophysiologic process in stroke (see Chapter 31), is usually involved in the development of a thrombosis and is often implicated in strokes caused by emboli. (The role that atherosclerosis plays in the development of thrombosis and emboli is shown in Fig. 31-4.) Initially an abnormal infiltration of lipids occurs in the intima of the arteries. This fatty streak may develop into an atherosclerotic plaque. These plaques often develop where there is increased turbulence in the blood, as at the bifurcation of an artery or a tortuous area (Fig. 55-2). Turbulence may later damage the atherosclerotic plaque, resulting in a loss of intimal continuity or ulceration. Platelets and fibrin aggregate on the roughened surface. Parts of the plaque may break off and travel to a narrower distal artery. Cerebral infarction occurs at the point where the blood supply is cut off.

Types of Strokes

Strokes may be classified as either *ischemic* or *hemorrhagic* on the basis of their underlying pathophysiology (Table 55-1). Ischemic strokes result from a decreased blood flow to the brain secondary to partial or complete occlusion of an artery. They occur much more frequently than hemorrhagic strokes. The most common types of ischemic stroke are *thrombotic* and *embolic.* Hemorrhagic strokes are generally the result of spontaneous bleeding into the brain tissue itself (intracerebral or intraparenchymal hemorrhage) or into the subarachnoid space or the ventricles (subarachnoid hemorrhage).

Thrombosis. Thrombosis is the formation of a blood clot or coagulum that results in the narrowing of the lumen of a blood vessel with eventual occlusion. It is the most common cause of cerebral infarction.[12] Two thirds of the strokes caused by thrombosis are associated with hypertension or diabetes mellitus, both of which are conditions that accelerate the atherosclerotic process. Thrombosis may be preceded by prodromal warnings, such as *paresthesias* (abnormal sensations), *paresis* (decreased strength and mobility of an extremity), and *aphasia* (disturbance of language function). These transient periods of neurologic deficit, called *transient ischemic attacks* (TIAs), can signal a developing lesion.

A stroke caused by thrombosis usually occurs during or after a period of repose or sleep. It is characterized by intermittency or erratic progression of signs and symptoms. The resultant ischemia leads to edema and congestion of the affected area. The manifestations usually peak within 72 hours and are often secondary to the developing edema. The degree of involvement depends on the rapidity of onset, the size of the lesion, and the presence of collateral circulation. As edema subsides, some improvement is usually apparent within 2 weeks. In most cases, maximal improvement is

Table 55-1 Types of Stroke

Type	Gender/Age	Warning	Time of Onset	Course/Prognosis
Ischemic				
Thrombotic	Men more than women, oldest median age	TIA (30-50% of cases)	During or after sleep	Stepwise progression, usually some improvement, recurrence in 20-25% of survivors
Embolic	Men more than women	TIA (uncommon)	Lack of relationship to activity, sudden onset	Single event, usually some improvement, recurrence common without aggressive treatment of underlying disease
Hemorrhagic				
Intracerebral	Slightly higher in women	Headache (25% of cases)	Activity (often)	Progression over 24 hr; poor prognosis, fatality more likely with presence of coma
Subarachnoid	Slightly higher in women, youngest median age	Headache (common)	Activity (often), sudden onset Most commonly related to head trauma	Single sudden event usually, fatality more likely with presence of coma

TIA, Transient ischemic attack.

attained in 12 to 24 weeks, although some patients continue to show improvement as long as 2 years after the stroke.

Embolism. Cerebral embolism is the occlusion of a cerebral artery by an embolus, resulting in necrosis and edema of the area supplied by the involved blood vessel. Embolism is the second most common cause of stroke. The majority of emboli originate in the endocardial (inside) layer of the heart, with plaques or tissue breaking off from the endocardium and entering the circulation. The embolus lodges at the point where an artery becomes too narrow for it to pass and causes ischemic infarction. Cardiac diseases or situations that contribute to the development of emboli include chronic atrial fibrillation, myocardial infarction, valvular disease, valve replacements, rheumatic heart disease, and infective bacterial endocarditis. Atherosclerotic plaques in the extracranial arteries are a second source of emboli. The emboli from the heart or extracranial arteries usually travel up through the carotid system and lodge in the middle cerebral artery or in one of its branches. Emboli are increasingly being implicated in TIAs.

The clinical picture of an embolic stroke is more varied than that of a thrombotic stroke. It can affect any age group. An embolic stroke secondary to rheumatic heart disease may involve young to middle-aged adults. An embolus arising from an atherosclerotic plaque is more common in older adults. A prodromal warning is less common than with thrombosis. The onset of the stroke is usually sudden and unrelated to activity. The patient usually maintains consciousness, although a headache may develop on the side where the embolus is lodged. Prognosis is related to the amount of brain tissue deprived of its blood supply. For example, if the embolus lodges in the main stem of the middle cerebral artery, most of the lateral cerebral hemisphere suffers ischemic damage and the prognosis is poor. More frequently, however, the embolus breaks apart, sending smaller particles to lodge downstream in smaller branches of the arterial tree. This phenomenon accounts for the pronounced improvement frequently seen after embolic stroke. However, recurrence of embolic stroke is common unless the underlying cause is aggressively treated.

Intracerebral Hemorrhage. Intracerebral hemorrhage, or bleeding into the brain tissue itself, can occur spontaneously in patients with hypertension or atherosclerosis of the intracranial blood vessels. These conditions cause degenerative changes in the walls of the arteries, resulting in rupture and subsequent hemorrhage. As a result of this type of hemorrhage, the escaping blood creates a mass that compresses and displaces the brain. In a large hemorrhage, herniation of the brain tissue may occur, usually resulting in coma and death. The prognosis for survival is worse for hemorrhagic than for ischemic strokes. Mortality rates as high as 50% to 60% have been reported for intracerebral hemorrhage. The outlook has improved with the increased use of computed tomography (CT) scanning with resultant earlier diagnosis and more definitive treatment. The prognosis for survival and recovery is related to the extent and location of the hemorrhage.

Subarachnoid Hemorrhage. A subarachnoid hemorrhage caused by the rupture of an intracranial aneurysm may occur after trauma or physical exertion but usually happens during normal daily activities. Approximately one third of subarachnoid hemorrhages occur during sleep. The first symptom is usually a sudden severe headache. Loss of consciousness may occur and is associated with a poor prognosis for recovery. Unlike other types of stroke, a massive subarachnoid hemorrhage may cause sudden death. Signs of meningeal irritation, such as nuchal rigidity and

Kernig's and Brudzinski's signs, are usually present. Fever is common. Focal signs, such as hemiparesis or aphasia, may not be seen.

Initially a clot forms at the site of a ruptured aneurysm. As the clot begins to dissolve and vasospasm subsides, the chance of renewed bleeding increases. Reduced activity and the prevention of straining are critical parts of the management of a ruptured aneurysm to decrease the possibility of clot disruption.

Temporal Development

The classification of the temporal development of CVAs includes TIA, reversible ischemic neurologic deficit, stroke-in-evolution or progressing stroke, and completed stroke (stable stroke).[13] Knowledge of this classification is useful in planning nursing care.

Transient Ischemic Attack. A TIA is a brief episode of neurologic deficit that passes without apparent residual effects. The deficits usually last less than 30 minutes but may last for up to 24 hours. There is no sign of permanent neurologic deficit between attacks. Of persons who have one TIA, about one third will have no further TIAs, about one third will have more than one TIA and not have a completed stroke, and about one third will eventually have a completed stroke.[13] A widely held hypothesis is that TIAs are caused by microemboli breaking off from atherosclerotic plaques in the extracranial arteries and temporarily interrupting cerebral oxygenation.[5] Although embolic occurrence is most common, a TIA may be caused by decreased cerebral blood flow.[14] A TIA is considered a warning signal and is usually a sign of advanced atherosclerotic disease of the cerebral arteries. A patient with symptoms of TIA should seek medical care promptly.

A TIA must be differentiated from other causes of cerebral ischemia, such as a developing subdural hematoma or an increasing tumor mass. Cardiac monitoring and tests often reveal an underlying cardiac condition that is responsible for the clot formation. Medications that prevent platelet aggregation, such as aspirin, dipyridamole (Persantine), and anticoagulant medications may be prescribed for long-term therapy after a TIA.

The signs and symptoms vary according to the part of the brain affected. The anatomic location of the neurologic deficit can be identified on the basis of clinical manifestations. If the carotid system is involved, the patient may report a temporary loss of vision in one eye, a transient hemiparesis, or a sudden inability to speak. Common symptoms of TIA related to vertebrobasilar insufficiency are tinnitus, vertigo, darkened or blurred vision, diplopia, ptosis, dysarthria, dysphagia, and unilateral or bilateral numbness or weakness.

Reversible Ischemic Neurologic Deficit. The term reversible ischemic neurologic deficit is sometimes used if the neurologic deficit remains after 24 hours but leaves no residual signs or symptoms after days to weeks. This is considered by some to be a completed stroke with minimal to no residual deficit.

Stroke-in-Evolution. A stroke-in-evolution, or a progressing stroke, develops for a period of hours or days. This pattern of progression is most characteristic of an enlarging intraarterial thrombus. A stepwise or intermittent progression of deteriorating neurologic findings is common. However, any stroke may have a gradual progression of manifestations for up to 72 hours after the infarct. The progression of manifestations correlates with the degree of edema secondary to the inflammatory process.

Completed Stroke. When the neurologic deficit remains unchanged over a 2- to 3-day period, the stroke is called a completed stroke (stable stroke). An embolic stroke may demonstrate this characteristic from the onset. With the exception of stroke secondary to a ruptured aneurysm, a completed stroke signals readiness for more aggressive rehabilitative treatment. If a ruptured aneurysm is the suspected cause, activity may be restricted for as long as 3 to 4 weeks to reduce the possibility of additional hemorrhage.

CLINICAL MANIFESTATIONS

The concept of stroke evokes a common mental picture. However, this picture varies greatly from patient to patient. The manifestations of stroke depend on (1) the anatomic site of the lesion, (2) the rate of onset, (3) the size of the lesion, and (4) the presence of collateral circulation. Table 55-2 lists signs and symptoms seen when specific cerebral arteries are involved, regardless of whether the CVA is due to thrombosis, embolus, or hemorrhage. The physical disabilities are usually easy to identify. The language and spatial-perceptual problems are more subtle and difficult to recognize; consequently, these problems are often ignored or misunderstood. Figure 55-3 illustrates the manifestations of right-sided and left-sided stroke.

Neuromotor Function

Motor deficits are the most obvious manifestations of stroke. These symptoms are caused by the destruction of motor neurons in the pyramidal pathway. This destruction can result in the loss of skilled voluntary movements (akinesia), impairment of integration of movements, and alterations in muscle tone and reflex activity. The hyporeflexia that initially occurs with the stroke progresses to hyperreflexia for most patients.

These losses follow characteristic patterns. Because the pyramidal pathway decussates at the lower end of the medulla, a stroke in the right hemisphere of the brain causes paralysis of the left side. The upper and lower extremities of the involved side may be affected to different degrees, depending on the part of the cerebral circulation that was compromised. The middle cerebral artery distribution is the most common site for cortical strokes, leading to greater weakness in the upper extremity than in the lower extremity. The shoulder tends to rotate internally and the hip rotates externally. The foot is plantar flexed and inverted. A period of flaccidity (hypotonia) may last for a few days to several weeks. Flaccidity is usually followed by spasticity (hypertonia). During the spastic stage the deep tendon reflexes are exaggerated. The Babinski reflex is present.

Problems with motor control may affect nutrition and respiration, as well as mobility. In addition to experiencing

Table 55-2 Clinical Manifestations: Specific Cerebral Artery Involvement

Middle Cerebral Artery Involvement
- Blockage of main stem
  - Contralateral paralysis (hemiplegia)
  - Contralateral anesthesia; loss of proprioception, fine touch, localization (hemiparesis)
  - Dominant hemisphere: aphasia
  - Nondominant hemisphere: neglect of opposite side, dysmetria
  - Homonymous hemianopsia, conjugate gaze paralysis

Anterior Cerebral Artery Involvement
- Occlusion of stem*
- Occlusion distal to anterior to communicating artery
  - Contralateral sensory and motor deficits of foot and leg
  - Contralateral weakness of proximal upper extremity
  - Urinary incontinence (possibly unrecognized by patient)
  - Contralateral grasp and sucking reflexes may be present
  - Apraxia
  - Personality change: flat affect, loss of spontaneity, distractibility
  - Possible cognitive impairment

Posterior Cerebral Artery Involvement†
- Thalamogeniculate branch occlusion
  - Contralateral sensory loss
  - Temporary hemiparesis
  - Homonymous hemianopsia
- Paramedian branch occlusion: central midbrain and subthalamus
  - Weber's syndrome: oculomotor nerve palsy and contralateral hemiplegia
- Cortical occlusion: temporal and occipital lobes
  - Incomplete homonymous hemianopsia
  - Dominant hemisphere: dysphasia, anomia
  - Nondominant hemisphere: disorientation
- Upper basilar occlusion (bilateral)
  - Visual disturbances (blindness, homonymous hemianopsia, visual hallucinations, apraxia of ocular movements)
  - Anomia: objects and inability to count
  - Possible memory loss

Vertebrobasilar Artery Involvement
- Bilateral motor and sensory deficits of all extremities
- Ipsilateral Horner's syndrome: miosis, ptosis, decreased sweating
- Hoarseness
- Dysphagia
- Nystagmus, diplopia, blindness
- Nausea, vomiting
- Ataxia

*There is usually no problem if the stem is occluded near the anterior communicating artery because perfusion from the opposite side is maintained.

†The site of occlusion, the origin of the basilar arteries, and the arrangement of the Circle of Willis are involved in the type of deficit seen. This can occur from a thrombus or embolus.

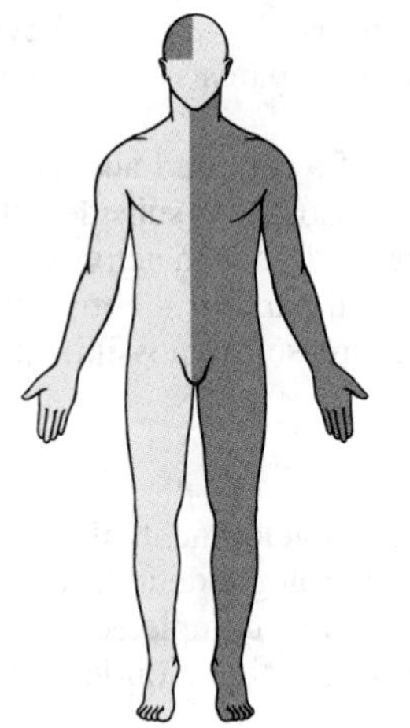

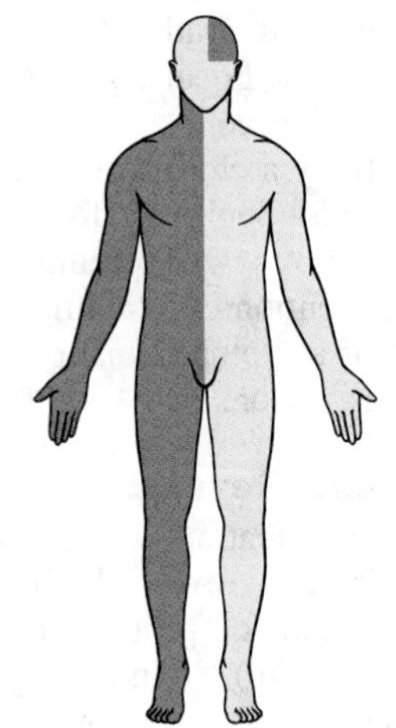

Right brain damage	Left brain damage
• Paralyzed left side	• Paralyzed right side
• Spatial-perceptual deficits	• Speech-language deficits (if left brain dominant)
• Behavioral style: quick, impulsive	• Behavioral style: slow, cautious
• Memory deficits: peformance	• Memory deficits: language
• Indifference to the disability	• Distress and depression in relation to the disability

Fig. 55-3 Manifestations of right-sided and left-sided stroke.

difficulty with self-feeding, the patient may have impairment of swallowing (dysphagia) because of weakness of the mouth and throat muscles. The swallow reflex may also be diminished or absent. This problem is generally more severe with a brainstem stroke (bulbar dysphagia), but it may also be seen with a cortical stroke (pseudobulbar dysphagia). The patient may be unable to swallow secretions and consequently is susceptible to aspiration pneumonia.

Problems related to the motor control of elimination are more complex. Fortunately such problems are usually transient. When the stroke is confined to one hemisphere, the prognosis for return to normal bladder function is excellent. The reflex arc remains intact, a partial sensation of bladder filling remains, and the patient maintains partial voluntary control over urination.[1] Initially, the patient may experience frequency, urgency, and incontinence. Bladder training is facilitated if started immediately. Because a retention catheter may interfere with this process, it should be used only during the most acute period of the stroke if absolutely necessary. Motor control of the bowel is usually not a problem. However, the patient is prone to constipation. This is attributed to immobility, weakened abdominal muscles, decreased oral intake, inability to communicate the need to defecate, and lack of response to the defecation reflex.

Communication

The left hemisphere is dominant for language in all right-handed persons and in the majority of left-handed persons. When the stroke occurs in the dominant hemisphere, the patient may experience communication difficulties or *aphasia.*[1] Language disorders involve the expression and the comprehension of written or spoken words. When the lesion involves Wernicke's area of the brain, the patient experiences *receptive* aphasia; neither the sounds of speech nor its meaning can be distinguished, and comprehension of both written and spoken language is impaired. The lesion causing *expressive* aphasia affects Broca's area, the motor area for speech. This patient has difficulty in speaking and writing. Aphasias may be classified as either nonfluent or fluent (Fig. 55-4). In *nonfluent* aphasia the patient speaks little and produces speech slowly and with obvious effort. In *fluent* aphasia the patient may speak, but the phrases have little meaning because of impaired comprehension. Conduction aphasia is a type of fluent aphasia in which the lesion is in the pathway between Broca's and Wernicke's areas. Most aphasias are mixed, with some impairment of both expression and understanding. A massive lesion may result in *global* aphasia, in which virtually all language function is lost.

Another communication problem that many stroke patients experience is *dysarthria*, or slurred speech. Dysarthria results from a disturbance in muscular control and produces impairment of pronunciation, articulation, and phonation. Dysarthria does not result in any disturbance of language function itself. However, an occasional stroke patient may be unfortunate enough to have both aphasia and dysarthria.

Affective Function

Patients with a stroke may demonstrate loss of control of their emotions. Their emotional responses may be exaggerated or unpredictable. This is compounded by the depression experienced with the change in body image and the frustration related to communication problems. It may be difficult to determine whether the patient is crying because of emotional lability or depression.

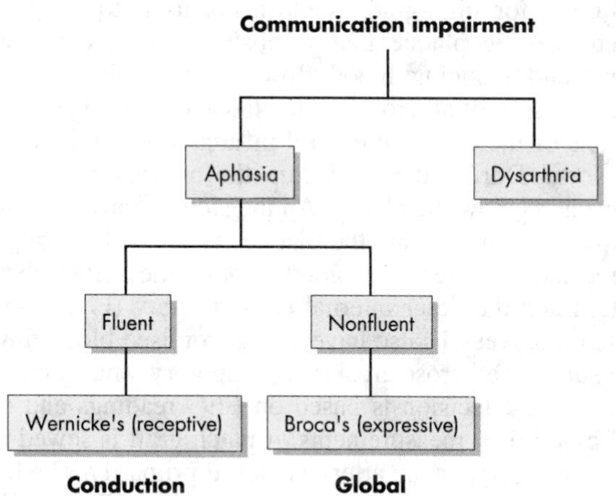

Fig. 55-4 Types of communication impairment common after stroke.

Intellectual Function

Both memory and judgment may be impaired as a result of stroke. These impairments are experienced in right-sided and left-sided lesions. A left-sided lesion is more likely to result in memory problems related to language; a right-sided lesion usually causes problems related to spatial-perceptual content. The patient with a left-sided lesion tends to be overly cautious in matters of judgment. In contrast, the patient with a right-sided lesion may be quick and impulsive. Both may experience difficulty in making generalizations, which interferes with the ability to learn.

Spatial-Perceptual Alterations

A stroke in the right hemisphere is more likely to cause deficits in spatial-perceptual orientation, although they can occur with damage to the left hemisphere as well. These spatial-perceptual deficits may be divided into four categories. The first relates to the patient's erroneous perception of self and illness. This deficit follows lesions of the parietal lobe. Patients may deny their illnesses or their own body parts. The second category concerns the patient's erroneous perception of self in space. The patient may neglect all input from the affected side. This may be compounded by homonymous hemianopsia, in which blindness occurs in the corresponding halves of the visual fields of both eyes. In addition, the patient has difficulty with spatial orientation, such as judgment of distances. The third spatial-perceptual deficit is *agnosia*, the inability to recognize an object by sight, touch, or hearing. The fourth deficit is *apraxia,* the inability to carry out learned sequential movements on command.

DIAGNOSTIC STUDIES

After a stroke, various diagnostic studies are carried out in an effort to determine the cause of the stroke and as a basis for decisions about therapeutic or surgical treatment (Table 55-3). A CT scan is the primary diagnostic test used after a stroke. It can indicate the size and location of the lesion. CT testing is also useful in differentiating between infarction and hemorrhage. Serial CT scans are often used to determine the effectiveness of treatment and to evaluate the course of healing.

Certain neurodiagnostic tests such as skull x-rays, brain scan, lumbar puncture, and electroencephalogram (EEG) that were formerly used in the diagnosis of stroke are currently used much less. Although the skull x-ray is usually normal after a stroke, there may be a pineal shift with a massive infarction. A brain scan shows increased uptake of radioactive media in infarction.

A lumbar puncture, although not performed routinely, may show a transient increase in leukocytes in the cerebrospinal fluid (CSF). The presence of blood in the CSF is indicative but not diagnostic of hemorrhage. A lumbar puncture is usually not done in the presence of increased

Table 55-3 Diagnostic Tests for Suspected Cerebrovascular Accident

Diagnosis of CVA, Including Extent of Involvement
- CT scan
- Magnetic resonance imaging
- Electroencephalogram
- Radionuclide scan (brain scan)
- Angiography
- Cerebrospinal fluid analysis
- Positron emission tomography
- Digital subtraction angiography

Evaluation of Etiology of CVA
- Cerebral Blood Flow
  - Doppler ultrasonography
    - Transcranial Doppler (TCD)
    - Carotid duplex
  - Carotid angiography
- Cardiac Assessment
  - Electrocardiogram
  - Cardiac enzymes
  - Echocardiography
  - Holter monitor (evaluation for dysrhythmias)

CT, Computed tomography; *CVA*, cerebrovascular accident.
*For cerebrospinal fluid testing, a lumbar puncture is avoided if elevation of intracranial pressure is suspected.

ICP because of the danger of herniation from a sudden decrease in pressure. An EEG may show low-voltage, slow waves in ischemic infarction. If hemorrhage is the cause of the stroke, the EEG may show high-voltage slow waves. Arteriography can demonstrate areas of cervical and cerebrovascular occlusion, atherosclerotic plaques, and malformation of vessels. If the suspected cause of the stroke includes emboli from the heart, cardiac diagnostic tests should be done (see Table 55-3).

Other diagnostic tests used in some medical centers to aid in the diagnosis of stroke include magnetic resonance imaging (MRI), positron emission tomography (PET), and digital subtraction angiography (DSA). MRI uses a magnetic field instead of radiation to produce a picture of the brain that is superficially similar to that of a CT scan. MRI is considered by some to be the best imaging method to differentiate hemorrhagic from nonhemorrhagic infarcts. The use of MRI in the diagnosis of stroke has increased significantly in recent years. PET shows the chemical activity of the brain and provides an excellent depiction of the extent of tissue damage after a stroke. Less active or diseased tissue appears darker than healthy, active cells. Major research efforts are aimed at perfecting this technique to aid in the diagnosis and treatment of brain disease.[13]

DSA involves the intravenous (IV) or arterial injection of a contrast agent to produce good visualization of neck vessels and the large vessels of the Circle of Willis. Intraarterial injection of contrast material has almost completely replaced IV DSA because the arterial approach requires a smaller bolus of contrast fluid and produces superior results.[13] It is considered safer than cerebral angiography because less vascular manipulation is required. However, conventional intraarterial angiography is still needed for examination of intracranial arteries. Because angiography is potentially dangerous as a result of the possibility of dislodging an embolus or of causing vasospasm or further hemorrhage, it is used only when no other, safer test can provide the needed information.

Transcranial Doppler (TCD) ultrasonography measures the velocity of blood flow in the cerebral arteries. TCD has been shown to be effective in detecting microemboli and vasospasm.

THERAPEUTIC MANAGEMENT

Prevention

Once a stroke has occurred, the impact of therapeutic management on modifying the extent of brain tissue damage is limited. The priority of therapy is therefore prevention—both the prevention of infarction in the patient with a TIA and the prevention of recurrence in the patient who has had a stroke. Patients with known risk factors, such as diabetes, hypertension, or cardiac dysfunction, should be followed closely. Measures designed to prevent the development of a thrombus or embolus are used. The administration of aspirin (ASA) or dipyridamole (Persantine) has decreased the incidence of stroke. A newer platelet aggregation inhibitor, ticlopidine hydrochloride (Ticlid), has been shown to be more effective than aspirin in reducing stroke for both women and men in studies in Canada and the United States.[5] Anticoagulants are also used for patients with TIAs, although the possibility of hemorrhage must be considered.

The most common surgical procedures used to reduce the frequency of TIAs and the danger of impending stroke are carotid endarterectomy and extracranial-intracranial (EC-IC) bypass. Transluminal angioplasty is a third surgical procedure currently being studied. These procedures are designed to maintain cerebral blood flow and must be performed before an infarction occurs, or the hazards outweigh the benefits. An endarterectomy, an effective treatment for high-grade stenosis, is used to remove an atherosclerotic plaque that is obstructing an extracranial artery and reducing blood flow to the brain. The most common sites of atherosclerotic plaque development are the regions of the common carotid bifurcation and the arch of the aorta. During the procedure the arteries are clamped above and below the plaque. An incision slightly larger than the plaque is made, and the plaque is removed. During this period the brain receives blood through the vertebrobasilar system and the other internal carotid artery (Fig. 55-5). If these blood vessels also have a compromised blood flow as a result of atherosclerosis, a temporary shunt may be placed. This decision is based on EEG readings and cerebral blood flow measurements. A patch graft is sewed in to close the artery, or the artery is closed primarily. The blood pressure during surgery is maintained above 170 mm Hg to maintain critical perfusion pressure.

EC-IC bypass is used for intracranial problems when the obstruction cannot be removed directly. Although there are

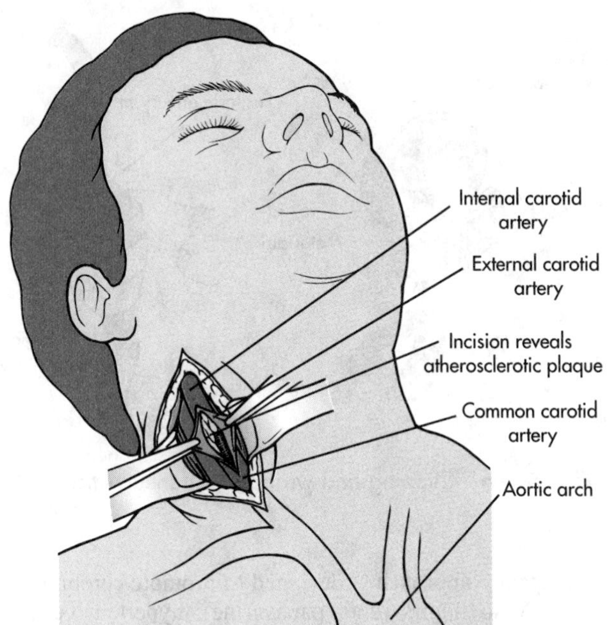

Fig. 55-5 Carotid endarterectomy. The atherosclerotic plaque in the internal carotid artery is removed to prevent impending cerebral infarction.

a number of variations, the procedure usually involves anastomosing a branch of an extracranial artery to an intracranial artery just beyond the obstruction. Branches of the middle cerebral artery are most commonly used. A burr hole is drilled in the skull and is used to connect the extracranial artery to the involved intracranial artery. In this way an intracranial occlusion is bypassed.

Percutaneous transluminal angioplasty has been used to treat patients with symptoms related to stenosis in the vertebrobasilar or carotid arteries and their major branches. This procedure carries with it the risk of dislodging emboli that can travel to the brain or retina. Further investigation of angioplasty in the treatment of strokes is ongoing. (Angioplasty for the treatment of coronary artery disease is discussed in Chapter 31.)

Acute Management

The focus of therapeutic management of the stroke patient is preservation of life, prevention of additional brain damage, and lessening of disability. The diagnostic tests used to determine the cause of the stroke are the same for all types of stroke; the treatment differs according to type of stroke and whether the aim of treatment is prevention, management during the acute phase, or long-term rehabilitation (Table 55-4).

The first goal of therapeutic management is to maintain a patent airway, which may be compromised because of a decreased consciousness.[15] Interventions to accomplish this goal must be initiated at the scene of the stroke to prevent cerebral anoxia and permanent brain damage. Table 55-5 outlines emergency management of the patient with a cerebrovascular accident. Oxygen, an artificial airway, or

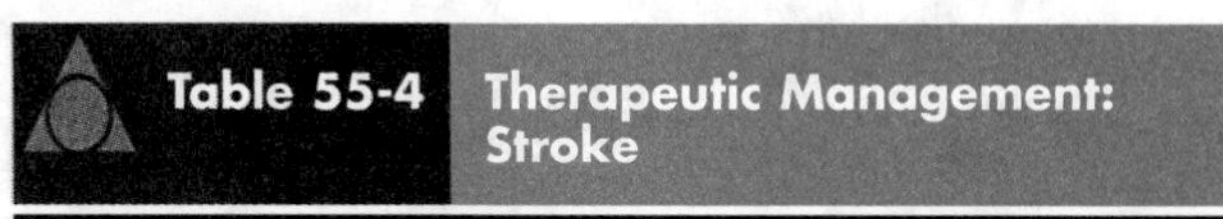

Table 55-4 Therapeutic Management: Stroke

Prevention
- Thrombotic stroke
  - Control of hypertension
  - Control of diabetes mellitus
- Embolic stroke of cardiogenic origin
  - Anticoagulation therapy for patients with atrial fibrillation
  - Treatment of underlying condition
- Intracerebral hemorrhage
  - Control of hypertension
- Surgical intervention for patients with aneurysms at risk of bleeding

Treatment in Acute Phase
- Thrombotic TIAs
  - Anticoagulation
  - Antiplatelet aggregation
  - Endarterectomy
  - EC-IC bypass
- Progressing stroke (stroke-in-evolution)
  - Anticoagulation (not hemorrhagic strokes)
- Completed stroke with mixed neurologic deficit
  - Treatment of brain edema
- Embolic stroke of cardiogenic origin
  - Treatment of underlying cause
- Intracerebral hemorrhage
  - Treatment of brain edema, surgical decompression, if indicated
- Subarachnoid hemorrhage
  - Surgical extirpation (dependent on size and location of hemorrhage)

EC-IC, Extracranial-intracranial; *TIA*, transient ischemic attack.

possibly intubation and mechanical ventilation may be indicated.

The patient is monitored closely for signs of increasing neurologic deficit. Therapeutic, surgical, and pharmacologic interventions may be appropriate, depending on the reason for the increasing deficit.

Because of cerebral edema, the fluid and electrolyte balance must be carefully controlled. Initially the patient retains fluids because of the stress response (increased antidiuretic hormone and aldosterone). Inappropriate secretion of antidiuretic hormone may occur. This may be partially offset by the patient's inability to drink or by hyperosmolar tube feedings. All factors must be considered before fluids are ordered.

The physician usually tries to keep the patient slightly dehydrated yet provide enough fluids to prevent capillary sludging. Adequate fluid intake during the acute phase is usually 1500 to 2000 ml per day. When the period of acute stress is over, the fluid requirements increase as diuresis starts. If the patient is unable to eat within 5 days, parenteral nutrition or tube feedings are instituted.

Three therapeutic approaches have been used with varying success to prevent additional brain damage. The first and most effective is the use of measures designed to

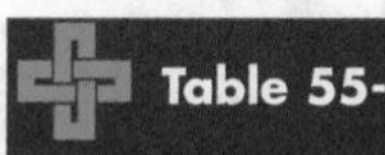

Table 55-5 Emergency Management: Stroke

Possible Etiology

Sudden vascular compromise causing disruption of blood flow to the brain, which can be caused by thrombosis, trauma, aneurysm, embolism, or hemorrhage

Possible Assessment Findings

Alteration in level of consciousness
Weakness, numbness, paralysis of portion of body
Speech or visual disturbances
Severe headache
Increased or decreased pulse rate
Respiratory distress
Unequal pupils
Hypertension
Drooping facial features on affected side, difficulty swallowing
Seizures
Loss of bladder or bowel control
Nausea and vomiting

Management

- Monitor airway; have airway equipment available including suction and intubation supplies; anticipate need to intubate if gag reflex is absent.
- Remove dentures, bridges.
- Administer oxygen via nasal cannula or nonrebreather mask (100%) and monitor for respiratory distress; if patient is not breathing, ventilate with bag valve mask.
- Establish intravenous access with one large-bore catheter (14 or 16 gauge) with normal saline; avoid fluid overloading.
- Remove patient's clothing and maintain patient warmth using warm blankets, warm intravenous fluids, overhead warming lights, warm humidified oxygen.
- Monitor vital signs, including level of consciousness, O_2 saturation, cardiac rhythm, Glasgow Coma Scale score, pupil size.
- Position head midline and head of bed elevated 30 degrees if no symptoms of shock.
- Institute seizure precautions; pad side rails, suction at bedside.

reduce cerebral edema, which interferes with metabolism of the viable cells. This interference, although a temporary phenomenon, may result in the death of additional cells or even of the person. Hyperosmotic agents, such as mannitol, may be employed. A hyperosmotic agent tends to draw fluid from the extravascular spaces into the vascular system. The second approach used to prevent additional brain damage involves measures designed to reduce the metabolic needs of the brain. Hypothermia and barbiturate therapy are among the treatments that have been attempted for this purpose, although neither has proved effective. The third

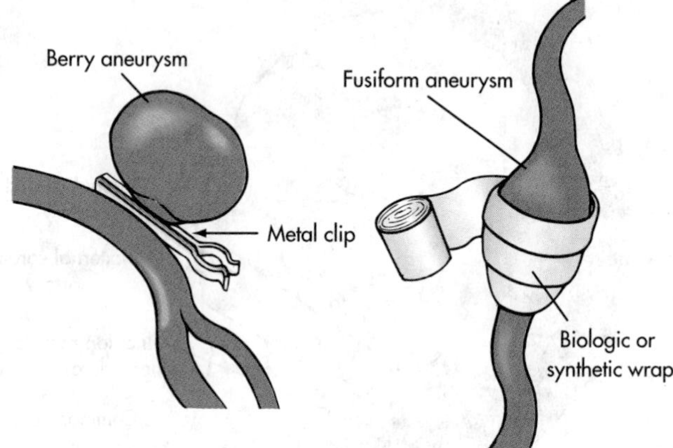

Fig. 55-6 Clipping and wrapping of aneurysms.

therapeutic approach is designed to promote cerebral blood flow. Vasodilators (e.g., papaverine), hypertensive agents (treatment to increase blood pressure), and hyperventilation therapy have all been attempted but have been of little documented value.

When a cerebral hemorrhage is the result of rupture of an aneurysm, surgical intervention may be appropriate. Early surgery to decrease the danger of rebleeding and to facilitate management of vasospasm has become more widely accepted.[16] Clips may be placed on either side of the aneurysm. The aneurysm may be wrapped or reinforced with muscle (Fig. 55-6).

If the patient's condition or the location of the aneurysm indicates that internal repair is inadvisable, external repair may be attempted. This involves clamping of the common carotid artery, a procedure that requires perfusion of the affected hemisphere by circulation from the opposite side. The adequacy of this circulation is determined by angiogram and isotope blood flow studies.

Chronic Management

After the stroke has stabilized for 12 to 24 hours, therapeutic management shifts from the preservation of life to the lessening of disability. At this point the patient may be evaluated by a physiatrist, a physician who specializes in physical medicine and rehabilitation. Depending on the available resources and the patient's estimated rehabilitation potential, the physiatrist may recommend that the patient be transferred to a rehabilitation unit. Other possible approaches may be to initiate various rehabilitation treatments in the acute-care setting, have the patient participate in rehabilitation therapy on an outpatient basis, or set up a home care rehabilitation program in which therapists treat the patient in the patient's home.

As part of the long-term therapeutic management after a stroke, various members of the health care team may be involved in the effort to return the patient to optimal functioning. The exact composition of the team depends on the needs of the patient and the resources of the involved institution (Fig. 55-7).

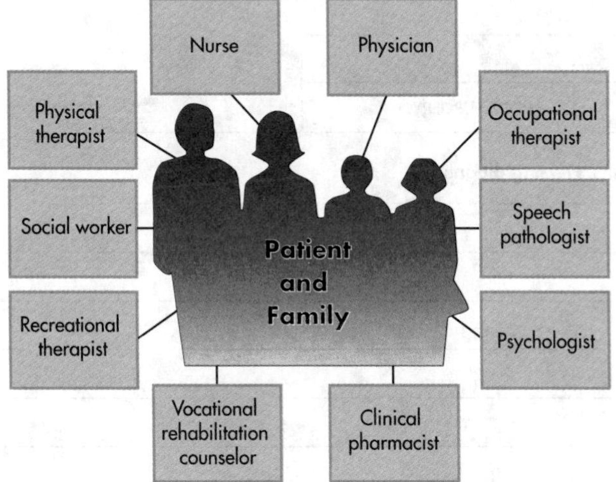

Fig. 55-7 Representative membership of the rehabilitation team.

Pharmacologic Management

Hyperosmotic Agents. When the cerebral edema accompanying a stroke threatens to cause herniation, a dehydrating agent is used. IV mannitol is the drug of choice. This hyperosmotic agent reduces the ICP caused by edema. It must be used with caution in patients with renal dysfunction because the increased circulatory volume may compromise damaged kidneys. Side effects of mannitol include fever, angina, pulmonary congestion, headache, and blurred vision.

Anticoagulants. Heparin is used as an anticoagulant in the treatment of TIAs, thrombotic strokes, and strokes in evolution. It exerts its effect by the activation of plasma antithrombin and the subsequent inactivation of thrombin. Heparin is used as the first step in anticoagulation. It is most effective when administered by continuous IV infusion at a rate of 1000 U per hour or until the partial thromboplastin time is 1.5 to 2 times normal. The duration of treatment is usually 7 to 10 days. Complications include bleeding and easy bruising. Because its effectiveness in the treatment of stroke syndromes is controversial, the risk of bleeding has to be weighed against potential benefits.

Long-term anticoagulation is accomplished by the oral administration of warfarin (Coumadin, Panwarfin), which inhibits prothrombin synthesis and decreases the vitamin K-dependent clotting factors. The usual dosage is 5 to 10 mg per day. A prothrombin time of 1.5 to 2 times normal is desirable. The duration of treatment in stroke syndromes is 3 to 6 months. Excessive bleeding is the primary complication. (Table 35-14 lists the nursing implications related to anticoagulant therapy and patient education.)

A patient taking warfarin on a long-term basis needs to know the following:

1. Signs of anticoagulant overdosage
2. Drugs with which warfarin interacts
3. Rationale for avoiding modifications in diet
4. Importance of avoiding trauma
5. Importance of a Medic-Alert bracelet
6. Need for routine blood testing

Platelet Aggregation Inhibitors. Platelet aggregation inhibitors, which interfere with platelet function, are used in the management of TIAs and symptoms of progressing stroke. Aspirin, dipyridamole, and ticlopidine are three such agents.

Acetylsalicylic acid (aspirin, ASA) is used to prevent platelet aggregation at the site of an atherosclerotic plaque. The optimum dosage is currently unclear; recommendations vary from a low of 75 mg per day to a high of 1300 mg per day administered orally. The complications of gastrointestinal (GI) bleeding are increased with higher doses and may be reduced by administering the aspirin with meals. There is some research evidence that low dosages and high dosages of aspirin are similar in efficacy.[17] Aspirin is contraindicated in patients with peptic ulcer disease and must be used with caution when anticoagulants are also being taken. The duration of treatment is indefinite.

Dipyridamole (Persantine) also inhibits platelet aggregation. It is used alone or with aspirin in the treatment of TIAs. It is administered orally in doses of 50 to 75 mg four times per day (or three times per day with aspirin). Complications include nausea and vomiting, which can be managed by administration of the drug with meals. Duration of treatment is indefinite.

Ticlopidine hydrochloride (Ticlid) is a new platelet aggregation inhibitor that has been shown in multicenter, randomized trials to be beneficial in reducing strokes compared with both placebo and aspirin. The usual dosage of ticlopidine is 250 mg twice daily administered orally with food. The most common side effects of ticlopidine have been diarrhea and reversible neutropenia.[18]

Thrombolytic Therapy. Reperfusion of acutely occluded intracranial arteries has great appeal for treatment of acute ischemic strokes. Fibrinolytic therapy is being used for the treatment of acute myocardial infarction (see Chapter 31). In stroke therapy tissue plasminogen activator (tPA) is the primary fibrinolytic therapy in use and under study. The lytic action of tPA occurs as plasminogen is converted to plasmin (fibrinolysin), whose enzymatic action digests fibrin and fibrinogen, lysing the clot. Although a major side effect is hemorrhage, if tPA is used within the first few hours after a stroke, the risk of bleeding is decreased. Continued research is needed on the safety, optimal dose, timing, and efficacy of tPA.

Nutritional Management

After the acute phase, the dietitian can assist in determining the appropriate daily caloric intake based on the patient's overall size, weight, and activity level. Residual physical problems (e.g., paralysis of the dominant arm) and psychosocial problems (e.g., depression) must also be considered in relation to a nutritional plan.

If the patient is unable to take in an adequate diet orally, tube feeding may be initiated, usually by the nasogastric

(Text continued on p. 1738.)

Clinical Pathway for Cerebrovascular Accident

SERVICE		PHYSICIAN	
PRIMARY NURSE		PRIMARY NURSE	
DISCHARGE DATE	ADMISSION DATE		DATE OF SURGERY

Problem Number	Patient problems/Nursing diagnoses
#1	Lack of knowledge
#2	Impaired verbal communication
#3	Self-care deficit bathing/hygiene
#4	Feeding, toileting
#5	Impaired physical mobility
#6	Altered nutrition

Problem number		Day 1	Day 2	Day 3	Day 4
#2 #4 #6 #7	Assessment/ monitoring	Assess for fall prevention Assess ability to communicate Assess for skin breakdown (Braden scale) Assess neurologic status and information processing VS q4hr ×1 ×2 ×3 ×4 ×5 ×6 I & O q8hr ×1 ×2 ×3 Patient is able to convey needs to others	Assess for skin breakdown Assess neurologic status and information processing VS q4hr ×1 ×2 ×3 ×4 ×5 ×6 I & O q8hr ×1 ×2 ×3 Skin integrity is maintained	Assess for skin breakdown Assess neurologic status and information processing VS q8hr ×1 ×2 ×3 DC I & O	Assess for skin breakdown Assess neurologic status and information processing VS q8hr ×1 ×2 ×3
#1 #3 #4 #5	Consults	PT OT Speech pathologist—communication disorders and swallowing disorders	Evaluation complete within 24 hr Evaluation complete within 24 hr *MBS evaluation completed within 24 hr		
#7	Procedure/test	CT—Head (usually done in ER) ECG CXR Echo Holter Carotid studies CBC PT/PTT SMA6	*Dobhoff placed PT/*PTT CVA is diagnosed	All test results charted PT/*PTT	PT/*PTT

continued

CLINICAL PATHWAY FOR CEREBROVASCULAR ACCIDENT—cont'd

Care Path CVA 400

CNS	DIETARY	RT
HOME HEALTH	OT	OTHER
PT	SW	OTHER

Problem number	Patient problems/Nursing diagnoses
#7	Alteration in cerebral tissue perfusion

Day 5	Day 6	Day 7	Day 8	Discharge outcomes
				Neurologic deficits have stabilized or improved **Patient is able to convey needs to others**
Assess for skin breakdown Assess neurologic status and information processing VS q8hr ×1 ×2 ×3	Assess for skin breakdown	Assess for skin breakdown	Assess for skin breakdown	**Skin remains intact with no evidence of breakdown** **Oriented ×3 or disorientation is minimized**
*LTR evaluation completed		Home health/outpatient for speech pathology		
PT/*PTT				**CVA is diagnosed** **Anticoagulation is at therapeutic level as indicated by PT/*PTT**

continued

Clinical Pathway for Cerebrovascular Accident—cont'd

Problem number		Day 1	Day 2	Day 3	Day 4
#3 #4 #5 #7	**Treatment**	IV fluids *TEDS *Air support mattress/bed *NG tube *Foley catheter *O_2	IV Fluids *TEDS DC NG	DC IVs *TEDS off DC Foley catheter SP—functional communication established, swallowing protocol initiated	Communication goals addressed, swallowing continues
#7	**Activity**	Bed rest	Chair bid ×1 ×2	*PT—to satellite for Rx ×1 *OT—to satellite ×1 to begin ADLs	*To PT—to satellite bid ×1 ×2 *To OT satellite bid ×1 ×2
#7	**Meds/IVs**	Heparin drip	Heparin drip	Heparin gtt Start PO anticoagulant	DC heparin Continue oral anticoagulant
#3 #5	**Nutrition**	Diet as tolerated LoChol/NAS Maintain hydration	*TF Able to tolerate diet	*TF	*TF
#1 #7	**Patient/family education**	Orient to unit and medical condition, Dx procedures and anticoag safety (Heparin)		Discuss disease process, anticoag safety (coumadin) Patient/family understands med and activity restrictions	Begin D/C teaching: Nutrition OT/ADLs PT/activity Nsg/Meds
#1 #2 #3 #4 #5 #6 #7	**Discharge planning**	Patient/family verbalize understanding of Care Path Plan of care has been mutually set with patient and family	SW HR screening and initiate assessment of discharge needs	SW coordinates with other disciplines re: discharge planning needs	
#1	**Psychosocial/emotional needs**	*SW for crisis intervention PC assess family dyamics related to CVA	HR screening to assess counseling needs	Permit patient/family to express concerns and offer support PC with family, construct a value of hope that is appropriate to patient's condition	Explore discharge options with patient/family and provide resource information
Signatures					

continued

Clinical Pathway for Cerebrovascular Accident—cont'd

Day 5	Day 6	Day 7	Day 8	
Communication goals addressed, swallowing continues	Specific communication goals and swallow plan confirmed with MD and caretaker			
*To PT satellite bid ×1×2 *To OT satellite bid ×1×2	Establish equipment needs			**Able to function with assistance in ADLs and mobility**
Continue PO anticoag				
*TF				**Able to tolerate adequate diet and maintain hydration**
	Begin PT/OT DC inst: home exercise ADLs	SP begin DC inst.		**Patient/family verbalize understanding/able to return demonstrate DC teaching: nutrition home exercise program ADLs medications communication *swallowing protocol**
SW complete evaluation of DC planning needs DC plan is established	LTR DC orders completed by MD	SW complete referrals for DC destination (equipment HH)	Review and finalize DC plans	**Patient/family is ready for DC and has information necessary for care**
Develop on-going recovery and support plan congruent with patient's values and beliefs		SW assess patient/family understanding of DC plans		**Patient/family have understanding as to how CVA may be viewed in harmony with their world view. Patient/family is able to access feelings related to diagnosis and are aware of support systems and resources available**

Developed by Barnes Hospital, St. Louis, MO. Licensed by Center for Case Management, South Natick, MA.
ADLs, Activities of daily living; *bid,* twice a day; *CBC,* complete blood count; *CNS,* central nervous system; *CT,* computed tomography; *CVA,* cerebrovascular accident; *CXR,* chest x-ray; *DC,* discharge; *Dx,* diagnostic; *ECG,* electrocardiogram; *ER,* emergency room; *gtt,* drop or drip; *HH/OP,* home health outpatient; *HR,* heart rate; *I & O,* intake and output; *NAS,* no salt added; *NG,* nasogastric; *OT,* occupational therapy; *PC,* pastoral care; *PO,* by mouth; *PT,* prothrombin time; *PTT,* partial thromboplastin time; *RT,* respiratory therapy; *Rx,* prescription; *SMA-6,* blood chemistry; *SP,* speech pathologist; *SW,* social worker; *TF,* tube feeding; *VS,* vital signs.

route. Most commercially prepared formulas provide about 100 calories per 100 ml. Sustagen, Isocal, and Ensure are examples of complete nutritional formulas. The latter two are also low in lactose and residue. Because tube feedings tend to be hyperosmotic, they may dehydrate the patient. When intermittent feedings are administered, they should be preceded and followed by water. Cramping and diarrhea are side effects of tube feedings. These can usually be controlled by administration of small, frequent, less concentrated feedings at room temperature. It may also be helpful to use a formula that contains fiber (e.g., Enrich). (Tube feedings are discussed in Chapter 37.)

Although the patient may experience diarrhea from the tube feedings, more commonly the patient who has had a stroke tends to be constipated. The following dietary measures aid in the prevention of constipation:

1. Fluid intake of 2500 to 3000 ml daily unless contraindicated
2. Prune juice (120 ml) or stewed prunes daily
3. Cooked fruit three times daily
4. Cooked vegetables three times daily
5. Whole-grain cereal or bread three to five times daily

These dietary measures are effective in preventing constipation. Other measures to prevent constipation include a regular schedule, privacy, a footstool to increase abdominal pressure, and exercise.

NURSING MANAGEMENT

STROKE

Nursing Assessment

Subjective and objective data that should be obtained about a person who has had a stroke are presented in Table 55-6 on p. 1742. The subjective data include examples of questions asked of the patient or persons who are familiar with the patient. These questions help the nurse determine the patient's experience of the stroke from the patient's personal perspective. The objective data include specific physical assessment findings commonly associated with stroke (e.g., hemiparesis, dysphagia, aphasia).

Nursing Diagnoses

Nursing diagnoses are determined when the problem and etiologic factors are supported by clinical data. Nursing diagnoses related to stroke include, but are not limited to, those presented in the nursing care plan for the stroke patient on p. 1739.

Planning

The overall goals are that the patient who has experienced a stroke will (1) maintain a stable or improved level of consciousness, (2) attain maximum physical functioning and self-care activities, (3) avoid complications of immobility, (4) maintain stable body functions such as bladder control and acceptable weight, (5) maximize remaining communication abilities, and (6) maintain effective coping (patient and family).

Nursing Implementation

Health Promotion and Maintenance. To reduce the incidence of stroke, the nurse should focus teaching efforts toward stroke prevention for persons with known risk (e.g., patients with TIAs, hypertension, or diabetes mellitus).[8] The significance of other potentially modifiable risk factors for the occurrence of stroke is unclear. However, control of risk factors implicated in coronary artery disease may indirectly help prevent stroke. (For the nurse's role in management of these risk factors, see Table 31-4.) In any health care setting and for the population as a whole, nurses can play a major role in the promotion of a healthy lifestyle. An overall program to prevent events such as stroke includes the recognition that people are responsible to some degree for their own health and for the health of future generations.[19]

Acute Intervention

Respiratory system. During the acute phase of a stroke the nursing priority is management of respiratory function. Stroke patients are particularly vulnerable to respiratory problems. Advancing age and immobility make them particularly susceptible to atelectasis. With dysphagia or coma, aspiration pneumonia may develop. In coma the tongue tends to fall back and obstruct the airway. This problem requires that the patient be positioned in a side-lying position.

An oropharyngeal airway may be used during the first 24 to 48 hours. This airway holds the tongue in place, preventing airway obstruction and providing access for suctioning. If the patient is unable to breathe without an airway after 48 hours, a tracheostomy is performed. A suction machine should be available in the room. Coughing and deep breathing are helpful to the patient who has had a stroke. However, because these activities increase ICP, they should not be used in a hemorrhaging patient or when the possibility of herniation is imminent. In most patients who have had a stroke, an obstructed airway is more harmful than increased ICP secondary to coughing.

Neurologic system. The patient's neurologic status must be monitored closely to detect stroke in evolution or increased ICP. The level of consciousness, mental status, pupillary responses, movement and strength of extremities, and vital signs are checked at regular intervals. The frequency of neurologic checks (see Chapter 53) depends on the condition of the patient. A decreasing level of consciousness, the earliest and most sensitive sign of increasing ischemia in the brain, should prompt the nurse to check the patient more frequently. Such a change should be reported promptly to the attending physician.

Cardiovascular system. Nursing goals for the cardiovascular system are designed to maintain homeostasis. Because of advancing age or heart problems, many patients have decreased cardiac reserve after a stroke. Fluids are retained because of increased production of antidiuretic hormone and aldosterone secondary to stress. Fluid retention plus overhydration can result in fluid overload. It can also increase cerebral edema. The nurse therefore should closely monitor intake and output. IV therapy is also carefully regulated. In the initial stages, fluids may be

NURSING CARE PLAN Patient with a Stroke

Planning: Outcome Criteria	Nursing Interventions and Rationales
➤ NURSING DIAGNOSIS	Impaired physical mobility *related to* generalized weakness, muscle atrophy, or paralyzed extremities *as manifested by* decreased physical activity, limited range of motion, decreased muscle strength or control
Transfer and ambulate at maximal level of ability.	Assess and document range of motion, transfer abilities, and positioning ability *to determine extent of problem and plan appropriate interventions.* Administer passive or active range-of-motion exercises to affected extremities at least tid *to prevent unnecessary muscle atrophy and contractures.* Position correctly with support pillows according to procedures; teach and assist family and patient with positioning techniques; document progress *to prevent contractures.* Encourage as much self-mobility as possible *to maintain physical activity to highest degree possible and to promote patient's sense of control.*
➤ NURSING DIAGNOSIS	Impaired verbal communication *related to* residual aphasia *as manifested by* refusal or inability to speak, word-finding problems, use of inappropriate words, inability to follow verbal directions
Demonstrate ability to communicate effectively.	Assess exact communication deficits and strengths *to determine extent of problem and plan appropriate interventions.* Intervene as appropriate. Use short, simple questions that elicit "yes" and "no" answers; speak slowly and allow adequate time for response *to avoid overwhelming patient with verbal stimuli.* Use gestures *to support verbal cues.* Treat the patient as an adult regardless of degree of impairment *to avoid frustration and anger, which can worsen the problem.* Discuss problem and strategies with family *to gain cooperation from patient's support system.*
➤ NURSING DIAGNOSIS	Self-care deficit (partial to total) *related to* motor weakness, paralysis, and loss of ability to effectively perform activities of daily living (ADLs) *as manifested by* observation or valid report of inability to eat, bathe, use toilet, dress, or groom independently
Perform ADLs by self or with assistance from family or staff; have needs met.	Assess and document level of self-care *to determine extent of problem and plan appropriate interventions.* Encourage independence, providing supervision or assistance as needed *to avoid the development of dependency.* Follow through with techniques for ADLs recommended by occupational or physical therapist *to help patient incorporate teaching from specialists into daily life and activities.* Observe and coach family and attendants in performing ADLs with patient *so patient's needs are met on a regular basis.*
➤ NURSING DIAGNOSIS	Sensory/perceptual alteration: visual deficit *related to* visual field cut, diplopia, and ptosis secondary to decreased circulation to brain *as manifested by* behavioral evidence or verbal report of inability to see objects in affected area of visual field
Bring objects into field of vision; scan with eyes; express satisfaction with vision.	Assess and document amount of visual field impairment *to determine extent of problem and plan appropriate interventions.* Teach patient to turn head and scan environment. Early in care, approach patient on unaffected side; place objects in patient's field of vision; give physical and verbal cues to aid in path finding *to compensate for visual field deficits.* Later in care, approach patient on affected side *to encourage patient to turn head.* Provide visual stimulation *to promote use of full range of visual capabilities.* Place objects on involved side *to assess ability to compensate.* Use an eye patch *to prevent diplopia.* If corneal reflex is absent, protect affected eye to prevent injury.

continued

NURSING CARE PLAN Patient with a Stroke—cont'd

Planning: Outcome Criteria	Nursing Interventions and Rationales
➤ **NURSING DIAGNOSIS**	Altered pattern of urinary elimination: incontinence *related to* impaired impulse to void or inability to reach toilet or manage tasks of voiding *as manifested by* flow of urine at unpredictable times, urination before reaching appropriate receptacle, nocturia
Have no urinary tract infection; satisfactory control by natural or artificial method.	Assess and record patient's continent and incontinent voidings *to determine patterns and plan appropriate interventions.* Note color and character of urine daily and as needed *to ensure early detection of urinary tract infection and to prevent very concentrated urine.* Provide fluid intake of 2000 ml/day unless contraindicated *to foster adequate elimination of dilute urine.* If indwelling catheter is used, give catheter care and clean perineum every shift and as needed *to avoid infection and ensure uninterrupted urinary flow.* Offer urinal or commode q2hr and as needed *to aid in establishing regular voiding pattern.* Assure patient of your willingness to assist with urinary problem *to avoid embarrassment and to demonstrate a caring attitude.*
➤ **NURSING DIAGNOSIS**	Constipation *related to* immobility, inadequate fiber or bulk intake, and impaired defecation impulse *as manifested by* changes in usual pattern in frequency or amount of stool, sensation of rectal fullness or pressure or abdominal discomfort, decreased bowel sounds, distended abdomen
Have regular formed stool at least every other day with no fecal incontinence.	Discuss previous bowel habits with family and patient and establish program; involve patient and family in making appropriate changes *so patient and support system can cooperate with treatment approach.* Teach patient and family about high-fiber foods to include in diet *because this will increase fecal bulk and aid in regular bowel movements.* If patient has dentures, instruct to insert them at mealtime *so patient can eat high-roughage foods.* Provide privacy for bowel program *because embarrassment can cause inhibition of defecation response.* Give suppository or stool softeners (if needed) *to encourage regular elimination.* Document results of bowel program *so plan can be revised if necessary.*
➤ **NURSING DIAGNOSIS**	Risk of ineffective airway clearance *related to* inability to raise secretions
Be able to expectorate secretions; have no respiratory distress.	Assess for weak, ineffective cough; bronchial congestion; adventitious breath sounds; changes in color, amount, and consistency of sputum *to determine if risk factors are present.* Observe for increase in pulmonary secretions, changes in color of secretions, and temperature elevation *as indicators of infection.* Auscultate lungs for diminished breath sounds daily and as needed *to determine adequacy of respiratory excursion.* Suction as needed *to remove accumulated secretions.* Instruct patient and family in feeding program and emergency measures *to prevent aspiration and resultant respiratory distress.*
➤ **NURSING DIAGNOSIS**	Impaired swallowing *related to* weakness or paralysis of affected muscles *as manifested by* drooling, difficulty in swallowing, choking
Have no signs or symptoms of aspiration; be able to tolerate foods and fluids without choking.	Assess patient *to determine ability to swallow and presence of gag reflex.* Have patient sit upright for meals and 30 min afterward *to use gravity to prevent aspiration.* Teach patient to take small bites in unaffected side of mouth, keep chin down, and stroke throat *to stimulate swallowing.* After patient has eaten, check mouth for pocketed food and teach patient and family this technique *to prevent collection and putrefaction of food and resultant risk of infection.* Give thick shakes, foods with texture, and cold foods *to facilitate swallowing and minimize danger of choking.* If problem with sputum and saliva production, avoid milk products, *which increase production of mucus and saliva.* Give oral care after meals *to promote comfort and oral health.* Notify dietitian of need to change food texture or fluids. Provide quiet environment and supervision as needed *to make mealtime as pleasant as possible for the patient.* If choking occurs, do not interfere unless difficulty in breathing develops; then use back blows, abdominal thrusts, and suction as needed *to allow patient opportunity to deal with problem so confidence in self-care is enhanced.*

continued

NURSING CARE PLAN Patient with a Stroke—cont'd

Planning: Outcome Criteria	Nursing Interventions and Rationales
➤ **NURSING DIAGNOSIS**	Altered nutrition: less than body requirements *related to* difficulty or inability to feed self, inadequate food and fluid intake, immobility, and possible depression *as manifested by* weight loss, altered taste sensation, fatigue, listlessness, thirst, dry skin, decreased skin turgor, weakness
Have adequate intake of food and fluids; stable weight or weight change as recommended by dietitian.	Weigh patient on admission and every other day as needed *to have baseline data so changes over time can be evaluated.* Request nutritious snacks between meals and at bedtime if indicated, assist with eating *to increase intake over 24-hr period.* Evaluate previous eating patterns and food preferences *to enhance appetite.* Perform interventions for choking and aspiration *to prevent emergency situation from developing.* Assess for dehydration *so appropriate plan can be initiated if present.* Measure intake and output for 3 days or until satisfactory balance is achieved; monitor adequate fluid intake *to prevent dehydration.*
➤ **NURSING DIAGNOSIS**	Self-esteem disturbance *related to* actual or perceived loss of function *as manifested by* refusal to touch or look at affected body parts, increasing dependence on others, refusal to participate in self-care
Verbalize feelings and concerns; participate in appropriate socialization with family and staff; set realistic goals.	Encourage patient to verbalize feelings *to assess effect of stroke sequelae on self-esteem.* Spend time with patient using good listening techniques *to show a caring, concerned attitude, which fosters confidence in a relationship.* Establish achievable goals; explain all procedures and involve patient in planning goals; offer praise for every success and step of progress; involve patient as soon as possible in rehabilitation program *to promote sense of satisfaction and control and reduce frustration.* Refer for counseling or medical-psychiatric evaluation if indicated *so patient can have expert help with serious problems.*
➤ **NURSING DIAGNOSIS**	Risk of ineffective management of therapeutic regimen *related to* functional, cognitive, or communication limitations
Patient or family will make satisfactory arrangements to have patient's needs met on a daily basis.	Assess degree of functional, cognitive, or communication limitations patient is experiencing *to determine teaching plan and arrange appropriate interventions.* Teach patient and family how to treat, prevent, and monitor for problems *so early intervention is ensured.* Evaluate plan *to determine if regimen is being followed or must be revised based on changing patient status or circumstances.*

limited to 1500 to 2000 ml per day or approximately 63 to 83 ml per hour. Every effort must be made to ensure a constant flow rate and to avoid a sudden rush of IV fluid. Manifestations of fluid overload are crackles, dyspnea, shortness of breath, and coughing. In addition, the nurse should regularly assess for other cardiovascular problems, such as hypertension and dysrhythmias.

After a stroke the patient is at risk for thrombophlebitis and deep-vein thrombosis in the weak or paralyzed lower extremity. This risk is related to both immobility and decreased muscle pumping activity in the extremity. The most effective prevention is to keep the patient moving. Active range-of-motion exercises should be taught if the patient has any voluntary movement in the affected extremity. For the patient with hemiplegia, passive range-of-motion exercises should be done at least several times a day. Additional measures often used to prevent thrombophlebitis include positioning to minimize the effects of dependent edema and the use of elastic compression gradient stockings or support hose. Intermittent pneumatic compression stockings may be ordered for long-term bedridden patients.

Musculoskeletal system. The nursing goal for the musculoskeletal system is to maintain function. This is accomplished by the prevention of joint contractures and muscular atrophy. In the acute phase, range-of-motion exercises and positioning are important nursing interventions. Passive range-of-motion exercise is begun on the first day of hospitalization. If the stroke is due to a cerebral hemorrhage, the movements are limited to the limbs. The patient is taught to actively exercise the affected limbs as soon as possible. Muscle atrophy secondary to lack of innervation and to inactivity can develop in as little as 1 month.

The paralyzed side needs special attention when the patient is positioned. Each joint should be positioned higher than the joint proximal to it. Specific deformities on the

Table 55-6 Nursing Assessment: Stroke

Subjective Data

Important health information

Past health history: Hypertension; previous stroke, TIA(s), aneurysm, cardiac disease (including recent myocardial infarction), dysrhythmias, congestive heart failure, valvular disease, infective endocarditis; alcohol abuse, smoking, hyperlipidemia, diabetes, gout

Medications: Use of oral contraceptives, use of and compliance with antihypertensive and anticoagulant agents

Functional health patterns

Health perception–health management: Positive family history; easy fatigability

Nutritional-metabolic: Anorexia, nausea, vomiting; dysphagia, disturbances in taste and smell

Elimination: Change in bladder and bowel patterns

Activity-exercise: Loss of movement and sensation; syncope; tingling, numbness, weakness on one side; generalized weakness

Cognitive-perceptual: Loss of memory; alteration in speech, language, problem solving; pain; headache, possibly sudden and severe (hemorrhage); visual disturbances

Objective Data

General

Emotional lability, lethargy, apathy or combativeness, fever

Respiratory

Loss of cough reflex, labored or irregular respirations, tachypnea, rhonchi (aspiration), airway occlusion (tongue), apnea

Cardiovascular

Hypertension, tachycardia, carotid bruit

Gastrointestinal

Loss of gag reflex, bowel incontinence, decreased or absent bowel sounds

Urinary

Incontinence

Neurologic

Contralateral motor and sensory deficits, including weakness, paresis, paralysis, anesthesia; unequal pupils, hand grasps; akinesia, aphasia (expressive, receptive, global), agnosias, apraxia, visual deficits, perceptual or spatial disturbances, altered level of consciousness (drowsiness to deep coma) and Babinski sign, decreased followed by increased deep tendon reflexes, flaccidity followed by spasticity, amnesia, ataxia, personality change, nuchal rigidity, seizures

Possible findings

Polycythemia, positive CT and MRI scans showing size and location of lesion, positive Doppler ultrasonography and cerebral angiography

CT, Computed tomography; *MRI,* magnetic resonance imaging; *TIA,* transient ischemic attack.

affected side of the patient with hemiplegia that nurses must be aware of are shoulder adduction; flexion contractures of the hand, wrist, and elbow; external rotation of the hip; and plantar flexion of the foot. Subluxation of the shoulder on the affected side is common and not preventable. However, careful positioning and moving of the affected arm may prevent the development of a painful shoulder condition. Immobilization of the affected upper extremity may precipitate a painful shoulder-hand syndrome.

Use of a footboard is not recommended for positioning a stroke patient in bed. Rather than preventing *plantar flexion* (foot drop), the sensory stimulation of a footboard against the bottom of the foot increases plantar flexion. A trochanter roll should be used to prevent external rotation of the hip when the patient is in the supine position. However, even therapeutic interventions can be detrimental if the patient is allowed to remain in any position for too long.

Integumentary system. The skin of the patient who has had a stroke is particularly susceptible to breakdown because of loss of sensation and diminished circulation. These deficits are caused by interference with the nerve supply to the blood vessels of the affected side. The problem is compounded by the age of the patient and possible incontinence. Pressure points should be examined and massaged with each turning. If an area of redness develops, the patient should be turned more frequently. The patient should not be left in any position for longer than 2 hours. Time spent lying on the paralyzed side should be limited to 30 minutes at a time. In addition, the skin must be kept clean and dry. An emollient may be beneficial for the older adult or dehydrated patient. Special mattresses that are filled with water or air or that provide alternating pressure may help in relieving pressure areas. If an area of redness develops and does not return to normal color within 15 minutes after pressure is relieved, the epidermis and dermis are damaged and should not be massaged because massage will cause greater damage. Control of pressure is the single most important factor in the prevention and treatment of skin breakdown. Vigilance is required for pressure sores to be prevented.

Gastrointestinal system. The stress of illness contributes to a catabolic state that can interfere with recovery. Although neurologic and respiratory problems take priority in the acute phase of stroke, nutritional requirements should be addressed as soon as the patient is medically stable. The patient may be maintained for 5 to 7 days on IV fluids. Facial weakness on the affected side and dysphagia (difficulty swallowing) present special problems. If the patient is conscious, oral feeding should be considered.

The first oral feeding should be approached with caution because the gag reflex may be impaired. Before initiation of feeding, the gag reflex may be assessed by gently stimulating the back of the throat with a tongue blade. If a gag reflex is present, the patient will gag spontaneously. If it is absent, the feeding should be deferred and exercises to stimulate swallowing should be started. The speech therapist or the occupational therapist is usually responsible for designing this program.[20] However, the nurse may be called on to develop the program in some clinical settings. To assess swallowing ability, the nurse should elevate the head of the bed to an upright position (unless contraindicated) and give the patient a small amount of crushed ice or ice water to swallow. If the gag reflex is present and the patient is able to swallow safely, the nurse may proceed with the feeding. Mouth care before feeding helps stimulate sensory awareness and salivation and can facilitate swallowing. The patient should remain in a high Fowler's position, preferably in a chair with the head flexed forward for the feeding and for 30 minutes after the feeding. Foods should be easy to swallow and provide enough texture, temperature (fairly hot or fairly cold), and flavor to stimulate a swallow reflex. Pureed foods are not usually the best choice because they are often bland and too smooth and at room temperature by the time the patient is fed. Thin liquids are often difficult to swallow and may promote coughing. Milk products should be avoided because they tend to increase the viscosity of mucus and increase salivation. Food should be placed on the unaffected side of the mouth. The nurse should ensure that the atmosphere is unrushed and nonstressful. Each feeding must be followed by scrupulous oral hygiene because food tends to collect on the affected side of the mouth.

The most common bowel problem is constipation. The patient should be checked every 2 days for impaction. Because diet, fluids, and exercise are limited during the acute phase of stroke, a laxative or a stool softener may have to be used. It is often the responsibility of the nurse to request these medications. Suppositories may be necessary to relieve constipation. Enemas are used only if suppositories and digital stimulation are ineffective, because they cause vagal stimulation and increase ICP.

Urinary system. In the acute stage of stroke, the primary urinary problem is poor bladder control, resulting in incontinence. Efforts should be made to promote normal bladder function and avoid the use of an indwelling catheter. If an indwelling catheter is used initially, it should be removed as soon as the patient is medically and neurologically stable. Long-term use of an indwelling catheter promotes the development of a urinary tract infection and prolongs bladder retraining. An intermittent catheterization program may be used for patients with urinary retention. An adequate fluid intake is critical for bladder retraining. A commode, bedpan, or urinal should be offered every 2 hours. A condom catheter may be used for men.

Communication. During the acute stage the nurse's role in meeting the psychologic needs of the patient is primarily supportive. An alert patient is usually anxious because of lack of understanding of what has happened and inability to communicate. Extensive evaluation and treatment of language and communication deficits are usually done after the patient's condition has stabilized. In the acute phase the patient's response to one or two simple questions should give the nurse a guideline for structuring explanations and instructions. If the patient cannot understand words, gestures may be used to support the verbal cues. It may help to speak slowly and calmly and to use relatively simple words (Table 55-7). The stroke patient with aphasia may be easily overwhelmed by verbal stimuli.

Table 55-7 Communicating with a Patient Who Has Aphasia

- Treat the patient as an adult.
- Present one thought or idea at a time.
- Keep questions simple or ask questions that can be answered with "yes" or "no."
- Organize the patient's day by preparing and following a schedule (the more familiar the routine, the easier it will be for the person with aphasia).
- Make use of gestures or demonstration as an acceptable alternative form of communication. Encourage this by saying "Show me. . ." or "Point to what you want."
- Speak with normal volume and tone.
- Allow body contact (e.g., the clasp of a hand or touching) as much as possible. Realize that touching may be the only way the patient can express feelings.
- Give the patient time to process information and generate a response before repeating a question or statement.
- Decrease environmental stimuli that may be distracting and disrupting to communication efforts.

Sensory-perceptual alterations. *Homonymous hemianopsia* (blindness in the same half of each visual field) is a common problem after a stroke (Fig. 55-8). Persistent disregard of objects in part of the visual field should alert the nurse to this possibility. The patient must learn to compensate for these deficits. Initially, the nurse compensates for the perceptual problem by arranging the environment within the patient's perceptual field. Later the patient is instructed to consciously attend to the neglected side. The

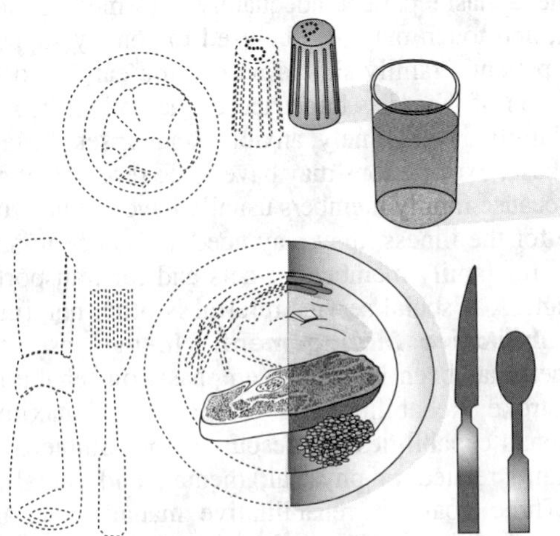

Fig. 55-8 Spatial and perceptual deficits in stroke. Perception of a patient with homonymous hemianopsia shows that food on the left side is not seen and thus ignored.

position of the affected arm or leg in space must be checked by the patient to prevent unfelt trauma.

In the clinical situation it is often difficult to distinguish between a visual field cut and a neglect syndrome. Both problems may occur with strokes affecting either the right side or the left side of the brain. A person may be unfortunate enough to have both homonymous hemianopsia and a neglect syndrome, which increase the inattention to the affected side. A neglect syndrome results in decreased safety awareness and puts the patient at considerable risk of injury. Immediately after the stroke the nurse must anticipate potential safety hazards and provide protection from injury. This involves the use of careful observation while the patient is awake or the use of side rails and soft vest restraints. The use of restraints is sometimes contraindicated if their use agitates the patient.

Other visual problems may include diplopia, loss of the corneal reflex, and ptosis, particularly if the stroke is in the vertebrobasilar distribution (see Table 55-2). Diplopia is often treated with the use of an eye patch. If the corneal reflex is absent, the patient is at risk of a corneal abrasion and should be observed closely and protected against eye injuries. There are no definitive nursing interventions to use for ptosis, and the problem is usually not severe after a stroke.

Coping. A stroke is usually a sudden, extremely stressful event for both the patient and close family members. If the patient is married, it is often as if the stroke had happened to the couple. An older couple may perceive the stroke as a very real threat to life and to their accustomed lifestyle. Reactions to this threat vary considerably but may involve fear and apprehension, denial of the severity of the stroke, depression, and anger. During the acute phase of caring for the stroke patient and the family, nursing intervention designed to facilitate coping involves providing information and emotional support.

Explanations to the patient about what has happened and about diagnostic and therapeutic procedures should be clear and understandable. It will be particularly challenging to keep the aphasic patient adequately informed. Tone, demeanor, and touch may also be used to convey support.

The patient's family should be given a careful, detailed explanation of what has happened to the patient. However, if the family is extremely anxious and upset during the acute phase, explanations may have to be repeated at a later time. Because family members usually have not had time to prepare for the illness, they may need assistance in arranging care for family members or pets and for transportation and finances. A social service referral is often helpful.

Rehabilitative Management. In the past several years there has been increasing emphasis on rehabilitation after a stroke. Rehabilitation is the process of maximizing the patient's capabilities and resources to promote optimal functioning related to physical, mental, and social well-being. Three goals of rehabilitative management are to prevent deformity, maintain function, and restore function.[4,21] Work toward the first two goals begins at the time the patient enters the health care system. For example, on admission the nurse attempts to prevent deformity in the hemiplegic patient by proper positioning and range-of-motion exercises. In addition, measures to maintain the function of the respiratory and GI systems are implemented. With physiologic stabilization of the patient, the focus shifts to restoration of function. During this stage the patient begins to relearn and to regain control over bodily actions and functions that are deficient or lost because of the stroke. These activities may focus on speech, walking, bowel and bladder control, and activities of daily living.

Because no member of the health team has all the knowledge and skills necessary for rehabilitation, a team approach is usually used. The rehabilitation team works together to achieve the patient's goals. This requires a great deal of communication and coordination. The nurse is in a good position to facilitate this process and is often the key person in successful rehabilitation efforts. The patient's participation in decision making during the rehabilitative phase is essential to goal achievement after a stroke. In addition to patient and family, nurse, and physiatrist, members of the rehabilitation team may include representatives from the following disciplines: physical therapy, occupational therapy, speech pathology, recreational therapy, social service, psychology, clinical pharmacy, pastoral care, and vocational counseling. Physical therapists focus on mobility, progressive ambulation, transfer techniques, and equipment needed for mobility. The main emphasis of occupational therapy is on retraining for activities of daily living, such as eating, dressing, hygiene, and other activities that involve fine motor skills. Occupational therapists also perform cognitive and perceptual evaluation and retraining.

The long-term management of the stroke patient is focused on rehabilitation. The problems the stroke patient has are caused by or are a response to a neurologic deficit. Many of the nursing interventions outlined in the nursing care plan for the patient with a stroke are initiated in the acute phase and continued throughout the rehabilitation phase of care.

Musculoskeletal system. In the rehabilitation of the musculoskeletal system the nurse initially emphasizes the functions the patient needs to eat, toilet, and walk around the room. Before the initiation of any intervention the nurse should assess the stage of recovery of muscle function. If the muscles are still flaccid after several weeks, the prognosis for regaining function is poor and the focus of care is on preventing additional loss. Most patients begin to show signs of spasticity with exaggerated reflexes within 48 hours. This actually denotes progress. As improvement continues, small voluntary movements of the hip or shoulder may be accompanied by involuntary movements in the rest of the extremity (synergy). In the final stage of recovery the patient acquires voluntary control of isolated muscle groups.

Balance training is an initial rehabilitative effort and begins with the patient sitting up in bed or on the edge of the bed. The nurse must be alert for dizziness or syncope as a result of vasomotor instability.

Next the patient needs to learn to transfer from the bed to an armchair or a wheelchair. The chair is placed next to the bed on the patient's unaffected side. The patient rises to a standing position facing the chair. When the patient is stable in the standing position, the unaffected hand is placed on the far arm of the chair. The patient turns and sits down. The nurse may provide minimal assistance by standing at the patient's weak side, supporting the affected arm and blocking the affected knee to keep it from buckling. In some rehabilitation settings a Bobath approach (neurodevelopmental treatment) is used in work with stroke patients. The goal of a Bobath approach is to help the patient gain control over patterns of spasticity by inhibiting abnormal reflex patterns. Therapists and nurses who use a Bobath approach focus on encouraging normal muscle tone, and movement, and promoting bilateral functions.[22] If therapists and nurses are using a Bobath approach, transfers are taught to unaffected and affected sides to facilitate more normal, bilateral functioning.

Support or assistive devices, such as canes, walkers, or leg braces, may eventually be needed but are not used unless absolutely necessary. If they are used, the physical therapist usually selects the most appropriate ones for the patient. The nurse should incorporate physical therapy activities into the daily routine of the patient for additional practice and repetition of the rehabilitative efforts.

Gastrointestinal system. Inability to self-feed and lack of bowel regularity are two common GI problems after a stroke. The inability to feed oneself is frustrating and may result in malnutrition. The easiest solution is to have the patient switch hands for eating. The unaffected hand may be clumsy at first, but the end result is usually better than can be achieved with assistive devices. However, eating with only one hand is still a challenge. Assistive devices, such as a rocker knife, a plate guard, and a nonslip mat to keep the plate from sliding, are particularly useful eating aids (Fig. 55-9). Removal of unnecessary items from the tray or table can reduce spills and resulting embarrassment and decrease sensory overload and distraction. Careful attention to aesthetic and environmental details is an important nursing consideration related to improving appetite.

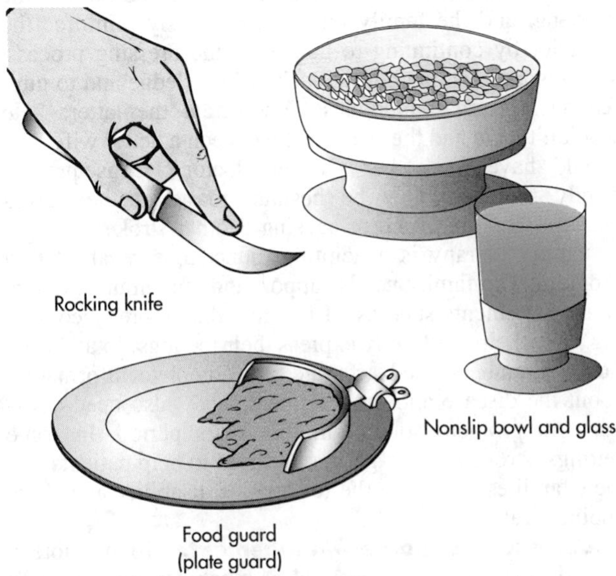

Fig. 55-9 Assistive devices for eating.

Problems with bowel control may be alleviated by implementation of a bowel-training program. A high-fiber diet (see Table 40-9) and adequate fluid (2000 to 3000 ml/day), as well as the selected dietary inclusions, should be given unless contraindicated. The patient should be placed on a bedpan, assisted to a bedside commode, or walked to the bathroom at a regular time each day to assist with reestablishment of bowel regularity. For most individuals, sitting up on a toilet or commode promotes the most effective bowel elimination. A good time to establish this pattern is within 30 minutes after breakfast each day, which takes advantage of the gastrocolic reflex. If the patient's usual bowel habits differ from this pattern, efforts should be made to adhere to the individual timing. Stool expanders and stool softeners are often used in addition to diet and habit retraining.

If these techniques are ineffective in reestablishing bowel regularity, a glycerin suppository may be inserted 15 to 30 minutes before the usual evacuation time. This stimulates the anorectal reflex and can often be discontinued when a regular pattern is reestablished. A suppository that produces chemical stimulation (e.g., bisacodyl [Dulcolax]) is used only if a glycerin suppository is ineffective. Bisacodyl may cause uncomfortable abdominal cramping in older individuals.

Urinary system. If the patient is unable to monitor urination, the nurse should assist with this activity. An indwelling catheter is not practical for long-term use because of the likelihood of urinary tract infection and later problems with reestablishing bladder control. Incontinence often results from the patient's inability to make elimination needs known. Nursing measures aimed at maintaining urinary continence include palpating the bladder regularly to assess for bladder distention and offering the commode, bedpan, or urinal every 2 hours during waking hours and every 3 to 4 hours at night. In addition, the nurse should ensure that the patient maintains a high fluid intake during the day. Assumption of the usual position for urination (standing for a man and sitting for a woman) and application of pressure over the bladder area often aid in urination.

The use of fluid restriction or incontinent briefs or keeping of a urinal in place at all times are temporary measures to reduce the occurrence or effects of incontinence. Long-term use of these measures discourages continence and can lead to dehydration and skin problems. Intermittent catheterization or external devices may be used for short periods until bladder retraining can be attempted.

If the patient is unable to regain bladder control, a serious care problem develops. A coordinated retraining program by all members of the nursing staff is a major nursing responsibility. Until bladder and bowel control are attained, further rehabilitation efforts are hampered.

Sexual function. A patient who has had a stroke may be concerned about loss of sexual function. Many patients are comfortable in expressing their fears if the nurse provides an atmosphere in which sexuality can be discussed.[23] The nurse sometimes has to initiate the conversation. Fear that sexual activity will bring on another stroke, alternative positions for intercourse, and the possibility of impotence are common concerns. Impotence, if it occurs, is more likely to result from psychologic factors than neurologic deficits.

Communication. Speech and language deficits constitute one of the most difficult problems for the social system to handle. Speech therapy is only a partial answer. The nurse should be a role model for the patient's family when communicating with the patient with aphasia (see Table 55-7). The patient needs frequent, meaningful, verbal stimulation. A common phenomenon is the patient who does not read the cue cards with *dog* and *cat* written on them but can read a menu. The patient perceives this well-meaning intervention as a childish game and refuses to play. A better approach for the nurse and the patient's family is to talk about the activities of daily living that are familiar to the patient. The patient should always be allowed sufficient time to answer. A relaxed atmosphere should be maintained, and the patient should not be pressured to respond. Reinforcing the use of simple responses such as "yes" or "no" may give the patient enough confidence to tackle more difficult communication.

Sensory-perceptual. Patients who have had strokes often exhibit emotional reactions that are not appropriate to the situation, as well as perceptual deficits. The type of response depends on the location of the stroke. Patients with a stroke on the right side of the brain are more likely to have difficulty judging position, distance, and rate of movement. Moreover, they tend to deny these difficulties and are assertive in tackling unfamiliar tasks. Patients may appear apathetic or unduly cheerful. They may fail to correlate spatial-perceptual problems with their inability to perform certain activities, such as getting the wheelchair through a wide doorway. They should be supervised in all activities before being allowed to pursue them independently. Directions should be given verbally and broken down into small steps. Distracting clutter in the environment should be reduced, and rooms should be kept well lighted and free of obstacles. A mirror may help orient the patient in relation to the environment. One-sided neglect is more common with left hemiplegia. The nurse may need to remind the patient to care for the affected side.

A stroke in the left hemisphere often results in depression, inappropriate or exaggerated mood swings, or both. This emotional lability is upsetting and embarrassing to both the patient and the family. The patient may be unable to control emotions and may burst into tears or laughter. The behavior is out of context and often unrelated to the underlying emotional state of the patient. Inappropriate behavior can be alleviated by distraction. The patient is usually uncomfortable with this lack of control and will appreciate the intervention. The family should be counseled that inappropriate behavior is not a purposeful act by the patient. Punitive acts such as shaming, scolding, or embarrassing the patient are to be avoided.

Coping. In addition to the psychologic problems secondary to neurologic deficits, the patient with a stroke may need to be assisted to cope with permanent loss of function secondary to the stroke. Patients often go through all the stages associated with grief and mourning. Many patients are plagued by long-term depression, which may manifest itself with symptoms of anxiety; loss of energy, weight, and appetite; and sleep disturbances.[24,25] Inability to resume prestroke role tasks is often a cause of depression. In addition, the time and energy required to perform previously simple tasks can result in anger and frustration.

The family and friends of a patient who has had a stroke also need assistance from the nurse. The poststroke physical, mental, and emotional capabilities of the patient may differ greatly from those of the prestroke person. Family members must understand the true significance of residual stroke damage so that they can make realistic plans regarding both their own and the patient's welfare.

It is a nursing responsibility to instruct the caregivers regarding the patient's exercise, diet, activity, bowel and bladder activities, skin care, and oral hygiene. A public health referral promotes continuity of care and provides a support system for the family.

In their communication with the patient and in the rest of their relationships, family members tend to develop patterns of interaction. These are sometimes detrimental to the long-term health of the patient. For example, family members may respond by keeping the patient in the dependent sick role. At the opposite extreme, family members may reject the patient's illness because they expect prestroke behavior. The preferred solution is a compromise between these two ends of the continuum.

Family members have to cope with three aspects of the patient's behavior. First, they must recognize those changes that are secondary to neurologic deficits and that cannot be changed. Second, they must cope with the patient's response to the losses at the same time that they are dealing with their own response. Third, they must deal with behavior that they have reinforced in the early stages of the illness. For example, the patient may be reluctant to resume dressing, and the family may unconsciously reinforce the behavior by continuing to help with the dressing process. This response is due both to lack of knowledge and to guilt feelings. Internal dialogues demonstrate the latter: "He wouldn't have had the stroke if I had been a better wife," "I should have made her see the doctor." Consequently, family members may be hesitant to assert themselves because they are afraid of causing another stroke.

Family therapy is a helpful adjunct to a rehabilitation program. The family needs support and reassurance. Open-ended statements such as "I imagine this is pretty confusing" may help the family express their feelings. In addition, family members need accurate and complete information about the disease and the treatment. They also need assistance in problem solving in this crisis period. In some settings, stroke support groups are used to help patients and their families deal with the realities of disability and share coping strategies.[26]

Chronic and Home Management. To promote a smooth transition from hospital or rehabilitation setting to an intermediate-care or long-term care facility or to home

RESEARCH

IMPLICATIONS FOR NURSING PRACTICE

INTERVENTIONS FOR OLDER ADULTS WHO HAVE HAD STROKES

Citation Folden SL: Effect of a supportive-educative nursing intervention on older adults' perceptions of self-care after a stroke, *Rehabil Nurs* 18:162-167, 1993.

Purpose To test the effects of a supportive-educative nursing intervention directed at helping the patient make decisions regarding self-care goals.

Methods A quasi-experimental design used a convenience sample of 68 individuals participating in stroke rehabilitation programs. The study tested the effects of an individually focused, guided decision-making intervention on individuals' perception of self-care ability following a stroke. Pretesting and posttesting were done using a revised version of the Exercise of Self-Care Agency scale.

Results and Conclusions Findings indicated the potential effectiveness of this intervention in significantly increasing individuals' perceptions of their self-care ability after a stroke. The short-term and long-term goals expressed by patients were realistic in relation to their present and projected future functional ability.

Implications of Nursing Practice Stroke rehabilitation focuses on teaching self-care skills to help individuals cope with their functional disabilities. However, when stroke rehabilitation focuses only on physical skills and fails to integrate individual goals, patients may be dissatisfied with rehabilitation efforts. Patients' participation in self-care will increase their confidence and make them feel an integral part of the rehabilitation team.

and community, discharge planning should begin as early as possible during hospitalization. Once hospital care is no longer required the family may need assistance in arranging transfer to an intermediate-care facility. This transfer may be temporary or permanent, depending on the condition of the patient and the situation of the primary care provider.

The care provider needs instruction and practice in necessary areas of care while the patient is hospitalized. This allows for support and encouragement, as well as opportunities for feedback. Adjustments in the home environment, such as removal of a door to accommodate a wheelchair, can be made before discharge.

Specific areas for instruction related to home care of the stroke patient include exercise and ambulation techniques; dietary requirements; recognition of signs indicating the possibility of another stroke, such as headache, vertigo, numbness, and visual disturbances; understanding of emotional lability and the possibility of depression; medication routine; and time, place, and frequency of follow-up activities, such as occupational therapy and physical therapy. To assist the primary care provider to stay healthy after the

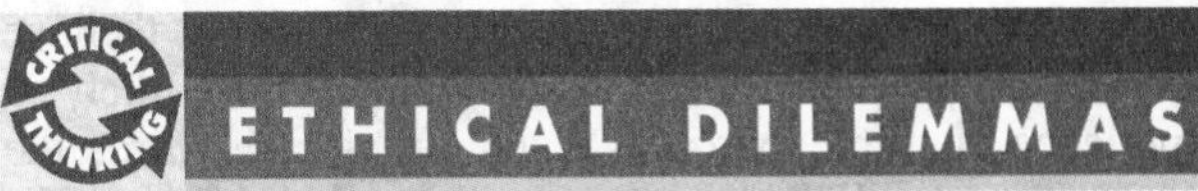

RIGHT TO DIE

Situation A 93-year-old woman has had three strokes in the last 20 months. They have left her partially paralyzed and in need of full-time care. She has repeatedly told her home care nurse that she would not want to live like this. She is now hospitalized for another stroke and her prognosis is the complete loss of physical functioning. She has tried to remove the feeding tube, which causes her discomfort. Responding to repeated questions of both the nurse and physician about whether she wants them to stop treatment and let her die, she has consistently answered yes.

Discussion Patients with severe life-threatening diseases or physical conditions may express concerns about not being kept alive. Providers should document these and encourage patients to execute advance directives while they are still able to do so. This patient had no advance directives but has witnesses to her repeated statements about not wanting to live like this. Competent adults have the right to refuse treatment, even if by doing so they hasten their own death. If the health care providers determined that she is competent and then asked several differently worded questions to clarify the patient's desire to die, consistent responses would constitute the patient's desire to cease treatment, including artificial hydration and nutrition, in order to die.

ETHICAL AND LEGAL PRINCIPLES

- Competent adults have the legal right to choose to forego life-sustaining treatment, even if by doing so they hasten their death.
- The American Medical Association and other medical and nursing organizations support the ethical appropriateness of not imposing unwanted treatment on competent adults.
- By virtue of its delivery mechanism, artificial hydration and nutrition are considered to be medical treatments rather than simply the provision of food and water. The invasive nature of feeding tubes can be the grounds on which a patient refuses to continue this treatment.

patient is discharged home, it is important to plan for respite or time away from caregiving activities on a regular basis. Caregivers may become overburdened with caregiving and not realize what has happened until they become ill themselves.

Community integration. Traditionally, successful return to the community following a stroke has been measured by the extent of physical functioning and return to work. There are several reasons why these measures may not be as useful now and in the future as they were in the past. First, an individual who functions well physically may experience persistent subtle problems related to cognition and coping that significantly interfere with individual and family quality of life. Second, as the population continues to age, stroke survivors will be older, will be likely to have more severe poststroke deficits, and will be more likely to experience multiple chronic health problems. Third, the impact of technologic advances will result in more individuals surviving severe strokes and also having the potential to function more effectively despite their disabilities. The determination of success of poststroke recovery includes a combination of more objective measures such as physical functioning and performance of self-care activities and more subjective perceptions held by patient and family about quality of life.

Community resources can be an asset to patients and their families. The National Stroke Association provides information, resources, and referral services, as well as a quarterly newsletter on stroke (see under Organizations in the section bibliography). The American Heart Association has information about stroke, hypertension, diet, exercise, and assistive devices. It also sponsors self-help groups in many locales. The Easter Seal Society may provide wheelchairs and other assistive devices. Other local groups are often available to aid with meals and transportation. Referral to a community health nurse promotes continuity of care.

Gerontologic Considerations

Strokes are among the primary causes of death and disability in older people. Although the incidence of stroke has decreased over the past decade, it is definitely a disease of older adults with the incidence increasing with age.

A stroke is a profound disruption in the lives of older adults. The magnitude of disability and profound changes in both physical and mental function can lead patients to question whether they can regain any part of their old selves. Daily life has to be reorganized to bear some resemblance to the previous life. When the older patient returns home, it can be traumatic. The patient must face a world where they previously lived with physical, emotional, and cognitive impairments. These experiences reinforce the sense of loss.[27]

The nursing management of the older person who has a stroke is a challenge. Skilled nursing care is obviously needed in the acute phase. However, the more demanding nursing challenge occurs in the rehabilitative phase in assisting the older patient to deal with the residual deficits of stroke as well as aging. These patients may become fearful and depressed because they think they may have another attack or die. The fear can become immobilizing and prevent effective rehabilitation.

There may be changes in the patient-spouse relationships. The dependency resulting from a stroke may be threatening to a previously stable marriage. The spouse may also have chronic medical problems that may affect the ability to take care of the patient with the stroke.

One of the most difficult tasks in home management is helping the spouse or significant other who has to take care of the stroke patient. Living with these demands can be challenging for a younger person and can be even more so for the older spouse. The spouse may experience guilt if others try to help with care. The patient may not want anyone other than the spouse to provide care.

Nursing care should focus on the supportive spouse as well as the person who has the stroke. The spouse should be provided opportunities to get away from the home and the responsibilities of care of the stroke patient. (Special care needs of older adults are addressed in Chapter 3.)

CRITICAL THINKING EXERCISES

CASE STUDY

ACUTE STROKE

Patient Profile

Earl, a 61-year-old man, had a left hemisphere thrombotic stroke 4 days ago.

Subjective Data

- Has weakness on the right side of the body
- Was diagnosed with hypertension 10 years ago

Objective Data

Physical Examination

- Sensory impairment
- Mild aphasia consisting primarily of word-finding difficulty
- Homonymous hemianopsia

Critical Thinking Questions

1. What is the relationship between stroke and hypertension?
2. How can a recurrence of Earl's stroke be prevented?
3. What behavioral style is anticipated with a stroke in the left hemisphere of the brain?
4. How can the nurse assist Earl and his wife to cope with their situation?
5. What nursing measures may be used to help Earl compensate for the visual field cut?
6. What factors should be considered in evaluation of Earl's potential to benefit from transfer to an intensive inpatient rehabilitation setting? When should he be transferred to the rehabilitation setting?
7. Based on the assessment data presented, write one or more nursing diagnoses. Are there any collaborative problems?

NURSING RESEARCH ISSUES

1. Determine patient characteristics associated with compliance with antiplatelet aggregation therapy.
2. Examine the relationship between quality of life and functional abilities in patients after a stroke.
3. Determine the effectiveness of a bowel program composed of high-fiber diet and regular toileting on episodes of constipation and fecal impaction in poststroke patients.
4. Determine the effectiveness of an intervention program focused on reducing blood pressure in decreasing episodes of TIA.
5. Examine factors that contribute to caregiver burden and distress of caregivers of stroke patients.

REVIEW QUESTIONS

The number of the question corresponds to the same-numbered objective at the beginning of the chapter.

1. Which of the following patients is most likely to have a stroke?
  a. An African-American 65-year-old man with hypertension
  b. A Caucasian 20-year-old woman on oral contraceptives
  c. An obese 15-year-old Native American
  d. An Asian-American 35-year-old woman who smokes

2. Which of the following is the *most* potent regulator of cerebral blood flow?
  a. Oxygen
  b. Carbon dioxide
  c. Bicarbonate
  d. Lactic acid

3. A stroke caused by thrombosis
  a. is associated with hypertension.
  b. occurs following activity.
  c. is usually fatal within 4 to 6 weeks.
  d. is associated with cardiac dysfunction.

4. A right-sided hemiplegia may be caused by a lesion in the
  a. lateral spinothalamic tract.
  b. motor area of the left frontal lobe.
  c. medial superior area of the paracentral lobule.
  d. posterolateral nucleus of the thalamus.

5. In the diagnosis of stroke, arteriography is used to determine the
  a. site and size of the infarction.
  b. patency of the cerebrovascular system.
  c. presence of increased ICP.
  d. presence of blood in the CSF.

6. For a patient with a TIA the goal of therapy is the
  a. prevention of stroke.
  b. reduction of disability.
  c. reduction of cerebral edema.
  d. prevention of complications.

7. For a stroke patient with hemiplegia the nurse positions each joint
  a. higher than the proximal joint.
  b. lower than the proximal joint.
  c. at the same level as the proximal joint.
  d. at the same level as the distal joint.

8. Bowel training after a stroke includes all of the following interventions *except*

a. adequate fluid intake.
b. assisting patient to toilet or commode at regular time daily.
c. an enema every other day.
d. a high-fiber diet.

9. The most common response of the stroke patient to the change in body image is

a. denial.
b. depression.
c. disassociation.
d. intellectualization.

REFERENCES

1. Bronstein KS, Popovich JM, Stewart-Amidei C: *Promoting stroke recovery: a research-based approach for nurses,* St Louis, 1991, Mosby.
2. Nowak TJ, Handford AG: *Essentials of pathophysiology,* Dubuque, IA, 1994, Brown.
3. Petrasovits A, Nair C: Epidemiology of stroke in Canada, *Health Rep* 6:39, 1994.
4. Garrison SJ, Rolak LA: Rehabilitation of the stroke patient. In DeLisa JA, Gans BM, editors: *Rehabilitation medicine principles and practice,* ed 2, Philadelphia, 1993, Lippincott.
5. Feinberg WM: Guidelines for the management of transient ischemic attacks, *Heart Dis Stroke* 3:275, 1994.
6. Donnan GA and others: Hypertension and stroke, *J Hypertens* 12:865, 1994.
7. Price DW: The hypertensive patient in family practice, *J Am Board Fam Pract* 7:403, 1994.
8. Kelly-Hayes M: A preventive approach to stroke, *Nurs Clin North Am* 26:931, 1991.
9. Klag MJ, Whelton PK: The decline in stroke mortality: an epidemiologic perspective, *Ann Epidemiol* 3:571, 1993.
10. Biller J, Love BB: Diabetes and stroke, *Med Clin North Am* 77:95, 1993.
11. Love BB: Stroke in women, *Hawaii Med J* 53:258, 1994.
12. Langhorne P, Dennis MS: Management of thrombosis in stroke, *Br Med Bull* 50:911, 1994.
13. Whisnant JP: Classification of cerebrovascular diseases, III, *Stroke* 21:637, 1990.
14. Fode NC: Carotid endarterectomy: nursing care and controversies, *J Neurosci Nurs* 22:25, 1990.
15. Pryse-Phillips W, Yegappan MC: Management of acute stroke: ways to minimize damage and maximize recovery, *Postgrad Med* 96:75, 1994.
16. Barnett HJ, Eliasziw M, Meldrum HE: Drugs and surgery in the prevention of ischemic stroke, *N Engl J Med* 332:238, 1995.
17. Easton JD: Antiplatelet therapy in the prevention of stroke, *Drugs* 42 (suppl 5):39, 1991.
18. Miller CA: The nurse's role in preventing "brain attack," *Geriatr Nurs* 15:227, 1994.
19. Barnett HJ: Progress in stroke prevention: an overview, *Health Rep* 6:132, 1994.
20. Emick-Herring B, Wood P: A team approach to neurologically based swallowing disorders, *Rehabil Nurs* 15:126,1990.
21. McCourt A, editor: *The specialty practice of rehabilitation nursing: a core curriculum,* ed 3, Evanston, IL, 1993, Rehabilitation Nursing Foundation.
22. Borgman MF, Passarella PM: Nursing care of the stroke patient using Bobath principles: an approach to altered movement, *Nurs Clin North Am* 26:1019, 1991.
23. Burgener S, Logan G: Sexuality concerns of the post-stroke patient, *Rehabil Nurs* 14:178, 1989.

*24. Whitney FW and others: Depression in stroke survivors: the relationship of laterality in right and left hemisphere damage, *Rehab Nurs Res* 3:130, 1994.

25. Bruckbauer EA: Recognizing poststroke depression, *Rehabil Nurs* 16:34, 1991.
26. Pasquarello MA: Developing, implementing and evaluating a stroke recovery group, *Rehabil Nurs* 15:26, 1990.
27. Becker G: Continuity after a stroke: implications of life-course disruption in old age, *Gerontologist* 33:148, 1993.

*Nursing research-based articles.

Chapter 56

NURSING ROLE IN MANAGEMENT

Chronic Neurologic Problems

Judith M. Ozuna

Learning Objectives

1. Explain the potential impact of chronic neurologic disease on physical and psychologic well-being.
2. Compare and contrast tension-type, migraine, and cluster headaches in terms of etiology, clinical manifestations, and therapeutic and nursing management.
3. Describe the etiology, clinical manifestations, diagnostic studies, and management of epilepsy, multiple sclerosis, Parkinson's disease, and myasthenia gravis.
4. Explain the nursing role in the acute and chronic management of a patient with a chronic neurologic disease.
5. Describe the clinical manifestations and management of amyotrophic lateral sclerosis and Huntington's chorea.
6. Identify common physical complications in a patient who is immobilized by chronic neurologic disease.
7. Outline the major goals of treatment for the patient with a chronic, progressive neurologic disease.

Management of chronic neurologic diseases can be challenging for both the patient and the health care provider. Many neurologic disorders involve progressive deterioration in physical or mental capabilities, which can be devastating to the patient and the family. The patient may experience psychologic upheaval in the form of depression, fear, anxiety, anger, or withdrawal. This is compounded by changes in body image and self-esteem. In addition, the physical disabilities that result from degenerative diseases necessitate varying and sometimes extreme alterations in lifestyle, which add to the emotional trauma of the patient. Families are torn between their sense of obligation to care for the ill patient and the need to lead their own lives. They are simultaneously pushed and pulled by feelings of guilt, love, despair, hope, resentment, and empathy.

The challenge of chronic neurologic illness is equally great for health care providers. Many of these diseases have no cure, so health care professionals can only attempt to alleviate physical symptoms, prevent complications, assist patients in maximizing self-care abilities in the face of neurologic deficits, and help them in the difficult task of adjusting to their illness. Nurses can and should greatly influence these aspects of management.

Reviewed by Hiliary Lipe, RN, MN, Research Nurse Practitioner in Neurology, VA Medical Center, Seattle, WA, and Sally A. Weiss, RN, MSN, Associate Professor, Broward Community College, Pembroke Pines, FL.

HEADACHE

Headache is probably the most common type of pain experienced by humans. Of all persons with headache, the majority have *functional* headaches, such as benign migraine or tension-type; the remainder have *organic* headaches caused by significant intracranial or extracranial disease.

Not all tissues of the cranium are sensitive to pain. The pain-sensitive structures in the head include the venous sinuses, the dura (at the base of the brain near large blood vessels), cranial blood vessels, the three divisions of the trigeminal nerve (CN V), the facial nerve (CN VII), the glossopharyngeal nerve (CN IX), the vagus nerve (CN X), and the first three cervical nerves. Thus, headache pain can arise from both intracranial and extracranial sources.[1]

Headaches are classified based on the characteristics of the headache and the facial pain. The primary classifications include tension-type, migraine, and cluster headaches. Characteristics of these headaches are shown in Table 56-1. A patient may have more than one type of headache. The history and neurologic examination are diagnostic keys to determining the type of headache.

Tension-Type Headache

Tension-type headache has been called *muscle-contraction, tension, psychogenic,* and *rheumatic* headache. It is the most common type of headache and is also considered the most difficult to treat.

Pathophysiology. It was originally thought that tension-type headache was the result of sustained and painful contraction of the muscles of the scalp and the neck.

Table 56-1 Comparison of Tension-Type, Migraine, and Cluster Headaches

Pattern	Tension-type	Migraine	Cluster
Site	Bilateral, bandlike pressure at base of skull, in face, or in both	Unilateral (in 60%), may switch sides, commonly anterior	Unilateral, radiating up or down from one eye
Quality	Constant, squeezing tightness	Throbbing, synchronous with pulse	Severe, bone-crushing
Frequency	Cycles for several years	Periodic; cycles of several months to years	May have months or years between attacks; attacks occur in clusters: one to three times a day over a period of 4-8 wk
Duration	Intermittent for months or years	Continuous for hours or days	30 to 90 min
Time and mode of onset	Not related to time	May be preceded by prodrome; onset after awakening; gets better with sleep	Nocturnal; commonly awakens patient from sleep
Associated symptoms	Palpable neck and shoulder muscles, stiff neck, tenderness	Nausea or vomiting, edema, irritability, sweating, photophobia, prodrome of sensory, motor, or psychic phenomena; family history (in 65%)	Vasomotor symptoms such as facial flushing or pallor, unilateral lacrimation, ptosis, and rhinitis

Recent evidence, however, does not support this mechanism in all patients with tension-type headaches, and it is currently thought that this type of headache is related to abnormal neuronal sensitivity and pain facilitation at the level of the brainstem.[1] The exact etiology still remains obscure.

Clinical Manifestations. There is no *prodrome* (early manifestation of impending disease) in tension-type headache. The pain is usually bilateral, occurring most often in the back of the neck. It usually does not interfere with sleep. The pain is often described as a tight, squeezing, bandlike pressure. It is sustained, chronic, dull, and persistent. The headaches may occur intermittently for weeks, months, or even years. Many patients can have a combination of migraine and tension-type headaches, with features of both headaches occurring simultaneously. Patients with migraine headaches may experience tension-type headaches between migraine attacks.

Diagnostic Studies. Careful history taking is probably the most important diagnostic tool for tension-type headache. Electromyography (EMG) may reveal sustained contraction of the neck, scalp, or facial muscles, but many patients may not show increased muscle tension with this test, even when the test is done during the actual headache. Conversely, patients with diagnosed migraine headaches may show increased muscle tension on EMG. If tension-type headache is present during physical examination, increased resistance to passive movement of the head and tenderness of the head and neck may be present.

Migraine Headache

For some individuals *migraine headaches* begin in childhood or adolescence. A family history of migraine can be found in 65% of patients with migraine. A recent study estimates that 8.7 million women and 2.6 million men in the United States suffer from migraine headache, with moderate to severe disability.[2] Although migraine headaches have often been associated with patients who are high achievers and who suppress expressions of aggression and hostility, no single personality type describes all patients who experience migraine headache.

Pathophysiology. In the past it was thought that migraine headaches had a vascular origin and involved the intracranial and extracranial arteries of the head. The classic theory of migraine headaches is that the prodromal or aural phase is associated with vasoconstriction and decreased blood flow. The headache phase is associated with vasodilatation and increased blood flow. Although the exact etiology of migraine headaches is not known, recent evidence suggests that neurologic, vascular, and chemical factors are involved. Sterile inflammation of the arterial vessels by endogenous monoamines (serotonin), peptides (substance P), estrogen, or diet (alcohol) may be responsible for migraine headaches. Serotonin, in particular, appears to play an important role in migraine headache progression. Levels of serotonin increase during the prodromal phase and decrease during the headache phase. A neurogenic mechanism in which there is a primary derangement of brain function may be involved.[3]

A mechanism other than vasoconstriction may also account for the prodromal phase of the migraine headache. The *aura* of migraine is associated with "spreading depression," a wave of *oligemia* (diminished cerebral blood flow) beginning in the occipital lobe and spreading forward in the brain at a rate of 2 to 3 mm per minute. This continues into the headache phase. During the headache phase, substance P and other polypeptides are released by the perivascular nerve endings.[3] Substance P causes vasodilatation, increased capillary permeability, perivascular inflammation, and stimulation of afferent fibers.

Clinical Manifestations. There are two major types of migraine headaches: migraine without aura (formerly called common migraine) and migraine with aura (formerly called classic migraine). *Migraine without aura* is the most common type of migraine headache. The prodrome is not sharply defined, and it can involve psychic disturbances, gastrointestinal upset, and changes in fluid balance. The prodrome may precede the headache phase by several hours or several days. The headache itself may last several hours or days.

Migraine with aura occurs in only 10% of migraine headache episodes. The sharply defined aura may last for 10 to 30 minutes before the start of the headache and may include sensory dysfunction (e.g., visual field defects, tingling or burning sensations, or paresthesias), motor dysfunction (e.g., weakness, paralysis), dizziness, confusion, and even loss of consciousness. The classic preheadache symptom is perception of flashing lights in one quadrant of the visual field, often referred to as *scintillating scotomata.* This type of migraine headache usually peaks in 1 hour and may last several hours.

Clinical manifestations that occur in migraine with and without aura are generalized edema, irritability, pallor, nausea and vomiting, and sweating. During the headache phase, patients with migraine tend to "hibernate"; that is, they seek shelter from noise, light, odors, people, and problems. The headache is described as a steady, throbbing pain that is synchronous with the pulse. Although the headache is usually unilateral, it may switch to the opposite side in another episode. The diagnosis of migraine headache is usually made from the history. The neurologic and other diagnostic examinations are often normal.

Migraine headaches, in many cases, have no known precipitating events. However, for other patients, the headache may be precipitated by stress, excitement, bright lights, menstruation, alcohol, or certain foods such as chocolate or cheese.

Cluster Headache

Cluster headache is one of the most severe forms of head pain known to man.[4] Cluster headache occurs less frequently than migraine (the cluster headache to migraine frequency is 1:10) and is more frequent in men than in women by a ratio of 5:1. The onset is usually between 30 and 60 years of age.

Pathophysiology. Neither the cause nor the pathophysiology of cluster headache is fully known. The vasodilatation that occurs in the affected part of the face is extracranial. The trigeminal nerve is implicated in the production of pain. Activation of this nerve causes release of substance P and other vasoactive substances that cause vasodilatation, stimulation of afferent pain fibers, and neurogenic inflammation with extravasation of protein and platelets in the perivascular areas. The periodicity and the clocklike regularity of cluster headache indicate a dysfunction of the biologic clock mechanisms of the hypothalamus.[5] These headaches can also be triggered by alcohol ingestion.

Clinical Manifestations. The headache has an abrupt onset, usually without a prodrome. It peaks in 5 minutes and lasts 30 to 90 minutes. It is not uncommon for this type of headache to start at night, awakening the patient after a few hours of sleep. They may recur several times a day over a period of several days, with each cluster lasting 2 to 3 months. It usually affects the upper face, the periorbital region, and the forehead on one side of the face and the head. The headache may not recur for months or years. The patient may also exhibit conjunctivitis, increased lacrimation (tearing), and nasal congestion on the side of the headache. Sweating may occur on the forehead of the affected side. A partial *Horner's syndrome* (constriction of the pupil and *ptosis* [drooping] of the eyelid on the affected side) may be seen. The headache is described as deep, steady, and penetrating but not throbbing.

Unlike the patient with migraine, who seeks isolation and quiet, the patient with a cluster headache paces the floor, cries out, does bizarre things, and resents being touched. The patient with a cluster headache does not experience the systemic manifestations that accompany a migraine headache, such as nausea or vomiting. As with migraine headaches, there are usually no complications.

Diagnostic Studies. The diagnosis of cluster headache is primarily based on the history. However, computed tomography (CT) scan with contrast dye and cerebral angiography may be performed to rule out an aneurysm, tumor, or infection.

Other Types of Headaches

Although tension, migraine, and cluster headaches are by far the most common types of headaches, other types of headache can also occur. These headaches may be the first symptom of a more serious illness. Headache can accompany subarachnoid hemorrhage, brain tumors, other intracranial masses, arteritis, vascular abnormalities, trigeminal neuralgia (tic douloureux), diseases of the eyes, nose, and teeth, and systemic illness (e.g., bacteremia, carbon monoxide poisoning, mountain sickness, polycythemia vera). The symptoms vary greatly. Because of the variety of causes of headache, clinical evaluation must be thorough. It should include an evaluation of personality, life adjustment, environment, and family situation as well as a comprehensive evaluation of physical status.

Therapeutic Management of Headaches

If no systemic underlying disease is found, therapy is directed toward the functional type of headache. Table 56-2 outlines the general workup for a patient with headache to rule out any intracranial or extracranial disease. Table 56-3 summarizes the current therapies for symptomatic and therapeutic relief of common headaches. These therapies include meditation, yoga, biofeedback, and muscle relaxation training.

Biofeedback involves the use of physiologic monitoring equipment to give the patient information regarding muscle tension and peripheral blood flow (skin temperature of the hand). The patient is trained to relax the muscles and raise the hand temperature and is given reinforcement (operant conditioning) in accomplishing these physiologic alterations.

Acupuncture, acupressure, and hypnosis are successful innovative therapies that work well in some patients with headaches. Some patients can benefit from psychotherapy that is aimed at helping them recognize conflicts and deal with them more effectively. Treatments for tension-type headache include physical therapy (e.g., massage, hot packs, cervical collar), injection of local anesthetic into spastic muscles, and correction of faulty posture.

Table 56-2 Diagnostic Workup for Patient with Headache

- Complete health history
- Clinical examination (often negative)
  - Inspection for local infections
  - Palpation for tenderness, hardened arteries, bony swellings
  - Auscultation for bruits over major arteries
- Routine laboratory studies to rule out underlying causes of headache
  - CBC
  - Electrolytes
  - Urinalysis
  - Serologic studies
- X-ray study of sinuses
- Special studies (e.g., CT scan, angiography, EMG, electroencephalography, MRI) for structural disease

CBC, Complete blood count; *CT*, computed tomography; *EMG*, electromyography; *MRI*, magnetic resonance imaging.

Pharmacologic Management

Tension-type headache. Drug treatment for tension-type headache usually involves a nonnarcotic analgesic (e.g., aspirin, acetaminophen) used alone or in combination with a sedative, a muscle relaxant, a tranquilizer, or codeine. However, many of these drugs have potentially dangerous side effects. The patient should be cautioned about the long-term use of aspirin and aspirin-containing drugs because they can cause gastric bleeding and coagulation abnormalities in susceptible patients. Long-term use of Fiorinal should be avoided because in addition to aspirin it contains a barbiturate, which may be habit forming. Drugs containing acetaminophen (Tylenol, Phenaphen, Midrin) can cause liver and kidney damage with chronic use. Daily use of nonsteroidal antiinflammatory drugs (NSAIDs) can cause chronic daily headaches. Narcotics and benzodiazepines can cause addiction and habituation. Discontinuing an overused medication too abruptly can lead to withdrawal symptoms (analgesic rebound).

Migraine headache. Drug treatment of the acute migraine attack is aimed at treating all the components of the acute attack and preventing escalation of the headache.[6] Ergotamine is the symptomatic treatment of choice for migraine when simple analgesics do not relieve headache.[5] Ergotamine inhibits the reuptake of neuronally liberated norepinephrine into storage sites of the postganglionic nerve terminal of the sympathetic nervous system. This allows more norepinephrine to attach to alpha-adrenergic

Table 56-3 Therapeutic Management: Headache

	Tension-type Headache	Migraine Headache	Cluster Headache
Diagnostic	History of neck and head tenderness, resistance to movement, EMG	History	History, thermography
Therapeutic			
▪ Symptomatic	Nonnarcotic analgesics (aspirin, acetaminophen, ibuprofen) Analgesic combinations (Fiorinal) Muscle relaxants	Nonnarcotic analgesics (aspirin, acetaminophen) Serotonin receptor agonist (sumatriptan) Alpha-adrenergic blockers (ergotamine tartrate) Vasoconstrictors (isometheptene) Corticosteroids (dexamethasone)	Alpha-adrenergic blockers (ergotamine tartrate) Vasoconstrictors Oxygen
▪ Prophylactic	Tricyclic antidepressants (doxepin, amitriptyline) Beta-adrenergic blockers (propranolol) Biofeedback Muscle relaxation training Psychotherapy	Beta-adrenergic blockers (propranolol) Serotonin antagonists* (methysergide) Antidepressants (amitriptyline, imipramine) Calcium channel blockers Biofeedback Yoga Meditation Electric counterstimulation	Alpha-adrenergic blockers (ergotamine tartrate) Serotonin antagonists (methysergide) Corticosteroids (prednisone) Lithium Calcium channel blockers (nifedipine)

EMG, Electromyography.
*Only for patients suffering from one or more severe headaches per week.

sites on smooth muscle in the artery wall, thereby causing prolonged vasoconstriction of cranial vessels. Ergotamine can be administered orally, sublingually, parenterally, rectally, or by inhalation. The usual dosage is 1 to 2 mg (oral or rectal) at the onset of the headache, followed by 2 mg within 1 hour. No more than 6 mg is given for any single attack. Other drugs that may relieve migraine headache include Fiorinal, Midrin, aspirin, acetaminophen (Tylenol, Datril), meperidine (Demerol), and codeine.

Drugs that affect serotonin have also been found to be beneficial in the treatment of migraine headaches. Sumatriptan succinate (Imitrex), which is selective for vascular serotonin receptors, produces vasoconstriction and is used for the management of acute migraine headaches. Sumatriptan is given subcutaneously and can be self-administered. Methysergide (Sansert) is an ergot alkaloid that competitively blocks serotonin receptors in the central and peripheral nervous system. This drug has been found to be effective in the prevention of migraine headaches. However, because of side effects including fibrotic complications, it is recommended that a patient take a break ("drug holiday") every 4 to 6 months.

A variety of drugs are used to prevent further tension-type and migraine attacks. These drugs are taken daily or during the interval between attacks rather than during the actual headache. Beta blockers (e.g., propranolol), tricyclic antidepressants, calcium channel blockers, carbamazepine, clonidine, thiazides, and other antihypertensive drugs may be used prophylactically for very severe or very frequent migraine headaches.

Cluster headache. Because cluster headaches occur suddenly, often at night, and are not long lasting, pharmacologic management is not as useful as it is for the other types of headache. Inhalation of pure oxygen will abort the headache in approximately 50% of the patients.[6] Ergotamine and methysergide may be used prophylactically when the cluster headache recurs at a known time. However, because of its adverse side effects, methysergide is not used on a long-term basis for chronic cluster headaches. Sumatriptan (Imitrex) has been shown to shorten cluster headaches in 70% to 75% of patients studied.[7]

NURSING MANAGEMENT

HEADACHES

Nursing Assessment

Subjective and objective data that should be obtained from a patient with headache are presented in Table 56-4. Because the history provides the key to assessment of headache, it should include specific details of the headache itself, such as the location and type of pain, the onset, the frequency, the duration, the relation to events (emotional, psychologic, physical), and the time of day of the occurrence. Information about previous illnesses, surgery, trauma, allergies, family history, and response to medication should also be obtained. The nurse can suggest that the patient keep a diary of headache episodes with specific details. This type of record can be of great help in determining the type of headache as well as the precipitating events.

Table 56-4 Nursing Assessment: Headaches

Subjective Data

Important health information

Past health history: Hypertension, seizures, cancer, recent fall, trauma, cranial infection, craniotomy; cerebrovascular accident; asthma or allergies; mental illness; relationship of headache to overwork, menstruation, exercise, travel, bright lights, other noxious environmental stimuli; ingestion of alcohol, caffeine, cheese, chocolate, monosodium glutamate, lunch meats, sausage, hot dogs, onions, avocados

Medications: Hydralazine, bromides, nitroglycerin, ergotamine (withdrawal), indomethacin (Indocin), oral contraceptives, over-the-counter or prescription remedies

Functional health patterns

Health perception–health management: Positive family history; fatigue, malaise

Nutritional-metabolic: Fever; anorexia, nausea, vomiting (migraine prodrome); projectile vomiting (brain tumor); unilateral lacrimation (cluster)

Activity-exercise: Nuchal rigidity (meningeal, tension-type); nasal congestion and discharge (sinusitis); vertigo

Sleep-rest: Insomnia

Cognitive-perceptual:

- Migraine: Unilateral, severe, throbbing (possible switching of side) headache; visual disturbances; photophobia
- Cluster: Unilateral and severe, nocturnal headache
- Tension-type: Bilateral, bandlike, dull and persistent, base of skull headache
- Sinus: Frontal and facial, gradual onset, worsening in morning, dull pain and pressure headache
- Posttraumatic: Severe, chronic, localized or generalized headache; increases with coughing, position changes, emotional disturbances
- Meningeal: Severe and generalized, radiation-to-neck headache; photophobia
- Temporal arteritis: Severe, throbbing, burning, temporal-area headache
- Brain tumor: Generalized, intense, and steady headache; associated with neurologic deficits; visual disturbances

Self-perception–self-concept: Depression

Coping–stress tolerance: Stress, anxiety

Objective Data

General

Anxiety, apprehension

Integumentary

Cluster: diaphoresis, pallor, facial flushing with cheek edema; migraine prodrome: generalized edema

Cardiovascular

Carotid bruits

Neurologic

Brain tumor: papilledema, gait disturbances; meningeal: paresthesias, confusion, decreased level of consciousness; cluster: Horner's syndrome

Possible findings

Evidence of disease, deformity, or infection may be obained after MRI, cerebral arteriography, lumbar puncture, electroencephelography, EMG, skull x-ray examination; CT findings nonspecific

CT, Computed tomography; *EMG,* electromyography; *MRI,* magnetic resonance imaging.

NURSING CARE PLAN Patient with Headache

Planning: Outcome Criteria	*Nursing Interventions and Rationales*
➤ **NURSING DIAGNOSIS**	Acute pain *related to* headache *as manifested by* complaints of steady, throbbing, or severe crushing pain
Have reduced pain; state satisfaction with pain relief.	Assess pain intensity, characteristics, location, and duration *to determine appropriate interventions.* Encourage patient to keep a log of headaches and associated or precipitating factors *to provide patient some control in identifying and controlling factors that may precipitate headaches.* Encourage patient to use alternative therapies such as meditation, yoga, biofeedback, and muscle-relaxation techniques *to supplement drug therapy and provide the patient with some sense of control over pain.* Support patient's use of counseling or psychotherapy *to enhance conflict resolution and stress reduction.* Administer drugs as ordered *to reduce pain.* Monitor patient after pain medication administration *to assess efficacy and identify adverse effects.* Provide a quiet, dimly lit environment *to reduce stimuli that may trigger headaches.* Massage head-neck-shoulder area as tolerated *to relieve muscle tension and promote relaxation.*
➤ **NURSING DIAGNOSIS**	Anxiety *related to* lack of knowledge of etiology and treatment of headache and uncertainty of occurrence of headache *as manifested by* increased heart rate, insomnia, trembling, feeling of helplessness, inability to concentrate
Report increased psychologic comfort and decreased anxiety; use effective coping mechanisms to manage anxiety.	Assess level of anxiety *to determine appropriate interventions.* Encourage patient to verbalize concerns *as this reduces anxiety.* Teach relaxation techniques *to foster muscle relaxation and reduce anxiety.* Explain etiology of patient's specific headache type *to reduce patient's fear of unknown.* Reinforce physician's explanation of diagnostic tests *to relieve concerns about cause and seriousness of headache.* Discuss the physiologic dynamics of tension and anxiety *as knowledge about how these factors influence headache can help with management.*
➤ **NURSING DIAGNOSIS**	Risk for ineffective individual coping *related to* chronic pain behavior
Demonstrate appropriate actions in response to headache; identify personal strengths.	Assess for isolation, verbalization of inability to cope with the pain, and inability to continue usual self-care behaviors *to determine presence and severity of problem.* Assess patient's functional capacity *as acute or chronic pain can interfere with coping ability.* Discuss patient's usual coping methods *to identify positive or maladaptive behaviors.* Encourage expression of feelings *as this enables patient to recognize feelings in relation to pain.* Discuss how headaches interfere with work and social activities *to communicate empathy and assist patient in making lifestyle adjustments.*
➤ **NURSING DIAGNOSIS**	Hopelessness *related to* chronic pain, alteration of lifestyle, and ineffective treatment modalities *as manifested by* expressions of extreme apathy and listlessness, lack of interest in doing usual activities
Express confidence in ability to function in spite of headaches; demonstrate increased activity.	Assess patient's degree of hopelessness *to enable appropriate planning.* Explore patient's self-treatment of pain and alterations in lifestyle *to identify appropriateness and make necessary adjustments.* Promote verbalization of fears and concerns *to convey empathy and correct patient's misconceptions.* Assist patient in identifying support systems which can be used *to bolster hopefulness.* Initiate referrals as indicated for counselor or spiritual leader *to continue work on feeling of hopelessness.*
➤ **NURSING DIAGNOSIS**	Sleep pattern disturbance *related to* pain *as manifested by* inability to maintain usual sleep pattern
Use new strategies to get to sleep; report feeling rested.	Assess patient's usual sleep pattern *to determine appropriate interventions.* Reduce external stimuli *to provide a calm environment conducive to sleep.* Use massage or relaxation techniques *to facilitate relaxation and sleep.* Schedule analgesia administration *so maximum effect for headache relief will coincide with bedtime.* Medicate for pain if patient awakens with headache pain *to foster return to sleep and pain-free awakening.*

Nursing Diagnoses

Nursing diagnoses are determined when the problem and the etiologic factors are supported by clinical data. Nursing diagnoses related to headaches may include, but are not limited to, those presented in the nursing care plan for the patient with a headache on p. 1756.

Planning

The overall goals are that the patient with a headache will (1) have reduced or no pain, (2) experience increased comfort and decreased anxiety, (3) understand triggering events and treatment strategies, and (4) use positive coping strategies to deal with chronic pain.

Nursing Implementation

Patients with chronic headache present a great challenge to health care providers. Headaches may result from an inability to cope with daily stresses. The most effective therapy may be to help patients examine their lifestyle, recognize stressful situations, and learn to cope with them more appropriately. Precipitating factors can be identified, and ways of avoiding them can be developed. Daily exercise, relaxation periods, and socializing can be encouraged, since each can help decrease the recurrence of headache. The nurse can suggest alternative ways of handling the pain of headache through techniques such as relaxation, meditation, yoga, and self-hypnosis.

In addition to using analgesics and analgesic combination drugs for the symptomatic relief of headache, the patient should be encouraged to use relaxation techniques because they are effective in tension-type and migraine headaches. The migraine sufferer often needs a quiet, dimly lit environment. Massage and moist hot packs to the neck and head can help a patient with tension-type headaches. The patient should learn about the medications prescribed for prophylactic and symptomatic treatment of headache and should be able to describe the purpose, action, dosage, and side effects of the medication. To prevent accidental overdose, the patient should make a written note of each dose of medication or headache remedy.

For the patient whose headaches are triggered by food, dietary counseling may be provided. The patient is encouraged to eliminate foods which may provoke headaches (e.g., vinegar, chocolate, onions, alcohol [particularly red wine], excessive caffeine, cheese, fermented or marinated foods, monosodium glutamate, aspartame). Active challenge and provocative testing with specific foods may be necessary to determine the specific causative agents.[8]

SEIZURE DISORDERS AND EPILEPSY

A *seizure* is a sudden alteration in normal brain activity that causes distinctive changes in behavior and body function. Seizures are frequently symptoms of an underlying illness. They may accompany a variety of disorders, or they may occur spontaneously without any apparent cause. Seizures resulting from systemic and metabolic disturbances are not considered epilepsy if the seizures cease when the underlying problem is corrected. In the adult, metabolic disturbances that cause seizures include acidosis, electrolyte imbalances, hypoglycemia, hypoxia, alcohol and barbiturate withdrawal, dehydration, and water intoxication. Extracranial disorders that can cause seizures are heart, lung, liver, and kidney disease, systemic lupus erythematosus, diabetes, hypertension, and septicemia.

Epilepsy connotes spontaneously recurring seizures. There are an estimated 1 to 2 million patients with epilepsy in the United States. The incidence rates are very high during the first year of life, decline through childhood and adolescence, plateau in middle age, and rise sharply again among the elderly.[9]

Etiology

The most common causes of epilepsy during the first 6 months of life are severe birth injury, congenital defects involving the central nervous system (CNS), infections, and inborn errors of metabolism. In patients between 2 and 20 years of age, the primary factors are birth injury, infection, trauma, and genetic factors. In individuals between 20 to 30 years of age, epilepsy usually occurs as the result of structural lesions, such as trauma, brain tumors, or vascular disease. After 50 years of age the primary causes of epilepsy are cerebrovascular lesions and metastatic brain tumors. Although many causes of epilepsy have been identified, three fourths of all epilepsy cases cannot be attributed to a specific cause and are termed *idiopathic*.

The role of heredity in the etiology of epilepsy has been difficult to determine because of the problem of separating hereditary from environmental or acquired influences. However, pedigree analysis suggests that in some instances, a predisposition to epilepsy is inherited in a Mendelian fashion (i.e., controlled by a single genetic locus).[10] In addition, some families carry a predisposition to epilepsy in the form of an inherently low threshold to seizure-producing stimuli, such as trauma, disease, and high fever. For example, an inherently low seizure threshold may explain the reason some patients develop seizures after a head injury or similar insult, whereas others do not.

Pathophysiology

Seizures are paroxysmal, uncontrolled electric discharges of neurons in the brain that interrupt normal function. The specific clinical manifestations of a seizure are determined by the site of the electric disturbance. Seizures can result from a variety of physical alterations. Because the brain transmits information by electric and chemical processes, anything that disrupts these processes can cause a seizure.

In recurring seizures (epilepsy) a group of abnormal neurons (*seizure focus*) seems to undergo spontaneous firing. This firing spreads by physiologic pathways to involve adjacent or distant areas of the brain. If this activity spreads to involve the whole brain, a generalized seizure occurs. The factor that causes this abnormal firing is not clear. Any stimulus that causes the cell membrane of the neuron to depolarize induces a tendency to spontaneous firing. Often the area of the brain from which the epileptic activity arises is found to have scar tissue (*gliosis*). The scarring is thought to interfere with the normal chemical and structural environment of the brain neurons, making them more likely to fire abnormally.

Repetitive electric discharges from an epileptic focus in experimental animals can produce long-lasting and possibly permanent changes in neuron excitability, both locally and in distant areas of the brain.[11] This effect is called *kindling,* and it presents an interesting and important implication for epilepsy in humans: seizures can beget more seizures. Clinical experience indicates that the longer a patient goes without good seizure control, the lower the likelihood that the seizures will be controllable. Therefore a vigorous attempt must be made to control recurring seizures.

Clinical Manifestations

The preferred method of classifying seizures is the International Classification System proposed by Gastaut in 1970 and revised in 1981 (Table 56-5).[12,13] This system is based on the clinical and electroencephalographic manifestations of seizures. In this system, seizures are divided into two major classes, *generalized* and *partial.* Depending on the type, a seizure may progress through several phases, which include (1) the *prodromal* phase with signs or activity, which precede a seizure, (2) the *aural* phase with a sensory warning, (3) the *ictal* phase with full seizure, and (4) *postictal* phase, which is the period of recovery after the seizure.

Table 56-5 International Classification of Epileptic Seizures

Generalized Seizures (bilaterally symmetric and without local onset)
- Absence seizures, atypical absence seizures
- Myoclonic seizures
- Clonic seizures
- Tonic seizures
- Tonic-clonic seizures
- Atonic seizures

Partial Seizures (local onset)
- Simple partial seizures (no impairment of consciousness)
  - With motor symptoms
  - With somatosensory or special sensory symptoms
  - With autonomic symptoms
  - With psychic symptoms
- Complex partial seizures (impairment of consciousness)
  - Simple partial seizures with progression to impairment of consciousness
    - With no other features
    - With features of simple partial seizures
    - With automatisms
  - Impairment of consciousness at onset
    - With no other features
    - With features of simple partial seizures
    - With automatisms

Unclassified Epileptic Seizures (inadequate or incomplete data)

Modified from Commission on Classification and Terminology of the International League against Epilepsy: Proposal for revised clinical and electroencephalographic classification of epileptic seizures, *Epilepsia* 22:489, 1981.

Generalized Seizures. Generalized seizures are characterized by bilateral synchronous epileptic discharge in the brain from the onset of the seizure. Because the entire brain is affected at the onset of the seizures, there is no warning or aura. In most cases, the patient loses consciousness for a few seconds to several minutes.

Tonic-clonic seizures. The most common generalized seizure is the generalized tonic-clonic, or *grand mal,* seizure. This seizure is characterized by loss of consciousness and falling to the ground if the patient is upright, followed by stiffening of the body (tonic phase) for 10 to 20 seconds and subsequent jerking of the extremities (clonic phase) for another 30 to 40 seconds. Cyanosis, excessive salivation, tongue or cheek biting, and incontinence may accompany the seizure.

In the postictal phase the patient usually has muscle soreness, is very tired, and may sleep for several hours. Some patients may not feel normal for several hours or days after a seizure. The patient has no memory of the seizure activity.

Typical absence seizures. The absence (petit mal) seizure usually occurs only in children and rarely continues beyond adolescence. This type of seizure may cease altogether as the child matures, or it may evolve into another type of seizure. The typical clinical manifestation is a brief staring spell that lasts only a few seconds, so it often occurs unnoticed. There may be an extremely brief loss of consciousness. When untreated, the seizures may occur up to 100 times a day.

The electroencephalogram (EEG) demonstrates a 3-Hz (cycles per second) spike-and-wave pattern that is unique to this type of seizure. Absence seizures can often be precipitated by hyperventilation and flashing lights.

Atypical absence seizures. Another type of generalized seizure is the staring spell accompanied by other signs and symptoms, including brief warnings, peculiar behavior during the seizure, or confusion after the seizure. The EEG demonstrates atypical spike-and-wave patterns, usually greater or less than 3 Hz.

Other types of generalized seizures. Other generalized seizures are *myoclonic* and *akinetic* seizures. A myoclonic seizure is characterized by a sudden, excessive jerk of the body or extremities. The jerk may be forceful enough to hurl the person to the ground. These seizures are very brief and may occur in clusters. The terms *akinetic* (arrest of movement), *atonic* (loss of tone), and *astatic* (loss of balance) have been used interchangeably to describe drop attacks or falling spells. This type of seizure involves either a tonic episode or a paroxysmal loss of muscle tone and begins quite suddenly with the person falling to the ground. Consciousness usually returns by the time the person hits the ground, and normal activity can be resumed immediately. Patients with this type of seizure are at a great risk of head injury and often have to wear protective helmets. A less severe akinetic seizure involves brief loss of muscle tone without falling.

Partial Seizures. Partial (focal) seizures are another major class of the International Classification System. Partial seizures begin in a specific region of the cortex, as indicated by the EEG and usually by the clinical manifestations. For example, if the discharging focus is located in the medial aspect of the postcentral gyrus, the patient may experience paresthesias and tingling or numbness in the leg on the side opposite the focus. If the discharging focus is located in the part of the brain that governs a particular function, sensory, motor, cognitive, or emotional manifestations may occur.

Partial seizures may be confined to one side of the brain and remain partial or focal in nature, or they may spread to involve the entire brain, culminating in a generalized tonic-clonic seizure. Any tonic-clonic seizure that is preceded by an aura or warning is a partial seizure that generalizes secondarily. Many tonic-clonic seizures that appear to be generalized from the outset may actually be secondary generalized seizures, but the preceding partial component may be so brief that it is undetected by the patient, the observer, or even on the EEG. Unlike the primary generalized tonic-clonic seizure, the secondary generalized seizure may result in a transient residual neurologic deficit postictally. This is referred to as *Todd's paralysis* (focal paresis), which resolves after varying lengths of time.

Partial seizures are further divided into those with simple motor or sensory phenomena and those with complex symptoms (also called *psychomotor* seizures). Simple partial seizures with elementary symptoms do not involve loss of consciousness and rarely last longer than 1 minute. They may involve motor, sensory, or autonomic phenomena or a combination of these. The terms *focal motor, focal sensory,* and *Jacksonian* have been used to describe seizures of the simple partial type.

Partial seizures with complex symptoms can involve a variety of behavioral, emotional, affective, and cognitive functions. The location of the discharging focus is usually in the temporal lobe; hence the term *temporal lobe seizure.* These seizures usually last longer than 1 minute and are frequently followed by a period of postictal confusion. Partial complex seizures are distinct from simple partial (focal motor, focal sensory) seizures in that they involve some alteration in consciousness. The sole manifestation of partial complex seizures may be clouding of consciousness or a confused state without any motor or sensory components. This type of attack is sometimes called *temporal lobe absence.* There is rarely the complete loss of consciousness that is typical of the generalized absence attack; nor does the patient snap back to the preseizure state as does the patient who has had a generalized absence attack.

The most common complex partial seizure involves lip smacking and *automatisms* (repetitive movements that may not be appropriate). These are often called *psychomotor seizures.* The patient may continue an activity that was initiated before the seizure, such as counting out change or picking items from a grocery shelf but, after the seizure, does not remember the activity performed during the seizure. Other automatisms are less organized, such as picking at clothing, fumbling with objects (real or imaginary), or simply walking away.

A variety of psychosensory symptoms may occur during a partial complex seizure, including distortions of visual or auditory sensations and vertigo. There may be alterations in memory, such as a feeling of having experienced an event before (*deja vu*), or alterations in thought processes. Alterations in sexual functioning can vary from hyposexuality to hypersexuality. Many patients with temporal lobe seizures have decreased sexual drive or erectile dysfunction. However, some may experience sexual sensations during their seizures. This is because the abnormal electrical activity arises from the brain centers responsible for these sensations. Some experience increased sexual drive just after a seizure. In addition, some antiepileptic medications can cause a decrease in sexual drive because of sedation. Others can cause erectile dysfunction.

Complications

Physical. *Status epilepticus* is the most serious complication of epilepsy. This is a state in which seizures recur in rapid succession and the patient does not regain consciousness or normal function between seizures. Status epilepticus can involve any type of seizure. During repeated seizures the brain uses more energy than can be supplied. Neurons become exhausted and cease to function. Permanent brain damage may result. Tonic-clonic status epilepticus is the most dangerous because it can cause ventilatory insufficiency, hypoxemia, cardiac dysrhythmias, hyperthermia, and systemic acidosis, all of which can be fatal.

Another complication of epilepsy is severe injury and even death from trauma suffered during a seizure. Patients who lose consciousness during a seizure are at greatest risk. Death can result from head injury incurred in a fall, from drowning in the bathtub, or from severe burns.

Psychosocial. Perhaps the most common complication of epilepsy is the effect it has on a patient's lifestyle. Although attitudes have improved in recent years, epilepsy still carries a social stigma. It used to be associated with supernatural powers, possession by the devil, and insanity. Today the stigma probably exists because the characteristics of seizures are in direct conflict with modern societal values of self-control, conformity, and independence. The patient with epilepsy may experience discrimination in employment and educational opportunities. Transportation may be difficult because of legal sanctions against driving in some states. The patient may develop ineffective methods of coping.

Diagnostic Studies

The most useful diagnostic tools are accurate and comprehensive description of the seizures and the patient's health history (Table 56-6). The EEG is a useful diagnostic adjuvant to the history but only if it shows abnormalities. Abnormal findings help to determine the type of seizure and to pinpoint the seizure focus. Unfortunately, only a small percentage of patients with epilepsy have abnormal findings on the EEG the first time the test is done. EEGs need to be repeated often before abnormalities are detected.

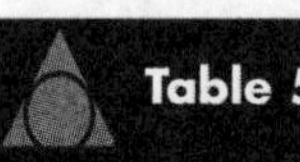

Table 56-6 Therapeutic Management: Seizures

Diagnostic
- Complete history and physical examination
  - Birth and development history
  - Significant illnesses and injuries
  - Family history
  - Febrile seizures
  - Comprehensive neurologic assessment
- Seizure history
  - Precipitating factors
  - Antecedent events
  - Seizure description (including onset, duration, frequency, postictal state)
- Diagnostic studies
  - CBC, urinalysis, electrolytes, blood urea nitrogen, fasting blood glucose
  - Lumbar puncture
  - CT scan, MRI
  - Electroencephalography

Therapeutic
- Antiepileptic medication*
- Surgery†
- Psychosocial counseling

CBC, Complete blood count; *CT*, computed tomography; *MRI*, magnetic resonance imaging.
*See Table 56-9.
†See Table 56-8.

Abnormal discharges may not occur during the 30 to 40 minutes of sampling during EEG, and the test may never indicate an abnormality. It is not a foolproof test. Some patients who do not have epilepsy have abnormal patterns on their EEGs, whereas many patients with epilepsy have normal EEGs.

A complete blood count, standard blood chemistries, studies of liver and kidney function, and urinalysis should be done initially. Plain skull x-ray studies; CT, MRI, and radionuclide brain scans; cerebral angiography; and positron emission tomography are also used in selected clinical situations.

Therapeutic Management

Most seizures do not require professional emergency medical care because they are self-limiting and rarely cause bodily injury. However, if status epilepticus occurs, if significant bodily harm occurs, or if the event is a first-time seizure, medical care should be sought immediately. Table 56-7 summarizes emergency care of the patient with a generalized tonic-clonic seizure, the seizure most likely to warrant professional emergency medical care.

The diagnostic and therapeutic management of seizure disorders is summarized in Table 56-6. Epilepsy is treated primarily with antiepileptic medication. Therapy is aimed at preventing seizures, because cure is not possible. Medications generally act by stabilizing nerve cell membranes and preventing spread of the epileptic discharge. Alternative therapies for epilepsy are surgical removal of the epileptic focus and biofeedback or operant conditioning in selected cases.

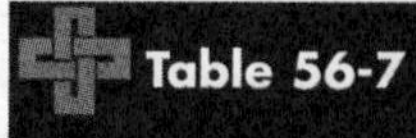

Table 56-7 Emergency Management: Tonic-Clonic Seizures

Possible Etiologies
Idiopathic, head trauma, traumatic birth injury, drug overdose, hypertensive crisis, stroke, meningitis, cardiac arrest, fluid and electrolyte imbalance, hypoglycemia, septicemia, brain tumors, psychiatric disorders, high fevers, medical disorders (e.g., heart, liver, lung, or kidney disease; systemic lupus erythematosus)

Possible Assessment Findings
- Aura hallucinations, peculiar sensations that precede seizure
- Loss of consciousness
- Tonic phase—continuous muscle contractions
- Hypertonic phase—extreme muscular rigidity lasting 5-15 sec
- Clonic phase—ridigity and relaxation alternate in rapid succession
- Postictal phase—lethargy, alteration in level of consciousness
- Loss of bowel and bladder control
- Increased pulse rate
- Postseizure stupor
- Confusion and headache

Management
- Establish and maintain an adequate airway. Anticipate need for intubation if gag reflex absent.
- Do not force an airway between a patient's clenched teeth.
- Assist with ventilations if patient does not breathe spontaneously after seizure.
- Suction as needed.
- Stay with patient until seizure has passed.
- Protect patient from injury during hypertonic, clonic, and tonic phases.
- Monitor vital signs, including level of consciousness, O_2 saturation, Glasgow coma scale, pupil size.
- Establish an intravenous infusion with large-gauge needle following seizure.
- Remove or loosen any tight clothing.
- Do not restrain the patient.
- Protect the patient's privacy.
- Reassure and reorient the patient after seizure.
- Attempt to determine underlying cause.

In about 70% of the patients epilepsy is controlled by medication. Of the remaining 30%, a significant number are candidates for surgical intervention (Table 56-8). Surgery may be considered to control intractable seizures, prevent cerebral degeneration from repeated seizures, prevent toxic

Table 56-8 Surgical Procedures for Epilepsy

Type of Seizure	Surgical Procedure	Results
Complex partial seizure of temporal lobe origin	Resectioning of epileptogenic tissue	Absence of seizures 5 yr postoperatively in 55-70% of patients
Partial seizures of frontal lobe origin	Resectioning of epileptogenic tissue (if in resectable area)	Absence of seizures 5 yr postoperatively in 30-50% of patients
Generalized seizures (Lennox-Gastaut syndrome or drop attacks)	Sectioning of corpus callosum	Persistence of seizures, less violent, less frequent, less disabling events
Intractable unilateral multifocal epilepsy associated with infantile hemiplegia	Hemispherectomy or callosotomy	Reduction in seizure frequency and type, improvement in behavior

syndromes from long-term use of antiepileptic drugs, and improve the quality of life.[14]

Not all types of epilepsy benefit from surgery. The benefits of surgery include cessation or reduction in frequency of the seizures. An extensive preoperative evaluation is important, including continuous EEG monitoring and other specific tests to ensure precise localization of the focal point. Before surgery is performed, three requirements must be met: (1) the diagnosis of epilepsy must be confirmed; (2) there must have been an adequate trial with drug therapy without satisfactory results; and (3) the electroclinical syndrome must be defined.[14]

Biofeedback to control seizures is aimed at teaching the patient to maintain a certain brain-wave frequency that is refractory to seizure activity. This method is still in the experimental stage.

Pharmacologic Management. The primary goal of antiepileptic drug therapy is to obtain maximum seizure control with a minimum of toxic side effects. The principle of drug management is to begin with a single drug and increase the dosage until seizures are controlled or toxic side effects occur. Serum levels of the drug should be monitored regularly. The therapeutic range for each drug indicates the serum level above which most patients experience toxic side effects and below which most continue to have seizures. Therapeutic ranges are only guides for therapy. If the patient's seizures are well controlled with a subtherapeutic level, the drug dose need not be increased. Likewise, if a drug level is above the therapeutic range and the patient has good seizure control without toxic side effects, the drug dose need not be decreased. If seizure control is not achieved with a single drug, a second drug is added.

The primary drugs for treatment of generalized tonic-clonic and partial seizures are phenytoin (Dilantin), carbamazepine (Tegretol), phenobarbital, primidone (Mysoline), and divalproex (Depakote). The primary drugs for treatment of absence, akinetic, and myoclonic seizures are ethosuximide (Zarontin), divalproex (Depakote), and clonazepam (Klonopin). Three new antiepileptic drugs have recently been approved by the Food and Drug Administration (FDA). Felbamate (Felbatol) is indicated for partial seizures, secondary generalized seizures, and Lennox-Gastaut syndrome. However, because felbamate use has been associated with aplastic anemia, its use is limited to those patients whose seizure disorder is refractory to other medications. Gabapentin (Neurontin) and lamotrigine (Lamictal) are indicated for partial seizures and for secondary generalized seizures. These drugs are currently used as adjunctive therapy. (Table 56-9 summarizes the known interactions of the major antiepileptic drugs.) Because many of these drugs (e.g., phenytoin, phenobarbital, ethosuximide) have a long half-life, they can be given in once- or twice-daily doses. This increases the patient's compliance with taking medication by simplifying the drug regimen and avoiding the need to take medication at work or school. Antiepileptic drugs should not be discontinued abruptly because this can precipitate seizures.

Toxic side effects of antiepileptic drugs involve the CNS and include diplopia, drowsiness, ataxia, and mental slowing. Neurologic assessment for dose-related toxicity involves testing the eyes for nystagmus. Mild nystagmus confirms that the drug is being taken. If it is associated with diplopia, the dosage may have to be decreased. Hand and gait coordination should be assessed as well as cognitive functioning and general alertness.

Idiosyncratic side effects involve organs outside the CNS, including the skin (rashes), gingivae (hypertrophy), bone marrow (blood dyscrasias), liver, and kidneys. Nurses should be knowledgeable about these side effects so that patients can be informed and proper treatment can be instituted. A common idiosyncratic side effect of phenytoin is hypertrophy of the gingivae, especially in children and young adults. This can be limited by good dental hygiene, including regular toothbrushing and flossing. If gingival hypertrophy is extensive, the hypertrophied tissue may have to be surgically removed (gingivectomy), and phenytoin may have to be replaced by another antiepileptic drug.

NURSING MANAGEMENT
SEIZURES
Nursing Assessment

Subjective and objective data that should be obtained from a patient with a seizure disorder are presented in Table

Table 56-9 Antiepileptic Drugs and Drug Interactions

Drug	Known Drug Interactions
Generalized Tonic-Clonic and Partial Seizures	
Phenytoin (Dilantin)	Aspirin, benzodiazepines, bishydroxycoumarin, carbamazepine, cimetidine, clonazepam, coumarin, chloramphenicol, dexamethasone, disulfiram, ethosuximide, ethanol, isoniazid, methylphenidate, phenothiazines, phenylbutazone, valproic acid, propoxyphene, phenobarbital, tolbutamide, trazodone, birth control pills
Carbamazepine (Tegretol)	Phenytoin, ethosuximide, erythromycin, propoxyphene, primidone, divalproex, birth control pills, calcium channel blockers
Phenobarbital	Bishydroxycoumarin, clonazepam, diazepam, dextropropoxy-phene, carbamazepine, chlorpromazine, desipramine, phenothiazines, phenylbutazone, phenytoin, divalproex, birth control pills
Divalproex (Depakote)	Clonazepam, phenytoin, phenobarbital, ethosuximide, carbamazepine, aspirin, antacids
Primidone (Mysoline)	Isoniazid, same as phenobarbital interactions
Felbamate (Felbatol)	Phenytoin, carbamazepine, valproate
Gabapentin (Neurontin)	None
Lamotrigine (Lamictal)	Phenobarbital, carbamazepine, divalproex, primidone
Absence, Akinetic, and Myoclonic Seizures	
Ethosuximide (Zarontin)	None
Divalproex (Depakote)	Same as above
Clonazepam (Klonopin)	Divalproex
Phenobarbital	Same as above

56-10. Data related to a specific seizure episode can be obtained from a witness.

Nursing Diagnoses
Nursing diagnoses are determined when the problem and the etiologic factors are supported by clinical data. Nursing diagnoses related to seizures may include, but are not limited to, those presented in the nursing care plan for the patient with seizures on p. 1764.

Planning
The overall goals are that the patient with seizures will (1) be free from injury during a seizure, (2) have optimal mental and physical functioning while taking antiepileptic medication, and (3) have satisfactory psychosocial functioning.

Nursing Implementation
Health Promotion and Maintenance. Many cases of epilepsy can be prevented by promotion of general safety measures, such as the wearing of helmets in situations involving risk of head injury. Improved perinatal, labor, and delivery care have reduced fetal trauma and hypoxia and thereby, have reduced brain damage leading to epilepsy. Children with fever should be treated quickly to avoid high temperatures, which may cause seizures.

The patient with epilepsy should practice good general health habits (e.g., maintaining a proper diet, getting adequate rest, and exercising). The patient should be helped to identify events or situations that precipitate the seizures and should be given suggestions for avoiding them or handling them better. Excessive alcohol intake, fatigue, and loss of sleep should be avoided, and the patient should be helped to handle stress constructively.

Acute Intervention. The nurse caring for a hospitalized epileptic patient or a patient who has had seizures as a result of metabolic factors has several responsibilities, including observation and treatment of the seizure, education, and psychosocial intervention. The nursing care for the patient with seizures summarizes many of these interventions.

When a seizure occurs, the nurse should carefully observe and record details of the event because the diagnosis and subsequent treatment often rest solely on the seizure description. All aspects of the seizure should be noted. What events preceded the seizure? When did the seizure occur? How long did each phase (aural [if any], ictal, postictal) last? What occurred during each phase?

Both subjective data (usually the only type of data in the aural phase) and objective data are important. Objective data should include the exact onset of the seizure (which body part was affected first and how), the course and nature of the seizure activity (loss of consciousness, tongue biting, automatisms, stiffening, jerking, total lack of muscle tone), the body parts involved and their sequence of involvement, and the presence of autonomic signs such as dilated pupils, excessive salivation, altered breathing, cyanosis, flushing, diaphoresis, or incontinence. Assessment of the postictal period should include a detailed description of the level of consciousness, vital signs, memory loss, muscle soreness, speech disorders (aphasia, dysarthria), weakness or paralysis, sleep period, and the duration of each sign or symptom.

During the seizure it is important to maintain a patent airway. This may involve supporting and protecting the head, turning the patient to the side, loosening constrictive clothing, or easing the patient to the floor, if seated. After the seizure the patient may require suctioning and oxygen may be needed.

A seizure can be a frightening experience for the patient and for others who may witness it. The nurse should assess the level of their understanding and provide information about how and why the event occurred. This is an excellent opportunity for the nurse to dispel many common misconceptions about seizures.

Chronic and Home Management. Prevention of recurring seizures is the major goal in the treatment of epilepsy. Because epilepsy cannot be cured, medication must be taken regularly and continuously, often for a lifetime. The nurse should ensure that the patient knows this, as well as the specifics of the medication regimen and what to do if a dose is missed. Usually the dose should be made up if the omission is remembered within 24 hours. The patient should be cautioned not to adjust medications without professional guidance because this can increase seizure frequency and even cause status epilepticus. The patient should be encouraged to report any medication side effects and to keep regular appointments with the health care provider.

Nurses should teach family members and significant others the first-aid treatment of tonic-clonic seizures. They should be reminded that it is not necessary to call an ambulance or send a person to the hospital after a single seizure unless the seizure is prolonged, another seizure immediately follows, or extensive injury has occurred.

Patients with epilepsy also experience concerns or fears related to recurrent seizures, incontinence, or loss of self-control. The nurse provides support for the patient through education and by helping to identify coping mechanisms.

Perhaps the greatest challenge that epilepsy presents to the patient is adjusting to the personal limitations imposed by the illness. Discrimination in employment is the most serious problem facing the person with epilepsy. Patients can be informed that the Rehabilitation Act of 1973 was designed to protect handicapped persons (including those with epilepsy) from discrimination in employment. For issues relating to job discrimination, patients can be referred to the State Human Rights Commission or the State Department of Vocational Rehabilitation.

A variety of other resources can be offered to the patient with epilepsy who has a specific problem. If the nurse believes that associating with others who have epilepsy would be beneficial, the patient can be referred to the local chapter of the Epilepsy Foundation of America (EFA), a voluntary agency that offers a variety of services to patients with epilepsy. The patient who is an eligible veteran can be referred to a Department of Veterans Affairs Medical Center that provides comprehensive care.

The patient should be informed that medical-alert bracelets, necklaces, and identification cards are available through

S…

Impo…

Past he…
injuries, …
infections; hy…
metabolic disord…
and carbon monoxid…
fever; pregnancy; systemic lupus ery…

Medications: Compliance with antiseizure me… barbiturate or alcohol withdrawal; use and ove… of cocaine, amphetamines, lidocaine, theophylline, penicillin, lithium, phenothiazines, tricyclic antidepressants

Functional health patterns

Health perception–health management: Positive family history; fatigue

Nutritional-metabolic: Nausea, vomiting; diarrhea

Cognitive-perceptual: Headaches, muscle pain (postictal), abdominal pain; aura; mood or behavioral changes before seizure; mentation changes

Objective Data

General

Precipitating factors, including severe metabolic acidosis or alkalosis, hyperkalemia, hypoglycemia, dehydration or water intoxication

Integumentary

Bitten tongue, soft-tissue damage, cyanosis, diaphoresis (postictal)

Cardiovascular

Hypertension, tachycardia (ictal)

Gastrointestinal

Incontinence, gingival hyperplasia from phenytoin (Dilantin), excessive salivation

Urinary

Incontinence

Neurologic

Generalized

Tonic-clonic: Loss of consciousness and postural tone, dilated pupils, hyperventilation, then apnea; possible airway occlusion; postictal phase

Absence: Altered consciousness (5-30 sec), minor facial motor activity

Partial

Complex: Altered consciousness with inappropriate behaviors, automatisms, amnesia of event

Simple: Aura, consciousness, focal sensory, motor, cognitive, or emotional phenomena (focal motor); unilateral "marching" motor seizure (Jacksonian)

Musculoskeletal

Paresthesia or paralysis (postictal)

Possible findings

Positive toxic screen and high alcohol level; altered serum electrolytes, acidosis or alkalosis, very low blood glucose level, elevated blood urea nitrogen, serum creatinine, liver function tests, ammonia; abnormal CT scan or MRI of head, lumbar puncture; seizure activity on EEG

CNS, Central nervous system; *CT,* computed tomography; *EEG,* electroencephalogram; *MRI,* magnetic resonance imaging.

NURSING CARE PLAN Patient with Seizures

Planning: Outcome Criteria	Nursing Interventions and Rationales
➤ **NURSING DIAGNOSIS**	Ineffective breathing pattern *related to* neuromuscular impairment secondary to prolonged tonic phase of seizure or during postictal period *as manifested by* abnormal respiratory rate, rhythm, or depth; nasal flaring; change in pulse (rate, rhythm, quality); dyspnea, shortness of breath; cyanosis, pallor, diaphoresis; absence of or abnormal breath sounds
Have clear breath sounds, appropriate rate, rhythm, and depth of respirations.	Loosen constricting clothing *to avoid restricting breathing.* Assess breathing pattern, observing for labored respiration, tachypnea, bradypnea, dyspnea, apnea, and cyanosis *to determine presence and extent of problem and initiate appropriate interventions.* Provide manual ventilation or oxygen when necessary; be prepared to assist with endotracheal intubation *to maintain adequate oxygenation and prevent hypoxia.* Insert oral airway (if indicated) only after seizure activity has ceased *to prevent mouth and teeth injury from forcing airway between clamped teeth.* Be prepared to obtain arterial blood gases *to evaluate adequacy of oxygenation.*
➤ **NURSING DIAGNOSIS**	Ineffective airway clearance *related to* tracheobronchial obstruction *as manifested by* ineffective cough, inability to remove secretions, absence of or abnormal breath sounds, abnormal respiratory rate, rhythm, or depth
Have no airway obstruction; clear breath sounds.	Observe for signs of airway constriction *to determine extent of problem and to plan appropriate interventions.* If vomiting occurs, turn patient's head gently to side and remove as much vomitus as possible after the seizure *to prevent aspiration of vomitus and subsequent interference with breathing.* Suction airway if necessary *to remove accumulated secretions.* Establish and maintain patent airway *to ensure adequate oxygenation.*
➤ **NURSING DIAGNOSIS**	Risk for injury *related to* seizure activity and subsequent impaired physical mobility secondary to postictal weakness or paralysis
Have no injury; verbalize knowledge of potential for injury during seizure; plan to arrange environment to minimize risk for injury.	Assess for trauma to mouth, cheek, tongue, and lips, abrasions, bruises, broken bones, and burns *as these injuries may occur during seizure activity.* Assess for weakness, paralysis of one side of body (Todd paralysis), ataxia, fatigue, lethargy *as potential postictal risks for injury to plan appropriate interventions.* Do not permit smoking in bed *to prevent the patient from being burned by a bed fire if a seizure occurs.* If patient has experienced frequent seizures recently, take axillary rather than oral temperature *to prevent mouth trauma from a broken thermometer.* If patient anticipates a seizure may occur, assist to a safe location or position; use seizure precautions as appropriate; remove potentially harmful objects from surrounding area; gently guide arm or leg movements *to prevent injury during a seizure.* Refrain from moving or restraining patient during a seizure *to prevent bone or soft tissue injury.* Assist in determining whether operation of a motor vehicle or dangerous machinery is appropriate for patient *to help direct patient in making informed choice about driving.* Assist with activities of daily living as necessary after a seizure *so patient needs are met.* Encourage mobility as tolerated *to prevent stiffness and depression.* Provide information about the hazards of immobility *to motivate patient to maintain mobility.*
➤ **NURSING DIAGNOSIS**	Impaired verbal communication *related to* transient aphasia secondary to postictal state *as manifested by* aphasia or dysphasia, dysarthria, confusion
Have evidence of adequate communication.	Assess verbal skills *to determine appropriate interventions.* Explain possible transient aphasia to patient and family *to decrease anxiety regarding this event.* Communicate in slow simple statements in postictal state *to promote understanding and reduce frustration.* Document effective communication techniques *so appropriate interventions will be carried out by all caregivers.*

continued

NURSING CARE PLAN Patient with Seizures—cont'd

Planning: Outcome Criteria	Nursing Interventions and Rationales
➤ **NURSING DIAGNOSIS**	Ineffective individual coping *related to* perceived loss of control, denial of diagnosis, or misconceptions regarding disease *as manifested by* verbalizations about not having epilepsy, lack of truth-telling regarding seizure frequency, noncompliant behavior (driving or other high-risk behaviors in face of frequent seizures)
Accept disorder as evidenced by using word *epilepsy* to describe illness; acknowledge that a seizure has occurred; be knowledgeable about disease.	Explore reasons for denial *to determine extent of problem and to plan appropriate interventions.* Implement and individualize teaching plan about causes and mechanisms of seizures, effectiveness of drugs in controlling seizures, inaccuracy of myths about epilepsy, avoidance of precipitating factors, state law regarding driving, pros and cons of medical identification tags, moderation in drinking and eating, exposure to stress, and avoidance of hazardous activities *to promote effective coping by providing facts.*
➤ **NURSING DIAGNOSIS**	Self-concept disturbance *related to* diagnosis of epilepsy *as manifested by* anxiety, fear, social isolation, depression, role disturbance, altered family dynamics
Share feelings about diagnosis; identify positive aspects about self; have appropriate interactions with others; attain and maintain high self-concept.	Develop long-term plan to deal with developmental issues *to minimize self-concept problems.* Discuss patient's views about self in relation to seizures *to clarify effect of disease on self-concept.* Provide information about possible overprotection, community resources, and social stigmas that may be encountered *to improve self-concept by increasing sense of control.* Assist patient with explaining seizures and management to friends, school personnel, and employers *so these people can provide support and acceptance.* Advise patient about employment counseling and job retraining *as gainful employment usually improves self-concept.* Determine effect of seizures on daily activities and other activities important to patient *as major interference will likely affect self-concept.* Encourage patient to focus on positive aspects of life *to avoid putting self down because of restrictions or limitations.* Provide information on referral to a neuropsychologist, psychologist, or social worker if indicated *so expert help can assist patient with self-concept problems.*
➤ **NURSING DIAGNOSIS**	Ineffective management of therapeutic regimen *related to* lack of knowledge about management of epilepsy *as manifested by* verbalization of deficiency in knowledge or skill, inaccurate perception of health status, failure to correctly perform desired or prescribed health behaviors, noncompliance with prescribed health behavior, exhibition or expression of psychologic alteration (e.g., anxiety, depression) resulting from misinformation or lack of information
Patient and family will demonstrate knowledge of health maintenance activities related to epilepsy; patient will have optimal seizure control, therapeutic drug levels; comply with appointments and other recommendations.	Provide education to patient and family about seizure activity and therapeutic management including diagnosis and treatment, lifestyle adjustments, and community resources *so patient and family can make necessary lifestyle modifications to manage a chronic disease.*

the EFA, local pharmacies, or companies specializing in identification devices. However, the use of these medical identification tags is optional. Some patients have found them beneficial, but others have found them to be more a burden than a help because they prefer not to be identified as having epilepsy.

Social workers and welfare agencies can help with financial problems and living arrangements. State services for individuals with developmental disabilities include assistance with job training, and placement for patients whose seizures are not well controlled. Sheltered housing and funding for special needs, such as medical and psychologic evaluation and transportation are also offered. State agencies specializing in vocational rehabilitation services can offer vocational assessment, counseling, funding for training, and assistance with job placement. They can also offer financial assistance for transportation and medical costs that are necessary for vocational rehabilitation or job maintenance. If intensive psychologic counseling is needed, the nurse can refer the patient to a community mental health center.

The patient should be encouraged to learn more about epilepsy through self-education materials. The EFA provides several information pamphlets. Many agencies that offer services to epileptic patients, as well as local chapters of EFA, have these available as teaching aids.

MULTIPLE SCLEROSIS

Significance

Multiple sclerosis (MS) is a chronic, progressive, degenerative disorder of the CNS. In the United States, this autoimmune disease affects 36 per 100,000 persons in areas south of the 37th parallel and 55 to 80 per 100,000 persons in the northern United States and Canada.[15,16] It is considered a disease of young adults, with the onset usually being between 15 and 50 years of age. Women are affected more often than men.

MS primarily affects white persons of northern European descent, which means that the disease is associated with certain environmental and familial factors. Incidence is highest in the temperate zones of the globe (between 45 and 65 degrees of latitude), especially northern Europe, Canada, and the northern United States. It is also associated with the place of birth. An individual born and raised in one of the regions listed above who moves to a warmer climate (nearer the equator) after 15 years of age carries the same risk of developing MS as do others in the country of origin. African-Americans and Asians have a lower incidence of MS than do Caucasians.

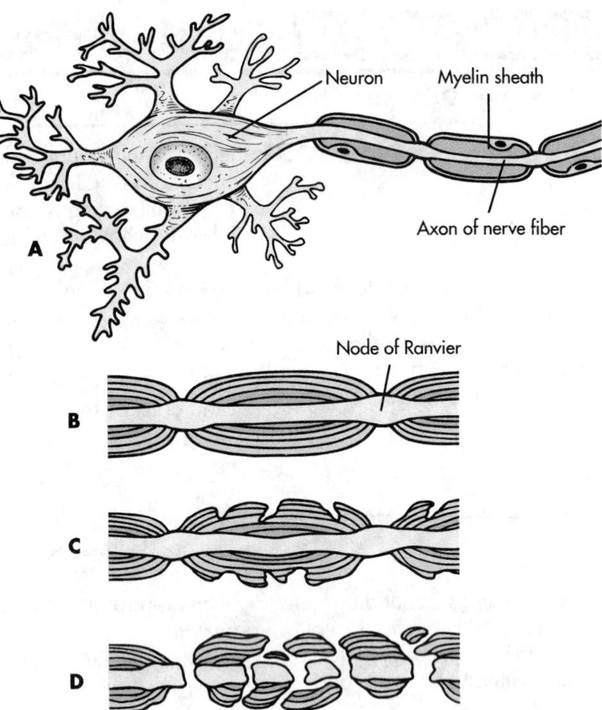

Fig. 56-1 ***A,*** Normal nerve cell with myelin sheath. ***B,*** Normal axon. ***C,*** Myelin breakdown. ***D,*** Myelin totally disrupted; axon not functioning.

Etiology

The cause of MS is unknown, although research findings suggest MS is related to infectious (viral), immunologic, and genetic factors and is perpetuated as a result of intrinsic factors (e.g., faulty immunoregulation). The susceptibility to MS appears to be inherited. First-, second-, and third-degree relatives of patients with MS are at a slightly increased risk. Multiple unlinked genes confer susceptibility to MS.

The role of precipitating factors such as exposure to pathogenetic agents in the etiology of MS is controversial. It is possible that their association with MS is random and that there is no cause and effect relationship. Possible precipitating factors include infection, physical injury, emotional stress, excessive fatigue, pregnancy, and a poorer state of health.

Pathophysiology

MS is characterized by demyelination in the CNS. The primary neuropathologic condition is an immune-mediated inflammatory demyelinating process which some believe may be triggered by a virus in genetically susceptible individuals. Activated T cells responding to environmental triggers (e.g., infection) enter the CNS in increased numbers. These T cells, in conjunction with astrocytes, disrupt the blood-brain barrier, thereby promoting the entry of other immune mediators into the CNS. These factors, in combination, damage oligodendrocytes (cells that make myelin), resulting in demyelination. Macrophages are recruited and cause further cell damage.[15] The process consists of loss of myelin, disappearance of oligodendrocytes, and the proliferation of astrocytes. These changes result in characteristic plaque formation, or *sclerosis,* with plaques scattered throughout *multiple* regions of the CNS.

Initially the myelin sheaths of the neurons in the brain and spinal cord are attacked (Fig. 56-1, *A* and *B*). Early in the disease the myelin sheath is damaged, but the nerve fiber is not affected and nerve impulses are still transmitted (Fig. 56-1, *C*). At this point the patient may complain of a noticeable impairment of function (e.g., weakness). However, the myelin can regenerate and the symptoms disappear, resulting in a remission.

As the disease progresses, the myelin is totally disrupted, and the axon becomes involved (Fig. 56-1, *D*). Myelin is replaced by glial scar tissue, which forms hard, sclerotic plaques in multiple regions of the CNS. Without myelin, nerve impulses slow down, and with destruction of nerve axons, impulses are totally blocked, resulting in permanent loss of function. In many chronic lesions, demyelination continues with progressive loss of nerve function.

Clinical Manifestations

Because the onset is often insidious and gradual, with vague symptoms that occur intermittently over months or years, the disease may not be diagnosed until long after the onset of the first symptom. Because the disease process has a spotty distribution in the CNS, the signs and symptoms vary over time. The disease is characterized by chronic, progressive deterioration in some persons and by remis-

RESEARCH

Implications for Nursing Practice

COGNITIVE CHANGES IN MULTIPLE SCLEROSIS PATIENTS

Citation Jansen DA and Cimprich B: Attentional impairment in persons with multiple sclerosis, *J Neurosci Nurs* 26:95-102, 1994.

Purpose To assess the ability of multiple sclerosis (MS) patients to inhibit competing and distracting stimuli while processing information from the environment.

Methods A one-group descriptive correlational design using 33 MS patients who had relapsing-remitting MS with minimal physical disability was used. The capacity to direct attention (CDA) and inhibit distracting stimuli was determined using a Digit Span Backward and Forward and Symbol Digit Modalities Test. The Functional Independence Measure was used to assess physical ability.

Results and Conclusions The MS patients had attentional deficits of varying severity in spite of the presence of only a few symptoms. These deficits were unrelated to depressive symptoms.

Implications for Nursing Practice The findings indicate that MS patients with very mild physical deficits can experience cognitive problems. Nurses need to consider attentional problems even in the most early disease states. Measures to maintain attentional capacities through supportive and restorative nursing interventions need to be explored in patients with MS.

sions and exacerbations in others. With repeated exacerbations, however, progressive scarring of the myelin sheath occurs, and the overall trend is progressive deterioration in neurologic function. The clinical manifestations vary according to the areas of the CNS involved. Some patients have severe, long-lasting symptoms early in the course of the disease. Others may experience only occasional and mild symptoms for several years after onset.

Common signs and symptoms include motor, sensory, cerebellar, and emotional phenomena. Motor symptoms include weakness or paralysis of the limbs, trunk, or head, diplopia, scanning speech, and spasticity of the muscles that are chronically affected. Sensory symptoms include numbness and tingling and other paresthesias, patchy blindness (*scotomas*), blurred vision, vertigo, tinnitus, and decreased hearing. Cerebellar signs include nystagmus, ataxia, dysarthria, and dysphagia.

Bowel and bladder function can be affected if the sclerotic plaque is located in areas of the CNS that control elimination. Problems with defecation usually involve constipation rather than fecal incontinence. Urinary problems are variable. A common problem in MS patients is a *spastic* (uninhibited) bladder. This indicates a lesion above the second sacral nerve, which cuts off suprasegmental inhibiting influences on bladder contractility. As a result, the bladder has a small capacity for urine, and its contractions are unchecked. This is accompanied by urinary urgency and frequency and results in dribbling or incontinence. A *flaccid* (hypotonic) bladder indicates a lesion in the reflex arc governing bladder function. The bladder has a large capacity for urine because there is no sensation or desire to void, no pressure, and no pain. Generally, there is urinary retention, but urgency and frequency may also occur with this type of lesion. Urinary problems cannot be adequately diagnosed and treated unless urodynamic studies are done.

Sexual dysfunction occurs in many persons with MS.[15] Physiologic impotence may result from spinal cord involvement in men. Women may experience decreased libido, difficulty with orgasmic response, painful intercourse, and decreased vaginal lubrication. Diminished sensation can prevent a normal sexual response in both sexes. The emotional effects of chronic illness and the loss of self-esteem also contribute to loss of sexual response.

Women with MS who become pregnant often experience remission or an improvement in their symptoms during the gestation period. The hormonal changes associated with pregnancy appear to affect the immune system. However, during the postpartum period women are at greater risk for exacerbation of the disease.[17]

Although intellectual functioning generally remains intact, emotional stability may be affected. Persons may experience anger, depression, or euphoria. Signs and symptoms of MS are aggravated or triggered by physical and emotional trauma, fatigue, and infection.

The average life expectancy after the onset of symptoms is more than 25 years. Death usually occurs because of infective complications (e.g., pneumonia) of immobility, or because of unrelated disease; occasionally, suicide is a cause.[15]

Diagnostic Studies

Because there is no definitive diagnostic test for MS, diagnosis is based primarily on history and clinical manifestations (Table 56-11). Certain laboratory tests are currently used as adjuncts to the clinical examination. In some patients, cerebrospinal fluid (CSF) analysis may show an increase in oligoclonal immunoglobulin G (IgG). The CSF also contains a high number of lymphocytes and monocytes. Sensory-evoked responses are often delayed in persons with MS because of decreased nerve conduction from the eye and the ear to the brain. CT and MRI may be helpful, because sclerotic plaques as small as 3 to 4 mm in diameter can be detected. Characteristic white-matter lesions scattered through the brain or spinal cord are evident on such scans.

Therapeutic Management

Because there is no cure for MS, therapeutic management is aimed at treating the disease process and providing symptomatic relief (Table 56-11). The disease process is treated with drugs, and the symptoms are controlled with a variety of medications and other forms of therapy. Spasticity is primarily treated with antispasmodic drugs. However, sur-

Table 56-11 Therapeutic Management: Multiple Sclerosis

Diagnostic
- History and physical examination
- CSF analysis
- Evoked response testing
- CT scan
- MRI

Therapeutic
Pharmacologic
- Antiinflammatory
- Immunosuppressive
- Anticholinergic
- Cholinergic
- Antispasmodic
- Immunomodulatory

Surgical
- Thalamotomy (unmanageable tremor)
- Neurectomy, rhizotomy, cordotomy (unmanageable spasticity)

CSF, Cerebrospinal fluid; *CT*, computed tomography; *MRI*, magnetic resonance imaging.

gery (e.g., neurectomy, rhizotomy, cordotomy) or dorsal-column electrical stimulation may be required. Intention tremor that becomes unmanageable with medication is sometimes treated by stereotactic surgery on the thalamus. This involves selective destruction of the ventrolateral nucleus in the thalamus. Neurologic dysfunction sometimes improves with physical therapy, speech therapy, and hypothermia, which normalizes body temperature if it is above normal.

Pharmacologic Management. Adrenocorticotropic hormone (ACTH), methylprednisolone, and prednisone are helpful in treating acute exacerbations of the disease, probably by reducing edema and acute inflammation at the site of demyelination. Recent evidence suggests that intravenous steroids (methylprednisolone) are more effective for acute relapses than are oral corticosteroid preparations.[18] However, these medications do not necessarily affect the ultimate outcome or degree of residual neurologic impairment from the exacerbation. Immunosuppressive drugs, such as azathioprine (Imuran), cyclosporine, and cyclophosphamide (Cytoxan), have been shown to produce some beneficial effects in patients with severe and relapsing MS. However, the potential benefits of these drugs in patients with MS needs to be counterbalanced against the potentially serious side effects.[18] Table 56-12 summarizes the drugs that are commonly used for symptomatic treatment of MS.

Beta-interferon (Betaseron) was approved by the FDA in 1993 for ambulatory patients with exacerbating and remitting MS. Clinical trials with subcutaneous injections every other day have shown that the drug decreased the number of exacerbations and the number of new lesions seen on an MRI scan.[19] Studies evaluating Copolymer I as an immunomodulating agent are underway. It is a synthetic analog of myelin basic protein, a component of CNS myelin.

Nutritional Management. Various nutritional measures that have been advocated in the management of MS include megavitamin therapy (vitamin B_{12}, vitamin C) and diets consisting of low-fat and gluten-free food and raw vegetables. These particular dietary measures have not come into widespread use because of lack of proof of their effectiveness.

A nutritious, well-balanced diet is essential. Although there is no standard prescribed diet, a high-protein diet with supplementary vitamins is often advocated. A diet high in roughage may help relieve the problem of constipation. Vitamins are merely supplemental and not curative.

NURSING MANAGEMENT

MULTIPLE SCLEROSIS

Nursing Assessment

Subjective and objective data that should be obtained from a person with multiple sclerosis are presented in Table 56-13.

Nursing Diagnoses

Nursing diagnoses are determined when the problem and the etiologic factors are supported by clinical data. Nursing diagnoses related to MS may include, but are not limited to, those presented in the nursing care plan for the patient with MS on p. 1772.

Planning

The overall goals are that the patient with MS will (1) maximize neuromuscular function, (2) maintain independence in activities of daily living for as long as possible, and (3) optimize psychosocial well-being.

Nursing Implementation

Health Promotion and Maintenance. The patient should be aware of triggers that may cause exacerbations or worsening of the disease. Exacerbations of MS are triggered by exogenous events including infection (especially upper respiratory infections), trauma, immunization, delivery after pregnancy, stress, and climactic changes. Of these the best documented are upper respiratory infections, delivery, and head trauma.[20] Each person responds differently to these triggers. The nurse should help the patient identify particular triggers and develop ways to avoid them or minimize their effects.

Acute Intervention. The most common reasons for hospitalization of the patient with MS are for a diagnostic workup and treatment of an acute exacerbation. During the diagnostic phase the patient needs reassurance that even though there is a tentative diagnosis of MS, certain diagnostic studies must be done to rule out other neurologic disorders. The nurse needs to assist the patient in dealing with the anxiety caused by a diagnosis of disabling illness. The patient with recently diagnosed MS may need assistance with the grieving process.

During an acute exacerbation the patient may be immobile and confined to bed for 2 to 3 weeks. The focus of nursing intervention at this phase is to prevent major com-

Table 56-12 Drugs for Symptomatic Treatment of Multiple Sclerosis

Drug	Symptoms Relieved	Precautions	Side Effects	Educational Needs
Corticosteroids				
ACTH Prednisone Methylprednisolone	Exacerbations	Widespread effects on many enzymes and metabolic processes, few adverse effects with use for <1 mo at a time	Edema, mental changes (euphoria), weight gain, redistribution of body fat*	Restrict salt intake. Do not abruptly stop therapy. Know drug interactions
Immunomodulators				
Beta-interferon (Betaseron)	Exacerbations	Monitor CBC, blood chemistries, and liver function tests every 3 mo	Flulike symptoms, local skin reactions, depression	Learn self-injection techniques, report side effects
Cholinergics				
Bethanecol (Urecholine) Neostigmine (Prostigmine)	Urinary retention (flaccid bladder)	History of hypotension, cardiac dysfunction, allergies, hyperthyroidism, stomach and intestinal problems; contraindication with adrenergic drugs (antiasthmatic drugs) because of possible induction of serious asthma attack (Urecholine only)	Hypotension, diarrhea, diaphoresis, salivation, muscle weakness	Consult physician before using other drugs.
Anticholinergics				
Propantheline (Pro-Banthine) Oxybutynin (Ditropan)	Urinary frequency† and urgency (spastic bladder)	History of glaucoma, prostatic hypertrophy, cardiac dysfunction, intestinal obstruction	Dry mouth, blurred vision, constipation, hypertension, flushing, urinary retention (too high of dose)	Consult physician before using other drugs, especially sleeping aids, antihistamines (possibly leading to potentiated effect).
Muscle Relaxants				
Diazepam (Valium)	Spasticity	History of narrow-angle glaucoma	Drowsiness, ataxia, fatigue	Avoid driving and similar activities because of CNS-depressant effects. Be aware of addictive potential; avoid long-term use. Avoid concomitant use of phenothiazines, narcotics, barbiturates, MAO inhibitors, other antidepressants.

continued

plications of immobility, such as respiratory and urinary tract infections and decubitus ulcers. The nursing care plan for a patient with MS presents appropriate nursing interventions (see p. 1772).

Chronic and Home Management. Chronic and home management is aimed at (1) helping the patient adjust to the illness, (2) teaching how to avoid factors that precipitate exacerbations, (3) maximizing self-care in light of current neurologic deficits, and (4) meeting the needs for activities of daily living. The main goal is to keep the patient active and maximally functional.

Physical therapy is important in keeping the patient as functionally active as possible. The purpose of therapy is to relieve spasticity, increase coordination, and train the patient to substitute unaffected muscles for impaired ones. An especially beneficial type of physical therapy is water exercise (see Fig. 56-2 on p. 1774). Water gives buoyancy to the body and allows the patient to perform activities that

Table 56-12 Drugs for Symptomatic Treatment of Multiple Sclerosis—cont'd

Drug	Symptoms Relieved	Precautions	Side Effects	Educational Needs
Baclofen (Lioresal)	Spasticity	History of hypersensitivity and renal damage, contraindication in pregnancy, possible exacerbation of seizures in patients with epilepsy	Drowsiness	Do not abruptly stop therapy (possibly leading to hallucinations). Avoid driving and similar activities because of sedative effect. Avoid use with other CNS depressants; take with food or milk.
Dantrolene (Dantrium)	Spasticity	History of respiratory or cardiac dysfunction, possible induction of abnormal liver function or hepatitis, contraindication with estrogen therapy because of predisposition of hepatotoxicity	Drowsiness, dizziness, malaise, fatigue, diarrhea	Avoid driving. Avoid use with tranquilizers and alcohol (possibly causing photosensitivity).

ACTH, Adrenocorticotropic hormone; *CBC*, complete blood count; *CNS*, central nervous system; *MAO*, monoamine oxidase.
*See Chapter 47 for effects of long-term corticosteroid therapy.
†Urodynamic studies must be done before institution of therapy because patients with MS have multiple lesions and type of bladder dysfunction cannot be diagnosed from symptoms alone.

would normally be impossible. In water, a patient experiences more control over the body.

Patient education should focus on building general resistance to illness, including avoiding fatigue, extremes of heat and cold, and exposure to infection. The last measure involves avoiding exposure to cold climates and to people who are sick, as well as vigorous and early treatment of infection when it does occur. It is important to teach the patient to (1) achieve a good balance of exercise and rest, (2) eat nutritious and well-balanced meals, and (3) avoid the hazards of immobility (contractures and pressure sores). Patients should know their treatment regimens, the side effects of medications and how to watch for them, and drug interactions with over-the-counter medications. The patient should consult a health care provider before taking nonprescription medications.

Bladder control is a major problem for many patients with MS. While anticholinergics may be beneficial for some patients to decrease spasticity, other patients may need to be taught self-catheterization (see Chapter 43). Bowel problems, particulary constipation, occur frequently in patients with MS. Increasing the dietary fiber may help some patients achieve regularity in bowel habits.

The patient with MS and the family must make many emotional adjustments because of the unpredictability of the disease, the need to change lifestyles, and the challenge of avoiding or decreasing precipitating factors. The National Multiple Sclerosis Society and its local chapters can offer a variety of services to meet the needs of patients with MS.

PARKINSON'S DISEASE

Parkinsonism is a syndrome that consists of a slowing down in the initiation and execution of movement (*bradykinesia*), increased muscle tonus (*rigidity*), tremor, and impaired postural reflexes. Parkinson's disease, a form of parkinsonism, is named after James Parkinson, who, in 1817, wrote a classic essay on "shaking palsy," a disease whose cause is still unknown today. Many other disorders resemble this disease, but their causes are known. These include drug-induced parkinsonism, postencephalitic parkinsonism, and arteriosclerotic parkinsonism. The pathophysiology of these disorders, with the exception of drug-induced parkinsonism, is the same. Damage or loss of the dopamine-producing cells of the substantia nigra in the midbrain leads to depletion, in the basal ganglia, of dopamine that influences the initiation, modulation, and completion of movement and regulates unconscious autonomic movements (see Chapter 53). In cases of drug-induced parkinsonism the dopamine receptors in the brain are blocked.

Significance

About 500,000 persons in the United States have Parkinson's disease. About 1% of the population over 50 years of age is affected.[21] The disease shows no gender, socioeconomic, or cultural preference, and symptoms most commonly occur after 50 years of age. In Canada, however, men have a higher prevalence than women.[22] The average age of the patient with Parkinson's disease is 65 years. There is no apparent genetic cause and no known cure. The disease rarely occurs in African-Americans.

Etiology and Pathophysiology

There are many causes of parkinsonism. Encephalitis lethargica, or Type A encephalitis, has been clearly associated with the onset of parkinsonism. However, the incidence of postencephalitic parkinsonism has dwindled since the 1920s, when there was a large outbreak of this infectious illness.

Table 56-13 Nursing Assessment: Multiple Sclerosis

Subjective Data

Important health information

Past health history: Recent or past viral infections or vaccinations, residence in cold or temperate climates, recent physical or emotional stress, pregnancy, infections, exposure to heat

Medications: Use of and compliance in taking corticosteroids (e.g., ACTH, prednisone), immunosuppressants, anticholinergics, muscle relaxants

Functional health patterns

Health perception–health management: Positive family history; fatigue aggravated by heat

Nutritional-metabolic: Weight loss; difficulty in chewing; dysphagia

Elimination: Urinary frequency, urgency, or retention; constipation

Activity-exercise: Generalized muscle weakness; tingling and numbness

Cognitive-perceptual: Eye, back, leg, joint pain; painful muscle spasms; vertigo; blurred or lost vision; diplopia

Sexuality-reproductive: Impotence, decreased libido

Objective Data

General

Apathy, inattentiveness

Integumentary

Pressure sores

Neurologic

Scanning speech, nystagmus, ataxia, tremor, spasticity, hyperreflexia, tinnitus and decreased hearing, poor coordination

Musculoskeletal

Muscular weakness, paresis, paralysis, spasms, foot dragging, dysarthria

Possible findings

Reduction in T-suppressor cells, demyelinating lesions on CT and MRI scans, increased IgG or oligoclonal banding in cerebrospinal fluid

ACTH, Adrenocorticotropic hormone; *CT,* computed tomography; *MRI,* magnetic resonance imaging.

Parkinsonism-like symptoms have occurred after intoxication with a variety of chemicals, including carbon monoxide and manganese (among copper miners) and an analogue of meperidine (MPTP). Drug-induced parkinsonism can follow reserpine, methyldopa, haloperidol, and phenothiazine therapy. Although patients with cerebrovascular disease may have parkinsonism-like symptoms, there is little evidence that parkinsonism is caused by arteriosclerosis. Distinguishing arteriosclerosis from true Parkinson's disease is important for prognostic purposes. Patients with arteriosclerosis do not respond as well to treatment and are more likely to experience side effects of drug therapy. Most patients with parkinsonism have the degenerative or idiopathic form, for which the term *Parkinson's disease* is usually reserved.

The pathology of Parkinson's disease is associated with the degeneration of the dopamine-producing neurons in the substantia nigra of the midbrain (see Fig. 56-3 on p. 1775). It is hypothesized that there is normally a balance between acetylcholine (ACh) and dopamine (DA) in the basal ganglia. Any shift in the balance of activity (an increase in ACh or a decrease in DA) seems to lead to parkinsonism-like symptoms. Dopamine is a neurotransmitter that is essential for normal functioning of the extrapyramidal motor system, including control of posture, support, and voluntary motion. In Parkinson's disease the levels of DA-synthesizing enzymes and metabolites are reduced, and postmortem analysis of cross sections of the midbrain shows loss of the normal melanin pigment in the substantia nigra and loss of neurons. In addition, deficient amounts of γ-aminobutyric acid (GABA), serotonin, and norepinephrine have been found in basal ganglia and in the substantia nigra.

Clinical Manifestations

The onset of Parkinson's disease is gradual and insidious, with a gradual progression and a prolonged course. In the beginning stages, only a mild tremor, a slight limp, or a decreased arm swing may be evident. Later in the disease the patient may have a shuffling, propulsive gait with arms flexed and loss of postural reflexes. In some patients there may be a slight change in speech patterns. None of these alone is sufficient evidence for a diagnosis of the disease.

Because there is no specific diagnostic test for Parkinson's disease, the diagnosis is based solely on the history and the clinical features. A firm diagnosis can be made only when there are at least two of the three characteristic signs of the classic triad: tremor, rigidity, and bradykinesia (slow or retarded movement). Although dementia occurs in up to 40% of patients with Parkinson's disease, intellectual impairment does not occur in the majority of patients.[23,24] The ultimate confirmation of Parkinson's disease is a positive response to antiparkinsonian medication.

Tremor. Tremor, often the first sign, may be minimal initially, so the patient is the only one who notices it. This tremor can affect handwriting, causing it to trail off, particularly toward the end of words. Parkinsonian tremor is more prominent at rest and is aggravated by emotional stress or increased concentration. The hand tremor is described as "pill rolling" because the thumb and forefinger appear to move in a rotary fashion as if rolling a pill, coin, or other small object. Tremor can involve the diaphragm, tongue, lips, and jaw but rarely causes shaking of the head. Unfortunately, in many people a benign essential tremor has mistakenly been diagnosed as Parkinson's disease. Essential tremor occurs during voluntary movement, has a more rapid frequency than parkinsonian tremor, and is often familial.

Rigidity. Rigidity, the second sign of the triad, is the increased resistance to passive motion when the limbs are moved through their range of motion. Parkinsonian rigidity is typified by a jerky quality, as if there were intermittent catches in the movement of a cogwheel, when the joint is moved. This is called *cogwheel rigidity.* The rigidity is caused by sustained muscle contraction and consequently elicits a complaint of muscle soreness, feeling tired and achy, or pain in the head, upper body, spine, or legs.

NURSING CARE PLAN Patient with Multiple Sclerosis

Planning: Outcome Criteria	Nursing Interventions and Rationales
➤ NURSING DIAGNOSIS	Ineffective airway clearance *related to* impaired ability to cough *as manifested by* inability to remove secretions, abnormal breath sounds, dyspnea, shortness of breath
Have absence of respiratory infections, clear breath sounds, effective cough.	Assess respiratory status *to determine extent of problem and to plan appropriate interventions.* Monitor respiratory parameters *to evaluate effect of interventions.* Encourage and assist with coughing and deep breathing q4hr while patient is awake *to maintain patent airway and prevent respiratory complications.* Turn patient at least q2hr *to prevent stasis of pulmonary secretions.* Protect from infectious illnesses of patients, staff, and family *as infection may trigger an exacerbation of MS or worsen an existing problem.* Have patient in upright position with head flexed toward sternum for eating *to prevent aspiration.*
➤ NURSING DIAGNOSIS	Impaired physical mobility *related to* muscle weakness or paralysis and muscle spasticity *as manifested by* inability to ambulate, intermittent muscle spasms, pain associated with muscle spasms, ataxia
Demonstrate use of adaptive devices to increase mobility and minimize potential for injury; maintain or increase strength of unaffected limbs; decrease duration of muscle spasms.	Use assistive devices as indicated *to decrease fatigue and to enhance independence, comfort, and safety.* Do active range-of-motion exercises at least 2 times per day *to prevent contractures and minimize muscle atrophy.* Encourage and assist with ambulation and transfer as indicated *to maintain mobility, promote independence, and provide for safety.* Change position of patient (if bedridden) at least q2hr *to prevent pressure ulcers and circulatory problems.* Administer medication as ordered *to reduce spasticity or to treat inflammatory response.* Perform stretching exercises q6-8hr *to relieve spasms and contracted muscles.*
➤ NURSING DIAGNOSIS	Self-care deficit *related to* muscle spasticity and uncompensated neuromuscular deficits *as manifested by* inability to perform some or all activities of daily living
Have maximum level of functioning; manage activities of daily living independently or with assistance.	Assess self-care problems *to plan appropriate interventions to meet care needs.* Promote use of appropriate assistive devices *so patient can maximally participate in self-care activities with minimum fatigue.* Counsel regarding need for homemaker services *to assist in meeting patient's needs, conserving energy, and promoting independence.* Perform or assist with activities of daily living only as indicated *to promote patient's independence.* Encourage independence when appropriate *to promote patient's sense of autonomy and control.*
➤ NURSING DIAGNOSIS	Risk for impaired skin integrity *related to* immobility, sensorimotor deficits, and inadequate nutrition
Have intact skin free of redness.	On every shift assess skin for redness and irritation *to monitor changes in skin integrity and make appropriate plan for interventions.* Turn patient at least q2hr *to prevent pressure ulcers from developing.* Use circular massage of unreddened bony prominences with each turning *to improve circulation to these areas.* (This is avoided in patients who do not have fat pads over bones.) Provide high-protein diet *to promote healthy skin that is resistant to breakdown.* Cleanse back and buttocks if patient is incontinent *to prevent skin irritation.*
➤ NURSING DIAGNOSIS	Sensory or perceptual alteration *related to* visual disturbances *as manifested by* blurred vision, decreased visual acuity, visual field defects, diplopia
Have satisfactory visual function for activities of daily living; adjust care to prevent injury when visual problems are present.	Orient patient to environment *to promote safety and to compensate for visual disturbances.* Patch alternate eyes q4-24hr *to alleviate diplopia.* Assess visual acuity monthly *to monitor increase or decrease in vision.* Maintain safe environment (e.g., side rails up, bed in low position) *to prevent injury.* Indicate visual impairment on chart, on care plan, and over bed *to communicate visual problems to health team and foster continuity of care.*

continued

NURSING CARE PLAN Patient with Multiple Sclerosis—cont'd

Planning: Outcome Criteria	Nursing Interventions and Rationales
➤ **NURSING DIAGNOSIS**	Altered patterns of urinary elimination (retention) *related to* sensorimotor deficits or inadequate fluid intake *as manifested by* posturination residual urine >50 ml, dribbling, bladder distention
Have residual urine <50 ml; absence of dribbling and distention.	Administer cholinergic medications as ordered *to improve the muscle tone of bladder and facilitate emptying.* Follow intermittent catheterization protocol *to prevent distention or dribbling.* Use Credé maneuver or reflex stimulation (manual stimulation) *as an alternative method of emptying bladder.* (Credé is used only if there is no sphincter dysenergia.) Maintain fluid intake of 3000 ml/day *to dilute urine and reduce risk of UTI.* Teach patient signs and symptoms of UTI *to ensure early identification and treatment.*
➤ **NURSING DIAGNOSIS**	Altered patterns of urinary elimination (incontinence) *related to* sensorimotor deficits or possible UTI *as manifested by* incontinence, urgency, frequency
Have urinary continence.	Administer anticholinergic medications as ordered *to reduce urinary frequency and urgency.* Initiate bladder-training program *to help restore adequate bladder function.* Provide incontinence briefs *to ensure that patient is protected and will not be embarrassed by incontinence.* Assess for urinary tract infection *to ensure diagnosis and treatment.* Maintain fluid intake of 3000 ml/day *to promote urinary output and aid in preventing infection.*
➤ **NURSING DIAGNOSIS**	Constipation *related to* immobility, inadequate fluid intake, improper diet, and neuromuscular impairment *as manifested by* hard stool, decreased bowel sounds, infrequent or absent bowel movements, feelings of rectal fullness, straining and pain on defecation, palpable impaction
Have or develop satisfactory bowel habits.	Turn patient regularly; maintain activity according to individual tolerance *as mobility enhances peristalsis.* Maintain fluid intake (3000 ml/day) *to promote normal stool consistency.* Use prune juice at same time of day *as dihydroxyphenyl isatin in prune juice has a laxative effect.* Encourage high-residue diet *to improve stool consistency and promote evacuation.* Administer stool softeners and suppositories as ordered *to promote regularity by improving stool consistency.* Initiate and maintain bowel program *to foster regular bowel elimination.*
➤ **NURSING DIAGNOSIS**	Sexual dysfunction *related to* uncompensated neuromuscular deficits *as manifested by* impotence, verbalization of problem, dissatisfaction with sex role, limitations with sexual performance, decreased libido
Verbalize satisfaction with expression of sexuality.	Initiate sexual counseling if indicated *as not all nurses have the advanced education required for this type of counseling.* Suggest alternative methods of achieving sexual gratification *as sexual intercourse may not be possible because of neuromuscular deficits.*
➤ **NURSING DIAGNOSIS**	Self-concept disturbance *related to* prolonged debilitating condition *as manifested by* feelings of inadequacy, depression, fatigue, withdrawal
Maintain realistic self-concept in relation to disease.	Focus on remaining abilities and maintaining independence *because a major part of self-concept is the ability to perform one's role functions.* Assist patient in grieving process *as progressive losses or changes in body function may interfere with resolution of grieving process.* Encourage patient to discuss effect of MS on self-concept *to clarify issues and identify coping behaviors.* Discuss importance of maintaining social interactions *to prevent social isolation, withdrawal, and negative self-concept.*

continued

NURSING CARE PLAN Patient with Multiple Sclerosis—cont'd

Planning: Outcome Criteria	Nursing Interventions and Rationales
➤ **NURSING DIAGNOSIS**	Altered family processes *related to* changing family roles, potential financial problems, and fluctuating physical condition *as manifested by* strained family relations, ineffective communication, verbalization of financial concerns
Family will have open communication with patient, seek outside assistance when indicated, maintain adequate care of ill member.	Facilitate open communication among family members *to help family understand behaviors that may be triggered by emotional or physical effects of MS.* Promote problem solving *to enable them to handle the issues of long-term illness.* Refer for family and financial counseling (if indicated) *to provide additional help in coping with a chronic debilitating disease.* Educate family regarding fluctuating nature of disease *as lack of knowledge about MS affects ability to cope with the changes.*
➤ **NURSING DIAGNOSIS**	Risk for ineffective management of therapeutic regimen *related to* compromised functioning
Express confidence in ability to manage regimen and fluctuating health status.	Discuss patient's concerns regarding ability to make necessary lifestyle changes *because disease-related functional changes may make self-care progressively difficult.* Teach patient how to manage regimen *to increase confidence in ability to manage or supervise part or all of required care.* Assist patient to make plans for care when patient is unable *to ensure patient needs are met and to relieve patient's anxiety.*

MS, Multiple sclerosis; *UTI,* urinary tract infection.

Another consequence of rigidity is slowness of movement, because it inhibits the alternating of contraction and relaxation in opposing muscle groups (e.g., the biceps and triceps).

Bradykinesia. Bradykinesia is particularly evident in the loss of automatic movements, which is secondary to the physical and chemical alteration of the basal ganglia and related structures in the extrapyramidal portion of the CNS. In the unaffected patient, automatic movements are involuntary and occur subconsciously. They include blinking of the eyelids, swinging of the arms while walking, swallowing of saliva, self-expression with facial and hand movements, and minor movement of postural adjustment. The patient with Parkinson's disease does not execute these movements, and there is a lack of spontaneous activity. This accounts for the stooped posture, *masked facies* ("deadpan" expression), drooling of saliva, and shuffling gait (*festination*) that are characteristic of a person with this disease. In addition, there is difficulty in initiating movement. Movements such as getting out of a chair cannot be executed unless they are consciously willed.

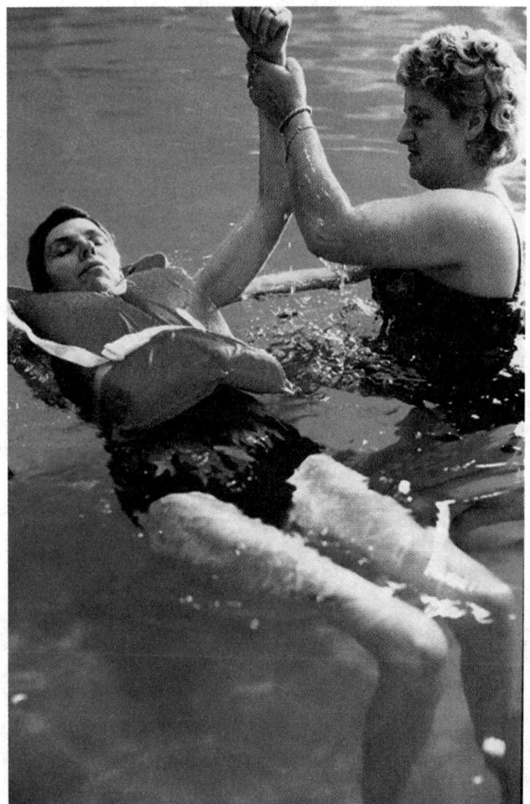

Fig. 56-2 Water therapy provides exercise and recreation for the patient with a chronic neurologic disease.

Complications

Many of the complications of Parkinson's disease are caused by the deterioration and loss of spontaneity of movement. Swallowing may become very difficult (dysphagia) in severe cases, leading to malnutrition or aspiration. General debilitation may lead to pneumonia, urinary tract infections, and skin breakdown. Mobility is greatly decreased. The gait slows, and turning is especially difficult. The gait usually consists of rapid, short, shuffling ministeps. The posture is

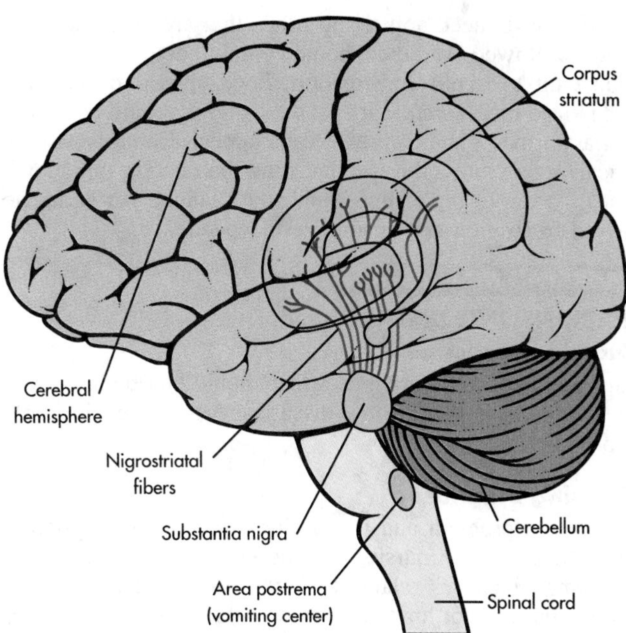

Fig. 56-3 Left-sided view of the human brain showing the substantia nigra and the corpus striatum (*shaded area*) lying deep within the cerebral hemisphere. Nerve fibers extend upward from the substantia nigra, divide into many branches, and carry dopamine to all regions of the corpus striatum.

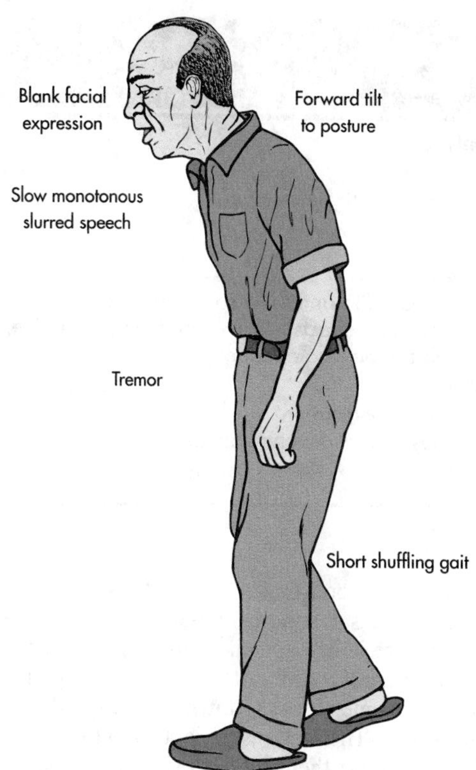

Fig. 56-4 Characteristic appearance of a patient with Parkinson's disease.

that of the "old man" image, with the head and trunk bent forward and the legs constantly flexed (Fig 56-4). The lack of mobility may lead to constipation, ankle edema, and, more seriously, contractures.

Orthostatic hypotension may occur in some patients, and along with loss of postural reflexes, may result in falls or other injury. Bothersome complications include *seborrhea* (increased oily secretion of the sebaceous glands of the skin), dandruff, excessive sweating, conjunctivitis, difficulty in reading, insomnia, incontinence, and depression.

Many of the apparent complications of Parkinson's disease are the result of side effects of medication, particularly levodopa. Dyskinesias (e.g., athetosis of the neck) and weakness and akinesia (total immobility) may cause problems. These complications become apparent after prolonged levodopa therapy when the therapeutic index decreases.

Therapeutic Management

Because there is no cure for Parkinson's disease, therapeutic management (Table 56-14) is aimed at relieving the symptoms. Antiparkinsonian drugs either enhance the release or supply of DA (dopaminergic) or antagonize or block the effects of the overactive cholinergic neurons in the striatum (anticholinergic) (Table 56-15).

The only other treatment for Parkinson's disease is cryothalamectomy or stereotaxic thalamotomy or pallidotomy for correction of severe unilateral tremor. Surgical treatment is most effective in younger patients. The greater risk of complications and residual neurologic deficits preclude the use of this treatment in older patients with more severe disease. Because the long-term benefits of surgery vary, the role of surgical intervention is limited.

Transplantation of adrenal tissue into the caudate nucleus in an attempt to provide viable dopamine-producing cells to the brain has had disappointing results.[25] The use of fetal tissue for this same purpose holds promise and more studies of the benefit of this procedure should be forthcoming, with the lifting of the ban on the use of federal funds for research involving fetal tissues.[26]

Pharmacologic Management. Pharmacotherapy of Parkinson's disease is aimed at correcting an imbalance of neurotransmitters within the CNS, characterized by a relative deficiency of DA and an excess of ACh in the corpus striatum. Levodopa with carbidopa (Sinemet), is often the first drug to be used. Levodopa is a precursor of dopamine

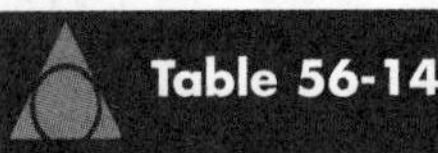

Table 56-14 Therapeutic Management: Parkinson's Disease

Diagnostic
- History
- Physical examination
  - Tremor
  - Rigidity
  - Bradykinesia
- Positive response to antiparkinson medication*
- Ruling out of side effects of phenothiazines, reserpine, benzodiazepines, haloperidol

Therapeutic
- Antiparkinson medication*
- Surgical destruction of ventrolateral nucleus of the thalamus

*See Table 56-15.

and can cross the blood-brain barrier. It is converted to dopamine in the basal ganglia. Sinemet is the preferred medication because it also contains carbidopa, an agent that inhibits the enzyme dopa-decarboxylase in the peripheral tissues. This enzyme breaks down levodopa before it reaches the brain. The net result is that more levodopa reaches the brain, and therefore less drug is needed. Bromocriptine is a DA agonist that activates DA receptors. It may be used as an adjuvant drug along with Sinemet.

Anticholinergic drugs are also used to manage Parkinson's disease. These drugs act by decreasing the activity of ACh and thus providing balance between cholinergic and dopaminergic actions. Antihistamines (e.g., diphenhydramine [Benadryl]) with anticholinergic properties are sometimes used to relieve tremor and rigidity. The antiviral agent amantadine (Symmetrel) is also an effective antiparkinsonian drug. Although its exact mechanism of action is not known, amantadine promotes the release of DA from neurons. Selegiline (L-deprenyl) is a monoamine oxidase (MAO) inhibitor which is sometimes used in combination with Sinemet. By inhibiting MAO, the degradative enzyme for DA, the levels of DA are increased. Although there is some evidence to suggest that selegiline may have some neuroprotective activity in early stages of Parkinson's disease, clinical trials have failed to demonstrate major differences.[27]

Table 56-15 summarizes the drugs commonly used in Parkinson's disease, the symptoms they relieve, and their common side effects. The use of only one drug is preferred, since there are fewer side effects and the medication is easier to adjust than when several drugs are used. Excessive amounts of dopaminergic drugs can lead to paradoxical intoxication (aggravation rather than relief of symptoms). Anticholinergic drugs can cause impaired erection and failure of ejaculation.

Nutritional Management. Diet is of major importance to the patient with Parkinson's disease because malnutrition and constipation can be serious consequences of inadequate nutrition. Patients who have dysphagia and bradykinesia need appetizing foods that are easily chewed and swallowed. The diet should contain adequate roughage and fruit to avoid constipation. Food should be cut into bite-sized pieces *before* it is served, and it should be served on a warmed plate to preserve its appeal. Eating six small meals a day may be less exhausting than eating three large meals a day. Ample time should be planned for eating to avoid frustration and encourage independence.

NURSING MANAGEMENT

PARKINSON'S DISEASE

Nursing Assessment

Subjective and objective data that should be obtained from a person with Parkinson's disease are presented in Table 56-16.

Nursing Diagnoses

When the problem and the etiologic factors are supported by clinical data, nursing diagnoses can be determined. Nursing diagnoses related to Parkinson's disease may include, but are not limited to, those presented in the nursing care plan for the patient with Parkinson's disease on p. 1779.

Planning

The overall goals are that the patient with Parkinson's disease will (1) maximize neurologic function, (2) maintain independence in activities of daily living for as long as possible, and (3) optimize psychosocial well-being.

Nursing Implementation

Promotion of physical exercise and a well-balanced diet are major concerns for nursing care. Exercise can limit the consequences of decreased mobility, such as muscle atrophy, contractures, and constipation. The American Parkinson's Disease Association publishes a booklet, *Home Exercises for Patients with Parkinson's Disease,* that illustrates a variety of exercises; it can be used by family members as well as health professionals.

A physical therapist may be consulted to design a personal exercise program aimed at strengthening specific muscles. Overall muscle tone as well as specific exercises to strengthen the muscles involved with speaking and swallowing should be included. Although exercise will not halt the progress of the disease, it will bring the patient's motor function to an optimal level.

Because Parkinson's disease is a chronic degenerative disorder with no acute exacerbations, nurses should note that health teaching and nursing care are directed toward maintenance of good health, encouragement of independence, and avoidance of complications such as contractures.

Problems secondary to bradykinesia can be alleviated by relatively simple measures. The following are helpful hints for patients who tend to "freeze" while walking: consciously think about stepping over imaginary or real lines on the floor, drop rice kernels and step over them, rock from side to side, lift the toes when stepping, take one step backward and two steps forward. The patient should be

Table 56-15 Drugs for Symptomatic Treatment of Parkinsonism

Drug	Symptoms Relieved	Side Effects and Precautions
Dopaminergic		
Levodopa (L-dopa)	Bradykinesia, tremor, rigidity	Nausea, dyskinesia, hypotension, palpitations, dysrhythmias; agitation, hallucinations, confusion (in older patient); avoidance of vitamin pills and diet high in vitamin B_6 (reversal of effect of levodopa); contraindicated in narrow-angle glaucoma
Levodopa/ carbidopa (Sinemet)	Bradykinesia, tremor, rigidity	Less nausea but greater chance of dyskinesia, confusion, hallucinations; periodic check of BUN, AST, WBCs, Hct; contraindicated in melanoma, narrow-angle glaucoma, combination with MAO inhibitors, reserpine, methyldopa, guanethidine, antipsychotics
Bromocriptine mesylate (Parlodel)	Bradykinesia, tremor, rigidity	Orthostatic hypotension, nausea, vomiting, toxic psychosis, limb edema, phlebitis, dizziness, headache, insomnia
Pergolide (Permax)	Same as above	Same as above
Amantadine (Symmetrel)	Rigidity, akinesia	Nervousness, insomnia, confusion, hallucinations, dry mouth, nausea, edema, orthostatic hypotension
Anticholinergic		
Trihexyphenidyl (Artane) Cycrimine (Pagitane) Procyclidine (Kemadrin) Benztropine Mesylate (Cogentin) Biperiden (Akineton)	Tremor	Dry mouth, blurred vision, constipation, delirium, anxiety, agitation, hallucinations; avoidance of drugs with similar actions, including over-the-counter drugs containing scopolamine or antihistamines (e.g., Sominex), antispasmodics (e.g., Donnatal, Bellergal), tricyclic antidepressants (Tofranil, Elavil, Norpramin, Vivactil)
Antihistamine		
Diphenhydramine (Benadryl) Orphenadrine (Disipal) Chlorphenoxamine (Phenoxene) Phenindamine (Thephorin)	Tremor, rigidity	Sedation, same precautions as for anticholinergic drugs
Monoamine Oxidase-B Inhibitor		
Selegiline (Eldepryl)	Bradykinesia, rigidity, tremor	Similar to dopaminergic drugs

AST, Aspartate aminotransferase; *BUN,* blood urea nitrogen; *Hct,* hematocrit; *MAO,* monoamine oxidase; *WBCs,* white blood cells.

assessed for the possibility of levodopa overdose because it is a common cause of akinesia "freezing." A brief period of dyskinesia, usually athetosis of the neck, should alert the nurse to this possibility.

Getting out of a chair can be facilitated by using an upright chair with arms and placing the back legs on small (2 inch) blocks. Other aspects of the environment can be altered. Rugs and excess furniture can be removed to avoid stumbling. An ottoman can be used to elevate the legs and avoid dependent ankle edema. Clothing can be simplified by the use of slip-on shoes and velcro hook and loop fasteners or zippers on clothing, instead of buttons and hooks. An elevated toilet seat can facilitate getting on and off the toilet. The nurse should work closely with the patient's family in exploring creative adaptations that allow maximum independence and self-care.

MYASTHENIA GRAVIS

Myasthenia gravis (MG) is a disease of the neuromuscular junction characterized by the fluctuating weakness of certain skeletal muscle groups. The prevalence is estimated to be from 43 to 84 persons per million. The peak age at onset in women is 20 to 30 years. Women are affected slightly more often than are men, although among patients with both thymoma and myasthenia gravis (15% of all persons with MG), the majority are men over the age of 50.

Etiology and Pathophysiology

MG is caused by an autoimmune process that results in production of antibodies directed against the acetylcholine (ACh) receptors and a reduction in the number of ACh receptor sites at the neuromuscular junction. This prevents ACh molecules from attaching and stimulating muscle

Table 56-16 Nursing Assessment: Parkinson's Disease

Subjective Data

Important health information

Past health history: CNS trauma, cerebrovascular disorders, syphilis, exposure to metals and carbon monoxide, encephalitis

Medication: Use of potent tranquilizers, especially haloperidol (Haldol) and phenothiazines, reserpine, methyldopa

Functional health patterns

Health perception–health management: Fatigue

Nutritional-metabolic: Excessive salivation, dysphagia; excessive sweating; weight loss

Elimination: Constipation

Activity-exercise: Difficulty in initiating movements; frequent falls; loss of dexterity; micrographia (handwriting deterioration)

Cognitive-perceptual: Diffuse pain in legs, shoulders, neck, back and hips; muscle soreness and cramping

Self-perception–self-concept: Depression; mood swings

Objective Data

General

Blank (masked) facies, slow and monotonous speech, infrequent blinking

Integumentary

Seborrhea

Cardiovascular

Postural hypotension

Gastrointestinal

Drooling

Neurologic

Tremor at rest, first in hands (pill-rolling), later in legs, arms, face, and tongue; aggravation of tremor with anxiety, absence in sleep; shuffling gait; poor coordination; subtle dementia

Musculoskeletal

"Cogwheel" rigidity, dysarthria, bradykinesia, contractures, stooped posture

Possible findings

Lack of specific tests, diagnosis on basis of history and physical findings

CNS, Central nervous system.

contraction. Anti-ACh receptor antibodies are detectable in the serum of 70% to 85% of patients with MG. As a result of this process there is loss of muscle strength. Thymic tumors are found in about 15% of patients. Although a viral infection is suspected as precipitating an attack, a single specific cause for all cases of MG has not been found.

Clinical Manifestations

The primary feature of MG is easy fatigability of skeletal muscle during activity. Strength is usually restored after a period of rest. The muscles most often involved are those used for moving the eyes and eyelids, chewing, swallowing, speaking, and breathing. The cell bodies of the neurons for these muscles are located in the brainstem. The muscles are generally the strongest in the morning and become exhausted with continued activity. Consequently, by the end of the day, muscle fatigue is prominent.

In more than 90% of the cases, the eyelid muscles or extraocular muscles are involved. Facial mobility and expression can be impaired. There may be difficulty in chewing and swallowing food. Speech is affected, and the voice often fades after a long conversation. The muscles of the trunk and limbs are less often affected. Of these, the proximal muscles of the neck, shoulder, and hip are more often affected than the distal muscles. No other signs of neural disorder accompany MG; there is no sensory loss, reflexes are normal, and muscle atrophy is rare.

The course of this disease is highly variable. Some patients may have short-term remissions, others may stabilize, and others may have severe, progressive involvement. Restricted ocular myasthenia, usually seen only in men, has a good prognosis. Exacerbations of MG can be precipitated by emotional stress, pregnancy, menses, secondary illness, trauma, temperature extremes, hypokalemia, ingestion of drugs with neuromuscular blocking properties, and surgery. In some cases the onset of MG occurs after one of these events.

Complications

The major complications of MG result from muscle weakness in areas that affect swallowing and breathing. Aspiration, respiratory insufficiency, and respiratory infection are the major complications. An acute exacerbation of this type is sometimes called *myasthenic crisis.*

Diagnostic Studies

The simplest diagnostic test for myasthenia gravis is to have the patient look upward for 2 to 3 minutes. If the problem is MG, there will be an increased droop of the eyelids, so that the person can barely keep the eyes open. After a brief rest the eyes can open again. Other tests may be used if the diagnosis is still in doubt. EMG may show a decrementing response to repeated stimulation of the hand muscles, indicative of muscle fatigue. Use of pharmacologic agents may also aid in the diagnosis. The Tensilon test in a patient with MG reveals improved muscle contractility after intravenous (IV) injection of the anticholinesterase agent edrophonium chloride (Tensilon chloride). This test also aids in the diagnosis of cholinergic crisis (secondary to overdose of neostigmine). In this condition, Tensilon does not improve muscle weakness but may actually increase it. Atropine should be readily available to counteract Tensilon effects when it is used diagnostically.

Therapeutic Management

The major forms of therapy for MG are anticholinesterase drugs, alternate-day corticosteroids, immunosuppressants, and plasmapheresis (Table 56-17). Because the presence of the thymus gland in the patient with MG appears to enhance the production of ACh receptor antibodies, removal of the thymus gland results in improvement in 85% of patients. Thymectomy is indicated for almost all patients with thymoma, for a variable subset of patients with generalized MG

NURSING CARE PLAN Patient with Parkinson's Disease

Planning: Outcome Criteria	***Nursing Interventions and Rationales***
➤ **NURSING DIAGNOSIS**	Impaired physical mobility *related to* rigidity, tremor, bradykinesia, and akinesia *as manifested by* cogwheeling, difficulty in initiation of volitional movements, shuffling gait
Have maximal safe ambulation; maintain joint mobility.	Assist with ambulation *to assess degree of impairment and to prevent injury.* Perform active ROM exercises to all extremities *to maintain joint motility, prevent atrophy, and strengthen muscles.* Consult physical therapist or occupational therapist for aids *to facilitate activities of daily living and safe ambulation.* Evaluate tremor in relation to medication *to monitor patient's response and identify possible overdose.* Assist with fine and gross motor activities as needed *to reduce patient's frustration.* Teach techniques to assist with mobility by instructing patient to step over imaginary line, rock from side to side to initiate leg movements *as these are helpful in dealing with "freezing" (akinesia) while walking.* Remove environmental barriers *to prevent injury.*
➤ **NURSING DIAGNOSIS**	Self-care deficit *related to* parkinsonian symptoms *as manifested by* inability to perform activities of daily living, need for assistive devices
Have optimal independence in ADLs; have daily needs met by self or others.	Encourage ADLs within limits of mobility *to prolong patient's independence.* Arrange patient's room *to facilitate optimal self-care.* Plan sufficient time for patient to perform self-care *as rigidity causes slowness of movement.* Provide assistance as needed *so patient needs are met and frustration is reduced.* Arrange occupational therapy consultation *to teach additional strategies for achieving ADLs and to minimize complications such as contractures.* Offer emotional support *to bolster patient's effort in coping with a chronic degenerative disease.*
➤ **NURSING DIAGNOSIS**	Impaired verbal and written communication *related to* dysarthria and tremor or bradykinesia *as manifested by* decreased amount of communication, slow and slurred speech, inability to move facial muscles, decreased tongue mobility, micrographia, inability to write
Develop methods of communication to meet needs.	Allow sufficient time for communication *to reduce patient's frustration.* Assist with diaphragmatic speech. Encourage deep breaths before speaking. Consult speech therapist *to provide specialized guidance in care of the patient.* Provide alternative communication methods such as picture books or flash cards because muscle involvement has impaired writing and speaking ability. Massage patient's facial and neck muscles *to foster relaxation which can facilitate speech.*
➤ **NURSING DIAGNOSIS**	Constipation *related to* immobility *as manifested by* hardened stool, decreased bowel sounds, reported discomfort, nausea, decreased appetite
Maintain regular bowel evacuation.	Increase fluid intake to 3000 ml/day *to maintain soft stool.* Increase fiber in diet with every meal *to provide bulk to stool.* Increase mobility to tolerance *as mobility stimulates peristalsis.* Give stool softeners, laxatives, suppositories as needed *to ensure regular bowel evacuation.*

continued

without thymoma, and occasionally for selected patients with disabling ocular myasthenia.[28]

Plasmapheresis as a therapy for MG was first reported in 1976. This procedure involves separation of plasma from blood by a machine called a cell separator, which is connected to the patient by a vascular cannula. This process removes anti-ACh receptor antibodies. Plasmapheresis can yield a short-term improvement in symptoms and is indicated for patients in crisis or in preparation for surgery when corticosteroids need to be avoided. (Plasmapheresis is discussed in Chapter 10.)

Pharmacologic Management. Anticholinesterase drugs are used in the management of MG. Acetylcholinesterase is the enzyme responsible for the breakdown of ACh in the synaptic cleft. Thus, inhibition of this enzyme by an anticholinesterase inhibitor will prolong the action of ACh and facilitate transmission of impulses at the neuromuscular junction. Neostigmine (Prostigmin) and pyridostigmine

NURSING CARE PLAN Patient with Parkinson's Disease—cont'd

Planning: Outcome Criteria	*Nursing Interventions and Rationales*
➤ **NURSING DIAGNOSIS**	Sleep pattern disturbance *related to* medication side effects (e.g., hallucinations), anxiety, rigidity, and muscle discomfort *as manifested by* poor sleep history, inability to sleep uninterrupted, nightmares, vivid dreams or hallucinations, anxiety, rigidity, or muscle discomfort
Verbalize feeling rested on awakening.	Provide quiet environment *to promote uninterrupted sleep.* Turn and position patient for comfort *as muscle soreness and inability to make minor postural changes because bradykinesia may interfere with sleep.* Provide passive ROM exercises to extremities *to alleviate rigidity which may interfere with sleep.* Provide daytime stimulus to maintain wakefulness *to avoid excess napping which prevents quality nighttime sleep.* Offer support if hallucinations are present *to decrease anxiety since levodopa may produce hallucinations.* Give sleep medications as ordered *to facilitate sleep.*
➤ **NURSING DIAGNOSIS**	Altered nutrition: less than body requirements *related to* dysphagia *as manifested by* difficulty in swallowing and chewing, inadequate secretion clearance, drooling, decreased gag reflex
Maintain satisfactory body weight.	Carefully monitor swallowing ability during medication administration and mealtime *to evaluate patient's level of impairment and minimize risk of aspiration.* Report any difficulty to physician *so that medications may be adjusted.* Provide soft-solid and thick-liquid diet *as these consistencies are more easily swallowed.* Massage patient's facial and neck muscles before meals *to reduce rigidity and enhance ability to chew and swallow.* Maintain patient in upright position for all meals *to reduce risk of aspiration.* Consult speech therapist and dietitian *as these experts can provide specific plans to improve swallowing and intake.* Maintain calorie counts and weekly weights *to evaluate patient's nutritional status and adjust plan if indicated.* Have tonsil tip suction available *to remove pooled secretions and prevent choking and aspiration.*
➤ **NURSING DIAGNOSIS**	Diversional activity deficit *related to* inability to perform usual recreational activities *as manifested by* boredom, lack of participation, restlessness, depression, hostility
Engage in satisfying diversional activities; express acceptance of diminished capabilities.	Assess patient's activity *to determine physical and emotional response to difficulties.* Determine preferred diversional activities *so individual needs are considered.* Adapt difficult activities when possible *so patient is able to continue performing.* Initiate new activities within patient's capabilities *such as reading to replace activities patient can no longer perform.* Encourage patient to discuss emotional response to decreasing capabilities *to provide opportunity to solve problems and demonstrate a caring attitude.*

ADLs, Activities of daily living; *ROM,* range of motion.

(Mestinon) are the most successful drugs of this group. Tailoring the dose to avoid a myasthenic or a cholinergic crisis often presents a clinical challenge. Because of the autoimmune nature of the disorder, corticosteroids (specifically prednisone) are used to suppress immunity. Cytotoxic drugs such as azathioprine (Imuran) and cyclophosphamide (Cytoxan) may also be used for immunosuppression.

Many drugs are contraindicated or must be used with caution in patients with MG. Classes of drug that should be cautiously evaluated before use include anesthetics, antidysrhythmics, antibiotics, quinine, antipsychotics, barbiturates and sedative-hypnotics, cathartics, diuretics, narcotics, muscle relaxants, thyroid preparations, and tranquilizers.

NURSING MANAGEMENT

MYASTHENIA GRAVIS

Nursing Assessment

The nurse can assess the severity of MG by asking the patient about fatigability, what body parts are affected, and how severely they are affected. The patient's coping abilities and understanding of the disorder should also be assessed. Some patients become so fatigued that they are no longer able to work or even ambulate.

Objective data should include respiratory rate and depth, arterial blood gas analyses, pulmonary function tests, and evidence of respiratory distress in patients with acute myasthenic crisis. Muscle strength of all face and limb

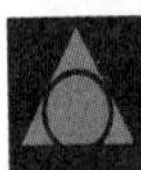

Table 56-17 Therapeutic Management: Myasthenia Gravis

Diagnostic
- History
- Physical examination
  - Fatigability with prolonged upward gaze (2-3 min)
  - Muscle weakness
- EMG
- Tensilon test

Therapeutic
- Drugs
  - Anticholinesterase agents
  - Corticosteroids
  - Immunosuppressive agents
- Surgery (thymectomy)
- Plasmapheresis

EMG, Electromyography.

muscles should be assessed, as should swallowing, speech (volume and clarity), and cough and gag reflexes.

Nursing Diagnoses

Nursing diagnoses specific to the patient with MG include, but are not limited to, the following:

- Ineffective breathing patterns related to intercostal muscle weakness
- Ineffective airway clearance related to intercostal muscle weakness and impaired cough and gag reflex.
- Impaired verbal communication related to weakness of the larynx, lips, mouth, pharynx, and jaw
- Altered nutrition: less than body requirements related to impaired swallowing, weakness, and inability to prepare food or feed self
- Sensory or perceptual visual alterations related to ptosis, decreased eye movements, and dysconjugate gaze
- Activity intolerance related to muscle weakness and fatigability
- Body-image disturbance related to inability to maintain usual lifestyle and role responsibilities.

Planning

The overall goals are that the patient with MG will (1) have a return of normal muscle endurance, (2) avoid complications, and (3) maintain a quality of life appropriate to disease progression.

Nursing Implementation

The patient with MG who is admitted to the hospital usually has a respiratory tract infection or is in an acute myasthenic crisis. Nursing care is aimed at maintaining adequate ventilation, continuing drug therapy, and watching for side effects of therapy. The nurse must be able to distinguish cholinergic from myasthenic crisis (Table 56-18), because the causes and treatment of the two conditions differ greatly.

As with other chronic illnesses, care focuses on the neurologic deficits and their impact on daily living. A balanced diet with food that can be chewed and swallowed easily should be prescribed. Semisolid foods may be easier to eat than solids or liquids. Scheduling doses of medication so that peak action is reached at mealtime may make eating less difficult. Diversional activities that require little physical effort and match the interests of the patient should be arranged. Education should focus on the importance of following the medical regimen, potential adverse reactions to specific drugs, planning activities of daily living to avoid fatigue, the availability of community resources, and the complications of the disease and therapy (crisis conditions) and what to do about them. Contact with the MG Society or an MG support group may be very helpful and should be explored.

ALZHEIMER'S DISEASE

Alzheimer's disease is a type of dementia that is characterized by progressive deterioration in memory and other

Table 56-18 Comparison of Myasthenic Crisis and Cholinergic Crisis

	Myasthenic Crisis	Cholinergic Crisis
▪ Causes	Exacerbation of myasthenia following precipitating factors or failure to take medication as prescribed or dose of medication too low	Overdose of anticholinesterase drugs resulting in increased ACh at the receptor sites, remission (spontaneous or after thymectomy).
▪ Differential Diagnosis	Improved strength after IV administration of anticholinesterase drugs; increased weakness of skeletal muscles manifesting as ptosis, bulbar signs (e.g., difficulty in swallowing, difficulty in articulating words), or dyspnea.	Weakness within 1 hr after ingestion of anticholinesterase; increased weakness of skeletal muscles manifesting as ptosis, bulbar signs, dyspnea; effects on smooth muscle include pupillary miosis, salivation, diarrhea, nausea or vomiting, abdominal cramps, increased bronchial secretions, sweating, or lacrimation

ACh, Acetylcholine; *IV,* intravenous.

aspects of cognition. The term dementia of the Alzheimer type (DAT) is used to identify this type of dementia, regardless of age. DAT is increasingly recognized as one of the major health problems in the United States, particularly for persons over 65 years of age. It accounts for more than half of the cases of dementia (about 1 to 2 million cases). The major causes of progressive dementia are listed in Table 56-19.

Etiology and Pathophysiology

Although no single cause for DAT has been found, there are several hypotheses regarding the etiology, including disordered immune function, viral infection, and genetic factors.[29] Major research efforts are currently under way to further explore the possible causes of DAT. Cellular changes associated with DAT include neurofibrillary tangles and β-amyloid plaques in the cerebral cortex and hippocampus. There is also an excessive loss of cholinergic neurons, particularly in regions essential for memory and cognition.

There has been much research on the possible genetic etiology of DAT. Genes on chromosome 21 (the site of abnormality for patients with Down syndrome) have been linked to a predisposition to DAT. In the familial form of DAT, the age of onset is younger (50 to 60 years of age) and the severity of the dementia is greater than in nonfamilial cases.

Clinical Manifestations

An initial sign of DAT is a subtle deterioration in memory. Inevitably this progresses to more profound memory loss that interferes with the patient's ability to function. Recent events and new information cannot be recalled. Some patients develop psychotic symptoms. Personal hygiene deteriorates, as does the ability to maintain attention. Later in the disease, long-term memories cannot be recalled, and patients lose the ability to recognize family members. Eventually the ability to communicate and to perform activities of daily living is lost. The progression of the deterioration, which eventually leads to death, varies but can last as long as 20 years.

DAT must be distinguished from depression, a clinically similar condition, because depression is potentially reversible and often responds to appropriate treatment. A careful assessment can distinguish the two clinical conditions (see Table 56-20).

Diagnostic Studies

The diagnosis of DAT is a diagnosis of exclusion. When all other possible conditions that can cause mental impairment have been ruled out and the manifestations of dementia persist, the diagnosis of DAT can be made. A CT scan or an MRI scan may show brain atrophy and enlarged ventricles in the later stages of the disease, although this finding occurs in other diseases and can also be seen in normal persons. Neuropsychologic testing can help document the degree of cognitive dysfunction in the early stages. The definitive diagnosis of DAT can be made only at autopsy, when the presence of neurofibrillary tangles is observed.

Therapeutic and Pharmacologic Management

The therapeutic management of DAT is aimed at controlling the undesirable symptoms that the patient may exhibit. Table 56-21 details the manifestation of symptoms, the usual pharmacologic management, and the possible side

Table 56-19 Major Causes of Progressive Dementia

Cause	%
Senile dementia, Alzheimer type	50%
Multiinfarct (arteriosclerotic)	10%
Combination of senile dementia and multiinfarct	15%
Communicating hydrocephalus Alcoholic or posttraumatic dementia Huntington's chorea Intracranial mass lesions	15%
Uncommon or in combination with other causes Chronic drug use, Creutzfeldt-Jakob disease, metabolic disease (thyroid, liver), nutritional deficits, degenerative disease (spinocerebellar, amyotrophic lateral sclerosis, parkinsonism, multiple sclerosis, Pick's disease, Wilson's disease, epilepsy), AIDS dementia, static postanoxic dementia	10%

AIDS, Acquired immunodeficiency syndrome.
Modified from Andreoli TE and others: *Cecil essentials of medicine,* ed 3, Philadelphia, 1994, Saunders.

Table 56-20 Differentiation of Depression and Dementia of the Alzheimer's Type

Characteristic	Depression	Dementia
Onset	Abrupt (weeks)	Insidious
Psychiatric history	Previous depression common	Usually no history
Mental status	Pervasive dysphoria	Flattening of affect
	Normal or impaired cognition	Impaired cognition
	Variable performance	Stable performance
	Variable memory disturbance	Serious effects on memory
Sleep disturbance	Initial and early-morning insomnia	Frequent awakenings
Somatic complaints	Often multiple	Often none
Self-image	Poor	Normal
Suicidal ideation	Present	Present early in disease, then absent
Treatment	High effectiveness of antidepressants	Very limited usefulness of antidepressants
Weight loss	Yes, with appetite disturbance	Not until late in disease

effects of the prescribed drugs. It is important to be aware that these drugs do not alter the course of the disease.

Many other forms of drug therapy, such as hyperbaric oxygen, routine and megadose vitamins, herbs, algae in the form of manna, and chelation, have been used. None have proved beneficial. Drugs which inhibit the breakdown of acetylcholine in the brain have been studied. In 1993, the drug tacrine, an acetylcholinesterase inhibitor, was approved for DAT. Although it may delay deterioration in cognitive function, its long-term efficacy remains to be determined.[30]

NURSING MANAGEMENT

ALZHEIMER'S DISEASE

Nursing Assessment

Subjective and objective data that should be obtained from a person with Alzheimer's disease are presented in Table 56-22.

Nursing Diagnoses

Nursing diagnoses are determined when the problem and the etiologic factors are supported by clinical data. Nursing diagnoses for Alzheimer's disease may include, but are not limited to, those presented in the nursing care plan for the patient with Alzheimer's disease on p. 1785.

Planning

The overall goals are that the patient with Alzheimer's disease will (1) maintain functional ability for as long as possible, (2) be maintained in a safe environment with a minimum of injuries, and (3) have personal care needs met.

Nursing Implementation

Although there is no current effective treatment for DAT, there is a need for ongoing monitoring of both the patient with DAT and the patient's caregiver. An important nursing responsibility is to work collaboratively with the patient's physician to manage symptoms effectively as they change over time. (See the nursing care plan for the patient with Alzheimer's disease on p. 1785.) The nurse is often responsible for teaching the caregiver to perform the many tasks that are required by this type of patient. The nurse must consider both the patient with DAT and the caregiver as patients with overlapping but unique problems. To aid in identifying the many problems of the caregiver, a nursing care plan for the caregiver of a person with DAT is presented.

Adult day care is one of the options available to the caregivers of a person with DAT. Although programs vary in size, structure, physical environment, and degree of experience of staff, the common goals of all day care programs are to provide respite for the family and a protective environment for the patient.

The middle stage of the disease is probably the most beneficial time for adult day care when the person with DAT can still benefit from stimulating activities that encourage independence and decision making in a protective environment. The patient returns home tired, content, less frustrated, and ready to be with the family. The respite from the demands of care allows the family to be more responsive to the patient's needs.

Although adult day care may delay the transition, the demands on the caregiver eventually exceed the resources, and the person with DAT may be placed in an institutional setting. Special units to care for persons with DAT are becoming increasingly common in long-term care settings. The nursing care needs of the patient with DAT change as the disease progresses, emphasizing the need for regular assessment, monitoring, and support. Regardless of the setting, the severity of the symptoms and the amount of care required intensify over time.

Table 56-21 Pharmacologic Management of Alzheimer's Disease

Manifestation	Drugs	Side Effects
Depression	Tricyclic antidepressants (e.g., nortriptyline [Aventyl, Pamelor], amitriptyline [Elavil], imipramine [Tofranil], doxepin [Sinequan])	Orthostatic hypotension, sedation, dry mouth, constipation, urinary retention, blurry vision
	Nontricyclic antidepressant (e.g., trazodone [Desyrel])	Dry mouth, sedation, confusion
Psychoses and behavioral disturbances	Neuroleptics or antipsychotics (e.g., loxapine [Loxapac], haloperidol [Haldol])	Sedation, extrapyramidal effects, orthostatic hypotension, tardive dyskinesia
	Benzodiazepines (e.g., oxazepam [Serax], diazepam [Valium])	Sedation, confusion, disinhibition with paradoxical agitation, unsteady gait, dysarthria, incoordination
Anxiety	Benzodiazepines	Same as in psychoses and behavioral disturbances
Sleep disturbances	Benzodiazepines, neuroleptics	Same as in psychoses and behavioral disturbances
Decreased memory and cognition	Tacrine (Cognex)	Liver toxicity, nausea and vomiting

Table 56-22 Nursing Assessment: Alzheimer's Disease

Subjective Data

Important health information

Past health history: Repeated head trauma, exposure to metals (especially aluminum), previous CNS infection

Medication: Use of any drug to mitigate symptoms (e.g., tranquilizers, hypnotics, antidepressants)

Functional health patterns

Health perception–health management: Positive family history; fatigue; emotional lability

Cognitive-perceptual: Forgetfulness, inability to cope with complex situations, difficulty with problem solving (early signs)

Objective Data

General

Advanced—Poor hygiene, inability to perform activities of daily living, anorexia, malnutrition, weight loss, incontinence

Neurologic

Early—Loss of recent memory; disorientation to date and time; flat affect; lack of spontaneity; impaired abstraction, cognition, and judgment; loss of remote memory; restlessness and agitation; inability to recognize family and friends; nocturnal wandering; repetitive behavior; loss of social graces; stubbornness, paranoia, belligerence

Advanced—Aphasia, agnosia, alexia (inability to understand written language), seizures

Possible findings

Diagnosis by exclusion, cerebral cortical atrophy on CT scan, poor scores on mental status tests, hippocampal atrophy on MRI scan

CNS, Central nervous system; *CT,* computed tomography; *MRI,* magnetic resonance imaging.

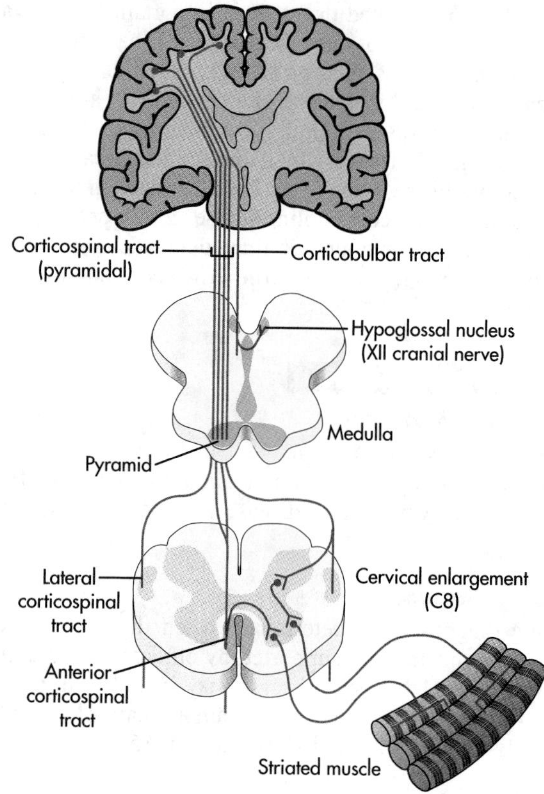

Fig. 56-5 Pathogenesis of amyotrophic lateral sclerosis. This disease is characterized by degeneration of the pyramidal tract and the motor cells in the anterior gray horns. In cases with corticobulbar involvement, the motor nuclei of cranial nerves V, VII, IX, X, XI, and XII also undergo degeneration.

Patients with DAT are subject to acute and other chronic illnesses. Their inability to communicate health symptoms and problems places the responsibility for assessment and diagnosis on caregivers and health professionals. Hospitalization of the patient with DAT can be a traumatic event for both the patient and the caregiver and can precipitate a crisis. Hospitalization often taxes the limited reserve resources of the patient with DAT to the point where adaptation is no longer possible, and the disease seems to worsen quickly.

DAT is a devastating disease that disrupts all aspects of personal and family life. Support groups have been formed throughout the United States to provide an atmosphere of understanding and to give current information about the disease itself and related topics such as safety, legal, ethical, and financial issues. Nurses often receive personal and professional satisfaction in participating in such support groups.

OTHER NEUROLOGIC DISORDERS

Amyotrophic Lateral Sclerosis

Loss of motor neurons is the major morphologic change in *amyotrophic lateral sclerosis* (ALS), a rare progressive neurologic disease that usually leads to death in 2 to 6 years. This disease became known as Lou Gehrig's disease when the famous baseball player was stricken with it in the early 1940s. The onset is between 40 and 70 years of age, and two times as many men as women are affected.

For unknown reasons, motor neurons in the brainstem and spinal cord gradually degenerate in ALS (Fig. 56-5). The dead motor neuron cannot produce or transport vital signals to muscle. Consequently, electrical and chemical messages originating in the brain do not reach the muscles to activate them.

The primary symptoms are weakness of the upper extremities, dysarthria, and dysphagia. Muscle wasting and fasciculations result from the denervation of the muscles and lack of stimulation and use. Death usually results from respiratory infection secondary to compromised respiratory function. Unfortunately, there is no cure and no treatment for ALS. This illness is devastating because the patient remains cognitively intact while wasting away. The challenge of nursing care is to support the patient's cognitive and emotional functions by facilitating communication, providing diversional activities such as reading and human companionship, and helping the person and family with anticipatory grieving related to loss of motor function and ultimate death.

NURSING CARE PLAN Patient with Alzheimer's Disease

Planning: Outcome Criteria	Nursing Interventions and Rationales
➤ **NURSING DIAGNOSIS**	Total self-care deficit *related to* memory deficit, neuromuscular impairment, inability to recognize function of grooming equipment, and inability to distinguish appropriate from inappropriate patterns of dressing, grooming, eating, and toileting *as manifested by* inability to independently and appropriately dress, bathe, groom, or toilet
Be clean and exhibit adequate hygiene; dress and groom appropriately; eat adequate amounts of nutritious foods; establish satisfactory toileting routine.	Assess self-care deficits and determine probable causes *to plan interventions specific to patient's unique problems.* Verbally remind (cue) patient of appropriate activity; demonstrate use of equipment (e.g., toothbrush, hairbrush, washcloth); lay out clothing daily *as memory loss impairs patient's ability to plan and complete specific sequential activities.* Continue to assess self-care capabilities and deficits intervening when necessary *as self-care abilities fluctuate and interventions need to be revised regularly.* Toilet and change incontinence brief as scheduled *to prevent discomfort and skin irritation and promote regularity.* Direct patient to feed self or feed patient if necessary *to ensure adequate food and fluid intake.*
➤ **NURSING DIAGNOSIS**	Sleep pattern disturbance *related to* physical discomfort, environmental changes, excessive napping secondary to inability to initiate activities, and lack of physical activity *as manifested by* erratic sleep patterns, nighttime wandering, daytime sleepiness
Have reasonable periods of uninterrupted rest at appropriate times.	Monitor patient's sleep pattern or get report from caregiver *to plan appropriate interventions.* Ensure that patient's physical needs are met related to bedtime (e.g., patient is toileted, room temperature is comfortable, environment is quiet) *to prevent physical discomfort from interfering with quality sleep.* Adapt usual nightly habits such as bedtime, night lights, warm milk *to provide as much continuity as feasible.* Reassure wakened patient and reorient in soft, soothing tone (e.g., "It's nighttime. It is time to go back to bed") *to avoid development of anxiety and fear.* Prevent patient from taking excessive naps *to promote nighttime tiredness.* Identify and initiate appropriate daytime diversional activities; plan and implement periods of physical activity during the day *to prevent napping and foster nighttime tiredness.*
➤ **NURSING DIAGNOSIS**	Altered health maintenance *related to* impaired communication ability, short-term memory deficit, and cognitive impairment *as manifested by* inability to monitor health status
Have prompt diagnosis and treatment of acute illness; have optimal physical health status.	Complete physical assessment on initial contact *to determine physical status for baseline data and to plan appropriate interventions.* Monitor physical status *to evaluate plan of care and make revisions as necessary.* Assess any acute changes in behavior promptly and refer for adequate workup *as patient is unable to report health problems and must rely on staff to note and follow-up problems.* Use simple questions requiring "yes" or "no" answers when questioning patient *to avoid confusing patient by questions requiring complex answers.* Point directly to body parts when attempting to ascertain site of discomfort or pain *to increase patient's understanding and likelihood of accurate response.*
➤ **NURSING DIAGNOSIS**	Risk for injury *related to* impaired judgment, possible gait instability, muscle weakness, and sensory or perceptual alteration
Have no accidental injuries.	Assess regularly for bruises, abrasions, broken bones, and burns *to determine presence of injury.* Monitor activity; maintain environment free from safety hazards, such as cluttered walkways, slippery floors, matches, high water temperatures, medications, possibility of wandering *to decrease or prevent occurrence of injury.* Assess and record extent of physical limitation (if any) *so appropriate adjustments can be made in care routine and environment.* Provide assistance when necessary *so patient's needs are met.* Incorporate ambulation into care plan *to prevent problems associated with immobility.* Plan and implement periods of safe activity during the day *to provide mental stimulation and foster sleep.*

continued

NURSING CARE PLAN Patient with Alzheimer's Disease—cont'd

Planning: Outcome Criteria	Nursing Interventions and Rationales
➤ **NURSING DIAGNOSIS**	Risk for violence *related to* sensory overload, misinterpretation of environmental stimuli, lack of appropriate coping mechanisms, and unfamiliar environment
Have no self-directed or other-directed physical trauma.	Monitor for risk factors such as acting out behavior, verbal threats, and agitation *to identify possibility of violent behavior and initiate appropriate nursing plan.* Prevent sensory overload; avoid giving patient tasks that prove frustrating *to avoid triggering violent behavior.* Ensure adequate sleep and rest periods *as tiredness and exhaustion can provoke violence.* Provide opportunities for patient to vent anxiety and frustration *to prevent these emotions from escalating to a catastrophic reaction.* Observe and document in detail any catastrophic reaction and precipitating events *so interventions can be incorporated into care plan to prevent recurrence.*
➤ **NURSING DIAGNOSIS**	Ineffective individual coping *related to* depression in response to diagnosis of Alzheimer's disease *as manifested by* depression, withdrawal, fatigue, social isolation
Have feeling of value as individual.	Assess for possibility and extent of depression *to develop appropriate interventions.* Provide opportunity for patient to verbalize feelings *to help clarify issues and show a caring attitude.* Facilitate communication between patient and family *to foster mutual understanding about relevant issues.* Provide appropriate diversional activities *to provide pleasurable activities to relieve depression.* Allow patient to make decisions regarding self-care and environment when possible *to increase sense of worth and control.* Refer for further evaluation and counseling if indicated.
➤ **NURSING DIAGNOSIS**	Risk for ineffective management of therapeutic regimen *related to* decreasing level of cognitive functioning and memory
Have care and treatment needs met by self or others as condition deteriorates.	Discuss with patient the need to make plans for care as condition deteriorates *to ensure patient's wishes are respected and health needs are met.* Assist patient to make lifestyle adjustments such as labeling items and ceasing driving *to compensate for changing cognitive status and live independently as long as possible.*
➤ **NURSING DIAGNOSIS**	Altered thought processes *related to* effects of dementia *as manifested by* loss of memory and cognitive deficits
Participate in care discussions and social activities to maximum level of ability.	Assess extent of cognitive deficits by direct contact with patient and information from family *to plan appropriate interventions.* Plan strategies to promote communication, increase self-esteem, and provide stimulation *to maximize patient's cognitive abilities.* Avoid confusion by such means as reality orientation (early) and adhering to a schedule; do not challenge patient by asking questions patient cannot answer *to decrease patient's stress and prevent a catastrophic reaction.*

NURSING CARE PLAN Caregiver of the Patient with Alzheimer's Disease

Planning: Outcome Criteria	*Nursing Interventions and Rationales*
➤ **NURSING DIAGNOSIS**	Ineffective individual coping *related to* unrelieved caregiving responsibilities, inadequate support systems, perceived powerlessness, fatigue secondary to interrupted sleep pattern, and lack of knowledge regarding coping strategies and strategies for behavioral management and relaxation techniques *as manifested by* fatigue; verbalization of inability to cope; inability to meet needs, make decisions, or ask for help; frequent illness or accidents; inappropriate defense mechanisms
Verbalize confidence in ability to cope effectively with long-term caregiving responsibilities.	Assess health status of caregiver *to determine if health planning is needed.* Refer for medical evaluation when appropriate. Instruct in relaxation and effective coping strategies; assess knowledge of Alzheimer's disease process and management techniques; assist caregiver in defining problem areas and assist with problem-solving techniques *to bolster caregiver's ability to cope.* Instruct in management of problem behaviors referring for medical management when indicated *to reduce stress-producing situations.* Evaluate caregiver's readiness and motivation to use community resources *as caregivers are often reluctant to relinquish care responsibilities.*
➤ **NURSING DIAGNOSIS**	Social isolation *related to* diminishing social relationships secondary to unrelieved caregiving responsibilities, behavioral problems of patient with Alzheimer's disease, and underdeveloped social support system *as manifested by* feelings of abandonment and uselessness, behavior changes (irritability, hypoactivity, depression, withdrawal), eating changes, inability to make decisions or concentrate
Have satisfactory contact with significant others or members of a support group.	Assess past social network and diversional activities *to determine size and scope of network and personal interests.* Assess social support system of family and willingness and ability to participate in care *to develop care alternatives.* Assist in planning respite care through this system or formal community resources *to enable caregiver to continue with important activities and social contacts.* Refer to social services *for realistic appraisal of financial resources for respite care and for linkage to community resources.* Provide information regarding available support groups (e.g., Alzheimer's Disease and Related Disorders Association) *as these groups can help meet socialization, recreational, and educational needs of caregiver.*
➤ **NURSING DIAGNOSIS**	Anxiety *related to* uncertain outcome, perceived powerlessness, possible change in role functioning, erratic behavioral patterns of the person with Alzheimer's disease, high risk for injury secondary to possible violent reactions of patient, and financial insecurity *as manifested by* autonomic changes (e.g., tachycardia, hypertension), apprehension, helplessness, fear, irritability, cognitive changes (e.g., forgetfulness, inability to concentrate)
Have decreased anxiety; has sense of control of situation.	Assess past roles of patient with Alzheimer's disease and of caregiver *to determine extent of role changes required of caregiver.* Document changes in role expectations and refer to community resources or provide instruction as needed; assess knowledge of behavioral management techniques and instruct as appropriate; assist caregiver in problem-solving techniques; assist in looking at possible causes of catastrophic reactions as well as indications of agitation which may indicate their onset *to ensure that caregiver has skills to manage changing roles and patient status.* Refer to social services as indicated for complete list of community resources and possible sources of financial aid *to relieve anxiety related to financial insecurity.*
➤ **NURSING DIAGNOSIS**	Risk for altered health maintenance *related to* unrelieved caregiving responsibilities, fatigue, and chronic stress *as manifested by* failure to care for self
Have optimal health; practices appropriate health practices for age and sex.	Assess physical and emotional health status of caregiver *to determine if problem is present and to plan appropriate interventions.* Collaborate with caregiver in planning interventions in major identified problem areas *to prevent further deterioration of health.* Refer for additional evaluation if indicated. Assist with planning of continued care of patient *so that caregiver's personal health needs can be pursued.* Stress need for maintaining own health *to avoid increasing the complexity of the caregiving situation.*

continued

NURSING CARE PLAN Caregiver of the Patient with Alzheimer's Disease—cont'd

Planning: Outcome Criteria	Nursing Interventions and Rationales
➤ **NURSING DIAGNOSIS**	Risk for ineffective family coping *related to* chronic and deteriorating nature of Alzheimer's disease, feelings of helplessness and hopelessness, increasing financial hardship, and disappearing support systems *as manifested by* verbalization of lack of help and hope in caring for family member, concern over finances, deteriorating emotional and physical health of caregiver.
Have no evidence of destructive coping behaviors.	Encourage family to discuss caregiving situation with one another *so consensus can be reached regarding plan of care.* Provide information on community resources such as day care, support groups, counseling, and respite care *to relieve stress and facilitate coping.* Encourage and support family in their caregiving efforts *to bolster persons involved in a difficult situation.* Refer for assistance with financial concerns. Provide information on nature and course of Alzheimer's disease *so appropriate plans can be made for the patient based on accurate information.*

Huntington's Disease

Huntington's disease is a genetically transmitted, autosomal dominant disorder that affects both men and women of all races. The offspring of a person with this disease have a 50% risk of inheriting it. The diagnosis often occurs after the affected individual has had children. In the United States, approximately 25,000 persons have Huntington's disease and another 150,000 have a 50-50 chance of developing it.[31] Diagnosis is based on family history, clinical symptoms, and the detection of the characteristic DNA pattern from blood samples.

Like Parkinson's disease, the pathology of Huntington's disease involves the basal ganglia and the extrapyramidal motor system. However, instead of a deficiency of DA, Huntington's disease involves a deficiency of the neurotransmitters ACh and GABA. The net effect is an excess of DA, which leads to symptoms that are the opposite of those of parkinsonism. The clinical manifestations, the onset of which is between 35 and 45 years of age, are characterized by abnormal and excessive involuntary movements (chorea). These are writhing, twisting movements of the face, limbs, and body. The movements get worse as the disease progresses. Facial movements involving speech, chewing, and swallowing are affected and may cause aspiration and malnutrition. The gait deteriorates, and ambulation eventually becomes impossible. Perhaps the most devastating deterioration is in mental functions, which include intellectual decline, emotional lability, and psychotic behavior. Death usually occurs 10 to 20 years after the onset of symptoms.

Because there is no cure, therapeutic management is palliative. Antipsychotic, antidepressant, and antichorea medications are prescribed and have some effect. However, they do not alter the course of the disease. This disease presents a great challenge to health care professionals. The goal of nursing management is to provide the most comfortable environment possible for the patient and the family by maintaining physical safety, treating the physical symptoms, and providing emotional and psychologic support. Because of the choreic movements, caloric requirements are high. Patients may require as high as 4000 to 5000 calories per day to maintain body weight. As the disease progresses, meeting caloric needs becomes a greater challenge when the patient has difficulty swallowing and holding the head still. Depression and mental deterioration can also compromise nutritional intake. Genetic counseling is very important.

CRITICAL THINKING EXERCISES

CASE STUDY

MULTIPLE SCLEROSIS

Patient Profile

Ms. S., a 32-year-old Caucasian woman, born and raised in Minneapolis, was diagnosed with multiple sclerosis after a 2-year history of deteriorating health.

Subjective Data

- Has difficulty seeing out of the right eye
- Has numbness and tingling on the left side that worsens in hot weather
- Tires easily
- Has used all sick days at work. Concerned about losing her job and ability to care for 3-year-old son

Objective Data

Physical Examination

- Crying softly during interview
- Tense and anxious

Diagnostic Studies

- Prolonged visual evoked response in right eye
- MRI scan of head shows several plaques in white matter

Critical Thinking Questions

1. What is the pathogenesis of multiple sclerosis?
2. What precipitating factors for multiple sclerosis are present in Ms. S's life?
3. Why did it take so long for a definitive diagnosis to be made for Ms. S?
4. What teaching plan should be developed for Ms. S?
5. What treatment would be appropriate for Ms. S?
6. Write one or more appropriate nursing diagnoses based on the assessment data presented. Are there any collaborative problems?

NURSING RESEARCH ISSUES

1. What are the most effective nonpharmacologic methods of relieving migraine headaches?
2. How can caregivers of patients with Alzheimer's disease be helped to deal with their situation?
3. What are the most effective ways to assist patients with chronic neurologic problems to maintain a positive self-esteem?
4. Do patients with chronic neurologic disorders who are actively involved in an exercise program have an improved self-concept?
5. What is the quality of life for patients with epilepsy?

REVIEW QUESTIONS

The number of the question corresponds to the same-numbered objective at the beginning of the chapter.

1. Chronic neurologic disease often involves
   a. decreased nutritional requirements.
   b. progressive physical deterioration.
   c. only the elderly.
   d. a surgical cure.

2. Which behaviors are typical of a patient with migraine headaches?
   a. Seeking shelter from stimuli
   b. Seeking company of others
   c. Pacing the floor
   d. Acting out

3. The triad of symptoms common in Parkinson's disease is
   a. diplopia, tremor, bradykinesia.
   b. tremor, rigidity, bradykinesia.
   c. spasticity, diplopia, tremor.
   d. ataxia, drowsiness, dysarthria.

4. Nursing interventions for the patient with MS are aimed at management of
   a. incontinence, depression, spasticity.
   b. incontinence, hallucinations, tremor.
   c. bradykinesia, rigidity, tremor.
   d. rigidity, incontinence, diplopia.

5. The most common cause of death in ALS is
   a. cerebral infarction.
   b. renal failure.
   c. pulmonary embolus.
   d. respiratory infection.

6. Common physical complications of a patient who is immobilized by a chronic neurologic disease are
   a. constipation, skin breakdown, pneumonia.
   b. cerebral infarction.
   c. diarrhea.
   d. spasticity.

7. A major goal of treatment for the patient with a chronic, progressive neurologic disease is
   a. continuation of usual lifestyle.
   b. cure.
   c. adjustment by patient and family to the disease.
   d. total remission of the disease.

REFERENCES

1. Silberstein S: Advances in understanding the pathophysiology of headache, *Neurology* 42(Suppl 2):6, 1992.
2. Stewart WF and others: Prevalence of migraine headache in the United States, *JAMA* 267:64, 1992.
3. Solomon S: Migraine: current approaches to diagnosis and management, *Hosp Pract* 26:141, 1991.
4. Mathew NT: Cluster headache, *Neurology* 42(Suppl 2):22, 1992.
5. Schulman EA, Silberstein SD: Symptomatic and prophylactic treatment of migraine and tension type headache, *Neurology* 42(Suppl 2):16, 1992.
6. Edmeads J: Headache and facial pain. In Stein JH, editor: *Internal medicine,* ed 4, St Louis, 1994, Mosby.
7. Plosker GL, McTavish D: Sumatriptan: a reappraisal of its pharmacology and therapeutic efficacy in the acute treatment of migraine and cluster headache, *Drugs* 47:622, 1994.
8. Trotsky MB: Neurogenic vascular headaches, food and chemical triggers, *Ear Nose Throat J* 73:228, 1994.
9. Anngeners JF: The epidemiology of epilepsy. In Wyllie E, editor: *The treatment of epilepsy: principles and practice,* Philadelphia, 1993, Lea & Febiger.
10. Trieman L, Trieman DM: Genetic aspects of epilepsy. In Wyllie E, editor: *The treatment of epilepsy: principles and practice,* Philadelphia, 1993, Lea & Febiger.
11. Mody I: The molecular basis of kindling, *Brain Pathol* 3:395, 1993.
12. Gastaut H: Clinical and electroencephalographical classification of epileptic seizures, *Epilepsia* 11:102, 1970.
13. Commission on Classification and Terminology of the International League Against Epilepsy: Proposal for the revised clinical and electroencephalographic classification of epileptic seizures, *Epilepsia* 22:249, 1981.
14. National Institutes of Health Consensus Conference: Surgery for epilepsy, *JAMA* 264:729, 1990.
15. Matthews WB and others: *McAlpine's multiple sclerosis,* Edinburgh, 1991, Churchill-Livingstone.
16. Dean G: How many people in the world have multiple sclerosis? *Neuroepidemiology* 13:1, 1994.
17. Abramsky O: Pregnancy and multiple sclerosis, *Ann Neurol* 36:S38, 1994.
18. Wolinsky J: Multiple sclerosis, *Curr Neurol* 13:167, 1993.
19. The INFB Multiple Sclerosis Study Group: Interferon beta 1b is effective in relapsing-remitting multiple sclerosis, *Neurology* 43:655, 1993.
20. Panitch HS: Influence of infection on exacerbation of multiple sclerosis, *Ann Neurol* 36:S25. 1994.
21. Adams RA, Victor M: *Principles of neurology,* ed 5, New York, 1993, McGraw-Hill.
22. Svenson L: Regional disparities in the annual prevalence rates of Parkinson's disease in Canada, *Neuroepidemiology* 10:205, 1991.
23. Calne DB: Diagnosis and treatment of Parkinson's disease, *Hosp Pract* 30:83, 1995.
24. Scharre DW, Mahler ME: Parkinson's disease: making the diagnosis, selecting drug therapies, *Geriatrics* 49:14, 1994.
25. Diamond SG and others: Four year follow-up of adrenal-to-brain transplants in Parkinson's disease, *Arch Neurol* 51:559,1994.
26. Remond DE and others: Neural transplantation for neurodegenerative diseases: past, present and future, *Ann NY Acad Sci* 695:258, 1993.
27. Ahlskog JE: Treatment of Parkinson's disease: from theory to practice, *Postgrad Med* 95:52, 1994.
28. Lanska DJ: Indications for thymectomy in myasthenia gravis, *Neurology* 40:1828, 1990.
29. Cummings JL, Benson DF: *Dementia: a clinical approach,* ed 2, Boston, 1992, Butterworth-Heinemann.
30. Davis KL and others: A double-blind, placebo-controlled multicenter study of tacrine for Alzheimer's disease, *N Engl J Med* 327:1253, 1992.
31. France JK: Huntington's disease: helping the patient retain function, *Am J Nurs* 93:62, 1993.

Chapter 57

NURSING ROLE IN MANAGEMENT

Peripheral Nerve and Spinal Cord Problems

Diane H. Michalec   Connie A. Walleck

Learning Objectives

1. Explain the etiology, clinical manifestations, and therapeutic and nursing management of trigeminal neuralgia and Bell's palsy.
2. Explain the etiology, clinical manifestations, and treatment of Guillain-Barré syndrome, botulism, tetanus, and neurosyphilis.
3. Identify the population at risk for spinal cord injuries.
4. Describe the classification of spinal cord injuries and associated manifestations.
5. Describe the clinical manifestations and therapeutic and nursing management of spinal cord shock.
6. Correlate the clinical manifestations of spinal cord injury with the level of disruption and rehabilitation potential.
7. Describe the nursing management of the major physical and psychologic problems of the patient with a spinal cord injury.
8. Explain the types, clinical manifestations, and therapeutic and nursing management of spinal cord tumors.

CRANIAL NERVE DISORDERS

Cranial nerve disorders are commonly classified as peripheral neuropathies. The 12 pairs of cranial nerves are considered the peripheral nerves of the brain. The disorders usually involve the motor or sensory (or both) branches of a single nerve (*mononeuropathies*). Causes of cranial nerve problems include tumors, trauma, infections, inflammatory processes, and idiopathic (unknown) causes. Two common cranial nerve disorders are trigeminal neuralgia (tic douloureux) and acute peripheral facial paralysis (Bell's palsy).

Trigeminal Neuralgia

Pathophysiology. *Trigeminal neuralgia* (tic douloureux) is a relatively common cranial nerve disorder with an overall yearly incidence rate of 4.3 per 100,000 persons.[1] It is more commonly seen in women and usually begins in the fifth or sixth decade of life. The trigeminal nerve is the fifth cranial nerve (CN V) and has both motor and sensory branches. Only the sensory branches are involved in trigeminal neuralgia, primarily the maxillary and mandibular branches[2] (Fig. 57-1).

Reviewed by Richard Buhrer, RN, MN, CRRN, Veterans Administration Medical Center, Seattle, WA; and Sally A. Weiss, RN, MSN, Associate Professor, Broward Community College, Pembroke Pines, FL.

Although no specific cause has been identified, nerve compression by tortuous arteries of the posterior fossa blood vessels, demyelinating plaques, herpes virus infection, infection of teeth and jaw, and a brainstem infarct have been suggested as initiating pathologic events.[3] The effectiveness of antiepileptic drug therapy in shortening or suppressing the duration of an attack suggests a cell membrane defect similar to that in epilepsy.

Clinical Manifestations. The classic feature of trigeminal neuralgia is an abrupt onset of paroxysms of excruciating pain described as a burning, knifelike, or lightninglike shock in the lips, upper or lower gums, cheek, forehead, or side of the nose. Intense pain, twitching, grimacing, and frequent blinking and tearing of the eye occur during the acute attack (giving rise to the term *tic*). The attacks are usually brief, lasting seconds to 2 or 3 minutes, and are generally unilateral. Recurrences are unpredictable; they may occur several times a day or weeks or months apart. After the refractory (pain-free) period, a phenomenon known as *clustering* can occur that is characterized by a cycle of pain and refractoriness that continues for hours.

The painful episodes are usually initiated by a triggering mechanism of light cutaneous stimulation at a specific point (*trigger zone*) along the distribution of the nerve branches. Precipitating stimuli include chewing, teeth brushing, a hot or cold blast of air on the face, washing the face, yawning,

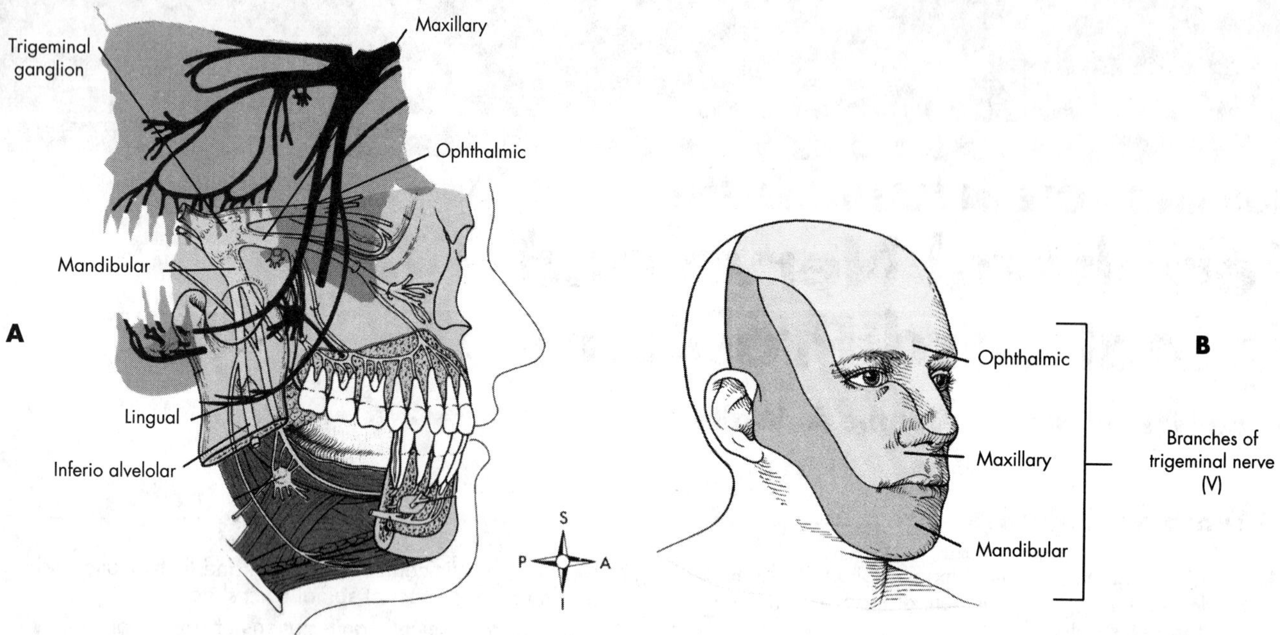

Fig. 57-1 ***A,*** Trigeminal (fifth cranial nerve) and its three main divisions, the ophthalmic, maxillary, and mandibular nerves. ***B,*** Cutaneous innervation of the head.

or even talking. Touch and tickle seem to predominate as causative triggers rather than pain or changes in temperature. As a result, the patient may not eat properly, neglect hygienic practices, wear a cloth over the face, and withdraw from interaction with other individuals. The patient may sleep excessively as a means of coping with the pain.

Although this condition is considered benign, the severity of the pain and the disruption of lifestyle can result in almost total physical and psychologic dysfunction or even suicide.

Therapeutic Management. The physician must rule out other problems with similar manifestations such as other forms of facial and cephalic neuralgias and pain arising from the sinuses, teeth, and jaws. A complete neurologic assessment is done, although results are usually normal. Once the diagnosis is made, the goal of treatment is relief of pain either medically or surgically (Tables 57-1 and 57-2). The majority of patients obtain adequate relief through antiepileptic drugs such as diphenylhydantoin (Dilantin) and carbamazepine (Tegretol). These drugs may prevent an acute attack or promote a remission of symptoms, although the mechanism by which they work is not known. These drugs may cause bone marrow suppression, leading to blood abnormalities, and routine complete blood cell (CBC) counts are required. Unfortunately, these drugs may lose their effectiveness and are not a permanent solution. Some patients may seek help repeatedly by numerous visits to otolaryngologists or from therapies such as acupuncture and megavitamins.

Nerve blocking with local anesthetics is another treatment possibility. Local nerve blocking results in complete anesthesia of the area supplied by the injected branches. Relief of pain is temporary, lasting from 6 to 18 months. This treatment is usually tolerated well by older adults.

Biofeedback is another strategy for pain management. For patients who are alert enough to understand the simple equipment and who can learn to use biofeedback to regulate one physiologic parameter such as heart rate, biofeedback offers an innovative approach to the control of the pain. In addition to controlling the pain, the patients also experience a strong sense of personal control by mastering the technique and altering certain body functions.

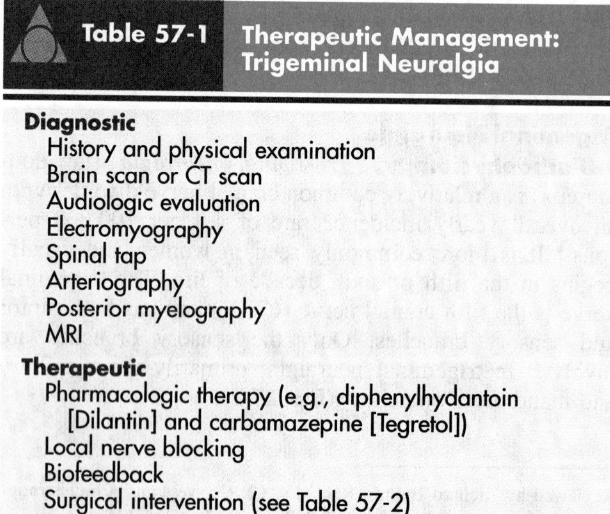

Table 57-1 Therapeutic Management: Trigeminal Neuralgia

Diagnostic
- History and physical examination
- Brain scan or CT scan
- Audiologic evaluation
- Electromyography
- Spinal tap
- Arteriography
- Posterior myelography
- MRI

Therapeutic
- Pharmacologic therapy (e.g., diphenylhydantoin [Dilantin] and carbamazepine [Tegretol])
- Local nerve blocking
- Biofeedback
- Surgical intervention (see Table 57-2)

CT, Computed tomography; *MRI,* magnetic resonance imaging.

Table 57-2 Surgical Interventions for Trigeminal Neuralgia

Procedure	Technique	Benefit
Peripheral		
Glycerol injection into one or more branches of the trigeminal nerve	Chemical ablation	Total pain relief with sparing of touch and corneal reflex
Intracranial		
Retrogasserian rhizotomy	Temporal craniotomy (sectioning of sensory root in middle cranial fossa)	Permanent anesthesia (with adeptness, corneal reflex, touch)
Suboccipital craniotomy	Sectioning of sensory root of posterior fossa	Permanent anesthesia
Percutaneous radiofrequency rhizotomy	Destruction of sensory fibers by low-voltage current	Total pain relief, sparing of touch and corneal reflex (increased risk for sensory changes)
Microvascular decompression (Jannetta procedure)	Lifting of artery pressing on nerve root in posterior fossa with wedge of sponge, leading to removal of pressure at nerve-root entry zone.	Permanent pain relief without loss of sensation

Surgical interventions. If a conservative approach is not effective, surgical therapy is available (Table 57-2). *Percutaneous radiofrequency rhizotomy* (electrocoagulation) and *microvascular decompression* afford the greatest relief of pain. Percutaneous radiofrequency rhizotomy consists of placing a needle into the trigeminal rootlets that are adjacent to the pons and destroying the area by means of a radiofrequency current. This can result in anesthesia of the face (although some degree of sensation may be retained) or trigeminal motor weakness. Irritation or inadvertent destruction of the ophthalmic branches of the nerve can result in loss of the corneal reflex. This procedure is easily performed with minimal risk to the patient. It is tolerated well by older adults and avoids a major operative procedure in the high-risk patient.[4] *Glycerol rhizotomy* has become more popular in the last 10 years and is preferred over percutaneous radiofrequency rhizotomy. Glycerol rhizotomy consists of an injection of glycerol through the foramen ovale into the trigeminal cistern (Fig. 57-2). Glycerol rhizotomy is a more benign procedure with less sensory loss and fewer sensory aberrations than radiofrequency rhizotomy and with comparable or better pain relief.[5]

Microvascular decompression of the trigeminal nerve is accomplished by displacing and repositioning blood vessels that appear to be compressing the nerve at the root-entry zone where it exits the pons. This procedure relieves pain without residual sensory loss but is potentially dangerous, as is any surgery near the brainstem. Microvascular decompression may be poorly tolerated in older adults because manipulation of the brainstem may result in blood pressure fluctuations. Such fluctuations can be dangerous if the cardiovascular system is already compromised.

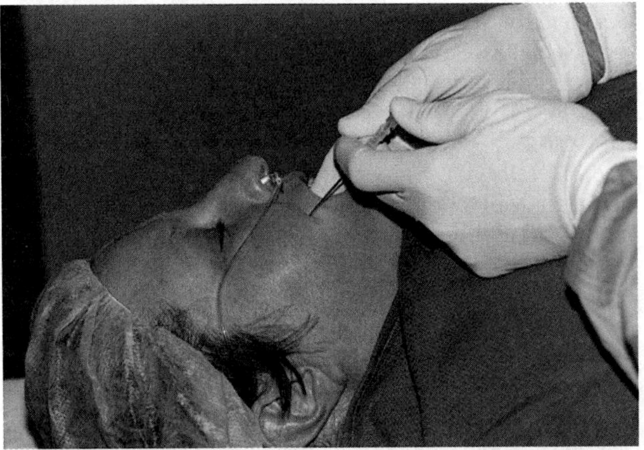

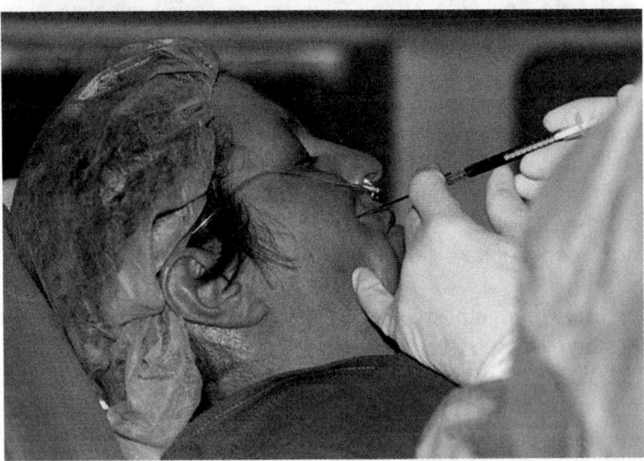

Fig. 57-2 ***A,*** Patient with trigeminal neuralgia having needle placed. ***B,*** Physician injecting glycerol.

NURSING MANAGEMENT

TRIGEMINAL NEURALGIA

Nursing Assessment

Assessment of the attacks, including the triggering factors, characteristics, frequency, and pain management techniques, helps the nurse plan for patient care. The nursing assessment should include the patient's nutritional status, hygiene (especially oral), and behavior (including withdrawal). Evaluation of the degree of pain and its effects on the patient's lifestyle, drug history, emotional state, and suicidal tendencies are other important factors.

Nursing Diagnoses

Nursing diagnoses specific to the patient with trigeminal neuralgia include, but are not limited to, the following:

- Pain related to inflammation or compression of the trigeminal nerve
- Altered nutrition: less than body requirements related to fear of eating causing pain
- Anxiety related to uncertainty of timing and initiating event of pain and uncertainty regarding effectiveness of pain-relieving treatments
- Risk for altered oral mucous membranes related to unwillingness to practice oral hygiene measures secondary to potential for initiating pain
- Social isolation related to anxiety over pain attacks and desire to maintain nonstimulating environment

Planning

The overall goals are that the patient with trigeminal neuralgia will (1) be free of pain, (2) maintain adequate nutritional and oral hygiene status, (3) have minimal to no anxiety, and (4) return to normal or previous socialization and occupational activities.

Nursing Implementation

Acute Intervention Pain relief is primarily obtained by the administration of the recommended drug therapy. The nurse should monitor the patient's response to therapy and note any side effects. Strong narcotics such as morphine should be used cautiously because of the potential for addiction over time. Moderate use of propoxyphene (Darvon) or pentazocine (Talwin) is acceptable. Alternative pain relief measures, such as biofeedback, should be explored for the patient who is not a surgical candidate and whose pain is not controlled by other therapeutic measures. Careful assessment of pain, including history, pain relief, and drug dependency, can assist in selecting appropriate interventions.

Environmental management is essential during an acute period to lessen triggering stimuli. The room should be kept at an even, moderate temperature and free of drafts. A private room is preferred during an acute period. The nurse must use care to avoid touching the patient's face or jarring the bed. Many patients prefer to carry out their own care, fearing that they will be inadvertently injured by someone else.

The nurse should instruct the patient about the importance of nutrition, hygiene, and oral care, conveying understanding if previous neglect is apparent. The nurse should provide lukewarm water and soft cloths or cotton saturated with solutions not requiring rinsing for cleansing the face. A small, very soft bristled toothbrush or a warm mouthwash assist in promoting oral care. Hygiene activities are best carried out when analgesia is at its peak.

The patient will probably not engage in extensive conversation during the acute period. Alternative communication methods such as paper and pencil should be provided.

Food should be high in protein and calories and easy to chew. It should be served lukewarm and offered frequently. The diet should be individualized according to personal, cultural, and religious preferences. When oral intake is sharply reduced and the patient's nutritional status is compromised, a nasogastric tube is inserted on the unaffected side for nasogastric feedings.

The nurse is responsible for instruction related to diagnostic studies to rule out other problems, such as acoustic neuroma and neoplasms, and preoperative teaching if surgery is planned. The nurse may also need to reinforce the surgeon's instructions related to postoperative expectations; appropriate teaching of postoperative activities depends on whether a craniotomy or a local procedure is planned. The patient needs to know that he will be awake during local procedures so that he can cooperate when corneal and ciliary reflexes and facial sensations are checked.

After the operation the patient's pain is compared with the preoperative level. The corneal reflex, extraocular muscles, hearing, sensation, and facial nerve function are evaluated frequently (see Chapter 53). General postoperative nursing care after a craniotomy is appropriate if intracranial surgery is performed. Diet and ambulation should be increased according to the patient's progress or specific orders.

After a radiofrequency percutaneous electrocoagulation procedure, an ice pack is applied to the jaw on the operative side for 3 to 5 hours. To avoid injuring the mouth, the patient should not chew on the operative side until sensation has returned.

Chronic and Home Management. Regular follow-up care should be planned. The patient needs instruction regarding the dosage and side effects of medications. Although relief of pain may be complete, the patient should be encouraged to keep environmental stimuli to a moderate level and to use stress reduction methods. Herpes simplex infection (cold sores) can occur from manipulation of the gasserian ganglion. Treatment consists of topical antiviral agents such as acyclovir (see Chapter 20).

Long-term management after surgical intervention depends on the residual effects of the type of procedure. If anesthesia is present or the corneal reflex is altered, the patient should be taught to (1) chew on the unaffected side; (2) avoid hot foods or beverages, which can burn the mucous membranes; (3) check the oral cavity after meals to remove food particles; (4) practice meticulous oral hygiene and continue with semiannual dental visits; (5) protect the face against extremes of temperature; (6) use an electric razor; and (7) wear a protective eye shield.

The patient may have developed protective practices to prevent pain and may need counseling or psychiatric assistance in the readjustment, especially in reestablishing personal relationships. Some patients grieve the loss of the pain, especially if it had a special significance such as relieving guilt or anxiety. Occasionally patients may have used their pain to manipulate family members and friends and may not adjust after successful relief of pain. Careful management in the rehabilitative period can prevent the patient from claiming continual pain for secondary gain (see Chapter 6).

Bell's Palsy

Pathophysiology. *Bell's palsy* (peripheral facial paralysis, acute benign cranial polyneuritis) is a disorder characterized by a disruption of the motor branches of the facial nerve (CN VII) on one side of the face in the absence of any other disease such as a stroke. It can affect any age group, but it is more commonly seen in the 20- to 60-year age range. The cause is still unknown, but current theories suggest that the herpes simplex virus may cause inflammation and demyelination of the nerve.

The onset of Bell's palsy is often accompanied by an outbreak of herpes vesicles in or around the ear. Bell's palsy is considered benign, with full recovery after 3 to 4 months in about 85% of patients, especially if treatment is instituted immediately. A small number of patients may have some residual effects. Failure to show spontaneous recovery after 6 months indicates that the problem is probably not Bell's palsy.

Clinical Manifestations and Complications. The paralysis of the motor branches of the facial nerve typically results in a flaccidity of the affected side of the face, with drooping of the mouth accompanied by drooling (Fig. 57-3). An inability to close the bottom eyelid, with an upward movement of the eyeball when closure is attempted, is also evident. A widened palpebral fissure (the opening between the eyelids), flattening of the nasolabial fold, and inability to smile, frown, or whistle are also common. Unilateral loss of taste is common. Decreased muscle movement may alter chewing ability, and although some patients may experience a loss of tearing, many patients complain of excessive tearing. The muscle weakness causes the lower lid to turn out, allowing overflow of normal tear production. Pain may be present behind the ear on the affected side, especially before the onset of paralysis.

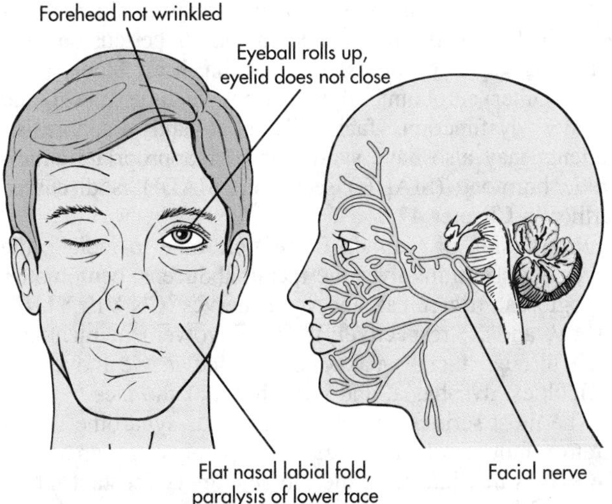

Fig. 57-3 Bell's palsy: facial characteristics.

Interventions are primarily supportive until the patient has a return of function. Complications can include psychologic withdrawal because of changes in appearance, malnutrition and dehydration, mucous membrane trauma, muscle stretching, and facial spasms and contractures.

Therapeutic Management. The diagnosis of Bell's palsy and its prognosis are indicated by observation of the typical pattern of onset and signs and testing of percutaneous nerve excitability. Corticosteroids, especially prednisone, are started immediately, and the best results are obtained if corticosteroids are initiated before paralysis is complete. When the patient improves to the point that the corticosteroids are no longer necessary, they should be tapered off over a 2-week period. Usually the steroid treatment decreases the edema and pain, but mild analgesics can be used if necessary. Other methods of treatment include moist heat, gentle massage, and electrical stimulation of the nerve. Stimulation may maintain muscle tone and prevent atrophy. Care is primarily focused on relief of symptoms and prevention of complications.

NURSING MANAGEMENT

BELL'S PALSY

Nursing Assessment

Early recognition of the possibility of Bell's palsy is important. Because herpes simplex is a possible etiologic factor, any person who is prone to herpes simplex should be alerted to seek health care if pain occurs in or around the ear. Assessment of facial muscles for any signs of weakness should also be done (see Chapter 53). Careful recording of assessment data provides information related to the progress of the syndrome.

Nursing Diagnoses

The nursing diagnoses specific to the patient with Bell's palsy include, but are not limited to, the following:

- Pain related to the inflammation of CN VII (facial)
- Altered nutrition: less than body requirements related to inability to chew secondary to muscle weakness
- Risk for trauma to the eye (corneal abrasion) related to inability to blink
- Body-image disturbance related to change in facial appearance secondary to facial muscle weakness

Planning

The overall goals are that the patient with Bell's palsy will (1) be pain free or have pain controlled, (2) maintain adequate nutritional status, (3) not experience injury to the eye, (4) return to normal or previous perception of body image, and (5) be optimistic about disease outcome.

Nursing Implementation

Mild analgesics can relieve pain. Hot wet packs can reduce the discomfort of herpetic lesions and aid circulation and relieve pain. The face should be protected from cold and drafts because trigeminal hyperesthesia may accompany the syndrome. Maintenance of good nutrition is important. The patient should be taught to chew on the unaffected side of the mouth to avoid trapping food and to enjoy the taste of food. Thorough oral hygiene must be carried out after each meal to prevent the development of parotitis, caries, and periodontal disease from accumulated residual food.

Dark glasses may be worn for protective and cosmetic reasons. Artificial tears (methylcellulose) should be instilled frequently during the day to prevent drying of the cornea. The eye should be inspected for the presence of eyelashes. Ointment and an impermeable eye shield can be used at night to retain moisture. In some patients taping the lids closed at night may be effective.

A facial sling may be helpful to support affected muscles, improve lip alignment, and facilitate eating. The facial sling is usually made and fitted by a physical or occupational therapist. Vigorous massage can break down tissues, but gentle upward massage has psychologic benefits even if physical effects other than the maintenance of circulation are questionable. When function begins to return, active facial exercises are performed several times a day.

The change in physical appearance as a result of Bell's palsy can be devastating. The patient must be reassured that a stroke did not occur and that chances for a full recovery are good. The patient's need for privacy should be respected, especially during meals, but the nurse's assistance in the patient's adjustment to the physical changes should not be delayed. Enlisting support from family and friends is important.

POLYNEUROPATHIES

Guillain-Barré Syndrome

Pathophysiology. *Guillain-Barré syndrome* (Landry-Guillain-Barré-Strohl syndrome, postinfectious polyneuropathy, ascending polyneuropathic paralysis) is an acute, rapidly progressing, and potentially fatal form of polyneuritis. It affects the peripheral nervous system and results in loss of myelin (a segmental demyelination) and in edema and inflammation of the affected nerves, causing a loss of neurotransmission to the periphery. With adequate supportive care, 85% of these patients will recover completely from this disorder.[6]

The etiology of this disorder is unknown, but it is believed to be a cell-mediated immunologic reaction directed at the peripheral nerves. The syndrome is frequently preceded by immune system stimulation from a viral infection, trauma, surgery, viral immunizations, or lymphoproliferative neoplasms. These stimuli are thought to cause an alteration in the immune system, resulting in sensitization of T lymphocytes to the patient's myelin, causing myelin damage. Demyelination occurs and the transmission of nerve impulses are stopped or slowed down. The muscles innervated by the damaged peripheral nerves undergo denervation and atrophy. In the recovery phase, remyelination occurs slowly and returns in a proximal to distal pattern. The lymphocytes are basically normal and return to complete functioning after the illness.

The syndrome affects both genders equally and is more commonly seen in adults 20 to 50 years of age, although it is observed in all age groups.[3] Some evidence has associated the occurrence of Guillain-Barré syndrome with the swine flu vaccine.[7] During the mass screening against the swine flu in 1976 an 8 to 10 times greater incidence of the syndrome occurred in individuals who were immunized. It is not known whether this increase was attributed to the specific vaccine or whether the increase would also have occurred with other vaccines. However, there have been no other links between flu vaccines and the disease.

A chronic form of Guillain-Barré syndrome has been described in which the paralysis evolves more slowly. An apparent relapsing of symptoms occurs, with no involvement of respiratory function or cranial nerves. The patient with this type of polyneuritis generally does not have a full recovery.[8]

Clinical Manifestations and Complications. Symptoms of Guillain-Barré syndrome usually develop 1 to 3 weeks after an upper respiratory or gastrointestinal infection. Weakness of the lower extremities (evolving more or less symmetrically) occurs over hours to days to weeks, usually peaking about the fourteenth day. Distal muscles are more severely affected. *Paresthesia* (numbness and tingling) is frequent, and paralysis usually follows in the extremities. Hypotonia and areflexia are common, persistent symptoms. Objective sensory loss is variable, with deep sensitivity more affected than superficial sensations.

Autonomic nervous dysfunction results from alterations in both the sympathetic and parasympathetic nervous systems. Autonomic disturbances are usually seen in patients with severe muscle involvement and respiratory muscle paralysis. The most dangerous autonomic dysfunctions include orthostatic hypotension, hypertension, and abnormal vagal responses (bradycardia, heart block, asystole). Other autonomic dysfunctions include bowel and bladder dysfunction, facial flushing, and diaphoresis.[7] Patients may also have syndrome of inappropriate antidiuretic hormone (SIADH) secretion. SIADH is discussed further in Chapter 47.

Progression of Guillain-Barré syndrome to include the lower brainstem involves the facial, abducens, oculomotor, hypoglossal, trigeminal, and vagus nerves (CN VII, VI, III, XII, V, and X, respectively). This involvement manifests itself through facial weakness, extraocular eye movement difficulties, dysphagia, and paresthesia of the face.

The most serious complication of this syndrome is respiratory failure, which occurs as the paralysis progresses to the nerves that innervate the thoracic area. Constant monitoring of the respiratory system by checking respiratory rate, depth, forced vital capacity, and negative inspiratory force provides information about the need for immediate intervention. Approximately 20% of the patients with Guillain-Barré syndrome require ventilatory support, and as many as 5% to 10% die from respiratory failure or dysrhythmias.[8] Respiratory or urinary tract infections may occur. Fever is generally the first sign of infection, and treatment is directed at the infecting organism. Immobility from the paralysis can cause problems such as paralytic ileus, muscle atrophy, deep vein thrombosis, pulmonary emboli, skin breakdown, orthostatic hypotension, and nutritional deficiencies.

Pain is a common symptom in the patient with Guillain-Barré syndrome. The pain can be categorized as paresthesias, muscular aches and cramps, and hyperesthesias. Pain appears to be worse at night. Narcotics may be indicated for those experiencing severe pain. Pain may lead to a decrease in appetite and may interfere with sleep.

Diagnostic Studies and Therapeutic Management. Diagnosis is based primarily on the patient's history and clinical signs. Cerebrospinal fluid is normal or has a low protein content initially, but after 7 to 10 days shows a greatly elevated protein level to 700 mg/dl (7 g/L) (normal protein is 15 to 45 mg/dl [0.15 to 0.45 g/L]). Electromyographic (EMG) and nerve conduction studies are markedly abnormal (reduced nerve conduction velocity) in the affected extremities.

Therapeutic management is aimed at supportive care, particularly ventilatory support, during the acute phase. Plasmapheresis is being used for severe Guillain-Barré syndrome that involves the respiratory muscles. It is an attempt to remove antibodies that may be present and shorten the course of the disease. Plasmapheresis appears to be more effective in younger than in older patients and when administered early (first 2 weeks) in the course of the disease.[1] (Plasmapheresis is discussed in Chapter 10.) Corticosteroids and ACTH are used to suppress the immune response but appear to have little effect on the prognosis or duration of the disease.

Monitoring blood pressure and cardiac rate and rhythm is also important during the acute phase because transient cardiac dysrhythmias have been reported. Autonomic dysfunction is common and usually takes the form of bradycardia. Orthostatic hypotension secondary to muscle atony may occur in severe cases. Vasopressor agents and volume expanders may be needed to treat the low blood pressure.

Nutritional Management

Nutritional intake is compromised in the patient with Guillain-Barré syndrome. During the acute phase the patient may experience difficulty swallowing because of cranial nerve involvement. Mild dysphagia can be managed by placing the patient in an upright position and flexing the head forward during feeding. For more severe dysphagia, tube feedings may be required. Later in the course of the disease motor paralysis or weakness will affect the ability to self-feed. The patient's nutritional status, including body weight, serum albumin levels, and calorie counts, must be evaluated at regular intervals.

NURSING MANAGEMENT

GUILLAIN-BARRÉ SYNDROME

Nursing Assessment

Assessment of the patient is the most important aspect of nursing care during the acute phase. The nurse must monitor the ascending paralysis, assess respiratory function, monitor arterial blood gases (ABGs), and assess the gag, corneal, and swallowing reflexes during the routine assessment.

Nursing Diagnoses

Nursing diagnoses specific to the patient with Guillain-Barré syndrome include, but are not limited to, the following:

- Risk for respiratory distress related to progression of disease process resulting in respiratory muscle paralysis
- Risk for aspiration related to dysphagia
- Pain related to paresthesias, muscle aches and cramps, and hyperesthesias
- Impaired verbal communication related to intubation or paralysis of the muscles of speech
- Fear related to uncertain outcome and seriousness of the disease
- Total self-care deficit related to inability to use muscles to accomplish activities of daily living

Planning

The overall goals are that the patient with Guillain-Barré syndrome will (1) maintain adequate ventilation, (2) be free from aspiration, (3) be pain free or have pain controlled, (4) maintain an acceptable method of communication, (5) maintain adequate nutritional intake, and (6) return to usual physical functioning.

Nursing Implementation

The objective of therapy is to support body systems until the patient recovers. Respiratory failure and infection are serious threats. Monitoring the vital capacity and ABGs is essential. If the vital capacity drops to less than 800 ml or the ABGs deteriorate, a tracheostomy may be done so that the patient can be mechanically ventilated (see Chapter 61). Meticulous suctioning technique is needed to prevent infection whether the patient has an endotracheal tube or tracheostomy. Thorough bronchial hygiene and chest physiotherapy help clear secretions and prevent respiratory deterioration. If fever develops, sputum cultures should be obtained to identify whether the respiratory tract is the source of the pathogen. Appropriate antibiotic therapy is then initiated.

A communication system must be established with the use of the patient's available abilities. This is extremely difficult if the disease progresses to involvement of the cranial nerves. At the peak of a severe episode the patient may be incapable of communicating. The nurse must explain all procedures before doing them and reassure the patient that muscle function will return to some part of the body so that needs and desires can be communicated.

Urinary retention is common for a few days. Intermittent catheterization is preferred to an indwelling catheter to avoid urinary tract infections. However, for the acutely ill patient receiving a large volume of fluids (>2.5 L/day) indwelling catheterization may be safer to reduce overdistention of a temporarily flaccid bladder and to prevent vesicoureteral reflux. Physiotherapy is indicated early to help prevent problems related to immobility. Passive range-of-motion exercises and attention to body position help maintain function and prevent contractures. Nutritional needs must be met in spite of possible problems associated with delayed gastric emptying, paralytic ileus, and potential for aspiration if the gag reflex is lost. In addition to checking for the gag reflex, nurses should note drooling and other difficulties with secretions, which may be more indicative of an inadequate gag reflex. Initially tube feedings or parenteral nutrition may be used to ensure adequate caloric intake. Fluid and electrolyte therapy must be monitored carefully to prevent electrolyte imbalances.

Throughout the course of the illness, the nurse should provide support and encouragement to the family and patient. Because residual problems and relapses are uncommon except in the chronic form of the disease, complete recovery can be anticipated even though it is generally a slow process that takes months or years if axonal degeneration occurs.

Botulism

Pathophysiology. *Botulism* is the most serious type of food poisoning. It is caused by GI absorption of the neurotoxin produced by *Clostridium botulinum.* This organism is found in the soil, and the spores are difficult to destroy. It can grow in any food contaminated with the spores. Improper home canning of foods is often the cause. It is thought that the neurotoxin destroys or inhibits the neurotransmission of acetylcholine at the myoneural junction, resulting in disturbed muscle innervation. Symptoms are usually nausea, vomiting, and abdominal cramps, generally within 12 to 36 hours after consumption of the contaminated food. Neurologic manifestations develop rapidly over 2 to 4 days. They include difficulty in convergence of the eyes, photophobia, ptosis, paralysis of extraocular muscles, blurred vision, diplopia, dry mouth, sore throat, and difficulty in swallowing. Other manifestations include paralytic ileus, mild muscle weakness, and respiratory symptoms that can rapidly deteriorate to respiratory arrest.

Because botulism is a reportable disease, local, state, and federal health agencies, particularly the Centers for Disease Control in Atlanta, must be notified.

Therapeutic Management. The initial treatment of botulism is intravenous (IV) administration of botulinum antitoxin. Before administration of the antitoxin, an intradermal test dose for sensitivity to horse serum is given. If there are no reactions, the test dose is followed by daily doses of 50,000 units of botulism antitoxin intramuscularly until improvement begins.[1]

The GI tract is purged by laxatives, high colonic enemas, and gastric lavage to decrease the absorption of the toxin. Prophylactic penicillin may be ordered to halt the release of toxin in the gastrointestinal tract.

NURSING MANAGEMENT
BOTULISM

Health Promotion and Maintenance

Primary prevention is the goal of nursing management through educating consumers to be alert to situations that may result in botulism. Particular attention should be given to foods with a low acid content, which support germination and the production of botulin, a deadly poison. These foods include fish, vichyssoise, and peppers. All varieties of spores are destroyed by boiling for 10 minutes or maintaining a temperature of 176° F (80° C) for 30 minutes. Specific suggestions related to the preparation, storage, and use of food include the following:[9]

1. In home canning, the equipment manufacturer's directions should be followed. Only fresh fruits and vegetables with questionable spots removed should be used. All containers and utensils must be cleansed, and the seal on the can or jar must be airtight. Canned foods should be stored properly in a cool, dry place.
2. A can with a swollen end should never be used; the swelling may be caused by gases from *Clostridium botulinum.*
3. If the food is forcefully expelled when a container is opened, it should be discarded immediately and the contents should not be tasted.
4. If the contents of a can look or smell bad after opening, the can should be discarded without tasting of the contents.

Lye should be added to suspicious materials, and they should be stored for 24 hours before burying to destroy bacteria and toxins to prevent further contamination. Materials may be flushed down the toilet or disposed of in the garbage disposal if a large amount of water is used.

Acute Intervention

Nursing care during the acute illness is similar to that for Guillain-Barré syndrome. Supportive nursing interventions include rest, activities to maintain respiratory function, adequate nutrition, and prevention of loss of muscle mass. Because the recovery process is slow, the patient may develop problems related to a feeling of helplessness, boredom, and low morale.

Tetanus

Pathophysiology. *Tetanus* is an extremely severe polyradiculitis and polyneuritis affecting spinal and cranial nerves. It results from the effects of a potent neurotoxin released by the anaerobic bacillus *Clostridium tetani.* The toxin interferes with the function of the reflex arc by blocking of inhibitory transmitters at the presynaptic sites in the spinal cord and brainstem.[1] The spores of the bacillus are present in soil, garden mold, and manure. Thus *Clostridium tetani* enters the body through a traumatic or suppurative wound that provides an appropriate low-oxygen environment for the organisms to mature and produce toxin. Other possible sources include dental infection, injections of heroin, human and animal bites, frostbite, compound fractures, and gunshot wounds. The incubation period is usually 7 days but can range from 1 to 54 days, with symptoms frequently appearing after the original wound is healed. In general, the longer the incubation period, the milder the illness and the better the prognosis.

Worldwide the number of cases per year is estimated to be 1 million. Most victims are neonates born to unimmunized mothers in developing countries. In the United States the incidence rate of tetanus is about 1 case per 1 million of population per year.[12] Of those reported cases the majority of patients are over the age of 59, suggesting inadequate immunization among older adults.[10] Mortality rates vary according to age, with infants and persons more than 60 years of age most seriously affected. Overall mortality rates range from 45% to 55%.

Clinical Manifestations. Manifestations of generalized tetanus include a feeling of stiffness in the jaw (*lockjaw*) or neck, slight fever, and other symptoms of general infection. Generalized tonic spasms occur because of the lack of reciprocal innervation. As the disease progresses, the neck muscles, back, abdomen, and extremities become progressively rigid. In severe forms, continuous tonic convulsions may occur with *opisthotonos* (extreme arching of the back and retraction of the head). Laryngeal and respiratory spasms cause apnea and anoxia. Additional effects are manifested by overstimulation of the sympathetic nervous system, including profuse diaphoresis, labile hypertension, episodic tachycardia, hyperthermia, and dysrhythmias.[11] The slightest noise, jarring motion, or bright light can set off the convulsion. These convulsions are agonizingly painful. Mortality is almost 100% in the severe form. Death is usually attributable to asphyxia or heart failure, the result of constantly recurring spasms. Residual injury, such as vertebral fracture, muscle contracture, and brain damage secondary to hypoxia, may be long-term consequences.

Therapeutic Management. The therapeutic management of tetanus includes administration of tetanus toxoid booster (Td) and tetanus immune globulin (TIG) before the onset of symptoms to neutralize circulating toxins (see Table 62-6).

Serum electrolytes, CBC count, albumin, clotting factors, glucose, and ABGs are monitored. Cardiac function is monitored by electrocardiogram (ECG) and auscultation. As increasing numbers of nerve cells become involved, their inhibitory control over muscle activity decreases and symptoms develop. Control of spasms is essential and is managed by deep sedation, usually with diazepam (Valium), barbiturates, or chlorpromazine (Thorazine). A 10-day course of penicillin is recommended.

Because of laryngospasm, a tracheostomy is usually performed early and the patient is maintained on mechanical ventilation. If sedation does not control seizures, skeletal muscle–paralyzing drugs such as d-tubocurarine (curare) are used. Pain is relieved by means of codeine or meperidine, often with the addition of promethazine (Phenergan). Any recognized wound should be debrided or an abscess drained. Antibiotics may be given to prevent secondary infections. Nutrition is maintained through parenteral or nasogastric feeding. Even with the best of care, the mortality rate is 50%. Those who recover have a long convalescence that includes extensive physiotherapy.

NURSING MANAGEMENT

TETANUS

Health teaching is aimed at ensuring tetanus prophylaxis, which is the most important factor influencing the incidence of this disease. Tetanus prevention and immunization protocols are summarized in Table 62-6. The patient should be taught that immediate, thorough cleansing of all wounds with soap and water is important in the prevention of tetanus. If an open wound occurs and the patient has not been immunized within 10 years, the primary care provider should be contacted so that a tetanus booster can be given.

If equine tetanus antitoxin is to be used, the patient should be tested for sensitivity. Administration of equine antitoxin is not recommended if sensitivity occurs; anaphylactic shock is potentially life threatening and desensitization is ineffective. The side effects of routine administration of the antitoxin are mild and include a sore arm, swelling at the site, and itching. Serious side effects rarely occur. Routine administration of a booster shot to an adequately immunized patient can cause arm swelling and lymphadenopathy.

Every patient should receive a written record of immunizations and be encouraged to complete the active immunization schedule. The patient's immunization history should be accurately recorded to protect the patient and care providers.

The acute nursing management of the patient with tetanus is aimed at supportive care based on the treatment of clinical manifestations. The patient should be placed in a quiet, darkened room insulated against noise. Judicious sedation should be given. Nursing care should be administered with the utmost caution to avoid triggering spasms. For example, the nurse should avoid unnecessary touching, use firm touching when necessary, avoid the use of linens to cover the patient, and maintain a slightly higher than normal ambient temperature. Nursing care related to tracheostomy and mechanical ventilation is given as appropriate. An indwelling bladder catheter may be used to prevent bladder distention and urinary reflux in the presence of spasms in the muscles of the pelvic floor. Attention must also given to skin care. The patient needs emotional support during the acute phase because the fear of death is real. The family also needs support and explanations.

Neurosyphilis

Neurosyphilis (tertiary syphilis) is an infection of any part of the nervous system by the organism *Treponema pallidum.* It is the result of untreated or inadequately treated syphilis (see Chapter 50). The organism can invade the central nervous system (CNS) within a few months of the original infection. Except for causing some changes in the cerebrospinal fluid, including increased white blood cells (WBCs) and protein and positive serologic reaction, the organism lies dormant for years. Untreated neurosyphilis, although not contagious, can be fatal. Penicillin therapy is effective for syphilitic meningitis, but the neurologic deficits remain.

Late neurosyphilis results from degenerative changes in the spinal cord (tabes dorsalis) and brainstem (general paresis). *Tabes dorsalis* (progressive locomotor ataxia) is characterized by vague, sharp pains in the legs; ataxia; "slapping" gait; loss of proprioception and deep tendon reflexes; and zones of hyperesthesia. *Charcot's joints,* which are characterized by enlargement, bone destruction, and hypermobility, also occur as a result of joint effusion and edema.

Dementia paralytica is an ongoing spirochetal meningoencephalitis that causes a general dissolution of mental and physical capabilities. It may mimic a number of major or minor psychoses. Management includes treatment with penicillin, symptomatic care, and protection from physical injury.

SPINAL CORD TRAUMA

Significance

The manifestations of spinal cord injury are generally the direct result of trauma that causes cord compression, ischemia, edema, and possible cord transection. Before World War II, the life expectancy for the person with a spinal cord injury ranged from months to 10 years from the onset of injury. The leading causes of death were renal failure and sepsis. Today, with improved treatment strategies (specifically, intermittent catheterization), even the very young patient with a spinal cord injury can anticipate a long life. The prognosis for life is generally only about 5 years less than for persons of the same age without spinal cord injury. The cause of premature death in the patient with quadriplegia is usually related to compromised respiratory function.

Health care providers often consider spinal cord disability to be one of the most devastating of physical disabilities. However, patients with spinal cord injury are remarkably resourceful, with impressive resilience and an ability to work out new patterns of living and coping.[12] Staff members often underestimate the patient's potential for independence. Misplaced sympathy and overidentification can compromise the nurse's attempt to give the involved and complex care required by the injured person for optimal rehabilitation. Recovery is prolonged, and nurses must learn to gauge progress in inches rather than miles. Skilled, persistent care draws on every known nursing intervention until the patient achieves a maximal level of independence.

The disruption of individual growth and development, altered family dynamics, economic loss in terms of absence from work, and the high cost of rehabilitation or maintenance make spinal cord trauma a devastating problem. About 250,000 people in the United States today had traumatic spinal cord injuries and 8000 to 10,000 people are newly injured each year.[10] The economic impact of spinal cord injuries in the United States is estimated to be at $4 billion per year.[13,14]

Although many patients with spinal cord injuries can care for themselves with minimal assistance, a larger number are confined to nursing homes, care centers, and rehabilitation units. The loss to the workforce in terms of human potential is enormous.

Etiology

The risk population for spinal cord injury is primarily young adult men between the ages of 15 and 30 and those who are impulsive or risk takers in daily living. A history of numerous injuries before the cord injury is common. A high correlation exists between alcohol and drug abuse and spinal cord injury. Individuals at risk for spinal cord injury include motorcyclists, sky divers, football players, police officers, divers, and military personnel. The causes of spinal cord injury include motor vehicle accidents, falls, acts of violence, and sports injuries.[13] The resulting spinal cord injury can be due to cord compression by bone displacement, interruption of blood supply to the cord, or traction resulting from pulling on the cord.

Classification

Spinal cord injuries are classified by the mechanism of injury, level of injury, or degree of injury. The major mechanisms of injury are flexion, hyperextension, flexion-rotation, extension-rotation, and compression (Fig. 57-4). The flexion injury that includes dislocation is the most unstable of all injuries because the ligamentous structures that stabilize the spine are torn. This injury is most often implicated in severe neurologic deficits.

The level of injury may be cervical, thoracic, or lumbar. Cervical and lumbar injuries are most common because

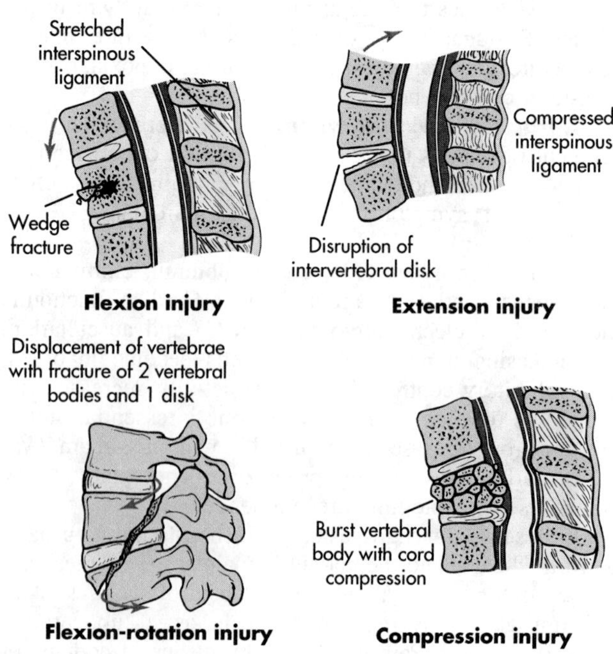

Fig. 57-4 Mechanisms of spinal injury.

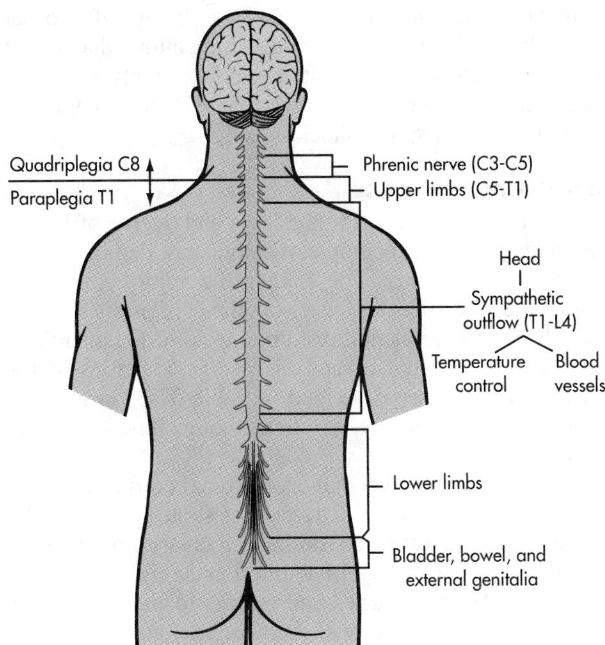

Fig. 57-5 Symptoms, degree of paralysis, and potential for rehabilitation depend on the level of the lesion.

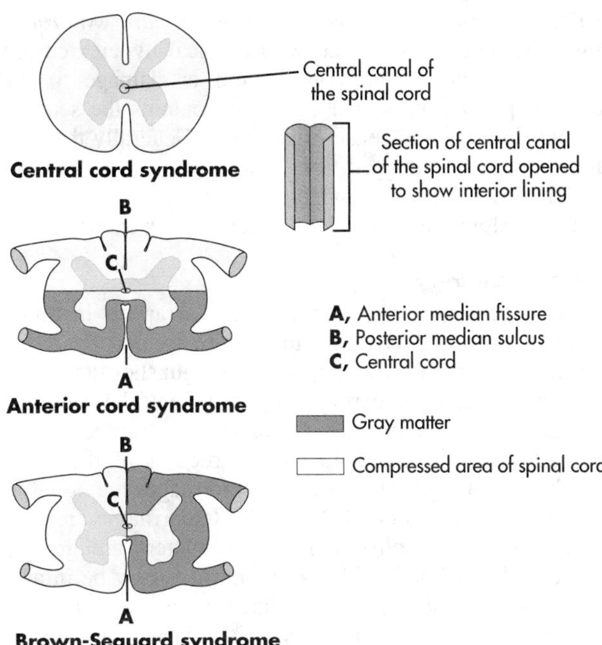

Fig. 57-6 Three syndromes associated with incomplete cord lesions.

these levels are associated with the greatest flexibility and movement.

The degree of spinal cord involvement may be either *complete* or *incomplete* (partial). Complete cord involvement results in flaccid paralysis and total loss of sensory and motor function below the level of the lesion (injury). If the cervical cord is involved, paralysis of all four extremities (particularly the hands and forearms) occurs, resulting in quadriplegia. However, even with a cervical injury the arms are rarely completely paralyzed. If the thoracic or lumbar cord is damaged, the result is paraplegia. Figure 57-5 shows affected structures and functions at different levels of cord injury.

Incomplete cord lesion involvement (partial transection) results in a mixed loss of voluntary motor activity and sensation and leaves some tracts intact. The degree of sensory and motor loss varies depending on the level of the lesion and reflects the specific nerve tracts damaged and those spared. Four syndromes are associated with incomplete lesions: central cord syndrome, anterior cord syndrome, Brown-Sequard syndrome, and posterior cord syndrome.

Damage in the cervical central cord is termed *central cord syndrome,* which is characterized by microscopic hemorrhage, edema of the central spinal cord, and compression on anterior horn cells (Fig. 57-6). Central cord syndrome is more common in older adults. Motor weakness is present in both the upper and lower extremities, but the weakness is much greater in the upper extremities than in the lower ones. It may change to a progressive lesion. Sensory dysfunction varies according to the site of injury or lesion. Bladder dysfunction is common. This syndrome is frequently a result of hyperextension of an osteoarthritic spine. The extent of recovery depends on the resolution of edema and the intactness of the spinal cord tracts.

Anterior cord syndrome is characterized by injury resulting in an acute compression of the anterior portion of the spinal cord, often a flexion injury (Fig. 57-6). The spinal cord lesion is in the anterior two thirds of the cord. Compression is usually caused by a disk or bony fragment; it may also be caused by actual destruction of the anterior cord by an anterior spinal artery occlusion caused by ischemia or thrombus. Manifestations include immediate, complete motor paralysis from the site of the injury and below. *Hypoesthesia* (decreased sensation), decreased pain sensation, and loss of temperature occur below the level of injury. Because the posterior cord tracts are not injured, sensations of touch, position, vibration, and motion remain intact. Dorsal column function is preserved. If the syndrome is caused by the compression of the anterior cord from bony fragments, surgical decompression is indicated.

Brown-Sequard syndrome is a result of transection or lesion of one half of the spinal cord (Fig. 57-6). Brown-Sequard syndrome is usually caused by penetrating injuries, such as a gunshot wound or knife or possibly an acute ruptured disk. This syndrome is characterized by a loss of motor function (paralysis) and position and vibratory sense, as well as vasomotor paralysis on the same side (ipsilateral) and below the hemisection. The opposite (contralateral) side of the hemisection has loss of pain and temperature sensation below the level of the lesion or hemisection. Fibers that carry pain and temperature cross to the opposite side of the cord immediately after entering the cord and ascend, which accounts for the described symptoms.

Less commonly seen is the *posterior cord syndrome.* This syndrome is associated with cervical hyperextension trauma. It results from compression or damage to the posterior part of the spinal cord that contains the sensory neurons and position-sense capabilities. Generally the dorsal columns are damaged, resulting in loss of proprioception. However, pain, temperature sensation, and motor function below the level of the lesion remain intact.

Pathophysiology

Initial Injury. The spinal cord is wrapped in tough layers of dura and is rarely torn or transected by direct trauma. Penetrating trauma, such as gunshot and stab wounds, can result in tearing and transection. The complete cord dissolution (previously thought to be transection) in severe trauma is related to autodestruction of the cord. Shortly after the injury, petechial hemorrhages are noted in the central gray matter of the cord. Hemorrhagic areas in the center of the spinal cord (gray matter) are grossly visible within 1 hour. Within 4 hours there may be infarction in the gray matter.[15] Hemorrhage, edema, and metabolites act together to produce ischemia, which progresses to necrotic destruction of the cord. The resulting hypoxia reduces the oxygen tension below the level that meets the metabolic needs of the cord. Lactate metabolites and a gross increase in norepinephrine are noted. At high levels, norepinephrine causes vasospasms, hypoxia, and subsequent necrosis. Unfortunately, the spinal cord has minimal ability to adapt to vasospasm by means of increased flow from anastomotic areas.

By 24 hours permanent damage has occurred because of the development of edema. Edema secondary to the inflammatory response is particularly harmful because of lack of space for tissue expansion. Therefore resultant compression of the cord and extension of edema above and below the injury increase the ischemic damage. The end result is the same as mechanical severance of the cord.

The hemorrhagic necrosis causes the lesion to be complete after 48 hours, and any function of nerves that arise in and pass through this level is lost. Because additional edema extends the level of injury beyond the immediate level of destruction for 72 hours to 1 week, the exact extent of injury cannot be determined before that time.

Spinal Shock. In addition to the discrete damage at the trauma site, the entire cord below the level of the lesion fails to function, resulting in spinal shock characterized by hypotension, bradycardia, and warm, dry extremities. Spinal shock usually occurs at the time of injury in response to severe damage to the cord and results in immediate depression of all cord functions. The onset of spinal shock causes the patient to have a complete loss of motor and sensory activity below the level of the lesion. Loss of sympathetic innervation causes peripheral vasodilatation, venous pooling, and a decreased cardiac output. These effects are generally associated with a cervical or high thoracic injury. With spinal shock there is also flaccid paralysis below the level of injury. This affects musculoskeletal, bowel, and bladder function.

Spinal shock generally lasts for 7 to 10 days after onset but can last from weeks to months. Indications that spinal shock has ended include spasticity, reflex emptying of the bladder, and hyperreflexia. Active rehabilitation may begin in the presence of spinal shock.

Clinical Manifestations

Manifestations are related to the level and degree of injury. The patient with an incomplete lesion may demonstrate a mixture of symptoms. The higher the injury, the more serious the sequelae because of the proximity of the cervical cord to the medulla and brainstem. Movement and rehabilitation potential related to specific locations of the spinal cord injury are described in Table 57-3. In general, sensory function closely parallels motor function at all levels.

The types of accidents that cause spinal cord trauma can also result in head injury. The patient should therefore be assessed for signs of concussion and increased intracranial pressure (see Chapter 54). In addition, a careful assessment for musculoskeletal injuries and trauma to internal organs should be performed. Because there are no muscle, bone, or visceral sensations, the only clue to internal trauma with hemorrhage may be a rapidly falling hematocrit level. Urinary output is examined for hematuria, which is also indicative of internal injuries.

Complications

Immediate postinjury problems include maintaining a patent airway, adequate ventilation, and adequate circulating blood volume; and preventing extension of cord damage.

Respiratory System. Cervical injury or fracture above the level of C4 presents special problems because of the total loss of respiratory muscle function. Mechanical ventilation is required to keep the patient alive. At one time the majority of these patients died at the scene of the injury, but with improved Emergency Medical Services more of these patients are surviving the initial events of their spinal cord injury. Injury or fracture below the level of C4 results in diaphragmatic breathing if the phrenic nerve is functioning. Even if the injury is below C4, spinal cord edema and hemorrhage can affect the function of the phrenic nerve and cause respiratory insufficiency. Hypoventilation almost always occurs with diaphragmatic respirations because of the decrease in vital capacity and tidal volume.

Cervical fractures or severe injuries cause a paralysis of abdominal musculature and frequently intercostal musculature; therefore the patient cannot cough effectively enough to remove secretions, leading to atelectasis and pneumonia. An artificial airway provides direct access for pathogens, and bronchial hygiene and chest physiotherapy are extremely important. In multiple trauma a neurogenic pulmonary edema may result from the sudden changes in thoracic pressure at the time of the injury. Pulmonary edema may also be due to fluid overload.

Cardiovascular System. Any cord transection above the level of T5 greatly decreases the influence of the sympa-

Table 57-3 Functional Level of Spinal Cord Disruption and Rehabilitation Potential

Autonomic	Movement Remaining	Rehabilitation Potential
Quadriplegia		
C1-C3		
Usually fatal injury, vagus nerve domination of heart, respiration, blood vessels, all organs below injury	Movement in neck and above, loss of innervation to diaphragm, absence of independent respiratory function	Ability to drive electric wheelchair equipped with portable respirator by using chin control or mouth stick, headpiece to stabilize head, lack of bowel and bladder control
C4		
Vagus nerve domination of heart, respirations, and all vessels and organs below injury	Sensation and movement above neck	Ability to drive electric wheelchair by using chin control or mouth stick, lack of bowel and bladder control
C5		
Vagus nerve domination of heart, respirations, and all vessels and organs below injury	Full neck, partial shoulder, back, biceps; gross elbow, inability to roll over or use hands; decreased respiratory reserve	Ability to drive electric wheelchair with mobile hand supports, ability to use powered hand splints (in some patients), lack of bowel and bladder control, feed self with setup and adaptive equipment
C6		
Vagus nerve domination of heart, respirations, and all vessels and organs below injury	Shoulder and upper back abduction and rotation at shoulder, full biceps to elbow flexion, wrist extension, weak grasp of thumb, decreased respiratory reserve	Ability to assist with transfer and perform some self-care, feed self with hand devices, push wheelchair on smooth, flat surface; lack of bowel and bladder control
C7-C8		
Vagus nerve domination of heart, respirations, and all vessels and organs below injury	All triceps to elbow extension, finger extensors and flexors, good grasp with some decreased strength, decreased respiratory reserve	Ability to transfer self to wheelchair, roll over and sit up in bed, push self on most surfaces, perform most self-care; independent use of wheelchair; ability to drive car with powered hand controls (in some patients); lack of bowel and bladder control
Paraplegia		
T1-T6		
Sympathetic innervation to heart, vagus nerve domination of all vessels and organs below injury	Full innervation of upper extremities, back, essential intrinsic muscles of hand; full strength and dexterity of grasp; decreased trunk stability, decreased respiratory reserve	Full independence in self-care and in wheelchair, ability to drive car with hand controls (in most patients), ability to use full body brace for exercise but not for functional ambulation, lack of bowel and bladder control
T6-T12		
Vagus nerve domination only of leg vessels, GI and genitourinary organs	Full, stable thoracic muscles and upper back; functional intercostals, resulting in increased respiratory reserve	Full independent use of wheelchair; ability to stand erect with full body brace, ambulate on crutches with swing (though gait difficult); inability to climb stairs; lack of bowel and bladder control
L1-L2		
Vagus nerve domination of leg vessels	Varying control of legs and pelvis, instability of lower back	Good sitting balance, full use of wheelchair
L3-L4		
Partial vagus nerve domination of leg vessels, GI and genitourinary organs	Quadriceps and hip flexors, absence of hamstring function, flail ankles	Completely independent ambulation with short leg braces and canes, inability to stand for long periods, bladder and bowel continence

GI, Gastrointestinal.

thetic nervous system. Bradycardia occurs as a result of the unopposed effect of the parasympathetic nervous system on the heart, and vasodilatation results in hypotension. Close cardiac monitoring is necessary. In marked bradycardia, appropriate medications to increase the heart rate and prevent hypoxemia are necessary. The peripheral vasodilatation reduces the venous return of blood to the heart and subsequently decreases cardiac output, resulting in hypotension. IV fluids may resolve the problem, or vasopressor drugs may be required.

Urinary System. Urinary retention is a common development in acute spinal cord injuries and spinal shock. While the patient is in spinal shock the bladder is atonic and will become overdistended. An indwelling catheter is inserted to drain the bladder. In the postacute phase the bladder can be hyperirritable, with a loss of inhibition of reflex from the brain. Consequently, the patient urinates small amounts frequently. The bladder becomes distended because of inadequate emptying. Urinary retention increases the chance of infection. In addition, urinary calculi are likely to develop in a distended bladder retaining urine. Catheterization is usually indicated. The indwelling catheter should be removed as early as possible, and intermittent catheterization should begin when spinal shock has resolved.

Gastrointestinal System. If the cord transection has occurred above the level of T5, the primary gastrointestinal problems are related to hypomotility. Decreased gastrointestinal motor activity will contribute to the development of paralytic ileus and gastric distention. A nasogastric tube for intermittent suctioning may relieve the gastric distention, and standard treatment is used for paralytic ileus. The development of stress ulcers is common because of excessive release of hydrochloric acid in the stomach. Histamine H_2 receptor blockers (e.g., ranitidine) are frequently used to prevent the occurrence of these ulcers during the initial phase. Antacids can also be used. Intraabdominal bleeding may occur and is difficult to diagnose because no subjective signs such as pain, tenderness, and guarding are observed. Continued hypotension in spite of vigorous treatment may be the only indication of bleeding. Expanding girth of the abdomen may also be noted. Additional gastrointestinal problems include gallstone formation, constipation, and fecal impaction.

Integumentary System. A major consequence of lack of movement is the potential for tissue breakdown in the area of denervation, which can occur quickly and can lead to major infection or sepsis. A certain degree of muscle atrophy occurs during the flaccid paralysis state, whereas contractures tend to occur during the spastic state.

Poikilothermism is the adjustment of the body temperature to the room temperature. This occurs in spinal cord injuries because the interruption of the sympathetic nervous system prevents temperature sensations from reaching the hypothalamus. Another factor is the reduction in heat generation because of minimal movement. With spinal cord disruption there is also decreased ability to sweat, which will also affect the ability to regulate body temperature.

Metabolic Needs. Correcting an existing acid-base disturbance and maintaining acid-base balance promote the functions of other body systems. Nasogastric suctioning may lead to metabolic alkalosis, and decreased tissue perfusion may lead to acidosis. Electrolyte levels, including sodium and potassium, can be altered by gastric suctioning and must be monitored until suctioning is discontinued and a normal diet is resumed. A positive nitrogen balance and a high-protein diet help prevent skin breakdown and infections and help decrease the rate of muscle atrophy.

Peripheral Vascular Problems. Deep vein thrombosis (DVT) is a common problem accompanying spinal cord injury. Retrospective studies have shown a 12.5% to 17% incidence of DVT and 3% to 15.3% for pulmonary embolism.[16] Pulmonary embolism is one of the leading causes of death in patients with spinal cord injury. Techniques for assessment of DVT include Doppler exam, impedance plethysmography, and measuring leg and thigh girth.

Therapeutic Management

Emergency Management. The initial goals for the patient with a spinal cord injury are to sustain life and prevent further cord damage. Table 57-4 outlines the emergency management of the patient with a spinal cord injury. Systemic and spinal cord shock must be treated. For injury at the cervical level, all body systems must be maintained until the full extent of the damage can be evaluated. Treatment of a spinal cord injury may be medical or surgical. Therapeutic management for the patient with a cervical injury is described in Table 57-5. The systemic support required by the patient is less intense for spinal cord injuries of the thoracic and lumbar vertebrae. Respiratory care is not as intense, and bradycardia is not a problem. Specific problems are treated symptomatically.

After stabilization at the accident scene the person is transferred to a medical facility. A thorough assessment is done to specifically evaluate the degree of deficit and to establish the level and degree of injury. A history is obtained, with emphasis on how the accident occurred and the degree of disruption as perceived by the patient immediately after the accident. Assessment involves testing muscle groups rather than individual muscles. Muscle groups should be tested with and against gravity, alone and against resistance, and on both sides of the body. Spontaneous movement should be noted. The patient should be asked to move legs and then hands, spread fingers, extend wrists, and shrug shoulders. After assessment of motor status, a sensory examination including touch and pain as tested by pinprick should be carried out, starting at the toes and working upward. If time and conditions permit, position sense and vibration can also be assessed.

An x-ray is done to document the injury. The patient must be handled carefully before and during the x-ray procedure to prevent further injury. Respiratory, cardiac, urinary, and gastrointestinal functions should be monitored closely. The patient may go directly to surgery following initial immobilization and stabilization or to the intensive care unit (ICU) for monitoring and management.

Surgical Interventions. The decision to perform surgery on a patient with a spinal cord injury often depends on

Table 57-4 Emergency Management: Spinal Cord Injury

Possible Etiologies
Compression, flexion, extension, or rotational injuries from motor vehicle collisions, falls, or diving; penetrating injuries caused by gunshot and stab wounds causing a stretched, torn, crushed, or lacerated spinal cord

Possible Assessment Findings
Pain, tenderness, deformities, or muscle spasms adjacent to the vertebral column
Numbness, paresthesias
Alterations in sensation: temperature, light touch, deep pressure, proprioception
Weakness or heaviness in limbs
Weakness, paralysis, or flaccidity of muscles
Cuts, bruises, open wounds over head, face, neck, or back
Signs and symptoms of neurogenic shock (e.g., hypotension, bradycardia, dry, flushed skin)
Bowel and bladder incontinence or urinary retention
Difficulty breathing
Priapism

Management
- Monitor airway; have airway equipment available, including suction and intubation supplies; anticipate need for intubation if gag reflex absent.
- Maintain cervical spine precautions.
- Administer oxygen via nasal cannula or non-rebreather mask (100%) and monitor for respiratory distress.
- If patient is not breathing or needs assistance, ventilate with bag valve mask.
- Establish intravenous access with one large-bore catheter (14 or 16 gauge); if multiple trauma, use two large-bore catheters and normal saline.
- Assess for other injuries and control external bleeding.
- Monitor vital signs, including level of consciousness, O_2 saturation, cardiac rhythm.
- Obtain history and attempt to determine underlying cause (e.g., assault, fall, motor vehicle accident).
- Keep warm.

the preference of a particular clinician. Surgery is necessary when there is continued compression of the spinal cord by extrinsic forces. Surgery stabilizes the spinal column. In general, accepted criteria for early surgery include (1) evidence of cord compression, (2) progressive neurologic deficit, (3) compound fracture of the vertebra, (4) bony fragments (may dislodge and penetrate the cord), and (5) penetrating wounds of the spinal cord or surrounding structures.[17]

The more common surgical procedures include decompression laminectomy by anterior cervical and thoracic approaches with fusion, posterior laminectomy with the use of acrylic wire mesh and fusion, and insertion of stabilizing

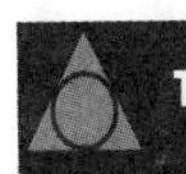

Table 57-5 Therapeutic Management: Cervical Cord Injury

Diagnostic
Complete neurologic examination
ABGs
Electrolytes, glucose, hemoglobin, and hematocrit levels
Urinalysis
Anteroposterior, lateral, and odontoid spinal x-ray studies
CT scan
Myelography
MRI
EMG to measure evoked potentials

Therapeutic

Acute
Immobilization of vertebral column by skeletal traction
Maintenance of heart rate (e.g., atropine) and blood pressure (e.g., dopamine)
Methylprednisone therapy to reduce edema
Insertion of nasogastric tube and attachment to suction
Intubation (if indicated by ABGs)
Oxygen by high humidity mask
Indwelling urinary catheter
Administration of IV fluids with moderate fluid restriction the first 72 hr

Chronic
Stress ulcer prophylaxis
Physical therapy (range-of-motion exercises)
Occupational therapy (splints, activities of daily living training)

ABGs, Arterial blood gases; *CT*, computed tomography; *EMG*, electromyelogram; *IV*, intravenous; *MRI*, magnetic resonance imaging.

rods (e.g., Harrington rods for the correction and stabilization of thoracic deformities). (Specific surgical and nursing interventions for these techniques are discussed in Chapter 59.)

Experimental Treatments. The management of spinal cord injury has changed dramatically in recent years. Although many experimental methods are used, the prognosis for the patient with indirect trauma has improved. An astonishing variety of treatments have been claimed to be beneficial for spinal cord injury in the past decade. In the early 1980s hypothermia and steroids were the only treatments being considered for clinical trials. In 1985 naloxone and thyroid-releasing hormone were being investigated. These drugs counteract the self-destructive pathophysiologic process by blocking the chemical endorphin. In 1991 lipid peroxidation inhibitors were studied for their effects in treating spinal cord injuries. Regeneration therapy is currently being investigated and involves the transplantation of fetal tissue into the injured spinal cord.[18]

Pharmacologic Management. Vasopressor agents employed in the acute phase are useful adjuvants to treatment. Dopamine is the drug of choice. The goal is to maintain the mean arterial pressure at a level greater than 80 to 90 mm Hg so that perfusion to the spinal cord is improved.

The most recent advancement in treating spinal cord injuries pharmacologically is methylprednisolone (MP). MP, a blocker of lipid peroxidation by-products, has been found to improve blood flow and reduce edema in the spinal cord.[20] MP produces a number of effects that may account for the overall improvement noted in the spinal cord–injured patient, including reduction of posttraumatic spinal cord ischemia, improvement of energy balance, restoration of extracellular calcium, improvement of nerve impulse conduction, and repression of the release of free fatty acids from spinal cord tissues.[19] The National Acute Spinal Cord Injury Study II (NASCIS II) reported that patients treated with MP within 8 hours of injury showed an increased recovery of neurologic function. As a result of this study, MP is now administered IV to spinal cord–injured patients.[20]

Pharmacologic properties and drug metabolism are altered in spinal cord injury; therefore drug interactions may occur. For example, propoxyphene (Darvon) is believed to enhance vasodilatation and possibly aggravate orthostatic hypotension, as well as act as an analgesic. The result may aggravate existing problems in the neurologically disabled patient. Drug-induced sedation can also mask a decreasing level of consciousness.

Pharmacologic agents are used to treat specific autonomic dysfunctions such as gastrointestinal hyperactivity, bleeding, bradycardia, orthostatic hypotension, inadequate emptying of the bladder, and autonomic dysreflexia. The nurse must observe the response to these drugs and provide specific interventions when adverse reactions are seen.

Table 57-6 Nursing Assessment: Spinal Cord Injury

Subjective Data

Important health information

Past health history: Motor vehicle accident, sports injury, industrial accident, gunshot or stabbing injury, falls

Medications: Use of alcohol or recreational drugs

Functional health patterns

Activity-exercise: Loss of strength, movement, and sensation below level of injury; dyspnea, inability to breathe adequately

Cognitive-perceptual: Presence of pain at or above level of injury; numbness, tingling, burning, twitching of extremities; fear

Objective Data

General

Depression, anger, denial, anxiety, poikilothermia

Integumentary

Pallor or cyanosis, cool skin, lack of perspiration below level of lesion

Respiratory

Lesions at C1 to C3: apnea, inability to cough; lesions at C4: poor cough, diaphragmatic breathing, hypoventilation; lesions at C5 to T6: decreased respiratory reserve, cyanosis possible

Cardiovascular

Lesions above T5: bradycardia, hypotension, postural hypotension, absence of vasomotor tone

Gastrointestinal

Decreased or absent bowel sounds (for paralytic ileus in lesions above T5), abdominal distention, constipation, fecal incontinence, fecal impaction

Urinary

Retention (for lesions between T1, L2); flaccid bladder (in acute stages)

Reproductive

Priapism, loss of sexual function

Neurologic

Complete: flaccid paralysis and anesthesia below level of injury resulting in quadriplegia (for lesions above C8) or paraplegia (for lesions below C8), hyperactive deep tendon reflexes, bilaterally positive Babinski's test; *Incomplete:* mixed loss of voluntary motor activity and sensations

Musculoskeletal

Muscle atony (in flaccid state), contractures (in spastic state)

Possible findings

Location of level and type of bony involvement on spinal x-ray: lesion, edema, compression on CT and MRI scans; positive finding on myelogram

CT, Computed tomography; *MRI,* magnetic resonance imaging.

NURSING MANAGEMENT

SPINAL CORD INJURY

Nursing Assessment

Subjective and objective data that should be obtained from a patient with a spinal cord injury are presented in Table 57-6.

Nursing Diagnoses

Nursing diagnoses for the patient with a spinal cord injury depend on the severity of the injury and the level of dysfunction. The nursing diagnoses presented in the nursing care plan on p. 1807 are for a patient with a complete cervical cord injury.

Planning

The overall goals are that the patient with a spinal cord injury will (1) maintain optimal level of neurologic functioning, (2) have minimal or no complications of immobility, and (3) return to home and the community at an optimal level of functioning.

Nursing Implementation

Health Promotion and Maintenance. Nursing interventions include identification of risk populations, counseling, and education. Support of local legislation related to seat-belt use in cars, helmets for motorcyclists and bicyclists, child-safety seats, and tougher penalties for drunk-driving offenses are a professional responsibility. A coordinated community program for the training of emergency personnel is essential.

Acute Intervention. High cervical injury caused by flexion-rotation is the most complex spinal cord injury and will be discussed in this section. Interventions for this type

NURSING CARE PLAN Patient with a Spinal Cord Injury*

Planning: Outcome Criteria	Nursing Interventions and Rationales
➤ **NURSING DIAGNOSIS**	Impaired gas exchange *related to* muscle fatigue and retained secretions *as manifested by* decreased oxygen content, increased carbon dioxide concentration, cyanosis, fatigue, diminished breath sounds
Have ABGs within normal limits; normal chest x-ray; clear lungs on auscultation; absence of respiratory distress.	Maintain a patent airway *to prevent respiratory arrest.* Assess all respiratory parameters initially and at least q2hr *to determine extent of problem and plan appropriate interventions.* Monitor ABGs. Provide aggressive pulmonary toilet, including chest physical therapy and quad-assist coughing q4hr *to facilitate the raising of secretions.* Assess strength of cough at least q4hr *to determine adequacy for raising secretions.* Provide rest periods *to prevent fatigue.* Suction as necessary *to remove accumulated secretions.* Note skin color *because cyanosis is an indicator of inadequate ventilation.*
➤ **NURSING DIAGNOSIS**	Decreased cardiac output *related to* venous pooling of blood and immobility *as manifested by* hypotension, tachycardia, restlessness, oliguria, decreased central venous and pulmonary artery pressures
Have adequate cardiac output as measured by thermodilution technique; stable blood pressure and pulse; absence of cyanosis and dysrhythmias; have no complications such as venous thrombosis or pulmonary emboli.	Monitor blood pressure and pulse at least q2hr initially; monitor cardiac rhythm *as indicators of cardiac status.* Administer dopamine or other vasopressor agents *to maintain mean blood pressure >80 mm Hg.* Apply pneumatic compression devices to calves or compression gradient stockings *to prevent venous pooling and thromboemboli.* Perform range-of-motion exercises to all extremities at least q8hr *to cause muscle contractions, which aid in venous return.* Measure pulmonary capillary wedge pressure and cardiac output as ordered *to evaluate circulatory status.*
➤ **NURSING DIAGNOSIS**	Impaired skin integrity *related to* immobility and poor tissue perfusion *as manifested by* reddened skin over bony prominences and pin and tong sites
Have intact skin with no obvious pressure areas.	Inspect all skin areas, especially over bony prominences, at least q2hr; observe area around pins or tongs for signs of breakdown or infection at least every shift *so intervention can be initiated promptly if a problem develops.* Turn patient at least q2hr; use low air-loss bed, kinetic treatment table, or other specialty care devices as needed *to prevent development of pressure areas.* Ensure adequate nutritional intake *to maintain healthy skin resistant to breakdown.* Wash and dry patient's skin thoroughly *to prevent moisture from macerating tissue.*
➤ **NURSING DIAGNOSIS**	Constipation *related to* the injury, inadequate fluid intake, diet low in roughage, and immobility *as manifested by* lack of bowel movement for more than 2 days, decreased bowel sounds, palpable impaction, hard stool or stool incontinence
Have bowel program established, bowel movement at least every other day.	Auscultate bowel sounds at least q4hr; monitor abdominal distention *to determine if peristalsis is present.* Note any nausea and vomiting *as possible indicators of paralytic ileus.* Administer stool softeners *to soften stool for easier elimination.* Begin bowel program as soon as bowel sounds return and include suppository every other day *to establish a bowel routine as quickly as possible.* Check rectum daily *to prevent impaction.* Teach patient and family the bowel program *to ensure continuity of the program and foster a sense of usefulness by family.* Ensure appropriate food and fluid intake *because bulk, fiber, and fluids are necessary to the success of a bowel program.*

continued

NURSING CARE PLAN Patient with a Spinal Cord Injury*—cont'd

Planning: Outcome Criteria	Nursing Interventions and Rationales
➤ **NURSING DIAGNOSIS**	Altered patterns of urinary elimination: retention *related to* injury and limited fluid intake *as manifested by* lack of urine output, bladder distention, involuntary emptying of bladder (after spinal shock)
Have no urinary retention or infection; be able to perform catheterization or Credé maneuver to empty bladder.	Palpate bladder every shift *because loss of autonomic and reflex control of bladder and sphincter can cause distention.* Insert indwelling catheter during acute phase *to ensure continuous flow of urine, preventing kidney reflux or possible bladder rupture.* Begin intermittent catheterization program when appropriate; teach patient and family intermittent catheterization using a clean technique *to avoid long-term use of indwelling catheter with high potential for infection.* Maintain accurate intake and output records *to evaluate fluid balance.* Encourage fluids (2-4 L/day) *to maintain high volume of dilute urine, which aids in preventing infection.* Send urine for culture at least once a week *to monitor for infection.* Monitor BUN and serum creatinine levels, and WBC count *to monitor kidney function and presence of infection.* Measure urine specific gravity and pH *because an acidic urine discourages bacterial growth.* Teach Credé maneuver *to manually supplement intermittent catheterization or use alone for more complete emptying of the bladder.*
➤ **NURSING DIAGNOSIS**	Impaired physical mobility *related to* spinal cord injury, vertebral column instability, or forced immobilization by traction *as manifested by* inability to move purposefully, limited muscle strength, impaired coordination, impaired perception of position or presence of body parts
Have no or minimal complications of immobility.	Check traction to ensure that frames are secure and properly aligned and that weights are hanging freely *to ensure maintenance of vertebral column stability.* Promote good pulmonary function *because pulmonary complications are a common sequelae of immobility.* Turn patient as ordered *to prevent prolonged pressure, which can lead to pressure ulcers.* Perform full range-of-motion exercises to all extremities several times a day *to promote circulation and prevent contractures.* Use splints as appropriate *to prevent contractures and promote functional positioning.* Assess motor and sensory function at least q4hr initially *to promptly detect deterioration of neurologic status.* Mobilize patient as quickly as appropriate *to prevent hazards of immobility and provide encouragement to patient.*
➤ **NURSING DIAGNOSIS**	Acute pain *related to* muscle spasm *as manifested by* report of pain, actions and facies indicative of pain
Have minimal complaints of discomfort; satisfactory control of muscle spasms.	Assess type, location, and degree of pain *to plan appropriate interventions.* Change patient's position as appropriate *to relieve pain and show a caring attitude.* Medicate with antispasmodic agents as ordered and analgesics as needed. Use relaxation therapy *to assist in decreasing spasms.* Avoid sudden movements *to avoid producing spasms.*
➤ **NURSING DIAGNOSIS**	Self-care deficit: total *related to* paralysis *as manifested by* varying ability to perform activities of daily living
Have all care needs met; be rehabilitated to maximal self-care potential.	Perform all activities of daily living as needed t*o ensure that the patient's daily needs are met.* Encourage independence as appropriate *to give patient a sense of control and provide encouragement.* Give frequent rest periods after activity *because patient is easily fatigued by even mild activity.*

continued

NURSING CARE PLAN Patient with a Spinal Cord Injury*—cont'd

Planning: Outcome Criteria	Nursing Interventions and Rationales
➤ **NURSING DIAGNOSIS**	Risk for dysreflexia *related to* reflex stimulation of sympathetic nervous system secondary to loss of automatic control after resolution of spinal shock
Have no occurrence of dysreflexia; receive immediate and appropriate nursing or medical interventions if dysreflexia occurs.	Assess for hypertension, bradycardia, severe headache, sweating, blurred vision, flushed feeling, nasal congestion *as signs of dysreflexia.* Reduce or eliminate noxious stimuli such as fecal impaction, urinary retention, tactile stimulation, and skin lesions by appropriate interventions *to prevent occurrence of autonomic dysreflexia.* Teach patient and family to recognize and treat dysreflexia *to reverse occurrence and prevent occurrence of status epilepticus, stroke, and possible death.* If nursing interventions do not reverse symptoms, notify physician so immediate medical interventions can be initiated *to prevent a life-threatening situation from developing.*
➤ **NURSING DIAGNOSIS**	Altered nutrition: less than body requirements *related to* paralytic ileus, need for increased intake of nutrients, and inability to eat independently *as manifested by* weight loss >5.5 lb (2.5 kg) of admission weight, decreased serum albumin
Have weight loss <10 lb (4.5 kg) of admission weight.	Assess nutritional status on admission *to provide baseline data.* Ensure enteral feedings given as ordered during acute phase *so nutrient intake is not interrupted.* If patient is eating, encourage high-protein, high-carbohydrate, high-calorie diet with high bulk *to counteract the severe catabolism that occurs with spinal cord injury and to promote bowel function.* Allow patient to select foods *to encourage maximum intake and foster patient's sense of control.* Encourage family to bring in foods patient likes *to provide maximal intake and satisfaction with food.* Take time when feeding patient *to prevent decreased intake caused by feeling of "being a bother" or being rushed.* Keep a caloric count and weigh patient at least weekly *to evaluate nutritional plan and continue or revise as necessary.*
➤ **NURSING DIAGNOSIS**	Sexual dysfunction *related to* inability to achieve erection or perceive pelvic sensations and lack of knowledge of alternative means of achieving sexual satisfaction *as manifested by* inability to achieve erection or perceive pelvic sensation, verbalization of lack of knowledge of how to achieve sexual satisfaction
Express satisfaction with sexual activities; know about variety of ways to achieve sexual expression.	Establish an honest, caring relationship with patient and sexual partner *to encourage open discussion of sexual concerns.* Provide accurate information about effects of spinal cord injury on sexual functioning; encourage questions; suggest alternative methods and use of assistive devices to achieve sexual satisfaction *to provide important information to patient.* Discuss reflexogenic erection with men and vaginal lubrication techniques with women *as means of enhancing sexual satisfaction.* Suggest that patient discuss possibility of penile prosthesis with physician. Encourage patient to be relaxed and unhurried during sexual activity *because stress decreases probability of a satisfactory sexual experience.* Refer for sexual counseling if indicated.
➤ **NURSING DIAGNOSIS**	Risk for injury *related to* sensory deficit and lack of self-protective abilities
Have no injuries related to spinal cord injury.	Assess environment for potentially injurious situations *to plan appropriate adjustments.* Use side rails; pad side rails; turn and transfer patient carefully with adequate assistance *as means of preventing patient injury.* Assess skin every shift *to determine presence of irritation and injury.* Answer call light promptly; anticipate patient's needs *to prevent patient from attempting potentially dangerous activities unassisted.*

continued

NURSING CARE PLAN Patient with a Spinal Cord Injury*—cont'd

Planning: Outcome Criteria	Nursing Interventions and Rationales
➤ **NURSING DIAGNOSIS**	Altered family processes *related to* change in function of ill family member *as manifested by* poor communication patterns among family members, use of ineffective coping techniques (e.g., shouting, blaming, isolation), unwillingness of family members to assist with patient care
Family will maximize individual and collective strengths and meet patient's needs.	Assess family dynamics related to roles and responsibilities *to determine problematic areas and strengths.* Encourage open communication among family members regarding long-term planning to meet patient's needs, including financial aspects, *so ideas and concerns of all involved family members are considered.* Assist family members to understand patient's feelings *to strengthen patient's feeling of worth and support.* Assist family members to develop an action plan to meet patient's needs *to reduce sense of frustration and helplessness.* Make referral for counseling as appropriate.
➤ **NURSING DIAGNOSIS**	Risk for ineffective individual coping *related to* loss of control over bodily functions and altered lifestyle secondary to quadriplegia
Verbalize ability to cope with effects of spinal cord injury; use appropriate problem-solving techniques; be active participant in planning of care.	Assess for prolonged use of inappropriate defense mechanisms, inability to accept permanence of prognosis, refusal to use available support services *to determine presence of risk factors for ineffective coping.* Listen to patient, noting tone of voice and facial expression *as clues to how patient is coping with injury.* Offer support and acceptance of feelings; assist patient with problem solving *to bolster patient's confidence in ability to cope.* Teach patient relaxation techniques *because these techniques are positive coping mechanisms.* Encourage use of support systems *to discuss concerns.* Provide information *because knowledge of expectations can help patient cope with the future.* Teach patient healthy coping behaviors to *prevent patient from practicing ineffective behaviors such as smoking, drinking, or angry outbursts.*
➤ **NURSING DIAGNOSIS**	Body-image disturbance *related to* quadriplegia *as manifested by* expression of anger or other negative feelings, refusal to discuss changes in function, participate in social contacts, or look at body
Express feelings about self; work through feelings to adaptation; begin to accept altered physical abilities.	Establish a trusting relationship *so patient will feel comfortable discussing personal concerns.* Encourage discussion of feelings *to aid patient in venting and clarifying feelings.* Allow patient to grieve *because spinal cord injury results in a real loss that requires adjustment through grieving.* Provide accurate information about altered body functions *so patient knows what to expect and can have accurate body image.* Maintain privacy as necessary *because altered body appearance and function may be embarrassing to the patient.* Encourage social interaction *to foster sense of returning normalcy to life.* Assist family members in supporting patient *to enhance patient's sense of worth and value as a person.* Make referral for counseling as needed.

ABGs, Arterial blood gases; *BUN,* blood urea nitrogen; *WBC,* white blood cell.
*This care plan is suitable for a patient with a high cervical injury caused by flexion-rotation. It can be modified for patients with less severe problems.

of injury can be modified for patients with less severe problems.

Immobilization. Proper immobilization of the neck involves the maintenance of a neutral or extension position. Sandbags can be used to stabilize the neck to prevent lateral rotation of the cervical spine. The body should always be correctly aligned and turning should be performed so that the patient is moved as a unit to prevent movement of the spine. For cervical injuries, skeletal traction is usually provided by Crutchfield (Fig. 57-7), Vinke (Fig. 57-8), or other types of skull tongs. Traction is provided by a rope that is extended from the center of the tongs over a pulley and has weights attached at the end. Traction must be maintained at all times. One disadvantage of skull tongs is that the skull pins can be displaced. If this occurs, the head should be held in a neutral or extended position and help should be summoned. Sandbags can be positioned to stabilize the head while the physician reinserts the tongs.

Infection at the sites of tong insertion is another potential problem. Preventive care includes cleansing the sites twice a day with normal saline solution and applying an antibiotic ointment that acts as a mechanical barrier to the entrance of bacteria. The preventive care of insertion sites may vary depending on individual hospital standards of care.

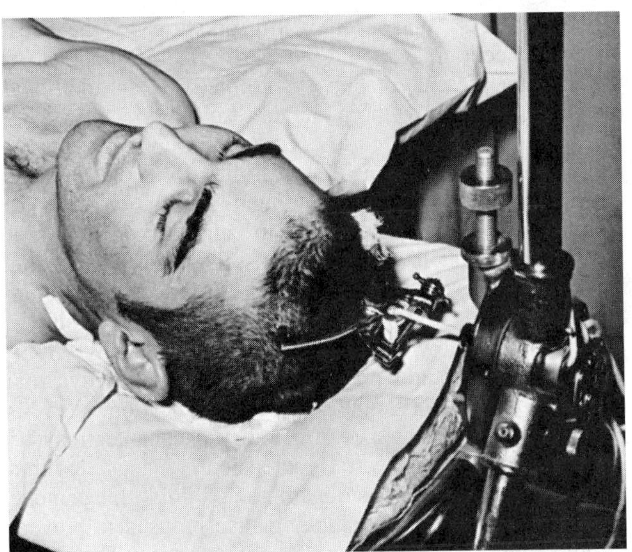

Fig. 57-7 Cervical traction is attached to tongs inserted in the skull.

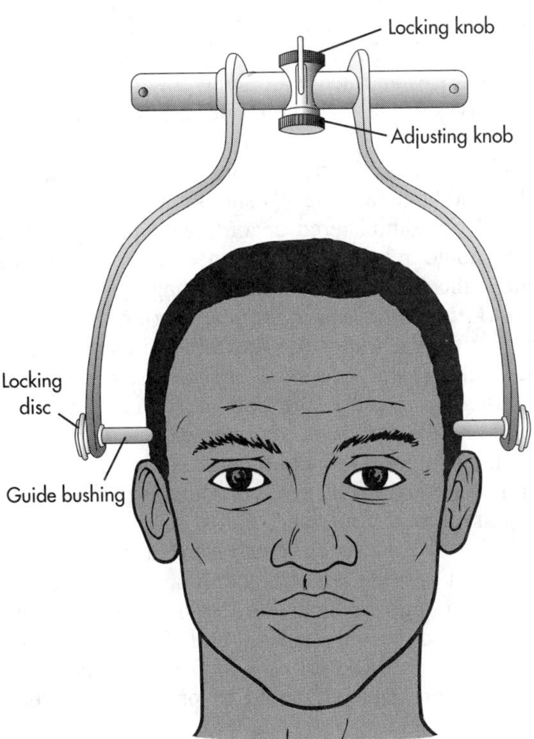

Fig. 57-8 Vinke tongs for cervical immobilization.

Special frames and beds are often used in the management of the patient with a spinal cord injury. Equipment includes the Stryker frame and the kinetic therapy Rotorest bed (Fig. 57-9). The Stryker frame was developed in 1939 and was the first bed that afforded some benefits of mobilization. The Stryker frame bed uses a side-to-side lateral turn. The kinetic therapy Rotorest bed uses a con-

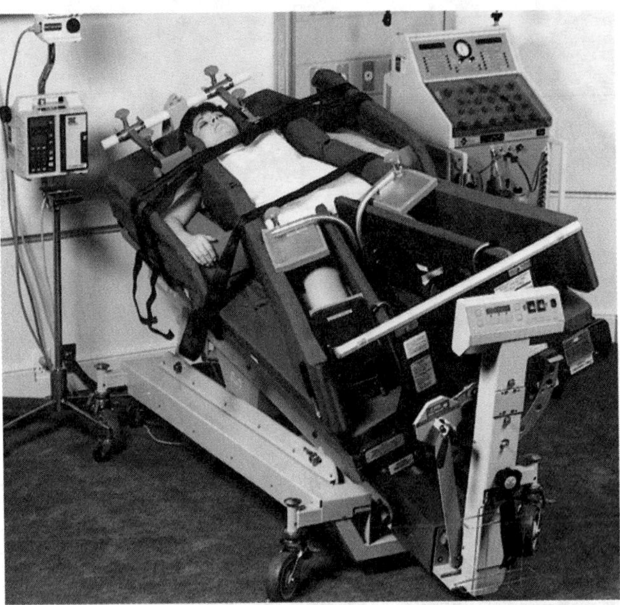

Fig. 57-9 Kinetic therapy treatment table (Rotorest bed).

tinual side-to-side slow rotation with the patient in constant motion. The bed allows a frequency of turns of greater than 200 times per day. The bed is used to decrease the likelihood of pressure sores and cardiopulmonary complications. However, in some patients the turning can induce motion sickness and fear of falling out of bed when turned to the extremes.

Depending on the type of injury and therapeutic interventions, the tongs and traction may be removed 2 to 4 weeks after injury. In a stable injury, halo traction may be applied in the Emergency Department. The removal of traction and application of a collar or halo traction device allows the patient to be more mobile and to begin active rehabilitation. The halo apparatus applies cervical traction by means of a jacketlike arrangement that allows greater mobility and wheelchair activity than other traction systems (Fig. 57-10).

Immobilization of the neck of the patient with a spinal cord injury prevents further injury, but the effects of immobility are profound. The decrease or lack of neural stimulation and any movement greatly increases catabolism and produces dysfunction in body organs. The paralysis and accompanying psychologic stress cause a lifelong problem related to nitrogen balance.

Meticulous skin care is critical because decreased sensation and circulation make the patient particularly susceptible to skin breakdown. Patients should be removed from backboards as soon as possible and cervical collars properly fitted or replaced with other forms of immobilization to prevent coccygeal and occipital area skin breakdown.

Respiratory dysfunction. During the first 48 hours after injury, edema may increase the level of dysfunction and respiratory distress may occur. If the patient is exhausted from labored breathing or ABGs deteriorate (indicating inadequate oxygenation), endotracheal intubation or tra-

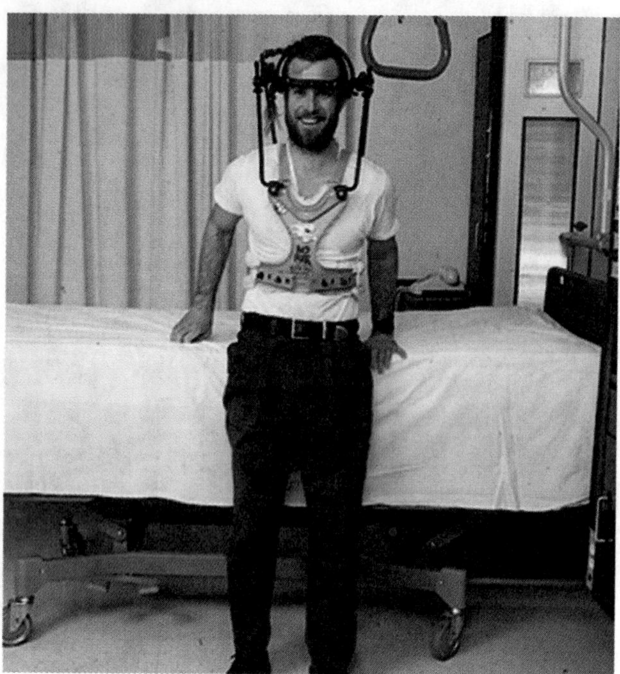

Fig. 57-10 Halo vest. Note the rigid shoulder straps and encompassing vest. Various vest sizes are available prefabricated. The halo ring, superstructure, and vest are magnetic resonance imaging (MRI)-compatible.

cheostomy and mechanical ventilation should be initiated. Respiratory arrest is a possibility that requires careful monitoring of the respiratory system and prompt action should it occur. Pneumonia and atelectasis are potential problems because of the loss of vital capacity and the loss of intercostal and abdominal muscle function, resulting in diaphragmatic breathing, pooled secretions, and an ineffective cough. Nasal stuffiness and bronchospasms are also problems.

The nurse should regularly assess (1) breath sounds, (2) ABGs, (3) tidal volume, (4) vital capacity, (5) skin color, (6) breathing patterns (especially the use of accessory muscles), (7) subjective comments about the ability to breathe, and (8) the amount and color of sputum. A PaO_2 (partial pressure of oxygen in arterial blood) above 60 mm Hg and a $PaCO_2$ (partial pressure of carbon dioxide in arterial blood) below 45 mm Hg are acceptable values in a patient with uncomplicated quadriplegia. The nurse should note the effect of the prone position because it can significantly reduce vital capacity and result in respiratory arrest. A patient who is unable to count to 10 out loud without taking a breath needs immediate attention.

In addition to monitoring activities, the nurse can intervene in maintaining ventilation. Oxygen is administered until ABGs stabilize. Chest physiotherapy and quad-assist coughing facilitate the raising of secretions. Quad-assist coughing stimulates the action of the ineffective abdominal muscles during the expiratory phase of a cough. The nurse places a fist or the heel of a hand between the umbilicus and xiphoid process and exerts firm pressure to the area. Tracheal suctioning should be performed if crackles or rhonchi are present. Incentive spirometry is an additional technique to improve the patient's respiratory status.

Cardiovascular instability. Because of unopposed vagal response, the heart rate is slowed, often to below 60 beats per minute. Any increase in vagal stimulation such as turning or suctioning can result in cardiac arrest. Loss of sympathetic tone in peripheral vessels results in chronic low blood pressure with potential postural hypotension. Lack of muscle tone to aid venous return can result in sluggish blood flow and predispose the patient to DVT.

Vital signs should be assessed frequently. If bradycardia is symptomatic, an anticholinergic medication such as atropine is administered. A temporary pacemaker may be inserted in some instances. Hypotension is managed with a vasopressor agent such as dopamine and fluid replacement.

Compression gradient stockings can be used to prevent thromboemboli and to promote venous return. The stockings must be removed every 8 hours for skin care. The use of pneumatic compression devices for the calves is advocated, and they need to be applied as soon as possible after admission and maintained throughout the hospitalization. Venous duplex studies may be performed before applying compression devices. The nurse should also perform range-of-motion exercises and heel-cord stretching regularly. The thighs and calves of the legs should be assessed every shift for signs of DVT.

If blood loss has occurred from other injuries, the hemoglobin and hematocrit levels should be monitored and blood should be administered according to protocol. The nurse also should monitor the patient for indications of hypovolemic shock secondary to hemorrhage.

Fluid and nutritional maintenance. During the first 48 to 72 hours after the injury the gastrointestinal tract may stop functioning (paralytic ileus) and a nasogastric tube must be inserted. Because the patient cannot have oral intake, fluid and electrolyte needs must be carefully monitored. Specific solutions and additives are ordered based on individual requirements. Once bowel sounds are present or flatus is passed, oral food and fluids can gradually be introduced. Because of severe catabolism, a high-protein, high-calorie diet is necessary for energy and tissue repair. In patients with high cervical cord injuries, swallowing must be evaluated before starting oral feedings. If the patient is unable to resume eating within 3 to 4 days, total parenteral nutrition may be started to provide nutritional support.

Increased roughage should be included to promote bowel function. Some patients experience anorexia, which can be due to psychologic depression, boredom with institutional food, or discomfort at being fed (often by a hurried nurse). Some patients have a normally small appetite. Occasionally, refusal to eat is used as a means of maintaining control over the environment because of diminished or absent body control. If the patient is not eating adequately, the cause should be thoroughly assessed. On the basis of this assessment, a contract may be made with the patient regarding the diet that uses mutual goal setting. This gives the patient increased control of the situation and often results in improved nutritional intake. General measures such as providing a pleasant eating environment, allowing adequate time to eat (including any self-feeding the patient can achieve), encouraging the family to bring in special foods, and planning social rewards for eating may be useful. A calorie count should be kept and the patient's daily weight recorded as a means of evaluating progress. If feasible, the patient should participate in recording calorie intake. The nurse should avoid allowing the patient's nutritional intake to become a basis for a power struggle.

Bowel and bladder management. Urine is retained because of the loss of autonomic and reflex control of the bladder and sphincter. Because there is no sensation of fullness, overdistention of the bladder can result in reflux into the kidney with eventual kidney failure. Bladder overdistention may even result in rupture of the bladder. Consequently an indwelling catheter is usually inserted as soon as possible after injury. Its patency must be ensured by frequent inspection and irrigation if warranted. In some institutions a physician's order is required for this procedure. Strict aseptic technique for catheter care is essential to avoid introducing infection. After the patient is stabilized, the best means of managing long-term urinary function is assessed. Usually the patient is started on an intermittent catheterization program. The patient is usually maintained on a fluid restriction of 1800 to 2000 ml per day to facilitate a bladder training program. Urinary output is monitored closely.

Urinary tract infections are a common problem. A large fluid intake and the liberal use of juices such as cranberry, grape, and apple are used to prevent infections. When used in large quantities, these juices leave an acid ash in the urine, which discourages bacterial growth. Citrus juices are used sparingly. Ascorbic acid and a urinary antiseptic such as methenamine mandelate (Mandelamine) are sometimes given. The pH of the urine should be tested daily to evaluate acidity. If the appearance or odor of the urine is suspicious, a specimen is sent for culture.

Constipation is generally a problem during spinal shock because no voluntary or involuntary evacuation of the bowels occurs. Suppositories are used in combination with a laxative to assist in bowel evacuation. Enemas are used only if absolutely necessary because they can overdistend the rectum and create problems for initiating an effective bowel program.

Temperature control. Because there is no vasoconstriction, piloerection, or heat loss through perspiration below the level of injury, temperature control is largely external to the patient. Therefore the nurse monitors the environment closely to maintain an appropriate temperature. Body temperature is monitored regularly. The patient is not overloaded with covers or unduly exposed (such as during bathing). If an infection develops, more extensive means of temperature control such as a cooling blanket may be necessary.

Stress ulcers. Stress ulcers are a problem for the patient with a spinal cord injury because of the physiologic response to severe trauma, psychologic stress, and high-dose corticosteroids. Peak incidence is 6 to 14 days after injury. Stool and gastric content are tested daily for blood, and the hematocrit is observed for a slow drop. When corticosteroids are given, they should be accompanied by antacids or food. Histamine H_2 receptor antagonists such as ranitidine (Zantac) and famotidine (Pepcid) may be given prophylactically to decrease the secretion of hydrochloric acid. Gastrointestinal bleeding may also predispose to aspiration pneumonia.

Sensory deprivation. The nurse must compensate for the patient's absent sensations to prevent sensory deprivation. This is done by stimulating the patient above the level of injury. Conversation, music, strong aromas, and interesting flavors should be a part of the nursing care plan. Prism glasses are provided so that the patient can read and watch television. Every effort should be made to prevent the patient from withdrawing from the environment.

Patients with spinal cord injury often report altered sensorium and vivid dreams during the acute phase of their treatment. Whether this is due to drugs used to manage pain and anxiety is not known. Patients may also experience disrupted sleep patterns as a result of the hospital environment or posttraumatic stress disorder.

Reflexes. Once spinal cord shock is resolved, the return of reflexes may complicate rehabilitation. Lacking control from the higher brain centers, reflexes are inappropriate and often excessive. Erections can occur from a variety of stimuli, causing embarrassment and discomfort. Spasms ranging from mild twitches to convulsive movements below the level of the lesion may also occur. This reflex activity may be interpreted by the patient or family as a return of function, and the nurse must tactfully explain the reason for the activity. The patient may be informed of the positive use of these reflexes in sexual, bowel, and bladder retraining. Spasms may be relieved with the use of warm baths, whirlpool treatments, antispasmodics, and muscle relaxants. Peak spasticity occurs after 2 years, and if it is severe, destruction of the reflexes (cordotomy) may be necessary. This procedure compromises retraining and should only be done as a last resort.

Autonomic dysreflexia. Autonomic dysreflexia (hyperreflexia) is a massive uncompensated cardiovascular reaction mediated by the sympathetic division of the autonomic nervous system. It occurs in response to visceral stimulation once spinal shock is resolved in patients with spinal cord lesions above T7. The condition is a life-threatening situation that requires immediate resolution. If resolution does not occur, this condition can lead to status epilepticus, stroke, and even death.

The most common precipitating cause is a distended bladder or rectum, although any sensory stimulation may cause autonomic dysreflexia. Contraction of the bladder or rectum, stimulation of the skin, or stimulation of the pain receptors may also cause autonomic dysreflexia. Manifestations include hypertension (up to 300 mm Hg systolic), blurred vision, throbbing headache, marked diaphoresis above the level of the lesion, bradycardia (30 to 40 beats/min), piloerection (erection of body hair) as a result of pilomotor spasm, nasal congestion, and nausea. It is important to measure blood pressure when a patient with a spinal cord injury complains of a headache.

The pathology of autonomic dysreflexia involves the stimulation of sensory receptors below the level of the cord lesion. The intact autonomic system below the level of the lesion responds to the stimulation with a reflex arteriolar vasoconstriction that increases blood pressure. Baroreceptors in the carotid sinus and the aorta sense the hypertension and stimulate the parasympathetic system. This results in a decrease in heart rate, but the visceral and peripheral vessels do not dilate because efferent impulses cannot pass through the cord lesion.

Nursing interventions in this serious emergency are elevation of the head of the bed 45 degrees, notification of the physician, and assessment to determine the cause. The most common cause is bladder irritation. Immediate catheterization to relieve the distention may be necessary. Catheter irrigation performed slowly and gently may open a plugged catheter, or a new catheter may be inserted. A digital rectal examination should be performed only after application of an anesthetic ointment to decrease rectal stimulation and to prevent an increase of symptoms. The nurse should remove all skin stimuli such as constrictive clothing and tight shoes. If symptoms persist after the source has been relieved, an α-adrenergic blocker or an arteriolar vasodilator may be given. Careful monitoring must continue until the vital signs stabilize.

Patient and family must be taught the causes and symptoms of autonomic dysreflexia. They must understand the life-threatening nature of this dysfunction and must know how to relieve the cause.

Chronic and Home Management. The physiologic and psychologic rehabilitation of the person with spinal cord injury is complex and involved. With physical and psychologic care and intensive and specialized rehabilitation, the patient with a spinal cord injury learns to function at the highest level of wellness. Special rehabilitation centers are available, but patients must demonstrate adequate motivation for self-care to be admitted.

Many of the problems identified in the acute period become chronic and continue throughout life. Rehabilitation focuses on refined retraining of physiologic processes. Braces, electronic wheelchairs, and mechanical devices are used to maximize the patient's remaining function (Fig. 57-11). The patient with high cervical spinal cord injury has greatly increased mobility with phrenic nerve stimulators or electronic diaphragmatic pacemakers. Diaphragmatic pacemakers may allow the patient to become independent of mechanical ventilation. Generally these devices are used after neurologic recovery is complete (at least 1 year after injury). Today, ventilators are also reasonably portable, and ventilator-dependent quadriplegic patients can be mobile and somewhat independent. Although rehabilitation and the special equipment required are costly, many programs are funded by the state or federal governments.

If the patient can be successfully brought through the acute period, the patient's life can be fuller and richer than previously believed possible. Like other persons who have been close to death, some patients find that their lives are richer and more meaningful than before the injury. Unfortunately, other patients may not have such a positive future outlook. The nurse has a pivotal role in the coordinated efforts of the health team to influence a positive outcome.

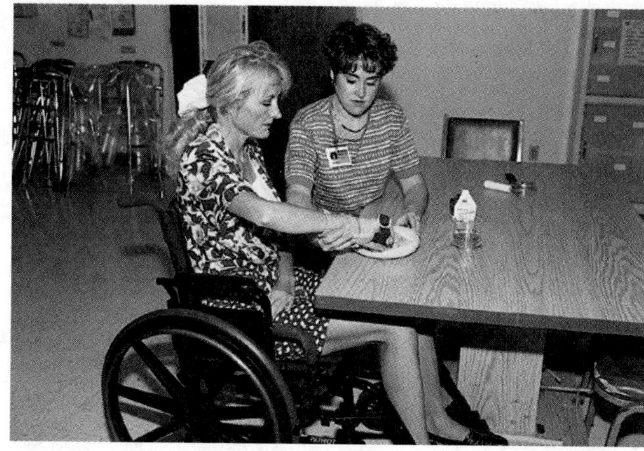

Fig. 57-11 A patient participating in occupational therapy using mobile arm supports and upper-extremity orthotics.

Neurogenic bladder. Once spinal cord shock and the resulting bladder atony are resolved, the bladder is neurogenic. A neurogenic bladder is any type of bladder dysfunction related to abnormal or absent bladder innervation. It may lead to problems with residual urine, stone formation (urolithiasis), or infection and is often associated with progressive renal deterioration and urinary incontinence. The network of fibers of the detrusor muscle forms the muscular wall of the bladder. The trigone is a small rectangular area near the bladder neck sometimes called the *internal sphincter.* The urogenital diaphragm or baseplate encircles the urethral opening completely and is sometimes called the *external sphincter.* Depending on the lesion, a neurogenic bladder may have no reflex detrusor contractions (*areflexic, flaccid*) or may have hyperactive reflex detrusor contractions (*hyperreflexic, spastic*). Common symptoms of a neurogenic bladder include urgency, frequency, incontinence, inability to void, and characteristics of obstruction.

Neurogenic bladder can be classified according to reflex detrusor activity, intravesical filling pressure, and continence function. Types of neurogenic bladder are outlined in Table 57-7. Diagnostic and therapeutic management of neurogenic bladder are described in Table 57-8.

The patient with a spinal cord injury and a neurogenic bladder requires a comprehensive program to manage bladder function. The program should include the following:

1. *Diagnostic evaluation:* after the patient's overall condition is stable with evidence of neurologic reflexes, a cystometrogram, an IV pyelogram, and a urine culture are taken.
2. *Pharmacologic:* drugs to increase the strength of bladder contractions (detrusor), acidify the urine, and relax the urethral sphincter are administered.

Table 57-7 Types of Neurogenic Bladders

Type	Characteristics	Cause	Clinical Manifestations
■ Uninhibited	No inhibitions influence time and place of voiding	Corticospinal tract lesion; observed in CVA, multiple sclerosis, brain tumor, brain trauma	Incontinence, increased frequency, urgency
■ Reflex	Bladder behaves as part of spinal reflex arc with no connection to brain	Lesion of motor and sensory fibers; occasionally seen in multiple sclerosis, pernicious anemia	Incontinence, urinary frequency, lack of sensation of bladder filling
■ Autonomous	Bladder behaves autonomously, as if it were cut off from brain and spinal cord	Lesions of cauda equina, pelvic nerves, spina bifuda	Incontinence, difficulty initiating micturition
■ Motor paralysis	Bladder acts as if there were paralysis of all motor functions	Lower motor neuron lesion caused by trauma involving S2-S4	If sensory function intact, feels bladder distention and hesitancy; no control of micturition, resulting in overdistention of bladder and overflow incontinence
■ Sensory paralysis	Bladder acts as if there were paralysis of all sensory modalities	Damage to sensory limb of bladder spinal reflex arc; seen in multiple sclerosis, diabetes mellitus, pernicious anemia	Poor bladder sensation, infrequent voiding, large residual volume

CVA, Cerebrovascular accident.

3. *Nutrition:* a low-calcium diet (1 g/day) is advocated to reduce the possibility of kidney and bladder stones.

4. *Fluids:* a fluid intake of 1800 to 2000 ml per day must be maintained to prevent stone formation and to ensure adequate urine flow.

5. *Urine drainage:* the method used for urinary drainage depends on the condition of the patient; the preference of the physician, nursing staff, and patient; and the policy of the institution. Numerous drainage methods are possible, including reflex training, indwelling catheter, intermittent catheterization, urinary diversion surgery, and artificial sphincter.

Many factors are considered when selecting a bladder management strategy. These include upper extremity function, caregiver burden, and lifestyle choices.

With the return of the reflex arc, bladder function may be a reflex. However, because of the interruption in the pathways to the brain, the patient has no control over urination, which results in a bladder with a small capacity, hyperirritable detrusor muscle and sphincter, and loss of inhibition of the reflex by the brain. The patient or the nurse can use techniques such as the Credé and Valsalva maneuvers or a rectal stretch to facilitate complete emptying of the bladder. The Credé maneuver involves the exertion by the nurse or patient of downward pressure over the bladder with a pumping motion. This maneuver is only used in those patients with a lower motor neuron pattern bladder and may require a physician's order in some settings because

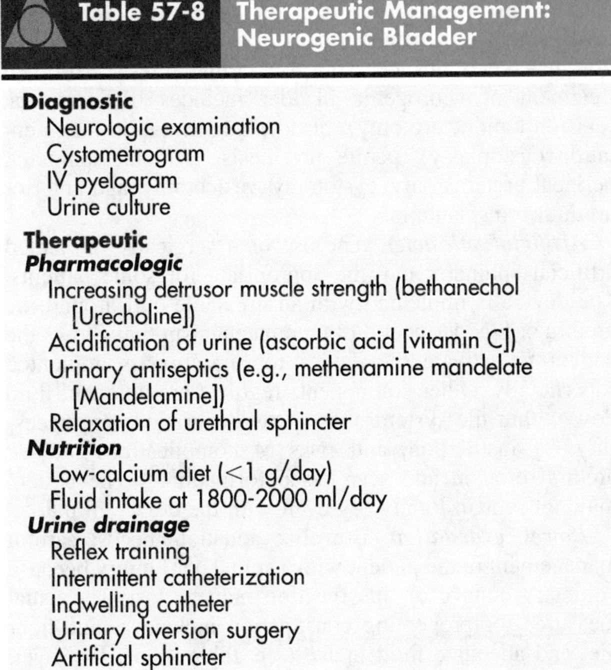

Table 57-8 Therapeutic Management: Neurogenic Bladder

Diagnostic
- Neurologic examination
- Cystometrogram
- IV pyelogram
- Urine culture

Therapeutic

Pharmacologic
- Increasing detrusor muscle strength (bethanechol [Urecholine])
- Acidification of urine (ascorbic acid [vitamin C])
- Urinary antiseptics (e.g., methenamine mandelate [Mandelamine])
- Relaxation of urethral sphincter

Nutrition
- Low-calcium diet (<1 g/day)
- Fluid intake at 1800-2000 ml/day

Urine drainage
- Reflex training
- Intermittent catheterization
- Indwelling catheter
- Urinary diversion surgery
- Artificial sphincter

IV, Intravenous.

it has the potential of stimulating autonomic dysreflexia in the patient with upper motor neuron disease. In the Valsalva maneuver, the patient inhales deeply, holds his or her breath, and bears down. The rectal stretch is the insertion of a gloved finger into the rectum, gently pulling to exert pressure on the sphincter to cause relaxation of the perineal floor. Combining the Valsalva maneuver with rectal stretch results in more complete emptying of the bladder. The patient should be regularly assessed for residual urine after reflex bladder emptying. It may take up to 3 to 5 days before residual urine is less than 100 ml. Many drugs affect urinary retention and thus should be assessed for their effects on residual volume. The ultimate goal for this technique is for the patient to not need a catheter.

The long-term use of an indwelling catheter should be carefully evaluated because of the associated high incidence of urinary tract infection, fistula formation, and diverticula. Adequate fluid intake and patency of the catheter should be ensured. The frequency of catheter changing ranges from 1 week to 1 month, depending on the type of catheter used and agency policy.

Intermittent catheterization is the recommended method of bladder management (see Chapter 43). Nursing assessment is important in selecting the time interval between catheterizations. Initially, catheterization is done every 4 hours. If less than 200 ml of urine is drained, the time interval may be extended. If 500 ml or more of urine is obtained, the time interval is shortened. An overdistended bladder can cause ischemia, which may predispose tissues to bacterial invasion and infection. Patients often experience diuresis at a regular time during a 24-hour period, which may necessitate an extra catheterization. The number of intermittent catheterizations per day is usually five or six.

Urinary diversion surgery may be necessary if the patient has repeated urinary tract infections with renal involvement or repeated stones or if therapeutic intervention has been unsuccessful (see Table 43-15). Surgical treatment of neurogenic bladder includes bladder neck revision (sphincterotomy), bladder augmentation (augmentation cystoplasty), penile prosthesis, artificial sphincter, perineal ureterostomy, cystotomy, vesicotomy, and anterior urethral transplantation.

Artificial sphincter. The use of a surgically implanted artificial sphincter may be appropriate for some patients. The device is implanted with an inflatable cuff around the urethra or bladder neck. A pump mechanism that allows the patient to activate the device for urination is implanted superficially. Other components regulate pressure and fluid flow within the system. One or two operations are necessary for instillation, and risks of complications include urethral erosion and scar tissue formation.[21] The patient may not remain totally dry even with the device in place.

Bowel evacuation. Bowel evacuation needs careful management in the patient with a spinal cord injury because voluntary control of this function may be lost. The usual measures for preventing constipation include a high-fiber diet and adequate fluid intake (see Table 40-9). However, these measures by themselves may not be adequate to stimulate emptying. In addition, suppositories or digital stimulation by the nurse or patient may be necessary. In the patient with an upper motor neuron lesion, digital stimulation is necessary to promote emptying. Small-volume enemas and agents such as docusate sodium, bisacodyl, and glycerine may also be used. Valsalva and manual stimulation are useful in patients with lower motor neuron lesions. The Valsalva maneuver requires intact abdominal muscles, so it is used in those patients with injuries below T12.

In general, a bowel movement every other day is considered adequate. However, preinjury patterns should be considered. Incontinence can result from too much stool softener or a fecal impaction. Careful recording of bowel movements, including amount, time, and consistency, is important to the overall success of the program.

Sexuality. Because the majority of patients with spinal cord injuries are men between 18 and 35 years of age, sexual rehabilitation is a major issue. It is important to remember that sexuality is an important issue regardless of the patient's age. To work with these patients, the nurse must have an awareness and an acceptance of personal sexuality, as well as knowledge of human sexual responses.

RESEARCH

Implications for Nursing Practice

NO-TOUCH CATHETERIZATION IN THE SPINAL CORD–INJURED PATIENT

Citation Charbonneau-Smith R: No-touch catheterization and infection rates in a select spinal cord injured population, *Rehabil Nurs* 18:296-305, 1993.

Purpose To evaluate a no-touch catheter as compared with a traditional straight intermittent catheter relative to their effect on urinary tract infections.

Methods Retrospective analysis comparing two intermittent catheterization techniques used with spinal cord–injured patients. Charts were reviewed for 92 patients with traumatic spinal cord injuries who were on intermittent catheterization, and the incidence of urinary tract infection was determined. A convenience sample of 18 patients participated in a prospective study using a no-touch method of catheterization for 7 months.

Results The retrospective analysis of charts of patients using standard intermittent catheterization indicated an infection rate of nearly 80%. In the experimental group the infection rate was 44%. The no-touch method reduced the total number of infections and the duration of infection. A nurse satisfaction questionnaire revealed that the nursing staff preferred this method of intermittent catheterization to the traditional method.

Implications for Nursing Practice Intermittent catheterization is the treatment of choice for patients who are unable to empty their bladders completely. In spite of this study's limitations, it does indicate that the no-touch method of catheterization can minimize urinary tract infections in spinal cord–injured patients.

Table 57-9 Potential for Sexual Activity in Men with Spinal Cord Injuries

Erection	Ejaculation	Orgasm
Upper Motor Neuron		
Complete		
Frequent (93%), reflexogenic only	Rare	Absent
Incomplete		
Most frequent (99%), reflexogenic (80%), reflexogenic and psychogenic (19%)	Less frequent (32%), after reflexogenic erection (74%), after psychogenic erection (26%)	Present (if ejaculation occurs)
Lower Motor Neuron		
Complete		
Infrequent (26%)	Infrequent (18%)	Present (if ejaculation occurs)
Incomplete		
Psychogenic and reflexogenic	Frequent (70%), after psychogenic and reflexogenic erections	Present (if ejaculation occurs)

When discussing sexual potential, the nurse should use scientific terminology rather than slang whenever possible. Knowledge of the level of the lesion is needed to understand the patient's potential for orgasm, erection, and fertility and the patient's capacity for sexual satisfaction (Table 57-9). All patients with spinal cord injuries generally lack perineal sensation during intercourse regardless of the type of lesion.

Reflex sexual function capability is possible if the patient has an upper motor neuron lesion. The presence of tone in the external rectal sphincter indicates an upper motor lesion. The absence of external rectal sphincter tone, bulbocavernosus reflex, or both indicates that the patient has lower motor neuron involvement and may be capable of psychogenic erection but not reflex erection. If ejaculation occurs, it may be retrograde into the bladder.

The type of lesion determines the physical sexual response. Men with upper motor neuron lesions may have reflexogenic erections that are produced by reflex activity or external stimuli or that occur spontaneously. These spontaneous erections are often short lived and uncontrolled and cannot be maintained or summoned at the time of coitus. Orgasm and ejaculation are usually not possible for men with a complete upper motor neuron lesion.

Most patients with a complete lower motor neuron lesion are unable to have either psychogenic or reflexogenic erections. Patients with incomplete lower motor neuron lesions have the highest possibility of successful psychogenic erection with ejaculation, and up to 10% of these patients are fertile.

The woman of childbearing age with a spinal cord injury usually remains fertile, although orgasmic ability is lost. The injury does not affect the ability to become pregnant or to deliver through the normal birth canal.

Sexual rehabilitation for both men and women should begin informally after the acute phase of the injury has passed. Questions such as "Have you had an erection since your accident?" and "Have your menstrual periods continued since the accident?" are nonthreatening ways to introduce the topic of sexual functioning. The male patient may pose a question such as, "Can I ever be a man again?"

Open discussion with the patient is essential. This important aspect of rehabilitation should be handled by someone specially trained in sexual counseling. Unless this type of training has occurred the nurse should not attempt to direct the plan for sexual rehabilitation.

The properly trained nurse works with the patient and partner to provide support during new relationships, with the emphasis on open communication. The nurse's educational role requires respect for every couple's personal standards of religious and cultural beliefs. Alternative methods of obtaining sexual satisfaction such as oral-genital sex (cunnilingus and fellatio) may be suggested. Explicit films (e.g., *Touching*) may also be used. This film demonstrates the sexual activities of a patient with paraplegia and a nondisabled partner. Graphics should be used cautiously because they may be too limiting or focus too much on the mechanics of sex rather than on the relationship.

Sexual activities may require more planning and be less spontaneous than before the injury. For example, an attendant may have to undress the patient and remove equipment.

Care should be taken not to dislodge the indwelling catheter during sexual activity. If a Texas catheter is used, it should be removed before sexual activity and the patient should refrain from fluids. The bowel program should include evacuation the morning of sexual activity. The partner should be informed that an accident is always possible. Illustrations for teaching management of urinary equipment are available.[22] The woman may need a water-soluble lubricant to supplement diminished vaginal secretions and facilitate vaginal penetration.

Menses may cease for as long as 6 months. If sexual activity is resumed, protection against an unplanned pregnancy is necessary. A normal pregnancy may be complicated by urinary tract infections, anemia, and autonomic dysreflexia. Because uterine contractions are not felt, a precipitous delivery is always a danger. In men, fertility is reduced because of decreased number and motility of sperm and retrograde ejaculation of sperm into the bladder. For male patients desiring children, alternative methods include sperm harvesting and concentrating, adoption, and artificial insemination.

A relaxed atmosphere with music and perfume creates an attractive environment. Ample time for caressing, fondling, and kissing is essential. The partners should be encouraged to explore each other's erogenous areas, such as the lips, neck, and ears, which can arouse psychogenic erection or orgasm. Few demands should be made initially.

Grief. Patients with spinal cord injuries are aware of the extent of injury but also feel an overwhelming sense of loss. They are no longer in control but must depend on others for activities of daily living and for life-sustaining measures. Patients may believe that they are useless and burdens to their families. At a stage when independence is often of the greatest importance developmentally, they are totally dependent on others.

The patient's response and recovery differ in some important aspects from those experiencing loss from amputation or terminal illness. First, regression can and does occur at different stages. The usual 2-year period for healthy adjustment to loss cannot be applied to the patient with spinal cord injury. Working through grief is a difficult, lifelong process with which the patient needs support and encouragement. With recent advances in rehabilitation, it is usual for the patient to be independent physically and discharged from the rehabilitation center before completion of the grief process. Another phenomenon involves that of triggering experiences, including new experiences such as marriage, that may recall earlier unresolved difficulties. Depending on the success of previous grief work, the new demand for grief work may be shortened or prolonged. The goal of recovery is related more to adjustment than to acceptance. Adjustment implies the ability to go on with living with certain limitations. Although the patient who is cooperative and accepting is easier to treat, the nurse should expect a wide fluctuation of emotions from a patient with a spinal cord injury. Depression may not be a component of the recovery process. Societal norms allow depression after severe loss and almost impose it on those confronted with death or radical lifestyle changes. However, every patient may not experience depression.

The nurse's role in grief work is to allow mourning as a component of the rehabilitation process. Table 57-10 summarizes the mourning process and appropriate nursing interventions. During the shock and denial stage the nurse reassures the patient and stresses the expertise of the entire health care team. During the anger stage, the nurse assists the patient in achievement of control over the environment, particularly by allowing the patient's input into the plan of care. The nurse should not respond to anger or manipulation or become involved with a power struggle with the patient. As self-care abilities increase, the patient's independence increases.

The patient's family also requires counseling to avoid promoting dependency in the patient through guilt or misplaced sympathy. The family is also experiencing an intense grieving process. A support group of family members and friends of patients with spinal cord injury can help increase family members' knowledge and participation in the grieving process, physical difficulties, rehabilitation plan, and the meaning of the disability in society.

During the stage of depression, the nurse must be patient, persistent, and maintain a sense of humor. Sympathy is not helpful. The patient should be treated in an adult manner and involved in decision making about care, but the nurse must insist that the care be performed. A primary

Table 57-10 Mourning Process and Nursing Interventions in Spinal Cord Injury

Patient Behavior	Nursing Intervention
Shock and Denial	
Struggle for survival, complete dependence, excessive sleep, withdrawal, fantasies, unrealistic expectations	Use of meticulous nursing care. Be honest. Use simple diagrams to explain injury. Encourage patient to begin long road to recovery.
Anger	
Refusal to discuss paralysis, decreased self-esteem, manipulation, hostile and abusive language	Coordinate care with patient and encourage self-care. Support family members; prevent alleviation of guilt by supporting dependency. Use humor liberally. Allow patient outbursts. Do not allow fixation on injury.
Depression	
Sadness, pessimism, anorexia, nightmares, insomnia, agitation, psychomotor retardation, "blues," suicidal preoccupation, refusal to participate in any self-care activities	Encourage family involvement and resources. Plan graded steps in rehabilitation to give success with minimal opportunity for frustration. Give cheerful and willing assistance with activities of daily living. Avoid sympathy. Use firm kindness.
Adjustment	
Planning for future, active participation in therapy, finding of personal meaning in experience and continuation of growth, return to premorbid personality	Remember that patients with spinal cord injuries have individual personalities. Balance support systems to encourage independence. Set goals with patient input. Emphasize potentials as achieved by others. Avoid use of clichés.

nurse relationship is helpful, but the nurse needs some relief from the intense stress of continual interaction with the patient. Staff planning and sessions in which staff members can express their feelings are helpful in providing consistency of care. To achieve the stage of adjustment, the patient needs continual support throughout the rehabilitation in the forms of acceptance, affection, and caring. The nurse must be attentive when the patient needs to talk and sensitive to needs at the various stages of the grief process.

SPINAL CORD TUMORS

Pathophysiology

Tumors that affect the spinal cord account for 0.5% to 1% of all neoplasms. These tumors are classified as primary (arising from some component of cord, dura, nerves, or vessels), secondary (caused by intraspinal extension from the vertebrae, neck, or thoracic abdominal tumors), and metastatic (from primary growths in the breast, thyroid, lung, kidney, and other sites). The thoracic and lumbar spine, including the sacrum, are the most commonly affected areas. Spinal cord tumors are further classified as extradural, subdural, intradural-extramedullary, and intradural-intra medullary tumors (Fig. 57-12, Table 57-11). Neurofibromas, meningiomas, gliomas, and hemangiomas are the most frequently occurring neoplasms.

Because many of these tumors are slow growing, their symptoms stem from the mechanical effects of slow compression and irritation of nerve roots, displacement of the cord, or gradual obstruction of the vascular supply. The slowness of growth does not cause autodestruction as in traumatic lesions. Therefore complete functional restoration is possible when the tumor is removed, except with the intradural-intramedullary tumors.

Most metastatic tumors are extradural lesions.[23] Tumors that commonly metastasize to the spinal epidural space are those that spread to bone, such as carcinomas of the breast, lung, prostate, and kidney.

Clinical Manifestations

The most common early symptom of a spinal cord tumor outside the cord is pain in the back with radiations simulating intercostal neuralgia, angina, or herpes zoster. The location of the pain depends on the level of compression. The pain worsens with activity, coughing, straining, and lying down. Sensory disruption is later manifested by coldness, numbness, and tingling in an extremity or in several extremities, slowly progressing upward until it reaches the level of the lesion. Impaired sensation of pain, temperature, and light touch precedes a deficit in vibration and position sense that may progress to complete anesthesia. Motor weakness accompanies the sensory disturbances and consists of slowly increasing clumsiness, weakness, and spasticity. The sensory and motor disturbances are ipsilateral to the lesion. Bladder disturbances are marked by urgency with difficulty in starting the flow and progressing to retention with overflow incontinence.

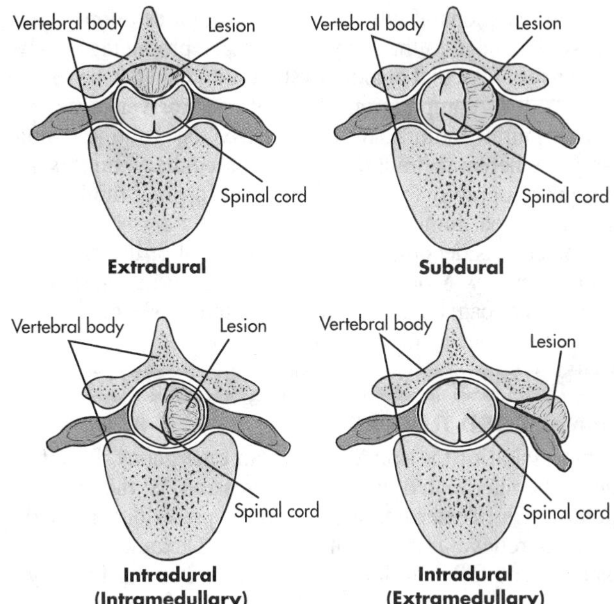

Fig. 57-12 Types of spinal cord tumors.

Table 57-11 Classification of Spinal Cord Tumors

Type	Incidence	Treatment	Prognosis
▪ Extradural (from bones of spine, in extradural space, or in paraspinal tissue)	20-50% of all intraspinal tumors, mostly malignant metastatic lesions	Relief of cord pressure by surgical laminectomy, radiation, chemotherapy, or combination approach	Poor
▪ Intradural extramedullary (within dura mater outside cord)	Most frequent of intradural tumors (40%), mostly benign meningiomas and neurofibromas	Complete surgical removal of tumor (if possible), partial removal followed by radiation	Usually very good if lack of damage to cord from compression
▪ Intradural intramedullary	Least frequent of intradural tumors (5-10%)	Partial surgical removal, radiation therapy (resulting in only temporary improvement)	Very poor

Manifestations of intradural spinal tumor develop as progressive damage to the long spinal tracts, producing paralysis, sensory loss, and bladder dysfunction. Pain can be severe as a result of compression of spinal roots or vertebrae.

Extradural tumors are seen early on routine spinal x-rays, whereas intradural and intramedullary tumors require myelography for detection. Cerebrospinal fluid analysis may reveal tumor cells.

The cord is decompressed after removal of the tumor by a laminectomy. More than 85% of primary neoplasms are benign and can be completely resected; 90% of patients recover without residual problems.

THERAPEUTIC AND NURSING MANAGEMENT

SPINAL CORD TUMORS

Compression of the spinal cord is an emergency. Relief of the ischemia related to the compression is the goal of therapy. Corticosteroids are generally prescribed immediately to relieve tumor-related edema. Dexamethasone is usually used, often in large doses (up to 100 mg initially).

Treatment for nearly all spinal cord tumors is surgical removal. The exception is the metastatic tumor that is sensitive to radiation and that has caused only minimal neurologic deficits in the patient.[23] In general, tumors of the extradural or intradural-extramedullary group can be completely removed surgically. Intramedullary tumors offer a less favorable prognosis; however, exploration and removal is usually attempted.

Radiation therapy after the operation is fairly effective. Maximum permissible tissue dose is given over 6 to 8 weeks. Chemotherapy has also been used in conjunction with radiation therapy.

Relief of pain and return of function are the ultimate goals of treatment. Nurses must be aware of the neurologic status of the patient before and after treatment. Ensuring that the patient receives pain medication as needed is an important nursing responsibility. Depending on the amount of neurologic dysfunction exhibited, the patient may need to be cared for as though recovering from a spinal cord injury.

CRITICAL THINKING EXERCISES

CASE STUDY

SPINAL CORD INJURY

Patient Profile

Charles B., an 18-year-old male, is admitted to the emergency department following a motor vehicle accident.

Subjective Data

- Was unrestrained driver of car at time of accident
- Experienced loss of consciousness at the scene
- Is not oriented
- Is upset and asking why he cannot move his legs
- Has complaints of neck pain

Objective Data

Physical Examination

- Weak bicep strength bilaterally
- No tricep movement
- No movement in lower extremities
- Decreased sensation from shoulders down
- No bladder or bowel control
- BP 100/60; pulse 52; respirations 30 and labored

Diagnostic Studies

- X-rays revealed C5 fracture dislocation

Therapeutic Management

- Admitted to intensive care unit
- Placed in tongs with traction
- Started on methylprednisolone

Critical Thinking Questions

1. What nursing activities would be a priority upon Charles B.'s arrival in the intensive care unit?
2. What physiologic problems are causing Charles B. to have hypotension and bradycardia?
3. What would the first line of treatment be for Charles B.'s hypotension and bradycardia?
4. Within 48 hours what interventions might Charles B. require secondary to effects of spinal cord edema?
5. What can the nurse do to decrease Charles B.'s anxiety?
6. Based on the assessment data provided, write one or more nursing diagnoses. Are there any collaborative problems?

NURSING RESEARCH ISSUES

1. Compare the effectiveness of the Rotorest bed with the Stryker frame bed in preventing skin breakdown.
2. What nursing interventions enhance self-care activities in the spinal cord–injured patient?
3. What factors predispose the spinal cord–injured patient to pulmonary infections?
4. What is the best method of preventing deep vein thrombosis in the spinal cord–injured patient?
5. When is the best time to begin physical therapy in the spinal cord–injured patient?
6. What is the most effective method of skeletal traction pin care to prevent infection?

REVIEW QUESTIONS

The number of the question corresponds to the same-numbered objective at the beginning of the chapter.

1. The classic paroxysms of excruciating facial pain associated with trigeminal neuralgia are due to which of the following?

a. Cerebrospinal fluid infection
b. Nerve compression by tortuous arteries of the posterior fossa
c. Migraine headaches
d. Ear infections

2. During routine assessment of a patient with Guillain-Barré syndrome the nurse finds the patient to be short of breath. The patient's respiratory distress is caused by

a. immobility caused by ascending paralysis.
b. paralysis ascending to the nerves that stimulate the thoracic area.
c. elevated protein levels in the cerebrospinal fluid.
d. corticosteroid therapy.

3. The person most likely to sustain a spinal cord injury is a

a. 60-year-old woman with multiple sclerosis.
b. 35-year-old male tennis player.
c. 75-year-old man with heart disease.
d. 18-year-old man who rides a motorcycle.

4. A patient is admitted to the ICU with a C7 spinal cord injury and diagnosed with Brown-Sequard syndrome. Which of the following would most likely be found on physical examination?

a. Upper extremity weakness only
b. Loss of position sense and vibration in both lower extremities
c. Ipsilateral motor loss and contralateral sensory loss below C7
d. Complete motor and sensory loss below C7

5. Which of the following statements is true about the pathophysiology of indirect spinal cord trauma?

a. The cord is delicate and is readily transected by indirect trauma.
b. Hemorrhage and edema produce ischemia and necrosis.
c. Oxygen tension in the cord is usually normal.
d. The injury process starts in the white matter.

6. A patient with an injury at the C5 level will be able to

a. assist with transfer activities.
b. drive an electric wheelchair.
c. feed self with hand devices.
d. control bowel and bladder functions.

7. Autonomic dysreflexia could occur in a patient with a

a. T10 spinal cord injury.
b. C5 spinal cord injury 1 week after injury.
c. C2 spinal cord injury in spinal shock.
d. C7 spinal cord injury 1 year after injury.

8. The most common early symptom of a spinal cord tumor is

a. urinary incontinence.
b. back pain that worsens with activity.
c. paralysis below the level of injury.
d. foot drop.

REFERENCES

1. Adams RD, Victor M, editors: *Principles of neurology,* ed 5, New York, 1993, McGraw-Hill.
2. Fromm GH: Trigeminal neuralgia and related disorders, *Crit Care Clin* 7:305, 1989.
3. Andreoli TE and others, editors: *In Cecil essentials of medicine,* ed 3, Philadelphia, 1993, Saunders.
4. McConaghy DJ: Trigeminal neuralgia: a personal review and nursing implications, *J Neurosci Nurs* 26:85, 1994.
5. Jannetta PJ: Treatment of trigeminal neuralgia by microoperative decompression. In Youmans JR, editor: *Neurologic surgery: a comprehensive guide to the diagnosis and management of neurosurgical procedures,* ed 3, Philadelphia, 1990, Saunders.
6. Koski CL: Guillain-Barré syndrome and chronic inflammatory demyelinating polyneuropathy: pathogenesis and treatment, *Semin Neurol* 14:123, 1994.
7. Morgan SP: A passage through paralysis, *Am J Nurs* 91:70, 1991.
8. Hughes R: The management of Guillain-Barré syndrome, *Hosp Pract* 27:107, 1992.
9. Hui YH and others, editors: *Foodborne disease handbook,* New York, 1994, Marcel Dekker.
10. Gilbert DN: Clostridial infections. In Stein JH, editor: *Internal medicine,* ed 4, St Louis, 1994, Mosby.
11. Chamberlain C: Admission diagnoses: rule out tetanus, *Focus Crit Care* 16:473, 1989.
12. Dunnum L: Life satisfaction and spinal cord injury: the patient perspective, *J Neurosci Nurs* 22:43, 1990.
13. Walker MD: Acute spinal cord injury, *N Engl J Med* 26:324, 1991.
14. Harvey C and others: New estimates of the direct cost of traumatic spinal cord injuries: results of a nationwide survey, *Paraplegia* 30: 834, 1992.
15. Hickey JV: *The clinical practice of neurological and neurosurgical nursing,* ed 3, Philadelphia, 1992, Lippincott.
16. Merli GJ and others: Etiology, incidence, and prevention of deep vein thrombosis in acute spinal cord injury, *Arch Phys Med Rehabil* 74:1199, 1993.
17. Bergman TA, Seljeskog EL: Management of thoracolumbar and lumbar spine injuries. In Youmans JR, editor: *Neurological surgery,* ed 3, Philadelphia, 1990, Saunders.
18. Young W: Clinical trials and experimental therapies of spinal cord injury. In *Handbook of clinical neurology: spinal cord trauma,* Amsterdam, 1992, Elsevier Science.
19. Nayduch D, Lee A, Butler D: High-dose methylprednisolone after acute spinal cord injury, *Crit Care Nurse* 14:69, 1994.
*20. Hilton G, Frei J: High-dose methylprednisolone in the treatment of spinal cord injuries, *Heart Lung* 20:675, 1991.
21. Strawbridge LR and others: Augmentation cystoplasty and the artificial genitourinary sphincter, *J Urol* 142:297, 1989.
22. Spica MM: Sexual counseling standards for the spinal cord injured, *J Neurosci Nurs* 21:56, 1989.
23. Simeone FA: Spinal cord tumors in adults. In Youmans JR, editor: *Neurological surgery,* ed 3, Philadelphia, 1990, Saunders.

*Nursing research-based articles.

Chapter 58

NURSING ASSESSMENT

Musculoskeletal System

Susan C. Ruda

Learning Objectives

1. Describe the gross anatomic and microscopic composition of bone.
2. Explain the classification system of joints and movements at synovial joints.
3. Describe the types and structure of muscle tissue.
4. Describe the functions of cartilage, muscles, ligaments, tendons, fascia, and bursae.
5. Describe age-related changes in the musculoskeletal system and differences in assessment findings.
6. Identify the significant subjective and objective data related to the musculoskeletal system that should be obtained from a patient.
7. Describe the appropriate techniques used in the physical assessment of the musculoskeletal system.
8. Differentiate normal from abnormal findings of a physical assessment of the musculoskeletal system.
9. Describe the purpose, significance of results, and nursing responsibilities related to diagnostic studies of the musculoskeletal system.

The ability to perform complex and precise movements permits human beings to interact and adapt to the environment. Proper functioning of the musculoskeletal system makes such movements possible. The musculoskeletal system is the largest organ system of the human body. It consists of bones, muscles, joints, cartilage, ligaments, tendons, fascia, and bursae.

The musculoskeletal system is particularly vulnerable to external forces. These forces can cause alteration in the structure of bone or soft connective tissue, resulting in functional disruption. The consequences may be deformity, alteration of body image, alteration in mobility, pain, or permanent disability. These problems may produce long-term health problems that interfere with activities of daily living and quality of life.

STRUCTURES AND FUNCTIONS OF THE MUSCULOSKELETAL SYSTEM

Bone

Function. The main functions of the musculoskeletal system are support, protection of vital organs, movement, blood cell production, and mineral storage.[1] Bone forms the body's supporting framework. Without this support, the body would collapse. Bone also allows the body to bear weight. The musculoskeletal system is important in protecting underlying vital organs and tissues. For example, the skull protects the brain, the vertebrae protect the spinal cord, and the rib cage protects the lungs and heart. Bones serve as a point of attachment for muscles; muscles are anchored to bones by tendons. Bone acts as a lever for muscles, and joints serve as fulcrums. Movement occurs as a result of muscle contractions applied to these levers. Bone also serves as a site for storage of inorganic minerals such as calcium and phosphorus. Cancellous bone contains hematopoietic tissue for production of blood cells and platelets.

Gross Structure. Bone is a dynamic tissue that changes form and substance continually. It is composed of organic (collagen) and inorganic material (calcium, phosphate). Internal and external growth and remodeling are continuous processes.

Bone is classified according to structure as *compact* (dense) or *cancellous* (spongy). In compact bone, haversian systems fit closely together, giving a dense consistency to the bone structure. In cancellous bone there are many open spaces between thin processes and networks of bone tissue that are filled with either red or yellow marrow.

The anatomic structure of bone can best be visualized by the typical long bone (e.g., femur) (Fig. 58-1). Each long bone consists of an epiphysis, articular cartilage, a diaphysis, periosteum, and a medullary (marrow) cavity.

The *epiphysis* is located at each end of a long bone and is composed of cancellous bone. It is the location for muscle attachment and provides stability for the joint. *Articular*

Reviewed by Mary Rodts, MS, RN, ONC, Orthopedics and Scoliosis, Ltd.; and Assistant Professor, Rush College of Nursing, Chicago, IL.

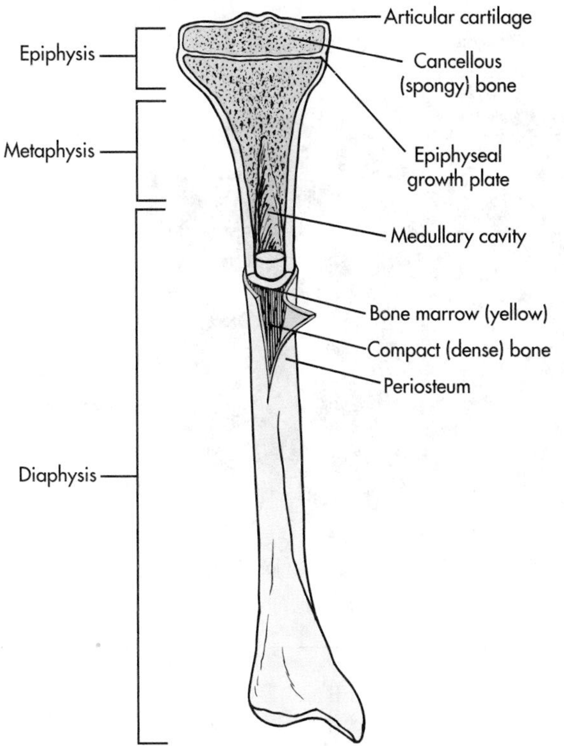

Fig. 58-1 Anatomic structure of a typical long bone.

cartilage covers the ends of the bone and provides smooth surfaces for joint movement.

The *diaphysis* is the main shaft of bone. It provides the bone with structural support and is composed of compact bone. The *metaphysis* is the flared area between the epiphysis and the diaphysis. During bone development it contains the growth zones. In the adult the metaphysis is joined to the epiphysis. The *epiphyseal plate*, or growth zone, is the cartilaginous area that actively produces bone and results in longitudinal growth in children. Injury to the epiphyseal plate in a growing child can cause significant problems, such as altered growth of the extremity. In the adult, this plate hardens to mature bone, and longitudinal growth ceases.

The *periosteum* is fibrous connective tissue that covers the bone. Musculotendinous fibers attach to the outer layer of the periosteum. The inner layer of the periosteum contains osteoblasts (bone-forming cells), which are essential for transverse bone growth and fracture repair.

The *medullary* (marrow) *cavity* is in the center of the diaphysis. In the adult the medullary cavity of long bones contains yellow bone marrow, which is mainly adipose tissue. In the growing child, red bone marrow in the medullary cavity is actively involved in hematopoiesis. In the adult, hematopoiesis normally occurs only in the red bone marrow of the skull, ribs, sternum, pelvis, vertebrae, and proximal ends of the humerus and femur.

Microscopic Structure. The three types of bone cells are osteoblasts, osteocytes, and osteoclasts. *Osteoblasts* synthesize organic bone matrix (collagen) and are the basic bone-forming cells. *Osteocytes* are the mature bone cells. *Osteoclasts* are involved in resorption of bone tissue and participate in bone remodeling. Bone remodeling is the removal of old bone by osteoclasts and the deposition of new bone by osteoblasts. The inner layer of bone is primarily made up of osteoblasts with a few osteoclasts.

Bone is a special kind of connective tissue in which organic matter (collagen) has become mineralized. The structural unit of compact bone is the haversian system (Fig. 58-2). It consists of lamellae, which are concentric layers of calcified collagen matrix that enclose a long canal (haversian system). The main function of the haversian system is to transport blood to bone tissue. Blood vessels from the periosteum travel through Volkmann's canals to the blood vessels of the haversian system.

Osteocytes (mature bone cells) lie in small spaces called *lacunae* between lamellae. *Canaliculi* (tiny canals) extend from lacunae to connect the osteocytes to one another and to the haversian system.

Types. The skeleton consists of 206 named bones. These bones are classified according to shape as long, short, flat, or irregular.

Long bones are characterized by a central shaft (diaphysis) and two epiphyseal ends (see Fig. 58-1). Examples include the femur, humerus, and radius. *Short bones* are characterized by cancellous bone covered by a thin layer of compact bone. Examples include the carpals and tarsals.

Flat bones are characterized by two layers of compact bone separated by a layer of cancellous bone. Examples include the ribs, skull, scapula, and sternum. The spaces in the cancellous bone contain bone marrow. *Irregular bones* have a variety of shapes and sizes. Examples include the vertebrae, sacrum, and mandible.

Joints

A *joint* (articulation) is a place where two bones come together. Joints hold bones firmly together while permitting movement between them. Joints are commonly classified according to their degree of movement (Fig. 58-3).

The *diarthrodial* (synovial) type, the most common joint, consists of a cavity between the articular surfaces of the bones that make up the joint (Fig. 58-4). The ends of the bone are covered with articular (hyaline) cartilage. A capsule of connective tissue called the *fibrous* or *joint capsule* joins the two bones together, forming a cavity. The capsule is lined by a synovium, or synovial membrane, which secretes a thick synovial fluid to lubricate the joint and reduce friction. Types of diarthrodial joints are shown in Fig. 58-5.

Cartilage

Cartilage is a rigid connective tissue that functions to support soft tissue and provides the articular surfaces for joint movement. It protects underlying tissues. The cartilage that makes up the epiphyseal plate is also essential for the growth of long bones before physical maturity is reached.

Cartilage is avascular and therefore is nourished by the diffusion of material from capillaries in adjacent connective

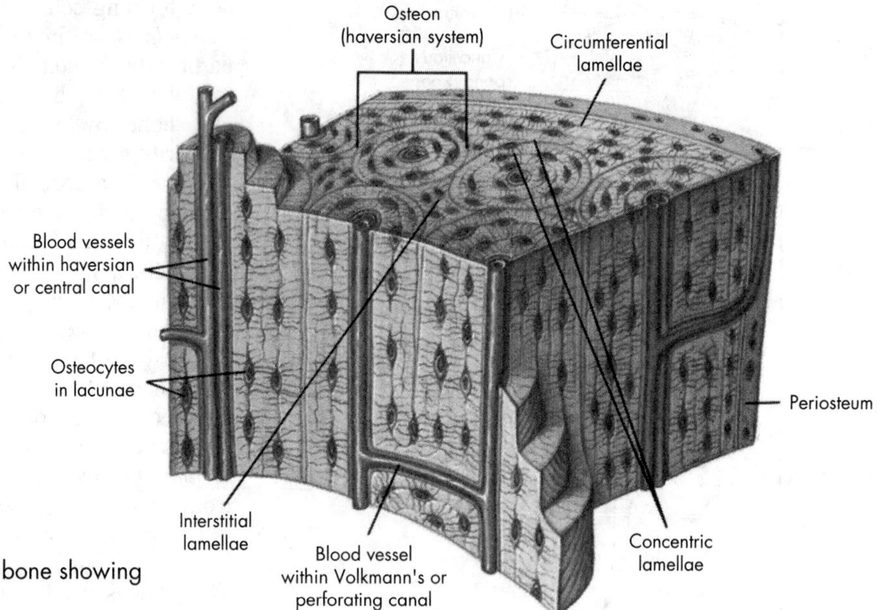

Fig. 58-2 Structure of compact bone showing haversian system.

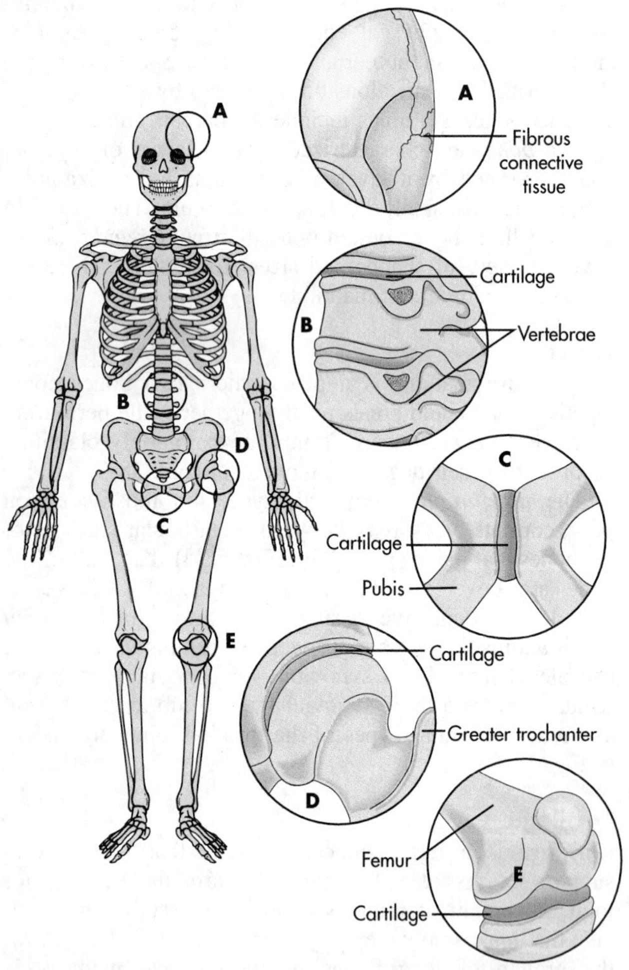

Fig. 58-3 Classification of joints. ***A, B, C,*** Synarthrotic (immovable) and amphiarthrotic (slightly movable) joints. ***D, E,*** Diarthrotic (freely movable) joints.

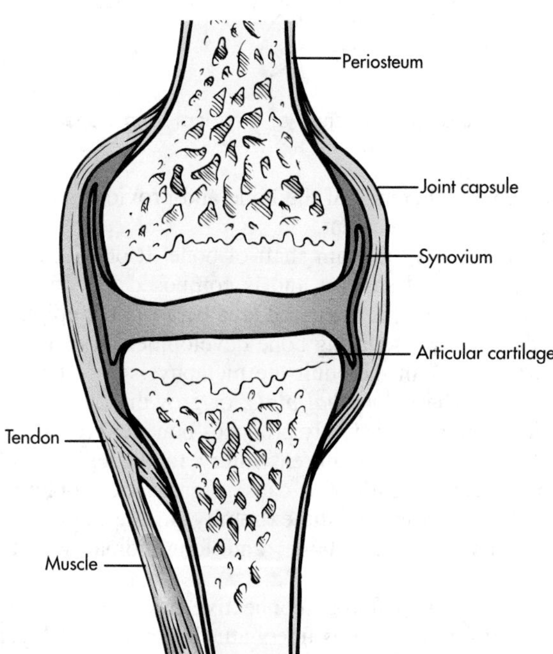

Fig. 58-4 Normal diarthrodial (synovial) joint of the knee.

tissue. Cartilage cells are slow to reproduce because of the lack of a direct blood supply, which explains why damaged cartilage heals slowly.

The three types of cartilage tissue are hyaline, elastic, and fibrous. *Hyaline cartilage*, the most common, contains a moderate amount of collagen fibers. It is found in the trachea, bronchi, nose, and articular surfaces of bones. *Elastic cartilage*, which contains collagen and elastic fibers, is more flexible than hyaline cartilage. It is found in the ear, epiglottis, and larynx. *Fibrocartilage*, which consists mostly of collagen fibers, is a tough tissue that often

Joint	Movement	Examples	Illustration
Hinge joint	Flexion, extension	Elbow joint (shown), interphalangeal joints, knee joint	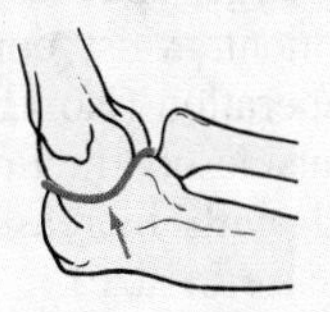
Ball and socket (spheroidal)	Flexion, extension; adduction, abduction; circumduction	Shoulder (shown), hip	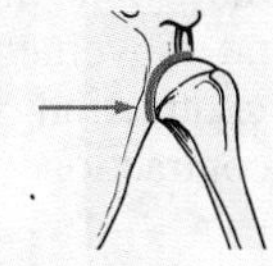
Pivot (rotary)	Rotation	Atlas-axis, proximal radioulnar joint (shown)	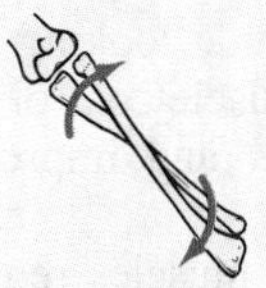
Condyloid	Flexion, extension; abduction, adduction; circumduction	Wrist joint (between radial and carpals) (shown)	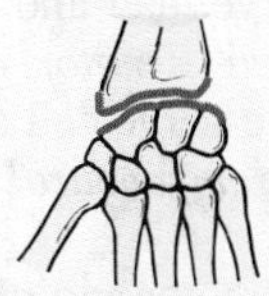
Saddle	Flexion, extension; abduction, adduction; circumduction, thumb-finger opposition	Carpometacarpal joint of thumb	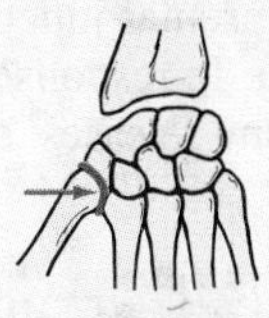
Gliding	One surface moves over another surface	Between tarsal bones, sacroiliac joint, between articular processes of vertebrae, between carpal bones (shown)	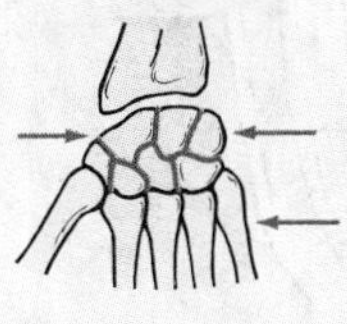

Fig. 58-5 Types of diarthrodial joints.

functions as a shock absorber. It is found between vertebral disks and in the knee. Fibrocartilage also forms a protective cushion between the bones of the pelvic girdle.

Muscle

Types. The three types of muscle tissue are *cardiac, smooth* (nonstriated), and *skeletal* (striated) muscle. Cardiac muscle is found in the heart. Its contractions provide the major force for propelling blood through the circulatory system. Smooth muscle is found in the walls of hollow structures such as airways, the gastrointestinal (GI) tract, urinary bladder, uterus, and blood vessels. Cardiac muscle contracts spontaneously. Skeletal muscle requires neuronal stimulation. Smooth muscle contraction is modulated by neuronal and hormonal influences. Skeletal muscle composes the largest mass of tissue in the body and is the focus of the following dicussion.

Structure. Muscle is composed of cells called fibers. The structural unit of muscle is the muscle cell, which is also called a muscle fiber. Skeletal muscle fibers are multinucleated cylinders that range in length from several millimeters to several centimeters. Muscle fibers are composed of myofibrils, which in turn are made up of contractile filaments.

Under a microscope, skeletal muscle shows alternating banding, which accounts for the striated appearance.[2] This appearance is due to a repeating pattern of filaments seen in the myofibrils. The sarcomere is the contractile unit of the myofibrils. Each sarcomere contains myosin (thick) filaments and actin (thin) filaments. The arrangement of the thin and thick filaments accounts for the banding. As thick and thin filaments slide past each other, the sarcomeres shorten and muscle shortens.

Contractions. Skeletal muscle contractions are responsible for the functions of posture, movement, and facial expressions. *Isometric* contractions increase the tension within a muscle but do not produce movement. Repeated isometric contractions make muscles grow larger and stronger. *Isotonic* contractions produce movement. Most contractions are a combination of tension generation (isometric) and shortening (isotonic). Without muscle contraction there is *atrophy* (decrease in size) and with increased muscle activity there is *hypertrophy* (increase in size).

Skeletal muscle produces other types of contractions that have little to do with functional posture and movement. They are a *twitch* contraction—a quick, contraction in response to a single stimulus; and a *tetanic* contraction—a more sustained twitch.

The types of skeletal muscle contractions help explain the major benefits of exercise. These include looking and feeling better, improved posture, greater muscle control and strength, better muscle tone, less fatigue, and improved heart and lung function.

Neuromuscular Junction. Skeletal muscles require a nerve supply in order to contract. The nerve fiber and the skeletal muscle fibers it supplies are called a *motor end plate*.[3] The junction between the axon of the nerve cell and the muscle cell it supplies is called the *myoneural* or neuromuscular junction (Fig. 58-6).

When acetylcholine is released from the motor end plate of the neuron, it diffuses across the neuromuscular junction and binds with receptors on the muscle fiber. In response to this stimulation, the sarcoplasmic reticulum releases calcium ions into the cytoplasm. The presence of these ions triggers the contraction in the myofibrils.

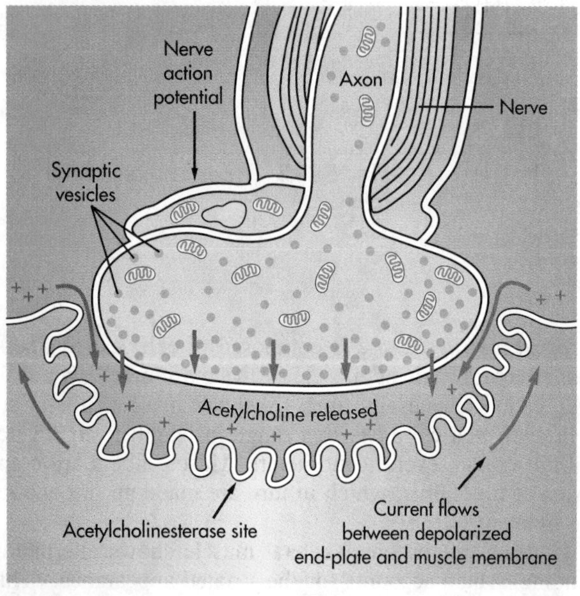

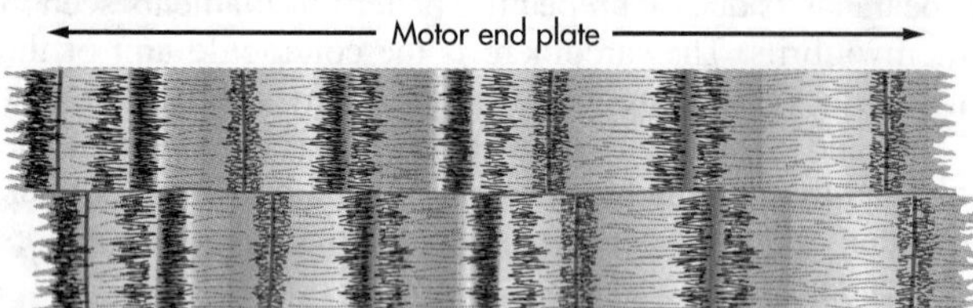

Fig. 58-6 Neuromuscular junction.

Energy Source. The energy source used in muscle fiber contractions comes from adenosine triphosphate (ATP). ATP is synthesized by cellular oxidative metabolism in numerous mitochondria located close to the myofibrils. A second energy source is creatine phosphate, which supplies phosphate to rephosphorylate ATP. Creatine phosphate is synthesized and stored in muscle tissue.

Ligaments and Tendons

Ligaments and *tendons* are both composed of dense, fibrous connective tissue. This type of connective tissue contains large numbers of collagen fibers that are closely packed. Tendons attach muscles to bones. They are an extension of the muscle sheath that attaches to the periosteum. Ligaments connect bones to bones at joints (e.g., the knee joint). They permit movement while providing stability.

Fibrous connective tissue has a relatively poor blood supply. Although the tissue can repair itself after injury, it is usually a slow process. For example, a sprain may require a long time to heal despite the minor nature of the injury.

Fascia

Fascia is the term used for layers of connective tissue. It is classified as either superficial or deep. *Superficial fascia* is the loose connective tissue located immediately under the skin. *Deep fascia* (dense, fibrous connective tissue) is found surrounding muscle, between muscles, and surrounding the bundles that bind nerves and blood vessels together.

Fascia separates one muscle from another to permit independent muscle action. It allows gliding of one muscle over another. In addition, fascia provides strength to muscle tissues.

Bursae

Bursae are small sacs of connective tissue lined with synovial membrane and synovial fluid. They are commonly located at joints. Bursae function as cushions to relieve pressure between the moving parts and prevent friction. They are found between the patella and the skin (prepatellar bursa), between the olecranon process and the skin (olecranon bursa), between the head of the humerus and the acromion process (subacromial bursa), and between the lower portion of the gluteus maximus muscle and the bony ischial tuberosity (submuscular bursa) (Fig. 58-7). *Bursitis* (inflammation of the bursa) may be caused by mechanical injury to the bursa or excessive use of a joint.

Gerontologic Considerations

Many of the functional problems of older adults are due to changes of the musculoskeletal system. Many of these changes begin in early adulthood, but obvious signs of musculoskeletal impairment may not appear until later in adulthood. These changes can alter posture, function, gait, and body image. They affect the older adult's lifestyle and activities of daily living, ranging from discomfort and decreased ability to perform activities of daily living to severe, chronic pain and immobility.[4] Many musculoskeletal problems are a result of deconditioning rather than aging.

In addition to the usual musculoskeletal assessment with a particular emphasis on exercise practices, the nurse should determine the impact of age-related changes of the musculoskeletal system on the functional status of the older patient. Functional limitations that are accepted by older adults as a normal part of aging can often be halted or reversed with appropriate preventive strategies (Table 58-1). Table 58-2 lists age-related changes of the musculoskeletal system and differences in assessment findings.

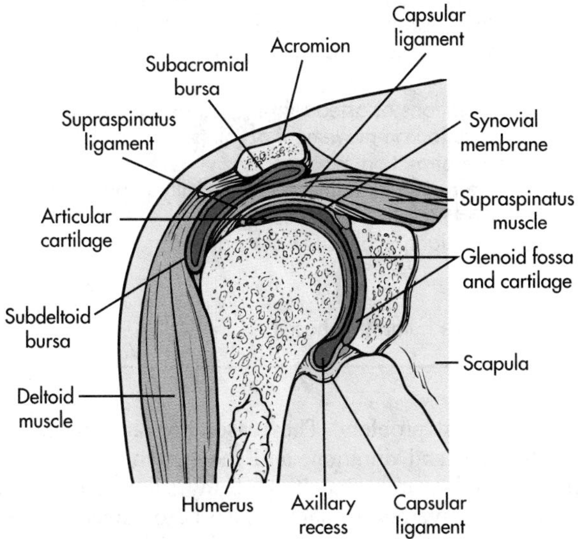

Fig. 58-7 Bursae of the shoulder joint.

ASSESSMENT OF THE MUSCULOSKELETAL SYSTEM

Correct diagnosis depends on an accurate patient history and a thorough examination. A musculoskeletal assessment can be made on a specific body part, as part of a general physical examination, or as an examination in itself. Judgment must be used in selecting all or part of the components of the musculoskeletal history and physical examination on the basis of the patient's problem. Accidents often result in trauma to the musculoskeletal system and require a thorough assessment. If the injury is serious or life-threatening, only pertinent information related to the accident is obtained, and a complete assessment is deferred.

Complaints that should alert the nurse to obtain subjective and objective data related to the musculoskeletal system include joint or muscle pain, joint swelling, decreasing strength or function, change in size of an extremity or muscle, deformity, spasms, crepitation, changes in sensation, stiffness, and changes in gait.

Subjective Data

Important Medical Information

Past health history. Certain illnesses are known to affect the musculoskeletal system either directly or indi-

Table 58-1 Prevention of Age-Related Musculoskeletal Problems

Action	Rationale
Use of ramps in buildings and at street corners instead of steps	Stair-walking motion may create enough stress on fragile bones to cause a hip fracture. Use of ramps may prevent falls.
Elimination of scatter rugs in the home	These are notorious for causing falls and fractures.
Response to pain and discomfort of osteoarthritis	
Resting in reclining position	Osteoarthritis is seen on x-ray of most persons over the age of 50 and causes pain. Rest is the most useful way to decrease its discomfort.
Use of plain or enteric-coated aspirin or ibuprofen	Aspirin and other antiinflammatory drugs (as prescribed by physician) diminish inflammation of joints and hence reduce pain.
Use of a walker or cane to help with walking	Assistance decreases stress on inflamed joints and thus decreases discomfort. Use may prevent falls.
Eating amount and kind of foods to prevent excess weight gain	Obesity adds stress to bones, which may predispose patient to osteoarthritis.
Regular and frequent exercise	
Activities of daily living	Activities of daily living provide range-of-motion exercise, which should be done four times a day; 100% range of motion is not as critical as the ability to perform usual and preferred activities.
Hobbies (e.g., jigsaw puzzles, needlework, model building)	These exercise distal joints and prevent stiffness.
Walking short distances daily with shoes that give good support	Some weight-bearing exercise is essential and should be done two or three times daily. Good shoes provide for safety and promote comfort.
Gradual initiation of all activities	Starting gradually promotes optimal coordination. When a patient rises slowly to a standing position, dizziness and hence falls and fractures can be prevented.

Table 58-2 Gerontologic Differences in Assessment: Musculoskeletal System

Changes	Differences in Assessment Findings
Muscle	
Decreased number and diameter of muscle cells, replacement of muscle cells by fibrous connective tissue	Decreased muscle strength and bulk, abdominal protrusion, muscle flabbiness
Loss of elasticity in ligaments and cartilage	Decreased fine motor activity, decreased agility
Decrease in oxidate activity from reduction in glycolytic enzymes	Slowed reaction times, slowing of most muscle reflexes, slowing of impulse conduction along motor units, easy fatigability
Joints	
Erosion of articular cartilage, possible direct contact between bone ends	Manifestations of osteoarthritis, joint stiffness, possible crepitation on movement of joints, pain with range-of-motion movements
Overgrowth of bone around joint margins (osteophytes)	Heberden's nodes in fingers (especially in women), limited mobility in affected joints
Loss of water from disks between vertebrae, narrowing of joint vertebral spaces	Loss of height, kyphosis, back pain
Bone	
Decrease in bone mass	Dowager's hump (kyphosis)

ectly. The patient should be questioned specifically about a history of tuberculosis, poliomyelitis, diabetes mellitus, gout, inflammatory and degenerative arthritis, rickets, osteomalacia, scurvy, osteomyelitis or soft tissue infection, fungal infection of the bones or joints, and neuromuscular disabilities. If the patient has a history of any of these problems, a detailed account of the illness should be obtained (see Chapter 4). In addition, the patient should be questioned about possible sources of secondary bacterial infections, such as ears, tonsils, teeth, sinuses, or genitourinary tract, which can result in osteomyelitis.

Medications. The patient should be questioned carefully regarding prescription and over-the-counter drugs used to treat a musculoskeletal problem. Information on the reason for taking the medication, its name, the dose and frequency, length of time it was taken, its effect, and any side effects should be obtained. Specific inquiry should be made related to skeletal muscle relaxants, antirheumatoid agents, antiinflammatory agents, narcotics, and systemic corticosteroids. The patient should be questioned about GI distress or a bleeding ulcer if antiinflammatory agents have been taken.

In addition to drugs taken for treatment of a musculoskeletal problem, the patient should be questioned about drugs that can have detrimental effects on this system. These drugs include anticonvulsants (osteomalacia), phenothiazines (gait disturbances), corticosteroids (abnormal fat distribution, avascular necrosis, decreased bone mass, and muscle weakness), and potassium-depleting diuretics (cramps and muscle weakness). Amphetamines and caffeine intake can cause a generalized increase in motor activity. Older women should be questioned about their menopausal status, the use of hormone replacement therapy, and calcium supplementation.

Surgery or other treatments. Information should be obtained about hospitalizations that were necessitated by a musculoskeletal problem. The reason for the hospitalization, the date and duration, and the treatment should be carefully documented. Specifics of any surgical procedure and postoperative course should also be obtained. If there was a period of prolonged immobilization, the possible development of osteoporosis and muscle atrophy should be considered. The patient should also be questioned about emergency treatment related to musculoskeletal disorders and injuries.

Functional Health Patterns. The use of functional health patterns aids the nurse in organizing the data and formulating diagnoses based on data collected about the musculoskeletal system. Table 58-3 summarizes the questions to ask in relation to functional health patterns.

Health perception–health management pattern. The nurse asks about the patient's health practices related to the musculoskeletal system such as maintenance of a normal body weight, avoidance of excessive stress on muscles and joints, and use of proper body mechanics when lifting objects.

The patient should be specifically questioned about immunizations related to tetanus and polio. The most current date and reaction to a tuberculin skin test should also be obtained.

Food or contact allergies are of little consequence in relation to musculoskeletal problems. However, the general malaise often associated with allergic reactions may manifest in musculoskeletal stiffness and lethargy. Allergic reactions to drugs used to treat musculoskeletal problems can interfere with therapy, and an alternative treatment may have to be employed if the allergic reaction is severe.

The list of minor and major injuries of the musculoskeletal system can be extensive in the patient who is a good historian. It includes documentation of fractures, sprains, strains, and dislocations. The information should be recorded chronologically and should include the following:

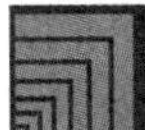

Table 58-3 Key Questions: Patient with a Musculoskeletal Problem

Health Perception–Health Management Pattern
Describe your usual daily activities.
Do you experience any difficulties performing these activities?* Describe what you do when you experience difficulty in dressing, feeding yourself, performing basic hygiene, or maintaining your home.
Do you use any mechanical assistive devices?* Do you have to lift heavy objects? If so, describe how you do this.
Describe any specialized equipment you use or wear when you work or exercise that helps to protect you from injury.
What type of safety precautions do you take?
Do you take any medications to manage your musculoskeletal problem? If so, what is/are the name(s) of the medication? When did you have your last tetanus and polio immunization? When were you last tested for tuberculosis?

Nutritional-Metabolic Pattern
Give a 24-hr diet recall. Do you take supplemental vitamins or minerals (ask specifically about calcium supplements)?
What is your weight? Have you had a recent change in your weight?*

Elimination Pattern
Does your musculoskeletal problem make it difficult for you to the reach the toilet in time?* Do you experience constipation related to immobility?
Do you need any assistive devices or equipment to achieve satisfactory toileting?*

Activity-Exercise Pattern
Do you have any limitations in your activities of daily living because of a musculoskeletal problem?*
Describe your usual exercise pattern. Do you experience symptoms related to your musculoskeletal system when exercising?*
Are you able to move all your joints comfortably through full range of motion? Describe any limitations in mobility.
Do you require assistance in moving or in doing activities of daily living?*
Do you use any prosthetic devices?*

Sleep-Rest Pattern
Do you experience any difficulty sleeping because of a musculoskeletal problem?* Do you require frequent position changes at night? Why?
Do you wake up at night because of musculoskeletal pain?*

Cognitive-Perceptual Pattern
Describe any musculoskeletal pain you experience. How do you manage your pain?

Self-Perception–Self-Concept Pattern
Describe how changes in your musculoskeletal system (posture, walking, muscle strength) or the ability to do certain things have affected how you feel about yourself. How have these changes affected your lifestyle?

Role-Relationship Pattern
Do you live alone?
Describe how your family or others assist you with your musculoskeletal problems.
Describe the effect of your musculoskeletal problem on your work and on your social relationships.

Sexuality-Reproductive Pattern
Describe the effect of your musculoskeletal problem on your sexual activity. How do you feel about this?

Coping-Stress Tolerance Pattern
Describe how you deal with the problems such as pain or immobility that have resulted from your musculoskeletal problem.

Value-Belief Pattern
Describe any cultural or religious beliefs that may influence the treatment of your musculoskeletal problem.

*If yes, describe.

1. Mechanism of the injury (twist, crush, stretch)
2. Circumstances related to the injury
3. Diagnostic evaluations
4. Methods of treatment
5. Duration of treatment
6. Current status related to the injury
7. Need for assistive devices
8. Interference with activities of daily living

A three-generation family history should be obtained related to rheumatoid arthritis, degenerative joint disease, gout, osteoporosis, and scoliosis because these problems have a familial predisposition.

Safety practices can play a role in the patient's predisposition for certain injuries and illnesses. Specific questions should be asked about safety practices of the patient as they relate to the job environment, recreation, and exercise. For example, if the patient is a jogger, the type of shoes worn and the jogging surface used should be investigated. The high incidence of trauma to the musculoskeletal system requires a careful investigation in the area of safety practices. Identification of problems in this area will direct the plan for patient education.

Nutritional-metabolic pattern. The patient's recounting of a typical day's diet can provide clues to areas of nutritional concern in relation to the musculoskeletal system. Obesity predisposes people to ligamentous instability, particularly in the lower back region. It also adds stress to weight-bearing joints such as the knees and hips. The maintenance of normal weight is an important patient goal.

Abnormal nutritional states can also predispose individuals to specific musculoskeletal problems such as osteoporosis, osteomalacia, and rickets. Adequate amounts of vitamins C and D, calcium, and protein are essential for a healthy, intact musculoskeletal system.

Elimination pattern. The patient's ability to ambulate adequately to reach a toileting facility should be assessed. A musculoskeletal problem could be an etiologic factor in functional incontinence of bladder and bowel. Also, immobility secondary to a musculoskeletal problem can result in constipation. The patient should be asked if an assistive device such as an elevated toilet seat or grab bar is necessary to accomplish toileting.

Activity-exercise pattern. A detailed account of the type, duration, and frequency of activities related to exercise and recreation should be obtained and assessed regarding adequacy and predisposition to musculoskeletal problems. This information can be obtained when the patient recounts a typical day. Daily, weekend, and seasonal patterns should be compared because occasional or sporadic exercise can be more problematic than regular exercise. Many musculoskeletal problems can affect the patient's activity-exercise pattern. The nurse should question the patient about limitations of movement, pain, weakness, clumsiness, crepitus, or any change in the bones or joints that interfere with daily activities.

Extremes of activity related to occupation can affect the musculoskeletal system. A sedentary occupation does not allow for maintaining muscle flexibility and strength. Jobs that require extreme effort and use of the body for heavy lifting and pushing can result in damage to the joints and supporting structures of the body. The nurse should inquire about job-related injuries to the musculoskeletal system, the amount of time lost from work, and the treatments used.

Sleep-rest pattern. Musculoskeletal disorders might require frequent position changes at night. Discomfort may also interfere with a normal sleep pattern. The patient should be questioned about sleep patterns and how they have been altered. If the patient recounts that a musculoskeletal problem is interfering with sleep, further inquiry should be made related to the type of bedding, pillows used, sleeping partner, and sleeping positions.

Cognitive-perceptual pattern. Any pain experienced by the patient as a result of a musculoskeletal problem should be fully explored and documented. Pain assessment conducted over time can assist in determining the effectiveness of the treatment plan. Other complaints that could cause a problem either directly or indirectly through pain include joint swelling, decreasing strength, and changes in sensation.

Self-perception–self-concept pattern. Many musculoskeletal problems are chronic and deforming. Such changes can have a serious impact on the patient's body image and sense of personal worth. An account of how the patient feels about these changes should be addressed by the nurse.

Role-relationship pattern. Musculoskeletal problems that affect mobility or result in a chronic pain syndrome can seriously affect the patient's roles and responsibilities, such as spouse, parent, worker. Also, such problems can affect the ability to seek and maintain meaningful social and personal relationships. These problems should be assessed and documented during the history.

If the patient lives alone, the possibility of maintaining this living arrangement in the future should be assessed in light of the problem and rehabilitation potential. The degree of assistance from family, friends, and organized caregivers should also be determined.

Sexuality-reproductive pattern. Musculoskeletal problems and the resulting pain or potential for pain can greatly affect the patient's sexual satisfaction. This area must be sensitively assessed so the patient feels comfortable in relating sexual problems related to movement and positioning.

Coping–stress tolerance pattern. Mobility limitations and pain, both acute and chronic, can be serious stressors that affect the patient's coping ability. The nurse must recognize the potential for ineffective coping and gather adequate data to determine if a musculoskeletal problem is causing a coping problem.

Objective Data

Physical Examination. The primary methods used in the physical examination of the musculoskeletal system include inspection and palpation. The data gathered from a careful health history will provide the nurse with clues about areas on which to concentrate the examination.

Inspection. Inspection begins during the nurse's initial contact with the patient. The nurse should observe the patient for any apparent asymmetry and for sitting and standing posture, gait, general body build, and configuration of the muscles. The nurse should be particularly aware of limitations in the patient's ability to perform normal activities such as dressing, toileting, and eating.

The condition of the skin is observed for general color, scars, or overt signs of previous injury or operations. A systematic inspection is performed starting at the head and neck and proceeding to the upper extremities, the lower extremities, and the back. Although the order is not of great importance, the regular use of a systematic approach is important to avoid missing important aspects of the examination. The nurse should specifically inspect for joint motion and asymmetry of movement, swelling, deformity, masses, and evidence of limb-length or muscle-size discrepancies. The patient's opposite body part is used for comparison when an abnormality is suspected.

Palpation. Any area that has aroused concern because of a subjective complaint or has been noted on inspection should be carefully palpated. The examiner's hands should be warm to prevent muscle spasm, which can interfere with identification of essential landmarks or soft-tissue structures. Palpation of the soft tissues, including muscles and joints, enables the examiner to evaluate skin temperature, local tenderness, swelling, and crepitation. It is important to establish the relationship of adjacent structures and to evaluate the general contour, abnormal prominences, and local landmarks. The usual sequence is to begin at the neck and proceed cephalopedally (head to toe) to examine the neck, shoulders, elbows, wrists, hands, back, hips, knees, ankles, and feet. Both superficial and deep palpation are usually performed consecutively.

Movement. When examining joint movement, the nurse must carefully evaluate passive and active range of joint motion. Normally the active and passive joint motions are similar. There are three range-of-motion categories: passive, active, and functional. *Passive range of motion* occurs when someone else moves the patient's joints through their range of motion. Caution is required when testing passive joint motion because of the possibility of injury to the underlying soft-tissue structures. Manipulation must cease immediately if pain or resistance is encountered. *Active range of motion* means the patient actively moves his own joints through their normal range of motion. *Functional range of motion* is assessed by asking the patient if the activities of daily living, such as eating and bathing independently, are performed with assistance, or not at all. The patient may require an assistive device such as a splint, wheelchair, or walker, which should be noted.

Joint motion is most accurately measured by a goniometer, which measures the amount of bending or angles of the joints (Fig. 58-8). Specific degrees of range of motion of all joints are usually not measured unless a musculoskeletal problem has been identified. A less accurate but nevertheless valuable method is to compare the range of motion of one extremity with the range of motion on the opposite side. The common movements at synovial joints and the description of the movement are listed in Table 58-4.

Measurement. Limb length and circumferential measurement of muscle mass are often obtained when subjective problems or length discrepancies are noted. For example, leg length measurements are obtained when gait disorders are observed. Limb length is measured between two bony prominences and compared with the similar measurement of the opposite extremity. Muscle mass is measured circumferentially at the largest area of the mass.

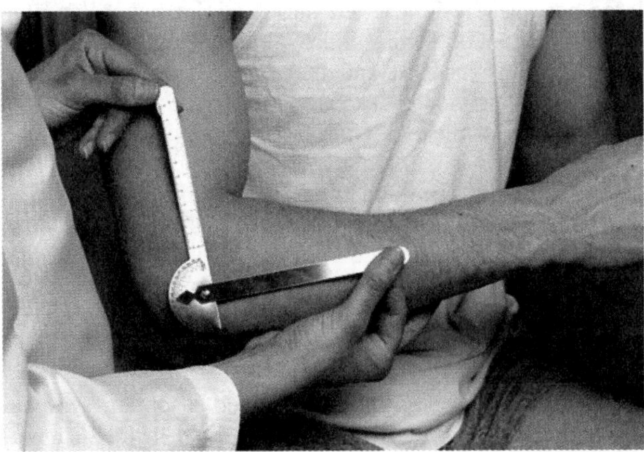

Fig. 58-8 Measurement of joint motion with a goniometer.

When recording measurements, the nurse should record the exact location at which the measurements were obtained (e.g., the quadriceps muscle is measured 15 cm above the patella). This informs the next examiner of the exact area to be measured and ensures consistency in future examinations.

Muscle-strength testing. The strength of individual muscles or groups of muscles is graded in performance of movements during contraction against applied resistance (Table 58-5). The examiner should instruct the patient to apply resistance to the force exerted by the examiner. For example, the examiner tries to pull the bent arm down while the patient tries to raise it. Muscle strength should also be compared to the strength of the opposite extremity. Subtle variations in muscle strength may be noted when comparing the patient's dominant side to the nondominant side.

Table 58-4 Movement at Synovial Joints

Movement	Description
Flexion	Bending of joint that decreases angle between two bones, shortening of muscle length
Extension	Bending of joint that increases angle between two bones
Hyperextension	Extension in which angle exceeds 180 degrees
Abduction	Movement of part away from midline
Adduction	Movement of part toward midline
Pronation	Turning of palm downward or sole outward
Supination	Turning of palm upward or sole inward
Circumduction	Combination of flexion, extension, abduction, and adduction resulting in circular motion of body part
Rotation	Movement about longitudinal axis
Inversion	Turning of sole inward toward midline
Eversion	Turning of sole outward away from midline

Table 58-5 Muscle Strength Scale

0—No detection of muscular contraction
1—A barely detectable flicker or trace of contraction
2—Active movement of body part with elimination of gravity
3—Active movement against gravity
4—Active movement against gravity and some resistance
5—Active movement against full resistance without evident fatigue (normal muscle strength)

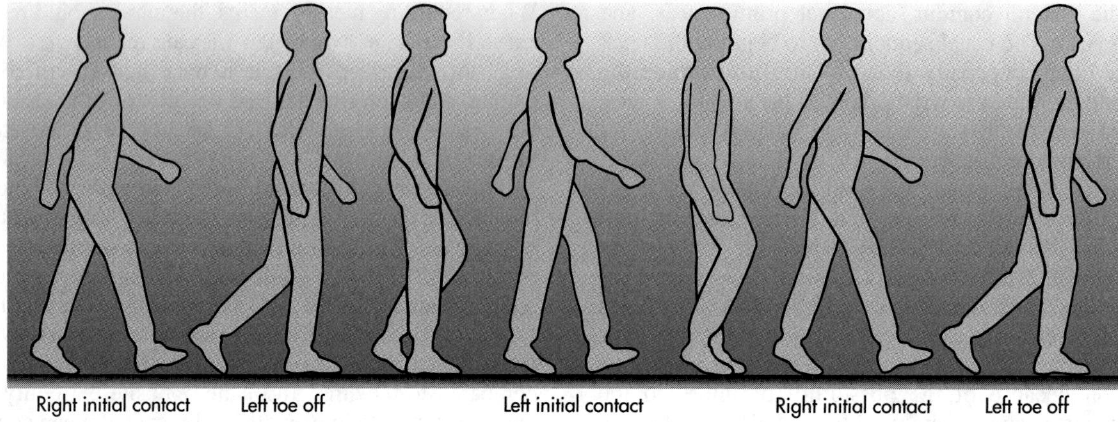

Fig. 58-9 Phases of gait.

Gait. The nurse assesses gait by having the patient walk across the room and back. The normal gait is divided into two separate phases, the stance phase and the swing phase (Fig. 58-9). The two occur simultaneously: while one limb is in stance phase, the other is in swing phase. Musculoskeletal and neurologic problems can result in gait abnormalities.

Other. Assessment of reflexes is discussed in Chapter 53. Table 58-6 is an example of how to record a normal physical assessment of the musculoskeletal system. Common abnormal assessment findings of the musculoskeletal system are presented in Table 58-7.

Diagnostic Studies. Diagnostic studies provide important information to the nurse in monitoring the patient's condition and planning appropriate interventions. These studies are considered to be objective data. Table 58-8 contains diagnostic studies common to the musculoskeletal system.

DIAGNOSTIC STUDIES

Radiologic Studies

The most common diagnostic study used to assess musculoskeletal problems is an *x-ray examination.* Radiologic studies are important to establish the presence of a musculoskeletal problem and to follow its progress and the effectiveness of treatment.

A standard x-ray study is a film produced by the action of x-rays emitted from a cathode tube diphotosensitive surface. X-rays can be thought of as shadows of structures, particularly bony structures. Bones are more dense than other tissues and do not allow the x-ray to penetrate. The standard x-ray develops dense areas as white.

The anteroposterior and lateral views are the most commonly used standard x-ray perspectives. Because disk and cartilage structures are not visible on standard x-rays special x-rays (diskograms, arthrograms) involving the use of contrast media can be used to visualize them.

Table 58-6 Normal Physical Assessment of Musculoskeletal System

Full range of motion of all joints
No joint swelling, deformity, or crepitation
Normal spinal curvatures
No tenderness on palpation of spine
No muscle atrophy or asymmetry
Muscle strength of 5

Magnetic Resonance Imaging

Magnetic resonance imaging (MRI) is a diagnostic study that is useful in diagnosing numerous musculoskeletal disorders. Radiowaves and magnetic fields are used to construct soft tissue and bone images. It is advantageous in determining soft tissue disorders, including cartilage and ligament tears and herniated disks, but it also can be helpful in diagnosing bone disorders such as avascular necrosis, tumors, and multiple myeloma.

Arthroscopy

Endoscopy of the joints involves the use of an arthroscope for direct visualization of the interior of a joint cavity. It is performed in the operating room under sterile conditions. After local or general anesthesia has been administered, a large-bore needle is inserted into the joint pouch, and the joint is distended with saline solution (Fig. 58-10). The arthroscope is inserted and the joint cavity is examined. Photographs or videotapes can be made through the scope, and a biopsy of the synovium or cartilage can be obtained. The procedure is particularly useful in the diagnosis of disorders of the knee and shoulder. It can also be used in procedures involving other joints, such as the wrist, elbow, and ankle. Minor tears in cartilage and other repairs can be made through the arthroscope, thus eliminating the need for a more extensive incision and surgical procedure.

Arthrocentesis and Synovial Fluid Analysis

An arthrocentesis is usually performed to obtain synovial fluid for examination. It may also be used to instill medications and remove fluid to relieve pain. After the skin has been cleaned, a local anesthetic is instilled. An 18-gauge or

Table 58-7 Common Assessment Abnormalities: Musculoskeletal System

Finding	Description	Possible Etiology and Significance
Ankylosis	Scarring within a joint leading to stiffness or fixation	Chronic joint inflammation
Atrophy	Wasting of muscle, characterized by decrease in circumference and flabby appearance and resulting in decrease in function and muscle tone	Prolonged disuse, contraction, immobilization, muscle denervation
Contracture	Resistance to movement of muscle or joint as result of fibrosis of supporting soft tissues	Shortening of muscle or ligament structure, tightness of soft tissue, immobilization, incorrect positioning
Crepitation	Crackling sound or grating sensation as result of friction between bones	Fracture, chronic inflammation, dislocation
Effusion	Escape of fluid into body part, possibly with swelling and pain	Trauma, especially to knee
Felon	Abscess occurring in pulp space (tissue mass) of distal phalanx of finger as a result of infection	Minor hand injury, puncture wound, laceration
Ganglion	Small, fluid-filled cyst usually on dorsal surface of wrist and foot	Degeneration of connective tissue close to tendons and joints leading to formation of small cysts
Hypertrophy	Increase in size of muscle as result of enlargement of existing cells	Exercise, increased androgens, increased stimulation or use
Kyphosis (round back)	Anteroposterior or forward bending of spine with convexity of curve in posterior direction, common at thoracic and sacral levels	Poor posture, tuberculosis, chronic arthritis, growth disturbance of vertebral epiphysis, osteoporosis
Lordosis	Deformity of spine resulting in anteroposterior curvature with concavity in posterior direction; common in lumbar spine	Secondary to other deformities of spine, muscular dystrophy, obesity, flexion contracture of hip, congenital dislocation of hip
Pes planus	Flatfoot	Congenital condition, muscle paralysis, mild cerebral palsy, early muscular dystrophy
Scoliosis	Deformity resulting in lateral curvature of spine	Idiopathic or congenital condition, fracture or dislocation, osteomalacia, functional condition
Subluxation	Partial dislocation of joint	Instability of joint capsule and supporting ligaments (e.g., from trauma, arthritis)
Valgus	Angulation of bone away from midline	Alteration in gait, pain, abnormal erosion of articular cartilage
Varus	Angulation of bone toward midline	Alteration in gait, pain, abnormal erosion of articular cartilage

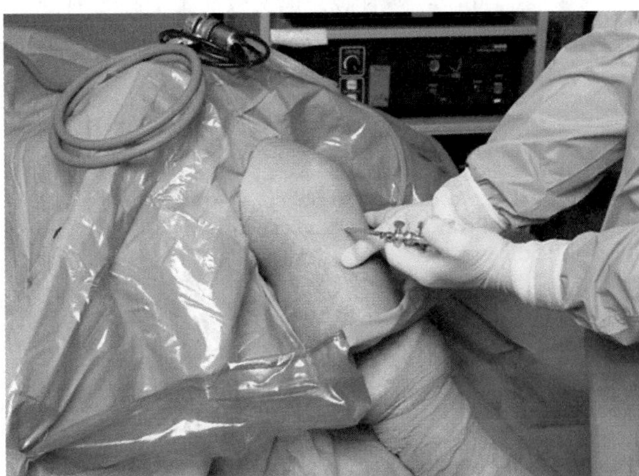

Fig. 58-10 Arthroscopy of a joint.

larger needle is inserted into the joint, and fluid is aspirated. The appropriate container must be readily available for laboratory analysis of the aspirated fluid.

The fluid is examined grossly for volume, color, clarity, viscosity, and mucin clot formation. Normal synovial fluid is clear, light yellow, and scanty (1 to 3 ml). Fluid from a septic joint may be purulent and thick, or gray and thin. In gout the fluid may be whitish yellow. Blood may be aspirated if there is hemarthrosis because of injury. The mucin clot test indicates the character of the protein portion of the synovial fluid. Normally a white, ropelike mucin clot is formed. In an inflammatory process the clot breaks apart easily and fragments.

The fluid is examined microscopically for cell count and identification of the cells. The normal white blood cell (WBC) count is less than 200 cells/μl with fewer than 25% neutrophils and no bacteria. The WBC count and protein are increased in an inflammatory process. The presence of uric acid crystals may indicate gout.

(Text continued on p. 1838.)

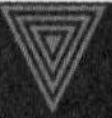

Table 58-8 Diagnostic Studies: Musculoskeletal System

Study	Description and Purpose	Nursing Responsibility
Radiologic		
Standard x-ray	An x-ray is taken to determine density and texture of bone. Study evaluates structural or functional changes of bones and joints. In anteroposterior view, x-ray beam passes from front to back, allowing one-dimensional view; lateral position provides two-dimensional view.	Avoid excessive exposure of patient and self. Before procedure, remove any radiopaque objects that can interfere with results. Explain procedure to patient.
Arthrogram	Study involves injection of contrast medium or air into joint cavity, which permits visualization of joint structures. Joint movement is followed with series of x-rays.	Assess patient for possible allergy to contrast medium. Explain procedure. Prepare area to be injected aseptically.
Diskogram	An x-ray of cervical or lumbar intervertebral disk is done after injection of contrast dye into nucleus pulposus. Study permits visualization of intervertebral disk abnormalities.	Same as for arthrogram.
Sinogram	An x-ray is taken after injection of contrast dye into sinus tract (deep draining wound). Study visualizes course of sinus and tissues involved.	Same as for arthrogram.
Tomogram	Multiple x-ray views of body region are focused at successively deeper layers of tissue lying in predetermined planes. Study focuses on certain tissues, eliminating or blurring surrounding structures. Technique is useful in locating bone destruction, small body cavities, foreign bodies, and lesions overshadowed by opaque structures.	Explain procedure to patient.
Computed tomography (CT) scan	An x-ray beam is used with a computer to provide a three-dimensional picture. It is used to identify soft-tissue abnormalities, bony abnormalities, and various musculoskeletal trauma.	Explain procedure to patient. Inform patient that procedure is painless. Inform patient of importance of remaining still during procedure.
Magnetic resonance imaging (MRI)	Radiowaves and magnetic field are used to view soft tissue. Study is especially useful in the diagnosis of avascular necrosis, disk disease, tumors, osteomyelitis, ligament tears, cartilage tears. Patient is placed inside scanning chamber. Gadolinium may be injected into a vein to enhance visualization of the structures.	Explain procedure to patient. Inform patient that it is painless. Be aware that it is contraindicated in patient with aneurysm clips, metallic implants, pacemakers, electronic devices, hearing aids, shrapnel, and extreme obesity. Ensure that patient has no metal on clothing (e.g., snaps, zippers, jewelry, credit cards). Convert IV to heparin lock. Inform patient of importance of remaining still throughout examination. Inform patients who are claustrophobic that they may experience symptoms during examination. Administer antianxiety agent (if indicated and ordered).
Bone Mass Measurements		
Radiogrammetry, radiodensitometry	Study evaluates bone mass of metacarpals. A very low dose of radiation is used.	Explain procedure to patient. Inform patient that procedure is painless.
Single-photon absorptiometry (SPA)	Low-dose radiation scanner measures mostly peripheral cortical bone at distal radius or midradius. Study is not useful for follow-up because of slow changes in cortical bone.	Same as above.
Dual-photon absorptiometry (DPA)	Technique measures mixed trabecular and cortical bones at sites such as hip and lumbar spine. It can be used to calculate total body calcium concentration.	Same as above.

continued

Table 58-8 Diagnostic Studies: Musculoskeletal System—cont'd

Study	Description and Purpose	Nursing Responsibility
Bone Mass Measurements—cont'd		
Dual-energy x-ray absorptiometry (DEXA)	Technique measures bone mass of spine, femur, forearm, and total body. Considered to be fast and precise with low dose of radiation.	Same as above.
Computed tomography scan	Scan measures almost pure trabecular bone. High radiation dose and higher errors of measurement are disadvantages. It is useful for following up effects of treatment.	Same as above.
Radioisotope Studies		
Bone scan	Technique involves injection of radioisotope (usually sodium pertechnate) that is taken up by bone. Camera scans entire body (front and back), and recording is made on paper. Degree of uptake is related to blood flow to bone. Increased uptake is seen in osteomyelitis, osteoporosis, and primary and metastatic malignant lesions of bone and with certain fractures.	Explain procedure to patient. Give calculated dose of radioisotope 2 hr before procedure. Ensure that bladder is emptied before scan. Inform patient that procedure requires 1 hr while patient lies supine and that no pain or harm will result from isotopes. Be aware that no follow-up scans are required.
Endoscopy		
Arthroscopy	Study involves insertion of arthroscope into joint (usually knee) for visualization of structure and contents. It can be used for exploratory surgery (removal of loose bodies and biopsy) and for diagnosis of abnormalities of meniscus, articular cartilage, ligaments, or joint capsule. Other structures that can be visualized through the arthroscope include the shoulder, elbow, and ankle.	Explain procedure to patient. Inform patient that procedure is performed in OR with strict asepsis and that either local or general anesthesia is used. After procedure, cover wound with sterile dressing. Wrap leg from midthigh to midcalf with compression dressing for 24 hr for knee arthroscope. Instruct patient to limit activity for a few days.
Mineral Metabolism		
Alkaline phosphatase	This enzyme, produced by osteoblasts of bone, is needed for mineralization of organic bone matrix. Elevated levels are found in healing fractures, bone cancers, osteoporosis, osteomalacia, and Paget's disease. *Normal:* 20-90 U/L (0.3-1.5 μkat/L)	Explain procedure to patient. Obtain blood samples by venipuncture. Observe venipuncture site for bleeding or hematoma formation. Inform patient that procedure does not require fasting.
Calcium	Bone is primary organ for calcium storage. Calcium provides bone with rigid consistency. Decreased serum level is found in osteomalacia, renal disease, and hypoparathyroidism; increased level is found in hyperparathyroidism, bone tumors, and osteoporosis. *Normal:* 9-11 mg/dl (2.3-2.7 mmol/L).	Explain procedure to patient. Observe venipuncture site for bleeding or hematoma formation. Inform patient that procedure does not require fasting.
Phosphorus	Amount present is directly related to calcium metabolism. Decreased level is found in osteomalacia; increased level is found in chronic renal disease, healing fractures, osteolytic metastatic tumor. *Normal:* 2.8-4.5 mg/dl (0.9-1.5 mmol/L).	Explain procedure to patient. Observe venipuncture site for bleeding or hematoma formation. Inform patient that procedure does not require fasting.

continued

Table 58-8 Diagnostic Studies: Musculoskeletal System—cont'd

Study	Description and Purpose	Nursing Responsibility
Serologic		
Rheumatoid factor (RF)	Study assesses presence of autoantibody (rheumatoid factor) in serum. Factor is not specific for rheumatoid arthritis and is seen in other connective tissue diseases as well as small percentage of normal population. *Normal:* negative or titer <1:20.	Explain procedure to patient. Observe venipuncture site for bleeding or hematoma formation. Inform patient that procedure does not require fasting.
Erythrocyte sedimentation rate (ESR)	Study is nonspecific index of inflammation. Study measures rapidity with which red blood cells settle out of unclotted blood in 1 hr. Results are influenced by physiologic factors as well as diseases. Elevated levels are seen with any inflammatory process (especially rheumatoid arthritis, rheumatic fever, bone infections, and respiratory infections). *Normal:* <20 mm/hr.	Explain procedure to patient. Observe venipuncture site for bleeding or hematoma formation. Inform patient that procedure does not require fasting.
Lupus erythematosus cells	Lupus erythematosus cells are seen in about 80% of cases of lupus erythematosus. Normally no lupus erythematosus cells are present.	Obtain blood from patient and have blood smear made on slide.
Antinuclear antibody (ANA)	Study assesses presence of antibodies capable of destroying nucleus of body's tissue cells. Finding is positive in 95% of patients with lupus erythematosus and may also be positive in individuals with scleroderma or rheumatoid arthritis and in small percentage of normal population.	Explain procedure to patient. Observe venipuncture site for bleeding or hematoma formation. Inform patient that procedure does not require fasting.
Anti-DNA antibody	Study detects serum antibodies that react with DNA. It is the most specific test for systemic lupus erythematosus.	Explain procedure to patient. Observe venipuncture site for bleeding or hematoma formation. Inform patient that procedure does not require fasting.
Complement	Complement, a normal body protein, is essential to both immune and inflammatory reactions. Complement components used up in these reactions are depleted. Subsequent test applied to serum yields little or no serum complement components. Complement depletions may be found in patients with rheumatoid arthritis or systemic lupus erythematosus.	Explain procedure to patient. Observe venipuncture site for bleeding or hematoma formation. Inform patient that procedure does not require fasting.
Uric acid	End product of purine metabolism is normally excreted in urine. Although not specific, levels are usually elevated in gout. *Normal:* male 4.5-6.5 mg/dl (268-387 μmol/L); female 2.5-5.5 mg/dl (149-327 μmol/L).	Explain procedure to patient. Observe venipuncture site for bleeding or hematoma formation. Inform patient that procedure does not require fasting.
C-reactive protein (CRP)	Study is used to diagnose inflammatory diseases, infections, and active widespread malignancy. CRP is synthesized by the liver and is present in large amounts in serum 18-24 hr after onset of tissue damage. *Normal:* negative.	Explain procedure to patient. Observe venipuncture site for bleeding or hematoma formation. Inform patient that procedure does not require fasting.
Human leukocyte antigen (HLA)-B27	Antigen present in disorders such as ankylosing spondylitis and variants of rheumatoid arthritis. *Normal:* negative.	Explain procedure to patient. Observe venipuncture site for bleeding or hematoma formation. Inform patient that procedure does not require fasting.

continued

Table 58-8 Diagnostic Studies: Musculoskeletal System—cont'd

Study	Description and Purpose	Nursing Responsibility
Muscle Enzymes		
Creatine kinase (CK)	Highest concentration is found in skeletal muscle. Increased values are found in progressive muscular dystrophy, polymyositis, and traumatic injuries. *Normal:* men 5-55 U/L (0.1-0.9 μkat/L); women 5-35 U/L (0.01-0.6 μkat/L).	Explain procedure to patient. Observe venipuncture site for bleeding or hematoma formation. Inform patient that procedure does not require fasting.
Aldolase	Study is useful in monitoring muscular dystrophy and dermatomyositis. *Normal:* 1.0-7.5 U/L (16.7-125 nkat/L).	Explain procedure to patient. Observe venipuncture site for bleeding or hematoma formation. Inform patient that procedure does not require fasting.
Aspartate aminotransferase (AST) or serum glutamic oxaloacetic transaminase (SGOT)	Enzyme is found in skeletal muscle but is primarily an enzyme of cardiac and hepatic cells. *Normal:* 15-45 U/L (0.12-0.67 μkat/L).	Explain procedure to patient. Observe venipuncture site for bleeding or hematoma formation. Inform patient that procedure does not require fasting.
Invasive Procedures		
Arthrocentesis	Incision or puncture of joint capsule is done to obtain samples of synovial fluid from within joint cavity or to remove excess fluid. Local anesthesia and aseptic preparation are used before needle is inserted into joint and fluid aspirated. Study is useful in diagnosis of joint inflammation.	Explain procedure to patient. Inform patient that procedure is usually done at bedside or in examination room. Send samples of synovial fluid to laboratory for examination (if indicated). After procedure apply compression dressing and have patient rest joint for 8-24 hr. Observe for leakage of blood or fluid on dressing.
Electromyogram	Study evaluates electrical potential associated with skeletal muscle contraction. Long, small-gauge needles are inserted into certain muscles. Needle probes are attached to leads that feed information to electromyogram machine. Recordings of electrical activity of muscle are traced on audiotransmitter as well as on oscilloscope and recording paper. Study is useful in providing information related to lower motor neuron dysfunction and primary muscle diseases.	Inform patient that procedure is usually done in electromyogram laboratory while patient lies supine on special table. Keep patient awake to cooperate with voluntary movement. Inform patient that procedure involves some discomfort from needle insertion. Avoid administration of stimulants and sedatives 24 hr before procedure.
Miscellaneous		
Thermography	Technique uses infrared detector, which measures degree of heat radiating from skin surface. Study is useful in investigation of cause of inflamed joints and in following up patient's response to antiinflammatory drug therapy.	Inform patient that procedure is painless and noninvasive.
Plethysmography	Study records variations in volume and pressure of blood passing through tissues. Test is nonspecific and quantitative.	Inform patient that procedure is painless and noninvasive.
Somatosensory evoked potential (SSEP)	Study evaluates evoked potential of muscle contractions. Electrodes are placed on skin and provide recordings of electrical activity of muscle. Study useful in identifying subtle dysfunction of lower motor neuron and primary muscle disease. SSEP measures nerve conduction along pathways not accessible by electromyogram. Transcutaneous or percutaneous electrodes are applied to the skin and help identify neuropathy and myopathy.	Explain procedure to the patient. Inform patient that procedure is similar to electromyogram but does not involve needles. Electrodes are applied to the skin.

IV, Intravenous; *OR,* operating room.

Muscle Enzymes

Muscle enzymes are released from injured or dead muscle cells. Determinations of muscle enzyme values are used to distinguish between muscle weakness that is due to nerve innervation problems and dystrophic disease of the muscle itself. The level of enzymes reflects the progress of the disorder and the effectiveness of treatment. Aspartate aminotransferase (AST) (also known as serum glutamic-oxaloacetic transaminase [SGOT]) levels are the least sensitive indicators of muscle disease, and creatine kinase (CK) levels are the most sensitive.

Serologic Studies

Approximately 85% of people with rheumatoid arthritis and related diseases have an autoantibody known as *rheumatoid factor* in their serum. This autoantibody is usually of the IgM class, although it may be IgG. The test used to determine the presence of this factor is the latex fixation test. Latex particles are coated with aggregated immunoglobulin G. If serum containing rheumatoid factor is mixed with these latex particles, it reacts with the latex particles and causes agglutination. An estimation of the titer is obtained by performing serial dilutions of the serum.

Other diagnostic studies of the musculoskeletal system are summarized in Table 58-8.

REVIEW QUESTIONS

The number of the question corresponds to the same-numbered objective at the beginning of the chapter.

1. The bone cells that synthesize organic bone matrix are called
 a. osteocytes.
 b. osteoclasts.
 c. osteoblasts.
 d. osteoids.

2. What type of joint is the knee joint?
 a. Hinge joint
 b. Saddle joint
 c. Ball-and-socket joint
 d. Gliding joint

3. Which type of muscle can be controlled voluntarily?
 a. Cardiac
 b. Smooth
 c. Skeletal
 d. Nonstriated

4. The function of bursae is to
 a. separate muscle from muscle.
 b. connect bone to bone.
 c. secrete synovial fluid.
 d. relieve pressure between moving parts.

5. Loss of elasticity in ligaments and cartilage in older adults results in
 a. decreased agility.
 b. Heberden's nodes.
 c. decreased muscle bulk.
 d. slowed reaction time.

6. Which of the following musculoskeletal problems has a familial predisposition?
 a. Osteomyelitis
 b. Fractures
 c. Rheumatoid arthritis
 d. Low back pain

7. When grading muscle strength, a score of 5 indicates
 a. active movement against full resistance without evident fatigue.
 b. no detection of muscular contraction.
 c. active movement against gravity.
 d. barely detectable flicker of contraction.

8. Which of the following is considered a normal assessment finding?
 a. A lateral curvature of the spine
 b. Angulation of bone toward midline
 c. Muscle strength of 3
 d. Simultaneous occurrence of stance and swing phase of gait

9. The study that evaluates the electrical potential associated with skeletal muscle contraction is the
 a. electromyogram.
 b. dual-photon absorptiometry.
 c. magnetic resonance imaging.
 d. aldolase muscle enzyme.

REFERENCES

1. Seeley RA, Stephens TD, Tate P: *Anatomy and physiology*, ed 2, St Louis, 1992, Mosby.
2. Guyton AC: *Human physiology and mechanisms of disease*, ed 5, Philadelphia, 1992, Saunders.
3. Guyton AC: *Textbook of medical physiology*, ed 8, Philadelphia, 1991, Saunders.
4. Carnevali DL, Patrick M, editors: *Nursing management for the elderly*, ed 3, Philadelphia, 1993, Lippincott.

Chapter 59

NURSING ROLE IN MANAGEMENT

Musculoskeletal Problems

Susan Ruda

Learning Objectives

1. Explain the pathophysiology, clinical manifestations, and management of soft-tissue injuries, including strains, sprains, dislocations, subluxations, bursitis, carpal tunnel syndrome, repetitive strain injury, and muscle spasms.
2. Describe the sequential events involved in fracture healing.
3. Explain common complications associated with fracture injury and fracture healing.
4. Differentiate among open reduction, closed reduction, traction, and cast immobilization regarding purpose, complications, and nursing management.
5. Explain the neurovascular assessment of an injured extremity.
6. Describe the therapeutic and nursing management of patients with specific fractures.
7. Describe the pathophysiologic basis for the management of osteomyelitis.
8. Describe the indications and therapeutic and nursing management for an amputation.
9. Describe the types, pathophysiology, clinical manifestations, and treatment of bone cancer.
10. Differentiate between the causes and characteristics of acute and chronic low back pain.
11. Describe the conservative and surgical treatments of low back pain.
12. Describe the postoperative nursing management of a patient who has undergone spinal surgery.
13. Explain the causes and management of common foot disorders.
14. Describe the pathophysiology, clinical manifestations, and management of metabolic bone disorders.

The most common cause of musculoskeletal problems is injury from accidents resulting in fracture, dislocations, and associated soft-tissue injuries. Although most of these injuries are not fatal, the cost in terms of pain, disability, medical expense, and lost wages is enormous. For all ages, accidents are exceeded only by heart disease, cancer, and strokes as a cause of death. Accidents are the leading cause of death in children and young adults.

The nurse has an important role in educating the public in the basic principles of safety and accident prevention. The morbidity associated with accidents can be significantly reduced if people are aware of environmental hazards, use existing safety equipment, and apply safety and traffic rules. In the industrial setting, the nurse should educate employees and employers about the use of proper safety equipment and avoidance of hazardous working situations.

In the home environment, falls account for many musculoskeletal injuries. Preventive education should be directed toward the importance of wearing shoes with functional soles and heels, avoidance of wet or slippery surfaces, careful placement of throw rugs, and removal of obstacles from the pathway of high-risk individuals such as persons with gait instability or visual or cognitive impairment.

Reviewed by Mary F. Rodts, MS, RN, ONC, Orthopedics and Scoliosis, Ltd.; and Assistant Professor, Rush College of Nursing, Chicago, IL.

SOFT-TISSUE INJURIES

Soft-tissue injuries include sprains, strains, dislocations, and subluxations. These common injuries are usually caused by trauma. The increase in the number of people who have committed themselves to maintaining a regular fitness program or participate in sports is believed to contribute to the increased incidence of soft-tissue injuries and inflammatory responses of the musculoskeletal system.[1] Common sports-related injuries are summarized in Table 59-1.

Sprains and Strains

Sprains and strains are the two most common types of injury affecting the musculoskeletal system. These injuries are usually associated with abnormal stretching forces, which may occur during vigorous activities.

A *sprain* is classified according to the amount of ligament fibers torn. A first-degree sprain involves tears of only

Table 59-1 Common Sports-Related Injuries

Injury	Definition	Treatment
■ Impingement syndrome	Entrapment of soft-tissue structures under coracoacromial arch of the shoulder	NSAIDs; rest until symptoms decrease and then gradual range-of-motion and strengthening exercises
■ Rotator cuff tear	Tear within muscle or ligaments of shoulder	If minor tear, rest, NSAIDs, and gradual mobilization with range-of-motion and strengthening exercises
■ Shin splints	Inflammation along tibial shaft from tearing away of tendons caused by improper shoes, overuse, or running on hard pavement	Rest, ice, NSAIDs, proper shoes; gradual increase in activity; if pain persists, x-ray should be done to rule out stress fracture of tibia
■ Tendinitis	Inflammation of tendon in upper or lower extremity as a result of overuse or incorrect use	Rest, ice, NSAIDs; gradual return to sport activity; protective brace may be necessary if symptoms recur
■ Ligament injury	Tearing or stretching of ligament; usually occurs as a result of direct blow; characterized by sudden pain, swelling, and instability	Rest, ice, NSAIDs; protection of affected extremity by use of brace; if symptoms persist, surgical repair may be necessary
■ Meniscal injury	Cartilage injury to the knee characterized by popping, clicking, or tearing sensation, swelling	Rest, ice, NSAIDs; gradual return to regular activities; if symptoms persist, surgical arthroscopy to diagnose and repair meniscal injury may be necessary

NSAIDs, Nonsteroidal antiinflammatory drugs.

a few fibers resulting in mild tenderness and slight swelling. A second-degree sprain is partial disruption of the involved tissue with more swelling and tenderness. A third-degree sprain is a complete tearing of the tissues. A gap in the muscle may be apparent or felt through the skin if the muscle is torn. Because these areas are rich in nerve endings, the injury can be quite painful. The most common areas where sprains occur are the ankle and wrist. A *strain* is a stretching of a muscle and its fascial sheath.

Minor sprains and strains are usually self-limiting, with full function returning within 3 to 6 weeks. A severe sprain can result in an avulsion fracture, in which the ligament pulls loose a fragment of bone. Alternatively, the joint structure may become unstable and result in dislocation. At the time of injury, *hemarthrosis* (bleeding into a joint space or cavity) or disruption of the synovial lining may occur. An acute strain may involve partial or complete rupture of a muscle.

X-rays of the affected part are usually taken to rule out a fracture or widening of the joint structure. Surgical repair may be necessary if the injury is significant enough to produce severe disruption of ligamentous or muscle structures, fracture, or dislocation.

NURSING MANAGEMENT

SPRAINS AND STRAINS

Nursing Assessment

The clinical manifestations of sprains and strains are similar and include pain, edema, decrease in function, and bruising. Pain aggravated by continued use is common. Edema develops in the injured area because of minute hemorrhages within the disrupted tissues and the ensuing inflammatory response. Usually, the patient will recount a history of traumatic injury, possibly of a twisting nature or recent exercise activity.

Nursing Diagnoses

Nursing diagnoses for the patient with a sprain or strain include, but are not limited to, the following:

- Pain related to edema, muscle spasm, and ineffective pain relief or comfort measures
- Impaired physical mobility related to pain, activity restriction, or an immobilization device

Planning

The overall goals are that the patient with a sprain or strain will (1) return to normal movement and function and (2) have satisfactory relief of pain and discomfort until healing is complete.

Nursing Implementation

Health Promotion and Maintenance. The use of elastic support bandages or adhesive tape wrapping before beginning a vigorous activity is thought to reduce the occurrence of sprains. However, some physicians do not support preventive wrapping or taping because it may predispose the athlete to injury. Stretching and warm-up exercises before vigorous activity also help prevent strains.

Preconditioning exercise protects an inherently weak joint because slow stretching is tolerated better by biologic tissues than is quick stretching. Warm-up exercises "prelengthen" potentially strained tissues by avoiding the quick

Table 59-2 Emergency Management: Acute Soft-Tissue Injury

Possible Etiologies

Falls, direct blows, forced flexion, hyperextension, rotation from motor vehicle collisions, sports injuries

Possible Assessment Findings

Swelling
Ecchymosis
Pain, tenderness
Decreased sensation if severe swelling
Decreased pulse, movement, and capillary refill
Pallor
Shortening or rotation of extremity (dislocation)
Loss of use or inability to bear weight (if lower extremity involved)
Muscle spasms

Management

- Assess neurologic and circulatory status of involved limb.
- Elevate involved limb.
- Apply compression bandage (unless dislocation).
- Apply ice packs to affected area.
- Immobilize affected extremity.
- *Do not* allow weight bearing of the involved limb (if lower extremity involved).
- Anticipate need for x-rays of injured extremity.
- Give analgesia as necessary.

stretch often encountered in sports. Warm-up exercises also increase the temperature of muscle, which increases the speed of cell metabolism and the speed of nerve impulse transmission. The increased metabolism contributes to better oxygenation of muscle fiber during work. Stretching is also thought to improve kinesthetic awareness, thus lessening the chance of uncoordinated movement.

Acute Intervention. If an injury occurs, the immediate care focuses on rest and limitation of movement, application of ice to the injured area, compression of the involved extremity, elevation of the extremity, and analgesia as necessary (Table 59-2). Movement should be limited and the extremity rested as soon as pain is felt. Unless the injury is severe, prolonged rest is usually not necessary. Cold in several forms can be used to produce hypothermia to the involved part. Physiologic changes that occur in soft tissue as a result of the use of cold include vasoconstriction, reduction in transmission of nerve impulses, and reduction in conduction velocity.[2] These changes result in analgesia and anesthesia, reduction of muscle spasm without changes in muscular strength or endurance, reduction of local edema and inflammation, and reduction of local metabolic requirements. Few unwanted side effects accompany the use of cold to treat a soft-tissue injury. Cold is most useful when applied immediately after the injury has occurred. Ice applications should not exceed 20 to 30 minutes per application, with a "warm-down" time of 10 to 15 minutes between applications.

Compression also helps limit swelling, which, if left uncontrolled, could lengthen healing time. A compression bandage can be wrapped around the injured part. The bandage is too tight if numbness is felt in the area or if there is cramping or additional pain or swelling beyond the edge of the bandage. The bandage can be left in place for 30 minutes, then removed for 15 minutes to ease circulation.

The injured part should be elevated above heart level to help drain excess fluid from the area and decrease further edema. The part should be elevated even during sleep. Mild analgesia such as aspirin, ibuprofen, or acetominophen may be necessary to manage patient discomfort.

After the acute phase (usually lasting 24 to 48 hours), warm, moist heat can be applied to the affected part to reduce swelling and provide comfort. Heat applications should not exceed 20 to 30 minutes, allowing a "cool-down" time between applications. The patient is encouraged to use the limb provided that the joint is protected from assuming the position of injury by means of casting, taping, or splinting. Movement of the joint surfaces maintains cartilage nutrition, and muscle contraction speeds circulation and resolution of the hematoma.

Chronic and Home Management. With the exception of treatment in the emergency department following the injury, sprains and strains are treated in the outpatient setting. The patient should be instructed in the use of ice to reduce edema and the use of mild analgesics to promote comfort. Use of an elastic wrap may provide added support during activity. To prevent reinjury, the patient should learn proper measures of prevention.

The physical therapist may help provide added comfort by means of specialized techniques. The therapist may also teach the patient exercises to perform to strengthen shortened muscles.

Dislocation and Subluxation

A *dislocation* is a severe injury of the ligamentous structures that surround a joint. It results in the complete displacement or separation of the articular surfaces of the joint. A *subluxation* is a partial or incomplete displacement of the joint surface. The clinical manifestations of a subluxation are similar to those of a dislocation but are less severe. Treatment of subluxation is similar to that of a dislocation, but subluxation requires less healing time.

Dislocations characteristically result from overwhelming forces transmitted to the joint that cause a disruption of the soft tissues of the joint. The joints most frequently dislocated in the upper extremity include the thumb, elbow, and shoulder. In the lower extremity, the hip is vulnerable to dislocation caused by severe trauma, often associated with motor vehicle accidents (Fig. 59-1).

X-ray studies are performed to determine the extent of shifting of the involved structures. The joint may also be aspirated to determine the presence of fat cells. If fat cells from the exposed marrow are found in the synovial fluid, an intraarticular fracture is present.

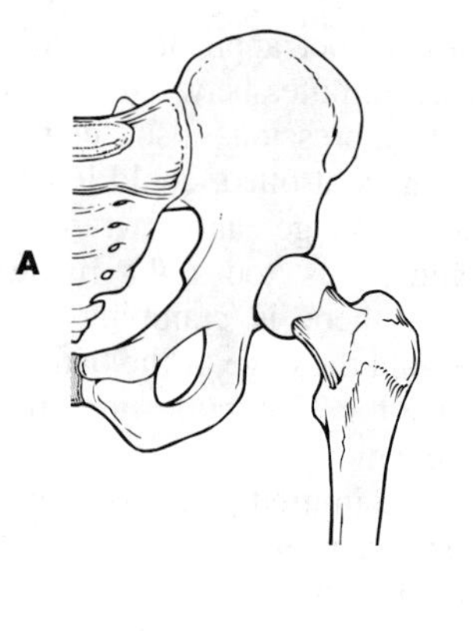

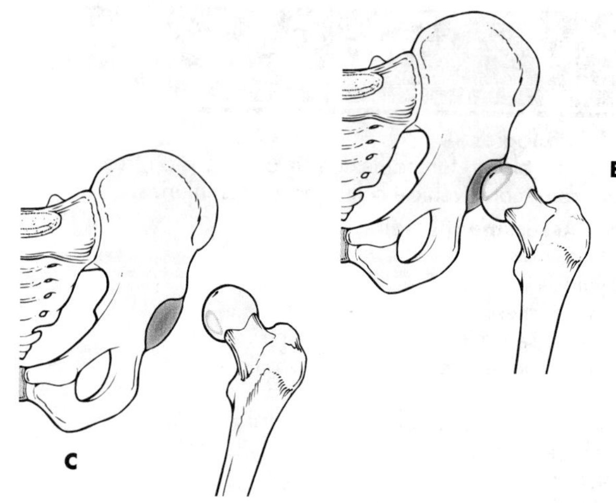

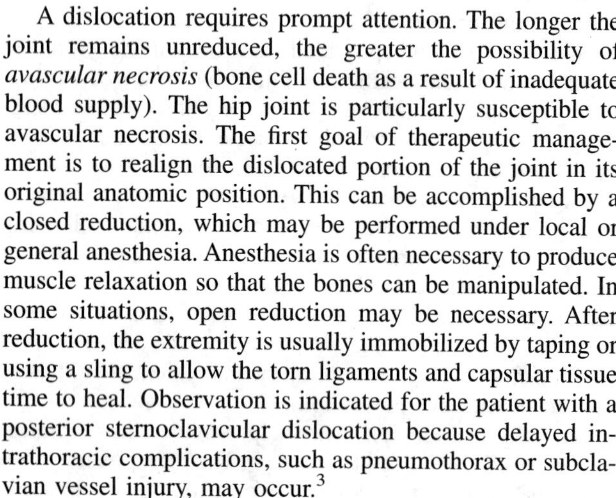

Fig. 59-1 Soft-tissue injury of the hip. ***A,*** Normal. ***B,*** Subluxation. ***C,*** Dislocation.

A dislocation requires prompt attention. The longer the joint remains unreduced, the greater the possibility of *avascular necrosis* (bone cell death as a result of inadequate blood supply). The hip joint is particularly susceptible to avascular necrosis. The first goal of therapeutic management is to realign the dislocated portion of the joint in its original anatomic position. This can be accomplished by a closed reduction, which may be performed under local or general anesthesia. Anesthesia is often necessary to produce muscle relaxation so that the bones can be manipulated. In some situations, open reduction may be necessary. After reduction, the extremity is usually immobilized by taping or using a sling to allow the torn ligaments and capsular tissue time to heal. Observation is indicated for the patient with a posterior sternoclavicular dislocation because delayed intrathoracic complications, such as pneumothorax or subclavian vessel injury, may occur.[3]

NURSING MANAGEMENT

DISLOCATIONS

Nursing Assessment

The most obvious clinical manifestation of a dislocation is asymmetry of the musculoskeletal contour. For example, if a hip is dislocated, the limb is shorter on the affected side. Additional manifestations include local pain, tenderness, loss of function of the injured part, and swelling of the soft tissues in the region of the joint. The major complications of a dislocated joint are open joint injuries, intraarticular fractures, fracture dislocation, and damage to adjacent neurovascular tissue.

Nursing Diagnoses

Nursing diagnoses for the patient with dislocation or subluxation include, but are not limited to, the following:

- Pain related to edema, muscle spasm, ineffective pain or comfort measures
- Impaired physical mobility related to pain, activity restrictions, or immobilization device

Planning

The overall goals are that the patient with a subluxation or dislocation will (1) have satisfactory relief of pain and discomfort, (2) have realignment of the articular joint surfaces as quickly as possible, and (3) return to preinjury function.

Nursing Implementation

Nursing care is directed toward symptomatic relief of pain and support and protection of the injured joint. After the joint has been immobilized, motion is usually restricted. A carefully regulated rehabilitation program can prevent the formation of contractures. The patient should not stretch the joint beyond its limits because the torn capsule and ligament heal in a shortened position with fibrous scar tissue that is not as strong as the original tissue. An exercise program slowly and methodically restores the joint to its original range of motion without causing another dislocation. The patient will gradually return to normal activities.

A patient who has dislocated a joint may be at greater risk to experience chronic dislocation events because the joint has been weakened by shortened ligaments and scar tissue at the joint surface. Activity restrictions of the affected joint may be imposed to decrease the risk of dislocating the joint on a chronic basis.

Carpal Tunnel Syndrome

Carpal tunnel syndrome is a condition caused by compression of the median nerve beneath the transverse carpal ligament within the narrow confines of the carpal tunnel located at the wrist (Fig. 59-2). This condition is frequently due to pressure from trauma or edema caused by inflammation of a tendon (tenosynovitis), neoplasm, rheumatoid synovial disease, or soft-tissue masses such as ganglia. Carpal tunnel syndrome occurs most frequently in middle-aged or postmenopausal females and persons who are employed in occupations that require continuous wrist movement (e.g., butchers, secretaries, carpenters, computer operators).

Therapeutic management is directed toward relieving the underlying cause of the nerve compression. The early symp-

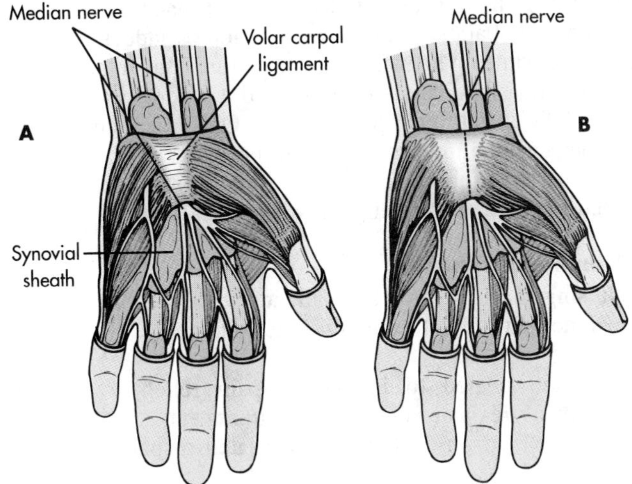

Fig. 59-2 ***A,*** Wrist structures involved in carpal tunnel syndrome. ***B,*** Decompression of median nerve.

toms associated with carpal tunnel syndrome can usually be relieved by placing the hand and wrist at rest by immobilizing them in a hand splint. If the cause is inflammation, injection of hydrocortisone directly into the carpal tunnel may provide relief. If the problem continues, the median nerve may have to be surgically decompressed by longitudinal division of the transverse carpal ligament under regional anesthesia. Endoscopic carpal tunnel release is a new procedure in which the decompression is done through a small puncture site.

NURSING MANAGEMENT

CARPAL TUNNEL SYNDROME

Nursing Assessment

The clinical manifestations of carpal tunnel syndrome are weakness, pain and numbness of the hand, impaired sensation in the distribution of the median nerve, and clumsiness in performing fine hand movements. Numbness and tingling may be present and may awaken the patient at night. Holding the wrist in acute flexion for 60 seconds will produce tingling and numbness over the distribution of the median nerve, the palmar surface of the thumb, the index finger, the middle finger, and part of the ring finger. This is known as a positive *Phalen's sign.* In late stages there is atrophy of thenar muscles. This syndrome can result in recurrent pain and eventual dysfunction of the hand.

Nursing Diagnoses

Nursing diagnoses for the patient with carpal tunnel syndrome include, but are not limited to, the following:

- Pain related to ineffective pain or comfort measures or nerve compression
- Impaired physical mobility related to pain and weakness
- Risk for injury related to impaired sensation and clumsiness of the involved hand

Planning

The overall goals are that the patient with carpal tunnel syndrome will (1) not experience an injury as a result of impaired sensation, (2) have relief from associated discomfort, and (3) have satisfactory mobility of the hands.

Nursing Implementation

Prevention of carpal tunnel syndrome involves educating employees and employers to identify risk factors. Adaptive devices such as wrist splints may be worn to relieve pressure on the median nerve. Special keyboard pads are available for computer operators to help prevent carpal tunnel syndrome or a worsening of symptoms if present. Comfort should be maintained by use of medication and splints to relieve pain and protect the area. The patient's sensation may be impaired. Therefore the patient should be instructed to avoid hazards such as extreme heat because of the risk of thermal injury. Nursing care of the patient with carpal tunnel syndrome usually occurs in the office or outpatient setting. The patient may be required to consider occupational changes because of discomfort and sensory and functional changes.

If surgery is performed, the neurovascular status of the hand should be evaluated regularly. The patient should be instructed in the appropriate assessments to perform at home because the surgery is done on an outpatient basis.

Repetitive Strain Injury

Repetitive strain injury (RSI) is defined as a cumulative trauma disorder resulting from prolonged, forceful, or awkward hand movements. These movements cause strain on the tendons and muscles and reduce circulation. These stresses also cause tiny tears in the muscles and tendons, which become inflamed. If the tissues are not given time to heal properly, scarring can occur. Blood vessels of the arms and hands may become constricted, depriving tissues of vital nutrients and causing an accumulation of toxins. Without intervention, tendons and muscles can deteriorate and nerves can become hypersensitive. At this point even the slightest hand movement can cause pain.

In addition to the repetitive movements, other factors related to RSI include poor posture and positioning, ill-fitting furniture, a badly designed keyboard, and a heavy workload. The result is damage to the muscles, tendons, and nerves of the neck, shoulder, forearm, and hand. Symptoms of RSI include pain, weakness, numbness, or impairment of motor function. Persons most often affected by RSI include musicians, dancers, and, most commonly, keyboard operators.

RSI is becoming a serious public health problem. It costs businesses $20 billion a year.[4] The average compensation of an RSI patient is $29,000. It accounts for 60% of all job-related injuries. It is expected that the number of cases of RSI will continue to increase as computers become more commonplace.

RSI can be prevented through education, ergonomics (consideration of interaction of the human being and the work environment), and appropriate job design. Once diagnosed, the treatment of RSI consists of avoidance of the precipitating activity, physical therapy, and careful use of analgesia. In most cases, the muscle and tendon damage associated with RSI cannot be surgically repaired.

Meniscus Injury

Meniscus injuries are closely associated with ligament sprains commonly occurring in athletes engaged in sports such as basketball, rugby, football, soccer, and hockey. These activities produce a rotational stress when the knee is in a flexed position and the foot is fixed. A blow to the knee can cause the meniscus to be trapped between the femoral condyles and the plateau of the tibia, resulting in a torn meniscus (Fig. 59-3). A causal relationship exists between occupations that require working in a squatting or kneeling position and meniscus injuries.

An arthrogram or arthroscopy can diagnose knee problems. Magnetic resonance imaging (MRI) is beneficial in confirming the diagnosis before arthroscopy is used. It has eliminated the use of an arthrogram as a diagnostic tool in many cases. In addition to precision diagnosis, arthroscopy can be performed to surgically remove damaged intraarticular structures or to repair structures such as the meniscus or cruciate ligament through miniature incisions.[5]

Initial treatment includes exercises aimed at strengthening the stability of the knee, such as straight leg raises. The knee may also be unlocked by manipulation, followed by the use of a removable splint. If conservative treatment is not effective in relieving symptoms, surgical excision of the meniscus (*meniscectomy*) may be necessary.

NURSING MANAGEMENT

MENISCUS INJURY

Nursing Assessment

Meniscus injuries alone do not usually cause chronic edema because cartilage is avascular and aneural. However, a torn meniscus may be suspected when local tenderness or pain is reported. Pain is elicited by abduction or adduction of the leg at the knee. The usual clinical picture is a feeling by the patient that the knee is unstable and a report that the knee may click and lock periodically. Quadricep atrophy is evident if the injury has been present for some time. Degenerative joint disease can occur if a damaged, roughened meniscus is not surgically removed.

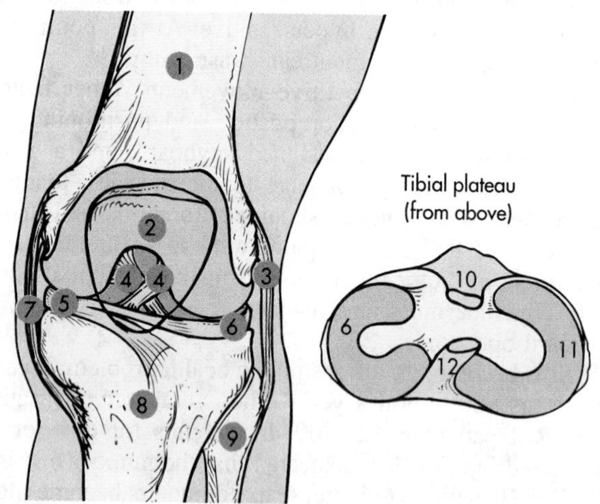

Fig. 59-3 Front view of injured knee with torn medial meniscus. ***1,*** Femur; ***2,*** patella; ***3,*** lateral collateral ligament; ***4,*** cruciate ligaments; ***5,*** medial meniscus; ***6,*** lateral meniscus; ***7,*** ruptured medial collateral ligament; ***8,*** tibia; ***9,*** fibula; ***10,*** anterior cruciate ligament; ***11,*** torn medial meniscus; ***12,*** posterior cruciate ligament.

Nursing Diagnoses

Nursing diagnoses for the patient with a meniscus injury include, but are not limited to, the following:

- Pain related to ineffective pain relief or comfort measures and failure to seek treatment
- Impaired physical mobility related to pain and knee instability

Planning

The overall goals are that the patient with a meniscus injury will have (1) satisfactory pain relief, (2) return of knee stability, and (3) resumption of preferred activities.

Nursing Implementation

Because most meniscal injuries are caused by sports-related activity, athletes should be educated about warm-up activities. Proper stretching may make the patient less prone to meniscal injury when a fall or twisting occurs. Examination of the acutely injured knee should occur within 24 hours of injury. Initial care of this type of injury involves application of ice, immobilization, and protected weight bearing.[1] Most meniscal injuries are treated in an outpatient setting. The patient should be allowed to ambulate as tolerated. Crutches may be necessary. Use of an immobilizer during the first few days protects the knee. After acute pain has decreased, gradual increases in flexion and strengthening help return the patient to full functioning. Physical therapy may be needed to help the patient strengthen muscles before returning to sport activities. Treatment by arthroscopy may be necessary to repair meniscal tears.

Bursitis

Bursae are closed sacs that are lined with synovial membrane and contain a small amount of synovial fluid. They are located beneath the skin at sites of friction, (e.g., between tendons, bones, and overlying joints). A bursa may become inflamed (*bursitis*) from repeated or excessive trauma or friction, gout, rheumatoid arthritis, or infection. The primary clinical manifestations of bursitis are pain and swelling as a result of edema in the affected part. Sites at which bursitis commonly occurs include the hand, knee, trochanter, shoulder, and elbow.

Attempts are made to determine and correct the cause of the bursitis. Rest is often the only treatment needed. The affected part may be immobilized in a compression dressing or plaster splint. Aspiration of the bursal fluid and injection of hydrocortisone may be necessary. If the bursa wall has become thickened and continues to interfere with normal joint function, surgical excision (bursectomy) may be necessary. For example, subacromial bursal thickening causes pain and loss of range of motion on abduction of the shoulder. Septic bursae usually require surgical drainage.

Muscle Spasms

Local muscle spasms are a common condition often associated with overdoing everyday activities and sports activities. Injury to a muscle stimulates free nerve endings, resulting in muscle excitation and spasm. The spasms produce additional pain, and a repetitive cycle is established. The clinical manifestations of muscle spasm of local origin include local pain, palpable muscle mass in spasm, tenderness, diminished range of motion of the affected site, and limitation of daily activities.

A careful history should be taken and physical examination performed to rule out central nervous system (CNS) problems. Muscle spasms can be managed with drug therapy, physical therapy, or both. A physical therapy program might include the use of heat, supervised exercise, massage, hydrotherapy, local heat-producing applications, ultrasound (deep heat), manipulation, and bracing. Drugs used for treatment of local muscle spasm include analgesics, tranquilizers, and skeletal muscle relaxants.

FRACTURES

Classification

A fracture is a disruption or break in the continuity of the structure of bone. Traumatic injuries account for the majority of fractures, although some fractures are secondary to a disease process (pathologic fractures). Fractures are described and classified according to (1) type (Fig. 59-4), (2) communication or noncommunication with the external environment (Fig. 59-5), and (3) location of fracture (Fig. 59-6). Fractures are also described as stable or unstable. A *stable fracture* occurs when some of the periosteum is intact across the fracture and either external or internal fixation has rendered the fragments stationary. Stable fractures are usually transverse, spiral, or greenstick. An *unstable fracture* is grossly displaced during injury and is a site of poor fixation. Unstable fractures are usually comminuted or oblique.

Clinical Manifestations

The patient's history indicates injury associated with numerous signs and symptoms, including immediate localized pain, decreased function, and inability to use the affected part (Table 59-3). The patient guards and protects the part against movement. The fracture may not be accompanied by obvious bone deformity. If a fracture is suspected, the affected part should be immobilized. Unnecessary movement increases soft-tissue damage and may convert a closed fracture to an open fracture. Careful management is particularly important for fractures through the epiphyseal place in children. If fixation is not solid, the entire long bone may cease its longitudinal growth at all areas or in part of the epiphyseal plate.

Fracture Healing

It is important to understand the principles of fracture healing (see Fig. 59-7 on p. 1848) to provide appropriate therapeutic interventions. Bone goes through a remarkable reparative process of self-healing (called *union*) that occurs in the following stages:

1. *Fracture hematoma.* When a fracture occurs, bleeding and edema precede the development of a hematoma, which surrounds the ends of the fragments. The hematoma is extravasated blood that changes from a liquid to a semisolid clot.
2. *Granulation tissue.* During this stage active phagocytosis absorbs the products of local necrosis. The hematoma changes into new tissue known as granulation tissue. Granulation tissue (consisting of young blood vessels, fibroblasts, and osteoblasts) produces a new bone substance called *osteoid.*
3. *Callus formation.* As minerals are deposited in the osteoid, it forms an unorganized network of bone that is woven about the fracture parts. Callus is primarily composed of cartilage, osteoblasts, calcium, and phosphorus. It usually begins to appear by the end of the first week after injury. Evidence of callus formation can be verified by x-ray.
4. *Ossification.* Ossification of the callus begins within 2 to 3 weeks after the fracture and continues until the fracture has healed. This stage is marked by ossification of the callus that is sufficient to prevent movement at the fracture site when the bones are gently stressed. However, the fracture is still evident on x-ray. During this stage of clinical union the patient can be converted from skeletal traction to a cast or the cast can be removed to allow mobility.
5. *Consolidation.* As callus continues to develop, the distance between bone fragments diminishes and eventually closes. This stage is called consolidation, and ossification continues. It can be equated with radiographic union.
6. *Remodeling.* Excess cells are absorbed in the final stage of bone healing, and union is completed. Gradual return of the injured bone to its preinjury structural strength and shape occurs. Remodeling of bone is enhanced as it responds to physical stress. Initially, stress is provided through exercise. Weightbearing is gradually introduced. New bone is deposited in sites subjected to stress and resorbed at areas where there is little stress. Radiographic union occurs when there is x-ray evidence of complete bony union.

Many factors, such as age, initial displacement of the fracture, site of the fracture, and blood supply to the area, influence the time required for fracture healing to be complete. Fracture healing may not occur in the expected time (*delayed union*) or may not occur at all *(nonunion).* The ossification process is arrested by causes such as inadequate immobilization and reduction, excess movement, infection, and poor nutrition. Healing time for fractures increases with age. For example, an uncomplicated midshaft fracture of the femur heals in 3 weeks in a newborn and requires 20 weeks in an adult. Table 59-4 (on p. 1849) summarizes complications of fracture healing.

Electrical stimulation is used successfully to stimulate bone healing in situations of nonunion or delayed fusion. The electric current acts by modifying cell behavior, causing bone remodeling.[6] The underlying mechanism for elec-

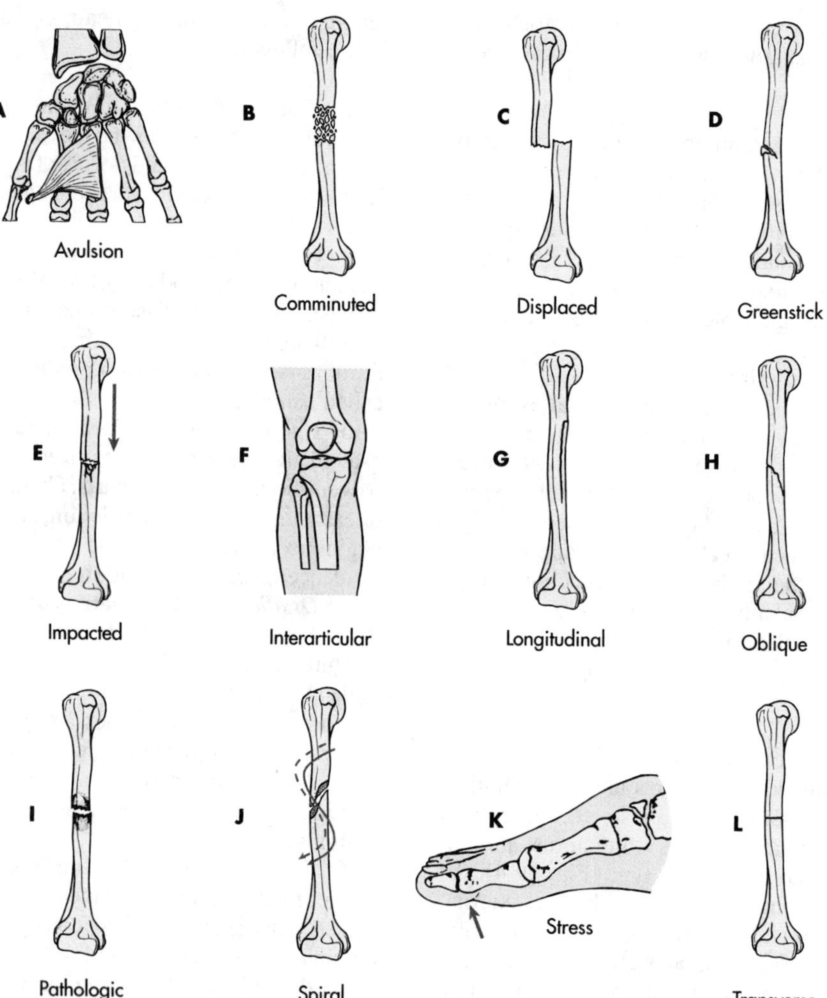

Fig. 59-4 Types of fractures. ***A,*** An avulsion is a fracture of bone resulting from the strong pulling effect of tendons or ligaments at the bone attachment. ***B,*** A comminuted fracture is a fracture with more than two fragments. The smaller fragments appear to be floating. ***C,*** A displaced (overriding) fracture involves a displaced fracture fragment that is overriding the other bone fragment. The periosteum is disrupted on both sides. ***D,*** A greenstick fracture is an incomplete fracture with one side splintered and the other side bent. The periosteum is not torn away from the bone. ***E,*** An impacted fracture is a comminuted fracture in which more than two fragments are driven into each other. ***F,*** An interarticular fracture is a fracture extending to the articular surface of the bone. ***G,*** A longitudinal fracture is an incomplete fracture in which the fracture line runs along the axis of the bone. The periosteum is not torn away from the bone. ***H,*** An oblique fracture is a fracture in which the line of the fracture extends in an oblique direction. ***I,*** A pathologic fracture is a spontaneous fracture at the site of a bone disease. ***J,*** A spiral fracture is a fracture in which the line of the fracture extends in a spiral direction along the shaft of the bone. ***K,*** A stress fracture is a fracture that occurs in normal or abnormal bone that is subject to repeated stress, such as from jogging, running, or striking a lever. ***L,*** A transverse fracture is a fracture in which the line of the fracture extends across the bone shaft at a right angle to the longitudinal axis.

trically induced bone remodeling remains unknown. The electrodes are semiinvasive, noninvasive, or surgically implanted. Patient motivation and adherence to prescribed stimulator use must be high because the treatment takes up to 10 hours a day for 3 to 6 months.[1]

Therapeutic Management

The overall goals of fracture treatment are (1) anatomic realignment of bone fragments, (2) immobilization to maintain realignment, and (3) restoration of function of the part. Table 59-5 summarizes the therapeutic management of fractures.

Fracture Reduction

Manipulation or closed reduction. Manipulation is a nonsurgical, manual realignment of bones to their previous anatomic position. Traction and countertraction are manually applied to the bone fragments to restore position, length, and alignment. Closed reduction is usually performed under local or general anesthesia. After reduction or manipulation the injured part is immobilized by casting or traction to maintain alignment until healing occurs.

Open reduction. Open reduction is the correction of bone alignment through a surgical incision. It may include internal fixation of the fracture with the use of wire, screws,

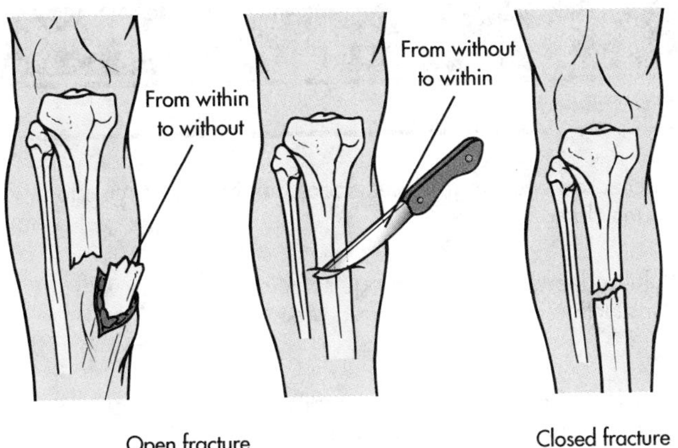

Fig. 59-5 Fracture classification according to communication.

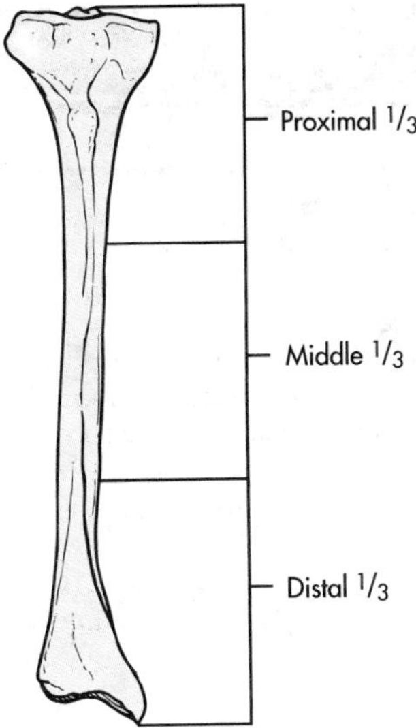

Fig. 59-6 Fracture classification according to location.

pins, plates, intramedullary rods, or nails. The type and location of the fracture, as well as the result of attempted closed reduction by means of traction, influence the decision to use open reduction. The chief disadvantages of this form of treatment are the possibility of infection and the complications associated with anesthesia.

If open reduction and internal fixation are used, early initiation of range of motion of the joint is indicated. Machines that provide continuous passive motion to various joints are now available. Use of such machines can result in prevention of intraarticular adhesions, faster reconstruction of the subchondral bone plate, and possibly better healing of the articular cartilage. If open reduction is used, early ambulation may be initiated in some instances for patients with lower-extremity fractures. Early ambulation decreases the risk of complications related to prolonged immobility.

Traction. Traction devices apply a pulling force on the fractured extremity and result in realignment. The two most common types of traction are *skin traction* and *skeletal traction*. Skin traction is generally used for short-term treatment (48 to 72 hours) until skeletal traction or surgery is possible. Tape, boots, or slings are applied directly to the skin to maintain alignment, assist in reduction, and help diminish muscle spasms in the injured part. The traction weights are usually limited to 5 to 10 pounds (2.3 to 4.5 kg). Skeletal traction, generally in place for longer periods of time, is used to align injured bones and joints. It provides a long-term pull that keeps the injured bones and joints aligned. To establish skeletal traction, the physician inserts a nail, pin, wire, or pair of tongs into the bone, either partially or completely, to align and immobilize the injured body part. The traction weights are usually 5 to 45 pounds (2.3 to 20.4 kg).[7]

When traction is used to treat fractures, the forces are usually exerted on the distal fragment in order to obtain alignment with the proximal fragment. Several types of traction are used for this purpose (see Table 59-6 on p. 1850). Fracture alignment depends on the correct positioning and alignment of the patient while the traction forces remain constant. For extremity traction to be effective, forces must be pulling in the opposite direction (*countertraction*) to prevent the patient from sliding to the end of the bed. Countertraction may be achieved by elevating the end of the bed 8 to 12 inches, which allows the weight of the patient's own body to be used.

Fracture Immobilization

External fixation. External fixation of fractures is achieved by a cast or an external fixator. Casting is a common treatment after closed reduction has been performed. It allows the patient to perform many normal activities of daily living while providing sufficient immobilization to ensure stability. Major cast materials include fiberglass, plaster of Paris, polyurethane, thermoplastic resins, and thermolabile plastic.

Plaster of Paris, after immersion in water, is wrapped and molded around the affected part (see Fig. 59-8 on p. 1852). It is anhydrous calcium sulfate embedded in a gauze roll. The strength of the cast is determined by the number of layers of plaster bandage and the technique of application. As the cast dries, it recrystallizes and hardens. Heat is generated during the drying process. Increased edema from increased circulation may occur as a result of heat produced by the drying cast. After the cast is completely dry, it is strong and firm and can withstand stresses. The plaster is hard within 15 minutes, so the patient can move around without problems. However, it is not strong enough for weightbearing until it is dry (after about 24 to 48 hours).

Thermolabile plastic (Orthoplast) and *thermoplastic resins* (Hexcelite) are molded to fit the torso or extremity after being heated in warm water. Polyurethane, which is formed from polyester and cotton fabric impregnated with a chemical, is water activated by immersing in cool water to start the chemical process. Casts made of this fiberglass tape are frequently used because they are lightweight and relatively waterproof and support earlier mobilization. They are ap-

Table 59-3 Clinical Manifestations of Fracture

Manifestation	Significance
Edema and Swelling	
Disruption of soft tissues or bleeding into surrounding tissues	Unchecked swelling in closed space can occlude circulation and damage nerves.
Pain and Tenderness	
Muscle spasm as result of involuntary reflex action of muscle, direct tissue trauma, increased pressure on sensory nerve, movement of fracture parts	Pain and tenderness encourage splinting of fracture with reduction in motion of injured area.
Muscle Spasm	
Protective response to injury and fracture	Muscle spasms may displace nondisplaced fracture or prevent it from reducing spontaneously.
Deformity	
Abnormal position of bone as result of original forces of injury and action of muscles pulling fragment into abnormal position	Deformity is cardinal sign of fracture; if uncorrected, it may result in problems with bony union and restoration of function of injured part.
Ecchymosis	
Discoloration of skin as result of extravasation of blood in subcutaneous tissues	Ecchymosis usually appears several days after injury and may appear distal to injury. The nurse should reassure patient that process is normal.
Loss of Function	
Disruption of bone, preventing functional use	Fracture must be managed properly to ensure restoration of function.
Crepitation	
Grating or crunching together of bony fragments, producing palpable or audible crunching sensation	Examination of crepitation may increase chance for nonunion if bone ends are allowed to move excessively.

propriate in cases in which severe edema is not present or when multiple cast changes are not anticipated.

An *external fixator* is a metallic device used to compress fracture fragments and to immobilize reduced fragments when the use of a cast or traction is not appropriate. The external gear holds fracture fragments in place, similar to surgically implanted internal devices. The external fixator is attached directly to the bones by percutaneous pins (see Fig. 59-9 on p. 1853). Assessment for pin loosening and infection is critical. Infection signaled by exudate, redness, tenderness, and pain may require removal of the device. An external fixator used to treat fractures with associated soft-tissue trauma facilitates wound care.

External fixator devices can also be used as part of a limb-lengthening process for patients who have a significant leg length discrepancy. The pins connected to these fixators are turned regularly as part of a prescribed regimen.

TYPES OF CASTS (SEE FIG. 59-8). Immobilization of an acute fracture or soft-tissue injury of the upper extremity is frequently accomplished by use of (1) the sugar-tong splint, (2) the short arm cast, or (3) the long arm cast. The *sugar-tong splint* is typically used for acute wrist injuries. Multiple layers of plaster splints are applied to the padded forearm, beginning at the phalangeal joints of the hand and extending up the dorsal aspect of the forearm around the distal humerus and then extending down the volar aspect of the forearm to the distal palmar crease. The splinting material is wrapped with either elastic bandage or bias stocking. The major advantage of the sugar-tong cast is avoidance of the circumferential effects of a nonelastic cylinder.

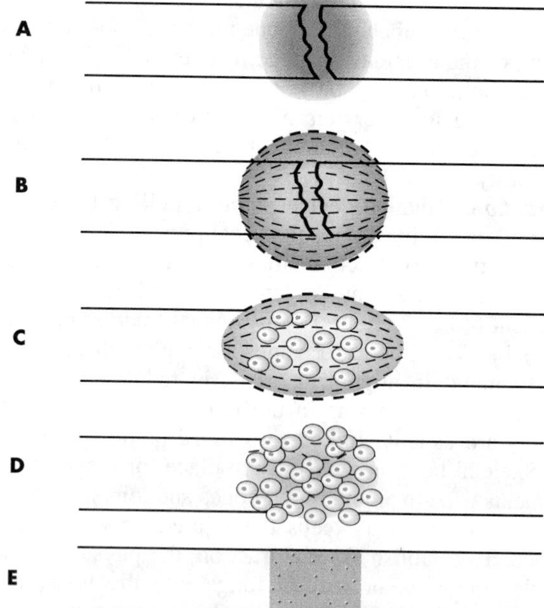

Fig. 59-7 Bone healing (schematic representation). ***A,*** Bleeding at broken ends of the bone with subsequent hematoma formation. ***B,*** Organization of hematoma into fibrous network. ***C,*** Invasion of osteoblasts, lengthening of collagen strands, and deposition of calcium. ***D,*** Callus formation: new bone is built up as osteoclasts destroy dead bone. ***E,*** Remodeling is accomplished as excess callus is reabsorbed and trabecular bone is laid down.

Table 59-4 Complications of Fracture Healing

Problem	Description
Delayed union	Fracture healing progresses more slowly than expected; healing eventually occurs.
Nonunion	Fracture fails to heal properly despite treatment, resulting in fibrous union or pseudoarthrosis.
Malunion	Fracture heals in expected time but in unsatisfactory position, possibly resulting in deformity or dysfunction.
Angulation	Fracture heals in abnormal position in relation to midline of structure (type of malunion).
Pseudoarthrosis	This type of malunion occurs at fracture site in which false joint is formed on shaft of long bones. It is a fracture site that failed to fuse (neoarthrosis). Each bone end is covered with fibrous scar tissue.
Posttraumatic osteoporosis	This condition represents loss of mineral (bone substance) as result of immobilization or disuse.
Refracture	New fracture occurs through original fracture site.
Myositis ossificans	This condition is a response to muscle hemorrhage caused by trauma. The hematoma ossifies. Response may occur in arm, elbow, and thigh.

The *short arm cast* is frequently used for the treatment of stable wrist or metacarpal fractures. An aluminum finger splint can be fabricated into the short arm cast for treatment of phalangeal injuries. The short arm cast is a circular cast extending from the distal palmar area to the proximal forearm. This cast provides wrist immobilization and permits unrestricted elbow motion.

The *long arm cast* is commonly used for stable forearm or elbow fractures and unstable wrist fractures. It is similar to the short arm cast but extends to the proximal humerus, restricting motion in the wrist and elbow. Nursing measures should be directed toward supporting the extremity and reducing the effects of edema by maintaining extremity elevation with a sling. When a sling is used, the nurse must ensure that the axillary region is well padded to prevent skin maceration associated with direct skin-to-skin contact. Placement of the sling should not put undue stress on the neck. Movement of the fingers should be encouraged to enhance the pumping action of veins to decrease edema. The nurse should also encourage the patient to actively move nonimmobilized joints of the upper extremity to prevent stiffness and contractures.

Table 59-5 Therapeutic Management: Fractures

Diagnostic
- History and physical examination
- X-ray examination

Therapeutic

Fracture reduction
- Manipulation
- Open reduction
- Closed reduction
- Traction devices
  - Skin traction
  - Skeletal traction

Fracture immobilization
- External casting or external fixation
- Internal fixation devices
- Maintenance traction

Open fractures
- Surgical debridement
- Tetanus immunization
- Prophylactic antibiotic therapy
- Immobilization

The *body jacket cast* is frequently used for immobilization and support for stable spine injuries of the thoracic or lumbar spine. This cast is applied around the chest and abdomen and extends from above the nipple line to the pubis. After application of the cast, the nurse must assess the patient for the development of a *cast syndrome*. This condition occurs if the body cast is applied too tightly and the cast compresses the superior mesenteric artery against the duodenum. The patient generally complains of abdominal pain, abdominal pressure, nausea, and vomiting. Treatment includes gastric decompression with a nasogastric tube and suction. The cast may have to be removed or split. Nursing assessment also includes observation of respiratory status, bowel and bladder function, and areas of pressure over the bony prominences, especially the iliac crest. During the time required for the cast to dry, the nurse should reposition the patient every 2 to 3 hours to promote even cast drying and to relieve pressure and discomfort.

The *hip spica* cast is commonly used in treating femoral fractures. The purpose of the hip spica cast is to immobilize the affected extremity and the trunk securely. It includes two separate casts joined together: (1) the body jacket and (2) the long leg cast. The location of the femoral fracture will determine whether the unaffected extremity will have to be immobilized to restrict rotation of the pelvis and possible hip motion on the side of the femur fracture. The hip spica cast extends from above the nipple line to the base of the foot (single spica) and may include the opposite extremity up to an area above the knee (spica and a half) or both extremities (double spica). The nurse should assess the patient for the same problems associated with the body jacket cast. During the initial drying stage the patient should not be placed in the prone position because the cast

Table 59-6 Common Types of Traction

Type	Indications	Nursing Implications
Skin		
Buck's	Used for many conditions affecting hip, femur, knee, or back. It is generally used for temporary immobilization and stabilization of fractured hips or fractures of the femoral shaft. It can be unilateral or bilateral.	Assess for nerve and circulatory disturbances caused by circumferential bandages, especially over bony prominences, and for skin necrosis, an allergic reaction to the adhesive material, rotation of the extremity, and constant traction and countertraction forces. 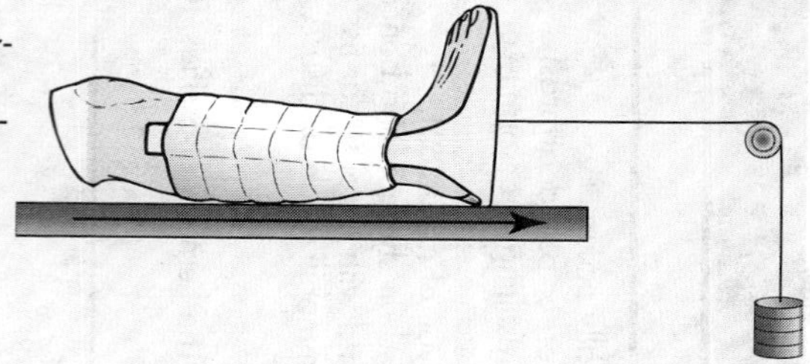
Russell's	Used for fractures of femur, hip, and certain knee problems.	Same as above. Assess knee sling for smoothness and an overly tight edge. Because the arrangement of this traction may vary, be aware of initial set-up and maintain it. 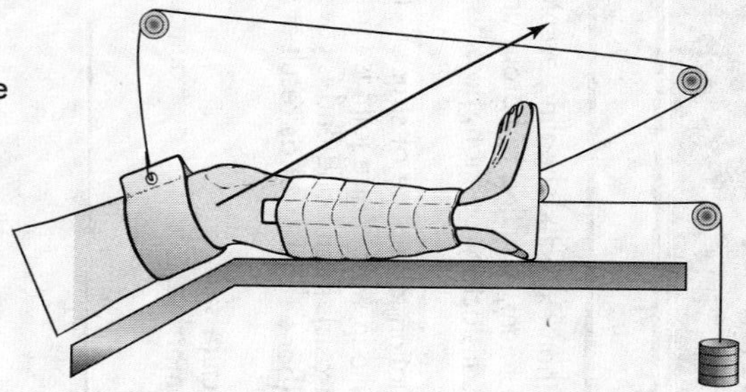
Bryant's	Used for fractures of the femur, fractures in small children, and stabilization of hip joints in children under 2 yr or 30 lb (14 kg) in weight.	Be aware that with traction in place, buttocks should just clear the mattress. Check for undue pressure over the outer head and neck of fibula, dorsum of foot, Achilles tendon, scapulae, and shoulders. Check that bandages or boot has not slipped. Be aware that these are usually removed for skin care and assessment q8hr. 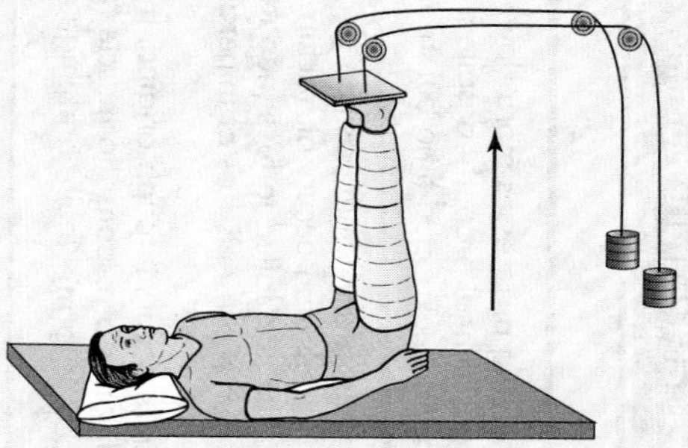
Pelvic	Used for sciatica, muscle spasms (low back), and minor fractures of the lower spine.	Check for security of the pelvic belt. Check frequently for skin irritation over iliac crests. Use measures to prevent skin breakdown. Check and adjust pelvic belt straps so that they are unrestricted and equal in length. Secure the straps with adhesive tape. Use a footboard to prevent foot drop. Maintain the correct angle of pull of the traction. Be aware that the physician orders the type of countertraction. 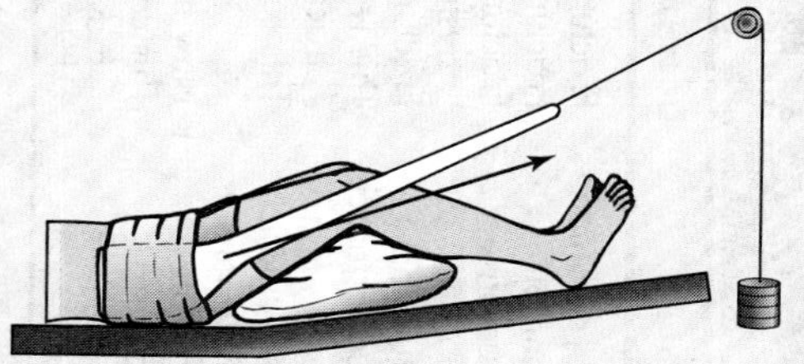

continued

Table 59-6 Common Types of Traction—cont'd

Type	Indications	Nursing Implications
Circumferential		
Head halter	Used for soft-tissue disorders and degenerative disk disease of the cervical spine. It is not commonly used for unstable fractures of the cervical spine.	Assess for alignment with trunk, areas of local pressure under the chin and occipital area, and pain or dysfunction in the temporomandibular joint. 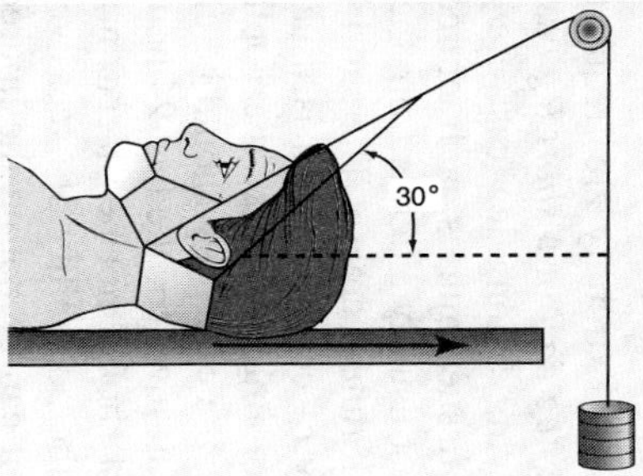
Skeletal		
Overhead arm (90°-90°)	Commonly used for immobilization of fractures and dislocations of the upper arm and shoulder.	Be aware that the shoulder and elbow joint are maintained at 90° angles. 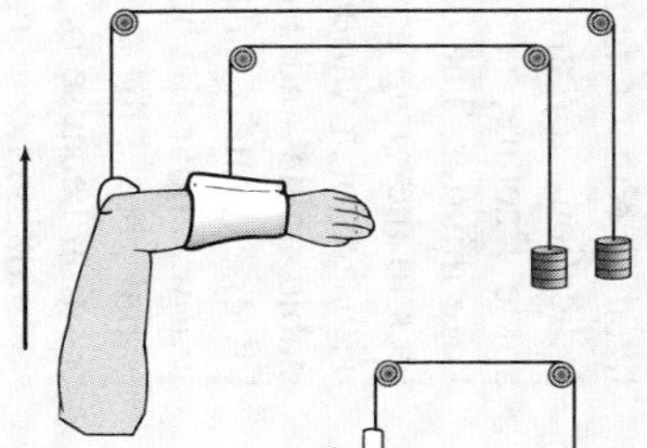
Lateral arm	Commonly used in immobilization of fractures and dislocations of the upper arm and shoulder.	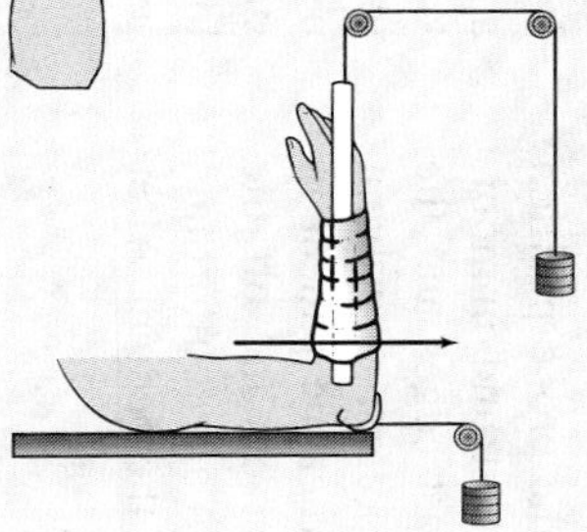
Balanced suspension traction	Used for injury or fracture of the femoral shaft of the femur, acetabulum, hip, lower leg, or any combination of these.	Be aware that this traction uses half-ring Thomas splint *(1)* and Pearson attachment *(2)* and that suspension of the extremity *(A)* and direct skeletal traction *(B)* are applied. Be aware that type allows raising of the buttocks off the bed for bedpan use and skin care without altering the line of traction. Use nursing assessments so that countertraction is maintained (e.g., position patient high in bed so that feet do not press on foot of bed, do not elevate the head of the bed >25° if it causes continual movement toward foot of the bed). Encourage self-help in patient's performance of activities of daily living, movement in bed with help of trapeze, and flexion and extension of affected foot to prevent foot drop. Assess and care for skin of the groin (ischial) area, sacrum, and scapulae. Inspect the pin site and perform pin site care according to hospital policy. 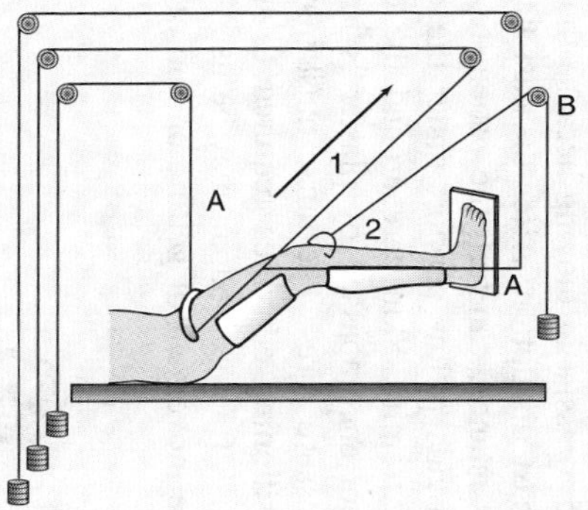

may break. The patient should be slightly turned from side to side and supported with pillows. When the patient is repositioned, the support bar joining the thighs must never be used to assist in moving because the bar can break and cause cast disruption. After the cast has dried, the nurse, with assistance, can turn the patient to the prone position and provide pillow support under the chest and immobilized extremity. Skin care around the cast edges and the areas not encompassed by plaster is important to prevent any pressure sores. The nurse must instruct the patient in the positioning activities required to get on and off the bedpan. A fracture bedpan may be used to aid comfort and ease the movement of getting on and off the bedpan. After

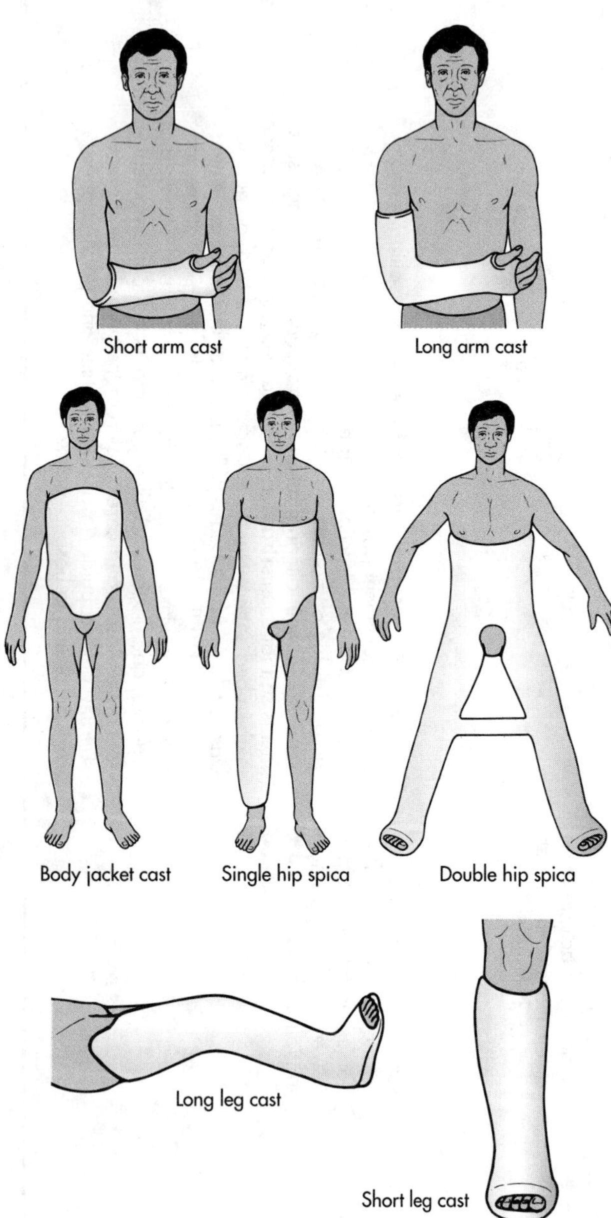

Fig. 59-8 Common casts used in treatment of disorders of the musculoskeletal system.

the hip spica cast has dried sufficiently, the patient is instructed in ambulation techniques by the physical therapist.

Injuries to the lower extremity are frequently immobilized by either a *long leg cast* or a *short leg cast*. The usual indications for applying a long leg cast are an unstable ankle fracture, soft-tissue injuries, a fractured tibia, and knee injuries. The cast usually extends from the base of the toes to the groin and gluteal crease. The short leg cast can be used for a variety of conditions but is usually used for stable ankle and foot injuries. After the application of a lower-extremity cast, the extremity should be elevated with pillows above the heart level for the first 24 hours. After the initial phase, the cast should not be placed in a dependent position because of the possibility of excessive edema.

Initially, no weight can be put on the injured extremity. Later, a walking heel or cast shoe may be added to the cast if the patient will be allowed to bear weight and walk on the affected leg. The nurse should observe for signs of pressure, especially in the regions of the fibular head and malleoli.

Internal fixation. Internal fixation devices are surgically inserted at the time of realignment. Examples of internal fixation devices include pins, plates, and screws. They are biologically inert devices used to realign and maintain bony fragments. Proper alignment is evaluated by x-ray studies at regular intervals.

Maintenance traction. Maintenance traction is initiation or continuation of traction and countertraction. A continuous pulling force can be applied directly to bone with wires and pins (*skeletal traction*), or it can be applied indirectly by weights that are attached to the skin with adhesive straps or boots (*skin traction*). Skin traction is usually applied directly to the extremity by adhesive material that is wrapped circumferentially with a bandage or a special garment that is attached to a rope with a weight. Skin traction is applied for a short time and usually consists of not more than 7 to 10 pounds (3.2 to 4.5 kg) of traction weight because of skin intolerance to pressure. Skeletal traction is usually indicated when the traction forces are expected to exceed 10 pounds (4.5 kg) or when traction will be used for a long time. Use of too much weight to maintain traction can result in delayed union or nonunion. The major disadvantages of skeletal traction are infection in the area of bone where the skeletal pin has been inserted and the consequences of prolonged immobility necessitated by skeletal traction.

Open fracture. Tetanus prevention should be ensured with use of tetanus toxoid or tetanus antitoxin for a patient with an open fracture who has not been immunized. A broad-spectrum antibiotic is usually used prophylactically. A decision on whether to close the wound or leave it open is based on the degree of contamination and the time elapsed before initiation of treatment. Infection is the greatest risk of an open fracture.

The overall long-term goal of treatment is the correction of the fracture and return of the patient to the preinjury level of functioning as soon as possible. Discharge planning should include referral to the appropriate human service agency for assistance in the transition to the home environment.

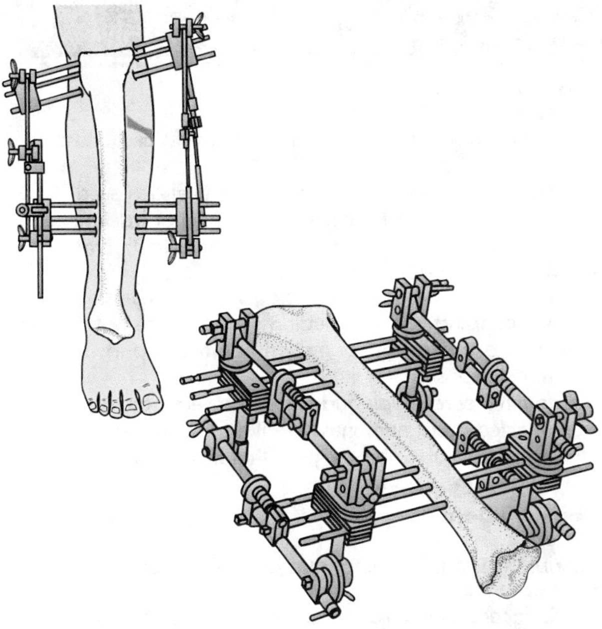

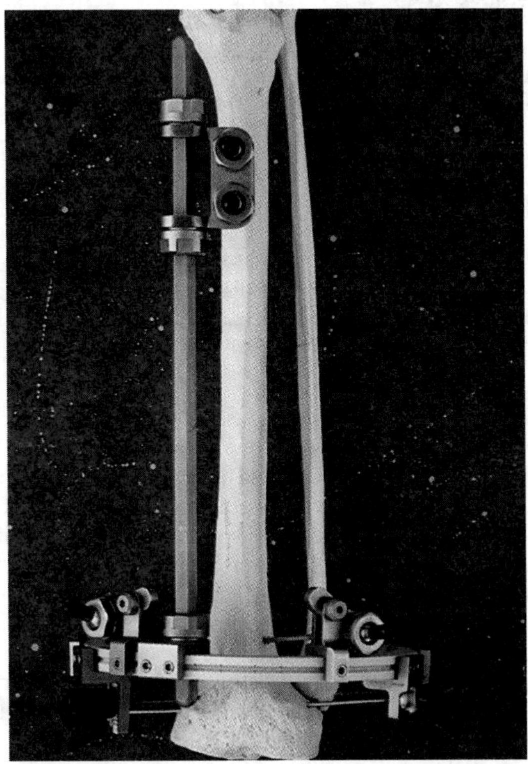

Fig. 59-9 External fixator attached to bones of lower extremity. Note open wound with external fixator in place.

Pharmacologic Management

Patients with fractures often experience varying degrees of pain associated with muscle spasms. These spasms are caused by involuntary reflexes that result from the muscle injury. Medications such as muscle relaxants are often prescribed for relief of pain associated with muscle spasms.

Medications used primarily as muscle relaxants include carisoprodol (Rela, Soma), chlorphenesin carbamate (Maolate), chlorzoxazone (Paraflex), dantrolene sodium (Dantrium), cyclobenzaprine (Flexeril), metaxalone (Skelaxin), methocarbamol (Robaxin), mephenesin (Atensin), orphenadrine (Disipal), and stryamate (Sinaxar). Medications that combine sedative action with muscle relaxant properties include chlormezanone (Trancopal), diazepam (Valium), meprobamate (Equanil, Miltown), and tybamate (Solacen, Tybatran).

Common side effects associated with muscle relaxants are drowsiness, lassitude, headache, weakness, fatigue, blurred vision, ataxia, and gastrointestinal upset. Hypersensitivity reactions include skin rash and pruritus. Ingestion of large doses of muscle relaxants may cause hypotension, tachycardia, or respiratory depression. The possible habituating effects associated with long-term use and the potential for abuse must be carefully considered.

Some physicians do not advocate the use of muscle relaxants for relief of muscle spasms. Their rationale is that the reflex spasm will continue as long as the precipitating pain persists. If the pain is controlled by use of appropriate analgesia, the muscle spasms will cease.

Nutritional Management

Proper nutrition is an essential component of the reparative process in injured tissue. An adequate energy source is needed to promote muscle strength and tone, build endurance, and enhance ambulation and gait-training skills. The patient's dietary requirements must include ample protein (e.g., 1 g per kilogram of body weight), vitamins (especially B and C), and calcium to ensure optimal soft-tissue and bone healing. Low serum protein levels and vitamin C deficiencies interfere with tissue healing. Immobility and callus formation increase calcium needs. Three well-balanced meals a day usually provide the necessary nutrients. The well-balanced meal should be supplemented by a fluid intake of 2000 to 3000 ml per day to promote optimal bladder and bowel function. Adequate fluid and a high-fiber diet will prevent constipation associated with immobility. If immobilized in a body jacket or hip spica bandage, the patient should be instructed not to overeat to avoid abdominal pressure and cramping.

NURSING MANAGEMENT

FRACTURES

Nursing Assessment

A brief history of the accident, mechanism of injury, and the position in which the victim was found can be obtained from the patient or witnesses. As soon as possible, the patient should be transported to an emergency department, where thorough assessment and treatment can be initiated

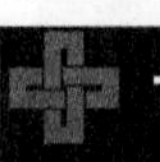

Table 59-7 Emergency Management: Fractured Extremity

Possible Etiologies

Falls, direct blows, forced flexion or hyperextension, twisting forces, pathologic conditions, violent muscle contractions (seizures)

Possible Assessment Findings

Deformity or unnatural position of affected limb
Swelling and discoloration (ecchymosis)
Muscle spasm
Tenderness and pain
Loss of use
Numbness, tingling, loss of distal pulses
Grating and crepitus
Open wound over injured site, exposure of bone

Mangement

- Treat any life-threatening injury.
- Assess airway, breathing, and circulation.
- Assess patient for any bleeding sites.
- Control external bleeding with sterile pressure dressing.
- Immobilize joints above and below fracture site by splinting extremity.
- Check pulses distal to injury before and after splinting.
- Elevate injured limb (if possible).
- *Do not* attempt to straighten fractured or dislocated joints.
- *Do not* manipulate protruding bone ends.
- Apply ice packs to affected area.
- Anticipate need for x-rays.
- Monitor for signs and symptoms of compartment syndrome (e.g., excessive pain with passive stretch) and fat embolism (dyspnea, chest pain).

Table 59-8 Nursing Assessment: Fracture

Subjective Data

Important health information

Past health history: Long-term repetitive forces (cause of stress fracture)
Medications: Use of analgesics and relief achieved
Surgery and other treatments: Treatment of fracture before emergency department or hospital treatment

Functional health patterns

Health perception–health management: Circumstances surrounding injury, including sudden force or trauma
Activity-exercise: Loss of motion of affected part; muscle spasms
Cognitive-perceptual: Sudden and severe pain in affected area; numbness, tingling, loss of sensation distal to injury; chronic pain that increases with activity (in stress fracture)

Objective Data

General

Apprehension, bleeding, guarding of injured site

Integumentary

Skin lacerations, color changes, bleeding into soft tissues (ecchymosis)

Cardiovascular

Reduced or absent pulse distal to injury, edema, delayed capillary refill, pallor, hematoma

Musculoskeletal

Restricted or lost function of affected part, local deformities, abnormal angulation, shortening, rotation, crepitation, muscle weakness

Neurologic

Paresthesias, decreased sensation

Possible findings

Location and extent of fractures on x-ray, bone scans, tomograms, CT or MRI scans

CT, Computed tomography; *MRI,* magnetic resonance imaging.

(Table 59-7). Subjective and objective data that should be obtained from an individual with a fracture are presented in Table 59-8.

Special emphasis must be focused on the region distal to the site of injury. The involved extremity should be compared with the uninvolved extremity. Clinical findings must be documented before fracture treatment is initiated to avoid doubts about whether a problem discovered later was missed during the original examination or was caused by the treatment. Misdiagnosis may result from failure to consider clinical procedures as the cause of a patient's complaints.

Neurovascular Assessment. Many musculoskeletal injuries have the potential of causing neurovascular injuries. Such events as the original trauma, application of a cast or constrictive dressing, or poor positioning can cause nerve or vascular damage, usually distal to the injury. One method to use for a neurovascular assessment is to consider the five *P*'s: pain, pulses, paresthesia, pallor, and paralysis.[8]

The nurse should carefully assess the location, quality, and intensity of the *pain* of the affected extremity. Pain unrelieved by medication could be an early sign of compartment syndrome. The *pulses* on both the unaffected and injured extremity should be compared to identify differences in rate or quality. A diminished or absent pulse distal to the injury can indicate vascular insufficiency.

Paresthesia (subjective sensation experienced as numbness or tingling) can be evaluated by comparing the patient's sensations above and below the injury. Comparison of the sensations felt between the injured and uninjured extremity should also be made. Changes in sensation such as decreased sensation, hypersensation, numbness, tingling, or loss of sensation may be reported by the patient.

Next, color (*pallor*) and temperature changes in the area of nerve distribution of the affected extremity should be assessed. Pallor or a cold extremity below the injury could indicate arterial insufficiency. A warm, bluish extremity could indicate venous stasis. Capillary refill should also be checked. A compressed nailbed should return to its original color within 3 seconds. Comparisons should be made between the injured and uninjured extremities.

The final assessment of a neurovascular assessment is to check for *paralysis*. Range of motion and strength can be compared between the two extremities. Reduced motion or strength in the injured extremity may indicate problems with the motor portion of the involved nerves.

Nursing Diagnoses

Nursing diagnoses are determined when the problem and etiologic factors are supported by clinical data. Nursing diagnoses related to fractures include, but are not limited to, those presented in the nursing care plan for the patient with a fracture on p. 1856.

Planning

The overall goals are that the patient with a fracture will (1) have no associated complications, (2) obtain satisfactory pain relief, and (3) achieve maximal rehabilitation potential.

Nursing Implementation

Health Promotion and Maintenance. The public should be educated to take appropriate safety precautions to prevent injuries while at home, at work, when driving, or when participating in sports. The nurse should be a vocal advocate for personal actions known to reduce injuries, such as regular use of seat belts, driving within posted speed limits, and not combining drinking and driving.

Acute Intervention. The patient with a fracture may be treated in an emergency department or physician's office and released to home care, or the patient may require hospitalization. (Specific nursing measures depend on the type of treatment used and the setting in which the patient is treated.)

Preoperative management. If surgical intervention is required to treat the fracture, the patient will need preoperative preparation. In addition to the usual preoperative nursing measures (see Chapter 14), the nurse should inform patients of the type of immobilization device that will be used and the expected activity limitations. The patient must be assured that all needs will be met by the nursing staff until the patient can again meet his or her own needs. Assurance that pain medication will be available if needed is often beneficial.

Proper skin preparation is an important part of preoperative preparation. The protocol for skin preparation varies among agencies and may be the responsibility of the nurse. The aim of skin preparation is to clean the skin and remove debris and hair to reduce the possibility of infection. Careful attention to this preoperative treatment can influence the postoperative course.

Postoperative management. In general, postoperative nursing care and management are directed toward monitoring vital signs and applying the general principles of postoperative nursing care (see Chapter 16). Frequent neurovascular assessments of the affected extremity are necessary to detect subtle changes. Any limitations of movement or activity related to turning, positioning, and extremity support should be monitored closely. Pain and discomfort can be minimized through proper alignment and positioning. Dressings or casts should be carefully observed for any overt signs of bleeding or drainage. Increases in bleeding can be monitored by drawing a circle on the cast around an area of drainage, noting the date and time. A significant increase in size of the drainage area should be reported. If a wound-drainage system is in place, the patency of the system and the volume of drainage should be assessed at least once each shift. Whenever the contents of a drainage system are measured or emptied, the nurse should use sterile technique to avoid contamination. Additional nursing responsibilities depend on the type of immobilization used. A blood salvage and reinfusion system that allows for recovery and reinfusion of the patient's own blood may be used. The blood is retrieved from a joint space or cavity and the patient receives this blood in the form of an autotransfusion.[9]

Cast care. Immediately after a cast is applied, there is a short period of exothermic reaction, during which heat is released from the plaster. The patient should be alerted to this occurrence because it can increase edema. Evaporation of water and dissipation of heat from the cast can be hastened by exposing the cast to room air. A fresh cast should never be covered with a blanket because air cannot circulate and heat builds up in the cast. The patient should be turned every 2 hours to reduce continuous pressure and promote even drying of the cast. The drying process is usually complete within 24 to 72 hours. During the drying period the cast should not be subjected to any wetness, soiling, or abnormal stresses that can cause weakening or a break in the cast. It should be carefully handled by the palms of the hands rather than with the fingertips to avoid indentations that will dry and become potential pressure areas. Once the cast is thoroughly dry, the edges may have to be finished if the cast is rough to avoid skin irritation from rough spots (Fig. 59-10).

Regardless of the type of material of which it is made, a cast can interfere with circulation and nerve function from being applied too tightly or because of excessive edema after application. Thus frequent neurovascular assessments of the immobilized extremity are critical. The patient should be educated about signs of cast complication so that they can be reported promptly. Elevation of the extremity above the level of the heart to promote venous return and applications of ice to control or prevent edema are measures frequently used during the initial phase of immobilization. The nurse should instruct the patient to exercise joints above and below the cast. Pulling out cast padding and scratching or placing foreign objects inside the cast is forbidden because it predisposes the patient to skin breakdown and infection within the cast.

If the patient is immobilized as a result of the fracture, the nurse must plan care to prevent the occurrence of constipation and renal calculi. Constipation can be prevented by maintenance of a high fluid intake and a diet high in bulk and roughage. If these measures are not effective in maintaining the patient's normal bowel pattern, stool softeners, laxatives, or suppositories may be necessary. Maintaining a regular time for elimination despite bed rest is effective in promoting regularity.

Renal calculi can develop as a result of bone demineralization caused by immobilization. The resulting hypercal-

NURSING CARE PLAN Patient with a Fracture

Planning: Outcome Criteria	Nursing Interventions and Rationales
➤ **NURSING DIAGNOSIS**	Risk for peripheral neurovascular dysfunction *related to* nerve compression
Have normal neurovascular status on examination.	Assess for signs and symptoms of peripheral neurovascular dysfunction such as pain in affected extremity that is unrelieved by medication, paresthesias, pallor, diminished pulse *to ensure early recognition and intervention.* Elevate extremity above heart level *to reduce edema by promoting return circulation to heart.* Apply ice compresses as ordered *because ice reduces edema by constriction and provides comfort by localized anesthetic effects.* Assess nerve and vascular status of affected extremity q15-30 min initially then q2hr *to ensure early identification if problem develops.* Instruct patient to notify nurse if pain is unrelieved by medication or unusual sensations in affected extremity are experienced *because a neurovascular dysfunction may be present.* Notify physician immediately if patient complains of increasing pain that is unrelieved by medication *because this may indicate neurovascular impairment, which can result in paralysis if unrelieved.*
➤ **NURSING DIAGNOSIS**	Pain *related to* edema, movement of bone fragments and muscle spasms *as manifested by* pain descriptors, guarding; altered time perception; behaviors indicative of pain, such as moaning, crying, restlessness, altered muscle tone, autonomic responses, decreased activity
Verbalize tolerable or no pain; be satisfied with plan for pain relief.	Gently and correctly position fractured extremity *to minimize pain and prevent bone displacement.* Assess site for constriction or pressure caused by immobilization apparatus *to prevent skin or neurovascular injury.* Give patient analgesics or muscle relaxants as indicated *to relieve pain and promote muscle relaxation.* Elevate and support affected extremity *to reduce edema and promote comfort.*
➤ **NURSING DIAGNOSIS**	Risk for infection *related to* disruption of skin integrity and presence of environmental pathogens secondary to open fracture or external fixation pins
Have no evidence of wound infection.	Assess fracture or pin insertion points for blistering, discoloration, and frothy or foul-smelling drainage *as indicators of infection.* Use sterile technique when providing pin or wound care or when performing dressing change *to prevent cross-contamination and possible introduction of infection.* Obtain culture of wound if infection is suspected *to identify infective organism.* Administer antibiotics as ordered *to provide prophylaxis or treatment of diagnosed infection.* Monitor temperature q2hr *because fever may reflect developing sepsis.* Isolate patient *to prevent dissemination of pathogen or cross-contamination of wound, if indicated.*
➤ **NURSING DIAGNOSIS**	Activity intolerance *related to* prolonged immobility *as manifested by* verbal reports of fatigue or weakness, abnormal physiologic responses to activity
Have normal physiologic responses to activity; report no problems associated with activity.	Encourage active range-of-motion exercise of joints not immobilized *to maintain muscle strength and joint range of motion.* Perform resistance exercises of unaffected extremities *to put stress on bones to reduce demineralization.* Plan rest periods between activities *to allow a period of recuperation.* Encourage patient participation in activities of daily living and exercises *to foster independence, increase activity, and decrease fatigue.* Monitor vital signs during activity *to evaluate patient's response and guide planning of rest periods.*

continued

cemia causes a rise in urine pH and stone formation resulting from the precipitation of calcium. Unless contraindicated, a fluid intake of 2100 to 2800 ml per day is recommended. Cranberry juice is often recommended to acidify the urine and discourage the development of calcium stones.

Rapid deconditioning of the circulatory system can occur as a result of bed rest. Unless contraindicated, these effects can be diminished by permitting the patient to sit on the side of the bed, allowing the patient's lower limbs to dangle over the bedside, and by performing standing transfers. When the patient is allowed to increase activity,

NURSING CARE PLAN Patient with a Fracture—cont'd

Planning: Outcome Criteria	Nursing Interventions and Rationales
➤ **NURSING DIAGNOSIS** Risk for impaired skin integrity *related to* immobility and presence of cast	
Have no evidence of skin breakdown.	Examine potential pressure areas regularly *to provide data on condition of skin.* Petal cast edges *to prevent skin abrasion.* Turn patient q2hr *to reduce pressure over bony prominences.* Keep bed free of wrinkles and crumbs *to reduce risk of skin abrasions, tears, and irritation.* Assess exposed skin areas of traction sites for signs of infection or irritation *because improper positioning of traction devices can cause localized skin breakdown.* Seek medical attention if cast becomes loose *to prevent rotation, flexion, or skin abrasion.* Instruct patient not to insert items into cast such as hangers or forks *because these may cause tissue injury.*
➤ **NURSING DIAGNOSIS:** Ineffective management of therapeutic regimen *related to* lack of knowledge regarding muscle atrophy, exercise program, and cast care *as manifested by* questioning of long-term effect of casting and cast care, activity restrictions	
Have minimal loss of muscle bulk of affected extremity; verbalize confidence in ability to follow prescribed discharge plan; demonstrate mobility with assistive device.	Instruct patient on home care measures related to exercise, cast care, and prevention of complications *so patient can carry out prescribed discharge plan.* Plan for follow-up care with physician *to evaluate correct alignment and healing of fracture.* Explain factors that contribute to atrophy; emphasize relationship of activity to muscle atrophy *so patient will exercise involved extremity to maximum allowed and will not be alarmed at appearance of extremity when cast is removed.* Teach gait-training principles to patient (non–weight-bearing gait status unless otherwise ordered by physician): sit with feet over edge of bed, stand with no weight on affected extremity, measure and adjust crutches *to promote mobility according to patient's abilities.* Start gait training on parallel bars *because this increases patient's confidence.* Ensure that gait is compatible with weight-bearing status *to prevent malalignment.* Cooperate with physical therapist regarding exercise and gait-training *to reinforce plan and to provide unified approach to patient.* Explain importance of activity of affected extremity as tolerated *to minimize muscle atrophy and loss of function.* Reinforce exercise program as prescribed by physician *so patient receives encouragement to continue.*

COLLABORATIVE PROBLEMS

Nursing Goals	Nursing Interventions and Rationales
➤ **POTENTIAL COMPLICATION** Fat embolism *related to* fracture of a long bone	
Monitor for embolic phenomena, report abnormal findings, and carry out appropriate medical and nursing interventions.	Monitor for changes in mental status caused by hypoxemia; symptoms of acute respiratory distress syndrome, such as chest pain, tachypnea, cyanosis, dyspnea, apprehension, tachycardia, and decreased PaO_2; and petechiae on upper trunk and axillae *to enable prompt identification and reporting to physician.* Immobilize long bone fractures *to reduce the occurrence of fat embolism.* Be alert to patient's verbalization of a feeling of impending doom *because this is frequently a premonitory sign.* Provide emergency respiratory support as needed *to prevent respiratory arrest.*

careful evaluation should be made to assess for orthostatic hypotension.

Chronic and Home Management. Because many fractures are casted in an outpatient setting, the patient often requires only a short hospitalization or none at all. Therefore, patient education is an important nursing responsibility to prevent complications. In addition to specific instructions for cast care and recognition of complications, the nurse should encourage the patient to contact the clinic or care provider should questions arise. Table 59-9 summarizes patient instructions for cast care. The nurse should validate the patient's understanding of these instructions before discharge from the clinic or hospital.

Traction. The nurse is responsible for patient comfort and safety while traction is used and for ensuring proper functioning of the traction equipment. The equipment should be regularly examined for frayed ropes, loose knots, ropes out of the groove of the pulley, pulley clamps not

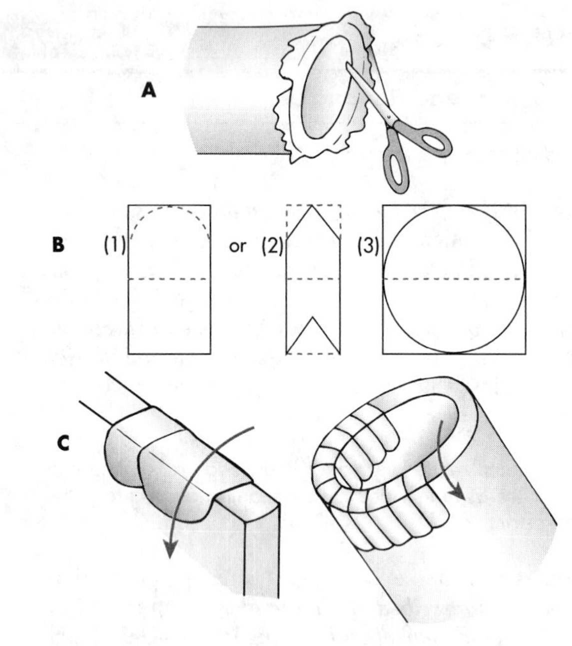

A

B (1) or (2) (3)

C

Fig. 59-10 Finishing edges of cast with waterproof adhesive strips. ***A,*** The cast must be thoroughly dry. The nurse trims the excess sheet wadding and stretches the stockinette over the cast edge (when possible). ***B,*** Several strips (petals) of waterproof adhesive tape (2-inch-wide strips for wide areas and 1-inch-wide strips for small areas, each 1 inch long) are made in advance. ***C,*** The uncut end of the tape is placed beneath the cast edge. Each succeeding petal overlaps the previous one by ½ inch, ensuring a smooth cast edge. A family member can help, and this can be done at home as needed.

Table 59-9 Patient Instructions for Cast Care

Do Not
- Get cast wet*
- Remove any padding
- Insert any foreign object inside cast
- Bear weight on new cast for 48 hr
- Cover cast with plastic for prolonged periods

Do
- Apply ice directly over fracture site for first 24 hr (avoid getting cast wet by keeping ice in plastic bag and protecting cast with cloth)
- Check with physician before getting cast wet
- Dry cast thoroughly after exposure to water†
  - Blot dry with towel
  - Use hair dryer on low setting until cast is thoroughly dry
- Elevate extremity above level of heart for first 48 hr
- Move joints above and below cast regularly
- Report signs of possible problems to health care provider
  - Increasing pain
  - Swelling associated with pain and discoloration of toes or fingers
  - Pain during motion
  - Burning or tingling under cast
- Keep appointment to have fracture and cast checked

*Plaster of Paris cast.
†Synthetic cast.

fastened firmly to the bed frame, and weights not hanging freely.

When slings are used with traction, the nurse should inspect the skin area that is exposed in and near the sling regularly. Pressure over a bony prominence or a wrinkled area can impair blood flow, causing injury to the peripheral neurovascular structures. Skeletal traction pin sites must be observed for signs of infection. Pin-site care varies according to the preference of the physician but usually includes regular removal of exudate with peroxide, rinsing pin sites with sterile saline, drying of the area with sterile gauze, and application of antibiotic ointment. External rotation of the hip can occur when skin traction is used on the lower extremity. The nurse can correct this position by placing a pillow, sandbag, or rolled-up drawsheet along the outer aspect of the femur. Whenever traction is used, the nurse should ensure that the patient's body is always correctly aligned. Generally the patient should be in the center of the bed in a supine position. Misalignment can result in increased pain, nonunion, or malunion.

To offset some of the problems associated with prolonged immobility, the nurse should discuss specific patient activity with the physician. If exercise is permitted, the nurse should encourage participation by the patient in a simple exercise regimen within activity restrictions. Activities that the patient should participate in include frequent position changes, range-of-motion exercises of unaffected joints, deep-breathing exercises, isometric exercises, and use of the trapeze bar (if permitted) to raise oneself off the bed for linen changes and use of the bedpan. These activities should be performed several times each day.

Active exercises that move joints through the range of motion are the preferred activity, if allowed. Frequent exercise of the trunk and extremities is an excellent stimulus to deep breathing.

Rehabilitation Management of Fractures

Psychosocial problems. Short-range rehabilitative goals are directed toward the transition from dependence to independence in performing simple activities of daily living and preserving or increasing strength and endurance. Long-range rehabilitative goals are aimed at preventing problems associated with musculoskeletal injury (Table 59-10). An important part of nursing care during the rehabilitative phase is assisting the patient to adjust to any problems caused by the injury (e.g., separation from family, financial impact of medical care, loss of income from inability to work). The nurse must exhibit gentleness, support, and encouragement and should actively listen to the patient's fears.

Ambulation. The physical therapist often assumes primary responsibility for directing the patient during the strengthening phase of care. The nurse must know the overall goals of physical therapy in relation to the patient's

Table 59-10 Problems Associated with Injury of the Musculoskeletal System

Problem	Description	Nursing Considerations
Muscle atrophy	Decreased muscle mass normally occurs as a result of disuse following prolonged immobilization.	An isometric muscle-strengthening exercise regimen within the confines of the immobilization device assists in reducing the amount of atrophy. Muscle atrophy interferes with and prolongs the rehabilitation process.
Contracture	Caused by improper support and positioning of a joint. This results from an imbalance of muscle or ligament, which adaptively adjusts to a shortened position in the region of a joint.	This condition can be prevented by frequent position change, correct body alignment, and active-passive range-of-motion exercises several times a day. Contracture of a joint immobilized for a long time with a cast is common. Intervention requires gradual and progressive stretching of the muscles or ligaments in the region of the joint.
Foot drop	Plantar-flexed position of the foot (foot drop) occurs when the Achilles tendon in the foot shortens because it has been allowed to assume an unsupported position. This may signify damage to the peroneal nerve.	Nursing management of the patient with long-term injuries must include preventive measures by supporting the foot in dorsiflexion. Once foot drop has developed, ambulation and gait training may be significantly hindered.
Pain	Frequently associated with fractures, edema, and muscle spasm; pain varies in intensity from mild to severe and is usually described as aching, dull, burning, throbbing, sharp, or deep.	Important causal factors of pain include incorrect positioning and alignment of the extremity, incorrect support of the extremity, sudden movement of the extremity, and immobilization device that is applied too tightly or in an incorrect position, constrictive dressings, motion occurring at the fracture site, and psychosocial factors. Pain is a valuable assessment parameter, and the underlying causes should be determined so that corrective nursing action can be taken before analgesics are administered.
Muscle spasms	Caused by involuntary muscle contraction after fracture and may last as long as several weeks. Pain associated with muscle spasms is often intense. The duration varies from several seconds to several minutes.	Nursing measures to reduce the intensity of the muscle spasms are similar to the corrective actions for pain control. The area involved in muscle spasms should not be massaged.

abilities, needs, and tolerance. Mobility training and instruction in the use of assistive aids constitute one of the major areas of responsibility of the physical therapist. The patient with lower-extremity dysfunction is usually started in mobility training when able to sit in bed and dangle the feet over the side. This activity should be done two or three times per day for 10 to 15 minutes, with the nurse assisting as necessary. As endurance increases, the patient is instructed in the techniques of transferring from bed to chair. Progressive ambulation is usually started with parallel bars and progresses to ambulatory assistive devices. When the patient begins to ambulate, the nurse must know the weight bearing allowed for the affected extremity and the correct technique if the patient is using an assistive device. There are different degrees of weight-bearing ambulation: (1) non–weight-bearing ambulation, (2) partial–weight-bearing ambulation, and (3) full–weight-bearing ambulation.

Assistive devices. Devices for ambulation range from a cane, which can relieve up to 40% of the weight normally borne by a lower limb, to a walker or crutches, which allow complete non–weight-bearing ambulation. The decision about which device is appropriate for a patient involves weighing the need for maximum stability and safety versus maneuverability, which is required in small spaces such as bathrooms and buses. The decision is made more easily by discussing with patients the requirements of their lifestyles and determining the device with which each patient feels most secure and independent.

The technique for using assistive devices varies. The involved limb is usually advanced at the same time or immediately after the advance of the device. The uninvolved limb is advanced last. In almost all cases, canes are held in the hand opposite the involved extremity.

The common gait patterns with assistive devices are as follows:

- *Two-point gait:* crutch on one side advances simultaneously with the opposite foot; also used with cane ambulation

- *Four-point gait:* slower version of the two-point gait; each "point" is advanced separately
- *Swing-to gait:* both crutches are advanced together, followed by the lifting of both lower limbs to the same place; also used with walkers.
- *Swing-through gait:* similar to the swing-to gait, but the patient swings body past the crutches.

A belt can be placed around the patient's waist to provide stability during the learning stages. The nurse should discourage the patient from reaching for furniture or relying on another person for support. When there is inadequate upper-limb strength or poorly fitted crutches, the patient bears weight at the axilla rather than at the hands, endangering the neurovascular bundle that passes across the axilla. If verbal coaching does not correct the problem, the patient should be kept from further ambulation until strength is adequate.

The patient who must ambulate without weight bearing requires sufficient upper-limb strength to lift the patient's own weight at each step. Because the muscles of the shoulder girdle are not accustomed to this work, they require vigorous and diligent training in preparation for this task. Push-ups, pull-ups using the overhead trapeze bar, and lifting weights develop the triceps and biceps. Straight leg raises and quadriceps-setting exercises strengthen the quadriceps.

Counseling and referrals. During the rehabilitative process the patient's family assumes an important role in the provision and follow-through of long-term care plans. The family must be instructed in the techniques of strength and endurance exercises, assistance with mobility training, and promoting activities that enhance the quality of daily living. Sexual counseling should be included in discharge planning. Unless the nurse has specific preparation for sexual health counseling, the nurse should remember that wrong answers may be more harmful than no answers. For referral purposes the nurse must know whether sexual activity is compatible with the degree of injury, whether any restrictions are imposed, and whether any immobilization or support devices are necessary.

Complications

The majority of fractures heal without complications. If death occurs after a fracture, it is usually the result of damage to underlying organs and soft tissue or of certain complications of the fracture. Complications of fractures may be either direct or indirect. Direct complications include problems with bone union, avascular necrosis, and bone infection. Indirect complications of fractures are associated with blood vessel and nerve damage resulting in conditions such as compartment syndrome, venous thrombosis, fat embolism, and traumatic or hypovolemic shock. Although most musculoskeletal injuries are not life threatening, open fractures or fractures accompanied by severe blood loss and fractures that damage vital organs are medical emergencies requiring immediate attention.

Infection. Open fractures and soft-tissue injuries have a high incidence of infection. An open fracture usually results from the impact of severe external forces. The soft-tissue injury often has more serious consequences than the fracture. Devitalized and contaminated tissue is an ideal medium for many common pathogens, including gas-forming bacilli. Treatment of infections is costly in terms of extended nursing and medical care and treatment and loss of patient income. Infection may be present for a long time.

Therapeutic management. Open fractures require surgical intervention. The wound is cleaned by extensive irrigation, usually with sterile normal saline, and any gross contaminants are mechanically removed. Contused, contaminated, and devitalized tissue such as muscle, subcutaneous fat, skin, and fragments of bone are surgically excised (*debridement*). The extent of the soft-tissue damage determines whether the wound will be closed at the time of surgery, whether closed suction drainage will be used, and whether skin grafting will be necessary. Depending on the location and extent of the fracture, reduction may be maintained by a cast or by traction. During surgery the open wound may be irrigated with antibiotic solution. During the postoperative phase the patient may have antibiotics administered intravenously, intramuscularly, or orally, usually for 7 to 10 days. Antibiotics, in conjunction with aggressive surgical management, have greatly reduced the occurrence of infection.

Compartment Syndrome. Compartment syndrome is the compression of structures within closed compartments of the upper and lower extremities formed by fascial walls. The closed compartment may be created by an externally applied circumferential dressing, splint, or cast on the patient's skin or fascia.[10] Normally there is some increase in edema as a result of soft-tissue injury in the general region of the injury. If edema continues, there may be an increase of pressure within the closed spaces of the tissue compartments formed by the nonelastic fascia. This can create sufficient pressure to obstruct venous circulation and cause arterial occlusion, resulting in inadequate circulation to the extremity or ischemia. As ischemia continues, muscle and nerve cells are destroyed and fibrotic tissue replaces the healthy tissue. Contracture and loss of function can occur. Untreated compartment syndrome can result in permanent hyperesthesia and motor weakness.[11]

Compartment syndrome is associated with fractures or extensive soft-tissue damage in an extremity. The forearm or lower leg are the most common sites of compartment syndrome. Fractures of the distal humerus and proximal tibia are the most common fractures associated with compartment syndrome. In the upper extremity this condition is referred to as *Volkmann's contracture* (Fig. 59-11) and in the lower extremity as *anterior compartment syndrome*, although the underlying pathophysiology is similar.

Clinical manifestations. Early recognition and treatment of compartment syndrome is essential to avoid permanent damage to muscles and nerves. This can occur within 4 to 12 hours after onset. The earliest sign of a developing compartment syndrome is progressive pain distal to the injury that is not relieved by the usual analgesics. The overlying skin may appear normal because surface vessels are not occluded. In addition to inability to actively

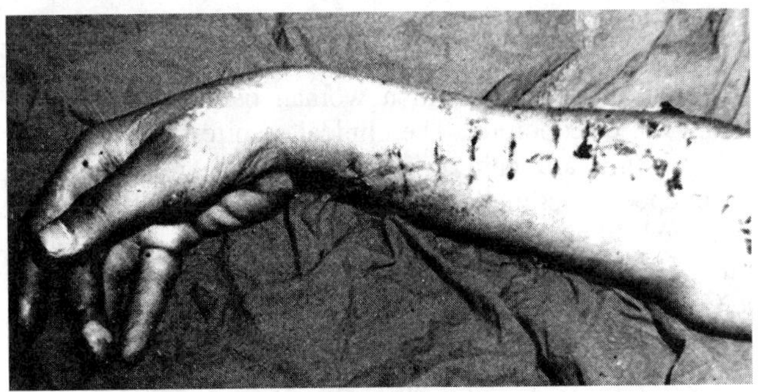

Fig. 59-11 Volkmann's ischemic contracture of the forearm secondary to a supracondylar fracture of the humerus. Note the incision line of an unsuccessful fasciotomy.

extend the digits, pain results from passive extension of the digits. Other symptoms that develop as the condition progresses include numbness and tingling, tenseness of the compartment envelope, pain on passive stretch of muscle traveling through the compartment, loss of sensation, loss of function, pallor, coolness of the extremity, and diminished or absent peripheral pulses. Absence of a peripheral pulse is an ominous sign that indicates severe disturbance of circulation. Regular neurovascular assessments should be performed on all patients with injury of the distal humerus or proximal tibia or soft-tissue disruption in these areas. Infection as a result of tissue necrosis is the most common complication. It can be due to delayed decompression, inadequate release of the wound, or delayed closure of a fasciotomy.

Because of the possibility of muscle damage, urine output should be assessed. Myoglobin, released from damaged muscle cells, can be trapped in renal tubules because of its high molecular weight. Common signs of myoglobinuria are (1) dark urine associated with a positive benzidine test in the absence of hematuria and (2) the manifestations associated with acute renal failure (see Chapter 44).

Therapeutic management. Prompt, accurate diagnosis of compartment syndrome is critical. Prevention or early recognition is the key. The extremity should be elevated and ice should be applied to enhance venous return and decrease edema. It may also be necessary to remove or loosen the bandage or cast or to reduce poundage on traction to prevent edema formation. It may also be necessary to relieve compression and restore blood supply by surgically incising the fascia (*fasciotomy*). If compartment syndrome goes untreated, amputation may be necessary to combat sepsis. Death may result if compartment syndrome progresses.[11]

Venous Thrombosis. The veins of the lower extremities and pelvis are highly susceptible to thrombus formation after fracture injury. Precipitating factors are venous stasis caused by incorrectly applied casts or traction, local pressure on a vein, or prolonged bed rest. Venous stasis is aggravated by inactivity of the muscles that normally assist in the pumping action of venous return of blood in the extremities. In addition to wearing compression gradient stockings and using mechanical compression devices, the patient should be instructed to move the fingers or toes of the affected extremity against resistance and to perform range-of-motion exercises on all unaffected extremities. Because of the risk of venous thrombosis in the immobile patient, prophylactic anticoagulant medication such as aspirin, warfarin, or heparin may be ordered. Low molecular weight heparin (enoxaparin) has recently been shown to be more effective in preventing venous thrombosis as compared with warfarin.[12] Because it has a predictable dose response, there is no need to provide follow-up monitoring of prothrombin time. Assessment and management of venous thrombosis are discussed in Chapter 35.

Fat Embolism. Fat emboli occur in 0.5% to 2% of patients with fractures of long bones and up to 10% of patients with multiple fractures associated with pelvic injuries.[13] They are a contributory factor in many deaths associated with fractures. The fractures that most frequently cause fat embolism are those of the femur, ribs, tibia, and pelvis with only minor associated injuries. There are two theories related to the origin of fat emboli. One theory suggests that fat is released from the marrow of injured bone. It is driven out by an increase in intramedullary pressure and enters the circulation through draining veins traveling to pulmonary capillaries, where it lodges. Some fat droplets traverse the capillary bed to enter systemic circulation and embolize to other sites. The other theory postulates that catecholamines released at the time of trauma mobilize free fatty acids from the adipose tissue, which causes loss of chylomicron emulsion stability.[14] The chylomicrons form large fat globules that lodge in the lungs. This is possibly due to some biochemical change initiated by injury. The tissues of the lungs, brain, heart, kidneys, and skin are most frequently affected.

Clinical manifestations. Early recognition of fat embolus is crucial in preventing a potentially lethal course. Initial manifestations usually occur 12 to 72 hours after injury.[15] The fat globules transported to the lungs cause a hemorrhagic interstitial pneumonitis that produces symptoms of acute respiratory distress syndrome, such as chest pain, tachypnea, cyanosis, dyspnea, apprehension, tachycardia, and decreased partial pressure of arterial oxygen (PaO_2). All of these symptoms are caused by poor oxygen exchange. The changes in the mental state as a result of hypoxemia are important to recognize. Memory loss, restlessness, confusion, elevated temperature, and headache prompt further investigation so that CNS involvement is not mistaken for alcohol withdrawal or acute head injury. The continued change in level of consciousness and petechiae located around the neck, anterior chest wall, axilla, buccal membrane of the mouth, and conjunctiva of the eye help distinguish fat emboli from other problems. Petechiae result from intravascular thromboses caused by decreased oxygenation.

The clinical course of a fat embolus may be brief and acute. Frequently the patient expresses a feeling of impending disaster. In a short time, skin color changes from pallor to cyanosis, and the patient may become comatose. No specific laboratory examinations are available to aid in the diagnosis. However, certain diagnostic abnormalities may be present. These include fat cells in the blood, urine, or sputum; a decrease of the PaO_2 to less than 60 mm Hg; ST segment changes on ECG; a decrease in the platelet count and hematocrit levels; and a prolonged prothrombin time.[15] A chest x-ray may reveal areas of pulmonary infiltrate or multiple areas of consolidation. This is sometimes referred to as the *snowstorm effect*.

Therapeutic management. Treatment for fat embolism is directed at prevention. Careful immobilization of a long bone fracture is probably the most important factor in the prevention of fat embolism. Adequate hydration washes the irritating fatty acids through the system. Use of steroids to prevent or treat fat embolism is controversial.[10] Oxygen is administered to treat hypoxia. Intubation or intermittent positive-pressure breathing may be considered if a satisfactory PaO_2 cannot be obtained with supplemental oxygen alone. Management is essentially symptom related and supportive. It includes maintaining adequate fluid intake, correction of acidosis, and replacement of any blood loss. Coughing and deep breathing should be encouraged. The patient should be repositioned as little as possible before fracture immobilization or stabilization because of the danger of dislodging more fat droplets into the general circulation. Some patients may develop pulmonary edema, acute respiratory distress syndrome, or both, leading to an increased mortality.

Types of Fractures

Colles' Fracture. A Colles' fracture is a fracture of the distal radius and is one of the most common fractures in adults. The styloid process of the ulna may be involved as well. The injury usually occurs when the patient attempts to break a fall with an outstretched hand. This type of fracture most frequently occurs in a woman over age 50 whose bones are osteoporotic. The clinical manifestations of Colles' fracture are pain in the immediate area of injury, pronounced swelling, and dorsal displacement of the distal fragment (dinner-fork deformity). This may appear as a bump on the wrist. The major complication associated with a Colles' fracture is vascular insufficiency as a result of edema.

A Colles' fracture is usually managed by closed manipulation of the fracture and immobilization by either a sugar-tong splint or a long arm cast. The elbow must be immobilized to prevent wrist supination and pronation. Nursing management should include measures to prevent or reduce edema and accurate neurovascular assessment. Support and protection of the extremity should be provided, along with encouragement of active movement of the thumb and fingers. This type of movement helps reduce edema and increases venous return. The patient should be instructed to perform active movements of the shoulder to prevent stiffness or contracture.

Fracture of the Humerus. Fractures involving the shaft of the humerus are a common injury among young and middle-aged adults. The prominent clinical manifestations are an obvious displacement of the humerus shaft, shortened extremity, abnormal mobility, and pain (Fig. 59-12). The major complications associated with fracture of the humerus are radial nerve injury and vascular injury to the brachial artery as a result of laceration, transection, or spasm.

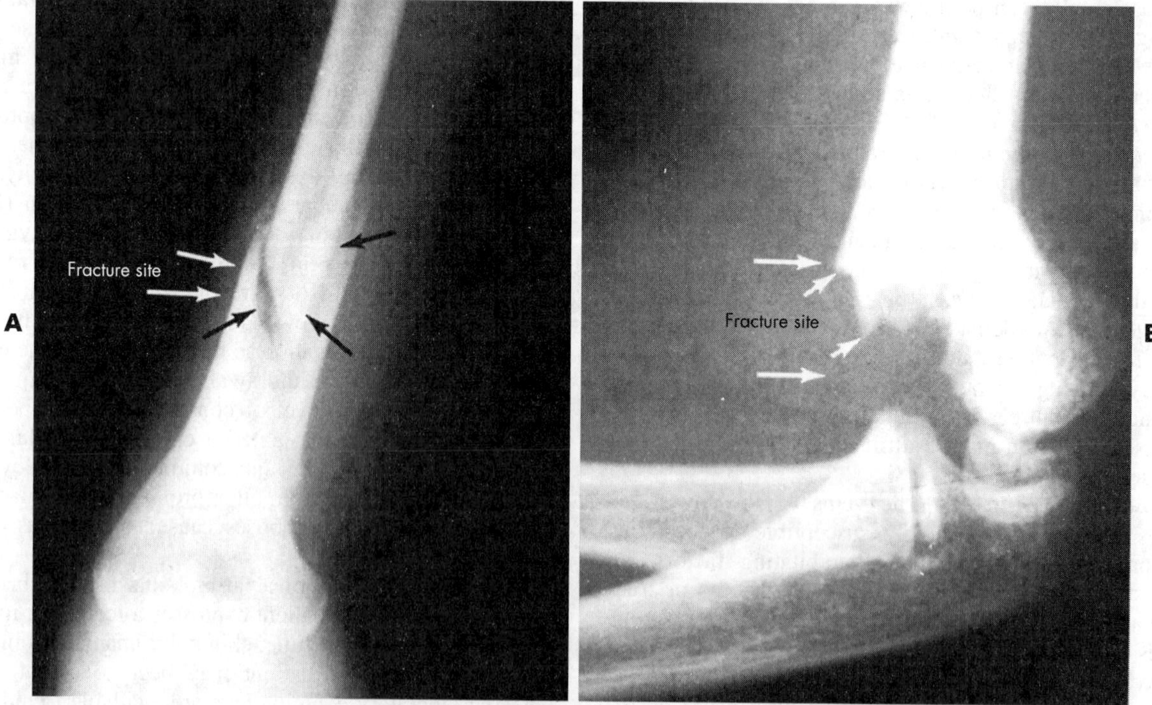

Fig. 59-12 ***A,*** Supracondylar fracture of the humerus. This type of injury results in the formation of a large hematoma. ***B,*** Fracture of distal shaft of humerus.

The treatment for a fracture of the humerus depends on the location and displacement of the fracture. Treatment may include a hanging arm cast or the sling and swathe, which is a type of immobilization that prevents glenohumeral movement. The swathe encircles the trunk and humerus as an additional binder. It is often used for surgical repairs and shoulder dislocation.

When these devices are used, the head of the bed should be elevated to assist gravity in reducing the fracture. The arm should be allowed to hang when the patient is sitting and standing. Nursing care should include measures to protect the axilla and prevent skin maceration. Skin or skeletal traction may also be used for purposes of reduction and immobilization.

During the rehabilitative phase an exercise program geared toward improving strength and motion of the injured extremity is extremely important. This should include assisted motion of the hand and fingers. The shoulder can also be exercised to prevent stiffness if the fracture is stable.

Fracture of the Pelvis. Pelvic fractures are usually caused by vehicular accidents. Older adult patients may sustain this injury from a fall. Although only 3% of all fractures are pelvic fractures, this type of injury accounts for 5% to 20% of the mortality from fractures. Preoccupation with associated injuries at the time of an accident may result in neglect of pelvic injuries. Pelvic fractures may cause serious intraabdominal injury, such as colon laceration, paralytic ileus, hemorrhage, and rupture of the urethra or bladder.

Physical examination demonstrates local swelling, tenderness, deformity, and ecchymosis. The neurovascular status of the lower extremities and manifestations of associated injuries should be assessed. Pelvic fractures are diagnosed and classified by x-ray study. They may range from simple undisplaced fractures to more serious fracture dislocations with the potential for serious complications.

Treatment of a pelvic fracture depends on the severity of the injury. Bed rest for stable pelvic fractures is maintained for a few days to 6 weeks. More complex fractures may be treated with pelvic slings, skeletal traction, hip spica casts, open reduction, or a combination of these methods. Internal fixation of a pelvic fracture may be necessary if the fracture is displaced. Extreme care in handling or moving the patient is important to prevent serious injury from a displaced fracture fragment. Because a pelvic fracture can damage other organs, appropriate assessments are important early nursing activities for this patient.

The patient should be turned only when specifically ordered by the physician. Back care is provided while the patient is raised from the bed either by independent use of the trapeze or with adequate assistance. Weight bearing on the affected side should be avoided until healing is complete. If the pelvic fracture is undisplaced, the patient is usually allowed to ambulate using a walker or crutches to distribute the weight bearing between the upper and lower extremities. Elimination needs may require the use of an indwelling catheter in female patients if a pelvic sling is used.

Fracture of the Hip. Hip fractures are a common trauma in older adults. There are more than 250,000 hip fractures annually. A hip fracture may be expected to occur more frequently in women than in men older than 65 years because of osteoporosis. It is estimated that 30% of patients who experience a hip fracture die within 1 year of injury because of medical complications caused by the fracture or resulting immobility.[12] Thirty percent to 50% of the survivors never regain their prefracture functional status.[16]

Fractures that occur within the capsule are called *intracapsular* fractures. Intracapsular fractures are further identified by a name taken from their specific location: (1) subcapital, (2) transcervical, and (3) basilar neck. These fractures are often associated with osteoporosis and minor trauma. *Extracapsular* fractures occur below the capsule and are termed *intertrochanteric* if they occur in a region between the greater and lesser trochanter. They are termed *subtrochanteric* if they occur in the region below the trochanter (Fig. 59-13). Extracapsular fractures are usually caused by severe direct trauma or a fall.

Clinical manifestations. The clinical manifestations of a hip fracture are external rotation, shortening of the affected extremity, and severe pain and tenderness in the region of the fracture site. Displaced femoral neck fractures cause serious disruption of the blood supply to the femoral head, which can result in avascular necrosis.

Therapeutic management. Surgical repair is the preferred method of managing intracapsular and extracapsular hip fractures. Surgical treatment permits the patient to be out of bed sooner and decreases the major complications associated with immobility. In contrast, treatment with traction requires 12 to 16 weeks of immobilization for healing to occur, even if the blood supply to the region is intact. Initially the affected extremity may be temporarily immobilized by either Buck's or Russell's traction until the patient's physical condition is stabilized and surgery can be

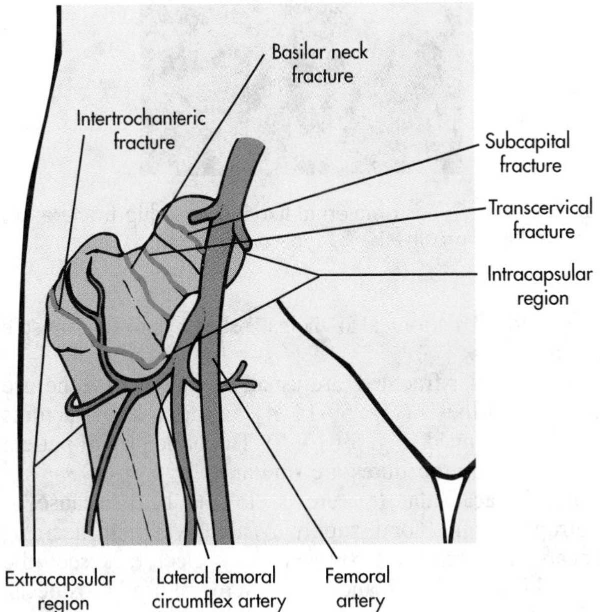

Fig. 59-13 Femur with location of various types of fracture.

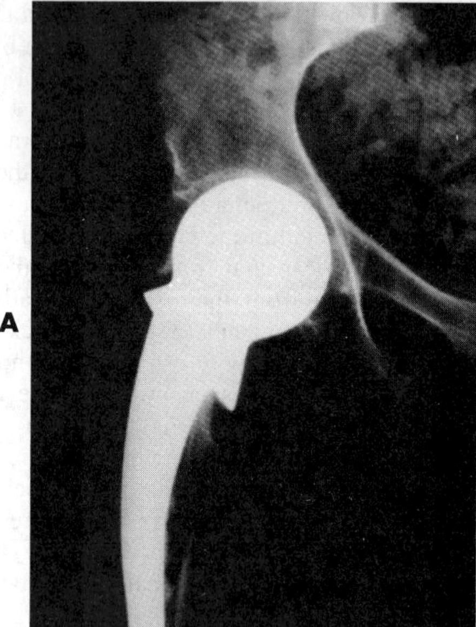

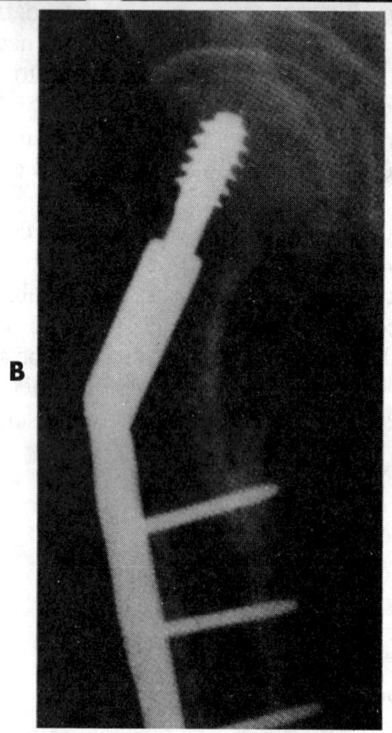

Fig. 59-14 Types of internal fixation for a hip fracture. ***A,*** Femoral head prosthesis. ***B,*** Type of hip nail.

performed. Traction also helps relieve painful muscle spasms.

Intracapsular fractures are usually repaired with the use of a hip prosthesis (Fig. 59-14, *A*). Extracapsular fractures are usually pinned (Fig. 59-14, *B*). The principles of patient care for these procedures are similar.

The intracapsular fracture is slow to heal because of interruptions in blood supply. When avascular necrosis appears imminent, the surgeon may elect to resect the femoral head and neck and insert a femoral head prosthesis. A variety of devices in the forms of compression screws and plates, nails, and pins are available to the surgeon for the purpose of repairing a hip fracture by pinning.

NURSING MANAGEMENT

HIP FRACTURE

Acute Intervention

Preoperative Management. Because older adults are most prone to hip fractures, chronic health problems must often be considered when planning treatment. Diabetes mellitus, hypertension, cardiac decompensation, and arthritis are chronic problems that may complicate clinical status. Surgery may be delayed for a brief time until the patient's general health improves.

Before surgery, severe muscle spasms can increase pain. These spasms are managed by appropriate medications, comfortable positioning unless contraindicated, and properly adjusted traction if it is being used.

Careful preoperative patient teaching can affect future mobility. The patient should know the method and frequency for exercising the unaffected leg and both arms. The patient should also be shown how to use the trapeze bar and opposite side rail to assist in changing positions. Practice in getting out of bed and transferring to a chair should be discussed and demonstrated before surgery. The family should be informed about the patient's weight-bearing status after surgery. Plans for discharge should be discussed, and arrangements should be initiated well before the actual discharge date.

Postoperative Management. The initial postoperative management of a patient following surgical repair of hip fracture is similar to that for any older surgical patient: the nurse monitors vital signs and intake and output, supervises respiratory activities such as deep breathing and coughing, administers pain medication cautiously, and observes the dressing and incision for signs of bleeding and infection. Specific nursing interventions for the patient with a fracture of the hip are described in the nursing care plan on p. 1865.

In the early postoperative period there is a potential for impairment of circulation, movement, and sensation. The nurse should assess the patient's toes for (1) ability to move, (2) warmth and pink color, (3) numbness or tingling, and (4) edema. Edema, which may develop after the patient is out of bed, is alleviated by elevation of the leg whenever the patient is in a chair. The pain resulting from poor alignment of the affected extremity can be prevented by keeping pillows (or an abductor splint) between the knees when the patient is turning to either side. Sandbags and pillows are also used to prevent external rotation.

The physical therapist usually supervises active assistance exercises for the affected extremity and ambulation when the surgeon permits it. Ambulation usually begins the first or second postoperative day. The nurse should monitor the patient's ambulation status for proper crutch walking or use of the walker. The patient must be able to use crutches or a walker before discharge.

Complications associated with femoral neck fracture include nonunion, avascular necrosis, and degenerative

NURSING CARE PLAN Patient with Fracture of the Hip

Planning: Outcome Criteria	*Nursing Interventions and Rationales*
➤ **NURSING DIAGNOSIS**	Pain *related to* edema, movement of bone fragments, muscle spasms, and ineffective pain relief or comfort measures *as manifested by* pain descriptors, guarding, altered time perception; behaviors indicative of pain such as moaning, crying, restlessness; altered muscle tone, autonomic responses; lack of mobility
Have decrease in or absence of pain; express satisfaction with pain relief.	Align and position extremity and patient correctly *to reduce pressure on nerves and tissue.* Use gentleness when positioning or turning *to prevent muscle spasm and malalignment of bone fragments.* Maintain constant traction forces *to reduce muscle spasm and maintain alignment of bone.* Administer analgesics as indicated *to reduce pain and muscle spasms.*
➤ **NURSING DIAGNOSIS**	Risk for disuse syndrome *related to* immobility secondary to fractured hip
Have no skin breakdown, no evidence of pulmonary infection or restriction of joint motion, adequate circulation, satisfactory elimination pattern, adequate urinary output, maintain orientation and alertness.	Assess for abnormal findings related to all body systems *to determine presence of risk factors.* Foster activity to tolerance *to promote maximum activity.* Provide adequate hydration, nutrition, diversion *to prevent complications of immobility such as urinary tract infection or stones, negative nitrogen balance, constipation, and boredom.* Plan passive and active range-of-motion and deep-breathing exercises *to maintain joint function and muscle strength and prevent systemic pulmonary complications associated with prolonged immobility.* Turn patient q2hr *to reduce pressure on bony prominences and improve ventilation.*
➤ **NURSING DIAGNOSIS**	Impaired physical mobility *related to* decreased muscle strength, presence of immobilizing device, such as a cast, pin, or traction *as manifested by* inability to purposefully move within physical environment, limited joint range of motion, decreased muscle strength, mobility restrictions, inability to bear weight, inability to ambulate with proper, safe technique
Have sufficient muscle strength to participate in gait-training program, restoration of optimal mobility, optimal level of function with ambulatory assistive device.	Cooperate with physical therapist in muscle-strengthening program *to maximize patient's progress in rehabilitation.* Teach and assist patient in exercise program; include resistive strengthening exercises of uninvolved lower and both upper limbs, elbow extension, shoulder depressors, and knee and hip extension *to develop strength in all extremities preparatory to initiation of ambulation.* Increase activities as tolerated *to gradually increase strength.* Assist patient in standing at side of bed using non–weight-bearing support on affected leg *to increase mobility.* Encourage quadriceps exercises, arm-strengthening exercises, and abdominal and gluteal contraction exercises *to develop muscle strength, which will help with rehabilitation.* Instruct patient about ambulatory training program *to promote effective rehabilitation.* Be aware that non–weight-bearing status of involved extremity must be maintained unless changed by an order from physician *because soft tissue surrounding the hip requires about 3-5 mo of healing to sufficiently stabilize the prothesis.* Get patient out of bed and into chair, usually within 24-48 hr after surgery, *to reduce the complications associated with immobility.* Instruct and assist patient with transfer from bed to chair *to prevent accidental falling and improper movements, which could cause prosthesis displacement or hip malalignment.* Instruct and assist patient in use of ambulatory assistive devices with non–weight-bearing gait *to ensure safe ambulation.*
➤ **NURSING DIAGNOSIS**	Risk for wound infection *related to* exposure to environmental pathogens and surgical procedure
Have no evidence of wound infection, normal temperature.	Monitor patient's immune status, extent of trauma, and environmental exposure to pathogens *to identify risk factors for infection and plan appropriate interventions if present.* Assess wound site for erythema and drainage; monitor temperature *to identify signs of possible infection and initiate appropriate interventions.* Obtain wound culture if indicated *to identify infecting organism.* Administer antibiotics as ordered *for prophylaxis or to treat infection.* Use sterile technique when changing dressings or providing wound care *to minimize the risk of cross-contamination.*

continued

NURSING CARE PLAN Patient with Fracture of the Hip—cont'd

Planning: Outcome Criteria	Nursing Interventions and Rationales
➤ **NURSING DIAGNOSIS**	Ineffective management of therapeutic regimen *related to* injury, surgery, unavailable support system, and lack of knowledge of postdischarge care *as manifested by* verbalization of concern by unavailable support system, patient or caregiver regarding ability to care for patient after discharge, observation of lack of knowledge regarding postdischarge care
Verbalize confidence in ability to manage postdischarge care by patient and family.	Assess home environment *to identify needed modifications such as elevated toilet seat, height of shelves, steps.* Teach patient and family about proper ambulation, diet, medications, wound care, and physician follow-up *to reduce risk of injury, promote proper wound healing, and foster effective rehabilitation.* Inform about symptoms to report to physician such as fever, severe pain, cognitive changes *because these are indicators of complications that require prompt treatment.* Teach patient and family positions and activities to avoid such as putting on shoes and socks, crossing legs while seated, sitting on low seats *because these may cause dislocation of prosthesis.* Refer for home care as needed *because this resource can provide additional therapy and other assistance.*
➤ **NURSING DIAGNOSIS**	Self-esteem disturbance *related to* uncertain future, perceived helplessness, and possible self-care deficits *as manifested by* expressions of hopelessness, despair; inability to concentrate on reading, writing, conversation; misdirected anger; extreme dependency on others
Maintain optimistic attitude about recovery.	Ambulate patient as prescribed and tolerated *to increase mobility and provide encouragement about ability to resume self-care or previous life situation.* Allow as much independence and decision making as possible *to foster independence.* Talk about future activities with a positive attitude *to build confidence.* Involve patient and family in planning care *because this increases self-esteem and provides knowledge of realistic abilities.* Plan for discharge needs *to meet home care and rehabilitation requirements.*
➤ **NURSING DIAGNOSIS**	Altered thought processes *related to* pain medication, change of environment, bed rest, social isolation, and decreased vision or hearing *as manifested by* impairment of ability to recall previous events, attention span, perception, judgment, and decision-making ability
Maintain orientation and other cognitive funtions to preinjury level.	Orient patient to place and reason for hospitalization *to help patient maintain contact with reality.* Encourage visits by family and friends *to provide familiar contacts.* Keep side rails up if a family or staff member is not present; keep light on at night *to prevent injury and minimize disorientation.* Minimize pain *as pain can cause disorientation, especially in elderly patients.* Give careful explanation of procedures *as anxiety over the unknown can increase confusion.* Reinforce instructions as necessary *as confusion impairs memory.*
➤ **NURSING DIAGNOSIS**	Risk for impaired physical mobility *related to* flexion contracture of the hip secondary to prolonged flexed position
Have no flexion contracture of the hip.	Monitor for equal leg length and flexed position of affected leg at the hip *to identify muscle shortening and flexion contracture.* Avoid placing patient in flexed position >45 degrees for more than 1 hr *because this position encourages development of flexion contracture.* Place patient in a prone position at least once a day *to encourage full extension of the hips.*

COLLABORATIVE PROBLEMS

Nursing Goals	Nursing Interventions and Rationales
➤ **POTENTIAL COMPLICATION**	Thromboembolic phenomenon *related to* immobility
Monitor for thromboembolic phenomena, report abnormal findings, and carry out appropriate medical and nursing interventions.	Monitor for altered circulation, edema, redness, calf pain, dyspnea, tachycardia, chest pain, petechiae *to detect signs of thromboembolism.* Apply elastic compression gradient stockings to unaffected lower extremity *to promote venous return and reduce venous stasis.* Teach resistive range-of-motion exercises of unaffected extremities, especially ankle plantar flexion against footboard, *to facilitate venous return from lower extremity.* With assistance, change patient's position by using trapeze bar or opposite side rail q1-2hr *to prevent venous pooling.*

arthritis. As a result of an intertrochanteric fracture, the affected leg may be shortened.

Chronic and Home Management

If the hip fracture has been treated by insertion of a femoral-head prosthesis, measures to prevent dislocation must always be used (Table 59-11). The patient and family must be fully aware of positions and activities that predispose the patient to dislocation (extreme flexion, adduction, or internal rotation). Many daily activities may reproduce these positions (e.g., putting on shoes and socks, crossing the legs or feet while seated, assuming the side-lying position incorrectly, standing up or sitting down while the body is flexed relative to the chair, sitting on low seats). Until the soft tissue surrounding the hip has healed sufficiently to stabilize the prosthesis these activities must be avoided, usually for at least 6 weeks. Sudden severe pain and extreme external rotation indicate prosthesis dislocation. This requires a closed or open reduction to realign the femoral head in the acetabulum.

In addition to teaching the patient and family how to prevent prosthesis dislocation, the nurse should (1) place a large pillow between the patient's legs when turning, (2) keep leg abductor splints on the patient except when bathing, (3) avoid extreme hip flexion, and (4) avoid turning the patient on the affected side until approved by the surgeon.

If the hip fracture is treated by pinning, dislocation precautions are not necessary. The patient is usually encouraged to be out of bed on the first postoperative day. Weight bearing on the involved extremity may be restricted until x-ray examination indicates adequate healing, usually within 3 to 5 months.

Table 59-11 Patient Instructions for Femoral-Head Prosthesis

Do Not
- Force hip into more than 90 degrees of flexion*
- Force hip into adduction
- Force hip into internal rotation
- Cross legs
- Put on own shoes or stockings until 8 wk after surgery
- Sit on chairs without arms to aid rising to a standing position*

Do
- Use toilet elevator on toilet seat*
- Place chair inside shower or tub and remain seated while washing
- Use pillow between legs for first 8 wk after surgery when lying on "good" side or when supine*
- Keep hip in neutral, straight position when sitting, walking, or lying*
- Notify surgeon if severe pain, deformity, or loss of function occurs*
- Inform dentist of presence of prosthesis before dental work so that prophylactic antibiotics can be given

*These precautions also apply after a hip pinning.

The nurse must assist both the patient and the family in adjusting to the restrictions and dependence imposed by the hip fracture. Depression can easily occur, but creative nursing care and awareness of the problem can do much to prevent it. The patient and family should be informed about community referral services that can assist in the postdischarge rehabilitation phase. Hospitalization averages 5 to 7 days. Regular follow-up care after discharge should be arranged.

Gerontologic Considerations

Factors that contribute to the occurrence of a hip fracture in older adults include a propensity to fall, inability to correct

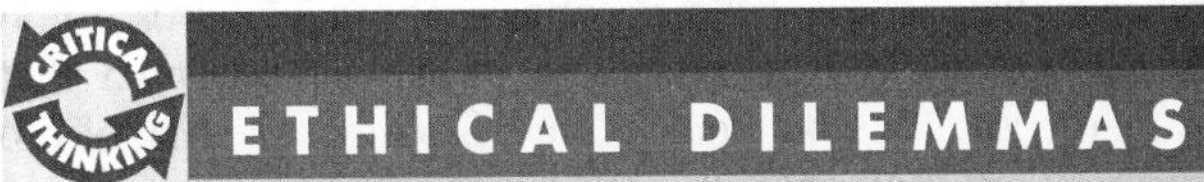

ETHICAL DILEMMAS

PREMATURE DISCHARGE OF PATIENT

Situation

An 83-year-old male patient with a total hip replacement is to be discharged from the hospital because of diagnostic review group standards for the number of days in the hospital. The nurse knows that the patient lives alone, has no relatives to care for him, and is unable to manage at this stage in his recovery with the limited home care available to him. Should the nurse request that the patient not be discharged at this time?

Discussion Third-party payer procedures for determining reimbursement for medical care are a means to determine reimbursement and *not* medical diagnoses. They are based on standards of medical care and pooled patient information rather than individual patients' histories and their physicians' orders. In his current condition this patient does not seem to have access to appropriate home care. If discharge planning is unable to find suitable care or to arrange transfer to an intermediate nursing facility, it would be unethical to discharge him. Both the physician and the administrator of the hospital should be involved in the plans for this patient in order to guarantee that appropriate care will be extended beyond the hospital. If it is not, the hospital might be liable for any medical consequences of the patient's inadequate care.

ETHICAL AND LEGAL PRINCIPLES

- Medicare began basing payment for short-term hospitalization on a diagnostic review group system in 1983, but not all facilities receiving Medicare reimbursement are covered under this system.
- Facilities may extend the length of stay beyond the diagnostic review group allotted time, but the reimbursement for the patient will be reduced for the additional days.
- Medical decisions may not be ethically or legally made based on profit or reimbursement concerns. Concerns about reimbursement procedures and social policy should not be expressed in individual patient care contexts.

a postural imbalance, side-orientation of the fall, inadequate local tissue shock absorbers, and underlying skeletal weakness.[17]

Several factors have been identified in older persons that increase their risk of falling. These include gait and mobility problems, leg and foot dysfunction (including balance problems), and medication use.[18] A fall to the side, the most common type in the frail elderly, is more likely to result in a hip fracture than is a forward fall.

Two important factors influencing the amount of force imposed on the hip include the presence of energy-absorbing soft tissue over the greater trochanter and the state of leg muscle contraction at the time of the fall. Because many elderly persons are thin and have poor muscle tone, these factors are important in the severity of a fall. Finally, elderly women often have osteoporosis and accompanying low bone density. It has been shown that women with low bone density have 8.5 times the risk of hip fracture than women with high bone density.[19]

The use of targeted interventions to reduce hip fractures in the elderly include a variety of strategies. Calcium supplementation, vitamin D supplementation, estrogen replacement, and calcitonin have been shown to increase bone density and decrease the likelihood of fracture. External hip pads have been shown to reduce hip fractures in the elderly, but compliance is poor.[20] Nurses must be vigilant in planning interventions for the elderly that are known to reduce the incidence of hip fracture.

Femoral Shaft Fracture

Femoral shaft fracture is a common injury, particularly in young adults. Severe direct force is required to produce this injury, because the femur can bend approximately 2 inches (0.8 cm) before actual fracture occurs. The force exerted to cause the fracture frequently causes damage to the adjacent soft-tissue structures. These injuries may be more serious than the bone injury. Displacement of the fracture fragments frequently results in open fracture and increased soft-tissue damage. This can result in considerable blood loss.

The clinical manifestations of a fracture of the femoral shaft are usually obvious. They include pronounced deformity and angulation, shortening of the extremity, inability to move either the hip or knee, and pain. The common complications associated with fracture of the femoral shaft include fat embolism, nerve and vascular injury, and problems associated with union, open fracture, and soft-tissue damage.

Initial management is directed toward stabilization of the patient and immobilization of the fracture. Treatment may consist of tibial pinning with balanced skeletal traction. Traction continues for 8 to 12 weeks. The nurse must encourage the patient to perform exercises and range-of-motion activities for the uninvolved extremities and joints. The physician determines when active exercise can be instituted on the affected extremity. When there is sufficient clinical evidence of bone union, a hip spica cast may be applied.

Internal fixation is another way to manage a femoral fracture. It is carried out with an intramedullary rod or compression plate. Internal fixation is frequently the preferred treatment because it reduces hospital stay and the complications associated with prolonged bed rest. Other indications for internal fixation are failure to obtain satisfactory reduction by nonsurgical methods and multiple associated injuries. In some instances the surgically repaired femur may be supported by suspension traction for 3 to 4 days to prevent excessive movement of the extremity and to control rotation; non–weight-bearing gait training is then begun.

Promotion and maintenance of strength in the affected extremity usually include gluteal and quadriceps exercises. It is important to ensure performance of range-of-motion and strengthening exercises for all uninvolved extremities in preparation for ambulation. The patient may be immobilized in a hip spica cast and gradually progress to an articulating cast brace or may be allowed to begin non–weight-bearing activities with an ambulatory assistive device. Full weight-bearing is usually restricted until there is x-ray evidence of bony union of the fracture fragments.

Fracture of the Tibia

The tibia is vulnerable to injury because it lacks anterior muscle covering, but strong force is required to produce a fractured tibia. As a result, soft-tissue damage, devascularization, and open fracture are frequent. Other problems associated with tibial fractures are compartment syndrome, fat embolism, problems associated with bony union, and possible infection associated with open fracture.

The recommended management for closed tibial fracture is closed reduction followed by immobilization in a long leg cast. Open reduction may be achieved with a compression plate. With either method of reduction, emphasis is placed on maintaining the strength of the quadriceps, because delayed union is frequent.

The neurovascular status of the affected extremity must be assessed at least every 2 hours during the first 48 hours. Patients are instructed to perform active range-of-motion exercises with all uninvolved extremities and exercises for the upper extremities to build the strength required for crutch walking. When the physician has determined that the patient is ready for gait training, the patient is instructed in the principles of crutch walking. The patient may be restricted to non–weight-bearing activities for 6 to 12 weeks depending on healing. When fracture healing has progressed sufficiently, a walking heel is applied to the cast and full weight-bearing is allowed.

Stable Vertebral Fractures

A stable fracture of the vertebral column is usually caused by motor vehicle accidents, falls, diving, or athletic injuries. A stable fracture is one in which the fracture or the fragment is not likely to move or cause spinal cord damage. This type of injury is frequently confined to the anterior element (vertebral body) of the spinal column in the lumbar region. It involves the cervical and thoracic regions less frequently. The vertebral bodies are usually protected from displacement by the intact spinal ligaments.

Most patients with spinal fractures have stable fractures and experience only brief periods of disability. If the ligamentous structures are significantly disrupted, however, dislocation of the vertebral structures may occur, resulting in instability and injury to the spinal cord (unstable fracture). These injuries may require surgery. The most serious complication of vertebral fractures is fracture displacement, which can cause damage to the spinal cord (see Chapter 57). Although stable vertebral fractures are not associated with abnormal spinal cord pathology, all spinal injuries should initially be considered unstable and potentially serious until diagnostic tests and the physician determine that the fracture is stable.

The most common injury to the vertebral body is the compression type of fracture caused by excessive vertical load, such as a severe fall on the buttocks or injury resulting from sudden flexion that forces the spine beyond its normal range of motion. The patient usually complains of pain and tenderness in the affected region of the spine. Compression fractures are associated with a gibbous deformity (flexion angulation localized to one vertebral level). This deformity may be noted during the physical examination. Bowel and bladder dysfunction may be an indication of a temporary interruption of the sympathetic nervous system or injury to the spinal cord.

The overall goal in management of stable fractures of a vertebral body is to keep the spine in good alignment until union has been accomplished. Many nursing implementations are aimed at assessing the possibility of spinal cord trauma. Vital signs and bowel and bladder function should be evaluated regularly, as should the motor and sensory status of the peripheral nerves distal to the injured region. Any deterioration in the patient's neurovascular status should be promptly reported.

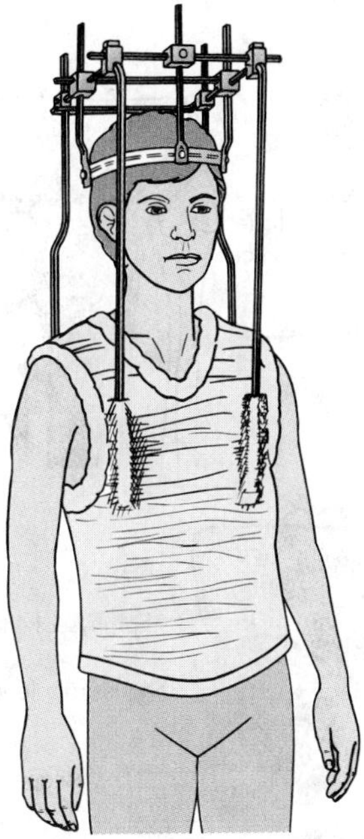

Fig. 59-15 Halo apparatus attached to a body cast. It may also be attached to a brace. A halo vest can be used in treatment of a cervical spine injury or following cervical spine surgery.

Treatment includes support, heat, and traction. The patient is usually placed in a standard hospital bed with firm support from the mattress or a bedboard. The aim is to support the spinal cord, relax muscles, and release any compression on nerve roots. Heat and traction may be used to relieve muscle spasms resulting from the fracture. Traction may also be used to reduce and immobilize fracture fragments. A trapeze is not usually allowed because its use disrupts spinal alignment. Upright position and turning of the torso are prohibited. When turning, the patient should be taught to keep the spine straight by turning the shoulders and pelvis together. Nursing assistance is necessary for the patient to learn how to turn in this "logrolling" fashion.

Several days after the initial injury, the physician may apply a specially constructed orthotic device, a jacket cast, or a removable corset if there is no evidence of neurologic deficit. If the fracture is in the cervical spine, a cervical collar may be worn by the patient. Some cervical fractures are immobilized by use of a halo vest (Fig. 59-15). This consists of a plastic jacket or cast fitted about the chest and attached to a halo, which is held in place by skeletal pins inserted into the cranium. These devices immobilize the spine in the fracture area but allow patient mobility. The patient is discharged after regaining ambulation skills, learning care of the cast or orthotic device, and learning how to cope with interferences in safety and security imposed by injury and treatment.

Facial Fractures

Any bone of the face can be fractured as a result of trauma. The primary concern after facial injury is to establish and maintain a patent airway and to provide adequate ventilation by removal of foreign material and blood. Suctioning may be necessary. An artificial airway (tracheostomy) may be needed if a patent airway cannot be maintained. Hemorrhage is controlled by pressure packing. Table 59-12 describes the clinical manifestations of more common facial fractures.

Concurrent soft-tissue injury often makes assessment of a facial injury difficult. Oral and maxillofacial examinations should be performed after the patient has been stabilized and any life-threatening situations have been treated.

Table 59-12 Clinical Manifestations of Facial Fractures

Fracture	Clinical Manifestation
Frontal bone	Rapid edema that may mask underlying fractures
Periorbital	Possible frontal sinus involvement
Nasal	Displacement of nasal bones, epistaxis
Zygomatic arch	Depression of zygomatic arch
Maxilla	Segmental motion of maxilla
Mandible	Dental fractures, bleeding, limited motion of mandible

An x-ray documents the extent of the injury. Computed tomography (CT) imaging is most valuable for midface injuries. The CT scan can demonstrate air or hemorrhage in the cranium, orbits, and soft tissues.[21]

Injury to the eye must be suspected when a facial injury occurs, particularly if the injury is near the orbit. Unless a global rupture is suspected (because the globe is soft to palpation) the eyes should be measured for intraocular pressure.[22] If the intraocular pressure is elevated or uneven, the patient should be evaluated by an ophthalmologist.

Specific treatment of a facial fracture depends on the site and extent of the fracture and the associated soft-tissue injury. Immobilization or stabilization may be necessary. (Mandibular fractures are discussed in Chapter 38.)

The patient who sustains a facial fracture requires sensitive nursing care because alteration in appearance after the trauma may be drastic. Edema and discoloration subside with time, but concurrent soft-tissue injuries may result in permanent scarring. Attention to maintenance of a patent airway and adequate nutrition are ongoing concerns of the nurse throughout the recovery period.

OSTEOMYELITIS

Etiology and Pathophysiology

Osteomyelitis is an infection of bone by direct or indirect invasion by an organism. In children long bones are most commonly affected, whereas in adults the vertebrae are more commonly affected. Direct entry results from contamination as a result of an open fracture or surgical implementation. Indirect inoculation results from a blood-borne infection from a distant site such as teeth, infected tonsils, or furuncles. The most common infecting organism is *Staphylococcus aureus*. Aerobic gram-negative bacteria alone or mixed with gram-positive organisms are often found.[23] The course and virulence of osteomyelitis are influenced by the blood supply to the affected bone. The widespread use of antibiotics in conjunction with surgical treatment has significantly reduced the mortality associated with osteomyelitis. The incidence and morbidity remain relatively unchanged, however, because new, drug-resistant strains of organisms have developed.

Indirect-entry (also called *hematogenous*) osteomyelitis most frequently affects growing bone in boys and is associated with local trauma. The most common sites of indirect-entry osteomyelitis are the long bones of the leg, although any bone can be involved.

Direct-entry osteomyelitis can occur at any age when there is an open wound. After gaining entrance to the bone by way of arterial supply, the bacteria lodge in an area of bone in which circulation slows, usually the metaphysis. The locus of bacteria grows, resulting in an increase in pressure because of the nonexpanding container of tubular bone. This increasing pressure eventually leads to ischemia and vascular compromise. Once ischemia occurs, the bone dies. The area of devitalized bone eventually separates from the surrounding living bone, forming *sequestra*. These sequestra form havens for bacteria, and chronic osteomyelitis develops.

Once formed, a sequestrum continues to be an infected island of bone, surrounded by pus and unreachable by any blood-borne antibiotics or leukocytes. It enlarges and serves as a source of bacteria for metastasis to other sites, including the lungs and brain. Two situations are possible. The sequestrum may extrude through a defect in tubular bone; however, this is hindered by the formation of new bone laid down by the elevated periosteum called *involucrum* (Fig. 59-16). Once outside the bone, the sequestrum may revascularize and undergo removal by normal defense processes. The other possibility is surgical removal. Unless resolved naturally or surgically, the necrotic sequestrum may develop a sinus tract, resulting in chronic wound drainage.

Wound culture determines the causative organism. A bone or tissue biopsy may also be necessary to determine the causative agent. The patient's blood cultures are frequently positive. An elevated leukocyte count and sedimentation rate may also be present. Radiologic signs suggestive of osteomyelitis usually do not appear until 10 days to 2 weeks after the appearance of clinical symptoms, by which time the disease will have progressed. Radionuclide bone scans can establish the diagnosis within 24 to 72 hours.[24] MRI may be used to help identify the boundaries of the infection.

Acute osteomyelitis refers to the initial infection or an infection of less than 1 month in duration. *Chronic osteomyelitis* refers to a bone infection that persists for longer than 4 weeks or an infection that has failed to respond to the initial course of antibiotic therapy.

Chronic osteomyelitis can represent either a continuous, persistent problem or a process of exacerbations and quiescence. Pus accumulates, causing ischemia of the bone. Over time, granulation tissue turns to scar tissue. This avascular

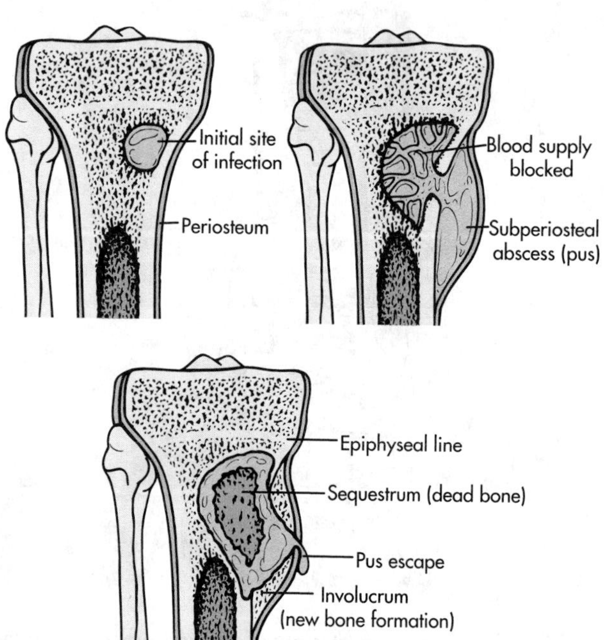

Fig. 59-16 Development of osteomyelitis infection with involucrum and sequestrum.

scar tissue provides an ideal site for bacterial growth and is impenetrable to antibiotics.

Therapeutic Management

Vigorous antibiotic therapy is the treatment of choice for acute osteomyelitis, as long as ischemia has not yet occurred. Wound cultures should be taken before antibiotic therapy is initiated so that the specific antibiotic therapy can be determined by sensitivity studies. If antibiotic therapy is not started early in the course of the illness, surgical debridement and decompression are necessary to relieve pressure within the bone and prevent ischemia. Some type of immobilization for the affected part is usually indicated. IV or oral antibiotic therapy is usually continued for 4 to 8 weeks after discharge.

The most serious, and potentially fatal, complication of osteomyelitis is the development of overwhelming sepsis from metastasis of bacteria to other sites. Pathologic fractures may occur because of weakened, devitalized bone. Soft tissue and bone healing occur slowly in the presence of infection, and subsequent deformity of the extremity may develop.

Treatment for chronic osteomyelitis includes surgical removal of poorly vascularized tissue and dead bone and extended use of antibiotics. After surgical debridement of devitalized and infected tissue, the wound may be closed, and a suction irrigation system for removal of any devitalized tissues remaining in the wound area is inserted. Regional perfusion involving constant irrigation of the affected bone with antibiotics may be initiated. Hyperbaric oxygen therapy may be used as an adjunctive therapy where available.[25]

Treatment for chronic osteomyelitis previously involved an extended hospital stay for intravenous (IV) antibiotic treatment or stabilization of the patient and discharge with IV antibiotics. Oral antibiotics have limited success rate because of poor penetration into organic bone. Currently, ciprofloxacin (Cipro) is being used successfully to treat osteomyelitis and has good bone penetration. Usually the patient is started on IV doses of this medication and switched to oral medication after 1 to 2 weeks.[23] Enoxacin is an investigational drug awaiting approval by the Food and Drug Administration.

Surgical removal of the infection may be necessary. Skin and bone grafting may be necessary if destruction is extensive. Antibiotic-impregnated bead chains may be surgically implanted at the time of debridement to combat the infection.[26] Infection may occur in the presence of a foreign body such as an implant or an orthopedic device such as a plate or a total joint. It may be necessary to remove the device to effectively treat the infection. Infection and bone destruction may be so extensive that amputation of the extremity is necessary to preserve life.

NURSING MANAGEMENT

OSTEOMYELITIS

The nursing management of the patient with osteomyelitis is challenging and demanding. Often a prolonged hospital or long-term care facility stay is required to ensure that adequate remission has been achieved.

Nursing Assessment

The clinical manifestations of osteomyelitis are both systemic and local. Subjective and objective data that should be obtained from an individual with osteomyelitis are presented in Table 59-13.

Nursing Diagnoses

Nursing diagnoses are determined when the problem and etiologic factors are supported by clinical data. Nursing diagnoses related to osteomyelitis include, but are not limited to, those presented in the nursing care plan for the patient with osteomyelitis on p. 1872.

Planning

The overall goals are that the patient with osteomyelitis will (1) have satisfactory pain and fever control, (2) have no transmission of infection to other areas of the body, (3) not experience any complications associated with osteomyelitis, (4) cooperate with the treatment plan, and (5) maintain a positive outlook on the outcome of the disease.

Table 59-13 Nursing Assessment: Osteomyelitis

Subjective Data

Important health information

Past health history: Bone trauma, open fracture, open or puncture wounds, other acute infections (e.g., streptococcal sore throat, bacterial pneumonia, sinusitis, skin or tooth infection, chronic urinary tract infection)

Medications: IV drug abuse, use of analgesics or antibiotics

Surgery and other treatments: Bone surgery

Functional health patterns

Health perception–health management: Malaise

Nutritional-metabolic: Fever, chills, anorexia, weight loss

Activity-exercise: Weakness, muscle spasms around affected bone

Cognitive-perceptual: Increase in pain with movement of affected bone

Objective Data

General

Restlessness, irritability; high, spiking temperatures

Integumentary

Diaphoresis, erythema over infected bone

Musculoskeletal

Local tenderness, edema, warmth; restricted movement; wound drainage; spontaneous fractures

Possible findings

Leukocytosis, positive blood and wound cultures, elevated erythrocyte sedimentation rate; rarefaction with presence of sequestrum and involucrum on x-rays and radionuclide bone scans

IV, Intravenous.

NURSING CARE PLAN Patient with Osteomyelitis

Planning: Outcome Criteria	Nursing Interventions and Rationales
➤ **NURSING DIAGNOSIS**	Pain *related to* inflammatory process secondary to infection *as manifested by* pain descriptors, guarding; altered time perception; behaviors indicative of pain, such as moaning, crying, restlessness; altered muscle tone, autonomic responses; decreased activity
Have decrease in or absence of pain; be satisfied with pain relief.	Assess location, severity, and success of pain-relieving measures *to plan appropriate interventions.* Avoid activities that increase circulation, such as exercise or application of heat *to prevent increasing edema and subsequent pain.* Use gentle handling and support when moving extremity *to reduce pain and prevent pathologic fractures.* Maintain patient's body in correct alignment and positioning *to prevent unusual position or muscle stretching from increasing pain.* Restrict ambulation or teach patient to use assistive device (e.g., crutches) *to prevent pathologic fracture, pain, and increased stress on bone.* Avoid jarring bed *to prevent pain.* Use bed cradle *to reduce discomfort caused by weight of covers.* Give analgesics as indicated *to relieve pain.*
➤ **NURSING DIAGNOSIS**	Altered comfort: fever *related to* infection *as manifested by* elevated temperature, restlessness, diaphoresis, chills, altered time perception, confusion
Have normal temperature, minimal discomfort, absence of chilling or dehydration, evidence of effective antibiotic therapy.	Take temperature q4hr *to determine presence of elevated temperature and to monitor patient's response to treatment.* Provide cool environment, light clothing and bedding, antipyretic drugs as ordered, and sponge bath or tub bath *to increase patient's comfort and reduce temperature.* Offer fluids every hour *to prevent dehydration from insensible fluid loss.* Observe skin turgor and moistness of mucous membranes *because delayed rebound and dry mucous membranes indicate dehydration.*
➤ **NURSING DIAGNOSIS**	Edema of effected part *related to* inflammatory process and immobility *as manifested by* increase in size, redness, warmth in affected area
Have decrease in or absence of edema in affected extremity.	Measure circumference of affected extremity daily *to have quantitative data on degree of edema and evaluate effectiveness of treatment.* Elevate affected extremity unless contraindicated *to assist venous return to heart.* Assess peripheral pulse of affected extremity every shift *because diminished pulse can indicate impaired circulation with resultant increase in edema.*
➤ **NURSING DIAGNOSIS**	Risk for infection transmission *related to* contaminated wound drainage
Have absence of transmission of infection.	Observe for open, draining wound; inadequate asepsis by health care providers *to make appropriate plans to reduce these risk factors.* Follow hospital procedures for isolation techniques if indicated *to prevent cross-contamination.* Use proper technique for dressing changes and disposal of soiled dressings *to prevent spread of infection to other patients.*

continued

Nursing Implementation

Health Promotion and Maintenance. Although there is no method of preventing osteomyelitis, patients with artificial implants such as a total joint replacement or metallic bone implants should be educated about methods to prevent osteomyelitis. Some physicians recommend prophylactic doses of antibiotics for procedures such as teeth cleaning, colonoscopy, or vaginal exams.

Acute Intervention. The involved extremity should be handled carefully to avoid excessive manipulation, which increases pain and could possibly cause pathologic fracture. Various types of sterile dressings are used to contain the exudate from draining wounds. Besides protecting the wound area, dressings are also used as adjuncts in the mechanical debridement of devitalized tissue from the wound site when they are removed. Types of dressings used include dry, sterile dressings, dressings saturated in saline or antibiotic solution, and wet-to-dry dressings. Soiled dressings should be handled carefully to prevent cross-contamination of the wound or spread of the infection to other patients. When the dressing is changed, sterile technique is essential; it should always include sterile dressing sets, gloves, and surgical cap, gown, and mask to reduce wound contamination from external sources.

NURSING CARE PLAN Patient with Osteomyelitis—cont'd

Planning: Outcome Criteria	Nursing Interventions and Rationales
➤ **NURSING DIAGNOSIS**	Ineffective individual coping *related to* isolation, hospitalization, immobility, perceived powerlessness, and uncertain outcome *as manifested by* expressions of hopelessness; inability to concentrate on writing, reading, conversation; continual questioning of self-worth, withdrawal from others; misdirected anger; irritability; extreme dependency on others
Have optimistic attitude toward recovery; demonstrate effective coping strategies.	Assess coping skills *to determine adequacy or need to learn new skills.* Allow patient and family to participate in care and decision making *to increase their sense of control and ability to cope.* Encourage patient to verbalize concerns *to enable patient to recognize feelings and begin problem solving.* Keep patient informed of treatment plans and progress *to bolster coping by providing accurate information.* Teach healthy coping behaviors *so patient is better able to participate in decisions and cooperate in treatment plans.* Visit patient frequently and provide diversion *because recovery involves prolonged bed rest or limited activity, resulting in boredom.*
➤ **NURSING DIAGNOSIS**	Impaired physical mobility *related to* limited use of affected extremity secondary to pain and edema *as manifested by* inability or unwillingness to move purposefully within environment
Have consistent increase in mobility and range of motion with minimal pain or discomfort.	Assist patient as needed *to reduce patient's frustration with impaired mobility and prevent injury.* Increase mobility as ordered and tolerated *to maintain muscle function and strength.* Provide support and encouragement *to assist in coping with extended recovery.*
➤ **NURSING DIAGNOSIS**	Ineffective management of therapeutic regimen *related to* lack of knowledge regarding long-term management of osteomyelitis *as manifested by* verbalization of concern regarding home care by patient or family members, need to learn new knowledge or skills for home management
Verbalize confidence in self or caregiver's ability to carry out home management routine; demonstrate ability to perform necessary procedures such as sterile dressing changes.	Provide information and instruction regarding wound care, aseptic technique, and dressing disposal *to reduce risk of cross-contamination and encourage wound healing.* Review medication regimen, including schedule, name, dosage, purpose, and side effects, *because long-term antibiotic therapy is required.* Stress importance of proper diet, rest, physician follow-up, and physical rehabilitation *to facilitate wound healing and reduce risk of chronic osteomyelitis.*

COLLABORATIVE PROBLEMS

Nursing Goals	Nursing Interventions and Rationales
➤ **POTENTIAL COMPLICATION**	Pathologic fracture of involved bone *related to* presence of weakened necrotic bone
Monitor and report occurrence of pathologic fracture and initiate appropriate medical and nursing interventions.	Monitor patient for signs of pathologic fracture such as loss of function, increased pain, or abnormal positioning of involved bone *to determine appropriate interventions.* Administer antibiotics as ordered *to treat underlying osteomyelitis.* Provide patient with assistive device such as crutches if indicated *to relieve weight-bearing if lower extremity involved.* Maintain patient on bed rest if ordered *to decrease risk of pathologic fracture from ambulation activities.* Provide assistance with activities of daily living if indicated *to decrease use of involved extremity.*

IV, Intravenous.

Good body alignment and frequent position changes prevent complications associated with immobility and promote comfort. Flexion deformity, especially of the hip or knee, is a common sequela of osteomyelitis of the lower extremity because the patient frequently positions the affected extremity in a flexed position to promote comfort. This can cause the development of contracture, which may progress to a deformity. Foot drop can develop quickly in the lower extremity if the foot is not correctly supported. A splint is frequently applied to the involved extremity in an attempt to maintain immobilization, support, and comfort. The patient should be instructed to avoid any activities such as exercise or heat application that increase circulation and serve as stimuli to the spread of infection.

Patients are frightened and discouraged because of the serious nature of the disease, systemic symptoms, pain, and the length and cost of treatment. Continued psychologic support is an integral part of nursing management.

Chronic and Home Management. With the introduction of various intermittent venous access devices, IV antibiotics can be administered to the patient in a nursing home or home setting. If at home, the patient and family must be instructed on the proper care and management of the venous access device. They must also be taught how to administer the antibiotic. Periodic home nursing visits provide the family with a resource on correct technique, which relieves anxiety. If there is an open wound, dressing changes may be necessary. The patient may require supplies and instruction on the technique.

If the osteomyelitis becomes chronic, patients need physical and psychologic support for a prolonged period. They may become suspicious and hostile toward the care providers when treatment plans do not effect a cure. Well-informed patients are better able to participate in decisions and cooperate in treatment plans.

AMPUTATION

During the past 20 years, major advances have been made in surgical amputation techniques, prosthetic design, and rehabilitation programs. These advances are enabling amputees to return to productive and satisfying social roles. There are an estimated 400,000 amputees in the United States, with an annual increase of 20,000. The middle and older age groups have the highest incidence of amputation because of the effects of peripheral vascular disease, especially atherosclerosis and diabetes mellitus. Traumatic injury is the usual cause for amputation in the younger adult. Amputation is required more often in persons engaged in hazardous occupations. The incidence in men is greater, because men are more often involved in such occupations.

Clinical Indications

The clinical features that indicate the need for an amputation depend on the underlying diseases or traumas. Common indications for amputation include circulatory impairment resulting from a peripheral vascular disorder, traumatic and thermal injuries, malignant tumors, uncontrolled or widespread infection of the extremity, and congenital disorders. These conditions may manifest as loss of sensation, inadequate circulation, pallor, sweating, and local or systemic infection. Although pain is often present, it is not usually the primary reason for an amputation. The underlying problem dictates whether the amputation is performed as elective or emergency surgery.

Therapeutic Management

The types of diagnostic studies done depend on the underlying problem that makes the amputation necessary (Table 59-14). An elevated white blood cell (WBC) count is indicative of infection. Vascular studies such as arteriography provide information about circulatory status of the extremity. The potential for revascularization surgery rather than amputation can be assessed on the basis of vascular studies. If the amputation is considered to be "elective," the patient's general health is carefully monitored. Chronic illnesses and infection are monitored closely. The patient and family should be helped to understand the need for the amputation and be assured that rehabilitation can result in an active, useful life. If the amputation is done on an emergency basis as a result of trauma, the management is physically and emotionally more complicated.

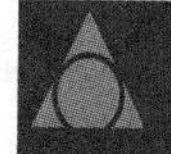

Table 59-14 Therapeutic Management: Amputation

Diagnostic
- Physical examination
  - Physical appearance of soft tissues
  - Skin temperature
  - Sensory function
  - Presence of peripheral pulses
- Arteriography
- Thermography
- Plethysmography
- Transcutaneous ultrasonic Doppler recordings

Therapeutic

Medical
- Appropriate management of underlying disease process
- Stabilization of trauma victim

Surgical
- Appropriate type of amputation, leaving as long a stump as possible
- Stump management
  - Immediate prosthetic fitting
  - Delayed prosthetic fitting

Rehabilitation
- Coordination of prosthesis-fitting and gait-training activities
- Coordination of muscle-strengthening and physical therapy regimens

The goal of amputation surgery is to preserve extremity length and function, while removing all infected or ischemic tissue. This improves the possibility of good prosthetic, cosmetic, and functional satisfaction. (Levels of amputation of upper and lower extremities are illustrated in Fig. 59-17.) The type of amputation depends on the reason for the surgery. A *closed amputation* is performed to create a weight-bearing stump; an anterior skin flap with dissected soft-tissue padding covers the bone stump. The skin flap is sutured posteriorly so it will not be positioned in a weight bearing area. Special care is necessary to prevent the accumulation of drainage, which can produce pressure and harbor infection. *Disarticulation* is an amputation performed through a joint. A Symes amputation is a form of disarticulation at the ankle.

An *open amputation* leaves a stump surface that is not covered with skin. This type of surgery is generally indicated for control of actual or potential infection. The wound

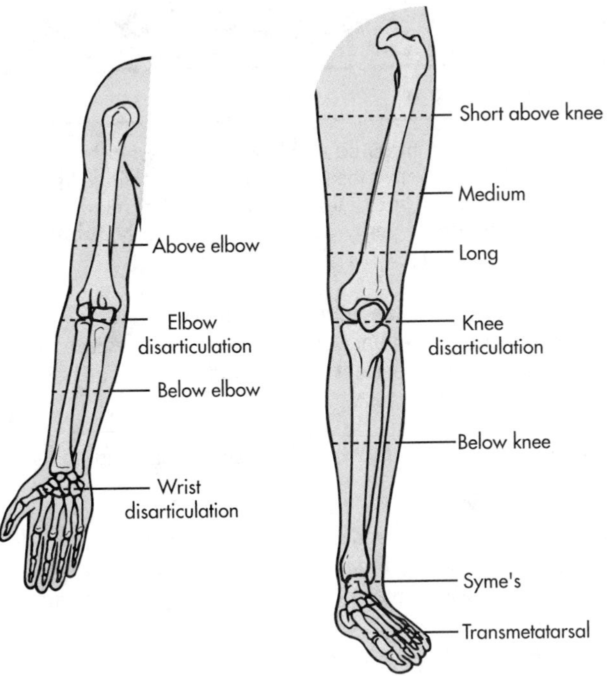

Fig. 59-17 Location and description of amputation sites of the upper and lower extremities.

is usually closed later by a second surgical procedure or closed by skin traction surrounding the stump. This type of amputation is often referred to as a *guillotine amputation.*

NURSING MANAGEMENT

AMPUTATION

Nursing Assessment

Preexisting illnesses must be adequately assessed because most amputations are performed because of neurologic and vascular problems. Assessment of the neurologic and vascular status is an important part of this assessment process (see Chapters 29 and 53).

Nursing Diagnoses

Nursing diagnoses are determined when the problem and etiologic factors are supported by clinical data. Nursing diagnoses related to the patient with an amputation include, but are not limited to, those presented in the nursing care plan for the patient with an amputation on p. 1876.

Planning

The overall goals are that the patient with an amputation will (1) have relief from the underlying health problem, (2) have satisfactory pain control, (3) reach maximal rehabilitation potential with the use of a prosthesis (if indicated), (4) cope with the body-image changes, and (5) make satisfying lifestyle adjustments.

Nursing Implementation

Health Promotion and Maintenance. Most lower-limb amputations result from peripheral vascular disease, and most upper-limb amputations result from severe trauma. This knowledge directs patient education related to prevention of amputation. Control of causative illnesses such as peripheral vascular disease, diabetes mellitus, chronic osteomyelitis, and skin ulcers can eliminate or delay the need for amputation. The patient with these problems must be taught to carefully examine the lower extremities daily for signs of potential problems. If the patient cannot assume this responsibility, a family member should be instructed in the procedure. The patient and family should be instructed to report problems such as change in skin color or temperature, decrease or absence of sensation, tingling, pain, or the presence of a lesion to the health care provider.

Instruction in proper safety precautions in recreation and in the performance of hazardous work is a nursing responsibility of major importance. Preventing limb mutilation and subsequent amputation is one of the serious consequences of trauma avoided through such instruction.

Acute Intervention. The nurse must recognize the tremendous psychologic and social implications of a lower-limb amputation for the patient. The disruption in body image caused by an amputation often causes a patient to go through psychologic stages similar to the grieving process of death. Allowing the patient to go through a period of depression and recognizing it as a normal consequence of the amputation may do much to aid the patient's acceptance of the amputation. The patient's family must also be helped to work through the process to arrive at a realistic and positive attitude about the future. The reasons for an amputation and the rehabilitation potential depend on age, diagnosis, occupation, personality, resources, and support systems.

Preoperative care. Before surgery, the nurse should reinforce information the patient and family have received about the reasons for the amputation, the proposed prosthesis, and the mobility training program. In addition to the usual preoperative instructions, the patient undergoing an amputation has special education needs. To meet these needs, the nurse must know the level of amputation, the type of postsurgical dressing to be applied, and the type of prosthesis planned. The patient should receive instruction in the performance of upper-extremity exercises such as push-ups in bed or in the wheelchair to promote arm strength. This is essential for later crutch walking and gait training. If possible, the nurse should instruct the patient in the technique of crutch walking and the type of gait that will be used after surgery and during gait training with the prosthesis. General postoperative nursing care should be discussed, including positioning, support, and stump care. If a compression bandage is to be used after surgery the patient should be instructed about its purpose and how it will be applied. If an immediate prosthesis is planned, the general ambulation program should be discussed.

The patient should be warned that there may be a feeling that the amputated limbs are still present after surgery. This *phantom sensation* (a sensation of aching, tingling, or itching of the amputated limb) usually disappears but may cause the patient grave concern unless there is a forewarning. If pain was present in the affected limb preoperatively,

NURSING CARE PLAN Patient with an Amputation

Planning: Outcome Criteria	Nursing Interventions and Rationales
➤ **NURSING DIAGNOSIS**	Body-image disturbance *related to* amputation and impaired mobility *as manifested by* verbalization of concerns about change in lifestyle, negative feelings about body, feelings of helplessness, hopelessness, powerlessness; change in social involvement or social relationships; preoccupation with loss of body part; refusal to verify actual change in body; refusal to touch or look at involved area
Accept changed body image; integrate changes into lifestyle.	Assess impact of amputation on body image to plan appropriate interventions. Provide psychologic support, active listening, and encouragement *to assist patient in integrating loss of limb into body image.* Assist patient to be as independent as possible *to prevent feelings of helplessness and dependence.*
➤ **NURSING DIAGNOSIS**	Risk for impaired skin integrity *related to* immobility, improperly fitting prosthesis, and underlying disease process
Have no evidence of skin breakdown.	Assess for signs of impaired skin integrity such as reddened skin area, verbalization of pain, discomfort, or altered sensation in area *to determine extent of problem and plan interventions.* Examine potential pressure areas regularly *to note development of pressure areas so prompt treatment can be initiated.* Use proper technique when wrapping stump *to foster shaping and modeling for eventual prosthesis fitting.* Turn and reposition q2hr and massage bony prominences *to prevent prolonged pressure on tissues and to increase circulation.*
➤ **NURSING DIAGNOSIS**	Pain *related to* phantom limb sensation, surgical procedure, and ineffective comfort measures *as manifested by* complaints of pain in amputated limb and at surgical site; altered time perception, behaviors indicative of pain such as moaning, crying, restlessness; altered muscle tone, autonomic responses
Have reduction or absence of pain; express satisfaction with pain relief.	Assess pain for location and severity *to plan appropriate interventions.* Administer analgesics as ordered *to relieve pain.* Apply transcutaneous electrical nerve stimulation unit *for relief of phantom limb pain.* Encourage position changes *to promote circulation and reduce edema and muscle spasm, which cause increase in pain.* Provide opportunities for distraction—direct attention to something away from the pain *to help patient cope with the pain.* Explain phantom limb sensation to patient *to reduce fears caused by sensation of aching, tingling, or itching in amputated limb.*
➤ **NURSING DIAGNOSIS**	Impaired physical mobility *related to* amputation of lower limb and decreased muscle strength secondary to immobility and surgery *as manifested by* inability to move purposefully within physical environment, limited joint range of motion, decreased muscle strength, mobility restrictions
Will become mobile within limitations imposed by site of amputation and state of health.	Assess patient's general health, coordination,and arm strength *to determine plan for mobility.* Teach gait-training principles *to enable safe crutch walking.* Adjust prosthesis as needed *to prevent irritation of the stump.* Teach patient upper-extremity exercises *to promote arm strength essential for later crutch walking and gait training.* Perform active or passive range-of-motion exercises on all joints *to maintain joint flexibility and prevent contractures.* Assist with exercises to increase strength in remaining extremities *to prepare and strengthen muscles for ambulation.*

continued

the patient may experience *phantom limb pain* postoperatively. The patient may have feelings of coldness and heaviness or cramping, shooting, burning, or crushing pain. Often the patient may be extremely anxious about this pain because the patient knows the limb is gone but still feels pain in it. Usually phantom limb pain goes away in time, although it can become chronic. The pain is a real sensation to the patient and interventions should be provided for relief. As recovery and ambulation progress, phantom limb sensation usually subsides.

NURSING CARE PLAN Patient with an Amputation—cont'd

Planning: Outcome Criteria	Nursing Interventions and Rationales
➤ **NURSING DIAGNOSIS**	Activity intolerance *related to* prolonged immobility, weakness, and fatigue *as manifested by* verbal reports of fatigue or weakness, abnormal physiologic responses to activity; reluctance to attempt ambulation
Have normal physiologic response to activity; express satisfaction with progression of activity.	Monitor patient's response to activity *to determine presence of abnormal response and plan appropriate interventions.* Encourage active range-of-motion exercise of joints *to maintain muscle strength and joint flexibility.* Perform resistive exercises for unaffected extremities *to develop strength and to learn balance of the altered body.* Plan progressive increase in activity with frequent rest periods *so patient is eventually able to resume preamputation activities.* Monitor vital signs during activity *as indicators of physiologic response to activity.* Encourage active participation in activities of daily living and exercises *to promote independence and improve strength.* Provide positive support *to build confidence and promote healthy coping.*
➤ **NURSING DIAGNOSIS**	Risk for impaired physical mobility *related to* joint contractures secondary to prolonged flexed position and immobility
Have full range of motion of extremities.	Assess for malaligned stump, inability to move stump through full range of motion; improper positioning *to identify risk for contractures and plan interventions.* Plan regular range-of-motion exercises; perform passive or active exercises *to increase muscle strength and joint flexibility.* Position stump in correct alignment *to maintain joint flexibility and prevent contractures.* Instruct patient in exercise techniques *to foster cooperation, good technique, and regularity of exercise regimen.* Do not place stump on pillow after 24 hr postoperatively *to prevent hip or other joint contracture.* Assist patient to assume prone position 3-4 times/day with hip in extension position *to prevent hip flexion contracture.*
➤ **NURSING DIAGNOSIS**	Risk for trauma from falling *related to* change in center of balance, physical weakness, and impaired mobility secondary to amputation
Have no falls or other incidents of trauma.	Monitor for risks of falling such as impaired judgment, previous trauma, lack of safety precautions, inability to adapt to loss of limb *to determine extent of problem and plan interventions.* Teach patient gait-training principles *to allow safe mobility.* Offer assistance as needed *to encourage independence while providing safety.* Provide safe environment *to reduce risk of injury.* Teach muscle-strengthening exercises *to improve balance and strengthen muscles.*
➤ **NURSING DIAGNOSIS**	Ineffective individual coping *related to* effects of amputation on lifestyle *as manifested by* verbalization of inability to cope, anxiety, fear, anger, irritability, tension; inability to meet role expectations; altered social participation; ineffective or inappropriate use of defense mechanisms; change in usual communication patterns; excess food intake, alcohol consumption, smoking; digestive, appetite disturbance; chronic fatigue or disturbance in sleep pattern
Not develop chronic sick-role behavior; use positive coping strategies.	Explain factors that may contribute to development of maladaptive coping behavior *to assist patient in learning effective coping skills.* Describe and role-play use of therapeutic coping skills *to enhance self-esteem and social interaction.*
➤ **NURSING DIAGNOSIS**	Ineffective management of therapeutic regimen *related to* prolonged rehabilitation and care needs *as manifested by* frequent questioning or inaccurate knowledge about care for stump and ambulation plan.
Have uneventful postdischarge recovery; have no problems with healing stump.	Teach patient to assess stump site daily *to detect developing problems;* report problems to physician *so treatment can be initiated promptly.* Teach patient proper stump and stocking care *to prevent skin breakdown.* Advise patient to discontinue use of prosthesis if redness or skin irritation develops at stump site *to prevent further skin breakdown*; advise regular fit check and prothesis check by prosthetist *to ensure proper fit.* Provide instruction to patient and family regarding ambulation, prevention of contractures, and exercise *to promote satisfactory long-term rehabilitation.*

Postoperative care. General postoperative care for the patient who has had an amputation depends largely on the patient's general state of health, the reason for the amputation, and the patient's age. Nursing care must be individualized on the basis of these factors. For example, an older adult patient needs particularly careful monitoring of respiratory status; a victim of a motor vehicle accident may need careful neurologic monitoring.

Prevention or detection of complications are important nursing responsibilities during the postoperative period. Careful monitoring of the patient's vital signs and dressing can alert the nurse to hemorrhage in the operative area. Careful attention to sterile technique during dressing changes reduces the potential for wound infection and subsequent interruption of rehabilitation.

If an immediate postoperative prosthesis has been applied, the nurse must monitor vital signs carefully because the surgical site is heavily covered and may not be visible. A surgical tourniquet must always be available for emergency use. If hemorrhage occurs, the surgeon should be notified immediately and efforts to control the hemorrhage should begin at once.

The surgeon must decide the type of prosthetic fitting that will be used after surgery. An *immediate prosthetic fitting*, often called the *immediate postsurgical fitting* or the *immediate postoperative fitting*, is done in the operating room after the amputation (Fig. 59-18). A rigid plastic bandage can be applied around the closed stump with prosthetic pylon and ankle-foot assembly. While the patient is still anesthetized, the prosthetic pylon and ankle-foot assembly are aligned and adjusted to provide smooth gait and to avoid excessive pressure on the stump area. A strap is placed on the proximal anterior surface of the rigid plaster bandage and attached to a waistband to prevent slippage. The main advantages of this device are reduction of edema and the psychologic benefit of early ambulation. A disadvantage is the inability to directly see the surgical site.

The *delayed prosthetic fitting* may be the best choice for certain patients. Patients who have had amputations above the knee or below the elbow, older adults, debilitated individuals, and those with infection usually have delayed prosthetic fittings. The appropriate time for use of a prosthesis depends on satisfactory healing of the stump and the general condition of the patient. A temporary prosthesis may be used for partial weightbearing once the sutures are removed. Barring any problems the patient can bear full weight on a permanent prosthesis by approximately 3 months after amputation.

Not all patients are candidates for a prosthesis. It is important that the surgeon discuss ambulation possibilities frankly with the patient and family. The seriously ill or debilitated patient may not have the energy required to use a prosthesis. Mobility with a wheelchair may be the most realistic goal for this type of patient.

Therapeutic management also includes the direction and coordination of the rehabilitation program for the amputee. Success depends on the physical and emotional health of the patient. Chronic illness and debilitation complicate aggressive rehabilitation efforts.

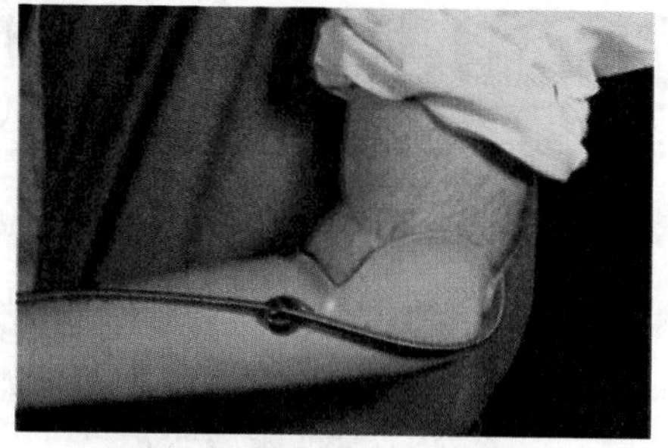

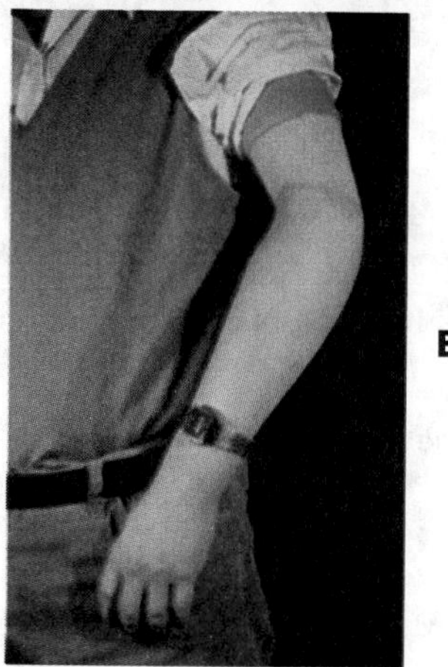

Fig. 59-18 Two types of prosthesis. ***A,*** Traditional fiberglass. ***B,*** New materials and techniques have made possible fabrication of prosthetic sockets that are light, soft, flexible, and secure.

Flexion contractures may delay the rehabilitation process. The most common and debilitating contracture is hip flexion. Hip adduction contracture is rare. Patients should avoid sitting in a chair with hips flexed or having pillows under the surgical extremity for long intervals to prevent flexion contractures. Unless specifically contraindicated, patients should lie on their abdomens for 30 minutes three to four times each day and position the hip in extension while prone.

Proper stump bandaging fosters shaping and modeling for eventual prosthesis fitting (Fig. 59-19). The physician usually orders a compression bandage to be applied immediately after surgery to support the soft tissues, reduce edema, hasten healing, minimize pain, and promote stump shrinkage and maturation. This bandage may be an elastic roll applied to the stump or a stump shrinker—an elastic stocking that fits over the stump and lower trunk area.[27] The compression bandage is initially worn at all times except during physical therapy and bathing. The bandage is taken off and reapplied several times daily, and care is taken so that it is applied snugly but not so tight as to interfere with circulation. Shrinker bandages should be washed and changed daily. After the stump has matured, it is bandaged only when the patient is not wearing the prosthesis. The patient should be instructed to avoid dangling the stump over the bedside to minimize edema formation.

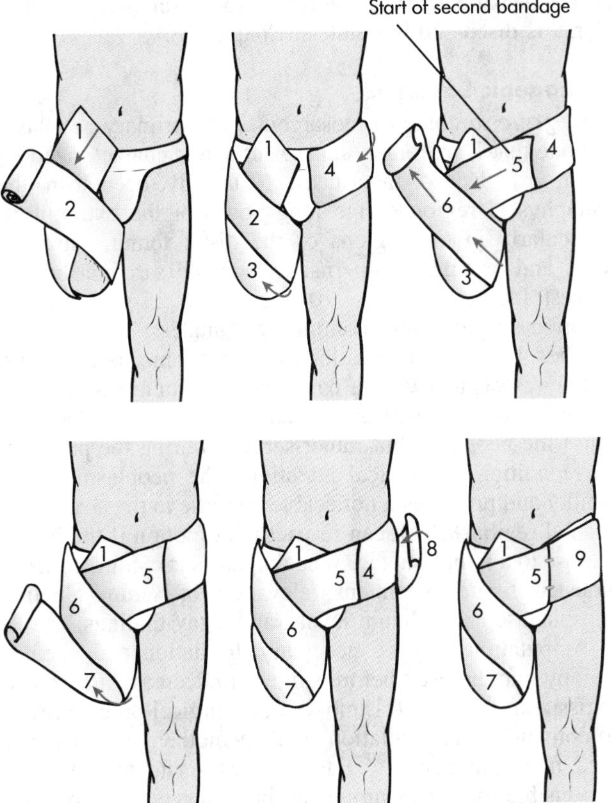

Fig. 59-19 Stump bandaging for the above-the-knee stump. Figure-eight style covers progressive areas of stump. Two bandages are required.

As the patient's overall condition improves, the nurse begins instruction in the principles and techniques of transferring from bed to chair and back. Active exercises and conditioning are essential in developing ambulation skills. The exercise regimen is normally started under the supervision of the physician and the physical therapist. The nurse must have a clear understanding of the exercise regimen to reinforce it and ensure that the exercises are performed correctly. Active range-of-motion exercises of all joints should be started as soon after surgery as the patient's pain level and medical status permit. In preparation for mobility, the patient should increase triceps strength, shoulder depressors, and lower-limb support and should learn balance of the altered body. The loss of the weight of a limb requires adaptation of the patient's proprioceptive mechanisms to prevent falls and frustration.

Crutch walking is started as soon as the patient is physically able. If the patient has had immediate postsurgical fitting, orders related to weightbearing must be carefully followed to avoid disruption of the skin flap and delay of the training process. Initial periods of ambulation should not exceed 5 minutes to prevent dependent edema.

Before discharge, the patient and family need careful instruction related to stump care, ambulation, prevention of contractures, recognition of complications, exercise, and follow-up care. Table 59-15 outlines appropriate stump care.

Table 59-15 Patient Instruction for Stump Care

- Inspect the stump daily for signs of skin irritation, especially redness.
- Discontinue use of the prosthesis if an irritation develops. Have the area checked before resuming use of the prosthesis.
- Wash thoroughly each night with warm water and a bacteriostatic soap. Rinse thoroughly and dry gently. Expose the stump to air for 20 min.
- Do not use any substance such as lotions, alcohol, powders, or oil unless prescribed by the physician.
- If a stump sock is worn, wear only the one supplied by the prosthetist. Change daily. Launder in a mild soap, squeeze, and lay flat to dry.

Rehabilitative Management. When the stump has healed satisfactorily and is well molded, the patient is ready for a prosthesis fitting. Matching a patient with a suitable prosthesis involves many factors, including age, general health, intelligence, motivation, occupation, and finances. After the physician makes the recommendation, the patient is referred to a prosthetist, who initially makes a mold of the stump and measures landmarks for the fabrication of the prosthesis. The molded stump socket allows the stump to fit snugly into the prosthesis. The stump is covered with a stump sock to ensure good fit and prevent skin breakdown. The stump may continue to shrink, causing a loose fit, in which case a new socket has to be fabricated. The patient may need to have the prosthesis adjusted to prevent rubbing and friction between the stump and the socket. Excessive movement of a loose prosthesis can cause severe skin irritation and breakdown.

The prosthesis is fitted by the prosthetist, who may also train the amputee to use it. It is important for the nurse to be familiar with the training program to encourage and assist the patient. Learning to use a prosthesis is frustrating, and the patient may easily become discouraged. The nurse must continually offer support until the patient is able to manage alone.

Artificial limbs become an integral part of the patient's body image. Proper care ensures their long life and useful functioning. The patient should be instructed to clean the prosthesis socket daily with a mild soap and rinse thoroughly to remove irritants. The leather and metal parts of the prosthesis should not get wet. The patient should be encouraged to have regular maintenance of the prosthesis. Consideration of the condition of the shoe is also necessary. A badly worn shoe alters the gait and may cause damage to the prosthesis.

Chronic and Home Management. The long-term goal of returning to normal activity will not be achieved in the hospital setting. Referral to a community health nurse can foster optimal physical and emotional adjustment. The family should be instructed on ambulation, transfer techniques, and proper stump care.

Gerontologic Considerations

If a lower-limb amputation has been performed on an older adult, the patient's previous ability to ambulate may affect the extent of recovery. Use of a prosthesis requires a significant amount of energy for ambulation. An older adult whose general health is weakened by disorders such as cardiac or pulmonary problems may not be a candidate for prosthesis use. This patient's ability to ambulate will be very limited. If possible, this should be discussed with the patient and family before surgery so that realistic expectations can be set.

Special Considerations in Upper-Limb Amputation

The emotional implications of an upper-limb amputation are often more devastating than those for lower-limb amputation. The enforced dependency brought about by one-handedness is both frustrating and humiliating to many patients. Because most upper-extremity amputations result from trauma, the patient has also not had the opportunity to adjust psychologically to an amputation or to participate in the decision-making process.

Both immediate and delayed prosthetic fittings are possible for the below-the-elbow amputee. Prosthetic fitting is delayed for the above-the-elbow amputee. The usual functional prosthesis is the arm and hook. A cosmetic hand is available but has limited functional value. As with the lower-limb prosthesis, patient motivation and endurance are major factors in a satisfactory outcome.

BONE CANCER

Primary malignant bone neoplasms are rare in adults and account for less than 1% of all deaths attributed to cancer. They are characterized by their rapid metastasis and bone destruction. Primary neoplasms occur most frequently during childhood through young adulthood.

Multiple Myeloma

In adults, multiple myeloma (plasma cell myeloma) is the most frequently occurring primary tumor arising in bone. It is a malignant neoplasm of plasma cells causing widespread infiltration and destruction of bone marrow and cortex, which produces osteolytic lesions throughout the skeletal system. The most commonly involved bones are those with active marrow, such as the axial skeleton, sternum, ribs, spine, clavicles, skull, pelvis, and long bones.[28]

Back pain, anemia, thrombocytopenia, and bleeding tendencies are common. The diagnosis of multiple myeloma is confirmed by biopsy or bone marrow aspiration. The overall prognosis is poor because by the time diagnosis has been confirmed, the disease has usually invaded the axial skeleton. Chemotherapeutic treatment of multiple myeloma has limited usefulness; it is primarily directed toward suppressing plasma cell growth. Steroids are commonly used in conjunction with melphalen and cyclophosphamide and increase the patient's susceptibility to infection. (Multiple myeloma is discussed in detail in Chapter 28.)

Osteogenic Sarcoma

Osteogenic sarcoma (osteosarcoma) is a primary neoplasm of bone that is extremely malignant and is characterized by rapid growth and metastasis. It usually occurs in the metaphyseal region of the long bones of the extremities, particularly in the regions of the distal femur, proximal tibia, and proximal humerus. Osteogenic sarcoma has its highest incidence in the 10-year-old to 25-year-old age group and occurs most commonly in males.

The clinical manifestations of osteogenic sarcoma are usually associated with a past history of minor injury and gradual onset of pain and swelling. The injury does not cause the neoplasm but rather serves to bring the preexisting condition to medical attention. The neoplasm grows rapidly and produces a noticeable increase in the size of the general region, which can restrict joint motion if the lesion is close to a joint structure. The diagnosis is confirmed from biopsied tissue specimens, elevation of serum alkaline phosphatase and calcium levels, and x-ray findings.

Amputation may be necessary. Radiation and chemotherapy may be used before surgery to decrease tumor size or tissue involvement. Limb-salvage surgical procedures in combination with radiation and chemotherapy are being used more frequently.[29] Early metastasis to the lungs is responsible for a poor prognosis and a survival rate of 15% to 20%.

Osteoclastoma

True *osteoclastoma* (giant cell tumor) is a malignant, destructive neoplasm that arises in the cancellous ends of long bones in young adults. Some variant giant cell tumors that have been put in this class of neoplasm are usually benign. Giant cell tumors most commonly occur between the ages of 20 and 35. The common sites are the distal ends of the femur, proximal tibia, and distal radius. The giant cell tumor is a locally destructive lesion, the growth of which extends from a few months to several years. The clinical manifestations are usually swelling, local pain, and some disturbances in joint function. X-ray evidence of giant cell tumor is variable but usually reveals local areas of bone destruction and eventual expansion of the bone ends. Treatment initially includes biopsy to establish the diagnosis, followed by surgical curettage of the lesion with bone grafting. After treatment there is a greater than 50% chance of recurrence. Recurrent giant cell tumors may subsequently make amputation necessary. Advances in chemotherapy have improved the rate of survival.

Ewing's Sarcoma

Ewing's sarcoma is the third most common primary malignant neoplasm of bone, occurring most frequently in male patients under age 30. This neoplasm is characterized by rapid growth within the medullary cavity of long bone, especially the femur, pelvis, tibia, and ribs, and early metastasis. The most frequent site of metastasis is the lungs. Ewing's sarcoma has a poor prognosis, with a survival rate estimated at only 5%. Common manifestations are progressive local pain, swelling, palpable soft-tissue mass, noticeable increase in size of the affected part, fever, and leukocytosis. Initially, x-rays show periosteal bone destruction. Treatment usually involves radiation therapy and surgical resection or amputation. Chemotherapeutic agents commonly used are cyclophosphamide (Cytoxan), dactinomycin, vincristine (Oncovin), methotrexate, ifosfamide, and doxorubicin (Adriamycin). New chemotherapeutic drugs hold promise of improvement in survival rates. Surgical resection of the tumor may also help decrease the rate of recurrence.

Metastatic Lesions

The most common type of malignant bone tumor occurs as a result of metastasis from a primary tumor. Common sites for the primary tumor include the breast, intestinal tract, lungs, prostate, kidney, ovary, and thyroid. The metastatic lesion is commonly found in the spine, pelvis, femur, humerus, or ribs. Pathologic fractures at the site of metastasis are common because of weakening of the involved bone.

Once a primary lesion has been identified, bone scans are often done to detect the presence of metastatic lesions before they are visible on x-ray. Treatment is palliative and consists of pain management and radiation. Prognosis is poor.

NURSING MANAGEMENT

CANCER OF THE BONE

Nursing Assessment

The patient with bone cancer should be assessed for the location and severity of pain. Weakness caused by anemia and increased debility may also be noted. Swelling at the involved site and decreased joint function, depending on the tumor site, should also be monitored.

Nursing Diagnoses

Nursing diagnoses related to the patient with bone cancer include, but are not limited to, the following:

- Pain related to disease process, inadequate pain or comfort measures
- Impaired physical mobility related to disease process, pain, weakness and debility
- Body-image disturbance related to possible amputation, deformity, swelling, effects of chemotherapy
- Anticipatory grieving related to poor prognosis of the disease
- Risk for injury: pathologic fracture related to disease process and inadequate handling or positioning of affected body part

Planning

The overall goals are that the patient with cancer of the bone will (1) have satisfactory pain relief, (2) maintain preferred activities as long as possible, (3) accept body image changes resulting from chemotherapy, radiation, and surgery, (4) be free from injury, and (5) have a realistic idea of disease progression and prognosis.

Nursing Implementation

Health Promotion and Maintenance. The nurse should teach the public to recognize the warning signs of bone cancer, including swelling, bone pain of unexplained origin, limitation of joint function, and changes in skin temperature. As with all forms of cancer, health promotion should stress the importance of periodic health examinations.

Acute Intervention. Nursing care of the patient with a malignant bone neoplasm does not differ significantly from the care given to the patient with a malignant disease of any other body system. However, special attention is required to reduce the complications associated with prolonged bed rest and to prevent pathologic fractures. The patient is often reluctant to participate in therapeutic activities because of weakness and fear of pain. Regular rest periods should be provided between activities. Careful handling of the affected extremity is important to prevent pathologic fractures.

Chronic and Home Management. The nurse must be able to assist the patient in accepting the guarded prognosis associated with neoplasms of the bone. Inability to accomplish age-specific developmental tasks can increase the frustrations with this condition. General principles related to cancer nursing are applicable (see Chapter 12). Special attention is necessary for the problems of pain and dysfunction, chemotherapy, and specific surgery such as spinal cord decompression or amputation.

LOW BACK PAIN

Etiology and Pathogenesis

Low back pain is common and has probably affected every adult at least once. In industry, low back pain is responsible for more lost working hours than any other medical condition and represents one of the nation's costliest health problems. Each year about 18 million visits are made to physicians for treatment of this condition.

Several risk factors are associated with low back pain, including smoking, low educational level, and tension and anxiety. Jobs that require repetitive heavy lifting, vibration (such as a jackhammer operator), and extended periods of driving are also associated with low back pain.[30]

Pain in the lumbar region is a common problem because this area (1) bears most of the weight of the body, (2) is the most flexible region of the spinal column, (3) contains nerve roots that are vulnerable to injury or disease, and (4) has an inherently poor biomechanical structure.

Low back pain is most often caused by a musculoskeletal problem. However, other causes, such as metabolic, circulatory, gynecologic, urologic, or psychologic problems, which may refer pain to the lower back, must not be overlooked. The causes of low back pain of musculoskeletal origin include (1) acute lumbosacral strain, (2) instability of lumbosacral bony mechanism, (3) osteoarthritis of the lumbosacral vertebrae, (4) intervertebral disk degeneration, and (5) herniation of the intervertebral disk. Of these, the most common cause is mechanical strain of paravertebral muscles. Herniation of the nucleus pulposus is another common cause of low back pain.

Acute Low Back Pain

Acute low back pain is usually associated with some type of activity that causes undue stress on the tissues of the lower back. Often symptoms do not appear at the time of injury but develop later because of gradual buildup of paravertebral muscle spasms. Few definitive diagnostic abnormalities are present with paravertebral muscle strain. The straight-leg-raise test may produce pain in the lumbar area without radiation along the sciatic nerve.

Therapeutic Management. If the muscle spasms are not severe, the patient may be treated on an outpatient basis with a combination of the following: (1) analgesics, (2) nonsteroidal antiinflammatory drugs (NSAIDs), (3) muscle relaxants, and (4) use of a corset.[31] A corset prevents rotation, flexion, and extension of the lower back.

If the spasms and pain are severe, a period of hospitalization may be necessary. Because paravertebral muscle spasms are worse when the patient is upright, bed rest is the prime treatment for acute low back pain. Bathroom privileges are usually allowed. Bed rest is maintained until the patient can move and turn from side to side with minimal discomfort. At this time, activity is gradually increased. Bed rest may last for 5 to 10 days. When the patient is comfortable on oral pain medication, the patient is discharged to continue bed rest and activity restrictions at home.

If conservative treatment is ineffective and the cause of the pain is nerve root irritation, an *epidural steroid injection* may be performed. A needle is inserted into the epidural space under fluoroscopy and steroid and a local anesthetic are injected. Epidural steroids have been shown to decrease pain, speed return of function, and improve objective neurologic signs. These injections are most effective in patients with acute rather than chronic pain and patients with radicular pain who are not candidates for surgery. Epidural injections typically consist of a series of one to three injections over a span of several days to several weeks.

NURSING MANAGEMENT

ACUTE LOW BACK PAIN

Nursing Assessment

Subjective and objective data that should be obtained from the patient with low back pain are summarized in Table 59-16.

Table 59-16 Nursing Assessment: Low Back Pain

Subjective Data

Important health information

Past health history: Acute or chronic lumbosacral strain, osteoarthritis, degenerative disk disease, obesity, occupational risk factors

Medications: Use of analgesics, muscle relaxants, nonsteroidal antiinflammatory drugs, corticosteroids, over-the-counter remedies

Surgery: Previous back surgery, epidural injections

Functional health patterns

Activity-exercise: Poor posture; muscle spasms; activity restrictions; relationship of pain to activity

Cognitive-perceptual: Pain in back, buttocks, or leg associated with walking, turning, straining, coughing, leg raising; numbness or tingling of legs, feet, toes

Objective Data

General

Guarding

Neurologic

Depressed or absent Achilles tendon reflex

Musculoskeletal

Tense, tight paravertebral muscles on palpation, decreased range of motion of spine

Possible findings

Localization of site of lesion on myelogram and CT scan, determination of muscular disorder on electromyography

CT, Computed tomography.

Nursing Diagnoses

Nursing diagnoses are determined when the problem and etiologic factors are supported by clinical data. Nursing diagnoses related to low back pain include, but are not limited to, those presented in the nursing care plan for the patient with low back pain on p. 1884.

Planning

The overall goals are that the patient with low back pain will (1) have satisfactory pain relief, (2) avoid constipation secondary to medication and immobility, (3) learn back-sparing practices, and (4) return to previous level of activity within prescribed restrictions.

Nursing Implementation

Health Promotion and Maintenance. The nurse is a significant role model and teacher for patients with low back problems. As a role model, the nurse should use proper body mechanics at all times. This should be a primary consideration when teaching patients and care providers transfer and turning techniques. The nurse should assess the patient's use of body mechanics and offer advice when activities that could produce back strain are used (Table 59-17).

Some physicians refer patients with back pain to a program called "Back School." It is a formal program usually taught by health professionals such as physicians, nurses, and physical therapists. It is designed to teach the patient how to minimize back pain and avoid repeat episodes of low back pain. The five keys to prevention of back injury advocated by the Back School are listed in Table 59-18.

Patients are also advised to maintain appropriate weight. Excess body weight places extra stress on the lower back and weakens the abdominal muscles that support the lower back.

The position assumed while sleeping is also important in preventing low back pain. Sleeping in a prone position should be avoided because it produces excessive lumbar lordosis, placing excessive stress on the lower back. A firm

Table 59-17 Patient Instructions for Low Back Problems

Do Not

- Lean forward without bending knees
- Lift anything above level of elbows
- Stand in one position for prolonged time
- Sleep on abdomen or on back or side with legs out straight
- Exercise without consulting health care provider if patient has severe pain
- Exceed prescribed amount and type of exercises without consulting health care provider

Do

- Prevent lower back from straining forward by placing a foot on a step or stool during prolonged standing
- Sleep in a side-lying position with knees and hips bent
- Sleep on back with a lift under knees and legs or on back with 10-inch-high pillow under knees to flex hips and knees
- Sit in a chair with knees higher than hips and support arms on chair or knees
- Exercise 15 min in the morning and 15 min in the evening regularly; begin exercises with a 2- or 3-min warm-up period by moving arms and legs, by alternately relaxing and tightening muscles; exercise slowly with smooth movements as directed by a physical therapist
- Avoid chilling during and after exercising
- Maintain appropriate body weight
- Use a lumbar roll or pillow for sitting

Table 59-18 Five Keys to Prevention of Back Injury

1. **Posture**
   The reason for most strains and sprains to the back is overstretching of the supportive structures. Stretching occurs when the lower back is bowed out. In order to prevent strain, the lower back must maintain its normal position or posture at all times.
2. **Lifting**
   Most back injuries occur while lifting. Mastering the proper techniques will prevent this type of injury.
3. **Body Mechanics**
   Reaching and staying in one position for prolonged period are dangerous for the spine. Learning how to hold the spine properly reduces the danger of these activities.
4. **Rest**
   Proper rest is vital to the maintenance and function of a healthy back.
5. **Exercise**
   Proper exercise is an important part of the prevention of back injury, with the goal of maintaining mobility and strength in the back. Daily exercise should be a lifelong routine activity.

Modified from *Back Facts*, American Back School, PO Box 193, Ashland, KY 41105-1193.

mattress is recommended. The patient should sleep in either a supine or side-lying position with the knees and hips flexed to prevent unnecessary pressure on support muscles, ligamentous structures, and lumbosacral joints.

Acute Intervention. The primary nursing responsibilities in acute low back pain are to assist the patient to maintain bed rest, promote comfort, and educate the patient about the disease process. Whether the patient is at home or hospitalized, measures to ensure bed rest should be enforced. Other nursing interventions are summarized in the care plan. Use of analgesics, nonsteroidal antiinflammatory agents, and muscle relaxants to promote comfort is incorporated into the plan of care.

Muscle-strengthening exercises may be part of the management plan. Although the actual exercises are often taught by the physical therapist, it is the nurse's responsibility to ensure that the patient understands the type and frequency of exercise prescribed, as well as the rationale for the program.

Chronic and Home Management. The goal of management is to make an episode of acute low back pain an isolated incident. If the lumbosacral mechanism is unstable, repeated episodes can be anticipated. The lumbosacral spine may be unable to meet the demands placed on it without strain because of factors such as obesity, poor posture, poor muscular support, advancing age, or local trauma. Intervention is aimed at strengthening the supporting muscles by exercise and use of a corset to limit extremes of movement. In addition, weight reduction decreases the mechanical demands on the lower back.

Persistent use of poor body mechanics may result in repeated episodes of low back pain. If the strain is work-related, occupational counseling may be necessary. The frustration, pain, and disability imposed on the patient with low back pain require emotional support and understanding care by the nurse.

Chronic Low Back Pain

Pathophysiology. The causes of chronic low back pain include degenerative disk disease, lack of physical exercise, obesity, structural and postural abnormalities, and systemic disease. Structural degeneration of the intervertebral disk results in degenerative disk disease manifested by low back pain. This degeneration can also occur in the cervical spine area. The degeneration results in intervertebral narrowing and a lessening of the efficiency of the intervertebral disks in acting as shock absorbers. This inefficiency causes small tears in the annulus fibrosis, which predisposes the patient to herniated nucleus pulposus. As the stresses on the degenerated disk continue and eventually exceed the strength of the disk, herniation of the intervertebral disk may result. Nuclear material from the intervertebral disk herniates, causing compression or tension on a lumbar or sacral spinal nerve root (Fig. 59-20).

NURSING CARE PLAN Patient with Low Back Pain

Planning: Outcome Criteria	Nursing Interventions and Rationales
ACUTE MANAGEMENT	
➤ **NURSING DIAGNOSIS**	Acute pain *related to* specific physical problem, muscle spasms, and ineffective comfort measures *as manifested by* verbalization of back pain on movement; guarded movements; altered time perception; behaviors indicative of pain such as moaning, crying, restlessness; altered muscle tone, autonomic responses; palpable muscle spasm; decreased physical activity
Have reduction or absence of pain and muscle spasms; express satisfaction with pain relief.	Assess location, severity, and circumstances of pain *to plan appropriate interventions.* Enforce bed rest *to reduce paravertebral muscle spasms and resulting pain.* Keep head of bed elevated 20 degrees and knee of bed flexed *to promote comfort by relaxing back muscles.* Maintain pelvic traction, correctly aligned, as ordered *to reduce muscle spasm.* Examine skin for pressure over iliac crest *because the belt for pelvic traction rests on iliac crests and can cause skin breakdown and pain.* Apply moist heat to lower back *to reduce pain and muscle spasm.* Administer analgesics or muscle relaxants as ordered; document effect *to promote comfort and evaluate effectiveness.*
➤ **NURSING DIAGNOSIS**	Impaired physical mobility *related to* pain and muscle spasms *as manifested by* limited active joint range of motion, movement restrictions
Have unrestricted gait; ambulate within normal limits; resume previous level of mobility.	Have patient perform range-of-motion and muscle-strengthening exercises daily *to strengthen the supporting muscles and maintain all joints in normal range of motion.* Start ambulation program and progress with assistance *to promote gradual and progressive return to previous mobility level.* Avoid having patient bend, sit, or lift *to prevent back strain and increased pain.* Report leg or back pain and change in sensation *because these are indicators of severe lumbosacral intravertebral pressure and sciatic nerve involvement.*
➤ **NURSING DIAGNOSIS**	Constipation *related to* immobility, inadequate fluids and fiber, and pain medications *as manifested by* reduced frequency of bowel movement, hard stools, decrease in quantity, palpable rectal mass, report of feeling of pressure on rectum, abdominal cramps, impaired appetite, nausea
Have regular bowel movements, no pain associated with straining.	Assess bowel regularity and character of stools *to determine extent of problem and plan appropriate interventions.* Provide high-bulk, high-fiber diet *to promote peristalsis and increase fecal mass.* Administer stool softeners as ordered *to promote soft stool by permitting water to be absorbed by fecal matter in bowel.* Monitor bowel movements *to evaluate patient's response to treatment.* Maintain adequate hydration; monitor fluid intake *to ensure adequate intake to provide soft stools.* Encourage ambulation as allowed *to stimulate peristalsis.*
CHRONIC MANAGEMENT	
➤ **NURSING DIAGNOSIS**	Chronic pain *related to* progression of problem to chronic state *as manifested by* verbal report or evidence of pain >6 mo in duration, fear of reinjury, physical and social withdrawal, altered ability to continue previous activities, weight changes, anorexia, changes in sleep pattern
Develop effective methods of managing pain; express satisfaction with pain control measures.	Assess variety and effectiveness of pain management techniques *to determine extent of problem and develop appropriate interventions.* Instruct patient and family about home care and alternative methods of pain control, including use of heat, transcutaneous electrical nerve stimulation, and massage *to provide information about supplementary methods of pain management.* Avoid strenuous activities *that increase pain.* Assist in identifying activities that exacerbate pain *to make adjustments in lifestyle so that pain is reduced.*

continued

NURSING CARE PLAN Patient with Low Back Pain—cont'd

Planning: Outcome Criteria	Nursing Interventions and Rationales
➤ **NURSING DIAGNOSIS**	Ineffective individual coping *related to* effects of chronic pain on lifestyle *as manifested by* verbalization of inability to cope, anxiety, fear, anger, irritability, tension; inability to meet role expectations; altered participation in social events; ineffective or inappropriate use of defense mechanisms; change in usual communication patterns; excess food intake, alcohol consumption, smoking; digestive, bowel, appetite disturbances; chronic fatigue or sleep-pattern disturbance
Not develop chronic sick-role behavior.	Explain factors that may contribute to development of maladaptive coping behavior *to communicate information and a caring attitude.* Explain how to develop therapeutic coping skills and activities that enhance self-esteem and social interaction *to foster effective coping behaviors and adjustment to chronic-pain condition.* Discuss chronic nature of pain and need for lifestyle adjustments with patient *to avoid repeated and demoralizing attempts to eliminate pain.*
➤ **NURSING DIAGNOSIS**	Ineffective management of therapeutic regimen *related to* lack of knowledge regarding posture, body mechanics, and weight reduction *as manifested by* lack of necessary knowledge to participate in treatment plan, inadequate understanding or inaccurate follow-through of previous instructions
Use of proper body mechanics at all times; maintain weight within normal limits; maintain activity and ambulation appropriate to age and state of health.	Assess body mechanics *to identify incorrect techniques and intervene appropriately.* Instruct patient on proper body mechanics and use of firm mattress or bedboard *to reduce risk of reinjury, provide back support, and maintain proper body alignment.* Assess for development of joint contracture or instability and decreasing muscle strength *to identify complications and modify care plan.* Refer to physical therapist for low back exercises *to develop abdominal and paravertebral muscle strength to provide increased support.* Encourage activity and ambulation within limitations *to maintain physical mobility and minimize sick-role behaviors.* Maintain patient's position of correct anatomic alignment *to reduce muscle spasm and strain.* Teach about weight reduction if indicated *because increased abdominal weight puts strain on low back.*
➤ **NURSING DIAGNOSIS**	Body-image disturbance *related to* impaired mobility and chronic pain *as manifested by* concern about change in lifestyle, negative feelings about body, change in social involvement or relationships; feelings of helplessness, hopelessness, powerlessness
Have positive self-concept and positive attitude about self; continue participation in meaningful activities.	Provide psychologic support, active listening, and encouragement *to prevent development of negative body image.* Assist patient in becoming as independent as possible *to prevent assumption of sick-role behavior.*

Clinical Manifestations. The most characteristic feature of a lumbar herniated intervertebral disk is back pain with associated buttock and leg pain along the distribution of the sciatic nerve. (Specific manifestations based on the level of lumbar disk herniation are summarized in Table 59-19.) The straight-leg-raise test may be positive. Back or leg pain may be reproduced by raising the leg and flexing the foot at 90 degrees. Low back pain from other causes may not be accompanied by leg pain.

Reflexes may be depressed or absent, depending on the spinal nerve root involved, and numbness or tingling in the toes and feet may be felt by the patient. If the disk ruptures in the cervical area, the clinical manifestations are stiff neck, shoulder pain radiating to the hand, and paresthesias and sensory disturbances of the hand.

Diagnostic Studies. Plain x-rays are done to note any structural defects. A myelogram, MRI, or CT scan is helpful in localizing the site of herniation. A diskogram may be necessary if other methods of diagnosis are unsuccessful. An electromyogram (EMG) of the lower extremities can be performed to determine the severity of nerve irritation caused by herniation (see Table 59-19). Low back pain from other causes may not be accompanied by leg pain.

Therapeutic Management. Degenerative disk disease is managed conservatively with pelvic traction, rest,

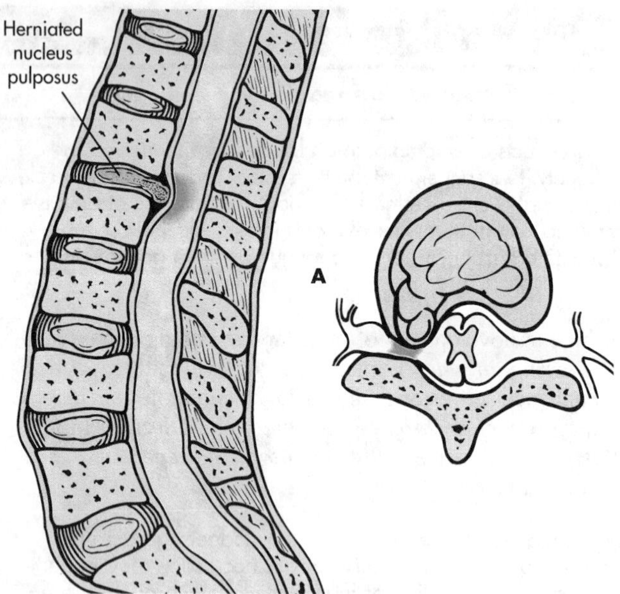

Fig. 59-20 Compression of spinal cord caused by herniation of nucleus pulposus into spinal cord. ***A,*** Pressure on nerves as they leave the spinal canal.

limitation of extremes of spinal movement (corset), local heat, ultrasound, transcutaneous electrical nerve stimulation, and NSAIDs.[31] If herniation of the disk occurs, more aggressive treatment is indicated (Table 59-20). Conservative treatment sometimes results in a healing over of the herniated area with a decrease in the pain of nerve-root irritation. Complete bed rest is often encouraged during this phase. Traction may be used to decrease muscle spasms. Once the symptoms subside, back-strengthening exercises are begun. The patient should be educated in principles of good body mechanics. Extremes of flexion and torsion are strongly discouraged. Most patients with herniated disks recover with a conservative treatment plan. However, if conservative treatment is unsuccessful, surgery may be indicated.

Surgical interventions. A *percutaneous diskectomy* is a surgical procedure using a tube that is passed through the retroperitoneal soft tissues to the lateral border of the disk with the aid of fluoroscopy. The herniated portion of the disk is shaved and removed in small portions.[32,33] No incision is made, only small stab wounds, and minimal blood loss occurs during a percutaneous diskectomy. The long-term effects of this procedure are being investigated.

A *diskectomy* is another type of surgical procedure that may be performed to decompress the nerve root. It involves the partial removal of the lamina. *Microsurgical diskectomy* is a version of the standard diskectomy in which the surgeon uses a microscope to allow better visualization of the disk and disk space during surgery to aid in the removal of the herniated portion.[31]

The traditional and most common procedure performed is a *laminectomy*. It involves the surgical excision of part of the posterior arch of the vertebra (referred to as the *lamina*) to gain access to part or all of the protruding disk to remove it. A laminectomy may be performed in combination with a diskectomy.

A *spinal fusion* may be performed if an unstable bony mechanism is present. The spine is stabilized by creating an ankylosis (fusion) of contiguous vertebrae with a bone graft from the patient's fibula or iliac crest or donated bone. If vertebral instability exists, metal fixation with rods, plates, or screws may be implanted at the time of spinal surgery to provide more stability and decrease vertebral motion.

RESEARCH

IMPLICATIONS FOR NURSING PRACTICE

REDUCTION OF BACK INJURY IN HEALTH CARE WORKERS

Citation Owen BD, Garg A: Back stress isn't part of the job, *Am J Nurs* 93:48-51, 1993.

Purpose To determine if reducing the physical demands of a job by altering the environment can reduce back stress.

Methods Phase 1 of the study analyzed the sources of back strain among 38 nurses' aids in a nursing home. Phase 2 of the study had the nurses' aids rate their perception of exertion/stress on the lower back using eight different techniques to reduce back stress.

Results and Conclusions Transferring wheelchair patients to and from the bed, the toilet, and the chair scale was rated as most stressful to the lower back. Using the different techniques to aid in transfers, the average rating of physical exertion dropped almost in half. Average compression force fell within the range of safety for most workers. There were significant decreases in back-injury rate following teaching of the interventions.

Implications for Nursing Practice Use of techniques such as a walking belt, patient hoist, and a wheelchair-ramp scale can greatly reduce back stress associated with common nursing activities such as transferring or bathing a patient. Teaching back care and body mechanics can further reduce back injury and subsequent pain and lost days at work.

NURSING MANAGEMENT

SPINAL SURGERY

Acute Intervention

Patients who have undergone spinal surgery require vigilant postoperative care. Nursing implementation is aimed at maintaining proper alignment of the spine at all times until healing has occurred. Flat bed rest may be maintained for 1 to 2 days depending on the extent of surgery. Logrolling patients when turning is essential to maintain proper body alignment. Pillows can be used under the thighs of each leg when supine and between the legs when in side-lying positions to provide comfort and ensure alignment.

Table 59-19 Neurologic Assessment of Lumbar Disk Herniation*

Intervertebral Level	Subjective Pain	Affected Reflex	Motor Function	Sensation
L3-L4	Back to buttocks to posterior thigh to inner calf	Patellar	Quadriceps, anterior tibialis	Inner aspect of lower leg, anterior part of thigh
L4-L5	Back to buttocks to dorsum of foot and big toe	None	Anterior tibialis, extensor halucis longus, gluteus medius	Dorsum of foot and big toe
L5-S1	Back to buttocks to sole of foot and heel	Achilles	Gastrocnemius, hamstring, gluteus maximus	Heel and lateral foot

*A disk herniation is occasionally so extensive that pressure on more than one nerve root results.

Severe muscle spasms in the surgical area can be managed with medication and with correct turning and positioning. The patient often fears turning or any movement that increases pain by straining the surgical area. The nurse must offer reassurance to the patient that proper technique is being used to maintain body alignment. Sufficient staff should be available to move the patient without undue pain or strain on staff members or the patient.

Because the spinal canal may be unintentionally entered during surgery, there is potential for spinal fluid leakage. Severe headache or leakage of spinal fluid should be reported immediately. Cerebrospinal fluid appears clear on the dressing. It has a high glucose concentration and will be positive for glucose when a dipstick test is done. The amount and characteristics of drainage should be noted by the nurse.

Frequent monitoring of neurologic signs is a routine postoperative nursing responsibility after spinal surgery. Movement of arms and legs and responses to tests of sensation should be unchanged when compared to the preoperative status. Table 59-21 summarizes a lumbar laminectomy check appropriate for the patient who has undergone back surgery. This check is repeated every 2 to 4 hours during the first 48 hours after surgery, and findings are compared with the preoperative assessment. Sensations such as numbness and tingling may not be relieved immediately after surgery. Any new muscle weakness or paresthesias should be documented and reported to the surgeon immediately.

Table 59-20 Therapeutic Management: Herniated Intervertebral Disk

Diagnostic
- History
- Physical examination with emphasis on neurologic deficits and straight leg raising
- CT scan
- MRI
- Myelogram
- Diskogram
- EMG
- Somatosensory evoked potential

Therapeutic

Conservative
- Absolute bed rest
- Medication
  - Analgesics
  - Antiinflammatory agents
  - Muscle relaxants
- Diathermy and local heat
- Pelvic traction

Surgical
- Laminectomy with or without spinal fusion
- Diskectomy
- Percutaneous lateral diskectomy
- Spinal fusion with or without instrumentation

CT, Computed tomography; *EMG,* electromyelogram; *MRI,* magnetic resonance imaging.

Table 59-21 Postoperative Assessment Following Lumbar Surgery

Sensation*
- Assess sensation of extremities.
- Assess for feelings of numbness and tingling.

Movement*
- Assess ability to move all extremities.

Muscle Strength*
- Assess for any motor weakness of the extremities.

Circulation
- Assess patient's extremities for pulse, warmth, color.

Wound
- Assess dressing for drainage and note amount, color, characteristics.

Pain
- Document location of the pain.
- Ask patient to rate the pain on a scale of 1 to 10, with *1* being no pain and *10* being worst pain.
- Evaluate pain after analgesia has been administered.

*Postoperative findings should be compared with preoperative assessments. It is not unusual for the patient to continue to experience these symptoms after surgery. Symptoms gradually decrease over several months.

Interference with bowel function may occur for several days and requires careful monitoring to prevent constipation and distention. Paralytic ileus can be evaluated by noting whether the patient is passing flatus, is nauseated, has a flat, soft abdomen, and has bowel sounds.

Adequate bladder emptying may be altered because of activity restrictions, narcotics, or anesthesia. It may require the use of a bedpan or urinal. If allowed by the surgeon, men should be encouraged to dangle or stand to urinate. Patients should use the commode or ambulate to the bathroom when allowed to promote adequate emptying of the bladder. The nurse should ensure that privacy is maintained. It is necessary to clarify whether the patient can be allowed up to the bathroom without the corset or brace. Intermittent catheterization or an indwelling catheter may be necessary for patients who have difficulty urinating.

Loss of sphincter tone or bladder tone may indicate nerve damage. Incontinence or difficulty evacuating the bowel or bladder must be monitored closely and reported to the surgeon.

Activity prescriptions vary with surgeons, but the patient who has had spinal surgery usually ambulates early in the postoperative period. It is a nursing responsibility to know the specific orders related to activity for any given patient.

In addition to the nursing care appropriate for a patient who has had a laminectomy, there are other nursing responsibilities if the patient has also had a spinal fusion. Because a bone graft is involved, the postoperative healing time is prolonged compared with that of a laminectomy. Immobilization over an extended time may be necessary. A rigid orthosis (thoracic-lumbar-sacral orthosis or chair-back brace) is often used during the period of immobilization. Some surgeons require that the patient be taught to put it on and take it off by logrolling in bed, whereas others allow their patients to apply the brace in a sitting or standing position. The nurse should verify the preferred method before initiating this activity. The extended immobilization required by a spinal fusion carries with it all the potential problems related to this inactive state.

In addition to the primary surgical site, the donor site for the bone graft must be regularly assessed. The donor site may cause greater postoperative pain than the fused area. The donor site is bandaged with a pressure dressing to prevent excessive bleeding. If the donor site is the fibula, neurovascular assessment of the extremity is a postoperative nursing responsibility.

Table 59-18 summarizes principles that should be reviewed with the patient before discharge from the hospital. Any restrictions on activity such as exercise should be clarified with the physician.

As the bone graft heals, the patient must adjust to the permanent immobility at the graft or fusion site. Instruction in proper body mechanics is essential and should be completed during the hospital stay.

Chronic and Home Management

The patient should be instructed to avoid sitting or standing for prolonged periods. Activities that should be encouraged include walking, lying down, and shifting weight from one foot to the other when standing. The patient should learn to mentally think through an activity before starting any potentially injurious task such as bending, lifting, or stooping. The thighs and knees, rather than the back, should be used to absorb the shock of activity and movement. A firm mattress or bedboard is essential.

NECK PAIN

Causes of neck pain are similar to those of low back pain. Patients have symptoms of neck pain and possible pain radiating into the arm and hand or numbness or tingling. Diagnosing the cause of neck pain is done by x-ray, MRI, CT scan, and myelogram. An EMG of the upper extremities is done to confirm cervical radiculopathy.

Types of surgery done on the neck are similar to those done on the lower back. These include a diskectomy, laminectomy, and a spinal fusion. If surgery is done on the cervical spine, the nurse must be alert for symptoms of cord edema such as respiratory distress and a worsening neurologic status of the upper extremities. After surgery, the patient's neck is immobilized in either a soft or hard cervical collar.

COMMON FOOT PROBLEMS

The foot is the platform that provides support for the weight of the body and absorbs considerable shock in ambulation. It is a complicated structure composed of bony structures, muscles, tendons, and ligaments. It can be affected by (1) congenital conditions, (2) structural weakness, (3) traumatic injuries, and (4) systemic conditions such as diabetes mellitus and rheumatoid arthritis.

Abnormalities of the foot affect over 80 million persons in the United States. Much of the pain, deformity, and disability associated with foot disorders can be directly attributed to or accentuated by improperly fitting shoes, which cause crowding and angulation of the toes and inhibition of the normal movement of foot muscles. The purpose of footwear is to provide support, foot stability, shock absorption, and a foundation for orthoses; increase friction with the walking surface; and treat foot abnormalities. (Table 59-22 summarizes common foot problems and their treatment.)

NURSING MANAGEMENT

COMMON FOOT PROBLEMS

Heath Promotion and Maintenance

Well-constructed and properly fitted shoes are essential for healthy, pain-free feet. Fashion styles, especially for women, often influence selection of footwear instead of considerations of comfort and support. Patient education should stress the importance of having a shoe that conforms to the foot rather than to current fashion trends. The shoe must be long enough and wide enough to prevent crowding of the toes and forcing of the great toe into a position of hallux valgus. At the metatarsal head the width of the shoe should be sufficient to allow free movement of the foot muscles and permit bending of the toes. The shank of the shoe should be rigid enough to give optimal support. The

Table 59-22 Common Foot Problems

Disorder	Definition	Treatment
Common Disorders		
Forefoot		
Hallux valgus (bunion)	Painful deformity of large toe consisting of lateral angulation of large toe toward second toe, bony enlargement of medial side of first metatarsal head, and formation of bursa or callus over bony enlargement	Conservative treatment includes wearing shoes with wide forefoot or "bunion pocket" and use of bunion pads to relieve pressure on bursal sac. Surgical treatment is removal of bursal sac and bony enlargement and correction of lateral angulation of large toe.
Hallux rigidus	Painful stiffness of first metatarsophalangeal joint due to osteoarthritis or local trauma	Conservative treatment includes intraarticular corticosteroids and passive manual stretching of first metatarsophalangeal joint. A shoe with a stiff sole decreases pain in the joint during walking. Surgical treatment is joint fusion or arthroplasty with silicone rubber implant.
Hammertoe	Deformity of second toe, including dorsiflexion of metatarsophalangeal joint, plantar flexion of proximal interphalangeal joint and callus on dorsum of proximal interphalangeal joint and end of involved toe; complaints related to hammertoe include burning on bottom of foot and pain and difficulty in walking when wearing shoes	Conservative treatment consists of passive manual stretching of proximal interphalangeal joint and use of metatarsal arch support. Surgical correction consists of resection of base of middle phalanx and head of proximal phalanx and bringing raw bone ends together. Kirschner wire maintains straight position.
Morton's neuroma (Morton's toe or plantar neuroma)	Neuroma in web space between third and fourth metatarsal heads, causing sharp, sudden attacks of pain and burning sensations	Surgical excision is the usual treatment.
Midfoot		
Pes planus (flatfoot)	Breakdown or lowering of metatarsal arch causing pain in foot or leg or referred pain to other parts of body	Symptoms are relieved by use of resilient longitudinal arch supports. Surgical treatment consists of triple arthrodesis, fusion of subtalar joint.
Pes cavus	Elevation of longitudinal arch of foot resulting from contracture of plantar fascia or bony deformity of arch	Treatment is manipulation and casting (in patients younger than 6 yr of age); surgical correction is necessary if it interferes with ambulation (in patients older than 6 yr of age).
Hindfoot		
Painful heels	Complaint of heel pain with weight bearing, common cause of plantar bursitis or calcaneal spur in adult	Corticosteroids are injected locally into inflamed bursa and sponge rubber heel cushion is used; surgical excision of bursa or spur is peformed.
Local Problems		
Corn	Localized thickening of skin caused by continual pressure over bony prominences, especially metatarsal head, frequently causing localized pain	Corn is softened with warm water or preparations containing salicylic acid and trimmed with razor blade or scalpel. Pressure on bony prominences caused by shoes is relieved.
Soft corn	Painful lesion caused by bony prominence of one toe pressing against adjacent toe; usual location in web space between toes; softness caused by secretions keeping web space relatively moist.	Pain is relieved by placing cotton between toes to separate them. Surgical treatment is excision of projecting bone spur.
Callus	Similar formation to corn but covering of wider area and usual location on weight-bearing part of foot	Same as for corn.
Plantar wart	Painful papillomatous growth caused by virus that may occur on any part of skin on sole of foot	Excision with electrocoagulation or surgical removal is done; ultrasound may also be used.

height of the heel should be realistic in relation to the purpose for which the shoe is worn. Ideally, the heel of the shoe should not rise more than 1 inch higher than the forefoot support.

Acute Intervention

Many foot problems require surgery. When surgery is performed, the foot is usually immobilized by a bulky dressing, short leg cast, slipper (plastic) cast, or a platform "shoe" that fits over the dressing and has a rigid sole. The foot should be elevated with the heel off the bed to help reduce discomfort and prevent edema. The neurovascular status should be assessed frequently during the immediate postoperative period. Depending on the type of surgery, pins or wires may extend through the toes, or a protective splint that extends over the end of the foot may be in place. Care must be taken not to jar these devices and cause pain. The devices may interfere with or preclude assessment for movement. The nurse should be aware that sensation may be difficult to evaluate, because postoperative pain can interfere with the patient's ability to differentiate pain caused by the surgical procedure from pain resulting from nerve pressure or circulatory impairment.

The type and extent of surgery determine the degree of ambulation allowed. Crutches may be necessary. The patient may experience pain or a throbbing sensation when starting ambulation. The nurse should reinforce instructions given by the physical therapist and ensure that the patient does not develop a faulty gait pattern such as walking on the heels in an attempt to avoid excessive pain or pressure. The nurse must reinforce the importance of walking with an erect posture and with proper weight distribution. Dysfunction of gait or continued pain should be reported to the physician. The nurse should instruct the patient on the importance of frequent rest periods with the feet elevated.

Chronic and Home Management

Foot care should include daily hygienic care and the wearing of clean stockings. Stockings should be long enough to avoid wrinkling and the development of pressure areas. Trimming toenails straight across helps prevent ingrown toenails and reduces the possibility of infection. Persons with impaired circulation or diabetes mellitus require detailed instruction to prevent serious complications associated with blisters, pressure areas, and infections (see Table 46-21).

Gerontologic Considerations

The older adult is prone to developing foot problems because of poor circulation in the lower extremities. Sensation may also be altered. A patient may develop a sore but not feel it because of altered sensation. This may be the result of peripheral vascular disease or diabetic neuropathy. Older adults should be instructed to inspect their feet daily and report any sores or breaks in the skin to their physician. If left untreated, sores may become infected and require surgical debridement. If infection becomes widespread, amputation may be necessary.

METABOLIC DISEASE OF BONE

Normal bone metabolism depends on adequate intake, absorption, and use of calcium, phosphorus, protein, and vitamins. When there is dysfunction in one of these critical factors, generalized reduction of bone mass may result.

Osteomalacia

Osteomalacia is an uncommon disorder of adult bone associated with vitamin D deficiency, resulting in decalcification and softening of bone. This disease is the same as rickets in children except that the epiphyseal growth plates are closed in the adult. Vitamin D is required for the absorption of calcium from the intestines. Insufficient vitamin D intake can interfere with the normal mineralization of bone, causing failure or insufficient calcification of bone, which results in softening of bone and deformities. Etiologic factors in the development of osteomalacia include lack of exposure to ultraviolet rays, gastrointestinal malabsorption, chronic diarrhea, pregnancy, and kidney disease.

The most common clinical feature of osteomalacia is persistent skeletal pain, especially while bearing weight. Other clinical manifestations include low back pain, progressive muscular weakness, weight loss, and progressive deformities of the spine (kyphosis) or extremities. Fractures are common and demonstrate delayed healing.

Laboratory findings commonly associated with osteomalacia are decreased serum calcium and phosphorus levels and elevated serum alkaline phosphatase. X-ray examination may demonstrate the effects of generalized bone demineralization, especially loss of calcium in bones of the pelvis and the presence of associated bone deformity. Looser's transformation zones (ribbons of decalcification in bone found on x-ray) are diagnostic of osteomalacia. Significant osteomalacia may exist without demonstrable x-ray changes.

Therapeutic management of osteomalacia is directed toward correction of the underlying cause. Vitamin D is usually supplemented, and the patient often shows dramatic response. Calcium and phosphorus intake may also be supplemented.

Osteoporosis

Osteoporosis is a condition in which there is a decrease in total bone mass. A crippling, painful bone disease, it is the major cause of fractures in postmenopausal women and older adults in general.[34] Osteoporosis is increasing in incidence because more people are surviving to an older age. The loss of bone substance causes the bone to become mechanically weakened and prone to either spontaneous fractures or fractures from minimal trauma. At least 15 million persons in the United States have some degree of osteoporosis. In the United States, the total cost of osteoporosis in terms of medical care, nursing home fees, and loss of income was estimated to exceed $14 billion.[35] Demographic risk factors for osteoporosis are female gender, increasing age, Caucasian and Asian race, oophorectomy, prolonged immobility, and insufficient dietary calcium. Increased risk is associated with cigarette smoking and alcoholism, and decreased risk is associated with adequate physical activity and fluoride and vitamin D ingestion.

CULTURAL & ETHNIC
Considerations

OSTEOPOROSIS

- Caucasian women have a higher incidence of osteoporosis than African-American women.
- African-American women have 10% more bone mass than Caucasian women.
- Postmenopausal women are at the highest risk regardless of cultural background or ethnic group.

Peak bone mass is determined by a combination of four major factors: genetic makeup, nutrition, exercise, and hormone function. Bone loss from midlife (age 35 to 40 years) onward is inevitable, but the rate of loss varies. From age 40 to menopause, women lose approximately 0.3% to 0.5% of their cortical bone per year; this accelerates to 2% to 3% per year immediately after menopause with reduced rates after 8 to 10 years.[36] When bone loss (resorption) exceeds bone formation and bones fracture under common, everyday stress, the condition becomes known as *osteoporosis.* Although resorption affects the entire skeletal system, osteoporosis occurs most commonly in the bones of the spine, hips, and wrists. Over time, wedging and fractures of the vertebrae produce gradual loss of height and a humped back known as *dowager's hump* or *kyphosis.* The usual first signs are back pain or spontaneous fractures.

This disease often goes unnoticed because it cannot be detected by conventional x-ray until more than 25% to 40% of calcium in the bone is lost; it is usually evident when the patient is 60 to 65 years of age. Serum calcium, phosphorus, and alkaline phosphatase levels remain normal, although alkaline phosphatase may be elevated after a fracture.

Osteoporosis is eight times more common in women than in men for several reasons: (1) women tend to have lower calcium intake than men throughout their lives (men between 15 to 50 years of age consume twice as much calcium as women); (2) women have less peak bone mass because of their generally smaller frame size; (3) resorption begins at an earlier age in women and is accelerated at menopause; (4) pregnancy and breast-feeding deplete a woman's skeletal reserve unless calcium intake is adequate; (5) longevity increases the likelihood of osteoporosis, and women live longer than men.

Specific diseases associated with osteoporosis include intestinal malabsorption, kidney disease, rheumatoid arthritis, advanced alcoholism, cirrhosis of the liver, and diabetes mellitus. Many medications are known to decrease calcium retention, including glucocorticoids, aluminum-containing antacids, caffeine, nicotine, and tetracycline. At the time a medicine is prescribed, the patient should be informed of this possible side effect. When a glucocorticoid is taken, there is a disproportionate loss of trabecular bone. Medical management of patients receiving steroids includes prescribing the lowest possible dose of steroid, calcium and vitamin D supplementation, estrogen replacement in postmenopausal women, and thiazide administration for renal calcium loss.[37] If osteopenia is evident on bone densitometry, treatment with agents such as calcitonin or a bisphosphonate may be considered.[38]

Recently, a gene associated with the development of osteoporosis has been identified.[39] A genetic marker, the vitamin D receptor (VDR) gene has been linked to bone density. The VDR gene is responsible for constructing the receptors that help cells use vitamin D, a vitamin important to bone and calcium metabolism. Persons with a specific gene combination have significantly lower bone density. Identification of persons with this gene combination will allow targeted interventions at an early age for persons genetically at risk for the development of osteoporosis.

Prevention of osteoporosis focuses on adequate calcium intake (1000 mg/day in premenopausal women and postmenopausal women taking estrogen and 1500 mg/day in postmenopausal women who are not receiving supplemental estrogen) and regular exercise to strengthen bones. If dietary intake of calcium is inadequate (Table 59-23), supplemental calcium should be taken. Calcium supplementation decreases age-related bone loss; however, no new bone is formed. Foods that are high in calcium include whole and skim milk, yogurt, turnip greens, cottage cheese, ice cream, sardines, and spinach.

Estrogen replacement therapy after menopause is used to prevent osteoporosis. Although the exact mechanism for the protective function of estrogen is not known, it is believed that estrogen attaches to specific receptors on bone cells, leading to decreased bone resorption. Estrogen replacement continues to have significant beneficial effects for 5 to 10 years after menopause. Transdermal estrogen treatment has been found to be effective in the treatment of postmenopausal women with established osteoporosis.[40] (See Chapter 51 for further discussion of estrogen replacement therapy.)

Calcitonin treatment acts by blocking effects of parathyroid hormone on bone resorption. It is available in injectable form of 50 to 100 IU three to seven times weekly. The medication is costly. Preliminary studies are being done with calcitonin in a nasal spray form.

Etidronate disodium (Didronel), a bisphosphonate, inhibits osteoclast-mediated bone resorption. Intermittent cyclical therapy with etidronate significantly increases vertebral bone mass and decreases the rate of vertebral fracture in women with postmenopausal osteoporosis.[41]

The same measures used to prevent osteoporosis, such as weight-bearing exercise and adequate calcium intake, are also beneficial in treating osteoporosis. Although loss of bone cannot be significantly reversed, further loss can be prevented if the three-part program (i.e., estrogen replacement, exercise, calcium) is followed.

Efforts are made to keep patients with osteoporosis ambulatory to prevent further loss of bone substance as a result of immobility. Treatment also involves protecting areas of potential pathologic fractures; for example, a corset can be used to prevent vertebral collapse.

Table 59-23 Sources of Calcium

Food	Calcium (mg)
1 cup milk	
Buttermilk	285
Chocolate	284
Whole	291
Low-fat	300
Skim	302
Half and half	254
Evaporated, canned	657
Egg nog	330
1 oz cheese	
American	174
Blue	150
Brie	52
Camembert	110
Cheddar	130
Cottage	130
Mozzarella	207
Parmesan	390
Swiss	272
8 oz yogurt	415
1 cup ice cream	176
Soft serve	272
3 oz seafood	
Salmon	167
Sardines with bones	372
Shrimp	98
Oysters	113
1 med stalk cooked broccoli	158
1 cup cooked spinach	200
1 cup cooked mustard greens	193
1 cup turnip greens	252
1 cup cooked collard greens with stems	289
1 cup bok choy	250
1 cup kale	206
Bonus Sources	
1 cup almonds	304
1 cup hazelnuts	240
1 tbs blackstrap molasses	137
Poor Sources	
Egg	28
1 cup cabbage	44
1 oz cream cheese	23
3 oz beef, pork, poultry	10
Apple, banana	10
½ grapefruit	20
1 med potato	14
1 med carrot	14
¼ head lettuce	27

Paget's Disease

Paget's disease (osteitis deformans) is a skeletal bone disorder in which there is excessive bone resorption followed by replacement of normal marrow by vascular, fibrous connective tissue. It occurs most often after the fourth decade of life and most commonly in men. It is characterized by deformities of bone caused by unexplained abnormal remodeling and resorption of bone, fibrotic changes, and remodeling with structurally uneven bone. The regions of the skeleton commonly affected are the pelvis, long bones, spine, ribs, and cranium. The cause of Paget's disease is unknown.

In milder forms of Paget's disease, patients may remain free of symptoms, and the disease may be discovered incidentally on x-ray. The initial clinical manifestations are usually insidious development of skeletal pain (which may progress to severe intractable pain), complaints of fatigue, and progressive development of bowlegs. Patients may complain that they are becoming shorter or that their heads are becoming larger. Serum alkaline phosphatase levels are greatly elevated in advanced forms of the disease. X-ray examination reveals that the normal contour of the affected bone is curved and the bone cortex is thickened, especially the weight-bearing bones and cranium. Pathologic fracture is the most common complication of Paget's disease and may be the first indication of the disease. Other complications include malignant osteosarcoma, chondrosarcoma, and fibrosarcoma. Therapeutic management of Paget's disease is usually limited to symptomatic and supportive care and correction of secondary deformities by either surgical implementation or braces. Bone resorption, relief of acute symptoms, and lowering the serum alkaline phosphatase levels may be significantly influenced by the administration of calcitonin, which inhibits osteoclastic activity. Resistance to calcitonin therapy may occur after about 2 years of use. Diphosphonates and their derivatives also inhibit the activity of Paget's disease. Radiation therapy and local surgical procedures such as periosteal stripping may be used for the control of the patient's pain.

NURSING MANAGEMENT

METABOLIC BONE DISEASES

A firm mattress should be used to provide back support and to relieve pain. The patient may be required to wear a corset or light brace to relieve back pain and provide support when in the upright position. The patient should be proficient in the correct application of such devices and know how to regularly examine areas of the skin for friction damage. Activities such as lifting and twisting should be discouraged. Good body mechanics are essential. Analgesics and muscle relaxants may be administered to relieve pain. A properly balanced nutritional program is important in the management of metabolic disorders of bone, especially pertaining to vitamin D, calcium, and protein, which are necessary to ensure the availability of the components for bone formation. Prevention measures such as patient education, use of an assistive device, and environmental changes should be actively pursued to prevent falls and subsequent fractures.

Gerontologic Considerations

Osteomalacia, osteoporosis, and Paget's disease are common in older adults. Patients should be instructed in proper nutritional management to prevent further bone loss such as that occurring from osteomalacia and osteoporosis.

CRITICAL THINKING EXERCISES

CASE STUDY

LOW BACK PAIN

Patient Profile

Howard is a 38-year-old truck driver who slipped on a wet floor at work and landed on his buttocks.

Subjective Data

- Experienced immediate, severe lower back pain, with pain radiating into his right buttock
- Had worsening of pain in 3 days, with pain radiating down his entire leg into his foot
- Experienced tingling of his toes
- Rested at home for 2 weeks without relief
- Smokes 1 pack of cigarettes a day

Objective Data

- Is 5′8″ tall, weights 253 lb

Diagnostic Studies

- MRI revealed large herniated disk at L4-5 level

Therapeutic Management

- Had microdiskectomy at L4-5
- Discharged 2 days after surgery

Critical Thinking Questions

1. What risk factors made Howard prone to low back pain?
2. What measures can be taken to relieve pain while at home?
3. What preoperative teaching should be done for Howard?
4. What postoperative activity restrictions will Howard have to follow?
5. What postoperative nursing assessments will be done while Howard is hospitalized?
6. What discharge teaching plan will the nurse initiate?
7. Based on the assessment data presented, write one or more nursing diagnoses. Are there any collaborative problems?

NURSING RESEARCH ISSUES

1. How effective is epidural analgesia in relieving postoperative pain for the patient who has had an open reduction with internal fixation of the hip?
2. What is the best technique of providing pin care for a patient in skeletal traction?
3. How successful is "Back School" in the prevention of episodes of low back pain?
4. What degree of obesity causes problems related to low back pain?
5. What factors are important for the nurse to address in helping a person with an amputation of an upper extremity adjust to the loss? Of a lower extremity?

Because metabolic bone disorders increase the possibility of pathologic fractures, the nurse must use extreme caution when the patient is turned or moved. It is important to keep the patient as active as possible to retard demineralization of bone resulting from disuse or extended immobilization. A supervised exercise program is an essential part of the treatment program. If the patient's condition permits, ambulation without causing fatigue must be encouraged.

REVIEW QUESTIONS

The number of the question corresponds to the same-numbered objective at the beginning of the chapter.

1. An ankle sprain may occur when a person
   a. has finished running a 10-mile race and has ankle pain.
   b. is hit by another soccer player on the field.
   c. has a twisting injury while running the bases during a softball game.
   d. drops a 10-lb weight on his foot at the health club.

2. A healed fracture is indicated by
   a. complete union of bone.
   b. callus formation.
   c. formation of hematoma at fracture site.
   d. presence of granulation tissue.

3. An indication of compartment syndrome as compared with a healing fracture is
   a. pain.
   b. swelling.
   c. extremity pallor.
   d. itching.

4. Open reduction for a fracture is indicated when
   a. adequate alignment cannot be obtained by other methods.
   b. a cast would be too uncomfortable.
   c. the patient cannot tolerate the discomfort of a closed reduction.
   d. the patient is at risk for problems from having anesthesia.

5. A neurovascular problem is indicated when
a. pain is uncontrolled by ordinary pain measures.
b. pain is decreased.
c. extremity movement is exaggerated.
d. sensation remains unchanged.

6. A patient with a pelvic fracture should be monitored for
a. changes in pain sensation.
b. sudden decrease in blood pressure.
c. changes in urinary output.
d. sudden thirst.

7. The most common infecting organism associated with osteomyelitis is
a. streptococci.
b. *Escherichia coli.*
c. *Staphylococcus aureus.*
d. *Proteus* organism.

8. During the postoperative period the patient with a lower-extremity amputation should be instructed that the amputated extremity should not be positioned in a flexed position because
a. this position promotes thrombosis formation.
b. unnecessary movement of the extremity can cause wound separation.
c. the flexed position can promote flexion contracture.
d. this position increases pain and edema.

9. Clinical manifestations of osteogenic sarcoma include all of the following except
a. pain following an injury to the extremity.
b. soft-tissue swelling in the area of the lesion.
c. pathologic fracture.
d. draining lesion.

10. Which patient is at greatest risk for low back pain?
a. A 100-lb aerobics instructor
b. A 62-year-old widow who walks daily
c. A 25-year-old newborn-nursery nurse
d. A long-distance truck driver

11. Which treatment is indicated for a patient who has had a single episode of low back pain?
a. Percutaneous diskectomy
b. Rest,with gradual increase in activity as symptoms subside
c. Increased activity
d. Use of a halo brace

12. Important nursing intervention after a spinal fusion include all of the following *except*
a. maintenance of proper body alignment.
b. prevention of constipation and distention.
c. assessing for paralytic ileus.
d. prolonged bed rest.

13. Lateral angulation of the great toe in relation to the first metatarsal head is a condition of the foot known as
a. hallux rigidus.
b. hallux varus.
c. hallux valgus.
d. hammertoe.

14. Which measure(s) should be taken to decrease the risk of osteoporosis?
a. Eat a high-protein diet
b. Avoid skim milk
c. Reduce activity
d. Stop smoking

REFERENCES

1. Maher AB, Salmond SW, Pellino TA, editors: *Orthopaedic nursing,* Philadelphia, 1994, Saunders.
2. Weston M and others: Changes in local blood volume during cold gel pack application to traumatized ankles, *J Orthop Sports Phys Ther* 19:197, 1994.
3. DeLee JC, Drez D, editors: *Orthopedic sports medicine: principles and practice,* Philadelphia, 1994, Saunders.
4. Pascarelli E, Quilter D: *Repetitive strain injury,* New York, 1994, Wiley.
5. Whittington CF, Carlson CA: Anterior cruciate ligament injuries, *Nurs Clin North Am* 26:149, 1991.
6. Barden RM, Sinkora GL: Bone stimulators for fusions and fractures, *Nurs Clin North Am* 26:89, 1991.
7. Webber JE and others: Managing traction, *Nursing* 24:66, 1994.
8. Dykes PC: Minding the five Ps of neurovascular assessment, *Am J Nurs* 93:38, 1993.
9. Arlington RG, Costigan KA, Aievoli CP: Postoperative blood salvage and reinfusion, *Orthop Nurs* 11:30, 1992.
10. Slye DA: Orthopedic complications: compartment syndrome, fat embolism, and venous thromboembolism, *Nurs Clin North Am* 26:113,1991.
11. Mravic PJ, Massey DM: Compartment syndrome, *J Vasc Nurs* 10:9, 1992.
12. Gerhart TN and others: Low-molecular-weight heparinoid compared with warfarin for prophylaxis of deep-vein thrombosis in patients who are operated on for fracture of the hip, *J Bone Joint Surg* 73A:494, 1991.
13. Reed LJ, Keegan MJ: Fat embolism syndrome: a complication of trauma, *Crit Care Nurse* 13:33, 1993.
14. Rippe JM and others, editors: *Intensive care medicine,* ed 2, Boston, 1991, Little, Brown, & Co.
15. Browner BD and others, editors: *Skeletal trauma,* Philadelphia, 1992, Saunders.
16. Liscum B: Osteoporosis: the silent disease, *Orthop Nurs* 11:24, 1992.
17. Kiel DP: New strategies to prevent hip fracture, *Hosp Pract* 29:47, 1994.
18. Cummings SR, Nevitt MC: A hypothesis: the causes of hip fractures, *J Gerontol* 44:M107, 1989.
19. Cummings SR and others: Bone density at various sites for prediction of hip fractures, *Lancet* 341:72, 1993.
20. Lauritzen JB, Petersen MM, Lund B: Effect of external hip protectors on hip fractures, *Lancet* 341:11, 1993.
21. Moore EE, Mattox KL, Feliciano DV, editors: *Trauma,* ed 2, Norwalk, CT, 1991, Appleton & Lange.
22. Shingleton BJ, Hersch PS, Kenyan KR, editors: *Eye trauma,* St Louis, 1991, Mosby.
23. Mader JT, Landon GC, Calhoun J: Antimicrobial treatment of osteomyelitis, *Clin Orthop* 295;87, 1993.
24. Mader JT, Calhoun J: Long-bone osteomyelitis diagnosis and management, *Hosp Pract* 29:71,1994.
25. Calhoun JH, Cobos JA, Mader JT: Does hyperbaric oxygen have a place in the treatment of osteomyelitis? *Orthop Clin North Am* 22:467, 1991.

26. Klemm KW: Antibiotic bead chains, *Clin Orthop* 295:63, 1993.
27. Crenshaw AH, editor: *Campbell's operative orthopaedics,* ed 8, St Louis, 1992, Mosby.
28. Simon MA, Finn HA: Diagnostic strategy for bone and soft-tissue tumors, *J Bone Joint Surg* 75A:622, 1993.
29. Piasecki P: Update in orthopaedic oncology, *Orthop Nurs* 11:36, 1992.
30. Dvorkin ML: *Office orthopaedics,* Norwalk, CT, 1993, Appleton & Lange.
31. Salmond SW, Mooney NE, Verdisco LA, editors: *Core curriculum for orthopaedic nursing,* ed 2, Pitman, NJ, 1991, Anthony J Jannetti.
32. Jerva MJ: Automated percutaneous lumbar discectomy: a review, *Orthop Nurs* 12:27, 1993.
33. Sherk HH and others: Laser diskectomy, *Orthopedics* 16:573, 1993.
34. Wilson JD, Foster DW, editors: *Williams textbook of endocrinology,* ed 8, Philadelphia, 1992, Saunders.
35. Bauer RL: Assessing osteoporosis, *Hosp Pract* 26:23, 1991.
36. Notelovitz M: Osteoporosis: screening, prevention, and management, *Fertil Steril* 59:707, 1993.
37. Levis R: Osteoporosis: prevention is key to management, *Geriatrics* 48:18, 1993.
38. Metlak BH, Nussbaum SR: Diagnosis and treatment of osteoporosis, *Annu Rev Med* 44:265, 1993.
39. Anonymous researchers discover genetic clue, *Osteoporos Rep* 10:1, 1994.
40. Lulkin EG and others: Treatment of postmenopausal osteoporosis with transdermal estrogen, *Ann Intern Med* 117:1, 1992.
41. Harris ST: Osteoporosis: pharmacologic treatment strategies, *Adv Intern Med* 38:303, 1993.

Chapter 60

NURSING ROLE IN MANAGEMENT

Arthritis and Other Rheumatic Disorders

Gayle Ziegler Casterline

Learning Objectives

1. Describe the pathophysiology, clinical manifestations, and therapeutic management of osteoarthritis, rheumatoid arthritis, gout, systemic lupus erythematosus, and systemic sclerosis.
2. Describe the clinical manifestations and management of juvenile rheumatoid arthritis, HLA-associated rheumatic diseases, septic arthritis, polymyositis, dermatomyositis, and fibromyalgia.
3. Describe the sequence of events leading to joint destruction in osteoarthritis and rheumatoid arthritis.
4. Compare osteoarthritis with rheumatoid arthritis related to clinical manifestations, treatment, and prognosis.
5. Identify the nursing management of arthritis and related rheumatic disorders.
6. Describe the types of reconstructive surgery associated with arthritis and related rheumatic disorders.
7. Identify the preoperative and postoperative teaching and management of the patient having reconstructive surgery associated with arthritis and related rheumatic disorders.
8. Describe the pharmacologic management and related nursing considerations associated with arthritis and related rheumatic disorders.
9. Identify psychologic and sociocultural issues of the patient with rheumatic disease and the appropriate nursing strategies that meet these needs.
10. Identify the importance of the interdisciplinary team approach to comprehensive management of rheumatic disease.

OSTEOARTHRITIS

Osteoarthritis (OA), also known as *degenerative joint disease* (DJD), is a slowly progressive disorder of mobile joints, particularly weight-bearing articulations, and is characterized by degeneration of articular cartilage. The damage from OA is confined to the joints and surrounding tissues. Clinical symptoms include joint pain, stiffness, and limited range of motion (ROM). Radiographically, the disease is characterized by joint-space narrowing, subchondral sclerosis, and osteophyte formation. The spectrum of severity is wide, ranging from annoying and uncomfortable symptoms to significantly disabling disease.[1] OA may occur as a primary idiopathic or secondary disorder. The cause of primary OA is unknown. Although both are influenced by multiple factors (e.g., metabolic, mechanical, genetic, and chemical), secondary OA has an identifiable precipitating event, such as previous trauma, fractures, infection, or congenital deformities, that is believed to predispose the person to later degenerative changes.

Significance

The most significant risk factor for OA is age. It is estimated that nearly one third of all adults have x-ray evidence of degenerative joint disease, with increasing incidence to 60% to 80% by age 60. Because only one half of these adults experience significant symptoms, joint pain and functional disability should not be considered a normal finding in aging persons. Under 55 years of age, men and women are affected equally. In older individuals, OA of the hips is more common in men and OA of interphalangeal joints and thumb base is more common in women.[2]

Etiology and Pathophysiology

Degenerative changes over time cause the normally smooth, white, translucent joint cartilage to become yellow and opaque, with rough surfaces and areas of *malacia* (softening). As the layers of cartilage become thinner, bony surfaces are drawn closer together. As the cartilage breaks down, fissures may appear and fragments of cartilage become

Reviewed by Janice Smith Pigg, MS, RN, Nurse Consultant Rheumatology, Director, Program Development and Research, Columbia Musculoskeletal Institute, Columbia Hospital, Milwaukee, WI.

CULTURAL & ETHNIC Considerations

ARTHRITIS AND CONNECTIVE TISSUE DISORDERS

- Systemic lupus erythematosus is more common among African-American women than Caucasian women.
- Ankylosing spondylitis is more common and disease presentation is more severe in Caucasians than in non-Caucasians.
- Sarcoidosis is 10 times more common among African-Americans than Caucasians.
- Degenerative joint disease is more common in Native Americans than Caucasians.

loose. Secondary inflammation of the synovial membrane may follow. As the articular surface becomes totally denuded of cartilage, subchondral bone increases in density and becomes sclerotic (*eburnated*). New bone (*osteophyte*) is formed at joint margins and at the attachment sites of ligaments and tendons.

There are several theories concerning the cause of cartilage deterioration. The enzyme hyaluronidase, which is normally found in the synovial fluid, may be responsible for digestion of proteoglycans through cracks in the surface layer of articular cartilage. Another theory suggests that inadequate nutrition of the cartilage may result in cartilage degeneration. Because cartilage is avascular, nutrients are provided by the synovial fluid. It has been demonstrated that deterioration of cartilage is an active process. DNA synthesis, which is normally absent in adult articular cartilage, is active in OA tissue and appears to be directly proportional to disease severity.[3]

Specific predisposing factors such as excessive use of or stress on a joint have been identified as accelerating osteoarthritic changes (e.g., in the knees of football players and the feet and ankles of ballet dancers). Genetic factors influence the development of Heberden's nodes, which involve a single autosomal gene, dominant in women and recessive in men.

Other factors that influence the development of OA include congenital structural defects (e.g., Legg-Calvé-Perthes disease, genu varum), metabolic disturbances (e.g., diabetes mellitus, acromegaly), repeated intraarticular hemorrhage (e.g., hemophilia), neuropathic arthropathies, and inflammatory and septic arthritis.

Clinical Manifestations

Systemic. Constitutional symptoms such as fatigue or fever are not present in OA. Other organ involvement is absent as well, which is an important differentiation between OA and inflammatory joint disorders such as rheumatoid arthritis.

Joints. Articular manifestations are related to the particular joint involved. The patient has pain on motion and weight bearing that is generally relieved by rest. In advanced disease sleep may be disrupted by night pain. As cartilage (which does not contain nerve endings) is worn away, direct irritation and pressure occur on the nerves of subchondral bones. Pain is most often caused by swelling and stretching of soft tissue structures surrounding the joint, not by the arthritic joint itself.[4] Increasing pain is accompanied by progressive loss of function. Overall body coordination and posture may be affected as a result of the pain and loss of mobility.

Unlike pain, which is typically provoked by activity, joint stiffness occurs after periods of rest or static position. The symptoms are often aggravated by rising humidity and falling barometric pressure. *Crepitation* (grating sensation caused by the rubbing together of abnormal synovial surfaces) on joint motion and malalignment of the extremity may be noted on physical examination. Advanced disease is complicated by gross deformity and *subluxation* (partial dislocation) caused by deterioration of cartilage, collapse of subchondral bone, and extensive bony overgrowth.

Joints are usually affected asymmetrically. The joints most frequently involved are the distal interphalangeal joints of the fingers, first carpometacarpal joint, hips, knees, first metatarsophalangeal joint, and lower lumbar and cervical vertebrae (Fig. 60-1). Degenerative changes are rarely seen in metacarpophalangeal joints, wrists, elbows, or shoulders.

Nodules. *Heberden's nodes* are another common manifestation of OA, particularly in women with primary OA. These nodes are reactive bony overgrowths located at the distal interphalangeal joints (Fig. 60-2). Heberden's nodes are palpable protuberances that are often associated with flexion and lateral deviation of the distal phalanx, occur more frequently in women, and tend to appear in families. *Bouchard's nodes*, seen less commonly in OA, involve the proximal interphalangeal joints.

Heberden's nodes and Bouchard's nodes may present with redness, swelling, tenderness, and aching. They often begin in one finger and spread to others. Although there is usually no significant loss of function caused by the bony enlargements, the patient is often distressed by the resulting disfigurement of the hands. Little can be done to prevent the occurrence of these nodes.

Hips. OA of the hips (malum coxae senilis) may be extremely disabling. Congenital or structural abnormalities are frequent causes. This problem occurs more frequently in men than in women and may be unilateral or bilateral. Hip pain may be perceived as pain in the groin, buttock, or medial side of the thigh or knee, so the patient may find it difficult to localize the problem correctly. Pain on motion or on weight bearing may become progressively severe, and pain on rest may ensue. Sitting down is difficult, as is rising from a chair when the hips are lower than the knees. The patient learns to sit in a high seat with firm support and arm rests. Eventually, loss of ROM is significant, with pronounced limitation of extension and internal rotation.

Knees. Softening of the posterior surface of the patella (chondromalacia patellae) is seen most commonly in young people. Degeneration of the weight-bearing surfaces

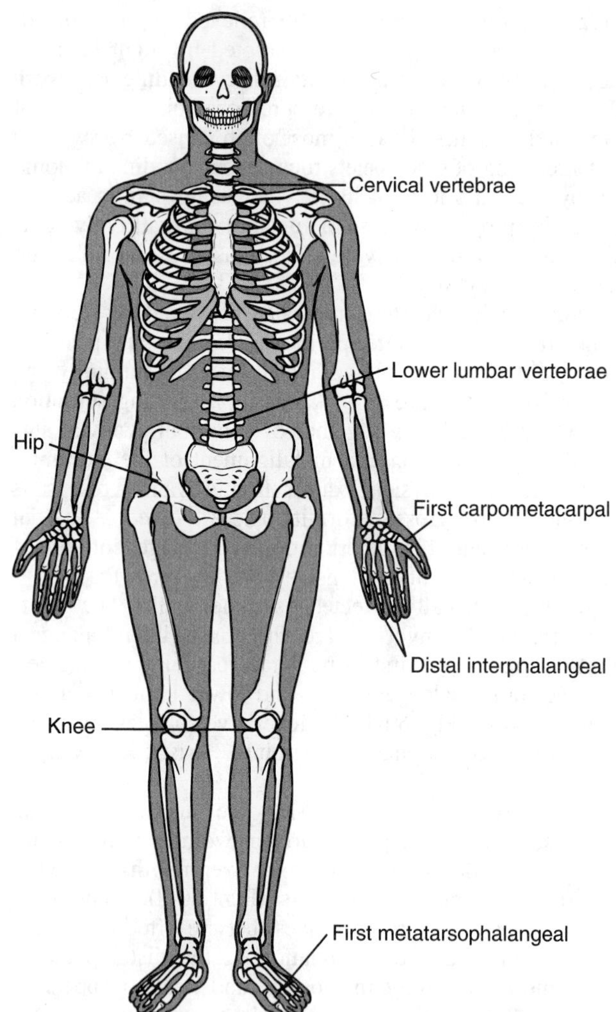

Fig. 60-1 Joints most frequently involved in osteoarthritis.

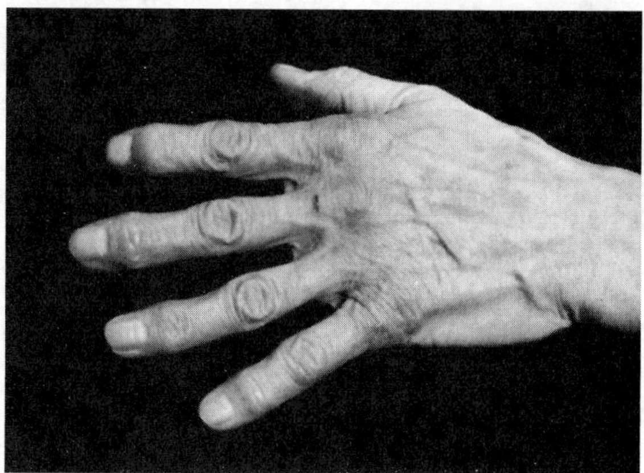

Fig. 60-2 Osteoarthritis and Heberden's nodes.

of the femoral and tibial condyles is usually seen in older women and is associated with limitation of motion, crepitus, and flexion deformity. Obesity has been implicated in OA of the knee in women, possibly the result of mechanical stress or the metabolic effects on cartilage by excess fat.

Vertebral Column. OA in the spine may produce localized symptoms of stiffness and pain. Degenerative disease of the intervertebral disks results as the nucleus pulposus deteriorates, becoming brittle and inelastic. Herniation of the degenerating nucleus most often occurs posteriorly or laterally, compressing a nerve root and causing muscle spasm or radicular pain. Another type of OA of the vertebral column involves development of degenerative disease of the intervertebral (apophyseal) joints, which generally follows disk disease by a number of years. Marginal osteophytes (spurs) also appear at vertebral attachments of the anulus, periosteum, and longitudinal ligaments. These osteophytes may fuse and limit ROM, or they may press against intervertebral foramina, producing symptoms of nerve root compression. Osteophyte formation in the posterior aspect of the cervical spine may rarely produce vascular compression and insufficiency, resulting in intermittent dizziness, visual disturbances, headaches, and ataxia.

Diagnostic Studies

In late disease, x-rays show joint space narrowing, bony sclerosis, spur formation, and in some cases subluxation. X-ray changes do not always correlate with the degree of pain experienced by the patient. The patient may be completely free of symptoms, despite significant radiologic joint space narrowing. Conversely, some patients have severe pain with only moderate x-ray changes. No specific laboratory abnormalities are useful in the diagnosis of OA. The erythrocyte sedimentation rate (ESR) is normal except in instances of erosive OA, when moderate elevation may be noted. Synovial fluid aspirated from an involved joint may be increased in volume but is clear yellow and viscous. Analysis of the fluid reveals little or no sign of inflammation.

Therapeutic Management

There are no specific therapies for the management of OA. Therapy is aimed at pain control, prevention of progression and disability, and restoration of joint function (Table 60-1). Once the diagnosis is confirmed, the patient should be assured that OA is likely to remain confined to a few joints and does not generally cause crippling. However, if joint destruction is extensive and pain is severe, surgery may be an option.

Pharmacologic Management. Aspirin is the most commonly used drug for the treatment of OA. It is generally prescribed in larger than usual doses and is given on a regular basis. In addition to relieving pain, aspirin reduces inflammation and consequently reduces swelling, stiffness, and possibly joint damage. Aspirin taken in the effective dosage range may cause ringing in the ears (tinnitus) and slight deafness. These symptoms disappear if the dosage is reduced. Gastrointestinal (GI) problems related to aspirin can be alleviated by taking the drug with meals, by the use of antacids, or by taking enteric-coated aspirin or aspirin combined with an antacid preparation. Because drug ab-

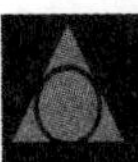

Table 60-1 Therapeutic Management: Osteoarthritis

Diagnostic
- Complete history and physical examination
- X-ray of involved joints
- Erythrocyte sedimentation rate
- Synovial fluid analysis

Therapeutic
- Rest and joint protection
- Heat, cold, exercise
- Mild analgesia
- Assistive devices
- Stress management
- Orthopedic surgery
  - Debridement
  - Arthrodesis
  - Arthroplasty
  - Osteotomy
  - Total joint replacement

sorption is slowed when taken with food, the dose of aspirin may have to be increased to be effective.

Nonsteroidal antiinflammatory drugs (NSAIDs) are particularly beneficial for persons who are intolerant to aspirin or who do not respond adequately. Newer agents are available that offer the advantage of a once- or twice-daily regimen. The need to take fewer drugs during the day improves compliance (see Table 60-2 for a listing of drugs used in the management of OA). When given in equivalent antiinflammatory dosages, all NSAIDs are comparable. Individual responses and side effects are variable. Aspirin should not be used in combination with NSAIDs because both inhibit platelet function and prolong bleeding time. Intraarticular injections of corticosteroids are used to treat a symptomatic flare. Systemic use of corticosteroids should be avoided because it may accelerate the disease process. For some patients, analgesia through drugs such as acetaminophen achieve the same symptomatic benefits as NSAIDs, with fewer side effects and at a reduced cost.[5]

Nutritional Management. There is no specific diet for OA except one that maintains optimal health. If a patient is overweight, a weight-reduction program becomes an important part of the total treatment plan. Body weight is magnified five times through the hips and three times through the knees. The additional strain of extra pounds can greatly increase pain and loss of function in OA. In addition, heavy thighs lead to malalignment at the knee, increasing wear on the medial aspect. (Chapter 37 discusses ways to assist the patient in obtaining and maintaining a healthy body weight.)

NURSING MANAGEMENT

OSTEOARTHRITIS

Nursing Assessment

Nursing assessment of the patient with OA should include careful documentation of the nature, location, severity, and frequency of joint pain and stiffness. The extent to which these symptoms affect the patient's ability to perform activities of daily living should also be assessed. Successful and unsuccessful pain-relieving practices should be noted. Physical examination of the affected joint or joints includes assessment of tenderness, swelling, limitation of movement, and crepitation. It is useful to compare the involved joint with the same joint on the opposite side of the body if that joint is not affected.

Nursing Diagnoses

Nursing diagnoses specific to the patient with OA include, but are not limited to, the following:

- Pain related to physical activity and lack of knowledge of pain self-management techniques
- Sleep pattern disturbance related to pain
- Impaired physical mobility related to weakness, stiffness, or pain on ambulation
- Self-care deficit related to joint deformity and pain with activity
- Altered nutrition: more than body requirements related to intake in excess of energy output
- Self-esteem disturbance related to changing social and work roles

Planning

The overall goals are that the patient with OA will (1) balance rest and activity; (2) use joint protection measures to improve activity tolerance; (3) modify the home and work environment to include work-saving and joint-protecting assistive devices; (4) use pharmacologic and nonpharmacologic pain management techniques to achieve satisfactory pain control; and (5) perform ROM, muscle-strengthening, and aerobic exercise regularly.

Nursing Implementation

Health Promotion and Maintenance. Prevention of primary OA is not possible; however, preventive education may include elimination of excessive strain on joints by reduction of occupational and recreational hazards and nutritional counseling for weight reduction. Community education may include proper body mechanics of lifting and good posture. Athletic instruction and physical fitness programs should include safety measures that protect and reduce trauma to the joint structures. Congenital conditions, such as Legg-Calvé-Perthes disease, that are known to predispose to the development of OA should be treated promptly.

Acute Intervention. The person with OA is most troubled by pain, stiffness, limitation of function, and the frustration of coping with these physical difficulties on a daily basis. The older adult may believe that OA is an inevitable part of the aging process and that nothing can be done to ease the discomfort and related disability.

Usually a patient with OA is treated on an outpatient basis by a team of arthritis professionals including a personal physician or rheumatologist, a nurse, an occupational therapist, and a physical therapist. The goals of therapy are to relieve pain, protect joints from further

Table 60-2 Pharmacologic Management of Rheumatic Disorders

Drug	Mechanism of Action	Side Effects	Nursing Considerations
Salicylates			
Aspirin, salsalate (Disalcid) Choline salicylate (Arthropan) Choline magnesium trisalicylate (Trilisate) Diflunisal (Dolobid)	Antiinflammatory Analgesic Antipyretic effect Act by inhibiting the synthesis of prostaglandins	GI irritation (ulcer, gastritis, hemorrhage), hypersensitivity, salicylism (nausea, tinnitus, dizziness, hyperpnea), prolonged bleeding time	When drug is taken for antiinflammatory effect, discontinue if pain decreases. Administer drug with food, milk, antacids as prescribed, or full glass of water or use enteric-coated aspirin. Report signs of bleeding (e.g., tarry stool, bruising, petechiae, melena). Need for frequent dosing decreases compliance.
Nonsteroidal Antiinflammatory Drugs			
Ibuprofen (Motrin, Advil, Rufen) Naproxen (Naprosyn, Anaprox) Piroxicam (Feldene) Indomethacin (Indocin) Sulindac (Clinoril) Tolmetin (Tolectin) Diclofenac (Voltaren) Meclofenamate (Meclomen) and many others	Antiinflammatory Analgesic Antipyretic effect Act by inhibiting the synthesis of prostaglandins	GI irritation (dyspepsia, nausea, and vomiting), GI bleeding, dizziness, rash, headache, tinnitus, prolonged bleeding time, elevated serum transaminases, drug-induced nephrotoxicity, exacerbation of asthma	Report signs of bleeding, edema, skin rashes, persistent headaches, or visual disturbances.
Corticosteroids			
Intraarticular injections			
Methylprednisolone acetate (Depo-Medrol) Triamcinolone hexacetonide (Aritsopan)	Antiinflammatory Analgesic Act by inhibiting the synthesis of prostaglandins	Local osteoporosis or neuropathic arthropathy from repeated injection	Use strict aseptic technique as joint fluid is removed and steroids are injected. Inform patient that joint may feel worse immediately after injection. Inform patient that improvement lasts weeks to months after injection and that weight bearing should be minimized for 2-6 wk after injection.
Systemic			
Hydrocortisone sodium succinate (Solu-Cortef) Methylprednisolone succinate (Solu-Medrol) Dexamethasone (Decadron) Prednisone Triamcinolone (Aristocort)	Antiinflammatory Analgesic	Cushing's syndrome, including fluid retention, GI irritation, osteoporosis, hypertension, diabetes mellitus, acne, menstrual irregularities, hirsutism, risk of infection, bruising	Use only when symptoms persist with less potent antiinflammatory drugs or in life-threatening situations. Administer for limited time only, tapering dose slowly. Be aware that exacerbation of symptoms occurs with abrupt withdrawal. Monitor blood pressure, weight, CBC, and potassium. Limit sodium intake. Report signs of infection. Instruct patient to report corticosteroid use to surgeon or dentist to avoid postoperative adrenal insufficiency.

continued

Table 60-2 Pharmacologic Management of Rheumatic Disorders—cont'd

Drug	Mechanism of Action	Side Effects	Nursing Considerations
Immunosuppressive			
Azathioprine (Imuran)	Acts as an immunosuppressant by inhibiting purine metabolism and decreasing DNA, RNA, and protein synthesis	GI irritation and ulceration, alopecia, oral lesions, dermatitis, blood dyscrasia, bone marrow depression, general increase in susceptibility to infection	Be aware of teratogenic potential that cautions against use for children or adults of childbearing age. Monitor CBC and urinalysis values. Be aware that drug should be used with great caution in patients with hepatic or renal impairment and should not be used in patients with a history of malignant tumors.
Cyclophosphamide (Cytoxan)	Acts as an immunosuppressant by cross-linking DNA and RNA strands and inhibiting the synthesis of protein	GI irritation and ulceration, alopecia, oral lesions, dermatitis, blood dyscrasia, bone marrow depression, oncogenicity, hemorrhagic cystitis, sterility	Be aware that therapy is limited to patients not responsive to conventional therapy. Monitor CBC and urinalysis values. Be aware of teratogenic potential that cautions against use for children or adults of childbearing age. Inform patient that contraception should be used during therapy. Use usually limited to treatment of rheumatoid vasculitis.
Methotrexate	Acts as an immunosuppressant by inhibiting the metabolism of folic acid, thus inhibiting the synthesis of RNA and DNA	GI irritation, photosensitivity, oral lesions, hepatic toxicity, blood dyscrasia, infertility	Monitor CBC and liver enzyme values. Instruct patient to avoid alcoholic beverages and report signs of jaundice. Be aware of teratogenic potential that cautions against use for children or adults of childbearing age. Inform patient that contraception should be used during and 3 mo after treatment.
Disease-Modifying Agents			
Chrysotherapy			
Parenteral Gold sodium thiomalate (Myochrysine) Oral Aurothioglucose (Solganal) Auranofin (Ridaura)	Unknown inflammatory suppressive effect, possibly caused by inhibition of macrophage function, complement activation, prostaglandin synthesis	Parenteral: dermatitis, pruritus, stomatitis, blood dyscrasia, nephrotoxicity, diarrhea Oral: less toxic than parenteral; GI irritation, mucocutaneous, hematopoietic system, and kidney complications	Parenteral: test blood and urine regularly. Check urine for blood and protein before each dose and delay injection until negative. Mix drug well and give deep intramuscular injection in buttocks. Inform patient that symptomatic improvement is not expected for 3-6 mo and that therapy may be continued indefinitely. Oral: institute new oral therapy with bulking agents. Do not taper oral dosage; be aware that laboratory testing is less frequent with oral drug. Instruct patient to not become pregnant while receiving chrysotherapy. Less toxic and less effective than parenteral gold.

continued

stress, and restore mechanical function and alignment. Hospitalization is usually necessary only if joint surgery is planned.

Medications are administered for the relief of pain and inflammation, if present. Nonpharmacologic pain management includes massage, application of heat (thermal packs) and cold (ice packs), relaxation, and visual imagery. Once an acute flare has subsided, a physical therapist can provide valuable assistance in planning an exercise program.

The hospital or home health nurse should assist the patient with activities of daily living as necessary and help the patient plan rest periods during the day. The patient needs sufficient time to move stiff, painful joints, especially when arising in the morning or after any period of sustained

Table 60-2 Pharmacologic Management of Rheumatic Disorders—cont'd

Drug	Mechanism of Action	Side Effects	Nursing Considerations
Antimalarials			
Chloroquine (Aralen) Hydroxychloroquine (Plaquenil)	Unknown; has the ability to bind and alter DNA	Nausea, abdominal discomfort, rash, asymptomatic retinopathy, corneal opacity, headache, dizziness, blood dyscrasia	Inform patient that ophthalmologic examination including slit lamp studies is required every 3-6 mo. Instruct patient to take drug with meals, milk, or antacid as prescribed, to report all skin eruptions and visual disturbances, and to avoid excessive sun exposure. Be aware that drugs are contraindicated for patients with psoriasis. Monitor CBC and liver enzyme values periodically. Instruct patient to discuss condition with physician before pregnancy and breast-feeding.
Other			
Penicillamine (Cuprimine)	Unknown, disease-modifying effect	Blood dyscrasias, glomerulonephropathy, rashes, GI irritation, diarrhea	Give drug on empty stomach before meals (not with). Monitor CBC, urinalysis, and liver enzyme values. Report fever, sore throat, chills, bruising, or bleeding. Be aware that drug is contraindicated with gold therapy. Instruct patient to not become pregnant while taking drug.

CBC, Complete blood count; *GI*, gastrointestinal.

inactivity. Proper body alignment should be maintained at all times.

Patient education related to OA is an important nursing responsibility that should be carried out regardless of the care setting. Teaching should include information about the nature and treatment of the disease, pain management, correct posture and body mechanics, correct use of assistive devices such as a cane or walker, principles of joint protection and energy conservation (Table 60-3), and a therapeutic exercise program. Home management goals must be individualized to meet the patient's needs, and family and social supports should be included in goal setting and education.

Chronic and Home Management. After diagnosis of OA and the initial educational efforts have been completed, the nurse needs to assist the patient in developing long-term strategies in managing the disease. The patient should be assured that OA is a localized disease and that severe deforming arthritis is not the usual course.

Safety measures in the home and work environment are important. These measures include removing scatter rugs, providing rails at stairs and bathtub, using night-lights, and wearing well-fitting supportive shoes. Assistive devices such as canes, walkers, elevated toilet seats, and grab bars reduce joint load and promote safety.

Splints may be prescribed to rest and stabilize painful or inflamed joints. Soft collars or cervical traction may be used at home for cervical OA. Stiff, painful hands can be relieved by warm-water soaking, contrast baths, or paraffin. If swelling is more diffuse, stretch gloves can be worn at night to provide relief. Sexual counseling helps the patient and loved one to enjoy physical closeness by learning to adapt positions, alter timing, and increase awareness of partner's needs.

Management of the chronic pain and loss of function of affected joints continue to be a primary concern. Nonpharmacologic techniques such as meditation, relaxation, and transcutaneous electric nerve stimulation (TENS) are particularly suited to chronic pain management (see Chapter 6). The nurse should be open to helping the patient and family to develop creative new approaches to pain relief. Nursing interventions should assist the patient and family to overcome feelings of helplessness and encourage active participation in managing chronic symptoms. The correct combination of joint protection, exercise (range of motion, isotonic, and isometric), heat or cold therapy, and medication can restore self-esteem and improve physical functioning. The benefits of an aerobic exercise program such as walking or aerobic aquatics have been documented.[6]

RHEUMATOID ARTHRITIS

Rheumatoid arthritis (RA) is a chronic, systemic disease characterized by recurrent inflammation of the diarthrodial joints and related structures. It is frequently accompanied by a variety of extraarticular manifestations, such as rheumatoid nodules, arteritis, neuropathy, scleritis, pericarditis, lymphadenopathy, and splenomegaly.[7] RA is characterized by periods of remission and exacerbation of disease activity. The course of illness varies, ranging from episodes of illness separated by periods of remission to a more continu-

RESEARCH

Implications for Nursing Practice

FACTORS THAT INFLUENCE EXERCISE BEHAVIOR IN PATIENTS WITH ARTHRITIS

Citation Budesheim G and others: Determinants of exercise and aerobic fitness in outpatients with arthritis, *Nurs Res* 43:11-17, 1994.

Purpose To test the strength of eight variables in a theoretical model to predict the exercise behavior and aerobic fitness levels of adult outpatients with rheumatoid arthritis and osteoarthritis.

Methods Data were collected from 100 outpatients with rheumatoid arthritis and osteoarthritis related to perceived health status, benefits of and barriers to exercise, and impact of arthritis on health; demographic and biologic characteristics; and postexercise behavior. These data were entered into a theoretic model intended to predict exercise behavior and fitness levels. The variables in the model included age, education, income, body mass index, previous exercise, pain, duration of arthritis, and impact of arthritis on health status.

Results and Conclusions The theoretic model predicted 20% of the variance in composite exercise scores but none of the variance in aerobic fitness levels. Perceived benefits of exercise was a significant predictor of exercise participation.

Implications for Nursing Practice Knowledge of the predictors for exercise behavior among individuals with arthritis could provide the foundation for planning appropriate interventions for a population greatly in need of increased exercise. In particular, assessment of perceived benefits of exercise is important information for the nurse to obtain because it is a good indicator of exercise participation.

ous, progressive disease. The long-term outcome in RA is not as good as once thought.[8] Some studies done over the last decade have shown increased mortality rates in patients with RA and have shown that patients with severe forms of disease die 10 to 15 years earlier than expected.[9]

Significance

Of the approximately 6 million Americans who have RA, 75% are women. There are no geographic or racial predispositions. Although RA can occur at any age, it most often occurs in women of childbearing age.[10] In terms of its potential for chronic disability, RA is considered a significant national health problem.

Etiology

The cause of RA remains unknown. Whether a single causative factor is responsible or multiple factors are involved is unclear. Several etiologies are possible:

Table 60-3 Patient Education for Joint Protection and Energy Conservation

- Maintain good posture and proper body mechanics.
- Maintain normal weight.
- Use assistive devices, if indicated.
- Avoid positions of deviation and stress.
- Find less stressful ways to perform tasks.
- Avoid tasks that cause pain.
- Develop organizing and pacing techniques.
- Avoid forceful repetitive movements.

1. *Infection.* Research continues to probe the possibility of specific infectious pathogens, such as Epstein-Barr virus, parvovirus, and mycobacteria, which may trigger the process.
2. *Autoimmunity.* RA is characterized by the presence of autoantibodies against immunoglobulin G (IgG). Although no virus particles have been identified, it is likely that an antigenic stimulus such as a virus leads to the formation of the abnormal IgG. The autoantibodies to this altered IgG are known as *rheumatoid factors*, and they combine with IgG to form immune complexes that deposit in the joints, blood vessels, and pleura. Complement is activated and an inflammatory response results (see Chapter 9). Neutrophils are attracted to the site of inflammation and release proteolytic enzymes that can damage articular cartilage and basement membranes of blood vessels and pleura.

Joint changes are characterized by chronic inflammation with the presence of inflammatory cells and mediators that result in persistent immunologic activity. The infiltrating macrophages are activated and release a variety of cytokines, including interleukin-1 and interleukin-6; tumor necrosis factor, and colony-stimulating factor[11] (see Table 10-4). The activity of these cytokines accounts for many of the features of rheumatoid synovitis, including the synovial tissue inflammation, synovial proliferation, cartilage and bone damage, and systemic manifestations of RA.

3. *Genetic factors.* Certain familial factors may influence the expression of the disease. An increased prevalence of a human leukocyte antigen (HLA) known as the HLA-DR4 occurs in 65% of persons with RA. Persons in this group seem to experience a particularly crippling form of the disease. It is possible that the presence of this HLA-antigen and perhaps other genetic factors increase genetic susceptibility to an unidentified environmental antigen, such as a virus, initiate the disease process (see Chapter 10).
4. *Other factors.* Metabolic and biochemical abnormalities, nutritional and environmental factors, and occupational and psychosocial influences may play a part in the cause or expression of the disease, but their contribution is entirely speculative.

Table 60-4 Comparison of Rheumatoid Arthritis and Osteoarthritis

Parameter	Rheumatoid Arthritis	Osteoarthritis
Age	Young and middle-aged	Usually >40 yr of age
Gender	Female more often than male	Same incidence
Weight	Weight loss	Usually overweight
Illness	Systemic manifestations	Local joint manifestations
Affected joints	PIPs, MCPs, MTPs, wrists, elbows, shoulders, knees, hips, cervical spine Usually bilateral	DIPs, first CMCs, thumbs, first MTPs, knees, spine, hips; asymmetric, one or more joints
Effusions	Common	Uncommon
Nodules	Present	Heberden's nodes
Synovial fluid	Inflammatory	Noninflammatory
X-rays	Osteoporosis, narrowing, erosions	Osteophytes, subchondral cysts, sclerosis
Anemia	Common	Uncommon
Rheumatoid factor	Positive	Negative
Sedimentation rate	Elevated	Normal except in erosive osteoarthritis

CMC, Carpometacarpal; *DIP*, distal interphalangeal; *MCP*, metacarpophalangeal; *MTP*, metatarsophalangeal; *PIP*, proximal interphalangeal.

Pathophysiology

The pathogenesis of RA is more clearly understood than its etiology. If unarrested, the disease progresses through four stages:

1. *First stage.* The unknown etiologic factor initiates joint inflammation, or synovitis, with swelling of the synovial lining membrane and production of excess synovial fluid.
2. *Second stage. Pannus* (granulation inflammatory tissue) is formed at the juncture of synovium and cartilage. This extends over the surface of the articular cartilage and eventually invades the joint capsule and subchondral bone.
3. *Third stage.* Tough fibrous connective tissue replaces pannus, occluding the joint space. Fibrous ankylosis results in decreased joint motion, malalignment, and deformity.
4. *Fourth stage.* As fibrous tissue calcifies, bony ankylosis may result in total joint immobilization.

Clinical Manifestations

Joints. RA typically develops insidiously. Nonspecific manifestations such as fatigue, anorexia, weight loss, and generalized stiffness may precede the onset of arthritic complaints. The stiffness becomes more localized after weeks to months. Some patients report a history of a precipitating stressful event such as infection, work stress, physical exertion, childbirth, surgery, or emotional upset. However, no data correlate these events and the onset of RA.

Specific articular involvement is manifested clinically by pain, stiffness, limitation of motion, and signs of inflammation (heat, swelling, and tenderness). Joint symptoms are generally bilaterally symmetric and frequently affect small joints of the hands (proximal interphalangeal and metacarpophalangeal) and feet (metatarsophalangeal), as well as larger peripheral joints, including wrists, elbows, shoulders, knees, hips, ankles, and jaw. The cervical spine may be affected, but the axial spine is generally spared. Early shoulder involvement is common in the older adult. Table 60-4 compares the manifestations of RA and OA.

The patient characteristically has joint stiffness on arising in the morning and after periods of inactivity. This morning stiffness (gel phenomenon) may last for 30 minutes to several hours or more, depending on disease activity. Metacarpal and proximal interphalangeal joints are typically swollen. The fingers may become spindle shaped from synovial hypertrophy and thickening of the joint capsule (Fig. 60-3). Joints become tender, painful, and warm to the touch. The pain is more pronounced on motion, varies in intensity, and may not be proportional to the degree of inflammation. Tenosynovitis frequently affects the extensor and flexor tendons around the wrists, producing symptoms of carpal tunnel syndrome (see Chapter 59) and making it difficult to grasp objects.

As disease activity progresses, inflammation and fibrosis of the joint capsule and supporting structures may lead to deformity and disability. Atrophy of muscles and destruction of tendons around the joint cause one articular surface to slip past the other (subluxation). Typical deformities of the hand include "ulnar drift," "swan neck," and boutonniere deformities (Fig. 60-4). Metatarsal-head subluxation and hallux valgus (bunion) may cause pain and walking disability.

Extraarticular Manifestations. *Rheumatoid nodules* are present in 25% of all people with RA and are probably the most common extraarticular finding. Small-vessel vasculitis is considered to be the initiating event in the formation of these nodules. They appear subcutaneously as firm, nontender masses and are usually found on olecranon bursae or along the extensor surface of the forearm. Nodules at the base of the spine and back of the head are common in older adults as a result of longer periods at rest.

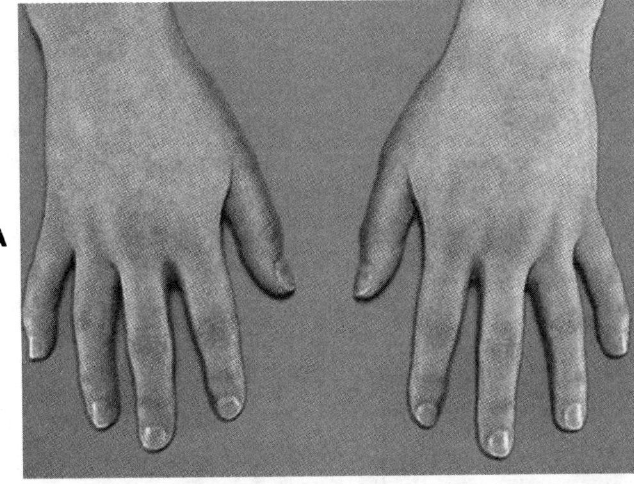

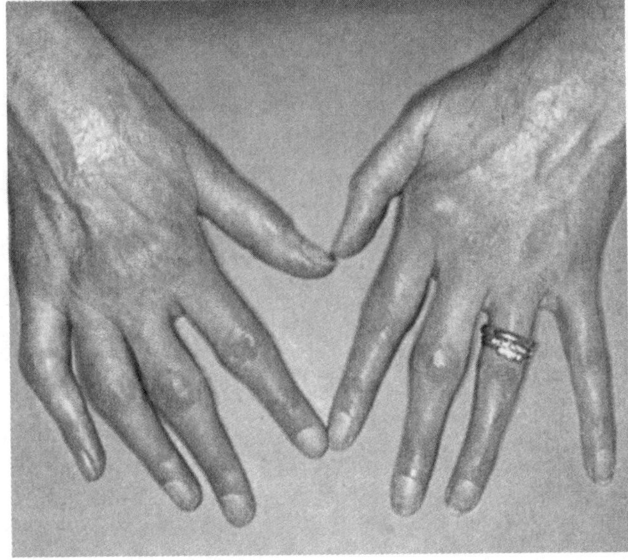

Fig. 60-3 Rheumatoid arthritis of the hand. ***A,*** Early stage. ***B,*** Moderate involvement.

Nodules develop insidiously and can persist or regress spontaneously. They are usually not removed unless they are significantly disabling because of the high probability of recurrence. Nodules may also appear on the eye or lungs; these indicate active disease and a poor prognosis.

Vasculitis (inflammation of blood vessels) may be responsible for a variety of systemic complications, including peripheral neuropathy, myopathy, cardiopulmonary involvement, and ischemic ulcerations of the skin. Figure 60-5 shows the variety of extraarticular manifestations of RA.

Complications

Potential complications include infection, osteoporosis, amyloidosis, and Sjögren's syndrome. Spinal cord compression may occur from instability of articulations in the cervical spine.

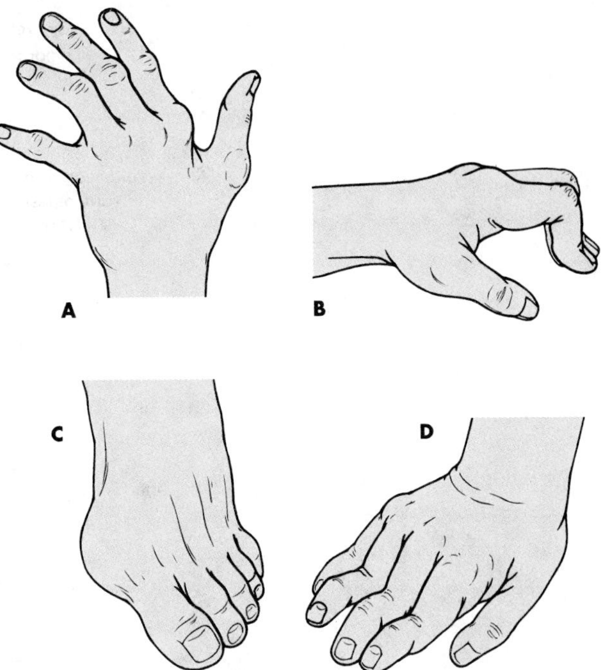

Fig. 60-4 Typical deformities of rheumatoid arthritis. ***A,*** Ulnar drift. ***B,*** Boutonniere deformity. ***C,*** Hallux valgus. ***D,*** Swan-neck deformity.

Diagnostic Studies

Although no single laboratory test is conclusive, several findings are helpful in diagnosing RA in conjunction with the history and physical examination.[12] Moderate anemia is common. The ESR is elevated in 85% of patients and is useful in monitoring the response to therapy. Serum rheumatoid factor is present in titers greater than 1:160 in nearly 80% of cases. Antinuclear antibody and lupus cell tests may be positive in a smaller percentage of patients.

Synovial fluid analysis may show increased volume and turbidity but decreased viscosity. The white blood cell (WBC) count is elevated (often as high as 30,000/μl [30×10^9/L]) and consists predominantly of polymorphonuclear leukocytes. Inflammatory changes in the synovium can be confirmed by tissue biopsy.

X-ray findings (which are not specifically diagnostic) may reveal only bone demineralization and soft-tissue swelling during the early months of the disease. Later, narrowing of the joint space, destruction of articular cartilage, erosion, subluxation, and deformity are present. Malalignment and ankylosis occur in advanced disease. Table 60-5 describes the anatomic stages of RA.

Therapeutic Management

Therapeutic management of RA begins with a comprehensive program of pharmacotherapy and education. Physical comfort is promoted by NSAIDs and rest. The patient and family are educated about the disease process and home management strategies. Responsible compliance with medi-

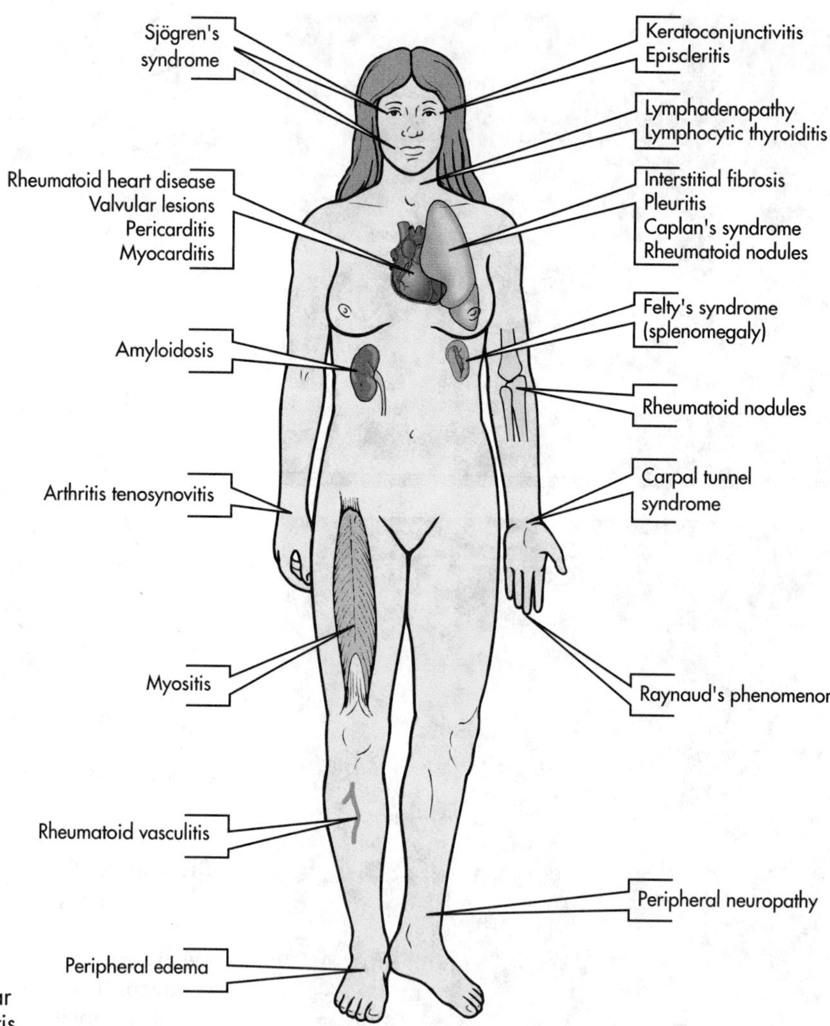

Fig. 60-5 Common extraarticular manifestations of rheumatoid arthritis.

cations includes correct administration, reporting of side effects, and frequent medical and laboratory follow-up visits. Physical therapy maintains joint motion and muscle strength. Occupational therapy develops upper-extremity function and encourages joint protection through the use of splinting, pacing techniques, and assistive devices.

An individualized treatment plan considers the nature of the disease activity, joint function, age, gender, family and social roles, and response to previous treatment (Table 60-6). Therapy emphasizes both the physical and the psychologic consequences of chronic arthritis. A caring, long-term relationship with an arthritis health care team promotes patient self-esteem and hope and discourages the use of unproven remedies, which waste money and time.

Pharmacologic Management. The concepts regarding the pharmacologic management of RA have changed considerably in recent years. In the past, patients were maintained on high doses of aspirin or NSAIDs for several years until there was x-ray evidence of characteristic bone erosions. Recent evidence that an erosive, destructive process begins within the first 2 years of disease, new data that RA shortens life, and knowledge that RA can profoundly alter a patient's functional status have made a more aggressive pharmacologic approach more common.

Many rheumatologists are now using a disease-modifying agent early in the course of the disease. A disease-modifying agent is a drug that has the potential to lessen the permanent effects of RA such as joint deformity. The crippling effects of the disease may be prevented or postponed by this plan. The exact time to introduce a disease-modifying drug varies among clinicians. Some start treatment when the patient has been symptomatic for only a few weeks. Others prefer to wait several months until the diagnosis is confirmed with a positive rheumatoid factor assay and sustained symptomatic arthritis. At this time, there is no way to differentiate patients with mild disease from the larger group whose disease may be relentlessly progressive.[13] The least toxic agent, alone or in combination, that is likely to be effective is usually the drug chosen for initial therapy. Table 60-2 lists drugs commonly used in the treatment of RA.

For patients with mild disease, hydroxychloroquine is often prescribed initially. It is one of the safest of the disease-modifying drugs. The most common side effects of

Table 60-5 American Rheumatism Association Anatomic Stages of Rheumatoid Arthritis

Stage I—Early
No destructive changes on x-ray, possible x-ray evidence of osteoporosis

Stage II—Moderate
X-ray evidence of osteoporosis, with or without slight bone or cartilage destruction, no joint deformities (although possibly limited joint mobility), adjacent muscle atrophy, possible presence of extraarticular soft tissue lesions (e.g., nodules, tenovaginitis)

Stage III—Severe
X-ray evidence of cartilage and bone destruction in addition to osteoporosis; joint deformity, such as subluxation, ulnar deviation, or hyperextension, without fibrous or bony ankylosis; extensive muscle atrophy; possible presence of extraarticular soft tissue lesions (e.g., nodules, tenosynovitis)

Stage IV—Terminal
Fibrous or bony ankylosis, criteria of stage III

Modified from Steinbrocker O, Traeger CH, Batterman RC: Therapeutic criteria in rheumatoid arthritis, *JAMA* 140:659, 1949.

this drug are nausea, abdominal discomfort, and rash. The possibility of rare, irreversible retinal degeneration caused by deposition of these drugs in the pigment layer of the retina requires ophthalmologic examination before therapy and at 4-month to 6-month intervals. Often, a low dose of prednisone is given with or instead of hydroxychloroquine.

Corticosteroid therapy can be used to achieve disease control. Intraarticular injections are administered for a flare in one or two joints. Pain in the joint may increase for 1 to 2 days after injection because of the irritation by the medication. Pain and swelling are usually relieved for 1 to 6 weeks.

Bridge therapy (5 mg orally of the prescribed corticosteroid for 4 to 6 weeks) is used until one of the longer-acting drugs, such as hydroxychloroquine, gold, or D-penicillamine, has been taken long enough to suppress disease activity. *Burst corticosteroid therapy* consists of high-dose (e.g., 60 mg) corticosteroid used for a severe articular flare, which is then quickly tapered in 10 to 14 days. *Pulse therapy* (Solu-Medrol, at dosages of no more than 1 g per day intravenously for 3 days) is used to achieve fast control of inflammation and results in fewer side effects over the long term as a result of taking a smaller daily dose. Regardless of the regimen, high-dose or long-term corticosteroid therapy carries a high risk of drug dependency and serious side effects (see Chapter 47).

For patients with moderate to severe disease with symmetric joint involvement and a positive rheumatoid factor assay, a more aggressive drug regimen may be initiated. Usually methotrexate is the first drug of choice.[14] The rapid antiinflammatory effect of methotrexate reduces clinical symptoms in days to weeks. Methotrexate therapy requires

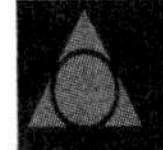

Table 60-6 Therapeutic Management: Rheumatoid Arthritis

Diagnostic
- Complete history and physical examination
- Laboratory studies
  - Complete blood cell count
  - Erythrocyte sedimentation rate
  - Rheumatoid factor
  - Antinuclear antibody levels
- Joint x-ray examination
- Synovial fluid analysis

Therapeutic
- General
  - Education, including disease process and management
  - Nutrition
  - General health measures
- Physical
  - Rest, including local joint, systemic, and emotional
  - Therapeutic exercise
  - Joint protection and energy conservation
- Pharmacotherapy
  - Nonsteroidal antiinflammatory drugs
  - Disease-modifying drugs such as hydroxychloroquine, gold, penicillamine
  - Intraarticular or systemic corticosteroids
  - Cytotoxic drugs (e.g., azathioprine, methotrexate, cyclophosphamide)
- Orthopedic surgery, especially reconstructive joint replacement

frequent laboratory follow-up. The duration of safe treatment and the possibility of long-term hepatic or lung disease must be monitored. Avoidance of alcohol is often advised.

Gold therapy may be considered for patients who do not respond to methotrexate. The exact mechanism for the effectiveness of gold in the treatment of RA is not known.[15] It is usually given in a weekly injection for 5 months, then biweekly or monthly to sustain the clinical effects. Although the serious side effects of proteinuria and cytopenia are uncommon, gold therapy often causes minor side effects, such as skin rashes, mouth sores, and gastrointestinal problems, particularly diarrhea.

Azathioprine or penicillamine may be used if the patient does not respond to either methotrexate or gold therapy. Azathioprine may cause mild pancytopenia. The high incidence of adverse reactions to penicillamine make patient compliance a problem.

Although new drug regimens are being used with increasing frequency, aspirin and NSAIDs are still commonly used. Aspirin is often used in high dosages of 4 to 6 g per day (10 to 18 tablets) in divided doses to obtain a blood level of 15 to 30 mg/dl. Enteric-coated aspirin is absorbed in the small intestine and is often used to prevent gastric irritation. Enteric-coated tablets have a special covering to prevent them from disintegrating in the stomach and may require higher doses. The ability to obtain serum salicylate levels, unavailable with other NSAIDs, is helpful in individualizing treatment programs and evaluating compliance.

NSAIDs have antiinflammatory, analgesic, and antipyretic properties. Although many NSAIDs are potent inhibitors of inflammation, they do not appear to alter the natural history of RA. Although some relief from NSAIDs may be noted within days of the start of treatment, it takes approximately 2 to 3 weeks for full effectiveness to be demonstrated. NSAIDs may be used when patients are intolerant to high doses of aspirin. NSAIDs that are taken only once or twice a day may improve patient compliance.

There are significant but subtle differences in mechanisms of action, effectiveness in different diseases, and other properties of NSAIDS. The unpredictable differences in effectiveness in different patients make it worthwhile to try a series of these drugs if the first drug does not work satisfactorily in a given patient. NSAIDs are often used in conjunction with disease-remittive drugs for their antiinflammatory effect.

Nutritional Management. There is no special diet for RA; however, balanced nutrition is important. The fatigue, pain, depression, limited endurance, and limitation of mobility that may accompany RA may interfere with the patient's appetite and ability to shop for and prepare food, resulting in weight loss. The occupational therapist may help the patient to modify the home environment and to use assistive devices to make food preparation easier. Patients are vulnerable to fad claims for improvement through health foods and vitamins even though there is no credible research evidence for their use.

Corticosteroid therapy or immobility secondary to pain may result in unwanted weight gain. A sensible weight loss program consisting of balanced nutrition and exercise reduces stress on arthritic joints. Limited sodium intake may help minimize weight gain caused by sodium retention. Steroids also increase the appetite, resulting in a higher caloric intake. Even the most compliant patient becomes distressed as Cushing's syndrome symptoms, such as moon face and redistribution of fatty tissue to the trunk, change the body's appearance. The patient must be encouraged to continue a balanced diet and not to alter corticosteroid dose or stop therapy abruptly. Weight slowly adjusts to normal several months after cessation of therapy.

Gerontologic Considerations

The prevalence of rheumatic disease in older adults is high, and the disease is accompanied by problems unique to this age group. The most problematic areas related to rheumatic disease in older adults include the following:

1. The high incidence of OA expected in older adults often keeps the clinician from considering the presence of other rheumatic diseases.
2. Age alone causes changes in serologic profiles, making interpretation of laboratory values such as rheumatoid factors more difficult.
3. Multidrug regimens common to the older adult can result in iatrogenic arthritis.
4. Nonorganic musculoskeletal pain syndromes and weakness may be related to depressive reactions and physical inactivity.
5. Rheumatic diseases that commonly manifest in younger adults can occur in older adults, but often in milder form.
6. Residual effects of rheumatic disease are present for long periods and must be managed.

Aging brings many physical and metabolic changes that may increase the older patient's sensitivity to both the therapeutic and toxic effects of some drugs. The use of NSAIDs with a shorter half-life requiring more frequent dosing may produce fewer side effects in the older patient with altered drug metabolism. The common occurrence of polypharmacy makes the use of multidrug therapy in RA particularly problematic in the older adult because of the increased likelihood of untoward drug interactions. Particular care should be taken when the older adult takes NSAIDs because of their increased propensity for side effects, particularly GI and renal toxicity. The frequency of taking medication and the complexity of the drug regimen should be simplified as much as possible to increase compliance in the older adult, particularly for the patient without regular assistance.

A major concern of treatment in the older patient relates to the use of corticosteroid therapy. Steroid-induced osteopenia adds to the problem of age-related and inactivity-related osteoporosis and can increase the occurrence of pathologic fractures, especially compression fractures of vertebrae. Steroid-induced myopathy can be minimized or prevented by an age-appropriate exercise program. Although important for all age groups, an adequate support system for the older adult is a critical factor in compliance with the management program, which should include nutritional planning, exercise, general health maintenance, and appropriate pharmacotherapy.

NURSING MANAGEMENT

RHEUMATOID ARTHRITIS

Nursing Assessment

Subjective and objective data that should be obtained from the patient with RA are presented in Table 60-7.

Nursing Diagnoses

Nursing diagnoses related to RA include, but are not limited to, those presented in the nursing care plan for the patient with rheumatoid arthritis on p. 1910.

Planning

The overall goals are that the patient with RA will (1) have satisfactory pain relief, (2) have minimal loss of functional ability of the affected joints, (3) participate in planning and carrying out the therapeutic regimen, (4) maintain a positive self-image, and (5) perform self-care to the maximum amount possible.

Table 60-7 Nursing Assessment: Rheumatoid Arthritis

Subjective Data

Important health information

Past health history: History of remissions and exacerbations, precipitating factors (e.g., emotional upset, infections, overwork, childbirth, surgery)

Medications: Use of aspirin, NSAIDs, corticosteroids, gold salts, penicillamine

Surgery and other treatments: Any joint surgery

Functional health patterns

Health perception–health management: Family history, fatigue, ability to comply with therapeutic regimen

Nutritional-metabolic: Weight loss; dry mucous membranes of mouth and pharynx; fever

Elimination: Melena

Activity-exercise: Morning stiffness and joint swelling, muscle weakness

Cognitive-perceptual: Paresthesias of hands and feet; numbness, tingling, loss of sensation; symmetric joint pain and aching that increases with motion or stress on joint

Objective Data

General

Lymphadenopathy

Integumentary

Keratoconjunctivitis; subcutaneous rheumatoid nodules on forearm, elbows; skin ulcers; shiny, taut skin over involved joints

Cardiovascular

Symmetric pallor and cyanosis of fingers (Raynaud's phenomenon)

Gastrointestinal

Splenomegaly (Felty's syndrome)

Musculoskeletal

Symmetric joint involvement with swelling, erythema, heat, tenderness, and deformities; Bouchard's nodes (enlargement of proximal phalangeal and metacarpophalangeal joints); limitation of joint movement; muscle contractures; osteoporosis, muscle atrophy

Possible findings

Positive rheumatoid factor, elevated ESR; soft tissue swelling on MRI; osteoporosis, joint space narrowing, and bony erosion on x-ray

ESR, Erythrocyte sedimentation rate; *MRI,* magnetic resonance imaging; *NSAIDs,* nonsteroidal antiinflammatory drugs.

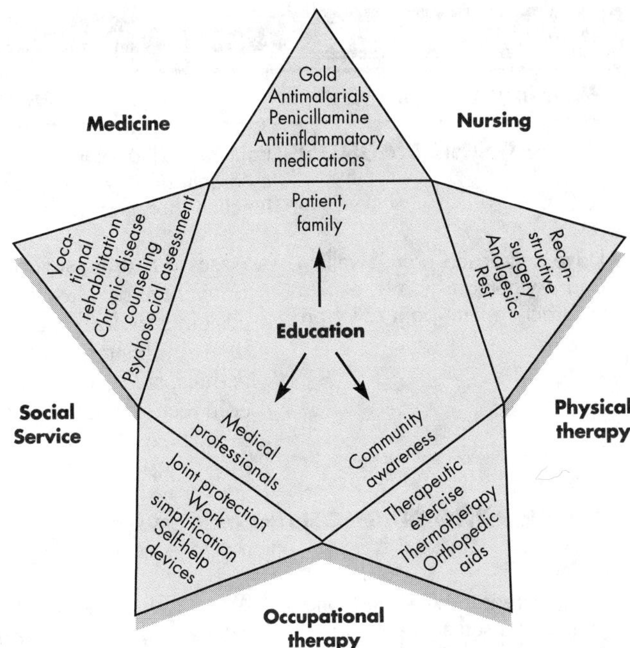

Fig. 60-6 Team approach to the management of rheumatoid arthritis.

Nursing Implementation

Health Promotion and Maintenance. Prevention of RA is not possible at this time. However, community education programs should include information concerning the symptoms of RA to promote early diagnosis and treatment. Many publications for the public are available through the Arthritis Foundation (see Organizations listed in Bibliography).

Acute Intervention. The primary objectives in the management of RA are reduction of inflammation, relief of pain, preservation of joint function, and prevention or correction of joint deformity. These may be approached by a comprehensive program of daily anti-inflammatory medication, rest, joint protection, therapeutic heat, exercise, and thorough patient and family education. The nurse is an integral member of the health team, working closely with the physician, physical and occupational therapists, and social worker to restore function and to help the patient make lifestyle adjustments to chronic illness (Fig. 60-6).

The newly diagnosed patient with RA may be hospitalized for control of acute inflammation, evaluation of systemic involvement, and comprehensive education by the health team. Hospitalization may also be necessary for patients with extraarticular complications or advanced disease requiring reconstructive surgery for disabling deformities.

Nursing intervention begins with a careful assessment of physical needs (joint pain, swelling, ROM, and general health status), psychosocial needs (family support, sexual satisfaction, emotional stress, financial constraints, vocation and career limitations), and environmental needs (transportation, home or work modifications). After the identification of problems and potential problems, a carefully planned program for rehabilitation and education can be coordinated by the nurse for the health care team.

Suppression of inflammation is most effectively achieved through the administration of antiinflammatory or disease-modifying agents. Careful attention to timing sustains the salicylate level and reduces early-morning stiffness. Education centers around the action and side effects of each drug prescribed and the importance of laboratory monitoring when necessary. Many patients with RA are taking many different drugs. The nurse must make the drug

NURSING CARE PLAN Patient with Rheumatoid Arthritis

Planning: Outcome Criteria	Nursing Interventions and Rationales
➤ NURSING DIAGNOSIS	Pain *related to* joint inflammation, overuse of joint, and ineffective pain or comfort measures *as manifested by* communication of pain descriptors, guarding behavior, and limited joint function; hot, swollen, painful joints; limited ROM
Have decreased pain, swelling, and erythema of joints; express satisfaction with pain relief program.	Assess location, severity, and precipitators of pain *to plan appropriate interventions.* Encourage decreased activity, increased rest, and supportive resting splints for affected joints *to decrease stress on joint and resulting pain during acute period.* Teach self-administration of antiinflammatory medications as prescribed, including names, actions, side effects, dose, and administration of prescribed drugs; use of heat and cold therapy; use of daily rest periods; protective techiques that limit stress to joints; avoidance of undue physical and emotional stress; and nonpharmacologic pain strategies (e.g., meditation, yoga) *to reduce pain and swelling.*
➤ NURSING DIAGNOSIS	Impaired physical mobility *related to* joint pain, stiffness, and swelling *as manifested by* limitation of joint motion, strength, and endurance; inability to perform routine activities of daily living
Have increased ROM and function, decreased stiffness, maximum mobility within limitations of disease activity.	Apply moist heat to affected joints (e.g., paraffin bath, hot packs, warm shower) *to relieve stiffness and increase mobility.* Encourage ROM exercises *to prevent unnecessary mobility restriction;* reduce frequency if pain and swelling are present *to prevent joint destruction if active disease is present.* Schedule morning care and procedures later in the day *after morning stiffness subsides.* Teach patient to use assistive devices *to promote independence.* Encourage aquatic exercise program or aerobic conditioning (e.g., stationary bicycle, walking) *to increase joint motion, flexibility, and endurance.*
➤ NURSING DIAGNOSIS	Fatigue *related to* exacerbation of disease activity, pain, anemia, drug side effects, muscle atrophy, sleep disturbance, or depression *as manifested by* weakness, decreased activity tolerance, poor sleep habits, reduced appetite, irritability, depression, hopelessness, poor posture
Have improved stamina and endurance, better-quality sleep and eating habits, positive affect.	Assess causative factors and degree of fatigue *to plan appropriate activities.* Balance activity with rest periods. Encourage regular general physical exercise such as walking, bicycling, or swimming to patient's level of tolerance *to prevent deconditioning and foster a positive attitude.* Review nutrition and sleep patterns *to determine if adjustments could prevent or alter negative effects of fatigue.* Refer for psychologic counseling and coping strategies *if a strong emotional component for fatigue is suspected.*
➤ NURSING DIAGNOSIS	Altered nutrition: less than body requirements *related to* fatigue, pain, treatment, loss of appetite, stomatitis, gastritis, dyspepsia, or self-care deficit *as manifested by* weight loss, anemia
Have weight at or close to ideal; have good appetite; enjoy food and eating experience.	Take diet history *to determine usual food intake and to identify barriers to good nutrition.* Assess medications and treatments *to determine if GI side effects are present.* Assess patient's ability to shop for and prepare food *because joint effects of rheumatoid arthritis may make these tasks difficult or impossible.* Use assistive devices *to make preparation and eating easier and less painful.*
➤ NURSING DIAGNOSIS	Joint deformity *related to* disease activity, noncompliance, and lack of knowledge of contracture prevention *as manifested by* ulnar deviation, muscle contracture, limited ROM
Have minimal deformity, optimal function, proper body alignment.	Instruct patient on correct application of resting splints, selection of properly fitting footwear, maintenance of proper posture and body alignment, and selection and use of assistive devices *to prevent joint deformity as much as possible.* Assist patient to develop less stressful ways to do tasks; encourage compliance with prescribed treatment and daily ROM exercises *to provide maximum joint protection.* Explore with patient reasons for not following prescribed treatment and daily ROM exercises *to assist in planning strategies to improve compliance.*

continued

NURSING CARE PLAN Patient with Rheumatoid Arthritis—cont'd

Planning: Outcome Criteria	Nursing Interventions and Rationales
➤ NURSING DIAGNOSIS	Body-image disturbance *related to* chronic disease activity, long-term treatment program, deformities, stiffness, and inability to perform usual activities *as manifested by* social withdrawal, flat affect, altered self-concept, reduced sexual interest, lack of social support
Accept body changes; maintain interest in life.	Allow patient to express feelings about disease *to determine extent of problem and plan appropriate interventions.* Offer psychologic support to patient and family *to prevent unnecessary or excessive emotional response to disease.* Assist patient to recognize need for regular therapeutic management and to resist false advertising and unproven remedies *so that only proven methods of treatment will be used on a consistent basis by qualified professionals.* Provide sexual counseling *because sexual problems and concerns can seriously affect body image.* Reassure patient of self-worth *so that a positive body image is fostered in spite of distressing physical manifestations.*
➤ NURSING DIAGNOSIS	Ineffective management of therapeutic regimen *related to* complexity of chronic health problem, pain, and fatigue *as manifested by* questioning management plan, self-doubt about management ability, pain descriptors, ability to perform activities for only short periods
Express increased confidence in ability to manage disease; recount correct treatment plan; and express satisfaction with pain and fatigue management.	Assess patient's knowledge of disease *to plan appropriate interventions.* Plan and initiate program of education on basis of patient readiness and need *to increase likelihood of learning taking place.* Include patient's family in discussion of disease management *to increase their sense of control and to increase patient's sense of support.* Evaluate patient's understanding through verbalization and demonstration *to ensure correct understanding of disease management.* Focus on patient's problems of pain and fatigue *because these are major deterrents to successful disease management.*
➤ NURSING DIAGNOSIS	Altered family processes *related to* patient's inability to function secondary to chronic illness and treatment regimen *as manifested by* changes in family, social, and occupational roles; dysfunctional family dynamics; loss of work status, economic resources
Patient and family will make successful adjustment to disease activity; have vocational rehabilitation or modification.	Help patient and family to identify appropriate coping strategies *to foster adjustment to changes in function and role responsibilities.* Refer patient to community vocational centers *for job modifications or retraining.* Encourage professional family counseling *because unresolved serious family problems can interfere with successful disease management.*
➤ NURSING DIAGNOSIS	Self-care deficit (partial to total) *related to* disease progression, weakness, and contracture *as manifested by* inability to perform one or more activities of daily living
Complete activities of daily living independently or with assistance; express satisfaction with way self-care needs are met.	Assess patient's ability to perform activities of daily living *to plan appropriate interventions.* Assist patient with activities of daily living as necessary *to ensure that all needs are met.* Provide assistive devices or refer to occupational therapist where appropriate *to compensate for contractures and weakness so patient can perform as many self-care activities as possible.* Encourage patient to pace activities *to foster maximum independence with minimal fatigue.*

GI, Gastrointestinal; *ROM,* range of motion.

regimen as clear and simple as possible. High-dose intravenous (IV) corticosteroids (pulse therapy) require careful observation for changes in blood pressure, peripheral edema, and signs of congestive heart failure.

Nonpharmacologic relief of pain includes the use of therapeutic heat and cold, rest, relaxation techniques, joint protection (see Tables 60-3 and 60-8), biofeedback, transcutaneous electrical nerve stimulation, and hypnosis. Assessment for individual differences and preference allows the nurse to help the patient and family set goals that promote optimal comfort.

Lightweight splints are sometimes used to rest an inflamed joint and prevent deformity from muscle spasms and contractures. These splints should be removed, skin care

Table 60-8 Patient Education for Protection of Small Joints

- Avoid positions of deformity.
  Press water from a sponge instead of wringing.
  Do not use pillows under knees.
- Use strongest joint available for any task.
  When rising from chair, push with palms rather than fingers.
  Carry laundry basket in both arms rather than with fingers.
- Distribute weight over many joints instead of stressing a few.
  Slide objects instead of lifting them.
  Hold packages close to body for support.
- Change positions frequently.
  Do not hold book or grip steering wheel for long periods without resting.
  Avoid grasping pencil or cutting vegetables with knife for extended periods.
- Avoid repetitious movements.
  Do not knit for long periods.
  Rest between rooms when vacuuming.
- Modify chores to avoid stress on joints.
  Avoid heavy tasks.
  Sit on stool instead of standing.

given, ROM exercises performed, and splints reapplied as prescribed. The occupational therapist may help identify self-help devices that can assist in activities of daily living.

Morning care and procedures should be planned around the patient's morning stiffness. Sitting or standing in a warm shower, sitting in a tub with warm towels around the shoulders, or simply soaking the hands in a basin of warm water may help relieve joint stiffness and allow the patient to comfortably perform activities of daily living. Careful skin care should be offered, particularly if the patient is confined to bed.

The professional nurse acts as liaison between the patient, family, and other members of the health team, coordinating services and evaluating the patient's understanding of the total home management program (see the nursing care plan for the patient with rheumatoid arthritis).

Chronic and Home Management

Rest. Regularly scheduled rest periods alternated with activity throughout the day help relieve fatigue and pain and minimize excessive weight bearing.[16] The amount of rest necessary varies according to the severity of the disease and each patient's limitations. Total bed rest is rarely necessary and should be avoided to prevent stiffness and immobility. Even a patient with mild disease may require daytime rest in addition to 8 to 10 hours of sleep at night. The nurse should help the patient identify ways to modify daily activities because overexertion can lead to fatigue and a flare-up in disease activity. For instance, the patient may tolerate meal preparation more easily if the patient sits on a high stool in front of the sink. Patients should rest before becoming exhausted. The nurse should assist the patient to pace activities and set priorities on the basis of realistic goals.

Good body alignment while resting is important. A firm mattress or bedboard should be used. Positions of extension should be encouraged, and positions of flexion should be avoided. Lying prone for half an hour twice daily is recommended. Pillows should never be placed under the knees. A small, flat pillow may be used under the head and shoulders. Splints and casts may be helpful in maintaining proper alignment and promoting rest, especially when joint inflammation is present.

Joint protection. Protecting joints from stress is an important part of the therapeutic regimen for RA. Nursing intervention includes helping the patient identify ways to modify tasks. Each patient must learn less stressful ways to accomplish routine activities, ways that put less stress on joints. The emphasis is on changing the way the task is done and on work-simplification techniques.

Energy conservation requires careful planning. Work should be done in short periods with scheduled rest breaks to avoid fatigue (pacing). Chores should be spread through the week rather than concentrated (e.g., all cleaning should not be done on the weekend). Activities should be organized to avoid running up and down stairs. Carts should be used to carry things. Materials used often should be stored in a convenient, easily reached area. Time-saving and joint-protective devices (e.g., electric can opener) should be used if possible. Chores should be delegated to other family members.

The nurse should instruct the patient with arthritis to protect the small joints from stress. Assessment of patient performance of tasks at work, in the hospital, and in the home identifies activities that must be revised. Joint-saving activities should be reinforced. Table 60-8 lists sample activities that protect small joints.

Patient independence may be increased by occupational therapy training with assistive devices that help simplify tasks, such as built-up utensils, buttonhooks, modified drawer handles, lightweight plastic dishes, and raised toilet seats. Wearing clothing with buttons or a zipper down the front instead of the back makes dressing easier. A cane or a walker offers support and relief of pain when walking. A platform-wheeled walker minimizes strain on the small joints of the hands and wrists. The *Arthritis Foundation Self-Help Manual* is an excellent resource for additional suggestions related to self-care.[17]

Daily heat and exercise. Heat and cold therapy help relieve stiffness, pain, and muscle spasm. Application of ice may be beneficial in an acute episode, and moist heat appears to offer better relief of chronic stiffness. Superficial heat sources such as heating pads, moist hot packs, paraffin baths, whirlpool baths, and warm baths or showers relieve stiffness before therapeutic exercises; the modality should be selected according to disease severity, ease of application, and cost. Cold therapy effectively relieves joint and muscle pain. Easy home applications include plastic bags of frozen vegetables (peas or corn), which can easily mold around the shoulder, wrists, or knees, or "icing" the skin proximally or distally to a painful joint with ice cubes or small paper cups of frozen water. Heat and cold can be used as often as desired as long as the heat application does not exceed 20 minutes at one time and the cold application does not exceed 10 minutes at one time.[18] The nurse should alert the patient to the possibility of a burn, especially if a heat-producing liniment is used with another external heat device.

Individualized exercise is an integral part of the treatment plan. This program is usually developed by a physical therapist and includes exercises to improve flexibility, strength, and endurance. The nurse should reinforce compliance with the program and ensure that the exercises are being done correctly. Inadequate joint movement can result in progressive joint immobility and muscle weakness; overaggressive exercise can result in increased pain, inflammation, and joint damage.

Gentle ROM exercises are usually done daily to keep the joints functional. The nurse should emphasize that usual daily activities do not provide adequate exercise to maintain joint motion. Careful adherence to the prescribed exercise program should be a prime goal of the teaching program. The patient should have the opportunity to practice the exercises with supervision. Warm-water (78° F to 83° F [25° C to 28° C]) aquatic exercises allow easier ROM because of the buoyancy of the water.[19] Aerobic conditioning programs have been shown to improve the physical fitness levels of patients with arthritis. During an acute inflammatory episode, exercise should be limited to one or two repetitions of ROM.

Psychologic support. Self-management and adherence to an individualized home program are contingent on a thorough understanding of RA, the nature and course of the disease, and the objectives of treatment. In addition, the patient's perception of the disease and value system must be considered. Chronic pain or loss of function may make the patient vulnerable to fad claims of false advertising and unproven remedies.

A treatment program tailored to individual problems and lifestyle increases adherence. The nurse can help the patient recognize common fears and concerns faced by all people living with a chronic illness. Evaluation of the family support system is important. The patient is constantly threatened by problems of limited function and fatigue, loss of self-esteem, altered body image, and fear of disability and deformity. Alterations in sexuality should be discussed. Financial planning may be necessary. Community resources such as a home care nurse, homemaker services, and vocational rehabilitation may be considered. Self-help groups are beneficial for some patients. Self-management classes are available in many communities.

JUVENILE RHEUMATOID ARTHRITIS

Juvenile rheumatoid arthritis (JRA), a major rheumatic disease of youth, is defined as RA beginning before 16 years of age. It may be classified on the basis of the type of onset: systemic, pauciarticular, or polyarticular.[20] The last form most closely resembles adult RA; the others may represent other types of arthritis with onset during childhood. Children as young as 6 months of age may be affected, with the peak ages at onset between 1 and 5 years and again between 9 and 12 years. Prognosis is generally favorable, with nearly 70% of children having few or no inflammatory symptoms by adulthood. Residual deformity, however, may be a severe problem for some patients.

JRA may occur with arthritis confined to one joint (*pauciarticular*) or several (*polyarticular*). Children most often do not complain of joint pain but may assume a position of flexion to minimize pain, carefully limit movement, or refuse to walk at all. A more constitutional variant known as *Still's disease* (systemic onset) presents with high-spiking fever, vague arthralgias, generalized rash, hepatosplenomegaly, lymphadenopathy, and pleuritis or pericarditis. Complications of JRA include retarded growth and development and chronic, asymptomatic (and at times vision-threatening) eye inflammation.

The criterion for the diagnosis of JRA is persistent arthritis of one or more joints for at least 6 consecutive weeks, provided certain other similar disorders are ruled out. High-spiking fever, rheumatoid rash, generalized lymphadenopathy, and splenomegaly are more common in children than in adults with RA. Leukocytosis is common, whereas rheumatoid factor is present in only 15% of those affected. Aspirin suppresses inflammation in the majority of cases. Chrysotherapy (treatment with gold salts) can be used for arthritis unresponsive to aspirin. Steroids are avoided when possible because of their effect on growth.

Nursing intervention requires an individualized written home program with emphasis on compliance. The family is best counseled about the course and prognosis of their child's arthritis according to the onset classification. Daily participation in a planned physical training program encourages full ROM and muscle strengthening and does not strain affected joints. Swimming, bicycling, and dance therapy are better than running, jumping, and kicking. Growth and development should be documented. Slit-lamp ophthalmologic examinations must be done routinely for those children at highest risk for developing ocular complications (pauciarticular group).

The school nurse should be involved in the child's care. Early-morning classes and stair climbing may be difficult for the child with arthritis. Parents are encouraged to treat the child as normally as possible, avoiding infantilizing or overprotecting. An experienced multidisciplinary health care team can help the child and family meet the challenges of social and personality development. A family-oriented rather than a child-oriented approach is critical for the optimal management of JRA.

DISEASES ASSOCIATED WITH HLA-B27

Tissue typing is used in organ transplantation because *histocompatibility antigens* are responsible for the acceptance or rejection of a donor organ. These antigens are on the cell surfaces of all nucleated cells and were first described on leukocytes; hence they were called *human leukocyte antigens*. It soon became apparent that there was an association between a number of autoimmune diseases and HLA antigens (see Table 10-16). An unusually high frequency of HLA-B27 is found in patients with ankylosing spondylitis, psoriatic arthritis, and Reiter's syndrome, known as the *seronegative spondyloarthritides*.[11] The unifying characteristics of the spondyloarthropathies are (1) predilection for involvement of sacroiliac joints and spine; (2) oligoarticular asymmetric arthritis; (3) enthesopathy (e.g., plantar fasciitis, Achilles tendinitis); (4) absence of rheumatoid factor and autoantibodies; (5) extraarticular disease in characteristic sites (eye, heart, skin, mucous membranes); (6) male predominance; and (7) a strong association with the HLA antigen B27.[22] Detection of this marker is an important aid to early diagnosis of these diseases.

Ankylosing Spondylitis

Ankylosing spondylitis (AS) is a chronic inflammatory disease that primarily affects the sacroiliac joints, apophyseal and costovertebral joints of the spine, and adjacent soft tissues. Approximately 90% of Caucasian patients with AS are positive for HLA-B27. The disease typically appears in adolescence or young adulthood.

AS is equally prevalent in both sexes, but progressive disease is more common in men. Because women tend to have more peripheral joint involvement, the diagnosis is often delayed or missed.[23] There appears to be a definite familial tendency, and the disease is unusual in African-Americans.

Etiology and Pathophysiology. The cause of AS is unknown. Genetic predisposition appears to play an important role in the disease pathogenesis, but the precise mechanisms are unknown. Environmental factors and infectious agents are also suspected. Inflammation in joints and adjacent tissue causes the formation of granulation tissue, eroding vertebral margins and resulting in spondylitis. Calcification tends to follow the inflammation process, leading to bony ankylosis.

Clinical Manifestations and Complications. The patient typically has lower back pain, stiffness, and limitation of motion that is worse during the night and in the morning but improves with mild activity. General constitutional features such as fever, fatigue, anorexia, and weight loss are rarely present. Other symptoms depend on the stage of the disease and include peripheral arthritis of the shoulders, hips, and knees and occasional ocular inflammation (iritis).

Involvement of costovertebral joints leads to a decrease in chest expansion. Advancing kyphosis leads to a bent-over posture, and compensating hip-flexion contractures may occur. There is pronounced impairment of neck motion in all directions. Extraskeletal involvement may include iritis, aortic valvular regurgitation, and apical pulmonary fibrosis.

Diagnostic Studies. Changes on x-rays may not become apparent for months to years after the onset of symptoms. When abnormalities are present, they include sacroiliac joints that show pseudowidening of the joint space and later obliteration with ankylosis. New bone formation (syndesmophytes) may be spotty or generalized (classic "bamboo spine"). ESR, alkaline phosphatase, and creatinine kinase levels are usually elevated. Tissue typing is positive for HLA-B27 in the majority of patients.

Therapeutic Management. Prevention of AS is not possible; however, families with diagnosed HLA-B27–positive rheumatic diseases should be alert to signs of lower back pain and arthritis symptoms so early treatment could be initiated.

Therapeutic management is aimed at maintaining maximal skeletal mobility. Proper posture is important in all activities. Although drugs do not halt the progression of the disease, NSAIDs, drugs such as phenylbutazone and indomethacin, can provide pain relief, which makes proper posture easier. Surgery to correct extreme flexion deformities may be performed in certain cases. A total hip replacement is done for patients with crippling hip ankylosis.

NURSING MANAGEMENT

ANKYLOSING SPONDYLITIS

Nursing responsibilities for the patient with AS include education about the nature of the disease and principles of therapy. A home management program consists of local heat and exercise and proper use of medications. Baseline ROM including chest expansion should be assessed by the nurse. Pain should be managed by appropriate medication, heat, massage, and gentle exercise. Application of moist heat should be followed by ROM exercises and daily chest expansion and deep-breathing exercises (Fig. 60-7). A continuing physical therapy program incorporating gentle, graded stretching and strengthening exercises preserves

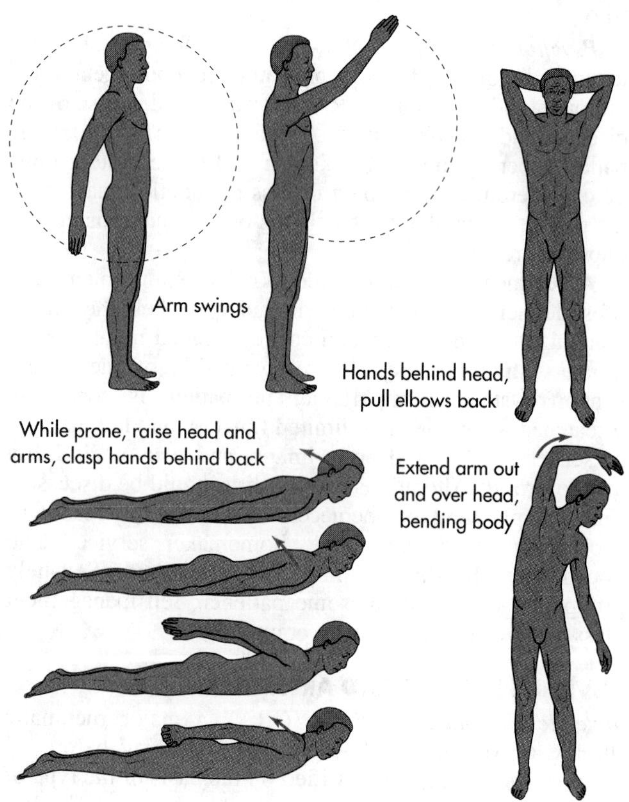

Fig. 60-7 Typical chest-cage stretching and deep chest breathing exercises for ankylosing spondylitis.

ROM and improves thoracolumbar flexion and extension. Excessive physical exertion during periods of active inflammation should be discouraged. Proper positioning at rest is essential. The mattress should be firm, and pillows must be avoided. The patient should sleep on the back and avoid positions that encourage flexion deformity. Postural training emphasizes avoiding forward flexion (e.g., leaning over a desk), heavy lifting, and prolonged walking, standing, or sitting. Sports that facilitate natural stretching, such as swimming and racquet games, should be encouraged. Family counseling and vocational rehabilitation are important.

Psoriatic Arthritis

Psoriatic arthritis (PsA) can be defined as an association of clinically apparent psoriasis with inflammatory polyarthritis (see Chapter 20). Psoriatic skin changes may precede or follow articular symptoms. Approximately 10% to 15% of persons with psoriasis have such an arthritis, which is generally mild, with intermittent flare-ups affecting only a few peripheral joints. However, a severe erosive form is also seen. Certain x-ray findings such as asymmetric distribution and resorption of tufts of the distal phalanges of hands, feet, and metatarsal bones help distinguish psoriatic arthritis from RA. Patients with psoriasis are subject to spondylitis, associated with an 80% frequency of HLA-B27 positivity. Hyperuricemia often accompanies the disease. Forms of treatment include splinting, joint protection, and physical therapy. Although gold has recently been used with success for the treatment of psoriatic arthritis, methotrexate continues to be one of the most effective agents for both cutaneous and articular manifestations.

Reiter's Syndrome

Reiter's syndrome is a self-limiting disease associated with arthritis, urethritis, conjunctivitis, and mucocutaneous lesions. Although the exact etiology is unknown, Reiter's syndrome appears to be a reactive arthritis after certain enteric (e.g., *Shigella*) or venereal (e.g., *Chlamydia trachomatis*) infections. The disease usually affects males, and 85% of patients with Reiter's syndrome are positive for HLA-B27, which provides evidence for a genetic predisposition. Few other laboratory abnormalities occur, although the ESR may be elevated.

The arthritis of Reiter's syndrome tends to be asymmetric, frequently involving the weight-bearing joints of the lower extremities and sometimes the lower part of the back. Arthralgias usually begin 1 to 3 weeks after the appearance of the initial infection. The full attack may be accompanied by fever and other constitutional complaints, including anorexia with considerable weight loss, and may prove highly debilitating. Soft-tissue manifestations commonly include Achilles tendinitis.

Prognosis is favorable, with most patients recovering after 2 to 16 weeks. Lesions heal without a trace, and many patients have complete remission with full joint function. About one half of the patients, however, have recurring acute attacks; others follow a chronic course, having continued synovitis and progression of x-ray changes closely resembling those of AS. Progressive disease may result in major disability. Treatment is symptomatic. Joint inflammation is treated with NSAIDs.

SEPTIC ARTHRITIS

Septic arthritis (infectious or bacterial arthritis) is caused by invasion of the joint cavity with microorganisms. Various bacteria are commonly responsible, including *Staphylococcus aureus, Streptococcus hemolyticus, Diplococcus pneumoniae*, and *Neisseria gonorrhoeae*. Factors increasing the risk of such infections include previous joint trauma or arthritic disease, diseases of decreased host resistance such as leukemia and diabetes mellitus, treatment with corticosteroids or immunosuppressive drugs, and serious chronic illness. Infants, young children, and older adults appear to be more frequently affected by the infectious arthritides, with the exception of gonococcal arthritis, which affects sexually active young adults. A site of active infection is often responsible for bacteremia (microorganisms reaching the bloodstream), leading to hematogenous seeding of joints.

Inflammation of the joint cavity causes severe pain, erythema, and swelling of one or several joints. Large joints, such as the knee and the hip, are most frequently involved. Fever or shaking chills often accompany articular symptoms because bacterial entry into a joint is most often by the hematogenous route from a primary site of infection. Precise diagnosis is made by aspiration of the joint and culture of the synovial fluid. Blood cultures for aerobic and anaerobic organisms should be obtained.

Septic arthritis is a medical emergency that requires prompt diagnosis and treatment to prevent joint destruction. Parenteral antibiotic administration is maintained until there are no clinical signs of active synovitis or inflammation in the joint fluid. Infections may respond to treatment within 2 weeks or take as long as 4 to 8 weeks, depending on the causative organism. Open surgical drainage may be required. Nursing intervention includes assessment and monitoring of joint inflammation, pain, and fever. Immobilization of affected joints to control pain is often achieved by resting splints or traction. Gentle ROM exercises should be done. Strict aseptic technique should be used during assistance with joint aspiration procedures. The necessity of antibiotics should be explained, and the importance of their continued use should be stressed. Support should be offered to the patient requiring repeated arthrocentesis or operative drainage. The extent of joint damage is generally related to the invading microorganism and the time between infection onset and initiation of effective treatment.

LYME DISEASE

Lyme disease is a spirochetal infection caused by *Borrelia burgdorferi* and transmitted by the bite of an infected tick, first identified in Lyme, Connecticut, after an unusual clustering of arthritis in children.[24] It is the most common vector-borne disease in the United States.[25] The tick is no bigger than a poppy seed and typically feeds on mice, dogs, cats, cows, horses, raccoons, deer, and humans. Wild animals do not exhibit the illness, but clinical Lyme disease does occur in domestic animals. The peak season for human infection is during the summer months.

The most characteristic clinical symptom is a skin lesion, *erythema migrans (EM)*, which occurs at the site of the tick bite in 80% of patients. This lesion begins as a red macule or papule that slowly expands to form a large round lesion with a bright red border and central clearing. The EM lesion is often accompanied by other acute symptoms, such as intermittent fever, headache, fatigue, stiff neck, and migratory joint and muscle pain. If not treated, Lyme disease can progress in several weeks or months to debilitating arthritis, atrioventricular conduction defects, bradycardia or myocarditis, and neurologic abnormalities including meningitis, facial palsy, and radiculoneuropathy.

Diagnosis is based on clinical manifestations, history of exposure in an endemic area, and a positive serologic test for *Borrelia burgdorferi*. Other illnesses are frequently misdiagnosed as Lyme disease, particularly chronic fatigue syndrome and fibromyalgia. Serologic testing is not standardized, and false-positive results are common. Most U.S. cases occur in three endemic areas: along the northeastern coast from Maryland to Massachusetts; in the midwestern states of Wisconsin and Minnesota; and along the northwestern coast of northern California and Oregon.[26]

Active lesions can be treated with antibiotic therapy. Oral doxycycline or amoxicillin is often effective in early-stage infection and in prevention of later stages of the disease. More diffuse infection may require 20 to 30 days of therapy. Intravenous ceftriaxone (Rocephen) is used for cardiac or neurologic abnormalities. Lyme arthritis usually responds to oral antibiotic therapy. However, in genetically susceptible persons, chronic arthritis of the knees may not respond to either oral or IV antibiotics. This presumably immune-mediated syndrome may be treatable with antiinflammatory agents. It usually resolves eventually, although it may take several years. Public education for the prevention of Lyme disease is outlined in Table 60-9.

Table 60-9 Patient Education for Prevention of Lyme Disease

- Avoid walking through tall grasses and low brush.
- Mow grass and remove brush along paths, buildings, and campsites.
- Move woodpiles and bird feeders away from house.
- Wear long pants or nylon tights of tightly woven, light-colored fabric so that ticks can be easily seen.
- Tuck pants into boots or long socks, tuck long-sleeved shirts into pants, and wear closed shoes when hiking.
- Check often for ticks crawling from legs to open skin.
- Thoroughly inspect and wash clothes.
- Spray insect repellent containing DEET on skin or permethrin on clothes, especially on lower extremities.
- Have pets wear tick collars, inspect them often, and do not allow them on furniture or beds.
- Remove attached ticks with tweezers (not fingers). Grasp tick's mouth parts as close to skin as possible and gently pull straight out. Do not twist or jerk.
- Dispose of tick in alcohol or flush down toilet. Do not crush with fingers.
- Wash bitten area with soap and water and apply antiseptic. Wash hands.
- See a doctor immediately if flulike symptoms or "bull's-eye" rash appears within a few weeks after removal of tick.

DEET, NN, Diethyl-M-Toluamide.

HUMAN IMMUNODEFICIENCY VIRUS INFECTION AND ARTHRITIS

A variety of inflammatory arthritis conditions have been reported in the presence of human immunodeficiency virus (HIV) infection.[27] The pathogenesis of these disorders is unknown. With suppression of the CD4 T lymphocytes, opportunistic organisms cause infectious arthritis, osteomyelitis, and pyomyositis. RA and SLE generally improve as immunodeficiency develops. However, rheumatic diseases associated with HLA-B27 appear to become more severe in HIV-infected patients; for example, progressive, erosive upper-extremity joint disease occurs in Reiter's syndrome, and psoriatic arthritis exhibits a generalized, pustular rash. A Sjögren's-type sicca syndrome, diffuse infiltrative lymphocytosis syndrome, has been identified as a response to HIV infection in children and adults with specific HLA typing. Vasculitis may be responsible for unexplained multisystem disease, arthritis, or fever of unknown origin in HIV-infected patients. Antirheumatic therapy may be effective for short periods but may impair cellular immunity and promote exacerbations of underlying infections.

Table 60-10 Associated Conditions Leading to Hyperuricemia

Obesity	Malignant disease
Diabetes mellitus	Sickle cell anemia
Hyperlipidemia	Cytotoxic drugs
Hypertension	Intrinsic renal disease
Atherosclerosis	Drug-induced renal impairment
Myeloproliferative disorders	Acidosis or ketosis

GOUT

Gout is characterized by recurrent attacks of acute arthritis in association with increased levels of serum uric acid. It may be classified as primary or secondary. In *primary gout* a hereditary error of purine metabolism leads to the overproduction or retention of uric acid. *Secondary gout* may be related to another acquired disorder (Table 60-10) or may be the result of medications known to inhibit uric acid excretion. Secondary gout may also be caused by medications that increase the rate of cell death, such as the chemotherapeutic agents used in treating leukemia.

Significance

Primary gout occurs predominantly (90%) in middle-aged men, with almost no incidence in premenopausal women. Frequency of hyperuricemia is increased in the families of patients with primary gout. Although some races have been identified as having a low incidence of gout, people of the same race living in another country may exhibit higher mean serum uric acid levels, indicating that both genetic and environmental factors contribute to the etiology.

Etiology and Pathophysiology

Uric acid represents the major end product of the catabolism of purines and is primarily excreted by the kidneys. Thus hyperuricemia may be the result of increased purine synthesis, decreased renal excretion, or both. About half the patients with primary gout can be shown to produce excessive amounts of uric acid. Folklore has long associated excesses of food and drink with acute attacks of gouty arthritis. Although high dietary intake of purine alone has relatively little effect on uric acid levels, it is clear that hyperuricemia may result from prolonged fasting or excessive drinking because of increased production of keto acids, which then inhibit normal renal excretion of uric acid.

Clinical Manifestations

In the acute phase, gouty arthritis may occur in one or more joints but usually less than four. Affected joints may appear dusky or cyanotic and are extremely tender. Inflammation of the great toe (*podagra*) is most commonly the initial involvement and occurs in 75% of all patients. Other joints affected are the midtarsal, ankle, knee, and wrist joints and the olecranon bursa. Acute gouty arthritis is usually precipitated by events such as trauma, surgery, alcohol ingestion, or systemic infection. Onset of symptoms is usually rapid, with swelling and pain peaking within several hours, often accompanied by low-grade fever. Individual attacks usually subside, treated or untreated, in 2 to 10 days. The affected joint returns entirely to normal, and patients are often free of symptoms between attacks.

Chronic gout is characterized by multiple joint involvement and deposits of sodium urate crystals (*tophi*). These are typically seen in the synovium, subchondral bone, olecranon bursa, and vertebrae; along tendons; and in the skin and cartilage (Fig. 60-8). Tophi are rarely present at the time of the initial attack and are generally noted only many years after the onset of disease.

The severity of gouty arthritis is variable. The clinical course may consist of infrequent mild attacks or multiple severe episodes associated with a slowly progressive disability. In general, the higher the serum uric acid level, the earlier the appearance of tophi and the greater the tendency toward more frequent and severe episodes of acute gout. An elevated serum uric acid alone does not indicate gout, even when joint symptoms are present, because high serum uric acid is found in a variety of diseases. Gout can be diagnosed unequivocally only when urate crystals are found in joint fluid.

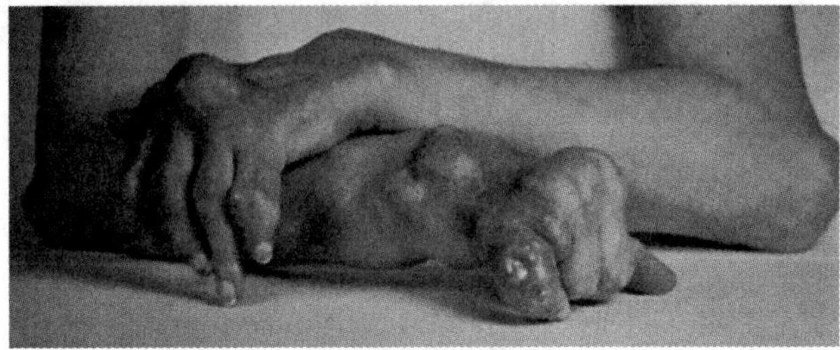

Fig. 60-8 Tophaceous gout.

Complications

Chronic inflammation may result in joint deformity. Destruction of the cartilage may predispose the joint to secondary OA. Tophaceous deposits may be large and unsightly and may perforate overlying skin, producing draining sinuses that often become secondarily infected. Excessive uric acid excretion may lead to kidney or urinary tract stone formation. Pyelonephritis associated with intrarenal sodium urate deposits and obstruction may contribute to renal disease.

Diagnostic Studies

The diagnosis can be established by finding monosodium urate monohydrate crystals in the synovial fluid of an inflamed joint or tophus. In another goutlike syndrome, referred to as *pseudogout*, nonurate (calcium pyrophosphate dihydrate) crystals are identified in synovial fluid analysis. Serum uric acid levels are almost always elevated to 8 mg/dl (476 μmol/L) or higher. Specimens for 24-hour urine uric acid levels are obtained to control for daily fluctuations in urate concentrations and are important in determining whether the patient undersecretes or overproduces uric acid. Hyperuricemia is not specifically diagnostic of gout because increased levels may be related to a variety of drugs or may exist as a totally asymptomatic abnormality in the general population.

Therapeutic Management

Therapeutic management of gout (Table 60-11) has several goals. The first is to terminate an acute attack. This is accomplished by the use of an anti-inflammatory agent such as colchicine. Future attacks are prevented by a maintenance dose of colchicine, weight reduction if necessary, avoidance of alcohol and high-purine foods, and the use of drugs to reduce the serum urate concentration. Treatment is also aimed at preventing the formation of uric-acid kidney stones and other associated conditions such as hypertriglyceridemia and hypertension.

Pharmacologic Management. Acute gouty arthritis is treated with one of three types of antiinflammatory agents: colchicine, NSAIDs, or corticosteroids. Corticosteroids should be reserved for cases in which colchicine or NSAIDs are contraindicated or ineffective.

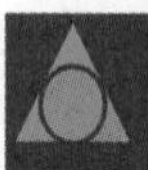

Table 60-11 Therapeutic Management: Gout

Diagnostic
- History and physical examination
- Family history of gout
- Presence of monosodium urate monohydrate crystals in synovial fluid
- Elevated serum uric acid levels
- Elevated 24-hr urine for uric acid levels

Therapeutic
- Bed rest and joint immobilization
- Local application of heat or cold
- Joint aspiration and intraarticular corticosteroids
- Nonsteroidal antiinflammatory drugs
- Drug therapy (e.g., colchicine, probenecid, allopurinol)

Although medication does not prevent recurrent attacks of gout, it can control its symptoms in 75% of gout attacks, particularly with prompt treatment. Oral administration of colchicine generally produces dramatic pain relief within 24 to 48 hours. Colchicine has diagnostic merit in that a good response to treatment gives further evidence for the diagnosis of gout. Prophylactic doses of colchicine reduce the frequency of attacks but do not alter the serum uric acid level.

For many years the standard therapy for hyperuricemia has been a uricosuric drug (e.g., probenecid), which acts by increasing urinary uric acid excretion by inhibiting tubular reabsorption of urates. Aspirin inactivates the effect of uricosurics, resulting in urate retention, and should be avoided while patients are taking probenecid and other uricosuric drugs. Acetaminophen can be used safely if analgesia is required.

Adequate urine volume must be maintained to prevent precipitation of uric acid in the renal tubules. Allopurinol (Zyloprim), which blocks the production of uric acid, may control the serum level and is particularly useful in patients with uric acid stones or renal impairment, in whom uricosuric drugs may be ineffective or dangerous. Regardless of which drug or combination of drugs is prescribed, it is essential that the concentration of serum uric acid be checked regularly to monitor the effectiveness of treatment.

Nutritional Management. Dietary restrictions may include limiting the use of alcohol and of foods high in purine (see Table 43-9). However, medication can generally control the situation without necessitating these limitations. Obese patients should be instructed in a carefully planned weight-reduction program.

NURSING MANAGEMENT

GOUT

Acute gouty arthritis may be prevented by maintenance of the serum uric acid at normal levels. Nursing intervention is directed at supportive care of the inflamed joints. Bed rest may be appropriate, with affected joints properly immobilized. The limitation of motion and degree of pain should be assessed. Treatment effectiveness should be documented. Special care is taken to avoid causing pain to an inflamed joint by careless handling. Involvement of a lower extremity may require use of a cradle or footboard to protect the painful area from the weight of bed clothes.

The patient and the family should understand that hyperuricemia and gouty arthritis are chronic problems that can be controlled with careful adherence to a treatment program.[28] Thorough explanations should be given concerning the importance of drug therapy and the need for periodic determination of blood uric acid levels. The patient should be able to demonstrate knowledge of precipitating factors that may cause an attack, including overindulgence in intake of calories, purines and alcohol, starvation (fasting), medication use (e.g., aspirin, diuretics), and major medical events (e.g., surgery, myocardial infarction).

SYSTEMIC LUPUS ERYTHEMATOSUS

Systemic lupus erythematosus (SLE) is a chronic multisystem inflammatory disease of connective tissue that often involves the skin, joints, serous membranes (pleura, pericardium), kidneys, hematologic system, and central nervous system (CNS).[29] SLE is characterized by its variability within and among persons, with a chronic unpredictable course of exacerbations of disease activity alternating with periods of remission. The clinical presentation of SLE ranges from a mild to a serious illness with a tendency to acute, occasionally fatal exacerbations precipitated by several factors. Individuals with SLE can now live a normal life span.

Significance

The true incidence of SLE is uncertain, but the rate appears to be increasing. It is unknown whether this increase is a reflection of heightened diagnostic awareness or a true increase in frequency.[30] The general prevalence of SLE is approximately 1 in 2100. Women have a higher incidence (about 5:1) than men. Women account for 78% to 96% of all cases in the United States and 85% of all cases in Canada.[31] The disease is observed three times more often in African-American than in Caucasian women.[32] Because of the difficulty in diagnosing SLE, the incidence and prevalence of the disease may be much higher than statistics show.

Etiology and Pathophysiology

The etiology of SLE is unknown. However, factors implicated in the etiology of SLE include genetic predisposition, sex hormones, race, environmental factors (e.g., ultraviolet radiation, drugs, chemicals), viruses and infections, stress, and immunologic abnormalities. SLE is a disorder of immune regulation. Pathophysiology depends on autoimmune reactions directed against constituents of the cell nucleus, particularly DNA. In SLE, autoantibodies are produced against nuclear antigens (DNA, histones, ribonucleoproteins, and nucleolar factors), cytoplasmic antigens (ribosomal and cardiolipin), and blood cell surface antigens (WBCs, red blood cells [RBCs], platelets, and granulocytes). When autoantibodies bind to their specific antigens, complement activation occurs. Accumulation of immune complexes within the blood vessel walls and subsequent complement activation leads to a condition called lupus vasculitis. The ensuing ischemia within the blood vessel walls gradually leads to the thickening of the internal cell lining, fibrinoid degeneration, and thrombus formation. The specific manifestations of SLE depend on which cell types or organs are involved.

The overaggressive antibody response is related to B-cell hyperactivity accompanied by multiple abnormalities in immunoregulation. Examples of this include decreased T-suppressor cells and diminished interleukin-2 production.[33]

The importance of heredity in the development and expression of SLE has been supported by recognition of familial clustering and the identification of genetic markers.[34] The major histocompatibility complexes HLA-DR2 and HLA-DR3 show significant associations with SLE.

Hormones are known to play a role in the etiology of SLE. There are a disproportionate number of females with SLE. In addition there is a propensity for the disease to worsen during pregnancy and the immediate postpartum period. Healthy women are more immunologically reactive than healthy men because estrogens enhance immune reactivity, whereas androgens suppress it. It is thought that estrogens produce their effect through their impact on suppressor T cells, which normally regulate B-cell reactivity. In the absence of the T-cell regulatory function, the antibody proliferation by the B cells ensues.[31] In addition, it has been determined that the type of lymphocytes vary between women and men. Women have slightly higher proportions of T helper cells (which increase immune reactivity) and lower T suppressor cells (which decrease immune reactivity) than men.[32] These factors may increase a woman's potential for acquiring autoimmune diseases. Onset or exacerbation of disease symptoms sometimes occurs after the onset of menarche, with the use of oral contraceptives, and during and after pregnancy.

SLE may also be precipitated or aggravated by certain drugs such as procainamide, hydralazine, and a number of antiepileptic anticonvulsant agents. Some antiinfective agents (e.g., penicillins, sulfonamide) and oral contraceptives may also aggravate the disease.

Clinical Manifestations and Complications

SLE is extremely variable in its severity, ranging from a relatively mild disorder to a rapidly progressive one affecting many organ systems (Fig. 60-9). There is no characteristic pattern of progressive organ involvement, nor is it predictable which systems may become affected. Theoretically, any organ can be affected by the accumulation of the circulating immune complexes. However, cutaneous and muscle tissue, the lining of the lungs, the heart, nervous tissue, and the kidneys are most commonly affected. SLE is characterized by alternating periods of remission and exacerbation. General constitutional complaints include fever, weight loss, arthralgia, and excessive fatigue and may precede an exacerbation of disease activity.

Dermatologic Manifestations. The most common cutaneous feature of SLE is an erythematous rash that can occur on the face, neck, and extremities. The classic butterfly rash, which is distributed across the bridge of the nose and cheeks, occurs in about 40% of patients (Fig. 60-10). The rash may appear as discoid (coinlike) lesions or as a diffuse maculopapular rash; it may occur anywhere on the body but is most frequently seen on the face and chest. A small group of patients have persistent lesions, photosensitivity, and mild systemic disease, and test positive for SS-A (Ro) antibodies. This syndrome is referred to as *subacute cutaneous lupus.*[35]

Exposure to sunlight and to other sources of ultraviolet radiation can cause a severe skin reaction and may precipitate a flare-up of disease activity in persons who are photosensitive. Ulcers of the oral or nasopharyngeal membranes occur in up to one third of patients with SLE. Transient diffuse or patchy hair loss (alopecia) is common, with or without underlying scalp lesions. The hair may grow back during remission. The scalp becomes dry, scaly, and atrophied because of deposits of immune complexes in the microcirculation.

Musculoskeletal Problems. Polyarthralgia with morning stiffness is often the patient's first complaint and may precede the onset of multisystem disease by many years. Arthritis occurs in 95% of all patients with SLE at some time in the disease course. Joint symptoms are typically migratory, producing pain without objective signs of inflammation. Lupus-related arthritis is generally nonerosive, but it may cause deformities such as swan neck, ulnar deviation, and subluxation with hyperlaxity of the joints. Only about 30% of SLE patients test positive for rheumatoid factor.[36]

Cardiopulmonary Problems. Pericarditis is present in nearly one fourth of patients with SLE and is usually associated with myocardial disease. Patients treated with corticosteroids have a higher incidence of atherosclerosis. Pleurisy with or without effusion is seen in nearly 50% of patients at some time during the illness, and pulmonary function studies are abnormal in 90%. Raynaud's phenomenon occurs in 20% of patients (see Chapter 35). Cardiovascular involvement is an ominous sign of advanced disease and contributes significantly to the morbidity and mortality seen in SLE.

Renal Problems. Clinical evidence of renal involvement is present in nearly one half of patients with SLE and includes microscopic hematuria, excessive cellular casts in the urine sediment, proteinuria, and elevation of serum creatinine level. Kidney involvement varies in degree but may eventually end in renal failure. Regardless of whether renal manifestations are evident, nearly all patients with SLE show renal histologic abnormalities in renal biopsy studies or autopsy results. Nephritis is the leading cause of death in SLE.[37]

Clinical factors, including blood pressure, urinalysis, serum creatinine levels, serum complement levels, and autoantibodies to DNA, should be monitored carefully and frequently over prolonged periods because renal involvement in the early stages is usually asymptomatic.

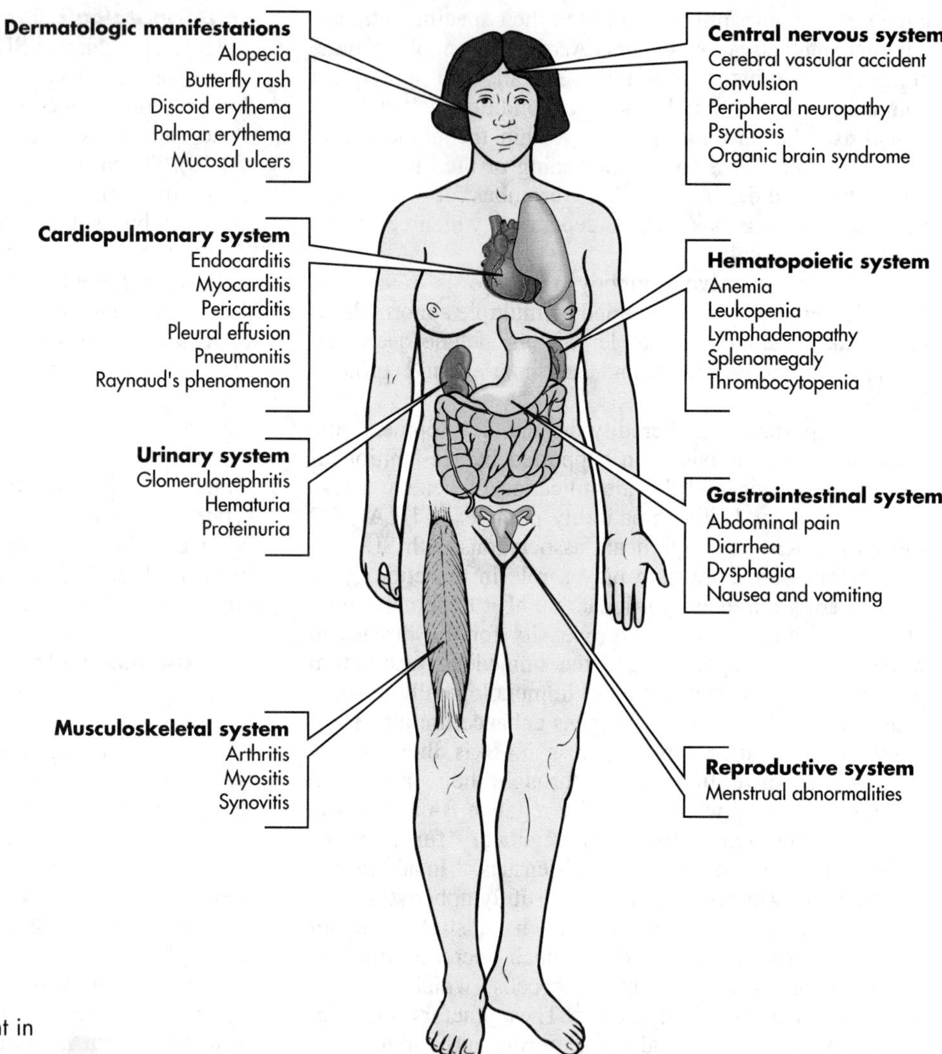

Fig. 60-9 Multisystem involvement in systemic lupus erythematosus.

Central Nervous System Problems. CNS involvement ranks close behind kidney disease and infection as a leading cause of death in SLE. Seizures are the most common neurologic manifestation and occur in as many as 15% of patients with SLE by the time of diagnosis. They may be of the grand mal, petit mal, or psychomotor type and are generally controlled by corticosteroids or anticonvulsant therapy.

Organic brain syndrome, another recognized CNS manifestation of SLE, may result from the deposition of immune complexes within brain tissue. It is characterized by disordered thought processes, disorientation, memory deficits, and psychiatric symptoms such as severe depression and psychosis. Recovery from organic brain disease is expected, although some residual impairment may result. Occasionally a cerebrovascular accident (stroke) or aseptic meningitis may be attributable to SLE. It is difficult to differentiate neuropsychiatric SLE from non-SLE neurologic problems.

Hematologic Problems. The formation of antibodies against blood cells such as erythrocytes, leukocytes, thrombocytes, and coagulation factors is one of the most common features of SLE. Anemia (98%), mild leukopenia (80%), thrombocytopenia (36%), and lupus anticoagulant (50%) are often present.[36] Some patients show a tendency to bleed whereas others show a tendency toward blood clots. In addition, SLE patients have positive antinuclear antibodies.

Infection. Patients with SLE appear to have increased susceptibility to infections, possibly related to defects in their ability to phagocytize invading bacteria, deficiencies in production of antibodies, and the immunosuppressive effect of many anti-inflammatory drugs. Infection, a major cause of death, has an incidence of 30%. Pneumonia is most common. Any fever should be considered serious because it may indicate an underlying infectious process rather than lupus activity alone.

Diagnostic Studies

The diagnosis of SLE is based on the history, physical examination, and laboratory findings (Table 60-12). A variety of abnormalities may be present in the blood, including

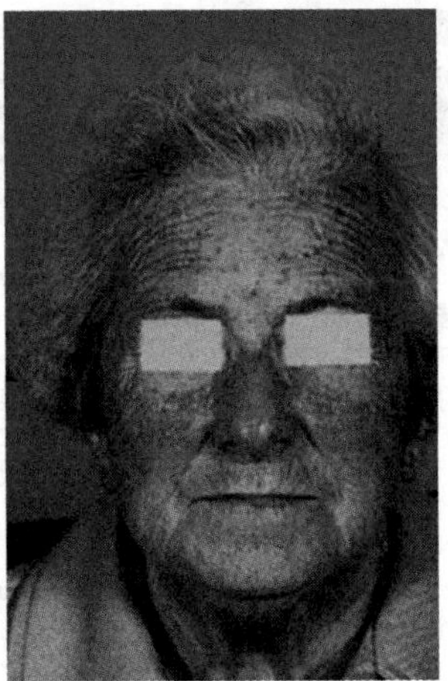

Fig. 60-10 Butterfly rash of systemic lupus erythematosus.

elevated ESR, increased γ-globulin levels, anemia, decreased WBC and platelet counts, electrocardiogram (ECG) or chest x-ray evidence of pericarditis or pleural effusion, and a false-positive serologic test for syphilis. Abnormalities in urine sediment (cellular casts, proteinuria), reduced serum complement, and tissue specimens demonstrating changes compatible with SLE are other confirmatory findings.

Autoantibodies directed against nuclear antigens (ANA) have been detected in 99% of persons with SLE. Although extremely sensitive, ANA is not specific for SLE because it is present in 5% of normal persons and 38% of all persons more than 60 years of age. Anti-DNA is found most commonly in SLE and is rarely seen in other rheumatic diseases. Anti-Sm antibody, an antibody to the Smith nuclear antigen, is a definitive serologic marker for SLE and is not demonstrated in other rheumatic diseases.[38]

Therapeutic Management

The rate of spontaneous remission in SLE is high. Corticosteroids remain the mainstay for treatment of severe illness. Their use should be reserved for acute generalized exacerbation or serious organ involvement, although a reduced maintenance dosage is sometimes used. Immunosuppressive drugs may be used for symptoms that are resistant to corticosteroid therapy (Table 60-13). Efficacy of treatment is most appropriately monitored by serial serum complement levels and anti-DNA titers.

An improving prognosis of SLE may be the result of earlier diagnosis, prompt recognition of serious organ involvement, and better therapeutic regimens. Survival is influenced by several factors, including age, race, gender, socioeconomic status, accompanying morbid conditions, and severity of disease. For example, childhood-onset SLE accounts for nearly 20% of all cases and has a higher incidence of nephritis (up to 80%) than in other age groups, adversely influencing prognosis.

Pharmacologic Management. Therapeutic programs for SLE are prescribed to suppress inflammation and the immune system and depend almost entirely on disease activity. Aspirin or other NSAIDs may reduce mild symptoms such as fever and arthritic complaints. GI upset and tinnitus should be reported. Antimalarial drugs such as hydroxychloroquine (Plaquenil) may be used to improve skin problems, but eye examinations must be scheduled periodically during this therapy because visual loss is a rare but serious side effect. Topical steroid preparations and intralesional steroid injections are effective treatments for skin lesions.

Table 60-12 Criteria for Diagnosis of Systemic Lupus Erythematosus*

Malar rash
Discoid rash
Photosensitivity
Oral ulcers
Arthritis: nonerosive, involvement of two or more joints
Serositis: pleuritis or pericarditis
Renal disorder: proteinuria or cellular casts in urine
Neurologic disorder: seizures or psychosis
Hematologic disorder: hemolytic anemia, leukopenia, lymphopenia, or thrombocytopenia
Immunologic disorder: positive lupus cell preparation; anti-DNA antibody or antibody to Sm nuclear antigen; false-positive serologic tests for syphilis
Antinuclear antibodies

*A person is classified as having SLE if four or more of the criteria are present, serially or simultaneously, during any interval of observation. Revised criteria by a subcommittee of the American College of Rheumatology are used for the purpose of *classification* in population surveys, *not* for the diagnosis of individual patients.

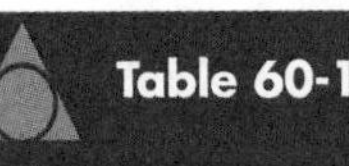

Table 60-13 Therapeutic Management: Systemic Lupus Erythematosus

Diagnostic
- History and physical examination
- Lupus cell preparation
- Antibodies
  - Anti-DNA antibody
  - Anti-Sm antibody
  - Antinuclear antibody (ANA)
- Complete blood cell count
- Urinalysis
- X-ray of affected joints
- Chest x-ray
- Complement levels (CH_{50}, C3)
- ECG

Therapeutic
- NSAIDs
- Antimalarials
- Corticosteroids for exacerbations and severe disease
- Immunosuppressive drugs (e.g., cyclophosphamide)

DNA, Deoxyribonucleic acid; *ECG*, electrocardiogram; *NSAIDs*, nonsteroidal antiinflammatory drugs; *Sm antibody*, Smith antibody.

Corticosteroids are potent antiinflammatory medications used for acute generalized exacerbations of SLE and for the treatment of serious involvement of vital organs, including hematologic abnormalities. As clinical and laboratory values improve, the dosages are gradually tapered.

Patient education must include indications for use and proper administration of steroids and possible side effects (see Chapter 47). The patient should understand that abrupt cessation may precipitate recurrence of disease activity. Immunosuppressive drug therapy such as azathioprine (Imuran) and cyclophosphamide (Cytoxan) is occasionally used in life-threatening situations for symptoms unresponsive to more conservative treatment.

NURSING MANAGEMENT

SYSTEMIC LUPUS ERYTHEMATOSUS

Nursing Assessment

As in the majority of rheumatic diseases, the chronic and unpredictable nature of SLE presents many challenges to the patient and family. The physical, psychologic, and sociocultural problems associated with the long-term management of SLE require the varied approaches and skills of the multidisciplinary health care team.

Subjective and objective data that should be obtained from a patient with SLE are presented in Table 60-14. The extent to which pain and fatigue influence activities of daily living must be evaluated. A developmental approach focuses on age-appropriate educational and counseling issues, such as personal relationships, family planning, occupational responsibilities, and recreational activities.

Table 60-14 Nursing Assessment: Systemic Lupus Erythematosus

Subjective Data

Important health information

Past health history: History of remissions and exacerbations; triggers, including overexposure to UV light, staphylococcal or viral infections, physical or psychological stress, x-ray exposure

Medications: Use of hydralazine, isoniazid, anticonvulsants (possibly causing symptoms of SLE), corticosteroids, NSAIDs

Functional health patterns

Health perception–health management: Family history; fatigue, malaise

Nutritional-metabolic: Weight loss, oral and nasal ulcers; xerostomia (salivary gland dryness), dysphagia; nausea and vomiting; photosensitivity with rash; frequent infections

Elimination: Hematuria, decreased urine output; diarrhea or constipation

Activity-exercise: Morning stiffness; joint pain and swelling

Sleep-rest: Insomnia

Cognitive-perceptual: Visual disturbances; vertigo; headache; polyarthralgia, chest pain (pericardial, pleuritic); abdominal pain; joint pain; depression

Sexuality-reproductive: Amenorrhea, irregular menstrual periods

Objective Data

General

Lymphadenopathy, periorbital edema, anxiety, mania

Integumentary

Alopecia, keratoconjunctivitis, malar "butterfly" rash, palmar or discoid erythema, urticaria, purpura or petechiae, leg ulcers

Respiratory

Pleural friction rub

Cardiovascular

Vasculitis, pericardial friction rub; hypertension, edema, dysrhythmias, murmurs, bilateral symmetric pallor and cyanosis of fingers (Raynaud's phenomenon)

Gastrointestinal

Painless oral and pharyngeal ulcers, hepatosplenomegaly

Neurologic

Facial weakness, peripheral neuropathies, papilledema, dysarthria, confusion, hallucination, disorientation, psychosis, seizures, aphasia, hemiparesis

Musculoskeletal

Myopathy, myositis, arthritis

Possible laboratory findings

Positive lupus cell preparation, elevated ANA titers, presence of anti-DNA and Sm-nuclear antibodies, decreased T-suppressor lymphocyte count

ANA, Antinuclear antibodies; *DNA*, deoxyribonucleic acid; *NSAIDs*, nonsteroidal antiinflammatory drugs; *SLE*, systemic lupus erythematosus; *UV*, ultraviolet.

Nursing Diagnoses

Nursing diagnoses related to SLE include, but are not limited to, those presented in the nursing care plan for the patient with SLE on p. 1923.

Planning

The overall goals are that the patient with systemic lupus erythematosus will (1) have satisfactory pain relief, (2) comply with therapeutic regimen to achieve maximum symptom management, (3) avoid activities that induce disease exacerbation, and (4) maintain a positive self-image.

Nursing Implementation

Acute Intervention. Prevention of SLE is not possible at this time. Education of health professionals and the community may promote a clearer understanding of the disease and earlier diagnosis and treatment.

During an exacerbation, patients may become abruptly and dramatically ill. Nursing intervention includes accurately recording the severity of symptoms and documenting response to therapy. Fever pattern, joint inflammation, limitation of motion, location and degree of discomfort, and fatigability should be specifically assessed. The patient's weight and fluid intake and output should be monitored because of the fluid-retention effect of steroids and the possibility of renal failure. Careful collection of 24-hour

NURSING CARE PLAN Patient with Systemic Lupus Erythematosus

Planning: Outcome Criteria	Nursing Interventions and Rationales
➤ **NURSING DIAGNOSIS**	Fatigue *related to* disease process *as manifested by* lack of energy, inability to maintain usual routine
Complete priority activities; practice pacing of activities; verbalize having more energy.	Analyze energy level patterns *to use in planning daily activities.* Assist patient to prioritize activities *to establish preferred daily routine.* Teach energy conservation techniques such as sitting at kitchen sink and enlisting aid of others *to accomplish as much as possible with a minimum of energy expenditure.** Include family in planning *to increase patient's sense of support and family understanding of fatigue problem.* Teach patient techniques such as meditation and yoga *to provide patient with stress-reducing strategies.* Encourage patient to rest regularly and as needed *to temporarily reverse effect of fatigue.*
➤ **NURSING DIAGNOSIS**	Pain *related to* disease process and inadequate comfort measures *as manifested by* complaints of joint pain, lack of relief from pain-relieving measures; reduction of activity to avoid exacerbating pain
Express satisfaction with pain relief measures; perform activities of daily living without pain.	Assess pain location and severity *to plan appropriate interventions.* Provide for periods of rest *to provide recuperation from exhaustion that results from pain.* Administer analgesia as ordered; monitor effect; teach joint protection measures; apply heat or cold *as individually determined effective to relieve pain.* Use nonpharmacologic pain interventions such as relaxation and visual imagery *to replace or supplement analgesics.*
➤ **NURSING DIAGNOSIS**	Body-image disturbance *related to* change in physical appearance *as manifested by* verbalization of dissatisfaction with physical appearance, lack of participation in hygiene and grooming practices, isolation, refusal to see friends and family
Have increased self-interest and participation in self-care; express positive comments about self.	Discuss realistic expectations of physical changes *to help patient make plans to maximize physical assets and minimize problematic areas.* Encourage interest in hygiene and grooming; teach ways to use cosmetics creatively *because these activities improve body image and sense of control.* Encourage discussion about feelings and positive attributes *to reduce patient's sense of isolation and poor body image and redirect self-focus to positive attributes.*
➤ **NURSING DIAGNOSIS**	Impaired skin integrity *related to* photosensitivity, skin rash, urticaria, and alopecia *as manifested by* rash anywhere on body, butterfly rash on face, alopecia, areas of ulceration on fingertips
Limit direct exposure to sun and use sunscreens; have no open skin lesions; plan strategies to cope with alopecia.	Assess and monitor location and progression of rash *to plan appropriate interventions.* Administer medications and apply ointments as ordered *to control skin manifestations.* Keep skin clean and dry *to avoid secondary infections.* Avoid unprescribed ointments *because these often exacerbate existing conditions.* Discuss need to limit direct sun exposure and use SPF 15 when outdoors *because sun exacerbates skin and systemic manifestations.*

continued

urine for protein may be required. The nurse should observe for signs of bleeding that result from drug therapy, such as pallor, skin bruising, petechiae, or tarry stools.

Careful assessment of neurologic status includes observation for visual disturbances, headaches, personality changes, and forgetfulness. Psychosis may indicate CNS disease or may be the effect of corticosteroid therapy. Irritation of the nerves of the extremities (peripheral neuropathy) may produce numbness, tingling, and weakness of the hands and feet. Less frequently a stroke may result.

The nurse must explain the nature of the disease and modes of therapy and prepare the patient for numerous diagnostic procedures. Emotional support for the patient and family is essential.

Chronic and Home Management. Nursing interventions must emphasize health teaching and home man-

NURSING CARE PLAN Patient with Systemic Lupus Erythematosus—cont'd

Planning: Outcome Criteria	*Nursing Interventions and Rationales*
➤ **NURSING DIAGNOSIS**	Activity intolerance *related to* arthralgia, weakness, and fatigue *as manifested by* inability or unwillingness to ambulate or engage in physical activity, dyspnea, abnormal response to activity (e.g., increased heart rate, respiratory rate)
Express satisfaction with activity pattern; participate in sufficient activities to avoid problems related to immobility; pace activities to level of tolerance.	Assess tolerance to activity *to plan appropriate interventions and modifications.* Pace activities and allow periods of rest between activities *to promote recuperation and to foster maximum participation in activities.** Encourage patient to assist in setting activity schedule *to allow patient a sense of control and foster cooperation with the plan.* Monitor vital signs when ambulating *because an increasing pulse and respiratory rate may indicate a need to allow patient to rest.* Provide bed rest during exacerbation *to conserve energy for vital activities.* Increase activities slowly *to allow patient to adjust to increased energy demands.* Provide range-of-motion exercises q4hr to unaffected joints *to prevent contractures and stiffness from developing.* Encourage use of assistive devices *to minimize energy expense.*
➤ **NURSING DIAGNOSIS**	Altered nutrition: less than body requirements *related to* anorexia, fatigue, oral ulcerations, nausea, vomiting, weakness, and immunosuppressive therapy *as manifested by* weight loss
Maintain weight; have intake of sufficient quantity and quality of food to meet daily needs; derive pleasure from meals.	Assess food preferences and include them in meal planning when possible *to promote adequate intake and patient's sense of control.* Offer small, frequent meals *to foster adequate intake by reducing fatigue and bloating associated with larger, less frequent meals.* Provide good oral hygiene before and after meals *to increase patient comfort and prevent causing or exacerbating oral ulcerations.* Monitor pertinent laboratory values such as hemoglobin, electrolytes, and protein levels *because lowered levels can indicate inadequate intake.* Encourage family to bring in favorite foods *to increase patient's intake and as a gesture of love and caring.*
➤ **NURSING DIAGNOSIS**	Ineffective management of therapeutic regimen *related to* lack of knowledge of long-term management of disease *as manifested by* questioning about SLE or incorrect answers to questions by patient or family, use of unproven remedies
Express confidence in ability to manage SLE over time and in home environment.	Teach patient about disease process, including chronic management *to increase probability of successful long-term management.* Include family in teaching activities *to provide caregivers during exacerbation and to increase their sense of involvement and control.* Discuss need to wear Medic-Alert bracelet *to alert uninformed health care providers in time of emergency.* Inform patient of availability of assistance from Lupus Foundation and Arthritis Foundation *to provide additional sources of information and sharing.*

COLLABORATIVE PROBLEMS

Nursing Goals	*Nursing Interventions and Rationales*
➤ **POTENTIAL COMPLICATION**	Increased inflammatory response *related to* exacerbation of disease process
Monitor for signs of increased inflammatory response of any associated body system, report deviations from acceptable parameters, and carry out appropriate medical and nursing interventions.	Assess and monitor body systems regularly through vital signs, physical examination, laboratory studies, and patient's subjective comments about health *to detect presence of problems associated with any affected body system* (e.g, edema, hypertension, seizures, mental status, pain and joint swelling, dyspnea, cyanosis, oral and skin lesions). Report alterations suggestive of a problem to physician; teach patient signs and symptoms to observe for and what to report to physician; encourage ongoing medical follow-up *to ensure early intervention.*

SLE, Systemic lupus erythematosus; *SPF,* sun protection factor.
*See Tables 60-3 and 60-8.

agement. The patient with a chronic illness must be taught to live *with* the disease, not *for* it.

The patient must understand that even perfect adherence to the treatment plan is not a guarantee against exacerbation because the course of the disease is unpredictable. However, a variety of factors may encourage exacerbation, such as fatigue, sun exposure, emotional stress, infection, drugs, and surgery. Nursing interventions should be directed toward assisting the patient and family to eliminate or minimize exposure to precipitating factors. Patient understanding and cooperation are important to this goal. Patient and family education should include the following:

1. Education on the disease process
2. Names of medications and actions, side effects, dosage, and administration
3. Energy-conservation and pacing techniques
4. Daily heat and exercise program (for arthralgia)
5. Avoidance of physical and emotional stress, overexposure to ultraviolet light, and unnecessary exposure to infection
6. Regular medical and laboratory follow-up
7. Marital counseling, if necessary
8. Referral resources to community and health care agencies

Lupus and pregnancy. For the best outcome for the female patient with SLE, pregnancy should be planned with the cooperation of the primary physician and obstetrician at a point when the disease activity is minimal.[39] Only women with serious renal, cardiac, or CNS involvement should be counseled against pregnancy. Exacerbation is common during the postpartum period. Therapeutic abortion offers the same risk of postdelivery exacerbation as carrying the fetus to term.

Fetal risks include increased rates of miscarriage, prematurity, and stillbirth. Neonatal lupus is an uncommon occurrence, characterized by rash, transient lupus antibodies, or congenital complete heart block. SS-A antibodies in the mother appear to be associated with complete heart block in the fetus. Antiphospholipid antibodies may be predictive of placental insufficiency and thrombosis and have been correlated with repeated miscarriage and intrauterine fetal death. Regular clinical and laboratory monitoring is essential for the pregnant woman with SLE.

Psychosocial issues. Many psychosocial issues confront the patient with SLE. Disease onset may be vague, and SLE is often undiagnosed for long periods of time. The nurse should counsel the patient and family that SLE has a good prognosis for the majority of persons. Men are often embarrassed that they have a "woman's disease." Families are anxious about hereditary aspects and want to know whether their children will also have SLE. Many young couples require pregnancy and sexual counseling. Young people making decisions about marriage and careers worry about how SLE will interfere with their plans. The nurse may have to educate teachers and work personnel.

The obvious physical effects of skin rashes, discoid lesions, and alopecia may cause social isolation for the patient with SLE, yet pain and fatigue are cited most frequently as interfering with quality living. Friends and relatives are confused by the patient's complaints of transient joint pain and overwhelming fatigue. Pacing techniques and relaxation therapy can help keep the patient actively involved. Daily planning should include recreational and occupational activities. Children and young adults find sun restrictions and physical limitations particularly difficult to follow. SLE also has a negative effect on the patient's self-esteem and body image.[40] Nursing interventions assist the patient in developing and accomplishing reasonable goals toward improving mobility, energy levels, and self-esteem.[41]

SYSTEMIC SCLEROSIS

Systemic sclerosis (SS), or *scleroderma*, is a disorder of connective tissue characterized by fibrotic, degenerative, and occasionally inflammatory changes in the skin, blood vessels, synovium, skeletal muscle, and internal organs. Skin thickening and tightening are the cardinal features. The disease may range from a diffuse cutaneous thickening with rapidly progressive and fatal visceral involvement to a more benign variant called CREST syndrome (*c*alcinosis, *R*aynaud's phenomenon, *e*sophageal hypomotility, *s*clerodactyly [skin change of the fingers], and *t*elangiectasia [macule-like angioma on the skin]).[42]

Significance

SS affects women three times more frequently than men, with the female to male ratio increasing to 15:1 during the childbearing years. SS has been reported in all races but is more common in African-Americans than Caucasians. Although symptoms may begin at any time, the usual age at onset is between 30 and 50 years. SS affects approximately 250,000 people in the United States.

The disease course of SS is variable. Persons with CREST syndrome have limited disability and the longest survival rates, although they are at higher risk for pulmonary arterial hypertension. Myocardial and renal involvement adversely affect the outcome in diffuse disease.

Etiology and Pathophysiology

The exact cause of SS remains unclear. Collagen, the protein that gives normal skin its strength and elasticity, is overproduced (Fig. 60-11). Widespread systemic disease may be the result of primary vessel injury or immune dysregulation. Disruption of the cell is followed by platelet aggregation, myointimal cell proliferation, and fibrosis. Proliferation of collagen disrupts the normal functioning of internal organs, such as the lungs, kidney, heart, and GI tract.

Clinical Manifestations

Raynaud's Phenomenon. Raynaud's phenomenon (paroxysmal vasospasm of the digits) occurs in nearly 98% of patients with SS and is the most common initial complaint in CREST syndrome. Patients have diminished blood flow to fingers and toes on exposure to cold (blanching or white phase), followed by cyanosis as hemoglobin releases

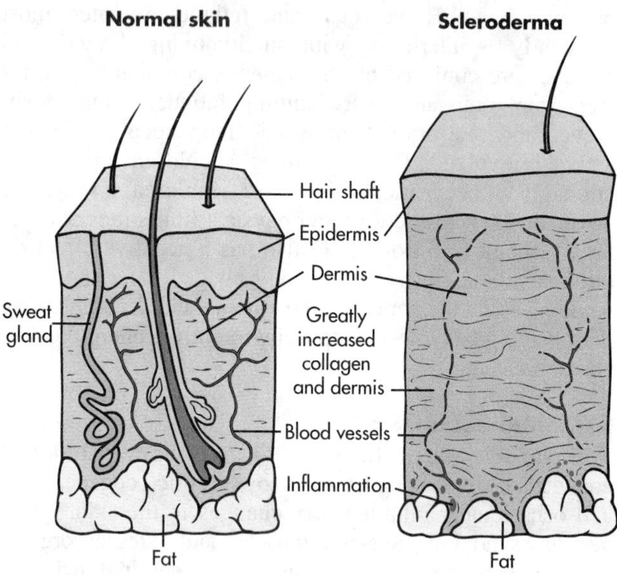

Fig. 60-11 Scleroderma skin changes.

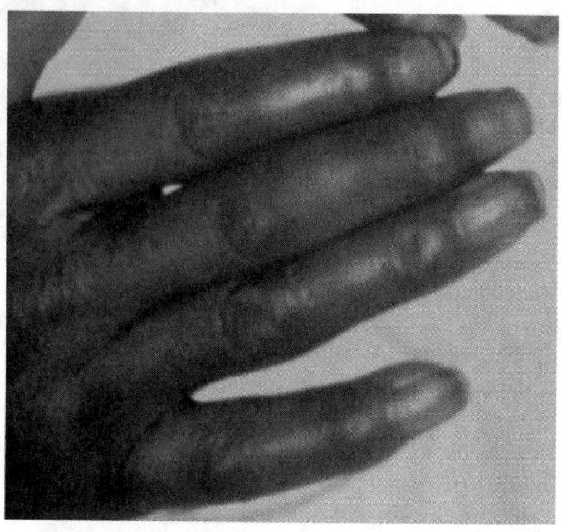

Fig. 60-12 Hand of a patient with systemic sclerosis.

oxygen to the tissues (blue phase), and then erythema on rewarming (red phase). The color changes are often accompanied by numbness and tingling. Raynaud's phenomenon may precede the onset of systemic disease by months, years, or even decades.

Skin and Joint Changes. Symmetric painless swelling or thickening of the skin of the fingers and hands may progress to diffuse scleroderma of the trunk. In CREST syndrome skin thickening is generally limited to the fingers and face. The skin loses elasticity and becomes taut and shiny, producing the typical expressionless facies with tightly pursed lips. Flexion contractures and atrophy of soft tissue may give the hands a clawlike appearance (Fig. 60-12). Polyarthralgias and morning stiffness may be early symptoms. Tendon friction rubs may be present.

Internal Organ Involvement. Esophageal hypomotility causes frequent reflux of gastric acid, causing heartburn, and substernal dysphagia for solid foods. If swallowing becomes difficult, the patient often decreases food intake and loses weight. GI complaints also include abdominal distention, diarrhea, malodorous floating stools (malabsorption syndrome) as a result of small-bowel disease, and constipation secondary to colonic involvement.

Lung involvement includes pleural thickening and pulmonary fibrosis on x-ray, as well as pulmonary function abnormalities. Pulmonary hypertension is seen almost exclusively in CREST syndrome.

Primary heart disease consists of pericarditis, pericardial effusion, and cardiac dysrhythmias. Myocardial fibrosis resulting in congestive failure occurs most frequently in those persons with diffuse SS.

Renal disease is a major cause of death in SS. Malignant arterial hypertension associated with rapidly progressive and irreversible renal insufficiency is often present. Recent improvements in dialysis, bilateral nephrectomy in patients with uncontrollable hypertension, and the advent of kidney transplantation have offered some hope to patients with renal failure.

Diagnostic Studies

Blood studies may reveal a mildly elevated ESR and occasionally hypergammaglobinemia. The presence of ANA is observed in almost all persons with SS. Autoantibody Scl-70 has been reported in diffuse SS; anticentromere antibody is associated with the CREST syndrome. Nail-bed capillary microscopy characteristically shows capillary loop dilatation with limited disease and dilatation with avascular areas in patients with diffuse disease.[43] If renal involvement is present, urinalysis may show proteinuria, microscopic hematuria, and casts. X-ray evidence of subcutaneous calcification, digital tuft resorption, distal esophageal hypomotility, or bilateral pulmonary fibrosis are diagnostic of SS. Pulmonary function studies reveal decreased vital capacity and diffusion capacity for carbon dioxide. Skin biopsy shows dermal collagen thickening, condensation, or homogenization.

Therapeutic Management

The therapeutic management of SS (Table 60-15) offers no specific treatment with long-range effect. It is directed toward attempts to prevent or treat secondary complications of involved organs. Various drugs such as anti-inflammatory agents, D- penicillamine, and colchicine have been used with varying degrees of success.

Physical therapy helps maintain joint mobility and preserve muscle strength. Occupational therapy assists the patient in maintaining functional abilities. Gastroesophageal reflux may be treated by antacids and periodic dilatation of the esophagus. Raynaud's phenomenon may be temporarily relieved by thoracic sympathectomy.

Pharmacologic Management. No specific drugs or combination of drugs has been proved effective as treatment for SS. Corticosteroids are generally reserved for patients with myositis or overlap syndromes (e.g., mixed connective tissue disease). Penicillamine (Cuprimine) increases the solubility of dermal collagen and may cause thinning of the skin, but it has many side effects. Colchicine is being used

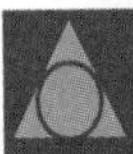

Table 60-15 Therapeutic Management: Systemic Sclerosis

Diagnostic
- History and physical examination
- Antinuclear antibody titers
- Nail-bed capillary microscopy
- X-rays of chest, hands, GI tract
- Skin or visceral biopsy
- Urinalysis (proteinuria, hematuria, casts)

Therapeutic
- Vasodilator and antihypertensive drugs
- Antiinflammatory agents (colchicine, D-penicillamine, NSAIDs)
- Physical therapy
- Antacids

GI, Gastrointestinal; *NSAIDs*, nonsteroidal antiinflammatory drugs.

to inhibit the accumulation of collagen, but evidence is still insufficient to prove its therapeutic worth. The use of immunosuppressive agents is under investigation.

Supportive measures include oral vasodilating drugs and intraarterial injections of reserpine. However, calcium channel blockers (nifedipine, diltiazem) are the treatment of choice for Raynaud's phenomenon. Infected ulcers of the fingertips may be treated by soaking with hyaluronidase and using bacterial antibiotic ointment. Joint symptoms may be relieved by aspirin and other NSAIDs. Antacids may be useful for heartburn. Combinations of antihypertensive medications, including hydralazine, minoxidil, captopril, propranolol, and methyldopa, have been used in the treatment of hypertension and renal failure.

NURSING MANAGEMENT

SYSTEMIC SCLEROSIS

Because prevention is not possible, nursing intervention often begins during a hospitalization for diagnostic purposes. Vital signs, weight, intake and output, respiratory function, and joint ROM should be assessed daily as indicated by specific symptoms to plan appropriate care. Emotional stress and a cold environment may aggravate Raynaud's phenomenon. Patients with SS should not have finger-stick blood testing done because of compromised circulation and poor digital healing. Diagnostic studies should be thoroughly explained. The nurse can help the patient resolve feelings of helplessness by providing information about the illness and encouraging active participation in planning care.

Health teaching is a major nursing concern as the patient and family begin to live with this unusual disease. Obvious changes in the face and hands lead to poor self-image and loss of mobility and function. The patient must actively carry out therapeutic exercises at home. The nurse should reinforce heat therapy, the use of assistive devices, and organization of activities to preserve strength and reduce disability.

Hands and feet should be protected from cold exposure and possible burns or cuts that might heal slowly. Smoking should be avoided because of its vasoconstricting effect. Signs of infection should be reported. Lotions may help alleviate skin dryness and cracking but must be rubbed in for an unusually long time because of the thickness of the skin. Dysphagia may be reduced by eating small, frequent meals, chewing carefully and slowly, and drinking fluids. Heartburn may be minimized by using antacids 45 to 60 minutes after each meal and by sitting upright for 30 to 45 minutes after eating. Using additional pillows or raising the head of the bed on blocks may help reduce nocturnal gastroesophageal reflux.

Job modifications are often necessary because stair climbing, typing, writing, and cold exposure may pose particular problems. The patient may become socially withdrawn as skin tightening alters the appearance of the face and hands. Some people must wear gloves to protect fingertip ulcers and to provide extra warmth. Sensitive areas on fingertips resulting from ulcers or calcinosis may require padded utensils or special assistive devices to reduce discomfort. Dining out may become a socially embarrassing event because the patient's small mouth, difficulty swallowing, and reflux make eating less enjoyable. Daily oral hygiene must be emphasized, or neglect may lead to increased tooth and gingival problems. The patient needs a dentist who is familiar with SS and can deal with a small oral aperture. Psychologic support reduces stress and may positively influence peripheral motor response. Biofeedback training and relaxation techniques have been reported to reduce tension, improve sleeping habits, and raise digital temperature.

Sexual dysfunction resulting from body changes, pain, muscular weakness, limited mobility, decreased self-esteem, and decreased vaginal secretions may require sensitive counseling by the nurse. Specific suggestions based on individual patient assessment should be offered.[44]

POLYMYOSITIS AND DERMATOMYOSITIS

Polymyositis and *dermatomyositis* are diffuse inflammatory myopathies of striated muscle, producing symmetric weakness usually most severe in the proximal muscles (e.g., the trunk, shoulders, and hips). They occur twice as frequently in women as in men, except for childhood dermatomyositis or myositis associated with neoplasia. Onset of the disease occurs most frequently in the fifth and sixth decades of life. The incidence is slightly greater than that of muscular dystrophy in adults. In cases of dermatomyositis, especially among older persons, the frequency of malignancy appears to be increased.

Etiology and Pathophysiology

The exact cause of polymyositis and dermatomyositis is unknown. Theories include presence of an infectious agent, a hypersensitivity response, and cell-mediated immune system abnormalities. Close association with neoplastic disease suggests an autoimmune reaction. Histopathologic study typically reveals the presence of inflammatory infiltrates, degeneration, regeneration, necrosis, and fibrosis of muscle fibers.

Clinical Manifestations and Complications

Muscular. The patient usually experiences an insidious onset of proximal muscle weakness over a period of several months, primarily of the shoulders, neck, and pelvic girdle. The patient may have difficulty rising from a chair or bathtub, climbing stairs, combing the hair, or reaching into a high cupboard. Neck muscles may become so weak that the patient is unable to raise the head from the pillow. Muscle discomfort or tenderness is uncommon. Muscle examination reveals an inability to move against resistance or even gravity. Weak pharyngeal muscles may produce dysphagia and dysphonia (nasal or hoarse voice).

Dermal. The typical skin rash appears as a dusky erythema of the face, neck, shoulders, anterior part of the chest, upper part of the back, and arms and occurs in nearly 40% of patients with muscular disease. A heliotrope (lavender hue) rash over the eyelids and periorbital edema are nearly pathognomonic for dermatomyositis.[45] The rash is prominent on the extensor surfaces of the forearms, elbows, knuckles, periungual areas, knees, and ankles. A scaly, red, often raised rash on the knuckles is the Goltron's rash of dermatomyositis, which may easily be confused with that of psoriasis or seborrheic dermatitis. Hyperemia and telangiectasias are often present at the nail beds.

Other. Nearly half of the patients with polymyositis have mild or transient arthritis or Raynaud's phenomenon. Cotton wool patches can occur in the retina. Calcinosis, contractures, and muscle atrophy may occur with advanced disease. Aspiration pneumonia may result from weak pharyngeal muscles. Childhood dermatomyositis appears to have a more progressive, crippling course. Dermatomyositis diagnosed in men older than 40 years of age is more frequently associated with concurrent malignant disease. In severe cases, deglutition impairment and cardiorespiratory complications, such as pulmonary fibrosis and conduction defects, contribute to mortality.

Diagnostic Studies

Elevations in serum muscle enzymes (creatine kinase, aldolase, and aspartate aminotransferase) are most valuable in determining diagnosis and response to treatment. Circulating autoantibodies designated anti-Jo (antibodies to histidyl tRNA synthetase) are now recognized to be highly disease specific in patients with inflammatory myopathies.[38] Elevation of ESR is expected with active disease. The electromyogram (EMG) shows polyphasic, short-duration potentials, fibrillation, and positive-spike waves. Muscle biopsy reveals necrosis, degeneration, regeneration, and interstitial chronic inflammatory cell infiltration (primary lymphocytes).

Therapeutic Management

Polymyositis and dermatomyositis can be treated with some success by the use of corticosteroids and, occasionally, immunosuppressive drugs. Improvement is generally achieved with prompt institution of corticosteroid therapy, and dosage is usually reduced as clinical improvement is noted. Relapses are common. Topical steroids may be applied to the skin rash. Patients who respond poorly to corticosteroids may improve with immunosuppressives (e.g., intermittent IV or daily oral cyclophosphamide). Corticosteroid therapy may cause potassium, which is necessary for normal muscle contraction, to be released from damaged muscle cells and to be lost in the urine. Supplemental dietary potassium (e.g., from orange juice, bananas) is encouraged. Steroid-induced myopathy may complicate long-term therapy. Immunosuppressive agents such as methotrexate, azathioprine, and cyclophosphamide are used for their corticosteroid-sparing effect, allowing functional improvement with reduction in corticosteroid dosage.

Physical therapy can be helpful and should be tailored to the activity of the disease. Massage and passive movement are appropriate during active disease, with more aggressive exercises reserved for periods when disease activity is minimal, as evidenced by low serum enzyme levels.

A careful search for possible malignant lesions should be undertaken for the patient more than 40 years of age. If malignant disease is found, it should be treated appropriately (see Chapter 12). Complete remission of dermatomyositis may occur if the malignant lesion is removed.

NURSING MANAGEMENT

POLYMYOSITIS AND DERMATOMYOSITIS

Although prevention is not possible, greater recognition of polymyositis and its insidious onset resembling muscular dystrophy may favorably influence prognosis by more rapid diagnosis and institution of therapy.

Nursing interventions should include assessment of muscular weakness and limitation of motion. The nurse promotes bed rest and assists the patient with activities of daily living when extreme weakness is present. Special attention is provided at mealtime to prevent aspiration. The nature of the disease and modes of therapy should be thoroughly reviewed, and the diagnostic tests should be explained. Understanding that the benefits of therapy are often delayed is important; for example, weakness may increase during the first few weeks of corticosteroid therapy.

The patient should have a thorough understanding of the chronic nature of this disorder, the usefulness and the side effects of all prescribed medications, and the importance of regular medical care and serial laboratory testing. The nurse should provide guidelines for conserving energy by means of organizing activities and pacing techniques. Daily ROM exercises are encouraged to prevent contractures. When active inflammation is not evident, muscle-strengthening (repetitive) exercises may be started. Home care will be necessary during the acute phase of polymyositis because profound muscle weakness renders the patient unable to carry out activities of daily living. Homemaker services, visiting nurses, and family caregivers are needed to assist the patient in routine hygiene, meal preparation and eating, and ambulation.

Overlapping Forms of Connective Tissue Disease

Patients having a combination of clinical features of several rheumatic diseases are described as having *overlapping* or *mixed connective tissue disease*. Although this combination was believed to be a distinct clinical disorder, follow-up revealed evolution primarily to SLE or SS. This early undifferentiated or transitional form of connective tissue disease has a typical serologic pattern, including high titer of speckled pattern of ANA (a type of ANA), high levels of antibody to ribonuclease-sensitive extractable nuclear antibody, and autoantibodies to ribonucleoprotein.

SJÖGREN'S SYNDROME

Sjögren's syndrome is characterized by autoantibodies to two protein-RNA complexes termed *SS-A/Ro* and *SS-B/La*. The manifestations are caused by inflammation and dysfunction of the exocrine glands, particularly the salivary and lacrimal glands.[46]

More than 90% of the patients are women, and half have RA or another connective tissue disease. Dry mouth can complicate the differential diagnosis in older women. Decreased tearing leads to a "gritty" sensation in the eyes, burning, and photosensitivity. Dry mouth produces buccal membrane fissures, dysphagia, and frequent dental caries. Dry nasal and respiratory passages are common and can result in a cough. Often the parotid glands are enlarged. Other exocrine glands may also be affected; for example, vaginal dryness may lead to dyspareunia.

Histologic study reveals lymphocyte infiltration of salivary and lacrimal glands, but the disease may become more generalized and involve lymph nodes, bone marrow, and visceral organs (pseudolymphoma). Extraglandular proliferation may become frankly malignant (e.g., lymphoma). Rheumatoid and antinuclear factors are present in the majority of patients. Anemia, leukopenia, hypergammaglobulinemia, and elevated ESR are usually found.

Ophthalmologic examination (Schirmer test), salivary flow rates, and lower lip biopsy of minor salivary glands confirm the diagnosis. The treatment is symptomatic, including (1) artificial tears instillation as often as necessary to maintain adequate hydration and lubrication, (2) surgical punctal occlusion, and (3) increased fluids with meals. Dental hygiene is important. Increased humidity at home may reduce respiratory infections. Vaginal lubrication with a water-soluble product such as K-Y jelly may increase comfort during intercourse. Corticosteroids and immunosuppressive drugs are indicated for treatment of pseudolymphoma.

FIBROMYALGIA

Fibromyalgia (FM) is a musculoskeletal chronic pain syndrome of unknown etiology.[47] It is characterized by tender joints, fatigue, stiffness, myalgias, arthralgias, headaches, irritable bowel syndrome, sleep disturbance, and feelings of hopelessness. There is a 70% association of FM and irritable bowel syndrome. FM is seen most commonly in women (3.5% of the female population) and occurs more frequently in older persons. The highest incidence of FM occurs in women between ages 60 and 79.[48]

Although the etiology and pathogenesis of FM is not known, clinicians have speculated that the syndrome is a result of referred pain from deep structures (pain amplification), a pain-spasm cycle, repetitive stress to the muscle, or reactivation of a latent virus. It is known that FM has a powerful stress-related component that needs attention for long-lasting resolution.

The diagnosis of FM is made by the presence of typical symptoms and the presence of *tender points*. Eighteen points, tender in normal people, have been identified that are hypersensitive in persons with FM. A major diagnostic criterion for FM is the presence of at least 11 consistent tender points.[49] FM may be localized to a specific region of the body or generalized with migratory tender points.

The treatment of FM is symptomatic and requires a high level of patient motivation. The nurse can play a key role in educating the patient to be an active participant in the therapeutic regimen. Pain, aching, and tenderness can be helped by rest and NSAIDs. Stress, fatigue, and sleep disturbances can be helped by low-dose tricyclic antidepressants (e.g., amitriptyline [Elavil], imipramine [Tofranil]), muscle relaxants, stress management and stress-reduction techniques, deep relaxation, and a high-energy, healthy diet. Participation in a safe, moderate exercise program (e.g., swimming, walking) is one of the most beneficial approaches for reducing symptoms. All parameters of FM except morning stiffness improve on cyclobenzaprine (Flexeril), a muscle relaxant that is a tricyclic derivative.

Because of the chronic nature of FM and the need to maintain an ongoing rehabilitation program, the patient with FM needs consistent support from the nurse and other members of the health care team. The most successful treatment approaches combine physical fitness, stress-reduction programs, and psychologic counseling (individual or group).

COMMON JOINT SURGICAL PROCEDURES

Surgery plays an important role in the treatment and rehabilitation of patients with various forms of arthritis, conditions related to trauma, and other painful conditions resulting in functional disability. Joint replacement surgery is the most common orthopedic operation performed on older adults. Significant advances in the field of reconstructive surgery have resulted in improvements in prosthetic design, materials, and surgical techniques that provide significant relief of pain and deformity and improve function and joint motion for patients with arthritis.

Indications

Surgery is aimed at relieving pain, improving joint motion, correcting deformity and malalignment, reducing vertical loads and shear stresses, and removing intraarticular causes of erosion. Pain is one of the primary reasons for joint surgery. In addition to the effects of chronic pain on the physical and emotional well-being of the patient, any movement of the painful joint is often avoided. If this lack of movement is not corrected, contraction with limitation of motion often occurs. Limitation of motion at any joint can be demonstrated on physical examination and by joint-space narrowing on radiologic examination.

There may also be a slow loss of cartilage in affected joints, which may be related to loss of motion. Synovitis can cause tendon damage, resulting in rupture or sublux-

(Text continued on p. 1935.)

Clinical Pathway for Total Hip Replacement

CARE PATH
800 Total Hip Replacement

SERVICE		PHYSICIAN
PRIMARY NURSE		PRIMARY NURSE
DISCHARGE DATE	ADMISSION DATE	DATE OF SURGERY

Problem number	Patient problems/Nursing diagnoses
#1	Impaired physical mobility
#2	Alteration in comfort
#3	Lack of knowledge
#4	Potential for injury

Problem number		PRE ADMIT	Day 1 (DOS)	Day 2 (POD 1)	Day 3 (POD 2)	Day 4 (POD 3)
#1 #4	Assessment/ monitoring		Telemetry Hip dressing dry HV patent to suction Monitor posterior precautions Assess for abdominal distention	D/C telemetry Hip dressing dry HV patent to suction Monitor posterior precautions No significant arrhythmias Assess for abdominal distention	Hip dressing dry HV patent to suction HV DC'd per HO Monitor posterior precautions No abdominal distention HV output ≤10 cc ×2 shifts	Incision dry, well approximated; 4 × 4 dressing over old HV site Monitor posterior precautions
#1	Consults	SW, OT, PT	SW, OT, PT			
#3		Prescreening				
#4	Procedure/test	Admit labs UA with micro, PT, PTT, CBC, SMA6, H & H, CXR, ECG	Postop CBC, SMA6, AP/ orthopelvic x-rays in OR	CBC, SMA6, PT (Maintain Hgb 9g/dl if history of cardiac problems or symptomatic)	CBC, SMA6, PT	PT, UA with micro, C & S (CVS if male, straight cath. if female)

continued

Clinical Pathway for Total Hip Replacement—cont'd

Problem number		PRE ADMIT	Day (1 DOS)	Day 2 (POD 1)	Day 3 (POD 2)	Day 4 (POD 3)
#1 #2 #4	**Treatment**		Indwelling catheter Softcare mattress Overhead frame with trapeze Abdominal pillow at all times Hemovac I/O IS, TCDB q2°hr ×1 ×2 ×3 ×4 ×5 ×6 ×7 ×8 ×9 ×10 ×12 Check hip dressing	D/C indwelling cath. before transfer to floor Abdominal pillow while in bed IS, TCDB q2°hr ×1 ×2 ×3 ×4 ×5 ×6 ×7 ×8 ×9 ×10 ×11 ×12 Check hip dressing	Abdominal pillow while in bed; obtain walker and BSC from central D/C I & O ISq2°WA ×1 ×2 ×3 ×4 ×5 ×6 ×7 ×8 Check hip dressing I/O adequate	Regular pillow for abdomen during day if AO IS, q2°hr WA ×1 ×2 ×3 ×4 ×5 ×6 ×7 ×8
#1 #4	**Activity**		Bed rest Turn q2°hr ×1 ×2 ×3 ×4 ×5 ×6 ×7 ×8 ×9 ×10 ×11 ×12	Nursing: up to chair bid ×1 ×2 MD to determine weight-bearing status Stand with walker with PT Participate in ADLs	Nursing: up to chair bid ×1 ×2 Begin ambulation with walker and exercises with PT Increased participation in ADLs	Nursing: up to chair ×1 ×2 ×3 Up to BSC on days and evenings Continue PT bid ×1 ×2

continued

Clinical Pathway For Total Hip Replacement—cont'd

CNS	DIETARY	RT	
HOME HEALTH	OT	OTHER	
PT	RT	OTHER	

Problem number	Patient problems/nursing diagnoses

Day 5 POD 4	Day 6 POD 5	Day 7 POD 6	Day 8 POD 7	Discharge outcomes	*Posterior precautions
Incision dry, well-approximated, 4×4 dressing over old HV site Monitor posterior precautions Minimal HV site drainage	Incision line clean, dry, well approximated. Maintains posterior precautions	Incision line clean, dry, well approximated. Maintains posterior precautions No drainage from HV site	Staples/sutures removed per HO if not on prednisone. (If on prednisone, remove in 14 days in MDs office) Check walker/crutches to go home with patient for safety.	No signs or symptoms of infection. No evidence of dislocation.	Do not flex hip greater than 90 degrees. Do not adduct hip. Do not internally rotate. Do not lean or bend forward while sitting or standing. Do not cross legs. Do not reach to extremes across the body. Do not sit on low or soft surfaces. Avoid sitting in recliner without special measures.
	Home Health				
PT	PT, CBC	PT in AM, then D/C No coumadin on day of discharge		Wound clean and dry. Hb and Hct stable.	
IS, q2°hr WA ×1 ×2 ×3 ×4 ×5 ×6 ×7 ×8	IS, q4°hr WA ×1 ×2 ×3 ×4 Afebrile, lungs clear	IS, q4°hr WA ×1 ×2 ×3 ×4		Lungs clear or WNL	
↑ chair ×1 ×2 ×3 Up to bathroom with over-the-toilet adjustable commode PT ×1 ×2 Continue OT, ADL training ADL per pt with assistance	PT: Ambulate with walker/crutches ×1 ×2 Stair walking with PT ×1 Nursing: up to chair ×1 ×2 ×3 Ambulate to bathroom prn ADLs per patient with minimal assistance	PT: Ambulate with walker/crutches, steps ×1 ×2 Nursing: chair ×1 ×2 ×3 Ambulate to bathroom prn ADLs per patient with minimal assistance	PT: Ambulate with walker/crutches, with steady gait ×1 ×2. Nursing: chair ×1 ×2 ×3 Ambulate to bathroom prn ADLs per patient with minimal assistance	Able to ambulate independently with steady gait with walker/crutches. Able to correctly use ADL equipment and perform self-care activities.	

continued

Clinical Pathway for Total Hip Replacement—cont'd

			Day 1 (DOS)	Day 2 (POD 1)	Day 3 (POD 2)	Day 4 (POD 3)
#2	Meds/IVs		Ancef ×6 doses PCA with IVFs Coumadin 5 mg	Ancef ↓ IV to KVO for PCA PCA Coumadin per MD	Ancef D/C PCA → Heparin lock IV PO pain meds Coumadin per MD Pain controlled	Ancef discontinued per HO Incisions without drainage PO pain meds HL patent Coumadin per MD
	Nutrition		Clear liquid/full liquid	Advance to regular		
#3	Patient/family education	PA: Preop teaching Give teaching booklet incentive spirometer use Tour unit	Nursing: Reinforce preop teaching. Posterior precautions* (See last column) Instructions on PCA	PT and Nursing Instruct on bed-chair transfers	Nursing and PT: Reinforce gait training Reinforce posterior precautions* Instruct to ask for pain meds	Nursing and PT: Reinforce gait training Reinforce posterior precautions* Encourage PO pain meds 30 min before PT
#3	Discharge planning	SW & PA: Assess conditions at home	Patient/family verbalize understanding of Care Path; Plan of care has been mutually set with patient/family	High-risk screening SW	ADL equipment form OT-reacher, etc.	F/U with OT & PT regarding discharge plans ADL training with OT Initial evaluation of discharge by SW
#3	Psychosocial/ emotional needs	Provide emotional support			Give verbal praise for accomplishments	
Signatures						

continued

Clinical Pathway for Total Hip Replacement—cont'd

Day 5 (POD 4)	Day 6 (POD 5)	Day 7 (POD 6)	Day 8 (POD 7)	Discharge outcomes
PO pain meds D/C HL if Hct ≥28% Coumadin per MD	PO pain meds Coumadin per MD	PO pain meds Coumadin per MD	D/C Rx: ASA gr X po BID ×3 wk Rx: Pain meds per MD	Patient will be pain-free or pain controlled with oral analgesics
Nursing and PT: Reinforce gait training Reinforce posterior precautions*	Nursing: Reinforce posterior precautions, gait training, and use of OT equipment	Nursing and PT: Review discharge plan in the AM Reinforce posterior precautions for at home and gait training. PT: Instruct patient/family on home exercise program	Nursing: Review posterior precautions and wound care	Able to verbalize and demonstrate posterior precautions and correct weight-bearing status Able to verbalize understanding of home exercise program
Continue F/U with OT, PT, and SW Team assessment for discharge to home vs rehab. Continue ADL training with OT Demonstrates correct use of equipment ADL equipment from OT-reacher etc.	PT, OT, SW: Acquire equipment to go home with patient; continue F/U with OT, PT, and SW	PT to instruct on getting in and out of car SW to assess need for discharge transportation	Discharge patient with instructions, prescriptions, and abdominal pillow	Discharge to appropriate level of care with MD/clinic follow-up
	Patient accepting discharge plan and motivated to continue			Will demonstrate appropriate coping and emotional response

Developed by Barnes Hospital, St. Louis, MO. Licensed by Center for Case Management, South Natick, MA.

ADLs, Activities of daily living; *AO*, alert and oriented; *AP*, anterior-posterior; *bid*, twice a day; *BSC*, bedside commode; *C & S*, culture and sensitivity; *CBC*, complete bloot count; *CVS*, clear voided specimen; *CXR*, chest x-ray; *D/C*, discontinue; *DOS*, day of surgery; *ECG*, electrocardiogram; *F/U*, follow-up; *H & H*, hematocrit and hemoglobin; *HL*, heparin lock; *HO*, house officer; *HV*, Hemovac; *I & O*, intake and output; *IS*, incentive spirometer; *IVF*, intravenous fluids; *KVO*, keep vein open; *OT*, occupational therapy; *PA*, physician assistant; *PCA*, patient-controlled analgesia; *POD*, postoperative day; *PT*, prothrombin time; *PTT*, partial thromboplastin time; *RT*, respiratory therapist; *SS*, social service; *SW*, social worker; *WA*, while awake; *WNL*, within normal limits.

ation of the joint and subsequent loss of function. Continuing disease activity may cause loss of cartilage and bony surface and result in mechanical barriers to movement requiring surgical intervention.

Types of Joint Surgeries

Synovectomy. Synovectomy (removal of synovial membrane) is used as a prophylactic measure and as a palliative treatment of RA. Removal of synovial membrane, thought to be the location of the basic pathologic changes in joint destruction, helps prevent further progression of joint damage. A synovectomy is best performed early in the disease process to prevent serious destruction of joint surfaces. Removal of the thickened synovium prevents extension of the inflammatory process into the adjacent cartilage, ligaments, and tendons.

It is impossible to surgically remove all the synovium in a joint. The underlying disease process is still present and will again affect the regenerating synovium. However, the disease appears to be milder after synovectomy, and definite improvement in pain, weight bearing, and ROM can be expected. Common sites for this surgery include the elbow, wrist, and fingers. Synovectomy in the knee is done less frequently because of improved joint replacement techniques.

Osteotomy. An osteotomy is performed by removing a wedge or slice of bone to change its alignment and shift weight bearing, thereby correcting deformity and relieving pain. Cervical osteotomy may be used to correct deformity in some patients with ankylosing spondylitis. A halo and body jacket are worn until fusion occurs (3 or 4 months). Subtrochanteric or femoral osteotomy may provide some relief of pain and improve motion in selected patients with osteoarthritis, but it does not greatly improve the stability of the hip. It has proven ineffective in patients with inflammatory joint disease. Osteotomy (of the knee) provides limited relief of pain, and for this reason advanced joint destruction is usually corrected by joint replacement surgery. The postoperative care is similar to the treatment of an internal fixation of a fracture at a comparable site (see Chapter 59). The osteotomy is usually fixed by internal wires, screws and plates, bone grafts, or fixation material.

Debridement. Debridement is the removal of degenerative debris such as loose bodies, osteophytes, joint debris, and degenerated menisci from a joint. This procedure is usually performed on the knee or the shoulder using a fiberoptic endoscope called an arthroscope. A compression dressing is applied postoperatively. Weight bearing is permitted following knee arthroscopy. Nursing care includes assessment of peripheral pulses; color, temperature, sensation; pain; and swelling of the involved extremity. Patient education includes signs of infection, pain management, and restriction of excessive activity for 24 to 48 hours.

Arthroplasty. Arthroplasty is the reconstruction or replacement of a joint. This surgical procedure is performed to relieve pain, improve or maintain ROM, and correct deformity—conditions that can result from OA, RA, avascular necrosis, congenital deformities or dislocations, and other systemic problems. There are several types of arthroplasty, including replacement of part of a joint, surgical reshaping of the bones of the joints, and total joint replacement. Innovative procedures and prosthetic devices offer exciting possibilities for future reconstructive joint surgery (Fig. 60-13). Replacement arthroplasty is available for the elbow, shoulder, phalangeal joints of the fingers, hip, knee, ankle, and feet.

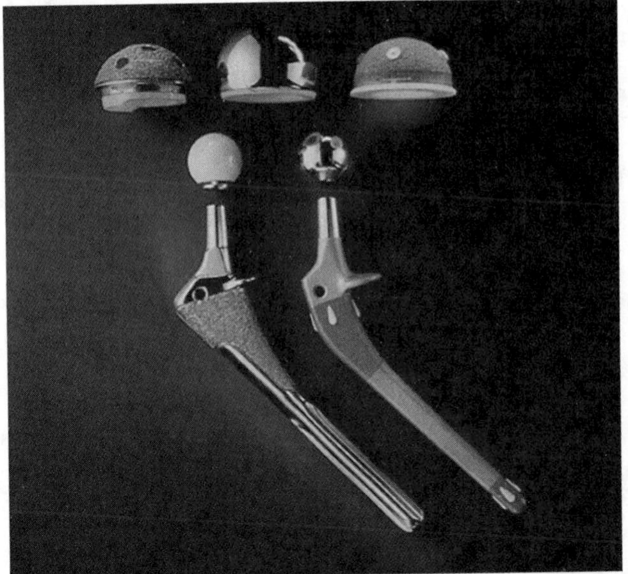

A

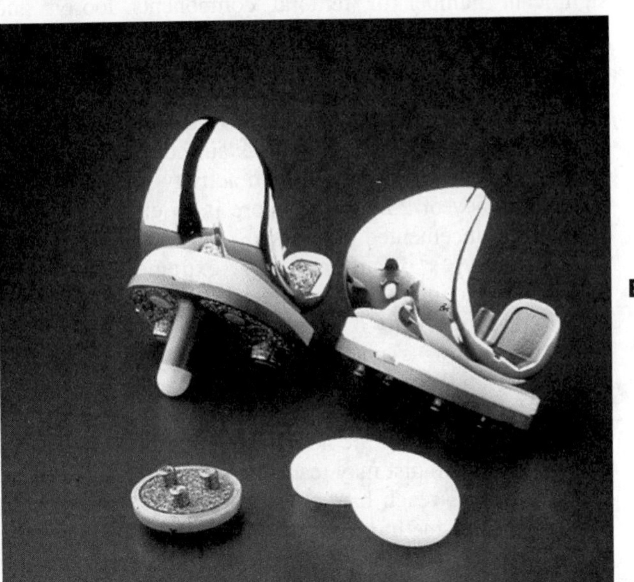

B

Fig. 60-13 Total joint replacements. ***A,*** Hip. ***B,*** Knee.

Hip. Total hip replacement is undoubtedly the most important advancement in reconstructive surgery of the twentieth century and has provided significant relief of pain and improvement of function for patients with arthritis. Hip reconstruction is frequently used in the treatment of patients with RA and OA, as well as for fractures of the hip.

Implants are "cemented" in place with polymethylmethacrylate, which bonds to the bone. With time, a

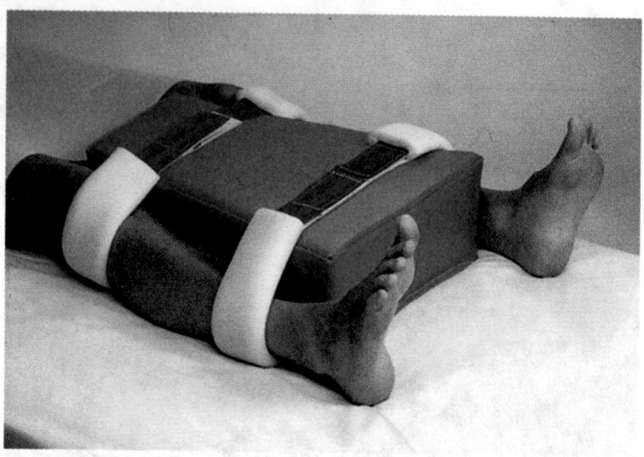

Fig. 60-14 Maintaining postoperative abduction following total hip replacement.

significant number of femoral components loosen and require revision. Because of this risk, total hip replacement is recommended for less active, older adults. More recently, "cementless" arthroplasties have been used. They provide long-term implant stability by facilitating biologic ingrowth of new bone tissue into the porous surface coating of the prosthesis.[50] A patient with a high activity potential and a life expectancy of 25 years or more is an excellent candidate for an uncemented prosthesis.

In both types of arthroplasties, extremes of internal rotation, adduction, and 90 degree flexion of the hip must be avoided for 4 to 6 weeks postoperatively. A foam abduction pillow is placed between the legs to prevent dislocation of the new joint (Fig. 60-14). Elevated toilet seats and platforms under chairs at home are necessary. Tub baths and driving a car are not allowed for 4 to 6 weeks. An occupational therapist may teach the patient to use assistive devices such as reach bars ("reachers") to avoid bending over to pick something off the floor, long-handled shoe horns, or sock pullers. The knees must be kept apart; the patient must never cross the legs or twist to reach behind. Physical therapy is initiated 1 day postoperatively with ambulation and weight bearing with a walker for cemented prosthesis and non–weight bearing on the operative side for uncemented prosthesis.

Exercises are designed to restore strength and muscle tone in the hip muscles essential to improved function and range of motion. These include quadriceps setting, gluteal muscle setting, leg raises in supine and prone positions, and abduction exercises (swinging the leg out but never crossing midline) from supine and standing positions.

Home care management includes nursing assessment of anticoagulation status, pain management, and monitoring for infection. Periodic dressing changes are made. The incision may be closed with metal staples, which are removed at the surgeon's office. Prothrombin times will be drawn weekly and anticoagulation adjusted accordingly. The patient should be instructed to use prophylactic antibiotics before dental appointments or procedures that might put the patient at risk for bacteremia.

A physical therapist will assess range of motion, ambulation, and compliance with the exercise regimen. The patient will gradually increase the number of repetitions of exercises, add weights to ankles, swim, and may eventually use a stationary bicycle to tone quadriceps and improve cardiovascular fitness.[51] High-impact exercises and sports, such as jogging and tennis, may loosen the implant and should be avoided. The elderly adult may require rehabilitation at an extended care facility until able to function independently.

Knee. Unremitting pain and instability as a result of severe destructive deterioration of the knee joint is the main indication for knee arthroplasty. The presence of osteoporosis may necessitate bone grafting to augment defects and to correct bone deficiencies. Either part or all of the knee joint may be replaced with a metal and plastic prosthetic device. A compression dressing is used to immobilize the knee in extension immediately after the operation. This is removed before discharge and replaced with a knee immobilizer or posterior plastic shell, which maintains extension during ambulation and at rest for about 4 weeks.

Great emphasis is placed on postoperative exercising, and dislocation is not a problem. Isometric quadricep-setting begins the first day after surgery. The patient progresses to straight leg raises and gentle ROM to increase muscle strength and obtain 90-degree knee flexion. Active flexion exercises through the use of a passive-motion machine postoperatively promotes earlier joint mobility and shortens hospitalization. Partial weight bearing is begun before discharge. An active home exercise program involves progressive ROM, muscle strengthening, and stationary bicycle exercising.

Finger joints. A silicone rubber arthroplastic device is used to help restore function in the fingers of the patient with RA. The goal of hand surgery is primarily to restore function related to grasp, pinch, stability, and strength rather than to correct cosmetic deformity. The metacarpophalangeal and proximal interphalangeal joints are most commonly involved. Ulnar deviation is often present, which results in severe functional limitations of the hand. Before surgery the patient is instructed in hand exercises, including flexion, extension, abduction, and adduction of the fingers. Postoperatively, the hand is kept elevated with a bulky dressing in place. The operative area and the hand should be checked for sensation, temperature, pulse, and signs of infection. Once the dressing is removed, a guided splinting program is initiated. The success of the surgery depends largely on the postoperative treatment plan, which is often carried out under the direction of an occupational therapist. The patient is discharged with splints to use while sleeping and hand exercises to perform for 10 to 12 weeks at least three to four times a day. The patient is also instructed to avoid lifting heavy objects.

Elbows and shoulders. Although available, total replacement of elbow and shoulder joints is not as common as other forms of arthroplasty. Shoulder replacements are used in patients with severe pain because of RA, OA, necrosis, or an old trauma. The shoulder replacement is usually considered if the patient has adequate surrounding muscle strength and bone stock. If joint replacement is necessary for both elbow and shoulder, the elbow is usually done first because a severely painful elbow interferes with the shoulder rehabilitation program.

Significant pain relief has been achieved in all diagnostic groups, with 90% of patients having no pain at rest or minimal pain with activity. Functional improvements have resulted in better hygiene and increased ability to perform activities of daily living in most patients. Rehabilitation is longer and more difficult than with other joint surgeries.

Arthrodesis. Arthrodesis is the surgical fusion of a joint. This procedure is indicated only if articular surfaces are too severely damaged or infected to allow joint replacement or for reconstructive surgery failures. Arthrodesis relieves pain and provides a stable but immobile joint. The fusion is usually accomplished by removal of the articular hyaline cartilage and the addition of bone grafts across the joint surface. The affected joint must be immobilized until bone healing has occurred. Common areas of fusion are the wrist, ankle, cervical spine, and lumbar spine.

Complications

Deep infection is a serious complication of joint surgery, particularly joint replacement surgery. The most common causative organisms are gram-positive aerobic streptococci and staphylococci. Infection almost always leads to pain and septic loosening, generally requiring extensive surgery. Efforts to reduce the incidence of deep infection include the use of specially designed hypersterile operating rooms with laminar air flow and prophylactic antibiotic administration.

Deep vein thrombosis is another potentially serious complication after selected joint surgeries, particularly those involving the lower extremities. Prophylaxis such as aspirin, warfarin, or pneumatic compression of the legs is usually instituted. Patients may be followed postoperatively with venous plethysmography to detect proximal deep vein thrombosis, the source of most pulmonary emboli. The peak incidence of pulmonary embolus is on the fourth postoperative day.

Therapeutic Management

Preoperative Management. As surgical techniques and care improve, more patients with chronic diseases such as RA are being considered as surgical candidates. The primary goal of preoperative assessment is to identify risk factors associated with postoperative complications so that nursing strategies can be implemented that promote optimal positive outcomes. A careful history will include previous medical diagnosis and complications such as diabetes and thrombophlebitis, pain tolerance and management preferences, current functional status and expectations following surgery, and level of social support and home care needs after discharge. The patient should be free from evidence of infection and acute joint inflammation. If lower-extremity surgery is planned, upper-extremity muscle strength and joint function are assessed to determine the type of assistive devices needed postoperatively for ambulation and activities of daily living. Preoperative education informs the patient and family of the expected hospital course and postoperative management at home and readies them for a lifestyle that is compatible with the intrinsic capabilities of the prosthetic components so that prosthesis longevity can be maximized.

Postoperative Management. Postoperatively, a neurovascular assessment of the affected extremity is done to assess nerve function and circulatory status. Anticoagulation therapy, analgesia, and parenteral antibiotics are administered. In general, the affected joint is exercised and ambulation is encouraged as early as possible to prevent complications of immobility. Specific protocols vary according to patient, type of prosthesis, and surgeon preference.

NURSING MANAGEMENT

JOINT SURGERY

The nursing management of the patient undergoing joint surgery begins with preoperative education and realistic goal setting. It is important that the patient understands and accepts the limitations of the proposed surgery and realizes that it will not remove the underlying disease process. Postoperative procedures such as turning, coughing, and deep breathing, use of bedpan and bedside commode, and use of abductor pillows should be explained and opportunities for practice provided. The patient should be reassured that pain relief will be available. A preoperative visit from a physical therapist allows rehearsal of postoperative exercises and measurement for crutches or other assistive devices. The spirit of respect and cooperation displayed between the physical therapist and the nurse can do much to reassure an anxious patient.

Discharge planning begins immediately. The duration of the hospital stay and the expected postoperative events should be discussed so that the patient and family can plan ahead. The home environment should be assessed for safety (e.g., presence of scatter rugs and electric cords) and accessibility. (Are the bathroom and bedroom on the first floor? Are doorframes wide enough to accommodate a walker?) Social support must be assessed. Is a friend or family member available to assist the patient in the home? Will the patient require homemaker or meal services? The elderly patient may need the rehabilitation services of an extended care facility for a few weeks postoperatively to progressively develop independent living skills. Specific nursing interventions related to joint surgery are summarized in the nursing care plan for the patient undergoing joint surgery on p. 1938.

Patient education includes instructions on reporting complications, including infection (e.g., fever, increased pain, and drainage) and dislocation of the prosthesis (pain, loss of function, shortening or malalignment of an extremity). The home care nurse acts as the liaison between the patient and the surgeon, monitoring for postoperative complications, assessing comfort and ROM, and facilitating improvements in functional performance.

NURSING CARE PLAN Patient Undergoing Joint Surgery

Planning: Outcome Criteria	Nursing Interventions and Rationales
➤ **NURSING DIAGNOSIS**	Impaired physical mobility *related to* pain, stiffness, and surgical procedure *as manifested by* difficulty in ambulating; reluctance, unwillingness, or inability to participate in physical rehabilitation; guarded movement; expression of fear about ambulating
Have functional ROM of operated joint.	Assess effect of surgery on patient's mobility *to plan appropriate interventions.* Begin exercise program as directed *to minimize mobility impairment and stiffness.* Cooperate with physical therapist *to increase patient compliance and continuity of exercise.* Give pain medication before exercise *to decrease discomfort from exercise and increase patient cooperation.*
➤ **NURSING DIAGNOSIS**	Risk for infection *related to* exposure of joint during surgery, presence of environmental pathogens, and ineffective prophylaxis
Have no evidence of infection (e.g., fever, increased pain, drainage).	Assess for fever, purulent drainage and redness at wound site, increased pain, elevated WBC count *as indicators of infection.* Monitor vital signs and dressing for amount and character of drainage q4hr *because regular assessment ensures early detection of infection.* Assess level of pain *because infection can increase local pain.* Use strict aseptic technique for dressing changes *to prevent introducing infection or cross-contaminating wound.* Give antibiotics as ordered *as prophylaxis or treatment of infection.*
➤ **NURSING DIAGNOSIS**	Risk for injury: falls *related to* weakness, fatigue, orthostatic hypotension, pain, gait instability, and use of assistive device
Experience no falls; ambulate safely.	Assess for predisposing factors such as unsteady gait, weakness, light-headedness, improper use of assistive device when upright *to determine presence of risk factors.* Assess patient's readiness to ambulate *to prevent premature initiation of ambulation and subsequent falls.* Assist as necessary with ambulation; assess environment for fall potential and alter as indicated *to prevent falling.* Schedule pain medication administration *to maximize effectiveness during ambulation.* Provide supervised practice with assistive devices *to ensure proper use.*
➤ **NURSING DIAGNOSIS**	Self-care deficit *related to* restrictions imposed by joint surgery, pain, weakness *as manifested by* inability or unwillingness to perform part or all of activities of daily living
Have activities of daily living met satisfactorily by patient or caregivers.	Assess patient's ability to perform activities of daily living *to plan appropriate assistance.* Assist as necessary *to ensure that all basic needs are met.* Assure patient of your willingness to assist with activities of daily living postoperatively *to relieve anxiety related to feelings of helplessness.* Assure patient that self-care abilities will be resumed with time *to decrease anxiety over dependency.*
➤ **NURSING DIAGNOSIS**	Ineffective management of therapeutic regimen *related to* lack of knowledge of follow-up care *as manifested by* expression of concern with ability to care for self after discharge, frequent questioning about follow-up care, lack of plan for follow-up care
Express confidence in ability to manage self-care after discharge and to make necessary lifestyle changes.	Instruct patient on usual follow-up protocol, including activity limitations, medications, follow-up visit, and signs to observe related to infection and dislocation *to prepare patient for self-care and decision making.* Make clear to patient that joint surgery does not alter underlying disease process *to avoid patient having unrealistic expectations about surgical outcome.* Assist patient to identify activities that require modification *so appropriate modification can be made.* Refer for vocational counseling *so expert guidance is available if necessary.* Initiate a nurse referral *to monitor the long-term exercise program at home.*

continued

NURSING CARE PLAN Patient Undergoing Joint Surgery—cont'd

Planning: Outcome Criteria	Nursing Interventions and Rationales
➤ NURSING DIAGNOSIS Risk for ineffective individual coping *related to* unrealistic expectations, limited physical activity, and inadequate support system	
Accept and adjust limitations of function and strength, use positive coping mechanisms.	Assess for risk factors such as expression of inability to cope; use of inappropriate coping mechanisms such as anger, crying, withdrawal, isolation; high anxiety level; inadequate support system *to determine if inadequate or inappropriate coping is a problem.* Discuss realistic postoperative expectations with patient *to avoid disappointment.* Identify possible areas requiring adjustments *so appropriate interventions can be planned.* Assess support system and enhance if necessary *so patient can use this system for coping.* Teach patient replacement coping techniques if indicated. Encourage realistic appraisal of present situation and attempt to problem solve *to assist patient to practice positive coping strategies.* Initiate home health nurse referral *if patient needs to do additional work on effective coping strategies and to ease the transition from hospital to home.*
➤ NURSING DIAGNOSIS Risk for peripheral neurovascular dysfunction *related to* edema and dislocated prosthesis	
Have palpable peripheral pulses, warm extremities, brisk capillary refill.	Assess nerve and circulatory status q1hr first 24 hr, then q2-4hr *to determine if problem is present so treatment can be initiated promptly.* Notify surgeon immediately if abnormalities are noted *so interventions are started without delay.* Initiate measures such as cold packs *to minimize edema.* Carry out measures to prevent dislocation *because this can be a cause of neurovascular dysfunction.* Encourage movement of unaffected limbs *to promote circulation in affected extremity.* Teach patient to report signs of neurovascular dysfunction such as anesthesia, paresthesia, coldness, pallor, excessive pain, swelling of affected extremity or body area *so treatment is not delayed.*

COLLABORATIVE PROBLEMS

Nursing Goals	Nursing Interventions and Rationales
➤ POTENTIAL COMPLICATION Dislocation of prosthesis *related to* improper movement or activity and infection	
Monitor and report signs of joint dislocation, and carry out appropriate medical and nursing interventions.	Monitor for pain in affected joint, loss of function, shortening or malalignment of extremity *to determine if dislocation has occurred.* Instruct patient on safe positions and activities; use assistive devices (e.g., raised toilet seat) as indicated *to avoid extremes of movement, which can cause dislocation.* Reinforce instructions of physical therapists *to foster confidence in plan and prevent misunderstanding.* Teach signs of dislocation to report (e.g., pain, loss of function, deformity) *so treatment is initiated promptly.*
➤ POTENTIAL COMPLICATION Thrombophlebitis *related to* surgery and immobilization	
Monitor and report signs of thrombosis, and carry out appropriate medical and nursing interventions.	Apply support stockings, gradient compression stockings, and instruct patient to perform isotonic exercises such as quadriceps setting, ankle rolling, and pushing on foot board *to promote circulation and prevent clot formation.* Monitor for redness, swelling, and tenderness of the extremity *to recognize and report thrombus formation.* Provide adequate parenteral and oral fluids *to prevent dehydration and increased blood coagulability.* Instruct the patient on the importance of home exercise *to prevent venous stasis.* Instruct the patient and caregivers in the proper administration and follow-up of oral anticoagulation medications *to prevent side effects of undercoagulation or overanticoagulation.* Avoid rubbing extremity *to prevent dislodging thrombus.*

ROM, Range of motion; *WBC,* white blood cell.

CRITICAL THINKING EXERCISES

CASE STUDY

SYSTEMIC LUPUS ERYTHEMATOSUS

Patient Profile

Madeline is a 28-year-old, married female who is admitted to the rheumatology clinic following a recent vacation to Hawaii.

Subjective Data

- Works in a delicatessen
- Complains of migratory joint pain, overwhelming fatigue, and a facial rash
- Is 3 months pregnant
- Has Raynaud's phenomenon when she restocks the freezer at work
- Had episode of pleurisy at age 19
- Fears she is going to die
- Is afraid to take medication because of pregnancy

Objective Data

Physical Examination

- Malar rash
- Swelling of third and fourth metacarpophalangeal joints of both hands
- Pain on motion of both wrists, shoulders, and knees with no obvious swelling

Diagnostic Studies

- 4000 μl (4×10^9/L)
- Platelets 150,000/μl (150×10^9 /L)
- Complement (C_3) is 60 mg/dl (0.6 g/L)
- Positive ANA and antiphospholipid antibodies

Therapeutic Management

- Diagnosed with systemic lupus erythematosus
- Started on prednisone 10 mg daily

Critical Thinking Questions

1. How might the nurse explain the pathophysiology of systemic lupus erythematosus to Madeline?
2. How might the vacation have influenced the symptoms that she is currently experiencing?
3. What are some home and work modifications that the nurse can suggest to Madeline that will reduce her symptoms?
4. Discuss the types of prenatal and postpartal considerations essential in caring for Madeline.
5. What other sources of information regarding systemic lupus erythematosus might the nurse suggest to Madeline and her family?
6. Based on the assessment data presented, write one or more nursing diagnoses. Are there any collaborative problems?

NURSING RESEARCH ISSUES

1. What is the relationship between social support systems and quality of life for people with arthritis?
2. Does the level of aerobic conditioning influence the subjective perception of fatigue in women with systemic lupus erythematosus?
3. Is gender a factor in the experience of arthritis pain?
4. Does cultural diversity affect compliance with arthritis home management programs?
5. How do environmental stressors trigger exacerbation of disease activity in rheumatic disease?

REVIEW QUESTIONS

The number of the question corresponds to the same-numbered objective at the beginning of the chapter.

1. The pathophysiology of SLE includes

a. hyperuricemia as a result of increased purine synthesis, decreased renal excretion, or both.
b. autoimmune disorder directed against constituents of the cell DNA.
c. chronic inflammation and cytokine activity, which results in synovial proliferation and cartilage and bone damage.
d. autoimmune reaction resulting in degeneration, necrosis, and fibrosis of muscle fibers.

2. All of the following are true about ankylosing spondylitis (AS) *except*

a. 90% of Caucasians with AS are HLA-B27 positive.
b. patient education includes therapeutic exercise, which helps preserve ROM and prevent deformity.
c. AS may be a reactive arthritis following enteric or venereal infection.
d. complications of AS include decreased chest expansion.

3. The pathogenesis of rheumatoid arthritis (RA) includes

a. the development of Heberden's nodes.
b. cartilage deterioration by hyaluronidase.
c. the familial effects of HLA-B27.
d. invasion of pannus into the joint capsule and subchondral bone.

4. Which of the following assessment data indicate degenerative joint disease?

a. Symmetric swelling of metacarpophalangeal joints
b. Progressive joint pain with activity
c. Significant morning stiffness
d. Elevated ESR

5. Education of the patient with arthritis includes all of the following *except*

a. teaching a balance between activity and rest.
b. use of pharmacologic and nonpharmacologic methods of pain management.
c. use of assistive devices for joint protection.
d. encouraging inactivity to preserve joint surfaces.

6. The purpose of an arthroplasty is to

a. prevent further joint damage.
b. fuse a joint and reduce pain.
c. assess the extent of cartilage damage.
d. replace the joint and improve function.

7. All of the following are important instructions for patients recovering from total hip arthroplasty *except*

a. avoid hip flexion greater than 90 degrees.
b. maintain position of adduction at night.
c. use elevated chairs and toilet seats.
d. lie prone for 20 minutes a day.

8. Correct nursing knowledge related to antiinflammatory medications includes all of the following *except*

a. blood levels cannot be determined for salicylates.
b. enteric-coated tablets have a sparing effect on GI mucosa.
c. a clinical response to gold therapy is noted in several weeks.
d. high-dose corticosteroids should be stopped as soon as inflammation is controlled.

9. Adherence to a treatment program can be enhanced by all of the following nursing interventions *except*

a. discouraging talk of fears and concerns.
b. encouraging usual lifestyle preferences.
c. discussing sexual concerns.
d. evaluating family support system.

10. The most effective way to manage the health care needs of the patient with arthritis is to

a. provide round-the-clock nursing care.
b. let the family take over the patient's work load.
c. endorse the skills of a multidisciplinary health care team.
d. explore the patient's spiritual response to pain.

REFERENCES

*1. Burke M, Flaherty MJ: Coping strategies and health status of elderly arthritic women, *J Adv Nurs* 18:7, 1993.

2. Brandt KD: Osteoarthritis. In Isselbacker K and others, editors: *Harrison's principles of internal medicine,* ed 13, New York, 1994, McGraw-Hill.

3. Moskowitz RW, Pun Y, Haqqi TM: Genetics and osteoarthritis, *Bull Rheum Dis* 41:4, 1992.

4. de Bock GH and others: Osteoarthritis pain assessment in family practice, *Arthritis Care Res* 7:40, 1994.

5. Brandt KD: NSAIDs in the treatment of osteoarthritis, *Bull Rheum Dis* 42:1, 1993.

*6. Dexter PA: Joint exercises in elderly persons with symptomatic osteoarthritis of the hip or knee: performance patterns, medical support patterns, and the relationship between exercising and medical care, *Arthritis Care Res* 5:36, 1992.

7. Zvaifler NJ: Etiology and pathogenesis of rheumatoid arthritis. In McCarty DJ, editor: *Arthritis and allied conditions,* ed 12, Philadelphia, 1993, Lea & Febiger.

8. *Bull Rheum Dis,* 42:1, 1993.

9. Shumacher W, editor: *Primer on the rheumatic diseases,* ed 10, Atlanta, 1993, Arthritis Foundation.

10. Medsger TA, Masi AT: Epidemiology of the rheumatic diseases. In McCarty DJ, editor: *Arthritis and allied conditions,* ed 12, Philadelphia, 1993, Lea & Febiger.

11. Tirestein G, Zvaifler N: The pathogenesis of rheumatoid arthritis, *Rheum Dis Clin North Am* 13:447, 1987.

12. Arnett FC and others: The American Rheumatism Association 1987 revised criteria for the classification of RA, *Arthritis Rheum* 31:315, 1988.

13. McGuire JL, Ridgway WM: Aggressive drug therapy for rheumatoid arthritis, *Hosp Pract* 28:45, 1993.

*14. Hawley DJ, Wolfe F: Sensitivity to change of the Health Assessment Questionnaire (HAQ) and other clinical and health status measures in rheumatoid arthritis, *Arthritis Care Res* 5:130, 1992.

15. Kuhn MA: Antiinflammatory agents. In Mathewson-Kuhn M, editor: *Pharmacotherapeutics: a nursing process approach,* ed 3, Philadelphia, 1994, Davis.

16. Yocum D: Rheumatoid arthritis: immunopathogenesis and implications for therapy, *Consultant* 31:39, 1991.

17. *Guide to independent living for people with arthritis,* Atlanta, 1988, Arthritis Foundation.

18. Mirabelli L: Caring for patients with rheumatoid arthritis, *Nursing* 20:67, 1990.

19. Gerber LH, Hicks JE: Exercise in rheumatic disease. In Basmajian JV, Wolf SL, editors: *Therapeutic exercise,* ed 5, Baltimore, 1990, Williams & Wilkins.

20. Cassidy JT and others: A study of classification criteria for a diagnosis of juvenile rheumatoid arthritis, *Arthritis Rheum* 29:274, 1986.

21. Hooker RS: Clinical characteristics of the seronegative spondyloarthropathies, *J Am Acad Physician Assistants* 5:110, 1992.

22. Inman RD: Reiter's syndrome and reactive arthritis. In Paget SA, Fields TR, editors: *Summaries in clinical practice: rheumatic disorders,* Boston, 1992, Andover Medical.

23. Bluestone R: Atypical ankylosing spondylitis, *Hosp Pract* 24:88, 1989.

24. Powell MA: Lyme disease, *J Am Acad Nurse Pract* 5:40, 1993.

25. Steere AC: Current understanding of Lyme disease, *Hosp Pract* 28:37, 1993.

26. Schulze TL, Taylor RC, Bosler EM: Lyme disease: a proposed ecological index to assess areas of risk in the northeastern United States, *Am J Public Health* 81:714, 1991.

27. Calabrese LH: Human immunodeficiency virus (HIV) infection and arthritis, *Rheum Dis Clin North Am* 19:477, 1993.

28. Yeomans AC: Assessment and management of gouty arthritis, *Nurse Pract* 16:18, 1991.

29. Lahita RG: The early diagnosis of systemic lupus erythematosus, *J Women's Health* 1:117, 1992.

30. Masi AT, Medsger TA Jr: Epidemiology of the rheumatic diseases. In McCarty DJ, editor: *Arthritis and allied conditions,* ed 11, Philadelphia, 1989, Lea & Febiger.

31. Lash AA: Why so many women? Part 1: systemic lupus erythematosus, *Medsurg Nurs* 2:259, 1993.

32. Kimberly RP: Systemic lupus erythematosus. In Paget SA, Fields TR, editors: *Summaries in clinical practice: rheumatic disorders,* Boston, 1992, Andover Medical.

33. Bizzaro A and others: Influence of testosterone therapy on clinical and immunological features of autoimmune diseases associated with Klinefelter's syndrome, *J Clin Endocrinol Metab* 64:32, 1987.
34. Harley JB and others: Systemic lupus erythematosus: considerations for a genetic-approach, *J Invest Dermatol* 103:1445, 1994.
35. Hess EV, Farhey Y: Epidemiology, etiology, and environmental relationships of systemic lupus erythematosus, *Curr Opin Rheumatol* 6:474, 1994.
36. Lash AA: Systemic lupus erythematosus. Part 2: diagnosis, treatment modalities, and nursing management, *Medsurg Nurs* 2:375,1993.
37. Hahn BH: Lupus nephritis: therapeutic decisions, *Hosp Pract* 25:89, 1990.
38. Reichlin M: Antibodies to defined antigens in the systemic rheumatic diseases, *Bull Rheum Dis* 42:4, 1993.
39. Harvey CJ, Verklan T: Systemic lupus erythematosus: obstetric and neonatal implications, *NAACOG's Clin Iss Perinatal and Women's Health Nurs* 1:177, 1990.
*40. Cornwell CJ, Schmitt MH: Perceived health status, self-esteem and body image in women with rheumatoid arthritis of systemic lupus erythematosus, *Res Nurs Health* 13:99, 1990.
41. Braden CJ, McGlone K, Pennington F: Specific psychosocial and behavioral outcomes from the systemic lupus erythematosus self-help course, *Health Educ Q* 20:29, 1993.
42. Larabee JH: Progressive systemic sclerosis: part I—the disease and medical management, *ANNA J* 16:489, 1990.
43. Leryo EC: The spectrum of scleroderma. In Paget SA, Fields TR, editors: *Summaries in clinical practice: rheumatic disorders,* Boston, 1992, Andover Medical.
44. Leroy EC, Medsger TA: *The spectrum of scleroderma-related syndromes, primer on the rheumatic diseases,* ed 10, Atlanta, 1993, Arthritis Foundation.
45. Plotz PH: New understanding of myositis, *Hosp Prac* 27:33, 1992.
46. Andreoli TE and others: *Cecil essentials of medicine,* ed 2, Philadelphia, 1990, Saunders.
47. Boisset-Pioro MH, Esdaile JM, Fitzcharles MA: Sexual and physical abuse in women with fibromyalgia syndrome, *Arthritis Rheum* 38:235, 1995.
48. Wolfle F and others: The prevalence and characteristics of fibromyalgia in the general population, *Arthritis Rheum* 38:19, 1995.
49. Stein JH, Hutton JJ: *Internal medicine,* ed 3, Boston, 1990, Little, Brown.
50. Gorab RS, Covino BM, Borden LS: The rationale for cementless revision total hip replacement with contemporary technology, *Orthop Clin North Am* 24:627, 1993.
51. Brandler VA, Stulberg SD, Chang RW: Life after total hip arthroplasty, *Bull Rheum Dis* 42:1, 1993.

SECTION XI BIBLIOGRAPHY

Books

Adams R, Victor M: *Principles of neurology,* ed 5, New York, 1993, McGraw-Hill.

Browner BD and others, editors: *Skeletal trauma,* Philadelphia, 1992, WB Saunders.

Bryne TN, Waxman SG: *Spinal cord compression: diagnosis and principles of management,* Philadelphia, 1990, FA Davis.

Chapman MW, editor: *Operative orthopaedics,* ed 2, Philadelphia, 1993, JB Lippincott.

Cohen GD: *The brain in human aging,* New York, 1990, Springer.

Crenshaw AH, editor: *Campbell's operative orthopaedics,* ed 8, St Louis, 1992, Mosby.

DeLee JC, Drez D, editors: *Orthopedic sports medicine: principles and practice,* Philadelphia, 1994, WB Saunders.

Dvorkin ML: *Office orthopaedics,* Norwalk, CT, 1993, Appleton & Lange.

Ellert G: *Arthritis exercise book,* Chicago, 1990, Contemporary Books.

Errico TJ, Bauer RD, Waugh T, editors: *Spinal trauma,* Philadelphia, 1991, JB Lippincott.

Gumnit RJ: *The epilepsy handbook: the practical management of seizure,* ed 2, New York, 1995, Raven Press.

Hamdy RC and others: *Alzheimer's disease: a handbook for caregivers,* ed 2, St Louis, 1994, Mosby.

Hertling D, Kessler RM: *Management of common musculoskeletal disorders: physical therapy principles and methods,* ed 2, Philadelphia, 1990, JB Lippincott.

Hogstel MO: *Clinical manual of gerontological nursing,* St Louis, 1992, Mosby.

Kelly WN: *Textbook of rheumatology,* ed 4, Philadelphia, 1993, WB Saunders.

Lahita RG: Systemic lupus erythematosus, ed 2, New York, 1992, Churchill-Livingstone.

Lechtenberg R: *Seizure recognition and treatment,* New York, 1990, Churchill-Livingstone.

Lorig K: *Arthritis helpbook,* ed 3, Reading, Mass, 1990, Addison-Wesley.

Maher AB, Salmond SW, Pellion TA, editors: *Orthopaedic nursing,* Philadelphia, 1994, WB Saunders.

McCarty DJ, editor: *Arthritis and allied conditions: a textbook of rheumatology,* ed 12, Philadelphia, 1993, Lea & Febiger.

Moore EE, Mattox KL, Feliciano DV, editors: *Trauma,* ed 2, Norwalk, CT, 1991, Appleton & Lange.

Mourad LA: *Orthopedic disorders,* St Louis, 1991, Mosby.

Prentice WE: *Rehabilitation techniques in sports medicine,* St Louis, 1990, Mosby.

Reckling FW, Reckling JB, Mohn MP, editors: *Orthopaedic anatomy and surgical approaches,* St Louis, 1990, Mosby.

Rippe JM and others, editors: *Intensive care medicine,* ed 2, Boston, 1991, Little, Brown.

Salcman M, editor: *Neurological emergencies: recognition and management,* ed 2, New York, 1990, Raven Press.

Salmond SW, Mooney NE, Verdisco LA, editors: *Core curriculum for orthopaedic nursing,* ed 2, Pitman, NJ, 1991, Anthony J Jannetti.

Sherman OH, Minkoff J, editors: *Arthroscopic surgery,* Baltimore, 1990, Williams & Wilkins.

Sledge, CG: *Arthritis surgery,* Philadelphia, 1993, WB Saunders.

Snell RS: *Clinical neuroanatomy,* ed 3, Boston, 1992, Little, Brown.

Wallace DJ, Dubois EJ, editors: *Dubois' lupus erythematosus,* ed 4, Philadelphia, 1993, Lea & Febiger.

Umphred DA, editor: *Neurological rehabilitation,* ed 2, St Louis, 1990, Mosby.

Zuckerman JC, editor: *Comprehensive care of orthopaedic injuries in the elderly,* Baltimore, 1990, Urban & Schwarzenberg.

Journals

Acorn S, Andersen S: Depression in multiple sclerosis: critique of the research literature, *J Neurosci Nurs* 22:209, 1990.

*Adkins ER: Quality of life after stroke: exposing a gap in nursing literature, *Rehabil Nurs* 18:144, 1993.

Ailinger RL, Dear MR: Self-care agency in persons with rheumatoid arthritis, *Arthritis Care Res* 6:134, 1993.

Alexander MP: Stroke rehabilitation outcome. A potential use of predictive variables to establish levels of care, *Stroke* 25:128, 1994.

Ammons AM: Cerebral injuries and intracranial hemorrhages as a result of trauma, *Nurs Clin North Am* 25:23, 1990.

Arlington RG, Costigan KA, Aievoli CP: Postoperative blood salvage and reinfusion, *Orthop Nurs* 11:30, 1992.

*Nursing research-based articles.

Arthur V: Nursing care of patients with rheumatoid arthritis, *Br J Nurs* 3:325, 1994.

Barden RM, Sinkora GL: Bone stimulators for fusions and fractures, *Nurs Clin North Am* 26:89, 1991.

Bauer RL: Assessing osteoporosis, *Hosp Pract* 26:23, 1991.

Belinsky JD: Acetabular fracture: ORIF, *Orthop Nurs* 12:42, 1993.

*Bell JC, Matthews SD: Results of a clinical investigation of four pressure-reduction replacement mattresses, *J ET Nurs* 20:204, 1993.

*Belza BL and others: Correlates of fatigue in older adults with rheumatoid arthritis, *Nurs Res* 42:93, 1993.

Berg E: Anterior shoulder dislocation, *Orthop Nurs* 12:51, 1992.

Bertino LS: The bite of a wolf: systemic lupus erythematosus, *Rehabil Nurs* 18:173, 1993.

Braden CJ: Description of learned response to chronic illness: depressed versus nondepressed self-help class participants, *Public Health Nurs* 9:103, 1992.

Brewer CC, Storms BS: The final phase of rehabilitation: work hardening, *Orthop Nurs* 12:9, 1993.

*Bridges-Parlet S, Knopman D, Thompson T: A descriptive study of physically aggressive behavior in dementia by direct observation, *J Am Geriatr Soc* 42:192, 1994.

Buelow JM, Jamieson D: Potential for altered nutritional status in the stroke patient, *Rehabil Nurs* 15:260, 1990.

*Burckhardt CS, Clark SR, Bennett RM: A comparison of pain perceptions in women with fibromyalgia and rheumatoid arthritis: relationship to depression and pain extent, *Arthritis Care Res* 5:216, 1992.

Calhoun JH, Cobos JA, Mader JT: Does hyperbaric oxygen have a place in the treatment of osteomyelitis? *Orthop Clin North Am* 22:467, 1991.

Calne S: Examining causes and care of idiopathic parkinsonism, *Nurs Times* 90:38, 1994.

Carroll P: Deep venous thrombosis: implications for orthopaedic nursing, *Orthop Nurs* 12:33, 1993.

Charbonneau-Smith R: No-touch catheterization and infection rates in a select spinal cord injured population, *Rehabil Nurs* 18:296, 1993.

*Clough DH: The effects of cognitive distortion and depression on disability in rheumatoid arthritis, *Res Nurs Health* 14:439, 1991.

*Danner C and others: Cognitively impaired elders. Using research findings to improve nursing care, *J Gerontol Nurs* 19:5, 1993.

Davis E: The diagnostic puzzle and management challenge of Raynaud's syndrome, *Nurse Pract* 18:18, 1993.

Davis P: Managing brachial plexus injuries, *Nurs Stand* 8:31, 1994.

*DeVivo MJ and others: A cross-sectional study of the relationship between age and current health status for persons with spinal cord injuries, *Paraplegia*, 30:820, 1992.

*Dillehay RC, Sandys MR: Caregivers for Alzheimer's patients: what we are learning from research, *Int J Aging Hum Dev* 30:263, 1990.

*Downe-Wamboldt B: Coping and life satisfaction in elderly women with osteoarthritis, *J Adv Nurs* 16:1328, 1991.

*Dunnum L: Life satisfaction and spinal cord injury: the patient perspective, *J Neurosci Nurs* 22:43, 1990.

*Edwards RM and others: Knowledge about aging and Alzheimer's disease among baccalaureate nursing students, *J Nurs Educ* 31:127, 1992.

Evans RL, Rubash HE, Albrecht SA: The efficacy of postoperative autotransfusion in total joint arthroplasty, *Orthop Nurs* 12:11, 1993.

Exum ME and others: Sundown syndrome: is it reflected in the use of PRN medications for nursing home residents? *Gerontologist* 33:756, 1993.

Falconer JA and others: Stroke inpatient rehabilitation: a comparison across age groups, *J Am Geriatr Soc* 42:39, 1994.

*Farkkila M, Penttila P: Plasma exchange therapy reduces the nursing care needed in Guillain-Barre syndrome, *J Adv Nurs* 17:672, 1992.

Feingold DJ and others: Complications of lumbar spine surgery, *Orthop Nurs* 10:39, 1991.

Fiatarone MA and others: Exercise training and nutritional supplementation for physical frailty in very elderly people, *N Engl J Med* 330:1769, 1994.

Finocchiaro DN, Herzfeld ST: Understanding autonomic dysreflexia, *Am J Nurs* 90:56, 1990.

Fitzsimmons B, Bunting LK: Parkinson's disease. Quality of life issues, *Nurs Clin North Am* 28:807, 1993.

*Folden SL: Effect of a supportive-educative nursing intervention on older adults' perceptions of self-care after a stroke, *Rehabil Nurs* 18:162, 1993.

Franssen EH and others: The neurologic syndrome of severe Alzheimer's disease. Relationship to functional decline, *Arch Neurol* 50:1029, 1993.

Fuller C, Hartley B: Systemic lupus erythematosus in adolescents, *J Pediatr Nurs* 6:251, 1991.

Gerhart TN and others: Low-molecular-weight heparinoid compared with warfarin for prophylaxis of deep-vein thrombosis in patients who are operated on for fracture of the hip, *J Bone Joint Surg Am* 73A:494, 1991.

Gibbon B: Implications for nurses in approaches to the management of stroke rehabilitation: a review of the literature, *Int J Nurs Stud* 30:133, 1993.

Gill KP, Ursic P: The impact of continuing education on patient outcomes in the elderly hip fracture population, *J Contin Educ Nurs* 25:181, 1994.

Giuffre M and others: Postoperative joint replacement pain: description and opioid requirement, *J Post Anesth Nurs* 6:239, 1991.

Grinspun D: Bladder management for adults following head injury, *Rehabil Nurs* 18:300, 1993.

Guin P: Standardized nursing care plans for acute care SCI: improved documentation, *SCI Nurs* 7:4, 1990.

Gwynn M: tPA in acute stroke—risk or reprieve? *J Neurosci Nurs* 25:180, 1993.

Hall GR: Caring for people with Alzheimer's disease using the conceptual model of progressively lowered stress threshold in the clinical setting, *Nurs Clin North Am* 29:129, 1994.

Halverson PB, Holmes SB: Systemic lupus erythematosus: medical and nursing treatments, *Orthop Nurs* 11:17, 1992.

Hart K: Using the Ilizarov external fixator in bone transport, *Orthop Nurs* 13:35, 1994.

Held JL, Peahota A: Nursing care of the patient with spinal cord compression, *Oncol Nurs Forum* 20:1507, 1993.

Hubsky EP, Sears JH: Fatigue in multiple sclerosis: guidelines for nursing care, *Rehabil Nurs* 17:176, 1992.

Hughes MC: Critical care nursing for the patient with a spinal cord injury, *Crit Care Nurs Clin North Am* 2:33, 1990.

Jansen DA, Cimprich B: Attentional impairment in persons with multiple sclerosis, *J Neurosci Nurs* 26:95, 1994.

Jerva MJ: Automated percutaneous lumbar discectomy: a review, *Orthop Nurs* 12:27, 1993.

Kaplan H, Weinblatt ME, Wilder RL: Drug therapy in rheumatoid arthritis, *Patient Care* 26:111, 1992.

*Kasper CE and others: Alterations in skeletal muscle related to impaired physical mobility: an empirical model, *Res Nurs Health* 16:265, 1993.

Kelley CL, Smeltzer SC: Betaseron: the new MS treatment, *J Neurosci Nurs* 26:52, 1994.

Kerr ME, Brucia J: Hyperventilation in the head-injured patient: an effective treatment modality? *Heart Lung* 22:516, 1993.

Kerr ME and others: Head-injured adults: recommendations for endotracheal suctioning, *J Neurosci Nurs* 25:86, 1993.

Killen JM: Role stabilization in families after spinal cord injury, *Rehabil Nurs* 15:19, 1990.

King CA, Myers LC: Head trauma. Perioperative nursing implications, *Todays OR Nurse* 15:15, 1993.

Kirkevold M: Caring for stroke patients: heavy or exciting? *Image J Nurs Sch* 22:79, 1990.

Klemm KW: Antibiotic bead chains, *Clin Orthop Related Res* 295:63, 1993.

Larese F, Fiorito A: Musculoskeletal disorders in hospital nurses: a comparison between two hospitals, *Ergonomics* 37:1205, 1994.

Leisifer D: Monitoring pain control and charting, *Crit Care Clin* 6:283, 1990.

Lipsitz LA and others: Muscle strength and fall rates among residents of Japanese and American nursing homes: an international cross-cultural study, *J Am Geriatr Soc* 42:953, 1994.

*Lisanti P, Verdisco LA: Perceived body space and self-esteem in adult females with chronic low back pain, *Orthop Nurs* 13:55, 1994.

Lugger KE: Dysphagia in the elderly stroke patient, *J Neurosci Nurs* 26:78, 1994.

Mac HL and others: Comparison of autotransfusion and standard drainage systems in total joint arthroplasty patients, *Orthop Nurs* 12:19, 1993.

Mader JT, Landon GC, Calhoun J: Antimicrobial treatment of osteomyelitis, *Clin Orthop Related Res* 295:87, 1993.

McConnell EA: Providing cast care, *Nursing* 23:19, 1993.

McPherson ML: Medication management of rheumatoid arthritis, *J Home Health Care Pract* 4:34, 1992.

Miller CM: Trajectory and empowerment theory applied to care of patients with multiple sclerosis, *J Neurosci Nurs* 25:343, 1993.

Mravic PJ, Massey DM: Compartment syndrome, *J Vasc Nurs* 10:9, 1992.

Nance DK, Mardjetko SM: Technical aspects and nursing considerations of limb lengthening, *Orthop Nurs* 13:21, 1994.

Negus E: Stroke-induced dysphagia in hospital: the nutritional perspective, *Br J Nurs* 3:263, 1994.

Nelson AL: Patients' perspectives of a spinal cord injury unit, *SCI Nurs* 7:44, 1990.

Neuberger GB and others: Promoting self-care in clients with arthritis, *Arthritis Care Res* 6:141, 1993.

Oldham J and others: Rehabilitation of muscle function, part 2, *Nurs Stand* 6:37, 1992.

Oldham J and others: Rehabilitation: objective assessment of muscle function, *Nurs Stand* 6:37, 1992.

Olson B, Ustanko L: Self-care needs of patients in the halo brace, *Orthop Nurs* 9:27, 1990.

Pallett PJ: A conceptual framework for studying family caregiver burden in Alzheimer's-type dementia, *Image J Nurs Sch* 22:52, 1990.

Paxquarello MA: Developing, implementing and evaluating a stroke recovery group, *Rehabil Nurs* 15:26, 1990.

Peck SA: Crush syndrome: pathophysiology and management, *Orthop Nurs* 9:33, 1990.

Piasecki P: Update in orthopaedic oncology, *Orthop Nurs* 11:36, 1992.

Poole JL, Steen VD: The use of the health assessment questionnaire (HAQ) to determine physical disability in systemic sclerosis, *Arthritis Care Res* 4:27, 1991.

Printz-Feddersen V: Group process effect on caregiver burden, *J Neurosci Nurs* 22:164, 1990.

Richmond TS: Spinal cord injury, *Nurs Clin North Am* 25:57, 1990.

*Richmond TS and others: Powerlessness in acute spinal cord injury patients: a descriptive study, *J Neurosci Nurs* 24:146, 1992.

Romito D: A critical path for CVA patients, *Rehabil Nurs* 15:153, 1990.

Roth EJ and others: The older adult with a spinal cord injury, *Paraplegia* 30:520, 1992.

St. George CL: Spasticity. Mechanisms and nursing care, *Nurs Clin North Am* 28:819, 1993.

Sherk HH and others: Laser diskectomy, *Orthopedics* 16:573, 1993.

Simon MA, Finn HA: Diagnostic strategy for bone and soft-tissue tumors, *J Bone Joint Surg* 75A:622, 1993.

Slye DA: Orthopedic complications. Compartment syndrome, fat embolism, and venous thromboembolism, *Nurs Clin North Am* 26:113, 1991.

Stenger KM: Surveillance of spinal cord motor and sensory function, *Nurs Clin North Am* 28:783, 1993.

Thapa PB and others: Comparison of clinical and biomechanical measures of balance and mobility in elderly nursing home residents, *J Am Geriatr Soc* 42:493, 1994.

Tinetti ME, Liu WL, Claus EB: Predictors and prognosis of inability to get up after falls among elderly persons, *JAMA* 269:65, 1993.

*Tutuarima JA, de Haan RJ, Limburg M: Number of nursing staff and falls: a case-control study on falls by stroke patients in acute-care settings, *J Adv Nurs* 18:1101, 1993.

Ulmer DB: Special needs of the young spinal cord injured patient in a nursing home, *SCI Nurs* 7:27, 1990.

*Watson R: Measuring feeding difficulty in patients with dementia: developing a scale, *J Adv Nurs* 19:257, 1994.

Weiler K: Legal aspects of nursing documentation for the Alzheimer's patient, *J Gerontol Nurs* 20:31, 1994.

Wetherbee LL: Caring for the client with arthritis: an overview, *Home Health Nurse* 12:13, 1994.

Whitney F: Drug therapy for acute stroke, *J Neurosci Nurs* 26:111, 1994.

Whittington CF, Carlson CA: Anterior cruciate injuries, *Nurs Clin North Am* 26:149, 1991.

Wild D: Stroke: a nursing rehabilitation role, *Nurs Stand* 8:36, 1994.

Wilde AH and others: Symposium: advances in the prevention of venous thromboembolic disease in orthopaedics. The introduction of LMWH, *Contemp Orthop* 27:551, 1993.

Wilkinson MM: Small intestinal complications in progressive systemic sclerosis, *Gastroenterol Nurs* 15:50, 1992.

Organizations

Academy of Aphasia (AA)
Boston Veterans Administration
Medical Center 116B
150 So. Huntingdon Avenue
Boston, MA 02130
617-495-4342

Alzheimer's Disease and Related Disorders Association
4709 Golf Road, Suite 1015
Skokie, IL 60076
708-933-1000

American Association of Biofeedback Clinicians
2424 Demster Street
Des Plaines, IL 60016
312-827-0440

The American Association of Cardiovascular and Pulmonary Rehabilitation (AACVPR)
53 Park Place
New York, NY 10007

American Association of Neuroscience Nurses
218 North Jefferson Street, #204
Chicago, IL 60606
312-993-0043

*Nursing research-based articles.

American Association for Rehabilitation Therapy (AART)
P.O. Box 6412
Gulfport, MS 39506

American Association of Spinal Cord Injury Nurses (AASCIN)
75-20 Astoria Boulevard
Jackson Heights, NY 11370-1177
718-803-3782
FAX: 718-803-0414

American Congress of Rehabilitation Medicine
5700 Old Orchard Road
Skokie, IL 60077
708-966-0095

American Paralysis/Spinal Cord Hotline
800-526-3456
800-638-1733 (in MD)

American Speech, Language, Hearing Association
10801 Rockville Pike
Rockville, MD 20852
301-897-5700

Amyotrophic Lateral Sclerosis Association
21021 Ventura Blvd., Suite 321
Woodland Hills, CA 91364
818-990-2151

Arthritis Foundation
1314 Spring Street, NW
Atlanta, GA 30309

Association of Rehabilitation Nurses
5700 Old Orchard Road, 1st floor
Skokie, IL 60077
708-966-8673
FAX: 708-966-9418

Association of Rheumatology Health Professionals
P.O. Box 102295
Atlanta, GA 30368-9990

Epilepsy Foundation of America
4351 Garden City Drive, 5th floor
Landover, MD 20785
301-459-3700

Guillain Barre Syndrome Foundation International
P.O. Box 262
Wynnewood, PA 19096
215-667-0131

Independent Living for the Handicapped
1301 Belmont Street, NW
Washington, DC 20009
202-797-9803

Information Center for Individuals with Disabilities
Fort Point Place, 1st floor
27-43 Wormwood Street
Boston, MA 02210-1606
617-727-5540

The Library of Congress
Division of the Blind and Physically Handicapped
1291 Taylor Street, NW
Washington, DC 20542
202-707-5100

Lupus Foundation of America, Inc.
4 Research Place, Suite 180
Rockville, MD 20850-3226

National Association of Orthopaedic Nurses, Inc.
East Holly Avenue
Box 56
Pitman, NJ 08071
609-256-2310
FAX: 609-589-7463

National Easter Seal Society
70 E. Lake Street
Chicago, IL 60601
312-726-6200

National Foundation March of Dimes
1275 Mamaroneck Avenue
White Plains, NY 10605
914-428-7100

National Head Injury Foundation
333 Turnpike Road
Southborough, MA 01772
508-485-9950

National Headache Foundation
5252 North Western Avenue
Chicago, IL 60625
800-843-2256
FAX: 312-907-6278

National Institute of Neurological and Communicative Disorders and Stroke
Building 31, Room 8A52
9000 Rockville Pike
Bethesda, MD 20892
301-496-9746

National Institute of Neurological Disorders and Stroke (NINDS)
Office of Scientific and Health Reports
Building 31, Room 8A16
9000 Rockville Pike
Bethesda, MD 20892
301-496-5751

National Institute of Neurological Disorders and Stroke (NINDS)
Division of Stroke and Trauma (grant applications)
Federal Building, Room 1016
7550 Wisconsin Avenue
Bethesda, MD 20892
301-496-4188

National Multiple Sclerosis Society
205 E. 42nd Street, 3rd floor
New York, NY 10017
212-986-3240

National Parkinson Foundation
Bob Hope Road
Miami, FL 33136

National Rehabilitation Information Center
8455 Colesville Road, Suite 935
Silver Spring, MD 20910
301-588-9284

National Spinal Cord Injury Association
600 W. Cummings Park, Suite 2000
Woburn, MA 01801
617-935-2722

National Stroke Association
300 East Hampden Avenue, Suite 240
Englewood, CO 80110-2654
303-762-9922

Paralyzed Veterans of America
801 18th Street NW
Washington, DC 20006
202-872-1300

Parkinson's Disease Foundation
William Black Medical Research Building
Columbia Presbyterian Medical Center
650 West 168th Street
New York, NY 10032
212-923-4700

Rehabilitation Services Administration
Department of Human Services
Room 101M
605 G Street, NW
Washington, DC 20001
202-727-3211

Stroke Clubs International
805 12th Street
Galveston, TX 77550
409-762-1022

Nursing Care *in* Specialized Settings

Section Twelve

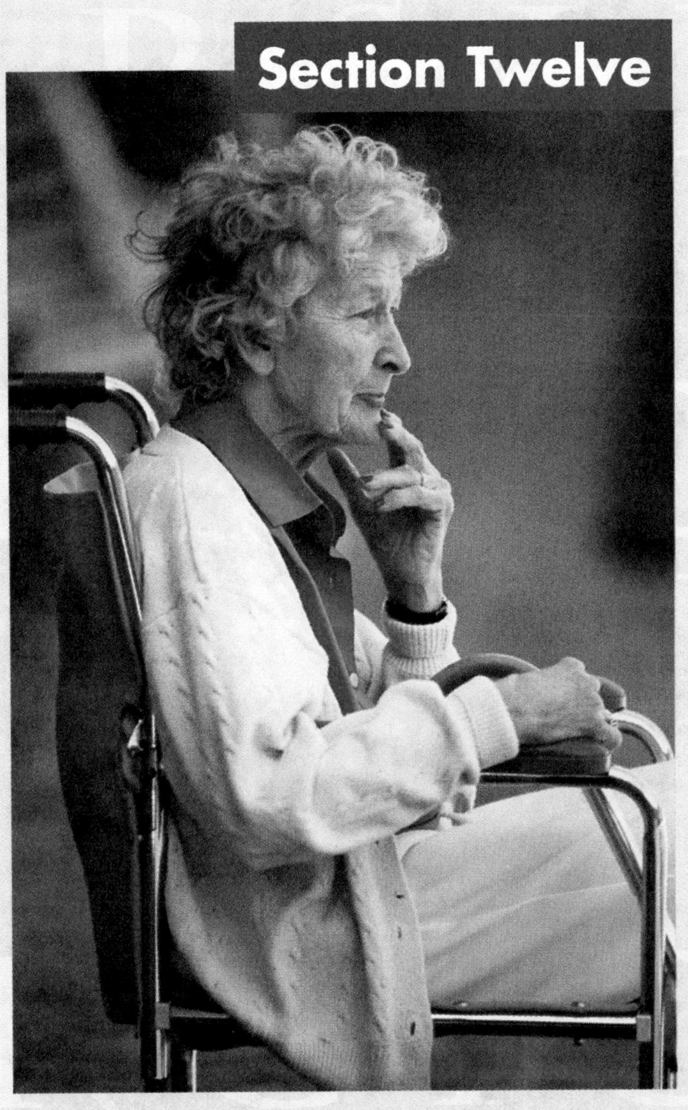

MEDICAL
SURGICAL
NURSING
MEDICAL
SURGICAL
NURSING
MEDICAL
SURGICAL
NURSING
MEDICAL
SURGICAL

Chapter 61

NURSING ROLE IN MANAGEMENT

Critical Care

Eleanor F. Bond

Learning Objectives

1. Describe the critical care environment.
2. Identify common problems and needs of patients in critical care units and related nursing management.
3. Identify common problems and needs of families of patients in critical care units and related nursing management.
4. Describe the principles of hemodynamic monitoring and related nursing management.
5. Describe the purpose and function of intraaortic balloon pumping and related nursing management.
6. Describe the types, potential complications, and nursing management of artificial airways.
7. Describe the indications for mechanical ventilation, modes of mechanical ventilation, and related nursing management.
8. Describe the principles of intracranial pressure monitoring.
9. Identify strategies for management of patients with increased intracranial pressure.
10. Describe the pathophysiology and clinical manifestations of systemic inflammatory response syndrome, sepsis, and multiple organ dysfunction syndrome.
11. Describe the therapeutic and nursing management of the patient with systemic inflammatory response syndrome, sepsis, or multiple organ dysfunction syndrome.

CRITICAL CARE NURSING

Critical Care Units

Critical care units or intensive care units were designed to meet the special needs of acutely and critically ill patients. The concept of clustering the most acutely ill is not new. Florence Nightingale recommended grouping acutely ill patients together.[1] During poliomyelitis and tuberculosis pandemics earlier this century, special units were established, equipped with technical apparatus to manage the airway and ventilate the patient and staffed by specialized care providers. During World War II and the Vietnam War trauma units were developed for battle casualties.

In the 1960s technical developments allowed for more accessible monitoring of electrocardiogram (ECG), arterial and central venous pressures, and arterial blood gases. Coronary care units were developed for patients with acute myocardial infarction. In these units patients were continually monitored for cardiac dysrhythmias and nurses were trained to identify and aggressively manage dysrhythmias. By the 1970s the intensive care unit (ICU) was a standard component of most general hospitals. Since that time, technologic advances have continued at a rapid pace, bringing improved monitoring capabilities and new strategies to manage life-threatening problems.

The term *critical care nursing* is often used interchangeably with the term *ICU nursing*. The critical care nurse is responsible for diagnosing life-threatening conditions and instituting appropriate treatment. Today the technology and equipment available in the ICU are extensive and continually evolving. In ICUs the capability exists to continuously monitor ECG, blood pressure, cardiac output, ventilation, intracranial pressure, oxygenation, and temperature. More advanced monitoring devices allow for the measurement of stroke volume, ejection fraction, end tidal carbon dioxide, and oxygen consumption. Patients may be receiving continual support from the ventilator, cardiac assist devices, or dialysis machines. A typical critical care patient unit is illustrated in Fig. 61-1.

Critical Care Nurse

The critical care nurse cares for patients and the families of patients with acute and unstable physiologic problems in an environment equipped for technically advanced methods of assessing and managing patient problems. The American Association of Critical-Care Nurses (AACN) defines critical care nursing as that specialty dealing with human responses to life-threatening problems. The specialty requires knowledge of physiology, pathophysiology, pharma-

Reviewed by Susan B. Stillwell, RN, MSN, Consultant, Critical Care Nursing, Shaker Heights, OH.

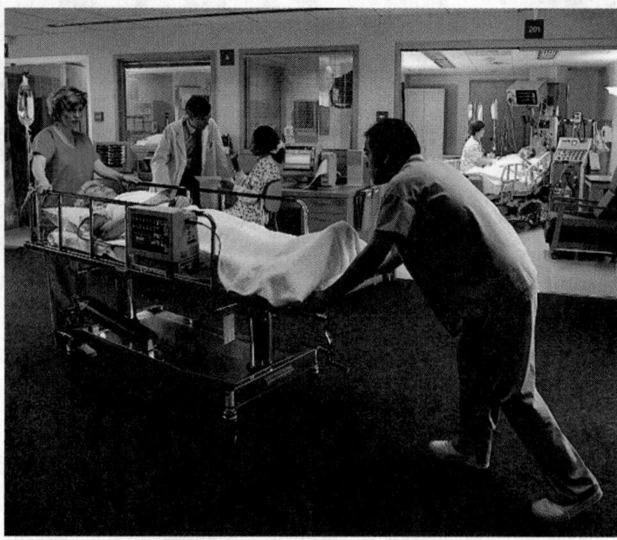

Fig. 61-1 Typical intensive care unit.

cology, and the ability to use advanced technology to accurately measure physiologic parameters. It is important that the nurse understand the assumptions on which measurements depend and determine if those assumptions are correct for each specific patient. The nurse provides ongoing assessment and early recognition and management of complications while fostering healing and recovery. Appropriate actions by an astute nurse can prevent complications. The nurse must be able to provide psychologic support to the patient and the family. To be effective the critical care nurse must be able to communicate clearly and work as a team member.

Nursing practice in the ICU often follows a primary care model with the patient cared for by a limited group of nurses who become intensely familiar with the patient's condition and needs and the needs of the patient's family. That primary care nurse spends most working hours near the patient's bedside. Specialization in ICU nursing usually requires formal training and mentored clinical practice, followed by an internship. Training takes place in a variety of settings. Only a small percentage of baccalaureate nursing programs include critical care as a separate course, often with a minimal clinical component.[2] The number of associate degree programs offering critical care content is unknown. Many clinical institutions offer ICU preparation, as do continuing education agencies.

Certification in critical care nursing (CCRN) is offered by AACN Certification Corporation. The designation requires clinical experience and successful completion of a written test. Additional experience and testing or education are required for recertification. CCRN certification designates competency and not advanced practice. It does not require a master's degree and is not a basis for prescriptive authority.

Advanced practice critical care nurses generally have a graduate (master's or doctorate) degree. These nurses are employed as patient and staff educators, consultants, administrators, researchers, or practitioners. The *critical care clinical nurse specialist* role traditionally includes aspects of each of these role components. An important emerging role is the *acute care nurse practitioner.* These master's-prepared nurses provide advanced, comprehensive, risk-appropriate care to selected critically ill patients and their families. The acute care nurse practitioner is prepared to conduct comprehensive health assessments, order and interpret diagnostic tests, diagnose and treat health problems and disease-related symptoms, prescribe and evaluate drugs and treatments, and coordinate care during transitions in settings. They may practice independently (e.g., providing comprehensive care to the chronically critically ill), or collaboratively (e.g., providing symptom management in conjunction with physician specialists).

Table 61-1 Common Intensive Care Unit Admission Diagnoses

Diagnosis	Admissions (%)
Postoperative management	16.2
Ischemic heart disorder	16.1
Respiratory insufficiency or failure	14.6
Heart failure	5.8
Neurologic dysfunction	4.9
Dysrhythmia	4.0
Sepsis	4.0
Trauma	3.2
Gastrointestinal hemorrhage	3.0
Multiple organ dysfunction syndrome	2.1
Hemodynamic abnormality	1.5
Metabolic or electrolyte abnormality	1.5
Burn	1.4
Renal insufficiency or failure	1.3
Intoxication or drug overdose	1.2
Shock	0.8

From Groeger JS and others: Descriptive analysis of critical care units in the United States: patient characteristics and intensive care unit utilization, *Crit Care Med* 21:279, 1993.

Critical Care Patient

A patient is generally admitted to the ICU for one of three reasons. First, the patient may be *physiologically unstable,* requiring advanced and sophisticated clinical judgments by the nurse or physician. Second, the patient may be *at risk for serious complications* and require frequent and often invasive physical assessment. Third, the patient may be stable but *require intensive and complicated nursing support,* including ventilation, hemodynamic monitoring, feeding, turning, wound care, and hygiene.

ICUs may serve a variety of patients or specialize in a disease condition (e.g., neurology) or age group (e.g., pediatrics). ICU patients are sometimes clustered by acuity (e.g., acute and unstable versus technology dependent but stable). The patient with myocardial ischemia or infarction or respiratory distress is commonly treated in the ICU, as is the patient with acute neurologic impairment, after cardiac surgery, or after major organ transplantation (Table 61-1). Trauma ICUs treat the critically injured. The patient with a medical emergency (e.g., sepsis; diabetic ketoacidosis; drug overdoses; poisonings; thyroid, adrenal, or hematologic crises) is often treated in a medical ICU. The patient with a serious underlying condition may be monitored in the ICU while receiving care for unrelated conditions. The patient who is not expected to recover is not treated in an ICU. The ICU should not be used to treat the patient in a persistent vegetative state, nor should ICU care be used to prolong the natural process of death.

Common Problems of the Critical Care Patient. The patient admitted into the ICU is at risk for complications and special problems. Invasive devices carry a risk of infection, particularly in the patient with a compromised immunologic status. Sepsis and multiple organ dysfunction syndrome may follow. These complications are discussed later in the chapter. Other special problems for ICU patients include anxiety, dependency, impaired communication, sensory-perceptual problems, and sleep difficulties.

Anxiety. Patients commonly find the ICU frightening. Frequently patients are at risk of dying and fear death. Many patients and families feel uncomfortable in the ICU environment with its equipment, high noise and light levels, and intense pace of activity. The nurse can assist the patient and family with their feelings of anxiety by encouraging them to express concerns, ask questions, and state their needs. The nurse should explain equipment and procedures. The nurse may be able to structure the patient's surrounding environment in a way that may decrease anxiety. For example, family members can be encouraged to bring in photographs and personal items.

Dependency. Patients in the ICU commonly are unable to perform self-care activities such as eating, bathing, and oral hygiene. The patient may lack control over bodily functions such as elimination and breathing. The patient is frequently dependent on the nursing staff for access to food, liquids, the bedpan, and other needed items. In addition, the ICU patient is frequently connected to equipment and placed on bed rest. The degree of dependency experienced by an ICU patient can be distressing. Although the highest priority is the safety of the patient, the nurse should provide as much autonomy as the patient's condition allows. Family members can be taught to assist the patient with activities of daily living.

Impaired communication. Inability to communicate can be a distressing problem for the patient who may be unable to speak because of the use of paralyzing drugs or an endotracheal tube. As part of any procedure the nurse should explain what will happen or is happening to the patient. When the patient cannot speak, the nurse should explore alternative methods of communication, including the use of devices such as picture boards, magic slates, or computer keyboards. When speaking with the patient, the nurse should look directly at the patient and use hand gestures when appropriate. Nonverbal communication is important. The ICU is characterized by high levels of procedure-related touch and decreased affection-related or comfort-related touch. Patients have different levels of tolerance for being touched, possibly related to cultural background and personal history. It may be appropriate to provide comforting touch with ongoing evaluation of the patient's response.

Sensory-perceptual problems. Transient sensory-perceptual changes are common in ICU patients. Approximately 50% of patients treated in the ICU experience decreased orientation and impaired cognition.[3-5] The combination of changes in mentation (e.g., hallucinations, delusions) and behavior (e.g., shouting, hitting) has been called *ICU psychosis*. Patients with ICU psychosis or delirium may demonstrate confusion, irritability, and inappropriate behavior. Factors predisposing the patient to sensory-perceptual changes include sleep deprivation, anxiety, sensory overload, stress, and many drugs. Physical conditions such as hypoxemia and electrolyte disturbances can produce similar symptoms, including confusion and irritability. Potassium, calcium, and magnesium imbalances are common in the critically ill patient, and each can result in altered cognition.

The task of the ICU nurse is to identify predisposing factors, whether they be physiologic, psychologic, or environmental, and attempt to improve the patient's mental clarity and cooperation with therapy. The use of clocks and calendars may help the patient remain oriented. Although symptoms may be managed pharmacologically with a sedative, hypnotic, or a psychotropic (e.g., haloperidol [Haldol]) medication, these drugs may decrease the patient's ability to interact with family members. This may deprive patients and families of what may be the short and precious time remaining to discuss intimate and important issues.

Sensory overload can also result in patient distress and anxiety. Noise levels are particularly high in the ICU.[6] The "meaning" of a noise may determine its stressfulness. For example, meaningful noise is less stressful. The nurse can limit noise and assist the patient in understanding noises that cannot be prevented. Conversation is a particularly stressful noise, especially when the discussion concerns the patient and is conducted in the presence of, but without participation from, the patient. The nurse can restructure the environment to eliminate this source of stress by identifying better places for discussing the patient or by including the patient in the discussion. The nurse can also limit noise levels directly by muting phones, setting alarms appropriate to the patient's condition, and eliminating unnecessary alarms. For example, the nurse should silence the blood pressure alarms while balancing, calibrating, and flushing lines and reactivate the alarms when the procedures are complete. Similarly, ventilator alarms should be transiently silenced during endotracheal suctioning procedures. Overhead paging should be limited in patient care areas. Music should be played only if it comforts the patient.

Sleep problems. Nearly all ICU patients experience serious *sleep disturbances*.[7] Patients may have difficulty falling asleep or have disrupted sleep because of frequent monitoring or treatment procedures.[8,9] Drugs such as sedatives and hypnotics result in disturbed sleep patterns, including reductions in slow wave and rapid eye movement (REM) sleep. Sleep disturbance is a significant stressor in the ICU, contributing to impaired cognition and possibly affecting recovery. The ICU nurse can structure the environment to promote patient sleep. Strategies include clustering activities, scheduling rest, making physiologic measurements without changing the patient's position (when appropriate), limiting noise, and promoting comfort and relaxation.

Issues Related to Family Members

The experience of having a friend or family member in the ICU is physically and emotionally difficult. Families of the critically ill are usually anxious about the patient's condition and prognosis. They have concerns regarding the patient's pain and other discomforts. They may question the quality of care that the patient is receiving. In addition, it is common for families to experience anxiety regarding the financial issues related to planning and providing care in the next phases of the illness. The family will typically be experiencing disruption of their daily routines in order to support the patient. They may be far from their own home, routines, and supportive friends and family members. During these difficult times, they are often asked to make critical decisions.

Lack of information is a source of anxiety for families. The nurse should assess the family's understanding of the patient's status, goals, treatments, and prognosis and provide information as appropriate. The first time the family member visits it is important for the nurse to prepare the visitor for the experience by briefly describing the patient's appearance, condition, treatments, tubes, and equipment. Families should be told what to expect regarding the environment (sounds, noise, odors). It is helpful if the nurse can accompany the family members as they enter the room. They should be encouraged to touch, hug, and speak with the patient. Chairs should be provided whenever possible. The nurse should observe the responses of both patient and family to the visit. The patient may be fatigued by the visitors yet unwilling to ask them to leave. The visitors might have a difficult time dealing with a sick loved one and may need help and support. Rather than a rigid open or closed visiting policy, each patient should have a plan tailored to the patient's and family's needs.

The family needs information about the way in which the patient's care is managed and decisions are made. They should have the opportunity to affect decision making. The family should be invited to meet the health care team members, including physicians, dietitian, respiratory therapist, social worker, and physical therapist. The nurse should evaluate the appropriateness of including family members in multidisciplinary care conferences. Family members are able to enhance care by sharing information regarding the patient's preferences, skills, and deficits. It may help family members to accept and cope with problems if they observe that providers are caring and competent, that decisions are deliberate, and that they themselves have the opportunity to help shape the course of care.

The nurse should assess the family to determine the appropriate extent of their involvement in care. In some cases this might be limited to sitting with the patient and holding the patient's hand during quiet periods. Other family members might welcome the opportunity to participate in physical care such as shaving or oral hygiene. The nurse should encourage such activity. Other contributions include assisting with procedures, ambulation, and feeding. Family involvement should be included in the plan of care.

While working with families, the ICU nurse should assess the response of the family to the stress. Their feelings should be acknowledged and accepted. They should be supported in their decisions. Institutional support systems such as chaplains, social workers, and psychologists may be helpful in assisting the family and patient to adjust. The extent to which the family is involved and supported will in turn affect the patient's clinical course in the ICU.

RESEARCH

Implications for Nursing Practice

FAMILY VISITATION IN CRITICAL CARE UNITS

Citation Lazure LLA, Baun MM: Increasing patient control of family visiting in the coronary care unit, *Am J Crit Care* 4:157-164, 1995.

Purpose To determine if patient control of the timing of family visitation would minimize undesired psychophysiologic effects of coronary care unit (CCU) visiting.

Methods Study involved a two-group, repeated-measures experimental design. Subjects (n = 60) were randomly assigned to a control or experimental group. The experimental group used a visitor control device to communicate whether they wanted to restrict or allow visitation. Dependent variables were heart rate and rhythm, premature ventricular contractions, blood pressure, salivary cortisol, and finger temperature.

Results and Conclusions Repeated-measures analyses showed that over time perceived control of visits and rest between visits were greater, and heart rate and diastolic blood pressure were lower for the patients with the visitor control device. Based on positive comments, increased perceived control over visiting, and decreased blood pressure, the visitor control device was judged beneficial.

Implications for Nursing Practice The importance of control of visits by CCU patients should be acknowledged by family and staff members. Family and critical care nurses may show initial resistance in allowing the patient to exert control over visits but if incorporated into a consistent plan encompassing a variety of environmental concerns, use of such a device might be well received by all concerned.

HEMODYNAMIC MONITORING

Hemodynamic monitoring refers to measurement of pressure, flow, and oxygenation of blood within the cardiovascular system. Both invasive (internally placed devices) and noninvasive (external devices) measurements are made in the ICU. Values commonly measured include systemic and pulmonary arterial pressures, central venous pressure (CVP), pulmonary capillary wedge pressure (PCWP), cardiac output, and oxygen saturation of the hemoglobin of arterial and mixed venous blood. From these measurements the clinician calculates several values, including the resistance of the systemic and pulmonary arterial vasculature and oxygen content, delivery, and consumption. When these data are integrated with clinical assessment, the nurse can derive a detailed and accurate picture of the patient's problem and the effect of therapy. It is important that all measures be made with attention to technical aspects. False or inaccurate data are potentially misleading and thus dangerous.

Hemodynamic Terminology

Cardiac Output. Cardiac output is the volume of blood pumped by the heart in 1 minute. Although minor beat-to-beat changes may occur, generally the left and right ventricles pump the same volume. The volume pumped with each heartbeat is the *stroke volume*. Stroke volume times heart rate equals cardiac output. *Blood pressure,* the force exerted by blood on the vessel wall, is determined by cardiac output and the forces opposing blood flow. The opposition to blood flow offered by the vessels is called *systemic vascular resistance* or *pulmonary vascular resistance*. Stroke volume (and thus cardiac output and blood pressure) is determined by preload, afterload, and contractility (see Chapter 29). Understanding these concepts and relationships is essential for the ICU nurse. In addition, the nurse must understand the effects of manipulation of each of these variables. Normal values for hemodynamic variables are given in Table 61-2.

Preload. Preload is the pressure within a cardiac chamber at the end of diastole. Preload of the left ventricle is called *left ventricular end-diastolic pressure*. If there is no mitral valve regurgitation or stenosis, left atrial pressure is equivalent to left ventricular end-diastolic pressure. PCWP also reflects left ventricular end-diastolic pressure if there are no mitral valve problems. CVP, measured in the right atrium or in the vena cava close to the heart, is the right ventricular preload or *right ventricular end-diastolic pressure* when there is no tricuspid valve pathology. The effects of preload are based on tissue length. The greater the stretch of the heart muscle at the end of diastole, the greater the force of the next contraction. As preload increases, force generated in the following contraction increases, thus stroke volume and cardiac output increase. The greater the preload, the greater the chamber stretch and the greater the oxygen requirement of the myocardium. Hence, increases in cardiac output via increased preload require increased delivery of oxygen to cardiac tissue.

In the clinical setting myocardial fiber length cannot be measured, so pressure is measured as a reflection of length. However, the nurse should remember that the therapeutic effect of preload is related directly to cardiac tissue length (volume) and only indirectly to pressure.

Table 61-2 Hemodynamic Parameters at Rest

Indicators	Normal Range
Preload	
Right atrial pressure (RAP) or central venous pressure (CVP)	2-8 mm Hg
Pulmonary capillary wedge pressure (PCWP) or left atrial pressure (LAP)	6-12 mm Hg
Pulmonary artery diastolic pressure	4-12 mm Hg
Afterload	
Pulmonary vascular resistance (PVR) = (mean pulmonary artery pressure [PAP] − mean pulmonary capillary wedge pressure [PCWP]) × 80/cardiac output	<250 dyne sec/cm^5
Pulmonary vascular resistance index (PVRI) × 80 = pulmonary vascular resistance (PVR) × body surface area	160-380 dyne sec m^2/cm^5
Systemic vascular resistance (SVR) = (mean arterial pressure − central venous pressure) × 80/cardiac output	800-1200 dyne sec/cm^5
Systemic vascular resistance index (SVRI)=(systemic vascular resistance) × body surface area	1970-2390 dyne sec m^2/cm^5
Mean arterial pressure (MAP) = diastolic blood pressure + ⅓ pulse pressure	70-105 mm Hg
Mean pulmonary artery pressure (PAP) = pulmonary artery diastolic pressure + ⅓ pulmonary artery pulse pressure	10-20 mm Hg
Other	
Stroke volume = (cardiac output × 1000)/heart rate	60-180 ml/beat
Stroke volume index = (cardiac index × 1000)/heart rate	30-65 ml/beat/m^2
Heart rate	60-100 beats/min
Cardiac output = stroke volume × heart rate	4-8 L/min
Cardiac index = cardiac output/body surface area	2.2-4.0 L/min/m^2
Arterial hemoglobin oxygen saturation	92-99%
Mixed venous hemoglobin oxygen saturation	60-80%

Compliance. Compliance is the change in volume divided by the change in pressure. As the volume of the heart chamber increases and there is greater stretch on the muscle, compliance decreases. In a "stiff" noncompliant heart, small volume increments result in large increases in preload. Cardiac compliance decreases with scarring (e.g., following myocardial infarction). An aneurysm can produce increased compliance. Clinically, one cannot readily measure compliance. However, the nurse monitors the CVP and PCWP as indicators of preload. Compliance is low (i.e., the heart is stiff) if these measures increase dramatically following saline bolus administration.

Afterload. Afterload refers to the forces opposing ventricular ejection. The pressure in the aorta, the resistance offered by the aortic valve, and the mass and density of the blood to be moved contribute to afterload. Clinically, although the measures fail to include all the components of afterload, *systemic vascular resistance* and *arterial pressure* are indices of left ventricular afterload. Similarly, *pulmonary vascular resistance* and *pulmonary arterial pressure* are indices of right ventricular afterload. Increased afterload results in decreased cardiac output. Cardiac output can be increased by decreasing afterload (i.e., decreasing forces opposing contraction). When afterload is reduced, myocardial oxygen needs are decreased. Thus cardiac output is increased and myocardial oxygen requirements are decreased. Therapies directed at reducing afterload are used in the management of heart failure (see Chapter 32).

Contractility. Contractility describes the strength of contraction. Increased contractility occurs when preload is not changed, yet the heart contracts more forcefully. Contractility is increased by epinephrine, norepinephrine, isoproterenol, dopamine, dobutamine, digitalis-like drugs, amrinone, and milrinone. These agents are called *positive inotropes*. Contractility is diminished by *negative inotropes*, such as acidosis and certain drugs (e.g., barbiturates, alcohol, procainamide, calcium channel blockers, β-blockers). Increased contractility results in increased stroke volume and increased myocardial oxygen requirements. There are no direct clinical measures of cardiac contractility. To indirectly determine contractility, the ICU nurse measures the patient's preload (PCWP) and cardiac output and graphs the results. If preload, heart rate, and afterload have remained constant, yet cardiac output changes, contractility is altered. Contractility is diminished in the failing heart.

Vascular Resistance. *Systemic vascular resistance* (SVR) is the resistance of the systemic vascular bed. *Pulmonary vascular resistance* (PVR) is the resistance of the pulmonary vascular bed. SVR and PVR are calculated as indicated in Table 61-2.

Principles of Invasive Pressure Monitoring

Invasive lines are commonly used in the ICU to measure systemic and pulmonary blood pressures. Components of a typical invasive arterial pressure monitoring system are illustrated in Fig. 61-2. Catheter, pressure tubing, flush system, and usually the transducer are disposable.

To accurately measure pressure, equipment must be balanced, calibrated, and tested for signal distortion. These procedures are performed routinely every 4 hours and each time a major component in the monitoring system is changed, the recording system is moved, or unusual readings are obtained. *Balancing* establishes an accurate zero reference so that when pressure within the system is zero, the equipment reads zero. The port of the stopcock nearest the transducer is usually the zero reference for the transducer. *Calibrating* ensures that applied pressures are accurately read.

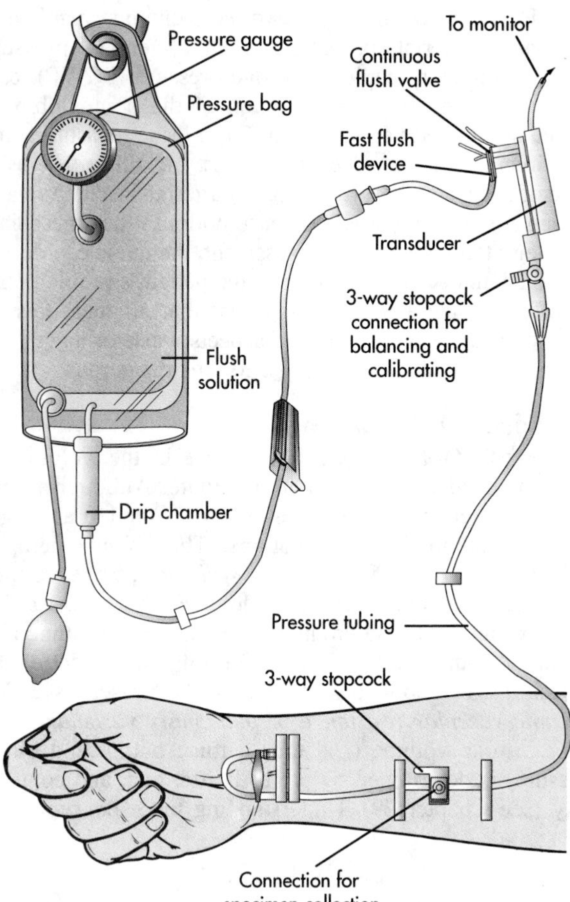

Fig. 61-2 Components of a pressure monitoring system. The cannula, shown entering the radial artery, is connected via pressure (nondistensible) tubing to the transducer. The transducer converts the pressure wave into an electronic signal. The transducer is wired to the electronic monitoring system, which amplifies, conditions, displays, and records the signal. Stopcocks are inserted into the line for specimen withdrawal and for balancing and calibrating procedures. A flush system, consisting of a pressurized bag of intravenous fluid, tubing, and a flush device is inserted into the line. The flush system provides continuous slow (1 to 3 ml hourly) flushing, and provides a mechanism for fast flushing of lines. All items except the electronic monitoring system are commonly disposable equipment.

To read pressures accurately the zero reference for the transducer is placed level with the left atrium. The position of the left atrium is determined through the use of an

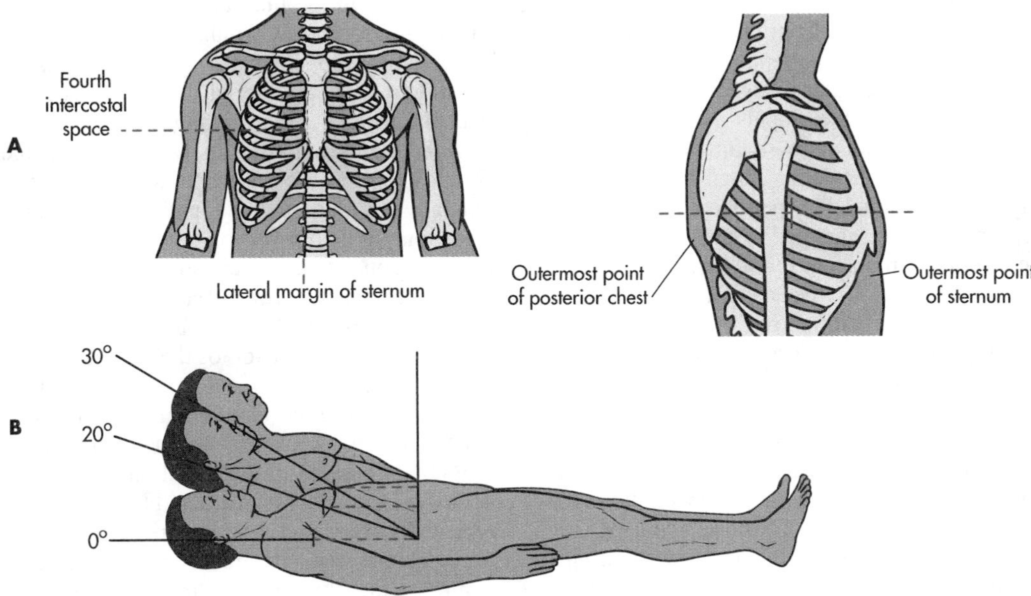

Fig. 61-3 Identification of the phlebostatic axis. ***A,*** The phlebostatic axis is an external landmark used to identify the level of the left atrium in the supine patient. The phlebostatic axis is defined as the intersection of a plane drawn transversely through the fourth intercostal space at the sternum and a frontal plane drawn through the mid chest, halfway between the outermost anterior and outermost posterior points of the chest. ***B,*** As the backrest of the supine patient is elevated, the phlebostatic axis remains at the same anatomic location, becoming progressively elevated from the floor. The zero-reference point must be repositioned with changes in backrest elevation, in order to keep it at the phlebostatic level.

external landmark, the *phlebostatic axis*. To identify the *phlebostatic axis*, two imaginary planes are drawn with the patient supine (see Fig. 61-3). One plane is midchest, halfway between the outermost anterior and posterior surfaces. The second plane is transverse through the fourth intercostal space at the sternum. The phlebostatic axis is the intersection of the two planes. Once the phlebostatic axis is identified, it is marked on the patient's chest with a permanent marker. The port of the stopcock nearest the transducer is positioned level with the phlebostatic axis.

Steps in measuring pressure with an invasive line are given in Table 61-3. Pressure measurements can be obtained from both digital and printed analog outputs. However, pressures are most accurately read from a printed pressure tracing at the end-expiration point. Initial readings are made with the patient flat. Unless the patient's blood pressure is extremely sensitive to orthostatic change, values at modest degrees of backrest elevation (up to 30°) are generally equivalent to measurements with the patient flat. After confirming that values are similar whether the patient is flat or slightly elevated, subsequent measurements can be made with the backrest slightly elevated. Thus it is not necessary to reposition the patient for each pressure reading. However, it is necessary to move the zero reference stopcock to keep it positioned at the phlebostatic axis. It is difficult to identify consistent landmarks for the left atrium when the patient is lying on the side; thus it is difficult to measure pressures accurately in side-lying positions.

Table 61-3 Measurement of Blood Pressure with Invasive Lines

1. Explain the procedure to the patient.
2. Inactivate the high-pressure and low-pressure alarms for the duration of the procedure.
3. Identify and mark the phlebostatic axis on the patient's chest (mid–anterior-posterior chest at the fourth intercostal space [see Fig. 61-3]).
4. Position the patient supine and flat, or if appropriate, elevated up to 30°.
5. Confirm that the system has been appropriately balanced and calibrated within 4 hr of the measurement and following all equipment changes.
6. Confirm that the zero reference (port of the stopcock nearest the transducer) is placed at the level of the phlebostatic axis. It may be helpful to use a carpenter's level.
7. Observe the monitor trace and assess the quality of the trace.
8. Obtain an analog printout, if available, and measure the pressures of interest at end expiration. If no printout is available, freeze the trace on the oscilloscope screen and use the cursor to measure the pressures at end expiration.
9. Reset the high-pressure and low-pressure alarms.
10. Record the pressure measurements promptly, including (if available) the printout marked to identify the points read.

Types of Invasive Pressure Monitoring

Arterial Blood Pressure. Continuous arterial pressure monitoring is indicated for patients experiencing hypotension or increased intracranial pressure, receiving vasoactive drugs (e.g., nitroprusside, dopamine), or requiring frequent arterial blood sampling (e.g., for arterial blood gases [ABGs]). A 20-gauge, 1.5-inch (3.8-cm) plastic catheter is typically used to cannulate a peripheral artery such as the radial, brachial, dorsalis pedis, or femoral. The catheter can be inserted percutaneously or via cutdown. It is important that the insertion site be stabilized by an arm board so that the line is not being moved.

Measurements. The nurse can use the arterial line to obtain accurate systolic, diastolic, and mean blood pressure (see Fig. 61-4). The arterial waveform provides useful information. In heart failure, the systolic upstroke is slower. In volume depletion, systolic pressure varies greatly with mechanical ventilation, diminishing during inspiration. In severe congestive heart failure, systolic amplitude does not vary with ventilation. With dysrhythmias it is useful to observe simultaneous ECG and pressure tracings. Dysrhythmias that significantly diminish arterial pressure are more urgent than those that cause only a slight decrease in systolic amplitude.

Complications. Arterial lines carry the risk of hemorrhage, infection, thrombus formation, and distal circulatory occlusion. *Hemorrhage* is most likely to occur when the catheter becomes dislodged or the line becomes disconnected. To avoid this serious complication, the nurse twists a luer-lock and tapes all connections and always activates (and records activation of) the low-pressure alarm. Thus, if the pressure in the line falls (as it usually would when the line is disconnected), an alarm sounds immediately, allowing prompt repair of the problem. Pressure is always monitored when an arterial line is in place, even if the line was placed for ABG sampling.

Infection is a risk with any invasive line. The nurse should inspect the insertion site for inflammation and exudate and monitor the patient for signs of systemic infection. When infection occurs, the catheter, tubing, flushing apparatus, and transducers must be changed.

Circulatory impairment can result from formation of a thrombus around the catheter, release of an embolus, spasm, or from occlusion of the circulation by the catheter. Before inserting a line into the radial artery, it must be confirmed that ulnar circulation is sufficient to sustain the hand. This is checked with the *Allen test.* In this test, pressure is applied to the radial and ulnar arteries simultaneously. The patient is instructed to open and close the hand repeatedly. The hand should blanch. The nurse then releases the pressure over the radial artery while continuing to compress the ulnar artery. Pinkness should return within 6 seconds. The procedure is repeated, releasing the ulnar artery while compressing the radial artery. If pinkness fails to return within 6 seconds, the ulnar artery is insufficient, indicating that the radial artery should not be used for line insertion. The nurse should evaluate the circulation distal to the arterial insertion site at least hourly. The limb with compromised arterial flow will appear cool and pale, with capillary refill greater than 3 seconds. There may be symptoms of neurologic impairment, such as tingling or paresthesia. Circulatory impairment can result in loss of a

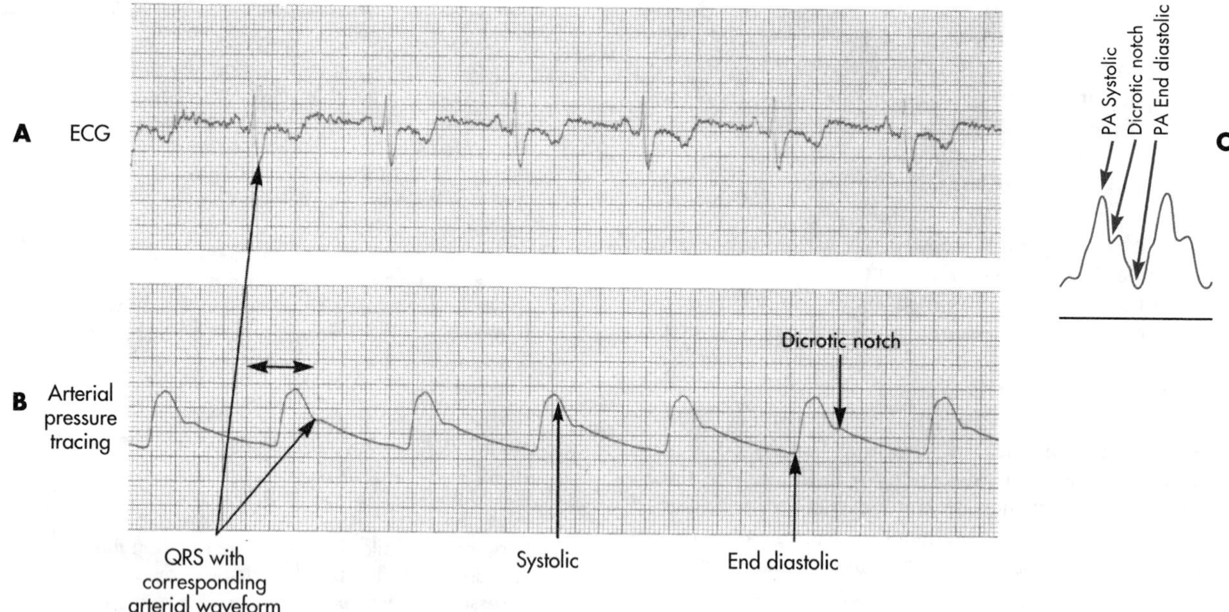

Fig. 61-4 ***A,*** Simultaneously recorded electrocardiogram (ECG) tracing, and ***B,*** typical arterial pressure trace. ***C,*** Systolic pressure is the peak value. Ventricular relaxation (diastole) begins with a slow descent in pressure. The dicrotic notch indicates aortic valve closure. Diastolic pressure is the lowest value before contraction. Mean pressure is the average pressure over time calculated by the equipment (see Table 61-2). *PA,* Pulmonary artery.

limb and is an emergency. The nurse routinely (every hour) monitors circulation distal to arterial lines and maintains continuous irrigation of lines via the flush system.

Pulmonary Artery Flow-Directed Catheter. Pulmonary artery (PA) pressure monitoring is used to guide acute phase management in patients with complicated cardiac and intravascular volume problems (Table 61-4). PA diastolic (PAD) pressure and PCWP are sensitive indicators of fluid volume status. PAD pressure and PCWP increase in fluid volume overload and decrease with volume deficit. Fluid therapy based on PA pressure allows restoration of fluid balance while avoiding overcorrection of the problem. Monitoring PA pressures can allow precise therapeutic manipulation of preload, which allows cardiac output to be maintained without placing the patient at risk for pulmonary edema. PA pressure monitoring is common in ICUs.

A PA flow-directed catheter (e.g., Swan-Ganz) is used to measure PA pressures, including PCWP. The standard PA catheter is No. 7 French, 43 inches (110 cm) long, with four lumina (Fig. 61-5). When properly positioned, the distal lumen is within the pulmonary artery (Fig. 61-6). This lumen is used to monitor PA pressures, withdraw mixed venous blood specimens (e.g., to evaluate oxygen saturation), and deliver fluids. The distal lumen is surrounded by a balloon connected to an external valve via a second lumen. Balloon inflation has two purposes: to allow moving blood to float the catheter forward and to allow PCWP measurement. The third and fourth lumina are proximal, with exit ports in the right atrium. These are used for measurement of CVP, infusion of fluid and drugs, injection of fluid for cardiac output determination, and withdrawal of blood specimens. The larger of the two proximal lumina is used for blood specimen collection. Often, when the patient is receiving total parenteral nutrition, the smaller proximal lumen is reserved for that infusion and is not interrupted for blood testing or injections. A thermistor located near the distal tip is wired to an external connector. The thermistor allows monitoring of core temperature and is used in the thermodilution method of measuring cardiac output.

In addition to these relatively standard and common features of the PA flow-directed catheter, modifications include an atrial electrode, useful in recording the atrial ECG or pacing the heart. The distal tip is often equipped

Table 61-4 Clinical Indications for Pulmonary Artery Catheterization

- Acute respiratory distress syndrome
- Acute respiratory failure in patients with chronic obstructive pulmonary disease
- Cardiac tamponade
- Cardiogenic or noncardiogenic pulmonary edema
- Complex fluid imbalance (burns, sepsis)
- Evaluation of circulatory syndromes (mitral valve regurgitation and intraventricular shunts)
- Intraaortic balloon support
- Myocardial infarction with left ventricular failure or cardiogenic shock
- Perioperative fluid imbalance in high-risk patients
- Septic and hypovolemic shock
- Vasoactive pharmacologic support

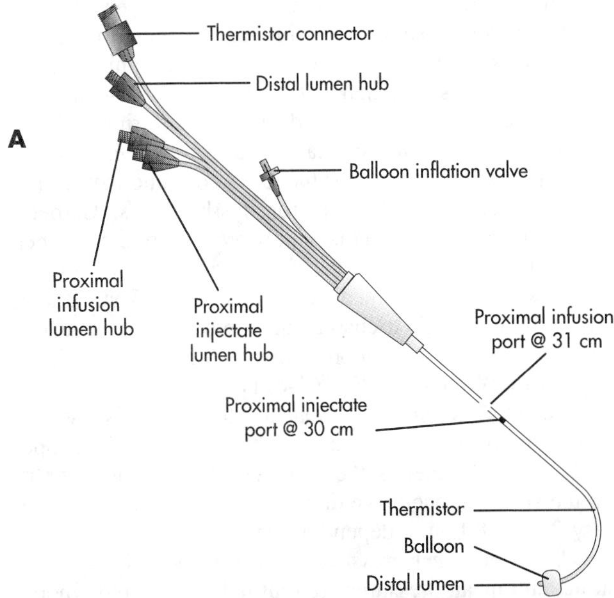

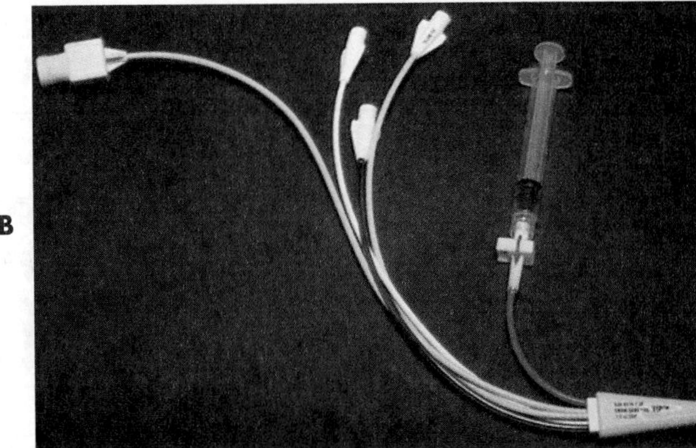

Fig. 61-5 Venous infusion port pulmonary artery (PA) catheter. ***A,*** The illustrated catheter has 4 lumina. When properly positioned, the distal lumen exit port is in the PA and the proximal lumina ports are in the right atrium. The distal and one of the proximal ports are used to measure PA and central venous pressures, respectively. A balloon surrounds the catheter near the distal end. The balloon inflation valve is used to inflate the balloon with air for up to 4 respiratory cycles to allow reading of the pulmonary capillary wedge pressure. A thermistor located near the distal tip senses PA temperature and is used to measure thermodilution cardiac output when solution cooler than body temperature is injected into a proximal port. ***B,*** Actual catheter.

with a fiberoptic sensor to detect mixed venous oxygen saturation. Another type of catheter provides continuous measurement of right ventricular volume and ejection fraction. A fifth lumen, the venous infusion port, is useful to administer intravenous fluids.

Pulmonary artery catheter insertion. The PA catheter is inserted into a deep peripheral vein using surgical asepsis. Although a cutdown may be necessary, percutaneous insertion is more common. Internal or external jugular, subclavian, antecubital, or femoral veins are acceptable insertion sites. Before catheter insertion, the nurse notes the patient's electrolyte, acid-base, oxygenation, and coagulation status. Imbalances such as hypokalemia, hypomagnesemia, hypoxemia, or acidosis can make the heart more irritable and increase the risk of ventricular dysrhythmia during catheter insertion. Coagulopathy increases the risk of hemorrhage.

It is necessary to monitor the ECG continuously during insertion because of the risk for dysrhythmias. Catheter insertion is guided by the distal port pressure tracing. When the distal tip is placed in the right atrium, the balloon is inflated with the recommended volume of air. The catheter is floated through the tricuspid valve into the right ventricle and then through the pulmonic valve and into the PA. Once a typical PCWP tracing (Fig. 61-6) is observed, the balloon is deflated. Following insertion, a chest x-ray is used to confirm the position. To maintain the catheter in its proper position, the catheter is then sutured at its point of entry into the skin. An occlusive dressing is applied and changed every 24 to 48 hours, depending on unit protocol.

Pulmonary artery pressure measurements. Systolic, diastolic, and mean pressures are routinely monitored when a PA line is in place. PA systolic is the peak pressure and PA diastolic is the lowest pressure point. Mean PA pressure is the time-weighted average. Because PA ports are in the chest, intrathoracic pressures alter PA pressure. To produce consistent data, PA measurements are obtained at end expiration.

The measurement of PCWP is obtained by slowly inflating the balloon with air up to the prescribed maximum volume while observing the distal lumen pressure tracing. When the tracing changes from arterial to atrial, the catheter is said to be "wedged" and PCWP is measured (see Fig. 61-6). The balloon should be inflated for less than four respiratory cycles. As with other hemodynamic pressures, PCWP varies with ventilation and is read at the end-expiration point. If possible, readings should be acquired from an analog strip pressure recording, and the strip should be placed into the patient's record.

Central venous pressure measurement. CVP is a measurement of right ventricular preload. It can be measured with a PA catheter using one of the proximal lumen. Occasionally a CVP line may be placed. CVP is measured as a mean pressure at end expiration. Although the PA diastolic pressure and PCWP are more sensitive indicators of fluid volume status, CVP also reflects fluid volume problems. CVP provides information regarding right ventricular function.

Thermodilution cardiac output measurement. Cardiac output is frequently monitored in patients with hemodynamic instability. The PA catheter is commonly used to measure cardiac output via thermodilution technique. Normal resting cardiac output is 4 to 8 L per minute and varies with body size. *Cardiac index* is cardiac output divided by body surface area. Cardiac index can be compared among

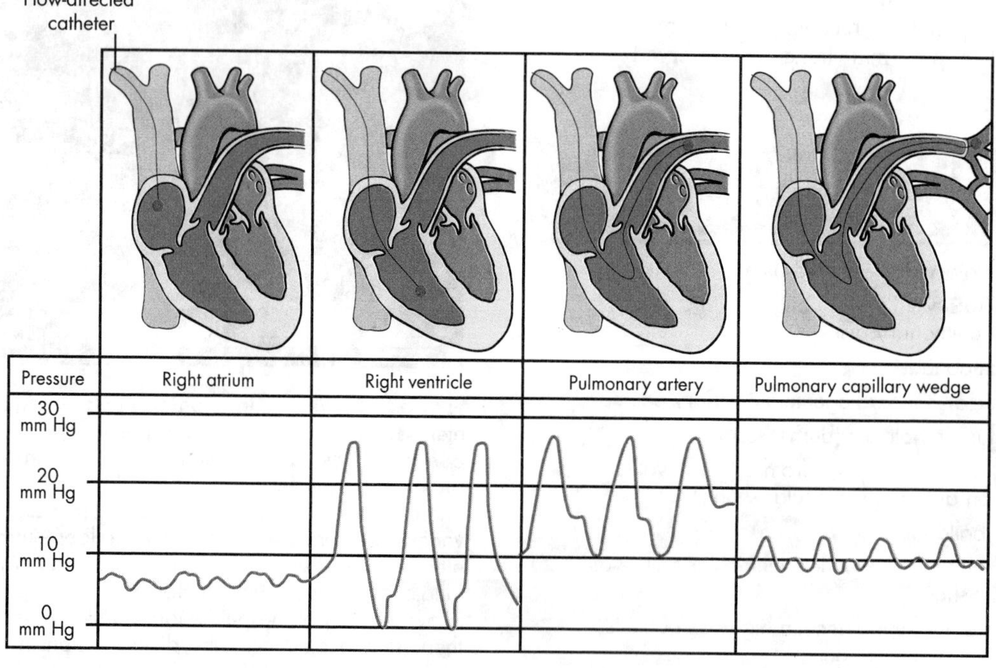

Fig. 61-6 Position of the pulmonary artery flow directed catheter during progressive stages of insertion with corresponding pressure waveforms.

individuals of varying body sizes. The normal cardiac index is 2.2 to 4.0 L per min/m^2. The cardiac output is decreased in conditions such as hemorrhagic or cardiogenic shock and heart failure. Under normal conditions, cardiac output increases with exercise. Increases in cardiac output at rest may indicate fever or sepsis.

SVR can be calculated each time cardiac output is measured. The formula for calculating SVR is shown in Table 61-2. Normal SVR is 800 to 1200 dynes/sec/cm^{-5}. Increased SVR may indicate the presence of fever, shock, stress (e.g., increased release or administration of epinephrine or norepinephrine), or left ventricular failure. A low SVR (less than 600 dynes/sec/cm^{-5}) may occur during sepsis, septic shock, neurogenic shock, or with drugs that reduce afterload.

***Mixed venous oxygen saturation* (SvO_2).** PA catheters can include sensors to measure oxygen saturation of hemoglobin of PA blood (termed mixed venous blood). This value (SvO_2), when considered in conjunction with the arterial oxygen saturation, is useful in analyzing hemodynamic status and response to treatments or activities (Table 61-5). Normal SvO_2 at rest is 60% to 80%. Sustained increases and decreases in SvO_2 must be analyzed carefully. Decreased SvO_2 may indicate decreased arterial oxygenation. If arterial oxygenation as measured by pulse oximetry or ABG analysis is unchanged, decreased SvO_2 indicates a change in the balance between oxygen supply and tissue demand. Oxygen consumption may have increased (e.g., increased metabolic rate or exercise) without a comparable increase in cardiac output, causing more oxygen to be extracted from blood. Another possibility is that cardiac output has diminished while oxygen consumption has remained constant. Increased SvO_2 may also indicate a clinical change (e.g., improved arterial saturation) or problems (e.g., sepsis). In sepsis cardiac output increases greatly. The same amount of oxygen might be consumed by the body or perhaps slightly more as temperature and metabolic rate increase. However, the increase in the cardiac output is larger, resulting in increased mixed venous oxygen saturation. The nurse might note that the patient's heart rate increased moderately during ambulation to a chair but that the SvO_2 remained stable. In this case the nurse might conclude that the position change was tolerated and continue to monitor the patient during activity progression. If the heart rate increased and the SvO_2 fell, the nurse would conclude that the activity was not well tolerated.

In many cases as activity or metabolism increases, heart rate and cardiac output increase and SvO_2 remains constant.

Table 61-5 Clinical Interpretation of SvO_2 Measurements

SvO_2 Measurement	Physiologic Basis for Change in SvO_2	Clinical Diagnosis and Rationale
High SvO_2 (80-95%)	Increased oxygen supply	Patient receiving more oxygen than required by clinical condition
	Decreased oxygen demand	Anesthesia, which causes sedation and decreased muscle movement
		Hypothermia, which lowers metabolic demand (e.g., with cardiopulmonary bypass)
		Sepsis caused by decreased ability of tissues to use oxygen at a cellular level and increased cardiac output
		False high-positive because pulmonary artery catheter is wedged in a pulmonary capillary
Normal SvO_2 (60-80%)	Normal oxygen supply and metabolic demand	Balanced oxygen supply and demand
Low SvO_2 (<60%)	Decreased oxygen supply caused by	
	Low hemoglobin (Hb)	Anemia or bleeding with compromised cardiopulmonary system
	Low arterial saturation (SaO_2)	Hypoxemia resulting from decreased oxygen supply or lung disease
	Low cardiac output	Cardiogenic shock caused by left ventricular pump failure
	Increased oxygen consumption	Metabolic demand exceeds oxygen supply in conditions that increase muscle movement and increase metabolic rate, including such physiologic states as shivering, exercise, seizures, and hyperthermia and such nursing interventions as obtaining bed-scale weight and turning

From Thelan LA and others, editors: *Critical care nursing: diagnosis and management,* ed 2, St Louis, 1994, Mosby.

In this case, heart rate and cardiac output are more sensitive clinical indicators of patient status. However, it is not uncommon for critically ill patients to have conditions that prevent substantial increases in cardiac output. For example, this could occur in the patient with heart failure, preexisting tachycardia, complete heart block, or cardiac transplantation. In these cases, SvO_2 can provide a useful indicator of the balance between oxygen consumption and perfusion.

Complications with pulmonary artery catheters. Like arterial lines, PA lines are associated with an increased risk of *thrombus* and *embolus* formation. Lines are continuously flushed to prevent thrombus formation. If a thrombus begins to form, the waveform appears blunted or the pressures drift.

Infection and *sepsis* are serious problems associated with PA lines. Careful surgical asepsis for insertion and maintenance of the line is mandatory to prevent infection. The skin is cleaned according to unit procedure, usually with an iodine preparation. Lines are covered with an occlusive dressing. The nurse should monitor the patient for local and systemic signs of infection (e.g., redness and exudate at site, fever, increased WBC count). The line should be removed if there are local or systemic signs of infection. To reduce the risk of infection, PA catheters should not be left in place any longer than necessary.

Air embolus caused by balloon rupture is another risk associated with PA catheters. The nurse decreases this risk by never injecting more than the recommended volume of air. Because the catheter lumens are in the chest, line disconnection could cause life-threatening air embolization. The negative pressure generated within the chest during inspiration is transmitted through the PA line, and there is an increased risk for air to be sucked into the catheter.

Several factors put the patient with a PA catheter at risk for *pulmonary infarction*, including the following: (1) the balloon may rupture, releasing fragments that could embolize; (2) balloon inflation may obstruct blood flow; (3) the catheter may advance into a wedge position, obstructing blood flow; and (4) a thrombus could embolize. To reduce the risk of pulmonary infarction, the balloon must never be left inflated for more than four breaths once it has been positioned. PA pressure waveforms are monitored continuously for early indications of catheter occlusion and dislocation. If the PA catheter advances and becomes lodged in the smaller vessels, the waveform appearance changes from arterial (i.e., with a systolic peak, dicrotic notch, and diastolic descent) to atrial (i.e., lower amplitude and with a, c, and v waves reflecting left atrial pressure).

Ventricular *dysrhythmias* can occur during PA catheter insertion or removal or if the tip migrates back from the PA to the right ventricle. The catheter should be repositioned, usually by the physician.

Noninvasive Arterial Oxygenation Monitoring. A noninvasive and continuous method of determining arterial oxygenation is *pulse oximetry*. The principle underlying pulse oximetry is that the absorption of light differs between oxyhemoglobin and reduced hemoglobin (deoxyhemoglobin). Arterial hemoglobin is normally 95% to 100% saturated with oxygen. As hemoglobin binds oxygen, its color changes. This change in color is detected by the oximetry probe. To decrease the interference of other tissues that may absorb light, the probe is usually placed on the earlobe or finger. However, improved technology has allowed for greater flexibility with respect to probe placement.

A common use for pulse oximetry is the determination of the effectiveness of oxygen therapy. By continuously monitoring arterial oxygenation, there is less need for ABG sampling. A decreased arterial saturation indicates inadequate oxygenation of the blood in the lung, which may be corrected by increasing the fraction of inspired oxygen. Continuous monitoring of oxygenation is also useful to the nurse. The nurse can monitor effects of activities, changes in position, and treatments. For example, the nurse might note that arterial saturation falls when the patient is positioned in a left lateral recumbent position. The nurse could then plan position changes that pose less risk for the patient.

The nurse should remember that both the PA oximeter and the pulse oximeter have been proven accurate in the normal, healthy, young individual. Accuracy in the patient with hypotension, anemia, and peripheral vasoconstriction is not proven.

NURSING MANAGEMENT

HEMODYNAMIC MONITORING

Assessment of hemodynamic status requires integration of data from many sources and comparison of the data over time. Observations begin with the patient's general appearance. Does the patient appear weak, tired, exhausted? There may be too little cardiac reserve to sustain minimum activity. Changing skin color or temperature may indicate diminished cardiac output. If shock is developing, blood pressure and even heart rate might be relatively stable, yet the patient may become increasingly pale and cool because of vasoconstriction of the peripheral circulation. The nurse can confirm suspicion of impending shock by noting the SVR, which would increase in these circumstances. Conversely, the patient may remain warm and pink yet develop tachycardia and blood pressure instability. These features are characteristic of septic shock. The suspicion can be confirmed with measurements of cardiac output, which would increase with septic shock, and of SVR, which would progressively decrease.

The heart rate is often a useful indicator of the hemodynamic state. As tissue perfusion becomes compromised, heart rate increases. Although heart rates of 100 beats per minute are common among stressed, compromised, critically ill patients, further increases in heart rate may herald compromised perfusion. In patients in whom heart rate cannot increase, such as those with atrioventricular block, the SvO_2 can be a useful indicator of impending compromise.

In addition to high-technology measurements available to the ICU nurse, simple observations may provide useful insights into the patient's hemodynamic status. Mental clarity reflects cerebral perfusion. Urine output reflects renal perfusion. The patient with diminished gastrointestinal perfusion may develop hypoactive or absent bowel sounds and may have nausea and vomiting when gastrointestinal motility is impaired by a lack of perfusion. By carefully monitoring the patient, the astute nurse is able to recognize early cues and manage problems before they escalate.

CIRCULATORY ASSIST DEVICES

Mechanical circulatory support devices, including the intraaortic balloon pump (IABP) and left ventricular assist devices (VADs), have been used to stabilize and maintain patients with heart failure. The type of device used depends on the extent and nature of the myocardial problem and the capabilities of the institution and staff. Circulatory assist devices are used to support the patient for a period of time in three types of situations: (1) the left ventricle requires time to recover from acute injury; (2) the heart requires surgical repair (e.g., a ruptured septum) and time is needed to stabilize the patient and prepare for the procedure; and (3) the patient in end-stage heart failure awaits cardiac transplantation. All circulatory support devices decrease left ventricular workload, increase myocardial perfusion, and augment circulation. Because the most commonly used device is the IABP and thus most ICU nurses encounter patients receiving IABP support, this device is described in this chapter. Several types of VADs are available, and additional devices are under development. VADs are discussed in Chapter 32.

Intraaortic Balloon Pump

The IABP provides temporary circulatory assistance to the compromised heart by reducing afterload (via reduction in systolic pressure) and augmenting the aortic diastolic pressure. Table 61-6 lists clinical conditions for which the IABP is used. The IABP consists of a sausage-shaped balloon, a pump that inflates and deflates the balloon, control devices for synchronizing the balloon inflation to cardiac contraction, and fail-safe devices (Figs. 61-7, 61-8). The balloon is inserted percutaneously or surgically into the femoral artery, advanced toward the heart, and positioned in the descending thoracic aorta just below the left subclavian artery, but above the renal arteries. A pneumatic device cyclically fills the balloon with helium during diastole and deflates it during systole. The ECG is used to trigger deflation on the R wave and inflation on the T wave. The arterial wave is used to refine timing so that inflation occurs at the arterial dicrotic notch and deflation occurs just before systole. IABP support is referred to as *counterpulsation* because the timing of balloon inflation is opposite ventricular contraction.

Effects of Counterpulsation. The balloon is rapidly inflated at the start of diastole, immediately after aortic valve closure, partially occluding the aorta. Displaced blood is forced forward into the extremities and back into the coronary arteries and main branches of the aortic arch. Diastolic arterial pressure rises (diastolic augmentation), increasing perfusion of vital organs and coronary artery perfusion pressure. The rise in coronary artery perfusion pressure usually causes an increase in blood flow to the myocardium and may increase development of coronary artery collateral circulation. The balloon is rapidly deflated just before systole. The suddenly created vacuum causes aortic pressure to drop. With aortic resistance to left ventricular ejection reduced (reduced afterload), the left ventricle empties more easily and completely. As with other types of afterload reduction, the stroke volume increases, yet the myocardial oxygen consumption decreases. Hemodynamic effects of the IABP are summarized in Table 61-7.

Table 61-6 Indications and Contraindications for the Intraaortic Balloon Pump

Indications
- Preinfarction, accelerating, or crescendo angina (when conventional modes of therapy, such as bed rest, nitrates, β-blockers, and calcium channel blockers have failed)
- Severe cardiac disease (when undergoing cardiac catheterization or noncardiac surgery)
- Acute myocardial infarction with any of the following:*
  - Ventricular aneurysm accompanied by ventricular dysrhythmias
  - Acute ventricular septal defect
  - Acute mitral valve regurgitation
  - Cardiogenic shock
  - Continuing chest pain
- Preoperative, intraoperative, and postoperative open heart surgery (e.g., aneurysectomy, revascularization, or valve replacement); often used to wean from cardiopulmonary bypass
- Cardiogenic shock

Contraindications
- Irreversible brain damage
- Terminal or untreatable diseases of any major organ system
- Ruptured or dissecting aortic or thoracic aneurysm
- Generalized peripheral vascular disease (may prevent placement of balloon)
- Insufficient aortic valve (considered an *absolute* contraindication)

*Allows time for emergency angiography and corrective cardiac surgery to be performed.

Complications with Intraaortic Balloon Pumps. Complications are common with the IABP. Patients receiving an IABP are prone to infections. Insertion site infection or sepsis caused by an unknown source necessitates catheter removal. Vascular injuries such as dislodging of plaque, arterial dissection, and compromised distal extremity circulation are common, with an incidence reported as high as 10% to 35%.[10-12] Thrombus and embolus formation add to the risk of distal circulation compromise. Peripheral nerve damage can occur, particularly when a cutdown is performed for insertion. To reduce these risks, hourly neurovascular assessment is necessary. Because the balloon pumping can cause physical destruction of platelets, thrombocytopenia is common and coagulation status indicators must be monitored. Displacement of the balloon can occlude the left subclavian, renal, or mesenteric arteries.

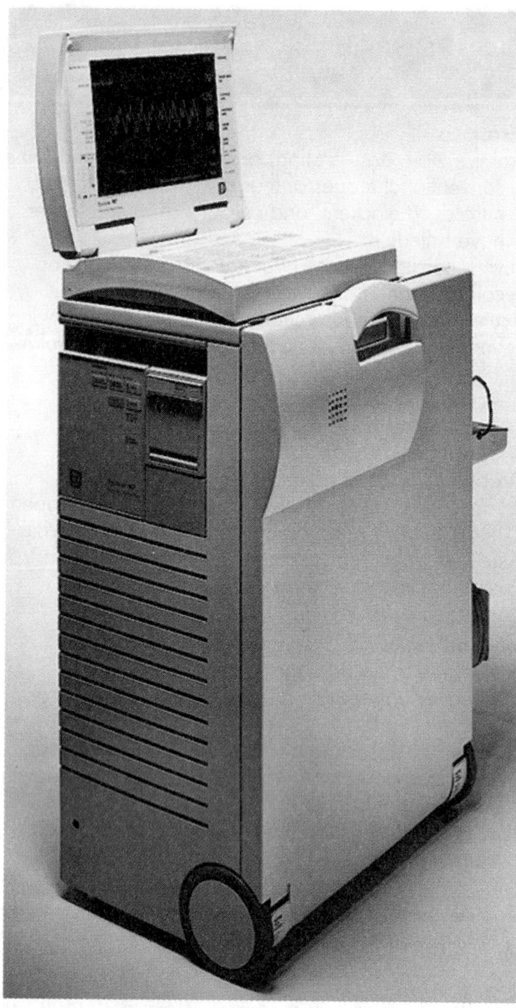

Fig. 61-7 Intraaortic balloon pump machine.

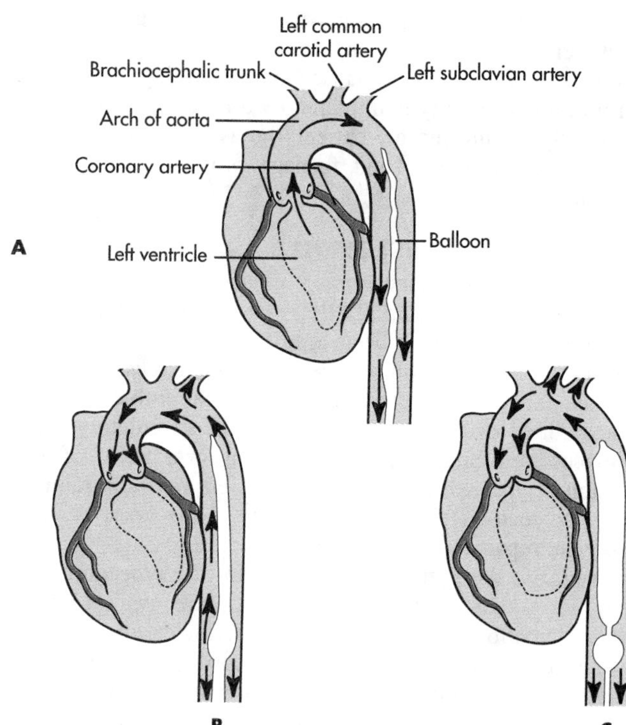

Fig. 61-8 ***A,*** During systole the balloon is deflated, which facilitates ejection of the blood into the periphery where systemic arterial resistant vessels are perfused. ***B,*** In early diastole, the balloon begins to inflate. ***C,*** In late diastole, the balloon is totally inflated, which augments aortic pressure and increases the coronary perfusion pressure with the end results of increased coronary and cerebral blood flow.

Mechanical complications are rare but may occur. Improper timing of balloon inflation may occur and is generally corrected by the nurse according to unit protocol. If the balloon develops a leak, the catheter must be changed immediately to avoid a gas embolus. Signs of a leak include less effective augmentation and blood backing up into the catheter. A malfunction of the balloon or console triggers fail-safe alarms and automatic unit shutdown.

The patient with an IABP is relatively immobile, limited to side-lying or supine positions with the head of the bed elevated no more than 15 degrees. The leg in which the catheter is inserted must not be flexed at the hip. The patient may be receiving ventilatory support and will likely have multiple invasive lines that increase the challenge of comfortable positioning. Skin care and comfort measures are required.

As the patient improves, the patient is "weaned" from IABP; that is, circulatory support provided by the IABP is gradually reduced. Weaning involves moving balloon inflation later into diastole or reducing the pumping to every second or third beat until the IABP cannula is removed. Even if the patient is stable without IABP, pumping is usually continued every third or fourth beat until the line is removed. This reduces the risk of thrombus formation around the catheter. Detailed, frequent hemodynamic assessment continues to be required during the weaning phase.

NURSING MANAGEMENT

INTRAAORTIC BALLOON PUMP

Initiating, maintaining, and terminating the IABP require highly skilled nurses. Detailed cardiovascular assessment, including measurement of vital signs, hemodynamic pressures, cardiac output, cardiac auscultation, and cardiac rhythm evaluation, is performed every 10 to 60 minutes. Assessments of myocardial ischemia (indicated by T-wave inversion, ST segment changes), chest pain, skin color and temperature, mentation, urine output, and bowel sounds are also performed at regular intervals. It is expected that with continuing IABP treatment these parameters should improve. X-ray confirmation of tube placement should be performed before balloon inflation. Nursing management of IABP complications is covered in Table 61-8.

Table 61-7 Hemodynamic Effects of Intraaortic Balloon Pumps

Effects of Inflation During Diastole
- Increased diastolic pressure (may exceed systolic pressure)
- Increased pressure in the aortic root during diastole
- Increased coronary perfusion pressure
- Improved oxygen delivery to the myocardium
  - Decreased angina pain
  - Decreased ECG evidence of ischemia
  - Decreased ventricular ectopy

Effects of Deflation During Systole
- Decreased afterload
- Decreased peak systolic pressure
- Decreased myocardial oxygen consumption
- Increased stroke volume, possibly associated with
  - Improved sensorium
  - Warmed skin
  - Increased urine output
  - Decreased heart rate
- Increased forward flow of blood, decreasing preload
  - Decreased PA pressures, including PCWP
  - Decreased crackles

ECG, Electrocardiogram; *PA,* pulmonary artery; *PCWP,* pulmonary capillary wedge pressure.

ARTIFICIAL AIRWAYS*

The patient in the ICU often requires mechanical assistance to maintain airway patency. An artificial airway is created by inserting a tube into the trachea, bypassing upper airway and laryngeal structures. *Intubation* is the process of tube insertion, and *extubation* is the process of tube removal. A patient with an endotracheal tube in place is said to be "intubated." Artificial airways are usually required for persons receiving mechanical ventilation. Other indications include obstruction relief, airway protection (e.g., after general anesthesia until cough and other protective mechanisms return), and facilitation of secretion removal. There are two types of artificial airways: *endotracheal tube* (ET) and *tracheostomy*. An ET tube may be inserted via the mouth (orotracheal) or nose (nasotracheal). Chapter 23 reviews types of endotracheal tubes, indications for use, and routine care procedures for assessing and managing patients with ET tubes.

Complications of Endotracheal Intubation

The major complications of ET intubation result from injury to the hypopharynx, larynx, and trachea and are related to the pressure exerted on upper airway structures

*Trisch Van Sciver contributed much of the content for this section in previous editions.

Table 61-8 Nursing Management of Potential Complications of the Intraaortic Balloon Pump

Potential Complication	Nursing Management
Wound infection caused by multiple lines into cardiovascular system	Use strict aseptic technique for insertion and dressing changes for all lines. Cover all insertion sites with occlusive dressings. Administer prescribed prophylactic antibiotic for entire course of therapy.
Respiratory infection caused by immobilization	Reposition patient q2hr, being careful not to displace balloon. When performing physical therapy of the chest, avoid introducing an ECG artifact.
Arterial trauma caused by insertion or displacement of balloon	Evaluate and mark peripheral pulses before insertion of balloon to use as baseline for assessing pulses after insertion. After insertion of balloon, evaluate perfusion to both extremities every hour. Measure urine output every hour (occlusion of renal arteries causes severe decrease in urine output). Observe arterial waveforms for sudden changes. Do not elevate head of bed higher than 15 degrees or flex cannulated leg at the hip. Restrain cannulated leg to prevent flexion.
Thromboembolism caused by trauma, balloon obstruction of blood flow distal to catheter	Administer prophylactic heparin if ordered. Evaluate pulses, urine output every hour. Evaluate level of consciousness every hour. Do not allow balloon to be deflated for more than 30 min. Manually inflate and deflate balloon if console malfunctions.
Hematologic complications caused by platelet aggregation along the balloon (decrease in platelets possible)	Administer Rheomacrodex (low-molecular-weight dextran) if ordered. Monitor coagulation status, hematocrit, and platelet count.

ECG, Electrocardiogram.

Table 61-9 Complications of Endotracheal Tubes and Nursing Management

Complications	Causes	Prevention/Treatment
▪ Tube obstruction	Patient biting tube Tube kinking during repositioning Cuff herniation Dried secretions, blood, or lubricant Tissue from tumor Trauma Foreign body	*Prevention:* Place bite block. Sedate patient prn. Suction prn. Humidify inspired gases. *Treatment:* Replace tube.
▪ Tube displacement	Movement of patient's head Movement of tube by patient's tongue Traction on tube from ventilator tubing Self-extubation	*Prevention:* Secure tube to upper lip. Restrain patient's hands. Sedate patient prn. Ensure that only 2 in of tube extend beyond lip. Support ventilator tubing. *Treatment:* Replace tube.
▪ Sinusitis and nasal injury	Obstruction of paranasal sinus drainage Pressure necrosis of nares	*Prevention:* Avoid nasal intubations. Cushion nares from tube and tape/ties. *Treatment:* Remove all tubes from nasal passages. Administer antibiotics.
▪ Tracheoesophageal fistula	Pressure necrosis of posterior tracheal wall resulting from overinflated cuff and rigid nasogastric tube	*Prevention:* Inflate cuff with minimal amount of air necessary. Monitor cuff pressures q8hr. *Treatment:* Position cuff of tube distal to fistula. Place gastrostomy tube for enteral feedings. Place esophageal tube for secretion clearance proximal to fistula.
▪ Mucosal lesions	Pressure at tube and mucosal interface	*Prevention:* Inflate cuff with minimal amount of air necessary. *Treatment:* May resolve spontaneously. Perform surgical intervention.
▪ Laryngeal or tracheal stenosis	Injury to area from end of tube or cuff, resulting in scar tissue formation and narrowing of airway	*Prevention:* Inflate cuff with minimal amount of air necessary. Monitor cuff pressures q8hr. Suction area above cuff frequently. *Treatment:* Perform tracheostomy. Place laryngeal stent. Perform surgical repair.
▪ Cricoid abscess	Mucosal injury with bacterial invasion	*Prevention:* Inflate cuff with minimal amount of air necessary. Monitor cuff pressures q8hr. Suction area above cuff frequently. *Treatment:* Perform incision and drainage of area. Administer antibiotics.

From Thelan LA and others, editors: *Critical care nursing: diagnosis and management,* ed 2, St Louis, 1994, Mosby.

by the tube and cuff. Improper tube placement, aspiration, oral and nasal pressure sores, and accidental extubation are also potential problems. Table 61-9 summarizes complications seen in patients with ET tubes.

Oral, Nasal, and Pharyngeal Damage. Nasotracheal intubation may cause erosion and necrosis of the nasal septum and turbinates and sinusitis by blockage of the ostia. Injury to the lips, teeth, tongue, and posterior pharynx may occur with oral intubation. Measures to prevent these complications include proper tube positioning and stabilizing so that the tube does not put pressure on the sides of the nose or mouth, and daily changes in the position of the oral ET tube from one side of the mouth to the other. The mouth and nose should be inspected every 4 to 8 hours for pressure areas and ulceration and to check the condition of mucosa, gums, and teeth. Because the patient's mouth is always open when an oral ET tube is in place, lips and mouth should be moistened with saline or water swabs to prevent mucosal drying. Mouth care, including cleaning of teeth and gums, should be performed every 4 to 8 hours as a comfort measure and to prevent injury to the gums and loss of teeth resulting from plaque accumulation. Mouthwash containing alcohol should not be used because these preparations dry the mucosa, predisposing it to cracking and thus creating sites for infection. Paranasal sinusitis occurs in many nasally intubated patients. Sinusitis should be suspected when there is unexplained fever or sepsis, purulent nasal drainage, or sinus tenderness.

Laryngeal and Tracheal Damage. Laryngeal injury from ET tubes is common. A cuff usually surrounds the tube and is inflated with air to prevent movement of air and fluid around the outside of the tube (see Chapter 23). The tissue adjacent to the cuff is the most common site of tracheal injury because of the direct pressure of the cuff on the tissue. Movement of the patient or tube during inspiration contributes to laryngeal and tracheal injury. The development of vocal cord congestion or a membranous glottis is common even when the patient is intubated for less than 30 hours. Patients with laryngeal damage can exhibit stridor or symptoms of upper airway obstruction, which may indicate laryngospasm. Other postextubation symptoms of laryngeal damage include hoarseness, sore throat, cough, sputum, and hemoptysis. Upper airway injury sites usually heal rapidly, with complete resolution of symptoms in most cases within 3 to 6 months. The incidence of serious laryngeal and tracheal damage increases with the duration of intubation. Ulceration of the tracheal mucosa, tracheal stenosis, tracheomalacia, tracheoesophageal fistulas, and tracheainnominate bleeding have greatly decreased in incidence and severity with the use of low-pressure cuffs.

Tracheal stenosis is a stricture or narrowing of the airway caused by the healing process, resulting in scarring of the trachea. *Tracheomalacia*, a destruction or softening of the tracheal cartilages, results in collapse of the trachea during inspiration. Stenosis may occur alone, although malacia and stenosis often occur together. Tracheomalacia may be present if increasing volumes of air are required to seal the cuff or if a large air leak persists around the cuff. An increase in the cuff/tube width ratio seen on a chest x-ray may also be a clue to the presence of tracheomalacia. Tracheal stenosis should be suspected if decreasing volumes of air are required to seal the ET tube cuff.

Development of a *tracheoesophageal fistula* may occur with prolonged use of both ET and hard plastic, large-bore nasogastric tubes. A hard plastic nasogastric tube resting against the posterior esophageal wall and an ET tube resting in the trachea may both exert pressure on the anterior esophagus. This continuous pressure may lead to weakness in the posterior tracheal and anterior esophageal wall, with fistula development. Thus tube feedings should be administered with a small-diameter (size 8 Fr) soft feeding tube for the patient receiving long-term ventilatory support. Tracheoesophageal fistulas may be detected or tested for by adding food coloring to tube feeding and observing for the presence of the color in suctioned secretions. Suctioned secretions can be tested with a dipstick for glucose. Normally, tracheal secretions should be negative for glucose. If tube feeding formula is present, the secretions will test positive for glucose.

A rare but catastrophic artificial airway complication is *innominate artery rupture* from erosion of the ET tube or cuff into the anterior tracheal wall. This is usually a fatal event, heralded by blood gushing from the ET tube. Rapidly overinflating the cuff on the ET tube may help tamponade the bleeding vessel until more definitive treatment is obtained.

Laryngeal and tracheal injuries may be minimized by the following procedures:

1. Using the smallest-diameter ET tube that permits ventilation without undue added resistance
2. Minimizing traction on the airway by using swivel connectors and flexible tubing
3. Stabilizing the airway
4. Supporting the patient's head and tubes when turning; avoiding unnecessary head motion
5. Using proper cuff inflation; using low-pressure cuffs
6. Using a small-bore, soft, flexible tube when enteral feedings are required on an intubated patient

Laryngeal and tracheal problems often become evident after extubation. Patients must be observed closely for manifestations of airway obstruction after extubation. Symptoms include hoarseness, cough, aspiration, swallowing difficulties, sore throat, inspiratory stridor, and respiratory distress. Inspiratory stridor can be assessed by placing the stethoscope diaphragm at the neck and listening for a high-pitched, musical sound on inspiration. Inspiratory stridor is a cardinal clinical manifestation of glottic edema. If it is heard immediately after extubation, the patient should be treated aggressively with racemic epinephrine nebulization and corticosteroids. Usually hoarseness, cough, and sore throat end after several days. If these manifestations persist, they must be investigated. Intubation and tracheostomy trays should be kept nearby in case reintubation becomes necessary.

Improper Tube Placement and Accidental Extubation. Improper tube placement is another potential hazard of ET intubation. It is possible for the ET tube to be inserted into the esophagus or to slip so that it extends into the right mainstem bronchus and ventilates only the right lung. Positioning of the distal tube orifice against the carina or tracheal wall may cause airway obstruction. The ET tube might kink when the patient moves the head, and this could cause airway obstruction. Use of a bite block or placement of an oral airway will prevent the patient from biting on the ET tube. There are also ready-made orotracheal tube holders that help stabilize the tube.

A chest x-ray should be taken immediately after intubation and at any time there is a question of improper ET tube placement. The tube should be repositioned as needed by a provider able to reintubate if necessary. The ET tube tip should be seen on chest x-ray at least 2 cm above the carina. Chest auscultation should be done immediately after intubation and before securing the tube to determine the presence of bilateral equal breath sounds. Auscultation of breath sounds is performed regularly at least every 4 hours. The tube must be well secured to prevent slipping or accidental extubation. Accidental extubation can be prevented in the patient who is not fully mentally alert (e.g., after anesthesia, during heavy sedation) by the use of soft wrist restraints. It is wise to mark the tube with india ink at the lip or nose level or note the centimeter mark closest to the lip or nose level and chart it on the care plan or flowchart. This mark provides a quick reference point to check proper tube placement.

The ET tube should not extend more than 1.5 to 3 inches (3.8 to 7.6 cm) out of the patient's nose or mouth because this can add to pressure exerted on structures. Once ET position has been verified by chest x-ray, the tube can be cut and the adapter reapplied. It is important to chart that the tube has been cut. In some units the cut portion is taped on the wall at the head of the bed as a reminder.

Aspiration. Aspiration is a potential hazard for the patient with an ET tube. Oral secretions accumulate above the cuff, and when the cuff is deflated secretions move into the lungs. For this reason the posterior pharynx should be suctioned before cuff deflation. Oral intubation increases salivation, so the mouth should be suctioned frequently. Patients often can be instructed to use a Yankauer or tonsil suction. Other factors causing aspiration include cuff leak, tracheal distention, and tracheoesophageal fistula.

Tracheostomy Tubes

Tracheostomy tubes are the preferred artificial airway for long-term intubation (see Chapter 23). Upper airway damage is minimized and patient comfort maximized if a tracheostomy is performed early in the course of treatment. The patient may be able to eat and to speak with some types of tracheostomy tubes. There is debate regarding when to perform a tracheotomy in the patient with an oral or nasotracheal ET tube. With the use of ET tube cuffs that minimize the pressure against the tracheal mucosa and the use of techniques to maintain low cuff pressures, ET tubes can be left in place longer. The situation varies with the patient, physician, and institution. The span of time ranges from 72 hours to 2 to 3 weeks; some institutions use ET intubation in patients for up to 6 weeks without harmful sequelae. (Types of tracheostomy tubes are listed in Table 23-5.)

NURSING MANAGEMENT

ARTIFICIAL AIRWAY

Routine care of the patient with an ET or tracheostomy tube is discussed in Chapter 23. Procedures for suctioning and inflating and deflating the cuff are described (see Table 23-4, Table 23-5, and Fig. 23-8). The following discussion focuses on complications seen in the critically ill patient. Nursing care for the patient with an artificial airway is presented in the nursing care plan on p. 1967.

Cuff Problems. ET and tracheostomy tubes inserted on an acute or emergent basis usually have a cuff that creates a seal between the airway and tube. The cuff prevents gas from the ventilator from escaping around the tube and minimizes the risk of aspiration of gastric or oral contents into the lungs.

Overinflation of the cuff is a common cause of problems. A cuff inflated to seal during peak inspiration is overinflated during exhalation. Cuff overinflation results in tracheal dilatation. A vicious cycle sometimes occurs, in which the cuff is overinflated, the trachea becomes dilated, and the cuff no longer seals. The care provider might exacerbate the problem by adding more air to the cuff. Tracheal dilatation may lead to esophageal compression, causing aspiration and swallowing difficulty. This problem is prevented by using the minimal occlusive volume cuff inflation technique and by maintaining the cuff pressures at less than 25 cm H_2O (18 to 20 mm Hg) (see Chapter 23).

A rare problem peculiar to some low-pressure cuffs is ballooning of the cuff over the tube lumen, resulting in airway obstruction. This can occur with cuff overinflation. Cuff-related obstruction should be suspected if there is an increase in peak airway pressure, decrease in exhaled tidal volume, increased resistance during bag ventilation, difficulty in passing a suction catheter, and an abnormal musical sound associated with inhalation. If this problem is suspected, the cuff should be totally deflated, airway patency checked, and the cuff slowly reinflated.

Other cuff problems include ineffective sealing caused by cuff rupture or inadequate cuff inflation. A decrease in exhaled tidal volume, problems maintaining positive end-expiratory pressure (PEEP), noisy gurgling on inspiration, and aspiration of saliva, vomitus, or ingested materials may signal these events. The quickest and easiest method to verify a cuff leak is to deflate the cuff with a syringe (after suctioning the oropharynx) and measure the volume of air. If air cannot be withdrawn by this method, a cuff leak or rupture is probably present. If air can be withdrawn, the cuff should be reinflated and the volume of air noted. The amount of air withdrawn should be compared with the amount of air instilled. Differences in these amounts may indicate a cuff leak. Air should be aspirated from the cuff before air is instilled to prevent overinflation. If the balloon remains deflated, a new tube is indicated.

NURSING CARE PLAN Patient with an Artificial Airway*

Planning: Outcome Criteria	*Nursing Interventions and Rationales*
➤ **NURSING DIAGNOSIS**	Ineffective airway clearance *related to* accumulation of secretions in airways, inability to mobilize secretions, drying of mucous membranes, and prolonged immobility *as manifested by* presence of abnormal breath sounds (crackles), frequent or absent cough, presence of thick or copious secretions, high peak inspiratory pressures on ventilator, frequent high-pressure alarm sounds on ventilator
Have normal breath sounds, thin and easily removed secretions, lungs clear to auscultation.	Use effective suctioning technique (see Table 61-10) *to prevent tissue damage.* Suction only when auscultory data support need. If able, have patient attempt to expel secretions by coughing and bringing into proximal airway for suctioning. Observe for blood streaks or tissue particles in suctioning aspirate, *which would indicate mucosal damage.* Use blunt ring-tipped catheters *to diminish trauma to trachea and bronchi.* Use catheter with diameter less than half the tube diameter *to allow space for air to move in or out around the catheter and prevent lung collapse.* Limit negative suction pressure (−80 to −120 mm Hg) *to prevent excess buildup of negative pressure.* Use postural drainage, vibration, and percussion maneuvers when indicated *to help move secretions into larger airways.* Encourage mobility; change patient's position at least q2hr as tolerated *to prevent pooling of secretions.* Keep ventilator tubing cleared of condensed water *to eliminate a source of infection and to maximize oxygenation.* Empty ventilator tubing before position changes and as needed *to prevent accidental spillage of condensate into patient's lungs.* Assess need for other measures *to facilitate secretion, liquefication, and mobilization.* Keep patient well hydrated. Provide warm (98.6° F [37° C]) humidified gases for ventilation. Administer antibiotics and rhDNases as prescribed *to treat infection and liquefy secretions.* Administer aerosolized bronchodilators (if indicated) *to treat bronchospasm and reduce bronchial narrowing.*
➤ **NURSING DIAGNOSIS**	Risk for respiratory infection *related to* exposure to pathogens, loss of normal protective barrier to infection, and possible decreased resistance to infection secondary to debilitated state, prolonged immobility, and inadequate nutrition
Have no evidence of infection, negative sputum cultures.	Observe for change in color, quantity, odor, and viscosity of sputum; difficulty in suctioning secretions; increase in cough; fever; chills; diaphoresis; increase in respiratory rate with spontaneous ventilation; abnormal breath sounds (e.g., crackles, wheezing); tachycardia; deterioration of ABGs; flushing of skin; elevated WBC count; evidence of infiltrate or atelectasis on chest x-ray; positive sputum cultures; decrease in lung compliance *to determine if infection is present or developing.* Obtain sputum culture and order sensitivity test if secretions become purulent or tenacious, change color, or become odorous *to diagnose infectious agent.* Ensure that ventilator tubing is changed at least q24hr *to remove a source of infection.* Change manual resuscitation bag and tubing q24hr *because these may be a source of infection.* Use sterile technique with suctioning (see Table 61-10) *to reduce the risk of infection.* Provide mouth care *to promote hygiene and comfort.* Provide adequate nutritional and fluid intake *to promote patient's health and resistance to infection.*

continued

Suctioning

Suctioning an ET or tracheostomy tube should be performed as needed and not routinely. Dyspnea, increased ventilator peak-inspiratory pressures, activation of the ventilator pressure alarm, noisy or gurgling respirations, and coarse rhonchi may indicate the presence of airway secretions. The recommended procedure for suctioning is presented in Table 23-4. For the patient receiving mechanical ventilation, two procedures are described in Table 61-10 (on p. 1970). Complications associated with suctioning include hypoxemia, dysrhythmias, mucosa damage, pneumothorax, contamination and infection, retained secretions, discomfort, and anxiety. Hypoxemia occurs when oxygen-enriched gas is sucked from the lungs along with secretions. Other causes

NURSING CARE PLAN Patient with an Artificial Airway*—cont'd

Planning: Outcome Criteria	Nursing Interventions and Rationales
➤ **NURSING DIAGNOSIS**	Risk of injury *related to* improper suctioning, right mainstem intubation, esophageal intubation, accidental extubation, mechanical obstruction or kinking of ET tube, cuff herniation over tip of ET tube, and irritation secondary to presence of artificial airway
Maintain tube alignment; have no accidental extubation, no aspiration, no gastric contents in trachea, no tracheal trauma.	Assess for progressive hypoxemia, tachycardia, tachypnea, increase in blood pressure, cyanosis, absent or unilateral breath sounds, dyspnea *to identify signs of ineffective ventilation.* Monitor for inability to ventilate patient with ventilation bag, inability to introduce suction catheter into ET tube, misplacement of ET tube on chest x-ray, high peak airway pressures and frequent high airway pressure alarms, aspiration of gastric contents, positive methylene blue test, frequent suctioning *to determine the presence of indicators of ineffective respirations.* Use bite block or oral airway *to keep patient from biting tube and obstructing tube opening.* Stabilize and secure tube. Move patient with care if connected to ventilator *to avoid traction on ET tube from ventilator tubing.* Support patient's head and airway. Mark tube with india ink or indelible marker at lip or nose insertion point *as indicator of proper positioning.* Cut off excess ET tube beyond 1-3 in (2.2-6.7 cm) from oral insertion point once in correct position *to prevent inadvertent insertion of extra tubing.* Note on chart that tube has been cut. Use rolled towel or sheet *to support ET tube/mechanical ventilator manifold connection.* Auscultate breath sounds immediately after intubation, q4hr, and as needed *to ensure correct placement and effective ventilation.* Ensure that chest x-ray is done immediately after intubation and whenever serious question of tube position arises *to validate correct placement.* Place patient in sniffing position (head hyperextended) and attempt to pass catheter *if there is a question of mechanical obstruction.* Deflate cuff totally and try again *if catheter will not pass.* Oxygenate and ventilate patient after cuff has been slowly reinflated *to ensure adequate oxygenation.* Suction posterior pharynx and mouth before cuff deflation *to prevent aspiration of secretions that may collect on top of the cuff.*
➤ **NURSING DIAGNOSIS**	Risk of aspiration *related to* presence of artificial airway
Have no occurrence of aspiration.	Elevate head of bed and inflate cuff during tube feedings *to prevent aspiration.* Use small-bore feeding tubes for enteral nutrition *to minimize pressure on esophagus.* Observe consistency of suctioned tracheal aspirate *to assess aspiration of gastric contents.* Add food coloring to feedings *to make identification of aspiration easier.* If suspicious of esophageal fistula, perform methylene blue test. Inject methylene blue diluted in water into feeding tube. If blue (positive), test secretions with dipstick for glucose. If positive, aspirations or regurgitation may have occurred. If patient is eating, encourage anteflexion of head *to open esophagus wider.* Keep cuff inflated and elevate head of bed while patient is eating *to prevent aspiration.* Obtain order and administer antiemetics. Insert NG tube if patient feels nauseated and is apt to vomit *to decrease risk of aspiration.* Position patient in side-lying position (never flat on back) *if risk of aspiration is high.*
➤ **NURSING DIAGNOSIS**	Altered oral mucous membranes *related to* tissue trauma caused by presence of artificial airway, open mouth, dryness of mouth; dehydration; decreased salivary flow, increased oral secretions, frequent mechanical stimulation with suction catheter, and lack of humidity *as manifested by* presence of red, shiny, edematous mucosa of mouth; bleeding tendency of gingivae or mucosa of mouth; presence of stomatitis; coated or encrusted oral ulcers; red, dry, swollen tongue with white or brown coating
Have pink, moist, intact mucous membranes; absence of lesions, crusts, hard debris.	With bite block or oral airway removed, gently brush mouth and teeth with toothbrush, toothette, or swab with equal mixture of saline solution q4-8hr and as needed *to provide comfort and to maintain integrity of oral mucosa.* Rinse with saline solution. Brush tongue as tolerated. Clean bite block or oral airway with equal amounts of saline solution and hydrogen peroxide solution, rinse, and replace in mouth. Apply lubricant to lips with cotton applicators or gloved hands *to protect lips from drying.* Check temperature on ventilator thermostat and maintain at 98.6° F (37° C) *to ensure adequate humidity and warmth.* Check cascade water level on ventilator *to ensure that respiratory gases are continually humidified.*

continued

NURSING CARE PLAN Patient with an Artificial Airway*—cont'd

Planning: Outcome Criteria	*Nursing Interventions and Rationales*
➤ **NURSING DIAGNOSIS**	Risk for ineffective breathing pattern *related to* possible upper airway damage secondary to cuffed ET tube
Maintain normal integrity of upper airway structures; be able to phonate and swallow adequately within 1 wk after extubation.	Monitor for tachypnea, tachycardia, decreased breath sounds, inspiratory stridor, use of accessory muscles, inability to phonate, hoarseness, sore throat, cough, swallowing difficulties after extubation *to identify signs of ineffective breathing pattern.* Use smallest-diameter ET tube that will support effective ventilation *to minimize tracheal trauma.* Use only low-pressure cuffs for intubation *to minimize tracheal and laryngeal damage.* Use minimal leak or MOV technique and cuff pressures of <15-18 mm Hg (or 25 cm H_2O) to prevent tracheal dilatation, *which may lead to esophageal compression, causing aspiration and difficulty in swallowing.* Stabilize tube, tubing, and patient's head when turning *to promote patient comfort and decrease tracheal trauma.* Limit patient's head movements *to decrease tracheal trauma.* Use swivel adaptor connection between patient and ventilator *to increase patient's mobility.* Provide care of mouth and nares q4-8hr *to maintain healthy mucosa.* Inspect nares with flashlight and sides of mouth around oral ET tube *for areas of pressure or ulceration.* Change positions of oral ET tube at least once a day *to relieve localized pressure.* Secure tube firmly with tape or tube holder *to prevent displacement.* Assess chest x-rays *to determine tracheal size and relationship to tube.* Observe for clinical signs of aspiration *to allow for early intervention.* Record amount of air and pressure in cuff q8hr. Assess for cuff leak such as hissing or gurgling at mouth, decreased tidal volume *to identify ineffective seal of esophagus.* If patient is able to swallow or suction saliva, deflate cuff when mechanical ventilator is not required for ventilation *to relieve pressure on the trachea.* Immediately after extubation, monitor patient closely *for signs of respiratory distress secondary to laryngeal edema and other signs of upper airway damage.*
➤ **NURSING DIAGNOSIS**	Impaired verbal communication *related to* presence of artificial airway *as manifested by* inability to speak
Have effective method of communication; be able to communicate needs.	Provide patient with paper and pencil, magic slate, alphabet board, symptom board or computer *to have an alternate means of communication.* Learn to read patient's body language, facial expression, and signals *to ease patient's efforts to communicate.* Attempt to anticipate patient's needs *to decrease frustration.* Provide easily accessible call light or bell *to enable patient to call for assistance.* Explain temporary nature of problem and that patient will have no vocalization with ET tube in place and will be hoarse after intubation *to inform patient and relieve anxiety.* Acknowledge that inability to speak can be frustrating *to empathize with patient.* Instruct family in effective strategies for communication with patient.
➤ **NURSING DIAGNOSIS**	Altered nutrition: less than body requirements *related to* possible inability to take nourishment orally, increased caloric demands secondary to clinical condition, and need for mechanical ventilation. See nursing care plan for the patient with acute respiratory failure (Chapter 26) for nursing interventions related to this diagnosis

ABGs, Arterial blood gases; *ET,* endotracheal tube; *MOV,* minimal occlusive volume; *WBC,* white blood cell.
*Nursing care plan for the patient with a tracheostomy is presented in Chapter 23.

of hypoxemia include irritation-induced bronchospasm and microatelectasis resulting from aspiration of intrapulmonary air. Arterial oxygen tension may be reduced by 10 to 39 mm Hg with ET suctioning.[13]

Hypoxemia is prevented by preoxygenation, postoxygenation, and hyperinflation and by limiting each suction pass to 10 to 15 seconds. If a PA catheter is in place, the mixed venous oxygen level can be monitored. Similarly, if pulse oximetry is used, the arterial oxygen level can be assessed throughout the suctioning procedure. During suctioning, the patient must be observed for tachycardia, dysrhythmias, hypertension, diaphoresis, and pallor or graying of mucous membranes. If these occur, the patient should be ventilated with a manual resuscitation bag

Table 61-10 Suctioning Procedure for a Patient on a Mechanical Ventilator

General Measures

1. Wash hands.
2. Explain procedure, purpose, and sensations to patient.
3. Prepare all equipment:
   Check negative suction pressure (usual range between −80 and −120 mm Hg).
   Pour sterile normal saline solution into sterile container.
   Turn on O_2 flow to bag ventilator to 15 L.
   Place bag ventilator on bed.
   Open suction catheter and glove packages. Suction catheter should be no wider than half the diameter of artificial airway.

One-Person Method

1. Pause ventilator alarms.
2. Disconnect patient from ventilator.
3. Preoxygenate with 100% O_2* and hyperventilate patient with manual resuscitation bag or ventilator breaths 3-6 times (done before and after suctioning).
4. Connect patient to ventilator.
5. Put on sterile glove and pick up catheter with sterile hand.
6. Connect catheter to suction tubing, using sterile hand for catheter and nonsterile hand for suction tubing.
7. Disconnect patient from ventilator.
8. Using nonsterile hand, stabilize artificial airway and hold catheter suction regulator (patient may turn head to right with chin up to attempt to place catheter in left mainstem bronchus).
9. Insert catheter gently, swiftly, and without suction with sterile hand.
10. When resistance is met, pull back catheter 1-2 cm without suction.
11. Begin depressing suction vacuum regulator in an on-off (intermittent) fashion with nonsterile hand while rotating catheter in sterile hand between thumb and forefinger.
12. Swiftly remove catheter. Each suctioning pass should not exceed 15 sec.
13. Rinse catheter in sterile saline between suctioning passes as necessary.
14. With nonsterile hand, reconnect patient to ventilator.
15. Depress manual breath or sigh button (if activated) on ventilator to hyperventilate or ventilate patient.†
16. Let patient equilibrate for 30 sec to 1 min or as needed.
17. Rinse catheter with sterile normal saline solution.
18. Repeat procedure as needed.
19. Place patient back on ventilator.
20. Suction oropharynx.
21. Discard catheter.
22. Hyperventilate and oxygenate via manual resuscitation bag or ventilator for three to six breaths.
23. Assess patient's tolerance to suctioning (continuous observation of the patient during entire suctioning procedure is necessary).
24. Confirm that ventilator alarms are reactivated.

Two-Person Method

1. First person hyperventilates and preoxygenates before, between, and after suctions; stabilizes airway.
2. Second person suctions as in one-person method.

*Use O_2 concentration of 60% or less for patients with chronic hypercapnia who are breathing spontaneously.
†As nurse becomes more adept at suctioning, bag ventilation may be done with nonsterile hand between suctioning passes. Ideally, it is better for two persons to be present during suctioning so one person can bag ventilate the patient while the other person does the suctioning. (One nurse with one hand on the bag ventilator can generate up to 800 ml and with two hands up to 1000 ml.)

(MRB) or placed back on the ventilator until equilibration occurs before another suction pass is attempted. In spontaneously breathing patients with chronic hypercapnia (e.g., patients with chronic obstructive pulmonary disease [COPD]) an MRB with 35% to 60% oxygen should be used, and the patient should be assessed for spontaneous ventilatory activity after the suctioning procedure.

Ideally two persons should perform the suctioning procedure. One person can use both hands to bag-ventilate the patient (Fig. 61-9). This is important because hyperinflation with volumes 1.5 times the tidal volume ensures adequate preoxygenation. The ventilator can be used to hyperinflate the patient, but the nurse must know the specific ventilator's characteristic lag time between adjusting the oxygen concentration and actual delivery. Generally the delay is 1 to 2 minutes before the ventilator delivers the increased concentration of oxygen. If the ventilator oxygen concentration is increased, it must be returned to the presuctioning level after suctioning. Some ventilators have a purge mechanism for instantaneous delivery of an altered concentration and some automatically return to the preset oxygen level after 2 minutes. There is some evidence that patients are more stable hemodynamically when ventilator-delivered preoxygenation is used.[13]

A

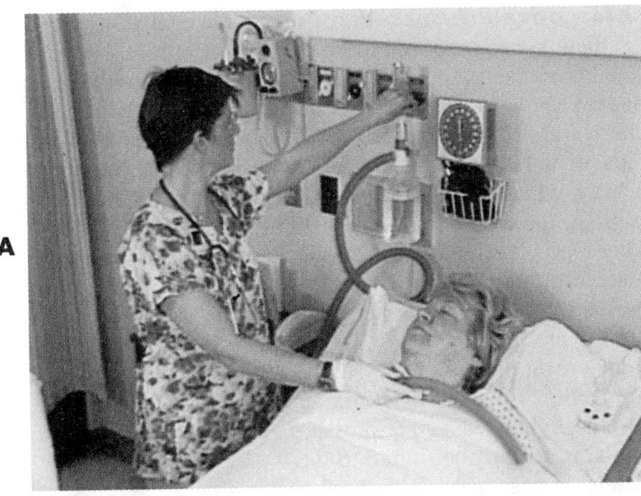

B

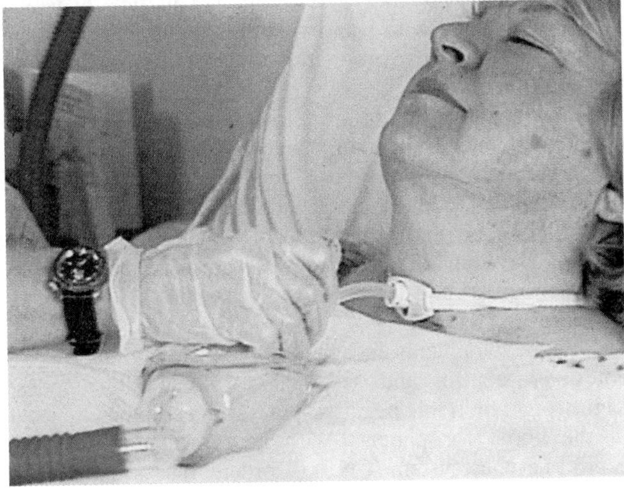

Fig. 61-9 A, Nurse ensuring adequate oxygen to patient before suctioning. **B,** Tracheostomy care.

Causes of cardiac dysrhythmias during suctioning include hypoxemia (thus myocardial hypoxia), vagal stimulation caused by tracheal irritation, and sympathetic nervous system stimulation caused by anxiety or discomfort. Dysrhythmias include tachycardia; bradycardia; premature atrial, junctional, or ventricular beats; and asystole. Suctioning should be halted if serious dysrhythmias develop. The patient should be slowly ventilated via MRB with 100% oxygen until the dysrhythmia subsides. Excessive suctioning should be avoided in patients with hypoxemia or bradycardia.

Tracheal mucosal damage may occur because of excessive suction pressures, overly vigorous catheter insertion, and the characteristics of the suction catheter itself. The presence of blood streaks or tissue shreds in aspirated mucus indicates that mucosal damage has occurred. Mucosal damage increases the risk of infection. Trauma to the mucosa can be prevented by the following precautions:

1. Use blunt or ring-tipped catheters with side holes.
2. Limit negative suction to −80 to −120 mm Hg.
3. Insert the catheter gently and quickly without suction.
4. Withdraw the catheter 1 to 2 cm before applying suction (prevents adhering to mucosa).
5. Lubricate the catheter tip with sterile saline solution.
6. Apply intermittent suction as the catheter is removed.
7. Stabilize the ET tube.
8. Gently rotate the catheter during removal.

Although rare, pneumothorax can occur when a large catheter is inserted into a small-diameter artificial airway. If there is inadequate space for air to move in or out around the catheter, the lung may collapse or microatelectasis may occur when vacuum is applied. To prevent this, the suction catheter should not occupy more than half the internal diameter of the tube being suctioned. Suction should be maintained at −80 to −120 mm Hg. Intermittent suction should be used when removing the catheter.

Secretions may be thick and difficult to suction because of inadequate hydration, inadequate humidification, infection, or inaccessibility of the left mainstem bronchus or lower airways. Chest physiotherapy and having the patient turn and cough before suctioning may help move secretions into larger airways.[14] If the patient is inadequately hydrated, oral or IV fluids should be administered. If the airway is inadequately humidified, the inspired gases should be prewarmed to body temperature and hydrated with sterile water. If infection causes thick mucus, the patient should be placed on appropriate antibiotics. The drug rhDNase reduces viscoelasticity of mucus. It is delivered as an aerosol and is used in patients with cystic fibrosis or COPD patients with acute infections. The use of angle-tipped, directional tip, or coudé catheters may increase the possibility of entering the left mainstem bronchus. Turning the patient's head to the right may make access to the left mainstem bronchus easier.

The patient may experience anxiety during suctioning because of the inability to breathe, choking, or not knowing what to expect. An explanation should precede each suctioning. The patient should be told that breathing will be impossible for a short period but that the patient will soon be connected to oxygen and receive ventilation. The patient should be told that suctioning often stimulates coughing. If the patient has severe coughing during suctioning, ventilation should be done with slow, small-volume breaths using the MRB. Large volumes of air are avoided because they may overdistend the lungs and reflexly stimulate further coughing episodes. The nurse should assume a calm, assured manner and allow patients to participate by bag ventilating themselves if possible.

Closed tracheal suction systems (CTSS), in which a suction catheter is enclosed in a plastic sleeve connected directly to the patient's artificial airway and ventilator, is used in many ICUs (Fig. 61-10). With CTSS, suctioning can be accomplished without disconnecting the ventilator or opening the system. This closed system reduces cross-contamination and reduces the risk of hypoxemia. However, there may be an increased risk of tissue trauma because the tubing is somewhat heavy and tends to cause extra pulling on the airway. Another problem with the

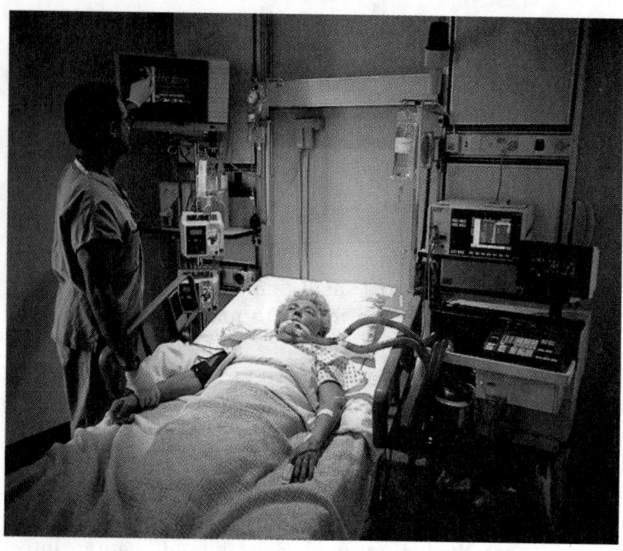

Fig. 61-10 Patient receiving mechanical ventilation with an oral endotracheal tube.

system is difficulty in assessing how far down the catheter has been inserted. When a nurse is adept in the system's use, the feeling of control over the catheter placement increases. The entire system is changed every 24 hours.

MECHANICAL VENTILATION*

Mechanical ventilation is the process in which air or oxygen-enriched air is moved into and out of the lungs mechanically. Mechanical ventilation is not curative. It is a means of supporting patients until they recover the ability to breathe independently. Indications for mechanical ventilation are listed in Table 61-11.

Mechanical ventilation is not usually initiated in cases in which disease reversibility is not possible (e.g., end-stage respiratory failure in patients with severe COPD). Patients with chronic pulmonary disease and their families who are managed by pulmonary health care specialists on a continuous, long-term basis should be given the opportunity to decide the issue of mechanical ventilation before terminal respiratory disease develops. Other patients with chronic disease should also be encouraged to discuss the subject. It is much easier for the physician, patient, and family to decide not to institute ventilatory support initially than it is to remove the support system once it has been initiated. The decision to use mechanical ventilation must be made carefully, respecting the informed wishes of the patient and family.

Types of Mechanical Ventilators

There are two major types of mechanical ventilators: negative-pressure and positive-pressure ventilators.

Negative-Pressure Ventilators. Negative-pressure ventilators are composed of chambers that encase the chest or body and surround it with intermittent subatmospheric or negative pressure. Intermittent negative pressure around the chest wall causes the chest to be pulled outward. This reduces intrathoracic pressure. Air rushes in via the upper airway, which is outside the sealed chamber. Expiration is passive; the machine cycles off, allowing chest retraction. This type of ventilation is similar to normal ventilation in that inspiration is produced by decreased intrathoracic pressures and expiration is passive. An artificial airway is not required.

The iron lung, formerly used to treat patients with poliomyelitis, is an example of a negative-pressure ventilator. Another type of negative-pressure ventilator is the cuirass, which is a rigid shell fitted to the thorax and connected by a flexible hose to a pump that generates negative pressure. The device must be individually fitted. This type of ventilator is associated with skin irritation around areas contacting the shell. Another problem is that volume per breath is not controlled.

Other negative-pressure ventilators include the Poncho (Puritan Bennett, Emerson) and Pulmowrap (Lifecare). These ventilators are made of a flexible nylon cover that fits over the head, ties at the neck with drawstrings, and fastens to the arms or wrists and upper legs with elastic (Fig. 61-11). The Poncho and Pulmowrap are more comfortable than the cuirass and less likely to cause pressure injury to the skin.

New developments in negative-pressure ventilation enable both control and assist-control ventilation modes. Lightweight, portable negative-pressure ventilators are used in the home for patients with neuromuscular diseases, central nervous system (CNS) disorders, diseases and fractures of the spinal cord, and severe COPD. Negative-pressure ventilators are not used for acutely ill patients. With these ventilators, it is more difficult to observe the patient without interrupting the negative intrapleural pressure, thus interfering with ventilation.

Positive-Pressure Ventilators. Positive-pressure ventilation is the primary method used with acutely ill patients. During inspiration the ventilator forces air into the lungs under positive pressure. Unlike spontaneous ventilation, intrathoracic pressure is raised during lung inflation rather than lowered. Expiration occurs passively as in normal expiration. Positive pressure may be added during expiration, but expiration remains passive. The three types of positive-pressure ventilators are (1) time-cycled or time-limited, (2) pressure-cycled or pressure-limited, and (3) volume-cycled or volume-limited ventilators. Each type is classified by the physical parameter that ends the inspiratory cycle. An example of a mechanical ventilator is illustrated in Fig. 61-12.

Time-cycled or time-limited ventilators. Time-cycled ventilators terminate inspiration and switch to expiration at a preset time. The tidal volume is regulated by adjusting inspiratory duration and flow rate of the pressurized gas. The tidal volume and inspiratory pressure delivered to the

*Trisch Van Sciver contributed much of the content for this section in previous editions.

Table 61-11 Indications for Mechanical Ventilation and Weaning

	Measurement and Significance	Normal Values*	Mechanical Ventilation Indicated*	Weaning Feasible*
Tests of Ventilatory Reserve or Mechanical Ability				
V_T	Amount of air exchanged during normal breathing at rest	7-9 ml/kg	<5 ml/kg	>5 ml/kg
Respiratory rate per minute		12-20		12-20
Forced vital capacity	Maximal inspiration and then measurement of air during maximal forced expiration; determination of whether patient can sigh deeply enough to avoid atelectasis; best indicator of ventilatory reserve; patient's cooperation necessary	65-75 ml/kg	<10 or >35 <10–15 ml/kg	>10-15 ml/kg
Peak inspiratory pressure, negative inspiratory force	Complete occlusion of anaeroid manometer attached to airway or mouth for 10-20 sec while negative inspiratory efforts of patient noted; useful index of neuromuscular strength; less patient cooperation necessary	−75 to −100 cm H_2O	>−25 cm H_2O	<−20 cm H_2O
Forced expiratory volume in 1 sec	Volume of air measured in first second of exhalation of forced vital capacity maneuver; use in patients with COPD to determine degree of obstruction	50-60 ml/kg	<10 ml/kg	>16 ml/kg
Resting minute ventilation	Multiplication of tidal volume by respiratory rate for 1 min, general indication of patient's total ventilation	5-10 L/min	>10 L/min	<10 L/min
V_D/V_T	Estimation from V_T; accurate calculation requiring $PaCO_2$ and partial pressure of CO_2 in mixed expired gas; measurement of portion of each breath that does not participate in gas exchange; indication of lungs' efficiency in removing CO_2	0.25-0.40	>0.6	<0.5-0.6
$PaCO_2$	Indication of lungs' efficiency in removing CO_2 and reflection of body's acid-base status	35-45 mm Hg	>55 mm Hg	<45 mm Hg
Tests of Oxygenation Capability				
Q_s/Q_T	Determination of amount of cardiac output shunted (Q_s) in relation to amount of total cardiac output (Q_T); indication of extent of shunt expressed as a percentage of cardiac output	<5%	>30%	<20%
$D(A-a)O_2$, $P(A-a)O_2$	Calculation from PaO_2, PAO_2, and respiratory quotient on FIO_2 of 1.0; indication of lung's ability to oxygenate blood; index of extent of $\dot{V}/\dot{Q}$ mismatch, diffusion defect, or shunt	25-65 mm Hg	>450 mm Hg	<300-350 mm Hg
PAO_2	Provision of evidence of lung's ability to oxygenate arterial blood; PaO_2 of 60 mm Hg necessary to saturate Hb by 90% for adequate tissue oxygenation	80-110 mm Hg (altitude dependent)	<60 mm Hg with FIO_2 >0.6	>60-80 mm Hg with FIO_2 ≤0.5

COPD, Chronic obstructive pulmonary disease.
*These parameters are only guidelines and must be related to the individual patient's status (e.g., patients with severe COPD may have a normal $PaCO_2$ of 60 mm Hg and values lower than normal for FEV_1, VC, MV, and maximal voluntary ventilation).

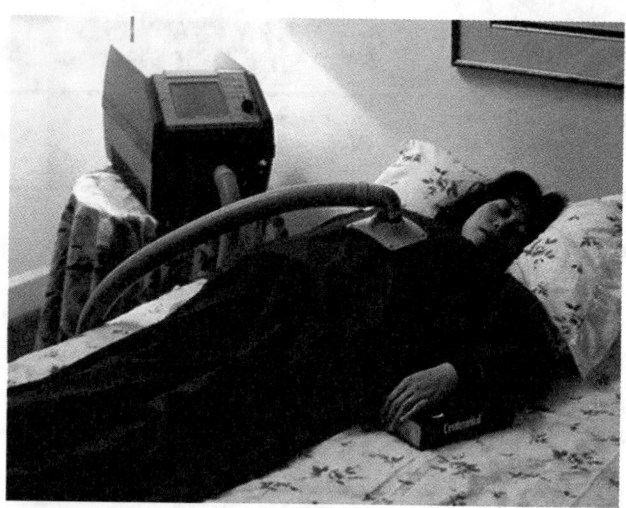

Fig. 61-11 Negative-pressure ventilator.

patient may vary from breath to breath. Time-cycled ventilators (e.g., Veriflo CV 200) are used primarily for neonates and infants. The Siemans 900-C is an example of a time-cycled ventilator for adults. Time-cycled ventilators have fail-safe pressure limits beyond which the ventilator ceases to push gas into the lungs, thus preventing lung overdistention and barotrauma.

Pressure-cycled or pressure-limited ventilators. Pressure-cycled ventilators terminate inspiration when a preselected airway pressure is achieved. The volume of gas delivered to the patient and duration of delivery vary according to airway resistance, pulmonary compliance, and ventilator circuit integrity. For example, increased airway resistance could result when thick secretions are coughed into the upper airway. Secretions increase resistance to air and ventilatory pressure rises. The volume of ventilator gas delivered before the presence of secretions is larger than the volume with secretions present. Pressure-limited ventilators are typically not able to deliver precisely controlled levels of oxygen. Pressure-cycled ventilators are not used as often as time-cycled or volume-cycled ventilators for acutely ill patients. They are used predominantly for treatments, home therapy, short-term ventilation, or in a patient whose lungs are relatively free of diseases involving altered resistance and compliance. An example of a pressure-cycled ventilator is the Bennett PR-1. Pressure-cycled ventilators can be used with a mask, mouthpiece, or artificial airway.

Volume-cycled or volume-limited ventilators. Volume-cycled ventilators are the most common type used for intubated adults and older children. Inspiration is terminated when a preset volume of gas is delivered into the ventilator circuit. Volume-cycled ventilators have built-in pressure-limiting valves to prevent excess pressure in the lungs. Once the pressure limit is reached, the remainder of the tidal volume is vented to the outside air. With volume-cycled ventilators, volume delivery remains constant despite lung resistance and compliance changes (unlike pressure-cycled ventilators). Inspired oxygen concentration remains consistent. An example is the Siemens Servo 900. Some ventilators (e.g., Monoghan 225) can be adapted to function as pressure cycled, time cycled, or volume cycled.

Generally an ET or tracheostomy tube is required for volume-cycled ventilation. When mechanical ventilation is required but intubation is undesirable, nocturnal nasal positive-pressure ventilation (NNPPV) can be used to deliver a preset volume of air at a preset pressure (see Chapter 26).

Settings of Mechanical Ventilators

Mechanical ventilator settings regulate the rate, depth, and other characteristics of ventilation (Table 61-12). Settings are based on the patient's status (ABGs, body weight, level of consciousness, muscle strength). The ventilator is tuned as finely as possible to match the patient's ventilatory pattern. Settings are evaluated and adjusted frequently until the patient achieves optimal ventilation. Some settings serve as a fail-safe, alerting staff to problems with ventilation. It is important that the nurse ensure and document that all ventilator alarms are turned on at all times. Alarms sense potentially dangerous situations of mechanical malfunction, apnea, or patient asynchrony with the ventilator. On many ventilators the alarms can be temporarily bypassed or silenced for up to 2 minutes for suctioning or testing. After that period of time, the alarm system automatically becomes functional again.

Modes of Volume-Cycled Ventilation

Mode refers to the manner in which the breath is initiated and the volume controlled, either by the mechanical ventilator or the patient. Mode is selected based on the patient's ventilatory status, including respiratory drive and ABGs. The four basic modes of mechanical ventilation are (1) controlled mechanical ventilation (CMV), (2) assist-control ventilation (ACV), (3) intermittent mandatory ventilation (IMV), and (4) synchronized intermittent mandatory ventilation (SIMV). These modes are compared in Table 61-13.

Controlled Mechanical Ventilation. With CMV, breaths are delivered regularly and independent of the patient's ventilatory efforts. CMV is usually used when the patient has no drive to breathe (e.g., the anesthetized patient, drug overdose), is unable to breathe spontaneously (e.g., the paralyzed patient), or requires deliberate hyperventilation (e.g., the patient with elevated intracranial pressure). With CMV the normal processes of regulation of ventilation are not operating, thus the patient's ability to adjust ventilation to changing demands has been lost. The patient receiving CMV must be carefully monitored with frequent ABG assessments.

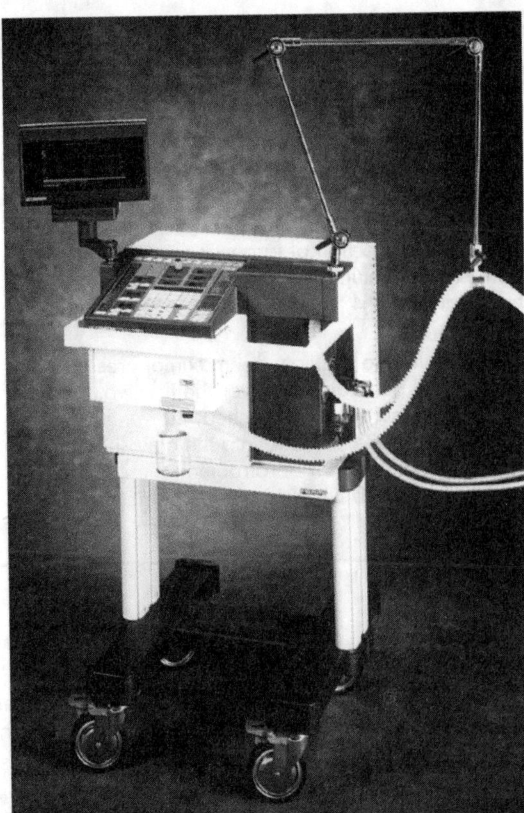

Fig. 61-12 Typical postive-pressure ventilator.

Patients receiving CMV who are not apneic usually require some type of sedation (e.g., propofol) or paralyzing agent (e.g., pancuronium) to facilitate optimal ventilation. Before initiating anesthesia or paralysis in the mechanically ventilated patient who is agitated, it is important to assess for the cause of agitation. Common problems that can result in patient agitation include ET tube malposition, pain, hypoxemia, pulmonary embolism, drug reaction, and emotional distress. The treatment should be explained to the patient. If the patient is paralyzed, the nurse should remember that the patient can hear, see, think, and feel. Sedative and pain medications should be administered appropriately. Close monitoring is essential. In particular, patients on CMV require frequent ABG analysis to allow prompt recognition and correction of hyperventilation and hypoventilation.

Assist-Control Mechanical Ventilation. With ACV, the ventilator is set similarly to CMV in that it delivers a preset tidal volume at a preset frequency. However, unlike CMV the patient is able to initiate a breath by attempting to inhale. The ventilator senses a decrease in intrathoracic pressure and then delivers the preset tidal volume. The patient can ventilate faster than the preset rate but not slower. This mode has the advantage of allowing the patient some control over ventilation while providing support. ACV is used in patients with a variety of conditions, including neuromuscular disorders (e.g., Guillain-Barré syndrome), pulmonary edema, and acute respiratory distress syndrome. The patient with ACV mode has the potential for hypoventilation and hyperventilation. If the volume and minimum rate are set too high, the patient will be hyperventilated. If the volume or minimum rate is set low and the patient is apneic or weak, the patient will be hypoventilated. Thus these patients require vigilant assessment and monitoring of ventilatory status, including ABGs. It is important that the amount of negative pressure required to initate a breath is appropriate to the patient's condition. If it is too difficult to initiate a breath, the work of breathing is increased. If it is too easy, the patient will be at risk for overventilation and respiratory alkalosis.

Intermittent Mandatory Ventilation. With IMV, the ventilator delivers a preset tidal volume at a preset frequency either at regular intervals (IMV) or in synchrony with the patient's spontaneous breathing (SIMV). Between ventilator-delivered breaths, the patient is able to breathe spontaneously through the ventilator circuit. Thus the patient receives the preset inspired oxygen concentration during the spontaneous breaths but self-regulates the rate and depth of those breaths. These modes of ventilation differ from ACV, in which all breaths are of the same preset volume. SIMV is the most common mode of ventilatory support. IMV and SIMV are used during continuous ventilation and during weaning from the ventilator. Potential benefits of IMV and SIMV include avoidance of respiratory alkalosis, minimizing the patient "fighting" the ventilator, lower mean airway pressure, more uniform intrapulmonary gas distribution, and prevention of muscle atrophy.[15]

IMV and SIMV have advantages over other modes with respect to cardiovascular effects. Spontaneous inspiration decreases intrathoracic pressure, reduces mean intrathoracic pressure, and enhances venous blood return to the heart. Thus the patient with an extracellular fluid volume deficit is better able to maintain the cardiac output. Because of the lower mean intrathoracic pressure, higher levels of PEEP may be used with IMV and SIMV than with other modes of volume-controlled ventilation.

Weaning patients from ventilators can be accomplished using IMV and SIMV. Instead of abruptly removing patients from ventilators and letting them breathe totally on their own, these modes allow a smooth transition to spontaneous ventilation by gradually decreasing the ventilator rate as patients assume an increasing percentage of the total work of breathing.

There are disadvantages with IMV and SIMV. If spontaneous breathing decreases when the rate is low, ventilation might not be adequately supported. Low-rate IMV or SIMV should be used only in patients with regular, spontaneous breathing. Weaning with IMV or SIMV demands close monitoring and may take longer because the rate of breathing is gradually reduced. Patients being weaned with IMV or SIMV may become fatigued, especially during the night.

Table 61-12 Settings of Mechanical Ventilation

Respiratory Rate
Number of breaths the ventilator will deliver per minute

Tidal Volume (VT)
Volume delivered to patient during a normal ventilator breath. Usual volume selected is 10 to 15 ml/kg.

Oxygen Concentration (FIO_2)
Selects delivery of oxygen between 21% and 100%

I:E Ratio
Ratio of inspiratory time to expiratory time. Determined by adjusting the inspiratory flow rate. Usually 1:2, unless inverse ratio ventilation is in use.

Inspiratory Flow Rate (Peak Flow)
Flow of tidal volume delivery.

Sensitivity
Control that adjusts the ventilatory response to patient's respiratory effort. It determines the amount of effort the patient must generate to initiate a breath.

Sighs
Allows periodic selection of larger-than-normal tidal volume. Usual volume is 1½ to 2 times tidal volume, and usual rate is 4 to 5 times an hour.

Pressure Limits
Adjustable setting to regulate the maximal pressure the machine can generate to deliver the tidal volume. Once the pressure limit is reached, the ventilator will spill the undelivered volume into the atmosphere to protect the patient from barotrauma. The limit is usually set at 10 to 20 cm H_2O above the normal peak pressure.

From Thelan LA and others, editors: *Critical care nursing: diagnosis and management*, ed 2, St Louis, 1994, Mosby.

Other Ventilatory Maneuvers

Positive End-Expiratory Pressure. PEEP is a ventilatory maneuver in which positive pressure is applied to the airway during exhalation. Normally during exhalation airway pressure drops to zero, and exhalation occurs passively. With PEEP exhalation remains passive, but pressure falls to a preset level greater than zero, often 3 to 20 cm H_2O. With PEEP lung volume during expiration and between breaths is greater than normal. Thus PEEP increases functional residual capacity (FRC). This often improves oxygenation. The mechanisms by which PEEP increases FRC and oxygenation include increased distention of already patent alveoli, prevention of alveolar collapse, and aeration of previously collapsed alveoli.[15] PEEP often allows the fraction of inspired oxygen (FIO_2) to be reduced, thus lowering the risk of oxygen toxicity.

PEEP is prescribed in increments of 2 to 5 cm H_2O. The amount of PEEP selected is determined by the amount that improves oxygenation without decreasing blood pressure and cardiac output. This is called best or optimal PEEP. Often 5 cm H_2O PEEP (so-called physiologic PEEP) is used prophylactically to replace the glottic mechanism and help maintain a normal FRC and prevent alveolar collapse. Clinical studies vary regarding the benefits of physiologic PEEP. PEEP of 5 cm H_2O is also used for patients with a history of alveolar collapse during weaning. PEEP has demonstrated improvements in gas exchange, vital capacity, and inspiratory force when used during weaning.

Inspiratory pressure increases when expiratory pressure is added. When PEEP is applied during CMV or ACV, the term *continuous positive-pressure ventilation* may be used. The most common mode of PEEP delivery is with IMV or SIMV. The decreased mean airway pressure that occurs during spontaneous breathing is enough to prevent some of the adverse effects produced by the increased pressures.

In general, the major purpose of PEEP is to maintain adequate oxygenation while limiting risk of oxygen toxicity. PEEP is also used to prevent atelectasis. PEEP is useful in pulmonary edema, providing a counterpressure opposing fluid extravasation. It has been proposed that PEEP may assist in healing damaged lungs by maintaining airway stability and improving surfactant production or distribution. PEEP is indicated in lungs with diffuse disease, severe hypoxemia unresponsive to FIO_2 greater than 0.5, and loss of compliance or stiffness. The classic indication for PEEP therapy is acute respiratory distress syndrome (ARDS) in which the FRC is reduced. PEEP is generally contraindicated or used with extreme caution in patients with highly compliant lungs (e.g., COPD), unilateral or nonuniform disease, hypovolemia, and low cardiac output. In these situations the adverse effects of PEEP may outweigh any benefits.

Continuous Positive Airway Pressure. Continuous positive airway pressure (CPAP) is the use of PEEP in a spontaneously breathing patient. With CPAP there is a constant flow of gas at a rate greater than the patient's spontaneous inspiratory flow rate. Thus the patient's airway pressure never falls to zero. For example, if CPAP is 5 cm H_2O, during exhalation airway pressure is 5 cm H_2O; during inspiration, 1 to 2 cm H_2O of negative pressure is generated, reducing airway pressure to 3 or 4 cm H_2O. The patient receiving IMV with PEEP receives CPAP when breathing spontaneously. CPAP is often used in infants. It is commonly used in the treatment of obstructive sleep apnea. CPAP can be administered by a tight-fitting mask or an ET or tracheal tube. CPAP increases work of breathing because the patient must forcibly exhale against the CPAP.

Pressure Support Ventilation. With pressure support ventilation (PSV), positive pressure is applied to the airway only during inspiration. Similar to CPAP, PSV is

Table 61-13 Modes of Mechanical Ventilation

Description	Advantages	Disadvantages	Uses
Controlled Mechanical Ventilation (CMV)			
Machine delivers preset number of breaths/min at preset volume. Patient cannot trigger breathing.	Breathing is totally controlled by ventilator.	Does not allow patient to initiate breathing or respiratory rate to change with varying patient needs. Airway pressure always positive during inspiration, compromising venous return. Provides limited use of respiratory muscles.	Apnea secondary to brain damage, respiratory muscle paralysis, drug overdose, sedation
Assist-Control Ventilation (ACV)			
Delivery of breath is triggered by inspiratory effort of patient after preselected time interval has elapsed. If patient fails to initiate breathing, ventilator cycles as in controlled ventilation.	Patient can initiate own breathing, use respiratory muscles, and alter respiratory rate according to need. Intrathoracic pressure decreases transiently before inspiratory phase, decreasing the venous return and suppression of cardiac output.	Problems of overventilation and underventilation are possible and can occur in anxious patients or in those with low lung compliance.	Wide range of situations in which patients are spontaneously breathing but have ventilatory failure or gas exchange inefficiency
Intermittent Mandatory Ventilation (IMV)			
Patient breathes spontaneously at own VT and rate. At preset frequency, ventilator delivers a breath.	Ventilator breaths are not synchronized to patient's respiratory pattern. Machine breath can be given during patient's exhalation or peak inhalation.	Allows maintenance of even minor spontaneous excursions. Respiratory muscles remain in use. Ventilator augments patient's own efforts.	Wide range of situations in which patients need ventilatory support, method of weaning
Synchronized Intermittent Mandatory Ventilation (SIMV)			
Ventilation method is modification of IMV. Ventilator is synchronized to patient's ventilatory rate. Machine set to give certain number of breaths and is triggered by patient's inspiration.	Ventilator does not compete with patient's breathing.	At low rate levels, patient may not be adequately ventilated. Low volume and rate alarms need to be set when low levels are used.	Same as above.

used in conjunction with the patient's spontaneous respirations. A preset level of positive airway pressure is selected so that the gas flow rate is greater than the patient's inspiratory flow rate. As the patient initiates a breath, the machine senses the spontaneous effort and supplies a rapid flow of gas, supporting the inspiratory effort. With PSV the patient determines inspiratory length, flow rate, and respiratory rate. Tidal volume depends on the pressure level and airway compliance. PSV can be used with continuous ventilation or during weaning. PSV is rarely used as a sole ventilatory support during acute respiratory failure in patients with unstable respiratory drive, secretions, bronchospasm, pain, or anxiety because of the risk of hypoventilation.[15] Advantages to PSV include increased patient comfort, decreased work of breathing (because inspiratory efforts are augmented), decreased oxygen consumption (because inspiratory work is reduced), and increased endurance conditioning (because the patient is exercising respiratory muscles).[16]

Inverse-Ratio Ventilation. With inverse-ratio ventilation (IRV) inspiration is prolonged and expiration shortened. The I/E ratio is the ratio of duration of inspiration (I) to the duration of expiration (E). This value is normally less than one. With IRV the I/E ratio approaches or exceeds 1. With IRV a prolonged positive pressure is applied during inspiration. IRV progressively expands collapsed alveoli.

The short expiratory time has a PEEP-like effect, preventing alveolar collapse. Because IRV imposes a nonphysiologic breathing pattern, the patient requires sedation or paralysis. IRV is indicated for patients with ARDS who continue to have refractory hypoxemia despite a PEEP of 15 cm H_2O or more. Not all patients with poor oxygenation respond to IRV.

High-Frequency Ventilation. High-frequency ventilation (HFV) involves delivery of a small tidal volume (usually 1 to 5 ml/kg body weight) at rapid respiratory rates (100 to 300 breaths/min). HFV can minimize some complications attributed to conventional mechanical ventilation because mean airway pressure is lower. Use of HFV is limited to high-risk, severely ill patients. HFV is used in patients with bronchopleural fistulas because lower peak airway pressures can prevent worsening of this condition. Some patients with ARDS and acute respiratory failure may benefit from HFV, although results of trials do not indicate many advantages or improvement in mortality rates over conventional forms of mechanical ventilation.[16] HFV is more commonly used in neonatal patients and in patients with smoke inhalation.

Complications of Mechanical Ventilation

Although mechanical ventilation may be essential to maintain ventilation and oxygenation, it can cause adverse effects. It is often difficult to distinguish complications of mechanical ventilation from the underlying disease.

Cardiovascular System. Positive-pressure mechanical ventilation can cause circulatory problems due to transmission of increased mean airway pressure to the thoracic cavity. With increased intrathoracic pressure, thoracic vessels are compressed. This results in decreased venous return to the heart, decreased left ventricular end-diastolic volume (preload), decreased cardiac output, and lowered blood pressure. Mean airway pressure is further increased with PEEP.

If the lungs are noncompliant (as in ARDS), airway pressures are not as easily transmitted to the heart and blood vessels. Thus effects of mechanical ventilation on cardiac output are reduced. Conversely, with compliant lungs (e.g., emphysema), there is increased danger of transmission of high airway pressures and cardiac output may decrease.

Compromise of venous return by positive-pressure ventilation is exaggerated by hypovolemia (e.g., hemorrhage, multiple trauma) and decreased venous tone (e.g., sepsis, spinal shock). Restoration and maintenance of the circulating blood volume is important in minimizing cardiovascular complications.

Some studies have found improved cardiac performance after the initiation of mechanical ventilation in patients with poor left ventricular function.[17] It is postulated that positive-pressure ventilation decreases right-sided heart preload by its increase in intrathoracic pressure. Also the increased airway pressure may restrict left ventricular filling by mechanical compression. These effects may improve the failing left ventricle by optimizing ventricular end-diastolic volume.

Sodium and Water Balance. Progressive fluid retention often occurs after 48 to 72 hours of mechanical ventilation. Fluid retention can lead to pulmonary edema. Positive-pressure ventilation, especially with PEEP, is associated with decreased urinary output and increased sodium retention. Fluid balance changes may be due to decreased cardiac output, which in turn results in diminished renal perfusion. Renin release is stimulated, which increases aldosterone secretion and subsequent sodium and water retention. It is also possible that pressure changes within the thorax are associated with decreased release of atrial natriuretic peptide, also causing sodium retention. Mild water retention is also associated with mechanical ventilation. There is less insensible water loss via the airway, because inspired gases are saturated with water at body temperature. In addition, as with all stressed patients, release of antidiuretic hormone may be increased, causing water retention.

Pulmonary System

Barotrauma. As lung inflation pressures increase, risk of pneumothorax, pneumomediastinum, and subcutaneous emphysema increases. Patients with compliant lungs (e.g., COPD) are at greater risk because the increased airway pressure readily distends the lungs and may rupture alveoli or emphysematous blebs. Patients with stiff lungs (e.g., ARDS), who require high inspiratory pressures and high levels of PEEP, and patients with suppurative lung abscesses resulting from necrotizing organisms (e.g., staphylococci) are also susceptible to barotrauma.

Air can escape into the pleural space from alveoli or interstitium, accumulate, and become trapped. Pleural pressure increases and collapses the lung, causing *pneumothorax*. (Clinical manifestations of pneumothorax are discussed in Chapter 24.) The lung receives air during inspiration but cannot expel it during expiration. Respiratory bronchioles are larger on inspiration than expiration. They may close on expiration, and air becomes trapped. With positive-pressure breathing, a simple pneumothorax can become a life-threatening tension pneumothorax. With tension pneumothorax, the mediastinum and contralateral lung are compressed, compromising cardiac output. Immediate chest tube insertion is required.

Pneumomediastinum usually begins with rupture of alveoli into the lung interstitium; progressive air movement then occurs into the mediastinum and subcutaneous neck tissue. This is commonly followed by pneumothorax. Occurrence of new, unexplained subcutaneous air is indication for immediate chest x-ray. Pneumomediastinum and subcutaneous emphysema in the neck may be too small to be detected radiographically or clinically before the development of a pneumothorax.

Subcutaneous emphysema may occur after a tracheotomy as a result of leakage of air around the surgical site, or it may occur around the site of a chest tube for pneumothorax. In the latter case, subcutaneous emphysema is usually caused by the passage of gas from the pleural space into the chest tube wound, indicating that the space is not being adequately drained. Chest tube patency must be maintained to prevent a further increase in the pneumothorax.

Alveolar hypoventilation. Hypoventilation can be caused by inappropriate ventilator settings, leakage of air from the ventilator tubing or around the ET tube or tracheostomy cuff, lung secretions or obstruction, and low ventilation-perfusion ratio. Low tidal volume or respiratory rate decreases minute ventilation, causing hypoventilation. A leaking cuff or tubings that are not secured may cause air leakage, lowering the delivered tidal volume. Too low an IMV or SIMV rate in a patient who is unable to produce adequate spontaneous ventilation causes hypoventilation, respiratory acidosis, and problems related to acidosis such as cardiac dysrhythmias. Lung secretions can cause hypoventilation. This can be prevented by turning the patient every 1 to 2 hours, providing chest physiotherapy to lung areas with increased secretions, encouraging deep breathing and coughing, and suctioning as needed. Low ventilation-perfusion ratio is a cause of hypoxemia. Use of mechanical ventilation can exaggerate ventilation-perfusion mismatch because pressurized ventilator gas tends to flow to areas of low resistance and high compliance. Thus collapsed alveoli may not be ventilated, producing atelectasis and low ventilation-perfusion ratio. Use of large tidal volumes, small increments of PEEP, and sighing of the patient lessens the likelihood of atelectasis. Frequent position change also helps. Major clinical indicators of atelectasis are decreased breath sounds over the area and a drop in arterial oxygenation.

Alveolar hyperventilation. It is easy to overventilate a patient on mechanical ventilation. Particularly at risk is the patient with chronic alveolar hypoventilation and CO_2 retention (e.g., the COPD patient). This patient may have a chronic arterial CO_2 elevation and compensatory bicarbonate retention by the kidneys. When the patient is ventilated, the patient's "normal" rather than standard normal values should be the therapeutic goal. If the COPD patient is returned to a standard normal arterial CO_2 tension, the patient will develop alkalosis because of the retained bicarbonate. Such a patient would move from compensated acidosis to serious metabolic alkalosis. The presence of alkalosis makes weaning from the ventilator difficult. Alkalemia, especially if the onset is abrupt, can have additional serious consequences, including hypokalemia, predisposing the patient to dysrhythmias. Alkalemia shifts the oxygen-hemoglobin dissociation curve to the left, making oxygen release to the tissues more difficult. Neuromuscular irritability, seizures, coma, and death can occur.

To prevent alkalosis, mechanical ventilation should be initiated and remain at a level that will not dramatically lower the arterial CO_2 level. ABGs must be assessed 15 to 30 minutes after mechanical ventilation begins and after each ventilator change, serially thereafter, and whenever changes in the patient's clinical status occur. Arterial CO_2 tension should be gradually lowered only to the patient's baseline (before acute illness) level. Usually patients with COPD on the ventilator do better with a short inspiratory and longer expiratory time.

Respiratory alkalosis can occur if the rate or tidal volume is set too high (mechanical overventilation) or if the patient receiving assisted ventilation is hyperventilating. Hyperventilation means that the arterial CO_2 tension is less than 35 mm Hg. The patient or the ventilator is blowing off CO_2 too rapidly. Decreasing the respiratory rate or tidal volume or both can help correct the respiratory alkalosis. However, if the current rate and volume are necessary to prevent atelectasis, mechanical dead space may be added to increase arterial CO_2 tension.

If the hyperventilation is spontaneous, it is important to determine the cause and treat it. Causes might include hypoxemia, pain, fear, anxiety, or compensation for metabolic acidosis. Patients who fight the ventilator or breathe out of synchrony may be anxious or in pain. Secretion accumulation or movement or kinking of the ET tube in the airway may also cause this problem. If the patient is anxious and fearful, sitting with the patient and verbally coaching the patient to breathe with the ventilator may help. If these measures fail, manually bagging the patient slowly with the manual rebreathing bag (MRB) connected to an oxygen source may slow breathing enough to bring it in synchrony with the ventilator. The patient may require morphine, diazepam, or other sedatives. However, sedation must be administered with extreme caution in patients on IMV or SIMV at low rates because respiratory drive may be significantly depressed.

Pulmonary infection. Pulmonary infection is common with mechanical ventilation. Because normal upper airway defenses have been bypassed by the ET or tracheostomy tube, the patient is at increased risk of infection. In addition, poor nutritional state, immobility, and the underlying disease process (e.g., immunosuppression, organ failure) make the patient more prone to infection.

In patients receiving prolonged mechanical ventilation, sputum cultures often grow gram-negative bacteria such as *Pseudomonas, Serratia*, and *Klebsiella*. These are abundant in the hospital environment and the patient's digestive tract. Organisms can spread in a number of ways, including contaminated respiratory equipment, inadequate hand washing, adverse environmental factors such as poor room ventilation and high traffic flow, and decreased patient ability to cough and clear secretions. Colonization of the upper respiratory tract by aspiration of gram-negative organisms is a predisposing factor in the development of gram-negative pneumonia.

Infection can be minimized by using strict aseptic technique while suctioning or handling the artificial airway. Frequent hand washing is imperative. The ventilator humidifier and tubing provide a warm, moist environment conducive to the growth of organisms. Ventilator tubing should be changed at least every 24 to 48 hours. When water has condensed in the tubing, it should be drained, especially before repositioning the patient. This measure will prevent the patient from aspirating the water. Corrugated ventilator tubings must be pulled gently to remove water that has condensed in the folds. Chest physiotherapy, adequate humidification of inspired gases, and sterile suctioning may help prevent infection by eliminating secretion accumulation. The MRB (e.g., Ambu bag) and oxygen tubing kept at the patient's bedside also must be replaced and cleaned periodically (at least every 24 to 48 hours).

Clinical evidence suggesting pulmonary infection includes fever, elevated WBC count, purulent sputum, sputum odor, auscultation that reveals crackles or rhonchi, and pulmonary infiltrates noted on chest x-ray. The patient is treated with antibiotics after appropriate cultures are taken by tracheal suctioning or bronchoscopy and when infection is evident. Aerosolized rhDNase may be used to decrease the viscoelasticity of the mucus in the patient with cystic fibrosis and COPD.

Neurologic System. In patients with head injury, positive-pressure ventilation, especially with PEEP, can impair cerebral blood flow. This is related to increased intrathoracic positive pressure impeding venous drainage from the head, as evidenced by jugular venous distention. As a result of the impaired venous return and increase in cerebral volume, the patient may exhibit increases in intracranial pressure. Positioning the patient with the head midline may facilitate venous drainage from the brain and decrease intracranial pressure.

Gastrointestinal System. Patients receiving mechanical ventilation are often stressed because of serious illness, immobility, and discomforts associated with the ventilator. Thus the ventilated patient is at risk for developing stress ulcers and gastrointestinal (GI) bleeding. Patients with preexisting ulcer or those receiving corticosteroid therapy are at an especially increased risk. Direct visualization of the stomach via gastroscopy demonstrates that gastric mucosal changes occur in many critically ill patients. Any kind of circulatory compromise, including reduction of cardiac output caused by mechanical ventilation, may contribute to ischemia of the intestinal mucosa and thus increase the risk of translocation of GI bacteria.

Prophylactic administration of antacids to maintain a gastric pH greater than 5 reduces the occurrence of upper GI bleeding. Specially designed feeding tubes with a pH-sensitive probe allow for the measurement of gastric pH. Other methods of assessment include checking the pH of gastric aspirates. Early and frequent nasogastric feedings have also been successfully used to decrease gastric ulcers and bleeding. Prophylactic use of histamine H_2 receptor blockers cimetidine (Tagamet) and ranitidine (Zantac), administered intravenously or orally, decrease gastric acidity and diminish the risk of stress ulcer and hemorrhage.

Gastric and bowel dilatation may occur as a result of gas accumulation in the GI tract. Gas may escape around the ET tube cuff or may be swallowed into the stomach. The irritation of an artificial airway may cause excessive air swallowing and subsequent gastric dilatation. Gastric or bowel dilatation may put pressure on the vena cava, decrease cardiac output, and prohibit adequate diaphragmatic excursion during spontaneous breathing. Elevation of the diaphragm as a result of paralytic ileus or bowel dilatation leads to compression of the lower lobes of the lungs, which may cause atelectasis and compromise respiratory function. Decompression of the stomach can be accomplished by the insertion of a nasogastric tube. Some clinicians routinely insert nasogastric tubes prophylactically when mechanical ventilation is initiated. A nasogastric tube may also be inserted to prevent aspiration if the patient is in danger of vomiting.

Immobility, sedation, circulatory impairment, decreased oral intake, use of opioid pain medications, and stress contribute to decreased peristalsis. The patient's inability to exhale against a closed glottis may make defecation difficult. As a result the ventilated patient is predisposed to constipation.

Musculoskeletal System. Maintenance of muscle strength and prevention of the problems associated with immobility are important. Exercise tolerance is enhanced by adequate analgesia and adequate nutrition. Progressive ambulation of patients receiving long-term ventilation can be attained without interruption of mechanical ventilation. The ventilator can be pushed around the room, or the patient can be ventilated with an oxygenated MRB while ambulating. Passive and active exercises, consisting of movements to maintain muscle tone in the upper and lower extremities, should be done in bed. Simple maneuvers such as leg lifts, knee bends, quadriceps setting, or arm circles are appropriate. Prevention of contractures, pressure areas, decubitus ulcers, foot drop, and external rotation of the hip and legs by proper positioning is important.

Psychologic Effects. The patient receiving mechanical ventilation may experience physical and emotional stress. Vital functions have been altered. The patient is unable to speak, eat, move, or breathe normally. Tubes and machines may cause fear and anxiety. Ordinary functions such as eating, elimination, or coughing are complicated. Death may seem inevitable. The patient's productive role in society and in the family is temporarily suspended. Being unable to participate fully in family matters may cause feelings of inadequacy, overwhelming helplessness, and frustration. These problems are compounded by sensory overload. Ringing alarms, constant lights, and frequent interruptions by personnel are stressful.

The patient must be given a means to communicate. A computer, paper and pencil, an alphabet, word or picture boards, or magic slate might be provided. In some instances tracheostomy tubes that allow speech can be used. The nurse should be attuned to the patient's body language and facial expressions, but this should not be allowed to substitute for providing the patient an opportunity for verbal expression.

Measures to make the ventilated patient's environment more restful include efficient scheduling of care to reduce interruptions and a calm, reassuring approach. Sedation may enhance sleep. The patient receiving long-term ventilation should be moved to an area with a window, to appreciate better night and day, and the outside world. Even if the patient is unable to converse, the patient should be addressed. The nurse should discuss the patient's interests and explain in simple terms what the different tubes and equipment are and what progress is being made. Reassuring the patient honestly about progress and allowing the patient as much control as possible may ease the frustration of dependence. Deciding when to bathe or wash hair, which direction to turn, or what to eat may be the patient's only way of maintaining control.

Machine Malfunction or Disconnection. Mechanical ventilators may malfunction or become disconnected. When turned on and operative, alarms alert the nurse to problems. Most deaths from accidental ventilator disconnections occur while the alarm is turned off, and most accidental disconnections in critical care settings are discovered by alarm activation. The most frequent site for disconnection is between the tracheal tube and the adapter. Disconnection is more likely with a tracheostomy tube than with a nasal or oral ET tube. The nurse should ascertain that alarms are set at all times and should chart that this is the case. Alarms should be paused (not inactivated) during suctioning or removal from the ventilator. Each assessment of the patient should include verification that alarms are set appropriately. The patient should be provided a call bell, so that the patient can bring attention to problems. Connections, particularly to tracheostomy tubes, should be pushed together and then twisted to secure them more tightly. The patient's bedside should be arranged so that an MRB with tubing sufficient to reach the patient is set up and functional at all times. Before placing the patient in a chair, the nurse should make sure that the MRB is accessible and functional and that the tubing will reach the patient in the event of an emergency. Although most institutions have emergency generators in the event of a power failure, the nurse should always consider the possibility that power will fail and have a plan for manually ventilating all the patients who are dependent on a ventilator.

Nutritional Management of the Patient Receiving Mechanical Ventilation

Mechanical ventilation, immobility, and the physical and emotional stresses of critical illness can contribute to poor nutrition. Presence of an ET tube eliminates the normal route for eating. Although patients who are nasotracheally intubated may be allowed liquid and semiliquid feedings orally, it is difficult to ingest sufficient calories, protein, and fat. A patient with a tracheostomy can eat normally once the wound has healed. When a tracheostomy tube is present, the cuff is usually inflated and the patient should tilt the head slightly forward to facilitate swallowing and to prevent aspiration. Often, soft foods (e.g., puddings, ice cream) are more easily swallowed than liquids.

Patients likely to be without food for 3 to 5 days should have a nutritional program initiated. Inadequate nutrition makes the patient receiving prolonged mechanical ventilation more prone to poor oxygen transport secondary to anemia and to poor tolerance of minimal exercise. Disuse of respiratory muscles and poor nutrition result in decreased respiratory muscle strength. In addition, caloric expenditure is elevated in the presence of fever, anxiety, pain, and the increased work of breathing. Serum protein levels (e.g., transferrin, prealbumin) are usually decreased. Inadequate nutrition can delay weaning, decrease the speed of recovery, and decrease resistance to infection. Total parenteral nutrition with intravenous fat emulsion or enteral feeding should be considered.

A concern regarding the nutritional support of patients on mechanical ventilation is the carbohydrate content of the diet. Metabolism of carbohydrates results in high levels of CO_2 production. The resulting CO_2 load results in a higher required minute ventilation. This in turn can cause an unnecessary increased effort to breathe. Decreasing carbohydrate content in the diet lowers CO_2 production. Preparations such as Pulmocare, which are high in protein and fat but low in carbohydrate content, may be beneficial in ventilated patients. A dietitian can provide useful consultation for the ventilated patient.

The intubated patient receiving nasogastric feedings should have the ET cuff inflated and the head of the bed elevated. A soft, flexible, small-bore, and easily positioned feeding tube should be used. When the tube is initially placed, the position of the tube is verified by x-ray. (Procedures for tube feedings are discussed in Chapter 37.)

Tube feedings should be stopped if the patient is in a head-down postural drainage position (for at least 30 minutes before treatment), if bowel sounds are absent, or if regurgitation occurs. The patient must be observed closely for signs of hypoglycemia if the tube feedings are discontinued for long periods of time. Food coloring in the feedings can help identify the presence of feedings in secretions suctioned from the trachea. The presence of a positive glucose reaction on a dipstick of tracheal secretions may indicate aspiration of feedings into the trachea. If there is evidence that aspiration may have occurred, the tube feeding should be stopped immediately and the physician notified.

Manual Resuscitation Bag and Suction Equipment

All patients receiving mechanical ventilation should have an MRB attached to oxygen and suctioning equipment ready and available at the bedside. There are two basic types of bags: the *anesthesia bag* and the *self-inflatable bag*. The anesthesia bag is used by the anesthesiologist in surgery to ventilate the patient. It delivers 100% oxygen. Self-inflatable bags vary in the concentration of oxygen delivered. Bags containing reservoir tubings or other devices to sequester oxygen deliver oxygen concentrations of 90% to 95%. The slower the bag is deflated and inflated, the higher the oxygen concentration that will be delivered. The Ambu (air mask bag unit) is the best known self-inflatable bag. This unit consists of a bag fitted to a face mask or a tracheal tube attachment.

Weaning from Mechanical Ventilation

The process of reducing ventilator support and resuming spontaneous ventilation is known as "weaning." Weaning may be of varying length, ranging from hours in postoperative open heart patients to weeks in the patient with chronic respiratory disease. Patients likely to require prolonged mechanical ventilation generally are those with underlying lung disease who develop respiratory failure because of surgical procedure, trauma, or infection. Preparations for weaning begin when the patient initially receives ventilation. These preparations include maintaining nutrition, exercise, fluid-electrolyte and acid-base balances, cardiac output, intracranial pressure, pulmonary, and psychologic status.

Readiness for weaning depends on many factors[18] (see Table 61-11). Criteria vary, depending on prior lung status and ventilatory reserve. For weaning to be successful, the patient should be as stable as possible. Respiratory parameters should demonstrate a patent airway, adequate ventilatory muscle strength, and an effective cough. Arterial oxygenation should be adequate, evidenced by a stable oxygen tension of at least 60 mm Hg, achieved with an FIO_2 of less than 0.5. The lungs should be reasonably clear on auscultation and chest x-ray. It is important to have an alert, well-rested patient relatively free from pain who will readily take deep breaths to obtain optimum alveolar ventilation and to prevent atelectasis. This does not mean complete withdrawal from sedatives or analgesics. Instead, medications should be titrated to relieve pain without causing excessive drowsiness.

Three weaning methods are commonly used. The patient might be placed on IMV or SIMV with ventilator breath frequency gradually reduced as the patient's ventilatory status permits. A second method uses pressure-support ventilation. Pressure amplitude is slowly decreased (e.g., 5 cm H_2O/hr, 5 cm H_2O/shift, etc.) until the patient is able to breathe spontaneously without pressure support. In a third method the patient is transferred periodically from assisted mechanical ventilation or IMV or SIMV to humidified oxygen through a T-piece or Briggs' adapter. The patient might be allowed spontaneous ventilation for 10 minutes each hour and receive ventilator support for 50 minutes, with the ratio of spontaneous ventilation to ventilation support gradually increasing. With all methods, patients usually require a 10% increase in FIO_2 to maintain arterial oxygen tension. This is because tidal volume usually drops with spontaneous respiration, and carbon dioxide tension may increase. Weaning is usually carried out during the day, with the patient ventilated at night until there is sufficient spontaneous ventilation without excess fatigue. Rest is important, regardless of the weaning technique used.

The patient being weaned should be provided continuing psychologic support. The weaning process should be explained and the patient informed of progress. The patient should be placed in a sitting or semirecumbent position and made comfortable. Respiratory parameters are measured to provide a baseline with which serial determinations can be compared. The tidal volume, negative inspiratory force, and vital capacity are measured. ABGs are drawn at baseline and at specified intervals during weaning. The cuff may be deflated totally or partially during weaning unless it is needed to prevent aspiration because the cuff may add to airway resistance.

The patient must be monitored closely for signs of respiratory distress, including shallow breathing, use of accessory respiratory muscles, restlessness, tiring, somnolence, tachycardia, decrease or increase in blood pressure, tachypnea or bradypnea, ECG changes, pallor or graying of mucous membranes, and secretion buildup with a need for frequent suctioning. Statements from the patient regarding weaning tolerance must be considered. The use of continuous oximetry is helpful during weaning.

When the patient is ready for extubation, the mouth should be thoroughly suctioned and the cuff deflated. An oxygen mask or cannula should be set up and ready for use. The patient should be told to expect to cough when the tube is removed. The nurse should be prepared to manage copious secretions. Once the patient has been extubated and stabilized with oxygen delivered by mask or cannula, care of the mouth and nares should be provided. ABGs are obtained 20 to 30 minutes after extubation. The patient must be monitored for respiratory distress caused by the underlying lung problems and also because laryngeal or tracheal edema may develop. Manifestations of laryngeal and tracheal edema include symptoms of acute upper airway obstruction. Measures to ensure pulmonary toilet (e.g., coughing, deep breathing, turning, and suctioning [if necessary]) must be continued.

Home Mechanical Ventilation

Mechanical ventilators are no longer limited to the ICU, but are now a part of home health care. Families can be taught to care for the person receiving mechanical ventilation as an alternative to prolonged hospitalization.[19-20] The emphasis on controlling hospital health care costs has increased the early discharge of patients and the need to provide highly technical care such as mechanical ventilation in home settings.

Home mechanical ventilation has several advantages. Having the patient in the home eliminates the strain that the hospital setting may impose on family dynamics. The feeling of helplessness by family members when they first hear about the necessity for long-term mechanical ventilation is frequently countered by the ability of the family to participate fully in the patient's care in the home setting. At home the patient may be able to participate more in activities of daily living around a more individualized schedule and, because of the smaller size of the home ventilator, be more mobile.[21] Another advantage of home mechanical ventilation is the reduction in the patient's risk of nosocomial infection. Disadvantages include problems related to reimbursement, equipment, caregiving, and the complex needs of these patients.[21] Ventilated patients are usually dependent, requiring extensive nursing care. In one study it was found that an average of 8 hours of care per day was required.[19] Disposable products may be nonreimbursable. Financial resources must be carefully assessed when arranging home mechanical ventilation. Another disadvantage of home mechanical ventilation is its potential impact on the family. Family members may seem enthusiastic about caring for their loved one in the home but may be motivated by guilt. They may lack understanding of the potential sacrifices they may have to make financially and in time and commitment.

Both negative-pressure and positive-pressure (volume) ventilators can be used in the home. Negative-pressure ventilators are frequently the ventilator of choice because they do not require an artificial airway and are less complicated to use. Small, portable volume ventilators that can be attached to a wheelchair or placed on a bedside table are available. Settings and alarms on these ventilators are similar to the larger ones used in ICUs. Some home ventilators have IMV capability.

NURSING MANAGEMENT

MECHANICAL VENTILATION

Nursing management of the patient receiving mechanical ventilation is outlined in the nursing care plan on p. 1984.

INTRACRANIAL PRESSURE MONITORING

Intracranial pressure (ICP) is the hydrostatic force measured in the brain cerebrospinal fluid (CSF) compartment. ICP may become elevated because of head trauma, stroke, subarachnoid hemorrhage, brain tumor, or other cause of brain tissue damage (Table 61-14). Any patient who becomes acutely unconscious, regardless of the cause, is managed as if there were actual or potential increased ICP. Patients with or at risk for elevated ICP are usually cared for in an ICU and often receive invasive ICP monitoring. As with other invasive ICU measures, ICP monitoring is provided to those who may benefit from treatment and in whom the underlying process is thought to be self-limiting. Patients with irreversible pathology or advanced neurologic decline caused by primary or metastatic lesions usually do not receive ICP monitoring. Nursing management goals in elevated ICP include preservation of function, early identification of neurologic changes, and prevention of complications. Patients may require intensive physical care and emotional support.

Pathophysiology and Clinical Manifestations

Important Variables. ICP is important because it influences *cerebral perfusion*. When evaluating cerebral perfusion, it is important to consider blood pressure, ICP, blood flow, vascular resistance, and blood volume. Mean arterial pressure (MAP) provides the driving force for brain blood flow. ICP, reflecting the pressure within the brain tissue and CSF, opposes blood flow. Thus *cerebral perfusion pressure* (CPP), which equals MAP minus ICP, is the clinically relevant variable that must be considered. *Cerebral blood flow*, expressed in milliliters of blood per minute, must be maintained at a relatively high rate because of the high and continuing metabolic needs of brain tissue. *Cerebral vascular resistance*, generated by the arterioles within the cranium, links CPP and blood flow as follows: CPP = flow × resistance. The volume of blood within the cranium (*intracranial blood volume*) is important because it affects ICP, as outlined later. Intracranial blood volume is contained primarily in the veins.

Normally, ICP remains low and changes in MAP occur without causing major changes in the blood flow to the brain. This is because as MAP increases, cerebral vascular resistance increases. As MAP decreases, cerebral vascular resistance decreases. In each case cerebral blood flow is relatively constant despite changes in perfusion pressure. Thus brain blood flow is said to be *autoregulated.*

Under normal conditions, the cranium contains brain tissue (80% of total volume), blood (10%), and CSF (10%). Because the skull is not distensible, any increase in volume of one of these components causes a decrease in volume of another component, an increase in ICP, or both. This is called the *Monro-Kellie doctrine*. For example, an increase in cranial volume occurs because of brain tissue swelling; early response might include reductions in CSF volume and blood volume in the cranium. CSF would shift from cranial spaces to the spinal subarachnoid space. Subarachnoid villi would absorb more CSF, thus reducing the amount of circulating CSF. Venous blood volume would decrease and venous return to the heart increase. As a result ICP and CPP would change little. However, decreases in CSF and blood volume are both limited responses. With more swelling, ICP would begin to increase.

The rate at which ICP increases with increased cranial volume is called *stiffness* (change in pressure/change in volume). *Compliance* is the inverse of stiffness (change in volume/change in pressure). A typical stiffness curve is illustrated in Fig. 61-13 (on p. 1987). In the normal volume range, small volume increases result in slight ICP increases. However, as ICP increases, the same small volume change results in larger ICP increases. The cranium is said to be stiff, or noncompliant. When the cranium is noncompliant, small decreases in cranial volume can result in large ICP decreases. Therapies are based on this observation. For example, CSF volume can be reduced by removing CSF via ventriculostomy, and this reduces ICP. Hyperventilation reduces carbon dioxide tension, which reduces intracranial blood flow and blood volume, in turn reducing ICP (see Table 61-15 on p. 1987).

Factors Affecting Cerebral Blood Flow. Normally vascular resistance changes so that cerebral blood flow is autoregulated, remaining fairly constant with changes in MAP. However, when MAP is extremely high, cerebral blood flow increases; when MAP is extremely low it decreases. Several factors (e.g., carbon dioxide and oxygen tension, sympathetic stimulation) modify the relationship between MAP and cerebral blood flow. Thus, even within

Table 61-14 Conditions Associated with Cerebral Edema

Head trauma	**Vascular insult**
Hemorrhage	Infarct (thrombotic or embolic)
Contusion (hematomas)	Ischemia and anoxia
Posttraumatic brain edema	**Toxic or metabolic**
Neurosurgery	Lead or arsenic
Involves tissue manipulation	Renal or liver failure
Mass lesions	Reye's syndrome
Neoplasm (primary or secondary)	**Infectious**
Abscess	Meningitis
Intracerebral and extracerebral hemorrhage	Encephalitis

NURSING CARE PLAN Patient on Mechanical Ventilation

Planning: Outcome Criteria	Nursing Interventions and Rationales
➤ **NURSING DIAGNOSIS**	Risk for injury *related to* possible machine malfunction, accidental disconnection, inability to breathe unassisted, asynchrony with ventilator, and settings unsuitable to maintain adequate ventilation
Have ABGs within normal range for patient; have early detection of signs and symptoms of decreased PaO_2 and increased $PaCO_2$; breathe synchronously with ventilator; have early detection, correction, or prevention of complications associated with mechanical malfunction or disconnection.	Monitor for risk factors such as hypoxemia, hypercapnia, tachycardia, tachypnea, increase in blood pressure, agitation, confusion, headache, lethargy, cyanosis; respiratory pattern asynchronous with machine's pattern of ventilation; machine malfunction or disconnection *to determine presence of risk factors and plan for interventions.* Begin mechanical ventilation slowly (especially in patients with COPD); lower $PaCO_2$ only to patient's baseline level *to prevent alkalosis, especially in patient with compensated respiratory acidosis.* ABGs should be drawn approximately 20 min after each ventilator change, serially thereafter, and whenever there are changes in patient's clinical status *to assess ventilatory status.* Assess patient for other possible causes of hyperventilation such as retained secretions, hypoxemia, pain, fear, and anxiety. Check ventilator settings (FIO_2, respiratory rate, tidal volume, O_2 flow rate, PEEP, airway pressure, thermistor temperature, and I/E ratio) *to determine if appropriate to clinical situation.* Keep manual resuscitation bag ventilator connected to O_2 source at bedside *for use in case of an emergency.* If patient is fighting ventilation, slowly bag for 3-6 breaths *to help synchronize them with ventilator.* Determine cause of asynchrony. Try verbally coaching patient to breathe with ventilator *to synchronize breathing.* Sedate with propofol, diazepam, or haloperidol as necessary *if pain or anxiety is identified as the cause.* Determine if patient receiving PEEP is pulling subatmospheric or negative airway pressures on inspiration *because this interferes with the effect of the treatment.* Turn all alarms on; pause but do not turn off alarms during suctioning and disconnections. Respond immediately to alarm *because potentially dangerous situations of mechanical malfunction or patient asynchrony with the ventilator may be present.* One person should bag ventilate patient while another person checks ventilator tubing for disconnections, leaks, and sticky bellows *so ventilation is not interrupted while the system is assessed.* When connecting ventilator circuit to artificial airway (especially tracheostomy), twist connection rather than pushing it together *to ensure secure connection.* Check cuff for leaks *to prevent loss of ventilation gas and to prevent aspiration of oral secretions.* Monitor weaning of patient carefully *to identify deterioration in status.* Monitor ventilator tubing q1-2hr for condensed water and drain when water present *to prevent aspiration of accumulated fluid.*
➤ **NURSING DIAGNOSIS**	Altered tissue perfusion and decreased cardiac output *related to* compromised venous return by positive-pressure ventilation *as manifested by* decreased blood pressure, increased heart rate, decreased cardiac output, decreased urine output, presence of dysrhythmias, mental confusion
Have blood pressure and cardiac output within normal range, no evidence of decreased tissue perfusion, adequate urinary output.	Monitor vital signs q2-4hr. Observe and monitor for clinical manifestations of decreased cardiac output *to identify decreased venous return to the heart, decreased left ventricular end-diastolic volume, decreased cardiac output, and lowered blood pressure.* Monitor direct measurement of cardiac output by thermodilution, especially when >10 cm H_2O PEEP is used, *to identify need for plasma expanders, vasopressors, and IV fluids as ordered because hemodynamic complications of decreased venous return induced by positive-pressure ventilation are exaggerated by hypovolemia.*
➤ **NURSING DIAGNOSIS**	Ineffective airway clearance *related to* presence of artificial airway, problems with positioning, accumulation of secretions, and immobility *as manifested by* presence of abnormal breath sounds, frequent or absent cough, presence of thick or copious secretions, high peak airway pressures, or frequent high-pressure alarm sounds on ventilator
Have normal breath sounds, thin and easily removed secretions.	Use large tidal volumes (12-15 ml/kg) *to increase mean airway pressures and decrease the risk of atelectasis.* Change patient's position q2hr *to prevent pooling of secretions in the lungs.* Have patient cough and, if feasible, deep breathe q2hr *to remove secretions and to prevent hypoventilation.* Auscultate breath sounds q2-4hr *to monitor effectiveness of interventions.*

continued

NURSING CARE PLAN Patient on Mechanical Ventilation—cont'd

Planning: Outcome Criteria	Nursing Interventions and Rationales
➤ **NURSING DIAGNOSIS**	Risk for respiratory infection *related to* exposure to environmental pathogens, presence of artificial airway, decreased resistance secondary to debilitated state, prolonged immobility, and inadequate nutrition*
➤ **NURSING DIAGNOSIS**	Altered nutrition: less than body requirements *related to* inability to take in nourishment orally and increased caloric demands secondary to clinical condition and need for mechanical ventilation†
➤ **NURSING DIAGNOSIS**	Impaired physical mobility *related to* restricted movement secondary to prolonged mechanical ventilation and clinical condition *as manifested by* inability to perform active range-of-motion exercises, presence of signs of pressure areas
Have normal range of motion of joints, no evidence of pressure sores or thromboemboli; be able to get out of bed for short periods of time if condition permits.	Provide progressive ambulation for patients receiving long-term ventilation *to prevent "pulmonary crippling."* Perform active and passive range-of-motion exercises (e.g., leg lifts, knee bends, quadriceps settings, arm circles) *to maintain patient's joint and muscle functioning and improve circulation.* Prevent contractures and external rotation of hips by proper positioning *to prevent musculoskeletal complications resulting from bed rest.* Observe for pressure areas *to ensure early detection and treatment of pressure sores.* Turn frequently *to prevent pressure areas.* Use footboard, high-top sneakers, and frequent foot flexion *to prevent foot drop.* Sit patient in chair as soon as medically feasible *to prevent the occurrence of complications associated with immobility.* Use pneumatic antiembolism stockings and prophylactic heparin as ordered *to reduce occurrence of thromboembolism.*
➤ **NURSING DIAGNOSIS**	Anxiety *related to* clinical condition, possible machine malfunction or disconnection, inability to communicate, environmental factors, possibility of death, and fear of suffocation and choking *related to* oral airway *as manifested by* expression of feelings of anxiety, anxious appearance, rigid body posture
Communicate feelings and anxieties; have absent or manageable anxiety level.	Assess patient's behavior of handling stressful situation *to determine a plan for interventions.* Be available to family and offer support *to lessen their anxiety and increase their cooperation.* Assure patient of continuous monitoring by well-trained staff *to increase ability to relax.* Give simple, honest explanations regarding care and progress *to foster a hopeful attitude and help patient make informed decisions.* Offer positive reinforcement for patient's behaviors that demonstrate improvement *to encourage patient further.* When possible, allow patient to make decisions regarding all aspects of care *to increase patient's sense of control.* Provide periods of privacy for patient and significant others *to demonstrate respect for the patient.* Converse with patient and family members about their interests. Provide diversion and occupational therapy as needed and tolerated *to relieve anxiety.* Schedule care to allow frequent rest periods *so patient does not become fatigued.* Encourage family to bring patient's personal items to bedside *to reduce patient's sense of isolation.* Provide calendar and clock *to promote patient orientation.* Refer to psychiatric liaison, clinical nurse specialist, psychiatrist, or hospital chaplain when appropriate *to offer additional counseling and support.*
➤ **NURSING DIAGNOSIS**	Sleep pattern disturbance *related to* anxiety, depression, and unfamiliar environmental factors *as manifested by* insomnia, restlessness, irritability, disorientation, morning headaches, psychotic behavior, awake frequently
Be rested on awakening; have no evidence of sleep disturbance; have minimal number of awakenings by caregivers for treatments.	Perform bedtime preparations (e.g., wash patient's face and hands, rub back, provide oral care) *to promote relaxation and facilitate sleep.* Turn off lights at night *to preserve usual sleep-wake cycle.* Provide pharmacologic intervention as ordered *to promote sleep.* Move patient to a room with window (if available) *to help with orientation to day and night.* Orient patient to person, place, and time. Provide relaxation techniques and tapes *to promote relaxation.* Schedule activities so that patient gets at least 2 hr of uninterrupted time to sleep. Schedule caregiving activities, family and friend visits *to allow for uninterrupted rest periods.* Consider allowing family members or friends to sit at bedside *to promote relaxation.*

continued

NURSING CARE PLAN Patient on Mechanical Ventilation—cont'd

Planning: Outcome Criteria	*Nursing Interventions and Rationales*
➤ NURSING DIAGNOSIS	Dysfunctional ventilatory weaning response *related to* inadequate nutrition, too-rapid pacing of the weaning process, insufficient knowledge of the weaning process, and anxiety *as manifested by* restlessness, tiring, somnolence, shallow breathing, use of accessory muscles, tachycardia, increased blood pressure, tachypnea, skin color changes (e.g., pallor or cyanosis)
Achieve progressive weaning goals; remain extubated; communicate increased comfort during weaning; be less tired from work of weaning.	Assess respiratory parameters (e.g., inspiratory effort, minute ventilation, vital capacity, effective cough) *to determine patient's weaning ability.* Explain the weaning process *so patient understands what is expected.* Prepare patient psychologically *to relieve anxiety and increase self-confidence.* Jointly negotiate progressive weaning goals *to involve patient in establishing the plan.* Adopt a weaning pace that will ensure success and minimize setbacks *to maintain patient confidence.* Provide regular rest periods *to reduce negative effects of anxiety and fatigue.* Draw ABGs at specified periods during the weaning *to monitor patient's ventilatory status.* Deflate cuff totally or partially during weaning *because tracheal tubes add to airway resistance.* Monitor for respiratory distress and place patient back on ventilator if observed *to ensure adequate ventilation.* If the weaning process is discontinued, explain rationale and revised plan to patient *to minimize frustration and disappointment and enhance cooperation.*

COLLABORATIVE PROBLEMS

Nursing Goals	*Nursing Interventions and Rationales*
➤ POTENTIAL COMPLICATION	Gastric distention *related to* improper tube placement, GI bleeding, or paralytic ileus
Perform abdominal assessment; identify gastric distention and institute appropriate diagnostic and therapeutic procedures.	Assess for abdominal distention, tympany, and bowel sounds and measure abdominal girth *to detect signs of bowel dilatation.* Test stools and gastric drainage for occult blood *because the patient is at risk of developing stress ulcers and GI bleeding.* Monitor postural vital signs and hematocrit *to detect blood loss.* Assess patient's complaints of pain, fullness, bloated feeling, or need for laxative *to evaluate bowel status.* Maintain adequate bowel evacuation program *because patient may have difficulty defecating as a result of being unable to exhale against a closed glottis.* Check for gastric air on chest x-ray. Administer antacids, H_2-receptor blocker, and tube feedings as ordered *to reduce the occurrence of GI bleeding and to decrease the acidity of gastric secretions.* If abdominal distention is present, elevate head of bed *to allow for optimal diaphragmatic excursion.* Obtain order and place nasogastric tube or, if present, confirm patency by irrigating to relieve gastric tension. Confirm correct position of nasogastric tube *to prevent aspiration and the accumulation of GI fluids.*
➤ POTENTIAL COMPLICATION	Pneumothorax or pneumomediastinum secondary to barotrauma caused by positive-pressure ventilation
Monitor for signs of pneumothorax; report positive findings; and carry out appropriate medical and nursing interventions.	Observe for manifestations of pneumothorax such as sudden increase (by 5 cm H_2O or more) in peak inspiratory pressure, sudden patient agitation or coughing, frequent activation of high-pressure alarm, decrease in static and effective compliance, palpable subcutaneous emphysema over neck and anterior chest areas, deterioration in ABGs and blood pressure, decrease or absence of breath sounds, hyperresonance on percussion; pneumothorax on chest x-ray. If pneumothorax is suspected, obtain chest x-ray *to confirm.* Bag ventilate with O_2 using tidal volume *to reduce airway pressures until a chest tube can be inserted.* Notify physician and set up for chest tube insertion immediately *because pneumothorax can convert to a life-threatening tension pneumothorax.* Check and record ventilator settings q4hr. Record level of peak inspiratory pressure *to establish baseline data to evaluate changes in lung compliance.*‡

ABGs, Arterial blood gases; *COPD,* chronic obstructive pulmonary disease; *GI,* gastrointestinal; *I/E,* inspiration/expiration; *PEEP,* positive end-expiratory pressure.

*Interventions for this nursing diagnosis are presented in the nursing care plan for the patient with an artificial airway (earlier this chapter).

†Interventions for this nursing diagnosis are presented in the nursing care plan for the patient with acute respiratory failure (Chapter 26).

‡This assessment is especially important in patients receiving PEEP because they are at risk for barotrauma.

Table 61-15 Factors Altering Intracranial Blood Volume

Increased Blood Volume*	Decreased Blood Volume
Increased arterial CO_2 tension Hypoxemia Sympathetic blockade (decreases sensitivity to CO_2 tension) Valsalva maneuver Positive end-expiratory pressure Halothane anesthesia Isometric exercise Neck flexion	Decreased arterial CO_2 tension Elevated arterial O_2 tension Sympathetic stimulation (sensitizes to CO_2 tension)

*Increased blood volume can be associated with increased intracranial pressure.

the normal range of MAP, there can be variation in cerebral blood flow (Fig. 61-14).

When MAP falls (while ICP is normal and constant), cerebral resistance falls. Arterioles dilate, keeping blood flow constant. Locally released factors contribute to this dilatation. As MAP falls below 60 mm Hg, arteriolar dilatation is limited. Therefore blood flow decreases and ischemia develops. The patient with elevated ICP would be more vulnerable to ischemia with low MAP. When MAP increases (assuming normal ICP), vascular resistance increases. Arterioles constrict and blood flow remains constant. This process is limited. With high MAP (e.g., exceeding 160 mm Hg), flow increases as pressure increases. Increased flow may bring increased blood volume, elevating ICP.

Arterial CO_2 tension is the most potent regulator of cerebral blood flow. Reducing CO_2 tension by hyperventilation diminishes cerebral blood flow. This may be associated with a decreased blood volume and may contribute to lowering ICP. A patient with elevated ICP may be deliberately overventilated to reduce ICP. Elevated CO_2 tension (e.g., hypoventilation) increases cerebral blood flow, possibly increasing blood volume and ICP. Thus, respiratory status is carefully monitored in the patient with an actual or potential ICP problem. It is likely that the effect of CO_2 is mediated via changes in the pH of CSF, with acidosis causing arteriolar dilatation. Chronic metabolic acidosis, which lowers the pH of CSF, results in increased cerebral blood flow. Patients with diabetic coma have a high cerebral blood flow. Chronic alkalosis decreases cerebral blood flow.

Arterial O_2 tension has an effect opposite that of CO_2 tension: diminished O_2 tension increases blood flow. There is a sharp increase in cerebral blood flow with arterial O_2 tension less than 50 to 60 mm Hg. Because increased flow may be associated with increased blood volume, and thus elevations in ICP, the patient with increased ICP is monitored carefully to avoid hypoxemia. Cerebral blood flow is constant within the normal range of oxygen tensions.

Sympathetic stimulation modifies cerebral blood flow responses, causing vasoconstriction. However, the blood-brain barrier prevents circulating catecholamines from altering cerebral circulation.

Venous outflow obstruction can dramatically increase ICP. Obstructing the veins increases intracranial blood

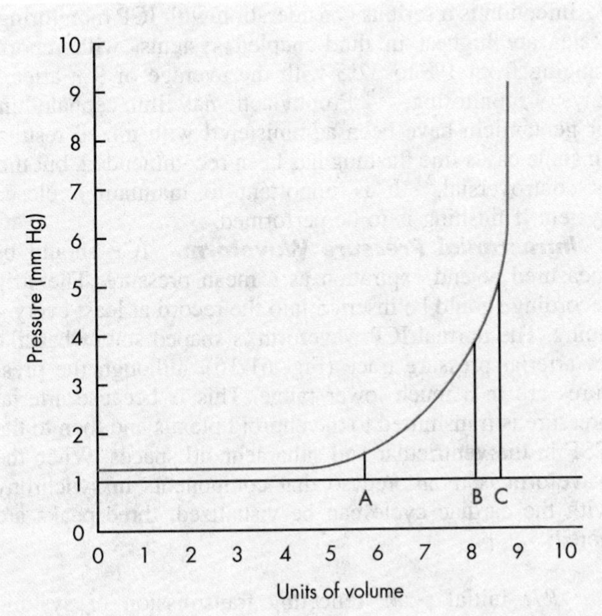

Fig. 61-13 Intracranial volume-pressure curve. ***A,*** Pressure is normal, and increases in intracranial volume are tolerated with little increase in intracranial pressure. ***B,*** Increases in volume cause moderate increases in pressure. ***C,*** Small increases in volume cause large increases in pressure.

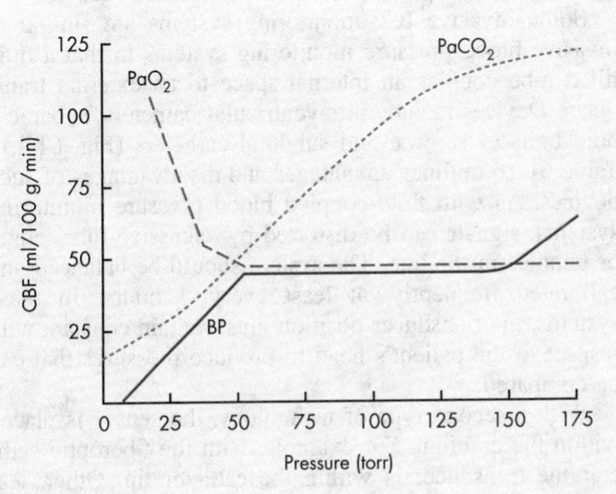

Fig. 61-14 Effects of independent changes in arterial blood pressure, oxygen, or carbon dioxide on cerebral blood flow (CBF).

volume. In the noncompliant brain, such an increase dramatically increases the ICP. The jugular vein can be obstructed by rotation of the head to either side. Thus, the patient with potential ICP elevation is positioned with the head midline.

Clinical Applications. Elevated ICP is clinically significant because it diminishes CPP, causing brain ischemia or infarction. Also, brain structures can be compressed and damaged or irreversibly destroyed. Death can occur. High ICP causes *herniation* of brain tissue, that is, extrusion into abnormal spaces. Cerebral hemispheres can shift across the midline. Brain stem and cerebral hemispheres can herniate through the tentorium cerebelli. The cerebellum can herniate through the foramen magnum ("tonsillar herniation"). These complications are generally fatal.

A slow increase in ICP, as with an enlarging brain tumor, is tolerated better than a rapid increase, as in primary brain injury. If an elevated pressure is evenly distributed throughout the brain, it is better tolerated. Crucial to preservation of tissue is preservation of cerebral blood flow. With slower, distributed rises, blood flow tends to be preserved.

CPP is useful in evaluating brain blood flow. Normal CPP is 70 to 100 mm Hg. At least 50 to 60 mm Hg is necessary for adequate cerebral perfusion. CPP less than 30 to 40 mm Hg is associated with ischemia and neuronal death. It is of paramount importance to maintain blood pressure when ICP is elevated. It should be remembered that CPP might not reflect perfusion pressure in all parts of the brain. There may be local areas of swelling and compression. Thus tissue damage may occur even with an adequate CPP.

Intracranial Pressure Measurement and Line Management

Technical Apparatus. In 1960 a technique was refined for continuous ICP monitoring using a ventricular catheter.[22] Since that time, technology for monitoring ICP has greatly improved. ICP monitoring is used regularly to guide therapy in patients with suspected increased ICP.

Some invasive ICP monitoring systems are similar to invasive blood pressure monitoring systems in that a fluid filled tube couples an internal space to an external transducer. Devices include intraventricular catheters, subarachnoid bolts or screws, and subdural catheters (Fig. 61-15). Table 61-16 outlines advantages and disadvantages of such devices. As with fluid-coupled blood pressure monitoring systems, signals can be distorted by excessive tube length or bubbles in the line. The system should be balanced and calibrated frequently, at least every 4 hours. In these systems, the transducer position must remain constant with respect to the patient's head to produce pressures that can be compared.

With a second type of technology, the sensor is placed within the cranium. For example, with the fiberoptic catheter the transducer is within the catheter tip. Other, less commonly used transducers include pneumatic systems, or intracranial strain gauges. These systems produce excellent quality waveforms and do not require repositioning with

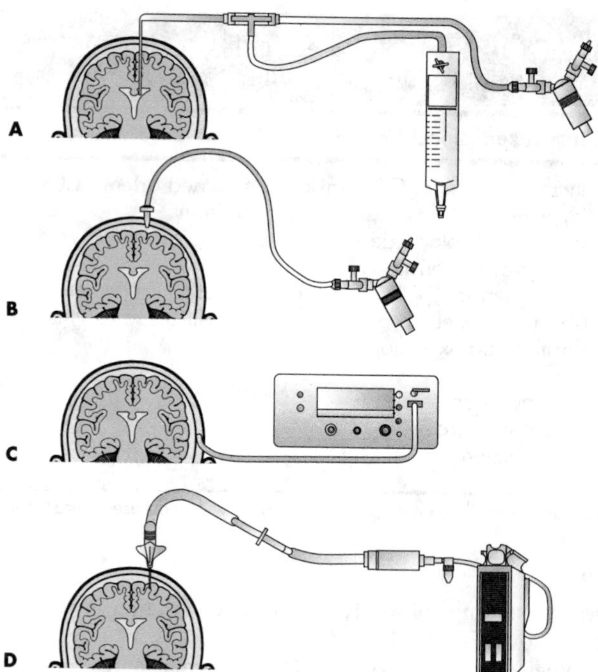

Fig. 61-15 ***A,*** Ventricular pressure monitoring system. ***B,*** Subarachnoid pressure monitoring system. ***C,*** Epidural pressure monitoring system. ***D,*** Intraparenchymal pressure monitoring system.

patient movement. They usually cannot be rebalanced and recalibrated.

Infection is a serious consideration with ICP monitoring. Rates are highest in fluid-coupled systems, with reports ranging from 1% to 22% with the average of 9% after 5 days of monitoring.[23,24] Prophylactic nafcillin, cephalothin, or gentamicin have been administered with mixed results. In some cases line flushing has been recommended, but this is controversial.[24] It is important to maintain a closed system if flushing is to be performed.

Intracranial Pressure Waveform. ICP should be measured at end expiration as a mean pressure. The strip recording should be inserted into the record at least every 4 hours. The normal ICP waveform is shaped somewhat like an arterial pressure trace (Fig. 61-16), although the pressures are in a much lower range. This is because arterial pressure is transmitted to the choroid plexus and then to the CSF in the ventricular and subarachnoid spaces. When the waveform is monitored so that components in synchrony with the cardiac cycle can be visualized, three peaks are noted:

- *P1:* initial peak, reflecting transmission of systolic arterial pressure from the choroid plexus
- *P2:* (the "tidal wave") reflects venous pressure; ends in the dicrotic notch
- *P3:* third wave, follows the dicrotic notch; also may reflect venous pressure

Table 61-16 Comparison of Intracranial Pressure Monitoring Systems

System	Description	Advantages	Disadvantages
Ventricular Catheter	External transducer system; soft, radiopaque Silastic tube inserted via stylet, usually through a twist drill hole into anterior horn of lateral ventricle of nondominant hemisphere	Accurate (can balance, calibrate) CSF can be tapped to reduce ICP and sample CSF Compliance can be tested Contrast media can be inserted for diagnostic tests	Infection risk Hemorrhage risk Difficult to place in patient with small ventricles or intracranial shift Transducer must be repositioned with head movement
Subarachnoid Screw or Bolt	External transducer system; hollow metal shaft or screw, threaded at one end; threaded end is inserted through a hole drilled into bone through dura into subarachnoid space; placed over frontal area of nondominant hemisphere so that same site can be used for subsequent placement of ventricular catheter if needed.	Simple insertion procedure Useful if ventricle is small or shifted No disruption of neuron tissue of brain Less risk of infection, hemorrhage	Leaks can limit accuracy Obstruction by blood or brain tissue can distort readings Some risk of infection (less than ventriculostomy) Intact skull is required Not useful for draining CSF Not useful for compliance testing If made of metal, patient cannot have MRI performed Transducer must be repositioned with head motion
Fiberoptic Devices	Intracranial transducer system; catheter consists of a mobile mirrored diaphragm; fiberoptic signal is bounced off diaphragm and sensed by another fiberoptic cable within the same catheter; usually has CSF sampling port; can be placed into ventricle, subdural, subarachnoid space, or brain parenchyma	Versatile regarding site Insertion possible through subarachnoid bolt Irrigation not necessary Detailed, artifact-free waveform produced If intraventricular, CSF can be tapped to reduce ICP and sample CSF No need to modify equipment with head movement	Catheter fragile Once positioned, rebalancing and calibration not possible Unique monitoring system required (but couples to most oscilloscopes) Expensive

CSF, Cerebrospinal fluid; *ICP,* intracranial pressure; *MRI,* magnetic resonance imaging.

Three types of pathologic waves might be seen when ICP is elevated. Visualization of these requires monitoring with a slowly moving strip recorder.

- *A:* "Plateau waves," seen with ICP elevations of 50 to 100 mm Hg; last 5 to 20 min; associated with a fall in CPP to less than 40 mm Hg; associated with severe cerebral ischemia; signal a neurologic emergency and must be treated promptly to avoid irreversible brain damage
- *B:* sharp, rhythmic pressure elevations of 20 to 40 mm Hg; frequency of 1 per 30 to 120 seconds; seen with changes in the respiratory pattern; may be precursors of A waves
- *C:* transient rhythmic pressure elevations of less than 20 mm Hg; frequency of one every 4 to 8 minutes; significance not determined

It is important that the nurse monitor ICP waveform, as well as mean pressure. It has been noted that when the height of P2 is higher than P1, the intracranial space may be noncompliant and the patient is at risk for development of elevated ICP.[25] The patient must be monitored for pathologic waves. In addition to noting pressure measurements and waveform morphology, it is important to consider the rate at which changes occur and the patient's clinical condition. It is important to note that neurologic deterioration might not occur until ICP elevation is pronounced and sustained.[26] If A or B waves are noted, the physician must be informed immediately.

In fluid-coupled systems, the waveform should be inspected for damping, which could indicate the presence of bubbles in the line or that the line is obstructed with tissue blood clots. Inaccurate ICP readings can be caused by CSF leaks around the monitoring device, obstruction of the intraventricular catheter or bolt, difference in the height of the bolt and the transducer, kinks in the tubing, and the Valsalva maneuver.

Cerebrospinal Fluid Drainage. With the ventricular catheter and certain fiberoptic systems, it is possible to control ICP by removing CSF. To do this, a Y-connector is inserted in the line. A closed system should be used to decrease infection risk. ICP and drainage volume are

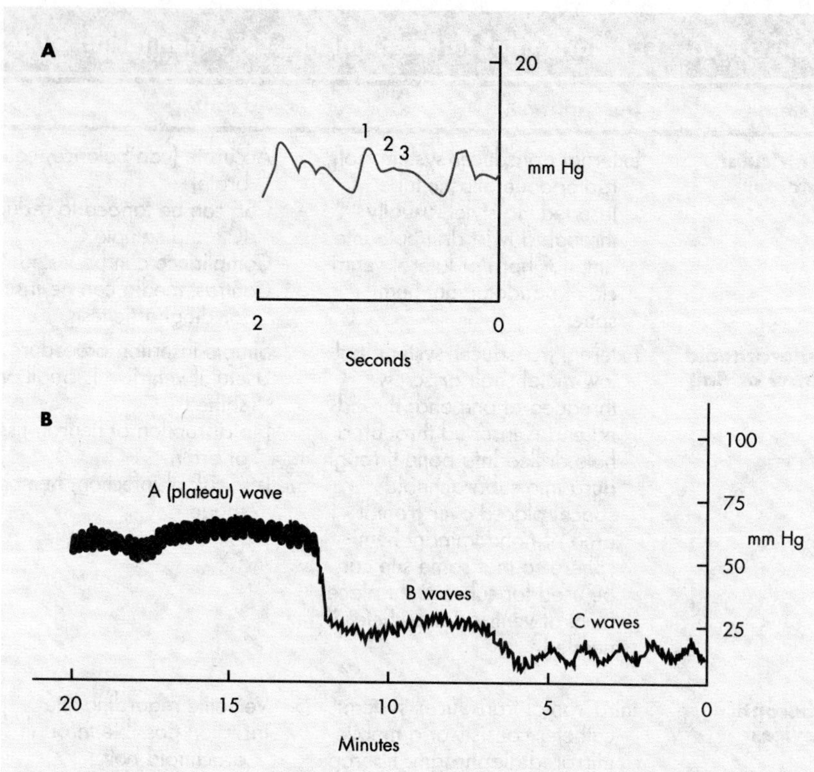

Fig. 61-16 ***A,*** Intracranial pressure (ICP) waveform as noted on a fast time scale recording. 1, 2, 3 indicate P1, P2, P3 (see text). ***B,*** Pathologic ICP waves as noted on a slow time scale recording.

controlled by the height of the drainage bag or drip chamber relative to the patient reference point. Typically, a point 15 cm above the ear canal is selected. Raising the system diminishes drainage (ICP becomes higher); lowering the system increases drainage volume (ICP becomes lower). Careful monitoring of volume of CSF drained is essential, keeping in mind that normal adult CSF production is about 20 to 30 ml per hour, with a total CSF volume of 90 to 150 ml within the ventricles and subarachnoid space. The amount of fluid to be drained, the height of the highest point in the system, and other details of the drainage should be ordered by the physician.

Ventricular collapse, a major complication of this type of drainage system, occurs when fluid is removed too rapidly. Another complication of rapid decompression is development of a subdural hematoma. A common technique to ensure that fluid is not removed too rapidly is the use of intermittent drainage. With this method the line would typically be opened to drain 4 times per hour.

THERAPEUTIC AND NURSING MANAGEMENT

INCREASED INTRACRANIAL PRESSURE

Care of the patient with actual or potential increased ICP is similar to that described for the patient with primary brain injury or the unconscious patient (see Chapter 54). Specific therapies to decrease intracranial volume and ICP may be indicated. Therapies include hyperventilation, oxygenation, osmotic diuresis, nonosmotic diuresis, fluid restriction, CSF removal, corticosteroids, blood pressure control, positioning, and environmental restructuring. Intensive monitoring is required, including vital signs, heart rate and rhythm, ventilation, oxygenation, fluid balance, mental status and level of consciousness, ICP, cranial nerve function, peripheral movement, and sensation.

Hyperventilation and Oxygenation. Iatrogenic hyperventilation is often prescribed to reduce cerebral blood flow and thus cerebral blood volume. CO_2 tension of 25 mm Hg has been recommended, with tensions less than 20 mm Hg to be avoided.[27] Arterial pH should not exceed 7.6. The impact of this therapy is greatest in the initial 24 to 48 hours; it then diminishes as the pH of CSF normalizes. Rather than ceasing treatment abruptly, overventilation should be gradually decreased. Oxygenation should be maintained; arterial oxygen tensions greater than 100 mm Hg are recommended. Many patients with brain injury spontaneously hyperventilate. Overventilation may require sedation, intubation, and mechanical ventilation.

Hyperventilation is used when ICP monitoring has documented pressure elevation and in conditions commonly characterized by ICP elevation, such as head injury, Reye's syndrome, and fulminant hepatic failure. Hyperventilation is contraindicated in patients with focal ischemia or stroke because the resulting diminished blood flow can further impair circulation to the affected area, increasing ischemia. Hyperventilation is contraindicated in subarachnoid hemorrhage because it can increase vasospasm, causing further injury.[28]

If the patient requires ET intubation, the tube must be secured without ties around the neck. Neck ties impede venous return, thus elevating ICP. In patients with normal

ICP, ET suctioning is usually well tolerated. In patients with elevated ICP, suctioning can be dangerous. Three factors associated with suctioning might contribute to ICP elevation: hypercapnia, hypoxemia, and stress. Suctioning should be performed in patients with elevated ICP only when auscultatory examination confirms that suctioning is necessary.[29] The patient should be hyperinflated and preoxygenated before and after the procedure.

PEEP may be necessary to maintain oxygenation. However, PEEP increases mean intrathoracic pressure, so it may impede venous return and increase ICP. It is anticipated that suppression of venous return would be greatest in the patient with extracellular fluid volume deficit and in the patient with a highly compliant chest. Whenever intrathoracic pressures are changed, the effect on the ICP should be evaluated. Elevation of the bed 30 degrees can improve oxygenation, so the patient requires less PEEP. Similarly, relief of abdominal distention via a nasogastric tube can promote lung expansion and improve oxygenation.

Osmotic Diuresis, Nonosmotic Diuresis, and Fluid Restriction

Osmotic diuresis is prescribed to pull fluid from brain cells, diminishing brain volume. This therapy requires an intact blood-brain barrier because the osmotic agent must remain restricted in the vascular space, pulling water into that space. Mannitol (20% solution) is commonly used. It can be administered as a bolus (peak effect in approximately 20 minutes, lasts 4 to 6 hours) or as a continuous infusion. Serum osmolality should be monitored and maintained at 305 to 310 mOsm/kg (normal 285 to 295 mUsm/kg). Serum osmolality greater than 310 to 320 mOsm/kg can be dangerous. Complications of osmotic diuresis include hypernatremia, hypervolemia, and renal failure. Osmotic therapy is used cautiously in patients with potential cardiac failure. Rebound increases in ICP can occur. Furosemide and acetazolamide (nonosmotic diuretics) are useful because they diminish the rate of CSF production. The effects of furosemide and mannitol are additive, thus the drugs are often combined. Osmotic therapy may be combined with free water restriction, contributing to the reduction of intracellular volume and increasing the hyperosmolar state. Both saline and free water should be administered with extreme caution in patients with ICP problems.

Other Therapies

CSF removal may be prescribed to lower CSF volume and thus ICP. Because the patient with elevated ICP often has a noncompliant brain, removal of several millileters of CSF can substantially lower ICP. CSF removal is always performed cautiously, slowly, and against a counterpressure to avoid ventricular collapse. As noted previously, infection is a serious risk.

Corticosteroids are commonly administered in acute brain injury with the goal of diminishing the inflammatory response. Although steroid effectiveness is well established in treating edema associated with intracranial tumors, efficacy in acute brain injury is not proven. Studies demonstrate that corticosteroids do not reduce ICP, improve neurologic outcome, or improve mortality after head injury, intracerebral hemorrhage, nor cerebral infarction. Complications of corticosteroid administration include infection, sepsis, and hyperglycemia.

The blood pressure must be high enough to sustain a CPP greater than 50 mm Hg. Thus, as ICP rises, a rise in blood pressure maintains cerebral perfusion. The higher blood pressure should not be treated.

It is routine to elevate the bed 30 to 45 degrees when a patient has increased ICP. The head should be maintained midline to prevent venous outflow obstruction. The patient should be told to avoid Valsalva maneuvers and isometric exercise because these increase ICP. The patient may require assistance in turning to prevent the effects of isometric exercise with moving in bed. The patient should cross both arms on the chest during repositioning, rather than attempting to assist. An overhead trapeze should *not* be provided because the patient is to avoid this type of exercise. Patients are instructed to exhale while being turned. Stool softeners should be routinely administered to avoid the Valsalva manuever during bowel evacuation.

There is some evidence that restructuring the patient's environment to limit stress is potentially important. Conversations about the patient's condition within the patient's hearing can be associated with increased ICP, even in the apparently comatose. The presence of family members and provision of comfort measures such as gentle stroking can cause ICP to fall.

SYSTEMIC INFLAMMATORY RESPONSE AND MULTIPLE ORGAN DYSFUNCTION SYNDROMES

Significance

Sepsis, septic shock, systemic inflammatory response syndrome (SIRS), and multiple organ dysfunction syndrome (MODS) are common, serious, and interrelated complications in ICU patients. (See definitions in Table 61-17.) Sepsis is the thirteenth leading cause of death in the United States and the most common cause of death in noncoronary critical care units.[30] Sepsis is the most common cause of death in trauma patients, causing about 75% of deaths in non–head-injured trauma cases. It is estimated that more than 400,000 patients develop sepsis annually and that gram-negative organisms are responsible for approximately one half of these cases of sepsis.[31] Despite improved critical care, the mortality rates from severe sepsis and related shock have changed little over the past decades. Septic shock has a mortality rate of 40% to 60%[31] The mortality rate for patients with ARDS is 50% to 70%, with most of those dying from sepsis and MODS.[32,33] A variety of factors cause an increased susceptibility to sepsis, SIRS, and MODS (Table 61-18).

A paradoxic dilemma faces the health care provider. The ICU may be the only environment where a critically ill patient can be sustained, yet it is an environment in which there is high risk for infection. In addition, there is a high prevalence of multiresistant microorganisms. It is a major nursing responsibility to institute the highest standards of asepsis in caring for immunocompromised patients who are vulnerable to infection.

Table 61-17 Definition of Terms

Term	Definition
▪ Systemic inflammatory response syndrome (SIRS)	Abnormal host response characterized by generalized inflammation in organs remote from patient's initial insult. Can be caused by infectious or noninfectious insults. Characterized by acute development of two or more of the following: fever or hypothermia, tachycardia, tachypnea, leukocytosis or leukopenia, or the presence of >10% immature polymorphonuclear cells.
▪ Multiple organ dysfunction syndrome (MODS)	Progressive failure of two or more organ systems. Failure may or may not be related to initial injury.
Primary MODS	Occurs early and results from well-defined insult.
Secondary MODS	Results from uncontrolled systemic inflammation with resultant organ dysfunction. Develops latently after several insults.
▪ Bacteremia	Presence of viable bacteria in the blood. Demonstrated by positive culture.
▪ Sepsis	Presence of SIRS associated with an infectious process.
▪ Septic shock	Sepsis with hypotension, circulatory collapse, and decreased tissue perfusion (see Chapter 7).

Table 61-18 Risk Factors Related to Sepsis, Systemic Inflammatory Response Syndrome, and Multiple Organ Dysfunction Syndrome

Advanced age	Invasive catheters and monitoring devices
Burns	Major trauma
Diabetes mellitus	Malignancy
Hepatic failure	Malnutrition
HIV infection	Prolonged hospital stay
Hyposplenism	Underlying chronic illness
Immunosuppression	

HIV, Human immunodeficiency virus.

Pathophysiology

The pattern and causes of the clinical and physiologic changes in SIRS and MODS are beginning to be better understood. Transition from the hypermetabolic state of SIRS to clinically defined MODS does not occur in a clear-cut manner. This may be because these two entities represent a continuum. In addition, it is difficult to measure organ dysfunction at its earliest stage. One way to describe these syndromes is to use an *activator-mediator-responder organ* framework.

Activators. Activators are substances initiating systemic inflammatory responses. The initial insult that stimulates SIRS can come from a variety of sources (see Fig. 61-17). Bacteria are common activators, including staphylococci, meningococci, *Salmonella,* malaria, *Escherichia coli, Klebsiella,* and *Pseudomonas*. Sepsis associated with gram-negative organisms tends to have the worst prognosis. Other microorganisms causing sepsis include fungi, virus, rickettsia, protozoa, and mycobacterium. The most common sites of infection include the genitourinary tract, GI tract, respiratory tract, wounds, vascular access sites, and nasal sinuses. Microorganisms release toxins that serve as activators and elicit the release of systemic mediators. Exotoxins are released from certain bacteria (e.g., *Staphylococcus aureus* and *Clostridium perfringens*). Endotoxins originate from the cell walls of gram-negative bacteria (e.g., *E. coli, Pseudomonas*). These substances often have direct toxic effects and can activate cellular and humoral immune responses, and ultimately cause sepsis, SIRS, or MODS.

Other activators include dead or injured tissue (resulting from trauma or impaired perfusion), resolving hematomas (especially of the peritoneum or pelvis), and antigen-antibody reactions. Because these substances may stimulate release of the same mediators as invading microorganisms, it may be difficult to distinguish the patient with sepsis from the patient with SIRS caused by a noninfectious agent.

Mediators. Mediators are substances released by the body in response to activators. Whatever the stimulus, the cause of SIRS and MODS seems to be an uncontrollable systemic inflammatory response where the interaction and effects of multiple mediator systems and their by-products are important (Table 61-19, Fig. 61-18).

When the inflammatory process is not controlled, consequences may occur that can lead to SIRS and MODS. These include activation of inflammatory cells and release of mediators, direct damage to the vascular endothelium, hypermetabolism, and maldistribution of blood flow to organs.[34] During SIRS endothelial cells are common targets for WBC-derived mediators, which cause endothelial destruction and vascular permeability. Inflammatory mediators causing endothelial damage include endotoxin, tumor necrosis factor (TNF), interleukin-1 (IL-1), platelet activating factor (PAF), and many others (Table 61-19).

Responding Systems. Responding systems include the respiratory, cardiovascular, GI, renal, hepatic, neuro-

Table 61-19 Mediators of Sepsis, Systemic Inflammatory Response Syndrome, and Multiple Organ Dysfunction Syndrome

Mediator	Action
Endotoxin (component of gram-negative bacterial cell wall)	Stimulation of monocytes, macrophages, and neutrophils to produce cytokines
Interleukin-1	Vasodilatation, increased capillary permeability
Tumor necrosis factor	Vasodilatation, increased capillary permeability
Hageman factor	Activation of intrinsic clotting system
Prekallikrien	Production of bradykinin
Bradykinin	Arteriolar vasodilatation, increased capillary permeability, leukocyte chemotaxis
Complement components C3a, C5a	Neutrophil aggregation, release of toxic oxygen products, histamine release, vasodilatation, increased capillary permeability
Prostaglandins	Vasodilatation, decreased platelet aggregation
Platelet activating factor	Decreased renal perfusion, decreased coronary blood flow, decreased cardiac output
Histamine	Vasodilatation, increased capillary permeability
Catecholamines	Inotropic stimulation, altered regional blood flow
Cortisol	Gluconeogenesis, hyperglycemia
Myocardial depressant factor	Decreased cardiac contractility and output

logic, and hematologic systems. The lungs are highly vulnerable to mediator-induced injury and are generally the first organ system affected in MODS. Acute lung injury manifests as ARDS and generally occurs 1 to 3 days after the initial injury (ARDS is discussed in Chapter 26). ARDS is frequently accompanied by a hypermetabolic response.[35]

Cardiovascular changes include vasodilatation and venodilatation. Vasodilatation results in decreased systemic vascular resistance (decreased afterload) and decreased blood pressure. The baroreceptor reflex causes release of inotropic (increasing force of contraction) and chronotropic (increasing heart rate) factors that enhance cardiac output. For a while, blood pressure may be maintained but at a higher heart rate and cardiac output. Venodilatation decreases preload, thus limiting cardiac output. Increases in capillary permeability result in shifting of albumin and fluid from the vascular space, which further diminishes preload. The patient is warm and tachycardic with a high cardiac output and a low systemic vascular resistance. Mixed venous oxygen saturation may be abnormally high because the patient is perfusing areas not consuming much oxygen (e.g., skin, nonworking muscle). Eventually, perfusion of vital organs becomes insufficient and their function is compromised.

Mental changes are common with sepsis and SIRS. Acute alteration in mental status can be an early sign of SIRS. The patient may become confused and agitated, combative, disoriented, lethargic, or comatose. These changes may be due to hypoxemia or impaired perfusion. Mediators may damage neuronal tissue directly or indirectly via capillary leakage and related tissue damage.

Renal failure may result from prerenal causes (impaired perfusion) or from direct damage to renal tubular cells (acute tubular necrosis [ATN]). The frequent use of nephrotoxic drugs (see Table 42-2) for critically ill patients also increased the risk of ATN.

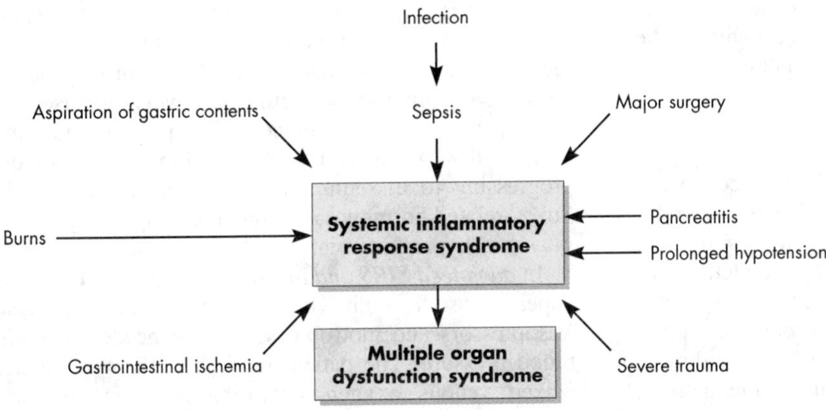

Fig. 61-17 Causes of systemic inflammatory response syndrome and multiple organ dysfunction syndrome.

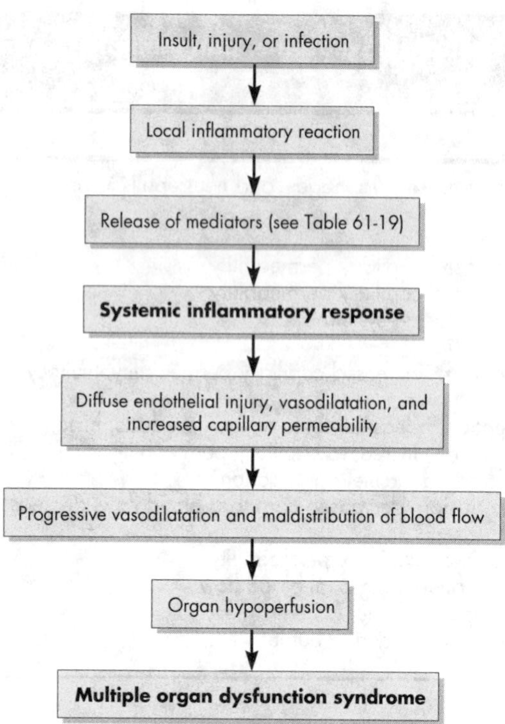

Fig. 61-18 Pathophysiology of systemic inflammatory response syndrome and multiple organ dysfunction syndrome.

The GI system is extremely vulnerable to ischemia. Impaired GI circulation may diminish motility, causing paralytic ileus. The most fragile tissue of the GI tract is mucosal epithelium. Following injury the potential for translocation of GI luminal bacteria into the systemic circulation is increased. This mechanism may be a source of additional activators (bacteria) of the septic process. Mucosal ischemia results in an increased incidence of gastric and duodenal ulcer formation. The patient is also at risk for GI bleeding.

Initially *leukocytosis* (increased white blood cell count) generally occurs. This is especially true if the activator is a microorganism. However, in time hematopoiesis is impaired, causing anemia, leukopenia, and thrombocytopenia. There is also an increased risk for internal bleeding.

Liver dysfunction may result in clinical evidence of bleeding, jaundice, hypoglycemia, and lactic acidosis. The patient develops hypoproteinemia because of a shift in the liver activity toward production of acute phase proteins. The serum level of liver enzymes is increased.

Metabolic changes are pronounced. Mediators such as catecholamines and glucocorticoids result in hyperglycemia. If hepatic insufficiency is severe, hypoglycemia occurs. Initially, glucose oxidation is high. There is a relatively high ratio of CO_2 production to oxygen consumption. As fat becomes the dominant fuel, CO_2 production decreases. Lipolysis is impaired, causing lipemia, hyperlipidemia, and hypertriglyceridemia. Serum protein and albumin levels are generally low because of hemodilution, leakage of these substances across capillary membranes, and altered liver production. Serum lactate and lactate/pyruvate ratio are elevated. Metabolic responses result in increased carbon dioxide production. The patient becomes tachypneic. If ventilation is impaired, hypercapnia may develop. Eventually the patient develops hypoxemia.

Electrolyte imbalances, which are common, are related to hormonal and metabolic changes and fluid shifts. These changes exacerbate mental status changes, neuromuscular dysfunction, and cardiac dysrhythmias. Antidiuretic hormone results in water retention and hyponatremia. Aldosterone increases urinary potassium loss, and the patient becomes hypokalemic. Catecholamines cause potassium to move into the cell, increasing hypokalemia. Hypokalemia is associated with dysrhythmias and muscle weakness. Metabolic acidosis results from impaired tissue perfusion, hypoxemia, and a shift to anaerobic metabolism with a related increase in hydrogen ion production. Progressive renal dysfunction also causes an increase in metabolic acidosis. Hypocalcemia, hypomagnesemia, and hypophosphatemia are common.

Clinical Manifestations

Patients with sepsis or SIRS have at least two of the following clinical and laboratory findings: fever or hypothermia, tachypnea, tachycardia, and elevated or left-shifted white blood cell counts (see Table 61-17). The patient may also demonstrate hypotension, confusion, hyperglycemia, and thrombocytopenia. Manifestations range from mild signs and symptoms to circulatory collapse.

Early signs and symptoms vary widely. Most patients initially have mild restlessness or confusion, hyperthermia, tachycardia, some increase in fluid requirements, tachypnea with mild respiratory alkalosis, oliguria with reduced responsiveness to diuretics, abdominal distention, and hyperglycemia or increased glucose requirements.

In *fully developed sepsis or SIRS* the patient appears acutely sick and unstable. Confusion worsens to lethargy or stupor. Cardiac output is greatly increased, the heart rate is rapid, and the skin is warm. Although large volumes of fluid are required to maintain preload, it tends to be low. Maintaining blood pressure requires volume expansion and vasoactive and cardiotonic drugs. Mixed venous oxygen saturation may be increased because of failure to efficiently distribute blood to working organs. The patient is tachypneic, hypocapneic, and hypoxemic. ARDS may develop. There is oliguria progressing to renal failure. The GI tract, especially the stomach and colon, is adynamic and enteral feedings are not tolerated. Stress ulceration may occur. As the liver is compromised, bilirubin levels increase and the patient may appear jaundiced. The prothrombin time is prolonged. The patient may develop thrombocytopenia progressing to disseminated intravascular clotting (DIC). Stress-related hormones are high, resulting in high catabolic rates and hyperglycemia.

In *advanced SIRS and MODS*, the patient is unstable and appears close to death. The patient may lose consciousness. Vasopressors and inotropic agents are needed to maintain blood pressure. The patient may have edema or anasarca. Mixed venous oxygen saturation may rise because of

Table 61-20 Modified Apache II Criteria for Organ System Failure

Cardiovascular Failure (presence of one or more of the following)
- Heart rate <54 beats/min
- Mean arterial pressure ≤49 mm Hg (systolic pressure ≤60 mm Hg)
- Occurrence of ventricular tachycardia or ventricular fibrillation
- Serum pH ≤7.24 with a $PaCO_2$ of ≤40 mm Hg

Respiratory Failure (presence of one or more of the following)
- Respiratory rate ≤5 breaths/min or ≥49 breaths/min
- $PaCO_2$ ≥50 mm Hg
- Alveolar-arterial oxygen difference ≥350 mm Hg (calculate as follows, at sea level: (713 × % oxygen in inspired gas) − $PaCO_2$ − PaO_2
- Dependent on ventilator or CPAP on the second day

Renal Failure (presence of one or more of the following)
- Urine output ≤479 ml/24 hr or ≤159 ml/8 hr
- Serum BUN ≥100 mg/dl (35.7 mmol/L)
- Serum creatinine ≥3.5 mg/dl (309 μmol/L)

Hematologic Failure (presence of one or more of the following)
- WBC count ≤1000/μl (1 × 10^9/L)
- Platelets ≤20,000/μl (20 × 10^9/L)
- Hematocrit ≤20%

Neurologic Failure
- Glasgow coma score ≤6 (in absence of sedation)

Hepatic Failure (presence of both of the following)
- Serum bilirubin ≥6 mg%
- Prothrombin time ≥4 sec over control in the absence of systemic anticoagulation

From Knaus WA, Wagner DP: Multiple systesm organ failure: epidemiology and prognosis, *Crit Care Clin* 5:221, 1989.
CPAP, Continuous positive airway pressure; *BUN,* blood urea nitrogen; *WBC,* white blood cell.

problems with tissue oxygen delivery or may fall if the patient has severe arterial hypoxemia. The patient may be hypercapneic despite aggressive ventilation and have a combined metabolic and respiratory acidosis. The patient may become anuric and require dialysis. Liver enzyme and bilirubin levels increase. Lactic acidosis worsens. Coagulopathy becomes impossible to correct.

Multiple organs can fail. The modified Apache II criteria for organ system failure are presented in Table 61-20. A prototype progression of MODS is presented in Table 61-21.

THERAPEUTIC AND NURSING MANAGEMENT

SYSTEMIC INFLAMMATORY RESOPONSE SYNDROME AND MULTIPLE ORGAN DYSFUNCTION SYNDROME

The goals of therapy for sepsis, SIRS, and MODS can be divided into three categories: (1) limit activators, (2) control mediators, and (3) protect responding organs. Because the prognosis of SIRS and MODS is poor, the most important goal is to prevent its development. An important component of the nursing role is vigilant assessment for signs of deterioration or organ dysfunction.

Table 61-21 Progression of Multiple Organ Dysfunction Syndrome*

1-4 Days after precipitating event or insult
- Low-grade fever
- Tachycardia
- Dyspnea
- Altered mental status
- Hyperdynamic/hypermetabolic state
- Lungs first to fail—acute respiratory distress syndrome

6-10 Days after precipitating event or insult
- Hyperdynamic/hypermetabolic state increases
- Bacteremia
- Signs of liver and renal failure

10-14 Days after precipitating event or insult
- Liver and renal failure more severe
- Gastrointestinal system fails
- Cardiovascular collapse

15-21 Days after precipitating event or insult
- Multiple organ dysfunction syndrome

21-28 Days after precipitating event or insult
- Death

*This is a possible prototype sequence.

Aggressive avoidance, early detection, and prompt treatment of infection may be the most effective means to *limit activators.* Prompt treatment of infection, hemorrhage, trauma, inadequate O_2 delivery, and isolated organ injury is of critical importance.[36] If there is an infection, it is important to quickly diagnose it. Sometimes infections may be difficult to identify. Known infections should be treated with specific agents. If the organism is not known, therapy should begin with broad-spectrum antibiotics and then changed to indicated antibiotics when the organism is identified. Early, aggressive surgery is recommended to remove necrotic tissue (e.g., early debridement of burn tissue). Aggressive pulmonary management, including early ambulation, can decrease infection. Strict asepsis can limit infections via invasive lines.

Patients may become infected even when infection control procedures are stringent. In some cases such infections are thought to be due to systemic invasion by GI bacteria, which are able to penetrate the mucosal barrier following ischemia of the GI tract. Decontamination of the GI tract and pharynx have been found to reduce infection rates but do not alter the death rate from MODS.[37] Another approach to the same problem is to institute early enteral feedings, which may enhance perfusion of the GI tract and decrease bacteria and endotoxin translocation.

Therapies to *control mediators* include metabolic support, maintenance of positive nitrogen and caloric balance, and control of sleep and pain. Monoclonal antibodies have been developed against a number of different mediators, including TNF, endotoxin, and IL-1. Preliminary results have not been encouraging. Thus continued research with this approach will be necessary before effective clinical therapy becomes available.[35]

Treatments to *protect responding organs* include maintaining airway patency, ventilation, and oxygenation; expanding intravascular volume; providing inotropic support; and providing adequate nutrition. With SIRS and MODS much of the care is supportive. Many patients require mechanical ventilation. These patients have greater O_2 needs and decreased O_2 supply to the tissues. Interventions that decrease O_2 demand and increase O_2 delivery are essential. Decreasing O_2 demand may be accomplished by sedation, mechanical ventilation, and rest. Oxygen delivery may be increased by maintenance of a normal hematocrit and PaO_2, by PEEP, by increasing preload or myocardial contractility to enhance cardiac output, or by reducing afterload to increase cardiac output. Throughout treatment, the ICU nurse must assess the intensity of symptoms, stability of the patient, and potential for recovery. The nurse should discuss the treatment progress with the patient and family.

The induction and maintenance of enteral feedings for patients with intestinal dysfunction (paralytic ileus or diarrhea) may improve the GI mucosal barrier and decrease the incidence of bacterial and endotoxin translocation. Selected bowel decontamination (gentamicin, polymycin) also decreases the incidence of bacterial translocation and decreases the incidence of gram-negative sepsis. However, neither therapy has been demonstrated to improve the clinical outcome.[28,37]

Protein-calorie malnutrition is one of the primary manifestations of hypermetabolism and MODS. Total energy expenditure is increased 1.5 to 2 times the normal metabolic rate. Plasma transferrin and prealbumin levels are monitored to indicate hepatic protein synthesis.

OTHER CRITICAL CARE CONTENT

Table 61-22 lists additional critical care content presented in other chapters of this text.

Table 61-22 Cross-Reference to Other Critical Care Content

Topic	Discussed in Chapter
Acute myocardial infarction	31
Acute respiratory distress syndrome	26
Advanced cardiac life support	33
Artificial heart	32
Burns	21
Cardiac dysrhythmias	33
Cardiac pacemakers	33
Cardiac surgery	32
Cardiopulmonary resuscitation	33
Emergencies	62
Head injury	54
Noninvasive blood pressure monitoring	30
Oxygen delivery	24
Renal dialysis	44
Shock and sepsis	7
Total parenteral nutrition	37
Tracheostomy	23
Trauma	62

CRITICAL THINKING EXERCISES

CASE STUDY

SHOCK

Patient Profile

Mr. Y. is a 26-year-old man who was just admitted to the ICU with a fractured left femur caused by a motor vehicle accident. A flow-directed pulmonary artery catheter is placed to monitor his cardiovascular and fluid volume status.

Subjective Data

- Appears to be in acute distress
- Complains of feeling anxious about condition
- Complains of pain at fracture site

Objective Data

- BP 80/44; heart rate 138 bpm, regular; respiratory rate 38/min
- CVP is 1 mm Hg
- PCWP is 4 mm Hg
- Cardiac output is 4 L/min
- SvO_2 is 40%
- SVR is 2000 dynes/sec/cm^{-5}
- Left leg is ecchymotic and swollen

Critical Thinking Questions

1. What are the possible reasons for the objective data?
2. Based on his cardiovascular values, what are appropriate nursing interventions for Mr. Y.?
3. What collaborative management strategies will likely be instituted for Mr. Y.?
4. Mr. Y.'s family wants to know what is happening. What would you tell them?
5. Based on the assessment data presented, write one or more nursing diagnoses. Are there any collaborative problems?

REVIEW QUESTIONS

The number of the question corresponds to the same-numbered objective at the beginning of the chapter.

1. Certification in critical care nursing by the American Association of Critical Care Nurses requires
   a. a master's degree in nursing.
   b. a minimum of 5 years of clinical experience in a critical care unit.
   c. clinical experience and passing a written examination.
   d. a baccalaureate degree in nursing.

2. Which of the following is a manifestation of delirium (ICU psychosis) in an ICU patient?
   a. Hallucinations
   b. Hypoxemia
   c. Hypokalemia
   d. Decreased arousal

3. Which of the following is correct regarding visiting by friends and family of an ICU patient?
   a. A structured visiting policy allowing visits 5 minutes of every hour is ideal.
   b. Open unrestricted visiting is most likely to promote patient comfort.
   c. Individually devised visiting policies based on assessment of patient and family's needs.
   d. Visitors should not be allowed in the ICU.

4. Which of the following are correct regarding hemodynamic monitoring?
   a. Pressure monitoring systems should be zeroed to the level of the catheter tip.
   b. Pressure monitoring systems should be zeroed to the level of the left atrium, identified as the phlebostatic axis.
   c. Pressure monitoring systems should be zeroed to the level of the left atrium, identified as the midaxillary line.
   d. Cardiac output monitoring systems must be zeroed to the level of the left ventricle.

5. Which of the following patients would *not* be a candidate for intraaortic balloon pump treatment?
   a. 26-year-old man with shock caused by hemorrhage
   b. 48-year-old man with an acute myocardial infarction and cardiogenic shock
   c. 62-year-old woman who is difficult to wean from cardiopulmonary bypass following coronary bypass grafting
   d. 35-year-old woman who is awaiting the arrival of a donor heart

6. Which of the following is *not* true regarding the nursing management of a patient with an artificial airway?
   a. Patient with a nasal endotracheal tube should be monitored for sinusitis.
   b. Patient with an orotracheal tube requires frequent oral care because of risk for drying of oral mucosa.
   c. Patient with a cuffed endotracheal tube is monitored for tracheal damage caused by cuff pressure.
   d. Patient with an artificial airway should be routinely suctioned at least every 2 hours.

7. All of the following are true regarding the nursing management of a patient with positive pressure mechanical ventilation *except*
   a. the patient must be monitored for signs of cardiovascular insufficiency because pressure in the chest impedes venous return.
   b. positive pressure ventilation is associated with increased urinary output and sodium depletion.
   c. the patient must be monitored for pneumothorax because the pressure can damage lung tissue.
   d. the patient must be monitored for signs of pulmonary infection because some of the tracheal protective mechanisms are bypassed.

8. Which of the following are normal ICP waveforms?
   a. Plateau waves
   b. A P3 wave following the dicrotic notch
   c. Sharp, rhythmic elevations of 20 to 40 mm Hg, lasting 30 seconds to 2 minutes
   d. Rhythmic pressure elevations of less than 20 mm Hg, at a frequency of one every 4 to 8 minutes

9. Which of the following is true regarding nursing management of the patient with elevated ICP?
   a. Hypoxemia decreases cerebral blood volume and ICP.
   b. Overventilation used to decrease the $PaCO_2$ decreases cerebral blood volume and ICP.
   c. The head is flexed to the right to facilitate venous return from the head.
   d. A regimen of increased fluids is instituted.

10. Which of the following statements is correct regarding clinical manifestations and pathophysiology of SIRS?
   a. SIRS is always the result of an infectious process.
   b. SIRS occurs only in patients with compromised immune function.
   c. SIRS is the most common cause of death in ICU patients.
   d. SIRS prolongs ICU recoveries but rarely leads to death or disability.

11. Which of the following is *not* correct regarding management of the patient with SIRS?
   a. The first line of treatment is generally focused on elimination of the source of the infection or inflammation.
   b. Infection can occur despite rigorous aseptic technique, possibly because of bacterial contamination from the gastrointestinal tract.
   c. SIRS can lead to the multiple organ dysfunction syndrome.
   d. All invasive lines should be removed and not replaced when the patient has SIRS.

REFERENCES

1. Nightingale F: *Notes on hospitals*, ed 3, Longman, 1863, Roberts-Green.
2. Alspach JG: Should baccalaureate programs include critical care nursing? *Crit Care Nurse* 10:12, 1990.

*3. Wilson VS: Identification of stressors related to patients' psychological responses to the surgical intensive care unit, *Heart Lung* 16:267, 1987.

*4. Easton C, Mackenzie F: Sensory-perceptual alterations: delirium in the intensive care unit, *Heart Lung* 17:229, 1988.

5. Tess MM: Acute confusional states in critically ill patients: a review, *J Neurosci Nurs* 23:398, 1991.
6. Balogh D and others: Noise in the ICU, *Intensive Care Med* 19:343, 1993.
*7. Fontaine DK: Measurement of nocturnal sleep patterns in trauma patients, *Heart Lung* 18:402, 1989.
8. Meyer TJ and others: Adverse environmental conditions in the respiratory and medical ICU settings, *Chest* 105:1211, 1994.
*9. Richards KC, Bairnsfather L: A description of night sleep patterns in the critical care unit, *Heart Lung* 17:35, 1988.
10. Tatar H and others: Vascular complications of intraaortic balloon pumping: unsheathed versus sheathed insertion, *Ann Thorac Surg* 55:1518, 1993.
11. Eltchanioff H, Dimas AP, Whitlow PL: Complications associated with percutaneous placement and use of intraaortic balloon counterpulsation, *Am J Cardiol* 71:328, 1993.
12. Mackenzie DJ and others: Vascular complications of the intraaortic balloon pump, *Am J Surg* 164:517, 1992
*13. Stone KS: Ventilator versus manual resuscitation bag as the method for delivering hyperoxygenation before endotracheal suctioning, *AACN Clin Iss Crit Care Nurs* 1:289, 1990.
14. Panacek EA and others: Selective left endobronchial suctioning in the intubated patient, *Chest* 95:885, 1989.
15. Sassoon CS: Positive pressure ventilation: alternate modes, *Chest* 100:1421, 1991.
16. Burns SM: Advances in ventilator therapy, *Focus Crit Care* 17:227, 1990.
17. Wright SE, Heffner JE: Positive pressure mechanical ventilation augments left ventricular function in acute mitral regurgitation, *Chest* 102:1625, 1992.
*18. Goodnough-Hanneman SK and others: Weaning from short-term mechanical ventilation: a review, *Am J Crit Care* 3:421, 1994.
*19. Sevick MA and others: Home-based ventilator-dependent patients: measurement of the emotional aspects of home caregiving, *Heart Lung* 23:269, 1994.
*20. Smith CE and others: Caregiver learning needs and reactions to managing home mechanical ventilation, *Heart Lung* 23:157, 1994.
21. Plummer AL, O'Donohue WJ, Petty TL: Consensus conference on problems in home mechanical ventilation, *Am Rev Respir Dis* 140:555, 1989.
22. Lundberg N: Continuous recording and control of ventricular fluid pressure in neurosurgical practice, *Acta Psychiatr Neurolog Scand* 36(suppl 149):1, 1960.
23. Winfield JA and others: Duration of intracranial pressure monitoring does not predict daily risk of infectious complications, *Neurosurgery* 33:424, 1993.
24. Hickman KM, Mayer BL, Muwaswes M: Intracranial pressure monitoring: review of risk factors associated with infection, *Heart Lung 19:84, 1990.*
25. Germon K: Interpretation of ICP pulse waves to determine intracerebral compliance, *J Neurosci Nurs* 20:344, 1988.
26. Doyle DJ, Mark PWS: Analysis of intracranial pressure, *J Clin Monit* 8:81, 1992.
27. Hayek DA, Veremakis C: Physiologic concerns during brain resuscitation. In Civetta JM, Taylor RW, Kirby RR, editors: *Critical care,* ed 2, Philadelphia, 1992, Lippincott.
28. Kerr ME, Brucia J: Hyperventilation in the head injured patient: an effective treatment modality? *Heart Lung* 22:516, 1993.
29. Kerr ME and others: Head-injured adults: recommendations for endotracheal suctioning, *J Neurosc Nurs* 25:86, 1993.
30. Hazinski MF and others: Epidemiology, pathophysiology, and clinical presentation of gram-negative sepsis. *Am J Crit Care* 2:224, 1994.
31. Centers for Disease Control: Increase in national hospital discharge survey rates for septicemia in the United States 1979-1987, *MMWR* 39:31, 1991.
32. Suchyta MR and others: The adult respiratory distress syndrome: a report of survival and modifying factors, *Chest* 101:1074, 1992.
33. Sloane PJ and others: A multicenter trial of patients with acute respiratory distress syndrome: physiology and outcome, *Am Rev Resp Dis* 146:419, 1992.
34. Fitzsimmons L: Consequences of trauma: systemic inflammation and multiple organ dysfunction, *Crit Care Nurs Q* 17:74, 1994.
35. St John RC, Dorinsky PM: An overview of multiple organ dysfunction syndrome, *J Lab Clin Med* 124:478, 1994.
36. Murray MJ, Coursin DB: Multiple organ dysfunction syndrome, *Yale J Biol Med* 66:501, 1993.
37. Stoutenbeek CP, Van Saene HK: Prevention of pneumonia by selective decontamination of the digestive tract, *Intensive Care Med* 18(suppl 1):S18, 1992.

*Nursing research-based articles.

Chapter 62

NURSING ROLE IN MANAGEMENT

Emergency Care Situations

Kristi Vaughn

Learning Objectives

1. Describe the purpose of the Emergency Medical Service system.
2. Explain the role of the nurse in emergency situations.
3. Describe the sequential steps in assessing a patient in an emergency situation.
4. Explain the pathophysiology, assessment, and management of selected environmental emergencies related to thermoregulatory emergencies, near drowning, animal bites, and poisonings.

OVERVIEW OF EMERGENCY CARE

Military conflicts have been the training grounds for the advancement of emergency care. Field resuscitation, transportation of the wounded, and rapid evacuation by trained personnel saved many lives during the Korean and Vietnam wars. In the 1970s bystander cardiopulmonary resuscitation (CPR), technologic advances, organized prehospital care, and emergency training programs decreased the morbidity and mortality rates of emergency victims. Advances in medical technology and medical equipment development (e.g., cardiac monitoring, Heimlich valves, orthopedic devices) tailored to be used in emergency situations have done much to improve the care of emergency victims. Care delivery protocols have standardized prehospital patient care management. Paraprofessionals such as the emergency medical technician (EMT) and paramedic (EMT-P) are specially trained to deliver prehospital emergency care. Transportation systems, including helicopters and small planes, ensure rapid emergency transport to hospitals so patients can receive definitive treatment.

Health care reform is pressuring emergency facilities to reduce costs while maintaining quality care. The Consolidated Omnibus Budget Reconciliation Act (COBRA) of 1989 requires that all persons requesting care in emergency facilities have a medical screening exam, regardless of the ability to pay.[1] Visits to emergency departments have increased significantly because of lack of health insurance, increased violence, and inability to access health care.

Emergencies are often divided into medical and traumatic emergencies. *Medical emergencies* are acute physiologic crises that are not directly caused by a traumatic impact to the body. *Traumatic emergencies* are physiologic crises that are directly caused by blunt or penetrating impact to the body. Specific emergency care for patients with various medical and traumatic emergencies are presented throughout this book where the disorders are discussed (Table 62-1).

This chapter discusses assessment, management, ongoing evaluation, and education of the emergency trauma patient. The concepts of trauma care can also be utilized for persons with medical emergencies. This chapter also discusses the Emergency Medical Service system, the role of the emergency nurse, and selected environmental emergencies.

Emergency Medical Service System

The *Emergency Medical Service* (EMS) *system* is an organized and coordinated system of prehospital providers, ground and air ambulances, and hospital emergency departments (EDs). *Prehospital care* is care rendered before entry into the hospital. In 1966 the Highway Safety Act developed guidelines and channeled funds to states to develop EMS systems. The 1973 EMS Systems Act provided funding for communities to access and develop regional EMS systems, known as 911. EMS systems provide training for EMS professionals and public education in first aid. In 1981 the Omnibus Reconciliation Act ended federal leadership in EMS. Responsibility, direction, and control of EMS systems is now with state and local governments.

The purpose of an EMS system is to integrate the use of personnel, facilities, and equipment for the coordinated delivery of emergency care over specific geographic areas.

Reviewed by Darlene T. Schelper, RN, MSN, CEN, Clinical Nurse Educator, Emergency Services, Hershey Medical Center, Hershey, PA; and Eileen Grass, RN, MSN, Staff Nurse, Trauma-Surgical Intensive Care Unit, University of New Mexico Hospital, Albuquerque, NM.

Table 62-1 Emergency Management Tables

These systems are mandated to provide for individual emergency care and care required during natural and other large-scale disasters. EMS systems join resources including physicians, nurses, paramedics, police officers, fire fighters, government agencies, and hospitals to provide emergency care.

Emergency Nursing

Emergency nursing is one of the most challenging nursing specialties. This specialty requires that the nurse, whether in the hospital emergency department or prehospital setting, use a scientific knowledge base, effective communication, clinical skills, and the nursing process to care for the physiologic and emotional needs of patients and families.[2] Crisis intervention and the use of emergency skills are important to the patient and family during stressful emergency situations. Rapid assessment, history taking, appropriate intervention, and emotional support for the family and patient must occur in a short period of time.

The emergency nurse promotes health by teaching patients about accident prevention and basic emergency care in the home. Explanations in lay terms are used to explain procedures and first aid. Public education, including initial treatment measures, taught by emergency nurses can greatly reduce morbidity and mortality. The nurse must actively listen to patients and families to determine their learning needs. Emergency nurses must have a wide knowledge of health problems to address the educational needs of all age groups.[3]

The emergency nurse should be aware of patients who regularly or consistently return to the hospital with injuries. They may be accident prone, victims of abuse, or have an alcohol or drug problem. Abuse includes both domestic violence and elderly abuse. Domestic abuse involves children, mentally disabled, intimate partner, and elder abuse. Although victims of domestic abuse are usually women, men can also be abused. Frequent visits to the ED by an older patient should raise an index of suspicion for abuse. The emergency nurse must be aware of agencies to which to refer abuse victims. The emergency nurse must also be knowledgeable of agencies for referral of substance abuse patients.

RESEARCH

Implications for Nursing Practice

DOMESTIC ABUSE

Citation Grunfeld AF and others: Detecting domestic violence against women in the emergency department: a nursing triage model, *J Emerg Nurs* 20:271-274, 1994.

Purpose To determine the disclosure rate for abuse in an emergency department setting.

Methods Cross-sectional survey of women (n = 252) assessed for triage in the emergency department of a large hospital. Nursing triage was used to determine disclosure rates for abuse.

Results and Conclusions Of the women in the study, 16 (6%) disclosed abuse and one half of these asked for help. A brief nursing triage question appears to be an efficient way of detecting abuse among women seen in the emergency department. Few patients expressed offense or embarrassment, and many appreciated the concern.

Implications for Nursing Practice Emergency departments could identify many battered women simply by asking them about abuse history during triage. A safe, private, confidential area is the logical place to address problems of patient safety and mobilization of resources. To uncover abuse, start by asking.

CARE OF THE EMERGENCY PATIENT

Recognition of a life-threatening illness or injury is one of the most important aspects of emergency care. Before a diagnosis can be determined, the recognition of dangerous clinical signs and symptoms and the initiation of actions to reverse or prevent a crisis are mandatory.

Triage

Triage is a French word meaning to "sort." Triage is a system to deal with large numbers of patients with various complaints. Prompt identification of patients requiring immediate treatment and determination of the appropriate treatment area are essential in a busy ED. A triage system identifies and categorizes patients so that the most critically ill are treated first. The triage nurse must have excellent assessment and interview skills to prioritize care. Within minutes of encountering emergency victims in the ED or a prehospital situation, the triage nurse is responsible for obtaining the chief complaint, determining patient acuity, and performing diagnostic tests and first aid. A good triage nurse is flexible, tracks patient flow, and communicates with families and health care providers.

Urgency Categories. Patients are triaged based on acuity into the following categories: emergent, urgent, and nonurgent. *Emergent* refers to life-threatening disorders that require immediate medical attention and intervention. These include cardiopulmonary arrest, pulmonary edema, seizure, gastrointestinal bleeding, and multisystem trauma. These patients should be taken immediately to a treatment area. *Urgent* complaints are those who require treatment as soon as possible (e.g., from 20 minutes to 2 hours). Generally these patients have stable vital signs. If treatment is delayed, some impairment may occur. Urgent problems include simple lacerations, fever, uncomplicated extremity fractures, abdominal pain, or other significant pain. *Nonurgent* problems refer to those situations that would not be significantly affected by a delay in treatment, such as sore throats, rash, chronic back pain, strains, and sprains. Nonurgent patients can wait for several hours to days to be treated without serious sequelae. Urgent care centers or fast tracks have been set up as independent medical offices or in EDs to care for patients with nonemergency health problems.

Disaster. The ED provides a critical interface between a disaster scene and the hospital. Disaster is defined as an occurrence of severity and magnitude that goes beyond the scope of what normally can be handled through routine procedures and resources.[4] In other words, a disaster exceeds human and material resources. A disaster can be either natural, such as a fire or an earthquake, or human-made, such as a chemical spill or an airplane crash. The emergency nurse must have a good understanding of the hospital and community disaster plan. A hospital disaster plan includes a chain of command, activation process, patient management plan, and communication plan.

Triage categories change during disaster management. Patients are tagged according to acuity. A red tag indicates a hyperacute situation; treatment must focus on airway, breathing, and circulation. First priority is given to patients who have life-threatening problems. Red, yellow, green, and black tag injuries are described in Table 62-2. The triage nurse's role during a disaster is to tag patients according to acuity, register the patient with a number system, assign the patient to a care area, monitor patient flow, and communicate with the disaster flow officer.[5]

Table 62-2 Disaster Triage Color Codes

Tag Color	Injury Severity and Examples
Red	**Hyperacute: first priority** Treatable life-threatening respiratory problem Severe blood loss, controllable hemorrhage Unconsciousness Severe shock
Yellow	**Serious: second priority** Moderate blood loss Conscious head injuries Spinal cord injury Extensive burns without respiratory compromise
Green	**Walking injured: third priority** Minor lacerations Minor fractures Minor burns
Black	Deceased, cardiopulmonary arrest, or other injuries exceeding available resources

Assessment of Emergency Patient

Because emergency patients require rapid intervention, physical assessment must occur during history taking. A primary and secondary survey must be done quickly to identify actual or potential life-threatening problems. Assessment is a continual process that is repeated at regular intervals to detect any changes in the patient's status. The principles of assessment can be applied to any emergency patient.

Primary Survey. Emergency assessment begins with the primary survey: airway, breathing, and circulation (Table 62-3). The initial assessment should take approximately 2 minutes. During the primary survey all life-threatening problems are identified and appropriate interventions started immediately.

A = *Airway with cervical spine immobilization.* Nearly all immediate trauma deaths occur because of airway obstruction. Saliva, bloody secretions, vomitus, direct trauma, laryngeal trauma, facial trauma, fractures, and the tongue can obstruct the airway. Medical patients at risk for airway compromise include those who have seizures, near drowning, anaphylaxis, foreign body obstruction, or are in cardiopulmonary arrest. If an airway is not maintained, obstruction of air flow occurs and hypoxia, acidosis, and death result.

Clinical manifestations of a compromised airway are respiratory distress, cough, stridor, cyanosis, and inability to speak. Airway maintenance should progress rapidly from the least to the most invasive method. Treatment includes suctioning of secretions, jaw thrust maneuver (avoiding hyperextension of the neck) (Fig. 62-1), insertion of a nasopharyngeal or oropharyngeal airway (will cause gag if patient is conscious), forward sitting position if no cervical spine injuries are present, and intubation. If unable to intubate because of airway obstruction, an emergency surgical cricothyroidotomy or tracheotomy should be performed (see Chapter 23).

Any patient with significant upper torso injuries or face, head, or neck trauma should always be suspected of cervical

Table 62-3 Primary Survey of an Emergency Patient

Assessment	Intervention
Airway with cervical spine Clear and open airway Assess for obstructed airway Assess for respiratory distress	Suction Jaw thrust avoiding hyperextension of neck Nasal or oral airway, endotracheal tube, cricothyroidotomy Cervical spine immobilization using collar, backboard, soft rolls, tape forehead
Breathing Assess ventilation Look for chest movements associated with breathing Listen for air being expired through nose and mouth Feel for air being expired Observe and count respiratory rate Note color of nail beds, mucous membranes, skin Auscultate lungs	If respirations absent, ventilate with bag valve mask with 100% O_2 Prepare to intubate if respiratory arrest Have suction available Give supplemental oxygen via appropriate delivery system If head trauma, hyperventilate with 100% O_2 If absent breath sounds, perform needle thoracostomy and prepare for chest tube insertion
Circulation Check carotid or femoral pulse Assess color, temperature, and moisture of skin Assess level of consciousness Check capillary refill Assess for external bleeding	If absent pulse, begin chest compressions If shock symptoms or hypotensive, start at least two large-bore (14-16 gauge) intravenous lines with normal saline or lactated Ringer's solution Administer blood products if ordered Consider autotransfusion if isolated chest trauma Obtain blood samples for type and crossmatch Control bleeding with direct pressure
Disability Assess level of consciousness Assess response to verbal and painful stimuli Assess extremity movement (all four limbs) Perform Glasgow Coma Scale (see Table 54-11) Check pupil response to light	Periodically reassess level of consciousness
Expose Assess for any injuries or illnesses	Remove all clothing for adequate examination

spine trauma. The cervical spine must be kept in alignment and immobilized during assessment of the airway. The cervical spine is immobilized with a stiff immobilization collar, soft rolls are taped to a backboard on either side of the head, and the patient's forehead is taped to the backboard. Sandbags should not be used because the weight of the bags could move the head if the patient must be turned.

B = *Breathing*. Adequate air flow through the upper airway does not ensure adequate ventilation. Breathing alterations are caused by many conditions, including fractured ribs, pneumothorax, penetrating injury, allergic reactions, pulmonary emboli, and asthma attacks. Every injured or ill patient has an increased metabolic and oxygen demand and should have supplemental oxygen. Life-threatening conditions such as tension pneumothorax, open pneumothorax, and flail chest can compromise ventilation. Treatment for a nonbreathing patient includes bag valve mask ventilation with 100% oxygen, intubation, and treatment of the underlying cause.

A *tension pneumothorax* can compress the heart vessels and the unaffected lung if untreated (Fig. 62-2, Table 24-23). Signs and symptoms are dyspnea; hypotension; tachycardia; cool, clammy skin; tracheal deviation toward unaffected side; decreased breath sounds on the affected side; distant heart sounds; and distended neck veins. Diagnostic and treatment measures include 100% oxygen, chest x-ray examination, pulse oximetry, arterial blood gases, and chest tube placement or needle thoracostomy. In an open pneumothorax any *sucking* chest wounds should be covered with an occlusive dressing on three sides to allow air to escape but not enter the chest. Patients with open chest wounds should be closely monitored for a tension pneumothorax and the dressing removed immediately if the patient becomes symptomatic. (Pneumothorax is discussed in Chapter 24.)

A *flail chest* is defined as two or three rib fractures occurring in more than one place (see Table 24-23 and Fig. 24-10). A flail chest can affect ventilation because of paradoxical movement of the chest wall resulting in pain,

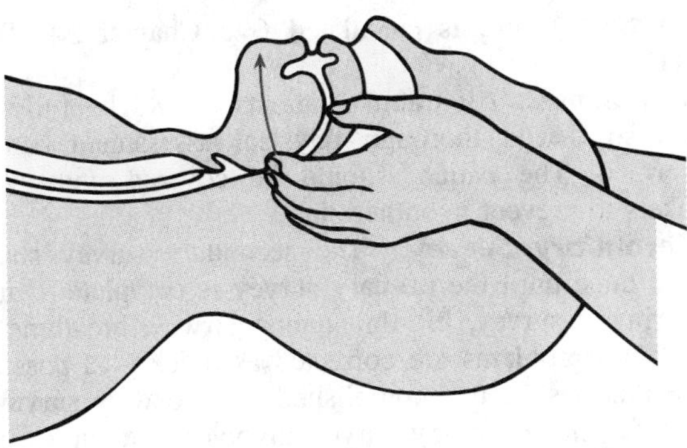

Fig. 62-1 Jaw-thrust maneuver is the only widely recommended procedure for use on an unconscious patient with possible neck or spinal injuries. The patient should be lying supine with the rescuer kneeling at the top of the head. The rescuer should carefully reach forward and gently place one hand on each side of the patient's chin at the lateral angles of the lower jaw. The patient's head should be stabilized with the rescuer's forearms, then the jaw pushed forward while pressure is applied with the index fingers.

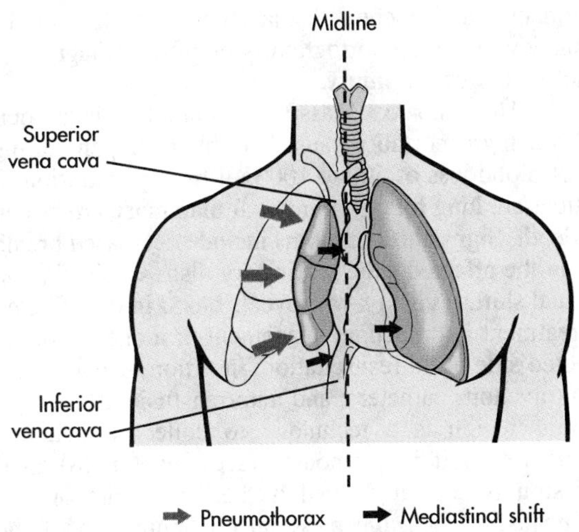

Fig. 62-2 Tension pneumothorax. As pleural pressure on the affected side increases, mediastinal displacement ensues with resultant respiratory and cardiovascular compromise.

atelectasis, hypoxia, and hypercapnia. Significant assessment findings include chest wall asymmetry; uncoordinated chest movement with respiration; crepitus; rapid, shallow respirations; and cyanosis. Treatment consists of oxygenation, analgesia, and alleviation of anxiety. If the cervical spine is not affected, the patient is placed on the affected side. A chest x-ray and arterial blood gases should be obtained and fluid replacement closely monitored. The patient should be continuously monitored for signs and symptoms of respiratory compromise, including tachycardia, breathing difficulty, confusion, agitation, increased or decreased respiratory rate and effort, and decreased oxygen saturation.

C = *Circulation with hemorrhage control.* An effective circulatory system includes the heart, intact blood vessels, and adequate blood volume. The patient's carotid or femoral pulse should be checked because peripheral pulses may be absent as a result of direct injury or vasoconstriction. Delayed capillary refill (longer than 3 seconds) and altered mental status are the most significant signs of shock. Care must be taken when evaluating capillary refill in cold environments because cold delays refill. Uncontrolled bleeding places a person at risk for hemorrhagic shock. During the assessment of circulation, pericardial tamponade, traumatic aortic dissection, other large vessel injuries, massive hemothorax, gastrointestinal bleeding, and cardiac insufficiency must be ruled out.

Intravenous lines are inserted into veins in the upper extremities unless contraindicated, such as in a massive fracture or an injury that affects limb circulation. Two large-gauge intravenous catheters should be inserted and aggressive fluid resuscitation initiated using lactated Ringer's solution or normal saline. Direct pressure with a sterile dressing should be applied to obvious bleeding sites. Blood samples are obtained for a type and crossmatch; electrolyte, glucose, blood urea nitrogen, and creatinine levels; complete blood cell count; and coagulation studies. Blood samples may also be obtained for alcohol or drug levels or liver or cardiac enzyme levels. The patient should be monitored by electrocardiogram (ECG) for dysrhythmias. Type-specific packed red blood cells should be administered if needed.

Pericardial Tamponade. Pericardial tamponade is defined as blood filling the pericardium from the heart or great vessels secondary to blunt or penetrating trauma. Leakage of blood into the sac increases intrapericardial pressure, restricting blood flow into the heart and decreasing ventricular filling and cardiac output. Clinical manifestations include dyspnea, increased central venous pressure, muffled heart tones, hypotension, pulsus paradoxus, cyanosis, tachycardia, and restlessness. A chest x-ray will reveal an enlarged heart and enlarged mediastinal space. Decreased voltage may appear on a 12-lead electrocardiogram. Treatment of pericardial tamponade is a *pericardiocentesis* (see Fig. 34-6) or thoracotomy to relieve the intrapericardial pressure.

Great Vessel Injury. Blunt or penetrating trauma to the great vessels has a high mortality rate because of rapid exsanguination into the chest. Many fatality victims in motor vehicle collisions die from an aortic dissection. The aorta is mobile in the chest, and sudden impact causes shearing of the innominate artery. The heart is displaced laterally by blunt force. The ascending aorta rotates and shears away from the heart, disrupting the aortic valve. Important clues to this type of injury include a history of blunt trauma or an acceleration/deceleration injury. Clinical manifestations include chest pain, back pain, severe shortness of breath, hemoptysis, systolic murmur, signs of shock, a difference in blood pressure between the left and right arm, and absent lower extremity pressures. A chest x-ray reveals a widened mediastinum, depressed left mainstem bronchus, and tracheal displacement with loss of the aortic shadow. An arch aortogram is helpful in diagnosing the exact nature of the injury.

MASSIVE HEMOTHORAX. Massive hemothorax is associated with a high mortality caused by blunt or penetrating trauma. A blood loss of 500 to 1000 ml from penetration of the aortic arch, lung hilum, or internal mammary artery can lead to death. Signs and symptoms include decreased breath sounds on the affected side, respiratory distress, shock, and mediastinal shift. A chest x-ray reveals blood in the affected lung. Treatment is immediate placement of a chest tube on the affected side, fluid resuscitation, insertion of two large-gauge intravenous catheters, and autotransfusion.

Autotransfusion is a technique to collect a patient's blood and return it intravenously (see Chapter 28). Autotransfusion is contraindicated if there is an abdominal injury because of possible bacterial contamination of the blood. Other risks include coagulopathies and air embolism. Some EDs add citrate phosphate dextrose (CPD) to the collection chamber to prevent clotting. If a facility protocol requires CPD, care must be taken to monitor the patient for coagulopathies, cardiac depression, and hyperkalemia. Phosphate binds with calcium, thus decreasing the circulating calcium. If coagulopathies occur, fresh frozen plasma may need to be administered. High flow oxygen, fluids, and blood should be administered. The amount of drainage must be monitored and documented.

UNCONTROLLED HEMORRHAGE. Uncontrolled hemorrhage is an acute loss of circulating blood volume. It accounts for 30% to 40% of all trauma deaths. Penetrating trauma to a major artery results in hypovolemic shock. External bleeding should be controlled as quickly as possible via direct pressure to the wound with a sterile dressing. Tourniquets should be avoided if possible. Large, bleeding head wounds can be controlled with scalp clips.

Pneumatic antishock garments (PASGs) or *military antishock trousers* (MASTs) were used in the military to control hemorrhage, but their use is currently controversial. PASGs initially were used to shunt blood away from the extremities to the body core. They make evaluation of abdominal and leg injuries difficult, take time and skill to put on, and should not replace initial resuscitation efforts. They have been used effectively to stabilize pelvic and long bone fractures for long ground transports to the hospital. PASGs should never be cut off because they are expensive and dramatic hypotension can result if PASGs are not deflated properly. To deflate them, the patient's blood pressure must be closely monitored. The abdominal compartment should be deflated first and then each leg slowly deflated, stopping if the patient's blood pressure drops more than 5 mm Hg. Fluid volume replacement is essential during deflation. (PASGs are discussed in Chapter 7.)

D = *Disability.* A brief neurologic exam should follow the primary survey. Level of consciousness and pupil size and reactivity to light should be assessed. A simple mnemonic to remember is AVPU: *A* = alert, *V* = responds to verbal stimuli, *P* = responds to painful stimuli, and *U* = unresponsive. Extremities should be observed for spontaneous movement and assessed for sensation. A Glasgow Coma Scale score is calculated (see Chapter 54, Table 54-11).

E = *Expose.* All trauma patients should be fully exposed so that a thorough physical assessment can be performed. The patient should be covered with warm blankets to prevent hypothermia.

Secondary Survey. The secondary survey should not be done until the primary survey is complete. During the primary survey, life-threatening airway, breathing, or circulation problems are corrected as quickly as possible. Once this has been accomplished, a secondary survey is initiated. The secondary survey involves obtaining a history, identifying all injuries, and performing a head-to-toe assessment, including evaluation of the patient's back (Table 62-4).

F = *Fahrenheit.* The patient is kept warm with warm intravenous fluids, warm blankets, and overhead warming lights. Trauma patients and ill medical patients are at risk for hypothermia caused by increased metabolism, hypovolemia, and environmental exposure.

G = *Get vitals.* A complete set of vital signs, including blood pressure, heart rate, respiratory rate, temperature, and oxygen saturation, should be obtained after the patient is exposed. The patient's heart rate and rhythm should be monitored.

H = *History and head-to-toe assessment*

HISTORY. The history of the incident, accident, or illness provides clues to the cause of the crisis and suggests specific assessment needs. The patient may be unable to give a history, but family, friends, and witnesses can frequently provide information. An experienced ED team can complete a history within 5 minutes of the patient's arrival. If the patient is emergently ill, a thorough history is obtained from the friends or family after the patient is taken to the treatment area. The history should include the following questions:

1. What is the chief complaint? What caused the person to seek attention?
2. How long ago did the accident or incident occur? How long ago did the patient become ill?
3. Where did the accident or incident occur? Where did the patient become ill?
4. Describe the accident, incident, or illness. How did it happen? Details of the incident are extremely important because the mechanism can indicate specific injuries. Table 62-5 lists important questions to ask the patient, paramedics, and witnesses. For example, a front seat passenger with a lap belt may have a head injury from hitting the windshield; knee, femur, or hip fractures or dislocation from striking the dashboard; and an abdominal injury from the lap belt. If other victims were dead at the scene, the patient has a high chance of significant injury.

Patients who jump from buildings or bridges may have bilateral calcaneal fractures, bilateral wrist fractures, and lumbar spine compression fractures and are at risk for aortic tears. Older patients who have climbed ladders and fallen may have had a cerebral vascular accident or myocardial infarction, which led to the fall.

Table 62-4 Secondary Survey of an Emergency Patient

Parameter	Assessment
Fahrenheit	Keep warm with warm blankets, warmed intravenous fluids, overhead lights
Get Vitals	Blood pressure Pulse, cardiac rhythm Respiratory rate and effort Temperature Oxygen saturation
History and Head-to-Toe Assessment	
History	Length of time since incident occurred Accident location Description of accident, incident, or illness (see Table 62-5) Allergies Medications Past health history, pregnancy status Last meal Events leading to accident, incident, or illness
Head, neck, face	Examination of face and scalp for lacerations, bone or soft tissue deformity, tenderness, bleeding, and foreign objects Examination of eyes, ears, nose, and mouth for bleeding, foreign bodies, drainage, pain, deformity, ecchymosis, lacerations Examination of head for depressions of cranial or facial bones, contusions, hematomas, areas of softness Examination of neck for stiffness, pain in cervical vertebrae, tracheal deviation, distended neck veins, bleeding or edema, difficulty swallowing, bruising
Chest	Anterior and posterior chest wall movements External signs of injury: petechiae, bleeding, cyanosis, bruises, abrasions, old scars
Abdomen and pelvis	Symmetry of external abdominal wall and bony structures External signs of injury: bruising, abrasions, lacerations, punctures Type and location of pain Bowel sounds Rigidity or distention of abdomen Genitalia for swelling, bruising, bleeding, lacerations Rectal bleeding, tone
Extremities	Signs of external injury: deformity, ecchymosis, abrasions, lacerations, swelling Pain Movement and strength in arms and legs Sensation in each limb Color of skin Presence and quality of peripheral pulses
Back	Log roll and inspect back for deformity, bleeding, lacerations, bruising

Bullets can ricochet in the body if they strike bone. It is essential to determine the number of shots fired and to look for entry and exit wounds. A patient shot in the abdomen may have a bullet lodged in the right shoulder. The bullet trajectory may have gone through the liver and lung en route to the shoulder.

5. What has happened since the onset of the illness or injury?
   a. Has the patient been moved?
   b. What emergency care was started at the scene of the incident?
   c. What are the patient's subjective complaints?
   d. What are witnesses' (if any) descriptions of the patient's behavior since the onset?
   e. What are the details of the EMS report?
6. What is the patient's health care history? The mnemonic AMPLE assists the nurse in remembering what to ask:

   A—Allergies
   M—Medications (current medications that the patient is taking)
   P—Past health history (especially cardiac and respiratory conditions and diabetes), pregnancy status
   L—Last meal
   E—Events preceding illness or injury

HEAD, NECK, AND FACE. The patient should be assessed for general appearance, skin color, and temperature. The eyes should be evaluated for extraocular movements. A discon-

Table 62-5 Mechanism of Injury and History Taking

Type of Accident	Questions
Motor vehicle collision	Driver or passenger? Seat belt, lap belt, shoulder harness? Hit steering wheel, windshield, or dashboard? Loss of consciousness? Speed of vehicle? Vehicle hit stationary or moving object? Damage to vehicle and impact location? Distance thrown? Condition of passengers? Treatment at the scene? Location of pain?
Falls	Distance of fall? What precipitated the fall? Underlying medical conditions? Type of surface struck? Loss of consciousness? Treatment at the scene? Location of pain?
Gunshot wounds or stab wounds	How long ago occurred? Number of shots fired? Number of stab wounds? Type of gun? Length of knife? Direction bullet or knife entered body? Location of pain?

jugate gaze is an indication of neurologic damage. Raccoon eyes or periorbital ecchymosis is usually caused by a basilar skull fracture. The tympanic membranes and external canal are checked for blood and cerebrospinal fluid. Drainage from the ear should not be stopped.

The throat and airway are assessed for bruising, foreign bodies, bleeding, edema, loose or missing teeth, difficulty swallowing, movement of the palate, and ability to open the mouth. Neck examination includes palpation and visualization of the trachea to determine that it is in the midline. A deviated trachea may signal a life-threatening tension pneumothorax. Subcutaneous emphysema may indicate laryngotracheal disruption. A stiff or painful cervical spine area may signify a fracture of a cervical vertebra. The cervical spine *must* be protected using a rigid collar, backboard, towel rolls, or other soft rolls on either side of the head, and the forehead should be taped to the backboard.

CHEST. The chest is examined for paradoxic chest movements and large sucking chest wounds. The sternum, clavicles, and ribs are palpated for deformity and point tenderness. The chest is assessed for pain on palpation, respiratory distress, decreased breath sounds, distant heart sounds, and distended neck veins. The ECG should be observed for dysrhythmias (e.g., bradycardia). In addition to tension pneumothorax and open pneumothorax, the patient should be evaluated for rib fractures, pulmonary contusion, myocardial contusion, and simple pneumothorax. In addition to the initial interventions, a 12-lead ECG should be obtained, particularly on an older patient or a patient with suspected heart disease.

ABDOMEN AND PELVIS. The abdomen is more difficult to assess. Frequent evaluation for subtle changes in the abdominal exam is essential. Blunt trauma can be caused by motor vehicle collisions and assaults. Penetrating trauma tends to injure specific organs. Decreased bowel sounds may indicate a temporary ileus. Bowel sounds in the chest may indicate a diaphragmatic rupture. The abdomen is percussed for gastric distention and peritoneal irritation. A dull sound indicates blood or fluid. The pelvis is gently palpated. If pain is elicited, it may indicate a pelvic fracture. The genitalia are inspected for bleeding and obvious injuries. A rectal exam is performed to check for blood in the vault, a high-riding prostate, and loss of sphincter tone.

EXTREMITIES. The upper and lower extremities are assessed (see Table 62-4). Injured extremities are splinted above and below the injury to decrease further soft tissue injury and pain. Grossly deformed, pulseless extremities should be realigned and splinted. Pulses are checked before and after movement of an extremity. The extremities are palpated for point tenderness, crepitus, and abnormal movements. Injured extremities should be elevated and ice packs applied. Prophylactic antibiotics are administered for open fractures. Patients with fractures should receive analgesia.

BACK. The trauma patient should always be turned (using spinal precautions) to inspect the back. The back is inspected for ecchymosis, abrasions, puncture wounds, cuts, and obvious deformities. The entire spine is palpated for misalignment, deformity, and pain.

Intervention and Evaluation

Regardless of the patient's chief complaint, a thorough assessment and an accurate history are critical in an emergency situation. Once the secondary survey is complete, all findings are recorded. Additional interventions include placement of a nasogastric tube to decrease gastric distention. The contents of the nasogastric drainage should be checked for blood. A nasogastric tube should not be placed in the nares in a patient suspected of having a basilar skull fracture because the tube might enter the brain; rather, it should be placed orally. An indwelling catheter is inserted and urinary output monitored. Urine output should be at least 0.5 ml/kg per hour. An indwelling catheter should not be inserted if a urethral tear is suspected. Patients with pelvic injuries, blood at the meatus, or men with high-riding prostates are at risk for a urethral tear. A urethrogram should be obtained before a catheter is inserted. The urine should be checked for blood and a urine pregnancy test performed on women. All trauma patients should receive tetanus prophylaxis if the tetanus status is unknown (Table 62-6).

Depending on the patient's injuries, the patient is transported for diagnostic tests such as a CT scan, x-ray, or MRI,

Table 62-6 Prophylaxis Against Tetanus in Wound Management

History of Tetanus Toxoid (Doses)	Type of Wound			
	Tetanus-Prone Wound		Non–Tetanus-Prone Wound	
	Td	TIG[*]	Td	TIG
Unknown to fewer than three	Yes	Yes	Yes	No
Three or more[†]	No[‡]	No	No[§]	No

Td, Tetanus and diphtheria toxoid absorbed (for adult use); *TIG,* tetanus immunoglobulin (human).
*When TIG and Td are administered concurrently, separate sites and syringes must be used.
†If only three doses of fluid toxoid have been received, a fourth dose of toxoid, preferably absorbed toxoid, should be given.
‡Yes, if more than 5 years since last dose.
§Yes, if more than 10 years since last dose.

or admitted to a general or intensive care unit. The emergency nurse is responsible for monitoring the trauma patient during transport and notifying the trauma team should the patient's condition change from baseline.

Death in the Emergency Department

Unfortunately, there are a number of emergency patients who do not benefit from the skill, expertise, and technology available in the ED. It is important for the emergency nurse to be able to deal with feelings about sudden death so that the nurse can help families and significant others begin the grieving process.

The emergency nurse should recognize the importance of certain hospital rituals in preparing the bereaved to grieve, such as collecting the belongings, arranging for an autopsy, viewing the body, and making mortuary arrangements. The death must seem real so that the significant others can begin to grieve and accept the death. The emergency nurse cannot afford to forget the surviving loved ones after a death in the ED. Family members may benefit from observing resuscitation of a loved one. Should a family member request to be present, it is essential that a member of the team explain care rendered and be available to answer questions.

ENVIRONMENTAL EMERGENCIES

Care of patients who have an environmental emergency is challenging because of the inability to control the environment and time constraints, especially if the patient's life is in jeopardy. It is extremely important to rapidly identify the primary problem, understand its pathology, and develop a plan of care to quickly treat the patient.

Emergency personnel often care for patients with specific environmental emergencies that occur because of exposure to extremes of cold or heat. Greater interest in recreational activities (especially for older adults), competitive athletic events, and winter and underwater exploration have increased the potential for environmental emergencies.

Cold-Related Emergencies

Cold-related emergencies vary in the degree of threat to life and depend on a multitude of factors such as age, duration

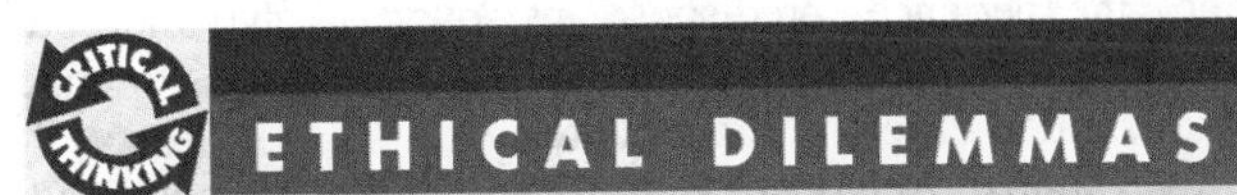

BRAIN DEATH

Situation The emergency nurse receives a radio call from the emergency medical technicians about a young male motorcycle accident victim. Because of flooding, the ambulance was unable to reach the scene until an hour after the call was received. The patient, who wore no helmet, has acute head trauma and appears to be dead. The ambulance crew asks if they should initiate life support. What should the nurse advise?

Discussion The degree of trauma and extent of brain damage cannot be assessed until the patient is carefully examined. If the patient is brain dead, there is total and irreversible brain damage. This patient may have extensive damage to just the cortex and no damage to the brainstem. In that case, he would be diagnosed as being in a persistent or permanent vegetative state. If he is brain dead, the hospital may choose to provide support in hopes of harvesting organs for transplantation purposes. A hospital is not obligated to continue futile medical care for a brain-dead patient who cannot survive even *with* mechanical intervention.

ETHICAL AND LEGAL PRINCIPLES

- The definition of brain death was orginally made in 1968 by a Harvard Medical School ad hoc committee in response to technology that kept the heart and lungs functioning even without brainstem activity and the growing need for organs that could be harvested for transplantation.
- Even if a patient is kept biologically alive, brain death will eventually cause the heart and lungs to cease functioning. Continuing to treat a brain-dead patient is medically futile.
- Brain death criteria do not address the problems of the lack of neocortical functioning (e.g., patients in a permanent vegetative state) or anencephalic infants because their brainstems are sufficient to keep them alive.

of exposure, temperature, preexisting conditions, medications, and alcohol level.

Predisposing Factors to Cold-Related Emergencies

Age. Older adults are less mobile and tend to have diminished energy reserves. Older adults have a decreased metabolic rate and decreased shivering response. They may have decreased sensory perception and chronic medical conditions, and they may take medications that alter body defenses. They can be misdiagnosed because hypothermia mimics other conditions such as cerebral or metabolic disturbances, ataxia, confusion, and withdrawal.

Activity. Hypothermia can occur in cases of near drowning (discussed later in this chapter). Water is 20 times more absorbant than air and will cause rapid, deep hypothermia. People who engage in winter sports or become lost in wilderness areas where night temperatures are low are also susceptible to hypothermia. Freezing temperatures, cold winds, wetness, physical exhaustion, inadequate clothing, and inexperience predispose persons to hypothermia. Homeless people may not have sufficient resources to cope with sudden drops in temperature.

Accidents. Accident victims are often immobilized, trapped, and exposed for long periods of time before they are extricated. Hypovolemia and acidosis complicate hypothermia. ED staff remove the patient's clothing, expose the patient, and may give unwarmed fluids, which can further compromise the patient's condition.

Alcohol and drugs. Drugs with depressant properties such as alcohol cause peripheral vasodilatation, increased warmth sensation, and depressed shivering, which lead to the loss of core heat. Other drugs that suppress shivering include psychotherapeutic agents, antiemetics, heroin, and narcotics.

Hypothermia. Hypothermia is defined as a decrease in body temperature with a continuum of symptoms of progressive severity as core temperature falls. Hypothermia occurs when the heat produced by the body is less than the amount of body heat lost to the environment. Exposure or accidental hypothermia is a core temperature less than 95° F (35° C). Heat is lost as radiant energy from the body in large amounts through the head and thorax and through breathing. As heat is lost, peripheral vasoconstriction occurs in an attempt to conserve heat. If clothing is wet, evaporation speeds heat loss. Wind also speeds heat loss by lowering the environmental temperature through conduction. The body gets its heat from caloric consumption. As cold temperatures persist, shivering and movement are the body's only mechanisms for producing heat. The lowest survivable recorded temperature is 62° F (17° C). Persons may appear dead; be pulseless, apneic, areflexia; and have fixed and dilated pupils, but they can survive. All severely hypothermic patients must be rewarmed before they are pronounced dead.

Any core temperature below 87° F (31° C) is considered severe and potentially life threatening. Possible assessment findings in hypothermia are variable and depend on the core temperature (Table 62-7). Patients with *mild hypothermia* (90°-95° F [33°-35° C]) have the following signs and symptoms: shivering, lethargy, confusion, rational to irrational behavior, and minor cardiac rate changes. Shivering disappears at temperatures less than 92° F (32° C). *Moderate hypothermia* (87°-90° F [31°-33° C]) results in rigidity, bradycardia, slowed respiratory rate, an irritable myocardium, blood pressure obtainable only by doppler, metabolic and respiratory acidosis, and hypovolemia. Movement of the patient should be avoided to prevent ventricular fibrillation. Persons with *profound hypothermia* (less than 87° F

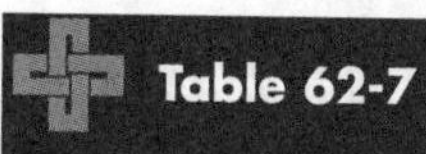

Table 62-7 Emergency Management: Hypothermia

Possible Etiologies

Prolonged exposure to cold, prolonged immersion, excessive perspiration, inadequate clothing relative to environmental temperature, any situation in which the body loses more heat than it produces (e.g., cold IV fluids, inadequate warming in the ED or OR)

Possible Assessment Findings

Shivering
Sleepiness
Apathy
Listlessness, areflexia
Unconsciousness, cyanosis
Decreased respiratory rate, pulse rate, temperature, blood pressure
Blue, white, or frozen extremities
Dysrhythmias (e.g., bradycardia, asystole, ventricular fibrillation)
Intoxication, history of exposure

Management

- Control scene; remove patient from cold environment.
- Monitor airway; have airway equipment available, including suction and intubation supplies; anticipate need for intubation if gag reflex is absent.
- Administer oxygen via nasal cannula or non-rebreather mask (100%) and monitor for respiratory distress; if patient is not breathing, ventilate with bag valve mask.
- Establish IV access with two large-bore catheters (14-16 gauge) and normal saline, and obtain blood samples.
- Assess for other injuries.
- Apply external warming materials (e.g., warm blankets, warm IV fluids, warm humidified oxygen); consider active rewarming if severely hypothermic (e.g., warm gastric lavage, open thoracotomy, cardiac bypass, bladder lavage).
- Transport immediately and avoid rewarming extremities if unable to keep warm during long-distance transport to hospital.
- Monitor vital signs, including level of consciousness, oxygen saturation, cardiac rhythm, temperature.
- Anticipate need for defibrillation and medications.
- Avoid rubbing body parts if frostbite suspected.

ED, Emergency department; *IV,* intravenous; *OR,* operating room.

[31° C]) appear dead on presentation. Signs and symptoms include comatose appearance, cyanosis, apnea, areflexia, fixed and dilated pupils, and no obtainable vital signs. The cardiac rhythm will show profound bradycardia, asystole, or ventricular fibrillation. Death can be pronounced only after the patient has been warmed to at least 90° F (32° C). The cause of death is usually from refractory ventricular fibrillation.

Cooling causes physiologic changes that complicate resuscitation. Intravascular volume decreases, resulting in an increased hematocrit, sludging of the blood, and thrombotic complications putting persons at risk for stroke, myocardial infarction, pulmonary edema, acute tubular necrosis, and renal failure. Decreased blood flow results in lactic acid accumulation from anaerobic metabolism and subsequent metabolic acidosis.

Hypothermia must be assessed with the use of core temperature measurements, arterial blood gases, ECG, and vital signs. Core temperature is closely monitored with an esophageal, rectal, or indwelling urinary catheter thermometer. Serial monitoring and careful handling is especially important. Hypothermic patients should have a central line, peripheral line, indwelling urinary catheter, and cardiac monitor. Core temperature should be increased at a rate of no faster than 1.5° F per hour. Fluid overload should be avoided because these patients are at risk for pulmonary edema and have decreased cardiac and renal function. Arterial blood gases help monitor oxygenation and acid-base status. Blood pH may be falsely low. PaO_2 and $PaCO_2$ may be elevated unless the laboratory corrects to the patient's temperature. Lab tests should include a complete blood count; serum levels of glucose, electrolytes, blood urea nitrogen, creatinine, and amylase; and urine myoglobin. Chest x-rays should be obtained on all hypothermic patients because pulmonary edema and aspiration pneumonia can occur.

Emergency management. Treatment of hypothermia is aimed at rewarming the patient, correcting the dehydration and acidosis, maintaining clear upper and lower airways, and treating cardiac dysrhythmias (see Table 62-7). *Passive rewarming* is the least invasive and labor intensive method to rewarm mildly hypothermic patients. The patient should be moved to a warm, dry environment and should be handled and stimulated as little as possible. Damp clothing should be removed and warm blankets should be placed around the patient.

Active rewarming is needed when the patient's internal reserves are not adequate. Heat must be added to assist rewarming. Thermal blankets, hot water bottles, and hot water baths are useful methods, but they decrease the ability to monitor the patient. *Active core rewarming* refers to heat applied directly to the core, warming the heart and brain first. It is invasive and labor intensive and requires an experienced team. Active core rewarming includes heated, humidified oxygen at 105° to 115° F (40.5°-46.1° C), heated intravenous fluids, heated bladder lavage, heated gastric lavage, heated peritoneal dialysis, hemodialysis, heart-lung bypass, and mediastinal lavage via thoracotomy. These patients should be carefully intubated and a nasogastric tube inserted. The nasogastric tube can be irrigated with warm crystalloid 200 to 400 ml, clamped for 5 minutes, drained, and suctioned. Active core rewarming depends on the severity of the situation, expertise of the team, and availability of equipment.

A patient with a temperature less than 85° F (29° C) is difficult to defibrillate. Therefore it is important not to inadvertently put the patient into fibrillation by moving the patient unnecessarily. Drugs are not metabolized and may accumulate to toxic levels. Care should be taken when administering drugs to hypothermic patients. Lidocaine has not been shown to be beneficial during cold fibrillation. Fluid resuscitation should be guided by central venous pressure monitoring and urine output to avoid fluid overload. Rewarming should not be too rapid.

Before discharge, the nurse should teach the patient how to avoid future problems. People should not travel to high elevations or venture out into cold temperatures unless they are prepared with extra clothing that is suitable for cold environments. They should carry high-carbohydrate foods for extra calories and have a plan for survival if an accident occurs. Homeless people need to be sheltered until fully recovered. Sending a homeless person back into a cold environment places him at great risk for becoming hypothermic again, and death may result.

Frostbite. Frostbite is caused by tissue damage secondary to peripheral vasoconstriction, which results in decreased blood flow (Fig. 62-3). *Frostnip* is a superficial form of frostbite in which the peripheral extremities feel tingling and burning. Rapid cooling results in the formation of ice crystals, increased intracellular sodium and chloride, cell membrane destruction, and damage to the organelles. The ears, nose, fingers, and toes are the most susceptible. Signs and symptoms vary depending on the person, previous exposure, and severity of the exposure. Length of exposure, degree of protection, previous injury, attempts to rewarm, chronic medical problems, and tetanus immunity

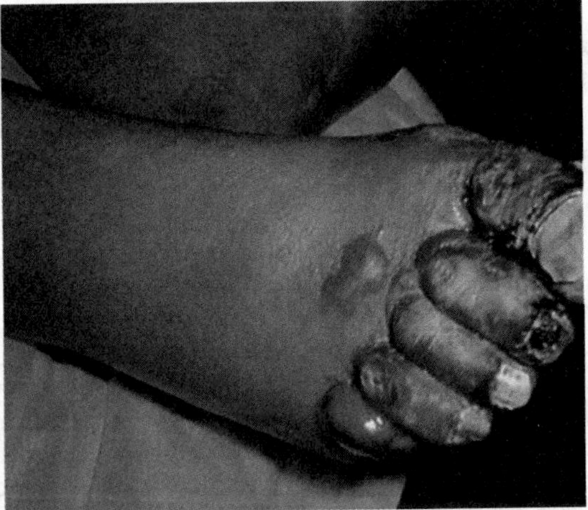

Fig. 62-3 Third-degree frostbite of the foot. Because vessels to the toes are protected by little subcutaneous tissue, these digits became ischemic and eventually required amputation.

need to be determined. On physical examination the skin appears pale and waxy. The affected tissues feel crunchy, and great care must be taken to prevent further damage. Frostbitten tissues should not be squeezed.

Emergency management. Emergency management of frostbite requires gentle handling and rewarming of the affected part by submersion of the extremity in a water bath at approximately 105° to 115° F (40.5°-46.1° C). The extremity should never be rewarmed near a flame or reexposed to a cold environment. Rewarming is extremely painful, and analgesia should be administered. Residual pain may last up to weeks or years, and the patient may have future temperature intolerance. Massage or scrubbing should be avoided because of the potential for tissue damage. All clothes and jewelry that constrict the frozen extremity should be removed. Pale blisters should be debrided and a sterile dressing applied. The patient should be evaluated for systemic hypothermia and the core temperature carefully monitored. The patient's tetanus status should be evaluated and tetanus toxoid administered as indicated (see Table 62-6). If there is a large amount of necrosis, tetanus immunoglobulin should be given.

Once the frostbitten limb has been rewarmed, treatment consists of 24 to 48 hours of hospital observation, bed rest, elevation of the injured part, and prophylactic antibiotics if infection is suspected. Significant edema may begin after 3 hours and blistering in 6 hours to days. If left untreated or if treatment is not successful, the affected part may have to be amputated to prevent further infection. Patients should be educated about how to prevent further cold-related injuries. Cessation of smoking should be recommended, and future cold-weather exposure should be avoided.

Heat-Related Emergencies

Heat-related emergencies are a failure of the heat mechanism to dissipate heat relative to the demands. The body is more efficient with dissipating than retaining heat. The core attempts to keep the body temperature at 100° F (37.8° C). Temperature regulation is discussed in Chapter 9.

Heat illness often occurs because of strenuous activities in hot or humid environments, the wearing of clothing that interferes with perspiration, high fevers, endocrine problems, and obesity. The basic mechanisms of heat illness are increased heat production, perspiration, and salt and water evaporation. These mechanisms increase the metabolic rate and muscle activity. Heat stress increases cardiac output to compensate for increased peripheral blood flow. Dehydration occurs because of increased sweating and evaporation of sweat that results in loss of salt and water.

Predisposing Factors to Heat-Related Emergencies. Heat-related emergencies are common during periods of prolonged heat and high humidity. The onset may be gradual or rapid. Older adults and individuals with diabetes mellitus or chronic renal, cardiovascular, or pulmonary disease are particularly vulnerable. Patients on certain drug therapies are at a greater risk of experiencing heat emergencies. Phototoxic drugs such as phenothiazines, antihistamines, and certain antibiotics increase the risk of heat emergencies. Alcohol increases metabolic heat production and causes impaired judgment, placing the user at greater risk during periods of high temperatures.

Heat Edema. Heat edema is swelling of the hands, feet, and ankles. Older people or individuals not acclimated to the environment may have pitting edema. The patient with heat edema will not have other signs and symptoms. The physical findings are due to heat-induced hyperaldosteronism. Treatment includes elevating the legs and reassurance (Table 62-8). Diuretics should not be used to treat heat edema.

Heat Cramps. Heat cramps are brief, intermittent, severe painful muscle cramps occurring in large muscle groups that are fatigued by heavy work. The cramps tend to occur while the patient is resting after exercise or heavy labor. They are usually seen in athletes who are acclimated, in good health, and have good fluid intake. These patients sweat profusely and replace lost fluid with salt-poor solutions. Heat cramps seem to be related to salt deficiency and are rapidly relieved by administration of oral or intravenous crystalloid salt solutions. Additional treatment includes elevation, gentle massage, and analgesia (Table 62-8). Education of the patient should emphasize including salt replacement during heavy exercise in a hot environment.

Heat Exhaustion. Heat exhaustion is due to prolonged heat exposure, resulting in volume and electrolyte depletion (Table 62-8). It is characterized by fatigue, lightheadedness, nausea, vomiting, diarrhea, and feelings of impending doom. The patient will be tachypneic, hypotensive, tachycardic, and will have a moderately elevated body temperature. The patient has dilated pupils, is mildly confused with impaired judgment, appears ashen, sweats profusely, and complains of a headache. Heat exhaustion is usually seen in people who have engaged in sports or strenuous exercise in hot, humid weather but it can also occur in sedentary people.

Treatment includes undressing the patient, intravenous normal saline solution, cooling, and bed rest. Often patients do not require much fluid because of vascular dilatation. Fluid and electrolyte replacement depends on the electrolyte laboratory results, blood urea nitrogen, and hematocrit. Older or chronically ill patients should be admitted to the hospital.

Heat Stroke. Heat stroke, or *hyperthermia,* is the most serious heat-related emergency and results in death if left untreated.[5] A core temperature greater than 103° to 106° F (39.4°-41.1° C) without sweating and with altered mentation is a true medical emergency. Prognosis is related to age, health, and length of exposure. Older adults and physiologically impaired individuals with diabetes mellitus or chronic renal, cardiovascular, or pulmonary disease are particularly vulnerable. Heat stroke is common during periods of prolonged heat for greater than 3 days with accompanying high humidity. Fluid and electrolytes become depleted and blood vessels dilate, which results in the need for increased cardiac output. Eventually the sweat glands stop functioning. When sweating ceases, the core temperature increases rapidly. The patient has hot, dry skin; a greatly elevated temperature; an altered level of consciousness; ashen skin; and cardiac collapse.

Table 62-8 Clinical Manifestations of Heat Edema, Heat Cramps, Heat Exhaustion, and Heat Stroke

Clinical Manifestations	Treatment
Heat Edema Swelling of hands, feet, ankles, pitting edema	Cool environment Elevate limbs
Heat Cramps Severe pain and cramps in lower-extremity muscles and abdomen, faintness, dizziness, weakness, profuse sweating	Increase sodium intake by giving salty liquids Intravenous crystalloid salt solution Encourage rest Move to cool environment Analgesia
Heat Exhaustion Pale skin, profuse sweating, nausea, vomiting, rapid weak pulse, lowered blood pressure, dilatation of pupils, confusion with impaired judgment, transient loss of consciousness, malaise, total body weakness	Place in cool environment Loosen clothing Apply cool compresses Elevate legs Intravenous crystalloid salt solution
Heat Stroke Elevated temperature (103°-106° F [39.4°-41.1° C]); reddish, flushed, hot, dry skin; initial elevation of blood pressure; bounding pulse; rapid and irregular respirations; agitation; weakness; dizziness; nausea and vomiting; decreased level of consciousness; coma	Provide oxygen Intravenous crystalloid salt solution Reduce body temperature rapidly Monitor core temperature Elevate head of bed Insert indwelling catheter and monitor urine output Draw blood samples

Treatment of heat stroke requires rapid initial assessment and aggressive treatment. Airway management includes administration of 100% oxygen to compensate for the hypermetabolic state, intubation if necessary, and ventilation with a bag valve mask. Intravenous fluids are initiated, and a central venous pressure or pulmonary artery catheter is inserted to monitor fluid status. Blood samples are drawn for arterial blood gases, electrolytes, coagulation studies, complete blood count, blood urea nitrogen, creatinine, serum glucose, and liver function tests, and a urinalysis is obtained. An indwelling catheter and nasogastric tube should be inserted. All clothing is removed and cooling methods initiated such as tepid water mist, fans, and ice packs to the head, groin, axillae, and neck. Shivering should be prevented because it generates muscle heat. Ice baths, alcohol rubs, and antipyretics are avoided. If conventional cooling methods are not successful, more aggressive treatment can include ice water lavage, cold water peritoneal dialysis, and cardiopulmonary bypass. Aggressive temperature reduction should continue until the patient's temperature reaches 101° F (38° C). If shivering occurs, diazepam (Valium) or other muscle relaxants may be administered.

Heat stroke carries a high risk of mortality and morbidity. All patients should be admitted to an intensive care unit for monitoring. Discharge teaching must be aimed at preventing recurrence of the emergency. Patients who are taking phototoxic drugs (e.g., phenothiazines, tetracycline) should be warned that these drugs make them more susceptible to heat emergencies.

Drowning and Near Drowning

Drowning accounts for approximately 8000 deaths each year in the United States. The majority of these deaths occur in swimming pools and are related to substance abuse. Drowning is the fourth leading cause of death in children. The highest incidence of drowning occurs in adolescents. Drowning is five times higher in men than women.[6]

Drowning is death from suffocation after submersion in water or some other fluid medium. *Near drowning* is survival for at least 24 hours after suffocation by submersion in water. *Immersion syndrome* is sudden death from vagally induced dysrhythmias that occur from sudden immersion in cold water.

As drowning victims hold their breath, carbon dioxide builds up, and hypoxia progresses, followed by air hunger and panic. Gasping inspirations cause either aspiration of fluid or laryngospasm, resulting in acute asphyxia. Laryngeal spasm may prevent aspiration of water. Victims who do not aspirate water have a better prognosis because fluid and acid-base imbalances are less severe.

Signs and symptoms of near drowning include progressive dyspnea, auscultatory wheezes, crackles, rhonchi, tachycardia, cyanosis, and a cough with pink frothy sputum (Table 62-9). The patient's temperature may be slightly elevated or below normal depending on the water temperature. The patient may experience chest pain, mental confusion, seizures, and increased muscle tone or may be in full cardiopulmonary arrest.

Near-drowning victims have recovered with no long-term effects after having been submerged in cold water for up to 40 minutes.[7] Aggressive resuscitation efforts and the mammalian diving reflex can improve survival. Cold water lowers the body's metabolic rate and oxygen demand. The mammalian diving reflex causes apnea, bradycardia, and peripheral vasoconstriction and further decreases metabolic rate. Blood flow is redistributed to the heart, lungs, and brain.

Table 62-9 Emergency Management: Near-Drowning Patient

Possible Etiologies

Exhaustion while swimming, loss of control or support in water, entrapment or entanglement by objects in water

Possible Assessment Findings

Panic
Ineffective breathing, dyspnea
Respiratory distress, respiratory arrest
Crackles, rhonchi
Exhaustion
Tachycardia
Cough with pink, frothy sputum
Loss of consciousness
Cardiac arrest

Management

- Control scene; place backboard under patient in the water and maintain cervical spine precautions, then remove patient from water.
- Initiate CPR in water if not breathing; clear airway of water, vomitus, debris.
- Monitor airway; have airway equipment available, including suction and intubation supplies; anticipate need for intubation if gag reflex is absent.
- Administer oxygen via nasal cannula or non-rebreather mask (100%) and monitor for respiratory distress; if patient is not breathing, ventilate with bag valve mask.
- Establish IV access with two large-bore catheters (14-16 gauge) and normal saline and obtain blood samples; avoid fluid overload.
- Assess for other injuries.
- Apply warming materials (e.g., warm blankets, warm IV fluids, warm humidified oxygen); consider active rewarming if severely hypothermic (e.g., warm gastric lavage, open thoracotomy, cardiac bypass, warm bladder lavage).
- Determine type of water involved (e.g., salt versus fresh) and temperature.
- Monitor vital signs, including level of consciousness, oxygen saturation, cardiac rhythm.
- Anticipate need for defibrillation and medications.

CPR, Cardiopulmonary resuscitation; *IV*, intravenous.

The osmotic gradient of aspirated fluid causes fluid imbalances in the body. Hypotonic *fresh water* is rapidly absorbed into the circulatory system through the alveoli. Fresh water can be contaminated with chlorine, mud, and algae, which cause lung surfactant breakdown, fluid seepage, and pulmonary edema. Hypertonic *salt water* draws fluid from the circulation into interstitial tissue and the alveoli, causing hemoconcentration and hypovolemia. Fluid is frequently swallowed by near-drowning victims. Large amounts of fresh water are rapidly absorbed via the GI system, causing hypervolemia, hyponatremia, interstitial edema, and swelling of cells. The most important life-threatening consequence of near-drowning is hypoxia. Pulmonary edema, pneumonia, respiratory failure, and acute respiratory disease syndrome (ARDS) follow near-drowning incidents and are a result of fluid-filled and poorly ventilated alveoli (Fig. 62-4).

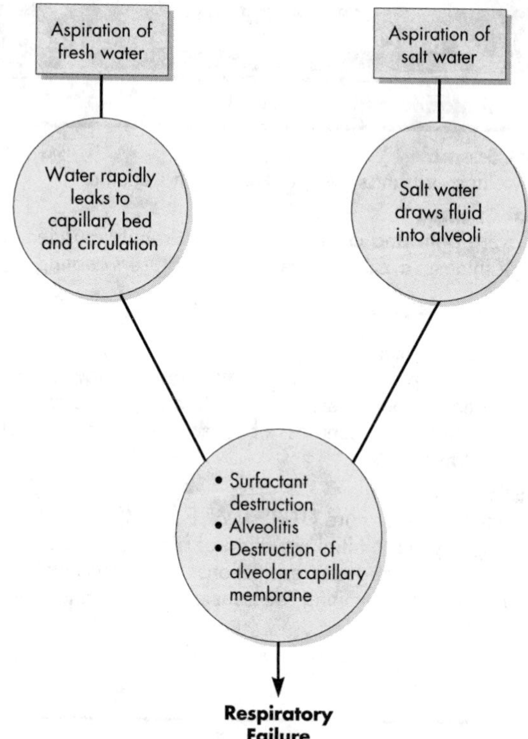

Fig. 62-4 Pulmonary effects of water aspiration.

The body attempts to compensate for hypoxia by shunting blood to the lungs, resulting in increased pulmonary pressures and shunted volume. Hypoxemia worsens as blood continues to be shunted through alveoli that are not oxygenated. Metabolic acidosis results from anaerobic metabolism.

Emergency Management. Treatment is directed at correcting hypoxia, acid-base imbalances, and fluid imbalances; supporting basic physiologic functions; and moderate rewarming (if severe hypothermia is present). Initial evaluation involves assessment of airway, cervical spine, breathing, and circulation. A cervical spine injury is always assumed. Cervical spine precautions are taken, the airway is cleared of secretions, and the jaw thrust maneuver is used. If the patient is in respiratory arrest, the patient should be ventilated with a bag valve mask on 100% oxygen and intubated. A 14- or 16-gauge intravenous catheter with lactated Ringer's or normal saline solution should be started for the delivery of emergency medications, and all patients should be monitored carefully for life-threatening dysrhythmias. Care must be taken not to overload the patient with fluid, and a central venous or pulmonary artery catheter should be considered. If the patient was submerged in cold water, core temperature should be monitored. Additional interventions include getting a chest x-ray, obtaining blood samples (including arterial blood gases), inserting a nasogastric tube to prevent aspiration of gastric contents, and inserting an indwelling catheter to monitor urine output.

If pulmonary edema is present or if alveolar collapse occurs, mechanical ventilation with positive end-expiratory pressure or continuous positive airway pressure may be used to improve gas exchange across the alveolar-capillary membrane. Ventilation and oxygenation are the primary means of treating acidosis. Mannitol or furosemide may be given to decrease the amount of free water and to treat cerebral edema.

Deterioration in neurologic status may indicate cerebral edema, increased hypoxia, or profound acidosis. Near-drowning victims may also have head injuries that may cause prolonged alterations in the level of consciousness. All victims of near drowning should be brought to the hospital for at least 4 to 6 hours of observation. Delayed pulmonary edema, pneumonia, and cerebral edema are common complications.

Education should be directed toward locking swimming pool gates, using pool covers, using life jackets, and getting swimming lessons. Individuals should be taught the dangers of combining substance abuse and swimming.

Animal Bites

Insect Bites (Hymenoptera). Insect bites, especially from bees, yellow jackets, hornets, and wasps, can cause a wide variety of reactions, from mild discomfort to anaphylactic shock (see Chapter 10). The stinger of the insect is often left in the skin after the bite and continues to release venom. The stinger should be removed by a scraping motion with a fingernail, knife, or needle; tweezers may cause more venom to be released by squeezing the stinger.

Signs and symptoms vary from stinging, burning, swelling, and itching to extremity edema, headache, fever, syncope, malaise, nausea, vomiting, wheezing, bronchospasm, laryngeal edema, and hypotension. Treatment depends on the severity of the reaction and consists of elevation; cool compresses; antipruritic lotions; oral, intramuscular, or IV antihistamines (diphenhydramine [Benadryl]); subcutaneous epinephrine (0.3-0.5 ml 1:1000); and corticosteroids. Rings, watches, and restrictive clothing should be removed. In severe cases an intravenous catheter should be inserted and the patient monitored closely for airway obstruction. Education should focus on persons known to be allergic to insects and the use of emergency insect-bite kits that contain epinephrine. (Allergic reactions and anaphylaxis are discussed in Chapter 10.)

Snakebite. Snakes fall into three major categories in the United States: Crotalids, Elapids, and Colubrids. Crotalids (rattlesnakes, copperheads, moccasins, cottonmouths, pit vipers) have moveable front fangs; Elapids (cobra, coral, sea snake krait) have fixed front fangs; and Colubrids (garter, king, lyre, hognose, and night snakes) have hind fangs (Fig. 62-5). Crotalids puncture and inject venom that is neurotoxic, cardiotoxic, hemotoxic, and cytotoxic. Elapids release a neurotoxin and must chew tissue to sequester the toxin. Colubrids are not venomous. It is important for the nurse to become familiar with the types and identifying characteristics of poisonous snakes in the region of the country in which the emergency facility is located.

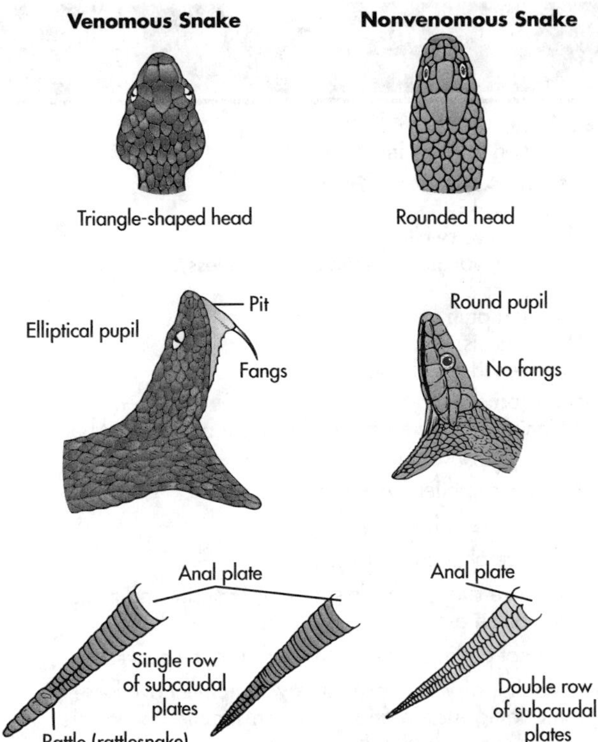

Fig. 62-5 Venomous and nonvenomous snakes.

Approximately 20% to 25% of snakebites are "dry," which means venom was not injected. To determine *envenomation* (injection of venom), pain, puncture, erythema, and edema should be noted after the bite. If swelling does not occur 30 minutes after the bite, envenomation is unlikely. Toxic reactions from snake venom include nausea and vomiting, dizziness, tachycardia, muscle fasciculation, GI bleeding, and respiratory problems. Envenomation by a coral snake may have neurotoxic manifestations, including drowsiness, weakness, muscle fasciculation, and muscle paresis.

Emergency management. Treatment in the field is focused on preventing the spread of the venom and decreasing panic (Table 62-10). Rings, watches, and restrictive clothing should be removed. The affected limb is splinted. Incision of the wound is controversial. If the affected person is greater than 1 hour away from the hospital, a vertical cut 0.125 inch (0.3 cm) deep is made and the venom is sucked out of the wound. If this is done within 3 minutes of the bite, 30% to 40% of the venom can be removed. Constricting bands are also controversial. If used, the band should be loose and moved proximally if edema spreads. Ice should never be used because it can cause tissue necrosis.

Immediate hospital care includes assessing airway, breathing, and circulation; administering oxygen if localized edema or breathing difficulties are present; inserting two

Table 62-10 Emergency Management: Snakebite

Etiology
Injection of toxin into blood stream

Possible Assessment Findings
Fang marks
Progressive swelling
Nausea, vomiting, headache, dizziness
Paresthesia
Burning pain
Ecchymosis, erythema
Decreased distal pulses

Management
- Control scene; remove patient from area; avoid being bitten by snake.
- Reassure patient, decrease panic.
- Immobilize affected part.
- Reduce physical activity.
- Remove rings, bracelets, or other constricting items on the bitten extremity.
- Do not put injured part in ice or use ice packs.
- Monitor airway; have airway equipment available, including suction and intubation supplies; anticipate need for intubation if gag reflex absent.
- Administer oxygen via nasal cannula or non-rebreather mask (100%) and monitor for respiratory distress; if patient is not breathing, ventilate with bag valve mask.
- Establish IV access with two large-bore catheters (14 or 16 gauge) and normal saline, and obtain blood samples; place catheters in unaffected extremity.
- Monitor vital signs, including level of consciousness, oxygen saturation, cardiac rhythm.
- Anticipate need for medications (e.g., antivenin, prophylactic antibiotics, tetanus toxoid).
- Complete blood count, electrolytes, blood glucose, blood urea nitrogen, creatinine, urine myoglobin, coagulation screen, urinalysis, type and crossmatch.
- Attempt to identify snake type.
- Monitor extremity size and color, pulses.

IV, Intravenous.

large-bore IV catheters; assessing the bite area for the degree of envenomation; and obtaining laboratory studies for blood typing and crossmatching, complete blood count, urinalysis, coagulation studies, blood urea nitrogen, creatinine, blood glucose, and serum electrolytes. Other measures include measuring and recording the circumference of the injured extremity every 30 to 60 minutes; skin testing for antivenin sensitivity; and administering tetanus prophylaxis, prophylactic antibiotics, and intravenous antivenin (Table 62-11).

Ongoing evaluation includes monitoring vital signs, urine output, respiratory status, level of consciousness, and cardiac rhythm. Emergency airway equipment, antihistamines, and epinephrine should be at the bedside.

Table 62-11 Antivenin Snakebite Treatment

Envenomation	Signs and Symptoms	Number of Vials of Antivenin*
None	Fang marks No local swelling or hemorrhage	None Tetanus prophylaxis, observation
Minimal	Fang marks Limited local swelling No systemic reactions	3-5 vials
Moderate	Swelling progressing rapidly beyond bite Systemic reactions	6-10 vials
Severe	Pronounced and rapidly progressive local and systemic reactions	15 + vials

*Depends on type of snakebite, body surface area, and age. Skin testing should be done before injection of antivenin.

Follow-up care of a snakebite may require debridement or fasciotomy. Most venomous snake bites become infected from contamination that occurs in the field (e.g., dirt, human oral flora, or contamination from the snake because snakes eat their prey live, and the prey may defecate in the snake's mouth). Education should be directed toward avoidance of snake-infested areas.

Spider Bites (Arachnid). Venomous spider bites most commonly occur by the *black widow spider* or the *brown recluse spider*.

Black widow spider. Black widow spiders are found in damp, cool places under rocks, in woodpiles, or in outhouses. They have black bodies and a bright red hourglass-shaped marking on their abdomens. Signs and symptoms of a black widow bite include a painful sting, tiny red bite, nausea, vomiting, elevated temperature, diaphoresis, respiratory distress, hypertension, headache, syncope, weakness, chest and abdominal pain, seizures, and shock. The venom is neurotoxic, and abdominal rigidity may develop if one is bitten in the lower half of the body. Chest, back, and shoulder rigidity and spasms may develop if one is bitten in the upper half of the body. Because the bite is not prominent, patients are often thought to have a perforated ulcer, appendicitis, pancreatitis, or another abdominal emergency.

Symptomatic treatment includes cooling the area, muscle relaxants, cleaning the wound, and tetanus prophylaxis. Antivenin is used if the symptoms are severe. Calcium gluconate or methocarbamol (Robaxin) is sometimes given to treat muscle spasms. The symptoms run their course in several hours, although mild recurrences are common. The patient usually recovers in a week with no complications. Young children and older adults should be closely monitored for respiratory difficulties, cardiac abnormalities, and altered level of consciousness.

Brown recluse spider. Brown recluse spiders inhabit the southeastern, southcentral, and southwestern United States in dark areas such as garages, closets, and boxes. They are light brown with a dark fiddle-shaped mark on their backs. Brown recluse spiders inject a venom that can cause skin necrosis and severe hemolysis. Signs and symptoms include stinging, burning, itching, pain, bleb (blister), and erythema formation that can eventually develop into necrotic lesions. Systemic manifestations include fever, myalgia, rash, hemolysis, coagulopathies, joint pain, seizures, shock, hemorrhage, and pulmonary edema. Hemolysis may lead to hemoglobinuria, renal failure, and death.

Treatment depends on the severity of the bite. If the patient is relatively free of symptoms, no treatment is necessary. If bleb or bullae formation, intense pain, and signs of rapidly progressive ischemia and necrosis are present, treatment is necessary. Treatment measures include cool compresses, analgesics, tetanus prophylaxis, elevation of the affected extremity, surgical debridement, antihistamines, corticosteroids, and antibiotics for prevention of a secondary infection. Patients with systemic manifestations should be hospitalized and monitored for signs of hemolysis, disseminated intravascular clotting, and acute renal failure.

Tick Bites. Ticks inhabit various parts of the country, in particular the Rocky Mountain region and the Northwest. Ticks may cause tick fever, Rocky Mountain spotted fever, and flaccid paralysis as a result of neurotoxins contained in their venom. Signs and symptoms include a history of a tick bite, paresthesias, pain, elevated temperature, headache, nuchal rigidity, seizures, and respiratory failure secondary to paralysis. Interventions include symptomatic treatment, removal of the tick (care must be exercised to remove the entire body and head), and monitoring respiratory status. Education about protection from bites and how to remove ticks should be given to campers and to others engaging in outdoor activities. (Lyme disease is discussed in Chapter 60.)

Human Bites. Human bites are the most serious bites because they carry a high risk of infection from the injection of oral bacterial flora, most commonly *Staphylococcus aureus* and streptococci. The hands, fingers, and nose are the most common sites of human bites. Infections occur in approximately 50% of all reported cases in which victims have not sought medical intervention within 24 hours of the injury.[8] If the human bite is deep, there can be significant damage to the tissue, with hematoma formation and deep invasion of oral flora. When a human bite occurs, there is usually a retraction of skin with edema that causes a trapping of organisms of the oral flora and results in a serious infection.

Treatment includes cleaning the wound, debridement, prophylactic antibiotics, and tetanus prophylaxis. Depending on the location of the human bite, x-rays may be indicated. The extremity should be kept elevated and the patient admitted to the hospital for intravenous antibiotic therapy. Wounds over joints should be splinted and suturing avoided except for facial wounds.

Dog, Cat, and Rodent Bites. Approximately 500,000 to 2 million animal bites are reported each year in the United States. Most of these bites are dog bites (80%) and cat bites (8% to 15%). Rodents, monkeys, and squirrels account for less than 10%.[8] Children are the most at risk for bites. The most significant problems associated with animal bites are infection and the mechanical destruction of skin, muscle, tendons, blood vessels, and bone. The bite injury may be a simple laceration, a crush injury, a puncture wound, or a tearing or avulsion of the tissue.

There is a greater incidence of infection from cat bites as compared with dog bites. *Cat bites* may involve the tendons and joint capsules because cat teeth are pointed and sharp. This can lead to complications such as septic arthritis, osteomyelitis, and tenosynovitis. Cats often come into contact with rodents and carry bacteria on their teeth and claws. *Pasteurella multocida* can be cultured in 75% of cat bite wounds.

Treatment of an animal bite is the same as that for any type of emergency, including the maintenance of an adequate airway, especially if the bite is near or on the neck or face. Control of bleeding with maintenance of adequate circulation is important. The wound is inspected for tissue integrity and location of nerves, tendons, blood vessels, ligaments, joints, and organs that may be affected by the bite. The wound should be irrigated with saline solution, antibiotics should be administered, and tetanus prophylaxis given.

The people at highest risk of developing infection are infants, older adults, immunosuppressed patients, alcoholics, diabetics, and people taking corticosteroids. Wounds from bites on the hand are most likely to get infected.

One of the most important considerations in the treatment of animal bites is whether rabies prophylaxis is indicated. Although rabies rarely affects human beings in the United States, every year approximately 25,000 persons receive rabies prophylaxis.[9] Rabies is transmitted when the neurotoxic virus is introduced into open cuts or wounds. If rabies is known to be present or is suspected of being present, the animal should be captured. Any animal exhibiting abnormal behavior or suspected of being rabid should be killed, and the brain should be examined. Rabies prophylaxis may involve passive immunization with rabies immune globulin or active immunization with antirabies vaccine. Indications for rabies prophylaxis include (1) a bite from a wild animal, (2) an unprovoked attack by a dog that cannot be examined for rabies for 10 days, and (3) a bite from an animal observed to develop signs of rabies.

POISONINGS

A poison is any chemical that harms the body. In the United States there are more than 1 million cases of poisoning annually. Poisonings may be accidental or purposeful, as in the case of suicide attempts. Many poison histories are not accurate. The history should include the type of poisoning present, the amount of toxin exposure, the length of time since the exposure occurred, symptoms that have appeared since the poisoning, and health history (including allergies and present medications being taken by the patient). If

Table 62-12 Common Poison Substances

Poison	Manifestations	Treatment
▪ Acetaminophen (Tylenol)	Nausea and vomiting, anorexia, malaise, diaphoresis, liver abnormalities	Activated charcoal, *N*-acetylcysteine
▪ Acids and alkalis *Acids:* toilet bowl cleaners, antirust compounds; *alkalis:* drain cleaners, dishwashing detergents, ammonia	Excess salivation, dysphagia, epigastric pain, pneumonitis, burns of mouth, esophagus, and stomach	Immediate dilution (water, milk), corticosteroids (for alkali burns), contraindication for gastric emptying
▪ Aspirin and aspirin-containing medications	Increased respiratory rate, respiratory alkalosis, headache, vertigo, tinnitus, sweating, nausea, electrolyte imbalances	Gavage, activated charcoal, alkaline diuresis, supportive care
▪ Bleaches	Irritation of lips, mouth, and eyes, superficial injury to esophagus; chemical pneumonia and pulmonary edema	Washing of exposed skin and eyes, dilution with water and milk, gastric lavage, prevention of vomiting and aspiration
▪ Carbon monoxide	Dyspnea, headache, tachypnea, confusion, impaired judgment, cyanosis, respiratory depression	Removal from source, administration of 100% oxygen
▪ Cyanide	Headache, faintness, vertigo, tachycardia, hypertension, nausea and vomiting, almond odor to breath	Amyl nitrate, sodium nitrate, sodium thiosulfate, oxygen
▪ Ethylene glycol	Sweet aromatic odor to breath, nausea and vomiting, slurred speech, ataxia, lethargy, respiratory depression	Gastric lavage, activated charcoal, supportive care
▪ Iron	Vomiting (often bloody), diarrhea (often bloody), fever, hyperglycemia, lethargy, hypotension, seizures, coma	Ipecac-induced vomiting, gastric lavage, chelation therapy (deferoxamine)
▪ Nonsteroidal antiinflammatory drugs	Gastroenteritis, abdominal pain, drowsiness, nystagmus, hepatic damage	Induced emesis, activated charcoal, cathartics
▪ Tricyclic antidepressants (e.g., amitriptyline, imipramine)	In low doses: anticholinergic effects, agitation, hypertension, tachycardia; in high doses: central nervous system depression, respiratory depression, seizures, hypotension	Activated charcoal, gastric lavage, supportive care, contraindication for induced emesis
▪ Alcohol, barbiturates, benzodiazepines, cocaine, hallucinogens, stimulants	See Chapter 8	See Chapter 8

contact is made with patients before their arrival in the ED, they should be instructed to bring the poison container to the hospital.

Poisonings may be inhaled, ingested, injected, or absorbed through the skin. The effect and extent of damage caused by a poison depends on the poison type, its concentration, and the way it enters the body. Common poison substances are presented in Table 62-12.

Surface Toxins

Surface or topical poisons may damage the skin. Most are corrosives or irritants that are slowly absorbed into body tissues and the bloodstream. Included in this group are many of the commonly used insecticides (e.g., malathion) and agricultural chemicals. Initially the corrosive chemicals may damage only the skin. Then they continue to damage tissues and are absorbed by the body, causing widespread damage. Treatment includes removing the patient from the exposure area and protecting others from exposure. A hazardous material team is best equipped to do this. Patients should be brought to community-designated decontamination centers. Patients should not be brought directly into the ED; they should be brought to a designated detoxification area. Most surface toxins must be washed from the patient with copious amounts of water as soon as possible, except for mustard gas. The use of water with mustard gas will cause a chemical reaction and would release chlorine gas into the air. Mustard gas should be brushed off of the patient. Special attention must be given to those body areas that serve as pockets collecting the toxin, such as the ears and the navel. All contaminated clothes should be removed, and the affected areas should be washed again. Clothing and the water used to wash the patient must be collected in specially designated containers and disposed of properly by the hazardous materials team. Interventions are directed toward maintaining the patient's airway, breathing, and circulation. The local poison center should be contacted regarding specific antidotes. Emergency nurses must be aware of industries that produce and use poisons in their area and have continuing education on how to decontaminate victims with potential exposures.

Inhaled Toxins

Inhaled toxins take the form of gases, vapors, and sprays. Many of these substances are in common use in homes, industry, and agriculture. These poisons include carbon monoxide (from car exhaust, wood-burning stoves, and furnaces), ammonia, chlorine, gases produced from volatile liquid chemicals (including many industrial solvents), and insect sprays. Inhaled toxins are difficult to treat and may result in hoarseness, chemical pneumonitis, and pulmonary edema. Appropriate treatment includes removing victims from the toxin source, protecting rescue personnel from exposure, administering oxygen, and observing for respiratory distress.

Ingested Toxins

Ingested toxins are common and may range from an overdose of medication to food poisoning. Some toxins require immediate induction of vomiting; others contraindicate this action. Induction of vomiting is controversial. The local poison control center should be called if one is available. In general, induction of vomiting is contraindicated in the following circumstances: (1) ingestion of strong bases or acids (e.g., drain cleaners, ammonia, toilet bowl cleaners) or low-viscosity petroleum products (e.g., kerosene, gasoline) because vomiting can cause aspiration and severe damage to the esophagus; (2) absence of gag reflex; (3) unconsciousness; and (4) seizures.

If none of these conditions exists, vomiting may be induced or gastric lavage used to remove toxic substances. Vomiting can be induced by giving the adult victim 30 ml syrup of ipecac by mouth, followed by 600 to 900 ml of oral fluid if ingestion occurred less than 1 hour previously. It is essential that the patient drink oral fluids after ipecac administration. Another method of removing the toxin is by inserting a large-bore oral-gastric tube into the patient's stomach and lavaging with at least 3 L of saline solution. The patient's airway must be carefully monitored during gastric lavage. The patient should be maintained in a left-sided Trendelenberg position to enhance irrigation and reduce the chance of aspiration.

Treatment of the poison victim is directed toward removing the toxin from the body, supporting the body systems, and administering an antidote if the poison is known and if a specific antidote to it exists. Frequently the specific poison is not known. Supportive care must be given regardless of whether an antidote is available. If the patient has ingested strong bases or acids or petroleum products, one or two glasses of milk or water can be drunk unless directed otherwise. Dilution is contraindicated when the patient has ingested medicinal substances because water can actually speed absorption.

Because many ingested poisons can be absorbed in the lower GI tract, an alert patient may become comatose and critically ill at a later time. Cathartics and activated charcoal are used to decrease the possibility of GI absorption. Activated charcoal is given orally or through a large oral-gastric tube. Activated charcoal can absorb a number of poisons from the GI tract. Activated charcoal does not absorb ethanol, alkali, iron, boric acid, lithium, methanol, or cyanide.

Cathartics are used to decrease toxicity by moving poisons through the GI system rapidly, thereby reducing absorption. Magnesium-containing cathartics are contraindicated in pesticide poisonings. It is important to instruct the patient that black to brown diarrhea may occur after receiving activated charcoal and cathartics.

Food poisoning is also a type of poison ingestion (see Chapter 38). Frequently a large number of people become ill after the ingestion of the same contaminated food. This can help speed identification of the toxic agent. Food poisoning may be caused by chemicals in the food or by bacterial toxins. These poisons cause GI symptoms that develop within a few minutes to 2 hours. Bacterial sources of food poisoning include *Clostridium botulinum* (found in improperly canned vegetables and preserved meat and fish), salmonellae (found in food contaminated by rat feces, the housefly, and human carriers), and staphylococci (found in contaminated milk, mayonnaise, and cream).

Treatment of food poisoning is supportive and directed toward relief of symptoms. Botulism is the most severe form and causes respiratory paralysis and death if untreated (see Chapter 57). Salmonellae and staphylococci poisoning cause severe GI distress (nausea, vomiting, and diarrhea).

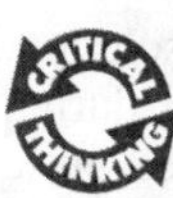

CRITICAL THINKING EXERCISES

CASE STUDY

TRAUMA

Patient Profile

A 42-year-old male trauma patient is brought to the ED via ambulance. He was the driver in a motor vehicle collision and was not wearing a seat belt. The passenger in the car was dead at the scene. The paramedics stated that there was significant damage to the car on the passenger side.

Subjective Data

- Is awake
- Complains of shortness of breath and abdominal pain

Objective Data

Physical Examination

- 4-cm head laceration
- Badly deformed right lower leg without pulses
- Unequal pupils
- Decreased breath sounds on left side of chest
- Asymmetric chest movement
- Vital signs: BP 90/40, HR 130, respiratory rate 36/min.
- O_2 saturation 82%

Critical Thinking Questions

1. What life-threatening injury does this patient probably have?
2. What is the priority of care?
3. What intervention is needed immediately?
4. What other interventions should the nurse consider?
5. How should the nurse deal with the family?
6. Based on the assessment data presented, write one or more nursing diagnoses. Are there any collaborative problems?

REVIEW QUESTIONS

The number of the question corresponds to the same-numbered objective at the beginning of the chapter.

1. Which of the following is *not* part of the EMS system?
   a. Public information campaign
   b. Transportation system
   c. Disaster preparedness
   d. Rehabilitative care facility

2. An important principle of history taking in emergency situations is to
   a. obtain history after giving emergency care.
   b. record history before giving care.
   c. verify history with family members or friends.
   d. ask leading questions to facilitate the process.

3. Which patient should be triaged first?
   a. A 2-year-old child with a head laceration who is awake and crying
   b. An 85-year-old woman with crushing chest pain who is diaphoretic and pale
   c. A 32-year-old complaining of a recent onset of a fever, aches, and chills after a camping trip
   d. A 16-year-old with a swollen ankle that he injured while playing basketball

4. An older male arrives at the ED disoriented and breathing rapidly. His skin is hot and dry. Your priority of treatment is to
   a. determine what kind of insurance he has before treating him.
   b. assess his airway, breathing, and circulation.
   c. look for his family and obtain a detailed medical history.
   d. make him wait in the waiting room because you have a patient with a broken arm to check in.

REFERENCES

1. Consolidated Omnibus Budget Reconciliation Act (COBRA), Amended Dec 19, 1989. Pub No 101-239, 62211 HR 3299.
*2. Moore KW, Schwartz KS: Psychosocial support of trauma patients in the emergency department by nurses, as indicated by communication, *J Emerg Nurs* 19:297, 1993.
3. Kitt S, Kaiser J: *Emergency nursing, a physiologic and clinical perspective*, Philadelphia, 1990, Saunders.
4. Sheehy SB: *Emergency nursing principles and practice*, ed 3, St Louis, 1992, Mosby.
*5. Simon HB: Hyperthermia and heatstroke, *Hosp Pract* 29:65, 1994.
6. Glankler DM: Caring for the victim of near drowning, *Crit Care Nurse* 13:25, 1993.

7. Siebake H and others: Survival after 40 minutes submersion without cerebral sequelae, *Lancet* 1:1275, 1975.
8. Auerbach P, Geehr E: *Management of wilderness and environmental emergencies,* ed 2, St Louis, 1989, Mosby.
9. Moore EE and others: *Early care of the injured patient,* ed 4, Philadelphia, 1990, Decker.

SECTION XII BIBLIOGRAPHY

Books

Cardona VC and others, editors: *Trauma nursing: from resuscitation through rehabilitation,* ed 2, Philadelphia, 1994, WB Saunders.

Fishman RA: *Cerebrospinal fluid in diseases of the nervous system,* ed 2, Philadelphia, 1992, WB Saunders.

George R and others: *Chest medicine essentials of pulmonary medicine,* ed 2, New York, 1990, Williams & Wilkins.

Hudak CM and others: *Critical care nursing: a holistic approach,* ed 6, Philadelphia, 1994, JB Lippincott.

Journals

*Christie J: Does the use of an assessment tool in the accident and emergency department improve the quality of care? *J Adv Nurs* 18:1758, 1993.

Cone M and others: Cardiopulmonary support in the intensive care unit, *Am J Crit Care* 1:98, 1992.

Corcoran E: President's message: scoping out our emergency nursing practice, *J Emerg Nurs* 19:474, 1993.

Daffurn K and others: Do nurses know when to summon emergency assistance? *Intensive Crit Care Nurs* 10:115, 1994.

*Evans RJ and others: Telephone advice in the accident and emergency department: a survey of current practice, *Arch Emerg Med* 10:216, 1993.

Goldstein G, Luce JM: Pharmacologic treatment of the adult respiratory distress syndrome, *Clin Chest Med* 11:773, 1990.

Heffner J: Airway management in the critically ill patient, *Crit Care Clin* 6:533, 1990.

*Johnson RI, Childress SE, Herron HL: Regulation of prehospital nursing practice: a national survey, *J Emerg Nurs* 19:437, 1993.

Liggins K: Inappropriate attendance at accident and emergency departments: a literature review, *J Adv Nurs* 18:1141, 1993.

Matthay MA: The adult respiratory distress syndrome, *Clin Chest Med* 11:575, 1990.

Niederman M, Fein A: Sepsis syndrome, the adult respiratory distress syndrome, and nosocomial pneumonia: a common clinical sequence, *Clin Chest Med* 11:633, 1990.

Rice M: Emergency nursing at a crossroads. Health care reform, hospital redesign, and other trends figure to transform the specialty. But emergency nurses know how to handle crises, *Am J Nurs* 94:65, 1994.

Rinaldo J, Christman J: Mechanisms and mediators of the adult respiratory distress syndrome, *Clin Chest Med* 11:621, 1990.

Smith C: Career developments in accident and emergency nursing, *Br J Nurs* 3:362, 1994.

Villar J and others: Nonconventional techniques of ventilatory support, *Crit Care Clin* 6:579, 1990.

White KM and others: The physiologic basis for continuous mixed venous oxygen saturation monitoring, *Heart Lung* 19:548, 1990.

Organizations

American Association of Critical-Care Nurses (AACN)
101 Columbia
Aliso Viejo, CA 92656
800-899-2226
714-362-2000
FAX: 714-362-2020

Emergency Nurses Association
216 Higgins Road
Park Ridge, IL 60068
708-698-9400
FAX: 708-698-9406

*Nursing research-based articles.

Appendix A

Nursing Diagnoses

Grouped by Functional Health Patterns

HEALTH PERCEPTION–HEALTH MANAGEMENT PATTERN

Altered Health Maintenance
Altered Protection
Effective Management of Therapeutic Regimen: Individual
Energy Field Disturbance
Health-Seeking Behaviors (Specify)
Ineffective Management of Therapeutic Regimen: Individuals
Ineffective Management of Therapeutic Regimen: Community
Ineffective Management of Therapeutic Regimen: Families
Noncompliance (Specify)
Risk for Infection
Risk for Injury
Risk for Perioperative Positioning Injury
Risk for Poisoning
Risk for Suffocation
Risk for Trauma

NUTRITIONAL-METABOLIC PATTERN

Altered Nutrition: Less than Body Requirements
Altered Nutrition: More than Body Requirements
Altered Nutrition: Potential for More than Body Requirements
Altered Oral Mucous Membrane
Effective Breast feeding
Fluid Volume Deficit
Fluid Volume Excess
Hyperthermia
Hypothermia
Impaired Skin Integrity
Impaired Swallowing
Impaired Tissue Integritiy
Ineffective Breastfeeding
Ineffective Infant Feeding Pattern
Ineffective Thermoregulation
Interrupted Breastfeeding
Risk for Altered Body Temperature
Risk for Aspiration
Risk for Fluid Volume Deficit
Risk for Impaired Skin Integrity

ELIMINATION PATTERN

Altered Urinary Elimination
Bowel Incontinence
Colonic Constipation
Constipation
Diarrhea
Functional Incontinence
Perceived Constipation
Reflex Incontinence
Stress Incontinence
Total Incontinence
Urge Incontinence
Urinary Retention

ACTIVITY-EXERCISE PATTERN

Activity Intolerance
Altered Growth and Development
Altered Tissue Perfusion (Specify Type)
(Renal, cerebral, cardiopulmonary, gastrointestinal, peripheral)
Bathing/Hygiene Self-Care Deficit
Decreased Cardiac Output
Disorganized Infant Behavior
Diversional Activity Deficit
Dressing Self-Care Deficit
Dysfunctional Ventilatory Weaning Response (DVWR)
Dysreflexia
Feeding Self-Care Deficit
Fatigue
Impaired Gas Exchange
Impaired Home Maintenance Management
Impaired Physical Mobility
Inability to Sustain Spontaneous Ventilation
Ineffective Airway Clearance
Ineffective Breathing Pattern
Potential for Enhanced Organized Infant Behavior
Risk for Activity Intolerance
Risk for Disorganized Infant Behavior
Risk for Disuse Syndrome
Risk for Peripheral Neurovascular Dysfunction

Modified from *NANDA nursing diagnosis: definitions and classifications 1995-1996,* North American Nursing Diagnosis Association; and Gordon M: *Manual of nursing diagnoses,* St Louis, 1995, Mosby.

SLEEP-REST PATTERN

Sleep Pattern Disturbance

COGNITIVE-PERCEPTUAL PATTERN

Acute Confusion
Altered Thought Processes
Chronic Confusion
Chronic Pain
Decisional Conflict (Specify)
Decreased Adaptive Capacity: Intracranial
Impaired Environmental Interpretation Syndrome
Impaired Memory
Knowledge Deficit (Specify)
Pain
Sensory-Perceptual Alterations
Unilateral Neglect

SELF-PERCEPTION–SELF-CONCEPT PATTERN

Anxiety
Body Image Disturbance
Chronic Low Self-Esteem
Fear (Specify Focus)
Hopelessness
Personal Identity Disturbance
Powerlessness
Risk for Loneliness
Risk for Self-Mutilation
Self-Esteem Disturbance
Situational Low Self-Esteem

ROLE-RELATIONSHIP PATTERN

Altered Family Processes
Altered Family Process: Alcoholism
Altered Parenting
Altered Role Performance
Anticipatory Grieving
Caregiver Role Strain
Dysfunctional Grieving
Impaired Social Interaction
Impaired Verbal Communication
Parental Role Conflict
Relocation Stress Syndrome
Risk for Altered Parent/Infant/Child Relationship
Risk for Altered Parenting
Risk for Caregiver Role Strain
Risk for Violence: Self-directed or directed at others
Social Isolation

SEXUALITY-REPRODUCTIVE PATTERN

Altered Sexuality Patterns
Rape-Trauma Syndrome
Rape-Trauma Syndrome: Compound Reaction
Rape-Trauma Syndrome: Silent Reaction
Sexual Dysfunction

COPING–STRESS TOLERANCE PATTERN

Defensive Coping
Family Coping: Potential for Growth
Impaired Adjustment
Ineffective Community Coping
Ineffective Coping (Individual)
Ineffective Denial
Ineffective Family Coping: Compromised
Ineffective Family Coping: Disabling
Posttrauma Response
Potential for Enhanced Community Coping

VALUE-BELIEF PATTERN

Potential for Enhanced Spiritual Well-Being
Spiritual Distress

Alphabetical Listing

Activity Intolerance
Activity Intolerance, Risk for
Adaptive Capacity, Intracranial, Decreased
Adjustment, Impaired
Airway Clearance, Ineffective
Anxiety
Aspiration, Risk for
Body Image Disturbance
Body Temperature, Risk for Altered
Bowel Incontinence
Breastfeeding, Effective
Breastfeeding, Ineffective
Breastfeeding, Interrupted
Breathing Patterns, Ineffective
Caregiver Role Strain
Caregiver Role Strain, Risk for
Communication, Impaired Verbal
Community Coping, Ineffective
Community Coping, Potential for Enhanced
Confusion, Acute
Confusion, Chronic
Constipation
Constipation, Colonic
Constipation, Perceived
Decisional Conflict (Specify)
Decreased Cardiac Output
Defensive Coping
Denial, Ineffective
Diarrhea
Disorganized Infant Behavior
Disorganized Infant Behavior, Risk for
Disuse Syndrome, Risk for
Diversional Activity Deficit
Dysfunctional Ventilatory Weaning Response
Dysreflexia
Energy Field Disturbance
Environmental Interpretation Syndrome, Impaired

Family Coping, Compromised, Ineffective
Family Coping: Disabling, Ineffective
Family Coping: Potential for Growth
Family Process: Alcoholism, Altered
Fatigue
Fear
Fluid Volume Deficit
Fluid Volume Deficit, Risk for
Fluid Volume Excess
Gas Exchange, Impaired
Grieving, Anticipatory
Grieving, Dysfunctional
Growth and Development, Altered
Health Maintenance, Altered
Health-Seeking Behaviors (Specify)
Home Maintenance Management, Impaired
Hopelessness
Hyperthermia
Hypothermia
Incontinence, Bowel
Incontinence, Functional
Incontinence, Reflex
Incontinence, Stress
Incontinence, Total
Incontinence, Urge
Individual Coping, Ineffective
Infant Feeding Pattern, Ineffective
Infection, Risk for
Knowledge Deficit (Specify)
Loneliness, Risk for
Management of Therapeutic Regimen: Community, Ineffective
Management of Therapeutic Regimen: Families, Ineffective
Management of Therapeutic Regimen: Individual, Effective
Management of Therapeutic Regimen: Individual, Ineffective
Memory, Impaired
Noncompliance (Specify)
Nutrition: Less than Body Requirements, Altered
Nutrition: More than Body Requirements, Altered
Nutrition: Potential for More than Body Requirements, Altered
Oral Mucous Membrane, Altered
Organized Infant Behavior, Potential for Enhanced
Pain
Pain, Chronic
Parent/Infant/Child Attachment, Risk for Altered
Parental Role Conflict
Parenting, Altered
Parenting, Risk for Altered
Perioperative Positioning Injury, Risk for
Peripheral Neurovascular Dysfunction, Risk for
Personal Identity Disturbance
Physical Mobility, Impaired
Poisoning, Risk for
Post-trauma Response
Powerlessness
Protection, Altered
Rape-Trauma Syndrome
Rape-Trauma Syndrome: Compound Reaction
Rape-Trauma Syndrome: Silent Reaction
Relocation Stress Syndrome
Role Performance, Altered
Self-Care Deficit
- Bathing/Hygiene
- Dressing/Grooming
- Feeding
- Toileting

Self-Esteem, Chronic Low
Self-Esteem, Situational Low
Self-Esteem Disturbance
Self-Mutilation, Risk for
Sensory/Perceptual Alterations (Specify) (Visual, auditory, kinesthetic, gustatory, tactile, olfactory)
Sexual Dysfunction
Sexuality Patterns, Altered
Skin Integrity, Impaired
Skin Integrity, Risk for Impaired
Sleep Pattern Disturbance
Social Interaction, Impaired
Social Isolation
Spiritual Distress
Spiritual Well-Being, Potential for Enhanced
Suffocation, Risk for
Sustain Spontaneous Ventilation, Inability to
Swallowing, Impaired
Thermoregulation, Ineffective
Thought Processes, Altered
Tissue Integrity, Impaired
Tissue Perfusion, Altered (Specify Type) (Renal, cerebral, cardiopulmonary, gastrointestinal, peripheral)
Trauma, Risk for
Unilateral Neglect
Urinary Elimination, Altered
Urinary Retention
Violence, Risk for: Self-directed or directed at others

Appendix B

Laboratory Values

Cecilia C. Dail **Sally D. Sperry** **John Scariano**

The tables in this appendix list some of the most common tests, their normal values, and possible etiologies of abnormal values. Laboratory values may vary with different techniques or different laboratories. Possible etiologies are presented in alphabetic order. Abbreviations appearing in the tables are defined as follows:

< = less than
> = greater than
L = liter
mEq = milliequivalent
ml = milliliter
dl = deciliter
mm Hg = millimeter of mercury
fl = femtoliter
mm = millimeter
g = gram
mg = millogram (10^{-3})
μg = microgram (one millionth of a gram) (10^{-6})
ng = nanogram (one billionth of a gram) (10^{-9})
pg = picogram (one trillionth of a gram) (10^{-12})
μU = microunit
μl = microliter
IU = international unit
mOsm = milliosmole
U = unit
μmol = micromole
nmol = nanomole
mmol = millimole
pmol = picomole
kPa = kilopascal
μkat = microkatal

Table B-1 Serum, Plasma, and Whole Blood Chemistries

Test	Normal Values		Possible Etiology	
	Conventional Units	SI Units	Higher	Lower
Acetone			Diabetic acidosis, high fat diet, low-carbohydrate diet, starvation	
Quantitative	0.3-2.0 mg/dl	52-344 μmol/L		
Qualitative	Negative	Same as conventional units		
Albumin	3.5-5.0 g/dl	507-725 μmol/L	Dehydration	Chronic liver disease, malabsorption, malnutrition, nephrotic syndrome, pregnancy
Aldolase	1.0-7.5 U/L	Same as conventional units	Skeletal muscle disease	Renal disease
α-1-Antitrypsin	200-400 mg/dl	2.0-4.0 g/L	Acute and chronic inflammation, arthritis, stress syndrome	Chronic lung disease (early onset), malnutrition, nephrotic syndrome
α-1-Fetoprotein	<25 ng/ml	<25 μg/L	Cancer of testes and ovaries, carcinoma of liver	
Ammonia	30-70 μg/dl	17.6-41.1 μmol/L	Severe liver disease	
Amylase	0-130 U/L (method dependent)	0-2.17 μkat/L	Acute and chronic pancreatitis, mumps (salivary gland disease), perforated ulcers	Acute alcoholism, cirrhosis of liver, extensive destruction of pancreas
Ascorbic acid	0.4-2.0 mg/dl	23-114 μmol/L	Excessive ingestion of vitamin C	Connective tissue disorders, hepatic disease, renal disease, rheumatic fever, vitamin C deficiency
Bicarbonate	20-30 mEq/L	20-30 mmol/L	Compensated respiratory acidosis, metabolic alkalosis	Compensated respiratory alkalosis, metabolic acidosis
Bilirubin			Biliary obstruction, impaired liver function, hemolytic anemia, pernicious anemia, prolonged fasting	
Total	0.2-1.3 mg/dl	3.4-22.0 μmol/L		
Indirect	0.1-1.0 mg/dl	1.7-17 μmol/L		
Direct	0.1-0.3 mg/dl	1.7-5.1 μmol/L		
Blood gases*				
Arterial pH	7.35-7.45	Same as conventional units	Alkalosis	Acidosis
Venous pH	7.35-7.45	Same as conventional units		
Arterial PCO_2	35-45 mm Hg	4.67-6.00 kPa	Compensated metabolic alkalosis	Compensated metabolic acidosis
Venous PCO_2	42-52 mm Hg	5.60-6.93 kPa	Respiratory acidosis	Respiratory alkalosis
Arterial PO_2	75-100 mm Hg	10.0-13.33 kPa	Administration of high concentration of oxygen	Chronic lung disease, decreased cardiac output
Venous PO_2	30-50 mm Hg	4.0-6.67 kPa		
Calcium	9-11 mg/dl (4.5-5.5 mEq/L)	2.25-2.74 mmol/L	Acute osteoporosis, hyperparathyroidism, vitamin D intoxication, multiple myeloma	Acute pancreatitis, hypoparthyroidism, liver disease, malabsorption syndrome, renal failure, vitamin D deficiency

continued

Table B-1 Serum, Plasma, and Whole Blood Chemistries—cont'd

Test	Normal Values		Possible Etiology	
	Conventional Units	SI Units	Higher	Lower
Calcium, ionized	4-4.6 mg/dl (2-2.3 mEq/L	1.0-1.15 mmol/L		
Carbon dioxide (CO_2 content)	20-30 mEq/L	20-30 mmol/L	Same as bicarbonate	
Carotene	50-200 μg/dl	0.93-3.70 μmol/L	Cystic fibrosis, hypothyroidism, pancreatic insufficiency	Dietary deficiency, malabsorption disorders
Chloride	95-105 mEq/L	95-105 mmol/L	Cardiac decompensation, metabolic acidosis, respiratory alkalosis, steroid therapy, uremia	Addison's disease, diarrhea, metabolic alkalosis, respiratory acidosis, vomiting
Cholesterol	140-200 mg/dl (age dependent)	3.6-5.2 mmol/L	Biliary obstruction, hypothyroidism, idiopathic hypercholesterolemia, renal disease, uncontrolled diabetes	Extensive liver disease, hyperthyroidism, malnutrition, steroid therapy
HDL (high-density lipoproteins)				
Male	>45 mg/dl	>1.2 mmol/L		
Female	>55 mg/dl	>1.4 mmol/L		
LDL (low-density lipoproteins)	<130 mg/dl	<3.4 mmol/L		
Cholinesterase (RBC)	0.65-1.00 pH 4-10 U/L	Same as conventional units	Exercise	Acute infections, insecticide intoxication, liver disease, muscular dystrophy
Pseudocholinesterase (plasma)		Same as conventional units		
Copper	80-150 μg/dl	12.6-23.6 μmol/L	Cirrhosis, female on contraceptives	Wilson's disease
Cortisol	8 AM: 5-25 μg/dl 8 PM: <10 μg/dl	0.14-0.69 μmol/L <0.28 μmol/L	Cushing's, syndrome, pancreatitis, stress	Adrenal insufficiency, panhypopituitary states
Creatine	0.2-1.0 mg/dl	15.3-76.3 μmol/L	Active rheumatoid arthritis, biliary obstruction, hyperthyroidism, renal disorders, severe muscle disease	Diabetes mellitus
Creatine kinase (CK)			Musculoskeletal injury or disease, myocardial infarction, severe myocarditis, exercise, numerous intramuscular injections, brain damage	
Male	<160 U/L	<2.67 μkat/L		
Female	<130 U/L (method dependent)	<2.17 μkat/L		
Creatinine	0.5-1.5 mg/dl	44-133 μmol/L	Severe renal disease	
Ferritin (serum)	20-300 ng/ml	20-300 μg/L	Siderablastic anemia, Anemia of chronic disease (infection, inflammation, liver disease)	Iron deficiency anemia
Folic acid (folate)	3-25 ng/ml	7-57 nmol/L	Hypothyroidism	Alcoholism, hemolytic anemia, inadequate diet, malabsorption syndrome, megaloblastic anemia
Gamma-glutamyl transpeptidase (GGT)	0-30 U/L	0-0.5 μkat/L		Liver disease, infectious mononucleosis

continued

Table B-1 Serum, Plasma, and Whole Blood Chemistries—cont'd

Test	Normal Values		Possible Etiology	
	Conventional Units	SI Units	Higher	Lower
Glucose, fasting	70-120 mg/dl	3.89-6.66 mmol/L	Acute stress, cerebral lesions, Cushing's disease, diabetes mellitus, hyperthyroidism, pancreatic insufficiency	Addison's disease, hepatic disease, hypothyroidism, insulin overdosage, pancreatic tumor, pituitary hypofunction, postgastrectomy dumping syndrome
Glucose tolerance (GTT)			Diabetes mellitus	Hyperinsulinism
Fasting	70-120 mg/dl	3.89-6.66 mmol/L		
30 min	30-60 mg/dl above fasting	1.67-3.33 mmol/L		
60 min	20-50 mg/dl above fasting	1.11-2.78 mmol/L		
120 min	5-15 mg/dl above fasting	0.28-0.83 mmol/L		
180 min	Fasting level or lower	Fasting level or lower		
Haptoglobin	70-200 mg/dl	0.7-2.0 g/L	Infectious and inflammatory processes, malignant neoplasms	Hemolytic anemia, mononucleosis, toxoplasmosis, chronic liver disease
Insulin	4-24 μU/ml	29-172 pmol/L	Acromegaly, adenoma of islet cells, untreated mild case of type II diabetes	Diabetes mellitus, obesity
Iron, total	50-150 μg/dl	9.0-26.9 μmol/L	Excessive RBC destruction	Iron-deficiency anemia, anemia of chronic disease
Iron-binding capacity	250-410 μg/dl	45-73 μmol/L	Iron-deficient state, oral contraceptives, polycythemia	Cancer, chronic infections, pernicious anemia, uremia
Lactic acid	5-20 mg/dl	0.56- 2.2 mmol/L	Acidosis, congestive heart failure, shock	
Lactic dehydrogenase (LDH)	50-150 U/L	0.83-2.5 μkat/L	Congestive heart failure, hemolytic disorders, hepatitis, metastatic cancer of liver, myocardial infarction, pernicious anemia, pulmonary embolus, skeletal muscle damage	
Lactic dehydrogenase isoenzymes				
LDH_1	20-35%	0.20-0.35	Myocardial infarction, pernicious anemia	
LDH_2	30-40%	0.30-0.40	Pulmonary embolus, sickle cell crisis	
LDH_3	15-25%	0.15-0.25	Malignant lymphoma, pulmonary embolus	
LDH_4	0-10%	0-0.10	Lupus erythematosus, pulmonary infarction	
LDH_5	4-12%	0.04-0.12	Congestive heart failure, hepatitis, pulmonary embolus and infarction, skeletal muscle damage	

continued

Table B-1 Serum, Plasma, and Whole Blood Chemistries—cont'd

Test	Normal Values		Possible Etiology	
	Conventional Units	SI Units	Higher	Lower
Lipase	0-160 U/L	0-2.66 μkat/L	Acute pancreatitis, hepatic disorders, perforated peptic ulcer	
Magnesium	1.5-2.5 mEq/L	0.75-1.25 mmol/L	Addison's disease, hypothyroidism, renal failure	Chronic alcoholism, hyperparathyroidism, hyperthyroidism, hypoparathyroidism, severe malabsorption
Osmolality	285-295 mOsm/kg	Same as conventional units	Chronic renal disease, diabetes mellitus	Addison's disease, diuretic therapy
Oxygen saturation (arterial)	95-98%	0.95-0.98 saturated	Polycythemia	Anemia, cardiac decompensation, respiratory disorders
pH	See blood gases			
Phenylalanine	0-2 mg/dl	0-121 μmol/L	Phenylketonuria	
Phosphatase, acid	0.11-0.60 U/L (method dependent)	Same as conventional units	Advanced Paget's disease, cancer of prostate, hyperparathyroidism	
Phosphatase, alkaline	30-120 U/L (method and age dependent)	Same as conventional units	Bone diseases, marked hyperparathyroidism, obstruction of biliary system, rickets	Excessive vitamin D ingestion, hypothyroidism, milk-alkali syndrome
Phosphorus, inorganic	2.8-4.5 mg/dl	0.90-1.45 mmol/L	Healing fractures, hypoparathyroidism, renal disease, vitamin D intoxication	Diabetes mellitus, hyperparathyroidism, vitamin D deficiency
Potassium	3.5-5.5 mEq/L	3.5-5.5 mmol/L	Addison's disease, diabetic ketosis, massive tissue destruction, renal failure	Cushing's syndrome, diarrhea (severe), diuretic therapy, gastrointestinal fistula, pyloric obstruction, starvation, vomiting
Prostate-specific antigen	<4 ng/mL	<4 μg/L	Prostate cancer	
Proteins				
Total	6.0-8.0 g/dl	60-80 g/L	Burns, cirrhosis (globulin fraction), dehydration	Congenital agammaglobulinemia, liver disease, malabsorption
Albumin	3.5-5.0 g/dl	35-50 g/L		
Globulin	2-3.5 g/dl	20-35 g/L		
Albumin/globulin ratio	1.5:1-2.5:1	Same as conventional units	Multiple myeloma (globulin fraction), shock, vomiting	Malnutrition, nephrotic syndrome, proteinuria, renal disease, severe burns
Renin			Renal hypertension, volume decrease (e.g., hemorrhage)	Increased salt intake, primary aldosteronism
Supine position	1.4-2.9 ng/ml/hr	0.39-0.81 ng/L•sec		
Upright position	0.4-4.5 ng/ml/hr	0.11-1.25 ng/L•sec		
Sodium	135-145 mEq/L	135-145 mmol/L	Dehydration, impaired renal function, primary aldosteronism, steroid therapy	Addison's disease, diabetic ketoacidosis, diuretic therapy, excessive loss from gastrointestinal tract, excessive perspiration, water intoxication

continued

Table B-1 Serum, Plasma, and Whole Blood Chemistries—cont'd

Test	Normal Values: Conventional Units	Normal Values: SI Units	Possible Etiology: Higher	Possible Etiology: Lower
Testosterone				Hypofunction of testes
Male	400-1200 ng/dl	13.9-41.6 nmol/L		
Female	25-90 ng/dl	0.87-3.1 nmol/L	Polycystic ovary, virilizing tumors	
T_4 (thyroxine), total	5-12 μg/dl	64-154 nmol/L	Hyperthyroidism, thyroiditis	Cretinism, hypothyroidism, myxedema
T_4 (thyroxine), free	0.8-2.3 μg/dl	10-30 pmol/L		
T_3 uptake	25-35%	0.25-0.35	Hyperthyroidism, metastatic neoplasms	Hypothyroidism, pregnancy
T_3 (triiodothyronine)	110-230 ng/dl	1.7-3.5 nmol/L	Hyperthyroidism	
Thyroid-stimulating hormone (TSH)	0.3-5.4 μU/ml	0.3-5.4 mU/L	Myxedema, primary hypothyroidism, Graves' disease	Secondary hypothyroidism
Transaminases				
Serum glutamicoxaloacetic (SGOT) or aspartate aminotrans ferase (AST)	7-40 U/L	0.12-0.67 μkat/L	Liver disease, myocardial infarction, pulmonary infarction, acute hepatitis	
Serum glutamicpyruvic (SGPT) or alanine aminotrans ferase (ALT)	5-36 U/L	0.08-0.6 μkat/L	Liver disease, shock	
Triglycerides	40-150 mg/dl	0.45-1.69 mmol/L	Diabetes mellitus, hyperlipidemia, hypothyroidism, liver disease	Malnutrition
Urea nitrogen (BUN)	10-30 mg/dl	1.8-7.1 mmol/L	Increase in protein catabolism (fever, stress), renal disease, urinary tract infection	Malnutrition, severe liver damage
Uric acid			Gout, gross tissue destruction, high-protein weight reduction diet, leukemia, renal failure, eclampsia	Administration of uricosuric drugs
Male	4.5-6.5 mg/dl	149-327 μmol/L		
Female	2.5-5.5 mg/dl	268-387 μmol/L		
Vitamin A	15-60 μg/dl	0.52-2.09 μmol/L	Excess ingestion of vitamin A	Vitamin A deficiency
Vitamin B_{12}	200-1000 pg/ml	148-738 pmol/L	Chronic myeloid leukemia	Strict vegetarianism, malabsorption syndrome, pernicious anemia, total or partial gastrectomy
Zinc	50-150 μg/dl	7.6-22.9 μmol/L		Alcoholic cirrhosis

RBC, Red blood cell.
*Because arterial blood gases are influenced by altitude, the value for PO_2 decreases as altitude increases. The lower value is normal for an altitude of 1 mile.

Table B-2 Hematology

Test	Normal Values		Possible Etiology	
	Conventional Units	SI Units	Higher	Lower
Bleeding time (Ivy) (Simplate)	1-6 min 3.0-9.5 min	60-360 sec 180-570 sec	Defective platelet function, thrombocytopenia, von Willebrand disease, aspirin ingestion, vascular disease	
Activated partial thromboplastin time (APTT)	30-45 sec*	Same as conventional units	Deficiency of factors I, II, V, VIII, IX and X, XI, XII; hemophilia, liver disease, heparin therapy	
Prothrombin time (Protime, PT)	10-14 sec*	Same as conventional units	Warfarin therapy, deficiency of factors I, II, V, VII, and X, vitamin K deficiency, liver disease	
Fibrinogen	200-400 mg/dl	2.0-4.0 g/L	Burns (after first 36 hr), inflammatory disease	Burns (during first 36 hr), DIC, severe liver disease
Fibrin split (degradation) products	<10 μg/ml	Same as conventional units	Acute DIC, massive hemorrhage, primary fibrinolysis	
D-Dimer	negative	Same as conventional units	DIC, myocardial infarction, deep vein thrombosis, unstable angina	
Erythrocyte count† (altitude dependent)			Dehydration, high altitudes, polycythemia vera, severe diarrhea	Anemia, leukemia, posthemorrhage
Male	$4.5\text{-}6.0 \times 10^6/\mu L$	$4.5\text{-}6.0 \times 10^{12}/L$		
Female	$4.0\text{-}5.0 \times 10^6/\mu L$	$4.0\text{-}5.0 \times 10^{12}/L$		
Mean corpuscular volume (MCV)	82-98 fl	Same as conventional units	Macrocytic anemia	Microcytic anemia
Mean corpuscular hemoglobin (MCH)	27-33 pg	Same as conventional units	Macrocytic anemia	Microcytic anemia
Mean corpuscular hemoglobin concentration (MCHC)	32-36%	0.32-0.36	Spherocytosis	Hypochromic anemia
Erythrocyte sedimentation rate (ESR), Westergren			Moderate increase: acute hepatitis, myocardial infarction; rheumatoid arthritis; marked increase: acute and severe bacterial infections, malignancies, pelvic inflammatory disease	Malaria Severe liver disease Sickle cell anemia
Male <50 yr >50 yr	<15 mm/hr <20 mm/hr	Same as conventional units		
Female <50 yr >50 yr	<20 mm/hr <30 mm/hr	Same as conventional units		

continued

Table B-2 Hematology—cont'd

Test	Normal Values: Conventional Units	Normal Values: SI Units	Possible Etiology: Higher	Possible Etiology: Lower
Hematocrit (altitude dependent)†			Dehydration, high altitudes, polycythemia	Anemia, hemorrhage, overhydration
Male	40-51%	0.40-0.51		
Female	38-44%	0.38-0.44		
Hemoglobin (altitude dependent)†				
Male	13.5-18.0 g/dl	135-180 g/L	COPD, high altitudes, polycythemia	Anemia, hemorrhage
Female	12.0-16.0 g/dl	120-160 g/L		
Hemoglobin, glycosylated	2.2-4.8%	Same as conventional units	Poorly controlled diabetes mellitus	Sickle cell Chronic renal failure Pregnancy
Red cell distribution width (RDW)	10.2-14.5%	Same as conventional therapy		Anisocytosis, macrocytic anemia, microcytic anemia
Platelet count (thrombocytes)	150-400 × $10^3/\mu l$	150-400 × 10^9/L	Acute infections, chronic granulocytic leukemia, chronic pancreatitis, cirrhosis, collagen disorders, polycythemia, postsplenectomy	Acute leukemia, DIC, thrombocytopenic purpura
Reticulocyte count (manual)	0.5-1.5% of RBC	0.005-0.015 of RBC	Hemolytic anemia, polycythemia vera	Hypoproliferative anemia, macrocytic anemia, microcytic anemia
White blood cell count†	4.0-11.0 × $10^3/\mu l$	4.0-11.0 × 10^9/L	Inflammatory and infectious processes, leukemia	Aplastic anemia, side effects of chemotherapy and irradiation
WBC Differential				
Segmented neutrophils	50-70%	0.50-0.70	Bacterial infections, collagen diseases, Hodgkin's disease	Aplastic anemia, viral infections
Band neutrophils	0-8%	0-0.08	Acute infections	
Lymphocytes	20-40%	0.20-0.40	Chronic infections, lymphocytic leukemia, mononucleosis, viral infections	Adrenocortical steroid therapy, whole body irradiation
Monocytes	4-8%	0.04-0.08	Chronic inflammatory disorders, malaria, monocytic leukemia, acute infections, Hodgkin's disease	
Eosinophils	0-4%	0-0.04	Allergic reactions, eosinophilic and chronic granulocytic leukemia, parasitic disorders, Hodgkin's disease	Steroid therapy
Basophils	0-2%	0-0.02	Hyperthyroidism, ulcerative colitis, myeloproliferative diseases	Hyperthyroidism, stress
Sickle cell solubility test	Negative	Same as conventional units	Sickle cell anemia	

COPD, Chronic obstructive pulmonary disease; *DIC*, disseminated intravascular coagulation; *RBC*, red blood cell.
*Values depend on reagent and instrumentation used.
†Components of complete blood count (CBC).

Table B-3 Serology-Immunology

Test	Normal Values		Possible Etiology	
	Conventional Units	SI Units	Higher	Lower
Antinuclear antibody (ANA)	Negative or titer <1:10	Same as conventional units	Chronic hepatitis, rheumatoid arthritis, scleroderma, systemic lupus erythematosus	
Anti-DNA antibody	Negative or titer <1:10 or <20% binding	Same as conventional units	Systemic lupus erythematosus	
Anti-RNP	Negative	Same as conventional units	Mixed connective tissue disease, rheumatoid arthritis, systemic lupus erythematosus, Sjögren's syndrome, scleroderma	
Anti-Sm	Negative	Same as conventional units	Systemic lupus erythematosus	
Antistreptolysin-O (ASO)	≤166 Todd units	Same as conventional units	Acute glomerulonephritis, rheumatic fever, streptococcal infection	
C-reactive protein (CRP)	Negative or ≤1.2 mg/dl	Same as conventional units	Acute infections, any inflammatory condition, widespread malignancy	
Carcinoembryonic antigen (CEA)	≤2.5 ng/ml	Same as conventional units ≤2.5 μg/L	Carcinoma of colon, liver, pancreas; chronic cigarette smoking; inflammatory bowel disease; other cancers	
Complement components				
C1q	11-21 mg/dl	0.11-0.21 g/L		Acute glomerulonephritis, systemic lupus erythematosus, rheumatoid arthritis, subacute bacterial endocarditis, serum sickness
C3	80-180 mg/dl	0.8-1.8 g/L		
C4	15-50 mg/dl	0.15-0.5 g/L		
Direct antihuman globulin test (DAT) or direct Coombs	Negative	Same as conventional units	Acquired hemolytic anemia, hemolytic disease of the newborn, drug reactions, transfusion reactions	
Fluorescent treponemal antibody (FTA-ABS)	Nonreactive	Same as conventional units	Syphilis	

continued

Table B-3 Serology-Immunology—cont'd

Test	Normal Values		Possible Etiology	
	Conventional units	SI Units	Higher	Lower
Hepatitis A antibody (IgM)	Negative	Same as conventional units	Hepatitis A	
Hepatitis B surface antigen (HB_sAg)	Negative	Same as conventional units	Hepatitis B	
Hepatitis C	Negative	Same as conventional units	Hepatitis C	
Immunoglobulin				
IgA	90-400 mg/dl	0.9-4.0 g/L	IgA myeloma, chronic liver disease, chronic infection, rheumatoid arthritis, autoimmune disorders	Burns, hereditary telangiectasia, malabsorption syndromes
IgD	0.5-12 mg/dl	5-120 mg/L	Chronic infection, connective tissue disease	
IgE	<1 mg/dl	<10 mg/L	Anaphylactic shock, atopic disease (allergies), parasite infections	
IgG	650-1800 mg/dl	6.5-18.0 g/L	Infections—acute and chronic, hepatitis, IgG monoclonal gammopathy, systemic lupus erythematosus	Congenital deficiencies, acquired deficiencies, nephrotic syndromes, burns, immunosuppression
IgM	55-300 mg/dl	0.5-3.0 g/L	Acute infections, rheumatoid arthritis, liver disease	Congenital and acquired antibody deficiencies, lymphocytic leukemia, protein-losing enteropathies
Monospot or monotest	Negative	Same as conventional units	Infectious mononucleosis	
Rheumatoid factor (RA factor)	Negative or titer <1:20	Same as conventional units	Rheumatoid arthritis, Sjögren's syndrome, systemic lupus erythematosus	
RPR	Nonreactive	Same as conventional units	Syphilis, systemic lupus erythematosus, rheumatoid arthritis, leprosy, malaria, febrile diseases, IV drug abuse	
VDRL	Nonreactive	Same as conventional units	Syphilis	
Thyroid antibodies	≤1:10 titer	Same as conventional units	Hashimoto's thyroiditis, thyroid carcinoma, early hypothyroidism, pernicious anemia, systemic lupus erythematosus, Graves' disease	

CSF, Colony-stimulating factor; *RNP,* ribonuclear protein; *RPR,* rapid plasma reagin test; *VDRL,* Venereal Disease Research Laboratory test.

Table B-4 Urine Chemistry

Test	Specimen	Normal Values: Conventional Units	Normal Values: SI Units	Possible Etiology: Higher	Possible Etiology: Lower
Acetone	Random	Negative	Same as conventional units	Diabetes mellitus, high-fat and low-carbohydrate diets, starvation states	
Aldosterone	24 hr	2-26 μg/day	5.5-72.1 nmol/day	Primary aldosteronism: adrenocortical tumors; secondary aldosteronism: cardiac failure, cirrhosis, large dose of ACTH, salt depletion	ACTH deficiency, Addison's disease, corticosteroid therapy
Amylase	24 hr	1-17 U/day	Same as conventional units	Acute pancreatitis	
Bence Jones protein	Random	Negative	Same as conventional units	Multiple myeloma, biliary duct obstruction	
Bilirubin	Random	Negative	Same as conventional units	Hepatitis	
Calcium	24 hr	100-250 mg/day	2.5-6.3 mmol/day	Bone tumor, hyperparathyroidism, milk-alkali syndrome	Hypoparathyroidism, malabsorption of calcium and vitamin D
Catecholamines	24 hr			Pheochromocytoma, progressive muscular dystrophy	
Epinephrine		<20 μg/day	<118 nmol/day		
Norepinephrine		<100 μg/day	<591 nmol/day		
Chloride	24 hr	110-250 mEq/day	110-250 mmol/day	Addison's disease	Burns, excess perspiration, vomiting, diarrhea, menstruation
Copper	24 hr	<30 μg/day	<0.5 μmol/day	Cirrhosis, Wilson's disease	
Coproporphyrin	24 hr	50-200 μg/day	76-305 nmol/day	Lead poisoning, oral contraceptive use, poliomyelitis	
Creatine	24 hr	<100 mg/day	<763 μmol/day	Carcinoma of liver, hyperthyroidism, diabetes, Addison's disease, infections, burns, muscular dystrophy, skeletal muscle atrophy	Hypothyroidism
Creatinine	24 hr	0.8-2.0 g/day	7.1-17.7 mmol/day	Anemia, leukemia, muscular atrophy, salmonellae	Renal disease
Creatinine clearance	24 hr	85-135 ml/min	1.42-2.25 ml/sec		Renal disease
Estrogens	24 hr				
Female				Gonadal or adrenal tumor	Agenesis of ovaries, endocrine disturbance, ovarian dysfunction
Ovulation peak		28-100 μg/day	104-370 nmol/day		
Luteal peak		22-80 μg/day	81-296 nmol/day		
Pregnancy		Up to 45,000 μg/day	Up to 166,455 nmol/day		
Menopause		1.4-19.6 μg/day	5.2-72.5 nmol/day		
Male		5-18 μg/day	18-67 nmol/day		
Glucose	Random	Negative	Same as conventional units	Diabetes mellitus, low renal threshold for glucose resorption, physiologic stress, pituitary disorders	

continued

Table B-4 Urine Chemistry—cont'd

Test	Specimen	Normal Values: Conventional Units	Normal Values: SI Units	Possible Etiology: Higher	Possible Etiology: Lower
Hemoglobin	Random	Negative	Same as conventional units	Extensive burns, glomerulonephritis, hemolytic anemias, hemolytic transfusion reaction	
5-Hydroxyindoleacetic 24 hr acid (5-HIAA)		2-9 mg/day	10.5-47.1 μmol/day	Malignant carcinoid syndrome	
Ketone bodies	24 hr	20-50 mg/day	0.34-0.86 mmol/day	Marked ketonuria	
Lead	24 hr	<100 μg/day	<0.48 μmol/day	Lead poisoning	
Metanephrine	24 hr	<1.3 mg/day	<7.1 μmol/day	Pheochromocytoma	
Myoglobin	Random	Negative	Same as conventional units	Crushing injuries, electric shock, extreme physical exertion	
pH	Random	4.0-8.0	Same as conventional units	Chronic renal failure, compensatory phase of alkalosis, salicylate intoxication, vegetable diet	Compensatory phase of acidosis, dehydration, emphysema
Phenylpyruvic acid	Random	Negative	Same as conventional units	Phenylketonuria	
Phosphorus, inorganic	24 hr	0.9-1.3 g/day	29-42 mmol/day	Fever, hypoparathyroidism, nervous exhaustion, rickets, tuberculosis	Acute infections, nephritis
Porphobilinogen	Random	Negative	Same as conventional units	Acute intermittent porphyria, liver disorders	
Protein (dipstick)	Random	Negative	Same as conventional units	Congestive heart failure, nephritis, nephrosis, physiologic stress	
Protein (quantitative)	24 hr	<150 mg/day	<0.15 g/day	Cardiac failure, inflammatory processes of urinary tract, nephritis, nephrosis, toxemia of pregnancy	
Sodium	24 hr	40-250 mEq/day	40-250 mmol/day	Acute tubular necrosis	Hyponatremia
Specific gravity	Random	1.003-1.030	Same as conventional units	Albuminuria, dehydration, glycosuria	Diabetes insipidus
Titratable acidity	24 hr	20-50 mEq/day	Same as conventional units	Metabolic acidosis	Metabolic alkalosis
Uric acid	24 hr	250-750 mg/day	1.5-4.5 mmol/day	Gout, leukemia	Nephritis

continued

Table B-4 Urine Chemistry—cont'd

Test	Specimen	Normal Values: Conventional Units	Normal Values: SI Units	Possible Etiology: Higher	Possible Etiology: Lower
Urobilinogen	24 hr Random	0.5-4.0 mg/day <1.0 Erhlich unit	0.8-6.8 μmol/day Same as conventional units	Hemolytic disease, hepatic parenchymal cell damage, liver disease	Complete obstruction of bile duct
Uroporphyrins	Random	Negative	Same as conventional units	Porphyria	
Vanillylmandelic acid	24 hr	1-8 mg/day 1.5-7 μg/mg creatine	5-40 μmol/day	Pheochromocytoma	

ACTH, Adrenocorticotropic hormone.

Table B-5 Gastric Analysis

Test	Normal Values: Conventional Units	Normal Values: SI Units	Possible Etiology: Higher	Possible Etiology: Lower
Basal				
Free hydrochloric acid	0.30 mEq/L	Same as conventional units	Hypermotility of stomach	Pernicious anemia
Total acidity	15-45 mEq/L	Same as conventional units	Gastric and duodenal ulcers	Gastric carcinoma
Combined acidity	10-15 mEq/L	Same as conventional units	Zollinger-Ellison syndrome	Severe gastritis
Poststimulation				
Free hydrochloric acid	10-130 mEq/L	Same as conventional units		
Total acidity	20-150 mEq/L	Same as conventional units		

Table B-6 Fecal Analysis

Test	Normal Values		Possible Etiology	
	Conventional Units	SI Units	Higher	Lower
Fecal fat	<6 g/24 hr	Same as conventional units	Chronic pancreatic disease, obstruction of common bile duct, malabsorption syndrome	
Urobilinogen	30-220 mg/100 g of stool	51-372 μmol/100 g of stool	Hemolytic anemias	Complete biliary obstruction
Mucus	Negative	Same as conventional units	Mucous colitis, spastic constipation	
Pus	Negative	Same as conventional units	Chronic bacillary dysentery, chronic ulcerative colitis, localized abscesses	
Blood*	Negative	Same as conventional units	Anal fissures, hemorrhoids, malignant tumor, peptic ulcer, ulcerative colitis	
Color				
Brown			Various color depending on diet	
Clay			Biliary obstruction or presence of barium sulfate	
Tarry			More than 100 ml of blood in gastrointestinal tract	
Red			Blood in large intestine	
Black			Blood in upper gastrointestinal tract or iron medication	

*Ingestion of meat may produce false-positive results. Patient may be placed on a meat-free diet for 3 days before the test.

Table B-7 Cerebrospinal Fluid Analysis

Test	Normal Values		Possible Etiology	
	Conventional Units	SI Units	Higher	Lower
Pressure	60-150 mm	Same as conventional units	Hemorrhage, intracranial tumor, meningitis	Head injury, spinal tumor, subdural hematoma
Blood	Negative	Same as conventional units	Intracranial hemorrhage	
Cell count (age dependent)				
WBC	0-5 cells/μl	0.5×10^6/L	Inflammation or infections of CNS	
RBC	0	0×10^6/L		
Chloride	100-130 mEq/L	100-130 mmol/L	Uremia	Bacterial infections of CNS (meningitis, encephalitis)
Glucose	45-75 mg/dl	2.5-4.2 mmol/L	Diabetes mellitus, viral infections of CNS	Bacterial infections and tuberculosis of CNS
Protein				
Lumbar	15-45 mg/dl	0.15-0.45 g/L	Guillain-Barré syndrome, poliomyelitis, traumatic tap	
Cisternal	15-25 mg/dl	0.15-0.25 g/L	Syphilis of CNS	
Ventricular	5-15 mg/dl	0.05-0.15 g/L	Acute meningitis, brain tumor, chronic infections, multiple sclerosis	

CNS, Central nervous system; *RBC*, red blood cell; *WBC*, white blood cell.

Table B-8 Toxicology of Common Drugs

Drug	Therapeutic Level		Toxic Level	
	Conventional Units	SI Units	Conventional Units	SI Units
Acetaminophen (Tylenol)	1-2 mg/dl	66-132 μmol/L	>5 mg/dl	>330 μmol/L
Barbiturates				
Short acting	1-2 mg/dl	Dependent on composition of mixture	>5 mg/dl	
Intermediate acting	1-5 mg/dl		>10 mg/dl	
Long acting	15-35 mg/dl		>40 mg/dl	
Carbon monoxide (carboxyhemoglobin)				
Normal values	<5% saturation of hemoglobin	<0.05	Symptoms with >20% saturation	>0.20
Urban nonsmokers	<5% saturation of hemoglobin	<0.05		
Rural nonsmokers	0.5-2% saturation of hemoglobin	0.005-0.02		
Smokers	5-9% saturation of hemoglobin	0.05-0.09		
Heavy smokers	>9% saturation of hemoglobin	>0.09		
Chlordiazepoxide (Librium)	0.05-5.0 mg/L	2-17 μmol/L	>10 μg/ml	>33 μmol/L
Chlorpromazine (Thorazine)	0.5 μg/ml	1.6 μmol/L	>2.0 μg/ml	>6.3 μmol/L
Diazepam (Valium)	0.10-0.25 mg/L	0.35-0.88 μmol/L	>1.0 mg/L ≥2.0 mg/L (lethal)	>3.5 μmol/L
Digitalis preparations				
Digoxin	0.8-2.4 ng/ml	1.0-3.1 nmol/L	>2.5 ng/ml	>2.6 nmol/L
Digitoxin	14-30 ng/ml	18-39 nmol/L	>30 ng/ml	>39 nmol/L
Dilantin	10-20 mg/L	40-80 μmol/L	>30 mg/ml	>120 μmol/L
Gentamicin (Garamycin)				
Peak	4-10 mg/L	9-22 μmol/L	>10 mg/L	>22 μmol/L
Trough	<2 mg/L	<4 mmol/L	>2 mg/L	>4 μmol/L
Meperidine (Dermerol)	20-200 μg/dl	2.83-8.09 μmol/L	>200 g/dl	>8.09 μmol/L
Propranolol (Inderal)	50-100 ng/ml	192-386 nmol/L	>200 ng/ml	>771 nmol/L
Salicylates	15-20 mg/dl	1.09-1.45 mmol/L	>20 mg/dl >60 mg/dl (lethal)	>1.45 mmol/L >4.34 mmol/L
Alcohol (ethanol)*				

*See Table 60-14.

Appendix C

Answer Key to Review Questions

CHAPTER 1

1. c
2. d
3. c
4. a
5. a
6. b
7. a
8. c
9. a
10. c

CHAPTER 2

1. c
2. b
3. c
4. d
5. d
6. b
7. d

CHAPTER 3

1. b
2. d
3. c
4. a
5. b
6. d
7. c
8. c
9. d
10. a
11. d
12. c
13. a
14. b

CHAPTER 4

1. b
2. c
3. b
4. b
5. d
6. a

CHAPTER 5

1. b
2. c
3. c
4. a
5. a
6. d
7. b
8. c

CHAPTER 6

1. a
2. b
3. c
4. d
5. b
6. b
7. b

CHAPTER 7

1. c
2. d
3. b
4. a
5. b
6. b

CHAPTER 8

1. a
2. a
3. b
4. c
5. c
6. a
7. c
8. a
9. c
10. a
11. b
12. c
13. d

CHAPTER 9

1. a
2. c
3. b
4. c
5. d
6. b
7. d
8. a
9. c
10. c

CHAPTER 10

1. d
2. d
3. b
4. a
5. d
6. c
7. d
8. c
9. b
10. b
11. a

CHAPTER 11

1. a
2. d
3. c
4. a
5. c
6. b
7. b
8. c

CHAPTER 12

1. d
2. a
3. c
4. a
5. c
6. b
7. d
8. c
9. d
10. b
11. d
12. a
13. d
14. a
15. c

CHAPTER 13

1. c
2. a
3. b
4. d
5. a
6. d
7. a
8. b
9. b

CHAPTER 14

1. b
2. c
3. b
4. a
5. b
6. a
7. d
8. d

CHAPTER 15

1. b
2. a
3. d
4. c
5. a
6. a
7. b
8. d
9. a

CHAPTER 16

1. b
2. b
3. d

4. c
5. c
6. c

CHAPTER 17

1. b
2. a
3. a
4. c
5. b
6. b
7. c

CHAPTER 18

1. c
2. a
3. c
4. a
5. c
6. c
7. b
8. a
9. a
10. b
11. a

CHAPTER 19

1. c
2. b
3. d
4. b
5. d
6. a
7. b
8. b
9. d

CHAPTER 20

1. d
2. a
3. d
4. d
5. d
6. c
7. b
8. b
9. d
10. e
11. d

CHAPTER 21

1. c
2. b
3. a
4. c
5. b
6. c
7. c
8. a
9. b
10. b
11. d
12. c

CHAPTER 22

1. c
2. a
3. d
4. a
5. c
6. d
7. b
8. c
9. c
10. a
11. c

CHAPTER 23

1. c
2. d
3. a
4. a
5. d
6. b
7. b
8. d
9. a
10. c

CHAPTER 24

1. c
2. a
3. c
4. d
5. c
6. a
7. b
8. a
9. a
10. a
11. d
12. d
13. c
14. a
15. d

CHAPTER 25

1. b
2. b
3. b
4. a
5. c
6. b

CHAPTER 26

1. d
2. a
3. b
4. b

CHAPTER 27

1. c
2. a
3. b
4. c
5. c
6. c
7. a
8. a

CHAPTER 28

1. c
2. a
3. a
4. c
5. a
6. c
7. d
8. a
9. b
10. a
11. b
12. c
13. c
14. c
15. a
16. a
17. b

CHAPTER 29

1. c
2. b
3. a
4. d
5. c
6. a
7. b
8. a
9. b
10. c
11. d

CHAPTER 30

1. b
2. a
3. a
4. c
5. b
6. d
7. c
8. a

CHAPTER 31

1. b
2. d
3. a
4. a
5. c
6. d
7. c
8. d
9. c
10. c

CHAPTER 32

1. d
2. b
3. c
4. a
5. a
6. d
7. c
8. a

CHAPTER 33

1. b
2. d
3. b
4. d
5. b
6. c
7. c
8. d

CHAPTER 34

1. a
2. a
3. a
4. c
5. b
6. d
7. a
8. a
9. c
10. d

CHAPTER 35

1. a
2. d
3. b
4. d
5. d
6. d
7. a
8. b
9. c
10. b
11. a
12. a

CHAPTER 36

1. a
2. d
3. a

4. b
5. b
6. c
7. c
8. a
9. b

CHAPTER 37

1. d
2. a
3. c
4. b
5. c
6. a

CHAPTER 38

1. a
2. a
3. d
4. b
5. c
6. d
7. b
8. c
9. b
10. a
11. a

CHAPTER 39

1. c
2. b
3. b
4. a
5. a
6. d

CHAPTER 40

1. b
2. c
3. a
4. c
5. a
6. d
7. a
8. d
9. b
10. a
11. a
12. a
13. a
14. a
15. d

CHAPTER 41

1. b
2. c
3. a
4. c
5. b
6. a
7. c
8. a
9. a
10. d
11. b

CHAPTER 42

1. b
2. c
3. c
4. a
5. d
6. c
7. c
8. b

CHAPTER 43

1. b
2. b
3. c
4. c
5. b
6. b
7. a
8. a
9. d
10. d
11. c
12. c

CHAPTER 44

1. b
2. b
3. c
4. c
5. a
6. c
7. d
8. a
9. c
10. d
11. a

CHAPTER 45

1. d
2. a
3. a
4. c
5. d
6. c
7. b
8. d
9. b

CHAPTER 46

1. c
2. d
3. a
4. d
5. d
6. c
7. c

CHAPTER 47

1. a
2. b
3. b
4. d
5. b
6. d
7. a
8. c
9. c

CHAPTER 48

1. c
2. d
3. b
4. c
5. a
6. b
7. b
8. c

CHAPTER 49

1. b
2. b
3. c
4. c
5. b
6. c
7. d
8. c

CHAPTER 50

1. c
2. c
3. b
4. a
5. d
6. c
7. b

CHAPTER 51

1. d
2. c
3. c
4. b
5. b
6. c
7. a
8. b
9. a
10. c
11. a
12. d
13. b
14. d
15. d

CHAPTER 52

1. a
2. c
3. d
4. b
5. b
6. d
7. c

CHAPTER 53

1. c
2. a
3. b
4. a
5. d
6. a
7. b
8. a
9. b
10. d
11. a

CHAPTER 54

1. a
2. c
3. b
4. a
5. b
6. c
7. d
8. b
9. d
10. a
11. a
12. d
13. c
14. d

CHAPTER 55

1. a
2. b
3. a
4. b
5. b
6. a
7. a
8. c
9. b

CHAPTER 56

1. b
2. a
3. b
4. a
5. d

6. a
7. c

CHAPTER 57

1. b
2. b
3. d
4. c
5. b
6. b
7. d
8. b

CHAPTER 58

1. c
2. a
3. c
4. d
5. a
6. c
7. a
8. d
9. a

CHAPTER 59

1. c
2. a
3. c
4. a
5. a
6. b
7. c
8. c
9. d
10. d
11. b
12. d
13. c
14. d

CHAPTER 60

1. b
2. c
3. d
4. b
5. d
6. d
7. b
8. c
9. a
10. c

CHAPTER 61

1. c
2. a
3. c
4. b
5. a
6. d
7. b
8. b
9. b
10. c
11. d

CHAPTER 62

1. d
2. c
3. b
4. b

CREDITS

Chapter 1 1-2, From Potter P, Perry A: *Basic nursing*, ed 3, St Louis, 1995, Mosby.

Chapter 2 2-1, 2-3, 2-7, 2-8, 2-9, Courtesy CLG Photographics, St Louis; 2-4, from Potter P, Perry A: *Basic nursing*, ed 3, St Louis, 1995, Mosby; 2-6, courtesy Caroline E. Brown, Hershey, PA.

Chapter 3 3-1, US Bureau of Census; 3-2, 3-5, 3-6, 3-7, Courtesy CLG Photographics, St Louis; 3-3, from Wilson SF, Thompson JM: *Respiratory disorders*, St Louis, 1995, Mosby; 3-4, redrawn from Bezon J: Approaching drug regimens with a therapeutic dose of suspicion, *Geriatr Nurs*, 12:4, 1991, p. 1813.

Chapter 4 4-1, From Potter P, Perry A: *Basic nursing*, ed 3, St Louis, 1995, Mosby; 4-2, 4-3, from Seidel H: *Mosby's guide to physical examinations,* ed 3, St Louis, 1995, Mosby; 4-4, from Carpenito LJ and others: *Nursing diagnoses: application to clinical practice*, Philadelphia, 1989, JB Lippincott, p. 54.

Chapter 6 6-17, 6-18, 6-19, Courtesy CLG Photographics, St Louis.

Chapter 8 8-4, Courtesy The Stock Market, New York.

Chapter 9 9-1, Christine Oleksyk; 9-4, courtesy Cameron Bangs, MD; 9-12, from Habif T: *Clinical dermatology*, ed 2, St Louis, 1992, Mosby.

Chapter 11 11-1, 11-2, 11-4, Redrawn from Gottfried SS: *Human biology*, St Louis, 1993, Mosby; 11-5, 11-6, from Grimes DE, Grimes RM: *AIDS and HIV infection*, St Louis, 1994, Mosby; 11-7, 11-8, redrawn from Grimes DE, Grimes RM: *AIDS and HIV infection*, St Louis, 1994, Mosby; 11-9, from the Centers for Disease Control, courtesy Jonathan WM Gold, MD, New York.

Chapter 12 12-19, Printed with permission from the American Cancer Society from: Krakoff: Cancer chemotherapeutic and biologic agents, *CA*, 41:268, 1991; 12-22, Courtesy Pharmacia Deltec, Inc., St Paul, MN; 12-23*B,* Strato Infusaid, Inc.

Chapter 14 14-1, 14-3, 14-4, Courtesy Rush Presbyterian St Luke's Medical Center, Chicago; 14-2, courtesy Swedish American Hospital, Rockford, IL; 14-5, courtesy St Joseph Hospital, Albuquerque, NM.

Chapter 15 15-1, Courtesy Greg McVicar; 15-2, from Potter P, Perry A: *Basic nursing*, ed 3, St Louis, 1995, Mosby; 15-3, courtesy SpaceLabs Medical.

Chapter 16 16-1, Courtesy Rush Presbyterian St Luke's Medical Center, Chicago.

Chapter 17 17-1, Marcia J Dohrmann; 17-3, from Thibodeau G, Patton K: *Anatomy and physiology*, ed 3, St Louis, 1993, Mosby; 17-8, Marcia J Dohrmann; 17-9, from Seidel H and others: *Mosby's guide to physical examination*, ed 3, St Louis, 1995, Mosby; 17-11, courtesy Medical Records Subcommittee of the University of Iowa Hospitals and Clinics, Iowa City, IA.

Chapter 18 18-8, 18-10, CLG Photographics, St Louis.

Chapter 19 19-1, From Thibodeau G, Patton K: *Anatomy and physiology*, ed 2, St Louis, 1993, Mosby; 19-3, 19-4, 19-5, redrawn from Habif T: *Clinical dermatology: a color guide to diagnosis and therapy,* ed 2, St Louis, 1990, Mosby.

Chapter 20 20-1, From Hill MJ: *Skin Disorders*, St Louis, 1994, Mosby; 20-2, 20-3, 20-7, 20-8, from Habif T: *Clinical dermatology: a color guide to diagnosis and therapy*, ed 2, St Louis, 1990, Mosby; 20-5, 20-6, US Centers for Disease Control; 20-10, from Tardy ME: *Facial aesthetic surgery*, St Louis, 1994, Mosby; 20-13, from Potter P, Perry A: *Basic nursing*, ed 3, St Louis, 1995, Mosby.

Chapter 22 22-1, Redrawn from Price S, Wilson L: *Pathophysiology: clinical concepts of disease processes*, ed 5, St Louis, 1996, Mosby; 22-2, from Thompson JM and others: *Clinical nursing*, ed 3, St Louis, 1993, Mosby; 22-3, Rolin Graphics; 22-4*A,* from Bone RC and others, editors: *Pulmonary and critical care medicine*, vol 1, St Louis, 1993, Mosby; 22-4*B,* Staub NC, Albertine KH: The structure of the lungs relative to their principal function, in Murray JF, Nadel JA, editors: *Textbook of respiratory medicine*, Philadelphia, 1988, WB Saunders; 22-8, redrawn from *Principles of pulse oximetry*, Nellcor Inc, Haywood, CA; 22-9, redrawn from Hayden RA: Trend-spotting with an SvO_2 monitor, *Am J Nurs* 93:31, 1993; 22-10, redrawn from Wilkins RL and others: *Clinical assessment in respiratory care,* ed 3, St Louis, 1994, Mosby; 22-12, modified from Thompson J and others: *Clinical nursing*, ed 3, St Louis, 1993, Mosby; 22-15, from Dib HR and others: Malignant thymoma, *Chest* 105:941, 1994; 22-16*A,* courtesy Olympus America, Melville, NY; 22-16*B,* from Meduri GU and others: Protected bronchoalveolar lavage, *Am Rev Respir Dis* 143:855, 1991; 22-17, redrawn from du Bois RM, Clarke SW: *Fiberoptic bronchoscopy in diagnosis and management,* Orlando, 1987, Grune & Stratton; 22-18; courtesy of Sherwood Medical, St Louis.

Chapter 23 23-4, From Middleton E and others: *Allergy principles and practice*, vol 2, ed 4, St Louis, 1993, Mosby; 23-5, from Smolley LA: How to help patients with obstructive sleep apnea, *J Respir Dis* 11: 723-732, 1990; 23-6, courtesy Respironics, Murrysville, PA; 23-11, from *Tracheostomy tube adult home care guide,* Sorin Biomedical Inc, 1992, Irvine, CA; 23-13, courtesy Passy-Muir, Inc, Irvine, CA; 23-16, from the American Cancer Society; 23-18, courtesy CLG Photographics, St Louis.

Chapter 24 24-1, 24-3, 24-9, Redrawn from Price S, Wilson L: *Pathophysiology: clinical concepts of disease processes*, ed 4, St Louis, 1992, Mosby; 24-2, McCance KL, Huether SE: *Pathophysiology: the biological basis for disease in adults and children*, ed 2, St Louis, 1994, Mosby; 24-6, CLG Photographics, St Louis; 24-13, courtesy Deknatel, Inc, Fall River, MA.

Chapter 25 25-3, 25-9, 25-10, Redrawn from Price S, Wilson L: *Pathophysiology: clinical concepts of disease processes*, ed 5, St Louis, 1996, Mosby; 25-4, 25-8, redrawn from McCance KL, Huether SE: *Pathophysiology: the biological basis for disease in adults and children*, ed 2, St Louis, 1994, Mosby; 25-5, courtesy Lovelace Medical Center, Albuquerque, NM; 25-6, from Teach your patients about asthma: a clinician's guide, National Asthma Education Program. NIH Publication No. 92-2737, October 1992; 25-7, Potter P, Perry A: *Basic nursing*, ed 3, St Louis, 1995, Mosby; 25-12, modified from Eubanks DH, Bone RC: *Comprehensive respiratory care: a learning system*, ed 2, St Louis, 1990, Mosby; 25-14, modified from Cherniak RM: *Current therapy of respiratory disease*, ed 3, St Louis, 1989, Mosby.

Chapter 27 27-2, 27-3, From McCance KL, Heuther SE: *Pathophysiology: the biological basis for disease in adults and children*, ed 2, St Louis, 1994, Mosby.

Chapter 28 28-4, Redrawn from Raven PH, Johnson GB: *Biology*, ed 2, St Louis, 1991, Mosby; 28-5, redrawn from McCance KL, Heuther SE: *Pathophysiology: the biological basis for disease in adults and children*, ed 2, St Louis, 1994, Mosby; 28-8, Bingham BJG, Hawke M, Kwok P: *Atlas of clinical otolaryngology*, St Louis, 1992, Mosby-Europe; 28-12, 28-13, reprinted from Groenwald SL, Frogge MH, Goodman M, editors: *Cancer nursing: principles and practice*, Boston, 1993, Jones & Bartlett.

Chapter 29 29-1, 29-3, 29-13, Modified from Price S, Wilson L: *Pathophysiology: clinical concepts of disease processes*, ed 4, St Louis, 1992, Mosby; 29-5, 29-9, modified from Kinney M and others: *Comprehensive cardiac care*, ed 7, St Louis, 1991, Mosby; 29-12, 29-16, from Kinney M and others: *Comprehensive cardiac care,* ed 7, St Louis, 1991, Mosby.

Chapter 30 30-1, Redrawn from West JB: *Physiological basis of medical practice*, ed 12, Baltimore, 1991, Williams & Wilkins; 30-3, from Kissane JM: *Anderson's pathology*, ed 9, St Louis, 1990, Mosby; 30-4, redrawn from McKenry LM, Salerno E: *Pharmacology in nursing*, ed 19, St Louis, 1995, Mosby; 30-5, from US Department of Health and Human Services: The fifth report of the Joint National Committee on Detection, Evaluation, and Treatment of High Blood Pressure (JNC-V), Washington DC, 1993, National Institutes of Health.

Chapter 31 31-1, 31-2, From 1993 Heart and Stroke Facts Statistics, 1992, copyright American Heart Association; 31-5, 31-12, 31-13, 31-14, 31-15, courtesy Mayo Clinic, Rochester, MN; 31-8, modified and reprinted with permission from Matrisciano L, Alspach JG: Unstable angina: an overview, *Crit Care Nurs* 12:31, 1992; 31-10, from *Heart Disease and Stroke* 2:199, 1993, copyright American Heart Association; 31-11, from *Heart Disease and Stroke* 2:201, 1993, copyright American Heart Association.

Chapter 32 32-1, Redrawn from McCance KL, Huether SE: *Pathophysiology: the biological basis for disease in adults and children*, ed 2, St Louis 1994, Mosby; 32-2, 32-3, 32-7, redrawn from Thelan LA and others: *Textbook of critical care nursing: diagnosis and management*, ed 2, St Louis, 1994, Mosby; 32-4, from Kissane JM: *Anderson's pathology*, ed 9, St Louis, 1990, Mosby; SpaceLabs Medical, Redmond, WA; 32-6, courtesy Mayo Clinic, Rochester, MN.

Chapter 33 33-2, From Goldberger AL, Goldberger E: *Clinical electrocardiography: a simplified approach*, ed 4, St Louis, 1990, Mosby; 33-4, 33-7, 33-10, 33-12 from Thelan LA and others: *Textbook of critical care nursing: diagnosis and management*, ed 2, St Louis, 1994, Mosby; 33-6, 33-11, 33-13, 33-14, 33-15, 33-19, 33-20, from Conover MB: *Understanding electrocardiograph, arrhythmias, and the 12-lead ECG*, ed 6, St Louis, 1992, Mosby; 33-21, 33-29 courtesy Physio-Control Corporation, Redmond, WA; 33-24*A*; 33-25, courtesy Medtronic, Inc., Minneapolis.

Chapter 34 34-2, From Kissane JM: *Anderson's pathology*, ed 9, St Louis, 1990, Mosby; 34-4, from Anderson WAD, Scotti TM: *Synopsis of pathology*, ed 10, St Louis, 1980, Mosby; 34-5, from Guzzetta CE, Dossey BM: *Cardiovascular nursing: holistic practice*, St Louis, 1992, Mosby; 34-6, redrawn from Lorell BH, Braunwald E: *Pericardial disease in heart disease: a textbook of cardiovascular medicine,* ed 3, Philadelphia, 1988, WB Saunders; 34-9, redrawn from Block PC: Balloon valvuloplasty, *Cardiol Consult* 9:4, 1988; 34-10, from Nichols L and others: Percutaneous Aortic Valvuloplasty Procedure and Implications for Nursing, *Heart Lung* 18:357, 1989; 34-13*A*, courtesy St Jude Medical Inc., St Paul, MN; 34-13*B,* courtesy Medtronic Inc., Irvine, CA; 34-13*C,* redrawn from Emery RW, Arom KV: *The aortic valve*, Philadelphia, 1991, Hanley & Belfus, Inc.

Chapter 35 35-2, Courtesy Jo Menzoian, Boston; 35-7, courtesy FW LoGerfo, Boston; 35-8, 35-9, from Kamal A, Brockelhursts JC: *Color atlas of geriatric medicine*, ed 2, St Louis, 1991, Mosby-Europe; 35-11, from Lofgren KA: Varicose veins. In Haimovici H, editor: *Vascular surgery: principles and techniques*, New York, 1976, McGraw-Hill; 35-12, from Habif T: *Clinical dermatology*, ed 2, St Louis, 1990, Mosby.

Chapter 36 36-1, 36-2, 36-3, From Thibodeau GA, Patton KT: *Anatomy and physiology,* ed 2, St Louis, 1992, Mosby; 36-8, 36-9, from Doughty DB, Jackson DB: *Mosby's clinical nursing series: gastrointestinal disorders*, St Louis, 1993, Mosby.

Chapter 37 37-1, From Human nutrition information service: making health food choices, Washington, DC, 1993, USDA; 37-2, redrawn from Mahan LK, Arlin M: *Krause's food, nutrition & diet therapy*, ed 4, Philadelphia, 1992, WB Saunders; 37-4, from Bray G: Obesity: Definition, Diagnosis and Disadvantages, *Med J Aust* 142, 1985.

Chapter 38 34-1, David J Mascaro & Associates; 38-3, from Murray PR and others: *Medical microbiology*, St Louis, 1990, Mosby; 38-5, courtesy R Doberneck, Albuquerque, NM; 38-6, courtesy RA Weinstein, Denver; 38-7, 38-11, modified from Price S, Wilson L: *Pathophysiology: clinical concepts of disease process*, ed 5, St Louis, 1996, Mosby; 38-9, from Doughty DB, Jackson DB: *Gastrointestinal disorders*, St Louis, 1993, Mosby.

Chapter 39 39-2, 39-5, redrawn from Price S, Wilson L: *Pathophysiology: clinical concepts of disease process*, ed 5, St Louis, 1996, Mosby.

Chapter 40 40-8, Redrawn from Gruendemann BJ, Meeker MH: *Alexander's care of the patient in surgery*, ed 9, St Louis, 1991, Mosby; 40-9, redrawn from Hampton BG, Bryant RA: *Ostomies and continent diversions*, St Louis, 1992, Mosby.

Chapter 41 41-1, From Kamal A, Brockelhursts JC: *Color atlas of geriatric medicine*, ed 2, St Louis, 1991, Mosby-Europe; 41-5, adapted from Doughty DB, Jackson DB: *Gastrointestinal disorders*, St Louis, 1993, Mosby; 41-8, courtesy Davol Rubber Company, Providence, RI.

Chapter 42 42-7, From Brundage DJ: *Renal disorders*, St Louis, 1992, Mosby; 42-8, from Price S, Wilson L: *Pathophysiology: clinical concepts of disease process*, ed 5, St Louis, 1996, Mosby.

Chapter 43 43-3, 43-5, Courtesy Harborview Medical Center, University of Washington, Seattle; 43-6, from Brundage DJ: *Renal disorders*, St Louis, 1992, Mosby; 43-9, 43-11, 43-12, courtesy Lynda Brubacher, Virginia Mason Hospital, Seattle.

Chapter 44 44-3, From United States Data System, Washington, DC, 1993, Department of Health and Human Services; 44-7, 44-8, 44-9, 44-10, copyright 1994 Baxter Healthcare Corp.; 44-12*A,* courtesy Quinton Instrument Co, Bothell, WA; 44-14, modified from Thelan L, Davie JK, Urden JD: *Textbook of critical care nursing: diagnosis and management*, ed 2, St Louis, 1994, Mosby; 44-15, courtesy Fresenius, USA, Walnut Creek, CA.

Chapter 45 45-1, From Thibodeau G, Patton K: *Anatomy and physiology*, ed 2, St Louis, 1993, Mosby; 45-9, Carlyn Iverson; 45-10, Sigler BA, Schuring LT: *Ear, nose, and throat disorders*, St Louis, 1994, Mosby.

Chapter 46 46-3, From Diabetes mellitus, Indianapolis, Eli Lilly, Inc; 46-4, 46-5, from American Diabetes Association, 1994; 46-10, 46-12, redrawn from McCance KL, Heuther SE: *Pathophysiology: the biological basis for disease in adults and children*, ed 2, St Louis, 1994, Mosby; 46-13, from Thelan L, Davie JK, Urden JD: *Textbook of critical care nursing: diagnosis and management*, ed 2, St Louis, 1994, Mosby.

Chapter 47 47-1, Courtesy Linda Haas, Seattle; 47-2, 47-3, 47-4, redrawn from Thelan L, Davie JK, Urden JD: *Textbook of critical care nursing: diagnosis and management*, ed 2, St Louis, 1994, Mosby; 47-5, courtesy of Paul W Ladenson, MD, Johns Hopkins University and Hospital, Baltimore, MD; 47-6, LV Bergman and Associates, Cold Spring, NY; 47-7, from Williams GH, Dluhy RG: Diseases of the Adrenal Cortex. In Isselbacker K and others, editors: *Harrison's principles of internal medicine*, ed 13, New York, 1994, McGraw-Hill.

Chapter 48 48-1, Ronald J Ervin; 48-3, from Thibodeau G, Patton K: *Anatomy and physiology*, ed 2, St Louis, 1993, Mosby; 48-5, Kevin A Sommerville; 48-6, David J Mascaro & Associates; 48-8, from Seeley R, Stephens T, Tate P: *Anatomy and physiology*, ed 3, St Louis, 1995, Mosby.

Chapter 49 49-5, Courtesy Michael Leadbetter, Cincinnati.

Chapter 50 50-1, From Centers for Disease Control, Atlanta, 1994; 50-2, from Centers for Disease Control: Sexually transmitted disease surveillance, 1991, Atlanta, July 1991; 50-3, from Centers for Disease Control, 1991; 50-4, 50-5, 50-6, courtesy USPHS, Washington, DC.

Chapter 51 51-2, From Govan ADT, Hodge C, Callander R: *Gynecology illustrated*, ed 3, New York, 1985, Churchill Livingstone; 51-4, from Bobak I, Jensen M, Zalar M: *Maternity and gynecologic care*, ed 5, St Louis, 1993, Mosby; 51-6, from Herbst A and others: *Comprehensive gynecology*, ed 2, St Louis, 1992, Mosby; 51-7, from Phipps W and others: *Medical-surgical nursing concepts and clinical practice*, St Louis, 1995, Mosby; 51-9*A,* from Green T: *Gynecology: essentials of clinical practice,* ed 3, Boston, 1977, Little, Brown & Co; 51-10, from Seidel HM and others; *Mosby's guide to physical examination*, ed 3, St Louis, 1995, Mosby.

Chapter 52 52-5, from Seidel HM and others: *Mosby's guide to physical examination*, ed 3, St Louis, 1995, Mosby; 52-7, courtesy of Mayo Clinic Health Letter with permission from Mayo Foundation for Medical Education and Research, Rochester, MN.

Chapter 53 53-1, 53-6, 53-10, Scott Bodell; 53-11, Barbara Cousins; 53-13*A,* David J Mascaro & Associates; 53-13*B-D,* Karen Waldo; 53-14, 53-15, from Thibodeau G, Patton K: *Anatomy and physiology*, ed 2, St Louis, 1993, Mosby.

Chapter 54 54-1, From Wong J, Wong S, Dempster JK: Care of the unconscious patient: a problem-oriented approach, *Am Assoc Neurosci Nurses* 16:145, 1984; 54-5, redrawn from McCance KL, Huether SE: *Pathophysiology: biological basis for disease in adults and children*, ed 2, St Louis, 1994, Mosby; 54-7, redrawn from Thelan LA and others: *Critical care nursing*, ed 2, St Louis, 1994, Mosby; 54-8, redrawn from Kinney MR and others, editors:

AACN's clinical reference for critical care nursing, St Louis, 1993, Mosby; 54-11, redrawn from Barker E: *Neuroscience nursing*, St Louis, 1994, Mosby; 54-12; from Bingham BJG, Hawke M, Kwok P: *Atlas of clinical otolaryngology*, St Louis, 1992, Mosby; 54-13, Price S, Wilson L: *Pathophysiology: clinical concepts of disease processes*, ed 5, St Louis, 1996, Mosby; 54-14, from Okazaki H, Scheithauer BW: *An atlas of neuropathology*, London, 1988, Gower Medical Publishing; 54-17, redrawn from Perkin GD and others: *Atlas of clinical neurology*, ed 2, St Louis, 1993, Mosby.

Chapter 55 55-1, Redrawn from Barker E: *Neuroscience nursing*, St Louis, 1994, Mosby; 55-6, redrawn from Chipps E and others: *Neurologic disorders*, St Louis, 1992, Mosby.

Chapter 56 56-4, Redrawn from Rudy E: *Advanced neurologic and neurosurgical nursing*, St Louis, 1984, Mosby; 56-5, redrawn from Barker E: *Neuroscience nursing*, St Louis, 1994, Mosby.

Chapter 57 57-1, David J Mascaro & Associates; 57-2, Joe Rothrock; 57-3, redrawn from Chipps E, Clanin N, Campbell V: *Neurologic disorders*, St Louis, 1992, Mosby; 57-7, courtesy Orthopedic Frame Company, Kalamazoo, MI; 57-9, courtesy Kinetic Concepts Company; 57-10, courtesy Acromed Corporation, Cleveland, OH; 57-11, CLG Photographics, St Louis; 57-12, redrawn from Barker E: *Neuroscience nursing*, St Louis, 1994, Mosby.

Chapter 58 58-2, John V. Hagen; 58-4, redrawn from Price SL, Wilson L: *Pathophysiology: clinical concepts of disease processes*, ed 5, St Louis, 1996, Mosby; 58-6, 58-7, redrawn from Thompson J and others: *Mosby's manual of clinical nursing*, ed 3, St Louis, 1993, Mosby; 58-8, 58-10, from Mourad LA: *Orthopedic disorders*, St Louis, 1991, Mosby; 58-9, modified from DeLisa J, Gans B: *Rehabilitation medicine principles*, ed 2, Philadelphia, 1993, JB Lippincott.

Chapter 59 59-1, Redrawn from Price SL, Wilson L: *Pathophysiology: clinical concepts of disease processes*, ed 5, St Louis, 1996, Mosby; 59-2, redrawn from Thompson J and others: *Mosby's manual of clinical nursing*, ed 3, St Louis, 1993, Mosby; 59-3, courtesy Eli Lilly, Indianapolis; 59-7, redrawn from Long BC, Phipps WJ, Cassmeyer VL: *Medical-surgical nursing: a nursing process approach*, St Louis, 1993, Mosby; 59-9, courtesy Zimmer, Inc, Warsaw, IN; 59-14, from Thompson J and others: *Mosby's manual of clinical nursing*, ed 3, St Louis, 1993, Mosby; 59-16, redrawn from Mourad L: *Orthopedic disorders*, St Louis, 1992, Mosby; 59-18, from Hunter JM and others: *Rehabilitation of the hand*, ed 3, St Louis, 1990, Mosby.

Chapter 60 60-3, From Shipley M: *A colour atlas of rheumatology*, ed 3, London, 1993, Mosby-Europe; 60-8, from Seidel HM and others: *Mosby's guide to physical examination*, ed 3, St Louis, 1995, Mosby; 60-10, from Lamey P, Lewis, MAO: *Pocket picture guide to oral medicine*, London, 1988, Gower Medical Publishing; 60-12, Zitelli BJ, Davis HW: *Atlas of pediatric physical diagnosis*, ed 2, London, 1992, Gower Medical Publishing; 60-13, 60-14, courtesy Zimmer, Inc, Warsaw, IN.

Chapter 61 61-1, Courtesy SpaceLabs Medical, Redmond, WA; 61-2, redrawn from Gardner PE: *Hemodynamic pressure monitoring*, SpaceLabs Medical, Redmond, WA, 1994; 61-3, 61-8, redrawn from Flynn JBM, Bruce NP: *Introduction to critical care skills*, St Louis, 1993, Mosby; 61-4, 61-6, from Thelan and others: *Critical care nursing: diagnosis and management*, ed 2, St Louis, 1994, Mosby; 61-5, from Edwards Critical care division, Baxter Healthcare Corporation, Santa Ana, CA; 61-7, courtesy Datascope System, Montvale, NJ; 61-10, courtesy SpaceLabs Medical, Redmond, WA; 61-11, courtesy LIFECARE Pulmo-Wrap; 61-12, courtesy Puritan-Bennett; 61-15, courtesy Camino Laboratories, San Diego, CA.

Chapter 62 62-3, From Grossman JA: *Atlas of minor injuries*, London, 1993, Gower Medical Publishing; 62-4, from Auerbach P, Geehr E: *Management of wilderness and environmental emergencies*, ed 3, St Louis, 1995, Mosby; 62-5, redrawn from Rosen P and others: *Emergency medicine*, vol 1, ed 2, St Louis, 1988, Mosby.

INDEX

A

Note: Entries and page numbers in **bold face** indicate main disorder discussions; page numbers followed by *f*, *t*, and *b* indicate figures, tables, and boxed material, respectively.

Note: Entries and page numbers in **bold face** indicate main disorder discussions; page numbers followed by *f, t,* and *b* indicate figures, tables, and boxed material, respectively.

Note: Entries and page numbers in **bold face** indicate main disorder discussions; page numbers followed by *f*, *t*, and *b* indicate figures, tables, and boxed material, respectively.

Note: Entries and page numbers in **bold face** indicate main disorder discussions; page numbers followed by *f*, *t*, and *b* indicate figures, tables, and boxed material, respectively.

Note: Entries and page numbers in **bold face** indicate main disorder discussions; page numbers followed by *f*, *t*, and *b* indicate figures, tables, and boxed material, respectively.

B

Note: Entries and page numbers in **bold face** indicate main disorder discussions; page numbers followed by *f*, *t*, and *b* indicate figures, tables, and boxed material, respectively.

Note: Entries and page numbers in **bold face** indicate main disorder discussions; page numbers followed by *f, t,* and *b* indicate figures, tables, and boxed material, respectively.

C

Note: Entries and page numbers in **bold face** indicate main disorder discussions; page numbers followed by *f, t,* and *b* indicate figures, tables, and boxed material, respectively.

Note: Entries and page numbers in **bold face** indicate main disorder discussions; page numbers followed by *f*, *t*, and *b* indicate figures, tables, and boxed material, respectively.

Note: Entries and page numbers in **bold face** indicate main disorder discussions; page numbers followed by *f*, *t*, and *b* indicate figures, tables, and boxed material, respectively.

Note: Entries and page numbers in **bold face** indicate main disorder discussions; page numbers followed by *f, t,* and *b* indicate figures, tables, and boxed material, respectively.

Note: Entries and page numbers in **bold face** indicate main disorder discussions; page numbers followed by *f, t,* and *b* indicate figures, tables, and boxed material, respectively.

D

Note: Entries and page numbers in **bold face** indicate main disorder discussions; page numbers followed by *f*, *t*, and *b* indicate figures, tables, and boxed material, respectively.

Note: Entries and page numbers in **bold face** indicate main disorder discussions; page numbers followed by *f*, *t*, and *b* indicate figures, tables, and boxed material, respectively.

E

Note: Entries and page numbers in **bold face** indicate main disorder discussions; page numbers followed by *f, t,* and *b* indicate figures, tables, and boxed material, respectively.

Note: Entries and page numbers in **bold face** indicate main disorder discussions; page numbers followed by *f*, *t*, and *b* indicate figures, tables, and boxed material, respectively.

F

Note: Entries and page numbers in **bold face** indicate main disorder discussions; page numbers followed by *f, t,* and *b* indicate figures, tables, and boxed material, respectively.

G

Note: Entries and page numbers in **bold face** indicate main disorder discussions; page numbers followed by *f, t,* and *b* indicate figures, tables, and boxed material, respectively.

H

Note: Entries and page numbers in **bold face** indicate main disorder discussions; page numbers followed by *f, t,* and *b* indicate figures, tables, and boxed material, respectively.

Note: Entries and page numbers in **bold face** indicate main disorder discussions; page numbers followed by *f*, *t*, and *b* indicate figures, tables, and boxed material, respectively.

Note: Entries and page numbers in **bold face** indicate main disorder discussions; page numbers followed by *f, t,* and *b* indicate figures, tables, and boxed material, respectively.

Note: Entries and page numbers in **bold face** indicate main disorder discussions; page numbers followed by *f, t,* and *b* indicate figures, tables, and boxed material, respectively.

I

Note: Entries and page numbers in **bold face** indicate main disorder discussions; page numbers followed by *f*, *t*, and *b* indicate figures, tables, and boxed material, respectively.

Note: Entries and page numbers in **bold face** indicate main disorder discussions; page numbers followed by *f, t,* and *b* indicate figures, tables, and boxed material, respectively.

J

K

L

Note: Entries and page numbers in **bold face** indicate main disorder discussions; page numbers followed by *f*, *t*, and *b* indicate figures, tables, and boxed material, respectively.

M

Note: Entries and page numbers in **bold face** indicate main disorder discussions; page numbers followed by *f*, *t*, and *b* indicate figures, tables, and boxed material, respectively.

Note: Entries and page numbers in **bold face** indicate main disorder discussions; page numbers followed by *f, t,* and *b* indicate figures, tables, and boxed material, respectively.

N

Note: Entries and page numbers in **bold face** indicate main disorder discussions; page numbers followed by *f, t,* and *b* indicate figures, tables, and boxed material, respectively.

Note: Entries and page numbers in **bold face** indicate main disorder discussions; page numbers followed by *f*, *t*, and *b* indicate figures, tables, and boxed material, respectively.

Note: Entries and page numbers in **bold face** indicate main disorder discussions; page numbers followed by *f, t,* and *b* indicate figures, tables, and boxed material, respectively.

O

Note: Entries and page numbers in **bold face** indicate main disorder discussions; page numbers followed by *f*, *t*, and *b* indicate figures, tables, and boxed material, respectively.

P

Note: Entries and page numbers in **bold face** indicate main disorder discussions; page numbers followed by *f*, *t*, and *b* indicate figures, tables, and boxed material, respectively.

Note: Entries and page numbers in **bold face** indicate main disorder discussions; page numbers followed by *f*, *t*, and *b* indicate figures, tables, and boxed material, respectively.

Note: Entries and page numbers in **bold face** indicate main disorder discussions; page numbers followed by *f, t,* and *b* indicate figures, tables, and boxed material, respectively.

Note: Entries and page numbers in **bold face** indicate main disorder discussions; page numbers followed by *f, t,* and *b* indicate figures, tables, and boxed material, respectively.

Q

R

Note: Entries and page numbers in **bold face** indicate main disorder discussions; page numbers followed by *f*, *t*, and *b* indicate figures, tables, and boxed material, respectively.

Note: Entries and page numbers in **bold face** indicate main disorder discussions; page numbers followed by *f*, *t*, and *b* indicate figures, tables, and boxed material, respectively.

S

Note: Entries and page numbers in **bold face** indicate main disorder discussions; page numbers followed by *f, t,* and *b* indicate figures, tables, and boxed material, respectively.

Note: Entries and page numbers in **bold face** indicate main disorder discussions; page numbers followed by *f, t,* and *b* indicate figures, tables, and boxed material, respectively.

Note: Entries and page numbers in **bold face** indicate main disorder discussions; page numbers followed by *f*, *t*, and *b* indicate figures, tables, and boxed material, respectively.

Note: Entries and page numbers in **bold face** indicate main disorder discussions; page numbers followed by *f*, *t*, and *b* indicate figures, tables, and boxed material, respectively.

T

Note: Entries and page numbers in **bold face** indicate main disorder discussions; page numbers followed by *f, t,* and *b* indicate figures, tables, and boxed material, respectively.

Note: Entries and page numbers in **bold face** indicate main disorder discussions; page numbers followed by *f*, *t*, and *b* indicate figures, tables, and boxed material, respectively.

U

Note: Entries and page numbers in **bold face** indicate main disorder discussions; page numbers followed by *f, t,* and *b* indicate figures, tables, and boxed material, respectively.

V

Note: Entries and page numbers in **bold face** indicate main disorder discussions; page numbers followed by *f*, *t*, and *b* indicate figures, tables, and boxed material, respectively.

W

Z

Note: Entries and page numbers in **bold face** indicate main disorder discussions; page numbers followed by *f*, *t*, and *b* indicate figures, tables, and boxed material, respectively.

Nutritional Management

Key Questions to Ask

Therapeutic Management